Williams
Obstetrics

21ST EDITION

Williams
Obstetrics

21ST EDITION

F. Gary Cunningham, MD

*Professor and Chairman, Department of Obstetrics &
Gynecology
Jack A. Pritchard Professor of Obstetrics & Gynecology
Beatrice & Miguel Elias Distinguished Chair
in Obstetrics & Gynecology
The University of Texas Southwestern Medical Center
at Dallas
Chief of Obstetrics & Gynecology,
Parkland Memorial Hospital
Dallas, Texas*

Norman F. Gant, MD

*Professor, Department of Obstetrics & Gynecology
The University of Texas Southwestern Medical Center
at Dallas
Executive Director, American Board of Obstetrics &
Gynecology
Attending Staff, Parkland Memorial Hospital
Dallas, Texas*

Kenneth J. Leveno, MD

*Gillette Professor, Department of Obstetrics & Gynecology
Vice-Chair for Maternal-Fetal Medicine
The University of Texas Southwestern Medical Center
at Dallas
Chief of Obstetrics, Parkland Memorial Hospital
Dallas, Texas*

Larry C. Gilstrap III, MD

*Professor and Chairman, Department of Obstetrics,
Gynecology, and Reproductive Sciences
Emma Sue Hightower Professor of Obstetrics & Gynecology
The University of Texas—Houston Medical School
Houston, Texas*

John C. Hauth, MD

*Professor and Interim Chairman,
Department of Obstetrics & Gynecology
J. Marion Sims Endowed Chair in Obstetrics & Gynecology
University of Alabama at Birmingham
Birmingham, Alabama*

Katharine D. Wenstrom, MD

*Professor, Department of Obstetrics & Gynecology
Co-Director, Division of Maternal-Fetal Medicine
University of Alabama at Birmingham
Birmingham, Alabama*

McGRAW-HILL
Medical Publishing Division

*New York   Chicago   San Francisco   Lisbon   London   Madrid   Mexico City
Milan   New Delhi   San Juan   Seoul   Singapore   Sydney   Toronto*

McGraw-Hill

A Division of The McGraw·Hill Companies

1234567890   DOW   DOW   0987654321

ISBN 0-8385-9647-9 (domestic)

This book was set in New Times Roman by The PRD Group, Inc.
The editors were Andrea Seils, Susan R. Noujaim, and
Karen Davis.
The production supervisor was Richard Ruzycka.
The text designer was Joan O'Connor.
The cover designer was Mary McKeon.
The index was prepared by Coughlin Indexing Services, Inc.
RR Donnelley & Sons was printer and binder.

This book is printed on acid-free paper.

Library of Congress Cataloging-in-Publication Data

Williams obstetrics / F. Gary Cunningham . . . [et al.].—21st ed.
    p. ; cm.
    Includes bibliographical references and index. [ADJUST 008?]
    ISBN 0-8385-9647-9 (alk. paper)
    1. Obstetrics. I. Title: Obstetrics. II. Cunningham, F. Gary. III.
Williams, J. Whitridge (John Whitridge), 1866–1931. Obstretrics.
    [DNLM: 1. Obstetrics. WQ 100 W7283 2001]
RG524.W7 2001
618.2—dc21
                                                          2001030497

ISBN 0-07-112195-1 (international)
Exclusive rights by The McGraw-Hill Companies, Inc., for manufacture and export. This book cannot be re-exported from the country to which it is consigned by McGraw-Hill. The International Edition is not available in North America.

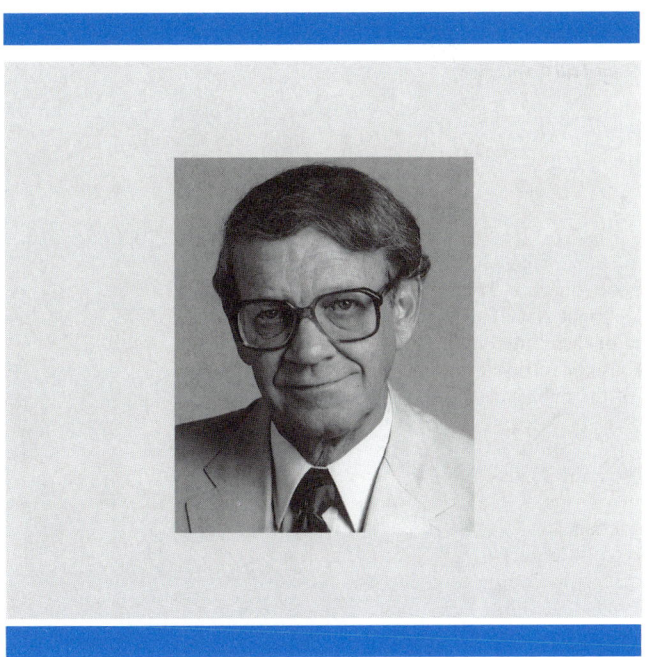

It is with sadness and pride that we dedicate this 21st Edition of *Williams Obstetrics* to Dr. Paul C. MacDonald. The sadness is because of his death on November 25, 1997. The pride comes from our association with him and his career which culminated at the time of his death as Professor of Obstetrics & Gynecology at The University of Texas Southwestern Medical Center at Dallas as well as the Cecil H. and Ida Green Distinguished Chair in Reproductive Biology and Director of the Cecil H. and Ida Green Center for Reproductive Biology Sciences.

After his residency training at Parkland Hospital, Paul MacDonald was a member of an elite group of young obstetrician-gynecologists who studied steroid biochemistry with Dr. Seymour Lieberman at Columbia University. After his return to Dallas, Dr. MacDonald rapidly earned a reputation as an astute clinician, a gifted teacher, and a brilliant investigator. His distinguished career was spent wedding the basic sciences with obstetrics, gynecology, and human reproduction. His earliest scientific discoveries included elucidation of the origin and metabolism of gonadal and adrenal steroid hormones in children, women, and men. While he served as Chairman of Obstetrics & Gynecology at UT Southwestern from 1970 to 1977, he developed a close relationship with the well-known philanthropists, Mr. and Mrs. Cecil H. Green. Mr. Green, a co-founder of Texas Instruments, endowed the Cecil H. and Ida Green Center for Reproductive Sciences headed by Dr. MacDonald as the Green Distinguished Chair in Reproductive Biology. The accomplishments of Dr. MacDonald and his team of clinicians and scientists included biochemical and molecular foundations of the initiation of human parturition; pathophysiology of pregnancy-induced hypertension; physiology and pathophysiology of endometrium; extraglandular estrogen formation in postmenopausal women and its relationship to obesity, age, and endometrial cancer; dehydroepiandrosterone sulfate as the precursor of placental estrogen in human pregnancy; and human fetal lung development and the respiratory distress syndrome of newborns.

For over 25 years, there were many clinician-scientists and postdoctoral fellows who trained with Dr. MacDonald and who subsequently served as division chiefs, departmental chairs, and deans of medical schools. He held numerous distinguished appointments including study sections, peer-review committees, and task forces for the National Institutes of Health and the March of Dimes. He was elected to the Institute of Medicine in 1987 and to the American Academy of Arts and Sciences in 1997. One particularly cherished honor was the Paul C. MacDonald Professorship in Obstetrics & Gynecology established by his trainees in conjunction with other national academics as well as community obstetricians-gynecologists. Shortly following his death, these same individuals tripled the endowment to that of the Paul C. MacDonald Distinguished Chair in Obstetrics & Gynecology.

A tireless worker, Dr. MacDonald always found time to offer help and to stimulate young clinicians and scientists. He demanded perfection of himself as well as those with whom he worked, but he always gave full credit to the entire team for their successes. He will be fondly remembered for his provocative insights into human reproduction and for his remarkable humanity.

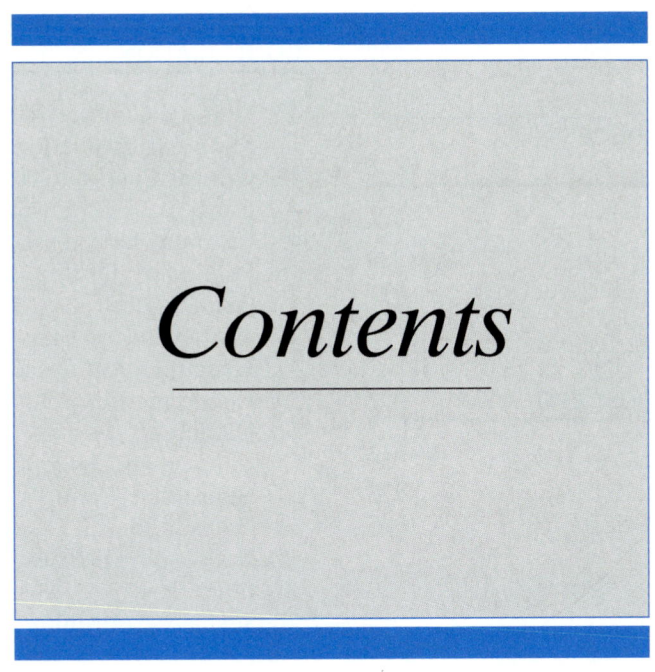

Contents

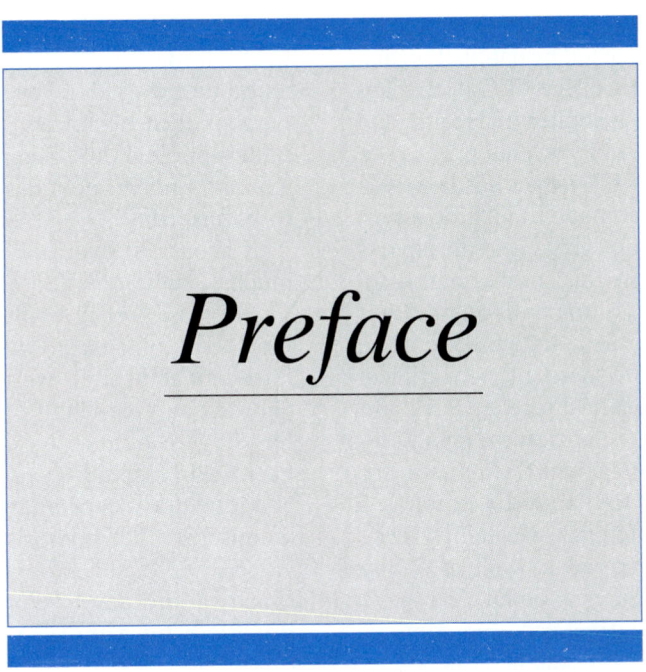

Preface

As *Williams Obstetrics* nears its 100th year of active service, we are again reminded of this excerpt from the preface in the First Edition:

> *In the following pages I have attempted to set forth with thoroughness the scientific basis for the practical application of the obstetrical art.... At the same time I have endeavored to present the more practical aspects of obstetrics in such a manner as to be of direct service to the obstetrician at the bedside.*
>
> JOHN WHITRIDGE WILLIAMS (1903)

This philosophy did not change in nineteen editions of this text that followed during the 20th century. The evolution of obstetrics as a clinical specialty was largely accomplished through the first half of the 1900s. Beginning then, academic leaders in our specialty demanded scientific verification of principles that underlie obstetrical practice. Thus, through the leadership of a relatively small number of "giants" in our field, scientific underpinnings of obstetrics began to assume a role of primary importance after the mid-20th century. Extensive research into maternal and fetal physiology, as well as endocrinology, infectious diseases, ultrasonography, and genetics paved the way for the birth of the subspecialty of Maternal-Fetal Medicine in the 1970s. Subsequently, genomic research and development of molecular techniques allowed opening of vistas in obstetrical research that likely will keep us busy much of the 21st century.

In addition to research to provide scientific proof of clinical practices, the demand for evidence-based medicine and documentation of clinical outcomes has been a major driving force in clinical medicine for the past two decades. Although there is no doubt that medicine remains an art, it is also a science, and many of these changes were long overdue.

For all of these reasons, our mandate to chronicle scientific and medical advances in this textbook, along with their clinical application to the care of mother and fetus, has assumed monumental proportions. With all of these caveats, is it possible for a single obstetrical textbook to be "everything to all"? Although the obvious answer may appear to be *no*, we have endeavored to provide to the practitioner of obstetrics and of maternal-fetal medicine scientific and clinical data that underlie recommendations for clinical practice. To help achieve this goal, we have sought new talent. Two new editors from the University of Alabama at Birmingham bring with them special expertise in the field of evidence-based clinical medicine and state-of-the-art application of clinical and molecular genetics as they pertain to obstetrics. Because of our participation in the Maternal-Fetal Medicine Units Network, we also draw heavily from the experiences of this multi-center collaborative to elucidate important problems that plague the mother and fetus. Careful consideration of the discoveries highlighted each year at the annual meetings of the Society for Maternal-Fetal Medicine and Society for Gynecologic Investigation also provides contemporaneous data. Finally, and as before, we continue to emphasize clinical practice recommendations that are promulgated by national organizations to include the American College of Obstetricians and Gynecologists, the National Institutes of Health, and the Centers for Disease Control and Prevention.

The 21st edition of *Williams Obstetrics* has been extensively revised and an attempt made to include a synopsis of the burgeoning literature relevant to all aspects of our specialty. To accomplish this, more than 4000 new references have been cited along with an addition of over 250 new figures and tables. As we have done for the past seven editions, we cite frequently our clinical experiences from the Obstetrical Service at Parkland Hospital. To our sometimes vocal critics, we again emphasize that these clinical management schemata are not the only acceptable ones that may be employed to obtain excellent clinical outcomes. Certainly these management guidelines have served us well in caring for over 400,000 indigent pregnant women. We have also cited time-honored clinical practices used contemporaneously at the University of Texas at Houston as well as the University of Alabama at Birmingham, and we again emphasize that these may be only one of several acceptable methods of management.

We are fortunate to have a large number of vitally important people who have helped us complete this work. At The University of Texas Southwestern, we are especially indebted to Dr. Linette Casey for her expertise in basic physiology and endocrinology of human reproduction, placental development and function, fetal development, and the science of parturition. Drs. George Wendel and Jeanne Sheffield provided valuable insight into infections and sexually transmitted diseases, Dr. Barry Schwarz for contraceptive and sterilization techniques, and Dr. David Miller for trophoblastic disease. Drs. Diane Twickler, Rigoberto Santos, and Jodi Dashe generously supplied ultrasonographs as well as other types of maternal and fetal imaging. Drs. Shiv Sharma and Donald Wallace provided input into the subject of obstetrical anesthesia. Finally, Dr. Don McIntire was essential for provision of demographic and prevalence statistics cited throughout many chapters. Importantly, much of the stimulus to determine why, when, and how tenets evolve in obstetrics was provided by our Maternal-Fetal Medicine fellows who were unre-

lenting! These include Drs. Nicole Yost, Jeanne Sheffield, Gerda Zeeman, and Julie Lo. Finally, the massive amount of work done by our residents, nurses, and other personnel in obstetrics and gynecology should not be underappreciated. Their dedication to the care of women, and in most cases indigent women, continues to be inspiring.

It is easy to overlook administrative duties when so much time is devoted to the creation of a textbook. To this end, many of the administrative duties at the University of Texas Southwestern Medical Center and Parkland Hospital were carried out by Dr. Barry Schwarz as Vice-Chair of Obstetrics & Gynecology and Dr. Steve Bloom as Associate Director of Obstetrics at Parkland Hospital.

Meticulous coordination of this multi-institutional manuscript that comprised over 4500 pages was provided by Marsha Congleton and Connie Utterback. Much of the day-to-day production was provided by Beverly King, Minnie Tregaskis, Melinda Epstein, Cynthia Allen, Barbara Smith, Leticia Varela, Lynne McDonnell, Julie Thompson, Jeanette Cogburn, Dina Trujillano, and Ellen Watkins in Dallas; Carol Durham and Grace Lopez at the University of Texas at Houston; and Belinda Rials and Rhonda Scott at the University of Alabama at Birmingham. As she had in the previous two editions, Nancy Marshburn lent her considerable artistic experience to the development of new and revised figures.

After almost 100 years, *Williams Obstetrics* has a new publisher. In the very short time we have known and worked with them, Andrea Seils, Susan Noujaim, Karen Davis, and Marty Wonsiewicz of McGraw-Hill have proven to be excellent colleagues as well as good friends. Happily, joining the new McGraw-Hill team from Appleton & Lange is John Williams, who has ably served as production editor the last three volumes. To all of these people, as well as to many, many more not cited, we as always are grateful.

Finally, our families have made contributions to this text in a number of ways, perhaps the most apparent being less time that we could spend with them. Thus, to Deann Gant, Marjorie Leveno, JoEllen Gilstrap, and Dr. Dwight Rouse, we offer our thanks for their unwavering support.

I

Human Pregnancy

1

Obstetrics in Broad Perspective

Publication of this 21st edition of *Williams Obstetrics* is conspicuously coincidental with the beginning of the 21st century. Indeed, the first 20 editions of this textbook have encompassed the 20th century and chronicled dramatic advances in obstetrics. As shown in Table 1–1, healthier mothers and babies ranks as one of the 10 great public health achievements in the United States between 1900 and 1999. At the beginning of the century, almost 1 in every 100 women giving birth in this country died of pregnancy-related complications, and nearly 1 of 10 infants died before age 1 year (Centers for Disease Control, 1999b). As shown in Figures 1–1 and 1–2, by the end of the 20th century, infant mortality had declined more than 90 percent to 7.2 per 1000 live births in 1997, and the maternal mortality rate declined almost 99 percent to 7.7 deaths per 100,000 live births in 1997.

This chapter provides a synopsis of the current state of maternal and newborn health in the United States. Following this is a perspective on the forces affecting obstetrics as we begin what we hope will become another successful century of *Williams Obstetrics*.

VITAL STATISTICS

The vital statistics of the United States are collected and published through a decentralized, cooperative system (Tolson and colleagues, 1991). Responsibility for the registration of births, deaths, fetal deaths, marriages, divorces, annulments, and induced terminations of pregnancy is vested in the individual states and certain separate governmental entities. The system comprises 57 registration areas: each state, the District of Columbia, New York City, American Samoa, Guam, the Northern Mariana Islands, Puerto Rico, and the Virgin Islands.

The first standard certificates for the registration of live births and deaths were developed in 1900. An act

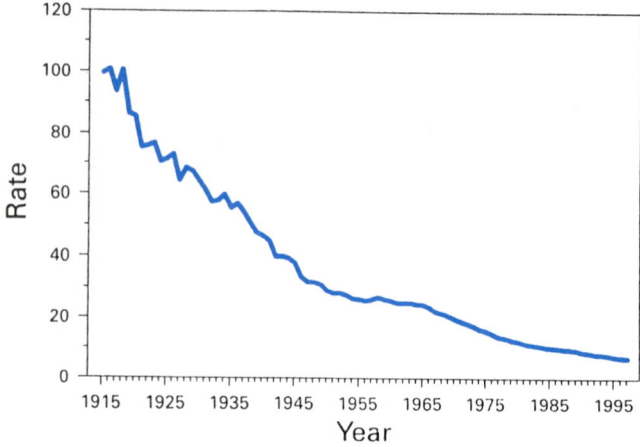

FIGURE 1–1. Infant mortality rate per 1000 live births, United States 1915–1997. (From the Centers for Disease Control, 1999a.)

of Congress in 1902 established the Bureau of the Census to develop a system for the annual collection of vital statistics. The overall objective was to develop and maintain a system for registration that is uniform in such matters as forms, procedures, and statistical methodology. The Bureau retained the authority for producing national vital statistics until 1946, when the function was transferred to the United States Public Health Service. It is presently assigned to the Division of Vital Statistics of the National Center for Health Statistics. The standard certificate of live birth was substantially revised in 1989 to include much more information on medical and lifestyle risk factors and also obstetrical care practices. Currently, more than 99 percent of births in the United States are registered (Ventura and colleagues, 2000). According to Dr. Stephanie Ventura of the National Center for Health Statistics, another revision of the birth certificate is planned for 2003. Changes

TABLE 1–1. Ten Great Public Health Achievements in the United States—1990–1999

Vaccination
Motor-vehicle safety
Safer workplaces
Control of infectious diseases
Decline in deaths from coronary heart disease and stroke
Safer and healthier foods
Healthier mothers and babies
Family planning
Fluoridation of drinking water
Recognition of tobacco use as a health hazard

From the Centers for Disease Control (1999b).

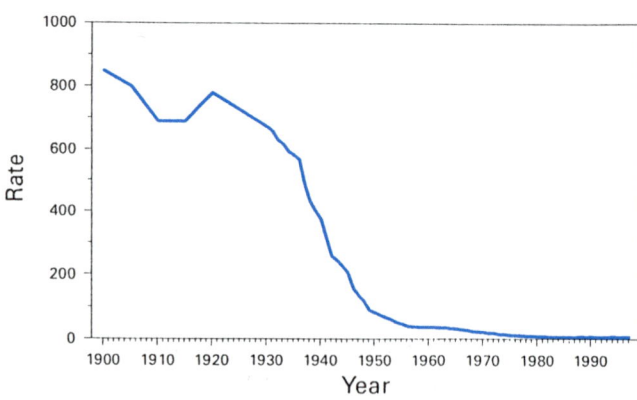

FIGURE 1–2. Maternal mortality rate per 100,000 live births by year—United States, 1900–1997. (From the Centers for Disease Control, 1999a.)

will include a format conducive to electronic processing, more explicit demographic data on the parents, and an improved selection of information regarding antepartum and intrapartum complications. Some examples of new data to be collected include labor progress, uterine rupture, blood transfusions, and pregnancy resulting from infertility treatment.

DEFINITIONS. To allow comparison of data from not only one state or region of the country to another, but from one country to another, uniform use of standard definitions is encouraged by the World Health Organization as well as the American Academy of Pediatrics and the American College of Obstetricians and Gynecologists (1997). It is recommended that United States statistics include all fetuses and infants born weighing at least 500 g, whether alive or dead. It should be clarified, however, that the states are not uniform in their reporting requirements for fetal deaths. For example, 28 states stipulate that fetal deaths beginning at 20 weeks' gestation should be recorded, eight states report all products of conception as fetal deaths, and still others use birthweights of 350 g, 400 g, or 500 g or greater to identify fetal deaths.

Definitions recommended by the National Center for Health Statistics and the Centers for Disease Control and Prevention are as follows:

- **Perinatal period.** This includes all births weighing 500 g or more and ends at 28 completed days after birth. When perinatal rates are based on gestational age, rather than birthweight, it is recommended that the perinatal period be defined to commence at 20 weeks.
- **Birth.** The complete expulsion or extraction from the mother of a fetus, irrespective of whether the umbilical cord has been cut or the placenta is attached. Fetuses weighing less than 500 g are usually not considered as births, but rather are termed abortuses for purposes of vital statistics.
- **Birthweight.** The weight of a neonate determined immediately after delivery or as soon thereafter as feasible. It should be expressed to the nearest gram.
- **Birthrate.** This is the number of live births per 1000 population.
- **Fertility rate.** This is the number of live births per 1000 females 15 through 44 years of age.
- **Live birth.** Whenever the infant at or sometime after birth breathes spontaneously, or shows any other sign of life such as a heartbeat or definite spontaneous movement of voluntary muscles, it is recorded as a live birth. Heartbeats are to be distinguished from transient cardiac contractions, and respirations are to be distinguished from fleeting respiratory efforts or gasps.
- **Stillbirth (fetal death).** No signs of life are present at or after birth.

- **Neonatal death.** Early neonatal death refers to death of a live-born infant during the first 7 days after birth. Late neonatal death refers to death after 7 days, but before 29 days.
- **Stillbirth rate (fetal death rate).** The number of stillborn infants per 1000 infants born, including live births and stillbirths.
- **Neonatal mortality rate.** The number of neonatal deaths per 1000 live births.
- **Perinatal mortality rate.** The number of stillbirths plus neonatal deaths per 1000 total births.
- **Infant death.** Includes all deaths of live-born infants from birth through 12 months of age.
- **Infant mortality rate.** The number of infant deaths per 1000 live births.
- **Low birthweight.** The first newborn weight obtained after birth is less than 2500 g.
- **Very low birthweight.** The first newborn weight obtained after birth is less than 1500 g.
- **Extremely low birthweight.** The first newborn weight obtained after birth is less than 1000 g.
- **Term infant.** An infant born anytime after 37 completed weeks of gestation and up until 42 completed weeks of gestation (260 to 294 days) is considered to be a term infant.
- **Preterm infant.** An infant born before 37 completed weeks (259th day).
- **Postterm infant.** An infant born anytime after completion of the 42nd week beginning with day 295.
- **Abortus.** A fetus or embryo removed or expelled from the uterus during the first half of gestation (20 weeks or less), weighing less than 500 g.
- **Induced termination of pregnancy.** The purposeful interruption of an intrauterine pregnancy with the intention other than to produce a live-born infant, and which does not result in a live birth. This definition excludes retention of products of conception following fetal death.
- **Direct maternal death.** This includes death of the mother resulting from obstetrical complications of pregnancy, labor, or the puerperium, and from interventions, omissions, incorrect treatment, or a chain of events resulting from any of these factors. An example is maternal death from exsanguination from rupture of the uterus.
- **Indirect maternal death.** This includes a maternal death not directly due to an obstetrical cause, but resulting from previously existing disease, or a disease that developed during pregnancy, labor, or the puerperium, but which was aggravated by maternal physiological adaptation to pregnancy. An example is maternal death from complications of mitral stenosis.
- **Nonmaternal death.** Death of the mother resulting from accidental or incidental causes not related to pregnancy are classified as nonmaternal deaths. An

example is death from an automobile accident or con-current malignancy.

- **Maternal mortality ratio.** The number of maternal deaths that result from the reproductive process per 100,000 live births. Used more commonly, but less accurately, are the terms *maternal mortality rate* or *maternal death rate*. The term ratio is more accurate because it includes in the numerator the number of deaths regardless of pregnancy outcome—for example, live births, stillbirths, ectopic pregnancies—while the denominator includes the number of live births.

PREGNANCY IN THE UNITED STATES

Pregnancy, and by extension obstetrics, has a major impact on the health of the nation. Data from diverse sources have been used to provide the following snapshot of pregnancy during the last years of the 20th century in the United States.

In 1998, the population of the United States was 269 million people and the fertility rate for women 15 to 44 years of age was 67 live births per 1000 women (National Center for Health Statistics, 2000). There were 3.94 million live births in 1998 which, when offset by 2.34 million deaths, resulted in a net increase in the population of 1.6 million people. Life expectancy for those born in 1998 was 76.5 years (Anderson, 1999).

The number of births in 1998 increased by 2 percent, and this was the first annual increase in the United States after a 7-year decline between 1990 and 1997 (U.S. News and World Report, 2000). American women average 3.2 pregnancies over their lifetimes, and 1.8 of these were considered wanted pregnancies (Ventura and colleagues, 1999). As shown in Figure 1–3, unwanted pregnancies are related to lesser amounts of education in the mother. About 1 percent of infants born to never-married women were relinquished for adoption in 1995, which is down from 9 percent of births before 1979 (Chandra and associates, 1999). After exclusion of fetal losses and induced terminations, American women on average deliver 2.0 live births in a lifetime.

Using 1996 as an example, there were 6.24 million pregnancies in the United States (Table 1–2 and Fig. 1–4); 62 percent ended with live births, 22 percent ended by induced terminations, and 16 percent were spontaneous miscarriages. Notable changes with regard to the setting and timing of births as well as in the birth attendant have taken place in the United States (Curtin and Park, 1999). Osteopaths and midwives are delivering an increasing share of births, but nearly all of these increases have been for in-hospital births. The use of electronic fetal monitoring, ultrasound, and labor induction and stimulation all increased, with the most dramatic change being the doubling in the number of births that

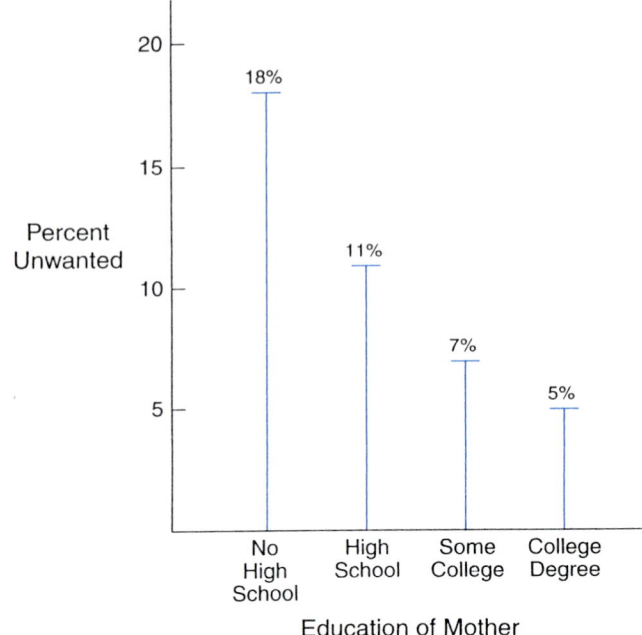

FIGURE 1–3. Proportion of births unwanted by the mother as compared with education status—United States, 1995. (Data from Ventura and colleagues, 1999.)

were induced. Partly as a result of the rise in inductions, there are more births on weekdays. The highest number of births occur in the summer months, with births most likely to occur on Tuesday throughout the year.

Pregnancy care is a major component of the American health care scene. In 1998, delivery was the second leading cause for hospitalization behind heart disease (Hall and Popovic, 2000). The average length of hospital stay for all deliveries was 2.5 days. Prenatal care was the fourth leading reason for office visits to physicians and accounted for nearly 23 million visits in 1997 (Woodwell, 1999). In 1991 and 1993 there were approximately 720,000 non–delivery-related hospitalizations for pregnancy complications, amounting to hospitalization for one in five pregnancies (Bennett and co-authors, 1998). Nondelivery hospitalizations have decreased substantially since the late 1980s, presumably due to managed care efforts to minimize expenditures. The leading indication for hospitalization unrelated to delivery was preterm labor. Nicholson and co-workers (2000) have estimated that the total national cost, in 1996 dollars, for hospitalization for preterm labor that did not eventuate in delivery was $360 million. This number increased to $820 million when those women with preterm labor and who actually delivered early, were added.

The magazine *OBG Management* (1999) surveyed approximately 1 percent of obstetricians-gynecologists in the United States in an effort to assess the state of obstetrics at the turn of the 20th century. The average

TABLE 1–2. Fetal and Neonatal Mortality in the United States—1950–1998

Year	Fetal Mortality Rate[a]	Neonatal Mortality Rate[b]
1950	18.4	20.5
1960	15.8	18.7
1970	14.0	15.1
1980	9.1	8.5
1985	7.8	7.0
1990	7.5	5.8
1991	7.3	5.6
1992	7.4	5.4
1993	7.1	5.3
1994	7.0	5.1
1995	7.0	4.9
1996	6.9	4.8
1997	6.8	4.8
1998	6.7	4.8

[a]Fetal deaths of 20 weeks or more.
[b]Infant deaths of less than 29 days per 1000 live births.
(Data from Murphy, 2000.)

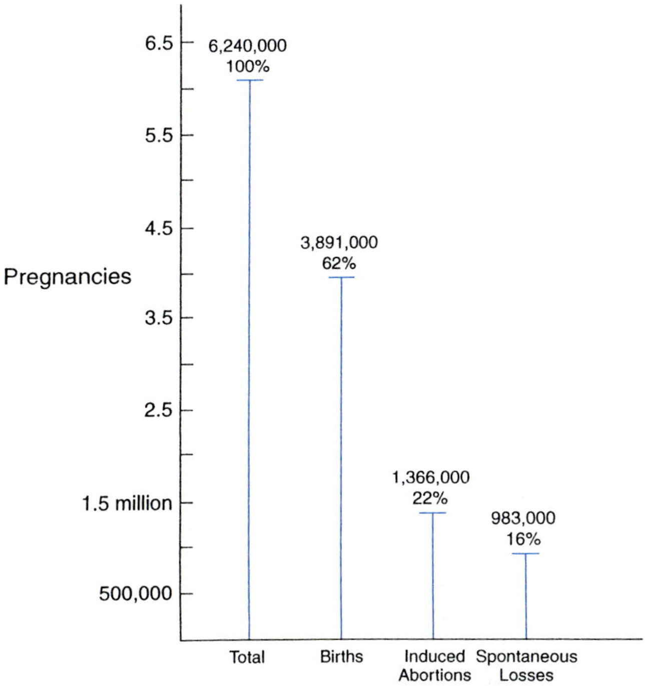

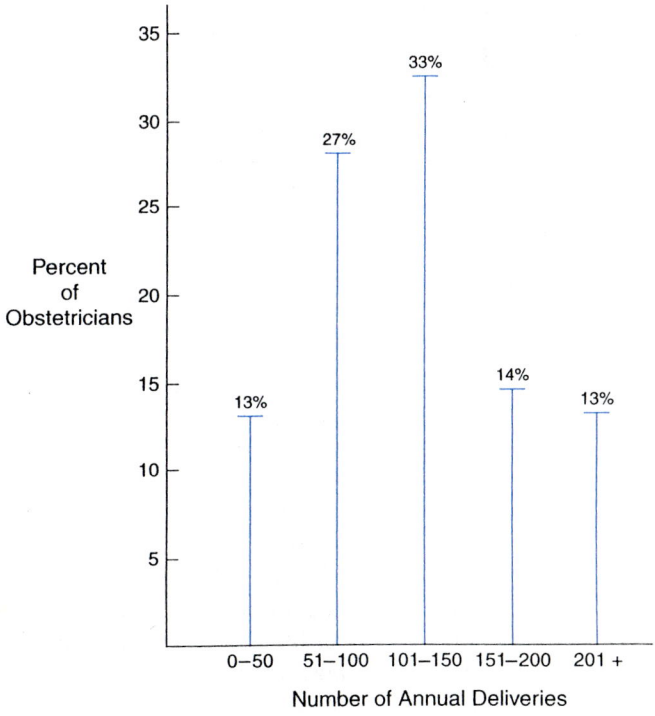

FIGURE 1–4. Results of 6,240,000 pregnancies in the United States, 1996. (Data from Ventura and colleagues, 1999.)

number of deliveries in 1998 was 140 per obstetrician (Fig. 1–5). More than 80 percent of those who responded to the survey reported that they continued to practice obstetrics as well as gynecology. Those who gave a reason for discontinuing their obstetrics practice cited medicolegal concerns, professional-liability premiums, and declining reimbursement as the reasons they stopped. Among those who still practice obstetrics, about 40 percent anticipated that their obstetrical caseload would increase in 1999.

HEALTHY PEOPLE 2010

In 1991, the United States Public Health Service issued a report titled *Healthy People 2000,* which proposed goals for improving the health of mothers and infants by the year 2000. Of the 17 maternal and infant health objectives included in *Healthy People 2000,* progress was made in eight objectives. In five objectives, however, movement was away from the target. Notable gains were made in the areas of infant death, fetal death, cesarean delivery (particularly repeat cesareans), breast feeding, early use of prenatal care, hospitalization for pregnancy complications, abstinence from tobacco use during pregnancy, and screening for fetal abnormalities and genetic disorders. For the remaining objectives, changes were neither positive or negative. These included maternal death, fetal alcohol syndrome, and low birthweight.

FIGURE 1–5. Number of annual deliveries by obstetricians-gynecologists in 1998. (From OBG Management, 1999.)

TABLE 1–3. Some Goals for Mothers and Infants for 2010

Outcome	1997 Baseline	2010 Goal
Fetal deaths before 20 weeks	6.8/1000	4.1/1000
Neonatal deaths through 28 days	4.8/1000	2.9/1000
Maternal deaths	8.4/100,000	3.3/100,000

From Healthy People 2010, Centers for Disease Control and Prevention and the Health Resources and Services Administration (2000).

New objectives for maternal and infant health have been promulgated for this decade as *Healthy People 2010.* Some of these goals are shown in Table 1–3, using 1997 data for a baseline. There were 27,968 infant deaths in 1997, and as shown in Figure 1–6, two thirds of these were within the first month of life. When analyzed by

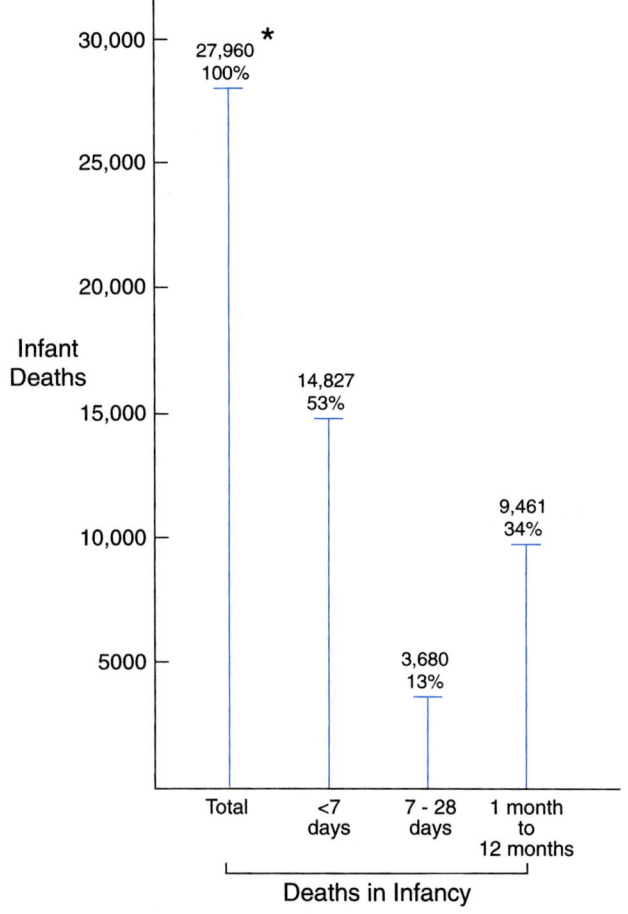

FIGURE 1–6. Infant deaths from birth through 12 months—United States, 1997. (Data from MacDorman and Atkinson, 1999.)

* Birthweight not stated for 333 infants

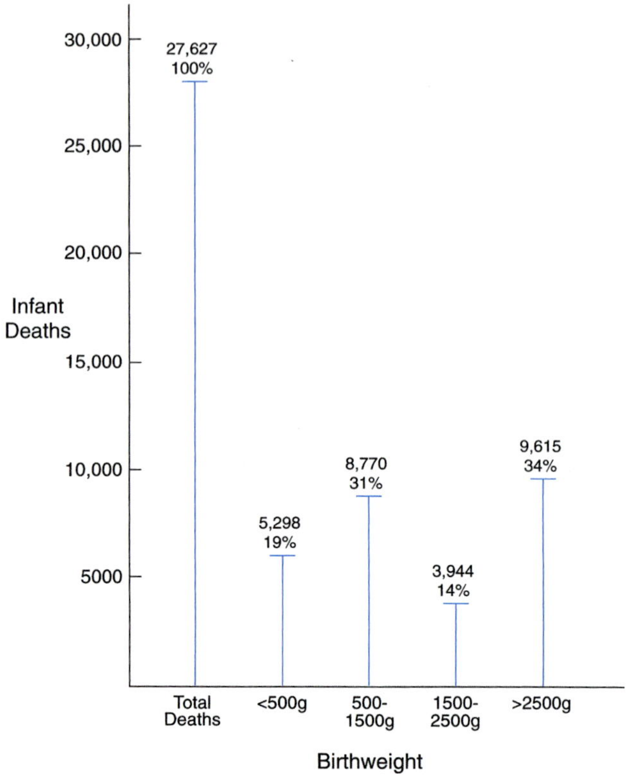

FIGURE 1–7. Infant deaths from birth through 12 months according to birthweight—United States, 1997. (Data from MacDorman and Atkinson, 1999.)

birthweight, two thirds of infant deaths were in low-birthweight infants (Fig. 1–7). Of particular interest are those births less than 500 g where neonatal intensive care is now often offered. In 1997 there were 5994 live births weighing less than 500 g and 87 percent of these died during the first 28 days of life. Of the 784 who survived the first 28 days of life, 696—12 percent of all births less than 500 g—survived infancy. St. John and associates (2000) have estimated the total cost of initial care in this country for all newborn infants was $10.2 billion annually. Almost 60 percent of this expenditure is attributed to preterm births before 37 weeks, and 12 percent is spent on infants born between 24 and 26 weeks.

In addition to deaths during infancy, the effect of pregnancy and childbirth on women's health is an important indicator of national health. In 1997, a total of 327 maternal deaths were identified by vital statistics (Hoyert and colleagues, 1999). It should be emphasized, however, that it is estimated that more than half of maternal deaths are not ascertained (Koonin and colleagues, 1997). As shown in Figure 1–8, there is considerable disparity in maternal mortality when analyzed according to race. Pregnancy-related mortality for black

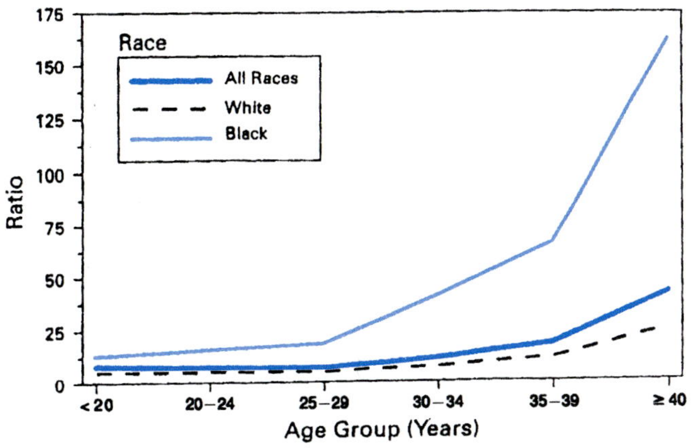

FIGURE 1–8. Pregnancy-related mortality ratio (deaths per 100,000 live births) by age group and race—United States, 1987–1990. (From Koonin and colleagues, 1997.)

women is three to four times higher than for white women. The maternal death differential between African-Americans and whites is highest for those pregnancies that did not end in birth of an infant. These include ectopic pregnancy, spontaneous and induced abortions, and gestational trophoblastic disease (Centers for Disease Control and Prevention, 1995). Shown in Table 1–4 are the causes of maternal death according to the outcome of pregnancy. Hemorrhage and infection are prominent causes of death in ectopic pregnancies and abortions, whereas hypertension, embolism, hemorrhage, and infection are the leading causes of maternal death in women delivered after midpregnancy.

PERSPECTIVES ON OBSTETRICS

Medical writers have recently turned to the opening line of Charles Dickens's *A Tale of Two Cities* to describe

TABLE 1–4. Percentage of Pregnancy-Related Maternal Deaths by Cause and Outcome of Pregnancy—United States, 1987–1990

| | Pregnancy Outcome | | | | |
Cause of Death	Live Birth	Still-Birth	Ectopic	Abortion	Molar
Hemorrhage	21	27	95	19	17
Embolism	23	11	1	11	—
Pregnancy hypertension	24	26	—	1	—
Infection	12	19	1	49	—
Cardiomyopathy	6	3	—	—	—
Anesthesia	3	0	2	9	—
Other	11	14	—	11	83

From Koonin and colleagues (1997).

these prevailing times in medicine and obstetrics as "the best of times. . . the worst of times. . ." (Grumbach, 1999; Morrison, 2000). Why are these times at once the best and worst of times for obstetrics? There are many reasons for this, and some are now considered.

BEST OF TIMES. The chronicle of maternal and infant mortality during the 20th century described earlier should suggest that much is good in the health care of women and their infants—indeed, better than it has ever been. "Better than ever" should be read here as previously unparalleled rather than unsurpassable because continual improvement must inevitably remain the goal in obstetrics.

These times could be the best of times for many other reasons. Just to mention a few would include the ascendance of evidence-based medicine. There have been striking developments in the study of the molecular basis for many diseases. In fact, gene therapy was recently first reported successful to "cure" severe combined immunodeficiency disease (Cavazzana-Calvo and colleagues, 2000). There has been completion of the mapping of the human genome. Importantly, the swelling ranks of women in obstetrics and gynecology is expected to reach parity with men by 2014 (American College of Obstetricians and Gynecologists, 1999b).

The National Institutes of Health is leading the current emphasis on outcomes-based research. In obstetrics, the National Institute of Child Health and Human Development has formed two clinical networks that are crucial to the study of obstetrical outcomes. The Maternal–Fetal Medicine Units Network and the Neonatal Units Network are multicenter groups that conduct investigations to study some of the more vexing and important problems in obstetrics and neonatal medicine. Not surprisingly, preterm labor and delivery as well as preeclampsia are in the foreground of these efforts.

The year 2000 marks the 50th anniversary of the American College of Obstetricians and Gynecologists (Pearse, 2000). Originally formed to promote continuing education, in 1975 the college became involved in legislative initiatives in a number of important arenas to include regionalization of perinatal care, maternal and child health, patient education, and most recently, to provide uninterrupted access of women to the obstetrician-gynecologist as their primary care physician.

In the 20th edition of *Williams Obstetrics* we offered the cartoon shown in Figure 1–9 to highlight the effects of for-profit managed care on obstetrics. We could use this same cartoon to highlight in this 21st edition the tempering of the effects of HMOs that has transpired in the last 5 years. Notably, mandatory early discharge was curtailed by federal legislation through the Newborns' and Mothers' Health Protection Act that went

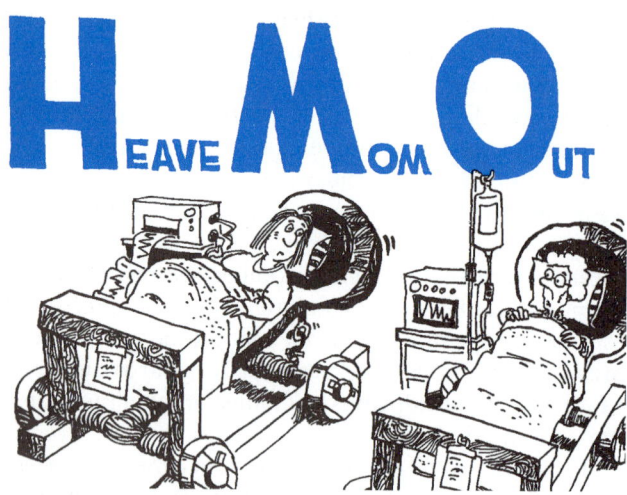

FIGURE 1–9. This 1995 editorial cartoon was shown in *Williams Obstetrics,* 20th edition, to give a new meaning to the acronym, HMO. (From Wasserman, 1995, Copyright, 1995, Boston Globe. Distributed by Los Angeles Times Syndicate. Reprinted by permission.)

into effect in January 1998 (Bragg and colleagues, 1997). Because of this, it is no longer legally possible to "heave mom out" before 48 hours. Because this is a victory of sorts, the cartoon is republished. If so much is fundamentally good in obstetrics, why the ambiguous contradiction that these are also the worst of times?

WORST OF TIMES. Among the most pressing challenges facing obstetrics and gynecology is that of epidemic *human immunodeficiency viral infection* (HIV). But there is even some good news here. Specifically, in 1995, according to the Centers for Disease Control and Prevention (1996), HIV infection was the leading cause of death in women 25 to 44 years old. By 1998, however, HIV-infection had dropped to the fifth leading cause of death in all 25- to 44-year-old Americans (Martin and colleagues, 1999). It unfortunately remained the number one cause of mortality for African-American men in this age group.

There are a number of other indicators from the National Center for Health Statistics and the Centers for Disease Control and Prevention that indicate African-American women are at a significant reproductive disadvantage. Although as shown in Figure 1–8, appreciable progress has been made in decreasing the maternal mortality ratio in both races, a disparate fourfold mortality rate endures in black women compared with whites. Not shown are data indicating that Hispanic women also have higher mortality ratios compared with white women, although the disparity is not as great as for African-American women (Hopkins and co-authors, 1999). Federal agencies reporting these statistics continue to emphasize that much of the disparity in mortal-

ity results from poor availability of medical care for minority women. This is even more apparent in deaths from ectopic pregnancy (Chap. 34, p. 886).

Unplanned pregnancy, especially among teenagers, is also a best and worst of times contradiction. According to the Centers for Disease Control and Prevention (2000a), the birth rate for teenagers in the United States has continually declined during the 1990s, and in 1998 was near the 1986 low record (Fig. 1–10). While this is good news, there still were 173,252 births recorded in 1998 to 15- to 17-year-old teenagers. These accounted for 4.5 percent of all births in the nation.

Obesity continues to increase in America. Results from the 1997 National Health Interview Survey indicate that half of adults are overweight and 20 percent are frankly obese (Centers for Disease Control and Prevention, 2000). The impact of this in current pregnancy is considered in Chapter 48 (p. 1298), and its impact on future generations in Chapter 29 (p. 757).

Domestic violence is a large problem in our country where nearly 5 million adult women experience physical

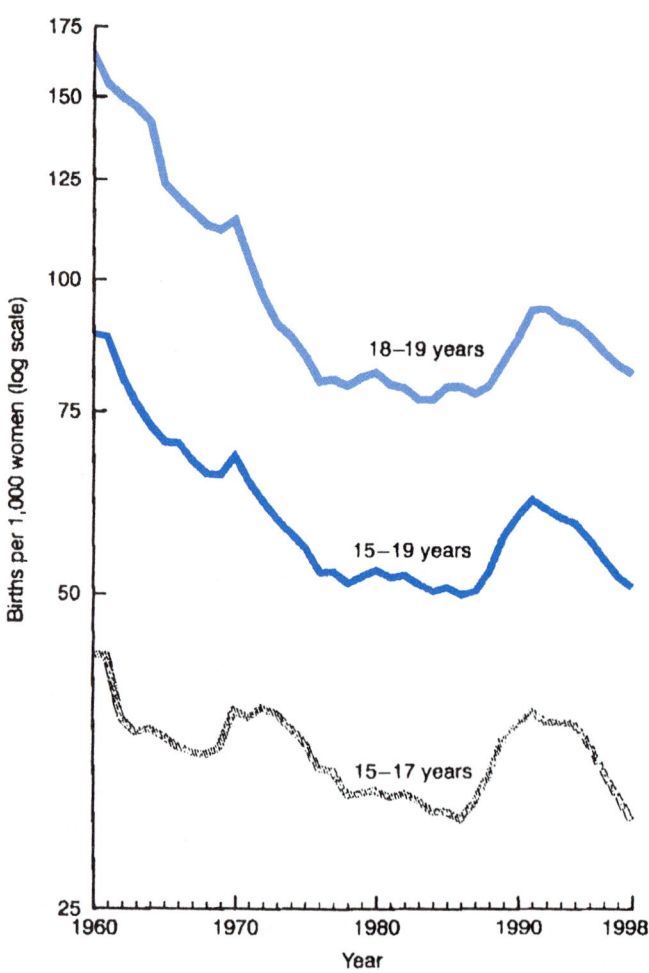

FIGURE 1–10. Birth rates for teenagers by age—United States, 1960–1998. (From Ventura and colleagues, 1999.)

abuse each year (American College of Obstetricians and Gynecologists, 1999a). As discussed in Chapter 43 (p. 1171), such abuse does not stop with pregnancy, and indeed, it may be exacerbated.

Other pressing problems include the erosion of health-care safety nets for the uninsured by for-profit plans that all too often quickly abandon the most vulnerable patients when profits are in jeopardy (Bodenheimer, 1997). There is evidence that the shifting of uninsured patients to for-profit medicine has substantially reduced the capacity to deliver the uncompensated care that is essential for the medically indigent (Lu and colleagues, 2000; Smith, 1997). It has also put minority communities at further risk for inferior health care and widened their already tragic disparity in health status (Murray-Garcia, 1997).

Another profound effect of transferring health care to the custody of the for-profit sector is the overwhelmingly negative effect that this has on the infrastructure that provides for teaching the coming generations of health-care providers. There is a similar deleterious effect on efforts to conduct the research necessary to move obstetrics forward (Weissman and colleagues, 1999). As Kuttner (1998) aptly described the situation, there are ". . . too many promoters, marketers, attorneys, underwriters, consultants, reviewers, and shareholders—all taking too big a cut of the premium dollar. . . ."

PORK BELLIES VERSUS PEOPLE. Dr. Marcia Angell, editor emeritus of the *New England Journal of Medicine,* summarized the current state of American health care in 1999: "The hallmark of the system is its reliance on the private market to deliver and, to a lesser extent, to fund health care. Accordingly, health care is treated as a commodity . . . other developed countries . . . consider it a social service, not a commodity." Hence the subtitle that juxtaposes pork bellies and people. Undoubtedly, the force most greatly affecting obstetrics as we begin the 21st century is the transformation for-profit medicine is forcing upon medicine.

The cost for medical malpractice—insurance premiums, attorney fees, and settlements and awards also continues to erode the health-care dollar. Tort reform has also had the best and worst of times in the recent decade. The *Daubert standard,* used in federal and most state courts, demands scientific evidence to support some of these claims of wrongdoing (Sturner and colleagues, 2000). Thus, in at least some cases, an "expert" with a degree and an opinion for sale cannot be heard without peer-reviewed evidence to support (frequently ludicrous) opinions. According to Mohr (2000), contingent fees are one of three legal factors that have helped to sustain malpractice litigation for 150 years. The contingency-fee system continues to offer personal injury attorneys the perverse incentive that encourages men-

dacity and promotes the "sleaze factor." Nowhere in obstetrics is this more prevalent than in "birth injury" litigation (Chap. 39, p. 1048). According to Collins (2000), in such cases it is not uncommon that obstetricians are expected to prove that their (in)actions did not cause neurological injury.

Attempts to mitigate some of these contentious issues have been only partially successful because of watered-down versions of legislations engineered by the plaintiffs bar. For example, Florida's Birth-Related Neurological Injury Compensation Plan was an experiment in no-fault compensation for brain-damaged babies. A RAND Corporation study by Studdert and associates (2000) found that within the first 10 years of the experiment, "bad baby" litigation continued unfettered in Florida. In fact, many plaintiff attorneys have pursued judgments both under the plan as well as in the courts! There can be no doubt that neurological impairment in a child is horrific and devastating, and as Brennan and colleagues (1996) have reported, it is the severity of injury that dictates payment, not the occurrence of an adverse event, even if due to negligence. Indeed, Cassidy and co-authors (2000) have shown that elimination of pain and suffering from insurance claims actually speeds recovery!

The impact of for-profit managed care was first addressed in the 20th edition of *Williams Obstetrics.* Much that has happened since that time gives us reason for optimism that these worst of times when health care is bought, sold, and traded like pork bellies, has perhaps run its course. Since our last writing, there has been an intense backlash from both the profession and the American health-care "consumer" (sic patient). For example, more than 89 articles on managed care—mostly on the abuses wrought by for-profit medicine—have appeared in the *New England Journal of Medicine* and the *Journal of the American Medical Association.* Shown in Table 1–5 is a selection of these articles that each serve to cross-section the unsavory effects for-profit medicine is having on health care as a profession and, more importantly, as a service to patients. The titles are self-explanatory.

SUMMARY OF THE STATE OF OBSTETRICS

Dr. Arnold Relman, editor emeritus of the *New England Journal of Medicine,* warned in 1980 that "The most important health-care development of the day is the recent, relatively unheralded use of a new industry that supplies health-care services for profit. Closer attention from the public and the profession, and careful study are necessary to ensure that the *medical-industrial complex* puts the interests of the public before those of the stockholders." At the 2000 Annual Clinical Meeting of the

TABLE 1–5. A Selection of Recent Articles on Managed Care in the Two Most Widely Subscribed National Journals

Topic of Article	Author and Source
A national bill of patients' rights.	Annas; *New England Journal of Medicine,* 1998.
The Medicare–HMO revolving door—the healthy go in and the sick go out.	Morgan and co-authors; *New England Journal of Medicine,* 1997
For our patients, not for profits—a call to action.	Himmelstein; *Journal of the American Medical Association,* 1997
Managed care and merger mania.	Fuchs; *Journal of the American Medical Association,* 1997
Who should determine when health care is medically necessary?	Rosenbaum and co-authors; *New England Journal of Medicine,* 1999
Bringing market medicine to professional account.	Emanuel; *Journal of the American Medical Association,* 1997
How large employers are shopping the health care marketplace.	Bodenheimer and Sullivan; *New England Journal of Medicine,* 1998
Primary care physicians' experience of financial incentives in managed-care systems.	Grumbach and co-authors; *New England Journal of Medicine,* 1999
The uncertain future of managed care.	Ginzberg; *New England Journal of Medicine,* 1999

American College of Obstetricians and Gynecologists, Relman gave an interim report: "Our present medical care system, which is largely based on investor owned managed care firms, is fatally flawed and will not survive in its present condition much longer." He also reported that while the current investor-owned managed care system has succeeded in squeezing out excess costs, and for a time also held down premiums, these savings have benefited the managed care industry rather than patients. Relman reported that the number of uninsured in the United States had reached 44 million and continues to climb annually. At the same time, teaching hospitals and community clinics have been crippled. His comments that the cause of the current "worst of times" may be ending was received with applause.

There is room for optimism. Recalling the 20th edition: "As obstetrics enters the 21st century, what needs reform is the new managed for-profit obstetrics." It seems such reform is now possible and we therefore cautiously look forward to the "best of times."

REFERENCES

American Academy of Pediatrics and the American College of Obstetricians and Gynecologists. Guidelines for Perinatal Care, 4th ed. Washington, DC, 1997

American College of Obstetricians and Gynecologists: ACM News, post meeting edition. San Francisco, May 22–24, 2000

American College of Obstetricians and Gynecologists: Domestic violence. Educational Bulletin No. 257, December, 1999a

American College of Obstetricians and Gynecologists: Ways to increase the role of women in the college. ACOG Clin 3(6):1, 1999b

Anderson RN: United States life tables, 1997. National Vital Statistics Reports, Vol 47, No. 28. Hyattsville, MD: National Center for Health Statistics, 1999

Angell M: The American Health Care System Revisited—A New Series. N Engl J Med 340:48, 1999

Bennett TA, Kotelchuck M, Cox CE, Tucker MJ, Nadeau DA: Pregnancy-associated hospitalizations in the United States in 1991 and 1992: A comprehensive view of maternal morbidity. Am J Obstet Gynecol 178:346, 1998

Bodenheimer T: The Oregon Health Plan—Lessons for the nation: Second of two parts. N Engl J Med 337:720, 1997

Bragg EJ, Rosenn BM, Khoury JC, Miodovnik M, Siddiqi TA: The effect of early discharge after vaginal delivery on neonatal readmission rates. Obstet Gynecol 89:930, 1997

Brennan TA, Sox CM, Burstin HR: Relation between negligent adverse events and the outcomes of medical-malpractice litigation. N Engl J Med 335:1963, 1996

Cassidy JD, Carroll LJ, Cote P, Lemstra M, Berglund A, Nygren A: Effect of eliminating compensation for pain and suffering on the outcome of insurance claims for whiplash injury. N Engl J Med 342:1179, 2000

Cavazzana-Calvo M, Hacein-Bey S, de Saint Basile G, Gross F, Yvon E, Nusbaum P, Selz F, Hue C, Certain S, Casanova JL, Bousso P, Deist FL, Fischer A: Gene therapy of human severe combined immunodeficiency (SCID)-X1 disease. Science 288:669, 2000

Centers for Disease Control and Prevention: National and state-specific pregnancy rates among adolescents. MMWR 49:605, 2000a

Centers for Disease Control and Prevention: National Center for Health Statistics: Prevalence of overweight and obesity among adults in the United States. September, 2000b, http://www.cdc.gov/nchs/releases

Centers for Disease Control and Prevention: Achievements in Public Health, 1990–1999. MMWR 48:1141, 1999a

Centers for Disease Control and Prevention: Achievements in Public Health, 1900–1999, Vol 48, No. 38. October 1, 1999b

Centers for Disease Control and Prevention: Maternal, infant, and child health. In: Healthy People 2010, conference ed. Atlanta, GA, CDC, November 30, 1999c

Centers for Disease Control and Prevention: Update: Mortality attributable to HIV infection among persons aged 25 to 44 years—United States, 1994. MMWR 45:121, 1996

Centers for Disease Control and Prevention: Differences in maternal mortality among black and white women, United States. MMWR 44:1, 1995

Centers for Disease Control and Prevention and Health Resources and Service Administration: Maternal, infant, and child health. In: Healthy People 2010, conference ed. Atlanta, GA, CDC, 2000

Chandra A, Abama J, Maza P, Bachrach C: Adoption, adoption seeking, and relinquishment for adoption in the United States. Advance Data from Vital and Health Statistics, No. 306. Hyattsville, MD: National Center for Health Statistics, 1999

Collins D: Why do patients sue their obstetrician/gynecologists? Contemp OB/Gyn 45:15, 2000

Curtin SC, Park MM: Trends in the attendant, place, and timing of births, and in the use of obstetric interventions: United States, 1989–97. National Vital Statistics Report, Vol 47, No. 27. Hyattsville, MD: National Center for Health Statistics, 1999

Grumbach K: Primary care in the United States—The best of times, the worst of times. N Engl J Med 341:2008, 1999

Hall MJ, Popovic JR: 1998 Summary: National Hospital Discharge Survey. Advance Data from Vital and Health Statistics, No. 316. Hyattsville, MD: National Center for Health Statistics, 2000

Hopkins FW, MacKay AP, Koonin LM, Berg CJ, Irwin M, Atrash HK: Pregnancy-related mortality in Hispanic women in the United States. Obstet Gynecol 94:747, 1999

Hoyert DL, Kochanek KD, Murph SL: Deaths: Final data for 1997. National Vital Statistics Report, Vol 47, No. 19. Hyattsville, MD: National Center for Health Statistics, 1999

Koonin LM, MacKay AP, Berg CJ, Atrash HK, Smith JC: Pregnancy-related mortality surveillance—United States, 1987–1990. MMWR 46:127, 1997

Kuttner R: Must good HMOs go bad? Second of two parts: The search for checks and balances. N Engl J Med 338:1635, 1998

Lu MC, Lin YG, Prietto NM, Garite TJ: Elimination of public funding of prenatal care for undocumented immigrants in California: A cost/benefit analysis. Am J Obstet Gynecol 182:233, 2000

Mohr JC: American medical malpractice litigation in historical perspective. JAMA 283:1731, 2000

Morrison JC: It was the best of times, it was the worst of times: Medicine in the 1990s: Presidential address. Am J Obstet Gynecol 182:1442, 2000

Murphy SL: Deaths: Final data for 1998. Natl Vital Stat Rep 48:1, 2000

Murray-Garcia J: Professionalism vs. commercialism in managed care: The need for a national council on medical care: Letters. JAMA 278:20, 1997

National Center for Health Statistics: Birth, marriages, divorces, and deaths: Provisional data for June 1999. National Vital Statistics Report, Vol 48, No. 8, 2000

Nicholson WK, Frick KD, Powe NR: Economic burden of hospitalizations for preterm labor in the United States. Obstet Gynecol 96:95, 2000

OBG Management Editorial Staff: The State of Obstetrics, 1999. December, 1999, p 38

Pearse WH: History of the American College of Obstetricians and Gynecologists. The past quarter century, 1975–2000. Washington, DC, American College of Obstetricians and Gynecologists, 2000

Relman AS: The new medical-industrial complex. N Engl J Med 303:963, 1980

St. John EB, Nelson KG, Cliver SP, Bishnoi RR, Goldenberg RL: Cost of neonatal care according to gestational age at birth and survival status. Am J Obstet Gynecol 182:170, 2000

Smith BM: Trends in health care coverage and financing and their implications for policy. N Engl J Med 337:1000, 1997

Studdert DM, Fritz LA, Brennan TA: The jury is still in: Florida's birth-related neurological injury compensation plan after a decade. J Health Polit Law 25:499, 2000

Sturner WQ, Herrmann MA, Boden C, Scaritt TP Jr, Sherman RE, Harmon TS, Woods KB: The Frye hearing in Florida: An attempt to exclude scientific evidence. J Forensic Sci 45:908, 2000

Tolson GC, Barnes JM, Gay GA, Kowaleski JL: The 1989 revision of the US Standard Certificates and Reports. Monthly Vital Statistics Report 40:1, 1991

U.S. Department of Health and Human Services. Healthy People 2000. DHHS Publications No. HRSA-M-CH-91-2. Washington, DC: 1991

U.S. News and World Report, April 10, 2000, p 54.

Ventura SJ, Mosher WD, Curtin SC, Abma JC, Henshaw S: Highlights of trends in pregnancies and pregnancy rates by outcome: Estimates for the United States, 1976–96. National Vital Statistics Report, Vol 47, No. 29. Hyattsville, MD: National Center for Health Statistics, 1999

Ventura SJ, Martin JA, Curtin SC, Mathews TJ, Park MM: Births: Final data for 1998. National Vital Statistics Report, Vol 48, No. 3. National Center for Health Statistics, 2000

Wasserman D: Heave Mom Out. Boston Globe, 1995

Weissman JS, Saglam D, Campbell EG, Causino N, Blumenthal D: Market forces and unsponsored research in academic health centers. JAMA 281:1093, 1999

Woodwell DA: National Ambulatory Medical Care Survey: 1997 Summary. Advance Data from Vital and Health Statistics, No. 305. Hyattsville, MD: National Center for Health Statistics, 1999

2

Pregnancy

OVERVIEW, ORGANIZATION, AND DIAGNOSIS

The clinical and basic sciences of obstetrics are concerned with all aspects of human reproduction and the health of women and their fetuses. These aspects include sexual maturation, gonadal function, gamete release and transport, ovum fertilization, zygote cleavage, blastocyst transport and implantation, embryo development, sexual differentiation of the embryo-fetus, pregnancy adaptations, fetal development, parturition, puerperal adaptation, lactation and breast feeding, and gonadal senescence. Any number of abnormalities can affect each of these processes.

OVERVIEW OF HUMAN REPRODUCTIVE FUNCTION

All physicians should be aware of the impact that reproductive biological processes may have on the physical and mental well-being of nonpregnant women. As is true of the female of all mammals, women are the limiting resource in human reproduction, but the physiological expenditures involuntarily obliged in women to ensure the perpetuation of humankind are enormous. In other mammalian species, including subhuman primates, the adult female experiences periodic episodes of estrus, usually during a defined time of the year (the breeding season). In women, however, spontaneous, cyclical ovulation at 25- to 35-day intervals continues throughout the year and from menarche to menopause, that is, for about 38 years. For the woman who does not use contraception, there are approximately 500 opportunities for pregnancy, which may occur with sexual intercourse on any one of 1500 days (the day of, and 2 days preceding, ovulation; see Chap. 5). Consequently, all physicians must be constantly vigilant and sensitive to the possibility that women of reproductive age, irrespective of their presenting complaint, may be pregnant. For the woman who chooses not to be pregnant, this means 500 ovarian cycles, with massive progesterone secretion/withdrawal, and then menstruation, occur for no physiological purpose. Many women choose to use some form of contraception, but most select a method that necessitates continued cyclical uterine bleeding because safe and effective methods for producing amenorrhea and infertility have not been developed.

HUMAN REPRODUCTION TODAY. From one vantage point, the success of human reproduction is the cause of one of the greatest problems of humankind—that is, overpopulation—which is a worldwide tragedy that is worsening each day. This is considered by many scholars, with considerable justification, to be the greatest hazard to the health and the environmental and economical future of humankind. One of the momentous social problems in the United States today is the high

and increasing number of unwanted pregnancies among teenage girls. Acquired immune deficiency syndrome (AIDS), a sexually transmitted disease, threatens the world with a horrific, deadly epidemic. From one perspective, human reproduction is little encumbered by the use of contraceptive methods or protection against sexually transmitted disease.

From another vantage point, the problem of human reproduction that haunts many women and men (and their physicians) is relative infertility, which may affect 20 percent of couples. This major cause of human reproductive failure is coupled with a living newborn pregnancy success rate for in vitro fertilization and embryo transfer of less than 25 percent in most clinics. To compound this dilemma, pregnancy failure caused by embryonic or fetal wastage can occur at every possible step of human reproduction. Commencing with failure of oocyte fertilization, and proceeding through failure of zygote cleavage and blastocyst implantation, embryonic losses are appreciable; and fetal losses from spontaneous abortion, fetal malformations, and preterm birth are major problems. From this perspective, it may be concluded that difficulty will be encountered in maintaining the human race, either quantitatively or qualitatively.

BIOLOGICAL AND INTELLECTUAL EVOLUTIONARY PERSPECTIVE. For physicians, researchers, demographers, anthropologists, all those interested in the reproductive biology sciences, and those entrusted with the health care of women, it would be helpful if a theoretical norm could be defined—one of human reproduction uncluttered by social, religious, or pharmacological intervention. To gain such a view, a vision of the natural history of human reproduction is required. But such an understanding is difficult to attain because of social customs.

According to Short (1980), the reproductive variables that ordinarily would lead to some sort of reproductive equilibrium include:

1. Age of puberty.
2. Frequency of embryonic and fetal death.
3. Neonatal (perinatal) mortality.
4. The duration of lactational amenorrhea, that is, breast feeding–induced anovulation or infertility.

But in humans, these constraints have been modified, even if unwittingly, such that the natural history of reproduction in our species has been diverted by social overlay (Short, 1976a). Three examples follow.

REPRODUCTION IN OTHER PRIMATES. To remove some of the social overlay that obscures our view of natural human reproduction, examination of reproduction in closely related primates living in the wild is valuable. Among female chimpanzees in the jungle, for example, the interval between births is almost 6 years; but this interval is shortened by infant death, suggesting that the long time between successive chimpanzee births normally is the result of lactation-induced infertility (anovulation and amenorrhea). Chimpanzees in the wild suckle their young several times per hour, secrete a milk similar to that of humans, and sleep with the infant at their breast during the night (Short, 1984). Menstruation is a phenomenon confined to only a few primates—the great apes, Old World monkeys, and women—and no other mammals (Chap. 4). Chimpanzees experience menstruation at intervals similar to women, but in those animals living in the wild, menstruation is rare because of repeated pregnancy and prolonged lactation-induced anovulation with amenorrhea.

Is it possible that the same would be true of ovulation and menstruation in women were it not for their advanced intellectual development—a development that has enabled women to choose infertility and to limit the duration of breast feeding? The social evolution of human reproduction did, indeed, involve the changing practices of breast feeding. Before modern times, its duration usually was dictated by the availability of soft foods for infants. Women today have the choice of ovulation and menstruation and infant formula feeding instead of near-continuous pregnancy and prolonged lactation.

REPRODUCTION IN PRIMITIVE SOCIETIES. In previous editions of this textbook, the reproductive success of the primitive nomadic hunter-gatherer !Kung tribe was described in detail and contrasted to their relatives who have become farmers. Simply stated, the nomadic branch of the tribe has fewer infants per woman when compared with the farmers. This likely is due to later childbearing in the nomads because of lean body mass, which is associated with delayed menarche. Also, their prolonged lactation, dictated by their mobility, prohibits quick return to ovulation. By contrast, the farmer tribe women can limit lactation because of increased availability of soft food and animal milk for their infants (Kolata, 1974; Short, 1976a, 1976b, 1984).

REPRODUCTION IN NORTH AMERICAN HUTTERITES. The Hutterites are a religious sect with an exceptionally high rate of fertility. The mean age of marriage for Hutterite women is 22.0 years of age (Eaton and Mayer, 1953). Reproduction is encouraged, but premarital sex is forbidden and rarely practiced. The 25 to 29 age-specific nuptial fertility rate among Hutterite women is 498—that is, there are 498 births per year for each 1000 married women in that age group. Stated differently, there is one birth per woman every 2 years, and the average completed family size of Hutterite women is 10.6 children.

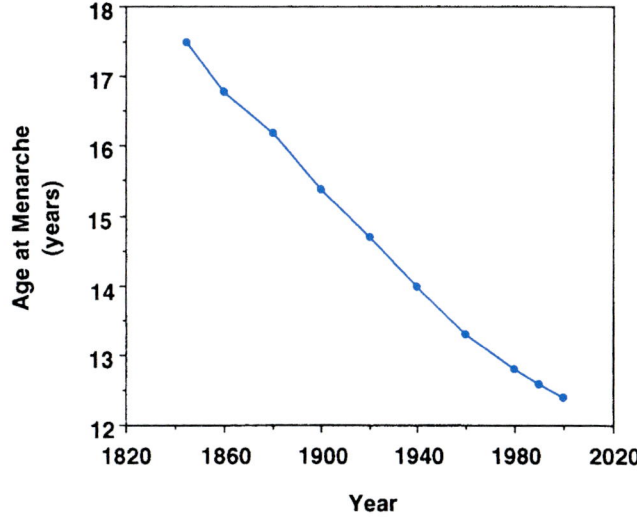

FIGURE 2–1. Age of menarche from 1830 to 1990.

Compared with the nomadic !Kung women, Hutterite women experience earlier puberty and ovulation, suckle their children on a rigid schedule, and choose to supplement breast feeding with soft foods earlier. Based on the reproductive history of the Hutterite women, the population doubling time of this group has been estimated to be 16 years (Eaton and Mayer, 1953; Short, 1984).

REPRODUCTION IN MODERN WOMEN. It seems reasonable to conclude that the sedentary, agrarian way of life of the past few centuries has contributed to a change in body composition and mass that favors earlier menarche and ovulation. Menarche in women in the United States today occurs at about 12½ years of age (Fig. 2–1); and whereas anovulation is more common immediately after menarche than later in reproductive life, most young postmenarchal girls are ovulatory and, therefore, potentially fertile. Most women today who choose to breast feed their newborns will do so for no more than a few weeks or at most a few months, and will suckle the baby no more than eight times per 24 hours compared with 48 times per 12 hours of daylight for !Kung women.

Therefore, two major factors have affected the natural course of human reproduction. These factors are nutrition and women's advanced intellectual capacity, which permits women the choice of infertility. Nutritional advances have led to:

1. Earlier menarche (and ovulation).
2. Artificial feeding of the newborn, resulting in decreased duration of lactation with associated anovulation and amenorrhea after childbirth.
3. More frequent and longer infant survival.

Because women in the United States today, on average, choose to have two pregnancies and to breast feed for only a few weeks, no more than 20 ovarian (menstrual) cycles are eliminated by pregnancy and the anovulation/amenorrhea of lactation. In the absence of pharmacological or surgical intervention, therefore, modern women experience nearly 500 ovulatory cycles, each of which is accompanied by massive progesterone secretion/withdrawal intervals and attendant menstruation, because of their intellectual capacity to choose infertility (MacDonald and colleagues, 1991).

OVULATION IS THE CARDINAL FUNCTION OF THE OVARY.

The endocrine changes of the ovarian cycle are optimized to create a hormonal environment that promotes ovulation. The endocrine milieu that evolves during the ovarian cycle also is optimal for the regeneration of endometrium after completion of a failed fertility cycle (menstruation) to prepare this tissue for the next pregnancy (implantation) opportunity.

Follicular estrogen (synthesized in granulosa cells) is produced in a cyclical manner that regulates ovarian–brain–pituitary function and follicular maturation, eventuating in ovulation. But the somatic effects of estrogen, such as those on bone density, must be accepted as coincidental benefits. There is no currently recognized physiological mechanism in place whereby somatic tissues can act to regulate the rate of ovarian estrogen secretion. Except for ovary and brain–pituitary, this is true of all estrogen-responsive tissues, including breast, uterus, bone, skin, vagina, and liver. For metabolic processes, other than those directly involved in reproduction, there also is no apparent advantage provided by the wide fluctuations in the levels of estrogen that are characteristic of the ovarian cycle. These considerations are important not only to an understanding of reproductive processes but for the development of rational therapeutic practices of estrogen replacement. Specifically, there is no merit in attempting to pharmacologically recreate the cyclical fluctuations in estrogen of the ovarian cycle in hypogonadal, castrate, or postmenopausal women.

It seems reasonable to deduce that repetitive, cyclical ovulation and menstruation are not the biological evolutionary norm. The relatively uncommon occurrence of menstruation among female chimpanzees living in the wild and among hunter-gatherer !Kung and Hutterite women is more likely to be representative of the biological norm. Recurrent ovulation and menstruation are the consequence of the more rapid intellectual than biological evolution of humans. Infertility can be chosen; but the physiological result, and the endocrinopathies that may accrue in women from this choice, is appreciable.

PREGNANCY ORGANIZATION: THE FETAL–MATERNAL COMMUNICATION SYSTEM

DEVELOPMENT OF THE FETAL–MATERNAL COMMUNICATION SYSTEM.

Ovulation is dependent upon brain–pituitary–ovarian interactions. After conception, the establishment and maintenance of human pregnancy is driven by the blastocyst and then the embryonic-fetal and extraembryonic tissues. A biomolecular communication system is established between the zygote-blastocyst-embryo-fetus and the mother that is operative from before nidation and continues through parturition and beyond. By way of breast feeding, this communication persists during infancy; and through maternal–infant bonding, a communication system between mother and child, in some form, may be created that is lifelong.

In the past, this communication system was believed to be unidirectional, delivering nutritive supplies from mother to fetus. It was presumed that the mother provided nutrients that were effectively taken up by the trophoblasts and transferred to the embryo-fetus. It is now known that numerous fetal messages are sent toward the mother in this bidirectional communication system.

The fetal–maternal communication system is essential for the success of blastocyst implantation, maternal recognition of pregnancy, immunological acceptance of the conceptus, the maintenance of pregnancy, maternal adaptations to pregnancy, fetal nutrition and maturation, and perhaps for the initiation of parturition. These physiological processes evolve primarily from embryonic-fetal tissue–directed modifications of maternal responses.

There are two major anatomical and functional arms of the fetal–maternal communication system. One is the **placental arm,** the functional components of which include nutritive, endocrine, and immunological processes. The other is the **paracrine arm,** the functional components of which include pregnancy maintenance, immunological acceptance, amnionic fluid volume homeostasis, and physical protection of the fetus (Fig. 2–2).

The placental arm of the fetal–maternal communication system is established by two factors. The first is the supply of maternal blood to the placental intervillous space via the endometrial/decidual spiral arteries. Maternal blood leaves these vessels and directly bathes the villous syncytiotrophoblast. The second factor is the fetal blood, which is confined within the capillaries that traverse within the intervillous spaces of the placental villi.

The paracrine arm of the communication system is established by direct cell-to-cell contact and biomolecu-

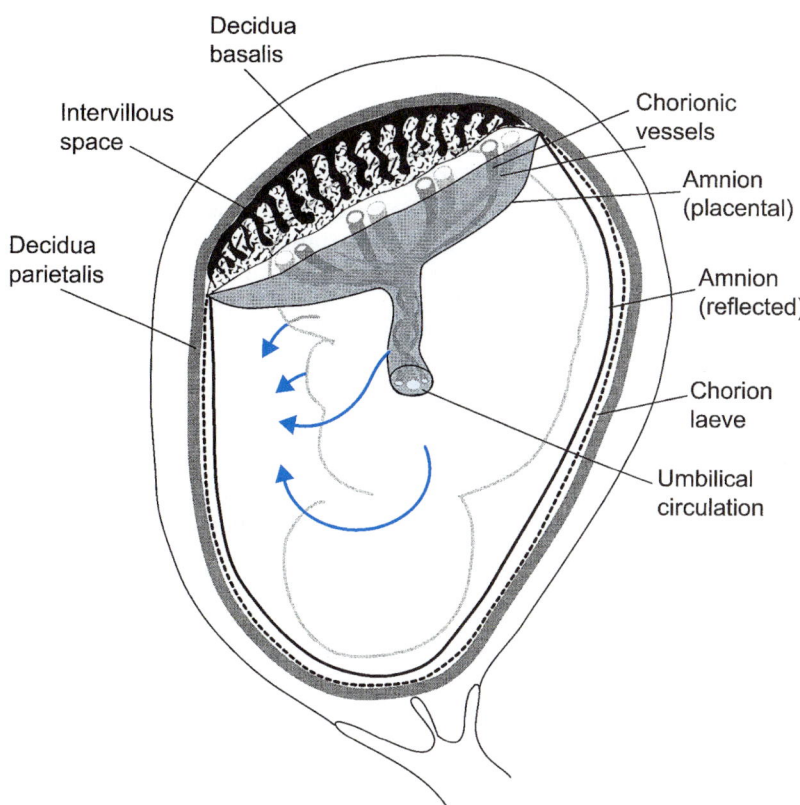

FIGURE 2–2. The fetal–maternal communication system. The proximal anatomical parts of the two arms of this system, the placental arm and the paracrine arm, are depicted. Fetal blood perfuses the placenta by way of the fetal villous capillaries. Maternal blood directly bathes the trophoblasts. Amnionic fluid, composed in large measure of fetal urine, and containing secretions from fetal lung and skin, bathes the avascular amnion, which is contiguous with avascular chorion laeve. The chorion laeve and decidua vera (parietalis) are in direct cell-to-cell contact. A trophoblastic "shell" separates the embryo-fetus from maternal cells and blood at all anatomical sites.

lar trafficking between fetal membranes (chorion laeve) and maternal decidua parietalis. In turn, the amnion, the innermost avascular fetal membrane, which is contiguous with the chorion laeve on the outer surface and bathed by the amnionic fluid on the inner surface, also is a component of this paracrine system. Amnionic fluid is rich in fetal excretions (kidney) and secretions (lung, skin), and provides for a unique but direct signal transmission system between the fetus and mother.

ORGANIZATION OF THE FETAL–MATERNAL COMMUNICATION SYSTEM. At the very commencement of pregnancy, at the time of blastocyst implantation, there is only one anatomically distinguishable communication link between blastocyst and mother. This is established between the trophectoderm of the blastocyst and the uterine endometrium (decidua) and then maternal blood. Even this early, the functional progenitors of the two mature arms of the communication system have begun.

PLACENTAL ARM: NUTRIENT TRANSFER AND ENDOCRINE SYSTEM. The placenta (villous trophoblast; syncytium) becomes the principal site of nutrient transfer between mother and fetus. The placenta also is the principal endocrine tissue of pregnancy, albeit one that is highly dependent upon the provision of blood-borne,

preformed maternal and fetal precursors for placental steroid hormone formation (Chap. 6). The proximal anatomical parts of the placental arm (nutrient transfer and endocrine function) of the fetal–maternal communication system are the fetal blood, the syncytium, and the maternal blood. Human placentation is hemochorioendothelial. The microvillar surface of the syncytiotrophoblast is bathed directly by maternal blood, but fetal blood is contained within fetal capillaries located in the villi of the placenta. Therefore, fetal blood is separated from the syncytiotrophoblast by the wall of the fetal capillaries, the mesenchyme in the villous space, and the cytotrophoblasts (Chap. 5). Importantly, fetal and maternal blood do not come into direct contact except in abnormal conditions.

PARACRINE ARM: FETAL MEMBRANES AND DECIDUA PARIETALIS. As the embryo and extraembryonic tissues grow, the amnion and chorion laeve develop as tough, avascular membranous structures that will come to lie adjacent to the entire surface of the decidua parietalis, that portion of decidua that is not occupied by the placenta (Chap. 5). This anatomical arrangement gives rise to the paracrine arm of the fetal–maternal communication system. The proximal anatomical parts of the paracrine arm of the fetal–maternal communication system are the amnionic fluid, amnion, chorion laeve, and decidua parietalis. Communication between fetus and mother through this paracrine arm is possible through constituents of amnionic fluid such as fetal urine and fetal lung secretions. In the reverse direction, decidual products as well as some maternal blood constituents enter amnionic fluid, and these products then can enter the fetus by fetal "inspiration" and swallowing of amnionic fluid. Some decidual products, such as prolactin (Chap. 5), preferentially enter the amnionic fluid. In addition, potent vasoactive peptides and growth factors are synthesized in the amnion, enter amnionic fluid, and are available to the fetus.

DYNAMIC ROLE OF THE FETUS IN PREGNANCY. In the past, the fetus was envisioned as a passive passenger of the pregnancy unit; but nothing could be further from the truth. It is important to recognize that whereas the embryo-fetus enjoys a position of protection from the external environment that is never to be experienced again in life, it is the dynamic force in the orchestration of its own destiny. The chemical impetus for implantation is provided by the trophoblasts and blastocyst products; invasion of the maternal endometrium and blood vessels is under the active direction of bioactive products synthesized in the trophoblasts; the maternal recognition of pregnancy is brought about by way of signals generated by the trophoblasts that act upon the maternal ovary; the immunological acceptance of the semiallogenic tissues of the conceptus is modulated by the regulation of human lymphocyte antigen (HLA) expression by trophoblasts; the maintenance of pregnancy is directed by fetal contributions to steroid hormone formation in the trophoblast; the maternal physiological changes of pregnancy are promoted by products formed and secreted by the placenta; and, indeed, it even is possible that the fetus initiates parturition at term (Chap. 11). From these multiple interactions, molecular trafficking and signal transmission/response between tissues of the fetus and its mother are clear (Fig. 2–3).

IMPLANTATION. Fertilization of the human ovum by a spermatozoan occurs in the fallopian tube within a short time (minutes to at most a few hours) after ovulation. By 6 days after fertilization, the blastocyst begins to implant in the endometrium. Clearly, the endometrium is not essential to implantation. The blastocyst sometimes is implanted in the fallopian tube, ovary, peritoneal cavity, or even in the spleen; and in experimental studies, it can be implanted successfully into many tissues, including the testis.

Thus, it is the blastocyst (trophoblast) that is the driving force in implantation. There are neoplastic and inflammatory processes involved in blastocyst implantation; the blastocyst produces or else provokes the formation of prostaglandins, platelet-activating factor, and

plasminogen activator. In fact, complete decidualization of endometrium in human pregnancy takes place only after blastocyst implantation. The trophoblasts produce metalloproteinases that effect degradation of the endometrial extracellular matrix proteins in a manner similar to that of metastasizing neoplastic cells. Selected cytotrophoblasts (Langhans cells) express an unusual monomeric class I (HLA-G) antigen (Chap. 5, p. 90).

FETAL-INDUCED MATERNAL RECOGNITION OF PREGNANCY. Among the early physiological arrangements provided by the fetal–maternal communication system is one referred to by Short (1969) as the maternal recognition of pregnancy. This is an extraordinarily important concept in mammalian pregnancy physiology. This arrangement, however, likely should be redesignated, as the fetal-induced maternal recognition of pregnancy. There is no doubt that there is maternal recognition of pregnancy, but this recognition is evoked by fetal signals.

The maternal recognition of pregnancy encompasses a series of processes that culminate in:

1. Prolongation of the life span of the corpus luteum with continued progesterone secretion.
2. Modifications of the trophoblast expression of major histocompatibility complex (HLA) antigens to facilitate maternal tissue acceptance of the fetal graft (Bazer and colleagues, 1986).

Chorionic gonadotropin (hCG), produced by trophoblasts, acts to **"rescue" or maintain the corpus luteum,** to promote continued progesterone formation by the ovary until such time as the placenta is able to synthesize sufficient amounts of progesterone to maintain pregnancy (Chaps. 6 and 11).

There also is appreciable evidence, largely based on findings in sheep, that mammalian blastocysts and embryos produce agents, called trophoblast proteins—with similarities to interferons—that effect **decidual quiescence,** thus facilitating the maintenance of pregnancy (Godkin and co-workers, 1984; Hansen and colleagues, 1985; Imakawa and associates, 1987; Li and Roberts, 1994).

CORPUS LUTEUM AND PREGNANCY. The duration of corpus luteum function during early pregnancy has been the subject of many investigations. During infertile ovarian cycles, the corpus luteum produces progesterone in prodigious amounts for only about 1 week. Thereafter, in the next 5 to 6 days of infertile ovarian cycles, the rate of secretion of progesterone by the corpus luteum declines, reaching a nadir about 12 to 14 days after ovulation.

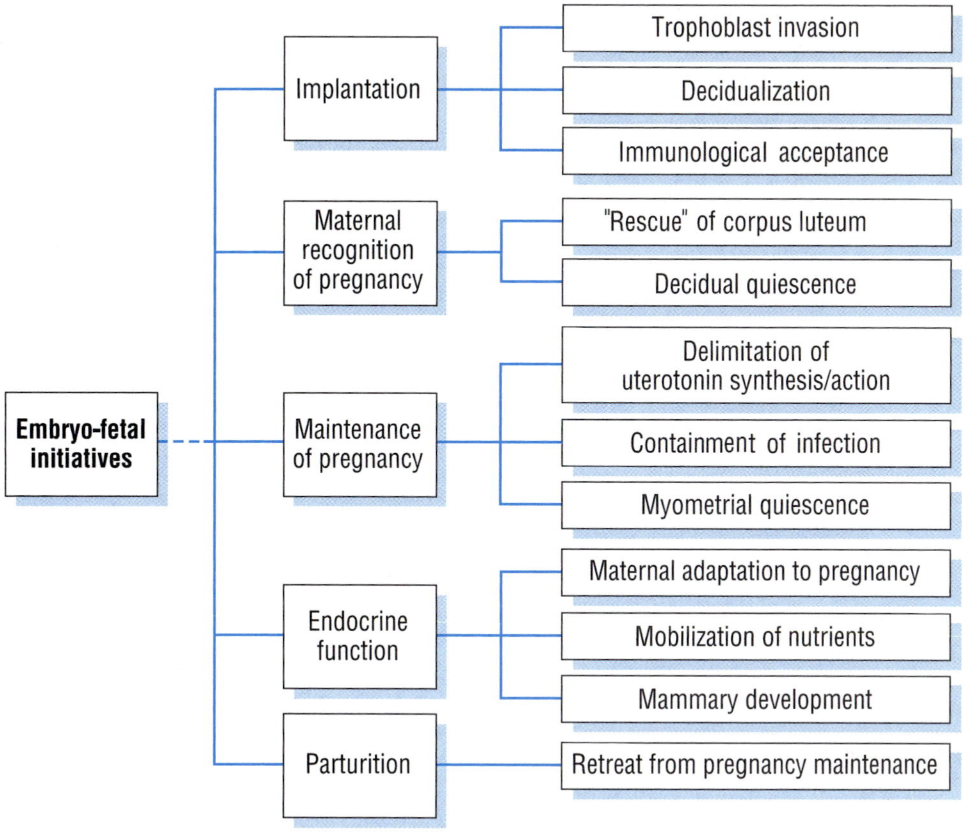

FIGURE 2–3. Fetal contributions to the maintenance of pregnancy. The fetus and extraembryonic fetal tissues are the dynamic, driving force in the establishment and maintenance of pregnancy. Fetal contributions include processes essential to implantation and maternal recognition of pregnancy; but more than this, the physiological and metabolic accommodations in the maternal organism that contribute to successful pregnancy are orchestrated by fetus-directed biomolecular initiatives.

PROGESTERONE SECRETION. With blastocyst implantation, the corpus luteum of menstruation is "rescued" by the action of hCG (and probably other factors originating in the blastocyst). As a result, progesterone synthesis is continued, but for only a relatively short time in the human. It is generally agreed that progesterone produced by the corpus luteum during the first 8 weeks (menstrual age) of human gestation is important for the **maintenance of pregnancy.** Thereafter, progesterone synthesis in the syncytiotrophoblast becomes dominant, as progesterone secretion by the corpus luteum declines between 6 and 8 weeks. Sometimes, however, with removal of the corpus luteum—usually because of bleeding from this structure—from the ovary prior to 10 weeks, pregnancy can still be maintained with intramuscular injection of 17-hydroxyprogesterone caproate (150 mg). This agent is chosen because:

1. The duration of action is predictable.
2. Rarely, if ever, does such treatment lead to virilization of a female fetus.
3. It can be given intramuscularly.

Between 8 and 10 weeks, the progestin is administered only at the time of surgery. Between 6 and 8 weeks, there may be some merit in a second injection of the progestin 1 week after surgery.

FETAL CONTRIBUTIONS TO MATERNAL ACCEPTANCE OF THE SEMIALLOGENIC FETAL GRAFT. Just after, or at about the time of blastocyst implantation, the expression of major histocompatibility complex (HLA) antigens is suppressed in extraembryonic fetal tissues (trophoblasts)—that is, in tissues that directly contact maternal tissues. This may be the most critical mechanism by which the blastocyst and embryo-fetus gain immunological acceptance by maternal tissues. As described in Chapter 5, the trophoblasts form an uninterrupted shell around the embryo such that, normally, maternal tissues never come into direct contact with blood or other tissues of the embryo-fetus.

FETAL CONTRIBUTIONS TO THE ENDOCRINOLOGY OF PREGNANCY. The hormonal changes of human pregnancy—in breadth and amount—are monumental and unmatched in endocrinology and endocrinopathology. Without exception, the endocrine changes of human pregnancy evolve as the consequence of embryonic-fetal–placental function, either directly or indirectly; thus, the conceptus is also responsible for the endocrine milieu of human pregnancy. The formation of estrogens during pregnancy takes place by way of the placental aromatization (the enzymatic reaction essential for estrogen synthesis) of C_{19}-steroids, which in turn are produced primarily in the fetal adrenal glands. Progesterone also is produced in the syncytium in massive quantities, but by way of the use of maternal plasma low-density lipoprotein (LDL) cholesterol. Indeed, the rate of trophoblast consumption of maternal plasma LDL for progesterone formation at term is so great in some pregnancies that it is equivalent to the total daily turnover of LDL in nonpregnant women (Chap. 6). But even in capturing LDL cholesterol, the fetus is aggressive and efficient. Placental hydrolysis of the LDL cholesteryl esters yields essential fatty acids, and the hydrolysis of the LDL apoprotein gives free amino acids, including essential amino acids.

Progesterone secreted by syncytium is converted to deoxycorticosterone, a potent mineralocorticosteroid, in extraadrenal maternal and fetal tissues. Placental progesterone, secreted into the maternal compartment, also serves indirectly, by way of increased angiotensin II formation, as the stimulus for increased maternal adrenal aldosterone secretion to a rate 20 times or more than that in men and nonpregnant women. Increased mineralocorticosteroid formation (aldosterone and deoxycorticosterone) is essential for normal blood volume expansion (Chap. 8). All of these endocrine changes, and many more, are effected by way of fetal tissue–produced or fetal tissue hormone–induced endocrine changes of normal human pregnancy (Chap. 6).

PLACENTAL SEQUESTRATION OF NUTRIENTS. Fetal villous syncytiotrophoblast is remarkably efficient in extracting and sequestering essential nutrients from maternal circulation (Chap. 7). In pregnant women with profound iron-deficiency anemia, for example, the iron stores of the fetus are normal; in pregnant women with severe folic acid deficiency causing severe anemia, the fetal hematocrit is normal. The fetus is a demanding and efficient parasite! We have long been fascinated by the observation that the amount of calcium assembled into the shell of the egg of the chicken in a period of 18 hours is equivalent to the amount of calcium contained in the entire bony skeleton of the hen. Thus, even in the avian, a species that arguably is never pregnant (no implantation), the demands of the embryo are met at whatever cost to the maternal organism.

FETAL RETREAT FROM PARTICIPATION IN PREGNANCY MAINTENANCE: INITIATION OF PARTURITION. The fetus also may be in control of its own destiny with respect to the timely onset of parturition. This may come about by way of fetal-induced retreat from the continued maintenance of the remarkable uterine quiescence that characterizes the first 90 to 95 percent of normal pregnancy (phase 0 of parturition; see Chap. 11). The importance of the fetus in the maintenance of pregnancy and in the initiation of parturition can be

understood by the natural outcome of many pregnancies after fetal death. After the fetus has died, labor may not immediately ensue; pregnancy may continue for days, weeks, or even months before spontaneous labor begins. It has been observed that with fetal death caused by Rh isoimmunization before 35 weeks, 50 percent of these pregnancies remain undelivered, in the absence of intervention, for up to 5 weeks (Townsend and Shelton, 1964). After removal of the fetus in rhesus monkey pregnancy, with the placenta left in situ, the placenta does not deliver spontaneously until sometime well after the expected due date of the pregnancy (Nathanielsz and associates, 1992). It seems that in response to death or removal of the fetus, there is no built-in mechanism for emptying the uterus through processes independently initiated within the maternal compartment. Spontaneous delivery in these circumstances may come about only with "progesterone withdrawal," which may eventuate with degeneration of the placenta after prolonged absence of fetal–placental blood flow.

FETAL AND NEWBORN CONTRIBUTIONS TO LACTATION AND MILK LET-DOWN. During pregnancy, estrogen and progesterone, together with prolactin and cortisol, act on maternal mammary tissues to induce optimal morphological and biochemical maturational processes that prepare the breasts for lactation. Progesterone also acts, however, to prevent lactogenesis itself; but with progesterone withdrawal after delivery of the placenta, lactogenesis promptly commences. Thereafter, newborn suckling induces episodic oxytocin secretion from the maternal neurohypophysis–posterior pituitary; and oxytocin acts on the myoepithelial cells of the breast ducts to cause milk let-down. Clearly, the fetus-infant acts to ensure its own survival.

These are but a few examples to indicate unambiguously that the embryo-fetus, extraembryonic fetal tissues, or both, direct the orchestration of the physiological adaptations of pregnancy. The maternal organism passively responds—even at times to her own detriment. Each of these arrangements will be referred to frequently: acceptance of the fetal semiallogenic graft (Chap. 5), the endocrinology of pregnancy (Chap. 6), fetal growth and development (Chap. 7), the physiological adaptations of maternal systems to pregnancy (Chap. 8), and the initiation of parturition (Chap. 11). The embryo-fetus–extraembryonic tissue initiatives that promote the success of pregnancy are summarized in Figure 2–3.

DIAGNOSIS OF PREGNANCY

Pregnancy is a physiological state, but the importance of the diagnosis of pregnancy cannot be overstated.

In the life of women, few diagnoses are more important than that of pregnancy. There are few life experiences that can evoke emotions of such absolute joy or else such pains of profound despair. Moreover, for all physicians entrusted with the medical management of women of reproductive age, knowledge of the existence of pregnancy is crucial to the proper diagnosis and treatment of all disease processes. Every physician who assumes the responsibility for the medical care of women of reproductive age, irrespective of the nature of the physician's practice or special interest, must always consider the question: Is she pregnant? Failure to do so may lead to incorrect diagnoses, inappropriate treatments, and, at times, medicolegal embroilment.

Many of the manifestations of the normal physiological adaptations of pregnancy are easily recognized and constitute important clues to the diagnosis of pregnancy and the evaluation of pregnancy progress. Some of these pregnancy changes are predictable with sufficient timeliness to constitute important milestones that verify the gestational age of the fetus. Meanwhile, the woman physiologically accommodates to the growth, maturation, and function of the uterus and conceptus.

The diagnosis of pregnancy is ordinarily very easy to establish; but unfortunately, this is not always the case. On occasion, pharmacological or pathophysiological processes may induce endocrine or anatomical changes that mimic those of pregnancy, causing confusion for the woman and sometimes the physician. At times, therefore, the diagnosis of pregnancy is not easy to make; but rarely is it impossible if appropriate clinical and laboratory tests are carefully conducted and evaluated.

Ordinarily, the woman is aware of the likelihood, or at least the possibility, of pregnancy when she consults a physician, although she may not volunteer this information unless questioned specifically. Mistakes in diagnosis of pregnancy are made most frequently in the first several weeks of pregnancy, while the uterus is still a pelvic organ. Although it is possible to mistake the enlarged uterus of pregnancy, even at term, for a tumor of some nature, such errors commonly are the result of a hasty or incomplete examination.

The endocrinological, physiological, and anatomical alterations that accompany pregnancy give rise to symptoms and signs that provide evidence that pregnancy exists. These symptoms and signs are classified into three groups: presumptive evidence, probable signs, and positive signs of pregnancy.

PRESUMPTIVE EVIDENCE OF PREGNANCY. Presumptive evidence of pregnancy is based largely on subjective symptoms that include:

1. Nausea with or without vomiting.
2. Disturbances in urination.
3. Fatigue.
4. The perception of fetal movement.

Presumptive signs include:

1. Cessation of menses.
2. Changes in the breasts.
3. Discoloration of the vaginal mucosa.
4. Increased skin pigmentation and the development of abdominal striae.
5. Especially important, does the woman believe that she is pregnant?

SYMPTOMS OF PREGNANCY. There are a number of symptoms that frequently alert the parous woman to an early pregnancy.

NAUSEA WITH OR WITHOUT VOMITING. Pregnancy is commonly characterized by disturbances of the digestive system, manifested particularly by nausea and vomiting. This so-called morning sickness of pregnancy usually commences during the early part of the day but passes in a few hours, although occasionally it persists longer and may occur at other times. This disturbing symptom usually begins about 6 weeks after the commencement (first day) of the last menstrual period, and ordinarily disappears spontaneously 6 to 12 weeks later. The cause of this disorder is unknown but seems to be associated with higher levels of selected forms of hCG (variations in glycosylation) with the greatest thyroid-stimulating capacity. Chorionic gonadotropin, especially isoforms with relatively diminished amounts of sialic acid, act via the thyroid-stimulating hormone (TSH) receptor to accelerate iodine uptake (Chap. 6).

DISTURBANCES IN URINATION. During the first trimester, the enlarging uterus, by exerting pressure on the urinary bladder, may cause frequent micturition. As pregnancy progresses, the frequency of urination gradually diminishes as the uterus rises up into the abdomen. The symptom of frequent urination reappears near the end of pregnancy, however, when the fetal head descends into the maternal pelvis, impinging upon the volume capacity of the bladder.

FATIGUE. Easy fatigability is such a frequent characteristic of early pregnancy that it provides a noteworthy diagnostic clue.

PERCEPTION OF FETAL MOVEMENT. Sometime between 16 and 20 weeks (menstrual age), the pregnant woman becomes conscious of slight fluttering movements in the abdomen, and these movements gradually increase in intensity. These sensations are caused by fetal movements, and the day that these are first recognized by the pregnant woman is designated as **quickening,** or the perception of life. This sign provides only corroborative evidence of pregnancy, however, and in itself is of little diagnostic value. Quickening is, nonetheless, a milestone of the progress of pregnancy that, if dated accurately, can provide corroborative evidence in establishing the duration of gestation.

SIGNS OF PREGNANCY. There are a number of clinical findings that frequently herald pregnancy.

CESSATION OF MENSES. The abrupt cessation of menstruation in a healthy reproductive-age woman who previously has experienced spontaneous, cyclical, predictable menses is highly suggestive of pregnancy. There is appreciable variation in the length of the ovarian (and thus menstrual) cycle among women, and even in the same woman. It is not until 10 days or more after the time of expected onset of the menstrual period, therefore, that the absence of menses is a reliable indication of pregnancy. When a second menstrual period is missed, the probability of pregnancy is much greater.

Although cessation of menstruation is an early and important indication of pregnancy, conception may occur without prior menstruation, that is, in a girl before menarche. In certain Asian countries, where girls marry at a very early age, and in sexually promiscuous groups, pregnancy sometimes commences before menarche. Nursing mothers, who usually sustain amenorrhea during lactation because of lactation-induced hypogonadism and anovulation, sometimes ovulate and conceive at that time; and more rarely, women who believe they have passed the menopause may ovulate again after a few months of anovulation/amenorrhea and become pregnant.

Uterine bleeding somewhat suggestive of menstruation occurs occasionally after conception. One or two episodes of bloody discharge, somewhat reminiscent of and sometimes misinterpreted as menstruation, are not uncommon during the first half of pregnancy. Almost always, however, such bleeding is brief and scant. In a series of 225 consecutive pregnant women who did not abort, Speert and Guttmacher (1954) observed that macroscopical vaginal bleeding, which occurred between the time of conception and the 196th day of pregnancy, was reported by 22 percent of these women. In the absence of cervical lesions, bleeding began on or before the 40th day of pregnancy in 8 percent. These investigators interpreted these bleeding episodes to be "physiological," that is, the consequence of blastocyst implantation. Bleeding during pregnancy was three times more frequent among multiparas than among primigravidas. Of 83 multiparas, 25 percent experienced bleeding. Alleged instances of women having "menstru-

ated" every month throughout pregnancy are incorrect; true uterine bleeding during pregnancy is undoubtedly the result of some abnormality of the reproductive organs. Bleeding per vagina at any time during pregnancy must be regarded as abnormal and portends an increased likelihood of serious pregnancy complications.

Cessation of menstruation can be caused by a number of conditions other than pregnancy. The most common cause of a delay in the time of onset of the expected next menstrual period (other than pregnancy) is anovulation. This, in turn, may be the consequence of a number of factors that include severe illness and physiological aberrations induced by emotional disorders, including the fear of pregnancy. Environmental changes as well as a variety of chronic disease processes also may suppress menstruation by causing anovulation. Delays in the onset of menstruation also have been attributed to persistent function of a cystic corpus luteum; but the evidence for such an entity is not convincing. Most, if not all, instances of prolonged function of the corpus luteum, we believe, are caused by a pregnancy episode, even though the pregnancy may be unrecognized, as in the case of early missed or incomplete abortion or undiagnosed ectopic pregnancy.

CHANGES IN CERVICAL MUCUS. If cervical mucus is aspirated, spread on a glass slide, allowed to dry for a few minutes, and examined microscopically, characteristic patterns can be discerned that are dependent on the stage of the ovarian cycle and the presence or absence of pregnancy, that is, on progesterone secretion in large amounts. From about the 7th to about the 18th day of the menstrual cycle, a fernlike pattern of dried cervical mucus is seen (Fig. 2–4). It is sometimes called a process of arborization or the palm leaf pattern. After approximately the 21st day, this fern pattern does not develop, but rather there is a quite different pattern that forms, giving a beaded or cellular appearance (Fig. 2–5). This pattern also is usually encountered in pregnancy. The crystallization of the mucus, which is necessary for the production of the fern, or arborized pattern, is dependent upon the concentration of electrolytes, principally sodium chloride, in the secretion. In general, a concentration of sodium chloride of 1 percent is required for the full development of a fern pattern; below that concentration, either a beaded pattern or an atypical or incomplete arborization is seen.

The concentration of sodium chloride, and in turn the presence or absence of the fern pattern, is determined by the response of the cervix to hormonal action. Whereas the cervical mucus is relatively rich in sodium chloride when estrogen, but not progesterone, is being produced, the secretion of progesterone (even without a reduction in the rate of secretion of estrogen) promptly acts to lower the sodium chloride concentration to levels at

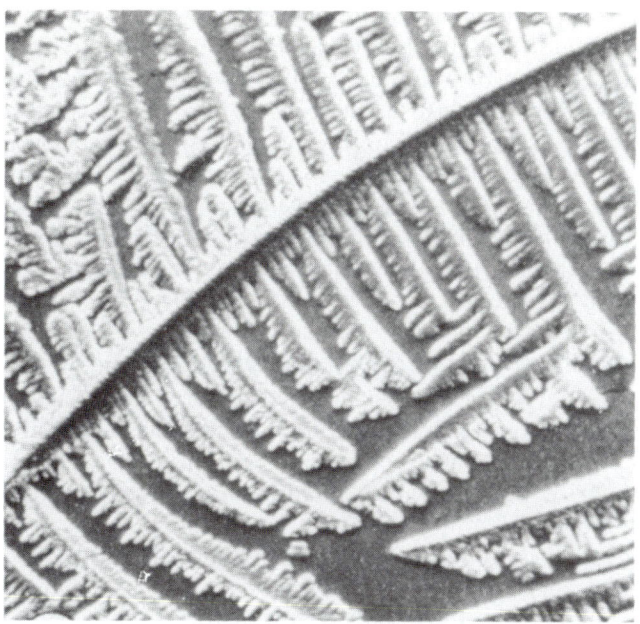

FIGURE 2–4. Scanning electron microscopy of cervical mucus obtained on day 11 of the menstrual cycle. (From Zaneveld and associates, 1975.)

which ferning will not occur. During pregnancy, progesterone usually exerts a similar effect, even though the amount of estrogen produced is enormous compared with that produced during a normal ovarian cycle.

If copious thin mucus is present and if a fern pattern develops on drying, early pregnancy is very unlikely,

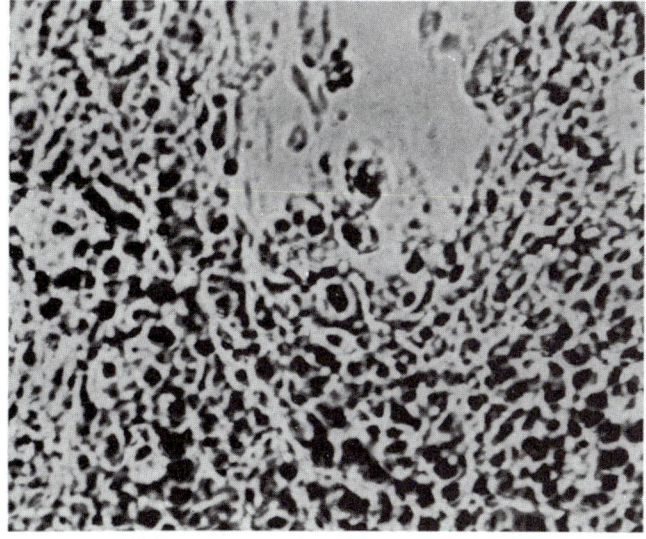

FIGURE 2–5. Photomicrograph of dried cervical mucus obtained from the cervical canal of a woman pregnant at 32 to 33 weeks. The beaded pattern is characteristic of progesterone action on the endocervical gland mucus composition. (Courtesy of Dr. J.C. Ullery.)

and the woman almost certainly will experience uterine bleeding after treatment with and withdrawal of progestin. If relatively little cervical mucus is present and a highly cellular pattern forms, she may or may not be pregnant. If not pregnant, she may or may not sustain uterine bleeding after receiving progestin, depending upon her own supply of endogenous progesterone. Moreover, there is fear that progestins are potential teratogens (Chap. 38, p. 1017). Therefore, progestins should not be administered to women who are believed to be pregnant except in unusual circumstances, such as that discussed earlier concerning surgical removal of the corpus luteum before completion of 8 weeks.

CHANGES IN THE BREASTS. Generally, the anatomical changes in the breasts that accompany pregnancy are quite characteristic in primiparas. These are less obvious in multiparas, whose breasts may contain a small amount of milky material or colostrum for months or even years after the birth of their last child, especially if breast feeding was chosen. Occasionally, changes in the breasts similar to those caused by pregnancy are found in women with prolactin-secreting pituitary tumors, and in women taking prescribed drugs such as most commonly prescribed anxiolytic agents like benzodiazepines, which induce hyperprolactinemia. Instances of similar breast changes in women with spurious or imaginary pregnancy also have been reported as discussed subsequently.

DISCOLORATION OF THE VAGINAL MUCOSA. During pregnancy, the vaginal mucosa usually appears dark bluish or purplish-red and congested; this is the so-called **Chadwick sign** (Chadwick, 1886). This appearance is presumptive evidence of pregnancy, but it is not conclusive. Similar changes in the appearance of the vaginal mucosa may be induced by any condition that causes intense congestion of the pelvic organs.

INCREASED SKIN PIGMENTATION AND APPEARANCE OF ABDOMINAL STRIAE. These cutaneous manifestations are common to, but not diagnostic of pregnancy. They may be absent during pregnancy; conversely, these changes can occur with the ingestion of estrogen–progestin contraceptives.

PROBABLE EVIDENCE OF PREGNANCY. The probable signs of pregnancy include:

1. Enlargement of the abdomen.
2. Changes in the shape, size, and consistency of the uterus.
3. Anatomical changes in the cervix.
4. Braxton Hicks contractions.
5. Ballottement.

6. Physical outlining of the fetus.
7. Presence of chorionic gonadotropin in urine or serum.

ENLARGEMENT OF THE ABDOMEN. By 12 weeks, the uterus usually is palpable through the abdominal wall as a tumor just above the symphysis; thereafter, the uterus gradually increases in size until the end of pregnancy. Any enlargement of the abdomen in women during the childbearing period is strongly suggestive of pregnancy. Abdominal enlargement in nulliparous women may be less pronounced than in multiparous women, in whom some of the abdominal muscle tone was lost during previous pregnancies. Indeed, the abdominal wall in some multiparous women is so flaccid that the uterus sags forward and downward, producing a pendulous abdomen. This difference in abdominal tone between first and subsequent pregnancies is sometimes so obvious that women in the latter part of a second pregnancy commonly suspect a twin pregnancy because of the apparent greater size of their abdomen, as compared with their previous pregnancy. The abdomen of the pregnant woman also undergoes significant changes in shape depending on the woman's body position. The uterus is much less prominent, of course, when the pregnant woman is in the supine position.

CHANGES IN SIZE, SHAPE, AND CONSISTENCY OF THE UTERUS. During the first few weeks of pregnancy, the increase in size of the uterus is limited principally to the anteroposterior diameter, but a little later in gestation, the body of the uterus is almost globular; an average uterine diameter of 8 cm is attained by 12 weeks. On bimanual examination, the body of the uterus during pregnancy feels doughy or elastic and sometimes becomes exceedingly soft. At about 6 to 8 weeks after the onset of the last menstrual period, the **Hegar sign** becomes evident. With one hand of the examiner on the abdomen and two fingers of the other hand placed in the vagina, the still-firm cervix is felt, with the elastic body of the uterus above the compressible soft isthmus, which is between the two. Occasionally, the softening at the isthmus is so marked that the cervix and the body of the uterus seem to be separate organs. At this time in pregnancy, the inexperienced examiner may mistakenly conclude that the cervix is a small uterus, and that the softened body of the fundus is an adnexal mass. This sign is not, however, positively diagnostic of pregnancy, because occasionally it may be present when the walls of the uterus of a nonpregnant woman are excessively soft for reasons other than pregnancy.

CHANGES IN THE CERVIX. By 6 to 8 weeks, the cervix usually is considerably softened. In primigravidas, the consistency of cervical tissue that surrounds the external os is more similar to that of the lips of the mouth than to that of the nasal cartilage, which is characteristic of the cervix in nonpregnant women. Other conditions, however, may cause softening of the cervix, such as estrogen–progestin contraceptives. As pregnancy progresses, the cervical canal may become sufficiently patulous to admit the fingertip. In certain inflammatory conditions, as well as with carcinoma, the cervix may remain firm during pregnancy, yielding only with the onset of labor, if at all.

BRAXTON HICKS CONTRACTIONS. During pregnancy, the uterus undergoes palpable but ordinarily painless contractions at irregular intervals from the early stages of gestation. These contractions, referred to as Braxton Hicks contractions, may increase in number and amplitude when the uterus is massaged. These are not, however, positive signs of pregnancy, because similar contractions are sometimes observed in uteri of women with hematometra and occasionally in the uterus in which there are soft myomas, especially those of the pedunculated, submucous variety. The detection of Braxton Hicks contractions, however, may be helpful in excluding the existence of an ectopic abdominal pregnancy. In the last few days of pregnancy, the frequency of contractions increases, especially during nighttime hours. This is associated with uterine preparedness for labor, that is, phase 1 of parturition (Chap. 11, p. 265).

BALLOTTEMENT. Near midpregnancy, the volume of the fetus is small compared with that of amnionic fluid. Consequently, sudden pressure exerted on the uterus may cause the fetus to sink in the amnionic fluid and then rebound to its original position; the tap produced (ballottement) is felt by the examining fingers.

OUTLINING THE FETUS. In the second half of pregnancy, the outlines of the fetal body may be palpated through the maternal abdominal wall, and the outlining of the fetus becomes easier the nearer that term is approached. Occasionally, subserous myomas may be of such a size and shape as to simulate the fetal head, small parts, or both, thus causing serious diagnostic errors. Therefore, a positive diagnosis of pregnancy cannot be made from this sign alone.

DETECTION OF CHORIONIC GONADOTROPIN. The presence of chorionic gonadotropin (hCG) in maternal plasma and its excretion in urine provides the basis for the endocrine tests for pregnancy. This hormone can be identified in body fluids by any one of a variety of immunoassay or bioassay techniques.

Chorionic gonadotropin is important for maternal recognition of pregnancy because it acts to "rescue" the corpus luteum, the principal site of progesterone formation during the first 6 weeks. It prevents corpus luteum involution. It also is a luteinizing hormone (LH)–like agent that acts as a surrogate in responsive tissues, such as the ovary (corpus luteum) and testis (Leydig cells). Specifically, hCG acts by way of the plasma membrane LH receptor.

As discussed in Chapter 6 (p. 110), hCG is a glycoprotein with a high carbohydrate content; the molecule is a heterodimer composed of two dissimilar subunits, designated α and β, which are noncovalently linked. These subunits have been separated and isolated in pure form, the primary structure of each has been characterized, and the genes encoding these subunits have been analyzed in appreciable detail.

LEVELS OF hCG IN PREGNANCY. The hormone is produced exclusively by the syncytiotrophoblast, not by cytotrophoblast. Production begins very early in pregnancy, almost certainly by the day of implantation. Thereafter, hCG levels in maternal plasma and urine rise very rapidly. With a sensitive test, it can be detected in maternal plasma or urine by 8 to 9 days after ovulation. The doubling time of plasma hCG concentration is 1.4 to 2.0 days (Chartier and colleagues, 1979). Levels increase from the day of implantation to reach peak levels at about 60 to 70 days. Thereafter, the concentration declines slowly until a nadir is reached at about 100 to 130 days (Fig. 2–6).

PREGNANCY TESTS. There are a number of inexpensive, commercially available kits for pregnancy testing. They can be completed in 3 to 5 minutes, with high accuracy and, with certain precautions, high precision. Many different test systems are available in kit form; each, however, is dependent upon the same principle: recognition of hCG (or a subunit) by an antibody to the hCG molecule or epitopes of the β-subunit. Nearly 15 years ago, Bandi and colleagues (1987) reported that there were 39 commercially available kits for *urine* pregnancy tests. By 1991, Cole and Kardana (1992) observed that there were more than 50 commercial kits for *serum* measurement.

With the recognition that LH and hCG were composed of an α- and a β-subunit, that the two subunits of each molecular species could be separated and purified, and that the β-subunits of each were structurally distinct, antibodies were developed with high specificity for the β-subunit of hCG. These have little or no discernible cross-reactivity against LH. They have been raised by immunization of animals (polyclonal antibodies) or by hybridoma techniques (monoclonal antibodies) against recognition sites on the β-subunit of hCG. Immunogenicity of gonadotropin subunits is very great, and vaccines that prevent pregnancy have been developed using human β-hCG as a heterospecies dimer with the α-subunit of ovine LH (Talwar and co-workers, 1994).

IMMUNOASSAYS WITHOUT RADIOISOTOPES. In many immunoassay procedures, the principle of **agglutination inhibition** is used. This involves prevention of flocculation of hCG-coated particles, such as latex, to which hCG is covalently bound. The commercially available kits contain two reagents. One is a suspension of latex particles coated with or covalently bound to hCG, and the other contains a solution of hCG antibody. To test for hCG, one drop of urine is mixed with one drop of the antibody-containing solution on a black glass slide. If hCG is not present in the test sample, antibody will remain available to agglutinate the hCG-coated latex particles, which are added subsequently. Agglutination of the latex particles can be easily observed. If hCG were present in the urine, it would bind to the antibody and thus prevent antibody-induced agglutination of the hCG-coated latex particles. Therefore, the pregnancy test is positive if no agglutination occurs; the pregnancy test is negative when agglutination occurs.

The **enzyme-linked immunosorbent assay (ELISA)** is useful for quantification of extremely small amounts of hormone. The ELISA test uses a monoclonal antibody bound to a solid-phase support (usually plastic), which binds the hCG in the test sample. A second antibody is added to "sandwich" the test sample hCG. It is the second antibody to which an enzyme, such as alkaline phosphatase, is linked. When substrate for this enzyme is added, a blue color develops, the intensity of which is proportional to the amount of enzyme and thus

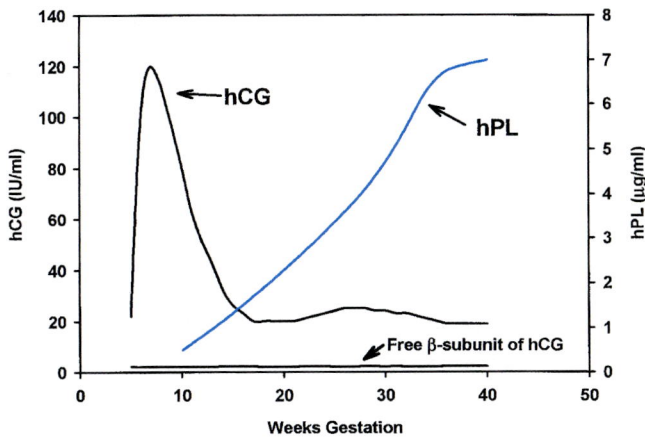

FIGURE 2–6. Mean concentration of chorionic gonadotropin (hCG) and placental lactogen (hPL) in serum of women throughout normal pregnancy. The free β-subunit of hCG is in low concentration or else undetectable throughout pregnancy. The concentration of free α-subunit of hCG in serum increases gradually during pregnancy in a manner similar to that of hPL, albeit in much smaller amounts. (Data from Ashitaka and colleagues, 1980; Selenkow and co-workers, 1971.)

to the amount of second antibody bound. This, in turn, is a function of the amount of hCG in the test sample. The sensitivity of ELISA for hCG in serum is 50 mIU per mL.

The **immunoflurometric assay (IFMA)** uses photon emission from a fluorescent label to provide sensitivity almost comparable with that of radioimmunoassay. The assays are sufficiently sensitive to detect hCG, presumably of anterior pituitary origin, in serum of postmenopausal women (Tyrey, 1995).

IMMUNOASSAYS OF hCG USING RADIOISOTOPES. In the classical **radioimmunoassay (RIA),** [125I] iodo-hCG is used as the radiolabeled ligand for antibodies against hCG. This assay is dependent upon displacement of, or competition with, the radiolabeled ligand by non-radiolabeled hCG in the biological sample tested. In radioimmunoassays, "free" and "bound" [125I] iodo-hCG are separated and the unbound radioactivity is assayed. By construction of standard curves, hCG is quantified with great accuracy and sensitivity.

The **immunoradiometric assay (IRMA)** is characterized by the use of antibody (binding sites) in excess as the radiolabeled material, rather than the ligand (hCG). One approach is the use of two antibodies that recognize separate epitopes on the hCG. One antibody, connected to a solid support, is used to capture the hCG from the sample. The second antibody is the radiolabeled probe and functions to quantify the captured ligand. Immuno-radiometric assays also can be specific for the β-subunit of hCG.

ACCURACY. In a multicenter collaborative study sponsored by the National Institutes of Health, Jova-novic and associates (1987) found that laboratories conducting routine clinical tests could detect hCG accurately at the time of first "missed" menses, but not necessarily before this time.

QUANTIFICATION OF hCG. Precise quantification of hCG in biological fluids is important in the management of some conditions. These include pregnancy monitoring to exclude ectopic pregnancy and to evaluate the course and treatment of neoplastic trophoblastic disease. By use of very sensitive radioimmunoassays, hCG can be detected even in many normal persons, presumably because this small amount of hCG arises by pituitary secretion.

HOME PREGNANCY TESTS. A number of relatively inexpensive over-the-counter pregnancy test kits are available. In several, the principle of hemagglutination inhibition using sheep erythrocytes and antibodies to hCG is used to test a urine sample. Home pregnancy-testing kits are one-step tests. Essential features are the use of:

1. An absorbent wick that is held in contact with a porous membrane, which contains three separate zones of antibody.
2. The principles of immunochromatography.

The first zone of antibody is deposited so as to be mobilizable; it consists of colored latex particles sensitized with monoclonal antibodies to the β-subunit of hCG, which is immobilized in the membrane. If the urine contains hCG, it will react with the anti–β-hCG on the latex, and this will be trapped by the second, anti–β-subunit hCG zone antibody, causing the formation of a colored line in the large window (May, 1991).

In early studies, the false-negative rate was about 25 percent (Valanis and Perlman, 1982). Later, Lee and Hart (1990) showed that while tests were capable of 97 percent accuracy, this was only when done by trained technologists. Bastian and colleagues (1998) evaluated published results of 16 kits, of which only five met their inclusion criteria. If testing was done by volunteers, a mean 91-percent sensitivity was obtained. Importantly, however, actual patients only obtained 75 percent sensitivity.

ECTOPIC PREGNANCY. Because hCG is present in plasma and urine of all women with ectopic pregnancies, its measurement has become indispensable as part of modern clinical management of these. This subject is discussed in detail in Chapter 34.

POSITIVE SIGNS OF PREGNANCY. The three positive signs of pregnancy are:

1. Identification of fetal heart action separately and distinctly from that of the pregnant woman.
2. Perception of active fetal movements by the examiner.
3. Recognition of the embryo and fetus any time in pregnancy by sonographic techniques or of the more mature fetus radiographically in the latter half of pregnancy.

FETAL HEART ACTION. Hearing or observing the pulsations of the fetal heart assures the diagnosis of pregnancy. Fetal heart contractions can be identified by auscultation with a special fetoscope, by use of the Doppler principle with ultrasound, and by sonography.

The fetal heartbeat can be detected by auscultation with a stethoscope by 17 weeks, on average, and by 19 weeks in nearly all pregnancies in non-obese women (Jimenez and co-workers, 1979). The fetal heart rate at this stage and beyond ranges from 120 to 160 bpm and is heard as a double sound resembling the tick of a watch under a pillow. It is not sufficient merely to "hear" the "fetal" heart; it must be different from that of the maternal pulse. During much of pregnancy, the fetus moves freely in amnionic fluid, and consequently, the site on the maternal abdomen where fetal heart sounds can be heard best will vary.

Several instruments are available that make use of the Doppler principle to detect the action of the fetal heart. Ultrasound is directed toward moving fetal blood. The sound reflected by moving blood undergoes a frequency shift, the echo of which is detected by a receiving crystal immediately adjacent to the transmitting crystal. Because of the difference in heart rates, pulsatile flow in the fetus is easily differentiated from that of the mother unless there is severe fetal bradycardia or significant maternal tachycardia. Fetal cardiac action can be detected almost always by 10 weeks with appropriate Doppler equipment.

Echocardiography can be used to detect fetal heart action as early as 48 days after the first day of the last normal menses. Real-time sonography with a vaginal probe can detect fetal heart action as early as 5 weeks of amenorrhea.

In the later months of pregnancy, the examiner may often hear sounds other than those produced by fetal heart action. The most common of these are:

1. The funic (umbilical cord) souffle.
2. The uterine souffle.
3. Sounds resulting from fetal movement.
4. Maternal pulse.
5. Gurgling sounds produced by gas or liquid propulsion through the maternal intestine.

The funic souffle is caused by the rush of blood through the umbilical arteries. It is a sharp, whistling sound that is synchronous with the fetal pulse. It is inconstant, sometimes being recognizable distinctly at the time of one examination, but not found in the same pregnancy on other occasions.

The uterine souffle is heard as a soft, blowing sound that is synchronous with the maternal pulse. It is usually heard most distinctly during auscultation of the lower portion of the uterus. This sound is produced by the passage of blood through the dilated uterine vessels and is characteristic not only of pregnancy but of any condition in which the blood flow to the uterus is greatly increased. Accordingly, a uterine souffle may be heard in nonpregnant women with large uterine myomas or large ovarian tumors.

Frequently, the maternal pulse can be heard distinctly by auscultation of the abdomen; and in some women, the pulsation of the aorta is unusually loud. Occasionally during examination, the pulse of the mother may become so rapid as to simulate the fetal heart sounds.

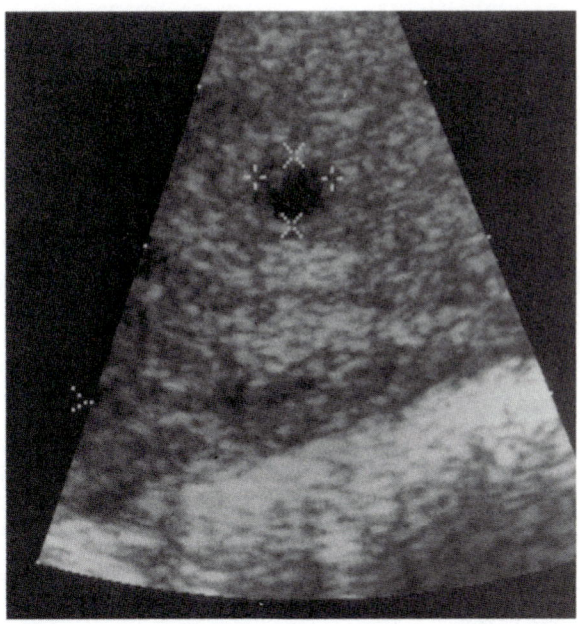

FIGURE 2–7. Abdominal sonogram in which a gestational sac at 4 to 5 weeks' gestational (menstrual) age is demonstrated. (Courtesy of Dr. Diane Twickler.)

PERCEPTION OF FETAL MOVEMENTS. Detection by the examiner of fetal movements can occur after about 20 weeks. Fetal movements vary in intensity from a faint flutter early in pregnancy to brisk motions at a later period; the latter are sometimes visible as well as palpable. Occasionally, somewhat similar sensations may be produced by contractions of the abdominal muscles or intestinal peristalsis, although these should not deceive an experienced examiner.

ULTRASONIC RECOGNITION OF PREGNANCY. The use of transvaginal sonography has revolutionized imaging of early pregnancy and its growth and development. A gestational sac may be demonstrated by abdominal sonography after only 4 to 5 weeks' menstrual age (Fig. 2–7). By 35 days, all normal sacs should be visible, and after 6 weeks, a heartbeat should be detectable (American College of Obstetricians and Gynecologists, 1995). By 8 weeks, the gestational age can be estimated quite accurately (see Table 41–3). Up to 12 weeks, the crown–rump length is predictive of gestational age within 4 days. This measurement is discussed in detail in Chapter 41 (p. 1114).

REFERENCES

American College of Obstetricians and Gynecologists: Gynecologic ultrasonography. ACOG Technical Bulletin No. 215, November 1995

Ashitaka Y, Nishimura R, Takemori M, Tojo S: Production and secretion of hCG and hCG subunits by trophoblastic tissue. In Segal S (ed): Chorionic Gonadotropins. New York, Plenum, 1980, p 151

Bandi ZL, Schoen I, DeLara M: Enzyme-linked immunosorbent urine pregnancy tests: Clinical specificity studies. Am J Clin Pathol 87:236, 1987

Bastian LA, Nanda K, Hasselblad V, Simel DL: Diagnostic efficiency of home pregnancy test kits. A meta-analysis. Arch Fam Med 7:465, 1998

Bazer RW, Vallet JL, Roberts RM, Sharp DC, Thatcher WW: Role of conceptus secretory products in establishment of pregnancy. J Reprod Fertil 76:841, 1986

Chadwick JR: Value of the bluish coloration of the vaginal entrance as a sign of pregnancy. Trans Am Gynecol Soc 11:399, 1886

Chartier M, Roger M, Barrat J, Michelon B: Measurement of plasma chorionic gonadotropin (hCG) and CG activities in the late luteal phase: Evidence of the occurrence of spontaneous menstrual abortions in infertile women. Fertil Steril 31:134, 1979

Cole LA, Kardana A: Discordant results in human chorionic gonadotropin assays. Clin Chem 38:263, 1992

Eaton JW, Mayer AJ: The social biology of very high fertility among the Hutterites: The demography of a unique population. Hum Biol 25:206, 1953

Godkin JD, Bazer FW, Roberts RM: Ovine trophoblast protein, 1. An early secreted blastocyst protein binds specifically to uterine endometrium and affects protein synthesis. Endocrinology 114:120, 1984

Hansen PJ, Anthony RV, Bazer RW, Baumbach GA, Roberts RM: In vitro synthesis and secretion of ovine trophoblast protein-1 during the period of maternal recognition of pregnancy. Endocrinology 117:1424, 1985

Imakawa K, Anthony RV, Kazemi M, Marotti KR, Polites HG, Roberts RM: Interferon-like sequence of ovine trophoblast protein secreted by embryonic trophectoderm. Nature 330:377, 1987

Jimenez JM, Tyson JE, Santos-Ramos R, Duenhoelter JH: Comparison of obstetric and pediatric evaluation of gestational age. Pediatr Res 13:498, 1979

Jovanovic L, Singh M, Saxena BB, Mills JL, Tulchinsky D, Holmes LB, Simpson JL, Metzger BE, Labarbera A, Aarons J, Van Allen MI: NICHD-DIEP Study Group: Verification of early pregnancy tests in a multicenter trial. Proc Soc Exp Biol Med 184:201, 1987

Kolata GB: !Kung hunter-gatherers: Feminism, diet and birth control. Science 185:932, 1974

Lee C, Hart LL: Accuracy of home pregnancy tests. DICP 24:712, 1990

Li J, Roberts RM: Interferon-tau and interferon-alpha interact with the same receptors in bovine endometrium. Use of a readily iodinatable form of recombinant interferon-tau for binding studies. J Biol Chem 269:13544, 1994

MacDonald PC, Dombroski RA, Casey ML: Recurrent secretion of progesterone in large amounts: An endocrine/metabolic disorder unique to young women? Endocr Rev 12:372, 1991

May K: Home tests to monitor fertility. Am J Obstet Gynecol 165:2000, 1991

Nathanielsz PW, Figueroa JP, Honnebier MB: In the rhesus monkey placental retention after fetectomy at 121 to 130 days' gestation outlasts the normal duration of pregnancy. Am J Obstet Gynecol 166:1529, 1992

Selenkow HA, Varina K, Younger D, White P, Emerson K Jr: Patterns of serum immunoreactive human placental lactogen (IR-HPL) and chorionic gonadotropin (IR-HCG) in diabetic pregnancy. Diabetes 20:696, 1971

Short RV: Breast feeding. Sci Am 250:35, 1984

Short RV: The origins of human sexuality. In Austin CR, Short RV (eds): Reproduction in Mammals: Human Sexuality. Cambridge, Cambridge University Press, 1980, p 2

Short RV: Definition of the problem: The evolution of human reproduction. In Short RV, Baird DT (eds): Contraceptives of the Future. Cambridge, University Printing House, 1976a, p 3

Short RV: The evolution of human reproduction. Proc Roy Soc Lond 195:3, 1976b

Short RV: Maternal recognition of pregnancy. In Wolstenhome GEW, O'Connor M (eds): Foetal Autonomy. London, Churchill, 1969, p 2

Speert H, Guttmacher AF: Frequency and significance of bleeding in early pregnancy. JAMA 155:172, 1954

Talwar GP, Singh O, Pal R, Chatterjee N, Sahai P, Dhall K, Kaur J, Das SK, Suri S, Buckshee K, Saraya L, Saxena BN: A vaccine that prevents pregnancy in women. Proc Natl Acad Sci USA 91:8532, 1994

Townsend L, Shelton JG: Intrauterine death due to fetal erythroblastosis. Aust NZ J Obstet Gynaecol 4:84, 1964

Tyrey L: Human chorionic gonadotropin: Properties and assay methods. Semin Oncol 22:121, 1995

Valanis BG, Perlman CS: Home pregnancy testing kits: Prevalence of use, false-negative rates, and compliance with instructions. Am J Public Health 72:1034, 1982

Zaneveld IJ, Tauber PF, Port C, Propping D: Scanning electron microscopy of cervical mucus crystallization. Obstet Gynecol 46:419, 1975

3

Anatomy of the Reproductive Tract

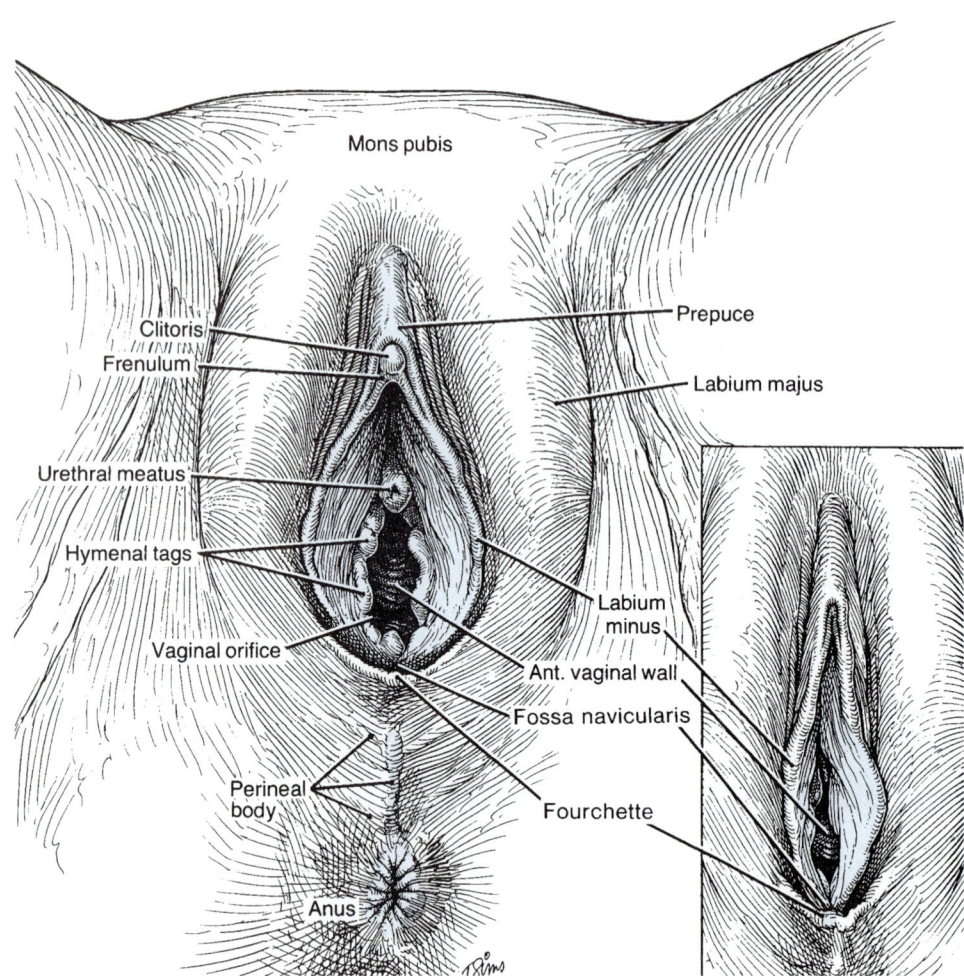

FIGURE 3–1. External organs of reproduction of women. The lower anterior vaginal wall is visible through the labia minora. In nulliparous women, the vaginal orifice is not so readily visible (inset) because of the close apposition of the labia minora.

The organs of reproduction of women are classified as either external or internal. There may be marked variation in anatomical structures in a given woman, and this is especially true for major blood vessels and nerves.

EXTERNAL GENERATIVE ORGANS

The *pudenda,* or the external organs of generation, are commonly designated the *vulva,* which includes all structures visible externally from the pubis to the perineum, that is, the mons pubis, labia majora and minora, clitoris, hymen, vestibule, urethral opening, and various glandular and vascular structures (Fig. 3–1).

MONS PUBIS. The mons pubis, or mons veneris, is the fat-filled cushion that lies over the symphysis pubis. After puberty, the skin of the mons pubis is covered by curly hair that forms the *escutcheon.* Generally, the distribution of pubic hair differs in the two sexes. In women, it is distributed in a triangular area, the base of which is formed by the upper margin of the symphysis, and a few hairs are distributed downward over the outer surface of the labia majora. In men, the escutcheon is not so well circumscribed.

LABIA MAJORA. The labia majora are two rounded folds of adipose tissue that are covered with skin, and that extend downward and backward from the mons pubis. Among adult women, these structures vary somewhat in appearance, principally according to the amount of fat that is contained within these tissues. Embryologically, the labia majora are homologous with the male scrotum. The round ligaments terminate at the upper borders of the labia majora. After repeated childbearing, the labia majora are less prominent, and in old age usually begin to shrivel. Ordinarily, these structures are 7 to 8 cm in length, 2 to 3 cm in width, and 1 to 1.5 cm in thickness, and are somewhat tapered at the lower extremities. In children and nulliparous women (Fig. 3–1), the labia majora usually lie in close apposition, and thereby completely conceal the underlying tissues; whereas in multiparous women, the labia majora may gape widely. The labia majora are continuous directly with the mons pubis above and merge into the perineum posteriorly, at a site where these structures are joined medially to form the *posterior commissure.*

Before puberty, the outer surface of the labia is similar to that of the adjacent skin, but after puberty they are covered with hair. In nulliparous women, the inner surface is moist and resembles a mucous membrane; whereas in multiparous women, the inner surface becomes more skinlike but is not covered with hair. The labia majora are richly supplied with sebaceous glands. Beneath the skin, there is a layer of dense connective tissue that is rich in elastic fibers and adipose tissue but is nearly void of muscular elements. Unlike the squamous epithelium of the vagina and cervix, there are epithelial appendages in parts of the vulvar skin. Beneath the skin, there is a mass of fat, which provides the bulk of the volume of the labium; this tissue is supplied with a plexus of veins that, as the result of injury, may rupture to create a hematoma.

LABIA MINORA. Two flat, reddish folds of tissue are visible when the labia majora are separated. These structures are the labia minora, or nymphae; structures that join at the upper extremity of the vulva. The labia minora vary greatly in size and shape. In nulliparous women, they usually are not visible behind the nonseparated labia majora, whereas in multiparous women, it is common for the labia minora to project beyond the labia majora.

Each labium minus is a thin fold of tissue that, when projected, is moist and reddish in appearance and is similar to that of a mucous membrane. These structures, however, are covered by stratified squamous epithelium into which numerous papillae project. There are no hair follicles in the labia minora, but there are many sebaceous follicles and, occasionally, a few sweat glands. The interior of the labial folds is comprised of connective tissue with many vessels and some smooth muscular fibers, as is the case in typical erectile structures. These structures are supplied with a variety of nerve endings and are extremely sensitive.

The tissues of the labia minora converge superiorly, where each is divided into two lamellae, the lower pair of which fuses to form the *frenulum of the clitoris,* and the upper pair of which merges to form the *prepuce* of the clitoris. Inferiorly, the labia minora extend to approach the midline as low ridges of tissue that fuse to form the *fourchette* in nulliparous women; in multiparous women the labia minora usually are imperceptibly contiguous with the labia majora.

CLITORIS. The clitoris is the homologue of the penis and is located near the superior extremity of the vulva. This erectile organ projects downward between the branched extremities of the labia minora. The clitoris is comprised of a glans, a body (corpus), and two crura. The glans is made up of spindle-shaped cells, and in the body there are two corpora cavernosa, in the walls of which are smooth muscle fibers. The long, narrow crura arise from the inferior surface of the ischiopubic rami and fuse just below the middle of the pubic arch to form the corpus.

Rarely does the clitoris exceed 2 cm in length, even in a state of erection (Verkauf and associates, 1992), and it is bent sharply by traction that is exerted by the labia minora. As a result, the free end of the clitoris is pointed downward and inward toward the vaginal opening. The glans, which rarely exceeds 0.5 cm in diameter, is covered by stratified squamous epithelium that is richly supplied with nerve endings and is, therefore, extremely sensitive. The vessels of the erectile clitoris are connected with the vestibular bulbs; the clitoris is the principal erogenous organ of women.

In the labia majora, as well as the labia minora and clitoris, Krantz (1958) reported that there is a delicate network of free nerve endings, the fibers of which terminate in small knoblike thickenings in or adjacent to the cells. These nerve endings are encountered more frequently in the papillae than elsewhere; moreover, tactile discs are also found in abundance in these areas. The number of genital corpuscles, which are considered the main structures that are mediators of erotic sensation, varies considerably. These structures are distributed sparsely and randomly in the labia majora deep in the corium, but are abundant in the labia minora and in the skin that overlies the glans clitoris.

VESTIBULE. The vestibule is an almond-shaped area that is enclosed by the labia minora laterally and extends from the clitoris to the fourchette. The vestibule is the functionally mature female structure of the urogenital sinus of the embryo; in the mature state it usually is perforated by six openings: the urethra, the vagina, the ducts of the Bartholin glands, and, at times, the ducts of the paraurethral glands, also called the Skene ducts and glands (Fig. 3–2). The posterior portion of the vestibule between the fourchette and the vaginal opening is called the *fossa navicularis,* and it is usually observed only in nulliparous women.

The *Bartholin glands* (Fig. 3–2) are a pair of small compound structures about 0.5 to 1 cm in diameter. Each is situated beneath the vestibule on either side of the vaginal opening and they are the *major vestibular glands.* The Bartholin glands lie under the constrictor muscle of the vagina and sometimes are found to be covered partially by the vestibular bulbs. The gland ducts are 1.5 to 2 cm long and open on the sides of the vestibule just outside the lateral margin of the vaginal orifice. The small gland lumen ordinarily admits only the finest of probes. At times of sexual arousal, mucoid

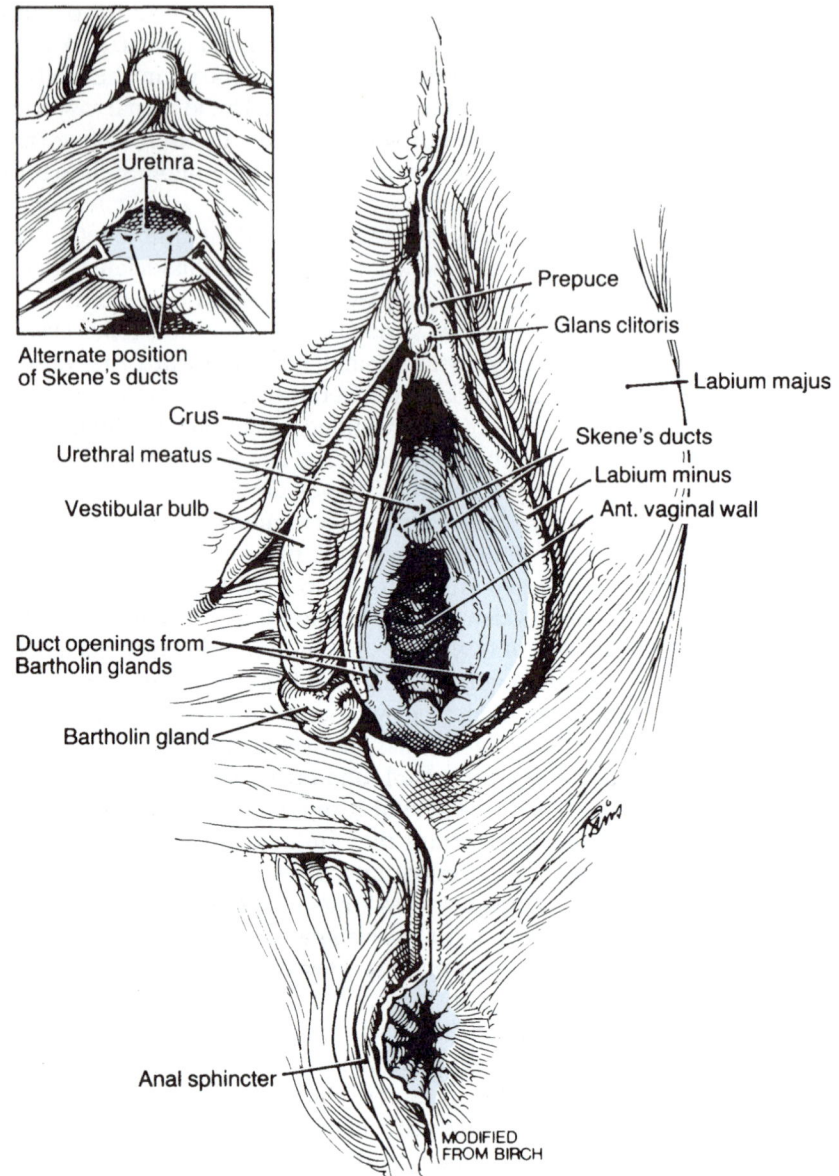

Urethra

Alternate position
of Skene's ducts

Crus

Urethral meatus

Vestibular bulb

Duct openings from
Bartholin glands

Bartholin gland

Anal sphincter

Prepuce

Glans clitoris

Labium majus

Skene's ducts

Labium minus

Ant. vaginal wall

MODIFIED
FROM BIRCH

FIGURE 3–2. The external genitalia with the skin and subcutaneous tissue removed from the right side.

material is secreted from these glands. These glands may harbor *Neisseria gonorrhoeae,* or other bacteria, which in turn may cause suppuration and a Bartholin gland abscess (Chap. 35, p. 921).

URETHRAL OPENING. The lower two thirds of the urethra lies immediately above the anterior vaginal wall. The urethral opening or meatus is in the midline of the vestibule, 1 to 1.5 cm below the pubic arch, and a short distance above the vaginal opening. The urethral orifice appears as a vertical slit, which can be distended to 4 or 5 mm in diameter. Ordinarily, the *paraurethral ducts,* also known as the Skene ducts, open onto the vestibule on either side of the urethra; but occasionally they open

on the posterior wall of the urethra just inside the meatus (Fig. 3–2). These ducts are about 0.5 mm in diameter, and of variable length.

VESTIBULAR BULBS. Beneath the mucous membrane of the vestibule on either side are the vestibular bulbs, which are almond-shaped aggregations of veins, 3 to 4 cm long, 1 to 2 cm wide, and 0.5 to 1 cm thick. These bulbs lie in close apposition to the ischiopubic rami and are partially covered by the ischiocavernosus and constrictor vaginae muscles. The lower terminations of the vestibular bulbs usually are at about the middle of the vaginal opening, and anteriorly, the vestibular bulbs extend upward toward the clitoris.

Embryologically, the vestibular bulbs correspond to the anlage of the corpus spongiosum of the penis. During childbirth, they usually are pushed up beneath the pubic arch; because the posterior ends partially encircle the vagina, however, these structures are liable to injury and rupture, which may result in a vulvar hematoma or hemorrhage.

VAGINAL OPENING AND HYMEN. The vaginal opening varies considerably in size and shape. In virginal women, it most often is hidden by the overlapping labia minora, and when exposed, it usually appears almost completely closed by the membranous hymen.

There also are marked differences in shape and consistency of the hymen, which is comprised mainly of elastic and collagenous connective tissue. Both the outer and inner surfaces are covered by stratified squamous epithelium. Connective tissue papillae are more numerous on the vaginal surface and at the free edge. There are no glandular or muscular elements in the hymen, and it is not richly supplied with nerve fibers.

In the newborn, the hymen is very vascular and redundant; in pregnant women, the epithelium is thick and the tissue is rich in glycogen; after menopause, the epithelium of the hymen is thin and focal cornification may develop. In adult virginal women, the hymen is a membrane of various thickness that surrounds the vaginal opening more or less completely, with an aperture varying in diameter from that of a pinpoint to a caliber that admits the tip of one or even two fingers. The hymenal opening usually is crescentic or circular, but occasionally may be cribriform, septate, or fimbriated. The fimbriated type of hymen in virginal women may be indistinguishable from one that has been penetrated during intercourse; thus, it is not possible to determine virginity by such an examination.

As a rule, the hymen is torn at several sites during first coitus, usually in the posterior portion. The edges of the torn tissue soon cicatrize, and the hymen becomes divided permanently into two or more portions that are separated by narrow sulci. The extent to which rupture occurs varies with the structure of the hymen and the extent to which it is distended. Although commonly it is believed that rupture of the hymen is accompanied by bleeding, this is not evident in all women. Occasionally with hymenal rupture, however, there may be profuse bleeding. Rarely, the hymenal membrane may be very resistant and incision of the tissue may be necessary before coitus can be accomplished.

The changes in the hymen that are brought about by coitus are occasionally of medicolegal importance, especially in instances of alleged sexual assault. Usually when nulliparous women are examined a few hours after an attack, the finding of fresh hymenal lacerations, abrasions, or bleeding points on the hymen constitutes corroborative evidence of recent vaginal penetration, possibly by intercourse. The absence of such findings is of no significance, however, because the hymen may not be lacerated even with repeated coitus in a short time period. In fact, many cases of pregnancy have been reported in women in whom the hymen did not appear to have been "ruptured."

As a rule, the changes produced in the hymen by childbirth are readily recognizable. After recovery from delivery, several cicatrized nodules of various sizes are formed, the tissue remnants of the hymen. *Imperforate hymen,* a rare lesion, is a condition in which the vaginal orifice is occluded completely, causing retention of the menstrual discharge.

VAGINA. The vagina is a tubular, musculomembranous structure that extends from the vulva to the uterus, interposed anteriorly and posteriorly between the urinary bladder and the rectum (Figs. 3–3 and 3–4). This organ has many functions: it is the excretory canal of the uterus, through which uterine secretions and menstrual flow escape; the female organ of copulation; and part of the birth canal. The upper portion of the vagina arises from the müllerian ducts, and the lower portion is formed from the urogenital sinus. Anteriorly, the vagina is in contact with the bladder and urethra, from which it is separated by connective tissue, often referred to as the vesicovaginal septum. Posteriorly, between the lower portion of the vagina and the rectum, there are similar tissues that together form the rectovaginal septum. Usually, the upper fourth of the vagina is separated from the rectum by the rectouterine pouch, also called the cul-de-sac of Douglas.

Normally, the anterior and posterior vaginal walls lie in contact with only a slight space that intervenes between the lateral margins. Thus, when not distended, the vaginal canal on transverse section is H-shaped (Fig. 3–5). The vagina can be distended markedly, a characteristic that is most evident during childbirth.

Vaginal length varies considerably; commonly, the anterior and posterior vaginal walls are, respectively, 6 to 8 cm, and 7 to 10 cm in length. The upper end of the vaginal vault is subdivided into the anterior, posterior, and two lateral fornices by the uterine cervix. Because the vagina is attached higher up on the posterior wall than on the anterior wall of the cervix, the depth of the posterior fornix is appreciably greater than the anterior. The lateral fornices are intermediate in depth. The fornices are of considerable clinical importance because the internal pelvic organs usually can be palpated through the thin walls of the fornices. Moreover, the posterior fornix usually provides ready surgical access to the peritoneal cavity.

Prominent longitudinal ridges project into the vaginal

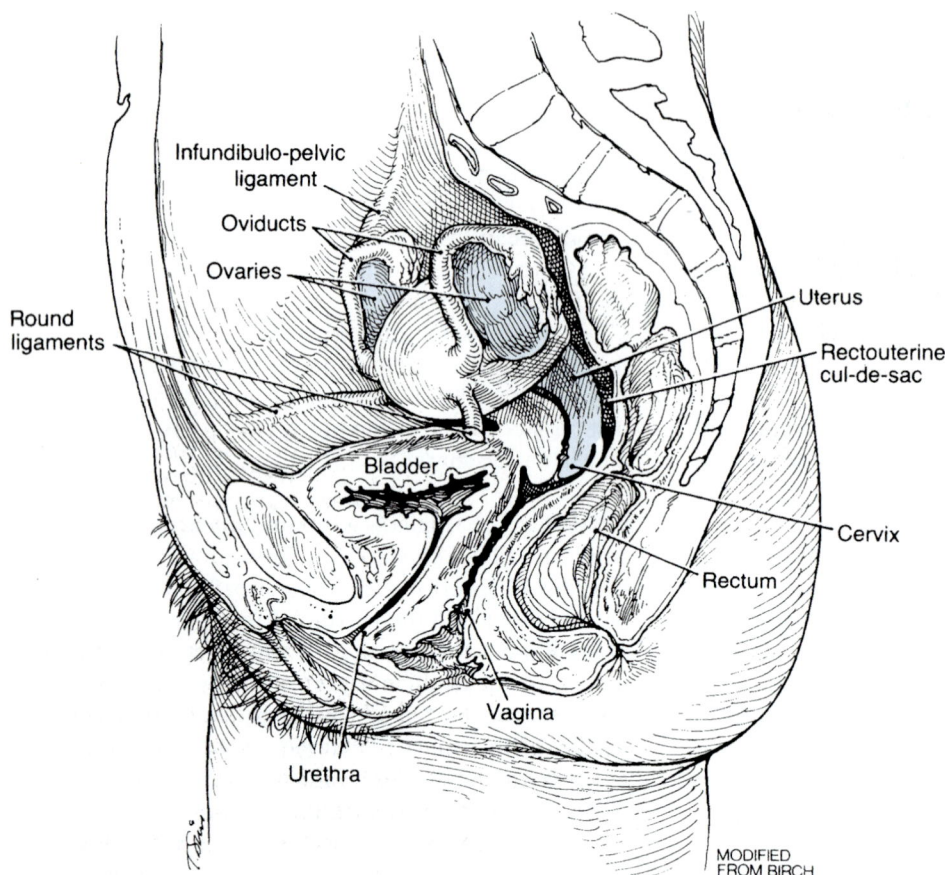

Infundibulo-pelvic ligament

Oviducts

Ovaries

Round ligaments

Uterus

Rectouterine cul-de-sac

Bladder

Cervix

Rectum

Vagina

Urethra

MODIFIED FROM BIRCH

FIGURE 3–3. Sagittal section of the pelvis of an adult woman showing relations of pelvic viscera.

lumen from the midlines of both the anterior and posterior walls. In nulliparous women, numerous transverse ridges, or *rugae,* extend outward from and almost at right angles to the longitudinal vaginal ridges. The rugae are such as to form a corrugated surface, which is not

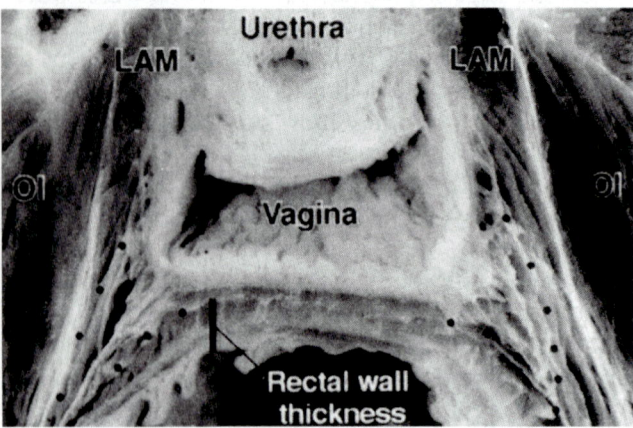

Urethra

LAM   LAM

OI   OI

Vagina

Rectal wall thickness

FIGURE 3–4. Macroscopic section of a 14-year-old nulliparous cadaver. Fibers of the endopelvic fascia that are outlined by dots attach to the lateral sulcus of the posterior vaginal wall. (LAM = levator ani muscle; OI = obturator internus muscle.) (From Delancey, 1999, with permission.)

present before menarche and is one that gradually becomes obliterated after repeated childbirth and after menopause. In elderly multiparous women, the vaginal walls often are smooth.

The vaginal mucosa is comprised of noncornified stratified squamous epithelium. Beneath the epithelium there is a thin fibromuscular coat, usually consisting of an inner circular layer and an outer longitudinal layer of smooth muscle. There is a thin layer of connective tissue beneath the mucosa and the muscularis; one that is rich in blood vessels, and one in which there are a few small lymphoid nodules. The mucosa and muscularis are attached very loosely to the underlying connective tissue. Some argument remains as to whether this connective tissue, often referred to as perivaginal endopelvic fascia, is a definite fascial plane in the strict anatomical sense.

Normally, glands are not present in the vagina. In parous women, however, fragments of stratified epithelium, which sometimes give rise to cysts, are occasionally embedded in the vaginal connective tissue. These *vaginal inclusion cysts* are not glands, but rather are remnants of mucosal tags that were buried during the healing or repair of vaginal lacerations after childbirth. Occasionally, other cysts may be found that are lined

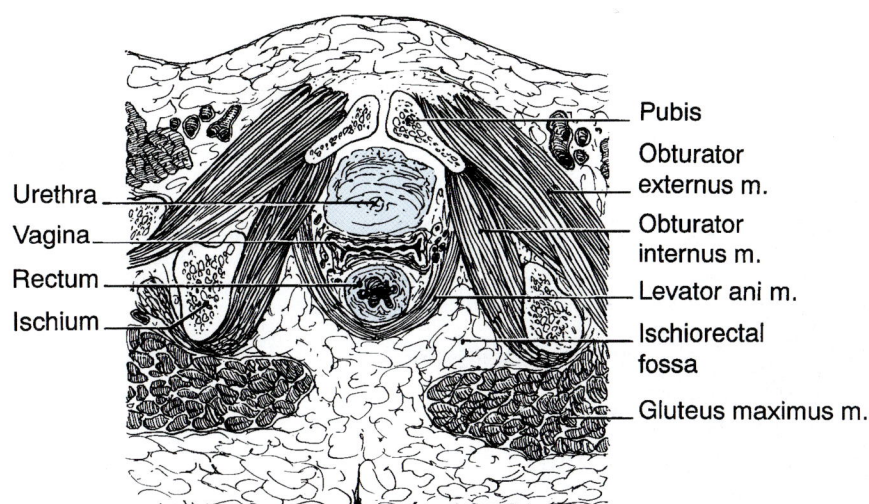

Pubis

Obturator
externus m.

Obturator
internus m.

Levator ani m.

Ischiorectal
fossa

Gluteus maximus m.

Urethra

Vagina

Rectum

Ischium

N. Marshburn

FIGURE 3–5. Cross section of the pelvis of an adult woman; the H-shaped lumen of the vagina is apparent. (m. = muscle.) (N. Marshburn after E. H. Brödel.)

by columnar or cuboidal epithelium and that are believed to be derived from embryonic remnants.

From early in infancy until after menopause, there is a considerable amount of glycogen in the superficial cells of the vaginal mucosa. By examination of cells that are exfoliated from the vaginal epithelium, one can identify the various hormonal events of the ovarian cycle.

In nonpregnant women, the vagina is kept moist by a small amount of secretion from the uterus. During pregnancy, there is copious, acidic vaginal secretion, which normally consists of a curdlike product of exfoliated epithelium and bacteria. *Lactobacillus* species are recovered from most pregnant women in higher concentrations than in nonpregnant women (Larsen and Galask, 1980; McGregor and French, 2000). These are the predominant bacteria of the vagina during pregnancy.

There is an abundant vascular supply to the vagina; the upper third is supplied by the cervicovaginal branches of the uterine arteries, the middle third by the inferior vesical arteries, and the lower third by the middle rectal and internal pudendal arteries. The vaginal artery may branch directly from the internal iliac artery. There is an extensive venous plexus that immediately surrounds the vagina, vessels that follow the course of the arteries; eventually, these veins empty into the internal iliac veins. For the most part, the lymphatics from the lower third of the vagina, along with those of the vulva, drain into the inguinal lymph nodes; those from the middle third drain into the internal iliac nodes; and those from the upper third drain into the iliac nodes. According to Krantz (1958), although the vagina is devoid of any special nerve endings (genital corpuscles), occasionally, free nerve endings are found in the papillae.

PERINEUM. The many structures that make up the perineum are illustrated in Figure 3–6. Most of the support of the perineum is provided by the pelvic and urogenital diaphragms. The *pelvic diaphragm* consists of the levator ani muscles plus the coccygeus muscles posteriorly and the fascial coverings of these muscles. The levator ani muscles form a broad muscular sling that originates from the posterior surface of the superior rami of the pubis, from the inner surface of the ischial spine, and between these two sites, from the obturator fascia. The muscle fibers are inserted in several locations as follows: around the vagina and rectum to form efficient functional sphincters for each; into a raphe in the midline between the vagina and rectum; into a midline raphe below the rectum; and into the coccyx. The *urogenital diaphragm* is positioned external to the pelvic diaphragm, that is, in the triangular area between the ischial tuberosities and the symphysis pubis. The urogenital diaphragm is made up of the deep transverse perineal muscles, the constrictor of the urethra, and the internal and external fascial coverings.

Of particular importance because they may be torn or cut with even normal delivery, are the *external* and *internal anal sphincter* muscles. The external sphincter is shown in Figure 3–6, where its proximity to the posterior vaginal fourchette is apparent. The relationship of the internal and external sphincter is shown in Figure 3–7. Damage to either sphincter increases the likelihood of rectal incontinence following vaginal delivery (Chap. 13, p. 328).

The major blood supply to the perineum is via the internal pudendal artery and its branches. Branches of the internal pudendal artery include the inferior rectal artery and posterior labial artery.

The innervation of the perineum is primarily via the

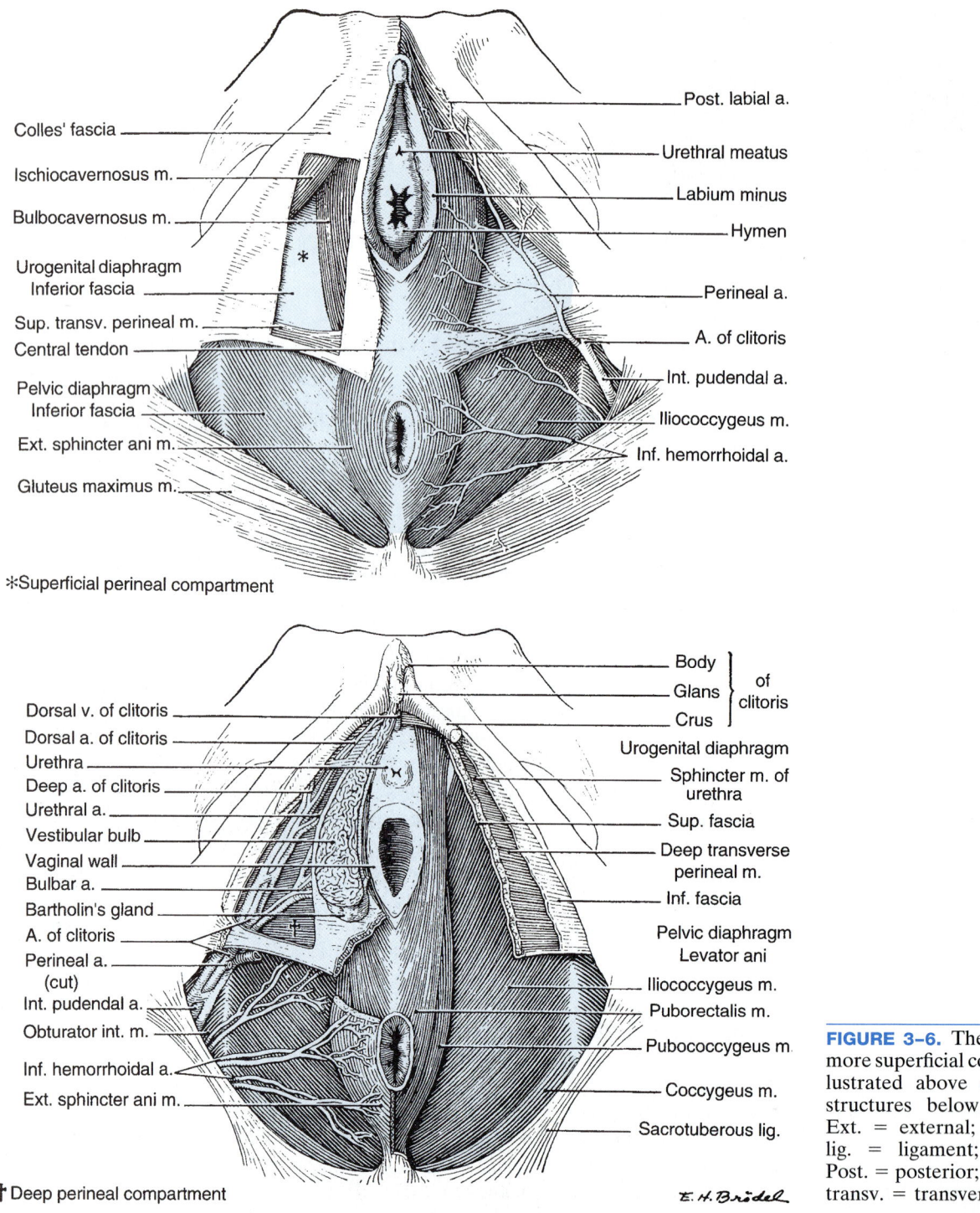

Post. labial a.

Colles' fascia

Ischiocavernosus m.

Bulbocavernosus m.

Urethral meatus

Labium minus

Hymen

Urogenital diaphragm
Inferior fascia

Sup. transv. perineal m.

Central tendon

Perineal a.

A. of clitoris

Pelvic diaphragm
Inferior fascia

Int. pudendal a.

Iliococcygeus m.

Ext. sphincter ani m.

Inf. hemorrhoidal a.

Gluteus maximus m.

✳Superficial perineal compartment

Dorsal v. of clitoris

Dorsal a. of clitoris

Urethra

Deep a. of clitoris

Urethral a.

Vestibular bulb

Vaginal wall

Bulbar a.

Bartholin's gland

A. of clitoris

Perineal a.
(cut)

Int. pudendal a.

Obturator int. m.

Inf. hemorrhoidal a.

Ext. sphincter ani m.

Body
Glans   of
Crus   clitoris

Urogenital diaphragm

Sphincter m. of
urethra

Sup. fascia

Deep transverse
perineal m.

Inf. fascia

Pelvic diaphragm
Levator ani

Iliococcygeus m.

Puborectalis m.

Pubococcygeus m.

Coccygeus m.

Sacrotuberous lig.

† Deep perineal compartment

E. H. Bridel

FIGURE 3–6. The perineum. The more superficial components are illustrated above and the deeper structures below. (a. = artery; Ext. = external; Int. = internal; lig. = ligament; m. = muscle; Post. = posterior; Sup. = superior; transv. = transverse.)

pudendal nerve and its branches. The pudendal nerve originates from the S_2, S_3, and S_4 portion of the spinal cord.

PERINEAL BODY. The median raphe of the levator ani, which is positioned between the anus and the vagina,

is reinforced by the central tendon of the perineum, on which converge the bulbocavernosus muscles, superficial transverse perineal muscles, and external anal sphincter. These structures, which contribute to the perineal body, provide much of the support for the perineum.

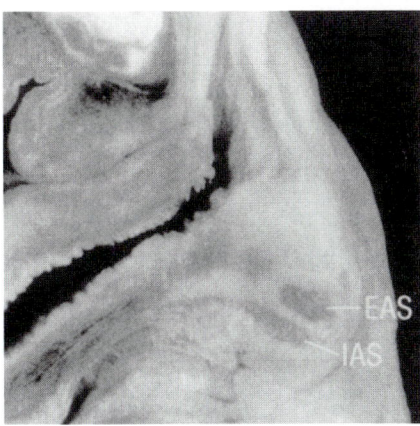

FIGURE 3-7. Photograph of a 35-year-old cadaver specimen showing the internal anal sphincter (IAS) and the external anal sphincter (EAS) between the vaginal lumen and the anal canal. (From Delancey and colleagues, 1997, with permission.)

INTERNAL GENERATIVE ORGANS

UTERUS. The uterus is a muscular organ that is covered, partially, by peritoneum, or serosa. The cavity of the uterus is lined by the endometrium.

ANATOMICAL RELATIONSHIPS. The uterus of the nonpregnant woman is situated in the pelvic cavity between the bladder anteriorly and the rectum posteriorly. Almost the entire posterior wall of the uterus is covered by serosa, or peritoneum, the lower portion of which forms the anterior boundary of the *recto-uterine cul-de-sac,* or pouch of Douglas. Only the upper portion of the anterior wall of the uterus is so covered (Fig. 3–8). The lower portion is united to the posterior wall of the

bladder by a well-defined but normally loose layer of connective tissue (Fig. 3–3).

SIZE AND SHAPE. The uterus is a structure that resembles a flattened pear in shape (Fig. 3–8). It consists of two major but unequal parts: an upper triangular portion, the *body,* or corpus; and a lower, cylindrical, or fusiform portion, the *cervix,* which projects into the vagina. The *isthmus* is that portion of the uterus between the internal cervical os and the endometrial cavity. It is of special obstetrical significance because it forms the lower uterine segment during pregnancy (Chap. 11, p. 254). The anterior surface of the body of the uterus is almost flat, whereas the posterior surface is distinctly convex. The oviducts, or fallopian tubes, emerge from the *cornua* of the uterus at the junction of the superior and lateral margins. The convex upper segment between the points of insertion of the fallopian tubes is called the *fundus.* Laterally, the portion of the uterus below the insertion of the fallopian tubes is not covered directly by peritoneum but is the site of the attachments of the broad ligaments.

The uterus varies widely in size and shape, and the age and parity of women influence this tremendously. Before puberty, the organ varies in length from 2.5 to 3.5 cm (Orsini and colleagues, 1984). The uterus of adult nulliparous women is from 6 to 8 cm in length as compared with 9 to 10 cm in multiparous women. Uteri of nonparous and parous women also differ considerably in weight, averaging from 50 to 70 g for the former, and 80 g or more for the latter (Langlois, 1970). The relationship between the length of the body of the uterus and that of the cervix likewise varies widely. In the premenarchal girl, the body of the uterus is only half as long as the cervix. In nulliparous women, the two are

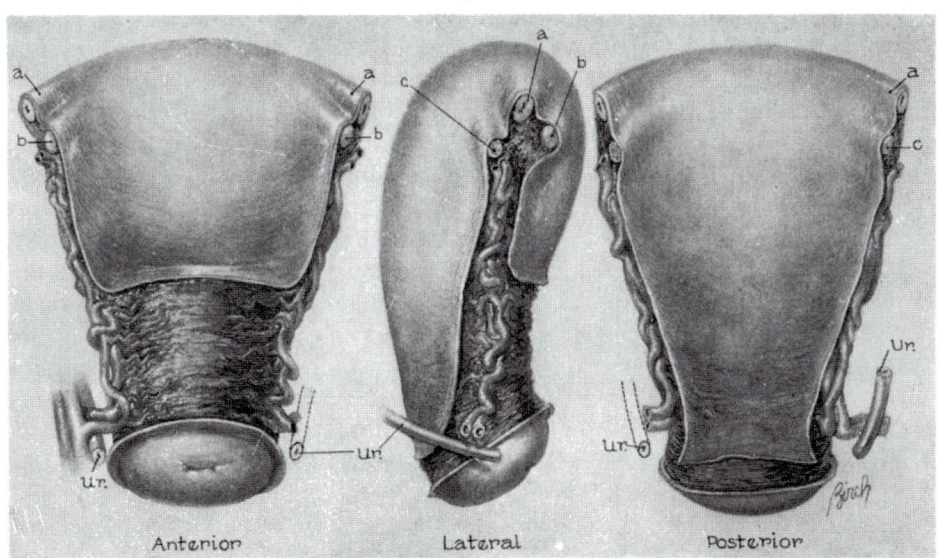

FIGURE 3-8. Anterior, right lateral, and posterior views of the uterus of an adult woman. (a, oviduct; b, round ligament; c, ovarian ligament; Ur. = ureter.)

about equal in length. In multiparous women, the cervix is only a little more than a third of the total length of the organ.

The bulk of the body of the uterus, but not the cervix, is comprised of muscle. The inner surfaces of the anterior and posterior walls of the uterus lie almost in contact; the cavity between these walls forms a mere slit. On frontal section, the cavity of the body of the uterus is triangular. The cervical canal is fusiform and is open at each end by small apertures, the *internal os* and the *external os.* The margins of parous uteri become concave instead of convex, and hence the triangular appearance of the uterine cavity is less pronounced.

After menopause, the size of the uterus decreases as a consequence of atrophy of both the myometrium and the endometrium. Congenital anomalies of müllerian fusion may give rise to a number of uterine abnormalities, detectable by hysterosalpingogram or magnetic resonance imaging (Carrington and co-workers, 1990). Obstetrical implications of such malformations are discussed in Chapter 35.

UTERUS DURING PREGNANCY. As described in Chapter 8 (p. 168), the uterus during pregnancy undergoes remarkable growth due to hypertrophy of muscle fibers. Its weight increases from 70 g in the nonpregnant state to about 1100 g at term. Its total volume averages about 5 L. As growth proceeds, the uterine fundus, a previously flattened convexity between tubal insertions, now becomes dome shaped (Fig. 3–9). The round ligaments now appear to insert at the junction of the middle and upper thirds of the organ. The fallopian tubes elongate, but the ovaries grossly appear unchanged.

UTERINE CERVIX. The cervix is the specialized portion of the uterus that is below the isthmus. Anteriorly, the upper boundary of the cervix, the internal os, corresponds approximately to the level at which the peritoneum is reflected upon the bladder. The cervix is divided by the attachment of the vagina into vaginal and supravaginal portions. The supravaginal segment on its posterior surface is covered by peritoneum. Laterally, it is attached to the cardinal ligaments, and anteriorly, it is separated from the overlying bladder by loose connective tissue. The external os is located at the lower extremity of the vaginal portion of the cervix, the *portio vaginalis.*

The external cervical os varies greatly in appearance. Before childbirth, it is a small, regular, oval opening; after childbirth, the orifice is converted into a transverse slit that is divided such that there are the so-called anterior and posterior lips of the cervix. If the cervix was torn deeply during delivery, it might heal in such a manner that it appears to be irregular, nodular, or stel-

late. These changes are sufficiently characteristic to permit an examiner to ascertain with some certainty whether a given woman has borne children by vaginal delivery (Fig. 3–10).

The cervix is composed predominantly of collagenous tissue plus elastic tissue and blood vessels, although it does contain some smooth muscle fibers. The transition from the primarily collagenous tissue of the cervix to the primarily muscular tissue of the body of the uterus, although generally abrupt, may be gradual, and may extend over as much as 10 mm. The results of studies by Danforth and colleagues (1960) suggest that the physical properties of the cervix are determined in large measure by the state of the connective tissue, and that during pregnancy and labor the remarkable ability of the cervix to dilate is the result of dissociation of collagen. Buckingham and co-workers (1965) quantified the amount of muscle and collagen in cervical tissue. In the normal cervix, the proportion of muscle is, on average, about 10 percent, whereas in women with an *incompetent cervix,* sometimes the proportion of muscle is appreciably greater. A number of clinically important structural abnormalities of both cervix and uterus have been described in women exposed in utero to *diethylstilbestrol* (Chap. 35, p. 918). These are often diagnosed by physical examination or magnetic resonance imaging, and may have important reproductive implications (Hricak and associates, 1990).

The mucosa of the cervical canal is composed of a single layer of very high, columnar epithelium that rests upon a thin basement membrane. The oval nuclei are situated near the base of the columnar cells, the upper portions of which appear to be rather clear because of content of mucus. These cells are supplied abundantly with cilia.

There are numerous cervical glands that extend from the surface of the endocervical mucosa directly into the subjacent connective tissue; because there is no submucosa as such, these glands furnish the thick, tenacious secretion of the cervical canal. If the ducts of the cervical glands are occluded, retention cysts, known as *Nabothian follicles* or *cysts,* are formed.

Normally, the squamous epithelium of the vaginal portion of the cervix and the columnar epithelium of the cervical canal form a sharp line of demarcation very near the external os, that is, the squamo-columnar junction. In response to inflammation or trauma, however, the stratified epithelium may extend gradually up the cervical canal and come to line the lower third, or occasionally even the lower half, of the canal. This change is more marked in multiparous women, in whom the lips of the cervix often are everted. Uncommonly, the two varieties of epithelium abut on the vaginal portion outside the external os, as in *congenital ectropion.*

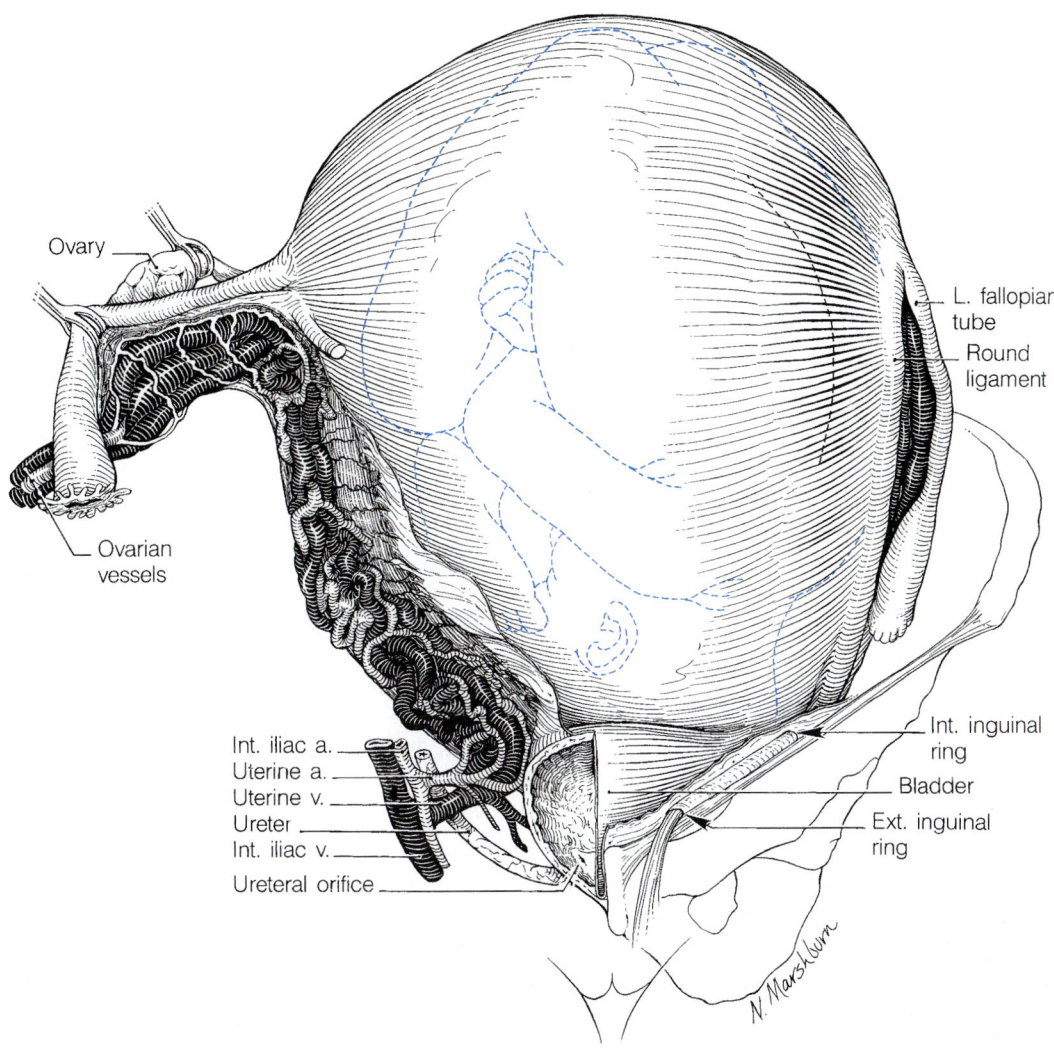

Ovary

Ovarian
vessels

Int. iliac a.
Uterine a.
Uterine v.
Ureter
Int. iliac v.
Ureteral orifice

L. fallopian
tube
Round
ligament

Int. inguinal
ring
Bladder
Ext. inguinal
ring

N. Marshburn

FIGURE 3–9. Uterus of near-term pregnancy. The fundus is now dome shaped and the tubes and round ligaments appear to insert in the upper middle portion of the uterine body. Note the markedly hypertrophied vascular supply. (a. = artery; Ext. = external; Int. = internal; v. = vein.)

BODY OF THE UTERUS. The wall of the body of the uterus is composed of serosal, muscular, and mucosal layers. The serosal layer is formed by the peritoneum that covers the uterus, and to which it is firmly adherent except at sites just above the bladder and at the lateral

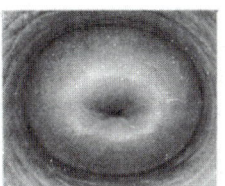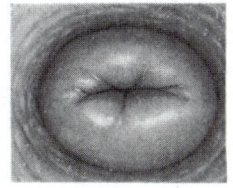

FIGURE 3–10. **A.** Cervical external os of a nonparous woman. **B.** Cervical external os of a parous woman.

margins where the peritoneum is deflected in a manner to form the broad ligaments.

ENDOMETRIUM. The endometrium is the mucosal layer that lines the uterine cavity in nonpregnant women. It is a thin, pink, velvet-like membrane, which on close examination is found to be perforated by a large number of minute openings; these are the ostia of the uterine glands. Because of the repetitive cyclical changes during the reproductive years, the endometrium normally varies greatly in thickness, and measures from 0.5 mm to as much as 5 mm. The endometrium is comprised of surface epithelium, glands, and interglandular mesenchymal tissue in which there are numerous blood vessels.

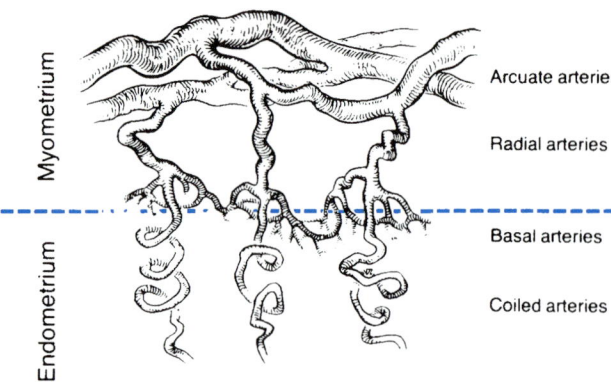

Myometrium

Endometrium

Arcuate arteries

Radial arteries

Basal arteries

Coiled arteries

FIGURE 3–11. Stereographic representation of myometrial and endometrial arteries in the macaque. Above, parts of myometrial arcuate arteries from which myometrial radial arteries course toward the endometrium. Below, the larger endometrial coiled arteries and the smaller endometrial basal arteries. (From Okkels and Engle, 1938.)

The epithelium of the endometrial surface is comprised of a single layer of closely packed, high columnar, ciliated cells. During much of the endometrial cycle, the oval nuclei are situated in the lower portions of the cells but not so near the base as in the endocervix. The ciliated cells are located in discrete patches, whereas secretory activity appears to be limited to nonciliated cells. The ciliary current in both the fallopian tubes and the uterus is in the same direction and extends downward from the fimbriated end of the tubes toward the external os.

The tubular *uterine glands* are invaginations of the epithelium, which in the resting state are reminiscent of the fingers of a glove. The glands extend through the entire thickness of the endometrium to the myometrium, which is occasionally penetrated for a short distance. Histologically, the inner glands resemble the epithelium of the surface and are lined by a single layer of columnar, partially ciliated epithelium that rests upon a thin basement membrane. The glands secrete a thin, alkaline fluid.

In the classical monograph of Hitschmann and Adler (1908), the endometrium was described as undergoing constant, hormonally controlled changes during each ovarian cycle. These three fundamental phases—*menstrual, proliferative* (*follicular*), and *secretory* (*luteal*)—are discussed in detail in Chapter 4 in the section on menstruation. After menopause, the endometrium is atrophic and the epithelium flattens. The glands gradually disappear, and the interglandular tissue becomes more fibrous.

The connective tissue of the endometrium, between the surface epithelium and the myometrium, is a mesenchymal stroma. Immediately after menstruation, the stroma is composed of closely packed cells with oval-

and spindle-shaped nuclei, around which there is very little cytoplasm. When separated by edema, the cells appear to be stellate, with cytoplasmic processes that branch to form anastomoses. These cells are packed more closely around the glands and blood vessels than elsewhere. Several days before menstruation, the stromal cells usually become larger and more vesicular, like decidual cells; and at the same time, there is a diffuse leukocytic infiltration.

The vascular architecture of the endometrium is of signal importance in the phenomena of menstruation and pregnancy. Arterial blood is transported to the uterus by way of the uterine and ovarian arteries. As the arterial branches penetrate the uterine wall obliquely inward and reach its middle third, these vessels ramify in a plane that is parallel to the surface; these vessels are therefore named the *arcuate arteries* (DuBose and colleagues, 1985). Radial branches extend from the arcuate arteries at right angles toward the endometrium. The endometrial arteries comprise *coiled* or *spiral arteries*, which are a continuation of the radial arteries, and *basal arteries*, which branch from the radial arteries at a sharp angle (Figs. 3–11 and 3–12). The coiled arteries supply most of the midportion and all of the superficial third of the endometrium. The walls of these vessels are responsive (sensitive) to the action of a number of hormones, especially by vasoconstriction, and thus probably serve an important role in the mechanism(s) of menstruation. The straight basal endometrial arteries are smaller in both caliber and length than are the coiled vessels. These vessels extend only into the basal layer

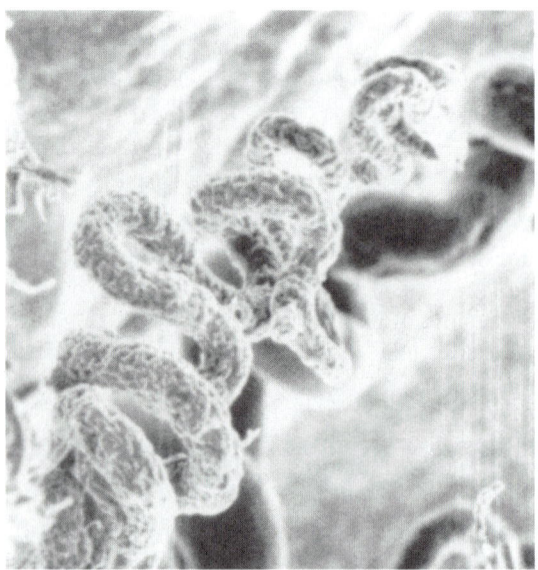

FIGURE 3–12. Corrosion cast of the complexly branching endometrial capillary network of the upper compact layer of a rhesus monkey on the 25th day of the menstrual cycle × 400. (From Ferenczy and Richart, 1974.)

of the endometrium, or at most a short distance into the middle layer, and are not responsive to hormonal action.

MYOMETRIUM. The myometrium, which makes up the major portion of the uterus, is composed of bundles of smooth muscle united by connective tissue in which there are many elastic fibers. According to Schwalm and Dubrauszky (1966), the number of muscle fibers of the uterus progressively diminishes caudally such that in the cervix, muscle comprises only 10 percent of the tissue mass. In the inner wall of the body of the uterus, there is relatively more muscle than in the outer layers; and in the anterior and posterior walls, there is more muscle than in the lateral walls. During pregnancy, the myometrium increases greatly via hypertrophy, with no significant change in the muscle content of the cervix (Chap. 8, p. 168).

LIGAMENTS. The *broad ligaments* are made up of two winglike structures that extend from the lateral margins of the uterus to the pelvic walls and thereby divide the pelvic cavity into anterior and posterior compartments. Each broad ligament consists of a fold of peritoneum, and there are superior, lateral, inferior, and medial margins. The inner two thirds of the superior margin form the *mesosalpinx,* to which the fallopian tubes are attached. The outer third of the superior margin of the broad ligament, which extends from the fimbriated end of the oviduct to the pelvic wall, forms the *infundibulopelvic ligament* (suspensory ligament of the ovary), through which the ovarian vessels traverse.

At the lateral margin of each broad ligament, the peritoneum is reflected onto the side of the pelvis. The base of the broad ligament, which is quite thick, is continuous with the connective tissue of the pelvic floor. The most dense portion—referred to as the *cardinal ligament,* transverse cervical ligament, or Mackenrodt ligament—is composed of connective tissue that medially is united firmly to the supravaginal portion of the cervix. In the base of the broad ligament, the uterine vessels and the lower portion of the ureter are enclosed.

A vertical section through the uterine end of the broad ligament is triangular, and the uterine vessels are found within its broad base (Fig. 3–13). In its lower part, it is widely attached to the connective tissues that are adjacent to the cervix, that is, the *parametrium.* The upper part is made up of three folds that nearly cover the oviduct, the utero-ovarian ligament, and the round ligament.

The *round ligaments* extend from the lateral portion of the uterus, arising somewhat below and anterior to that of the origin of the oviducts. Each round ligament is located in a fold of peritoneum that is continuous with the broad ligament and extends outward and downward to the inguinal canal, through which it passes to terminate in the upper portion of the labium majus. In nonpregnant women, the round ligament varies from 3 to 5 mm in diameter, and is comprised of smooth muscle cells that are continuous directly with those of the uterine wall and a certain amount of connective tissue. The round ligament corresponds, embryologically, to the gubernaculum testis of men. During pregnancy, the round ligaments undergo considerable hypertrophy and increase appreciably in both length and diameter.

Each *uterosacral ligament* extends from an attachment posterolaterally to the supravaginal portion of the cervix to encircle the rectum, and thence insert into the fascia over the second and third sacral vertebrae. The uterosacral ligaments are composed of connective tissue and some smooth muscle and are covered by peritoneum. These ligaments form the lateral boundaries of the rectouterine cul-de-sac, or pouch of Douglas.

POSITION. When a nonpregnant woman stands upright, the body of the uterus most often is almost horizontal, flexed somewhat anteriorly with the fundus resting upon the bladder, whereas the cervix is directed backward toward the tip of the sacrum with the external os approximately at the level of the ischial spines. The position of the body of the uterus is variable as a function of the degree of distension of the bladder, rectum, or both.

Normally, the uterus is a partially mobile organ; whereas the cervix is anchored, the body of the uterus is free to move in the anteroposterior plane. The posterior directed, or retroflexed uterus (that is, with the fundus resting on the rectum) is a normal variant and is encountered in many women.

BLOOD VESSELS. The vascular supply of the uterus is derived principally from the uterine and ovarian arteries. The uterine artery, a main branch of the internal iliac (hypogastric) artery, enters the base of the broad ligament, and makes its way medially to the side of the uterus. Immediately adjacent to the supravaginal portion of the cervix, the uterine artery is divided into two main branches. The smaller cervicovaginal artery supplies blood to the lower portion of the cervix and the upper portion of the vagina. The main branch turns abruptly upward and extends thereafter as a highly convoluted vessel that traverses along the margin of the uterus; a branch of considerable size extends to the upper portion of the cervix, and numerous other branches penetrate the body of the uterus. Just before the main branch of the uterine artery reaches the oviduct, it divides into three terminal branches: fundal, tubal, and ovarian. The ovarian branch of the uterine artery anastomoses with the terminal branch of the ovarian artery; the tubal branch makes its way through the mesosalpinx and supplies part of the oviduct; and the

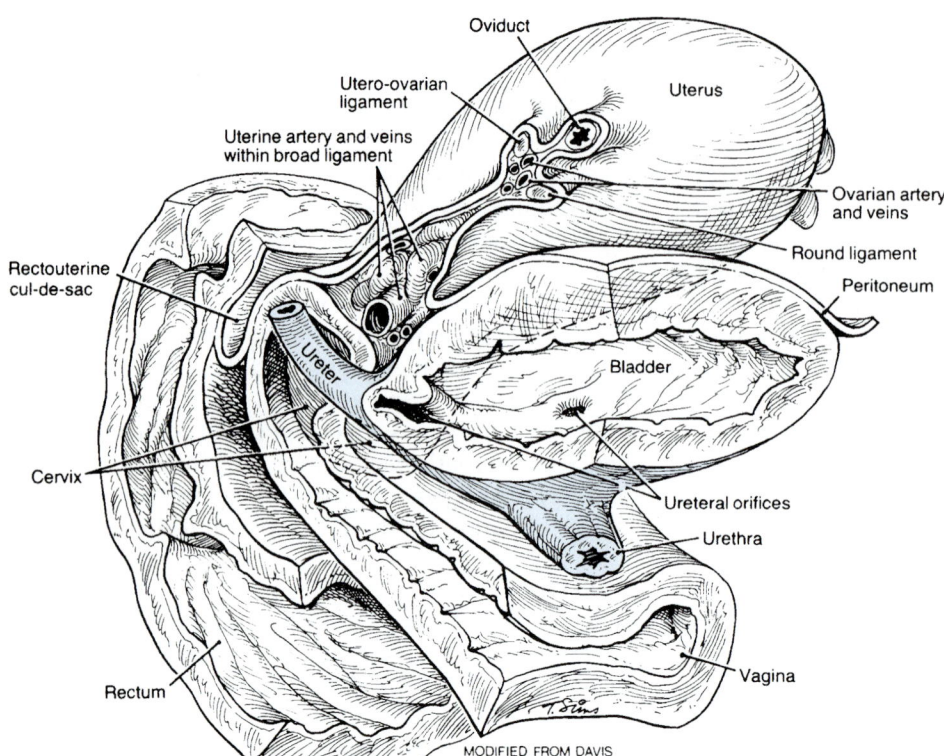

FIGURE 3–13. Vertical section through the uterine end of the right broad ligament.

fundal branch is distributed to the uppermost portion of the uterus.

About 2 cm lateral to the cervix, the uterine artery crosses over the ureter (Figs. 3–8 and 3–14). The proximity of the uterine artery and uterine vein to the ureter at this point is of great surgical significance because, during hysterectomy, the ureter may be injured or ligated in the process of clamping and ligating the uterine vessels.

A major portion of the blood supply to the pelvis is via the branches of the internal iliac artery, as shown in the arteriogram in Figure 3–15. In the past, this commonly was referred to as the hypogastric artery. Other branches of the anterior division of the internal iliac artery besides the uterine artery include the umbilical, middle and inferior vesical, middle rectal, obturator, internal pudendal, middle hemorrhoidal, vaginal, and inferior gluteal arteries. The branches of the posterior division of the internal iliac artery include the lateral sacral, superior gluteal, and iliolumbar arteries (Table 3–1).

The *ovarian artery,* a direct branch of the aorta, enters the broad ligament through the infundibulopelvic ligament. At the ovarian hilum, it is divided into a number of smaller branches that enter the ovary; whereas the main stem of the ovarian artery traverses the entire length of the broad ligament very near the mesosalpinx and makes its way to the upper portion of the lateral margin of the uterus, where it anastomoses with the ovarian branch of the uterine artery. There are numerous additional communications among the arteries on both sides of the uterus.

When the uterus is in a contracted state, its numerous venous lumens are collapsed; however, in injected specimens the greater part of the uterine wall appears to be occupied by dilated venous sinuses. On either side, the arcuate veins unite to form the *uterine vein,* which empties into the internal iliac vein and thence into the common iliac vein.

Some of the blood from the upper part of the uterus and blood from the ovary and upper part of the broad ligament is collected by several veins that, within the broad ligament, form the large *pampiniform plexus,* the vessels that terminate in the ovarian vein. The right ovarian vein empties into the vena cava, whereas the left ovarian vein empties into the left renal vein.

During pregnancy, there is marked hypertrophy of the blood supply to the uterus (Fig. 3–9). This accommodates uteroplacental blood flow estimated at 500 to 700 mL/min (Chap. 8, p. 169).

LYMPHATICS. The endometrium is abundantly supplied with lymphatics, but true lymphatic vessels are confined largely to the basal layer. The lymphatics of the underlying myometrium are increased in number toward the serosal surface and form an abundant lym-

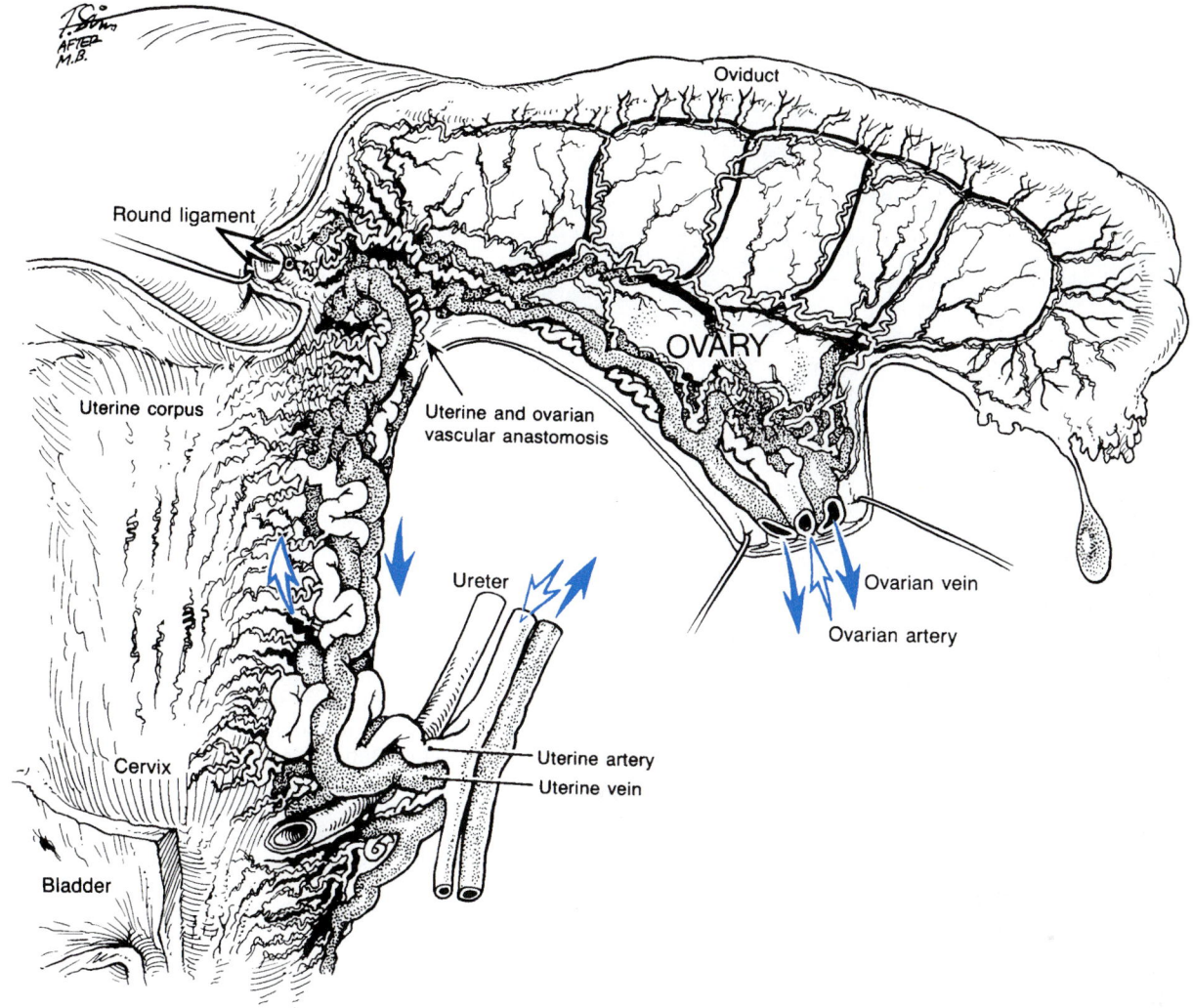

FIGURE 3–14. Blood supply to the left ovary, left oviduct, and the left side of the uterus. The ovarian and uterine vessels anastomose freely. Note the uterine artery and vein crossing over the ureter that lies immediately adjacent to the cervix.

phatic plexus just beneath it, especially on the posterior wall of the uterus and, to a lesser extent, on the anterior wall.

The lymphatics from the various segments of the uterus drain into several sets of lymph nodes. Those from the cervix terminate mainly in the hypogastric nodes, which are situated near the bifurcation of the common iliac vessels. The lymphatics from the body of the uterus are distributed to two groups of nodes. One set of vessels drains into the internal iliac nodes; the other set, after joining certain lymphatics from the ovarian region, terminates in the periaortic lymph nodes.

INNERVATION. The nerve supply is derived principally from the sympathetic nervous system, but also partly from the cerebrospinal and parasympathetic systems. The parasympathetic system is represented on either side by the pelvic nerve, which is comprised of a few fibers that are derived from the second, third, and fourth sacral nerves; it loses its identity in the cervical ganglion of Frankenhäuser. The sympathetic system enters the pelvis by way of the internal iliac plexus that arises from the aortic plexus just below the promontory of the sacrum. After descending on either side, it also enters the uterovaginal plexus of Frankenhäuser, which is made up of ganglia of various sizes, but particularly of a large ganglionic plate that is situated on either side of the cervix and just above the posterior fornix in front of the rectum.

Branches from these plexuses supply the uterus, bladder, and upper vagina. Some of these fibers terminate freely between the muscular fibers, whereas others accompany the arteries into the endometrium.

In the 11th and 12th thoracic nerve roots, there are

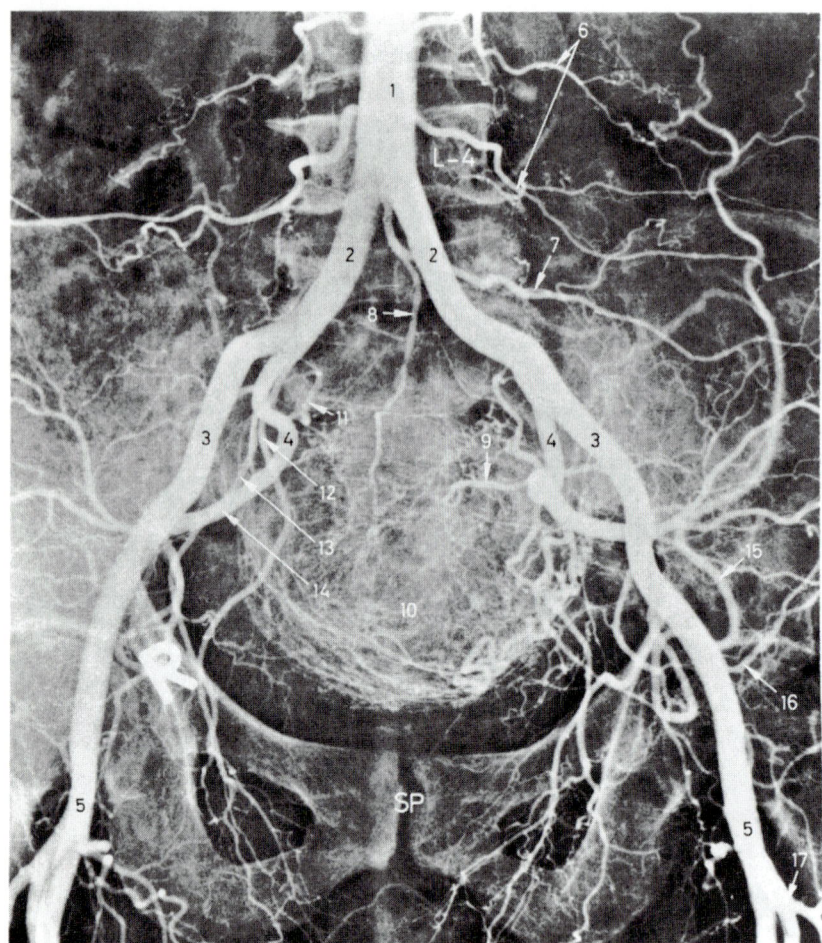

FIGURE 3–15. Iliac arteriogram. It can be seen that the bifurcation of the aorta (1) into the two common iliac arteries (2) occurs at the lower border of the body of the L-4 vertebra. The common iliac vessels branch into external (3) and internal (4) iliac arteries. The internal iliac artery (4) on each side serves a number of branches to the pelvis, perineum, and gluteal region, while the external iliac artery (3), after giving off the inferior epigastric (15) and deep circumflex iliac (16) arteries, becomes the femoral artery below the inguinal ligament. (Also shown: 5 = femoral artery; 6 = lumbar arteries; 7 = iliolumbar artery; 8 = median sacral artery; 9 = uterine artery; 10 = uterus; 11 = lateral sacral artery; 12 = obturator artery; 13 = internal pudendal artery; 14 = superior gluteal artery; 17 = deep femoral artery; L-4 = the lumbar vertebra; SP = symphysis pubis.) (From Wickee, 1982, with permission.)

sensory fibers from the uterus that transmit the painful stimuli of uterine contractions to the central nervous system. The sensory nerves from the cervix and upper part of the birth canal pass through the pelvic nerves to the second, third, and fourth sacral nerves, whereas those from the lower portion of the birth canal pass primarily through the pudendal nerve.

OVIDUCTS. The oviducts, or fallopian tubes, vary from 8 to 14 cm in length and are covered by peritoneum; their lumen is lined by mucous membrane. Each fallopian tube is divided into an *interstitial portion, isthmus, ampulla,* and *infundibulum.* The interstitial portion is embodied within the muscular wall of the uterus. Its approximate course is obliquely upward and outward from the uterine cavity. The isthmus, or the narrow portion of the tube that adjoins the uterus, passes gradually into the wider, lateral portion, or *ampulla.* The *infundibulum,* or fimbriated extremity, is the funnel-shaped opening of the distal end of the fallopian tube (Fig. 3–16). The oviduct varies considerably in thickness; the narrowest portion of the isthmus measures from 2 to 3 mm in diameter, and the widest portion of the ampulla measures from 5 to 8 mm. The oviduct is surrounded completely by peritoneum except at the attachment of the mesosalpinx.

The fimbriated end of the infundibulum opens into

TABLE 3–1. Branches of the Internal Iliac Artery

Anterior Division	Posterior Division
Uterine	Superior gluteal
Umbilical	Lateral sacral
Inferior vesical	Iliolumbar
Obturator	
Internal pudendal	
Inferior gluteal	
Middle vesical	
Middle rectal	
Vaginal	

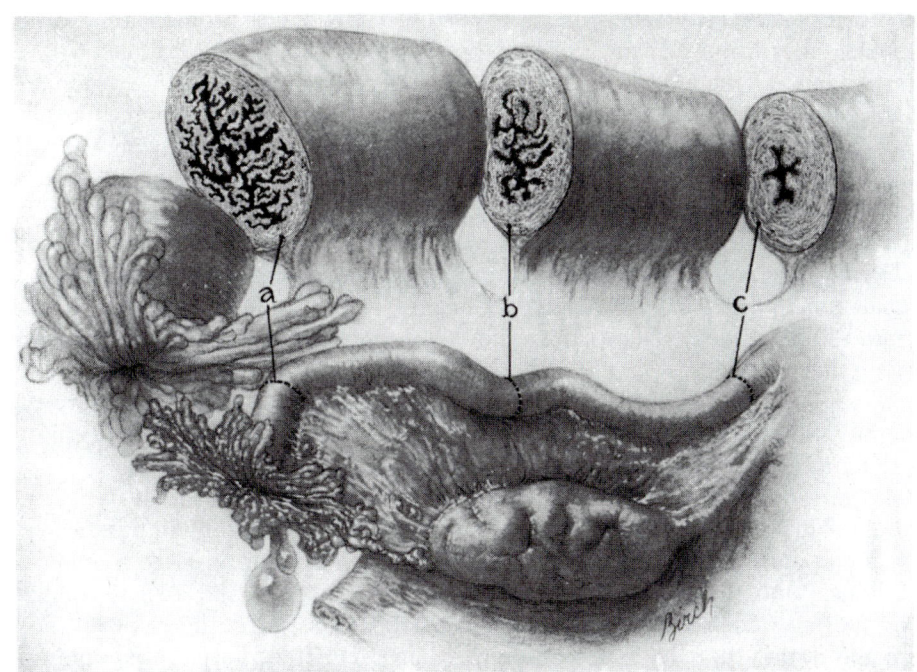

FIGURE 3–16. The oviduct of an adult woman with cross-sectioned illustrations of the gross structure of the epithelium in several portions: a, infundibulum; b, ampulla; c, isthmus.

the abdominal cavity. One projection, the *fimbria ovarica,* which is considerably longer than the other fimbriae, forms a shallow gutter that approaches or reaches the ovary.

The musculature of the fallopian tube is arranged in two layers, an inner circular and an outer longitudinal layer. In the distal portion of the oviduct, the two layers are less distinct and, near the fimbriated extremity, are replaced by an interlacing network of muscular fibers. The tubal muscularture undergoes rhythmic contractions constantly, the rate of which varies with the hormonal changes of the ovarian cycle. The greatest frequency and intensity of contractions is reached during transport of ova. Contractions are slowest and weakest during pregnancy.

The fallopian tube is lined by a single layer of columnar cells, some of them ciliated and others secretory. The ciliated cells are most abundant at the fimbriated extremity; elsewhere, these cells are found in discrete patches. There are differences in the proportions of these two types of cells in different phases of the ovarian cycle. Because there is no submucosa, the epithelium is in close contact with the underlying muscle. In the tubal mucosa, there are cyclical histological changes similar to, but much less striking than, those of the endometrium. The postmenstrual phase is characterized by a low epithelium that rapidly increases in height. During the follicular phase, the cells are taller; the ciliated elements are broad, with nuclei near the margin; and the nonciliated cells are narrow, with nuclei nearer the base. During the luteal phase, the secretory cells enlarge, pro-

ject beyond the ciliated cells, and the nuclei are extruded. During the menstrual phase, these changes are even more marked. Changes in the fallopian tubes during late pregnancy and in the puerperium include the development of a low mucosa, plugging of the capillaries with leukocytes, and a decidual reaction.

The mucosa of the oviducts is arranged in longitudinal folds that are more complex toward the fimbriated end. On cross sections through the uterine portion, four simple folds are found that form a figure that resembles a Maltese cross. The isthmus is more complex; in the ampulla, the lumen is occupied almost completely by the arborescent mucosa, which consists of very complicated folds (Fig. 3–16). The current produced by the tubal cilia is such that the direction of flow is toward the uterine cavity. Tubal peristalsis is believed to be an extraordinarily important factor in transport of the ovum.

The tubes are supplied richly with elastic tissue, blood vessels, and lymphatics. Sympathetic innervation of the tubes is extensive, in contrast to parasympathetic innervation. The role of these nerves in tubal function is poorly understood (Hodgson and Eddy, 1975).

Diverticula may extend occasionally from the lumen of the tube for a variable distance into the muscular wall and reach almost to the serosa. These diverticula may serve a role in the development of ectopic pregnancy (Chap. 34, p. 884). The gross anatomical, histological, and ultrastructural aspects of the human oviduct was summarized elegantly by Woodruff and Pauerstein (1969).

EMBRYOLOGICAL DEVELOPMENT OF THE UTERUS AND OVIDUCTS. The uterus and fallopian tubes arise from the müllerian ducts, which first appear near the upper pole of the urogenital ridge in the fifth week of embryonic development. This ridge is composed of the mesonephros, gonad, and associated ducts. The first indication of the development of the müllerian duct is a thickening of the coelomic epithelium at about the level of the fourth thoracic segment. This thickening becomes the fimbriated extremity of the fallopian tube, which invaginates and grows caudally to form a slender tube at the lateral edge of the urogenital ridge. In the sixth week of embryonic life, the growing tips of the two müllerian ducts approach each other in the midline and reach the sinus 1 week later. At that time, a fusion of the two müllerian ducts is begun at the level of the inguinal crest, or gubernaculum (primordium of the round ligament), to form a single canal. Thus, the upper ends of the müllerian ducts produce the oviducts and the fused parts give rise to the uterus. The uterine lumen from the fundus to the vagina is completed during the third month of fetal life. The vaginal canal is not patent throughout its entire length until the sixth month of fetal life (Koff, 1933).

OVARIES. The ovaries are almond-shaped organs, the functions of which are the development and extrusion of ova and the synthesis and secretion of steroid hormones. The ovaries vary considerably in size. During childbearing years, they are 2.5 to 5 cm in length, 1.5 to 3 cm in breadth, and 0.6 to 1.5 cm in thickness. After menopause, ovarian size diminishes remarkably.

Normally, the ovaries are situated in the upper part of the pelvic cavity and rest in a slight depression on the lateral wall of the pelvis between the divergent external and internal iliac vessels—the ovarian fossa of Waldeyer. The position of the ovaries is subject to marked variation, and it is rare to find both ovaries at exactly the same level.

The ovary is attached to the broad ligament by the *mesovarium.* The *utero-ovarian ligament* extends from the lateral and posterior portion of the uterus, just beneath the tubal insertion, to the uterine or lower pole of the ovary. Usually, it is several centimeters long and 3 to 4 mm in diameter. It is covered by peritoneum and is made up of muscle and connective tissue fibers that are continuous with those of the uterus. The *infundibulopelvic* or *suspensory ligament of the ovary* extends from the upper or tubal pole to the pelvic wall; through it course the ovarian vessels and nerves.

The exterior surface of the ovary varies in appearance with age. In young women, the organ is smooth, with a dull white surface through which glisten several small, clear follicles. As the woman grows older, the ovaries become more corrugated; in elderly women, the exterior surfaces may be convoluted markedly.

The ovary consists of two portions, the *cortex* and *medulla.* The cortex, or outer layer, varies in thickness with age and becomes thinner with advancing years. It is in this layer that the ova and graafian follicles are located. The cortex of the ovary is composed of spindle-shaped connective tissue cells and fibers, among which there are scattered primordial and graafian follicles that are in various stages of development. As the woman ages, the follicles become less numerous. The outermost portion of the cortex, which is dull and whitish, is designated as the *tunica albuginea;* on its surface, there is a single layer of cuboidal epithelium, the germinal epithelium of Waldeyer.

The medulla, or central portion, of the ovary is composed of loose connective tissue that is continuous with that of the mesovarium. There are a large number of arteries and veins in the medulla and a small number of smooth muscle fibers that are continuous with those in the suspensory ligament; the muscle fibers may be functional in movements of the ovary.

Both sympathetic and parasympathetic nerves are supplied to the ovaries. The sympathetic nerves are derived, in large part, from the ovarian plexus that accompanies the ovarian vessels; a few are derived from the plexus that surrounds the ovarian branch of the uterine artery. The ovary is richly supplied with nonmyelinated nerve fibers, which for the most part accompany the blood vessels. These are merely vascular nerves, whereas others form wreaths around normal and atretic follicles, and these give off many minute branches that have been traced up to, but not through, the membrana granulosa.

EMBRYOLOGY. At first, the changes in the gonads are the same in both sexes. The earliest sign of a gonad is one that appears on the ventral surface of the embryonic kidney at a site between the eighth thoracic and fourth lumbar segments at about 4 weeks. As illustrated in Figure 3–17, the coelomic epithelium is thickened, and clumps of cells are seen to bud off into the underlying mesenchyme. This circumscribed area of the coelomic epithelium often is called the *germinal epithelium.* By the fourth to sixth week, however, there are many large ameboid cells in this region that have migrated into the body of the embryo from the yolk sac; these cells have been recognized in this region as early as the third week. These *primordial germ cells* are distinguishable by a large size and certain morphological and cytochemical features. They react strongly in tests for alkaline phosphatase (McKay and associates, 1949), and are recognizable even after repeated divisions.

When the primordial germ cells reach the genital area, some enter the germinal epithelium and others

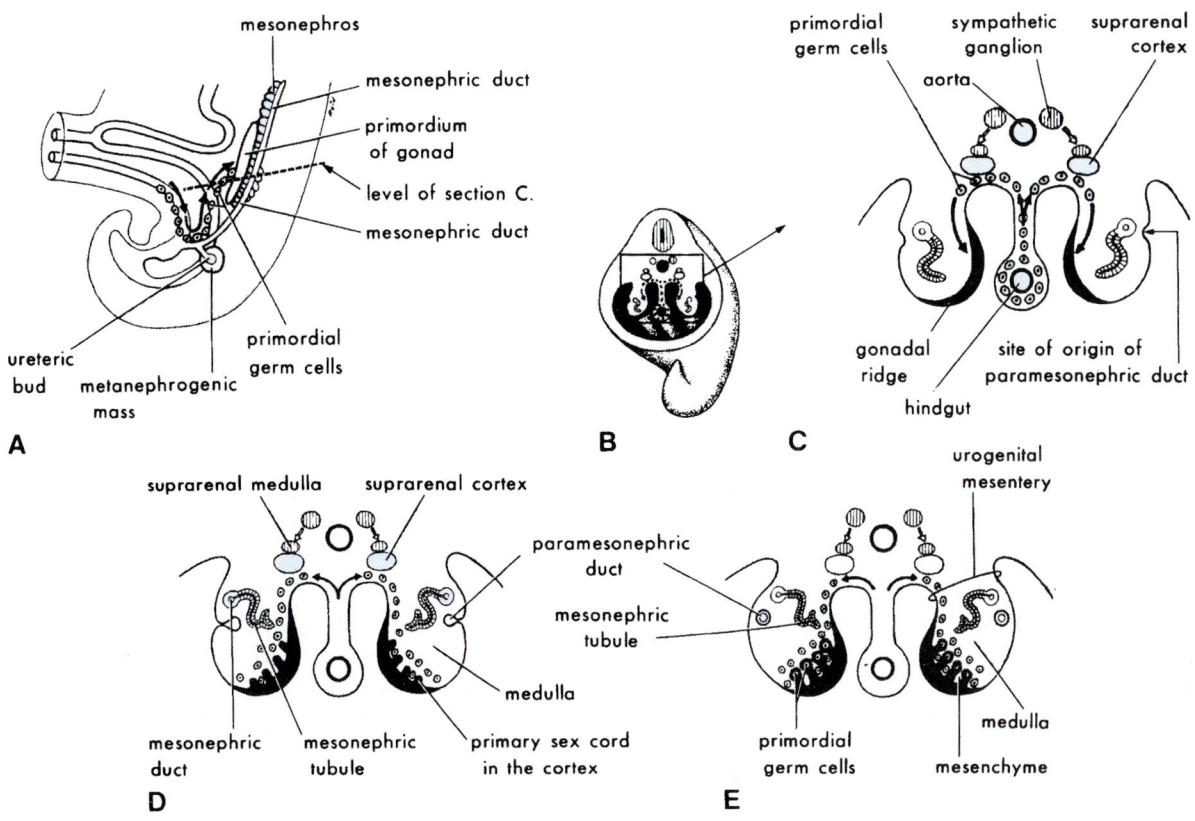

FIGURE 3–17. A. Sketch of 5-week embryo illustrating the migration of primordial germ cells. **B.** Three-dimensional sketch of the caudal region of a 5-week embryo showing the location and extent of the gonadal ridges on the medial aspect of the urogenital ridges. **C.** Transverse section showing the primordium of the adrenal glands, gonadal ridges, and migration of the primordial germ cells. **D.** Transverse section through a 6-week embryo showing the primary sex cords and developing paramesonephric ducts. **E.** Similar section at later stage showing the indifferent gonads and the mesonephric and paramesonephric ducts (From Moore, 1983.)

mingle with the groups of cells that proliferate from it or lie in the mesenchyme. By the end of the fifth week, rapid division of all these types of cells results in development of a prominent *genital ridge*. The ridge projects into the body cavity medially to a fold in which there are the mesonephric (wolffian) and the müllerian ducts (Fig. 3–18). Because the growth of the gonad at the surface is more rapid, it enlarges centrifugally. By the seventh week (Figs. 3–17 and 3–18), it is separated from the mesonephros except at the narrow central zone, the future hilum, where the blood vessels enter. At this time, the sexes can be distinguished, because the testes can be recognized by well-defined radiating strands of cells (sex cords). These cords are separated from the germinal epithelium by mesenchyme that is to become the tunica albuginea. The sex cords, which consist of large germ cells and smaller epithelioid cells derived from the germinal epithelium, develop into the seminiferous tubules and tubuli rete. The rete, probably derived from mesonephric elements, establishes connection with

the mesonephric tubules that develop into the epididymis (Fig. 3–18). The mesonephric ducts become the vas deferens.

In the female, the germinal epithelium continues to proliferate for a much longer time. The groups of cells thus formed lie at first in the region of the hilum. As connective tissue develops between them, these appear as sex cords. These give rise to the medullary cords and persist for variable times (Forbes, 1942). By the third month, medulla and cortex are defined (Fig. 3–18). The bulk of the organ is made up of cortex, a mass of crowded germ and epithelioid cells that show some signs of grouping, but there are no distinct cords as in the testis. Strands of cells extend from the germinal epithelium into the cortical mass, and mitoses are numerous. The rapid succession of mitoses soon reduces the size of the germ cells to the extent that these no longer are differentiated clearly from the neighboring cells; these cells are now called *oogonia*. Some of the oogonia in the medullary region are soon distinguishable by a series

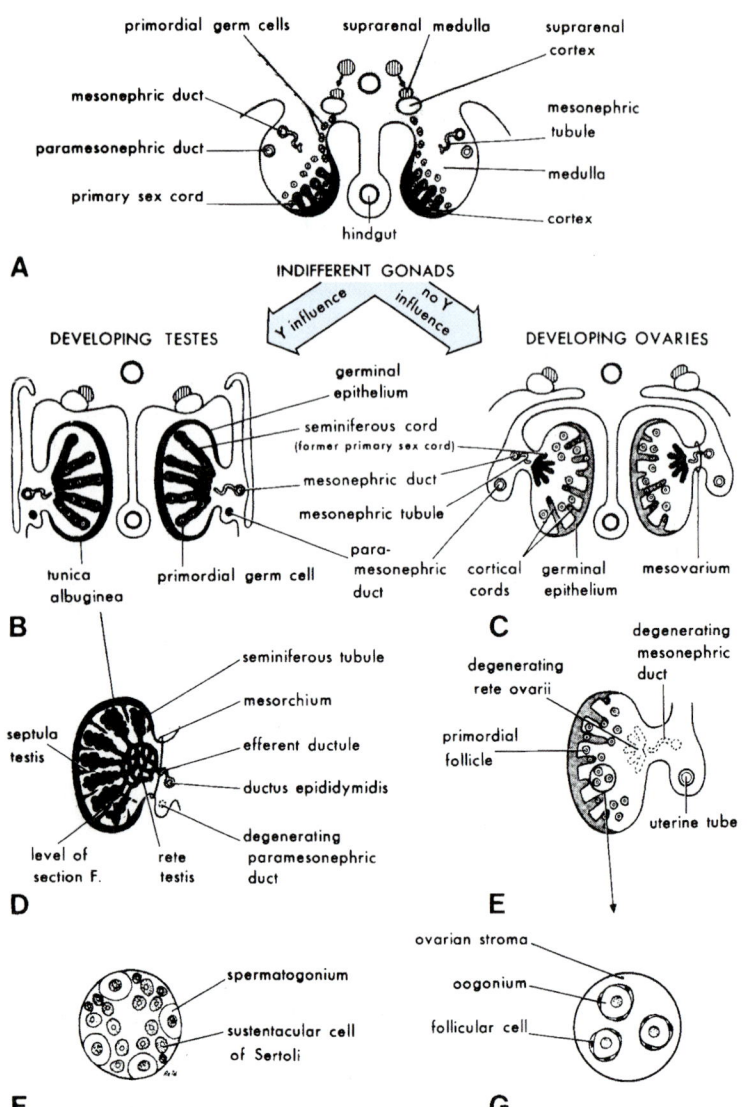

FIGURE 3–18. Schematic sections illustrating the differentiation of the indifferent gonads into testes or ovaries. **A.** Six weeks, showing the indifferent gonads that are composed of an outer cortex and an inner medulla. **B.** Seven weeks, showing testes developing under the influence of a Y chromosome. Note that the primary sex cords have become seminiferous cords and that they are separated from the surface epithelium by the tunica albuginea. **C.** Twelve weeks, showing ovaries beginning to develop in the absence of Y chromosome influence. Cortical cords have extended from the surface epithelium, where they form the rudimentary rete ovarii. **D.** Testis at 20 weeks, showing the rete testis and the seminiferous tubules derived from the seminiferous cords. An efferent ductule has developed from a mesonephric tubule, and the mesonephric tubule and duct are regressing. **E.** Ovary at 20 weeks, showing the primordial follicles formed from the cortical cords. The rete ovarii derived from primary sex cords and the mesonephric tubule and duct are regressing. **F.** Section of a seminiferous tubule from a 20-week fetus. Note that no lumen is present at this stage and that the seminiferous epithelium is composed of two kinds of cells. **G.** Section from the ovarian cortex of a 20-week fetus showing three primordial follicles. (From Moore, 1983.)

of peculiar nuclear changes. Large masses of nuclear chromatin appear, very different from the chromosomes of the oogonial divisions. This change marks the beginning of *synapsis,* which involves interactions between pairs of chromosomes that are derived originally from father and mother. Various stages of synapsis soon can be seen throughout the cortex; because similar changes occur in adjacent cells, groups or "nests" appear. During one stage of synapsis, the chromatin is massed at one side of the nucleus, and the cytoplasm becomes highly fluid. Unless the in vitro preservation is prompt and perfect, these cells appear to be degenerating.

By the fourth month, some germ cells, again in the medullary region, having passed through synapsis, begin to enlarge. These are called *primary oocytes* at the beginning of the phase of growth that continues until maturity is reached. During this period of cell growth, many oocytes undergo degeneration, both before and after

birth. The primary oocytes soon become surrounded by a single layer of flattened *follicle* cells that were derived originally from the germinal epithelium. These structures are now called *primordial follicles* and are first seen in the medulla and later in the cortex. Some follicles begin to grow even before birth and some are believed to persist in the cortex almost unchanged until menopause.

By 8 months of gestation, the ovary has become a long, narrow, lobulated structure that is attached to the body wall along the line of the hilum by the *mesovarium,* in which lies the *epoophoron.* At that stage of development, the germinal epithelium has been separated for the most part from the cortex by a band of connective tissue (tunica albuginea), which is absent in many small areas where strands of cells, usually referred to as cords of Pflüger, are in contact with the germinal epithelium. Among these cords are cells believed by many investigators to be oogonia that have come to resemble the other epithelial cells as a result of repeated mitoses. In the underlying cortex, there are two distinct zones. Superficially, there are nests of germ cells in synapsis, interspersed with Pflüger cords and strands of connective tissue. In the deeper zone, there are many groups of germ cells in synapsis, as well as primary oocytes, prospective follicular cells, and a few primordial follicles.

At term, the various types of ovarian cells in the human female fetus may still be found. In some cases, there are vesicular follicles in the medulla, which are all doomed to early degeneration.

HISTOLOGY. From the first stages of its development until after the menopause, the ovary undergoes constant change. The number of oocytes at the onset of puberty has been estimated variously at 200,000 to 400,000. Because only one ovum ordinarily is cast off during each ovarian cycle, it is evident that a few hundred ova suffice for purposes of reproduction.

Mossman and co-workers (1964), in an attempt to clarify the terminology of glandular elements of ovaries of adult women, distinguished interstitial, thecal, and luteal cells. The interstitial glandular elements are formed from cells of the theca interna of degenerating or atretic follicles; the thecal glandular cells are formed from the theca interna of ripening follicles; and the true luteal cells are derived from the granulosa cells of ovulated follicles and from the undifferentiated stroma that surround them.

The huge store of primordial follicles at birth is exhausted gradually during the time of sexual maturation. Block (1952) found that there is a gradual decline from a mean of 439,000 oocytes in girls under 15 years to a mean of 34,000 in women over the age of 36.

In the young girl, the greater portion of the ovary is composed of the cortex, which is filled with large numbers of closely packed primordial follicles. Those nearest the central portion of the ovary are at the most advanced stages of development. In young women, the cortex is relatively thinner but still contains a large number of primordial follicles, which are separated by bands of connective tissue cells in which there are spindle-shaped or oval nuclei. Each primordial follicle is made up of an oocyte and its surrounding single layer of epithelial cells, which are small and flattened, spindle-shaped, and somewhat sharply differentiated from the still smaller and spindly cells of the surrounding stroma.

The oocyte is a large, spherical cell in which there is clear cytoplasm and a relatively large nucleus located near the center of the ovum. In the nucleus, there is one large and several smaller nucleoli, and numerous masses of chromatin. The diameter of the smallest oocytes in the ovaries of adult women averages 33 μm, and that of the nuclei, 20 μm.

EMBRYOLOGICAL REMNANTS. The *parovarium*, which can be found in the scant loose connective tissue within the broad ligament in the vicinity of the mesosalpinx, comprises a number of narrow vertical tubules that are lined by ciliated epithelium. These tubules connect at the upper ends with a longitudinal duct that extends just below the oviduct to the lateral margin of the uterus, where ordinarily it ends blindly near the internal os; infrequently, it may extend laterally down the vagina to the level of the hymen. This canal, the remnant of the wolffian (mesonephric) duct in women, is called the *Gartner duct.* The parovarium, also a remnant of the wolffian duct, is homologous, embryologically, with the caput epididymis in men. The cranial portion of the parovarium is the *epoophoron,* or organ of Rosenmüller; the caudal portion, or *paroophoron,* is a group of vestigial mesonephric tubules that lie in or around the broad ligament. It is homologous, embryologically, with the paradidymis of men. Usually the paroophoron in adult women disappears, but on occasion macroscopic cysts are formed from these remnants.

SURGICAL ANATOMY. Shown in Figure 3–19 are illustrations of female pelvic surgical anatomy. The hysterectomy depicted is of a nonpregnant uterus. Refer to Figure 3–9 of the pregnant uterus for anatomical differences.

THE BONY PELVIS

In both women and men the pelvis forms the bony ring through which body weight is transmitted to the lower extremities, but in women it has a special form that adapts it to childbearing (Fig. 3–20). The pelvis is composed of four bones: the sacrum, coccyx, and two innominate bones. Each innominate bone is formed by the fusion of the ilium, ischium, and pubis. The innominate bones are joined to the sacrum at the sacroiliac synchondroses and to one another at the symphysis pubis.

PELVIC ANATOMY. The false pelvis lies above the linea terminalis and the true pelvis below this anatomical boundary (Fig. 3–20). The false pelvis is bounded posteriorly by the lumbar vertebrae and laterally by the iliac fossae, and in front the boundary is formed by the lower portion of the anterior abdominal wall.

The true pelvis is the portion important in childbearing. It is bounded above by the promontory and alae of the sacrum, the linea terminalis, and the upper margins of the pubic bones, and below by the pelvic outlet. The cavity of the true pelvis can be described as an obliquely truncated, bent cylinder with its greatest height posteriorly, because its anterior wall at the symphysis pubis measures about 5 cm and its posterior wall

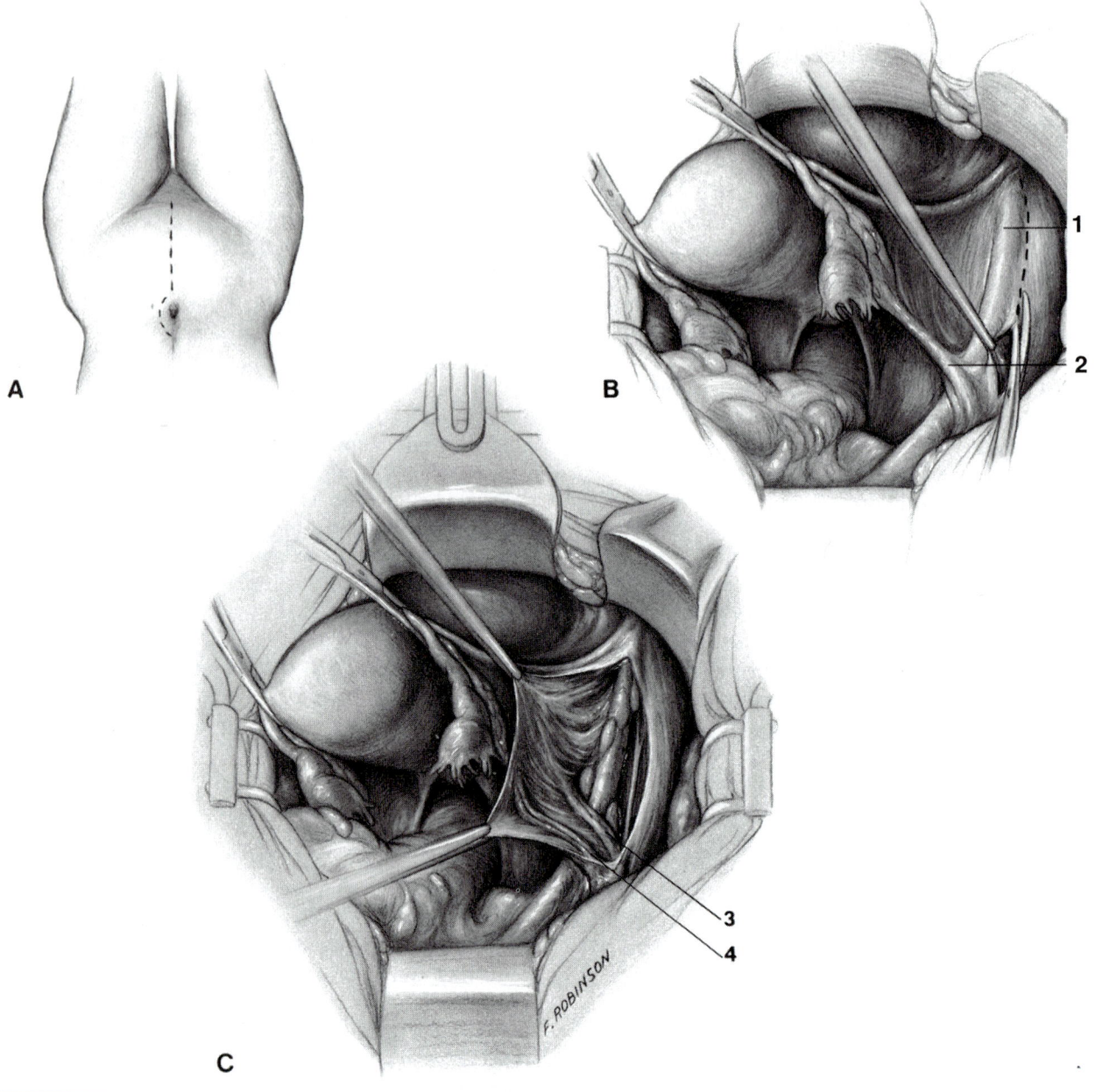

FIGURE 3–19. Illustrated are the pelvic viscera as seen through a long midline incision **(A)** made in the lower abdomen. **B.** Retractors have been placed to spread the abdominal incision. The small intestine and omentum that overlie the pelvic contents have been displaced from the operative field. The oviducts, utero-ovarian ligaments, and round ligaments have been clamped bilaterally at their origin immediately adjacent to the uterus. Peritoneum just lateral to the right external iliac artery (1) is incised and the right infundibulopelvic ligament (2) is tensed by pulling the uterus to the left. **C.** The right broad ligament has been opened laterally. The right ureter (3) is now visible as it crosses the iliac vessels at the pelvic brim and courses medially and downward toward the cervix and bladder. The right ovarian artery and vein (4) are visible after dissection of the infundibulopelvic ligament. **D.** The ovarian vessels have been clamped and are being severed. The uterus is retracted to the left and the external iliac is seen to the right. **E.** The round ligament (1) and the ovarian vessels (2) have been ligated and severed. More of the ureter is visible (3). **F.** The origin of the right uterine artery (4) from the internal iliac artery (5) is illustrated. Note the ureter (6) coursing beneath the uterine artery (4) just lateral to the junction of the cervix and body of the uterus. **G.** The operator's finger is in the paracervical ureteral tunnel through the right cardinal ligament just lateral to supravaginal portion of the cervix. The ureter is being retracted laterally. (From Nelson, 1977.)

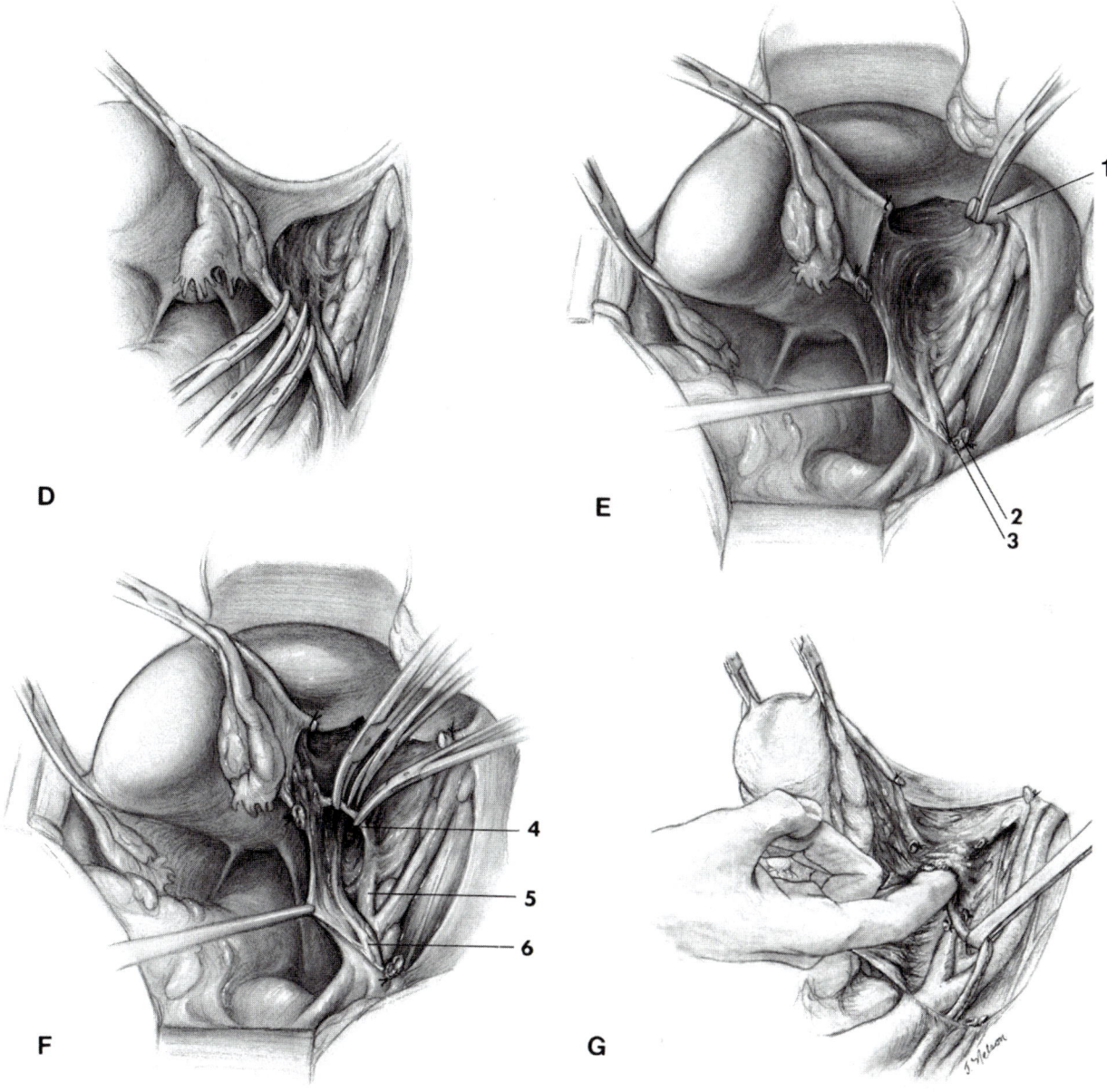

D

E

F

G

FIGURE 3–19. (continued)

about 10 cm (Figs. 3–21 and 3–22). With the woman upright, the upper portion of the pelvic canal is directed downward and backward, and its lower course curves and becomes directed downward and forward.

The walls of the true pelvis are partly bony and partly ligamentous. The posterior boundary is the anterior surface of the sacrum, and the lateral limits are formed by the inner surface of the ischial bones and the sacrosciatic notches and ligaments. In front the true pelvis is bounded by the pubic bones, the ascending superior rami of the ischial bones, and the obturator foramina.

The sidewalls of the true pelvis of the normal adult woman converge somewhat; therefore, if the planes of the ischial bones were extended downward, they would meet near the knee. Extending from the middle of the posterior margin of each ischium are the ischial spines. The ischial spines are of great obstetrical importance because the distance between them usually represents the shortest diameter of the pelvic cavity. They also serve as valuable landmarks in assessing the level to which the presenting part of the fetus has descended into the true pelvis (Chap. 12, p. 300).

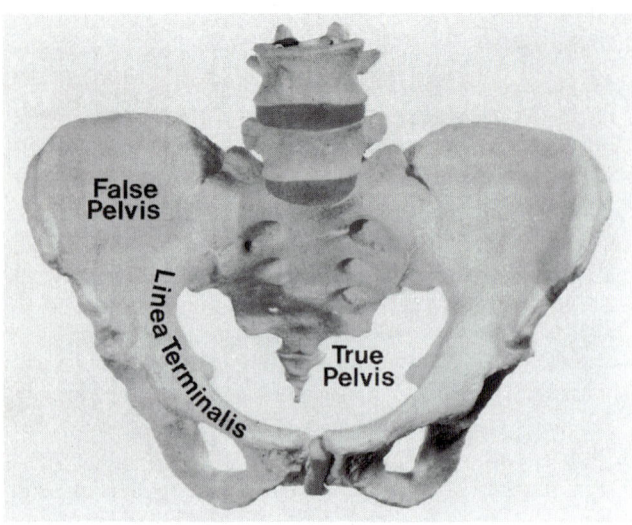

FIGURE 3–20. Normal female pelvis with the false and true pelvis identified.

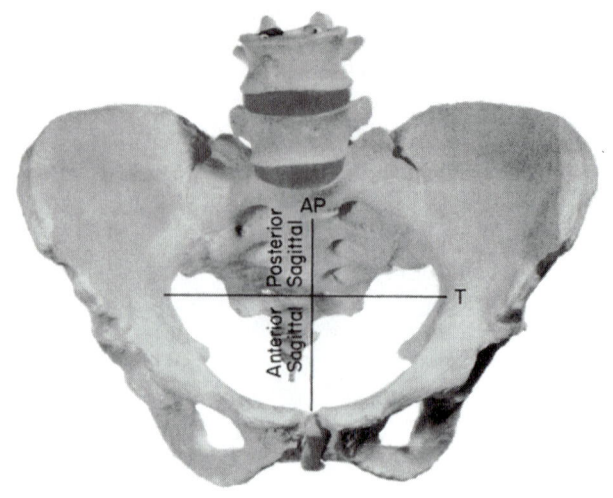

FIGURE 3–22. Adult female pelvis. Anteroposterior (AP) and transverse (T) diameters of the pelvic inlet are illustrated, as well as the posterior sagittal of the inlet.

The sacrum forms the posterior wall of the pelvic cavity. Its upper anterior margin corresponds to the body of the first sacral vertebra and is designated as the promontory. The promontory may be felt on vaginal examination in small pelves and can provide a landmark for clinical pelvimetry. Normally the sacrum has a marked vertical and a less pronounced horizontal concavity, which in abnormal pelves may undergo important variations. A straight line drawn from the promontory to the tip of the sacrum usually measures 10 cm, whereas the distance along the concavity averages 12 cm.

The descending inferior rami of the pubic bones unite at an angle of 90 to 100 degrees to form a rounded arch under which the fetal head must pass.

PELVIC JOINTS

SYMPHYSIS PUBIS. Anteriorly, the pelvic bones are joined together by the symphysis pubis. This structure consists of fibrocartilage and the superior and inferior pubic ligaments; the latter is frequently designated the *arcuate ligament of the pubis* (Fig. 3–23). The symphysis

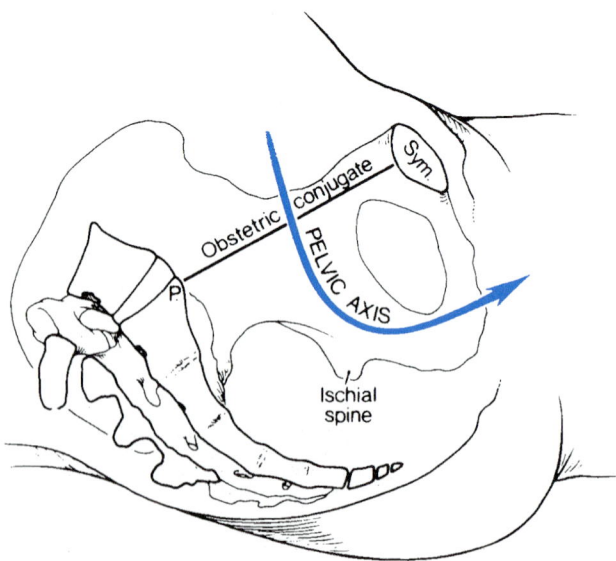

FIGURE 3–21. The cavity of the true pelvis is comparable to an obliquely truncated, bent cylinder with its greatest height posteriorly. Note the curvature of the pelvic axis.

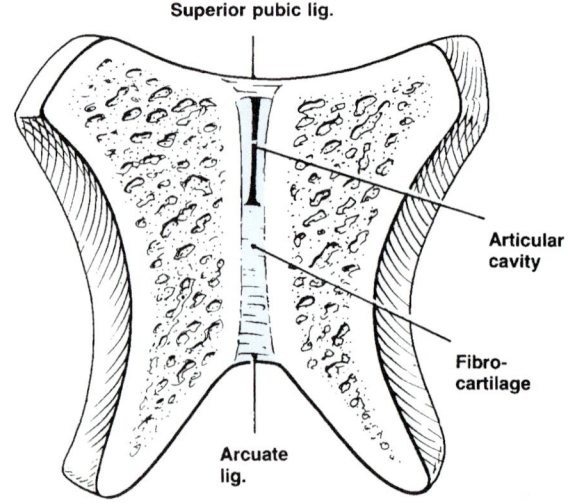

FIGURE 3–23. Frontal section through symphysis pubis. (lig. = ligament.) (Redrawn from Spalteholz, 1933.)

has a certain degree of mobility, which increases during pregnancy. This fact was demonstrated by Budin (1897), who reported that if a finger was inserted into the vagina of a pregnant woman and she then walked, the ends of the pubic bones could be felt moving up and down with each step.

SACROILIAC JOINTS. Posteriorly the pelvic bones are joined by the articulations between the sacrum and the iliac portion of the innominate bones (sacroiliac joints). These joints also have a certain degree of mobility.

RELAXATION OF THE PELVIC JOINTS. During pregnancy, relaxation of these joints likely results from hormonal changes. Abramson and co-workers (1934) observed that relaxation of the symphysis pubis commenced in women in the first half of pregnancy and increased during the last 3 months. These investigators reported that regression of relaxation began immediately after parturition and was completed within 3 to 5 months. The symphysis pubis also increases in width during pregnancy (more in multiparas than in primigravidas), and returns to normal soon after delivery. By careful radiographic studies, Borell and Fernstrom (1957) demonstrated that the rather marked mobility of the pelvis of women at term was caused by an upward gliding movement of the sacroiliac joint. The displacement, which is greatest in the dorsal lithotomy position, may increase the diameter of the outlet by 1.5 to 2.0 cm. **This is the main justification for placing a woman in this position for a vaginal delivery.** It should be noted, however, that the increase in the diameter of the pelvic outlet occurs only if the sacrum is allowed to rotate posteriorly, that is, *only* if the sacrum is not forced anteriorly by the weight of the maternal pelvis against the delivery table or bed (Russell, 1969, 1982). This is likely the reason that the McRoberts maneuver often is successful in releasing an obstructed shoulder in a case of shoulder dystocia (Chap. 19, p. 461). Gardosi and co-workers (1989) reported in a randomized controlled trial that a modified squatting position in the second stage of labor resulted in a shorter second stage and fewer perineal lacerations. However, there was an increase in labial lacerations. The authors attributed the "success" of the method to increasing the interspinous diameter and the diameter of the pelvic outlet (Russell, 1969, 1982) as well as to improving the "pushing efforts" of the laboring woman. Although these observations are unconfirmed, such a squatting position is assumed by many primitive women as the usual position for birth (Gardosi and associates, 1989; Russell, 1982).

PLANES AND DIAMETERS OF THE PELVIS. Because of its complex shape, it is difficult to describe the exact location of an object within the pelvis. For convenience, therefore, the pelvis is described as having four imaginary planes:

1. The plane of the pelvic inlet (superior strait).
2. The plane of the pelvic outlet (inferior strait).
3. The plane of the midpelvis (least pelvic dimensions).
4. The plane of greatest pelvic dimensions.

Because this last plane has no obstetrical significance, it is not considered further.

PELVIC INLET. The pelvic inlet (superior strait) is bounded posteriorly by the promontory and alae of the sacrum, laterally by the linea terminalis, and anteriorly by the horizontal rami of the pubic bones and symphysis pubis (Figs. 3–21, 3–22, 3–24, and 3–25). The configuration of the inlet of the human female pelvis typically is more nearly round than ovoid. Caldwell and co-workers (1934) identified radiographically a nearly round or *gynecoid* pelvic inlet in approximately 50 percent of the pelves of white women.

Four diameters of the pelvic inlet are usually described: anteroposterior, transverse, and two obliques. The obstetrically important anteroposterior diameter is the shortest distance between the promontory of the sacrum and the symphysis pubis, and is designated the *obstetrical conjugate* (Figs. 3–21, 3–22, and 3–24). Normally, the obstetrical conjugate measures 10 cm or more, but it may be considerably shortened in abnormal pelves.

The transverse diameter is constructed at right angles to the obstetrical conjugate and represents the greatest

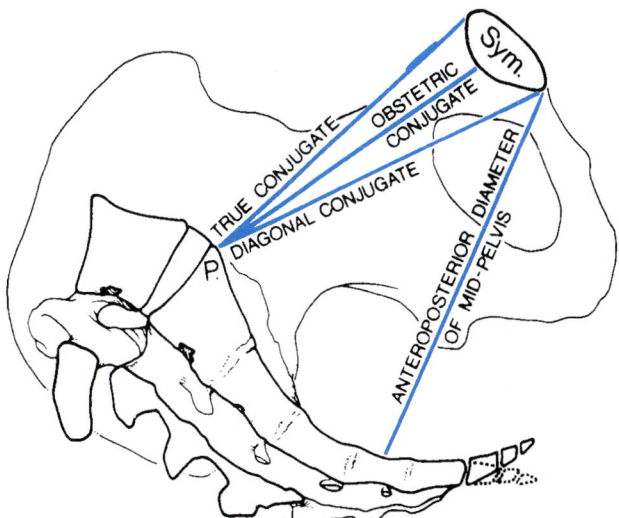

FIGURE 3–24. Three anteroposterior diameters of the pelvic inlet are illustrated: the true conjugate, the more important obstetrical conjugate, and the clinically measurable diagonal conjugate. The anteroposterior diameter of the midpelvis is also shown. (P = sacral promontory; Sym = symphysis pubis.)

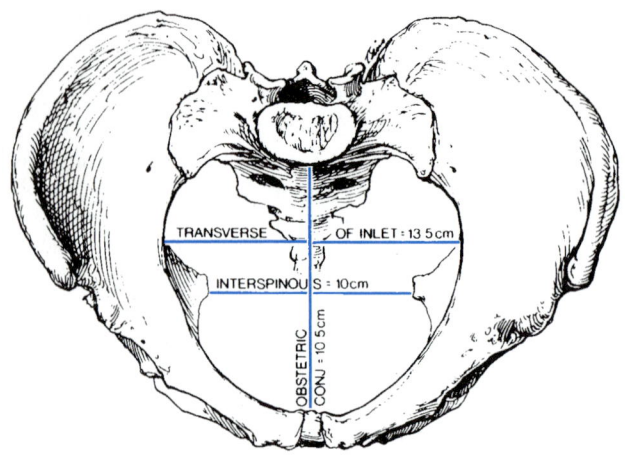

FIGURE 3–25. Adult female pelvis demonstrating anteroposterior and transverse diameters of the pelvic inlet and transverse (interspinous) diameter of the midpelvis. The obstetrical conjugate is normally greater than 10 cm.

distance between the linea terminalis on either side. It usually intersects the obstetrical conjugate at a point about 4 cm in front of the promontory (Fig. 3–22). The segment of the obstetrical conjugate from the intersection of these two lines to the promontory is designated the *posterior sagittal* diameter of the inlet.

Each of the oblique diameters extends from one of the sacroiliac synchondroses to the iliopectineal eminence on the opposite side of the pelvis. They average just under 13 cm and are designated right and left, according to whether they originate at the right or left sacroiliac synchondrosis.

The anteroposterior diameter of the pelvic inlet that has been identified as the *true conjugate* does not represent the shortest distance between the promontory of the sacrum and symphysis pubis (Fig. 3–24). The shortest distance is the *obstetrical conjugate,* which is the shortest anteroposterior diameter through which the head must pass in descending through the pelvic inlet (Figs. 3–21, 3–22, and 3–24).

The obstetrical conjugate cannot be measured directly with the examining fingers; therefore, various instruments have been designed in an effort to obtain such a measurement. Unfortunately, none of these instruments has proven to be reliable. For clinical purposes, it is sufficient to estimate the length of the obstetrical conjugate indirectly. This is accomplished by measuring the distance from the lower margin of the symphysis to promontory of the sacrum, that is, the *diagonal conjugate* (Fig. 3–24), and subtracting 1.5 to 2 cm from the result, according to the height and inclination of the symphysis pubis (see "Pelvic Size and Its Clinical Estimation" later in the chapter).

MIDPELVIS. The midpelvis at the level of the ischial spines (midplane, or plane of least pelvic dimensions) is of particular importance following engagement of the fetal head in obstructed labor. The interspinous diameter, 10 cm or somewhat more, is usually the smallest diameter of the pelvis. The anteroposterior diameter, through the level of the ischial spines, normally measures at least 11.5 cm. The posterior component (posterior sagittal diameter), between the sacrum and the line created by the interspinous diameter, is usually at least 4.5 cm.

PELVIC OUTLET. The outlet of the pelvis consists of two approximately triangular areas not in the same plane but having a common base, which is a line drawn between the two ischial tuberosities (Fig. 3–26). The apex of the posterior triangle is at the tip of the sacrum, and the lateral boundaries are the sacrosciatic ligaments and the ischial tuberosities. The anterior triangle is formed by the area under the pubic arch. Three diameters of the pelvic outlet usually are described: the anteroposterior, transverse, and posterior sagittal. The anteroposterior diameter (9.5 to 11.5 cm) extends from the lower margin of the symphysis pubis to the tip of the sacrum (Fig. 3–26). The transverse diameter (11 cm) is the distance between the inner edges of the ischial tuberosities. The posterior sagittal diameter extends from the tip of the sacrum to a right-angle intersection with a line between the ischial tuberosities. The normal *posterior sagittal diameter* of the outlet usually exceeds 7.5 cm (Fig. 3–26).

In obstructed labors caused by a narrowing of the midpelvis or pelvic outlet, the prognosis for vaginal delivery often depends on the length of the posterior sagittal diameter of the pelvic outlet (see Figs. 18–7 and 18–8).

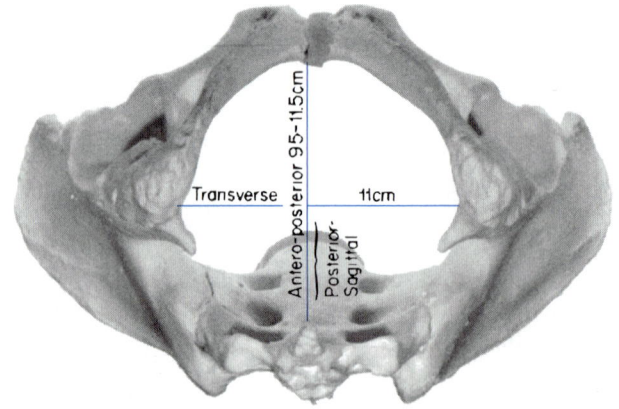

FIGURE 3–26. Pelvic outlet with diameters marked. Note that the anteroposterior diameter may be divided into anterior and posterior sagittal diameters.

PELVIC SHAPES. In the past, x-ray pelvimetry was used frequently in women with suspected cephalopelvic disproportion or fetal malpresentation. Pelvic radiography also was used as an aid in understanding the general architecture and configuration of the pelvis, as well as its size. Caldwell and Moloy (1933, 1934) developed a classification of the pelvis that is still used. The classification is based upon the shape of the pelvis, and familiarity with the classification helps the physician to understand the mechanisms of labor in normally and abnormally shaped pelves.

CALDWELL–MOLOY CLASSIFICATION. A line drawn through the greatest transverse diameter of the inlet divides it into anterior and posterior segments. The shapes of these segments are important determinants in this method of classification (Fig. 3–27). The character of the posterior segment determines the type of pelvis, and the character of the anterior segment determines the tendency. Many pelves are not pure but mixed types; for example, a gynecoid pelvis with an android tendency means that the posterior pelvis is gynecoid and the anterior pelvis is android in shape.

GYNECOID PELVIS. The posterior sagittal diameter of the inlet is only slightly shorter than the anterior sagittal. The sides of the posterior segment are well rounded and wide. Because the transverse diameter of the inlet is either slightly greater than or about the same as the anteroposterior diameter, the inlet is either slightly oval or round. The sidewalls of the pelvis are straight, the spines are not prominent, the pubic arch is wide, and the transverse diameter at the ischial spines is 10 cm or more. The sacrum is inclined neither anteriorly nor posteriorly. The sacrosciatic notch is well rounded and never narrow. Caldwell and co-workers (1939) ascertained the frequency of the four parent pelvic types by study of Todd's collection, and they reported that the gynecoid pelvis was found in almost 50 percent of women.

ANDROID PELVIS. The posterior sagittal diameter at the inlet is much shorter than the anterior sagittal, limiting the use of the posterior space by the fetal head. The sides of the posterior segment are not rounded but tend to form, with the corresponding sides of the anterior segment, a wedge at their point of junction. The anterior pelvis is narrow and triangular. The sidewalls are usually convergent, the ischial spines are prominent, and the subpubic arch is narrowed. The bones are characteristically heavy, and the sacrosciatic notches are narrow and highly arched. The sacrum is set forward in the pelvis and usually is straight, with little or no curvature, and the posterior sagittal diameter is de-

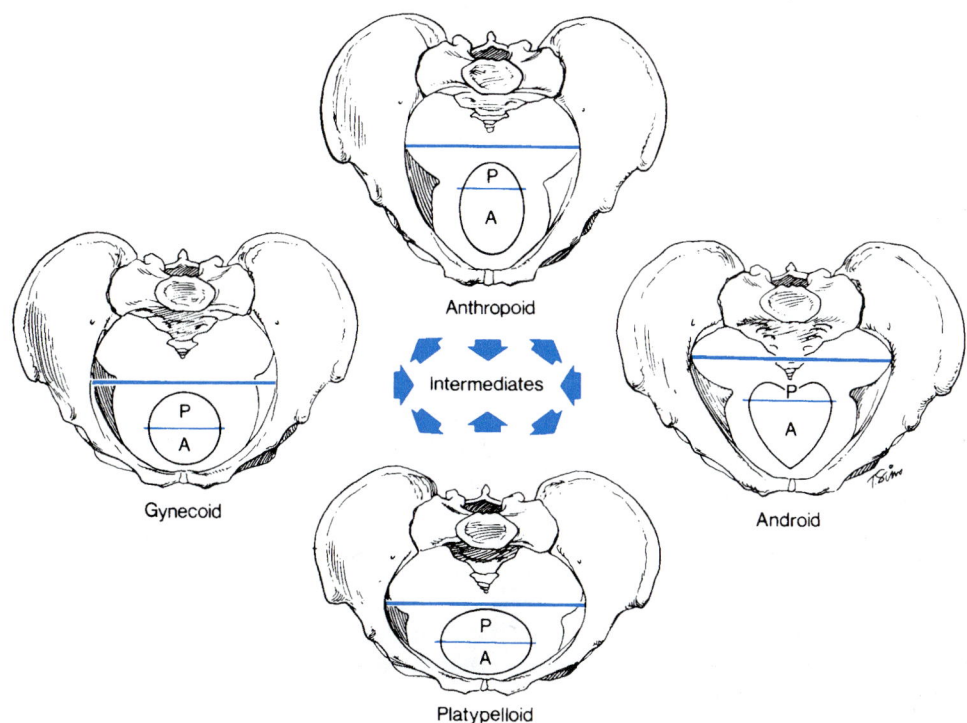

FIGURE 3–27. The four parent pelvic types of the Caldwell–Moloy classification. A line passing through the widest transverse diameter divides the inlet into posterior (P) and anterior (A) segments.

creased from inlet to outlet by the forward inclination of the sacrum. Not infrequently there is considerable forward inclination of the sacral tip.

The extreme android pelvis presages a poor prognosis for vaginal delivery. The frequency of difficult forceps operations increases substantively when there is a *small* android pelvis. Android-type pelves made up one third of pure-type pelves encountered in white women and one sixth in nonwhite women in the Todd collection.

ANTHROPOID PELVIS. The anteroposterior diameter of the inlet is greater than the transverse. This results in an oval anteroposteriorly, with the anterior segment somewhat narrow and pointed. The sacrosciatic notches are large, and the sidewalls often are convergent. The sacrum usually has six segments and is straight, making the anthropoid pelvis deeper than the other types.

The ischial spines are likely to be prominent. The subpubic arch frequently is narrowed but well shaped. Anthropoid-type pelves make up one fourth of pure-type pelves in white women and nearly one half of those in nonwhite women.

PLATYPELLOID PELVIS. The platypelloid pelvis has a flattened gynecoid shape, with a short anteroposterior and a wide transverse diameter. The latter is set well in front of the sacrum, as in the typical gynecoid pelvis. The angle of the anterior pelvis is very wide, and the anterior puboiliac and posterior iliac portions of the iliopectineal lines are well curved. The sacrum usually is well curved and rotated backward. Thus, the sacrum is short and the pelvis shallow, creating wide sacrosciatic notches. The platypelloid pelvis is the rarest of the pure varieties and is found in less than 3 percent of women.

INTERMEDIATE-TYPE PELVES. Intermediate or mixed types of pelves are much more frequent than pure types.

PELVIC SIZE AND ITS CLINICAL ESTIMATION

PELVIC INLET MEASUREMENTS

DIAGONAL CONJUGATE. In many abnormal pelves, the anteroposterior diameter of the pelvic inlet (the obstetrical conjugate) is considerably shortened. It is important therefore to determine its length, but this measurement can be obtained only by radiographic techniques. The distance from the sacral promontory to the lower margin of the symphysis pubis (the diagonal conjugate), however, can be measured clinically (Figs. 3–28 and 3–29). The examiner introduces two fingers into the vagina; before measuring the diagonal conjugate, the mobility of the coccyx is evaluated and the anterior surface of the sacrum is palpated. The mobility of the coccyx is tested by palpating it with the fingers

in the vagina and attempting to move it to and fro. The anterior surface of the sacrum is then palpated from below upward, and its vertical and lateral curvatures are noted. In normal pelves only the last three sacral vertebrae can be felt without indenting the perineum, whereas in markedly contracted pelves the entire anterior surface of the sacrum usually is readily accessible. Occasionally, the mobility of the coccyx and the anatomical features of the lower sacrum may be defined more easily by rectal examination.

Except in extreme degrees of pelvic contraction, in order to reach the promontory of the sacrum, the examiner's elbow must be depressed and, unless the examiner's fingers are unusually long, the perineum forcibly indented by the knuckles of the examiner's third and fourth fingers. The index and the second fingers, held firmly together, are carried up and over the anterior surface of the sacrum. By sharply depressing the wrist, the promontory may be felt by the tip of the second finger as a projecting bony margin. With the finger closely applied to the most prominent portion of the upper sacrum, the vaginal hand is elevated until it contacts the pubic arch; and the immediately adjacent point on the index finger is marked, as shown in Figure 3–28. The hand is withdrawn, and the distance between the mark and the tip of the second finger is measured. The diagonal conjugate is determined, and the obstetrical conjugate is computed by subtracting 1.5 to 2.0 cm, depending upon the height and inclination of the symphysis pubis, as illustrated in Figure 3–29. If the diagonal conjugate is greater than 11.5 cm, it is justifiable to assume that the pelvic inlet is of adequate size for vaginal delivery of a normal-sized fetus.

Transverse contraction of the inlet can be measured only by imaging pelvimetry (Chap. 18, p. 438). Such a contraction is possible even in the presence of an adequate anteroposterior diameter.

ENGAGEMENT. This refers to the descent of the biparietal plane of the fetal head to a level below that of the pelvic inlet (Figs. 3–30 and 3–31). When the biparietal, or largest, diameter of the normally flexed fetal head has passed through the inlet, the head is engaged. Although engagement of the fetal head usually is regarded as a phenomenon of labor, in nulliparas it commonly occurs during the last few weeks of pregnancy. When it does so, it is confirmatory evidence that the pelvic inlet is adequate for that fetal head. **With engagement, the fetal head serves as an internal pelvimeter to demonstrate that the pelvic inlet is ample for that fetus.**

Whether the head is engaged may be ascertained by rectal or vaginal examination or by abdominal palpation. After gaining experience with vaginal examination, it becomes relatively easy to locate the station of the lowermost part of the fetal head in relation to the level

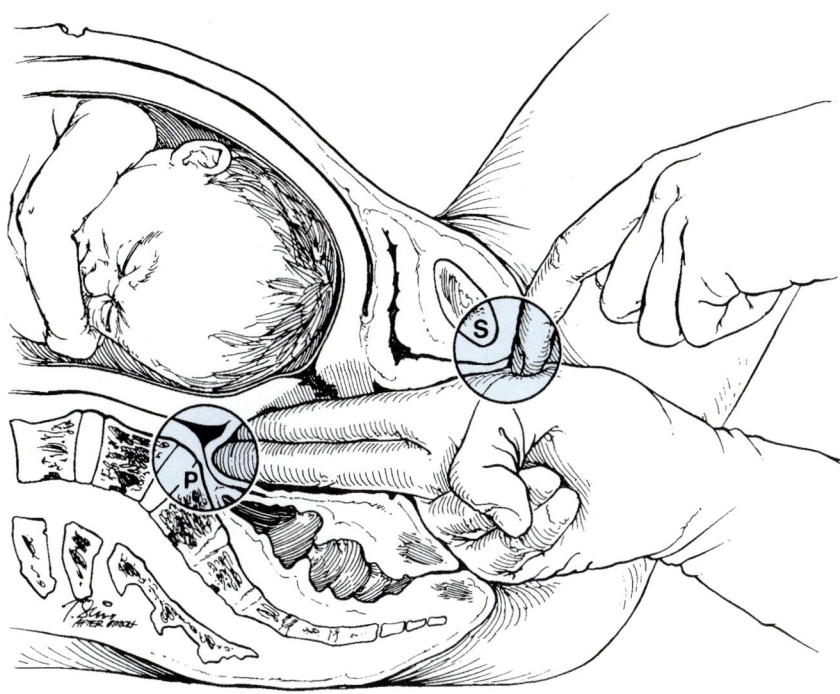

FIGURE 3–28. Vaginal examination to determine the diagonal conjugate. (P = sacral promontory; S = symphysis pubis.)

of the ischial spines. If the lowest part of the occiput is at or below the level of the spines, the head usually, but not always, is engaged, because the distance from the plane of the pelvic inlet to the level of the ischial spines is approximately 5 cm in most pelves, and the distance from the biparietal plane of the unmolded fetal head to the vertex is about 3 to 4 cm. Under these circumstances, the vertex cannot possibly reach the level of the spines unless the biparietal diameter has passed the inlet, or unless there has been considerable elongation of the fetal head because of molding and formation of a *caput succedaneum.*

Engagement may be ascertained less satisfactorily by abdominal examination. If the biparietal plane of a term-sized infant has descended through the inlet, the examining fingers cannot reach the lowermost part of the head. Thus, when pushed downward over the lower abdomen, the examining fingers will slide over that portion of the head proximal to the biparietal plane (nape of the neck) and diverge. Conversely, if the head is not engaged, the examining fingers can easily palpate the lower part of the head and will converge (the fourth Leopold maneuver; see Chap. 12, p. 257).

Fixation of the fetal head is its descent through the pelvic inlet to a depth that prevents its free movement in any direction when pushed by both hands placed over the lower abdomen. Fixation is not necessarily synonymous with engagement. Although a head that is

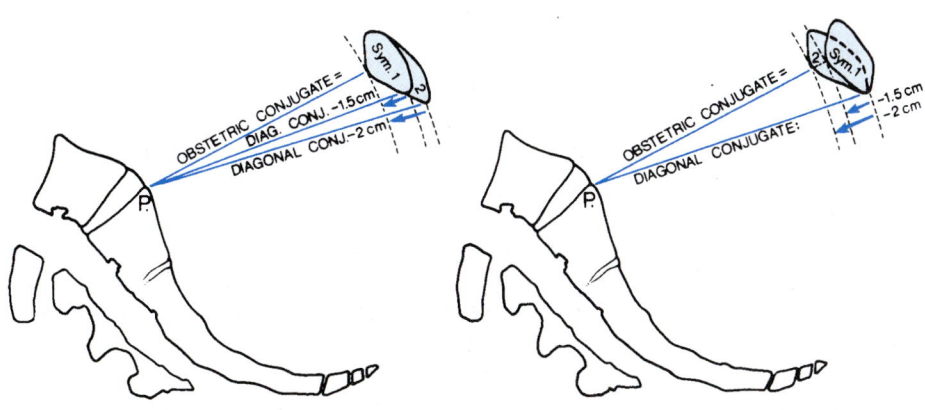

FIGURE 3–29. Variations in length of diagonal conjugate dependent on height and inclination of the symphysis pubis. (P = sacral promontory; Sym = symphysis pubis.)

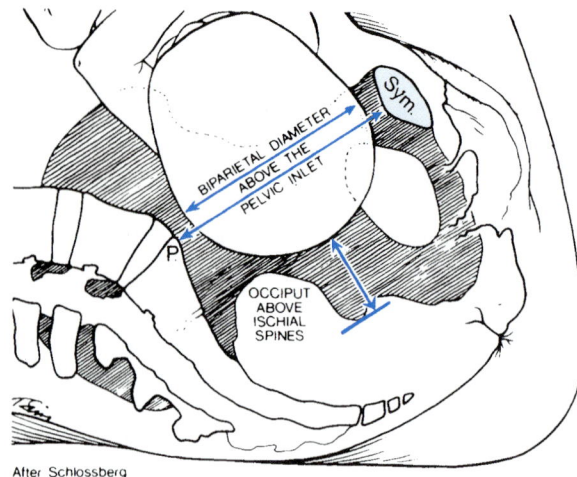

After Schlossberg

FIGURE 3–30. When the lowermost portion of the fetal head is above the ischial spines, the biparietal diameter of the head is not likely to have passed through the pelvic inlet and therefore is not engaged. (P = sacral promontory; Sym = symphysis pubis.)

freely movable on abdominal examination cannot be engaged, fixation of the head is sometimes seen when the biparietal plane is still 1 cm or more above the pelvic inlet, especially if the head is molded appreciably.

Although engagement is conclusive evidence of an adequate pelvic inlet for that fetal head, its absence is by no means always indicative of pelvic contraction.

PELVIC OUTLET MEASUREMENTS. An important dimension of the pelvic outlet that is accessible for clinical measurement is the diameter between the ischial tuber-

osities, variously called the *biischial diameter, intertuberous diameter,* and *transverse diameter of the outlet.* A measurement of over 8 cm is considered normal. The measurement of the transverse diameter of the outlet can be estimated by placing a closed fist against the perineum between the ischial tuberosities, after first measuring the width of the closed fist. Usually the closed fist is wider than 8 cm. The shape of the subpubic arch also can be evaluated at the same time by palpating the pubic rami from the subpubic region toward the ischial tuberosities.

MIDPELVIS ESTIMATION. Clinical estimation of midpelvis capacity by any direct form of measurement is not possible. If the ischial spines are quite prominent, the sidewalls are felt to converge, and the concavity of the sacrum is very shallow; if the biischial diameter of the outlet is less than 8 cm, then suspicion is aroused about a contraction in this region.

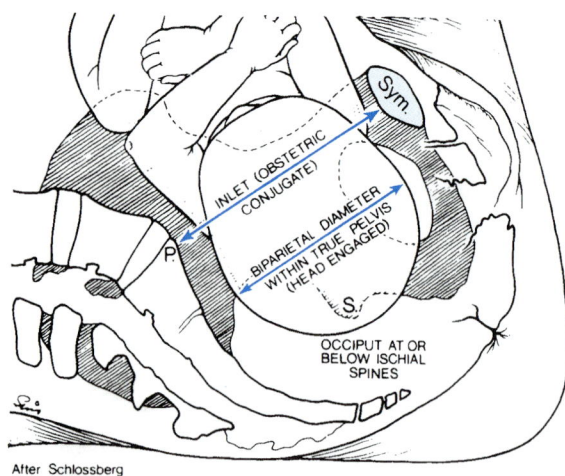

After Schlossberg

FIGURE 3–31. When the lowermost portion of the fetal head is at or below the ischial spines, it is usually engaged. Exceptions occur when there is considerable molding, caput formation, or both. (P = sacral promontory; S = ischial spine; Sym = symphysis pubis.)

REFERENCES

Abramson D, Roberts SM, Wilson PD: Relaxation of the pelvic joints in pregnancy. Surg Obstet Gynecol 58:595, 1934

Block E: Quantitative morphological investigation of the follicular system in women. Acta Anat 14:108, 1952

Borell U, Fernstrom I: Movements at the sacroiliac joints and their importance to changes in pelvic dimensions during parturition. Acta Obstet Gynecol Scand 36:42, 1957

Buckingham JC, Buethe RA Jr, Danforth DN: Collagen-muscle ratio in clinically normal and clinically incompetent cervices. Am J Obstet Gynecol 91:232, 1965

Budin RC: X-radiography of a Naegele pelvis. Obstetrique Par 2:499, 1897

Caldwell WE, Moloy HC: Anatomical variations in the female pelvis and their effect in labor with a suggested classification. Am J Obstet Gynecol 26:479, 1933

Caldwell WE, Moloy HC, D'Esopo DA: Further studies on the pelvic architecture. Am J Obstet Gynecol 28:482, 1934

Caldwell WE, Moloy HC, Swenson PC: The use of the roentgen ray in obstetrics, 1. Roentgen pelvimetry and cephalometry; technique of pelviroentgenography. Am J Roentgenol 41:305, 1939

Carrington BM, Hricak H, Nuruddin RN, Secaf E, Laros RK Jr, Hill C: Müllerian duct anomalies: MR imaging evaluation. Radiology 176:715, 1990

Danforth DN, Buckingham JC, Roddick JW Jr: Connective tissue changes incident to cervical effacement. Am J Obstet Gynecol 80:939, 1960

Delancey JOL: Structural anatomy of the posterior pelvic compartment as it relates to rectocele. Am J Obstet Gynecol 180:815, 1999

Delancey JOL, Toglia MR, Perucchini D: Internal and external anal sphincter anatomy as it relates to midline obstetric lacerations. Obstet Gynecol 90:924, 1997

DuBose TJ, Hill LW, Hennigan HW Jr, Nichols DH, Mezaraups GG, Porter L, Marley L, Butschek CM, Karnaze GC,

Walser E: Sonography of arcuate uterine blood vessels. J Ultrasound Med 4:229, 1985

Ferenczy A, Richart RM: Female Reproductive System: Dynamics of Scanning and Transmission Electron Microscopy. New York, Wiley, 1974

Forbes TR: On the fate of the medullary cords of the human ovary. Contrib Embryol 30:9, 1942

Gardosi J, Hutson N, Lynch CB: Randomised, controlled trial of squatting in the second stage of labour. Lancet 2:74, 1989

Hitschmann F, Adler L: The structure of the endometrium of the sexually mature woman. Monatschr Geburtsh Gynaek 27:1, 1908

Hodgson BJ, Eddy CA: The autonomic nervous system and its relationship to tubal ovum transport—a reappraisal. Gynecol Invest 6:161, 1975

Hricak H, Chang YC, Cann CE, Parer J: Cervical incompetence: Preliminary evaluation with MR imaging. Radiology 174:821, 1990

Koff AK: Development of the vagina in the human fetus. Contrib Embryol 24:59, 1933

Krantz KE: Innervation of the human vulva and vagina. Obstet Gynecol 13:382, 1958

Langlois PL: The size of the normal uterus. J Reprod Med 4:220, 1970

Larsen B, Galask RP: Vaginal microbial flora: Practical and theoretic relevance. Obstet Gynecol 55:100S, 1980

McGregor JA, French JI: Bacterial vaginosis in pregnancy. Obstet Gynecol Surv 55:S1, 2000

McKay DG, Robinson D, Hertig AT: Histochemical observations on granulosa cell tumors, thecomas and fibromas of the ovary. Am J Obstet Gynecol 58:625, 1949

Moore K: The Developing Human. Philadelphia, Saunders, 1983

Mossman HW, Koering MJ, Ferry D Jr: Cyclic changes in interstitial gland tissue of the human ovary. Am J Anat 115:235, 1964

Nelson JH: Atlas of Radical Pelvic Surgery, 2nd ed. New York, Appleton, 1977, p 133

Okkels H, Engle ET: Studies on the finer structure of the uterine blood vessels of the macacus monkey. Acta Pathol Microbiol Scand 15:150, 1938

Orsini LF, Salardi S, Pilu G, Bovicelli L, Cacciari E: Pelvic organs in premenarcheal girls: Real-time ultrasonography. Radiology 153:113, 1984

Russell JGB: The rationale of primitive delivery positions. Br J Obstet Gynaecol 89:712, 1982

Russell JGB: Moulding of the pelvic outlet. J Obstet Gynaecol Br Commonw 76:817, 1969

Schwalm H, Dubrauszky V: The structure of the musculature of the human uterus—muscles and connective tissue. Am J Obstet Gynecol 94:391, 1966

Spalteholz: Hand Atlas of Human Anatomy, vol 1. Philadelphia, Lippincott, 1933

Verkauf BS, Von Thron J, O'Brien WF: Clitoral size in normal women. Obstet Gynecol 80:41, 1992

Wicke L: Atlas of Radiologic Anatomy, 3rd ed. Baltimore, Urban & Schwarzenberg, 1982

Woodruff JD, Pauerstein CJ: The Fallopian Tube. Baltimore, Williams & Wilkins, 1969

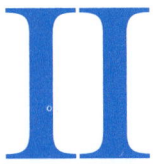

SECTION

Physiology
of
Pregnancy

4

The Endometrium and Decidua

MENSTRUATION AND PREGNANCY

Endometrium/decidua is the anatomical site of blastocyst apposition, implantation, and placental development. The endometrium is the mucosal lining of the uterine cavity and the decidua is the highly modified and specialized endometrium of pregnancy. From an evolutionary perspective, the human endometrium is highly developed in order to accommodate a hemochorioendothelial type of placentation. Endometrial development of a magnitude similar to that observed in women, that is with special spiral (or coiling) arteries, is restricted to only the catarrhine primates—such as humans, great apes, and Old World monkeys. Trophoblasts of the blastocyst invade these endometrial arteries during implantation and placentation to establish uteroplacental vessels.

The catarrhine primates are the only mammals that menstruate, a process of endometrial tissue shedding with hemorrhage that is dependent upon sex steroid hormone-directed changes in blood flow in the spiral arteries. With nonfertile, but ovulatory, ovarian cycles, menstruation effects desquamation of the endometrium. New endometrial growth and development must be initiated with each ovarian cycle, so that endometrial maturation corresponds rather precisely with the next pregnancy (implantation) opportunity. There seems to be a very narrow window of endometrial receptivity to blastocyst implantation in the human that corresponds approximately to menstrual cycle days 20 to 24.

MATERNAL TISSUES OF THE FETAL–MATERNAL COMMUNICATION SYSTEM

Direct cell-to-cell contact between blastocyst and maternal endometrium is first established 6 days after fertilization of the ovum. At this time, the blastocyst contacts the endometrial surface epithelium, a process called "blastocyst" apposition. For a brief time, the surface epithelium of the endometrium is the only maternal tissue in direct contact with the blastocyst; but even then, biological processes are occurring between the two. Soon after apposition, the blastocyst becomes adherent to the endometrium, and the process of implantation has begun. The fundamental components of immunological acceptance of the conceptus, maternal recognition of pregnancy, placental development, pregnancy maintenance, and fetal nutrition are quickly established.

THE CARDINAL FUNCTION OF THE UTERUS. Biologically, the single salutary function of the uterus is the accommodation of a conceptus (pregnancy). There is no known endocrine or other physiological function of the endometrium or myometrium, independent of pregnancy, that affects the metabolic homeostasis or the physical well-being of women. There is no evidence that the uncomplicated removal of the myometrium, endometrium, and cervix (hysterectomy) adversely affects the life span or general good health of women.

OVERVIEW OF ENDOMETRIAL FUNCTION. The growth and functional characteristics of the human endometrium are unique. The epithelial (glandular) cells, the stromal (mesenchymal) cells, and the blood vessels of the endometrium replicate cyclically in reproductive-age women at a rapid rate. The endometrium is regenerated during each endometrial (ovarian–menstrual) cycle. The superficial two thirds of the entire endometrium is shed and regenerated almost 500 times, on average, during the reproductive lifetime of most women. There is no other example in humans of the cyclical shedding and regrowth of an entire tissue.

To place repetitive menstruation in perspective, the lifetime cumulative blood loss associated with normal endometrial shedding is 10 to 20 liters or more, an amount of blood that contains at least three times the total body iron content of the average adult woman. The 38-year reproductive lifetime cumulative production of progesterone by corpora lutea and placenta in the woman who chooses two pregnancies but experiences 450 nonfertile ovarian cycles is about 150,000 mg (150 g), which is similar to the cumulative amount of cortisol secreted by the adrenal cortices during the same 38 years. This incredible investment in endometrial tissue growth provides for regular renewal of the functional portion of this tissue in preparation for the next pregnancy opportunity.

THE ACCOMMODATION OF PREGNANCY IS THE CARDINAL FUNCTION OF THE ENDOMETRIUM/DECIDUA. The single physiological and metabolic function of the endometrium/decidua is to serve as the maternal tissue interface of pregnancy. The endometrium is the optimal site for blastocyst implantation and embryo-fetal/placental development; but it cannot be claimed that this function of the endometrium/decidua is unique because of the known success, albeit limited, of ectopic pregnancies. "Decidualization" of tissues in which ectopic pregnancies implant is prominent.

There also may be a role for the endometrium in sperm capacitation; but again, it cannot be argued that this function is unique to this tissue, as evidenced by the success of sperm capacitation and fertilization of human ova in vitro.

The decidual cells are differentiated from the stromal cells of the endometrium under the influence of progesterone and other stimuli. In addition, there are many bone marrow–derived cells (a variety of lymphocytes and leukocytes) in normal endometrium and decidua.

The unique spiral arteries persist in one portion of the decidua (parietalis), but these arteries are invaded and modified by trophoblasts in the decidua (basalis) underlying the implantation site.

The implantation of the blastocyst on the surface of the endometrial cavity provides an anatomical site from which the fetus can be born. The decidua is continuous with the birth canal, that is, there is access from the surface of the endometrium/decidua through the cervical canal to the vagina. This anatomical arrangement also provides for the expulsion of the fetus, by the contractions of the myometrium, which effect dilatation of the cervix and descent of the fetus with childbirth.

The endometrium and decidua are specialized tissues that carry out multiple functions.

1. The hormonal responsiveness and phenotypic changes of the endometrial/decidual cells facilitates apposition and implantation of the blastocyst.
2. The decidua serves as an immunologically specialized tissue.
3. The endometrium/decidua and the spiral arteries accept trophoblast invasion, providing for embryo-fetal nutrition.
4. The decidua contributes cytokines and growth factors that promote placental growth, function, and the inhibition of (trophoblast) apoptosis.

The decidua, with its bone marrow-derived cells, also serves first to accept and then to limit trophoblast invasion into maternal tissues. Lastly, the decidua is a highly versatile endocrine tissue, producing prolactin, 1,25-dihydroxy-vitamin D_3, corticotropin-releasing hormone, parathyroid hormone–related protein, relaxin, prorenin, somatostatin, oxytocin, activin, inhibin, corticosteroid-binding globulin, insulin-like growth factor–binding protein(s), and multiple pregnancy-specific proteins (Popovici and associates, 2000). These functions of the endometrium were reviewed by Tang and co-workers (1994).

The role of the decidua in promoting as well as accommodating placental growth and function is a topic of great research interest. Many investigations are directed toward a definition of the role of cytokines and growth factors, produced in the decidua, in trophoblast replication and differentiation, or in modifying growth factor receptors in the trophoblasts. It seems likely that trophoblasts secrete agents that induce the decidua to produce factors that incite further growth and differentiation of trophoblasts in a paracrine arrangement. The specifics of this coordinated process are not fully defined, but there seems to be little doubt that trophoblasts are capable of enlisting maternal decidual tissue support to ensure placental growth, development, and survival.

SPECIALIZED FUNCTIONS OF THE DECIDUA. The decidua likely is endowed with capacities to respond to microbiological challenges without simultaneously mounting an immunological response that results in abortion or preterm labor. The endometrial cavity is anatomically open, potentially and functionally patent to the external environment. The same is true of the decidua during pregnancy, at least at the juncture of the lower pole of the amnionic sac with the decidua parietalis. There is, however, functional closure of the cervical canal during pregnancy that is effected by a mucus "plug" that has antimicrobial properties. Therefore, the decidua must function in an exceptionally successful manner to limit bacterial colonization at the lower pole of the chorion laeve–decidual interface. Many investigators have suggested that infections that originate by ascending spread of microorganisms from the cervix of vaginal fluid may constitute one cause of the onset of preterm labor (Chap. 11, p. 281).

ESTROGEN ACTION. Estradiol-17β, the biologically potent, naturally occurring estrogen, which is secreted by the granulosa cells of the dominant ovarian follicle, acts to promote responses of the endometrium in a manner that is classical for steroid hormone action. By use of estrogens of high specific radioactivity, Jensen and Jacobson (1962) demonstrated that nonmetabolized (radiolabeled) estradiol-17β is sequestered in estrogen-responsive tissues, notably the uterus. These research findings marked the beginning of the contemporary era of the study of the mechanisms of steroid action through specific steroid receptor proteins.

Estradiol-17β enters cells from blood by simple diffusion; but in estrogen-responsive cells, estradiol-17β is sequestered by binding to estrogen receptor protein molecules. The receptor is a macromolecule characteized by high affinity, but low capacity, for estradiol-17β and other biologically active (synthetic) estrogens. The estradiol-17β-receptor complex, after transformational changes, is a transcriptional factor that becomes associated with the estrogen response element of specific genes. This interaction brings about estrogen receptor-specific initiation of gene transcription, which promotes the synthesis of specific messenger RNAs, and thereafter the synthesis of specific proteins. Among the many proteins synthesized in most estrogen-responsive cells are additional estrogen receptors and other macromolecules characterized by high affinity for progesterone (progesterone receptors). Thus, estradiol-17β acts in the endometrium and in other estrogen-responsive tissues to promote the perpetuation of estrogen action and to promote the responsiveness of that tissue to progesterone.

The endometrial epithelial (glandular) cells are estrogen responsive but do not necessarily replicate as a result of the direct action of estradiol-17β on the epithelial cells. Estrogen, administered to castrate or postmenopausal women, promotes growth of the endometrium, especially the glandular epithelial cells. Replication of human endometrial epithelial cells in culture, however, is not increased appreciably, if at all, when estrogen is added to the medium. It seems more likely that estradiol-17β and other bioactive estrogens in vivo cause replication of the epithelium indirectly (probably through actions on the stromal cells). It has been suggested that estrogen acts on the endometrial stromal cells to promote the synthesis of an endometrial epithelial cell growth factor, which functions in a paracrine manner to cause replication of the adjacent epithelial cells. This type of arrangement may be commonplace in epithelial–mesenchymal interactions in hormone-responsive tissues.

PROGESTERONE ACTION. This hormone also enters cells by diffusion and in responsive tissues becomes associated with progesterone receptors with high affinity, but low capacity, for progestins. Commonly, the cellular content of progesterone receptors is dependent on previous estrogen action. The progesterone–receptor complex also promotes gene transcription, but the response to progesterone is strikingly different from that evoked by the estradiol-17β–estrogen receptor complex. Progesterone actions include a decreases in the synthesis of estrogen receptor molecules (Tseng and Gurpide, 1975). This is one means by which progesterone (and synthetic progestins) attenuates estrogen action. Tseng and Gurpide (1974) also found that progesterone acts to increase the rate of enzymatic inactivation of estradiol-17β through an increase in the activity of the enzyme, estradiol dehydrogenase. Progesterone also acts to increase sulfurylation of estrogens (estrogen sulfotransferase), another means of estrogen inactivation (Tseng and Liu, 1981).

Steroid hormones also may act by mechanisms other than the receptor-mediated, genomic process just described. For example, progesterone and some of its metabolites induce profound biological (cellular) responses through receptor-independent, nongenomic processes.

THE ENDOMETRIAL CYCLE OF OVULATORY WOMEN

In 1937, Rock and Bartlett suggested that the histological features of the endometrium were sufficiently characteristic to permit "dating" of the ovarian cycle of the woman from whom the endometrial tissue was obtained. The histological changes that occur in the endometrium during the nonfertile (but ovulatory) menstrual cycle are summarized in Figure 4–1 and Table 4–1.

HORMONE-INDUCED MORPHOLOGICAL CHANGES OF THE ENDOMETRIUM. The cyclical changes in endometrial histology are faithfully reproduced during each ovulatory ovarian cycle. These sex steroid hormone-induced modifications can be summarized as follows.

1. During the preovulatory, or follicular, phase of the cycle, estradiol-17β is secreted—principally by a single dominant follicle of one ovary—in increasing quantities until just before ovulation.
2. During the postovulatory, or luteal, phase of the cycle, progesterone is secreted by the corpus luteum in increasing amounts (up to 40 to 50 mg per day) until the midluteal phase.
3. Beginning about 7 to 8 days after ovulation, the rates of progesterone (and estrogen) secretion by the corpus luteum begin to decline and diminish progressively before menstruation.

In response to these cyclical changes in the rates of ovarian sex steroid hormone secretion, there are five main stages of the corresponding endometrial cycle:

1. Menstrual/postmenstrual reepithelialization.
2. Endometrial proliferation in response to stimulation (directly or indirectly) by estradiol.
3. Abundant glandular secretion, in response to the combined action of estrogen and progesterone.
4. Premenstrual ischemia, the result of endometrial tissue volume involution, which causes stasis of blood in the spiral arteries.
5. Menstruation, which is preceded and accompanied by severe vasoconstriction of the endometrial spiral arteries and collapse and desquamation of all but the deepest layer of the endometrium.

In the final analysis, menstruation is the consequence of the withdrawal of factors that maintain endometrial growth.

Commonly, the initiation of menstruation is attributed to "progesterone withdrawal," but this is probably a very oversimplified explanation. It is true that the administration of estrogen to castrate women and then treatment/withdrawal with progesterone will effect menstruation, even with continued estrogen treatment. Nonetheless, the heretofore dominant role attributed to progesterone in promoting pregnancy-favorable phenomena and the physiological importance of progesterone withdrawal in the initiation of menstruation seem to have been overestimated. Progesterone facilitates and permits decidualization of the endometrium and the maintenance of pregnancy; progesterone withdrawal may favor the initiation of menstruation, lactation, and parturition. There are, however, multiple other coordinated, interactive processes that are operative and essential for the success of each of these events (Chap. 11, p. 262).

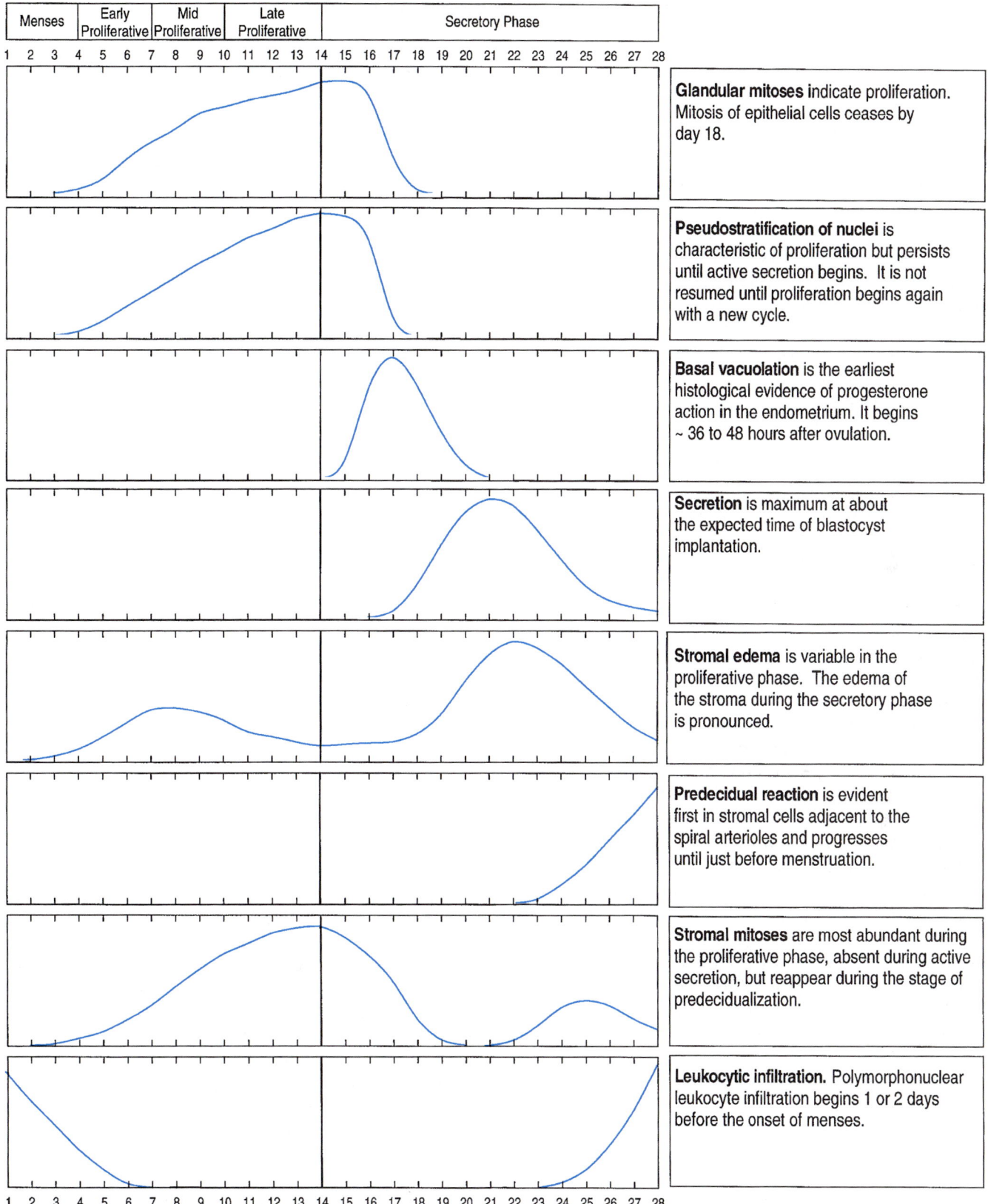

Menses	Early Proliferative	Mid Proliferative	Late Proliferative	Secretory Phase

1 2 3 4 5 6 7 8 9 10 11 12 13 14 15 16 17 18 19 20 21 22 23 24 25 26 27 28

Glandular mitoses indicate proliferation. Mitosis of epithelial cells ceases by day 18.

Pseudostratification of nuclei is characteristic of proliferation but persists until active secretion begins. It is not resumed until proliferation begins again with a new cycle.

Basal vacuolation is the earliest histological evidence of progesterone action in the endometrium. It begins ~ 36 to 48 hours after ovulation.

Secretion is maximum at about the expected time of blastocyst implantation.

Stromal edema is variable in the proliferative phase. The edema of the stroma during the secretory phase is pronounced.

Predecidual reaction is evident first in stromal cells adjacent to the spiral arterioles and progresses until just before menstruation.

Stromal mitoses are most abundant during the proliferative phase, absent during active secretion, but reappear during the stage of predecidualization.

Leukocytic infiltration. Polymorphonuclear leukocyte infiltration begins 1 or 2 days before the onset of menses.

1 2 3 4 5 6 7 8 9 10 11 12 13 14 15 16 17 18 19 20 21 22 23 24 25 26 27 28

FIGURE 4–1. Dating of the endometrium according to the day of the menstrual cycle during a hypothetical 28-day ovarian cycle. Correlation of typical morphological findings. (From Noyes and colleagues, 1950).

The follicular (preovulatory or proliferative) phase, and the postovulatory (luteal or secretory) phase of the ovarian/endometrial cycles, are customarily divided into early and late stages. The normal secretory phase of the endometrial (menstrual) cycle can be subdivided rather finely (almost day by day), by histological criteria, from shortly after ovulation until the onset of menstruation.

EARLY PROLIFERATLIVE PHASE ENDOMETRIUM.

About two thirds of the functional endometrium is fragmented and shed during menstruation; but, reepithelialization is in progress even before menstrual bleeding has ceased. By the fifth day of the endometrial cycle (first day of menses equals day 1), the epithelial surface of the endometrium has been restored and revascularization of the endometrium is in progress. During the early part of the proliferative phase, the endometrium is thin, usually less than 2 mm in thickness. The glands at this stage are narrow, tubular structures that pursue almost a straight and parallel course (one with the other) from the basal layer toward the surface of the endometrial cavity. Mitotic figures, especially in the glandular epithelium, are identified by the fifth day after the commencement of menstruation, and mitotic activity in both epithelium and stroma persists until 2 to 3 days after ovulation. Although blood vessels are numerous and prominent, there is no extravasated blood or leukocyte infiltration in the endometrium at this stage. Clearly, reepithelialization and angiogenesis are important to the cessation of endometrial bleeding at the end of menstruation, and these processes are dependent upon tissue regrowth.

LATE PROLIFERATRIVE PHASE ENDOMETRIUM.

In the late proliferative phase, the endometrium has become thicker, the result of both glandular hyperplasia and an increase in stromal ground substance (edema and proteinaceous material). The loose stroma is especially prominent, and the glands in the superficial portions of the endometrium (functional zone) are widely separated compared with those of the deeper zone, where the glands are crowded and tortuous and the stroma is more dense. At midcycle, as the time of ovulation is approached, the glandular epithelium has become taller and pseudostratified.

Day-by-day dating of the endometrium by histological criteria is not possible during the proliferative phase because of the considerable variation among women in the length of the follicular (preovulatory) phase of the cycle. The luteal or secretory (postovulatory) phase of the cycle among women is remarkably constant in duration (12 to 14 days), but the length of the proliferative or follicular (preovulatory) phase varies greatly. In apparently normal, fertile women, the follicular phase may be as short as 5 to 7 or as long as 21 to 30 days.

SPIRAL (COILED) ARTERIES OF THE ENDOMETRIUM AND DECIDUA.

Boyd and Hamilton (1970) emphasized the extraordinary importance of the spiraling or coiled arteries of the human endometrium, pointing out that William Hunter in 1774 referred to these vessels as the "curling" arteries. The endometrial spiral arteries arise from the arcuate arteries, which are branches of the uterine vessels (Chap. 3, p. 42). The morphological and functional properties of these vessels are unique and essential for establishing the changes in blood flow that permit menstruation. An important characteristic of the secretory-phase endometrium is the striking growth and development of these coiled arteries, which become much more tortuous at this time. Ovarian/endometrial cycle-specific modifications in the rate of blood flow in the spiral arteries are essential for:

1. The initiation of menstruation.
2. The limitation of blood loss with menses.

Pregnancy-induced modifications of these vessels result in the establishment of maternal blood flow to the syncytiotrophoblast, that is, the delivery of maternal blood to the intervillous space of the placenta. The spiral arteries branch, and the arterioles break up into capillaries within the compact layer of endometrium. Superficially, a capillary network forms near the endometrial surface, and these are the first vessels invaded by cytotrophoblasts of the implanting blastocyst.

POSTOVULATORY ENDOMETRIUM.

In the catarrhine primates the midluteal/secretory phase of the ovarian/endometrial cycle is a critical branch point in the development and differentiation of the endometrium (Fig. 4–2). This is the time of biochemical transition when (with blastocyst implantation) full decidualization commences, or else (in the absence of blastocyst implantation) the multiple changes in endometrium begin that are preparatory to menstruation (including predecidualizaton of stromal cells). It has been suggested that transforming growth factor-β acts in an autocrine/paracrine fashion to define the functional destiny of the endometrium at this critical branch point of development (Casey and McDonald, 1996).

With rescue of the corpus luteum and continued progesterone secretion after implantation, transforming growth factor-β facilitates decidualization. In the absence of implantation and a decline in progesterone secretion, transforming growth factor-β facilitates the complete abandonment of progesterone action, resulting in menstruation. The possibility that uterine leukocytes are instrumental in the decidualization/menstruation branch point has been reviewed by King (2000).

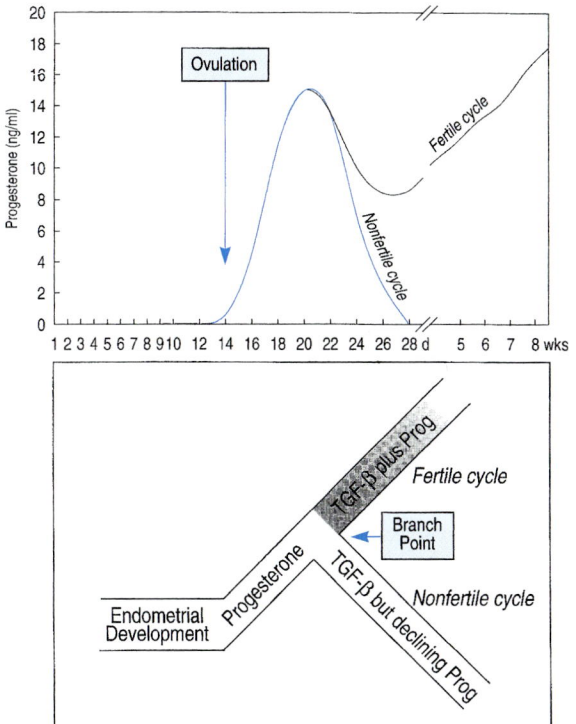

FIGURE 4–2. Endometrial development at the midluteal phase of the ovulatory cycle may proceed to decidualization with a fertile cycle or else become prepared for menstruation in the absence of implantation. This critical branch point in endometrial development may be dependent in part on the action of growth factors (for example, transforming growth factor-β [TGF-β]) with continued or else with declining progesterone (Prog) levels.

CHANGES IN ENDOMETRIAL SPIRAL ARTERY BLOOD FLOW. From observations made in a classical study, Markee (1940) described the tissue and vascular changes that occur in endometrium before menstruation. He observed cyclical alterations in endometrial tissue explants that he had transplanted to the anterior chamber of the eye of rhesus monkeys. At magnifications up to 150 $\times$, Markee studied 432 separate cycles (2 to 72 per animal) in pieces of endometrial tissue in each of 41 monkeys during an intense 9-year investigation, including each menstrual cycle of one monkey for 6 years! From many thousands of detailed observations, Markee deduced that the vascular changes that occur in endometrium are in response to growth cycles. He concluded that menstruation occurred during a phase of regression of endometrial growth (as estrogen and progesterone secretion by the corpus luteum decline).

Markee also surmised that there were marked changes in blood flow to the endometrium during the time of growth regression, and that these changes are essential for menstruation, that is, endometrial shedding with bleeding. He emphasized that the endometrium is supplied with blood by two types of vessels:

1. Straight arteries, which supply the basal one third of endometrium.
2. Coiled or spiral (curling) arteries, which supply the superficial two thirds of this tissue.

During and preceding menstruation, the straight arteries do not contract.

During the phase of endometrial growth, the spiral arteries lengthen at a rate that is appreciably greater than the rate of increase in endometrial tissue height or thickness (Fig. 4–3). This discordance in growth between the two tissues obliges even greater coiling of the already spiraling vessels. Perrot-Applanat and associates (1988) described progesterone and estrogen receptors in the smooth muscle cells of the uterine arteries, including the spiral arteries. It is likely, however, that specific angiogenic agents are produced by endometrial stromal (and epithelial) cells in response to estrogen (Zhang and colleagues, 1995).

As endometrial growth regresses, commencing concomitantly with the decline in corpus luteum function during nonfertile ovarian cycles, an even greater coiling of the spiral arteries is obliged. When the coiling of the spiral arteries becomes sufficiently severe, the resistance to blood flow in these vessels is increased strikingly, becoming so marked that profound stasis develops, causing hypoxia of the endometrium. Perhaps in response to hypoxia, vasodilatation at this time was sometimes observed (45 percent of cycles). Somewhat later, at 4 to 24 hours before bleeding into the endometrium began, there was, invariably, a period of intense vasoconstriction of the spiral arteries. Markee emphasized that the anemic appearance of the functional zone of the endometrium that results during this time of spiral artery vasoconstriction may be striking.

Markee also emphasized that the period of vasoconstriction preceding the onset of menstruation is the most striking and constant event of the menstrual cycle. Based on the sequence of vascular changes in endometrium, Markee reasoned that the intense vasoconstriction of the spiral arteries served to limit blood loss during menstruation. The reduction in spiral artery blood flow and resultant stasis before the time of vasoconstriction, however, was the primary cause of endometrial ischemia and then tissue degeneration.

Markee hypothesized that, immediately preceding menstruation, a substance is produced in the hypoxic endometrium that acts to induce severe vasospasm of the spiral arteries. His observations led him to surmise that what is now referred to as a paracrine mechanism was involved in the induction of the characteristic premenstrual vasoconstriction of the spiral arteries. Namely, he deduced that a vasoconstrictor was produced by endometrial stromal cells. Endothelin-1 is one candidate for the stromal cell vasoconstrictor that

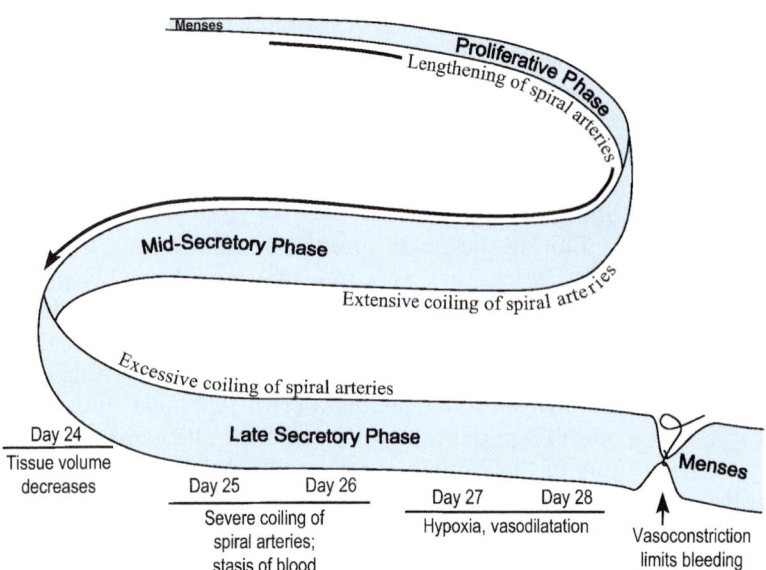

FIGURE 4–3. Modifications in the spiral arteries of the human endometrium during the ovulatory cycle. Changes in blood flow through these vessels facilitates endometrial growth, followed by excessive coiling and stasis in blood flow with regression of corpus luteum function and a decline in endometrial tissue volume. Just prior to the commencement of endometrial bleeding, intense spiral artery vasospasm serves to limit blood loss with menstruation.

Markee predicted (Casey and MacDonald, 1993, 1996; Economos and colleagues, 1992).

Markee also noted that when an individual coiled artery relaxed, after a period of constriction, hemorrhage occurred from that artery or its branches. Thereafter, in sequence, the arterioles of these constricted arteries relax and bleed; the succession of small hemorrhages from individual arterioles or capillaries continues for a variable but very short time (seconds to a few minutes). Although this sequence of vasoconstriction, relaxation, and hemorrhage appears to be well established, the mechanism(s) that actually brings about the escape of blood from the vessels is not certain. Perhaps damage to the walls of these vessels occurs during the period of intense vasoconstriction, favoring the rupture of these vessels once the constricted segment relaxes and blood flow is resumed.

LEUKOCYTE INFILTRATION OF ENDOMETRIUM. Another notable histological characteristic of the late premenstrual phase endometrium is the infiltration of the stroma by polymorphonuclear leukocytes, giving a pseudoinflammatory appearance to the tissue. The infiltration of neutrophils occurs primarily on the day or two immediately preceding the onset of menstruation. The endometrial stromal and epithelial cells produce interleukin-8 (IL-8), a chemotactic/activating factor for neutrophils (Arici and associates, 1993). IL-8 may be one of the agents that serves to recruit neutrophils to the endometrium just prior to the onset of menstruation. Similarly, the endometrium is capable of synthesizing monocyte chemotactic protein-1 (MCP-1), a potent chemoattractant for monocytes (Arici and colleagues, 1995). The rates of synthesis of IL-8 and MCP-1 in endometrial stromal cells appears to be modulated, in part, by sex steroid hormones and transforming growth factor-β (Arici and associates, 1996a,b).

Interleukin-15 (IL-15) is also expressed in endometrium and preferentially during the secretory phase (Okada and associates, 2000). Verma and associates (2000) demonstrated that IL-15 acts to induce proliferation of decidual natural killer cells. These findings are suggestive that IL-15 produced in situ may be involved in replication of natural killer cells that occurs in secretory endometrium.

VASOACTIVE AGENTS PRODUCED IN THE ENDOMETRIUM. Blood flow in the endometrium (spiral arteries) appears to be regulated in an endocrine manner by sex steroid hormone-induced modifications of a local (paracrine-mediated) vasoactive/peptide system.

PROSTAGLANDINS. These bioactive tissue autacoids are most commonly synthesized in the same cells in which these substances act or else in nearby cells. Thus, prostaglandins usually are autocrine- or paracrine-acting agents rather than endocrine (or humoral) hormones. Prostaglandins act through a host of separate but specific plasma membrane G-protein–linked receptors that also facilitate some degree of specificity of the actions of various prostaglandins. Prostaglandins are degraded rapidly in the tissues of origin such as endometrium, or in nearby tissues, and in more remote sites such as the lungs, in a reaction catalyzed by the enzyme prostaglandin dehydrogenase (Casey and associates, 1980, 1989).

A role for prostaglandins, especially PGF_2 (a vasoconstrictor), in the initiation of menstruation has been suggested by many investigators (Abel, 1985). Large amounts of prostaglandins are present in menstrual blood, and the administration of $PGF_{2\alpha}$ to women also gives rise to symptoms that mimic those of dysmenorrhea, which is commonly associated with normal ovulatory menses (menstruation after progesterone withdrawal), and likely caused by myometrial contractions and uterine ischsemia. The administration of $PGF_{2\alpha}$ to nonpregnant women also will cause menstruation; this response is believed to be mediated by $PGF_{2\alpha}$-induced vasoconstriction of the endometrial spiral arteries.

An alternative explanation is that prostaglandins are produced in endometrium at the time of menstruation in an accelerated fashion in response to inflammation, hypoxia, and trauma. Membrane glycerophospholipid hydrolysis is accelerated with tissue insult, causing the release of arachidonic acid, the precursor of prostaglandins, a major route by which arachidonic acid is metabolized. Prostaglandin formation in endometrium is obliged with hypoxia caused by stasis of blood in the highly coiled spiral arteries with regression of endometrial growth. Prostaglandin formation also may account, in part, for Markee's observation that vasodilatation oftentimes accompanied the stasis of blood flow in the spiral arteries. PGE_2 and PGI_2 (prostacyclin) both act to effect vasodilation. Consequently, accelerated prostaglandin formation in endometriums is most likely the result of, and not the cause of, tissue hypoxia and menstruation.

Prostaglandin dehydrogenase activity also is greater in early secretory endometrium than in endometrium before ovulation (Fig. 4–4). This enzyme activity, however, is localized primarily in the glandular epithelium and may be involved more intimately in implantation processes rather than in the initiation of menstruation (Casey and co-workers, 1980).

VASOACTIVE PEPTIDES. The actions of a number of peptides may explain a hormone-responsive paracrine system in the endometrium to regulate spiral artery blood flow. One is the endothelin/enkephalinase system (Casey and MacDonald, 1996). The endothelins (endothelin-1, -2, and -3) are small (21 amino acids) peptides. Endothelin-1 is a very potent vasoconstrictor, which was first identified as a product of vascular endothelial cells (Yanagisawa and colleagues, 1988).

The endothelins are degraded by the enzyme enkephalinase (membrane metalloendopeptidase), which also inactivates the enkephalins in brain cells; atrial natriuretic peptide in kidney; substance P in bronchial epithelium and intestine; and the endothelins in endometrium. Enkephalinase is localized in endometrial stromal cells, and its specific activity in these cells increases strikingly and in parallel with the increase in blood levels of progesterone after ovulation. As shown in Figure 4–4, the specific activity of enkephalinase in endometrium is highest during the midluteal phase of the ovarian cycle

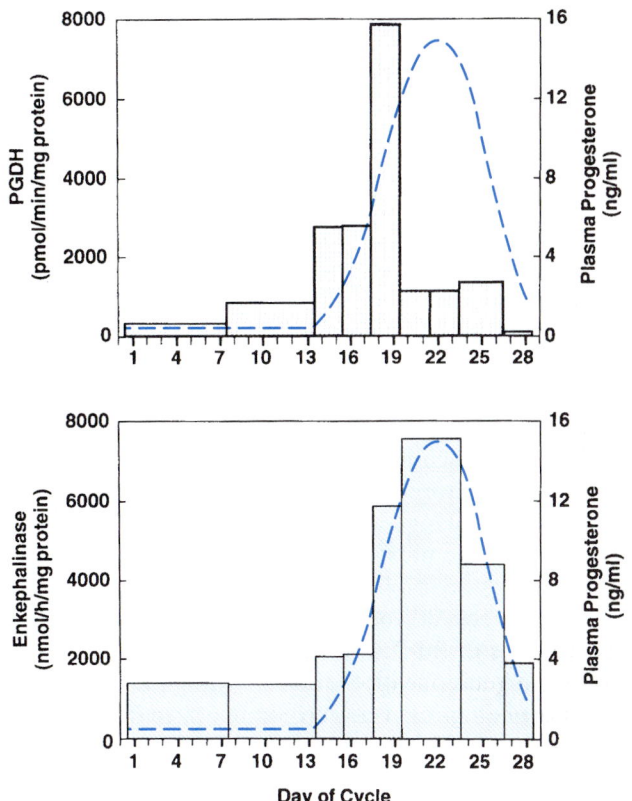

FIGURE 4–4. A. Specific activity (mean $\pm$ SEM) and NAD^+-dependent 15-hydroxyprostaglandin dehydrogenase (PGDH) in cytosolic fractions (bars) of human endometrial tissues obtained on various days of the menstrual cycle or from anovulatory women. **B.** Specific activity of enkephalinase in endometrial tissue (bars). Days of the menstrual cycle were idealized to that of a 28-day ovulatory cycle according to menstrual history, histological appearance of the endometrium, and serum progesterone concentrations on the day of endometrial sampling. (From Casey and associates, 1980).

and declines steadily thereafter as the plasma levels of progesterone decrease with regression of the corpus luteum (Casey and associates, 1991).

Parathyroid hormone–related protein (PTH-rP) is another vasoactive peptide demonstrated in human endometrial stromal cells (Casey and colleagues, 1992). PTH-rP and parathyroid hormone (PTH) act as vasorelaxants. Thus, an endothelin-1/enkephalinase/PTH-rP system may be operative in endometrial stroma cells to modulate endometrial spiral arterial blood flow in a local but hormonally responsive manner. The potential roles of PTH-rP in other reproductive processes and in placental function and fetal life are discussed in Chapters 6, 7, and 11.

ORIGIN OF MENSTRUAL BLOOD. Menstrual bleeding is of both arterial and venous origin, but arterial bleeding is, quantitatively, appreciably greater than venous. Endometrial bleeding appears to begin by rhexis of an arteriole of a coiled artery with consequent formation of a hematoma. On occasion, however, bleeding takes place by leakage through a spiral artery. When a hematoma forms, the superficial endometrium is distended and then ruptures. Subsequently, fissures develop in the adjacent functional layers, and blood, as well as fragments of tissue of various sizes, are detached. Although some tissue autolysis occurs, as a rule, fragments of endometrium can be identified in menstrual discharge collected from the vagina. Hemorrhage stops when the arterioles are again constricted. The changes that accompany partial tissue necrosis also serve to seal off the tip of the vessel; and in the superficial portion, often only the endothelium remains. The surface of the endometrium is restored, according to Markee (1940), by growth of the flanges, or collars, that form the everted free ends of the uterine glands. These flanges increase in diameter very rapidly, and the continuity of the epithelium is reestablished by the fusion of the edges of these sheets of thin, migrating cells.

The correlations of ovarian hormonal and endometrial morphological events are summarized in Table 4–1.

CLINICAL ASPECTS OF MENSTRUATION

Menstruation is the periodic discharge of blood, mucus, and cellular debris from the uterine mucosa. Menses occur at more or less regular, cyclical, and predictable intervals from menarche to menopause except during pregnancy, lactation, anovulation, or pharmacological intervention. It is convenient and more descriptive to use the term menstruation to refer to the bleeding that accompanies progesterone withdrawal after ovulation with nonfertile cycles, and to refer to other episodes of endometrial hemorrhage in nonpregnant women as uterine or endometrial bleeding.

MENARCHE AND PUBERTY. During the past two centuries, the age at which menstruation begins during puberty, menarche, has declined steadily until recent years (see Fig. 2–1). This decline in age of menarche in girls living in the United States, however, seems to have ceased. The average time at which menstruation begins is now between 12 and 13 years of age, but in a small proportion of apparently normal girls, menarche may occur as early as the 10th or as late as the 16th year. The term menarche refers specifically to the first menstruation, whereas puberty is a more general term that encompasses the entire process of sexual maturation in the transition from childhood to maturity. Menarche is just one sign of puberty; but when menarche is the consequence of ovulation (and attendant hormonal se-

cretion), the fundamental physiological events of puberty have been completed.

INTERVAL BETWEEN MENSES. The modal interval at which menstruation recurs is considered to be 28 days, but there is considerable variation among women in general, as well as in the cycle lengths of a given woman. Marked variation in the intervals between menstrual cycles is not necessarily indicative of infertility.

Arey (1939), who analyzed the findings of 12 separate studies comprising about 20,000 calendar records from 1500 women, concluded that there is no evidence of perfect menstrual cycle regularity. Gunn and co-workers (1937), in a study of 479 normal British women, found that the typical difference between the shortest and the longest cycle was 8 or 9 days. In 30 percent of women, it was more than 13 days, but it was never fewer than 2 days in any woman. Arey found that among average adult women, one third of menstrual cycles departed by more than 2 days from the mean of the lengths of all cycles. In Arey's analysis of 5322 cycles in 485 normal women, an average interval of 28.4 days was estimated; his finding for the average cycle length in pubertal girls was longer, 33.9 days. Chiazze and associates (1968) analyzed the intervals between 30,655 menstrual cycles of 2316 women. The mean for all cycles was 29.1 days. For cycle intervals that ranged from 15 to 45 days, the average length was 28.1 days. The degree of variability was such that only 13 percent of the women experienced cycles that varied by less than 6 days. Haman (1942) surveyed 2460 cycles in 150 housewives who attended a clinic where special attention was directed to recording accurately the length of the menstrual cycles. Arey's data and those of Haman, which are similar, and the distribution curve computed from averages of these data, are shown in Figure 4–5.

DURATION OF MENSTRUAL BLEEDING. The duration of menstrual flow also is variable, most commonly 4 to 6 days. Bleeding for 2 to 8 days may be normal for a given woman, but the duration of the menstrual flow is usually reasonably similar from cycle to cycle in the same woman.

MENSTRUAL BLOOD. Menstruation in ovulatory women (after progesterone withdrawal) is characterized by the extrusion of shed fragments of endometrium mixed with a variable quantity of blood. Usually the blood is liquid; but if the rate of hemorrhage is excessive, clots of various sizer may appear. The extrusion of clots with uterine bleeding, especially if bleeding is not cyclical or predictable, is suggestive of anovulation, that is, bleeding that occurs without benefit of progesterone action and withdrawal (Hahn, 1980).

Considerable research has been conducted to under-

TABLE 4–1. Important Milestones in the Correlation of Ovarian and Endometrial (Menstrual) Cycles (Idealized 28-Day Cycle)

	Phase					
Menstrual (1–5 days)	**Early Follicular** (6–8 days)	**Advanced Follicular** (9–13 days)	**Ovulation** (14 days)	**Early Luteal** (15–19 days)	**Advanced Luteal** (20–25 days)	**Premenstrual** (26–28 days)
Ovary Formation of corpus albicans from corpus luteum of preceding cycle. Recruitment of follicles.	Follicular maturation and development of the chosen or dominant follicle.		Ovulation and luteinization of granulosa cells in the ruptured follicle.	Vascularization of granulosa lutein cells and formation of corpus luteum. Follicular atresia.	Mature corpus luteum and continued follicular atresia.	Involution of corpus luteum and initiation of follicular recruitment for the next cycle.
Estrogen Low; derived principally from extraglandularly produced estrone; little estradiol-17β secretion by the ovary.	Estradiol-17β secretion, principally by granulosa cells of the dominant follicle, increases strikingly, maximal rates being attained just prior to the LH surge.		Immediately after, or coincident with, ovulation, there is an abrupt, indeed, precipitous decline in estradiol-17β secretion.	Gradual and progressive postovulatory rise in estradiol-17β secretion by the corpus luteum.	Maximal rates of postovulatory estradiol-17β secretion are attained; luteal phase estradiol-17β secretion rates, however, are not nearly as great as those observed in the immediate preovulatory phase.	Estradiol-17β secretion declines precipitously and, as during menstruation, the principal estrogen produced is estrone, which is formed in extra-glandular sites.
Progesterone Low secretion; there is little secretion of progesterone by the adrenal cortex and the corpus luteum of the preceding ovarian cycle has regressed.	During the follicular phase of the ovarian cycle, progesterone levels remain low. This is due to the fact that human granulosa cells cannot synthesize cholesterol, the obligate precursor of progesterone, but are dependent upon LDL cholesterol that can be obtained only from the blood after vascularization of the granulosa cells after ovulation.		Progesterone secretion increases steadily as the consequence of the availability of LDL and LH action to effect cholesterol side-chain cleavage.	Progesterone secretion remains high until the end of the advanced luteal phase.		Precipitous decline in progesterone secretion.
Endometrium Menstrual desquamation and early reorganization of endometrial glandular epithelium.	Proliferation of glandular epithelium with many mitoses.	Pseudostratification of nuclei—no secretion, early stromal changes.	Appearance of subnuclear vacuoles that are rich in glycogen.	Migration of vacuoles to the luminal surface; cessation of mitosis. The endometrial glands become very tortuous.	Vacuoles have been secreted and decidual-ization commences. Stromal edema and enlargement of stromal cells is prominent.	Disruption and disintegration of stromal cells. Leukocyte infiltration and interstitial hemorrhage.
Pituitary Secretion: FSH Continuing decline in FSH levels that had become modestly increased coincident with the decline in steroid secretion by the regressing corpus luteum of the preceding cycle.	FSH secretion is at all times pulsatile in nature, but during the proliferative phase of the ovarian cycle, prior to the time of the LH surge at midcycle, FSH levels remain low.		There is a significant surge of FSH secretion, albeit less prominent than that of LH, that heralds the commencement of the ovulatory process.	After the midcycle gonadotropin surge, FSH levels falls abruptly to levels similar to those found during the preovulatory phase of the cycle.		As steroid secretion by the regressing corpus luteum diminishes, there is a modest but significant increase in FSH.
Pituitary Secretion: LH The levels of LH are low and reasonably constant until just prior to ovu-lation.			Coincident with, or just after, the striking increase in estradiol-17β secretion by the dominant follicle, there is a striking increase in LH section—the "LH surge."	The levels of LH are low and reasonably con-stant until just prior to ovulation.		

FSH = follicle-stimulating hormone; LDL = low-density lipoprotein; LH = luteinizing hormone.

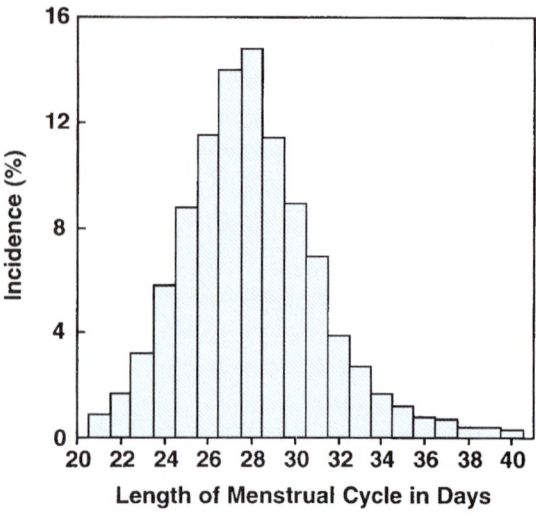

FIGURE 4–5. Duration of menstrual cycle. (Based on distribution data of Arey, 1939, and Haman, 1942.)

stand the incoagulability of menstrual blood. The most logical explanation is consistent with the conclusions of Whitehouse (1914) that the blood is coagulated as it is shed, but thereafter is liquefied by fibrinolytic activity. There are potent thromboplastic properties of endometrium that promptly initiate clotting, but there also are potent fibrinolytic properties that effect prompt lysis of the fibrin clots that are formed.

TISSUE FACTOR AND MENSTRUAL BLOOD CLOTTING.
Tissue factor is a plasma membrane–bound protein that is involved in the extrinsic coagulation pathway, which serves to effect clotting after vascular disruption. Ultimately, tissue factor is important in promoting the conversion of prothrombin to thrombin in the initiation of clotting. Lockwood and colleagues (1994) have shown that tissue factor is expressed in human endometrial stromal cells, and that progesterone acts indirectly to increase tissue factor (and plasminogen activator inhibitor 1) expression in these cells. This effect of progesterone requires activation of the epidermal growth factor receptor by epidermal growth factor or transforming growth factor-β. Plasminogen activator inhibitors act to inhibit plasminogen activator action directly, and therefore prevent fibrinolysis (Lockwood and associates, 1999).

FIBRINOLYSIS OF MENSTRUAL BLOOD CLOTS.
Serine proteinases (and their inhibitors) also are produced in endometrium in a cyclical manner suggestive of hormonal regulation. Among the proteinases, plasminogen activator is the enzyme believed to be important in the promotion of fibrinolysis. Plasmin is formed through the action of plasminogen activator (e.g., urokinase) produced in endometrium on blood-borne plasminogen.

BLOOD LOSS WITH MENSES.
The amount of blood lost during individual normal menstrual periods has been quantified by several groups of investigators who found the range to be from about 25 to 60 mL (Baldwin and associates, 1961; Hallberg and co-workers, 1966; Hytten and associates, 1964). With a normal hemoglobin concentration of 14 g per dL and a hemoglobin iron content of 3.4 mg per g, these volumes of blood contain from 12 to 29 mg of iron and represent blood loss equivalent to 0.4 to 1.0 mg of iron for every day of the cycle, or from 150 to 400 mg per year. Because the amount of iron that is absorbed from the diet usually is quite limited, this seemingly negligible iron loss is quantitatively important because it contributes further to the low iron stores of the majority of women (Scott and Pritchard, 1967).

The volume of blood lost with each menstruation is relatively small, especially considering that the surface area of the endometrium of normal uteri of nonpregnant women is 10 to 45 cm^2 (Chimbira and colleagues, 1980). Therefore, there must be an effective means of hemostasis in endometrium during menstruation. The control of blood loss likely is not induced by myometrial contractions to compress uterine vessels, as is the case after delivery of the fetus and placenta. Excessive blood loss with menstruation is common, however, in women with coagulation or platelet disorders. It is likely that hemostasis in endometrium is effected by:

1. Hemostatic plug formation as in other tissues (Christiaens and associates, 1985).
2. The intense vasoconstriction of the spiral arteries that commences immediately before and continues during menstruation (Markee, 1940).

PREMENSTRUAL SYNDROMES

A variety of maladies, sometimes disabling, beset many ovulatory women in a recurrent manner during the luteal phase of each ovarian cycle. Although the biological basis for this association is not defined, evidence points to a causal relationship between progesterone secretion and withdrawal and the development of these premenstrual syndromes (PMS). As reviewed by MacDonald and associates (1991), symptoms include disorders in mood, behavior, and physical well-being. Commonly, there is a characteristic cluster of the same symptoms in a given woman month after month.

RECURRENT PROGESTERONE SECRETION: AN ENDOCRINOPATHY?
It is important to recognize that the cyclical recurrence of PMS symptoms is restricted to women in whom endogenous progesterone is secreted in large amounts and then withdrawn, and that these

symptoms recur but are limited to the time of progesterone secretion and withdrawal. Specifically, these symptoms do not recur predictably in prepubertal, postmenopausal, anovulatory, or castrate women. Also, PMS-like symptoms do not recur in hypogonadal women treated with estrogen, whether given continuously or cyclically. Moreover, the symptoms of PMS can be relieved by treatment with gonadotropin-releasing hormone (GnRH) agonists, which arrest ovarian function, and by oophorectomy. All of these correlates are indicative of the obligatory involvement of ovulation and the secretion and withdrawal of progesterone in the biogenesis of PMS.

It has been generally assumed that (aside from pregnancy) cyclical ovulation and menstruation is the pinnacle of endocrinological normality in reproductive-age women. In several previous editions of this book, we emphasized, with great conviction, that such a history is highly suggestive of recurrent ovulation, corpus luteum formation, and progesterone secretion. Therefore, from the perspective of ovarian function, recurrent, cyclical, spontaneous menstruation is evidence of normal ovarian function.

Indisputably, the brain–pituitary–ovarian cycle that culminates in ovulation is a normal physiological event. Moreover, the sex hormone–induced biochemical and morphological antecedents of menstruation, eventuating in intense vasospasm of the endometrial spiral arteries, and culminating in the near-complete shedding of the endometrium, provide a unique physiological finale to this cycle. Nonetheless, and even though ovulation is the penultimate in ovarian physiological achievement, the repetition of this process at approximately monthly intervals (followed by menstruation) may not be considered the **evolutionary norm,** however universal these phenomena may be among young women (Chap. 2, p. 16).

PROGESTERONE AND PMS. Except for pregnancy, progesterone is produced in large amounts only during the luteal phase of each ovarian cycle. The rate of progesterone secretion at these times is greater, by a large margin, than that of any other steroid hormone produced in men or nonpregnant women (Fig. 4–6).

But, how can progesterone bring about PMS in some but not all women? There is no apparent difference in the rates of progesterone secretion by the corpus luteum in women who do and those who do not suffer from PMS. Until relatively recently, it was believed that progesterone action was mediated singularly by way of the progesterone receptor acting via the progesterone response element in selected genes. Based on this presumption, there were no known actions of progesterone that would clearly implicate this steroid in the biogenesis of PMS, let alone explain the striking differences among

women in the spectrum or severity of the multiple symptoms that characterize this disorder(s).

It has now been demonstrated that some of the bioactions of progesterone and its metabolites are mediated by progesterone receptor–independent cellular mechanisms. Progesterone acts at the level of the plasma membrane of selected cells by a nongenomic mechanism to inhibit the activation of adenylate cyclase, for example, in oocytes and in spermatozoa. Progesterone is metabolized, by extraadrenal 21-hydroxylation, to deoxycorticosterone, which acts by way of the mineralocorticosteroid receptor. Another metabolite, 5α-pregnan-3α-ol-20-one, acts in brain as an anesthetic/anxiolytic agent by binding to the gamma-aminobutyric acid $(GABA)_A$ receptor. GABA is an inhibitory neurotransmitter, an endogenously produced anxiolytic-like compound. The anesthetic/anxiolytic steroids act to increase GABA action.

To explain the role of progesterone in the development of PMS, the suggestion was made that (1) the extent of extrahepatic metabolism of progesterone to selected bioactive metabolites may be dissimilar among women, and (2) there may be a close correlation between the metabolic fate of progesterone in a given woman and the recurrence of luteal phase disabilities (MacDonald and associates, 1991). This theory evolved from the findings that (1) the fractional conversion of progesterone to deoxycorticosterone varies by 30-fold among women (but is constant in the same woman from time to time), and (2) selected 5α-reduced metabolites of progesterone are bioactive as anxiolytic/anesthetic agents.

The wide variation in the conversion of plasma progesterone to deoxycorticosterone among women is the reason for wide variations in the production rate of deoxycorticosterone during the luteal phase of the ovarian cycle. Deoxycorticosterone is produced from plasma progesterone in a manner that is not regulated by adrenocorticotropic hormone (ACTH) or angiotensin II.

It has been known for more than 50 years that selected metabolites of progesterone, administered to experimental animals or to humans, cause anesthesia. GABA-producing neurons and $GABA_A$ receptors are widely distributed in brain. Apparently the confirmational change of the $GABA_A$ receptor after anxiolytic steroid binding increases the affinity of GABA for this receptor. These steroids, therefore, are active only in the presence of GABA. The benzodiazepine class of drugs also act at the $GABA_A$ receptor in a manner analogous to that of the 5α-reduced metabolites of progesterone, namely to increase the affinity of the $GABA_A$ receptor for GABA.

Steroidal anesthetics were synthesized for use in humans; and many hundreds of cesarean deliveries have been performed in women in Great Britain with the

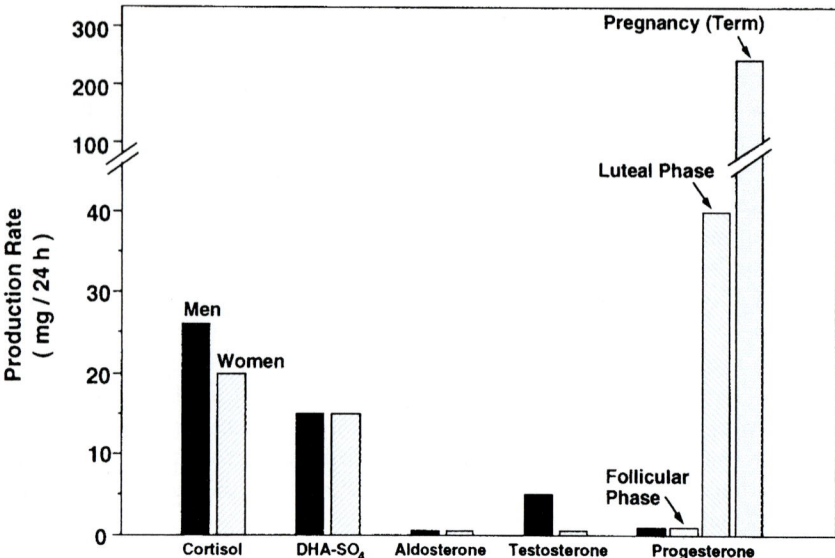

FIGURE 4-6. Steroid production rates in men and women. (From MacDonald and colleagues, 1991, with permission.)

steroid anesthetic *althesin*, or 11-keto-5α-pregnan-3α-ol-20-one. The endogenously produced anxiolytic metabolite of progesterone, 5α-pregnan-3α-ol-20-one (allopregnanolone), is formed in women during the luteal phase of the cycle when progesterone levels are high. A role for progesterone metabolite formation and withdrawal in the biogenesis of postpartum depression, a severe emotional disorder that develops during the early puerperium in some women has also been proposed (Chap. 53, p. 1420). Monteleone and associates (2000) found that the plasma levels of allopregnanolone in women with premenstrual syndrome are decreased. Given the benzodiazepine-like action of allopregnanolone, lower levels of this metabolite could lead to some symptoms of premenstrual syndrome.

PROGESTERONE METABOLISM. The potential importance of these bioactive progesterone metabolites in the biogenesis of PMS likely resides in the stereospecificity of their actions and in the potential for differences among women in the rates of formation of these compounds in extrahepatic tissues. It is now known that the majority (50 to 60 percent) of plasma progesterone is metabolized by initial 5 α-reduction, and much of this metabolism occurs in extrahepatic tissues (Chantilis and colleagues, 1996). Ultimately, the 5α-reduced metabolites of progesterone are transported to liver and there are preferentially sulfoconjugated and excreted in bile. In the intestine, these sulfoconjugates are acted upon by enzymes in intestinal bacteria to give products that have not been readily identifiable.

SAFE CONTRACEPTION, WITHOUT MENSTRUATION. It therefore may be that recurrent, cyclical progesterone secretion by the corpus luteum of women who choose not to be pregnant is not the **evolutionary norm.** In an evolutionary sense, menstruation may be viewed as the fail-safe, end result of fertility failure, whether the infertility was purposefully chosen or naturally occurring.

The development of safe and effective contraceptive agents, according to Baird (1985), who also referred to the writings of his father, Sir Dugald Baird, "has relieved [women] from the tyranny of excessive fertility—'the fifth freedom.' Because the social and physical demands of continuous [pregnancy and] breast-feeding, are unlikely to be acceptable to women of the 20th century," they have chosen menstruation as an alternative, "in the absence of a simple, safe means of inducing amenorrhea pharmacologically."

Clearly, it is vitally important to search for more acceptable means of effective and safe human contraception. As an intermediate goal, women should be able to choose an infertility-promoting method that may not oblige a possible endocrinopathy induced by recurrent secretion and withdrawal of progesterone. Safe, effective contraception that does not cause uterine bleeding or loss of the metabolic benefits of estrogen likely will be developed for use by women who would select such an alternative.

THE DECIDUA

This tissue is the specialized, highly modified endometrium of pregnancy. The transformation of secretory endometrium to decidua is dependent upon the action of estrogen and progesterone and other stimuli provided by the implanting blastocyst (or maternal platelets) during trophoblast invasion of the endometrium and its blood vessels. The special relationship that exists between the endometrium/decidua and the invading trophoblast seemingly defies the laws of transplantation immunology. The success of this unique autograft is not only a scientific curiosity but may involve processes that harbor insights into more successful transplantation surgery and perhaps the control of neoplasia as well. Some of the processes that appear to be fundamentally important in the immunological acceptance of the conceptus are considered in Chapter 5 (p. 89).

STRUCTURE. William Hunter, 19th-century British gynecologist, provided the first scientific description of the *membrana decidua.* According to Damjanov (1985), the term was coined in the best tradition of formal logic applied to scientific writing—*membrana,* denoting its gross appearance, while the qualifier, *decidua,* was added in analogy with deciduous leaves to indicate its ephemeral nature and the fact that it is shed from the rest of the uterus after childbirth. Wewer and associates (1985) provided evidence that decidua indeed qualifies to be called a membrane, not only because of its gross appearance but because it contains most if not all of the major basement membrane components.

Moreover, each mature decidual cell becomes surrounded by a membrane, indeed a pericellular membrane. Thus, the human decidual cells clearly build walls around themselves and possibly around the fetus. In fact, the pericellular matrix surrounding the decidual cells may provide for attachment of cytotrophoblasts through cellular adhesion molecules. This would provide the scaffolding for trophoblast attachment. The pericellular decidual cell membrane also may provide for protection of the decidual cell against selected proteinases of the cytotrophoblasts.

DECIDUAL REACTION. In human pregnancy, the decidual reaction is completed only with blastocyst implantation. Predecidual changes, however, commence first in endometrial stromal cells adjacent to the spiral arteries and arterioles, spreading thereafter in waves throughout the mucosa of the uterus and then from the site of implantation. The endometrial stromal cells enlarge to form polygonal or round, decidual cells. The nuclei become round and vesicular, and the cytoplasm becomes clear, slightly basophilic, and surrounded by a translucent membrane. In early pregnancy, the decidua begins to thicken, eventually attaining a depth of 5 to 10 mm. With magnification, furrows and numerous small openings, representing the mouths of uterine glands, can be detected. Later in pregnancy, as the fetus grows and the amnionic fluid expands, the thickness of the decidua decreases, presumably because of the pressure exerted by the expanding uterine contents.

The portion of the decidua directly beneath the site of blastocyst implantation is modified by trophoblast invasion and becomes the *decidua basalis;* that portion overlying the enlarging blastocyst, and initially separating it from the rest of the uterine cavity, is the *decidua capsularis* (Fig. 4–7). The decidua capsularis is most prominent during the second month of pregnancy, consisting of decidual cells covered by a single layer of flattened epithelial cells without traces of glands. Internally, this portion of the decidua contacts the avascular, extraembryonic fetal membrane, the *chorion laeve.* The remainder of the uterus is lined by *decidua parietalis,* sometimes called the *decidua vera* when decidual capsularis and decidua parietalis are joined.

During the early weeks of pregnancy, there is a space between the decidua capsularis and decidua parietalis because the gestational sac does not fill the entire uterine cavity. By 14 to 16 weeks, the expanding sac has enlarged enough to fill the uterine cavity; and with fusion of the decidua capsularis and parietalis, the uterine cavity is functionally obliterated.

The decidua parietalis and the decidua basalis, like the secretory endometrium, are each composed of three layers: a surface, or compact zone (zona compacta); a middle portion, or spongy zone (zona spongiosa), with remnants of glands and numerous small blood vessels; and a basal zone (zona basalis). The zona compacta and spongiosa together form the functional zone (zona functionalis). The basal zone remains after delivery and gives rise to new endometrium.

BLOOD SUPPLY. This is changed as a consequence of implantation. The blood supply to the decidua capsularis is lost as the embryo-fetus grows and expands into the uterine cavity. The blood supply to the decidua parietalis through the spiral arteries persists, as in the endometrium during the luteal phase of the cycle. The spiral arteries in the decidua parietalis retain a smooth muscle wall and endothelium and thereby remain responsive to vasoactive agents that act upon the smooth muscle or endothelial cells of these vessels.

The (spiral) arterial system supplying the decidua basalis directly beneath the implanting blastocyst, and ultimately the intervillous space surrounding the syncytiotrophoblast, however, are altered remarkably. These spiral arterioles and arteries are invaded by the cytotrophoblasts; during this process, the walls of these vessels are destroyed, leaving only a shell without smooth muscle or endothelial cells. In consequence, these vascular conduits of maternal blood—which become the uteroplacental vessels—are not responsive to vasoactive agents (Chap. 5, p. 92). By contrast, the fetal chorionic vessels, which transport blood between the placenta and the fetus, contain smooth muscle and do respond to vasoactive agents, as do the maternal spiral arteries.

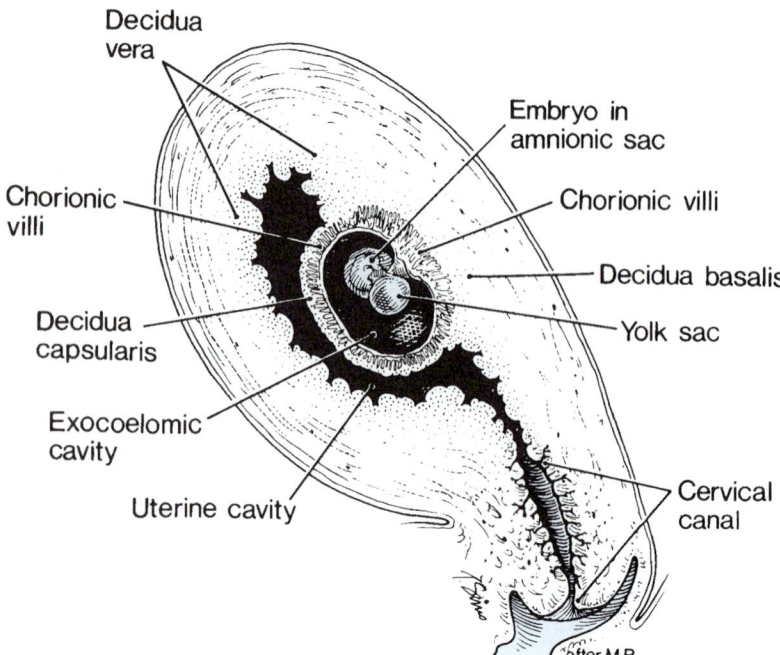

FIGURE 4–7. Decidualized endometrium covers the early embryo. Three portions of the decidua (basalis, capsularis, and parietalis, or vera) are also illustrated.

HISTOLOGY. The compact layer of the decidua consists of large, closely packed, epithelioid, polygonal, lightly staining cells with round vesicular nuclei. Many stromal cells appear stellate (particularly when the decidua is edematous) with long protoplasmic processes that anastomose with those of adjacent cells. Numerous small round cells, which contain very little cytoplasm, are scattered among the decidual cells, especially in early pregnancy. These are a particular type of natural-killer lymphocytes and are referred to as **uterine large granular lymphocytes,** in which a special and unusual phenotype has been defined. These are bone marrow–derived cells that at one time entered endometrium from peripheral blood; but thereafter, these large granular lymphocytes arise primarily by replication in the endometrium in situ at specific times in the cycle (Chap. 5, p. 90).

Early in pregnancy, the spongy layer of the decidua consists of large distended glands, often exhibiting marked hyperplasia but separated by minimal stroma. At first, the glands are lined by typical cylindrical uterine epithelium with abundant secretory activity. Presumably, the glandular secretion contributes to the nourishment of the blastocyst during its histotrophic phase, before the establishment of a placental circulation. As pregnancy progresses, the epithelium gradually becomes cuboidal or even flattened, later degenerating and sloughing to a greater extent into the lumens of the glands. Later in pregnancy, the glandular elements of the decidua largely disappear.

In comparing the decidua parietalis at 16 weeks' gestation with the early proliferative endometrium of a nonpregnant woman, it is clear that there is marked hypertrophy but only slight hyperplasia of the endometrial stroma during decidual transformation.

The decidua basalis contributes to the formation of the basal plate of the placenta, and differs histologically from the decidua parietalis in two important respects (Fig. 4–8). First, the spongy zone of the decidua basalis consists mainly of arteries and widely dilated veins; by term, the glands have virtually disappeared. Second, the decidua basalis is invaded by trophoblastic giant cells, which appear at the time of implantation. The number and depth of endometrial penetration of the giant cells varies greatly. Although generally confined to the decidua, these cells may penetrate the myometrium. In such circumstances, their number and invasiveness may be so extensive as to be suggestive of choriocarcinoma to the inexperienced observer.

AGING OF THE DECIDUA. Where invading trophoblasts meet the decidua, there is a zone of fibrinoid degeneration, **Nitabuch layer.** Whenever the decidua is defective, as in placenta accreta (Chap. 25, p. 632), the Nitabuch layer is usually absent. There also is an inconstant deposition of fibrin, **Rohr stria,** at the bottom of the intervillous space and surrounding the fastening villi. McCombs and Craig (1964) found that decidual necrosis is a normal phenomenon in the first and probably the second trimester. The presence of necrotic decidua obtained through curettage after spontaneous abortion in the first trimester should not, therefore, nec-

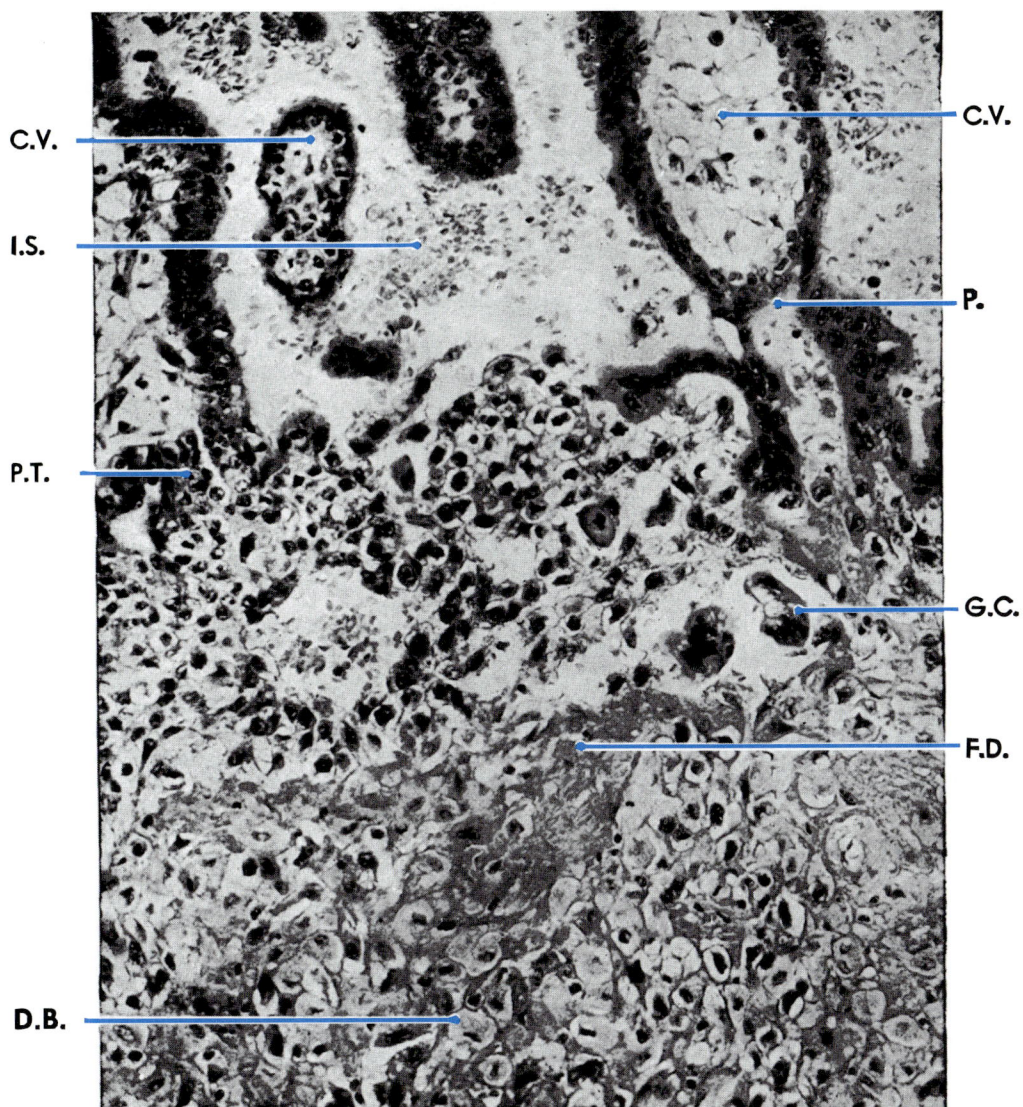

C.V.

I.S.

P.T.

D.B.

C.V.

P.

G.C.

F.D.

FIGURE 4–8. Section through junction of chorion and decidua basalis at fourth month of gestation. (C. V. = chorionic villi; D. B. = decidua basalis; F. D. = fibrinoid degeneration; G. C. = giant cell; I. S. = intervillous space containing maternal blood; P. = fastening villus; P. T. = proliferating trophoblast.)

essarily be interpreted as either a cause or an effect of the abortion.

PROLACTIN IN THE DECIDUA. Convincing evidence was presented by Riddick and co-workers (1979) and Golander and associates (1978) that the decidua is a source of prolactin, which is present in enormous amounts in the amnionic fluid during human pregnancy. Decidual prolactin is not to be confused with placental lactogen (hPL), which is produced only by the syncytio-trophoblast (Chap. 6, p. 113). Rather, decidual prolactin is a product of the same gene that encodes for prolactin that is secreted by the anterior pituitary.

The levels of prolactin in amnionic fluid during the 20th to 24th week of pregnancy may reach 10,000 ng per mL (Tyson and co-workers, 1972). As described in Chapter 8 (p. 191), the concentration of prolactin in amnionic fluid is extraordinarily high compared with the highest levels of prolactin in fetal (up to about 350 ng/mL) or maternal plasma (up to about 150 to 200 ng/mL). Prolactin produced in decidua preferentially enters amnionic fluid and little or none enters maternal blood. This is the classical example of the peculiar trafficking of molecules between maternal and fetal tissues of the paracrine arm of the fetal–maternal communication system.

The factors that regulate prolactin secretion in decidua are not clearly defined. Most of the agents known to affect, either negatively or positively, the rate of secretion of prolactin by the anterior, pituitary—for example, dopamine and dopamine agonists and thyrotropin-releasing hormone—do not alter the rate of decidual prolactin secretion (either in vivo or in vitro). Brosens and colleagues (2000) demonstrated that progestin (namely, medroxyprogesterone acetate) acts synergistically with cyclic AMP on human endometrial stromal cells in culture to increase the expression of prolactin. The findings of these investigators are indicative that the decidualization process, as marked by prolactin production, is determined by the level of progesterone receptor. It has been reported that arachidonic acid, but not $PGF_{2\alpha}$ or PGE_2, attenuates the rate of decidual prolactin secretion (Handwerger and colleagues, 1981). In addition, a variety of cytokines, including interleukin-1 and interleukin-2, act to decrease decidual prolactin secretion, as does endothelin-1 (Chao and colleagues, 1994; Frank and co-workers, 1995; Kanda and colleagues, 1999). Blithe and associates (1991) found that "free alpha" molecules stimulate prolactin synthesis and the secretion of prolactin by human decidual cells. By "free" alpha is meant the common α-subunit of several glycoprotein hormones including hCG, follicle-stimulating hormone (FSH), luteinizing hormone (LH), and thyroid-stimulating hormone (TSH). Free α-subunit is produced by placenta (Chap. 6, p. 111), and the levels of free α-subunit in maternal blood increase as pregnancy advances. In part, this is the case because the synthesis of the β-subunit of hCG (but not the α-subunit) is limiting in the syncytiotrophoblast formation of complete hCG.

The physiological role of prolactin produced in decidua is not known. Because all (or most) of prolactin produced in decidua enters amnionic fluid, it has been speculated that there may be a role for this hormone in solute and water transport across the chorioamnion, and thus in the maintenance of amnionic fluid volume homeostasis. It also has been shown, however, that prolactin receptors are present in a number of bone marrow–derived immune cells, and that prolactin acts on bone cells to modify selected immune functions (Pellegrini and colleagues, 1992). Recall that many bone marrow–derived lymphocytes are present in endometrium and decidua throughout pregnancy, and the function of these immune cells is modified appreciably in this tissue site. Therefore, prolactin produced in decidua may act in regulating immunological functions in this tissue during pregnancy. Various other roles for prolactin have been suggested, but presently these must be considered as speculative.

REFERENCES

Abel MH: Prostanoids and menstruation. In Baird DT, Michie EA (eds): Mechanisms of Menstrual Bleeding. New York, Raven, 1985, p 139

Arey LB: The degree, of normal menstrual irregularity: An analysis of 20,000 calendar records from 1,500 individuals. Am J Obstet Gynecol 37:12, 1939

Arici A, Head JR, MacDonald PC, Casey ML: Regulation of interleukin-8 gene expression in human endometrial cells in culture. Mol Cell Endocrinol 94:195, 1993

Arici A, MacDonald PC, Casey ML: Modulation of the levels of interleukin-8 messenger ribonucleic acid and interleukin-8 protein synthesis in human endometrial stromal cells by transforming growth factor-beta 1. J Clin Endocrinol Metab 81:3004, 1996a

Arici A, MacDonald PC, Casey ML: Progestin regulation of interleukin-8 mRNA levels and protein synthesis in human endometrial cells by transforming growth factor-beta 1. J Steroid Biochem Mol Biol 58:71, 1996b

Arici A, MacDonald PC, Casey ML: Regulation of monocyte chemotactic protein-1: gene expression in human endometrial cells in cultures. Mol Cell Endocrinol 107:189, 1995

Baird DT: Preface. In Baird DT, Michie EA (eds): Mechanisms of Menstrual Bleeding. New York, Raven, 1985

Baldwin RM, Whalley PJ, Pritchard JA: Measurements of menstrual blood loss. Am J Obstet Gynecol 81:739, 1961

Blithe DL, Richards RG, Skarulis MC: Free alpha molecules from pregnancy stimulate secretion of prolactin from human decidual cells: A novel function for free alpha in pregnancy. Endocrinology 129:2257, 1991

Boyd JD, Hamilton WJ: The Human Placenta. Cambridge, England, Heffer, 1970

Brosens JJ, Hayashi N, White JO: Progesterone receptor regulates decidual prolactin expression in differentiating human endometrial stromal cells. Eur J Endocrinol 142:269, 2000

Casey ML, Delgadillo M, Cox KA, Niesert S, MacDonald PC: Inactivation of prostaglandins in human decidua vera (parietalis) tissue: Substrate specificity of prostaglandin dehydrogenase. Am J Obstet Gynecol 160:3, 1989

Casey ML, Hemsell DL, MacDonald PC, Johnston JM: NAD⁺-dependent 15-hydroxyprostaglandin dehydrogenase activity in human endometrium. Prostaglandins 19:115, 1980

Casey ML, MacDonald PC: The endothelin-parathyroid hormone-related protein vasoactive peptide system in human endometrium: Modulation by transforming growth factor-β. Hum Reprod, Suppl 2:62, 1996

Casey ML, MacDonald PC: Modulation of endometrial flood flow: Regulation of endothelin-1 biosynthesis and degradation in human endometrium. In Alexander NJ, d'Arcangues C (eds): Steroid Hormones and Uterine Bleeding. Washington, DC, AAAS Press, 1993, pp 209-227

Casey ML, Mibe M, Erk A, MacDonald PC: Transforming growth-β stimulation of parathyroid hormone-related protein expression in human uterine cells in culture: mRNA levels and protein secretion. J Clin Endocrinol Metab 74:950, 1992

Casey ML, Smith JW, Nagai K, Hersh LB, MacDonald PC: Progesterone-regulated cyclic modulation of membrane metalloendopeptidase (enkephalinase) in human endometrium. J Biol Chem 266:23041, 1991

Chantilis S, Dombroski R, Shackleton CH, Casey ML, MacDonald PC: Metabolism of 5α-dihydroprogesterone in women and men: 3α- and 3α, 6α-dihydroxy-5α-pregnan-20-ones are major urinary metabolites. J Clin Endocrinol Metab 81:3644, 1996

Chao HS, Poisner AM, Poisner R, Handwerger S: Endothelin-1 modulates renin and prolactin release from human decidua by different mechanisms. Am J Physiol 267:E842, 1994

Chiazze L, Brayer FT, Macisco JJ, Parker MP, Duffy BJ: The length and variability of the human menstrual cycle. JAMA 203:377, 1968

Chimbira TH, Anderson ABM, Turnbull AC: Relation between measured menstrual blood loss and patient's subjective assessment of loss, duration of bleeding, number of sanitary towels used, uterine weight and endometrial surface area. Br J Obstet Gynaecol 87:603, 1980

Christiaens GCML, Sixma JJ, Haspels AA: Vascular and haemostatic changes in menstrual endometrium. In Baird DT, Michie EA (eds): Mechanism of Menstrual Bleeding. Serono Symposia, vol 25. New York, Raven, 1985, p 27

Damjanov I: Editorial: Vesalius and Hunter were right: Decidua is a membrane. Lab Invest 53:597, 1985

Economos K, MacDonald PC, Casey ML: Endothelin-1 gene expression and protein biosynthesis in human endometrium. Potential modulator of endometrial blood flow. J Clin Endocrinol Metab 74:14, 1992

Frank GR, Brar AK, Jikihara H, Cedars MI, Handwerger S: Interleukin-1 beta and the endometrium: An inhibitor of stromal cell differentiation and possible autoregulator of decidualization in humans. Bio Reprod 52:184, 1995

Golander A, Hurley T, Barret J, Hizi A, Handwerger S: Prolactin synthesis by human chorion decidual tissue: A possible source of prolactin in the amniotic fluid. Science 202:311, 1978

Gunn DL, Jenkin PM, Gunn AL: Menstrual periodicity: Statistical observations on a large sample of normal cases. J Obstet Gynaecol Br Emp 44:839, 1937

Hahn L: Composition of menstrual blood. In Diczfalusy E, Fraser is, Webb FTG (eds): Endometrial Bleeding and Steroidal Contraception. Proceedings of Symposium on Steroid Contraception and Mechanism of Menstrual Bleeding. Bath, England, Pitman Press, 1980, p 107

Hallberg L, Hogdahl AM, Nilsson L, Rybo G: Menstrual blood loss, a population study: Variation at different ages and attempts to define normality. Acta Obstet Gynecol Scand 45:320, 1966

Haman JO: The length of the menstrual cycle: A study of 150 normal women. Am J Obstet Gynecol 43:870, 1942

Handwerger S, Barry S, Barrett J, Markoff E, Zeitler P, Cwikel B, Siegel M: Inhibition of the synthesis and secretion of decidual prolactin by arachidonic acid. Endocrinology 109:2016, 1981

Hytten FE, Cheyne GA, Klopper AI: Iron loss at menstruation. J Obstet Gynaecol Br Commonw 71:255, 1964

Jensen EV, Jacobson HI: Basic guides to the mechanism of estrogen action. Recent Prog Horm Res 18:387, 1962

Kanda Y, Jikihara H, Markoff E, Handwerger S: Interleukin-2 inhibits the synthesis and release of prolactin from human decidual cells. J Clin Endocrinol Metab 84:677, 1999

King A: Uterine leukocytes and decidualization. Hum Reprod Update 6:28, 2000

Lockwood CJ, Krikun G, Papp C, Toth-Pal E, Markiewicz L, Wang EY, Kerenyi T, Zhou X, Hausknecht V, Papp Z, Schatz F: The role of progestationally regulated stromal cell tissue factor and type-1 plasminogen activator inhibitor (PAI-1) in endometrial hemostasis and menstruation. Ann NY Acad sci 734:57, 1994

Lockwood CJ, Krikun G. Schatz F: The decidua regulates hemostasis in human endometrium. Semin Reprod Endocrinol 17:45, 1999

MacDonald PC, Dombroski RA, Casey ML: Recurrent secretion of progesterone in large amounts: An endocrine/metabolic disorder unique to young women? Endocrine Rev 12:372, 1991

Markee JE: Menstruation in intraocular endometrial transplants in the rhesus monkey. Contrib Embryol 28:219, 1940

McCombs HL, Craig MJ: Decidual necrosis in normal pregnancy. Obstet Gynecol 24:436, 1964

Monteleone P, Luisi S, Tonetti A, Bernardi F, Genazzani AD, Luisi M, Petraglia F, Genazzani AR: Allopregnanolone concentrations and premenstrual syndrome. Eur J Endocrinol 142:269, 2000

Noyes RW, Hertig AT, Rock J: Dating the endometrial biopsy. Fertil Steril 1:3, 1950

Okada S, Okada H, Sanezumi M, Nakajima T, Yasuda D, Kanzaki H: Expression of interleukin-15 in human endometrium and decidua. Mol Hum Reprod 6:1, 2000

Pellegrini I, Lebrun JJ, Ali S, Kelly PA: Expression of prolactin and its receptor in human lymphoid cells. Mol Endocrinol 6:1023, 1992

Perrot-Applanat M, Groyer-Picard MT, Garcia E, Lorenzo F, Milgrom E: Immunocytochemical demonstration of estrogen and progesterone receptors in muscle cells of uterine arteries in rabbits and humans. Endocrinology 123:1511, 1988

Riddick DH, Luciano AA, Kusmik WF, Maslar IA: Evidence for a nonpituitary source of amniotic fluid prolactin. Fertil Steril 31:35, 1979

Rock J, Bartlett M: Biopsy studies of human endometrium. JAMA 108:2022, 1937

Scott DE, Pritchard JA: Iron deficiency in healthy young college women. JAMA 199:897, 1967

Tang B, Guller S, Gurpide E: Mechanism of human endometrial stromal cells decidualization. Ann NY Acad Sci 734:19, 1994

Tseng L, Gurpide E: Effects of progestins on estradiol receptor levels in human endometrium. J Clin Endocrinol Metab 41:402, 1975

Tseng L, Gurpide E: Estradiol and 20α-dihydroprogesterone dehydrogenase activities in human endometrium during the menstrual cycle. Endocrinology 94:419, 1974

Tseng L, Liu HC: Stimulation of acylsulfotransferase activity by progestins in human endometrium in vitro. J Clin Endocrinol Metab 53:418, 1981

Tyson JE, Hwang P, Guyda H, Friesen HG: Studies of prolactin secretion in human pregnancy. Am J Obstet Gynecol 113:14, 1972

Verma S, Hiby SE Loke YW, King A: Human decidual natural killer cells express the receptor for and respond to the cytokine interleukin 15. Biol Reprod 62:959, 2000

Wewer UM, Faber M, Liotta LA, Albrechtsen R: Immunochemical and ultrastructural assessment of the nature of the pericellular basement membrane of human decidual cells. Lab Invest 53:624, 1985

Whitehouse HB: Pathological uterine haemorrhage. Lancet 1:951, 1914

Yanagisawa M, Kurihara H, Kimura S, Tomobe Y, Kobayashi M, Mitsui Y, Yazaki Y, Goto K, Masaki T: A novel potent vasoconstrictor peptide produced by vascular endothelial cells. Nature 332:411, 1988

Zhang L, Rees MC, Bicknell R: The isolation and long-term culture of normal human endometrial epithelium and stroma. Expression of mRNAs for angiogenic polypeptides basally and on oestrogen and progesterone challenges. J Cell Sci 108:323, 1995

5

The Placenta and Fetal Membranes

The development of the human placenta is as uniquely intriguing as the embryology of the fetus. The placenta is a fascinating organ, especially when its function is considered. During its brief intrauterine existence, the fetus is dependent upon the placenta as its lung, liver, and kidneys. The organ serves these purposes until sufficient maturation of the fetus allows it to survive ex utero as an air-breathing organism.

Despite its unassailable role in human fetal development, study of the placenta has lagged behind that of the fetus. A number of anatomists and embryologists worked through the 1980s to provide some basic knowledge. It has not been until recently that clinicians have appreciated the plethora of knowledge that can be gained by microscopic study of the placenta. This latter enlightenment has transposed through the efforts of placental pathologists such as Benirschke, Driscoll, Fox, and Naeye. Their work, as well as that of many of their colleagues, has shown that careful examination of the placenta may frequently shed light on the etiopathogenesis of a number of maternal–fetal disorders (Benirschke, 2000; Benirschke and Kauffman, 2000). Abnormal placentation, placental pathology, and their effects on pregnancy outcome, as well as adverse placental effects from maternal diseases, are considered in Chapters 31 and 32.

Boyd and Hamilton (1970) presented a marvelous account of the history of placental research. A summary of this history was presented in Chapter 5 (p. 95) of the 20th edition of *Williams Obstetrics.* The interested reader is referred to this summary or to the treatise of Boyd and Hamilton (1970).

FETAL TISSUES OF THE FETAL–MATERNAL COMMUNICATION SYSTEM

The two arms of the fetal–maternal communication system of human pregnancy were described in Chapters 2 and 4 (see Fig. 2–2). The extravillous and villous trophoblasts are the embryonic-fetal tissues of the anatomical interface of the placental arm; the avascular fetal membranes—the amnion and chorion laeve—are the fetal tissues of the anatomical interface of the paracrine arm of this system.

The placental arm of this system links the mother and fetus as follows: maternal blood (spurting out of the uteroplacental vessels) directly bathes the syncytiotrophoblast, the outer surface of the trophoblastic villi; fetal blood is contained within fetal capillaries, which traverse within the intravillous spaces of the villi. This is a hemochorioendothelial type of placenta. The paracrine arm of this system links the mother and fetus through the anatomical and biochemical juxtaposition of (extraembryonic) chorion laeve and (maternal uterine) decidua parietalis tissue.

Therefore, at all sites of direct cell-to-cell contact, maternal tissues (decidua and blood) are juxtaposed to extraembryonic cells (trophoblasts) and not to embryonic cells or fetal blood. This is an extraordinarily important arrangement for communication between fetus and mother and for maternal (immunological) acceptance of the conceptus.

The role of the placenta in nidation and in the transfer of nutrients from mother to embryo-fetus has longed fueled interest in this unique organ. Subsequently, the enormous diversity of form and function of the placenta was recognized as the incredible metabolic, endocrine, and immunological properties of its trophoblasts were discovered.

EARLY HUMAN DEVELOPMENT

The definitions that follow are taken from Moore (1973, 1988).

- **Zygote:** The cell that results from the fertilization of the ovum by a spermatozoan.
- **Blastomeres:** Mitotic division of the zygote (cleavage) yields daughter cells called blastomeres.
- **Morula:** The solid ball of cells formed by 16 or so blastomeres.
- **Blastocyst:** After the morula reaches the uterus, a fluid-filled cavity is formed, converting the morula to a blastocyst.
- **Embryo:** The embryo-forming cells, grouped together as an inner cell mass, give rise to the embryo, which usually is so designated when the bilaminar embryonic disc forms. The embryonic period extends until the end of the seventh week, at which time the major structures are present.
- **Fetus:** After the embryonic period, the developing conceptus is referred to as the fetus.
- **Conceptus:** This term is used to refer to all tissue products of conception—embryo (fetus), fetal membranes, and placenta. The conceptus includes all tissues, both embryonic and extraembryonic, that develop from the zygote.

FERTILIZATION OF THE OVUM AND CLEAVAGE OF THE ZYGOTE. Few, if any, naturally occurring phenomena are of greater importance to humankind than the union of egg and sperm. Fertilization occurs in the fallopian tube; and it is generally agreed that fertilization of the ovum must occur within minutes or no more than a few hours after ovulation. Consequently, spermatozoa must be present in the fallopian tube at the time of ovulation. Most all pregnancies occur when intercourse occurs during the 2 days preceding or on the day of ovulation. If intercourse takes place on the day after ovulation, pregnancy probably will not result.

After fertilization in the fallopian tube, the mature ovum becomes a zygote—a diploid cell with 46 chromosomes—that then undergoes segmentation, or cleavage, into blastomeres. The first typical mitotic division of the segmentation nucleus of the zygote results in the formation of two blastomeres (Fig. 5–1). The zygote undergoes slow cleavage for 3 days while still within the fallopian tube; fertilized human ova that are recovered from the uterine cavity may be composed of only 12 to 16 blastomeres. As the blastomeres continue to divide, a solid mulberry-like ball of cells, referred to as the *morula,* is produced. The morula enters the uterine cavity about 3 days after fertilization. The gradual accumulation of fluid between blastomeres within the morula results in the formation of the *blastocyst* (Fig. 5–2). The compact mass of cells at one pole of the blastocyst, called the *inner cell mass,* is destined to be the embryo. The outer mass of cells is destined to be the trophoblasts.

THE EARLY HUMAN ZYGOTE. Hertig and co-workers (1954) found in the two-cell zygote that the blastomeres and the polar body are free in the perivitelline fluid and are surrounded by a thick zona pellucida (Fig. 5–1A). In a 58-cell blastocyst, the outer cells which are progenitors of the trophoblasts can be distinguished from the inner cells that form the embryo (Fig. 5–2B). The 107-cell blastocyst was found to be no larger than the earlier cleavage stages, despite the accumulated fluid (Fig. 5–1C). It measured 0.153 by 0.155 mm in diameter before fixation and after the disappearance of the zona pellucida. The eight formative or embryo-producing cells were surrounded by 99 trophoblastic cells.

IMPLANTATION. Just before implantation, the zona pellucida disappears and the blastocyst touches the endometrial surface; at this time of apposition, the blastocyst is composed of 107 to 256 cells. The blastocyst adheres to the endometrial epithelium, and implantation occurs most commonly on the endometrium of the upper part and on the posterior wall of the uterus. After gentle erosion between epithelial cells of the surface endometrium, the invading trophoblasts burrow deeper into the endometrium, and the blastocyst becomes totally encased within the endometrium, being covered over by the endometrium.

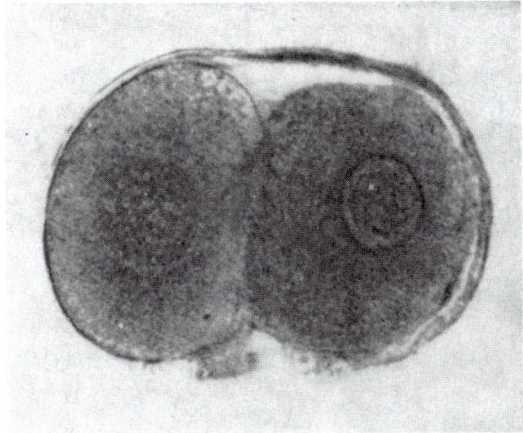

A

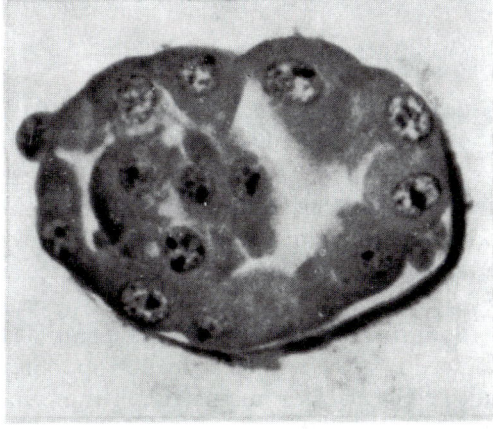

B

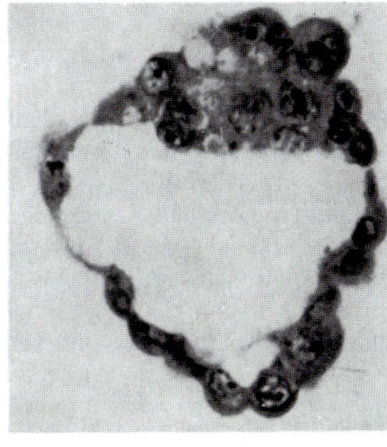

C

FIGURE 5–1. Human preimplantation stages. **A.** Two-cell stage. Intact fertilized ovum surrounded by zona pellucida, photographed after fixation. Washed from fallopian tube about 1 1/2 days after conception. Nuclei shimmer through granular cytoplasm and the polar body is seen in the perivitelline space. (Carnegie Collection no. 8698; × 500.) **B.** A 58-cell blastula with intact zona pellucida found in uterine cavity 3 to 4 days after conception. Thin section showing outer (probably trophoblastic) and inner (embryo-forming) cells and beginning segmentation cavity. (Carnegie Collection no. 8794; × 600). **C.** A 107-cell blastocyst found free in uterine cavity about 5 days after conception. There is a shell of trophoblastic cell enveloping fluid-filled blastocele and inner cell mass consisting of embryo-forming cells. (Carnegie Collection no. 8663; × 600. (From Hertig and associates, 1954.)

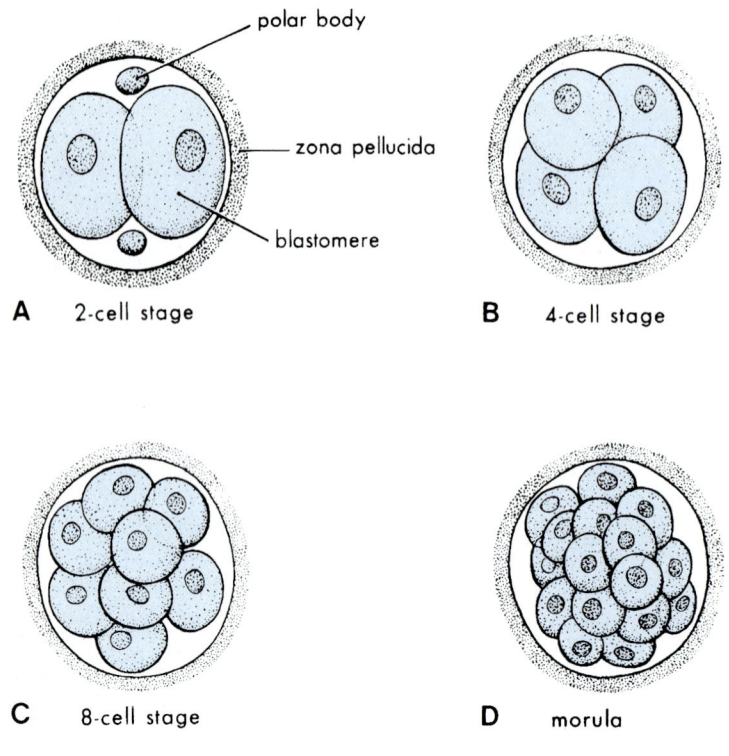

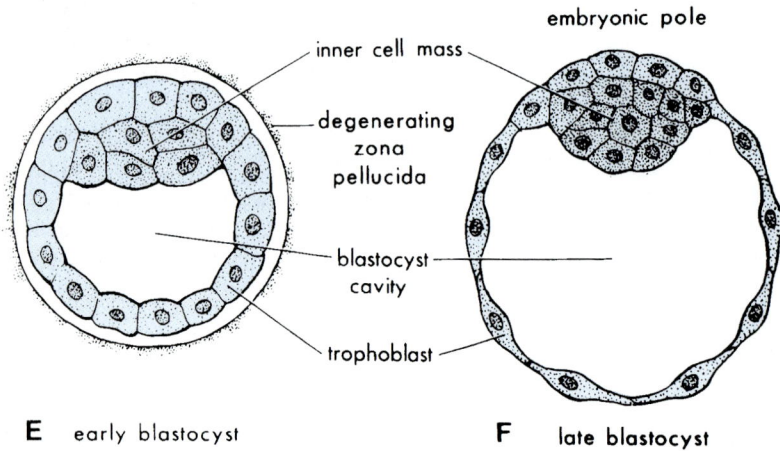

FIGURE 5–2. Cleavage of the zygote and formation of the blastocyst. **A** to **D** show various stages of cleavage. The period of the morula begins at the 12- to 16-cell stage and ends when the blastocyst forms, which occurs when there are 50 to 60 blastomeres present. **E** and **F** are sections of blastocysts. The zona pellucida has disappeared by the late blastocyst stage (5 days). The polar bodies shown in **A** are small, nonfunctional cells that soon degenerate. (From Moore, 1988.)

BIOLOGY OF THE TROPHOBLAST. Of all placental components, the trophoblast is the most variable in structure, function, and development. Its invasiveness provides for attachment of the blastocyst to the decidua of the uterine cavity; its role in nutrition of the conceptus is reflected in its name; and its function as an endocrine organ in human pregnancy is essential to maternal physiological adaptations and to the maintenance of pregnancy.

DIFFERENTIATION. Morphologically, trophoblasts are either **cellular** or **syncytial,** and may appear as uni-

nuclear cells or multinuclear giant cells. At implantation, some of the innermost cytotrophoblasts or *Langhans cells* that are contiguous with and invading the endometrium, coalesce to become an amorphous, multinucleated, continuous membrane that is uninterrupted by intercellular spaces, the syncytium. There are no individual cells, only a continuous lining; therefore it is the singular "syncytiotrophoblast" or syncytium. The true syncytial nature of the human syncytiotrophoblast has been confirmed by electron microscopy. The mechanism of syncytial growth, however, was a mystery in view of the discrepancy between an increase in the number of nuclei in the syncytiotrophoblast and equivocal evidence (at best) of intrinsic nuclear replication. Mitotic figures are completely absent from the syncytium, being confined to the cytotrophoblasts.

FORMATION OF THE SYNCYTIUM. Ulloa-Aguirre and co-workers (1987) elegantly demonstrated the conversion of cytotrophoblasts to a morphologically and functionally characteristic syncytium in vitro. They established that at least part of this differentiation process involves the action of cyclic adenosine monophosphate (cAMP). Based on their methods of isolation and characterization of human cytotrophoblasts, others developed systems to evaluate blastocyst implantation in vitro (Kliman and associates, 1986; Ringler and Strauss, 1990). Isolated cytotrophoblasts, placed in serum-containing medium, migrate toward one another and form aggregates. Ultimately, the aggregates fuse and syncytium is produced during 3 to 4 days. The syncytium also is formed in the absence of serum, provided that extracellular matrix components are present to serve as a lattice for cytotrophoblast migration. The syncytium produced in vitro is covered by microvilli, as it is in vivo. Cytotrophoblast aggregation is dependent upon protein synthesis, and involves a calcium-dependent cell adhesion molecule, *E-cadherin,* for aggregation. Desmosomes develop between the cells; and as the cytotrophoblasts fuse, the expression of E-cadherin diminishes.

The cytotrophoblast is the germinal cell; the syncytium, or the secretory component, is derived from cytotrophoblasts. Therefore, the cytotrophoblasts are the cellular progenitors of the syncytiotrophoblast. Well-demarcated borders and a single, distinct nucleus characterize each cytotrophoblast; and there are frequent mitoses among the cytotrophoblasts. These characteristics are lacking, however, in the syncytium, in which the cytoplasm is amorphous, without cell borders, and the nuclei are multiple and diverse in size and shape. The absence of cell borders in the syncytium obliges transport across this structure. Hence, the control of transport is not dependent on the participation of individual cells.

Coutifaris and Coukos (1994) presented a succinct and informative review of the processes of human implantation. They point out that after apposition and adherence of the trophectoderm of the blastocyst to the endometrial epithelial cells, implantation commences by intrusion of cytotrophoblasts between endometrial epithelial cells. This process of trophoblast invasion is facilitated by degradation of the extracellular matrix of the endometrium/decidua, catalyzed by urokinase-type plasminogen activator, urokinase plasminogen activator receptor, and metalloproteinases that are produced by selected cytotrophoblasts at various stages of implantation/placentation. **These functions of cytotrophoblasts invading the endometrium are indistinguishable from those of metastasizing malignant cells.** As the cytotrophoblasts move through the decidua, selected populations of these cells bind to various extracellular matrix components of the decidual stromal cells. This facilitates migration and thence the establishment of placental anchors to the decidua.

IMMUNOLOGICAL ACCEPTANCE OF THE CONCEPTUS

Over the last half century, many attempts to explain the survival of the semiallogenic fetal graft have been proposed. One of the earliest explanations was based on the theory of antigenic immaturity of the embryo-fetus. This was disproved by Billingham (1964) who showed that transplantation (HLA) antigens are demonstrable very early in embryonic life. The trophoblasts are the only cells of the conceptus in direct contact with maternal tissues or blood and these tissues are genetically identical with fetal tissues. Another explanation was based on diminished immunological responsiveness of the pregnant woman. There is, however, no evidence for this to be other than an ancillary factor. In a third explanation, the uterus (decidua) is proposed as an immunologically privileged tissue site. This would preclude well-documented advanced ectopic pregnancies discussed in Chapter 34. Clearly, transplantation immunity can be evoked and expressed in the uterus as in other tissues. Therefore, the acceptance and the survival of the conceptus in the maternal uterus must be attributed to an immunological peculiarity of the trophoblasts, not the decidua.

CURRENT STATUS OF RESEARCH. It still is enigmatic that maternal tissues accept and tolerate the grafted conceptus. Moreover, the placenta likely expresses "novel" genes (Dizon-Townson and colleagues, 2000). Several novel aspects of the expression of the HLA system in trophoblasts, together with a unique set of lymphocytes, may provide an explanation for this.

IMMUNOCOMPETENCY OF THE TROPHOBLASTS. Almost 50 years ago, Sir Peter Medawar (1953) suggested that the solution to the riddle of the fetal allograft might be explained by *immunological neutrality.* As early as 1932, Witebsky and Reich found that blood group antigens are lacking in human trophoblasts. Subsequently, many researchers focused on defining the expression of the *major histocompatibility complex (MHC)* antigens in trophoblasts. *Human leukocyte antigens,* or *HLA,* by international agreement, are the human analogue of the major histocompatibility complex (see also Chap. 52, p. 1384).

MHC class II antigens are absent from trophoblasts at all stages of gestation (Weetman, 1999). Before blastocyst implantation in the mouse, MHC class I antigens on the trophectoderm are expressed in low levels, but these antigens disappear at the time of implantation, not to reappear except later in selected subpopulations of trophoblasts in the mature placenta.

TROPHOBLAST HLA CLASS I EXPRESSION. King and Loke (1991) reasoned that normal implantation is dependent upon controlled trophoblastic invasion of maternal endometrium/decidua and the spiral arteries—a mechanism for permitting and then limiting trophoblast invasion. They suggested that such a system involves the uterine large granular lymphocytes (LGLs) and the unique expression (or absence thereof) of a specific monomeric HLA class I gene in trophoblasts.

HLA-I GENE EXPRESSION. The HLA genes are the products of multiple genetic loci of the MHC located within the short arm of chromosome 6 (Hunt and Orr, 1992). There are 17 HLA class I genes, which include three classical genes. The three classical genes—HLA-A, -B, and -C—which encode the major class I(a) transplantation antigens. Three other class I(b) genes, designated HLA-E, -F, and -G also encode class I HLA antigens. The remaining DNA sequences appear to be pseudogenes or partial gene fragments.

Class I antigen(s) in cytotrophoblasts is accounted for by the expression of a single gene for HLA-G. As HLA-G is monomorphic (or nearly so), this antigen is recognized as "self" and therefore should not evoke an immunological response by maternal immune cells against fetal trophoblasts expressing HLA-G (Kilburn and associates, 2000; Weetman, 1999). Its expression may be stimulated by hypoxias (Kilburn and associates, 2000). To elucidate HLA-G expression, it is important to understand the nature of the unusual lymphocyte population of the human decidua.

UTERINE LARGE GRANULAR LYMPHOCYTES (LGLs). These distinctive cells are believed to be lymphoid and of bone marrow origin and natural killer (NK) cell lineage. They are present in large numbers only at the midluteal phase of the cycle—at the expected time of implantation (Johnson and colleagues, 1999). These LGLs have a distinct phenotype characterized by a high surface density of CD56 or *neural cell adhesion molecule* (Loke and King, 1995).

Near the end of the luteal phase of nonfertile ovulatory cycles, the nuclei of the uterine LGLs begin to disintegrate. With blastocyst implantation, these cells persist in the decidua during the early weeks of pregnancy. At term, however, there are relatively few LGLs

in decidua. It is speculated that LGLs are involved in the regulation of trophoblast invasion. They secrete large amounts of granulocyte/macrophage-colony stimulating factor (GM-CSF), suggestive that the LGLs in first trimester decidua are in an activated state. This has led Jokhi and co-workers (1994) to speculate that GM-CSF may function primarily not to promote trophoblast replication but rather to forestall trophoblast apoptosis. According to this theory, LGLs rather than the T lymphocytes would bear the primary responsibility for immunosurveillance in decidua.

HLA-G EXPRESSION IN HUMAN TROPHOBLASTS. This hypothesis involves developmental modifications in HLA-G class I antigen expression on trophoblasts. HLA-G is expressed only in the human. Indeed, HLA-G antigen is identified only in extravillous cytotrophoblasts in the decidua basalis and in the chorion laeve (McMaster and colleagues, 1995). HLA-G is not present in villous trophoblasts, either in the syncytium or in the cytotrophoblasts. HLA-G is expressed in cytotrophoblasts that are contiguous with maternal tissues (decidual cells). A soluble major isoform, HLA-G2, is increased during pregnancy (Hunt and associates, 2000). It is hypothesized that HLA-G is immunologically permissive of the antigen mismatch between mother and fetus (LeBouteiller and co-workers, 1999). Indeed, Goldman-Wohl and colleagues (2000) have provided evidence for abnormal HLA-G expression in extravillous trophoblasts from women with preeclampsia.

HLA EXPRESSION IN THE HUMAN EMBRYO. As gestation progresses, cells from the inner cell mass of the blastocyst (those that form the embryo) gradually develop both class I and class II HLA antigens. Importantly, these tissues are not in direct contact with maternal tissues or blood.

IMPLANTATION AND INTEGRIN SWITCHING. The attachment of the trophectoderm of the blastocyst to the endometrial surface by apposition and adherence and then the intrusion and invasion of the endometrium/decidua by cytotrophoblasts (implantation) appears to be dependent upon two factors:

1. Trophoblast elaboration of specific proteinases that degrade selected extracellular matrix proteins of the endometrium/decidua.
2. A coordinated and alternating process referred to as *integrin switching,* which facilitates migration and then attachment of trophoblasts in the decidua.

The integrins, one of four families of cell adhesion molecules (CAMs), are cell-surface receptors that mediate the adhesion of cells to extracellular matrix proteins (Frenette and Wagner, 1996). Great diversity of cell binding to a host of different extracellular matrix proteins is possible by way of the integrin system.

Recall that the decidual cell becomes completely encased by a pericellular (extracellular matrix) membrane. This "wall" around the decidual cell provides the scaffolding for the attachment of the extravillous trophoblasts, the *anchoring cytotrophoblasts* (Chap. 4, p. 79). These cells first elaborate selected proteinases that degrade the extracellular matrix of decidua. Thereafter, the expression of a specific group of integrins enables the docking of these cells. By alternating between these two processes and by "integrin switching," the movement of cytotrophoblasts into the decidua is aggressive, but regulated. Specific decidual localization of the cytotrophoblasts to establish attachment of the placenta to the wall of the uterine cavity results. Craven and colleagues (2000) have provided evidence that a similar process is operative for trophoblastic invasion of uterine veins.

TROPHOBLAST ATTACHMENT IN DECIDUA: ONCO-FETAL FIBRONECTIN.

As described by Feinberg and colleagues (1991), oncofetal fibronectin (onfFN) molecules are characterized by a unique glycopeptide of the fibronectin molecule. They refer to onfFN as *trophouteronectin* or *trophoblast glue* to suggest a critical role for this protein in the migration and attachment of trophoblasts to maternal decidua. They localized onfFN to the junction of cytotrophoblast with extracellular matrix. Importantly, onfFN was localized to the extracellular matrix connecting extravillous cytotrophoblasts and cytotrophoblastic cell columns to the uterine decidua. As onfFN is formed by extravillous trophoblasts, including those of the chorion laeve, these investigators suggest that it may function to facilitate separation of the extraembryonic tissues from the uterus at delivery. More recently, Feinberg and associates (1994) have shown that transforming growth factor-β (TGF-β) promotes the synthesis of onfFN. This is consistent with the proposition that TGF-β is intimately involved in multiple aspects of implantation and decidualization.

Lockwood and colleagues (1991) and others evaluated cervical and vaginal secretions for the presence of onfFN in association with term and preterm labor. Their findings are discussed further in Chapter 27 (p. 702) concerning the usefulness of the identification of onfFN to predict preterm labor. Clearly the levels of onfFN are increased in cervical/vaginal fluids that are obtained during labor. One possibility is that this represents some type of separation (chemical, mechanical, or both) of chorion laeve (trophoblasts) from decidua parietalis. Feinberg and associates speculate that the "leakage" of onfFN is the result of enzymatic action to release the onfFN. This putative enzyme activity may be part of the parturitional process. Alternatively, separation of chorion laeve and decidua could be a mechanical consequence of labor, that is, the chorion laeve is pulled away from decidua by shear stress as labor progresses. Recent evidence is suggestive that digital cervical examination affects fetal fibronectin levels (McKenna and associates, 1999).

EMBRYONIC AND PLACENTAL DEVELOPMENT

EARLY BLASTOCYSTS. In a description of the earliest stages of the human blastocyst, the wall of the primitive blastodermic vesicle was characterized as consisting of a single layer of ectoderm (Fig. 5–1). As early as 72 hours after ovum fertilization, the 58-cell blastula had differentiated into 5 embryo-producing cells and 53 cells destined to form trophoblasts (Hertig, 1962). Although trophoblasts have not been distinguished before blastocyst implantation, both cytotrophoblasts and syncytiotrophoblast are present in the earliest implanted blastocyst of the monkey. Indeed, evidence has been presented that chorionic gonadotropin (hCG) is secreted by cells of the human blastocyst at the time of implantation (Chap. 6, p. 110).

Soon after blastocyst adherence to the endometrial epithelium, the cytotrophoblasts proliferate rapidly and begin to invade the surrounding decidua. The extravillous cytotrophoblasts that ultimately form the anchoring cells in the decidua remain as individual cells or cytotrophoblasts. As the blastocyst and its surrounding trophoblasts, which are completely covered by decidua, grow and expand, one pole of this mass extends toward the endometrial cavity and the other pole remains buried in the endometrium/decidua. The innermost pole enters into the formation of the placenta, that is, the anchoring cytotrophoblasts and the villous trophoblasts. The trophoblasts of the villus are the outer layer of syncytium and an inner layer of cytotrophoblasts. The pole developing toward the endometrial cavity is covered by the chorion frondosum, which at this time is covered by decidua (capsularis). As the growth of embryonic and extraembryonic tissues continues, the blood supply of the chorion facing the endometrial cavity is restricted, and consequently the villous nature of this tissue and its blood supply are lost. This portion of the chorion becomes the avascular fetal membrane that touches the decidua parietalis, that is, the chorion laeve or smooth chorion. With continued expansion of the embryo-fetus, the chorion laeve becomes contiguous with the entire maternal decidua (parietalis) that is not occupied by the placenta. The chorion laeve is comprised of cytotrophoblasts and fetal mesodermal (mesenchymal) cells that survive in a relatively low oxygen atmosphere.

As the fetus grows, the decidua capsularis merges with the decidua parietalis. The decidua capsularis, however, is largely lost by pressure and the attendant loss of blood supply. The area of decidua where decidua capsularis and decidua parietalis merge, is referred to as the decidua vera.

One of the earliest implanting blastocysts discovered by Hertig and Rock (1944) is shown in Figure 5–3. It measured only 0.36 by 0.31 mm, and it was believed to have been in the process of penetrating the endometrium, with the thin outer wall of the blastocyst still within the uterine cavity. An implanting blastocyst at a similar stage of development, 9 days after fertilization, is shown in Figure 5–4. It appears to have been flattened in the process of penetrating the uterine epithelium; the enlargement and multiplication of the trophoblasts in contact with the endometrium are alone responsible for the increase in size of the implanted blastocyst as compared with the free blastocyst.

EMBRYONIC DEVELOPMENT AFTER IMPLANTATION.

At 9 days of development (Fig. 5–4), the wall of the blastocyst that faces toward the uterine lumen is a single layer of flattened cells. The opposite, thicker wall comprises two zones, the trophoblasts and the embryo-forming inner cell mass. As early as 7 1/2 days after fertilization, the inner cell mass, referred to as the embryonic disc, is differentiated into a thick plate of primitive ectoderm and an underlying layer of endoderm. Some small cells appear between the embryonic disc and the trophoblast, and enclose a space that will become the amnionic cavity.

As the embryo enlarges, more maternal tissue (decidua basalis) is invaded, and the walls of the superficial decidual capillaries are eroded. As a consequence, maternal blood leaks into the lacunae. With deeper burrowing and blastocyst invasion into the decidua, the strands of trophoblasts branch to form the solid primitive villi that traverse the lacunae. The villi that were located over the entire blastocyst surface later disappear except over the most deeply implanted portion, the site destined to form the placenta.

The embryonic mesenchyme first appears as isolated cells within the cavity of the blastocyst. When the cavity is completely lined with mesoderm, it is termed the chorionic vesicle, and its membrane, now called the chorion, is composed of trophoblasts and mesenchyme. The mesenchymal cells within the cavity are most numerous about the embryo, where these eventually condense to form the body stalk, which serves to join the embryo to the nutrient chorion and later develops into the umbilical cord.

The syncytiotrophoblast of the chorionic shell is permeated by a system of intercommunicating channels of trophoblastic lacunae that contain maternal blood. At the same time, the decidual reaction intensifies in the surrounding stroma, which is characterized by enlargement of the decidual stromal cells and glycogen storage.

CYTOTROPHOBLAST INVASION OF DECIDUAL VESSELS.

The capillary network of the most superficial portion of the endometrium is invaded by cytotrophoblasts. Subsequently, the arterioles and then the spiral arteries are invaded, and the walls of these vessels are destroyed. This phenomenon will be considered in some detail because of its special importance to an under-

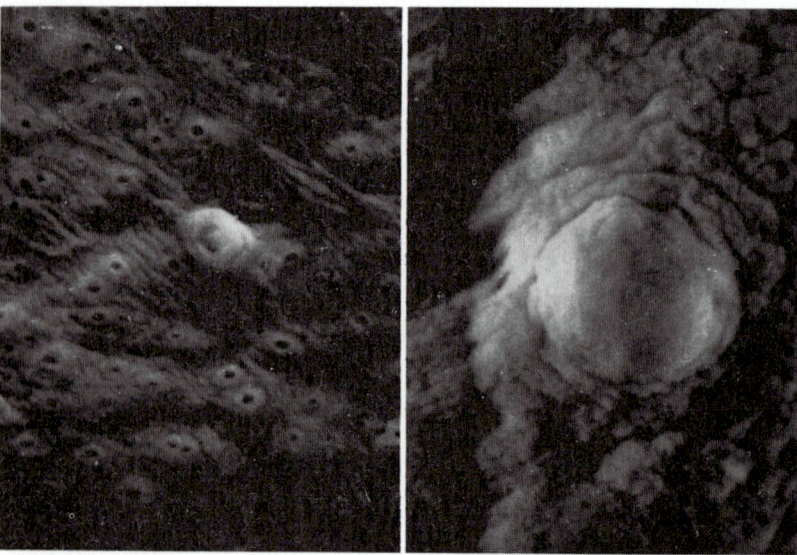

FIGURE 5–3. Low- and high-power photomicrographs of surface view of an early implanted blastocyst obtained on day 22 of the endometrial cycle, fewer than 8 days after conception. Site was slightly elevated and measured 0.36 × 0.31 mm. Mouths of uterine glands appear as dark spots surrounded by halos. (Carnegie Collection no. 8225.) (From Hertig and Rock, 1944.)

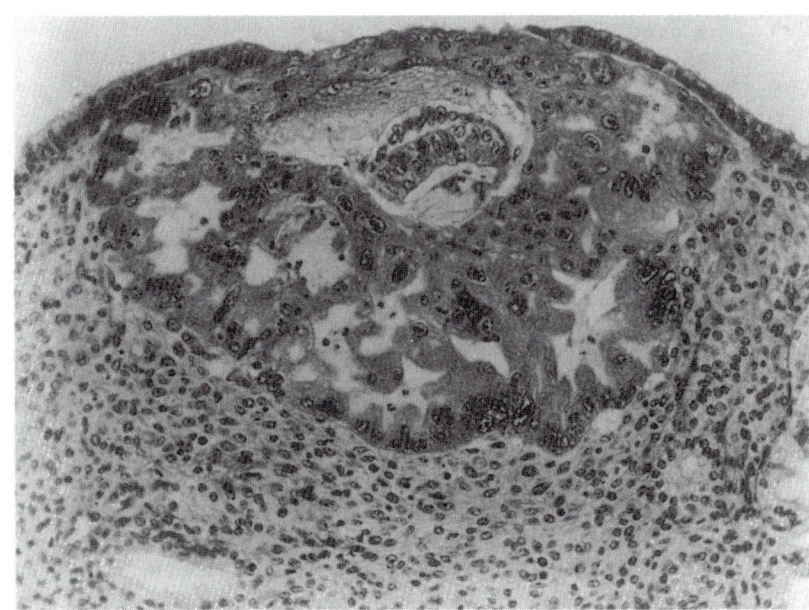

FIGURE 5–4. Section through middle of an implanting embryo at about 9 days. Regeneration of the endometrial epithelium is taking place. Lacunae appear as clear spaces in the large mass of syncytiotrophoblast. The bilaminar embryonic disk is seen. (From Hertig and Rock, 1945).

standing of human uteroplacental blood flow. Hamilton and Boyd (1966) give credit to Friedlander (1870) for the first description of the striking structural changes of the spiral arteries of the decidua basalis during human placentation. During implantation, the spiral arteries acquire a lining of cells within the endothelium that is derived from the invading cytotrophoblasts. During this vascular invasion, degenerative changes occur in the arterial wall, affecting all layers of these vessels. The most striking change involves the vascular smooth muscle, which becomes nonrecognizable.

The cytotrophoblasts that invade the spiral arteries can pass several centimeters along the vessel lumen; indeed, Hamilton and Boyd observed cytotrophoblasts in myometrial portions of these vessels. They also emphasize that these vascular changes are not observed in the decidua parietalis—that is, in decidual sites removed from the invading cytotrophoblasts. The intraluminal trophoblastic cells diminish in number near term. In midtrimester pregnancy, however, trophoblasts are present in all of the spiral arteries of the decidua at the placental site.

Hamilton and Boyd took special notice of several curious features of these observations:

1. The cytotrophoblasts in the vessel lumens do not appear to replicate.
2. Oddly, these cells are not readily dislodged by the flow of blood.
3. In fact, these cytotrophoblasts appear to migrate against arterial flow and pressure.
4. There is no obvious adhesion of these cells one to the other.

5. The invasion of maternal vascular tissues by trophoblasts involves only the decidual spiral arteries, not the decidual veins.

Maternal blood enters the intervillous space from the spiral arteries in fountain-like bursts. Thus, maternal blood that is propelled outside of the maternal vessels sweeps over and directly bathes the syncytiotrophoblast. The maternal surface of the syncytiotrophoblast consists of a complex microvillus structure that undergoes continual shedding and reformation during pregnancy.

As endometrial invasion by trophoblasts progresses, decidual spiral arteries are tapped to form lacunae, which are soon filled with maternal blood. The term **hemochorioendothelial** used to describe human placentation is derived as follows: *hemo* refers to maternal blood, which directly bathes the syncytiotrophoblast; *chorio* is for chorion-placenta, which in turn is separated from fetal blood by the *endothelial* wall of the fetal capillaries that traverse the intravillous space. The characteristics of this type of placentation are illustrated in Figures 5–5 and 5–6. As the lacunae join, a complicated labyrinth is formed that is partitioned by solid cytotrophoblastic columns. The trophoblast-lined labyrinthine channels and the solid cellular columns form the intervillous space and primary villous stalks, respectively.

GERM LAYERS. The amnion and yolk sac, with both epithelial and mesenchymal components, are illustrated in Figures 5–5 and 5–6. The body stalk, from which the

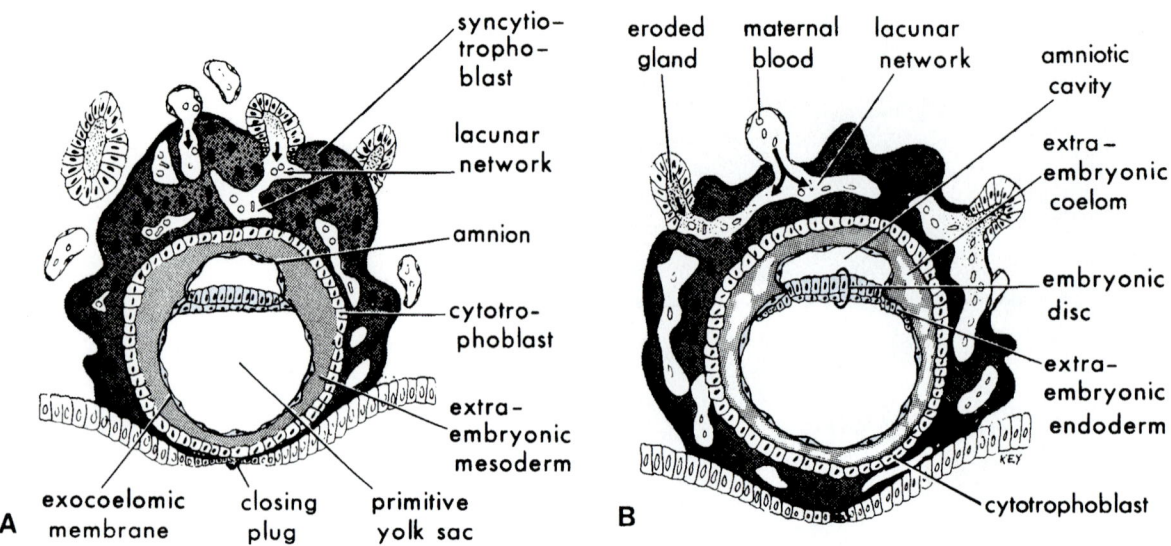

FIGURE 5-5. Drawing of sections through implanted blastocysts. **A.** At 10 days. **B.** At 12 days after fertilization. The stage of development is characterized by the intercommunication of the lacunae filled with maternal blood. Note in **B** that large cavities have appeared in the extraembryonic mesoderm, forming the beginning of the extraembryonic coelom. Also note that extraembryonic endodermal cells have begun to form on the inside of the primary yolk sac. (From Moore, 1988.)

caudal end of the embryo arises, can also be recognized at this stage.

ORGANIZATION OF PLACENTA

TROPHOBLAST ULTRASTRUCTURE. From the electron microscopic studies of Wislocki and Dempsey (1955), data were provided that permitted a functional interpretation of the fine structure of the placenta. There are prominent microvilli on the syncytial surface, corresponding to the "brush border" described by light microscopy (Fig. 5–7). Associated pinocytotic vacuoles and vesicles are related to the absorptive and secretory placental functions. The inner layer of the villi—the cytotrophoblasts—persists to term, although often compressed against the trophoblastic basal lamina, and retains its ultrastructural simplicity (Fig. 5–8).

CHORIONIC VILLI. Villi can first be distinguished easily in the human placenta on about the 12th day after fertilization. When a mesenchymal cord, presumably derived

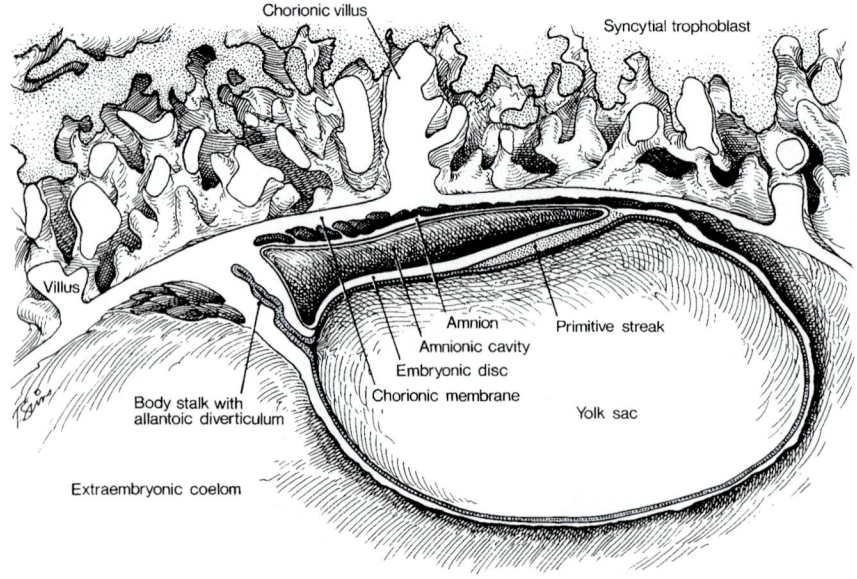

FIGURE 5-6. Median view of a drawing of a wax reconstruction of Mateer embryo, showing the amnionic cavity and its relations to chorionic membrane and yolk sac (× 500). (After Streeter, 1920.)

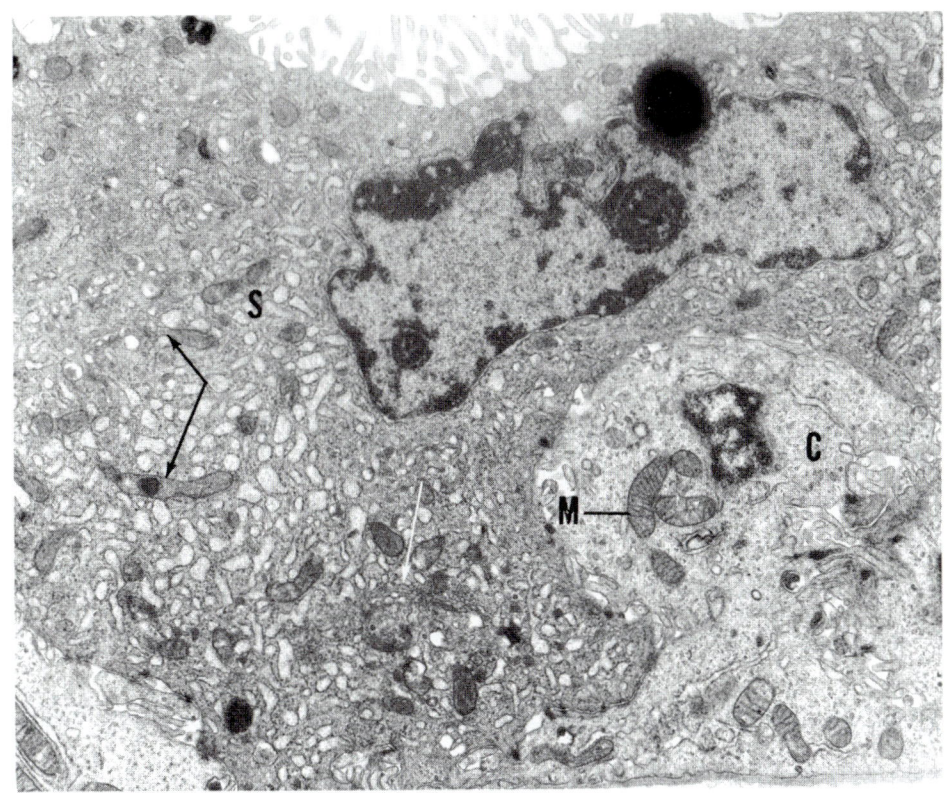

FIGURE 5–7. Electron micrograph of first-trimester human placenta showing well-differentiated syncytiotrophoblast (S) with numerous mitochondria (*black arrows*) and Golgi complexes (*white arrow*). Cytotrophoblast (C) has large mitochondria (M) but few other organelles. At the top, there is a prominent border of microvilli arising from the syncytium (S).

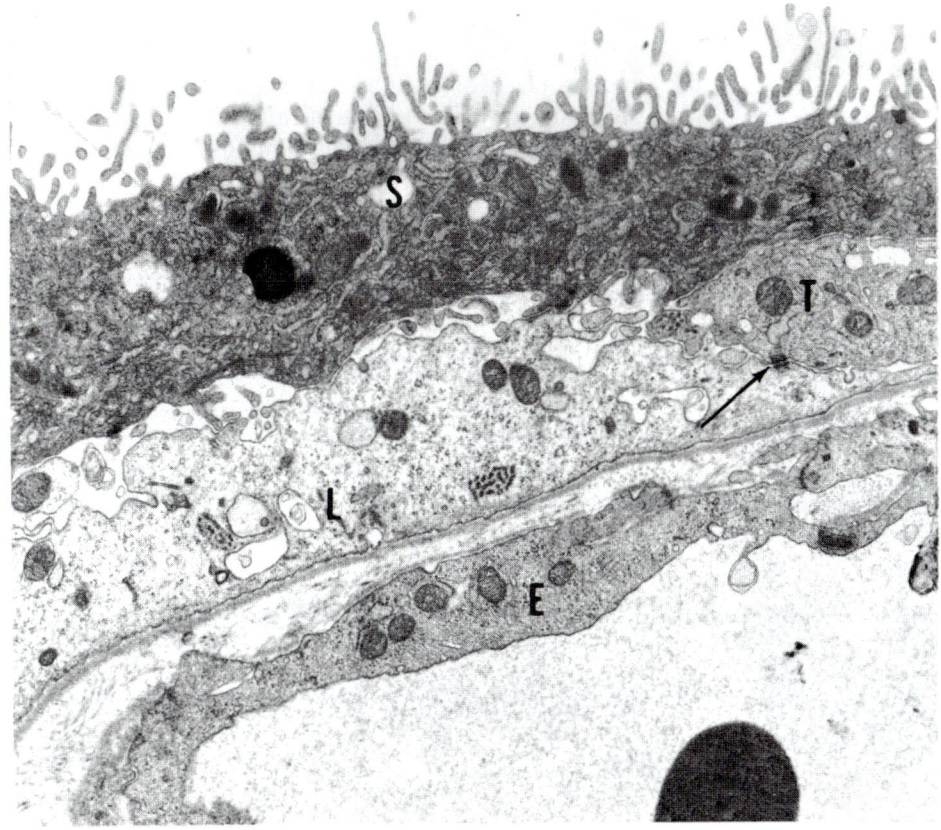

FIGURE 5–8. Term human placenta showing electron-dense syncytium (S), Langhans cells (cytotrophoblasts) (L), transitional cytotrophoblast (T), and capillary endothelium (E). Arrow points to desmosome. (Courtesy of Dr. Ralph M. Wynn.)

from cytotrophoblasts, invades the solid trophoblast column secondary villi are formed. After angiogenesis occurs from the mesenchymal cores in situ, the resulting villi are termed tertiary. Maternal venous sinuses are tapped early in the implantation process, but until the 14th or 15th day after fertilization, maternal arterial blood does not enter the intervillous space. By about the 17th day, fetal blood vessels are functional, and a placental circulation is established. The fetal–placental circulation is completed when the blood vessels of the embryo are connected with the chorionic blood vessels. Some villi, in which failure of angiogenesis results in a lack of circulation, become distended with fluid and form vesicles. A striking exaggeration of this process is characteristic of the development of hydatidiform mole (Chap, 32, 836).

Proliferation of cellular cytotrophoblasts at the tips of the villi produces the trophoblastic cell columns, which are not invaded by fetal mesenchyme but are anchored to the decidua at the basal plate. Thus, the floor of the intervillous space (maternal-facing side) consists of cytotrophoblasts from the cell columns, the peripheral syncytium of the trophoblastic shell, and decidua of the basal plate. The floor of the chorionic plate, consisting of the two layers of trophoblasts externally and fibrous mesoderm internally, forms the roof of the intervillous space.

In early pregnancy, the villi are distributed over the entire periphery of the chorionic membrane. A blastocyst dislodged from the endometrium at this stage of development appears shaggy (Fig. 5–9). The villi in contact with the decidua basalis proliferate to form the leafy chorion, or chorion frondosum, the fetal component of the placenta; the villi in contact with the decidua capsularis cease to grow and degenerate to form the

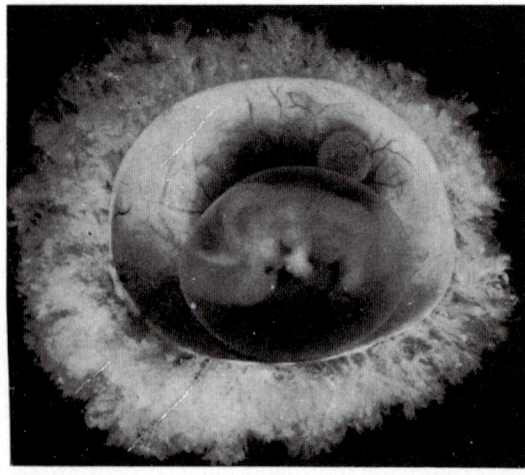

FIGURE 5–9. Human chorionic vesicle at ovulatory age of 40 days. (Carnegie Collection no. 8537.)

chorion laeve. The chorion laeve is generally more nearly translucent than the amnion even though rarely exceeding 1 mm in thickness. The chorion laeve contains ghost villi, and decidua clings to its surface.

Until near the end of the third month, the chorion laeve is separated from the amnion by the exocoelomic cavity. Thereafter, the amnion and chorion are in intimate contact. In the human, the chorion laeve and amnion form an avascular amniochorion, but these two structures are important sites of molecular transfer and metabolic activity. They constitute the paracrine arm of the fetal–maternal communication system.

PLACENTAL COTYLEDONS. Certain villi of the chorion frondosum extend from the chorionic plate to the decidua and serve as *anchoring villi.* Most villi, however, arboresce and end freely in the intervillous space without reaching the decidua (Fig. 5–10). As the placenta matures, the short, thick, early stem villi branch repeatedly, forming progressively finer subdivisions and greater numbers of increasingly small villi (Fig. 5–11). Each of the main stem (truncal) villi and their ramifications (rami) constitute a placental cotyledon (lobe). Each cotyledon is supplied with a branch (truncal) of the chorionic artery; and for each cotyledon, there is a vein, constituting a 1:1:1 ratio of artery to vein to cotyledon.

BREAKS IN THE PLACENTAL "BARRIER." The placenta does not maintain absolute integrity of the fetal and maternal circulations. This is evidenced by numerous findings of the passage of cells between mother and fetus in both directions. This situation is best exemplified clinically by erythrocyte D-antigen isoimmunization and the occurrence of *erythroblastosis fetalis* (Chap. 39, p. 1061). Typically, a few fetal blood cells are found in maternal blood; but on extremely rare occasions, the fetus exsanguinates into the maternal circulation. Fetal leukocytes may replicate in the mother and leukocytes bearing a Y chromosome have been identified in women for up to 5 years after giving birth to a son (Ciaranfi and colleagues, 1977). Desai and Creger (1963) labeled maternal leukocytes and platelets with atabrine and found that the atabrine-labeled cells crossed the placenta from mother to fetus.

PLACENTAL SIZE AND WEIGHT. Crawford (1959) suggested that the total number of cotyledons remains the same throughout gestation. Individual cotyledons continue to grow, although less actively in the final weeks. Placental weights vary considerably, depending upon how the placenta is prepared. If the fetal membranes and most of the cord are left attached and adherent maternal blood clot is not removed, the weight may be

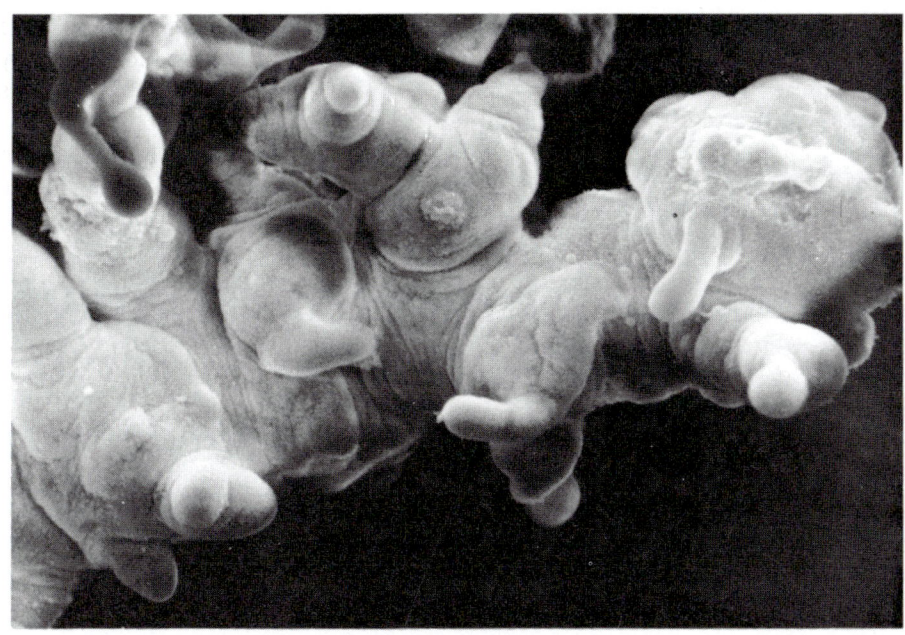

FIGURE 5–10. Scanning electron micrograph of placental villi at 10 to 14 weeks' gestation. Note the larger stem villi and the small syncytial sprouts at various stages of formation. Furrows or creases on the surface also are evident, especially at the bases of larger villi ($\times$ 289). (From King and Menton, 1975.)

greater by nearly 50 percent (Thomson and co-workers, 1969).

THE PLACENTA AT TERM. According to Boyd and Hamilton (1970), the placenta at term is, on average, 185 mm in diameter and 23 mm in thickness, with an average volume of 497 mL, and weight of 508 g; but these measurements vary widely. There are multiple shapes and forms of the human placenta and a variety of types of umbilical cord insertions, which are discussed in Chapter 32. Viewed from the maternal surface, the number of slightly elevated convex areas called lobes (or if small, lobules) varies from 10 to 38. These lobes are separated, albeit incompletely, by grooves of variable depth, the *placental septa*. The lobes are also referred to as *cotyledons*.

PLACENTAL AGING. As the villi continue to branch and the terminal ramifications become more numerous and smaller, the volume and prominence of cytotrophoblasts decrease. As the syncytium thins and forms knots, the vessels become more prominent and lie closer to the surface. The stroma of the villi also exhibits changes associated with aging. In placentas of early pregnancy, the branching connective tissue cells are separated by an abundant loose intercellular matrix. Later, the stroma becomes denser and the cells more spindly and more closely packed.

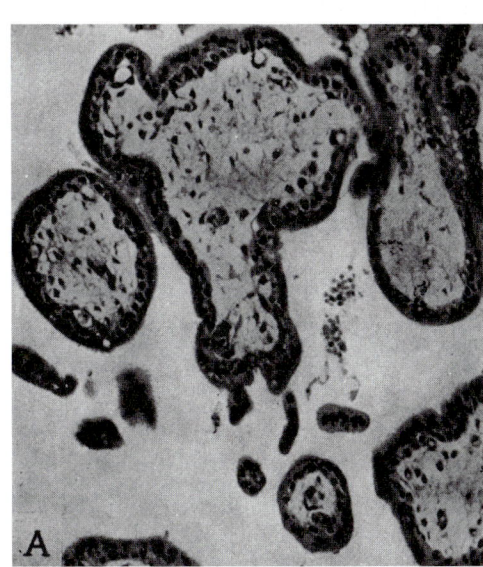
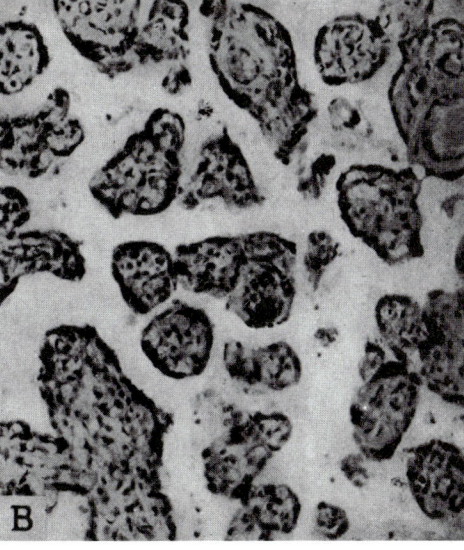

FIGURE 5–11. Comparison of chorionic villi in early and late pregnancy. **A.** About 8 weeks' gestation. Note inner Langhans cells (cytotrophoblasts) and outer syncytial layer. **B.** Term placenta. Syncytial layer is obvious, but Langhans cells (cytotrophoblasts) are difficult to recognize at low magnification in light micrographs.

Another change in the stroma involves the *Hofbauer cells,* which likely are fetal macrophages. These cells are nearly round with vesicular, often eccentric nuclei and very granular or vacuolated cytoplasm. These cells are characterized histochemically by intracytoplasmic lipid and are readily distinguished from plasma cells.

Certain of the histological changes that accompany placental growth and aging are suggestive of an increase in the efficiency of transport and exchange to meet increasing fetal metabolic requirements. Among these changes are a decrease in thickness of the syncytium, partial reduction of cytotrophoblastic cells, decrease in the stroma, and an increase in the number of capillaries and the approximation of these vessels to the syncytial surface. By 4 months, the apparent continuity of the cytotrophoblasts is broken, and the syncytium forms knots on the more numerous smaller villi. At term, the covering of the villi may be focally reduced to a thin layer of syncytium with minimal connective tissue; and

the fetal capillaries seem to abut the trophoblast. The villous stroma, Hofbauer cells, and cytotrophoblasts are markedly reduced, and the villi appear filled with thin-walled capillaries.

Other changes, however, are suggestive of a decrease in the efficiency for placental exchange. These changes include thickening of the basement membranes of the trophoblast capillaries, obliteration of certain fetal vessels, and fibrin deposition on the surface of the villi in the basal and chorionic plates as well as elsewhere in the intervillous space.

BLOOD CIRCULATION IN THE MATURE PLACENTA

Because the placenta functionally represents a rather intimate association of the fetal capillary bed to maternal blood, its gross anatomy primarily concerns vascular

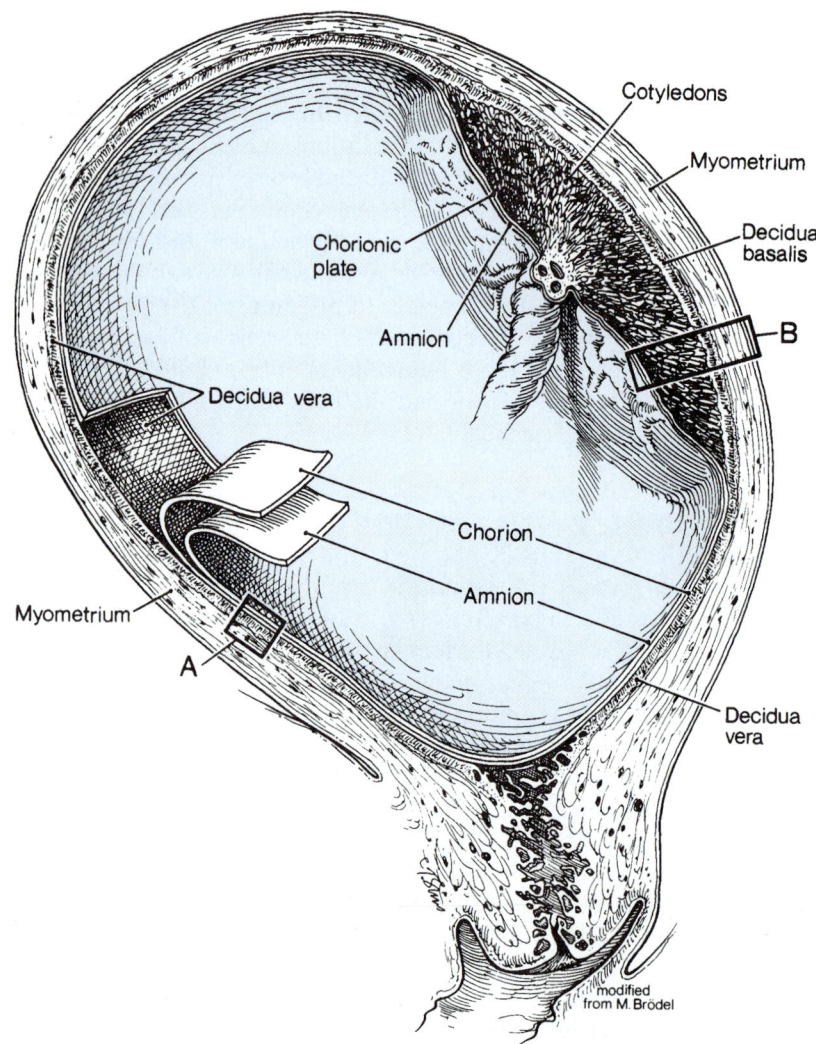

Cotyledons

Myometrium

Chorionic plate

Decidua basalis

Amnion

B

Decidua vera

Chorion

Amnion

Myometrium

A

Decidua vera

modified from M. Brödel

FIGURE 5–12. Uterus of pregnant woman showing normal placenta in situ. **A.** Location of section shown in Figure 5–13. **B.** Location of section shown in Figure 5–14.

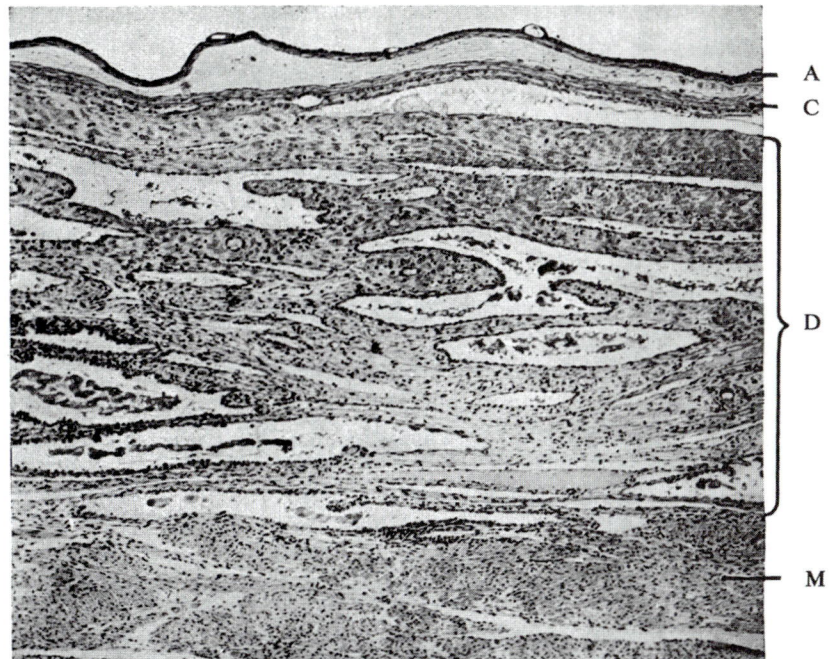

A
C

D

M

FIGURE 5–13. Section of fetal membranes and uterus opposite placental site at **A** in Figure 5–12. (A = amnion; C = chorion laeve; D = decidua parietalis; M = myometrium.)

relations. The fetal surface of the placenta is covered by the transparent amnion beneath which the fetal chorionic vessels course. A section through the placenta in situ (Figs. 5–12 to 5–14) includes amnion, chorion, chorionic villi and intervillous spaces, decidual plate, and myometrium. The maternal surface of the placenta (Fig. 5–15) is divided into irregular lobes by furrows produced by septa, which consist of fibrous tissue with sparse vessels confined mainly to their bases. The broad-based septa ordinarily do not reach the chorionic plate, thus providing only incomplete partitions.

FETAL CIRCULATION. Fetal deoxygenated, or "venous-like," blood flows to the placenta through the two umbilical arteries. At the juncture of the umbilical cord with the placenta, the umbilical vessels branch repeatedly beneath the amnion and again within the dividing villi, finally forming capillary networks in the terminal divisions (Fig. 5–16). Blood, with significantly higher oxygen content, returns from the placenta to the fetus through a single umbilical vein.

The branches of the umbilical vessels that traverse along the fetal surface of the placenta (the chorionic plate) are referred to as the placental surface or chorionic vessels. These vessels are responsive to vasoactive substances; but anatomically, morphologically, histologically, and functionally, these are curious vessels. The chorionic arteries always cross over the chorionic veins. Identification of chorionic artery and vein is most readily recognized by this interesting relationship because, as Benirschke points out, it is nearly impossible to distin-

guish the two by histological criteria. Immediately before or just after entering the chorionic plate, the two umbilical arteries are joined by a transverse connection, the *Hyrtl anastomosis,* which is rarely missing. The two umbilical arteries separate at the chorionic plate to supply branches to the cotyledons. There are two different patterns of chorionic artery branching: disperse (63 percent) and magistral (37 percent). The pattern of distribution in the disperse type is that of a fine network of vessels that traverse from the site of insertion of the umbilical cord to the various cotyledons. The magistral pattern is characterized by arteries that traverse to the edge of the placenta without an appreciable decrease in the diameter of the vessel. The arteries are end arteries, supplying one cotyledon, as the branch turns downward to pierce the chorionic plate.

The truncal arteries are the perforating branches of the surface arteries that pass through the chorionic plate. Each truncal artery supplies one cotyledon. There is a decrease in smooth muscle of the vessel wall and an increase in the caliber of the vessel as it penetrates through the basal plate; the loss in smooth muscle continues as the truncal arteries branch into the rami; the same is true of the vein walls.

At about 10 postconceptional weeks, the pattern of umbilical blood velocity waveforms changes abruptly (Fisk and colleagues, 1988; Loquet and associates, 1988). Before this time, there are no "end-diastolic frequencies." Later in gestation, this finding would be considered abnormal. Maulik (1996) provided an excellent review of these findings.

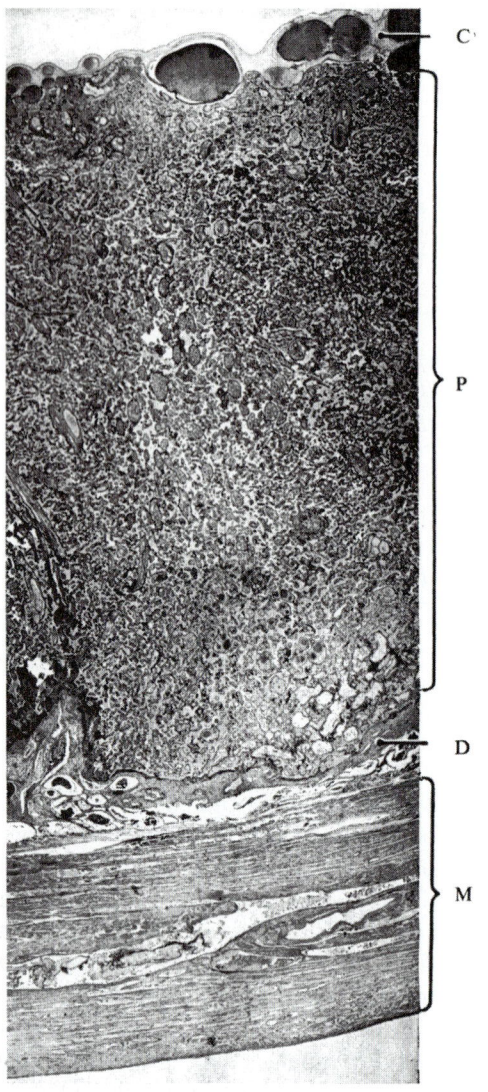

FIGURE 5–14. Section of placenta and uterus through **B** in Figure 5–12. (C = chorionic plate with fetal blood vessels; D = decidua basalis; M = myometrium; P = placental villi.)

The "definitive" chorionic plate also is formed by 8 to 10 weeks as the amnionic and primary chorionic plate mesenchyme fuse with each other. This is accomplished by expansion of the amnionic sac, which also surrounds the connective stalk and the allantois and joins these structures to form the umbilical cord (Kaufmann and Scheffen, 1992). There is another curious feature of the chorionic vessels; the thickness of the wall of these vessels is asymmetric, being much thinner on the side contiguous with the amnion (the fetal side).

MATERNAL CIRCULATION. Fetal homeostasis is dependent on an efficient maternal–placental circulation. Consequently investigators have sought to define the factors that regulate the flow of blood into and from the intervillous space. An adequate theory must explain how (1) blood can leave the maternal circulation; (2) flow into an amorphous space (lined by trophoblast syncytium, rather than capillary endothelium; and (3) return through maternal veins without producing arteriovenous-like shunts that would prevent maternal blood from remaining in contact with the villi long enough for adequate exchange. It was not until the studies of Ramsey and co-workers (1963, 1966) that a physiological explanation of the placental circulation, consistent with both experimental and clinical findings, was available (Fig. 5–16). These investigators discarded the crude corrosion technique of previous researchers, and proved, by careful, slow injections of radiocontrast material under low pressure, which avoided disruption of the circulation, that the arterial entrances as well as the venous exits are scattered at random over the entire base of the placenta.

The physiological particulars of the maternal–placental circulation are as follows. Maternal blood enters through the basal plate and is driven high up toward the chorionic plate by the head of maternal arterial pressure before lateral dispersion occurs (Fig. 5–16). After bathing the external microvillus surface of chorionic villi, the maternal blood drains back through venous orifices in the basal plate and enters the uterine veins. Therefore, maternal blood traverses the placenta randomly without performed channels, propelled by the maternal arterial pressure. Generally the spiral arteries are perpendicular to, but the veins are parallel to, the uterine wall, an arrangement that facilitates closure of the veins during a uterine contraction and prevents squeezing of essential maternal blood from the intervillous space. According to Brosens and Dixon (1963), there are about 120 spiral arterial entries into the intervillous space of the human placenta at term, discharging blood in spurts that displace the adjacent villi, as described by Borell and co-workers (1958).

Ramsey's concept is supported by the findings of numerous arteriographic studies. Clearly, the spiral arterial spurts are associated with the "lakes," and the closure of uteroplacental veins is affected by pressure produced at the beginning of uterine contractions. She found that with myometrial contractions there is a slight delay in the appearance of contrast medium in the veins of the uterine wall with injection during a strong contraction. The pressure in the intervillous space may be decreased sufficiently so that blood cannot be expressed against the prevailing myometrial pressure. Ramsey provided further evidence of independent activity of the uteroplacental (spiral) arteries, as indicated by the appearance of spurts in different locations even when injections were performed under conditions of minimal myometrial pressure. Not all endometrial spiral arteries are continuously patent, nor do all spiral arteries neces-

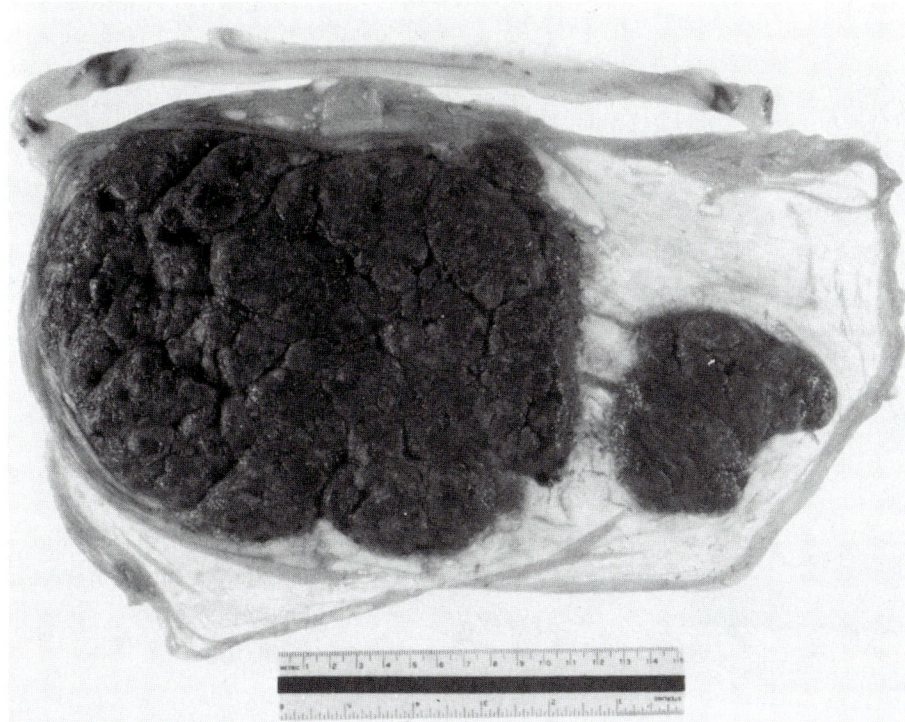

FIGURE 5–15. Maternal surface of term placenta. Variably discrete, irregularly shaped adjacent lobes are evident plus a large separate (succenturiate) lobe.

sarily discharge blood into the intervillous space simultaneously.

In summary, Ramsey found that maternal blood enters the intervillous space in spurts produced by the maternal blood pressure. The *vis a tergo* forces blood in discrete streams toward the chorionic plate until the head of pressure is reduced. Lateral spread then occurs. The continuing influx of arterial blood exerts pressure on the contents of the intervillous space, pushing the blood toward exits in the basal plate, from which it is drained through uterine veins. During uterine contractions, both inflow and outflow are curtailed, although the volume of blood in the intervillous space is maintained, thus providing for continual, albeit reduced, exchange.

Bleker and associates (1975) used serial sonography during normal labor and found that the length, thickness, and surface of the placenta increased during contractions. They attributed these changes to distension of the intervillous spaces by blood as the consequence of relatively greater impairment of venous outflow compared with arterial inflow. During contractions, therefore, a somewhat larger volume of blood is available for exchange even though the rate of flow is decreased. Subsequently, by use of Doppler velocimetry, it was shown that diastolic flow velocity in spiral arteries is diminished during uterine contractions. Therefore, the principal factors regulating blood flow in the intervillous space are arterial blood pressure, intrauterine pressure,

the pattern of uterine contractions, and factors that act specifically upon the arteriolar walls.

Ramsey and Donner (1980) presented a summary of anatomical studies of the uteroplacental vasculature. Cytotrophoblastic elements are initially confined to the terminal portions of the uteroplacental arteries. By the 16th week, cytotrophoblasts are found in many of the arteries of the inner layer of myometrium. The accumulation of trophoblasts may ultimately stop circulation through some of these vessels. The number of arterial openings into the intervillous space is gradually reduced by cytotrophoblasts and by breaching of the walls of the more proximal parts of the arteries by deeply penetrating trophoblasts. After the 30th week, a prominent venous plexus separates the decidua basalis from the myometrium (Fig. 5–16), thus participating in providing a plane of cleavage for placental separation.

THE AMNION

The amnion at term is a tough and tenacious but pliable membrane. It is the innermost fetal membrane and is contiguous with the amnionic fluid. This particular avascular structure occupies a role of incredible importance in human pregnancy. In many obstetrical populations, preterm premature rupture of the fetal membranes is the single most common antecedent of preterm delivery (Chap. 11, p. 281). The amnion is the tissue that provides

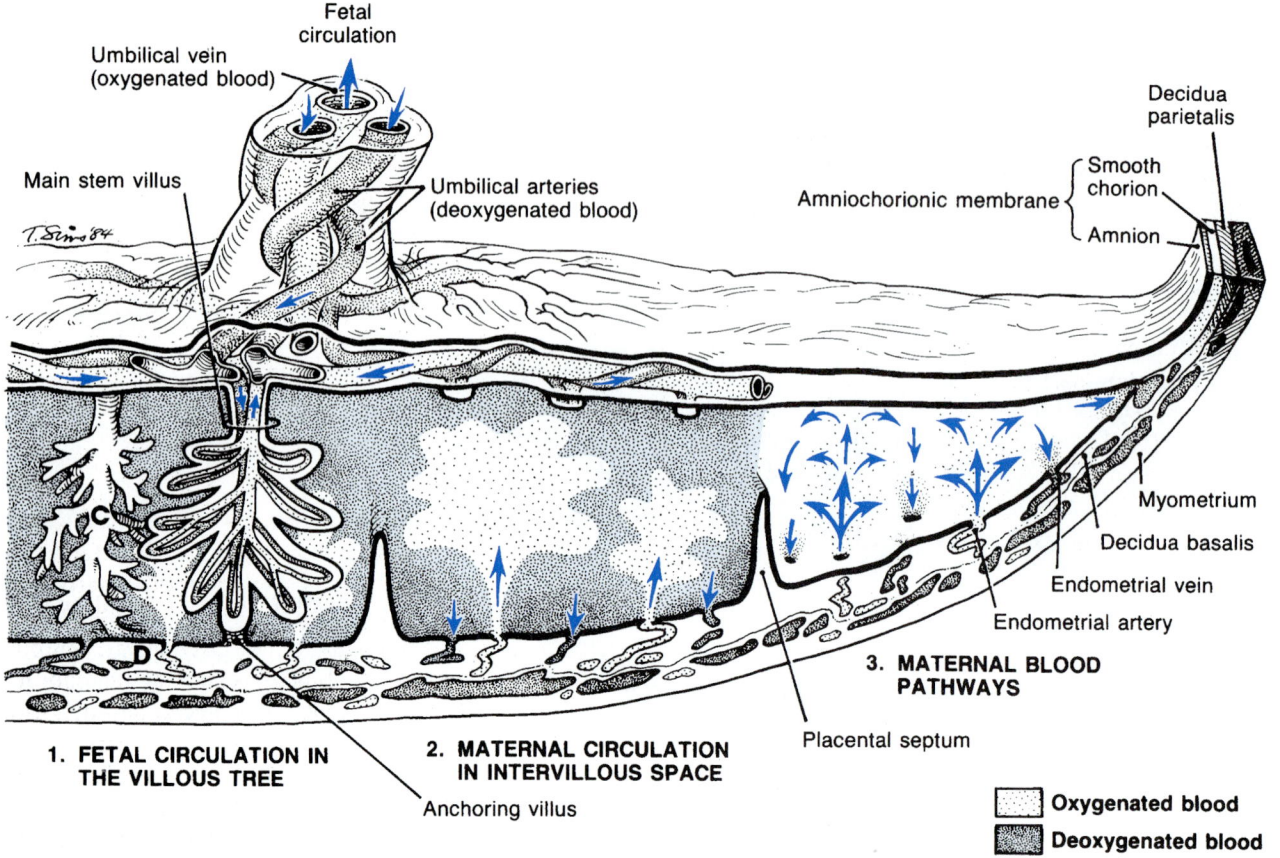

FIGURE 5–16. Schematic drawing of a section through a full-term placenta: **1.** The relation of the villous chorion (C) to the decidua basalis (D) and the fetal–placental circulation. **2.** The maternal blood flows into the intervillous spaces in funnel-shaped spurts, and exchanges occur with the fetal blood as the maternal blood flows around the villi. **3.** The inflowing arterial blood pushes venous blood into the endometrial veins, which are scattered over the entire surface of the decidua basalis. Note also that the umbilical arteries carry deoxygenated fetal blood to the placenta and that the umbilical vein carries oxygenated blood to the fetus. The cotyledons are separated from each other by placental (decidual) septa. Each cotyledon consists of two or more mainstem villi and their many branches. (Based on Moore, 1988.)

almost all of the tensile strength of the fetal membranes. Therefore, the development of the component(s) of the amnion that protects against rupture or tearing is vitally important to successful pregnancy outcome.

STRUCTURE. Bourne (1962) described five separate layers of amnion tissue. The inner surface, which is bathed by the amnionic fluid, is an uninterrupted, single layer of cuboidal epithelial cells, believed to be derived from embryonic ectoderm. This epithelium is attached firmly to a distinct basement membrane that is connected to the acellular compact layer, which is composed primarily of interstitial collagens I, III, and V. On the outer side of the compact layer, there is a row of fibroblast-like mesenchymal cells (which are widely dispersed at term). These cells are probably derived from mesoderm of the embryonic disc. There also are a few fetal macrophages in the amnion. The outermost layer

of amnion is the relatively acellular zona spongiosa, which is contiguous with the second fetal membrane, the chorion laeve. The important "missing" elements of human amnion are smooth muscle cells, nerves, lymphatics, and importantly, blood vessels.

DEVELOPMENT. Early in the process of implantation, a space develops between the embryonic cell mass and adjacent trophoblasts (Fig. 5–5). Small cells that line this inner surface of trophoblasts have been called amniogenic cells, the precursors of the amnionic epithelium. The human amnion is first identifiable about the seventh or eighth day of embryo development. Initially, a minute vesicle (Fig. 5–5), the amnion, develops into a small sac that covers the dorsal surface of the embryo. As the amnion enlarges, it gradually engulfs the growing embryo, which prolapses into its cavity (Benirschke and Kaufman, 2000).

Distension of the amnionic sac eventually brings it into contact with the interior surface of the chorion laeve. Apposition of the mesoblasts of chorion laeve and amnion near the end of the first trimester then causes an obliteration of the extraembryonic coelom. The amnion and chorion laeve, though slightly adherent, are never intimately connected, and usually can be separated easily, even at term.

AMNION CELL HISTOGENESIS. It is now generally accepted that the epithelial cells of the amnion are derived from fetal ectoderm of the embryonic disc. They do not arise by delamination from trophoblasts. This is an important consideration from both the embryological and the functional perspectives. For example, HLA class I gene expression in amnion is more akin to that in cells of the embryo than that in trophoblasts.

In addition to the epithelial cells that line the innermost (amnionic fluid) side of the amnion, there is a layer of fibroblast-like (mesenchymal) cells, which also are likely derived from embryonic mesoderm. Early in human embryogenesis, the mesenchymal cells of the amnion lie immediately adjacent to the basilar surface of the epithelium. At this time, therefore, the amnion surface is a two cell–layer structure with approximately equal numbers of epithelial and mesenchymal cells. Simultaneously with growth and development, interstitial collagens are deposited between these two layers of cells. This marks the commencement of the formation of the compact layer of the amnion, which also brings about a distinct separation of the two layers of amnion cells. As the amnionic sac expands to envelop the placenta and then the chorion frondosum at about 10 to 14 weeks, there is a progressive reduction in the compactness of the mesenchymal cells. These cells continue to separate and in the process become rather sparsely distributed. It appears that early in pregnancy the epithelial cells of the amnion replicate at a rate appreciably faster than the mesenchymal cells. At term, the epithelial cells form a continuous uninterrupted epithelium on the fetal surface of the amnion. The mesenchymal cells, however, are widely dispersed, being connected by a fine lattice network of extracellular matrix with the appearance of long slender fibrils.

AMNION EPITHELIAL CELLS. Epithelial cells line the entire inner (amnionic fluid) side of all portions of the amnionic membrane. These are the cells usually referred to and those studied most commonly in investigations of amnion function. The apical surface of the epithelial cells is replete with highly developed microvilli, consistent with a major site of transfer between amnionic fluid and amnion (Fig. 5–17). They also are active metabolically; for example, these epithelial cells of amnion are the site of preferential synthesis of tissue inhibitor of metalloproteinase-1 (Rowe and associates, 1997).

AMNION MESENCHYMAL CELLS. The mesenchymal cells of the fibroblast layer of amnion are responsible for major amnion functions. The synthesis of interstitial collagens that make up the compact layer of the amnion, the source of the majority of tensile strength of this membrane, takes place in mesenchymal cells (Casey and MacDonald, 1996). These cells also are highly capable of synthesizing cytokines to include interleukin (IL)-6, IL-8, and monocyte chemoattractant protein-1 (MCP-1). Their synthesis is increased in response to bacterial toxins and interleukin-1. This functional capacity of amnion mesenchymal cells is an important consideration in the study of amnionic fluid for evidence of labor-associated accumulation of inflammatory mediators (Garcia-Velasco and Arici, 1999).

ANATOMY. Reflected amnion is fused to the chorion laeve. Placental amnion covers the fetal surface of the placenta, and thereby is in contact with the adventitial surface of the chorionic vessels, which traverse the chorionic plate and branch into the cotyledons. Umbilical amnion covers the umbilical cord. In the conjoined portion of the membranes of diamnionic–dichorionic twin placentae, the fused amnions are separated by fused chorion laeve; and aside from the small area of the fetal membranes immediately over the cervical os, this is the only site at which the reflected chorion laeve is not contiguous with decidua. With diamnionic–monochorionic placentae, there is no intervening tissue between the fused amnions of each twin.

TENSILE STRENGTH. More than 125 years ago, Matthew Duncan (1868) examined the nature of the forces involved in fetal membrane rupture. During tests of tensile strength—resistance to tearing and rupture—he found that the decidua and then the chorion laeve gave way long before the amnion ruptured. Indeed, the membranes are quite elastic and can expand to twice normal size during pregnancy (Benirschke and Kauffman, 2000). The amnion provides the major strength of the membranes. Moreover, the tensile strength of amnion resides almost exclusively in the compact layer, which is comprised of cross-linked interstitial collagens I, III, and lesser amounts of V and VI.

INTERSTITIAL COLLAGENS. Collagens are the major macromolecules of most connective tissues and the most abundant proteins in the body. Collagen I is the major interstitial collagen in tissues characterized by great tensile strength such as bone and tendon. In other tissues, collagen III is believed to make a unique contribution to tissues integrity, serving to increase tissue extensibility as well as tensile strength. For example, the ratio of collagen III to collagen I in the walls of a number of highly extensible tissues—amnionic sac, blood ves-

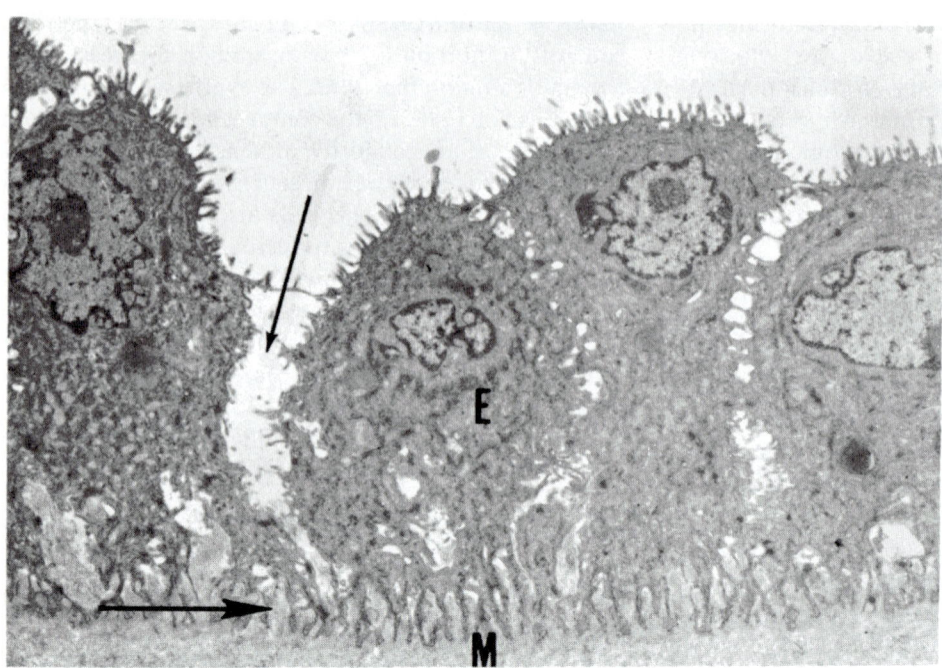

FIGURE 5–17. Electron micrograph of human amnion at term. Epithelium (E) and mesenchyme (M) are shown. Thin arrow indicates intercellular space. Thick arrow points to specializations of basal plasma membranes. (Courtesy of Dr. Ralph M. Wynn.)

sels, urinary bladder, bile ducts, intestine, and gravid uterus—is greater than that in nonelastic tissues. There is a high percentage of collagen III relative to collagen I in fetal skin, and as the proportion of collagen III decreases with fetal and newborn age, there is a parallel decrease in skin extensibility. Because there is little elastin in amnion, it is likely that collagen III provides the extensibility of this membrane. Another unique structural feature of interstitial collagens important to amnion integrity is resistance to proteolytic degradation (Jeffrey, 1991).

COLLAGEN SYNTHESIS IN AMNION. Interstitial amnionic collagens—types I and III—are produced primarily in mesenchymal cells (Casey and MacDonald, 1996, 1997). Epithelial cells, conversely, produce primarily basement membrane proteins such as procollagen IV, fibronectin, and laminin. The finding that metallothionein, a protein with high affinity for Cu^{2+}, is expressed in high amounts in amnion epithelial cells led to the hypothesis that decreased collagen synthesis may occur in women who smoke (King and colleagues, 1997). This is the proposed mechanism leading to the increased risk for prematurely ruptured membranes. Cadmium, inhaled in cigarette smoke, enters amnionic fluid and will act on amnion epithelial cells to induce high levels of metallothionein. As a result, Cu^{2+} deficiency may limit the activity of lysyl oxidase and hence the capacity of mesenchymal cells to form cross-linked collagens.

McLaren and associates (1999) and McParland and colleagues (2000) have identified unique changes in the morphology of the fetal membranes at the site of rupture. They found that modifications in the differentiation of cells in the chorion laeve in this specific area may weaken the fetal membranes. Whether these changes involve interstitial collagen content is not known.

METABOLIC FUNCTIONS. The amnion is clearly more than a simple avascular membrane that functions to contain amnionic fluid. It is metabolically active, involved in solute and water transport to maintain amnionic fluid homeostasis, and produces a variety of interesting bioactive compounds, including vasoactive peptides, growth factors, and cytokines.

VASOACTIVE PEPTIDES. A number of investigators have demonstrated the capacity of amnion to synthesize the vasoconstrictor endothelin-1 as well as vasorelaxant parathyroid hormone–related protein (Casey and associates, 1991, 1992; Germain and co-workers, 1992). Amnion epithelium also produces brain natriuretic peptide (BNP) and corticotropin-releasing hormone (CRH), and these two peptides also are smooth muscle relaxants (Itoh and associates, 1993, 1994; Riley and co-workers, 1991; Warren and Silverman, 1995). Thus, the vasoactive peptides produced in amnion may gain access to the adventitial surface of the chorionic vessels. These findings suggest that the placental amnion could become involved in modulating chorionic vessel tone and blood flow.

The amnion vasoactive peptides also function in other tissues in diverse physiological processes, including the promotion of cell replication and calcium metabolism. After secretion from the amnion, these bioactive agents can enter amnionic fluid and thereby are available to the fetus by swallowing and fetal thoracic movements.

AMNIONIC FLUID. The normally clear fluid that collects within the amnionic cavity increases in quantity as pregnancy progresses until near term, when there is a decrease in amnionic fluid volume in many normal pregnancies. An average volume of about 1000 mL is found at term, although this may vary widely from a few milliliters to many liters in abnormal conditions (oligohydramnios and polyhydramnios or hydramnios). The origin, composition, circulation, and function of the amnionic fluid are discussed further in Chapters 11 and 31.

UMBILICAL CORD AND RELATED STRUCTURES

DEVELOPMENT. The yolk sac and the umbilical vesicle into which it develops are quite prominent early in pregnancy. At first, the embryo is a flattened disc interposed between amnion and yolk sac (Fig. 5–6). Because the dorsal surface grows faster than the ventral surface, in association with the elongation of the neural tube, the embryo bulges into the amnionic sac and the dorsal part of the yolk sac is incorporated into the body of the embryo to form the gut. The allantois projects into the base of the body stalk from the caudal wall of the yolk sac or, later, from the anterior wall of the hindgut.

As pregnancy advances, the yolk sac becomes smaller and its pedicle relatively longer. By about the middle of the third month, the expanding amnion obliterates the exocoelom, fuses with the chorion laeve, and covers the bulging placental disc and the lateral surface of the body stalk, which is then called the umbilical cord, or funis. Remnants of the exocoelom in the anterior portion of the cord may contain loops of intestine, which continue to develop outside the embryo. Although the loops are later withdrawn, the apex of the midgut loop retains its connection with the attenuated vitelline duct. The duct terminates in a crumpled, highly vascular sac 3 to 5 cm in diameter lying on the surface of the placenta between amnion and chorion or in the membranes just beyond the placental margin, where occasionally it may be identified at term.

The cord at term normally has two arteries and one vein. The right umbilical vein usually disappears early during fetal development, leaving only the original left vein. Sections of any portion of the cord frequently reveal, near the center, the small duct of the umbilical vesicle, lined by a single layer of flattened or cuboid epithelial cells. In sections just beyond the umbilicus, but never at the maternal end of the cord, another duct representing the allantoic remnant is occasionally found. The intra-abdominal portion of the duct of the umbilical vesicle, which extends from umbilicus to intestine, usually atrophies and disappears, but occasionally it remains patent, forming a Meckel diverticulum. The most common vascular anomaly is the absence of one umbilical artery (Chap. 32, p. 832).

STRUCTURE AND FUNCTION. The umbilical cord, or funis, extends from the fetal umbilicus to the fetal surface of the placenta or chorionic plate. Its exterior is dull white, moist, and covered by amnion, through which three umbilical vessels may be seen. Its diameter is 0.8 to 2.0 cm, with an average length of 55 cm and a range of 30 to 100 cm. Generally, cord length less than 30 cm is considered abnormally short (Benirschke and Kauffman, 2000). Folding and tortuosity of the vessels, which are longer than the cord itself, frequently create nodulations on the surface, or false knots, which are essentially varices. The extracellular matrix, which is a specialized connective tissue, consists of Wharton jelly (Figs. 5–18 and 5–19). After fixation, the umbilical vessels appear empty, but Figure 5–19 more accurately is representative of the situation in vivo, when the vessels are not emptied of blood. The two arteries are smaller in diameter than the vein. When fixed in their normally distended state, the umbilical arteries exhibit transverse intimal *folds of Hoboken* across part of their lumens (Chacko and Reynolds, 1954). The mesoderm of the cord, which is of allantoic origin, fuses with that of the amnion.

Blood flows from the umbilical vein by two routes—the ductus venosus, which empties directly into the infe-

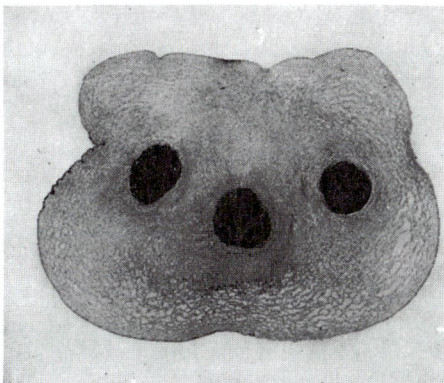

FIGURE 5–18. Cross section of umbilical cord fixed after blood vessels had been emptied. The umbilical vein, carrying oxygenated blood to the fetus, is in the center; on either side are two umbilical arteries carrying deoxygenated blood from the fetus to the placenta. (From Reynolds, 1954.)

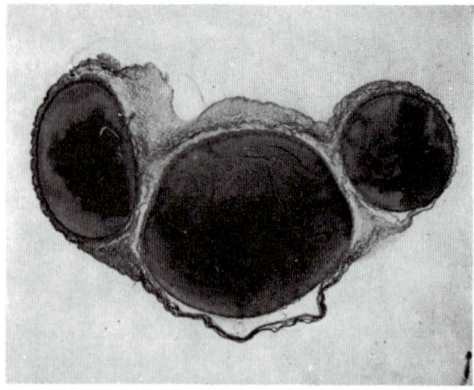

FIGURE 5–19. Cross section of the same umbilical cord shown in Figure 5–18, but through a segment from which the blood vessels had not been emptied. This photograph represents more accurately the conditions in utero. (From Reynolds, 1954.)

rior vena cava, and numerous smaller openings into the fetal hepatic circulation—and then into the inferior vena cava by the hepatic vein. The blood takes the path of least resistance through these alternate routes. Resistance in the ductus venosus is controlled by a sphincter situated at the origin of the ductus at the umbilical recess and innervated by a branch of the vagus nerve.

Anatomically, the umbilical cord can be regarded as a fetal membrane. The vessels contained in the cord are characterized by spiraling or twisting. The spiraling may occur in a clockwise (dextral) or anticlockwise (sinistral) direction. The anticlockwise spiral is present in 50 to 90 percent of cases. It is believed that the spiraling serves to attenuate "snarling," which occurs in all hollow cylinders subjected to torsion. Boyd and Hamilton (1970) note that these twists are not really spirals, but rather they are cylindrical helices in which a constant curvature is maintained equidistant from the central axis. Benirschke and Kauffman (2000) reported that 11 is the average number of helices in the cord.

REFERENCES

Benirschke K: Timing fetal injury: The role of the placenta. OBG Management, p. 72, March, 2000

Benirschke K, Kaufman P: Pathology of the Human Placenta, 4th ed. New York, Springer, 2000

Billingham RE: Transplantation immunity and the maternal-fetal relation. N Engl J Med 270:667, 1964

Bleker OP, Kloosterman GJ, Mieras DJ, Oosting J, Salle HJA: Intervillous space during uterine contractions in human subjects: An ultrasonic study. Am J Obstet Gynecol 123:697, 1975

Borell U, Fernstrom I, Westman A: An arteriographic study of the placental circulation. Geburtshilfe Frauenheilkd 18:1, 1958

Bourne GL: The Human Amnion and Chorion. Chicago, Year Book, 1962

Boyd JD, Hamilton WJ: The Human Placenta. Cambridge, England, Heffer, 1970

Brosens I, Dixon HG: The anatomy of the maternal side of the placenta. Br J Obstet Gynaecol 73:357, 1963

Casey ML, MacDonald PC: Lysyl oxidase (*ras* recision gene) expression in human amnion: Ontogeny and cellular localization. J Clin Endocrinol Metab 82:167, 1997

Casey ML, MacDonald PC: Interstitial collagen synthesis and processing in human amnion: A property of the mesenchymal cells. Biol Reprod 55:1253, 1996

Casey ML, Mibe M, Erk A, MacDonald PC: Transforming growth factor-β stimulation of parathyroid hormone-related protein expression in human uterine cells in culture: mRNA levels and protein secretion. J Clin Endocrinol Metab 74:950, 1992

Casey ML, Word RA, MacDonald PC: Endothelin-1 gene expression and regulation of endothelin mRNA and protein biosynthesis in avascular human amnion. J Biol Chem 266:5762, 1991

Chacko AW, Reynolds SRM: Architecture of distended and nondistended human umbilical cord tissues, with special references to the arteries and veins. Contrib Embryol 35:135, 1954

Ciaranfi A, Curchod A, Odartchenko N: Survie de lymphocytes foetaux dans de sang maternal postpartum. Schweiz Med Wschr 107:134, 1977

Coutifaris C, Coukos G: Fertilization and implantation. In Bruner JP (ed): Endocrinology of Pregnancy. In Diamond MP, Decherney AH (eds): Infertility and Reproductive Medicine Clinics of North America, Vol XV. Philadelphia, Saunders, 1994, p 571

Craven CM, Zhao L, Ward K: Lateral placental growth occurs by trophoblast cell invasion of decidual veins. Placenta 21:160, 2000

Crawford JM: A study of human placental growth with observations on the placenta in erythroblastosis foetalis. Br J Obstet Gynaecol 66:855, 1959

Desai RG, Creger WP: Maternofetal passage of leukocytes and platelets in man. Blood 21:665, 1963

Dizon-Townson DS, Lu J, Morgan TK, Ward KJ: Genetic expression by fetal chorionic villi during the first trimester of human gestation. Am J Obstet Gynecol 183:706, 2000

Feinberg RF, Kliman HJ, Lockwood CJ: Is oncofetal fibronectin a trophoblast glue for human implantation? Am J Pathol 138:537, 1991

Feinberg RF, Kliman HJ, Wang CL: Transforming growth factor-beta stimulates trophoblast oncofetal fibronectin synthesis in vitro: Implications for trophoblast implantation in vivo. J Clin Endocrinol Metab 78:1241, 1994

Fisk NM, Maclachlan N, Ellis C, Tannirandorm Y, Tonge HM, Rodeck CH: Absent endodiastolic flow in first trimester umbilical artery. Lancet 2:1256, 1988

Frenette PS, Wagner DD: Adhesion molecules—part I. N Engl J Med 334:1526, 1996

Garcia-Velasco JA, Arici A: Chemokines and human reproduction. Fertil Steril 71:983, 1999

Germain AM, Attaroglu H, MacDonald PC, Casey ML: Parathyroid hormone-related protein mRNA in avascular human amnion. J Clin Endocrinol Metab 75:1173, 1992

Goldman-Wohl DS, Ariel I, Greenfield C, Hochner-Celnikier D, Cross J, Fisher S, Yagel S: Lack of human leukocyte antigen-G expression in extravillous trophoblasts is associated with peeclampsia. Mol Hum Reprod 6:88, 2000

Hamilton WJ, Boyd JD: Trophoblast in human utero-placental arteries. Nature 212:906, 1966

Hertig AT: The placenta: Some new knowledge about an old organ. Obstet Gynecol 20:859, 1962

Hertig AT, Rock J: Two human ova of the pre-villous stage, having a developmental age of about seven and nine days respectively. Contrib Embryol 31:65, 1945

Hertig AT, Rock J: On the development of the early human ovum, with special reference to the trophoblast of the pre-villous stage: A description of 7 normal and 5 pathologic human ova. Am J Obstet Gynecol 47:149, 1944

Hertig AT, Rock J, Adams EC, Mulligan WJ: On the preimplantation stages of the human ovum. Contrib Embryol 35:199, 1954

Hunt JS, Jadhav L, Chu W, Geraghty DE, Ober C: Soluble HLA-G circulates in maternal blood during pregnancy. Am J Obstet Gynecol 183:682, 2000

Hunt JS, Orr HT: HLA and maternal-fetal recognition. FASEB J 6:2344, 1992

Itoh H, Sagawa N, Hasegawa M, Inamori K, Ueda H, Kitagawa K, Nanno H, Ihara Y, Kobayashi F, Mori T, Suga S, Yoshimasa T, Itoh H, Nakao K: Transforming growth factor-beta stimulates, and glucocorticoids and epidermal growth factor inhibit, brain natriuretic peptide scretion from cultured human amnion cells. J Clin Endocrinol Metab 79:176, 1994

Itoh H, Sagawa N, Hasegawa M, Okagaki A, Inamori K, Ihara Y, Mori T, Ogawa Y, Suga S, Mukoyama M, Nakao K, Imura H: Brain natriuretic peptide is present in the human amniotic fluid and is secreted from amnion cells. J Clin Endocrinol Metab 76:907, 1993

Jeffrey JJ: Collagen and collagenase: Pregnancy and parturition. Semin Perinatol 15:118, 1991

Johnson PM, Christmas SE, Vince GS: Immunological aspects of implantation and implantation failure. Hum Reprod 2:26, 1999

Jokhi PP, King A, Loke YW: Production of granulocyte-macrophage colony-stimulating factor by human trophoblast cells and by decidual large granular lymphocytes. Hum Reprod 9:1660, 1994

Kaufmann P, Scheffen I: Placental development. In Polin RA, Fox WW (eds): Fetal and Neonatal Physiology. Philadelphia, Saunders, 1992, p 47

Kilburn BA, Wang J, Duniec-Dmuchkowski ZM, Leach RE, Romero R, Armant DR: Extracellular matrix composition and hypoxia regulate the expression of HLA-G and integrins in a human trophoblast celline. Biol Reprod 62:739, 2000

King A, Loke YW: On the nature and function of human uterine granular lymphocytes. Immunol Today 12:432, 1991

King BF, Menton DN: Scanning electron microscopy of human placental villi from early and late in gestation. Am J Obstet Gynecol 122:824, 1975

King LA, MacDonald PC, Casey ML: Regulation of metallothionein expression in human amnion epithelial and mesenchymal cells. Am J Obstet Gynecol 177:1496, 1997

Kliman HJ, Nestler JE, Sermasi E, Sanger JM, Strauss JF: Purification, characterization, and in vitro differentiation of cytotrophoblasts from human term placenta. Endocrinology 118:1567, 1986

LeBouteiller P, Solier C, Proll J, Aguerre-Girr M, Fournel S, Lenfant F: Placental HLA-G protein expression in vivo: Where and what for? Hum Reprod Update 5:223, 1999

Lockwood CJ, Senyei AE, Dische MR, Casal D, Shah KD, Thung SN, Jones L, Deligdisch L, Garite TJ: Fetal fibronectin in cervical and vaginal secretions as a predictor of preterm delivery. N Engl J Med 325:669, 1991

Loke YM, King A: In: Human Implantation. Cell Biology and Immunology. Cambridge, England, Cambridge University Press, 1995, p 82

Loquet P, Broughton-Pipkin F, Symonds EM, Rubin PC: Blood velocity waveforms and placental vascular formation. Lancet 2:1252, 1988

Maulik D: Doppler ultrasound in obstetrics. Williams Obstetrics, 19th ed (Suppl 16). Stamford, CT, Appleton & Lange, 1996, p 1

McKenna DS, Chung K, Iams JD: Effect of digital cervical examination on the expression of fetal fibronectin. J Reprod Med 44:796, 1999

McLaren J, Malak TM, Bell SC: Structural characteristics of term human fetal membranes prior to labour: Identification of an area of altered morphology overlying the cervix. Hum Reprod 14:237, 1999

McMaster MT, Librach CL, Zhou Y, Lim KH, Janatpour MJ, DeMars R, Kovats S, Damsky C, Fisher SJ: Human placental HLA-G expression is restricted to differentiated cytotrophoblasts. J Immunol 154:3771, 1995

McParland PC, Taylor DJ, Bell SC: Myofibroblast differentiation in the connective tissues of the amnion and chorion of term human fetal membranes: Implications for fetal membrane rupture and labour. Placenta 21:44, 2000

Medawar PB: Some immunological and endocrinological problems raised by the evolution of viviparity in vertebrates. Symp Soc Exp Biol 44:320, 1953

Moore KL: The Developing Human: Clinically Oriented Embryology, 4th ed. Philadelphia, Saunders, 1988

Moore KL: The Developing Human: Clinically Oriented Embryology, 1st ed. Philadelphia, Saunders, 1973

Ramsey EM, Davis RW: A composite drawing of the placenta to show its structure and circulation. Anat Rec 145:366, 1963

Ramsey EM, Donner MW: Placental Vascular and Circulation. Philadelphia, Saunders, 1980

Ramsey EM, Harris JWS: Comparison of uteroplacental vasculature and circulation in the rhesus monkey and man. Contrib Embryol 38:59, 1966

Reynolds SRM: Hemodynamic characteristics of the fetal circulation. Am J Obstet Gynecol 68:69, 1954

Riley SC, Walton JC, Herlick JM, Challis JR: The localization and distribution of corticotropin-releasing hormone in the human placenta and fetal membranes throughout gestation. J Clin Endocrinol Metab 72:1001, 1991

Ringler GE, Strauss III JF: In vitro systems for the study of human placental endocrine function. Endocr Rev 11:105, 1990

Rowe TF, King LA, MacDonald PC, Casey ML: Tissue inhibitor of metalloproteinase-1 and tissue inhibitor of metalloproteinase-2 expression in human amnion mesenchymal and epithelial cells. Am J Obstet Gynecol 176:915, 1997

Streeter GL: A human embryo (Mateer) of the presomite period. Contrib Embryol 9:389, 1920

Thomson AM, Billewicz WZ, Hytten FE: The weight of the placenta in relation to birthweight. Br J Obstet Gynaecol 76:865, 1969

Ulloa-Aguirre A, August AM, Golos TG, Kao LC, Sakuragi N, Kliman HJ, Strauss JF: 8-Bromo-adenosinc 3′,5′-monophosphate regulates expression of chorionic gonadotropin and fibronectin in human cytotrophoblasts. J Clin Endocrinol Metab 64:1002, 1987

Warren WB, Silverman AJ: Cellular localization of cortico-trophin releasing hormone in the human placenta, fetal membranes and decidua. Placenta 16:147, 1995

Weetman AP: The immunology of pregnancy. Thyroid 9:643, 1999

Wislocki GB, Dempsey EW: Electron microscopy of the human placenta. Anat Rec 123:133, 1955

Witebsky ES, Reich H: Zur gruppenspezifischen Differenzierung der Placentarorgan. Klin Wochenschr 11:1960, 1932

6

The Placental Hormones

The production of steroid and protein hormones by human trophoblasts is greater in amount and diversity than that of any endocrine tissue known in all of mammalian physiology. In a few species, for example, the horse, during pregnancy, estrogen but not progesterone formation, is high. In others, for example, rat and mouse, progesterone production is relatively high but estrogen is not. A variety of protein hormones of the prolactin–growth hormone–placental lactogen family are synthesized in the placenta of most mammals, including humans. But incredible amounts of chorionic gonadotropin are produced in the syncytium only in primates and equids.

A unique and obligatory relationship was discovered between the incredible hyperestrogenic state of human pregnancy and the fetal adrenal secretion of very large quantities of C_{19}-steroids which serve as plasma-borne precursors for estrogen synthesis. An interactive system also has been identified by which human syncytiotrophoblast takes up maternal plasma low-density lipoprotein (LDL)-cholesterol for use in progesterone biosynthesis.

A compendium of the average production rates for various steroid hormones in nonpregnant and in near-term pregnant women is given in Table 6–1. It is readily apparent that the alterations in steroid hormone production that accompany normal human pregnancy are incredible.

The human placenta also synthesizes an enormous amount of protein and peptide hormones: approximately 1 gram of placental lactogen (hPL) each 24 hours, massive quantities of chorionic gonadotropin (hCG),

chorionic adrenocorticotropin (ACTH) as well as other products of proopiomelanocortin, chorionic thyrotropin, growth hormone variant, parathyroid hormone–related protein (PTH-rP), calcitonin, and relaxin; and a variety of hypothalamic-like releasing and inhibiting hormones, including thyrotropin-releasing hormone (TRH), gonadotropin-releasing hormone (GnRH), corticotropin-releasing hormone (CRH), somatostatin, and growth hormone–releasing hormone (GHRH). The human placenta also produces inhibins, activins, and atrial natriuretic peptide.

It is understandable, therefore, that yet another remarkable feature of human pregnancy is the success of the physiological adaptations of pregnant women to a most unusual endocrine milieu (Chap. 8). The anatomical parts of the endocrine system of the placental arm of the fetal–maternal communication system are illustrated in Figure 6–1.

HUMAN CHORIONIC GONADOTROPIN (hCG)

The "pregnancy hormone" is a glycoprotein with biological activity very similar to luteinizing hormone (LH), both of which act via the plasma membrane LH/hCG receptor. HCG is produced almost exclusively in the placenta, but is synthesized in fetal kidney, and a number of fetal tissues produce the β-subunit or intact hCG molecule (McGregor and associates, 1981, 1983).

A variety of malignant tumors also produce hCG, sometimes in reasonably large amounts—especially neoplastic trophoblasts. HCG is produced in very small amounts in tissues of men and nonpregnant women, perhaps primarily in the anterior pituitary gland. Nonetheless, the detection of hCG in blood or urine is almost always indicative of pregnancy (Chap. 2, p. 26).

CHEMICAL CHARACTERISTICS. HCG is a glycoprotein (M_r about 36,700) with the highest carbohydrate (30 percent) content of any human hormone. The carbohydrate component, and especially the terminal sialic acid, protects the molecule from catabolism. The plasma half-life of intact hCG (24 hours) is much longer than that of LH (2 hours).

The hCG molecule is composed of two dissimilar subunits, designated α (92 amino acids) and β (145 amino acids), which are noncovalently linked. They are held together by electrostatic and hydrophobic forces that can be separated in vitro. There is no intrinsic LH-like biological activity of either separated subunit because neither subunit binds to the LH receptor.

HCG is related structurally to three other glycoprotein hormones—LH, follicle-stimulating hormone (FSH), and thyroid-stimulating hormone (TSH). The amino acid sequence of the α-subunits of these four

TABLE 6–1. Steroid Production Rates in Nonpregnant and Near-Term Pregnant Women

Steroid[a]	Production Rates (mg/24 hr)	
	Nonpregnant	Pregnant
Estradiol-17β	0.1–0.6	15–20
Estriol	0.02–0.1	50–150
Progesterone	0.1–40	250–600
Aldosterone	0.05–0.1	0.250–0.600
Deoxycorticosterone	0.05–0.5	1–12
Cortisol	10–30	10–20

[a]Estrogens and progesterone are produced by placenta. Aldosterone is produced by the maternal adrenal glands in response to the stimulus of angiotensin II. Deoxycorticosterone is produced in extraglandular tissue sites by way of the 21-hydroxylation of plasma progesterone. Cortisol production during pregnancy is not increased, even though the blood levels are elevated because of decreased clearance caused by increased cortisol-binding globulin.

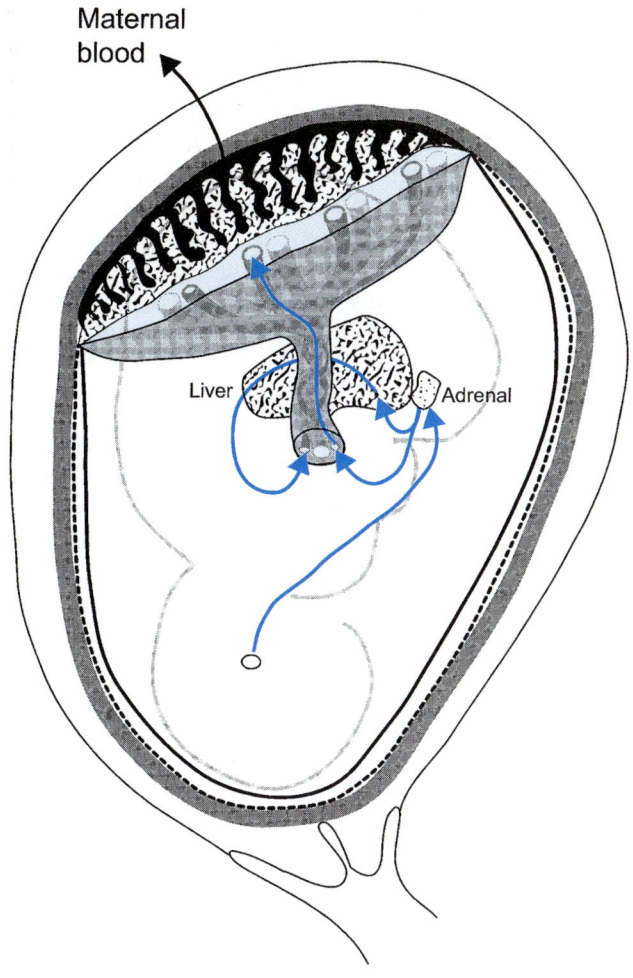

Maternal blood

Liver

Adrenal

FIGURE 6–1. Anatomical parts of the endocrine component of the placental arm of the fetal–maternal communication system. Adrenocorticotropin hormone (ACTH) from the fetal pituitary gland stimulates fetal adrenal steroidogenesis. Fetal adrenal dehydroepiandrosterone sulfate and 16α-OH-dehydroepiandrosterone sulfate are transported to the placenta and converted to estradiol-17β and estriol, respectively (Fig. 6–3). Fetal liver is the major site of production of low-density lipoprotein (LDL) cholesterol, the principal precursor for fetal adrenal steroidogenesis. Cholesterol, derived from LDL in maternal plasma, serves as the precursor for progesterone biosynthesis in placenta.

glycoproteins is identical; but the β-subunits of FSH and TSH, as well as those of hCG and LH, while sharing certain similarities, are characterized by distinctly different amino acid sequences. Recombination of an α- and a β-subunit of the four glycoprotein hormones gives a molecule with biological activity characteristic of the hormone from which the β-subunit was derived.

BIOSYNTHESIS. The synthesis of the α- and β-chains of hCG is regulated separately. A single gene—on chromosome 6 at q12–q21—codes for the α-subunit of all four glycoprotein hormones. There are eight separate genes on chromosome 19 for the β-hCG/β-LH family. Seven of these genes code for β-hCG and one for β-LH, but only three of the β-hCG genes are expressed. Both the α- and β-subunits of hCG are synthesized as larger molecular weight precursors which are cleaved by microsomal endopeptidases. Once intact hCG is assembled, the molecule is rapidly released from the cell but its regulation is not understood.

The rate of synthesis of the β-subunit of hCG is believed to be limiting in the formation of the complete molecule. Trophoblasts of normal placenta and those of hydatidiform mole and choriocarcinoma tissues secrete free α- and β-subunits as well as intact hCG; but there is an excess of hCG α-subunits in placenta and in plasma. The hCG free β-subunit, however, is present in plasma in only small quantities.

CELLULAR SITES OF ORIGIN. The complete hCG molecule is synthesized primarily in the syncytiotrophoblast. It has been demonstrated, however, that immunoreactive hCG is present in cytotrophoblasts before 6 weeks. Thereafter, hCG is localized almost exclusively in the syncytium. A similar cellular distribution for immunoreactive hPL in early pregnancy also has been reported (Maruo and associates, 1992).

REGULATION OF hCG SUBUNIT BIOSYNTHESIS. The amounts of mRNA for both the α- and β-subunits of hCG in syncytiotrophoblast from the first trimester are greater than at term. This may be an important consideration in the measurement of hCG in plasma as a screening procedure to identify abnormal fetuses. The finding of mRNA for the α- and β-subunits of hCG in cytotrophoblasts or in intermediate trophoblasts is suggestive that the genes for hCG are expressed before full differentiation of the trophoblasts. Cytotrophoblasts begin to disappear from the placenta at the end of the first trimester; but in some abnormal pregnancies in which there is a reappearance of cytotrophoblasts, as with D-antigen isoimmunization and gestational diabetes, plasma levels of hCG may be increased.

MOLECULAR FORMS OF hCG IN PLASMA AND URINE. There are multiple forms of hCG in maternal plasma and urine. Some of these arise as the result of enzymatic degradation, and others are accounted for by modifications during the normal cellular sequence of synthesis/processing of the hCG molecule. The multiple forms of hCG vary enormously in bioactivity and immunoreactivity.

FREE SUBUNIT. As cited, the levels of the β-subunit in plasma are very low or undetectable throughout human pregnancy (see Fig. 2–6). In part, this finding is the result of the rate-limiting synthesis of the β-subunit.

Free α-subunits that do not combine with the β-subunit are found in placenta and maternal plasma. The increased size of the oligosaccharides of free α-subunits prevent dimerization with β-hCG. The plasma levels of free α-subunits increase gradually, but steadily, until about 36 weeks, when a plateau is attained that is maintained for the remainder of pregnancy. This pattern is similar to that of hPL in plasma (see Fig. 2–6). Thus, the secretion of α-hCG roughly corresponds to placental mass, whereas the rate of secretion of the complete hCG molecule is maximal at 8 to 10 weeks. The plasma concentration of α-hCG, however, is always much less (10 percent or less) than that of intact hCG.

NICKS IN THE hCG MOLECULE. During the past 10 years, it has been shown that many of the hCG molecules in serum and urine contain nicks, or missing peptide linkages. This is true of purified standard preparations and of individual samples from serum and urine as well. These nicks occur primarily between β-subunit amino acids 44–45 and 47–48. The extent of nicking in standard preparations from pooled urine is 10 to 20 percent, but in individual samples it varies from 0 to 100 percent. The origin of these nicks is believed to be through enzymatic action on the molecule that occurs near the cellular site of synthesis of the β-subunit. One example is that these reactions are catalyzed by leukocyte elastase. The biological importance of these nicked molecules is unknown, but the bioactivity of nicked hCG is diminished to about 20 percent and the immunoreactivity to monoclonal antibodies may be severely attenuated but variable (Cole and associates, 1991). This can be an issue of some concern when monitoring changes in the hCG levels if assays are conducted with different antibodies.

CONCENTRATIONS OF hCG IN SERUM AND URINE. The intact hCG molecule is detectable in plasma of pregnant women about 7 1/2 to 9 1/2 days after the midcycle surge of LH that precedes ovulation. Thus, it is likely that hCG enters maternal blood at the time of blastocyst implantation (Chap. 2, p. 27). Blood levels increase rapidly thereafter, with maximal levels being attained at about 8 to 10 weeks. Appreciable fluctuations in the levels of plasma hCG are observed on the same day, and evidence has accrued that the trophoblast secretion of protein hormones is episodic.

Maternal urine concentration is closely parallel to that in plasma, which is approximately 1 IU/mL by 6 weeks after the commencement of the last menstrual period, increasing to an average value of about 100 IU/mL between the 60th and 80th days after the last menses (see Fig. 2–6). The levels of hCG in plasma of pregnant women may reach 15 mg/mL. Beginning at about 10 to 12 weeks, the levels of hCG in maternal plasma begin to decline, a nadir being reached by about 20 weeks. The levels of hCG in plasma are maintained at this lower level for the remainder of pregnancy.

The pattern of appearance of hCG in fetal blood (as a function of gestational age) is similar to that in the mother, but the levels of hCG in fetal plasma are only about 3 percent of those in maternal plasma. The concentration of hCG in amnionic fluid early in pregnancy is similar to that in maternal plasma; but as pregnancy progresses, the concentration of hCG in amnionic fluid declines, so that near term, the levels are only a fifth those in maternal plasma.

ELEVATED OR DEPRESSED hCG LEVELS IN MATERNAL PLASMA OR URINE. Significantly higher plasma levels of hCG are sometimes found in pregnancies with multiple fetuses, and with a single erythroblastotic fetus resulting from maternal D-antigen isoimmunization. The levels of hCG in plasma and urine may be increased strikingly in women with hydatidiform mole or choriocarcinoma. Relatively higher levels of plasma hCG may be found at midtrimester with Down syndrome. The reason for this is not clear, but it has been speculated that the placenta in these pregnancies is less mature compared with those with normal fetuses. Relatively lower levels of hCG in plasma are found with ectopic pregnancies and impending spontaneous abortion.

REGULATION OF hCG SYNTHESIS. Placental GnRH is likely involved in the regulation of hCG formation. A role for placental inhibin in regulation of hCG also has been proposed. A large number of compounds act to increase hCG secretion by trophoblasts in vitro. Among these are derivatives of cyclic AMP, hypothalamic-like hormones (GnRH, CRH), some cytokines, various growth factors, colony-stimulating factors, and thyroid hormones. From this brief compilation, it is evident that the in vivo regulation of hCG synthesis is not yet clearly understood.

METABOLIC CLEARANCE OF hCG. The renal clearance of hCG accounts for 30 percent of metabolic clearance and the remainder is cleared by other pathways, likely by metabolism in liver and kidney (Nishula and Wehmann, 1980). Clearances of β-subunit and α-subunit are about 10-fold and 30-fold, respectively, greater than that of intact hCG. By contrast, renal clearance of subunits is considerably lower than that of dimeric hCG.

ASSAY OF hCG. The methods for detecting hCG in urine or blood are of considerable importance, because these assays form the basis for the vast majority of pregnancy tests (Chap. 2, p. 27).

BIOLOGICAL FUNCTIONS OF hCG. Both subunits of hCG are required for normal binding to the LH/hCG receptor. There are LH/hCG receptors in a variety of tissues other than the corpus luteum and the testis (Chap. 11, p. 272).

RESCUE OF THE CORPUS LUTEUM. The best known biological function of hCG is the "rescue" and maintenance of function of the corpus luteum—that is, continued progesterone production. Bradbury and colleagues (1950) found that the progesterone-producing life span of the corpus luteum of menstruation could be prolonged perhaps for 2 weeks by the administration of hCG to nonpregnant women. This action provides only an incomplete explanation for the physiological role of hCG in pregnancy. The maximum plasma hCG concentrations are attained at a time in gestation that is well after hCG-stimulated corpus luteum secretion of progesterone has ceased. Specifically, progesterone synthesis by the corpus luteum begins to decline at about 6 weeks despite continued and increasing hCG production.

HCG STIMULATION OF FETAL TESTIS. Fetal testicular secretion of testosterone is maximum at approximately the same time in gestation when the maximal levels of hCG are attained. Thus, at a critical time in sexual differentiation of the male fetus, hCG, entering fetal plasma from syncytiotrophoblast, acts as an LH surrogate, stimulating the replication of fetal testicular Leydig cells and testosterone synthesis to promote male sexual differentiation (Chap. 7, p. 158). Before about 110 days of human pregnancy, there is no vascularization of the fetal anterior pituitary from the hypothalamus, and thus little LH secretion from the pituitary. HCG acts as LH before this time. Thereafter, as hCG levels fall, pituitary LH maintains a lower level of fetal testicular stimulation.

HCG STIMULATION OF THE MATERNAL THYROID. In many women with hydatidiform mole or choriocarcinoma, biochemical and clinical evidence of hyperthyroidism sometimes develops (Chap. 32, p. 840). For a time it was believed that the formation of chorionic thyrotropins by the neoplastic trophoblasts was the cause of the hyperthyroid-like findings in these women. Later, however, it was shown that some forms of hCG bind to the TSH receptors of thyroid cells. Treatment of normal men with hCG increases thyroid activity. The thyroid-stimulatory activity in plasma of first-trimester pregnant women varies appreciably from sample to sample. Modifications in the oligosaccharides of hCG seem to be important in establishing the capacity of hCG to stimulate thyroid function. Some of the acidic isoforms of hCG stimulate thyroid activity, and some more basic

forms also stimulate iodine uptake (Kraiem and co-workers, 1994; Tsuruta and colleagues, 1995; Yoshimura and associates, 1994). There also is preliminary evidence that the LH/hCG receptor is expressed in the thyroid (Tomer and co-workers, 1992). Thus, the possibility exists that hCG stimulates thyroid activity via the LH/hCG receptor and by the TSH receptor as well.

OTHER PROPOSED FUNCTIONS. HCG acts in vivo to promote relaxin secretion by the corpus luteum. LH/hCG receptors are found in myometrium and in uterine vascular tissue, and it has been hypothesized that hCG may act to promote uterine vascular vasodilation and myometrial smooth muscle relaxation (Chap. 11).

HUMAN PLACENTAL LACTOGEN

Prolactin-like activity in the human placenta was first described by Ehrhardt in 1936. The protein responsible for this activity was isolated from extracts of human placenta and retroplacental blood and partially purified by Ito and Higashi (1961) and by Josimovich and MacLaren (1962). Because of the potent lactogenic and growth hormone-like bioactivity (and an immunochemical resemblance to human growth hormone), it was first called human placental lactogen or chorionic growth hormone. This hormone also has been referred to as chorionic somatomammotropin. Recently, most authors have used the original name, human placental lactogen (hPL). Grumbach and Kaplan (1964) found, by immunofluorescence studies, that this hormone, like hCG, was concentrated in the syncytiotrophoblast. HPL is detected in the trophoblast as early as the second or third week after fertilization of the ovum. It was originally believed that hPL in placenta was localized exclusively in the syncytiotrophoblast, indicating that the genes for hPL are expressed only in the fully differentiated trophoblast. This, however, does not appear to be the case; as with hCG, hPL is identified in cytotrophoblasts from before 6 weeks in pregnancy (Maruo and associates, 1992).

CHEMICAL CHARACTERISTICS. HPL is a single nonglycosylated polypeptide chain with a molecular weight of 22,279 d, which is derived from a precursor of 25,000 d that contains a 26 amino-acid signal sequence. There are 191 amino acid residues in placental lactogen, compared with 188 in human growth hormone; the amino acid sequence in each hormone is strikingly similar, with 96 percent homology. HPL also is structurally similar to human prolactin (hPRL), with about 67 percent amino-acid sequence homology. For these reasons, it has been suggested that the genes for hPL, hPRL, and hGH evolved from a common ancestral gene (probably PRL) by repeated gene duplication (Ogren and Talamantes, 1994).

HPL production is not restricted to the trophoblast. The hormone has been detected by direct radioimmunoassay in sera from men and women with various malignancies other than those originating in trophoblast or gonad, including bronchogenic carcinoma, hepatoma, lymphoma, and pheochromocytoma (Weintraub and Rosen, 1970).

GENE STRUCTURE AND EXPRESSION. There are five genes in the prolactin–growth hormone–placental lactogen gene family; these genes are linked and located on chromosome 17. Two of these genes, hCS-A and hCS-B, both code for hPL, and the amount of mRNA in the term placenta is similar for each. The gene for hPRL (prolactin) is located on chromosome 6 (Owerbach and co-workers, 1980, 1981).

SECRETION AND METABOLISM. HPL accounts for 7 to 10 percent of the proteins synthesized by placental ribosomes at term. In fact, 5 percent of the mRNA of term placenta is hPL mRNA. The production rate of hPL near term, about 1 g/day, is the greatest (by far) of any known hormone in humans.

SERUM CONCENTRATION. HPL is demonstrable in placenta within 5 to 10 days after conception and hPL can be detected in serum as early as 3 weeks after fertilization. Maternal plasma concentration rises steadily until about 34 to 36 weeks, it is approximately proportional to placental mass. The serum concentration reaches higher levels in late pregnancy (5 to 15 μg/mL) than those of any other known protein hormone (see Fig. 2–6). The half-life of hPL in maternal plasma is between 10 and 30 minutes (Walker and associates, 1991).

Very little hPL is detected in fetal blood or in the urine of the mother or newborn; the concentration of hPL in amnionic fluid is somewhat lower than that in maternal plasma. Because hPL is secreted primarily into the maternal circulation, with only very small amounts in cord blood, it appears that the role of the hormone in pregnancy, if any, is mediated through actions in maternal rather than in fetal tissues. Nonetheless, there is continuing interest in the possibility that hPL in the fetus serves select functions in fetal growth.

REGULATION OF hPL BIOSYNTHESIS. The levels of mRNA for hPL in syncytiotrophoblast remain relatively constant throughout pregnancy. This finding is supportive of the idea that the rate of hPL secretion is proportional to placental mass. There are very high levels of hCG in the blood of women with neoplastic trophoblas-

tic disease, but only low levels of hPL in these same women.

Prolonged maternal starvation in the first half of pregnancy leads to an increase in the plasma concentration of hPL. Short-term changes in plasma glucose or insulin, however, have relatively little effect on plasma levels of hPL. The synthesis of hPL is stimulated by insulin and cAMP. PGE_2 and $PGF_{2\alpha}$ seem to inhibit the secretion of hPL.

METABOLIC ACTIONS. HPL has putative actions in a number of important metabolic processes. These include:

1. Lipolysis and an increase in the levels of circulating free fatty acids—thereby providing a source of energy for maternal metabolism and fetal nutrition.
2. An anti-insulin action, leading to an increase in maternal levels of insulin, which favors protein synthesis and provides a mobilizable source of amino acids for transport to the fetus.

OTHER PLACENTAL PROTEIN HORMONES

CHORIONIC ADRENOCORTICOTROPIN. A protein similar to adrenocorticotropic hormone (ACTH) has been isolated from placental tissue. Odagiri and colleagues (1979) found that ACTH, lipotropin, and β-endorphin are recovered in placental extracts and presumably are derived from the same or a similar 31-kd precursor molecule, proopiomelanocortin (POMC). Liotta and colleagues (1977) also found that ACTH is produced by dispersed placental cells. Dexamethasone treatment of pregnant women does not alter the levels of bioactive or immunoreactive ACTH in placental tissue. Finally, evidence comes from radiolabeled amino acid uptake into peptides that characterize ACTH.

The physiological role of placental ACTH is unclear. ACTH plasma levels at all times in pregnancy (before labor) are lower than those in men and nonpregnant women; nonetheless, the concentration increases as pregnancy advances (Carr and colleagues, 1981). The placenta may produce ACTH that is secreted into the mother or fetus during pregnancy, but ACTH does not cross the placenta (i.e., from mother to fetus). The administration of dexamethasone to pregnant women does not cause suppression of urinary free cortisol levels as effectively as it does in men and nonpregnant women.

Corticotropin-releasing hormone stimulates the synthesis and release of chorionic ACTH in vitro (p. 115).

CHORIONIC THYROTROPIN. There is evidence that the placenta produces a chorionic thyrotropin, but a significant biological role for this peptide in normal human pregnancy has not been established. The neoplastic trophoblasts of hydatidiform mole and choriocarcinoma may produce a family of chorionic thyrotropins, but the increased thyroid-stimulating activity in women with neoplastic trophoblastic disease is believed to be attributable primarily to the thyroid-stimulating properties of hCG (p. 113).

RELAXIN. Expression of relaxin has been demonstrated in human corpus luteum, decidua, and placenta (Bogic and colleagues, 1995). This peptide is synthesized as a single 105 amino-acid preprorelaxin molecule that gives rise to two chains (A and B) by cleavage of the preprorelaxin. Relaxin is structurally similar to insulin and nerve growth factor. There are two relaxin genes (H1 and H2), but only H2 is transcribed in the corpus luteum. Other tissues, including decidua, placenta, and fetal membranes, also express H1. Relaxin acts on myometrial smooth muscle to stimulate adenylyl cyclase and to promote uterine relaxation (Chap. 11, p. 272). An understanding of relaxin synthesis and action, however, is far from complete.

PARATHYROID HORMONE–RELATED PROTEIN (PTH-rP). The chemical relationships between PTH and PTH-rP were described in Chapters 4 and 5. Since PTH-rP was identified, many potential functions have been suggested. The synthesis of PTH-rP has been demonstrated in a number of normal adult tissues, especially in reproductive organs of men and women, including the uterus (myometrium and endometrium), corpus luteum, and lactating mammary tissue. Recall that PTH-rP is not produced in the parathyroid glands of normal adults.

A number of fetal tissues also synthesize PTH-rP, including the fetal parathyroid, kidney, and placenta. Because immunoreactive PTH is not readily detected in fetal blood, and because PTH-rP is produced by several fetal tissues, it has been suggested that PTH-rP may serve as the parathyroid of the fetus. The findings of recently conducted studies are supportive of this view. The rate of PTH secretion by the adult parathyroid is modulated by plasma Ca^{2+} concentration. PTH-rP secretion from other tissues is not regulated by calcium concentration except in the placenta. Hellman and associates (1992) found that PTH-rP secretion by trophoblasts is responsive to extracellular Ca^{2+}.

GROWTH HORMONE-VARIANT (hGH-V). There is a gene which encodes a growth hormone variant that is expressed in the placenta, but not in the pituitary. The gene is located in the growth hormone–prolactin gene cluster. The variant of hGH, sometimes referred to as placental growth hormone, is a 191-amino acid protein that differs in 15 amino acid positions from the sequence

for hGH. hGH-V is synthesized in placenta, presumably in the syncytium, but the pattern of synthesis of hGH-V secretion with gestation is not precisely known because antibodies available against hGH-V cross-react with hGH. It is believed that hGH-V is present in maternal plasma by 21 to 26 weeks, increasing in concentration to about 36 weeks, and remaining relatively constant thereafter. There is a correlation between the levels of hGH-V in maternal plasma and those of insulin growth factor-1, and the secretion of hGH-V by trophoblasts in vitro is inhibited by glucose in a dose-dependent manner (Patel and colleagues, 1995). The biological activity profile of hGH-V is similar to that of hPL.

HYPOTHALAMIC-LIKE RELEASING HORMONES

For each of the known hypothalamic-releasing or -inhibiting hormones described—GnRH, TRH, CRH, GHRH, and somatostatin—there is an analogous hormone produced in human placenta (Petraglia and colleagues, 1992; Siler-Khodr, 1988). Their role in trophoblasts, however, has not been completely resolved. Many investigators have proposed that the presence of these substances in placental tissue is indicative of a hierarchy of control of the synthesis of chorionic trophic agents.

GONADOTROPIN-RELEASING HORMONE (GnRH). There is a reasonably large amount of immunoreactive gonadotropin-releasing hormone (GnRH) in placenta (Siler-Khodr, 1988; Siler-Khodr and Khodr, 1978). Interestingly, these investigators also found that immunoreactive GnRH was present in cytotrophoblasts, but not in the syncytiotrophoblast. Siler-Khodr (1983) has referred to chorionic GnRH as hCG-releasing hormone. Gibbons and co-workers (1975) and Khodr and Siler-Khodr (1980) demonstrated that the human placenta can synthesize both GnRH and TRH (thyrotropin-releasing hormone) in vitro.

CORTICOTROPIN-RELEASING HORMONE (CRH). Attempts to isolate and identify corticotropin-releasing hormone (CRH) from the hypothalamus took some 40 years. The same CRH gene (long arm of chromosome 8) expressed in hypothalamic tissues is also expressed in trophoblasts, amnion, chorion laeve, and decidua. In nonpregnant women, the plasma level of CRH is about 15 pg/mL. This increases to about 250 pg/mL in the early third trimester and to 1000 to 2000 pg/mL abruptly during the last 5 to 6 weeks (Goland and associates, 1988). After labor begins, maternal plasma levels of CRH increase further by about two- to threefold (Petraglia and colleagues, 1989, 1990).

The biological function of CRH synthesized in placenta (and fetal membranes/decidua) is not so clear. Receptors for CRH are present in many tissues: placenta, adrenal, sympathetic ganglia, lymphocytes, gastrointestinal tract, pancreas, gonads, and myometrium. The finding that only very small amounts of placental CRH enter the fetal umbilical circulation mitigates against a role for placental CRH in fetal adrenal steroidogenesis. Large amounts of CRH from trophoblast enter the maternal blood, but there also is a large concentration of a specific CRH-binding protein in maternal plasma, and the bound CRH seems to be biologically inactive and targeted for degradation. Other proposed biological roles include the induction of smooth muscle relaxation (vascular and myometrial) and immunosuppression. The physiological reverse, the induction of myometrial contractions (i.e., the initiation of parturition by CRH) has also been suggested (Wadhwa and associates, 1998). Prostaglandin formation in placenta, amnion, chorion laeve, and decidua is increased by treatment with CRH (Jones and Challis, 1989).

As described in Chapter 50 (p. 1351), a few cases have been reported of Cushing syndrome that developed during pregnancy with spontaneous resolution after delivery (Aron and co-workers, 1990). It would be interesting to know if the abnormality in some of these women resided in a deficiency in the formation of CRH-binding protein such that placental CRH stimulated pituitary ACTH formation.

Glucocorticosteroids act in the hypothalamus to inhibit *CRH release*, but in the trophoblast, glucocorticosteroids *stimulate* the expression of the CRH gene, with two- to fivefold increases in CRH mRNA and protein after treatment of human trophoblasts in culture (Robinson and associates, 1988). Therefore, the possibility of a positive feedback loop has been considered in placenta that involves placental CRH stimulation of placental ACTH formation, placental ACTH stimulation of glucocorticosteroid formation, and glucocorticosteroid stimulation of placental CRH expression (Riley and colleagues, 1991).

THYROTROPIN-RELEASING HORMONE (cTRH). The synthesis of chorionic thyroid-releasing hormone (cTRH) in placenta has been demonstrated, but relatively little is known of its regulation synthesis or biological role.

GROWTH HORMONE-RELEASING HORMONE (GHRH). This is also known as **somatocrinin**. It is expressed in selected human tumors and is implicated in the development of acromegaly in persons with such tumors. The mRNA for GHRH has been identified in human placenta, (Berry and co-workers, 1992). The function of placental GHRH is not known.

OTHER PLACENTAL PEPTIDE HORMONES

NEUROPEPTIDE-Y (NPY) This small 36-amino-acid peptide is widely distributed in brain. It also is found in sympathetic neurons innervating the cardiovascular, respiratory, gastrointestinal, and genitourinary systems. Neuropeptide-Y (NPY) has been isolated from placenta and localized in cytotrophoblasts (Petraglia and colleagues, 1989). Receptors for NPY have been demonstrated in placenta, and treatment of placental cells with NPY causes the release of CRH.

INHIBIN AND ACTIVIN. Inhibin is a glycoprotein hormone that acts preferentially to inhibit FSH release by the pituitary. It is produced by human testis and by the granulosa cells of the ovary, including the corpus luteum. Inhibin is a heterodimer with dissimilar α- and β-subunits. The inhibin β-subunit is composed of one of two distinct peptides, βA or βB. Activin is closely related to inhibin and is formed by the combination of two β-subunits. The placenta produces inhibin α-, βA-, and βB-subunits with the greatest levels present at term (Petraglia and colleagues, 1991). Inhibin, produced in placenta, in conjunction with the large amounts of sex steroid hormones produced in human pregnancy, may serve to inhibit FSH secretion and thereby preclude ovulation during pregnancy. Petraglia and colleagues (1994) found that serum activin A levels decline rapidly after delivery. It is not detectable in fetal blood before labor but is present in umbilical cord blood after labor began. The receptor for activin is expressed in placenta and amnion. Inhibin may act via GnRH to regulate hCG synthesis/secretion in placenta (Petraglia and associates, 1987). Chorionic activin and inhibin may serve functions in placental metabolic processes other than GnRH synthesis, but these functions have not been established.

ATRIAL NATRIURETIC PEPTIDE (ANP). This 28-amino-acid peptide acts to effect natriuresis, diuresis, and vasorelaxation. It normally is produced in atrial myocytes, and also is synthesized in placental cytotrophoblast-like cells (Lim and Gude, 1995). Atrial natriuretic peptide (ANP) receptors are found in placenta myometrial tissues (Chap. 11, p. 273).

ESTROGENS

The placenta produces huge amounts of estrogens as well as progesterone. Steroid biosynthesis in human syncytium, however, is dependent upon blood-borne steroidal precursors. Near term, normal human pregnancy is a hyperestrogenic state of major proportions. The amount of estrogen produced each day by syncytiotrophoblast during the last few weeks of pregnancy is equivalent to that produced in one day by the ovaries of no fewer than 1000 ovulatory women. By way of another analogy, more estrogen is produced by the placenta during the course of one normal pregnancy than is secreted by the ovaries of 200 ovulatory women during the same 40 weeks. The hyperestrogenic state of human pregnancy is one of continually increasing magnitude as pregnancy progresses, terminating abruptly after delivery.

During the first 2 to 4 weeks of pregnancy, relatively small amounts of estrogen are produced by the maternal ovaries. The levels of urinary estrogens were not reduced, however, after bilateral oophorectomy conducted as early as the 78th day of pregnancy (Diczfalusy and Borell, 1961). Similar results were obtained in several studies of urinary estrogen levels in pregnant women after surgical removal of the corpus luteum. As early as the seventh week of human pregnancy, more than 50 percent of estrogen entering the maternal circulation is produced in placenta (MacDonald, 1965; Siiteri and MacDonald, 1963, 1966b).

PLACENTAL ESTROGEN BIOSYNTHESIS. The pathways of estrogen synthesis in human placenta differ from those in the ovarian follicle (granulosa cells) of nonpregnant women. Estrogen is produced in the ovary de novo, from acetate or cholesterol. Specifically, androstenedione, synthesized in ovarian theca cells, is transferred into the follicular fluid, from which it is taken up by the granulosa cells for estradiol-17β synthesis. Conversely, progesterone synthesis in the human corpus luteum (luteinized granulosa cells) is accomplished by use of preformed cholesterol taken up in LDL particles from plasma.

In human placenta (trophoblast), neither acetate nor cholesterol, nor even progesterone, can serve as precursor for estrogen biosynthesis. A crucial enzyme necessary for sex steroid synthesis—steroid 17α-hydroxylase/17,20-desmolase, encoded by the CYP17 gene—is not expressed in the human placenta. Consequently, the conversion of C_{21}-steroids to C_{19}-steroids, the latter being the immediate and obligatory precursors of estrogens, is not possible. Ryan (1959a) found that there was an exceptionally high capacity of placenta to convert appropriate C_{19}-steroids to estrone and estradiol-17β. These C_{19}-steroids are dehydroepiandrosterone, androstenedione, and testosterone, which are converted to estrone, estradiol-17β, or both. These findings were crucial to the design of investigations conducted later in which the role of plasma-borne, preformed C_{19}-steroids in estrogen biosynthesis in trophoblast was defined.

PLASMA C_{19}-STEROIDS AS ESTROGEN PRECURSORS. Amoroso (1960) first suggested that the placenta might,

through its abundant enzymatic activity, bring about the formation of active agents by converting inactive materials derived from the fetus. Frandsen and Stakemann (1961) found that the levels of urinary estrogens in women pregnant with an anencephalic fetus were only about a tenth of those in urine of women pregnant with a normal fetus. Because of the characteristic absence of the fetal zone of the adrenal cortex in anencephalic fetuses, they reasoned that the glands might provide a substance(s) that serves to promote placental estrogen formation. The adrenal glands of anencephalic fetuses are atrophic because of the absence of hypothalamic–pituitary function, which precludes ACTH stimulation of the fetal adrenal glands.

In subsequent studies, radiolabeled dehydroepiandrosterone sulfate infused into pregnant women was converted to radioactive urinary estrogens in high yield (Baulieu and Dray, 1963; Siiteri and MacDonald, 1963). Other radiolabeled unconjugated C_{19}-steroids—dehydroepiandrosterone, androstenedione, and testosterone—also were converted to estrogens. The large amounts of dehydroepiandrosterone sulfate in plasma and its much longer half-life uniquely qualified it as the principal circulating precursor for placental estradiol-17β synthesis. The presentation as a sulfate ester does not preclude its use because the placenta normally is a rich source of sulfatase activity (Pulkkinen, 1961; Warren and Timberlake, 1962). By the 30th week, 30 to 40 percent of dehydroepiandrosterone sulfate secreted by the maternal adrenal glands is converted to estradiol-17β. Conversely, little (less than 0.1 percent) is normally converted to estrogen in men or nonpregnant women (Siiteri and MacDonald, 1963, 1966b).

PLACENTAL AROMATASE ENZYME. Estrogen formation from androstenedione is catalyzed by an enzyme complex referred to as aromatase, which is composed of a specific cytochrome P-450 monooxygenase, aromatase cytochrome P-450 (P-450$_{AROM}$; P-450$_{XIX}$, the product of the CYP19 gene), and a flavoprotein, NADPH-cytochrome P-450 reductase. The principal cellular location of P-450$_{AROM}$ in the placenta is in the syncytiotrophoblast (Bonenfant and colleagues, 2000). It is found in the ovary in granulosa cells. CYP19 is also expressed in much lower levels in adipose tissue stromal cells, Sertoli and Leydig cells of the testis, hypothalamus, fetal (but not adult) liver, but not normal endometrium.

SECRETED ESTROGENS. The product estrogen in tissues in which aromatase activity is present is dependent on the nature of the substrate available and on the particular 17β-hydroxysteroid dehydrogenase (17βHSD) isozyme in that tissue. Estradiol-17β is the product hormone secreted by the ovary and testis. In the ovary, for example, the aromatization of androstenedione gives estrone, which is converted (by 17β-hydroxysteroid dehydrogenase type 1) to estradiol-17β before secretion by the granulosa cells. In adipose tissue, however, androstenedione is converted to estrone, and the estrone formed (without conversion in situ to estradiol-17β) is the product that enters the blood. Testosterone is converted to estradiol-17β directly in all tissue sites of aromatization.

In human placenta, estradiol-17β is one estrogen secretory product; but in addition, 16α-hydroxyandrostenedione is converted to 16α-hydroxyestrone, which in turn is converted to estriol before secretion by trophoblast. Therefore, the syncytiotrophoblast secretes two estrogens, estradiol-17β and estriol.

METABOLISM OF DEHYDROEPIANDROSTERONE SULFATE. Gant and co-workers (1971) found that there is a 10- to 20-fold increase in the metabolic clearance rate (MCR) of plasma dehydroepiandrosterone sulfate in normally pregnant women at term compared with that in men and nonpregnant women. As a consequence, there is a progressive decrease in its plasma concentration (Milewich and colleagues, 1978; Siiteri and Mac-Donald, 1966a).

The increase in the MCR of plasma dehydroepiandrosterone sulfate in pregnant women appears to be attributable primarily to:

1. Removal through conversion to estradiol-17β in the syncytium.
2. Accelerated 16α-hydroxylation (probably in maternal liver) with 30 to 40 percent converted near term to 16α-hydroxydehydroepiandrosterone sulfate (Madden and associates, 1976, 1978).

The maternal adrenal glands do not produce sufficient amounts of dehydroepiandrosterone sulfate during pregnancy to account for more than a small fraction of placenta estrogen biosynthesis. **The fetal adrenal glands are the quantitatively important source of placental estrogen precursors in human pregnancy.**

FETAL ADRENAL GLANDS

Morphologically, functionally, and physiologically, the human fetal adrenal glands are remarkable organs. Compared with adult organs, the adrenal cortex is the largest organ of the fetus. At term, they weigh the same as adrenal glands of the adult (Fig. 6–2). More than 85 percent of the fetal gland is normally composed of a peculiar fetal zone, which is not found in adults.

The daily production of steroids by the fetal adrenal glands near term is estimated to be 100 to 200 mg per day. Steroid secretion in resting adults rarely exceeds

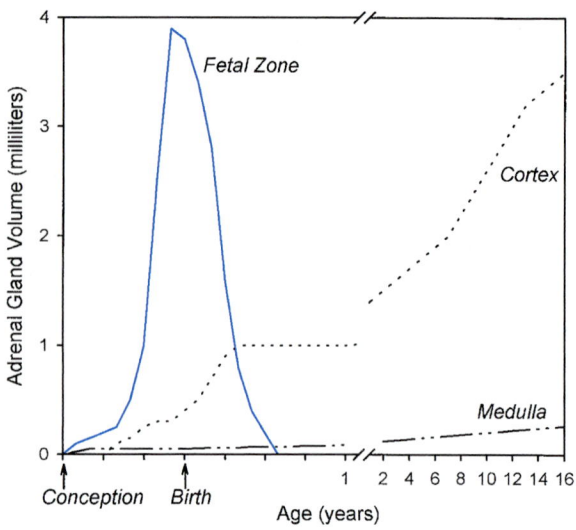

FIGURE 6–2. Size of the adrenal gland and its component parts in utero, during infancy, and during childhood. (Adapted from Bethune, 1974.)

30 to 40 mg/day; thus, the human fetal adrenal gland is a truly prodigious steroidogenic tissue.

The adrenal cortex begins a process of involution commencing immediately after birth. The weight of the adrenal glands decreases strikingly during the first few weeks of life, and the size attained by the fetal glands just before birth is not achieved again until late in adolescence or early adult life.

CONTRIBUTION TO PLACENTAL ESTROGEN FORMATION. As discussed earlier, women pregnant with an anencephalic fetus excrete little urinary estrogen. This together with the finding of high levels of dehydroepiandrosterone sulfate in cord blood of normal newborns, were suggestive that fetal adrenal cortices are the principal source of placental estrogen precursors. The finding that dehydroepiandrosterone sulfate in maternal plasma is converted to estrogen in placenta established this concept. Confirmation was provided by Bolté and co-workers (1964a, 1964b), who demonstrated that radiolabeled dehydroepiandrosterone sulfate perfused through the placenta was converted to estradiol-17β.

Near term, about half of estradiol-17β produced in placenta arises from maternal and half from fetal plasma dehydroepiandrosterone sulfate (Siiteri and MacDonald, 1966b). These findings alone, however, did not provide an explanation for the inordinately large amount of estriol in blood and urine of pregnant women.

PLACENTAL ESTRIOL SYNTHESIS. In nonpregnant women, the estrogen secreted by the granulosa cells of the "chosen" follicle is estradiol-17β; the estrogen formed from plasma androstenedione in extraglandular tissues is estrone. These two primary estrogens give rise to all metabolites of estrogen, including estriol. In nonpregnant women, the ratio of the concentration of urinary estriol to that of estrone plus estradiol-17β is approximately one. This ratio increases to 10 or more near term; thus there is a striking and disproportionate increase in estriol formation during pregnancy. This could not be accounted for by a pregnancy-associated change in metabolism of estrone or estradiol-17β to favor estriol (Brown, 1956). Moreover, neither estrone nor estradiol-17β is converted to estriol in the placenta.

Ryan (1959b) and MacDonald and Siiteri (1965b) found that the 16α-hydroxylated C_{19}-steroids—16α-hydroxydehydroepiandrosterone, 16α-hydroxy-androstenedione, and 16α-hydroxytestosterone—also were converted to estriol by placental tissue. In addition, large amounts of 16α-hydroxydehydroepiandrosterone sulfate were found in umbilical cord blood (Colas and co-workers, 1964). Thus, the disproportionate increase in estriol formation during pregnancy is accounted for by placental synthesis of estriol principally from plasma-borne 16α-hydroxydehydroepiandrosterone sulfate. This compound is synthesized by the fetal adrenal and by 16α-hydroxylation of plasma dehydroepiandrosterone sulfate in the fetal liver (Fig. 6–3). **Near term, the fetus is the source of 90 percent of the placental estriol precursor in normal human pregnancy**. Maternal plasma dehydroepiandrosterone sulfate is converted in maternal liver to 16α-hydroxydehydroepiandrosterone sulfate, which is then converted to estriol by the placenta (Madden and colleagues, 1976, 1978).

FETAL ADRENAL DEVELOPMENT. Early in embryonic life, the adrenal cortex is composed of cells that resemble those that, later in fetal development, comprise the fetal zone. These cells proliferate rapidly prior to the time that vascularization of the pituitary gland by the hypothalamus is complete. This is suggestive that early development of the fetal adrenal glands is under trophic influences that do not conform to those of the adult (Mulchahey and colleagues, 1987). ACTH does not cross the placenta; therefore, it is likely that during the first weeks of pregnancy, ACTH is secreted by the fetal pituitary gland in the absence of hypothalamic corticotropin-releasing hormone (CRH) stimulation, or else ACTH (or CRH) arises from a source other than the fetal pituitary gland, such as chorionic ACTH (or CRH), which is synthesized in syncytiotrophoblasts from early in gestation (p. 115).

FETAL ADRENAL GROWTH. The cortex continues to grow throughout gestation; and during the last 5 to 6 weeks of pregnancy, there is a very rapid increase in adrenal size. Relative to body weight, the fetal adrenal glands at term are 25 times larger than those of adults.

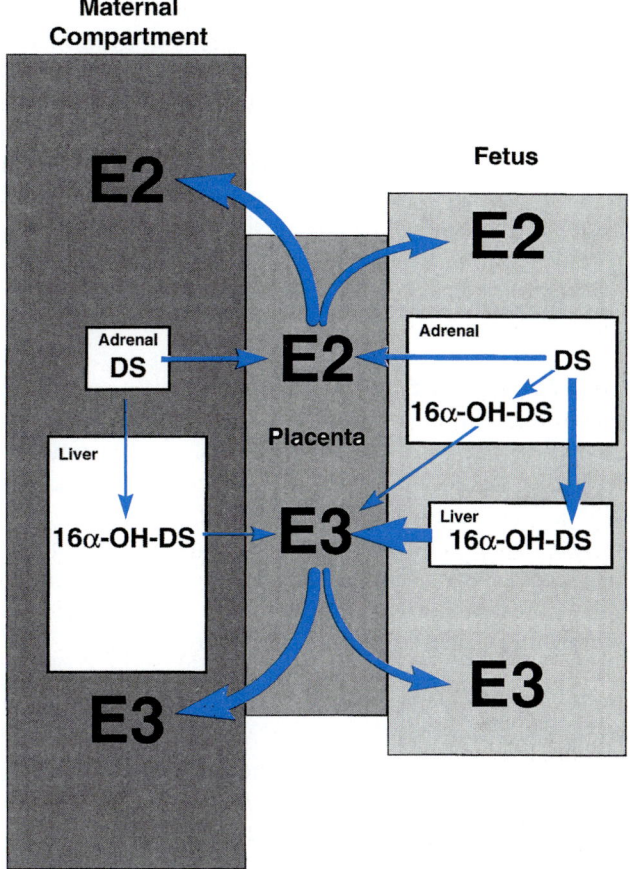

FIGURE 6–3. Schematic presentation of the biosynthesis of estrogen in the human placenta. Dehydroepiandrosterone sulfate (DS), secreted in prodigious amounts by the fetal adrenal glands, is converted to 16α-hydroxydehydroepiandrosterone sulfate (16α-OH-DS) in fetal adrenal glands and liver. These steroids, DS and 16α-OH-DS, are converted in the placenta to estrogens, namely, estradiol-17β (E2) and estriol (E3). Near term, half of E2 is derived from fetal adrenal DS and half from maternal DS. On the other hand, 90 percent of E3 in the placenta arises from fetal 16α-OH-DS and only 10 percent from all other sources. Most (80 to 90 percent) of steroids produced in the placenta are secreted into the maternal blood.

Because of the enormous size and their very great capacity for steroid synthesis, many investigators have surmised that in addition to ACTH, there must be other growth stimuli for these glands. Indeed, there is a continual decrease in the concentration of immunoreactive ACTH in human fetal plasma as pregnancy progresses, and the fetal adrenal glands are growing at a rapid rate (Winters and associates, 1974). Generally, ACTH acts to promote hypertrophy, but not hyperplasia, of adrenal cells.

It now seems most likely that the rate of growth of the fetal adrenal glands is determined by growth factors that may not affect the rate of steroidogenesis directly. There is sufficient ACTH in the fetal circulation at all stages of gestation to ensure adequate activity of the cholesterol side-chain cleavage enzyme, the rate-limiting step in adrenal steroidogenesis. The stimulation of fetal adrenal growth (cell replication) leading to an increased mass of functional cells would result in an increase in the capacity of the gland for steroid formation even if the putative growth factor did not act directly to increase steroidogenesis. This would account for the continued growth of the fetal adrenal glands throughout gestation, but rapid involution immediately after birth.

ENZYMATIC CONSIDERATIONS. There is a severe deficiency in the expression of the microsomal enzyme 3β-hydroxysteroid dehydrogenase, Δ^{5-4}-isomerase (3βHSD) in the fetal zone cells (Doody and associates, 1990). This limits the conversion of pregnenolone to progesterone and of 17α-hydroxypregnenolone to 17α-hydroxyprogesterone, an obligatory step in cortisol biosynthesis. There is, however, very active steroid sulfotransferase activity in the fetal adrenal glands. As a consequence, the principal secretory products of the fetal adrenal glands are pregnenolone sulfate and dehydroepiandrosterone sulfate. Comparatively, cortisol, which likely arises primarily in the neocortex of the fetal adrenal glands and not in the fetal zone, is a minor secretory product of the fetal adrenal.

FETAL ADRENAL STEROID PRECURSOR. The precursor for fetal adrenal steroidogenesis is cholesterol. The rate of steroid biosynthesis in the fetal adrenal is so great that its steroidogenesis alone is equivalent to a fourth of the total daily LDL cholesterol turnover in adults.

The fetal adrenal glands can synthesize cholesterol from two-carbon fragments, that is, acetate. The rate of de novo cholesterol synthesis by fetal adrenal tissue, however, is insufficient to account for more than a small part of the steroids produced by these glands. Therefore, cholesterol must be assimilated from the fetal circulation. Plasma cholesterol and its esters are present in the form of lipoproteins designated according to density as determined by ultracentrifugation: very-low-density lipoprotein (VLDL), low-density lipoprotein (LDL), and high-density lipoprotein (HDL).

Simpson, Carr, and their co-workers (1979) ascertained that human fetal adrenal glands take up lipoproteins as a source of cholesterol for steroidogenesis. HDL was much less effective than LDL, and VLDL was devoid of stimulatory activity. They also evaluated the relative contribution of cholesterol synthesized de novo and that of cholesterol derived from LDL uptake. They confirmed that the fetal adrenal glands are highly dependent upon circulating LDL as a source of cholesterol for optimum steroidogenesis (Carr and colleagues, 1980,

1982; Carr and Simpson, 1981b). A model of cholesterol metabolism in the fetal adrenal glands as described by Carr and Simpson is shown in Figure 6–4.

REGULATION OF FETAL CHOLESTEROL LEVELS. The majority of fetal plasma cholesterol arises by de novo synthesis in the fetal liver (Carr and Simpson, 1984). The low level of LDL cholesterol in fetal plasma is not the consequence of impaired fetal LDL synthesis, but instead, it is the result of the rapid use of LDL by the fetal adrenal glands for steroidogenesis. Early in human pregnancy, fetal plasma levels of LDL cholesterol are similar to those of the adult. As pregnancy progresses, however, levels of LDL cholesterol in fetal plasma decline as the fetal adrenal glands grow. In the normal term newborn, the concentration of LDL cholesterol is only about 30 mg/dL (Parker and associates, 1980, 1983). In the anencephalic newborn in whom the adrenal glands are atrophic, the levels of LDL cholesterol in umbilical cord plasma are high.

ESTROGEN PRODUCTION IN PREGNANCY: CLINICAL CONSIDERATIONS. A schematic representation of the pathways of estrogen formation in the placenta is presented in Figure 6–3.

FETAL CONDITIONS THAT AFFECT ESTROGEN PRODUCTION. A number of conditions affecting the fetus may alter the rate of steroid synthesis in placenta.

FETAL DEATH. It has been known for many decades that death of the human fetus is followed by a striking reduction in the levels of urinary estrogens. Moreover, it was demonstrated that after ligation of the umbilical cord with the fetus and placenta left in situ, there was an abrupt and striking decrease in the production of placental estrogens (Cassmer, 1959). The findings of this classical study were subject to at least two interpretations. The first was that maintenance of the fetal placental circulation is essential to the functional integrity of the placenta. This explanation was unlikely to be correct, however, because in Cassmer's study, the placental production of progesterone was maintained after occlusion of the umbilical cord. A second explanation for the marked decrease in urinary estrogens was that after umbilical cord ligation, an important source of precursors of placental estrogen (but not progesterone) biosynthesis was eliminated—that is, the fetus.

FETAL ANENCEPHALY. In the absence of the fetal zone of the adrenal cortex, as in anencephaly, the rate of formation of placental estrogens (especially estriol) is severely limited because of limited availability of C_{19}-steroid precursors. Verification of the diminished levels of precursors in anencephalic fetuses was pro-

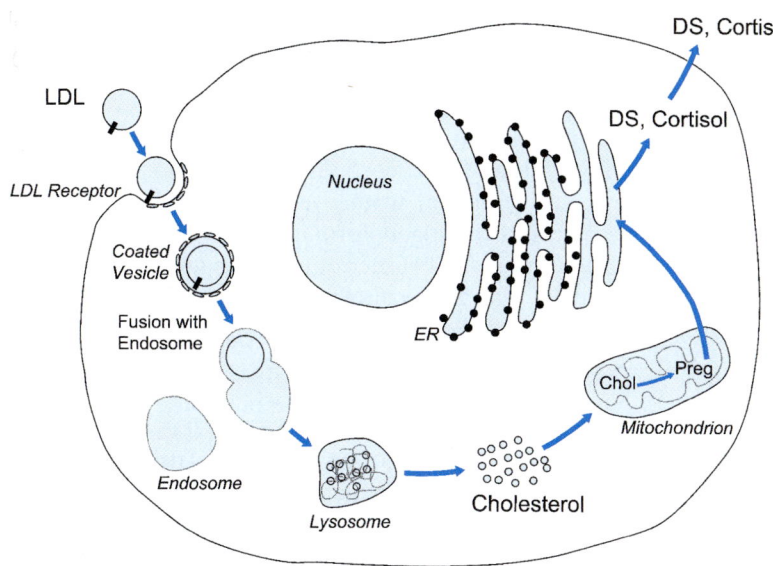

FIGURE 6–4. A model proposed for the regulation of fetal adrenal steroidogenesis, low-density lipoprotein (LDL) use, and cholesterol (chol) metabolism in the human fetal gland. (DS = dehydroepiandrosterone sulfate; Preg = pregnenolone). DS is produced in the fetal zone and cortisol primarily in the neocortex of the fetal adrenal glands.

vided by the finding of low levels of dehydroepiandrosterone sulfate in cord blood of such newborns (Nichols and co-workers, 1958). Therefore, almost all of the estrogens produced in women pregnant with an anencephalic fetus arise by the placental use of maternal plasma dehydroepiandrosterone sulfate. Furthermore, in such pregnancies the production of estrogens can be increased by the administration (to the mother) of ACTH, which stimulates the rate of dehydroepiandrosterone sulfate secretion by the maternal adrenal (ACTH does not cross the placenta). Finally, placental production of estrogens is decreased in women pregnant with an anencephalic fetus during the administration of a potent glucocorticosteroid, which suppresses ACTH secretion and thus decreases the rate of secretion of dehydroepiandrosterone sulfate from the maternal adrenal cortex (MacDonald and Siiteri, 1965a, 1965b). Estriol formation is disproportionally decreased in pregnancies with an anencephalic fetus because the fetal adrenal at term normally provides 90 percent of placental estriol precursor.

FETAL ADRENAL HYPOPLASIA. A rare disorder of human pregnancy involves adrenal hypoplasia in an otherwise normal fetus. Estrogen formation in pregnancies with such a fetus also is very limited because of the absence of fetal adrenal C_{19}-precursors for placental estrogen formation.

PLACENTAL SULFATASE DEFICIENCY. Estrogen formation in placenta is generally regulated by the availability of C_{19}-steroid prohormones in fetal and maternal plasma. Specifically, there is no rate-limiting enzymatic reaction in the placental pathway from C_{19}-steroids to estrogen biosynthesis. Moreover, aside from minor al-

terations in placental aromatase induced by xenobiotics, the excess of placental enzymatic machinery for estrogen formation is large. An exception to this generalization was found by France and Liggins (1969), who were the first to establish that placental sulfatase deficiency is a cause of very low estrogen levels in otherwise normal (except possibly for dysfunctional labor) pregnancies. Sulfatase deficiency precludes the hydrolysis of C_{19}-steroid sulfates, the first enzymatic step in the placental use of these circulating prehormones for estrogen biosynthesis. This is an X-linked disorder (all affected fetuses are male) associated with the development of ichthyosis in the affected males later in life (Bradshaw and Carr, 1986).

PLACENTAL AROMATASE DEFICIENCY. There are a few well-documented examples of (placental) aromatase deficiency (Shozu and colleagues, 1991). Fetal adrenal dehydroepiandrosterone sulfate, which is produced in large quantities, is converted in placenta to androstenedione, but because of the aromatase deficiency, androstenedione could not be converted to estradiol-17β. Rather, metabolites of dehydroepiandrosterone produced in placenta, including androstenedione and testosterone, are secreted into the maternal and fetal circulations, causing virilization of the mother and the female fetus (Harada and colleagues, 1992).

Pregnancies with aromatase deficiency and a male fetus are uneventful. In these estrogen-deficient males, however, epiphyseal closure does not occur properly during puberty, and in consequence, the affected men continue to grow during adulthood, becoming very tall and with deficient mineralization of bone (Morishima and associates, 1995).

DOWN SYNDROME. In the conduct of second-trimester pregnancy screening of maternal blood for levels of hCG and alpha-fetoprotein, it was discovered that serum unconjugated estriol levels were low in pregnancies with a Down syndrome fetus (Chap. 37, p. 984). The reason for diminished levels of estrogen are not established, but the best possibility would be inadequate formation of C_{19}-steroids in the adrenal glands of these trisomic fetuses. (Newby and colleagues, 2000).

DEFICIENCY IN FETAL LDL CHOLESTEROL BIOSYNTHESIS. A successful pregnancy in a woman with beta-lipoprotein deficiency has been described (Parker and colleagues, 1986). The absence of LDL in the maternal plasma led to little or no progesterone formation in the corpus luteum and restricted the amount of placental progesterone formation. In addition, the levels of estriol were also lower than normal. Presumably, the diminished estrogen production was the result of decreased LDL formation in the fetus, who was heterozygous for the LDL deficiency. Decreased fetal LDL formation will limit fetal adrenal production of dehydroepiandrosterone sulfate and thereby reduce the availability of precursor for placental estrogen synthesis. The fetal adrenal glands are dependent upon plasma LDL as well as the de novo synthesis of cholesterol as precursor for steroidogenesis (Carr and Simpson, 1981a; Mason and Rainey, 1987).

FETAL ERYTHROBLASTOSIS. In some cases of severe fetal D-antigen isoimmunization, the levels of estrogens in maternal plasma are elevated above normal for gestational age. This is likely due to an increased placental weight (hypertrophy) which occurs in such pregnancies.

DECREASED FETAL ADRENAL USE OF LDL. The most common cause of decreased placental estrogen formation (aside from fetal death) is an acquired reduction in fetal adrenal use of plasma LDL. This leads to a reduction in the rate of formation of dehydroepiandrosterone sulfate and thereby a reduction in placental estrogen precursor availability. This sequence of events is observed most commonly in pregnancies complicated by hypertension or more severe forms of diabetes (Parker and associates, 1984, 1987). As noted before, the final consequence may be as follows: Placental estrogen formation is decreased and estrogen levels in maternal blood and urine are decreased. The levels of dehydroepiandrosterone sulfate in umbilical venous blood are decreased, but the levels of LDL are increased. At the same time, because of a redistribution of placental estrogens, the levels of estriol in umbilical venous blood may be increased.

MATERNAL CONDITIONS THAT AFFECT PLACENTAL ESTROGEN FORMATION

GLUCOCORTICOSTEROID TREATMENT. The administration of glucocorticosteroids, in moderate to high doses, to pregnant women causes a striking reduction in placental estrogen formation. Glucocorticosteroids act to inhibit ACTH secretion by the maternal and fetal pituitary glands, resulting in decreased maternal and fetal adrenal secretion of placental estrogen precursor, dehydroepiandrosterone sulfate.

MATERNAL ADRENAL DYSFUNCTION. In pregnant women with Addison disease, maternal urinary estrogen levels are reduced (Baulieu and co-workers, 1956). The decrease principally affects estrone and estradiol-17β, because the fetal adrenal contribution to the synthesis of estriol, particularly in the latter part of pregnancy, is quantitatively much more important.

MATERNAL OVARIAN ANDROGEN-PRODUCING TUMORS. The extraordinary efficiency of the placenta in the aromatization of C_{19}-steroids may be exemplified by two considerations. First, Edman and associates (1981) found that the placental clearance of maternal plasma androstenedione to estradiol was very similar to estimated placental blood flow. Thus, virtually all of the androstenedione entering the intervillous space is taken up by syncytium and converted to estradiol-17β and none of this C_{19}-steroid escapes into the fetus. Second, it is relatively rare that a female fetus is virilized in a pregnant woman who is known to have an androgen-secreting ovarian tumor. This finding also indicates that the placenta efficiently converts aromatizable C_{19}-steroids—including bioactive testosterone—to estrogens, thereby precluding transplacental passage. Indeed, it may be that virilized female fetuses of women with an androgen-producing tumor are cases in which a nonaromatizable C_{19}-steroid androgen is produced by the tumor (e.g., 5α-dihydrotestosterone), or else testosterone is produced very early in pregnancy in amounts that exceed the capacity of placental aromatase.

MATERNAL RENAL DISEASE. Lower levels of estriol in urine of pregnant women with pyelonephritis may be observed. Presumably this is the consequence of diminished renal clearance, as the levels of estrogen in serum are normal in such pregnancies.

MATERNAL HYPERTENSIVE DISORDERS AND DIABETES. With disorders of the mother associated with decreased uteroplacental blood flow, fetal adrenal formation of dehydroepiandrosterone is impaired (p. 118). Therefore, the primary reason for diminished estrogen formation with these maternal disorders is not a decrease in placental function.

GESTATIONAL TROPHOBLASTIC DISEASE. In the case of complete hydatidiform mole or choriocarcinoma, there is no fetal adrenal source of C_{19}-steroid precursor for trophoblast estrogen biosynthesis. Consequently, estrogen formation in placenta is limited to the use of C_{19}-steroids in the maternal plasma, and therefore the estrogen produced is principally estradiol-17β (MacDonald and Siiteri, 1964, 1966). Great variation is observed in the rates of both estradiol-17β and progesterone formation in molar pregnancies; however, that is not necessarily related to the volume of neoplastic trophoblastic tissue. There is variable disruption of large masses of molar tissue from the uterine wall by blood clots. Consequently, variable amounts of trophoblastic tissue are separated from the maternal blood supply of precursors for estradiol-17β and progesterone formation (MacDonald and Siiteri, 1964, 1966).

PROGESTERONE

After the first few (6 to 7) weeks of human gestation, very little progesterone is produced in the ovary (Diczfalusy and Troen, 1961). Surgical removal of the corpus luteum or even bilateral oophorectomy conducted during the 7th to 10th weeks of pregnancy does not cause a decrease in the rate of excretion of urinary pregnanediol, the principal urinary metabolite of progesterone. There is a gradual increase in the levels of plasma progesterone as well as those of estradiol and estriol in normal human pregnancy, as shown in Figure 6–5.

PROGESTERONE PRODUCTION RATES. Isotope dilution techniques for the measurement of the rates of endogenous hormone production in humans were first applied to the study of progesterone in pregnancy. The results of these studies, conducted by Pearlman in 1957, gave daily production of progesterone in late normal, singleton pregnancies of about 250 mg. The findings of studies in which other methods have been employed since then are in agreement with this value. In some pregnancies with multiple fetuses, however, the daily progesterone production rate may exceed 600 mg per day.

SOURCE OF CHOLESTEROL FOR PLACENTAL PROGESTERONE BIOSYNTHESIS. Progesterone is synthesized from cholesterol in a two-step enzymatic reaction. First, cholesterol is converted, in mitochondria, to the steroid intermediate, pregnenolone, in a reaction catalyzed by cytochrome P_{450} cholesterol side-chain cleavage

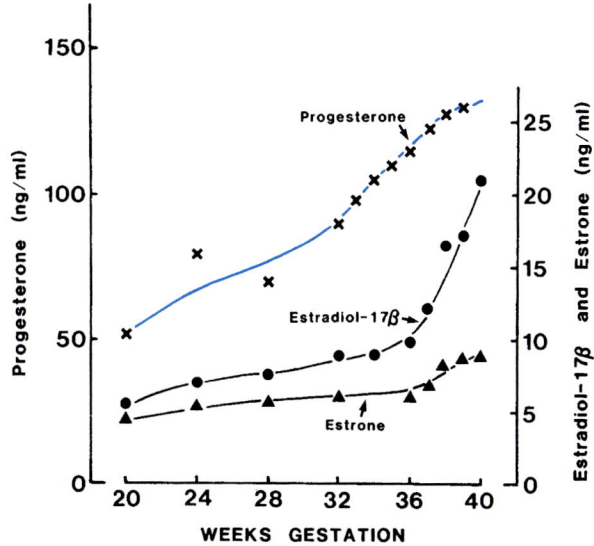

FIGURE 6–5. Mean plasma levels of progesterone, unconjugated estradiol, and unconjugated estriol in 33 normal women during the last 9 weeks before delivery. (Adapted from Tungsubutra and France, 1978.)

enzyme. Pregnenolone is converted to progesterone, in microsomes, by 3β-hydroxysteroid dehydrogenase, Δ^{5-4}-isomerase.

The human placenta produces a prodigious amount of progesterone; nonetheless, there is a limited capacity for the biosynthesis of cholesterol in trophoblast. The rate of incorporation of radiolabeled acetate into cholesterol by placental tissue proceeds very slowly, and the activity of the rate-limiting enzyme in cholesterol biosynthesis, 3-hydroxy-3-methylglutaryl coenzyme A (HMG CoA) reductase, in placental tissue microsomes is small.

Thus, the placenta must rely on exogenous cholesterol for progesterone formation. Bloch (1945) and Werbin and co-workers (1957) found that after the intravenous administration of radiolabeled cholesterol to pregnant women, the specific activity of urinary pregnanediol was similar to that of plasma cholesterol. Hellig and associates (1970) also found that maternal plasma cholesterol was the principal precursor (up to 90 percent) of progesterone biosynthesis in human pregnancy. These findings are consistent with the conclusion that the de novo synthesis of cholesterol in trophoblast is minimal. Placental HMG CoA reductase in trophoblast is inhibited by the high levels of LDL in blood, causing inhibition of its synthesis. With LDL deficiency, de novo cholesterol synthesis in trophoblast is appreciable, albeit much less than sufficient to meet the needs of placenta for both membrane synthesis and normal progesterone synthesis.

**PLACENTAL USE OF MATERNAL PLASMA LDL CHOLES-
TEROL.** In studies similar to those described by use of
fetal adrenal tissue, Simpson and associates (1979, 1980)
demonstrated that the trophoblast preferentially uses
LDL cholesterol for progesterone biosynthesis. Thus,
the formation of placental progesterone occurs through
the uptake and use of a circulating precursor. But unlike
estrogens, which are formed principally from fetal adrenal precursors, placental progesterone biosynthesis proceeds by using a maternal precursor, LDL cholesterol.
This subject was reviewed by Casey and colleagues
(1992).

These findings provide insights into not only the biochemical mechanism for placental progesterone formation but perhaps also into other aspects of maternal–
placental–fetal physiology. The rate of progesterone
biosynthesis is largely dependent on the number of LDL
receptors on the plasma membrane of the trophoblasts,
and thereby primarily independent of uteroplacental
blood flow.

Simpson and Burkhart (1980) also found that progesterone, in concentrations similar to those found in human placental tissue, inhibits the activity of the enzyme
that catalyzes cholesterol esterification. This physiological event may serve to ensure a supply of cholesterol
for progesterone biosynthesis by preventing the sequestration of cholesterol into a nonusable storage form,
cholesterol esters, and may protect the liberated essential fatty acids from reesterification with cholesterol.

TROPHOBLAST LDL RECEPTORS. The LDL receptors
are localized in coated pits on the microvillous membranes of syncytium and are demonstrable as early as
4 weeks after conception. The affinity of these receptors
for LDL remains constant throughout human pregnancy
and similar to that in other tissues. The trophoblast is
unique in that two mRNA species for the LDL receptor
are found in human trophoblast, the usual 5.3-kb mRNA
and an additional 3.7-kb mRNA. Furuhashi and colleagues (1989) proposed that the differential use of
splicing sites may give rise to the smaller LDL receptor
mRNA. The expression of LDL receptor gene in
trophoblast is highest in the first trimester; this high level
of expression may be important in trophoblast growth
at this time of pregnancy as well as in provision of
progesterone precursor. There is a decrease in the 5.3-kb
mRNA for the LDL receptor as pregnancy progresses.

PROGESTERONE SYNTHESIS AND FETAL WELL-BEING.
The relationships that exist between fetal well-being
and the placental production of estrogen cannot be demonstrated in the case of progesterone. Fetal death, ligation of the umbilical cord with the fetus and placenta
remaining in situ, and anencephaly are all conditions
associated with very low maternal plasma levels and

urinary excretion of estrogens. In these circumstances,
however, there is no concomitant decrease in the plasma
levels of progesterone to anywhere near the same extent
as those of estrogen until some indeterminate time after
fetal death. Thus, placental endocrine function, including the formation of protein hormones such as hCG, and
progesterone biosynthesis, may persist for long periods
(weeks) after fetal death.

PROGESTERONE METABOLISM DURING PREGNANCY.
The metabolic clearance rate of progesterone in pregnant women is similar to that found in men and nonpregnant women. This is an important consideration in evaluating the role of progesterone in the initiation of
parturition (Chap. 11, p. 263).

During pregnancy, there is a disproportionate increase in the plasma concentration of 5α-dihydro-
progesterone. Thus the ratio of the concentration of
this progesterone metabolite to the concentration of
progesterone is increased in pregnant women (Milewich
and co-workers, 1975). The mechanisms for this are not
defined completely, but may be relevant to the resistance to pressor agents that normally develop in pregnant women (Everett and associates, 1978; see also
Chap. 8, p. 184). Progesterone also is converted to the
potent mineralocorticosteroid deoxycorticosterone in
pregnant women and in the fetus. The concentration of
deoxycorticosterone is increased strikingly in both the
maternal and fetal compartments. The extra-adrenal
formation of deoxycorticosterone from circulating progesterone accounts for the vast majority of its production in human pregnancy (Casey and MacDonald,
1982a, 1982b).

**DIRECTIONAL SECRETION OF STEROIDS FROM SYN-
CYTIOTROPHOBLAST.** Estrogens synthesized in syncytium preferentially enter the maternal circulation. Gurpide and co-workers (1966) reported that more than 90
percent of estradiol-17β and estriol formed in syncytiotrophoblast enters maternal plasma. The same is true
of progesterone formed in the syncytium. Gurpide and
co-workers (1972) also found that 85 percent or more
of placental progesterone enters maternal plasma, and
very little maternal plasma progesterone crosses the
placenta to the fetus.

The placental estrogens that enter the maternal compartment are estradiol-17β and estriol. Somewhat surprisingly, estrone as well as estradiol-17β enter the fetus,
and there is preferential entry of estrone rather than
estradiol-17β into the fetal plasma (Gurpide and co-
workers, 1982; Walsh and McCarthy, 1981). They emphasized that this might be attributed to extratropho-
blastic conversion of estradiol-17β to estrone in fetal
tissues or erythrocytes.

Estriol synthesized in trophoblasts enters both fetal

and maternal plasma, but most (90 percent) enters the mother.

TRANSFER OF STEROIDS FROM SYNCYTIOTROPHO-BLASTS INTO MATERNAL AND FETAL BLOOD.

The placental arm of the fetal–maternal communication system of human pregnancy is established by way of hemochorioendothelial placentation. Therefore, steroids secreted from the syncytiotrophoblast enter maternal blood directly. There is no evidence of specific estrogen binding within the trophoblast; therefore, net transfer between trophoblast and intervillous space favors entry into maternal blood, which rapidly enters the general maternal circulation.

Steroids that leave the syncytium toward the fetal compartment, however, do not enter fetal blood directly. First, steroids traveling toward the fetus must traverse the cytotrophoblasts and then enter the intravillous space. Steroids in this space can reenter the syncytium. Second, steroids that escape the intravillous space toward the fetus must then traverse the wall of the fetal capillaries to reach fetal blood. Steroids in the fetal capillaries of the intravillous space then can reenter the intravillous space and then the syncytium.

The net result of this hemochorioendothelial arrangement is that there is substantially greater entry of steroids formed in syncytium into the maternal circulation compared with the amount that enters the fetal blood.

An interesting phenomenon exists in the distribution of steroids formed in syncytium to the maternal and fetal compartments in pregnancies in which there is decreased uteroplacental blood flow. In newborns of women with pregnancy-induced hypertension, chronic hypertension, and severe diabetes, the umbilical cord plasma levels of estrogens and progesterone are significantly greater than in newborns of normal women. Initially, this was a surprise, because with decreased uteroplacental blood flow, estrogen production in placenta is decreased, as are the levels of estrogen in the maternal compartment. These seemingly discordant findings can be interpreted as follows: As uteroplacental blood flow is reduced, there is relative stasis of maternal blood in the intervillous space. This results in a redistribution of steroids formed in syncytium in favor of the fetal compartment. In particular, there is a decrease in the net exit of steroids into the maternal circulation, probably because of stasis of intervillous blood and thereby greater reentry of steroids from the intervillous space back into the syncytium. This favors a relative increase in the transfer of steroids from the syncytiotrophoblast into the fetal compartment. There is therefore an increase in the concentration of steroids formed in trophoblast in the umbilical vein. This occurs even in the face of a decrease in total placental estrogen formation and, in consequence, a decrease in estrogen levels in the maternal compartment. This is an important concept that may be pertinent in evaluations of the role(s) of steroids produced in the placenta in fetal development, as with lung maturation, which may be accelerated in fetuses of pregnancies in which uteroplacental blood flow is believed to be reduced (Parker and associates, 1987; see also Chap. 7).

REFERENCES

Amoroso EC: Comparative aspects of the hormonal functions. In Villee CA (ed): The Placenta and Fetal Membranes. Baltimore, Williams & Wilkins, 1960, p 3

Aron DC, Schnall AM, Sheeler LR: Spontaneous resolution of Cushing syndrome after pregnancy. Am J Obstet Gynecol 162:472, 1990

Baulieu EE, Bricaire H, Jayle MF: Lack of secretion of 17-hydroxycorticosteroids in a pregnant woman with Addison's disease. J Clin Endocrinol 16:690, 1956

Baulieu EE, Dray F: Conversion of ^{3}H-dehydroepiandrosterone (3β-hydroxy-Δ^5-androstene-17-one) sulfate to ^{3}H-estrogens in normal pregnant women. J Clin Endocrinol 23:1298, 1963

Berry SA, Srivastava CH, Rubin LR, Phipps WR, Pescovitz OH: Growth hormone releasing hormone-like messenger ribonucleic acid and immunoreactive peptide are present in human testis and placenta. J Clin Endocrinol Metab 75:281, 1992

Bethune JE: The Adrenal Cortex, A Scope Monograph. Kalamazo, MI, Upjohn, 1974, p 11

Bloch K: The biological conversion of cholesterol to pregnandiol. J Biol Chem 157:661, 1945

Bogic LV, Mandel M, Bryant-Greenwood GD: Relaxin gene expression in human reproductive tissues by in situ hybridization. J Clin Endocrinol Metab 80:130, 1995

Bolté E, Mancuso S, Eriksson G, Wiqvist N, Diczfalusy E: Studies on the aromatization of neutral steroids in pregnant women, 1. Aromatization of C-19 steroids by placenta perfused in situ. Acta Endocrinol 35:535, 1964a

Bolté E, Mancuso S, Eriksson G, Wiqvist N, Diczfalusy E: Studies on the aromatization of neutral steroids in pregnant women, 2. Aromatization of dehydroepiandrosterone and of its sulphate administered simultaneously into a uterine artery. Acta Endocrinol 45:560, 1964b

Bonenfant M, Provost PR, Drolet R, Termblay Y: Localization of type 1 17beta-hydroxysteroid dehydrogenase mRNA and protein in syncytiotrophoblasts and invasive cytotrophoblasts in the human term villi. J Endocrinol 165:217, 2000

Bradbury JT, Brown WE, Guay LA: Maintenance of the corpus luteum and physiologic action of progesterone. Recent Prog Horm Res 5:151, 1950

Bradshaw KD, Carr BR: Placental sulfatase deficiency and X-linked ichthyosis. Obstet Gynecol Surv 41:401, 1986

Brown JB: Urinary excretion of oestrogens during pregnancy, lactation, and the reestablishment of menstruation. Lancet 1:704, 1956

Carr BR, Ohashi M, Simpson ER: Low density lipoprotein binding and de novo synthesis of cholesterol in the neocortex and fetal zones of the human fetal adrenal gland. Endocrinology 110:1994, 1982

Carr BR, Parker CR Jr, Madden JD, MacDonald PC, Porter JC: Maternal plasma adrenocorticotropin and cortisol relationships throughout human pregnancy. Am J Obstet Gynecol 139:416, 1981

Carr BR, Porter JC, MacDonald PC, Simpson ER: Metabolism of low density lipoprotein by human fetal adrenal tissue. Endocrinology 107:1034, 1980

Carr BR, Simpson ER: Cholesterol synthesis by human fetal hepatocytes: Effect of lipoproteins. Am J Obstet Gynecol 150:551, 1984

Carr BR, Simpson ER: De novo synthesis of cholesterol by the human fetal adrenal gland. Endocrinology 108:2154, 1981a

Carr BR, Simpson ER: Lipoprotein utilization and cholesterol synthesis by the human fetal adrenal gland. Endocr Rev 2:306, 1981b

Casey ML, MacDonald PC, Simpson ER: Endocrinologic changes in pregnancy. In Foster DW, Wilson JD (eds): Williams Textbook of Endocrinology. Philadelphia, Saunders, 1992, p 977

Casey, ML, MacDonald PC: Extraadrenal formation of a mineralcorticosteroid: Deoxycorticosterone and deoxycorticosterone sulfate biosynthesis and metabolism. Endocr Rev 3:396, 1982a

Casey ML, MacDonald PC: Metabolism of deoxycorticosterone and deoxycorticosterone sulfate in men and women. J Clin Invest 70:3112, 1982b

Cassmer O: Hormone production of the isolated human placenta. Acta Endocrinol (Suppl) 32:45, 1959

Colas A, Heinrichs WL, Tatum HJ: Pettenkofer chromogens in the maternal and fetal circulations: Detection of 3α, 16α-dihydroxyandrost-5-en-17-one in umbilical cord blood. Steroids 3:417, 1964

Cole LA, Kardana A, Ying FC, Birken S: The biological and clinical significance of nicks in human chorionic gonadotropin and its free β-subunit. Yale J Biol Med 64:627, 1991

Diczfalusy E, Borell U: Influence of oophorectomy on steroid excretion in early pregnancy. J Clin Endocrinol 21:1119, 1961

Diczfalusy E, Troen P: Endocrine functions of the human placenta. Vitam Horm 19:229, 1961

Doody KM, Carr BR, Rainey WE, Byrd W, Murry BA, Strickler RC, Thomas JL, Mason JI: 3β-Hydroxysteroid dehydrogenase activity in glandular and extraglandular human fetal tissues. Endocrinology 126:2487, 1990

Edman CD, Toofanian A, MacDonald PC, Gant NF: Placental clearance rate of maternal plasma androstenedione through placental estradiol formation: An indirect method of assessing uteroplacental blood flow. Am J Obstet Gynecol 141:1029, 1981

Everett RB, Worley RJ, MacDonald PC, Gant NF: Modification of vascular responsiveness to angiotensin II in pregnant women by intravenously infused 5α-dihydroprogesterone. Am J Obstet Gynecol 131:555, 1978

France JT, Liggins GC: Placental sulfatase deficiency. J Clin Endocrinol 29:138, 1969

Frandsen VA, Stakemann G: The site of production of oestrogenic hormones in human pregnancy: Hormone excretion in pregnancy with anencephalic foetus. Acta Endocrinol 38:383, 1961

Furuhashi M, Seo H, Mizutani S, Narita O, Tomoda Y, Matsui N: Expression of low density lipoprotein receptor gene in human placenta during pregnancy. Mol Endocrinol 3:1252, 1989

Gant NF, Hutchinson HT, Siiteri PK, MacDonald PC: Study of the metabolic clearance rate of dehydroisoandrosterone sulfate in pregnancy. Am J Obstet Gynecol 111:555, 1971

Gibbons JM, Mitnick M, Chieffo V: In vitro biosynthesis of TSH-and LH-releasing factors by human placenta. Am J Obstet Gynecol 121:127, 1975

Goland RS, Wardlaw SL, Blum M, Tropper PJ, Stark RI: Biologically active corticotropin-releasing hormone in maternal and fetal plasma during pregnancy. Am J Obstet Gynecol 159:884, 1988

Grumbach MM, Kaplan SL: On placental origin and purification of chorionic growth hormone prolactin and its immunoassay in pregnancy. Trans NY Acad Sci 27:167, 1964

Gurpide E, Marks C, de Ziegler D, Berk PD, and Brandes JM: Asymmetric release of estrone and estradiol derived from labeled precursors in perfused human placentas. Am J Obstet Gynecol 144:551, 1982

Gurpide E, Schwers J, Welch MT, VandeWiele RL, Lieberman S: Fetal and maternal metabolism of estradiol during pregnancy. J Clin Endocrinol Metab 26:1355, 1966

Gurpide E, Tseng L, Escarcena L, Fahning M, Gibson C, Fehr P: Fetomaternal production and transfer of progesterone and uridine in sheep. Am J Obstet Gynecol 113:21, 1972

Harada N, Ogawa H, Shozu M, Yamada K, Suhara K, Nishida E: Biochemical and molecular genetic analyses on placental aromatase. J Biol Chem 267:4781, 1992

Hellig HD, Gattereau D, Lefèvre Y, Bolté E: Steroid production from plasma cholesterol, 1. Conversion of plasma cholesterol to placental progesterone in humans. J Clin Endocrinol Metab 30:624, 1970

Hellman P, Ridefelt P, Juhlin C, Akerstrom G, Rastad J, Gylfe E: Parathyroid-like regulation of parathyroid hormone-related protein release and cytoplasmic calcium in cytotrophoblast cells of human placenta. Arch Biochem Biophys 293:174, 1992

Ito Y, Higashi K: Studies on prolactin-like substance in human placenta, 2. Endocrinol Jpn 8:279, 1961

Jones SA, Challis JRG: Local stimulation of prostaglandin production by corticotropin-releasing hormone in human fetal membranes and placenta. Biochem Biophys Res Commun 159:192, 1989

Josimovich JB, MacLaren JA: Presence in human placenta and term serum of highly lactogenic substance immunologically related in pituitary growth hormone. Endocrinology 71:209, 1962

Khodr GS, Siler-Khodr TM: Placental luteinizing hormone-releasing factor and its synthesis. Science 207:315, 1980

Kraiem Z, Sadeh O, Blithe DL, Nisula BC: Human chorionic gonadotropin stimulates thyroid hormone secretion, iodide uptake, organification, and adenosine 3, 5-monophosphate formation in cultured human thyrocytes. J Clin Endocrinol Metab 79:595, 1994

Lim AT, Gude NM: Atrial natriuretic factor production by the human placenta. J Clin Endocrinol Metab 80:3091, 1995

Liotta A, Osathanondh R, Ryan KJ, Krieger DT: Presence of corticotropin in human placenta: Demonstration of in vitro synthesis. Endocrinology 101:1552, 1977

MacDonald PC: Placental steroidogenesis. In Wynn RM (ed): Fetal Homeostasis, Vol I. New York, New York Academy of Sciences, 1965, p 265

MacDonald PC, Siiteri PK: The in vivo mechanisms of origin of estrogen in subjects with trophoblastic tumors. Steroids 8:589, 1966

MacDonald PC, Siiteri PK: The conversion of isotope-labeled dehydroisoandrosterone and dehydroisoandrosterone sulfate to estrogen in normal and abnormal pregnancy. In Paulsen CA (ed): Estrogen Assays in Clinical Medicine. Seattle, University of Washington Press, 1965a, p 251

MacDonald PC, Siiteri PK: Origin of estrogen in women pregnant with an anencephalic fetus. J Clin Invest 44:465, 1965b

MacDonald PC, Siiteri PK: Study of estrogen production in women with hydatiform mole. J Clin Endocrinol Metab 24:685, 1964

Madden JD, Gant NF, MacDonald PC: Studies of the kinetics of conversion of maternal plasma dehydroisoandrosterone sulfate to 16α-hydroxydehydroisoandrosterone sulfate, estradiol and estriol. Am J Obstet Gynecol 132:392, 1978

Madden JD, Siiteri PK, MacDonald PC, Gant NF: The pattern and rates of metabolism of maternal plasma dehydroisoandrosterone sulfate in human pregnancy. Am J Obstet Gynecol 125:915, 1976

Maruo T, Ladines-Llave CA, Matsuo H, Manalo AS, Mochizuki M: A novel change in cytologic localization of human chorionic gonadotropin and human placental lactogen in first-trimester placenta in the course of gestation. Am J Obstet Gynecol 167:217, 1992

Mason JI, Rainey WE: Steroidogenesis in the human fetal adrenal: A role for cholesterol synthesized de novo. J Clin Endocrinol Metab 64:140, 1987

McGregor WG, Kuhn RW, Jaffe RB: Biologically active chorionic gonadotropin: Synthesis by the human fetus. Science 220:306, 1983

McGregor WG, Raymoure WJ, Kuhn RW, Jaffe RB: Fetal tissue can synthesize a placental hormone: Evidence for chorionic gonadotropin β-subunit synthesis by human fetal kidney. J Clin Invest 68:306, 1981

Milewich L, Gomez-Sanchez CE, Madden JD, Bradfield DJ, Parker PM, Smith SL, Carr BR, Edman CD, MacDonald PC: Dehydroisoandrosterone sulfate in peripheral blood of premenopausal, pregnant, and postmenopausal women and men. J Steroid Biochem 9:1159, 1978

Milewich L, Gomez-Sanchez CE, Madden JD, MacDonald PC: Isolation and characterization of 5α-pregnane-3, 20-dione and progesterone in peripheral blood of pregnant women: Measurement throughout pregnancy. Gynecol Invest 6:291, 1975

Morishima A, Grumbach MM, Simpson ER, Fisher C, Qin K: Aromatase deficiency in male and female siblings caused by a novel mutation and the physiological role of estrogens. J Clin Endocrinol Metab 80:3689, 1995

Mulchahey JJ, DiBlasio AM, Martin MC, Blumenfeld A, Jaffe RB: Hormone production and peptide regulation of the human fetal pituitary gland. Endocr Rev 8:406, 1987

Newby D, Aitken DA, Howatson AG, Connor JM: Placental synthesis of oestriol in Down's syndrome pregnancies. Placenta 21:263, 2000

Nichols J, Lescure OL, Migeon CJ: Levels of 17-hydroxycorticosteroids and 17-ketosteroids in maternal and cord plasma in term anencephaly. J Clin Endocrinol 18:444, 1958

Nishula BC, Wehmann R: Distribution, metabolism, and excretion of human chorionic gonadotropin and its subunits in man. In Segal S (ed): Chorionic Gonadotropin. New York, Plenum, 1980, p 199

Odagiri E, Sherrill BJ, Mount CD, Nicholson WE, Orth DN: Human placental immunoreactive corticotropin, lipotropin, and β-endorphin: Evidence for a common precursor. Proc Natl Acad Sci USA 16:2027, 1979

Ogren L, Talamantes F: The placenta as an endocrine organ: Polypeptides. In Knobil E, Neill JD (eds): The Physiology of Reproduction. New York, Raven, 1994, p 875

Owerbach D, Martial JA, Baxter JD, Rutter WJ, Shows TB: Genes for growth hormone, chorionic somatomammotropin, and growth hormone-like gene on chromosome 17 in humans. Science 209:289, 1980

Owerbach D, Rutter WJ, Cooke NE, Martial JA, Shows TB: The prolactin gene is located on chromosome 6 in humans. Science 212:815, 1981

Parker CR Jr, Carr BR, Simpson ER, MacDonald PC: Decline in the concentration of low-density lipoprotein-cholesterol in human fetal plasma near term. Metabolism 32:919, 1983

Parker CR Jr, Hankins GDV, Carr BR, Leveno KJ, Gant NF, MacDonald PC: The effect of hypertension in pregnant women on fetal adrenal function and fetal plasma lipoprotein-cholesterol metabolism. Am J Obstet Gynecol 150:263, 1984

Parker CR Jr, Hankins GDV, Guzick DS, Rosenfeld CR, MacDonald PC: Ontogeny of unconjugated estriol in fetal blood and the relation of estriol levels at birth to the development of respiratory distress syndrome. Pediatr Res 21:386, 1987

Parker CR Jr, Illingworth DR, Bissonnette J, Carr BR: Endocrinology of pregnancy in abetalipoproteinemia: Studies in a patient with homozygous familial hypobetalipoproteinemia. N Engl J Med 314:557, 1986

Parker CR Jr, Simpson ER, Billheimer DW, Leveno KJ, Carr BR, MacDonald PC: Inverse relation between low-density lipoprotein-cholesterol and dehydroisoandrosterone sulfate in human fetal plasma. Science 208:512, 1980

Patel N, Alsat E, Igout A, Baron F, Hennen G, Porquet D: Glucose inhibits human placenta GH secretion, in vitro. J Clin Endocrinol Metab 80:1743, 1995

Pearlman WH: [16-³H] Progesterone metabolism in advanced pregnancy and in oophorectomized-hysterectomized women. Biochem J 67:1, 1957

Petraglia F, Calza L, Giardino L, Sutton S, Marrama P, Rivier J, Genazzani AR, Vale W: Identification of immunoreactive neuropeptide- (gamma) in human placenta: Localization, secretion, and binding sites. Endocrinology 124: 2016, 1989

Petraglia F, Gallinelli A, De-Vita D, Lewis K, Mathews L, Vale W: Activin at parturition: Changes of maternal serum levels and evidence for binding sites in placenta and fetal membranes. Obstet Gynecol 84:278, 1994

Petraglia F, Garuti GC, Calza L, Roberts V, Giardino L, Genazzani AR, Vale W, Meunier H: Inhibin subunits in human placenta: Localization and messenger ribonucleic acid levels during pregnancy. Am J Obstet Gynecol 165:750, 1991

Petraglia F, Giardino L, Coukos G, Calza L, Vale W, Genazzani AR: Corticotropin-releasing factor and parturition: Plasma and amniotic fluid levels and placental binding sites. Obstet Gynecol 75:784, 1990

Petraglia F, Sawchenko P, Lim AT, Rivier J, Vale W: Localization, secretion, and action of inhibin in human placenta. Science 237:187, 1987

Petraglia F, Woodruff TK, Botticelli G, Botticelli A, Genazzani AR, Mayo KE, Vale W: Gonadotropin-releasing hormone, inhibin, and activin in human placenta: Evidence for a common cellular localization. J Clin Endocrinol Metab 74:1184, 1992

Pulkkinen MO: Arylsulphatase and the hydrolysis of some steroid sulphates in developing organism and placenta. Acta Physiol Scand (Suppl) 180:52, 1961

Riley SC, Walton JC, Herlick JM, Challis JRG: The localization and distribution of corticotropin-releasing hormone in the human placenta and fetal membranes throughout gestation. J Clin Endocrinol Metab 72:1001, 1991

Robinson BG, Emanuel RL, Frim DM, Majzoub JA: Glucocorticoid stimulates expression of corticotropin-releasing hormone gene in human placenta. Proc Natl Acad Sci USA 85:5244, 1988

Ryan KJ: Biological aromatization of steroids. J Biol Chem 234:268, 1959a

Ryan KJ: Metabolism of C-16-oxygenated steroids by human placenta: The formation of estriol. J Biol Chem 234: 2006, 1959b

Shozu M, Akasofu K, Harada T, Kubota Y: A new cause of female pseudohermaphroditism: Placental aromatase deficiency. J Clin Endocrinol Metab 72:560, 1991

Siiteri PK, MacDonald PC: The origin of placental estrogen precursor: During human pregnancy. Excerpta Medica Int Cong Ser 132:726, 1966a

Siiteri PK, MacDonald PC: Placental estrogen biosynthesis during human pregnancy. J Clin Endocrinol Metab 26: 751, 1966b

Siiteri PK, MacDonald PC: The utilization of circulating dehydroisoandrosterone sulfate for estrogen synthesis during human pregnancy. Steroids 2:713, 1963

Siler-Khodr TM: Chorionic peptides. In McNellis D, Challis JRG, MacDonald PC, Nathanielsz PW, Roberts JM (eds): The Onset of Labor: Cellular and Integrative Mechanisms. An NICHD Workshop. Ithaca, Perinatology Press, 1988, p 213

Siler-Khodr TM: Hypothalamic-like peptides of the placenta. Semin Reprod Endocrinol 1:321, 1983

Siler-Khodr TM, Khodr GS: Content of luteinizing hormone-releasing factor in the human placenta. Am J Obstet Gynecol 130:216, 1978

Simpson ER, Burkhart M: Acyl CoA: Cholesterol acyl transferase activity in human placental microsomes: Inhibition by progesterone. Arch Biochem Biophys 200:79, 1980

Simpson ER, Carr BR, Parker CR, Milewich L, Porter JC, MacDonald PC: The role of serum lipoproteins in steroidogenesis by the human fetal adrenal cortex. J Clin Endocrinol Metab 49:146, 1979

Tomer Y, Huber GK, Davies TF: Human chorionic gonado- tropin (hCG) interacts directly with recombinant human TSH receptors. J Clin Endocrinol Metab 74:1477, 1992

Tsuruta E, Tada H, Tamaki H, Kashiwai T, Asahi K, Takeoka K, Mitsuda N, Amino N: Pathogenic role of asialo human chorionic gonadotropin in gestational thyrotoxicosis. J Clin Endocrinol Metab 80:350, 1995

Tungsbutra GV, France JT: Steroid levels in pregnancy. Aust NZ J Obstet Gynaecol 18:97, 1978

Wadhwa PD, Porto M, Garite TJ, Chicz-DeMet A, Sandman CA: Maternal corticotropin-releasing hormone levels in the early third trimester predict length of gestation in human pregnancy. Am J Obstet Gynecol 179:1079, 1998

Walker WH, Fitzpatrick SL, Barrera-Saldana HA, Resendez-Perez D, Saunders GF: The human placental lactogen genes: Structure, function, evolution and transcriptional regulation. Endocr Rev 12:316, 1991

Walsh SW, McCarthy MS: Selective placental secretion of estrogens into fetal and maternal circulations. Endocrinology 109:2152, 1981

Warren JC, Timberlake CE: Steroid sulfatase in the human placenta. J Clin Endocrinol 22:1148, 1962

Weintraub D, Rosen SW: Ectopic production of human chorionic somatomammotropin (HCS) in patients with cancer. Clin Res 18:375, 1970

Werbin H, Plotz EJ, LeRoy GV, David ME: Cholesterol: A precursor of estrone in vivo. J Am Chem Soc 79:1012, 1957

Winters AJ, Oliver C, Colston C, MacDonald PC, Porter JC: Plasma ACTH levels in the human fetus and neonate as related to age and parturition. J Clin Endocrinol Metab 39:269, 1974

Yoshimura M, Pekary AE, Pang XP, Berg L, Goodwin TM, Hershman JM: Thyrotropic activity of basic isoelectric forms of human chorionic gonadotropin extracted from hydatidiform molar tissues. J Clin Endocrinol Metab 78:862, 1994

7

Fetal Growth and Development

The high purposes of obstetrics are to maintain the health of the pregnant woman and to ensure the optimal well-being of the newborn. To this end, contemporary obstetrical research focuses on the physiology and pathophysiology of the fetus, its development, and its environment.

An important direct result of this research is that the status of the fetus has been elevated to that of a patient who, in large measure, can be given the same meticulous care that obstetricians provide for pregnant women. In the course of these studies it has become apparent that the conceptus is the dynamic force in the pregnancy unit. In general, the maternal organism responds passively to signals emanating from embronic-fetal and extraembryonic tissues. The contributions of the conceptus to implantation, maternal recognition of pregnancy, immunological acceptance, endocrine function, nutrition, and parturition are enormous, and absolutely essential for successful pregnancy (see Fig. 2–3).

Normal fetal development is considered in this chapter. In Chapters 36, 37, 40, and 41, techniques used to evaluate fetal well-being, or fetal health, are presented in some detail. Anomalies, injuries, and diseases that affect the fetus and newborn are addressed in detail in Chapter 39.

DETERMINATION OF GESTATIONAL AGE

Several different terms are used to define the duration of pregnancy, and thus fetal age, but these are somewhat confusing. Gestational age or menstrual age is the time elapsed since the first day of the last menstrual period, a time that actually precedes conception. This starting time, which is usually about 2 weeks before ovulation and fertilization and nearly 3 weeks before implantation of the blastocyst, has traditionally been used because most women know when their last period was but not when they last ovulated, although the increasing use of infertility therapy has changed this somewhat. Embryologists, however, describe embryo-fetal development in days or weeks from the time of ovulation (ovulation age) or conception (postconceptional age), the latter two being nearly identical.

Obstetricians customarily calculate gestational age as menstrual age of a given pregnancy. About 280 days, or 40 weeks, elapse on average between the first day of the last menstrual period and the birth of the fetus; 280 days correspond to 9 1/3 calendar months, or 10 units of 28 days each. The unit of 28 days has been referred to, commonly but imprecisely, as a lunar month of pregnancy; actually, the time from one new moon to the next is 29 1/2 days. A quick estimate of the due date of a pregnancy based on menstrual cycle can be made as follows: add 7 days to the first day of the last menstrual

period and subtract 3 months. For example, if the first day of the last menses was June 8, the due date of this pregnancy is 06 08 + 7 (days) minus 3 (months) = 03 15, or March 15 of the following year. As noted in Chapter 41 (p. 116), however, many women now undergo first or early second trimester ultrasound examination to confirm gestational age, and the sonographic estimate is usually a few days later than that determined by the last period. To rectify this inconsistency—and to reduce the number of pregnancies diagnosed as postterm—some authorities suggest assuming that the average pregnancy is actually 283 days long instead of 280, and thus adding 10 days to the last menses instead of 7 (Olsen and Clausen, 1998).

The period of gestation can also be divided into three units of three calendar months each, or three trimesters, because important obstetrical milestones can be designated conveniently by trimesters. The possibility of spontaneous abortion, for example, is limited principally to the first trimester, whereas the likelihood of survival of the infant born preterm is increased greatly in pregnancies that reach the third trimester.

MORPHOLOGICAL GROWTH

OVUM, ZYGOTE, AND BLASTOCYST. During the first 2 weeks after ovulation, several successive phases of development can be identified:

1. Ovulation.
2. Fertilization of the ovum.
3. Formation of free blastocyst.
4. Implantation of the blastocyst (Fig. 7–1).

Primitive chorionic villi are formed soon after implantation. With the development of chorionic villi, it is conventional to refer to the products of conception not as a fertilized ovum, or zygote, but as an embryo. The early stages of preplacental development, and formation of the placenta, are described in Chapter 5.

EMBRYO. The embryonic period commences at the beginning of the third week after ovulation/fertilization, which coincides in time with the expected day that the next menstruation would have started. Most pregnancy tests that measure human chorionic gonadotropin (hCG) use are positive by this time (Chap. 2, p. 26), and the embryonic disc is well defined. The body stalk is differentiated; the chorionic sac is approximately 1 cm in diameter (Figs. 7–2 and 7–3). There is a true intervillous space that contains maternal blood and villous cores in which angioblastic chorionic mesoderm can be distinguished.

By the end of the fourth week after ovulation, the

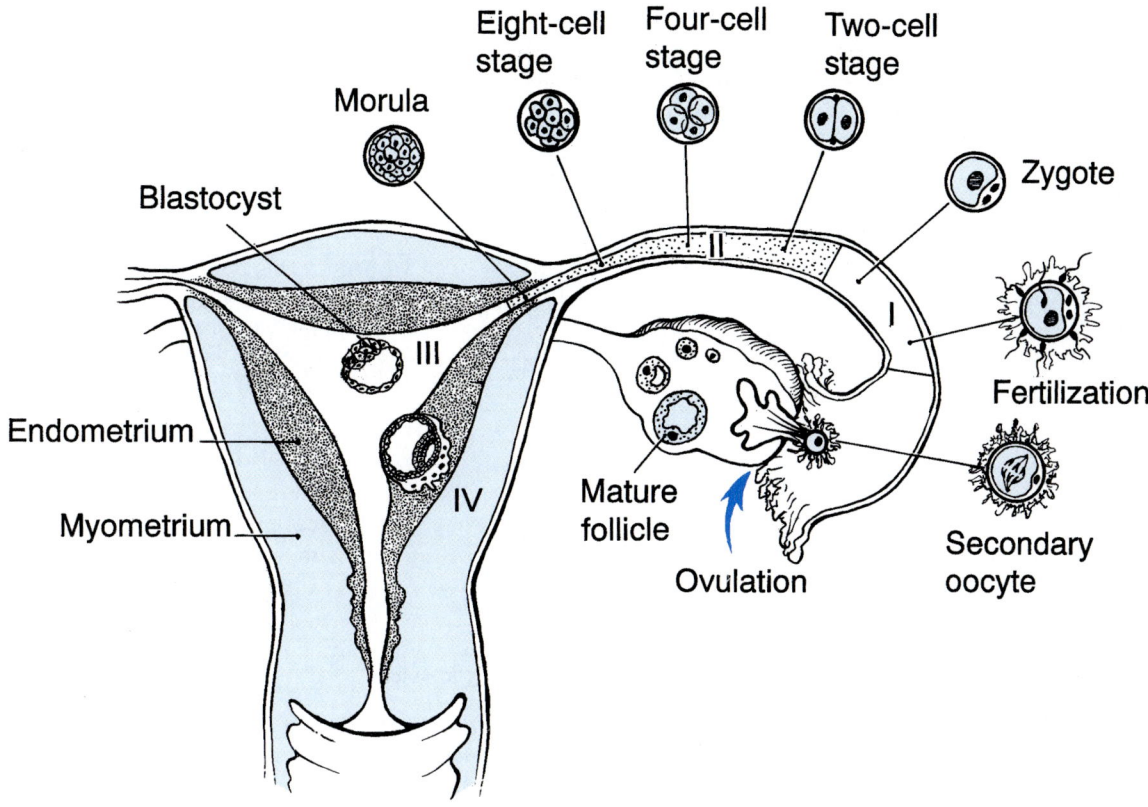

FIGURE 7–1. Diagrammatic summary of the ovarian cycle, fertilization, and human blastocyst development during the first week. (Adapted from Moore, 1988, with permission.)

chorionic sac is 2 to 3 cm in diameter, and the embryo is about 4 to 5 mm in length (Fig. 7–4). Partitioning of the primitive heart begins in the middle of the fourth week. Arm and leg buds are present, and the amnion is beginning to unsheathe the body stalk, which thereafter becomes the umbilical cord.

At the end of the sixth week after fertilization, the embryo is 22 to 24 mm in length, and the head is quite large compared with the trunk. The heart is completely formed. Fingers and toes are present, and the arms bend at the elbows. The upper lip is complete and the external ears form definitive elevations on either side of the head.

FETUS. The end of the embryonic period and the beginning of the fetal period is arbitrarily designated by most embryologists to occur 8 weeks after fertilization, or 10 weeks after the onset of the last menstrual period. At this time, the embryo-fetus is nearly 4 cm long. The major portion of lung development is yet to occur, but few other new major body structures are formed after

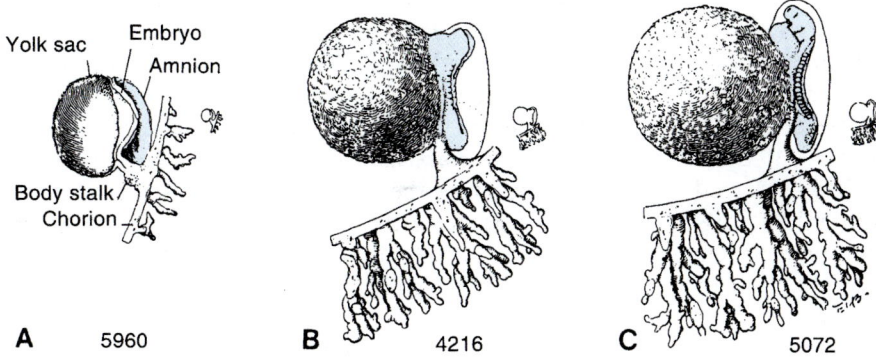

A   5960   **B**   4216   **C**   5072

FIGURE 7–2. Early human embryos. Only the chorion adjacent to the body stalk is shown. Small outline to right of each embryo gives its actual size. Ovulation ages: **A.** 19 days (presomite). **B.** 21 days (7 somites). **C.** 22 days (17 somites). (After drawings and models in the Carnegie Institute.)

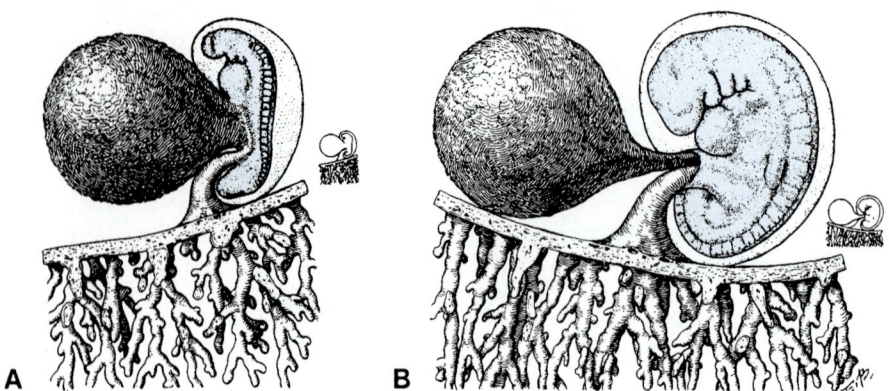

FIGURE 7–3. Early human embryos. Small outline to right of each embryo gives its actual size. Ovulation ages: **A.** 22 days. **B.** 23 days. (After drawings and models in the Carnegie Institute.)

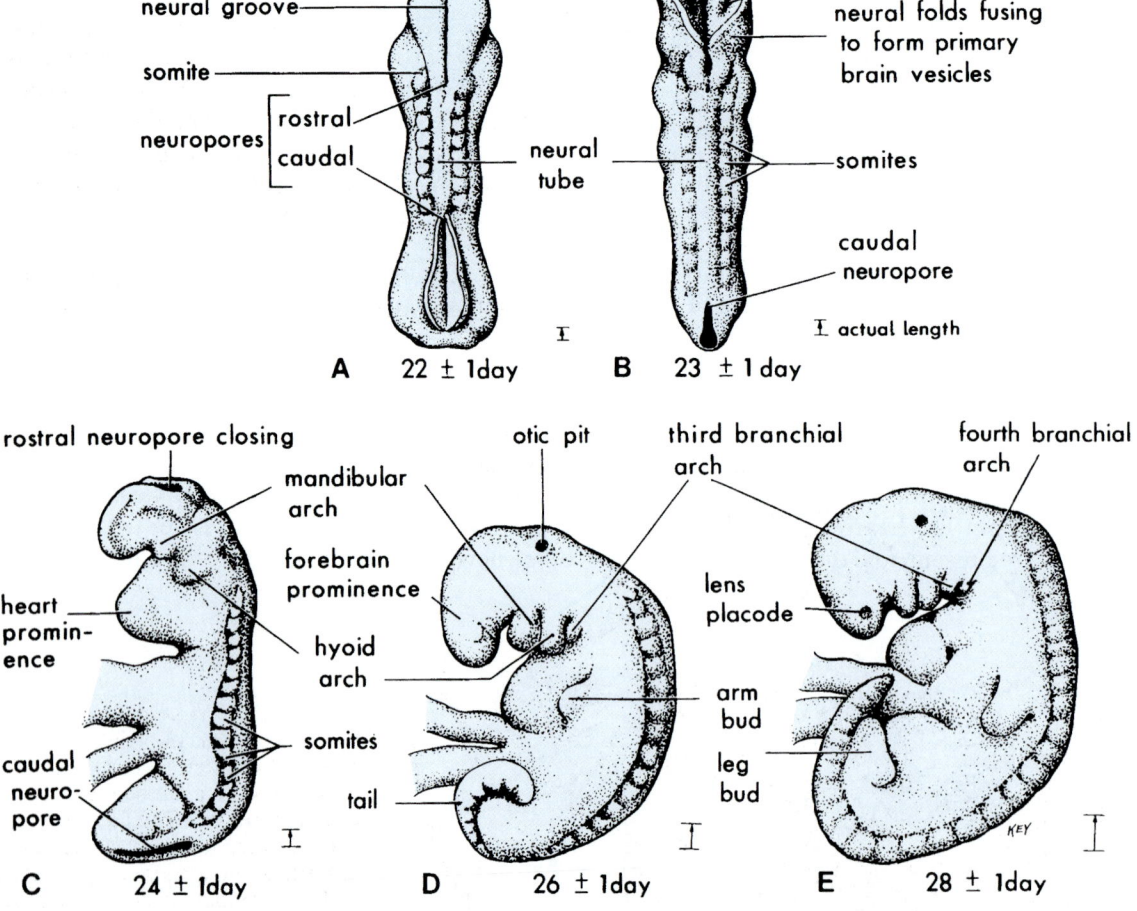

FIGURE 7–4. Three-to four-week-old embryos. **A, B.** Dorsal views of embryos during about 22 to 23 days of development showing 8 and 12 somites, respectively. **C–E.** Lateral views of embryos during 24 to 28 days, showing 16, 27, and 33 somites, respectively. (From Moore, 1988, with permission.)

this time. Development during the fetal period of gestation consists of growth and maturation of structures that were formed during the embryonic period.

12 GESTATIONAL WEEKS. By the end of the 12th week of pregnancy, when the uterus usually is just palpable above the symphysis pubis, the crown-rump length of the fetus is 6 to 7 cm (Fig. 7–5). Centers of ossification have appeared in most of the fetal bones, and the fingers and toes have become differentiated. Skin and nails have developed and scattered rudiments of hair appear; the external genitalia are beginning to show definitive signs of male or female gender. The fetus begins to make spontaneous movements.

16 GESTATIONAL WEEKS. By the end of the 16th week, the crown-rump length of the fetus is 12 cm, and the weight is 110 g. Gender can be correctly determined by experienced observers by inspection of the external genitalia by 14 (menstrual) weeks.

20 GESTATIONAL WEEKS. The end of the 20th week is the midpoint of pregnancy as estimated from the beginning of the last normal menstrual period. The fetus now weighs somewhat more than 300 g, and the weight begins to increase in a linear manner. The fetal skin has become less transparent, a downy lanugo covers its entire body, and some scalp hair has developed.

24 GESTATIONAL WEEKS. By the end of the 24th week, the fetus weighs about 630 g. The skin is characteristically wrinkled, and fat deposition begins. The head is still comparatively quite large; eyebrows and eyelashes are usually recognizable. The canalicular period of lung development, during which the bronchi and bronchioles enlarge and alveolar ducts develop, is nearly completed. A fetus born at this period will attempt to breathe, but most will die because the terminal sacs, required for gas exchange, have not yet formed.

28 GESTATIONAL WEEKS. By the end of the 28th week, a crown-rump length of about 25 cm is attained and the fetus weighs about 1100 g. The thin skin is red and covered with vernix caseosa. The pupillary membrane has just disappeared from the eyes. An infant born at this time moves the limbs quite energetically and cries weakly. The otherwise normal infant of this age has a 90 percent chance of intact survival.

32 GESTATIONAL WEEKS. At the end of 32 gestational weeks, the fetus has attained a crown-rump length of about 28 cm and a weight of about 1800 g. The surface of the skin is still red and wrinkled. Barring other complications, infants born at this period usually survive intact.

36 GESTATIONAL WEEKS. At the end of 36 weeks gestation, the average crown-rump length of the fetus is about 32 cm and the weight is about 2500 g. Because of the deposition of subcutaneous fat, the body has become more rotund, and the previous wrinkled appearance of the face has been lost. Infants born at this time have an excellent chance of survival with proper care.

40 GESTATIONAL WEEKS. Term is reached at 40 weeks from the onset of the last menstrual period. At this

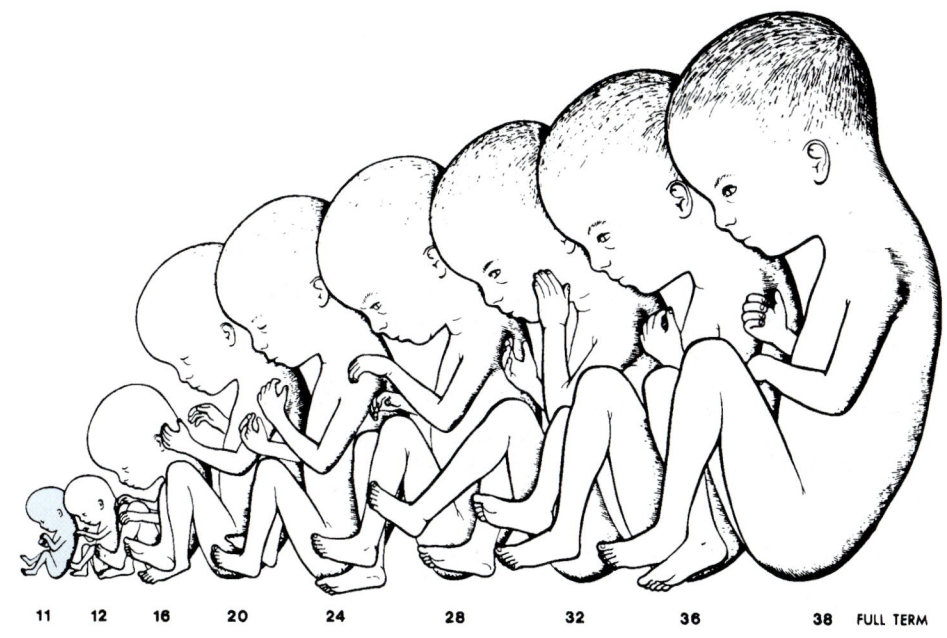

FIGURE 7–5. The embryonic period ends after the eighth week after fertilization; by this time, the beginnings of all essential structures are present. The fetal period, extending from the ninth week until birth, is characterized by growth and differentiation of structures. Gender is clearly distinguishable by postconceptional age 12 weeks. (From Moore, 1988, with permission.)

11 12 16 20 24 28 32 36 38 FULL TERM

time, the fetus is fully developed, with the characteristic features of the newborn infant to be described here. The average crown-rump length of the fetus at term is about 36 cm, and the weight is approximately 3400 g, with variations to be discussed subsequently.

LENGTH OF FETUS. Because of the variability in the length of the legs and the difficulty of maintaining them in extension, measurements corresponding to the sitting height (crown-to-rump) are more accurate than those corresponding to the standing height. The average sitting height and weight of the fetus at the end of each lunar month were determined by Streeter (1920) from 704 specimens. These values are similar to those found more recently and shown in Table 7–1. Such values are approximate, but generally, length is a more accurate criterion of gestational age than weight.

WEIGHT OF THE NEWBORN. The average term infant in the United States at birth weighs about 3000 to 3600 g, depending upon race, parental economic status, size of the parents, parity of the mother, and altitude, with boys about 100 g (3 oz) heavier than girls. During the second half of pregnancy, the fetal weight increases in a linear manner with time until about the 37th week of gestation, and then the rate slows variably. The principal determinants of fetal growth late in pregnancy are related, in large part, to factors influenced by the socioeconomic status of the mother, such as diet, smoking, or substance abuse. In general, the greater the socioeconomic deprivation, the slower the rate of fetal growth late in pregnancy.

Birthweights over 5000 g occur occasionally (Chap. 29, p. 757), but many tales of huge babies vastly exceeding this figure are based on hearsay or inaccurate measurements at best. Presumably, the largest baby recorded in the medical literature is that described by Belcher (1916), a stillborn female weighing 11,340 g (25 lb). Term infants, however, frequently weigh less than 3200 g, and sometimes as little as 2250 g (5 lb) or even less. It was customary in the past, when the birthweight was 2500 g or less, to classify the infant as preterm even though in some cases the low birthweight was not the consequence of preterm birth but rather the result of restricted growth.

FETAL HEAD. From an obstetrical viewpoint, the size of the fetal head is important because an essential fea-

TABLE 7–1. Criteria for Estimating Age During the Fetal Period

Age (wk)		Crown-Rump Length (mm)[a]	Foot Length (mm)[a]	Fetal Weight (g)[b]	Main External Characteristics
Menstrual	Fertilization				
11	9	50	7	8	Eyes closing or closed. Head more rounded. External genitalia still not distinguishable as male or female. Intestines are in the umbilical cord.
12	10	61	9	14	Intestines in abdomen. Early fingernail development.
14	12	87	14	45	Sex distinguishable externally. Well-defined neck.
16	14	120	20	110	Head erect. Lower limbs well developed.
18	16	140	27	200	Ears stand out from head.
20	18	160	33	320	Vernix caseosa present. Early toenail development.
22	20	190	39	460	Head and body (lanugo) hair visible.
24	22	210	45	630	Skin wrinkled and red.
26	24	230	50	820	Fingernails present. Lean body.
28	26	250	55	1000	Eyes partially open. Eyelashes present.
30	28	270	59	1300	Eyes open. Good head of hair. Skin slightly wrinkled.
32	30	280	63	1700	Toenails present. Body filling out. Testes descending.
34	32	300	68	2100	Fingernails reach fingertips. Skin pink and smooth.
38	36	340	79	2900	Body usually plump. Lanugo hairs almost absent. Toenails reach toe tips.
40	38	360	83	3400	Prominent chest; breast protrudes. Testes in scrotum or palpable in inguinal canals. Fingernails extend beyond fingertips.

[a]These measurements are averages and so may not apply to specific cases; dimensional variations increase with age.
[b]These weights refer to fetuses that have been fixed for about 2 weeks in 10 percent formalin. Fresh specimens usually weigh about 5 percent less.
From Moore, 1977, with permission.

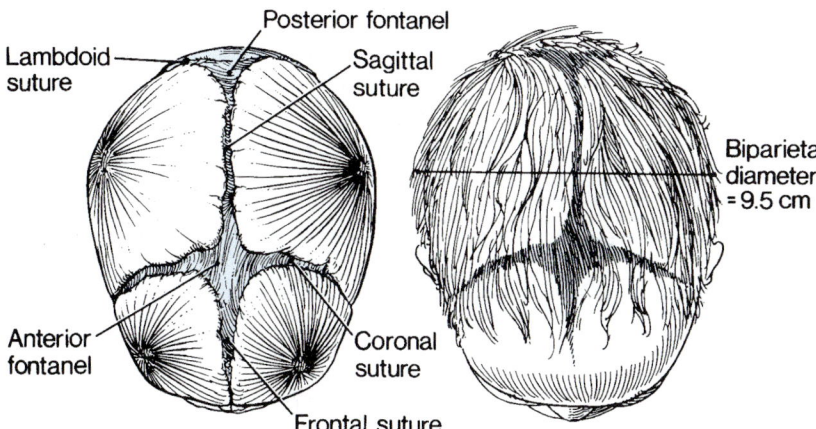

FIGURE 7–6. Fetal head at term showing fontanels, sutures, and the biparietal diameter.

ture of labor is the adaptation between the fetal head and the maternal bony pelvis. Only a comparatively small part of the head at term is represented by the face; the rest is composed of the firm skull, which is made up of two frontal, two parietal, and two temporal bones, along with the upper portion of the occipital bone and the wings of the sphenoid.

These bones are not united rigidly, but rather are separated by membranous spaces, called sutures (Fig. 7–6). The most important sutures are the frontal, between the two frontal bones; the sagittal, between the two parietal bones; the two coronal, between the frontal and parietal bones; and the two lambdoid, between the posterior margins of the parietal bones and upper margin of the occipital bone. With a vertex presentation, all of the sutures are palpable during labor except the temporal sutures, which are situated on either side between the inferior margin of the parietal and upper margin of the temporal bones, covered by soft parts, and cannot be felt in the living fetus.

Where several sutures meet, an irregular space forms, which is enclosed by a membrane and designated as a fontanel (Fig. 7–6). The three most clinically important fontanels are the greater, the lesser, and the temporal fontanels. The greater or anterior fontanel is a lozenge-shaped space that is situated at the junction of the sagittal and the coronal sutures. The lesser or posterior fontanel is represented by a small triangular area at the intersection of the sagittal and lambdoid sutures. Both can be palpated readily during labor. The localization of these fontanels gives important information concerning the presentation and position of the fetus. The temporal, or casserian fontanels, situated at the junction of the lambdoid and temporal sutures, have no diagnostic significance.

It is customary to measure certain critical diameters and circumferences of newborn head (Fig. 7–7). The diameters most frequently used, and the average lengths thereof, are as follows:

1. The *occipitofrontal* (11.5 cm), which follows a line extending from a point just above the root of the nose to the most prominent portion of the occipital bone.
2. The *biparietal* (9.5 cm), the greatest transverse diameter of the head, which extends from one parietal boss to the other.
3. The *bitemporal* (8.0 cm), the greatest distance between the two temporal sutures.
4. The *occipitomental* (12.5 cm), from the chin to the most prominent portion of the occiput.
5. The *suboccipitobregmatic* (9.5 cm), which follows a line drawn from the middle of the large fontanel to the undersurface of the occipital bone just where it joins the neck (Figs. 7–6 and 7–7).

The greatest circumference of the head, which corresponds to the plane of the occipitofrontal diameter, averages 34.5 cm, a size too large to fit through the pelvis without flexion. The smallest circumference, corresponding to the plane of the suboccipitobregmatic diameter, is 32 cm. As a rule, white infants have larger heads than nonwhite infants; boys, somewhat larger than girls; and the infants of multiparas, larger heads than those of nulliparas. The bones of the cranium are normally connected only by a thin layer of fibrous tissue which allows considerable shifting or sliding of each bone to accommodate the size and shape of the maternal pelvis. This intrapartum process is termed *molding*. Because of the varying mobility of the bones of the skull and varying presentations of the fetal head relative to the pelvis, a variety of newborn head shapes are possible. The head position and degree of skull ossification result in a spectrum of cranial plasticity from minimal to great and, in some cases, undoubtedly contributes to fetopelvic disproportion, a leading indication for cesarean delivery (Chap. 18, p. 440).

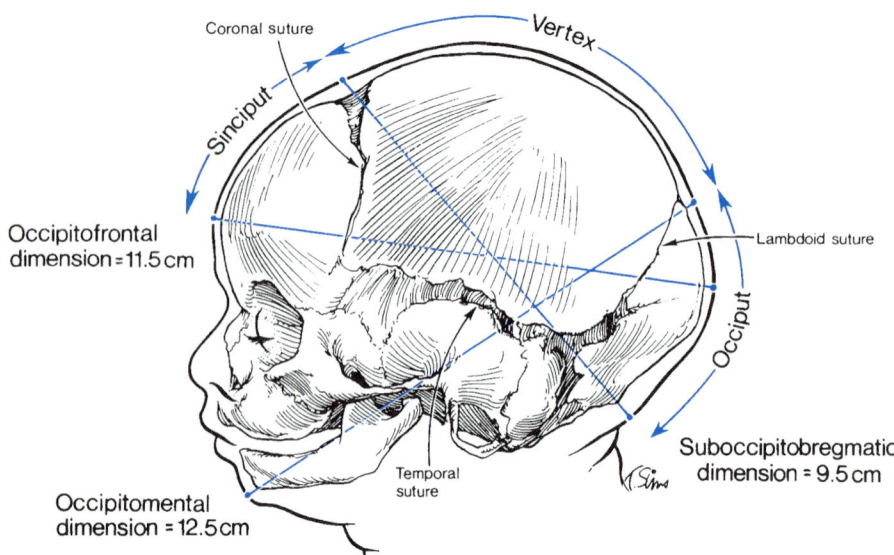

FIGURE 7–7. Diameters of the fetal head at term.

FETAL BRAIN. There is a steady gestational age-related change in the appearance and function of the fetal brain (Fig. 7–8). It is therefore possible to identify fetal age rather precisely from its external appearance (Dolman, 1977). Myelination of the ventral roots of the cerebrospinal nerves and brainstem begins at approximately 6 months, but the major portion of myelination occurs after birth. The lack of myelin and the incomplete ossification of the fetal skull permit the structure of the brain to be seen with ultrasound throughout gestation.

THE FETAL–MATERNAL COMMUNICATION SYSTEM: PLACENTAL ARM

The transfer of oxygen and a great variety of nutrients from the mother to the fetus, and conversely the transfer of carbon dioxide and other metabolic wastes from fetus to mother, is accomplished by way of the nutritive component of the placental arm of the fetal–maternal communication system (see Fig. 2–3). The placenta is the organ of transfer between mother and fetus. The placenta, and to a limited extent the attached membranes, supply all materials required for fetal growth and energy production while removing products of fetal catabolism.

There are no direct communications between the fetal blood, which is contained in the fetal capillaries in the intravillous space of the chorionic villi, and the maternal blood, which remains in the intervillous space. The one exception to this dictum is the occasional development of breaks in the chorionic villi, permitting the escape of fetal erythrocytes and leukocytes, in various numbers, into the maternal circulation. This leakage is the mechanism by which some D-negative women become sensi-

tized by the erythrocytes of their D-positive fetus (Chap. 39, p. 1057). Aside from these occasional leaks, however, there is no gross intermingling of the macromolecular constituents of the two circulations. The transfer of substances from mother to fetus and from fetus to mother, therefore, depends primarily on the processes that permit or facilitate the transport of such substances through the syncytiotrophoblast of the intact chorionic villi.

THE INTERVILLOUS SPACE: MATERNAL BLOOD. The intervillous space is the primary biological compartment of maternal–fetal transfer. Maternal blood in this extravascular compartment directly bathes the trophoblasts. Substances transferred from mother to fetus first enter the intervillous space and are then transported to the syncytiotrophoblast. Substances transported from the fetus to the mother are transferred from the syncytium into the same space. This process of transfer supplies the fetus with oxygen as well as nutrients and provides for elimination of metabolic waste products. Thus the chorionic villi and the intervillous space, together, function for the fetus as lung, gastrointestinal tract, and kidney.

Although renal function develops gradually, fetal urination begins early in pregnancy, and fetal urine comprises the major portion of the amnionic fluid after 16 weeks. At 22 weeks, an average of 2.2 mL/h is produced, increasing to 10 mL/h at 30 weeks and 50 mL/h at term (Kurjak and associates, 1981).

The circulation of maternal blood within the intervillous space is described in Chapter 5 (p. 100). The residual volume of the intervillous space of the term placenta measures about 140 mL; the normal volume of the intervillous space before delivery, however, may be twice this value (Aherne and Dunnill, 1966). Uteroplacental

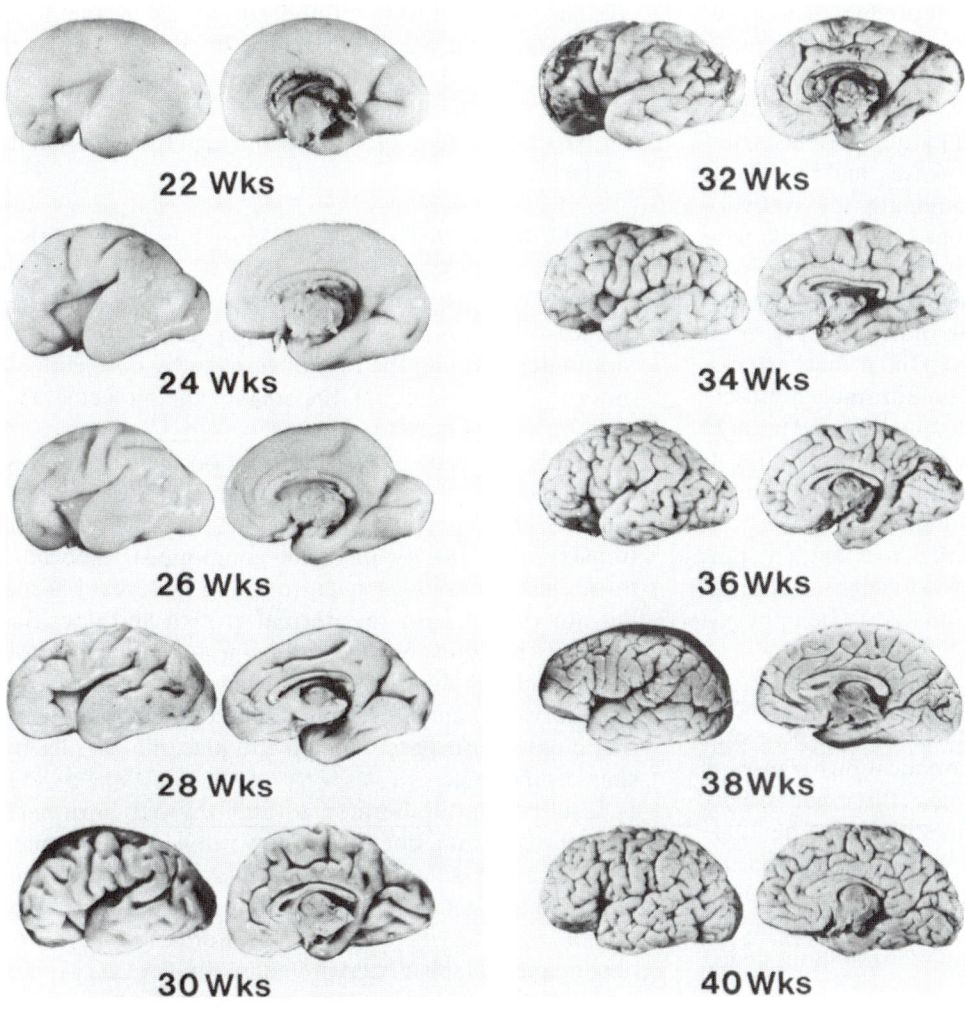

22 Wks

24 Wks

26 Wks

28 Wks

30 Wks

32 Wks

34 Wks

36 Wks

38 Wks

40 Wks

FIGURE 7–8. Characteristic configuration of fetal brains from 22 to 40 weeks of gestation at 2-week intervals. (From Dolman, 1977, with permission.)

blood flow near term has been estimated to be about 700 to 900 mL/min, with most of the blood apparently going to the intervillous space.

The forceful uterine contractions of active labor cause a reduction in blood flow into the intervillous space, the degree of reduction depending in large measure upon the intensity of the contraction. Blood pressure within the intervillous space is significantly less than the uterine arterial pressure, but somewhat greater than uterine venous pressure. Uterine venous pressure, in turn, varies depending upon several factors, including maternal position. When supine, for example, pressure in the lower part of the inferior vena cava is elevated; consequently, in this position, pressure in the uterine and ovarian veins, and in turn in the intervillous space, is increased. An even greater increase in intervillous pressure is likely when the pregnant woman is standing.

FETAL CAPILLARIES OF THE INTRAVILLOUS SPACE: FETAL BLOOD. The hydrostatic pressure in the fetal capillaries that traverse the chorionic villi is probably not appreciably different from that in the intervillous space. During normal labor, the rise in fetal blood pressure must be parallel to the pressure in the amnionic fluid and the intervillous space. Otherwise, the capillaries in the chorionic villi would collapse and fetal blood flow through the placenta would cease.

PLACENTAL TRANSFER

CHORIONIC VILLUS. Substances that pass from maternal blood to fetal blood must traverse (1) syncytiotrophoblast, (2) stroma of the intravillous space, and (3) fetal capillary wall. Although this histological barrier separates the blood in the maternal and fetal circulations, it does not behave in a uniform manner like a simple physical barrier. Throughout pregnancy, syncytiotrophoblast actively or passively permits, facilitates, and adjusts the amount and rate of transfer of a wide range of substances to the fetus. After midpregnancy, the number of Langhans cells, or cytotrophoblasts, lining the innermost layer of villi decreases, and the villous epithelium then consists predominantly of syncytiotrophoblast. The walls of the villous capillaries likewise become thinner, and the relative number of fetal vessels increases in relation to the villous connective tissue. It is important to recall that the walls of the fetal placental surface vessels, after branching from the truncal arteries of the chorionic vessels, do not contain smooth muscle cells (Chap. 5, p. 99). Several attempts have been made to estimate the total surface area of chorionic villi in the human placenta at term. From the planimetric measurements made by Aherne and Dunnill (1966) of the villous surface area of the placenta, it is evident that there is a close correlation with fetal weight. The total surface area at term has been estimated to be approximately 10 m².

REGULATION OF PLACENTAL TRANSFER.

The syncytiotrophoblast is the fetal tissue interface of the placental arm of the fetal–maternal (communication) transport system. The maternal-facing surface of this tissue is characterized by a complex microvillus structure. The fetal-facing (basal) cell membrane of the trophoblast is the site of transfer to the intravillous space through which the fetal capillaries traverse. The fetal capillaries are an additional site for transport from the intravillous space into fetal blood, or vice versa.

In determining the effectiveness of the human placenta as an organ of transfer, at least 10 variables are important:

1. The concentration of the substance under consideration in the maternal plasma, and in some instances the extent to which it is bound to another compound, such as a carrier protein.
2. The rate of maternal blood flow through the intervillous space.
3. The area available for exchange across the villous trophoblast epithelium.
4. If the substance is transferred by diffusion, the physical properties of the tissue barrier interposed between blood in the intervillous space and in the fetal capillaries.
5. For any substance actively transported, the capacity of the biochemical machinery of the placenta for effecting active transfer, for example, specific receptors on the plasma membrane of the trophoblast.
6. The amount of the substance metabolized by the placenta during transfer.
7. The area for exchange across the fetal capillaries in the placenta.

8. The concentration of the substance in the fetal blood, exclusive of any that is bound.
9. Specific binding or carrier proteins in the fetal or maternal circulation.
10. The rate of fetal blood flow through the villus capillaries.

MECHANISMS OF TRANSFER.

Most substances with a molecular mass less than 500 d diffuse readily through the placental tissue interposed between the maternal and fetal circulations. Molecular weight is clearly important in determining the rate of transfer by diffusion; all other things being equal, the smaller the molecule, the more rapid the transfer rate.

Simple diffusion, however, is by no means the only mechanism of transfer of low molecular weight compounds. The syncytiotrophoblast actively facilitates the transfer of a variety of small compounds, especially those that are in low concentration in maternal plasma but are essential for the normal growth and development of the fetus. Simple diffusion appears to be the mechanism involved in the transfer of oxygen, carbon dioxide, water, and most (but not all) electrolytes. Anesthetic gases also pass through the placenta rapidly by simple diffusion.

Insulin, steroid hormones, and thyroid hormones cross the placenta, but at very slow rates. The hormones synthesized in situ in the trophoblasts enter both the maternal and fetal circulations, but not equally (Chap. 6). For example, concentrations of chorionic gonadotropin and placental lactogen in fetal plasma are very much lower than in maternal plasma. Substances of very high molecular weight usually do not traverse the placenta, but there are important exceptions, such as immune gamma globulin G—with an M_r of about 160,000—which is transferred by way of a specific trophoblast receptor–mediated mechanism.

TRANSFER OF OXYGEN AND CARBON DIOXIDE.

In their excellent account of placental transport, Morriss and associates (1994) recall that Mayow, in 1674, suggested that the placenta served as the fetal lung. Erasmus Darwin, in 1796, only 22 years after the discovery of oxygen, observed that the color of blood passing through lungs and gills became bright red. He deduced that from the structure as well as the position of the placenta, that it appeared to be a respiratory organ by which the fetus becomes oxygenated.

The transfer of carbon dioxide across the placenta is diffusion limited. The transfer of oxygen, however, is blood-flow limited, and there are other limitations. The placenta supplies about 8 mL O_2/min/kg of fetal weight, and because fetal blood oxygen stores are sufficient for only 1 to 2 minutes, this supply must be continuous (Longo, 1991). Normal values for oxygen, carbon diox-

TABLE 7–2. Normal Values for Oxygen, Carbon Dioxide, and pH in Human Maternal and Fetal Blood

	Uterine		Umbilical	
	Artery	Vein	Vein	Artery
P_{O_2} (mm Hg)	95	40	27	15
O_2Hb (% saturation)	98	76	68	30
O_2 content (mL/dL)	15.8	12.2	14.5	6.4
Hemoglobin (g/dL)	12.0	12.0	16.0	16.0
O_2 capacity (mL O_2/dL)	16.1	16.1	21.4	21.4
P_{CO_2} (mm Hg)	32	40	43	48
CO_2 content (mM/L)	19.6	21.8	25.2	26.3
HCO_3 (mM/L)	18.8	20.7	24.0	25.0
pH	7.40	7.34	7.38	7.35

From Longo, 1987, with permission.

ide, and pH in maternal and fetal blood, are presented in Table 7–2. Because of the continuous passage of oxygen from the maternal blood in the intervillous space to the fetus, the oxygen saturation of this blood resembles that in the maternal capillaries. The average oxygen saturation of intervillous space blood is estimated to be 65 to 75 percent, with a partial pressure (P_{O_2}) of about 30 to 35 mm Hg. The oxygen saturation of umbilical vein blood is similar, but with an oxygen partial pressure somewhat lower.

Despite the relatively low P_{O_2}, the fetus normally does not suffer from lack of oxygen. The human fetus probably behaves like the lamb fetus, and therefore has a cardiac output considerably greater per unit of body weight than does the adult. The high cardiac output, the increased oxygen-carrying capacity of fetal hemoglobin, and, late in pregnancy, a higher hemoglobin concentration than in adults, compensate effectively for the low oxygen tension (see p. 146). Additional evidence that the fetus normally does not experience lack of oxygen is provided by measurements of the lactic acid content of fetal blood, which is only slightly higher than that of the mother (Morriss and associates, 1994).

In general, transfer of fetal carbon dioxide is accomplished by diffusion. The placenta is highly permeable to carbon dioxide, which traverses the chorionic villus more rapidly than oxygen. Near term, the partial pressure of carbon dioxide (P_{CO_2}) in the umbilical arteries is estimated to average about 48 mm Hg, or about 5 mm Hg more than in the maternal intervillous blood. Fetal blood has less affinity for carbon dioxide than does maternal blood, thereby favoring the transfer of carbon dioxide from the fetus to the mother. Also, mild hyperventilation by the pregnant woman results in a fall in P_{CO_2} favoring a transfer of carbon dioxide from the fetal compartment into maternal blood.

SELECTIVE TRANSFER AND FACILITATED DIFFUSION. While simple diffusion is an important method of placental transfer, the trophoblast and chorionic villus unit demonstrate enormous selectivity in transfer. This results in different concentrations of a variety of metabolites on the two sides of the villus.

The concentrations of a number of substances which are not synthesized by the fetus are several times higher in fetal than in maternal blood. Ascorbic acid is a good example of this phenomenon. This relatively low molecular weight substance resembles the pentose and hexose sugars and might be expected to traverse the placenta by simple diffusion. The concentration of ascorbic acid, however, is two to four times higher in fetal plasma than in maternal plasma (Morriss and associates, 1994). The unidirectional transfer of iron across the placenta provides another example of transport and sequestration of selected agents. Typically, iron is present in the plasma of the pregnant woman at a lower concentration than in her fetus; and at the same time, the iron-binding capacity of maternal plasma is much greater. Nonetheless, iron is transported actively from maternal to fetal plasma; and in the human fetus, the amount transferred appears to be independent of maternal iron status.

Infections of the fetus caused by viruses, bacteria, and protozoa are occasionally encountered (Chap. 39). Many viruses, including rubella, varicella, cytomegalovirus, and human immunodeficiency virus may cross the placenta and infect the fetus. A number of bacteria, notably treponemes and tuberculosis; as well as protozoans like toxoplasma and plasmodium also may cause fetal infection. With protozoal and bacterial—but not necessarily viral—infections, there is almost always histological evidence of placental involvement.

Rarely, malignant cells arising in neoplasias in the pregnant woman are transferred to the placenta, the fetus, or both (Gilstrap and Cunningham, 1996). As discussed in Chapter 32 (p. 848), most such cases are limited to the placenta, but occasionally malignant melanomas or hematopoietic cell malignancies can metastasize to the fetus origin.

NUTRITION OF THE FETUS

During the first 2 months of pregnancy, the embryo consists almost entirely of water; later in fetal development, relatively more solids are added. The amounts of water, fat, nitrogen, and certain minerals in the fetus at successive weeks of gestation are given in Table 7–3. Because of the small amount of yolk in the human ovum, growth of the embryo-fetus from the very early stage of development is dependent on nutrients obtained from the mother. During the first few days after implantation, the nutrition of the blastocyst comes from the interstitial

TABLE 7–3. Total Amounts of Fat, Nitrogen, and Minerals in the Body of the Developing Fetus

Body Weight (g)	Approx. Fetal Age (wk)	Water (g)	Fat (g)	N (g)	Ca (g)	P (g)	Mg (g)	Na (mEq)	K (mEq)	Cl (mEq)	Fe (mg)	Cu (mg)	Zn (mg)
30	13	27	0.2	0.4	0.09	0.09	0.003	3.6	1.4	2.4	—	—	—
100	15	89	0.5	1.0	0.3	0.2	0.01	9	2.6	7	5.1	—	—
200	17	177	1.0	2.8	0.7	0.6	0.03	20	7.9	14	10	0.7	2.6
500	23	440	3.0	7.0	2.2	1.5	0.10	49	22	33	28	2.4	9.4
1000	26	860	10	14	6.0	3.4	0.22	90	41	66	64	3.5	16
1500	31	1270	35	25	10	5.6	0.35	125	60	96	100	5.6	25
2000	33	1620	100	37	15	8.2	0.46	160	84	120	160	8.0	35
2500	35	1940	185	49	20	11	0.58	200	110	130	220	10	43
3000	38	2180	360	55	25	14	0.70	240	130	150	260	12	50
3500	40	2400	560	62	30	17	0.78	280	150	160	280	14	53

From Widdowson, 1968, with permission.

fluid of the endometrium and the surrounding maternal tissue. Within the next week, the forerunners of the intervillous space are formed. In the beginning, these are simply lacunae that are filled with maternal blood, but during the third week after fertilization the fetal blood vessels in the chorionic villi appear. During the fourth week, a cardiovascular system has formed, and thereby a true circulation is established both within the embryo and between the embryo and the chorionic villi.

Ultimately, the maternal diet provides all nutrients supplied to the fetus. Ingested foodstuff is translated into storage forms that are made available continuously, in an orderly fashion, to meet the demands for energy, tissue repair, and new growth, including maternal needs for pregnancy. Three major maternal storage depots, the liver, muscle, and adipose tissue and the storage hormone insulin, are intimately involved in the metabolism of the nutrients absorbed from the maternal gut. Maternal insulin is released in response to various compounds liberated during digestion and absorption. Insulin secretion is sustained by increased serum levels of glucose and amino acids. The net effect is storage of glucose as glycogen primarily in liver and muscle, retention of some amino acids as protein, and storage of the excess as fat. Storage of maternal fat peaks in the second trimester, and then declines as fetal demands increase in late pregnancy (Pipe and colleagues, 1979).

During times of fasting, glucose is released from glycogen, but maternal glycogen stores are not large and cannot provide an adequate amount of glucose to meet requirements for maternal energy and fetal growth. Cleavage of triacylglycerols, stored in adipose tissue, however, provides the mother with energy in the form of free fatty acids. Lipolysis is activated, directly or indirectly, by a number of hormones, including glucagon, norepinephrine, placental lactogen (hPL), glucocorticosteroids, and thyroxine.

GLUCOSE AND FETAL GROWTH. The fetus is not exposed to a constant supply of glucose, and maternal plasma levels may vary by up to 75 percent. Although the fetus is quite dependent on the mother for nutrition, the fetus is not a passive parasite and actively participates in providing for its own nutrition. At midpregnancy, fetal glucose concentration is independent of and may exceed maternal levels (Bozzetti and colleagues, 1988).

Glucose is a major nutrient for fetal growth and energy. It is thus logical that mechanisms exist during pregnancy to minimize maternal glucose use so that the limited maternal supply is available to the fetus. It is believed that placental lactogen (hPL), a hormone normally present in abundance in the mother but not the fetus, blocks the peripheral uptake and use of glucose while promoting the mobilization and use of free fatty acids by maternal tissues (Chap. 6, p. 114). It does not appear however, that hPL, nor placental growth hormone, are absolutely required for a normal pregnancy outcome.

GLUCOSE TRANSPORT. The transfer of D-glucose across cell membranes is accomplished by a carrier-mediated, stereospecific, nonconcentrating process of facilitated diffusion. Six separate glucose transport proteins (GLUT) have been discovered. They belong to the 12-transmembrane segment transporter superfamily and are characterized further by tissue-specific distribution (Chap. 29, p. 745). Transporter proteins for D-glucose, GLUT-1, and GLUT-3, have been identified in the plasma membrane (the microvilli) of human syncytiotrophoblast. GLUT-1 expression is prominent in human placenta, increases as pregnancy advances, and is induced by almost all growth factors (Sakata and colleagues, 1995). GLUT-3 is also expressed prominently in placenta, being localized in human syncytiotrophoblast (Hahn and associates, 1995).

A great deal of investigative effort continues to be focused on maternal nutrition and its effect on fetal growth and development. Fetal size is a function not only of fetal age, but of the efficiency of nutrient transport, nutrient availability, and a number of cofactors. For example, in women with maternal diabetes with no significant maternal vascular disease, the fetus may be larger than normal because of high maternal glucose levels and efficient transfer. Conversely, if severe maternal vascular disease is a complication of the diabetes, the fetus may be appreciably smaller than normal because transport is impaired (Chap. 29, p. 751).

GLUCOSE, INSULIN, AND FETAL MACROSOMIA. The precise biomolecular events in the pathophysiology of fetal macrosomia are not defined. Nonetheless, it seems clear that fetal hyperinsulinemia is one driving force (Schwartz and colleagues, 1994). As discussed in Chapter 29 (p. 744), insulin-like growth factor (IGF-I), as well as fibroblast-growth factor (FGF-2), also are involved (Guidice and associates, 1995; Hill and colleagues, 1995). Therefore, a hyperinsulinemic state with increased levels of selected growth factors, together with increased expression of GLUT proteins in syncytiotrophoblast, may promote excessive fetal growth.

LACTATE. This substance also is transported across the placenta by facilitated diffusion. By way of co-transport with hydrogen ions, lactate is probably transported as lactic acid.

FREE FATTY ACIDS AND TRIGLYCERIDES. Among mammalian neonates, the human newborn has a large proportion of fat, specifically 15 percent of body weight on average (Kimura, 1991). This is indicative that late in pregnancy, a substantial part of substrate transferred to the human fetus is stored as fat. Neutral fat (triacylglycerols) does not cross the placenta, but glycerol does. It is likely that most fatty acids cross the placenta by simple diffusion. Moreover, fatty acids are also synthesized in the placenta. Lipoprotein lipase is present on the maternal but not on the fetal side of the placenta. This arrangement should favor hydrolysis of triacylglycerols in the maternal intervillous space while preserving these neutral lipids in fetal blood. Fatty acids transferred to the fetus can be converted to triacylglycerols in the fetal liver.

The placental uptake and use of low-density lipoprotein (LDL) was cited in Chapter 6 (p. 123) as an alternate mechanism for fetal assimilation of essential fatty acids and amino acids. The LDL particles from maternal plasma bind to specific LDL receptors in the coated-pit regions of the microvilli on the maternal-facing side of the syncytiotrophoblast. The large (about 250,000 d) LDL particle is taken up by a process of receptor-mediated endocytosis. The apoprotein and cholesterol esters of LDL are hydrolyzed by lysosomal enzymes in the syncytium to give:

1. Cholesterol for progesterone synthesis.
2. Free amino acids—including essential amino acids.
3. Essential fatty acids, primarily linoleic acid.

Indeed, the concentration of arachidonic acid, which is synthesized from linoleic acid in fetal plasma, is greater than that in maternal plasma. Linoleic acid (and/or arachidonic acid) must be assimilated from maternal dietary intake.

AMINO ACIDS. In addition to the hydrolysis of LDL, the placenta is known to concentrate a large number of amino acids intracellularly (Lemons, 1979). Neutral amino acids from maternal plasma are taken up by trophoblasts by at least three specific processes. Presumably, amino acids are concentrated in the syncytiotrophoblasts, and thence transferred to the fetal side by diffusion. Based upon data from cordocentesis blood samples, the concentration of amino acids in cord umbilical plasma is greater than in maternal venous or arterial plasma (Morriss and associates, 1994).

PROTEINS. Generally, there is very limited transfer of larger proteins across the placenta. There are important exceptions; for example, immunoglobulin G (IgG) crosses the placenta in large amounts. Another exception is retinol-binding protein.

Near term, IgG is present in approximately the same concentrations in cord and maternal sera, but IgA and IgM in cord serum are considerably lower. Although IgA and IgM of maternal origin are effectively excluded from the fetus, IgG crosses the placenta with considerable efficiency (Gitlin and colleagues, 1972). Fc receptors are present on trophoblasts; the transport of IgG is accomplished by way of these receptors through a classical process of endocytosis. Increased amounts of IgM are found in the fetus only after the fetal immune system has been provoked into antibody response by infection in the fetus.

IONS AND TRACE METALS. Iodide transport across the placenta is clearly attributable to a carrier-mediated, energy-requiring active process; indeed, the placenta concentrates iodide. The concentrations of zinc in the fetal plasma also are greater than those in maternal plasma. Conversely, copper levels in fetal plasma are less than those in maternal plasma. This is of particular interest because important copper-requiring enzymes are required for fetal development.

PLACENTAL SEQUESTRATION OF HEAVY METALS. The heavy metal–binding protein, metallothionein-1, is expressed in human syncytiotrophoblast. This protein binds (sequesters) a host of heavy metals including zinc, copper, lead, and cadmium.

The most common source of cadmium in the environment is cigarette smoke. Cadmium levels in maternal blood and placenta are increased with maternal smoking, but there is no increase in cadmium transfer into the fetus. The cadmium concentration in cord blood is less than that in maternal blood, and there is little or no cadmium in fetal liver or kidney. Presumably, the low levels of cadmium in the fetus are attributable to the sequestration (binding) of cadmium by metallothionein(s) in trophoblast. This comes about because cadmium acts to increase the transcription of the metallothionein gene(s); and cadmium-induced increases in trophoblast metallothionein levels result in placenta cadmium accumulation (sequestration). Metallothionein also binds (sequesters) copper (Cu^{2+}) in placenta, thus accounting for the low levels of Cu^{2+} in cord blood. A number of mammalian enzymes require Cu^{2+}, and its deficiency results in inadequate collagen cross-linking and, in turn, diminished tensile strength of tissues.

The concentration of cadmium in amnionic fluid is similar to that in maternal blood. The incidence of preterm premature rupture of the fetal membranes (amnion) is increased in women who smoke. It is possible that cadmium provokes metallothionein synthesis in amnion, causing sequestration of Cu^{2+} and a pseudocopper deficiency.

CALCIUM AND PHOSPHORUS. These also are actively transported from mother to fetus. A calcium-binding protein is present in placenta. Parathyroid hormone–related protein (PTH-rP), as the name implies, acts as a surrogate PTH in many systems, including the activation of adenylate cyclase and the movement of Ca^{2+}. The history and selected special actions proposed for PTH-rP in endometrium/decidua are described in Chapter 4 (p. 73). The production of PTH-rP in placenta is addressed in Chapter 6 (p. 115), and the potential role of this agent in myometrium is cited in Chapter 11 (p. 272). PTH-rP is not produced in normal adult parathyroid glands, but is produced in the fetal parathyroid and in the placenta and other fetal tissues, especially the fetal kidney. Moreover, PTH is not demonstrable in human fetal plasma, but PTH-rP is present. For those reasons, some refer to PTH-rP as

the fetal parathormone (Abbas and associates, 1990). There is a Ca^{2+}-sensing receptor in trophoblast as there is in the parathyroid glands (Juhlin and colleagues, 1990). The expression of PTH-rP in cytotrophoblasts is modulated by the extracellular concentration of Ca^{2+} (Hellman and co-workers, 1992). It seems possible, therefore, that PTH-rP synthesized in decidua, placenta, and other fetal tissues is important in fetal calcium transfer and homeostasis.

VITAMINS. The concentration of *vitamin A* (*retinol*) is greater in fetal than in maternal plasma. Vitamin A in fetal plasma is bound to retinol-binding protein and to prealbumin. Retinol-binding protein is transferred from the maternal compartment across the syncytium. The transport of *vitamin C* (*ascorbic acid*) across the placenta from mother to fetus is accomplished by an energy-dependent, carrier-mediated process. The levels of the principal *vitamin D* (*cholecalciferol*) metabolites, including 1,25-dihydroxycholecalciferol, are greater in maternal plasma than are those in fetal plasma. The 1α-hydroxylation of 25-hydroxyvitamin D_3 is known to take place in placenta and in decidua.

PHYSIOLOGY OF THE FETUS

AMNIONIC FLUID. In early pregnancy, amnionic fluid is an ultrafiltrate of maternal plasma. By the beginning of the second trimester, it consists largely of extracellular fluid which diffuses through the fetal skin, and thus reflects the composition of fetal plasma (Gilbert and Brace, 1993). After 20 weeks, however, the cornification of fetal skin prevents this diffusion and amnionic fluid is composed largely of fetal urine. The fetal kidneys start producing urine at 12 weeks' gestation, and by 18 weeks are producing 7 to 14 mL per day. Fetal urine contains more urea, creatinine, and uric acid than plasma, as well as desquamated fetal cells, vernix, lanugo, and various secretions. Because these are hypotonic, the net effect is decreasing amionic fluid osmolality with advancing gestation. Pulmonary fluid contributes a small proportion of the amnionic volume, and fluid filtering through the placenta accounts for the rest.

The volume of amnionic fluid at each week of gestation is quite variable. In general, the volume increases by 10 mL per week at 8 weeks and increases up to 60 mL per week at 21 weeks, then declines gradually back to a steady state by 33 weeks (Brace and Wolf, 1989). The usual amnionic fluid volume thus increases from 50 mL at 12 weeks to 400 mL at midpregnancy and 1000 mL at term (Gillibrand, 1969).

Amnionic fluid serves to cushion the fetus, allowing

musculoskeletal development and protecting it from trauma. It also maintains temperature and has a minimal nutritive function. Epidermal growth factor (EGF) and EGF-like growth factors, such as transforming growth factor-α, are present in amnionic fluid. Ingestion of amnionic fluid into the lung and gastrointestinal tract may promote growth and differentiation of these tissues by inspiration and swallowing amnionic fluid. PTH-rP and endothelin-1 also are present in amnionic fluid, and it has been proposed that these peptides may be involved in fetal development. Both act as growth factors in selected cells, and PTH-rP promotes surfactant synthesis cells in type II pneumonocytes in vitro (Rubin and co-workers, 1994).

A more important function, however, is to promote the normal growth and development of the lungs and gastrointestinal tract. Animal studies have shown that pulmonary hypoplasia can be produced by draining off amnionic fluid, by banding the trachea to prevent "inhalation" of fluid into the lungs, by chronically draining pulmonary fluid through the trachea, and by physically preventing the prenatal chest excursions that mimic breathing (Adzick and associates, 1984; Alcorn and colleagues, 1977). Thus the formation of intrapulmonary fluid and, at least as important, the alternating egress and retention of fluid in the lungs by breathing movements, are essential to normal pulmonary development. Clinical implications of oligohydramnios and pulmonary hypoplasia are discussed in Chapter 31 (p. 822).

FETAL CIRCULATION. This differs fundamentally from that of the adult. For example, because fetal blood does not need to enter the pulmonary vasculature to be oxygenated, the major portion of the right ventricular output bypasses the lungs. Oxygen and nutrient materials required for fetal growth and maturation are delivered to the fetus from the placenta by the single umbilical vein, and thus do not need to be absorbed through the gastrointestinal tract (Fig. 7–9). Additionally, the chambers of the fetal heart work in parallel, not in series, which effectively supplies the brain and heart with more highly oxygenated blood than the rest of the body. The fetal circulation is unique, and functions smoothly until the moment of birth, when it is required to change dramatically.

Oxygenated blood is brought to the fetus by the umbilical vein, which enters the abdomen through the umbilical ring and ascends along the anterior abdominal wall toward the liver. The vein then divides into the ductus venosus and the portal sinus. The ductus venosus is the major branch of the umbilical vein, and traverses the liver to enter the inferior vena cava directly. Because it does not supply oxygen to the intervening tissues, it carries well-oxygenated blood directly to the heart. In contrast, the portal sinus carries blood to the hepatic veins primarily on the left side of the liver, where oxygen is extracted. The relatively deoxygenated blood from the liver then flows back into the inferior vena cava, which also receives less oxygenated blood returning from the lower body. Blood flowing to the fetal heart from the inferior vena cava, therefore, consists of an admixture of arterial-like blood that passes directly through the ductus venosus and less well-oxygenated blood that returns from most of the veins below the level of the diaphragm. The oxygen content of blood delivered to the heart from the inferior vena cava is thus lower than that which leaves the placenta.

In contrast to postnatal life, the ventricles of the fetal heart work in parallel, not in series. Well-oxygenated blood enters the left ventricle, which supplies the heart and brain, and less oxygenated blood enters the right ventricle, which supplies the rest of the body. The two separate circulations are maintained by the structure of the right atrium, which effectively directs entering blood to either the left atrium or the right ventricle, depending on its oxygen content. This separation of blood according to its oxygen content is facilitated by the pattern of blood flow in the inferior vena cava. The well-oxygenated blood tends to course along the medial aspect of the inferior vena cava and the less oxygenated blood stays along the lateral vessel wall, facilitating their shunting into opposite sides of the heart. Once this blood enters the atrium, the configuration of the upper interatrial septum, called the crista dividens, is such that it preferentially shunts the well-oxygenated blood from the medial side of the inferior vena cava and the ductus venosus through the foramen ovale into the left heart and then to the heart and brain (Dawes, 1962). After these tissues have extracted needed oxygen, the resulting less oxygenated blood returns to the right heart through the superior vena cava.

The less oxygenated blood coursing along the lateral wall of the inferior vena cava enters the right atrium and is deflected through the tricuspid valve to the right ventricle. The superior vena cava courses inferiorly and anteriorly as it enters the right atrium, ensuring that less well-oxygenated blood returning from the brain and upper body will also be shunted directly to the right ventricle. Similarly, the ostium of the coronary sinus lies just superior to the tricuspid valve so that less oxygenated blood from the heart also returns to the right ventricle. As a result of this blood flow pattern, blood in the right ventricle is 15 to 20 percent less saturated than blood in the left ventricle.

The major portion (87 percent) of blood exiting the right ventricle is then shunted through the ductus arteriosus to the descending aorta. The high pulmonary vascular resistance and the comparatively lower resistance in the ductus arteriosus and the umbilical–placental vasculature ensure that only approximately 13 percent of right

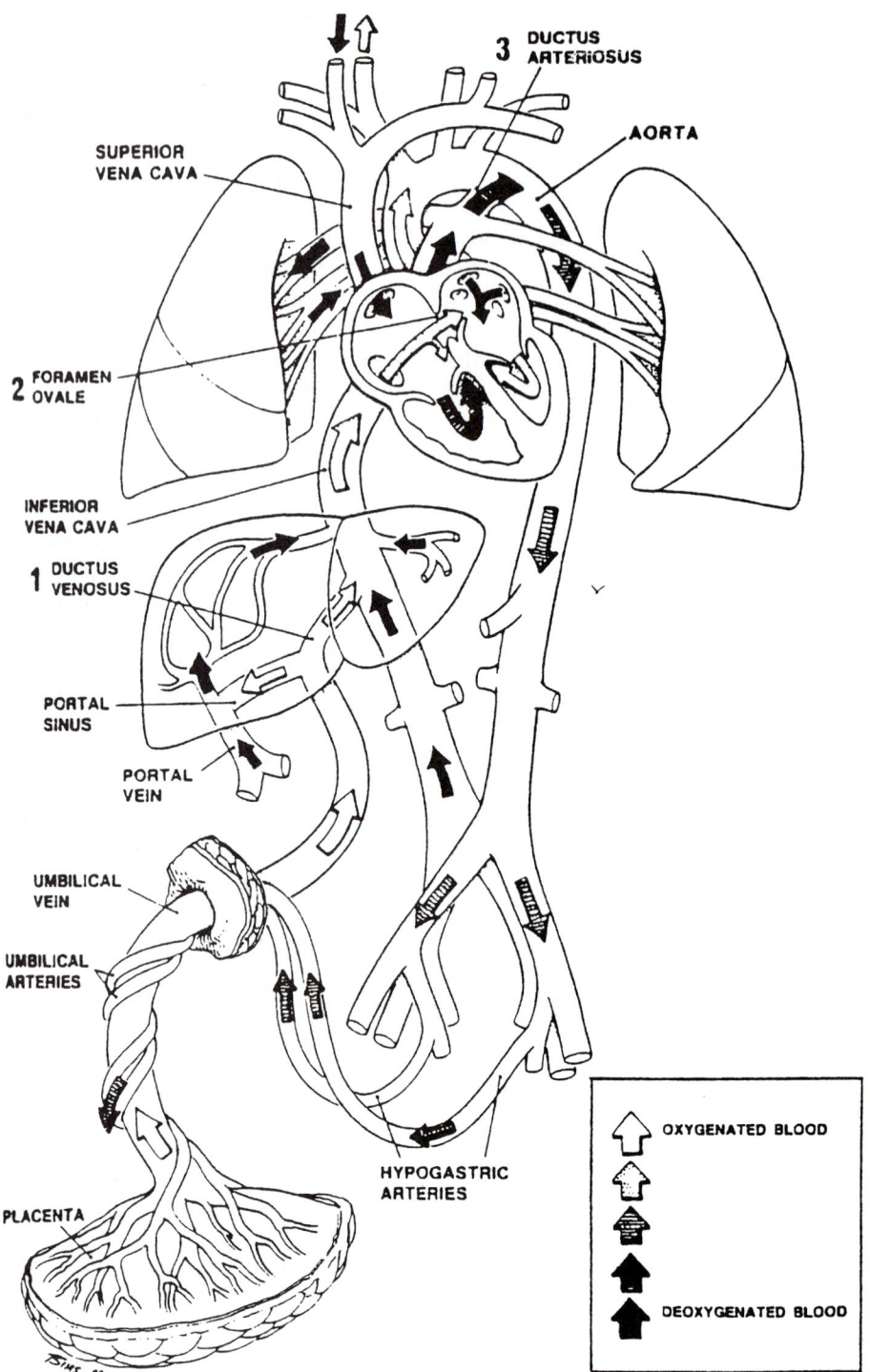

FIGURE 7–9. The intricate nature of the fetal circulation is evident. The degree of oxygenation of blood in various vessels differs appreciably from that in the postnatal state as the consequences of oxygenation being provided by the placenta rather than the lungs and the presence of three major vascular shunts: **1.** Ductus venosus. **2.** Foramen ovale. **3.** Ductus arteriosus.

ventricular output (8 percent of the combined ventricular output) goes to the lungs (Teitel, 1992). One third of the blood passing through the ductus arteriosus is delivered to the body, and the remaining right ventricular output returns to the placenta through the two hypogastric arteries, which distally become the umbilical arteries. In the placenta, this blood picks up oxygen and other nutrients, and is then recirculated back through the umbilical vein.

After birth, the umbilical vessels, ductus arteriosus, foramen ovale, and ductus venosus normally constrict or collapse. With the functional closure of the ductus arteriosus and the expansion of the lungs, blood leaving the right ventricle preferentially enters the pulmonary vasculature to become oxygenated before it returns to the left heart. Virtually instantaneously, the ventricles which had worked in parallel in fetal life now effectively work in series. The more distal portions of the hypogastric arteries, which course from the level of the bladder along the abdominal wall to the umbilical ring and into the cord as the umbilical arteries, undergo atrophy and obliteration within 3 to 4 days after birth. These become the umbilical ligaments while the intra-abdominal remnants of the umbilical vein form the ligamentum teres. The ductus venosus constricts by 10 to 96 hours after birth and is anatomically closed by 2 to 3 weeks, resulting in the formation of the ligamentum venosum (Clymann and Heymann, 1981).

ANIMAL STUDIES. The lamb fetus has been studied intensively by several groups of investigators who have concluded that the circulatory function of the mature lamb fetus is similar (in many respects) to that of the mature human fetus. Attempts to measure cardiac output in the lamb fetus have yielded somewhat variable results. Assali and associates (1968) found a mean output of about 225 mL/kg/min, but with considerable individual variation. Paton and co-workers (1973) found very similar values in baboon fetuses. Such a high fetal cardiac output, which per unit of body weight is about three times that of an adult at rest, would serve to compensate for the low oxygen content of fetal blood. The high cardiac output is accomplished, in part, by the fast heart rate of the fetus and a low systemic (peripheral) resistance.

It is estimated that in the fetal lamb, about half the combined output of the two ventricles goes to the placenta. By injecting isotopically labeled plastic microspheres into the fetal lamb circulation at various sites, the distribution of cardiac output during the last third of gestation was determined to be approximately as follows: placenta, 40 percent; carcass, 35 percent; brain, 5 percent; heart, 5 percent; gastrointestinal tract, 5 percent; lungs, 4 percent; kidneys, 2 percent; spleen, 2 percent; and liver (hepatic artery only), 2 percent (Rudolph and Heymann, 1968).

Clamping of the umbilical cord and expansion of the fetal lungs, either through spontaneous breathing or artificial respiration, promptly induce a variety of hemodynamic changes in sheep (Assali and associates, 1968). The systemic arterial pressure initially falls slightly, apparently the result of the reversal in the direction of blood flow in the ductus arteriosus, but it soon recovers and then rises above the control value. These investigators concluded that several factors served to regulate the flow of blood through the ductus arteriosus. One is the difference in pressure between the pulmonary artery and aorta, and another is the oxygen tension of the blood passing through the ductus arteriosus. They were able to influence flow through the ductus arteriosus by altering the P_{O_2} of the blood. When the lungs were ventilated with oxygen and the P_{O_2} rose above 55 mm Hg, ductus flow dropped, but ventilation with nitrogen, initially at least, returned the ductus flow to the original pattern.

The effects of variations in the oxygen tension of blood flowing through the ductus arteriosus are believed to be mediated through the actions of prostaglandins on the ductus. Prostaglandin E_2 dilates the constricted ductus arteriosus and is intimately involved in maintaining normal patency in utero. Inhibitors of prostaglandin synthase, when given to the mother, may lead to premature closure of the ductus arteriosus (Chap. 27, p. 716; Chap. 38, p. 1027). These drugs also can be used pharmacologically to close a symptomatic patent ductus arteriosus postnatally (Brash and associates, 1981).

FETAL BLOOD

HEMOPOIESIS. In the very early embryo, hemopoiesis is demonstrable first in the yolk sac. The next major site of erythropoiesis is the liver, and finally the bone marrow. The contributions made by each site throughout the growth and development of the embryo and fetus are demonstrated graphically in Figure 7–10. Erythropoiesis is regulated primarily by erythropoietin, which increases along with gestational age (Thomas and colleagues, 1983).

The first erythrocytes released into the fetal circulation are nucleated and macrocytic. The mean cell volume is at least 180 fL in the embryo and normally decreases to 105 to 115 fL at term. The erythrocytes of aneuploid fetuses generally do not undergo this maturation and maintain high mean cell volumes, 130 fL on average (Sipes and associates, 1991). As fetal development progresses, more and more of the circulating erythrocytes are smaller and nonnucleated. As the fetus grows, not only does the volume of blood in the common fetoplacental circulation increase, but hemoglobin con-

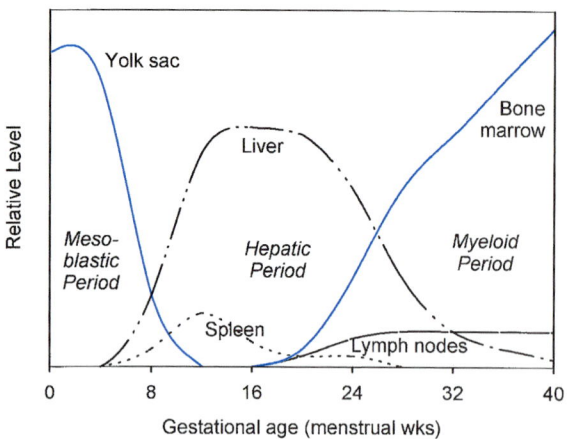

FIGURE 7–10. Sites of hemopoiesis synthesized at various stages of fetal development (From Brown, 1968, with permission.)

centration rises as well (see Fig. 39–13, p. 1065). Hemoglobin content of fetal blood rises to the level of about 12 g/dL at midpregnancy. By term, it is about 18 g/dL, a hemoglobin concentration that is high by maternal standards (Walker and Turnbull, 1953).

Fetal erythrocytes have a short life span. The life span of nucleated red blood cells is shorter in immature fetuses and progressively lengthens to approximately 90 days at term (Pearson, 1966). As a consequence, red cell production is increased. Reticulocytes are initially present at high levels, but decrease to about 4 to 5 percent of the total at term. The erythrocytes of the fetus differ structurally and metabolically from those of the adult. Fetal erythrocytes are more deformable, which serves to offset their higher viscosity, and contain several enzymes with appreciably different activities (Smith and co-workers, 1981).

ERYTHROPOIESIS. This process is controlled primarily by erythropoietin made by the fetus. Maternal erythropoietin does not cross the placenta. Fetal erythropoietin production is apparently under fetal control and is not influenced by maternal factors (Stockman and deAlarcon, 1992). It is produced in response to hypoxic stress such as that associated with bleeding, labor, or isoimmunization (Stangenberg and associates, 1993; Widness and colleagues, 1984). The concentration of erythropoietin correlates inversely with the hemoglobin concentration in fetuses of D-antigen–sensitized pregnancies. Erythropoietin production is influenced by testosterone, estrogen, prostaglandins, thyroid hormone, and lipoproteins (Stockman and deAlarcon, 1992). Erythropoietin levels increase with fetal maturity as do the numbers of erythrocytes responsive to it. The exact site of erythropoietin production is disputed, but the fetal liver appears to be an important source until renal production begins.

There is a close correlation between the concentration of erythropoietin in amnionic fluid and that in umbilical venous blood obtained by cordocentesis. After birth, erythropoietin normally may not be detectable for up to 3 months.

FETAL BLOOD VOLUME. Precise measurements of human fetoplacental volume are lacking. Usher and associates (1963), however, have measured blood volume of term normal infants very soon after birth and found an average of 78 mL/kg when immediate cord-clamping was conducted. Gruenwald (1967) found the volume of blood of fetal origin contained in the placenta after prompt cord-clamping to average 45 mL/kg of fetus. Thus, fetoplacental blood volume at term is approximately 125 mL/kg of fetus.

FETAL HEMOGLOBIN. Hemoglobin is a tetramer composed of two copies each of two different peptide chains. The identity of the two peptide chains determines the type of hemoglobin produced; α and β chains make up normal adult hemoglobin A. During embryonic and fetal life, a variety of α and β chain precursors are produced, resulting in the serial production of several different embryonic hemoglobins. The genes that direct production of the various embryonic versions of these chains are arranged in the order in which they are activated on chromosome 11 (β-type chains) and 16 (α-type chains). This sequence is shown in Figure 7–11 and each of these genes is turned on and then off during fetal life, until the α and β genes, which direct the production of hemoglobin A, are permanently activated.

Interestingly, the timing of the production of each of these early hemoglobin versions corresponds to changes in the site of hemoglobin production. As Figure 7–10 illustrates, fetal blood is first produced in the yolk sac, where hemoglobins Gower 1, Gower 2, and Portland are made. Erythropoiesis then moves to the liver, where hemoglobin F (fetal hemoglobin) is produced. When hemopoiesis finally moves to the bone marrow at around 11 weeks, normal hemoglobin A appears in fetal red cells and is present in progressively greater amounts as the fetus matures (Pataryas and Stamatoyannopoulos, 1972).

The final adult version of the α chain is produced exclusively by 6 weeks—after this there are no functional alternative versions. If an α gene mutation or deletion occurs, there is thus no alternate α type chain which could substitute to form functional hemoglobin. In contrast, at least two versions of the β chain, delta and gamma, remain in production throughout fetal life and beyond. In the case of a β gene mutation or deletion, these two other versions of the β chain often continue to be produced resulting in hemoglobin A_2 or hemoglobin F, which substitute for the abnormal or missing hemoglobin.

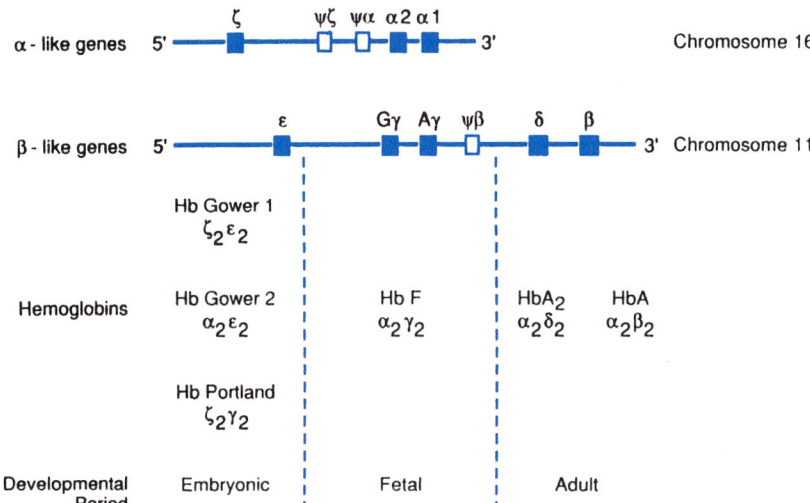

FIGURE 7–11. Schematic drawing of the arrangement of the α and β gene precursors on chromosomes 11 and 16, and the types of hemoglobin made from them. (From Thompson and colleagues, 1991, with permission.)

The mechanism by which genes are turned off is methylation of the control region (Chap. 36, p. 963). Thus the switch from the various embryonic hemoglobins to hemoglobin A likely is associated with methylation of the early globin genes. In some situations, methylation does not occur, and in newborns of diabetic women there may be persistence of hemoglobin F from hypomethylation of the γ-gene (Perrine and associates, 1988). With sickle cell anemia, the γ-gene remains unmethylated, and large quantities of fetal hemoglobin continue to be produced (Chap. 49. p. 1319).

There is a functional difference between hemoglobin A and F. At any given oxygen tension and at identical pH, fetal erythrocytes that contain mostly hemoglobin F bind more oxygen than do erythrocytes that contain nearly all hemoglobin A (see Fig. 43–4, p. 1166). The major reason for this is that hemoglobin A binds 2,3-diphosphoglycerate (2,3-DPG) more avidly than does hemoglobin F and this lowers the affinity of hemoglobin A for oxygen (De Verdier and Garby, 1969). The increased oxygen affinity of the fetal erythrocyte results from a lower concentration of 2,3-DPG compared with that of the maternal erythrocyte in which the 2,3-DPG level is increased during pregnancy.

The amount of hemoglobin F in fetal erythrocytes falls somewhat during the latter weeks of pregnancy. At term, about three fourths of the total hemoglobin normally is hemoglobin F. During the first 6 to 12 months of life, the proportion of hemoglobin F continues to decrease, eventually to reach the low level found in erythrocytes of normal adults. One factor that appears to mediate the switch from fetal to adult hemoglobin is the action of glucocorticosteroids, the effect of which is irreversible (Zitnik and associates, 1995).

COAGULATION FACTORS IN THE FETUS. There are no embryonic forms of the various hemostatic proteins. With the exception of fibrinogen, the fetus starts producing normal, adult-type, procoagulant, fibrinolytic, and anticoagulant proteins by about 12 weeks, but at appreciably reduced levels. The fetus does not benefit from the higher levels of these proteins found in maternal blood, as they do not cross the placenta. The concentrations of several coagulation factors at birth are thus markedly below the levels that develop within a few weeks of life (Corrigan, 1992). Factors that are low in cord blood are II, VII, IX, X, XI, XII, XIII, and fibrinogen. Without prophylactic vitamin K treatment, K-dependent coagulation factors usually decrease even further during the first few days after birth, especially in breast-fed infants, and may lead to hemorrhage in the newborn (see Chap. 39, p. 1071).

Fetal fibrinogen, which appears as early as 5 weeks, has the same amino acid composition as adult fibrinogen, but has different properties (Klagsburn and colleagues, 1988). It forms a less compressible clot and the fibrin monomer has a lower degree of aggregation (Heimark and Schwartz, 1988). For reasons unknown, the time for conversion of fibrinogen in plasma to fibrin clot when thrombin is added (thrombin time) is somewhat prolonged compared with that of older children and adults. Fibrinogen levels at birth are somewhat less than in nonpregnant adults.

Functional factor XIII (fibrin-stabilizing factor) levels in plasma are significantly reduced compared with those in normal adults (Henriksson and co-workers, 1974). Severe deficiencies of factor VIII, IX, XI, or XIII are usually suspected after observing a continuous "ooze" from the umbilical stump. Nielsen (1969) described low levels of plasminogen and somewhat increased fibrinolytic activity in cord plasma compared with maternal plasma. Platelet counts in cord blood are in the normal range for nonpregnant adults.

Despite this relative reduction in protein factors necessary for coagulation, the fetus seems to be protected from hemorrhage, and fetal bleeding is a rare event. Excessive bleeding does not usually occur even after invasive fetal procedures like cordocentesis. Ney and colleagues (1989) have shown that amnionic fluid thromboplastins and some factor in Wharton jelly combine to facilitate coagulation at the umbilical cord puncture site.

A variety of thrombophilias such as protein C, S, or antithrombin III deficiency, or the Leiden (factor V) mutation may cause thromboses and pregnancy complications in adults (Chap. 49, p. 1332). If the fetus inherits one of these mutations, thrombosis and infarction can develop. Thorarensen and colleagues (1997) described three neonates with ischemic infarction or hemorrhagic stroke who were heterozygous for factor V Leiden mutation. One had multiple thromboses in the placental vasculature. Similarly, Tharakan and co-workers (1993) described a stillbirth followed by maternal pulmonary embolism associated with protein S deficiency.

FETAL PLASMA PROTEINS. Liver enzymes and other plasma proteins are produced by the fetus, and these levels do not correlate with maternal levels (Weiner and colleagues, 1992). Concentrations of plasma protein, albumin, lactic dehydrogenase, aspartate aminotransferase, γ-glutamyl transpeptidase, and alanine transferase all increase with gestational age. At birth, the mean total plasma protein and albumin concentrations in fetal blood are similar to maternal levels (Foley and associates, 1978).

ONTOGENY OF THE FETAL IMMUNE RESPONSE. Infections in utero have provided an opportunity to examine some of the mechanisms for immune response by the human fetus. Evidence of immunological competence has been reported as early as 13 weeks. Altshuler (1974) described infection of the placenta and fetus by cytomegalovirus with characteristic severe inflammatory cell proliferation as well as viral inclusions. Fetal synthesis of complement late in the first trimester has been demonstrated by Kohler (1973) and confirmed by Stabile and co-workers (1988). All components of complement are produced at an early stage of fetal development. In cord blood at or near term, the average level for most components is about half of the adult value (Adinolfi, 1977).

IMMUNOCOMPETENCE OF THE FETUS. In the absence of a direct antigenic stimulus, such as infection, the immunoglobulins in the fetus consist almost totally of immune globulin G (IgG) synthesized in the maternal compartment and subsequently transferred across the placenta by receptor-mediated processes in syncytiotrophoblast, as described later. Therefore, antibodies in the fetus and the newborn infant are most often reflective of maternal immunological experiences.

IMMUNOGLOBULIN G. IgG transport from mother to fetus begins at about 16 weeks and increases thereafter. The bulk of IgG is acquired by the fetus from the mother during the last 4 weeks of pregnancy (Gitlin, 1971). Accordingly, preterm infants are endowed relatively poorly with maternal antibodies. Newborns begin to produce IgG, but slowly and, adult values are not attained until 3 years of age. In certain situations, the transfer of IgG antibodies from mother to fetus can be harmful rather than protective to the fetus. The classical example is hemolytic disease of the fetus and newborn resulting from D-antigen isoimmunization (Chap. 39, p. 1057).

IMMUNOGLOBULIN M. In the adult, production of immune globulin M (IgM) in response to antigen is superseded in a week or so predominantly by production of IgG. In contrast, the IgM response is dominant in the fetus and remains so for weeks to months in the newborn. IgM is not transported from mother to fetus; therefore, any IgM in the fetus or newborn is that which it produced. Very little IgM is produced by normal, healthy fetuses and that which is produced may include antibody to maternal T lymphocytes (Hayward, 1983). Increased levels of IgM are also found in newborns with congenital infection such as rubella, cytomegalovirus, or toxoplasmosis. Serum IgM levels in umbilical cord blood and identification of specific antibodies may be useful in the diagnosis of intrauterine infection. Adult levels of IgM are normally attained by 9 months of age.

IMMUNOGLOBULIN A. Differing from many animals, the human newborn infant does not acquire much in the way of passive immunity from the absorption of humoral antibodies ingested in colostrum. Nevertheless, immunoglobulin A (IgA) ingested in colostrum provides mucosal protection against enteric infections. This is likely also true for IgA ingested with amnionic fluid before delivery.

LYMPHOCYTES. The immune system begins to mature early in fetal life. B lymphocytes appear in liver by 9 weeks and are present in blood and spleen by 12 weeks. T lymphocytes begin to leave the thymus at about 14 weeks (Hayward, 1983). Despite this, the newborn responds poorly to immunization, and especially poorly to bacterial capsular polysaccharides. This immaturity of response may be due to either deficient response of newborn B cells to polyclonal activators, or lack of T cells that proliferate in response to specific stimuli (Hayward, 1983).

MONOCYTES. In the newborn, monocytes are able to process and present antigen when tested with maternal antigen-specific T cells.

NERVOUS SYSTEM AND SENSORY ORGANS. The spinal cord extends along the entire length of the vertebral column in the embryo, but after that it grows more slowly. By 24 weeks, the spinal cord extends only to S_1, at birth to L_3, and in the adult to L_1. Myelination of the spinal cord begins in the middle of gestation and continues through the first year of life. Synaptic function is sufficiently developed by the eighth week to demonstrate flexion of neck and trunk (Temiras and co-workers, 1968). At 10 weeks, local stimuli may evoke squinting, opening the mouth, incomplete finger closure, and plantar flexion of the toes. Complete finger closure is achieved during the fourth lunar month. Swallowing begins at about 10 weeks and respiration is evident at 14 to 16 weeks (Miller, 1982). Rudimentary taste buds are present at 7 weeks, and mature receptors are present by 12 weeks (Mistretta, 1975). The ability to suck is not present until at least 24 weeks (Lebenthal and Lee, 1983). During the third trimester, integration of nervous and muscular function proceeds rapidly.

The internal, middle, and external components of the ear are well developed by midpregnancy. The fetus apparently hears some sounds in utero as early as 24 to 26 weeks. By 28 weeks, the eye is sensitive to light, but perception of form and color is not complete until long after birth.

GASTROINTESTINAL TRACT. Swallowing begins at 10 to 12 weeks, coincident with the ability of the small intestine to undergo peristalsis and transport glucose actively (Koldovsky and colleagues, 1965; Miller, 1982). Much of the water in swallowed fluid is absorbed, and unabsorbed matter is propelled as far as the lower colon (Fig. 7–12). It is not clear what stimulates swallowing, but the fetal neural analog of thirst, gastric emptying, and change in the amnionic fluid composition are potential factors (Boyle, 1992). The fetal taste buds may play a role because saccharin injected into amnionic fluid increases swallowing, while injection of a noxious chemical inhibits it (Liley, 1972). Fetal swallowing appears to have little effect on amnionic fluid volume early in pregnancy, because the volume swallowed is small compared with the total volume. Late in pregnancy, however, the volume of amnionic fluid appears to be regulated substantially by fetal swallowing, for when swallowing is inhibited, hydramnios is common (Chap. 31, p. 817). Term fetuses reportedly swallow between

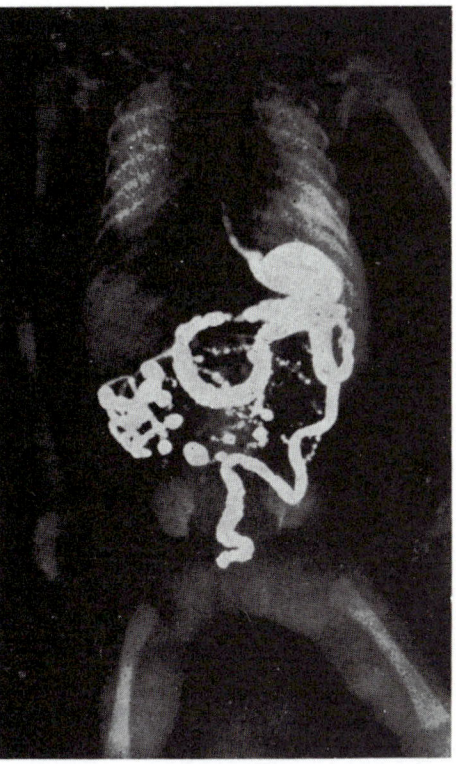

FIGURE 7–12. X-ray of 115-g fetus in which radiopaque dye is present in the lungs, esophagus, stomach, and entire intestinal tract after injection into the amnionic cavity 26 hours before delivery. This is illustrative not only of intrauterine "respiration" by the fetus but also active swallowing of amnionic fluid. (From Davis and Potter, 1946, with permission.)

200 and 760 mL per day—an amount comparable with the neonate (Pritchard, 1966).

In late pregnancy, swallowing serves to remove some of the insoluble debris that is normally shed into the amnionic sac and sometimes abnormally excreted into it. Hydrochloric acid and some adult digestive enzymes are present in the stomach and small intestine in very small amounts in the early fetus. Intrinsic factor is detectable by 11 weeks, and pepsinogen by 16 weeks. In the preterm infant, however, transient deficiencies of these enzymes are often present depending upon the gestational age when born (Lebenthal and Lee, 1983).

Stomach emptying appears to be stimulated primarily by volume. Movement of amnionic fluid through the gastrointestinal system may enhance growth and development of the alimentary canal and condition the fetus for alimentation after birth. Other regulatory factors may be involved, however, as anencephalic fetuses, in whom swallowing is limited, often have normal amnionic fluid volumes and normal appearing gastrointestinal tracts. The undigested portions of the swallowed debris can be identified in meconium. The amnionic fluid swallowed probably contributes little to the caloric requirements of the fetus but may contribute essential nutrients. Gitlin (1974) demonstrated that late in pregnancy about 0.8 g of soluble protein, approximately half albumin, appears to be ingested by the fetus each day.

Several anomalies can affect normal fetal gastrointestinal function. *Hirschsprung disease*, or *congenital aganglionic megacolon*, prevents the bowel from undergoing parasympathetic-mediated relaxation and thus emptying normally (Watkins, 1992). It may be recognized prenatally by grossly enlarged bowel on sonography. Obstructions such as duodenal atresia, megacystis/microcolon syndrome, or imperforate anus can also prevent the bowel from emptying normally. Meconium ileus, commonly found with fetal cystic fibrosis, is bowel obstruction caused by thick, viscid meconium which blocks the distal ileum.

MECONIUM. This consists not only of undigested debris from swallowed amnionic fluid, but to a larger degree, of various products of secretion such as glycerophospholipids from the lung, desquamated fetal cells, lanugo, scalp hair, and vernix. The dark greenish-black appearance is caused by pigments, especially biliverdin. Meconium passage can occur as the result of normal bowel peristalsis in the mature fetus or as the result of vagal stimulation due to cord compression. It can also occur when hypoxia stimulates arginine vasopressin (AVP) release from the fetal pituitary gland. AVP stimulates the smooth muscle of the colon to contract, resulting in intra-amnionic defecation (DeVane and co-workers, 1982; Rosenfeld and Porter, 1985).

Small bowel obstruction may lead to vomiting in utero (Shrand, 1972). Fetuses who suffer from congenital chloride diarrhea may have diarrhea in utero, which leads to hydramnios and preterm delivery (Holmberg and associates, 1977).

LIVER. Hepatic function in the fetus differs, in several ways, from that of the adult. As discussed earlier, fetal liver enzyme levels increase with gestational age, but are present in reduced amounts compared with those in later life. The liver has a very limited capacity for converting free bilirubin to bilirubin diglucuronoside (Chap. 39, p. 1067). The more immature the fetus, the more deficient the system for conjugating bilirubin.

Because the life span of fetal erythrocytes is shorter than that of adult erythrocytes, relatively more bilirubin is produced. Most of the bilirubin is transferred to the maternal circulation through the placenta (Bashore and colleagues, 1969). The fetal liver conjugates only a small fraction, which is excreted through the biliary tract into the intestine and ultimately oxidized to biliverdin. Unconjugated bilirubin, however, is excreted into the amnionic fluid after 12 weeks and is then transferred across the placenta. Placental transfer, however, is bidirec-

tional. To illustrate, a pregnant woman with sickle cell anemia who was isoimmunized as the result of red cell transfusions could not be evaluated with amnionic fluid ΔOD_{450} measurements because maternal bilirubin readily passed into the amnionic fluid (Goepfert and colleagues, personal communication). Conjugated bilirubin is not exchanged to any significant degree between mother and fetus.

Most of the cholesterol in the fetus is produced in fetal liver. Indeed, the large demand for LDL cholesterol by the fetal adrenal glands is met primarily by fetal hepatic synthesis.

Glycogen is present in low concentration in fetal liver during the second trimester, but near term there is a rapid and marked increase to levels two to three times those in adult liver. After birth, glycogen content falls precipitously.

PANCREAS. The discovery of insulin by Banting and Best (1922) came from its extraction from the fetal calf pancreas. Insulin-containing granules can be identified in the human fetal pancreas by 9 to 10 weeks, and insulin in fetal plasma is detectable at 12 weeks (Adam and associates, 1969). The fetal pancreas responds to hyperglycemia by increasing plasma insulin (Obenshain and colleagues, 1970). Although the precise role of insulin of fetal origin is not clear, fetal growth must be determined to a considerable extent by the amounts of basic nutrients from the mother with anabolism through the action of fetal insulin. Serum insulin levels are high in newborns of diabetic mothers and in other large-for-gestational-age infants, but insulin levels are low in infants who are small-for-gestational age (Brinsmead and Liggins, 1979). This relationship is discussed further in Chapter 29.

Glucagon has been identified in the fetal pancreas at 8 weeks. Induced hypoglycemia and infused alanine cause an increase in maternal glucagon levels in the rhesus monkey, yet similar stimuli to the fetus do not. Within 12 hours of birth, however, the infant is capable of responding (Chez and co-workers, 1975). Fetal pancreatic α-cells are capable of responding to L-dopa (Epstein and associates, 1977). Therefore, α-cell nonresponsiveness to hypoglycemia is likely the consequence of failure of glucagon release rather than inadequate production. This is consistent with findings of the developmental expression of pancreatic genes in the fetus (Mally and associates, 1994).

Most pancreatic enzymes are present by 16 weeks. Trypsin, chymotrypsin, phospholipase A, and lipase are present in the 14-week fetus at low levels, and they increase with gestational age (Werlin, 1992). Amylase has been identified in amnionic fluid at 14 weeks (Davis, 1986).

The exocrine function of the fetal pancreas is limited.

Physiologically important secretion occurs only after stimulation by a secretogogue such as acetylcholine, which is released locally after vagal stimulation (Werlin, 1992). Cholecystokinin is normally released only after ingestion of protein, and thus would not ordinarily be found in the fetus. Its release, however, can be stimulated experimentally. Pritchard (1965) injected radioiodine-labeled albumin into the amnionic sac where it was swallowed by the fetus, digested, and absorbed from the fetal intestine. Evidence of digestion and absorption was provided by the prompt excretion of the iodine in the maternal urine.

URINARY SYSTEM. Two primitive urinary systems, the pronephros and the mesonephros, precede the development of the metanephros. The pronephros has involuted by 2 weeks and the mesonephros is producing urine at 5 weeks and degenerates by 11 to 12 weeks. Failure of these two structures either to form or to regress may result in anomalous development of the definitive urinary system. Between 9 and 12 weeks, the ureteric bud and the nephrogenic blastema interact to produce the metanephros. By week 14 the loop of Henle is functional and reabsorption occurs (Smith and associates, 1992). New nephrons continue to be formed until 36 weeks, however, and their formation continues after birth in preterm infants.

Although the fetal kidneys produce urine, their ability to concentrate and modify the pH of urine is quite limited even in the mature fetus. Fetal urine is hypotonic with respect to fetal plasma and has low concentrations of electrolytes. In the human fetus, the kidneys receive between 2 and 4 percent of the cardiac output, compared with 15 and 18 percent in the newborn (Gilbert, 1980). Renal vascular resistance is high and the filtration fraction is low compared with later life (Smith, 1992). Fetal renal blood flow and thus urine production are controlled or influenced by the renin-angiotensin system, the sympathetic nervous system, prostaglandins, kallikrein, and atrial natriuretic factor. The glomerular filtration rate is low in the fetus, but increases with gestational age from less than 0.1 mL/min at 12 weeks to 0.3 mL/min at 20 weeks. In later gestation, the glomerular filtration rate remains constant when corrected for fetal weight (Smith and colleagues, 1992). Hemorrhage or hypoxia generally results in a decrease in renal blood flow, glomerular filtration rate, and urine output.

Urine is usually found in the bladder even in small fetuses. The fetal kidneys start producing urine at 12 weeks' gestation. By 18 weeks they are producing 7 to 14 mL/day, and at term this increases to 27 mL/hr or 650 mL/day (Wladimiroff and Campbell, 1974). Maternally administered diuretics (furosemide) increase fetal urine formation, and uteroplacental insufficiency and other types of fetal stress decrease it. Kurjak and associates (1981) found that fetal glomerular filtration rates and fetal tubular water reabsorption were decreased in 33 percent of growth-restricted infants and in 17 percent of infants of diabetic mothers. All values were normal in anencephalic infants and in cases of polyhydramnios.

Obstruction of the urethra, bladder, ureters, or renal pelves can damage renal parenchyma and distort fetal anatomy; the bladder may become sufficiently distended that it ruptures or dystocia results. Kidneys are not essential for survival in utero, but are important in the control of the composition and volume of amnionic fluid. Furthermore, abnormalities that cause chronic anuria are usually accompanied by oligohydramnios and hypoplasia of the lungs. Pathological correlates and prenatal therapy of urinary tract obstruction are discussed in Chapter 37 (p. 995).

PULMONARY SYSTEM. As discussed in Chapter 39 (p. 1042), the timetable of lung maturation and the identification of biochemical indices of functional fetal lung maturity are of considerable importance (and concern) to the obstetrician. Morphological or functional immaturity of the lung at birth leads to the development of the respiratory distress syndrome, and complicates the course and treatment of other neonatal disorders.

The presence of a sufficient amount of surface-active materials in the amnionic fluid is usually taken as evidence of fetal lung maturity. As Liggins (1994) emphasized, however, the structural and morphological maturation of fetal lung also is extraordinarily important to proper lung function in newborns. It is also important to the choice of therapeutic agents used to hasten fetal lung maturation when preterm delivery seems likely or mandated. Therefore, two separate but complementary aspects of fetal lung maturation must be considered. These are anatomical and morphological development and the capacity of fetal lung for surfactant formation.

ANATOMICAL MATURATION OF THE FETAL LUNG. Like the branching of a tree, lung development proceeds along an established timetable that apparently cannot be hastened by antenatal or neonatal therapy. The limits of viability, therefore, appear to be determined by the usual process of pulmonary growth. There are three essential stages of lung development as described by Moore (1983). During the *pseudoglandular stage*, which entails the growth of the intrasegmental bronchial tree between the fifth and 17th weeks, the lung looks microscopically like a gland. This period is followed by the *canalicular stage*, from 16 to 25 weeks, during which the bronchial cartilage plates extend peripherally. Each terminal bronchiole gives rise to several respiratory bronchioles, and each of these in turn divides into multiple saccular ducts. The final stage is the *terminal sac stage*, during which the alveoli give rise to the primitive pulmonary alveoli, called the terminal sacs. Simultaneously, an extracellular matrix develops from proximal to distal lung segments until term, an extensive capillary network develops, the lymph system forms, and the type II cells start to produce surfactant. At birth, only about 15 percent of the adult number of alveoli are present, and thus the lung continues to grow, adding more alveoli, from late fetal life up to about 8 years.

Various insults can upset this process, and the timing of the insult determines the outcome. With renal agenesis, for example, no amnionic fluid is present from the beginning of lung growth, and major defects occur in all three stages. The fetus with membrane rupture before 20 weeks usually exhibits nearly normal bronchial branching and cartilage development but has immature alveoli. Membrane rupture occurring after 24 weeks may have little long-term effect on pulmonary structure.

SURFACTANT. After birth, the terminal sacs must remain expanded despite the pressure imparted by the tissue-air interface within them; surfactant keeps them from collapsing. There are more than 40 cell types in the lung, but surfactant is formed specifically in the type II pneumonocytes that line the alveoli (Fig. 7–13). The type II cells are characterized by multivesicular bodies which produce the lamellar bodies in which surfactant is assembled. During late fetal life, at a time when the alveolus is characterized by a water-to-tissue interface, the intact lamellar bodies are secreted from the lung and swept into the amnionic fluid during fetal respiratory-like movements, that is, fetal breathing.

At birth, with the first breath, an air-to-tissue interface is produced in the lung alveolus. This permits surfactant to uncoil from the lamellar bodies; the surface tension–lowering material then spreads to line the alveolus and thereby prevents alveolar collapse during expiration. Therefore, it is the capacity for fetal lungs to produce surfactant, and not the actual laying down of this material in the lungs in utero, that establishes lung maturity before birth.

SURFACTANT COMPOSITION. The principal surface-active component of surfactant is a specific lecithin, or dipalmitoylphosphatidylcholine. From the work of Gluck and associates (1967, 1970, 1972) and Hallman and co-workers (1976), it is now known that about 90 percent of surfactant (dry weight) is lipid. Proteins account for the other 10 percent of surfactant mass.

Approximately 80 percent of the glycerophospholipids are phosphatidylcholines (lecithins), of which disaturated lecithin, accounts for nearly 50 percent (Fig. 7–14). Phosphatidylglycerol, the second most surface-active glycerophospholipid component of surfactant, accounts for 8 to 15 percent (Keidel and Gluck, 1975). Phosphatidylglycerol is capable of reducing surface tension in the alveolus, but its precise role is unclear. Infants born with a "mature" L/S ratio, but without phosphatidylglycerol, usually do well.

SURFACTANT SYNTHESIS. Surfactant biosynthesis takes place in the type II cells of the lung. The apoproteins are produced in the endoplasmic reticulum and

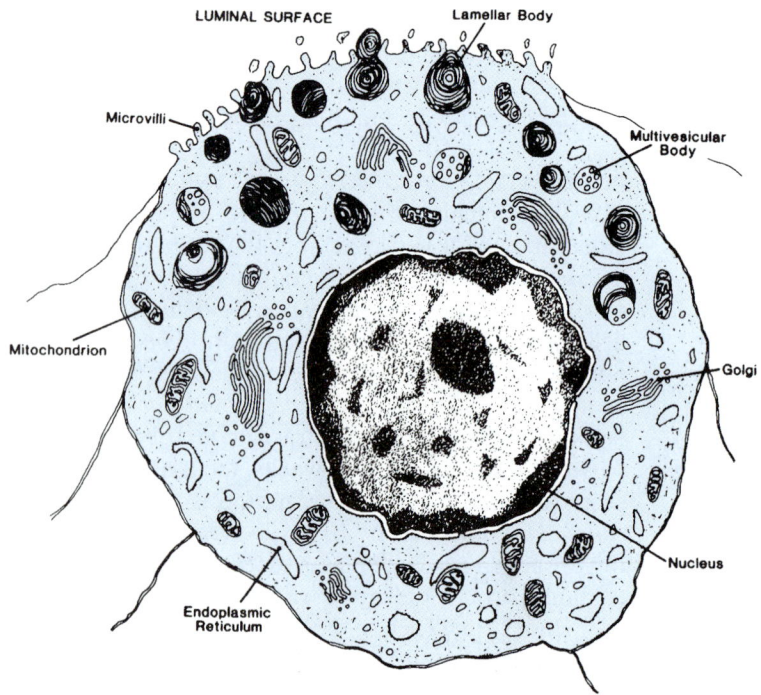

LUMINAL SURFACE   Lamellar Body

Microvilli

Multivesicular Body

Mitochondrion

Golgi

Nucleus

Endoplasmic Reticulum

FIGURE 7–13. Drawing of lung type II pneumonocyte. Prominent microvilli on the apical surface are identifiable. Many multivesicular bodies (rich in surfactant) that are migrating toward the luminal surface prior to extrusion into the alveolar space, are illustrated.

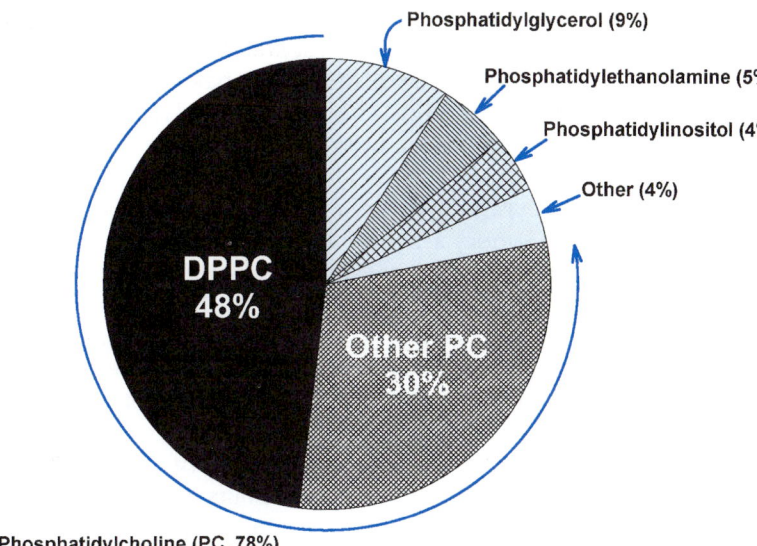

FIGURE 7–14. Glycerophospholipid composition of "mature" surfactant. Surfactant is especially enriched in lecithin (phosphatidylcholine) and, in particular, the surface-active dipalmitoylphosphatidylcholine (DPPC, 48 percent). The phosphatidylglycerol content of surfactant (8 to 15 percent) also is very high.

the glycerophospholipids are synthesized by cooperative interactions of several cellular organelles. Phospholipid is the primary surface tension–lowering component of surfactant, while the surfactant apoproteins serve to facilitate the forming and re-forming of a surface film in the alveoli during respiration.

The surface properties of the surfactant phospholipids are determined by the composition and degree of saturation of the long chain fatty acids, the presence and identity of minor lipids and proteins, and the temperature. The regulation of phosphatidylglycerol synthesis is especially important. Hallman and co-workers (1976) have shown that increased surfactant concentrations of phosphatidylglycerol, together with decreased concentrations of phosphatidylinositol, also herald lung maturation (Fig. 7–15).

Three surfactant-associated proteins are known: surfactant proteins A, B, and C (Whitsett, 1992). The major apoprotein is surfactant A (SP-A), a glycoprotein (M_r about 28,000 to 35,000). It is synthesized in the type II cells, and increased synthesis is related temporally to increased surfactant formation in maturing fetal lungs. The amnionic fluid content of SP-A also increases, as does the L/S ratio, as a function of gestational age and fetal lung maturity. Synthesis of SP-A is known to be increased by treatment of fetal lung tissue with cyclic AMP (analogs) and by epidermal growth factor and triiodothyronine. SP-A seems to be important in the structural transformation of the secreted lamellar body into tubular myelin within the lumen of the alveolus. SP-A also may be involved in the endocytosis and recycling of secreted surfactant by the type II cells.

There are also a number of smaller molecular weight apoproteins (M_r about 5000 to 18,000). SP-B and SP-C

are believed to be important in optimizing the surface-active properties of surfactant. Deletions in the surfactant SP-B gene have been discovered. Newborns with this abnormality do not survive despite the production of large amounts of surfactant lipids. In addition, SP-A, after being taken back into the type II cells by receptor-mediated endocytosis, acts to inhibit surfactant glycerophospholipid synthesis and secretion.

Increases in surfactant apoprotein synthesis precede the increase in surfactant glycerophospholipid synthesis (Mendelson and associates, 1986). SP-A gene expression is not detectable at 16 to 20 weeks, but is demonstrable at 29 weeks (Snyder and colleagues, 1988). More

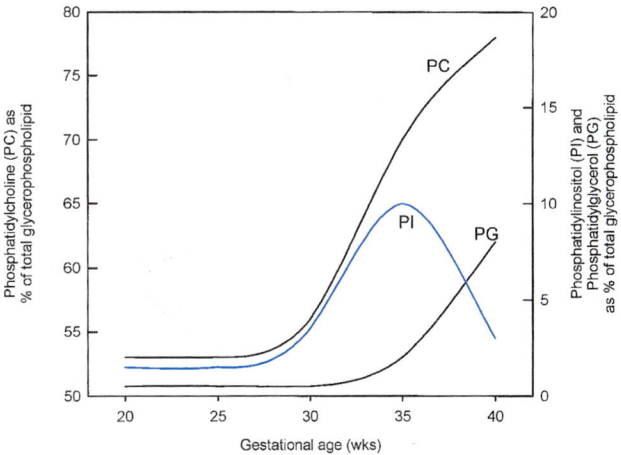

FIGURE 7–15. Relation between the levels of lecithin (dipalmitoylphosphatidylcholine [PC]), phosphatidylinositol (PI), and phosphatidylglycerol (PG) in amnionic fluid as a function of gestational age.

recently it has been demonstrated that there are two separate SP-A genes (SP-A1 and SP-A2), and that the regulation of synthesis of these two genes (chromosome 10) is distinctive and different. McCormick and Mendelson (1994) found that the two SP-A genes are differentially regulated. Cyclic AMP is more important in SP-A2 expression (11-fold), whereas dexamethasone caused a decrease in SP-A2 expression.

CORTICOSTEROIDS AND FETAL LUNG MATURATION.

Liggins (1969) observed that there appeared to be accelerated lung maturation in lambs delivered preterm that had been treated with glucocorticosteroids prior to birth. Since that time, many investigators have suggested that cortisol, produced in the fetal adrenal glands, is the natural stimulus for lung maturation and augmented surfactant synthesis. Corticosteroids may not be the only stimulus for augmented surfactant formation in the maturing human fetal lung. Respiratory distress syndrome is not necessarily observed in human neonates in whom the capacity to secrete cortisol is limited, such as those with anencephaly, adrenal hypoplasia, or congenital adrenal hyperplasia. There is now appreciable evidence that glucocorticosteroids administered in large amounts to the woman at certain critical times during gestation effect an increase in the rate of fetal lung maturation. In addition, the advent of neonatal surfactant therapy, given alone or after prenatal corticosteroid treatment, has significantly reduced the incidence of respiratory disease. The use of betamethasone to accelerate fetal lung maturity followed by surfactant therapy as needed is widely accepted, as discussed in Chapters 27 (p. 708) and 39 (p. 1040).

OTHER THERAPIES USED FOR FETAL LUNG MATURATION.

Buoyed by the success of betamethasone, or perhaps dismayed by its side effects, investigators have searched for other pharmacological means to hasten fetal pulmonary maturity. Animal studies suggested that administration of *thyroxine* to fetuses at various stages of gestation was associated with accelerated lung maturation and an early appearance of osmophilic lamellar inclusions within the type II pneumonocytes (Rooney and colleagues, 1974; Wu and associates, 1971, 1973). Others found that thyroxine had no effect on the activities of the enzymes involved in surfactant synthesis or surfactant concentration (Mason, 1973; Rooney and associates, 1974). Others have tested maternally administered *aminophylline, prolactin, cAMP*, and *thyroidreleasing hormone* (Ballard and colleagues, 1992; DiRenzo and associates, 1989; O'Brien, 1991). One multicenter randomized trial compared betamethasone alone to betamethasone plus thyrotropin-releasing hormone in 190 women in preterm labor, and found no difference in outcome between the two groups (Collabo-

rative Santiago Surfactant Group, 1998). None of the studies to date have documented significant additional benefit from therapies other than betamethasone given to the mother 24 to 48 hours before delivery followed by neonatal surfactant therapy.

RESPIRATION. Within a very few minutes after birth, the respiratory system must be able to provide oxygen as well as eliminate carbon dioxide. Respiratory muscles develop early and movements of the fetal chest wall have been detected by ultrasonic techniques as early as 11 weeks (Boddy and Dawes, 1975). From the beginning of the fourth month, the fetus is capable of respiratory movement sufficiently intense to move amnionic fluid in and out of the respiratory tract. In the radiograph in Figure 7–12, obtained 26 hours after injection of radiopaque dye into the amnionic sac, the contrast medium is present in fetal lung.

VAGITUS UTERI.

Crying in utero is a rare phenomenon. After rupture of the membranes, air may gain access to the amnionic cavity and be inspired by the fetus. Thiery and associates (1973) described three cases in which fetal crying was heard during vaginal examination, amnioscopy, or application of a clip electrode to the fetus. Fetal hiccuping is a more common phenomenon, and frequently the movement produced by the fetus is appreciated by the mother.

ENDOCRINE GLANDS

PITUITARY GLAND.

The fetal endocrine system is functional for some time before the central nervous system reaches a state of maturity competent to perform many functions associated with homeostasis (Mulchahey and co-workers, 1987). The endocrine system of the fetus does not necessarily mimic that of the adult, but nonetheless may be one of the first homeostatic systems to develop. The fetal pituitary develops from two different sources. The adenohypophysis develops from the oral ectoderm—Rathke pouch; and the neurohypophysis develops from the neuroectoderm.

ANTERIOR PITUITARY. The adenohypophysis, or anterior pituitary, differentiates into five cell types which secrete six protein hormones: (1) lactotropes, producing prolactin (PRL); (2) somatotropes, producing growth hormone (GH); (3) corticotropes, producing corticotropin (ACTH); (4) thyrotropes, producing thyroid-stimulating hormone (TSH); and (5) gonadotropes, producing luteinizing hormone (LH) and follicle-stimulating hormone (FSH). ACTH is first detected in the fetal pituitary gland at 7 weeks, and before the end of the 17th week the fetal pituitary gland is able to synthesize and store all pituitary hormones. GH, ACTH, and LH have been identified by 13 weeks. Moreover, the fetal pituitary is responsive to hypophysiotropic hormones and is capable of secreting these hormones from early in gestation (Grumbach and Kaplan, 1974).

The levels of immunoreactive growth hormone are rather high in cord blood, although its role in fetal growth and development is not clear. Anencephalic fetuses, with little pituitary tissue, are not remarkably different in weight from normal fetuses. The fetal pituitary produces and releases β-endorphin in a manner separate from maternal plasma levels (Browning and colleagues, 1983). Furthermore, cord blood levels of β-endorphin and β-lipotropin were found to decrease with declining fetal pH but correlate in a positive manner with fetal P_{CO_2}.

NEUROHYPOPHYSIS. This is well developed by 10 to 12 weeks, and oxytocin and arginine vasopressin (AVP) are demonstrable. In addition, the neurohypophyseal hormone of submammalian vertebrates, arginine vasotocin (AVT), is present in fetal pituitary and pineal glands. AVT is present only in fetal life in humans (Fisher, 1986). It is probable that oxytocin as well as AVP function in the fetus to conserve water by actions largely at the level of lung and placenta rather than kidney. Levels of AVP in umbilical cord plasma are increased strikingly compared with the maternal levels (Chard and associates, 1971; Polin and co-workers, 1977). AVP in cord and fetal blood appears to be elevated with fetal stress (DeVane and Porter, 1980; DeVane and co-workers, 1982).

INTERMEDIATE PITUITARY GLAND. There is a well-developed intermediate lobe in the pituitary gland of the human fetus. The cells of this structure begin to disappear before term and are absent from the pituitary of adults. The principal secretory products of the intermediate lobe cells are α-melanocyte–stimulating hormone (α-MSH) and β-endorphin. The levels of fetal α-MSH decrease progressively with gestation.

THYROID. The pituitary–thyroid system is functional by the end of the first trimester (Table 7–4). The thyroid gland is able to synthesize hormones by 10 to 12 weeks, and TSH, thyroxine, and thyroid-binding globulin have been detected in fetal serum as early as 11 weeks (Ballabio and colleagues, 1989). The placenta actively concentrates iodide on the fetal side and, by 12 weeks and throughout pregnancy, the fetal thyroid concentrates iodide more avidly than does the maternal thyroid. Thus, administering either radioiodide or appreciable amounts of ordinary iodide to the mother is hazardous after this time. Normal fetal levels of free T_4, free T_3, and thyroxin-binding globulin increase steadily throughout gestation (Ballabio and associates, 1989). Fetal serum

TABLE 7–4. Phases of Thyroid Maturation in the Human Fetus and Newborn Infant

Phase	Events	Gestational Age
I	Embryogenesis of pituitary–thyroid axis	2–12 weeks
II	Hypothalamic maturation	10–35 weeks
III	Development of neuroendocrine control	20 weeks to 4 weeks after birth
IV	Maturation of peripheral monodeiodination systems	30 weeks to 4 weeks after birth

From Fisher (1979).

concentrations of TSH are higher than the adult level and total and free T_3 concentrations are lower than the adult level, while the T_4 concentration is similar to that in adults by 36 weeks. This suggests that the fetal pituitary may not become sensitive to feedback until late in fetal life (Thorpe-Beeston and co-workers, 1991; Wenstrom and colleagues, 1990).

Fetal thyroid hormone plays a role in the normal development of virtually all fetal tissues, but especially the brain. Its influence is illustrated by congenital hyperthyroidism, which occurs when maternal thyroid-stimulating antibody crosses the placenta to stimulate the fetal thyroid. These fetuses develop tachycardia, hepatosplenomegaly, hematological abnormalities, craniosynostosis, and growth restriction. As children they have perceptual motor difficulties, hyperactivity, and reduced growth (Wenstrom and colleagues, 1990).

Placental tissue and membranes appear to prevent substantial passage of maternal thyroid hormones to the fetus by rapidly deiodinating maternal T_4 and T_3 to reverse -T_3, a relatively inactive form (Vulsma and colleagues, 1989). However, the long-acting thyroid stimulators, LATS and LATS-protector, and thyroid-stimulating immunoglobulin cross the placenta readily when present in high concentrations in the mother (Chap. 50, p. 1341).

Maternal thyroid hormones cross the placenta to a very limited degree, as illustrated by congenital hypothyroidism. The latter results in a variety of neonatal problems, including neurological abnormalities, respiratory difficulties, dysmorphic facies, lethargy and hypotonia, and myxedema of the larynx and epiglottis. These problems typically develop only after birth, and can be avoided with prompt thyroid replacement. Although it was previously thought that normal fetal growth and development provided evidence that the thyroid was not essential for fetal growth, it is now known that this proceeds normally without fetal thyroid hormone because small quantities of maternal T_4 reach the fetus and prevent antenatal cretinism. Vulsma and colleagues

(1989) studied fetuses who were markedly hypothyroid because of thyroid agenesis or because they had congenital absence of thyroid peroxidase, an enzyme necessary for iodination of thyroglobulin. They found that fetal levels of T_4 were very low and represented maternal hormone that crossed the placenta.

Immediately after birth, there are major changes in thyroid function and metabolism. Atmospheric cooling evokes sudden and marked increase in thyrotropin secretion, which in turn causes a progressive increase in serum T_4 levels maximal 24 to 36 hours after birth. There are nearly simultaneous elevations of serum T_3 levels. Failure of these changes to occur, such as when the fetus is congenitally hypothyroid, causes multiple problems including cretinism, a form of mental retardation resulting from postnatal brain injury.

ADRENAL GLANDS. These are much larger in relation to total body size than in adults. The bulk of the enlargement is made up of the inner or so-called *fetal zone* of the adrenal cortex. The normally hypertrophied fetal zone involutes rapidly after birth. It is scant to absent in rare instances where the fetal pituitary gland is congenitally absent. The function of the fetal adrenal glands and the control of fetal adrenal steroidogenesis (dehydroepiandrosterone sulfate and cortisol) are discussed in detail in Chapter 6 (p. 118).

The fetal adrenal glands also synthesize aldosterone. In one study, aldosterone levels in cord plasma near term exceeded those in maternal plasma, as did renin and renin substrate (Katz and colleagues, 1974). The renal tubules of the newborn, and presumably the fetus, appear relatively insensitive to aldosterone (Kaplan, 1972).

FETAL GENDER

The establishment of the primary sex ratio in humans is impractical, for it would require the recovery and assignment of sex to zygotes that fail to cleave, blastocysts that fail to implant, and early pregnancy losses. Carr (1963) suggested that the primary sex ratio in humans may be unity. The secondary sex ratio, however, that is, the sex ratio of fetuses that reach viability is usually quoted as approximately 106 males to 100 females. Studies from industrialized nations more recently suggest that the proportion of male births is dropping. Davis and colleagues (1998) report a significant decline in male births since 1950 in Denmark, Sweden, the Netherlands, the United States, Germany, Norway, and Finland. Allan and co-workers (1997) reviewed the male:female ratio for all live births in Canada and found that since 1970, the proportion of males has dropped by 2.2

male births per 1000 live births. In the Atlantic region, the decline was 5.6 male births per 1000!

Although theoretically there should be as many Y-bearing as X-bearing sperm, and thus a primary sex ratio of one at the time of fertilization, recent data dispute this. Many factors, such as differential susceptibility to toxins and other environmental exposures and concomitant medical disorders, have been shown to contribute to the sex at conception. Parental age appears to influence the primary sex ratio and Manning (1997) reported that couples with a large age discrepancy have an excess of male offspring. James (1986) theorizes that this may be due to high stress in urbanized society which may increase corticotropin secretion that stimulates maternal adrenal androgen secretion that favors male conceptions. If this is not the case, the unbalanced secondary sex ratio can only be explained by the loss of more female than male embryo-fetuses during the early months of pregnancy.

GENDER ASSIGNMENT AT BIRTH. The first thing that parents in the delivery room want to know is the sex of their infant. If the external genitalia of the newborn are ambiguous, the obstetrician faces a profound dilemma. Griffin and Wilson (1986) state that it is no exaggeration to say that the detection of sexual ambiguity in the newborn constitutes a true medical emergency. An incorrect assignment of gender portends grave psychological and social problems for the baby and family. Furthermore, several endocrinological causes of sexual ambiguity are associated with profound blood pressure instability and serious metabolic abnormalities.

It is no longer believed that the proper functional sex assignment for newborns with genital ambiguity can be made in the delivery room. Assignment to one sex or the other requires knowledge of the karyotypic sex, gonadal sex, hormonal milieu to which the fetus was exposed, anatomy, and all possibilities for surgical correction. In the past, many physicians simply assigned all infants with a small or likely insufficient phallus to the female gender. Based on what is now known of the role of fetal exposure to hormones in establishing sexual preference and behavior, it can be seen why such a policy caused gender identity disorder (Slijper and colleagues, 1998). Thus, the best approach is to tell the parents that the baby appears healthy, but to honestly admit that the sex will need to be determined by a series of tests. In order to develop a plan by which to determine the cause of ambiguous genitalia, the mechanisms of normal and abnormal sexual differentiation must be considered.

SEXUAL DIFFERENTIATION OF THE EMBRYO-FETUS. Ultimate gender differentiation is determined by chromosomal make-up, acting in conjunction with gonad development; together they result in phenotypic gender.

CHROMOSOMAL SEX. Genetic sex, XX or XY, is established at the time of fertilization of the ovum. For the first 6 weeks thereafter, however, the development of male and female embryos is morphologically indistinguishable. The differentiation of the primordial gonad into testis or ovary heralds the establishment of gonadal sex (Fig. 7–16).

GONADAL SEX. Primordial germ cells originate in the endoderm of the yolk sac and migrate to the genital ridge to form the indifferent gonad (Simpson, 1997). If a Y chromosome is present, at about 6 weeks after conception the gonad begins developing into a testis. Testes development is directed by a gene located on the short arm of Y, namely *testis-determining factor (TDF)*, also called *sex-determining region (SRY)*. This gene encodes a transcription factor that acts to modulate the rate of transcription of a number of genes involved in gonadal differentiation. The SRY gene is specific to the Y chromosome and is expressed in the human single-cell zygote immediately after ovum fertilization. It is not expressed in the spermatozoa (Fiddler and co-workers, 1995; Gustafson and Donahoe, 1994).

In addition, testis development requires a *dose-dependent sex reversal (DDS)* region on the X chromosome, as well as yet unidentified autosomal genes. It is not clear how these genes, or the Y chromosome, direct the biomolecular events involved in gonadal differentiation into testis.

The contribution of chromosomal sex to gonadal sex is illustrated by several paradoxical conditions. The incidence of 46,XX phenotypic human males is estimated to be about 1 in 20,000 male births. These apparently result from translocation of the Y chromosome fragment containing TDF to the X chromosome during meiosis of male germ cells (George and Wilson, 1988). Similarly, individuals with XY chromosomes can appear phenotypically female if they carry a mutation in the TDF (SRY) gene. There is evidence that genes on Xp are capable of suppressing testicular development, despite the presence of the SRY gene. Indeed, this accounts for a form of X-linked recessive gonadal dysgenesis.

The existence of autosomal sex-determining genes is supported by several genetic syndromes in which disruption of an autosomal gene causes, among other things, gonadal dysgenesis. For example, camptomelic dysplasia, localized to chromosome 17, is associated with XY sex reversal. Similarly, male pseudohermaphroditism has been associated with a mutation in the Wilms tumor suppressor gene on chromosome 11.

PHENOTYPIC SEX. After establishment of gonadal sex, phenotypic sex develops very rapidly. It is clear that male phenotypic sexual differentiation is directed by the function of the fetal testis. In the absence of the testis, female differentiation ensues irrespective of the genetic sex.

The development of urogenital tracts in both sexes of human embryos is indistinguishable before 8 weeks. Thereafter, development (differentiation) of the internal and external genitalia to the male phenotype is dependent upon testicular function. The fundamental experiments to determine the role of the testis in male sexual differentiation were conducted by the French anatomist, Alfred Jost. Ultimately, he established that the induced-phenotype is male and that secretions from

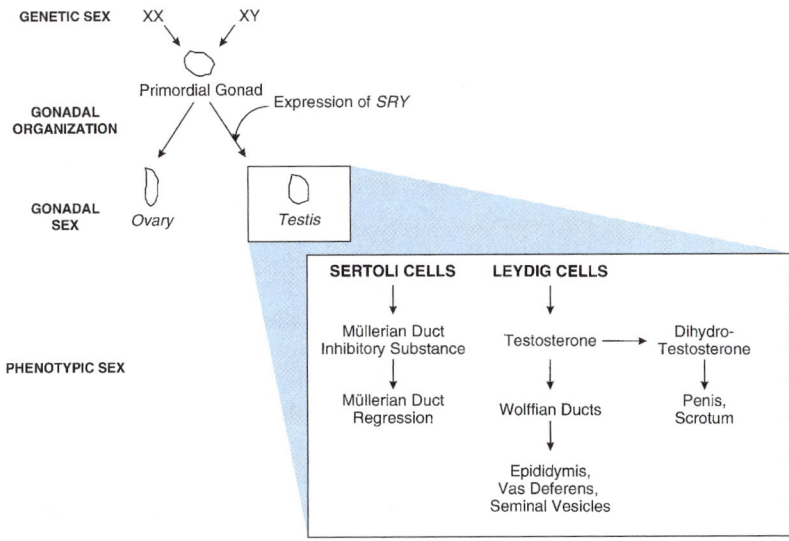

FIGURE 7–16. Sexual differentiation. Genetic sex is established at the time of fertilization of the ovum. At a time thereafter, the primordial gonad differentiates to testis if the SRY gene is expressed. The fetal testicular secretions effect male phenotypic sex differentiation.

the gonads are not necessary for female differentiation. Specifically, the fetal ovary is not required for female sexual differentiation.

Jost and associates (1973) found that if castration of rabbit fetuses was conducted before differentiation of the genital anlagen, all newborns were phenotypic females with female external and internal genitalia. Thus, the müllerian ducts developed into uterus, fallopian tubes, and upper vagina.

If castration of fetuses was conducted before differentiation of the genital anlagen, and thereafter a testis was implanted on one side in place of the removed gonad, the phenotype of all fetuses was male. Thus, the external genitalia of such fetuses was masculinized. On the side of the testicular implant, the wolffian duct developed into the epididymis, vas deferens, and seminal vesicle. On the side of the testicular implant, müllerian structures, including the uterine horn and fallopian tube, were not present. On the side without the implant, the müllerian duct did develop (with castration) but the wolffian duct did not.

In another experiment, these investigators found that if after castration of the fetus at the sexually indifferent stage, an androgen pellet was implanted on one side—in the site of a removed gonad—that the external genitalia masculinized. So did the wolffian duct on the side of the androgen pellet. The müllerian duct, however, did not regress; that is, the uterine horn and fallopian tube developed in spite of the androgen implant.

Wilson and Gloyna (1970) and Wilson and Lasnitzki (1971) demonstrated that testosterone action was amplified by conversion to 5α-dihydrotestosterone. All of these observations form the basic framework of our understanding of the mechanisms of sexual differentiation of the human embryo-fetus. These investigators demonstrated convincingly that in most androgen-responsive tissues, testosterone is converted to 5α-dihydrotestosterone in a reaction catalyzed by the enzyme(s) 5α-reductase. This hormone acts primarily (almost exclusively) in the genital tubercle and labioscrotal folds.

PHYSIOLOGICAL AND BIOMOLECULAR BASIS OF SEXUAL DIFFERENTIATION. Based on these observations, the physiological basis of sexual differentiation can be summarized as follows: Genetic sex is established at fertilization. Gonadal sex is determined primarily by factors encoded by genes on the Y chromosome, such as the SRY gene. In a manner not yet understood, differentiation of the primitive gonad into a testis is accomplished.

FETAL TESTICULAR CONTRIBUTIONS TO MALE SEXUAL DIFFERENTIATION. The fetal testis secretes a proteinaceous substance called *müllerian-inhibiting substance*, a dimeric glycoprotein (M_r about 140,000). It acts

locally as a paracrine factor to cause regression of the müllerian duct. Thus, it prevents the development of uterus, fallopian tube, and upper vagina. Fetal testes secrete testosterone, which acts to cause virilization of the external and internal genital anlagen.

Müllerian-inhibiting substance is produced by the Sertoli cells of the seminiferous tubules. Importantly, these tubules appear in fetal gonads before differentiation of Leydig cells, which are the cellular site of testosterone synthesis. Thus, müllerian-inhibiting substance is produced by Sertoli cells even before differentiation of the seminiferous tubules, and is secreted as early as 7 weeks. Müllerian duct regression is completed by 9 to 10 weeks, which is before testosterone secretion has commenced. Because it acts locally near its site of formation, if a testis were absent on one side, the müllerian duct on that side would persist and the uterus and fallopian tube would develop on that side.

Secretion of müllerian-inhibiting substance continues throughout fetal life and after birth, but the expression of its receptor is very brief in embryonic life. The levels of müllerian-inhibiting substance in serum of young boys remains high (10 to 50 ng/mL) before declining to baseline values of 1 to 5 ng/mL at puberty. Müllerian-inhibiting substance also is produced in granulosa cells of the ovary, but not during fetal or postnatal life until near the expected time of puberty. Serum levels of müllerian-inhibiting substance, however, may be distinctly elevated in women with granulosa cell tumors of the ovary (Gustafson and Donahoe, 1994).

FETAL TESTOSTERONE SECRETION. Apparently through stimulation initially by chorionic gonadotropin (hCG), and later by fetal pituitary LH, the fetal testes secrete testosterone. Some investigators are of the view that early embryo-fetal testosterone synthesis is gonadotropin independent. Testosterone acts directly on the wolffian duct to effect the development of the vas deferens, epididymidis, and seminal vesicles. Testosterone also enters fetal blood and acts on the anlagen of the external genitalia. In these tissues, however, testosterone is converted to 5α-dihydrotestosterone, which amplifies the androgen action of testosterone to cause virilization of the external genitalia.

GENITAL AMBIGUITY OF THE NEWBORN. This ambiguity is the result of either excessive androgen action in an embryo-fetus that was destined to be female, or inadequate androgen representation for one destined to be male. Rarely, genital ambiguity indicates true hermaphroditism. **If the neonate is a phenotypic male with bilateral cryptorchidism, or if the genitalia are completely ambiguous, congenital adrenal hyperplasia is diagnosed and the neonate treated until appropriate tests confirm or rule it out.** This obtains because, of all the causes of genital ambiguity, only congenital adrenal hyperplasia can be life threatening. If not treated immediately, adrenal failure provokes nausea, vomiting, diarrhea, dehydration, and shock (Speroff and co-workers, 1994).

The human abnormalities of sexual differentiation causing genital ambiguity can be assigned to one of four clinically defined categories:

1. Female pseudohermaphroditism.
2. Male pseudohermaphroditism.
3. Dysgenetic gonads, including true hermaphroditism.
4. (Rarely) true hermaphroditism.

CATEGORY 1. FEMALE PSEUDOHERMAPHRODITISM. In this condition:

1. Müllerian-inhibiting substance is not produced.
2. Androgen exposure of the embryo-fetus is excessive, but variable, for a fetus destined to be female.
3. The karyotype is 46,XX.
4. Ovaries are present.

Therefore, by genetic and gonadal sex, all subjects of this category are destined to be female, and the basic abnormality is androgen excess. Because müllerian-inhibiting substance is not produced, the uterus, fallopian tubes, and upper vagina develop in these subjects. If affected fetuses were exposed to a small androgen excess reasonably late in fetal development, the only genital abnormality will be slight to modest clitoral hypertrophy, with an otherwise normal female phenotype. With somewhat greater androgen exposure, clitoral hypertrophy will be more pronounced and posterior labial fusion will develop. With progressively increasing androgen excess somewhat earlier in embryonic development, progressively more severe virilization can occur. This includes formation of labioscrotal folds, development of a urogenital sinus (in which the vagina empties into the posterior urethra), and even to the development of a penile urethra with scrotal formation (the empty scrotum syndrome).

The androgenic excess in fetuses with female pseudohermaphroditism most commonly arises as the result of congenital adrenal hyperplasia. These defects in steroidogenic enzymes in the synthesis of cortisol from cholesterol cause increased secretion of androgenic prehormones by the fetal adrenal cortex. With impaired cortisol synthesis, pituitary ACTH secretion is not inhibited and excessive ACTH stimulation of the fetal adrenal glands leads to the secretion of large amounts of cortisol precursors, including androgenic prehormones. These prehormones, for example, androstenedione, are converted to testosterone in extra-adrenal fetal tissues. The enzyme deficiency may involve any of several enzymes, but the most common are steroid 21-hydroxylase, 11-β-hydroxylase, or 3-β-hydroxysteroid dehydrogenase. Deficiency of 3-β-hydroxysteroid hydrogenase prevents synthesis of virtually all steroid hormones. Deficiency of either 17-β-hydroxylase or 11-β-hydroxylase results in the increased production of deoxycorticosterone, which causes hypertension and hypokalemic acidosis. These forms of congenital adrenal hyperplasia thus constitute medical emergencies.

Another cause of androgen excess in the female embryo-fetus is the transfer of androgen from the maternal compartment. Excess maternal androgen secretion may arise from the ovaries with hyperreactio luteinalis or theca lutein cysts or tumors such as luteomas, arrhenoblastomas (Sertoli/Leydig cell tumors), or hilar cell tumors. In most of these, however, the female does not become virilized. This is because during most of pregnancy, the fetus is protected from excess maternal androgen by the extraordinary capacity of the syncytiotrophoblast to convert most C_{19}-steroids (including testosterone) to estradiol-17β. The only exception to this generalization is that with fetal aromatase deficiency there is both maternal and fetal virilization (Chap. 6, p. 121). Drugs ingested in pregnancy can also cause female fetal androgen excess. Most commonly, the drugs implicated are synthetic progestins or anabolic steroids (Chap. 38, p. 1051).

Importantly, all subjects with female pseudohermaphroditism, except those with aromatase deficiency, can be normal, fertile women if the proper diagnosis is made and appropriate and timely treatment is initiated.

CATEGORY 2. MALE PSEUDOHERMAPHRODITISM. These subjects are characterized by:

1. Production of müllerian-inhibiting substance.
2. Incomplete but variable androgenic representation for a fetus destined to be male.
3. A 46,XY karyotype.
4. The presence of testes or else no gonads.

Incomplete masculinization of the fetus destined to be male is caused by inadequate production of testosterone by the fetal testis. It also may arise from diminished responsiveness of the genital anlagen to normal quantities of androgen, which includes failure of the in situ formation of 5α-dihydrotestosterone in androgen-responsive tissue. Because testes were present, at least at some time in embryonic life, müllerian-inhibiting substance is produced during embryonic life. Thus, the uterus, fallopian tubes, and upper vagina do not develop.

Deficient fetal testicular testosterone production may occur if there is an enzymatic defect of steroidogenesis that involves any one of four enzymes in the biosynthetic pathway for testosterone synthesis. Impaired fetal testicular steroidogenesis can also be caused by an abnormality in the LH/hCG receptor and by Leydig cell hypoplasia.

With embryonic testicular regression, the testes regress during embryonic or fetal life, and there is no testosterone production thereafter (Edman and associates, 1977). These subjects have a spectrum of phenotypes that varies from a normal female with absent uterus, fallopian tubes, and upper vagina, to normal male phenotype with anorchia.

Androgen resistance, or deficiencies in androgen responsiveness, are caused by an abnormal (or absent) androgen receptor protein, or else by failure of conversion of testosterone to 5α-dihydrotestosterone in such tissues because of deficient enzyme activity (Wilson and MacDonald, 1978).

ANDROGEN INSENSITIVITY SYNDROME. This formerly was called testicular feminization and it is the most extreme form of the androgen resistance syndrome. These individuals have no tissue responsiveness to androgen. Affected subjects have a female phenotype with a short, blind-ending vagina, no uterus or fallopian tubes, and no wolffian duct structures. At the expected time of puberty, testosterone levels in affected women increase to values similar to normal men. Nonetheless, virilization does not occur, and even pubic and axillary hair do not develop because of end-organ resistance. Presumably, because of androgen resistance at the level of the brain and pituitary, LH levels also are elevated. In response to high concentrations of LH, there is also increased testicular secretion of estradiol-17β compared with that in normal men (MacDonald and colleagues, 1979). Increased estrogen secretion, and absence of androgen responsiveness, act in concert to cause feminization (breast development).

Individuals with *incomplete androgen insensitivity* are slightly responsive to androgen. They ordinarily have modest clitoral hypertrophy at birth; but at the expected time of puberty, pubic and axillary hair develop although virilization does not occur. These women also develop feminine breasts, presumably through the same endocrine mechanisms as in women with the complete form of the disorder (Madden and co-workers, 1975).

Another group has been referred to as *familial male pseudohermaphroditism, type I* (Walsh and colleagues, 1974). It also is commonly referred to as *Reifenstein syndrome,* but constitutes a spectrum of incomplete genital virilization that can vary from a phenotype similar to that of women with incomplete androgen insensitivity to that of a male phenotype with only a bifid scrotum, infertility, and gynecomastia. In these subjects, androgen resistance is demonstrated by demonstrating diminished 5α-dihydrotestosterone–binding capacity in fibroblasts grown in culture from genital skin biopsies.

The gene encoding the androgen receptor is located on the X chromosome. More than 100 different mutations of this gene have been demonstrated. This accounts for the wide variability in androgen responsiveness among persons in whom the androgen receptor protein is absent or abnormal, and for the many different mutations associated with one disorder (McPhaul and associates, 1991; Patterson and co-workers, 1994).

An alternate form of androgen resistance is caused by 5α-reductase deficiency in androgen-responsive tissues. Because androgen action in the external genitalia anlagen is mediated by 5α-dihydrotestosterone, persons with this enzyme deficiency have external genitalia that are female (modest clitoral hypertrophy). But because androgen action in the wolffian duct is mediated directly by testosterone, there are well-developed epididymides, seminal vesicles, and vas deferens, and the male ejaculatory ducts empty into the vagina (Walsh and associates, 1974).

Andersson and co-workers (1991) have demonstrated that there are two genes that encode for steroid 5α-reductase. The type 1 gene is expressed in many tissues and the enzyme encoded by this gene functions primarily as the initial reaction in testosterone metabolism by the liver. The type 2 gene is expressed primarily in androgen-responsive tissues and abnormal expression causes male pseudohermaphroditism. A composite photograph of the external genitalia of subjects with each of four types of androgen resistance is shown in Figure 7–17.

CATEGORY 3: DYSGENETIC GONADS. This category includes abnormalities of sexual differentiation that have in common several features:

1. Müllerian-inhibiting substance is not produced.
2. Fetal androgen exposure is variable.
3. The karyotype varies among subjects and is commonly abnormal.
4. Neither normal ovaries nor testes are present—rarely, both ovarian and testicular tissues are found. The uterus, fallopian tubes, and upper vagina are present in all of the subjects of this category.

In the majority of subjects of category 3, the gonads are dysgenetic. With the most common form of gonadal dysgenesis, *Turner syndrome (46X),* the phenotype is female, but secondary sex characteristics do not develop at the time of expected puberty, and sexual infantilism persists. In some persons with dysgenetic gonads, the genitalia are ambiguous, a finding indicating that an abnormal gonad produced androgen, albeit in small amounts, during embryo-fetal life. Generally, there is mixed gonadal dysgenesis in these subjects, and an example is a dysgenetic gonad on one side and an abnormal testis or dysontogenetic tumor on the other side.

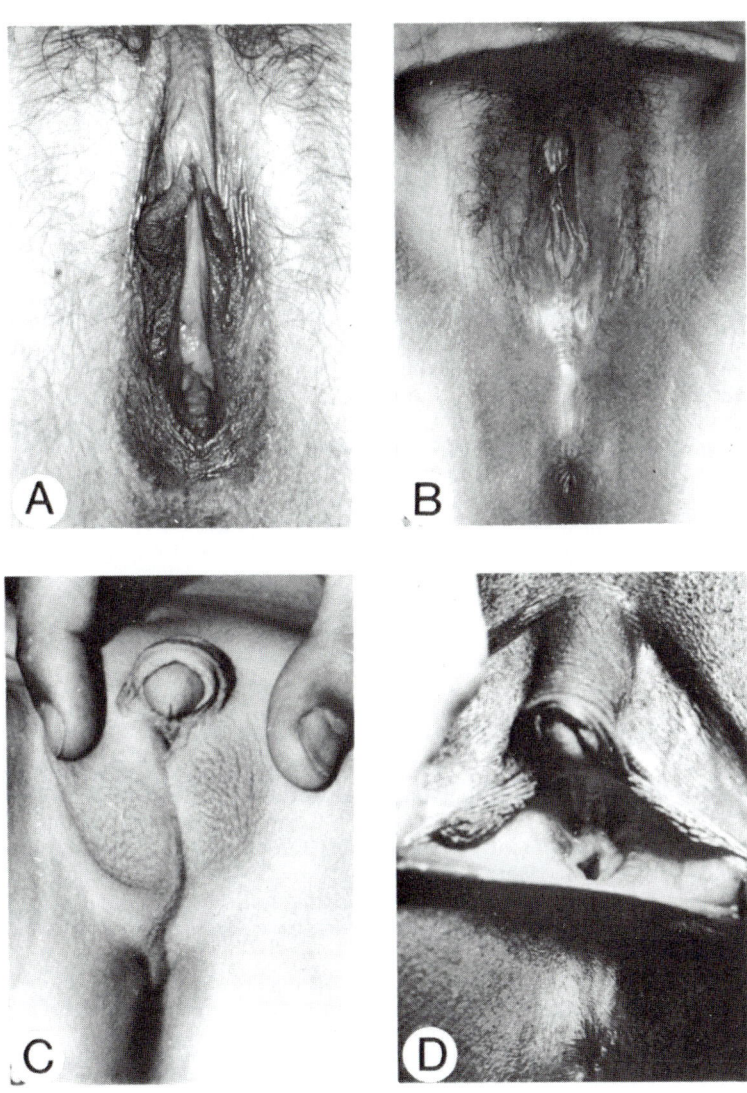

FIGURE 7–17. External genitalia of representative subjects with male pseudohermaphroditism due to androgen resistance. **A.** Testicular feminization (androgen receptor defect). **B.** Incomplete testicular feminization (androgen receptor defect). **C.** Familial male pseudohermaphroditism, type I (Reifenstein syndrome, androgen receptor defect). **D.** 5α-reductase deficiency (5α-reductase type 2 gene mutation). (From Wilson and MacDonald, 1978, with permission.)

CATEGORY 4: TRUE HERMAPHRODITISM. In most subjects with true hermaphroditism, the guidelines for category 3 are met. In addition, true hermaphrodites have both ovarian and testicular tissues, and in particular, germ cells (ova and sperm) of both sexes are found in the abnormal gonads.

PRELIMINARY DIAGNOSIS OF THE CAUSE OF GENITAL AMBIGUITY. A *preliminary* diagnosis of the etiology and pathogenesis of genital ambiguity can be made at the time of birth of an affected child. By physical and ultrasonic examination of the newborn, the experienced examiner can ascertain important findings. These include whether gonads are palpable, and if so, where they are; phallus length and diameter; position of the urethral meatus; degree of labioscrotal fold fusion; and whether there is a vagina, vaginal pouch, or urogenital sinus (Speroff and associates, 1994). If the uterus is present, the diagnosis must be female pseudohermaph-

roditism, testicular or gonadal dysgenesis, or true hermaphroditism. A family history of congenital adrenal hyperplasia is helpful. If the uterus is not present, the diagnosis is male pseudohermaphroditism. Androgen resistance and enzymatic defects in testicular testosterone biosynthesis are often familial.

REFERENCES

Abbas SK, Pickard DW, Illingworth D, Storer J, Purdie DW, Moniz C, Dixit M, Caple IW, Ebeling PR, Rodda CP, Martin TJ, Care AD: Measurement of PTH-rP protein in extracts of fetal parathyroid glands and placental membranes. J Endocrinol 124:319, 1990

Adam PAJ, Teramo K, Raiha N, Gitlin D, Schwartz R: Human fetal insulin metabolism early in gestation: Response to acute elevation of the fetal glucose concentration and placental transfer of human insulin-I-131. Diabetes 18:409, 1969

Adinolfi M: Human complement: Onset and site of synthesis during fetal life. Am J Dis Child 131:1015, 1977

Adzick NS, Harrison MR, Glick PL, et al: Experimental pulmonary hypoplasia and oligohydramnios: Relative contributions of lung fluid and fetal breathing movements. J Pediatr Surg 19:658, 1984

Aherne W, Dunnill MS: Morphometry of the human placenta. Br Med Bull 22:1, 1966

Alcorn D, Adamson TM, Lambert TF, Maloney JE, Ritchie BC, Robinson PM: Morphological effects of chronic tracheal ligation and drainage in the fetal lamb lung. J Anat 3:649, 1977

Allan BB, Brant R, Seidel JE, Jarrell JF: Declining sex ratios in Canada. CMAJ 156:37, 1997

Altshuler G: Immunologic competence of the immature human fetus. Obstet Gynecol 43:811, 1974

Andersson S, Berman DM, Jenkins EP, Russell DW: Deletion of steroid 5 alpha-reductase 2 gene in male pseudohermaphroditism. Nature 354:159, 1991

Assali NS, Bekey GA, Morrison LW: Fetal and neonatal circulation. In Assali NS (ed): Biology of Gestation, Vol II. The Fetus and Neonate. New York, Academic Press, 1968

Ballabio M, Nicolini U, Jowett T, Ruiz de Elvira MC, Ekins RP, Rodeck CH: Maturation of thyroid function in normal human foetuses. Clin Endocrinol 31:565, 1989

Ballard PL, Ballard RA, Creasy RK, Padbury J, Polk DH, Bracken M, Moya FR, Gross I: Plasma thyroid hormones and prolactin in premature infants and their mothers after prenatal treatment with thyrotropin-releasing hormone. Ped Research 32:673, 1992

Banting FG, Best CH: Pancreatic extracts. J Lab Clin Med 1:464, 1922

Bashore RA, Smith F, Schenker S: Placental transfer and disposition of bilirubin in the pregnant monkey. Am J Obstet Gynecol 103:950, 1969

Belcher DP: A child weighing 25 pounds at birth. JAMA 67:950, 1916

Boddy K, Dawes GS: Fetal breathing. Br Med Bull 31:3, 1975

Boyle JT: Motility of the upper gastrointestinal tract in the fetus and neonate. In Polin RA, Fox WW (eds): Fetal and Neonatal Physiology. Philadelphia, Saunders, 1992, p 1028

Bozzetti P, Ferrari MM, Marconi AM, Ferrazzi E, Pardi G, Makowski EL, Battaglia FC: The relationship of maternal and fetal glucose concentrations in the human from midgestation until term. Metabolism 37:358, 1988

Brace RA, Wolf EJ: Normal amniotic fluid volume changes throughout pregnancy. Am J Obstet Gynecol 161:382, 1989

Brash AR, Hickey DE, Graham TP, Stahlman MT, Oates JA, Cotton RB: Pharmacokinetics of indomethacin in the neonate: Relation of plasma indomethacin levels to response of the ductus arteriosus. N Engl J Med 305:67, 1981

Brinsmead MW, Liggins, GC: Somadomedin-like activity, prolactin, growth hormone and insulin in human cord blood. Aust NZ J Obstet Gynecol 19:129, 1979

Brown AK: Bilirubin metabolism in the developing liver. In Assali NS (ed): Biology of Gestation, Vol II. The Fetus and Neonate. New York, Academic Press, 1968, p 361

Browning AJF, Butt WR, Lynch SS, Shakespear RA: Maternal plasma concentrations of β-lipotropin, β-endorphin and γ-lipotrophin throughout pregnancy. Br J Obstet Gynaecol 90:1147, 1983

Carr D: Chromosome studies in abortuses and stillborn infants. Lancet 2:603, 1963

Chard T, Hudson CN, Edwards CRW, Boyd NRH: Release of oxytocin and vasopressin by the human foetus during labour. Nature 234:352, 1971

Chez RA, Mintz DH, Reynolds WA, Hutchinson DL: Maternal-fetal plasma glucose relationships in late monkey pregnancy. Am J Obstet Gynecol 121:938, 1975

Clymann RI, Heymann MA: Pharmacology of the ductus arteriosus. Pediatr Clin North Am 28:77, 1981

Collaborative Santiago Surfactant Group: Collaborative trial of prenatal thyrotropin-releasing hormone and corticosteroids for prevention of respiratory distress syndrome. Am J Obstet Gynecol 178:33, 1998

Corrigan JJ Jr: Normal hemostasis in the fetus and newborn: Coagulation. In Polin RA, Fox WW (eds): Fetal and Neonatal Physiology. Philadelphia, Saunders, 1992, p 1368

Davis DL, Gottlieb MB, Stampnitzky JR: Reduced ratio of male to female births in several industrial countries: A sentinel health indicator? JAMA 279:1018, 1998

Davis ME, Potter EL: Intrauterine respiration of the human fetus. JAMA 131:1194, 1946

Davis MM, Hodes ME, Munsick RA, Ulbright TM, Goldstein DJ: Pancreatic amylase expression in human pancreatic development. Hybridoma 5:137, 1986

Dawes GS: The umbilical circulation. Am J Obstet Gynecol 84:1634, 1962

DeVane GW, Naden RP, Porter JC, Rosenfeld CR: Mechanism of arginine vasopressin release in the sheep fetus. Pediatr Res 16:504, 1982

DeVane GW, Porter JC: An apparent stress-induced release of arginine vasopressin by human neonates. J Clin Endocrinol Metab 51:1412, 1980

De Verdier CH, Garby L: Low binding of 2,3-diphosphoglycerate to hemoglobin F. Scand J Clin Lab Invest 23:149, 1969

DiRenzo GC, Anceschi MM, Cosmi EV: Lung surfactant enhancement in utero. Eur J Obstet Gynecol Reprod Biol 32:1, 1989

Dolman CL: Characteristic configuration of fetal brains from 22 to 40 weeks gestation at two week intervals. Arch Pathol Lab Med 101:193, 1977

Edman CD, Winters AJ, Porter JC, Wilson J, MacDonald PC: Embryonic testicular regression. A clinical spectrum of XY agonadal individual. Obstet Gynecol 49:208, 1977

Epstein M, Chez RA, Oakes GK, Mintz DH: Fetal pancreatic glucagon responses in glucose-intolerant nonhuman primate pregnancy. Am J Obstet Gynecol 127:268, 1977

Fiddler M, Abdel-Rahman B, Rappolee DA, Pergament E: Expression of SRY transcripts in preimplantation human embryos. Am J Med Genet 55:80, 1995

Fisher DA: The unique endocrine milieu of the fetus. J Clin Invest 78:603, 1986

Fisher DA: Ross Conference on Obstetrical Decisions and Neonatal Outcome, San Diego, 1979

Foley ME, Isherwood DM, McNicol GP: Viscosity, hematocrit, fibrinogen and plasma proteins in maternal and cord blood. Br J Obstet Gynaecol 85:500, 1978

George FW, Wilson JD: Sex determination and differentiation. In Knobil E, Neill J (eds): The Physiology of Reproduction. New York, Raven, 1988, p 3

Gilbert RD: Control of fetal cardiac output during changes in blood volume. Am J Physiol 238:H80, 1980

Gilbert WM, Brace RA: Amniotic fluid volume and normal flows to and from the amniotic cavity. Sem Perinatol 17:150, 1993

Gillibrand PN: Changes in amniotic fluid volume with advancing pregnancy. J Obstet Gynaecol Br Commonw 76:527, 1969

Gilstrap LC, Cunningham FG: Cancer in pregnancy. Williams Obstetrics, 19th ed (suppl 17). Stamford, CT, Appleton & Lange, February/March 1996

Gitlin D: Protein transport across the placenta and protein turnover between amnionic fluid, maternal and fetal circulation. In Moghissi KS, Hafez ESE (eds): The Placenta. Springfield, IL, Thomas, 1974

Gitlin D: Development and metabolism of the immune globulins. In Kaga BM, Stiehm ER (eds): Immunologic Incompetence. Chicago, Year Book, 1971

Gitlin D, Kumate J, Morales C, Noriega L, Arevalo N: The turnover of amniotic fluid protein in the human conceptus. Am J Obstet Gynecol 113:632, 1972

Giudice LC, de-Zegher F, Gargosky SE, Dsupin BA, de las Fuentes L, Crystal RA, Hintz RL, Rosenfeld RG: Insulin-like growth factors and their binding proteins in the term and preterm human fetus and neonate with normal and extremes of intrauterine growth. J Clin Endocrinol Metab 80:1548, 1995

Gluck L, Kulovich MV, Eidelman AI, Cordero L, Khazin AF: Biochemical development of surface activity in mammalian lung, 4. Pulmonary lecithin synthesis in the human fetus and newborn and etiology of the respiratory distress syndrome. Pediatr Res 6:81, 1972

Gluck L, Landowne RA, Kulovich MV: Biochemical development of surface activity in mammalian lung, 3. Structural changes in lung lecithin during development of the rabbit fetus and newborn. Pediatr Res 4:352, 1970

Gluck L, Motoyama EK, Smits HL, Kulovich MV: The biochemical development of surface activity in mammalian lung, 1. The surface-active phospholipids; the separation and distribution of surface-active lecithin in the lung of the developing rabbit fetus. Pediatr Res 1:237, 1967

Griffin JE, Wilson JD: Disorders of sexual differentiation. In Walsh PC, Gittes RF, Perlmutter AD, Stamey RA (eds): Campbell's Urology. Philadelphia, Saunders, 1986, p 1819

Gruenwald P: Growth of the human foetus. In McLaren A (ed): Advances in Reproductive Physiology. New York, Academic Press, 1967

Grumbach MM, Kaplan SL: Fetal pituitary hormones and the maturation of central nervous system regulation of anterior pituitary function. In Gluck L (ed): Modern Perinatal Medicine. Chicago, Year Book, 1974

Gustafson ML, Donahoe PK: Male sex determination: Current concepts of male sexual differentiation. Annu Rev Med 45:505, 1994

Hahn T, Hartmann M, Blaschitz A, Skofitsch G, Graf R, Dohr G, Desoye G: Localisation of the high affinity facilitative glucose transporter protein GLUT 1 in the placenta of human, marmoset monkey (Callithrix jacchus) and rat at different developmental stages. Cell Tissue Res 280:49, 1995

Hallman M, Kulovich MV, Kirkpatrick E, Sugarman RG, Gluck L: Phosphatidylinositol and phosphatidylglycerol in amniotic fluid: Indices of lung maturity. Am J Obstet Gynecol 125:613, 1976

Hayward AR: The human fetus and newborn: Development of the immune response. Birth Defects 19:289, 1983

Heimark R, Schwartz S: Cellular organization of blood vessels in development and disease. In Ryan U (ed): Endothelial Cells, Vol II. Boca Raton, FL, CRC Press, 1988, p 103

Hellman P, Ridefelt P, Juhlin C, Akerstrom G, Rastad J, Gylfe E: Parathyroid-like regulation of parathyroid hormone-related protein release and cytoplasmic calcium in cytotrophoblast cells of human placenta. Arch Biochem Biophys 293:174, 1992

Henriksson P, Hedner V, Nilsson IM, Boehm J, Robertson B, Lorand L: Fibrin-stabilization factor XIII in the fetus and the newborn infant. Pediatr Res 8:789, 1974

Hill DJ, Tevaarwerk GJ, Caddell C, Arany E, Kilkenny D, Gregory M: Fibroblast growth factor 2 is elevated in term maternal and cord serum and amniotic fluid in pregnancies complicated by diabetes: Relationship to fetal and placental size. J Clin Endocrinol Metab 80:2626, 1995

Holmberg C, Perheentupa J, Launiala K, Hallman N: Congenital chloride diarrhea. Arch Dis Child 52:255, 1977

James WH: Hormonal control of sex ratio. J Theor Biol 118:427, 1986

Jost A, Vigier B, Prepin J: Studies on sex differentiation in mammals. Recent Prog Horm Res 29:1, 1973

Juhlin C, Lundgren S, Johansson H, Lorentzen J, Rask L, Larsson E, et al: 500-Kilodalton calcium sensor regulating cytoplasmic Ca^{2+} in cytotrophoblast cells of human placenta. J Biol Chem 265:8275, 1990

Kaplan S: Disorders of the endocrine system. In Assali NS (ed): Pathophysiology of Gestation, Vol III. Fetal and Neonatal Disorders. New York, Academic Press, 1972

Katz FH, Beck P, Makowski EL: The renin-aldosterone system in mother and fetus at term. Am J Obstet Gynecol 118:51, 1974

Keidel W, Gluck L: Lipid biochemistry and biochemical development of the lung. In Scarpelli E (ed): Pulmonary Physiology of the Fetus, Newborn, and Child. Philadelphia, Lea & Febiger, 1975, p 96

Kimura RE: Lipid metabolism in the fetal-placental unit. In Cowett RM (ed): Principles of Perinatal-Neonatal Metabolism. New York, Springer-Verlag, 1991, p 291

Klagsbrun M: Angiogenesis factors. In Ryan U (ed): Endothelial Cells, Vol II. Boca Raton, FL, CRC Press, 1988, p 37

Kohler PF: Maturation of the human complement system. J Clin Invest 52:671, 1973

Koldovsky O, Heringova A, Jirsova U, Jirasek JE, Uher J: Transport of glucose against a concentration gradient in everted sacs of jejunum and ileum of human fetuses. Gastroenterology 48:185, 1965

Kurjak A, Kirkinen P, Latin V, Ivankovic D: Ultrasonic assessment of fetal kidney function in normal and complicated pregnancies. Am J Obstet Gynecol 141:266, 1981

Lebenthal E, Lee PC: Interactions of determinants of the ontogeny of the gastrointestinal tract: A unified concept. Pediatr Res 1:19, 1983

Lemons JA: Fetal placental nitrogen metabolism. Semin Perinatol 3:177, 1979

Liggins GC: Fetal lung maturation. Aust NZ J Obstet Gynaecol 34:247, 1994

Liggins GC: Premature delivery of fetal lambs infused with glucocorticoids. J Endocrinol 45:515, 1969

Liley AW: Disorders of amniotic fluid. In Assali NS (ed): Pathophysiology of Gestation. New York, Academic Press, 1972

Longo LD: Respiration in the fetal–placental unit. In Cowett RM (ed): Principles of Perinatal-Neonatal Metabolism. New York, Springer-Verlag, 1991, p 304

Longo LD: Respiratory gas exchange in the placenta. In Fishman AP, Farhi LE, Tenney SM (eds): Handbook of Physiology, section 3. The Respiratory System, Vol IV. Gas Exchange. Washington, DC, American Physiological Society, 1987, p 351

MacDonald PC, Madden JD, Brenner PF, Wilson JD, Siiteri PK: Origin of estrogen in normal men and in women with testicular feminization. J Clin Endocrinol Metab 49:905, 1979

Madden JD, Walsh PC, MacDonald PC, Wilson JD: Clinical and endocrinological characterization of a patient with syndrome of incomplete testicular feminization. J Clin Endocrinol 41:751, 1975

Mally MI, Otonkoski T, Lopez AD, Hayek A: Developmental gene expression in the human fetal pancreas. Pediatr Res 36:537, 1994

Manning JT, Anderton RH, Shutt M: Parental age gap skews child sex ratio. Nature 389:344, 1997

Mason RJ: Disaturated lecithin concentration of rabbit tissues. Am Rev Respir Dis 107:678, 1973

McCormick SM, Mendelson CR: Human SP-A1 and SP-A2 genes are differentially regulated during development and by cAMP and glucocorticoids. Am J Physiol 266:367, 1994

McPhaul MJ, Marcelli M, Tilley WD, Griffin JE, Wilson JD: Androgen resistance caused by mutations in the androgen receptor gene. FASEB J 5:2910, 1991

Mendelson CR, Chen C, Boggaram V, Zacharias C, Snyder JM: Regulation of the synthesis of the major surfactant apoprotein in fetal rabbit lung tissue. J Biol Chem 261:9938, 1986

Miller AJ: Deglutition. Physiol Rev 62:129, 1982

Mistretta CM, Bradley RM: Taste and swallowing in utero. Br Med Bull 31:80, 1975

Moore KL: The Developing Human: Clinically Oriented Embryology, 4th ed. Philadelphia, Saunders, 1988

Moore KL: Before We Are Born. Basic Embryology and Birth Defects, 2nd ed. Philadelphia, Saunders, 1983

Moore KL: The Developing Human, 2nd ed. Philadelphia, Saunders, 1977

Morriss FH Jr, Boyd RDH, Manhendren D: Placental transport. In Knobil E, Neill J (eds): The Physiology of Reproduction, Vol II. New York, Raven, 1994, 813

Mulchahey JJ, DiBlasio AM, Martin MC, Blumenfeld Z, Jaffe RB: Hormone production and peptide regulation of the human fetal pituitary gland. Endocr Rev 8:406, 1987

Ney JA, Fee SC, Dooley SL, Socol ML, Minogue J: Factors influencing hemostasis after umbilical vein puncture in vitro. Am J Obstet Gynecol 160:424, 1989

Nielsen NC: Coagulation and fibrinolysin in normal women immediately postpartum and in newborn infants. Acta Obstet Gynecol Scand 48:371, 1969

O'Brien WF: Use of TRH in the fetus to advance lung maturity. Adv Exp Med Biol 299:243, 1991

Obenshain SS, Adam PAJ, King KC, Teramo K, Raivio KO, Raiha N, Schwartz R: Human fetal insulin response to sustained maternal hyperglycemia. N Engl J Med 283:566, 1970

Olsen O, Clausen JA: Determination of the expected day of delivery—ultrasound has not been shown to be more accurate than the calendar method. Ugeskr Laeger 160:2088, 1998

Pataryas HA, Stamatoyannopoulos G: Hemoglobins in human fetuses: Evidence for adult hemoglobin production after the 11th gestational week. Blood 39:688, 1972

Paton JB, Fisher DE, DeLannoy CW, Behram RE: Umbilical blood flow, cardiac output, and organ blood flow in the immature baboon fetus. Am J Obstet Gynecol 117:560, 1973

Patterson MN, MJ McPhaul, IA Hughes: Androgen insensitivity syndrome. Bailleres Clin Endocrinol Metab 8:379, 1994

Pearson HA: Recent advances in hematology. J Pediatr 69:466, 1966

Perrine SP, Greene MF, Cohen RA, Faller DV: A physiological delay in human fetal hemoglobin switching is associated with specific globin DNA hypomethylation. FEBS Lett 228:139, 1988

Pipe NGJ, Smith T, Halliday D, Edmonds CJ, Williams C,

Coltart TM: Changes in fat, fat-free mass and body water in human normal pregnancy. Br J Obstet Gynaecol 86:929, 1979

Polin RA, Husain MK, James LS, Frantz AG: High vasopressin concentrations in human umbilical cord blood—lack of correlation with stress. J Perinat Med 5:114, 1977

Pritchard JA: Fetal swallowing and amniotic fluid volume. Obstet Gynecol 28:606, 1966.

Pritchard JA: Deglutition by normal and anencephalic fetuses. Obstet Gynecol 25:289, 1965

Rooney SA, Gross I, Motoyama EK, Warshaw JB: Effects of cortisol and thyroxine on fatty acid and phospholipid biosynthesis in fetal rabbit lung. Physiologist 17:323, 1974

Rosenfeld CR, Porter JC: Arginine vasopressin in the developing fetus. In Albrecht ED, Pepe GJ (eds): Research in Perinatal Medicine, 4. Perinatal Endocrinology. Ithaca, NY, Perinatology Press, 1985, p 91

Rubin LP, Kifor O, Hua J, Brown EM, Torday JS: Parathyroid hormone (PTH) and PTH-related protein stimulate surfactant phospholipid synthesis in rat fetal lung, apparently by a mesenchymal-epithelial mechanism. Biochim Biophys Acta 1223:91, 1994

Rudolph AM, Heymann MA: The fetal circulation. Annu Rev Med 19:195, 1968

Sakata M, Kurachi H, Imai T, Tadokoro C, Yamaguchi M, Yoshimoto Y, Oka Y, Miyake A: Increase in human placental glucose transporter-1 during pregnancy. Eur J Endocrinol 132:206, 1995

Schwartz R, Gruppuso PA, Petzold K, Brambilla D, Hiilesmaa V, Teramo KA: Hyperinsulinemia and macrosomia in the fetus of the diabetic mother. Diabetes Care 17:640, 1994

Shrand II: Vomiting in utero with intestinal atresia. Pediatrics 49:767, 1972

Simpson JL: Diseases of the gonads, genital tract, and genitalia. In Rimoin DL, Connor JM, Pyeritz RE (eds): Emery and Rimoin's Principles and Practice of Medical Genetics, Vol. I, 3rd ed. New York, Churchill Livingstone, 1997, p 1477

Sipes SL, Weiner CP, Wenstrom KD, Williamson RA, Grant SS: The association between fetal karyotype and mean corpuscular volume. Am J Obstet Gynecol 165:1371, 1991

Slijper FM, Drop SL, Molenaar JC, de Muinck Keizer-Schrama SM: Long-term psychological evaluation of intersex children. Arch Sex Behav 27:125, 1998

Smith CM II, Tukey DP, Krivit W, White JG: Fetal red cells (FC) differ in elasticity, viscosity, and adhesion from adult red cells (AC). Pediatr Res 15:588, 1981

Smith FG, Nakamura KT, Segar JL, Robillard JE: In Polin RA, Fox WW (eds): Fetal and Neonatal Physiology. Philadelphia, Saunders, 1992, p 1187

Snyder JM, Kwun JE, O'Brien JA, Rosenfeld CR, Odom MJ: The concentration of the 35 kDa surfactant apoprotein in aminotic fluid from normal and diabetic pregnancies. Pediatr Res 24:728, 1998

Speroff L, Glass RH, Kase NG: Clinical Gynecologic Endocrinology and Infertility, 5th ed. Baltimore, MD, Williams & Wilkins, 1994

Stabile I, Nicolaides KH, Bach A, Teisner B, Rodeck C, Westergaard JG, Grudzinskas JG: Complement factors in fetal and maternal blood and amniotic fluid during the second trimester of normal pregnancy. Br J Obstet Gynaecol 95:281, 1988

Stangenberg M, Legarth J, Cao HL, Lingman G, Persson B, Rahman F, Westgren M: Erythropoietin concentrations in amniotic fluid and umbilical venous blood from Rh-immunized pregnancies. J Perinat Med 21:225, 1993

Stockman JA III, deAlarcon PA: Hematopoiesis and granulopoiesis. In Polin RA, Fox WW (eds): Fetal and Neonatal Physiology. Philadelphia, Saunders, 1992, p 1327

Streeter GL: Weight, sitting height, head size, foot length, and menstrual age of the human embyro. Contrib Embryol 11:143, 1920

Teitel DF: Physiologic development of the cardiovascular system in the fetus. In Polin RA, Fox WW (eds): Fetal and Neonatal Physiology, Vol I. Philadelphia, Saunders, 1992, p 609

Temiras PS, Vernadakis A, Sherwood NM: Development and plasticity of the nervous system. In Assali NS (ed): Biology of Gestation, Vol VII. The Fetus and Neonate. New York, Academic Press, 1968

Tharakan T, Baxi LV, Diuguid D: Protein S deficiency in pregnancy: A case report. Am J Obstet Gynecol 168:141, 1993

Thiery M, Yo Le Sian A, Vrijens M, Janssens D: Vagitus uterinus. J Obstet Gynaecol Br Commonw 80:183, 1973

Thomas RM, Canning CE, Cotes PM, Linch DC, Rodeck CH, Rossiter CE, Huehns ER: Erythropoietin in cord blood haemoglobin and the regulation of fetal erythropoiesis. Br J Obstet Gynaecol 90:795, 1983

Thompson MW, McInnes RR, Willard HF: The hemoglobinopathies: Models of molecular disease. In Thompson MW, McInnes RR, Huntington FW (eds): Thompson and Thompson Genetics in Medicine, 5th ed. Philadelphia, Saunders, 1991, Chap. 11, pp 247

Thorarensen O, Ryan S, Hunter J, Younkin DP: Factor V Leiden mutation: An unrecognized cause of hemiplegic cerebral palsy, neonatal stroke, and placental thrombosis. Ann Neurol 42:372, 1997

Thorpe-Beeston JG, Nicolaides KH, Felton CV, Butler J, McGregor AM: Maturation of the secretion of thyroid hormone and thyroid-stimulating hormone in the fetus. N Engl J Med 324:532, 1991

Usher R, Shephard M, Lind J: The blood volume of the newborn infant and placental transfusion. Acta Paediatr 52:497, 1963

Vulsma T, Gons MH, De Vijlder JJM: Maternal-fetal transfer of thyroxine in congenital hypothyroidism due to a total organification defect or thyroid agenesis. N Engl J Med 321:13, 1989

Walker J, Turnbull EPN: Haemoglobin and red cells in the human foetus and their relation to the oxygen content of the blood in the vessels of the umbilical cord. Lancet 2:312, 1953

Walsh PC, Madden JD, Harrod MJ, Goldstein JL, MacDonald PC, Wilson JD: Familial incomplete male pseudohermaphroditism, type 2: Decreased dihydrotestosterone formation in pseudovaginal perineoscrotal hypospadias. N Engl J Med 291:944, 1974

Watkins JB: Physiology of the gastrointestinal tract in the fetus and neonate. In Polin RA, Fox WW (eds): Fetal and Neonatal Physiology. Philadelphia, Saunders, 1992, p 1015

Weiner CP, Sipes SL, Wenstrom K: The effect of fetal age upon normal fetal laboratory values and venous pressure. Obstet Gynecol 79:713, 1992

Wenstrom KD, Weiner CP, Williamson RA, Grant SS: Prenatal diagnosis of fetal hyperthyroidism using funipuncture. Obstet Gynecol 76:513, 1990

Werlin SL: Exocrine pancreas. In Polin RA, Fox WW (eds): Fetal and Neonatal Physiology. Philadelphia, Saunders, 1992, p 1047

Whitsett JA: Composition of pulmonary surfactant lipids and proteins. In Polin RA, Fox WW (eds): Fetal and Neonatal Physiology. Philadelphia, Saunders, 1992, p 941

Widdowson EM: Growth and composition of the fetus and newborn. In Assali NS (ed): Biology of Gestation, Vol II. The Fetus and Neonate. New York, Academic Press, 1968

Widness JA, Clemons GK, Garcia JF, Oh W, Schwartz R: Increased immunoreactive erythropoietin in cord blood after labor. Am J Obstet Gynecol 148:194, 1984

Wilson JD, Gloyna RE: The intranuclear metabolism of testosterone in the accessory organs of reproduction. Recent Prog Horm Res 26:309, 1970

Wilson JD, Lasnitzki I: Dihydrotestosterone formation in fetal tissues of the rabbit and rat. Endocrinology 89:659, 1971

Wilson JD, MacDonald PC: Male pseudohermaphroditism due to androgen resistance: Testicular feminization and related syndromes. In Stanbury JB, Wyngaarden JD, Frederickson DS (eds): The Metabolic Basis of Inherited Disease. New York, McGraw-Hill, 1978

Wladimiroff JW, Campbell S: Fetal urine-production rates in normal and complicated pregnancy. Lancet 1:151, 1974

Wu B, Kikkawa Y, Orzalesi MM, Motoyama EK, Kaibara M, Zigas CJ, Cook CD: The effect of thyroxine on the maturation of fetal rabbit lungs. Biol Neonate 22:161, 1973

Wu B, Kikkawa Y, Orzalesi MM, Motoyama EK, Kaibara M, Zigas CJ, Cook CD: Accelerated maturation of fetal rabbit lungs by thyroxine. Physiologist 14:253, 1971

Zitnik G, Peterson K, Stamatoyannopoulos G, Papayannopoulou T: Effects of butyrate and glucocorticoids on gamma- to beta-globin gene switching in somatic cell hybrids. Mol Cell Biol 15:790, 1995

8

Maternal Adaptations to Pregnancy

The anatomical, physiological, and biochemical adaptations to pregnancy are profound. Many of these changes begin soon after fertilization and continue throughout gestation, and most of these remarkable adaptations occur in response to physiological stimuli provided by the fetus. Equally astounding is that the woman who was pregnant is returned almost completely to her prepregnancy state after delivery and lactation. The understanding of these adaptations to pregnancy remains a major goal of obstetrics, and without such knowledge, it is almost impossible to understand the disease processes that can threaten women during pregnancy and the puerperium.

Because of these physiological adaptations, in some cases there are marked aberrations that would be perceived as abnormal in the nonpregnant state. For example, cardiovascular changes normally include substantive increases in blood volume and cardiac output, with hemodynamic adaptations that accompany them. This "high-output state" resembles thyrotoxicosis and other abnormal states. At the same time, underlying heart disease may lead to cardiac failure with these burdens.

Thus, physiological adaptations of normal pregnancy can be misinterpreted as disease, but they also may unmask or worsen preexisting disease. A number of laboratory values may appear abnormal, for example, pregnancy hypervolemia is accompanied by plasma volume expansion out of proportion to red cell mass increase. The result is so-called "physiological anemia" that is a major misnomer. The impact of these marked physiological changes on underlying disease, and vice versa, are considered in some detail in Section XII, which deals with medical and surgical complications of pregnancy.

GENITAL TRACT

UTERUS. In the nonpregnant woman, the uterus is an almost-solid structure weighing about 70 g and with a cavity of 10 mL or less. During pregnancy, the uterus is transformed into a relatively thin-walled muscular organ of sufficient capacity to accommodate the fetus, placenta, and amnionic fluid. The total volume of the contents at term averages about 5 L but may be 20 L or more, so that by the end of pregnancy the uterus has achieved a 500 to 1000 times greater capacity than in the nonpregnant state. There is a corresponding increase in uterine weight, and at term, the organ weighs approximately 1100 g.

During pregnancy, uterine enlargement involves stretching and marked hypertrophy of muscle cells, whereas the production of new myocytes is limited. The myometrial smooth muscle cells are surrounded by an irregular array of collagen fibrils. The force of contraction is transmitted from the contractile proteins of the myocytes to the surrounding connective tissue through the collagen reticulum.

Accompanying the increase in size of muscle cells is an accumulation of fibrous tissue, particularly in the external muscle layer, together with a considerable increase in elastic tissue. The network that is formed adds materially to the strength of the uterine wall. Concomitantly, there is a great increase in size and number of blood vessels and lymphatics. The veins that drain the placental site are transformed into large uterine sinuses, and there is hypertrophy of the nerves exemplified by the increase in size of the Frankenhäuser cervical ganglion.

During the first few months, uterine hypertrophy is probably stimulated chiefly by the action of estrogen and perhaps that of progesterone. It is apparent that early hypertrophy is not entirely in response to mechanical distention by the products of conception, because similar uterine changes are observed with ectopic pregnancy (Chap. 34, p. 890). But after about 12 weeks, the increase in uterine size is in large part related in some manner to the effect of pressure exerted by the expanding products of conception.

During the first few months of pregnancy, the uterine walls become considerably thicker, but as gestation advances the walls gradually thin. At term, the walls of the corpus are only about 1.5 cm or less in thickness. Early in pregnancy, the uterus loses the firmness and resistance characteristic of the nonpregnant organ. In the later months, the uterus is changed into a muscular sac with thin, soft, readily indentable walls, demonstrable by the ease with which the fetus usually can be palpated.

Uterine enlargement is not symmetrical, and it is most marked in the fundus. The differential growth is readily apparent by observing the relative positions of the attachments of the fallopian tubes and ovarian and round ligaments. In the early months of pregnancy, these structures attach only slightly below the apex of the fundus, whereas in the later months, they are located slightly above the middle of the uterus (see Fig. 3–9, p. 41). The position of the placenta also influences the extent of uterine hypertrophy, because the portion of the uterus surrounding the placental site enlarges more rapidly than does the rest.

ARRANGEMENT OF THE MUSCLE CELLS. The uterine musculature during pregnancy is arranged in three strata:

1. An external hoodlike layer, which arches over the fundus and extends into the various ligaments.
2. An internal layer, consisting of sphincter-like fibers around the orifices of the tubes and the internal os.

3. Lying between these two, a dense network of muscle fibers perforated in all directions by blood vessels.

The main portion of the uterine wall is formed by the middle layer, which consists of an interlacing network of muscle fibers between which extend the blood vessels. Each cell in this layer has a double curve, so that the interlacing of any two gives approximately the form of the figure eight. As a result of this arrangement, when the cells contract after delivery they constrict the penetrating blood vessels and thus act as ligatures.

The muscle cells composing the uterine wall in pregnancy, especially in its lower portion, overlap one another like shingles on a roof. One end of each fiber arises beneath the serosa of the uterus and extends obliquely downward and inward toward the decidua, forming a large number of muscular lamellae that are interconnected by short muscular processes.

UTERINE SIZE, SHAPE, AND POSITION. For the first few weeks the uterus maintains its original pear shape, but as pregnancy advances the corpus and fundus assume a more globular form, becoming almost spherical by 12 weeks. Subsequently, the organ increases more rapidly in length than in width and assumes an ovoid shape. **By the end of 12 weeks, the uterus has become too large to remain totally within the pelvis.** As the uterus continues to enlarge, it contacts the anterior abdominal wall, displaces the intestines laterally and superiorly, and continues to rise, ultimately reaching almost to the liver. As the uterus rises, tension is exerted upon the broad ligaments and upon the round ligaments.

With the pregnant woman standing, the longitudinal axis of the uterus corresponds to an extension of the axis of the pelvic inlet. The abdominal wall supports the uterus and, unless it is quite relaxed, maintains this relation between the long axis of the uterus and the axis of the pelvic inlet. When the pregnant woman is supine, the uterus falls back to rest upon the vertebral column and the adjacent great vessels, especially the inferior vena cava and the aorta.

With ascent of the uterus from the pelvis, it usually undergoes rotation to the right, and this *dextrorotation* likely is caused by the rectosigmoid on the left side of the pelvis.

CONTRACTILITY. From the first trimester onward, the uterus undergoes irregular contractions, which are normally painless. In the second trimester, these contractions may be detected by bimanual examination. Because attention was first called to this phenomenon in 1872 by J. Braxton Hicks, the contractions have been known by his name. Such contractions appear unpredictably and sporadically, are usually nonrhythmic, and their intensity varies between approximately 5 and 25

mm Hg (Alvarez and Caldeyro-Barcia, 1950). Until the last month of gestation, *Braxton Hicks contractions* are infrequent, but increase during the last week or two. At this time, the contractions may develop as often as every 10 to 20 minutes and may also assume some degree of rhythmicity. Late in pregnancy, these contractions may cause some discomfort and account for so-called *false labor* (Chap. 14, p. 355).

UTEROPLACENTAL BLOOD FLOW. The delivery of most substances essential for growth and metabolism of the fetus and placenta, as well as removal of most metabolic wastes, is dependent upon adequate perfusion of the placental intervillous space (Chap. 5, p. 98). Placental perfusion is dependent upon uterine blood flow through the uterine and ovarian arteries. There is a progressive increase in uteroplacental blood flow during pregnancy, and the reported values range from 450 to 650 mL/min late in pregnancy. Values must be viewed as approximations because of inherent errors in the methods of measurement as well as the appreciable changes in uterine blood flow that are likely induced by changes in position (Edman and associates, 1981; Kauppila and colleagues, 1980).

Assali and co-workers (1968), using electromagnetic flow meters, studied the effects of labor on uteroplacental blood flow in sheep and dogs at term. They found that uterine contractions, either spontaneous or induced, caused a decrease in uterine blood flow that was approximately proportional to the intensity of the contraction, and that a tetanic contraction caused a precipitous fall in uterine blood flow. Harbert and associates (1969) made similar observations in gravid monkeys.

Janbu and Nesheim (1987) studied normal women in labor and correlated Doppler waveforms with intrauterine pressure readings. They found an almost linear correlation between pressure and decreased velocity. With contractions generating 50 mm Hg pressure, velocity was decreased by 60 percent. Uterine contractions appear to affect fetal circulation much less, and Brar and colleagues (1988) reported no adverse effects on umbilical artery flow.

CONTROL OF UTEROPLACENTAL BLOOD FLOW. Increases in uterine blood flow occur progressively throughout gestation in both the human and sheep. In sheep, however, there is a definite redistribution of blood flow within the gravid uterus (Makowski and coworkers, 1968). Before pregnancy, uterine blood flow is divided equally among myometrium, endometrium, and future placental implantation sites. By the end of the first third of ovine pregnancy, endometrial blood flow is 50 percent of the total. By term, blood flow to the placental cotyledons accounts for approximately 90 percent of total uterine blood flow (Rosenfeld and associates, 1974).

It is not clear what induces the increase in uterine blood flow during the first two thirds of ovine pregnancy. It is in part the consequence of increasing placental size and number of blood vessels (Teasdale, 1976). The increase in maternal–placental blood flow principally occurs by means of vasodilation, whereas fetal–placental blood flow is increased by a continuing increase in placental vessels. Palmer and colleagues (1992) showed that uterine artery diameter doubled by 20 weeks and concomitant flow velocity was increased eightfold. It appears likely that this late-pregnancy vasodilation is at least in part the consequence of estrogen stimulation. Naden and Rosenfeld (1985) showed that estradiol-17β administration to nonpregnant sheep induced cardiovascular changes similar to those observed in pregnant animals. Using measurements of uterine resistance index, Jauniaux and associates (1994) found that both estradiol and progesterone contributed to the downstream fall in resistance to blood flow with advancing gestational age in humans.

CATECHOLAMINES. Both epinephrine and norepinephrine cause significant decreases in placental perfusion in sheep even in the absence of any change in blood pressure (Rosenfeld and co-workers, 1976; Rosenfeld and West, 1977). Such a response is likely the consequence of a greater sensitivity to catecholamines of the uteroplacental vascular beds when compared with the systemic vasculature.

ANGIOTENSIN II. Vascular refractoriness to the pressor effects of angiotensin II appears to be a normal response of both human and ovine pregnancy (Gant and co-workers, 1973; Rosenfeld and Gant, 1981). The initial increase in uteroplacental blood flow characteristic of normal pregnancy likely results as a consequence of a blunted uterine vascular resistance to angiotensin II, and possibly other pressor agents such as endothelin.

NITRIC OXIDE. This compound may have important implications for uteroplacental perfusion and setting of vascular tone or resistance in a number of tissue beds. Once called *endothelium-derived relaxing factor* (*EDRF*), nitric oxide is a potent vasodilator released by endothelial cells and it also inhibits platelet aggregation and adhesion to vascular endothelium (Hull and associates, 1994; Seligman and co-workers, 1994). *Nitric oxide synthase* (*NOS*) has been demonstrated in 97 percent of endothelial cells of the umbilical vein, but in only 7 percent of endothelial cells of umbilical arteries (Dikranian and colleagues, 1994). It is also found in the amnionic epithelium and in cells of Wharton jelly. Izumi and colleagues (1994) suggested that the amount of en-

dothelium-derived nitric oxide, as well as the sensitivity of smooth muscle to nitric oxide, both decrease as gestation advances.

CERVIX. During pregnancy, there is pronounced softening and cyanosis of the cervix, often demonstrable as early as a month after conception. The factors responsible for these changes are increased vascularity and edema of the entire cervix, together with hypertrophy and hyperplasia of the cervical glands. Although the cervix contains a small amount of smooth muscle, its major component is connective tissue. The cervix will undergo a rearrangement of its collagen-rich connective tissue, producing a 12-fold reduction in mechanical strength by term (Rechberger and colleagues, 1988).

As shown in Figure 8–1, the glands of the cervix undergo such marked proliferation that by the end of pregnancy they occupy approximately half of the entire cervical mass, rather than a small fraction as in the nonpregnant state. Moreover, the septa separating the glandular spaces become progressively thinner, resulting in the formation of a structure resembling a honeycomb, the meshes of which are filled with tenacious mucus. Soon after conception, a clot of very thick mucus obstructs the cervical canal. At the onset of labor, if not before, this so-called *mucus plug* is expelled, resulting in a *bloody show*. The glands near the external os proliferate beneath the stratified squamous epithelium of the portio vaginalis. These are customarily red and velvety in appearance and are covered by columnar

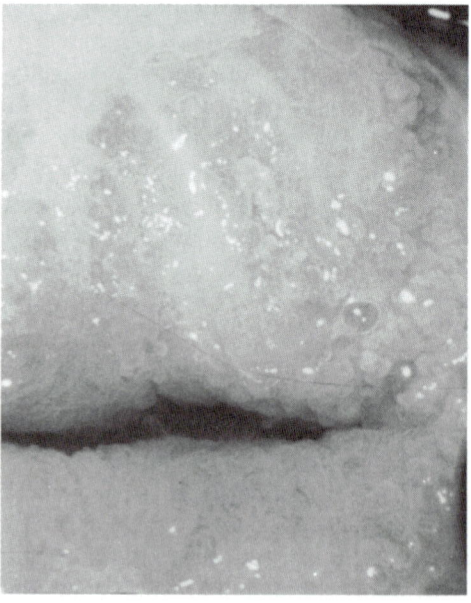

FIGURE 8–1. Cervical eversion of pregnancy as viewed through a colposcope. The eversion represents columnar epithelium on the portio of the cervix. (Courtesy of Dr. Phil DiSaia.)

epithelium. These normal pregnancy-induced changes represent an extension, or *eversion,* of the proliferating columnar endocervical glands. This tissue tends to be friable and bleeds even with minor trauma, such as with taking Pap smears.

There is a change in the consistency of the cervical mucus during pregnancy. In the great majority of pregnant women, cervical mucus, spread and dried on a glass slide, is characterized by fragmentary crystallization, or *beading,* typical of the effect of progesterone. In some women, arborization of the crystals, or *ferning,* is observed.

During pregnancy, basal cells near the squamocolumnar junction histologically are likely to be prominent in size, shape, and staining qualities. These changes are considered to be estrogen induced. The frequency of less-than-optimal Pap smears is increased in the pregnant woman (Kost and associates, 1993).

OVARIES. Ovulation ceases during pregnancy and the maturation of new follicles is suspended. Ordinarily, only a single corpus luteum of pregnancy can be found in the ovaries of pregnant women. This most likely functions maximally during the first 6 to 7 weeks of pregnancy (4 to 5 weeks postovulation), and thereafter, contributes relatively little to progesterone production. These observations have been confirmed in vivo by surgical removal of the corpus luteum before 7 weeks (5 weeks postovulation), which results in a rapid fall in maternal serum progesterone and then spontaneous abortion (Csapo and co-workers, 1973). After this time, however, corpus luteum removal ordinarily does not cause abortion or labor.

RELAXIN. Human relaxin is a protein hormone composed of nonidentical A and B chains of similar length. There are structural features of relaxin that are similar to insulin and insulin-like growth factors I and II. Its major biological action in mammals is remodeling of the connective tissue of the reproductive tract, allowing accommodation of pregnancy and successful parturition (Weiss and colleagues, 1993). Relaxin is secreted by the corpus luteum of pregnancy, the placenta, and by the decidua parietalis (Bogic and colleagues, 1995). The pattern of secretion is similar to that of chorionic gonadotropin.

Whereas 17α-hydroxyprogesterone and progesterone secretion by the corpus luteum declines to negligible rates by 7 to 8 weeks, appreciable relaxin secretion continues throughout pregnancy. Among 15 women between 8 and 13 weeks, the median concentration of relaxin was 1000 ng/L in maternal serum, 122 ng/L in coelomic fluid, and 9 ng/L in amnionic fluid (Johnson and colleagues, 1994a, 1994b). Between 10 and 12 weeks, relaxin levels correlated with the number of fetuses; however, levels did not fall with reduction of fetal number. They suggested that circulating levels of relaxin throughout pregnancy are determined by gonadotropin stimulation, and within the first 10 weeks by the luteotropic stimulus from the conceptus.

The role of relaxin during human pregnancy is not completely defined; however, it is known to have effects on the biochemical structure of the cervix (Bell and colleagues, 1993). The hormone also affects contractility of the myometrium that may be implicated in preterm birth (Weiss and colleagues, 1993). Although peripheral joint laxity increases during human pregnancy, this change does not correlate with serum relaxin levels (Schauberger and colleagues, 1996).

PREGNANCY LUTEOMA. In 1963, Sternberg described a solid ovarian tumor that developed during pregnancy that was composed of large acidophilic luteinized cells. Luteoma of pregnancy represents an exaggeration of the luteinization reaction of the ovary of normal pregnancy. Thus, while not true neoplasms, they may present as quite large abdominal masses (Fig. 8–2). The luteoma regresses after delivery, but may recur in subsequent pregnancies (Shortle and associates, 1987).

Even though maternal virilization may be prominent, the female fetus is usually not affected, presumably because of the protective role of the placenta through its high capacity to convert androgens and androgen-like steroids to estrogens (Edman and co-workers, 1979). Despite this, a female fetus can become virilized (Cohen and associates, 1982).

HYPERREACTIO LUTEINALIS. This is a second benign lesion of the ovary that causes maternal virilization during pregnancy. Although the cellular pattern is similar to that of a luteoma, the two tumors are different grossly. The luteoma is solid, and hyperreactio luteinalis is a cystic tumor. Additionally, hyperreactio luteinalis is commonly associated with extremely high serum chorionic gonadotropin levels (Muechler and colleagues, 1987). Bradshaw and co-workers (1986) described a nullipara who developed temporal balding, hirsutism, and clitoromegaly during the third trimester. Levels of androstenedione and testosterone were elevated massively in maternal serum but were normal in umbilical cord blood. Maternal serum levels of chorionic gonadotropin were twice the mean for normal late pregnancy. Bilateral multicystic ovarian masses obstructed fetal descent during labor and necessitated cesarean delivery. Increased ovarian responsiveness to gonadotropin was confirmed 8 weeks postpartum.

OTHER CHANGES. A *decidual* reaction on and beneath the surface of the ovaries, similar to that found in the endometrial stroma, is common in pregnancy and may

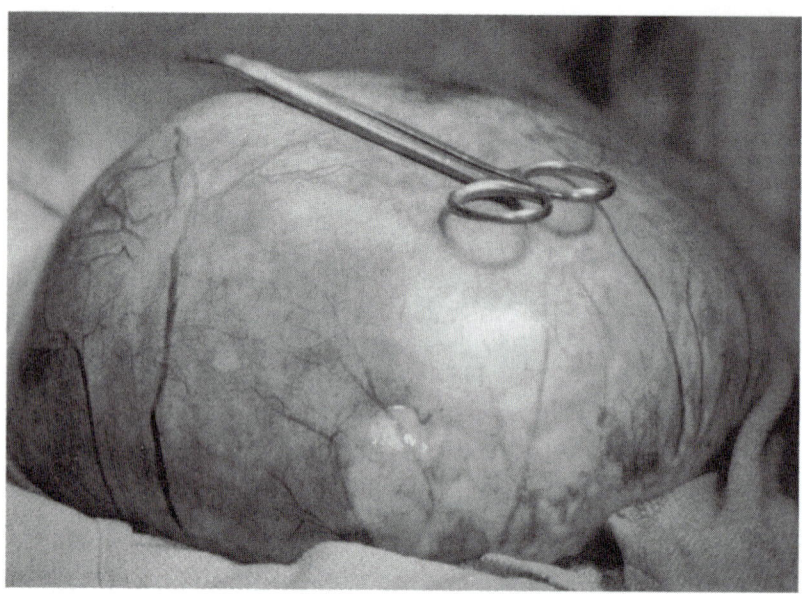

FIGURE 8–2. Large luteoma of pregnancy removed at laparotomy postpartum.

be observed at cesarean delivery. These elevated patches of tissue bleed easily and may, on first glance, resemble freshly torn adhesions. Similar decidual reactions are occasionally seen on the posterior uterine serosa and upon or within other pelvic or even extrapelvic abdominal organs.

The enormous caliber of the ovarian veins viewed at cesarean delivery is startling. Hodgkinson (1953) found that the diameter of the ovarian vascular pedicle increased during pregnancy from 0.9 cm to approximately 2.6 cm at term.

FALLOPIAN TUBES. The musculature of the fallopian tubes undergoes little hypertrophy during pregnancy. The epithelium of the tubal mucosa becomes flattened compared with the nonpregnant state. Decidual cells may develop in the stroma of the endosalpinx, but a continuous decidual membrane is not formed.

VAGINA AND PERINEUM. During pregnancy, increased vascularity and hyperemia develop in the skin and muscles of the perineum and vulva, and there is softening of the normally abundant connective tissue of these structures. Increased vascularity prominently affects the vagina. The copious secretion and the characteristic violet color of the vagina during pregnancy (*Chadwick sign*) result chiefly from hyperemia. The vaginal walls undergo striking changes seemingly in preparation for the distention that occurs during labor. There is considerable increase in thickness of the mucosa, loosening of the connective tissue, and hypertrophy of the smooth-muscle cells to nearly the same extent as in the uterus. These changes effect such an increase in length

of the vaginal walls that sometimes, in parous women, the lower portion of the anterior vaginal wall protrudes slightly through the vulvar opening. The papillae of the vaginal mucosa also undergo considerable hypertrophy, creating a fine, hobnailed appearance.

SECRETIONS. The considerably increased cervical and vaginal secretions during pregnancy consist of a somewhat thick, white discharge. Its pH is acidic, varying from 3.5 to 6, the result of increased production of lactic acid from glycogen in the vaginal epithelium by the action of *Lactobacillus acidophilus*.

HISTOPATHOLOGY. Early in pregnancy the vaginal epithelial cells are similar to those found during the luteal phase. As pregnancy advances, two patterns of response may be seen:

1. Small intermediate cells, called *navicular cells* by Papanicolaou, are found in abundance in small, dense clusters. These ovoid cells contain a vesicular, somewhat elongated nucleus.
2. Vesicular nuclei without cytoplasm, or so-called naked nuclei, are evident along with an abundance of *Lactobacillus*.

SKIN

ABDOMINAL WALL. In the later months of pregnancy, reddish, slightly depressed streaks commonly develop in the skin of the abdomen and sometimes in the skin over the breasts and thighs in about half of pregnant women. In multiparous women, in addition to the reddish striae of the present pregnancy, glistening, silvery lines that represent the cicatrices of previous striae frequently are seen.

Occasionally the muscles of the abdominal walls do not withstand the tension to which they are subjected, and the rectus muscles separate in the midline, creating a diastasis recti of varying extent. If severe, a considerable portion of the anterior uterine wall is covered by only a layer of skin, attenuated fascia, and peritoneum.

PIGMENTATION. In many women, the midline of the abdominal skin becomes markedly pigmented, assuming a brownish-black color to form the *linea nigra.* Occasionally, irregular brownish patches of varying size appear on the face and neck, giving rise to *chloasma* or *melasma gravidarum (mask of pregnancy).* There is also accentuation of pigment of the areolae and genital skin. Fortunately, this usually disappears, or at least regresses considerably after delivery (Chap. 54, p. 1430). Oral contraceptives may cause similar pigmentation in these same women. There is very little known of the nature of these pigmentary changes, although melanocyte-stimulating hormone, a polypeptide similar to corticotropin, has been shown to be elevated remarkably from the end of the second month of pregnancy until term (see also Chap. 6). Estrogen and progesterone are reported to have some melanocyte-stimulating effects. Vaughn Jones and Black (1999) attribute most changes to estrogen. These are considered in greater detail in Chapter 54.

VASCULAR CHANGES. Angiomas, called *vascular spiders,* develop in about two thirds of white women and approximately 10 percent of African-American women during pregnancy. These are minute, red elevations on the skin, particularly common on the face, neck, upper chest, and arms, with radicles branching out from a central body. The condition is often designated as nevus, angioma, or telangiectasis. *Palmar erythema* is encountered in pregnancy in about two thirds of white women and a third of black women. The two conditions are of no clinical significance and disappear in most women shortly after pregnancy. They are most likely the consequence of the hyperestrogenemia of pregnancy.

BREASTS

In the early weeks, the pregnant woman often experiences tenderness and tingling. After the second month, the breasts increase in size and delicate veins become visible just beneath the skin. The nipples become considerably larger, more deeply pigmented, and more erectile. After the first few months, a thick, yellowish fluid,

colostrum, can often be expressed from the nipples by gentle massage. At that time, the areolae become broader and more deeply pigmented. Scattered through the areolae are a number of small elevations, the so-called glands of Montgomery, which are hypertrophic sebaceous glands. If the increase in size of the breasts is very extensive, striations similar to those observed in the abdomen may develop. Interestingly, prepregnancy breast size and volume of milk production do not correlate (Hytten, 1995). Histological and functional changes of the breasts induced by pregnancy and lactation are further discussed in Chapter 17 (p. 407).

METABOLIC CHANGES

In response to the rapidly growing fetus and placenta and their increasing demands, the pregnant woman undergoes metabolic changes that are numerous and intense. Certainly no other physiological event in postnatal life induces such profound metabolic alterations.

WEIGHT GAIN. Most of the increase in weight during pregnancy is attributable to the uterus and its contents, the breasts, and increases in blood volume and extravascular extracellular fluid. A smaller fraction of the increased weight is the result of metabolic alterations that result in an increase in cellular water and deposition of new fat and protein, so-called *maternal reserves.* Hytten (1991) reported an average weight gain of 12.5 kg (Table 8–1). Maternal aspects of weight gain during pregnancy are considered in Chapter 10 (p. 231).

TABLE 8–1. Analysis of Weight Gain Based on Physiological Events during Pregnancy

Tissues and Fluids	Cumulative Increase in Weight (g) Up To:			
	10 Weeks	20 Weeks	30 Weeks	40 Weeks (Total)
Fetus	5	300	1500	3400
Placenta	20	170	430	650
Amnionic fluid	30	350	750	800
Uterus	140	320	600	970
Breasts	45	180	360	405
Blood	100	600	1300	1450
Extravascular fluid	0	30	80	1480
Maternal stores (fat)	310	2050	3480	3345
Total	650	4000	8500	12,500

Modified from Hytten (1991), with permission.

METABOLISM

WATER METABOLISM. Increased water retention is a normal physiological alteration of pregnancy. This is mediated, at least in part, by a fall in plasma osmolality of approximately 10 mOsm/kg induced by a resetting of osmotic thresholds for thirst and vasopressin secretion (Lindheimer and Davidson, 1995). As shown in Figure 8–3, this phenomenon is functioning by early pregnancy.

At term, the water content of the fetus, placenta, and amnionic fluid amounts to about 3.5 L. Another 3.0 L accumulates as a result of increases in the maternal blood volume and in the size of the uterus and the breasts. Thus, the minimum amount of extra water that the average women retains during normal pregnancy is about 6.5 L. Clearly demonstrable pitting edema of the ankles and legs is seen in a substantial proportion of pregnant women, especially at the end of the day. This accumulation of fluid, which may amount to a liter or so, is caused by an increase in venous pressure below the level of the uterus as a consequence of partial occlusion of the vena cava. A decrease in interstitial colloid osmotic pressure induced by normal pregnancy also favors edema late in pregnancy (Øian and co-workers, 1985).

Longitudinal studies of body composition have shown a progressive increase in total body water and fat mass during pregnancy. It has been known for decades that both initial maternal weight and the weight gained during pregnancy are highly associated with

birthweight. It is unclear, however, what role maternal fat or water have in fetal growth. Recent studies in well-nourished term women suggest that maternal body water, rather than fat, contributes more significantly to infant birthweight (Lederman and associates, 1999; Mardones-Santander and associates, 1998).

PROTEIN METABOLISM. The products of conception, as well as uterus and maternal blood, are relatively rich in protein rather than fat or carbohydrate. At term, the fetus and placenta together weigh about 4 kg and contain approximately 500 g of protein, or about half of the total pregnancy increase (Hytten and Leitch, 1971). The remaining 500 g is added to the uterus as contractile protein, to the breasts primarily in the glands, and to the maternal blood as hemoglobin and plasma proteins.

From nitrogen balance studies in pregnant women, it appears that actual nitrogen use is only 25 percent (Calloway, 1974). Therefore, daily requirements for protein intake during pregnancy are increased appreciably to correct for this. Equally important is the ingestion of adequate carbohydrates and fat. If these are not consumed in adequate amounts, energy requirements must be met by catabolism of maternal protein stores. Amino acids used for energy are not available for synthesis of maternal protein. With increasing intake of fat and carbohydrates as energy sources, less dietary protein is required to maintain positive nitrogen balance.

CARBOHYDRATE METABOLISM. Normal pregnancy is characterized by mild fasting hypoglycemia, postprandial hyperglycemia, and hyperinsulinemia (Fig. 8–4). The fasting plasma glucose concentration falls somewhat, possibly due to increased plasma levels of insulin. This cannot be explained by a change in the metabolism of insulin because its half-life during pregnancy is not changed (Lind and associates, 1977).

The increased basal level of plasma insulin observed in normal pregnancy is associated with several unique responses to glucose ingestion. For example, after an oral glucose meal, there is both prolonged hyperglycemia and hyperinsulinemia in pregnant women, with a greater suppression of glucagon (Phelps and associates, 1981). The purpose of such a mechanism is likely to ensure a sustained or maintained postprandial supply of glucose to the fetus. This response is consistent with a pregnancy-induced state of peripheral resistance to insulin, which is suggested by three observations:

1. Increased insulin response to glucose.
2. Reduced peripheral uptake of glucose.
3. Suppressed glucagon response.

The mechanism(s) responsible for insulin resistance is not completely understood. Progesterone and estrogen may act, directly or indirectly, to mediate this resistance.

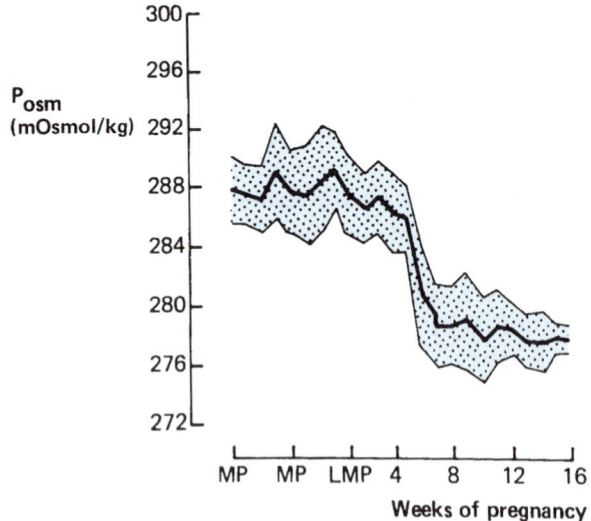

FIGURE 8–3. Mean values (±SD) for plasma osmolality measured at weekly intervals in nine women from before conception to 16 weeks. (LMP = last menstrual period; MP = menstrual period.) (From Davison and colleagues, 1981, with permission.)

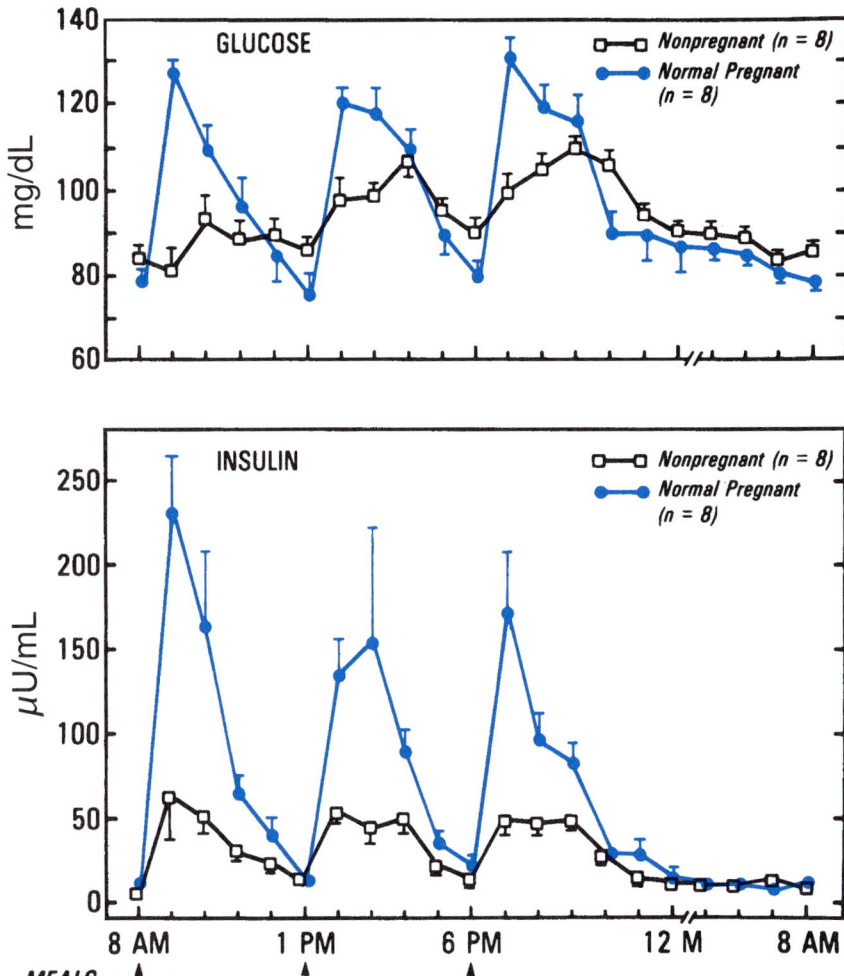

FIGURE 8-4. Diurnal changes in plasma glucose and insulin in normal late pregnancy. (From Phelps and colleagues, 1981, with permission.)

Plasma levels of placental lactogen increase with gestation, and this protein hormone is characterized by growth hormone–like action that may result in increased lipolysis with liberation of free fatty acids (Freinkel, 1980). The increased concentration of circulating free fatty acids also may facilitate increased tissue resistance to insulin.

The mechanisms cited ensure that a continuous supply of glucose is available for transfer to the fetus. The pregnant woman, however, changes rapidly from a postprandial state characterized by elevated and sustained glucose levels to a fasting state characterized by decreased plasma glucose and amino acids such as alanine. There also are higher plasma concentrations of free fatty acids, triglycerides, and cholesterol in the pregnant woman during fasting (Fig. 8–5). Freinkel and colleagues (1985) have referred to this pregnancy-induced switch in fuels from glucose to lipids as **accelerated starvation.** Certainly, when fasting is prolonged in the pregnant woman, these alterations are exaggerated and ketonemia rapidly appears.

Hornnes and Kuhl (1980) measured glucagon and insulin responses to a standard glucose stimulus late in normal pregnancy and again in the same women postpartum. The peak insulin response to glucose infusion was increased fourfold in late pregnancy. In contrast, plasma glucagon concentrations were suppressed, and the degree was similar in late pregnancy and the puerperium. These results are consistent with the view that β-cell sensitivity to a glucose challenge is increased significantly in normal pregnant women, but that the α-cell sensitivity to a glucose stimulus is unaltered.

FAT METABOLISM. The concentrations of lipids, lipoproteins, and apolipoproteins in plasma increase appreciably during pregnancy. Desoye and co-workers (1987) found that there were positive correlations between the concentrations of lipids shown in Figure 8–5 and those of estradiol, progesterone, and placental lactogen.

Plasma lipoprotein cholesterol levels also increase significantly. Low-density lipoprotein cholesterol (LDL-C) levels peak at approximately week 36, likely the

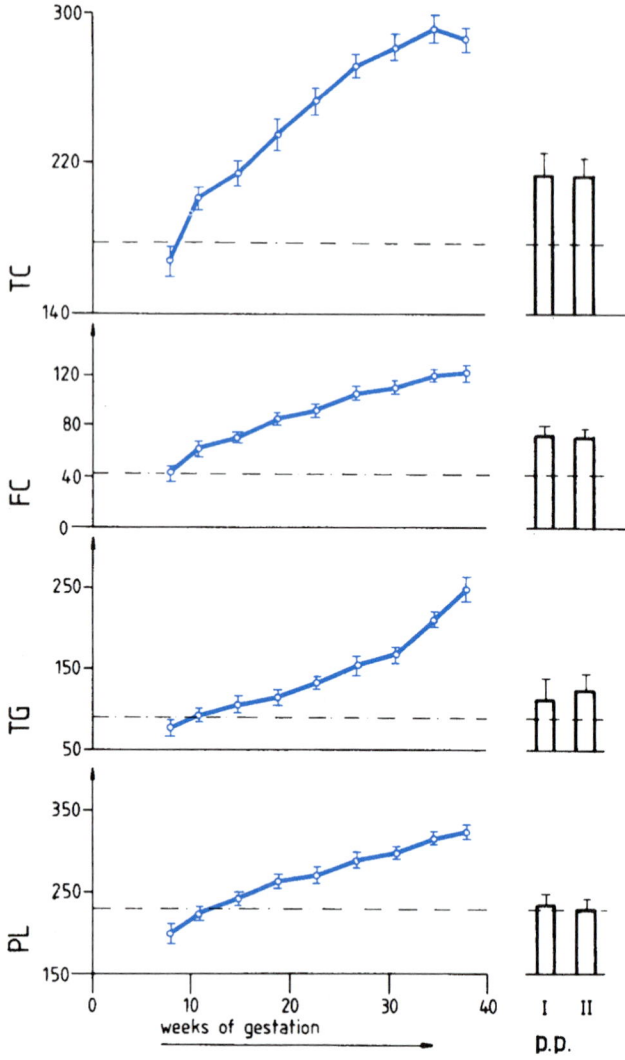

FIGURE 8–5. Mean (±SEM) plasma lipid concentrations (mg/dL) throughout gestation (n = 42) and during the luteal (I) and follicular (II) phases postpartum (p.p.; n = 23). The dashed lines represent the mean values of the control group (n = 24). (FC = free cholesterol; PL = phospholipids; TC = total cholesterol; TG = triglycerides.) (From Desoye and associates, 1987, with permission.)

consequence of the hepatic effects of estradiol and progesterone (Desoye and associates, 1987). High-density lipoprotein cholesterol (HDL-C) peaks at week 25, decreases until week 32, and remains constant for the remainder of pregnancy. The initial increase is believed to be caused by estrogen. High-density lipoprotein-2 and -3 cholesterol levels peak at approximately 28 weeks and remain unchanged throughout the remainder of pregnancy. Brizzi and colleagues (1999) have suggested that changes in the low-density lipoprotein (LDL) pattern during normal pregnancy might be used to identify those women who later in life may be predisposed to atherogenesis.

After delivery, the concentrations of these lipids, lipoproteins, and apolipoproteins decrease at different rates (Desoye and co-workers, 1987). Lactation increases the rate of decrease of many of these compounds (Darmady and Postle, 1982).

Hytten and Thomson (1968) and Pipe and co-workers (1979) concluded that storage of fat occurs primarily during midpregnancy. This fat is deposited mostly in central rather than peripheral sites. Later in pregnancy, as fetal nutritional demands increase remarkably, maternal fat storage decreases. Hytten and Thomson (1968) cited some evidence that progesterone may act to reset a *lipostat* in the hypothalamus, and at the end of pregnancy the lipostat returns to its previous nonpregnant level and the added fat is lost. Such a mechanism for energy storage, theoretically at least, might protect the mother and fetus during times of prolonged starvation or hard physical exertion.

MINERAL METABOLISM. The requirements for **iron** during pregnancy are considerable and often exceed the amounts available (p. 178). With respect to most other minerals, pregnancy induces little change in their metabolism other than their retention in amounts equivalent to those used for growth of fetal and, to a lesser extent, maternal tissues (Chaps. 7, p. 139 and 10, p. 235).

During pregnancy, **calcium** and **magnesium** plasma levels decline, the reduction probably reflecting for the most part the lowered plasma protein concentration and, in turn, the consequent decrease in the amount bound to protein. Bardicef and colleagues (1995), however, concluded that pregnancy is a state of magnesium depletion. They showed that total and ionized magnesium levels were significantly lower in normal pregnancy compared with nonpregnant women. Fogh-Andersen and Schultz-Larsen (1981) demonstrated a small but significant increase in free calcium ion concentration in late pregnancy by correcting for blood pH changes. Serum **phosphate** levels are within the nonpregnant range. The renal threshold for inorganic phosphate excretion is elevated in pregnancy due to increased calcitonin (Weiss and colleagues, 1998). Cole and co-workers (1987) reported that bone turnover was reduced during early pregnancy, returned toward normal during the third trimester, and increased in postpartum lactating women.

ACID–BASE EQUILIBRIUM. As discussed subsequently (p. 186), minute ventilation increases during pregnancy and this causes a respiratory alkalosis by lowering the P_{CO_2} of blood. A moderate reduction in plasma bicarbonate from 26 to about 22 mmol/L *partially* compensates for this. As a result, there is only a minimal increase in blood pH. This increase shifts the oxygen dissociation curve to the left and increases the affinity of maternal hemoglobin for oxygen (*Bohr effect*), thereby decreasing the oxygen-releasing capacity of maternal blood. Thus, the hyperventilation that results in a reduced maternal P_{CO_2} facilitates transport of carbon dioxide from the fetus to the mother but *appears to impair* release of oxygen from maternal blood to the fetus. The increase in blood pH, however, although minimal, stimulates an increase in 2, 3-diphosphoglycerate in maternal erythrocytes (Tsai and deLeeuw, 1982). This counteracts the Bohr effect by shifting the oxygen dissociation curve back to the right, facilitating oxygen release to the fetus.

PLASMA ELECTROLYTES. Despite large accumulations during pregnancy of sodium and potassium, the serum concentration of these electrolytes decreases. During normal pregnancy, nearly 1000 mEq of sodium and 300 mEq of potassium are retained (Lindheimer and colleagues, 1987). Despite that their glomerular filtration is increased, sodium and potassium excretion are unchanged during pregnancy (Brown and colleagues, 1986, 1988). Thus, their fractional excretion is decreased, and it has been postulated that progesterone counteracts the natriuretic and kaliuretic effects of aldosterone.

HEMATOLOGICAL CHANGES

BLOOD VOLUME. The maternal blood volume increases markedly during pregnancy. In studies of normal women, the blood volumes at or very near term averaged about 40 to 45 percent above their nonpregnant levels (Pritchard, 1965; Whittaker and associates, 1996). The degree of expansion varies considerably, in some women there is only a modest increase, while in others the blood volume nearly doubles. A fetus is not essential for the development of hypervolemia during pregnancy, for increases in blood volume have been demonstrated in some women with hydatidiform mole (Pritchard, 1965).

Pregnancy-induced hypervolemia has several important functions:

1. To meet the demands of the enlarged uterus with its greatly hypertrophied vascular system.
2. To protect the mother, and in turn the fetus, against the deleterious effects of impaired venous return in the supine and erect positions.
3. To safeguard the mother against the adverse effects of blood loss associated with parturition.

As shown in Figure 8–6, maternal blood volume starts to increase during the first trimester, expands most rapidly during the second trimester, and then rises at a much slower rate during the third trimester to plateau during the last several weeks of pregnancy.

Increased blood volume results from an increase in both plasma and erythrocytes. Although more plasma than erythrocytes is usually added to the maternal circulation, the increase in volume of erythrocytes is considerable, averaging about 450 mL, or an increase of about 33 percent (Pritchard and Adams, 1960). The importance of this increase in creating a demand for iron is discussed on page 178.

Moderate erythroid hyperplasia is present in the bone marrow, and the reticulocyte count is elevated slightly during normal pregnancy. This is almost certainly related to the increase in maternal plasma erythropoietin levels (Chap. 49, p. 1310). These levels increase after 20 weeks, corresponding to when erythrocyte production is most marked (Harstad and co-workers, 1992).

ATRIAL NATRIURETIC PEPTIDES. This group of biologically active peptides is synthesized and secreted by atrial myocytes. Three separate forms (α, β, Δ) have been isolated (Kangawa and co-workers, 1985). Atrial natriuretic peptide produces significant natriuresis and diuresis. It increases renal blood flow and glomerular filtration rate and decreases renin secretion. The actual mechanism(s) responsible for the natriuresis remains unclear, with evidence consistent for both a hemodynamically induced natriuresis and an inhibitory effect upon tubular sodium reabsorption (Wakitani and colleagues, 1985). Atrial natriuretic peptides also have been shown to reduce basal release of aldosterone from zona glomerulosa cells and to blunt corticotropin and angiotensin II–stimulated release of aldosterone as well (Atarashi and associates, 1984). Renin secretion is also inhibited by this peptide. Finally, atrial natriuretic peptides have a direct vasorelaxant action upon vascular smooth muscle stimulated by angiotesin II or norepinephrine.

Castro and associates (1994) summarized several studies done to evaluate plasma levels of atrial natriuretic peptide in normal and hypertensive pregnancy. The mean level rose by 40 percent over nonpregnant values by the third trimester and by 150 percent during the first week postpartum. These investigators hypothesized that atrial stretch receptors sense the expanded blood volume of pregnancy as normal to moderately increased. The marked rise in peptide levels during the first week postpartum is consistent with known hemodynamic changes and suggests that the hormone is involved in postpartum diuresis.

By comparison, Thomsen and colleagues (1994) investigated 10 healthy primigravid twin pregnancies and reported that all atrial natriuretic peptide levels during pregnancy were lower than values at 12 weeks postpar-

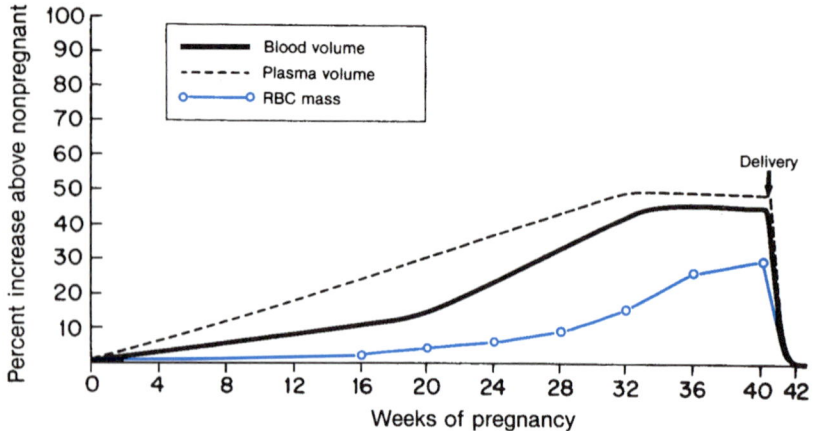

FIGURE 8–6. Blood volume changes during pregnancy. (From Scott, 1972, with permission.)

tum. At 20, 28, and 32 weeks, plasma peptide levels were lower in twin than in singleton pregnancies. These observations may serve to explain in part the relatively increased plasma volume characteristic of women with twins compared with those with singleton fetuses.

HEMOGLOBIN CONCENTRATION AND HEMATOCRIT.

In spite of augmented erythropoiesis, hemoglobin concentration and the hematocrit decrease slightly during normal pregnancy. As a result, whole blood viscosity decreases (Huisman and colleagues, 1987). Hemoglobin concentration at term averages 12.5 m/dL and in 6 percent of women it is below 11.0 g/dL (see Fig. 49–1 and Table 49–1). Thus, in most women, a hemoglobin concentration below 11.0 g/dL, especially late in pregnancy, should be considered abnormal and usually due to iron deficiency rather than to hypervolemia of pregnancy.

IRON METABOLISM

IRON STORES. Although the total body iron content averages about 4 g in men, in healthy young women of average size, it is probably half that amount. Commonly, iron stores of normal young women are only about 300 mg (Pritchard and Mason, 1964). As in men, heme iron in myoglobin and enzymes and transferrin-bound circulating iron together total only a few hundred milligrams. The total iron content of normal adult women ranges from 2.0 to 2.5 g.

IRON REQUIREMENTS. The iron requirements of normal pregnancy total about 1000 mg. About 300 mg are actively transferred to the fetus and placenta and about 200 mg are lost through various normal routes of excretion. These are obligatory losses and occur even when the mother is iron deficient. The average increase in the total volume of circulating erythrocytes of about 450

mL during pregnancy, when iron is available, uses another 500 mg of iron, because 1 mL of normal erythrocytes contains 1.1 mg of iron. Practically all of the iron for these purposes is used during the latter half of pregnancy. Therefore, the iron requirement becomes quite large during the second half of pregnancy, averaging 6 to 7 mg/day (Pritchard and Scott, 1970). Because this amount is not available from body stores in most women, the desired increase in maternal erythrocyte volume and hemoglobin mass will not develop unless exogenous iron is made available in adequate amounts. In the absence of supplemental iron, the hemoglobin concentration and hematocrit fall appreciably as the maternal blood volume increases. Hemoglobin production in the fetus, however, will not be impaired, because the placenta obtains iron from the mother in amounts sufficient for the fetus to establish normal hemoglobin levels even when the mother has severe iron-deficiency anemia.

The amount of iron absorbed from diet, together with that mobilized from stores, is usually insufficient to meet the demands imposed by pregnancy. This is true even though gastrointestinal tract iron absorption appears to be moderately increased during pregnancy (Hahn and associates, 1951). If the pregnant woman who is not anemic is not given supplemental iron, serum iron and ferritin concentrations decline during the second half of pregnancy (Fig. 8–7). The somewhat unexpected early pregnancy increases in serum iron and ferritin are thought to be due to minimal iron demands during the first trimester as well as to a positive iron balance because of amenorrhea. These values, summarized in Table 8–2, show that standard deviations for a given mean value are quite large. For example, in pregnant women with overt anemia and not given supplemental iron, serum ferritin levels can vary from 7 to 22 ng/mL during the third trimester. Also shown in Figure 8–7 is the increase in iron-binding capacity (transferrin)

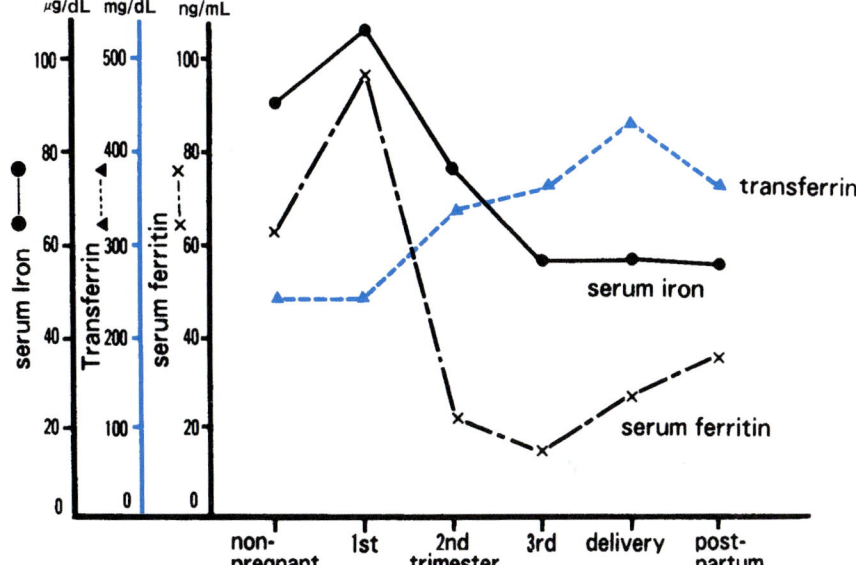

FIGURE 8–7. Indices of iron turnover during pregnancy in women without overt anemia but who were not given iron supplementation. (From Kaneshige, 1981, with permission.)

that occurs even when iron deficiency has been eliminated by oral iron supplementation.

BLOOD LOSS. Not all the iron added to the maternal circulation in the form of hemoglobin is necessarily lost from the mother. During normal vaginal delivery and through the next few days, only about half of the erythrocytes added to the maternal circulation during pregnancy are lost from the majority of women. These losses are by way of the placental implantation site, the placenta itself, the episiotomy or lacerations, and in the lochia. On the average, an amount of maternal erythrocytes corresponding to about 500 to 600 mL of predelivery blood is lost during and after vaginal delivery of a single fetus (Pritchard, 1965; Ueland, 1976). The average blood loss associated with cesarean delivery or with the vaginal delivery of twins is about 1000 mL, or nearly twice that lost with the delivery of a single fetus.

IMMUNOLOGICAL AND LEUKOCYTE FUNCTIONS. Pregnancy has been assumed to be associated with suppression of a variety of humoral and cellularly mediated immunological functions in order to accommodate the "foreign" semiallogeneic fetal graft (Chap. 2, p. 20). In fact, humoral antibody titers against several viruses— for example, herpes simplex, measles, and influenza A— decrease during pregnancy. The decrease in titers, however, is accounted for by the hemodilutional effect of pregnancy. The prevalence of a variety of autoantibodies is unchanged (Patton and colleagues, 1987). Furthermore, α-interferon, which is present in almost all fetal tissues and fluids, is most often absent in normally pregnant women (Chard and co-workers, 1986). There is evidence, as yet unexplained, that polymorphonuclear leukocyte chemotaxis and adherence functions are depressed beginning in the second trimester and continuing throughout pregnancy (Krause and associates,

TABLE 8–2. Concentrations of Hemoglobin, Serum Iron, Transferrin, and Serum Ferritin during Pregnancy in Women without Overt Anemia and Not Given Dietary Iron Supplementation

Concentration	Nonpregnant (n = 10)	1st Trimester (n = 17)	2nd Trimester (n = 26)	3rd Trimester (n = 17)	At Delivery (n = 33)	Postpartum (n = 27)
Hemoglobin (g/dL)	13.0 ± 0.6	12.2 ± 1.3	10.9 ± 0.8	11.0 ± 0.9	12.4 ± 1.0	11.5 ± 1.0
Serum iron (μg/dL)	90.0 ± 32.9	106.5 ± 24.5	75.3 ± 37.8	56.0 ± 31.0[a]	57.1 ± 31.2[a]	56.0 ± 21.8[a]
Transferrin (μg/dL)	242.1 ± 32.7	244.6 ± 52.7	336.2 ± 72.6[a]	362.8 ± 55.4[a]	438.2 ± 80.0[a]	363.4 ± 40.5[a]
Serum ferritin (ng/mL)	63.0 ± 34.7	97.4 ± 39.4[a]	22.2 ± 14.6[b]	14.7 ± 7.7[b]	27.6 ± 15.6[b]	36.0 ± 23.0[b]

Each value represents the mean ± standard deviation.
Significantly different from nonpregnant value:
[a] $P < .05$.
[b] $P < .005$.
From Kaneshige and associates (1981), with permission.

1987). It is possible that these depressed leukocyte functions of pregnant women account in part for the improvement observed in some with autoimmune diseases and the possibly increased susceptibility to certain infections. Thus, both function and absolute numbers of leukocytes appear to be important factors when considering the leukocytosis of normal pregnancy.

The leukocyte count varies considerably during normal pregnancy. Usually it ranges from 5000 to 12,000/μL. During labor and the early puerperium it may become markedly elevated, attaining levels of 25,000 or even more; however, the concentration averages 14,000 to 16,000/μL (Taylor and co-workers, 1981). The cause for the marked increase is not known, but the same response occurs during and after strenuous exercise. It probably represents the reappearance in the circulation of leukocytes previously shunted out of the active circulation. During pregnancy there is a neutrophilia that consists predominantly of mature forms; however, an occasional myelocyte is found.

Beginning quite early in pregnancy, the activity of **leukocyte alkaline phosphatase** is increased. Such elevated activity is not peculiar to pregnancy but occurs in a wide variety of conditions, including most inflammatory states. **C-reactive protein** is an acute-phase serum reactant. Serum concentrations rise rapidly to 1000-fold in response to tissue trauma or inflammation. Watts and colleagues (1991) measured C-reactive protein sequentially during 81 normal pregnancies to establish normal values. Median C-reactive protein values during pregnancy were higher than values for nonpregnant individuals, and these values were elevated further in labor. In women not in labor, 95 percent of values were 1.5 mg/dL or less, and gestational age did not affect serum levels. Another marker of inflammation, the **erythrocyte sedimentation rate** (ESR) is elevated in normal pregnancy due to elevated plasma globulins and fibrinogen (Hytten and Leitch, 1971). This test thus cannot be used to reliably diagnose inflammation during pregnancy. Complement factors C_3 and C_4 are significantly elevated during the second and third trimesters of pregnancy (Gallery and colleagues, 1981).

COAGULATION. In normal pregnancy, the coagulation cascade is in an activated state (Baker and Cunningham, 1999). Evidence of activation includes increased concentrations of all clotting factors except factors XI and XIII, with increased levels of high-molecular-weight fibrinogen complexes. Considering the substantive physiological increase in plasma volume in normal pregnancy, such increased concentrations represent a marked increase in production of these procoagulents. For example, plasma fibrinogen (factor I) in normal nonpregnant women averages about 300 mg/dL and ranges from about 200 to 400 mg/dL. During normal pregnancy, fibrinogen concentration increases about 50 percent to average about 450 mg/dL late in pregnancy, with a range from 300 to 600. The increase in the concentration of fibrinogen undoubtedly contributes greatly to the striking increase in the *erythrocyte sedimentation rate* discussed earlier (Ozanne and co-workers, 1983). The end-product of the coagulation cascade is fibrin formation.

High-molecular-weight soluble fibrin-fibrinogen complexes circulate in normal pregnancy and D-dimer levels increase with gestational age (Lee and associates, 1996; Nolan and colleagues, 1993). The clotting times of whole blood in either plain glass tubes (wettable surface) or silicone-coated or plastic tubes (nonwettable surface) do not significantly differ in normal pregnant women. Some of the pregnancy-induced changes in the levels of coagulation factors can be duplicated by the administration of estrogen plus progestin contraceptive tablets.

Normal pregnancy also involves changes in platelets (Baker and Cunningham, 1999). Although there is little change in platelet count in normal pregnancy, platelet width and volume increase. One explanation for these changes is increased platelet consumption leading to an increased proportion of younger, and therefore, larger platelets. Alterations such as these during normal pregnancy may be equated with continuing low-grade intravascular coagulation. In support of this concept, Tygart and associates (1986) interpreted these observations to represent an increased level of thrombocytopoiesis as a consequence of both dilutional and consumptive stimuli of normal pregnancy.

The end product of the coagulation cascade is fibrin formation, and the main function of the fibrinolytic system is to remove excess fibrin. The inactive precursor plasminogen is activated by serine proteases (plasminogen-activators) which convert plasminogen into plasmin. The activity of these plasminogen-activators is balanced by specific inhibitors present in plasma and platelets. The result of plasmin activity on fibrin is fibrinolysis producing fibrin degradation products such as D-dimers. Studies of the fibrinolytic system in pregnancy have produced conflicting results, although the majority of evidence suggests that fibrinolytic activity is actually reduced in normal pregnancy (Baker and Cunningham, 1999). It appears that plasminogen-activator inhibitors may be increased in normal pregnancy (Koh and co-authors, 1993). These potentially conflicting findings—that is, evidence of both increased and decreased fibrinolysis—may reflect the difficulty in interpreting measures of fibrinolysis.

REGULATORY PROTEINS. These are natural inhibitors of coagulation, and deficiencies of any of these factors is referred to as *thrombophilia*. Inherited hypercoagulable states such as protein C, protein S, and antithrombin

III deficiencies account for 15 to 20 percent of recurrent thromboembolic episodes (Chap. 49, p. 1330). Lockwood (1999) has recently reviewed coagulopathies in pregnancy arising from regulatory protein deficiencies.

Bremme and co-workers (1992) reported that **protein C** activity showed no significant trends and remained within normal reference ranges throughout pregnancy. Similarly, in a cross-sectional study of 91 normal pregnant women, Faught and associates (1995) found no significant change in antigenic or functional protein C levels. The discovery of the factor V Leiden mutation as causing **resistance to activated protein C** introduced new variables into thrombophilias. In affected women, measurement of this resistance during pregnancy is difficult and DNA testing is recommended.

Faught and colleagues (1995) also showed that total **protein S** levels remained unchanged, but free protein S levels fell significantly from the first to the second trimester (0.45 to 0.26 U/mL) and stayed depressed throughout gestation. Gatti and colleagues (1994) reported no change in protein S antigen; however, protein S activity decreased early and persisted throughout gestation. Bremme and associates (1992) found that the mean free protein S level significantly decreased from 0.26 U/mL in early pregnancy to 0.14 U/mL at 35 weeks. Oral contraceptives decrease these levels by about 20 percent, leading to speculation that the decrease is hormonally mediated.

Levels of **antithrombin III** are essentially unchanged during normal pregnancy (Weenink and co-workers, 1982). The levels of **thrombin-antithrombin III complexes,** however, progressively increase (de Boer and colleagues, 1989). This suggests coagulation activation as is consistent with some observations that fibrinopeptides A and B also are elevated.

CARDIOVASCULAR SYSTEM

During pregnancy and the puerperium there are remarkable changes involving the heart and the circulation. The most important changes in cardiac function occur in the first eight weeks of pregnancy (McLaughlin and Roberts, 1999). Cardiac output is increased as early as the fifth week of pregnancy and this initial increase is a function of reduced systemic vascular resistance and an increase in heart rate. Between weeks 10 and 20, notable increases in plasma volume occur such that preload is increased. Ventricular performance during pregnancy is influenced by both the decrease in systemic vascular resistance and changes in pulsatile arterial flow. Vascular capacity increases, in part, due to an increase in vascular compliance. As discussed in the following section, multiple factors contribute to these changes in overall hemodynamic function, allowing the cardiovas-

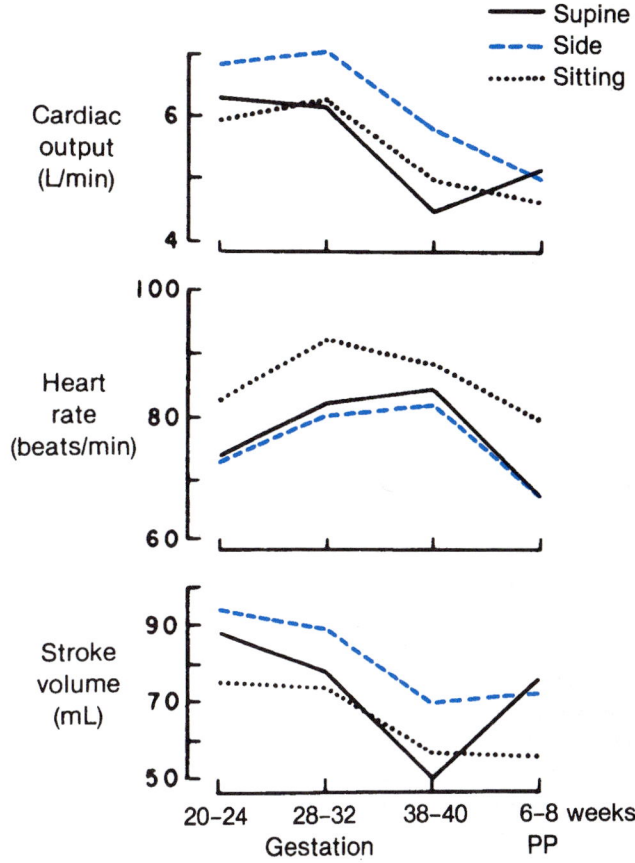

FIGURE 8–8. Effect of maternal posture on hemodynamics. (From Ueland and Metcalfe, 1975, with permission.)

cular system to adjust to the physiological demands of the fetus while maintaining maternal cardiovascular integrity. These changes during the last half of pregnancy are graphically summarized in Figure 8–8, which also shows the important effects of maternal posture on hemodynamic events during pregnancy.

HEART. The resting pulse rate increases about 10 bpm during pregnancy (Stein and co-workers, 1999). As the diaphragm becomes progressively elevated, the heart is displaced to the left and upward, while at the same time it is rotated somewhat on its long axis. As a result, the apex of the heart is moved somewhat laterally from its position in the normal nonpregnant state, and an increase in the size of the cardiac silhouette is found in radiographs (Fig. 8–9). The extent of these changes is influenced by the size and position of the uterus, toughness of the abdominal muscles, and configurations of the abdomen and thorax. Furthermore, normally pregnant women have some degree of benign pericardial effusion which may increase the cardiac silhouette (Enein and colleagues, 1987). Variability of these factors makes it

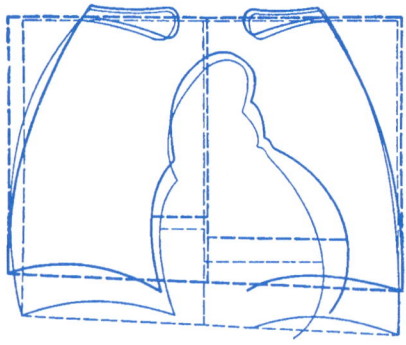

FIGURE 8–9. Change in cardiac outline that occurs in pregnancy. The light lines represent the relations between the heart and thorax in the nonpregnant woman, and the heavy lines represent the conditions existing in pregnancy. These findings are based on x-ray findings in 33 women. (From Klafen and Palugyay, 1927.)

difficult to identify precisely moderate degrees of cardiomegaly by simple x-ray studies.

Katz and co-workers (1978) studied left ventricular performance during pregnancy and the puerperium using echocardiography. Both left ventricular wall mass and end-diastolic dimensions increased during pregnancy, as did heart rate, calculated stroke volume, and cardiac output. The changes in stroke volume were directly proportional to end-diastolic volume, implying, at least, that there is little change in the inotropic state of the myocardium during normal pregnancy. Sadaniantz and associates (1996) reported that these changes are not cumulative in subsequent pregnancies. In multifetal pregnancies, however, cardiac output is increased predominantly by **increased inotropic effect** (Veille and co-workers, 1985). The increased heart rate and inotropic contractility imply that cardiovascular reserve is reduced.

During pregnancy, some of the cardiac sounds may be altered. Cutforth and MacDonald (1966) obtained phonocardiograms at varying stages of pregnancy in 50 normal women and documented the following changes:

1. An exaggerated splitting of the first heart sound with increased loudness of both components; no definite changes in the aortic and pulmonary elements of the second sound; and a loud, easily heard third sound.
2. A systolic murmur in 90 percent of pregnant women, intensified during inspiration in some or expiration in others, and disappearing very shortly after delivery; a soft diastolic murmur transiently in 20 percent; and continuous murmurs arising from the breast vasculature in 10 percent.

Normal pregnancy induces no characteristic changes in the *electrocardiogram,* other than slight deviation of

the electrical axis to the left as a result of the altered position of the heart.

CARDIAC OUTPUT. During normal pregnancy, arterial blood pressure and vascular resistance decrease while blood volume, maternal weight, and basal metabolic rate increase. Each of these events would be expected to affect cardiac output. It is now evident that cardiac output *at rest,* when measured in the lateral recumbent position, increases significantly beginning in early pregnancy (Duvekot and colleagues, 1993; Mabie and co-workers, 1994). It continues to increase and remains elevated during the remainder of pregnancy (Fig. 8–10). Typically, cardiac output in late pregnancy is appreciably higher when the woman is in the lateral recumbent position than when she is supine, because in the supine position the large uterus often impedes cardiac venous return. Ueland and Hansen (1969), for example, found cardiac output to increase 1100 mL (20 percent) when the pregnant woman was moved from her back onto her side. When she assumes the standing position after sitting, cardiac output in the pregnant woman falls to the same degree as in the nonpregnant woman (Easterling and associates, 1988).

During the first stage of labor, cardiac output increases moderately, and during the second stage, with vigorous expulsive efforts, it is appreciably greater (Fig. 8–10). After the substantively augmented cardiac out-

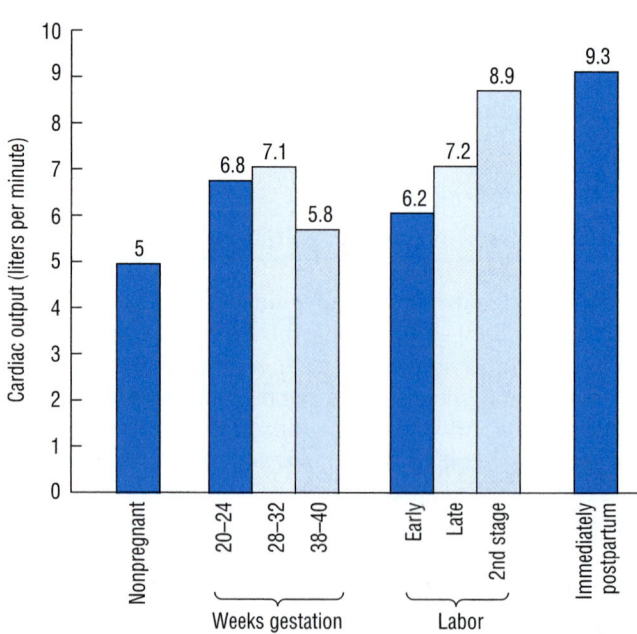

FIGURE 8–10. Cardiac output during three stages of gestation, labor, and immediately postpartum compared with values of nonpregnant women. All values were determined with women in the lateral recumbent position. (Adapted from Ueland and Metcalfe, 1975, with permission.)

TABLE 8–3. Central Hemodynamic Changes in 10 Normal Nulliparous Women between 35 and 38 Weeks' Gestation and Again When 11 to 13 Weeks' Postpartum

Factor	Pregnant[a]	Postpartum	Change
Mean arterial pressure (mm Hg)	90 ± 6	86 ± 8	No change
Pulmonary capillary wedge pressure (mm Hg)	8 ± 2	6 ± 2	No change
Central venous pressure (mm Hg)	4 ± 3	4 ± 3	No change
Heart rate (beats/min)	83 ± 10	71 ± 10	±17%
Cardiac output (L/min)	6.2 ± 1.0	4.3 ± 0.9	+43%
Systemic vascular resistance (dyne/sec/cm^{-5})	1210 ± 266	1530 ± 520	−21%
Pulmonary vascular resistance (dyne/sec/cm^{-5})	78 ± 22	119 ± 47	−34%
Serum colloid osmotic pressure (mm Hg)	18.0 ± 1.5	20.8 ± 1.0	−14%
COP–PCWP gradient (mm Hg)	10.5 ± 2.7	14.5 ± 2.5	−28%
Left ventricular stroke work index (g/m/m²)	48 ± 6	41 ± 8	No change

COP = colloid osmotic pressure; PCWP = pulmonary capillary wedge pressure.
[a] Made in lateral recumbent position.
Adapted from Clark and colleagues (1989), with permission.

put in the immediate puerperium, most of the pregnancy-induced increase is lost very soon after delivery.

HEMODYNAMIC VALUES FOR LATE PREGNANCY. Clark and colleagues (1989) conducted studies of maternal cardiovascular hemodynamics that serve to define normal values late in pregnancy (Table 8–3). Right heart catheterization was performed in 10 healthy nulliparous women at 35 to 38 weeks, and again at 11 to 13 weeks postpartum. Late pregnancy was associated with the expected increases in heart rate, stroke volume, and cardiac output. Systemic vascular and pulmonary vascular resistance both decreased significantly, as did colloid osmotic pressure. Pulmonary capillary wedge pressure and central venous pressure did not change appreciably between late pregnancy and the puerperium. These investigators concluded that normal late pregnancy is not associated with hyperdynamic left ventricular function as determined by Starling function curves (see Fig. 44–1, p. 1183).

FACTORS CONTROLLING VASCULAR REACTIVITY IN PREGNANCY. Gant and associates (1973) conducted a prospective study of vascular reactivity to angiotensin II throughout pregnancy. Normal nulliparas who remained normotensive were refractory to the pressor effects of infused angiotensin II. Conversely, those destined to become hypertensive lost this refractoriness. This clear divergence of sensitivity to angiotensin II was likely the result of significant alterations in a variety of physiological processes that serve to control vascular reactivity to angiotensin II.

RENIN, ANGIOTENSIN II, AND PLASMA VOLUME. The resin-angiotensin-aldosterone axis is intimately involved in renal control of salt and water balance. All components of this system are increased in normal pregnancy (Gallery and Lindheimer, 1999). Renin is produced both by the maternal kidney and the uteroplacental unit while increased renin substrate (angiotensinogen) is produced by both maternal and fetal liver. This increase in angiotensinogen is due in part to high levels of estrogen production during normal pregnancy. August and colleagues (1995) provided data from first-trimester pregnancies and showed that stimulation of the renin-angiotensin system was important in blood pressure maintenance. Gant and co-workers (1974) and Cunningham and associates (1975) found that various acute volume loads, including normal saline (1000 mL), dextran (500 mL), and packed red blood cells (950 mL), did not alter pressor responsiveness to angiotensin II in normotensive pregnant women. Therefore, the increased refractoriness to angiotensin II characteristic of normal pregnancy is likely the consequence of individual vessel refractoriness to angiotensin II. That is, in the woman destined to develop preeclampsia, or in the woman already acutely ill with preeclampsia, the increased sensitivity to angiotensin II was the result of an alteration in vessel wall refractoriness rather than the consequence of changes in blood volume or circulating renin-angiotensin levels.

PROSTAGLANDINS. Increased production of prostaglandins in normal pregnancy may well play a central role in control of vascular tone, blood pressure, and sodium balance (Gallery and Lindheimer, 1999). Prostaglandin E_2 synthesis in the renal medulla is markedly increased in late pregnancy and is presumed to be natriuretic. Prostacyclin, the principal prostaglandin of endothelium, is also increased in late pregnancy and functions in regulation of blood pressure as well as coagulation. Prostacyclin has also been implicated to be a factor in the angiotensin resistance characteristic of normal pregnancy (Friedman, 1988). There has also been considerable interest in the ratio of prostacyclin to thromboxane in maternal urine and blood as this relates to preeclampsia (Chap. 24, p. 586).

PROGESTERONE AND METABOLITES. A progestin-induced mechanism may modulate prostaglandin-mediated vascular responsiveness to the pressor effects of angiotensin II characteristic of normal human pregnancy. Normally pregnant women lose pregnancy-acquired vascular refractoriness to angiotensin II within 15 to 30 minutes after the placenta is delivered. Moreover, large amounts of intramuscular progesterone given during late labor delay this loss. Conversely, intravenously administered progesterone does not restore angiotensin II refractoriness to women with pregnancy-induced hypertension; however, the infusion of a major progesterone metabolite—5α-dihydroprogesterone—does. Similarly, infusion of this steroid into five normally pregnant women who had been rendered angiotensin II–sensitive by indomethacin also restored vascular refractoriness (Everett and associates, 1978a).

CYCLIC AMP. Administration of theophylline to angiotensin II–sensitive pregnant women with early-onset pregnancy-induced hypertension more than doubled the mean effective pressor dose of angiotensin II, restoring the vascular refractoriness characteristic of normal pregnancy (Everett and co-workers, 1978b). This effect of theophylline likely results from its inhibition of the enzyme *phosphodiesterase,* a principal regulator of intracellular cyclic nucleotide accumulation. Phosphodiesterase activity inhibition would promote the accumulation of cyclic adenosine monophosphate (cAMP) within vascular smooth muscle and should lead to the promotion of vascular smooth muscle relaxation.

CALCIUM ENTRY TO VASCULAR SMOOTH MUSCLE. Reductions in vascular refractoriness to infused angiotensin II have been reported in normal women and several different animals after the administration of various agents that act as calcium-channel blockers (Anderson, 1987; Hof, 1985; Pasanisi, 1985; and their co-workers).

ENDOTHELIN. The endothelins are a recently discovered family of 21-amino-acid peptides. Endothelin-1 is produced in endothelial cells and vascular smooth muscle and regulates local vasomotor tone by causing vasoconstriction (Levin, 1995). Endothelin-2 and -3 are produced within the kidney and intestine.

There are endothelin receptors in pregnant and non-pregnant myometrium and endothelins have also been identified in amnion, amnionic fluid, decidua, and placental tissue (Kubota and colleagues, 1992; Sagawa and associates, 1994). Their putative role in human parturition is discussed in detail in Chapter 11 (p. 279).

Endothelin-1 acts in a paracrine fashion and is the most potent vasoconstrictor substance yet identified. Its production is stimulated by angiotensin II, arginine vasopressin, and thrombin. Endothelins in turn stimulate secretion of atrial natriuretic peptide, aldosterone, and catecholamines. They reduce cardiac output, renal blood flow, and glomerular filtration. Endothelins bind to receptors (endothelin A and B), activate phospholipase C, and increase intracellular calcium concentration.

CIRCULATION. The posture of the pregnant woman affects *arterial blood pressure*. Blood pressure in the brachial artery varies when sitting or lying in the lateral recumbent supine position. Usually, arterial blood pressure decreases to a nadir at about midpregnancy and rises thereafter. Diastolic pressure decreases more than systolic (Fig. 8–11).

The antecubital *venous pressure* remains unchanged during pregnancy, but in the supine position the femoral venous pressure rises steadily, from 8 cm H_2O early in pregnancy to 24 cm H_2O at term (Fig. 8–12). Employing radiolabeled tracers, Wright and co-workers (1950) and others have demonstrated that blood flow in the legs is retarded during pregnancy except when the lateral recumbent position is assumed. This tendency toward stagnation of blood in the lower extremities during the latter part of pregnancy is attributable to the occlusion of the pelvic veins and inferior vena cava by pressure of the enlarged uterus. The elevated venous pressure returns to normal if the pregnant woman lies on her side and immediately after delivery (McLennan, 1943). From a clinical viewpoint, the retarded blood flow and increased lower extremity venous pressure are of great importance. These alterations contribute to the dependent edema frequently experienced by women as they approach term, and to the development of varicose veins in the legs and vulva, as well as hemorrhoids. They also predispose to deep-vein thrombosis as discussed in Chapter 46 (p. 1235).

SUPINE HYPOTENSION. In late pregnancy with the woman in the supine position, the large pregnant uterus rather consistently compresses the venous system that returns blood from the lower half of the body to the extent that cardiac filling may be reduced and cardiac output decreased. In about 10 percent of women, this causes significant arterial hypotension, sometimes referred to as the *supine hypotensive syndrome* (Kinsella and Lohmann, 1994). Bieniarz and associates (1968) observed that in the supine position, the large pregnant

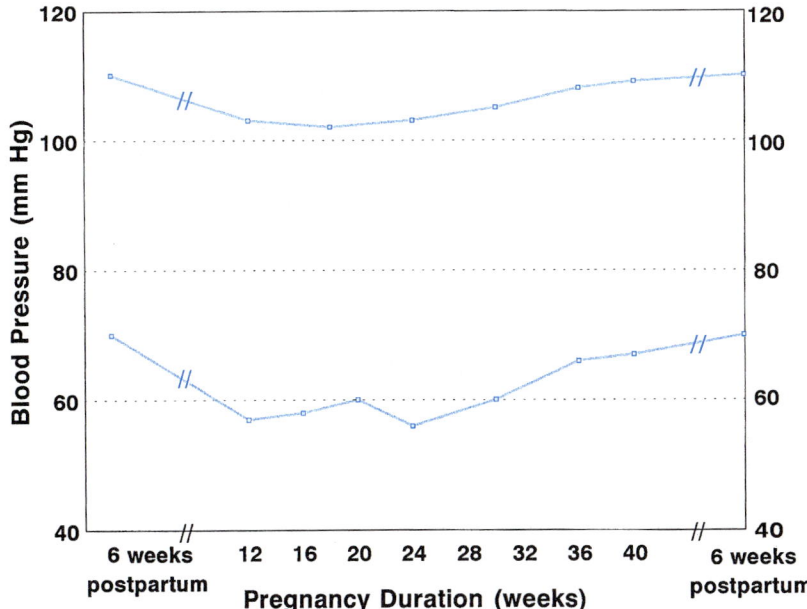

FIGURE 8–11. Blood pressure changes as a result of pregnancy. Pressures 6 weeks postpartum are shown before and after pregnancy. Values are means ± 1 SD. (Data from MacGillivray and colleagues, 1969.)

uterus may also compress the aorta sufficiently to lower arterial blood pressure below the level of compression. They demonstrated that the usual measurement of blood pressures in the brachial artery does not provide a reliable estimate of the pressure in the uterine or other arteries that lie distal to aortic compression. When the pregnant woman is supine, uterine arterial pressure is significantly lower than that in the brachial artery. In the presence of systemic hypotension, as occurs with spinal analgesia, the decrease in uterine arterial pressure is even more marked than in arteries above the level of aortic compression (Chap. 15, p. 372).

BLOOD FLOW IN SKIN. Increased cutaneous blood flow in pregnancy serves to dissipate excess heat generated by increased metabolism.

RESPIRATORY TRACT

The diaphragm rises about 4 cm during pregnancy (see Fig. 8–9). The subcostal angle widens appreciably as the transverse diameter of the thoracic cage increases about 2 cm. The thoracic circumference increases about 6 cm, but not sufficiently to prevent a reduction in the residual volume of air in the lungs created by the elevated diaphragm. Diaphragmatic excursion is actually greater during pregnancy than when nonpregnant.

PULMONARY FUNCTION. At any stage of normal pregnancy, the amount of oxygen delivered into the lungs by the increase in tidal volume clearly exceeds the oxygen need imposed by the pregnancy. Moreover, the amount of hemoglobin in the circulation, and in turn the total oxygen-carrying capacity, increases appreciably during normal pregnancy, as does cardiac output. As the consequence, *maternal arteriovenous oxygen* difference is decreased.

Hankins and colleagues (1999) used pulmonary and radial artery catheters to directly measure oxygen transport in 10 normal women during the third trimester

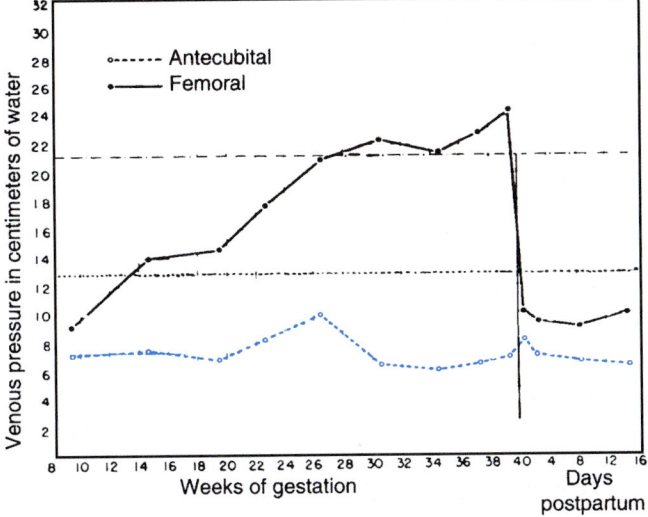

FIGURE 8–12. Serial changes in antecubital and femoral venous blood pressure throughout normal pregnancy and early puerperium. These measurements were made on women in the lateral recumbent position. (From McLennan, 1943.)

(36 to 38 weeks) and again 12 weeks postpartum. The oxygen content of arterial blood was significantly lower in the third trimester than in the postpartum period (16 and 12 mL/dL, respectively). Although cardiac output was significantly increased consistent with normal pregnancy, its effects on oxygen delivery were negated by a substantially lower hemoglobin content. Thus, the relative or physiological anemia of pregnancy accounted for the lower arterial oxygen content observed in this study.

The respiratory rate is little changed during pregnancy but the *tidal volume, minute ventilatory volume,* and *minute oxygen uptake* increase appreciably as pregnancy advances (Table 8–4). The *maximum breathing capacity* and *forced* or *timed vital capacity* are not altered appreciably. The *functional residual capacity* and the *residual volume* of air are decreased as the consequence of the elevated diaphragm. *Lung compliance* is unaffected by pregnancy. *Airway conductance* is increased and *total pulmonary resistance* is reduced, possibly as a result of progesterone action. The critical *closing volume,* or the lung volume at which airways in the dependent parts of the lung begin to close during expiration, has been considered to be higher in pregnancy by some investigators but not by others (DeSwiet, 1991).

An increased awareness of a desire to breathe is common even early in pregnancy (Milne and colleagues, 1978). This may be interpreted as dyspnea, which in turn suggests pulmonary or cardiac abnormalities when none exist. The mechanism of physiological dyspnea is thought to be increased tidal volume that lowers the blood P_{CO_2} slightly, which paradoxically causes dyspnea. The increased respiratory effort and in turn the reduction in P_{CO_2} during pregnancy is most likely induced in large part by progesterone and to a lesser degree estrogen. The site of progestin action appears to be central through a direct stimulatory effect on the respiratory center.

Although pulmonary function is not impaired by pregnancy, diseases of the respiratory tract may be more serious during gestation. Important factors are undoubtedly the increased oxygen requirements imposed by pregnancy and perhaps an increase in critical closing volume, especially when supine.

URINARY SYSTEM

KIDNEY. A remarkable number of changes are observed in the urinary system as a result of pregnancy (Table 8–5). *Kidney size* increases slightly during pregnancy. Bailey and Rolleston (1971), for example, found that the kidney was 1.5 cm longer during the early puerperium than when measured 6 months later. The *glomerular filtration rate* (*GFR*) and *renal plasma flow* (*RPF*) increase early in pregnancy, the former as much as 50 percent by the beginning of the second trimester, and the latter not quite so much (Chesley, 1963; Dunlop, 1981). As shown in Figure 8–13, elevated glomerular filtration has been found by most investigators to persist to term, and this is despite that renal plasma flow decrease during late pregnancy. *Kallikrein,* a tissue protease synthesized in cells of the distal renal tubule, is increased in several conditions associated with increased glomular perfusion in nonpregnant individuals. Platts and colleagues (2000) studied urinary kallikrein excretion rates during human pregnancy and found increased excretion at 18 and 34 weeks which returned to nonpregnant levels at term. The significance of these normal fluctuations in renal kallikrein excretion rates during pregnancy remains unknown.

Most studies of renal function conducted during pregnancy have been performed while the subjects were supine, a position that late in pregnancy may produce marked systemic hemodynamic changes that lead to

TABLE 8–4. Ventilatory Function in Pregnant Women Compared with the Postpartum Period

Factor	During Pregnancy			Postpartum 6–10 Weeks
	10 Weeks	24 Weeks	36 Weeks	
Respiratory rate	15–16	16	16–17	16–17
Tidal volume (mL)	600–650	650	700	550[a]
Minute ventilation (L)	—	—	10.5	7.5[a]
Vital capacity (L)	3.8	3.9	4.1	3.8
Inspiratory capacity (L)	2.6	2.7	2.9	2.5
Expiratory reserve volume (L)	1.2	1.2	1.2	1.3
Residual volume (L)	1.2	1.1	1.0	1.2[a]

[a] Significant increase or decrease compared with pregnant women.
From Spatling and colleagues (1992) and Gazioglu and associates (1970).

TABLE 8–5. Renal Changes in Normal Pregnancy

Alteration	Change	Clinical Relevance
Increased renal size	Renal length approximately 1 cm greater on x-rays	Postpartum decreases in size should not be mistaken for parenchymal loss
Dilation of pelves, calyces, and ureters	Resembles hydronephrosis on ultrasound or IVP (more marked on right)	Not to be mistaken for obstructive uropathy; retained urine leads to collection errors; upper urinary tract infections are more virulent; may be responsible for "distention syndrome"; elective pyelography should be deferred to at least 12 weeks postpartum
Increased renal hemodynamics	Glomerular filtration rate and renal plasma flow increase ~50 percent	Serum creatinine and urea nitrogen values decrease during normal gestation; > 0.8 mg/dL (> 72 μmol/L) creatinine already suspect; protein, amino acid, and glucose excretion all increase
Changes in acid–base metabolism	Renal bicarbonate threshold decreases; progesterone stimulates respiratory center	Serum bicarbonate and P_{CO_2} are 4–5 mEq/L and 10 mm Hg lower, respectively, in normal gestation; P_{CO_2} of 40 mm Hg already represents CO_2 retention
Renal water-handling	Osmoregulation altered: osmotic thresholds for AVP release and thirst decrease; hormonal disposal rates increase	Serum osmolality decreases 10 mOsm/L (serum Na ~ 5 mEq/L) during normal gestation; increased metabolism of AVP may cause transient diabetes insipidus in pregnancy

AVP = vasopressin; IVP = intravenous pyelography.
From Lindheimer and colleagues (2000).

alterations in several aspects of renal function. Late in pregnancy, for instance, urinary flow and sodium excretion average less than half the excretion rate in the supine position compared with the lateral recumbent position.

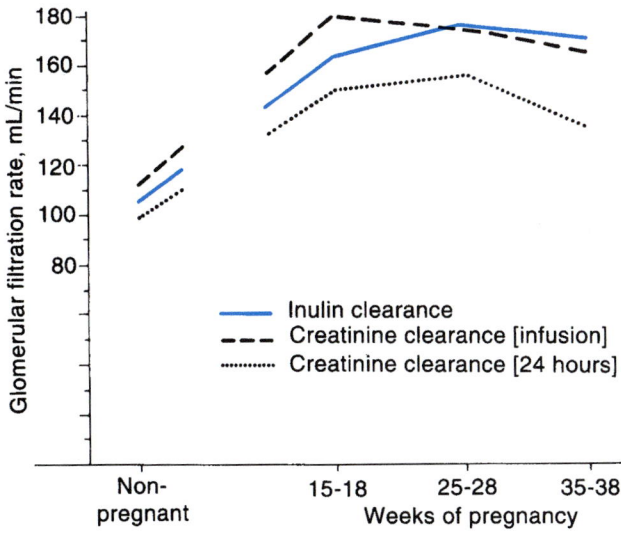

FIGURE 8–13. Mean glomerular filtration rate in healthy women over a short period with infused inulin (*solid line*), simultaneously as creatinine clearance during the inulin infusion (*broken line*), and over 24 hours as endogenous creatinine clearance (*dotted line*). (From Davison and Hytten, 1974.)

Although posture clearly affects sodium and water excretion in late pregnancy, its impact on glomerular filtration and renal plasma flow is much more variable. For example, Chesley and Sloan (1964) found both to be reduced when the pregnant woman was in the supine position, whereas Dunlop (1976) identified inconsequential reduction. Pritchard (1955) detected decreases while supine compared with lateral recumbency in some, but not most of women studied in late pregnancy. Ezimokhai and associates (1981) reported that the late pregnancy decrease in renal plasma flow is not due simply to a positional effect.

LOSS OF NUTRIENTS. One unusual feature of the pregnancy-induced changes in renal excretion is the remarkably increased amounts of various nutrients in the urine. Amino acids and water-soluble vitamins are lost in the urine of pregnant women in much greater amounts than in nonpregnant women (Hytten and Leitch, 1971).

TESTS OF RENAL FUNCTION. During pregnancy the plasma concentrations of creatinine and urea normally decrease as a consequence of their increased glomerular filtration. At times, the urea concentration may be so low as to suggest impaired hepatic synthesis, which sometimes occurs with severe liver disease.

Creatinine clearance is a useful test to estimate renal function in pregnancy provided that complete urine collection is made over an accurately timed period. *Urine concentration tests* may give results that are misleading (Davison and colleagues, 1981). During the day, pregnant women tend to accumulate water in the form of dependent edema; and at night, while recumbent, they mobilize this fluid and excrete it via the kidneys. This reversal of the usual nonpregnant diurnal pattern of urinary flow causes nocturia, and the urine is more dilute than in the nonpregnant state. Failure of a pregnant woman to excrete concentrated urine after withholding fluids for approximately 18 hours does not signify renal damage. In fact, the kidney in these circumstances functions perfectly normally by excreting mobilized extracellular fluid of relatively low osmolality.

URINALYSIS. *Glucosuria* during pregnancy is not necessarily abnormal. The appreciable increase in glomerular filtration, together with impaired tubular reabsorptive capacity for filtered glucose, accounts in most cases for the glucosuria (Davison and Hytten, 1975). Chesley (1963) calculated that for these reasons alone about one sixth of all pregnant women should spill glucose in the urine. Even though glucosuria is common during pregnancy, the possibility of diabetes mellitus should not be ignored when it is identified.

Proteinuria is normally not evident during pregnancy except occasionally in slight amounts during or soon after vigorous labor. Higby and associates (1994) measured protein excretion in 270 normal women throughout pregnancy. Their mean 24-hour excretion was 115 mg, and the upper 95 percent confidence limit was 260 mg/day. There were no significant differences by trimester (Fig. 8–14). They also showed that albumin excretion is minimal and ranges from 5 to 30 mg/day. Lopez-Espinoza and colleagues (1986) measured serial albumin excretion using a sensitive radioimmunoassay in 14 healthy pregnant women. There was a slight rise from a median of 7 to 18 mg/24 hours from early to late

pregnancy, however, albuminuria was not detected using conventional testing methods.

Hematuria, if not the result of contamination during collection, is compatible with a diagnosis of urinary tract disease (Chap. 47, p. 1259). Difficult labor and delivery, of course, can cause hematuria because of trauma to the lower urinary tract.

HYDRONEPHROSIS AND HYDROURETER. After the uterus rises completely out of the pelvis, it rests upon the ureters, compressing them at the pelvic brim. Increased intraureteral tonus above this level compared with that of the pelvic portion of the ureter has been identified (Rubi and Sala, 1968). Schulman and Herlinger (1975) found ureteral dilatation to be greater on the right side in 86 percent of pregnant women studied (Fig. 8–15). The unequal degrees of dilatation may result from a cushioning provided the left ureter by the sigmoid colon and perhaps from greater compression of the right ureter as the consequence of dextrorotation of the uterus. The right ovarian vein complex, which is remarkably dilated during pregnancy, lies obliquely over the right ureter and may contribute significantly to right ureteral dilatation.

Another possible mechanism causing hydronephrosis and hydroureter is from an effect of progesterone. Major support for this concept was provided by Van Wagenen and Jenkins (1939), who described further ureteral dilatation after removal of the monkey fetus but with the placenta left in situ. The relatively abrupt onset of dilatation in women at midpregnancy is more consistent with ureteral compression from an enlarging uterus rather than a hormonal effect.

Elongation accompanies distention of the ureter, which is frequently thrown into curves of varying size, the smaller of which may be sharply angulated. These so-called kinks are poorly named, because the term con-

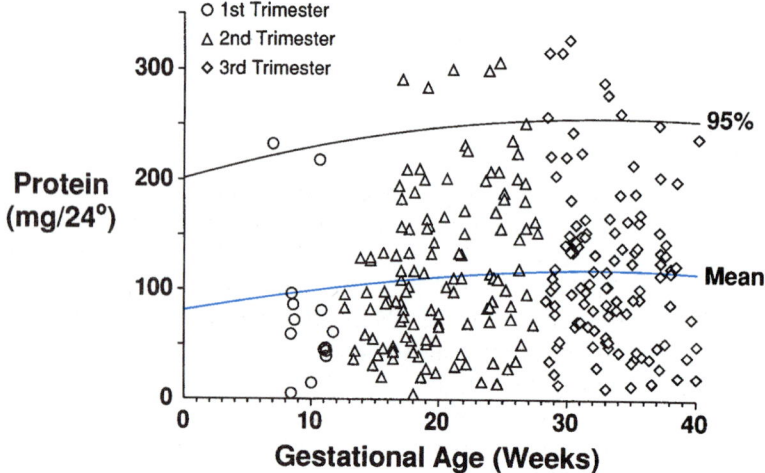

FIGURE 8–14. Scatter plot of all patients showing 24-hour urinary total protein excretion by gestational age. Mean and 95 percent confidence limits are outlined. (From Higby and colleagues, 1994, with permission.)

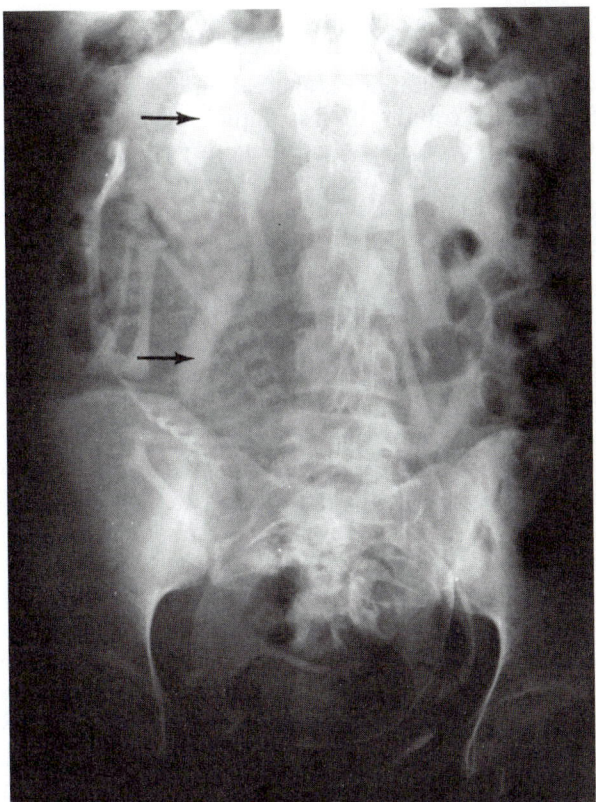

FIGURE 8–15. Normal intravenous pyelogram at 36 weeks. Pregnancy-induced hydronephrosis (*upper arrow*) and hydroureter (*lower arrow*) are more marked on the right. Elongation, dilation, and peristalsis of the ureter create the appearance of ureteral discontinuity.

notes obstruction. They are usually single or double curves, which when viewed in the radiograph taken in the same plane as the curve, appear as more or less acute angulations of the ureter (Fig. 8–15). Another exposure at right angles nearly always identifies them to be more gentle curves rather than kinks. The ureter undergoes not only elongation but frequently lateral displacement by the pressure of the enlarged uterus.

BLADDER. Thorp and colleagues (1999) studied 123 pregnant women throughout pregnancy and the puerperium and found that pregnancy was associated with an increase in urinary incontinence. When women were asked to compare urinary tract function week by week throughout their pregnancies, they reported a steady deterioration in perceived bladder function. Indeed, objective measures of urinary frequency and total daily urinary output increased throughout pregnancy.

There are few significant anatomical changes in the bladder before 12 weeks. From that time onward, however, the increased size of the uterus, together with the hyperemia that affects all pelvic organs, and the hyperplasia of the muscle and connective tissues, elevates the bladder trigone and causes thickening of its posterior, or intraureteric, margin. Continuation of this process to the end of pregnancy produces marked deepening and widening of the trigone. The bladder mucosa undergoes no change other than an increase in the size and tortuosity of its blood vessels.

Using urethrocystometry, Iosif and colleagues (1980) found that bladder pressure in primigravidas increased from 8 cm H_2O early in pregnancy to 20 cm H_2O at term. To compensate for reduced bladder capacity, absolute and functional urethral lengths increased by 6.7 and 4.8 mm, respectively. Finally, to preserve continence, maximal intraurethral pressure increased from 70 to 93 cm H_2O. Still, the majority of women will experience their initial episode of urinary incontinence during pregnancy. Indeed, loss of urine is always high in the differential diagnosis of the woman presenting with a question of ruptured membranes.

Toward the end of pregnancy, particularly in nulliparas in whom the presenting part often engages before labor, the entire base of the bladder is pushed forward and upward, converting the normal convex surface into a concavity. As a result, difficulties in diagnostic and therapeutic procedures are greatly increased. In addition, the pressure of the presenting part impairs the drainage of blood and lymph from the base of the bladder, often rendering the area edematous, easily traumatized, and probably more susceptible to infection. Both urethral pressure and length have been shown to be decreased in women following vaginal but not abdominal delivery (Van Geelen and co-workers, 1982). These investigators suggest that a weakness of the urethral sphincter mechanism due to pregnancy or delivery may play a role in the pathogenesis of urinary stress incontinence.

Normally there is little residual urine in nulliparas, but occasionally it develops in the multipara with relaxed vaginal walls and a cystocele. Incompetence of the ureterovesical valve may supervene, with the consequent probability of vesicoureteral reflux of urine.

GASTROINTESTINAL TRACT

As pregnancy progresses, the stomach and intestines are displaced by the enlarging uterus. As the result of the positional changes in these viscera, the physical findings in certain diseases are altered. The appendix, for instance, is usually displaced upward and somewhat laterally as the uterus enlarges, and at times it may reach the right flank (see Fig. 48–1, p. 1281).

Gastric emptying and intestinal transit times are delayed in pregnancy because of hormonal or mechanical factors. For example, this may be the result of progesterone or decreased levels of *motilin,* a hormonal peptide known to have smooth-muscle stimulating effects (Christofides and associates, 1982). Macfie and colleagues (1991) studied gastric emptying times using acetaminophen absorption and found these to be unchanged during each trimester and compared with nonpregnant women. During labor, however, and especially after administration of analgesic agents, *gastric-emptying time* is typically prolonged appreciably. A major danger of general anesthesia for delivery is regurgitation and aspiration of either food-laden or highly acidic gastric contents (Chap. 15, p. 366).

Pyrosis (heartburn) is common during pregnancy and is most likely caused by reflux of acidic secretions into the lower esophagus (Chap. 48, p. 1276). The altered position of the stomach probably contributes to its frequent occurrence; however, lower esophageal sphincter tone is also decreased. Intraesophageal pressures are lower and intragastric pressures higher in pregnant women. At the same time, esophageal peristalsis has lower wave speed and lower amplitude (Ulmsten and Sundström, 1978).

The gums may become hyperemic and softened during pregnancy and may bleed when mildly traumatized, as with a toothbrush. A focal, highly vascular swelling of the gums, the so-called *epulis* of pregnancy, develops occasionally but typically regresses spontaneously after delivery. Most evidence indicates that pregnancy does not incite tooth decay.

Hemorrhoids are fairly common during pregnancy. They are caused in large measure by constipation and the elevated pressure in veins below the level of the enlarged uterus.

LIVER. Although the liver in some animals increases remarkably in size during pregnancy, there is no evidence for such an increase during human pregnancy (Combes and Adams, 1971). Histological evaluation of liver biopsies, including examination with the electron microscope, have shown no distinct changes in liver morphology in normal pregnant women (Ingerslev and Teilum, 1946).

Some of the laboratory tests used to evaluate hepatic function yield appreciably different results during normal pregnancy. Moreover, some of those changes are similar to those in patients with liver disease. Total *alkaline phosphatase* activity in serum almost doubles during normal pregnancy, but much of the increase is attributable to heat-stable placental alkaline phosphatase isozymes. Serum aspartate transaninase (AST), alanine transaminase (ALT), gamma glutamyl transferase (GGT), and bilirubin levels are slightly lower during pregnancy compared with nonpregnant normal values (Girling and colleagues, 1997).

Mendenhall (1970) reconfirmed decreased *plasma al-*

bumin concentration, showing it to average 3.0 g/dL late in pregnancy compared with 4.3 g/dL in nonpregnant women. Total albumin is increased, however, because of a greater volume of distribution. The reduction in albumin concentrations, combined with a normal slight increase in plasma globulins, results in a decrease in the albumin-to-globulin ratio similar to that seen in certain hepatic diseases.

Plasma *cholinesterase* activity is reduced during normal pregnancy. The magnitude of the decrease is about the same as the decrease in the concentration of albumin (Kambam and associates, 1988; Pritchard, 1955). *Leucine aminopeptidase* activity is markedly elevated in serum from pregnant women. The increase results from the appearance of a pregnancy-specific enzyme (or enzymes) with distinct substrate specificities (Song and Kappas, 1968). Pregnancy-induced aminopeptidase has oxytocinase and vasopressinase activity.

GALLBLADDER. There is considerable alteration of gallbladder function during pregnancy. Braverman and co-workers (1980), using ultrasonography, found impaired gallbladder contraction and high residual volume. It has been suggested that progesterone impairs gallbladder contraction by inhibiting cholecystokinin-mediated smooth muscle stimulation, the primary regulator of gallbladder contraction. Impaired gallbladder contraction leads to stasis, and this, associated with the increased cholesterol saturation of pregnancy, at least partially explains the increased prevalence of cholesterol stones in women who have been pregnant many times.

The effects of pregnancy on maternal bile acid serum concentrations have been incompletely characterized despite the long-acknowledged propensity for pregnancy to cause intrahepatic cholestasis and pruritus gravidarum from retained bile salts (Chap. 48, p. 1283 and Chap. 54, p. 1431). Cholestasis has been linked to high circulating levels of estrogen, which inhibit intraductal transport of bile acids (Simon and colleagues, 1996). Leslie and associates (2000), however, compared circulating estrogen levels in normal pregnant women with those of women with cholestasis. They found the latter group to have significantly lower plasma estrogen levels as well as impaired fetal production of dehydroepiandrosterone (DHEA), which is the precursor to placental estrogen production. The significance of this recent finding is unclear.

ENDOCRINE SYSTEM

Some of the most important endocrine changes of pregnancy have been discussed elsewhere, especially in Chapter 6.

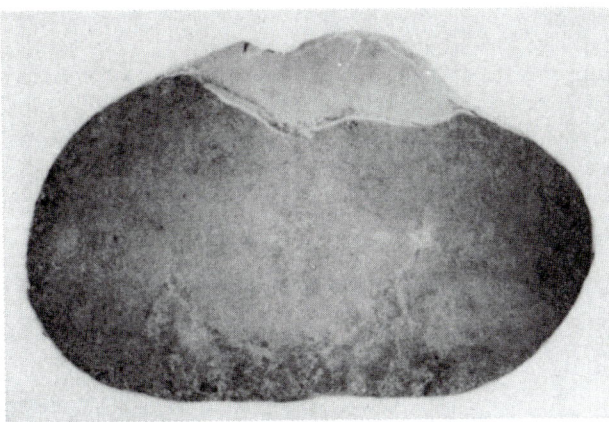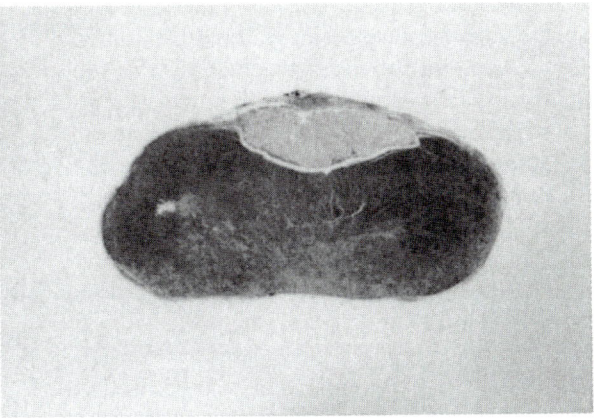

FIGURE 8–16. Photographs of pituitary glands showing normal hypertrophy during pregnancy on the left compared with normal gland size in a nonpregnant woman. Both pituitary glands magnified 6×. (From Scheithauer and colleagues, 1990.)

PITUITARY GLAND. As shown in Figure 8–16, the pituitary gland enlarges during pregnancy by approximately 135 percent compared with nonpregnant controls (Gonzalez and colleagues, 1988). Although there have been suggestions that it may increase sufficiently to compress the optic chiasma and reduce visual fields, visual changes during normal pregnancy are minimal. Scheithauer and colleagues (1990) have provided evidence that the incidence of pituitary prolactinomas is not increased during pregnancy. When these tumors are large before pregnancy—a macroadenoma is 10 mm or greater—then enlargement during pregnancy is more likely (Chap. 50, p. 1353).

The maternal pituitary gland is not essential for maintenance of pregnancy. A number of women have undergone hypophysectomy, completed pregnancy successfully, and have undergone spontaneous labor while receiving glucocorticoids along with thyroid hormone and vasopressin.

GROWTH HORMONE. During the first trimester, serum and amnionic fluid growth hormone concentrations are within nonpregnant values of 0.5 to 7.5 ng/mL (Kletzky and associates, 1985). Serum values increase slowly from approximately 3.5 ng/mL at 10 weeks to plateau after 28 weeks at approximately 14 ng/mL. Growth hormone in amnionic fluid peaks at 14 to 15 weeks and slowly declines thereafter to reach baseline values after 36 weeks. After delivery, growth hormone is elevated for some time but at levels lower than late pregnancy values (Spellacy and Buhi, 1969).

PROLACTIN. During the course of human pregnancy, there is a marked increase in the maternal plasma levels of prolactin. In fact, the levels increase 10-fold (to 150 ng/mL) at term compared with normal nonpregnant women. Paradoxically, after delivery, there is a decrease in plasma prolactin concentration even in women who are breastfeeding. During early lactation, there are pulsatile bursts of prolactin secretion apparently in response to suckling. The physiological cause of the marked increase in prolactin prior to parturition is not entirely certain. It is known, however, that estrogen stimulation increases the number of anterior pituitary lactotrophs and may stimulate the release of prolactin from these cells (Andersen, 1982). Thyroid-releasing hormone acts to cause an increased prolactin level in pregnant compared with nonpregnant women, but the response decreases as pregnancy advances (Andersen, 1982; Miyamoto, 1984). Serotonin also is believed to increase prolactin, and prolactin-inhibiting factor—dopamine—inhibits its secretion.

The principal function of maternal serum prolactin is to ensure lactation. Early in pregnancy, prolactin acts to initiate DNA synthesis and mitosis of glandular epithelial cells and the presecretory alveolar cells of the breast. Prolactin also increases the number of estrogen and prolactin receptors in these same cells. Finally, prolactin promotes mammary alveolar cell RNA synthesis, galactopoiesis, and production of casein and lactalbumin, lactose, and lipids (Andersen, 1982). Kauppila and co-workers (1987) found that a woman with an isolated prolactin deficiency failed to lactate after two pregnancies, establishing the absolute necessity of prolactin for lactation but *not* for successful pregnancy outcome.

Prolactin also is found in high concentration in the fetal plasma, attaining highest concentrations during the last 5 weeks of pregnancy (Winters and associates, 1975). Considerable evidence has accrued that prolactin in fetal plasma is of fetal pituitary origin.

Prolactin is present in amnionic fluid in high concentrations. Levels of up to 10,000 ng/mL are found at 20 to 26 weeks; thereafter, levels decrease and reach a nadir after 34 weeks. Several investigators have presented convincing evidence that the uterine decidua is the site of prolactin synthesis in amnionic fluid (Chap. 4, p. 81).

The function of amnionic fluid prolactin is not known. Some investigators have suggested that it impairs the transfer of water from the fetus into the maternal compartment, thus preserving fetal extracellular fluid and preventing fetal dehydration during late pregnancy when amnionic fluid is normally hypotonic.

THYROID GLAND. There are important changes in thyroidal economy during pregnancy that are due to three modifications in the regulation of thyroid hormones. First, pregnancy induces a marked increase in circulating levels of the major thyroxine transport protein, thyroxine-binding globulin, in response to high estrogen levels. Second, several thyroidal stimulatory factors of placental origin are produced in excess. Although it is well recognized that hyperthyroidism may develop in women with elevated chorionic gonadotropin due to trophoblastic disease, the role of this hormone in normal pregnancy is still debated. Evidence has accrued that the thyroid is under dual control of both thyrotropin and chorionic gonadotropin during normal and abnormal pregnancy (Kennedy and Darne, 1991). Third, pregnancy is accompanied by a decreased availability of iodide for the maternal thyroid. This is due to increased renal clearance and losses to the fetoplacental unit during late gestation, and it results in a relative iodine-deficiency state.

During pregnancy there is moderate enlargement of the thyroid caused by hyperplasia of glandular tissue and increased vascularity. Glinoer and colleagues (1990) assessed thyroid gland volume from 552 ultrasound examinations. Total gland volume increased from 12.1 mL in the first trimester to 15.0 mL at delivery. This increase was observed in the majority of women. Total volume also was found to be inversely proportional to serum thyrotropin concentrations. As emphasized by Levy and co-workers (1980), normal pregnancy does not typically cause significant thyromegaly, and any goiter in pregnancy should be investigated.

Glinoer and co-workers (1990) provided cross-sectional and longitudinal data of maternal thyroid function throughout pregnancy. As shown in Figure 8–17, thyroxine-binding globulin (TBG) increases beginning early in the first trimester, reaches its zenith at about 20 weeks, and stabilizes at approximately double baseline values for the remainder of pregnancy. Total (free and bound) serum thyroxine (T_4) increased sharply between 6 and 9 weeks, and thereafter only slowly, eventually reaching a plateau value at 18 weeks. Importantly, free serum T_4 levels return to normal after the first trimester.

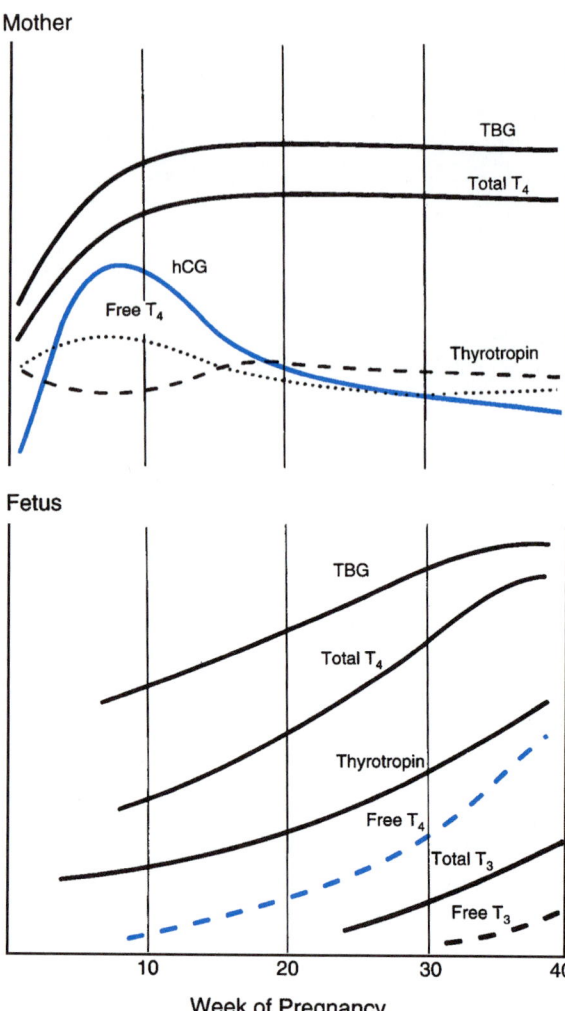

FIGURE 8–17. Relative changes in maternal and fetal thyroid function during pregnancy. Maternal changes include a marked and early increase in hepatic production of thyroxine-binding globulin (TBG) and placental production of chorionic gonadotropin (hCG). Increased thyroxine-binding globulin increases serum T_4 concentrations, and chorionic gonadotropin has thyrotropin-like activity and stimulates maternal T_4 secretion. The transient hCG-induced increase in serum from T_4 inhibits maternal secretion of thyrotropin. Except for minimally increased free thyroxine (free T_4) levels when hCG peaks, these levels are essentially unchanged. (From Burrow and colleagues, 1994, with permission.)

The rise in total triiodothyronine (T_3) is more pronounced up to 18 weeks; thereafter, it plateaus.

Glinoer and colleagues (1990) further observed that the adjustment of thyroidal output of T_4 and T_3 was not similar for all pregnant women. Specifically, in about a third of women, there was relative hypothyroxinemia, preferential T_3 secretion, and higher (albeit normal) serum thyrotropin levels. These results suggest considerable variability in thyroidal adjustments during normal pregnancy.

The modifications in serum thyroid-stimulating hormone and chorionic gonadotropin as a function of gestational age are also illustrated in Figure 8–17. There is an inverse relationship between the rise in chorionic gonadotropin and diminishing thyrotropin concentrations. Indeed, thyrotropin levels decrease in more than 80 percent of the women, even though levels are in the normal range for nonpregnant women. Thus, high serum chorionic gonadotropin levels are associated with thyroid stimulation, and this is consistent with a thyrotropin-like effect of chorionic gonadotropin.

These many complex alterations in thyroid regulation during pregnancy do not appear to alter maternal thyroid status as measured by metabolic studies. Although basal metabolic rate increases progressively during normal pregnancy by as much as 25 percent, most of this increase in oxygen consumption can be attributed to fetal metabolic activity. If fetal body surface area is considered along with that of the mother, the predicted and observed basal metabolic rates are quite similar.

THYROID-RELEASING HORMONE (TRH). This neurotransmitter is present throughout the brain but in highest concentrations in the hypothalamus. It stimulates synthesis and release of thyrotropin. It is not increased during normal pregnancy, but it does cross the placenta and may stimulate the fetal pituitary to secrete thyrotropin (Thorpe-Beeston and associates, 1991). Any role in fetal homeostasis is not clear.

FETAL THYROID GLAND. Changes in fetal thyroid physiology are also shown in Figure 8–17. These are discussed in detail in Chapter 7 (p. 155). As the fetal thyroid becomes autonomous about 10 weeks, there is gradual "maturation" that progresses to term. At least during the first trimester, the fetus is dependent on maternal thyroxine. Later, there is minimal transfer of thyroid hormones from the maternal into the fetal compartment (Burrow and colleagues, 1994). This is likely the consequence of placental thyroxine deiodination. Therefore, after development, fetal thyroid function appears to be independent of maternal thyroid status.

REVERSE TRIIODOTHYRONINE (RT₃). This hormone is formed from the monodeiodination of thyroxine. Its metabolic activity is much less than triiodothyronine. It is predominately a fetal hormone and its level in fetal blood and amnionic fluid is three to five times higher than in maternal blood (Roti and associates, 1983). This is likely because the conversion of thyroxine to reverse triiodothyronine takes place in fetal membranes and in the placenta.

PARATHYROID GLANDS. The regulation of calcium concentration is closely interrelated to magnesium, phosphate, parathyroid hormone, vitamin D, and calcitonin physiology. Any alteration of one of these factors is likely to change the others.

PARATHYROID HORMONE AND CALCIUM INTERRELATIONSHIPS. Acute or chronic decreases in plasma calcium or acute decreases in magnesium stimulate the release of parathyroid hormone, whereas increases in calcium and magnesium suppress parathyroid hormone levels. The action of this hormone on bone resorption, intestinal absorption, and kidney reabsorption is to increase extracellular fluid calcium and decrease phosphate.

Parathyroid hormone plasma concentrations decrease during the first trimester, and then increase progressively throughout the remainder of pregnancy (Pitkin and associates, 1985). Increased levels likely result from the lower calcium concentration in the pregnant woman. As discussed earlier, this is due to increase plasma volume, increased glomerular filtration rate, and maternal–fetal transfer of calcium. Ionized calcium is decreased only slightly and Reitz and co-workers (1977) suggest that during pregnancy there is a new "set point" between ionized calcium and parathyroid hormone. Estrogens also appear to block the action of parathyroid hormone on bone resorption, resulting in another mechanism to increase parathyroid hormone during pregnancy. The net result of these actions is a *physiological hyperparathyroidism* of pregnancy, likely to supply the fetus with adequate calcium.

The potential roles of parathyroid hormone–related peptide production in the fetus, placenta, and maternal tissues are discussed in Chapters 4 to 7.

CALCITONIN AND CALCIUM INTERRELATIONSHIPS. The calcitonin-secreting C cells are derived embryologically from the neural crest and are located predominantly in the perifollicular areas of the thyroid gland. Calcium and magnesium increase the biosynthesis and secretion of calcitonin. Various gastric hormones—gastrin, pentagastrin, glucagon, and pancreoxymin—and food ingestion also increase calcitonin plasma levels.

The known actions of calcitonin are generally considered to oppose those of parathyroid hormone and vitamin D to protect skeletal calcification during times of calcium stress. Pregnancy and lactation cause profound calcium stress, and during these times, calcitonin levels are appreciably higher than in nonpregnant women (Weiss and co-workers, 1998; Whitehead and associates, 1981).

VITAMIN D AND CALCIUM INTERRELATIONSHIPS. Vitamin D is a hormone synthesized in the skin or ingested, and it is converted into 25-hydroxyvitamin D₃ by the liver. This is then converted in the kidney, decidua, and placenta to 1,25-dihydroxyvitamin D_3 (Weisman and co-workers, 1979). This most likely is the biologically active compound, and it stimulates resorption of calcium from bone and absorption from the intestines.

Control and release of 1,25-dihydroxyvitamin D_3 production is unknown, but the conversion of 25-hydroxyvitamin D_3 to 1,25-dihydroxyvitamin D_3 is facilitated by parathyroid hormone and by low calcium and phosphate plasma levels and opposed by calcitonin. Levels of 1,25-dihydroxyvitamin D_3 are increased during normal pregnancy (Whitehead and associates, 1981).

ADRENAL GLANDS. In normal pregnancy, there is probably very little morphological change in the maternal adrenal glands.

CORTISOL. There is a considerable increase in the serum concentration of circulating cortisol, but much of it is bound by cortisol-binding globulin, or *transcortin.* The rate of adrenal cortisol secretion is not increased, and probably it is decreased compared with the nonpregnant state. The metabolic clearance rate of cortisol, however, is lower during pregnancy because its half-life is nearly twice as long as it is in nonpregnant women (Migeon and associates, 1957). Administration of estrogen, including most oral contraceptives, causes changes in levels of cortisol and transcortin similar to those of pregnancy.

In early pregnancy, the levels of circulating corticotropin (ACTH) are reduced strikingly. As pregnancy progresses, the levels of corticotropin and free cortisol rise. This apparent paradox is not understood completely. Nolten and Rueckert (1981) have presented evidence that the higher free cortisol levels observed in pregnancy are the result of a "resetting" of the maternal feedback mechanism to higher levels. They further propose that this might result from *tissue refractoriness* to cortisol. Thus, an elevated free cortisol would be needed during pregnancy to maintain homeostasis.

ALDOSTERONE. As early as 15 weeks, the maternal adrenal glands secrete considerably increased amounts of aldosterone. By the third trimester, about 1 mg/day is secreted. If sodium intake is restricted, aldosterone secretion is elevated even further (Watanabe and co-workers, 1963). At the same time, levels of renin and angiotensin II substrate are normally increased, especially during the latter half of pregnancy. This gives rise to increased plasma levels of angiotensin II, which by acting on the zona glomerulosa of the maternal adrenal glands, accounts for the markedly elevated aldosterone secretion. It has been suggested that the increased aldosterone secretion during normal pregnancy affords protection against the natriuretic effect of progesterone and

atrial natriuretic peptide. Progesterone administered to nonpregnant women is associated with a prompt increase in aldosterone excretion (Laidlaw and colleagues, 1962).

DEOXYCORTICOSTERONE. There is a striking increase in the maternal plasma levels of deoxycorticosterone (DOC) during pregnancy. Brown and co-workers (1972) found that in nonpregnant women and during the first two trimesters of pregnancy, the levels of plasma deoxycorticosterone are less than 100 pg/mL. During the last few weeks of pregnancy, these levels rise to 1500 pg/mL or more. The levels of deoxycorticosterone and its sulfate in fetal blood are appreciably higher than those in maternal blood, which suggests transfer of fetal deoxycorticosterone into the maternal compartment.

DEHYDROEPIANDROSTERONE SULFATE. As discussed in Chapter 6, the levels of *dehydroepiandrosterone sulfate* circulating in maternal blood and excreted in the urine are decreased during normal pregnancy. This is a consequence of increased metabolic clearance through extensive 16α-hydroxylation in the maternal liver and estrogen formation in the placenta.

ANDROSTENEDIONE AND TESTOSTERONE. Maternal plasma levels of these androgens are increased during pregnancy. This finding is not totally explained by alterations in their metabolic clearance. Maternal plasma androstenedione and testosterone are converted to estradiol in the placenta, which increases their clearance rates. Conversely, there is increased sex hormone–binding globulin in plasma of pregnant women which retards testosterone clearance. Thus, there is an increased plasma production rate of maternal testosterone and androstenedione during human pregnancy. The source of this increased C_{19}-steroid production is unknown but it likely originates in the ovary. Interestingly, little or no testosterone in maternal plasma enters the fetal circulation as testosterone. Even when massive testosterone levels are found in the circulation of pregnant women with androgen-secreting tumors, the testosterone level in umbilical cord venous plasma is likely to be too low to be detected. This finding is the result of the near complete conversion of testosterone to 17β-estradiol by the trophoblast (Edman and associates, 1979).

OTHER SYSTEMS

MUSCULOSKELETAL SYSTEM. Progressive *lordosis* is a characteristic feature of normal pregnancy. Compensating for the anterior position of the enlarging uterus, the lordosis shifts the center of gravity back over the lower extremities. There is increased mobility of the sacroiliac, sacrococcygeal, and pubic joints during pregnancy, presumably as a result of hormonal changes. Their mobility may contribute to the alteration of maternal posture, and in turn cause discomfort in the lower portion of the back, especially late in pregnancy. During late pregnancy, aching, numbness, and weakness are occasionally experienced in the upper extremities. This possibly is from the marked lordosis with anterior neck flexion and slumping of the shoulder girdle, which in turn produce traction on the ulnar and median nerves (Crisp and DeFrancesco, 1964).

EYES. Intraocular pressure decreases during pregnancy, attributed in part to increased vitreous outflow (Sunness, 1988). Corneal sensitivity is also decreased, with the greatest changes late in gestation. Most pregnant women demonstrate a measurable but slight increase in corneal thickness thought to be due to edema. Consequently, pregnant women may have difficulty with previously comfortable contact lenses. Brownish-red opacities on the posterior surface of the cornea—*Krukenberg spindles*—have also been observed with a higher than expected frequency during pregnancy. Hormonal effects are postulated as the cause of this increased pigmentation. Other than transient loss of accommodation reported with both pregnancy and lactation, visual function is unaffected by pregnancy.

CENTRAL NERVOUS SYSTEM. Women often report problems with attention, concentration, and memory throughout pregnancy and the early postpartum period. Systematic studies of memory in pregnancy, however, are limited and often anecdotal. Keenan and colleagues (1998) longitudinally investigated memory in pregnant women as well as a matched control group. They found a pregnancy-related decline in memory, which was limited to the third trimester. This decline was not attributable to depression, anxiety, sleep deprivation, or other physical changes associated with pregnancy. The observed decline in memory was transient and it quickly resolved following delivery.

Beginning as early as about 12 weeks, and extending through the first 2 months postpartum, women experience difficulty going to sleep, frequent awakenings, fewer hours of night sleep, and reduced sleep efficiency (Swain and colleagues, 1997; Lee and colleagues, 2000). The greatest disruption of sleep occurs postpartum and may contribute to postpartum "blues" and/or depression (Chap. 53, p. 1421).

REFERENCES

Alvarez H, Caldeyro-Barcia R: Contractility of the human uterus recorded by new methods. Surg Gynecol Obstet 91:1, 1950

Andersen JR: Prolactin in amniotic fluid and maternal serum during uncomplicated human pregnancy. Dan Med Bull 29:266, 1982

Anderson GH, Howland T, Domascek P, Streeten DHP: Effect of sodium balance and calcium channel blocking drugs on blood pressure responses. Hypertension 10:239, 1987

Assali NS, Dilts PV, Pentl AA, Kirschbaum TH, Gross SJ: Physiology of the placenta. In Assali NS (ed): Biology of Gestation, Vol I. The Maternal Organism. New York, Academic Press, 1968

Atarashi K, Mulrow PJ, Franco-Saenz R, Snajdar R, Rapp J: Inhibition of aldosterone production by an atrial extract. Science 224:992, 1984

August P, Mueller FB, Sealey JE, Edersheim TG: Role of renin–angiotensin system in blood pressure regulation in pregnancy. Lancet 345:896, 1995

Bailey RR, Rolleston GL: Kidney length and ureteric dilatation in the puerperium. J Obstet Gynaecol Br Commonw 78:55, 1971

Baker PN, Cunningham FG: Platelet and coagulation abnormalities. In Lindhemier ML, Roberts JM, Cunningham FG (eds): Chesley's Hypertensive Diseases in Pregnancy, 2nd ed. Stamford, CT, Appleton & Lange, 1999, p 349

Bardicef M, Bardicef O, Sorokin Y, Altura BM, Altura BT, Cotton DB, Resnick LM: Extracellular and intracellular magnesium depletion in pregnancy and gestational diabetes. Am J Obstet Gynecol 172:1009, 1995

Bell RJ, Permezel M, MacLennan A, Hughes C, Healy D, Brennecke S: A randomized, double-blind, placebo controlled trial of the safety of vaginal recombinant human relaxin for cervical ripening. Obstet Gynecol 82:328, 1993

Bieniarz J, Branda LA, Maqueda E, Morozovsky J, Caldeyro-Barcia R: Aortocaval compression by the uterus in late pregnancy, 3. Unreliability of the sphygmomanometric method in estimating uterine artery pressure. Am J Obstet Gynecol 102:1106, 1968

Bogic LV, Mandel M, Bryant-Greenwood GD: Relaxin gene expression in human reproductive tissues by in-situ hybridization. J Clin Endocrinol Metab 80:130, 1995

Bradshaw KD, Santos-Ramos R, Rawlins SC, MacDonald PC, Parker CR: Endocrine studies in a pregnancy complicated by ovarian thecalutein cysts and hyperreaction luteinalis. Obstet Gynecol 67:665, 1986

Brar HS, Platt LD, DeVore GR, Horenstein J, Medearis AL: Qualitative assessment of maternal uterine and fetal umbilical artery blood flow and resistance in laboring patients by Doppler velocimetry. Am J Obstet Gynecol 158:95, 1988

Braverman DZ, Johnson ML, Kern Jr F: Effects of pregnancy and contraceptive steroids on gallbladder function. N Engl J Med 302:362, 1980

Bremme K, Ostlund E, Almqvist I, Heinonen K, Blomback M: Enhanced thrombin generation and fibrinolytic activity in normal pregnancy and the puerperium. Obstet Gynecol 80:132, 1992

Brizzi P, Tonolo G, Esposito F, Puddu L, Dessole S, Maioli M, Milia S: Lipoprotein metabolism during normal pregnancy. Am J Obstet Gynecol 181:430, 1999

Brown MA, Gallery EDM, Ross MR, Esber RP: Sodium excretion in normal and hypertensive pregnancy: A prospective study. Am J Obstet Gynecol 159:297, 1988

Brown MA, Sinosich MJ, Saunders DM, Gallery EDM: Potassium regulation and progesterone-aldosterone interrelationships in human pregnancy: A prospective study. Am J Obstet Gynecol 155:349, 1986

Brown RD, Strott CA, Liddle GW: Plasma desoxycorticosterone in normal and abnormal human pregnancy. J Clin Endocrinol Metab 35:736, 1972

Burrow GN, Fisher DA, Larsen PR: Maternal and fetal thyroid function. N Engl J Med 331:1072, 1994

Calloway DH: Nitrogen balance during pregnancy. In Winick M (ed): Nutrition and Fetal Development, Vol II. New York, Wiley, 1974

Castro LC, Hobel CJ, Gornbein J: Plasma levels of atrial natriuretic peptide in normal and hypertensive pregnancies: A meta-analysis. Am J Obstet Gynecol 171:1642, 1994

Chard T, Craig PH, Menabawey M, Lee C: Alpha interferon in human pregnancy. Br J Obstet Gynaecol 93:1145, 1986

Chesley LC: Renal function during pregnancy. In Carey HM (ed): Modern Trends in Human Reproductive Physiology. London, Butterworth, 1963

Chesley LC, Sloan DM: The effect of posture on renal function in late pregnancy. Am J Obstet Gynecol 89:754, 1964

Christofides ND, Ghatei MA, Bloom SR, Borberg C, Gillmer MDG: Decreased plasma motilin concentrations in pregnancy. BMJ 285:1453, 1982

Clark SL, Cotton DB, Lee W, Bishop C, Hill T: Central hemodynamic assessment of normal term pregnancy. Am J Obstet Gynecol 161:1439, 1989

Cohen DA, Daughaday WH, Weldon VV: Fetal and maternal virilization associated with pregnancy. Am J Dis Child 136:353, 1982

Cole DEC, Gundberg CM, Stirk LJ, Atkinson SA, Hanley DA, Ayer LM, Baldwin LS: Changing osteocalcin concentrations during pregnancy and lactation: Implications for maternal mineral metabolism. J Clin Endocrinol Metab 65:290, 1987

Combes B, Adams RH: Pathophysiology of the liver in pregnancy. In Assali NS (ed): Pathophysiology of Gestation, Vol I. New York, Academic Press, 1971

Crisp WE, DeFrancesco A: The hand syndrome of pregnancy. Obstet Gynecol 23:433, 1964

Csapo AI, Pulkkinen MO, Wiest WG: Effects of hysterectomy and progesterone replacement in early pregnant patients. Am J Obstet Gynecol 115:759, 1973

Cunningham FG, Cox K, Gant NF: Further observations on the nature of pressor responsivity to angiotensin II in human pregnancy. Obstet Gynecol 46:581, 1975

Cutforth R, MacDonald CB: Heart sounds and murmurs in pregnancy. Am Heart J 71:741, 1966

Darmady JM, Postle AD: Lipid metabolism in pregnancy. Br J Obstet Gynaecol 89:211, 1982

Davison JM, Hytten FE: Glomerular filtration during and after pregnancy. J Obstet Gynaecol Br Commonw 81:558, 1974

Davison JM, Vallotton MB, Lindheimer MD: Plasma osmolality and urinary concentration and dilution during and after pregnancy: Evidence that lateral recumbency inhibits maximal urinary concentrating ability. Br J Obstet Gynaecol 88:472, 1981

De Boer K, ten Cate JW, Sturk A: Enhanced thrombin generation in normal and hypertensive pregnancy. Am J Obstet Gynecol 160:95, 1989

Desoye G, Schweditsch MO, Preiffer KP, Zechner R, Kostner GM: Correlation of hormones with lipid and lipoprotein levels during normal pregnancy and postpartum. J Clin Endocrinol Metab 64:704, 1987

DeSwiet M: The respiratory system. In Hytten FE, Chamberlain G (eds): Clinical Physiology in Obstetrics, 2nd ed. Oxford, Blackwell, 1991, p 83

Dikranian K, Trosheva M, Nikolov S, Bodin P: Nitric oxide synthase (NOS) in the human umbilical cord vessels. An immunohistochemical study. Acta Histochem 96:145, 1994

Dunlop W: Serial changes in renal haemodynamics during normal human pregnancy. Br J Obstet Gynaecol 88:1, 1981

Dunlop W: Investigations into influence of posture on renal plasma flow and glomerular filtration rate during late pregnancy. Br J Obstet Gynaecol 83:17, 1976

Duvekot JJ, Cheriex EC, Pieters FAA, Menheere PPCA, Peeters LLH: Early pregnancy changes in hemodynamics and volume homeostasis are consecutive adjustments triggered by a primary fall in systemic vascular tone. Am J Obstet Gynecol 169:1382, 1993

Easterling TR, Schmucker BC, Benedetti TJ: The hemodynamic effects of orthostatic stress during pregnancy. Obstet Gynecol 72:550, 1988

Edman CD, Devereux WP, Parker CR, MacDonald PC: Placental clearance of maternal androgens: A protective mechanism against fetal virilization. Abstract 112 presented at the 26th annual meeting of the Society for Gynecologic Investigation, San Diego, 1979. Gynecol Invest 67:68, 1979

Edman CD, Toofanian A, MacDonald PC, Gant NF: Placental clearance rate of maternal plasma androstenedione through placental estradiol formation: An indirect method of assessing uteroplacental blood flow. Am J Obstet Gynecol 141:1029, 1981

Enein M, Zina AAA, Kassem M, El-Tabbakh G: Echocardiography of the pericardium in pregnancy. Obstet Gynecol 69:851, 1987

Everett RB, Worley RJ, MacDonald PC, Gant NF: Modification of vascular responsiveness to angiotensin II in pregnant women by intravenously infused 5α-dihydroprogesterone. Am J Obstet Gynecol 131:352, 1978a

Everett RB, Worley RJ, MacDonald PC, Gant NF: Oral administration of theophylline to modify pressor responsiveness to angiotensin II in women with pregnancy-induced hypertension. Am J Obstet Gynecol 132:359, 1978b

Ezimokhai M, Davison JM, Philips PR, Dunlop W: Non-postural serial changes in renal function during the third trimester of normal human pregnancy. Br J Obstet Gynaecol 88:465, 1981

Faught W, Garner P, Jones G, Ivey B: Changes in protein C and protein S levels in normal pregnancy. Am J Obstet Gynecol 172:147, 1995

Fogh-Andersen N, Schultz-Larsen P: Free calcium ion concentration in pregnancy. Acta Obstet Gynecol Scand 60:309, 1981

Freinkel N: Banting lecture 1980: Of pregnancy and progeny. Diabetes 29:1023, 1980

Freinkel N, Dooley SL, Metzger BE: Care of the pregnant woman with insulin-dependent diabetes mellitus. N Engl J Med 313:96, 1985

Friedman SA: Preeclampsia: A review of the role of prostaglandins. Obstet Gynecol 71:122, 1988

Gallery EDM, Lindheimer MD. Alterations in volume homeostasis. In Lindhemier ML, Roberts JM, Cunningham FG (eds): Chesley's Hypertensive Diseases in Pregnancy, 2nd ed. Stamford, CT, Appleton and Lange, 1999, p 327

Gallery ED, Raftos J, Gyory AZ, Wells JV: A prospective study of serum complement (C_3 and C_4) levels during normal human pregnancy: Effect of the development of pregnancy-associated hypertension. Aust N Z J Med 11:243, 1981

Gant NF, Daley GL, Chand S, Whalley PJ, MacDonald PC:

The nature of pressor responsiveness to angiotensin II in human pregnancy. Obstet Gynecol 43:854, 1974

Gant NF, Daley GL, Chand S, Whalley PJ, MacDonald PC: A study of angiotensin II pressor response throughout primigravid pregnancy. J Clin Invest 52:2682, 1973

Gatti L, Tenconi PM, Guarneri D, Bertulessi C, Ossola MW, Bosco P, Gianotti GA: Hemostatic parameters and platelet activation by flow-cytometry in normal pregnancy: A longitudinal study. Int J Clin Lab Res 24:217, 1994

Gazioglu K, Kaltreider NL, Rosne M, Yu PN: Pulmonary function during pregnancy in normal women and in patients with cardiopulmonary disease. Thorax 25:445, 1970

Girling JC, Dow E, Smith JH: Liver function tests in preeclampsia: Importance of comparison with a reference range derived for normal pregnancy. Br J Obstet Gynaecol 104:246, 1997

Glinoer D, DeNayer P, Bourdoux P, Lemone M, Robyn C, Van Steirteghem A, Kinthaert J, Lejeune B: Regulation of maternal thyroid during pregnancy. J Clin Endocrinol Metab 71:276, 1990

Gonzalez JG, Elizondo G, Saldivar D, Nanez H, Todd LE, Villarreal JZ: Pituitary gland growth during normal pregnancy: An in vivo study using magnetic resonance imaging. Am J Med 85:217, 1988

Hahn PF, Carothers EL, Darby WJ, Martin M, Sheppard CW, Cannon RO, Beam AS, Densen PM, Peterson JC, McClellan GS: Iron metabolism in human pregnancy as studied with the radioactive isotope Fe^{59}. Am J Obstet Gynecol 61:477, 1951

Hankins GDV, Clark SL, Uckan E, Van Hook JW: Maternal oxygen transport variables during the third trimester of normal pregnancy. Am J Obstet Gynecol 180:406, 1999

Harbert GM, Cornell GW, Littlefield JB, Kayan JB, Thornton WN: Maternal hemodynamics associated with uterine contraction in gravid monkeys. Am J Obstet Gynecol 104:24, 1969

Harstad TW, Mason R, Cox SM: Serum erythropoietin quantitation in pregnancy using an enzyme-linked immunoassay. Am J Perinatol 9:231, 1992

Higby K, Suiter CR, Phelps JY, Siler-Khodr T, Langer O: Normal values of urinary albumin and fetal protein excretions during pregnancy. Am J Obstet Gynecol 171:984, 1994

Hodgkinson CP: Physiology of the ovarian veins in pregnancy. Obstet Gynecol 1:26, 1953

Hof RP: Modification of vasopressin- and angiotensin II-induced changes by calcium antagonists in the peripheral circulation of anaesthetized rabbits. Br J Pharmacol 85:75, 1985

Hornnes PJ, Kuhl C: Plasma insulin and glucagon responses to isoglycemic stimulation in normal pregnancy and postpartum. Obstet Gynecol 55:425, 1980

Huisman A, Aarnoudse JG, Heuvelmans JHA, Goslinga H, Fidler V, Huisjes HJ, Zijlstra WJ: Whole blood viscosity during normal pregnancy. Br J Obstet Gynaecol 94:1143, 1987

Hull AD, White CR, Pearce WJ: Endothelium-derived relaxing factor and cyclic GMP-dependent vasorelaxation in human chorionic plate arteries. Placenta 15:365, 1994

Hytten FE: Lactation. In: The Clinical Physiology of the Puerperium. London, Farrand Press, 1995, p 59

Hytten FE: Weight gain in pregnancy. In Hytten FE, Chamberlain G (eds): Clinical Physiology in Obstetrics, 2nd ed. Oxford, Blackwell, 1991, p 173

Hytten FE, Leitch I: The Physiology of Human Pregnancy, 2nd ed. Philadelphia, Davis, 1971

Hytten FE, Thomson AM: Maternal physiological adjustments. In Assali NS (ed): Biology of Gestation, Vol I. The Maternal Organism. New York, Academic Press, 1968

Ingerslev M, Teilum G: Biopsy studies on the liver in pregnancy, 2. Liver biopsy on normal pregnant women. Acta Obstet Gynecol Scand 25:352, 1946

Iosif S, Ingemarsson I, Ulmsten U: Urodynamic studies in normal pregnancy and the puerperium. Am J Obstet Gynecol 137:696, 1980

Izumi H, Garfield RE, Makino Y, Shirakawa K, Itoh T: Gestational changes in endothelium-dependent vasorelaxation in human umbilical artery. Am J Obstet Gynecol 170:236, 1994

Janbu T, Nesheim BI: Uterine artery blood velocities during contractions in pregnancy and labour related to intrauterine pressure. Br J Obstet Gynaecol 94:1150, 1987

Jauniaux E, Johnson MR, Jurkovic D, Ramsay B, Campbell S, Meuris S: The role of relaxin in the development of the uteroplacental circulation in early pregnancy. Obstet Gynecol 84:338, 1994

Johnson MR, Abbas AA, Allman AC, Nicolaides KH, Lightman SL: The regulation of plasma relaxin levels during human pregnancy. J Endocrinol 142:261, 1994a

Johnson MR, Jauniaux E, Jurkovic D, Sannino P, Campbell S, Nicolaides KH: Relaxin concentrations in exoembryonic fluids during the first trimester. Hum Reprod 9:1561, 1994b

Kambam JR, Perry SM, Entman S, Smith BE: Effect of magnesium on plasma cholinesterase activity. Am J Obstet Gynecol 159:309, 1988

Kaneshige E: Serum ferritin as an assessment of iron stores and other hematologic parameters during pregnancy. Obstet Gynecol 57:238, 1981

Kangawa K, Fukuda A, Matsuo H: Structural identification of β- and Δ-human atrial natriuretic polypeptides. Nature 313:397, 1985

Katz R, Karliner JS, Resnik R: Effects of a natural volume overload state (pregnancy) on left ventricular performance in normal human subjects. Circulation 58:434, 1978

Kauppila A, Chatelain P, Kirkinen P, Kivinen S, Ruokonen A: Isolated prolactin deficiency in a woman with puerperal alactogenesis. J Clin Endocrinol Metab 64:309, 1987

Kauppila A, Koskinen M, Puolakka J, Tuimala R, Kuikka J: Decreased intervillous and unchanged myometrial blood flow in supine recumbency. Obstet Gynecol 55:203, 1980

Keenan PA, Yaldro DT, Stress ME, Fuerst DR, Ginsburg KA: Explicit memory in pregnant women. Am J Obstet Gynecol 179:731, 1998

Kennedy RL, Darne J: The role of hCG in regulation of the thyroid gland in normal and abnormal pregnancy. Obstet Gynecol 78:298, 1991

Kinsella SM, Lohmann G: Supine hypotensive syndrome. Obstet Gynecol 83:774, 1994

Klafen, Palugyay: Vergleichende Untersuchungen über Lage und Ausdehnung von Herz und Lunge in der Schwangerschaft und im Wochenbett. Arch Gynaekol 131:347, 1927

Kletzky OA, Rossman F, Bertolli SI, Platt LD, Mischell DR: Dynamics of human chorionic gonadotropin, prolactin, and growth hormone in serum and amniotic fluid throughout normal human pregnancy. Am J Obstet Gynecol 151:878, 1985

Koh SC, Ananda-Kumar C, Montan S, Ratnam SS: Plasminogen activators, plasminogen activator inhibitors and markers of intravascular coagulation in preeclampsia. Gynecol Obstet Invest 35:214, 1993

Kost ER, Snyder RR, Schwartz LE, Hankins GDV: The "less

than optimal" cytology: Important in obstetric patients and in a routine gynecologic population. Obstet Gynecol 81:127, 1993

Krause PJ, Ingardia CJ, Pontius LT, Malech HL, LoBello TM, Maderazo EG: Host defense during pregnancy: Neutrophil chemotaxis and adherence. Am J Obstet Gynecol 157:274, 1987

Kubota T, Kamada S, Hirata Y, Eguchi S, Imai T, Marumo F, Aso T: Synthesis and release of endothelin-1 by human decidual cells. J Clin Endocrinol Metab 75:1230, 1992

Laidlaw JC, Ruse JL, Gornall AG: The influence of estrogen and progesterone on aldosterone excretion. J Clin Endocrinol 22:161, 1962

Lederman SA, Paxton A, Heymsfield SB, Wang J, Thornton J, Pierson RN: Maternal body fat and water during pregnancy: Do they raise infant birth weight? Am J Obstet Gynecol 180:235, 1999

Lee DH, Henderson PA, Blajchman MA: Prevalence of Factor V Leiden in a Canadian blood donor population. Can Med Assoc J 155:285, 1996

Lee KA, Zaffke ME, Mcenany G: Parity and sleep patterns during and after pregnancy. Obstet Gynecol 95:14, 2000

Leslie KK, Reznikov L, Simon FR, Fennessey PV, Reyes H, Ribalta J: Estrogens in intrahepatic cholestasis of pregnancy. Obstet Gynecol 95:372, 2000

Levin ER: Endothelins. N Engl J Med 333:356, 1995

Levy RP, Newman DM, Rejali LS, Barford DAG: The myth of goiter in pregnancy. Am J Obstet Gynecol 137:701, 1980

Lind T, Bell S, Gilmore E, Huisjes HJ, Schally AV: Insulin disappearance rate in pregnant and non-pregnant women, and in non-pregnant women given GHRIH. Eur J Clin Invest 7:47, 1977

Lindheimer MD, Davidson JM: Osmoregulation, the secretion of arginine vasopressin and its metabolism during pregnancy. Eur J Endocrinol 132:133, 1995

Lindheimer MD, Grünfeld J-P, Davison JM: Renal disorders. In Barran WM, Lindheimer MD (eds): Medical Disorders During Pregnancy, 3rd ed. St. Louis, Mosby, 2000, p 45

Lindheimer MD, Richardson DA, Ehrlich EN, Katz AI: Potassium homeostasis in pregnancy. J Reprod Med 32:517, 1987

Lockwood CJ: Heritable coagulopathics in pregnancy. Obstet Gynecol Surv 54:754, 1999

Lopez-Espinoza I, Dhar H, Humphreys S, Redman CWG: Urinary albumin excretion in pregnancy. Br J Obstet Gynaecol 93:176, 1986

Mabie WC, DiSessa TG, Crocker LG, Sibai BM, Arheart KL: A longitudinal study of cardiac output in normal human pregnancy. Am J Obstet Gynecol 170:849, 1994

Macfie AG, Magides AP, Richmond MN, Reilly CS: Gastric emptying in pregnancy. Br J Anaesth 67:54, 1991

MacGillivray I, Rose GA, Rowe B: Blood pressure survey in pregnancy. Clin Sci 37:395, 1969

Makowski EL, Meschia G, Droegemueller W, Battaglia FC: Distribution of uterine blood flow in the pregnant sheep. Am J Obstet Gynecol 101:409, 1968

Mardones-Santander FM, Salazar G, Rosso P, Villarroel L: Maternal body composition near term and birth weight. Obstet Gynecol 91:873, 1998

McLaughlin MK, Roberts JM: Hemodynamic changes. In Lindhemier ML, Roberts JM, Cunningham FG (eds): Chesley's Hypertensive Diseases in Pregnancy, 2nd ed. Stamford, CT, Appleton & Lange, 1999, p 69

McLennan CE: Antecubital and femoral venous pressure in normal and toxemic pregnancy. Am J Obstet Gynecol 45:568, 1943

Mendenhall HW: Serum protein concentrations in pregnancy,

1. Concentrations in maternal serum. Am J Obstet Gynecol 106:388, 1970

Migeon CJ, Bertrand J, Wall PE: Physiological disposition of 4-C[14] cortisol during late pregnancy. J Clin Invest 36:1350, 1957

Milne JS, Howie AD, Pack AI: Dyspnoea during normal pregnancy. Br J Obstet Gynaecol 85:260, 1978

Miyamoto J: Prolactin and thyrotropin responses to thyrotropin-releasing hormone during the periportal period. Obstet Gynecol 63:639, 1984

Muechler EK, Fichter J, Zongrone J: Human chorionic gonadotropin, estriol, and testosterone changes in two pregnancies with hyperreactio luteinalis. Am J Obstet Gynecol 157:1126, 1987

Naden RP, Rosenfeld CR: Systemic and uterine responsiveness to angiotensin II and norepinephrine in estrogen-treated nonpregnant sheep. Am J Obstet Gynecol 153:417, 1985

Nolan TE, Smith RP, DeVoe LD: Maternal plasma D-dimer levels in normal and complicated pregnancies. Obstet Gynecol 81:235, 1993

Nolten WE, Rueckert PA: Elevated free cortisol index in pregnancy: Possible regulatory mechanisms. Am J Obstet Gynecol 139:492, 1981

Øian P, Maltau JM, Noddeland H, Fadnes HO: Oedema-preventing mechanisms in subcutaneous tissue of normal pregnant women. Br J Obstet Gynaecol 92:1113, 1985

Ozanne P, Linderkamp O, Miller FC, Meiselman HJ: Erythrocyte aggregation during normal pregnancy. Am J Obstet Gynecol 147:576, 1983

Palmer SK, Zamudio S, Coffin C, Parker S, Stamm E, Moore LG: Quantitative estimation of human uterine artery blood flow and pelvic blood flow redistribution in pregnancy. Obstet Gynecol 80:1000, 1992

Pasanisi F, Elliott HL, Reid JL: Vascular and aldosterone responses to angiotensin II in normal humans: Effects of nicardipine. J Cardiovasc Pharmacol 7:1171, 1985

Patton PE, Coulam CB, Bergstralh E: The prevalence of autoantibodies in pregnant and nonpregnant women. Am J Obstet Gynecol 157:1345, 1987

Phelps RL, Metzger BE, Freinkel N: Carbohydrate metabolism in pregnancy, 17. Diurnal profiles of plasma glucose, insulin, free fatty acids, triglycerides, cholesterol, and individual amino acids in late normal pregnancy. Am J Obstet Gynecol 140:730, 1981

Pipe NGJ, Smith T, Halliday D, Edmonds CJ, Williams C, Coltart TM: Changes in fat, fat free mass and body water in human normal pregnancy. Br J Obstet Gynaecol 86:929, 1979

Pitkin RM, Reynolds WA, Williams GA, Hargis GK: Calcium metabolism in pregnancy: A longitudinal study. Am J Obstet Gynecol 151:99, 1985

Platts JK, Meadows P, Jones R, Harvey JN: The relation between tissue kallikrein excretion rate, aldosterone and glomerular filtration rate in human pregnancy. Br J Obstet Gynaecol 107:278, 2000

Pritchard JA: Changes in the blood volume during pregnancy and delivery. Anesthesiology 26:393, 1965

Pritchard JA: Plasma cholinesterase activity in normal pregnancy and in eclamptogenic toxemias. Am J Obstet Gynecol 70:1083, 1955

Pritchard JA, Adams RH: Erythrocyte production and destruction during pregnancy. Am J Obstet Gynecol 79:750, 1960

Pritchard JA, Mason RA: Iron stores of normal adults and

their replenishment with oral iron therapy. JAMA 190:897, 1964

Pritchard JA, Scott DE: Iron demands during pregnancy. In: Iron Deficiency-Pathogenesis: Clinical Aspects and Therapy. London, Academic Press, 1970, p 173

Rechberger T, Uldbjerg N, Oxlund H: Connective tissue changes in the cervix during normal pregnancy and pregnancy complicated by cervical incompetence. Obstet Gynecol 71:563, 1988

Reitz RE, Thomas AD, Woods JR, Weinstein RL: Calcium, magnesium, phosphorus, and parathyroid hormone interrelationships in pregnancy and newborn infants. Obstet Gynecol 50:701, 1977

Rosenfeld CR, Barton MD, Meschia G: Effects of epinephrine on distribution of blood flow in the pregnant ewe. Am J Obstet Gynecol 124:156, 1976

Rosenfeld CR, Gant NF Jr: The chronically instrumented ewe. A model for studying vascular reactivity to angiotensin II in pregnancy. J Clin Invest 67:486, 1981

Rosenfeld CR, Morriss FH Jr, Makowski EL, Meschia G, Battaglia FC: Circulatory changes in the reproductive tissues of ewes during pregnancy. Gynecol Invest 5:252, 1974

Rosenfeld CR, West J: Circulatory response to systemic infusion of norepinephrine in the pregnant ewe. Am J Obstet Gynecol 127:376, 1977

Roti E, Gnudi A, Braverman LE: The placental transport, synthesis and metabolism of hormones and drugs which affect thyroid function. Endocrinol Rev 4:131, 1983

Rubi RA, Sala NL: Ureteral function in pregnant women, 3. Effect of different positions and of fetal delivery upon ureteral tonus. Am J Obstet Gynecol 101:230, 1968

Sadaniantz A, Saint Laurent L, Parisi AF: Long-term effects of multiple pregnancies on cardiac dimensions and systolic and diastolic function. Am J Obstet Gynecol 174:1061, 1996

Sagawa N, Hasegawa M, Itoh H, Nanno H, Mori T, Yano J, Yoshimasa T, Nakao K: Current topic: The role of amniotic endothelin in human pregnancy. Placenta 15:565, 1994

Schauberger CW, Rooney BL, Goldsmith L, Shanton D, Silva PD, Schaper A: Peripheral joint laxity increases in pregnancy but does not correlate with serum relaxin levels. Am J Obstet Gynecol 174:667, 1996

Scheithauer BW, Sano T, Kovacs KT, Young WF Jr, Ryan N, Randah RV: The pituitary gland in pregnancy: A clinicopathologic and immunohistochemical study of 69 cases. Mayo Clin Proc 65:461, 1990

Schulman A, Herlinger H: Urinary tract dilatation in pregnancy. Br J Radiol 48:638, 1975

Scott DE: Anemia during pregnancy. Obstet Gynecol Ann 1:219, 1972

Seligman SP, Buyon JP, Clancy RM, Young BK, Abramson SB: The role of nitric oxide in the pathogenesis of preeclampsia. Am J Obstet Gynecol 171:944, 1994

Shortle BE, Warren MP, Tsin D: Recurrent androgenicity in pregnancy: A case report and literature review. Obstet Gynecol 70:462, 1987

Simon FR, Fortune J, Iwahashi M, Gartung C, Wolkoff A, Sutherland E: Ethinyl estradiol cholestasis involves alterations in expression of liver sinusoidal transporters. Am J Physiol 271:G1043, 1996

Song CS, Kappas A: The influence of estrogens, progestins and pregnancy on the liver. Vitam Horm 26:147, 1968

Spatling L, Fallenstein F, Huch A, Huch R, Rooth G: The variability of cardiopulmonary adaptation to pregnancy at rest and during exercise. Br J Obstet Gynaecol 18:99, 1992

Spellacy WN, Buhi WC: Pituitary growth hormone and placental lactogen levels measured in normal term pregnancy and at the early and late postpartum periods. Am J Obstet Gynecol 105:888, 1969

Stein PK, Hagley MT, Cole PL, Domitrovich PP, Kleiger RE, Rottman JN: Changes in 24-hour heart rate variability during normal pregnancy. Am J Obstet Gynecol 180:978, 1999

Sternberg WH: Non-functioning ovarian neoplasms. In Grady HG, Smith DE (eds): International Academy of Pathology monograph no. 3. The Ovary. Baltimore, Williams & Wilkins, 1963

Sunness JS: The pregnant woman's eye. Surv Ophthalmol 32:219, 1988

Swain AM, O'Hara MW, Starr KR, Gorman LL: A prospective study of sleep, mood, and cognitive function in postpartum and nonpostpartum women. Obstet Gynecol 90:381, 1997

Taylor DJ, Phillips P, Lind T: Puerperal haematological indices. Br J Obstet Gynaecol 88:601, 1981

Teasdale F: Numerical density of nuclei in the sheep placenta. Anat Rec 185:186, 1976

Thomsen JK, Fogh-Anderson N, Jaszczak P: Atrial natriuretic peptide, blood volume, aldosterone, and sodium excretion during twin pregnancy. Acta Obstet Gynecol Scand 73:14, 1994

Thorp JM, Norton PA, Wall LL, Kuller JA, Eucker B, Wells E: Urinary incontinence in pregnancy and the puerperium: A prospective study. Am J Obstet Gynecol 181:266, 1999

Thorpe-Beeston JG, Nicolaides KH, Snijders RJM, Butler J, McGregor AM: Fetal thyroid-stimulating hormone response to maternal administration of thyrotropin-releasing hormone. Am J Obstet Gynecol 164:1244, 1991

Tsai CH, deLeeuw NKM: Changes in 2,3-diphosphoglycerate during pregnancy and puerperium in normal women and in β-thalassemia heterozygous women. Am J Obstet Gynecol 142:520, 1982

Tygart SG, McRoyan DK, Spinnato JA, McRoyan CJ, Kitay DZ: Longitudinal study of platelet indices during normal pregnancy. Am J Obstet Gynecol 154:883, 1986

Ueland K: Maternal cardiovascular dynamics, 7. Intrapartum blood volume changes. Am J Obstet Gynecol 126:671, 1976

Ueland K, Hansen JM: Maternal cardiovascular dynamics, 2. Posture and uterine contractions. Am J Obstet Gynecol 103:1, 1969

Ueland K, Metcalfe J: Circulatory changes in pregnancy. Clin Obstet Gynecol 18:41, 1975

Ulmsten U, Sundström G: Esophageal manometry in pregnant and nonpregnant women. Am J Obstet Gynecol 132:260, 1978

Van Geelen JM, Lemmens WAJG, Eskes TKAB, Martin CB Jr: The urethral pressure profile in pregnancy and after delivery in healthy nulliparous women. Am J Obstet Gynecol 144:636, 1982

Van Wagenen G, Jenkins RH: An experimental examination of factors causing ureteral dilatation of pregnancy. J Urol 42:1010, 1939

Vaughan Jones SA, Black MM: Pregnancy dermatoses. J Am Acad Dermatol 40:233, 1999

Veille JC, Morton MJ, Burry KJ: Maternal cardiovascular adaptations to twin pregnancy. Am J Obstet Gynecol 153:261, 1985

Wakitani K, Cole BR, Geller DM, Currie MG, Adams SP, Fok KF, Needleman P: Atriopeptins: Correlation between renal vasodilatation and natriuresis. Am J Physiol 249:F49, 1985

Watanabe M, Meeker CI, Gray MJ, Sims EAH, Solomon S:

Secretion rate of aldosterone in normal pregnancy. J Clin Invest 42:1619, 1963

Watts DH, Krohn MA, Wener M, Escheubach DA: C-reactive protein in normal pregnancy. Obstet Gynecol 77:176, 1991

Weenink GH, Treffers PE, Kahle LH, ten Cate JW: Antithrombin III in normal pregnancy. Thromb Res 26:281, 1982

Weiss G, Goldsmith LT, Sachdev R, von Hagen S, Lederer K: Elevated first-trimester serum relaxin concentrations in pregnant women following ovarian stimulation predict prematurity risk and preterm delivery. Obstet Gynecol 82:821, 1993

Weiss M, Eisenstein Z, Ramot Y, Lipitz S, Shulman A, Frenkel Y: Renal reabsorption of inorganic phosphorus in pregnancy in relation to the calciotropic hormones. Br J Obstet Gynaecol 105:195, 1998

Weisman Y, Harell A, Edelstein S, David M, Spirer Z, Golander A: 1,25-Dihydroxyvitamin D_3 and 24,25-dihydroxyvitamin D in vitro synthesis by human decidua and placenta. Nature 281:317, 1979

Whitehead M, Lane G, Young O, Campbell S, Abeyasekera G, Hillyard CJ, MacIntyre I, Phang KG, Stevenson JC: Interrelations of calcium-regulating hormones during normal pregnancy. BMJ 283:10, 1981

Whittaker PG, MacPhail S, Lind T: Serial hematologic changes and pregnancy outcome. Obstet Gynecol 88:33, 1996

Winters AJ, Colston C, MacDonald PC, Porter JC: Fetal plasma prolactin levels. J Clin Endocrinol Metab 41:626, 1975

Wright HP, Osborn SB, Edmonds DG: Changes in rate of flow of venous blood in the leg during pregnancy, measured with radioactive sodium. Surg Gynecol Obstet 90:481, 1950

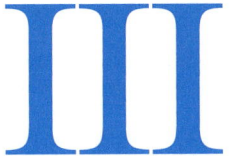

SECTION

Pregnancy Planning and Antepartum Management

9

Preconceptional Counseling

In the early part of the 20th century, women with medical problems were often unable to conceive or were advised not to. Medical breakthroughs such as the discovery of insulin and development of effective antihypertensive and other medications subsequently made it possible for such women to contemplate pregnancy. Obstetrical care of the women with medical problems during this time dealt almost exclusively with protecting maternal health, as little was known about pathological influences on fetal development. In the 1960s, research began to focus on the pathophysiology of pregnancy and perinatal outcome. As a result, prenatal care began to extend toward fetal concerns, and interest in perinatal research increased dramatically. Subsequently, the etiology of many pathological maternal and fetal conditions was elucidated, and intensive research clarified genetic origins of many diseases. At the same time, effective contraception was developed, and many women were now postponing pregnancy and limiting family size, while at the same time striving to optimize the outcome of each pregnancy. Thus, the focus of obstetrical care has changed once again, from treating maternal and fetal diseases to predicting and preventing them.

In 1990, the Public Health Service published *Healthy People 2000,* a guide for a nationwide preventive medicine program drafted by leading scholars and designed to address the highest priority health-care issues. The major goals of this program are to increase the span of healthy life, to reduce health disparities between individuals, and to improve access to preventive services. Preventive medicine for obstetrics figures prominently in this plan, and 3 of the 18 indicators selected for monitoring community health status reflect obstetrical care: infant mortality is number 1, low birthweight is number 14, and first-trimester prenatal care is number 16. A specific goal of the program is to increase to at least 60 percent the proportion of primary-care providers who provide preconceptional care and counseling.

Preconceptional counseling is preventive medicine for obstetrics. All factors that could potentially affect perinatal outcome are identified, the woman is advised of her risks, and a strategy is provided to reduce or eliminate the pathological influences made evident by her family, medical, or obstetrical history and/or specific testing. The 1989 Public Health Service Expert Panel on the Content of Prenatal Care stated that ''the preconceptional visit may be the single most important health care visit when viewed in the context of its effect on pregnancy.'' This chapter reviews a variety of data confirming that preconceptional counseling has a measurable positive impact on pregnancy outcome, describes the components of preconceptional counseling, and provides specific guidelines for the preconceptional management of a variety of medical, obstetrical, and genetic disorders.

BENEFITS OF PRECONCEPTIONAL COUNSELING

Randomized trials of the efficacy of preconceptional counseling are scarce; furthermore, in many cases, withholding such counseling would be considered unethical. Maternal and perinatal outcomes also are dependent upon the interaction of maternal, fetal, and environmental factors, and it is difficult to ascribe pregnancy outcome to one specific intervention. Nevertheless, there have been several prospective and case-control trials that clearly demonstrate that preconceptional counseling improves pregnancy outcomes.

UNINTENDED PREGNANCY. To be effective, counseling about potential pregnancy risks and strategies to prevent them must be provided before conception. By the time most women realize they are pregnant, 1 to 2 weeks after the first missed period, the fetal spinal cord has already formed and the heart is beating (Moore, 1983). Many prevention strategies, for example, folic acid to prevent neural-tube defects, are ineffective if initiated at this time. The Centers for Disease Control and Prevention (1999) estimates that up to half of all pregnancies are unplanned, and there is evidence that these may be at greatest risk.

Adams and colleagues (1993) conducted a population-based survey of almost 12,500 women in four states and found that women with unintended pregnancies were more likely than those with planned pregnancies to have an indication for preconceptional counseling. Hellerstedt and co-workers (1998) conducted a telephone survey of nearly 7200 pregnant women which showed that women with unintended pregnancies were more likely to have high-risk behaviors such as cigarette smoking and less likely to use vitamins daily. Jack and associates (1995) administered a comprehensive risk survey to 136 women at the time of a negative pregnancy test. The majority did not want to be pregnant, half reported a medical or reproductive risk that could adversely affect pregnancy, half reported a genetic risk, and a fourth reported risks for human immunodeficiency virus (HIV) infection and hepatitis B, as well as alcohol or recreational drug use.

An important measure of the effectiveness of preconceptional counseling is therefore its influence in reducing the number of unintended pregnancies. Moos and colleagues (1996) instituted a preconceptional care program for reproductive-age health department patients in 1985. Of 1378 women presenting for prenatal care, the 456 exposed to preconceptional counseling had a 50 percent greater likelihood of describing their pregnancies as intended when compared with 309 women who had health care but no counseling. They had a 65 percent greater likelihood when compared with women with no health care prior to pregnancy.

CHRONIC MEDICAL DISORDERS

DIABETES. Because maternal and fetal pathology associated with hyperglycemia is well known, diabetes is the prototype of a medical disorder for which preconceptional counseling is beneficial. Diabetes-associated risks to both mother and fetus are discussed in Chapter 51. Many of these complications can be avoided if conception occurs when glucose control is regulated (Jovanovic and colleagues, 1981). Such control requires that glucose control be either chronically well regulated—always a goal, but difficult to achieve—or that the woman make necessary changes before conceiving. Preconceptional counseling educates her about risks, and provides a program designed to reduce these risks before pregnancy.

PERINATAL MORBIDITY AND MORTALITY. The utility of preconceptional counseling in preventing diabetes-related complications at all stages of pregnancy has been confirmed. Figure 9–1 summarizes major studies in which the incidence of fetal anomalies in diabetic women who received preconceptional counseling are compared with the incidence in women who did not. Without exception, all studies showed that counseling is associated with fewer malformations.

Dunne and co-workers (1999) recently reviewed the impact of preconceptional counseling on diabetes-related neonatal morbidity other than birth defects. Women who received preconceptional counseling presented earlier for prenatal care, had lower hemoglobin A_{1c} levels, and were less likely to smoke during pregnancy. These women had no deliveries before 30 weeks compared with 17 percent in the uncounseled group; they had fewer macrosomic infants (25 versus 40 percent); had no growth-restricted infants (versus 8.5 percent); experienced no neonatal deaths (versus 6 percent); and their infants had 50 percent fewer admis-

sions to the intensive care nursery unit than diabetic women without counseling (17 versus 34 percent).

MATERNAL AND ECONOMIC MORBIDITY. Preconceptional counseling reduces obstetrical complications and health-care costs in diabetic women. In a prospective multicenter observational trial from five Michigan centers, Herman and colleagues (1999) confirmed these. Diabetics with counseling reported for prenatal care 3 weeks earlier than uncounseled women, had lower hemoglobin A_{1c} levels, were significantly less likely to require hospitalization for diabetes control during pregnancy (8 versus 68 percent), and required significantly fewer days of hospitalization (4.5 versus 15.7). They were also less likely to have hypoglycemic episodes, they had fewer episodes of diabetic ketoacidosis, they had no hypertensive complications, and their postpartum stay was 2 days shorter. These improved outcomes were associated with savings of $34,000 in direct medical costs per patient who had counseling.

EPILEPSY. Offspring of women with epilepsy are two to three times more likely to have structural anomalies than those of unaffected women; offspring exposed to anticonvulsants are at even higher risk (Chang and McAuley, 1998; Yerby, 1993). These risks are detailed in Chapter 38 (p. 1012). Preconceptional counseling usually includes the recommendation to switch to the least teratogenic drug regimen, or possibly even discontinue medication before conception. The American Academy of Neurology (1998) recommends that reproductive-age epileptic women undergo preconceptional counseling, and that they conceive while taking folic acid and the least teratogenic monotherapeutic antiseizure medication. Biale and Lewenthal (1984) performed a retrospective case-control study evaluating the effects of periconceptional folic acid supplementation in epileptic women taking anticonvulsants. They found that 10 of 66 (15 percent) unsupplemented pregnancies resulted in offspring with congenital malformations, whereas

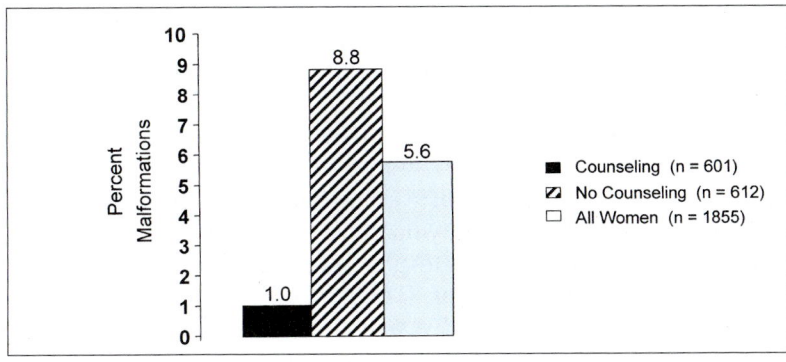

FIGURE 9–1. Major congenital anomalies in diabetic women according to whether they had preconceptional counseling. (Data from Gregory and Tattersall, 1992).

none of 33 neonates of supplemented women had anomalies.

OTHER CHRONIC DISEASES. Cox and co-workers (1992) reviewed subsequent pregnancy outcomes of 1075 couples who received preconceptional counseling. Pregnancy outcomes for 240 women with hypertension, renal disease, thyroid disease, asthma, and heart disease were significantly improved if they had received counseling. Indeed, 80 percent of those counseled gave birth to a normal infant in that pregnancy, compared with 40 percent in the previous gestation.

GENETIC DISEASES. Birth defects are currently the leading cause of infant mortality and account for 20 percent of all infant deaths. These can be avoided with primary, secondary, or tertiary prevention strategies (Czeizel, 1995). The preferred strategy is *primary prevention*—avoidance of causal factors—which is becoming possible for more congenital diseases as their etiologies are discovered. *Secondary prevention*—identifying and terminating affected pregnancies—is an alternate strategy for single-gene disorders and other defects that cannot be prevented. Benefits of preconceptional counseling are usually measured by comparing the incidence of new cases before and after the initiation of a counseling program. A few examples of congenital conditions clearly benefitted by counseling are provided.

NEURAL-TUBE DEFECTS. The incidence of these defects is 1 to 2 per 1000 live births, and they are second only to cardiac anomalies as the most frequent structural fetal malformation (Chap. 36, p. 958). Because some neural-tube defects are related to a specific mutation in the methylene tetrahydrofolate reductase gene (677C→T), the effects can be largely overcome by periconceptional folic acid supplementation (Ou and associates, 1996; van der Put and colleagues, 1995). The Medical Research Council on Vitamin Study Research Group (1991) conducted a randomized double-blind study at 33 centers in seven countries. The result showed that women with a previously affected child who took preconceptional folic acid reduced their recurrence risk by 72 percent. Czeizel and Dudas (1992) subsequently showed that supplementation reduced the *a priori* risk of a first occurrence.

PHENYLKETONURIA (PKU). This disorder is an inborn error of phenylalanine metabolism. It is an example of a disease in which the fetus is not at risk to inherit the disease, but may be damaged by the effects of maternal genetic disease. For such conditions, preconceptional counseling regarding strategies to improve the intrauterine environment constitutes primary prevention and may significantly reduce fetal morbidity. Affected individuals eating an unrestricted diet have abnormally high blood phenylalanine levels. This amino acid readily crosses the placenta to damage developing fetal organs, and neural tissue is particularly vulnerable (Chap. 36, p. 952). With preconceptional counseling, and adherence to a phenylalanine-restricted diet before pregnancy, the incidence of fetal malformations is dramatically reduced (Guttler and colleagues, 1990; Koch and associates, 1990). The Maternal Phenylketonuria Collaborative Study evaluated the effectiveness of preconceptional care in preventing PKU-related fetal defects (Rouse and co-workers, 1997). Almost 300 women with PKU were counseled and began a low phenylalanine diet before pregnancy. Compared with infants whose mothers had poor control, infants of women achieving good control had a lower incidence of microcephaly (6 versus 15 percent), neurological abnormalities (4 versus 14 percent), and cardiac defects (none versus 16 percent). The percentage of women treated preconceptionally increased from 7 to 51 from 1984 to 1994 (Platt and colleagues, 2000).

TAY SACHS DISEASE. This is a severe autosomal recessive neurodegenerative disorder leading to death in childhood. The effectiveness of preconceptional counseling in reducing genetic disease has been most clearly demonstrated in Tay Sachs disease. In the early 1970s, there were approximately 60 new cases in the United States each year, primarily in individuals of Jewish heritage. An intensive worldwide campaign was initiated to counsel Jewish people, to identify carriers through genetic testing, to provide prenatal testing for high-risk couples—secondary prevention, and even to help heterozygote carriers choose unaffected mates—primary prevention! The outcome of this preconceptional counseling initiative has been monitored by the National Tay-Sachs Disease and Allied Disorders Association (Kaback and colleagues, 1993). Within 8 years of its inception, nearly 1 million young adults around the world had been tested and counseled and the incidence of new Tay Sachs cases has plummeted to 3 to 5 new cases per year. Currently, most new cases are in the non-Jewish population.

THALASSEMIAS. Currently, 250 million people—4.5 percent of the world population—carry a gene for a hemoglobinopathy, and 300,000 affected infants are born each year (Angastiniotis and colleagues, 1995). Some of the more important thalassemia syndromes are discussed in Chapter 49 (p. 1321). Some of these could be avoided by both primary and secondary prevention (Fucharoen and associates, 1991; Wong, 1985). In endemic areas such as Mediterranean countries, counseling and other prevention strategies have reduced the incidence of new cases by at least 80 percent (Angastiniotis and Model, 1998). Mitchell and colleagues (1996) summarized experiences of a long-standing counseling program aimed at Montreal high school students at risk. Over 20 years, 25,274 students of Mediterranean origin were counseled and tested for β-thalassemia. Within a few years of initiation of the preconceptional program, all high-risk couples who requested prenatal diagnosis had already been counseled through the program, and no affected children have been born since that time.

PRECONCEPTIONAL COUNSELORS

Practitioners providing routine health maintenance for reproductive-age women have the best opportunity to provide preventive counseling. Gynecologists, internists, family practitioners, and pediatricians can provide counseling at the annual examination. The occasion of a negative pregnancy test is a good time for counseling. Jack and associates (1995) administered a comprehensive preconceptional risk survey to 136 women who had a negative pregnancy test in an ambulatory general practice clinic. Almost 95 percent of these women reported at least one problem which could affect a future pregnancy. Examples include medical or reproductive problems (52 percent), genetic risks (50 percent), risk for human immunodeficiency virus (30 percent), risk for hepatitis B and illegal substances (25 percent), alcohol risk (17 percent), and nutritional risk (54 percent).

Basic preconceptional advice regarding diet, alcohol use, smoking, illicit drug use, vitamin intake, exercise, and other influences can be provided by the primary-care provider, including the obstetrician-gynecologist. The counselor should be knowledgeable about relevant medical diseases or surgery, reproductive disorders, or genetic conditions. Medical records must be obtained if necessary, and the counselor must be able to interpret data provided by other specialists for both the woman and her future progeny. The practitioner who is uncomfortable providing counseling for a complex medical or genetic disorder should refer the woman or couple to a counselor with special expertise.

PATIENT HISTORY

Counseling begins with a thorough review of the medical, obstetrical, social, and family histories. Useful information is more likely obtained with specific questions about each aspect of the history. Such an interview may take 30 minutes to an hour. Some important information can be obtained by questionnaire, ideally at a routine prepregnancy visit. Questionnaires are commercially available which address medical and surgical history; reproductive history, including outcomes of each prior pregnancy; medication use and drug allergies; family history of medical or genetic diseases and reproductive abnormalities; racial or ethnic origin; social risk factors—alcohol, illicit drugs, smoking, high-risk sexual behavior, and spousal abuse; environmental risk factors—such as exposure to pesticides or dry-cleaning chemicals; and home environment and stress inducers. Answers are reviewed with the patient so that necessary follow-up is done by obtaining appropriate medical records or by consulting family members.

While most patients can provide some information regarding their history, their understanding may be limited. Maternal reports of familial genetic abnormalities may be especially inaccurate. Several studies have shown that women often fail to report a birth defect in the family or report it incorrectly. Romitti and associates (1997) interviewed 345 women who had a relative with a birth defect and 380 women without such a history. They verified their responses about family history by contacting relatives. Only 30 percent of all of these women correctly reported birth defects history. Rasmussen and colleagues (1990) used the Atlanta Birth Defects Registry to identify 4929 women whose child had a verified birth defect. When contacted, only 60 percent accurately reported the defect. It is thus important to verify the type of reported defect by reviewing pertinent medical records. The woman or couple is also asked to contact her affected relatives for additional information.

REPRODUCTIVE HISTORY. Reproductive history includes previous attempts at conception, any infertility, and abnormal pregnancy outcomes including miscarriage, ectopic pregnancy, or recurrent pregnancy loss. Reproductive history of first-degree relatives may also be helpful—for example, with recurrent pregnancy loss, other family members with the same history increases the risk of a familial translocation or another chromosome rearrangement. History suggesting incompetent cervix or uterine anomaly should prompt the appropriate evaluation.

The need for assisted reproductive technologies to become pregnant is noted. For example, as discussed in Chapter 36, preliminary data suggest that intracytoplasmic sperm injection (ICSI) is associated with certain poor outcomes (Bowen and colleagues, 1998). Cryopreservation of embryos may also slightly increase risks.

Risk factors for recurrent preterm delivery, preeclampsia, placental abruption, and repeat cesarean delivery are summarized elsewhere in this book, along with suggestions for their prevention.

SOCIAL HISTORY

MATERNAL AGE. At both ends of the reproductive years, maternal age impacts pregnancy outcome.

TEENAGE PREGNANCY. According to the National Center for Health Statistics (Smith and colleagues, 1999), women between ages 15 and 19 account for about 13 percent of all births. Teenagers are more likely to be anemic, and are at increased risk to have growth-restricted infants, preterm labor, and a higher infant mortality (Fraser and associates, 1995). Because most teen pregnancies are unplanned, they rarely present for preconceptional counseling. Counseling in early pregnancy can still be helpful. Teenagers are usually still growing and developing, and thus have greater caloric requirements than older women. The normal or underweight teenager should be advised to increase caloric intake by 400 kcal/day. Nonjudgmental questioning may elicit a history of substance abuse. As with all good prenatal care, common complications are reviewed.

PREGNANCY AFTER 35. Currently, about 10 percent of pregnancies occur in women in this age group. The older woman is more likely to request preconceptional counseling, either because she has postponed pregnancy and now wishes to optimize her outcome, or she does so prior to infertility treatment. In the past, the indelicate term *elderly gravida* was used to arbitrarily define women over 35. Although hopefully the term has been discarded, the occurrence of certain age-related adverse pregnancy outcomes do begin increasing at this age.

Early studies suggested that women over 35 are at increased risk for obstetrical complications as well as perinatal morbidity and mortality. For the older woman who has a chronic illness or who is in poor physical condition, these risks likely are valid. For the normal weight, physically fit woman without medical problems, however, the risks are much lower than previously reported.

The importance of socioeconomic and health status is illustrated by two studies of pregnancy outcome in different populations of older women. Berkowitz and co-workers (1990) described outcomes of almost 800 private-patient nulliparas over 35 whom they cared for at Mount Sinai Hospital in New York City. They reported only slightly increased risks for gestational diabetes, pregnancy-induced hypertension, placenta previa or abruption, and cesarean delivery. These women did not have an increased risk for preterm delivery, growth-restricted infants, or perinatal death. In contrast, our observations from Parkland Hospital (Cunningham and Leveno, 1995) of nearly 900 women over 35 showed a significantly increased incidence of hypertension, diabetes, abruption, preterm delivery, stillbirth, and placenta previa (Fig. 9–2). Not surprisingly, this group also had higher perinatal mortality rates. The disparate outcomes in these two groups of women likely is attributable to socioeconomic status, which influences access to health care and health status.

Some pregnancy outcomes in older women may be influenced by parity; for example, labor abnormalities are more common in older nulliparas. Bobrowski and Bottoms (1995) reviewed pregnancy outcomes in 8746 women and found that both age and parity influenced the incidence of diabetes, labor disorders, and cesarean delivery.

Maternal mortality is higher in women age 35 and older, but improved medical care may ameliorate this risk. Buehler and colleagues (1986) reviewed maternal deaths in the United States from 1974 through 1982. From 1974 through 1978, older women had a fivefold increased relative risk of maternal death compared with younger women. By 1982, however, the mortality rates for older women had decreased by 50 percent. They concluded that this was probably due to improvements in health care.

Maternal age-related fetal risks stem from iatrogenic preterm delivery required for some maternal complications that include hypertension and diabetes, from spontaneous preterm delivery, and from an increased incidence of aneuploidy. Although most researchers have found that maternal age significantly influences only the incidence of aneuploidy, our observations suggest otherwise. Hollier and colleagues (2000) studied 3885 infants with congenital malformations in nearly 103,000 pregnancies at Parkland Hospital. As shown in Figure 9–3, the risk for all nonchromosomal abnormalities increased significantly with maternal age. Club foot was increased significantly after 35 and heart disease after 40. In addition, increased paternal age is associated with increased birth defects due to new autosomal dominant mutations (Chap. 36, p. 951). Finally, while dizygotic twinning increases with maternal age, the most important cause of multiple gestation in these women currently is infertility treatment.

RECREATIONAL DRUGS AND SMOKING. Fetal risks associated with alcohol, marijuana, cocaine, amphetamines, and heroin are discussed in Chapter 38. Alcohol-related mental retardation is currently the only mental retardation syndrome amenable to primary prevention. The key to preventing this and other types of drug-related fetal damage is to have the woman provide an honest assessment of her usage. Questions should be nonjudgmental. The alcoholic can be identified by asking the well-studied TACE questions, which correlate with DSM-III-R criteria for lifetime alcohol diagnoses (Chang and associates, 1998). This is a series of four questions concerning: *tolerance* to alcohol, being *annoyed* by comments about their drinking, attempts to *cut down,* and a history of drinking early in the morning—the *eye opener.*

Smoking affects fetal growth in a dose-dependent

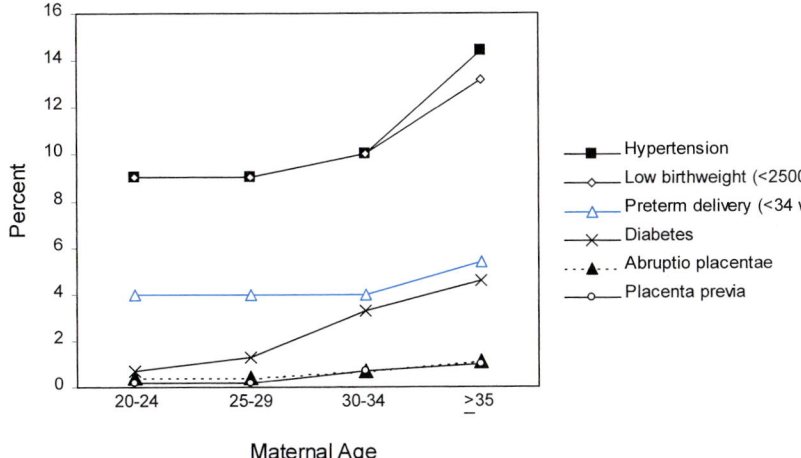

FIGURE 9–2. Incidence of some pregnancy complications in 20,525 women delivered at Parkland Hospital in 1987–1988. (Data from Cunningham and Leveno, 1995).

manner. It increases risks for preterm labor, fetal-growth restriction, and low birthweight as well as attention deficit hyperactivity disorder (ADHD) and behavioral and learning problems when school-age is reached (American College of Obstetricians and Gynecologists, 1999). It also increases the risk of pregnancy complications related to vascular insufficiency, such as uteroplacental insufficiency and placental abruption (Chap. 25, p. 621). The extent of cigarette use should be determined and the woman provided with a prepregnancy program to reduce or eliminate smoking.

ENVIRONMENTAL EXPOSURES. While everyone is exposed to environmental substances, only a few increase pregnancy risk. These exposures include infectious organisms—for example, neonatal nurses have potential exposure to cytomegalovirus or respiratory syncytial virus, and day-care workers may be exposed to parvovirus and rubella. Pregnant industrial workers may be exposed to chemicals such as heavy metals or organic solvents. Patients living in rural areas may be exposed to potentially harmful chemicals through pesticide use or contaminated well water. When harmful prenatal

exposure is likely, the woman planning conception should remove herself from the agent before conception and throughout gestation.

LIFESTYLE AND WORK HABITS. A number of personal and work habits and lifestyle issues may have an impact on pregnancy outcome.

DIET. Pica for ice, laundry starch, or clay and dirt is often associated with anemia. Many vegetarian diets are protein deficient, but can be corrected by increasing egg and cheese consumption. As discussed in Chapter 48 (p. 1298), **obesity** is associated with a number of maternal complications such as hypertension, preeclampsia, gestational diabetes, thrombophlebitis, labor abnormalities, postterm pregnancy, cesarean delivery, and operative complications (Wolfe, 1998). It is also associated with adverse fetal outcome. Cnattingius and co-workers (1998) evaluated 167,750 women in Sweden and found that those with a body mass index over 30 were at increased risk for late fetal death and preterm delivery before 32 weeks. Waller and colleagues (1994) have shown that offspring of obese women are at increased

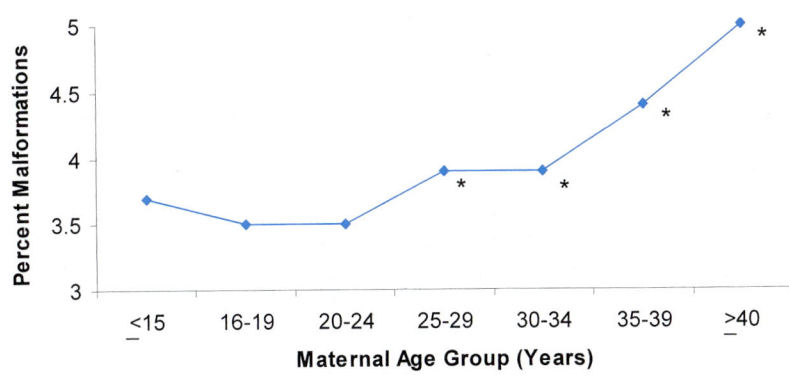

FIGURE 9–3. Rate of nonchromosomal abnormalities by maternal-age grouping in 102,728 pregnancies at Parkland Hospital. Data points with asterisk (*) are significantly different (P ≤ 0.03) from the referent 20 to 24 year age group. (Data from Hollier and colleagues, 2000).

risk for spina bifida, ventral wall defects, and intestinal malformations.

In addition to nutritional deficiencies, **anorexia** and **bulimia** increase the risk for associated problems such as electrolyte disturbances, cardiac arrhythmias, and gastrointestinal pathology (Becker and associates, 1999). In a study of 23 pregnancies in 15 women previously treated for anorexia nervosa or bulimia, Stewart and colleagues (1987) reported that those whose anorexia was not in remission at the time of conception had worsening of symptoms during pregnancy. They also gained less weight and had lighter infants.

EXERCISE. There are no data to suggest that exercise is deleterious during pregnancy. Most pregnant women can continue to exercise throughout gestation, although their prepregnancy routine may need to be altered. For example, pregnancy may cause balance problems and joint relaxation may predispose to orthopedic injury. The American College of Obstetricians and Gynecologists (1994) guidelines for exercise in pregnancy are shown in Table 9–1.

DOMESTIC ABUSE. Pregnancy can exacerbate interpersonal problems. There is increased risk from an abusive partner during pregnancy. As discussed in Chapter 43 (p. 1171), one in six women is abused during pregnancy (Eisenstat and Bancroft, 1999). The interviewer should inquire about risk factors for domestic violence, and should offer intervention as appropriate. Abuse is more likely in women whose partners abuse alcohol or drugs, are recently unemployed, and have a poor education or low income, and a history of arrest (Grisso and colleagues, 1999; Kyriacou and associates, 1999).

FAMILY HISTORY. The most thorough method for obtaining such a history is to construct a pedigree using symbols shown in Figure 9–4. The health and reproductive status of these "blood relatives" are reviewed for medical illnesses, mental retardation, birth defects, infertility, and pregnancy loss. Certain racial, ethnic, or religious backgrounds may indicate increased risk for certain recessive disorders. Family histories are not always accurate, but any concerns should be verified.

CHRONIC MEDICAL DISEASES

Preconceptional counseling should address historical risk factors for both mother and fetus. General questions to be answered include how pregnancy will affect maternal health, and how the high-risk condition will affect the fetus. Almost any medical, obstetrical, or genetic condition warrants some consideration prior to pregnancy. These conditions are discussed in general terms of maternal and fetal risk, suggestions for prepregnancy evaluation are offered, and counseling advice is provided. More detailed information on each disease, as well as other diseases not mentioned, are found elsewhere in this book.

DIABETES. Substantive risks to mother and fetus are increased with overt diabetes (Chap. 51). Maternal risks include retinal, renal, and cardiac damage, urinary infec-

---

TABLE 9–1. **Exercise Guidelines for Pregnancy and the Postpartum Period**

1. During pregnancy, women can continue to exercise and derive health benefit even from mild to moderate exercise routines. Regular exercise at least three times per week is preferable to intermittent activity.

2. Women should avoid exercise in the supine position. This position is associated with decreased cardiac output in most pregnant women because the remaining cardiac output is preferentially distributed away from splanchnic beds (including the uterus) during vigorous exercise. Prolonged periods of motionless standing should also be avoided.

3. Women should be aware of the decreased oxygen available for aerobic exercise during pregnancy. They should be encouraged to modify exercise intensity according to symptoms. Pregnant women should stop exercising when fatigued and not exercise to exhaustion. Weight-bearing exercises may under some circumstances be continued at intensities similar to those before pregnancy. Non–weight-bearing exercises, such as cycling or swimming, minimize the risk of injury and facilitate continuation of exercise.

4. Morphological changes in pregnancy should serve as a relative contraindication to types of exercise in which loss of balance could be detrimental to maternal or fetal well-being, especially in the third trimester. Any type of exercise involving the potential for even mild abdominal trauma should be avoided.

5. Pregnancy requires an additional 300 kcal/d to maintain metabolic homeostasis. Thus, women who exercise during pregnancy should be particularly careful to ensure an adequate diet.

6. Pregnant women who exercise in the first trimester should augment heat dissipation by ensuring adequate hydration, appropriate clothing, and optimal environmental surroundings.

7. Many of the physiological and morphological changes of pregnancy persist 4 to 6 weeks postpartum. Thus, prepregnancy exercise routines should be resumed gradually and based on physical capability.

Adapted from the American College of Obstetricians and Gynecologists (1994), with permission.

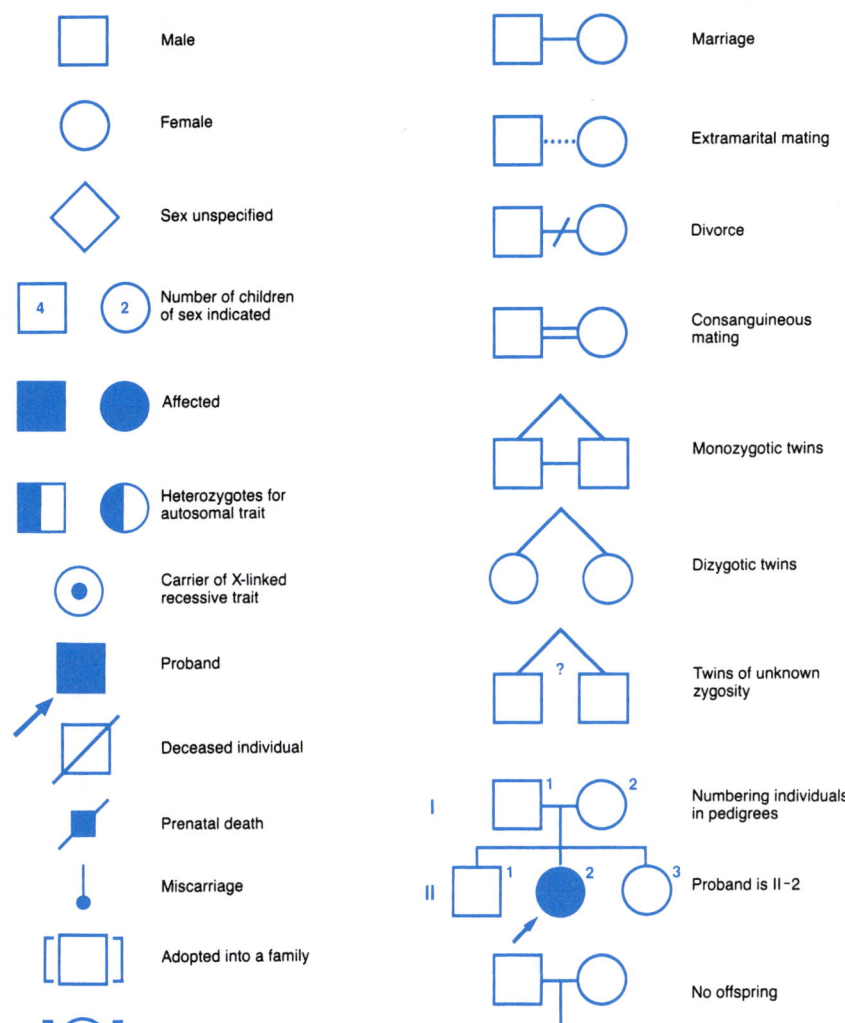

Male	Marriage
Female	Extramarital mating
Sex unspecified	Divorce
Number of children of sex indicated	Consanguineous mating
Affected	Monozygotic twins
Heterozygotes for autosomal trait	Dizygotic twins
Carrier of X-linked recessive trait	Twins of unknown zygosity
Proband	Numbering individuals in pedigrees
Deceased individual	Proband is II-2
Prenatal death	
Miscarriage	
Adopted into a family	No offspring
Adopted out of a family	

FIGURE 9–4. Symbols used for pedigree construction. (From Thompson and colleagues, 1991, with permission).

tions, diabetic ketoacidosis, and cesarean delivery. Hypertension is common and the diabetic woman with renal disease is at especially high risk for preeclampsia. Fetal risks include increased perinatal mortality, a variety of malformations, growth disturbances, iatrogenic preterm delivery, and neonatal metabolic instability. The embryo is particularly susceptible to teratogenic effects of hyperglycemia, and many malformations occur early before pregnancy is recognized (Reece and Hobbins, 1986). Neural-tube defects and cardiac and renal anomalies occur two to five times more often in diabetic pregnancies (American Diabetes Association, 1995). Sacral agenesis and holoprosencephaly are rare malformations that are seen commonly in the fetuses of severely diabetic women (Barr and colleagues, 1983; Passarge and co-workers, 1966).

Because poor glucose control early in pregnancy may be teratogenic, the prepregnancy visit should include a review of diabetic control and provocative factors.

Baseline glucose control and end-organ damage should be assessed to include renal and cardiac function and retinopathy. Counseling is provided concerning effects of poor control on fetal malformations as estimated from hemoglobin A_{1c} levels (Table 9–2). Pregnancy outcome risks in women with renal involvement are discussed later. In most cases of advanced renal insufficiency, pregnancy should be postponed until kidney transplantation.

The important elements of the preconceptional visit have been summarized by the American Diabetes Association (1996) and include an emphasis on patient education. Glucose control is achieved with diet, exercise, and insulin. Until very recently, oral hypoglycemic agents were not recommended and women planning pregnancy usually switch to insulin 2 to 3 months before conception. Folic acid in a dose of 400 μg/day should be ingested prior to conception, and if there is personal or family history of neural-tube defects then 4 mg/day is prescribed.

TABLE 9–2. Relationship of First-Trimester Glycosylated Hemoglobin to Major Congenital Anomalies in 320 Insulin-Dependent Diabetic Women

Glycohemoglobin (%)	Major Anomalies (%)
4.6–7.6	1.9
7.7–8.6	1.7
8.7–9.9	6.3
10–10.5	9.1
>10.6	25

From Kitzmiller and colleagues (1991).

RENAL DISEASE. Exacerbation of renoprival hypertension, along with superimposed preeclampsia, are concerns for women with any form of renal disease. As discussed in Chapter 47 (p. 1262), although controversial whether pregnancy increases renal damage or hastens permanent dysfunction, it appears more likely with severe disease. Jones and Hayslett (1996) analyzed 82 pregnancies in 67 women and found that a third of those whose serum creatinine was higher than 2 mg/dL had an accelerated decline in renal function during pregnancy. As shown in Table 9–3, there is evidence that some forms of renal disease have a worse prognosis for pregnancy. These are discussed in more detail in Chapter 47.

Regarding fetal risks, there may be associated vascular dysfunction that predisposes to growth restriction, preterm delivery, and perinatal mortality and morbidity. Worsening hypertension or superimposed preeclampsia increase the risk of iatrogenic preterm delivery. Angiotensin-converting enzyme inhibitors are associated with fetal renal tubular dysgenesis and renal failure (Chap. 38, p. 1014). The best predictor of perinatal outcome is the serum creatinine level (Table 9–4).

If pregnancy is planned, angiotensin-converting enzyme inhibitors should be discontinued and hypertension controlled with other drugs considered safe in pregnancy (Chap. 45, p. 1217). Women with severe or end-stage renal disease may choose to await renal transplantation before considering pregnancy.

HYPERTENSION. Although usually not as significant, risks for adverse pregnancy outcomes with chronic hypertension are similar to those for renal disease. Hypertension may worsen during pregnancy, with increased maternal morbidity. The need for additional drug therapy and iatrogenic preterm delivery also is increased. These risks generally parallel the degree of hypertension, and pregnancy-associated risks are discussed in Chapter 45 (p. 1212). In general, evaluation is done to search for obvious causes of hypertension. Renal and cardiac functions are assessed. Although most women have essential hypertension, a correctable cause will occasionally be discovered and ideally treated before conception. In many cases, obesity is a co-factor that can be altered by weight loss. Other benefits accrue

TABLE 9–3. Pregnancy Outcomes Associated with Specific Chronic Renal Diseases

Renal Disease	Effects
Chronic glomerulonephritis and focal glomerulosclerosis	There may be an increased incidence of hypertension late in gestation, but unusually no adverse affects if renal function is preserved and hypertension absent before gestation. Some disagree, believing that coagulation changes of pregnancy exacerbate these diseases, especially IgA nephropathy, focal glomerulosclerosis, and membranoproliferative glomerulonephritis.
Systemic lupus erythematosus	Expect more problems than most glomerular diseases, but prognosis is most favorable if disease is in remission for at least 6 months before conception.
Periarteritis nodosa and scleroderma	Associated with maternal deaths; reactivation of quiescent scleroderma can occur during pregnancy and postpartum; therapeutic abortion should be considered. Fetal prognosis is poor.
Diabetic nephropathy	Pregnancy does not accelerate functional loss; increased covert bacteriuria; high incidence of heavy proteinuria and hypertension late in gestation.
Chronic pyelonephritis (tubulointerstitial disease)	Bacteriuria in pregnancy may lead to acute exacerbations, but otherwise is well tolerated.
Polycystic disease	There is controversy concerning whether functional impairment, often minimal in childbearing years, is accelerated by pregnancy.
Urolithiasis	Ureteral dilatation and stasis do not seem to affect natural history; infections are more frequent; stents have been successfully placed during gestation.
Previous urological surgery	Depending on indication, other urogenital tract malformations may be present, urinary infections increase, and functional decrements have been observed. Cesarean delivery may be necessary to avoid disruption of the continence mechanism if artificial sphincters or neourethras are present.

From Lindheimer and colleagues (2000), with permission.

TABLE 9–4. Relationship of Chronic Renal Insufficiency with Pregnancy Outcome (in Percent)

Outcome	Serum Creatinine (mg/dL)		
	Mild (< 1.5)	Moderate (< 1.5–3.0)	Severe (≥ 3.0)
Preterm birth	13	50	100
Perinatal death	5	17	33
Fetal-growth restriction	10	20	100
Abortion[a]	11	21	25
Surviving infants	84	62	50

[a]Includes spontaneous miscarriage and induced abortion.
Data from Cunningham, 1990; Hou, 1985; Imbasciati, 1986; Jungers, 1986; Katz, 1980, and all their co-workers.

from weight loss, and in addition to reduced blood pressure, there is reduced ventricular mass, incidence of hyperinsulinemia, diabetes, and hypertriglyceridemia (Himeno and associates, 1999; Sjostrom and co-workers, 1999).

EPILEPSY. The most important pregnancy-associated risk to the epileptic woman is increased seizure activity. This is discussed in Chapter 53 (p. 1408). Most studies cite increased seizures in about a third of women during pregnancy. These may be related to reduced drug levels resulting from physiological changes of pregnancy with increased volume of distribution. The most important change appears to be increased drug clearance from induction of hepatic, plasma, and placental enzymes, along with significantly increased glomerular filtration rate. Moreover, nausea and vomiting causes skipped doses while pain and hyperventilation in labor lower the seizure threshold. A preventable cause of increased seizure activity is self-discontinuation of medication in the belief that the medication could harm the fetus. Counseling and preconceptional change in medication can prevent this. The woman is advised that seizures increase her risk of trauma. There is some evidence that uncontrolled seizures, often with associated hypoxia and hypotension, cause lesions in the cerebellum and hippocampus with degeneration of Purkinje cells, leading to the development of new seizure foci.

Offspring of epileptic women are at increased risk to have structural malformations. Although a portion of the risk is related to epilepsy itself, the majority of malformations are related to antiepileptic drugs as discussed in detail in Chapter 38 (p. 1012). Seizures during pregnancy may cause a transient reduction in uterine blood flow and fetal oxygenation. Maternal trauma during a seizure also increases fetal risk. Offspring of epileptic women are at increased risk to develop a seizure disorder (Annegers and co-workers, 1976). Women with fe-

brile convulsions as children are more likely to have children with that disorder. Finally, offspring of fathers with seizure disorders, however, are not at increased risk.

COUNSELING. The activity of the seizure disorder is assessed to determine whether antiepileptic medication is needed. If so, the lowest possible effective dose of the least teratogenic single agent is prescribed. In general, the woman taking monotherapy who has been free of seizures for at least 2 years is a candidate for discontinuing medication. A trial of stopping therapy is done in conjunction with a neurologist and is generally not recommended once the woman is pregnant. Up to two thirds of nonpregnant patients who stopped monotherapy remained seizure free for a mean of 35 months (Callaghan and colleagues, 1988).

CARDIAC DISEASE

CONGENITAL HEART DISEASE. With advances in neonatal care and surgical techniques, women with a wide variety of congenital cardiac abnormalities are surviving to reproductive age and many become pregnant. Individual anomalies and their effects on pregnancy are discussed in detail in Chapter 44. Counseling is addressed on a case-by-case basis. The risk of death should be estimated according to the nature of the cardiac disease and the functional cardiac status. Pregnancy-associated mortality correlates loosely with the type of cardiac lesion (see Table 44–3, p. 1184). Women with pulmonary hypertension of any etiology, complicated aortic coarctation, or Marfan syndrome with aortic involvement have a mortality risk sufficient to warrant recommendation against pregnancy.

CYANOTIC HEART DISEASE. These lesions pose the greatest risk in pregnancy of all congenital heart defects. Affected women are at increased risk to develop heart failure, thrombotic complications, arrhythmias, and infections. Maternal mortality and fetal morbidity and mortality rates are significantly increased. Sawhney and colleagues (1998) cited 14 percent stillbirths and 37 percent growth-restricted fetuses. Women with primary pulmonary hypertension or Eisenmenger syndrome have the highest mortality rate, which is 40 to 50 percent. Only 15 percent have liveborns at term (Weiss and Atanassoff, 1993; Yentis and co-workers, 1998).

Presbitero and colleagues (1994) reviewed 822 pregnancies in 416 women with cyanotic heart disease, excluding Eisenmenger syndrome. The perinatal prognosis with some of these lesions is summarized in Table 9–5. Only 43 percent of pregnancies resulted in live births and 37 percent of those were delivered preterm. Some important predictors of fetal outcome are also listed in Table 9–5.

TABLE 9–5. Predictors of Fetal Outcome in 816 Pregnancies Complicated by Maternal Cyanotic Heart Disease

Predictor	Specifics	Liveborn (%)
Lesion	Single ventricle and/or tricuspid atresia	31
	Tetralogy of Fallot or pulmonary atresia	33
	Ebstein anomaly, atrial septal defect	86
	Corrected TCA, VSD, and pulmonary stenosis	60
Hemoglobin (g/dL)	≤ 16	71
	17–19	45
	≥ 20	8
Arterial oxygen saturation (%)	≤ 85	12
	85–89	45
	≥ 90	92
Maternal age	≤ 23	35
	24–27	40
	≥ 28	45
Shunt	Yes	51
	No	35

TCA = tricuspid atresia; VSD = ventricular septal defect.
Adapted from Presbitero and colleagues (1994), with permission.

ABNORMALITIES REQUIRING ANTICOAGULATION. A number of cardiac conditions discussed in Chapter 44 require anticoagulation because of increased risk for thromboembolic events. The most common is mechanical valve placement. When the woman is not pregnant, warfarin anticoagulation is generally preferred; however, these derivatives are teratogenic (Chap. 38, p. 1014). If possible, the woman attempting pregnancy should be switched to heparin therapy. Excessive anticoagulation increases the risk for bleeding complications and failure to achieve adequate anticoagulation is associated with prosthetic valve thrombosis.

COUNSELING. Cardiac function is carefully evaluated with standard methods, including echocardiography and coronary angiography and radionuclide studies if necessary. Surgical records are reviewed, and all medications evaluated for fetal safety. If possible, warfarin is discontinued. In the case of a congenital defect, a pedigree should be obtained to define the fetal risk. Women with a significant risk of mortality should be advised to reconsider pregnancy. If the woman is a potential candidate for cardiac transplantation, she may wish to reconsider pregnancy until this is accomplished. In all cases, the condition is optimized, and cardiovascular training is instituted.

THROMBOEMBOLISM. There is an increased risk of recurrent thromboembolism during pregnancy (Chap. 46, p. 1240). An exact risk is difficult to provide, but it may be as high as 10 percent (American College of Obstetricians and Gynecologists, 2000; Tengborn and colleagues, 1985). Some factors modify the risk of thromboembolism. For example, women over age 35 have a twofold increased incidence compared with younger women (Greer, 1999). This may be related to the development of venous insufficiency after the first event (Bergqvist and colleagues, 1990). Older women who smoke more likely have cigarette-induced vascular damage. Older women are more likely obese and this too increases the risk for recurrence (McCall and co-workers, 1997). A risk factor of great importance is a family history of thromboembolic events which may suggest the possibility of hereditary thrombophilia as discussed next.

THROMBOPHILIAS. Most of these disorders are inherited anticoagulation deficiencies that include protein C or protein S deficiency, antithrombin III deficiency, activated protein C resistance (factor V Leiden mutation), hyperhomocystinemia (methylene tetrahydrofolate reductase mutation), and the prothrombin 20210G→A mutation. In addition, acquired coagulation defects include antiphospholipid antibodies to include the lupus anticoagulant and anticardiolipin antibodies. These are discussed in greater detail in Chapters 46 (p. 1234) and 52 (p. 1390).

Briefly, a wide variety of pregnancy complications may occur in these women. In addition to arterial and venous thromboembolism leading to pulmonary embolism and cerebral infarction, there is a greater risk of abortion, early preeclampsia, fetal-growth restriction, and stillbirth. The prevalence and risks for thromboem-

TABLE 9–6. Hereditary Thrombophilias

			Risk of Thromboembolism		
Abnormality	Prevalence	Relative Risk	Antepartum	Postpartum
Protein C deficiency	1/500 Heterozygote[a]	7.3	8–10%	7–19%
Protein S deficiency	Heterozygote	8.5	0–6%	7–22%
Antithrombin-III deficiency	1.5/1000 Heterozygote[a]	8.1	2–3%	
Activated protein C resistance (factor V Leiden)	3–5/1000 Tremendous regional and ethnic variation	2.2	14% symptomatic families	Probably > 14%
Prothrombin (20210G→A)	1.2–2.6/1000	—		

[a]Homozygosity is usually lethal.
Data from Greer (1999) and Martinelli and colleagues (1998).

bolism for some of these thrombophilias are listed in Table 9–6. This risk data should be considered preliminary because much of them were derived from high-risk families.

The woman with a history of thromboembolism and an associated inherited thrombophilia should be counseled considering her increased risk of recurrence, and that pregnancy may complicate attempts at prophylaxis. She is counseled also about lifelong risks and the possibility of chronic prophylaxis. Many nonpregnant women taking prophylaxis are given warfarin; as discussed earlier, this is teratogenic and heparin substituted if possible when pregnancy is attempted.

CONNECTIVE-TISSUE DISEASES. These disorders include systemic lupus erythematosus, rheumatoid arthritis, ankylosing spondylitis, Sjögren's syndrome, and scleroderma. They are autoimmune collagen-vascular disorders that are discussed in greater detail in Chapter 52. Pregnancy-associated risks for each disorder vary widely in severity and range from minimal to life threatening. For example, rheumatoid arthritis usually improves during pregnancy; however, 90 percent of women experience a relapse within 6 months of delivery (Ostensen, 1999). Women with ankylosing spondylitis often have increased back pain resulting from weight gain and lordosis, but otherwise do well. Lupus tends to be more serious and may have adverse effects on both mother and fetus.

Complications are higher for women with long-standing disease, nephritis, hypertension, antiphospholipid antibodies, and a previous pregnancy loss (Meng and Lockshin, 1999; Ostensen, 1999). Flares result in worsening hypertension and proteinuria. With scleroderma, symptoms from Raynaud phenomenon may improve during pregnancy, but esophageal reflux from hypomo-

tility usually gets worse. Women with diffuse scleroderma are at increased risk to have renal involvement and hypertension that is severe (Steen, 1999). Women with the lupus anticoagulant or anticardiolipin antibody have the worst outcomes. Anti-Ro antibody (anti SS-A) is associated with neonatal lupus—which generally resolves within the first year of life, and congenital heart block—which is permanent and has significant morbidity. If the woman has already had a child with congenital heart block, the recurrence risk approximates 15 percent (Meng and Lockshin, 1999). Maternal complications, especially severe hypertension and renal disease, increase the occurrence of adverse perinatal outcomes.

COUNSELING. The clinical course is carefully reviewed. Organ damage is assessed, specifically, renal function. The prognosis for women with significant renal disease is based on the degree of renal insufficiency as shown in Tables 9–3 and 9–4. Many medications commonly prescribed for collagen-vascular disorders, for example, corticosteroids, nonsteroidal anti-inflammatory agents, and analgesics, pose no increased fetal risk. In severe cases, potent immunosuppressive agents may be used, and although most are not believed to endanger the fetus, there are theoretical concerns about their safety (Chap. 38, p. 1029). Angiotensin-converting enzyme inhibitors may be teratogenic and are discontinued in the woman attempting pregnancy.

PSYCHIATRIC DISORDERS. Pregnancy can be stressful to any woman. It is not surprising that it increases the risk of relapse or return of dysphoric symptoms (Chap. 53, p. 1420). Some relapses are due to self-discontinuation of medication in the belief that it is harmful to the fetus. Symptoms also may be influenced by fluctuating hormone levels, increased stress, and disruption of eating and sleeping patterns as well as other normal activities. Inadequate prenatal care and co-existing substance abuse also play a role (Kelly and colleagues, 1999). The risk of severe postpartum depression or psychosis is especially increased in women with preexisting psychiatric disorders. Up to 15 percent of these women experience symptoms of depression in the first 3 months after delivery, and postpartum psychosis occurs in 1 to 2 per 1000 (Pederson, 1999). The incidence of postpartum psychosis in women with bipolar disorder is as high as 25 percent. Women who experienced postpartum psychosis in a previous pregnancy have a recurrence risk of 50 to 75 percent (Pederson, 1999). Women with a history of major depression, premenstrual syndrome, or previous *postpartum blues* are also at increased risk (Pariser and co-workers, 1997). Conversely, pregnancy does not appear to increase the risk of relapse in schizophrenia (Robinson and collaborators, 1999).

FETAL RISK. In general, the wide variety of psychiatric medications have not been associated with major birth defects or developmental fetal abnormalities (Chap. 38, p. 1026). Several types of mental illness are heritable. While the average lifetime risk of developing schizophrenia is 0.8 percent, children with one schizophrenic parent have a 12 percent risk; those with two schizophrenic parents have a 40 percent risk; siblings of schizophrenics have a 10 percent risk (Kinney, 1997). The average lifetime risk of bipolar disorder is estimated to be 0.5 to 1.0 percent (McInnis and DePaulo, 1997). If either parent has bipolar disorder, the risk for the offspring increases to 15 percent (McInnis and DePaulo, 1997). This may be higher if the mother was affected (McMahon and colleagues, 1995). Offspring of parents with affective disorders are also at risk for attention deficit hyperactivity disorder (Smith and co-workers, 1997).

COUNSELING. Close coordination with the psychiatric counselor is helpful when the woman with a major mental disorder wants to attempt pregnancy. The clinical course is reviewed, including an assessment of all medications. A pedigree may allow an assessment of fetal risk for mental illness. Confounding factors such as alcohol, drug, or cigarette abuse; social problems; or other medical illnesses are considered. When medication is needed, the woman is placed on the drug(s) with the fewest associated risks and at the lowest efficacious dose.

GENETIC DISEASES. Women whose ethnic background, race, or personal or family history place them at increased risk to have a fetus with a genetic disease should receive appropriate counseling. This includes the possibility of prenatal diagnosis (see Chapters 36 and 37). Women who have a genetic disease usually require

additional counseling about their own risks, as genetic conditions are often associated with unique medical problems which may be adversely affected by pregnancy or which can adversely affect pregnancy outcome. Such women should be counseled by someone knowledgeable about genetics and about the effects of pregnancy on the genetic disease in question. They often benefit from consultation with other specialists—for example, anesthesiologists, cardiologists, or surgeons. A variety of genetic resources can be accessed for detailed information about many inherited disorders.

IMMUNIZATIONS. Preconceptional counseling includes assessment of immunity to rubella and hepatitis B. Depending on health status, travel plans, and time of year, other immunizations may be in order (see Table 10–9, p. 92). Vaccines consist of either toxoids (tetanus); killed bacteria or viruses (influenza, pneumococcus, hepatitis B, meningococcus, rabies); or attenuated live viruses (measles, mumps, polio, rubella, chickenpox, yellow fever). Immunization during pregnancy with toxoids or killed bacteria or viruses has not been associated with adverse fetal outcomes (Chutivongse and colleagues, 1995; Czeizel and co-workers, 1999). Alternatively, live virus vaccines are not recommended during pregnancy, and should ideally be given at least 3 months before attempts to conceive. Women inadvertently given measles, mumps, rubella, or chickenpox vaccines during pregnancy, however, are not necessarily advised to seek pregnancy termination. Most reports indicate that immunizations to these agents pose only a theoretical risk to the fetus (Centers for Disease Control, 1989).

DIAGNOSTIC RADIATION EXPOSURE. Many women seek early postconceptional counseling because of inadvertent x-ray exposure. As discussed in Chapter 42 (p. 1150), there is no evidence that diagnostic radiation increases the risk of adverse outcomes for the fetus or for the child, including through adulthood (Boice and Miller, 1999; Doll and Wakeford, 1997).

ELECTROMAGNETIC ENERGY. There is no evidence in humans or animals that exposure to various electromagnetic fields such as high-voltage power lines, electric blankets, microwave ovens, and cellular phones causes adverse fetal effects (O'Connor, 1999; Robert, 1999). This is discussed further in Chapter 44.

REFERENCES

Adams MM, Bruce FC, Shulman HB, Kendrick JS, Brogan DJ, The Prams Working Group: Pregnancy planning and pre-conception counseling. Obstet Gynecol 82:955, 1993

American Academy of Neurology: Practice parameter: Management issues for women with epilepsy (summary statement). Report of the Quality Standards Subcommittee of the American Academy of Neurology. Epilepsia 39:1226, 1998

American College of Obstetricians and Gynecologists: Thromboembolism in pregnancy. ACDG Practice Bulletin No. 19, August 2000

American College of Obstetricians and Gynecologists: Psychosocial risk factors: Perinatal screening and interaction. ACOG Educational Bulletin No. 255, November 1999

American College of Obstetricians and Gynecologists: Exercise during pregnancy and the postpartum period. ACOG Technical Bulletin No. 189, February 1994

American Diabetes Association: Preconception care of women with diabetes. Diabetes Care 19:25, 1996

American Diabetes Association: Medical management of pregnancy complicated by diabetes, 2nd ed. [Jovanovic-Peterson L (ed)]. Alexandria, VA, ADA, 1995

Angastiniotis M, Modell B: Global epidemiology of hemoglobin disorders. Ann NY Acad Sci 850:251, 1998

Angastiniotis M, Modell B, Englezos P, Boulyjenkov V: Prevention and control of haemoglobinopathies. Bull World Health Organ 73:375, 1995

Annegers JF, Hauser WA, Elveback LR, Anderason VE, Kurland LT: Seizure disorders in offspring of parents with a history of seizures—a maternal-paternal difference? Epilepsia 17:1, 1976

Barr MB, Hanson JW, Currey K, Sharp S, Toriello H, Schmickel RD, Wilson GN: Holoprosencephaly in infants of diabetic mothers. J Pediatr 102:565, 1983

Becker AE, Grinspoon SK, Klibanski A, Herzog DB: Eating disorders. N Engl J Med 340:14, 1999

Bergqvist A, Bergqvist D, Lindhagen A, Matzsch J: Late symptoms alter pregnancy-related deep vein thrombosis. Br J Obstet Gynaecol 97:338, 1990

Berkowitz GS, Skovron ML, Lapinski RH, Berkowitz RL: Delayed childbearing and the outcome of pregnancy. N Engl J Med 322:659, 1990

Biale Y, Lewenthal H: Effect of folic acid supplementation on congenital malformations due to anticonvulsive drugs. Eur J Obstet Gynecol Reprod Biol 18:211, 1984

Bobrowski RA, Bottoms SF: Under appreciated risks of the elderly multipara. Am J Obstet Gynecol 172:1764, 1995

Boice JD Jr, Miller RW: Childhood and adult cancer after intrauterine exposure to ionizing radiation. Teratology 59:227, 1999

Bowen JR, Gibson FL, Leslie GI, Saunders DM: Medical and development outcome at 1 year for children conceived by intracytoplasmic sperm injection. Lancet 351:1529, 1998

Buehler JW, Kaunitz AM, Hogue CJR, Hughes JM, Smith HC, Rochat RW: Maternal mortality in women aged 35 years or older: United States. JAMA 255:53, 1986

Callaghan N, Garrett A, Goggin T: Withdrawal of anticonvulsant drugs in patients free of seizures for two years. N Engl J Med 318:942, 1988

Centers for Disease Control and Prevention: Insurance coverage of unintended pregnancies resulting in live-born infants. MMWR 48:1, 1999

Centers for Disease Control: Rubella vaccination during pregnancy—United States, 1971–1988. JAMA 261:3374, 1989

Chang S, McAuley JW: Pharmacotherapeutic issues for women of childbearing age with epilepsy. Ann Pharmacol 32:794, 1998

Chang G, Wilkins-Haug L, Berman S, Goetz MA, Behr H, Hiley A: Alcohol use and pregnancy: Improving identification. Obstet Gynecol 91:892, 1998

Chutivongse S, Wilde H, Benjavongkulchai M, Chomchey P, Punthawong S: Postexposure rabies vaccination during pregnancy: Effect on 202 women and their infants. Clin Infect Dis 20:818, 1995

Cnattingius S, Bergstrom R, Lipworth L, Kramer MS: Prepregnancy weight and the risk of adverse pregnancy outcomes. N Engl J Med 338:147, 1998

Cox M, Whittle MJ, Byrne A, Kingdon JCP, Ryan G: Prepregnancy counseling: Experience from 1075 cases. Br J Obstet Gynaecol 99:873, 1992

Cunningham FG, Cox SM, Harstad TW, Mason RA, Pritchard JA: Chronic renal disease and pregnancy outcome. Am J Obstet Gynecol 163:453, 1990

Cunningham FG, Leveno KJ: Childbearing among older women—the message is cautiously optimistic [editorial; comment]. N Engl J Med 333:1002, 1995

Czeizel AE: Primary prevention of birth defects by periconceptional care, including multivitamin supplementation [review]. Baillieres Clin Obstet Gynaecol 9:417, 1995

Czeizel AE, Dudas I: Prevention of the first occurrence of neural-tube defects by periconceptional vitamin supplementation. N Engl J Med 327:1832, 1992

Czeizel AE, Rockenbauer M: Tetanus toxoid and congenital abnormalities. Int J Gynaecol Obstet 64:253, 1999

Department of Commerce: Statistical Abstract of the United States, ed 111. Washington, DC, Government Printing Office, 1991

Doll R, Wakeford R: Risk of childhood cancer from fetal irradiation. Br J Radiol 70:130, 1997

Dunne FP, Brydon P, Smith T, Essex M, Nicholson H, Dunn J: Preconception diabetes care in insulin-dependent diabetes mellitus. QJM 92:175, 1999

Eisenstat SA, Bancroft L: Domestic violence. N Engl J Med 341:886, 1999

Fraser AM, Brockert JE, Ward RH: Association of young maternal age with adverse reproductive outcomes. N Engl J Med 332:1113, 1995

Fucharoen S, Winichagoon P, Thonglairoam V, Siriboon W, Siritanaratkul N, Kanokpongsakdi S, Vantanasiri C: Prenatal diagnosis of thalassemia and hemoglobinopathies in Thailand: Experience from 100 pregnancies. Southeast Asian J Trop Med Public Health 22:16, 1991

Greer IA: Thrombosis in pregnancy: Maternal and fetal issues. Lancet 353:1258, 1999

Gregory R, Tattersall RB: Are diabetic pre-pregnancy clinics worth while? Lancet 340:656, 1992

Grisso JA, Schwarz DF, Hirschinger N, Sammel M, Brensinger C, Santanna J, Lowe RA, Anderson E, Shaw LM, Bethel CA, Teeple L: Violent injuries among women in an urban area. N Engl J Med 341:1899, 1999

Guttler F, Lou H, Andresen J, Kok K, Mikkelsen I, Nielsen KB, Nielsen JB: Cognitive development in offspring of untreated and preconceptionally treated maternal phenylketonuria. J Inherit Metab Dis 13:665, 1990

Hellerstedt WL, Pirie PL, Lando HA, Curry SJ, McBride CM, Grothaus LC, Nelson JC: Differences in preconceptional and prenatal behaviors in women with intended and unintended pregnancies. Am J Public Health 88:663, 1998

Herman WH, Janz NK, Becker MP, Charron-Prochownik D: Diabetes and pregnancy: Preconception care, pregnancy outcomes, resource utilization and costs. J Reprod Med 44:33, 1999

Himeno E, Nishino K, Okazaki T, Nanri H, Ikeda M: A weight reduction and weight maintenance program with long-lasting improvement in left ventricular mass and blood pressure. Am J Hypertens 12:682, 1999

Hollier LM, Leveno KJ, Kelly MA, McIntire DD, Cunningham FG: Maternal age and malformations in singleton births. Obstet Gynecol 96:701, 2000

Hou SH, Grossman SD, Madias NE: Pregnancy in women with renal disease and moderate renal insufficiency. Am J Med 78:185, 1985

Imbasciati E, Pardi G, Capetta P, Ambroso G, Bozzetti P, Pagliari B, Ponticelli C: Pregnancy in women with chronic renal failure. Am J Nephrol 6:193, 1986

Jack BW, Campanile C, McQuade W, Kogan MD: The negative pregnancy test. An opportunity for preconception care. Arch Fam Med 4:340, 1995

Jones DC, Hayslett JP: Outcome of pregnancy in women with moderate or severe renal insufficiency. N Engl J Med 335:226, 1996

Jovanovic L, Druzin M, Peterson CM: Effect of euglycaemia on the outcome of pregnancy in insulin-dependent diabetic women as compared to normal control subjects. Am J Med 71:921, 1981

Jungers P, Forget D, Henry-Amar M: Chronic renal disease and pregnancy. Adv Nephrol 15:103, 1986

Kaback M, Lim-Steele J, Dabholkar D, Brown D, Levy N, Zieger K: Tay Sachs disease: Carrier screening, prenatal diagnosis, and the molecular era. JAMA 270:2307, 1993

Katz AL, Davison JM, Hayslett JP, Singson E, Lindheimer MD: Pregnancy in women with kidney disease. Kidney Int 18:192, 1980

Kelly RH, Danielsen BH, Golding JM, Anders TF, Gilbert WM, Zatzik DF: Adequacy of prenatal care among women with psychiatric diagnoses giving birth in California in 1994 and 1995. Psychiatr Serv 50:1584, 1999

Kinney DK: Schizophrenia. In Rimoin DL, Connor JM, Pyeritz RE (eds): Emery and Rimoin's Principles and Practice of Medical Genetics, 3rd ed. New York, Churchill Livingstone, p 1827, 1997

Kitzmiller JL, Gavin LA, Gin GD, Jovanovic-Peterson L, Main EK, Zigrang WD. Preconception care of diabetes. JAMA 265:731, 1991

Koch R, Hanley W, Levy H, Matalon R, Rouse B, Cruz FD, Azen C, Friedman EG: A preliminary report of the collaborative study of maternal phenylketonuria in the United States and Canada. J Inherit Metab Dis 13:641, 1990

Kyriacou DN, Anglin D, Taliaferro E, Stone S, Tubb T, Linden JA, Muelleman R, Barton E, Kraus JF: Risk factors for injury to women from domestic violence. N Engl J Med 341:1892, 1999

Lindheimer MD, Grünfeld J-P, Davison JM: Renal Disorders. Chapter 2. In Barron WM, Lindheimer MD (eds): Medical Disorders During Pregnancy, 3rd ed. St. Louis, Mosby, 2000, p 39

Martinelli I, Manucci P, DeStefano V: Different risks of thrombosis in four coagulation defects associated with inherited thrombophilia: A study of 150 families. Blood 92:2353, 1998

McCall M, Ramsay JE, Tait RC: Risk factors for pregnancy associated venous thromboembolism. Thromb Haemost 78:1183, 1997

McInnis MG, DePaulo JR Jr: Major mood disorders. In Rimoin DL, Connor JM, Pyeritz RE (eds): Emery and Rimoin's Principles and Practice of Medical Genetics, 3rd ed. New York, Churchill Livingstone, p 1843, 1997

McMahon FJ, Stine OC, Meyers DA, Simpson SG, DePaulo JR: Patterns of maternal transmission in bipolar affective disorder. Am J Hum Genet 56:1277, 1995

Medical Research Council on Vitamin Study Research Group: Prevention of neural tube defects: Results of the medical research council vitamin study. Lancet 338:131, 1991

Meng C, Lockshin M: Pregnancy in lupus. Curr Opin Rheumatol 11:348, 1999

Mitchell JJ, Capua A, Clow C, Scriver CR: Twenty-year outcome analysis of genetic screening programs for Tay-Sachs and beta-thalassemia disease carriers in high schools. Am J Hum Genet 59:793, 1996

Moore KL: Before We Are Born. Basic Embryology and Birth Defects, 2nd ed. Philadelphia, Saunders, 1983

Moos MK, Bangdiwala SI, Meibohm AR, Cefalo RC: The impact of a preconceptional health promotion program on intendedness of pregnancy. Am J Perinatol 13:103, 1996

O'Connor ME: Intrauterine effects in animals exposed to radiofrequency and microwave fields. Teratology 59:287, 1999

Ostensen M: Sex hormones and pregnancy in rheumatoid arthritis and systemic lupus erythematosus. Ann NY Acad Sci 876:131, 1999

Ou CY, Stevenson RE, Brown VK, Schwartz CE, Allen WP, Khoury MJ, Rozen R, Oakley GP, Adams MJ: 5, 10 Methylenetetrahydrofolate reductase genetic polymorphism as a risk factor for neural tube defects. Am J Med Gen 63:610, 1996

Pariser SF, Nasrallah HA, Gardner DK: Postpartum mood disorders: Clinical perspectives. J Womens Health 6:421, 1997

Passarge E, Lenz W: Syndrome of caudal regression in infants of diabetic mothers: Observations of further cases. Pediatrics 37:672, 1966

Pederson CA: Postpartum mood and anxiety disorders: A guide for the nonpsychiatric clinician with an aside on thyroid association with postpartum mood. Thyroid 9:691, 1999

Platt LD, Koch R, Hanley WB, Levy HL, Matalon R, Rouse B, Trefz F, de la Cruz F, Guttler F, Azen C. Friedman EG: The international study of pregnancy outcome in women with maternal phenylketonuria: Report of a 12-year study. Am J Obstet Gynecol 182:326, 2000

Presbitero P, Somerville J, Stone S, Aruta E, Spiegelhaalter D, Rabajoli F: Pregnancy in cyanotic congenital heart disease. Circulation 89:2673, 1994

Public Health Service: Healthy People 2000: National Health Promotion and Disease Prevention Objectives—full report, with commentary. Washington, DC, US Department of Health and Human Services, Public Health Service, 1990; DHHS publication no. (PHS) 91-50212

Public Health Service: Caring for the Future: The Content of Prenatal Care. Washington, DC, Department of Health and Human Services, 1989, p 26

Rasmussen SA, Mulinare J, Khoury MJ, Maloney EK: Evaluation of birth defect histories obtained through maternal interviews. Am J Hum Genet 46:478, 1990

Reece EA, Hobbins JC: Diabetic embryopathy: Pathogenesis, prenatal diagnosis and prevention. Obstet Gynecol Surv 41:325, 1986

Robert E: Intrauterine effects of electromagnetic fields (low frequency, mid-frequency RF, and microwave): Review of epidemiologic studies. Teratology 59:292, 1999

Robinson D, Woerner MG, Alvir JM, Bilder R, Goldman R, Geisler S, Koreen A, Sheitman B: Predictors of relapse following response from a first episode of schizophrenia or schizoaffective disorder. Arch Gen Psychiatry 56:241, 1999

Romitti PA, Burns TL, Murray JC: Maternal interview reports of family history of birth defects: Evaluation from a population-based case-control study of orofacial clefts. Am J Med Gen 72:422, 1997

Rouse B, Azen C, Koch R, Matalon R, Hanley W, Cruz FDL, Trefz F, Friedman E, Shifrin H: Maternal phenylketonuria collaborative study (MPKUCS) offspring: Facial anomalies, malformations, and early neurological sequelae. Am J Med Gen 69:89, 1997

Sawhney H, Suri V, Vasishta K, Gupta N, Devi K, Grover A: Pregnancy and congenital heart disease—maternal and fetal outcome. Aust NZ J Obstet Gynaecol 38:266, 1998

Sjostrom CD, Lissner L, Wedel H, Sjostrom L: Reduction in incidence of diabetes, hypertension and lipid disturbances after intentional weight loss induced by bariatric surgery: The SOS Intervention Study. Obes Res 7:477, 1999

Smith DS, Gilger JW, Pennington BF: Dyslexia and other specific learning disorders. In Rimoin DL, Connor JM, Pyeritz RE (eds): Emery and Rimoin's Principles and Practice of Medical Genetics, 3rd ed. New York, Churchill Livingstone, 1997, p 1781

Smith BL, Martin JA, Ventura SJ: Births and deaths: preliminary data for July 1997–June 1998. Natl Vital Stat Rep 47:1, 1999

Steen VD: Pregnancy in women with systemic sclerosis. Obstet Gynecol 94:15, 1999

Stewart DE, Raskin J, Garfinkel PE, MacDonald OL, Robinson GE: Anorexia nervosa, bulimia, and pregnancy. Am J Obstet Gynecol 157:1194, 1987

Tengborn L, Bergqvist D, Matzsh T, Bergquist A, Hedner U: Recurrent thromboembolism in pregnancy and puerperium. Am J Obstet Gynecol 28:107, 1985

Thompson MW, McInnes RR, Huntington FW (eds): Genetics in Medicine, 5th ed., Philadelphia, Saunders, 1991

van der Put NMJ, Steegers-Theunissen RPM, Frosst P, Trijbels FJM, Eskes TKAB, van den Heuvel LP, Mariman ECD, den Heyer M, Rozen R, Blom HJ: Mutated methylenetetrahydrofolate reductase as a risk factor for spina bifida. Lancet 345:1070, 1995

Walker R, Swartz CM: Electroconvulsive therapy during high-risk pregnancy. Gen Hosp Psychiatry 16:348, 1994

Waller DK, Mills JL, Simpson JL: Are obese women at higher risk for producing malformed offspring? Am J Obstet Gynecol 170:541, 1994

Weiss BM, Atanassoff PG: Cyanotic congenital heart disease and pregnancy: Natural selection, pulmonary hypertension, and anesthesia. J Clin Anesth 5:332, 1993

Wolfe H: High prepregnancy body-mass index—a maternal-fetal risk factor. N Engl J Med 338:191, 1998

Wong HB: Prevention of thalassaemias in South-East Asia. Ann Acad Med Singapore 14:654, 1985

Yentis SM, Steer PJ, Plaat F: Eisenmenger's syndrome in pregnancy: Maternal and fetal mortality in the 1990s. Br J Obstet Gynaecol 105:921, 1998

Yerby MS: Epilepsy and pregnancy. New issues for an old disorder. Neurol Clin 11:777, 1993

10

Prenatal Care

Organized prenatal care in the United States was introduced largely by social reformers and nurses (Merkatz and colleagues, 1990). In 1901, Mrs. William Lowell Putnam of the Boston Infant Social Service Department began a program of nurse visits to women enrolled in the home delivery service of the Boston Lying-in Hospital. This work was so successful that an outpatient prenatal clinic was established in 1911, and women were urged to enroll as early in pregnancy as possible. Former authors of *Williams Obstetrics* were early supporters of prenatal care. Nicholas J. Eastman credited the movement to organized prenatal care with having "done more to save mothers' lives in our time than any other single factor."

OVERVIEW OF PRENATAL CARE

By the end of the 20th century, prenatal care has become one of the most frequently used health services in the United States. In 1998, there were more than 41 million prenatal visits; the median number was 12.4 visits per pregnancy, and as shown in Figure 10–1, many women had 17 or more visits. The United States Public Health Service (1992) goal for the year 2000 was for at least 90 percent of American women to commence prenatal care in the first trimester. As shown in Table 10–1, 84 percent of American women had begun prenatal care in the first trimester by 1998. This measure of obstetrical care, after showing little improvement in the 1980s, has risen for nine consecutive years with a 10 percent total gain during the 1990s (Ventura and colleagues, 2000). In 1998, all but 1.2 percent of women received some prenatal care. Over the last decade, the largest gains in

TABLE 10–1. Live Births by Month Prenatal Care Began, for the United States, 1998

Month of Pregnancy Prenatal Care Began	Births	Percent[b]
Total live births[a]	3,753,920	100
1st trimester		
1st and 2nd mo	2,447,530	65
3rd mo	726,664	19
Total	3,174,194	84
4th–6th mo	508,373	14
7th–9th mo	149,645	3

[a] Total births with prenatal care stated on birth certificate.
[b] Total percent exceeds 100 due to rounding.
From Ventura and associates (2000).

timely prenatal care occurred among minority groups (Fig. 10–2), but disparity continues.

The number of women with significant obstetrical and medical risk factors or complications identifiable during prenatal care is summarized in Table 10–2. Almost a fourth have significant, identifiable, *treatable complications*. Kogan and colleagues (1998) analyzed prenatal care in 54 million live births between 1981 and 1995 in the United States and found a major increase in prenatal care use and especially in "intensive" prenatal care, defined as more than nine prenatal visits. They attributed this increase in intensive prenatal care to the expansion of Medicaid eligibility for pregnant women and to the development of maternal–fetal medicine as

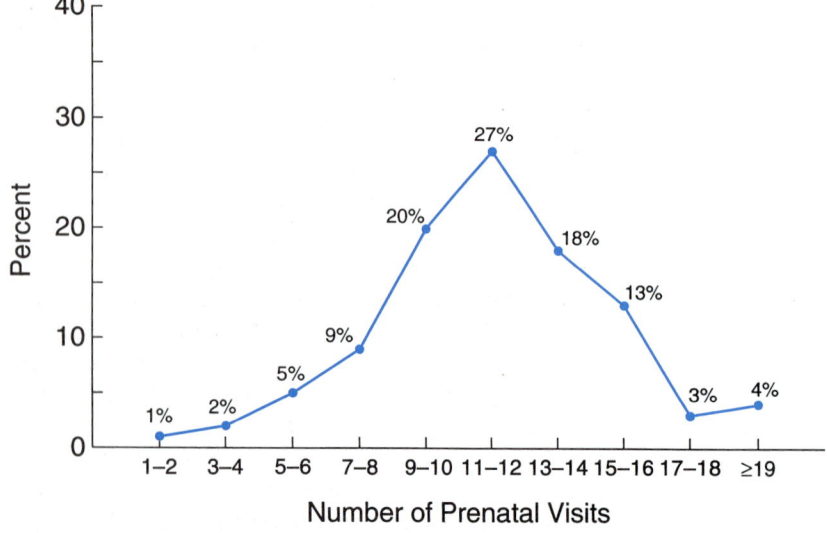

FIGURE 10–1. Frequency distribution for the number of prenatal visits for the United States in 1998. (Adapted from Ventura and associates, 2000.)

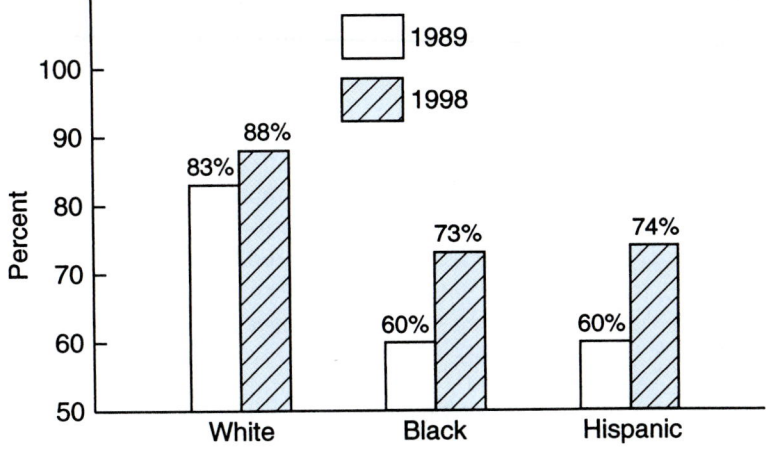

FIGURE 10–2. Percent of women with prenatal care beginning in the first trimester of pregnancy by race and Hispanic origin, United States, 1989 compared with 1998. (Adapted from Ventura and associates, 2000.)

a specialty coupled with widespread use of ultrasonography.

INADEQUATE PRENATAL CARE. The Centers for Disease Control and Prevention (2000a) analyzed 1989–1997 birth certificate data to examine the extent to which women received delayed or no prenatal care. They then used the 1997 Pregnancy Risk Assessment Monitoring System (PRAMS) data for 13 states to assess these same reasons. PRAMS is an ongoing, state-based surveillance system that randomly samples birth certificates and col-

lects information from mothers on pregnancy-related behaviors and experiences. They found that half of women with delayed or no prenatal care wanted to begin care earlier. Reasons for inadequate prenatal care varied by social/ethnic group, age, and method of payment. The most common reason was "I didn't know that I was pregnant." The second most common cited barrier was "I didn't have enough money or insurance to pay for my visits." The third was inability to get an appointment. Roberts and colleagues (1998) identified additional reasons that included problems finding child care, lack of transportation, and the tendency for parous women to ascribe less importance to prenatal care.

RECENT DEVELOPMENTS. In 1986, the Department of Health and Human Services convened an expert panel to review the content of prenatal care (Rosen, 1991). This was in response to a report by the Institute of Medicine and National Institutes of Health on the importance of prenatal care in reducing the incidence of low-birthweight infants as a national agenda. The panel concluded that many medical conditions (such as diabetes mellitus), as well as personal behaviors (alcohol abuse) associated with bad pregnancy outcomes could be identified and modified *prior to conception*. Because health during pregnancy depends on health before pregnancy, it is logical that preconceptional care should be an integral part of prenatal care (Chap. 9).

Systematic health care beginning long before pregnancy undoubtedly proves quite beneficial to the physical and emotional well-being of the prospective mother and her child-to-be. As the consequence of such a program, many acquired diseases and developmental abnormalities will be recognized before pregnancy. Thus, appropriate steps can be taken to eradicate these, or at least to minimize deleterious effects. A striking example is the diabetic women who can be advised of the benefits

TABLE 10–2. Nonemergent Obstetrical or Medical Risk Factors Detected During Prenatal Care in the United States, 1998

Risk Factor	Births	Percent
Total live births	3,941,553	100
Hypertension due to pregnancy	146,320	3.7
Diabetes	103,691	2.6
Anemia	84,795	2.2
Prior preterm or SGA infant	47,429	1.2
Acute or chronic lung disease	40,190	1.2
Genital herpes	32,969	.8
Chronic hypertension	27,442	.7
Rh sensitization	25,783	.7
Cardiac disease	20,528	.5
Renal disease	11,141	.3
Incompetent cervix	10,704	.3
Hemoglobinopathy	3,202	.1
Total with risk factors	554,194	14

SGA = small for gestational age.
Adapted from Ventura and co-workers (2000).

for the embryo-fetus to be achieved from near normalization of blood glucose levels before conception (Chap. 51, p. 1368).

The panel also recommended that the number of prenatal visits be reduced in women at no apparent risk. They suggested that such women would best be served by return visits targeted at specific times, for example, alpha-fetoprotein screening at 16 weeks. We have used such an approach for all pregnancies at Parkland Hospital since late 1988 (Table 10–3). Parous women with normal obstetrical histories are seen even less frequently. In this schedule, limited visits in the first 6 months are targeted to specific purposes. Kogan and colleagues (1994) studied over 9000 women with prenatal care given as recommended by the Expert Panel. They concluded that such care reduced the incidence of low-birthweight infants. Ward and associates (1996) found that such a scheme reduced routine visits, but the increase in urgent clinic visits offset this, so that the total number of visits was unchanged. As reviewed by Clement and co-workers (1999), there have been four randomized trials comparing different schedules of prenatal visits and all found reduced schedules to be safe in terms of the physical outcomes of the mothers and infants.

EFFECTIVENESS OF PRENATAL CARE. In an extensive review, Fiscella (1995) could not find conclusive evidence that prenatal care improved birth outcomes. Others have also raised concern about the effectiveness of prenatal care because during the 1980s and 1990s,

when utilization of prenatal care substantively increased, the rates of low birthweight and preterm birth in the United States worsened (Kogan and colleagues, 1998).

In counterpoint, however, should prenatal care be judged solely on the basis of its effect on birth outcomes? The impact of prenatal care on maternal health, a major focus of prenatal care when it was invented in the early years of the 20th century, has been dramatic. The recognition in the United States that maternal mortality was appallingly high was a slow process until about 1920 (Loudon, 1992). The maternal mortality rate in 1920 was 690 per 100,000 births and this had fallen to 50 per 100,000 by 1955, in association with many developments in health care for women and infants, of which prenatal care was but one component. The effectiveness of prenatal care cannot be gauged in isolation from the remainder of the obstetrical care system that has subsequently developed in this country and elsewhere. Indeed, and as the following statement from the 7th edition of *Williams Obstetrics* (1929) indicates, prenatal care was originally but one part of an organized health care program for pregnant women:

One of the few creditable achievements of American obstetrics consists in the development of so-called "Prenatal Care." The term has a wider application than the words imply, and may be defined as such supervision and care of the pregnant, parturient and puerperal woman as will enable her to pass through the dangers of pregnancy and labor with the least possible risk . . . the first step in such

TABLE 10–3. Prenatal Visit Schedule Used at Parkland Hospital for Nulliparous Women without Medical Risk Factors and Parous Women with Prior Normal Pregnancies[a]

Return Visit No.	Nulliparous Women	Parous Women[b]	Purpose of Visit
1	16 wk	16 wk	AFP screening; ultrasound if needed
2	19 wk	22 wk	Assess gestational age; FHT auscultated
3	26 wk	26 wk	Assess gestational age; gestational diabetes screening; anti-D immunoglobulin if needed
4	30 wk	30 wk	Assess fetal size; hematocrit, VDRL and syphilis serology
5	34 wk	36 wk	Assess fetal size, blood pressure
6	36 wk	38 wk	Blood pressure surveillance
7	37 wk	40 wk	Blood pressure surveillance
8	38 wk	41 wk	Blood pressure surveillance; schedule postterm induction for multiparas
9	39 wk		Blood pressure surveillance; Schedule postterm induction
10	40 wk		Blood pressure surveillance; Schedule postterm induction
11	41 wk		Blood pressure surveillance; Schedule postterm induction

AFP = alpha-fetoprotein; FHT = fetal heart tones; VDRL = Venereal Disease Research Laboratory test.
[a]Women with risk factors are seen more frequently, typically in specialized obstetrical complication clinics.
[b]18–34 years old and ≥ 1 prior normal pregnancies.

a program consists in organizing the obstetrical dispensary [sic, prenatal clinic] and indoor service [sic, intrapartum] as a single unit.

Thus, in this context, prenatal care was not an end in itself but a systematic *gateway* to coordinated intrapartum and postpartum care and often even beyond into a woman's later life.

Rooks (1998), using prevention of low birthweight as an example, emphasized that most of the risk factors for this outcome also require maternal behavior modification. The presumption is largely that psychosocial interventions during prenatal care have limited value in modifying maternal behavior. There are few systematic studies of behavior modification during pregnancy. Olds and colleagues (1997) have published a series of well-designed experiments examining the effects of psychosocial interventions during the prenatal period and the first 24 months of postnatal life (Earls, 1998). These studies have shown that such interventions can increase birthweight, prevent preterm birth, reduce child abuse and neglect, and also reduce antisocial behavior later in life (Olds and associates, 1986, 1997, 1998). Studies such as these suggest that the benefits and limitations of prenatal care should be measured not only in the context of immediate pregnancy outcomes, but also in the context that prenatal care can be a gateway to behavior modification for both mothers and their children. Put another way, measuring the effects of prenatal care should encompass more than counting the number of prenatal visits in relation to birth outcomes.

PROCEDURES FOR PRENATAL CARE

The American Academy of Pediatrics and the American College of Obstetricians and Gynecologists (1997) have defined prenatal care as follows: "A comprehensive antepartum care program that involves a coordinated approach to medical care and psychosocial support that optimally begins before conception and extends throughout the antepartum period." The content of such comprehensive care includes assessments during preconception, at initial presentation for pregnancy care, and during follow-up prenatal visits. Each of these components is discussed in the following section.

PRECONCEPTIONAL CARE. A comprehensive preconceptional care program has the potential to assist women who want to get pregnant by reducing risks, promoting healthy lifestyles, and improving readiness for pregnancy. In 1989, the Expert Panel on the Content of Prenatal Care suggested that the negative pregnancy test encounter was an opportunity for preconceptional care. This is discussed in detail in Chapter 9.

INITIAL PRENATAL EVALUATION. Prenatal care should be initiated as soon as there is a reasonable likelihood of pregnancy. This may be as early as a few days after a missed menstrual period, especially for the woman who desires pregnancy termination, but it should be no later than the second missed period for anyone. The major goals are:

1. To define the health status of the mother and fetus.
2. To determine the gestational age of the fetus.
3. To initiate a plan for continuing obstetrical care.

Components of the initial visit are summarized in Table 10–4. The initial plan for subsequent care may range from relatively infrequent routine visits to that of prompt hospitalization because of serious maternal or fetal disease.

PRENATAL RECORD. Use of a standardized prenatal record within a perinatal health care system greatly facilitates antepartum and intrapartum management. Such a record is used by the Parkland Hospital Obstetrics Service. The American Academy of Pediatrics and the American College of Obstetricians and Gynecologists (1997) have provided an excellent prototypical prenatal record.

DEFINITIONS. There are several definitions pertinent to establishment of an accurate prenatal record:

- **Primipara:** a woman who has been delivered only once of a fetus or fetuses who reached viability. Therefore, completion of any pregnancy beyond the stage of abortion (Chap. 33, p. 856) bestows parity upon the mother.
- **Multipara:** a woman who has completed two or more pregnancies to viability. It is the number of pregnan-

TABLE 10–4. Recommended Components of the Initial Prenatal Care Visit

Risk assessment to include genetic, medical, obstetrical, and psychosocial factors

Estimated due date

General physical examination

Laboratory tests: hematocrit (hemoglobin), urinalysis, urine culture, blood grouping, Rh, antibody screen, rubella status, syphilis screen, Pap smear, HbsAg testing; offer HIV testing

Patient education, e.g., use of seatbelts, avoidance of alcohol and tobacco

HbsAg = hepatitis B surface antigen; HIV = human immunodeficiency virus.
From the American Academy of Pediatrics and the American College of Obstetricians and Gynecologists (1997), with permission.

cies reaching viability, and not the number of fetuses delivered, that determines *parity*. Parity is not greater if a single fetus, twins, or quintuplets were delivered, nor lower if the fetus or fetuses were stillborn.

- **Nulligravida:** a woman who is not now, and never has been pregnant.
- **Gravida:** a woman who is or has been pregnant, irrespective of the pregnancy outcome. With the establishment of the first pregnancy, she becomes a primigravida, and with successive pregnancies a multigravida.
- **Nullipara:** a woman who has never completed a pregnancy beyond an abortion. She may or may not have been pregnant or have had a spontaneous or elective abortion(s).
- **Parturient:** a woman in labor.
- **Puerpera:** a woman who has just given birth.

In certain clinics it is customary to summarize past obstetrical history by a series of digits connected by dashes. The first digit refers to the number of term infants, the second to the number of preterm infants, the third to the number of abortions, and the fourth to the number of children currently alive. For example, a woman who is para 6–1–2–6 has had six term deliveries, one preterm delivery, two abortions, and she currently has six children alive.

NORMAL DURATION OF PREGNANCY. The mean duration of pregnancy calculated from the first day of the last normal menstrual period is very close to 280 days, or 40 weeks. Kortenoever (1950), in an analysis of 7504 pregnancies, found the average duration to be 282 days. A mean value of 281 days was calculated from the data of the Obstetrical Statistical Cooperative for 77,300 women who underwent spontaneous labor and whose infants weighed at least 2500 g.

It is customary to estimate the expected date of delivery by adding 7 days to the date of the first day of the last normal menstrual period and counting back 3 months (Naegele rule). For example, if the last menstrual period began on September 10, the expected date of delivery would be June 17. It is apparent that pregnancy is erroneously considered to have begun about 2 weeks before ovulation if the duration is so calculated. Nonetheless, clinicians conventionally calculate *gestational age* or *menstrual age* from the first day of the last menstrual period, to identify temporal events in pregnancy. Embryologists and other reproductive biologists more often employ *ovulatory age* or *fertilization age,* both of which are typically 2 weeks shorter. Bracken and Belanger (1989) tested the accuracy of various "pregnancy wheels" provided by three pharmaceutical companies and found that such devices were remarkably prone to error. Specifically, incorrect delivery dates were predicted in 40 to 60 percent of estimates, with a 5-day error being typical.

It has become customary to divide pregnancy into three equal *trimesters* of approximately 3 calendar months. Historically, the first trimester extended through the completion of 14 weeks, the second through 28 weeks, and the third included the 29th through 42nd weeks of pregnancy. Put another way, trimesters can be obtained by division of 42 into three periods of 14 weeks each. There are certain major obstetrical problems that cluster in each of these time periods. For example, most spontaneous abortions take place during the first trimester, whereas practically all cases of hypertensive disorders due to pregnancy become clinically evident during the third trimester.

The clinical use of trimesters to describe the duration of a specific pregnancy fosters imprecision and should be abandoned. For example, it is inappropriate in cases of uterine hemorrhage to categorize the problem temporally as "third-trimester bleeding." Appropriate management for the mother and her fetus will vary remarkably, depending upon whether the bleeding is encountered early or late in the third trimester (Chap. 25, p. 620). **Precise knowledge of the age of the fetus is imperative for ideal obstetrical management!** Therefore, expert attention must be given to this important measurement. The clinically appropriate unit of measure is *weeks of gestation completed.* Increasingly, clinicians designate gestational age using completed weeks and days, for example, 33 3/7 weeks for 33 completed weeks and 3 days.

HISTORY.   For the most part, the same essentials go into appropriate history-taking from the pregnant woman as elsewhere in medicine. The history is obtained unhurriedly in a private setting to establish the good rapport so necessary for a successful outcome. **Detailed information concerning past obstetrical history, if any, is crucial because many prior pregnancy complications tend to recur in subsequent pregnancies.**

The *menstrual history* is extremely important. The woman who spontaneously menstruates regularly every 28 days or so is most likely to ovulate at midcycle. Thus, the gestational age (menstrual age) becomes simply the number of weeks since the onset of the last menstrual period. If her menstrual cycles were significantly longer than 28 to 30 days, ovulation more likely occurred well beyond 14 days; or if the intervals were much longer and irregular, chronic anovulation is likely to have preceded some of the episodes of vaginal bleeding identified as menses. **Without regular, predictable, cyclic, spontaneous menses that suggest ovulatory cycles, accurate dating of pregnancy by physical examination is difficult.**

It is important to ascertain whether or not *steroidal contraceptives* were used before the pregnancy. It is now common, but not necessarily recommended, for women who sustain regularly recurring withdrawal bleeding while using oral contraceptives to cyclically stop their use and to conceive without any further menstrual-like bleeding. Ovulation, however, may not have resumed 2 weeks after the onset of the last withdrawal bleeding, but instead, it may have occurred at an appreciably later but highly variable date. Predicting the time of ovulation in this circumstance is difficult.

The possibility of the presence of an *intrauterine device* should be ascertained, because certain pregnancy complications are increased by its presence in utero (Chap. 58, p. 1539).

PSYCHOSOCIAL SCREENING. The American College of Obstetricians and Gynecologists (1999b) has reviewed the importance of psychosocial screening during prenatal care. The College concluded that addressing psychosocial issues is an essential step toward improving women's health and birth outcomes. Shown in Table 10–5 is a psychosocial screening tool developed by the Healthy Start Program of the Florida Department of Health and which is recommended for this purpose.

SMOKING DURING PREGNANCY. Except in teenagers, smoking has declined from 19.5 percent of pregnant women in 1989 to 12.9 percent in 1998 (Ventura and colleagues, 2000). As discussed in Chapter 38 (p. 1019), smoking cessation during pregnancy, including use of nicotine gum and transdermal nicotine patches has been reviewed by the American College of Obstetricians and Gynecologists (1997c). Cnattingius and co-workers (1999) studied the effects of smoking cessation on recurrent preterm birth in a population-based cohort of 243,858 Swedish women delivered between 1983 and 1993. Cessation of smoking between pregnancies was

---

TABLE 10–5. Psychosocial Prenatal Screening Questions

1. Do you have any problems that prevent you from keeping your health care appointments?
2. How many times have you moved in the past 12 months?
   0   1   2   3   > 3
3. Do you feel unsafe where you live?
4. Do you or any members of your household go to bed hungry?
5. In the past 2 months, have you used any form of tobacco?
6. In the past 2 months, have you used drugs or alcohol (including beer, wine, or mixed drinks)?
7. In the past year, has anyone hit you or tried to hurt you?
8. How do you rate your current stress level—low or high?
9. If you could change the timing of this pregnancy, would you want it earlier, later, not at all, or no change?

From Florida Department of Health (1997).

---

associated with reduction in the risk of recurrent preterm delivery.

ALCOHOL AND STREET DRUGS DURING PREGNANCY. Alcohol use is substantially underreported on the birth certificate; according to these data just 1.1 percent of women reported any alcohol use in 1998 (Ventura and colleagues, 2000). According to the Centers for Disease Control and Prevention, however, about 15 percent of women used alcohol during pregnancy in 1995 (Ebrahim and associates, 1998). This was down from 23 percent in 1988. The American College of Obstetricians and Gynecologists (1994b) has reviewed screening for alcohol abuse, as well as street drugs, during pregnancy (Chap. 38, p. 1030).

DOMESTIC VIOLENCE SCREENING. The term "domestic violence" usually refers to violence against adolescent and adult females within the context of family or intimate relationships (American College of Obstetricians and Gynecologists, 1999a). Such violence has been increasingly recognized as a major public health problem. Gazmararian and colleagues (1996) reported that the prevalence of domestic violence during pregnancy in most studies was 4 percent to 8 percent. The American College of Obstetricians and Gynecologists (1999a) has provided methods for screening for domestic violence, and recommends their use at the first prenatal visit, then again at least once per trimester, and again at the postpartum follow-up. The American College of Obstetricians and Gynecologists (1998b) concluded that mandatory reporting to governmental agencies cannot be justified at this time.

OBSTETRICAL EXAMINATION. The cervix is visualized employing a speculum lubricated with warm water. Bluish-red passive hyperemia of the cervix is characteristic, but not of itself diagnostic, of pregnancy. Dilated, occluded cervical glands bulging beneath the exocervical mucosa, so-called *nabothian cysts,* may be prominent. If the cervix is dilated appreciably, fetal membranes may be visualized through the cervical canal, implying at least that expulsion of the products of conception may be imminent. Next, in order to identify cytological abnormalities a Pap smear is obtained and specimens for identification of *Neisseria gonorrhoeae* and possibly *Chlamydia trachomatis* are obtained.

A moderate amount of white mucoid discharge is normal. The presence of foamy yellow liquid in the vagina is strongly suggestive of *Trichomonas,* whereas the presence of a curdlike discharge is consistent with *Candida* infection. Treatment of trichomoniasis and candidiasis is discussed on page 244.

The speculum is removed and the digital pelvic examination is completed by palpation, with special attention given to the consistency, length, and dilatation of the cervix; to the fetal presenting part, especially if late in pregnancy; to the bony architecture of the pelvis; and to any anomalies of the vagina and perineum, including cystocele, rectocele, and relaxed or torn perineum. The vulva and contiguous structures are also carefully inspected. All cervical, vaginal, and vulvar lesions are evaluated further by appropriate use of colposcopy, biopsy, culture, or dark-field examination. The perianal region should be visualized and digital rectal examination done to identify hemorrhoids or other lesions.

Between 18 and 32 weeks' gestation, there is good correlation between the gestational age of the fetus in weeks and the height of the uterine fundus in centimeters, when measured as the distance over the abdominal wall from the top of the symphysis pubis to the top of the fundus, with the bladder empty. It is important for the examiner to document the height of the fundus.

PHYSICAL EXAMINATION. The thorough physical examination should include evaluation of the teeth, so that repair of carious teeth can be undertaken promptly. When varicose veins are identified, frequent postural drainage should be urged and elastic support stockings provided.

LABORATORY TESTS. Recommended routine laboratory tests are shown in Table 10–4. The Institute of Medicine recommended that a national policy of universal screening be developed for human immunodeficiency virus (HIV) testing with patient notification, as a routine of prenatal testing. In a joint statement, the American College of Obstetricians and Gynecologists (1999c) and the American Academy of Pediatrics supported this recommendation. If a woman declines testing, this should be noted in the prenatal record. All pregnant women should also be screened for hepatitis B virus infection.

HIGH-RISK PREGNANCIES. There are major categories for increased risk that can be identified and given appropriate consideration in pregnancy management. These include:

1. Preexisting medical illness.
2. Previous poor pregnancy outcome, such as perinatal mortality, preterm delivery, fetal-growth restriction, malformations, placental accidents, or maternal hemorrhage.
3. Evidence of maternal undernutrition.

SUBSEQUENT PRENATAL VISITS

RETURN VISITS. Traditionally the timing of subsequent prenatal examinations has been scheduled at intervals of 4 weeks until 28 weeks, and then every 2 weeks until 36 weeks, and weekly thereafter (Table 10–6). As shown in Table 10–3, fewer visits are acceptable in uncomplicated pregnancies. Conversely, women with complicated pregnancies often require return visits at 1- to 2-week intervals.

FETAL HEART SOUNDS. In essentially all pregnancies, the fetal heart can first be heard between 16 and 19 weeks when carefully listened for with a DeLee fetal stethoscope (Chap. 2, p. 28). The ability to hear unamplified fetal heart sounds will depend upon several factors, including patient size and the examiner's hearing acuity. Herbert and co-workers (1987) reported that the fetal heart was audible by 20 weeks in 80 percent of women. By 21 weeks audible fetal heart sounds were present in 95 percent, and by 22 weeks in all.

FUNDAL HEIGHT. Measurement of the height of the uterine fundus above the symphysis can provide useful information. Jimenez and co-workers (1983) demonstrated that between 20 and 31 weeks the fundal height in centimeters equaled the gestational age in weeks. Quaranta and associates (1981) and Calvert and colleagues (1982) reported essentially identical observations up to 34 weeks' gestation. *The bladder must be emptied before making the measurement.* Worthen and Bustillo (1980), for example, demonstrated that at 17 to 20 weeks, fundal height was 3 cm higher with a full bladder.

GESTATIONAL AGE. One of the most important determinations at prenatal examinations is assessment of fetal age. Fortunately, it is possible to identify this with con-

TABLE 10–6. Recommended Components of Routine Prenatal Care after the First Visit

Visit intervals	Every 4 wk until 28 wk; then every 2–3 wk until 36 wk and weekly thereafter
Each visit	Assess blood pressure, weight, urine protein and glucose, uterine size, fetal heart rate, fetal movement, contractions, bleeding and membrane rupture; ultrasound is only used for specific indications
15–20 wk	Maternal serum alpha-fetoprotein screening
24–28 wk	Screen for gestational diabetes if indicated
28 wk	Test D-negative women for antibodies; give anti-D immune globulin if indicated

From the American Academy of Pediatrics and the American College of Obstetricians and Gynecologists (1997), with permission.

siderable precision through an appropriately timed, carefully performed clinical examination, coupled with knowledge of the time of onset of the last menstrual period. When this date and fundal height are repeatedly in temporal agreement, the duration of gestation can be firmly established. When gestational age cannot be clearly identified, sonography is of considerable value.

Later in pregnancy, precise knowledge of gestational age may be of considerable importance, because a number of pregnancy complications may develop, for which the optimal treatment will depend on fetal age. For example, with the development of preeclampsia at 38 weeks, very often delivery is most beneficial to both mother and fetus. If the duration of gestation is only 28 weeks when preeclampsia develops, however, attempts at conservative management and delay of delivery may be more beneficial.

UNIVERSAL ULTRASONOGRAPHY SCREENING. There is continuing controversy concerning the issue of universal screening of all pregnancies with ultrasonography (Chap. 41, p. 1113). Routine ultrasound is not currently recommended in low-risk pregnancies by the American College of Obstetricians and Gynecologists (1997b).

PRENATAL SURVEILLANCE. At each return visit steps are taken to determine the well-being of both the mother and her fetus. Certain information, obtained by history and examination, is especially important.

Fetal
• Heart rate(s).
• Size—actual and rate of change.
• Amount of amnionic fluid.
• Presenting part and station (late in pregnancy).
• Activity.

Maternal
• Blood pressure—actual and extent of change.
• Weight—actual and amount of change.
• Symptoms, including headache, altered vision, abdominal pain, nausea and vomiting, bleeding, fluid from vagina, and dysuria.
• Height in cm of uterine fundus from symphysis.
• Vaginal examination late in pregnancy often provides valuable information:
  • Confirmation of the presenting part.
  • Station of the presenting part (Chap. 13, p. 311).
  • Clinical estimation of pelvic capacity and its general configuration (Chap. 3, p. 58).
  • Consistency, effacement, and dilatation of the cervix.

SUBSEQUENT LABORATORY TESTS. If the initial results were normal, most of the procedures need not be repeated. Hematocrit (or hemoglobin) determination

and syphilis serology if it is prevalent in the population, should be repeated about 28 to 32 weeks.

Determination of maternal serum alpha-fetoprotein concentration at 16 to 18 weeks (15 to 20 weeks is acceptable) is recommended to screen for open neural-tube defects and some chromosomal anomalies. Precise knowledge of gestational age is paramount for accuracy of this screening test (Chap. 37, p. 979).

SPECIFIC PRENATAL NEEDS. A variety of needs or problems specific to individual women are discernible during the initial prenatal encounter if they have not already been addressed during preconceptional evaluation. Middle-school age adolescents (11 to 15 years old) are at increased risk for preterm birth as well as a variety of psychosocial problems. For example, Satin and colleagues (1994) in a study of 16,500 nulliparous women delivered at Parkland Hospital, found that preterm birth was increased significantly in 1622 pregnancies in these girls. Others have reported similar findings (Amini and associates, 1996).

ANCILLARY PRENATAL TESTS

GESTATIONAL DIABETES. For women at risk for gestational diabetes, screening is recommended between 24 and 28 weeks (Chap. 51, p. 1362).

CHLAMYDIA TRACHOMATIS. Universal testing of all pregnant women for chlamydial infection is not recommended (American Academy of Pediatrics and the American College of Obstetricians and Gynecologists, 1997). In high-risk women of low socioeconomic means, infection at 24 weeks was associated with a two- to threefold incidence of preterm birth (Andrews and colleagues, 2000).

BACTERIAL VAGINOSIS. Routine screening for bacterial vaginosis is not recommended (American College of Obstetricians and Gynecologists, 1998a). Carey and co-workers (2000b), in a study sponsored by the National Institute of Child Health and Human Development, randomized 1953 women from the general obstetrical population with asymptomatic bacterial vaginosis to receive two 2-g doses of metronidazole or placebo at 16 to 24 weeks' gestation. Treatment did not reduce preterm birth. In this same trial, metronidazole treatment increased the risk of preterm birth in women with asymptomatic trichomonal infection (Carey and co-workers, 2000a). Screening for bacterial vaginosis may be considered in women at high-risk for preterm labor (Chap. 27, p. 699).

FETAL FIBRONECTIN. Determination of this protein in vaginal fluid has been used to forecast preterm delivery in women with contractions (Chap. 27, p. 702). The Committee on Obstetric Practice of the American College of Obstetricians and Gynecologists (1997a) does not recommend the routine screening of the general obstetric population.

GROUP B STREPTOCOCCUS. Eradication of this organism during labor substantively decreases early-onset neonatal sepsis (Chap. 56, p. 1471). Currently, however, there is no clear consensus regarding screening cultures for streptococcal colonization. The American College of Obstetricians and Gynecologists Committee on Obstetrics (1996) and the Centers for Disease Control and Prevention (1996) recommend either of two strategies. The first is to treat pregnant women with chemoprophylaxis based solely on risk factors without screening cultures. The second is to perform screening cultures at 35 to 37 weeks, and to offer intrapartum treatment with penicillin if the culture is positive. At Parkland Hospital, women with risk factors for neonatal group B infection are given intrapartum intravenous ampicillin and all infants are administered aqueous penicillin G in the delivery room. This regimen has virtually eliminated neonatal group B infections (Wendel and colleagues, 2000).

SCREENING FOR GENETIC DISEASES. This screening can be offered based on family history or the ethnic or racial background of the couple (American College of Obstetricians and Gynecologists, 1995b). Examples include testing for Tay-Sachs disease for people of Eastern European Jewish or French Canadian ancestry; β-thalassemia for those of Mediterranean, Southeast Asian, Indian, Pakistani, or African ancestry; α-thalassemia for people of Southeast Asian or African ancestry; and sickle cell anemia for people of African, Mediterranean, Middle Eastern, Caribbean, Latin American, or Indian descent. Screening for cystic fibrosis may be offered to those with a family history of this disease. This is discussed in detail in Chapter 36.

NUTRITION

Meaningful studies of nutrition in human pregnancy are exceedingly difficult to design. For ethical reasons, experimental dietary deficiency must not be produced deliberately. In those instances in which severe nutritional deficiencies have been induced as a consequence of social, economic, or political disaster, coincidental events often have created many variables, the effects of which are not amenable to quantification. Some past experiences suggest, however, that in otherwise healthy women a state of near starvation is required to establish clear differences in pregnancy outcome.

During the severe European winter of 1944–1945, nutritional deprivation of known intensity prevailed in a well-circumscribed area of the Netherlands occupied by the German military (Stein and associates, 1972). At the lowest point, rations reached 450 kcal/day, with generalized undernutrition rather than selective malnutrition. Smith (1947) analyzed the outcomes of pregnancies that were in progress during this 6-month famine. Median infant birthweights decreased about 250 g and rose again after food became available. This indicated that birthweight can be significantly influenced by starvation during later pregnancy. The perinatal mortality rate, however, was not altered, nor was the incidence of malformations significantly increased. The frequency of pregnancy "toxemia" was found to decline during this "hunger winter."

Evidence of impaired brain development has been obtained in some animal fetuses whose mothers had been subjected to intense dietary deprivation. These studies stimulated interest in the subsequent intellectual development of young adults in the Netherlands whose mothers had been starved during pregnancy. The comprehensive study by Stein and co-workers (1972) was made possible because all males at age 19 underwent compulsory examination for military service. It was concluded that severe dietary deprivation during pregnancy caused no detectable effects on subsequent mental performance.

Maternal weight gain during pregnancy does influence birthweight of the infant. Abrams and Laros (1986) studied the effect of maternal weight gain on birthweight in 2946 pregnancies with term deliveries. Only eight women did not gain weight. Multiple regression analysis controlling for maternal age, race, parity, socioeconomic status, cigarette consumption, and gestational age was done. As shown in Figure 10–3, maternal weight gain affected birthweight; underweight women delivered smaller infants whereas the opposite was true for overweight women. The mean weight gain during pregnancy was 33 lb (15 kg). An important finding in this study was that weight gain does not appear requisite for fetal growth in obese women.

Information on maternal weight gain is collected on the birth certificate (Ventura and colleagues, 2000). In 1998, as shown in Figure 10–4, the majority of women (64 percent) gained 26 lb or more during pregnancy. The median weight gain was 30.5 lb. Maternal weight gain had a positive correlation with birthweight, and women with the greatest risk of delivering a low-birthweight infant (< 2500 g) were those with weight gains less than 16 lb. Indeed, 1 of 7 women who gained less than 16 lb delivered an infant weighing less than

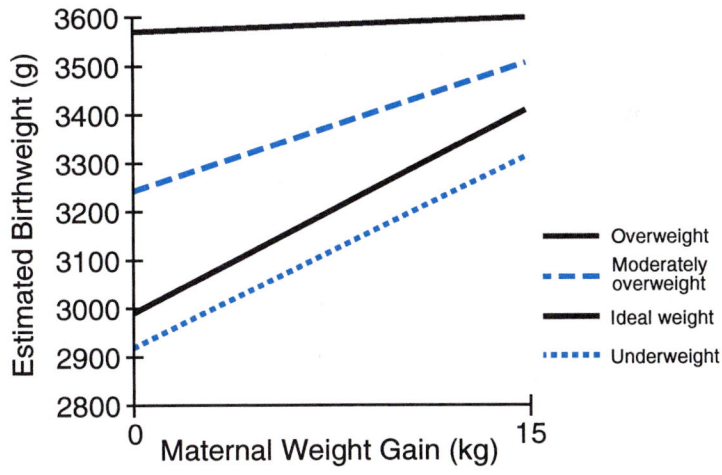

FIGURE 10–3. Birthweight of term infants according to pregnancy maternal body mass and weight gain, adjusted for confounding factors. (Modified from Abrams and Laros, 1986.)

2500 g. This incidence was 1 of 5 in African-American women.

RECOMMENDATIONS FOR WEIGHT GAIN. For the first half of the 20th century, it was recommended that weight gain during pregnancy be limited to less than 20 lb (9.1 kg). It was believed that such restriction would prevent pregnancy hypertensive disorders and fetal macrosomia resulting in operative deliveries. By the 1970s, however, women were encouraged to gain at least 25 lb (11.4 kg) to prevent preterm births and fetal growth restriction. In 1990, the Institute of Medicine recommended a weight gain of 25 to 35 lb (11.5 to 16 kg) for women with normal prepregnancy body mass index

(BMI). This index is easily calculated using the chart shown in Figure 48–8 (p. 1299). Weight gains recommended according to prepregnant body mass index categories are shown in Table 10–7. The American Academy of Pediatrics and the American College of Obstetricians and Gynecologists (1997) have endorsed these guidelines.

Feig and Naylor (1998) from Canada have challenged these recommendations for a population-wide strategy of liberal weight gain in industrial nations. They called this a potentially harmful policy that encourages women to overeat during pregnancy, and without addressing other causes of low-birthweight infants such as poor prenatal care, adolescent pregnancy, drug abuse, and

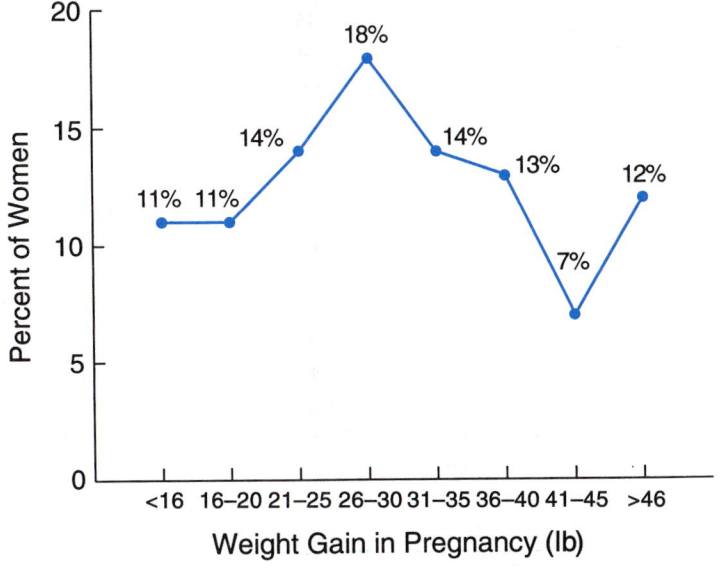

FIGURE 10–4. Maternal weight gain in the United States reported on the birth certificate in 1998. (From Ventura and colleagues, 2000.)

TABLE 10–7. Recommended Total Weight Gain Ranges for Pregnant Women with Singleton Pregnancies[a]

Prepregnancy BMI[b]	Recommended Total Gain	
	Pounds	Kilograms
Low (BMI < 19.8)	28–40	12.5–18
Normal (BMI 19.8–26)	25–35	11.5–16
High (BMI > 26–29)	15–25	7–11.5
Obese (BMI > 29)	< 15	< 7

[a]The range for women with twins is 35–45 lb (16–20 kg).
[b]BMI = body mass index prior to pregnancy.
From the Institute of Medicine (1992).

heavy smoking. They preferred the recommendation by the Committee on Medical Aspects of Food Policy in the United Kingdom, which a pregnant woman with a normal BMI should gain 15 to 25 lb during pregnancy (Report of the Panel on Dietary Reference Values, 1991).

Hytten (1991) reviewed data from over 20 years and observed that total weight gain throughout pregnancy in healthy primigravidas eating without restrictions is approximately 12.5 kg (27.5 lb). Normal physiological events cumulatively account for about 9 kg as fetus, placenta, amnionic fluid, uterine and breast hypertrophy, increased blood volume, and retained extracellular and extravascular fluid. The remainder of the 12.5 kg appears to be mostly maternal storage fat.

Hytten and Leitch (1971) examined the rate of weight gain during the second half of pregnancy in normal nulliparous women. The rate between 20 weeks and delivery was about 1 lb/wk, with a wide range (Fig. 10–5). Similar results were obtained by Petitti and co-workers (1991) in both African-American and white women who delivered infants with birthweights of 3000 g or more. In both groups, weight gain from 8 to 20 weeks was about 0.7 lb/wk and about 1 lb/wk from 20 weeks to delivery. Hickey and colleagues (1995) reported slightly higher values of 1 lb/wk in the second and third trimesters.

Several possible disadvantages of excessive weight gain as a consequence of the fetus-infant being heavier must be considered. Parker and Abrams (1992) examined the associations between maternal weight gain outside the recommendations of the Institute of Medicine in 6690 singleton births. The average prepregnancy weight was 57 kg (125 lb), and the average maternal weight gain was 15.2 ± 5.2 kg (33.4 ± 11.4 lb) in these predominantly Caucasian and Asian women. Less than half gained weight within the Institute's recommendations for their BMI. Weight gains within the recommendations reduced the risk of adverse outcomes studied. Conversely, low weight gains for a given habitus were associated with small-for-gestational age infants. There have been several other studies in which less weight gain than recommended was found to be associated with preterm or low-birthweight infants (Abrams and Selvin, 1995; Hickey and colleagues, 1995; Siega-Riz and associates, 1994). Parker and Abrams (1992) showed that excessive weight gains were linked to large-for-gestational age infants and correspondingly increased cesarean delivery rates (16 versus 22 percent). Witter and colleagues (1995) reported that the risk of cesarean delivery increases linearly with pregnancy weight gain, independent of birthweight. Johnson and Yancey (1996) emphasize that the consequences of the recommendations of the Institute of Medicine to increase pregnancy weight gain have been incompletely assessed.

Not all the weight put on during pregnancy is lost during and immediately after parturition (Hytten, 1991). The normal woman who gains 12.5 kg (27.5 lb) in pregnancy is about 4.4 kg (9 lb) above her prepregnant weight when she goes home postpartum. Schauberger and co-workers (1992) studied prenatal and postpartum weights in 795 women delivered in Wisconsin. Average weight gain was 13.0 ± 4.8 kg (28.6 ± 10.6 lb). As shown in Figure 10–6, the majority of maternal weight loss (about 5.5 kg or 12.1 lb) was at delivery and in the ensuing 2 weeks (about 4 kg or 8.8 lb). An additional 2.5 kg (5.5 lb) was lost between 2 weeks and 6 months postpartum. The average total weight loss was 12.2 ± 4.6 kg (26.8 ± 10.1 lb), resulting in an average retained weight of 1.4 ± 4.8 kg (3 ± 10.5 lb) due to pregnancy. Overall, the more weight gained during pregnancy, the more that was lost postpartum. Parous women retained more of their pregnancy weight, but the interval between pregnancies was not linked to long-term obesity. The effects of breast feeding on maternal weight loss was negligible.

SUMMARY OF WEIGHT GAIN. Perhaps the most remarkable finding about weight gain in pregnancy is that a wide range is compatible with good clinical outcomes and that departures from "normality" are very nonspecific for any adverse outcome in a given individual.

RECOMMENDED DIETARY ALLOWANCES. Periodically the Food and Nutrition Board of the National Research Council recommends dietary allowances for women, including those who are pregnant or lactating. Their latest recommendations are summarized in Table 10–8. Recommended daily allowances are not intended for application to individuals, but as guides to the needs of populations and groups, because individuals un-

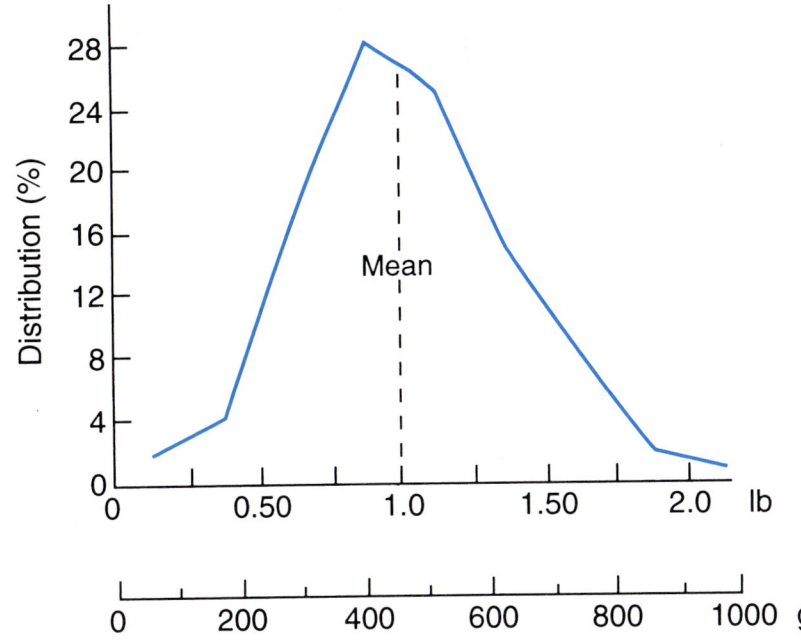

FIGURE 10–5. Distribution of weekly weight gain from 20 weeks to delivery in healthy young nulliparas. (From Hytten, 1991, with permission.)

doubtedly vary widely in their requirements. Certain prenatal vitamin–mineral supplements may lead to intakes well in excess of these allowances. This is not readily apparent to either the consumer or physician issuing the prescription, because label information is expressed in terms of the Food and Drug Administration (FDA) *U.S. Recommended Daily Allowances,* which are substantially different for several nutrients (Institute of Medicine, 1990). Moreover, the use of excessive supplements (for example, 10 times the recom-

mended daily allowances), which often are self-prescribed by a substantial portion of the general public, has led to concern about nutrient toxicities during pregnancy. Nutrients that can potentially exert toxic effects include iron, zinc, selenium, and vitamins A, B_6, C, and D. Vitamin and mineral intake more than twice the recommended daily dietary allowance shown in Table 10–8, should be avoided during pregnancy (American Academy of Pediatrics and the American College of Obstetricians and Gynecologists, 1997).

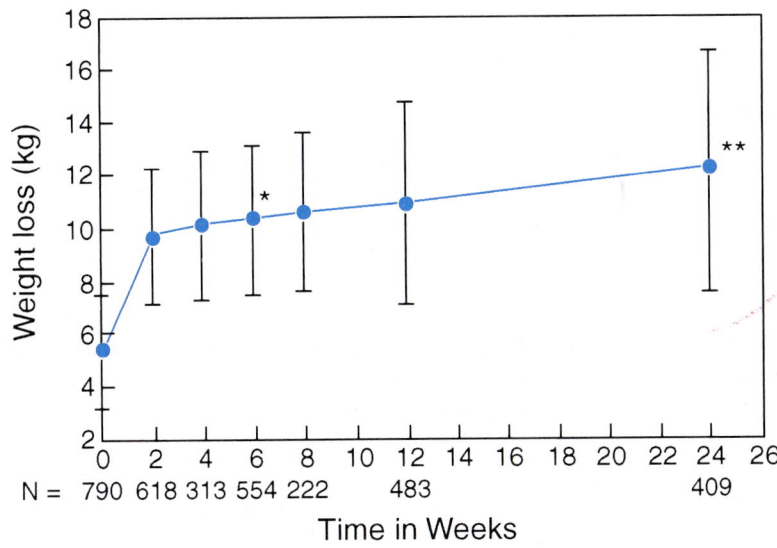

FIGURE 10–6. Cumulative weight loss from last antepartum visit to 6 months postpartum. *Statistically different from 2-week weight loss, **Statistically different from 6-week weight loss. (From Schauberger and co-workers, 1992, with permission.)

TABLE 10–8. National Research Council Recommended Daily Dietary Allowances for Women Before and During Pregnancy and Lactation

Nutrient	Nonpregnant[a]	Pregnant	Lactating
Kilocalories	2200	2500	2600
Protein (g)	55	60	65
Fat-soluble vitamins			
A (μg RE)[b]	800	800	1300
D (μg)	10	10	12
E (mg TE)[c]	8	10	12
K (μg)	55	65	65
Water-soluble vitamins			
C (mg)	60	70	95
Folate (μg)	180	400	280
Niacin (mg)	15	17	20
Riboflavin (mg)	1.3	1.6	1.8
Thiamine (mg)	1.1	1.5	1.6
Pyridoxine B_6 (mg)	1.6	2.2	2.1
Cobalamin B_{12} (μg)	2.0	2.2	2.6
Minerals			
Calcium (mg)	1200	1200	1200
Phosphorous (mg)	1200	1200	1200
Iodine (μg)	150	175	200
Iron (mg of ferrous iron)	15	30	15
Magnesium (mg)	280	320	355
Zinc (mg)	12	15	19

[a] For nonpregnant females ages 15–18.
[b] RE = retinol equivalent (1 RE = 1 μg retinol).
[c] TE = tocopherol equivalent.
From the National Research Council (1989).

PRENATAL VITAMIN AND MINERAL SUPPLEMENTATION. Up until the recommendation for folate supplementation to prevent neural-tube defects, iron was the only known nutrient for which requirements during pregnancy could not be met by diet alone (Institute of Medicine, 1990). A daily supplement of 30 mg of elemental iron is the recommended prophylaxis for iron deficiency in women at low risk for nutritional deficiency. Ingestion on an empty stomach will facilitate iron absorption for prophylaxis or treatment of iron-deficiency anemia (Chap. 49, p. 1309). In 1997, the FDA specified that iron preparations containing 30 mg or more of elemental iron per dosage had to be packaged as individual doses (e.g., blister packages). This regulation is targeted at preventing accidental iron poisoning in children.

Routine multivitamin supplementation is not recommended by the American Academy of Pediatrics and the American College of Obstetricians and Gynecologists (1997), unless the maternal diet is questionable or if she is at nutritional risk. The latter includes multiple gestation, substance abuse, complete vegetarians, epileptics, and women with hemoglobinopathies. In these high-risk women, daily multivitamin–mineral supplementation is recommended beginning in the second trimester. The suggested composition of this multivitamin–mineral supplement is 30 to 60 mg iron, 15 mg zinc, 2 mg copper, 250 mg calcium, 10 μg (400 IU) vitamin D, 50 mg vitamin C, 2 mg vitamin B_6, 300 μg folate, and 2 μg vitamin B_{12} (Institute of Medicine, 1992).

CALORIES. As shown in Figure 10–7, pregnancy requires an additional 80,000 kcal, which are accumulated primarily in the last 20 weeks. A daily caloric increase of 300 kcal throughout pregnancy is recommended by the National Research Council (1989). Calories are necessary for energy, and whenever caloric intake is inadequate, protein is metabolized for energy rather than being spared for its vital role in fetal growth and development. Total physiological requirements during preg-

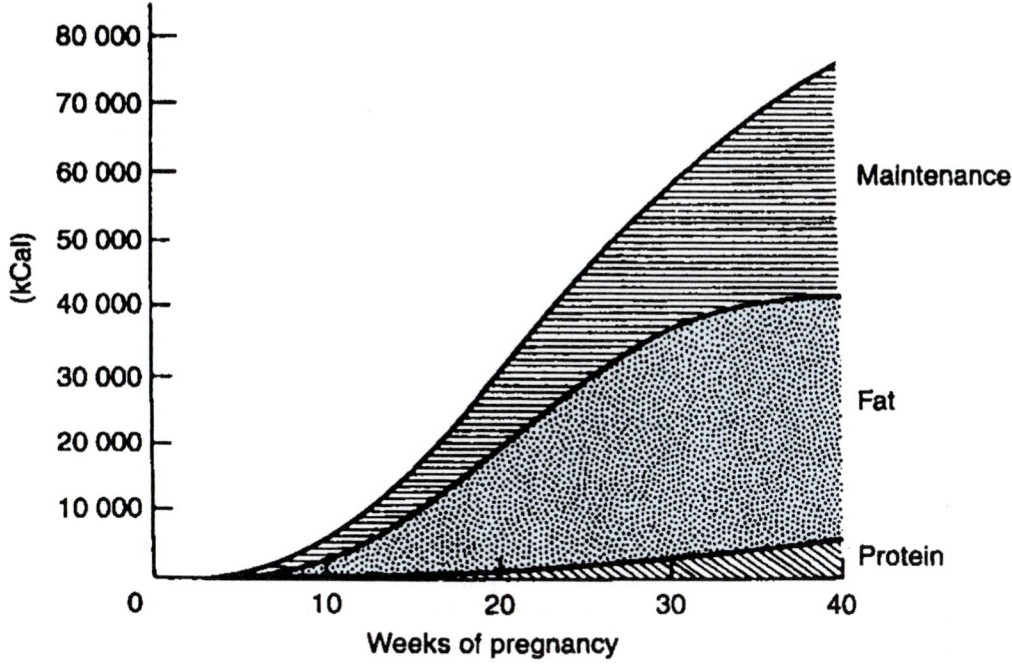

FIGURE 10–7. Cumulative kilocalories of energy required for pregnancy. (From Hytten and Chamberlain, 1991.)

nancy are not necessarily the sum of ordinary nonpregnant requirements plus those specific to pregnancy. For example, the additional energy required during pregnancy may be compensated in whole or in part by reduced physical activity (Hytten, 1991).

PROTEIN. To the basic protein needs of the nonpregnant woman are added the demands for growth and repair of the fetus, placenta, uterus, and breasts, and increased maternal blood volume. During the last 6 months of pregnancy, about 1 kg of protein is deposited, amounting to 5 to 6 g/day (Hytten and Leitch, 1971). Amino acids in maternal plasma have been incompletely studied other than to observe a marked fall in the concentrations of ornithine, glycine, taurine, and proline (Hytten, 1991). Exceptions during pregnancy are glutamic acid and alanine, which rise in concentration.

It is desirable that the majority of the protein be supplied from animal sources, such as meat, milk, eggs, cheese, poultry, and fish, because they furnish amino acids in optimal combinations. Milk and milk products have long been considered nearly ideal sources of nutrients, especially protein and calcium, for pregnant or lactating women.

MINERALS. The intakes recommended by the National Research Council (1989) for a variety of minerals are presented in Table 10–8. Practically all diets that supply sufficient calories for appropriate weight gain will contain enough minerals to prevent deficiency if iodized salt is used.

IRON. The reasons for increased iron requirements during pregnancy are discussed in Chapter 8 (p. 178). Of the approximately 300 mg of iron transferred to the fetus and placenta and the 500 mg incorporated, if available, into the expanding maternal hemoglobin mass, nearly all is used after midpregnancy. During that time, iron requirements imposed by pregnancy and maternal excretion total about 7 mg per day (Pritchard and Scott, 1970). Very few women have sufficient iron stores to supply this amount, and the diet seldom contains enough iron to meet this demand.

Iron supplementation is practiced commonly in the United States and elsewhere, although the merits of this practice continue to be questioned by some. Indeed, the U.S. Preventive Services Task Force (1993) takes a neutral stance, presumably because maternal anemia has not been proved to cause adverse pregnancy outcomes. This is illogical because it cannot be an advantage to enter a delivery in an anemic state when obstetrical hemorrhage is an ever-present threat.

Scott and co-workers (1970) established that as little as 30 mg of elemental iron supplied in the form of a simple iron salt such as ferrous gluconate, sulfate, or fumarate taken regularly once each day throughout the latter half of pregnancy, provided sufficient iron to meet the requirements of pregnancy and to protect any preexisting iron stores. This amount should also provide for the iron requirements of lactation. The pregnant woman may benefit from 60 to 100 mg of iron per day if she is large, has twin fetuses, is late in pregnancy, takes iron irregularly, or has a somewhat depressed hemoglobin level. The woman who is overtly anemic from iron deficiency responds well to 200 mg of iron per day in divided doses (Chap. 49, p. 1310).

Because iron requirements are slight during the first 4 months of pregnancy, it is *not* necessary to provide supplemental iron during this time. Withholding iron supplementation during the first trimester of pregnancy avoids the risk of aggravating nausea and vomiting. Ingestion of iron at bedtime also appears to minimize the possibility of an adverse gastrointestinal reaction. Iron-containing medication must be kept out of the reach of small children.

CALCIUM. The pregnant woman retains about 30 g of calcium, most of which is deposited in the fetus late in pregnancy (Pitkin, 1985). This amount of calcium represents only about 2.5 percent of total maternal calcium, most of which is in bone, and which can readily be mobilized for fetal growth. Moreover, Heaney and Skillman (1971) demonstrated increased calcium absorption by the intestine and progressive retention throughout pregnancy. According to Pitkin (1985), bound calcium levels, but not ionized calcium, fall slightly in maternal plasma as albumin concentration decreases (Chap. 8, p. 176).

PHOSPHORUS. The ubiquitous distribution of phosphorus ensures an adequate intake during pregnancy. Plasma levels of inorganic phosphorus do not differ appreciably from nonpregnant levels.

ZINC. Severe zinc deficiency may lead to poor appetite, suboptimal growth, and impaired wound healing. Profound zinc deficiency may cause dwarfism and hypogonadism. It may also lead to a specific skin disorder, *acrodermatitis enteropathica,* which is due to a rare, severe congenital zinc deficiency. Although zinc-deficient animal fetuses may have increased central nervous system malformations, the role of zinc in human pregnancy outcome is less clear (Goldenberg and associates, 1995).

Zinc in plasma is only about 1 percent of total body zinc. Moreover, plasma zinc is almost entirely bound to several plasma proteins and amino acids. Therefore, low plasma concentrations are generally the consequence of changes in concentration of the various binders in plasma rather than true zinc depletion (Swanson and King, 1983). Even though the concentration is reduced, the total zinc plasma pool of normally pregnant women is actually increased as the consequence of the large increase in pregnancy-induced plasma volume. Goldenberg and colleagues (1995) provided zinc supplementation (25 mg) in a randomized study of 580 indigent women beginning at a mean of 19 weeks. Plasma zinc levels were slightly and significantly higher in women supplemented. Infants born to zinc-supplemented women were slightly larger (mean 125 g) and had a slightly larger head circumference (mean increase 4 mm). Although the level of zinc supplementation that is safe for pregnant women has not been clearly established, recommended daily intake during pregnancy is 15 mg (Table 10–8).

IODINE. The use of iodized salt by all pregnant women is recommended to offset the increased need for fetal requirements and increased maternal renal losses. Iodine intake has been thought to be adequate in the United States, but it has declined substantially in the past 15 years (Utiger, 1999). Interest in increasing dietary iodine during pregnancy was heightened by a recent report linking subclinical maternal hypothyroidism to significant mental retardation in the children of such women (Haddow and colleagues, 1999).

Severe maternal iodine deficiency predisposes offspring to endemic cretinism, characterized by multiple severe neurological defects (Chap. 50, p. 1345). In parts of China and Africa where this condition is endemic, iodide supplementation very early in pregnancy prevents cretinism (Cao and colleagues, 1994). Iodine ingestion in pharmacological amounts during pregnancy may depress thyroid function and induce a sizable fetal goiter. The consumption of large amounts of seaweed by food faddists may do the same.

MAGNESIUM. Deficiency as the consequence of pregnancy has not been recognized. Undoubtedly, during prolonged illness with no magnesium intake, the plasma level might become critically low, as it would in the absence of pregnancy. We have observed magnesium deficiency during pregnancy complicated by the consequences of previous intestinal bypass surgery. Sibai and co-workers (1989) randomized 400 normotensive primigravid women to placebo tablets or 365 mg elemental magnesium supplementation from 13 to 24 weeks. Supplementation did not improve any measures of pregnancy outcome.

COPPER. Enzymes that contain copper, such as cytochrome oxidase, play key roles in many oxidative processes and hence in the production of most of the energy required for metabolism. Pregnancy has a major effect on maternal copper metabolism, with marked increases in serum ceruloplasmin and plasma copper. Copper deficiency has not been documented in humans during pregnancy. No studies of copper supplementation of pregnant women have been reported, although several prenatal supplements currently marketed provide 2 mg of copper per tablet.

SELENIUM. This is an essential component of the enzyme glutathione peroxidase, which catalyzes the conversion of hydrogen peroxide to water. Selenium is an important defensive component against free radical damage. Its deficiency has been identified in a large area of the People's Republic of China, where there is a severe geochemical deficiency. Deficiency is manifested by a frequently fatal cardiomyopathy in young children and women of childbearing age. Conversely, selenium toxicity due to oversupplementation has also been observed. There is no reported need to supplement selenium in American women during pregnancy.

CHROMIUM. Chromium is believed to play a physiological role as a co-factor for insulin, facilitating the initial attachment of the hormone to its peripheral receptors. The extent to which chromium is important in human nutrition remains uncertain, and there are no data suggesting that supplementation is advisable during pregnancy.

MANGANESE. This serves as a co-factor for enzymes such as the glycosyltransferases, which are necessary for the synthesis of polysaccharides and glycoproteins. Manganese deficiency has not been observed in human adults, and supplements are not indicated during pregnancy.

POTASSIUM. The concentration of potassium in maternal plasma decreases by about 0.5 mEq/L by midpregnancy (Brown and colleagues, 1986). Potassium deficiency develops in the same circumstances as when the woman is not pregnant. Prolonged nausea and vomiting may lead to hypokalemia and metabolic alkalosis. A previously rather common cause, the use of diuretics, has nearly disappeared.

SODIUM. Deficiency during pregnancy is most unlikely unless diuretics are prescribed or dietary sodium intake is reduced drastically. In general, salting food to taste will provide an abundance of sodium. Plasma sodium concentration normally decreases a few mEq during pregnancy; however, sodium excretion is unchanged, and averages 100 to 110 mEq/day (Brown and colleagues, 1986).

FLUORIDE. The value of supplemental fluoride during pregnancy has been questioned. Horowitz and Heifetz (1967) investigated the prevalence of caries in temporary and permanent teeth of children with the same postnatal exposure to optimally fluoridated water but

different patterns of prenatal exposure. They concluded that there were no additional benefits from maternal ingestion of fluoridated water if the offspring ingested such water from birth.

Glenn and associates (1982) reported a remarkably lower incidence (99 percent) of caries in children whose mothers ingested 2.2 mg of sodium fluoride daily during pregnancy, compared with those whose mothers used only fluoridated water. Fluoride supplementation during pregnancy has not been endorsed by the American Dental Association (Institute of Medicine, 1990).

Supplemental fluoride ingested by the lactating woman does not increase the fluoride concentration in her milk (Ekstrand, 1981).

VITAMINS. Most evidence concerning the importance of vitamins for successful reproduction has been obtained from animal experiments. Typically, severe deficiency has been produced in the animal by withholding the vitamin completely, beginning long before the time of pregnancy; or by giving a very potent vitamin antagonist. The administration of some vitamins in great excess to pregnant animals has been shown to exert deleterious effects on the fetus and newborn.

The increased requirements for vitamins during pregnancy shown in Table 10–8 in practically all circumstances can be supplied by any general diet that provides adequate amounts of calories and protein. The exception is folic acid during times of unusual requirements, such as pregnancy complicated by protracted vomiting, hemolytic anemia, or multiple fetuses.

FOLIC ACID. In the United States, approximately 4000 pregnancies are affected by neural-tube defects each year and more than half of these could be prevented with daily intake of 400 μg of folic acid throughout the periconceptional period (Centers for Disease Control and Prevention, 1999). Since 1992, the Public Health Service has recommended that all women capable of becoming pregnant consume 400 μg of folic acid daily throughout their childbearing years. The Food and Drug Administration (1996) later established standards fortifying cereal and grain products such as cereal, bread, rice, and pasta with folic acid. By putting 140 μg of folic acid into each 100 g of grain products, it was estimated that the folic acid intake of the average American woman of childbearing age would increase 100 μg per day.

There is evidence that this policy is contributing to a rise in serum folate levels (Lawrence and associates, 1999). There is also controversy over how much folic acid supplementation is enough to prevent neural-tube defects (Mills, 2000). Thus, it is unknown what lowest folic acid dose will prevent the estimated 50 percent of defects related to folic acid metabolism. Daly and colleagues (1997) contend that delivery of 200 μg daily by food fortification is effective against neural-tube defects and safer for the general population. The importance of a national food-fortification program is underscored by experiences in England and Wales where such a program is not used (Kadir and colleagues, 1999). Despite a large increase in sale of over-the-counter and prescription folic acid supplements in the 1990s in England and Wales, the rate of neural-tube defects has not changed. One explanation is that supplement sales likely do not represent the actual consumption of folic acid.

In 1997, the March of Dimes contracted the Gallup Organization to conduct a random-digit–dialed telephone survey of a national sample of 2001 women aged 15 to 45 years to assess knowledge about folic acid use (Centers for Disease Control and Prevention, 1999). Less than a third of women of childbearing age consume a daily supplement containing folic acid. Surprisingly, only 13 percent of women knew that folic acid helps prevent birth defects, and only 7 percent knew that folic acid should be taken before pregnancy. The March of Dimes will invest up to $10 million for a 3-year national folic acid education program.

VITAMIN A. Dietary intake of vitamin A in the United States appears to be adequate to meet the needs of most pregnant women (American College of Obstetricians and Gynecologists, 1998d). Routine supplementation during pregnancy is thus not recommended. A small number of case reports suggest an association with birth defects and very high doses of 10,000 to 50,000 IU daily during pregnancy. These malformations are similar to those produced by the vitamin A derivative isotretinoin (Accutane), which is a proven teratogen in humans (Chap. 38, p. 1015). Beta-carotene, the precursor of vitamin A found in fruits and vegetables, has not been shown to produce vitamin A toxicity.

VITAMIN B$_{12}$. The level of vitamin B$_{12}$ in maternal plasma decreases variably in otherwise normal pregnancies (Chap. 49, p. 1312). This is mostly from a reduction in plasma transcobalamins and is prevented only in part by supplementation. Vitamin B$_{12}$ occurs naturally only in foods of animal origin. It is now established that *strict vegetarians* may give birth to infants whose vitamin B$_{12}$ stores are low. Moreover, because breast milk of a vegetarian mother most likely contains little vitamin B$_{12}$, the deficiency may become profound in the breast-fed infant (Higginbottom and associates, 1978). Excessive ingestion of vitamin C can also lead to a functional deficiency of vitamin B$_{12}$.

VITAMIN B$_6$. Most clinical trials in pregnant women have failed to demonstrate any benefits of vitamin B$_6$ supplements (Institute of Medicine, 1990). For women at high risk for inadequate nutrition—e.g., substance abuse, adolescents, and those with multiple gestations—a daily supplement containing 2 mg is recommended.

VITAMIN C. The recommended dietary allowance for vitamin C during pregnancy is 70 mg/day, or about 20 percent more than when nonpregnant (Table 10–8). A reasonable diet should readily provide this amount. The maternal plasma level declines during pregnancy while the cord level is higher, a phenomenon observed with most water-soluble vitamins.

PRAGMATIC NUTRITIONAL SURVEILLANCE. Although the science of nutrition continues in its perpetual struggle to identify the ideal amounts of protein, calories, vitamins, and minerals for the pregnant woman and her fetus, those directly responsible for their care may best discharge their duties as follows:

- In general, advise the pregnant woman to eat what she wants in amounts she desires and salted to taste.
- Make sure that there is ample food to eat, especially in the case of the socioeconomically deprived woman.
- Ensure that she is gaining weight, with a goal of about 25 to 35 pounds in women with a normal body mass index.
- Periodically, explore the food intake by dietary recall. In this way, the occasional nutritionally absurd diet will be discovered.
- Give tablets of simple iron salts that provide at least 30 mg of iron daily. Give folate supplementation before and in the early weeks of pregnancy.
- Recheck the hematocrit or hemoglobin concentration at 28 to 32 weeks to detect any significant decrease.

COMMON CONCERNS

EXERCISE. In general, it is not necessary for the pregnant woman to limit exercise, provided she does not become excessively fatigued or risk injury to herself or her fetus. The current enthusiasm for jogging also has attracted a number of pregnant women. In fact, several women, even late in pregnancy, have run safely in marathons.

Clapp (1989) reported that 18 conditioned pregnant women actually improved their metabolic efficiency during exercise. Specifically, the amount of oxygen required to complete a treadmill exercise actually *decreased* during pregnancy! Pivarnik and co-workers (1990) used invasive hemodynamic monitoring and compared cardiovascular responses of seven healthy women to aerobic exercise (cycle or treadmill) during late pregnancy and again 3 months postpartum. Oxygen consumption, heart rate, stroke volume, and cardiac output all increased appropriately in response to exercise.

Pivarnik and associates (1994) later showed that pregnant women who exercised regularly had significantly larger blood volumes.

The effects have been described of maternal exercise on pregnancy outcomes, including spontaneous abortion, the course of labor, and birthweight (Clapp and Capeless, 1990; Clapp and Little, 1995). Continuation of aerobic exercise at intensities between 50 and 85 percent of their maximum capacity in 47 recreational runners and 40 aerobic dancers during the periconceptional period had no effect on the incidence of spontaneous abortion. Well-conditioned women who perform aerobics or run regularly were found to have shorter active labors and fewer cesarean deliveries, less meconium-stained amnionic fluid, and less fetal distress in labor. Continuation of regular aerobic or running exercise programs, however, did result in reduced birthweight (average 310 g) that primarily affected neonatal fat mass. Continuing regular exercise throughout pregnancy has even been observed to positively alter early neonatal behavior (Clapp and co-workers, 1999).

The American College of Obstetricians and Gynecologists (1994a) recommends that women who are accustomed to aerobic exercise before pregnancy should be allowed to continue this during pregnancy. They caution against starting new aerobic exercise programs or intensifying training efforts. For example, in women who were previously sedentary, aerobic activity more strenuous than walking is not recommended.

With some pregnancy complications, the mother and her fetus may benefit from a very sedentary existence. For example, women with hypertensive disorders due to pregnancy benefit from being sedentary (Chap. 24, p. 595), as do women pregnant with two or more fetuses (Chap. 30, p. 795), women suspected of having a growth-restricted fetus (Chap. 29, p. 755), and those with severe heart disease (Chap. 44, p. 1186).

EMPLOYMENT. The legal and social movements in the United States to provide equality of opportunity in the workplace have reached women who are or might become pregnant. Annas (1991) reviewed the legal issues involved with employment during pregnancy. Importantly, the United States Supreme Court buttressed the Pregnancy Discrimination Act of 1978 by ruling in 1991 that federal law prohibits employers from excluding women from job categories on the basis that they are or might become pregnant. More than 120 nations around the world currently provide paid maternity leave and health benefits by law, including most industrialized nations except the United States, Australia, and New Zealand (Luke and co-authors, 1999). Although the Family and Medical Leave Act (FMLA) was passed in 1993, a recent report to Congress found that because this leave is without pay, women eligible for leave did not take it for financial reasons. It is estimated that nearly half of women of childbearing age in the United States are in the labor force. Even larger proportions of socioeconomically less fortunate women are working.

Manshande and colleagues (1987) reported a sevenfold increased incidence of low-birthweight infants in women from Zaire who worked hard in the fields. Teitelman and co-workers (1990) evaluated maternal work activity and pregnancy outcome in 4186 women delivered at Yale-New Haven Hospital. Women were classified according to the type of jobs they held. *Standing* jobs, such as those of a cashier, bank teller, or dentist, required standing in the same position for more than 3 hours per day. *Active* jobs, such as physicians, waitresses, and real estate agents, involved continuous or intermittent walking. *Sedentary* jobs, such as librarian, bookkeeper, or bus driver, required less than an hour of standing per day. They found that pregnant women who work at jobs that require prolonged standing are at greater risk for preterm delivery, but it did not have any effect on fetal growth. Mozurkewich and colleagues (2000) reviewed 29 studies with over 160,000 pregnancies. They confirmed a 20 to 60 percent increase in preterm birth, fetal growth restriction, or hypertension with physically demanding work. Gabbe and Turner (1997) have reviewed work during pregnancy. Paul (1997) reviewed exposure to hazardous occupational agents during pregnancy.

Common sense dictates that any occupation that subjects the pregnant woman to severe physical strain should be avoided. Ideally, no work or play should be continued to the extent that undue fatigue develops. Adequate periods of rest should be provided during the working day. Women with previous pregnancy complications that are likely to be repetitive, such as low-birthweight infants, probably should minimize physical work. The American Academy of Pediatrics and the American College of Obstetricians and Gynecologists (1997) has concluded that women with uncomplicated pregnancies can usually continue to work until the onset of labor. A period of 4 to 6 weeks was recommended before return to work after delivery.

TRAVEL. Travel by the healthy woman has no harmful effect on pregnancy. Travel in properly pressurized aircraft offers no unusual risk, and American Airlines permits unrestricted travel as long as the woman feels well and is not within 7 days of her expected delivery date. Delta Airlines has no travel restrictions, but does recommend that the pregnant woman check with her physician if travel is scheduled after the "eighth month." At least every 2 hours, she should walk about. Perhaps the greatest risk with travel, especially international travel, is the development of a complication remote from facilities adequate to manage the complication.

The American College of Obstetricians and Gynecologists (1998c) has formulated guidelines for use of automobile passenger restraints during pregnancy. There is no evidence that safety restraints increase the chance of fetal injury. Indeed, the leading cause of fetal death in a motor accident is the death of the mother (Chap. 43, p. 1172). Therefore, pregnant women should be encouraged to wear properly positioned three-point restraints throughout pregnancy while riding in automobiles. The lap belt portion of the restraining belt should be placed under her abdomen and across her upper thighs. The belt should be as snug as comfortably possible. The shoulder belt also should be snugly applied and positioned between the breasts, although no serious harm appears to occur if the breast is compressed during a collision. There is little evidence concerning airbag use during pregnancy (Chap. 43, p. 1172). While some reports suggest their safety, we as well as others (Schultze and associates, 1998) have encountered stillbirths with their deployment.

BATHING. There is no objection to bathing during pregnancy or the puerperium. During the last trimester, the heavy uterus usually upsets the balance of the pregnant woman and increases the likelihood of her slipping and falling in the bathtub. For that reason, showers at the end of pregnancy may be preferable.

CLOTHING. It has generally been recommended that the clothing worn during pregnancy be comfortable and nonconstricting. According to fashion experts, however, pregnancy apparel has changed considerably in recent years (Morgan, 2000). One clothes designer stated: "It [sic, pregnancy] used to be about covering it up, and now its about showing it off. Today's maternity chic is body-hugging not body hiding."

The increasing mass of the breasts may make them pendulous and painful, and well-fitting supporting brassieres may be indicated for comfort. Constricting leg wear should be avoided.

BOWEL HABITS. Constipation is common, presumably because of prolonged transit time and compression of the lower bowel by the uterus or by the presenting part of the fetus (Chap. 48, p. 1277). In addition to the discomfort caused by the passage of hard fecal material, bleeding and painful fissures may develop in the edematous and hyperemic rectal mucosa. There is also greater frequency of *hemorrhoids* and, much less commonly, of prolapse of the rectal mucosa.

Women whose bowel habits are reasonably normal in the nonpregnant state may prevent constipation during pregnancy by close attention to bowel habits, taking sufficient quantities of fluid, and reasonable amounts of daily exercise, supplemented when necessary by a mild laxative, such as prune juice, milk of magnesia, bulk-producing substances, or stool-softening agents.

COITUS. Whenever abortion or preterm labor threatens, coitus should be avoided. Otherwise it has been generally accepted that in healthy pregnant women, sexual intercourse usually is not harmful before the last 4 weeks or so of pregnancy. In interviews with nearly 10,000 women enrolled in a prospective investigation, the Vaginal Infection and Prematurity Study Group found a significantly decreased frequency of sexual intercourse with advancing gestation (Read and Klebanoff, 1993). By 36 weeks, 72 percent reported intercourse less than once weekly. Bartellas and colleagues (2000) reported that this was due to decreased desire (58 percent) and fear of harm to the pregnancy (48 percent).

Risks from intercourse late in pregnancy have not been clearly delineated. Grudzinkas and co-workers (1979) found no association between gestational age at delivery and the frequency of coitus during the last 4 weeks of pregnancy. Naeye (1979), using data from the Collaborative Perinatal Project, reported that amnionic fluid infections and perinatal mortality were significantly increased if mothers had intercourse once or more weekly in the last month. In the large collaborative study described above by Read and Klebanoff (1993), there was no association with frequent intercourse and preterm delivery. Ekwo and colleagues (1993) interviewed over 1350 women and found that most sexual positions and activities were not associated with adverse outcomes. There was a twofold increased incidence of ruptured membranes with the male-superior position.

On occasion, sexual drive in the face of admonishment against intercourse late in pregnancy has led to sexual practices with disastrous consequences. Aronson and Nelson (1967) described a fatal cases of air embolism late in pregnancy as a result of air blown into the vagina during cunnilingus. Other near-fatal cases have been described (Bernhardt and associates, 1988).

CARE OF THE TEETH. Examination of the teeth should be included in the prenatal general physical examination. Pregnancy is rarely a contraindication to needed dental treatment. The concept that dental caries are aggravated by pregnancy is unfounded.

IMMUNIZATION. There has been some concern over the safety of various immunizations during pregnancy. Current recommendations are summarized in Table 10–9. Immunization in adults has been reviewed by Foley and Kopelman (1995) and Gardner and Schaffner (1993).

SMOKING. Since 1984 the Surgeon General has had warning labels on cigarette packages: "Smoking by pregnant women may result in fetal injury, premature birth,

TABLE 10–9. Recommendations for Immunization During Pregnancy

Live virus vaccines	Inactivated bacterial vaccines	Hyperimmune globulins
Measles—contraindicated	Pneumococcal—same as nonpregnant	Hepatitis B—postexposure prophylaxis: give along with hepatitis B vaccine initially, then vaccine alone at 1 and 6 mo
Mumps—contraindicated	Meningococcal—same as nonpregnant	Rabies—postexposure prophylaxis
Varicella-zoster—contraindicated	Hemophilus—same as nonpregnant	Tetanus—postexposure prophylaxis
Live bacterial vaccine	Cholera—risks vs benefits	Varicella—consider for postexposure within 96 h
Typhoid (Ty21a)—risks vs benefits		
Poliomyelitis—no longer recommended		
Yellow fever—high-risk areas only		
Inactivated virus vaccines	**Toxoids**	**Pooled immune serum globulins**
Influenza—after first trimester request	Tetanus–diphtheria—same as nonpregnant	Hepatitis A—postexposure prophylaxis
Rabies—same as nonpregnant		Measles—postexposure prophylaxis
Hepatitis A and B—same as nonpregnant		
Enhanced poliomyelitis (IPV-e)—risk of exposure		
Japanese encephalitis—weigh risks vs benefits		

Modified from the Association of Professors of Gynecology and Obstetrics (1999).

and low birthweight." Information on maternal smoking during pregnancy has been included on the birth certificate beginning in 1989. There has been a progressive decline in reported smoking during pregnancy from 20 percent in 1989 to 13 percent in 1998 (Ventura and colleagues, 2000). Similar results were observed using the Behavioral Risk Factor Surveillance System survey by the Centers for Disease Control and Prevention (Ebrahim and co-workers, 2000). It is noteworthy that the prevalence of cigarette smoking nationwide among high school students, in contrast to maternal smoking, increased during the 1990s (Centers for Disease Control and Prevention, 2000b).

A variety of adverse outcomes have been linked to smoking during pregnancy. Included are low birthweight due to either preterm delivery or fetal growth restriction, infant and fetal deaths, and placental abruption (Ananth and associates, 1996; Kleinman and colleagues, 1988; Lin and Santolaya-Forgas, 1998; Shah and Bracken, 2000; Ventura and co-workers, 2000). Suggested pathophysiological mechanisms for these adverse pregnancy effects include increased fetal carboxyhemoglobin levels, reduced uteroplacental blood flow, and fetal hypoxia (Jazayeri and colleagues, 1998; Monheit and co-workers, 1983). To put the smoking problem into a national perspective, in 1998, the 12 percent of American women who reported smoking during pregnancy accounted for one out of five infants weighing less than 2500 g at birth (Ventura and colleagues, 2000).

The American College of Obstetricians and Gynecologists (1997) has reviewed smoking cessation during pregnancy. The most successful efforts involved interventions that emphasize how to stop smoking. The Food and Drug Administration rates nicotine gum as category C (risk cannot be excluded) and transdermal systems are rated category D (positive evidence of risk). The American College of Obstetricians and Gynecologists (1997c) has concluded, however, that it is reasonable to use these nicotine medications during pregnancy if prior attempts to quit smoking have failed and the smoker is still using 10 to 15 cigarettes per day.

ALCOHOL. Ethanol is a potent teratogen (Chap. 38, p. 1011). Because alcohol use during pregnancy can cause the fetal alcohol syndrome, the Surgeon General recommends that women who are pregnant or considering pregnancy abstain from using any alcoholic beverages. The fetal alcohol syndrome is characterized by growth restriction, facial abnormalities, and central nervous system dysfunction. **From the evidence available, the best advice to the woman pregnant or about to become pregnant is to not consume alcohol.** It is hoped that the adverse effects of alcohol on pregnancy do not linger after the woman stops drinking.

CAFFEINE. In 1980, the Food and Drug Administration advised pregnant women to limit caffeine intake. The Fourth International Caffeine Workshop concluded shortly thereafter that there was no evidence that caffeine increased teratogenic or reproductive risk (Dews and colleagues, 1984). In small laboratory animals, caffeine is not a teratogen, but it does potentiate mutagenic effects of radiation and some chemicals if given in massive doses. When infused intravenously into sheep, it decreases uterine blood flow by 5 to 10 percent (Conover and colleagues, 1983).

Whether consumption of caffeine during pregnancy increases the risk of spontaneous abortion is controversial. Klebanoff and co-workers (1999) used a biological serum marker of caffeine consumption (paraxanthine) to estimate the dose of caffeine in 487 women with spontaneous abortions and in 2087 controls. Only extremely high serum paraxanthine concentrations were associated with abortion. Such high levels were equivalent to drinking more than 5 cups of coffee per day.

ILLICIT DRUGS. Chronic use during pregnancy of illicit drugs, including opium derivatives, barbiturates, and amphetamines, in large doses, is harmful to the fetus. Fetal distress, low birthweight, and serious compromise as the consequence of drug withdrawal soon after birth are well documented. Often the mother who uses hard drugs does not seek prenatal care, and even if she does, she may not admit to the use of such substances. Detection of scars from venipunctures may be the first clue. The management of pregnancy and delivery and successful care of the newborn infant may be extremely difficult.

The effects of a number of illicit drugs are considered in detail in Chapter 38, (p. 1030). The topic was also reviewed by the American College of Obstetricians and Gynecologists (1994b).

MEDICATIONS. Some drugs commonly ingested during pregnancy, and their possible adverse fetal effects, are considered in detail in Chapter 38. **With rare exception, any drug that exerts a systemic effect in the mother will cross the placenta to reach the embryo and fetus.** All physicians should develop the habit of ascertaining the likelihood of pregnancy before prescribing drugs for any woman, because a number of medications in common use can be injurious to the embryo and the fetus. Package inserts provided by pharmaceutical companies and approved by the FDA should be consulted before drugs are prescribed for pregnant women. If a drug is administered during pregnancy, the advantages to be gained must clearly outweigh any risks inherent in its use.

NAUSEA AND VOMITING. These are common complaints during the first half of pregnancy. Typically they commence between the first and second missed menstrual period and continue until about 14 weeks. Nausea and vomiting are usually worse in the morning, but may continue throughout the day. Lacroix and co-workers (2000) found that nausea and vomiting was reported by three fourths of pregnant women and lasted an average

of 35 days. Half of these had relief by 14 weeks' gestation, and 90 percent by 22 weeks. *Morning sickness* was a misnomer in this study because 80 percent of the women reported that nausea lasted all day.

The genesis of pregnancy-induced nausea and vomiting is not clear and it is discussed in Chapter 48 (p. 1275). While high levels of serum chorionic gonadotropin have been implicated, nausea is likely induced by estrogen levels that parallel gonadotropin levels. Flaxman and Sherman (2000) contend that nausea and vomiting during early pregnancy evolved to protect the developing fetus by encouraging its mother to avoid dangerous foods. There is no scientific evidence for this view.

Seldom is the treatment of nausea and vomiting of pregnancy so successful that the affected expectant mother is afforded complete relief. Fortunately, the unpleasantness and discomfort can usually be minimized. Eating small feedings at more frequent intervals but stopping short of satiation is of value. Because the smell of certain foods often precipitates or aggravates the symptoms, such foods should be avoided as much as possible. Very infrequently vomiting may be so severe that dehydration, electrolyte and acid–base disturbances, and starvation become serious problems. This is termed *hyperemesis gravidarum*, and its management is described in Chapter 48 (p. 1275).

CONSTIPATION. Constipation was discussed under "Bowel Habits" earlier in the chapter, and is covered extensively in Chapter 48 (p. 1277).

BACKACHE. Low back pain to some extent is reported in half of pregnant women. Minor degrees follow excessive strain or fatigue and excessive bending, lifting, or walking. Orvieto and associates (1994) studied 449 women and reported that back pain increased with duration of gestation. Prior low back pain and obesity were risk factors.

Back pain can be reduced by having women squat rather than bend over when reaching down, providing back support with a pillow when sitting down, and avoiding high-heeled shoes. Severe back pain should not be attributed simply to pregnancy until a thorough orthopedic examination has been conducted. Muscular spasm and tenderness, which often are classified clinically as acute strain or fibrositis, respond well to analgesics, heat, and rest. As discussed in Chapter 50 (p. 1349), some women with severe back and hip pain may have *pregnancy-associated osteoporosis* (Dunne and colleagues, 1993).

In some women, motion of the symphysis pubis and lumbosacral joints, and general relaxation of pelvic ligaments may be demonstrated. In severe cases the pregnant woman may be unable to walk or even remain comfortable without support furnished by a heavy girdle and prolonged periods of rest. Occasionally, anatomical, congenital, or traumatic defects are found. Pain caused by herniation of an intervertebral disc occurs during pregnancy with about the same frequency as at other times.

VARICOSITIES. These generally result from congenital predisposition, and are exaggerated by prolonged standing, pregnancy, and advancing age. Usually varicosities become more prominent as pregnancy advances, as weight increases, and as the length of time spent upright is prolonged. As discussed in Chapter 8 (p. 184), femoral venous pressure increases appreciably as pregnancy advances. The symptoms produced by varicosities vary from cosmetic blemishes on the lower extremities and mild discomfort at the end of the day to severe discomfort that requires prolonged rest with the feet elevated.

The treatment of varicosities of the lower extremities is generally limited to periodic rest with elevation of the legs, elastic stockings, or both. Surgical correction of the condition during pregnancy is generally not advised, although occasionally the symptoms may be so severe that injection, ligation, or even stripping of the veins is necessary in order to allow the pregnant woman to remain ambulatory. In general, these operations should be postponed until after delivery. Vulvar varicosities may be aided by application of a foam rubber pad suspended across the vulva by a belt of the type used with a perineal pad. Rarely, large varicosities may rupture, resulting in profuse hemorrhage.

Occasionally, *superficial thrombophlebitis* complicates preexisting varicose veins (Chap. 46, p. 1235).

HEMORRHOIDS. Varicosities of the rectal veins occasionally first appear during pregnancy. More often, pregnancy causes an exacerbation or recurrence of previous hemorrhoids. Their development or aggravation during pregnancy is undoubtedly related to increased pressure in the rectal veins caused by obstruction of venous return by the large uterus, and to the tendency toward constipation during pregnancy. Usually pain and swelling are relieved by topically applied anesthetics, warm soaks, and agents that soften the stool. Thrombosis of a rectal vein can cause considerable pain, but the clot can usually be evacuated by incising the wall of the involved vein with a scalpel under topical anesthesia.

HEARTBURN. This symptom is one of the most common complaints of pregnant women, and is caused by reflux of gastric contents into the lower esophagus. The increased frequency of regurgitation during pregnancy most likely results from the upward displacement and compression of the stomach by the uterus combined with relaxation of the lower esophageal sphincter. In most pregnant women, symptoms are mild and relieved by a regimen of more frequent but smaller meals and avoidance of bending over or lying flat. Antacid preparations may provide considerable relief. Aluminum hydroxide, magnesium trisilicate, or magnesium hydroxide, alone or in combination, should be used in preference to sodium bicarbonate. The pregnant woman who tends to retain sodium can become edematous as the result of ingestion of excessive amounts of sodium bicarbonate. Management for symptoms that do not respond to these simple measures is discussed in Chapter 48 (p. 1276).

PICA. There has been considerable historical interest in the alleged cravings (pica) of pregnant women for strange foods and, at times, nonfoods such as ice (pagophagia), starch (amylophagia), or clay (geophagia). The desire for dry lump starch, clay, chopped ice, or even refrigerator frost has been considered by some to be triggered by severe iron deficiency. Although some women crave these items, and although the craving is usually ameliorated after correction of iron deficiency, not all pregnant women with pica are necessarily iron deficient. Certainly, if strange "foods" dominate the diet, iron deficiency will be aggravated or it will develop eventually.

Golden (2000) reviewed the history of pica during pregnancy and traces its roots to medical legend beginning in the 16th century. For example, there is the legend of a 16th-century woman who craved a bite from the arm of a baker and refused all other food. To accommodate her pica, her husband paid the baker to permit the woman to take three bites. After enduring only two, he backed out of the agreement and she subsequently gave birth to triplets, and one was stillborn. This tale was cited up until the 1940s to support the popular belief that the longings of pregnant women should not be denied and that to refuse their demands was to put a child at risk.

We are of the view that pica is more legend than reality. For example, it is commonly believed that pregnant women crave pickles. In fact, during more than 25 years of observation of hospitalized pregnant women for various complications in the Parkland Hospital High-Risk Pregnancy Unit, only one woman demanded pickles be available at her bedside. It is probably time to end obstetrical credence for tales of unusual longings attributable to pregnancy.

PTYALISM. Women during pregnancy are occasionally distressed by profuse salivation. The cause of this ptyalism sometimes appears to be stimulation of the salivary glands by the ingestion of starch. This cause should be looked for and eradicated if found. Most cases are unexplained.

FATIGUE. Early in pregnancy, most women complain of fatigue and desire for excessive periods of sleep. The condition usually remits spontaneously by the fourth month of pregnancy and has no special significance. It may be due to the soporific effect of progesterone(s).

HEADACHE. This symptom is a frequent complaint early in pregnancy. A few cases may result from sinusitis or ocular strain caused by refractive errors. In the vast majority, however, no cause can be demonstrated. Treatment is largely symptomatic. By midpregnancy, most headaches decrease in severity or disappear. The pathological significance of headaches as the consequence of hypertensive disorders that develops later in pregnancy is considered in Chapter 24 (p. 570). Persistent or severe headaches of other origins, for example, migraine, are discussed in Chapter 53 (p. 1406).

LEUKORRHEA. Pregnant women commonly develop increased vaginal discharge, which in many instances is not pathological. Increased mucus formation by cervical glands in response to hyperestrogenemia is undoubtedly a contributing factor. If the secretion is troublesome, the woman may be advised to douche with water mildly acidified with vinegar.

Occasionally, troublesome leukorrhea is the result of an infection caused by *Trichomonas vaginalis* or *Candida albicans.*

TRICHOMONIASIS. In as many as 20 percent of women, *T. vaginalis* can be identified during prenatal examination. Symptomatic infection is much less prevalent, and vaginitis is characterized by foamy leukorrhea with pruritus and irritation. Trichomonads are demonstrated readily in fresh vaginal secretions as flagellated, pear-shaped, motile organisms that are somewhat larger than leukocytes.

Metronidazole has proved effective in eradicating *T. vaginalis.* The drug may be administered orally or vaginally. When ingested by the mother, metronidazole crosses the placenta and enters the fetal circulation. The possibility of teratogenicity from first-trimester exposure has been raised. As discussed in Chapter 38 (p. 1021) Rosa and colleagues (1987) found no increased frequency of birth defects in over 1000 women given metronidazole during early pregnancy. The drug is classified as category B by the manufacturer, but the Centers for Disease Control recommend against its use in early pregnancy.

CANDIDIASIS. *C. albicans* can be cultured from the vagina in about 25 percent of women approaching term. Asymptomatic vaginal candidiasis requires no treatment, but may sometimes cause an extremely profuse irritating discharge. Miconazole, clotrimazole, and nys-

tatin are effective for the treatment of candidiasis during pregnancy. Infection is likely to recur, thereby requiring repeated treatment during pregnancy; but it usually subsides at the end of gestation.

BACTERIAL VAGINOSIS. Not an infection in the ordinary sense, bacterial vaginosis is a maldistribution of bacterial populations that comprise normal vaginal flora. Lactobacilli are decreased, and overrepresented species tend to be anaerobic bacteria, including *Gardnerella vaginalis, Mobiluncus,* and some *Bacteroides* species. The Vaginal Infections and Prematurity Study Group (Hillier and colleagues, 1995) identified the condition in 16 percent of over 10,000 pregnant women studied at 23 to 26 weeks. Its prevalence during pregnancy varies from 10 to 30 percent (MacDermott, 1995). The issue of vaginosis causing preterm labor remains unresolved (Chap. 27, p. 699).

Treatment is reserved for symptomatic women who usually complain of a fishy-smelling malodorous discharge. Metronidazole, 500 mg twice daily orally for 7 days, will achieve cure in about 90 percent of cases.

REFERENCES

Abrams BF, Laros RK: Pre-prepregnancy weight, weight gain, and birthweight. Am J Obstet Gynecol 154:503, 1986

Abrams B, Selvin S: Maternal weight gain pattern and birth weight. Obstet Gynecol 86:163, 1995

American Academy of Pediatrics and American College of Obstetricians and Gynecologists: Guidelines for Perinatal Care, 4th ed. 1997

American College of Obstetricians and Gynecologists: Domestic Violence. Educational Bulletin No. 257, December, 1999a

American College of Obstetricians and Gynecologists: Psychosocial Risk Factors: Perinatal Screening and Intervention. Educational Bulletin No. 255, November, 1999b

American College of Obstetricians and Gynecologists: Statement of Policy in Human Immunodeficiency Virus Screening. May, 1999c

American College of Obstetricians and Gynecologists: Bacterial Vaginosis Screening for Prevention of Preterm Delivery. Committee Opinion No. 198, February, 1998a

American College of Obstetricians and Gynecologists: Mandatory Reporting of Domestic Violence. Committee Opinion No. 200, March, 1998b

American College of Obstetricians and Gynecologists: Obstetric Aspects of Trauma Management. Educational Bulletin No. 251, September, 1998c

American College of Obstetricians and Gynecologists: Vitamin A Supplemental During Pregnancy. Committee Opinion No. 196, January, 1998d

American College of Obstetricians and Gynecologists: Fetal Fibronectin Preterm Labor Risk Test. Committee Opinion No. 187, September, 1997a

American College of Obstetricians and Gynecologists: Routine Ultrasound in Low-risk Pregnancy. Practice Patterns No. 5, August, 1997b

American College of Obstetricians and Gynecologists: Smoking and Women's Health. Educational Bulletin No. 240, September, 1997c

American College of Obstetricians and Gynecologists Committee on Obstetrics: Prevention of Early-onset Group B Streptococcal Disease in Newborns. Committee Opinion No. 173, June, 1996

American College of Obstetricians and Gynecologists: Preconception Care. Technical Bulletin No. 205, May, 1995

American College of Obstetricians and Gynecologists: Exercise During Pregnancy and the Postpartum Period. Technical Bulletin No. 189, February, 1994a

American College of Obstetricians and Gynecologists: Substance Abuse in Pregnancy. Technical Bulletin No. 195, July, 1994b

Amini SB, Catalano PM, Dierker LJ, Mann LI: Births to teenagers: Trends and obstetric outcomes. Obstet Gynecol 87:668, 1996

Ananth CV, Savitz DA, Luther ER: Maternal cigarette smoking as a risk factor for placental abruption, placenta previa, and uterine bleeding in pregnancy. Am J Epidemiol 144:881, 1996

Andrews WW, Goldenberg RL, Mercer B, Iams J, Meis P, Moawad A, Das A, et al: The Preterm Prediction Study: Association of second-trimester genitourinary chlamydia infection with subsequent spontaneous preterm birth. Am J Obstet Gynecol 183:662, 2000

Annas GJ: Fetal protection and employment discrimination—the Johnson Controls case. N Engl J Med 325:740, 1991

Aronson ME, Nelson PK: Fatal air embolism in pregnancy resulting from an unusual sex act. Obstet Gynecol 30:127, 1967

Association of Professors of Obstetricians and Gynecologists: Immunization for women's health. APGO Education Series on Women's Health Issues. Washington, DC, Association of Professors of Obstetricians and Gynecologists, 1999

Bartellas E, Crane JMG, Daley M, Bennett KA, Hutchens D: Sexuality and sexual activity in pregnancy. Br J Obstet Gynaecol 107:964, 2000

Bernhardt TL, Goldmann RW, Thombs PA, Kindwall EP: Hyperbaric oxygen treatment of cerebral air embolism from urogenital sex during pregnancy. Crit Care Med 16:729, 1988

Bracken MB, Belanger K: Calculation of delivery dates. N Engl J Med 321:1483, 1989

Brown MA, Sinosich MJ, Saunders DM, Gallery ED: Potassium regulation and progesterone-aldosterone interrelationships in human pregnancy: A prospective study. Am J Obstet Gynecol 155:349, 1986

Calvert JP, Crean EE, Newcombe RG, Pearson JF: Antenatal screening by measurement of symphysis-fundus height. BMJ 285:846, 1982

Cao XY, Jiang XM, Dou ZH, Rakeman MA, Zhang ML, O'Donnell K, Ma T, Amette K, DeLong N, DeLong GR: Timing of vulnerability of the brain to iodine deficiency in endemic cretinism. N Engl J Med 331:1739, 1994

Carey JC, Klebanoff M, for the NICHD MFMU Network: Metronidazole treatment increased the risk of preterm birth in asymptomatic women with trichomonas. Am J Obstet Gynecol 182:513, 2000a

Carey JC, Klebanoff MA, Hauth JC, Hillier SL, Thom EA, Ernest JM, Heine RP, Nugent RP, Fischer ML, Leveno KJ, Wapner R, Varner M, Trout W, Moawad A, Sibai BM, Miodovnik M, Dombrowski M, O'Sullivan MJ, VanDorsten JP, Langer O, Roberts J, the National Institute of Child Health Human Development Network of Maternal–Fetal Medicine Units: Metronidazole to prevent preterm delivery

in pregnant women with asymptomatic bacterial vaginosis. N Eng J Med 342:534, 2000b

Centers for Disease Control and Prevention: Entry into prenatal care—United States, 1989–1997. MMWR 49:18, 2000a

Centers for Disease Control and Prevention: Tobacco use among middle and high school students—United States, 1999. MMWR 49:49, 2000b

Centers for Disease Control and Prevention: Knowledge and use of folic acid by women of childbearing age—United States 1995–1998. MMWR 48:16, 1999

Centers for Disease Control and Prevention: Prevention of perinatal group B streptococcal disease: A public health perspective. MMWR 45:1, 1996

Clapp JF III: Oxygen consumption during treadmill exercise before, during, and after pregnancy. Am J Obstet Gynecol 161:1458, 1989

Clapp JF III, Capeless EL: Neonatal morphometrics after endurance exercise during pregnancy. Am J Obstet Gynecol 163:1805, 1990

Clapp JF III, Little KD: The interaction between regular exercise and selected aspects of women's health. Am J Obstet Gynecol 173:2, 1995

Clapp JF III, Lopez B, Harcar-Sevcik R: Neonatal behavioral profile of the offspring of women who continued to exercise regularly throughout pregnancy. Am J Obstet Gynecol 180:91, 1999

Clement S, Candy B, Sikorski J, Wilson J, Smeeton N: Does reducing the frequency of routine antenatal visits have long term effects? Follow-up of participants in a randomized controlled trial. Br J Obstet Gynaecol 106:367, 1999

Cnattingius S, Granath F, Petersson G, Harlow BL: The influence of gestational age and smoking habits on the risk of subsequent preterm deliveries. N Engl J Med 341:943, 1999

Conover WB, Key TC, Resnik R: Maternal cardiovascular response to caffeine infusion in the pregnant ewe. Am J Obstet Gynecol 145:534, 1983

Daly S, Mills JL, Molloy AM, Conley M, Lee YJ, Kirke PN, Weir DG, Scott JM: Minimum effective dose of folic acid for food fortification to prevent neural-tube defects. Lancet 350:1666, 1997

Dews P, Grice HC, Neims A, Wilson J, Wurtman R: Report of Fourth International Caffeine Workshop, Athens, 1982. Food Chem Toxicol 22:163, 1984

Dunne F, Walter B, Marshall T, Heath DA: Pregnancy-associated osteoporosis. Clin Endocrinol 39:487, 1993

Earls F: Positive effects of prenatal and early childhood interventions. JAMA 280:1271, 1998

Ebrahim SH, Floyd RL, Merritt RK, Decoufle P, Holtzman D: Trends in pregnancy-related smoking rates in the United States, 1987–1996. JAMA 283:361, 2000

Ebrahim SH, Luman ET, Floyd RL: Alcohol consumption by pregnant women in the United States during 1988–1995. Obstet Gynecol 92:187, 1998

Ekstrand J, Boreus LO, de Chateau P: No evidence of transfer of fluoride from plasma to breast milk. BMJ (Clin Res Ed) 283:761, 1981

Ekwo EE, Gosselink CA, Woolson R, Moawad A, Long CR: Coitus late in pregnancy: Risk of preterm rupture of amniotic sac membranes. Am J Obstet Gynecol 168:22, 1993

Feig DS, Naylor CD: Eating for two: Are guidelines for weight gain during pregnancy too liberal? Lancet 351:1054, 1998

Fiscella K: Does prenatal care improve birth outcomes? A critical review. Obstet Gynecol 85:468, 1995

Flaxman SM, Sherman PW: Morning sickness: A mechanism for protecting mother and embryo. Q Rev Biol 75:113, 2000

Florida Department of Health: Healthy Start Prenatal Risk Screening Instrument. DH No. 3134, September, 1997

Foley KS, Kopelman JN: Immunizations in women. Prim Care Update Ob/Gyns 2:53, 1995

Food and Drug Administration. Food standards: Amendment of standards of identity for enriched grain products to require addition of folic acid. Fed Regist 61:8781, 1996

Gabbe SG, Turner LP: Reproductive hazards of the American lifestyle: Work during pregnancy. Am J Obstet Gynecol 176:826, 1997

Gardner P, Schaffner W: Immunization of adults. N Engl J Med 328:1252, 1993

Gazmararian JA, Lazorick S, Spitz AM, Ballard TJ, Saltzman LE, Marks JS: Prevalence of violence against pregnant women. JAMA 275:1915, 1996

Glenn FB, Glenn WD III, Duncan RC: Fluoride tablet supplementation during pregnancy for caries immunity: A study of the offspring produced. Am J Obstet Gynecol 143:560, 1982

Golden J: The woman who mistook her husband for a steak; the medical legends of morbid "longings." ACOG Clin Rev 5:12, 2000

Goldenberg RL, Tamura T, Neggers Y, Copper RL, Johnston KE, DuBard MB, Hauth JC: The effect of zinc supplementation on pregnancy outcome. JAMA 274:463, 1995

Grudzinskas JG, Watson C, Chard T: Does sexual intercourse cause fetal distress? Lancet 2:692, 1979

Haddow JE, Palomaki GE, Allan WC, Williams JR, Knight GJ, Gagnon J, O'Heir CE, Mitchell ML, Hermos RJ, Waisbren SE, Faix JD, Klein RZ: Maternal thyroid deficiency during pregnancy and subsequent neuropsychological development of the child. N Engl J Med 341:549, 1999

Heaney RP, Skillman TG: Calcium metabolism in normal human pregnancy. J Clin Endocrinol Metab 33:661, 1971

Herbert WNP, Bruninghaus HM, Barefoot AB, Bright TG: Clinical aspects of fetal heart auscultation. Obstet Gynecol 69:574, 1987

Hickey CA, Cliver SP, McNeal SF, Hoffman HJ, Goldenberg RL: Prenatal weight gain patterns and spontaneous preterm birth among nonobese black and white women. Obstet Gynecol 85:909, 1995

Higginbottom MC, Sweetman L, Nyhan WL: A syndrome of methylmalonic aciduria, homocystinuria, megaloblastic anemia and neurologic abnormalities in a vitamin B_{12}-deficient breast-fed infant of a strict vegetarian. N Engl J Med 299:317, 1978

Hillier SL, Nugent RP, Eschenbach DA, Krohn MA, Gibbs RS, Martin DH, Cotch MF, Edelman R, Pastorek JG, Rao AV, McNellis D, Regan JA, Carey C, Klebanoff MA: Association between bacterial vaginosis and preterm delivery of a low-birth-weight infant. N Eng J Med 333:1737, 1995

Horowitz HS, Heifetz SB: Effects of prenatal exposure to fluoridation on dental caries. Public Health Rep 82:297, 1967

Hytten FE: Weight gain in pregnancy. In Hytten FE, Chamberlain G (eds): Clinical Physiology in Obstetrics, 2nd ed. Oxford, Blackwell, 1991, p 173

Hytten FE, Chamberlain G: Clinical physiology in obstetrics. Oxford, Blackwell, 1991, p 152

Hytten FE, Leitch I: The Physiology of Human Pregnancy, 2nd ed. Oxford, Blackwell, 1971

Institute of Medicine: Nutrition during pregnancy and lactation: An implementation guide. Washington, DC, National Academy Press, 1992, p 14

Institute of Medicine: Nutrition During Pregnancy, 1. Weight Gain; 2. Nutrient Supplements. Washington, DC, National Academy Press, 1990

Jazayeri A, Tsibris JCM, Spellacy WN: Umbilical cord plasma erythropoietin levels in pregnancies complicated by maternal smoking. Am J Obstet Gynecol 178:433, 1998

Jimenez JM, Tyson JE, Reisch JS: Clinical measures of gestational age in normal pregnancies. Obstet Gynecol 61:438, 1983

Johnson JWC, Yancey MK: A critique of the new recommendations for weight gain in pregnancy. Am J Obstet Gynecol 174:254, 1996

Kadir RA, Sabin C, Whitlow B, Brockbank E, Economides D: Neural tube defects and periconceptional folic acid in England and Wales: Retrospective study. BMJ 319:92, 1999

Klebanoff MA, Levine RJ, DerSimonian R, Clemens JD, Wilkins DG: Maternal serum paraxanthine, a caffeine metabolite, and the risk of spontaneous abortion. N Engl J Med 341:1639, 1999

Klebanoff MA, Shiono PH, Carey JC: The effect of physical activity during pregnancy on preterm delivery and birthweight. Am J Obstet Gynecol 163:1450, 1990

Kleinman JC, Pierre MB, Madans JH, Land GH, Schramm WF: The effects of maternal smoking on fetal and infant mortality. Am J Epidemiol 127:274, 1988

Kogan MD, Alexander GR, Kotelchuck M, Nagey DA: Relation to the content of prenatal care to the risk of low birth weight. Maternal reports of health behavior advice and initial prenatal care procedures. JAMA 271:1340, 1994

Kogan MD, Martin JA, Alexander GR, Kotelchuck M, Ventura SJ, Frigoletto FD: The changing pattern of prenatal care utilization in the United States, 1981–1995, using different prenatal care indices. JAMA 279:1623, 1998

Kortenoever ME: Pathology of pregnancy: Pregnancy of long duration and postmature infant. Obstet Gynecol Surv 5:812, 1950

Lacroix R, Eason E, Melzack R: Nausea and vomiting during pregnancy: A prospective study of its frequency, intensity, and pattern of change. Am J Obstet Gynecol 182:931, 2000

Lawrence JM, Petitti DB, Watkins M, Umekubo MA: Trends in serum folate after food fortification. Lancet 354:915, 1999

Lin CC, Santolaya-Forgas J: Current concepts of fetal growth restriction: Part I. Causes, classification, and pathophysiology. Obstet Gynecol 92:1044, 1998

Loudon I: Death in Childbirth. New York, Oxford University Press, 1992, p 577

Luke B, Avni M, Min L, Misiunas R: Work and pregnancy: The role of fatigue and the "second shift" on antenatal morbidity. Am J Obstet Gynecol 181:1172, 1999

MacDermott RIJ: Bacterial vaginosis. Br J Obstet Gynaecol 102:92, 1995

Manshande JP, Eeckels R, Manshande-Desmet V, Vlietinck R: Rest versus heavy work during the last weeks of pregnancy: Influence on fetal growth. Br J Obstet Gynaecol 94:1059, 1987

Merkatz IR, Thompson JE, Walsh LV: History of prenatal care. In Merkatz IR, Thompson JE (eds): New Perspectives on Prenatal Care. New York, Elsevier, 1990, p 14

Mills JL: Fortification of foods with folic acid—how much is enough? N Engl J Med 342:1442, 2000

Monheit AG, Van Vunakis H, Key TC, Resnik R: Maternal and fetal cardiovascular effects of nicotine infusion in pregnant sheep. Am J Obstet Gynecol 145:290, 1983

Morgan K: Front and center. Dallas Morning News, June 7, 2000

Mozurkewich EL, Luke B, Avni M, Wolf EM: Working conditions and adverse pregnancy outcome: A meta-analysis. Obstet Gynecol 95:623, 2000

Naeye RL: Coitus and associated amniotic-fluid infections. N Engl J Med 301:1198, 1979

National Research Council: Recommended Dietary Allowances, 10th ed. Washington, DC, National Academy Press, 1989

Olds DL, Eckenrode J, Henderson CR, Kitzman H, Powers J, Cole R, Sidora K, Morris P, Pettitt LM, Luckey D: Long-term effects of home visitation on maternal life course and child abuse and neglect. JAMA 278:637, 1997

Olds DL, Henderson CR, Cole R, Eckenrode J, Kitzman H, Luckey D, Pettitt L, Sidora K, Morriss P, Powers J: Long-term effects of nurse home visitation on children's criminal and antisocial behavior. JAMA 280:1238, 1998

Olds DL, Henderson CR, Tatelbaum R, Chamberlin R: Improving the delivery of prenatal care and outcomes of pregnancy: A randomized trial of nurse home visitation. Pediatrics 77:16, 1986

Orvieto R, Achiron A, Ben-Rafael Z, Gelernter I, Achiron R: Low-back pain of pregnancy. Acta Obstet Gynecol Scand 73:209, 1994

Parker JD, Abrams B: Prenatal weight gain advice: An examination of the recent prenatal weight gain recommendations of the Institute of Medicine. Obstet Gynecol 79:664, 1992

Paul M: Occupational reproductive hazards. Lancet 349:1385, 1997

Petitti DB, Croughan-Minihane MS, Hiatt RA: Weight gain by gestational age in both black and white women delivered of normal-birth-weight and low-birth-weight infants. Am J Obstet Gynecol 164:801, 1991

Pitkin RM: Calcium metabolism in pregnancy and the perinatal period: A review. Am J Obstet Gynecol 151:99, 1985

Pivarnik JM, Lee W, Clark SL, Cotton DB, Spillman HT, Miller JF: Cardiac output responses of primigravid women during exercise determined by the direct Fick technique. Obstet Gynecol 75:954, 1990

Pivarnik JM, Mauer MB, Ayres NA, Kirshon B, Dildy GA, Cotton DB: Effects of chronic exercise on blood volume expansion and hematologic indices during pregnancy. Obstet Gynecol 83:265, 1994

Pritchard JA, Scott DE: Iron demands during pregnancy. In Hallberg L, Harwerth HG, Vannotti A (eds): Iron Deficiency: Pathogenesis, Clinical Aspects, Therapy. New York, Academic Press, 1970

Quaranta P, Currell R, Redman CWG, Robinson JS: Prediction of small-for-date infants by measurements of symphysial-fundal height. Br J Obstet Gynaecol 88:115, 1981

Read JS, Klebanoff MA: Sexual intercourse during pregnancy and preterm delivery: Effects of vaginal microorganisms. Am J Obstet Gynecol 168:514, 1993

Report of the Panel on Dietary Reference Values of the Committee on Medical Aspects of Food Policy: Dietary reference values for food, energy and nutrients for the United Kingdom. London, Department of Health, 1991, p 30

Roberts RO, Yawn BP, Wickes SL, Field CS, Garretson M, Jacobsen SJ: Barriers to prenatal care: Factors associated with late initiation of care in a middle class midwestern community. J Fam Pract 47:53, 1998

Rooks JP: Letter to the editor: Benefits and limitations of prenatal care. JAMA 280:2072, 1998

Rosa FW, Baum C, Shaw M: Pregnancy outcomes after first trimester vaginitis drug therapy. Obstet Gynecol 69:751, 1987

Rosen MG, Merkatz IR, Hill JG: Caring for our future: A report by the expert panel on the content of prenatal care. Obstet Gynecol 77:782, 1991

Satin AJ, Leveno KJ, Sherman ML, Reedy NJ, Lowe TW, McIntire DD: Maternal youth and pregnancy outcomes: Middle school versus high school age groups compared to women beyond the teen years. Am J Obstet Gynecol 171:184, 1994

Schauberger CW, Rooney BL, Brimer LM: Factors that influence weight loss in the puerperium. Obstet Gynecol 79:424, 1992

Schultze PM, Stamm CA, Roger J: Placental abruption and fetal death with airbag deployment in a motor vehicle accident. Obstet Gynecol 92:719, 1998

Scott DE, Pritchard JA, Saltin AS, Humphreyes SM: Iron deficiency during pregnancy. In Hallberg L, Harwerth HG, Vannotti A (eds): Iron Deficiency: Pathogenesis, Clinical Aspects, Therapy. New York, Academic Press, 1970

Shah NR, Bracken MB: A systematic review and meta-analysis of prospective studies on the association between maternal cigarette smoking and preterm delivery. Am J Obstet Gynecol 182:465, 2000

Sibai BM, Villar MA, Brayu E: Magnesium supplementation during pregnancy: A double-blind randomized controlled clinical trial. Am J Obstet Gynecol 161:115, 1989

Siega-Riz AM, Adair LS, Hobel CJ: Institute of Medicine maternal weight gain recommendations and pregnancy outcome in a predominantly Hispanic population. Obstet Gynecol 84:565, 1994

Smith CA: Effects of maternal undernutrition upon the newborn infant in Holland (1944–1945). Am J Obstet Gynecol 30:229, 1947

Stein Z, Susser M, Saenger G, Marolla F: Nutrition and mental performance. Science 178:708, 1972

Swanson CA, King JC: Reduced serum zinc concentration during pregnancy. Obstet Gynecol 62:313, 1983

Teitelman AM, Welch LS, Hellenbrand KG, Bracken MB: Effect of maternal work activity on preterm birth and low birthweight. Am J Epidemiol 131:104, 1990

United States Preventive Services Task Force: Routine iron supplementation during pregnancy. JAMA 270:2846, 1993

United States Public Health Service: Healthy People 2000, National Health Promotion and Disease Preventing Objectives.

Washington, DC, US Department of Health and Human Services, Public Health Service, 1992, p 381

Utiger RD: Maternal hypothyroidism and fetal development. N Engl J Med 341:601, 1999

Ventura SJ, Martin JA, Curtin SC, Mathews TJ, Park MM: Births: Final Data for 1998. National Vital Statistics Reports, Vol 48, No. 1. Hyattsville, MD, National Center for Health Statistics, 2000

Ward N, Bayer S, Calhour B: The impact of alternate prenatal care with reduced frequency of visits in residency teaching program. Am J Obstet Gynecol 174:339, 1996

Wendel GD, McIntire DD, Leveno KJ: Reducing neonatal group B streptococcal disease. N Engl J Med 342:1367, 2000

Williams Obstetrics, 7th ed. Stander HJ (ed). New York, Appleton-Century, 1929, p 278

Williams JW: The limitations and possibilities of prenatal care. JAMA 64:95, 1915

Witter FR, Caulfied LE, Stoltzfus RJ: Influence of maternal anthropometric status and birth weight on the risk of cesarean delivery. Obstet Gynecol 85:947, 1995

Worthen N, Bustillo M: Effect of urinary bladder fullness on fundal height measurements. Am J Obstet Gynecol 138:759, 1980

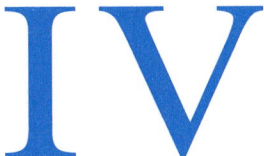

SECTION

Normal Labor and Delivery

11

Parturition

CLINICAL COURSE OF LABOR

The last few hours of human pregnancy are characterized by uterine contractions that effect dilatation of the cervix and force the fetus through the birth canal. Much energy is expended during this time; hence the use of the term *labor* to describe this process. The myometrial contractions of labor are painful, which is why the term *labor pains* is used to describe this process.

Before these forceful, painful contractions begin, however, the uterus must be prepared for labor. During the first 36 to 38 weeks of gestation, the myometrium is unresponsive; after this prolonged period of quiescence, a transitional phase is required during which myometrial unresponsiveness is suspended and the cervix is softened and effaced. Indeed, there are multiple functional states of the uterus that must be implemented during pregnancy and the puerperium; these are described later and categorized as the uterine phases of parturition.

Myometrial contractions that do not cause cervical dilatation may be observed at any time during pregnancy. These contractions are characterized by unpredictability in occurrence, lack of intensity, and brevity of duration. Any discomfort that they produce is usually confined to the lower abdomen and groin. Near the end of pregnancy, as the uterus undergoes preparation for labor, contractions of this type are more common, especially in multiparas, and sometimes are referred to as false labor. In some women, however, the forceful uterine contractions that effect cervical dilatation, fetal descent, and delivery of the conceptus begin suddenly, seemingly without warning.

MYOMETRIUM

ANATOMICAL AND PHYSIOLOGICAL CONSIDERATIONS. There are unique characteristics of myometrial muscle (and other smooth muscles) compared with skeletal muscle. Huszar and Walsh (1989) point out that these differences create a peculiar advantage for the myometrium in the efficiency of uterine contractions and the delivery of the fetus. First, the degree of shortening of smooth muscle cells with contractions may be one order of magnitude greater than that attained in striated muscle cells. Second, forces can be exerted in smooth muscle cells in any direction, whereas the contraction force generated by skeletal muscle is always aligned with the axis of the muscle fibers. Third, smooth muscle is not organized in the same manner as skeletal muscle; in myometrium, the thick and thin filaments are found in long, random bundles throughout the cells. This arrangement facilitates greater shortening and force-generating capacity of smooth muscle. Fourth, there is the advantage that multidirectional force gener-

ation in myometrial smooth muscle permits versatility in expulsive force directionality that can be brought to bear irrespective of the lie or presentation of the fetus.

BIOCHEMISTRY OF SMOOTH MUSCLE CONTRACTIONS. The interaction of myosin and actin is essential to muscle contraction. Myosin (M_r about 500,000) is comprised of multiple light and heavy chains and is laid down in thick myofilaments. The interaction of myosin and actin, which causes activation of ATPase, ATP hydrolysis, and force generation, is effected by enzymatic phosphorylation of the 20-kd light chain of myosin (Stull and colleagues, 1988, 1998). This phosphorylation reaction is catalyzed by the enzyme *myosin light chain kinase,* which is activated by Ca^{2+} (Fig. 11–1).

Ca^{2+} binds to calmodulin, a calcium-binding regulatory protein, which in turn binds to and activates myosin light chain kinase. In this manner, agents that act on myometrial smooth muscle cells to cause an increase in the intracellular cytosolic concentration of calcium ($[Ca^{2+}]_i$) promote contraction. Conditions that cause a decrease in $[Ca^{2+}]_i$ favor relaxation. Ordinarily, agents that cause an increase in the intracellular concentration of cyclic adenosine monophosphate (cAMP) or cyclic guanosine monophosphate (cGMP) promote uterine relaxation. It is believed that cAMP and cGMP act to cause a decrease in $[Ca^{2+}]_i$, although the exact mechanism(s) is not defined. The biochemistry and physiology of smooth muscle contractility have been reviewed by Barany and Barany (1990) and by Sanborn and colleagues (1994).

THE THREE STAGES OF LABOR. Active labor is divided into three separate stages. The first stage of labor begins when uterine contractions of sufficient frequency, intensity, and duration are attained to bring about effacement and progressive dilatation of the cervix. The first stage of labor ends when the cervix is fully dilated, that is, when the cervix is sufficiently dilated (about 10 cm) to allow passage of the fetal head. The first stage of labor, therefore, is the stage of cervical effacement and dilatation.

The second stage of labor begins when dilatation of the cervix is complete, and ends with delivery of the fetus. The second stage of labor is the stage of expulsion of the fetus.

The third stage of labor begins immediately after delivery of the fetus, and ends with the delivery of the placenta and fetal membranes. The third stage of labor is the stage of separation and expulsion of the placenta.

CLINICAL ONSET OF LABOR. A rather dependable sign of the impending onset of active labor (provided rectal or vaginal examinations have not been performed in the preceding 48 hours) is the discharge of a small amount of

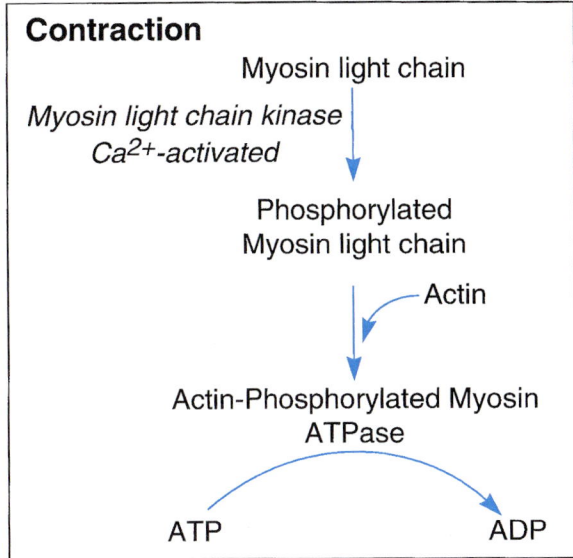

Contraction

Myosin light chain

Myosin light chain kinase
Ca²⁺-activated

Phosphorylated
Myosin light chain

— Actin

Actin-Phosphorylated Myosin
ATPase

ATP   ADP

Relaxation

1) Decreased intracellular Ca²⁺;
Ca²⁺ sequestration

2) Dephosphorylation of
myosin light chain

3) Inactivation of myosin light chain
kinase (*e.g.*, by cyclic AMP-
dependent phosphorylation)

FIGURE 11–1. Metabolic regulation of myometrial smooth muscle contraction and relaxation. An increase in intracellular, cytoplasmic, free Ca^{2+} activates myosin light chain kinase, which catalyzes the phosphorylation of the 20-kd light chain of myosin. Phosphorylated myosin interacts with actin and thereby activates ATPase; with the hydrolysis of ATP, force is generated and the muscle shortens. Relaxation is promoted by sequestration of Ca^{2+} in the sarcoplasmic reticulum, dephosphorylation of phosphorylated myosin by the action of phosphatase, and possibly by phosphorylation (inactivation) of myosin light chain kinase by a cAMP-dependent protein kinase.

blood-tinged mucus from the vagina. This represents the extrusion of the plug of mucus that had filled the cervical canal during pregnancy, and is referred to as "show" or "bloody show." This is a late sign, because commonly labor is already in progress or likely will ensue during the next several hours to few days. Normally, only a few drops of blood escape with the mucus plug; more substantial bleeding is suggestive of an abnormal cause.

UTERINE CONTRACTIONS CHARACTERISTIC OF LABOR. Unique among physiological muscular contractions, those of uterine smooth muscle of labor are painful. The cause of the pain is not known definitely, but several possibilities have been suggested:

1. Hypoxia of the contracted myometrium (as in angina pectoris).
2. Compression of nerve ganglia in the cervix and lower uterus by the interlocking muscle bundles.
3. Stretching of the cervix during dilatation.
4. Stretching of the peritoneum overlying the fundus.

Compression of nerve ganglia in the cervix and lower uterine segment by the contracting myometrium is an especially attractive hypothesis. Paracervical infiltration with a local anesthetic usually produces appreciable relief of pain during subsequent uterine contractions (Chap. 15, p. 371).

Uterine contractions are involuntary and, for the most part, independent of extrauterine control. Neural blockage from epidural analgesia does not diminish the frequency and intensity of uterine contractions. Moreover, the myometrial contractions in paraplegic women are normal, though painless, as in women after bilateral lumbar sympathectomy.

Mechanical stretching of the cervix enhances uterine activity in several species, including humans. This phenomenon has been referred to as the *Ferguson reflex* (1941). The exact mechanism by which mechanical dilatation of the cervix causes increased myometrial contractility is not clear. Release of oxytocin was suggested as the cause, but this is not proven. Manipulation of the cervix and "stripping" the fetal membranes is associated with an increase in the levels of prostaglandin $F_{2\alpha}$ metabolite (PGFM) in blood (see Chap. 20).

The interval between contractions diminishes gradually from about 10 minutes at the onset of the first stage of labor to as little as 1 minute or less in the second stage. Periods of relaxation between contractions, however, are essential to the welfare of the fetus. Unremitting contraction of the uterus compromises uteroplacental blood flow, and ultimately, fetal–placental flow, sufficiently to cause fetal hypoxemia. In the active phase of labor, the duration of each contraction ranges from 30 to 90 seconds, averaging about 1 minute. There is appreciable variability in the intensity of uterine contractions during apparently normal labor, as emphasized by Schulman and Romney (1970). They recorded the amnionic fluid pressures generated by uterine contractions during spontaneous labor; the average was about 40 mm Hg, but varied from 20 to 60 mm Hg (Chap. 14, p. 355).

DIFFERENTIATION OF UTERINE ACTIVITY. During active labor, the uterus is transformed into two distinct parts. The actively contracting upper segment becomes thicker as labor advances. The lower portion, comprising the lower segment of the uterus and the cervix, is relatively passive compared with the upper segment, and it develops into a much more thinly walled passage for the fetus. The lower uterine segment is analogous to a greatly expanded and thinned-out isthmus of the uterus of nonpregnant women, the formation of which is not solely a phenomenon of labor. The lower segment develops gradually as pregnancy progresses and then thins remarkably during labor (Figs. 11–2 and 11–3). By abdominal palpation, even before rupture of the membranes, the two segments can be differentiated during a contraction. The upper uterine segment is quite firm or hard, whereas the consistency of the lower uterine segment is much less firm. The former is the actively contracting part of the uterus; the latter is the distended, normally much more passive, portion.

If the entire wall of uterine musculature, including the lower uterine segment and cervix, were to contract simultaneously and with equal intensity, the net expulsive force would be decreased markedly. Herein lies the importance of the division of the uterus into an actively contracting upper segment and a more passive lower segment that differ not only anatomically but also physiologically. The upper segment contracts, retracts, and expels the fetus; in response to the force of the contractions of the upper segment, the softened lower uterine segment and cervix dilate and thereby form a greatly expanded, thinned-out muscular and fibromuscular tube through which the fetus can be extruded.

The myometrium of the upper uterine segment does not relax to its original length after contractions; rather, it becomes relatively fixed at a shorter length. The tension, however, remains the same as before the contraction. The upper portion of the uterus, or active segment, contracts down on its diminishing contents, but myometrial tension remains constant. The net effect is to take up slack, maintaining the advantage gained in the expulsion of the fetus, and keeping the uterine musculature in firm contact with the intrauterine contents. As the consequence of retraction, each successive contraction commences where its predecessor left off, so that the upper part of the uterine cavity becomes slightly smaller with each successive contraction. Because of the successive shortening of the muscular fibers with contractions, the upper active uterine segment becomes progressively thickened throughout the first and second stages of labor and tremendously thickened immediately after delivery of the fetus (Fig. 11–2). The phenomenon of retraction of the upper uterine segment is contingent upon a decrease in the volume of its contents. For the contents to be diminished, particularly early in labor when the entire uterus is virtually a closed sac with only a minute opening at the cervical os, the musculature of the lower segment must stretch. This permits increasingly more of the intrauterine contents to occupy the lower segment, and the upper segment retracts only to the extent that the lower segment distends and the cervix dilates.

The relaxation of the lower uterine segment is not a complete relaxation, but rather the opposite of retraction. The fibers of the lower segment become stretched with each contraction of the upper segment, after which these are not returned to the previous length but rather remain relatively fixed at the longer length; the tension, however, remains essentially the same as before. The musculature still manifests tone, still resists stretch, and still contracts somewhat on stimulation. The successive

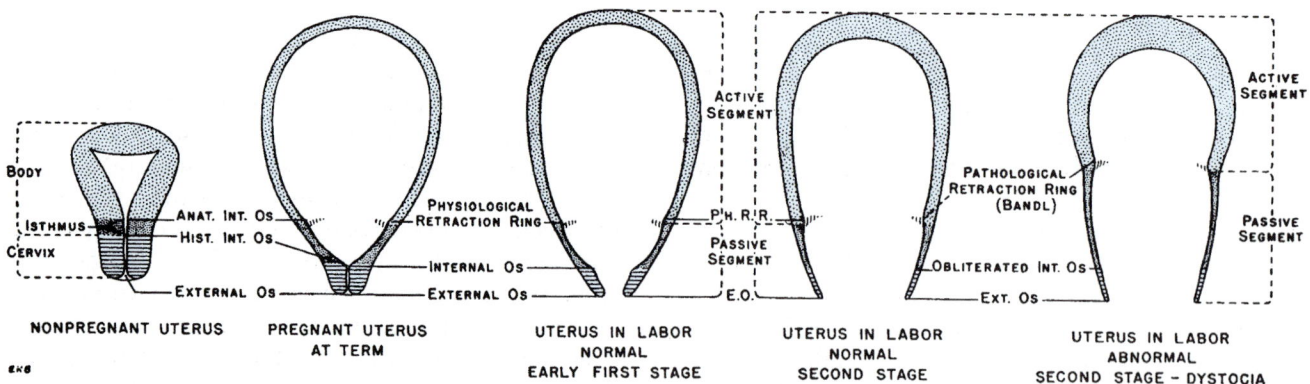

FIGURE 11–2. Sequence of development of the segments and rings in the uterus in pregnant women at term and in labor. Note comparison between the uterus of a nonpregnant woman, the uterus at term, and the uterus during labor. The passive lower segment of the uterine body is derived from the isthmus; the physiological retraction ring develops at the junction of the upper and lower uterine segments. The pathological retraction ring develops from the physiological ring. (Anat. Int. Os = anatomical internal os; E.O. = external os; Hist. Int. Os = histological internal os; Ph.R.R. = physiological retraction ring.)

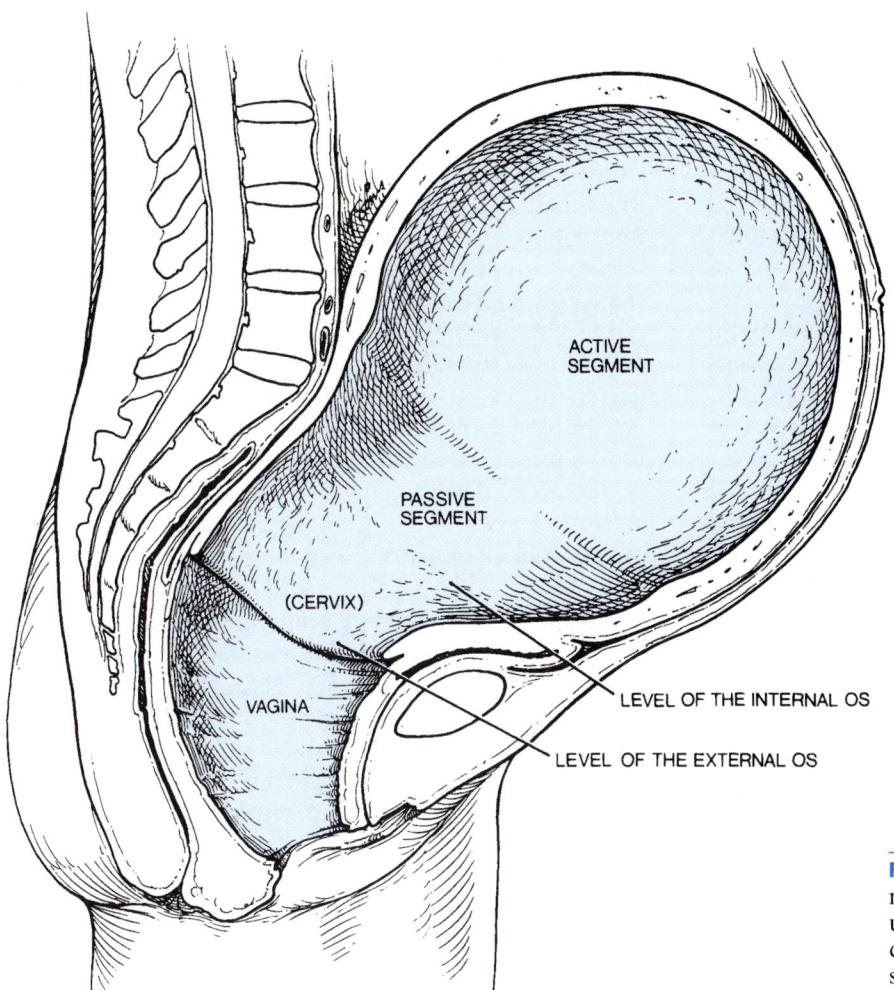

ACTIVE SEGMENT

PASSIVE SEGMENT

(CERVIX)

VAGINA

LEVEL OF THE INTERNAL OS

LEVEL OF THE EXTERNAL OS

FIGURE 11–3. The uterus at the time of vaginal delivery. The active upper segment of the uterus retracts about the fetus as the fetus descends through the birth canal. In the passive lower segment, there is considerably less myometrial tone.

lengthening of the muscular fibers in the lower uterine segment, as labor progresses, is accompanied by thinning, normally to only a few millimeters in the thinnest part. As a result of the thinning of the lower uterine segment and the concomitant thickening of the upper, the boundary between the two is marked by a ridge on the inner uterine surface, the **physiological retraction ring.** When the thinning of the lower uterine segment is extreme, as in obstructed labor, the ring is very prominent, forming a **pathological retraction ring.** This is an abnormal condition also known as **Bandl ring,** which is illustrated in Figure 11–2 and discussed further in Chapter 18 (p. 443). The existence of a gradient of diminishing physiological activity from fundus to cervix was established from measurements of differences in behavior of the upper and lower parts of the uterus during normal labor.

CHANGE IN UTERINE SHAPE. Each contraction produces an elongation of the uterine ovoid with a concomi-

tant decrease in horizontal diameter. By virtue of this change in shape, there are important effects on the process of labor. First, the decrease in horizontal diameter produces a straightening of the fetal vertebral column, pressing its upper pole firmly against the fundus of the uterus, whereas the lower pole is thrust farther downward and into the pelvis. The lengthening of the fetal ovoid thus produced has been estimated as between 5 and 10 cm. The pressure exerted in this fashion is known as the **fetal axis pressure.** Second, with lengthening of the uterus, the longitudinal fibers are drawn taut and because the lower segment and cervix are the only parts of the uterus that are flexible, these are pulled upward over the lower pole of the fetus. This effect on the musculature of the lower segment and on the cervix is an important factor in cervical dilatation.

ANCILLARY FORCES IN LABOR. After the cervix is dilated fully, the most important force in the expulsion of the fetus is that produced by increased maternal intra-abdominal pressure. This is created by contraction of the abdominal muscles simultaneously with forced respiratory efforts with the glottis closed. This is referred to as "pushing." The nature of the force produced is similar to that involved in defecation, but the intensity usually is much greater. The importance of intra-abdominal pressure in fetal expulsion is most clearly attested to by the labors of women who are paraplegic. Such women suffer no pain, although the uterus may contract vigorously. Cervical dilatation, in large measure the result of uterine contractions acting on a softened cervix, proceeds normally, but expulsion of the infant is accomplished more readily when the woman is instructed to bear down and can do so during a uterine contraction.

Although increased intra-abdominal pressure is required for the spontaneous completion of labor, it is futile until the cervix is fully dilated. Specifically, it is a necessary auxiliary to uterine contractions in the second stage of labor, but pushing accomplishes little in the first stage, except to produce fatigue. Intra-abdominal pressure also may be important in the third stage of labor, especially if the parturient is unattended. After the placenta has separated, its spontaneous expulsion is aided by the mother increasing intra-abdominal pressure.

CERVIX. Before the onset of labor, during the phase of uterine awakening and preparedness, the cervix is softened, which facilitates dilatation of the cervix once forceful myometrial contractions of labor begin.

CHANGES INDUCED IN THE CERVIX WITH LABOR. The effective force of the first stage of labor is the uterine contraction, which in turn exerts hydrostatic pressure through the fetal membranes against the cervix and lower uterine segment. In the absence of intact membranes, the fetal presenting part is forced directly against the cervix and lower uterine segment. As the result of the action of these forces, two fundamental changes—effacement and dilatation—take place in the already softened cervix. For the head of the average fetus at term to pass through the cervix, the cervical canal must dilate to a diameter of about 10 cm; at this time, the cervix is said to be completely (or fully) dilated. There may be no fetal descent during cervical effacement, but most commonly the presenting fetal part descends somewhat as the cervix dilates. During the second stage of labor, descent of the fetal presenting part typically occurs rather slowly but steadily in nulliparas. In multiparas, however, particularly those of high parity, descent may be very rapid.

CERVICAL EFFACEMENT. The "obliteration" or "taking up" of the cervix is the shortening of the cervical canal from a length of about 2 cm to a mere circular orifice with almost paper-thin edges. This process is referred to as effacement and takes place from above downward. The muscular fibers at about the level of the internal cervical os are pulled upward, or "taken up," into the lower uterine segment, as the condition of the external os remains temporarily unchanged. As illustrated in Figures 11–4 to 11–7, the edges of the internal os are drawn upward several centimeters to become a part (both anatomically and functionally) of the lower uterine segment. Effacement may be compared with a funneling process in which the whole length of a narrow cylinder is converted into a very obtuse, flaring funnel with a small circular orifice for an outlet. As the result of increased myometrial activity during uterine preparedness for labor, appreciable effacement of the softened cervix sometimes is accomplished before active labor begins. Effacement causes expulsion of the mucus plug as the cervical canal is shortened.

CERVICAL DILATATION. Compared with the body of the uterus, the lower uterine segment and the cervix are regions of lesser resistance. Therefore, during a contraction, these structures are subjected to distention, in the course of which a centrifugal pull is exerted on the cervix (Figs. 11–8 to 11–10). As the uterine contractions cause pressure on the membranes, the hydrostatic action of the amnionic sac in turn dilates the cervical canal like a wedge. In the absence of intact membranes, the pressure of the presenting part against the cervix and lower uterine segment is similarly effective. Early rup-

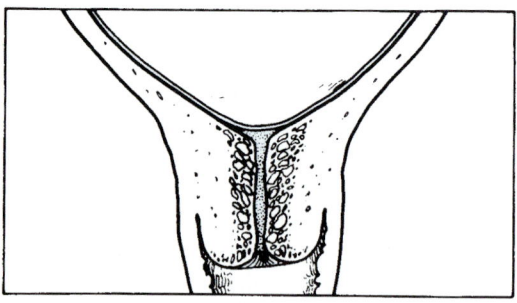

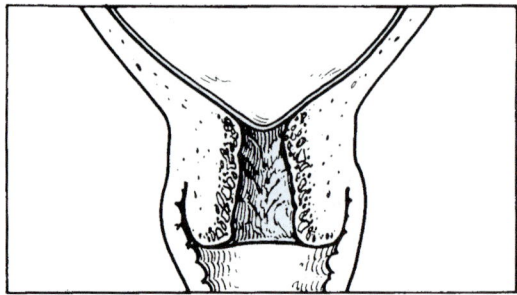

FIGURE 11–4. Cervix near the end of pregnancy but before labor. Top, primigravida; bottom, multipara.

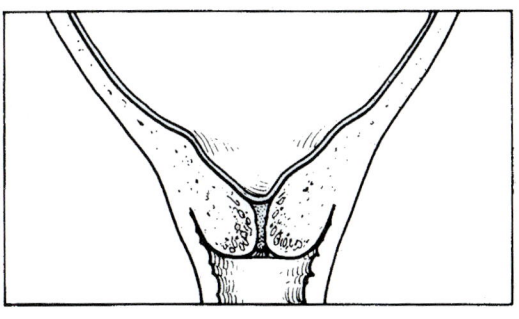

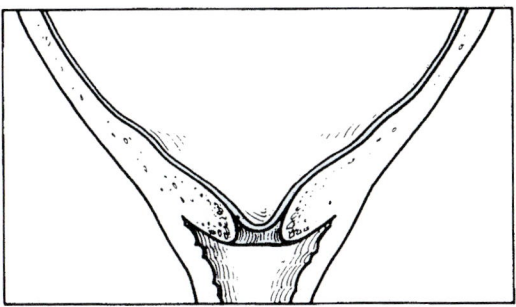

FIGURE 11–5. Beginning effacement of cervix. Note dilation of internal os and funnel-shaped cervical canal. Top, primigravida; bottom, multipara.

ture of the membranes does not retard cervical dilatation so long as the presenting part of the fetus is positioned to exert pressure against the cervix and lower uterine segment. The process of cervical effacement and dilatation causes the formation of the forebag of the amnionic fluid, which is later described in detail.

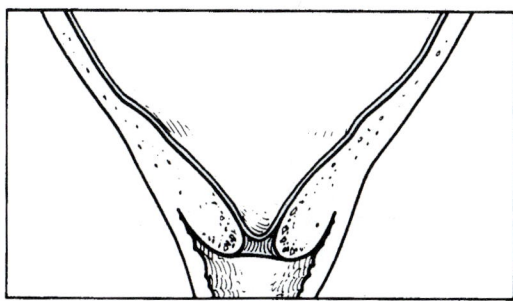

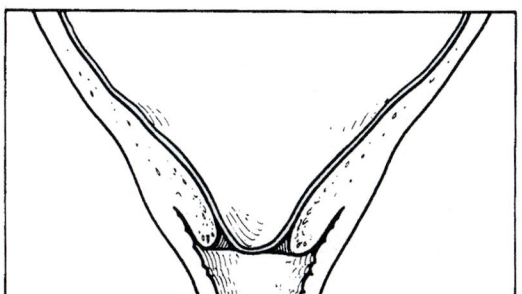

FIGURE 11–6. Further effacement of cervix. Top, primigravida; bottom, multipara.

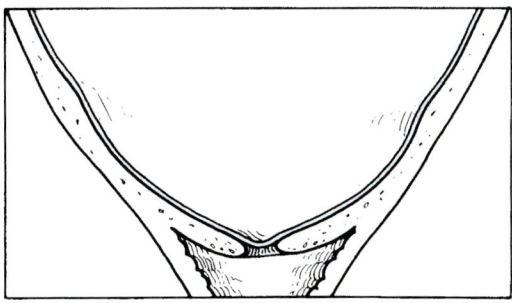

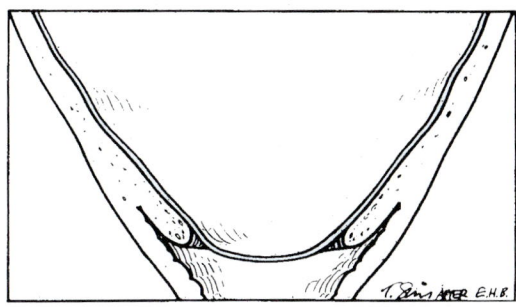

FIGURE 11–7. Cervical canal obliterated—that is, the cervix is completely effaced. Top, primigravida; bottom, multipara.

LABOR PATTERNS

PATTERN OF CERVICAL DILATATION. Friedman, in his treatise on labor (1978), stated that "the clinical features of uterine contractions—namely, frequency, intensity, and duration—cannot be relied upon as measures of progression in labor nor as indices of normality. . . . Except for cervical dilatation and fetal descent, none of the clinical features of the parturient. . . appears to be useful in assessing labor progression." The pattern of cervical dilatation that takes place during the course of normal labor takes on the shape of a sigmoid curve. As depicted in Figure 11–11, two phases of cervical dilatation are the latent phase and the active phase. The active phase has been subdivided further as the acceleration phase, the phase of maximum slope, and the deceleration phase (Friedman, 1978). The duration of the latent phase is more variable and subject to sensitive changes by extraneous factors and by sedation (prolongation of latent phase) and myometrial stimulation (shortening of latent phase). The duration of the latent phase has little bearing on the subsequent course of labor, whereas the characteristics of the accelerated phase are usually predictive of the outcome of a particular labor. Friedman considers the maximum slope as a "good measure of the overall efficiency of the machine," whereas the nature of the deceleration phase is more reflective of fetopelvic relationships. The completion of cervical dilatation during the active phase of labor is accomplished by cervical retraction about the pre-

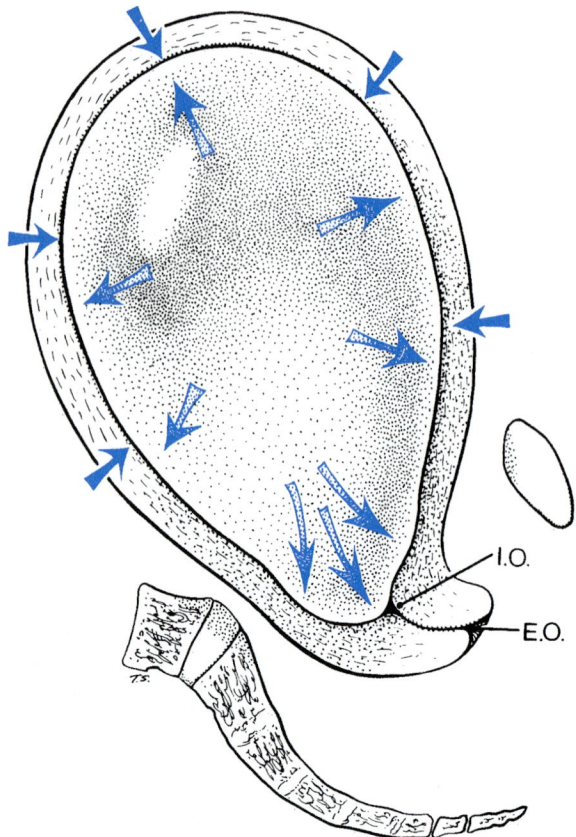

FIGURE 11–8. Hydrostatic action of membranes in effecting cervical effacement and dilatation. In the absence of intact membranes, the presenting part, applied to the cervix and forming the lower, uterine segments, acts similarly. In this and Figures 11–9 and 11–10, note changing relations of the external os (E.O.) and internal os (I.O.).

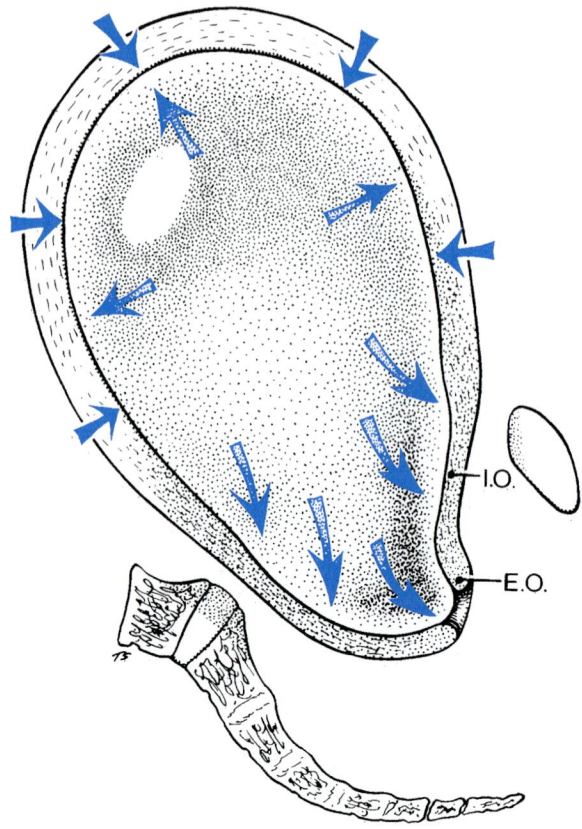

FIGURE 11–9. Hydrostatic action of membranes at completion of effacement.

senting part of the fetus. After complete cervical dilatation, the second stage of labor commences; thereafter, only progressive descent of the presenting fetal part is available to assess the progress of labor.

PATTERN OF FETAL DESCENT. In many nulliparas, engagement of the fetal head is accomplished before labor begins, and further descent does not occur until late in labor. In others in which engagement of the fetal head is initially not so complete, further descent occurs during the first stage of labor. In the descent pattern of normal labor, a typical hyperbolic curve is formed when the station of the fetal head is plotted as a function of the duration of labor. Active descent usually takes place after cervical dilatation has progressed for some time (Fig. 11–12). In nulliparas, increased rates of descent are observed ordinarily during the phase of maximum slope of cervical dilatation. At this time, the speed of descent increases to a maximum, and this maximal rate of descent is maintained until the presenting fetal part reaches the perineal floor (Friedman, 1978).

CRITERIA FOR NORMAL LABOR. Friedman also sought to select criteria that would delimit normal labor and thereby enable identification of significant abnormalities in labor. The limits, admittedly arbitrary, appear to be logical and clinically useful. The group of women studied were nulliparas and multiparas with no fetopelvic disproportion, no fetal malposition or malpresentation, no multiple pregnancy, and none were treated with heavy sedation or conduction analgesia, oxytocin, or operative intervention. All had a normal pelvis, were at term with a vertex presentation, and delivered average-sized infants. From these studies, Friedman developed the concept of three functional divisions of labor—preparatory, dilatational, and pelvic—to describe the physiological objectives of each division (Fig. 11–12). He found that the preparatory division of labor may be sensitive to sedation and conduction analgesia. Although little cervical dilatation occurs during this time, considerable changes take place in the extracellular matrix (collagen and other connective tissue components) of the cervix. The dilatational division of labor, during which time dilatation is occurring at the most rapid rate, is principally unaffected by sedation or conduction analgesia. The pelvic division of labor begins with the

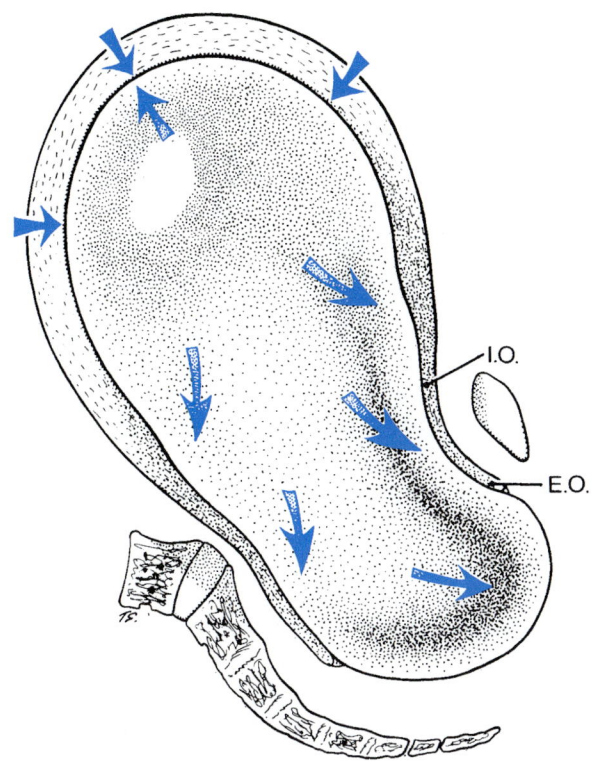

FIGURE 11-10. Hydrostatic action of membranes at full cervical dilatation.

deceleration phase of cervical dilatation. The classical mechanisms of labor, which involve the cardinal movements of the fetus, take place principally during the pelvic division of labor. The onset of the pelvic division is seldom clinically identifiable separate from the dilatational division of labor. Moreover, the rate of cervical dilatation does not always decelerate as full dilatation is approached; in fact, it may accelerate.

RUPTURE OF THE MEMBRANES. Spontaneous rupture of the membranes most often occurs sometime during the course of active labor. Typically, rupture is evident by a sudden gush of a variable quantity of normally clear or slightly turbid, nearly colorless fluid. Less frequently, the membranes remain intact until delivery of the infant. If by chance the membranes remain intact until completion of delivery, the fetus is born surrounded by them, and the portion covering the head of the newborn infant is sometimes referred to as the **caul.** Rupture of the membranes before the onset of labor at any stage of gestation is referred to as **premature rupture of the membranes.**

CHANGES IN THE VAGINA AND PELVIC FLOOR. The birth canal is supported and is functionally closed by a number of layers of tissues that together form the pelvic floor. Its most important structures are the levator ani muscle and the fascia covering its upper and lower surfaces, which for practical purposes may be considered as the pelvic floor (Chap. 3). This group of muscles closes the lower end of the pelvic cavity as a diaphragm and thereby a concave upper and a convex lower surface is presented (see Fig. 3-6). On either side, the levator ani consists of a pubococcygeus and iliococcygeus portion. The posterior and lateral portions of the pelvic floor, which are not filled out by the levator ani, are occupied by the piriformis and coccygeus muscles on either side.

The levator ani varies in thickness from 3 to 5 mm,

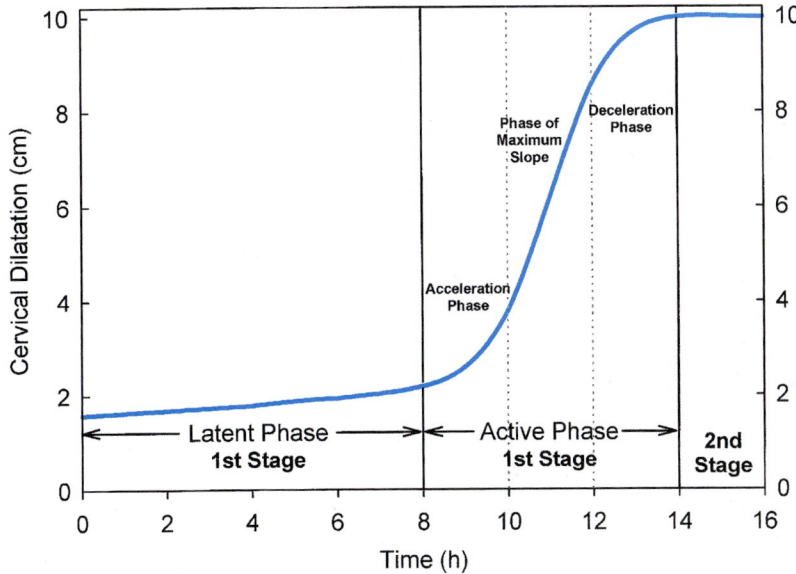

FIGURE 11-11. Composite of the average dilatation curve for nulliparous labor based on analysis of the data derived from the patterns traced by a large, nearly consecutive, series of gravidas. The first stage is divided into a relatively flat latent phase and a rapidly progressive active phase. In the active phase, there are three identifiable component parts: an acceleration phase, a linear phase of maximum slope, and a deceleration phase. (Illustration courtesy of Dr. L. Casey, redrawn from Friedman, 1978.)

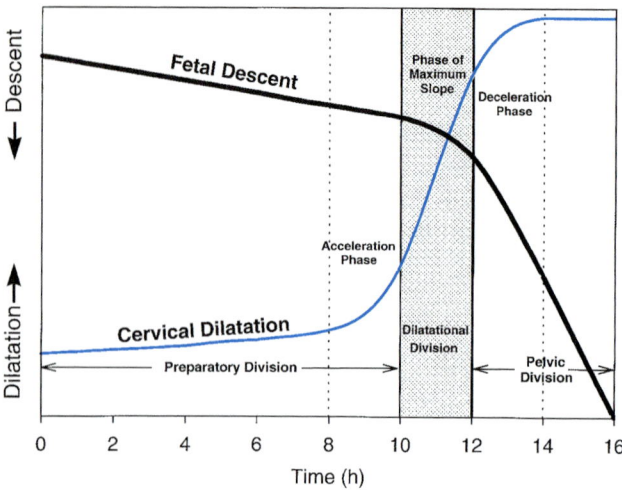

FIGURE 11–12. Labor course divided functionally on the basis of expected evolution of the dilatation and descent curves into (1) a preparatory division, including latent and acceleration phases; (2) a dilatational division, occupying the phase of maximum slope of dilatation; and (3) a pelvic division, encompassing both deceleration phase and second stage while concurrent with the phase of maximum slope of descent. (Illustration courtesy Dr. L. Casey, redrawn from Friedman, 1978.)

though its margins encircling the rectum and vagina are somewhat thicker. During pregnancy, the levator ani usually undergoes hypertrophy. By vaginal examination, the internal margin of this muscle can be felt as a thick band that extends backward from the pubis and encircles the vagina about 2 cm above the hymen. On contraction, the levator ani draws both the rectum and vagina forward and upward in the direction of the symphysis pubis and thereby acts to close the vagina. The more superficial muscles of the perineum are too delicate to serve more than an accessory function.

In the first stage of labor, the membranes and presenting part of the fetus serve a role in dilating the upper portion of the vagina. After the membranes have ruptured, however, the changes in the pelvic floor are caused entirely by pressure exerted by the fetal presenting part. The most marked change consists of the stretching of the fibers of the levator ani muscles and the thinning of the central portion of the perineum, which becomes transformed from a wedge-shaped mass of tissue 5 cm in thickness to (in the absence of an episiotomy) a thin, almost transparent membranous structure less than 1 cm in thickness. When the perineum is distended maximally, the anus becomes markedly dilated and presents an opening that varies from 2 to 3 cm in diameter and through which the anterior wall of the rectum bulges. The extraordinary number and size of the blood vessels that supply the vagina and pelvic floor effects a great increase in the amount of blood loss when these tissues are torn.

PLACENTAL SEPARATION. The third stage of labor begins immediately after delivery of the fetus and involves the separation and expulsion of the placenta. After delivery of the placenta and fetal membranes, active labor is completed. As the baby is born, the uterus spontaneously contracts down on its diminishing contents. Normally, by the time the infant is completely delivered, the uterine cavity is nearly obliterated and the organ consists of an almost solid mass of muscle, several centimeters thick above the thinner lower segment. The uterine fundus now lies just below the level of the umbilicus. This sudden diminution in uterine size is inevitably accompanied by a decrease in the area of the placental implantation site (Fig. 11–13). For the placenta to accommodate itself to this reduced area, it increases in thickness, but because of limited placental elasticity, it is forced to buckle. The resulting tension causes the weakest layer of the decidua—the spongy layer, or decidua spongiosa—to give way, and cleavage takes place at that site. Therefore, separation of the placenta results primarily from a disproportion created between the unchanged size of the placenta and the reduced size of the underlying implantation site. During cesarean delivery, this phenomenon may be directly observed when the placenta is implanted posteriorly.

Cleavage of the placenta is greatly facilitated by the nature of the loose structure of the spongy decidua, which may be likened to the row of perforations between postage stamps. As separation proceeds, a hematoma forms between the separating placenta and the remaining decidua. Formation of the hematoma is usually the result, rather than the cause, of the separation, because in some cases bleeding is negligible. The hematoma may, however, accelerate the process of cleavage. Because the separation of the placenta is through the spongy layer of the decidua, part of the decidua is cast off with the placenta, whereas the rest remains attached to the myometrium. The amount of decidual tissue retained at the placental site varies.

Placental separation ordinarily occurs within a very few minutes after delivery. Brandt (1933) and others, based on results obtained in combined clinical and radiographic studies, supported the idea that because the periphery of the placenta is probably the most adherent portion, separation usually begins elsewhere. Occasionally some degree of separation begins even before the third stage of labor, probably accounting for certain cases of fetal heart rate decelerations that occur just before expulsion of the infant.

SEPARATION OF AMNIOCHORION. The great decrease in the surface area of the cavity of the uterus simultaneously causes the fetal membranes (amniochorion) and the parietal decidua to be thrown into innumerable folds that increase the thickness of the layer from less than

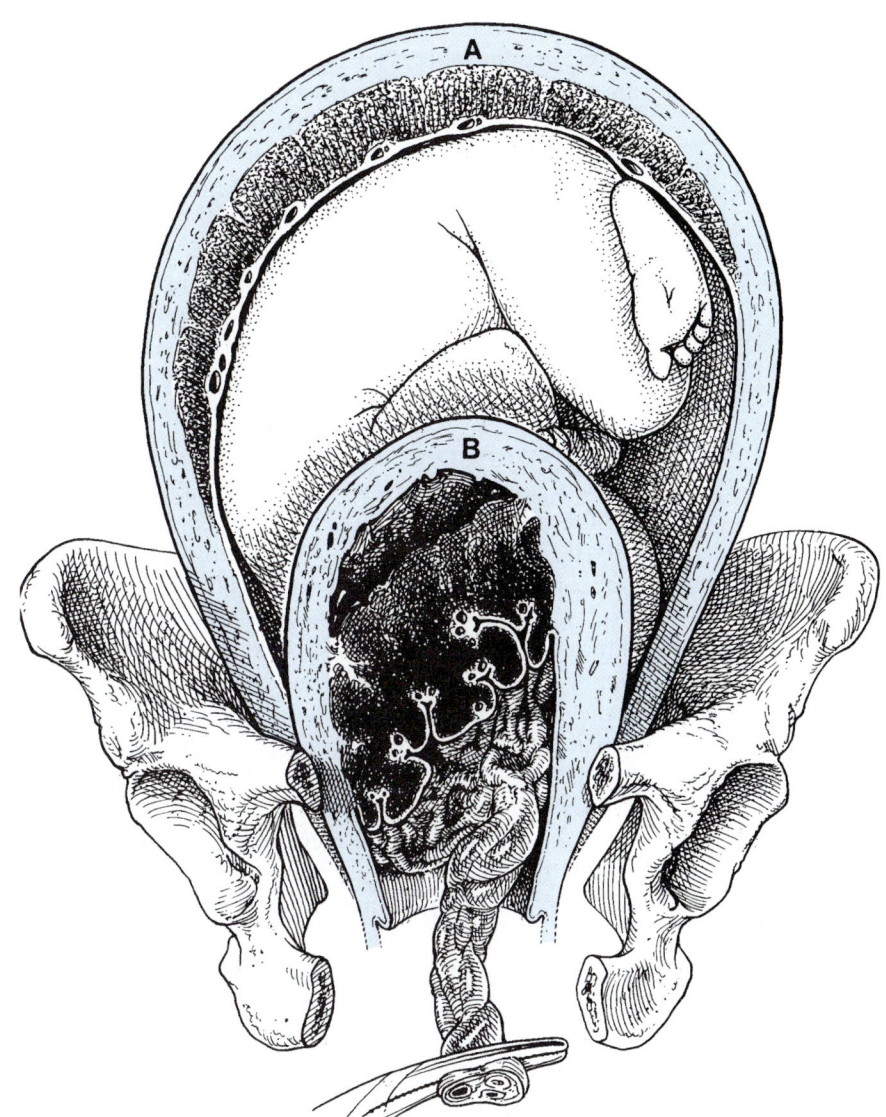

FIGURE 11–13. Diminution in size of placental site after birth of baby. **A.** Spatial relations before birth of the infant. **B.** Placental spatial relations after birth of the infant.

1 mm to 3 to 4 mm. The lining of the uterus early in the third stage indicates that much of the parietal layer of decidua parietalis is included between the folds of the festooned amnion and chorion laeve (Fig. 11–14). The membranes usually remain in situ until the separation of the placenta is nearly completed. These are then peeled off the uterine wall, partly by the further contraction of the myometrium and partly by traction that is exerted by the separated placenta, which lies in the thin lower uterine segment or in the upper portion of the vagina. The body of the uterus at that time normally forms an almost solid mass of muscle, the anterior and posterior walls of which, each measuring 4 to 5 cm in thickness, lie in close apposition such that the uterine cavity is almost obliterated.

PLACENTAL EXTRUSION. After the placenta has separated from its implantation site, the pressure exerted upon it by the uterine walls causes it to slide downward into the lower uterine segment or the upper part of the vagina. In some cases the placenta may be expelled from those locations by an increase in abdominal pressure, but women in the recumbent position frequently cannot expel the placenta spontaneously. An artificial means of completing the third stage is therefore generally required. The usual method employed is alternately to compress and elevate the fundus, while exerting minimal traction on the umbilical cord (Chap. 13).

MECHANISMS OF PLACENTAL EXTRUSION. When the central, or usual, type of placental separation occurs, the retroplacental hematoma is believed to push the placenta toward the uterine cavity, first the central portion and then the rest. The placenta, thus inverted and weighted with the hematoma, then descends. Because the surrounding membranes are still attached to the

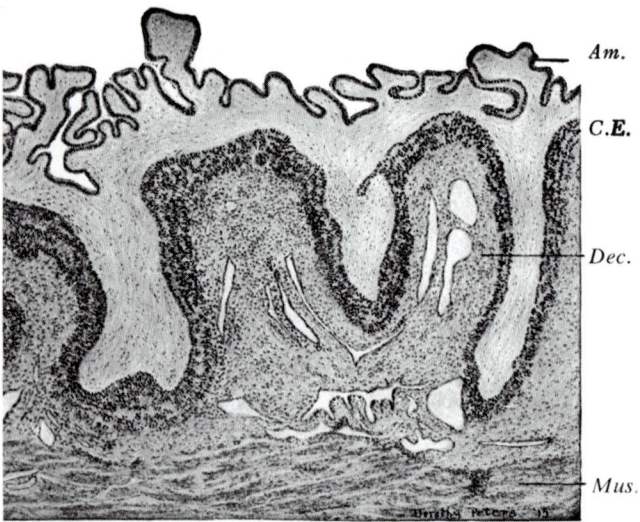

FIGURE 11–14. Folding of membranes as uterine cavity decreases in size. (Am. = amnion; C.E. = epithelium of chorion laeve; Dec. = decidua vera; Mus. = myometrium.)

decidua, the placenta can descend only by dragging the membranes along; the membranes then peel off its periphery. Consequently, the sac formed by the membranes is inverted, with the glistening amnion over the placental surface presenting at the vulva. The retroplacental hematoma either follows the placenta or is found within the inverted sac. In this process, known as the **Schultze mechanism** of placental expulsion, blood from the placental site pours into the inverted sac, not escaping externally until after extrusion of the placenta. The other method of placental extrusion is known as the **Duncan mechanism,** in which separation of the placenta occurs first at the periphery, with the result that blood collects between the membranes and the uterine wall and escapes from the vagina. In this circumstance, the placenta descends to the vagina sideways, and the maternal surface is the first to appear at the vulva.

PHYSIOLOGICAL AND BIOCHEMICAL PROCESSES OF PARTURITION

The physiological processes in human pregnancy that results in the initiation of parturition and the onset of labor are not defined. Until recently, it was generally accepted that successful pregnancy in all mammalian species was dependent upon the action of progesterone to maintain uterine quiescence until near the end of gestation. This assumption was supported by the finding that in the majority of mammalian pregnancies studied, **progesterone withdrawal** (whether naturally occurring or surgically or pharmacologically induced) precedes the initiation of parturition. In many of these species,

a decline, sometimes precipitous, in the levels of progesterone in maternal plasma normally begins after approximately 95 percent of pregnancy. Moreover, the administration of progesterone to these species late in pregnancy delays the onset of parturition.

In primate pregnancy (including humans), however, progesterone withdrawal does not precede the initiation of parturition. The levels of progesterone in the plasma of pregnant women increase throughout pregnancy, declining only after delivery of the placenta, the tissue site of progesterone synthesis in human pregnancy (Chap. 6).

PARTURITION THEORIES. Presently, there appear to be two general theorems. Viewed simplistically, these are the retreat from pregnancy maintenance hypothesis and the uterotonin induction of parturition theory. Several combinations of selected tenets of these two postulates are incorporated into the theorems of most investigators. Some researchers also speculate that the mature human fetus, in some undefined fashion, is the source of the initial signal for the commencement of the parturitional process. This has little direct experimental support in human parturition.

Other investigators suggest that one or another uterotonin, produced in increased amounts or in response to an increase in the population of its myometrial receptors, is the proximate cause of the initiation of human parturition. Indeed, an obligatory role for one or more uterotonins is included in most parturition theories, either as a primary or a secondary phenomenon in the final events of childbirth.

CONTEMPORARY HUMAN PARTURITION RESEARCH. Two independent sets of observations have influenced the direction of parturition research during the past 35 years. One was the identification of the mechanisms by which estrogen is synthesized in human pregnancy. By 1960, it was established that human pregnancy is a hyperestrogenic state (Chap. 6), and that the placenta is virtually the sole tissue site of estrogen formation. At that time, it also was known that the human placenta could not synthesize estrogens de novo, from acetate or cholesterol. In the late 1950s, human placental tissue was shown to convert C_{19}-steroids to estrogens. In the early 1960s, it was established that the fetal adrenal glands produce prodigious amounts of C_{19}-steroids, which are transported in fetal blood to the placenta. In syncytiotrophoblast, these fetal adrenal C_{19}-steroids are metabolized with great efficiency to estrogens. The human placenta, therefore, is an incomplete endocrine organ, at least in the case of estrogen biosynthesis. These several findings were assembled as one part of the concept of a fetal–maternal communication system of human pregnancy (Siiteri and MacDonald, 1963, 1966).

THE SHEEP MODEL OF PARTURITION. During this same decade, Liggins and associates (1967, 1968) demonstrated that in sheep pregnancy, the fetus provides the initial signal that leads to the timely commencement of parturition. They found that adrenalectomy or hypophysectomy of the sheep fetus in utero caused a delay in the initiation of parturition and delivery. Adrenalectomy or hypophysectomy of the ewe did not cause an alteration in the timing of parturition. Contrarily, the infusion of corticotropin, cortisol, or a synthetic glucocorticosteroid into the sheep fetus earlier in pregnancy caused preterm delivery. Liggins deduced that the sheep fetus provides a signal through interaction of brain–pituitary–adrenal glands, which provide another signal(s) that is transported in fetal blood, and acted upon by placental trophoblasts.

SHEEP FETAL ADRENAL CORTISOL SECRETION AND PLACENTAL STEROID SYNTHESIS. Liggins and colleagues (1968, 1973) as well as Challis and Lye (1994), identified and characterized many of the physiological phenomena of sheep parturition. Near the end of sheep pregnancy, a signal arising in the brain of the fetal sheep promotes the beginning of a coordinated sequence of endocrine phenomena that culminates in **progesterone withdrawal** (McDonald and Nathanielsz, 1991). The fetal brain parturition signal, presumably corticotropin-releasing hormone (CRH), is transmitted to the fetal pituitary gland via the hypophyseal–portal vessels to stimulate adrenocorticotropic hormone (ACTH) release from the anterior pituitary gland. An increase in ACTH secretion, together with augmented responsiveness of the fetal adrenal cortices that is acquired with maturation, causes increased fetal adrenal secretion of cortisol (Myers and colleagues, 1992). In response to increased fetal adrenal cortisol secretion, the expression of cytochrome P-450 17α-hydroxylase/17,20-lyase (P-450$_{17\alpha}$; CYP17) in sheep placenta is increased strikingly at the end of pregnancy. This enzyme catalyzes pregnenolone to eventually produce dehydroepiandrosterone, which in turn is aromatized to estrone. Thus, pregnenolone synthesized in placenta is diverted away from progesterone and toward estrogen.

PROGESTERONE WITHDRAWAL AND RETREAT FROM PREGNANCY MAINTENANCE IN SHEEP PREGNANCY. In some manner that is related to progesterone withdrawal, the continued maintenance of uterine quiescence in sheep pregnancy is withdrawn. Clearly, there is a transition period between the tranquil state of the uterus and the onset of labor in sheep parturition. Spe-

cifically, myometrial unresponsiveness is suspended and the uterus is awakened before labor begins.

DIVERGENCE OF ENDOCRINE PROCESSES IN SHEEP AND HUMANS. Crucial differences in key endocrine events in pregnant sheep and women are readily apparent.

1. Progesterone withdrawal marked by a decline in blood progesterone levels does not occur before the initiation of human parturition.
2. There is no profound increase in the levels of cortisol in the human fetus near term as there is in the sheep fetus.
3. The infusion of ACTH or cortisol into the human fetus does not bring about the premature initiation of parturition as it does in the sheep.
4. Glucocorticosteroid treatment in human pregnancy is associated with a pronounced decrease in estrogen formation by inhibiting fetal pituitary ACTH secretion and thus attenuating the supply of fetal adrenal C_{19}-steroid precursors for placental estrogen synthesis.
5. The sheep fetal adrenal glands are not the source of placental estrogen precursors as are the adrenal glands of the human fetus, and estrogen production in sheep pregnancy is small compared with that in humans.
6. The enzyme that diverts pregnenolone to estrogen (17α-hydroxylase/17,20-desmolase) is expressed in the sheep, but not human placenta.
7. Estrogen is produced very late in pregnancy in the sheep but throughout pregnancy in humans.
8. Plasma levels of progesterone in sheep pregnancy (about 10 ng/mL) are relatively small compared with those in the human (about 160 ng/mL).
9. Intrauterine prostaglandin formation during labor in sheep is at least 20 times that produced in human uterine tissues during labor (Casey and MacDonald, 1988a; Flower, 1977).

PROGESTERONE METABOLISM/PRODUCTION RATES AND HUMAN PARTURITION. Little and colleagues (1966) found that the metabolic clearance rate of plasma progesterone during human pregnancy is similar to that in men and nonpregnant women. Therefore, the plasma level of progesterone is directly proportional to its production rate.

RETREAT FROM PREGNANCY MAINTENANCE AND HUMAN PARTURITION. The mechanism whereby retreat from pregnancy maintenance occurs in human pregnancy, however, has not been identified. Searches for an alternative form of progesterone deprivation have produced no substantive evidence for alterations in progesterone metabolism, compartmentalization (sequestration) of progesterone, or alterations in progesterone-binding proteins or receptor numbers. Therefore, most investigators have concluded that progesterone withdrawal is not a fundamental component of the initiation of human parturition (Casey and MacDonald, 1988b).

INHIBITION OF PROGESTERONE ACTION. Progesterone treatment of women does not prevent, delay, or arrest labor at term or preterm (Casey and MacDonald, 1988b). This finding provides further support for the conclusion that a decrease in progesterone levels, even in specific tissue sites, is not involved in the initiation of human parturition. There is, however, another largely unexplored mechanism by which progesterone action could be subjugated near the end of pregnancy. Progesterone action may be interrupted by a specific agent(s) through a progesterone receptor–independent, gene-specific process (Casey and associates, 1993b; Casey and MacDonald, 1996). The very pinnacle of evolutionary development of systems for the withdrawal of progesterone could be the selective attenuation of some (but not all) progesterone effects, namely the interruption of progesterone action on specific genes. If only the actions of progesterone directly supportive of the maintenance of uterine quiescence were inhibited while other (salutary) actions of progesterone that are not involved directly in uterine contractile responsiveness, such as inhibition of lactogenesis, were preserved until delivery of the placenta, a much more sophisticated endocrine system for the initiation of parturition would have evolved.

Such a putative agent, however, must act in a cell-specific or gene-specific manner through a progesterone receptor–independent process. An endogenous selective agent that inhibits progesterone action could be targeted to alter the expression of specific genes—for example, by modifying progesterone-regulated gene transcription, mRNA stability, or protein function and stability. The specificity of progesterone antagonism could be mediated at:

1. The molecular level (use of specific promoters, by specificity of trans-acting factors).
2. The biochemical level (protein function, enzyme activity).
3. The cellular level (e.g., synthesis or activation of a putative antiprogestin or its receptor).

Such a gene-specific system for inhibiting progesterone action could provide for highly selective subjugation of selected progesterone actions consistent with an evolutionary hierarchy of humans in reproductive processes. Such a process would explain the failure of administered progesterone to delay or prevent the onset of human parturition at term or preterm. One candidate for this

role as selective, gene-specific antiprogestin has been identified, namely, transforming growth factor-β (TGF-β) (Casey and MacDonald, 1996).

IS PROGESTERONE ONLY ONE COMPONENT OF A REDUNDANT FAIL-SAFE SYSTEM OF PREGNANCY MAINTENANCE? The possibility also must be considered that the contractile unresponsiveness imposed on the uterus during most of human pregnancy is ensured by multiple processes that act independently and cooperatively to establish uterine quiescence. Progesterone is likely only one of several factors that contribute to the system that maintains myometrial contractile unresponsiveness. Because retreat from continued pregnancy maintenance near the end of pregnancy is pivotal to the preparation of the uterus for labor, an understanding of this phenomenon is central to the solution of the human parturition puzzle.

FETAL CONTRIBUTIONS TO INITIATION OF PARTURITION. It is intellectually satisfying to envision that the fetus, after appropriate maturation of vital organs, provides the initial signal that sets the parturitional process in motion. Teleologically, this seems to be the most logical manner by which parturition could begin in a timely fashion. A signal from the human fetus could be transmitted in one of several ways; but however this is accomplished, the end result must include the suspension of uterine quiescence. Regrettably, such a fetal signal has not been discovered. The fetal sheep signaling system that initiates the parturitional process is believed to proceed via the brain, pituitary gland, adrenal glands, and fetal blood to the placenta. The human fetus also may provide a signal through a fetal blood-borne agent that acts upon trophoblast. It is unlikely, however, that the initial signal for the initiation of parturition is a uterotonin such as oxytocin, prostaglandins, or endothelin-1. Rather, it is more likely that the uterus first must be prepared for labor before a uterotonin can be optimally effective (Casey and MacDonald, 1994).

FETAL ANOMALIES AND DELAYED PARTURITION. Anomalies of the brain of the fetal calf, fetal lamb, and sometimes the human fetus, delay the normal timing of parturition. With congenital absence of the pituitary gland in the bovine fetus, the gestation period is prolonged by several weeks. Adrenal hypoplasia in the bovine fetus is also associated with a delay in the onset of parturition. If early in pregnancy, the ewe grazes on *Veratrum californicum* or "skunk cabbage," the sheep fetus is characterized by a teratogen-induced cyclopean deformity. The brain anomalies of such a fetus include the absence of vascularization of the fetal pituitary gland from the hypothalamus. The fetal adrenal glands remain hypoplastic and pregnancy continues far beyond term (Challis and Lye, 1994; Thorburn, 1983).

In 1882, Speigelberg proposed that the signal for the initiation of human parturition also originated in the fetus (Thorburn, 1993). Rea (1898) observed an association between fetal anencephaly and prolonged human gestation. Malpas (1933) extended these observations and described a human pregnancy with an anencephalic fetus that went to 374 days (53 weeks). He concluded that the association between fetal anencephaly and prolonged human gestation seemed to be attributable to anomalous brain–pituitary–adrenal function in the anencephalic fetus. The adrenal glands of the anencephalic fetus are very small, and at term may be only 5 to 10 percent as large as those of a normal fetus. The smallness of the adrenal glands is caused by failure of development of the fetal zone that normally accounts for most of the human fetal adrenal mass and C_{19}-steroid biosynthesis (Chap. 6). Finally, in pregnancies in which the fetal adrenal glands are hypoplastic, the onset of labor may be delayed (Anderson and Turnbull, 1973). These findings were suggestive that in humans, as in sheep, the fetal adrenal glands are important for the timely onset of parturition.

THE HUMAN FETUS AND PARTURITION. There is fragmentary evidence that pregnancies in which there is relative hypoestrogenism—fetal anencephaly or adrenal hypoplasia, or placental sulfatase deficiency—are sometimes associated with prolonged gestation. However, while estrogen may facilitate the development of optimal parturitional processes by increasing the capacity of myometrium to contract and to respond to contractile agents, it is not the signal for the initiation of human parturition.

Other fetal abnormalities that prevent or severely reduce the entry of fetal urine (absence of fetal kidneys) or lung secretions (pulmonary hypoplasia) into amnionic fluid do not cause prolongation of human pregnancy. Thus, a signal from the fetus through the paracrine arm of the fetal–maternal communication system does not appear to be mandated for the initiation of parturition.

UTERINE PHASES OF PARTURITION. Parturition, the bringing forth of young, encompasses all physiological processes involved in birthing: the prelude to, the preparation for, the process of, and the parturient's recovery from childbirth. From the disparate nature of these physiological processes, it is evident that multiple transformations in uterine function must be accommodated in a timely manner during successful pregnancy and parturition. As shown in Figure 11–15, parturition can be arbitrarily divided into four uterine phases which correspond to the major physiological transitions of the myometrium and cervix during pregnancy (Casey and MacDonald 1993a, 1993c; MacDonald and Casey, 1996).

UTERINE PHASE 0 OF PARTURITION. Beginning even before implantation, a remarkably effective period of myometrial quiescence is imposed on the uterus. This phase of parturition is characterized by myometrial smooth muscle tranquility with maintenance of cervical structural integrity. This is the phase in which the inherent propensity of the myometrium to contract is harnessed. During this phase, which persists for about the first 95 percent of normal pregnancy, myometrial smooth muscle is rendered unresponsive to natural stimuli and relative contractile paralysis is imposed against a host of mechanical and chemical challenges that otherwise would promote emptying of the uterine contents. The myometrial contractile unresponsiveness of phase 0 is so extraordinary that near the end of pregnancy the myometrium must be awakened from this prolonged parturitional diapause in preparation for labor.

During phase 0 of parturition, as the myometrium is maintained in a quiescent state, the cervix must remain firm and unyielding. The maintenance of cervical anatomical and structural integrity is essential to the success of phase 0 of parturition. Premature cervical dilatation, structural incompetence, or both, portend an unfavorable pregnancy outcome that ends most often in preterm delivery (Chap. 27). Shortening of the cervix, when identified between 24 and 28 weeks of pregnancy, is indicative of increased risk of preterm delivery (Iams and colleagues, 1996).

UTERINE PHASE 1 OF PARTURITION. To prepare the uterus for labor, the uterine tranquility of phase 0 of parturition must be suspended; this is the time of uterine awakening. The morphological and functional changes in myometrium and cervix that prepare the uterus for labor may be the natural outcome of the suspension of uterine phase 0; but whatever the mechanism, the capacity of myometrial cells to regulate the concentration of cytoplasmic Ca^{2+} is restored; myometrial cell responsivity is reinstituted, uterotonin sensitivity develops, and intercellular communicability is established. As these functional capacities of myometrial smooth muscle to contract are implemented and the cervix is ripened, phase 1 of parturition merges into phase 2, active labor. Challis and Lye (1994) refer to the change in uterine functionality before labor as "activation."

UTERINE MODIFICATION DURING PHASE 1 OF PARTURITION. Specific modifications in uterine function evolve with the suspension of uterine phase 0:

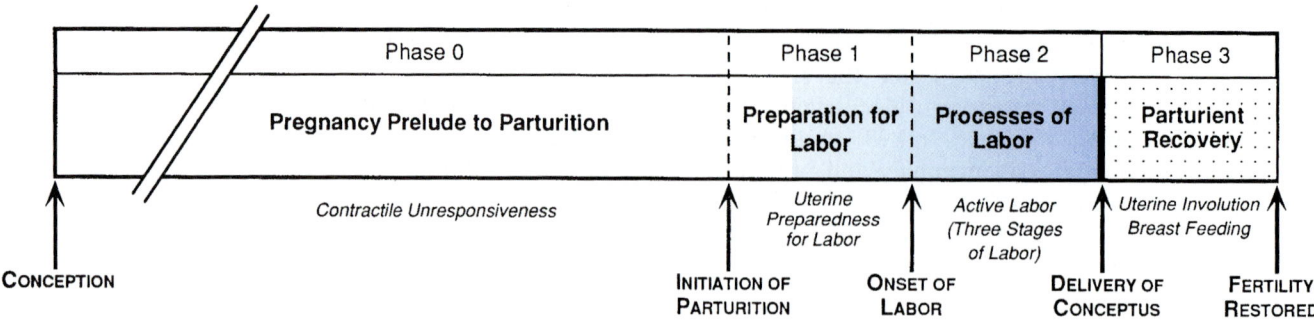

FIGURE 11–15. The initiation of parturition and the onset of labor.

1. A striking increase in myometrial oxytocin receptors.
2. An increase in gap junctions (number and surface area) between myometrial cells.
3. Uterine irritability.
4. Responsiveness to uterotonins.
5. Transition from a contractile state characterized predominantly by occasional painless contractions to one in which more frequent contractions develop.
6. Formation of the lower uterine segment.
7. Cervical softening.

With the development of a well-formed lower uterine segment, the fetal head oftentimes descends to or even through the maternal inlet of the pelvis, a distinctive event referred to as **lightening.** The abdomen of the pregnant woman commonly undergoes a change in shape, an event sometimes described by the mother as "the baby dropped." No doubt there are many other modifications of the uterus late in pregnancy during phase 1, some of which may be integral components of uterine preparedness for labor.

Late in pregnancy, at sometime during phase 1 of parturition, there is a striking—50-fold or more—increase in the number of oxytocin receptors in myometrium (Fuchs and associates, 1982). This coincides with the increase in uterine contractile responsiveness to oxytocin (Soloff and co-workers, 1979). Also, prolonged human gestation is associated with a delay in this increase in receptors (Fuchs and collaborators, 1984).

Also during phase 1, the number and size of gap junctions between myometrial cells increase before the onset of labor, continue to increase during labor, and then decrease quickly after delivery. This is true of spontaneous parturition, both at term and preterm (Garfield and Hayashi, 1981).

CERVICAL CHANGES OF PHASE 1 OF PARTURITION. The body of the uterus (the fundus) and the cervix, although parts of the same organ, must respond in quite different ways during pregnancy and parturition. On the one hand, it is essential that during most of pregnancy, the myometrium be dilatable but remain quiescent. On the other hand, the cervix must remain unyielding and reasonably rigid. Coincident with the initiation of parturition, however, the cervix must soften, yield, and become more readily dilatable. The fundus must be transformed from the relatively relaxed, unresponsive organ characteristic of most of pregnancy to one that will produce effective contractions that drive the fetus through the yielding (dilatable) cervix and on through the birth canal. Failure of a coordinated interaction between the functions of fundus and cervix portends an unfavorable pregnancy outcome. But despite the apparent reversal of roles between cervix and fundus from before to during labor, it is likely that the processes in both portions of the uterus are regulated by common agents.

COMPOSITION OF THE CERVIX. There are three principal structural components of the cervix: collagen, smooth muscle, and the connective tissue or ground substance. Constituents of the cervix important in cervical modifications at parturition are those in the extracellular matrix and ground substance, the glycosaminoglycans, dermatan sulfate and hyaluronic acid. The smooth muscle content of cervix is much less than that of the fundus, and varies anatomically from 25 to only 6 percent.

CERVICAL SOFTENING. The cervical modifications of phase 1 of parturition principally involve changes that occur in collagen, connective tissue, and its ground substance. Cervical softening is associated with two complementary changes:

1. Collagen breakdown and rearrangement of the collagen fibers.
2. Alterations in the relative amounts of the various glycosaminoglycans.

Hyaluronic acid is associated with the capacity of a tissue to retain water. Near term, there is a striking increase in the relative amount of hyaluronic acid in cervix, with a concomitant decrease in dermatan sulfate. The role for smooth muscle in the cervical softening process is not clear, but may be more important than previously believed. Rath and colleagues (1998) and Winkler and Rath (1999) have addressed this possibility in some detail.

Prostaglandin E_2 and $PGF_{2\alpha}$ applied directly to the cervix induce the maturational changes of cervical softening, that is, modification of collagen and alterations in the relative concentration of the glycosaminoglycans. Prostaglandin suppositories, placed intravaginally adjacent to the cervix, are used clinically to effect cervical softening and used to facilitate the induction of labor (Chap. 20, 470). In some species, these events can be induced in response to a decline in the levels of progesterone. Yet other compounds may serve as active participants in the activation or orchestration of these coordinated events. Relaxin, for example, acts to effect cervical softening while maintaining the uterus in a quiescent state. If a relaxin-mediated process were operative in human pregnancy, it would represent a very early functional modification of phase 1, and thereby relaxin could be regarded as a participant in implementing uterine phase 1. But despite the enormous importance of cervical softening to the success of parturition, relatively little is known of the precise sequence (or regulation) of the biochemical processes involved.

UTERINE PHASE 3 OF PARTURITION. Phase 2 is synonymous with active labor, that is, the uterine contractions that bring about progressive cervical dilatation and delivery of the conceptus. Phase 2 of parturition is customarily divided into the three stages of labor described earlier in the chapter. The onset of labor is the transition from uterine phase 1 to phase 2 of parturition.

UTERINE PHASE 3 OF PARTURITION. Phase 3 encompasses the events of the puerperium—maternal recovery from childbirth, maternal contributions to infant survival, and the restoration of fertility in the parturient. Immediately after delivery of the conceptus, and for about an hour or so thereafter, the myometrium must be held in a state of rigid and persistent contraction/retraction, which effects compression of the large uterine vessels and thrombosis of their lumens. In this coordinated fashion, fatal postpartum hemorrhage is prevented.

During the early puerperium, a maternal-type behavior pattern develops and maternal–infant bonding begins. The onset of lactogenesis and milk let-down in maternal mammary glands also is, in an evolutionary sense, crucial to the bringing forth of young. Finally, involution of the uterus, which restores this organ to the nonpregnant state, and the reinstitution of ovulation must be accomplished in preparation for the next pregnancy. Four to six weeks usually are required for complete uterine involution; but the duration of phase 3 of parturition is dependent on the duration of breast feeding. Infertility usually persists so long as breast feeding is continued because of lactation (prolactin)–induced anovulation and amenorrhea (Chap. 58, p. 1548).

A FAIL-SAFE SYSTEM TO MAINTAIN UTERINE QUIESCENCE. The myometrial quiescence of phase 0 of parturition is so remarkable (and ordinarily so successful) that it probably is induced by multiple independent and cooperative biomolecular processes. Individually, some of these processes may be redundant, that is, pregnancy may continue in the absence of one or more processes that normally contribute to the fail-safe system of pregnancy maintenance.

OVERCOMING THE INHERENT PROPENSITY OF THE MYOMETRIUM TO CONTRACT. The phasic myometrial smooth muscle is, inherently, a contractile tissue: strips of myometrium from uteri of nonpregnant women placed in an isotonic water bath contract in a rhythmical fashion without added stimuli, even in the presence of prostaglandin synthase inhibitors (Crankshaw and Dyal, 1994). Therefore, it is difficult to comprehend how the uterus can be expanded to accommodate a 3500 g fetus, 1 L of amnionic fluid, and 800 g of placenta and fetal membranes without erupting into powerful contractions. The volume capacity of the uterine cavity increases by several orders of magnitude during pregnancy. The uterus increases in size from an organ of about 50 to 70 g to one that weighs more than 1000 g at term. Knowing the incredible force that will be generated during labor, it is amazing that the intrauterine burden of human pregnancy is tolerated with such functional myometrial equanimity.

THE PHYSIOLOGICAL INVESTMENTS IN PHASE 0 OF PARTURITION. The physiological investments that must be made to sustain uterine phase 0 are enormous. It is likely that all manner of biomolecular systems (neural, endocrine, paracrine, and autocrine), calling upon multiple cell-signaling processes, are implemented and coordinated to impose a state of relative uterine unresponsiveness. Moreover, a complementary fail-safe system that protects the uterus against agents that could perturb the tranquil state of phase 0 also must be in place.

The actions of estrogen and progesterone via intracellular receptors; myometrial cell plasma membrane receptor-mediated increases in cyclic adenosine monophosphate (cAMP); the generation of cyclic guanosine monophosphate (cGMP); and other systems (modifications in myometrial cell ion channels) may all be opera-

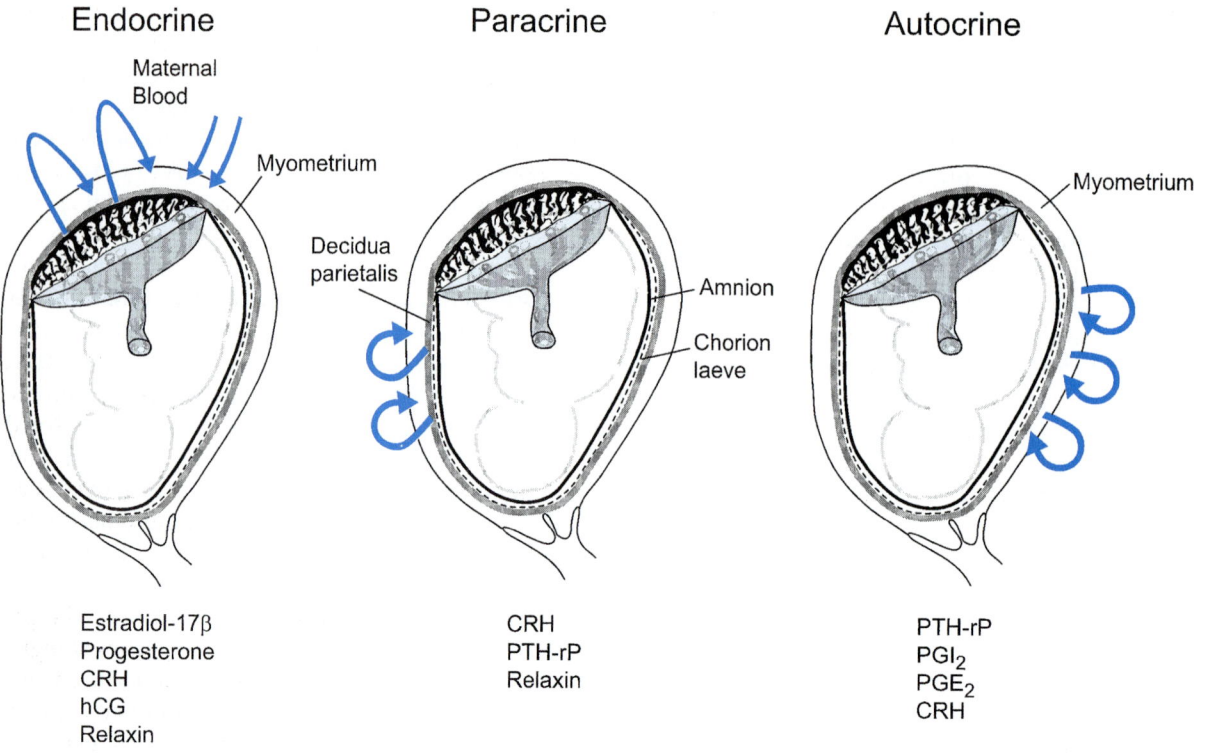

FIGURE 11–16. Theoretical fail-safe system involving endocrine, paracrine, and autocrine mechanisms for the maintenance of phase 0 of parturition, uterine quiescence. (CRH = corticotropin-releasing hormone; hCG = chorionic gonadotropin; PTH-rP = parathyroid hormone–related peptide.)

tive in phase 0 of human parturition. If this were the case, it also is possible that a defect (either naturally occurring or pharmacologically induced), however severe, in one component of this system might not necessarily preclude the successful maintenance of pregnancy to term (Fig. 11–16).

Redundant physiological processes in human pregnancy are well-known. For example, the formation of human placental lactogen (hPL), as well as placental growth-hormone variant, can be completely absent in an otherwise normal pregnancy (Chap. 6, pp. 113, 115). The near-complete absence of estrogen formation in human pregnancy caused by several different disorders does not preclude successful pregnancy and parturition. Even the administration of an antiprogestin to near-term pregnant women does not cause the onset of labor.

STEROID HORMONE CONTRIBUTIONS TO PHASE 0 OF PARTURITION. There is a commonly held belief that estrogen causes myometrial contractions and that progesterone attenuates contractile responsiveness. Partly because of this belief, reference is frequently made to the importance of "estrogen:progesterone ratios" (in blood or tissues) to uterine contractility. Most likely this is an oversimplification and quite possibly an incorrect interpretation of the role of these two sex steroid hormones in myometrial function. The plasma levels of estrogen and progesterone in normal human pregnancy are enormous; both are in great excess in terms of the affinity constants for the estrogen and progesterone receptors. For this reason, it is difficult to comprehend how relatively subtle changes in the ratio of the concentrations of these two steroids could modulate physiological processes during human pregnancy. The teleological reason for such high levels of estrogen and progesterone in human pregnancy is not known.

ESTROGEN. Acting directly or indirectly, estrogen promotes a variety of myometrial changes that enhance the capacity of the myometrium to generate powerful contractile force: myometrial cell hypertrophy, myometrial cell contractile potential, uterotonin receptors, and cell-to-cell communicability (Pepe and Albrecht, 1995). Estrogen does not act directly, however, to cause myometrial contractions; rather, estrogen promotes the capacity for forceful and coordinated contractions. Progesterone (directly or indirectly) seems to impose (probably in concert with other systems) contractile unresponsiveness. For example, estrogen may act to increase gap junctions between myometrial cells and L-type Ca^{2+} channels; but these junctions and channels must be opened to facilitate contractions.

Most likely, estrogen and progesterone act in concert to contribute to the effectiveness of phase 0 of parturition. Estrogen acts in part by promoting progesterone responsiveness. In many responsive tissues, the estrogen receptor—acting via the estrogen response element of the progesterone receptor gene—induces the synthesis of progesterone receptors.

PROGESTERONE. It has been presumed for decades that progesterone action is essential for the successful maintenance of pregnancy. Regrettably, however, neither the biomolecular particulars of this, nor the role of other agents in promoting this tolerant uterine state are clearly defined. Because of its action in other mammalian species, however, it is presumed that progesterone acts to establish and maintain uterine phase 0 of parturition.

STEROID HORMONES AND MYOMETRIAL CELL-TO-CELL COMMUNICATION. Communication is established between myometrial cells by gap junctions that facilitate the passage of current (electrical or ionic coupling) or metabolites (metabolite coupling). Gap junctions are transcellular membrane channels comprised of **connexons.** This is a hexameric assemblage of a specific connexin (the gap junction protein) joined in mirror symmetry with another connexon in the plasma membrane of an adjacent cell (Fig. 11–17). These pairs of connexons establish a conduit for the exchange of small molecules (M_r less than 1000) and ions between cells. Importantly for myometrial contractile function, both cAMP and Ca^{2+} are transported via these channels. In heart and myometrium, connexin43 (M_r about 43 kd) is the principal gap junction protein. The physiological importance of optimal numbers (area) of functional permeable gap junctions between myometrial cells is believed to be the establishment of electrical synchrony in the myometrium, which effects coordination of contractions and thereby greater force during labor.

Estrogen treatment promotes myometrial gap junction formation in some animals by increasing connexin43 synthesis. The simultaneous administration of antiestrogens prevents this (Burghardt and colleagues, 1984). Progesterone treatment also negates the stimulatory effect of estrogen on the development of gap junctions in some animals. Conversely, progesterone antagonists lead to the premature development of gap junctions and preterm labor and delivery (Chwalisz and colleagues, 1991).

In myometrial tissue obtained from pregnant women before labor when the number of gap junctions is small, a spontaneous increase in the number of gap junctions occurs in vitro (Hayashi and collaborators, 1985). This is suggestive that the excised tissue is relieved from a pregnancy endocrine milieu that prevented gap junction development in vivo. Chow and Lye (1994) found that the level of connexin43 mRNA in human myometrial tissues increased between 37 to 40 weeks before labor and increased further after labor began. Despite that connexin43 protein decreased, gap junctions increased during late pregnancy and labor. They suggested that gap junctional area is regulated by the level of connexin43 mRNA and connexon assembly.

Modifications in gap junctional permeability have been demonstrated in a variety of systems in response to various hormones, neurotransmitters, Ca^{2+}, cAMP, and phorbol esters. In animals, Cole and Garfield (1986) found that adenylyl cyclase activators caused a decrease in the permeability of gap junctions. Similar results were obtained using strips of human myometrial tissues (Sakai and co-workers, 1992). These findings are suggestive that intercellular myometrial communication via gap junctions may be regulated by the level (synthesis/degradation) of connexin43, the assembly of connexons, and the permeability of the gap junctions produced. These processes appear to be regulated in part by estrogen and progesterone.

STEROID HORMONES AND OXYTOCIN RECEPTORS. Most studies to evaluate the regulation of myometrial oxytocin receptor synthesis have been performed in the rat. Estradiol-17β treatment either in vivo or in myometrial explants causes an increase in myometrial oxytocin receptors. This action of estradiol-17β is prevented by simultaneous treatment with progesterone (Fuchs and colleagues, 1983). Progesterone also may act to increase oxytocin receptor degradation (Soloff and colleagues, 1983). Estradiol-17β treatment of sheep uterine tissue in vitro does not cause an increase in oxytocin receptors, but oxytocin and progesterone treatment lowers the level of these receptors (Sheldrick and Flick-Smith, 1993).

The human oxytocin receptor gene is a single-copy gene on chromosome 3 p26.2. An estrogen response element is not present in this gene. The level of oxytocin receptor mRNA in human myometrium tissues obtained at term is greater than that in uterine tissues of nonpregnant women. Thus, the increase in oxytocin receptor number in myometrium at term may be attributable to increased oxytocin gene transcription (Fuchs and associates, 1982).

Oxytocin receptors also are present in human endometrium and in decidua at term and these stimulate prostaglandin production (Fuchs and associates, 1981). Oxytocin receptors also are present in amnion and chorion–decidual tissues (Benedetto and associates, 1990).

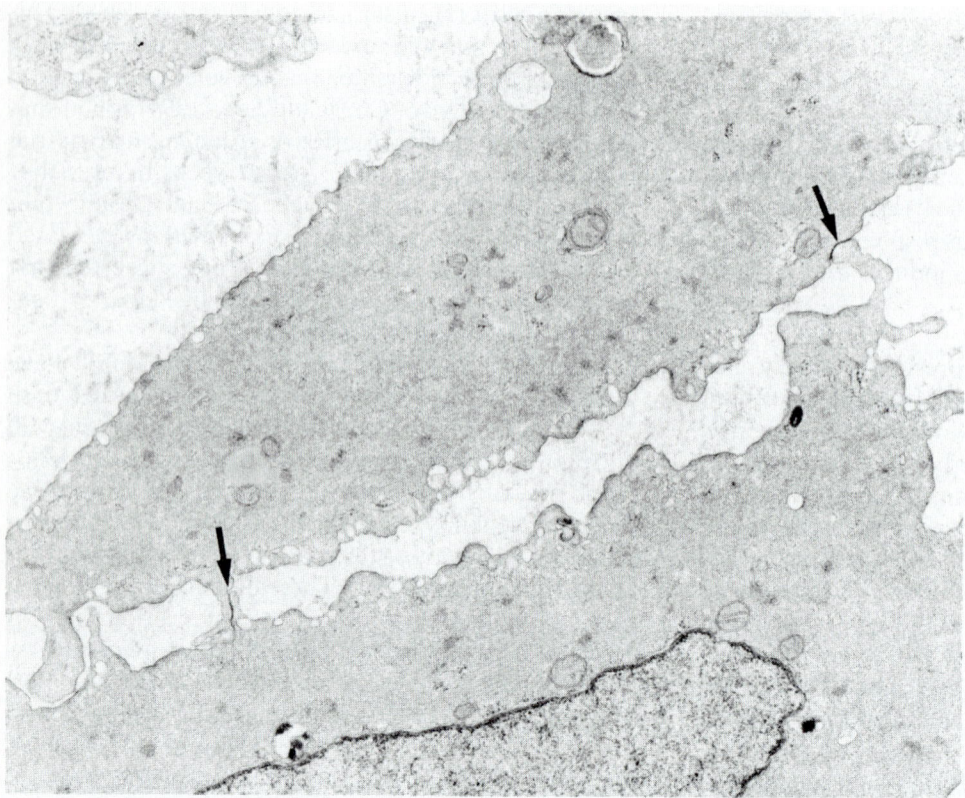

FIGURE 11–17. Electron photomicrograph of gap junctions in human myometrial cells. Tissue obtained after labor commenced. (Courtesy of Dr. R. Garfield.)

ABSENCE OF PROGESTERONE WITHDRAWAL BEFORE INITIATION OF PARTURITION IN PRIMATE PREGNANCY. Plasma progesterone levels do not decrease before labor in primates (Challis and Lye, 1994). Plasma levels decline only after delivery of the placenta. Nonetheless, the morphological and functional modifications that prepare the human uterus for labor occur in a timely manner in human pregnancy just as in those species in which progesterone withdrawal is a clearly demonstrable endocrine antecedent of parturition.

A successful human pregnancy has been observed in which the levels of progesterone in maternal plasma were low, particularly so early in pregnancy. Steroid hormone formation was evaluated in a woman homozygous for abetalipoproteinemia, a form of familial hypercholesterolemia caused by a defect in low-density lipoprotein (LDL) apoprotein synthesis (Parker and associates, 1986). Progesterone synthesis in the human corpus luteum is absolutely dependent upon the use of plasma LDL cholesterol. Most of progesterone synthesis in human placenta also is accomplished by the uptake and use of maternal plasma LDL, but limited cholesterol synthesis in syncytiotrophoblast is possible (Chap. 6). LDL is not available for uptake and use by steroidogenic tissues in persons with abetalipoproteinemia. Consequently, after spontaneous ovulation, there was no detectable progesterone in blood of the woman described, but the levels of estradiol-17β during the postovulatory phase, after the luteinizing hormone surge, were normal. This woman conceived, and her pregnancy progressed to term despite low levels of plasma progesterone, especially in early pregnancy.

PROGESTERONE ADMINISTRATION AND HUMAN PARTURITION. Progesterone administration to pregnant women does not delay the timely onset of parturition or arrest or prevent preterm labor. These findings are indicative that some "hidden" or unique form of progesterone deprivation is not the cause of the suspension of uterine phase 0 processes in human parturition. These observations, however, do not preclude the possibility that some progesterone actions are inhibited by a progesterone receptor-independent, selective antiprogestin-like mechanism during the initiation of parturition.

PROGESTERONE RECEPTOR ANTAGONISTS AND HUMAN PARTURITION. The steroidal antiprogestin RU-486 (mifepristone), administered to women during the latter phase of the ovarian cycle, induces menstruation prematurely and is quite effective in the induction of abortion during the first few weeks of human pregnancy. This compound is a classical steroid antagonist, acting at the level of the progesterone receptor. RU-486, however, is progressively less effective in inducing abortion or labor in women as pregnancy advances. Treatment of women near term with RU-486 may facilitate the induction of labor by oxytocin but is largely ineffective in independently causing labor (Frydman and colleagues, 1988). This is in contrast to the premature induction of labor by RU-486 in those species that normally experience progesterone withdrawal before labor.

PROGESTERONE AND UTERINE PHASE 0 OF PARTURITION: CONCLUSIONS. Based upon these several observations, an obligatory role for progesterone in the maintenance of human pregnancy can be neither established nor refuted. It seems most likely that the actions of estrogen and progesterone are involved as components of a broader-based fail-safe biomolecular system that implements and maintains phase 0 of human parturition.

CONTRIBUTION OF PLASMA MEMBRANE-MEDIATED MYOMETRIAL CELL-SIGNALING SYSTEMS TO PARTURITIONAL PROCESSES. In addition to intracellular receptor proteins, such as those that mediate the action of sex steroid hormones, myometrial cell signaling also is propagated by plasma membrane–associated receptors. There are three known classes of cell-surface receptors: G-protein linked, ion channel linked, and enzyme linked. Multiple examples of each class of these plasma membrane receptors have been identified in human myometrium, and all three of these cell membrane signaling mechanisms appear to be modified during phase 0 of parturition.

More than 100 heptahelical plasma membrane G-protein–linked receptors have been identified and characterized in the myometrium of pregnant and nonpregnant women. The ligands for the heptahelical receptors are neuropeptides, hormones, and autacoids. Some of these ligands are available to the myometrium during pregnancy in high concentration by several routes— from maternal blood (endocrine), contiguous tissues or adjacent cells (paracrine), or direct synthesis in the myometrial smooth muscle cells (autocrine) (Fig. 11–16). Most of these heptahelical receptors are associated with the activation of adenylyl cyclase. Other heptahelical receptors in myometrium, however, are more commonly associated with G-protein–mediated activation of phospholipase C.

THE G-PROTEINS. These guanine-binding proteins are heterotrimers composed of an alpha (α), beta (β), and gamma (γ) chain. The α-subunit binds GDP (guanine diphosphate) or GTP (guanine triphosphate) with high affinity. The active form (Gα-GTP) regulates effector proteins, namely plasma membrane–bound enzymes such as adenylyl cyclase and phospholipase C, and selected ion channels. Indeed, the hydrolysis of GTP to GDP serves as a "molecular switch" to regulate the activity of the G-protein (Linder and Gilman, 1992). Gα-subunits are classified into four major subfamilies Gα_s (stimulate adenylyl cyclase), Gα_I (inhibits adenylyl cyclase), Gα_q (activates phospholipase C), and Gα_{12} (regulate Na$^+$/K$^+$ exchange).

G-PROTEIN SIGNAL TRANSMISSION. The G-proteins are versatile, seemingly capable of more than one type of signal generation even by way of a single heptahelical receptor in the same cell. Consequently, there are multiple metabolic points that serve as regulatory intercepts. The heptahelical receptor–G-protein–effector phenotype of a cell is distinguished by:

1. Its complement of heptahelical receptors.
2. The α-, β-, and γ-subunits.
3. The G-protein–modulated effectors that a given cell expresses.

These phenotypic characteristics of a cell, however, can be modified during development or by metabolic/endocrine processes. It is conceivable, therefore, that the heptahelical receptor–G-protein–effector phenotype of myometrial smooth muscle may be an important determinant of the functional status of the myometrium, that is, the imposition of quiescence (activation of adenylyl cyclase) or the facilitation of contractions (activation of phospholipase C and increased [Ca^{2+}]$_i$).

Many G-protein-coupled receptors that participate in regulation of myometrial activity have been cloned. These were reviewed recently by Lopez Bernal and TambyRaja (2000).

HEPTAHELICAL RECEPTORS IN MYOMETRIUM THAT MEDIATE cAMP FORMATION. A number of heptahelical receptors that nominally are associated with Gα_s-mediated activation of adenylyl cyclase and increased levels of cAMP are present in myometrium. These receptors together with appropriate ligands may act (in concert with sex steroid hormones) as part of a fail-safe system to maintain uterine quiescence, phase 0 of parturition (Price and associates, 2000; Sanborn and colleagues, 1998).

β-ADRENORECEPTORS AND PHASE 0 OF PARTURITION. In studies of adenylyl cyclase and G-protein–linked receptor-mediated processes in the myometrium, the β-adrenergic adrenoreceptors have served as prototypes. Most commonly, the β-adrenergic receptors mediate Gα_s-stimulated increases in adenylyl cyclase, increased levels of cAMP, and myometrial cell relaxation.

The rate-limiting factor in the β-receptor system is likely the number of adenylyl cyclase enzyme units or the number of receptors. The number of G-proteins in most systems far exceeds the number of receptors and effector molecules. The role of β-adrenoreceptors in maintaining uterine quiescence in vivo, however, is difficult to evaluate.

LH/hCG RECEPTORS. The heptahelical receptor for LH/hCG has been demonstrated in a number of extragonadal tissues, including myometrial smooth muscle and blood vessels (Lei and co-workers, 1992; Ziecik and colleagues, 1992). Initially, their identification seemed quite aberrant considering the more commonly recognized tissue localization in the ovary and testis. The levels of the LH/hCG receptor in myometrium during pregnancy are greater before than during labor (Zuo and colleagues, 1994). Chorionic gonadotropin acts to activate adenylyl cyclase by way of a plasma membrane receptor–$G\alpha_s$-linked system. This causes a decrease in contraction frequency and force and a decrease in tissue-specific myometrial cell gap junctions (Ambrus and Rao, 1994; Eta and co-workers, 1994).

RELAXIN. This peptide hormone is a member of the insulin-like growth factor family of proteins, consisting of an A and B chain (Bogic and associates, 1995; Weiss, 1995). There are two separate human relaxin genes, designated H1 and H2. Relaxin in plasma of pregnant women is believed to originate exclusively by secretion from the corpus luteum. Plasma levels of relaxin are greatest (about 1 ng/mL) at between 8 and 12 weeks, and thereafter decline to lower levels that persist until term. The plasma membrane receptor for relaxin mediates the activation of adenylyl cyclase and promotes myometrial relaxation, but also cervical softening. Consequently, it has not been possible to envision a clear-cut role for this hormone in human parturition.

CORTICOTROPIN-RELEASING HORMONE (CRH). This heptahelical receptor is present in myometrium during pregnancy. There are multiple isoforms of the receptor in myometrium, and their affinity is modified late in pregnancy (Grammatopoulos and associates, 1994, 1995; Hillhouse and colleagues, 1993). CRH is synthesized in the placenta, amnion, decidua, and myometrium. As discussed in Chapter 6 (p. 115), plasma levels of CRH increase during early pregnancy, but during the final 6 to 8 weeks of normal pregnancy, they increase in dramatic fashion. Because of this, several investigators have suggested that CRH is involved in the initiation of human parturition. It is not immediately apparent, however, how CRH-induced parturition would come about because CRH acts to increase cAMP formation and it would be expected to promote myometrial smooth muscle relaxation (Jaffe, 1998).

PARATHYROID HORMONE-RELATED PROTEIN (PTH-rP). The PTH/PTH-rP receptor is a plasma membrane heptahelical receptor. Most often this receptor initiates $G\alpha_s$-mediated activation of adenylyl cyclase. PTH-rP is expressed in myometrium, decidua, amnion, and trophoblast. Estrogen and TGF-β treatment of human myometrial cells causes an increase in the levels of PTH-rP mRNA (Casey and associates, 1992; Paspalliaris and associates, 1995). PTH-rP expression in smooth muscle (including uterus) is also increased by stretching (Daifotis and associates, 1992; Yamamoto and colleagues, 1992). Whereas the function of PTH-rP in uterine physiology is not established, it may serve to maximize uterine blood flow during myometrial contractions by its vasorelaxant action (Thiede and colleagues, 1991a, 1991b). PTH-rP also may act on myometrial smooth muscle to facilitate the maintenance of uterine tranquility.

PROSTAGLANDINS. A number of prostaglandin receptors and subtypes, which belong to the large family of heptahelical plasma membrane G-protein–linked proteins, have been identified (Coleman and associates, 1994). The prostaglandin family of receptors is classified according to the specificity of binding of a given receptor to a particular prostaglandin. The receptors (and naturally occurring, preferred ligands) are TP (thromboxane A_2), DP (PGD_2), IP (PGI_2), FP ($PGF_{2\alpha}$), and EP (PGE_2).

PROSTAGLANDINS AND MYOMETRIAL RELAXATION. While prostaglandins most commonly have been considered as uterotonins, selected prostanoids are sometimes primarily muscle relaxants. Specifically, PGE_2, PGD_2, and PGI_2 cause relaxation of vascular smooth muscle and vasodilatation in many circumstances. Modifications in the relative expression of the various prostaglandin receptors in myometrium at various stages of gestation may account in part for many varied responses of human myometrial tissues to prostaglandins. For example, Breuiller and co-workers (1991) found that prostanoids stimulated adenylyl cyclase activity in myometrium obtained at 32 to 35 weeks, but not in tissue obtained at 39 to 40 weeks.

Yet another variable is caused by the lack of specificity of prostanoids via different receptors. For example, PGE_2 at low concentrations acts to stimulate $G\alpha_s$-induced adenylyl cyclase and smooth muscle relaxation. At higher concentrations, PGE_2 may act via $G\alpha_i$ or $G\alpha_q$ to inhibit adenylyl cyclase or activate phospholipase C, thereby causing increased myometrial contractions.

Therefore the net action of prostanoids is highly dependent upon multiple factors. It is entirely possible that prostanoids contribute to myometrial relaxation at one stage of pregnancy and to myometrial contractions after the initiation of parturition (Crankshaw and Dyal, 1994).

CYCLIC GMP (cGMP) IN MYOMETRIUM AND MYOMETRIAL RELAXATION.
The activation of guanylyl cyclase gives rise to increased intracellular levels of cGMP, which also promotes smooth muscle relaxation (Word and colleagues, 1993).

ATRIAL/BRAIN NATRIURETIC PEPTIDES.
Two forms of atrial natriuretic peptide (ANP)/brain natriuretic peptide (BNP) receptors are present in the myometrium during human pregnancy (Itoh and co-workers, 1994). These receptors express guanylyl cyclase activity and mediate an increase in the cellular levels of cGMP. Specifically, the ANP/BNP receptor molecule is a guanylyl cyclase. BNP is secreted by amnion in large amounts (Itoh and associates, 1993), and ANP is expressed in placenta (Lim and Gude, 1995).

NITRIC OXIDE SYNTHESIS AND cGMP.
The soluble form of guanylyl cyclase is activated by nitric oxide, which because of its very hydrophobic nature, readily penetrates the plasma membrane to enter cells. Nitric oxide reacts with iron in the active site of the soluble guanylyl cyclase enzyme, stimulating it to produce cGMP. Nitric oxide acts to cause myometrial relaxation (Izumi and colleagues, 1993). Nitric oxide is synthesized in decidua, myometrial blood vessels, and nerves (Yallampalli and colleagues, 1994a, 1994b). Whether nitric oxide gains access to the myometrium and how the synthesis and action of nitric oxide is regulated as it pertains to a potential contribution to uterine quiescence is not understood.

ACCELERATED UTEROTONIN DEGRADATION AND PHASE 0 OF PARTURITION.
In addition to pregnancy-induced compounds that stimulate myometrial cell refractoriness during phase 0, there are striking increases in the activities of enzymes that degrade or inactivate endogenously produced uterotonins. Some of these include prostaglandins—prostaglandin dehydrogenase (PGDH); endothelins—enkephalinase; oxytocin—oxytocinase; histamine—diamine oxidase; catecholamines—catechol-O-methyl transferase; angiotensin-II—angiotensinase(s); and, platelet-activating factor (PAF)—PAF-acetylhydrolase. The activities of several of these enzymes are increased by progesterone action (Bates and co-workers, 1979; Casey and associates, 1980, 1991; Germain and colleagues, 1994; Yasuda and Johnston, 1992).

A FAIL-SAFE SYSTEM TO ENSURE THE SUCCESS OF PHASE 2 OF PARTURITION

UTEROTONIN THEORIES OF THE INITIATION OF PARTURITION.
In part because progesterone withdrawal does not precede the initiation of parturition in human pregnancy, many researchers began to investigate the possibility that an increase in the formation of a uterotonin is the most likely cause of the initiation of parturition. Once phase 0 is suspended and uterine phase 1 processes are implemented, a number of uterotonins may be important to the success of phase 2, active labor. Just as multiple processes may contribute to the maintenance of the myometrial unresponsiveness of phase 0 of parturition, other processes may contribute jointly to a system to ensure the success of labor. Many uterotonins known to cause myometrial contractions of smooth muscle in vitro have been proposed: oxytocin, prostaglandins, serotonin, histamine, platelet-activating factor (PAF), angiotensin II, and many others. As opposed to the receptor-mediated $G\alpha_s$-adenylyl cyclase-linked systems of myometrium that may promote the accumulation of cAMP, other heptahelical receptors have been identified in human myometrium that more commonly activate $G\alpha_i$- or $G\alpha_q$-mediated processes that eventuate in increased myometrial cell $[Ca^{2+}]_i$.

MYOMETRIAL HEPTAHELICAL RECEPTORS AND PHASE 2 OF PARTURITION OXYTOCIN AND PHASE 2 OF PARTURITION.
Oxytocin means quick birth; and, oxytocin was the first uterotonin to be implicated in the initiation of parturition. In 1906, Sir Henry Dale discovered uterotonic bioactivity in extracts of the posterior pituitary gland. By 1909, the uterotonic property of these extracts was confirmed, and by 1911, they were in use in clinical obstetrics. In 1950, Pierce and Du Vigneaud determined the structure of oxytocin, the uterotonic agent of the posterior pituitary.

Oxytocin does not appear to cause the initiation of parturition. Once phase 1 of parturition is in place, however, oxytocin may be one of several participants in ensuring the effectiveness of active labor. In experimental animals, oxytocin acts by way of a heptahelical receptor which likely activates phospholipase (Ku and colleagues, 1995). Oxytocin appears to be a very important hormone of phase 3 of parturition.

BIOLOGY AND CHEMISTRY.
Oxytocin is a nanopeptide synthesized in the magnocellular neurons of the supraoptic and paraventricular neurons. The oxytocin prohormone is transported together with the carrier protein **neurophysin,** along the axons to the neural lobe of the posterior pituitary gland in membrane-bound vesicles for storage and later release. Oxytocin prohormone

is converted enzymatically to oxytocin during transport (Gainer and colleagues, 1988; Leake, 1990).

IS OXYTOCIN INVOLVED IN THE INITIATION OF HUMAN PARTURITION? There is a long history of the safe and successful induction of labor by oxytocin administration to near-term pregnant women. It was straightforward, therefore, to hypothesize that oxytocin was involved, physiologically, in the spontaneous initiation of parturition. Several lines of evidence were supportive of this premise. The effectiveness of oxytocin in inducing labor at term, the great potency of this uterotonin, and its natural occurrence in humans were sufficient reasons for suspecting that oxytocin might be involved in the initiation of parturition. More recent discoveries provide additional support for this theory:

1. There is a striking increase in the number of oxytocin receptors in myometrial and decidual tissues near the end of gestation.
2. Oxytocin acts upon endometrial (decidual) tissue to promote the release of prostaglandins.
3. Oxytocin is synthesized directly in decidual and extraembryonic fetal tissues or in the placenta (Chibbar and associates, 1993; Zingg and colleagues, 1995).

The synthesis of oxytocin in the "uterus," however, is apparently confined to the endometrium and has not been demonstrated in the myometrium. This is an important distinction that is not emphasized in reports or reviews on the tissue site(s) of origin of oxytocin.

There is evidence of increased fetal oxytocin secretion during human labor. Oxytocin levels are higher in umbilical arterial than venous plasma and higher after spontaneous labor than before parturition begins. There is no evidence, however, that oxytocin can escape placental degradation and enter the maternal circulation (Leake, 1990).

All of the evidence, examined critically, does not favor a role for oxytocin in the initiation of parturition. The levels of oxytocin in maternal blood do not increase before or during labor, at least not until the second stage of labor. While there is a striking increase in the concentration of oxytocin receptors in myometrium late in pregnancy, this occurs for some time before labor begins. Moreover, oxytocin does not act as an antiprogestin. There is no evidence that oxytocin is involved in the transition to phase 1 of parturition, specifically, it does not induce gap junction formation between myometrial cells, nor does it induce the synthesis of oxytocin receptors. Indeed, the infusion of oxytocin, even in relatively large amounts, is relatively ineffective in inducing labor in most human pregnancies except those near term.

OXYTOCIN AS THE PUERPERAL HORMONE OF PARTURITION. There is a large body of evidence in support of an important role for oxytocin during the second stage of labor and during the puerperium, phase 3 of parturition. There are increased maternal plasma levels of oxytocin during the second stage of labor (the end of phase 2 of parturition), in the early postpartum period, and during breast feeding (phase 3 of parturition) (Nissen and co-workers, 1995). This timing of increased oxytocin release is indicative of a role for oxytocin at the end of labor and during the puerperium.

Immediately after delivery of the fetus, placenta, and fetal membranes (completion of uterine phase 2), firm and persistent contraction and retraction of the uterus are essential for the prevention of postpartum uterine hemorrhage. Oxytocin likely causes persistent contraction of the uterus. Certainly, the levels of oxytocin in maternal plasma are increased at this time, and the increase in myometrial oxytocin receptors before the onset of labor favors this process.

UTERINE INVOLUTION. Oxytocin infusion in women promotes increased levels of mRNAs in myometrium of genes that encode proteins essential for uterine involution. These include interstitial collagenase, monocyte chemoattractant protein-1, interleukin-8 (IL-8), and urokinase plasminogen activator receptor (MacDonald and Casey, unpublished observations). Therefore, oxytocin action at the end of labor and during phase 3 of parturition may be involved in uterine involution.

OXYTOCIN AND MILK LET-DOWN. The oxytocin receptor population of the myoepithelial cells of the ducts of mammary tissue are increased in a fashion similar to that in the myometrial smooth muscle cells late in pregnancy. During the puerperium, oxytocin acts on these breast duct cells to effect milk let-down, a component of phase 3 of parturition.

PROSTAGLANDINS AND PHASE 2 OF PARTURITION. Many investigators have accepted and fostered the view that prostaglandins, particularly $PGF_{2\alpha}$ and PGE_2, are involved in the initiation of parturition at term. Several lines of evidence are supportive of this theory. First, the levels of prostaglandins (or their metabolites) in amnionic fluid, maternal plasma, and maternal urine are increased during labor (Keirse, 1979). Second, the treatment of pregnant women with prostaglandins, by any of several routes of administration, causes abortion or labor at all stages of gestation (Novy and Liggins, 1980). Third, it is commonly believed, although not rigorously established (Keirse, 1990), that the administration of PGH_2 synthase inhibitors to pregnant women will delay the time of onset of induced abortion or spontaneous labor and sometimes arrest preterm labor (Besinger and Neibyl, 1990). Fourth, prostaglandin treatment of myometrial smooth muscle tissues in vitro sometimes causes contraction, dependent upon the prostanoid tested and the physiological status of the tissue treated.

EVIDENCE AGAINST PROSTAGLANDIN INVOLVEMENT.
The findings of more recent studies have cast doubt on the preeminent role of autacoids in the initiation of parturition, either at term or preterm. As in the case of oxytocin, however, prostaglandins produced directly in myometrial tissue may contribute to the effectiveness of myometrial contractions of phase 2 (active labor) once parturition is initiated.

PROSTAGLANDINS IN AMNIONIC FLUID BEFORE LABOR.
Prostaglandins, primarily PGE_2 (but also $PGF_{2\alpha}$), are detected in amnionic fluid at all stages of gestation. Before labor begins, prostanoids in amnionic fluid originate by excretion in fetal urine and possibly skin, lungs, and umbilical cord (Casey and co-workers, 1983). As the fetus grows, the levels of prostaglandins in amnionic fluid increase gradually. There is, however, no increase in the levels of prostaglandins that can be related to or interpreted as a preparturition-related increase. In fact, the total amount of prostaglandins in amnionic fluid at term before labor begins (about 1 μg) is miniscule. Because the half-life of prostaglandins in amnionic fluid is very long (6 to 12 hours), the rate of entry of prostaglandins into amnionic fluid therefore is small.

PROSTAGLANDIN LEVELS IN AMNIONIC FLUID DURING LABOR.
The relationship between increased levels of prostaglandins in amnionic fluid and the initiation of parturition stood largely unquestioned for almost 30 years. It is now known, however, that the data in support of this relationship were misleading because prostaglandins that enter amnionic fluid at parturition are produced *after* labor begins (MacDonald and Casey, 1993, 1996).

THE FOREBAG OF THE AMNIONIC SAC.
To understand the experimental pitfalls in the evaluation of prostaglandins (and other mediators of inflammation) in amnionic fluid at parturition, the anatomical changes involving the fetal membranes during cervical dilatation must be envisioned. The lowermost pole of the fetal membranes is structurally modified in the formation of the forebag of the amnionic sac. Before labor, the fetal membranes are contiguous with and attached to the uterine decidua parietalis, which in the lower uterine segment of the uterus is thin and poorly developed. The slightest movement of the underlying uterine muscle during contractions causes the fetal membranes to be pulled away from

and then to slip back and forth over the decidua. As the lower pole of the amnionic sac is pulled away from the wall of the uterus, fragments of decidua parietalis are torn away but remain attached rather firmly to the outer surface of the chorion laeve (Fig. 11–18).

This normal phenomenon of early labor is complementary to successful cervical dilatation. Membranes that slide readily over the lower uterine segment and partly through the cervix are much more efficacious dilators. Provided the membranes are intact, the lower pole of the membranes, the forebag, becomes the leading wedge that facilitates cervical dilatation during early labor. This is the case prior to the time when the fetal presenting part has descended far enough into the maternal pelvis to assume this role (Figs. 11–8 to 11–10). Because the forebag is formed by the process of cervical effacement and dilatation, it comes into existence only after labor has begun—or with abnormal cervical dilatation or incompetence.

As the cervix is opened, the forebag presents through the cervix in the upper vagina, like the tip of a fluid-filled balloon under pressure being pushed through the enlarging diameter of a hollow cylinder. The surface area of the exposed forebag increases as cervical dilatation progresses during phase 2 of parturition. The innermost tissue of the forebag is the avascular amnion, which is bathed by the amnionic fluid on its epithelial surface. The outer surface of the amnion is adherent to the

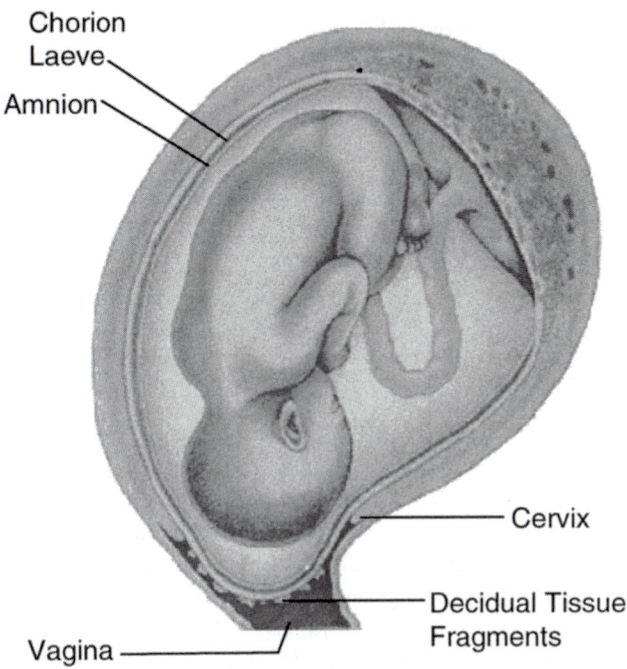

FIGURE 11–18. Sagittal view of the exposed forebag and attached decidual fragments after cervical dilatation during labor. (From MacDonald and Casey, 1996. Illustration by Michael Reingold.)

avascular chorion laeve. The traumatized, devascularized decidual tissue fragments that are torn away from the uterus form an irregular lining on the outer surface of the forebag, which presents in the vagina (Fig. 11–18).

Thereafter, the forebag tissues are bathed continuously by the vaginal fluid, which in all women (pregnant and nonpregnant) contains a large number and variety of microorganisms, bacterial toxins in large amounts, and prostaglandins and cytokines (Cox and associates, 1993b). Because of (1) trauma to decidual tissues in the formation of the forebag, (2) devascularization of the decidual fragments that are pulled away from the uterus, and (3) the action of the constituents of the vaginal fluids on these tissues, an inflammatory response in the decidual fragments of the forebag is obliged and readily demonstrable. The levels of pro-IL-1β mRNA in forebag decidua are much greater than those in decidua parietalis from the chorion laeve of the amnionic sac of the upper compartment during labor (MacDonald and associates, 1991). The forebag tissues secrete prostaglandin $F_{2\alpha}$ and cytokines IL-1β and IL-6 directly into the vagina. The quantity of the inflammatory mediators produced in forebag is large, but highly variable, dependent on the volume of decidual tissue that remains attached to the forebag (Cox and associates, 1993b). The prostaglandins synthesized in forebag tissues enter both the vagina and the forebag amnionic fluid (Fig. 11–19).

Recent findings of Rath and colleagues (1998) and Winkler and Rath (1999) are supportive of the possibility that inflammatory mediators facilitate cervical dilata-

tion. Products of extracellular matrix degradation, such as hyaluronic acid, induce the expression of IL-1 and tumor necrosis factor-α (TNF-α). In response to these cytokines, other prostaglandins and IL-6 and IL-8 induce further degradation of the extracellular matrix. It can be envisioned that these processes may effect the relatively rapid changes in the cervix that are characteristic of the parturitional process.

PROSTAGLANDINS IN AMNIONIC FLUID BEFORE AND DURING LABOR AT TERM.
To obviate anatomical sampling errors, amnionic fluid samples must be collected during labor either from the forebag compartment by direct needle aspiration or from the upper compartment either by transuterine amniocentesis at cesarean delivery conducted during labor. MacDonald and Casey (1993, 1996) used these techniques, and the levels of PGE_2, $PGF_{2\alpha}$, and PGFM in these amnionic fluids were determined. The data for amnionic fluids of both compartments and the levels of these autacoids as a function of cervical dilatation are shown in Figures 11–20 and 11–21. The concentrations of $PGF_{2\alpha}$, PGFM, and PGE_2 in the upper compartment of amnionic fluid early in labor (2.5 cm or less cervical dilatation) were no greater than those in amnionic fluid before labor began. The levels of prostaglandins in amnionic fluids obtained from the forebag during labor (collections commencing at 3 cm) were much greater than those in amnionic fluid before labor. Moreover, the levels and total content of $PGF_{2\alpha}$ in amnionic fluid of the forebag increased as cervical dilatation progressed.

Most importantly, the levels of prostaglandins in forebag amnionic fluid were much greater than those in the upper compartment at all stages of labor progress examined. The levels of prostaglandins in amnionic fluid of the upper compartment at 3 to 5 cm were significantly greater than those in amnionic fluid before labor began. Thereafter (5.5 to 7 cm), there was no further increase in the prostaglandin concentration in amnionic fluids of the upper compartment. As discussed in Chapter 19, cervical dilatation of 3 to 5 cm commonly is an important milestone in the progress of labor. At about this stage of labor progress, the presenting part of the fetus commonly has been engaged in the maternal pelvis, separating the amnionic fluid anatomically and functionally into two compartments. Before complete separation of the two compartments, constituents of the forebag amnionic fluid can mix with those in the upper compartment; but after complete separation of the amnionic fluid, the transfer of prostaglandins from the forebag to the upper compartment is attenuated or precluded.

The findings of this study also are indicative that the decidua parietalis lining the forebag is the principal site of formation of prostaglandins that enter forebag amnionic fluid. Specifically, $PGF_{2\alpha}$ and its stable

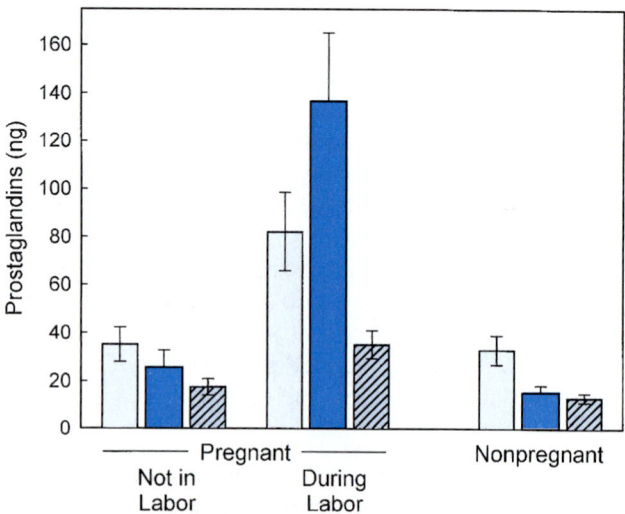

FIGURE 11–19. Prostaglandins recovered from vaginal fluid (by lavage) before and during labor. PGE_2 (open bar); $PGF_{2\alpha}$ (solid bar); PGFM (hatched bar). (From Cox and associates, 1993b, with permission.)

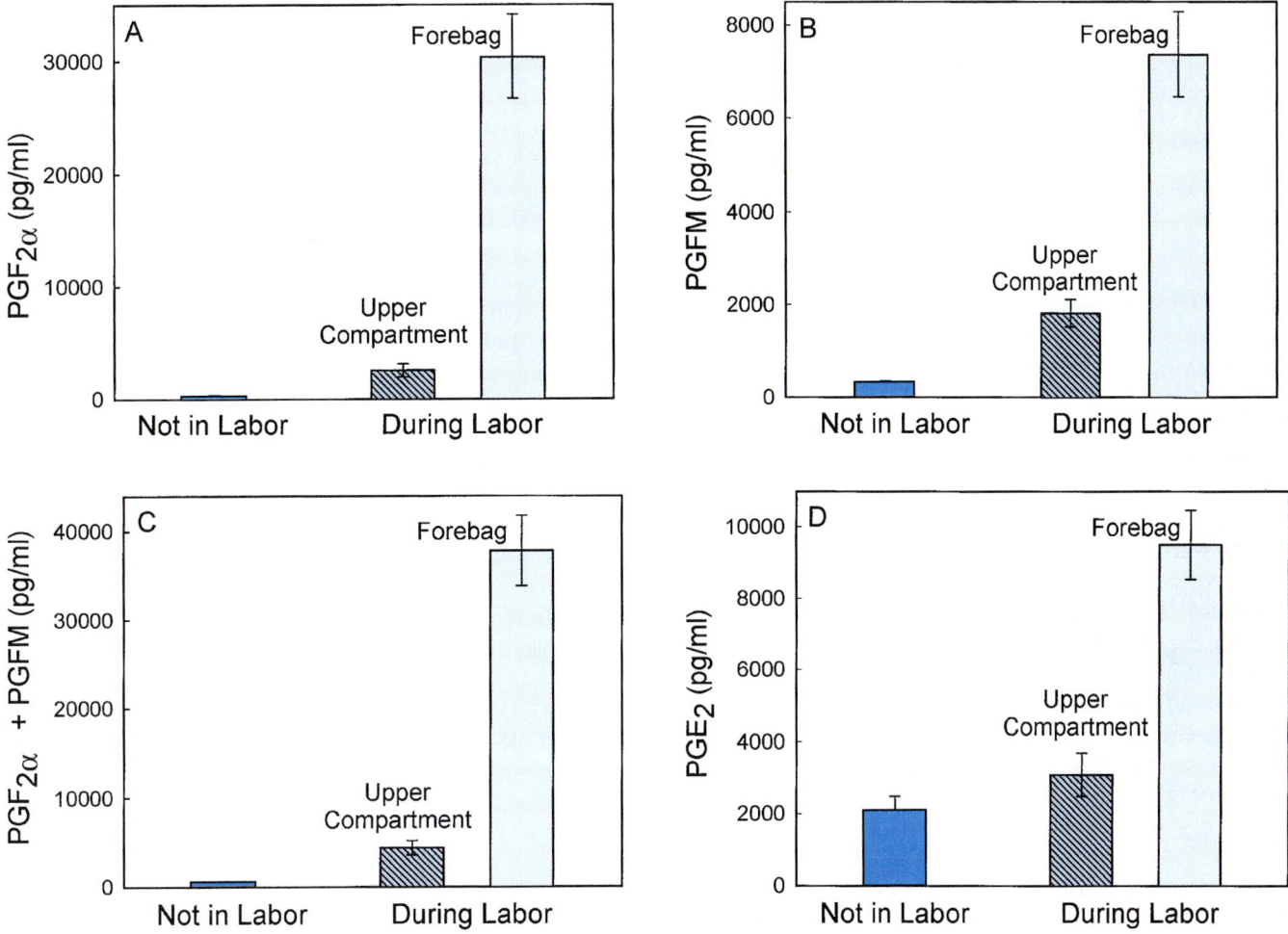

FIGURE 11–20. Mean values of $PGF_{2\alpha}$ (panel A), PGFM (panel B), $PGF_{2\alpha}$ + PGFM (panel C), and PGE_2 (panel D) in amnionic fluid at term before labor and in the upper and forebag compartments during labor. Values in labor = all stages of cervical dilatation. (From MacDonald and Casey, 1993, with permission.)

metabolite, PGFM, are present in the forebag amnionic fluid in much greater quantities than PGE_2. The decidua produces both $PGF_{2\alpha}$ and PGE_2, but amnion and chorion laeve produce primarily PGE_2 and very little $PGF_{2\alpha}$.

Thus, there are multiple lines of evidence that an increase in the levels of prostaglandins in amnionic fluid is not indicative of a role for these agents in the initiation of parturition.

1. There is no parturition-related increase in the levels of prostaglandins in amnionic fluid before labor begins.
2. The total amount of prostaglandins in amnionic fluid and the rate of entry of these autacoids into amnionic fluid before and during labor is miniscule compared with the amount required to induce labor.

3. The levels of prostaglandins in amnionic fluids obtained at the same stage of labor progress vary enormously (by 100-fold or more) among normal pregnancies (Fig. 11–22).
4. The concentrations of prostaglandins in the forebag compartment are correlated with the extent of cervical dilatation.
5. Prostaglandins are secreted at a brisk rate from the forebag into the vagina during labor.

While indeed these processes involved in parturition at term are similar to those of an inflammatory reaction, it is very unlikely that inflammatory processes initiate parturition. Rather, it is clear that the normal processes of labor beget inflammation, which includes increased prostaglandin synthesis.

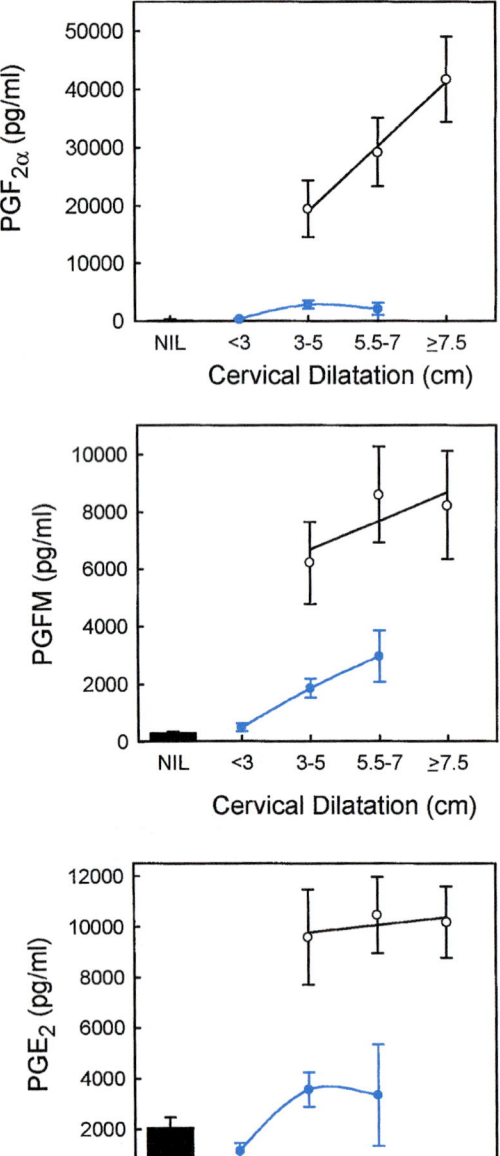

FIGURE 11–21. The levels of prostaglandins in amnionic fluid before labor and in the upper and forebag compartments during labor as a function of cervical dilatation. Top, $PGF_{2\alpha}$; middle, PGFM; bottom, PGE_2. (Modified from MacDonald and Casey, 1993, with permission; and MacDonald and Casey, 1996.)

INHIBITION OF PROSTAGLANDIN SYNTHESIS AND LABOR

INHIBITION OF PROSTAGLANDIN SYNTHESIS AND DELAYED ABORTION-INDUCTION TIME. Pretreatment of women with indomethacin, a prostaglandin syn-

thase inhibitor, causes a delay in the abortion-induction time after intra-amnionic instillation of hypertonic solutions during the midtrimester of pregnancy. This observation also has been cited as evidence for the involvement of prostaglandins in the initiation of parturition. A meaningful interpretation of these findings of delayed abortion-induction time by prostaglandin synthase inhibitors is, realistically, not possible because of the extremely large number of variables involved in such studies. Obviously, the entry of a hypertonic solution into the amnionic fluid is not a physiological feature of spontaneous parturition. Moreover, the maintenance of pregnancy at 12 to 16 weeks' gestation is not identical with that during the third trimester. For example, the administration of antiprogestins will effect abortion during early pregnancy, but the efficacy of these agents in promoting abortion or labor declines as pregnancy progresses. Near term, RU-486 treatment will not cause the onset of labor in human pregnancy. In addition, the effect of indomethacin and hypertonic solutions on the fetus may be important determinants of the outcome of such pregnancies.

INHIBITION OF PROSTAGLANDIN SYNTHESIS AND DELAYED PARTURITION AT TERM. There are few data to support the contention that the inhibition of prostaglandin synthesis delays the onset of parturition in human pregnancies at term. There are no properly conducted control studies to permit a definitive judgment concerning this possible relationship.

INHIBITION OF PROSTAGLANDIN SYNTHESIS AND PRETERM LABOR. Rigorous testing of the proposition that inhibitors of prostaglandin synthesis will prevent or arrest preterm labor has also not been conducted (Keirse, 1990). Fear of adverse effects on the fetus has prevented most investigators from conducting such studies. In monkeys, Sadowsky and colleagues (2000) showed that indomethacin blocked IL-1β-induced $PGF_{2\alpha}$ amnionic fluid levels.

PROSTAGLANDINS AND PHASE 2 OF PARTURITION: SUMMARY. The evidence in favor of a role for prostaglandins in the initiation of parturition is fragile. It is quite possible, perhaps probable, that prostaglandins and other uterotonins, such as oxytocin, are involved in the success of phase 2 of parturition after phase 0 is suspended and phase 1 processes are implemented. It is reasonable to surmise that a fail-safe system is operative to promote phase 2 of parturition, just as there probably is a fail-safe system that ensures the success of phase 0.

PLATELET-ACTIVATING FACTOR AND PHASE 2 OF PARTURITION. The platelet-activating factor (PAF) receptor also is a member of the heptahelical family of

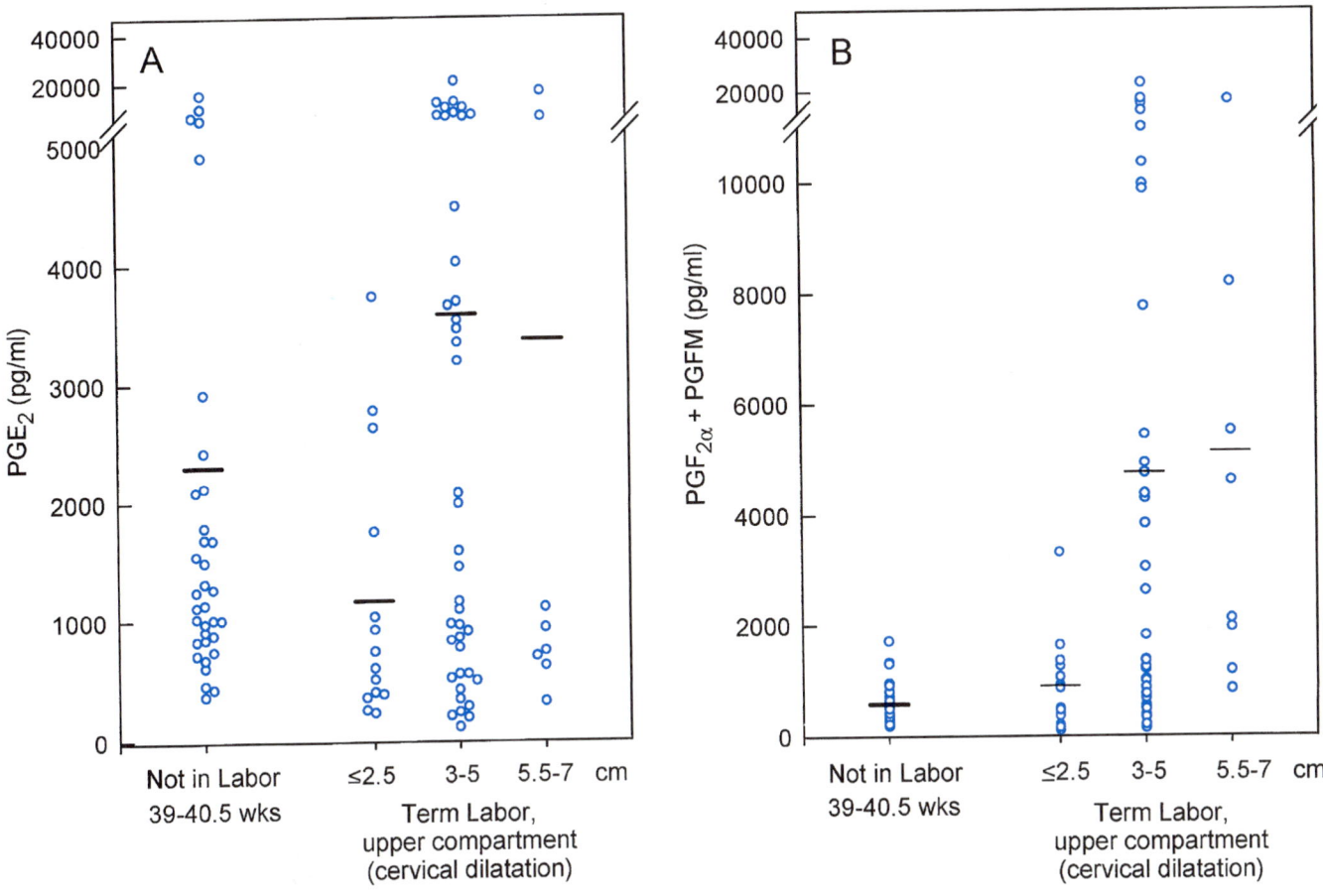

FIGURE 11–22. Wide range of values for PGE$_2$ (panel A) and PGF$_{2\alpha}$ + PGFM (panel B) in amnionic fluids before and in the upper compartment during labor at term. (From MacDonald and Casey, 1996.)

transmembrane receptors and acts to increase myometrial cell [Ca^{2+}]$_i$ and promote uterine contractions. The levels of PAF in amnionic fluid are increased during labor (Billah and colleagues, 1983; Nishihara and associates, 1984); and PAF treatment of myometrial tissue promotes contraction (Zhu and colleagues, 1992). It is likely that PAF, like prostaglandins, cytokines, and endothelin-1, is produced in leukocytes as a result of the inflammatory process that is obliged when cervical dilation brings about exposure of the traumatized forebag tissues to the vaginal fluids.

The transport of PAF from amnionic fluid to myometrium is uncertain but unlikely. PAF is inactivated enzymatically by PAF-acetylhydrolase; this enzyme is present in high specific activity in macrophages (Prescott and associates, 1990), which are present in large numbers in decidua. Thus, the myometrium may be protected from PAF action by PAF-acetylhydrolase in a manner similar to that for uterotonins: oxytocin and oxytocinase, endothelin-1 and enkephalinase, and prostaglandins and prostaglandin dehydrogenase.

ENDOTHELIN-1 AND PHASE 2 OF PARTURITION. The endothelins are very powerful inducers of myometrial smooth muscle contraction and endothelin receptors are demonstrable in myometrial tissue (Word and colleagues, 1990). The endothelin A receptor, preferentially expressed in smooth muscle cells, including the myometrium, acts to effect an increase in [Ca^{2+}]$_i$, apparently by linkage to both Gα_q- and Gα_i-subunits of the G-proteins. Endothelin-1 is produced in myometrium, but the exact cellular site of synthesis is not clearly established and the potential contribution of myometrial endothelin-1 to phase 2 of parturition is not defined.

Endothelin-1 is also synthesized in amnion. Like other uterotonins synthesized in amnion, it is unlikely that endothelin-1 can be transported from reflected amnion (or amnionic fluid), without degradation, to the myometrium (Eis and colleagues, 1992). One obstacle to endothelin-1 transport across the fetal membranes is the enzyme enkephalinase (membrane metalloendopeptidase), which is present in chorion laeve in high specific activity (Germain and associates, 1994). Enkephalinase catalyzes the degradation of endothelin-1 as well as several other small, bioactive peptides (e.g., the enkephalins, substance P, and atrial and brain natriuretic peptides).

MAST CELLS PRODUCTS AND PHASE 2 OF PARTURITION. The concentration of mast cells in the myometrium is very high and is increased further during pregnancy. The secretory products of mast cells (histamine and serotonin) act in vitro as uterotonins. Moreover, serotonin acts uniquely in myometrial cells to induce the expression of interstitial collagenase, membrane metalloproteinase-1, a major participant in postpartum uterine involution (Jeffrey and associates, 1991). Consequently, the products of mast cells, histamine and serotonin, also may promote the contractions of phase 2 of parturition.

ANGIOTENSIN II AND PHASE 2 OF PARTURITION. There are two heptahelical G-protein–linked angiotensin II receptors (AT1 and AT2) expressed in the uterus. In nonpregnant women, the AT2 receptor is predominant, but in myometrium of pregnant women, it is the AT1 receptor that is preferentially expressed (Cox and associates, 1993a). Most commonly, angiotensin II binding to the plasma membrane receptor on smooth muscle cells evokes contraction. During pregnancy, vascular smooth muscle, which expresses the AT2 receptor, is refractory to the pressor effects of angiotensin II (Chap. 8, p. 183). In myometrium near term, however, angiotensin II may be another component of the uterotonin system of phase 2 of parturition, acting to promote increased myometrial cell $[Ca^{2+}]_i$.

CRH, hCG, PTH-rP, AND PHASE 2 OF PARTURITION. There may be a late pregnancy modification in the CRH, LH/hCG, and/or PTH-rP receptor–G-protein phenotype in myometrium that favors a switch from cAMP formation to increased myometrial cell $[Ca^{2+}]_i$. Oxytocin acts to attenuate CRH-stimulated accumulation of cAMP in myometrial tissue, and CRH augments the contraction-inducing potency of a given dose of oxytocin in human myometrial strips (Quartero and colleagues, 1991, 1992). CRH also acts to increase myometrial contractile force in response to $PGF_{2\alpha}$ (Benedetto and associates, 1994). This was reviewed recently by Lockwood (1999).

HEPTAHELICAL RECEPTORS AND PHASE 2 OF PARTURITION: SUMMARY. Whereas multiple processes likely contribute to the success of phase 0 of parturition, it also is likely that multiple (possibly redundant) processes contribute to the success of phase 2 (active labor) once phase 0 is suspended and phase 1 of parturition is implemented. A variety of myometrial heptahelical receptors may promote uterine quiescence; but there is another group that should inhibit cAMP formation and/or activate phospholipase C. Perhaps the heptahelical receptor–G-protein–effector phenotype of the myometrial cells at various stages of pregnancy and under the influence of external signals contributes to the contractile response of the myometrium, that is, relaxation or contraction.

CONTRIBUTION OF INTRAUTERINE TISSUES TO PARTURITION. The potential role of amnion, chorion laeve, and decidua parietalis has been studied to define the participation, if any, of each tissue in promoting the initiation of parturition; but presently, an alternative role for these tissues appears to be more likely. The fetal membranes and decidua are part of an important tissue shell around the fetus that serves as a physical, immunological, and metabolic shield that protects against the untimely initiation of parturition.

AMNION. The amnion provides virtually all of the tensile strength (resistance to tearing and rupture) of the fetal membranes (Chap. 5, p. 103). The avascular human amnion is highly resistant to penetration by leukocytes, microorganisms, and neoplastic cells from the maternal compartment and constitutes a selective filter to prevent fetal squames as well as particulate-bound lung and skin secretions from reaching the maternal compartment. In this manner, maternal tissues are protected from constituents in the amnionic fluid that could adversely affect decidual or myometrial function or even maternal well-being, such as amnionic fluid embolism, which is discussed in Chapter 25 (p. 660).

A number of bioactive peptides and polypeptides, which are effective smooth muscle relaxants, are synthesized in amnion: PTH-rP, CRH, and brain natriuretic peptide. Specific receptors for these agents are present in myometrial tissue during pregnancy. A mechanism has not been established, however, whereby these vasoactive peptides can be transported from amnion to the myometrium without degradation. It is more likely that these agents act on contiguous tissues, such as the chorionic vessels of the placenta, or after inspiration or swallowing into the fetal lungs or gastrointestinal tract.

CHORION LAEVE AND PARTURITION. It is appreciably more difficult to work with isolated chorion laeve and its cytotrophoblastic cells than with isolated amnion and its epithelial cells or with decidua and isolated decidual cells. It is very difficult to separate chorion laeve tissue completely from tightly adherent fragments of decidua parietalis, and vice versa. After these technical problems are overcome, the chorion is similar to the amnion by serving primarily as a protective tissue—providing immunological acceptance—in the prevention of untimely parturition. In addition, the chorion laeve is enriched in enzymes that inactivate uterotonins such as prostaglandin dehydrogenase, oxytocinase, and enkephalinase (Germain and associates, 1994).

DECIDUA PARIETALIS AND PARTURITION. A metabolic contribution of decidua parietalis to the initiation of parturition has been an appealing possibility for a number of reasons, both anatomical and functional. The generation of uterotonins in decidua that act in a paracrine manner on contiguous myometrium is an interesting option. There are also several lines of evidence that decidual activation is an accompaniment of human parturition (Casey and MacDonald, 1988a, 1988b, 1990; MacDonald and colleagues, 1991). The central question, however, is whether decidual activation precedes or follows the onset of labor. The process of decidual activation appears to be localized to the exposed decidual fragments lining the forebag. Trauma, hypoxia, and exposure of forebag decidua to endotoxin lipopolysaccharide, microorganisms, and IL-1β in the vaginal fluids provokes an inflammatory reaction, which is an inevitable and consistent sequela of labor.

PRETERM LABOR

In a survey conducted by the Institute of Medicine of chairpersons of departments of obstetrics and gynecology in the United States and Canada, preterm birth was selected as the single most important clinical health problem encountered in the practice of obstetrics-gynecology (Townsend, 1992). As discussed in Chapter 27, preterm birth is one of the major health hazards of humans, being the greatest cause (other than congenital anomalies) of neonatal morbidity and mortality.

Preterm birth is not singularly the consequence of preterm labor. There are three major etiological factors that contribute to delivery before 34 weeks:

1. Preterm, premature rupture of the fetal membranes.
2. Spontaneous preterm labor in pregnancies with intact fetal membranes.
3. Complications of pregnancy that severely jeopardize fetal and sometimes maternal health and mandate delivery, usually because of a deteriorating intrauterine environment for the fetus (Goldenberg and colleagues, 2000).

PRETERM PREMATURE RUPTURE OF THE MEMBRANES. This term is used to denote spontaneous rupture of the fetal membranes before the onset of labor, whether at term or preterm. In some institutions, including Parkland Hospital, as many or more preterm deliveries are preceded by preterm premature rupture of the

membranes as by spontaneous preterm labor (Chap. 27, p. 704). The pathogenesis of premature rupture of the membranes is obscure; and unfortunately, new insights into the prevention of this serious pregnancy complication have not emerged.

MANDATED PRETERM DELIVERY INDEPENDENT OF LABOR: COMPROMISED FETAL, MATERNAL HEALTH. All too often, pregnancy complications oblige a clinical decision to effect preterm delivery rather than continue pregnancy in a deteriorating intrauterine environment for the fetus. A host of pregnancy disorders may mandate such a choice. Most commonly, these complications of pregnancy threaten fetal health so that a continued intrauterine existence will likely result in fetal death. Many examples may be cited, but the most common are maternal hypertension, severe diabetes mellitus, failure of fetal growth, and abruptio placenta. Each of these conditions is considered separately in great detail in other chapters.

PRETERM DELIVERY: SPONTANEOUS PRETERM LABOR. Pregnancies with intact fetal membranes and spontaneous preterm labor (for clinical as well as research purposes) must be distinguished from those in which there has been preterm premature rupture of the membranes.

Pregnancies complicated by spontaneous preterm labor, however, do not constitute a homogeneous group of pregnancies characterized singularly by the early initiation of parturition. Among the more common associated findings are preterm cervical dilatation; anatomical incompetence of the cervix; shortening of the cervix; uterine (fundal) abnormalities; fetal anomalies; multifetal pregnancies; severe maternal illness, including extrauterine infection such as appendicitis, peritonitis, pyelonephritis, and pneumonia; maternal thermal injury (body burns); autoimmune diseases; pregnancy-induced hypertension; and maternal systemic disorders. Setting aside uterine abnormalities, a common denominator among the fetal or maternal conditions that would provide a clue to the cause of the preterm onset of parturition has not been identified. If such a factor were found, many physiological processes of human parturition at term and preterm might become more understandable.

DOES INTRAUTERINE INFECTION CAUSE PRETERM LABOR? During the past few years, the most popular theory for one cause of preterm labor has been intrauterine infection. Many investigators suggest that preterm labor with intact fetal membranes is sometimes the result of ascending spread of bacteria from the vagina or cervical canal. It has been estimated that upwards of one third of preterm labor with intact membranes may be caused by intrauterine infection.

BACKGROUND. Among many obstetricians, there has been great suspicion that "silent" infection is a common accompaniment and cause of preterm labor. The term "silent" is used to describe a condition in which intrauterine infection exists but there is little or no clinical evidence of infection in the pregnant woman, and sometimes microorganisms cannot be cultured from the amnionic fluid (Iams and co-workers, 1987). The critical question, however, is whether infection—or an inflammatory process—precedes or follows the onset of labor (phase 2 of parturition). A distinction must be made between intrauterine infection as a cause of preterm labor and the development of inflammation in exposed tissues of the amnionic sac as a sequela of labor, at term and preterm.

THE IMPORTANCE OF THE PROBLEM. As MacDonald and Casey (1996) have cautioned, it is vitally important to establish or refute the validity of the theory that infection is a cause of the initiation of preterm parturition. If such an etiology were established, it also is crucial to determine the incidence of infection-induced preterm labor. If infection were a cause of preterm labor, this cause should be preventable. If, however, the evidence in favor of infection as a cause of preterm labor is artifactual, and the actual incidence of preterm labor caused by infection is very small, the widespread use of antibiotic treatment regimens to prevent preterm birth would be largely useless and unacceptable.

The evidence that infection causes preterm labor could be misinterpreted if based solely of the finding of mediators of the inflammatory response, including microorganisms and bacterial toxins, in amnionic fluids collected after labor is in progress. The inflammatory reaction that gave rise to these findings may not have begun until after labor started; the inflammatory response identified from studies of amnionic fluid could be the normal consequence of labor. Inflammation in the fragments of decidual tissue attached to the forebag of the amnionic sac is obliged during preterm labor as it is during spontaneous parturition at term (see p. 285). Mediators of the inflammatory response produced therein sometimes accumulate in the amnionic fluid during spontaneous labor both at term and preterm.

PROPOSED PATHOGENESIS OF INFECTION-INDUCED PRETERM LABOR

ANATOMICAL CONSIDERATIONS. The patency of the reproductive tract of women, although essential for the achievement of pregnancy and delivery of the fetus, is theoretically problematic during phase 0 of parturition. The lower pole of the fetal membrane–decidual junction embraces the orifice of the cervical canal, which anatomically is patent to the vagina. There is, of course, functional obliteration of the cervical canal during pregnancy by a mucus plug, and significant antimicrobial properties have been identified in the cervical mucus. Nonetheless, this anatomical arrangement could provide a passageway for the spread of microorganisms to intrauterine tissues. There are large numbers of microorganisms of a wide variety in the vaginal fluid of all women. Theoretically, microorganisms in the endocervical canal or vagina may, by ascending spread, colonize tissues at the lower pole of the fetal membranes and contiguous decidua.

Why is it, therefore, that all human pregnancies are not complicated by infection? It seems reasonable to surmise that the antimicrobial properties of the cervical glands and mucus are appreciable. In addition, the fetal membranes and amnionic fluid also must be highly capable of resisting invasion by most microorganisms. These factors, together with the antimicrobial properties of the resident leukocytes in the decidua, must be substantial in preventing ascending infection.

It has been suggested that selected microorganisms are more likely to be the pathogens that bring about preterm labor. But an association between specific microorganisms in the vaginal fluid or endocervix and an increased risk for preterm labor has not been established. A potential exception to this generalization, bacterial vaginosis, is considered separately (Chap. 27, p. 699).

BACKGROUND. It has been known for more than 50 years that the administration of bacterial endotoxin (lipopolysaccharide, or LPS) to pregnant animals causes abortion or preterm delivery, which is accompanied by decidual hemorrhage and necrosis (Zahl and Bjerknes, 1943). It was not until many years later, however, that the biomolecular particulars of the inflammatory response were defined in detail. These latter findings provided an attractive potential explanation whereby intrauterine infection might cause preterm labor. The inflammatory response elicited by bacterial toxins is mediated, in large measure, by specific receptors on mononuclear phagocytes. These cells release arachidonic acid, and PGE_2, in response to LPS. The primary cytokine, IL-1β, also is produced rapidly after LPS stimulation (Dinarello, 1986). IL-1β in turn acts to promote a series of responses that includes increased synthesis of other cytokines such as TNF-α, IL-6, IL-8, the proliferation, activation, and migration of leukocytes, modifications in extracellular matrix proteins, mitogenic and cytotoxic effects, fever, and the acute phase response (El-Bastawissi and colleagues, 2000). IL-1β also acts to promote prostaglandin formation in many tissues, including myometrium, decidua, and amnion (Romero and colleagues, 1989; Semer and associates, 1991).

INFECTION-INDUCED PRETERM LABOR: HYPOTHESIS.

Based on these insights into the inflammatory response, it was straightforward to construct a theory for the pathogenesis of infection-induced preterm labor. Namely, microorganisms, originating in the vagina or cervix, after ascending spread, colonize tissues (decidua and possibly the fetal membranes) and/or invade the amnionic sac. LPS (or other toxins) elaborated by these bacteria induce the formation of cytokines in mononuclear phagocytes of decidua or in monocytes recruited into the amnionic fluid. The cytokines, especially IL-1β, provoke prostaglandin release and thereby preterm labor (El-Bastawissi, 2000; MacDonald, 1988; Romero, 1998, and all their co-workers).

PRETERM LABOR: AMNIONIC FLUID CONSTITUENTS.

Many groups of investigators have evaluated amnionic fluids collected during preterm labor to identify and quantify mediators of inflammation. These have included microorganisms and bacterial products such as endotoxin and short-chain fatty acids; leukocyte number and type as well as leukocyte enzymes; prostaglandins; IL-1β, IL-1α, TNF-α, IL-6, IL-8, and other cytokines; and endothelin-1. Generally, the preterm labor pregnancies studied were less than 34 weeks' gestation with intact fetal membranes.

MICROORGANISMS IN AMNIONIC FLUID DURING PRETERM LABOR.

It is important to consider the potential mechanisms(s) whereby microorganisms may gain entrance into the amnionic fluid. The capacity for penetration of tissues (including the fetal membranes) by microorganisms varies appreciably among bacteria and among tissues. The likelihood of bacterial penetration of the amnionic sac may be dependent upon:

1. Exposure of these tissues to the microorganisms (cervical dilatation).
2. Metabolic integrity of the tissues (especially decidua parietalis).
3. The vaginal flora of a given woman.
4. Numbers of specific microorganisms.
5. Integrity of the fetal membranes.
6. The pH of the vaginal fluid.
7. Cooperative actions among microorganisms.

Most likely, the invasion of the amnionic sac by microorganisms occurs after labor begins, and the forebag tissues are exposed. Another factor in determining the likelihood of microbial invasion is the duration of exposure of the tissues in the vagina, that is, the duration of cervical dilatation.

Some microorganisms, for example, *Fusobacterium* species, are detected in amnionic fluid much more commonly than others. This finding was interpreted by some as presumptive evidence that specific microorganisms are more commonly involved as pathogens in the induction of preterm labor. Another interpretation, however, is that given direct access to the membranes (after cervical dilatation), selected microorganisms (such as fusobacteria) that are more capable of burrowing through these exposed tissues will do so. Fusobacteria are not commonly found in the vagina; nonetheless, they are the microorganisms most commonly isolated from amnionic fluid during preterm labor (Hill, 1993). Fusobacteria are found in the vaginal fluid of only 9 percent of women but in 28 percent of positive amnionic fluid cultures from preterm labor pregnancies with intact membranes (Chaim and Mazor, 1992).

Altshuler and Hyde (1988) found that fusobacteria burrow through amnion tissue rapidly and sometimes are present in amnion tissue in large numbers as if penetrating between the amnion epithelial cells. They also identified large numbers of fusobacteria in the Wharton jelly of the umbilical cord with intra-amnionic infections, suggesting a peculiar propensity for these microorganisms to penetrate amnion tissue, which also covers the umbilical cord. Fusobacteria produce a variety of toxins, some of which are extraordinarily potent in stimulating cytokine formation in mononuclear phagocytes. We interpret these data, and Hyde and Altshuler concur (personal communication), to mean that fusobacteria and possibly other microorganisms penetrate the fetal membranes **after** the tissues are exposed to these microorganisms in the cervical/vaginal fluid. This provides a reasonable explanation for the low incidence of fusobacteria in vaginal fluids but a much higher incidence in positive cultures of amnionic fluids.

MICROORGANISMS IN AMNIONIC FLUID DURING PRETERM AND TERM LABOR.

The incidence of positive cultures of amnionic fluid collected during **preterm labor** varies among studies from 10 to 40 percent, the average being about 13 percent (Romero and associates, 1988). In a study conducted by Gomez and co-workers (1995), the incidence of culture-positive amnionic fluids collected by amniocentesis during spontaneous **term labor** was 19 percent, which is similar to or greater than the incidence of culture-positive amnionic fluids during preterm labor identified by the same investigators. If the incidence of bacterial culture-positive amnionic fluids obtained during spontaneous labor at term was greater or equal to the incidence of positive cultures in amnionic fluids during preterm labor, the theory of infection-induced preterm labor must be reevaluated. Gomez and associates (1995) rationalized these findings by pointing to the sometimes larger number of microorganisms in amnionic fluid during preterm labor. This explanation is tenuous, however, because many cases of preterm labor have been in labor for a much longer time before amnionic fluid was collected, and therefore more time was available for microbial replication in the amnionic fluid in situ.

LEUKOCYTES IN AMNIONIC FLUID.
Macrophages are present in amnionic fluid in very small numbers before the onset of labor. Indeed, leukocytes do not readily penetrate normal fetal membranes either in vivo or in vitro. With inflammation of the exposed decidua of the tissues that form the forebag during preterm labor, however, maternal leukocytes are recruited into the amnionic fluid (presumably in response to chemoattractants). The same phenomenon is noted at term. Leukocyte activation is accelerated with inflammation, and activated leukocytes are able to penetrate the fetal membranes.

INTERLEUKIN-1β IN AMNIONIC FLUID.
It is convenient, in both the physiological context and in accordance with current nomenclature, to consider IL-1β as a primary cytokine. IL-1β is produced rapidly in response to infectious and immunological challenges and IL-1β acts in many cells to promote the synthesis of many other cytokines and other mediators of inflammation.

IL-1β is not detected in amnionic fluid of pregnancies with intact membranes before labor begins. The first extensive studies of amnionic fluid IL-1β during labor were conducted with samples collected during preterm labor. The results of these studies, from all laboratories reporting, have been virtually identical. Namely, IL-1β is present in amnionic fluid in approximately one third of preterm labor pregnancies (Romero and associates, 1987). The finding of IL-1β in amnionic fluid in these earlier studies was believed to constitute corroborative evidence of infection-induced preterm labor. It was hoped that confirmation for one cause of preterm labor had been obtained, supporting what many obstetricians had suspected for decades, that silent infection is a relatively common cause of preterm labor.

At the time of this interpretation, however, it was not realized that IL-1β was found with about equal frequency in amnionic fluid samples obtained from pregnancies during spontaneous labor at term. In about one third of pregnancies during spontaneous labor at term, there is readily measurable IL-1β in concentrations of about 100 to 5000 pg/mL (Romero and colleagues, 1990). Importantly, these amnionic fluids were collected by transabdominal or transuterine amniocentesis.

The finding of IL-1β in approximately equal proportions of amnionic fluids collected during spontaneous preterm and term labor also necessitated a reevaluation of the original hypothesis. Is the accumulation of a given agent in amnionic fluid indicative of a role for that compound in the initiation of parturition? Or does a particular agent accumulate in amnionic fluid as a natural consequence of the changes obliged during labor?

Parturition research often has been, and frequently continues to be, stifled by this dilemma. In part, this is because the initiation of parturition and the onset of labor have been taken as one and the same event.

ORIGIN OF IL-1β IN AMNIONIC FLUID.
As in the case of prostaglandins, IL-1β is produced in cells of the forebag decidua after labor-induced cervical dilatation exposes this tissue in the vagina. The distribution of IL-1β from forebag decidua into the vagina and amnionic fluid, however, is not comparable with the entry of prostaglandins produced in the forebag into these two spaces. First, IL-1β is a protein (M_r about 17,000). The transfer of IL-1β from decidua across the fetal membranes of the forebag into amnionic fluid appears to be severely limited. The rate of IL-1β secretion from forebag decidual tissue is great, but IL-1β is not detected in forebag amnionic fluid in two thirds of pregnancies during labor at term (Cox and colleagues, 1993b). Indeed, Kent and colleagues (1994) found that the transfer of radiolabeled IL-1β across the fetal membranes in vitro was negligible. The IL-1β in amnionic fluid does not arise from amnion tissue, fetal urine, or fetal lung secretions. Most likely, IL-1β in amnionic fluid is secreted by mononuclear phagocytes or neutrophils activated and recruited into the amnionic fluid after labor begins. Therefore, IL-1β in amnionic fluid likely is generated in situ from cells newly recruited into this space.

CHEMOATTRACTANTS.
There are very few leukocytes in the amnionic fluid of normal pregnancies before the onset of labor, but monocytes and neutrophils do enter amnionic fluid during labor in some pregnancies. There is a highly significant correlation between the presence of leukocytes and the concentration of IL-1β in amnionic fluid (Cox and colleagues, 1993b; Dr. Judith Head, personal communication). The amount of IL-1β in amnionic fluid may be determined by the number of leukocytes recruited, the activational status of these cells, or the effect of constituents of amnionic fluid on the rate of secretion of IL-1β by these leukocytes. The chemoattractants IL-8 (neutrophils) and monocyte chemoattractant protein-1 (monocytes/macrophages) are produced in amnion, and the synthesis of these chemoattractants in amnion cells is increased in response to LPS and IL-1 treatment. These chemoattractants may act to recruit leukocytes into the amnionic fluid from maternal decidual and fetal chorionic vessels.

OTHER CYTOKINES IN AMNIONIC FLUID.
A number of investigators also have cited the finding of very high levels of IL-6 or IL-8 (and many other cytokines) in amnionic fluid as evidence of an intrauterine infection-based cause of preterm labor. More recently, Athayde and associates (2000) found that the proinflammatory

IL-16 is a marker for microbial invasion of amnionic fluid. However, at least IL-6 and IL-8, unlike IL-1β, are present in amnionic fluid of normal pregnancies throughout most of gestation. These cytokines, again unlike IL-1β, are produced by amnion cells, and the production of IL-8 by amnion epithelial cells and IL-6 and IL-8 by amnion mesenchymal cells is increased strikingly by IL-1β (Casey and MacDonald, unpublished observations). It is not surprising, therefore, that the levels of IL-6 and IL-8 are increased in amnionic fluids in which IL-1β is present. Indeed, a very high correlation is found between the concentrations of IL-1β and IL-6 in amnionic fluids during labor at term and preterm (Cox and associates, 1997). Thus, increased levels of IL-6, and other cytokines, are to be expected whenever IL-1β formation is increased. IL-1β acts as a primary cytokine to promote the synthesis of other cytokines (MacDonald and Casey, 1996).

PRETERM LABOR AND HIGH LEVELS OF CYTOKINES IN AMNIONIC FLUID. In a small fraction of preterm labor pregnancies, the levels of cytokines in amnionic fluid are increased massively, that is, the levels are much greater than the highest levels in amnionic fluids collected during labor at term. Indeed, the levels of IL-1β in some preterm labor amnionic fluids may be 10 to 100 times the maximum values observed in IL-1β-positive fluids at term. These findings also have been cited as evidence of intrauterine infection as a cause of preterm labor.

To analyze this particular issue, it is important to recognize that there is a fundamental difference in the obstetrical management of labor in pregnancies at term compared with the management of preterm labor. In the former, efforts are directed toward effecting delivery in a safe and expedient manner. In the latter, management is commonly directed toward delaying delivery. In consequence, it is rare for labor to extend beyond 18 hours in term pregnancies. It is common, however, for the cervix to be dilated for more than 18 hours, sometimes for days during preterm labor. The very high levels of cytokines in amnionic fluid of preterm labor pregnancies are found primarily in those collected after very prolonged labor and dilatation of the cervix. The suggestion was made earlier that these prolonged preterm labor pregnancies also may be those in which the number of microorganisms is great.

PROSTAGLANDINS IN AMNIONIC FLUID DURING PRETERM LABOR. The infection-based theory of preterm labor has been anchored to the proposition that the proximate event in the onset of preterm labor is the accelerated production of prostaglandins. The levels of PGE$_2$ and PGF$_{2\alpha}$ in amnionic fluid during preterm labor are, however, not strikingly elevated (Fig. 11–23).

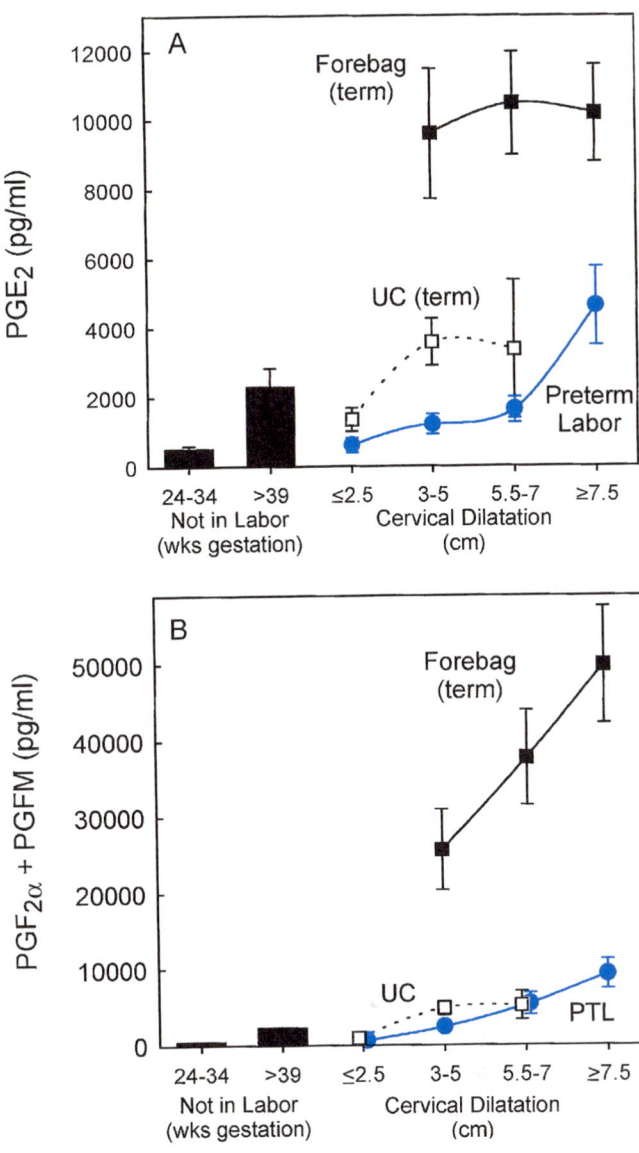

FIGURE 11–23. Comparison of the levels of PGE$_2$ (panel A) and PGF$_{2\alpha}$ + PGFM (panel B) in amnionic fluids of the forebag and upper compartment during labor at term and from single amnionic fluid compartment during preterm (less than 34 weeks) labor. (PTL = preterm labor; UC = upper compartment.) (Modified from MacDonald and Casey, 1996.)

Upon assessment of prostaglandins in amnionic fluid during preterm labor, many observers have been surprised to find that the levels usually are very low (Gomez and associates, 1995). Indeed, several groups of investigators have commented specifically on the surprisingly low levels of prostaglandins in amnionic fluid during preterm labor. The mean levels of prostaglandins in amnionic fluid during preterm labor, at comparable stages of labor progress, are similar to those in amnionic fluids of the upper compartment during labor at term

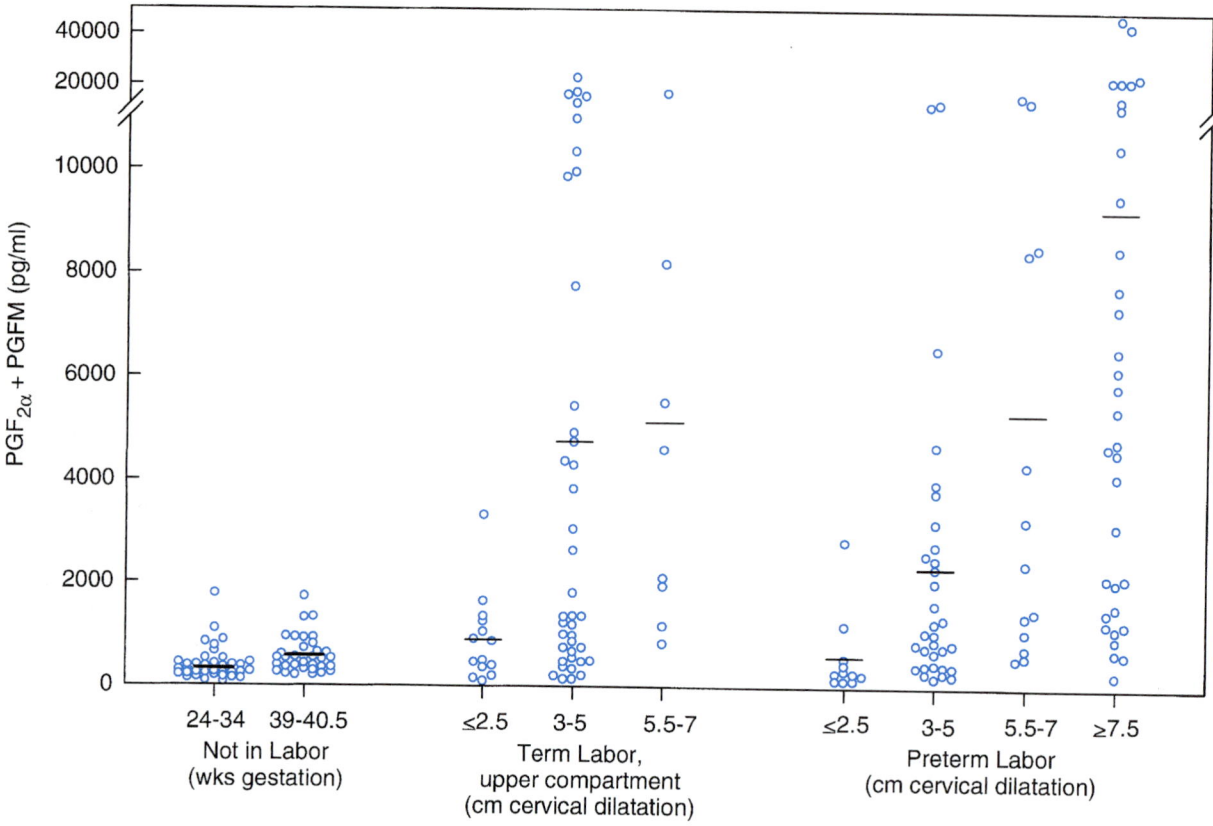

FIGURE 11–24. Wide range of values of PGE₂ (panel A) and PGF₂ₐ + PGFM (panel B) in amnionic fluids of different pregnancies before and during labor at term and preterm. Values are from amnionic fluids collected by amniocentesis (before labor and during preterm labor) and by transuterine amniocentesis (upper compartment) during labor at term. (From MacDonald and Casey, 1993, 1996).

(Fig. 11–23). In many cases of preterm labor, however, the levels of prostaglandins in amnionic fluids are no greater than those in amnionic fluids before labor began. The levels of prostaglandins in amnionic fluid during preterm labor also vary enormously among pregnancies at similar stages of labor progress (Fig. 11–24).

These findings are to be expected if the forebag tissues are the source of prostaglandins in amnionic fluid during preterm labor, as there is only a single amnionic fluid compartment in such pregnancies because the preterm fetal presenting part does not obstruct the maternal pelvis and separate amnionic fluid compartments are not formed.

It is clear that the prostaglandins that sometimes accumulate in amnionic fluid during labor, both at term and preterm, are produced as part of the inflammatory process in the forebag tissues that normally accompanies labor. The enormous variation in the levels of prostaglandins in amnionic fluids among pregnancies at similar stages of labor progress (at term and preterm) is likely

explained by variations in the amount of decidual tissue fragments attached to the forebag.

INFLAMMATORY MEDIATORS IN AMNIONIC FLUID: INTERPRETATION. Many of the bioactive agents that accumulate in amnionic fluid of some pregnancies during labor (both at term and preterm) are typical of the inflammatory mediators produced in other tissue sites with inflammation. The only unique feature of this response in intrauterine tissues is that several of the agents produced could serve as uterotonins: PGE₂, PGF₂ₐ, PAF, and endothelin-1 (Casey and co-workers, 1993a; Casey and MacDonald, 1993b). Nonetheless, these agents, produced in the forebag tissues exposed in the vagina, are formed after (not before) labor begins, and are largely unavailable to the myometrium because of sequestration in the amnionic fluid of the isolated forebag.

Inflammatory mediators (PGs and inflammatory cytokines) may be important in the process of cervical dilation and cervical extracellular matrix degradation (Rath and colleagues, 1998; Winkler and Rath, 1999).

REFERENCES

Altshuler G, Hyde S: Clinicopathologic considerations of fusobacteria chorioamnionitis. Acta Obstet Gynecol Scand 67:513, 1988

Ambrus G, Rao Ch V: Novel regulation of pregnant human myometrial smooth muscle cell gap junctions by human chorionic gonadotropin. Endocrinology 135:2772, 1994

Anderson ABM, Turnbull AC: Comparative aspects of factors involved in the onset of labor in ovine and human pregnancy. In Klopper A, Gardner J (eds): Endocrine Factors in Labour. London, Cambridge University Press, 1973, p 141

Athayde N, Romero R, Maymon E, Gomez R, Pacora P, Yoon BH, Edwin SS: Interleukin 16 in pregnancy, parturition, rupture of fetal membranes, and microbial invasion of the amniotic cavity. Am J Obstet Gynecol 182:135, 2000

Barany K, Barany M: Myosin light chain phosphorylation in uterine smooth muscle. In Carsten ME, Miller JD (eds): Uterine Function: Molecular and Cellular Aspects. Plenum, New York, 1990, p 71

Bates GW, Edman CD, Porter JC, MacDonald PC: Catechol-O-methyltransferase activity in erythrocytes of women taking oral contraceptive steroids. Am J Obstet Gynecol 133:691, 1979

Benedetto MT, DeCicco F, Rossiello F, Nicosia AL, Lupi G, Dell'Acqua S: Oxytocin receptor in human fetal membranes at term and during delivery. 35:205, 1990

Benedetto C, Petraglia F, Marozio L, Chiarolini L, Florio P, Genazzani AR, Massobrio M: Corticotropin-releasing hormone increases prostaglandin $F_{2\alpha}$ activity on human myometrium in vitro. Am J Obstet Gynecol 171:126, 1994

Besinger RE, Neibyl JR: The safety and efficacy of tocolytic agents for the treatment of preterm labor. Obstet Gynecol Surv 415, 1990

Billah MM, Johnston JM: Identification of phospholipid platelet-activating factor (1-0-alkyl-2-acetyl-sn-glycero-3-phosphocholine) in human amnionic fluid and urine. Biochem Biophys Res Commun 113:51, 1983

Bogic LV, Mandel M, Bryant-Greenwood GD: Relaxin gene expression in human reproductive tissues by in situ hybridization. J Clin Endocrinol Metab 80:130, 1995

Brandt ML: Mechanism and management of the third stage of labor. Am J Obstet Gynecol 25:662, 1933

Breuiller M, Doualla-Bell F, Litine MH, Leory MJ, Ferre F: Disappearance of human myometrial adenylate cyclase activation by prostaglandins at the end of pregnancy. Comparison with β-adrenergic response. Adv Prostaglandin Thromboxane Leukot Res 21b:811, 1991

Burghardt RC, Mitchell PA, Kurten RC: Gap junction modulation in rat uterus, II. Effects of antiestrogens on myometrial and serosal cells. Biol Reprod 30:249, 1984

Casey ML, Brown CEL, Peters M, MacDonald PC: Endothelin levels in human amniotic fluid at midtrimester and at term before and during spontaneous labor. J Clin Endocrinol Metab 76:1647, 1993a

Casey ML, Cox SM, Beutler B, Milewich L, MacDonald PC: Cachectin/tumor necrosis factor-α formation in human decidua: Potential role of cytokines in infection-induced preterm labor. J Clin Invest 83:430, 1989

Casey ML, Cutrer SI, Mitchell MD: Origin of prostanoids in human amniotic fluid: The fetal kidney as a source of amniotic fluid prostanoids. Am J Obstet Gynecol 147:547, 1983

Casey ML, Erk A, MacDonald PC: Parathyroid hormone and parathyroid hormone-related protein stimulate adenylate cyclase in human endometrial stromal cells. Ann NY Acad Sci 734:364, 1994

Casey ML, Hemsell DL, MacDonald PC, Johnston JM: NAD^+-dependent 15-hydroxyprostaglandin dehydrogenase activity in human endometrium. Prostaglandins 19:115, 1980

Casey ML, MacDonald PC: Transforming growth factor-beta inhibits progesterone-induced enkephalinase expression in human endometrial stromal cells. J Clin Endocrinol Metab 81:4022, 1996

Casey ML, MacDonald PC: Human parturition. In Bruner JP (ed): Infertility and Reproductive Medicine Clinics of North America. Philadelphia, Saunders, 1994, p 765

Casey ML, MacDonald PC: Human parturition: Distinction between the initiation of parturition and the onset of labor. In Ducsay CA (ed): Seminars in Reproductive Endocrinology. New York, Thieme, 1993a, p 272

Casey ML, MacDonald PC: Human parturition: Prostaglandins and cytokines are sequelae of labor. In Mornex C, Jaffiol C, Leclere J (eds): Progress in Endocrinology. Carnforth, England, Parthenon, 1993b, p 638

Casey ML, MacDonald PC: Transforming growth factor-β (TGF-β) acts as a gene-specific antiprogestin. Abstract presented at 40th annual meeting of Society for Gynecological Investigation, Toronto, 1993c

Casey ML, MacDonald PC: Biomolecular mechanisms in human parturition: Activation of uterine decidua. In d'Arcangues C, Fraser IS, Newton JR, Odlind V (eds): Contraception and Mechanisms of Endometrial Bleeding. Cambridge, England, Cambridge University Press, 1990, p 501

Casey ML, MacDonald PC: Biomolecular processes in the initiation of parturition: Decidual activation. Clin Obstet Gynecol 31:533, 1988a

Casey ML, MacDonald PC: The role of a fetal–maternal paracrine system in the maintenance of pregnancy and the initiation of parturition. In Jones CT (ed): Fetal and Neonatal Development. Ithaca, Perinatology, 1988b, p 521

Casey ML, Mibe M, Erk A, MacDonald PC: Transforming growth factor-β1 stimulation of parathyroid hormone–related protein expression in human uterine cells in culture: MRNA levels and protein secretion. J Clin Endocrinol Metab 74:950, 1992

Casey ML, Smith JW, Nagai K, MacDonald PC: Transforming growth factor-β inhibits enkephalinase (EC 3.4.24.11) gene expression in human endometrial stromal cells and sex skin fibroblasts in culture. J Clin Endocrinol Metab 77:144, 1993b

Chaim W, Mazor M: Intraamniotic infection with fusobacteria. Arch Gynecol Obstet 251:1, 1992

Challis JRG, Lye SJ: Parturition. In Knobil E, Neill JD (eds): The Physiology of Reproduction, 2nd ed, Vol II. New York, Raven, 1994, p 985

Chibbar R, Miller FD, Mitchell BF: Synthesis of oxytocin in amnion, chorion, and decidua may influence the timing of human parturition. J Clin Invest 91:185, 1993

Chow L, Lye SJ: Expression of the gap junction protein connexin-43 is increased in the human myometrium toward term and with the onset of labor. Am J Obstet Gynecol 170:788, 1994

Chwalisz K, Fahrenholz F, Hackenberg M, Garfield R, Elger W: The progesterone antagonist onapristone increases the effectiveness of oxytocin to produce delivery without changing the myometrial oxytocin receptor concentrations. Am J Obstet Gynecol 165:1760, 1991

Cole WC, Garfield RE: Evidence for physiological regulation of myometrial gap junction permeability. Am J Physiol 251:C411, 1986

Coleman RA, Smith WL, Narumiya S: Eighth International Union of Pharmacology. Classification of prostanoid receptors: Properties, distribution, and structure of the receptor and their subtypes. Pharmacol Rev 46:205, 1994

Cox BE, Ipson MA, Shaul PW, Kamm KE, Rosenfeld CR: Myometrial angiotensin II receptor subtypes change during ovine pregnancy. J Clin Invest 92:2240, 1993a

Cox SM, King MR, Casey ML, MacDonald PC: Interleukin-1 beta, -1 alpha, and -6 and prostaglandins in vaginal/cervical fluids of pregnant women before and during labor. J Clin Endocrinol Metab 77:805, 1993b

Cox SM, Casey ML, MacDonald PC: Accumulation of interleukin-1 beta and interleukin-6 in amniotic fluid: A sequela of labour at term and preterm. Hum Reprod Update 3:517, 1997

Crankshaw DJ, Dyal R: Effects of some occurring prostanoids and some cyclooxygenase inhibitors on the contractility of the human lower uterine segment in vitro. Can J Physiol Pharmacol 72:870, 1994

Daifotis AG, Weir EC, Dreyer BE, Broadus AE: Stretch-induced parathyroid hormone–related peptide gene expression in the rat uterus. J Biol Chem 267:23455, 1992

Dale HH: On some physiologic actions of ergot. J Physiol (Lond) 34:163, 1906

Eis AW, Mitchell MD, Myatt L: Endothelin transfer and endothelin effects on water transfer in human fetal membranes. Obstet Gynecol 79:411, 1992

El-Bastawissi AY, Williams MA, Riley DE, Hitti J, Krieger JN: Amniotic fluid interleukin-6 and preterm delivery: A review. Obstet Gynecol 95:1056, 2000

Eta E, Ambrus G, Rao CV: Direct regulation of human myometrial contractions by human chorionic gonadotropin. J Clin Endocrinol Metab. 79:1582, 1994

Ferguson JKW: A study of the motility of the intact uterus at term. Surg Gynecol Obstet 73:359, 1941

Flower RJ: The role of prostaglandins in parturition, with special reference to the rat. In Knight J, O'Connor M (eds): The Fetus and Birth. Ciba foundation symposium 47. Amsterdam, Elsevier, 1977, p 297

Friedman EA: Labor: Clinical Evaluation and Management, 2nd ed. New York, Appleton-Century-Crofts, 1978

Frydman R, Fernandez H, Pons JC, Ulmann A: Mifepristone (RU486) and therapeutic late pregnancy termination: A double-blind study of two different doses. Hum Reprod 3:803, 1988

Fuchs AR, Fuchs F, Husslein P, Soloff MS: Oxytocin receptors in the human uterus during pregnancy and parturition. Am J Obstet Gynecol 150:734, 1984

Fuchs AR, Fuchs F, Husslein P, Soloff MS, Fernström MJ: Oxytocin receptors and human parturition. A dual role for oxytocin in the initiation of labor. Science 215:1396, 1982

Fuchs AR, Husslein P, Fuchs F: Oxytocin and the initiation of human parturition, 2. Stimulation of prostaglandin production in human decidua by oxytocin. Am J Obstet Gynecol 141:694, 1981

Fuchs AR, Periyasamy S, Alexandrova M, Soloff MS: Correlation between oxytocin receptor concentration and responsiveness to oxytocin in pregnant rat myometrium: Effect of ovarian steroids. Endocrinology 113:742, 1983

Gainer H, Alstein M, Whitnall MH, Wray S: The biosynthesis and secretion of oxytocin and vasopressin. In Knobil E, Neill J (eds): The Physiology of Reproduction, Vol II. New York, Raven, 1988, p 2265

Garfield RE, Hayashi RH: Appearance of gap junctions in the myometrium of women during labor. Am J Obstet Gynecol 140:254, 1981

Germain A, Smith J, MacDonald PC, Casey ML: Human fetal membrane contribution to the prevention of parturition: Uterotonin degradation. J Clin Endocrinol Metab 78:463, 1994

Goldenberg RL, Hauth JC, Andrews WW: Intrauterine infection and preterm delivery. N Engl J Med 342:1500, 2000

Gomez R, Ghezzi F, Romero R, Munoz H, Tolosa JE, Rojas I: Premature labor and intra-amniotic infection. Clinical aspects and role of the cytokines in diagnosis and pathophysiology. Clin Perinatol 22:281, 1995

Grammatopoulos D, Milton NGN, Hillhouse EW: The human myometrial CRH receptor: G proteins and second messengers. Mol Cell Endocrinol 99:245, 1994

Grammatopoulos D, Thompson S, Hillhouse EW: The human myometrium expresses multiple isoforms of the corticotropin-releasing hormone receptor. J Clin Endocrinol Metab 80:2388, 1995

Hayashi RH, Garfield RE, Harper MJK: Regulation of human myometrial gap junctions: In vitro studies. In: The Physiological Development of the Fetus and Newborn. London, Academic Press, 1985, p 411

Hill GB: Investigating the source of amniotic fluid isolates of fusobacteria. Clin Infect Dis 16:S423, 1993

Hillhouse EW, Grammatopoulos D, Milton NGN, Quartero HWP: The identification of a human myometrial corticotropin-releasing hormone receptor that increases in affinity during pregnancy. J Clin Endocrinol Metab 76:736, 1993

Huszar G, Walsh MP: Biochemistry of the myometrium and cervix. In Wynn RM, Jollie WP (eds): Biology of the Uterus, 2nd ed. New York, Plenum, 1989, p 355

Iams JD, Clapp DH, Contox DA, Whitehurst R, Ayers LW, O'Shaughnessy RW: Does extraamniotic infection cause preterm labor? Gas-liquid chromatography studies of amniotic fluid in amnionitis, preterm labor, and normal controls. Obstet Gynecol 70:365, 1987

Iams JD, Goldenberg RL, Meis PJ, Mercer BM, Moawad A, Das A, Thom E, McNellis D, Copper RL, Johnson F, Roberts JM: The length of the cervix and the risk of spontaneous premature delivery. N Engl J Med 334:567, 1996

Itoh H, Sagawa N, Hasegawa M, Nanno H, Kobayashi F, Ihara Y, Mori T, Komatsu Y, Suga S, Yoshimasa T, Itoh H, Nakao K: Expression of biologically active receptors for natriuretic peptides in the human uterus during pregnancy. Biochem Biophys Res Commun. 203:602, 1994

Itoh H, Sagawa N, Hasegawa M, Okagaki A, Inamori K, Ihara Y, Mori T, Ogawa Y, Suga S, Mukoyama M, Nakao K, Imura H: Brain natriuretic peptide is present in the human amniotic fluid and is secreted from amnion cells. J Clin Endocrinol Metab 76:907, 1993

Izumi H, Yallampalli C, Garfield RE: Gestational changes in L-arginine-induced relaxation of pregnant rat and human myometrial smooth muscle. Am J Obstet Gynecol 169:1327, 1993

Jaffe RB, Mesiano S, Smith R, Coulter CL, Spencer SJ, Chakravorty A: The regulation and role of fetal adrenal development in human pregnancy. Endocr Res 24:919, 1998

Jeffrey JJ, Ehlich LS, Roswit WT: Serotonin: An inducer of collagenase in myometrial smooth muscle cells. J Cell Physiol 146:399, 1991

Keirse MJNC: Eicosanoids in human pregnancy and parturition. In M Mitchell (ed): Eicosanoids in Reproduction. Boca Raton, FL: CRC Press, 1990, p 199

Keirse MJNC: Prostaglandins in parturition. In Keirse M, Anderson A, Gravenhorst J (eds): Human Parturition. The Hague, Martinus Nijhoff, 1979, p 101

Kent AS, Sullivan MH, Elder MG: Transfer of cytokines through human fetal membranes. J Reprod Fertil 100:81, 1994

Ku CY, Qian A, Wen Y, Anwer K, Sanborn BM: Oxytocin stimulates myometrial guanosine triphosphatase and phospholipase-C activities via coupling to G alpha q/11. Endocrinology 136:1509, 1995

Leake RD: Oxytocin in the initiation of labor. In Carsten ME, Miller JD (eds): Uterine Function. Molecular and Cellular Aspects. New York, Plenum, 1990, p 361

Lei ZM, Reshef E, Rao CV: The expression of human chorionic gonadotropin/luteinizing hormone receptors in human endometrial and myometrial blood vessels. J Clin Endocrinol Metab 75:651, 1992

Liggins GC: Premature parturition after infusion of corticotrophin or cortisol into foetal lambs. J Endocrinol 42:323, 1968

Liggins GC, Fairclough RJ, Grieves SA, Kendall JZ, Knox BS: The mechanism of initiation of parturition in the ewe. Recent Prog Horm Res 29:111, 1973

Liggins GC, Kennedy PC, Holm LW: Failure of initiation of parturition after electrocoagulation of the pituitary of the fetal lamb. Am J Obstet Gynecol 98:1080, 1967

Lim AT, Gude NM: Atrial natriuretic factor production by the human placenta. J Clin Endocrinol Metab 80:3091, 1995

Linder ME, Gilman AG: G proteins. Sci Am 267:56, 1992

Little B, Tait JF, Tait SA, Erlenmeyer F: The metabolic clearance rate of progesterone in males and ovariectomized females. J Clin Invest 45:901, 1966

Lockwood CJ: Stress-associated preterm delivery: The role of corticotropin-releasing hormone. Am J Obstet Gynecol 180:S264, 1999

Lopez Bernal A, TambyRaja RL: Preterm labour. Baillieres Best Pract Res Clin Obstet Gynaecol 14:133, 2000

MacDonald PC, Casey ML: Preterm Birth. Sci Am 3:42, 1996

MacDonald PC, Casey ML: The accumulation of prostaglandins (PG) in amniotic fluid is an aftereffect of labor and not indicative of a role for PGE$_2$ and PGE$_{2\alpha}$ in the initiation of human parturition. J Clin Endocrinol Metab 76:1332, 1993

MacDonald PC, Cox SM, Casey ML: Infection-associated preterm labor as a model for parturition. In Genazzani AR, Petraglia F, Volpe A, Facchinetti F (eds): Advances in Gynecological Endocrinology, Vol I. Carnforth, UK, Parthenon, 1988, p 487

MacDonald PC, Koga S, Casey ML: Decidual activation in parturition: Examination of amniotic fluid for mediators of the inflammatory response. Ann NY Acad Sci 622:315, 1991

Malpas P: Postmaturity and malformation of the fetus. J Obstet Gynaecol Br Emp 40:1046, 1933

McDonald TJ, Nathanielsz PW: Bilateral destruction of the fetal paraventricular nuclei prolongs gestation in sheep. Am J Obstet Gynecol 165:764, 1991

Mitchell MD, Flint AP, Bibby J, Brunt J, Arnold JM, Anderson AB, Turnbull AC: Rapid increases in plasma prostaglandin concentrations after vaginal examination and amniotomy. BMJ 2:1183, 1977

Myers DA, McDonald TJ, Nathanielsz PW: Effect of bilateral lesions of the ovine fetal hypothalamic paraventricular nuclei at 118–122 days of gestation on subsequent adrenocor-

tical steroidogenic enzyme gene expression. Endocrinology 131:305, 1992

Nishihara J, Ishibashi T, Mai Y, Muramatsu T: Mass spectrometric evidence for the presence of platelet-activating factor (1-0-alkyl-2-sn-glycero-3-phosphocholine) in human amniotic fluid during labor. Lipids 19:907, 1984

Nissen E, Lilja G, Widstrom A-M, Uvnas-Moberg K: Elevation of oxytocin levels early post partum in women. Acta Obstet Gynecol Scand 74:530, 1995

Novy MJ, Liggins GC: Role of prostaglandin, prostacyclin, and thromboxanes in the physiologic control of the uterus and in parturition. Semin Perinatol 4:45, 1980

Parker CR Jr, Illingworth DR, Bissonnette J, Carr BR: Endocrine changes during pregnancy in a patient with homozygous familial hypobetalipoproteinemia. N Engl J Med 314:557, 1986

Paspalliaris V, Patersen DN, Thiede MA: Steroid regulation of parathyroid hormone–related protein expression and action in the rat uterus. J Steroid Biochem Mol Biol 53:259, 1995

Pepe GJ, Albrecht ED: Actions of placental and fetal steroid hormones in primate pregnancy. Endocr Rev 16:608, 1995

Pierce JG, du Vigneaud V: Studies on high potency oxytocic materials from beef posterior pituitary lobes. J Biol Chem 186:77, 1950

Prescott SM, Zimmerman GA, McIntyre TM: Platelet activating factor. J Biol Chem 265:17381, 1990

Price SA, Pochun I, Phaneuf S, Lopez Bernal A: Adenylyl cyclase isoforms in pregnant and nonpregnant human myometrium. J Endocrinol 164:21, 2000

Quartero HWP, Noort WA, Fry CH, Keirse MJNC: Role of prostaglandins and leukotrienes in the synergistic effect of oxytocin and corticotropin-releasing hormone (CRH) on the contraction force in human gestational myometrium. Prostaglandins 42:137, 1991

Quartero HWP, Strivatsa G, Gillham B: Role for cyclic adenosine monophosphate in the synergistic interaction between oxytocin and corticotrophin-releasing factor in isolated human gestational myometrium. Clin Endocrinol 36:141, 1992

Rath W, Winkler M, Kemp B: The importance of extracellular matrix in the induction of preterm delivery. J Perinatol Med 26:437, 1998

Rea C: Prolonged gestation, acrania, monstrosity and apparent placenta praevia in one obstetrical case. JAMA 30:1166, 1898

Romero R, Durum S, Dinarello CA, Oyarzun E, Hobbins JC, Mitchell MD: Interleukin-1 stimulates prostaglandin biosynthesis by human amnion. Prostaglandins 37:13, 1989

Romero R, Kadar N, Hobbins JC, Duff GW: Infection and labor: The detection of endotoxin in amniotic fluid. Am J Obstet Gynecol 157:815, 1987

Romero R, Mazor M, Wu YK, Sirtori M, Oyarzun E, Mitchell MD, Hobbins JC: Infection in the pathogenesis of preterm labor. Semin Perinatol 12:262, 1988

Romero R, Parvizi ST, Oyarzun E, Mazor M, Wu YK, Avila C, Athanassiadis AP, Mitchell MD: Amniotic fluid IL-1 in spontaneous labor at term. J Reprod Med 35:235, 1990

Sadowsky DW, Haluska GJ, Gravett MG, Witkin SS, Novy MJ: Indomethacin blocks interleukin-1 beta-induced myometrial contractions in pregnant rhesus monkeys. Am J Obstet Gynecol 183:173, 2000

Sakai N, Tabb T, Garfield RE: Modulation of cell-to-cell coupling between myometrial cells of the human uterus during pregnancy. Am J Obstet Gynecol 167:472, 1992

Sanborn BM, Anwer K, Wen Y, Stefani E, Toro L, Singh SP: Modification of Ca^{2+} regulatory systems. In Garfield RE,

Tabb TN (eds): Control of Uterine Contractility. Boca Raton, FL: CRC Press, 1994, p 105

Sanborn BM, Yue C, Wang W, Dodge KL: G protein signaling pathways in myometrium: Affecting the balance between contraction and relaxation. Rev Reprod 3:196, 1998

Schulman H, Romney SL: Variability of uterine contractions in normal human parturition. Obstet Gynecol 36:215, 1970

Semer D, Reisler K, MacDonald PC, Casey ML: Responsiveness of human endometrial stromal cells to cytokines. Ann NY Acad Sci 622:99, 1991

Sheldrick EL, Flick-Smith HC: Effect of ovarian hormones on oxytocin receptor concentrations in explants of uterus from ovariectomized ewes. J Reprod Fertil 97:241, 1993

Siiteri PK, MacDonald PC: Placental estrogen biosynthesis during human pregnancy. J Clin Endocrinol Metab 26:751, 1966

Siiteri PK, MacDonald PC: The utilization of circulating dehydroisoandrosterone sulfate for estrogen synthesis during human pregnancy. Steroids 2:713, 1963

Soloff MS, Alexandrova M, Fernström MJ: Oxytocin receptors: Triggers for parturition and lactation? Science 204:1313, 1979

Soloff MS, Fernström MA, Periyasamy S, Soloff S, Baldwin S, Wieder M: Regulation of oxytocin receptor concentration in rat uterine explants by estrogen and progesterone. Can J Biochem Cell Biol 61:625, 1983

Stull JT, Lin PJ, Krueger JK, Trewhella J, Zhi G: Myosin light chain kinase; functional domains and structural motifs. Acta Physiol Scand 164:471, 1998

Stull JT, Taylor DA, MacKenzie LW, Casey ML: Biochemistry and physiology of smooth muscle contractility. In McNellis D, Challis JRG, MacDonald PC, Nathanielsz P, Roberts J (eds): Cellular and Integrative Mechanisms in the Onset of Labor. An NICHD Workshop. Ithaca, Perinatology, 1988, p 17

Thiede MA, Harm SC, Hasson DM, Gardner RM: In vivo regulation of PTH-rP messenger ribonucleic acid in the rat uterus by 17β-estradiol. Endocrinology 128:2317, 1991a

Thiede MA, Harm SC, McKee RL, Grasser WA, Duong LT, Leach Jr RM: Expression of the PTH-rP gene in the avian oviduct. Endocrinology 129:1958, 1991b

Thorburn GD: Past and present concepts on the initiation of parturition. In MacDonald PC, Porter JC (eds): Initiation of Parturition: Prevention of Prematurity. Fourth Ross conference on obstetric research. Columbus, OH, Ross Laboratories, 1983, p 2

Thorburn GD: A speculative review of parturition in the mare. Equine Vet J Suppl 14:41, 1993

Townsend J, ed. Strengthening Research in Academic Ob/Gyn Departments. Washington, DC, Institute of Medicine, National Academy Press, 1992

Weiss G: Relaxin used to produce the cervical ripening of labor. Clin Obstet Gynecol 38:293, 1995

Winkler M, Rath W: Changes in the cervical extracellular matrix during pregnancy and parturition. J Perinatol Med 27:45, 1999

Word RA, Kamm KE, Stull JT, Casey ML: Endothelin increases cytoplasmic calcium and myosin phosphorylation in human myometrium. Am J Obstet Gynecol 162:1103, 1990

Word RA, Stull JT, Casey ML, Kamm KE: Contractile elements and myosin light chain phosphorylation in myometrial tissue from nonpregnant and pregnant women. J Clin Invest 92:29, 1993

Yallampalli C, Byam-Smith M, Nelson SO, Garfield RE: Steroid hormones modulate the production of nitric oxide and cGMP in the rat uterus. Endocrinology 134:1971, 1994b

Yallampalli C, Izumi H, Byam-Smith M, Garfield RE: An L-arginine-nitric oxide-cyclic guanosine monophosphate system exists in the uterus and inhibits contractility during pregnancy. Am J Obstet Gynecol 170:175, 1994a

Yamamoto M, Harm SC, Grasser WA, Thiede MA: Parathyroid hormone–related protein in the rat urinary bladder: A smooth muscle relaxant produced locally in response to mechanical stretch. Proc Natl Acad Sci USA 89:5326, 1992

Yasuda K, Johnston JM: The hormonal regulation of PAF-acetylhydrolase in the rat. Endocrinology 130:708, 1992

Zahl PA, Bjerknes C: Induction of decidua–placental hemorrhage in mice by the endotoxins of certain gram-negative bacteria. Proc Soc Exp Biol Med 54:329, 1943

Zhu YP, Word RA, Johnston JM: The presence of PAF binding sites in human myometrium and its role in uterine contraction. Am J Obstet Gynecol 166:1222, 1992

Ziecik AJ, Derecka-Reszka K, Rzucidlo SJ: Extragonadal gonadotropin receptors, their distribution and function. J Physiol Pharmacol 43:33, 1992

Zingg HH, Rozen F, Chu K, Larcher A, Arslan A, Richard S, Lefebvre D: Oxytocin and oxytocin receptor gene expression in the uterus. Recent Prog Horm Res 50:255, 1995

Zuo J, Lei ZM, Rao CV: Human myometrial chorionic gonadotropin/luteinizing hormone receptors in preterm and term deliveries. J Clin Endocrinol Metab 79:907, 1994

12

Mechanisms of Normal Labor

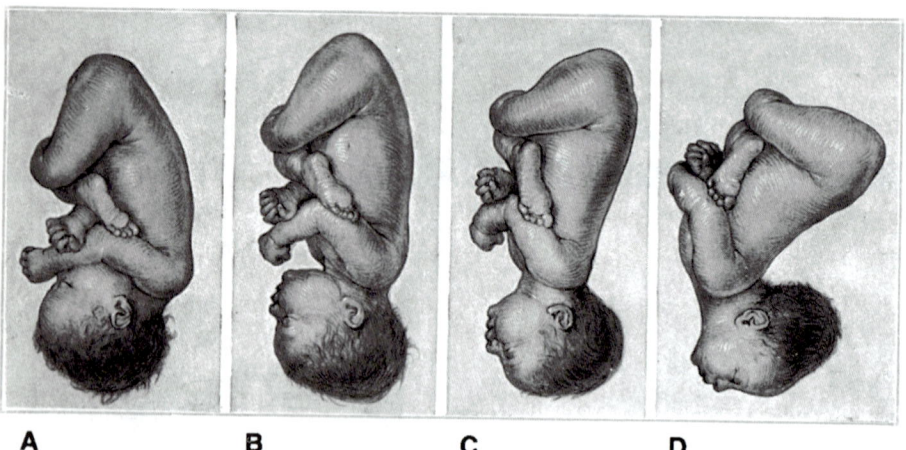

FIGURE 12-1. Longitudinal lie. Cephalic presentation. Differences in attitude of fetal body in **(A)** vertex, **(B)** sinciput, **(C)** brow, and **(D)** face presentations. Note changes in fetal attitude in relation to fetal vertex as the fetal head becomes less flexed.

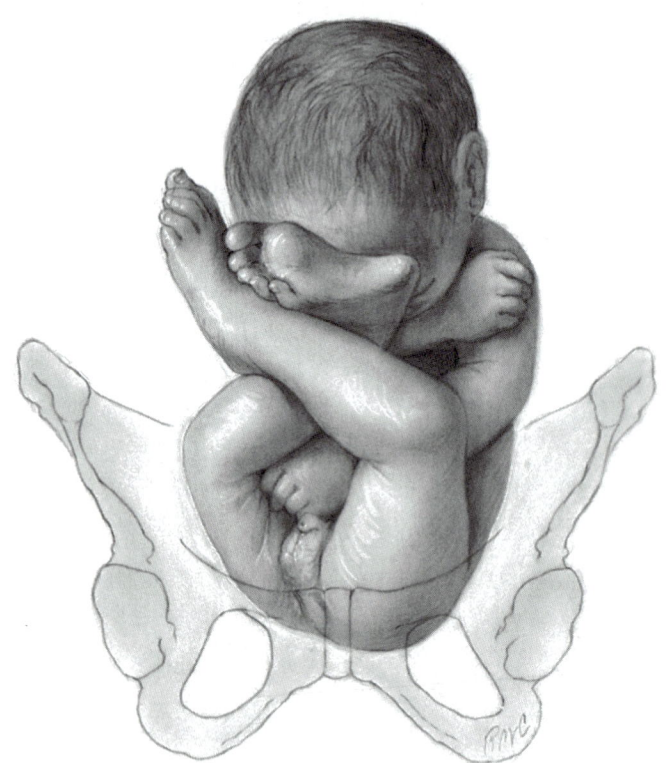

FIGURE 12-2. Longitudinal lie. Frank breech presentation.

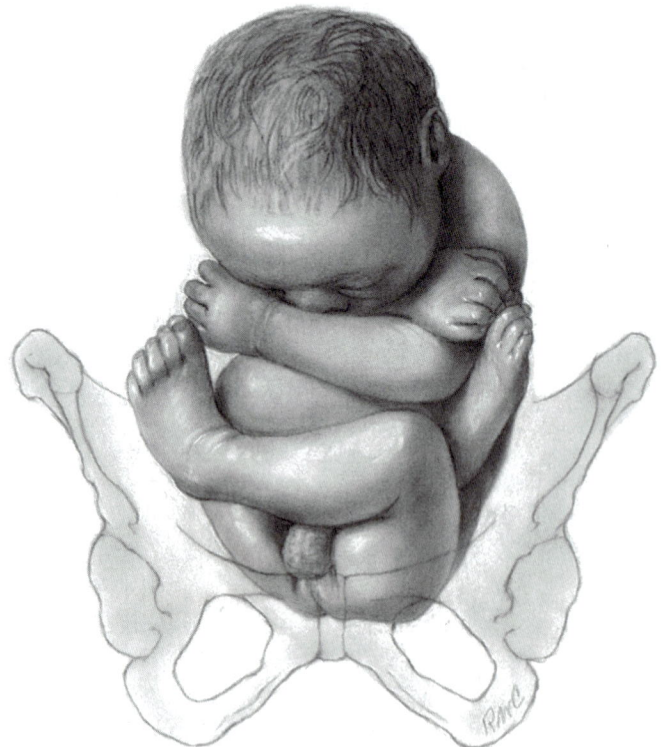

FIGURE 12-3. Longitudinal lie. Complete breech presentation.

At the onset of labor, the position of the fetus, with respect to the birth canal, is critical to the route of delivery. For example, if at the time of labor the fetus is transverse to the birth canal, either cesarean delivery or podalic version to a longitudinal lie are the only options for delivery of a viable infant. It is thus of paramount importance to know the fetal position within the uterine cavity at the onset of labor.

LIE, PRESENTATION, ATTITUDE, AND POSITION

By convention, fetal orientation is described with respect to fetal lie, presentation, attitude, and position. These can be established clinically by abdominal palpation, vaginal examination, and auscultation, or by technical means using sonography or x-ray. Clinical assessment is less accurate, or even sometimes impossible to perform and interpret in obese women.

FETAL LIE. The lie is the relation of the long axis of the fetus to that of the mother, and is either longitudinal or transverse. Occasionally, the fetal and the maternal axes may cross at a 45-degree angle, forming an oblique lie, which is unstable and always becomes longitudinal or transverse during the course of labor. Longitudinal lies are present in over 99 percent of labors at term. Predisposing factors for transverse lies include multiparity, placenta previa, hydramnios, and uterine anomalies (Gemer and Segal, 1994).

FETAL PRESENTATION. The presenting part is that portion of the body of the fetus that is either foremost within the birth canal or in closest proximity to it. The presenting part can be felt through the cervix on vaginal examination. The presenting part determines the presentation. Accordingly, in longitudinal lies, the presenting part is either the fetal head or breech, creating cephalic and breech presentations, respectively. When the fetus lies with the long axis transversely, the shoulder is the presenting part. Thus, a shoulder presentation is felt through the cervix on vaginal examination.

CEPHALIC PRESENTATION. These are classified according to the relation of the head to the body of the fetus (Fig. 12–1). Ordinarily the head is flexed sharply so that the chin is in contact with the thorax. In this circumstance, the occipital fontanel is the presenting part, and such a presentation is usually referred to as a vertex or occiput presentation. Actually, the vertex lies just in front of the occipital fontanel, and the occiput just behind the fontanel, as illustrated in Figure 7–7

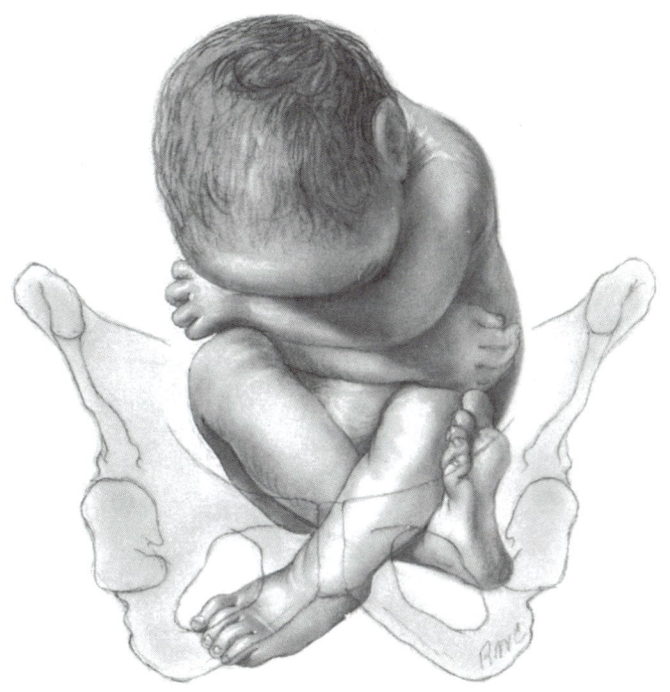

FIGURE 12–4. Longitudinal lie. Incomplete, or footling, breech presentation.

(p. 136). Much less commonly, the fetal neck may be sharply extended so that the occiput and back come in contact and the face is foremost in the birth canal—*face presentation*. The fetal head may assume a position between these extremes, partially flexed in some cases, with the anterior (large) fontanel, or bregma, presenting (*sinciput presentation*), or partially extended in other cases, with the brow presenting (*brow presentation*). These latter two presentations are usually transient. As labor progresses, sinciput and brow presentations are almost always converted into vertex or face presentations by flexion or extension, respectively.

BREECH PRESENTATION. When the fetus presents as a breech, there are three general configurations. When the thighs are flexed and the legs extended over the anterior surfaces of the body, this is termed a *frank breech presentation* (Fig. 12–2). If the thighs are flexed on the abdomen and the legs upon the thighs, this is a *complete breech presentation* (Fig. 12–3). If one or both feet, or one or both knees, are lowermost, then there is an *incomplete,* or *footling, breech presentation* (Fig. 12–4).

FETAL ATTITUDE OR POSTURE. In the later months of pregnancy the fetus assumes a characteristic posture described as attitude or habitus (Fig. 12–1). As a rule,

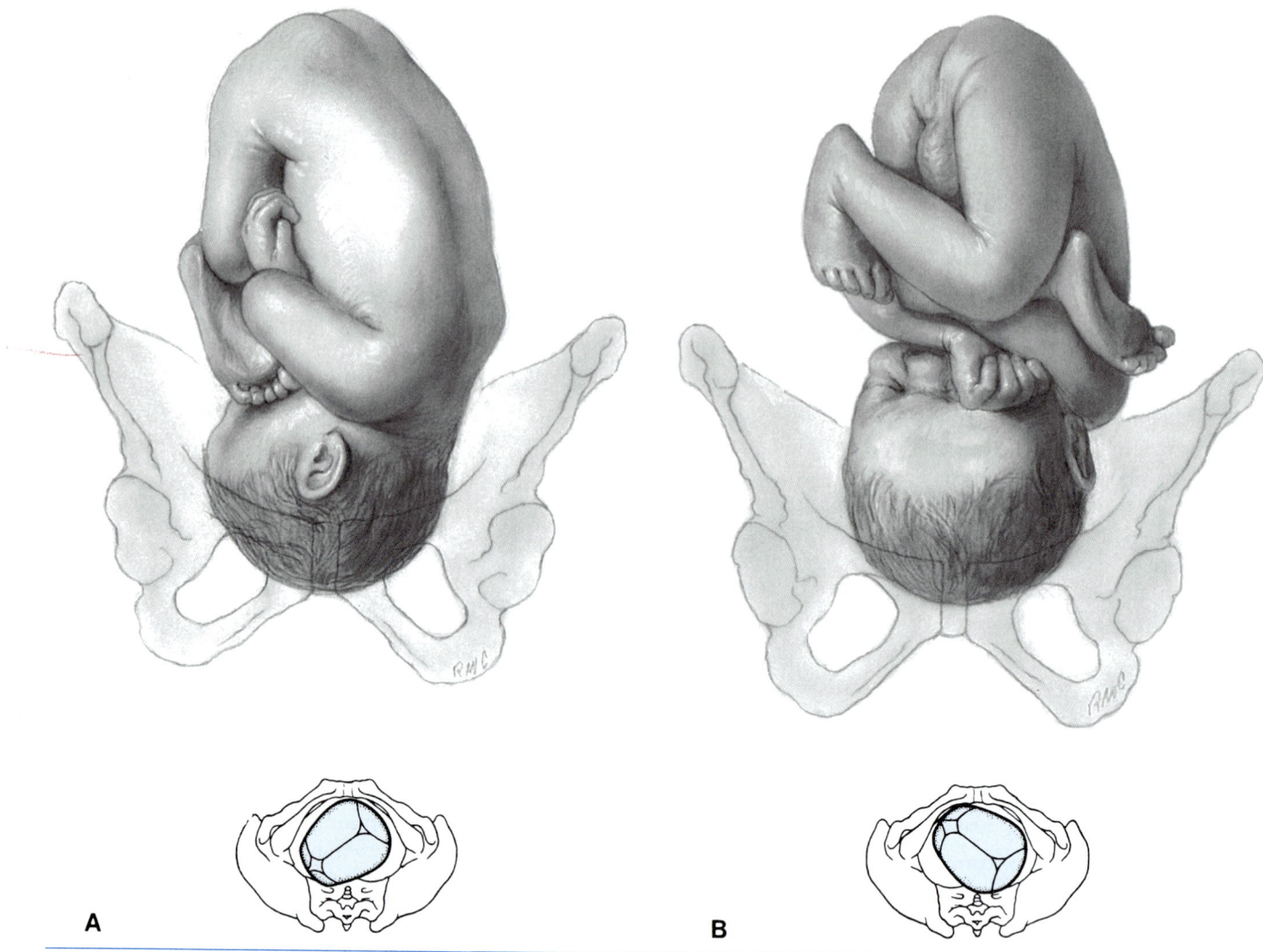

FIGURE 12–5. Longitudinal lie. Vertex presentation. **A.** Left occiput anterior (LOA). **B.** Left occiput posterior (LOP).

the fetus forms an ovoid mass that corresponds roughly to the shape of the uterine cavity. The fetus becomes folded or bent upon itself in such a manner that the back becomes markedly convex; the head is sharply flexed so that the chin is almost in contact with the chest; the thighs are flexed over the abdomen; the legs are bent at the knees; and the arches of the feet rest upon the anterior surfaces of the legs. In all cephalic presentations, the arms are usually crossed over the thorax or become parallel to the sides, and the umbilical cord lies in the space between them and the lower extremities. This characteristic posture results from the mode of growth of the fetus and its accommodation to the uterine cavity.

Abnormal exceptions to this attitude occur as the fetal head becomes progressively more extended from the vertex to the face presentation (Fig. 12–1D). This results in a progressive change in fetal attitude from a convex (flexed) to a concave (extended) contour of the vertebral column.

FETAL POSITION. Position refers to the relation of an arbitrarily chosen portion of the fetal presenting part to the right or left side of the maternal birth canal. Accordingly, with each presentation there may be two positions, right or left. The fetal occiput, chin (mentum), and sacrum are the determining points in vertex, face, and breech presentations, respectively (Figs. 12–5 to 12–8).

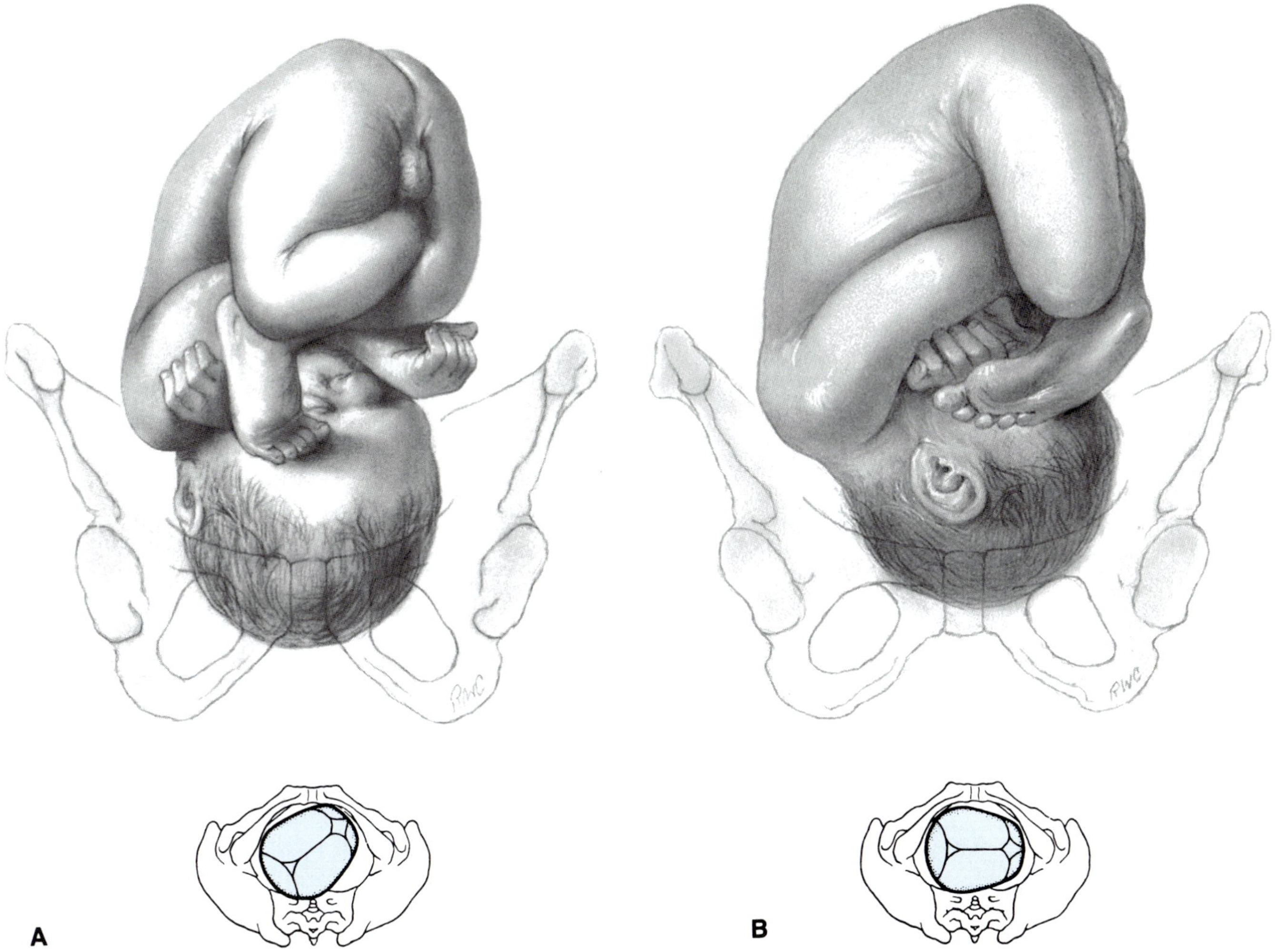

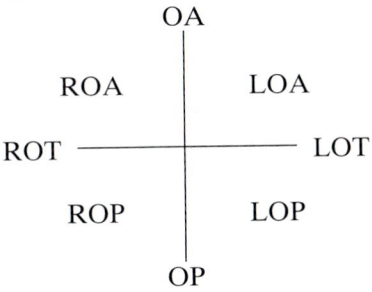

FIGURE 12–6. Longitudinal lie. Vertex presentation. **A.** Right occiput posterior (ROP). **B.** Right occiput transverse (ROT). (*Continued*)

VARIETIES OF PRESENTATION AND POSITION. For still more accurate orientation, the relation of a given portion of the presenting part to the anterior, transverse, or posterior portion of the maternal pelvis is considered. Because there are two positions, it follows that there must be three varieties for each position (either right or left), and six varieties for each presentation (three right and three left) (Figs. 12–5 to 12–8). Because the presenting part may be in either the left or right position, there are left and right occipital, left and right mental, and left and right sacral presentations, abbreviated as LO and RO, LM and RM, and LS and RS, respectively. Because the presenting part in each of the two positions may be directed anteriorly (A), transversely (T), or posteriorly (P), there are six varieties of each of these three presentations (Figs. 12–5 to 12–8). Thus, in an occiput

presentation, the presentation, position, and variety may be abbreviated in clockwise fashion as:

```
                    OA
         ROA                LOA
     ROT  ──────────────────  LOT
         ROP                LOP
                    OP
```

In shoulder presentations, the acromion (scapula) is the portion of the fetus arbitrarily chosen for orientation with the maternal pelvis. One example of the terminology sometimes employed for the purpose is illustrated

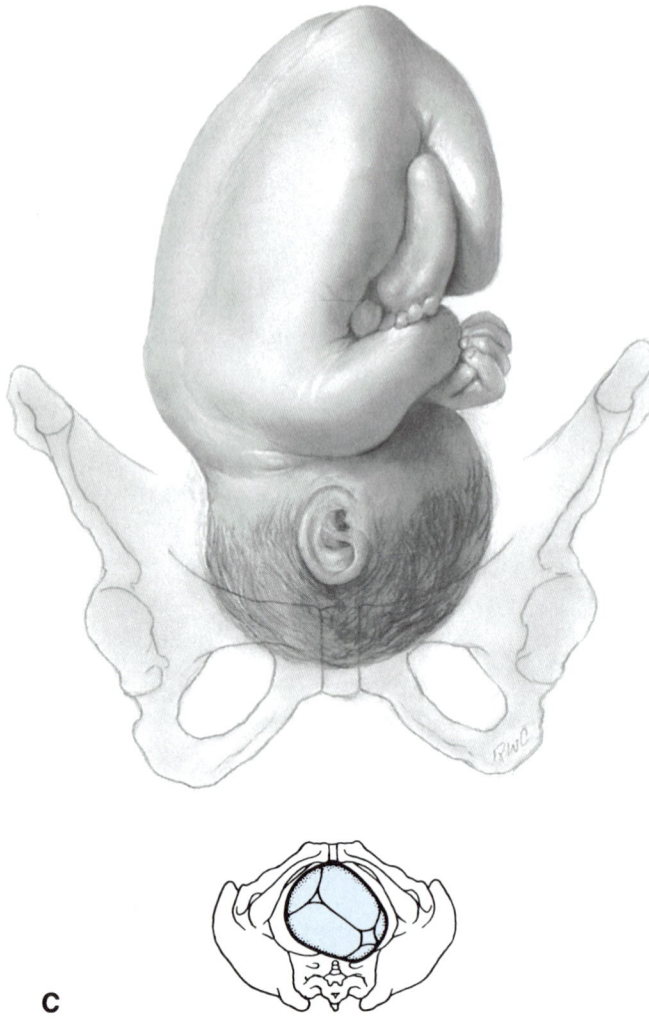

C

FIGURE 12–6 *(continued)* **C.** Right occiput anterior (ROA).

in Figure 12–9. The acromion or back of the fetus may be directed either posteriorly or anteriorly and superiorly or inferiorly (Chap. 19, p. 455). Because it is impossible to differentiate exactly the several varieties of shoulder presentation by clinical examination, and because such differentiation serves no practical purpose, it is customary to refer to all transverse lies simply as shoulder presentations. Another term used is transverse lie, with back up or back down.

FREQUENCY OF THE VARIOUS PRESENTATIONS AND POSITIONS

At or near term the incidence of the various presentations is approximately as follows: vertex, 96 percent; breech, 3.5 percent; face, 0.3 percent; and shoulder, 0.4 percent. About two thirds of all vertex presentations are in the left occiput position, and a third in the right.

Although the incidence of breech presentation is only a little over 3 percent at term (see Table 19–1), it is much greater earlier in pregnancy. Scheer and Nubar (1976), using ultrasonography, found the incidence of breech presentation to be 14 percent between 29 and 32 weeks' gestation. Subsequently, the breech converted spontaneously to vertex in increasingly higher percentages as term approached.

There are several explanations of why the term fetus usually presents by the vertex. The most logical is because the uterus is piriform shaped. Although the fetal head at term is slightly larger than the breech, the entire podalic pole of the fetus—that is, the breech and its flexed extremities—is bulkier and more movable than the cephalic pole. The cephalic pole is comprised of the fetal head only.

Until about 32 weeks, the amnionic cavity is large compared with the fetal mass, and there is no crowding of the fetus by the uterine walls. At approximately this time, however, the ratio of amnionic fluid volume to fetal mass becomes altered by relative diminution of amnionic fluid and by increasing fetal size. As a result, the uterine walls are apposed more closely to the fetal parts. The fetal lie then is more nearly dependent upon the piriform shape of the uterus. The fetus, if presenting by the breech, often changes polarity in order to make use of the roomier fundus for its bulkier and more movable podalic pole. The high incidence of breech presentation in hydrocephalic fetuses is in accord with this theory, because in this circumstance the cephalic pole of the fetus is larger than the podalic pole.

The cause of breech presentation may be some circumstance that prevents the normal version from taking place, for example, a septum that protrudes into the uterine cavity (Chap. 35, p. 914). A peculiarity of fetal attitude, particularly extension of the vertebral column as seen in frank breeches, may also prevent the fetus from turning. If the placenta implants in the lower uterine segment, normal intrauterine anatomy is distorted. Also, any condition contributing to an abnormality of fetal muscle tone or movement may predispose to persistent breech presentations.

DIAGNOSIS OF FETAL PRESENTATION AND POSITION

Several methods can be used to diagnose fetal presentation and position. These include abdominal palpation, vaginal examination, combined examination, auscultation, and in certain doubtful cases, imaging studies such as ultrasonography, computerized tomographic scans (CT), or magnetic resonance imaging (MRI) studies.

ABDOMINAL PALPATION—LEOPOLD MANEUVERS. Abdominal examination should be conducted systemat-

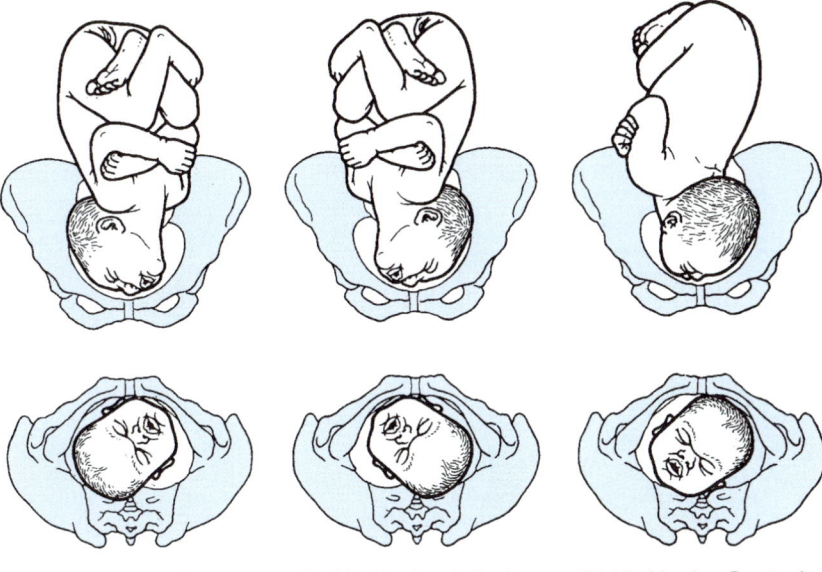

Left Mento-Anterior   Right Mento-Anterior   Right Mento-Posterior

FIGURE 12-7. Longitudinal lie. Face presentation. Left and right anterior and right posterior positions.

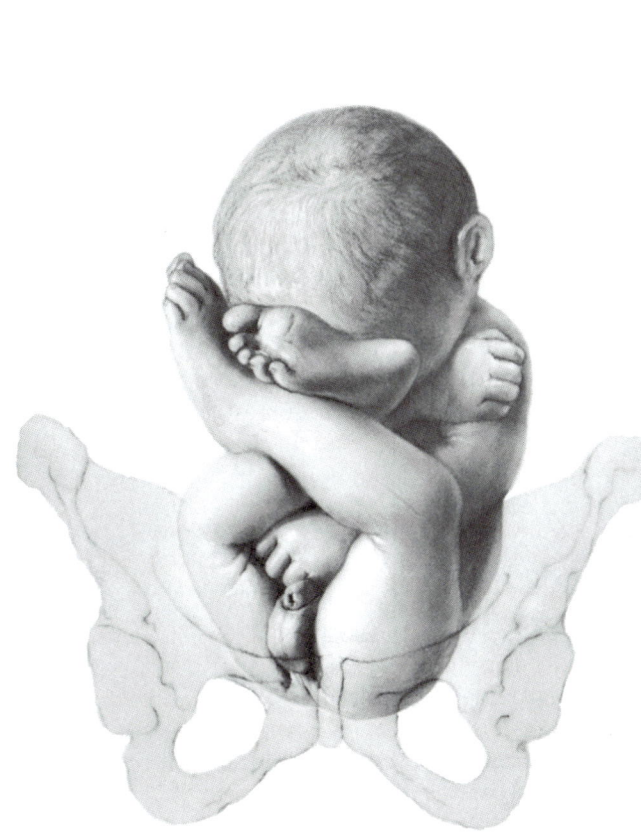

FIGURE 12-8. Longitudinal lie. Breech presentation. Left sacrum posterior positions (LSP).

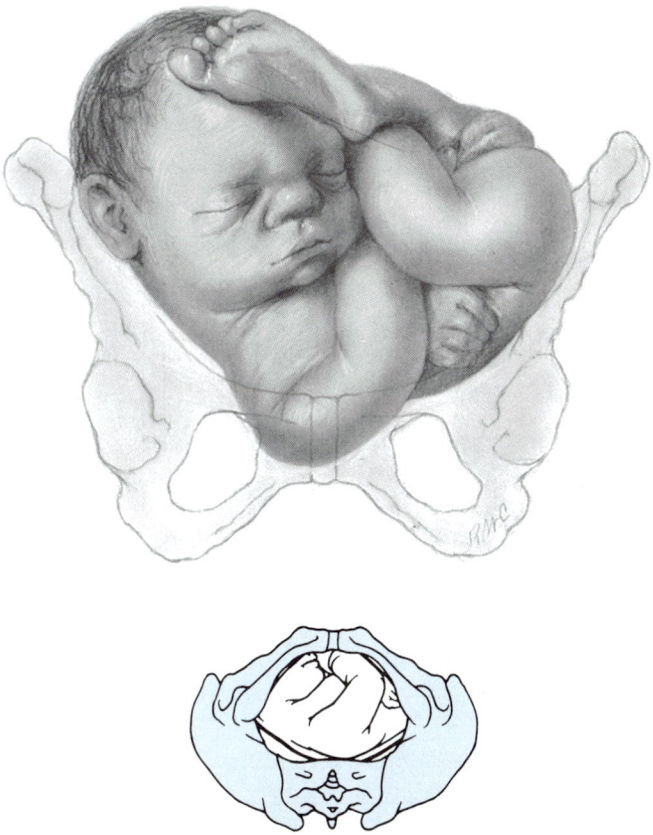

FIGURE 12-9. Transverse lie. Right acromiodorsoposterior position (RADP). The shoulder of the fetus is to the mother's right, and the back is posterior.

ically employing the four maneuvers described by Leopold and Sporlin in 1894. The mother should be supine and comfortably positioned with her abdomen bared. During the first three maneuvers, the examiner stands at the side of the bed that is most convenient and faces the patient; the examiner reverses this position and faces her feet for the last maneuver (Fig. 12–10). These maneuvers may be difficult if not impossible to perform and interpret if the patient is obese or if the placenta is anteriorly implanted.

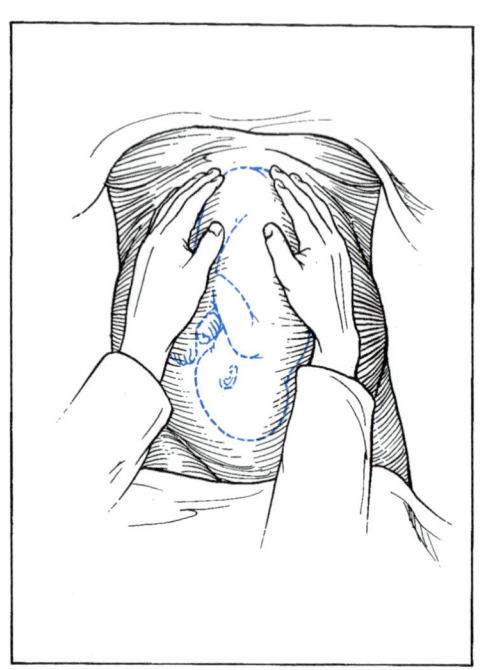

First maneuver

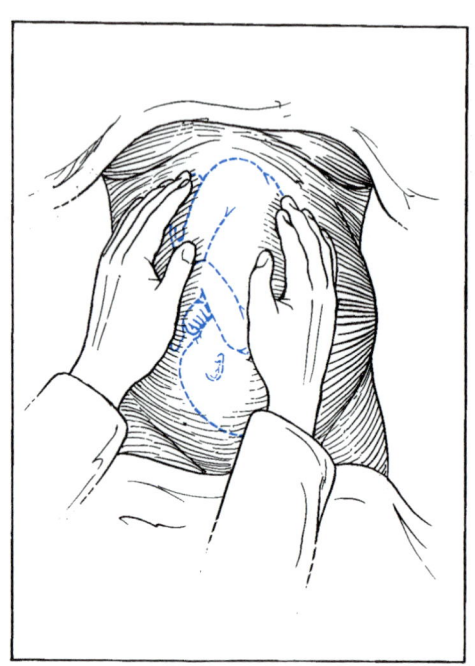

Second maneuver

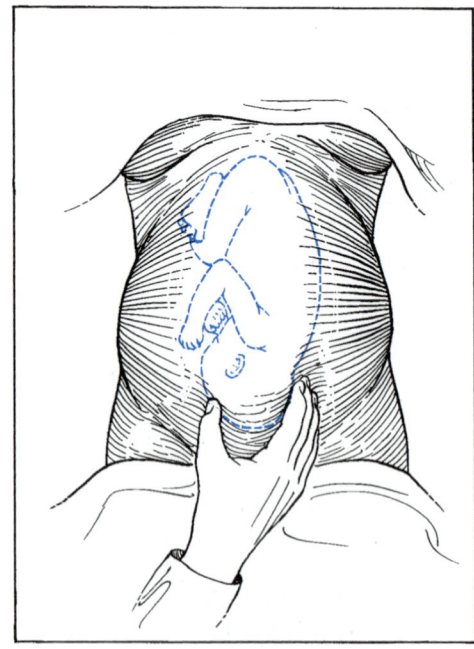

Third maneuver

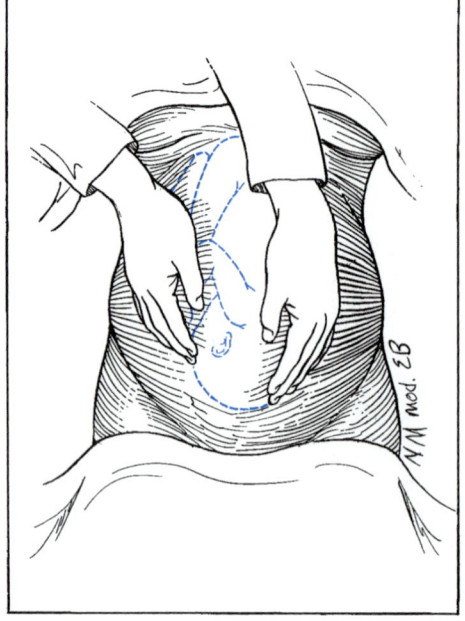

Fourth maneuver

FIGURE 12–10. Longitudinal lie. Palpation in left occiput anterior position (LOA) (Leopold maneuver).

FIRST MANEUVER. After outlining the contour of the uterus and ascertaining how nearly the fundus approaches the xiphoid cartilage, the examiner gently palpates the fundus with the tips of the fingers of both hands in order to define which fetal pole is present in the fundus. The breech gives the sensation of a large, nodular body, whereas the head feels hard and round and is more freely movable and ballottable.

SECOND MANEUVER. After determination of the pole that lies in the fundus, the palms are placed on either side of the abdomen, and gentle but deep pressure is exerted. On one side, a hard, resistant structure is felt, the back; and on the other, numerous small, irregular and mobile parts are felt, the fetal extremities. In women with a thin abdominal wall, the fetal extremities can often be differentiated, but in heavier women, only these irregular nodulations may be felt. In the presence of obesity or considerable amnionic fluid, the back is felt more easily by exerting deep pressure with one hand while counter-palpating with the other. By next noting whether the back is directed anteriorly, transversely, or posteriorly, a more accurate picture of the orientation of the fetus is obtained.

THIRD MANEUVER. Using the thumb and fingers of one hand, the lower portion of the maternal abdomen is grasped just above the symphysis pubis. If the presenting part is not engaged, a movable body will be felt, usually the head. The differentiation between head and breech is made as in the first maneuver. If the presenting part is not engaged, all that remains to be defined is the attitude of the head. If by careful palpation it can be shown that the cephalic prominence is on the same side as the small parts, the head must be flexed, and therefore the vertex is the presenting part. When the cephalic prominence of the fetus is on the same side as the back, the head must be extended. If the presenting part is deeply engaged, however, the findings from this maneuver are simply indicative that the lower fetal pole is fixed in the pelvis; the details are then defined by the last (fourth) maneuver.

FOURTH MANEUVER. The examiner faces the mother's feet and, with the tips of the first three fingers of each hand, exerts deep pressure in the direction of the axis of the pelvic inlet. If the head presents, one hand is arrested sooner than the other by a rounded body, the cephalic prominence, while the other hand descends more deeply into the pelvis. In vertex presentations, the prominence is on the same side as the small parts; and in face presentations, on the same side as the back. The ease with which the prominence is felt is indicative of the extent to which descent has occurred. In many instances, when the head has descended into the pelvis, the anterior shoulder may be differentiated readily by the third maneuver. In breech presentations, the information obtained from this maneuver is less precise.

Abdominal palpation can be performed throughout the latter months of pregnancy and during and between the contractions of labor. The findings provide information about the presentation and position of the fetus and the extent to which the presenting part has descended into the pelvis. For example, so long as the cephalic prominence is readily palpable, the vertex has not descended to the level of the ischial spines. The degree of cephalopelvic disproportion, moreover, can be gauged by evaluating the extent to which the anterior portion of the fetal head overrides the symphysis pubis. With experience, it is possible to estimate the size of the fetus, and even to map out the presentation of the second fetus in a twin gestation. According to Lydon-Rochelle and colleagues (1993), experienced clinicians accurately identify fetal malpresentation using Leopold maneuvers with a high sensitivity (88 percent), specificity (94 percent), positive predictive value (74 percent), and negative predictive value (97 percent).

VAGINAL EXAMINATION. Before labor, the diagnosis of fetal presentation and position by vaginal examination is often inconclusive, because the presenting part must be palpated through a closed cervix and lower uterine segment. With the onset of labor and after cervical dilatation, important information may be obtained. In vertex presentations, the position and variety are recognized by differentiation of the various sutures and fontanels. Face presentations are identified by the differentiation of the portions of the face. Breech presentations are identified by palpation of the sacrum and maternal ischial tuberosities.

In attempting to determine presentation and position by vaginal examination, it is advisable to pursue a definite routine, comprised of four maneuvers (Figs. 12–11 and 12–12):

1. After the woman is prepared appropriately, as described in Chapter 13 (p. 311), two fingers of either gloved hand are introduced into the vagina and carried up to the presenting part. The differentiation of vertex, face, and breech is then accomplished readily.
2. If the vertex is presenting, the fingers are introduced into the posterior aspect of the vagina. The fingers are then swept forward over the fetal head toward the maternal symphysis (Fig. 12–11). During this movement, the fingers necessarily cross the fetal sagittal suture. When it is felt, its course is outlined, with small and large fontanels at the opposite ends.
3. The positions of the two fontanels then are ascertained. The fingers are passed to the most anterior

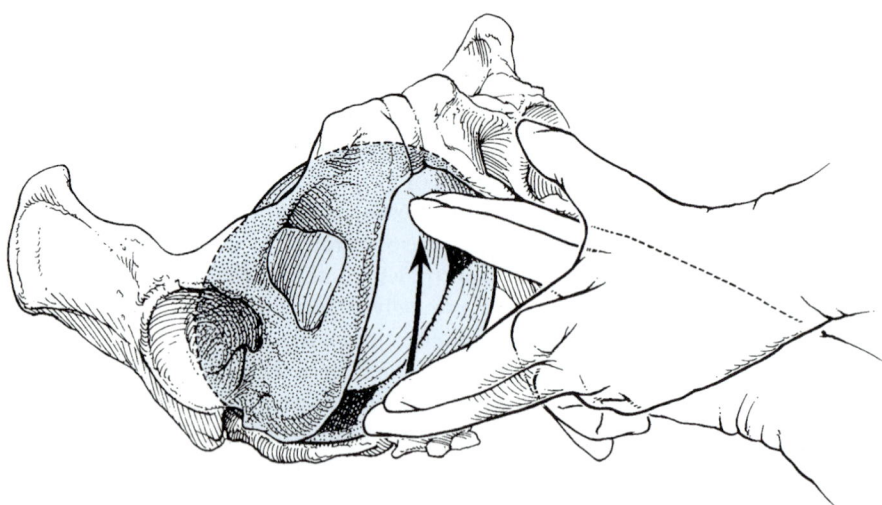

FIGURE 12–11. Locating the sagittal suture by vaginal examination.

extension of the sagittal suture, and the fontanel encountered there is examined carefully and identified; then by a circular motion, the fingers are passed around the side of the head until the other fontanel is felt and differentiated (Fig. 12–12).

4. The station, or extent to which the presenting part has descended into the pelvis, can also be established at this time (Chap. 3, p. 53).

Using these maneuvers, the various sutures and fontanels (Chap. 7, p. 135) are located readily, and the possibility of error is lessened considerably. In face and breech presentations, errors are minimized, because the various parts are distinguished more readily.

AUSCULTATION. While auscultation alone does not provide reliable information concerning fetal presentation and position, auscultatory findings sometimes reinforce results obtained by palpation. Ordinarily, fetal heart sounds are transmitted through the convex portion of the fetus that lies in intimate contact with the uterine wall. Therefore, fetal heart sounds are heard best through the fetal back in vertex and breech presentations, and through the fetal thorax in face presentations. The region of the abdomen in which fetal heart sounds are heard most clearly varies according to the presentation and the extent to which the presenting part has descended. In cephalic presentations, fetal heart sounds are best heard midway between the maternal umbilicus and the anterior superior spine of her ilium. In breech presentations, fetal heart tones are usually heard at or slightly above the umbilicus. In occipitoanterior positions, heart sounds usually are heard best a short distance from the midline; in the transverse varieties, they are heard more laterally; and in the posterior varieties, they are best heard well back in the flank.

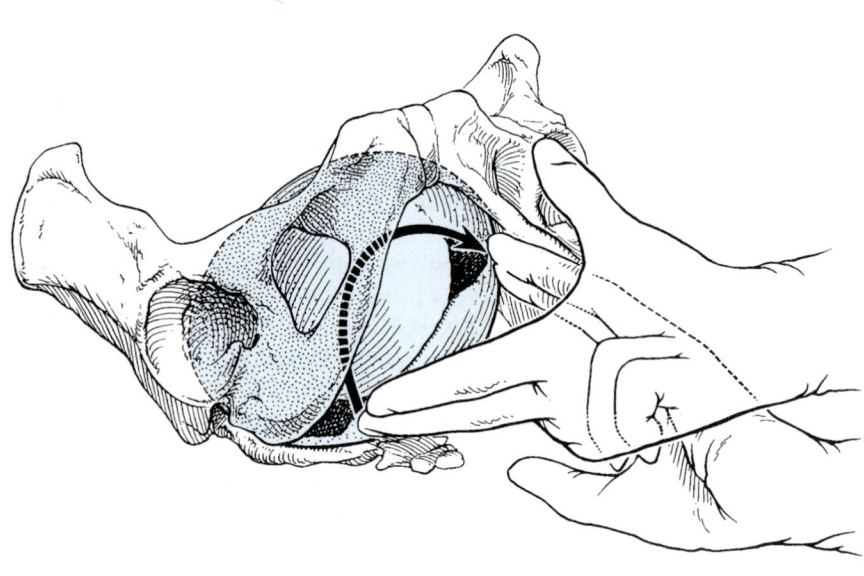

FIGURE 12–12. Differentiating the fontanels by vaginal examination.

SONOGRAPHY. Improvements in ultrasonic techniques have provided another diagnostic aid of particular value in doubtful cases. In obese women or in women whose abdominal walls are rigid, a sonographic examination may provide information to solve many diagnostic problems and lead to early recognition of a breech or shoulder presentation that might otherwise have escaped detection until late in labor. Employing ultrasonography, the fetal head and body can be located without the potential hazards of radiation. In some clinical situations, the information obtained radiographically far exceeds the minimal risk from a single x-ray exposure (Chap. 41, p. 1112).

LABOR WITH OCCIPUT PRESENTATIONS

The fetus is in the occiput or vertex presentation in approximately 95 percent of all labors. Presentation is most commonly ascertained by abdominal palpation and confirmed by vaginal examination sometime before or at the onset of labor. In the majority of cases, the vertex enters the pelvis with the sagittal suture in the transverse pelvic diameter (Caldwell and associates, 1934). The fetus enters the pelvis in the **left occiput transverse (LOT)** position in 40 percent of labors, compared with 20 percent in the **right occiput transverse (ROT)** position (Caldwell and associates, 1934). In **occiput anterior positions (LOA or ROA),** the head either enters the pelvis with the occiput rotated 45 degrees anteriorly from the transverse position, or subsequently does so. The mechanism of labor usually is very similar to that in occiput transverse positions.

In about 20 percent of labors, the fetus enters the pelvis in an **occiput posterior (OP)** position. The right occiput posterior (ROP) is slightly more common than the left (LOP) (Caldwell and associates, 1934). It appears likely from evidence obtained by radiographic studies that posterior positions are more often associated with a narrow forepelvis. They are also more commonly seen in association with anterior placentation (Gardberg and Tuppurainen, 1994a).

OCCIPUT ANTERIOR PRESENTATION. Because of the irregular shape of the pelvic canal and the relatively large dimensions of the mature fetal head, it is evident that not all diameters of the head can necessarily pass through all diameters of the pelvis. It follows that a process of adaptation or accommodation of suitable portions of the head to the various segments of the pelvis is required for vaginal delivery. These positional changes in the presenting part constitute the mechanisms of labor. The **cardinal movements of labor** are engagement, descent, flexion, internal rotation, extension, external rotation, and expulsion (Fig. 12–13).

For purposes of instruction, the various movements often are described as though they occurred separately and independently. In reality, the mechanism of labor consists of a combination of movements that are ongoing simultaneously. For example, as part of the process of engagement, there is both flexion and descent of the head. It is impossible for the movements to be completed unless the presenting part descends simultaneously. Concomitantly, uterine contractions effect important modifications in fetal attitude, or habitus, especially after the head has descended into the pelvis. These changes consist principally of a straightening of the fetus, with loss of dorsal convexity and closer application of the extremities to the body. As a result, the fetal ovoid is transformed into a cylinder, with the smallest possible cross section normally passing through the birth canal.

ENGAGEMENT. As discussed in Chapter 3 (p. 58), the mechanism by which the biparietal diameter, the greatest transverse diameter of the fetal head in occiput presentations, passes through the pelvic inlet is designated engagement. This phenomenon may take place during the last few weeks of pregnancy, or it may not occur until after the commencement of labor. In many multiparous and some nulliparous women, the fetal head is freely movable above the pelvic inlet at the onset of labor. In this circumstance, the head is sometimes referred to as "floating." A normal-sized head usually does not engage with its sagittal suture directed anteroposteriorly. Instead, the fetal head usually enters the pelvic inlet either in the transverse diameter or in one of the oblique diameters (Caldwell and colleagues, 1934).

ASYNCLITISM. Although the fetal head tends to accommodate to the transverse axis of the pelvic inlet, the sagittal suture, while remaining parallel to that axis, may not lie exactly midway between the symphysis and sacral promontory. The sagittal suture frequently is deflected either posteriorly toward the promontory or anteriorly toward the symphysis (Fig. 12–14). Such lateral deflection of the head to a more anterior or posterior position in the pelvis is called **asynclitism**. If the sagittal suture approaches the sacral promontory, more of the anterior parietal bone presents itself to the examining fingers, and the condition is called *anterior asynclitism*. If, however, the sagittal suture lies close to the symphysis, more of the posterior parietal bone will present, and the condition is called *posterior asynclitism*. At the extreme of posterior asynclitism, also called *Litzmann obliquity*, the posterior ear may be easily palpated.

Moderate degrees of asynclitism are the rule in nor-

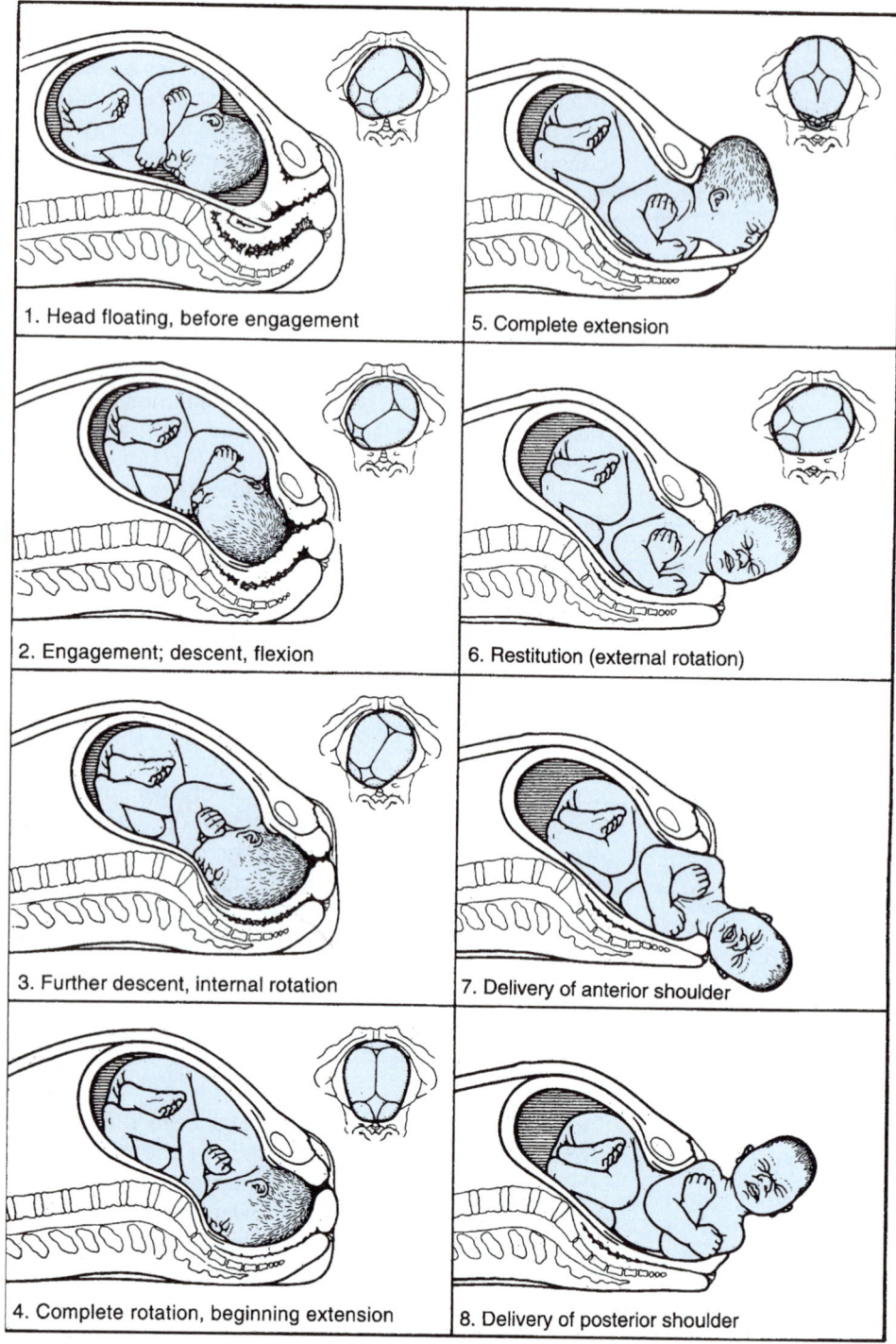

1. Head floating, before engagement

2. Engagement; descent, flexion

3. Further descent, internal rotation

4. Complete rotation, beginning extension

5. Complete extension

6. Restitution (external rotation)

7. Delivery of anterior shoulder

8. Delivery of posterior shoulder

FIGURE 12–13. Cardinal movements in the mechanism of labor and delivery, left occiput anterior position.

mal labor, but if severe, the asynclitism may lead to cephalopelvic disproportion even with an otherwise normal-sized pelvis. Successive changes from posterior to anterior asynclitism facilitate descent by allowing the fetal head to take advantage of the roomiest areas of the pelvic cavity.

DESCENT. This is the first requisite for birth of the infant. In nulliparas, engagement may take place before the onset of labor, and further descent may not follow until the onset of the second stage. In multiparous women, descent usually begins with engagement. Descent is brought about by one or more of four forces:

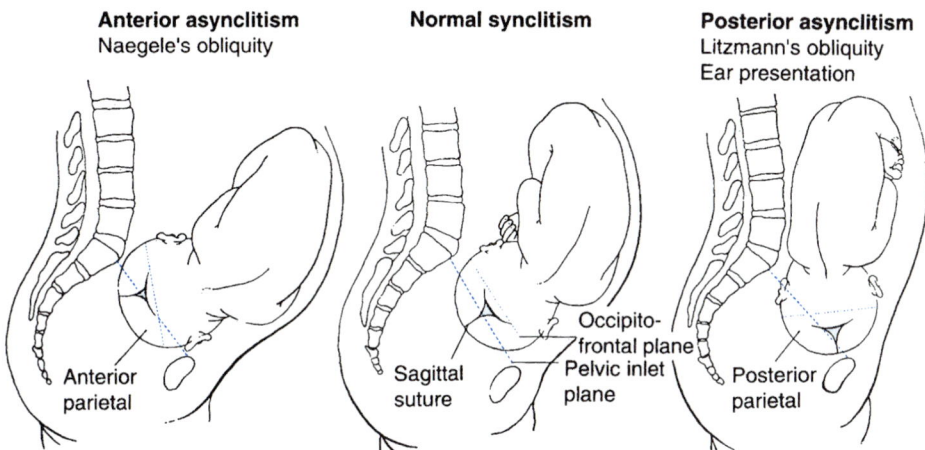

Anterior asynclitism
Naegele's obliquity

Anterior
parietal

Normal synclitism

Sagittal
suture

Occipito-
frontal plane
Pelvic inlet
plane

Posterior asynclitism
Litzmann's obliquity
Ear presentation

Posterior
parietal

FIGURE 12-14. Synclitism and asynclitism.

1. Pressure of the amnionic fluid.
2. Direct pressure of the fundus upon the breech with contractions.
3. Bearing down efforts with the abdominal muscles.
4. Extension and straightening of the fetal body.

FLEXION. As soon as the descending head meets resistance, whether from the cervix, walls of the pelvis, or pelvic floor, flexion of the head normally results. In this movement, the chin is brought into more intimate contact with the fetal thorax, and the appreciably shorter suboccipitobregmatic diameter is substituted for the longer occipitofrontal diameter (Figs. 12–15 and 12–16).

INTERNAL ROTATION. This is a turning of the head in such a manner that the occiput gradually moves from its original position anteriorly toward the symphysis pu-

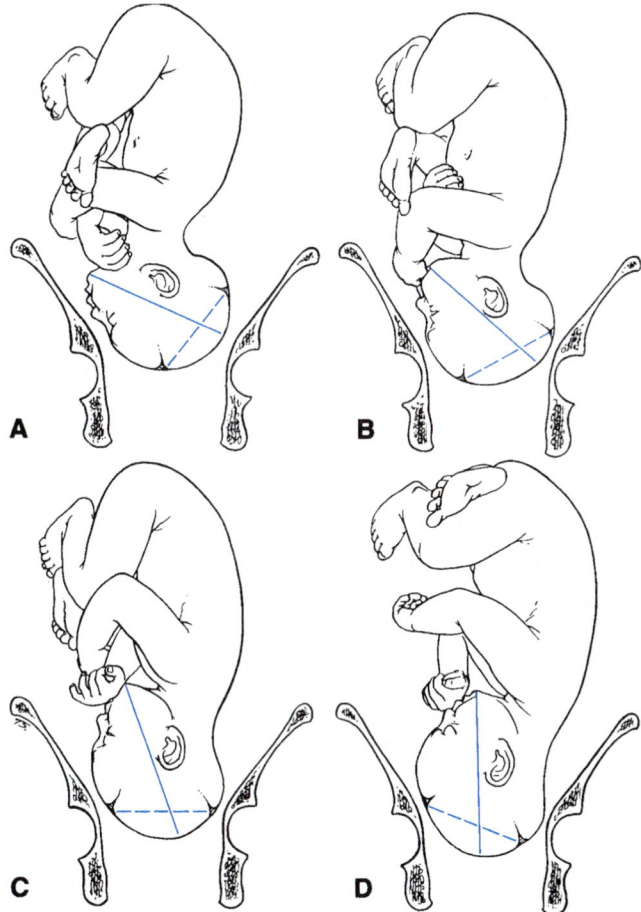

A   B

C   D

FIGURE 12-16. Four degrees of head flexion. Indicated by the solid line the occipitomental diameter; the broken line connects the center of the anterior fontanel with posterior fontanel: **A.** Flexion poor. **B.** Flexion moderate. **C.** Flexion advanced. **D.** Flexion complete. Note that with flexion complete the chin is on the chest, and the suboccipitobregmatic diameter, the shortest anteroposterior diameter of the fetal head, is passing through the pelvic inlet.

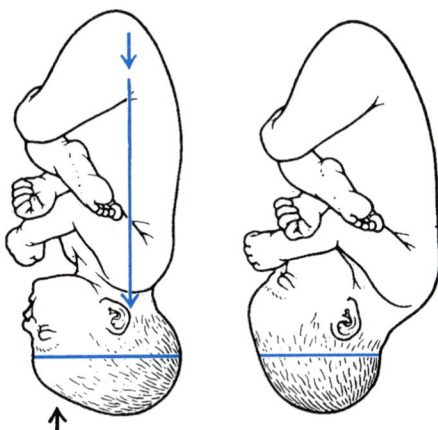

FIGURE 12-15. Lever action producing flexion of the head; conversion from occipitofrontal to suboccipitobregmatic diameter typically reduces the anteroposterior diameter from nearly 12 to 9.5 cm.

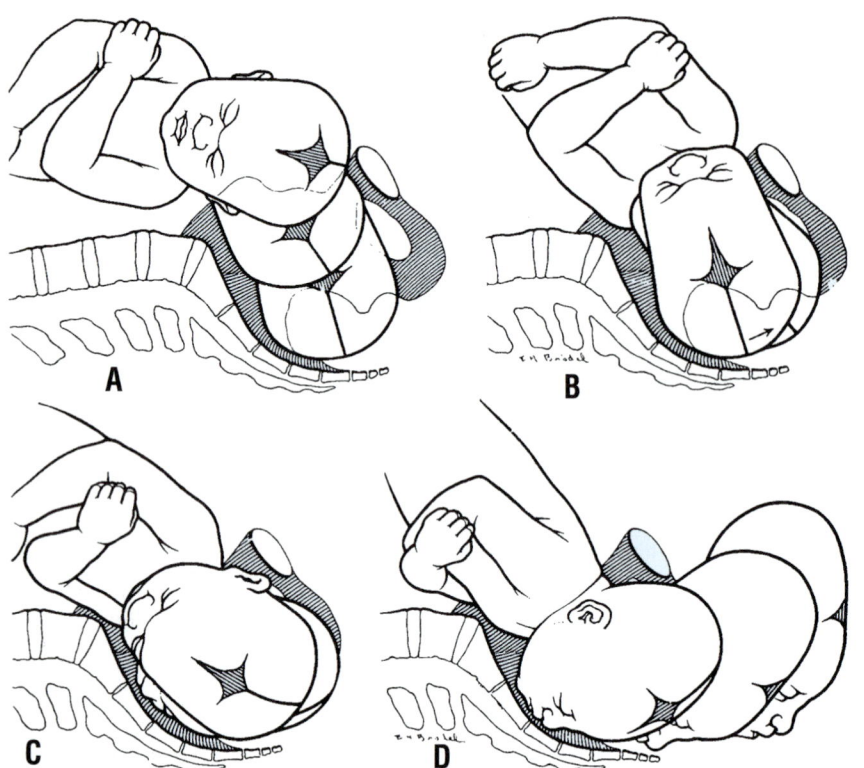

FIGURE 12–17. Mechanism of labor for the left occiput transverse position, lateral view. Posterior asynclitism **(A)** at the pelvic brim followed by lateral flexion, resulting in anterior asynclitism **(B)** after engagement, further descent **(C)**, rotation, and extension **(D)**.

bis or, less commonly, posteriorly toward the hollow of the sacrum (Figs. 12–17 to 12–19). Internal rotation is essential for the completion of labor, except when the fetus is unusually small. While it always is associated with descent, it usually is not accomplished until the head has reached the level of the spines and therefore is engaged.

Calkins (1939) studied more than 5000 women in labor to ascertain the time of internal rotation. He concluded that in approximately two thirds, internal rotation is completed by the time the head reaches the pelvic floor; in about a fourth, internal rotation is completed very shortly after the head reaches the pelvic floor; and in about 5 percent, anterior rotation does not take place.

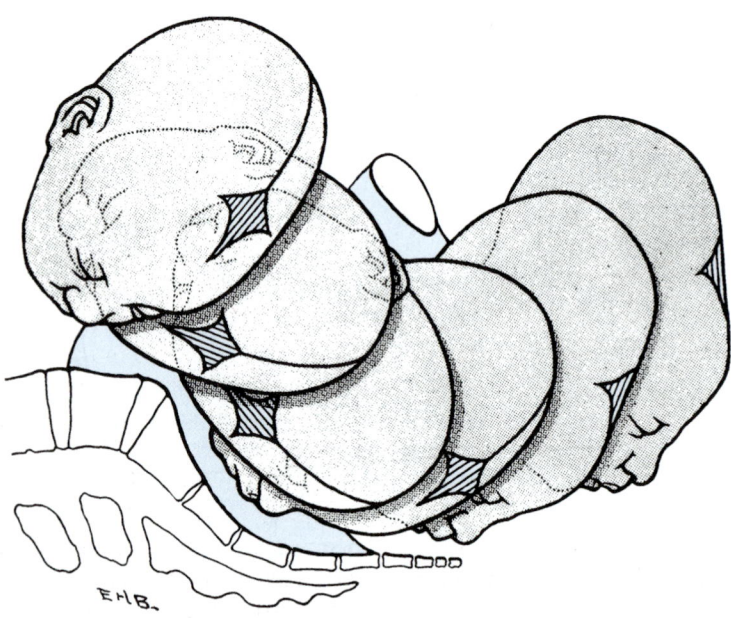

FIGURE 12–18. Mechanisms of labor for left occiput anterior position.

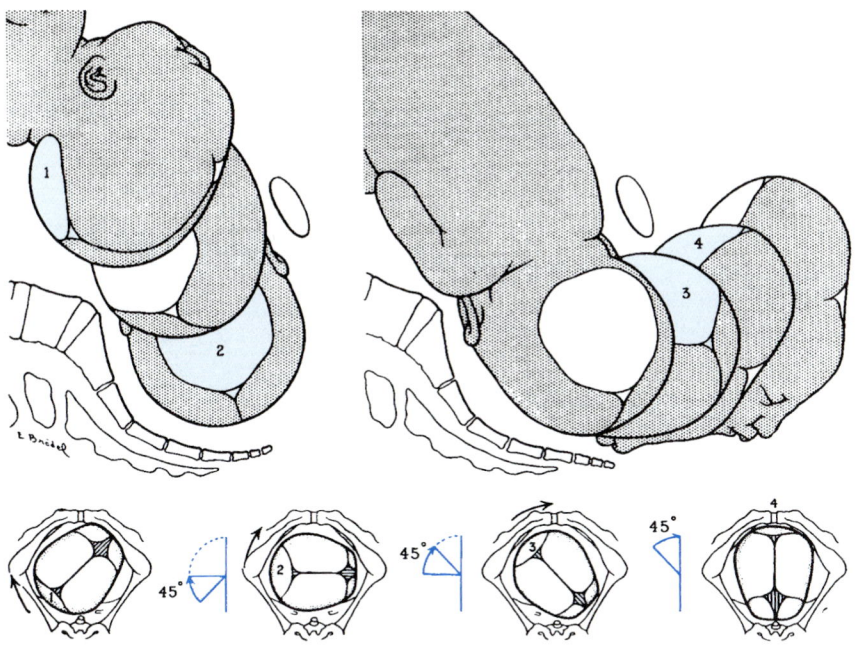

FIGURE 12–19. Mechanism of labor for right occiput posterior position, anterior rotation.

When rotation fails to occur until the head reaches the pelvic floor, it takes place during the next one or two contractions in multiparas; and in nulliparas, it occurs during the next three to five. He also found that rotation before the head reaches the pelvic floor is more frequent in multiparas than in nulliparas.

EXTENSION. When, after internal rotation, the sharply flexed head reaches the vulva, it undergoes extension which is essential to birth. This brings the base of the occiput into direct contact with the inferior margin of the symphysis pubis (Fig. 12–18). Because the vulvar outlet is directed upward and forward, extension must occur before the head can pass through it. If the sharply flexed head, on reaching the pelvic floor, did not extend but was driven farther downward, it would impinge upon the posterior portion of the perineum and would eventually be forced through the tissues of the perineum. When the head presses upon the pelvic gutter, however, two forces come into play. The first, exerted by the uterus, acts more posteriorly, and the second, supplied by the resistant pelvic floor and the symphysis, acts more anteriorly. The resultant vector is in the direction of the vulvar opening, thereby causing extension.

With progressive distention of the perineum and vaginal opening, an increasingly larger portion of the occiput gradually appears. The head is born by further extension as the occiput, bregma, forehead, nose, mouth, and finally the chin pass successively over the anterior margin of the perineum (Fig. 12–19). Immediately after its birth, the head drops downward so that the chin lies over the maternal anal region.

EXTERNAL ROTATION. The delivered head next undergoes restitution. If the occiput was originally directed toward the left, it rotates toward the left ischial tuberosity; if it was originally directed toward the right, the occiput rotates to the right. Restitution of the head to the oblique position is followed by completion of external rotation to the transverse position, a movement that corresponds to rotation of the fetal body, serving to bring its bisacromial diameter into relation with the anteroposterior diameter of the pelvic outlet. Thus, one shoulder is anterior behind the symphysis and the other is posterior. This movement is apparently brought about by the same pelvic factors that produced internal rotation of the head.

EXPULSION. Almost immediately after external rotation, the anterior shoulder appears under the symphysis pubis, and the perineum soon becomes distended by the posterior shoulder. After delivery of the shoulders, the rest of the body is quickly extruded.

OCCIPUT POSTERIOR POSITION. In the great majority of labors in the occiput posterior positions, the mechanism of labor is identical to that observed in the transverse and anterior varieties, except that the occiput has to rotate to the symphysis pubis through 135 degrees, instead of 90 and 45 degrees, respectively (Fig. 12–19).

With effective contractions, adequate flexion of the head, and a fetus of average size, the great majority of posteriorly positioned occiputs rotate promptly as soon as they reach the pelvic floor, and labor is not lengthened appreciably. In perhaps 5 to 10 percent of cases, however, these favorable circumstances do not occur (Gardberg and Tuppurainen, 1994b). For example, with poor contractions, faulty flexion of the head, or both, rotation may be incomplete or may not take place at all, especially if the fetus is large. Epidural analgesia, which diminishes abdominal muscular pushing as well as relaxing the muscles of the pelvic floor, also predisposes to incomplete rotation (Chap. 15, p. 376). If rotation is incomplete, transverse arrest results. If rotation toward the symphysis does not take place, the occiput may rotate to the direct occiput posterior position, a condition known as *persistent occiput posterior*. Both persistent occiput posterior and transverse arrest represent deviations from the normal mechanisms of labor and are considered further in Chapter 19.

Utilizing sonography in 408 women in labor at term, Gardberg and colleagues (1998) found that 68 percent of persistent occiput posterior positions resulted from malrotation during labor from an occipitoanterior position. Only approximately a third of persistent cases were in a posterior position at the onset of labor. In a review of 210 vaginal occiput posterior deliveries, Riethmuller and colleagues (1999) report that the overall prognosis for this presentation was good.

CHANGES IN SHAPE OF THE FETAL HEAD

CAPUT SUCCEDANEUM. In vertex presentations, the fetal head undergoes important characteristic changes in shape as the result of the pressures to which it is subjected during labor. In prolonged labors before complete cervical dilatation, the portion of the fetal scalp immediately over the cervical os becomes edematous, forming a swelling known as the *caput succedaneum* (Fig. 12–20). It usually attains a thickness of only a few millimeters, but in prolonged labors it may be sufficiently extensive to prevent the differentiation of the various sutures and fontanels. More commonly the caput is formed when the head is in the lower portion of the birth canal and frequently only after the resistance of a rigid vaginal outlet is encountered. Because it occurs over the most dependent area of the head, in LOT position it is found over the upper and posterior portion of the right parietal bone, and in ROT positions over the corresponding area of the left parietal bone. It follows that after labor the original position may often be ascertained by noting the location of the caput succedaneum.

MOLDING. Molding describes the change in fetal head shape from external compressive forces. Some molding occurs before labor, possibly related to Braxton Hicks contractions. Although taught in previous editions, most

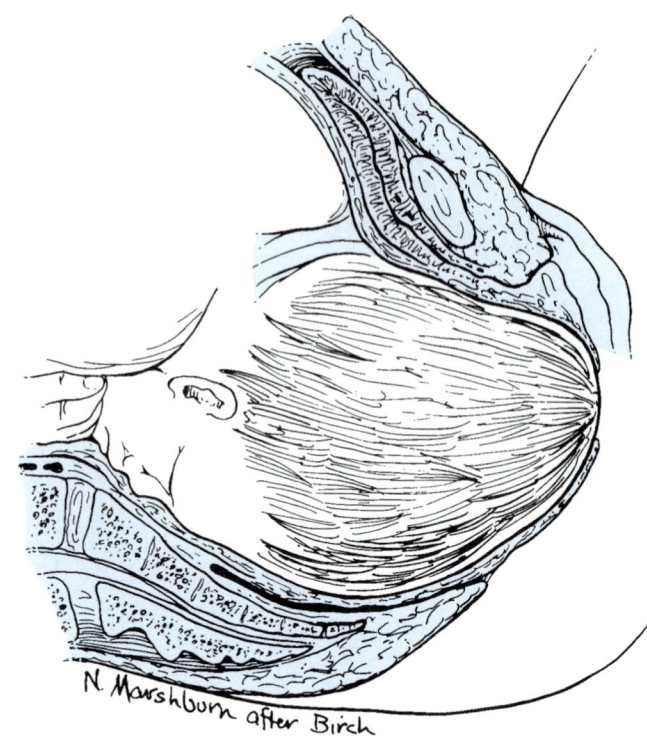

FIGURE 12–20. Formation of caput succedaneum.

studies indicate that there is seldom overlapping of the parietal bones. Instead, a "locking" mechanism at the coronal and lambdoidal connections prevents such overlapping (Carlan and colleagues, 1991). Molding is associated with a shortened suboccipitobregmatic diameter and a lengthening of the mentovertical diameter. These changes are of greatest importance in contracted pelves or asynclitic presentations. In these circumstances, the degree to which the head is capable of molding may make the difference between spontaneous vaginal delivery versus an operative delivery. Some older literature cited severe head molding as a cause for possible cerebral trauma. Because of the multitude of associated factors, for example, prolonged labor with fetal sepsis and acidosis, it is impossible to quantify the effects of molding with any alleged fetal or neonatal neurological sequelae.

REFERENCES

Caldwell WE, Moloy HC, D'Esopo DA: A roentgenologic study of the mechanism of engagement of the fetal head. Am J Obstet Gynecol 28:824, 1934

Calkins LA: The etiology of occiput presentations. Am J Obstet Gynecol 37:618, 1939

Carlan SJ, Wyble L, Lense J, Mastrogiannis DS, Parsons MT:

Fetal head molding: Diagnosis by ultrasound and a review of the literature. J Perinatol 11:105, 1991

Gardberg M, Laakkonen E, Salevaara M: Intrapartum sonography and persistent occiput posterior position: A study of 408 deliveries. Obstet Gynecol 91:746, 1998

Gardberg M, Tuppurainen M: Anterior placental location predisposes for occiput posterior presentation near term. Acta Obstet Gynecol Scand 73:151, 1994a

Gardberg M, Tuppurainen M: Persistent occiput posterior presentation—a clinical problem. Acta Obstet Gynecol Scand 73:45, 1994b

Gemer O, Segal S: Incidence and contribution of predisposing factors to transverse lie presentation. Int J Gynaecol Obstet 44:219, 1994

Leopold: Conduct of normal births through external examination alone. Arch Gynaekol 45:337, 1894

Lydon-Rochelle M, Albers L, Gorwoda J, Craig E, Qualls C: Accuracy of Leopold maneuvers in screening for malpresentation: A prospective study. Birth 20:132, 1993

Riethmuller D, Teffaud O, Eyraud JL, Sautiere JL, Schaal JP, Maillet R: Maternal and fetal prognosis of occipitoposterior presentation. J Gynecol Obstet Biol Reprod 28:41, 1999

Scheer K, Nubar J: Variation of fetal presentation with gestational age. Am J Obstet Gynecol 125:269, 1976

Steele KB, Javert CT: The mechanism of labor for transverse positions of the vertex. Surg Gynecol Obstet 75:477, 1942

13

Conduct of Normal Labor and Delivery

The ideal conduct of labor and delivery requires two potentially opposing accommodations on the part of obstetrical providers: first, that birthing be recognized as a normal physiological process that most women experience without complications, and second, that intrapartum complications can arise very quickly and unexpectedly. Thus, providers must simultaneously make the woman and her supporters feel comfortable, yet ensure safety for the mother and infant should complications suddenly develop. The American Academy of Pediatrics and the American College of Obstetricians and Gynecologists (1997) have collaborated in the development of *Guidelines for Perinatal Care*. These provide detailed information on the appropriate content of intrapartum care to include both personnel and facility requirements. Shown in Table 13–1 are the recommended nurse-to-patient ratios recommended for labor and delivery. Shown in Table 13–2 are the recommended room dimensions for these functions.

ADMISSION PROCEDURES

Pregnant women should be urged to report early in labor rather than to procrastinate until delivery is imminent for fear that they might be experiencing false labor. Early admittance to the labor and delivery unit is important; especially so if during antepartum care the woman, her fetus, or both have been identified as being at risk.

IDENTIFICATION OF LABOR. **One of the most critical diagnoses in obstetrics is the accurate diagnosis of labor.** If labor is falsely diagnosed, inappropriate interventions to augment labor may be made. Conversely, if labor is not diagnosed, the fetus-infant may be damaged by unexpected complications occurring in sites remote from medical personnel and adequate medical facilities.

TABLE 13–1. Recommended Nurse/Patient Ratios for Labor and Delivery

Nurse/Patient Ratio	Care Provided
1:2	Patients in labor
1:1	Patients in second-stage labor
1:1	Patients with medical or obstetrical complications
1:2	Oxytocin induction or augmentation of labor
1:1	Coverage for initiating epidural analgesia
1:1	Circulation for cesarean delivery

From the American Academy of Pediatrics and the American College of Obstetricians and Gynecologists, 1997, with permission.

TABLE 13–2. Recommended Minimum Room Dimensions for Labor and Delivery

Function	Net Floor Space
Labor	100–160 s.f.
LDR[a]	256 s.f.
Vaginal delivery	350 s.f.
Cesarean delivery	400 s.f.

[a]LDR = labor, delivery, and recovery.
From the American Academy of Pediatrics and the American College of Obstetricians and Gynecologists, 1997, with permission.

Although the differential diagnosis between false and true labor is difficult at times, it usually can be made on the basis of the contractions.

Contractions of True Labor
- Contractions occur at regular intervals
- Intervals gradually shorten
- Intensity gradually increases
- Discomfort is in the back and abdomen
- Cervix dilates
- Discomfort is not stopped by sedation

Contractions of False Labor
- Contractions occur at irregular intervals
- Intervals remain long
- Intensity remains unchanged
- Discomfort is chiefly in lower abdomen
- Cervix does not dilate
- Discomfort is usually relieved by sedation

In those instances when a diagnosis of labor cannot be established with certainty, it is often wise to observe the woman over a longer period of time. The general condition of mother and fetus should be ascertained accurately by history and physical examination, including blood pressure, temperature, and pulse. The frequency, duration, and intensity of the uterine contractions should be documented, and the time established when they first become uncomfortable. The degree of discomfort that the mother displays is noted. The heart rate, presentation, and size of the fetus should be determined and documented on admission. **The fetal heart rate should be checked, especially at the end of a contraction and immediately thereafter, to identify pathological slowing of the heart rate** (Chap. 14, p. 354). Inquiries are made about the status of the fetal membranes and whether there has been any vaginal bleeding. The questions of whether fluid has leaked from the vagina and, if so, how much and when the leakage first commenced are also addressed.

All Medicare-participating hospitals with emergency services must provide an appropriate medical screening examination for any pregnant women experiencing contractions who comes to the emergency department for evaluation. The definition of an emergency condition makes specific reference to a pregnant woman who is having contractions. Labor is defined as ". . . the process of childbirth beginning with the latent phase of labor continuing through delivery of the placenta. A woman experiencing contractions is in true labor unless a physician certifies that after a reasonable time of observation the woman is in false labor." A woman in true labor is considered "unstable" for inter-hospital transfer purposes until the child and placenta are delivered. An unstable woman may, however, be transferred at the direction of the patient or when a physician signs a written certification that benefits of treatment at another facility outweigh the risks of transfer. Physicians and hospitals violating these federal requirements are subject to civil penalties of up to $50,000, as well as termination from the Medicare program.

ELECTRONIC ADMISSION TESTING. Some investigators recommend that a nonstress test (NST) or contraction stress test (CST) be performed on all patients admitted to the labor and delivery unit, the so-called "fetal admission test" (Ingemarsson and associates, 1986). Such fetal surveillance is in reality an assessment of fetal heart rate accelerations or lack of the same with fetal movement (NST); or an assessment of fetal heart rate before, during, and following a uterine contraction if the patient is in labor (CST) (Freeman and colleagues, 1991). Fetal heart rate variability and variable decelerations also are used in these evaluations. It has been suggested that such tests of fetal well-being, alone or in combination with fetal acoustic stimulation, will identify unsuspected cases of fetal jeopardy (Ingemarsson and associates, 1988; Sarno and co-workers, 1990). Certainly, if the woman is to be discharged from the labor unit undelivered, this practice is reasonable to ensure, as nearly as possible, that fetal compromise is not identified at this time. At Parkland Hospital, external electronic monitoring is performed for at least one hour before discharging women with false labor.

VAGINAL EXAMINATION. Most often, *unless there has been bleeding in excess of bloody show*, a vaginal examination under aseptic conditions is performed. Careful attention to the following items is essential in order to obtain the greatest amount of information and to minimize bacterial contamination from multiple examinations.

1. *Amnionic fluid.* If there is a question of membrane rupture, a sterile speculum is carefully inserted, and fluid is sought in the posterior vaginal fornix. Any fluid is observed for vernix or meconium; if the source of the fluid remains in doubt, it is collected on a swab for further study, as described later.
2. *Cervix.* Softness, degree of effacement (length), extent of dilatation, and location of the cervix with respect to the presenting part and vagina are ascertained, as will be described. The presence of membranes with or without amnionic fluid below the presenting part often can be felt by careful palpation. The fetal membranes often can be visualized if they are intact and the cervix is dilated somewhat.
3. *Presenting part.* The nature of the presenting part should be positively determined and, ideally, its position as well, as described in Chapter 12.
4. *Station.* The degree of descent of the presenting part into the birth canal is identified, as will be described. If the fetal head is high in the pelvis (above the level of the ischial spines), the effect of firm fundal pressure on descent of the fetal head is tested.
5. *Pelvic architecture.* The diagonal conjugate, ischial spines, pelvic sidewalls, and sacrum are reevaluated for adequacy (Chap. 3, p. 51).

CERVICAL EFFACEMENT. The degree of cervical effacement is usually expressed in terms of the length of the cervical canal compared to that of an uneffaced cervix (Chap. 11, p. 256). When the length of the cervix is reduced by one half, it is 50 percent effaced; when the cervix becomes as thin as the adjacent lower uterine segment, it is completely, or 100 percent, effaced.

CERVICAL DILATATION. This is ascertained by estimating the average diameter of the cervical opening. The examining finger is swept from the margin of the cervix on one side to the opposite side, and the diameter traversed is expressed in centimeters. The cervix is said to be dilated fully when the diameter measures 10 cm, because the presenting part of a term-size infant usually can pass through a cervix this widely dilated.

POSITION OF THE CERVIX. The relationship of the cervical os to the fetal head is categorized as posterior, midposition, or anterior. A posterior position is suggestive of preterm labor.

STATION. The level of the presenting fetal part in the birth canal is described in relationship to the ischial spines, which are halfway between the pelvic inlet and the pelvic outlet. When the lowermost portion of the presenting fetal part is at the level of the ischial spines, it is designated as being at zero (0) station. In the past, the long axis of the birth canal above the ischial spines was arbitrarily divided into thirds. In 1988, the American College of Obstetricians and Gynecologists began using a classification of station that divides the pelvis above and below the spines into fifths. These divisions represent centimeters above and below the spines. Thus, as the presenting fetal part descends from the inlet toward the ischial spines, the designation is -5, -4, -3, -2, -1, then 0 station. Below the ischial spines, the presenting fetal part passes $+1$, $+2$, $+3$, $+4$, and $+5$ stations to delivery. Station $+5$ cm corresponds to the fetal head being visible at the introitus. An approximate correlation of the two methods of describing station is: $+2$ cm $= +1/3$ and $+4$ cm $= +2/3$ (American Academy of Pediatrics and the American College of Obstetricians and Gynecologists, 1997).

If the leading part of the fetal head is at 0 station or below, most often engagement of the head has occurred; that is, the biparietal plane of the fetal head has passed through the pelvic inlet. **If the head is unusually molded, or if there is an extensive caput formation, or both, engagement might not have taken place even though the head appears to be at 0 station.**

DETECTION OF RUPTURED MEMBRANES. The pregnant woman should be instructed during the antepartum period to be aware of leakage of fluid from the vagina and to report such an occurrence promptly. Rupture of the membranes is significant for three reasons. First, if the presenting part is not fixed in the pelvis, the possibility of prolapse of the umbilical cord and cord compression is greatly increased. Second, labor is likely to occur soon if the pregnancy is at or near term. Third, if delivery is delayed for 24 hours or more after membrane rupture, there is increasing likelihood of serious intrauterine infection.

A conclusive diagnosis of rupture of the membranes is made when amnionic fluid is seen pooling in the posterior fornix or clear fluid is passing from the cervical canal (American College of Obstetricians and Gynecologists, 2000). Although several diagnostic tests for the detection of ruptured membranes have been recommended, none is completely reliable. If the diagnosis remains uncertain, another method involves testing the pH of the vaginal fluid; the pH of vaginal secretions normally ranges between 4.5 and 5.5, whereas that of amnionic fluid is usually 7.0 to 7.5. The use of the indicator **nitrazine** for the diagnosis of ruptured membranes, first suggested by Baptisti (1938), is a simple and fairly reliable method. Test papers are impregnated with the dye, and the color of the reaction is interpreted by comparison with a standard color chart. The pH of the vaginal secretion is estimated by inserting a sterile cotton-tipped applicator deeply into the vagina, and then touching it to a strip of the nitrazine paper and comparing the color

of the paper with the chart supplied with the paper. A pH above 6.5 is consistent with ruptured membranes. False-positive tests occur with blood, semen, or bacterial vaginosis and false-negative tests with minimal fluid (American College of Obstetricians and Gynecologists, 2000).

Other tests have been used as markers for rupture of the membranes. Arborization or ferning of vaginal fluid suggests amnionic rather than cervical fluid. Detection of alpha-fetoprotein in the vaginal vault has been used to identify amnionic fluid (Yamada and colleagues, 1998). Unequivocal identification comes from injection of various dyes, including Evans blue, methylene blue, indigo carmine, or fluorescein, into the amnionic sac via abdominal amniocentesis.

VITAL SIGNS AND REVIEW OF PREGNANCY RECORD. The maternal blood pressure, temperature, pulse, and respiratory rate are checked for any abnormality, and these are recorded. The pregnancy record is promptly reviewed to identify complications. Any problems identified during the antepartum period, as well as any that were anticipated, should be displayed prominently in the pregnancy record.

PREPARATION OF VULVA AND PERINEUM. The woman is positioned to allow inspection and cleansing of the vulva and perineum. Scrubbing is directed from above, downward, and away from the introitus. Attention should be paid to careful cleansing of the vulvar folds. As the scrub sponge passes over the anal region, it is discarded. If hair on the lower half of the vulva or perineum is felt to interfere at the time of delivery, it can be clipped with scissors or a mini-shave prep can be performed. Routine shaving of the perineum is not performed at Parkland Hospital.

VAGINAL EXAMINATIONS. Ideally, after the vulvar and perineal regions have been properly prepared, and the examiner has donned sterile gloves, the thumb and forefinger of one hand are used to separate the labia widely to expose the vaginal opening and prevent the examining fingers from coming in contact with the inner surfaces of the labia. The index and second fingers of the other hand are then introduced into the vagina (Fig. 13–1). A precise routine of evaluation, as described earlier should be followed. It is important to avoid the anal region and not to withdraw the fingers from the vagina until the examination is completed. The number of vaginal examinations during labor does correlate with infectious morbidity, especially in cases of early membrane rupture.

ENEMA. Early in labor, a cleansing enema often is given to minimize subsequent contamination by feces,

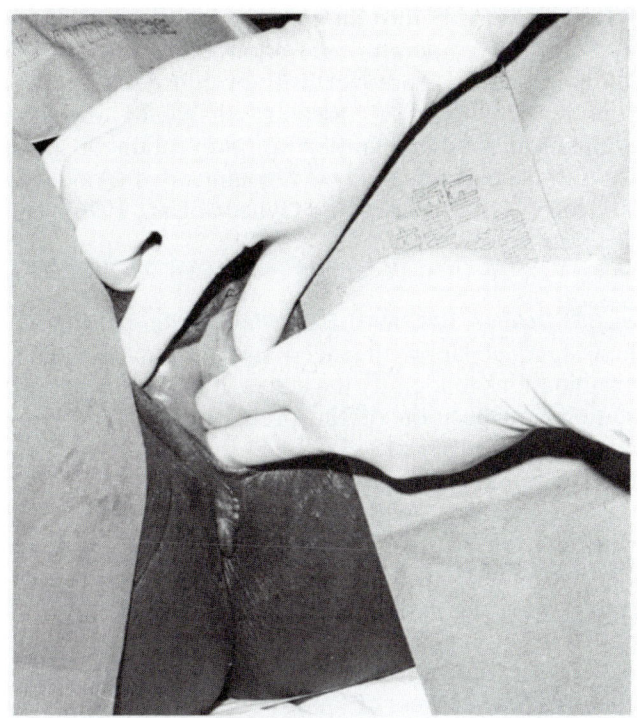

FIGURE 13–1. To perform vaginal examination, the labia have been separated with one hand and the first and second fingers of the other hand are carefully inserted into the introitus.

which otherwise may be a problem during the second stage of labor and delivery. A ready-to-use enema solution of sodium phosphate in a disposable container (Fleet enema) has proven satisfactory. Enemas are not routinely used at Parkland Hospital.

LABORATORY. When the woman is admitted in labor, most often the hematocrit, or hemoglobin concentration, should be rechecked. The hematocrit can be measured easily and quickly. Blood may be collected in a plain tube from which a heparinized capillary tube is filled immediately. By employing a small microhematocrit centrifuge in the labor-delivery unit, the value can be obtained in 3 minutes. A labeled tube of blood is allowed to clot and is kept on hand for blood type and screen, if needed, and another is used for routine serology. In some units, a voided urine specimen, as free as possible of debris, is examined for protein and glucose. We obtain a urine specimen for protein analysis only in hypertensive women. Patients who have had no prenatal care should be considered to be at risk for syphilis, hepatitis B, and human immunodeficiency virus (American Academy of Pediatrics and the American College of Obstetricians and Gynecologists, 1997). In unregistered patients, these laboratory studies as well as a blood type, Rh, and antibody screen for atypical antibodies should be performed. Some states, for exam-

ple Texas, now require routine testing for syphilis, hepatitis B, and human immunodeficiency virus in all women admitted to labor and delivery units.

MANAGEMENT OF FIRST STAGE OF LABOR

As soon as possible after admittance, the remainder of the general physical examination is completed. The physician can best reach a conclusion about the normalcy of the pregnancy when all examinations, including record and laboratory review, are completed. A rational plan for monitoring labor then can be established based on the needs of the fetus and the mother. If no abnormality is identified or suspected, the mother should be reassured. Although the average duration of the first stage of labor in nulliparous women is about 7 hours and in parous women about 4 hours, there are marked individual variations. Any precise statement as to the duration of labor, therefore, is unwise (Chap. 18, p. 427).

MONITORING FETAL WELL-BEING DURING LABOR.
It is mandatory for optimal pregnancy outcome that a well-defined program be established that provides careful surveillance of the well-being of both mother and fetus during labor. All observations must be appropriately recorded. The frequency, intensity, and duration of uterine contractions, and the response of the fetal heart rate to the contractions, are of considerable concern. These features can be promptly evaluated in logical sequence.

FETAL HEART RATE. The fetal heart rate may be identified with a suitable stethoscope or any of a variety of Doppler ultrasonic devices. Changes in the fetal heart rate that most likely are ominous almost always are detectable immediately after a uterine contraction. Therefore, it is imperative that the fetal heart be monitored by auscultation immediately after a contraction. To avoid confusing maternal and fetal heart rates, the maternal pulse should be counted as the fetal heart rate is counted. Otherwise, maternal tachycardia may be misinterpreted as a normal fetal heart rate.

Fetal jeopardy, compromise, or distress—that is, loss of fetal well-being—is suspected if the fetal heart rate immediately after a contraction is repeatedly below 110 bpm. Fetal jeopardy very likely exists if the rate is heard to be less than 100 per minute, even though there is recovery to a rate in the 110 to 160 bpm range before the next contraction. When decelerations of this magnitude are found after a contraction, further labor, if allowed, is best monitored electronically, as described in Chapter 14.

The American Academy of Pediatrics and American

College of Obstetricians and Gynecologists (1997) recommend that during the first stage of labor, in the absence of any abnormalities, the fetal heart should be checked immediately after a contraction at least every 30 minutes and then every 15 minutes during the second stage. If continuous electronic monitoring is used, the tracing is evaluated at least every 30 minutes during the first stage and at least every 15 minutes during second-stage labor. For women with pregnancies at risk, auscultation is performed at least every 15 minutes during the first stage of labor and every 5 minutes during the second stage. Continuous electronic monitoring may be used with evaluation of the tracing every 15 minutes during the first stage of labor, and every 5 minutes during the second stage.

UTERINE CONTRACTIONS. With the palm of the hand lightly on the uterus, the examiner determines the time of onset of the contraction. The intensity of the contraction is gauged from the degree of firmness the uterus achieves. At the acme of effective contractions, the finger or thumb cannot readily indent the uterus. Next, the time that the contraction disappears is noted. This sequence is repeated in order to evaluate the frequency, duration, and intensity of uterine contractions. It is best to quantify the contractions as regards the degree of firmness or resistance to indentation.

MATERNAL MONITORING AND MANAGEMENT DURING LABOR

MATERNAL VITAL SIGNS. Maternal temperature, pulse, and blood pressure are evaluated at least every 4 hours (Table 13–3). If fetal membranes have been ruptured

TABLE 13–3. Recommendations for Conduct of Normal First- and Second-Stage Labor in Women without Any Anesthetic, Medical, or Obstetrical Risk Factors

1. Maternal vital signs are checked at least every 4 hours.
2. Periodic vaginal examinations using sterile, water-soluble lubricants; avoid povidone–iodine and hexachlorophene antiseptics.
3. Sips of clear liquids, occasional ice chips, and lip moisturizers are permitted. Intravenous hydration is indicated when labor is lengthy.
4. The mother should have the option to stay out of bed during the early stages of labor.
5. Pain relief should depend on the needs and desires of the woman.

From the American Academy of Pediatrics and the American College of Obstetricians and Gynecologists, 1997, with permission.

for many hours before the onset of labor, or if there is a borderline temperature elevation, the temperature is checked hourly. Moreover, with prolonged membrane rupture—defined as greater than 18 hours—antimicrobial administration for prevention of group B streptococcal infections is recommended (American College of Obstetricians and Gynecologists, 1996). This is discussed in Chapter 56 (p. 1471).

SUBSEQUENT VAGINAL EXAMINATIONS. During the first stage of labor, the need for subsequent vaginal examinations to identify the status of the cervix and the station and position of the presenting part will vary considerably (Table 13–3). When the membranes rupture, an examination should be repeated expeditiously if the fetal head was not definitely engaged at the previous vaginal examination. The fetal heart rate should be checked immediately and during the next uterine contraction in order to detect an occult umbilical cord compression. At Parkland Hospital, periodic pelvic examinations are often performed at 2- to 3-hour intervals to evaluate the progress of labor (Chap. 18, p. 446).

ORAL INTAKE. Food should be withheld during active labor and delivery. Gastric emptying time is remarkably prolonged once labor is established and analgesics are administered. As a consequence, ingested food and most medications remain in the stomach and are not absorbed; instead, they may be vomited and aspirated (Chap. 15, p. 366). There is a trend toward giving liquids in moderation to laboring women (Table 13–3). Guyton and Gibbs (1994) cite studies in which 150 mL of fluids were given orally 2 hours before elective surgery. The incidence of aspiration was not affected. It is unclear whether these studies can be applied to women in labor, who are at risk for urgent cesarean delivery at all times.

INTRAVENOUS FLUIDS. Although it has become customary in many hospitals to establish an intravenous infusion system routinely early in labor, there is seldom any real need for such in the normally pregnant woman at least until analgesia is administered. An intravenous infusion system is advantageous during the immediate puerperium in order to administer oxytocin prophylactically, and at times therapeutically when uterine atony persists. Moreover, with longer labors, the administration of glucose, sodium, and water to the otherwise fasting woman at the rate of 60 to 120 mL/hr is efficacious to prevent dehydration and acidosis (Table 13–3).

MATERNAL POSITION DURING LABOR. The normal laboring woman need not be confined to bed early in labor. A comfortable chair may be beneficial psychologically and perhaps physiologically. In bed, the laboring woman should be allowed to assume the position she finds most comfortable, which will be lateral recumbency most of the time. She must not be restricted to lying supine. Bloom and colleagues (1998) conducted a randomized trial of walking during labor in over 1000 women with low-risk pregnancies. They found that walking neither enhanced nor impaired active labor and that it was not harmful.

ANALGESIA. As noted in Table 13–3, most often, analgesia is initiated on the basis of maternal discomfort. The kinds of analgesia, amounts, and frequency of administration should be based on the need to allay pain on the one hand and the likelihood of delivering a depressed infant on the other (Chap. 15, p. 363).

The timing, method of administration, and size of initial and subsequent doses of systemically acting analgesic agents are based to a considerable degree on the anticipated interval of time until delivery. A repeat vaginal examination is often appropriate before administering more analgesia. With the onset of symptoms characteristic of the second stage of labor, that is, an urge to bear down or "push," the status of the cervix and the presenting part should be reevaluated.

AMNIOTOMY. If the membranes are intact, there is a great temptation even during normal labor to perform amniotomy. The presumed benefits are more rapid labor, earlier detection of instances of meconium staining of amnionic fluid, and the opportunity to apply an electrode to the fetus and insert a pressure catheter into the uterine cavity. The advantages and disadvantages of amniotomy are discussed in Chapter 18 (p. 446). If amniotomy is performed, an aseptic technique should be used. Importantly, the fetal head must be well applied to the cervix and not be dislodged from the pelvis during the procedure; such an action invites prolapse of the umbilical cord.

URINARY BLADDER FUNCTION. Bladder distention should be avoided, because it can lead to obstructed labor and to subsequent bladder hypotonia and infection. During each abdominal examination, the suprapubic region should be visualized and palpated in order to detect a filling bladder. If the bladder is readily seen or palpated above the symphysis, the woman should be encouraged to void. At times she can ambulate with assistance to a toilet and successfully void, even though she could not void on a bedpan. If the bladder is distended and she cannot void, intermittent catheterization is indicated.

MANAGEMENT OF SECOND-STAGE LABOR

With full dilatation of the cervix, which signifies the onset of the second stage of labor, the woman typically begins to bear down, and with descent of the presenting part she develops the urge to defecate. Uterine contractions and the accompanying expulsive forces may last 1½ minutes and recur at times after a myometrial resting phase of no more than a minute.

DURATION. The median duration of the second stage is 50 minutes in nulliparas and 20 minutes in multiparas, but it can be highly variable. In a woman of higher parity with a relaxed vagina and perineum, two or three expulsive efforts after the cervix is fully dilated may suffice to complete the delivery of the infant. Conversely, in a woman with a contracted pelvis or a large fetus, or with impaired expulsive efforts from conduction analgesia or intense sedation, the second stage may become abnormally long (Chap. 18, p. 430).

FETAL HEART RATE. For the low-risk fetus, the heart rate should be auscultated during the second stage of labor at least every 15 minutes, whereas in those at high risk, 5-minute intervals are recommended (American Academy of Pediatrics and the American College of Obstetricians and Gynecologists, 1997). Slowing of the fetal heart rate induced by head compression is common during a contraction and the accompanying maternal expulsive efforts. If recovery of the fetal heart rate is prompt after the contraction and expulsive efforts cease, labor is allowed to continue. Not all instances of fetal heart rate slowing during second-stage labor are the consequence of head compression. The vigorous force generated within the uterus by its contraction and by maternal expulsive efforts may reduce placental perfusion appreciably. Descent of the fetus through the birth canal and the consequent reduction in uterine volume may trigger some degree of premature separation of the placenta, with further compromise of fetal well-being. Descent is more likely to tighten a loop or loops of umbilical cord around the fetus, especially the neck, sufficiently to obstruct umbilical blood flow. Prolonged, uninterrupted maternal expulsive efforts can be dangerous to the fetus in these circumstances. Maternal tachycardia, which is common during the second stage, must not be mistaken for a normal fetal heart rate.

MATERNAL EXPULSIVE EFFORTS. In most cases, bearing down is reflex and spontaneous during second-stage labor, but occasionally the woman does not employ her expulsive forces to good advantage and coaching is desirable. Her legs should be half-flexed so that she can push with them against the mattress. Instructions should be to take a deep breath as soon as the next uterine contraction begins, and with her breath held, to exert downward pressure exactly as though she were straining at stool. She should not be encouraged to "push" beyond the time of completion of each uterine contraction. Instead, she and her fetus should be allowed to rest and recover from the combined effects of the uterine contraction, breath holding, and considerable physical effort. Gardosi and associates (1989) have recommended a squatting or semi-squatting position using a specialized pillow. They claim that this shortens second-stage labor by increasing expulsive forces and by increasing the diameter of the pelvic outlet. Eason and colleagues (2000) performed an extensive review of positions and their effect on the incidence of perineal trauma. They found that the supported upright position had no advantages over the recumbent one.

Usually, bearing down efforts result in increasing bulging of the perineum—that is, further descent of the fetal head. The woman should be informed of such progress, for encouragement is very important. During this period of active bearing down, the fetal heart rate auscultated immediately after the contraction is likely to be slow, but should recover to normal range before the next expulsive effort.

As the head descends through the pelvis, feces is frequently expelled by the woman. As the head descends still farther, the perineum begins to bulge and the overlying skin becomes tense and glistening. Now the scalp of the fetus may be visible through the vulvar opening (Fig. 13–2). At this time, or before in instances where little perineal resistance to expulsion is antici-

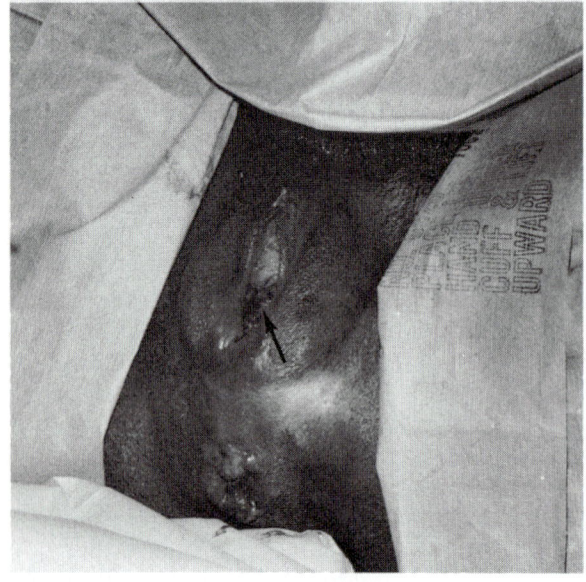

FIGURE 13–2. Scalp (*arrow*) appearing at vulva during a contraction.

pated, the woman and her fetus are prepared for delivery.

PREPARATION FOR DELIVERY. Delivery can be accomplished with the mother in a variety of positions. The most widely used and often the most satisfactory one is the dorsal lithotomy position in order to increase the diameter of the pelvic outlet. In many birthing rooms this is accomplished with the woman lying flat on the bed. For better exposure, leg holders or stirrups are used. In placing the legs in leg holders, care should be taken not to separate the legs too widely or place one leg higher than the other, as this will exert pulling forces on the perineum that might easily result in the extension of a spontaneous tear or an episiotomy into a fourth-degree tear. The popliteal region should rest comfortably in the proximal portion and the heel in the distal portion of the leg-holder. The leg should not be forced to conform to the preexisting setting. The legs are not strapped into the stirrups, thereby allowing quick flexion of the thighs back onto the abdomen should shoulder dystocia be encountered. Cramps in the legs may develop during the second stage in part because of pressure by the fetal head on nerves in the pelvis. Such cramps may be relieved by changing the position of the leg or by brief massage, but leg cramps should never be ignored.

Preparation for delivery entails vulvar and perineal cleansing. If desired, sterile drapes may be placed in such a way that only the immediate area about the vulva is exposed (Fig. 13–3). In the past, the major reason for care in scrubbing, gowning, and gloving was to protect the laboring woman from the introduction of infectious agents. Although these considerations remain valid, concern today also must be extended to the health-care providers, because of the threat of exposure to human immunodeficiency virus. Recommendations for protection of those who care for women during labor and delivery are summarized in Chapter 57 (p. 1498).

SPONTANEOUS DELIVERY

DELIVERY OF THE HEAD. With each contraction, the perineum bulges increasingly and the vulvovaginal opening becomes more dilated by the fetal head (Fig. 13–4), gradually forming an ovoid and finally an almost circular opening. With the cessation of each contraction, the opening becomes smaller as the head recedes. As the head becomes increasingly visible, the vaginal outlet and vulva are stretched further until they ultimately encircle the largest diameter of the fetal head (Fig. 13–5). This encirclement of the largest head diameter by the vulvar ring is known as crowning.

Unless an episiotomy has been made, as described

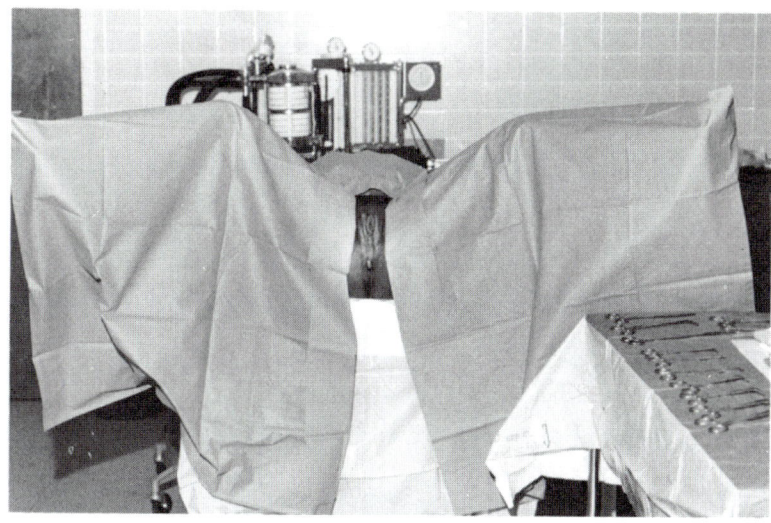

FIGURE 13–3. Following thorough scrubbing of the vulva, perineum, and adjacent regions, the field is sterile-draped in preparation for delivery.

later in the chapter, the perineum by now is extremely thin and, especially in the case of the nulliparous woman, may undergo spontaneous laceration. At the same time, the anus becomes greatly stretched and protuberant, and the anterior wall of the rectum may be easily seen through it. Over many years there has been considerable controversy concerning whether an episiotomy should be cut. We advocate individualization and do not routinely cut an episiotomy. It is now clear that an episiotomy will increase the risk of a tear into the external anal sphincter and/or the rectum. Conversely, anterior tears involving the urethra and labia are much more

common in women in whom an episiotomy is not cut. This is discussed in detail on page 325.

RITGEN MANEUVER. By the time the head distends the vulva and perineum (during a contraction) enough to open the vaginal introitus to a diameter of 5 cm or more, a towel-draped, gloved hand may be used to exert forward pressure on the chin of the fetus through the perineum just in front of the coccyx. At the same time, the other hand exerts pressure superiorly against the occiput (Fig. 13–6). Although this maneuver is simpler than that originally described by Ritgen (1855), it is

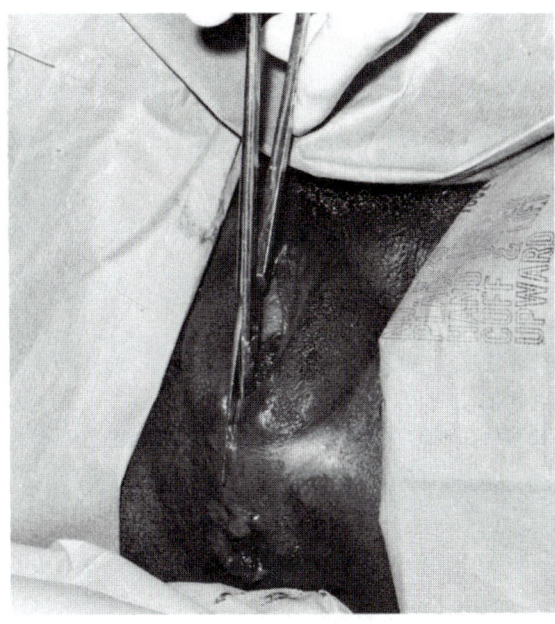

FIGURE 13–4. Vulva partially distended by fetal head. Midline episiotomy being made.

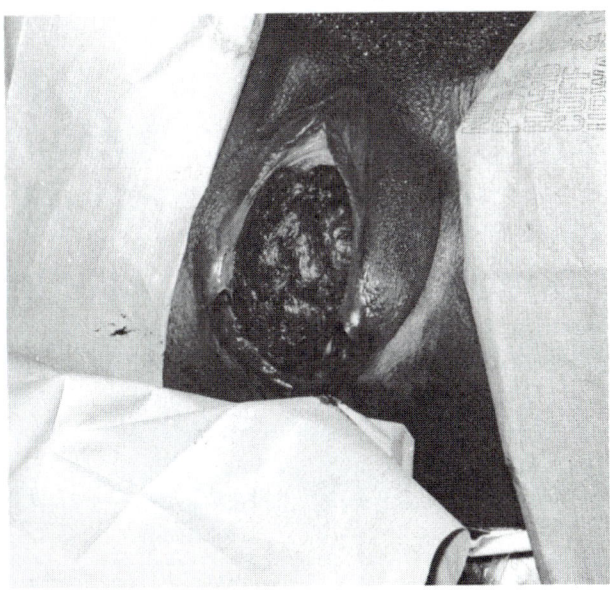

FIGURE 13–5. Birth of head. The occiput is being kept close to the symphysis by moderate pressure to the fetal chin at the tip of the maternal coccyx.

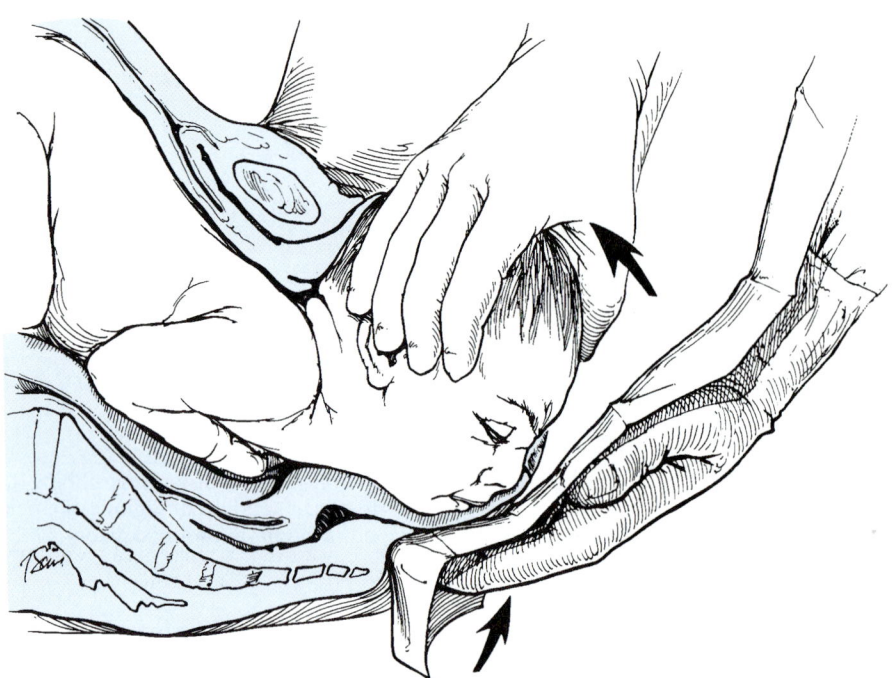

FIGURE 13–6. Near completion of the delivery of the fetal head by the modified Ritgen maneuver. Moderate upward pressure is applied to the fetal chin by the posterior hand covered with a sterile towel while the suboccipital region of the fetal head is held against the symphysis.

customarily designated the Ritgen maneuver, or the modified Ritgen maneuver. It allows control of the delivery of the head. It also favors extension, so that the head is delivered with its smallest diameters passing through the introitus and over the perineum (Fig. 13–7). The head is delivered slowly with the base of the occiput rotating around the lower margin of the symphysis pubis as a fulcrum, while the bregma (anterior fontanel), brow, and face pass successively over the perineum (Fig. 13–8).

DELIVERY OF SHOULDERS. After its birth, the head falls posteriorly, bringing the face almost into contact with the anus. As described in Chapter 12, the occiput

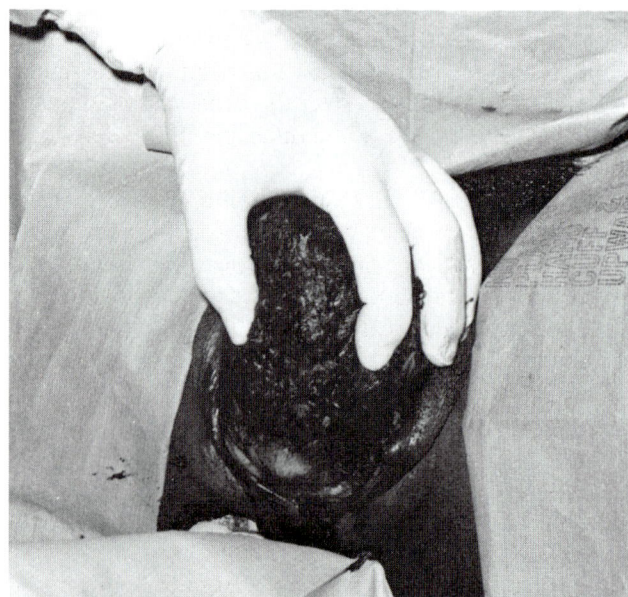

FIGURE 13–7. Pressure is applied through the towel covering the hand to the underside of the chin of the infant as soon as the occiput is beyond the symphysis. This extends the head. At the same time, the fingers of the other hand simultaneously elevate the scalp to help extend the head.

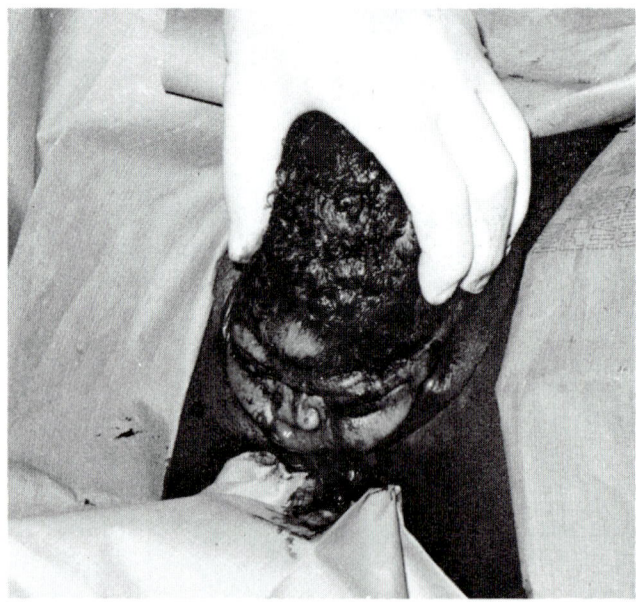

FIGURE 13–8. Birth of head; the mouth appears over the perineum.

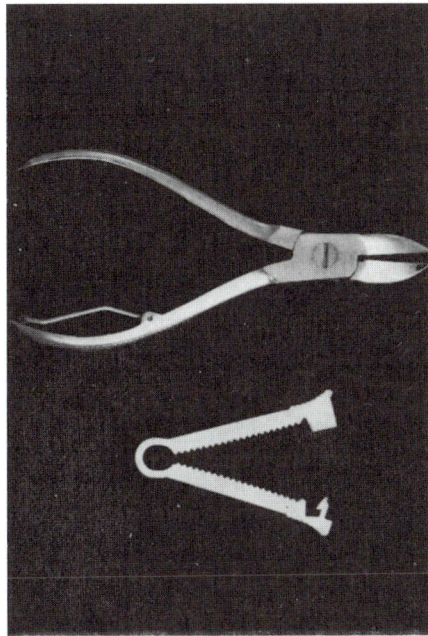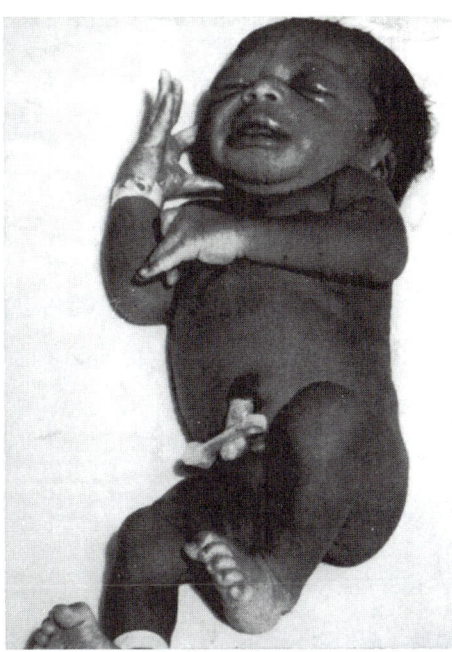

FIGURE 13–12. Plastic cord clamp. These clamps lock in place and cannot slip. They are removed on the second or third day simply by cutting the plastic at the loop, or they can be allowed to drop off with the cord.

separated is the usual practice. No massage is practiced; the hand is simply rested on the fundus frequently, to make certain that the organ does not become atonic and filled with blood behind a separated placenta.

SIGNS OF PLACENTAL SEPARATION. Because attempts to express the placenta prior to its separation are futile and possibly dangerous, it is most important that the following signs of placental separation be recognized:

1. The uterus becomes globular and, as a rule, firmer. This sign is the earliest to appear.
2. There is often a sudden gush of blood.
3. The uterus rises in the abdomen because the placenta, having separated, passes down into the lower uterine segment and vagina, where its bulk pushes the uterus upward.
4. The umbilical cord protrudes farther out of the vagina, indicating that the placenta has descended.

These signs sometimes appear within about 1 minute after delivery of the infant and usually within 5 minutes. When the placenta has separated, it should be ascertained that the uterus is firmly contracted. The mother may be asked to bear down, and the intra-abdominal pressure so produced may be adequate to expel the placenta. If these efforts fail, or if spontaneous expulsion is not possible because of anesthesia, and after ensuring that the uterus is contracted firmly, pressure is exerted with the hand on the fundus to propel the detached placenta into the vagina, as depicted and described in Figure 13–13. This approach has been termed physiological management, as later to be contrasted with "active management" of the third stage (Thilaganathan and colleagues, 1993).

DELIVERY OF THE PLACENTA. Placental expression should never be forced before placental separation lest the uterus be turned inside out. **Traction on the umbilical cord must not be used to pull the placenta out of the uterus.** *Inversion* of the uterus is one of the grave complications associated with delivery (Chap. 25, p. 642). As pressure is applied to the body of the uterus (Fig. 13–13), the umbilical cord is kept slightly taut. The uterus is lifted cephalad with the abdominal hand. This maneuver is repeated until the placenta reaches the introitus (Prendiville and associates, 1988b). As the placenta passes through the introitus, pressure on the uterus is stopped. The placenta is then gently lifted away from the introitus (Fig. 13–14). Care is taken to prevent the membranes from being torn off and left behind. If the membranes start to tear, they are grasped with a clamp and removed by gentle traction (Fig. 13–15). The maternal surface of the placenta should be examined carefully to ensure that no placental fragments are left in the uterus.

MANUAL REMOVAL OF PLACENTA. Occasionally, the placenta will not separate promptly. This is especially

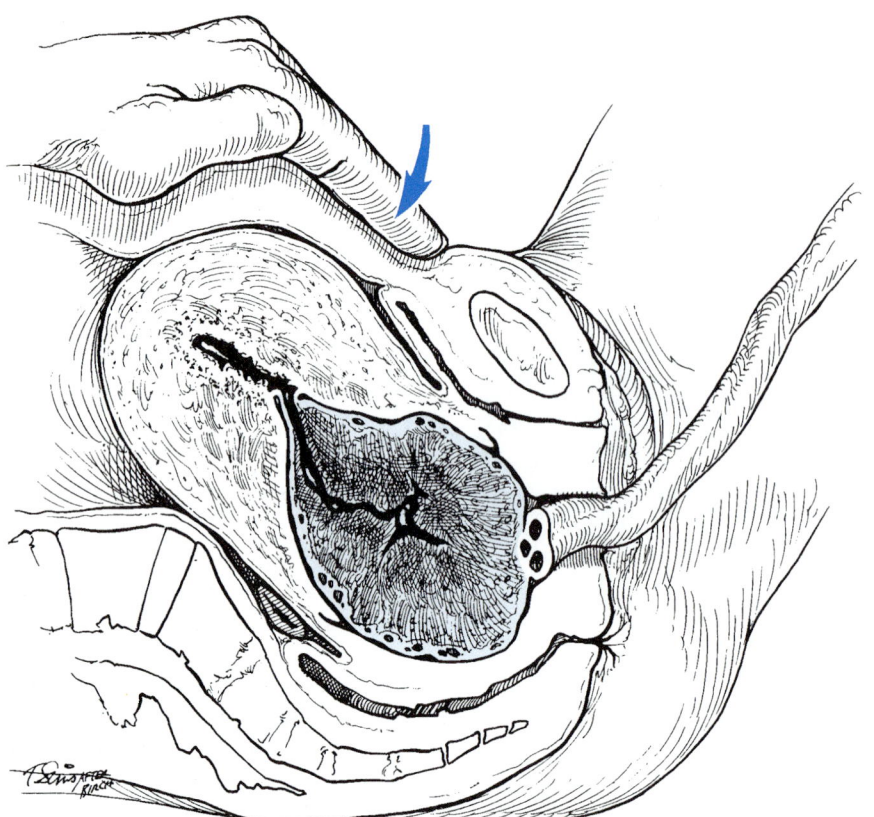

FIGURE 13-13. Expression of placenta. Note that the hand is *not* trying to push the fundus of the uterus through the birth canal! As the placenta leaves the uterus and enters the vagina, the uterus is elevated by the hand on the abdomen (*arrow*) while the cord is held in position. The mother can aid in the delivery of the placenta by bearing down. As the placenta reaches the perineum the cord is lifted, which, in turn, lifts the placenta out of the vagina. Adherent membranes are teased away from thin attachments so as to prevent their being torn off and retained in the birth canal.

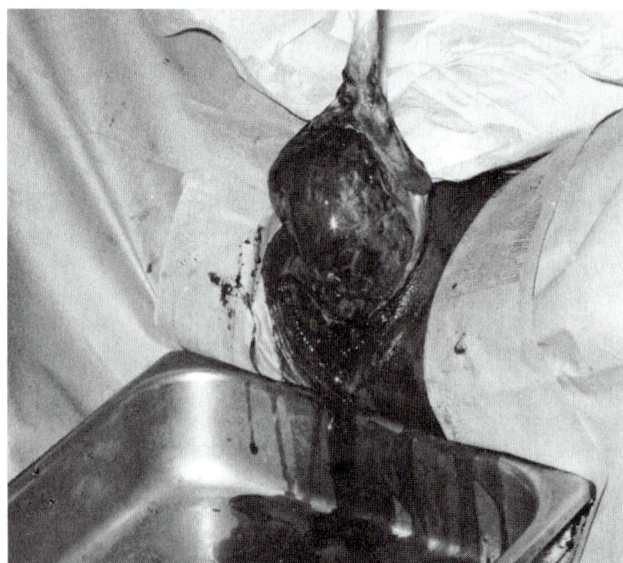

FIGURE 13-14. The placenta is removed from the vagina by lifting the cord.

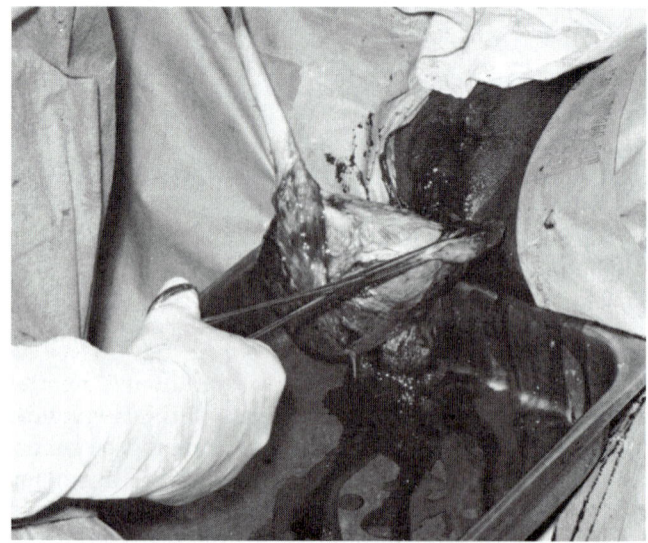

FIGURE 13-15. Membranes that were somewhat adherent to the uterine lining are separated by gentle traction with a ring forceps.

common in cases of preterm delivery (Dombrowski and colleagues, 1995). If at any time there is brisk bleeding and the placenta cannot be delivered by these techniques, manual removal of the placenta is indicated, using the safeguards described in Chapter 25 (p. 638 and Fig. 25–17). It is unclear as to the length of time that should elapse in the absence of bleeding before the placenta is manually removed. Manual removal of the placenta is rightfully practiced much sooner and more often than in the past. In fact, some obstetricians practice routine manual removal of any placenta that has not separated spontaneously by the time they have completed delivery of the infant and care of the cord in women with conduction analgesia. Proof of the benefits of this practice, however, has not been established, and most obstetricians await spontaneous placental separation unless bleeding is excessive.

ACTIVE MANAGEMENT OF THE THIRD STAGE. Thilaganathan and associates (1993) compared a regimen of active management with syntometrine (5 units of oxytocin with 0.5 mg of ergometrine) and controlled cord traction with one of physiological management wherein the cord was not clamped and the placenta was delivered by maternal efforts. Among 103 low-risk term deliveries, active management resulted in a reduction in the length of the third stage of labor, but no reduction in blood loss compared with physiological management. Mitchell and Elbourne (1993) found that syntometrine administered intramuscularly concurrent with delivery of the anterior shoulder was more effective than oxytocin (5 units intramuscularly) alone in the prevention of postpartum hemorrhage. Duration of the third stage of labor and need for manual removal of the placenta were similar. Side effects of nausea, vomiting, and blood pressure elevations with ergometrine prevented any recommendation for its routine usage.

"FOURTH STAGE" OF LABOR. The placenta, membranes, and umbilical cord should be examined for completeness and for anomalies, as described in Chapters 31 and 32. The hour immediately following delivery is critical and it has been designated by some as the "fourth stage of labor." Even though oxytocics are administered, postpartum hemorrhage as the result of uterine atony is more likely at this time. The uterus is frequently evaluated during this time. The perineum likewise is inspected frequently to detect excessive bleeding. The American Academy of Pediatrics and the American College of Obstetricians and Gynecologists (1997) recommend that maternal blood pressure and pulse should be recorded immediately after delivery and every 15 minutes for the first hour.

OXYTOCIC AGENTS

After the uterus has been emptied and the placenta has been delivered, the primary mechanism by which hemostasis is achieved at the placental site is vasoconstriction produced by a well-contracted myometrium. Oxytocin (Pitocin, Syntocinon), ergonovine maleate (Ergotrate), and methylergonovine maleate (Methergine) are employed in various ways in the conduct of the third stage of labor, principally to reduce blood loss by stimulating myometrial contractions (Phillips and Kinch, 1994; Prendiville and associates, 1988a).

OXYTOCIN. The synthetic form of the octapeptide oxytocin is commercially available in the United States as Syntocinon and Pitocin; 1 mg of oxytocin is equal to about 500 USP units. Each mL of injectable oxytocin contains 10 USP units, which is not effective by mouth. The half-life of intravenously infused oxytocin is approximately 3 minutes.

Before delivery, the spontaneously laboring uterus is very likely to be exquisitely sensitive to oxytocin. With an inappropriate dose of oxytocin, the pregnant uterus may contract so violently as to kill the fetus, rupture itself, or both (Chap. 20, p. 476). After delivery of the fetus, these dangers no longer exist. Nonetheless, at this time, there are other potentially grave dangers from inappropriate use of oxytocin.

CARDIOVASCULAR EFFECTS. Deleterious effects may on occasion follow the intravenous injection of a bolus of oxytocin. Hendricks and Brenner (1970) demonstrated with the rapid intravenous injection of 5 units (0.5 mL) of oxytocin that the uterus contracted tetanically for several minutes and maternal blood pressure decreased simultaneously. In one dramatic instance of hypotension from uterine bleeding following delivery of twins, they noted that a bolus injection of 5 units of oxytocin intravenously was promptly followed by a further decrease in blood pressure from 70/42 to 44/26 mm Hg (Fig. 13–16). After rapid administration of 500 mL of saline, the blood pressure increased and the mother again became responsive.

Secher and co-workers (1978) consistently observed that, even in healthy women, an intravenous bolus of 10 units of oxytocin caused a transient but marked fall in arterial blood pressure that was followed by an abrupt increase in cardiac output. They too concluded that these hemodynamic changes could be dangerous to women already hypovolemic from hemorrhage, or who had cardiac disease that limited cardiac output. The same danger is present for women with right-to-left cardiac shunts, as the decrease in systemic resistance would further increase the shunt. **Oxytocin should not**

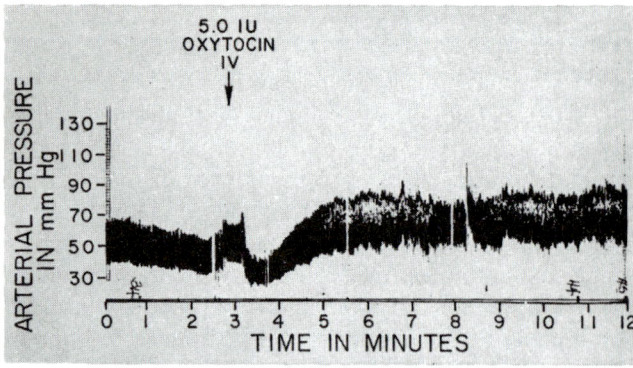

FIGURE 13–16. Adverse effect of the intravenous bolus of 5 units of oxytocin in a case of postpartum hemorrhage 18 minutes postdelivery. The hypotension worsened to a level of 44/26 mm Hg until saline was infused rapidly. (From Hendricks and Brenner, 1970).

be given intravenously as a large bolus, but rather as a much more dilute solution by continuous intravenous infusion, or be injected intramuscularly in a dose of 10 USP units. In cases of postpartum hemorrhage, direct injection into the uterus, either transvaginally or transabdominally, if following a vaginal birth, or directly if at cesarean delivery, has also proven effective. The use of nipple stimulation in the third stage of labor has also been shown to increase uterine pressures and to decrease the duration of the third stage of labor as well as blood loss (Irons and associates, 1994). Indeed, results were similar to those achieved using the combination of oxytocin (5 units) and ergometrine (0.5 mg).

ANTIDIURESIS. Although rare today, water intoxication causing maternal convulsions may result from the considerable antidiuretic action of oxytocin (Abdul-Karim and Assali, 1961). In women who are undergoing diuresis in response to the administration of water, the continuous intravenous infusion of 20 mU of oxytocin per minute usually produces a demonstrable decrease in urine flow. When the rate of infusion is raised to 40 mU/min, urinary flow is strikingly reduced. With doses of this magnitude, it is possible to produce water intoxication if the oxytocin is administered in a large volume of electrolyte-free aqueous dextrose solution (Eggers and Fliegner, 1979; Whalley and Pritchard, 1963). Schwartz and Jones (1978) described convulsions in both the mother and her newborn following the administration of 6.5 liters of 5 percent dextrose solution and 36 units of oxytocin predelivery. The concentration of sodium in cord plasma was 114 mEq/L.

In general, if oxytocin is to be administered in high doses for a considerable period of time, its concentration should be increased rather than increasing the rate of flow of a more dilute solution (see Chap. 20). Consideration should also be given to use of either normal saline or lactated Ringer solution in these circumstances.

ERGONOVINE AND METHYLERGONOVINE. Ergonovine is an alkaloid obtained from ergot, a fungus that grows on rye and some other grains, or it is synthesized in part from lysergic acid. Methylergonovine and ergonovine (also ergometrine or ergostetrine) are very similar alkaloids made from lysergic acid. The alkaloids are dispensed as the maleate (Ergotrate and Methergine) either in solution for parenteral use or in tablets for oral use.

EFFECTS. There is no convincing evidence of any appreciable difference in the actions of ergonovine and methylergonovine. Whether given intravenously, intramuscularly, or orally, ergonovine and methylergonovine are powerful stimulants of myometrial contraction, exerting an effect that may persist for hours. The sensitivity of the pregnant uterus to ergonovine and methylergonovine is very great. In pregnant women, an intravenous dose of as little as 0.1 mg, or an oral dose of only 0.25 mg, results in a tetanic uterine contraction that occurs almost immediately after intravenous injection of the drug and within a few minutes after intramuscular or oral administration. Moreover, the response is sustained with little tendency toward relaxation. The tetanic effect of ergonovine and methylergonovine is effective for the prevention and control of postpartum hemorrhage, but is very dangerous for the fetus and the mother prior to delivery.

The parenteral administration of these alkaloids, especially by the intravenous route, sometimes initiates transient but severe hypertension. Such a reaction is most likely when conduction analgesia is used for delivery and in women who are prone to develop hypertension. Browning (1974) described four instances of serious postdelivery side effects attributable to 0.5 mg of ergonovine administered intramuscularly. Two women promptly became severely hypertensive, the third became hypertensive and convulsed, and the fourth suffered a cardiac arrest. We have also seen an instance of such profound vasoconstriction from these compounds when given intravenously that all peripheral pulses were lost, and sodium nitroprusside was required to restore the peripheral circulation. Unfortunately, the mother sustained cerebral hypoxic ischemic injury. Because of the frequency of hypertension among our obstetrical population, we do not use these alkaloids routinely.

PROSTAGLANDINS. Prostaglandin compounds are not used routinely for management of the third stage of labor. Their use is restricted to the management of postpartum hemorrhage due to uterine atony, which is discussed in Chapter 25 (p. 637).

OXYTOCICS AFTER DELIVERY. Oxytocin, ergonovine, and methylergonovine are all employed widely in the conduct of the normal third stage of labor, but the timing of their administration differs in various institutions. Oxytocin, and especially ergonovine, given before delivery of the placenta will decrease blood loss somewhat (Prendiville and associates, 1988a). There is, however, a significant danger associated with this practice. The use of oxytocin, and especially ergonovine or methylergonovine, before delivery of the placenta may entrap an undiagnosed, undelivered second twin. This may prove injurious, if not fatal, to the entrapped fetus. In most cases following uncomplicated vaginal delivery, the third stage of labor can be conducted with reasonably small blood loss without using these agents before delivery of the placenta (Mitchell and Elbourne, 1993; Thilaganathan and associates, 1993).

If an intravenous infusion is in place, our standard practice has been to add 20 units (2 mL) of oxytocin per liter of infusate. This solution is administered after delivery of the placenta at a rate of 10 mL/min (200 mU/min) for a few minutes until the uterus remains firmly contracted and bleeding is controlled. The infusion rate then is reduced to 1 to 2 mL/min until the mother is ready for transfer from the recovery suite to the postpartum unit. At this time, the infusion is usually discontinued.

LACERATIONS OF THE BIRTH CANAL

Lacerations of the vagina and perineum are classified as first, second, third, or fourth degree. First-degree lacerations involve the fourchette, perineal skin, and vaginal mucous membrane but not the underlying fascia and muscle. Second-degree lacerations involve, in addition to skin and mucous membrane, the fascia and muscles of the perineal body but not the anal sphincter (Fig. 13–17). These tears usually extend upward on one or both sides of the vagina, forming an irregular triangular injury. Third-degree lacerations extend through the skin, mucous membrane, and perineal body, and involve the anal sphincter. A fourth-degree laceration extends through the rectal mucosa to expose the lumen of the rectum. Tears in the region of the urethra that may bleed profusely are also likely to occur with this type of laceration.

Because the repair of perineal tears is virtually the same as that of episiotomy incisions, albeit often less satisfactory because of irregular lines of tissue cleavage, the technique of repairing lacerations is discussed in the following section.

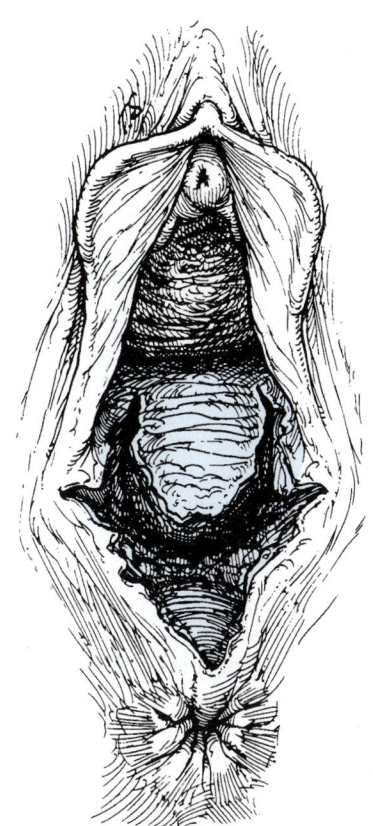

FIGURE 13–17. Deep second-degree laceration of perineum and vagina.

EPISIOTOMY AND REPAIR

In a strict sense, episiotomy is incision of the pudenda. Perineotomy is incision of the perineum. In common parlance, however, episiotomy is often used synonymously with perineotomy, a practice that will be followed here. The incision may be made in the midline (median or midline episiotomy), or it may begin in the midline but be directed laterally and downward away from the rectum (mediolateral episiotomy).

PURPOSES OF EPISIOTOMY. While still a common obstetrical procedure, the use of episiotomy has decreased remarkably over the past 20 years. Through the 1970s, it was common practice to cut an episiotomy for almost all women having their first delivery. This practice became controversial, and with the concept of evidence-based outcomes, a number of large studies have been carried out to address these controversies. The reasons for its popularity included substitution of a straight, neat surgical incision for the ragged laceration that otherwise might result. It is easier to repair, but the long-held beliefs that postoperative pain is less and healing improved with an episiotomy compared with a tear appeared not to be true (Larsson and colleagues, 1991).

Another commonly cited but unproven benefit of routine episiotomy was that it prevented pelvic relaxation, that is, cystocele, rectocele, and urinary incontinence. A number of observational studies and randomized trials showed that routine episiotomy is associated with an increased incidence of anal sphincter and rectal tears (Angioli, 2000; Argentine Collaborative Group, 1993; Eason, 2000; Henriksen, 1992; Thorp, 1987; Wilcox, 1989, and all their colleagues).

Carroli and Belizan (2000) reviewed the Cochrane Pregnancy and Childbirth Group trials registry. There were six randomized trials of nearly 5000 deliveries in which routine (73 percent rate) versus restrictive (28 percent rate) use of episiotomy was evaluated. There was less posterior perineal trauma, need for repair, and healing complications in the restrictive-use group. Alternatively, there was less anterior perineal trauma in the routine-use group. Along with these findings came the realization that while episiotomy did not protect the perineal body, it contributed to anal sphincter incontinence by increasing the risk of third- and fourth-degree tears. Signorello and associates (2000) reported that fecal and flatus incontinence were increased four- to sixfold in women with an episiotomy compared with a group delivered over an intact perineum. Even compared with spontaneous perineal lacerations, episiotomy tripled the risk of fecal incontinence and doubled it for flatus incontinence. Non-extension of the episiotomy did not lower this risk. Finally, even with recognition and repair of a third-degree extension, 30 to 40 percent of women have long-term anal incontinence (Gjessing and co-workers, 1998; Poen and colleagues, 1998).

It seems reasonable to conclude that episiotomy should not be performed routinely (Eason and Feldman, 2000). The procedure should be applied selectively for appropriate indications, some of which include fetal indications such as shoulder dystocia and breech delivery; forceps or vacuum extractor operations; occiput posterior positions; and in instances where it is obvious that failure to perform an episiotomy will result in perineal rupture. **The final rule is that there is no substitute for surgical judgment and common sense.**

The important variables if an episiotomy is to be used include when the incision is performed, the type of incision, and techniques for repair.

TIMING OF EPISIOTOMY. If episiotomy is performed unnecessarily early, bleeding from the incision may be considerable during the interim between the episiotomy and the delivery. If episiotomy is performed too late, lacerations will not be prevented. It is common practice to perform episiotomy when the head is visible during a contraction to a diameter of 3 to 4 cm (see Fig. 13–4).

When used in conjunction with forceps delivery, most practitioners perform an episiotomy after application of the blades (Chap. 21, p. 493).

MIDLINE VERSUS MEDIOLATERAL EPISIOTOMY. The advantages and disadvantages of the two types of episiotomies are summarized in Table 13–4. Except for the important issue of third- and fourth-degree extensions, midline episiotomy is superior. With proper selection of cases, it is possible to secure the advantages of midline episiotomy and at the same time reduce to a minimum this one disadvantage. In addition to a midline episiotomy, Combs and associates (1990) reported the following factors to be associated with an increased risk for third- and fourth-degree lacerations: nulliparity, second-stage arrest of labor, persistent occiput posterior position, mid- or low-forceps instead of a vacuum extractor, use of local anesthetics, and Asian race.

It is reasonable to use a mediolateral episiotomy when a third- or fourth-degree extension is likely, but to employ the midline incision otherwise. This policy was substantiated by Anthony and colleagues (1994), who presented data from the Dutch National Obstetric Database of over 43,000 deliveries. Indeed, many practitioners in the United States use midline episiotomy exclusively. Even with careful selection, however, the total number of third- and fourth-degree lacerations sustained with this policy is probably greater than with routine mediolateral episiotomy.

Venkatesh and colleagues (1989) reported a 5-percent incidence of third- and fourth-degree perineal tears in 20,500 vaginal deliveries. About 10 percent of these 1040 primary repairs had a wound disruption and 67 of the 101 required surgical correction. Goldaber and associates (1993) found that 21 of 390 (5.4 percent) women with fourth-degree lacerations experienced significant morbidity. There were 7 (1.8 percent) dehiscences, 11 (2.8 percent) infections with dehiscences, and 3 (0.8 percent) infections alone. Although administration of perioperative antibiotics (cefazolin sodium,

TABLE 13–4. Midline versus Mediolateral Episiotomy

Characteristic	Type of Episiotomy	
	Midline	*Mediolateral*
Surgical repair	Easy	More difficult
Faulty healing	Rare	More common
Postoperative pain	Minimal	Common
Anatomical results	Excellent	Occasionally faulty
Blood loss	Less	More
Dyspareunia	Rare	Occasional
Extensions	Common	Uncommon

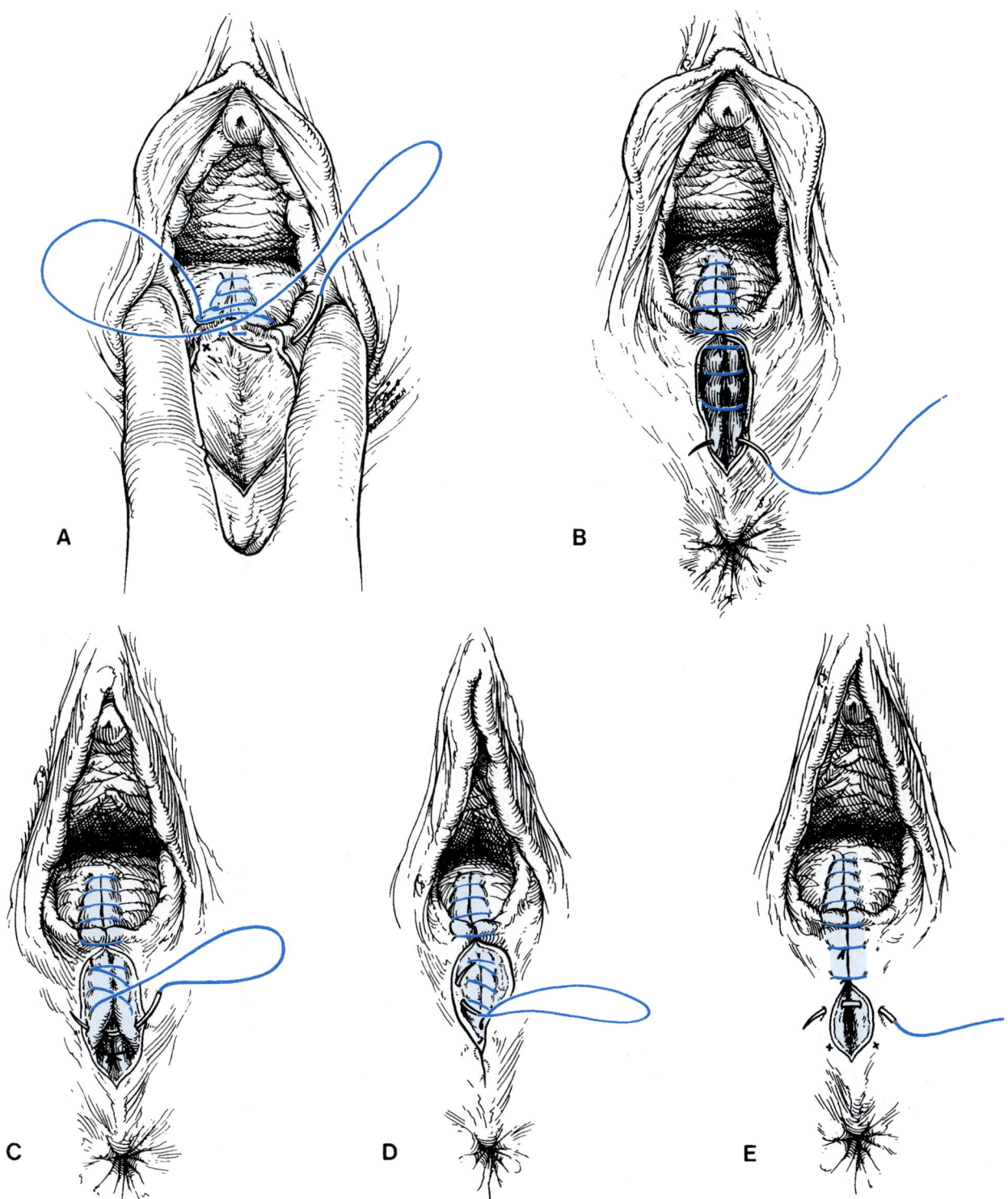

FIGURE 13–18. Repair of median episiotomy. **A.** Chromic 2-0 or 3-0 suture is used as a continuous suture to close the vaginal mucosa and submucosa. **B.** After closing the vaginal incision and reapproximating the cut margins of the hymenal ring, the suture is tied and cut. Next, three or four interrupted sutures of 2-0 or 3-0 chromic are placed in the fascia and muscle of the incised perineum. **C.** A continuous suture is carried downward to unite the superficial fascia. **D.** Completion of repair. The continuous suture is carried upward as a subcuticular stitch. (An alternative method of closure of skin and subcutaneous fascia is illustrated in E.) **E.** Completion of repair of median episiotomy. A few interrupted sutures of 3-0 chromic are placed through the skin and subcutaneous fascia and loosely tied. This closure avoids burying two layers of suture in the more superficial layers of the perineum.

2 g intravenously) reduced this morbidity, it was not totally eliminated.

TIMING OF THE REPAIR OF EPISIOTOMY. The most common practice is to defer episiotomy repair until the placenta has been delivered. This policy permits undivided attention to the signs of placental separation and delivery. Early delivery of the placenta is believed to decrease blood loss from the implantation site because it prevents the development of extensive retroplacental bleeding. A further advantage is that episiotomy repair is not interrupted or disrupted by the obvious necessity of delivering the placenta, especially if manual removal must be performed.

TECHNIQUE. There are many ways to close an episiotomy incision, but *hemostasis and anatomical restoration without excessive suturing are essential* for success with any method. A technique that commonly is employed is shown in Figure 13–18. The suture material ordinarily used is 3-0 chromic catgut, but Grant (1989) recommends suture composed of derivatives of polyglycolic acid. A decrease in postsurgical pain is cited as the major advantage of the newer materials despite the occasional need to remove some of the suture from the site of repair. It is important to distinguish that the repairs described by Grant involved predominantly mediolateral episiotomies and an entirely different closure, including transdermal sutures, than is usually employed for midline episiotomies, especially as done in the United States.

FOURTH-DEGREE LACERATION. The technique of repairing a fourth-degree laceration is shown in Figure 13–19. Various techniques have been recommended; but in all instances, it is essential to approximate the torn edges of the rectal mucosa with muscularis sutures placed approximately 0.5 cm apart. This muscular layer then is covered with a layer of fascia. Finally, the cut ends of the anal sphincter are isolated, approximated, and sutured together with three or four interrupted stitches. The remainder of the repair is the same as for an episiotomy. Stool softeners should be prescribed for a week, and enemas should be avoided. Prophylactic antimicrobials should be considered, as described by Goldaber and colleagues (1993).

Unfortunately, normal function is not always assured even with correct and complete surgical repair. Some women may experience continuing fecal incontinence due to injury to the innervation of the pelvic floor musculature (Roberts and co-workers, 1990).

PAIN AFTER EPISIOTOMY. Application of ice packs tends to reduce swelling and allay discomfort. Aerosol sprays containing a local anesthetic are helpful at times.

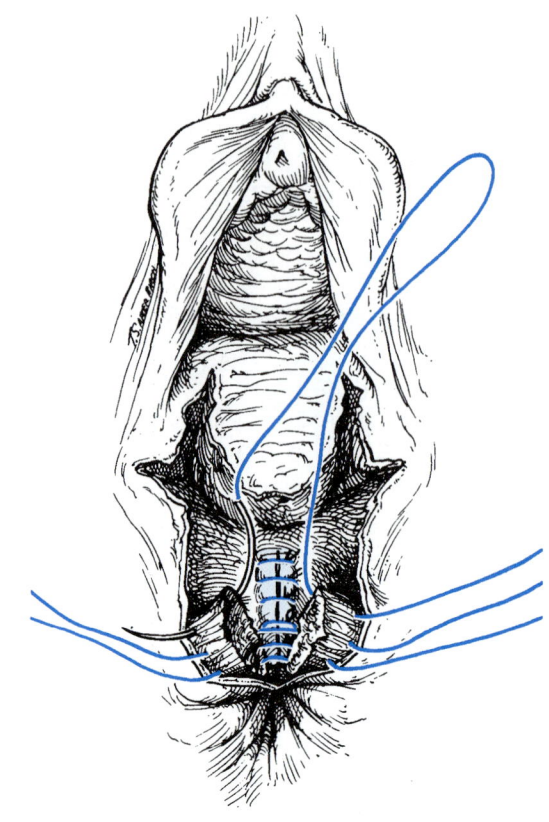

FIGURE 13–19. Repair of complete perineal tear. The rectal mucosa has been repaired with interrupted, fine (3-0 or 4-0) chromic sutures. The torn ends of the sphincter ani are next approximated with two or three interrupted chromic or Vicryl (2-0) sutures. The wound is then repaired, as in a second-degree laceration or an episiotomy.

Analgesics such as codeine give considerable relief. **Because pain may be a signal of a large vulvar, paravaginal, or ischiorectal hematoma or perineal cellulitis, it is essential to examine these sites carefully if pain is severe or persistent.** Management of these complications is discussed in Chapter 25.

REFERENCES

Abdul-Karim R, Assali NS: Renal function in human pregnancy, 5. Effects of oxytocin on renal hemodynamics and water and electrolyte excretion. J Lab Clin Med 57:522, 1961

American Academy of Pediatrics and the American College of Obstetricians and Gynecologists: Guidelines for Perinatal Care, 4th ed. 1997

American College of Obstetricians and Gynecologists: Precis, Obstetrics: An update in obstetrics and gynecology. Washington, D.C., American College of Obstetricians and Gynecologists, 2000

American College of Obstetricians and Gynecologists: Prevention of early-onset group B streptococcal disease in newborns. Committee Opinion no 173, June, 1996

Angioli R, Gomez-Marin O, Cantuaria G, O'Sullivan MJ: Severe perineal lacerations during vaginal delivery: The University of Miami experience. Am J Obstet Gynecol 182:1083, 2000

Anthony S, Buitendijk SE, Zondervan KT, Van Rijssel EJC, Verkerk PH: Episiotomies and the occurrence of severe perineal lacerations. Br J Obstet Gynaecol 101:1064, 1994

Argentine Episiotomy Trial Collaborative Group: Routine versus selective episiotomy: A randomized controlled trial. Lancet 342:1515, 1993

Baptisti A: Chemical test for the determination of ruptured membranes. Am J Obstet Gynecol 35:688, 1938

Bloom SL, McIntire DD, Kelly MA, Beimer HL, Burpo RH, Garcia MA, Leveno KJ: Lack of effect of walking on labor and delivery. N Engl J Med 339:76, 1998

Browning DJ: Serious side effects of ergometrine and its use in routine obstetric practice. Med J Aust 1:957, 1974

Carroli G, Belizan J: Episiotomy for vaginal birth. Cochrane Database Syst Rev 2:CD000081, 2000

Combs CA, Robertson PA, Laros RK: Risk factors for third-degree and fourth-degree perineal lacerations in forceps and vacuum deliveries. Am J Obstet Gynecol 163:100, 1990

Dombrowski MP, Bottoms SF, Saleh AAA, Hurd WW, Romero R: Third stage of labor: Analysis of duration and clinical practice. Am J Obstet Gynecol 172:1279, 1995

Eason E, Feldman P: Much ado about a little cut: Is episiotomy worthwhile? Obstet Gynecol 95:616, 2000

Eason E, Labrecque M, Wells G, Feldman P: Preventing perineal trauma during childbirth: A systematic review. Obstet Gynecol 95:464, 2000

Eggers TR, Fliegner JR: Water intoxication and syntocinon intoxication. Aust NZ J Obstet Gynaecol 19:59, 1979

Freeman K, Garite TJ, Nageotte MP: Pitfalls in intrapartum fetal monitoring. In Freeman K, Garite TJ, Nageotte MP (eds): Fetal Heart Rate Monitoring, 2nd ed. Baltimore, Williams & Wilkins, 1991, p 206

Gardosi J, Hutson N, Lynch CB: Randomised, controlled trial of squatting in the second stage of labour. Lancet 2:74, 1989

Gjessing H, Backe B, Sahlin Y: Third degree obstetric tears; outcome after primary repair. Acta Obstet Gynecol Scand 77:736, 1998

Goldaber KG, Wendel PJ, McIntire DD, Wendel GD: Postpartum perineal morbidity after fourth-degree perineal repair. Am J Obstet Gynecol 168:489, 1993

Grant A: The choice of suture materials and techniques for repair of perineal trauma: An overview of the evidence from controlled trials. Br J Obstet Gynaecol 96:1281, 1989

Guyton TS, Gibbs CP: Aspiration: Risk, Prophylaxis, and Treatment. In Chestnut DH (ed): Obstetric Anesthesia. Principles and Practice. St. Louis, Mosby, 1994, p 567

Hendricks CH, Brenner WE: Cardiovascular effects of oxytocic drugs used postpartum. Am J Obstet Gynecol 108:751, 1970

Henriksen TB, Bek KM, Hedegaard M, Secher NJ: Episiotomy and perineal lesions in spontaneous vaginal deliveries. Br J Obstet Gynaecol 99:950, 1992

Ingemarsson I, Arulkumaran S, Ingemarsson E, Tambyraja RL, Ratnam SS: Admission test: A screening test for fetal distress in labor. Obstet Gynecol 68:800, 1986

Ingemarsson I, Arulkumaran S, Paul RH, Ingemarsson E, Tambyraja RL, Ratnam SS: Fetal acoustic stimulation in early labor in patients screened with the admission test. Am J Obstet Gynecol 158:70, 1988

Irons DW, Sriskandabalan P, Bullough CH: A simple alternative to parental oxytocics for the third stage of labor. Int J Gynaecol Obstet 46:15, 1994

Larsson P, Platz-Christensen J, Bergman B, Wallstersson G: Advantage or disadvantage of episiotomy compared with spontaneous perineal laceration. Gynecol Obstet Invest 31:213, 1991

Mitchell GG, Elbourne DR: The Salford Third-stage Trial. Oxytocin plus ergometrine versus oxytocin alone in the active management of the third stage of labor. Online J Curr Clin Trials 83; 1993

Phillips CA, Kinch RA: Management of the third stage of labor: A survey of practice among Texas obstetricians. Tex Med 90:44, 1994

Poen AC, Felt-Bersma RJ, Strijers RL, Dekker GA, Cuesta MA, Meuwissen SG: Third-degree obstetric perineal tear: Long-term clinical and functional results after primary repair. Br J Surg 85:1433, 1998

Prendiville W, Elbourne D, Chalmers I: The effects of routine oxytocic administration in the management of the third stage of labour: An overview of the evidence from controlled trials. Br J Obstet Gynaecol 95:3, 1988a

Prendiville WJ, Harding JE, Elbourne DR, Stirrat GM: The Bristol third stage trial: Active versus physiological management of third stage of labour. Br Med J 297:1295, 1988b

Ritgen G: Concerning his method for protection of the perineum. Monatschrift für Geburtskunde 6:21, 1855. See English translation, Wynn RM: Am J Obstet Gynecol 93:421, 1965

Roberts PL, Coller JA, Schoetz DJ, Veidenheimer MC: Manometric assessment of patients with obstetric injuries and fecal incontinence. Dis Colon Rectum 33:16, 1990

Sarno AP, Ahn MO, Phelan JP, Paul RH: Fetal acoustic stimulation in the early intrapartum period as a predictor of subsequent fetal condition. Am J Obstet Gynecol 162:762, 1990

Schwartz RH, Jones RWA: Transplacental hyponatremia due to oxytocin. Br Med J 1:152, 1978

Secher NJ, Arnso P, Wallin L: Haemodynamic effects of oxytocin (Syntocinon) and methylergometrine (Methergin) on the systemic and pulmonary circulations of pregnant anaesthetized women. Acta Obstet Gynecol Scand 57:97, 1978

Signorello LB, Harlow BL, Chekos AK, Repke JT: Midline episiotomy and anal incontinence: Retrospective cohort study. BMJ 320:86, 2000

Thilaganathan B, Cutner A, Latimer J, Beard R: Management of the third-stage of labour in women at low risk of postpartum haemorrhage. Eur J Obstet Gynecol Reprod Biol 48:19, 1993

Thorp JM Jr, Bowes WA Jr, Brame RG, Cefalo R: Selected use of midline episiotomy: Effect of perineal trauma. Obstet Gynecol 70:260, 1987

Venkatesh KS, Ramanujam PS, Larson DM, Haywood MA: Anorectal complications of vaginal delivery. Dis Colon Rectum 32:1039, 1989

Whalley PJ, Pritchard JA: Oxytocin and water intoxication. JAMA 186:601, 1963

Wilcox LS, Strobino DM, Baruffi G, Dellinger WS: Episiotomy and its role in the incidence of perineal lacerations in a maternity center and a tertiary hospital obstetric service. Am J Obstet Gynecol 160:1047, 1989

Yamada H, Kishida T, Negishi H, Sagawa T, Fujimoto S: Silent premature rupture of membranes, detected and monitored serially by an AFP kit. J Obstet Gynaecol Res 24:103, 1998

Yao AC, Lind J: Placental transfusion. Am J Dis Child 127:128, 1974

14

Intrapartum Assessment

INTRAPARTUM FETAL ASSESSMENT

Internal Electronic Fetal Heart Rate Monitoring
External (Indirect) Electronic Fetal Heart Rate Monitoring
Fetal Heart Rate Patterns
Fetal Scalp Blood Sampling
Complications from Electronic Fetal Monitoring
Fetal Distress
Benefits of Electronic Fetal Heart Rate Monitoring

INTRAPARTUM SURVEILLANCE OF UTERINE ACTIVITY

Internal Uterine Pressure Monitoring
External Monitoring
Patterns of Uterine Activity

As safe methods were developed to intervene opera-tively during labor, various methods of intrapartum sur-veillance have been designed. Periodic auscultation with a fetoscope led to development of continuous electronic fetal heart rate monitoring, which is a marvelous inven-tion introduced into obstetrical practice during the late 1960s. No longer was the perception of fetal distress limited to heart sounds; the continuous graph paper portrayal of the fetal heart rate was potentially diagnos-tic in assessing pathophysiological events affecting the fetus. There were great expectations that:

1. Electronic fetal heart rate monitoring provided accu-rate information.
2. The information was of value in diagnosing fetal dis-tress.
3. It would be possible to intervene to prevent fetal death or morbidity.
4. Continuous electronic fetal heart rate monitoring was superior to intermittent methods.

When first introduced, electronic fetal heart rate monitoring was used primarily in complicated preg-nancies, but gradually it came to be used in most pregnancies. By 1978 it was estimated that nearly two thirds of American women were being monitored elec-tronically during labor (Banta and Thacker, 1979). In 1998, nearly 3.3 million American women, comprising 84 percent of all live births, underwent electronic fetal monitoring (Ventura and colleagues, 2000). Indeed, fe-tal monitoring was the most prevalent obstetrical proce-dure in the United States.

INTRAPARTUM FETAL ASSESSMENT

INTERNAL ELECTRONIC FETAL HEART RATE MONI-TORING. The fetal heart rate may be measured by at-taching a bipolar spiral electrode directly to the fetus (Fig. 14–1). The wire electrode penetrates the fetal scalp and the second pole is the metal wing on the electrode. Vaginal body fluids create a saline electrical bridge that completes the circuit and permits measurement of the voltage differences between the two poles. The electrical fetal cardiac signal—P wave, QRS complex, and T wave—is amplified and fed into a cardiotachometer for heart rate calculation. The peak R-wave voltage is the portion of the fetal electrocardiogram most reliably de-tected. The two wires of the bipolar electrode are attached to a reference electrode on the maternal thigh to eliminate electrical interference. Shown in Figure 14–2 is an example of the method of fetal heart rate processing employed when a scalp electrode is used. Time (t) in milliseconds between fetal R waves is fed into a cardiotachometer, where a new fetal heart rate

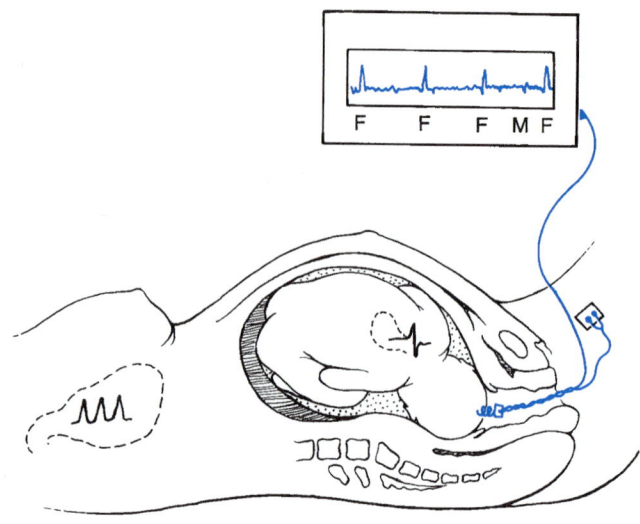

FIGURE 14–1. Schematic representation of bipolar electrode attached to fetal scalp for detection of fetal QRS complexes (F). Also shown is the maternal heart and corresponding electrical complexes (M). (Modified from Klavan and co-authors, 1977).

is set with the arrival of each new R wave. As shown in Figure 14–2, a premature atrial contraction is com-puted as a heart rate acceleration because the interval (t_2) is shorter than the preceding one (t_1). The phenom-ena of continuous R wave to R wave fetal heart rate

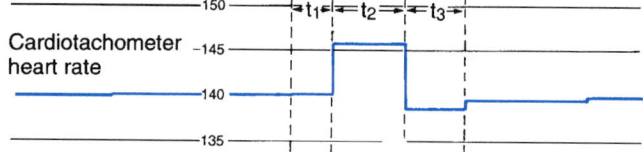

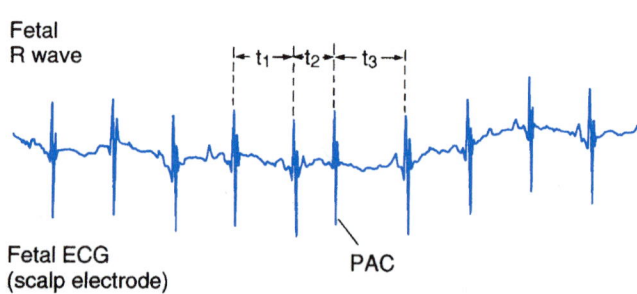

FIGURE 14–2. Schematic representation of fetal electrocar-diographic signals used to compute continuing beat-to-beat heart rate with scalp electrodes. Time intervals (t_1, t_2, t_3) in seconds between successive fetal R waves are used by car-diotachometer to compute instantaneous fetal heart rate. (PAC = premature atrial contraction.)

computation is known as *beat-to-beat variability*. The physiological event being counted, however, is not a mechanical event corresponding to a heartbeat but rather an electrical event.

Electrical cardiac complexes detected by the electrode include those generated by the mother. Although the maternal electrocardiogram (ECG) signal is approximately five times stronger than the fetal ECG, its amplitude is diminished when it is recorded through the fetal scalp electrode. In a live fetus, this low maternal ECG signal is detected but masked by the fetal ECG. If the fetus is dead, the weaker maternal signal will be amplified by the automatic gain control circuitry in the fetal monitor and displayed as "fetal" heart rate (Freeman and co-authors, 1991). Shown in Figure 14–3 are simultaneous recordings of maternal chest wall ECG signals and fetal scalp electrode ECG signals. This fetus is experiencing premature atrial contractions, which cause the cardiotachometer to rapidly and erratically seek new heart rates, resulting in the rate "spiking" shown in the standard fetal monitor tracing. Importantly, when the fetus is dead, the maternal R waves are still detected by the scalp electrode and are counted by the cardiotachometer as the next best signal (Fig. 14–4).

EXTERNAL (INDIRECT) ELECTRONIC FETAL HEART RATE MONITORING. The necessity for membrane rupture and uterine invasion may be avoided by use of external detectors to monitor fetal heart action and uterine activity. External monitoring does not provide the precision of fetal heart measurement or the quantification of uterine pressure afforded by internal monitoring.

The fetal heart rate is detected through the maternal abdominal wall using the *ultrasound Doppler principle* (Fig. 14–5). Ultrasonic waves undergo a shift in frequency as they are reflected from moving fetal heart valves and from pulsatile blood ejected during systole. The unit consists of a transducer that emits ultrasound and a sensor to detect a shift in frequency of the reflected sound. The transducer is placed on the maternal abdomen at a site where fetal heart action is best detected. A coupling gel must be applied because air conducts ultrasound poorly. The device is held in position by a belt. Care should be taken that maternal aortic pulsations are not confused with fetal cardiac motion.

Ultrasound Doppler signals are edited electronically before fetal heart rate data are printed onto the bedside monitor tracing paper. Reflected ultrasound signals from moving fetal heart valves are put through a micro-

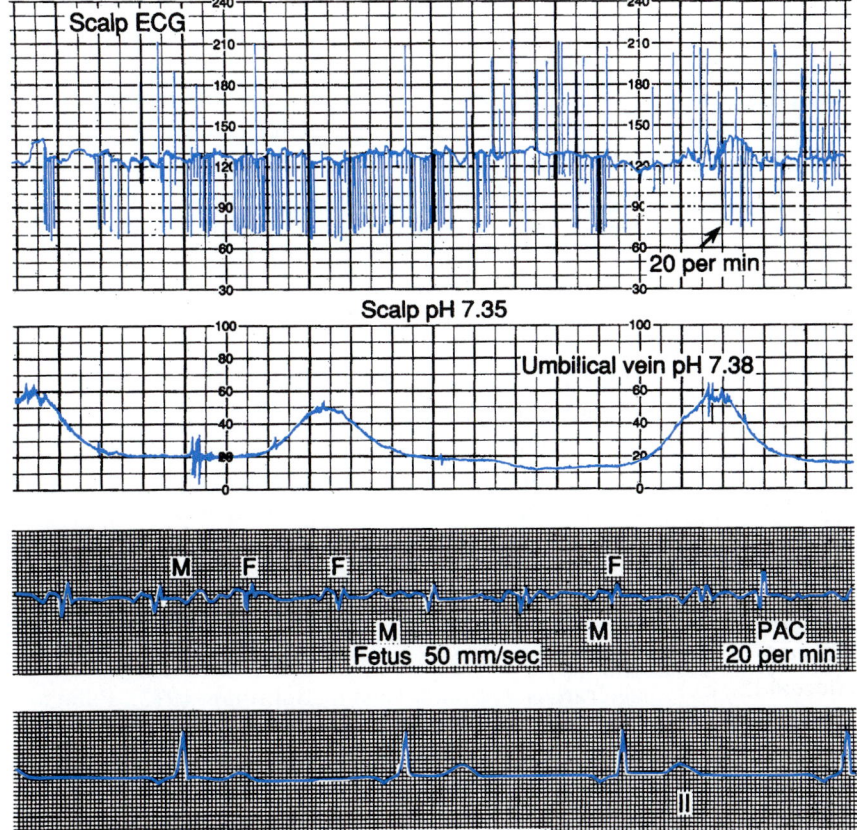

FIGURE 14–3. Standard fetal monitor tracing of heart rate using fetal scalp electrode shown at top. Bottom two tracings represent cardiac electrical complexes detected from fetal scalp and maternal chest wall electrodes. Spiking of the fetal rate in the monitor tracing is due to the premature atrial contractions. (F = fetus; M = mother; PAC = fetal premature atrial contraction.)

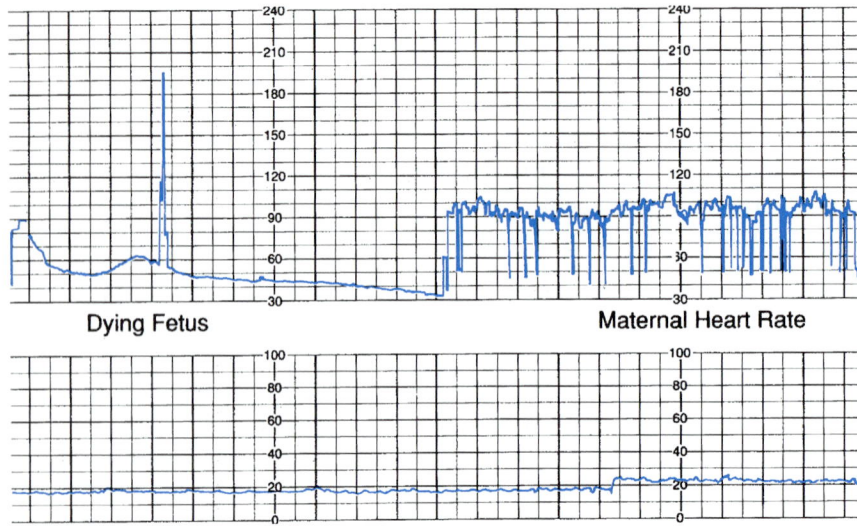

Dying Fetus   **Maternal Heart Rate**

FIGURE 14–4. Placental abruption: The fetal scalp electrode detected heart rate first of the dying fetus. After fetal death, the maternal ECG complex is detected and recorded.

processor that compares incoming signals with the most recent previous signal. This process, called *auto-correlation*, is based on the premise that the fetal heart rate has regularity whereas "noise" is random and without regularity. Several fetal heart motions must be deemed electronically acceptable by the microprocessor before the fetal heart rate is printed. Such electronic editing has greatly improved the tracing quality of externally recorded fetal heart rate.

FETAL HEART RATE PATTERNS. It is now generally accepted that interpretation of fetal heart rate patterns can be problematic because of the lack of agreement on definitions and nomenclature (Parer and Quilligan, 1996). The National Institute of Child Health and Hu-

man Development (NICHD) Fetal Monitoring Workshop (1997) brought together investigators with expertise in the field to propose standardized, unambiguous definitions for interpretation of fetal heart rate patterns during labor. The definitions proposed as a result of this workshop will be used in this chapter. It is important to recognize that interpretation of electronic fetal heart rate data is based upon the visual pattern of the heart rate as portrayed on chart recorder graph paper. Thus, the choice of vertical and horizontal scaling greatly affects the appearance of the fetal heart rate. Scaling factors recommended by the workshop are 30 bpm per vertical cm (range, 30 to 240 bpm) and 3 cm/min chart recorder paper speed. Fetal heart rate variation is falsely displayed at the slower 1 cm/min paper speed when compared with the smoother baseline recorded at 3 cm/min (Fig. 14–6). Thus, pattern recognition can be considerably distorted depending on the scaling factors used.

BASELINE FETAL HEART ACTIVITY. Baseline fetal heart activity refers to the modal characteristics that prevail apart from periodic accelerations or decelerations associated with uterine contractions. Descriptive characteristics of baseline fetal heart activity include *rate, beat-to-beat variability, fetal arrhythmia*, and distinct patterns such as *sinusoidal* or *saltatory* fetal heart rates.

RATE. With increasing fetal maturation, the heart rate decreases. This continues postnatally such that the average rate is 90 bpm by age 8 (Behrman, 1992). Pillai and James (1990) longitudinally studied fetal heart rate characteristics in 43 normal pregnancies. The baseline fetal heart rate decreased an average of 24 bpm between 16 weeks and term, or approximately 1 bpm/week. At 16 weeks the average baseline rate was about

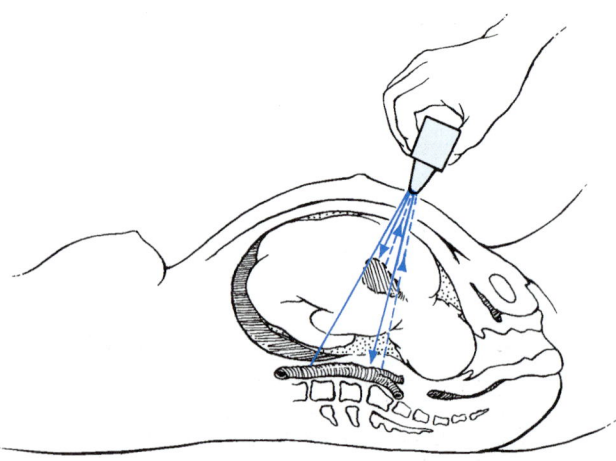

FIGURE 14–5. Ultrasound Doppler principle used externally to measure fetal heart motions. Pulsations of the maternal aorta may also be detected and counted. (Adapted from Klavan and co-authors, 1977, with permission.)

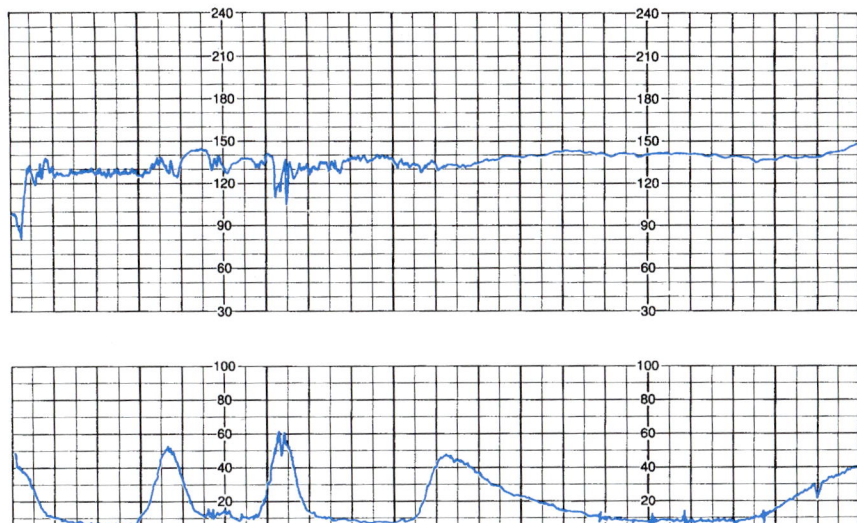

FIGURE 14-6. Fetal heart rate obtained by scalp electrode and recorded at 1 cm/min compared with 3 cm/min chart recorder paper speed.

160 bpm, which decreased to 150 at 40 weeks. It is postulated that this normal gradual slowing of the fetal heart rate corresponds to maturation of parasympathetic (vagal) heart control (Renou and co-workers, 1969).

The baseline fetal heart rate is the approximate mean rate rounded to increments of 5 bpm during a 10-minute tracing segment. In any 10-minute window the minimum interpretable baseline duration must be at least 2 minutes. If the baseline fetal heart rate is less than 110 bpm, it is termed **bradycardia;** if the baseline rate is greater than 160 bpm, it is termed **tachycardia.** The average fetal heart rate is considered to be the result of tonic balance between *accelerator* and *decelerator* influences on pacemaker cells. In this concept, the sympathetic system is the accelerator influence, and the parasympathetic system is the decelerator factor mediated via vagal slowing of heart rate (Dawes, 1985). Heart rate is also under the control of arterial chemoreceptors such that both hypoxia and hypercapnia can modulate rate. More severe and prolonged hypoxia, with a rising blood lactate level and severe metabolic acidemia, induces a prolonged fall of heart rate due to direct effects on the myocardium.

BRADYCARDIA. During the third trimester, the normal mean baseline fetal heart rate has generally been accepted to be between 120 and 160 bpm. The lower normal limit is disputed internationally with some investigators recommending 110 bpm (Manassiev, 1996). Pragmatically, a rate between 100 and 119 bpm, in the absence of other changes, is usually not considered to represent fetal compromise. Such low but potentially normal baseline heart rates have also been attributed to head compression from occiput posterior or transverse positions, particularly during second-stage labor

(Young and Weinstein, 1976). Such mild bradycardias were observed in 2 percent of monitored pregnancies and averaged about 50 minutes in duration. Moderate bradycardias are defined as 80 to 100 bpm, and severe bradycardias are less than 80 bpm, for 3 minutes or longer (Freeman and co-authors, 1991).

Other causes of fetal bradycardia include congenital heart block and serious fetal compromise. Figure 14–7 shows bradycardia in a fetus dying from placental abruption. Maternal hypothermia under general anesthesia for repair of a cerebral aneurysm or during maternal cardiopulmonary bypass for open-heart surgery can also cause fetal bradycardia (Chap. 44, p. 1187). Sustained

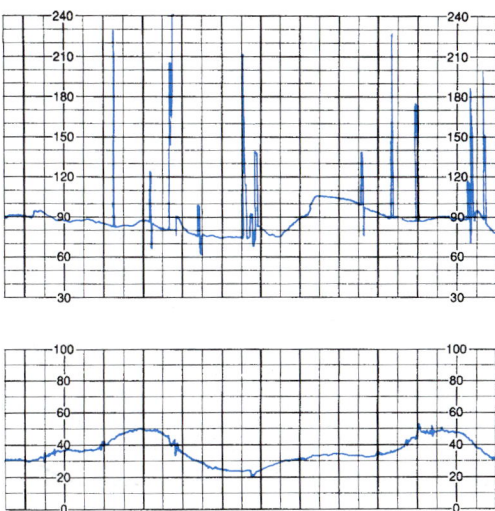

FIGURE 14-7. Fetal bradycardia measured with a scalp electrode in a pregnancy complicated by placental abruption and subsequent fetal death.

fetal bradycardia in the setting of severe pyelonephritis and maternal hypothermia has also been reported (Hankins and co-workers, 1997). These infants are apparently not harmed by several hours of such bradycardia.

TACHYCARDIA. This is considered by most as *mild* if the baseline rate is between 161 and 180 bpm and *severe* if 181 or more. The most common explanation for fetal tachycardia is maternal fever from amnionitis, although fever from any source can increase baseline fetal heart rate. Such infections have also been observed to induce fetal tachycardia before overt maternal fever is diagnosed (Gilstrap and associates, 1987). Fetal tachycardia caused by maternal infection is typically not associated with fetal compromise unless there are associated periodic heart rate changes or fetal sepsis.

Other causes of fetal tachycardia include fetal compromise, cardiac arrhythmias, and maternal administration of parasympathetic (atropine) or sympathomimetic (terbutaline) drugs. The key feature to distinguish fetal compromise in association with tachycardia seems to be concomitant heart rate decelerations. Prompt relief of the compromising event, such as correction of maternal hypotension caused by epidural analgesia, can result in fetal recovery.

BEAT-TO-BEAT VARIABILITY. Baseline variability is an important index of cardiovascular function and appears to be regulated largely by the autonomic nervous system (Kozuma and colleagues, 1997). That is, sympathetic and parasympathetic control via the sinoatrial node mediates moment-to-moment or beat-to-beat oscillation of the baseline heart rate. Such irregularity of the heart rate is defined as baseline variability. Variability is further divided into *short term* and *long term*.

Short-term variability reflects the instantaneous change in fetal heart rate from one beat (or R wave) to the next. This variability is a measure of the time interval between cardiac systoles (Fig. 14–8). *It can most reliably be determined to be normally present only when*

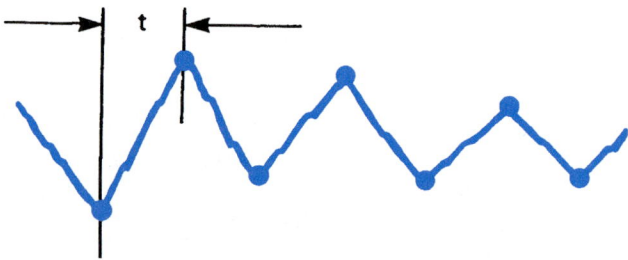

FIGURE 14–8. Schematic representation of short-term beat-to-beat variability measured by a fetal scalp electrode (t = time interval between successive fetal R waves). (From Klavan and co-authors, 1977.)

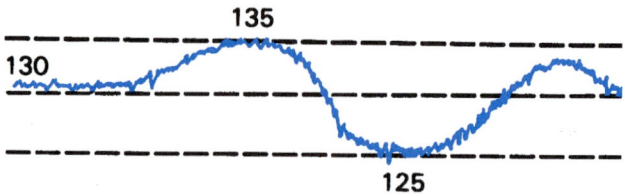

FIGURE 14–9. Schematic representation of long-term beat-to-beat variability of the fetal heart rate ranging between 125 and 135 bpm. (From Klavan and co-authors, 1977).

electrocardiac cycles are measured directly with a scalp electrode.

Long-term variability is used to describe the oscillatory changes that occur during the course of 1 minute and result in the waviness of the baseline (Fig. 14–9). The normal frequency of such waves is three to five cycles per minute (Freeman and co-authors, 1991).

It should be recognized that precise quantitative analysis of both short- and long-term variability presents a number of frustrating problems due to technical and scaling factors. For example, Parer and co-workers (1985) evaluated 22 mathematical formulas designed to quantify heart rate variability and most were unsatisfactory. Consequently, most clinical interpretation is based on visual analysis with subjective judgment of the smoothness or flatness of the baseline. The NICHD Fetal Monitoring Workshop (1997) did not recommend differentiating short-term variability and long-term variability because in actual practice they are visually determined as a unit.

The Workshop did, however, define baseline variability as those baseline fluctuations of two cycles per minute or greater. They recommended the criteria shown in Figure 14–10 for quantification of variability. Normal beat-to-beat variability was accepted to be 6 to 25 bpm.

Several physiological and pathological processes can affect or interfere with beat-to-beat variability. Dawes and co-workers (1981) described increased variability during **fetal breathing.** In healthy infants, short-term variability is attributable to respiratory sinus arrhythmia (Divon and co-workers, 1986). **Fetal body movements** also affect variability. Granat and co-investigators (1979) observed that fetuses exhibited 40- to 80-minute cycles of movements thought to correspond to fetal wakefulness. Van Geijn and co-workers (1980) analyzed electroencephalographic data in healthy term infants and observed 30- to 70-minute sleep cycles corresponding to fetal physical inactivity. Pillai and James (1990) reported increased baseline variability with **advancing gestation.** Up to 30 weeks, baseline characteristics were similar during both fetal rest and activity. After 30 weeks, fetal inactivity was associated with diminished baseline variability and, conversely, variability was in-

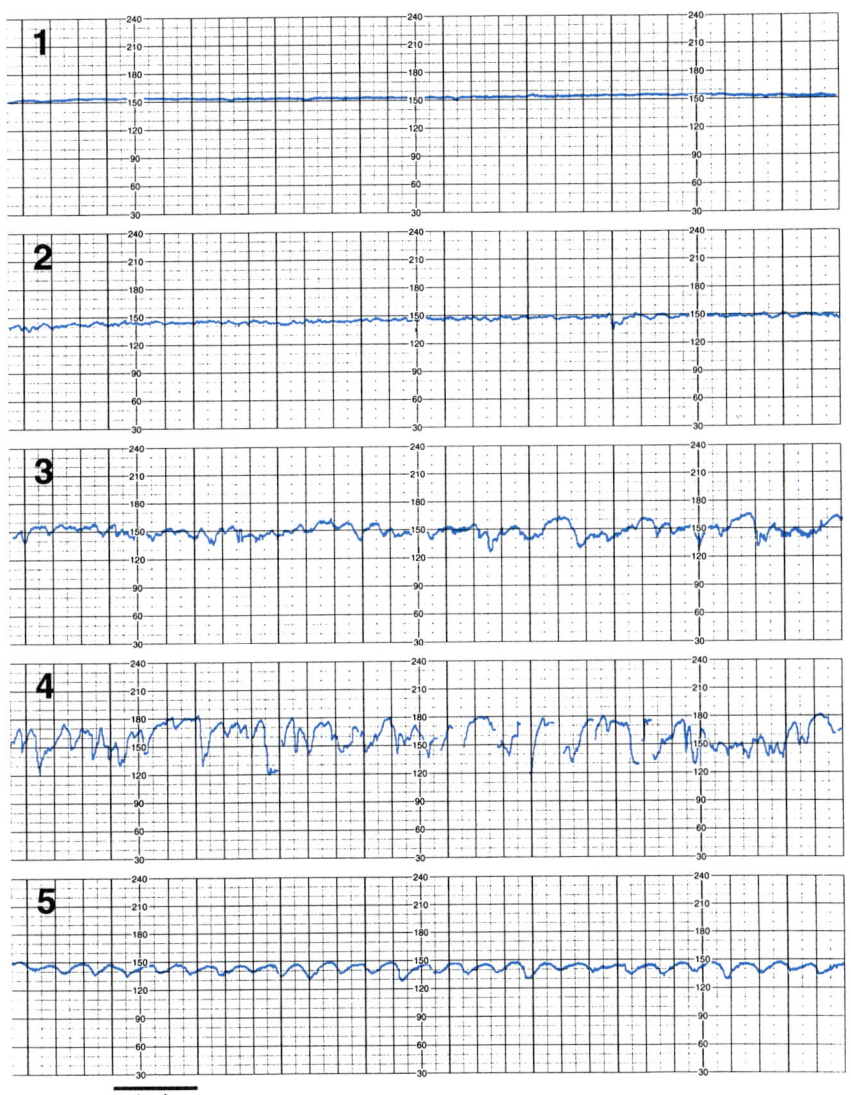

FIGURE 14–10. Grades of baseline fetal heart rate variability (irregular fluctuations in the baseline of 2 cycles per minute or greater) together with a sinusoidal pattern. The sinusoidal pattern differs from variability in that it has a smooth, sinelike pattern of regular fluctuation and is excluded in the definition of fetal heart rate variability. (1) Undetectable, absent variability; (2) minimal ≤ 5 bpm variability; (3) moderate (normal), 6 to 25 bpm variability; (4) marked, > 25 bpm variability; (5) sinusoidal pattern. (National Institute of Child Health and Human Development Fetal Monitoring Workshop, 1997.)

1 min

creased during fetal activity. Fetal gender does not affect heart rate variability (Ogueh and Steer, 1998).

It is important to recognize that the baseline fetal heart rate becomes more physiologically fixed (less variable) as the rate increases. Conversely, there is more instability or variability of the baseline at lower heart rates. This phenomenon presumably reflects less cardiovascular physiological wandering as beat-to-beat intervals shorten due to increasing heart rate.

Diminished beat-to-beat variability can be an ominous sign indicating a seriously compromised fetus. Paul and co-workers (1975) reported that loss of variability in combination with decelerations was associated with fetal acidemia. They analyzed variability in the 20 minutes preceding delivery in 194 pregnancies. Decreased variability was defined as 5 or fewer bpm excursion of the baseline (Fig. 14–10), whereas acceptable variability exceeded this range. Fetal scalp pH was measured 1119

times in these pregnancies, and mean values were progressively more acidemic when decreased variability was added to progressively intense heart rate decelerations. For example, mean fetal scalp pH was about 7.10 when severe decelerations were combined with 5 bpm or less variability, compared with a pH about 7.20 when greater variability was associated with similarly severe decelerations.

Severe **maternal acidemia** can also cause decreased fetal beat-to-beat variability, as shown in Figure 14–11 in a mother with diabetic ketoacidosis. The precise pathological mechanisms by which fetal hypoxemia results in diminished beat-to-beat variability are not totally understood.

Although loss of variability and its ominous significance are concepts familiar to most obstetricians, mild degrees of fetal hypoxemia have been reported to *increase* variability, at least at the outset of the hypoxic

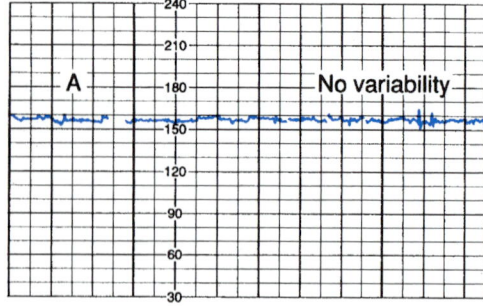

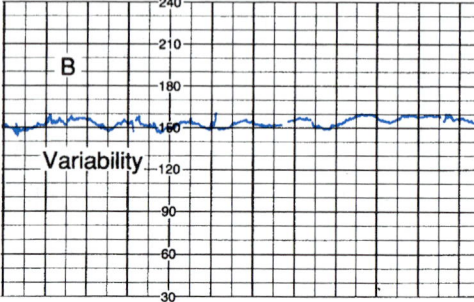

FIGURE 14–11. A. External fetal heart recording showing lack of long-term variability at 31 weeks during maternal diabetic ketoacidosis (pH 7.09). **B.** Recovery of fetal long-term variability after correction of maternal acidemia.

episode (Murotsuki and co-authors, 1997). According to Dawes (1985), it seems probable that the loss of variability is a result of metabolic acidemia that causes depression of the fetal brainstem or the heart itself. Thus, diminished beat-to-beat variability, when a reflection of compromised fetal condition, likely reflects acidemia rather than hypoxia.

A common cause of diminished beat-to-beat variability is analgesic drugs given during labor. A large variety of central nervous system depressant drugs can cause transient diminished beat-to-beat variability. Included are narcotics, barbiturates, phenothiazines, tranquilizers, and general anesthetics. Diminished variability occurs regularly within 5 to 10 minutes following intravenous meperidine administration, and the effects may last up to 60 minutes or longer depending on the dosage given (Petrie, 1993). Butorphanol given intravenously diminishes fetal heart rate reactivity (Schucker and colleagues, 1996). Reduced variability was observed by Viscomi and co-workers (1990) but not Hoffman and associates (1996) when fentanyl was administered epidurally for labor analgesia.

Magnesium sulfate, widely used in the United States for tocolysis as well as management of hypertensive women, has been arguably associated with diminished beat-to-beat variability. Hallak and colleagues (1999) randomized 34 normal, nonlaboring women to standard magnesium sulfate infusion versus isotonic saline. Magnesium sulfate was associated with statistically decreased variability only in the third hour of the infusion. However, the average decrease in variability was deemed clinically insignificant because the mean variability was 2.7 bpm in the third hour of magnesium infusion compared with 2.8 bpm at baseline. Magnesium sulfate also blunted the frequency of accelerations.

It is generally believed that reduced baseline heart rate variability is the single most reliable sign of fetal compromise. For example, Smith and co-workers (1988) performed a computerized analysis of beat-to-beat variability in growth-restricted fetuses *before* labor. They observed that diminished variability (4.2 bpm or less) that was maintained for 1 hour is diagnostic of developing acidemia and imminent fetal death. By contrast, Samueloff and associates (1994) evaluated variability as a predictor of fetal outcome during labor in 2200 consecutive deliveries. They concluded that variability by itself cannot be used as the only indicator of fetal well-being. Conversely, they also concluded that good variability should not be interpreted as necessarily reassuring.

In summary, beat-to-beat variability is affected by a variety of pathological and physiological mechanisms. Variability has considerably different meaning depending on the clinical setting. The development of decreased variability in the absence of decelerations is unlikely to be due to fetal hypoxia (Davidson and co-workers, 1992).

CARDIAC ARRHYTHMIA. When fetal cardiac arrhythmias are first suspected using electronic monitoring, findings can include baseline bradycardia, tachycardia, or most commonly in our experience, **abrupt baseline spiking** (Fig. 14–12). Intermittent baseline bradycardia is frequently due to congenital heart block. Documentation of an arrhythmia can only be accomplished, practically speaking, when scalp electrodes are used. Most fetal monitors can be adapted to output the scalp electrode signals into an electrocardiographic recorder. Because, only a single lead is obtained, this severely restricts interpretation of analysis of rhythm and rate disturbances.

Southall and co-authors (1980) studied antepartum fetal cardiac rate and rhythm disturbances in 934 normal pregnancies between 30 and 40 weeks. Arrhythmias and episodes of bradycardia less than 100 bpm, or tachycardia greater than 180 bpm, were encountered in 3 percent. Most supraventricular arrhythmias are of little significance during labor unless there is coexistent heart failure as evidenced by fetal hydrops. Many supraventricular arrhythmias disappear in the immediate neonatal period, although some are associated with structural cardiac defects. Simpson and Sharland (1998) retrospec-

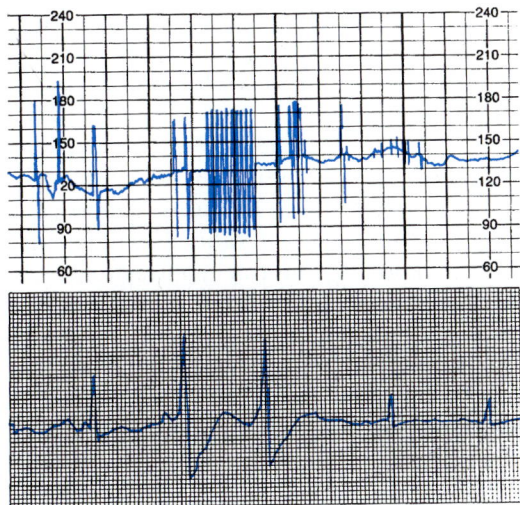

FIGURE 14–12. Internal fetal monitoring at term showed occasional abrupt beat-to-beat fetal heart rate spiking due to erratic extrasystoles shown in the superimposed fetal electrocardiogram. The normal infant was delivered spontaneously and had a normal cardiac rhythm in the nursery.

tively reviewed 127 consecutive fetuses with tachycardia. Echocardiography showed supraventricular tachycardia in 105 fetuses and atrial flutter in 22. Maternally administered drugs, to include digoxin, verapamil, and flecainide, were used to control the fetal arrhythmias. Almost all nonhydropic fetuses survived the neonatal period compared with only 73 percent in those with hydrops. Copel and co-authors (2000) used echocardiography to evaluate 614 fetuses referred for auscultated irregular heart rate without hydrops. Only 10 fetuses (2 percent) were found to have significant arrhythmias and all but one infant survived.

Other than ectopic systoles, which are as common in fetuses as in adults, ventricular arrhythmias are unusual in utero. As discussed in Chapter 52 (p. 1389), conduction defects, most commonly complete atrioventricular (AV) block, are usually found in association with connective-tissue diseases.

Although most fetal arrhythmias are of little consequence during labor when there is no evidence for fetal hydrops, such arrhythmias impair interpretation of intrapartum heart rate tracings. Ultrasonic survey of fetal anatomy as well as echocardiography may be useful. Some clinicians use fetal scalp sampling as an adjunct. Generally, in the absence of fetal hydrops, neonatal outcome is not measurably improved by pregnancy intervention. At Parkland Hospital, intrapartum fetal cardiac arrhythmias, especially in the presence of clear amnionic fluid, are managed conservatively. Deans and Steer (1994) have extensively reviewed interpretation of the fetal electrocardiogram during labor.

SINUSOIDAL HEART RATES. A true sinusoidal pattern such as that shown in panel 5 of Figure 14–10 may be observed with serious fetal anemia, whether from D-isoimmunization, ruptured vasa previa, fetomaternal hemorrhage, or twin-to-twin transfusion. Insignificant sinusoidal patterns have been reported following administration of meperidine, morphine, alphaprodine, and butorphanol (Angel, 1984; Egley, 1991; Epstein, 1982, and their associates). The pattern has also been described with amnionitis, fetal distress, and umbilical cord occlusion (Murphy and associates, 1991). Young and co-workers (1980a) and Johnson and colleagues (1981) concluded that intrapartum sinusoidal fetal heart patterns were not generally associated with fetal compromise.

Modanlou and Freeman (1982), based on their extensive review, proposed adoption of a strict definition:

1. Stable baseline heart rate of 120 to 160 bpm with regular oscillations.
2. Amplitude of 5 to 15 bpm (rarely greater).
3. Frequency of 2 to 5 cycles/min long-term variability.
4. Fixed or flat short-term variability.
5. Oscillation of the sinusoidal waveform above or below a baseline.
6. Absence of accelerations.

Although these criteria were selected to define a sinusoidal pattern that is most likely ominous, they observed that the pattern associated with alphaprodine is indistinguishable. Other investigators have proposed a classification of sinusoidal heart rate patterns into mild (amplitude 5 to 15 bpm), intermediate (16 to 24 bpm), and major (25 or more bpm) to quantify fetal risk (Murphy and colleagues, 1991; Neesham and co-workers, 1993).

Some investigators have defined intrapartum sine-wave–like baseline variation with periods of acceleration as *pseudosinusoidal*. Murphy and co-workers (1991) reported that pseudosinusoidal patterns were seen in 15 percent of monitored labors. Mild pseudosinusoidal patterns were associated with use of meperidine and epidural analgesia. Intermediate pseudosinusoidal patterns were linked to fetal sucking or transient episodes of fetal hypoxia caused by umbilical cord compression. In contrast, Egley and colleagues (1991) reported that 4 percent of fetuses demonstrated sinusoidal patterns transiently during normal labor. These authors observed patterns for up to 90 minutes in some cases and also in association with oxytocin and/or alphaprodine usage.

Shown in Figure 14–13 is a sinusoidal pattern seen with maternal meperidine administration. An important characteristic of this pattern when due to narcotics is the 6 cycles/min sine frequency.

The pathophysiology of sinusoidal patterns is unclear, in part due to various definitions. There seems to be general agreement that *antepartum* sine wave base-

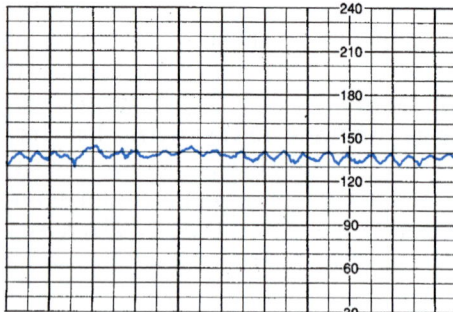

FIGURE 14–13. Sinusoidal fetal heart rate pattern associated with maternal intravenous meperidine administration. Sine waves are occurring at a rate of 6 cycles/min.

line undulation portends severe fetal anemia; however, few D-isoimmunized fetuses develop this pattern (Nicolaides, 1989). The sinusoidal pattern has been reported to develop or disappear after fetal transfusion (Del Valle and associates, 1992; Lowe and co-workers, 1984). Ikeda and colleagues (1999) have proposed, based upon studies in fetal lambs, that the sinusoidal fetal heart rate pattern is related to waves of arterial blood pressure, reflecting oscillations in the baroreceptor/chemoreceptor feedback mechanism for control of the circulation.

PERIODIC FETAL HEART RATE. The periodic fetal heart rate refers to deviations from baseline that are related to uterine contractions. **Acceleration** refers to an increase in fetal heart rate above baseline and **deceleration** to a decrease below baseline rate. The most commonly used system in the United States is based on the *timing* of the deceleration in relation to contractions— thus, **early, late,** or **variable** in onset compared with the corresponding uterine contraction. The waveform of these decelerations is also significant for pattern recognition. In early and late decelerations, the slope of fetal heart rate change is gradual, resulting in a curvilinear and uniform or symmetrical waveform. With variable decelerations, the slope of fetal heart rate change is abrupt and erratic, giving the waveform a jagged appearance. It has been proposed that decelerations be defined as *recurrent* if they occur with 50 percent or more of contractions in any 20-minute period (NICHD Fetal Monitoring Workshop, 1997).

Another system now used less often for description of decelerations is based on the pathophysiological events considered most likely to cause the pattern. In this system, early decelerations are termed *head compression,* late decelerations are termed *uteroplacental insufficiency,* and variable decelerations become *cord compression patterns.* The nomenclature of type I (early), type II (late), and type III (variable) "dips" proposed by Caldeyro-Barcia and co-workers (1973) is not used in the United States.

ACCELERATIONS. An acceleration is a visually apparent abrupt increase (defined as onset of acceleration to a peak in < 30 seconds) in the fetal heart rate baseline (NICHD Fetal Monitoring Workshop, 1997). According to Freeman and co-authors (1991), accelerations occur most commonly antepartum, in early labor, and in association with variable decelerations. Proposed mechanisms for intrapartum accelerations include fetal movement, stimulation by uterine contractions, umbilical cord occlusion, and fetal stimulation during pelvic examination. Fetal scalp blood sampling and acoustic stimulation also incite fetal heart rate acceleration (Clark and co-workers, 1982). Finally, acceleration can occur during labor without any apparent stimulus. Indeed, accelerations are common in labor and nearly always associated with fetal movement. These accelerations are virtually always reassuring and almost always confirm that the fetus is not acidemic at that time.

Accelerations seem to have the same physiological explanations as beat-to-beat variability in that they represent intact neurohormonal cardiovascular control mechanisms linked to fetal behavioral states. Krebs and co-workers (1982a) analyzed electronic heart rate tracings in nearly 2000 fetuses and found sporadic accelerations during labor in 99.8 percent. The presence of fetal heart accelerations during the first and/or last 30 minutes was a favorable sign for fetal well-being. The absence of such accelerations during labor, however, is not necessarily an unfavorable sign unless coincidental with other nonreassuring changes. There is about a 50 percent chance of acidemia in the fetus who fails to respond to stimulation in the presence of an otherwise nonreassuring pattern (Clark and colleagues, 1984; Smith and colleagues, 1986).

EARLY DECELERATION. Early deceleration of the fetal heart rate is a gradual decrease and return to baseline associated with a contraction (Fig. 14–14). *Early* deceleration of the fetal heart rate was first described by Hon (1958). He observed that there was a drop in heart rate with uterine contractions, and that this was related to cervical dilatation. He considered these physiological.

Freeman and co-authors (1991) defined early decelerations as those generally seen in active labor between 4 and 7 cm dilatation. In their definition, the degree of deceleration is generally proportional to the contraction strength and rarely falls below 100 to 110 bpm or 20 to 30 bpm below baseline. Such decelerations are uncommon during active labor and are not associated with baseline changes. Importantly, early decelerations are not associated with fetal hypoxia, acidemia, or low Apgar scores.

Head compression probably causes vagal nerve activation due to dural stimulation that mediates heart rate deceleration (Paul and co-workers, 1964). Ball and Parer (1992) concluded that fetal head compression is

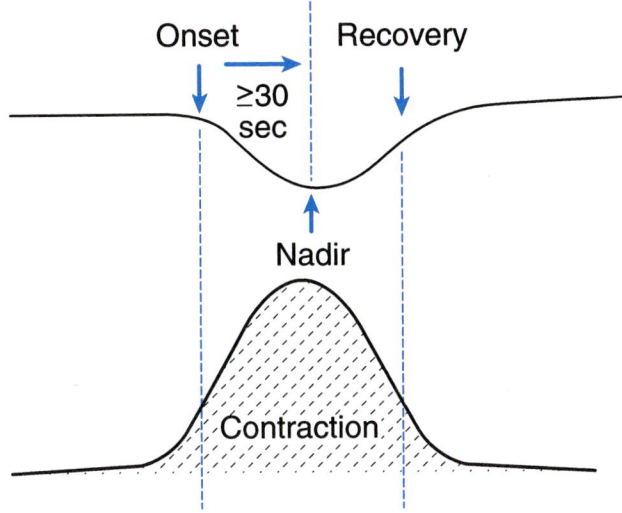

FIGURE 14–14. Features of early fetal heart rate deceleration. Characteristics include gradual decrease in the heart rate with both onset and recovery coincident with the onset and recovery of the contraction. The nadir of the deceleration is 30 seconds or more after the onset of the deceleration.

a likely cause not only for the deceleration shown in Figure 14–14 but also for those shown in Figure 14–15, which typically occur during second-stage labor. Indeed, they observed that head compression is the likely cause of many variable decelerations classically attributed to cord compression.

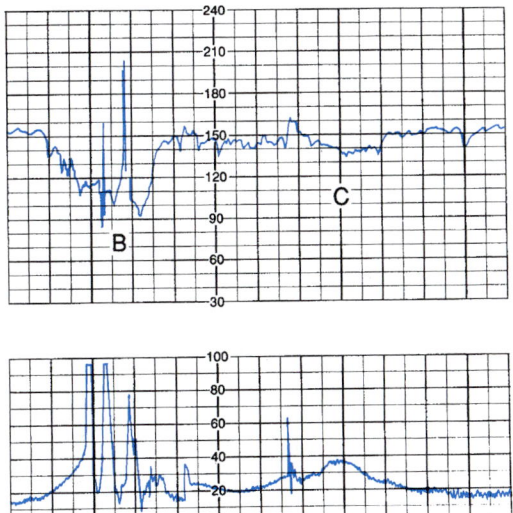

FIGURE 14–15. Two different fetal heart rate patterns during second-stage labor that are likely both due to head compression. Maternal bearing down efforts correspond to the spikes with uterine contractions. Fetal heart rate deceleration C is consistent with the pattern of head compression shown in Figure 14–14. Deceleration B, however, is "variable" in appearance because of its jagged configuration, and may also represent cord occlusion.

LATE DECELERATION. The fetal heart rate response to uterine contractions can be an index of either uterine perfusion or placental function. A late deceleration is a smooth, gradual symmetrical decrease in fetal heart rate beginning at or after the peak of the contraction and returning to baseline only after the contraction has ended (American College of Obstetrics and Gynecologists, 1995b). In most cases the onset, nadir, and recovery of the deceleration occur after the beginning, peak, and ending of the contraction, respectively (Fig. 14–16). The magnitude of late decelerations is rarely more than 30 to 40 bpm below baseline and typically not more than 10 to 20 bpm in intensity. Late decelerations are usually not accompanied by accelerations.

Myers and associates (1973) studied monkeys in which they compromised uteroplacental perfusion by lowering maternal aortic blood pressure. The time interval, or lag period from the onset of a contraction to the onset of a late deceleration, was directly related to basal fetal oxygenation. They demonstrated that the length of the lag phase was predictive of the fetal P_{O_2} but not fetal pH. The lower the fetal P_{O_2} prior to contractions, the shorter the lag phase to onset of late decelerations. This lag period reflected the time necessary for the fetal P_{O_2} to fall below a critical level necessary to stimulate arterial chemoreceptors which mediated decelerations.

Murata and co-workers (1982) also showed that a late deceleration was the first fetal heart rate consequence of uteroplacental induced hypoxia. During the course of progressive hypoxia that led to death over 2 to 13 days, the monkey fetuses invariably exhibited late decelerations before the development of acidemia. Variability of the baseline heart rate disappeared as acidemia developed.

A large number of clinical circumstances can result in late decelerations. Generally, any process that causes maternal hypotension, excessive uterine activity, or placental dysfunction can induce late decelerations. The two most common causes are hypotension from epidural analgesia and uterine hyperactivity due to oxytocin stimulation. Maternal diseases such as hypertension, diabetes, and collagen-vascular disorders can cause chronic placental dysfunction. A rare cause is severe chronic maternal anemia without hypovolemia. Placental abruption can cause acute and severe late decelerations (Fig. 14–17).

VARIABLE DECELERATIONS. The most common deceleration patterns encountered during labor are variable decelerations attributed to umbilical cord occlusion. Melchior and Bernard (1985) identified variable decelerations in 40 percent of over 7000 monitor tracings when labor had progressed to 5 cm dilatation and in 83 percent by the end of the first stage. Variable deceleration of the fetal heart rate is defined as a visually apparent *abrupt* decrease in rate. The onset of deceleration

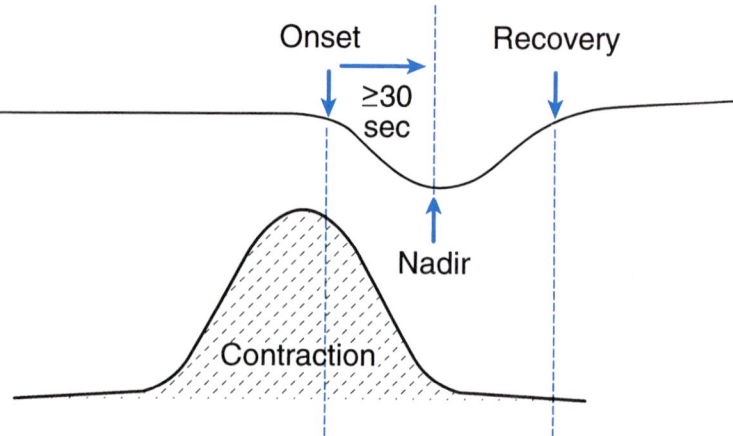

FIGURE 14–16. Features of late fetal heart rate deceleration. Characteristics include gradual decrease in the heart rate with the nadir and recovery occurring after the end of the contraction. The nadir of deceleration occurs 30 seconds or more after the onset of the deceleration.

commonly varies with successive contractions (Fig. 14–18). The duration is less than 2 minutes.

Very early in the development of electronic monitoring, Hon (1959) tested the effects of umbilical cord compression on fetal heart rate (Fig. 14–19). Similar complete occlusion of the umbilical cord in experimental animals produces abrupt, jagged-appearing deceleration of the fetal heart rate (Fig. 14–20). Concomitantly, fetal aortic pressure increases. Itskovitz and co-workers (1983) observed that variable decelerations in fetal lambs occurred only after umbilical blood flow was reduced by at least 50 percent.

Two types of variable decelerations are shown in Figure 14–21. The deceleration denoted by A is very

much like that seen with complete umbilical cord occlusion in experimental animals (Fig. 14–20). Deceleration B, however, has a different configuration because of the "shoulders" of acceleration before and after the deceleration component. Lee and co-workers (1975) proposed that the variation of variable decelerations was caused by differing degrees of partial cord occlusion. In this physiological scheme, occlusion of only the vein reduces fetal blood return, thereby triggering a baroreceptor-mediated acceleration. Subsequent complete occlusion results in fetal systemic hypertension due to obstruction of umbilical artery flow. This stimulates a baroreceptor-mediated deceleration. Presumably, the

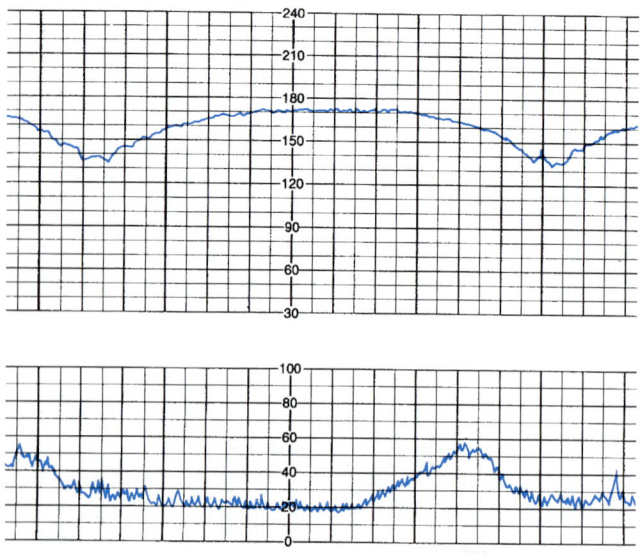

FIGURE 14–17. Late decelerations due to uteroplacental insufficiency resulting from placental abruption. Immediate cesarean delivery was performed. Umbilical artery pH was 7.05 and the P_{O_2} was 11 mm Hg.

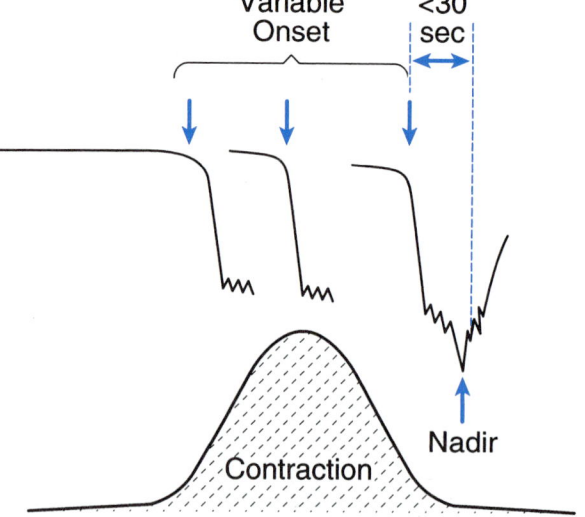

FIGURE 14–18. Features of variable fetal heart rate decelerations. Characteristics include abrupt decrease in the heart rate with onset commonly varying with successive contractions. The decelerations measure ≥ 15 bpm for 15 seconds or longer with an onset to nadir phase of less than 30 seconds. Total duration is less than 2 minutes.

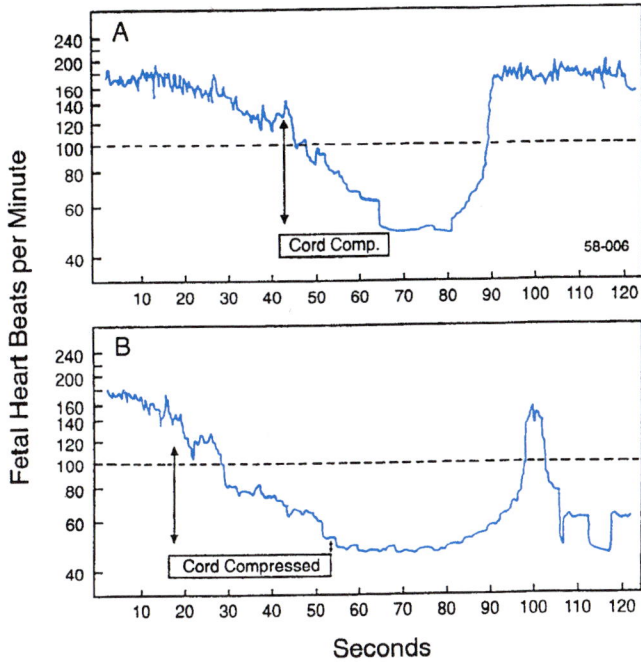

FIGURE 14-19. Fetal heart rate effects of manual compression of a prolapsed umbilical cord in a 25-week footling breech. **A** shows the effects of 25-second compression compared with 40 seconds in **B.** (Redrawn from Hon, 1959, with permission.)

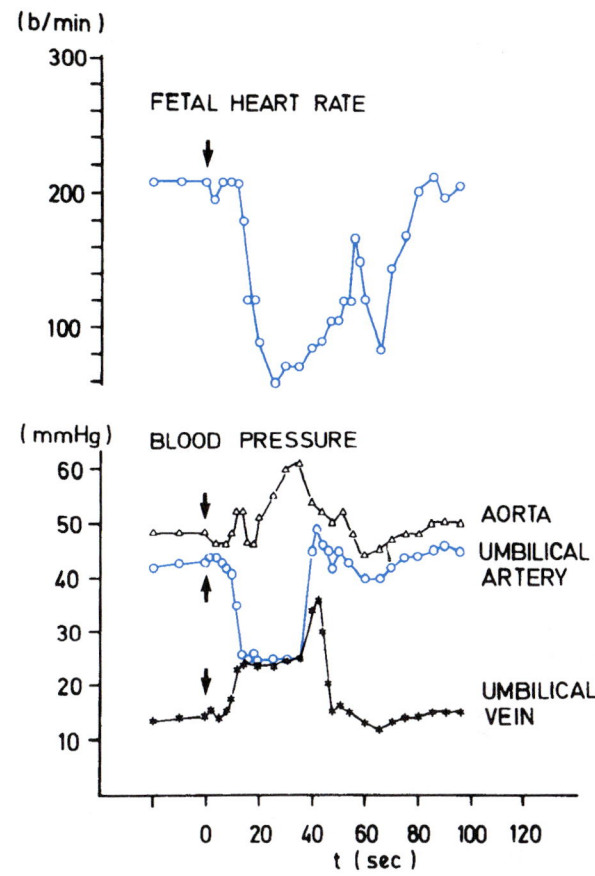

FIGURE 14-20. Total umbilical cord occlusion (*arrow*) in the sheep fetus is accompanied by increase in fetal aortic blood pressure. Blood pressure changes in the umbilical vessels are also shown. (From Kunzel, 1985, with permission.)

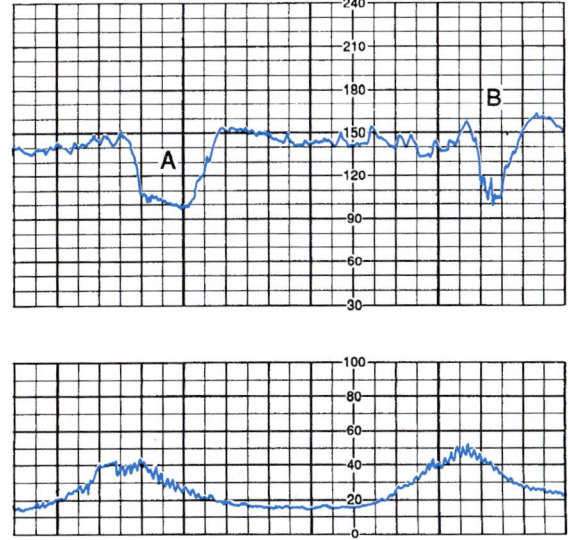

FIGURE 14-21. Varying (variable) fetal heart rate decelerations. Deceleration B exhibits "shoulders" of acceleration compared with deceleration A.

aftercoming shoulder of acceleration represents the same events occurring in reverse (Fig. 14–22).

Ball and Parer (1992) concluded that variable decelerations are vagally mediated and that the vagal response may be due to chemoreceptor or baroreceptor activity or both. Partial or complete cord occlusion (baroreceptor) produces afterload increase, hypertension, and decreases in fetal arterial oxygen content (chemoreceptor), both of which result in vagal activity leading to deceleration. In fetal monkeys the baroreceptor reflexes appear to be operative during the first 15 to 20 seconds of umbilical cord occlusion followed by decline in Po_2 at approximately 30 seconds, which then serves as a chemoreceptor stimulus (Mueller-Heubach and Battelli, 1982).

Thus, variable decelerations represent fetal heart rate reflexes that reflect either blood pressure changes due to interruption of umbilical flow or changes in oxygenation. It is likely that most fetuses have experienced brief but recurrent periods of hypoxia due to umbilical cord compression during gestation. The frequency and inevitability of cord occlusion has undoubtedly provided the fetus with these physiological mechanisms as a means of coping. The great dilemma for the obstetrician in managing variable fetal heart rate decelerations is determining when variable decelerations are pathological. The American College of Obstetricians and Gynecologists (1995b) has defined **significant** variable decel-

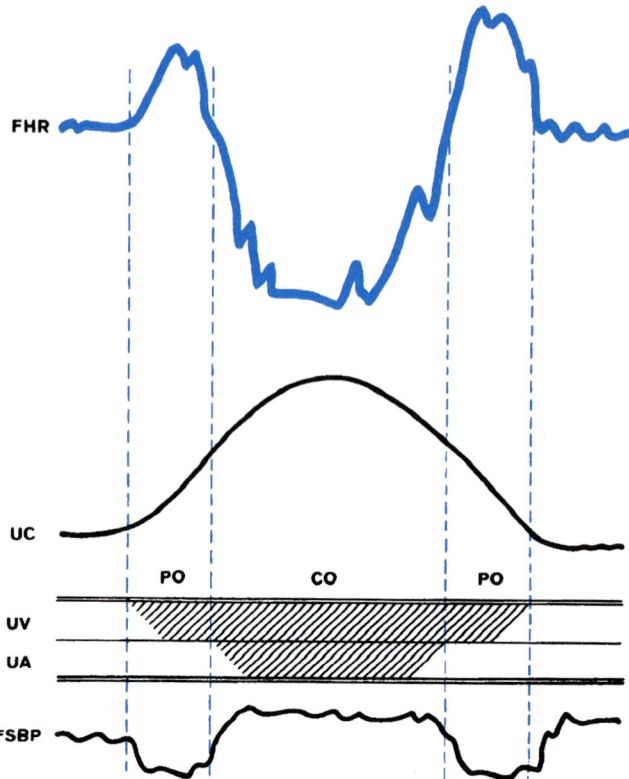

FIGURE 14–22. Schematic representation of the fetal heart rate (FHR) effects of partial occlusion (PO) and complete occlusion (CO) of the umbilical cord. (FSBP = fetal systemic blood pressure; UA = umbilical artery; UC = uterine contraction; UV = umbilical vein.) (From Lee and co-authors, 1975, with permission.)

erations as those decreasing to less than 70 bpm and lasting more than 60 seconds.

Other fetal heart rate patterns have been associated with umbilical cord compression. **Saltatory** baseline heart rate (Fig. 14–23) was first described by Hammacher and co-workers (1968) and linked to umbilical cord complications during labor. The pattern is considered due to rapidly recurring couplets of acceleration and deceleration causing relatively large oscillations of the baseline fetal heart rate. We also observed a relationship between cord occlusion and the saltatory pattern (Leveno and associates, 1984). In the absence of other fetal heart rate findings, these do not signal fetal compromise.

PROLONGED DECELERATION. Shown in Figure 14–24, these are defined as isolated decelerations lasting 2 minutes or longer, but less than 10 minutes from onset to return to baseline (NICHD Fetal Monitoring Workshop, 1997). Prolonged decelerations are difficult to interpret because they are seen in many different clinical situations. Some of the more common causes include

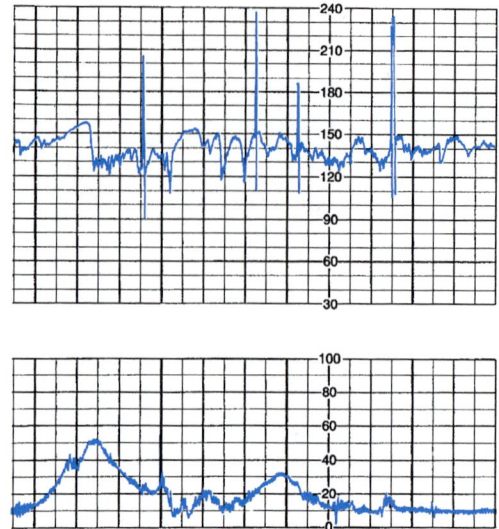

FIGURE 14–23. Saltatory fetal heart rate baseline showing rapidly recurring couplets of acceleration combined with deceleration.

cervical examination, uterine hyperactivity, cord entanglement, and maternal supine hypotension.

Epidural, spinal, or paracervical analgesia are frequent causes of prolonged deceleration of the fetal heart rate. For example, Eberle and colleagues (1998) reported that prolonged decelerations occurred in 4 percent of normal parturients given either epidural or intrathecal labor analgesia. Other causes of prolonged deceleration include maternal hypoperfusion or hypoxia due to any cause; placental abruption; umbilical cord

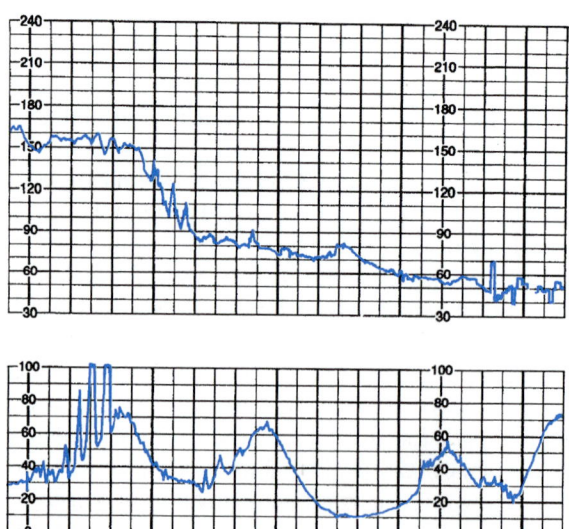

FIGURE 14–24. Prolonged fetal heart rate deceleration due to uterine hyperactivity. Approximately 3 minutes are shown, but the fetal heart rate returned to normal after uterine hypertonus resolved. Vaginal delivery later ensued.

knots or prolapse; maternal seizures including eclampsia and epilepsy; application of a fetal scalp electrode; impending birth; or even maternal Valsalva maneuver.

The placenta is very effective in resuscitating the fetus if the original insult does not recur immediately. Occasionally, such self-limited prolonged decelerations are followed by loss of beat-to-beat variability, baseline tachycardia, and even a period of late decelerations, all of which resolve as the fetus recovers. Freeman coauthors (1991) emphasize rightfully that the fetus may die during prolonged decelerations. Thus, management of prolonged decelerations can be extremely tenuous. Management of isolated prolonged decelerations is based on bedside clinical judgment, which will inevitably sometimes be imperfect given the unpredictability of these decelerations.

AMNIOINFUSION. Gabbe and co-workers (1976) showed in monkeys that removal of amnionic fluid produced variable decelerations and that replenishment of fluid with saline relieved the decelerations. Miyazaki and Taylor (1983) infused saline through the intrauterine pressure catheter in laboring women who had either variable decelerations or prolonged decelerations attributed to cord entrapment. They found that such therapy improved the heart rate pattern in half. Miyazaki and Nevarez (1985) subsequently randomized 96 pregnancies and found that nulliparous women in labor with cord compression patterns who were treated with amnioinfusion less often required cesarean delivery for fetal distress.

On the basis of these early reports, transvaginal amnioinfusion has been extended into three clinical areas:

1. Treatment of variable or prolonged decelerations.
2. Prophylactically in cases of known oligohydramnios, as with prolonged rupture of membranes.
3. In an attempt to dilute or wash out thick meconium (Chap. 39, p. 1044).

Many different amnioinfusion protocols have been reported, but most include a 500 to 800 mL bolus of warmed normal saline followed by a continuous infusion of approximately 3 mL per hour (Owen and co-workers, 1990; Pressman and Blakemore, 1996). Wenstrom and co-authors (1995) surveyed use of amnioinfusion in American teaching hospitals. The procedure was used in 96 percent of the 186 centers surveyed, and it was estimated that 3 to 4 percent of all women delivered at these centers received such infusion. Potential complications of amnioinfusion are summarized in Table 14–1.

TREATMENT OF ABNORMAL HEART RATE PATTERN. As previously mentioned, Miyazaki and Nevarez (1985) found that women in labor with cord compression patterns who were treated with amnioinfusion

TABLE 14–1. Complications Associated with Amnioinfusion from a Survey of 186 Obstetrical Centers

Complication	Centers Reporting No. (%)
Uterine hypertonus	27 (14)
Abnormal fetal heart rate tracing	17 (9)
Amnionitis	7 (4)
Cord prolapse	5 (2)
Uterine rupture	4 (2)
Maternal cardiac or respiratory compromise	3 (2)
Placental abruption	2 (1)
Maternal death	2 (1)

Adapted from Wenstrom and colleagues (1995), with permission.

less often required cesarean delivery for fetal distress. Spong and associates (1996) reported that relief of variable fetal heart rate decelerations was related to the amnionic fluid index (AFI) determined ultrasonically (Chap. 31, p. 816). For example, variable decelerations were relieved in 76 percent of women with AFI values 4 cm or less compared with 33 percent when the AFI was 8 cm or greater. In a randomized study, however, Owen and colleagues (1990) concluded that amnioinfusion was not beneficial in management of intrapartum variable decelerations.

PROPHYLACTIC AMNIOINFUSION FOR OLIGOHYDRAMNIOS. Amnioinfusion for oligohydramnios has been used prophylactically in an effort to avoid intrapartum fetal heart rate patterns from umbilical cord occlusion. Nageotte and co-workers (1991) found that such amnioinfusion resulted in significantly decreased frequency and severity of variable decelerations in labor. There was no improvement, however, in the cesarean delivery rate or condition of term infants. Macri and co-workers (1992) randomized prophylactic amnioinfusion in 170 term and postterm pregnancies complicated by both thick meconium and oligohydramnios. Amnioinfusion significantly reduced cesarean deliveries for fetal distress as well as meconium aspiration syndrome. In contrast, Ogundipe and associates (1994) randomly assigned 116 term pregnancies with an amnionic fluid index of less than 5 cm to receive prophylactic amnioinfusion or standard obstetrical care. There were no significant differences in overall cesarean delivery rates, deliveries for fetal distress, or umbilical gas studies.

AMNIOINFUSION FOR MECONIUM-STAINED AMNIONIC FLUID. Pierce and associates (2000) summarized the results of 13 prospective trials of intrapartum amnioinfusion in 1924 women with moderate to thick meconium-stained fluid. Infants born to women treated by amnioinfusion were significantly less likely to have meconium below the vocal cords and were less likely to develop meconium aspiration syndrome than infants not given amnioinfusion. The cesarean delivery rate was also lower in the amnioinfusion group. In contrast, at the University of Tennessee, amnioinfusion was found not feasible in half of women with moderate or thick meconium who were randomized to this treatment (Usta and colleagues, 1995). These investigators were also unable to demonstrate any improvement in neonatal outcomes. Spong and associates (1994) also concluded that, although prophylactic amnioinfusion did dilute meconium, it did not improve perinatal outcome.

SECOND-STAGE LABOR FETAL HEART RATE PATTERNS.

Decelerations are virtually ubiquitous. Melchior and Bernard (1985) reported that only 1.4 percent of over 7000 deliveries *did not* have fetal heart rate decelerations during second-stage labor. Both cord compression and fetal head compression have been implicated to cause decelerations and baseline bradycardia during second-stage labor. The high incidence of such patterns minimized their potential significance during early development of electronic monitoring. For example, Boehm (1975) described profound, prolonged fetal heart rate deceleration in the 10 minutes preceding vaginal delivery of 18 healthy infants. Subsequently, Herbert and Boehm (1981) reported another 18 pregnancies with similar prolonged decelerations during second-stage labor, but now associated with one stillbirth and one neonatal death. These experiences attest to the unpredictability of second-stage labor fetal heart rate. Spong and colleagues (1998) analyzed the characteristics of second-stage variable fetal heart rate decelerations in 250 deliveries and found that as the total number of decelerations to less than 70 bpm increased, the 5-minute Apgar score decreased. Put another way, the longer a fetus was exposed to variable decelerations, the lower the Apgar score at 5 minutes.

Picquard and co-workers (1988) analyzed heart rate patterns during second-stage labor in 234 women in an attempt to identify specific patterns to diagnose fetal compromise. Loss of beat-to-beat variability and baseline fetal heart rate less than 90 bpm were predictive of fetal acidemia. Krebs and co-workers (1981) also found that persistent or progressive baseline bradycardia, as well as baseline tachycardia, were associated with low Apgar scores. Gull and colleagues (1996) observed that abrupt fetal heart rate deceleration to less than 100 bpm, and associated with loss of beat-to-beat variability for 4 minutes or longer, was predictive of fetal acidemia. Thus, abnormal baseline heart rate—either bradycardia or tachycardia, absent beat-to-beat variability, or

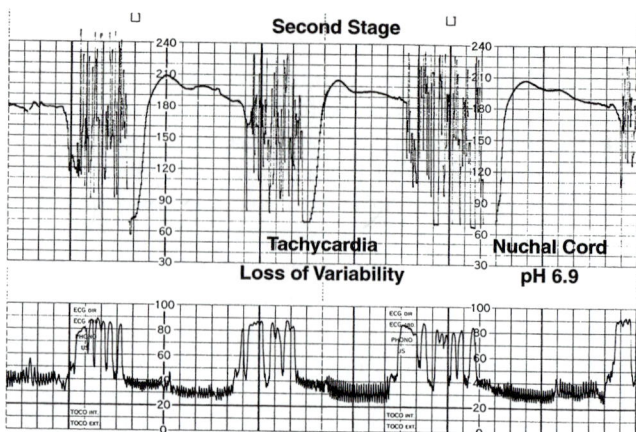

FIGURE 14-25. Cord compression fetal heart rate decelerations in second-stage labor associated with tachycardia and loss of variability. The umbilical cord arterial pH was 6.9.

both—in the presence of second-stage decelerations is associated with increased but not inevitable fetal compromise (Fig. 14-25).

FETAL SCALP BLOOD SAMPLING.

According to the American College of Obstetricians and Gynecologists (1995b), measurements of the pH in capillary scalp blood may help to identify the fetus in serious distress. The College also notes that the procedure is uncommonly used contemporaneously. An illuminated endoscope is inserted through the dilated cervix after ruptured membranes so as to press firmly against the fetal scalp (Fig. 14-26). The skin is wiped clean with a cotton swab and coated with a silicone gel to cause the blood to accumulate as discrete globules. An incision is made through the skin to a 2 mm depth with a special blade on a long handle. As a drop of blood forms on the surface, it is immediately collected into a heparinized glass capillary tube, and the pH of the blood is promptly measured.

The pH of fetal capillary scalp blood is usually lower than umbilical venous blood and approaches that of umbilical arterial blood. Zalar and Quilligan (1979) recommended the following protocol to try to confirm fetal distress: If the pH is greater than 7.25, labor is observed. If the pH is between 7.20 and 7.25, the pH measurement is repeated within 30 minutes. If the pH is less than 7.20, another scalp blood sample is collected immediately and the mother is taken to an operating room and prepared for surgery. Delivery is performed promptly if the low pH is confirmed. Otherwise, labor is allowed to continue and scalp blood samples are repeated periodically. The only benefits reported for scalp pH testing were estimates of fewer cesarean deliveries for fetal distress

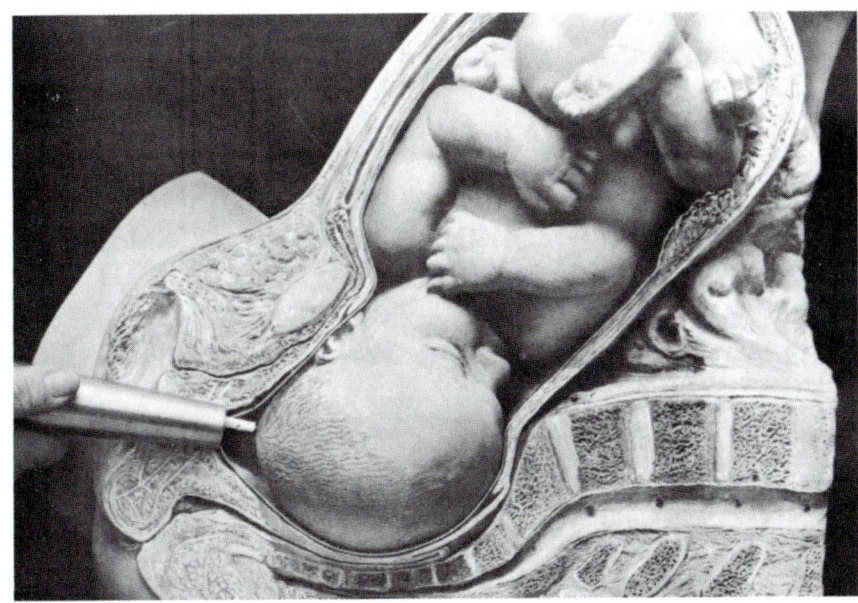

FIGURE 14–26. The technique of fetal scalp sampling utilizing an amnioscope. The end of the endoscope is displaced from the fetal vertex approximately 2 cm to show disposable blade against the fetal scalp before incision. (From Hamilton and McKeown, 1974.)

(Young and co-workers, 1980b). Goodwin and associates (1994), however, in a study of 112,000 deliveries, showed a fall in their scalp pH sampling rate from approximately 1.8 percent in the mid-1980s to 0.03 percent by 1992 with no increased delivery rate for fetal distress. They concluded that scalp pH sampling was unnecessary. Kruger and colleagues (1999) have advocated use of fetal scalp blood lactate concentration as an adjunct to pH.

SCALP STIMULATION. Clark and associates (1984) have suggested that scalp stimulation is an alternative to scalp blood sampling. An Allis clamp was used to pinch the fetal scalp just prior to obtaining scalp blood for pH measurement. Acceleration of the heart rate in response to pinching was invariably associated with a normal scalp blood pH. Conversely, failure to provoke acceleration was not uniformly predictive of fetal acidemia. Elimian and associates (1997) reported that of 58 cases in which the fetal heart rate accelerated 10 bpm or more after 15 seconds of gentle digital stroking of the scalp, 100 percent had a scalp pH of 7.20 or greater. Without an acceleration, however, only 30 percent had a scalp pH less than 7.20.

VIBROACOUSTIC STIMULATION. Fetal heart rate acceleration in response to vibroacoustic stimulation has been recommended as a substitute for scalp sampling (Edersheim and colleagues, 1987). The technique involves use of an electronic artificial larynx placed a centimeter or so from, or directly onto the maternal abdomen (Chap. 40, p. 1103). Response to vibroacoustic stimulation is considered normal if a fetal heart rate acceleration of at least 15 bpm for at least 15 seconds occurs within 15 seconds after the stimulation with prolonged fetal movements (Sherer, 1994). Lin and colleagues (1999) prospectively compared vibroacoustic stimulation with fetal scalp sampling in 113 women in labor and concluded that this technique can be used in lieu of measurement of scalp pH. In contrast, others have reported that although vibroacoustic stimulation in second-stage labor is associated with fetal heart rate reactivity, the quality of the response did not predict neonatal outcome or enhance labor management (Anyaegbunam and associates, 1994).

FETAL PULSE OXIMETRY. Using technology similar to that of adult pulse oximetry, instrumentation has been developed that may allow assessment of fetal oxyhemoglobin saturation once the membranes are ruptured. A unique padlike (Nellcor Puritan Bennett) sensor shown in Figure 14–27 is inserted through the cervix and positioned against the fetal face where it is held in place by the uterine wall. As reviewed by Yam and co-authors (2000), this device has been used extensively by many investigators and has been reported to reliably register fetal oxygen saturation in 70 to 95 percent of women throughout 50 to 88 percent of their labors. As shown in Figure 14–28, fetal oxygen saturation normally varies between approximately 30 percent and 70 percent throughout labor (Chua and colleagues, 1997). Based on these results, as well as those in experimental animals, the lower limit for normal oxygen saturation has been determined to be 30 percent (Yam and colleagues,

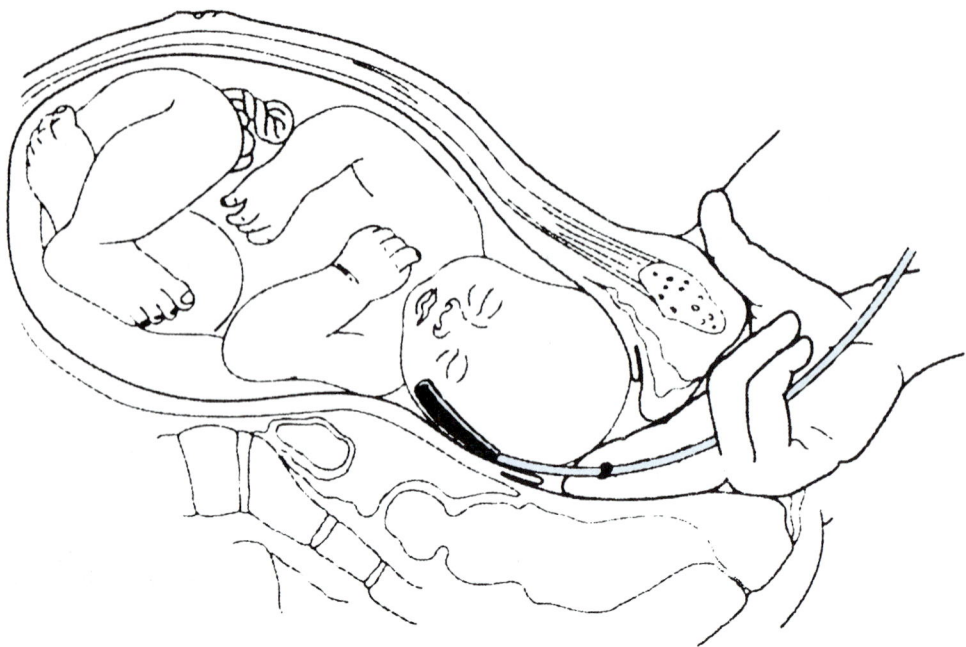

FIGURE 14–27. Schematic diagram of fetal pulse oximeter sensor placement (From Bloom and colleagues, 1999.)

2000). Bloom and colleagues (1999) reported that brief, transient fetal oxygen saturations below 30 percent were common during labor because such values were observed in 53 percent of fetuses with normal outcomes. Saturation values below 30 percent, however, when persistent for 2 minutes or longer, were associated with fetal compromise.

Garite and colleagues (2000) randomized 1010 women with term pregnancies, and who developed predefined abnormal fetal heart rate patterns, to either conventional fetal monitoring alone or fetal monitoring plus continuous fetal pulse oximetry. Cesarean delivery for fetal distress was done when pulse oximetry values remained less than 30 percent for the entire interval between two contractions or the fetal heart rate patterns met predefined guidelines. The use of fetal pulse oximetry significantly reduced the rate of cesarean delivery for nonreassuring fetal status from 10.2 percent to 4.5 percent. Alternatively, the cesarean delivery rate for dystocia significantly increased from 9 percent to 19 percent when pulse oximetry was used. There were no neonatal benefits or adverse effects associated with fetal pulse oximetry. In January 2000, the Obstetrics and Gynecology Devices Panel of the Medical Devices Ad-

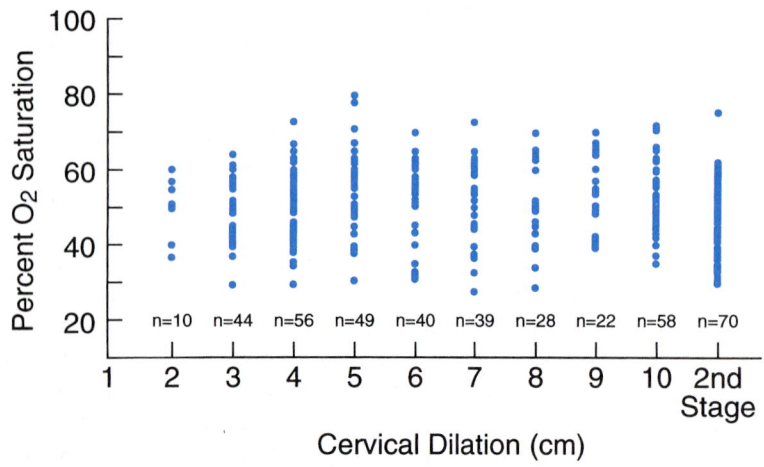

FIGURE 14–28. Fetal oxygen saturation at different maternal cervical dilations in 115 infants with normal outcomes. (Adapted from Chua and colleagues, 1997.)

visory Committee of the Food Drug Administration, based upon this randomized study, recommended marketing of the Nellcor N-400 Fetal Oxygen Monitoring System. The technique currently is being evaluated by the NICHD Maternal–Fetal Medicine Units Network.

FETAL ELECTROCARDIOGRAPHY. Concerns about the validity of continuous electronic fetal monitoring during labor have prompted searches for better methods of monitoring (Whittle, 2000). Because as fetal hypoxia worsens, there are changes in the ST segment and PR interval of the fetal ECG, several investigators have assessed the value of analyzing these as an adjunct to conventional fetal monitoring. Westgate and co-workers (1993) studied the benefits, if any, of monitoring ST-segment changes in a randomized trial of 2400 pregnancies. Infant outcomes were not improved compared with use of conventional fetal monitoring alone, although there was a reduction in cesarean births for fetal distress. Similarly, Strachan and co-workers (2000) found no benefit for adding PR-interval analysis to conventional monitoring.

INTRAPARTUM DOPPLER VELOCIMETRY. Doppler analysis of the umbilical artery has been studied as another potential adjunct to conventional fetal monitoring. Abnormal Doppler waveforms (Chap. 41, p. 1132), when present, may signify pathological umbilical–placental vessel resistance. Farrell and co-authors (1999) reviewed the literature on the use of intrapartum Doppler velocimetry and concluded that this technique was a poor predictor of adverse perinatal outcomes. They concluded that Doppler velocimetry had little, if any, role in the surveillance of fetal well-being during labor.

COMPLICATIONS FROM ELECTRONIC FETAL MONITORING. Injury to the fetal scalp or breech by the electrode is rarely a major problem, although application at some other site—such as the eye in case of a face presentation—can prove serious. A fetal vessel in the placenta may be ruptured by catheter placement (Trudinger and Pryse-Davies, 1978). Severe cord compression has been described from entanglement with the catheter. Penetration of the placenta, causing hemorrhage and uterine perforation during catheter insertion, has led to serious morbidity, as well as spurious recordings that resulted in inappropriate management.

Both the fetus and the mother may be at increased risk for *infection* as the consequence of internal monitoring. Scalp wounds from the electrode may become infected and cause osteomyelitis (McGregor and McFarren, 1989). Faro and associates (1990) observed puerperal infection to be increased from 12 percent in women externally monitored compared with 18 percent when an internal apparatus was used.

FETAL DISTRESS

DEFINITION. The term **fetal distress** is too broad and vague to be applied with any precision to clinical situations. Uncertainty about the diagnosis of fetal distress based upon interpretation of fetal heart rate patterns has given rise to use of descriptions such as *reassuring* or *nonreassuring*. "Reassuring" suggests a restoration of confidence by a particular pattern, whereas "nonreassuring" suggests inability to remove doubt. These patterns during labor are dynamic, such that they can rapidly change from reassuring to nonreassuring and vice versa. In this situation, obstetricians essentially experience surges of both confidence and doubt. Put another way, most diagnoses of fetal distress using heart rate patterns occur when obstetricians lose confidence or cannot assuage doubts about fetal condition. **These fetal assessments are entirely subjective clinical judgments inevitably subject to imperfection and must be recognized as such.**

Why is diagnosis of fetal distress based on heart rate patterns so tenuous? One explanation is that these patterns are more a reflection of fetal physiology than pathology. Physiological control of heart rate includes a variety of interconnected mechanisms that depend on blood flow as well as oxygenation. Moreover, the activity of these control mechanisms is influenced by the preexisting state of fetal oxygenation, as seen, for example, with chronic placental insufficiency. Importantly, the fetus is tethered by an umbilical cord, where blood flow is constantly in jeopardy, which demands that the fetus have a strategy for survival. Moreover, normal labor is a process of increasing acidemia (Rogers and colleagues, 1998). Thus, normal labor is a process of repeated fetal hypoxic events resulting inevitably in acidemia. Put another way, and assuming that "asphyxia" can be defined as hypoxia leading to acidemia, then normal parturition is an asphyxiating event for the fetus.

DIAGNOSIS. Identification of fetal distress based upon fetal heart rate patterns is imprecise and controversial. Experts in interpretation of these patterns so often disagree with each other that one organizer of the NICHD Fetal Monitoring Workshop (1997) lightheartedly compared the experts in attendance with marine iguanas of the Galapagos Islands—"all on the same beach but facing different directions and spitting at one another constantly" (Parer, 1997).

Ayres-de-Campos and colleagues (1999) investigated inter-observer agreement on interpretation of fetal heart rate patterns and found that agreement—or, conversely, disagreement—was related to whether the pattern was normal, suspicious, or pathological. Specifically, experts agreed on 62 percent of normal patterns, 42 percent of suspicious patterns, and only 25 percent

TABLE 14–2. **NICHD Fetal Monitoring Workshop (1997) Interpretations of Fetal Heart Rate Patterns**

Pattern	Workshop Interpretations
Normal	Baseline 110–160 bpm
	Variability 6–25 bpm
	Accelerations present
	No decelerations
Intermediate	No consensus
Severely abnormal	Recurrent late or variable decelerations with zero variability
	Substantial bradycardia with zero variability

of pathological patterns. Indeed, there is some consensus only about the definitions of fetal heart rate at the extremes of normal and severely abnormal patterns (Table 14–2).

There have been several recent research efforts aimed at testing the utility of well-defined fetal heart rate classification systems. Berkus and colleagues (1999) retrospectively analyzed fetal heart rate patterns during the last 30 minutes of labor in 1859 term pregnancies. The study was designed to determine if specific patterns, or combinations of patterns, predicted neonatal outcome. Indisputably normal fetal heart rate patterns were recorded within 30 minutes of delivery in only 26 percent of cases. Combinations of fetal heart rate patterns that indicated absence of accelerations *plus* severe variable or late decelerations, or prolonged bradycardia or tachycardia, were associated with an increased incidence of adverse infant outcomes. Low and colleagues (1999) analyzed fetal heart rate patterns of term infants born with significant metabolic acidemia (umbilical artery base deficit > 16 mmol/L). Such acidemia was rare, occurring in only 71 of 23,000 births. Patterns with absent baseline variability were the most specific, but identified only 17 percent of the acidemic fetuses. The sensitivity was 17 percent (true positive), and the specificity was 98 percent (true negative).

Dellinger and colleagues (2000) retrospectively analyzed intrapartum fetal heart rate patterns in 898 pregnancies using a classification system of their design. Fetal heart rate patterns during the hour before delivery were classified as "normal," "stress," or "distress." Fetal "distress" was diagnosed in 8 (1 percent) tracings and 70 percent were classified as "normal." Almost a third were intermediate patterns. Fetal "distress" was classified to include zero variability *plus* late or moderate-severe variable decelerations or baseline rate less than 110 bpm for 5 minutes or longer. Outcomes such as cesarean delivery, fetal acidemia, and admission to the neonatal intensive care nursery were significantly

related to the fetal heart rate pattern. The authors concluded that their classification system accurately predicted normal outcomes for fetuses as well as discriminating true fetal distress.

In summary, after more than 30 years of experience with interpretation of fetal heart rate patterns, there is finally emerging evidence that some combinations of fetal heart rate characteristics can be meaningfully used to identify normal and severely abnormal fetuses. True fetal distress patterns appear to be those where beat-to-beat variability is *zero* in conjunction with severe decelerations or persistent baseline rate changes or both. Fortunately, such fetal distress is rare. One explanation for the persistent failure to scientifically establish the benefits of fetal heart rate monitoring is the rarity of such fetal distress, effectively precluding sufficiently powerful clinical trials (Hornbuckle and colleagues, 2000).

MANAGEMENT. Clinical management for significantly variant fetal heart rate patterns consists of correcting the potential fetal insult, if possible. Measures suggested by the American College of Obstetricians and Gynecologists (1998) are shown in Table 14–3. Moving the mother to the lateral position, correcting maternal hypotension due to regional analgesia, and discontinuing oxytocin serve to improve uteroplacental perfusion. Examination to rule out prolapsed cord or impending delivery may be helpful.

TABLE 14–3. **Management Criteria for Nonreassuring Fetal Heart Rate Pattern: The Following Actions Should Be Documented in the Medical Record**

1. Repositioning of patient
2. Discontinuation of uterine stimulants and correction of uterine hyperstimulation
3. Vaginal examination
4. Correction of maternal hypotension associated with regional analgesia
5. Notification of anesthesia and nursing staff of the need for emergency delivery
6. Monitoring of fetal heart rate—by electronic fetal monitoring or auscultation—in the operating room prior to abdominal preparation
7. Request that qualified personnel be in attendance for newborn resuscitation and care[a]
8. Administration of oxygen to the mother

[a]Locally acceptable definitions of qualified personnel should be agreed upon by authorities at each institution.

TOCOLYSIS. A single intravenous or subcutaneous injection of 0.25 mg of terbutaline sulfate given to relax the uterus has been described as a temporizing maneuver in the management of nonreassuring fetal heart rate patterns during labor. The rationale for this is that inhibition of uterine contractions might improve fetal oxygenation, thus achieving in utero resuscitation. Cook and Spinnato (1994) described their experience with terbutaline tocolysis for fetal resuscitation in 368 pregnancies over a 10-year period. Such resuscitation improved fetal scalp blood pH values, although all of these women were delivered by cesarean. In their review, the investigators concluded that although the studies were small and rarely randomized, most reported favorable results with terbutaline tocolysis for nonreassuring patterns. Small intravenous doses of nitroglycerin (60 to 180 mg) have also been reported to be beneficial (Mercier and colleagues, 1997).

MECONIUM IN THE AMNIONIC FLUID. Obstetrical teaching throughout this century has included the concept that meconium passage is a potential warning of fetal asphyxia. J. Whitridge Williams, observed in 1903 that "a characteristic sign of impending asphyxia is the escape of meconium." He attributed meconium passage to "relaxation of the sphincter ani muscle induced by faulty aeration of the (fetal) blood." Obstetricians, however, have also long realized that the detection of meconium during labor is problematic in the prediction of fetal distress or asphyxia. In their review, Katz and Bowes (1992) emphasized the prognostic uncertainty of meconium by referring to the topic as a "murky subject." Indeed, although 12 to 22 percent of human labors are complicated by meconium, few such labors are linked to infant mortality. In a recent investigation from Parkland Hospital, meconium was found to be a "low-risk" obstetrical hazard because the perinatal mortality attributable to meconium was 1 death per 1000 live births (Nathan and co-workers, 1994).

Three theories have been suggested to explain fetal passage of meconium and may, in part, explain the tenuous connection between the detection of meconium and infant mortality. The pathological explanation proposes that fetuses pass meconium in response to hypoxia, and that meconium therefore signals fetal compromise (Walker, 1953). Alternatively, in utero passage of meconium may represent normal gastrointestinal tract maturation under neural control (Mathews and Warshaw, 1979). Third, meconium passage could also follow vagal stimulation from common but transient umbilical cord entrapment and resultant increased peristalsis (Hon and colleagues, 1961). Thus, fetal release of meconium could also represent physiological processes.

Ramin and co-authors (1996) studied almost 8000 pregnancies with meconium-stained amnionic fluid delivered at Parkland Hospital. Meconium aspiration syndrome was significantly associated with fetal acidemia at birth. Other significant correlates of aspiration included cesarean delivery, forceps to expedite delivery, intrapartum heart rate abnormalities, depressed Apgar scores, and need for assisted ventilation at delivery. Analysis of the type of fetal acidemia based on umbilical blood gases suggested that the fetal compromise associated with meconium aspiration syndrome was an acute event, because most acidemic fetuses had abnormally increased P_{CO_2} rather than the pure metabolic acidemia.

Interestingly, hypercarbia in fetal lambs has been shown to induce fetal gasping and resultant increased amnionic fluid inhalation (Dawes and co-workers, 1972). Jovanovic and Nguyen (1989) observed that meconium gasped into the fetal lungs caused aspiration syndrome only in asphyxiated animals. Ramin and co-authors (1996) hypothesized that the pathophysiology of meconium aspiration syndrome includes, but is not limited to, fetal hypercarbia, which stimulates fetal respiration leading to aspiration of meconium into the alveoli, and lung parenchymal injury secondary to acidemia-induced alveolar cell damage. In this pathophysiological scenario, meconium in amnionic fluid is a fetal environmental hazard rather than a marker of preexistent compromise. This proposed pathophysiological sequence is not exclusive, because it does not account for approximately half of cases of meconium aspiration syndrome in which the fetus was not acidemic at birth. It was concluded that the high incidence of meconium observed in the amnionic fluid during labor often represents fetal passage of gastrointestinal contents in conjunction with normal physiological processes. Such meconium, however, can become an environmental hazard when fetal acidemia supervenes. Importantly, fetal acidemia occurs acutely, and therefore meconium aspiration is unpredictable and likely unpreventable.

FETAL HEART RATE PATTERNS AND BRAIN DAMAGE. Attempts to correlate fetal heart rate patterns with brain damage have been based primarily on studies of infants identified as a result of medicolegal actions. For example, Rosen and Dickinson (1992) analyzed intrapartum fetal heart rate patterns in 55 such cases and found no specific pattern that was correlated with neurological injury.

Shields and Schifrin (1988) and Schifrin and associates (1994) described what they considered a unique fetal heart rate pattern characteristic of fetal brain damage. This pattern consisted of a normal baseline rate with persistently absent variability and mild variable decelerations with "overshoot." This pattern was frequently found in close proximity to what had been a reactive nonstress test. Other findings included postmaturity, meconium staining with fetal growth restriction, and reduced amnionic fluid volume. They concluded that such patterns most often represent chronic, intermittent cord compression from oligohydramnios resulting in repetitive antepartum central nervous system ischemia. Follow-up studies showed a high incidence of mental retardation, microcephaly, and seizure activity, in addition to cerebral palsy. Phelan and Ahn (1994) reported that among 48 fetuses later found to be neurologically impaired, a persistent nonreactive fetal heart rate tracing was already present at the time of admission in 70 percent; they concluded that fetal neurological injury occurred predominately prior to arrival to the hospital. When they looked retrospectively at heart rate patterns in 209 brain-damaged infants, only half were nonreactive at the time of admission (Ahn and co-workers, 1996). They concluded that there was not a single unique pattern that was associated with fetal neurological injury. Westgate and colleagues (1999) found that more than half of term infants with neonatal encephalopathy due to fetal acidemia were associated with events beyond the control of the obstetrician.

EXPERIMENTAL EVIDENCE. Fetal heart rate patterns necessary for perinatal brain damage have been studied in experimental animals. Myers (1972) described the effects of complete and partial asphyxia in rhesus monkeys in studies of brain damage due to perinatal asphyxia. Complete asphyxia was produced by total occlusion of umbilical blood flow that led to prolonged deceleration (Fig. 14–29). Fetal arterial pH did not reach 7.0 until about 8 minutes after complete cessation of oxygenation and umbilical flow. At least 10 minutes of such prolonged deceleration was required before there was evidence of brain damage in surviving fetuses.

Myers (1972) also produced partial asphyxia in rhesus monkeys by impeding maternal aortic blood flow. This resulted in late decelerations due to uterine and placental hypoperfusion. He observed that several hours of these late decelerations did not damage the fetal brain unless the pH fell below 7.0. Indeed, Adamsons and Myers (1977) reported subsequently that late decelerations were a marker of partial asphyxia long *before* brain damage occurred.

The most common fetal heart rate pattern during labor, due to umbilical cord occlusion, requires considerable time to significantly affect the fetus in experimental animals. Watanabe and associates (1992) showed that sequential complete occlusion of the umbilical cord for 40 seconds followed by 80 seconds of release for 30 minutes in sheep resulted in only moderate fetal acidemia. Similarly, Clapp and colleagues (1988) partially occluded the umbilical cord for 1 minute every 3 minutes in fetal sheep and observed brain damage after 2 hours. Ikeda and colleagues (1998, 2000) studied partial umbilical cord occlusion producing pH of less than 6.9 for 60 minutes in fetal sheep. Such profound asphyxia produced variable degrees of brain damage and multiorgan damage. Lesser durations, specifically, 10, 15, or 20 minutes of total cord occlusion, did not produce brain damage in fetal sheep (Keunen and colleagues, 1997).

Using fetal sheep, Matsuda and co-workers (1999) showed that similar brain injuries occurred with acute fetal hemorrhage. These investigators withdrew about a third of fetoplacental blood volume acutely which produced hypotension and subsequent periventricular white-matter changes.

HUMAN EVIDENCE. The contribution of intrapartum events to subsequent neurological handicaps has been greatly overestimated. Nelson and Grether (1998) performed a population-based study of children with disabling spastic cerebral palsy in which the intrapartum records of these children were compared with matched controls. Intrapartum fetal heart rate abnormalities did not distinguish between children with cerebral palsy and normal controls. Badawi and colleagues (1998) also per-

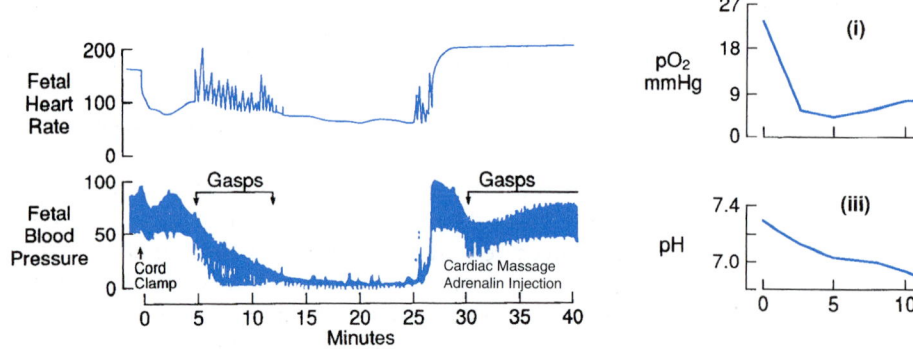

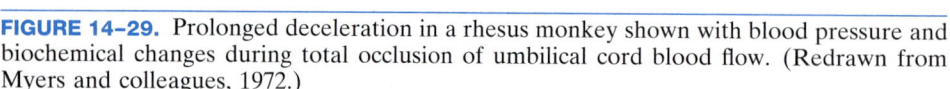

FIGURE 14–29. Prolonged deceleration in a rhesus monkey shown with blood pressure and biochemical changes during total occlusion of umbilical cord blood flow. (Redrawn from Myers and colleagues, 1972.)

formed a case-control population based study of infants with cerebral palsy in Western Australia. Only 5 percent of the brain-damaged infants had intrapartum factors, which led them to conclude that most cerebral palsy is unrelated to labor events.

Low and co-workers (1989) divided perinatal brain damage into three categories based on microscopic findings:

1. From 18 to 48 hours—neuronal necrosis with pyknosis or lysis of the nucleus in shriveled eosinophilic cells.
2. From 48 to 72 hours—more intense neuronal necrosis with macrophage response.
3. More than 3 days—all the preceding plus astrocyte response with gliosis and, in some, early cavitation.

Abnormal brain histopathology was not observed with acute, lethal asphyxia. Moreover, 43 percent of brain damage episodes occurred prior to labor and 25 percent were in the neonatal period. Similarly, in another investigation, Low and co-workers (1984) estimated that more than 1 hour of fetal hypoxia associated with profound metabolic acidemia (pH less than 7.0) was required before neurological abnormalities could be diagnosed at 6 to 12 months of age. Low and co-workers (1988) followed 37 term infants with profound metabolic acidemia at birth to 1 year and found major neurological deficits in 13 percent of the infants. Minor deficits were diagnosed in 10 infants, and the remaining 60 percent were normal. These investigators further observed that intrapartum fetal asphyxia with metabolic acidemia at delivery in both the term and preterm fetus was marked by severe complications not only of the central nervous system, but also of the respiratory and renal systems (Low and colleagues, 1994, 1995).

These observations further strengthen the position of the American College of Obstetricians and Gynecologists (1996) on birth asphyxia and cerebral palsy: In assessing a possible relationship between perinatal asphyxia and neurological deficit in an individual patient, all of the following criteria must be present before a plausible link can be made:

1. Profound umbilical artery metabolic or mixed acidemia (pH less than 7.00).
2. Persistence of an Apgar score of 0 to 3 for longer than 5 minutes.
3. Neonatal neurological sequelae (e.g., seizures, coma, or hypotonia).
4. Multiorgan system dysfunction (e.g., cardiovascular gastrointestinal, hematological, pulmonary, or renal).

Korst and colleagues (1999) have challenged this concept.

Clearly, for brain damage to occur, the fetus must be exposed to much more than a brief period of hypoxia.

Moreover, the hypoxia must cause profound, just barely sublethal metabolic acidemia. Fetal heart rate patterns consistent with these sublethal conditions are fortunately rare.

BENEFITS OF ELECTRONIC FETAL HEART RATE MONITORING. There are several fallacious assumptions behind expectations of improved perinatal outcome with electronic monitoring. One assumption is that fetal distress is a slowly developing phenomenon and that electronic monitoring makes possible early detection of the compromised fetus. This assumption is illogical, *viz*, how can all fetuses die slowly? Another presumption is that all fetal damage develops in the hospital. Only recently has attention focused on the reality that most damaged fetuses suffered insults before arrival to labor units. The very term "fetal monitor" implies that this inanimate technology in some fashion "monitors." The assumption is made that if a dead or damaged infant is delivered, the tracing strip must provide some clue, because this device was monitoring fetal condition. All of these assumptions led to great expectations and fostered the belief that all dead or damaged neonates were preventable. Parer and King (2000) reviewed reasons why fetal heart rate monitoring did not live up to its expectations. These unwarranted expectations have greatly fueled litigation in obstetrics. Indeed, Symonds (1994) reported that 70 percent of all liability claims related to fetal brain damage are based on reputed abnormalities seen in the electronic fetal monitor tracing.

Too many fetuses demonstrate fetal heart rate abnormalities during labor to permit accurate detection of those who are actually compromised. Indeed, most "fetal distress" does not represent an overtly compromised fetus. Importantly, debate continues about interpretation of many heart rate patterns. For example, Keith and co-workers (1995) asked each of 17 experts to review 50 tracings on two occasions, at least 1 month apart. About 20 percent changed their own interpretations, and approximately 25 percent did not agree with the interpretations of their colleagues.

By the end of the 1970s, questions about the efficacy, safety, and costs of electronic monitoring were being voiced from the Office of Technology Assessment, the United States Congress, and the Centers for Disease Control and Prevention. Banta and Thacker (1979) analyzed 158 reports and concluded that "the technical advances required in the demonstration that reliable recording could be done seems to have blinded most observers to the fact that this additional information will not necessarily produce better outcomes." They attributed the apparent lack of benefit to the imprecision of electronic monitoring to identify fetal distress. Moreover, increased usage was linked to more frequent cesarean delivery. They estimated that additional costs of childbirth in the United States, if half of labors had electronic monitoring, was approximately $400 million per year in 1979 dollars.

The National Institute of Child Health and Human Development (NICHD) appointed a task force to study these concerns, and a consensus report was published in 1979. After an exhaustive review of electronic monitoring literature, the group concluded that the evidence only suggested a trend toward improved infant outcome in complicated pregnancies. They emphasized that few scientifically conducted investigations had been done to address perinatal benefits. Almost 20 years later, the NICHD Fetal Monitoring Workshop (1997) once again formulated research recommendations intended to assess the reliability and validity of fetal heart rate patterns in the prevention of asphyxial brain damage.

PARKLAND HOSPITAL EXPERIENCE: SELECTIVE VERSUS UNIVERSAL MONITORING. In July 1982, an investigation began at Parkland Hospital to ascertain whether all women in labor should undergo electronic monitoring (Leveno and co-workers, 1986). In alternating months, universal electronic monitoring was rotated with selective heart rate monitoring, which was the prevailing practice. During the 3-year investigation, 17,410 labors were managed using universal electronic monitoring. No significant differences were found in any perinatal outcomes. There was a significantly small increase in cesarean delivery for fetal distress associated with universal monitoring. Thus, increased application of electronic monitoring at Parkland Hospital did not improve perinatal results, but it increased the frequency of cesarean delivery for fetal distress.

SUMMARY OF RANDOMIZED STUDIES. Thacker and co-authors (1995) identified 12 published randomized clinical trials of electronic fetal monitoring from 1966 to 1994. Total pregnancies included in these studies was 58,624. They concluded that the benefits once claimed for electronic monitoring are clearly more modest than believed, and appear to be primarily in the prevention of neonatal seizures. Long-term implications of this outcome, however, appear less serious than once believed. Abnormal neurological consequences were not consistently higher among children monitored by auscultation compared with electronic methods. They concurred with the current position of the American College of Obstetricians and Gynecologists (1995b) on intrapartum fetal surveillance.

CURRENT RECOMMENDATIONS. The methods most commonly used for intrapartum fetal heart rate monitoring include auscultation with a fetal stethoscope or a Doppler ultrasound device, or continuous electronic

TABLE 14–4. Guidelines for Intrapartum Fetal Heart Rate Surveillance

Surveillance	Low-Risk Pregnancies	High-Risk Pregnancies
Acceptable methods		
Intermittent auscultation	Yes	Yes
Continuous electronic monitoring (internal or external)	Yes	Yes
Evaluation intervals[a]		
First-stage labor (active)	30 min	15 min[b]
Second-stage labor	15 min	5 min[b]

[a]Following a uterine contraction.
[b]Includes tracing evaluation and charting with continuous electronic monitoring.
Adapted from the American College of Obstetricians and Gynecologists (1995b).

monitoring of the heart rate and uterine contractions. There is no scientific evidence that has identified the most effective method, including frequency or duration of fetal surveillance, that ensures optimum results. Table 14–4 gives current recommendations of the American College of Obstetricians and Gynecologists (1995b). Intermittent auscultation or continuous electronic monitoring are considered acceptable methods of intrapartum surveillance in both low- and high-risk pregnancies. The recommended interval between checking the heart rate, however, is longer in the uncomplicated pregnancy. When auscultation is used, it is recommended that it be performed after a contraction and for 60 seconds. It is also recommended that a 1-to-1 nurse–patient ratio be used if auscultation is employed.

INTRAPARTUM SURVEILLANCE OF UTERINE ACTIVITY

Analysis of electronically measured uterine activity permits some generalities concerning the relationship of certain contraction patterns to labor outcome. There is considerable normal variation, however, and caution must be exercised before judging true labor or its absence solely from study of a monitor tracing. Uterine muscle efficiency to effect delivery varies greatly. To use an analogy, 100-meter sprinters all have the same muscle groups yet cross the finish line at different times.

INTERNAL UTERINE PRESSURE MONITORING. Amnionic fluid pressure is measured between and during contractions by a fluid-filled plastic catheter with its distal tip located above the presenting part. The catheter is connected to a strain-gauge pressure sensor adjusted to the same level as the catheter tip in the uterus. The amplified electrical signal produced in the strain gauge by variation in pressure within the fluid system is recorded on a calibrated moving paper strip, simultaneously with fetal heart rate recording. Intrauterine pressure catheters are now available that have the pressure sensor in the catheter tip, which obviates the need for the fluid column.

EXTERNAL MONITORING. Uterine contractions can be measured by a displacement transducer in which the transducer button ("plunger") is held against the abdominal wall. As the uterus contracts, the button moves in proportion to the strength of the contraction. This movement is converted into a measurable electrical signal that indicates the *relative* intensity of the contraction—it does not give an accurate measure of intensity. External monitoring can give a good indication of the onset, peak, and end of the contraction.

PATTERNS OF UTERINE ACTIVITY. Caldeyro-Barcia and Poseiro (1960) from Montevideo, Uruguay, were pioneers who have done much to elucidate the patterns of spontaneous uterine activity throughout pregnancy. Their investigations were made possible by the development of electronic means of recording and quantifying uterine contractions before and during labor. Contractile waves of uterine activity were usually measured using intra-amnionic pressure catheters, but early in their studies as many as four simultaneous intramyometrial microballoons were also used to record uterine pressure. They also introduced the concept of **Montevideo units** to define uterine activity (Chap. 18, p. 441). By this definition, uterine performance is the product of the intensity—increased uterine pressure above baseline tone—of a contraction in mm Hg multiplied by contraction frequency per 10 minutes. For example, three contractions in 10 minutes, each of 50 mm Hg intensity, would equal 150 Montevideo units.

During the first 30 weeks, uterine activity is comparatively quiescent. Contractions are seldom greater than 20 mm Hg, and these have been equated with those first described in 1872 by John Braxton Hicks. Uterine activity increases gradually after 30 weeks and it is noteworthy that these *Braxton Hicks contractions* also increase in intensity and frequency. Further increases in uterine activity are typical of the last weeks of pregnancy, termed **prelabor.** During this phase, the cervix ripens, presumably as a consequence of increasing uterine contractions (Chap. 11, p. 257).

According to Caldeyro-Barcia and Poseiro (1960), clinical labor usually commences when uterine activity reaches values between 80 and 120 Montevideo units. This translates into approximately three contractions of 40 mm Hg every 10 minutes, or 120 Montevideo units. Importantly, there is no clear-cut division between pre-

labor and labor, but rather a gradual and progressive transition.

During first-stage labor, uterine contractions increase progressively in intensity from about 25 mm Hg at commencement of labor to 50 mm Hg at the end. At the same time, frequency increases from three to five contractions per 10 minutes, and uterine baseline tone from 8 to 12 mm Hg. Uterine activity further increases during second-stage labor, aided by maternal bearing down. Indeed, contractions of 80 to 100 mm Hg are typical, and occur as frequently as five to six per 10 minutes. Interestingly, the duration of uterine contractions—60 to 80 seconds—does not increase appreciably from early active labor extending through the second-stage (Pontonnier and colleagues, 1975). Presumably, this constancy of duration serves a fetal respiratory gas-exchange function. That is, functional fetal "breath holding" during a uterine contraction, which results in isolation of the intervillous space where respiratory gas exchange occurs, has a 60- to 80-second limit that remains relatively constant.

Caldeyro-Barcia and Poseiro (1960) also observed empirically that uterine contractions are clinically palpable only after their intensity exceeds 10 mm Hg. Moreover, until their intensity reaches 40 mm Hg, the uterine wall can readily be depressed by the finger. At greater intensity, it then becomes so hard that it resists easy depression. Uterine contractions are usually not associated with pain until their intensity exceeds 15 mm Hg, presumably because this is the minimum pressure required for distending the lower uterine segment and cervix. It follows that Braxton Hicks contractions exceeding 15 mm Hg may be perceived as uncomfortable because distention of the uterus, cervix, and birth canal is generally thought to elicit discomfort.

Hendricks (1968) observed that "the clinician makes great demands upon the uterus." The uterus is expected to remain well relaxed during pregnancy, to contract effectively but intermittently during labor, and then to remain in a state of almost constant contraction for several hours postpartum. Figure 14–30 demonstrates an example of normal uterine activity during labor. As also described by Caldeyro-Barcia and Poseiro (1960), uterine activity progressively and gradually increases from prelabor through late labor. Interestingly, as shown in Figure 14–30, uterine contractions after birth are identical to those resulting in delivery of the infant. Indeed, the pattern of uterine activity is one of gradual subsidence or reverse of that leading up to delivery. It is therefore not surprising that the uterus that performs poorly before delivery is also prone to atony and puerperal hemorrhage.

ORIGIN AND PROPAGATION OF CONTRACTIONS. The uterus has not been extensively studied in terms of its nonhormonal physiological mechanisms of function.

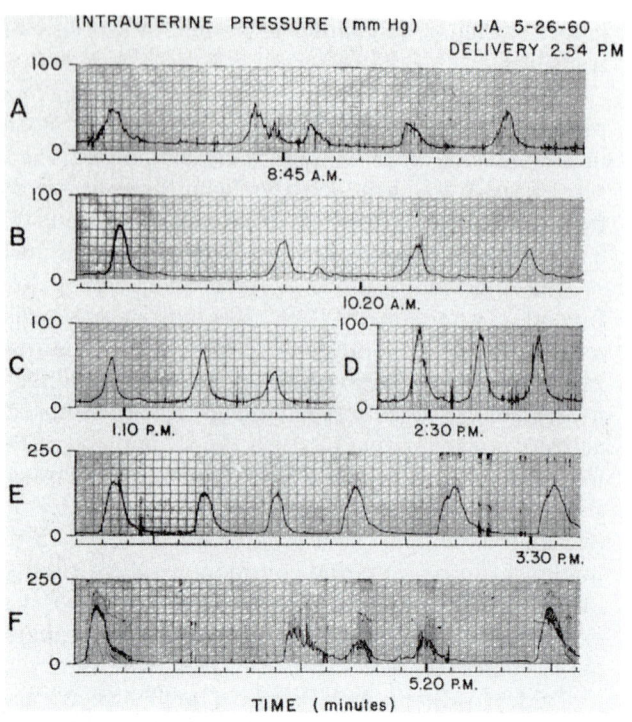

FIGURE 14–30. Intrauterine pressure recorded through a single catheter. **A.** Prelabor. **B.** Early labor. **C.** Active labor. **D.** Late labor. **E.** Spontaneous activity ½ hour postpartum. **F.** Spontaneous activity 2½ hours postpartum. (From Hendricks, 1968.)

contractile wave of the couplet. These small contractions alternating with larger ones appear to be typical of early labor, and indeed, labor may progress with such uterine activity, albeit at a slower pace. They also observed that labor would progress slowly if regular contractions were hypotonic—that is, contractions with intensity less than 25 mm Hg or frequency less than two per 10 minutes. Similar observations were made by Seitchik (1981) in a computer-aided analysis comparing women in active labor with those with arrested labor. Normal labor was characterized by a minimum of three contractions that averaged greater than 25 mm Hg and less than 4-minute intervals between contractions. A lesser amount of uterine activity was associated with arrest of active labor. Prospective diagnosis of hypotonic labor cannot be reliably based simply on a few uterine pressures.

Hauth and co-workers (1986) quantified uterine contraction pressures in 109 women at term who received oxytocin for labor induction or augmentation. Most of these women achieved 200 to 225 Montevideo units, and 40 percent had up to 300 units to effect delivery. They suggested that these levels of uterine activity should be sought before consideration of cesarean delivery for presumed dystocia—this recommendation was later endorsed by the American College of Obstetricians and Gynecologists (1995a).

The normal contractile wave of labor originates near the uterine end of one of the fallopian tubes; thus these areas act as "pacemakers" (Fig. 14–31). The right pacemaker usually predominates over the left and starts the great majority of contractile waves. Contractions spread from the pacemaker area throughout the uterus at 2 cm/sec, depolarizing the whole organ within 15 seconds. This depolarization wave propagates downward toward the cervix. Intensity is greatest in the fundus, and it diminishes in the lower uterus. This phenomenon is thought to reflect reductions of myometrial thickness from the fundus to the cervix. Presumably, this descending gradient of pressure serves to direct fetal descent toward the cervix as well as to efface the cervix. Importantly, all parts of the uterus are synchronized and reach their peak pressure almost simultaneously, giving rise to the curvilinear waveform shown in Figure 14–31.

The pacemaker theory also serves to explain the varying intensity of adjacent coupled contractions shown in panels A and B of Figure 14–30. Such coupling was termed **incoordination** by Caldeyro-Barcia and Poseiro (1960). A contractile wave begins in one cornual-region pacemaker, but does not synchronously depolarize the entire uterus. As a result, another contraction begins in the contralateral pacemaker and produces the second

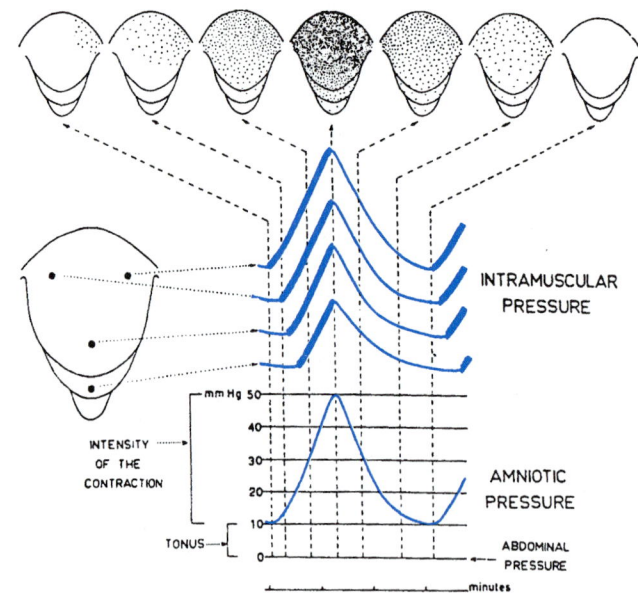

FIGURE 14–31. Schematic representation of the normal contractile wave of labor. Large uterus on the left shows the four points at which intramyometrial pressure was recorded with microballoons. Four corresponding pressure tracing are shown in relation to each other by shading on the small uteri. (From Caldeyro-Barcia and Poseiro, 1960.)

REFERENCES

Adamsons K, Myers RE: Late decelerations and brain tolerance of the fetal monkey to intrapartum asphyxia. Am J Obstet Gynecol 128:893, 1977

Ahn MO, Korst L, Phelan JP: Intrapartum fetal heart rate patterns in 209 brain damaged infants. Am J Obstet Gynecol 174:492, 1996

American College of Obstetricians and Gynecologists: Cesarean delivery for nonreassuring fetal status. Criteria Set no. 33, May, 1998

American College of Obstetricians and Gynecologists: Dystocia and the augmentation of labor. Technical Bulletin no. 218, December 1995a

American College of Obstetricians and Gynecologists: Fetal heart rate patterns: Monitoring, interpretation, and management. Technical Bulletin no. 207, July 1995b

American College of Obstetricians and Gynecologists: Use and abuse of the Apgar score. Committee Opinion no. 174, January 1996

Angel J, Knuppel R, Lake M: Sinusoidal fetal heart rate patterns associated with intravenous butorphanol administration. Am J Obstet Gynecol 149:465, 1984

Anyaegbunam AM, Ditchik A, Stoessel R, Mikhail MS: Vibroacoustic stimulation of the fetus entering the second stage of labor. Obstet Gynecol 83:963, 1994

Ayres-de-Campos D, Bernardes J, Costa-Pereira A, Pereira-Teite L: Inconsistencies in classification by experts of cardiotocograms and subsequent clinical decision. Br J Obstet Gynaecol 106:1307, 1999

Badawi N, Kurinczuk J, Keogh JM, Alessandri CM, O'Sullivan F, Burton PR, Penberton PJ, Stanley FJ: Intrapartum risk factors for newborn encephalopathy: The Western Australia case-control study. Br Med J 317:1554, 1998

Ball RH, Parer JT: The physiologic mechanisms of variable decelerations. Am J Obstet Gynecol 166:1683, 1992

Banta HD, Thacker SB: Assessing the costs and benefits of electronic fetal monitoring. Obstet Gynecol Surv 34:627, 1979

Behrman RE: The cardiovascular system. In Behrman RE, Kliegman RM, Nelson WE, Vaughn VC (eds): Nelson Textbook of Pediatrics, 14th ed. Philadelphia, Saunders, 1992, p 1127

Berkus MD, Langer O, Samueloff A, Xenakis EMJ, Field NT: Electronic fetal monitoring: What's reassuring? Acta Obstet Gynecol Scand 78:15, 1999

Bloom SL, Swindle RG, McIntire DD, Leveno KJ: Fetal pulse oximetry: Duration of desaturation and integration outcome. Obstet Gynecol 93:1036, 1999

Boehm FH: Prolonged end stage fetal heart rate deceleration. Obstet Gynecol 45:579, 1975

Caldeyro-Barcia R, Mendez-Bauer C, Poseiro JJ, Pose S: Fetal monitoring in labor. In Walloch HJ, Gold EM, Lis EF (eds): Maternal and Child Health Practices. Springfield, IL, Thomas, 1973, p 332

Caldeyro-Barcia R, Poseiro JJ: Physiology of the uterine contraction. Clin Obstet Gynecol 3:386, 1960

Chua S, Yeong SM, Razvi K, Arulkumaran S: Fetal oxygen saturation during labor. Br J Obstet Gynaecol 104:1080, 1997

Clapp JF, Peress NS, Wesley M, Mann LI: Brain damage after intermittent partial cord occlusion in the chronically instrumented fetal lamb. Am J Obstet Gynecol 159:504, 1988

Clark SL, Gimovsky ML, Miller FC: The scalp stimulation test: A clinical alternative to fetal scalp blood sampling. Am J Obstet Gynecol 148:274, 1984

Clark SL, Gimovsky ML, Miller FC: Fetal heart rate response to scalp blood sampling. Am J Obstet Gynecol 14:706, 1982

Clark SL, Paul RH: Fetal heart rate monitoring patterns. Am J Obstet Gynecol 155:914, 1986

Cook VD, Spinnato JA: Terbutaline tocolysis prior to cesarean section for fetal distress. J Matern Fetal Med 3:219, 1994

Copel JA, Liang RI, Demasio K, Ozeren S, Kleinman CS: The clinical significance of the irregular fetal heart rhythm. Am J Obstet Gynecol 182:813, 2000

Davidson SR, Rankin JH, Martin CB Jr, Reid DL: Fetal heart rate variability and behavioral state: Analysis by power spectrum. Am J Obstet Gynecol 167:717, 1992

Dawes GS: The control of fetal heart rate and its variability in counts. In Kunzel W (ed): Fetal Heart Rate Monitoring. Berlin, Springer-Verlag, 1985, p 188

Dawes GS, Fox HE, Leduc BM, Liggins GC, Richards RT: Respiratory movements and rapid eye movement sleep in the foetal lamb. J Physiol 220:119, 1972

Dawes GS, Visser GHA, Goodman JDS, Levine DH: Numerical analysis of the human fetal heart rate: Modulation by breathing and movement. Am J Obstet Gynecol 140:535, 1981

Deans AC, Steer PJ: The use of the fetal electrocardiogram in labour. Br J Obstet Gynaecol 101:9, 1994

Del Valle GO, Joffe GM, Izquierdo LA, Smith JF, Kasnic T, Gilson GJ, Chatterjee MS, Curet LB: Acute post traumatic fetal anemia treated with fetal intravascular transfusion. Am J Obstet Gynecol 166:127, 1992

Dellinger EH, Boehm FH, Crane MM: Electronic fetal heart rate monitoring: Early neonatal outcomes associated with normal rate, fetal stress, and fetal distress. Am J Obstet Gynecol 182:214, 2000

Divon MY, Winkler H, Yeh SY, Platt LD, Langer O, Merkatz IR: Diminished respiratory sinus arrhythmia in asphyxiated term infants. Am J Obstet Gynecol 155:1263, 1986

Dye T, Aubry R, Gross S, Artal R: Amnioinfusion and the intrauterine prevention of meconium aspiration. Am J Obstet Gynecol 171:1601, 1994

Eberle RL, Norris MC, Eberle AM, Naulty JS, Arkoosh VA: The effect of maternal position on fetal heart rate during epidural or intrathecal labor analgesia. Am J Obstet Gynecol 179:150, 1998

Edersheim TG, Hutson JM, Druzin ML, Kogut EA: Fetal heart rate response to vibratory acoustic stimulation predicts fetal pH in labor. Am J Obstet Gynecol 157:1557, 1987

Egley CC, Bowes WA, Wagner D: Sinusoidal fetal heart rate pattern during labor. Am J Perinatol 8:197, 1991

Elimian A, Figueroa R, Tejani N: Intrapartum assessment of fetal well-being: A comparison of scalp stimulation with scalp pH sampling. Obstet Gynecol 89:373, 1997

Epstein H, Waxman A, Gleicher N, Lauersen NH: Meperidine induced sinusoidal fetal heart rate pattern and reversal with naloxone. Obstet Gynecol 59:225, 1982

Faro S, Martens MG, Hammill HA, Riddle G, Tortolero G: Antibiotic prophylaxis: Is there a difference? Am J Obstet Gynecol 162:900, 1990

Farrell T, Chien PFW, Gordon A: Intrapartum umbilical artery Doppler velocimetry as a predictor of adverse perinatal outcome: A systematic review. Br J Obstet Gynaecol 106:783, 1999

Freeman RK, Garite TH, Nageotte MP: Fetal Heart Rate Monitoring, 2nd ed. Baltimore, Williams & Wilkins, 1991

Gabbe SG, Ettinger BB, Freeman RK, Martin CB: Umbilical cord compression associated with amniotomy: Laboratory observations. Am J Obstet Gynecol 126:353, 1976

Garite TJ, Dildy GA, McNamara H, Nageotte MP, Boehm FH, Dellinger EH, Knuppel RA, Porreco RP, Miller HS, Sunderji S, Varner MW, Swedlow DB: A multicenter controlled trial of fetal pulse oximetry in the intrapartum management of nonreassuring fetal heart rate patterns. Am J Obstet Gynecol 183:1049, 2000

Gilstrap LC III, Hauth JC, Hankins GDV, Beck AW: Second-stage fetal heart rate abnormalities and type of neonatal acidemia. Obstet Gynecol 70:191, 1987

Goodwin TM, Milner-Masterson L, Paul RH: Elimination of fetal scalp blood sampling on a large clinical service. Obstet Gynecol 83:971, 1994

Granat M, Lavie P, Cedar D, Sharf M: Short-term cycles in human fetal activity. Am J Obstet Gynecol 134:696, 1979

Gull I, Jaffa AJ, Oren M, Grisaru D, Peyser MR, Lessing JB: Acid accumulation during end-stage bradycardia in term fetuses: How long is too long? Br J Obstet Gynecol 103:1096, 1996

Hallak M, Martinez-Poyer J, Kruger ML, Hassan S, Blackwell SC, Sorokin Y: The effect of magnesium sulfate on fetal heart rate parameters: A randomized, placebo-controlled trial. Am J Obstet Gynecol 181:1122, 1999

Hamilton LA Jr, McKeown MJ: Biochemical and electronic monitoring of the fetus. In Wynn RM (ed): Obstetrics and Gynecology Annual, 1973. New York, Appleton-Century-Crofts, 1974

Hammacher K, Huter K, Bokelmann J, Werners PH: Foetal heart frequency and perinatal conditions of the fetus and newborn. Gynaecologia 166:349, 1968

Hankins GDV, Leicht TL, Van Houk JW: Prolonged fetal bradycardia secondary to maternal hypothermia in response to urosepsis. Am J Perinatol 14:217, 1997

Hauth JC, Hankins GV, Gilstrap LC, Strickland DM, Vance P: Uterine contraction pressures with oxytocin induction/augmentation. Obstet Gynecol 68:305, 1986

Hendricks CH: Uterine contractility changes in the early puerperium. In Anderson GV, Quilligan EJ (eds): Clinical Obstetrics and Gynecology, Thromboembolic Disorders, Physiology of Labor. New York, Harper & Row, 1968, p 125

Herbert CM, Boehm FH: Prolonged end-stage fetal heart deceleration: A reanalysis. Obstet Gynecol 57:589, 1981

Hicks JB: On the contractions of the uterus throughout pregnancy. Trans Obstet Soc Lond 13, 1872

Hoffman C III, Guzman E, Richardson M, Vintzileos A, Houlihan C, Benito C: The effects of narcotic and non-narcotic continuous epidural anesthesia on intrapartum fetal heart rate tracings as measured by computer analysis. Am J Obstet Gynecol 174:431, 1996

Hon EH: The fetal heart rate patterns preceding death in utero. Am J Obstet Gynecol 78:47, 1959

Hon EH: The electronic evaluation of the fetal heart rate. Am J Obstet Gynecol 75:1215, 1958

Hon EH, Bradfield AM, Hess OW: The electronic evaluation of the fetal heart rate. Am J Obstet Gynecol 82:291, 1961

Hornbuckle J, Vail A, Abrams KR, Thornton JG: Bayesian interpretation of trials: The example of intrapartum electronic fetal heart rate monitoring. Br J Obstet Gynaecol 107:3, 2000

Ikeda T, Murata Y, Quilligan EJ, Choi B, Parer JT, Doi S, Park SD: Physiologic and histologic changes in near-term fetal lambs exposed to asphyxia by partial umbilical cord occlusion. Am J Obstet Gynecol 178:24, 1998

Ikeda T, Murata Y, Quilligan EJ, Cifuentes P, Doi S, Park SD: Two sinusoidal heart rate patterns in fetal lambs undergoing extra corporeal membrane oxygenation. Am J Obstet Gynecol 180:462, 1999

Ikeda T, Murata Y, Quilligan EJ, Parer JT, Murayama T, Koono M: Histologic and biochemical study of the brain, heart, kidney, and liver in asphyxia caused by occlusion of the umbilical cord in near-term fetal lambs. Am J Obstet Gynecol 182:449, 2000

Itskovitz J, LaGamma EF, Rudoloph AM: Heart rate and blood pressure response to umbilical cord compression in fetal lambs with special reference to the mechanisms of variable deceleration. Am J Obstet Gynecol 147:451, 1983

Johnson TR Jr, Compton AA, Rotmeusch J, Work BA, Johnson JC: Significance of the sinusoidal fetal heart rate pattern. Am J Obstet Gynecol 139:446, 1981

Jovanovic R, Nguyen HT: Experimental meconium aspiration in guinea pigs. Obstet Gynecol 73:652, 1989

Katz VL, Bowes WA: Meconium aspiration syndrome: Reflections on a murky subject. Am J Obstet Gynecol 166:171, 1992

Keith RDF, Beckley S, Garibaldi JM, Westgate JA, Ifeachor EC, Greene KR: A multicentre comparative study of 17 experts and an intelligent computer system for managing labour using the cardiotocogram. Br J Obstet Gynaecol 102:688, 1995

Keunen H, Blanco CE, von Reempts JLH, Hasaart THM: Absence of neuronal change after umbilical cord occlusion of 10, 15 and 20 minutes mid gestational sheep. Am J Obstet Gynecol 176:515, 1997

Klavan M, Laver AT, Boscola MA: Clinical concepts of fetal heart rate monitoring. Waltham, MA, Hewlett-Packard, 1977

Korst LM, Phelan JP, Wang YM, Martin GI, Ahn MO: Acute fetal asphyxia and permanent brain injury: A retrospective analysis of current indications. J Matern-Fetal Med 8:101, 1999

Kozuma S, Watanabe T, Bennet L, Green LR, Hanson MA: The effect of carotid sinus denervation on fetal heart rate variation in normoxia, hypoxia and post-hypoxia in fetal sleep. Br J Obstet Gynaecol 104:460, 1997

Krebs HB, Petres RE, Dunn LJ: Intrapartum fetal heart rate monitoring, 5. Fetal heart rate patterns in the second stage of labor. Am J Obstet Gynecol 140:435, 1981

Krebs HB, Petres RE, Dunn LJ, Smith PJ: Intrapartum fetal heart rate monitoring, 6. Prognostic significance of accelerations. Am J Obstet Gynecol 142:297, 1982

Kruger K, Hallberg B, Blennow M, Kublickas M, Westgren M: Predictive value of fetal scalp blood lactate concentration and pH as markers of neurologic disability. Am J Obstet Gynecol 181:1072, 1999

Kunzel W: Fetal heart rate alterations in partial and total cord occlusion. In Kunzel W (ed): Fetal Heart Rate Monitoring: Clinical Practice and Pathophysiology. Berlin, Springer-Verlag, 1985, p 114

Lee CV, DiLaretto PC, Lane JM: A study of fetal heart rate acceleration patterns. Obstet Gynecol 45:142, 1975

Leveno KJ, Cunningham FG, Nelson S: Prospective comparison of selective and universal electronic fetal monitoring in 34,995 pregnancies. N Engl J Med 315:615, 1986

Leveno KJ, Quirk JG, Cunningham FG, Nelson SD, Santos R, Toofanian A, DePalma RT: Prolonged pregnancy: Observations concerning the causes of fetal distress. Am J Obstet Gynecol 150:465, 1984

Lin CC, Vassollo B, Mittendorf R: Intrapartum fetal heart rate responses to vibroacoustic stimulation versus fetal blood pH studies to predict outcome in labor. Am J Obstet Gynecol 180:S91, 1999

Low JA, Galbraith RS, Muir DW, Killen HL, Pater EA,

Karchmar EJ: Motor and cognitive deficits after intrapartum asphyxia in the mature fetus. Am J Obstet Gynecol 158:356, 1988

Low JA, Galbraith RS, Muir DW, Killen HL, Pater EA, Karchmar EJ: Factors associated with motor and cognitive deficits in children after intrapartum fetal hypoxia. Am J Obstet Gynecol 148:533, 1984

Low JA, Panagiotopoulos C, Derrick EJ: Newborn complications after intrapartum asphyxia with metabolic acidosis in the preterm fetus. Am J Obstet Gynecol 172:805, 1995

Low JA, Panagiotopoulos C, Derrick EJ: Newborn complications after intrapartum asphyxia with metabolic acidosis in the term fetus. Am J Obstet Gynecol 170:1081, 1994

Low JA, Robertson DR, Simpson LL: Temporal relationships of neuropathologic conditions caused by perinatal asphyxia. Am J Obstet Gynecol 160:608, 1989

Low JA, Victory R, Derrick J: Predictive value of electronic fetal monitoring for intrapartum fetal asphyxia with metabolic acidosis. Obstet Gynecol 93:285, 1999

Lowe TW, Leveno KJ, Quirk JG, Santos-Ramos R, Williams ML: Sinusoidal fetal heart rate patterns after intrauterine transfusion. Obstet Gynecol 64:215, 1984

Macri CJ, Schrimmer DB, Leung A, Greenspoon JS, Paul RH: Prophylactic amnioinfusion improves outcome of pregnancy complicated by thick meconium and oligohydramnios. Am J Obstet Gynecol 167:117, 1992

Manassiev N: What is the normal heart rate of a term fetus? Br J Obstet Gynaecol 103:1272, 1996

Mathews TG, Warshaw JB: Relevance of the gestational age distribution of meconium passage in utero. Pediatrics 64:30, 1979

Matsuda T, Okuyama K, Cho K, Hoshi N, Matsumoto Y, Kobayashi Y, Fujimoto S: Induction of antenatal periventricular leukomalacia by hemorrhagic hypotension in the chronically instrumented fetal sheep. Am J Obstet Gynecol 181:725, 1999

McGregor JA, McFarren T: Neonatal cranial osteomyelitis: A complication of fetal monitoring. Obstet Gynecol 73:490, 1989

Melchior J, Bernard N: Incidence and pattern of fetal heart rate alterations during labor. In Kunzel W (ed): Fetal Heart Rate Monitoring: Clinical Practice and Pathophysiology. Berlin, Springer-Verlag, 1985, p 73

Mercier FJ, Dounas M, Bouaziz H, Lhuisser C, Benhamou D: Intravenous nitroglycerin to relieve intrapartum fetal distress related to uterine hyperactivity: A prospective observation study. Anesth Analg 84:1117, 1997

Miyazaki FS, Nevarez F: Saline amnioinfusion for relief of repetitive variable decelerations: A prospective randomized study. Am J Obstet Gynecol 153:301, 1985

Miyazaki FS, Taylor NA: Saline amnioinfusion for relief of variable or prolonged decelerations. Am J Obstet Gynecol 146:670, 1983

Modanlou H, Freeman RK: Sinusoidal fetal heart rate pattern: Its definition and clinical significance. Am J Obstet Gynecol 142:1033, 1982

Mueller-Heubach E, Battelli AF: Variable heart rate decelerations and transcutaneous Po₂ (tc Po₂) during umbilical cord occlusion in the fetal monkey. Am J Obstet Gynecol 144:796, 1982

Murata Y, Martin CB, Ikenoue T, Hashimoto T, Taira S, Saqawa T, Sakata H: Fetal heart rate accelerations and late decelerations during the course of intrauterine death in chronically catheterized rhesus monkeys. Am J Obstet Gynecol 144:218, 1982

Murotsuki J, Bocking AD, Gagnon R: Fetal heart rate patterns in growth-restricted fetal sleep induced by chronic fetal placental embolization. Am J Obstet Gynecol 176:282, 1997

Murphy KW, Russell V, Collins A, Johnson P: The prevalence, aetiology and clinical significance of pseudo-sinusoidal fetal heart rate patterns in labour. Br J Obstet Gynaecol 98:1093, 1991

Myers RE: Two patterns of perinatal brain damage and their conditions of occurrence. Am J Obstet Gynecol 112:246, 1972

Myers RE, Mueller-Heubach E, Adamsons K: Predictability of the state of fetal oxygenation from a quantitative analysis of the components of late deceleration. Am J Obstet Gynecol 115:1083, 1973

Nageotte MP, Bertucci L, Towers CV, Lagrew DL, Modanlou H: Prophylactic amnioinfusion in pregnancies complicated by oligohydramnios: A prospective study. Obstet Gynecol 77:677, 1991

Nathan L, Leveno KJ, Carmody TJ, Kelly MA, Sherman ML: Meconium: A 1990s perspective on an old obstetric hazard. Obstet Gynecol 83:328, 1994

National Institute of Child Health and Human Development. Consensus Development Conference, 3. Predictors of intrapartum fetal distress. In: Antenatal Diagnosis. Bethesda, US Department of Health, Education and Welfare, Public Health Service, National Institutes of Health, 1979

National Institute of Child Health and Human Development Research Planning Workshop: Electronic fetal heart rate monitoring: Research guidelines for integration. Am J Obstet Gynecol 177:1385, 1997

Neesham DE, Umstad MP, Cincotta RB, Johnston DL, McGrath GM: Pseudo-sinusoidal fetal heart rate pattern and fetal anemia: Case report and review. Aust NZ J Obstet Gynecol 33:386, 1993

Nelson KB, Grether JK: Potentially asphyxiating conditions and cerebral palsy in infants of normal birth weight. Am J Obstet Gynecol 179:567, 1998

Nicolaides KH, Sadovsky G, Cetin E: Fetal heart rate patterns in red blood cell isoimmunized pregnancies. Am J Obstet Gynecol 161:351, 1989

Ogueh O, Steer P: Gender does not affect fetal heart rate variation. Br J Obstet Gynaecol 105:1312, 1998

Ogundipe OA, Spong CY, Ross MG: Prophylactic amnioinfusion for oligohydramnios: A re-evaluation. Obstet Gynecol 84:544, 1994

Owen J, Hanson BV, Hauth JC: A prospective randomized study of saline solution amnioinfusion. Am J Obstet Gynecol 162:1146, 1990

Parer J: NIH sets the terms for fetal heart rate pattern interpretation. OB/Gyn News, September 1, 1997

Parer JT, King T: Fetal heart rate monitoring: Is it salvageable? Am J Obstet Gynecol 182:982, 2000

Parer JT, Quilligan EJ: Lack of consistency in definitions of fetal heart rate (FHR) patterns. Am J Obstet Gynecol 174:698, 1996

Parer WJ, Parer JT, Holbrook RH, Block BSB: Validity of mathematical models of quantitating fetal heart rate variability. Am J Obstet Gynecol 153:402, 1985

Paul RH, Snidon AK, Yeh SY: Clinical fetal monitoring, 7. The evaluation and significance of intrapartum baseline FHR variability. Am J Obstet Gynecol 123:206, 1975

Paul WM, Quilligan EJ, MacLachlan T: Cardiovascular phenomena associated with fetal head compression. Am J Obstet Gynecol 90:824, 1964

Petrie RH: Dose/response effects of intravenous meperidine in fetal heart rate variability. J Matern Fetal Med 2:215, 1993

Phelan JP, Ahn MO: Perinatal observations in forty-eight neurologically impaired term infants. Am J Obstet Gynecol 171:424, 1994

Picquard F, Hsiung R, Mattauer M, Schaefer A, Haberey P: The validity of fetal heart rate monitoring during the second stage of labor. Obstet Gynecol 72:746, 1988

Pierce J, Gaudier FL, Sanchez-Ramos L: Intrapartum amnioinfusion for meconium-stained fluid: Meta-analysis of prospective clinical trials. Obstet Gynecol 95:1051, 2000

Pillai M, James D: The development of fetal heart rate patterns during normal pregnancy. Obstet Gynecol 76:812, 1990

Pontonnier G, Puech F, Grandjean H, Rolland M: Some physical and biochemical parameters during normal labour. Fetal and maternal study. Biol Neonate 26:159, 1975

Pressman EK, Blakemore KJ: A prospective randomized trial of two solutions for intrapartum amnioinfusion: Effects on fetal electrolytes, osmolality, and acid-base status. Am J Obstet Gynecol 175:945, 1996

Ramin KD, Leveno KJ, Kelly MS, Carmody TJ: Amnionic fluid meconium: A fetal environmental hazard. Obstet Gynecol 87:181, 1996

Renou P, Warwick N, Wood C: Autonomic control of fetal heart rate. Am J Obstet Gynecol 105:949, 1969

Rogers MS, Mongelli M, Tsang KH, Law KP: Lipid peroxidation in cord blood at birth: The effect of labour. Br J Obstet Gynaecol 105:739, 1998

Rosen MG, Dickinson JC: The incidence of cerebral palsy. Am J Obstet Gynecol 167:417, 1992

Samueloff A, Langer O, Berkus M, Fields N, Xenakis E, Ridgway L: Is fetal heart rate variability a good predictor of fetal outcome? Acta Obstet Gynecol Scand 73:39, 1994

Schifrin BS, Hamilton-Rubinstein T, Shields JR: Fetal heart rate patterns and the timing of fetal injury. J Perinatol 14:174, 1994

Schucker JL, Sarno AP, Egerman RS, Sibai BM: The effect of butorphanol on the fetal heart rate reactivity during labor. Am J Obstet Gynecol 174:491, 1996

Seitchik J: Quantitating uterine contractility in a clinical context. Obstet Gynecol 57:453, 1981

Sherer DM: Blunted fetal response to vibroacoustic stimulation associated with maternal intravenous magnesium sulfate therapy. Am J Perinatol 11:401, 1994

Shields JR, Schifrin BS: Perinatal antecedents of cerebral palsy. Obstet Gynecol 71:899, 1988

Simpson JM, Sharland GK: Fetal tachycardia: Management and outcome of 127 consecutive cases. Heart 79:576, 1998

Smith CV, Nguyen HN, Phelan JP, Paul RH: Intrapartum assessment of fetal well-being: A comparison of fetal acoustic stimulation with acid–base determinations. Am J Obstet Gynecol 155:726, 1986

Smith JH, Anand KJ, Cotes PM, Dawes GD, Harkness RA, Howlett TA, Rees LH, Redman CW: Antenatal fetal heart rate variation in relation to the respiratory and metabolic status of the compromised human fetus. Br J Obstet Gynaecol 95:980, 1988

Southall DP, Richards J, Hardwick RA, Shinebourne EA, Gibbens GL, Jones HT, DeSwiet M, Johnston PG: Prospective study of fetal heart rate and rhythm patterns. Arch Dis Child 55:506, 1980

Spong CY, McKindsey F, Ross MG: Amniotic fluid index (AFI) predicts the relief of variable decelerations following amnioinfusion bolus. Am J Obstet Gynecol 174:480, 1996

Spong CY, Ogundipe OA, Ross MG: Prophylactic amnioinfusion for meconium-stained amniotic fluid. Am J Obstet Gynecol 171:931, 1994

Spong CY, Rasul C, Collea JV, Eglinton GS, Ghidini A: Characterization and prognostic significance of variable decelerations in the second stage of labor. Am J Perinatol 15:369, 1998

Strachan BK, von Wijngaarden WJ, Sahota D, Chang A, James DK: Cardiotocography only versus cardiotocography plus PR-interval analysis in intrapartum surveillance: A randomized, multicenter trial. Lancet 355:456, 2000

Symonds EM: Fetal monitoring: Medical and legal implications for the practitioner. Curr Opin Obstet Gynecol 6:430, 1994

Thacker SB, Stroup DF, Peterson HB: Efficacy and safety of intrapartum electronic fetal monitoring: An update. Obstet Gynecol 86:613, 1995

Trudinger BJ, Pryse-Davies J: Fetal hazards of the intrauterine pressure catheter: Five case reports. Br J Obstet Gynaecol 85:567, 1978

Usta IM, Mercer BM, Aswad NK, Sibai BM: The impact of a policy of amnioinfusion for meconium-stained amniotic fluid. Obstet Gynecol 85:237, 1995

Van Geijn HP, Jongsma HN, deHaan J, Eskes TK, Prechtl HF: Heart rate as an indicator of the behavioral state. Am J Obstet Gynecol 136:1061, 1980

Ventura SJ, Martin JA, Curtin SC, Mathews TJ, Park MM: Births: Final Data for 1998. Monthly Vital Statistics Report 48, No 3. Hyattsville, MD, National Center for Health Statistics, 2000

Viscomi CM, Hood DD, Melone PJ, Eisenach JC: Fetal heart rate variability after epidural fentanyl during labor. Anesth Analg 71:679, 1990

Walker J: Foetal anoxia. J Obstet Gynaecol Br Commonw 61:162, 1953

Watanabe T, Okamura K, Tanigawara S, Shintaku Y, Akagi K, Endo H, Yajima A: Changes in electrocardiogram T-wave amplitude during umbilical cord compress is predictive of fetal condition in sheep. Am J Obstet Gynecol 166:246, 1992

Wenstrom K, Andrews WW, Maher JE: Amnioinfusion survey: Prevalence protocols and complications. Obstet Gynecol 86:572, 1995

Westgate JA, Gunn AJ, Gunn TR: Antecedents of neonatal encephalopathy with fetal acidemia at term. Br J Obstet Gynaecol 106:774, 1999

Westgate J, Harris M, Curnow JSH, Greene KR: Plymouth randomized trial of cardiotocogram only versus ST waveform plus cardiotocogram for intrapartum monitoring in 2400 cases. Am J Obstet Gynecol 169:1151, 1993

Whittle M: Is it time to abandon cardiotocographic ECG analysis? Lancet 355:422, 2000

Williams JW: Williams Obstetrics, 1st ed. New York, Appleton, 1903

Yam J, Chua S, Arulkumaran S: Intrapartum fetal pulse oximetry. Part I: Principles and technical issues. Obstet Gynecol Surv 55:163, 2000

Young BK, Katz M, Wilson SJ: Sinusoidal fetal heart rate, 1. Clinical significance. Am J Obstet Gynecol 136:587, 1980

Young BK, Weinstein HM: Moderate fetal bradycardia. Am J Obstet Gynecol 126:271, 1976

Young DC, Gray JH, Luther ER, Peddle LJ: Fetal scalp blood pH sampling: Its value in an active obstetric unit. Am J Obstet Gynecol 136:276, 1980b

Zalar RW, Quilligan EJ: The influence of scalp sampling on the cesarean section rate for fetal distress. Am J Obstet Gynecol 135:239, 1979

15

Analgesia and Anesthesia

361

Pain relief in labor presents unique problems. Labor begins without warning, and obstetrical anesthesia may be required within minutes of a full meal. Moreover, gastric emptying is delayed during pregnancy and prolonged even more during labor, especially after analgesics are given. Vomiting with aspiration of gastric contents is a constant threat and often a major cause of serious maternal morbidity and mortality. Finally, a host of disorders unique to pregnancy, such as preeclampsia, placental abruption, and chorioamnionitis, all superimposed on unique physiological adaptations of pregnancy, are directly affected by the choice of analgesia and anesthesia selected.

Data from the Pregnancy Mortality Surveillance Program of the Centers for Disease Control and Prevention from 1979 through 1990 include 155 maternal deaths caused by anesthesia-related complications (Hawkins and colleagues, 1997b). These represented 3.8 percent of a total of 4097 pregnancy-related deaths (Fig. 15–1). Over this 12-year surveillance, anesthesia-related mortality rates decreased from 4.3 to 1.7 per million live births. A similar trend has been reported for England and Wales (Hawkins and colleagues, 1997b; Hibbard and colleagues, 1994). The most common causes of anesthesia-related deaths in the United States from 1979 through 1990 are summarized in Table 15–1.

The most important single factor associated with anesthesia-related maternal mortality is the experience of the anesthetist (Breheny and McCarthy, 1982). Fifteen years ago, Gibbs and colleagues (1986) reported that less than half of the hospitals with fewer than 500 deliveries per year had general anesthesia for cesarean delivery provided by an anesthesiologist. In a recent survey supported by both the American Society of Anesthesiologists and the American College of Obstetricians and Gynecologists, Hawkins and colleagues (1997a) reported that fewer hospitals were providing obstetrical

care in 1992 compared with 1981. Most of the decrease was in hospitals with less than 500 deliveries. Although there was a significant increase in epidural analgesia, regional techniques were not available in 20 percent of the smallest hospitals. In 60 percent of the smallest hospitals, nurse anesthetists provided anesthesia for cesarean delivery. Almost 85 percent of women undergoing cesarean delivery received regional analgesia. Only 2 percent of labor epidural analgesia was provided by obstetricians compared with 30 percent in the 1981 survey.

GENERAL PRINCIPLES

OBSTETRICAL ANESTHESIA SERVICES. The American Academy of Pediatrics and the American College of Obstetricians and Gynecologists (1997) have published guidelines concerning anesthesia care for obstetrics. The American Society of Anesthesiologists Task Force on Obstetrical Anesthesia (1999) has also recently published practice guidelines for obstetrical anesthesia. Hospitals providing basic obstetrical care should be able to administer anesthesia on a 24-hour basis. A qualified person should be readily available to administer an appropriate anesthetic and to maintain support of vital functions in an obstetrical emergency. In larger facilities with complicated patients, 24-hour in-house anesthesia coverage is recommended. Moreover, hospitals providing obstetrical care should be capable of starting a cesarean delivery when necessary within 30 minutes from the time the decision is made. They also stressed the importance of properly trained individuals capable of managing anesthetic complications. Finally, they emphasize that certain risk factors should be communi-

TABLE 15–1. Causes of Anesthesia-related Maternal Deaths in the United States from 1979–1990: General Anesthesia versus Regional Analgesia

Complication	General Anesthesia (N = 67)	Regional Analgesia (N = 33)
Aspiration	33%	—
Intubation problems	22%	—
Inadequate ventilation	15%	—
Respiratory failure	3%	—
Cardiac arrest	22%	6%
Toxicity	—	51%
High spinal/epidural	—	36%
Unknown	5%	6%

Adapted from Hawkins and colleagues (1997b), with permission.

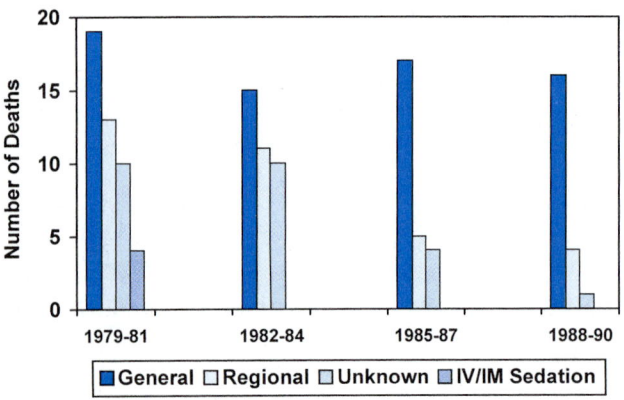

FIGURE 15–1. Anesthesia-related maternal deaths, by types of anesthesia. United States, 1979–1990. (From Hawkins and colleagues, 1997b, with permission.)

cated to the anesthesia-care provider in advance of delivery:

1. Marked obesity.
2. Severe edema or anatomical anomalies of the face and neck.
3. Protuberant teeth, small mandible, or difficulty in opening the mouth.
4. Short stature, short neck, or arthritis of the neck.
5. Large thyroid.
6. Asthma, chronic pulmonary disease, or cardiac disease.
7. Bleeding disorders.
8. Severe preeclampsia–eclampsia.
9. Previous history of anesthetic complications.
10. Other significant medical or obstetrical complications.

Bell and colleagues (2000) recently calculated the financial burden that may be incurred when trying to provide around-the-clock obstetrical analgesia. Given the average indemnity and Medicaid reimbursement for epidural analgesia during labor, they concluded that such coverage could not operate profitably at their tertiary referral institution. The American College of Obstetricians and Gynecologists (2000) has issued a joint statement with the American Society of Anesthesiology that reimbursement for regional analgesia should not be denied if given "only" for pain relief, that is, absence of other "medical indications."

PRINCIPLES OF PAIN RELIEF. Three essentials of obstetrical pain relief are simplicity, safety, and preservation of fetal homeostasis. The woman who is given any form of analgesia should be monitored closely. Risks vary according to the type of analgesia selected. Assiduous attention to monitoring after administration of spinal or epidural analgesia includes frequent measurement of blood pressure, anesthetic levels, and measurement of maternal oxygenation by pulse oximeter.

The obstetrician should become proficient in local and pudendal analgesia. Conduction analgesia also may be administered by the properly trained obstetrician in appropriately selected circumstances. In general, however, it is preferable for an anesthesiologist or anesthetist to provide this care, so that the obstetrician can focus attention on the obstetrical concerns. General anesthesia should be available immediately for laparotomy, but should be administered only by those with special training.

NONPHARMACOLOGICAL METHODS OF PAIN CONTROL. Fear and the unknown potentiate pain. A woman who is free from fear, and who has confidence in the obstetrical staff that cares for her, usually requires smaller amounts of analgesia.

Read (1944) emphasized that the intensity of pain during labor is related in large measure to emotional tension. He urged that women be well informed about the physiology of parturition and the various hospital procedures to which they will be subjected during labor and delivery. Lamaze (1970) subsequently described his psychoprophylactic method, which emphasized childbirth as a natural physiological process. Both taught that pain can be minimized by appropriate training in breathing and appropriate psychological support. These concepts have had a considerable impact on the reduction of potent analgesic, sedative, and amnestic drugs used during labor, as well as the reduced use of general anesthesia for delivery.

When motivated women have been prepared for childbirth, pain during labor has been found to be diminished by a third (Melzack, 1984). The presence of a supportive spouse or other family member, of conscientious labor attendants, and of a considerate obstetrician who instills confidence, contributes greatly to accomplishing this goal. In a study by Kennell and associates (1991), 412 nulliparous women in labor were randomized to two groups; one received continuous emotional support from an experienced companion, and the other was monitored only by an inconspicuous observer who did not interact with the laboring woman. The cesarean delivery rate was significantly lower in the continuous support group (8 versus 13 percent) as was the frequency of epidural analgesia for vaginal delivery (8 versus 23 percent).

ANALGESIA AND SEDATION DURING LABOR

When uterine contractions and cervical dilatation cause discomfort, pain relief with a narcotic such as meperidine, plus one of the tranquilizer drugs such as promethazine, is usually appropriate. The mother should rest quietly between contractions with a successful program of analgesia and sedation. In this circumstance, discomfort is usually felt at the acme of an effective uterine contraction, but the pain is generally not unbearable. Appropriate drug selection and administration should accomplish these objectives for the great majority of women in labor, without risk to them or their infants.

MEPERIDINE AND PROMETHAZINE. Meperidine, 50 to 100 mg, with promethazine, 25 mg, may be administered intramuscularly at intervals of 2 to 4 hours (American College of Obstetricians and Gynecologists, 1996). In general, a small dose given more frequently is preferable to a large one administered less often. Then, if delivery follows during the next hour or so after the injection, the neonate is less likely to be depressed by the medication. A more rapid effect is achieved by giving meperidine intravenously in doses of 25 to 50 mg every

1 to 2 hours. Whereas analgesia is maximal about 45 minutes after an intramuscular injection, it develops almost immediately following intravenous administration. The depressant effect in the fetus follows closely behind the peak analgesic effect in the mother. Meperidine readily crosses the placenta, and the half-life is approximately 2½ hours in the mother and 13 hours in the newborn (American College of Obstetricians and Gynecologists, 1996).

It is likely that these doses are insufficient for pain relief in many labors. In a randomized investigation of epidural analgesia from Parkland Hospital, patient-controlled intravenous analgesia (PCIA) with meperidine was found to be an inexpensive and effective method for labor analgesia (Sharma and colleagues, 1997). Women randomized to PCIA received 50 mg meperidine with 25 mg promethazine intravenously as an initial bolus, after which an infusion pump was set up to deliver 15 mg of meperidine every 10 minutes as needed until delivery. The mean and maximum total meperidine dosages were 140 and 500 mg, respectively. A fourth of the women received more than 200 mg of meperidine during their labors. Neonatal sedation, as measured by need for naloxone treatment in the delivery room, occurred in 3 percent.

OTHER DRUGS. The synthetic narcotic **butorphanol,** given in 1- to 2-mg doses, compares favorably with 40 to 60 mg of meperidine (Quilligan and colleagues, 1980). Neonatal respiratory depression is reported to be less than with meperidine, but care must be taken that the two drugs are not given contiguously because butorphanol antagonizes the narcotic effects of meperidine. Angel and colleagues (1984) and Hatjis and Meis (1986) described a sinusoidal fetal heart rate pattern following butorphanol administration. **Nalbuphine** is also a synthetic narcotic. When given in a dose of 15 to 20 mg intravenously, it does not cause neonatal depression (Wilson and associates, 1986). **Fentanyl** is a short-acting, very potent synthetic opioid. It is given in doses of 50 to 100 μg intravenously every hour if needed. Butorphanol provided better initial analgesia than fentanyl with fewer requests for more medication or for epidural anesthesia (Atkinson and associates, 1994).

Intravenous and intramuscular sedation is not without risks. Hawkins and colleagues (1997b) reported that 4 of 129 maternal anesthetic deaths were from such sedation—one from aspiration, two from inadequate ventilation, and one from overdosage.

NARCOTIC ANTAGONISTS. Meperidine or other narcotics used during labor may cause newborn respiratory depression. Newborn respiratory depression is most likely to occur 2 to 3 hours after meperidine administration (American College of Obstetricians and Gynecolo-

gists, 1996). **Naloxone** is a narcotic antagonist capable of reversing respiratory depression induced by opioid narcotics by displacing the narcotic from specific receptors in the central nervous system. Withdrawal symptoms may be precipitated in recipients who are physically dependent on narcotics. The suggested dose for newborns is 0.1 mg/kg injected into the umbilical vein (American College of Obstetricians and Gynecologists, 1996). This usually acts within 2 minutes with an effective duration of at least 30 minutes. The naloxone injection may have to be repeated in 3 to 5 minutes. In the absence of narcotics, naloxone exhibits no adverse effects on the newborn.

GENERAL ANESTHESIA

Without exception, all anesthetic agents that depress the maternal central nervous system cross the placenta and depress the fetal central nervous system. Another constant hazard with any general anesthetic is aspiration of gastric contents and particulate matter. Fasting before the time of anesthesia is not always an effective safeguard, because fasting gastric juice, even if free of particulate matter, is likely to be strongly acidic and thus can produce severe or even fatal aspiration pneumonitis. At the same time, tracheal intubation is valuable to ensure a satisfactory airway and minimize the risk of aspiration. Failed tracheal intubation fortunately is uncommon, but is still a major cause of anesthesia-related maternal deaths (Hawkins and colleagues, 1997b). Advances in technology, to include pulse oximetry and capnography, greatly facilitate timely diagnosis of failed intubation prompting corrective measures to restore ventilation. Even so, failure to be able to secure the airway with an endotracheal tube can, at best, be risky and at worst, be a disaster (Rasmussen and Malinow, 1994). In some cases an awake fiberoptic intubation may be necessary. Hawksworth and Purdie (1998) described such a case after failed spinal–epidural analgesia and failed asleep intubation.

With inhalation, the concentration of the anesthetic agent increases in the lungs of the pregnant woman somewhat more rapidly because the functional residual capacity and residual volume of her lungs are reduced. For the same reason, residual oxygen in the lung after expiration is appreciably less, a factor of importance when there is delay in intubation and oxygenation after injection of a muscle relaxant. Trained personnel and specialized equipment (including fiberoptic intubation) are mandatory for the safe use of general anesthesia.

INHALATION ANESTHESIA

GAS ANESTHETICS. Nitrous oxide (N_2O) may be used to provide pain relief during labor as well as at delivery.

This agent produces analgesia and altered consciousness, but by itself does not provide true anesthesia. Nitrous oxide does not prolong labor or interfere with uterine contractions. Self-administered nitrous oxide in a 50 percent mixture with 50 percent oxygen (Nitronox) can provide excellent pain relief during the second stage of labor.

Nitrous oxide is commonly also used as part of a balanced general anesthesia for cesarean delivery and some forceps deliveries. It is given along with the intravenous administration of a short-acting barbiturate (usually thiopental) and a muscle relaxant (usually succinylcholine) just prior to tracheal intubation.

VOLATILE ANESTHETICS. In doses that provide analgesia, volatile anesthetics are likely to cause unconsciousness and there is potential for aspiration with an unprotected airway. Halogenated hydrocarbons are used to supplement nitrous oxide during maintenance of general anesthesia. They cross the placenta readily and are capable of producing narcosis in the fetus. **Isoflurane** is the most commonly used volatile anesthetic in the United States. Both it and **halothane** are potent, nonexplosive agents that produce remarkable uterine relaxation when given in high, inhaled concentrations. Their use in high concentrations is restricted to those very uncommon situations in which uterine relaxation is a requisite rather than a hazard. They are used for internal podalic version of the second twin, breech decomposition, and replacement of the acutely inverted uterus. As soon as the maneuver has been completed, anesthetic administration should be stopped and immediate efforts made to promote myometrial contraction to minimize hemorrhage. Because of cardiodepressant and hypotensive effects, these agents may intensify the adverse effects of maternal hypovolemia. Halothane and isoflurane have occasionally been associated with hepatitis and massive hepatic necrosis (Gunarathnam and associates, 1995).

BALANCED GENERAL ANESTHESIA. Nitrous oxide and oxygen given for balanced general anesthesia have been associated with some degree of maternal awareness when these women were interviewed postpartum (Hodgkinson and colleagues, 1978). For this reason, as well as to be able to increase the inspired concentration of oxygen, many recommend the addition of one of the halogenated agents in concentrations of less than 1 percent (American College of Obstetricians and Gynecologists, 1996). Piggott and co-workers (1990) studied 200 women undergoing cesarean delivery and randomized them to either nitrous oxide (50 percent) and oxygen (50 percent) or oxygen (100 percent), both supplemented with isoflurane. There were no instances of awareness in either group, and infants of mothers who received 100 percent oxygen required less resuscitation and had higher Apgar scores.

The major concern regarding halogenated agents has been their association with increased blood loss (Combs and associates, 1991; Gilstrap and associates, 1987). Andrews and colleagues (1992) reported significantly lower postpartum hematocrit levels when general anesthesia with a halogenated agent was compared with regional techniques for women undergoing repeat cesarean delivery. Similarly, Maberry and colleagues (1992) evaluated blood loss in elective cesarean delivery using either general anesthesia with isoflurane or regional analgesia. They observed a postoperative decrease in hematocrit level of 5 volumes percent in 25 percent of women receiving general anesthesia compared with 7 percent of those given regional analgesia. None required transfusions. Conversely, a number of studies did not report such associations, especially if women at high risk for bleeding were excluded (Camann and Datta, 1991; Lamont and associates, 1988).

ANESTHETIC GAS EXPOSURE AND PREGNANCY OUTCOME. In some reports, the spontaneous abortion rate of female workers exposed to anesthetic gases was doubled and the minor malformation rate in children of exposed male workers was slightly greater. Although the exact fetal risk of chronic maternal exposure to waste anesthetic gas is unknown, available data suggest that there is not a substantial risk for either pregnancy loss or congenital anomalies (Cohen, 1994). This is discussed further in Chapter 38.

INTRAVENOUS DRUGS DURING ANESTHESIA

THIOPENTAL. This thiobarbituate given intravenously is widely used in conjunction with other agents for general anesthesia. The drug offers the advantages of ease and extreme rapidity of induction, ready controllability, and prompt recovery with minimal risk of vomiting. Thiopental and similar compounds are poor analgesic agents, and the administration of sufficient drug given alone to maintain anesthesia may cause appreciable newborn depression. Thus, thiopental is not used as the sole anesthetic agent, but in a dose that induces sleep, it is given along with a muscle relaxant, usually succinylcholine, and nitrous oxide plus oxygen.

KETAMINE. Given intravenously in low doses of 0.2 to 0.3 mg/kg, this drug is used to produce analgesia and sedation just prior to delivery. Doses of 1 mg/kg induce general anesthesia. It may prove useful in women with acute hemorrhage because, unlike thiopental, it is not associated with hypotension. In fact, it usually causes a rise in blood pressure, and thus it generally should be avoided in women already hypertensive. Unpleasant delirium and hallucinations are commonly induced by this agent.

ASPIRATION DURING GENERAL ANESTHESIA.
Pneumonitis from inhalation of gastric contents has in the past been the most common cause of anesthetic deaths in obstetrics. In its survey of over 4097 maternal deaths between 1979 and 1990, the Centers for Disease Control and Prevention (Hawkins and colleagues, 1997b) identified inhalation of gastric contents to be associated with 23 percent of 129 maternal anesthesia-related deaths (Table 15–1).

PROPHYLAXIS. Important to effective prophylaxis are the following measures:

1. Fasting from solids for at least 8 hours and preferably longer before anesthesia (American Society of Anesthesiologists Task Force on Obstetrical Anesthesia, 1999).
2. Use of agents to reduce gastric acidity during the induction and maintenance of general anesthesia.
3. Skillful tracheal intubation accompanied by pressure on the cricoid cartilage to occlude the esophagus—the *Sellick maneuver.*
4. After intubation, and during the surgery, passage of a nasogastric tube to empty the stomach of all contents. Additional antacids can be placed down the nasogastric tube. The stomach should again be emptied and the nasogastric tube (usually) pulled immediately before extubation.
5. Awake extubation with protective airway reflexes intact and without neuromuscular blockade and with the woman lying on her side with her head lowered.
6. Use of regional analgesia techniques when appropriate.

FASTING. There are insufficient data regarding fasting times for clear liquids and pulmonary aspiration during labor (American Society of Anesthesiologists Task Force on Obstetrical Anesthesia, 1999). Clear liquids such as water, clear tea, black coffee, carbonated beverages, and fruit juices without pulp may be allowed in uncomplicated laboring women. In a survey of 740 hospitals in the United States, Hawkins and colleagues (1998) reported that oral intake during labor is limited mostly to clear liquids. Women with complications such as diabetes and morbid obesity may need further restrictions of oral intake. Obvious solid foods should be avoided in laboring women. The Task Force also recommended that "a fasting period of 8 hours or more is preferable for uncomplicated parturients undergoing elective cesarean delivery." Despite these precautions, it should be assumed that any woman in labor has both gastric particulate matter as well as acidic contents.

ANTACIDS. The practice of administering antacids shortly before induction of anesthesia has probably done more to decrease mortality from general anesthesia than any other single practice. Gibbs and colleagues (1984) reported that 30 mL of sodium citrate with citric acid (Bicitra), given about 45 minutes before surgery, neutralized gastric contents (mean volume 70 mL) in nearly 90 percent of women undergoing cesarean delivery. For many years we have recommended administration of 30 mL of Bicitra within a few minutes of the anticipated time of anesthesia induction, either general or by major regional block. If more than 1 hour has passed between when the first dose was given and when anesthesia is induced, then a second dose is given.

H_2-antagonists, as well as antacids and dopamine antagonists, may be given prophylactically to decrease the risk of aspiration pneumonia (Rowe, 1997). **Cimetidine,** a histamine H_2-antagonist, given sometime before general anesthesia for delivery, has been recommended (Hodgkinson and colleagues, 1983). At least 60 minutes are required after parenteral administration to decrease gastric acidity to relatively safe levels. Therefore, in emergency situations, either an antacid or antacid plus cimetidine should be used. Thornburn and Moir (1987) studied 100 women undergoing emergency cesarean delivery who were given cimetidine, 200 mg intravenously, along with 30 mL of sodium citrate orally. The time interval from cimetidine administration to induction of general anesthesia was 5 to 208 minutes. None of the women had a gastric pH of less than 2.7, and all but one had a pH of 3.0 or higher.

A similar agent, **ranitidine,** can be given the night before surgery and will result in decreased gastric secretion through the next morning. This agent might prove useful when given along with a second dose on the morning of surgery for scheduled elective cesarean deliveries (Burchman, 1992). Yau and associates (1992) studied 49 women undergoing cesarean delivery who received ranitidine and sodium citrate. They reported that only one woman had an intragastric pH of less than 2.5 and a volume greater than 25 mL. In emergency cesarean delivery, co-administration of ranitidine and sodium citrate resulted in a smaller volume of gastric aspirate than in those women given antacid alone (Lim and Elegbe, 1992).

INTUBATION. Various positions have been tried to minimize aspiration before and during tracheal intubation and cuff inflation, but the disadvantages from positions other than supine outweigh any advantage. Cricoid pressure from the time of induction until intubation—the *Sellick maneuver*—should be performed by a trained associate. Intubation may be performed with the mother awake after adequate topical anesthesia is applied. Topical spray generally will not significantly depress the laryngeal reflex.

EXTUBATION. The tracheal tube may be safely removed only if the woman is conscious to a degree to follow commands and is capable of maintaining oxygen saturation with spontaneous respiration.

PATHOPHYSIOLOGY. Aspiration pneumonitis associated with obstetrical anesthesia was described by Mendelson in 1946. Teabeaut (1952) demonstrated experimentally that if the pH of aspirated fluid was below 2.5, severe chemical pneumonitis developed. In one study the pH of gastric juice of nearly half of women tested intrapartum without treatment was below 2.5 (Taylor and Pryse-Davies, 1966). The right mainstem bronchus usually offers the simplest pathway for aspirated material to reach the lung parenchyma, and therefore the right lower lobe is most often involved. In severe cases, there is bilateral widespread involvement.

The woman who aspirates may develop evidence for respiratory distress immediately or as long as several hours after aspiration, depending in part upon the material aspirated, the severity of the process, and the acuity of the attendants. Aspiration of a large amount of solid material causes obvious signs of airway obstruction. Smaller particles without acidic liquid may lead to patchy atelectasis and later to bronchopneumonia.

When highly acidic liquid is inspired, decreased oxygen saturation along with tachypnea, bronchospasm, rhonchi, rales, atelectasis, cyanosis, tachycardia, and hypotension are likely to develop. At the sites of injury, pulmonary capillary leakage results in protein-rich fluid containing numerous erythrocytes exuding from capillaries into the lung interstitium and alveoli to cause decreased pulmonary compliance, shunting of blood, and severe hypoxemia. Radiographic changes may not appear immediately and they may be quite variable, although the right lobe is most often affected. Therefore, chest x-ray alone should not be used to exclude aspiration.

TREATMENT. The methods recommended for treatment of aspiration have changed appreciably in recent years, indicating that previous therapy was not very successful. Suspicion of aspiration of gastric contents demands very close monitoring for evidence of any pulmonary damage. Attention to respiratory rate and oxygen saturation as measured by pulse oximetry are the most sensitive and earliest indicators of injury.

As much as possible of the inhaled fluid should be immediately wiped out of the mouth and removed from the pharynx and trachea by suction. Saline lavage may further disseminate the acid throughout the lung and is not recommended. If large particulate matter is inspired,

bronchoscopy may be indicated to relieve airway obstruction. There is no convincing clinical or experimental evidence that corticosteroid therapy or prophylactic antimicrobial administration is beneficial (Guyton and Gibbs, 1994). If clinical evidence of infection develops, however, then vigorous treatment is given.

When acute respiratory distress syndrome (ARDS) develops, mechanical ventilation with positive end-expiratory pressure may prove life saving (Chap. 43, p. 1164). Oxygen in increased concentration given by continuous positive pressure may be required to raise and maintain the arterial P_{O_2} at 60 mm Hg or higher.

FAILED INTUBATION. Failed intubation fortunately is uncommon, is often associated with aspiration, and is a major cause of anesthetic-related maternal mortality (Hawkins and colleagues, 1997b; Wallace and Sidawi, 1997). Hawkins and colleagues (1997b) reported that 22 percent of 67 maternal deaths associated with general anesthesia were secondary to induction or intubation problems (Table 15–1).

PREVENTION. History of previous difficulties with intubation as well as a careful assessment of anatomical features of the neck, maxillofacial, pharyngeal, and laryngeal structures may help predict a difficult intubation. Even in cases where the initial assessment of the airway was uneventful, edema may develop intrapartum and present considerable difficulties (Farcon and associates, 1994). Morbid obesity is a major risk factor for failed or difficult intubation. Of paramount importance is appropriate preoperative preparation to include the immediate availability of a short-handled laryngoscope, fiber-optic laryngoscope, and the liberal use of awake oral intubation techniques (Blass, 1991).

MANAGEMENT. An important principle is to start the operative procedure only after it has been ascertained that tracheal intubation has been successful and that adequate ventilation can be accomplished. Even with an abnormal fetal heart rate pattern, initiation of cesarean delivery will only serve to complicate matters if there is difficulty or failed intubation. Frequently, the woman must be allowed to awaken and a different technique used, such as an awake intubation or regional analgesia.

Following failed intubation, the woman is ventilated by mask and cricoid pressure is applied to reduce the chance of aspiration (Cooper and colleagues, 1994). Surgery may proceed with mask ventilation or the woman is allowed to awaken. In those cases where the woman has been paralyzed, and where an oral airway cannot be reestablished, a life-threatening emergency exists. Use of a fiber-optic laryngoscope may facilitate tracheal intubation. If not, a laryngeal mask airway is placed or needle cricothyroidotomy and jet ventilation is per-

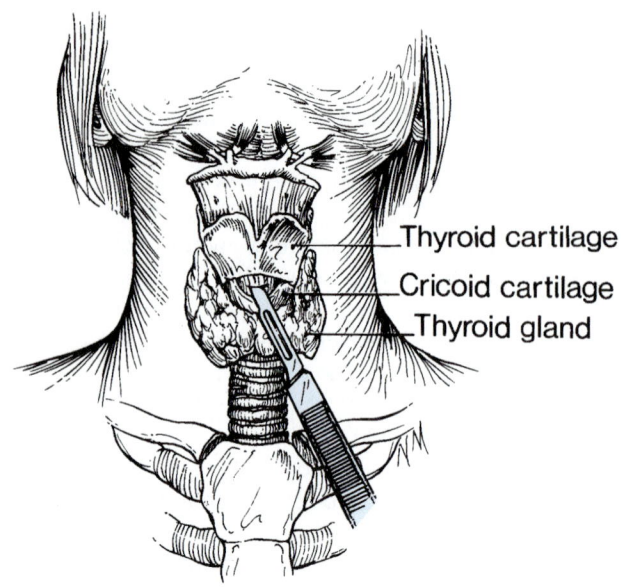

FIGURE 15–2. Use of a scalpel to puncture the cricothyroid membrane. Following insertion, the scalpel blade is rotated 90 degrees, thereby allowing a pediatric endotracheal tube to be inserted. (Redrawn from ATLS Student Manual, Committee of Trauma, American College of Surgeons.)

formed (American College of Obstetricians and Gynecologists, 1996). This can be accomplished with a 14- or 16-gauge needle connected to wall oxygen at a flow rate of 50 psi or 15 L/min. Alternatively, cricothyroidotomy can be performed using a size 10 scalpel blade and a pediatric endotracheal tube (Fig. 15–2).

REGIONAL ANALGESIA

A variety of nerve blocks have been developed over the years to provide pain relief for the woman in labor and at delivery. They are correctly referred to as regional analgesics.

SENSORY INNERVATION OF THE GENITAL TRACT

UTERINE INNERVATION. Pain in the first stage of labor is generated largely from the uterus. Visceral sensory fibers from the uterus, cervix, and upper vagina traverse through the Frankenhäuser ganglion, which lies just lateral to the cervix, into the pelvic plexus, and then to the middle and superior internal iliac plexuses. From there, the fibers travel in the lumbar and lower thoracic sympathetic chains to enter the spinal cord through the white rami communicantes associated with the 10th, 11th, and 12th thoracic and 1st lumbar nerves. Early in the first stage of labor, the pain of uterine contractions is transmitted predominantly through the 11th and 12th thoracic nerves.

The motor pathways to the uterus leave the spinal cord at the level of the seventh and eighth thoracic vertebrae. Theoretically, any method of sensory block that does not also block the motor pathways to the uterus can be used for analgesia during labor.

LOWER GENITAL TRACT INNERVATION. Pain with vaginal delivery arises from stimuli from the lower genital tract. These are transmitted primarily through the pudendal nerve, the peripheral branches of which provide sensory innervation to the perineum, anus, and the more medial and inferior parts of the vulva and clitoris. The pudendal nerve passes beneath the posterior surface of the sacrospinous ligament just as the ligament attaches to the ischial spine. The sensory nerve fibers of the pudendal nerve are derived from the ventral branches of the second, third, and fourth sacral nerves.

ANESTHETIC AGENTS. Some of the more commonly used local anesthetics, along with their usual concentrations, doses, and durations of action, are shown in Table 15–2. Some preparations suitable for epidural analgesia are not suitable for subarachnoid injection because the preservative may cause inflammation. Some contain dilute epinephrine to prolong the action of the anesthetic or to produce symptoms when a test dose is inadvertently given intravenously. The dose of each agent varies widely, and is dependent upon the particular nerve block and physical status of the woman. When the dose is increased, the onset, duration, and quality of analgesia are enhanced, but only incremental dosage of small-volume boluses allows safety through careful monitoring for early warning signs of toxicity. Administration of these agents must be followed by appropriate monitoring for adverse reactions, and equipment and personnel to manage these reactions must be immediately available.

Most often, serious toxicity follows injection of an anesthetic into a blood vessel, but it may also be induced by administration of excessive amounts. Because many of these agents are manufactured in more than one concentration and ampule size to be used for specific local or regional blocks, a thorough knowledge of the ones selected for use is essential for safety. Two manifestations of systemic toxicity from local anesthetics are those of the central nervous and cardiovascular systems.

CENTRAL NERVOUS SYSTEM TOXICITY. Symptoms include light-headedness, dizziness, tinnitus, bizarre behavior, slurred speech, metallic taste, numbness of the tongue and mouth, muscle fasciculation and excitation, generalized convulsions, and loss of consciousness. The convulsions should be controlled, an airway established, and oxygen delivered. Succinylcholine abolishes the peripheral manifestations of the convulsions and allows

TABLE 15–2. Some Local Anesthetic Agents Used in Obstetrics

Anesthetic Agent	Plain Solutions					
	Usual Concentration (%)	Usual Volume (mL)	Usual Dose (mg)	Onset	Average Duration (min)	Clinical Use
Amino-esters						
2-Chloroprocaine	1–2	20–30	400–600	Rapid	15–30	Local or pudendal block
	2–3	15–25	300–750		30–60	Epidural for cesarean
Tetracaine	0.2	—	4	Slow	75–150	Low spinal block/6% glucose
	0.5	—	7–10		75–150	Spinal for cesarean/5% glucose
Amino-amides						
Lidocaine	1	20–30	200–300	Rapid	30–60	Local or pudendal block
	2	15–30	300–450		60–90	Epidural for cesarean
	5	1–1.5	50–75		45–60	Spinal for cesarean or puerperal tubal ligation/7.5–8.25% glucose
	5	0.5–1	25–50		30–60	Spinal for vaginal delivery/7.5–8.25% glucose
Bupivacaine	0.5	15–20	75–100	Slow	90–150	Epidural for cesarean
	0.25	8–10	20–25		60–90	Epidural for labor
	0.75	1–1.5	7.5–11		60–120	Spinal for cesarean/8.25% glucose
Ropivacaine	0.5	15–20	75–100	Slow	90–150	Epidural for cesarean
	0.25	8–10	20–25		60–90	Epidural for labor

Courtesy of Dr. Shiv Sharma and Dr. Donald Wallace.

tracheal intubation. Thiopental or diazepam act centrally to inhibit convulsions. Magnesium sulfate, administered according to the regimen for eclampsia, also controls convulsions. Abnormal fetal heart rate patterns, such as late decelerations or persistent bradycardia, may develop from maternal hypoxia and lactic acidosis induced by convulsions. With arrest of the convulsions, administration of oxygen, and application of other supportive measures, the fetus likely will recover more quickly in utero than following immediate cesarean delivery. Moreover, maternal well-being is usually better served by waiting until the intensity of the hypoxia and the metabolic acidosis have diminished.

CARDIOVASCULAR TOXICITY. These manifestations do not always follow central nervous system involvement. Generally, they develop later than those from cerebral toxicity, because they are induced by higher blood levels of drug. The notable exception to this rule is bupivacaine, where neurotoxicity and cardiotoxicity develop at virtually identical serum drug levels. Like neurotoxicity, cardiovascular toxicity is characterized first by stimulation and then depression. Accordingly, there is hypertension and tachycardia, which soon is followed by hypotension and cardiac arrhythmias. Hypotension and arrhythmias contribute appreciably to impaired uteroplacental perfusion and fetal distress. Hypotension is initially managed by turning the woman onto either side to avoid aortocaval compression. A crystalloid solution is infused rapidly along with intravenously administered

ephedrine. Emergency cesarean delivery should be initiated if maternal vital signs have not been restored within 5 minutes of cardiac arrest (Chap. 43). As with convulsions, the fetus is likely to recover more quickly in utero once maternal cardiac output is reestablished.

LOCAL INFILTRATION. Local infiltration is of especial value in the following circumstances:

1. Before episiotomy and delivery.
2. After delivery into the site of lacerations to be repaired.
3. Around the episiotomy wound if there is inadequate analgesia.

From the standpoint of safety, local infiltration analgesia is preeminent in the aforementioned settings.

CESAREAN DELIVERY. A rare indication for local infiltration is the need to perform emergency cesarean section to save the life of the fetus in the absence of any anesthesia support. Local block might also be useful to augment an inadequate or "patchy" regional block that was given in an emergency.

TECHNIQUE. The skin is infiltrated in the line of the proposed incision, and the subcutaneous, muscle, and posterior rectus sheath layers as the abdomen is opened. A dilute solution of lidocaine (30 mL of 2 percent with 1:200,000 epinephrine diluted with 60 mL of normal saline) is prepared, and overall 100 to 120 mL is infil-

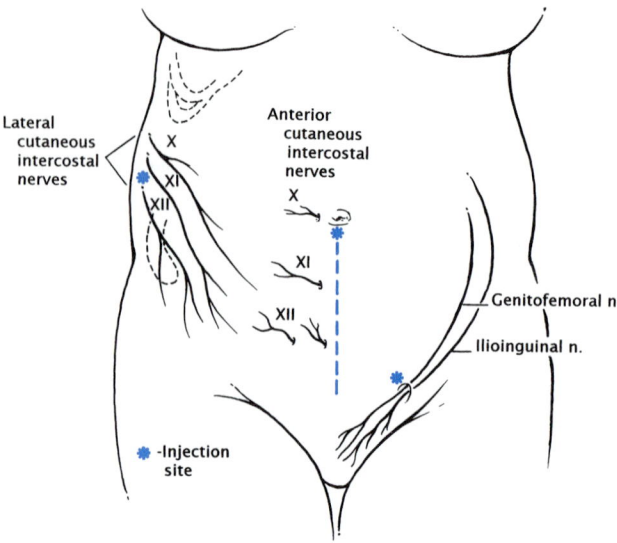

FIGURE 15–3. Local anesthetic block for cesarean delivery. The injection site is halfway between the costal margin and iliac crest in midaxillary line to block 10th, 11th, and 12th, intercostal nerves. The injection is along the line of proposed skin incision. The injection at the external inguinal blocks the genitofemoral and ilioinguinal nerves.

trated. Injection of large volumes into the fatty layers, which are relatively devoid of nerve supply, is avoided to limit total dose of local anesthetic needed. To minimize pain, nausea, and hypotension that may accompany intraperitoneal manipulations, each step is accomplished without haste.

Another technique involves a field block of the major branches supplying the abdominal wall, to include the 10th, 11th, and 12th intercostal nerves and the ilioinguinal and genitofemoral nerves (Busby, 1963). As shown in Figure 15–3, the former group of nerves is located at a point midway between the costal margin and the iliac crest in the midaxillary line. The latter group is found at the level of the external inguinal ring. Only one skin puncture is made at each of the four sites (right and left sides). At the intercostal block site, the needle is directed horizontally and injection is carried down to the transversalis fascia, avoiding injection of the subcutaneous fat. Approximately 5 to 8 mL of 0.5 percent lidocaine is injected. The procedure is repeated at a 45-degree angle cephalad and caudad at this site. The other side is then injected. At the ilioinguinal and genitofemoral sites, the injection is started at a site 2 to 3 cm from the pubic tubercle at a 45-degree angle. Finally, the skin overlying the planned incision is injected.

PUDENDAL BLOCK. A tubular director that allows 1.0 to 1.5 cm of a 15-cm 22-gauge needle to protrude beyond

its tip is used to guide the needle into position over the pudendal nerve (Fig. 15–4). The end of the director is placed against the vaginal mucosa just beneath the tip of the ischial spine. The needle is pushed beyond the tip of the director into the mucosa and a mucosal wheal is made with 1 mL of 1 percent lidocaine or an equivalent dose of another local anesthetic. Aspiration is attempted before this and all subsequent injections to guard against intravascular infusion. The needle is then advanced until it touches the sacrospinous ligament, which is infiltrated with 3 mL of lidocaine. The needle is advanced farther through the ligament, and as it pierces the loose areolar tissue behind the ligament, the resistance of the plunger decreases. Another 3 mL of the anesthetic solution is injected into this region. Next, the needle is withdrawn into the guide, the tip of the guide is moved to just above the ischial spine. The needle is inserted through the mucosa and the rest of 10 mL of solution is deposited. The procedure is then repeated on the other side.

Within 3 to 4 minutes of the time of injection, the successful pudendal block will allow pinching of the lower vagina and posterior vulva bilaterally without pain. It is often of benefit before pudendal block to infiltrate the fourchette, perineum, and adjacent vagina directly at the site where the episiotomy is to be made with 5 to 10 mL of 1 percent lidocaine solution. Then, if delivery occurs before pudendal block becomes effective, an episiotomy can be made without pain. By the time of the repair, the pudendal block usually has become effective.

Pudendal block usually works well and is an extremely safe and relatively simple method of providing analgesia for spontaneous delivery. It can also be used along with epidural analgesia given during labor. Pudendal block may not provide adequate analgesia for other than outlet forceps delivery or when delivery requires extensive manipulation. Moreover, analgesia limited to pudendal block is usually inadequate for women in whom complete visualization of the cervix and upper vagina, or manual exploration of the uterine cavity, are indicated.

COMPLICATIONS. Intravascular injection of a local anesthetic agent may cause serious systemic toxicity characterized by stimulation of the cerebral cortex leading to convulsions. Hematoma formation from perforation of a blood vessel may develop. This is most likely when there is defective coagulation such as that induced by heparin or by placental abruption. These are discussed in Chapter 25 (p. 657). Rarely, severe infection may originate at the injection site. The infection may spread posterior to the hip joint, into the gluteal musculature, or into the retropsoas space (Svancarek and associates, 1977).

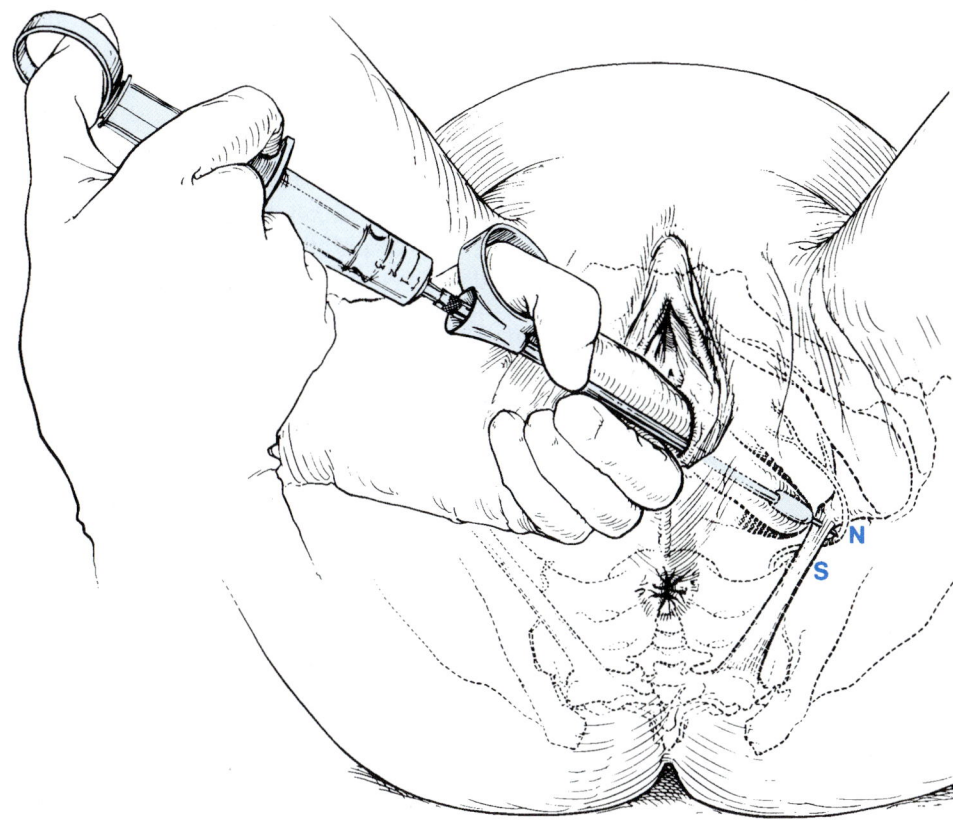

FIGURE 15-4. Local infiltration of the pudendal nerve. Transvaginal technique showing the needle extended beyond the needle guard and passing through the sacrospinous ligament (S) to reach the pudendal nerve (N).

PARACERVICAL BLOCK. This block usually provides good to excellent pain relief during the first stage of labor. Because the pudendal nerves are not blocked, however, additional analgesia is required for delivery. Usually lidocaine or chloroprocaine, 5 to 10 mL of a 1-percent solution, is injected at 3 and 9 o'clock. Because these anesthetics are relatively short acting, paracervical block may have to be repeated during labor.

COMPLICATIONS. Fetal bradycardia is a worrisome complication that has been reported in 10 to 70 percent of paracervical blocks. Bradycardia usually develops within 10 minutes and may last up to 30 minutes. Several investigators stress that bradycardia is not a sign of fetal asphyxia, because it usually is transient and the newborns are in most instances vigorous at birth. There are reports, however, in which fetal scalp blood pH and Apgar scores were sometimes found to be low, and a few fetuses have died. The effect may be the consequence of transplacental transfer of the anesthetic agent or its metabolites and, in turn, a depressant effect on the heart. Based on studies in pregnant ewes, Greiss (1976) and Fishburne (1979), and their associates, believe that fetal bradycardia results from decreased placental perfusion as the consequence of drug-induced uterine artery vasoconstriction and myometrial hypertonus. For

these reasons, paracervical block should not be used in situations of potential fetal compromise.

SPINAL (SUBARACHNOID) BLOCK. Introduction of a local anesthetic into the subarachnoid space to effect spinal block has long been used for delivery. Because of the smaller subarachnoid space during pregnancy, the same amount of anesthetic agent in the same volume of solution produces much higher blockade in parturients than in nonpregnant women. The smaller space is most likely the consequence of engorgement of the internal vertebral venous plexus.

VAGINAL DELIVERY. Low spinal block is a popular form of analgesia for forceps or vacuum delivery. The level of analgesia extends to the 10th thoracic dermatome, which corresponds to the level of the umbilicus. Blockade to this level provides excellent relief from the pain of uterine contractions.

Nearly all local anesthetic agents have been used for spinal analgesia. Lidocaine given in a hyperbaric solution produces excellent analgesia and has the advantage of a relatively short duration (Table 15–2). Tetracaine in a dose of 4 to 6 mg in a 6 percent dextrose solution provides satisfactory anesthesia in the lower vagina and the perineum for about an hour. Neither is administered for vaginal delivery until the cervix is fully dilated and all other criteria for safe forceps delivery have been fulfilled. Preanalgesic intravenous hydration with a liter of crystalloid solution will prevent hypotension in many cases.

CESAREAN DELIVERY. The level of spinal sensory blockade must extend at least to the eighth thoracic dermatome, which is just below the xiphoid process. Because a larger area is to be anesthetized, a larger dose of anesthetic agent is necessary, and this increases the frequency and intensity of toxic reactions. Depending upon maternal size, 8 to 10 mg of tetracaine, 12 mg of bupivacaine, or 50 to 75 mg of lidocaine are administered. The addition of 0.2 mg of morphine improves pain control during delivery and postoperatively.

COMPLICATIONS. A number of complications may ensue and close clinical monitoring of vital signs, including assessment of the level of analgesia, is imperative.

HYPOTENSION. This may develop very soon after injection of the local anesthetic agent. Defining hypotension as a 20 percent decrease from baseline, Hall and colleagues (1994) reported that 21 of 29 healthy women undergoing elective cesarean delivery developed hypotension. This is the consequence of vasodilatation from sympathetic blockade compounded by obstructed venous return from uterine compression of the vena cava and adjacent large veins. **In the supine position, even in the absence of maternal hypotension measured in the brachial artery, placental blood flow may still be significantly reduced.** As shown in Table 15–3, treatment of spinal block hypotension includes uterine displacement, intravenous hydration, and intravenous bolus injections of 10 to 15 mg of ephedrine (Morgan, 1994). Some prefer infusions of ephedrine at rates of 1 or 2 mg/min (Hall and colleagues, 1994).

Ramin and associates (1994) reported that prophylactic infusion of ephedrine was effective to prevent hypotension in healthy women undergoing elective cesarean delivery using spinal analgesia. The mean fetal umbilical arterial pH was lower, albeit of no clinical significance, in the ephedrine-treated group than in the controls. In a follow-up randomized study at Parkland Hospital, Morgan and colleagues (2000) found that the preferred strategy for prevention of maternal hypotension due to spinal analgesia for elective cesarean delivery was 1000 mL Ringer lactate infused over 20 minutes before spinal injection and 5 mg bolus of ephedrine as needed to maintain blood pressure. The mean umbilical artery blood pH with this approach was 7.26. In contrast, continuous prophylactic infusions with various dilate ephedrine solutions were associated with significant fetal acidemia (mean pH 7.11 to 7.13). Vercauteren and colleagues (2000) reported that a single intravenous dose of 5 mg ephedrine given to prehydrated women receiving "small-dose" spinal analgesia for cesarean delivery resulted in significantly less hypotension compared with women receiving placebo (25 percent versus 58 percent).

Although not specifically attributed to hypotension, Roberts and associates (1995) reported that 18 percent of infants exposed to regional analgesia had umbilical arterial blood pH values of 7.19 or less and 3 percent were 7.1 or less. The acidemia was exclusively respiratory, and more often associated with spinal than with epidural analgesia. In contrast, Valli and associates (1994) found no adverse effects on Apgar scores or umbilical arterial or venous blood acid–base status in women receiving either spinal or epidural analgesia.

TOTAL SPINAL BLOCKADE. Most often, total spinal blockade is the consequence of administration of an excessive dose of analgesic agent. This is certainly not always the case, as accidental total spinal block has even occurred following an epidural test dose (Palkar and associates, 1992). In complete spinal block, hypotension and apnea promptly develop and must be immediately treated to prevent cardiac arrest. In the undelivered woman, the uterus is displaced laterally to minimize aortocaval compression. Effective ventilation is established, preferably with tracheal intubation. Intravenous fluids and ephedrine are given to increase blood pressure.

SPINAL (POSTPUNCTURE) HEADACHE. Leakage of cerebrospinal fluid from the site of puncture of the meninges is thought to be the major factor in the genesis of spinal headache. When 22- or 24-gauge needles are used, about 1.5 percent of parturients develop postdural puncture headaches (Sears and co-workers, 1994). Presumably, when the woman sits or stands, the diminished volume of cerebrospinal fluid allows traction on pain-sensitive central nervous system structures. This complication can be reduced by using a small-gauge spinal

TABLE 15–3. Prophylaxis and Treatment for Complications Associated with Subarachnoid Block

Hypotension
Uterine displacement
Hydration with 500–1000 mL of a balanced salt solution
Ephedrine: 5–10 mg intravenously if hypotension persists

Total Spinal Block
Treat associated hypotension
Tracheal intubation
Ventilatory support

needle and avoiding multiple punctures. Sprotte or Whitacre needles with noncutting rounded tips are best (American College of Obstetricians and Gynecologists, 1996).

There is no good evidence that placing the woman absolutely flat on her back for several hours is very effective in preventing headache. Vigorous hydration may be of value, but also without compelling evidence to support its use. Abdominal support with a girdle or abdominal binder does seem to afford relief. Typically, the headache is remarkably improved by the third day and absent by the fifth. In severe cases, a blood patch is effective. A few mL of the woman's blood obtained aseptically without anticoagulant is injected into the epidural space at the site of the dural puncture. Relief is immediate and complications uncommon. Oh and Camann (1998) have reported severe meningeal irritation after a blood patch. Carter and Pasupuleti (2000) reported successful treatment with intravenous cosyntropin when blood patch had been unsuccessful.

CONVULSIONS. In rare instances, postdural puncture cephalgia is associated with blindness and convulsions. Shearer and colleagues (1995) described eight such cases associated with 19,000 regional analgesic procedures. It is presumed that these too are caused by cerebrospinal fluid hypotension.

BLADDER DYSFUNCTION. With spinal analgesia, bladder sensation is likely to be obtunded and bladder emptying impaired for the first few hours after delivery. As a consequence, bladder distention is a frequent postpartum complication, especially if appreciable volumes of intravenous fluid are given.

OXYTOCICS AND HYPERTENSION. Paradoxically, hypertension from ergonovine or methylergonovine injected following delivery is more common in women who have received a spinal or epidural block.

ARACHNOIDITIS AND MENINGITIS. Local anesthetics are no longer preserved in alcohol, formalin, or other toxic solutes, and disposable equipment is used by most. These practices coupled with aseptic technique, have made meningitis and arachnoiditis rarities. Still, these are occasionally documented (Harding and colleagues, 1994; Newton and associates, 1994).

CONTRAINDICATIONS TO SPINAL ANALGESIA. The most common serious complication from spinal block is hypotension. The supine position late in pregnancy predisposes to a reduction in return of blood from veins below the level of the large pregnant uterus and, in turn, a reduction in cardiac output. Moreover, sympathetic blockade from spinal analgesia is usually extensive, and

it leads to further pooling of blood in dilated blood vessels below the blockade. Obstetrical complications that are associated with maternal hypovolemia and hypotension are contraindications to the use of spinal block. Thus, severely decreased blood pressure can be predicted when subarachnoid analgesia is used in the presence of severe hemorrhage or severe preeclampsia. For these reasons, spinal block is felt by some obstetrical anesthesiologists to be contraindicated in severe preeclampsia (Reisner and Nichols, 1999). Conversely, others prefer spinal analgesia to general anesthesia for cesarean delivery in these women (Writer, 1994).

Hood and Curry (1999) retrospectively evaluated 138 women with severe preeclampsia undergoing cesarean delivery. They reported that the magnitude of decrease in blood pressure and maternal and fetal outcomes were similar after spinal or epidural analgesia. Wallace and colleagues (1995) randomized 80 women undergoing cesarean delivery with severe preeclampsia to general anesthesia or to either epidural or spinal–epidural analgesia. There were no differences in outcomes, but 30 percent of those given epidural analgesia and 22 percent of those given spinal–epidural blockage developed hypotension.

The cardiovascular effects of spinal block in the presence of acute blood loss, but in the absence of the hemodynamic effects of pregnancy, have been investigated by Kennedy and co-workers (1968). In 15 nonpregnant volunteers, spinal analgesia to the fifth thoracic sensory level was induced twice, the second time after a phlebotomy of 10 mL/kg. In the case of subarachnoid block without hemorrhage, the mean arterial blood pressure fell 10 percent while cardiac output rose slightly. In the case of hemorrhage without subarachnoid block, the mean blood pressure fell to the same degree and again the cardiac output rose slightly. With subarachnoid block after the modest hemorrhage, however, the mean arterial pressure fell nearly 30 percent and cardiac output fell 15 percent.

Disorders of coagulation and defective hemostasis preclude the use of spinal analgesia. Subarachnoid puncture is contraindicated when the skin or underlying tissue at the site of needle entry is infected. Neurological disorders are considered by many to be a contraindication, if for no other reason than exacerbation of the neurological disease might be attributed to the anesthetic agent (see Chap. 53). Other maternal conditions such as significant aortic stenosis or pulmonary hypertension are also contraindications to the use of spinal analgesia (Chap. 44, p. 1194). Akpek and colleagues (1999) reported a case of chronic subdural hematoma following spinal anesthesia for cesarean delivery.

EPIDURAL ANALGESIA. Relief from the pain of uterine contractions and delivery, vaginal or abdominal, can

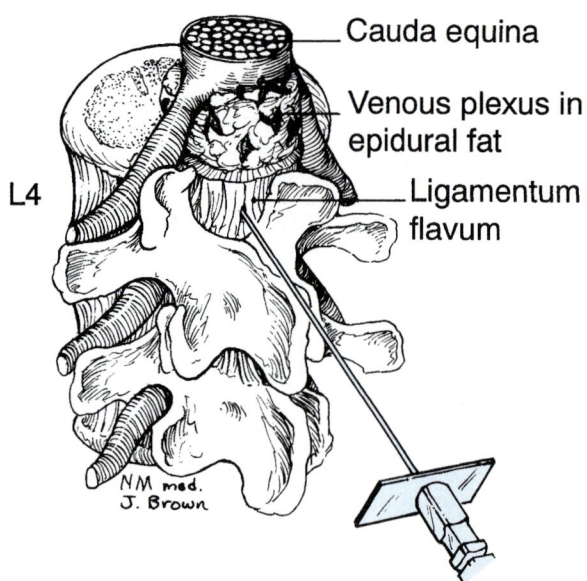

FIGURE 15–5. Midline approach for lumbar epidural nerve block which can be used for either single-injection or catheter insertion for continuous techniques. (Redrawn from Katz, 1994.)

be accomplished by injecting a suitable local anesthetic agent into the epidural or peridural space (Fig. 15–5). This is a potential space that contains areolar tissue, fat, lymphatics, and the internal venous plexus, which becomes engorged during pregnancy so that it appreciably reduces the volume of the space. The portal of entry for obstetrical analgesia is through either a lumbar intervertebral space for lumbar epidural analgesia, or through the sacral hiatus and sacral canal for caudal epidural analgesia. Although one injection may be used, much more often these are repeated through an indwelling catheter, or they are given by continuous infusion using a volumetric pump.

CONTINUOUS LUMBAR EPIDURAL BLOCK. Complete analgesia for the pain of labor and vaginal delivery necessitates a block from the 10th thoracic to the 5th sacral dermatomes. For abdominal delivery, the block is essential beginning at the eighth thoracic level and extending to the first sacral dermatome. The spread of the epidurally injected anesthetic agent will depend upon the location of the catheter tip; the dose, concentration, and volume of anesthetic agent used (Table 15–2); and whether position is head-down, horizontal, or head-up. The anatomy unique to each individual epidural space will also affect the block; for example, presence of synechiae may preclude establishment of a completely satisfactory block. It should also be recognized that the catheter tip may move from its original location during the course of labor.

Before any injection of the local anesthetic agent, a test dose is given and the woman observed for features of toxicity from intravascular injection and signs of spinal blockade from subarachnoid injection. Then a full dose is given carefully and analgesia is maintained by intermittent boluses of similar volume, or small volumes of the drug are delivered continuously by infusion pump. The addition of small doses of a short-acting narcotic, either fentanyl or sufentanil, has been shown to improve analgesic efficacy for labor or cesarean delivery (Chestnut and colleagues, 1988). The rationale for opiate use is to avoid motor block by allowing reduction in dose of local anesthetic.

When vaginal delivery is anticipated in 10 to 15 minutes, a rapidly acting agent is given through the epidural catheter to effect perineal analgesia.

TECHNIQUE. The sequential steps and techniques for performance of epidural anesthesia have been described by Glosten (1994) and are detailed in Table 15–4. It is again emphasized that appropriate resuscitation equipment and drugs must be available during administration of epidural analgesia.

COMPLICATIONS. Epidural analgesia for labor and delivery may provide most pleasant relief from the pain of labor. There are certain problems inherent in its use and, as with spinal blockade, it is imperative that close monitoring, including the level of analgesia, be performed by trained personnel. Table 15–5 summarizes the complications.

TOTAL SPINAL BLOCKADE. Dural puncture with inadvertent subarachnoid injection may cause total spinal block. Personnel and facilities must be immediately available to manage this complication as described under spinal block (p. 372). Postdural puncture headache is a less serious but troublesome complication of inadvertent entry.

INEFFECTIVE ANALGESIA. The extent to which pain relief during labor can be obtained with lumbar epidural analgesia varies, and establishment of effective pain relief with maximum safety takes time. Epidural analgesia for women of higher parity in rapid active labor is likely to prove not worth the risk and expense. Using currently popular continuous epidural infusions such as 0.125 percent bupivacaine with 2 μg/mL fentanyl, 90 percent of women rate their pain relief good to excellent and 95 percent express a desire for the same type of analgesia during a future delivery (Sharma and colleagues, 1997). Alternatively, these results also indicate that a few women find epidural analgesia to be inadequate. If the epidural analgesia is allowed to dissipate before another

TABLE 15–4. Technique for Labor Epidural Analgesia

1. Informed consent is obtained, and the obstetrician consulted.
2. Monitoring includes the following:
   - Blood pressure every 1–2 minutes for 15 minutes after giving a bolus of local anesthetic.
   - Continuous maternal heart rate monitoring during induction of anesthesia.
   - Continuous fetal heart rate monitoring.
   - Continual verbal communication.
3. Hydration with 500–1000 mL of lactated Ringer solution.
4. The woman assumes a lateral decubitus or sitting position.
5. The epidural space is identified with a loss-of-resistance technique.
6. The epidural catheter is threaded 3 cm into the epidural space.
7. A test dose of 3 mL of 1.5% lidocaine with 1:200,000 epinephrine or 3 mL of 0.25% bupivacaine with 1:200,000 epinephrine is injected after careful aspiration and after a uterine contraction (to minimize the chance of confusing tachycardia that results from pain with tachycardia secondary to intravenous injection of the test dose).
8. If the test dose is negative, one or two 5-mL doses of 0.25% bupivacaine are injected to achieve a cephalad sensory T_{10} level.
9. After 15–20 minutes, the block is assessed using loss of sensation to cold or pinprick. If no block is evident, the catheter is replaced. If the block is asymmetrical, the epidural catheter is withdrawn 0.5–1.0 cm and an additional 3–5 mL of bupivacaine is injected. If the block remains inadequate, the catheter is replaced.
10. The woman is positioned in the lateral or semi-lateral position to avoid aortocaval compression.
11. Subsequently, maternal blood pressure is recorded every 5–15 minutes. The fetal heart rate is monitored continuously.
12. The level of analgesia and intensity of motor block are assessed hourly.

From Glosten (1994), with permission.

TABLE 15–5. Complications of Epidural Analgesia

Immediate
  High or total spinal
  Hypotension
  Urinary retention
  Headache
  Postdural puncture seizures
  Meningitis
  Cardiorespiratory arrest
  Vestibulocochlear dysfunction
Long-term (epidural vs controls)
  Backache (19 vs 10%)
  Frequent headaches (4.6 vs 3%)
  Migraine headache (1.9 vs 1.1%)
  Neckache (2.4 vs 1.6%)
  Tingling in hands or fingers (3 vs 2.2%)

From the American College of Obstetricians and Gynecologists (1996); data from Hough and associates (1994), MacArthur and colleagues (1992), and Martin-Hirsch and Martin-Hirsch (1994).

injection of anesthetic drug, subsequent pain relief may be delayed, incomplete, or both.

At times, perineal analgesia for delivery is difficult to obtain, especially with the lumbar epidural technique. When this condition is encountered, a low spinal or pudendal block, or systemic analgesia is added.

HYPOTENSION. By blocking sympathetic tracts, epidurally injected analgesic agents may cause hypotension and decreased cardiac output. In normal pregnant women, hypotension induced by epidural analgesia can usually be prevented by rapid infusion of 500 to 1000 mL of crystalloid solution, or treated successfully as described for spinal analgesia. Danilenko-Dixon and associates (1996) showed that maintaining a lateral position minimized this compared with the supine position. Despite these precautions, hypotension is the most common side effect and occurs in a third of women (Sharma and colleagues, 1997).

CENTRAL NERVOUS STIMULATION. Convulsions are an uncommon but serious complication, the immediate management of which was described previously.

MATERNAL PYREXIA. Fusi and associates (1989) observed that the mean temperature in laboring women given epidural analgesia was significantly higher than in those given meperidine. Lieberman and colleagues (1997), in a study of 1657 nulliparous women, reported intrapartum fever in 15 percent of women receiving epidural analgesia versus only 1 percent of those without epidural analgesia. They also found that epidural analgesia was significantly associated with neonatal sepsis evaluation and antibiotic therapy. Dashe and co-workers (1999) studied placental histopathology in women delivered after labor epidural analgesia. Such analgesia was associated with intrapartum fever only in the presence of placental inflammation. This suggests that the fever reported with epidural analgesia is due to infection rather than the analgesia itself. Sharma (2000) has reviewed maternal fever associated with epidural analgesia. It appears that pyrexia is associated with a higher incidence of intrauterine infection from longer first-

TABLE 15–6. Progress of Labor in 715 Laboring Women According to Analgesia Method

Labor Progress[a]	Epidural Analgesia (n = 243)	Meperidine PCIA[b] (n = 259)	P Value
Cervical dilation at randomization (cm)	4 (3.5)	4 (3.5)	NS
Cervical dilation at initiation of analgesia (cm)	4 (4.5)	4.5 (4.5)	NS
Interval analgesia to complete dilation[c] (min)	260 ± 188	199 ± 171	< .001
Second stage of labor (min)	46.6 ± 68	36.4 ± 87	NS
Second stage ≥ 2 h (%)	15 (7)	12 (6)	NS
Oxytocin after analgesia (%)	80 (33)	40 (15)	< .0001
Temperature > 38°C in labor (%)	58 (24)	16 (6)	< .0001

[a] Data are median (first quartile, third quartile) or mean ± SD.
[b] PCIA = patient-controlled intravenous analgesia.
[c] Ten women in each group who underwent cesarean delivery did not achieve complete dilatation.
From Sharma and colleagues (1997), with permission.

stage labor (Halpern and co-workers, 1998; Mayer and associates, 1997; Sharma and colleagues, 1997).

BACK PAIN. Although an association of epidural analgesia and back pain has been reported by some, others have not found such an association (Breen, 1994; MacArthur, 1990, 1997; Russell, 1993, and all their colleagues). In a prospective cohort study, Butler and Fuller (1998) reported that postpartum back pain following epidural analgesia was common, but persistent or chronic back pain was uncommon.

EFFECT ON LABOR. The use of epidural analgesia during labor has greatly increased during the past two decades, coincident with a significant escalation in the maternal cesarean birth rate (Sachs and colleagues, 1999). As shown in Tables 15–6 and 15–7, epidural analgesia usually prolongs the first stage of labor, and increases the need for labor stimulation with oxytocin. It also increases the chance of an instrumental delivery due to

prolonged second-stage labor but with no adverse effects on the infant (Chestnut, 1999; Thorp and Breedlove, 1996). Investigators at Brigham and Women's Hospital observed that epidural analgesia is associated with an increase in the rate of severe perineal trauma because of the more frequent use of operative vaginal delivery (Robinson and associates, 1999).

A more contentious issue is whether epidural analgesia increases the risk of cesarean delivery. As reviewed by Sharma and Leveno (2000), several retrospective studies and a few randomized studies have suggested that epidural analgesia during labor is associated with increased cesarean deliveries.

Between 1993 and 1996, a total of 3276 women at Parkland Hospital with uncomplicated term pregnancies were randomized in three trials of various labor epidural analgesia techniques using dilute solutions of local anesthetic as well as methods for administration of meperidine intravenously. The results of all three of these trials, as pertains to cesarean deliveries, are shown

TABLE 15–7. Progress of Labor During Oxytocin Augmentation in 199 Women by Analgesia Method

Characteristic	Epidural (n = 126)	Meperidine (n = 73)	P Value
Cervical dilatation at oxytocin initiation (cm ± SD)	4.5 ± 1	4.0 ± 1	.02
Mean oxytocin infusion rate (mU/min ± SD)	12 ± 7	11 ± 7	NS
Maximum oxytocin infusion rate (mU/min ± SD)	23 ± 15	22 ± 14	NS
Duration of oxytocin infusion (h ± SD)	4.2 ± 0	3.4 ± 0	.03
Oxytocin dose per cm cervical dilatation (mU/min ± SD)	22 ± 26	16 ± 18	.009

From Alexander and colleagues (1998), with permission.

TABLE 15–8. Summary of Three Consecutive Randomized Trials of Labor Analgesia Conducted at Parkland Hospital in 3276 Women with Singleton Cephalic Gestations at Term in Spontaneous Labor, 1993–1996

Study	Epidural Analgesia		Narcotic Analgesia		Significance
	No.	Cesarean No. (%)	No.	Cesarean No. (%)	
Ramin et al (1995)					
All	664	43 (6)	666	37 (6)	NS
Multiparous	326	6 (2)	311	7 (2)	NS
Nulliparous	338	37 (11)	355	30 (9)	NS
Gambling et al (1998)					
All	616	39 (6)	607	34 (6)	NS
Multiparous	280	9 (4)	293	9 (3)	NS
Nulliparous	336	30 (10)	314	25 (9)	NS
Sharma et al (1997)					
All	358	13 (4)	357	16 (5)	NS
Multiparous	161	4 (3)	168	5 (3)	NS
Nulliparous	197	9 (5)	189	11 (6)	NS
Trials combined					
All	1638	95 (6)	1630	87 (5)	NS
Multiparous	763	19 (3)	769	21 (3)	NS
Nulliparous	875	76 (9)	861	66 (8)	NS

From Sharma and Leveno (2000), with permission.

in Table 15–8. Epidural analgesia did not significantly increase cesarean deliveries in either nulliparous or parous women in any individual trial or in their aggregate. These results are consistent with the belief of many investigators that the epidural administration of dilute solutions of local anesthetic is less likely to increase cesarean rates compared with concentrated solutions (Chestnut, 1997; Thompson and colleagues, 1998).

There have been several additional recent reports indicating that epidural analgesia is not associated with excess cesarean births. Halpern and colleagues (1998) performed meta-analysis of seven studies of 1183 women who received epidural analgesia versus 1186 who received opioids for labor pain. They reported no increase in the cesarean rate attributable to epidural analgesia. Yancey and co-workers (1999) published a remarkable report on the effects of introduction of an on-demand labor epidural analgesia service at Tripler Army Hospital in Hawaii. In late 1993, a policy change within the Department of Defense required the availability of on-demand labor epidural analgesia in military medical centers. As a result, the incidence of epidural analgesia during labor increased from 1 percent before the policy to 60 percent 2 years after the policy had been implemented. The primary cesarean rate was 13.4 percent before and 13.2 percent after this dramatic change in epidural usage.

In 1993, the American Society of Anesthesiologists and the American College of Obstetricians and Gynecologists issued the following joint statement: "There is no other circumstance where it is considered acceptable for a person to experience severe pain, amenable to safe intervention, while under a physician's care." This implies that all women should have access to effective pain relief during labor. We are of the view that the fear of increasing the risk of cesarean delivery should not preclude women from choosing epidural analgesia during labor.

TIMING OF EPIDURAL PLACEMENT. In a randomized trial, Chestnut and associates (1994) found no increase in either operative vaginal delivery or cesarean delivery with early—at or before 3 cm dilatation—administration of epidural analgesia compared with later administration. Similar results were reported by Rogers and co-workers (1999). In the Parkland Hospital trials described earlier in this section, epidural analgesia was not begun prior to 3 to 5 cm cervical dilatation, and this continues to be our practice unless labor is already being stimulated with oxytocin.

SAFETY. The relative safety of epidural analgesia is attested to by the extraordinary experiences reported by Crawford (1985) from the Birmingham Maternity Hospital in England. From 1968 through 1985, over 26,000 women were given epidural analgesia for labor, and there were no maternal deaths. The nine potentially life-threatening complications followed either inadvertent intravenous or intrathecal injections of lidocaine, bupivacaine, or both.

CONTRAINDICATIONS. As with spinal analgesia, contraindications to epidural analgesia include actual or anticipated serious maternal hemorrhage, infection at or near the sites for puncture, and suspicion of neurological disease. Rolbin and colleagues (1988) advise against epidural analgesia if the platelet count is below 100,000/μL. Conversely, Rasmus and associates (1989) found no cases in which bleeding was caused by regional analgesia in thrombocytopenic women. They recommended consideration of this method if the patient might be difficult to intubate or ventilate.

SEVERE PREECLAMPSIA–ECLAMPSIA. Ideal labor analgesia for women with severe preeclampsia has been controversial. This is discussed in Chapter 24. Obstetrical concerns centered on hypotension induced by sympathetic blockade, dangers from pressor agents given to correct hypotension, and potential for pulmonary edema following infusion of large volumes of crystalloid. Anesthesiologists are concerned that general anesthesia with tracheal intubation may result in severe, sudden hypertension further complicated by pulmonary or cerebral edema or intracranial hemorrhage.

Over the past two to three decades, most obstetrical anesthesiologists have come to favor epidural blockade for labor and delivery in women with severe preeclampsia (Cheek and Samuels, 1991; Gutsche, 1986). Indeed, the immense popularity and increasing availability of epidural analgesia for labor has led many anesthesiologists as well as obstetricians to develop the viewpoint that epidural analgesia is an important factor in the treatment of these women with severe disease (Chadwick and Easterling, 1991; Ramanathan, 1991). At the same time, many of these same authorities have criticized the use of general anesthesia. Although the ultimate decision for anesthetic management of cesarean delivery remains with the anesthesiologist, the obstetrician must approve the use of labor epidural analgesia, and both must be knowledgeable about the obstetrical effects of either method used for delivery.

There seems to be no argument that epidural analgesia for women with severe preeclampsia–eclampsia can be safely used when specially trained anesthesiologists and obstetricians are responsible for the woman and her fetus (American College of Obstetricians and Gynecologists, 1996; Cunningham and Leveno, 1995; Cunningham and Lindheimer, 1992; Moore and colleagues, 1985). In an evaluation of cesarean delivery for women with severe preeclampsia, Wallace and colleagues (1995) randomized 80 such women to receive general anesthesia, epidural analgesia, or combined spinal–epidural analgesia. Although no woman receiving general anesthesia required ephedrine for hypotension, this was necessary in 30 percent of those given epidural analgesia and 22 percent of those given spinal–epidural

analgesia. There were no significant differences in neonatal outcomes among the three groups. It was concluded that general anesthesia and regional analgesia are equally acceptable for cesarean delivery in women with severe preeclampsia.

Although epidural analgesia is widely used during labor in women with hypertensive disorders due to pregnancy, the effects of such analgesia in the mother and fetus are just coming under scrutiny. Lucas and colleagues (2001) randomized 738 women with hypertension and term pregnancies to epidural analgesia or patient-controlled intravenous analgesia during labor. It was concluded that it was safe to use epidural analgesia during labor in women with hypertensive disorders but that epidural analgesia should not be administered as a therapy for this obstetrical complication. In a retrospective analysis of 327 laboring women with severe hypertension, Hogg and colleagues (1999) found no difference in overall cesarean delivery rates (32 versus 28 percent) in women who received epidural analgesia compared with those who did not. The frequencies of pulmonary edema or renal failure were similar between the groups.

INTRAVENOUS FLUID PRELOADING. Most authorities recommend prehydration, usually with 500 to 1000 mL of crystalloid solution (Hogg and associates, 1999). Importantly, vasodilation produced by epidural blockade is usually less abrupt if the analgesia level is achieved slowly, thus allowing maintenance of blood pressure while simultaneously avoiding infusion of large volumes of crystalloid.

Newsome and colleagues (1986) demonstrated that lowered mean arterial pressure followed epidural blockade in women with severe preeclampsia. Despite this, cardiac index did not fall because vigorous intravenous crystalloid infusion caused elevation of pulmonary capillary wedge pressures as compared with women not given epidural analgesia and in whom fluids were restricted (Fig. 15–6). Although the intravascular volume of women with severe preeclampsia is not expanded as for normal pregnancy, total body water is increased. It is also generally recognized that there is a capillary leak with severe preeclampsia, and that this is manifested as pathological peripheral edema, proteinuria, and ascites. Aggressive volume replacement in these women increases their risk for pulmonary edema, especially in the first 72 hours postpartum (Clark and colleagues, 1985; Cotton and associates, 1986). Hogg and associates (1999) reported that 3.5 percent of women had pulmonary edema when pretreated with intravenous fluid without a protocol limitation to volume. By contrast, Lucas and colleagues (2001) reported no instances of pulmonary edema in 738 women in whom crystalloid preload was limited to 500 mL.

With vigorous intravenous crystalloid therapy, there

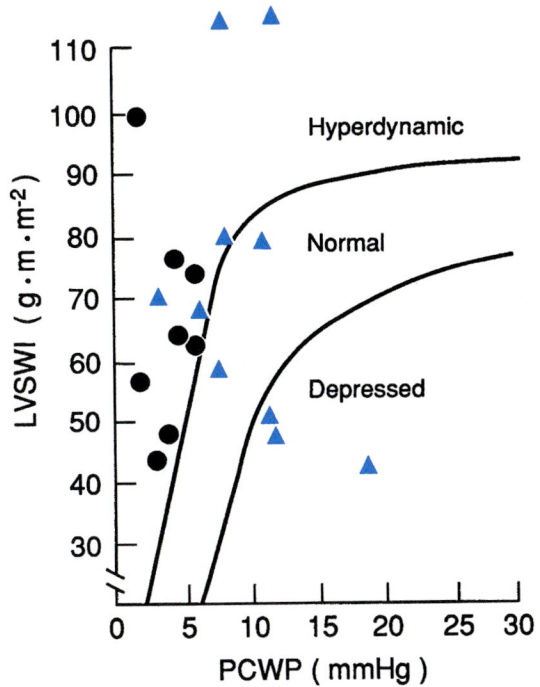

FIGURE 15–6. Comparison of ventricular function curves in women with severe preeclampsia. The solid circles represent values from women with eclampsia not given epidural analgesia and who were managed with fluid restriction. (Hankins and colleagues, 1984.) The triangles represent women given intravenous fluid preloading to prevent decreased cardiac output with epidural analgesia (LVSWI = left ventricular stroke work index; PCWP = pulmonary capillary wedge pressure). (Newsome and co-workers, 1986.)

is also concern for development of cerebral edema. Finally, Heller and co-workers (1983) demonstrated that the majority of cases of pharyngolaryngeal edema were related to aggressive volume therapy.

EPIDURAL OPIATE ANALGESIA. Injection of opiates into the epidural space to relieve pain from labor has become popular. Complications with this technique are less worrisome than those seen with epidural injection of local anesthetics alone. The mechanism of action of opiates given epidurally derives from their interaction with specific receptors in the dorsal horn and dorsal roots. Apparently both cerebral and spinal opioid receptors are stimulated by these narcotics (Ackerman and colleagues, 1992).

Opiates alone usually will not provide adequate analgesia, and they most often are given with a local anesthetic agent such as bupivacaine (American College of Obstetricians and Gynecologists, 1996). The major advantages of using such a combination are the rapid onset of pain relief, a decrease in shivering, and less dense motor blockade. Cohen and colleagues (1992), in a randomized study of epidural buprenorphine plus bupiva-

caine versus fentanyl plus bupivacaine, reported that both epidural opioids were equally efficacious. Steinberg and associates (1989) reported that sufentanil may provide adequate epidural analgesia when used alone. By comparison, a single lumbar intrathecal injection of 25 μg of fentanyl and 0.25 mg of morphine sulfate has been reported to result in a satisfactory level of pain relief without disrupting labor. Meister and colleagues (2000), in a randomized study of 50 laboring women, compared epidural analgesia with 0.125 percent ropivacaine and fentanyl to 0.125 percent bupivacaine and fentanyl. Both groups had similar labor analgesia, but the ropivacaine group had significantly less motor block.

Side effects are common (Herpelsheimer and Schretenthaler, 1994). They include pruritus (80 percent), urinary retention (55 percent), nausea and vomiting (45 percent), and headaches (10 percent). Rust and colleagues (1994) reported excellent pain relief (93 percent) using this technique, but again recorded a high incidence of pruritus and/or urinary retention. Immediate or delayed respiratory depression is worrisome (Ackerman and colleagues, 1992). Naloxone, given intravenously, will abolish these symptoms without affecting the analgesic action. Horta and colleagues (2000) reported a reduction in the incidence of pruritus with droperidol given in doses of up to 5 mg epidurally. This effect was dose-related and was not associated with other serious side effects. Hunt and colleagues (1989) reported a fetal sinusoidal heart rate pattern associated with maternal administration of epidural butorphanol and bupivacaine.

COMBINED SPINAL–EPIDURAL TECHNIQUES. The combination of spinal and epidural techniques may provide rapid and effective analgesia for labor or for cesarean delivery. Although neonatal complications are not increased, there is no consensus regarding maternal complications when comparing spinal or epidural analgesia with combined techniques (American Society of Anesthesiologists Task Force on Obstetrical Anesthesia, 1999). In a randomized trial of 110 laboring women, Van de Velde and associates (1999) compared epidural with combined spinal–epidural analgesia and reported that the combined method produced excellent immediate pain relief for labor. Side effects were similar between the two groups. Nickells and colleagues (2000) compared rapidity of onset of labor analgesia in 69 women given combined spinal–epidural versus 73 women given epidural analgesia. Onset of analgesia was only slightly faster for the combined technique (10.0 versus 12.1 minutes); however, it was associated with more side effects.

The largest study of the combined spinal–epidural technique performed in laboring women was conducted at Parkland Hospital (Gambling and co-workers, 1998). There were 1223 women with uncomplicated term pregnancies who were randomized to continuous spinal–epidural analgesia or boluses of intravenous meperidine. Emergency cesarean delivery for profound fetal tachycardia was performed in 9 of 616 women assigned to combined spinal–epidural analgesia compared with none of 607 in the meperidine groups ($P < .005$). Fetal bradycardia typically occurred within 30 minutes of the initiation of intrathecal analgesia and was defined as fetal heart rate less than 60 bpm lasting 60 seconds or longer. None of the cases responded to conservative measures such as changing maternal position, oxygen administration, or intravenous ephedrine. Interestingly, none of these cases were associated with maternal hypotension. Although, none of these infants suffered ill effects, we now avoid the combined spinal–epidural technique.

REFERENCES

Ackerman WE, Juneja M, Spinnato JA: Epidural opioids OB advantages. Contemp Obstet Gynecol 37:68, 1992

Akpek EA, Karaaslan D, Erol E, Caner H, Kayhan Z: Chronic subdural haematoma following caesarean section under spinal anaesthesia. Anaesth Intensive Care 27:206, 1999

Alexander JM, Lucas MJ, Ramin SM, McIntire DD, Leveno KJ: The course of labor with and without epidural analgesia. Am J Obstet Gynecol 178:516, 1998

American Academy of Pediatrics and American College of Obstetricians and Gynecologists: Guidelines for Perinatal Care, 4th ed. Washington, DC, 1997

American College of Obstetricians and Gynecologists: Obstetric anesthesia and analgesia. Technical Bulletin, No. 225, July 1996

American College of Obstetricians and Gynecologists, Committee on Obstetric Practice: Pain relief during labor. Committee Opinion No. 231, February 2000

American Society of Anesthesiologists Task Force on Obstetrical Anesthesia: Practice guidelines for obstetrical anesthesia. Anesthesiology 90:600, 1999

Andrews WW, Ramin SM, Wallace DH, Shearer V, Black S, Maberry MC, Dax JS: Effect of type of anesthesia on blood loss at elective repeat cesarean section. Am J Perinatol 9:197, 1992

Angel JL, Knuppel RA, Lake M: Sinusoidal fetal heart rate pattern associated with intravenous butorphanol administration: A case report. Am J Obstet Gynecol 149:465, 1984

Atkinson BD, Truitt LJ, Rayburn WF, Turnbull GL, Christensen HD, Wlodarer A: Double-blind comparison of intravenous butorphanol (Stadol) and fentanyl (Sublimaze) for analgesia during labor. Am J Obstet Gynecol 171:993, 1994

Bell ED, Penning DH, Cousineau EF, White WD, Hartle AJ, Gilbert WC, Lubarsky DA: How much labor is in a labor epidural? Manpower cost and reimbursement for an obstetric analgesia service in a teaching institution. Anesthesiology 92:851, 2000

Blass NH: The morbidly obese pregnant patient. In Datta S (ed): Anesthetic and Obstetric Management of High-risk Pregnancy. St Louis, Mosby-Year Book, 1991, p 59

Breen TW, Ransil BJ, Groves PA, Oriol NE: Factors associated with back pain after childbirth. Anesthesiology 81:29, 1994

Breheny F, McCarthy J: Maternal mortality. A review of maternal deaths over twenty years at the National Maternity Hospital, Dublin. Anaesthesia 37:561, 1982

Burchman CA: Maternal aspiration. In Ostheimer GW (ed): Manual of Obstetric Anesthesia, 2nd ed. New York, Churchill Livingstone, 1992, p 161

Busby T: Local anesthesia for cesarean section. Am J Obstet Gynecol 87:399, 1963

Butler R, Fuller J: Back pain following epidural anaesthesia in labour. Can J Anaesth 45:724, 1998

Camann WR, Datta S: Red cell use during cesarean delivery. Transfusion 31:12, 1991

Carter BL, Pasupuleti R: Use of intravenous cosyntropin in the treatment of postdural puncture headache. Anesthesiology 92:272, 2000

Chadwick HS, Easterling T: Anesthetic concerns in the patient with preeclampsia. Semin Perinatol 15:397, 1991

Cheek TG, Samuels P: Pregnancy induced hypertension. In Datta S (ed): Anesthesia and Management of High-Risk Pregnancy. St Louis, Mosby-Year Book, 1991

Chestnut DH: Effect on the progress of labor and method of delivery. In Chestnut DH (ed): Obstetric Anesthesia: Principles and Practice, 2nd ed. St Louis: Mosby-Year Book, 1999, p 408

Chestnut DH: Epidural analgesia and the incidence of cesarean section: Time for another close look. Anesthesiology 87:472, 1997

Chestnut DH, McGrath JM, Vincent RD Jr, Penning DH, Choi WW, Bates JN, McFarland C: Does early administration of epidural analgesia affect obstetric outcome in nulliparous women who are in spontaneous labor? Anesthesiology 80:1201, 1994

Chestnut DH, Owen CL, Bates JN, Ostman LG, Choi WW, Geiger MW: Continuous infusion epidural analgesia during labor: A randomized, double-blind comparison of 0.625% bupivacaine/0.0002% fentanyl versus 0.125% bupivacaine. Anesthesiology 68:754, 1988

Clark SL, Divon MY, Phelan JP: Preeclampsia/eclampsia: Hemodynamic and neurologic correlations. Obstet Gynecol 66:337, 1985

Cohen SE: Nonobstetric surgery during pregnancy. In Chestnut DL (ed): Obstetric Anesthesia: Principles and Practice. St Louis, Mosby-Year Book, 1994, p 273

Cohen SE, Amar D, Pantuck CB, Pantuck EJ, Weissman AM, Landa S, Singer N: Epidural patient-controlled analgesia after cesarean section: Buprenorphine—0.015% bupivacaine with epinephrine versus fentanyl—0.015% bupivacaine with and without epinephrine. Anesth Analg 74:226, 1992

Combs CA, Murphy EL, Laros RK Jr: Factors associated with hemorrhage in cesarean deliveries. Obstet Gynecol 77:77, 1991

Cooper SD, Benumof JL, Ozaki GT: Evaluation of the Bullard laryngoscope using the new intubating stylet: Comparison with conventional laryngoscopy. Anesth Analg 79:965, 1994

Cotton DB, Longmire S, Jones MM, Dorman KF, Tessem J, Joyce TH III: Cardiovascular alterations in severe pregnancy-induced hypertension: Effects of intravenous nitroglycerin coupled with blood volume expansion. Am J Obstet Gynecol 154:1053, 1986

Crawford JS: Some maternal complications of epidural analgesia for labour. Anesthesia 40:1219, 1985

Cunningham FG, Leveno KJ: Obstetrical concerns for anesthetic management of severe preeclampsia. Williams Obstetrics, 19th ed (Suppl 10). Norwalk, CT, Appleton & Lange, December 1994/January 1995

Cunningham FG, Lindheimer M: Hypertension in pregnancy. N Engl J Med 326:927, 1992

Danilenko-Dixon DR, Tefft L, Haydon B, Cohen RA, Carpenter MW: The effect of maternal position on cardiac output with epidural analgesia in labor. Am J Obstet Gynecol 174:332, 1996

Dashe JS, Rogers BB, McIntire DD, Leveno KJ: Epidural analgesia and integration fever: Placental findings. Obstet Gynecol 93:341, 1999

Farcon EL, Kim MH, Marx GF: Changing Mallampati score during labour. Can J Anaesth 41:50, 1994

Fishburne JI Jr, Greiss FC Jr, Hopkinson R, Rhyne AL: Response of the gravid uterine vasculature to arterial levels of local anesthetic agents. Am J Obstet Gynecol 133:753, 1979

Fusi L, Steer PJ, Maresh MJA, Beard RW: Maternal pyrexia associated with the use of epidural analgesia in labour. Lancet 1:1250, 1989

Gambling DR, Sharma SK, Ramin SM, Lucas MJ, Leveno KJ, Riley J, Sidawi JE: A randomized study of combined spinal–epidural analgesia versus intravenous meperidine during labor: Impact on cesarean delivery rate. Anesthesiology 89:1336, 1998

Gibbs CP, Banner TC: Effectiveness of Bicitra/Pr as a preoperative antacid. Anesthesiology 61:97, 1984

Gibbs CP, Krischer J, Pickham BM, Kirschbaum TH: Obstetric anesthesia: A national survey. Anesthesiology 65:298, 1986

Gilstrap LC, Hauth JC, Hankins DG, Patterson AR: Effect of type of anesthesia on blood loss at cesarean section. Obstet Gynecol 69:328, 1987

Glosten B: Local anesthetic techniques. In Chestnut DH (ed): Obstetric Anesthesia: Principles and Practice. St Louis, Mosby-Year Book, 1994, p 354

Greiss FC Jr, Still JG, Anderson SG: Effects of local anesthetic agents on the uterine vasculatures and myometrium. Am J Obstet Gynecol 124:889, 1976

Gunaratnam NT, Benson J, Gandolfi AJ, Chen M: Suspected isoflurane hepatitis in an obese patient with a history of halothane hepatitis. Anesthesiology 83:1361, 1995

Gutsche BB: The experts opine: The role of epidural anesthesia in preeclampsia. Surv Anesthesiol 30:304, 1986

Guyton TS, Gibbs CP: Aspiration: Risk, prophylaxis, and treatment. In Chestnut DH (ed): Obstetric Anesthesia: Principles and Practice. St Louis, Mosby-Year Book, 1994, p 565

Hall PA, Bennett A, Wilkes MP, Lewis M: Spinal anaesthesia for cesarean section: Comparison of infusions of phenylephrine and ephedrine. Br J Anaesth 73:471, 1994

Halpern SH, Leighton BL, Ohlsson A, Barrett JFR, Rice A: Effect of epidural vs parenteral opioid analgesia on the progress of labor. JAMA 280:2105, 1998

Hankins GDV, Wendel GW Jr, Cunningham FG, Leveno KJ: Longitudinal evaluation of hemodynamic changes in eclampsia. Am J Obstet Gynecol 150:506, 1984

Harding SA, Colis RE, Morgan BM: Meningitis after combined spinal–extradural anesthesia in obstetrics. Br J Anaesth 73:545, 1994

Hatjis CG, Meis PJ: Sinusoidal fetal heart rate pattern associated with butorphanol administration. Obstet Gynecol 67:377, 1986

Hawkins JL, Gibbs CP, Martin-Salvaj G, Orleans M, Beaty B: Oral intake policies on labor and delivery: A national survey. J Clin Anesthesia 10:449, 1998

Hawkins JL, Gibbs CP, Orleans M, Martin-Salvaj G, Beaty B: Obstetric anesthesia work force survey, 1981 versus 1992. Anesthesiology 87:135, 1997a

Hawkins JL, Koonin LM, Palmer SK, Gibbs CP: Anesthesia-related deaths during obstetric delivery in the United States, 1979–1990. Anesthesiology 86:277, 1997b

Hawksworth CRE, Purdie J: Failed combined spinal epidural then failed intubation at an elective cesarean section. Hospital Medicine 59:173, 1998

Heller PJ, Schneider EP, Marx GF: Pharyngo-laryngeal edema as a presenting symptom in preeclampsia. Obstet Gynecol 62:523, 1983

Herpolsheimer A, Schretenthaler J: The use of intrapartum intrathecal narcotic analgesia in a community-based hospital. Obstet Gynecol 84:931, 1994

Hibbard BM, Anderson MM, Drife JO, Tighe JR, Sykes K, Gordon G, Pinkerton JHM, Milner D, Botting B: Report on confidential enquiries into maternal deaths in the United Kingdom 1988–1990. London, Her Majesty's Stationery Office, 1994, p 80

Hodgkinson R, Bhatt M, Kim SS, Grewal G, Marx GF: Neonatal neurobehavioral tests following cesarean section under general and spinal anesthesia. Am J Obstet Gynecol 132:670, 1978

Hodgkinson R, Glassenberg R, Joyce TH, Coombs DW, Ostheimer GW, Gibbs CP: Comparison of cimetidine (Tagamet) with antacid for safety and effectiveness in reducing gastric acidity before elective cesarean section. Anesthesiology 59:86, 1983

Hogg B, Hauth JC, Caritis SN, Sibai BM, Lindheimer M, Van Dorsten JP, Klebanoff M, MacPherson C, Landon M, Paul R, Miodovnik M, Meis PJ, Thurnau GR, Dombrowski MP, McNellis D, Roberts JM: Safety of labor epidural anesthesia for women with severe hypertensive disease. National Institute of Child Health and Human Development Maternal–Fetal Medicine Units Network. Am J Obstet Gynecol 181:1096, 1999

Hood DD, Curry R: Spinal versus epidural anesthesia for cesarean section in severely preeclamptic patients: A retrospective survey. Anesthesiology 90:1276, 1999

Horta ML, Ramos L, Goncalves ZR: The inhibition of epidural morphine-induced pruritus by epidural droperidol. Anesth Analg 90:638, 2000

Hough MB, Bloor GK, Brighouse D: Cardiorespiratory arrest following combined spinal epidural anaesthesia. Anaesthesia 49:260, 1994

Hunt CO, Naulty JS, Malinow AM, Datta S, Ostheimer GW: Epidural butorphanol-bupivacaine for analgesia during labor and delivery. Anesth Analg 68:323, 1989

Katz J: Atlas of Regional Anesthesia, 2nd ed. Norwalk, CT, Appleton & Lange, 1994

Kennedy WF Jr, Bonica JJ, Akamatsu TJ, Ward RJ, Martin WE, Grinstein A: Cardiovascular and respiratory effects of subarachnoid block in the presence of acute blood loss. Anesthesiology 29:29, 1968

Kennell J, Klaus M, McGrath S, Robertson S, Hinkley C: Continuous emotional support during labor in a US hospital: A randomized controlled trial. JAMA 265:2197, 1991

Lamaze F: Painless Childbirth: Psychoprophylactic Method. Chicago, Henry Regnery, 1970

Lamont BJ, Pennant JH, Wallace DH, Jennings LW, Giesecke AH: Directly measured uterine tone and blood loss during anesthesia for cesarean section. Anesth Analg 67S:126, 1988

Lieberman E, Lang JM, Frigoletto F Jr, Richardson DK,

Ringer SA, Cohen A: Epidural analgesia, intrapartum fever, and neonatal sepsis evaluation. Pediatrics 99:415, 1997

Lim SK, Elegbe EO: Ranitidine and sodium citrate as prophylaxis against acid aspiration syndrome in obstetric patients undergoing cesarean section. Singapore Med 33:608, 1992

Lucas MJ, Sharma S, McIntire DD, Wiley J, Sidawi JB, Ramin SM, Leveno KJ, Cunningham FG: A randomized trial of labor analgesia in women with pregnancy-induced hypertension. Am J Obstet Gynecol 184:10, 2001

Maberry MC, Shearer V, Black S, Wallace DH: Effect of type of anesthesia on blood loss at elective repeat cesarean section. Am J Perinatol 9:197, 1992

MacArthur AJ, MacArthur C, Weeks SK: Is epidural anaesthesia in labour associated with chronic low back pain? A prospective cohort study. Anesth Analg 85:1066, 1997

MacArthur C, Lewis M, Knox EG: Investigation of long-term problems after obstetric epidural anaesthesia. BMJ 304:1279, 1992

MacArthur C, Lewis M, Knox EG, Crawford JS: Epidural anaesthesia and long-term backache after childbirth. BMJ 301:9, 1990

Martin-Hirsch DP, Martin-Hirsch PL: Vestibulocochlear dysfunction following epidural anaesthesia in labour. Br J Clin Pract 48:340, 1994

Mayer DC, Chescheir NC, Spielman FJ: Increased intrapartum antibiotic administration associated with epidural analgesia in labor. Am J Perinatol 14:83, 1997

Meister GC, D'Angelo R, Owen M, Nelson KE, Gaver R: A comparison of epidural analgesia with 0.125% ropivacaine with fentanyl versus 0.125% bupivacaine with fentanyl during labor. Anesth Analg 90:632, 2000

Melzack R: The myth of painless childbirth. Pain 19:321, 1984

Mendelson CL: The aspiration of stomach contents into the lungs during obstetric anesthesia. Am J Obstet Gynecol 52:191, 1946

Moore TR, Key TC, Reisner LS, Resnick R: Evaluation of the use of continuous lumbar epidural anesthesia for hypertensive pregnant women in labor. Am J Obstet Gynecol 152:104, 1985

Morgan D, Philip J, Sharma S, Gottumukkala V, Perez B, Wiley J: A neonatal outcome with ephedrine infusions with or without preloading during spinal anesthesia for cesarean section. Society of Anesthesiologists and Perinatologists, Montreal, Quebec, Canada. Anesthesiology (supplement): A5, 2000

Morgan P: The role of vasopressors in the management of hypotension induced by spinal and epidural anaesthesia. Can J Anaesth 41:404, 1994

Newsome LR, Bramwell RS, Curling PE: Severe preeclampsia: Hemodynamic effects of lumbar epidural anesthesia. Anesth Analg 65:31, 1986

Newton JA Jr, Lesnik IK, Kennedy CA: Streptococcus salivarius meningitis following spinal anaesthesia. Clin Infect Dis 18:840, 1994

Nickells JS, Vaughan DJ, Lillywhite NK, Loughnan B, Hasan M, Robinson PN: Speed of onset of regional analgesia in labour: A comparison of the epidural and spinal routes. Anaesthesia 55:17, 2000

Oh J, Camann W: Severe, acute meningeal irritative reaction after epidural blood patch. Anesth Analg 87:1139, 1998

Palkar NV, Boudreaux RC, Mankad AV: Accidental total spinal block: A complication of an epidural test dose. Can J Anaesth 39:1058, 1992

Piggott SWE, Bogod DG, Rosen M, Rees GA, Harmer M: Isoflurane with either 100% oxygen or 50% nitrous oxide in oxygen for cesarean section. Br J Anaesth 65:325, 1990

Quilligan EJ, Keegan KA, Donahue MJ: Double-blind comparison of intravenously injected butorphanol and meperidine in parturients. Int J Gynaecol Obstet 18:363, 1980

Ramanathan J: Anesthetic considerations in preeclampsia. Clin Perinatol 18:875, 1991

Ramin SM, Gambling DR, Lucas MJ, Sharma SK, Sidawi JE, Leveno KJ: Randomized trial of epidural versus intravenous analgesia during labor. Obstet Gynecol 86:783, 1995

Ramin SM, Ramin KD, Cox K, Magness RR, Shearer VE, Gant NF: Comparison of prophylactic angiotensin II versus ephedrine infusion for prevention of maternal hypotension during spinal anesthesia. Am J Obstet Gynecol 171:734, 1994

Rasmus KT, Rottman RL, Kotelko DM, Wright WC, Stone JJ, Rosenblatt RM: Unrecognized thrombocytopenia and regional anesthesia in parturients: A retrospective review. Obstet Gynecol 72:943, 1989

Rasmussen GE, Malinow AM: Toward reducing maternal mortality: The problem airway in obstetrics. Int Anesthesiol Clin 32:83, 1994

Read GD: Childbirth Without Fear. New York, Harper, 1944, p 192

Reisner LS, Nichols KP: Anesthetic considerations for complicated pregnancies. In Creasy RK, Resnick R (eds): Maternal-Fetal Medicine, 4th ed. Philadelphia, Saunders, 1999, p 1215

Roberts SW, Leveno KJ, Sidawi JE, Lucas MJ, Kelley MA: Fetal acidemia associated with regional anesthesia for elective cesarean delivery. Obstet Gynecol 85:79, 1995

Robinson JN, Norwitz ER, Cohen AP, Mcelrath TF, Lieberman ES: Epidural analgesia and third- or fourth-degree lacerations in nulliparas. Obstet Gynecol 94:259, 1999

Rogers R, Gilson G, Kammerer-Doak D: Epidural analgesia and active management of labor: Effects on length of labor and mode of delivery. Obstet Gynecol 93:995, 1999

Rolbin SH, Abbott D, Musclow E, Papsin F, Lie LM, Freedman J: Epidural anesthesia in pregnant patients with low platelet counts. Obstet Gynecol 71:918, 1988

Rowe TF: Acute gastric aspiration: Prevention and treatment. Semin Perinatol 21:313, 1997

Russell R, Groves P, Taub N, O'Dowd J, Reynolds F: Assessing long-term backache after childbirth. BMJ 306:1299, 1993

Rust LA, Waring RW, Hall GL, Nelson EI: Intrathecal narcotics for obstetric analgesia in a community hospital. Am J Obstet Gynecol 170:1643, 1994

Sachs BP, Castro MA, Frigoletto F: The risks of lowering the cesarean delivery rate. N Engl J Med 340:54, 1999

Sears DH, Leeman MI, Jassy LJ, O'Donnell LA, Allen SG, Reisner LS: The frequency of postdural headache in obstetric patients: A prospective study comparing the 24-gauge versus the 22-gauge Sprotte needle. J Clin Anesth 6:42, 1994

Sharma SK: Epidural analgesia during labor and maternal fever. Curr Opin Anesthesiology 13:257, 2000

Sharma SK, Leveno KJ: Update: Epidural analgesia during labor does not increase cesarean births. Current Anesthesiology Reports 2:18, 2000

Sharma SK, Sidawi JE, Ramin SM, Lucas MJ, Leveno KJ, Cunningham FG: Cesarean delivery: A randomized trial of epidural versus patient-controlled meperidine analgesia during labor. Anesthesiology 87:487, 1997

Shearer VE, Jhaveri HS, Cunningham FG: Puerperal seizures after postdural puncture headache. Obstet Gynecol 85:255, 1995

Steinberg RB, Powell G, Hu XH, Dunn SM: Epidural sufentanil for analgesia for labor and delivery. Reg Anesth 14:225, 1989

Svancarek W, Chirino O, Schaefer G Jr, Blythe JG: Retropsoas and subgluteal abscesses following paracervical and pudendal anesthesia. JAMA 237:892, 1977

Taylor G, Pryse-Davies J: The prophylactic use of antacids in the prevention of the acid pulmonary aspiration syndrome. Lancet 1:288, 1966

Teabeaut JR II: Aspiration of gastric contents: An experimental study. Am J Pathol 28:51, 1952

Thompson TT, Thorp JM, Mayer D, Kuller JA, Bowes WA Jr: Does epidural analgesia cause dystocia? J Clin Anesth 10:58, 1998

Thornburn J, Moir DD: Antacid therapy for emergency cesarean sections. Anaesthesia 42:352, 1987

Thorp JA, Breedlove G: Epidural analgesia in labor: An evaluation of risks and benefits. Birth 23:63, 1996

Valli J, Pirhonen J, Aantaa R, Erkkola R, Kanto J: The effects of regional anaesthesia for cesarean section on maternal and fetal blood flow velocities measured by Doppler ultrasound. Acta Anaesthesiol Scand 38:165, 1994

Van de Velde M, Mignolet K, Vandermeersch E, Van Assche A: Prospective, randomized comparison of epidural and combined spinal analgesia during labor. Acta Anaesthesiol Belg 50:129, 1999

Vercauteren MP, Coppejans HC, Hoffmann VH, Mertens E, Adriaensen HA: Prevention of hypotension by a single 5-mg dose of ephedrine during small-dose spinal anesthesia in prehydrated cesarean delivery patients. Anesth Analg 90:324, 2000

Wallace DH, Leveno KJ, Cunningham FG, Giesecke AH, Shearer VE, Sidawi JE: Randomized comparison of general and regional anesthesia for cesarean delivery in pregnancies complicated by severe preeclampsia. Obstet Gynecol 86:193, 1995

Wallace DH, Sidawi JE: Complications of obstetrical anesthesia. Williams Obstetrics, 20th ed (Suppl 3). Norwalk, CT, Appleton & Lange, June/July, 1997

Wilson SJ, Errick JK, Balkon J: Pharmacokinetics of nalbuphine during parturition. Am J Obstet Gynecol 155:340, 1986

Writer D: Hypertensive disorders. In Chestnut DL (ed): Obstetric Anesthesia: Principles and Management. St. Louis, Mosby, 1994, p 846

Yancey MK, Pierce B, Schweitzer D, Daniels D: Observations on labor epidural analgesia and operative delivery rates. Am J Obstet Gynecol 180:353, 1999

Yau G, Kan AF, Gin T, Oh TE: A comparison of omeprazole and ranitidine for prophylaxis against aspiration pneumonitis in emergency cesarean section. Anaesthesia 47:2, 1992

16

The Newborn Infant

ADAPTATION OF THE NEWBORN TO AIR BREATHING

At birth, the infant is subjected to rapid and profound physiological changes. Survival depends upon a prompt and orderly interchange of oxygen and carbon dioxide. For efficient interchange, the fluid-filled alveoli of the lungs must fill with air, the air must be exchanged by appropriate respiratory motion, and a vigorous micro-circulation must be established in close proximity to the alveoli.

INITIATION OF AIR BREATHING. Very soon after birth, the breathing pattern shifts from one of shallow episodic inspirations characteristic of the fetus to that of regular, deeper inhalations (Chap. 40, p. 1098). Aeration of the newborn lung is not the inflation of a collapsed structure, but instead, the rapid replacement of bronchial and alveolar fluid by air. In the lamb, and presumably in the human infant, residual alveolar fluid after delivery is cleared through the pulmonary circulation and, to a lesser degree, through pulmonary lymphatics (Chernick, 1978). Delay in removal of fluid from the alveoli probably contributes to the syndrome of **transient tachypnea of the newborn.** As fluid is replaced by air, there is considerable reduction in pulmonary vascular compression and, in turn, lowered resistance to blood flow. With the fall in pulmonary arterial blood pressure, the ductus arteriosus normally closes. Closure of the foramen ovale is more variable.

High negative intrathoracic pressures are required to bring about the initial entry of air into fluid-filled alveoli. Normally, from the first breath after birth, progressively more residual air accumulates in the lung, and with each successive breath, lower pulmonary opening pressure is required. In the mature normal infant, by about the fifth breath, pressure-volume changes achieved with each respiration are very similar to those of the adult.

ALVEOLAR SURFACE TENSION AND LUNG SURFAC-TANT. Surface-active material lowers surface tension in the alveoli and thereby prevents the collapse of the lung with each expiration. Lack of sufficient surfactant, common in preterm infants, leads to the prompt development of the **respiratory distress syndrome** (Chap. 39, p. 1040).

STIMULI TO BREATHE AIR. Normally, the newborn begins to breathe and cry almost immediately after birth, indicating the establishment of active respiration. All factors involved in the first breath of air have been difficult to elucidate, undoubtedly because many individually subtle stimuli contribute simultaneously. For example, *physical stimulation,* such as handling the infant during delivery, is believed to provoke respiration.

Compression of the thorax during the second stage of labor forces some fluid from the respiratory tract. Saunders (1978) found that considerable pressure is often produced by chest compression during vaginal delivery so that lung fluid is expelled equivalent to about a fourth of ultimate functional residual capacity. Thus, babies delivered by cesarean are likely to have more fluid and less gas in their lungs throughout the first 6 hours of life (Milner and colleagues, 1978). Thoracic compression incidental to vaginal delivery and the expansion that follows delivery may nevertheless be an auxiliary factor in initiation of respiration.

Deprivation of oxygen and accumulation of carbon dioxide also may stimulate respiration. Blood samples obtained from catheters implanted into vessels of experimental animal fetuses for prolonged periods of time, as well as cordocentesis in humans, contain a low P_{O_2} compared with adult standards. In animals, a further decrease in P_{O_2} diminishes or abolishes fetal respiratory motion, whereas an elevation of P_{CO_2} increases the frequency and magnitude of fetal breathing movements (Dawes, 1974). For the foregoing reasons, it seems that the fetus-infant most likely responds to hypoxia and to hypercapnia the same way in utero and after birth.

MANAGEMENT OF DELIVERY

IMMEDIATE CARE. With delivery of the head, either vaginally or by cesarean delivery, the face is immediately wiped and the mouth and nares are suctioned. A soft rubber syringe or its equivalent inserted with care is quite suitable. Before clamping and severing the cord, while the infant is still being held head down, it is beneficial to aspirate the mouth and pharynx again. Once the cord has been divided, the infant is placed supine with the head lowered and turned to the side in a heated unit that has appropriate thermal regulation and is equipped for immediate intensive care (Fig. 16–1). To minimize heat loss, the baby is wiped dry.

The individual who delivers the baby is responsible for immediate postdelivery care until another qualified person assumes this duty. An individual qualified to perform neonatal resuscitation should be immediately available in the hospital at the time of delivery.

INFANT EVALUATION. Before and during delivery, careful considerations must be given to the following determinants of neonatal well-being:

1. Health status of the mother.
2. Prenatal complications.
3. Labor complications.
4. Gestational age.
5. Duration of labor.
6. Duration of ruptured membranes.

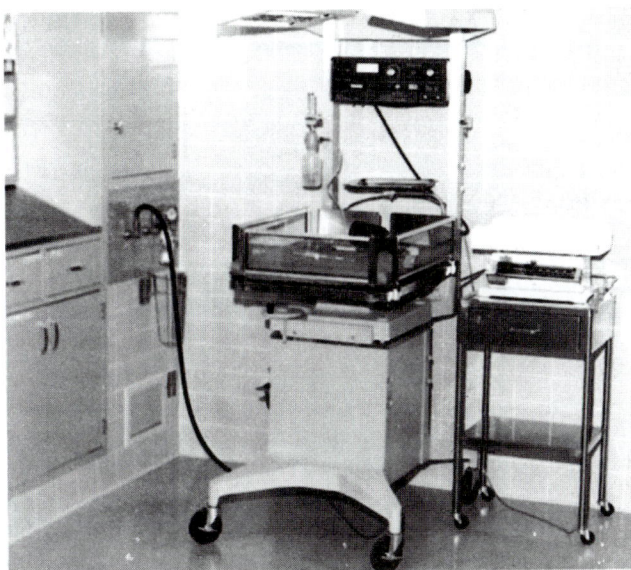

FIGURE 16–1. Thermostatically controlled infant care unit in delivery room.

7. Types, amounts, times, and routes of administration of medications.
8. Type and duration of anesthesia.
9. Any difficulty with delivery.

The infant is inspected for any visible abnormalities. The cord is cut and the infant then handed to a trained associate for further care.

The person immediately in charge of caring for the neonate should observe respirations closely and identify the heart rate. The heart rate can be determined by auscultation over the chest or by palpating the base of the umbilical cord. A readily discernible heartbeat of 100/min or more is acceptable. Persistent bradycardia requires prompt resuscitation. Next, the mouth, nares, and pharynx are suctioned carefully.

Most normal infants take a breath within a few seconds of birth and cry within half a minute. If respirations are infrequent, suction of the mouth and pharynx, followed by light slapping of the soles of the feet and rubbing of the back, usually together serve to stimulate breathing. Prolongation of these intervals beyond 1 and 2 minutes, respectively, indicates an abnormality. Continued lack of breathing demands active resuscitation.

LACK OF EFFECTIVE RESPIRATIONS. Important causes of failure to establish effective respirations include the following:

1. Fetal hypoxemia or acidosis from any cause.
2. Drugs administered to the mother.
3. Gross fetal immaturity.
4. Upper airway obstruction.
5. Pneumothorax.

6. Other lung abnormalities, either intrinsic (e.g., hypoplasia) or extrinsic (e.g., diaphragmatic hernia).
7. Aspiration of amnionic fluid grossly contaminated with meconium.
8. Central nervous system developmental abnormality.
9. Septicemia.

METHODS USED TO EVALUATE NEWBORN CONDITION

APGAR SCORE. A useful aid to evaluate the need for infant resuscitation is the Apgar scoring system applied at 1 minute and again at 5 minutes after birth (Table 16–1). The 1-minute Apgar score is used to identify the need for immediate resuscitation. Most infants at birth are in excellent condition, as indicated by Apgar scores of 7 to 10, and they require no aid other than perhaps simple nasopharyngeal suction. An Apgar score of 10 is in practice rarely assigned. An infant with a score of 4 to 6 at 1 minute demonstrates depressed respirations, flaccidity, and pale to blue color. Heart rate and reflex irritability, however, are good. Infants with scores of 0 to 3 usually have slow to inaudible heart rates and depressed or absent reflex responses. Resuscitation, including artificial ventilation, should be started immediately. Such infants are often easy to recognize. They may be flaccid, apneic, and often covered with meconium, and heart rates usually are below 100.

The Apgar score is a useful clinical tool used to identify those neonates who require resuscitation, as well as to indicate the effectiveness of any resuscitative measures. Unfortunately, attempts have also been made—without supporting data—to relate the Apgar score to antenatal events or to long-term outcomes. For reasons that are not entirely clear, erroneous definitions of asphyxia have been established, based upon the Apgar score alone. Because of these misconceptions, in 1986 the American College of Obstetricians and Gynecologists, and the American Academy of Pediatrics, issued a joint statement on the use and misuse of the Apgar score. This statement was reaffirmed most recently in 1996. Because of its importance, and with permission from the American College of Obstetricians and Gynecologists, it is reprinted here in its entirety.

USE AND MISUSE OF THE APGAR SCORE

The Apgar score, devised in 1952 by Dr. Virginia Apgar, is a quick method of assessing the state of the newborn infant (Apgar, 1953; Apgar and colleagues, 1958). Ease of scoring has led to its use in many studies of outcome. However, its misuse has led to an erroneous definition of asphyxia. Intrapartum asphyxia implies fetal hypercarbia and hypoxemia, which if prolonged will result in eventual

TABLE 16-1. Apgar Scoring System

Sign	0 Points	1 Point	2 Points
Heart rate	Absent	Below 100	Over 100
Respiratory effort	Absent	Slow, irregular	Good, crying
Muscle tone	Flaccid	Some flexion of extremities	Active motion
Reflex irritability	No response	Grimace	Vigorous cry
Color	Blue, pale	Body pink, extremities blue	Completely pink

From the American College of Obstetricians and Gynecologists (1996a), with permission.

metabolic acidemia. Because the intrapartum disruption of uterine or fetal blood flow is rarely, if ever, absolute, *asphyxia* is an imprecise, general term. Terms such as *hypercarbia, hypoxia,* and *metabolic, respiratory, or lactic acidemia* are more precise, both for immediate assessment of intrapartum management. Although the Apgar score continues to provide a convenient "shorthand" for reporting the status of the newborn and the effectiveness of resuscitation, the purpose of this statement is to place the Apgar score in its proper prospective.

The Apgar score comprises five components: heart rate, respiratory effort, muscle tone, reflex, irritability, and color, each of which is given a score of 0, 1, or 2 (Table 16–1). Reliable Apgar scores require assessment of individual components of the score by trained personnel.

Factors That May Affect Apgar Scores

Although rarely stated, it is important to recognize that elements of the Apgar score such as tone, color, and reflex irritability are partially dependent on the physiologic maturity of the infant. The healthy premature infant with no evidence of anoxic insult, acidemia, or cerebral depression may thus receive a low score only because of immaturity (Amon and associates, 1987; Catlin and co-workers, 1986).

A number of maternal medications and infant conditions may influence Apgar scores, including, but not limited to, neuromuscular or cerebral malformations that may decrease tone and respiratory effort. Cardiorespiratory conditions may also decrease the infant's heart rate, respiration, and tone. Infection may interfere with tone, color and response to resuscitative efforts. Additional information is required to interpret Apgar scores properly in infants receiving resuscitation. Thus, to equate the presence of a low Apgar score solely with asphyxia or hypoxia represents a misuse of the score.

Apgar Score and Subsequent Disability

A low 1-minute Apgar score does not correlate with the infant's future outcome. The 5-minute Apgar score, and particularly the change in the score between 1 and 5 minutes, is a useful index of the effectiveness of resuscitation efforts. However, even a 5-minute score of 0 to 3, although possibly a result of hypoxia, is limited as an indicator of the severity of the problem and correlates poorly with future neurologic outcome (Nelson and Ellenberg, 1981; Stanley, 1994). An Apgar score of 0 to 3 at 5 minutes is associated with an increased risk of cerebral palsy in term infants, but this increase is only from 0.3 percent to 1 percent (Nelson and Ellenberg, 1981; Stanley, 1994). A 5-minute Apgar score of 7 to 10 is considered "normal." Scores of 4, 5, and 6 are intermediate and are not markers of high levels of risk of later neurologic dysfunction. As previously mentioned, such scores are affected by physiologic immaturity, medication, the presence of congenital malformations, and other factors.

Because Apgar scores at 1 and 5 minutes correlate poorly with either cause or outcome, the scores alone should not be considered either evidence of or a consequence of substantial asphyxia. Therefore, a low 5-minute Apgar score alone does not demonstrate that later development of cerebral palsy was caused by perinatal asphyxia.

Correlation of the Apgar score with future neurologic outcome increases when the score remains 0 to 3 at 10, 15, and 20 minutes but still does not indicate the cause of future disability (Freeman and Nelson, 1988; Nelson and Ellenberg, 1981). The term *asphyxia* in a clinical context should be reserved to describe a combination of damaging acidemia, hypoxia, and metabolic acidosis. A neonate who has had "asphyxia" proximate to delivery that is severe enough to result in acute neurologic injury should demonstrate all of the following:

- Profound metabolic or mixed acidemia (pH < 7.0) on an umbilical cord arterial blood sample, if obtained.
- An Apgar score of 0–3 for longer than 5 minutes.
- Neonatal neurologic manifestations (e.g., seizures, coma, or hypotonia).
- Multisystem organ dysfunction (e.g., cardiovascular, gastrointestinal, hematologic, pulmonary, or renal system).

The Apgar score alone cannot establish hypoxia as the cause of cerebral palsy. A term infant with an Apgar score of 0 to 3 at 5 minutes whose 10-minute score improved to

4 or higher has a 99 percent chance of not having cerebral palsy at 7 years of age (Nelson and Ellenberg, 1981). Conversely, 75 percent of children with cerebral palsy had normal Apgar scores at birth (Nelson and Ellenberg, 1981).

Cerebral palsy is the only neurologic deficit clearly linked to perinatal asphyxia. Although mental retardation and epilepsy may accompany cerebral palsy, there is no evidence that they are caused by perinatal asphyxia unless cerebral palsy is also present, and even then a relationship is in doubt (Levene and collaborators, 1986; Paneth, 1993).

Conclusion

Apgar scores are useful in assessing the condition of the infant at birth. Their use in other settings, such as collection of a child's Apgar score upon entry to school, is inappropriate. Low Apgar scores may be indicative of a number of maternal and infant factors. Apgar scores alone should not be used as evidence that neurologic damage was caused by hypoxia that results in neurologic damage or by inappropriate intrapartum management. Hypoxia as a cause of acute neurologic injury and adverse neurologic outcome occurs in infants who demonstrate the four perinatal findings listed in this Committee Opinion and in whom other possible causes of neurologic damage have been excluded. In the absence of such evidence, subsequent neurologic deficiencies cannot be ascribed to perinatal asphyxia or hypoxia (Brann and Dykes, 1977; Nelson and Leviton, 1991).

UMBILICAL CORD BLOOD ACID–BASE STUDIES.

Blood taken from umbilical vessels is used for acid–base studies to examine the metabolic status of the fetus in the minutes and hours prior to birth. Fetal oxygenation and pH generally decline during the course of normal labor (Dildy and co-workers, 1994). Normal umbilical cord blood pH and blood gas values in term newborns are summarized in Table 16–2.

Using data from over 19,000 deliveries, the lower limits of normal pH in the newborn are from 7.04 to 7.10 (Boylan and Parisi, 1994). Thus, these values should be considered to define **neonatal acidemia.** Most fetuses will tolerate intrapartum acidemia with a pH as low as 7.00 without incurring neurological impairment (Freeman and Nelson, 1988; Gilstrap and associates, 1989). Goldaber and associates (1991) found that there were significantly more neonatal deaths and neurological dysfunction if a pH cutoff value of less than 7.00 was used (Table 16–3).

EFFECTS OF GESTATIONAL AGE ON APGAR SCORE AND pH.

Ramin and colleagues (1989) reported observations from 77 preterm and 1292 term neonates and found no significant difference in the frequency of acidemia based on gestational age. They also observed that preterm neonates had significantly lower Apgar scores than had been reported by other investigators (Catlin and associates, 1986; Goldenberg and colleagues, 1984). Using the erroneous International Classification of Disease (ICD-9-CM, 1980) coding for asphyxia based merely on a 1-minute Apgar score of less than 7 (see "Use and Misuse of the Apgar Score" earlier in the chapter), 36 percent of preterm infants in this latter study would have been labeled as having mild birth asphyxia (Apgar score of 6 or less) and 12 percent as having severe birth asphyxia (1-minute Apgar score of 3 or less). Conversely, only 8 percent of these infants

TABLE 16–2. Umbilical Cord Blood pH and Blood Gas Values in Normal Term Newborns

Value	Study (means ± 1 SD)			
	Yeomans et al, 1985[a] (n = 146)	Ramin et al, 1989[a] (n = 1292)	Riley and Johnson, 1993[b] (n = 3522)	Arikan et al, 2000 (n = 1281) (median and 2.5 centile)
Arterial Blood				
pH	7.28 (0.05)	7.28 (0.07)	7.27 (0.069)	7.25 (7.08)
Pco₂ (mm Hg)	49.2 (8.4)	49.9 (14.2)	50.3 (11.1)	50 (75, 97.5 centile)
HCO₃⁻ (mEq/L)	22.3 (2.5)	23.1 (2.8)	22.0 (3.6)	—
Base excess (mEq/L)	—	−3.6 (2.8)	−2.7 (2.8)	−4.3 (−11.1)
Venous Blood				
pH	7.35 (0.05)	—	7.34 (0.063)	—
Pco₂ (mm Hg)	38.2 (5.6)	—	40.7 (7.9)	—
HCO₃⁻ (mEq/L)	20.4 (4.1)	—	21.4 (2.5)	—
Base excess (mEq/L)	—	—	−2.4 (2)	—

[a] Infants of selected women with uncomplicated vaginal deliveries.
[b] Infants of unselected women with vaginal deliveries.

TABLE 16–3. Umbilical Arterial Blood pH Related to Neonatal Morbidity, Mortality, and Apgar Scores in Term Infants

Complication	Umbilical Artery pH			
	<7.00 (n = 85) No. (%)	7.00–7.04 (n = 95) No. (%)	7.05–7.09 (n = 290) No. (%)	7.10–7.14 (n = 798) No. (%)
Seizure	9 (11)	3 (3.2)	0	2 (0.3)
Neonatal deaths	7 (8)	2 (2.1)	0	3 (0.4)
Intensive care nursery	17 (21)	5 (5.3)	4 (1.4)	7 (0.9)
Intubated	32 (38)	3 (3.2)	9 (3.1)	10 (1.3)
Apgar scores ≤3				
1 min	23 (27)	6 (6.3)	12 (4.1)	19 (2.4)
5 min	9 (11)	0	5 (1.7)	0

From Goldaber and associates (1991), with permission.

had acidemia based on a high cutoff pH value of 7.20 or less. Thus, in the study by Ramin and associates (1989), it is apparent that a most important factor influencing the Apgar score is gestational age. Dickinson and colleagues (1992), in a larger study of the effect of preterm birth on umbilical cord blood gases, arrived at the same conclusion. This again emphasizes that an Apgar score of 7 in a preterm neonate may represent the upper normal value. **More importantly, umbilical cord gas indices may be of more value than Apgar scores in preterm infants.** Normal umbilical artery blood pH and blood gas values in preterm infants are shown in Table 16–4.

FETAL ACID–BASE PHYSIOLOGY. The fetus produces carbonic and organic acids. Carbonic acid (H_2CO_3) is formed by oxidative metabolism of CO_2. The fetus can rapidly clear CO_2 through the placental circulation; but when H_2CO_3 accumulates in fetal blood without an increase in organic acids, this is known as a **respiratory acidemia.** Organic acids primarily are formed by anaerobic metabolism and include lactic and β-hydroxybutyric

acids. These organic acids are cleared slowly from fetal blood, and when they accumulate without an increase in H_2CO_3, this results in a **metabolic acidemia.** With the development of metabolic acidemia, bicarbonate (HCO_3) decreases as it is used to buffer the organic acid. An increase in H_2CO_3 and an increase in the organic acid (seen as a decrease in HCO_3) is known as **a mixed respiratory–metabolic acidemia.**

In the fetus, respiratory and metabolic acidemia and ultimately tissue acidosis are most likely part of a progressively worsening continuum. This is different from the adult, in which there are distinct conditions that result in either respiratory (pulmonary disease) or metabolic (diabetes) acidemia. In the fetus, the placenta serves as both the lungs and, to a certain degree, the kidneys. One principal cause for developing acidemia in the fetus is a decrease in uteroplacental perfusion. This results in the retention of CO_2 (respiratory acidemia), and if protracted and severe enough, this ultimately leads to a mixed or metabolic acidemia.

The actual pH of blood is dependent upon the pro-

TABLE 16–4. Normal Umbilical Blood pH and Blood Gas Values in Preterm Infants

Value	Study (mean ± 1 SD)		
	Ramin et al, 1989[a] (n = 77)	Dickinson et al, 1992[b] (n = 949)	Riley and Johnson, 1993[b] (n = 1015)
pH	7.29 (0.07)	7.27 (0.07)	7.28 (0.089)
P_{CO_2} (mm Hg)	49.2 (9.0)	51.6 (9.4)	50.2 (12.3)
HCO_3^- (mEq/L)	23.0 (3.5)	23.9 (2.1)	22.4 (3.5)
Base excess (mEq/L)	−3.3 (2.4)	−3.0 (2.5)	−2.5 (3)

[a] Infants of selected women with uncomplicated vaginal deliveries.
[b] Infants of unselected women with vaginal deliveries.

portion of carbonic acid and organic acids as well as the amount of bicarbonate that is the major buffer in blood. This can best be illustrated by the Henderson–Hasselbach equation:

$$pH = pK + \log \frac{[base]}{[acid]} \text{ or } pH = pK + \log \frac{HCO_3}{H_2CO_3}$$

For clinical purposes, HCO_3 represents the metabolic component and is reported as HCO_3 in mEq/L. The H_2CO_3 concentration represents the respiratory component and is reported as the P_{CO_2} in mm Hg. Thus:

$$pH = pK + \log \frac{metabolic\ (HCO_3\ mEq/L)}{respiratory\ P_{CO_2}\ (mm\ Hg)}$$

Delta base is a calculated number used as a measure of the change in buffering capacity of bicarbonate (HCO_3). For example, bicarbonate will be decreased in concentration with a metabolic acidemia as it is consumed in order to maintain a normal pH. A **base deficit** occurs when HCO_3 concentration decreases to below normal levels, and a **base excess** occurs when HCO_3 values are above normal. It must be emphasized again that a large base deficit and a low HCO_3 (less than 12 mEq/L) associated with mixed respiratory–metabolic acidemia is more often associated with a depressed neonate than is a mixed acidemia with a minimal base deficit and a more nearly normal HCO_3 (American College of Obstetricians and Gynecologists, 1995; Gilstrap and Cunningham, 1994).

All of these considerations are based upon the assumption that maternal pH and blood gases are normal.

CLINICAL DIAGNOSIS OF SIGNIFICANT ACIDEMIA. In the fetus, metabolic acidemia develops when oxygen deprivation is of sufficient duration and magnitude to require anaerobic metabolism for fetal cellular energy needs. Metabolic acidosis, defined as an umbilical artery buffer base of less than 30 mmol/L, is rare; Low and associates (1994) described such acidosis in only 0.4 percent in a study of over 14,000 term births. They later proposed that the threshold for fetal acidosis is a base deficit of greater than 12 mmol/L (Low and co-workers, 1997). They considered a base deficit greater than 16 mmol/L to indicate severe fetal acidosis.

Metabolic acidemia is associated with a high rate of multiorgan dysfunction, and in rare cases such hypoxia-induced metabolic acidemia may be so severe as to cause subsequent neurological impairment. By definition, a fetus without such acidemia cannot have suffered recent hypoxic-induced injury. Even severe metabolic acidosis, however, is poorly predictive of subsequent neurological impairment in the term infant. Although more severe metabolic acidosis was associated with an increase in immediate neonatal complications in a group of infants with depressed 5-minute Apgar scores, Socol and col-

leagues (1994) found no difference in umbilical artery blood gas measurements among those individuals who developed cerebral palsy and those with subsequent normal neurological outcome. Such findings cast further doubt upon the relationship between intrapartum hypoxia and acidosis and subsequent cerebral palsy in term infants. In very-low-birthweight infants—those less than 1000 g—newborn acid–base status may be more closely linked to long-term neurological outcome (Gaudier and co-workers, 1994; Low and associates, 1995).

In contrast to metabolic acidemia, respiratory acidemia generally develops as a result of an acute interruption in placental gas exchange, with subsequent CO_2 retention. Transient umbilical cord compression is the most common antecedent factor in the development of fetal respiratory acidemia. In general, respiratory acidemia does not reflect an insult of potential harm to the fetus. Low and co-workers (1994) found no increase in newborn complications after respiratory acidosis. The degree to which pH is affected by P_{CO_2}, the respiratory component of the acidosis, can be calculated by the following relationship: 10 additional units of P_{CO_2} will lower the pH by 0.08 units (Eisenberg and colleagues, 1987). Thus in a mixed respiratory–metabolic acidemia, the benign respiratory component may be easily calculated:

> During labor, an acute cord prolapse occurred and the fetus was delivered by cesarean 20 minutes later. The umbilical artery pH at birth was 6.95, with a P_{CO_2} of 89 mm Hg. To calculate the degree to which the cord compression and subsequent impairment of CO_2 exchange affected the pH, the rules given earlier are applied: 89 mm Hg − 49 mm Hg (normal newborn P_{CO_2}) = 40 mm Hg (excess CO_2). To correct pH: (40 ÷ 10) × 0.08 = 0.32; 6.95 + 0.32 = 7.27. Therefore, the pH prior to cord prolapse was approximately 7.27, well within normal limits, thus confirming the clinical interpretation of the fetal heart rate record as reassuring prior to this unpredictable event.

As emphasized by the American College of Obstetricians and Gynecologists (1995), the term **birth asphyxia** is imprecise and should not be used. Furthermore, acidemia alone is not sufficient evidence to establish that there has been hypoxic injury. In order to establish that hypoxia near delivery was severe enough to cause hypoxic ischemic encephalopathy, all of the following must be present:

1. Umbilical artery metabolic or mixed respiratory–metabolic acidemia with pH less than 7.00.
2. A persistent Apgar score of 0 to 3 for more than 5 minutes.
3. Neonatal neurological sequelae, such as seizures, coma, or hypotonia.
4. Multiorgan system dysfunction.

UMBILICAL CORD BLOOD COLLECTION. A 10- to 20-cm segment of umbilical cord is clamped **immediately** following delivery with two clamps near the neonate and two clamps nearer the placenta. The importance of clamping the cord is underscored by the fact that delays of 20 to 30 seconds can alter both the P_{CO_2} and pH (Lievaart and deJong, 1984). The cord is then cut between the two proximal and two distal clamps. *Arterial blood* is drawn from the isolated segment of cord into a 1- to 2-mL commercially prepared plastic syringe containing lysophilized heparin or a similar syringe that has been flushed with a heparin solution containing 1000 U/mL. The needle is then capped, and the capped syringe is placed into a plastic sack containing crushed ice and immediately transported to the laboratory. There is little change in P_{CO_2} or pH in blood kept at room temperature for up to 60 minutes (Duerbeck and associates, 1992). Chauhan and associates (1994) developed mathematical models allowing reasonable prediction of birth acid–base status in properly collected cord samples analyzed as late as 60 hours after delivery.

RECOMMENDATIONS FOR CORD BLOOD GAS DETERMINATIONS. A cost-effectiveness analysis for universal cord blood gas measurements has not been conducted. In some centers, cord gas determination is made in all fetuses at the time of birth. The American College of Obstetricians and Gynecologists (1995) recommends that cord blood gas and pH analyses be used in select neonates with low Apgar scores to distinguish metabolic acidemia from hypoxia or other causes that might result in a low Apgar score. Although umbilical cord acid–base blood determinations have a low predictability for either immediate or long-term adverse neurological outcome, they are helpful to exclude intrapartum or birth events that may cause acidosis (Gilstrap and Cunningham, 1994).

ACTIVE RESUSCITATION

When infants become asphyxiated, either before or after birth, they demonstrate a well-defined sequence of events, leading to primary or secondary apnea (American Academy of Pediatrics and American Heart Association, 1994). Initial oxygen deprivation results in a transient period of rapid breathing. If such deprivation persists, breathing movements cease and the fetus-infant enters a stage of apnea known as **primary apnea.** This is accompanied by a fall in heart rate and loss of neuromuscular tone. Simple stimulation and exposure to oxygen will reverse primary apnea. If oxygen deprivation and asphyxia persist, the fetus-infant will develop deep gasping respirations, followed by **secondary apnea.** This is associated with a further decline in heart rate, falling

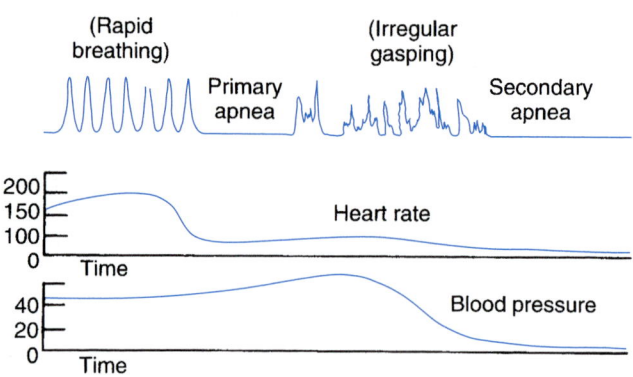

FIGURE 16–2. Physiological changes associated with primary and secondary apnea in the newborn. (From the American Academy of Pediatrics, 1994, with permission.)

blood pressure, and loss of neuromuscular tone. Infants in secondary apnea will not respond to stimulation and will not spontaneously resume respiratory efforts. Unless ventilation is assisted, death will occur (Fig. 16–2). Clinically, primary and secondary apnea are indistinguishable. For this reason, secondary apnea must be assumed, and resuscitation of the apneic infant must be started immediately.

The first rule of resuscitation is to recognize rapidly the neonate who requires these measures. Also, it should be remembered that suctioning of the mouth, nares, and trachea can result in significant vagal stimulation and reflex slowing of the heart rate; thus *unnecessary* or *overvigorous* suctioning of these areas should be avoided.

Successful active resuscitation requires:

1. Skilled personnel who are immediately available.
2. A suitably heated, well-lighted, appropriately large work area such as shown in Figure 16–1.
3. Equipment to deliver oxygen by intermittent positive pressure through a face mask and to carry out tracheal intubation with suction and positive-pressure oxygenation.
4. Drugs, syringes, needles, and catheters for possible intravenous administration of volume expanders (normal saline, Ringer lactate, blood, or 5 percent albumin), naloxone (Narcan), sodium bicarbonate, and epinephrine.

Equipment for resuscitation should be readily available, and the equipment should be checked often. A useful method to ensure that such supplies are available is a wall clipboard system arranged so that any missing equipment or drug is immediately apparent (Fig. 16–3).

RESUSCITATION PROTOCOL. Resuscitation will be most effective when an established protocol is followed. The following protocol for neonatal resuscitation is rec-

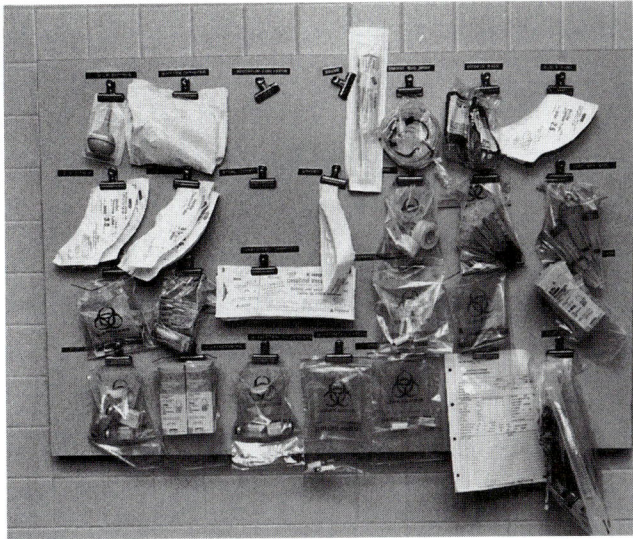

FIGURE 16–3. Wall clipboard system used to display equipment and drugs needed for neonatal resuscitation. As shown, a missing item can be identified at a glance and replaced between deliveries.

ommended by the American Academy of Pediatrics and the American Heart Association (1994):

1. **Prevent heat loss.** Place the infant in a radiant warmer on its back and dry off amnionic fluid.

2. **Open the airway.** The airway is opened by suctioning the mouth and nares if no meconium is present. If meconium is present, the trachea may require direct suctioning (Fig. 16–4).

3. **Evaluate the infant.** Observe for respirations, heart rate, and color to determine what further steps are necessary. These initial three steps should be performed in 20 seconds or less.

4. **Respiratory effort.** Evaluate respiratory effort first. If absent, positive pressure ventilation is carried out. If present, heart rate is evaluated.

5. **Heart rate.** Evaluate heart rate next. If the rate is less than 100 beats/min, positive pressure ventilation is instituted (skip to step 7). If the rate is greater than 100, infant color is evaluated next.

6. **Color.** Evaluate color last. If the infant is pink, or demonstrates only peripheral cyanosis, simple observation continues. If the infant exhibits central cyanosis, free-flowing oxygen is provided at concentrations of 80 to 100 percent. This is continued as long as the baby remains cyanotic.

7. **Heart rate (continued).** Heart rate is evaluated after 15 to 30 seconds of positive pressure ventilation. If the heart rate is now above 100, evaluate color, as in step 6. If the heart rate is 60 to 100 and increasing, ventilation is continued. If the heart rate is below

60, or below 80 and not increasing, ventilation is continued and chest compressions are begun. Under these circumstances, tracheal intubation should be considered.

8. **Chest compressions.** Initiate chest compressions at a rate of 2 per second with a 1/2-second pause every third compression for ventilation. Compression is stopped every 30 seconds for 6 seconds while the heart rate is checked. If the heart rate remains below 80 beats/min after 30 seconds of ventilation and chest compressions, chemical resuscitation is begun.

9. **Chemical resuscitation.** Chemical resuscitation consists of epinephrine, volume expansion, and possibly naloxone (Fig. 16–5). Epinephrine 1:10,000 is given rapidly, either intravenously or via the tracheal tube in a dose of 0.1 to 0.3 mL/kg. Volume expansion with 10 mL/kg whole blood, 5 percent albumin, normal saline, or Ringer lactate is given intravenously over 5 to 10 minutes in cases where hypovolemia is suspected. Sodium bicarbonate, 4.2 percent solution (0.5 mEq/mL) is given slowly, over at least 2 minutes (1 mEq/kg per min) in cases of prolonged arrest that do not respond to other therapy or if arterial blood gases are indicative of severe metabolic acidemia. Bicarbonate must only be given after effective ventilation has been established. Naloxone hydrochloride is indicated with marked respiratory depression and a maternal history of recent narcotic administration (American College of Obstetricians

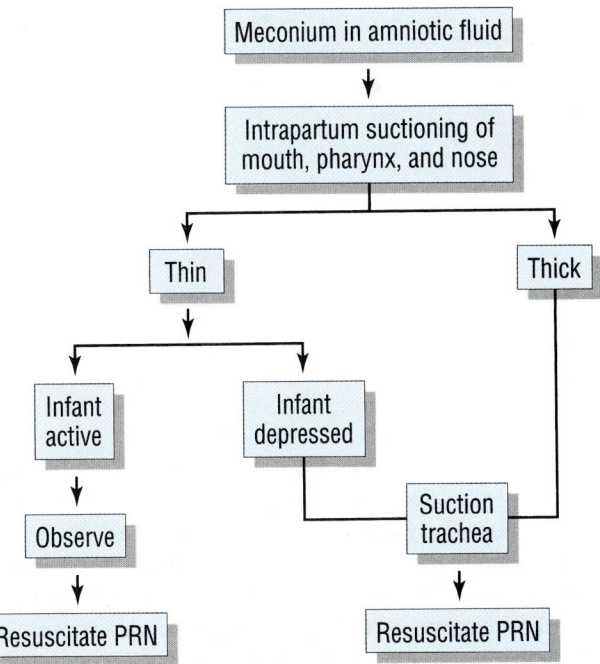

FIGURE 16–4. Protocol for dealing with meconium in the newborn. (From the American Academy of Pediatrics, 1994, with permission.)

Medications
  Epinephrine
  Volume expander
  Sodium bicarbonate

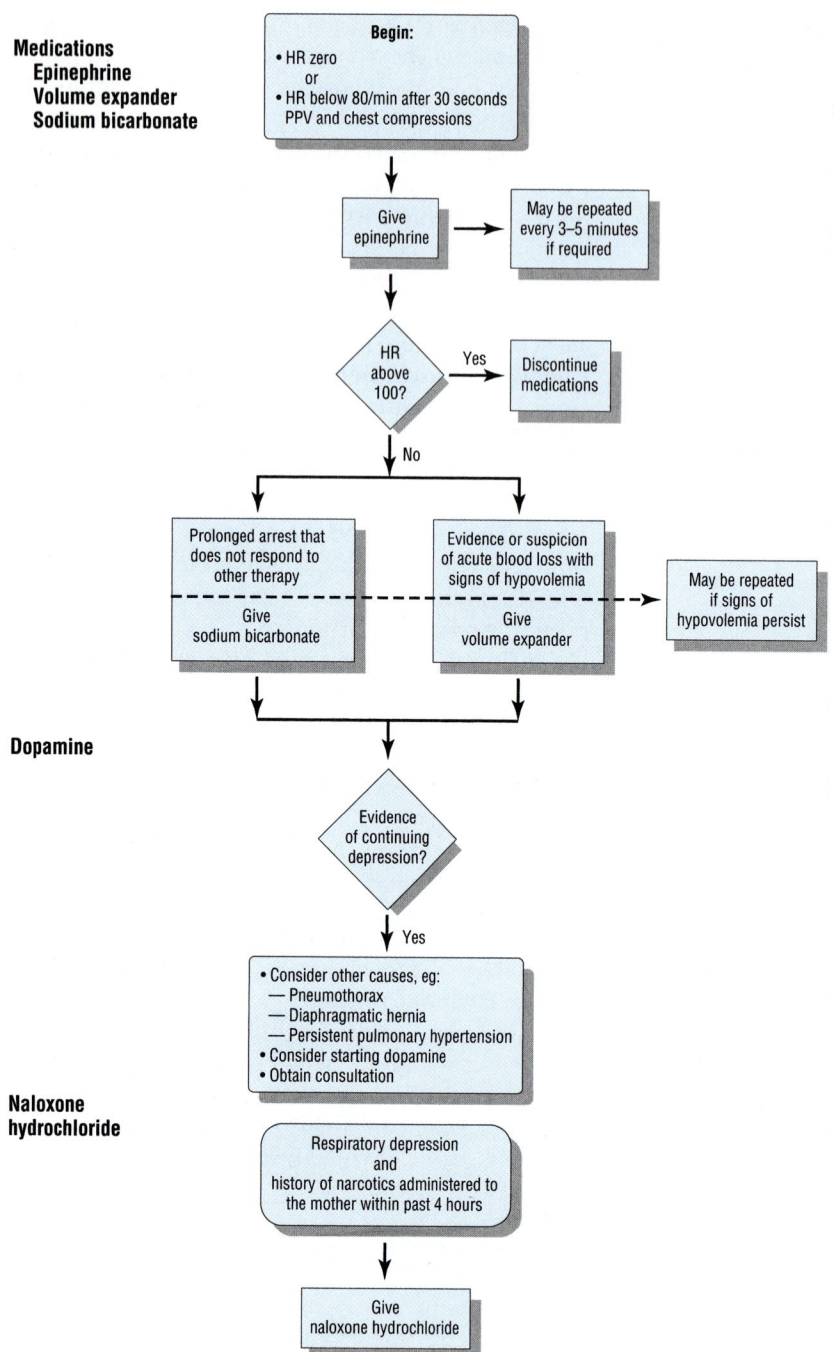

Dopamine

Naloxone hydrochloride

FIGURE 16–5. Chemical resuscitation of the depressed newborn. (HR = heart rate; PPV = positive pressure ventilation.) (From the American Academy of Pediatrics, 1994, with permission.)

and Gynecologists, 1996b). For either the preterm or term neonate, it is administered preferably intravenously or intratracheally at a dose of 0.1 mg/kg. Repeated doses are often necessary because the duration of action of some narcotics exceeds that of naloxone (1 to 4 hours). When given intramuscularly or subcutaneously, absorption may be delayed if the infant has vasoconstriction.

10. **Tracheal intubation.** Tracheal intubation is necessary in four circumstances: when prolonged positive

pressure ventilation is required, when bag and mask ventilation is ineffective, when tracheal suctioning is required, and when diaphragmatic hernia is suspected.

TECHNIQUE OF INTUBATION. The head of the supine infant is kept level. The laryngoscope is introduced into the right side of the mouth and then directed posteriorly toward the oropharynx (Fig. 16–6). The laryngoscope is next gently moved into the space between the base

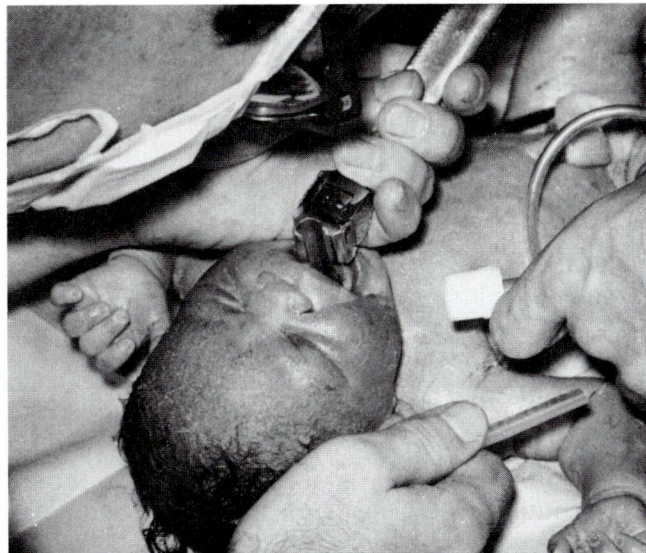

FIGURE 16–6. Use of laryngoscope to insert tracheal tube under direct vision. Oxygen is being delivered from curved tube held by an assistant.

of the tongue and the epiglottis. Gentle elevation of the tip of the laryngoscope will pick up the epiglottis and expose the glottis and the vocal cords. The endotracheal tube is introduced through the right side of the mouth and is inserted through the vocal cords until the shoulder of the tube reaches the glottis. It is essential that the appropriate-sized endotracheal tube be used (Table 16–5). Steps are taken to ensure that the tube is in the trachea and not the esophagus by listening for breath sounds or a gurgling sound if air is introduced into the stomach. Any foreign material encountered in the tracheal tube is immediately removed by suction. Meconium, blood, mucus, and particulate debris in amnionic fluid or in the birth canal may have been inhaled in utero or while passing through the birth canal.

The resuscitator, using an appropriate ventilation bag attached to the tracheal tube, should deliver puffs of oxygen-rich air into the tube at 1- to 2-second intervals

with a force adequate to lift the chest wall gently. Pressures of 25 to 35 cm H_2O are desired to expand the alveoli yet not cause pneumothorax or pneumomediastinum. If the stomach expands, the tube is almost certainly in the esophagus rather than in the trachea. Once adequate spontaneous respirations have been established, the tube can usually be removed safely.

COMMON ERRORS IN RESUSCITATION OF THE NEWBORN. If resuscitation efforts are not rapidly successful, the apparent failure may be the consequence of an easily correctable technical error. Even the most skilled and experienced operator can experience difficulties, and the possibility of technical errors should always be kept in mind when an infant fails to respond to resuscitation. Common errors include the following:

1. Failure to check resuscitation equipment beforehand:
   a. Damaged resuscitation bag.
   b. Laryngoscope with dull or flickering light.
2. Use of a cold resuscitation table.
3. Unsuccessful intubation:
   a. Hyperextension of neck.
   b. Inadequate suctioning.
   c. Excessive force.
   d. Use of an incorrect-sized endotracheal tube.
4. Inadequate ventilation:
   a. Improper head position.
   b. Improper application of mask.
   c. Placement of tracheal tube into esophagus or right mainstem bronchus.
   d. Failure to secure the tracheal tube.
5. Failure to detect and determine cause of poor chest movement or persistent bradycardia.
6. Failure to detect and treat hypovolemia.
7. Failure to perform cardiac massage.

ROUTINE NEWBORN CARE

ESTIMATION OF GESTATIONAL AGE. A rapid estimate of gestational age of the newborn between gestational weeks 32 to 40 may be made very soon after delivery by examining:

1. Sole creases.
2. Breast nodules.
3. Scalp hair.
4. Ear lobes.
5. For males, testes and scrotum (Table 16–6).

A more definitive estimate can be made in a few days with the help of neurological examination. Unfortunately, estimates of gestational age based upon physical and neurological examination are frequently unaccept-

TABLE 16–5. Appropriate-sized Endotracheal Tube Based upon Estimated Weight or Gestational Age

Tube Size, (inside diameter, mm)	Weight	Gestational Age
2.5	<1000	<28
3.0	1000–2000	28–34
3.5	2000–3000	34–38
3.5–4.0	>3000	>38

From the American Academy of Pediatrics and American Heart Association (1994), with permission.

TABLE 16-6. Rapid Estimation of Gestational Age of the Newborn

Sites	Gestational Age 36 Weeks or Less	37–38 Weeks	39 Weeks or More
Sole creases	Anterior transverse crease only	Occasional creases anterior two thirds	Sole covered with creases
Breast nodule diameter	2 mm	4 mm	7 mm
Scalp hair	Fine and fuzzy	Fine and fuzzy	Coarse and silky
Ear lobe	Pliable, no cartilage	Some cartilage	Stiffened by thick cartilage
Testes and scrotum	Testes in lower canal, scrotum small, few rugae	Intermediate	Testes pendulous, scrotum full, extensive rugae

ably inaccurate in preterm and growth-restricted infants (Spinnato and co-workers, 1984).

EYE INFECTION PROPHYLAXIS. Because of the possibility of neonatal eye infection during passage through the birth canal of a mother with gonorrhea, in 1884, Credé introduced the practice of instilling into each eye immediately after birth one drop of a 1 percent solution of silver nitrate, which was later washed out with saline. In most states, the use of an efficacious regimen as discussed subsequently is required by law. The efficacy of these regimens for gonococcal infection prophylaxis is less clear for chlamydial eye infections.

GONOCOCCAL OPHTHALMIA NEONATORUM. Fortunately, since the introduction of 1 percent silver nitrate solution, blindness due to neonatal infection from *Neisseria gonorrhoeae* has been largely eliminated. A variety of antibiotics have also proven to be effective in preventing gonococcal ophthalmia. These regimens shown in Table 16–7 are not 100 percent effective. Babl and colleagues (2000) described neonatal gonococcal arthritis despite a negative maternal genital screening culture and newborn eye prophylaxis. Current recommendations by the Centers for Disease Control and Prevention (1998) and by Smith and Finn (1999) include aqueous silver nitrate (1 percent), or erythromycin ophthlamic ointment (0.5 percent), or tetracycline ophthalmic ointment (1 percent).

For infants born to mothers with untreated gonorrhea, single dose ceftriaxone, 25 to 50 mg/kg is given intramuscularly or intravenously, not to exceed 125 mg.

CHLAMYDIAL CONJUNCTIVITIS/OPHTHALMIA NEONATORUM. The problem of providing adequate neonatal prophylaxis against chlamydial infection is much more complex. Although it is reasonable to expect that tetracycline and erythromycin ophthalmic ointments applied at birth should reduce the incidence of chlamydial conjunctivitis/ophthalmia, results with these agents and silver nitrate solution have been disappointing (Table 16–7). In a study from Kenya, Isenberg and colleagues (1995) showed that 2.5 percent povidone-iodine solution was superior to either 1 percent silver nitrate solution or 0.5 percent erythromycin ointment to prevent chlamydial conjunctivitis. Truly effective prophylaxis against chlamydial conjunctivitis/ophthalmia neonatorum is not available currently (Centers for Disease Control, 1998). Any case of conjunctivitis in an infant less than 30 days old should prompt consideration for chlamydial infection.

Perhaps the best method of preventing neonatal in-

TABLE 16-7. Incidence of Infection (Percent) Following Neonatal Eye Prophylaxis

Study	Silver Nitrate (1%) Ophthalmic Solution			Tetracycline (1%) Ophthalmic Ointment			Erythromycin (0.5%) Ophthalmic Ointment		
	GC	Chlam	Non	GC	Chlam	Non	GC	Chlam	Non
Laga et al (1988)	0.4	0.7	8.9	0.1	0.5	4.5	—	—	—
Buisman et al (1988)	0.9	1.8	2.9	—	—	—	—	—	—
Hammerschlag et al (1989)	0.008	—	—	0.02	—	—	0.03	—	—
Isenberg et al (1995)	0.4	10.5	6.6	—	—	—	1.0	7.4	6.8

Chlam = chlamydial conjunctivitis/ophthalmia neonatorum; GC = gonococcal ophthalmia neonatorum; Non = nongonococcal, nonchlamydial conjunctivitis/ophthalmia neonatorum.

fection is screening and treatment of women with chlamydial infection. These regimens are discussed in Chapter 57 and were reviewed recently by Brocklehurst and Rooney (2000).

PERMANENT INFANT IDENTIFICATION. A foolproof infant identification system must be operative at all hours. Except under unusual circumstances, mother and infant should not be separated until identification is complete. The system should provide a record easily recognized by the mother, such as an identification band. A permanent record should be kept on file at the hospital. Most hospitals today use footprints rather than fingerprints or palmprints in identifying infants, because the ridges in the feet are more pronounced and it is easier to obtain prints. Too often, however, the ridges are not discrete and therefore the print is of no value (Clark and associates, 1981). After discovering that identification by footprint was considered invalid by the Federal Bureau of Investigation, we discontinued this practice at Parkland Hospital in 1985.

SUBSEQUENT CARE

TEMPERATURE. The temperature of the infant drops rapidly immediately after birth. Thus, the infant must be cared for in a warm crib in which temperature control is regulated closely. During the first few days of life, the infant's temperature is unstable, responding to slight stimuli with considerable fluctuations above or below the normal level.

VITAMIN K. Routine administration of vitamin K is recommended, as described in Chapter 39 (p. 1072).

HEPATITIS B IMMUNIZATION. Routine immunization of all newborns against hepatitis B prior to hospital discharge was started about 10 years ago as recommended by the Centers for Disease Control (1991). Recently, there has been unsubstantiated evidence of a link with vaccination and susceptibility to a variety of autoimmune complications, including neurological syndromes similar to multiple sclerosis. United States Representative Daniel Burton of Indiana in 2000 is conducting hearings to ascertain the severity and magnitude of this issue. As of late 2000, the Centers for Disease Control and Prevention (2000) continues to recommend routine newborn vaccination. If the mother is hepatitis B surface-antigen positive, the neonate should also be passively immunized with hepatitis B immune globulin (see also Chap. 48, p. 1290).

UMBILICAL CORD. Loss of water from Wharton jelly leads to mummification of the cord shortly after birth. Within 24 hours it loses its characteristic bluish white, moist appearance and soon becomes dry and black. Gradually the line of demarcation appears just beyond the skin of the abdomen, and in a few days the stump sloughs, leaving a small, granulating wound, which after healing forms the umbilicus. Separation usually takes place within the first 2 weeks, with a range of 3 to 45 days (Novack and colleagues, 1988). The umbilical cord dries more quickly and separates more readily when exposed to the air; therefore, a dressing is not recommended.

Serious umbilical infections are sometimes encountered. The most likely offending organisms are *Staphylococcus aureus, Escherichia coli,* or group B *Streptococcus.* Because the umbilical stump in such cases may present no outward sign of infection, the diagnosis cannot be made with certainty except by autopsy. Strict aseptic precautions therefore should be observed in the immediate care of the cord. Most practitioners apply triple dye or bacitracin ointment. Gladstone and colleagues (1988) found that povidone-iodine applied daily was effective and acceptable.

Neonatal *tetanus* continues to kill infants in developing countries. Active immunization of the mother against tetanus with passage of antibody to the fetus, along with hygienic practices applied to the cutting and subsequent management of the umbilical cord, can serve to reduce this risk to the neonate.

SKIN CARE. Infants should be promptly patted dry to minimize heat loss caused by evaporation. Excess vernix, as well as blood and meconium, is gently wiped off. The remaining vernix is readily absorbed by the skin and disappears entirely within 24 hours. Newborns should not be washed until their temperature has stabilized, and handling of babies during this time should be minimized.

STOOLS AND URINE. For the first 2 or 3 days after birth, the contents of the colon are composed of soft, brownish-green *meconium,* which is composed of desquamated epithelial cells from the intestinal tract, mucus, and epidermal cells and lanugo (fetal hair) that have been swallowed along with amnionic fluid. The characteristic color results from bile pigments. During intrauterine life and for a few hours after birth, the intestinal contents are sterile, but bacteria soon gain access. The passage of meconium and urine in the minutes immediately after birth or during the next few hours indicates patency of the gastrointestinal and urinary tracts. Meconium stooling is seen in 90 percent of newborns within the first 24 hours; most of the rest do so within 36 hours. Voiding, although usually occurring shortly after birth, may not occur until the second day of life. Failure of the infant to stool or urinate after these times suggests a congenital defect, such as imperforate anus or a urethral valve.

After the third or fourth day, as the consequence of ingesting milk, meconium is replaced by light yellow homogenous feces with a characteristic odor. For the first few days, the stools are unformed, but soon thereafter they assume a cylindrical shape.

ICTERUS NEONATORUM. About a third of all babies, between the second and fifth day of life, develop so-called **physiological jaundice of the newborn.** Serum bilirubin levels at birth are 1.8 to 2.8 mg/dL. These levels increase during the next few days but with wide individual variation. Between the third and fourth day, the bilirubin in mature infants commonly reaches somewhat more than 5 mg/dL, the concentration at which jaundice usually becomes noticeable. Most of the bilirubin is free, or unconjugated. One cause is immaturity of the hepatic cells, resulting in less conjugation of bilirubin with glucuronic acid and reduced excretion in bile (Chap. 39, p. 1067). Reabsorption of free bilirubin as the consequence of the enzymatic splitting of bilirubin glucuronide by intestinal conjugase activity in the newborn intestine also appears to contribute significantly to the transient hyperbilirubinemia. In preterm infants, jaundice is more common and usually more severe and prolonged than in term infants, because of less hepatic enzymatic maturity. Increased erythrocyte destruction from any cause also contributes to hyperbilirubinemia.

INITIAL WEIGHT LOSS. Because most infants receive little nutriment for the first 3 or 4 days of life, they progressively lose weight until the flow of maternal milk or other feeding has been established. Preterm infants lose relatively more weight and regain their birthweight more slowly than do term infants. Infants that are small for gestational age but otherwise healthy regain their initial weight more quickly when fed than do preterm infants.

If the normal infant is nourished properly, birthweight is usually regained by the end of the 10th day. Subsequently, the weight typically increases steadily at the rate of about 25 g/day for the first few months, to double the birthweight by 5 months of age and to triple it by the end of the first year.

FEEDING. It is advisable to commence regular nursing within the first 12 hours postpartum. In many hospitals, infants begin breast feeding in the delivery room. Most term infants thrive best when fed at intervals of every 2 to 4 hours. Preterm or growth-restricted infants require feedings at shorter intervals. In most instances, a 3-hour interval is satisfactory. The proper length of each feeding depends on several factors, such as the quantity of breast milk, the readiness with which it can be obtained from the breast, and the avidity with which the infant nurses. It is generally advisable to allow the baby to remain at the breast for 10 minutes at first. Four to 5 minutes are sufficient for some infants; however, 15 to 20 minutes are required by others. It is satisfactory for the baby to nurse for 5 minutes at each breast for the first 4 days, or until the mother has a supply of milk. After the fourth day, the baby nurses up to 10 minutes on each breast. Breast feeding and formula choices are also discussed in Chapter 17 (p. 407).

CIRCUMCISION. The Committee on the Fetus and Newborn of the American Academy of Pediatrics recommended in 1971 that routine circumcision of newborn males not be performed. This was reaffirmed in their 1983 publication, *Guidelines for Perinatal Care.* These recommendations were widely adopted throughout the United States, and by 1987 only 61 percent of newborn males were circumcised (Poland, 1990).

In the 1992 *Guidelines for Perinatal Care* (American Academy of Pediatrics and American College of Obstetricians and Gynecologists), circumcision was no longer condemned, but it also was not recommended. This change likely resulted from the American Academy of Pediatrics Report of the Task Force on Circumcision (1989). The Task Force concluded that properly performed newborn circumcision prevented phimosis, paraphimosis, and balanoposthitis, and it decreased the incidence of penile cancer. The committee could not agree that circumcision resulted in a decreased incidence of urinary infections in babies because of the lack of well-designed studies. It cited an increased incidence of cervical cancer reported in sexual partners of uncircumcised men infected with human papillomavirus. The Task Force, however, could not agree on whether circumcision resulted in a decreased incidence of sexually transmitted diseases.

The Task Force concluded—without a recommendation—that newborn circumcision was generally a safe procedure when performed by an experienced operator, and should be an elective procedure performed in a healthy, stable neonate. Local anesthetic (dorsal penile nerve block) appeared to reduce the pain of the procedure, but the anesthetic was not without its own complications. The Task Force also concluded that circumcision has potential medical benefits and advantages as well as disadvantages and risks. They recommended that the benefits and risks be explained to the parents and informed consent obtained.

More recently, a similar conclusion was reached by the American Academy of Pediatrics Task Force on Circumcision (1999). It also concluded that there were not sufficient data to recommend routine circumcision because of potential benefits and risks. Thus, parents should determine what is in the best interest of the child and should make an informed choice after being given accurate and unbiased information. The Task Force considered it legitimate for parents to take into account cultural, religious, and ethnic traditions, in addition to medical factors, when making their decision. Similar conclusions were reached by the Canadian Paediatric Society (1996), which also concluded that newborn circumcision should not be routinely performed.

ANESTHESIA FOR CIRCUMCISION. Stang and colleagues (1988) reported that dorsal penile nerve block reduced behavioral distress and modified adrenocortical stress response in neonates undergoing circumcision. This observation was confirmed in subsequent clinical studies (Arnett and co-workers, 1990; Fontaine and Toffler, 1991).

A variety of techniques for pain relief have been described, including lidocaine-prilocaine topical cream, local analgesia infiltration, dorsal penile nerve block, and ring blocks. The results of these studies clearly favor the nerve block over topical analgesia and the ring block over both (Butler-O'Hara, 1998; Hardwick-Smith, 1998; Lander, 1997; Masciello, 1990; Taddio, 1997, and their colleagues). We agree with the view expressed by Maxwell and Yaster (1999) concerning analgesia—no more studies, just do it!

TECHNIQUE. The preferred technique of ring block is illustrated in Figure 16–7. After appropriate penile cleansing, the technique consists of placing a wheal of 1 percent lidocaine at the base of the penis and advancing the needle in a 180-degree arc around the base of the penis first to one side and then the other to achieve a circumferential ring of analgesia. The maximum dose of lidocaine is 1.0 mL. The addition of a buffering agent does not appear to offer a benefit (Newton and co-workers, 1999). **No vasoactive compounds such as epinephrine should ever be added to the local analgesic agent.**

COMPLICATIONS OF CIRCUMCISION. As with any surgical procedure, there is a risk of bleeding, infection, and hematoma formation. These risks, however, are low (Christakis and colleagues, 2000; Holman and colleagues, 1995). More unusual complications have been reported as isolated cases, including amputation of the distal penile glans during neonatal ritual circumcision (Neulander and colleagues, 1996), infection with human immunodeficiency virus-1 (HIV-1) and other sexually transmitted disease (Nicoll, 1997), postcircumcision meatal stenosis (Upadhyay and associates, 1998); denudation of the penis (Orozco-Sanchez and Neri-Vela, 1991), penile destruction with electrocautery (Gearhart

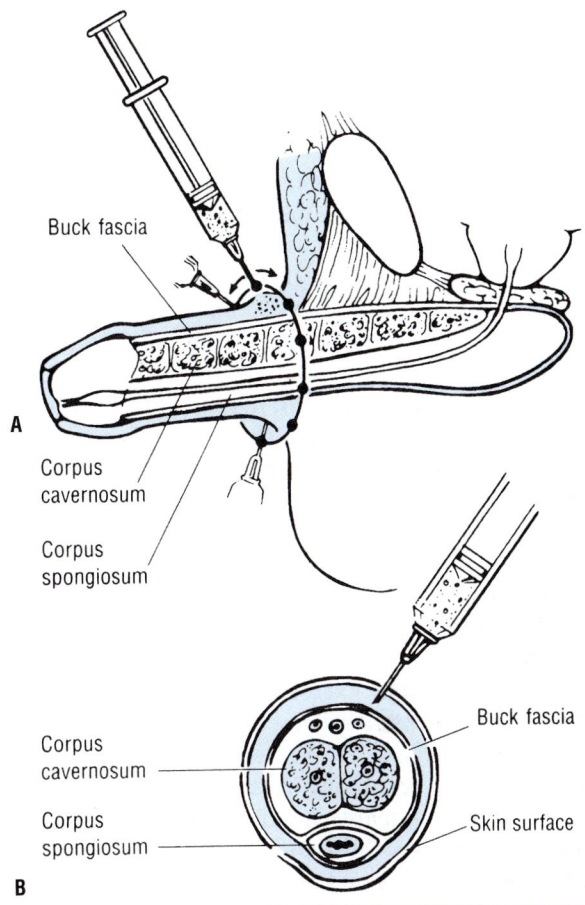

FIGURE 16–7. Subcutaneous ring block for circumcision. **A.** Needle is inserted at base of penis and subcutaneous bleb of lidocaine is placed. A 360-degree ring of anesthesia is completed around penis. **B.** Cross-section of penis at base showing paired dorsal nerves lateral to dorsal arteries and deep to Buck fascia. (Reproduced from Mattson, 1999, with permission.)

and Rock, 1989), and ischemia following the **inappropriate use of lidocaine with epinephrine** (Berens and Pontus, 1990).

It cannot be overemphasized that circumcision is an elective procedure. It should never be performed in a neonate with:

1. A family history of or a known clotting abnormality.
2. Ambiguous genitalia.
3. Hypospadias.
4. A febrile illness.

ROOMING-IN. In part, rooming-in stems from a trend to make all phases of childbearing as natural as possible and to foster proper mother–child relationships at an early date. By the end of 24 hours, the mother is generally fully ambulatory. Thereafter, with rooming-in, she can conduct for herself and her infant practically all routine care. An obvious advantage is her increased ability to assume full care of the baby when she arrives home.

HOSPITAL DISCHARGE. Traditionally, the newborn infant is discharged with its mother; in most cases, maternal stay has determined that of the child. In the past decade, the length of stay for the mother following uncomplicated vaginal delivery has declined. Currently, stays of 24 hours or less are common. Although it is clear that most newborns can also be safely discharged within 24 hours, this is not uniformly true. For example, using data from the Canadian Institute for Health Information, Liu and colleagues (2000) examined neonatal readmission rates in over 2.1 million discharges. As the length of hospital stay decreased from 4.2 days in 1990 to 2.7 days in 1997, the readmission rate increased from 27.3 to 38 per 1000 births. Dehydration and jaundice accounted for most of these readmissions. Danielsen and associates (2000) confirmed a similar association in statewide California births from 1992 to 1995. They did not, however, find an excessive rehospitalization due to early-infant discharge defined as an overnight stay. There was increased rehospitalization associated with same-day discharge. Using Washington state infant discharge data, Malkin and co-workers (2000) found about a fourfold increased 28-day mortality rate and a twofold increased 1-year mortality rate in infants discharged within 30 hours of birth. These practices need ongoing close scrutiny.

REFERENCES

American Academy of Pediatrics: Report of the Task Force on circumcision. Pediatrics 84:388, 1989

American Academy of Pediatrics: Task Force on circumcision: Circumcision policy statement. Pediatrics 103:686, 1999

American Academy of Pediatrics and the American College of Obstetricians and Gynecologists: Guidelines for Perinatal Care, 3rd ed. Washington, DC, 1992, pp 103, 109, 155

American Academy of Pediatrics and American Heart Association: Neonatal Resuscitation. Chicago, American Heart Association, 1994

American Academy of Pediatrics, Committee on Fetus and Newborn: Use and abuse of the Apgar score. Pediatrics 78:1148, 1986

American Academy of Pediatrics, Committee on the Fetus and Newborn: Standards and Recommendations for Hospital Care of Newborn Infants, 5th ed. Evanston, IL, American Academy of Pediatrics, 1971, p 110

American College of Obstetricians and Gynecologists: Committee on Obstetric Practice and American Academy of Pediatrics: Committee on Fetus and Newborn: Use and abuse of the Apgar score. Committee Opinion No. 174, July, 1996a

American College of Obstetricians and Gynecologists: Obstetric analgesia and anesthesia. ACOG Technical Bulletin No. 225, July, 1996b

American College of Obstetricians and Gynecologists: Umbilical artery blood acid–base analysis. Technical Bulletin No. 216, November, 1995

Amon E, Sibai BM, Anderson GD, Mabie WC: Obstetric variables predicting survival of the immature newborn (less than or equal to 1000 gm): A five-year experience in a single perinatal center. Am J Obstet Gynecol 156:1380, 1987

Apgar V: A proposal for a new method of evaluation of the newborn infant. Curr Res Anesth Analg 32:260, 1953

Apgar V, Holaday DA, James LS, Weisbrot IM, Berrien C: Evaluation of the newborn infant—second report. JAMA 168:1985, 1958

Arikan GM, Scholz HS, Petru E, Haeusler MC, Haas J, Weiss PA: Cord blood oxygen saturation in vigorous infants at birth: What is normal? Br J Obstet Gynaecol 107:987, 2000

Arnett RM, Jones JS, Horger EO III: Effectiveness of 1% lidocaine dorsal penile nerve block in infant circumcision. Am J Obstet Gynecol 163:1074, 1990

Babl FE, Ram S, Barnett ED, Rhein L, Carr E, Cooper ER: Neonatal gonococcal arthritis after negative prenatal screening and despite conjunctival prophylaxis. Pediatr Infec Dis J 19:346, 2000

Berens R, Pontus SP Jr: A complication associated with dorsal penile nerve block. Reg Anaesth 15:309, 1990

Boylan PC, Parisi VM: Fetal acid base balance. In Creasy RK, Resnik R (eds): Maternal–Fetal Medicine, 3rd ed. Philadelphia, Saunders, 1994

Brann AW Jr, Dykes FD: The effects of intrauterine asphyxia on the full-term neonate. Clin Perinatol 4:149, 1977

Brocklehurst P, Rooney G: Interventions for treating genital chlamydia trachomatis infection in pregnancy. Cochrane Database Syst Rev 2:CD000054, 2000

Buisman NJ, Abong Mwemba T, Garrigue G, Durand JP, Stilma JS, van Balen TM: Chlamydial ophthalmia neonatorum in Cameroon. Doc Ophthalmol 70:257, 1988

Butler-O'Hara M, LeMoine C, Guillet R: Analgesia for neonatal circumcision: A randomized controlled trial of EMLA cream versus dorsal penile nerve block. Pediatrics 101:691, 1998

Canadian Paediatric Society, Fetus and Newborn Committee: Clinical Practice Guidelines: Neonatal circumcision revisited. Can Med Assoc J 154:769, 1996

Catlin EA, Carpenter MW, Brann BS, Mayfield SR, Shaul PW, Goldstein M, Oh W: The Apgar score revisited: Influence of gestational age. J Pediatr 109:865, 1986

Centers for Disease Control and Prevention: National Center for Infectious Disease: Hepatitis B vaccine. www.cdc.gov/ncidod/diseases//hepatitis/b/faqbvax.htm, September, 2000.

Centers for Disease Control and Prevention: 1998 Guidelines for treatment of sexually transmitted diseases. MMWR 47:69, 1998

Centers for Disease Control and Prevention: Hepatitis B virus: A comprehensive strategy for eliminating transmission in the United States through universal childhood vaccination: Recommendations of the Immunization Practices Advisory Committee (ACIP). MMWR 40:1, 1991

Chauhan SP, Cowan BD, Meydrech EF, Magann EF, Morrison JC, Martin JN Jr: Determination of fetal acidemia at birth from a remote arterial blood gas analysis. Am J Obstet Gynecol 170:1705, 1994

Chernick V: Fetal breathing movements and the onset of breathing at birth. Clin Perinatol 5:257, 1978

Christakis DA, Harvey E, Zerr DM, Feudtner C, Wright JA,

Connell FA: A trade-off analysis of routine newborn circumcision. Pediatrics 105:246, 2000

Clark DA, Thompson J, Cahill J, Salisbury B: Footprinting the newborn—cost effective? Pediatr Res 15:552, 1981

Credé CSF: Die Verhütung der Augenenzündung der Neugeborenen. Berlin, Hirschwald, 1884

Danielsen B, Castles AG, Damberg CL, Gould JB: Newborn discharge timing and readmissions: California, 1992–1995. Pediatrics 106:31, 2000

Dawes GS: Breathing before birth in animals or man. N Engl J Med 290:557, 1974

Dickinson JE, Eriksen NL, Meyer BA, Parisi VM: The effect of preterm birth on umbilical cord blood gases. Obstet Gynecol 79:575, 1992

Dildy GA, van den Berg PP, Katz M, Clark SL, Jongsma HW, Nijhuis JG, Loucks CA: Intrapartum fetal pulseoximetry: Fetal oxygen saturation trends during labor in relationship to delivery outcome. Am J Obstet Gynecol 171:679, 1994

Duerbeck NB, Chaffin DG, Seeds JW: A practical approach to umbilical artery pH and blood gas determinations. Obstet Gynecol 79:959, 1992

Eisenberg MS, Cummins RO, Ho MT: Code blue: Cardiac arrest and resuscitation. Philadelphia, Saunders, 1987, p 146

Fontaine P, Toffler WL: Dorsal penile nerve block for newborn circumcision. Am Fam Physician 43:1327, 1991

Freeman JM, Nelson KB: Intrapartum asphyxia and cerebral palsy. Pediatrics 82:240, 1988

Gaudier FL, Goldenberg RL, Nelson KG, Peralta-Carcelen M, Johnson SE, DuBard MB, Roth TY, Hauth JC: Acid–base status at birth and subsequent neurosensory impairment in surviving 500 to 1000 gm infants. Am J Obstet Gynecol 170:48, 1994

Gearhart JP, Rock JA: Total ablation of the penis after circumcision with electrocautery: A method of management and long-term follow-up. J Urol 142:799, 1989

Gilstrap LC, Cunningham FG: Umbilical cord blood acid–base analysis. In Cunningham FG, MacDonald PC, Gant NF, Leveno KJ, Gilstrap LC (eds): Williams Obstetrics, 19th ed (suppl 4). Norwalk, CT, Appleton & Lange, 1994

Gilstrap LC, Leveno KJ, Burris J, Williams ML, Little BB: Diagnosis of birth asphyxia based on fetal pH, Apgar score, and newborn cerebral dysfunction. Am J Obstet Gynecol 161:825, 1989

Gladstone IM, Clapper L, Thorp JW, Wright DI: Randomized study of six umbilical cord care regimens. Comparing length of attachment, microbial control, and satisfaction. Clin Pediatr 27:127, 1988

Goldaber KG, Gilstrap LC, Leveno KJ, Dax JS: Pathologic fetal acidemia. Obstet Gynecol 78:1103, 1991

Goldenberg RL, Huddleston JF, Nelson KG: Apgar scores and umbilical arterial pH in preterm newborn infants. Am J Obstet Gynecol 149:651, 1984

Hammerschlag MR, Cummings C, Roblin PM, Williams TH, Delke I: Efficacy of neonatal ocular prophylaxis for the prevention of chlamydial and gonococcal conjunctivitis. N Engl J Med 320:769, 1989

Hardwick-Smith S, Mastrobattista JM, Wallace PA, Ritchey ML: Ring block for neonatal circumcision. Obstet Gynecol 91:930, 1998

Holman JR, Lewis EL, Ringler RL: Neonatal circumcision techniques. Am Fam Physician 52:511, 1995

Isenberg SJ, Apt L, Wood M: A controlled trial of povidone-iodine as prophylaxis against ophthalmia neonatorum. N Engl J Med 332:562, 1995

Laga M, Plummer FA, Piot P, Datta P, Namaara W, Ndinya-Achola JO, Nzanze H, Maitha G, Ronald AR, Pamba HO, Brunham RC: Prophylaxis of gonococcal and chlamydial ophthalmia neonatorum: A comparison of silver nitrate and tetracycline. N Engl J Med 318:653, 1988

Lander J, Brady-Fryer B, Metcalfe JB, Nazarali S, Muttitt S: Comparison of ring block, dorsal penile nerve block, and topical anesthesia for neonatal circumcision: A randomized controlled trial. JAMA 278:2157, 1997

Levene MI, Sands C, Grindulis H, Moore JR: Comparison of two methods of predicting outcome in perinatal asphyxia. Lancet 1:67, 1986

Lievaart M, deJong PA: Acid–base equilibrium in umbilical cord blood and time of cord clamping. Obstet Gynecol 63:44, 1984

Liu S, Wen SW, McMillan D, Trouton K, Fowler D, McCourt C: Increased neonatal readmission rate associated with decreased length of hospital stay at birth in Canada. Can J Public Health 91:46, 2000

Low JA, Lindsay BG, Derrick EJ: Threshold of metabolic acidosis associated with newborn complications. Am J Obstet Gynecol 177:1391, 1997

Low JA, Panagiotopoulos C, Derrick EJ: Newborn complications after intrapartum asphyxia with metabolic acidosis in the preterm fetus. Am J Obstet Gynecol 172:805, 1995

Low JA, Panagiotopoulos C, Derrick EJ: Newborn complications after intrapartum asphyxia with metabolic acidosis in the term fetus. Am J Obstet Gynecol 170:1081, 1994

Malkin JD, Garber S, Broder MS, Keeler E: Infant mortality and early postpartum discharge. Obstet Gynecol 96:183, 2000

Masciello AL: Anesthesia for neonatal circumcision: Local anesthesia is better than dorsal penile nerve block. Obstet Gynecol 75:834, 1990

Mattson SR: Routine anesthesia for circumcision: Two effective techniques. Post Grad Med 106:107, 1999

Maxwell LG, Yaster M: Analgesia for neonatal circumcision: No more studies, just do it. Arch Pediatr Adolesc Med 153:444, 1999

Milner AD, Saunders RA, Hopkins IE: The effect of delivery by caesarean section on lung mechanics and lung volume in the human neonate. Arch Dis Child 53:545, 1978

Nelson KB, Ellenberg JH: Apgar scores as predictors of chronic neurologic disability. Pediatrics 68:36, 1981

Nelson KB, Leviton A: How much of neonatal encephalopathy is due to birth asphyxia? Am J Dis Child 145:1325, 1991

Neulander E, Walfisch S, Kaneti J: Amputation of distal penile glans during neonatal ritual circumcision—a rare complication. Br J Urol 77:918, 1996

Newton CW, Mulnix N, Baer L, Bovee T: Plain and buffered lidocaine for neonatal circumcision. Obstet Gynecol 93:350, 1999

Nicoll A: Routine male neonatal circumcision and risk of infection with HIV-1 and other sexually transmitted diseases. Arch Dis Child 77:194, 1997

Novack AH, Mueller B, Ochs H: Umbilical cord separation in the normal newborn. Am J Dis Child 142:220, 1988

Orozco-Sanchez J, Neri-Vela R: Total denudation of the penis in circumcision. Description of a plastic technique for repair of the penis. Boll Med Hosp Infant Mex 48:565, 1991

Paneth N: The causes of cerebral palsy: Recent evidence. Clin Invest Med 16:95, 1993

Poland RL: The question of routine neonatal circumcision. N Engl J Med 322:1312, 1990

Ramin SM, Gilstrap LC, Leveno KJ, Burris JC, Little BB: Umbilical artery acid–base status in the preterm infant. Obstet Gynecol 74:256, 1989

Riley RJ, Johnson JWC: Collecting and analyzing cord blood gases. Clin Obstet Gynecol 36:13, 1993

Saunders RA: Pulmonary/volume relationships during the last phase of delivery and the first postnatal breaths in human subjects. J Pediatr 93:667, 1978

Smith J, Finn A: Antimicrobial prophylaxis. Arch Dis Child 80:388, 1999

Socol ML, Garcia PM, Riter S: Depressed Apgar scores, acid–base status, and neurologic outcome. Am J Obstet Gynecol 170:991, 1994

Spinnato JA, Sibai BM, Shaver DC, Anderson GD: Inaccuracy of Dubowitz gestational age in low birth weight infants. Obstet Gynecol 63:491, 1984

Stang JH, Gunnar MR, Snellman L, Condon LM, Kestenbaum R: Local anesthesia for neonatal circumcision. Effects on distress and cortisol response. JAMA 259:1507, 1988

Stanley FJ: Cerebral palsy trends: Implications for perinatal care. Acta Obstet Gynecol Scand 73:5, 1994

Taddio AN, Stevens B, Craig K, Rastogi R, Ben-David S, Stevan A, Mulligan P, Koren G: Efficacy and safety of lidocaine-prilocaine cream for pain during circumcision. N Engl J Med 336:1197, 1997

Upadhyay V, Hammodat HM, Pease PWB: Post circumcision meatal stenosis: 12 years' experience. N Z Med J 111:47, 1998

Yeomans ER, Hauth JC, Gilstrap LC III, Strickland DM: Umbilical cord pH, P_{CO_2} and bicarbonate following uncomplicated term vaginal deliveries. Am J Obstet Gynecol 151:798, 1985

17

The Puerperium

Puerperium is strictly defined as the period of confinement during and just after birth. By popular use, however, the meaning usually includes the 6 subsequent weeks during which normal pregnancy involution occurs (Hughes, 1972). Of course, and as described in Chapter 8, maternal adaptations to pregnancy do not necessarily all subside completely by 6 weeks postpartum.

CLINICAL AND PHYSIOLOGICAL ASPECTS OF THE PUERPERIUM

UTERINE CHANGES

CHANGES IN THE UTERINE VESSELS. Successful pregnancy requires a great increase in uterine blood flow. To provide for this, arteries and veins within the uterus, and especially to the placental site, enlarge remarkably, as do transport vessels to and from the uterus. Within the uterus, growth of new vessels also provides for the marked increase in blood flow. After delivery, the caliber of extrauterine vessels decreases to equal, or at least closely approximate, that of the prepregnant state.

Within the puerperal uterus, blood vessels are obliterated by hyaline changes, and vessels that are smaller replace them. Resorption of the hyalinized residue is accomplished by processes similar to those observed in the ovaries following ovulation and corpus luteum formation. Minor vestiges, however, may persist for years.

CHANGES IN THE CERVIX AND LOWER UTERINE SEGMENT. The outer cervical margin, which corresponds to the external os, is usually lacerated, especially laterally. The cervical opening contracts slowly, and for a few days immediately after labor it readily admits two fingers. By the end of the first week, it has narrowed. As the opening narrows, the cervix thickens, and a canal reforms. At the completion of involution, however, the external os does not resume its pregravid appearance completely. It remains somewhat wider, and typically, bilateral depressions at the site of lacerations remain as permanent changes that characterize the parous cervix. It should also be kept in mind that the cervical epithelium undergoes considerable remodeling as a result of childbirth. For example, Ahdoot and colleagues (1998) found that approximately 50 percent of women with high-grade squamous intraepithelial cells showed regression as a result of vaginal delivery.

The markedly thinned-out lower uterine segment contracts and retracts but not as forcefully as the body of the uterus. Over the course of a few weeks, the lower segment is converted from a clearly evident structure, large enough to contain most of the fetal head, into a barely discernible uterine isthmus located between the uterine corpus above and the internal cervical os below (Fig. 17–1).

INVOLUTION OF THE UTERINE CORPUS. Immediately after placental expulsion, the fundus of the contracted uterus is slightly below the umbilicus. The uterine body then consists mostly of myometrium covered by serosa and lined by basal decidua. The anterior and posterior walls, in close apposition, each measure 4 to 5 cm in thickness. Because its vessels are compressed by the contracted myometrium, the puerperal uterus on section appears ischemic when compared with the reddish-purple hyperemic pregnant organ. After the first 2 days, the uterus begins to shrink, so that within 2 weeks it has descended into the cavity of the true pelvis. It regains its previous nonpregnant size within about 4 weeks. The immediately postpartum uterus weighs approximately 1000 g. As the consequence of *involution,* 1 week later it weighs about 500 g, decreasing at the end of the second week to about 300 g, and soon thereafter to 100 g or less. The total number of muscle cells does not decrease appreciably; instead, the individual cells decrease markedly in size. The involution of the connective tissue framework occurs equally rapidly.

Because separation of the placenta and membranes involves the spongy layer, the decidua basalis remains in the uterus. The decidua that remains has striking variations in thickness, an irregular jagged appearance, and is infiltrated with blood, especially at the placental site.

AFTERPAINS. In primiparas the puerperal uterus tends to remain tonically contracted. Particularly in multiparas, the uterus often contracts vigorously at intervals, giving rise to *afterpains.* Occasionally these pains are severe enough to require an analgesic. Afterpains are noticeable particularly when the infant suckles, likely because of oxytocin release. Usually, they decrease in intensity and become mild by the third postpartum day.

LOCHIA. Early in the puerperium, sloughing of decidual tissue results in a vaginal discharge of variable quantity; this is termed *lochia.* Microscopically, lochia consists of erythrocytes, shreds of decidua, epithelial cells, and bacteria. Microorganisms are found in lochia pooled in the vagina and are present in most cases even when the discharge has been obtained from the uterine cavity.

For the first few days after delivery, blood in the lochia is sufficient to color it red—*lochia rubra.* After 3 or 4 days, lochia becomes progressively pale in color—*lochia serosa.* After about the 10th day, because of an admixture of leukocytes and reduced fluid content, lochia assumes a white or yellowish-white color—*lochia alba.*

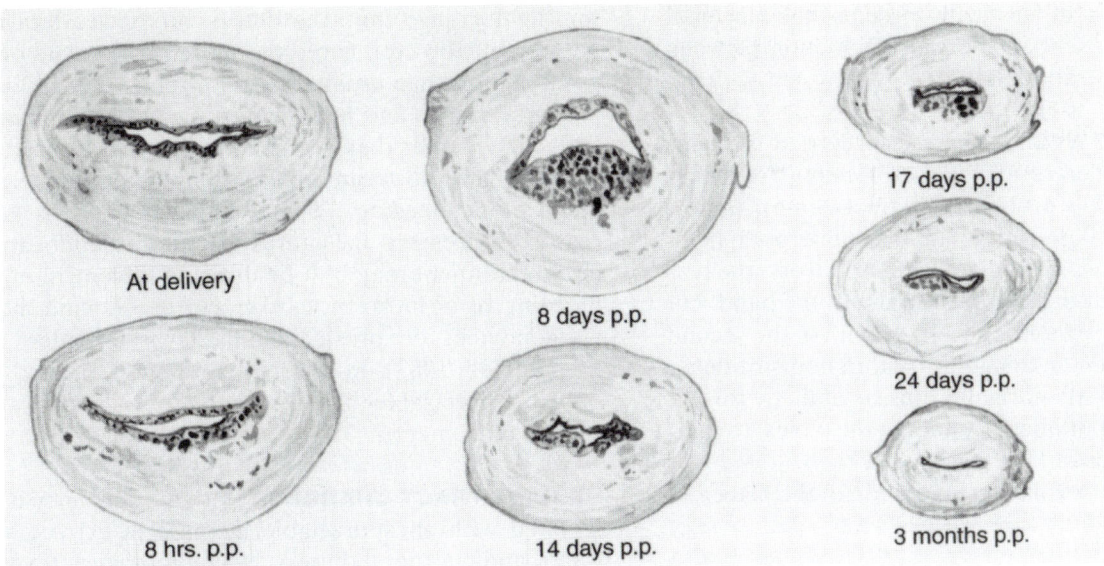

FIGURE 17–1. Cross-sections of uteri made at the level of the involuting placental site at varying times after delivery. (From Williams, 1931.)

Conventional obstetrical wisdom has for many years taught that lochia lasted for approximately 2 weeks after delivery. Recent studies, however, have indicated that lochia persists for up to 4 weeks and may stop and resume up to 56 days after delivery (Oppenheimer and colleagues, 1986; Visness and co-workers, 1997). Maternal age, parity, infant weight, and breast feeding do not influence the duration of lochia.

In some centers, it is routine to prescribe an oxytocic agent to hasten uterine involution by promoting uterine contractility. This also presumably diminishes bleeding complications. Newton and Bradford (1961), however, concluded that after the period immediately following delivery, routine administration of intramuscular oxytocin to normal women was of no value in decreasing blood loss or hastening uterine involution.

ENDOMETRIAL REGENERATION. Within 2 or 3 days after delivery, the remaining decidua becomes differentiated into two layers. The superficial layer becomes necrotic, and it is sloughed in the lochia. The basal layer adjacent to the myometrium remains intact and is the source of new endometrium. The endometrium arises from proliferation of the endometrial glandular remnants and the stroma of the interglandular connective tissue.

Endometrial regeneration is rapid, except at the placental site. Within a week or so, the free surface becomes covered by epithelium, and the entire endometrium is restored during the third week. Sharman (1953) identified fully restored endometrium in all biopsy specimens obtained from the 16th postpartum day onward. So-called endometritis identified histologically during the puerperium is only part of the normal reparative process. Similarly, in almost half of postpartum women, fallopian tubes, between 5 and 15 days, demonstrate microscopical inflammatory changes characteristic of acute salpingitis. This, however, is not infection, but only part of the involutional process (Andrews, 1951).

SUBINVOLUTION. This term describes an arrest or retardation of involution, the process by which the puerperal uterus is normally restored to its original proportions. It is accompanied by prolongation of lochial discharge and irregular or excessive uterine bleeding and sometimes by profuse hemorrhage. On bimanual examination, the uterus is larger and softer than normal for the particular period of the puerperium. Among the recognized causes of subinvolution are retention of placental fragments and pelvic infection. Because most cases of subinvolution result from local causes, they are usually amenable to early diagnosis and treatment. Ergonovine (Ergotrate) or methylergonovine (Methergine), 0.2 mg every 3 to 4 hours for 24 to 48 hours, is recommended by some clinicians, but its efficacy is questionable. On the other hand, metritis responds to oral antimicrobial therapy. Wager and colleagues (1980) reported that almost a third of cases of later postpartum uterine infection are caused by *Chlamydia trachomatis;* thus tetracycline therapy may be appropriate.

Andrew and colleagues (1989) described 25 cases of hemorrhage between 7 and 40 days postpartum associated with noninvoluted uteroplacental arteries. These abnormal arteries were characterized by no detectable endothelial lining and the vessels were filled with thrombi. Periauricular trophoblasts were also present in the walls of these vessels and the authors postulated that subinvolution, at least with regard to the placental vessels, may represent an aberrant interaction between uterine cells and trophoblast.

PLACENTAL SITE INVOLUTION. According to Williams (1931), complete extrusion of the placental site takes up to 6 weeks. This process is of great clinical importance, for when it is defective, late-onset puerperal hemorrhage may ensue. Immediately after delivery, the placental site is about the size of the palm of the hand, but it rapidly decreases thereafter. By the end of the second week, it is 3 to 4 cm in diameter. Within hours of delivery, the placental site normally consists of many thrombosed vessels that ultimately undergo the typical organization of a thrombus (Fig. 17–1).

Williams (1931) explained involution of the placental site as follows:

> Involution is not effected by absorption in situ, but rather by a process of exfoliation which is in great part brought about by the undermining of the implantation site by growth of endometrial tissue. This is affected partly by extension and downgrowth of endometrium from the margins of the placental site and partly by the development of endometrial tissue from the glands and stroma left in the depths of the decidua basalis after placental separation. Such exfoliation should be regarded as very conservative, and as a wise provision; otherwise great difficulty might be experienced in sloughing obliterated arteries and organized thrombi which, if they remained in situ, would soon convert a considerable part of the uterine mucosa and subjacent myometrium into a mass of scar tissue.

Anderson and Davis (1968) concluded that placental site exfoliation is brought about as the consequence of sloughing of infarcted and necrotic superficial tissues followed by a reparative process.

LATE POSTPARTUM HEMORRHAGE. Serious uterine hemorrhage occasionally develops 1 to 2 weeks into the puerperium. Hemorrhage most often is the result of abnormal involution of the placental site, but it may also be caused by retention of a portion of the placenta. Usually the retained piece of placenta undergoes necrosis with deposition of fibrin, and may eventually form a so-called *placental polyp*. As the eschar of the polyp detaches from the myometrium, hemorrhage may be brisk.

In a study by Lee and associates (1981) of 3822 women delivered during a 1-year period at Henry Ford Hospital, 27 women, or 0.7 percent, had significant uterine bleeding after the first 24 postpartum hours. In 20 of these women the uterus was judged to be empty by sonographic evaluation, and importantly, only one woman had retained placental tissue.

It has generally been accepted that with late postpar-

tum hemorrhage from the uterus, prompt curettage is necessary. However, curettage subsequent to late puerperal hemorrhage usually does not remove identifiable placental tissue, and hemorrhage frequently is intensified. Thus, rather than reducing hemorrhage, curettage is more likely to traumatize the implantation site and incite more bleeding. Especially where there is good reason to preserve the uterus for future childbearing, initial treatment may best be directed to control of the bleeding, using intravenous oxytocin, ergonovine, methylergonovine, or prostaglandins (Adrinopoulos and Mendenhall, 1983). In general, curettage is carried out only if appreciable bleeding persists or recurs after such management.

URINARY TRACT CHANGES. Normal pregnancy is associated with an appreciable increase in extracellular water, and puerperal diuresis is a physiological reversal of this process. Diuresis regularly occurs between the second and fifth days, even when intravenous fluids were not infused vigorously during labor and delivery. The fluid-retaining stimuli of pregnancy-induced hyperestrogenism and elevated venous pressure in the lower half of the body dissipate after delivery, and residual hypervolemia is lost. In preeclampsia, both retention of fluid antepartum and diuresis postpartum may be greatly increased (Chap. 24).

The puerperal bladder has an increased capacity and a relative insensitivity to intravesical fluid pressure. Overdistention, incomplete emptying, and excessive residual urine are common. The paralyzing effect of anesthesia, especially conduction analgesia, and the temporarily disturbed bladder neural function, are undoubtedly contributory factors. Residual urine and bacteriuria in a traumatized bladder, coupled with the dilated renal pelves and ureters, create optimal conditions for development of urinary infection. Dilated ureters and renal pelves return to their prepregnant state from 2 to 8 weeks after delivery (Chap. 8, p. 186).

Kerr-Wilson and colleagues (1984) studied the effect of labor on postpartum bladder function using urodynamic techniques. They concluded that, as long as prolonged labors were avoided and if catheterization was done promptly for bladder distention, there was no evidence for bladder hypotonia. Andolf and co-investigators (1994) used ultrasonography to measure residual bladder volumes 3 days after vaginal delivery in 539 unselected consecutive women. Only 12 (1.5 percent) had abnormal volumes and only four needed urinary catheters. Urinary retention was more common after instrumental delivery or epidural analgesia. These same women were rescanned 4 years later and a third had voiding difficulties.

Viktrup and colleagues (1992) followed 305 nulliparous women during pregnancy and postpartum and 7 percent developed stress incontinence after delivery. Obstetrical factors such as length of second-stage labor, infant head circumference, birthweight, and episiotomy were associated with the development of stress incontinence after delivery. Impaired muscle function in or around the urethra during vaginal delivery was proposed as the pathophysiology underlying puerperal incontinence. Most women returned to normal micturition by 3 months postpartum. **Careful attention to all postpartum women, with prompt catheterization for those who cannot void, will prevent most urinary problems.**

RELAXATION OF THE VAGINAL OUTLET AND PROLAPSE OF THE UTERUS. Early in the puerperium, the vagina and vaginal outlet form a capacious, smooth-walled passage that gradually diminishes in size but rarely returns to nulliparous dimensions. Rugae reappear by the third week. The hymen is represented by several small tags of tissue, which during cicatrization are converted into the *myrtiform caruncles.*

Extensive lacerations of the perineum during delivery are followed by relaxation of the vaginal outlet. Even when external lacerations are not visible, overstretching may lead to marked relaxation. Moreover, changes in the pelvic supports during parturition predispose to prolapse of the uterus and to urinary stress incontinence. In general, operative correction is postponed until childbearing is ended, unless, of course, serious disability, notably urinary stress incontinence, results in symptoms sufficient to require intervention.

PERITONEUM AND ABDOMINAL WALL. The broad and round ligaments are much more lax when nonpregnant, and they require considerable time to recover from the stretching and loosening that occurred during pregnancy.

As a result of the rupture of elastic fibers in the skin and the prolonged distention caused by the pregnant uterus, the abdominal wall remains soft and flabby. Return to normal for these structures requires several weeks, but recovery is aided by exercise. Except for silvery striae, the abdominal wall usually resumes its prepregnancy appearance. When muscles remain atonic, however, the abdominal wall also remains lax. There may be a marked separation, or diastasis, of the rectus muscles. In this condition, the abdominal wall in the vicinity of the midline is formed only by peritoneum, attenuated fascia, subcutaneous fat and skin.

BLOOD AND FLUID CHANGES. Rather marked leukocytosis and thrombocytosis occur during and after labor. The leukocyte count sometimes reaches $30,000/\mu L$, with the increase predominantly from granulocytes. There is also a relative lymphopenia and an absolute eosinopenia. Normally, during the first few postpartum days,

hemoglobin concentration and hematocrit fluctuate moderately. If they fall much below the levels present just prior to labor, a considerable amount of blood has been lost (Chap. 25, p. 635). By 1 week after delivery, the blood volume has returned nearly to its nonpregnant level. Robson and colleagues (1987) showed that cardiac output remains elevated for at least 48 hours postpartum. Most likely this is due to increased stroke volume from venous return, because the heart rate falls at the same time. By 2 weeks, these changes have returned to normal nonpregnant values.

Pregnancy-induced changes in blood coagulation factors persist for variable periods during the puerperium. Elevation of plasma fibrinogen and hence the sedimentation rate are maintained at least through the first week, and as a consequence, the elevated sedimentation rate normally found during pregnancy remains high.

WEIGHT LOSS. In addition to the loss of about 5 to 6 kg due to uterine evacuation and normal blood loss, there is usually a further decrease of 2 to 3 kg through diuresis. Chesley and co-workers (1959) demonstrated a decrease in sodium space of about 2 L, or 2 kg during the first week postpartum.

According to Schauberger and co-investigators (1992), most women approach their self-reported prepregnancy weight 6 months after delivery but still retain an average surplus of 1.4 kg (3 lbs). Factors that increased puerperal weight loss included weight gain during pregnancy, primiparity, early return to work outside the home, and smoking. Breast feeding, age, or marital status did not affect weight loss. Greene and colleagues (1988) analyzed data from the collaborative perinatal study, and found that prenatal weight gain in excess of 20 lbs was associated with postpartum weight retention.

MAMMARY GLANDS

BREAST ANATOMY. Anlagen of mammary glands are contained in ectodermal ridges that form on the ventral surface of the embryo and extend laterally from forelimb to hindlimb. The multiple pairs of buds normally disappear from the embryo except for one pair in the pectoral region that eventually develops into the two mammary glands (Fig. 17–2). At times, however, the buds elsewhere may not completely disappear, but instead they may participate to an amazing degree in the pattern of growth that characterizes the two normal mammary glands.

At midpregnancy, each of the two fetal mammary buds destined to form the breasts begins to grow and divide. This results in the formation of 15 to 25 secondary buds that provide the basis for the duct system in

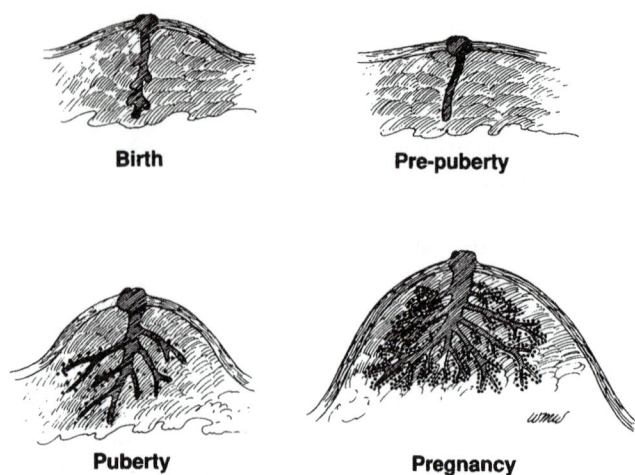

Birth **Pre-puberty** **Puberty** **Pregnancy**

FIGURE 17–2. Sequential growth of the mammary gland is illustrated from 8 weeks embryonic age through puberty and during pregnancy. (Courtesy of Dr. John C. Porter.)

the mature breast. Each secondary bud elongates into a cord, bifurcates, and differentiates into two concentric layers of cuboidal cells and a central lumen. The inner layer of cells eventually gives rise to the secretory epithelium, which synthesizes the milk. The outer cell layer becomes myoepithelium, which provides the mechanism for milk ejection (Fig. 17–3).

Thelarche is the onset of rapid breast growth that begins about the time of puberty when estrogen production rises. The previously infantile mammary glands respond to estrogen with growth and development of mammary ducts and fat deposition. With ovulation, progesterone stimulates development of the alveoli for future lactation.

Anatomically, each mature mammary gland is composed of 15 to 25 lobes that arose from the secondary buds described previously. The lobes are arranged radially and are separated from one another by varying amounts of fat. Each lobe consists of several lobules, which in turn are made up of large numbers of alveoli (Fig. 17–3). Every alveolus is provided with a small duct that joins others to form a single larger duct for each lobe. These lactiferous ducts open separately upon the nipple, where they may be distinguished as minute but distinct orifices. The alveolar secretory epithelium synthesizes the various milk constituents.

BREAST FEEDING

LACTATION. Colostrum is the deep lemon-yellow colored liquid secreted initially by the breasts. It usually can be expressed from the nipples by the second postpartum day.

COLOSTRUM. Compared with mature milk, colostrum contains more minerals and protein, much of which is globulin, but less sugar and fat. Colostrum nevertheless contains large fat globules in so-called colostrum corpuscles. These are thought by some investigators to be epithelial cells that have undergone fatty degeneration and by others to be mononuclear phagocytes containing fat. Colostrum secretion persists for about 5 days, with gradual conversion to mature milk during the ensuing 4 weeks. Antibodies are demonstrable in the colostrum, and its content of immunoglobulin A may offer protection for the newborn against enteric pathogens. Other host resistance factors, as well as immunoglobulins, are found in human colostrum and milk. These include complement, macrophages, lymphocytes, lactoferrin, lactoperoxidase, and lysozymes.

MILK. Human milk is a suspension of fat and protein in a carbohydrate-mineral solution. A nursing mother

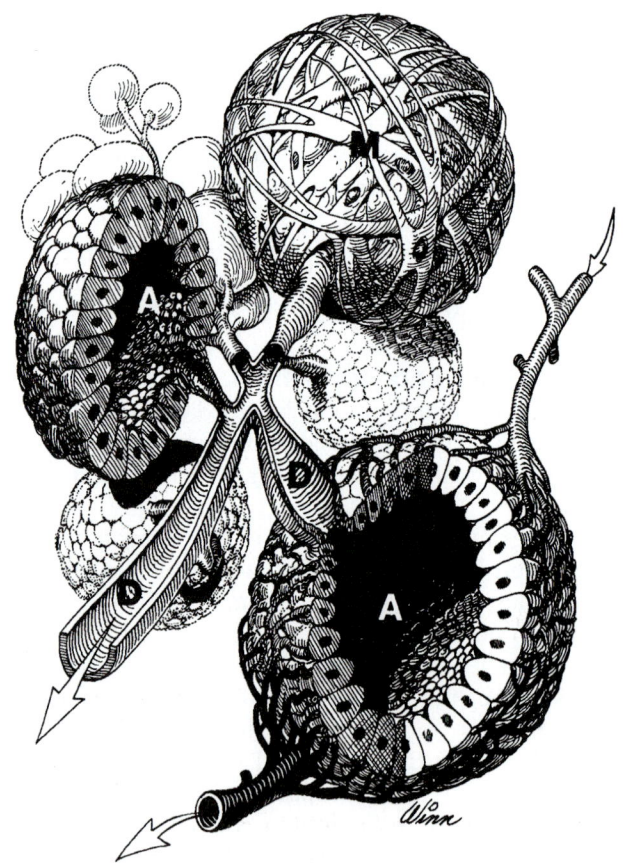

FIGURE 17–3. Graphic demonstration of alveolar and ductal system. Note the myoepithelial fibers (M) that surround the outside of the uppermost alveolus. The secretions from the glandular elements are extruded into the lumen of the alveoli (A) and ejected by the myoepithelial cells into the ductal system (D), which empties through the nipple. Arterial blood supply to the alveolus is identified by the upper right arrow and venous drainage by arrow beneath. (Courtesy of Dr. John C. Porter.)

easily makes 600 mL of milk per day. Milk is isotonic with plasma, with lactose accounting for half of the osmotic pressure. Major proteins, including α-lactalbumin, β-lactoglobulin, and casein, are also present. Essential amino acids are derived from blood, and nonessential amino acids are derived in part from blood or synthesized in the mammary gland. Most milk proteins are unique and not found elsewhere. Whey has been shown to contain large amounts of interleukin-6 (Saito and co-workers, 1991). Peak levels of this cytokine were found in colostrum, and there was a positive correlation between its concentration and the number of mononuclear cells in human milk. Additionally, interleukin-6 was associated closely with local immunoglobulin A production by the breast. Prolactin appears to be actively secreted into breast milk (Yuen, 1988). Epidermal growth factor (EGF) has also been identified in human milk (Koldovsky and associates, 1991; McCleary, 1991). Because this factor is not destroyed by gastric proteolytic enzymes, it may be absorbed orally and promote growth and maturation of intestinal mucosa.

There are major changes in milk composition by 30 to 40 hours postpartum, including a sudden increase of lactose concentration. Lactose synthesis from glucose in alveolar secretory cells is catalyzed by lactose synthase (Fig. 17–4). Some lactose enters the maternal circulation and is excreted by the kidney. This may be misinterpreted as glucosuria unless specific glucose oxidase is used in testing. Fatty acids are synthesized in the alveoli from glucose and are secreted by an apocrine-like process.

All vitamins except vitamin K are found in human milk, but in variable amounts, and maternal dietary supplementation increases the secretion of most of these (American Academy of Pediatrics, 1981). Vitamin K administration to the infant soon after delivery is required to prevent hemorrhagic disease of the newborn (Chap. 39, p. 1082).

Human milk contains a low iron concentration and maternal iron stores do not seem to influence the amount of iron in breast milk. Therefore, the use of supplemental iron-fortified infant formulas, or a weaning formula also fortified with iron, is recommended (American Academy of Pediatrics, 1997). Such formulas apparently have eliminated iron-deficiency anemia during childhood (Yip and associates, 1987). These formulas are well tolerated by most infants and there is no evidence that they impair absorption of zinc or copper (Nelson and associates, 1988; Yip and colleagues, 1985).

Mennella and Beauchamp (1991) documented what experienced nursing mothers have long known: breast-fed infants are aware of what their mothers eat and drink. They studied the effects of maternal ethanol ingestion equivalence to one can of beer. This caused the infants to suck more frequently during the first minute of feeding, but ultimately they consumed significantly less milk.

The mammary gland, like the thyroid gland, concentrates iodine and several other minerals, including gallium, technetium, indium, and possibly sodium. Radioactive isotopes of these minerals should not be given to nursing women because they rapidly appear in breast milk. The American Academy of Pediatrics (1997) recommends consultation with a nuclear medicine physician before performing a diagnostic study, so that a radionuclide with the shortest excretion time in breast milk can be used. They further recommend that the mother pump her breasts before the study and store enough milk in a freezer for feeding the infant. After the study, she should pump her breasts to maintain milk

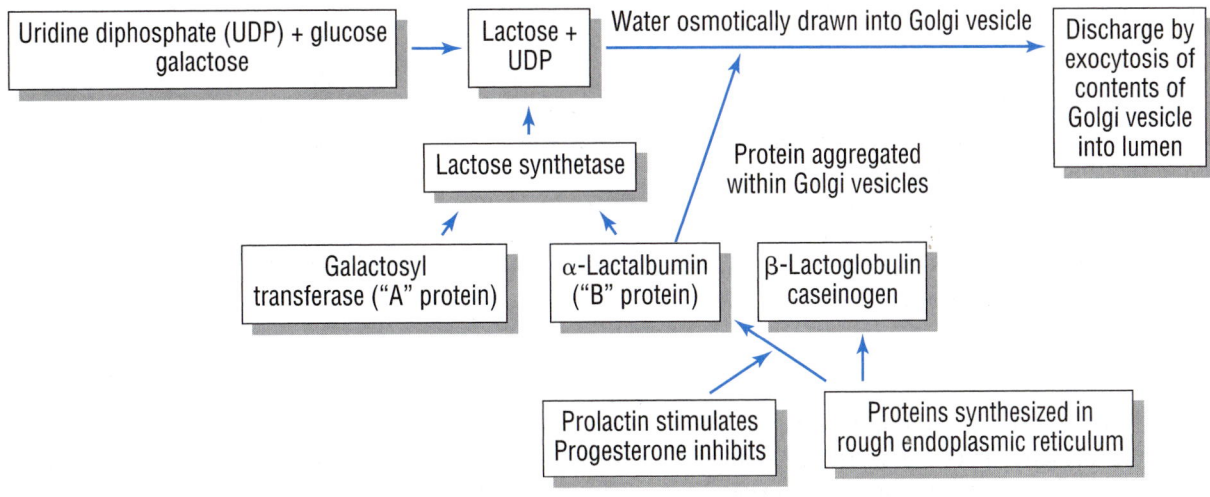

FIGURE 17–4. Relation of protein, lactose, and water secretion on lactation. Note that progesterone inhibits production of α-lactalbumin and prolactin stimulates its production. (Courtesy of Dr. John C. Porter.)

TABLE 17–1. Composition of Mature Human Milk, Cow Milk, and a Typical Formula Used for Term Infants

Composition Per 100 mL	Mature Breast Milk	Cow Milk	Formula with Iron
Calories	75	69	67
Protein	1.1	3.5	1.5
Lactalbumin (%)	80	18	60
Casein (%)	20	82	40
Water (mL)	87.1	87.3	90
Fat (g)	4.5	3.5	3.8
Carbohydrates	7.1	4.9	6.9
Ash (g)	0.21	0.72	0.34
Minerals (mg)			
Na	16	50	21
K	53	144	69
Ca	33	118	46
P	14	93	32
Mg	4	13	5.3
Fe	0.05	Trace	1.3
Zn	0.15	0.4	0.42
Vitamins			
A (IU)	182	140	210
C (mg)	5	1	5.3
D (IU)	2.2	42	42
E (IU)	0.18	0.04	0.83
Thiamine (mg)	0.01	0.04	0.04
Riboflavin (mg)	0.04	0.03	0.06
Niacin (mg)	0.2	0.17	0.7
pH	Alkaline	Acid	Acid
Bacterial content	Sterile	Nonsterile	Sterile

Modified from Avery and Fletcher (1987).

production, but discard all milk produced during the time that radioactivity is present. This ranges from 15 hours up to 2 weeks, depending upon the isotope used.

The approximate concentrations of the more important components of human colostrum, mature human milk, and cow milk are presented in Table 17–1. These concentrations vary depending upon maternal diet and when studied in the puerperium (Brasil and co-workers, 1991; Giovannini and colleagues, 1991; Ogunleye and associates, 1991). Gestational weight gain has little, if any, impact on the subsequent milk quantity or quality (Institute of Medicine, 1990).

ENDOCRINOLOGY OF LACTATION. The precise humoral and neural mechanisms involved in lactation are complex. Progesterone, estrogen, and placental lactogen, as well as prolactin, cortisol, and insulin, appear to act in concert to stimulate the growth and development of the milk-secreting apparatus of the mammary gland (Porter, 1974). With delivery, there is an abrupt and profound decrease in the levels of progesterone and estrogen, which removes the inhibitory influence of progesterone on the production of α-lactalbumin by the rough endoplasmic reticulum (Fig. 17–4). The increased α-lactalbumin serves to stimulate lactose synthase and ultimately increased milk lactose. Progesterone withdrawal also allows prolactin to act unopposed in its stimulation of α-lactalbumin production.

The intensity and duration of subsequent lactation are controlled, in large part, by the repetitive stimulus of nursing. Prolactin is essential for lactation; women with extensive pituitary necrosis, as in Sheehan syndrome, do not lactate. Although plasma prolactin falls after delivery to lower levels than during pregnancy, each act of suckling triggers a rise in levels (McNeilly and associates, 1983). Presumably a stimulus from the breast curtails the release of prolactin-inhibiting factor from the hypothalamus; this, in turn, transiently induces increased prolactin secretion.

The neurohypophysis, in pulsatile fashion, secretes oxytocin. This stimulates milk expression from a lactating breast by causing contraction of myoepithelial cells in the alveoli and small milk ducts. Milk ejection, or "letting down," is a reflex initiated especially by suckling, which stimulates the neurohypophysis to liberate oxytocin (McNeilly and associates, 1983). It may be provoked even by the cry of the infant or inhibited by fright or stress.

In women who continue lactating but who resume ovulation, there are acute alterations in breast milk composition 5 to 6 days before and 6 to 7 days following ovulation (Hartmann and Prosser, 1984). These changes are abrupt and characterized by increased concentrations of sodium and chloride, along with decreased potassium, lactose, and glucose concentrations. In women who become pregnant but who continue to breast feed, milk composition undergoes progressive alterations suggesting gradual loss of metabolic and secretory breast activity (Hartmann and Prosser, 1984).

IMMUNOLOGICAL CONSEQUENCES OF BREAST FEEDING. Antibodies are present in human colostrum and milk but are poorly absorbed, if at all, from the infant's gut. For example, no anti-D antibodies have been detected in the sera of infants fed milk containing a high titer of antibodies. This circumstance, however, does not lessen the importance of at least some of the antibodies in breast milk. The predominant immunoglobulin in milk is secretory IgA, a macromolecule that is important in antimicrobial processes in mucous membranes across which it is secreted. Milk contains secretory IgA antibodies against *Escherichia coli*, and it is known that breast-fed infants are less prone to enteric infections than bottle-fed babies (Cravioto and associates, 1991). It has been suggested that IgA exerts its action by preventing bacterial adherence to epithelial cells surfaces, thus preventing tissue invasion (Samra and associates, 1991). Moreover, human milk also provides protection against rotavirus infections, which cause up to 50 percent of cases of gastroenteritis among infants in the United States (Newburg and associates, 1998).

Much attention has been directed to an elucidation of the role of maternal breast milk lymphocytes in fetal immunological processes. Milk contains both the T and B lymphocytes, but the T lymphocytes appear to differ from those found in blood. Specifically, milk T lymphocytes are almost exclusively composed of cells that exhibit specific membrane antigens including the LFA-1 high-memory T-cell phenotype. These memory T cells appear to be another mechanism by which the neonate benefits from maternal immunological experience (Bertotto and associates, 1990). Lymphocytes in colostrum undergo blastoid transformation in vitro following exposure to specific antigens. In experimental animals, Beer and Billingham (1976) observed a transmission of viable lymphocytes from mother to infant through breast milk. As mentioned earlier, interleukin-6 is present in colostrum and appears to stimulate an increase in mononuclear cells in breast milk (Saito and co-workers, 1991).

NURSING. Between 1930 and the late 1960s, there was a dramatic decline in the percentage of American mothers who breast fed (Yaffe, 1994). The incidence declined from approximately 80 percent of children born between 1926 and 1930 to only 20 percent of births in 1972. At the present time in the United States, a number of surveys indicate that more than 60 percent of babies discharged from the hospital are breast fed, and the number is increasing (American College of Obstetricians and Gynecologists, 2000).

Human milk is ideal food for neonates. As reviewed by the American College of Obstetricians and Gynecologists (2000), it provides species- and age-specific nutrients for the infant. In addition to the right balance of nutrients, immunological factors, and antibacterial properties, human milk contains factors that act as biological signals for promoting cellular growth and differentiation. In 1997, the American Academy of Pediatrics published the policy statement on the infant benefits of nursing shown in Table 17–2. The United States Public Health Service goal for year 2010 is to increase the proportion of mothers who breast feed to 75 percent (American College of Obstetricians and Gynecologists, 2000).

In most instances, even though the supply of milk at first appears insufficient, it becomes adequate if suckling is continued. An exception is that 65 percent of women with augmentation mammoplasty have lactation insufficiency (Hurst, 1996). This depends on whether the implant incision was periaveolar or not (Chez and Fried-

TABLE 17–2. American Academy of Pediatrics Policy Statement on the Infant Benefits of Nursing

Research on Established and Potential Protective Effects of Human Milk and Breast Feeding on Infants

Research in the United States, Canada, Europe and other developed countries, among predominantly middle-class populations, provides strong evidence that human milk feeding decreases the incidence and/or severity of diarrhea, lower respiratory infection, otitis media, bacteremia, bacterial meningitis, botulism, urinary tract infection, and necrotizing enterocolitis. There are a number of studies that show a possible protective effect of human milk feeding against sudden infant death syndrome, insulin-dependent diabetes mellitus, Crohn's disease, ulcerative colitis, lymphoma, allergic diseases, and other chronic digestive diseases. Breastfeeding has also been related to possible enhancement of cognitive development.

From the American Academy of Pediatrics (1997), with permission.

mann, 2000). Nursing also accelerates uterine involution, because repeated stimulation of the nipples releases oxytocin, which contracts uterine muscle. **Aerobic exercise** performed four or five times per week beginning 6 to 8 weeks postpartum had no adverse effect on lactation and significantly improved the cardiovascular fitness of the mothers (Dewey and co-workers, 1994). Weight loss of approximately 0.5 kg per week in the first 3 months postpartum does not affect infant growth in exclusively breast feeding, overweight women (Lovelady and co-workers, 2000).

According to Chez and Friedmann (2000), a number of internet website resources are available for more information for breast feeding mothers; these include the American Academy of Pediatrics (www.aap.org) and LeLeche League International (www.laleche league.org).

LACTATION INHIBITION. Approximately 40 percent of American women currently elect to not breast feed, and many experience considerable breast pain and engorgement. Milk leakage, engorgement, and breast pain peak at 3 to 5 days postpartum (Spitz and associates, 1998). As many as 10 percent of women may report severe pain up to 14 days postpartum and a fourth to half of all women use analgesia for relief of puerperal breast pain.

In 1989, an advisory committee of the Food and Drug Administration, taking the view that there is no need for pharmacological therapy for lactation suppression, recommended that medicinals should no longer be used for lactation suppression. Bromocriptine, a commonly used drug for lactation inhibition, had been associated with strokes, myocardial infarctions, seizures, and psychiatric disturbances in puerperal women, although the evidence used to support these associations is tenuous (Morgans, 1995). Despite this, the manufacturer voluntarily removed lactation suppression in 1994 as an indication for bromocriptine (Food and Drug Administration, 1994).

The woman who does not desire to breast feed should be reassured that stopping milk production is not a major problem. During the stage of engorgement, the breasts become painful and should be supported with a well-fitting brassiere. Ice packs and oral analgesics for 12 to 24 hours may be required to relieve discomfort. Breast binders, rather than hormonal suppression of lactation, are routinely used at Parkland Hospital in women not desiring to nurse their infant.

CONTRACEPTION. There are many considerations, primarily theoretical, that govern recommendations for use of hormonal methods of contraceptions during lactation and the puerperium (Chap. 58). Contraception is not needed in the first 3 weeks postpartum because of a delay in return of ovulation in all women (American College of Obstetricians and Gynecologists, 2000). After this time, depending on individual biological variation as well as the intensity of breast feeding, ovulation may unpredictably resume in lactating women. Progestin-only contraceptives, including mini-pills, depot medroxyprogesterone, and levonorgestrel implants do not affect the quality of milk and increase, only very slightly, the volume of milk; therefore they are the contraceptives of choice for breast feeding women (American College of Obstetricians and Gynecologists, 2000). Recommendations for use of progestin-only contraceptives are shown in Table 17–3.

Estrogen–progestin contraceptives have been shown to reduce the quantity and quality of breast milk. Another concern is the predisposition puerperal women have to venous thrombosis, which could be increased by combination contraceptive pills. Accordingly, low-dose estrogen tablets (35 μg or lower) are preferred if combination hormonal contraceptives are to be used in lactating women (Table 17–3).

CONTRAINDICATIONS. Nursing is contraindicated in women who take street drugs or do not control alcohol use; have an infant with galactosemia; have HIV infection; have active, untreated tuberculosis; take certain medications; or are undergoing breast cancer treatment (American College of Obstetricians and Gynecologists, 2000). Cytomegalovirus and hepatitis B virus are excreted in milk, however, breast feeding is not contraindicated if hepatitis B immune globulin is given to infants of seropositive mothers.

Breast feeding has been recognized for over a decade as a mode of HIV transmission (Ziegler and colleagues, 1985). More recent data confirm that some mother-to-infant transmission occurs through breast feeding. Nduati and colleagues (2000) randomized 401 HIV-seropositive mother–infant pairs in Kenya to formula or breast feeding. The frequency of breast milk transmission of HIV was 16 percent. Use of breast milk substitutes prevented 44 percent of infant HIV infections during the first 2 years of life.

Women with active herpes simplex virus may suckle their infants if there are no breast lesions, and if particular care is directed to hand washing before nursing.

CARE OF THE BREASTS AND NIPPLES. The nipples require little attention in the puerperium other than cleanliness and attention to fissures. Because dried milk is likely to accumulate and irritate the nipples, cleaning of the areola with water and mild soap is helpful before and after nursing. Occasionally with irritated nipples it is necessary to use a nipple shield for 24 hours or longer. Inverted or retracted nipples may be troublesome; however, these can usually be teased out by gently pulling with the finger and thumb. This is best done during pregnancy to prepare the nipples for subsequent nursing.

Proper technique for positioning the mother and infant during nursing has been reviewed by the American College of Obstetricians and Gynecologists (2000). This includes proper techniques for "latch-on" of the infant during suckling.

DRUGS SECRETED IN MILK. Most drugs given to the mother are secreted in breast milk. Many factors influence their excretion, including the concentration of drugs in plasma, degree of protein binding, plasma and milk pH, degree of ionization, lipid solubility, and molecular weight. The amount of drug ingested by the infant typically is small. The ratio of drug concentrations

TABLE 17–3. ACOG Recommendations for Hormonal Contraception if Used by Breast Feeding Women

Progestin-only oral contraceptives prescribed or dispensed at discharge from the hospital to be started 2–3 weeks postpartum (e.g., the first Sunday after the newborn is 2 weeks old)

Depot medroxyprogesterone acetate initiated at 6 weeks postpartum[a]

Hormonal implants inserted at 6 weeks postpartum

Combined estrogen–progestin contraceptives, if prescribed, should not be started before 6 weeks postpartum, and only when lactation is well established and the infant's nutritional status is well-monitored.

[a]There are certain clinical situations in which earlier initiation might be considered.
From the American College of Obstetricians and Gynecologists (2000), with permission.

TABLE 17–4. Medications Contraindicated During Breast Feeding

Medication	Reason
Bromocriptine	Suppresses lactation
Cocaine	Cocaine intoxication
Cyclophosphamide	Possible immune suppression; unknown effect on growth or association with carcinogenesis; neutropenia
Cyclosporine	Possible immune suppression; unknown effect on growth or association with carcinogenesis
Doxorubicin[a]	Vomiting, diarrhea, convulsions (at doses used in migraine medications)
Lithium	One third to one half of therapeutic blood concentration in infants
Methotrexate	Possible immune suppression; unknown effect on growth or association with carcinogenesis; neutropenia
Phencyclidine	Potent hallucinogen
Phenindione	Anticoagulant; increased prothrombin and partial thromboplastin time in one infant; not used in United States
Radioactive iodine and other radiolabeled elements	Contraindications to breast feeding for various periods

[a]Medication is concentrated in human milk.
From the American Academy of Pediatrics and the American College of Obstetricians and Gynecologists (1997), with permission.

TABLE 17–5. Drugs of Choice for Breast Feeding Women

Drug Category	Drugs and Drug Groups of Choice
Analgesic drugs	Acetaminophen, flurbiprofen, ibuprofen, ketorolac, mefenamic acid, morphine, sumatriptan
Anticoagulant drugs	Acenocoumarol, heparin (regular and low-molecular-weight), warfarin
Antidepressant drugs	Sertraline, tricyclic antidepressant drugs
Antiepileptic drugs	Carbamazepine, phenytoin, valproic acid
Antihistamines (histamine H$_1$ blockers)	Loratadine
Antimicrobial drugs	Aminoglycosides, cephalosporins, macrolides, penicillins
β-Adrenergic antagonists	Labetalol, propranolol
Endocrine drugs	Insulin, levothyroxine, propylthiouracil
Glucocorticoids	Prednisolone and prednisone

Adapted from Ito (2000).

in breast milk to those in maternal plasma is called the milk-to-plasma drug-concentration ratio. Most drugs have a milk-to-plasma ratio of 1 or less; about 25 percent have ratios of more than 1, and about 15 percent have ratios greater than 2 (Ito, 2000).

The American Academy of Pediatrics and the American College of Obstetricians and Gynecologists (1997) have provided a list of drugs and other chemicals that are contraindicated during pregnancy (Table 17–4). Shown in Table 17–5 is a list of drugs of choice for breast feeding women.

BREAST FEVER. For the first 24 hours after the development of the lacteal secretion, it is not unusual for the breasts to become distended, firm, and nodular. These findings may be accompanied by a transient elevation of temperature. Puerperal fever from breast engorgement is common. Almeida and Kitay (1986) reported that 13 percent of all postpartum women had fever from this cause, and it ranged from 37.8 to 39°C. Fever seldom persisted for longer than 4 to 16 hours. The incidence and severity of breast engorgement, and fever associated with it, were lower if treatment was given for lactation suppression. Such fevers are particularly worrisome if infection cannot be excluded in women who have recently undergone cesarean delivery. **Other causes of fever, especially those due to infection, must be excluded.**

Treatment consists of supporting the breasts with a binder or brassiere, applying an ice bag, and an analgesic. Pumping of the breast or manual expression of milk may be necessary at first, but in a few days the condition is usually alleviated and the infant is able to nurse normally.

MASTITIS. Parenchymatous infection of the mammary glands is a rare complication antepartum but is occasionally observed during the puerperium and lactation. Stehman (1990) cited an incidence of 2 percent, which is much higher than our experiences. Symptoms of suppurative mastitis seldom appear before the end of the first week postpartum and, as a rule, not until the third or fourth week. Infection almost invariably is unilateral and marked engorgement usually precedes the inflammation, the first sign of which is chills or actual rigor, soon followed by fever and tachycardia. The breast becomes hard and reddened, and the woman complains of pain. About 10 percent of women with mastitis develop an abscess, and constitutional symptoms attending a mammary abscess are severe. The breast is somewhat harder than usual and more or less painful, but constitutional symptoms are either lacking or very slight. In such circumstances, the first indication of the true diagnosis often is afforded by the detection of fluctuation. Sonography may be helpful to detect an abscess.

ETIOLOGY. The most common offending organism is *Staphylococcus aureus,* and Matheson and colleagues (1988) cultured this organism from 40 percent of women with mastitis. Other commonly isolated organisms are coagulase-negative staphylococci and viridans streptococci. Rench and Baker (1989) reported an unusual case in which mother and male infant both developed mastitis and the mother a breast abscess caused by group B streptococcus. The immediate source of the organisms that cause mastitis is almost always the nursing infant's nose and throat. At the time of nursing, the organism enters the breast through the nipple at the site of a fissure or abrasion, which may be quite small. Whether the bacteria commonly cause mastitis simply by entering the lactiferous ducts of the breast with completely intact integument is not clear. In cases of true mastitis, the offending organism can usually be cultured from breast milk. Toxic shock syndrome has been reported in a woman with a puerperal breast abscess from which *S. aureus* was cultured (Demey and associates, 1989).

Suppurative mastitis among nursing mothers has at times reached epidemic levels. Such outbreaks most often coincide with the appearance of a new strain of antibiotic-resistant *Staphylococcus,* an example being methicillin-resistant *S. aureus* (MRSA). Typically, the infant becomes infected after contact with nursery personnel who are colonized. Attendants' hands are the major source of contamination of the newborn. The colonization of staphylococci in the infant may be totally asymptomatic or may locally involve the umbilicus or the skin. Occasionally the organisms cause a life-threatening systemic infection.

TREATMENT. Abscess formation is more common if *S. aureus* causes infection (Matheson and associates, 1988). Provided that appropriate therapy is started before suppuration begins, the infection usually resolves within 48 hours. Before initiating antimicrobial therapy, milk should be expressed from the affected breast onto a swab and cultured. By so doing, the organism can be identified and its antimicrobial sensitivities ascertained. Results of such cultures also provide information mandatory for a successful program for surveillance of nosocomial infections. The initial choice of antimicrobial will undoubtedly be influenced to a considerable degree by the current experiences with staphylococcal infections

at the institution. Many staphylococcal infections are caused by organisms sensitive to penicillin or a cephalosporin. Dicloxacillin (500 mg orally four times daily) may be started empirically (Hindle, 1994). Erythromycin is given to women who are penicillin sensitive. If the infection is caused by resistant, penicillinase-producing staphylococci, or if resistant organisms are suspected while awaiting the results of culture, an antimicrobial such as vancomycin, which is effective against methicillin-resistant staphylococci, should be given. Even though clinical response may be prompt and striking, treatment should be continued for about 7 to 10 days.

Marshall and colleagues (1975) demonstrated the importance of continued breast feeding. They reported that the only three abscesses that developed in 65 women with mastitis were in 15 women who chose to wean their infants. Thomsen and co-workers (1984) observed that vigorous milk expression was sufficient treatment alone in half of women with mastitis. Early therapy and continued lactation was successful in avoiding abscess formation in all 20 women described by Niebyl and co-investigators (1978). If the infected breast is too tender to allow suckling, gently pumping until nursing can be resumed is recommended. Sometimes the infant will not nurse on the inflamed breast. This is probably not related to any changes in the taste of the milk, but is secondary to engorgement and edema, which can make the areola harder to grip. Pumping can alleviate this. When nursing bilaterally, it is best to begin suckling on the uninvolved breast. This allows let-down to commence before moving to the tender breast.

BREAST ABSCESS. Clinical suspicion for abscess development is either from failure of defervescence within 48 to 72 hours or development of a palpable mass. Sonography may be helpful. Surgical drainage is essential and general anesthesia is usually required. The incision should be made corresponding to skin lines for a good cosmetic result (Stehman, 1990). In early cases, a single incision over the most dependent portion of the area of fluctuation is usually sufficient, but multiple abscesses require several incisions and a finger should be inserted to break up the walls of the locules. The resulting cavity is loosely packed with gauze, which should be replaced at the end of 24 hours by a smaller pack.

More recently, ultrasonic-guided aspiration using local anesthesia has been described. Karstrup and colleagues (1993) successfully treated 18 of 19 women with such an approach, and 10 were treated on an outpatient basis.

GALACTOCELE. Very exceptionally, as the result of the clogging of a duct by inspissated secretion, milk may accumulate in one or more lobes of the breast. The amount is ordinarily limited, but an excess may form a fluctuant mass that may give rise to pressure symptoms. They may resolve spontaneously or require aspiration.

SUPERNUMERARY BREASTS. One in every few hundred women has one or more accessory breasts (*polymastia*). The supernumerary breasts may be so small as to be mistaken for pigmented moles, or when without a nipple, for a lipoma. They rarely attain considerable size. They are likely to be situated in pairs on either side of the midline of the thoracic or abdominal walls, usually below the main breasts. They are also found in the axillae, and more rarely on other portions of the body such as the shoulder, flank, groin, or thigh. When arranged symmetrically, two or four are most common, although 10 have been described. Polymastia has no obstetrical significance, although occasionally the enlargement of supernumerary breasts in the axillae may result in considerable discomfort.

ABNORMALITIES OF THE NIPPLES. In some women, the lactiferous ducts open directly into a depression at the center of the areola. In marked cases of depressed nipple, nursing is out of the question. When the depression is not very deep, the breast may occasionally be made available by use of a breast pump.

More frequently, the nipple, although not depressed, is greatly inverted. In such a case, daily attempts should be made during the last few months of pregnancy to draw the nipple out, using traction with fingers.

Nipples that are normal in shape and size may become fissured. In such cases, the fissures almost invariably render nursing painful, sometimes with a deleterious influence upon the secretory function. Moreover, such lesions provide a convenient portal of entry for pyogenic bacteria. For these reasons, every effort should be made to heal such fissures, particularly by protecting them from further injury with a nipple shield and topical medication. If such measures are of no avail, the infant should not be permitted to nurse on the affected side. Instead, the breast should be emptied regularly with a suitable pump until the lesions are completely healed.

ABNORMALITIES OF SECRETION. There are marked individual variations in the amount of milk secreted, many of which are dependent not upon the general health and appearance of the woman but upon the development of the glandular portions of the breasts. Very rarely, there is complete lack of mammary secretion (*agalactia*). As a rule, it is possible to express a small amount from the nipple on the third or fourth day of the puerperium. Occasionally, the mammary secretion is excessive (*polygalactia*).

CARE OF THE MOTHER DURING THE PUERPERIUM

HOSPITAL CARE

ATTENTION IMMEDIATELY AFTER LABOR. For the first hour after delivery, blood pressure and pulse should be taken every 15 minutes, or more frequently if indicated. The amount of vaginal bleeding is monitored, and the fundus should be palpated to ensure that it is well contracted. If relaxation is detected, the uterus should be massaged through the abdominal wall until it remains contracted. Blood may accumulate within the uterus without external bleeding. This may be detected early by identifying uterine enlargement through frequent fundal palpation during the first few hours postpartum. Because the likelihood of significant hemorrhage is greatest immediately postpartum, even in normal cases, a trained attendant should remain with the mother for at least 1 hour after completion of the third stage of labor. Identification and management of postpartum hemorrhage is discussed in Chapter 25.

Following regional analgesia or general anesthesia, the mother should be observed in an appropriately equipped and staffed recovery area.

EARLY AMBULATION. Immediately after World War II, early ambulation became an accepted puerperal practice. Women are now out of bed within a few hours after delivery. The many advantages of early ambulation are confirmed by numerous well-controlled studies. Bladder complications and constipation are less frequent. Importantly, early ambulation has also reduced the frequency of puerperal venous thrombosis and pulmonary embolism (Toglia and Weg, 1996; see also Chap. 46). For at least the first ambulation, an attendant should be present if the woman should become syncopal.

CARE OF THE VULVA. The patient should be instructed to cleanse the vulva from anterior to posterior (vulva toward anus). An ice bag applied to the perineum may help reduce edema and discomfort during the first several hours after episiotomy repair. Beginning about 24 hours after delivery, moist heat as provided with warm sitz baths can be used to reduce local discomfort. Tub bathing after uncomplicated delivery is allowed.

BLADDER FUNCTION. Bladder filling after delivery may be quite variable. In most hospitals, intravenous fluids are infused during labor and for an hour after delivery. Oxytocin, in doses that have an antidiuretic effect, is commonly infused after placental delivery. As a consequence of infused fluid and the sudden withdrawal of the antidiuretic effect of oxytocin, rapid bladder filling is common. Moreover, both bladder sensation and its capability to empty spontaneously may be diminished by anesthesia, especially conduction analgesia, as well as by episiotomy, lacerations, or hematomas. It is not surprising, therefore, that urinary retention with bladder overdistention is a common complication of the early puerperium.

Prevention of overdistention demands observation after delivery to ensure that the bladder does not overfill and that with each voiding it empties adequately. The bladder may be palpated as a cystic mass suprapubically, or the enlarged bladder may be evident abdominally only indirectly as a consequence of elevating the uterine fundus above the umbilicus.

If the woman has not voided within 4 hours after delivery, it is likely that she cannot. The woman who has trouble voiding initially is likely to have further trouble. At times, an indwelling catheter is necessary to prevent overdistension. The likelihood of hematomas of the genital tract must be considered when the woman cannot void. Whenever the bladder becomes overdistended, an indwelling catheter should be left in place until the factors causing the retention have abated. Harris and colleagues (1977) reported that 40 percent of such women will develop bacteriuria; thus, a short course of antimicrobial therapy seems reasonable after catheter removal.

In cases of bladder overdistention, it usually is best to leave an indwelling catheter in place for at least 24 hours, so as to empty the bladder completely and prevent prompt recurrence as well as to allow recovery of normal bladder tone and sensation. When the catheter is removed, it is necessary subsequently to demonstrate ability to void appropriately. If the woman cannot void after 4 hours, she should be catheterized and urine volume measured. If there is more than 200 mL of urine, it is apparent that the bladder is not functioning appropriately. The catheter should be left in place and the bladder drained for another day. If less than 200 mL of urine is obtained, the catheter can be removed and the bladder rechecked subsequently as described.

BOWEL FUNCTION. At times, the lack of a bowel movement is no more than the expected consequence of an efficient cleansing enema administered before delivery. With both early ambulation and early feeding, constipation has become much less of a problem.

SUBSEQUENT DISCOMFORT. The discomfort from cesarean delivery, its causes, and its management are considered in Chapter 23. During the first few days after vaginal delivery, the mother may be uncomfortable for a variety of reasons, including afterpains, episiotomy and lacerations, breast engorgement, and at times, postspinal puncture headache. It is helpful to provide

codeine, 60 mg; aspirin, 600 mg; or acetaminophen, 500 mg, at intervals as frequent as every 3 hours during the first few days after delivery. Uterine contractions are commonly accentuated during nursing, giving rise at times to troublesome afterpains.

An episiotomy or lacerations may be uncomfortable, as discussed in Chapter 13 (p. 325). Early application of an ice bag may minimize swelling and discomfort. Most women also appear to obtain a measure of relief from the periodic application of a local anesthetic spray. Severe discomfort may indicate that a sizable hematoma has formed in the genital tract and warrants careful examination, especially whenever analgesics do not provide relief. The episiotomy incision normally is firmly healed and nearly asymptomatic by the third week.

MILD DEPRESSION. It is fairly common for a mother to exhibit some degree of depression a few days after delivery. The transient depression, or *postpartum blues,* most likely is the consequence of a number of factors. Prominent in its genesis are:

1. The emotional letdown that follows the excitement and fears that most women experience during pregnancy and delivery.
2. The discomforts of the early puerperium.
3. Fatigue from loss of sleep during labor and postpartum in most hospital settings.
4. Anxiety over her capabilities for caring for her infant after leaving the hospital.
5. Fears that she has become less attractive.

In the great majority of cases, effective treatment need be nothing more than anticipation, recognition, and reassurance.

This mild disorder is self-limited and usually remits after 2 to 3 days, although it sometimes persists for up to 10 days. Should postpartum blues persist, or worsen, then careful attention is given to searching for symptoms of depression, which may require prompt consultation (Chap. 53, p. 1421). In a preliminary study from Parkland Hospital, we found that symptoms of depression were actually present during pregnancy in 50 percent of women who developed postpartum depression. This raises the possibility that postpartum depression may be a manifestation of an underlying depressive disorder (Nielsen and colleagues, 2000).

ABDOMINAL WALL RELAXATION. An abdominal binder is unnecessary. It does not help restore the mother's figure. If the abdomen is unusually flabby or pendulous, an ordinary girdle is often satisfactory. Exercises to restore abdominal wall tone may be started any time after vaginal delivery and as soon as abdominal soreness diminishes after cesarean delivery.

DIET. There are no dietary restrictions for women who have been delivered vaginally. Two hours after a normal vaginal delivery, if there are no complications likely to necessitate an anesthetic, the woman should be given something to drink and eat if she desires. The diet of lactating women, compared with that consumed during pregnancy, should be increased in calories and protein, as recommended by the Food and Nutrition Board of the National Research Council (Chap. 8, p. 173). If the mother does not breast feed, her dietary requirements are the same as for a nonpregnant woman.

It is standard practice in our hospitals to continue iron supplementation for at least 3 months after delivery and to check the hematocrit at the first postpartum visit.

IMMUNIZATIONS. The D-negative woman who is not isoimmunized and whose baby is D-positive is given 300 μg of anti-D immune globulin shortly after delivery (Chap. 39, p. 1066). Women who are not already immune to rubella are excellent candidates for vaccination before discharge (Chap. 10, p. 240). Unless it is contraindicated, a diphtheria-tetanus toxoid booster injection may be administered at this time. Beginning in 1991, women delivered at Parkland Hospital have also been given measles (rubeola) immunization prior to postpartum discharge. This recommendation is based upon:

1. The failure of previously immunized persons to develop protective immunity (Centers for Disease Control, 1989).
2. Significant outbreaks of measles in the community.
3. Maternal morbidity and mortality due to measles pneumonitis.

TIME OF DISCHARGE. Following vaginal delivery, if there are **no complications,** hospitalization is seldom warranted for more than 48 hours. Before discharge, the woman should receive instructions concerning the anticipated normal physiological changes of the puerperium, including lochia patterns, weight loss due to diuresis, and when to expect milk let-down. She also should receive instructions concerning what to do if she becomes febrile, has excessive vaginal bleeding, or develops leg pain, swelling, or tenderness. Any shortness of breath or chest pains warrant immediate concern.

EARLY DISCHARGE. As discussed in Chapter 1, the issue of third-party payers dictating inappropriately short lengths of hospital stays following labor and delivery has been regulated by Federal law. In 2000, medical consensus recommends hospital stays of up to 48 hours following uncomplicated vaginal delivery and up to 96 hours following uncomplicated cesarean delivery (American Academy of Pediatrics and the American College of Obstetricians and Gynecologists, 1997). In 1980, the average stay for a vaginal delivery was 3.2 days. This had decreased to 1.7 days by 1995, but then increased to 2.1 days by 1997 (Neergaard, 1999). Despite this, in 1997, a fourth of new mothers (951,000) had a hospital stay of one day or less. This seems acceptable if this was indeed their choice and not forced upon these women. It is likely, however, that the timing of discharge has greater significance for the newborn infant.

CONTRACEPTION. During the hospital stay, a concerted effort should be made to provide family planning education. Steroidal contraception and its effects on lactation are discussed on page 412. Other forms of contraception are discussed in Chapters 58 and 59.

CARE AT HOME

COITUS. There is no definite time after delivery when coitus should be resumed. Resumption of intercourse **too soon** may prove to be unpleasant, if not frankly painful, due to incomplete uterine involution and incomplete healing of the episiotomy or lacerations. Glazener (1997) surveyed resumption of sexual activity in 1075 British women and found that 70 percent had intercourse within 8 weeks of delivery. The median interval between delivery and intercourse was 5 weeks but the range was 1 to 12 weeks. Difficulties frequently cited for not resuming intercourse included concern about perineal pain, bleeding, and fatigue.

In another survey, Barrett and colleagues (2000) reported that almost 90 percent of 484 primiparous women had resumed sexual activity by 6 months. Although 65 percent of these reported problems, only 15 percent discussed these with a professional.

The best rule to follow is one of common sense. After 2 weeks, coitus may be resumed *based upon the patient's desire and comfort.* The women should be advised that breast feeding will cause a prolonged period of suppressed estrogen production with a resulting vaginal atrophy and dryness. Such a physiological state results in decreased vaginal lubrication during sexual arousal.

INFANT FOLLOW-UP. Arrangements must be made to insure that the neonate receives appropriate follow-up care. Any neonate discharged early should be term, normal, and have stable vital signs. All laboratory studies should be normal, including direct Coombs test, bilirubin, hemoglobin and hematocrit, and blood glucose. The maternal serological test for syphilis and hepatitis B surface antigen should be nonreactive. Initial hepatitis B vaccine should be administered, and all screening tests required by law should be performed. These always include testing for phenylketonuria (PKU) and hypothyroidism. If subsequent phenylketonuria retesting is required after the neonate has consumed milk the mother

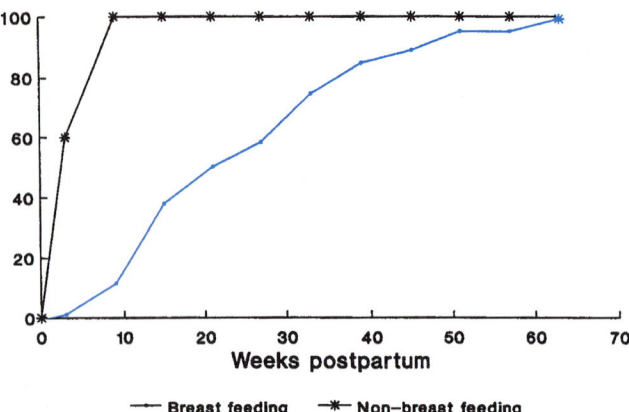

FIGURE 17–5. Cumulative proportion of breast feeding and non–breast feeding women who ovulated during the first 60 weeks of the puerperium. (From Campbell and Gray, 1993, with permission.)

must be so instructed. Finally, the importance of subsequent neonatal and well-baby care should be stressed and an emphasis placed on infant immunizations.

RETURN OF MENSTRUATION AND OVULATION. If the woman does not nurse her child, menses usually return within 6 to 8 weeks. At times, however, it is difficult clinically to assign a specific date to the first menstrual period after delivery. A minority of women bleed small to moderate amounts intermittently, starting soon after delivery. Menses may not appear so long as the infant is nursed, but great variations are observed. In lactating women, the first period may occur as early as the second or as late as the 18th month after delivery.

Sharman (1966), by means of histologic dating of the endometrium, identified ovulation as early as 42 days after delivery; Perez and associates (1972) did so as early as 36 days. Moreover, a corpus luteum has been observed 6 weeks after delivery at the time of sterilization. Thus, the necessity for instituting contraceptive techniques for sexually active women is obvious.

Ovulation is much less frequent in women who breast feed compared with those who do not. Nonetheless, pregnancy can occur with lactation. Campbell and Gray (1993) used daily urine specimens to determine ovulation in 92 women. This study is the first detailed description of the return of postpartum ovarian activity in breast feeding and non–breast feeding women in the United States. Shown in Figure 17–5 is the cumulative proportion of women spontaneously ovulating postpartum. Clearly, there is delayed resumption of ovulation with breast feeding, although as already mentioned, early ovulation is not precluded by persistent lactation. Other findings included the following:

1. Resumption of ovulation was frequently marked by return of normal menstrual bleeding.

2. Breast feeding episodes lasting 15 minutes seven times each day delayed resumption of ovulation.
3. Ovulation can occur without bleeding.
4. Bleeding can be anovulatory.

They estimated that the risk of pregnancy in breast feeding women was approximately 4 percent per year.

LATE MATERNAL MORBIDITY. Maternal morbidity after discharge is poorly characterized and underresearched. MacArthur and colleagues (1991), while studying the sequelae of labor epidural analgesia, uncovered a vast reservoir of previously unreported morbidity of considerable duration in puerperal women. Glazener and co-workers (1995), in an unprecedented investigation, surveyed health problems in 1249 British women after discharge and up to 18 months following delivery. Although only 3 percent of these women required readmission to the hospital within 8 weeks of delivery, 87 percent had lesser health problems during the first 8 weeks postpartum, and 76 percent of the women continued to have a variety of problems for up to 18 months (Table 17–6). Overall, the proportion of women with self-perceived health problems declined with time, indicating health did improve, although more slowly than generally assumed. Clearly, maternal morbidity following delivery is extensive and heretofore underrecognized. Glazener and co-authors (1995) called for a greater awareness of the needs of puerperal women as they convalesce from birthing.

TABLE 17–6. Morbidity (Percent) Reported by Puerperal Women After Hospital Discharge

Maternal Morbidity	Discharge–8 Weeks Postpartum	2–18 Months Postpartum
Tiredness	59	54
Breast problems	36	20
Anemia	25	7
Backache	24	20
Hemorrhoids	23	15
Headache	22	15
Tearfulness/depression	21	17
Constipation	20	7
Stitches breaking down	16	—
Vaginal discharge	15	8
Others[a]	2–7	1–8
At least one of the above	87	76

[a]Others include abnormal bleeding, urinary incontinence, hypertension, urinary infection, difficulty voiding, and epidural side effects.
From Glazener and co-workers (1995), with permission.

FOLLOW-UP CARE. By the time of discharge, women who had a normal delivery and puerperium can resume most activities, including bathing, driving, and household functions. Jimenez and Newton (1979) tabulated cross-cultural information on 202 societies from different international geographic regions. Postnatally, most societies did not restrict maternal work activity, and about half expected a return to full duties within 2 weeks. Tulman and Fawcett (1988) reported, however, that only half of women regained their usual level of energy by 6 weeks postpartum. Women who delivered vaginally were twice as likely to have normal energy levels at this time compared with those who had cesarean deliveries. Ideally, the care and nurturing received by the neonate should be provided by the mother with ample help from the father. For the mother to provide this care, her presence at home with the infant precludes her early return to full-time work or school.

Since 1969, puerperal women at Parkland Hospital have been given appointments for follow-up examination during the third postpartum week. This has proven quite satisfactory both to identify any abnormalities of the later puerperium as well as to initiate contraceptive practices. Estrogen plus progestin oral contraceptives started at this time have proven to be effective without increased morbidity. Moreover, the frequencies of uterine perforation, expulsions, and pregnancies when intrauterine devices were inserted during the third week postpartum were no greater than when the devices were inserted 3 months or more postpartum. Family planning techniques and follow-up care are further discussed in Chapters 58 and 59.

THROMBOEMBOLIC DISEASE. Thromboembolic disease traditionally was considered unique to the puerperium; however, this is no longer true. The frequency of deep-vein thrombosis complicating pregnancy and the puerperium has decreased in recent years, and now more cases are identified during the antepartum period (Gherman and colleagues, 1999). Deep-vein thrombosis and pulmonary embolism are discussed in Chapter 46 (p. 1235).

PELVIC VENOUS THROMBOSIS. During the puerperium, a thrombus may transiently form in any of the dilated pelvic veins, and possibly does so relatively often. Without associated thrombophlebitis, these thrombi likely do not incite clinical signs or symptoms unless the thrombosis is extensive or pulmonary embolism follows. Unfortunately, these vessels appear to be the source of many of the massive and fatal pulmonary emboli that develop without warning in the puerperium. As discussed in Chapter 26 (p. 681), symptomatic puerperal pelvic thrombosis is most commonly associated with uterine infection.

OBSTETRICAL PARALYSIS. Pressure on branches of the lumbosacral plexus during labor may be manifest by complaints of intense neuralgia or cramplike pains extending down one or both legs as soon as the head begins to descend the pelvis. In some instances, the pain continues after delivery and is accompanied by paralysis of the muscles supplied by the external popliteal nerve. These include the flexors of the ankles and the extensors of the toes, and result in weakened ankle dorsiflexion and footdrop. Less commonly, the femoral, obturator, or sciatic nerves may be involved. In some instances, the gluteal muscles are affected.

Separation of the symphysis pubis or one of the sacroiliac synchondroses during labor may be followed by pain and marked interference with locomotion.

REFERENCES

Adrinopoulos GC, Mendenhall HW: Prostaglandin $F_{2\alpha}$ in the management of delayed postpartum hemorrhage. Am J Obstet Gynecol 146:217, 1983

Ahdoot D, Van Nostrand KM, Nguyen NJ, Tewari DS, Kuraski T, DiSaia PJ, Rose GS: The effect of route of delivery on regression of abnormal cervical cytologic findings in the postpartum period. Am J Obstet Gynecol 178:1116, 1998

Almeida OD Jr, Kitay DZ: Lactation suppression and puerperal fever. Am J Obstet Gynecol 154:940, 1986

American Academy of Pediatrics, Committee on Nutrition: Nutrition and lactation. Pediatrics 68:435, 1981

American Academy of Pediatrics, Committee on Nutrition: Follow-up or weaning formulas. Pediatrics 83:1067, 1989

American Academy of Pediatrics, Work Group on Breastfeeding. Breastfeeding and the use of human milk. Pediatrics 100:1035, 1997

American Academy of Pediatrics and the American College of Obstetricians and Gynecologists: Guidelines for Perinatal Care, 4th ed. Washington, DC, 1997

American College of Obstetricians and Gynecologists: Breast feeding: Maternal and infant aspects. Education Bulletin No. 258, July, 2000

Anderson WR, Davis J: Placental site involution. Am J Obstet Gynecol 102:23, 1968

Andolf E, Iosif CS, Jörgensen, Rydhstrom H: Insidious urinary retention after vaginal delivery: Prevalence and symptoms at follow-up in a population-based study. Gynecol Obstet Invest 38:51, 1994

Andrew AC, Bulmer JN, Wells M, Morrison L, Buckley CH: Subinvolution of the uteroplacental arteries in the human placental bed. Histopathology 15:395, 1989

Andrews MC: Epithelial changes in the puerperal fallopian tube. Am J Obstet Gynecol 62:28, 1951

Avery GB, Fletcher AB: Nutrition. In Avery GB (ed): Neonatology, Pathophysiology and Management of the Newborn, 3rd ed. Philadelphia, Lippincott, 1987, p 1192

Barrett G, Pendry E, Peacock J, Victor C, Thakar R, Manyonda I: Women's sexual health after childbirth. BJOG 107:186, 2000

Beer AE, Billingham RE: The immunobiology of mammalian reproduction. Englewood Cliffs, NJ, Prentice-Hall, 1976, p 198

Bertotto A, Gerli R, Fabietti G, Crupi S, Arcangeli C, Scalis

F, Vaccaro R: Human breast milk T lymphocytes display the phenotype and functional characteristics of memory T cells. Eur J Immunol 20:1877, 1990

Brasil AL, Vitolo MR, Lopez FA, De Nobrega FJ: Fat and protein composition of mature milk in adolescents. J Adolesc Health 12:365, 1991

Campbell OMR, Gray RH: Characteristics and determinants of postpartum ovarian function in women in the United States. Am J Obstet Gynecol 169:55, 1993

Centers for Disease Control: Measles prevention: Recommendations of the Immunization Practice Advisory Committee. MMWR (suppl) 38:1, 1989

Chesley LC, Valenti C, Uichano L: Alterations in body fluid compartments and exchangeable sodium in early puerperium. Am J Obstet Gynecol 77:1054, 1959

Chez RA, Friedman AK: Offering effective breastfeeding advice. Contemp Ob/Gyn 45:32, 2000

Cravioto A, Tello A, Villafan H, Ruiz J, del Vedovo S, Neeser JR: Inhibition of localized adhesion of enteropathogenic Escherichia coli to HEp-2 cells by immunoglobulin and oligosaccharide fractions of human colostrum and breast milk. J Infect Dis 163:1247, 1991

Demey HE, Hautekeete MI, Buytaert P, Bossaert LL: Mastitis and toxic shock syndrome. A case report. Acta Obstet Gynecol Scand 68:87, 1989

Dewey KG, Lovelady CA, Nommsen-Rivers LA, McCrory MA, Lonnerdal B: A randomized study of the effects of aerobic exercise by lactating women on breast-milk volume and composition. N Engl J Med 330:449, 1994

Food and Drug Administration: Bromocriptine indication withdrawn. FDA Medical Bulletin, 24:2, 1994

Food and Drug Administration, Fertility and Maternal Health Drugs Advisory Committee: Summary minutes. Prevention of post-partum breast engorgement with sex hormones and bromocriptine. Washington, DC: US Food and Drug Administration, 1989

Gherman RB, Goodwin TM, Leung B, Byrne JD, Hethumumi R, Montoro M: Incidence, clinical characteristics, and timing of objectively diagnosed venous thromboembolism during pregnancy. Obstet Gynecol 94:730, 1999

Giovannini M, Agostoni C, Salari PC: The role of lipids in nutrition during the first months of life. J Int Med Res 19:351, 1991

Glazener CMA: Sexual function after childbirth: Women's experiences, persistent morbidity and lack of professional recognition. Br J Obstet Gynaecol 104:330, 1997

Glazener CM, Abdalla M, Stroud P, Naji S, Templeton, A, Russell IT: Postnatal maternal morbidity: Extent, causes, prevention and treatment. Br J Obstet Gynaecol 102:282, 1995

Greene GW, Smiciklas-Wright H, Scholl TO, Karp RJ: Postpartum weight change: How much of the weight gained in pregnancy will be lost after delivery? Obstet Gynecol 71:701, 1988

Harris RE, Thomas VL, Hui GW: Postpartum surveillance for urinary tract infection: Patients at risk of developing pyelonephritis after catheterization. South Med J 70:1273, 1977

Hartmann PE, Prosser CG: Physiological basis of longitudinal changes in human milk yield and composition. Fed Proc 43:2448, 1984

Hindle WH: Other benign breast problems. Clin Obstet Gynecol 37:916, 1994

Hughes EC: Obstetric-Gynecologic Terminology, 1st ed. American College of Obstetricians and Gynecologists. Philadelphia, Davis, 1972

Hurst NM: Lactation after augmentation mammoplasty. Obstet Gynecol 87:30, 1996

Institute of Medicine: Nutrition During Pregnancy. Washington, DC, National Academy of Science, 1990, p 202

Ito S: Drug therapy for breast-feeding women. N Engl J Med 343:118, 2000

Jimenez MH, Newton N: Activity and work during pregnancy and the postpartum period: A cross-cultural study of 202 societies. Am J Obstet Gynecol 135:171, 1979

Karstrup S, Solvin J, Nolsoe CP, Nilsson P, Khattar S, Loren I, Nilsson A, Court-Payen M: Acute puerperal breast abscesses. US-guided drainage. Radiology 188:807, 1993

Kerr-Wilson RH, Thompson SW, Orr JW, Davis RO, Cloud GA: Effect of labor on the postpartum bladder. Obstet Gynecol 64:115, 1984

Koldovsky O, Britton J, Grimes J, Schaudies P: Milk-borne epidermal growth factor (EGF) and its processing in developing gastrointestinal tract. Endocr Regul 25:58, 1991

Lee CY, Madrazo B, Drukker BH: Ultrasonic evaluation of the postpartum uterus in the management of postpartum bleeding. Obstet Gynecol 58:227, 1981

Lovelady CA, Garner KE, Moreno KL, Williams JP: The effect of weight loss in overweight, lactating women on the growth of their infant. N Engl J Med 342:449, 2000

MacArthur C, Lewis M, Knox EG: Health after childbirth. Br J Obstet Gynaecol 98:1193, 1991

Marshall BR, Hepper JK, Zirbel CC: Sporadic puerperal mastitis—An infection that need not interrupt lactation. JAMA 344:1377, 1975

Matheson I, Aursnes I, Horgen M, Aabø Ø, Melby K: Bacteriological findings and clinical symptoms in relation to clinical outcome in puerperal mastitis. Acta Obstet Gynecol Scand 67:723, 1988

McCleary MJ: Epidermal growth factor: An important constituent of human milk. J Hum Lact 7:123, 1991

McNeilly AS, Robinson ICA, Houston MJ, Howie PW: Release of oxytocin and prolactin in response to suckling. BMJ (Clin Res Ed) 286:257, 1983

Mennella JA, Beauchamp GK: The transfer of alcohol to human milk: Effects on flavor and the infants' behavior. N Engl J Med 325:981, 1991

Morgans D: Bromocriptine and postpartum lactation suppression. Br J Obstet Gynaecol 102:851, 1995

Nduati R, John G, Mbori-Hgacha D, Richardson B, Overbaugh J, Mwatha A, Ndinya-Achola J, Bwayo J, Onyango FE, Hughes J, Kreiss J: Effect of breastfeeding and formula feeding on transmission of HIV-1: A randomized clinical trial. JAMA 283:1167, 2000

Neergaard L: Longer stays for new moms. Abcnews.go.com/sections/living/dailynews/childbirth 990609, 1999

Nelson SE, Ziegler EE, Copeland AM, Edwards BB, Fomon SJ: Lack of adverse reactions to iron-fortified formula. Pediatrics 81:360, 1988

Newburg DS, Peterson JA, Ruiz-Palacias GM, Matson DO, Morrow AL, Shults J, Guerrero ML, Chaturvedi P, Newburg SO, Scallan CD, Taylor MR, Ceriani RL, Pickering LK: Role of human-milk lactadherin in protection against symptomatic rotavirus infection. Lancet 351:1160, 1998

Newton M, Bradford WM: Postpartal blood loss. Obstet Gynecol 17:229, 1961

Niebyl JR, Spence MR, Parmley TH: Sporadic (nonepidemic) puerperal mastitis. J Reprod Med 20:97, 1978

Nielsen-Forman D, Videbech P, Hedegaard M, Salvig J, Secher NJ: Postpartum depression: Identification of women at risk. BJOG 107:1210, 2000

Ogunleye A, Fakoya AT, Niizeki S, Tojo H, Sasajima I, Kobayashi M, Tateishi S, Yamaguchi K: Fatty acid composition of breast milk from Nigerian and Japanese women. J Nutr Sci Vitaminol (Tokyo) 37:435, 1991

Oppenheimer LW, Sherriff EA, Goodman JDS, Shah D, James CE: The duration of lochia. Br J Obstet Gynaecol 93:754, 1986

Perez A, Vela P, Masnick GS, Potter RG: First ovulation after childbirth: The effect of breastfeeding. Am J Obstet Gynecol 114:1041, 1972

Porter JC: Proceedings: Hormonal regulation of breast development and activity. J Invest Dermatol 63:85, 1974

Rench MA, Baker CJ: Group B streptococcal breast abscess in a mother and mastitis in her infant. Obstet Gynecol 73:875, 1989

Robson SC, Dunlop W, Hunter S: Haemodynamic changes during the early puerperium. BMJ (Clin Res Ed) 294:1065, 1987

Saito S, Maruyama M, Kato Y, Moriyama I, Ichijo M: Detection of IL-6 in human milk and its involvement in IgA production. J Reprod Immunol 20:267, 1991

Samra HK, Ganguly NK, Mahajan RC: Human milk containing specific secretory IgA inhibits binding of *Giardia lamblia* to nylon and glass surfaces. J Diarrhoeal Dis Res 9:100, 1991

Schauberger CW, Rooney BL, Brimer LM: Factors that influence weight loss in the puerperium. Obstet Gynecol 79:424, 1992

Sharman A: Ovulation in the post-partum period. Excerpta Medica International Congress Series, No. 133, 1966, p 158

Sharman A: Postpartum regeneration of the human endometrium. J Anat 87:1, 1953

Spitz AM, Lee NC, Peterson HB: Treatment for lactation suppression: Little progress in one hundred years. Am J Obstet Gynecol 179:1485, 1998

Stehman FB: Infections and inflammations of the breast. In Hindle WH (eds): Breast Disease for Gynecologists. Norwalk, CT, Appleton & Lange, 1990, p 151

Thomsen AC, Espersen T, Maigaard S: Course and treatment of milk stasis, noninfectious inflammation of the breast, and infectious mastitis in nursing women. Am J Obstet Gynecol 149:492, 1984

Toglia MR, Weg JG: Venous thromboembolism and pregnancy. N Engl J Med 335:108, 1996

Tulman L, Fawcett J: Return of functional ability after childbirth. Nurs Res 37:77, 1988

Viktrup L, Lose G, Rolff M, Barfoed K: The symptom of stress incontinence caused by pregnancy or delivery in primipara. Obstet Gynecol 79:945, 1992

Visness CM, Kennedy KI, Ramos R: The duration and character of postpartum bleeding among breast-feeding women. Obstet Gynecol 89:159, 1997

Wager GP, Martin DH, Koutsky L, Eschenbach DA, Daling JR, Chiang WT, Alexander ER, Holmes KK: Puerperal infectious morbidity: Relationship to route of delivery and to antepartum *Chlamydia trachomatis* infection. Am J Obstet Gynecol 138:1028, 1980

Williams JW: Regeneration of the uterine mucosa after delivery with especial reference to the placental site. Am J Obstet Gynecol 22:664, 1931

Yaffe SJ: Introduction. In Briggs GG, Freeman RK, Yaffe SJ (eds): Drugs in Pregnancy and Lactation, 4th ed. Baltimore, Williams & Wilkins, 1994

Yip R, Binkin NJ, Fleshood L, Trowbridge FL: Declining prevalence of anemia among low-income children in the United States. JAMA 258:1619, 1987

Yip R, Reeves JD, Lönnerdal B, Keen CL, Dallman PR: Does iron supplementation compromise zinc nutrition in healthy infants? Am J Clin Nutr 42:683, 1985

Yuen BH: Prolactin in human milk: The influence of nursing and the duration of postpartum lactation. Am J Obstet Gynecol 158:583, 1988

Ziegler JB, Cooper DA, Johnston RO, Gold J: Postnatal transmission of AIDS-associated retrovirus from mother to infant. Lancet 1:896, 1985

V

SECTION

Abnormal Labor

18

Dystocia
Abnormal Labor and Fetopelvic Disproportion

Dystocia literally means difficult labor and it is characterized by abnormally slow progress of labor. As a generalization, abnormal labor is common whenever there is disproportion between the presenting part of the fetus and the birth canal. It is the consequence of four distinct abnormalities that may exist singly or in combination:

1. Abnormalities of the expulsive forces—either uterine forces insufficiently strong or inappropriately coordinated to efface and dilate the cervix (uterine dysfunction), or inadequate voluntary muscle effort during the second stage of labor.
2. Abnormalities of the maternal bony pelvis—that is, pelvic contraction.
3. Abnormalities of presentation, position, or development of the fetus, which are presented in Chapter 19.
4. Abnormalities of soft tissues of the reproductive tract that form an obstacle to fetal descent, which are presented in Chapter 35.

The Greek antonym for *eutocia,* or normal labor, is *dystocia* to signify abnormal labor or difficult childbirth. Dystocia can result from several distinct abnormalities involving the cervix, uterus, fetus, maternal bony pelvis, or other obstructions in the birth canal. These abnormalities have been mechanistically simplified by the American College of Obstetricians and Gynecologists (1995a) into three categories:

1. Abnormalities of the *powers* (uterine contractility and maternal expulsive effort).
2. Abnormalities involving the *passenger* (the fetus).
3. Abnormalities of the *passage* (the pelvis).

Common clinical findings in women with these labor abnormalities are summarized in Table 18–1.

OVERDIAGNOSIS OF DYSTOCIA

Quite often combinations of abnormalities shown in Table 18–1 interact to produce dysfunctional labor. To-

TABLE 18–1. Common Clinical Findings in Women with Ineffective Labor

Inadequate cervical dilation or fetal descent
Protracted labor—slow progress
Arrested labor—no progress
Inadequate expulsive effort—ineffective "pushing"
Fetopelvic disproportion
Excessive fetal size
Inadequate pelvic capacity
Malpresentation or position of the fetus
Ruptured membranes without labor

day, expressions such as *cephalopelvic disproportion* and *failure to progress* are often used to describe ineffective labors when cesarean delivery is necessary.

The expression *cephalopelvic disproportion* came into use prior to the 20th century to describe obstructed labor due to disparity between the dimensions of the fetal head and maternal pelvis such as to preclude vaginal delivery. This term, however, originated at a time when the main indication for cesarean delivery was overt pelvic contracture due to rickets (Olah and Neilson, 1994). Such true disproportion is now rare, and most disproportions are due to malposition of the fetal head—asynclitism or extension of the bony diameters of the fetal head, or to ineffective uterine contractions. True cephalopelvic disproportion is a tenuous diagnosis because two thirds or more of women diagnosed as having this disorder and delivered by cesarean subsequently deliver even larger infants vaginally (Chap. 23, p. 541).

Failure to progress in either spontaneous or stimulated labor has become an increasingly popular description of ineffectual labor. This term is used to include lack of progressive cervical dilatation or lack of fetal descent.

Dystocia is the most common current indication for primary cesarean delivery. Gifford and colleagues (2000) reported that lack of progress in labor was the reason for 68 percent of unplanned cesarean deliveries in cephalic presentations. Notzon and associates (1994) found that 12 percent of American women without prior cesarean were diagnosed as having dystocia requiring abdominal delivery in 1990, and the rate had increased from 7 percent in 1980. A similar change was also reported in the United Kingdom (Leitch and Walker, 1998). Because many repeat cesareans are done in pregnancies subsequent to primary operations done for dystocia, an estimated 50 to 60 percent of all cesarean births in the United States may be attributable to this diagnosis (Gifford and colleagues, 2000).

It is generally agreed that dystocia leading to cesarean delivery is overdiagnosed in the United States and elsewhere. Factors leading to increased use of cesarean delivery for dystocia, however, are controversial. Those implicated have included incorrect diagnosis of dystocia, epidural analgesia (Thorp and colleagues, 1993a), fear of litigation, and even obstetrician convenience (Fraser and co-workers, 1987; Lieberman and co-workers, 1996; Savage and Francome, 1994).

Variability in the criteria for diagnosis is a major determinant of the increase in cesarean deliveries for dystocia. For example, Gifford and colleagues (2000) found that almost 25 percent of the cesarean deliveries performed annually in the United States for lack of progress were in women with cervical dilatation of only 0 to 3 cm (Fig. 18–1). According to Stephenson (2000), this practice is contrary to recommendations of the

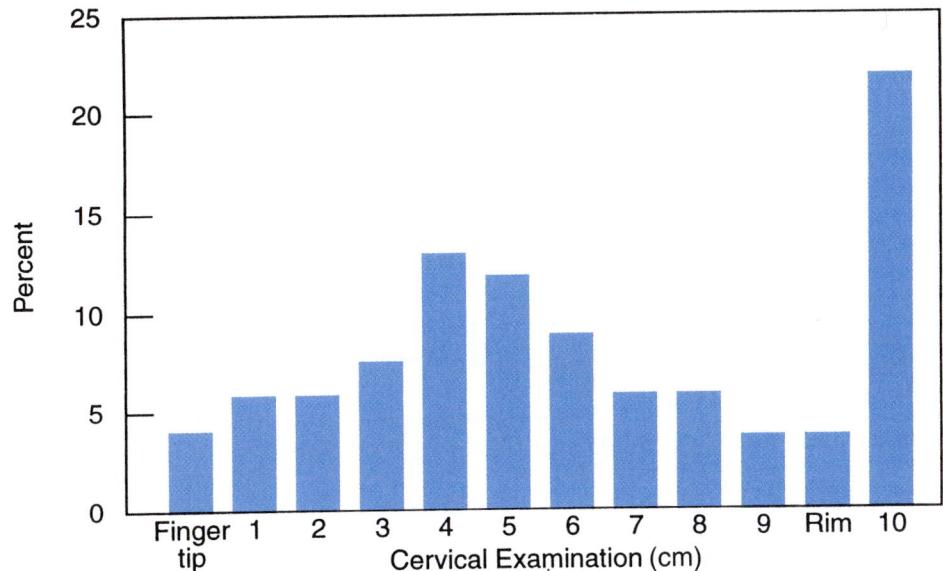

FIGURE 18–1. Distribution of cervical examinations at the time of cesarean delivery for dystocia. (From Gifford and colleagues, 2000, with permission.)

American College of Obstetricians and Gynecologists (1995a) that the cervix be dilated to 4 cm or more before a diagnosis is made. Thus, the diagnosis is often made before the active phase of labor and, therefore, before an adequate trial of labor. Another factor implicated in the increase in the diagnosis of dystocia is insufficient oxytocin stimulation of labor in women with slow labor (Rouse and colleagues, 1999). King (1993) found that cesareans for dystocia in private patients in the United Kingdom were related to office hours and surgery schedules, whereas the timing of procedures for fetal distress were evenly distributed throughout the day.

NORMAL LABOR

Dystocia is very complex, and although its definition—abnormal progress in labor—seems simple, there is no consensus as to what "abnormal progress" means. Thus, it seems prudent to attempt a better understanding of normal labor in order to determine departure(s) from normal.

The greatest impediment to understanding normal labor is recognizing its start. The strict definition of labor—*uterine contractions that bring about demonstrable effacement and dilatation of the cervix*—does not easily aid the clinician in determining when labor has actually begun, because this diagnosis is confirmed only after the event. Several options may be used to deal with this dilemma. One is to instruct the woman to quantify contractions for some specified period, and then define labor onset as the clock time when painful contractions become regular. This is very subjective and frequently causes considerable frustration for both obstetrician and patient. Indeed, uterine irritability that

causes discomfort, but that does not represent true labor, may develop at any time during pregnancy. As shown in Figure 18–2, contractions increase progressively during the third trimester, undoubtedly causing maternal uncertainty as to when labor has commenced. False labor often stops spontaneously, or it may proceed rapidly into effective contractions.

A second option is to define the onset of labor as beginning at the time of admission to the labor unit. At the National Maternity Hospital in Dublin, efforts have been made to codify admission criteria, following which labor management is disciplined (O'Driscoll and colleagues, 1993). These criteria at term require painful uterine contractions accompanied by any one of the following:

1. Ruptured membranes.
2. Bloody "show."
3. Complete cervical effacement.

In the Irish scheme, the duration of labor is determined based on time elapsed from admission to delivery.

In the United States, admission for labor is frequently based on the extent of dilatation accompanied by painful contractions. When the woman presents with intact membranes, cervical dilatation of 3 to 4 cm or greater is presumed to be a reasonably reliable threshold for diagnosis of labor. In this case, onset of labor commences with the time of admission. This presumptive method of diagnosing true labor obviates many of the uncertainties in diagnosing labor during earlier stages of cervical dilatation.

FIRST STAGE OF LABOR. Assuming that the diagnosis has been confirmed, then what are the expectations for

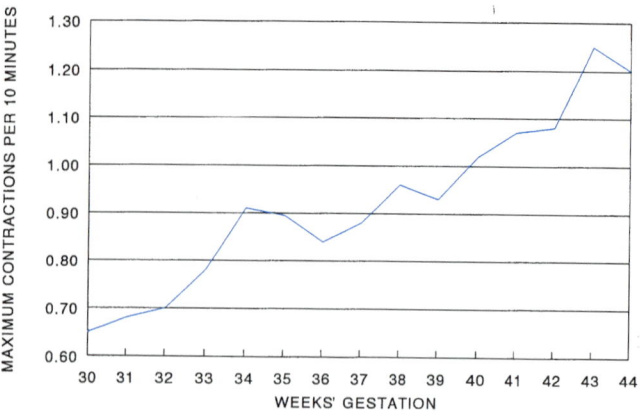

FIGURE 18-2. Increase in episodic maximum uterine contraction frequency with advancing gestation. (Modified from Nageotte and co-workers, 1988, with permission.)

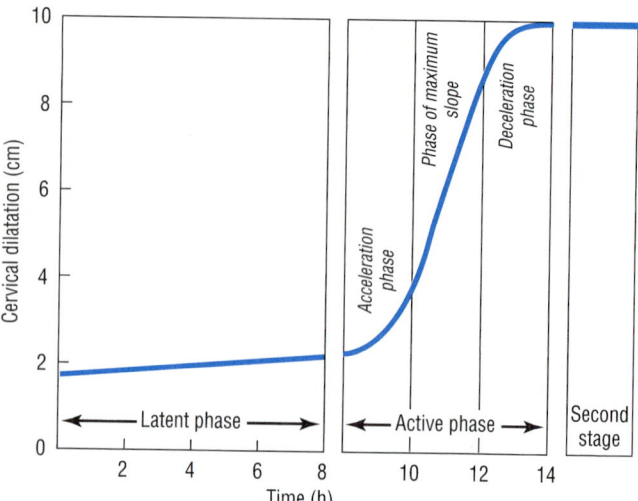

FIGURE 18-4. Composite of the average dilatation curve for nulliparous labor. The first stage is divided into a relatively flat latent phase and a rapidly progressive active phase. In the active phase, there are three identifiable component parts that include an acceleration phase, a linear phase of maximum slope, and a deceleration phase. (Illustration courtesy of Dr. L. Casey; redrawn from Friedman, 1978.)

progress of normal labor? Historically, this was usually described by simple elapsed time, with the realization that normal labor could be diagnosed only after the fact. A scientific approach was begun by Friedman (1954), who described a characteristic sigmoid pattern for labor when analyzed statistically and then graphing cervical dilatation against time (Chap. 11, p. 260). This graphic approach, based on statistical observations, eventually resulted in a change in labor management.

Friedman developed the concept of three functional divisions of labor to describe the physiological objectives of each division (Fig. 18–3). Although little cervical dilatation occurs during the **preparatory division,** con-

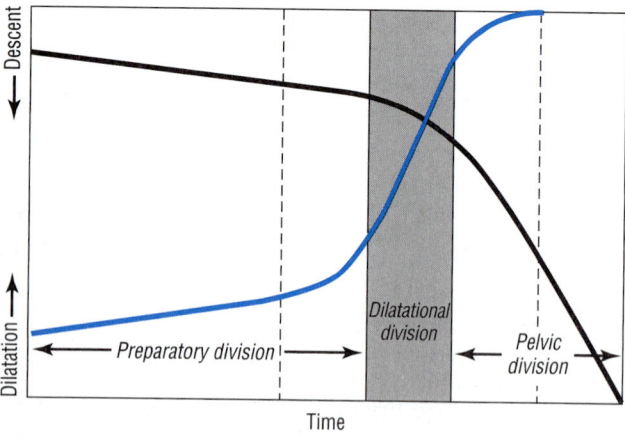

FIGURE 18-3. Labor course divided functionally on the basis of dilatation and descent curves into (1) a preparatory division, including latent and acceleration phases; (2) a dilatational division, occupying the phase of maximum slope of dilatation; and (3) a pelvic division, encompassing both deceleration phase and second stage concurrent with the phase of maximum slope of descent. (Illustration courtesy of Dr. L. Casey; redrawn from Friedman, 1978.)

siderable changes take place in the connective tissue components of the cervix. This division of labor may be sensitive to sedation and conduction analgesia. The **dilatational division,** during which time dilatation proceeds at its most rapid rate, is unaffected by sedation or conduction analgesia. The **pelvic division** commences with the deceleration phase of cervical dilatation. The classical mechanisms of labor that involve cardinal fetal movements in the cephalic presentation—engagement, flexion, descent, internal rotation, extension, and external rotation—take place principally during the pelvic division (Chap. 12, p. 301). In actual practice, however, the onset of the pelvic division is seldom clearly identifiable.

As shown in Figure 18–4, the pattern of cervical dilatation during the preparatory and dilatational divisions of normal labor is a sigmoid curve. Two phases of cervical dilatation are defined: the **latent phase** corresponds to the preparatory division and the **active phase** to the dilatational division. Friedman subdivided the active phase into the *acceleration phase,* the *phase of maximum slope,* and the *deceleration phase.*

LATENT PHASE. The onset of latent labor is defined according to Friedman (1972) as the point at which the mother perceives regular contractions. During this phase, orientation of uterine contractions takes place along with cervical softening and effacement. His minimum criteria for entry into the active phase are cervical dilatation rates of 1.2 cm/hr for nulliparas and

1.5 cm/hr for parous women. **These rates of cervical dilatation do not start at a specific dilatation.** For example, Peisner and Rosen (1986) found that 30 percent of women reached 5 cm dilatation before their dilatation rates conformed to active-phase labor. Conversely, other women dilated more rapidly and had active-phase dilatation rates at 3 cm. Thus, the latent phase commences with maternal perception of regular contractions that is accompanied by progressive, albeit slow, cervical dilatation, and ends at between 3 and 5 cm of dilatation. This threshold may be clinically useful, for it defines cervical dilatation limits beyond which active labor can be expected. Rosen (1990) recommended that all women be classified as "in active labor" when at a maximum of 5 cm dilatation, so that in the absence of progressive change, intervention should be considered.

Friedman and Sachtleben (1963) defined a **prolonged latent phase** to be greater than 20 hours in the nullipara and 14 hours in the parous woman. These are the 95th percentiles. In an earlier report, Friedman (1955) provided data on the duration of latent labor in nulliparas. Its mean duration was 8.6 hours (+2 SD 20.6 hours) and the range was 1 to 44 hours. Thus, the duration of latent phase of 20 hours for nulliparous and 14 hours for parous women represents a statistical maximum.

Factors that affect duration of the latent phase include excessive sedation or conduction analgesia, poor cervical condition (e.g., thick, uneffaced, or undilated), and false labor. Friedman claimed that either rest or oxytocin stimulation were equally efficacious and safe in correcting prolonged latent phases. Rest was preferable because unrecognized false labor was common. With strong sedatives, 85 percent of these women begin active labor. Another 10 percent cease contracting, and thus had false labor. Finally, 5 percent experience recurrence of an abnormal latent phase and require oxytocin stimulation. Amniotomy was discouraged because of the 10 percent incidence of false labor. Sokol and colleagues (1977) reported a 3 to 4 percent incidence of prolonged latent phase, regardless of parity. Friedman (1972) reported that prolongation of the latent phase did not adversely influence fetal or maternal morbidity or mortality, but Chelmow and co-workers (1993) disputed the long-held belief that prolongation of the latent phase is benign.

This concept of a latent phase has great significance in understanding normal human labor because labor is considerably longer when a latent phase is included. To better illustrate this, Figure 18–5 shows eight labor curves from nulliparas where labor was diagnosed beginning with admission, rather than with onset of regular contractions. When defined as such, there is remarkable similarity of individual labor curves. The principal difference between the labor curves, contingent upon when

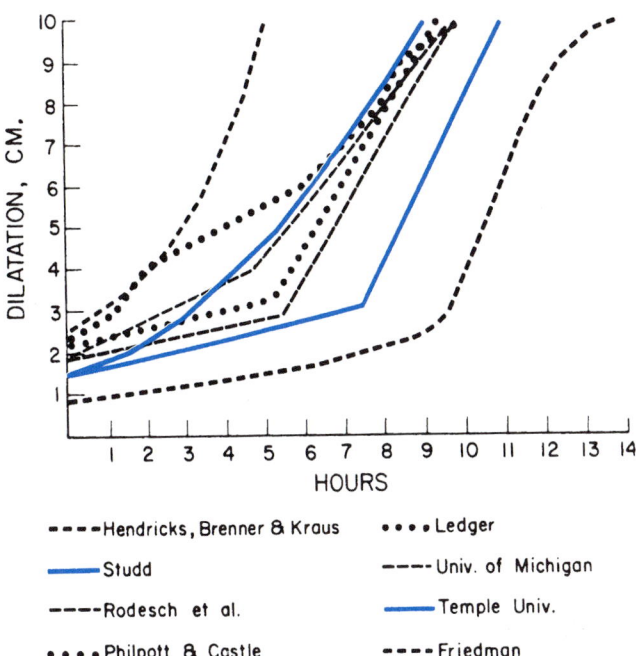

FIGURE 18–5. Progress of labor in primigravid women from the time of admission. When the starting point on the abscissa begins with admission to the hospital, there is no latent phase observed.

labor is defined to begin, is the presence or absence of a latent period.

ACTIVE LABOR. As shown in Figure 18–5, the progress of labor in nulliparous women has particular significance because these curves all reveal a rapid change in the slope of cervical dilatation between 3 and 4 cm. That is, the "active" phase of labor, in terms of most rapid rates of cervical dilatation, consistently begins when the cervix is 3 to 4 cm dilated. These rather remarkable similarities serve to define active labor and provide useful guideposts in management. **Thus, cervical dilatation of 3 to 4 cm or more, in the presence of uterine contractions, can be taken to reliably represent the threshold for active labor.** Similarly, these curves permit the clinician to ask, given that labor can be reliably diagnosed to have commenced, how much time should elapse in normal active labor?

Turning again to Friedman (1955), the mean duration of active phase labor in nulliparas was 4.9 hours. The standard deviation of 3.4 hours is quite large. Hence, the active phase was reported to have a statistical maximum of 11.7 hours (mean +2 SD) with considerable variation in the duration. Indeed, rates of cervical dilatation ranged from 1.2 to 6.8 cm/hr. Thus, when the rate of dilatation considered normal for active-phase labor in the nullipara is reported to be 1.2 cm/hr, this is the *minimum* normal rate, not the maximum. Multiparas progress somewhat faster in active-phase labor with a minimum normal rate of 1.5 cm/hour (Friedman, 1972).

Another feature shared by the several labor curves depicted in Figure 18–5 is the remarkable tendency for similar durations of active labor. Specifically, nulliparous women who enter the active phase at 3 to 4 cm can reliably be expected to reach 8 to 10 cm dilatation within 3 to 4 hours. This observation might have potential usefulness. For example, if cervical dilatation reaches 4 cm, the clinician could expect complete dilatation to be achieved in approximately 4 hours if spontaneous labor is "normal." Active labor phase abnormalities, however, are quite common. Sokol and co-workers (1977) reported that 25 percent of nulliparous labors were complicated by active-phase abnormalities while 15 percent of multigravidas developed this problem.

Understanding Friedman's analysis of active-phase labor is somewhat arduous because rates of fetal descent are considered in addition to cervical dilatation rates, and both of these are occurring concomitantly (Fig. 18–3). Descent begins in the later stage of active dilatation, commencing at about 7 to 8 cm in nulliparas and becoming most rapid after 8 cm. Friedman (1972) subdivided active-phase problems into **protraction** and **arrest** disorders. He defined protraction *as a slow rate* of cervical dilatation or descent, which for nulliparas was less than 1.2 cm dilatation per hour or less than 1 cm descent per hour. For multiparas, protraction was defined as less than 1.5 cm dilatation per hour or less than 2 cm descent per hour. He defined arrest as a *complete cessation* of dilatation or descent. **Arrest of dilatation** was defined as 2 hours with no cervical change, and **arrest of descent** as 1 hour without fetal descent. The prognosis for protraction and arrest disorders differed considerably, and he found that about 30 percent of women with protraction disorders had cephalopelvic disproportion, whereas this was diagnosed in 45 percent of women in whom an arrest disorder developed. Abnormal labor patterns, diagnostic criteria, and methods of treatment according to Cohen and Friedman (1983) are summarized in Table 18–2.

Other associations or factors contributing to both protraction and arrest disorders were excessive sedation, conduction analgesia, and fetal malposition such as persistent occiput posterior. In both protraction and arrest disorders, Friedman recommended fetopelvic examination to diagnose cephalopelvic disproportion. Recommended therapy for protraction disorders was expectant management, whereas oxytocin was advised for arrest disorders in the absence of cephalopelvic disproportion. The latter is not defined precisely in Friedman's 1955 report, other than to note that 8 of 39 diagnosed cases of disproportion had x-ray pelvimetry evidence of pelvic incapacity, and the remaining 31

women were considered to have "relative disproportion for a variety of reasons such as persistent occiput posterior." Remarkably, of the 500 women studied, only 2 percent had cesarean deliveries. Put another way, the great majority of active-phase disorders did not result in cesarean delivery. This fact must be kept in mind when considering the significance of Friedman's various labor abnormalities in the context of the current implication that cephalopelvic disproportion mandates cesarean delivery.

Hendricks and co-workers (1970) challenged Friedman's conclusions about the course of normal human labor. Their principal differences included:

1. Absence of a latent phase.
2. No deceleration phase.
3. Brevity of labor.
4. Dilatation at similar rates for nulliparas and multiparas after 4 cm.

They disputed the concept of a latent phase because they observed that cervical dilatation and effacement occurred slowly during the 4 weeks preceding labor. According to them, the "latent phase" actually occurred over several weeks. Hendricks and colleagues (1970) did observe that labor was relatively rapid; specifically, the average time from admission to complete dilatation was 4.8 hours for nulliparas and 3.2 hours for multiparas.

SECOND STAGE OF LABOR. This stage begins when cervical dilatation is complete and ends with fetal expulsion. Its median duration is 50 minutes for nulliparas and 20 minutes for multiparas, but it is also highly variable. In a woman of higher parity with a previously dilated vagina and perineum, two or three expulsive efforts after full cervical dilatation may suffice to complete delivery. Conversely, in a woman with a contracted pelvis or a large fetus, or with impaired expulsive efforts from conduction analgesia or intense sedation, the second stage may become abnormally long. Kilpatrick and Laros (1989) reported that average second-stage labor, prior to spontaneous fetal expulsion, was lengthened about 25 minutes by regional analgesia. As previously noted, the pelvic or fetal descent division of labor largely occurs following complete dilatation. Moreover, the second stage incorporates many of the cardinal movements necessary for the fetus to negotiate the birth canal (Chap. 12, p. 301). Given the mechanical requirements of these fetal movements, it is logical for disproportion of the fetus and pelvis to become apparent during the second stage. Indeed, in earlier times, cephalopelvic disproportion was diagnosed only after complete cervical dilatation had occurred and attempts to deliver the fetus with forceps had failed.

Until very recently, there have been unquestioned second-stage rules that limited its duration. The second

TABLE 18–2. Abnormal Labor Patterns, Diagnostic Criteria, and Methods of Treatment

Labor Pattern	Diagnostic Criteria		Preferred Treatment	Exceptional Treatment
	Nulliparas	*Multiparas*		
Prolongation Disorder (Prolonged latent phase)	> 20 hr	> 14 hr	Bed rest	Oxytocin or cesarean delivery for urgent problems
Protraction Disorders				
1. Protracted active phase dilatation	< 1.2 cm/hr	< 1.5 cm/hr	Expectant and support	Cesarean delivery for CPD
2. Protracted descent	< 1.0 cm/hr	< 2 cm/hr		
Arrest Disorders				
1. Prolonged deceleration phase	> 3 hr	> 1 hr	Oxytocin without CPD	Rest if exhausted
2. Secondary arrest of dilatation	> 2 hr	> 2 hr	Cesarean with CPD	Cesarean delivery
3. Arrest of descent	> 1 hr	> 1 hr		
4. Failure of descent	No descent in deceleration phase or second stage			

CPD = cephalopelvic disproportion.
Modified from Cohen and Friedman (1983).

stage in nulliparas was limited to 2 hours and extended to 3 hours when regional analgesia was used. For multiparas, 1 hour was the limit, extended to 2 hours with regional analgesia. At Parkland Hospital during 1999, only 6 percent of second-stage labors in nulliparas at term exceeded 2 hours.

The origin of the second-stage rule, which in essence limits its duration to 2 hours, cannot be assigned to any one individual (Hellman and Prystowsky, 1952). This rule seems to have been established fairly definitely in American obstetrics, however, by the turn of the century. The first edition of *Williams Obstetrics* in 1903 states that forceps are usually indicated if the second stage lasts more than 2 hours. This rule appears to have been derived from concerns about fetal health, and indeed, the concept of prophylactic forceps delivery to shorten the second stage was popular earlier in this century (Chap. 21, p. 490). This practice often led to the performance of difficult forceps operations, although the question was raised whether prolongation of the second stage until such a time as an easy forceps delivery might be accomplished would be of some advantage. This more conservative attitude is the contemporary practice.

Cohen (1977) investigated the fetal effects of second-stage labor length at Beth Israel Hospital during more modern times. He included 4403 term nulliparas in whom electronic fetal heart rate monitoring was performed. Infant mortality was not increased in women whose second-stage labor exceeded 2 hours. Epidural analgesia was used commonly, and this likely accounts for the large number of pregnancies with a prolonged second stage. These data influenced permitting an additional hour for the second stage when regional analgesia was used. This report also influenced the American College of Obstetricians and Gynecologists (1995a) to qualify the previous dictums about the duration of second-stage labor.

Menticoglou and colleagues (1995b) challenged the prevailing dictums on the duration of the second stage based on their experiences in Winnipeg. These dictums came under scrutiny at their hospitals because of grave neonatal injuries associated with forceps rotations to shorten second-stage labor (Menticoglou and colleagues, 1995a). As a result, they have allowed longer second stages in the hope that fewer vaginal operative deliveries would be necessary. Between 1988 and 1992, the second stage of labor exceeded 2 hours in a fourth of 6041 nulliparas at term. Labor epidural analgesia was used in 55 percent. As shown in Table 18–3, the length of the second stage, even in those lasting up to 6 hours or more, was not related to infant outcome. These good results were attributed to careful use of electronic monitoring and scalp pH measurements. They concluded that there is no compelling reason to intervene with a possibly difficult forceps or vacuum extraction because a certain number of hours has elapsed. They offered, however, an important caveat; after 3 hours in the second stage, delivery by cesarean or other operative method increased progressively such that by 5 hours the prospects for spontaneous delivery in the subsequent hour are only 10 to 15 percent.

TABLE 18–3. Relationship Between Infant Outcome and Duration of Second-Stage Labor in Nulliparous Women at Term and Delivered in Winnipeg, Canada, 1989–1992

Length of Second Stage	Births[a] No. (%)	5 min Apgar < 7 No. (%)	Infants Admitted to Intensive Care No. (%)	Infants with Seizures	Infant Deaths
0–1 hr	2622 (44)	33 (1)	26 (1)	3	0
1–2 hr	1805 (30)	21 (1)	18 (1)	1	0
2–3 hr	927 (15)	20 (2)	14 (2)	1	0
3–4 hr	379 (6)	7 (2)	6 (1)	0	0
4–5 hr	147 (2.4)	0	0	0	0
5–6 hr	79 (1.3)	5 (6)	2 (3)	0	0
> 6 hr	82 (1.3)	2 (2)	0	0	0
Total	6041 (100)	88 (2)	66 (1)	5	0

[a]Labor epidural analgesia used in 55 percent of all women.
Adapted from Menticoglou and colleagues (1995a), with permission.

DURATION OF LABOR. Our understanding of the normal duration of human labor may be clouded by the many clinical variables that affect conduct of labor in modern obstetrical units, and also by the complexities of the graphicostatistical labor curves discussed in the preceding sections. Specifically, how long is normal spontaneous labor and delivery?

Kilpatrick and Laros (1989) reported that the mean length of first- and second-stage labor was approximately 9 hours in nulliparous women without regional analgesia, and that the 95th percentile upper limit was 18.5 hours. Corresponding times for multiparous women were a mean of about 6 hours with a 95th percentile of 13.5 hours. They defined labor onset as the time when the woman recalled regular, painful contractions every 3 to 5 minutes, and leading to cervical change. Cervical dilatation at admission is not stated.

Spontaneous labor was analyzed in almost 25,000 women delivered at term at Parkland Hospital in the early 1990s. Almost 80 percent of women were admitted with dilatation of 5 cm or less. Labor and delivery times did not follow a normal distribution, indicating that use of parametric statistics (means) would falsely lengthen perceptions of labor duration. Parity (nulliparous versus multiparous) and cervical dilatation at admission were significant determinants of the length of spontaneous labor. The median time from admission to spontaneous delivery was 3.5 hours, and 95 percent of all women delivered within 10.1 hours. These results suggest that normal human labor is relatively short.

SUMMARY OF NORMAL LABOR. Labor is characterized by brevity, considerable biological variation, and less complexity than anticipated based on contemporary graphic statistical interpretations. Active labor can be

reliably diagnosed when cervical dilatation is 3 cm or more in the presence of uterine contractions. Once this cervical dilatation threshold is reached, normal progress to delivery can be expected, depending on parity, in the ensuing 4 to 6 hours or so. Anticipated progress during a 1- to 2-hour second stage is governed by rules intended to ensure fetal safety. Finally, most women in spontaneous labor, regardless of parity and if left unaided, will deliver within approximately 10 hours after admission for spontaneous labor. **When time breaches in normal labor boundaries are the only pregnancy complications, interventions other than cesarean delivery must be considered before resorting to this method of delivery for failure to progress.** Insufficient uterine activity is a common and correctable cause of abnormal labor progress.

INADEQUATE LABOR

According to Williams (1903) in the first edition of this text, and still true today (brackets cite corresponding chapter of the 21st edition):

Dystocia or difficult labour may be due to various aetiological factors, and is most commonly encountered in the following groups of cases: (1) those in which the expulsive forces [Chap. 18, uterine dysfunction] are subnormal and are not sufficiently strong enough to overcome the natural resistance offered to the birth of the child by the bony canal and maternal soft parts; (2) those in which, although the expulsive forces may be of normal strength, abnormalities in the structure or character of the birth canal offer an insuperable mechanical obstacle [Chap. 18, pelvic contracture] to the descent of the presenting part; (3) those in which the foetus, on account of faulty presentation

[Chap. 19] or excessive development [Chap. 18, excessive fetal size] cannot be extruded by the *vis a tergo* (sic, a force operating from behind or a propulsive force).

Figure 18–6, from the first edition of *Williams Obstetrics* (1903), is useful for conceptualizing the mechanical process of labor and the potential obstacles to successful pelvic passage of the fetal passenger. The cervix and lower uterus are shown at the end of pregnancy as well as at the end of labor. At the end of pregnancy, the fetal head, to traverse the birth canal, must encounter a relatively thicker lower uterine segment and undilated cervix, while the uterine fundus muscle is less developed and presumably therefore less powerful in its propulsive effectiveness. At this stage, uterine muscle contractions, cervical resistance, and the forward pressure exerted by the leading fetal head are factors influencing the progress of the first stage of labor (Chap. 13, p. 313).

After complete cervical dilatation (Fig. 18–6B), however, the mechanical relationship between fetal head size and position and pelvic capacity, or fetopelvic proportion, becomes clearer as the passenger (fetus) descends the pelvic passage unimpeded by the cervical obstacle. The uterine fundus muscle is much thicker, and thus more powerful in its propulsive effectiveness, which is undoubtedly enhanced by complete cervical dilatation. In regard to inadequate progress of labor, abnormalities in uterine function, viz., uterine dysfunction, likely predominate before complete cervical dilatation whereas abnormalities in fetopelvic proportions, viz., disproportion, likely become more apparent once the second stage is reached.

Possible explanations for malfunction of uterine muscle include overdistention due to excessive fetal size and/or uterine fatigue when labor is obstructed by inadequate pelvic capacity, excessive fetal size, or both. Thus, ineffective labor is generally accepted as a possible warning sign of fetopelvic disproportion. Such a simplistic understanding of labor abnormalities, divided into pure *uterine dysfunction* and *fetopelvic disproportion,* is incorrect because these two abnormalities are closely interlinked. For example, fetopelvic disproportion is most commonly manifest clinically as uterine dysfunction; however, most often, uterine dysfunction can be corrected with oxytocin and vaginal delivery can be safely accomplished (Chap. 20, p. 474). Indeed, according to the American College of Obstetricians and Gynecologists (1995a), the bony pelvis is not the factor, with rare exceptions, that limits vaginal delivery. Such a statement was not possible in the early decades of the 20th century when *rickets* was prevalent and deformed pelves were common—up to 15 percent of women were diagnosed to have *rachitic* pelves at the Johns Hopkins Hospital in 1924 (Williams, 1936).

Given the complex interrelationship between uterine dysfunction and fetopelvic disproportion, and in the absence of objective means of precisely distinguishing these two causes of labor failure, clinicians must rely on a *trial of labor* to determine if labor can be successful in effecting vaginal delivery. Defining the adequacy of a trial of labor is a priority, in our opinion, in moderating the primary cesarean delivery rate for dystocia in the United States.

UTERINE DYSFUNCTION. Propulsion and expulsion of the fetus is brought about by contractions of the uterus, reinforced during the second stage by voluntary or involuntary muscular action of the abdominal wall—"pushing." Either of these factors may be lacking in intensity and result in delayed or interrupted labor. The frequency and intensity of uterine contractions are informative. Uterine dysfunction, characterized by infrequent low-intensity contractions, is common with significant disproportion because the uterus does not often self-destruct when faced with mechanical obstruction. This cervical response to labor has great prognostic significance. In general, orderly spontaneous progression

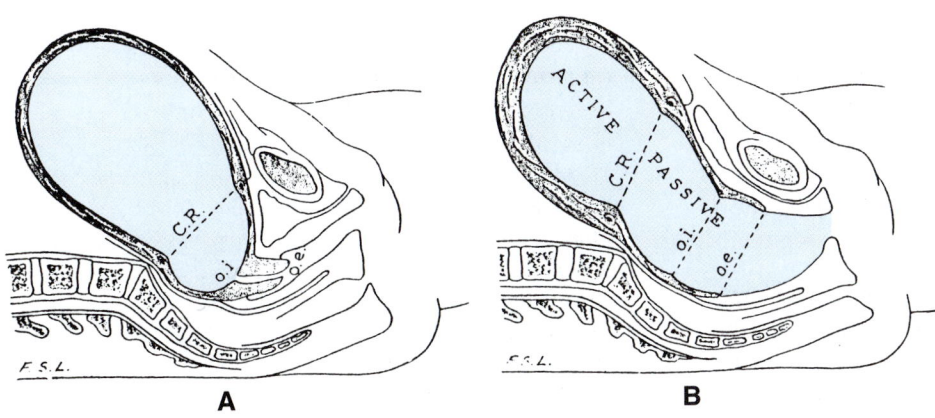

A   **B**

FIGURE 18–6. Diagrams of the birth canal at the end of pregnancy **(A)** and during the second stage of labor **(B),** showing formation of the birth canal. (From Williams, 1903.)

to full dilatation indicates that vaginal delivery most likely will be successful.

As described earlier, latent phase (*prodromal*) labor is usually several hours duration, during which time the cervix undergoes softening and effacement but only slight dilatation. This phase is characterized by uterine contractions of mild intensity, short duration, and variable frequency. The active phase, or phase of rapid dilatation, follows. During this time, in what has long been called simply labor, the cervix dilates more rapidly and there is descent of the presenting part through the birth canal (Fig. 18–3).

Descent normally begins well before the cervix reaches full dilatation and progresses until the presenting part reaches the perineum. **This pattern is highly variable.** The presenting part in nulliparous women may be at the +1 or even +2 station before the onset of labor, whereas in parous women, descent of the presenting part may not begin until the cervix nearly is dilated fully.

Uterine dysfunction in any phase of cervical dilatation is characterized by lack of progress, for one of the prime characteristics of normal labor is its progression. The diagnosis of uterine dysfunction in the latent phase is difficult and sometimes can be made only in retrospect. One of the most common errors is to treat women for uterine dysfunction who are not yet in active labor.

There have been three significant advances in the treatment of uterine dysfunction:

1. Realization that undue prolongation of labor may contribute to perinatal morbidity and mortality.
2. Use of dilute intravenous infusion of oxytocin in the treatment of certain types of uterine dysfunction.
3. More frequent use of cesarean delivery rather than difficult midforceps delivery when oxytocin fails or its use is inappropriate.

TYPES OF UTERINE DYSFUNCTION. Reynolds and co-workers (1948) emphasized that uterine contractions of normal labor are characterized by a gradient of myometrial activity, being greatest and lasting longest at the fundus (fundal dominance) and diminishing toward the cervix. Caldeyro-Barcia and colleagues (1950) from Montevideo inserted small balloons into the myometrium at various levels (Chap. 14, p. 355). With the balloons attached to strain-gauge transducers, they reported that in addition to a gradient of activity, there was a time differential in the onset of the contractions in the fundus, midzone, and lower uterine segments. Larks (1960) described the stimulus as starting in one cornu and then several milliseconds later in the other, the excitation waves then joining and sweeping over the fundus and down the uterus.

The Montevideo group also ascertained that the lower limit of contraction pressure required to dilate the cervix is 15 mm Hg. This figure is in agreement with the findings of Hendricks and co-workers (1959), who reported that normal spontaneous contractions often exert pressures of about 60 mm Hg. From these observations, it is possible to define two types of uterine dysfunction. In the more common **hypotonic uterine dysfunction,** there is no basal hypertonus and uterine contractions have a normal gradient pattern (synchronous), but the slight rise in pressure during a contraction is insufficient to dilate the cervix. In the other, **hypertonic uterine dysfunction** or **incoordinate uterine dysfunction,** either basal tone is elevated appreciably or the pressure gradient is distorted, perhaps by contraction of the midsegment of the uterus with more force than the fundus or by complete asynchronism of the impulses originating in each cornu, or a combination of these two.

REPORTED CAUSES OF UTERINE DYSFUNCTION. A variety of labor interventions have been implicated as causes of uterine dysfunction.

EPIDURAL ANALGESIA. It is important to emphasize that epidural analgesia can slow labor (Sharma and Leveno, 2000). For example, and as shown in Table 18–4, epidural analgesia has been associated with lengthening of both first- and second-stage labor as well as slowing of the rate of fetal descent.

CHORIOAMNIONITIS. Because of the association of prolonged labor with maternal intrapartum infection, some clinicians have suggested that infection itself plays a role in the development of abnormal uterine activity. Satin and co-workers (1992) studied the effects of chorioamnionitis on labor stimulation with oxytocin in 266 pregnancies. Chorioamnionitis diagnosed late in labor was found to be a marker of cesarean delivery for dystocia whereas this was not observed in women diag-

TABLE 18–4. Effect of Epidural Analgesia on the Progress of Labor in 199 Nulliparous Women Delivered Spontaneously at Parkland Hospital

Labor	Epidural Analgesia	Meperidine Analgesia	P Value
Cervical dilatation at analgesia, mean	4.1 cm	4.2 cm	NS
Active phase, mean	7.9 hr	6.3 hr	.005
Second stage, mean	60 min	48 min	.03
Fetal descent	4.2 cm/hr	7.9 cm/hr	.003

NS = not stated.
From Alexander and associates (1998).

nosed as having chorioamnionitis early in labor. Specifically, 40 percent of women developing chorioamnionitis after requiring oxytocin for dysfunctional labor later required cesarean delivery for dystocia. It is likely that uterine infection in this clinical setting is a consequence of dysfunctional and therefore prolonged labor rather than a cause of dystocia.

MATERNAL POSITION DURING LABOR. In the first edition of this textbook, Williams (1903) stated, "During the first stage of labour the patient usually prefers to move about her room, and frequently is more comfortable when occupying a sitting position. During this period, therefore, she should not be compelled to take to her bed unless she feels so inclined." Those early observations gave way to the opinion that recumbency should be the norm. This opinion, however, has been challenged on the grounds that recumbency impaired labor. Conversely, walking during labor has also been reported to shorten labor, decrease the need for augmentation with oxytocin, decrease the need for analgesia, and lower the frequency of instrumental vaginal delivery (Flynn and co-authors, 1978; Read and colleagues, 1981).

According to Miller (1983), uterine contractions occur more frequently but with less intensity with the mother in the supine position compared with lying on her side. Conversely, contraction frequency and intensity have been reported to increase with sitting or standing. Lupe and Gross (1986) concluded, however, that there is no conclusive evidence that upright maternal posture or ambulation improves labor. Without perturbations, women preferred to lie on their side or sit in bed. Few chose to walk, fewer to squat, and none wanted the knee-chest position. They tended to assume fetal positions in later labor. Most women enthusiastic about ambulating return to bed when active labor begins (Carlson and associates, 1986; Williams and co-workers, 1980).

Bloom and colleagues (1998) conducted a randomized trial to study the effects of walking during first-stage labor. In 1067 women with uncomplicated term pregnancies delivered at Parkland Hospital, they reported that ambulation neither improved nor delayed labor in nulliparous or parous women (Table 18–5). Walking during labor did not reduce the need for analgesia, nor was it harmful to the fetus-infant. Since these results provided no evidence for or against walking during labor, we now give women without complications the option of electing either recumbency or supervised ambulation during labor.

BIRTHING POSITION IN SECOND-STAGE LABOR. Considerable interest has been shown in alternative second-stage labor birth positions that might affect labor. Gupta and co-workers (1991) reported that several randomized controlled trials, with and without the use of specific birthing aids, have produced conflicting results and are confounded by observer bias. One reported advantage from avoiding the traditional lithotomy position is an increase in the dimensions of the pelvic outlet. Specifically, Russell (1969) described a 20 to 30 percent increase in the area of the pelvic outlet with squatting compared with the supine position. Gupta and co-workers (1991) compared the usual Western delivery position—recumbent with the head and shoulders up 30 degrees—with the squatting position and found no significant change in the dimensions of either the pelvic inlet or outlet. Crowley and associates (1991) randomized 634 women to deliver in an obstetrical birth chair and compared these with 596 women delivered in bed. There were no advantages with use of the birthing chair, but hemorrhage was increased in this group.

TABLE 18–5. Effects of Walking During Labor in Nulliparous and Parous Women Delivered at Parkland Hospital

	Nulliparous Women			Parous Women		
Outcome	*Walking Group (n = 272)*	*Usual Care Group (n = 272)*	*P Value*	*Walking Group (n = 264)*	*Usual Care Group (n = 259)*	*P Value*
Labor, hr						
First stage	7.6 ± 3.9[a]	7.3 ± 3.9	0.47	4.6 ± 2.4	4.7 ± 2.4	0.60
Second stage	1.0 ± 0.9	0.9 ± 0.8	0.46	0.2 ± 0.3	0.2 ± 0.3	0.42
Labor augmentation—no. (%)[b]	95 (35)	99 (36)	0.72	27 (10)	38 (15)	0.12
Forceps delivery—no. (%)	21 (8)	15 (6)	0.30	2 (1)	2 (1)	0.99
Cesarean birth—no. (%)	19 (7)	21 (8)	0.74	4 (2)	10 (4)	0.10

[a]Plus or minus values are means ± SD.
[b]Labor augmentation was defined as stimulation of labor with oxytocin because of inadequate uterine contractions.
From Bloom and colleagues (1998).

De Jong and co-workers (1997), in a randomized trial of 517 South African women, found no increase in hemorrhage with the sitting position. Obstetrical outcomes were not improved by enforcing the upright position for second-stage labor. The main benefits reported were less maternal pain and enhanced maternal satisfaction with the birthing experience. Babayer and co-authors (1998) cautioned that prolonged sitting or squatting during the second stage may cause peroneal neuropathy.

IMMERSION IN WATER. This has been advocated as a means of relaxation that may contribute to more efficient labor (Odent, 1983). Schorn and colleagues (1993) randomized 96 women at term to immersion in a hot tub with air jets or to their prevailing labor management. The women were permitted to stay in the tub as long as they desired, and most stayed 30 to 45 minutes. Water immersion did not alter the rate of cervical dilation, length of labor, route of delivery, or analgesia use. Robertson and associates (1998) reported that immersion was not associated with chorioamnionitis or endometritis. Kwee and co-workers (2000) studied the effects of immersion in 20 women and reported that maternal blood pressure decreased while fetal heart rate was unaffected.

FETOPELVIC DISPROPORTION. This arises from either diminished pelvic size, excessive fetal size, or more usually, a combination of both.

PELVIC CAPACITY. Any contraction of the pelvic diameters that diminishes the capacity of the pelvis can create dystocia during labor. There may be contractions of the pelvic inlet, the midpelvis, the pelvic outlet, or a generally contracted pelvis caused by combinations of these.

CONTRACTED PELVIC INLET. The pelvic inlet is usually considered to be contracted if its shortest anteroposterior diameter is less than 10.0 cm or if the greatest transverse diameter is less than 12.0 cm. The anteroposterior diameter of the pelvic inlet is commonly approximated by manually measuring the diagonal conjugate, which is about 1.5 cm greater. Therefore, inlet contraction is usually defined as a diagonal conjugate of less than 11.5 cm. The errors inherent in the use of this clinical measurement are discussed in Chapter 3 (p. 58).

Using clinical and, at times, imaging pelvimetry, it is important to identify the shortest anteroposterior diameter through which the fetal head must pass. Occasionally, the body of the first sacral vertebra is displaced forward so that the shortest distance may actually be between this false, or abnormal, sacral promontory and the symphysis pubis.

Prior to labor, the fetal biparietal diameter has been shown to *average* from 9.5 to as much as 9.8 cm. Therefore, it might prove difficult or even impossible for some fetuses to pass through an inlet with an anteroposterior diameter of less than 10 cm. Mengert (1948) and Kaltreider (1952), employing x-ray pelvimetry, demonstrated that the incidence of difficult deliveries is increased to a similar degree when either the anteroposterior diameter of the inlet is less than 10 cm or the transverse diameter is less than 12 cm. When both diameters are contracted, dystocia is much greater than when only one is contracted. The configuration of the pelvic inlet is also an important determinant of the adequacy of any pelvis, independent of actual measurements of these diameters and of calculated "areas" (see Fig. 3–28, and Caldwell-Moloy Classification, Chap. 3, p. 57).

A small woman is likely to have a small pelvis, but she is also likely to have a small infant. Thoms (1937) studied 362 nulliparas and found the mean birthweight of their offspring was significantly lower (280 g) in women with small pelves than in those with medium or large pelves. In veterinary obstetrics, it has frequently been observed that in most species maternal size rather than paternal size is the important determinant of fetal size.

Normally, cervical dilatation is facilitated by hydrostatic action of the unruptured membranes or, after their rupture, by direct application of the presenting part against the cervix. In contracted pelves, however, when the head is arrested in the pelvic inlet, the entire force exerted by the uterus acts directly upon the portion of membranes that overlie the dilating cervix. Consequently, early spontaneous rupture of the membranes is more likely to result.

After membrane rupture, the absence of pressure by the head against the cervix and lower uterine segment predisposes to less effective contractions. Hence, further dilatation may proceed very slowly or not at all. Cibils and Hendricks (1965) reported that the mechanical adaptation of the fetal passenger to the bony passage plays an important part in determining the efficiency of contractions. The better the adaptation, the more efficient are the contractions. Because adaptation is poor in the presence of a contracted pelvis, prolongation of labor often results. With degrees of pelvic contractions incompatible with vaginal delivery, the cervix seldom dilates satisfactorily. Thus, cervical response to labor provides a prognostic view of the outcome of labor in women with inlet contraction.

A contracted inlet plays an important part in the production of abnormal presentations. In normal nulliparas, the presenting part at term commonly descends into the pelvic cavity before the onset of labor. When the inlet is contracted considerably, however, descent usually does not take place until after the onset of labor, if at all. Cephalic presentations still predominate, but because the head floats freely over the pelvic inlet or rests more laterally in one of the iliac fossae, very slight influences may cause the fetus to assume other presentations. **In women with contracted pelves, face and shoulder presentations are encountered three times more frequently, and cord prolapse occurs four to six times more frequently.** Critchlow and colleagues (1994) have quantified the magnitude of risk for cord prolapse in women with cephalopelvic disproportion.

CONTRACTED MIDPELVIS. This is more common than inlet contraction. It is frequently a cause of transverse arrest of the fetal head, which can potentially lead to difficult midforceps operation or to cesarean delivery.

The obstetrical plane of the midpelvis extends from the inferior margin of the symphysis pubis, through the ischial spines, and touches the sacrum near the junction of the fourth and fifth vertebrae. A transverse line theoretically connecting the ischial spines divides the midpelvis into anterior and posterior portions. The former is bounded anteriorly by the lower border of the symphysis pubis and laterally by the ischiopubic rami. The posterior portion is bounded dorsally by the sacrum and laterally by the sacrospinous ligaments, forming the lower limits of the sacrosciatic notch.

Average midpelvis measurements are as follows: transverse (interspinous), 10.5 cm; anteroposterior (from the lower border of the symphysis pubis to the junction of the fourth and fifth sacral vertebrae), 11.5 cm; and posterior sagittal (from the midpoint of the interspinous line to the same point on the sacrum), 5 cm. Although the definition of midpelvic contractions has not been established with the same precision possible for inlet contractions, the midpelvis is likely contracted when the sum of the interischial spinous and posterior sagittal diameters of the midpelvis (normal, 10.5 plus 5 cm, or 15.5 cm) falls to 13.5 cm or below. This concept has been emphasized by Chen and Huang (1982) in evaluating possible midpelvic contraction. There is reason to suspect midpelvic contraction whenever the interischial spinous diameter is less than 10 cm. When it is smaller than 8 cm, the midpelvis is contracted.

The preceding definitions of midpelvic contraction do not imply that dystocia always develops in such a pelvis, but simply that it more likely will develop. Development of dystocia also depends upon the size and shape of the forepelvis and the size of the fetal head, as well as on the overall degree of midpelvic contraction.

Although there is no precise manual method of measuring midpelvic dimensions, a suggestion of contraction can sometimes be inferred if the spines are prominent, the pelvic sidewalls converge, or the sacrosciatic notch is narrow. Moreover, Eller and Mengert (1947) pointed

out that the relationship between the intertuberous and interspinous diameters of the ischium is sufficiently constant that narrowing of the interspinous diameter can be anticipated when the intertuberous diameter is narrow. A normal intertuberous diameter, however, does not always exclude a narrow interspinous diameter.

CONTRACTED PELVIC OUTLET. This is usually defined as diminution of the interischial tuberous diameter to 8 cm or less. The pelvic outlet may be roughly likened to two triangles with the interischial tuberous diameter constituting the base of both. The sides of the anterior triangle are the pubic rami, and its apex the inferior posterior surface of the symphysis pubis. The posterior triangle has no bony sides but is limited at its apex by the tip of the last sacral vertebra (not the tip of the coccyx). Floberg and associates (1987) reported that outlet contractions were found in almost 1 percent of over 1400 unselected term nulliparas.

Diminution in the intertuberous diameter with consequent narrowing of the anterior triangle must inevitably force the fetal head posteriorly (Fig. 18–7). Whether delivery can take place therefore partly depends on the size of the posterior triangle, or more specifically on the interischial tuberous diameter and the posterior sagittal diameter of the outlet. A contracted outlet may cause dystocia not so much by itself as through the often associated midpelvic contraction. *Outlet contraction without concomitant midplane contraction is rare.*

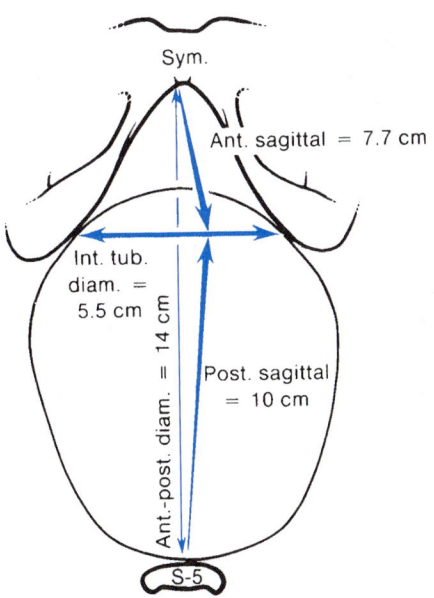

FIGURE 18–7. Diagram of pelvic outlet showing that even though the intertuberous diameter is quite narrow (5.5 cm), vaginal delivery is possible because of the long (10 cm) posterior sagittal diameter. (Int. tub. diam. = intertuberous diameter; Sym. = symphysis pubis; S-5 = fifth sacral vertebra.)

Even when the disproportion between the fetal head and the pelvic outlet is not sufficiently great to give rise to severe dystocia, it may play an important part in the production of perineal tears. With increasing narrowing of the pubic arch, the occiput cannot emerge directly beneath the symphysis pubis but is forced increasingly farther down upon the ischiopubic rami. In extreme cases, the head must rotate around a line joining the ischial tuberosities. The perineum, consequently, must become increasingly distended and thus exposed to greater danger of disruption.

PELVIC FRACTURES AND RARE CONTRACTURES.
Speer and Peltier (1972) reviewed experiences with pelvic fractures and pregnancy. Trauma from automobile collisions was the most common cause of pelvic fractures. With bilateral fractures of the pubic rami, compromise of birth canal capacity by callus formation or malunion was very common. A history of pelvic fracture warrants careful review of previous x-rays and possibly computed tomographic pelvimetry later in pregnancy. Descriptions and illustrations of rare pelvic contractions are discussed in the 10th through 17th editions of *Williams Obstetrics*.

ESTIMATION OF PELVIC CAPACITY. The techniques for clinical evaluation using digital examination of the bony pelvis during labor are described in detail in Chapter 3 (p. 58). Briefly, the examiner attempts to judge the anteroposterior diameter of the inlet (diagonal conjugate), the interspinous diameter of the midpelvis, and the intertuberous distances of the pelvic outlet. A narrow pelvic arch, less than 90 degrees, can signify a narrow pelvis. An unengaged fetal head can indicate either excessive fetal head size or reduced pelvic inlet capacity.

X-RAY PELVIMETRY. The prognosis for successful vaginal delivery in any given pregnancy cannot be established on the basis of x-ray pelvimetry alone, because the pelvic capacity is but one of several factors that determine the outcome (Mengert, 1948). Thus, x-ray pelvimetry is considered to be of limited value in the management of labor with cephalic presentations (American College of Obstetricians and Gynecologists, 1995b). If vaginal delivery is anticipated for a fetus presenting as a breech, however, x-ray pelvimetry still is used in many medical centers (Chap. 22, p. 512).

COMPUTED TOMOGRAPHIC SCANNING. An advantage of computed tomographic pelvimetry such as that shown in Figure 18–8 is a reduction in radiation exposure. The accuracy is greater than that of conventional x-ray pelvimetry, it is easier to perform, and costs are comparable. With either method, x-ray exposure is miniscule (Chap. 42, p. 1147). With conventional x-ray pel-

vimetry, the mean gonadal exposure is estimated to be 885 mrad by the Committee on Radiological Hazards to Patients (Osborn, 1963). Depending upon the machine and technique employed, fetal doses with computed tomography may range from 250 to 1500 mrad (Moore and Shearer, 1989).

MAGNETIC RESONANCE IMAGING (MRI). The advantages of MRI include the lack of ionizing radiation, accurate pelvic measurements, complete fetal imaging, as well as the potential for evaluating reasons for soft tissue dystocia (McCarthy, 1986; Stark and co-workers, 1985). Currently its use is limited because of expense, time involved for adequate imaging studies, and equipment availability.

Sporri and co-workers (1997) used magnetic resonance images postpartum to measure capacity at each level of the pelvis and ultrasound intrapartum to measure fetal head dimensions. In this study, "cephalic pelvic disproportion" was defined as arrest of labor for more than 4 hours in the presence of normal uterine contractions. "Failure to progress" was diagnosed when there was no labor progress and uterine activity was hypotonic. A fetal head volume exceeding measured pelvic capacity was a frequent finding in women with cephalopelvic disproportion, but not those with failure to progress. Clearly, use of MRI to measure pelvic capacity is investigational.

EXCESSIVE FETAL SIZE. It is interesting to review statements in previous editions of *Williams Obstetrics* concerning excessive fetal size as a cause of dystocia:

> 1st Edition (1903): Provided the pelvis is not contracted, it is very exceptional for a normally formed child, weighing less than 5000 g (10½ lbs) to give rise to dystocia by its mere size.

> 7th Edition (1936): Provided the pelvis is not contracted, it is very exceptional for a normally formed child, weighing less than 4500 g (10 lbs) to give rise to dystocia by its mere size.

> 13th Edition (1966): Provided the pelvis is not contracted, it is unusual for a normally formed child weighing less than 4500 g (10 lbs) to give rise to dystocia on the basis of its size alone.

The theme of these statements, although the fetal weight threshold decreased from 5000 g to 4500 g, has been that fetal size seldom is a suitable explanation for failed labor. The greatest obstetrical concern expressed in these earlier editions was not that the fetal head might fail to traverse the pelvic passage, but, rather, that the shoulders might not fit through the pelvic inlet or outlet (Chap. 19, p. 459). Remarkably, this is also the theme of contemporary statements about excessive fetal devel-

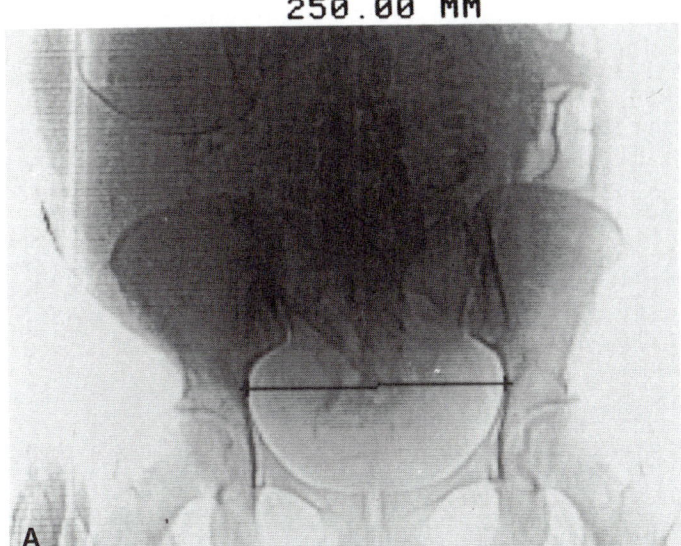

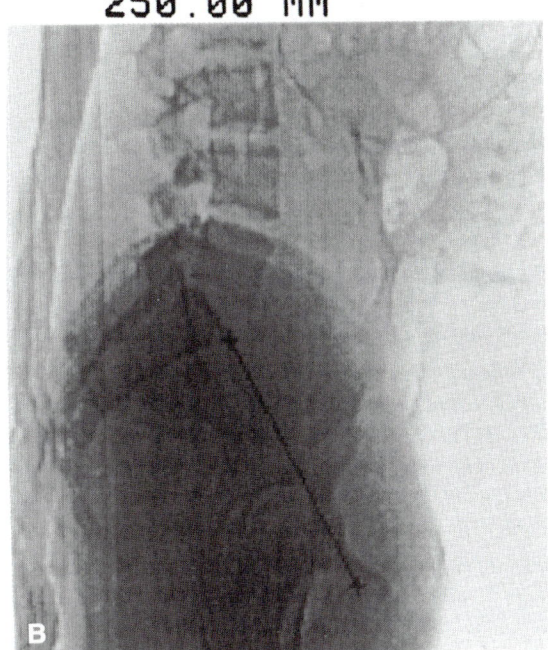

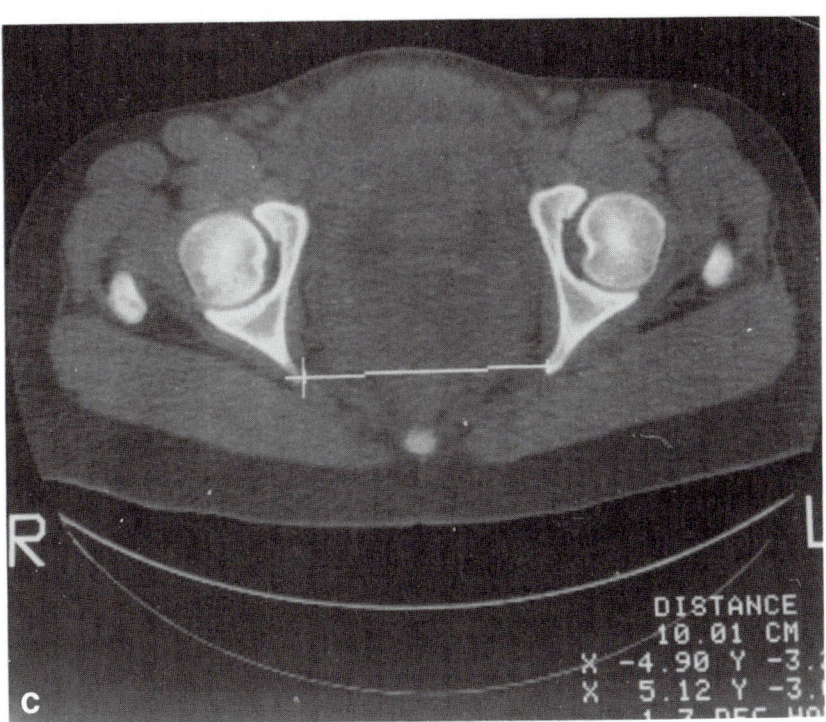

FIGURE 18–8. **A.** Anteroposterior view of digital radiograph. Illustrated is the measurement of the transverse diameter of the pelvic inlet using an electronic cursor. The fetal body is clearly outlined. The total fetal dose using the three exposures shown in parts **A** to **C** is approximately 250 mrad. **B.** Lateral view of digital radiograph. Illustrated are measurements of the anteroposterior diameters of the inlet and midpelvis measured using the electronic cursor. **C.** An axial computed tomographic section through the midpelvis. The level of the fovea of the femoral heads was ascertained from the anteroposterior digital radiograph because it corresponds to the level of the ischial spines. The interspinous diameter is measured using the electronic cursor.

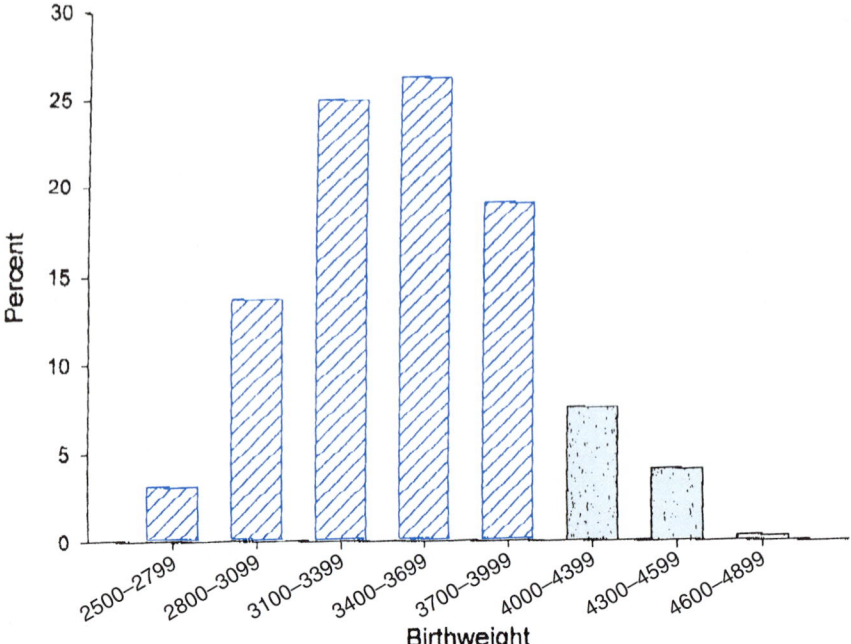

FIGURE 18–9. Birthweight distribution of 362 infants delivered by cesarean at Parkland Hospital (1989–1999) after a failed attempt to effect vaginal delivery with forceps. Only 12 percent (n = 44) of the infants weighed ≥ 4000 g (shaded bars).

opment (Chap. 29, p. 757). For example, the American College of Obstetricians and Gynecologists (1997a) has concluded that planned cesarean delivery, in an attempt to forego shoulder dystocia, is only a reasonable strategy for diabetic women with estimated fetal weights exceeding 4250 to 4500 g. Selection of a fetal size threshold to predict fetopelvic disproportion and, therefore, prevent obstructed labor, is not possible because most cases of disproportion occur in fetuses whose weight is well within the range of the general obstetrical population. As shown in Figure 18–9, two thirds of infants requiring cesarean delivery at Parkland Hospital after an attempt at forceps delivery failed, weighed less than 3700 g (8 lb 2 oz). Thus, fetopelvic disproportion usually is not associated with excessive fetal size.

ESTIMATION OF FETAL HEAD SIZE. Not only is there no definable fetal size threshold for predicting cephalopelvic disproportion, the methods for estimation of fetal head are also imprecise. Impression of the fetal head into the pelvis, as described by Müller (1880) and Hillis (1930), may provide useful information. In an occiput presentation, the brow and the suboccipital region are grasped through the abdominal wall with the fingers and firm pressure is directed downward in the axis of the inlet. Fundal pressure by an assistant usually is helpful. The effect of the forces on the descent of the head can be evaluated by concomitant vaginal examination. If no disproportion exists, the head readily enters the pelvis, and vaginal delivery can be predicted. Inability

to push the head into the pelvis, however, does not necessarily indicate that vaginal delivery is impossible. A clear demonstration of a flexed fetal head that overrides the symphysis pubis, however, is presumptive evidence of disproportion. Thorp and colleagues (1993b) performed a prospective evaluation of the *Mueller-Hillis maneuver* and concluded that there was no relation between dystocia and failure of descent of the head.

Measurements of fetal head diameters using plain radiographic techniques are not used because of parallax distortions. The biparietal diameter and head circumference can be measured by ultrasonic means. There have been attempts to use ultrasonic measurements of the fetus in the management of dystocia. Thurnau and colleagues (1991) used the fetal-pelvic index to identify labor complications. Unfortunately, the sensitivity of such measurements to predict of cephalopelvic disproportion is poor (Ferguson and associates, 1998). We are of the view that there is no currently satisfactory method for accurate prediction of fetopelvic disproportion due to excessive fetal head size.

RUPTURED MEMBRANES WITHOUT LABOR. Membrane rupture without spontaneous uterine contractions occurs in about 8 percent of term pregnancies. Until recently, management generally included stimulation of contractions when labor did not begin after 6 to 12 hours. This intervention evolved about 40 years ago because of maternal and fetal complications due to amnionitis (Calkins, 1952). Such routine intervention was the accepted practice until challenged by Kappy and co-workers (1979), who reported excessive cesarean delivery in term pregnancies with ruptured membranes managed with labor stimulation compared with those managed by expectant observation. Further interest in observation was stimulated by a randomized trial reported by Duff and colleagues (1984). In this study, 134 women with ruptured membranes without labor at term were randomly treated with observation or oxytocin. The cesarean rate was significantly lower in those women managed by observation.

Hannah and co-workers (1996) and Peleg and associates (1999) performed an international randomized investigation of 5042 pregnancies with ruptured membranes at term. They measured the effects of induction versus expectant management and also compared induction with intravenous oxytocin to prostaglandin E_2 gel. There were approximately 1200 pregnancies in each of the four study arms. They concluded that labor induction with intravenous oxytocin was the preferred management. This was based on significantly fewer intrapartum and postpartum infections in women whose labor was induced. There were no significant differences in cesarean delivery rates. Subsequent analysis by Hannah and colleagues (2000) indicated increased adverse outcomes when expectant management at home was compared with in-hospital observation. Similar conclusions were reached by Mozurkewich and Wolf (1997) after meta-analysis of reported trials on management of ruptured membrane at term.

In another analysis by Seaward and colleagues (1998) of the international randomized trial described earlier, clinical chorioamnionitis and maternal colonization with group B streptococcus were the most important predictors of subsequent neonatal infection. At Parkland Hospital, labor is stimulated with oxytocin when ruptured membranes are diagnosed at term.

DIAGNOSIS OF INADEQUATE LABOR

ACTIVE-PHASE DISORDERS. According to the American College of Obstetricians and Gynecologists (1995a), neither failure to progress nor cephalopelvic disproportion are precise terms. They concluded that a more practical classification is to divide labor abnormalities into either slower-than-normal (protraction disorder) or complete cessation of progress (arrest disorder). The woman must be in the active phase of labor (cervix dilated 3 to 4 cm or more) to diagnose either of these.

Handa and Laros (1993) diagnosed active-phase arrest (no dilatation for 2 hours or more) in 5 percent of term nulliparas. Interestingly, this incidence has not changed since the 1950s (Freidman, 1978). Inadequate uterine contractions, defined as less than 180 Montevideo units (Fig. 18–10), were diagnosed in 80 percent of women with active-phase arrest. Protraction disorders are less well described, probably because the time interval necessary before diagnosing slow progress is undefined. Said another way, how many hours must elapse before deciding that less than 1.2 cm/hr of cervical dilatation has occurred? The World Health Organization (1994) has proposed a labor management "partograph" in which protraction is defined as less than 1 cm/hr cervical dilatation *for a minimum of 4 hours.*

The current criteria recommended by the American College of Obstetricians and Gynecologists (1995a) for diagnosis of protraction and arrest disorders are shown in Table 18–6. These criteria are adapted from those of Cohen and Friedman (1983) shown in Table 18–2.

Hauth and co-workers (1986, 1991) reported that to effectively induce or augment labor with oxytocin, 90 percent of women achieve 200 to 225 Montevideo units, and 40 percent achieve at least 300 Montevideo units. These results suggest that there are certain minimums of uterine activity that should be achieved before performing cesarean delivery for dystocia. Accordingly, the American College of Obstetricians and Gynecologists (1989) has suggested that, before the diagnosis of arrest during first-stage labor is made, both of these criteria should be met:

1. The latent phase has been completed, with the cervix dilated 4 cm or more.
2. A uterine contraction pattern of 200 Montevideo units or more in a 10-minute period has been present for 2 hours without cervical change.

Rouse and colleagues (1999) have recently challenged the "2-hour rule" on the grounds that a longer time, i.e., at least 4 hours, is necessary before concluding that the active phase of labor has failed. We agree.

FETAL STATION AT ONSET OF ACTIVE LABOR. Descent of the fetal biparietal diameter to the level of the maternal pelvic ischial spines (O station) is defined as engagement (Chap. 13, p. 311). Friedman and Sachtleben (1965) reported that there was a significant association between higher station at the onset of labor and subsequent dystocia. They described both protraction and arrest labor disorders in women with fetal head stations above +1 cm and that the higher the station at the onset of labor in nulliparas, the more prolonged the labor (Friedman and Sachtleben, 1976). Handa and Laros (1993) found that fetal station at the time of arrested labor was also a risk factor for dystocia. Roshanfekr and associates (1999) analyzed fetal station in

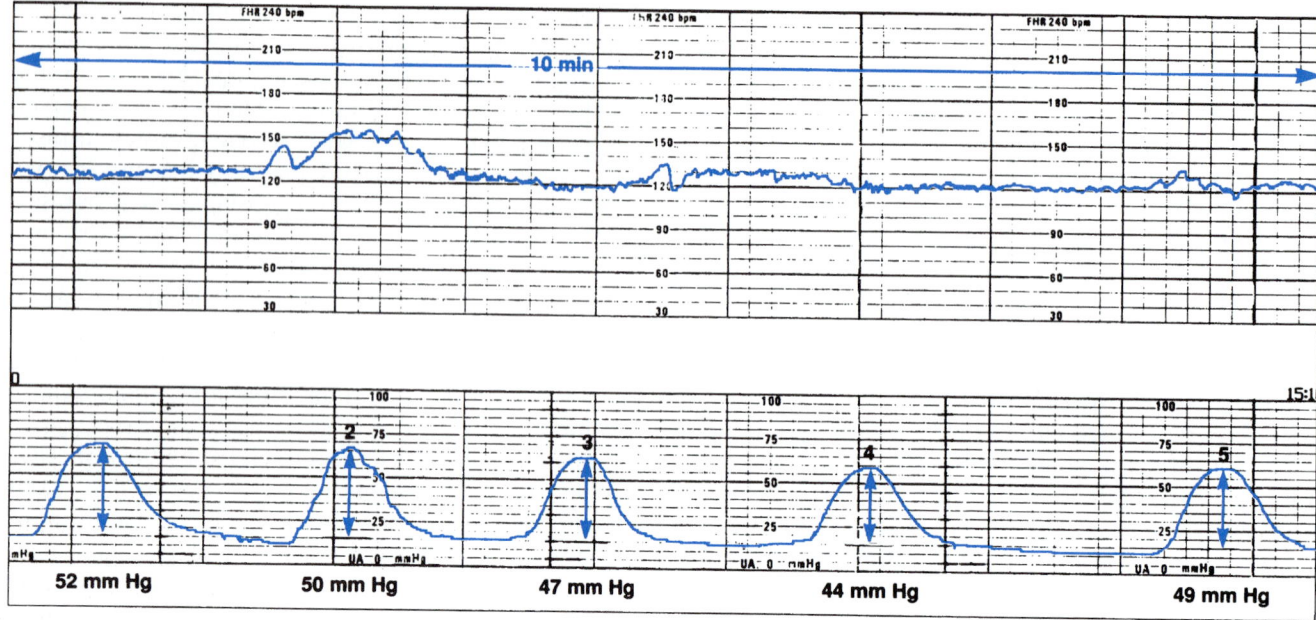

FIGURE 18–10. Montevideo units are calculated by subtracting the baseline uterine pressure from the peak contraction pressure for each contraction in a 10-minute window and adding the pressures generated by each contraction. In the example shown, there were five contractions, producing pressure changes of 52, 50, 47, 44, and 49 mm Hg, respectively. The sum of these five contractions is 242 Montevideo units. (From the American College of Obstetricians and Gynecologists, 1989, with permission.)

803 nulliparous delivered at term after active labor had been diagnosed. About 30 percent of these women presented to the hospital with the fetal head at or below 0 station, and the cesarean rate was 5 percent compared with 14 percent for those with higher fetal stations. The prognosis for dystocia, however, was not related to incrementally higher fetal head stations above the pelvic midplane (0 station). Importantly, 86 percent of nulliparous women without fetal head engagement at diagnosis of active labor delivered vaginally. Thus, lack of engagement at the onset of labor, although a statistical risk factor for dystocia, should not be assumed to necessarily predict fetopelvic disproportion. This is especially true for parous women because descent typically occurs relatively later in labor in these women.

SECOND-STAGE DISORDERS. With achievement of full cervical dilatation, the great majority of women cannot resist the urge to "bear down" or "push" each time the uterus contracts. Typically, the laboring woman inhales deeply, closes her glottis, and contracts her abdominal musculature repetitively with vigor to generate increased intra-abdominal pressure throughout the contractions. The combined force created by contractions of the uterus and abdominal musculature propels the fetus downward. Coaching women to push forcefully, compared with letting them follow their own urge to bear down, has been reported to offer no advantage (Parnell and associates, 1993; Vause and co-workers, 1998).

CAUSES OF INADEQUATE EXPULSIVE FORCES. At times, the magnitude of the force created by contractions of abdominal musculature is compromised sufficiently to prevent spontaneous vaginal delivery. Heavy sedation or conduction analgesia—lumbar epidural, caudal, or intrathecal—are likely to reduce the reflex urge to push, and at the same time may impair ability to contract the abdominal muscles sufficiently. In some

TABLE 18–6. Criteria for Diagnosis of Abnormal Labor Due to Arrest or Protraction Disorders

Labor Pattern	Nullipara	Multipara
Protraction disorder		
Dilation	< 1.2 cm/hr	< 1.5 cm/hr
Descent	< 1.0 cm/hr	< 2.0 cm/hr
Arrest disorder		
No dilation	> 2 hr	> 2 hr
No descent	> 1 hr	> 1 hr

From the American College of Obstetricians and Gynecologists (1995a), with permission.

instances, the inherent urge to push is overridden by the intensification of pain that is created by bearing down.

Careful selection of the kind of analgesia and the timing of its administration are important to avoid compromise of voluntary expulsive efforts. With rare exception, intrathecal analgesia or general anesthesia should not be administered until all conditions for a safe outlet forceps delivery have been met (Chap. 21, p. 490). With continuous epidural analgesia, it may be necessary to allow the paralytic effects to wear off so that the woman can generate intra-abdominal pressure sufficient to move the fetal head into position appropriate for outlet forceps delivery. The alternatives—a possibly difficult midforceps delivery or cesarean delivery—are unsatisfactory choices in the absence of any evidence of fetal distress.

For the woman who cannot bear down appropriately with each contraction because of great discomfort, analgesia is likely to be of considerable benefit. Perhaps the safest choice for both fetus and mother is nitrous oxide, mixed with an equal volume of oxygen and provided during the time of each uterine contraction (Chap. 15, p. 364). At the same time, appropriate encouragement and instruction are most likely to be of benefit.

MATERNAL–FETAL EFFECTS OF DYSTOCIA

Although maternal and fetal effects resulting from dystocia are divided arbitrarily in the following discussion, dystocia may result in serious consequences to either or both simultaneously.

INTRAPARTUM INFECTION. Infection is a serious danger to which mother and fetus are exposed in labors complicated by prolonged labor, especially in the setting of ruptured membranes. Bacteria in amnionic fluid traverse the amnion and invade decidua and chorionic vessels, thus giving rise to maternal and fetal bacteremia and sepsis. Fetal pneumonia, caused by aspiration of infected amnionic fluid is another serious consequence. Digital cervical examinations introduce vaginal bacteria into the uterus (Imseis and co-authors, 1999). These should be limited during labor, especially when dystocia is suspected. Maternal and fetal infections are discussed in Chapter 26 and Chapters 56 and 57, respectively.

UTERINE RUPTURE. Abnormal thinning of the lower uterine segment creates a serious danger during prolonged labor, particularly in women of high parity and in those with prior cesarean deliveries (Chap. 23, p. 542). When the disproportion between fetal head and pelvis is so pronounced that there is no engagement and descent, the lower uterine segment becomes increasingly stretched, and rupture may follow. In such cases, a **pathological retraction ring** may develop and may be felt as a transverse or oblique ridge extending across the uterus somewhere between the symphysis and the umbilicus. Whenever this condition is noted, immediate abdominal delivery is indicated.

PATHOLOGICAL RETRACTION RING. Very rarely, localized rings or constrictions of the uterus develop in association with prolonged labors. The most common type is the *pathological retraction ring of Bandl,* an exaggeration of the normal retraction ring described in Chapter 11 (p. 255). It is often the result of obstructed labor, with marked stretching and thinning of the lower uterine segment. In such a situation, the ring may be seen clearly as an abdominal indentation and signifies impending rupture of the lower uterine segment (see Fig. 19–7, p. 456). Localized uterine constrictions are rarely seen today because prolonged obstructed labor is unacceptable. These may still occur occasionally as hourglass constrictions of the uterus following birth of the first twin. In such a situation, they can sometimes be relaxed and delivery effected with appropriate general anesthesia, but occasionally prompt cesarean delivery offers a better prognosis for the second twin (Chap. 30, p. 797.

FISTULA FORMATION. When the presenting part is firmly weighed into the pelvic inlet but does not advance for a considerable time, portions of the birth canal lying between it and the pelvic wall may be subjected to excessive pressure. Because of impaired circulation, necrosis may result and become evident several days after delivery with the appearance of vesicovaginal, vesicocervical, or rectovaginal fistulas. Most often, pressure necrosis follows a very prolonged second stage of labor. Formerly, when operative delivery was deferred as long as possible, such complications were frequent, but today they are rarely seen except in undeveloped countries (Chap. 35, p. 923).

PELVIC FLOOR INJURY. A long held belief is that injury to the pelvic floor muscles or to their nerve supply or to the interconnecting fascia is an inevitable consequence of vaginal delivery, particularly if the delivery is difficult. During childbirth the pelvic floor is exposed to direct compression from the fetal head as well as downward pressure from maternal expulsive efforts. These forces stretch and distend the pelvic floor resulting in functional and anatomical alterations in the muscles, nerves, and connective tissues. There is accumulating concern that such effects on the pelvic floor during childbirth lead to urinary and anal incontinence, and pelvic organ prolapse (Leitch and Walker, 1998;

Sultan and Stanton, 1996). Due to these concerns, in a recent poll of English female obstetricians, 30 percent expressed preference for an elective cesarean delivery rather than vaginal delivery, and cited avoidance of pelvic floor injury as the explanation for their choice (Wagner, 2000).

There is a long obstetrical history of interventions intended to prevent pelvic floor injury. For example, in 1920 DeLee advocated childbirth with *prophylactic forceps* to reduce the muscular and nerve strain of second-stage labor and to protect the pelvic floor and adjacent fascia from overstretching (Chap. 21, p. 490). Obstetrical accomplishments, however, in the 20th century were largely focused on improving the prognosis for newborn infants and preventing maternal morbidity and mortality due to preeclampsia, infection, and obstetrical hemorrhage. Indeed, Brubaker (1998) characterized this period by observing that "birth injury" is currently used in the context of injury to the fetus-neonate, while earlier in the 20th century, "birth injury" indicated maternal injuries that resulted in urogynecological disorders manifest later in the lives of women.

A classic example of such childbirth injury are anal sphincter tears occurring at vaginal delivery and discussed in Chapter 13 (p. 328). Such tears occur in 3 to 6 percent of deliveries and approximately half of these women report subsequent fecal or gas incontinence (Zetterstrom and co-workers, 1999). Although childbirth undoubtedly plays a significant role in pelvic floor injury, the incidence and types of injuries reported vary widely between studies. Currently, there is uncertainty regarding the incidence of childbirth-associated pelvic floor injury, and there is insufficient information as to the relative roles of specific obstetrical antecedents (Samuellsson and associates, 1999).

FETAL EFFECTS. Prolonged labor itself may be deleterious. If the pelvis is contracted and there is associated prolonged membrane rupture and intrauterine infection, fetal and maternal risks are compounded. Intrapartum infection is not only a serious maternal complication but also an important cause of fetal and neonatal death. This obtains because bacteria in amnionic fluid traverse the amnion and invade decidua and chorionic vessels, thus giving rise to maternal and fetal bacteremia. Fetal pneumonia, caused by aspiration of infected amnionic fluid, is another serious consequence.

CAPUT SUCCEDANEUM. If the pelvis is contracted, during labor a large *caput succedaneum* frequently develops on the most dependent part of the fetal head. As shown in Figure 18–11, this may assume considerable size and lead to serious diagnostic errors. **The caput may reach almost to the pelvic floor while the head is still not engaged. An inexperienced physician may make premature and unwise attempts at forceps delivery.** Typically, even a large caput disappears within a few days after birth.

FETAL HEAD MOLDING. Under the pressure of strong uterine contractions, cranial plates overlap one another at the major sutures, a process referred to as *molding* (Fig. 18–11, see also Figs. 39–16 and 39–17, pp. 1074, 1075). As a rule, the median margin of the parietal bone that is in contact with the sacral promontory is overlapped by that of its fellow; the same result occurs with the frontal bones. The occipital bone, however, is pushed under the parietal bones. These changes are frequently accomplished without obvious detriment. Alternatively, when the distortion is marked, molding may

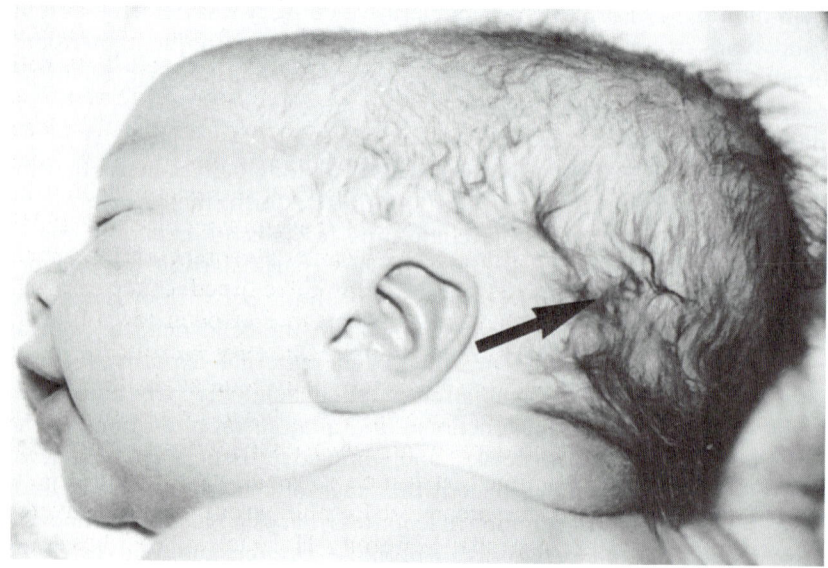

FIGURE 18–11. Considerable molding of the head and caput formation in a very recently delivered infant. The arrow is directed toward the caput succedaneum caused by appreciable scalp edema that overlies the occiput.

lead to tentorial tears, laceration of fetal blood vessels, and fatal intracranial hemorrhage.

Sorbe and Dahlgren (1983) measured fetal head diameters at birth and compared these with measurements obtained 3 days later. Molding was greatest in the subocciptobregmatic dimension and averaged 0.3 cm with a range up to 1.5 cm. The biparietal diameter was not affected by fetal head molding. Factors associated with molding included nulliparity, oxytocin labor stimulation, and delivery with a vacuum extractor. Carlan and colleagues (1991) described a locking mechanism by which the free edges of cranial bones are forced into one another, preventing further molding and presumably providing protection for the fetal brain. They also observed that severe fetal head molding could develop before labor. Holland (1922) observed that severe molding could lead to fatal subdural hemorrhage due to tears involving the dura mater septa, especially the tentorium cerebelli. Such tears were observed in both normal and complicated deliveries.

Coincidental with molding, the parietal bone, which was in contact with the promontory, may show signs of being subjected to marked pressure, sometimes even becoming flattened. Accommodation more readily oc-

curs when the bones of the head are imperfectly ossified. This important process may provide one explanation for the differences observed in the course of labor in two apparently similar cases in which the pelvis and the head present identical measurements. In one case, the head is softer and more readily molded, and spontaneous delivery results. In the other, the more ossified head retains its original shape and dystocia develops.

Characteristic pressure marks may form upon the scalp, covering the portion of the head that passes over the promontory of the sacrum. From their location, it is frequently possible to ascertain the movements that the head has undergone in passing through the inlet. Rarely, similar marks appear on the portion of the head that has been in contact with the symphysis pubis. Such marks usually disappear within a few days.

Skull fractures are occasionally encountered, usually following forcible attempts at delivery. As discussed in Chapter 39 (p. 1082), such fractures also may occur with spontaneous delivery or even with cesarean delivery (Skajaa and associates, 1987). The fractures are either a shallow groove or a spoon-shaped depression just posterior to the coronal suture (Fig. 18–12). The former is relatively common, but because it involves only the external bone plate, it is not very dangerous. The latter, however, if not surgically corrected, may lead to neonatal death, because it extends through the entire thickness of the skull and gives rise to inner surface projections that exert injurious pressure upon the brain. In these cases, it usually is advisable to elevate or remove the depressed portion of the skull.

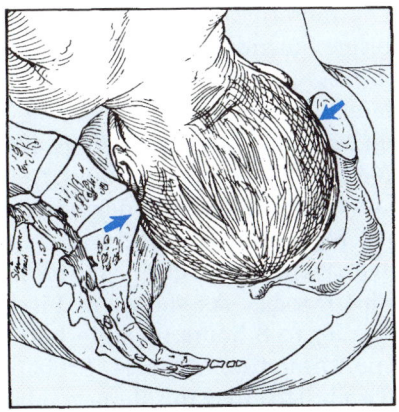

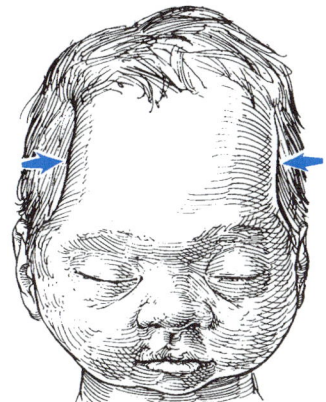

FIGURE 18–12. Depression of the skull (*arrows*) caused by labor with contracted pelvic inlet.

LABOR MANAGEMENT PROTOCOLS

O'Driscoll and colleagues (1984) at the National Maternity Hospital in Dublin pioneered the concept that a disciplined, standardized labor management protocol reduced cesarean deliveries for dystocia. Their overall cesarean rate was 5 percent in the 1970s and 1980s with such management. The approach is now referred to as *active management of labor*. Its components, or at least two of them—amniotomy and oxytocin—have been widely used, especially in English-speaking countries outside the United States (Thornton and Lilford, 1994). Recently, Impey and Boylan (1999) observed that active management was never intended to reduce the cesarean rate and that the rate had in fact been low (about 5 percent) at the National Maternity Hospital prior to implementation of active management. In their view, active management did serve, however, to prevent the escalation of cesarean deliveries in Dublin that occurred in the United States and elsewhere. More recently, however, the cesarean rate for nulliparous women delivered at the National Maternity Hospital in 1997 has more than doubled to 11.6 percent. This increase was attributed to induction of labor, cesarean delivery for breech presentation, and changing maternal attitudes.

ACTIVE MANAGEMENT OF LABOR. This phrase describes a codified approach to labor diagnosis and management only in nulliparous women. Labor is diagnosed when painful contractions are accompanied by complete cervical effacement, bloody "show," or ruptured membranes. Women with such findings are committed to delivery within 12 hours. Pelvic examination is performed each hour for the next 3 hours, and thereafter at 2-hour intervals. Progress is assessed for the first time 1 hour after admission. When dilatation has not increased by at least 1 cm, amniotomy is performed. Progress is again assessed at 2 hours and high-dose oxytocin infusion, described in Chapter 20 (p. 474), is started unless significant progress of 1 cm/hr is documented. Women are constantly attended by midwives.

If membranes rupture prior to admission, oxytocin is begun for no progress at the 1-hour mark. No special equipment is used, either to dispense oxytocin or monitor its effects, and electronic uterine contraction monitoring is not used. Oxytocin is dispensed by gravity regulated by a personal nurse. The solution contains 10 units of oxytocin in 1 liter of dextrose and water; the total dose may not exceed 10 units and the infusion rate may not exceed 60 drops/min or 30 to 40 mU/min (15 to 20 drops = 1 mL). In the Irish protocol, scalp blood sampling was used as the definitive test for fetal distress.

López-Zeno and colleagues (1992) prospectively compared active management with the "traditional" approach to labor management practiced at Northwestern Memorial Hospital in Chicago. They randomized, in an unblinded fashion, 705 uncomplicated nulliparas in spontaneous labor at term. The cesarean rate was 10.5 percent with active management and 14.1 percent with the "traditional" approach. Frigoletto and co-workers (1995) also reported a randomized trial of active management in 1934 nulliparous women delivered at Brigham and Women's Hospital in Boston. Although they found that such management somewhat shortened labor, it did not affect the cesarean rate. Similar results were reported by Rogers and colleagues (1997).

WORLD HEALTH ORGANIZATION PARTOGRAPH. A *partogram* was designed for use in developing countries (Dujardin and co-workers, 1992). Labor is divided into a latent phase, which should last no longer than 8 hours, and an active phase starting at 3 cm dilatation, the rate of which should be no slower than 1 cm/hr. A 4-hour wait (lag time) is recommended before intervention when the active phase is slow. Labor is graphed and analysis includes use of *alert* and *action* lines. The protocol has been found to be beneficial in Southeast Asia

(World Health Organization, 1994) and in Liverpool, England (Lavender and associates, 1998).

PARKLAND HOSPITAL LABOR MANAGEMENT PROTOCOL. During the 1980s, the obstetrical volume at Parkland Hospital doubled to approximately 15,000 births per year. In response, a second delivery unit designed for women with uncomplicated term pregnancies was developed. This provided a unique opportunity to implement and evaluate a standardized protocol for labor management. Its design was based upon the labor management approach that had evolved at our hospital up to that time, and which emphasized the implementation of specific, sequential interventions when abnormal labor was suspected. This approach is currently used in both complicated and uncomplicated pregnancies.

Women at term are admitted when active labor—defined as cervical dilatation of 3 to 4 cm or more in the presence of uterine contractions—is diagnosed or ruptured membranes confirmed. Management guidelines summarized in Figure 18–13 stipulate that pelvic examinations be performed approximately every 2 hours. Ineffective labor is suspected when the cervix does not dilate within about 2 hours of admission. Amniotomy is then performed and labor progress evaluated at the next 2-hour evaluation. In women whose labors do not progress, an intrauterine pressure catheter is placed to evaluate uterine function. Hypotonic contractions and no cervical progress after an additional 2 to 3 hours result in stimulation of labor using the high-dose oxytocin regimen described in Chapter 20 (p. 474). Uterine activity of 200 to 250 Montevideo units is expected for 2 to 4 hours before dystocia is diagnosed.

Dilatation rates of 1 to 2 cm/hr are accepted as evidence of progress after satisfactory uterine activity has been established with oxytocin. As shown in Figure 18–13, this can require up to 8 hours or more before cesarean delivery is performed for dystocia. Probably the cumulative time required to effect this stepwise management approach permits many women the time necessary to establish effective labor. This management protocol has been evaluated in more than 20,000 women with uncomplicated pregnancies. Cesarean delivery rates in nulliparous and parous women were 8.7 and 1.5 percent, respectively. Importantly, these labor interventions and the relatively infrequent use of cesarean delivery did not jeopardize the fetus-newborn infant.

PRECIPITATE LABOR AND DELIVERY

Not only can labor be too slow as described in this chapter, labor can also be abnormally rapid. Precipitate—that is, extremely rapid—labor and delivery may result from an abnormally low resistance of the soft

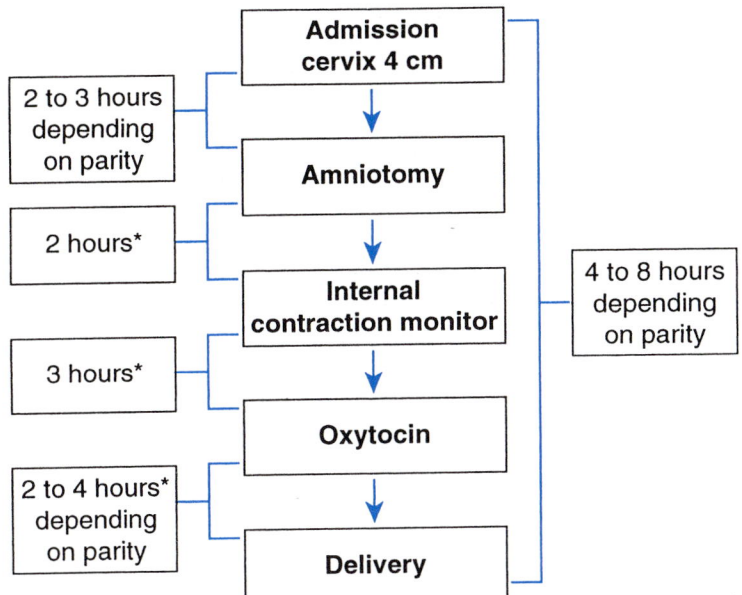

2 to 3 hours depending on parity	Admission cervix 4 cm	
2 hours*	Amniotomy	
3 hours*	Internal contraction monitor	4 to 8 hours depending on parity
2 to 4 hours* depending on parity	Oxytocin	
	Delivery	

*Depending on progress of cervical dilatation

FIGURE 18–13. Summary of labor management protocol in use at Parkland Hospital. The total admission-to-delivery times are shorter than the potential sum of the intervention intervals because not every woman requires every intervention.

parts of the birth canal, from abnormally strong uterine and abdominal contractions, or *very rarely,* from the absence of painful sensations and thus a lack of awareness of vigorous labor.

DEFINITION. According to Hughes (1972), precipitate labor terminates in expulsion of the fetus in less than 3 hours. Using this definition, 79,933 live births (2 percent) were complicated by precipitate labor in the United States during 1998 (Ventura and co-workers, 2000). Although so-defined precipitate labor is not rare, very little published information exists on its maternal and fetal effects. Mahon and colleagues (1994) described 99 pregnancies delivered within 3 hours of commencement of regular contractions. Short labors, defined as a rate of cervical dilatation of 5 cm/hr or faster for nulliparas and 10 cm/hr for multiparas, were associated with abruption (20 percent), meconium, postpartum hemorrhage, cocaine abuse, and low Apgar scores. Most (93 percent) of the women were multiparas and typically had uterine contractions more often than every 2 minutes.

MATERNAL EFFECTS. Precipitate labor and delivery are seldom accompanied by serious maternal complications if the cervix is effaced appreciably and easily dilated, the vagina has been stretched previously, and the perineum is relaxed. Conversely, vigorous uterine contractions combined with a long, firm cervix and a birth canal that resists stretch may lead to uterine rupture or extensive lacerations of the cervix, vagina, vulva, or perineum. It is in these latter circumstances that the

rare condition of *amnionic fluid embolism* most likely develops (Chap. 25, p. 660). **The uterus that contracts with unusual vigor before delivery is likely to be hypotonic after delivery, with hemorrhage from the placental implantation site as the consequence.** Postpartum hemorrhage from uterine atony is discussed in Chapter 25 (p. 637).

EFFECTS ON FETUS AND NEONATE. Perinatal mortality and morbidity from precipitate labor may be increased considerably for several reasons. The tumultuous uterine contractions, often with negligible intervals of relaxation, prevent appropriate uterine blood flow and fetal oxygenation. Another reason is that the resistance of the birth canal to expulsion of the head may cause intracranial trauma, although this must be rare. Acker and colleagues (1988) reported that Erb-Duchenne palsy was associated with such labors in a third of cases. Finally, during an unattended birth, the infant may fall to the floor and be injured or may need resuscitation that is not immediately available.

TREATMENT. Unusually forceful spontaneous uterine contractions are not likely to be modified to a significant degree by analgesia. The use of tocolytic agents such as magnesium sulfate is unproven in these circumstances. Use of general anesthesia with agents that impair uterine contractibility, such as halothane and isoflurane, is often excessively heroic. Certainly, any oxytocin agents being administered should be stopped immediately.

REFERENCES

Acker DB, Gregory KD, Sachs BP, Friedman EA: Risk factors for Erb-Duchenne palsy. Obstet Gynecol 71:389, 1988

Alexander JM, Lucas MJ, Ramin SM, McIntire DD, Leveno KJ: The course of labor with and without epidural analgesia. Am J Obstet Gynecol 178:516, 1998

American College of Obstetricians and Gynecologists. Shoulder dystocia. Practice Pattern No. 7, October, 1997a

American College of Obstetricians and Gynecologists. Utility of antepartum umbilical artery Doppler velocimetry in intrauterine growth restriction. Committee Opinion No. 18, October, 1997b

American College of Obstetricians and Gynecologists: Dystocia and the Augmentation of Labor. Technical Bulletin No. 218, December, 1995a

American College of Obstetricians and Gynecologists: Guidelines for diagnostic imaging during pregnancy. Committee Opinion No. 158, September, 1995b

American College of Obstetricians and Gynecologists: Dystocia. Technical Bulletin No. 137, December, 1989

Babayer M, Bodack MP, Creatura C: Common peroneal neuropathy secondary to squatting during childbirth. Obstet Gynecol 91:830, 1998

Bloom SL, McIntire DD, Kelly MA, Beimer HL, Burpo RH, Garcia MA, Leveno KJ: Lack of effect of walking on labor and delivery. N Engl J Med 339:76, 1998

Brubaker L: Vaginal delivery and the pelvic floor. Int Urogynecol J 9:363, 1998

Caldeyro-Barcia R, Alvarez H, Reynolds SRM: A better understanding of uterine contractility through simultaneous recording with an internal and a seven channel external method. Surg Obstet Gynecol 91:641, 1950

Calkins LA: Premature spontaneous rupture of the membranes. Am J Obstet Gynecol 64:871, 1952

Carlan SJ, Wyble L, Lense J, Mastrogiannis DS, Parsons MT: Fetal head molding. Diagnosis by ultrasound and a review of the literature. J Perinatol 11:105, 1991

Carlson JM, Diehl JA, Murray MS, McRae M, Fenwick L, Friedman EA: Maternal position during parturition in normal labor. Obstet Gynecol 68:443, 1986

Chelmow D, Kilpatrick SJ, Laros RK: Maternal and neonatal outcomes after prolonged latent phase. Obstet Gynecol 81:486, 1993

Chen HY, Huang SC: Evaluation of midpelvic contraction. Int Surg 67:516, 1982

Cibils LA, Hendricks CH: Normal labor in vertex presentation. Am J Obstet Gynecol 91:385, 1965

Cohen W: Influence of the duration of second stage labor on perinatal outcome and puerperal morbidity. Obstet Gynecol 49:266, 1977

Cohen W, Friedman EA (eds): Management of Labor. Baltimore, University Park Press, 1983

Critchlow CW, Leet TL, Benedetti TJ, Daling JR: Risk factors and infant outcomes associated with umbilical cord prolapse: A population-based case control study among births in Washington state. Am J Obstet Gynecol 170:613, 1994

Crowley P, Elbourne D, Ashurst H, Garcia J, Murphy D, Duigan N: Delivery in an obstetric birth chair: A randomized controlled trial. Br J Obstet Gynaecol 98:667, 1991

De Jong PR, Johanson RB, Baxen P, Adrians VD, vander Westhuisen S, Jones PW: Randomized trial comparing the upright and supine positions for the second stage of labour. Br J Obstet Gynaecol 104:567, 1997

DeLee JB: The prophylactic forceps operation. Am J Obstet Gynecol 1:34, 1920

Duff P, Huff RW, Gibbs RS: Management of premature rupture of membranes and unfavorable cervix in term pregnancy. Obstet Gynecol 63:697, 1984

Dujardin B, DeSchampheleire I, Sene H, Ndiaye F: Value of the alert and action lines on the partogram. Lancet 339:1336, 1992

Eller WC, Mengert WF: Recognition of mid-pelvic contraction. Am J Obstet Gynecol 53:252, 1947

Ferguson JE, Newberry YG, DeAngelis GA, Finnerty JJ, Agarwal S, Turkheimer E: The fetal-pelvic index has minimal utility in predicting fetal-pelvic disproportion. Am J Obstet Gynecol 179:1186, 1998

Floberg J, Belfrage P, Ohlsén H: Influence of pelvic outlet capacity on labor: A prospective pelvimetry study of 1429 unselected primi-paras. Acta Obstet Gynecol Scand 66:121, 1987

Flynn AM, Kelly J, Hollins G, Lynch PE: Ambulation in labour. BMJ 2:591, 1978

Fraser W, Usher RH, McLean FH, Bossenberry C, Thomson ME, Kramer MS, Smith LP, Power H: Temporary variation in rates of cesarean section for dystocia: Does "convenience" play a role? Am J Obstet Gynecol 156:300, 1987

Friedman EA: Labor: Clinical Evaluation and Management, 2nd ed. New York, Appleton-Century-Crofts, 1978

Friedman EA: An objective approach to the diagnosis and management of abnormal labor. Bull NY Acad Med 48:842, 1972

Friedman EA: Primigravid labor. A graphicostatistical analysis. Obstet Gynecol 6:567, 1955

Friedman EA: The graphic analysis of labor. Am J Obstet Gynecol 68:1568, 1954

Friedman EA, Sachtleben MR: Station of the fetal presenting part IV: Arrest of descent in nulliparas. Obstet Gynecol 47:129, 1976

Friedman EA, Sachtleben MR: Station of the fetal presenting part II: Effect on the course of labor. Am J Obstet Gynecol 93:530, 1965

Friedman EA, Sachtleben MR: Amniotomy and the course of labor. Obstet Gynecol 22:755, 1963

Frigoletto FD, Lieberman E, Lang JM, Cohen A, Barrs V, Ringer S, Datta S: A clinical trial of active management of labor. N Engl J Med 333:745, 1995

Gifford DS, Morton SC, Fiske M, Kefler JKE, Kahn KL: Lack of progress in labor as a reason for cesarean. Obstet Gynecol 95:589, 2000

Gupta JK, Glanville JN, Johnson N, Lilford RJ, Dunahm RJ, Walters JK: The effect of squatting in pelvic dimensions. Eur J Obstet Gynecol Reprod Biol 42:19, 1991

Handa VL, Laros RK: Active-phase arrest in labor: Predictors of cesarean delivery in a nulliparous population. Obstet Gynecol 81:758, 1993

Hannah ME, Hodnett ED, Willan A, Foster GA, DiCecco R, Helewa M, for the TermPROM Study Group: Prelabor rupture of the membranes at term: Expectant management at home or in hospital? Obstet Gynecol 96:533, 2000

Hannah M, Ohlsson A, Farine D, Hewson S, Hodnett E, Myhr T, Wang E, Weston J, Willan A: International Term PROM Trial: A RCT of induction of labor for prelabor rupture of membranes at term. Am J Obstet Gynecol 174:303, 1996

Hauth JC, Hankins GD, Gilstrap LC III: Uterine contraction pressures achieved in parturients with active phase arrest. Obstet Gynecol 78:344, 1991

Hauth JC, Hankins GD, Gilstrap LC III, Strickland DM,

Vance P: Uterine contraction pressures with oxytocin induction/augmentation. Obstet Gynecol 68:305, 1986

Hellman LM, Prystowsky H: The duration of the second stage of labor. Am J Obstet Gynecol 63:1223, 1952

Hendricks CH, Brenner WE, Kraus G: Normal cervical dilatation pattern in late pregnancy and labor. Am J Obstet Gynecol 106:1065, 1970

Hendricks CH, Quilligan EJ, Tyler AB, Tucker GJ: Pressure relationships between intervillous space and amniotic fluid in human term pregnancy. Am J Obstet Gynecol 77:1028, 1959

Hillis DS: Diagnosis of contracted pelvis by the impression method. Surg Gynecol Obstet 51:857, 1930

Holland E: Cranial stress in the foetus during labor. J Obstet Gynaecol Br Emp 29:549, 1922

Hughes EC: Obstetric-Gynecologic Terminology. Philadelphia, Davis, 1972, p 390

Impey L, Boylan P: Active management of labour revisited. Br J Obstet Gynaecol 106:183, 1999

Imseis HM, Trout WC, Gabbe SG: The microbiologic effect of digital cervical examination. Am J Obstet Gynecol 180:578, 1999

Kaltreider DF: Criteria of midplane contraction. Am J Obstet Gynecol 63:392, 1952

Kappy KA, Cetrulo C, Knuppel RA: Premature rupture of membranes: Conservative approach. Am J Obstet Gynecol 134:655, 1979

Kilpatrick SJ, Laros RK: Characteristics of normal labor. Obstet Gynecol 74:85, 1989

King JF: Obstetric intervention and the economic imperative. Br J Obstet Gynaecol 100:1063, 1993

Kwee A, Graziosi GCM, van Leeuwen JHS, van Venrooy FV, Bennink D, Mol BWJ, Cohlen BJ, Visser GHA: The effect of immersion on haemodynamic and fetal measures in uncomplicated pregnancies of nulliparous women. Br J Obstet Gynaecol 107:663, 2000

Larks SD: Electrohysterography. Springfield, IL, Thomas, 1960

Lavender T, Alfirevic Z, Walkinshaw S: Partogram action line study: A randomized trial. Br J Obstet Gynaecol 105:976, 1998

Leitch CR, Walker JJ: The rise in caesarean section rate: The same indications but a lower threshold. Br J Obstet Gynaecol 105:621, 1998

Lieberman E, Lang JM, Cohen A, D'Agostino R, Datta S, Frigoletto FD: Association of epidural analgesia with cesarean delivery in nulliparas. Obstet Gynecol 88:993, 1996

López-Zeno JA, Peaceman AM, Adashek JA, Socol ML: A controlled trial of a program for the active management of labor. N Engl J Med 326:450, 1992

Lupe PJ, Gross TL: Maternal upright posture and mobility in labor: A review. Obstet Gynecol 67:727, 1986

Mahon TR, Chazotte C, Cohen WR: Short labor: Characteristics and outcome. Obstet Gynecol 84:47, 1994

McCarthy S: Magnetic resonance imaging in obstetrics and gynecology. Magn Reson Imaging 4:59, 1986

Mengert WF: Estimation of pelvic capacity. JAMA 138:169, 1948

Menticoglou SM, Manning F, Harman C, Morrison I: Perinatal outcomes in relation to second-stage duration. Am J Obstet Gynecol 173:906, 1995a

Menticoglou SM, Perlman M, Manning FA: High cervical spinal cord injury in neonates delivered with forceps: Report of 15 cases. Obstet Gynecol 86:589, 1995b

Miller FC: Uterine motility in spontaneous labor. Clin Obstet Gynecol 26:78, 1983

Moore MM, Shearer DR: Fetal dose estimates for CT pelvimetry. Radiology 171:265, 1989

Mozurkewich EL, Wolf FM: Premature rupture of membranes at term: A meta-analysis of three management schemes. Obstet Gynecol 89:1035, 1997

Müller: On the frequency and etiology of general pelvic contraction. Arch Gynaek 16:155, 1880

Nageotte MP, Dorchester W, Port M, Keegan KA, Freeman RK: Quantitation of uterine activity preceeding preterm, term and postterm labor. Am J Obstet Gynecol 158:1254, 1988

Notzon FC, Cnattinguis S, Bergsjo P, Cole S, Taffel S, Irgens L, Daltveit AK: Cesarean section deliveries in the 1980s: International comparison by indication. Am J Obstet Gynecol 17:495, 1994

O'Connor TCF, Woods RE, Cavanaugh D: Indications for the simulation of labor. In Parke-Davis & Company: Oxytocin-induced Labor. Greenwich, CT, CPC Communications, 1976, p 10

Odent M: Birth under water. Lancet 2:1476, 1983

O'Driscoll K, Foley M, MacDonald D: Active management of labor as an alternative to cesarean section for dystocia. Obstet Gynecol 63:485, 1984

O'Driscoll K, Meagher D, Boylan P: Diagnosis of labor. Active Management of Labor, 3rd ed. London, Mosby-Year Book, 1993, p 43

Olah KSJ, Neilson J: Failure to progress in the management of labour. Br J Obstet Gynaecol 101:1, 1994

Osborn SB: The implications of the Committee on Radiological Hazards to Patients (Adrian Committee), 1. Variations in the radiation dose received by the patient in diagnostic radiology. Br J Radiol 36:230, 1963

Parnell C, Langhoff-Roos J, Iversen R, Damgaard J: Pushing method in the expulsive phase of labor: A randomized trial. Acta Obstet Gynecol Scand 72:31, 1993

Peisner DB, Rosen MG: Transition from latent to active labor. Obstet Gynecol 68:448, 1986

Peleg D, Hannah ME, Hodnett ED, Foster GA, Willan AR, Farine D: Predictors of cesarean delivery after prelabor rupture of membranes at term. Obstet Gynecol 93:1031, 1999

Read JA, Miller FC, Paul RH: Randomized trial of ambulation versus oxytocin for labor enhancement: A preliminary report. Am J Obstet Gynecol 139:669, 1981

Reynolds SRM, Heard OO, Bruns P, Hellman LM: A multichannel strain-gauge tokodynamometer: An instrument for studying patterns of uterine contractions in pregnant women. Bull Johns Hopkins Hosp 82:446, 1948

Robertson PA, Huang LJ, Croughan-Minihane MS, Kilpatrick SJ: Is there an association between water baths during labor and the development of chorioamnionitis or endometritis? Am J Obstet Gynecol 178:1215, 1998

Rogers R, Gilson GJ, Miller AC, Izquierdo LE, Curet LB, Quells CR: Active management of labor: Does it make a difference? Am J Obstet Gynecol 177:599, 1997

Rosen MG: Management of Labor. Physician Judgment and Patient Care. New York, Elsevier, 1990, p 52

Roshanfekr D, Blakemore KJ, Lee J, Hueppchen NA, Witter FR: Station at onset of active labor in nulliparous patients and risk of cesarean delivery. Obstet Gynecol 93:329, 1999

Rouse DJ, Owen J, Hauth JC: Active-phase labor arrest: Oxytocin augmentation for at least 4 hours. Obstet Gynecol 93:323, 1999

Russell JG: Moulding of the pelvic outlet. J Obstet Gynaecol Br Commonw 76:817, 1969

Samuelsson EC, Victor FTA, Tibblin G, Svardsudd KF: Signs of genital prolapse in a Swedish population of women 20 to 59 years of age and possible related factors. Am J Obstet Gynecol 180:299, 1999

Satin AJ, Maberry MC, Leveno KJ, Sherman ML, Kline DM: Chorioamnionitis: A harbinger of dystocia. Obstet Gynecol 79:913, 1992

Savage W, Francome C: British cesarean section rates: Have we reached a plateau? Br J Obstet Gynaecol 101:645, 1994

Schorn MN, McAllister JL, Blanco JD: Water immersion and the effect on labor. J Nurse Midwifery 38:336, 1993

Seaward PGR, Hannah ME, Myhr TL, Farine D, Ohlsson A, Wang EE, et. al: International multicenter term PROM study: Evaluation of predictors of neonatal infection in infants born to patients with premature rupture of membranes at term. Am J Obstet Gynecol 179:635, 1998

Sharma SK, Leveno KJ: Update: Epidural analgesia during labor does not increase cesarean births. Curr Anesthe Reports 2:18, 2000

Skajaa K, Hansen ES, Bendix J: Depressed fracture of the skull in a child born by cesarean section. Acta Obstet Gynecol Scand 66:275, 1987

Sokol RJ, Stojkov J, Chik L, Rosen MG: Normal and abnormal labor progress, 1. A quantitative assessment and survey of the literature. J Reprod Med 18:47, 1977

Sorbe B, Dahlgren S: Some important factors in the molding of the fetal head during vaginal delivery—a photographic study. Int J Gynaecol Obstet 21:205, 1983

Speer DP, Peltier LF: Pelvic fractures and pregnancy. J Trauma 12:474, 1972

Sporri S, Hanggi W, Brahetti A, Vock P, Schneider H: Pelvimetry by magnetic resonance imaging as a diagnostic tool to evaluate dystocia. Obstet Gynecol 89:902, 1997

Stark DD, McCarthy SM, Filly RA, Parer JT, Hricak H, Callen PW: Pelvimetry by magnetic resonance imaging. Am J Radiol 144:947, 1985

Stephenson J: An unkind cut? Health Agencies Update. JAMA 283:2514, 2000

Sultan AH, Stanton SL: Preserving the pelvic floor and perineum during childbirth: Elective cesarean-section? Br J Obstet Gynaecol 103:731, 1996

Thoms H: The obstetrical significance of pelvic variations: A study of 450 primiparous women. BMJ 2:210, 1937

Thornton JG, Lilford RJ: Active management of labour: Current knowledge and research issues. BMJ 309:366, 1994

Thorp JA, Hu DH, Albin RM, McNitt J, Meyer BA, Cohen GR, et al. The effect of intrapartum epidural analgesia on nulliparous labor: A randomized, controlled, prospective trial. Am J Obstet Gynecol 169:851, 1993a

Thorp JM Jr, Pahel-Short L, Bowes WA Jr: The Mueller-Hillis maneuver: Can it be used to predict dystocia? Obstet Gynecol 82:519, 1993b

Thurnau GR, Scates DH, Morgan MA: The fetal-pelvic index: A method of identifying fetal-pelvic disproportion in women attempting vaginal birth after previous cesarean delivery. Am J Obstet Gynecol 165:353, 1991

Vause S, Congdon HM, Thornton JG: Immediate and delayed pushing in the second stage of labour for nulliparous women with epidural analgesia: A randomized controlled trial. Br J Obstet Gynaecol 105:186, 1998

Ventura SJ, Martin JA, Curtin SC, Mathews TJ, Park MM: Births: Final data for 1998. National Vital Statistics Reports; Vol 48, No. 3. Hyattsville, MD, National Center for Health Statistics, 2000

Wagner M: Choosing caesarean section. Lancet 356:1677, 2000

Williams JW: Obstetrics, 7th ed. Stander HJ (ed). New York, Appleton-Century, 1936, p 971

Williams JW: Obstetrics: A Textbook for the Use of Students and Practitioners, 1st ed. New York, Appleton, 1903, p 282

Williams RM, Thom MH, Studd JW: A study of the benefits and acceptability of ambulation in spontaneous labor. Br J Obstet Gynaecol 87:122, 1980

World Health Organization: Partographic management of labour. Lancet 343:1399, 1994

Zetterstrom J, Lopez A, Auzen B, Normon M, Holmstrom B, Mellgren A: Anal sphincter tears at vaginal delivery: Risk factors and clinical outcome of primary repair. Obstet Gynecol 94:21, 1999

19

Dystocia

ABNORMAL PRESENTATION, POSITION, AND DEVELOPMENT OF THE FETUS

In nearly 97 percent of pregnancies, at the time of delivery, the fetus is entering the pelvis as a cephalic presentation (Table 19–1). In about 3 percent there is a breech presenting, and this is discussed in Chapter 22. In the remaining 0.5 percent, the fetus presents with the long axis either transverse or oblique, or the head may be extended to present the fetal face or brow.

FACE PRESENTATION

With a face presentation, the head is hyperextended so that the occiput is in contact with the fetal back and the chin (mentum) is presenting. The fetal face may present with the chin (mentum) anterior or posterior, relative to the maternal symphysis pubis. In term-size fetuses, labor progression is usually impeded with mentum posterior face presentations because the fetal brow (bregma) is compressed against the maternal symphysis pubis. This position precludes flexion of the fetal head necessary to negotiate the birth canal. In contrast, flexion of the head and vaginal delivery is typical with mentum anterior presentations. Many mentum posterior presentations convert spontaneously to anterior even in late labor (Duff, 1981).

INCIDENCE. Cruikshank and White (1973) reported an incidence of 1 in 600, or 0.17 percent. Among more than 70,000 singleton infants delivered at Parkland Hospital from 1995 through 1999, 36—or about 1 in 2000—were face presentations at delivery (Table 19–1).

DIAGNOSIS. Face presentation is diagnosed by vaginal examination and palpation of the distinctive facial features of the mouth and nose, malar bones, and particularly the orbital ridges. As discussed in Chapter 22 (p. 511), it is possible to mistake a breech for a face presentation, because the anus may be mistaken for the mouth and the ischial tuberosities for the malar prominences. The radiographic demonstration of the hyperextended

head with the facial bones at or below the pelvic inlet is quite characteristic (Fig. 19–1).

ETIOLOGY. Causes of face presentations are numerous, generally stemming from any factor that favors extension or prevents head flexion. In exceptional instances, marked enlargement of the neck or coils of cord about the neck may cause extension. Anencephalic fetuses naturally present by the face. Extended positions occur more frequently when the pelvis is contracted, or the fetus is very large. In a series of 141 face presentations studied by Hellman and co-workers (1950), the incidence of inlet contraction was 40 percent. This high incidence of pelvic contraction, as well as large infants, must be kept in mind when considering management.

In multiparous women, a pendulous abdomen may predispose to face presentation. It permits the back of the fetus to sag forward to laterally, often in the same direction in which the occiput points, thus promoting extension of the cervical and thoracic spine. High parity itself is a predisposing factor (Fuchs and colleagues, 1985).

TABLE 19–1. Fetal Presentation in 68,097 Singleton Pregnancies at Parkland Hospital, 1995–1999

Presentation	Percent	Incidence
Cephalic	96.8	—
Breech	2.7	1:36
Transverse	0.3	1:335
Compound	0.1	1:1000
Face	0.05	1:2000
Brow	0.01	1:10,000

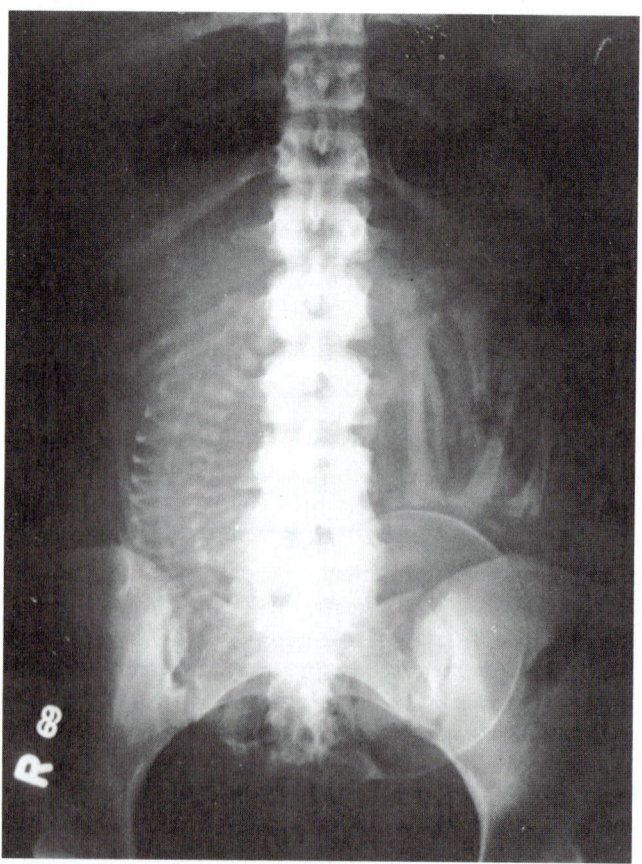

FIGURE 19–1. Radiograph showing face presentation. Note marked hyperextension of head and spine of fetus.

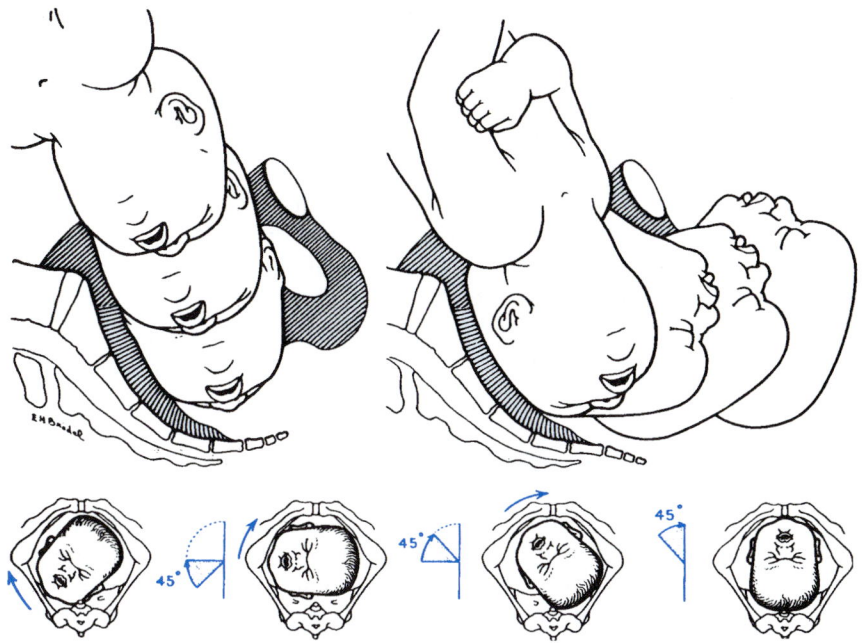

FIGURE 19-2. Mechanism of labor for right mentoposterior position with subsequent rotation of mentum anterior and delivery.

MECHANISM. Face presentations are rarely observed above the pelvic inlet. The brow generally presents, and it is usually converted into a face presentation after further extension of the head during descent. The mechanism of labor in these cases consists of the cardinal movements of descent, internal rotation, and flexion, and the accessory movements of extension and external rotation (Fig. 19–2). Descent is brought about by the same factors as in cephalic presentations. Extension results from the relation of the fetal body to the deflected head, which is converted into a two-armed lever, the longer arm of which extends from the occipital condyles to the occiput. When resistance is encountered, the occiput must be pushed toward the back of the fetus while the chin descends (Fig. 19–3).

The objective of internal rotation of the face is to bring the chin under the symphysis pubis. Only in this way can the neck subtend the posterior surface of the symphysis pubis. If the chin rotates directly posteriorly, the relatively short neck cannot span the anterior surface of the sacrum, which measures about 12 cm in length (Fig. 19–3). Hence, the birth of the head is impossible unless the shoulders enter the pelvis at the same time, an event that is impossible except when the fetus is extremely small or macerated. Internal rotation results from the same factors as in vertex presentations.

After anterior rotation and descent, the chin and mouth appear at the vulva, the undersurface of the chin presses against the symphysis, and the head is delivered by flexion (Fig. 19–2). The nose, eyes, brow (bregma), and occiput then appear in succession over the anterior margin of the perineum. After birth of the head, the occiput sags backward toward the anus. Next, the chin rotates externally to the side toward which it was originally directed, and the shoulders are born as in cephalic presentations.

Edema may sometimes significantly distort the face

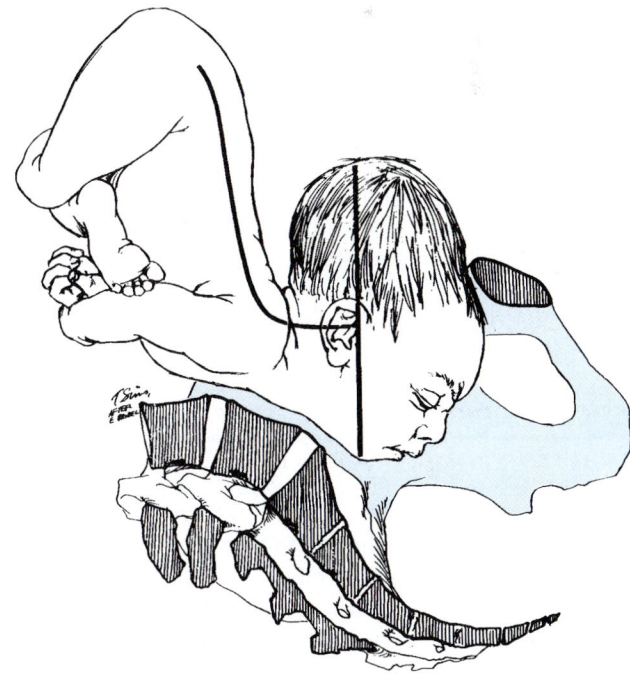

FIGURE 19-3. Face presentation. The occiput is the longer end of the head lever. The chin is directly posterior. Vaginal delivery is impossible unless the chin rotates anteriorly.

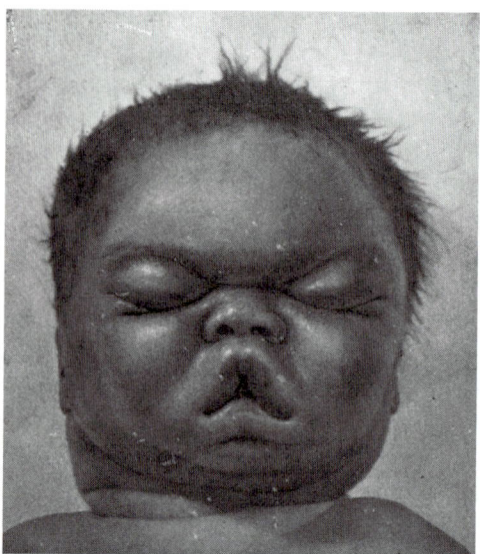

FIGURE 19–4. Edema in face presentation.

(Fig. 19–4). At the same time, the skull undergoes considerable molding, manifested by an increase in length of the occipitomental diameter of the head (Fig. 19–3).

MANAGEMENT. In the absence of a contracted pelvis, and with effective labor, successful vaginal delivery will usually follow. Fetal heart rate monitoring is probably better done with external devices to avoid damage to the face and eyes. Because face presentations among term-size fetuses are more common when there is some degree of pelvic inlet contraction, cesarean delivery is frequently indicated.

Attempts to convert a face manually into a vertex presentation, manual or forceps rotation of a persistently posterior chin to a mentum anterior position, and internal podalic version and extraction are dangerous and not attempted. Neuman and colleagues (1994) have described intrapartum bimanual conversion of mentoposterior to occipitoanterior presentations in 11 women who refused cesarean delivery.

BROW PRESENTATION

This is the rarest presentation (Table 19–1), and is diagnosed when that portion of the fetal head between the orbital ridge and the anterior fontanel presents at the pelvic inlet. As shown in Figure 19–5, the fetal head thus occupies a position midway between full flexion (occiput) and extension (mentum or face). Except when the fetal head is small or the pelvis is unusually large, engagement of the fetal head and subsequent delivery cannot take place as long as the brow presentation persists.

ETIOLOGY. The causes of persistent brow presentation are the same as those for face presentation. A brow presentation is commonly unstable and often converts to a face or an occiput presentation (Cruikshank and White, 1973).

DIAGNOSIS. The presentation may be recognized by abdominal palpation when both the occiput and chin can be palpated easily, but vaginal examination is usually necessary. The frontal sutures, large anterior fontanel, orbital ridges, eyes, and root of the nose can be felt on vaginal examination. Neither mouth nor chin is within reach, however (Fig. 19–5).

MECHANISM OF LABOR. With a very small fetus and a large pelvis, labor is generally easy. With a larger fetus, however, it is usually very difficult, because engagement is impossible until there is marked molding that shortens the occipitomental diameter or, more commonly, until there is either flexion to an occiput presentation or extension to a face presentation. The considerable molding essential for vaginal delivery of a persistent brow characteristically deforms the head. The caput succedaneum is over the forehead, and it may be so extensive that identification of the brow by palpation is impossible. In these instances, the forehead is prominent and squared, and the occipitomental diameter is diminished.

PROGNOSIS. In transient brow presentations, the prognosis depends upon the ultimate presentation. If the brow persists, prognosis is poor for vaginal delivery unless the fetus is small or the birth canal is huge.

MANAGEMENT. Principles are much the same as those for a face presentation. If, by chance, spontaneous labor is progressing without any evidence of distress in the closely monitored fetus, and without unduly vigorous uterine contractions, no interference is necessary.

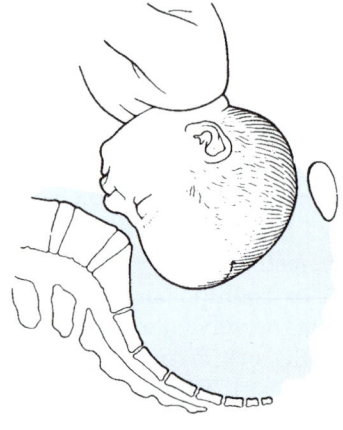

FIGURE 19–5. Brow posterior presentation.

TRANSVERSE LIE

This occurs when the long axis of the fetus is approximately perpendicular to that of the mother. When the long axis forms an acute angle, an **oblique lie** results. The latter is usually only transitory, because either a longitudinal or transverse lie commonly results when labor supervenes. For this reason, the oblique lie is called an *unstable lie* in Great Britain.

In transverse lies, the shoulder is usually over the pelvic inlet, with the head lying in one iliac fossa and the breech in the other. In such a **shoulder presentation,** the side of the mother toward which the acromion is directed determines the designation of the lie as right or left acromial. Moreover, because in either position the back may be directed anteriorly or posteriorly, superiorly or inferiorly, it is customary to distinguish varieties as dorsoanterior and dorsoposterior (Fig. 19–6).

INCIDENCE. Transverse lie occurred once in 322 singleton deliveries (0.3 percent) at both the Mayo Clinic and the University of Iowa Hospital (Cruikshank and White, 1973; Johnson 1964). At Parkland Hospital, transverse lie was encountered in about 1 in 335 singleton fetuses delivered over a 4-year period (Table 19–1).

ETIOLOGY. The common causes of transverse lie are:

1. Unusual relaxation of the abdominal wall resulting from high parity.
2. Preterm fetus.
3. Placenta previa.
4. Abnormal uterus.
5. Excessive amnionic fluid.
6. Contracted pelvis.

Women with four or more deliveries have a tenfold incidence of transverse lie compared with nulliparous women. Relaxation of the abdominal wall with a pendulous abdomen allows the uterus to fall forward, deflecting the long axis of the fetus away from the axis of the birth canal into an oblique or transverse position. Placenta previa and pelvic contraction act similarly. A transverse or oblique lie occasionally develops in labor from an initial longitudinal position.

DIAGNOSIS. This is usually made easily, often by inspection alone. The abdomen is unusually wide, whereas the uterine fundus extends to only slightly above the umbilicus. No fetal pole is detected in the fundus, and the ballottable head is found in one iliac fossa and the breech in the other. At the same time, the position of

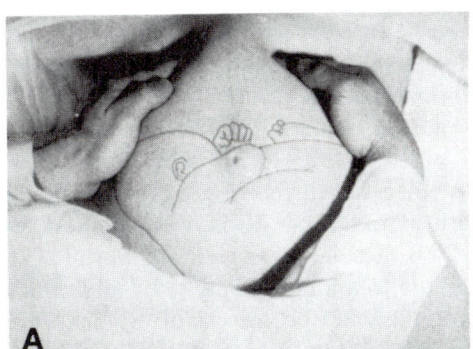
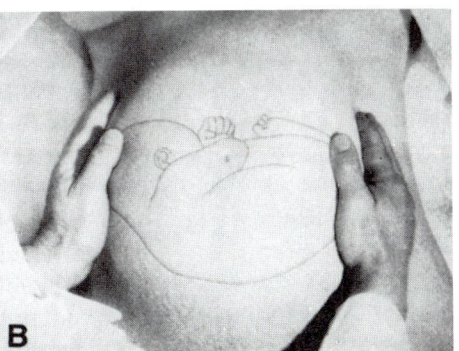
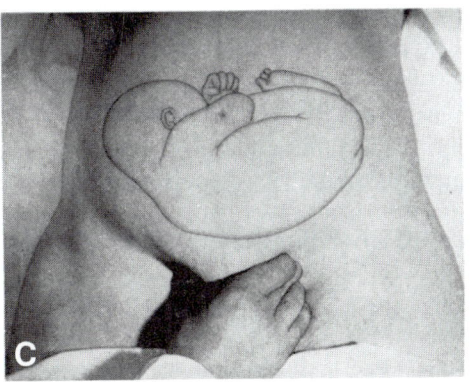
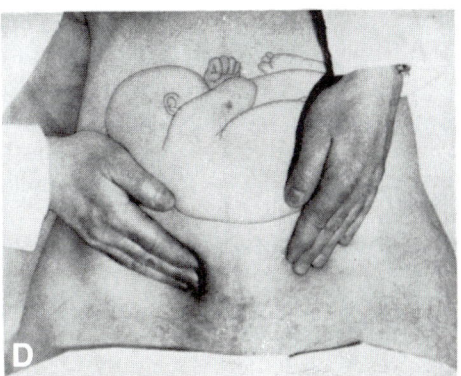

FIGURE 19–6. Palpation in transverse lie, right acromidorsoanterior position. **A.** First maneuver. **B.** Second maneuver. **C.** Third maneuver. **D.** Fourth maneuver.

the back is readily identified. When the back is anterior (Fig. 19–6), a hard resistance plane extends across the front of the abdomen; when it is posterior, irregular nodulations representing the small parts are felt in the same location.

On vaginal examination, in the early stages of labor, the side of the thorax, if it can be reached, may be recognized by the "gridiron" feel of the ribs. When dilatation is further advanced, the scapula and the clavicle are distinguished on opposite sides of the thorax. The position of the axilla indicates the side of the mother toward which the shoulder is directed. Later in labor, the shoulder will become tightly wedged in the pelvic canal, and a hand and arm frequently prolapse into the vagina and through the vulva (Fig. 19–7).

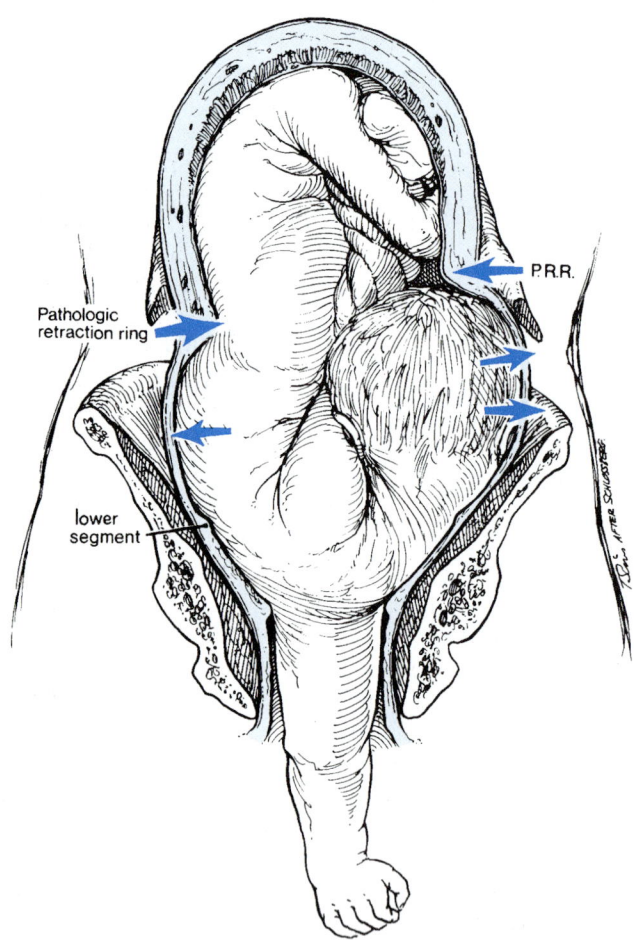

FIGURE 19–7. Neglected shoulder presentation. A thick muscular band forming a pathological retraction ring has developed just above the very thin lower uterine segment. The force generated during a uterine contraction is directed centripetally at and above the level of the pathological retraction ring. This serves to stretch further and possibly to rupture the very thin lower segment below the retraction ring. (P.R.R. = pathological retraction ring.)

COURSE OF LABOR. Spontaneous delivery of a fully developed infant is impossible with a persistent transverse lie. After rupture of the membranes, if labor continues, the fetal shoulder is forced into the pelvis, and the corresponding arm frequently prolapses (Fig. 19–7). After some descent, the shoulder is arrested by the margins of the pelvic inlet, with the head in one iliac fossa and the breech in the other. As labor continues, the shoulder is impacted firmly in the upper part of the pelvis. The uterus then contracts vigorously in an unsuccessful attempt to overcome the obstacle. After a time, a retraction ring rises increasingly higher and becomes more marked. The situation is referred to as a *neglected transverse lie.* If not promptly managed, the uterus eventually ruptures, and the mother and fetus die.

If the fetus is quite small (usually less than 800 g) and the pelvis is large, spontaneous delivery is possible despite persistence of the abnormal lie. The fetus is compressed with the head forced against the abdomen. A portion of the thoracic wall below the shoulder thus becomes the most dependent part, appearing at the vulva. The head and thorax then pass through the pelvic cavity at the same time, and the fetus, which is doubled upon itself (*conduplicato corpore*), is expelled.

PROGNOSIS. Labor with a shoulder presentation increases maternal risk and adds tremendously to fetal hazards. Most maternal deaths from neglected cases are from spontaneous or traumatic uterine rupture consequent upon late and ill-advised version and extraction. Even with the best of care, morbidity is increased because of the frequent association with placenta previa, increased likelihood of cord prolapse, and necessity for major operative interferences.

MANAGEMENT. In general, the onset of active labor in a woman with a transverse lie is an indication for cesarean delivery. Once labor is well established, attempts at conversion to a longitudinal lie by abdominal manipulation will likely not be successful. Before labor or early in labor, with the membranes intact, attempts at external version are worthy of a trial in the absence of other complications that indicate cesarean delivery. Phelan and co-workers (1986) recommend such an attempt only after 39 weeks because of the high (83 percent) spontaneous conversion to a longitudinal lie. If during early labor, the fetal head can be maneuvered by abdominal manipulation into the pelvis, it should be held there during the next several contractions in an attempt to fix the head in the pelvis. If these measures fail, cesarean delivery is performed.

Because neither the feet nor the head of the fetus occupy the lower uterine segment, a low transverse incision into the uterus may lead to difficulty in extraction of a fetus entrapped in the body of the uterus above the level of incision. Therefore, a vertical incision is likely to be indicated (Chap. 23, p. 550).

COMPOUND PRESENTATION

In a compound presentation, an extremity prolapses alongside the presenting part, with both presenting in the pelvis simultaneously (Fig. 19–8).

INCIDENCE AND ETIOLOGY. Goplerud and Eastman (1953) identified a hand or arm prolapsed alongside the head once in every 700 deliveries. Much less common was prolapse of one or both lower extremities alongside a cephalic presentation or a hand alongside a breech. We identified compound presentations in only 68 of more than 70,000 singleton fetuses delivered from 1995 through 1999, for an incidence of about 1 in 1000 (Table 19–1). Causes of compound presentations are conditions that prevent complete occlusion of the pelvic inlet by the fetal head, including preterm birth (Goplerud and Eastman, 1953).

PROGNOSIS AND MANAGEMENT. Perinatal loss is increased due to preterm delivery, prolapsed cord, and traumatic obstetrical procedures. In most cases, the prolapsed part should be left alone, because most often it will not interfere with labor. Goplerud and Eastman (1953) described 50 cases not associated with a prolapsed cord; in almost half, normal delivery ensued with loss of only one infant. If the arm is prolapsed alongside the head, the condition should be closely observed to ascertain whether the arm rises out of the way with descent of the presenting part. If it fails to do so and if it appears to prevent descent of the head, the prolapsed arm should be gently pushed upward and the head simultaneously downward by fundal pressure. Tebes and co-authors (1999) described a tragic outcome in an infant delivered spontaneously with the hand alongside the head. The child developed ischemic necrosis of the presenting forearm which required amputation.

PERSISTENT OCCIPUT POSTERIOR POSITION

Most often, occiput posterior positions undergo spontaneous anterior rotation followed by uncomplicated delivery. Although the precise reasons for failure of spontaneous rotation are not known, transverse narrowing of the midpelvis is undoubtedly a contributing factor. Gardberg and associates (1998) used ultrasonography to record the position of the fetal head in 408 term pregnancies at entry into labor (Fig. 19–9). Early in labor, about 15 percent of the fetuses were occiput posterior and 5 percent were in this position at delivery. Importantly, two thirds of occiput posterior deliveries were in those who were occiput anterior at the beginning of labor. Thus, most occiput posterior presentations at delivery are the result of malrotation of occiput anterior position during labor and most (87 percent) of occiput posterior presentations at the outset of labor spontaneously rotate anteriorly. Induction of labor and epidural analgesia were not factors linked to occiput posterior presentations in this study.

Labor and delivery need not differ remarkably from that with the occiput anterior. Progress may be ascertained by assessing cervical dilatation and descent of the head. In most instances, delivery can usually be accomplished without great difficulty once the head reaches the perineum. The possibilities for vaginal delivery are:

1. Await spontaneous delivery.
2. Forceps delivery with the occiput directly posterior.
3. Forceps rotation of the occiput to the anterior position and delivery.
4. Manual rotation to the anterior position followed by spontaneous or forceps delivery.

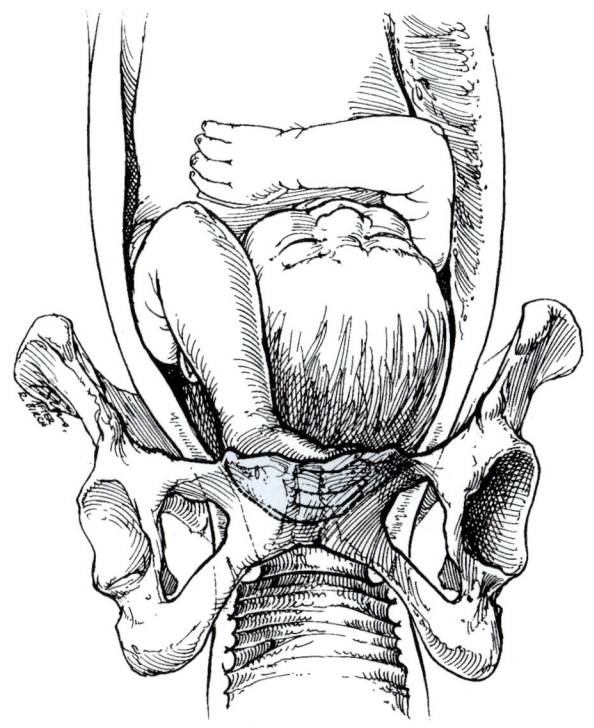

FIGURE 19–8. Compound presentation. The left hand is lying in front of the vertex. With further labor, the hand and arm may retract from the birth canal and the head may then descend normally.

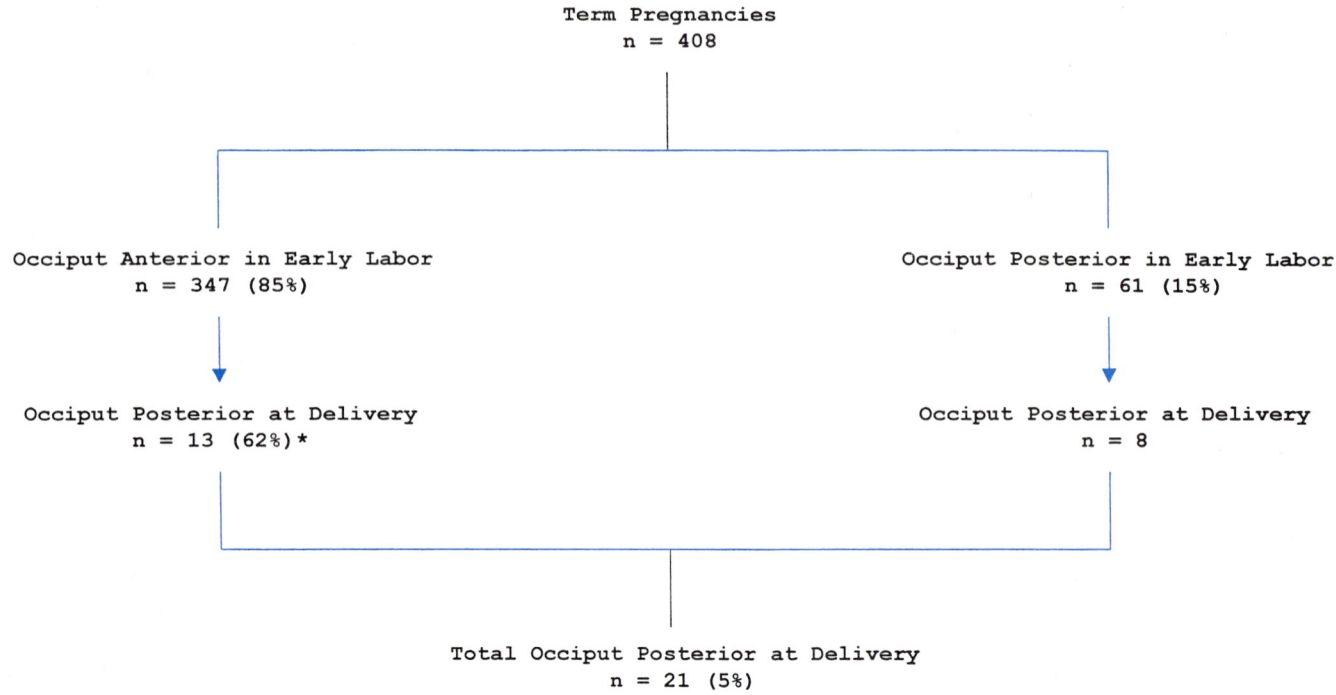

Term Pregnancies
n = 408

Occiput Anterior in Early Labor
n = 347 (85%)

Occiput Posterior in Early Labor
n = 61 (15%)

Occiput Posterior at Delivery
n = 13 (62%)*

Occiput Posterior at Delivery
n = 8

Total Occiput Posterior at Delivery
n = 21 (5%)

* 62% of occiput posterior presentations at delivery were occiput anterior
at the beginning of labor.

FIGURE 19–9. Occiput posterior presentation in early labor compared with presentation at delivery. Ultrasonography was used to determine position of the fetal head in early labor. (From Gardberg and associates, 1998.)

SPONTANEOUS DELIVERY. If the pelvic outlet is roomy and the vaginal outlet and perineum are somewhat relaxed from previous vaginal deliveries, rapid spontaneous delivery will often take place. If the vaginal outlet is resistant to stretch and the perineum is firm, late first stage or the second stage of labor, or both, may be appreciably prolonged. During each expulsive effort, with the occiput posterior, the head is driven against the perineum to a much greater degree than when anterior. Therefore, forceps delivery is often indicated. A generous episiotomy is usually needed.

FORCEPS DELIVERY AS AN OCCIPUT POSTERIOR. The need for more traction compared with forceps deliveries from the occiput anterior position can be minimized by making a larger episiotomy. The use of forceps and a large episiotomy warrant more complete analgesia than may be achieved with pudendal block and local perineal infiltration. The forceps are applied bilaterally along the occipitomental diameter, as described in Chapter 21 (p. 496).

It is important to identify the infrequent case in which protrusion of fetal scalp through the introitus is the consequence of marked elongation of the fetal head from molding combined with formation of a large caput. In this circumstance, the head may not even be engaged—that is, the biparietal diameter may not have passed through the pelvic inlet. Labor has characteristically been long in such a case and, in turn, descent of the head has been slow. Careful palpation above the symphysis may disclose the fetal head to be above the pelvic inlet. Prompt cesarean delivery is appropriate in such cases.

MANUAL ROTATION. The requirements for forceps rotation must be met before doing a manual rotation. When the hand is introduced to locate the posterior ear and thus confirm the posterior position, the occiput often rotates toward the anterior position. The head may be grasped with the fingers over the posterior ear and the thumb over the anterior ear and an attempt made to rotate the occiput to the anterior position (Chap. 21, p. 495).

FORCEPS ROTATION. If the head is engaged, the cervix fully dilated, and the pelvis adequate, forceps rotation may be attempted if the operator is sufficiently skilled. These circumstances are most likely to prevail when expulsive efforts of the mother during the second stage are ineffective, such as with continuous regional analgesia. Rotation with forceps is described in Chapter 21 (p. 497).

Menticoglou and co-workers (1995) reviewed the obstetrical features of 15 infants with birth-related high cervical spinal cord injuries in 13 Canadian hospitals between 1982 and 1994. All of these infants had in common cephalic delivery with forceps rotation of 90 degrees or more from occipitoposterior or occipitotransverse positions. They could not determine whether these serious—albeit rare—fetal injuries occurred as a result of mismanagement or as an intrinsic risk of properly performed forceps rotation. They estimated that this complication developed in less than 1 per 1000 forceps rotations.

OUTCOME. There are notable differences when persistent occiput posterior position is compared with the occiput anterior. Phillips and Freeman (1974) reported that labor was prolonged on the average 1 hour in parous women and 2 hours in nulliparous women. Episiotomy extension was increased appreciably. Gardberg and Tuppurainen (1994) later observed that both first- and second-stage labor were longer in persistent occiput posterior and that 65 percent required operative interventions. Johanson and co-workers (1993) found that both forceps and vacuum-assisted deliveries for occiput posterior positions more often failed compared with anterior presentations (24 versus 7 percent). With vaginal delivery, especially instrumental, accompanying severe perineal lacerations are associated with long-term morbidity, as discussed in Chapter 13 (p. 325).

At Parkland Hospital, either manual rotation to the anterior position followed by forceps delivery, or forceps delivery from the occiput posterior position, is used to effect delivery. When neither can be done with relative ease, cesarean delivery is performed.

PERSISTENT OCCIPUT TRANSVERSE POSITION

In the absence of a pelvic architecture abnormality, the occiput transverse position is most likely a transitory one as the occiput rotates to the anterior position. If hypotonic uterine dysfunction, either spontaneous or the consequence of regional analgesia, does not develop, spontaneous rotation is usually completed rapidly, thus allowing the choice of spontaneous delivery or delivery with outlet forceps.

DELIVERY. If rotation ceases because of lack of uterine action and in the absence of pelvic contraction, vaginal delivery can usually be accomplished readily in a number of ways. The occiput may be manually rotated anteriorly or posteriorly and forceps delivery carried out from either the anterior or posterior position. Another approach recommended by some is to apply forceps of the Kielland type to the head in the occiput transverse position (Chap. 21, p. 497), rotate the occiput to the anterior position, and then deliver the head with either the same forceps or with standard forceps. If failure of spontaneous rotation is caused by hypotonic uterine dysfunction *without cephalopelvic disproportion*, oxytocin may be infused with close monitoring.

The genesis of the occiput transverse position is not always so simple, or the treatment so benign. With the platypelloid (anteroposteriorly flat configuration) and the android (heart-shaped) pelves, there may not be adequate room for rotation of the occiput to either the anterior or the posterior position. With the android pelvis, the head may not even be engaged, yet the scalp may be visible through the vaginal introitus as the consequence of considerable molding and caput formation. This situation is fraught with danger to both the fetus and mother. If forceps are tried for delivery, it is imperative that undue force not be applied but, instead, cesarean delivery be accomplished.

SHOULDER DYSTOCIA

The incidence of shoulder dystocia varies greatly depending on the criteria used for diagnosis. For example, Gross and co-authors (1987) identified that 0.9 percent of almost 11,000 vaginal deliveries were coded for shoulder dystocia at the Toronto General Hospital. True shoulder dystocia, however, diagnosed because maneuvers were required to deliver the shoulders in addition to downward traction and episiotomy, was identified in only 24 births (0.2 percent). Significant infant trauma was observed only in shoulder dystocias requiring a maneuver to effect delivery. Current reports, where the diagnosis of shoulder dystocia is limited to those deliveries requiring a maneuver, cite an incidence that varies between 0.6 percent and 1.4 percent (American College of Obstetricians and Gynecologists, 2000; Baskett and Allen, 1995; McFarland and co-workers, 1995; Nocon and co-workers, 1993).

There is some evidence that the incidence of shoulder dystocia increased from 1960 to 1980 (Hopwood, 1982). This is likely due to increasing birthweight. Modanlou and co-workers (1982) showed that neonates experiencing shoulder dystocia had significantly greater shoulder-to-head and chest-to-head disproportions compared with equally macrosomic infants delivered without dystocia. It is also likely that the increased incidence of shoulder dystocia is due in part to increased attention to its appropriate documentation (Nocon and co-workers, 1993).

Use of maneuvers to define shoulder dystocia has been criticized (Beall and associates, 1998; Spong and colleagues, 1995). In deliveries in which shoulder dystocia is anticipated, one or more maneuvers may be used prophylactically, but no diagnosis of shoulder dystocia is recorded. In other cases, one or two maneuvers may be used with rapid resolution of shoulder dystocia and excellent outcome, and the diagnosis is not identified. Spong and colleagues (1995) attempted to more objectively define shoulder dystocia by witnessing 250 unselected deliveries and timing intervals from delivery of the head, to delivery of the shoulders, and to completion of the birth. The incidence defined by the use of obstetrical maneuvers was higher than previously reported (11 percent); however, only about half of these were diagnosed by the clinicians. The mean head-to-body delivery time in normal births was 24 seconds compared with 79 seconds in those with shoulder dystocia. They proposed that a head-to-body delivery time exceeding 60 seconds be used to define shoulder dystocia.

MATERNAL CONSEQUENCES. Postpartum hemorrhage, usually from uterine atony, but also from vaginal and cervical lacerations, is the major maternal risk (Benedetti and Gabbe, 1978; Parks and Ziel, 1978). Puerperal infection following cesarean delivery also remains a problem.

FETAL CONSEQUENCES. Shoulder dystocia may be associated with significant fetal morbidity and even mortality. Gherman and co-workers (1998) reviewed 285 cases of shoulder dystocia and 25 percent were associated with fetal injuries. Transient brachial plexus palsies were the most common injury, accounting for two thirds; 38 percent had clavicular fractures, and 17 percent sustained humeral fractures. There was one neonatal death, and four infants had persistent brachial plexus injuries. In this series, almost half of the cases of shoulder dystocia required a direct fetal manipulation such as the Woods maneuver, in addition to the McRoberts procedure, to effect release of the impacted shoulders. Direct fetal manipulation, however, when compared with use of the McRoberts procedure alone, was not associated with an increased rate of fetal injury.

BRACHIAL PLEXUS INJURY. Injury to the brachial plexus may be localized to the upper or lower part of the plexus (Chap. 39, p. 1080). It usually results from downward traction on the brachial plexus during delivery of the anterior shoulder. *Erb palsy* results from injury to the spinal nerves C_{5-6} and sometimes C_7. It consists of a paralysis of shoulder and arm muscles re-

sulting in a hanging upper arm that may be extended at the elbow. Involvement of the lower spinal nerves (C_7-T_1) always includes injury of the upper nerves and results in a palsy including the hand, which can cause a clawhand deformity. Hardy (1981) studied the prognosis of 36 infants with brachial plexus injuries. Interestingly, shoulder dystocia had been reported in only 10 of these, and two had been delivered abdominally. Nearly 80 percent of these children had complete recovery by 13 months, and none with residual defects had severe sensory or motor deficits in the hand. Jennett and associates (1992) and Gherman and colleagues (1999) have presented evidence that brachial plexus injuries may precede the delivery itself and may occur even prior to labor.

CLAVICULAR FRACTURE. Fractured clavicles are relatively common and have been diagnosed in 0.4 percent of infants delivered vaginally at Parkland Hospital (Roberts and co-workers, 1995). Such fractures, although at times associated with shoulder dystocia, often occur without any clinical events to suspect them. Investigators have concluded that isolated fractured clavicles are unavoidable, unpredictable, and are of no clinical consequence (Chez and co-authors, 1994; Roberts and co-workers, 1995).

PREDICTION AND PREVENTION OF SHOULDER DYSTOCIA. There has been considerable evolution in obstetrical thinking about the preventability of shoulder dystocia in the past two decades (Chap. 29, p. 758). During the 1970s, when the use of cesarean delivery was escalating rapidly, it was hoped that certain pregnancy risk factors could be used to identify women in whom cesarean delivery would avoid shoulder dystocia. During the 1980s it became apparent, however, that the rate of cesarean delivery was likely excessive. It also became obvious that predicting, and therefore preventing, shoulder dystocia was not simple. Although there are clearly several risk factors associated with shoulder dystocia, actual identification of individual instances before the fact has proven to be impossible.

RISK FACTORS. A variety of maternal, intrapartum, and fetal characteristics have been implicated in the development of shoulder dystocia (Baskett and Allen, 1995; Nesbitt and associates, 1998; Nocon and co-authors, 1993). Several maternal risk factors, including obesity, multiparity, and diabetes, all exert their effects because of associated increased birthweight. For example, Keller and co-workers (1991) identified shoulder dystocia in 7 percent of pregnancies complicated by gestational diabetes. Similarly, the association of postterm pregnancy with shoulder dystocia is likely because many fetuses continue to grow after 42 weeks (Chap. 28, p. 738).

Intrapartum complications associated with shoulder dystocia include midforceps delivery and prolonged first- and second-stage labor (Baskett and Allen, 1995; Nocon and co-authors, 1993). McFarland and co-workers (1995), however, using matched controls, found that first- and second-stage labor abnormalities were not useful clinical predictors of shoulder dystocia.

The common thread running through all current reports on risk factors for shoulder dystocia is increased birthweight (Nesbitt and colleagues, 1998). Table 19–2 gives the incidence of shoulder dystocia related to birthweight groupings at Parkland Hospital during 1994. Clearly, shoulder dystocia increases with greater birthweight; however, almost half of the births with shoulder dystocia weighed less than 4000 g. Indeed, Nocon and co-workers (1993) described shoulder dystocia with birth of a 2260-g infant. Despite this, some authors (O'Leary, 1992) advocate identification of macrosomia with ultrasound and liberal use of cesarean delivery to shoulder dystocia. Others have disputed the concept that cesarean delivery is indicated for identified large fetuses, even those estimated to weigh in excess of 4500 g. Rouse and Owen (1999) concluded that a prophylactic cesarean policy for macrosomic infants would require more than 1000 cesarean deliveries and millions of dollars to avert a single permanent brachial plexus injury. The American College of Obstetricians and Gynecologists (2000) has concluded that performing cesarean deliveries for all women suspected of carrying a macrosomic fetus is not appropriate, except possibly for estimated fetal weights over 5000 g in nondiabetic women and over 4500 g in those with diabetes.

PRIOR SHOULDER DYSTOCIA. Smith and colleagues (1994) identified recurrent shoulder dystocia in 5 of 42 (12 percent) women. Seven of these women had heavier infants in their subsequent pregnancy, but only two experienced recurrent shoulder dystocia. In contrast, Baskett and Allen (1995) found a much lower risk (1 to 2 percent) of recurrent shoulder dystocia.

TABLE 19–2. Incidence of Shoulder Dystocia According to Birthweight Grouping in Singleton Infants Delivered Vaginally in 1994 at Parkland Hospital

Birthweight Group	Births	Shoulder Dystocia (Percent)
≤ 3000 g	2953	0
3001–3500 g	4309	14 (0.3)
3501–4000 g	2839	28 (1.0)
4001–4500 g	704	38 (5.4)
> 4500 g	91	17 (19.0)
All weights	10,896	97 (0.9)

SUMMARY. The American College of Obstetricians and Gynecologists (1997, 2000) reviewed studies classified according to the evidence-based methods outlined by the United States Preventive Services Task Force. It concluded that the preponderance of current evidence is consistent with the view that:

1. Most cases of shoulder dystocia cannot be predicted or prevented because there are no accurate methods to identify which fetuses will develop this complication.
2. Ultrasonic measurements to estimate macrosomia have limited accuracy.
3. Planned cesarean delivery based on suspected macrosomia is not a reasonable strategy.
4. Planned cesarean delivery may be reasonable for the nondiabetic with an estimated fetal weight exceeding 5000 g or the diabetic whose fetus is estimated over 4500 g.

MANAGEMENT. Because shoulder dystocia cannot be predicted, the practitioner of obstetrics *must* be well versed in the management principles of this occasionally devastating complication. Reduction in the interval of time from delivery of the head to delivery of the body is of great importance to survival. An initial gentle attempt at traction, assisted by maternal expulsive efforts is recommended. Overly vigorous traction on the head or neck, or excessive rotation of the body, may cause serious damage to the infant.

Some have advocated performing a large episiotomy, and adequate analgesia is certainly ideal. The next step is to clear the infant's mouth and nose. Having completed these steps, a variety of techniques have been described to free the anterior shoulder from its impacted position beneath the maternal symphysis pubis:

1. Moderate **suprapubic pressure** is applied by an assistant while downward traction is applied to the fetal head.
2. The **McRoberts maneuver** was described by Gonik and associates (1983) and named for William A. McRoberts, Jr., who popularized its use at the University of Texas at Houston. The maneuver consists of removing the legs from the stirrups and sharply flexing them upon the abdomen (Fig. 19–10). Gherman and colleagues (2000) analyzed the McRoberts maneuver using x-ray pelvimetry. They found that the procedure caused straightening of the sacrum relative to the lumbar vertebrae, along with accompanying rotation of the symphysis pubis toward the maternal head and a decrease in the angle of pelvic inclination. While this does not increase pelvic dimensions, pelvic rotation cephalad tends to free the impacted anterior shoulder. Gonik and co-workers (1989) tested the McRoberts position objectively

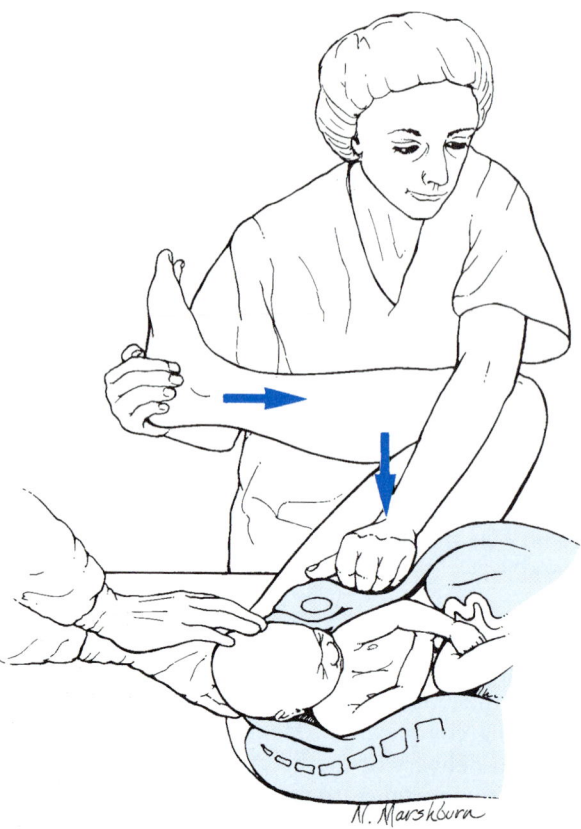

FIGURE 19–10. The McRoberts maneuver. The maneuver consists of removing the legs from the stirrups and sharply flexing the thighs upon the abdomen, as shown by the horizontal arrow. The assistant is also providing suprapubic pressure simultaneously (*vertical arrow*).

with laboratory models and found that the maneuver reduced fetal shoulder extraction forces.

3. Woods (1943) reported that, by progressively rotating the posterior shoulder 180 degrees in a corkscrew fashion, the impacted anterior shoulder could be released. This is frequently referred to as the **Woods corkscrew maneuver** (Fig. 19–11).

4. **Delivery of the posterior shoulder** consists of carefully sweeping the posterior arm of the fetus across the chest, followed by delivery of the arm. The shoulder girdle is then rotated into one of the oblique diameters of the pelvis with subsequent delivery of the anterior shoulder (Fig. 19–12).

5. Rubin (1964) recommended two maneuvers. First, the fetal shoulders are rocked from side to side by applying force to the abdomen. If this is not successful, the pelvic hand reaches the most easily accessible fetal shoulder, which is pushed toward the anterior surface of the chest. This most often results in abduction of both shoulders. This in turn produces a smaller shoulder-to-shoulder diameter

and displacement of the anterior shoulder from behind the symphysis pubis (Fig. 19–13).

6. Hibbard (1982) recommended that pressure be applied to the fetal jaw and neck in the direction of the maternal rectum, with strong fundal pressure applied by an assistant as the anterior shoulder is freed. Strong fundal pressure applied at the wrong time may result in even further impaction of the anterior shoulder. Gross and associates (1987) reported that fundal pressure in the absence of other maneuvers "**resulted in a 77 percent complication rate and was strongly associated with (fetal) orthopedic and neurologic damage.**"

7. Sandberg (1985) reported the **Zavanelli maneuver** for cephalic replacement into the pelvis and then cesarean delivery. The first part of the maneuver consists of returning the head to the occiput anterior or occiput posterior position if the head has rotated from either position. The second step is to flex the head and slowly push it back into the vagina, following which cesarean delivery is performed. Terbutaline (250 μg subcutaneously) is given to produce uterine relaxation. Sandberg (1999) has subsequently reviewed 103 reported cases in which the Zavanelli maneuver was used. This maneuver was successful in 91 percent of cephalic cases and in all cases of breech head entrapments. Fetal injuries were common in the desperate circumstances under which the Zavanelli maneuver was used; there were eight neonatal deaths, six stillbirths, and 10 neonates suffered brain damage. Uterine rupture was also reported.

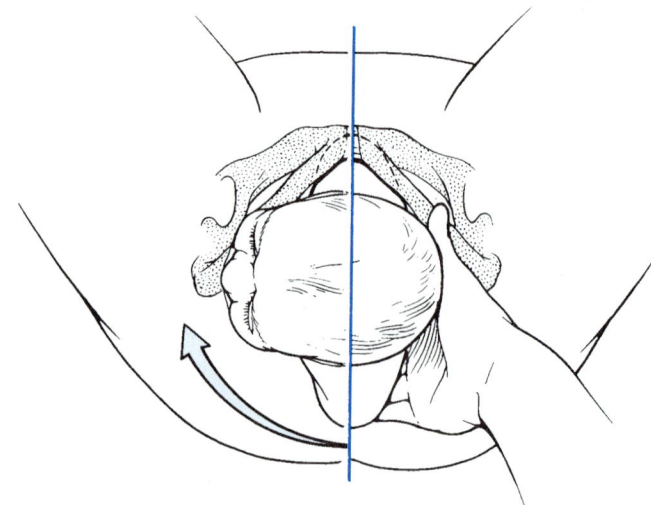

FIGURE 19–11. Woods maneuver. The hand is placed behind the posterior shoulder of the fetus. The shoulder is then rotated progressively 180 degrees in a corkscrew manner so that the impacted anterior is released.

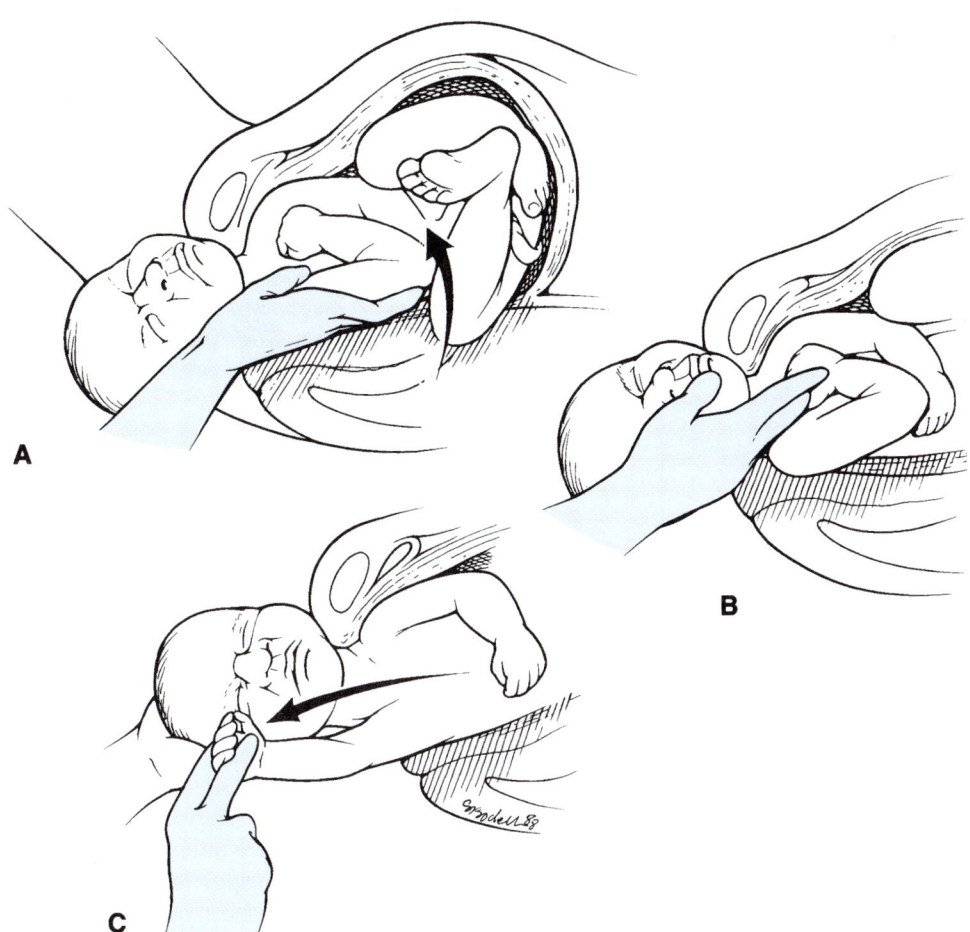

A

B

C

FIGURE 19–12. Shoulder dystocia with impacted anterior shoulder of the fetus. **A.** The operator's hand is introduced into the vagina along the fetal posterior humerus, which is splinted as the arm is swept across the chest, keeping the arm flexed at the elbow. **B.** The fetal hand is grasped and the arm extended along the side of the face. **C.** The posterior arm is delivered from the vagina.

8. Deliberate **fracture of the clavicle** by pressing the anterior clavicle against the ramus of the pubis can be done to free the shoulder impaction. In practice, however, it is difficult to deliberately fracture the clavicle of a large infant. The fracture will heal rapidly, and is not nearly as serious as a brachial nerve injury, asphyxia, or death.

9. **Cleidotomy** consists of cutting the clavicle with scissors or other sharp instruments, and is usually used on a dead fetus (Schramm, 1983).

10. **Symphysiotomy** also has been applied successfully as described by Hartfield (1986). Goodwin and colleagues (1997) reported three cases in which symphysiotomy was performed after the Zavanelli maneuver had failed—all three infants died and maternal morbidity was significant due to urinary tract injury.

Hernandez and Wendel (1990) suggested use of a *shoulder dystocia drill* to better organize emergency management of an impacted shoulder. The drill is a set of maneuvers performed sequentially as needed to complete vaginal delivery. The American College of Obstetricians and Gynecologists (1991) recommends

the following steps—their sequence will depend on the experience and preference of the individual operator:

1. Call for help—mobilize assistants, an anesthesiologist, and a pediatrician. At this time, an initial gentle attempt at traction is made. Drain the bladder if it is distended.

2. A generous episiotomy (mediolateral or episioproctotomy) may afford room posteriorly.

3. Suprapubic pressure is used initially by most practitioners because it has the advantage of simplicity. Only one assistant is needed to provide suprapubic pressure while normal downward traction is applied to the fetal head.

4. The McRoberts maneuver requires two assistants. Each assistant grasps a leg and sharply flexes the maternal thigh against the abdomen.

These maneuvers will resolve most cases of shoulder dystocia. If they fail, however, the following steps may be attempted:

5. The Woods screw maneuver.

6. Delivery of the posterior arm is attempted, but if it

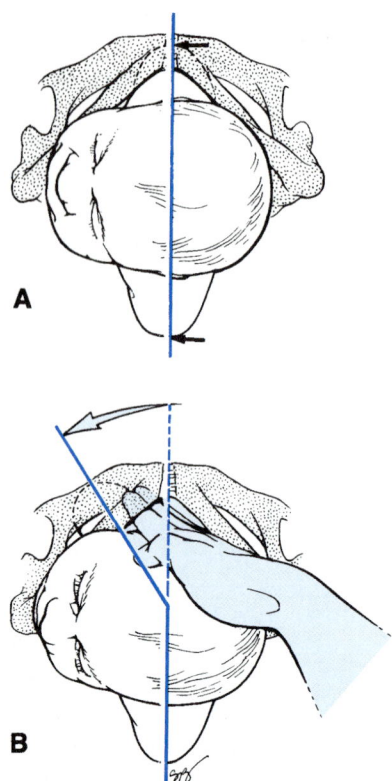

FIGURE 19–13. Rubin (second) maneuver. **A.** The shoulder-to-shoulder diameter is shown as the distance between the two small arrows. **B.** The more easily accessible fetal shoulder (the anterior is shown here) is pushed toward the anterior chest wall of the fetus. Most often, this results in abduction of both shoulders, reducing the shoulder-to-shoulder diameter and freeing the impacted anterior shoulder.

is in a fully extended position, this is usually difficult to accomplish.

7. Other techniques generally should be reserved for cases in which all other maneuvers have failed. These include intentional fracture of the anterior clavicle or humerus and the Zavanelli maneuver.

HYDROCEPHALUS AS A CAUSE OF DYSTOCIA

Hydrocephalus is an excessive accumulation of cerebrospinal fluid with consequent cranial enlargement. For a number of reasons, discussed in Chapter 41 (p. 1119), it is uncommon with births at term. Associated defects are common, especially neural-tube defects. Normal fetal head circumference at term ranges between 32 and 38 cm. With hydrocephalus, the circumference not infrequently exceeds 50 cm, and sometimes it reaches 80 cm. Fluid volume is usually between 500 and 1500 mL, but as much as 5 L may accumulate. Breech presentation

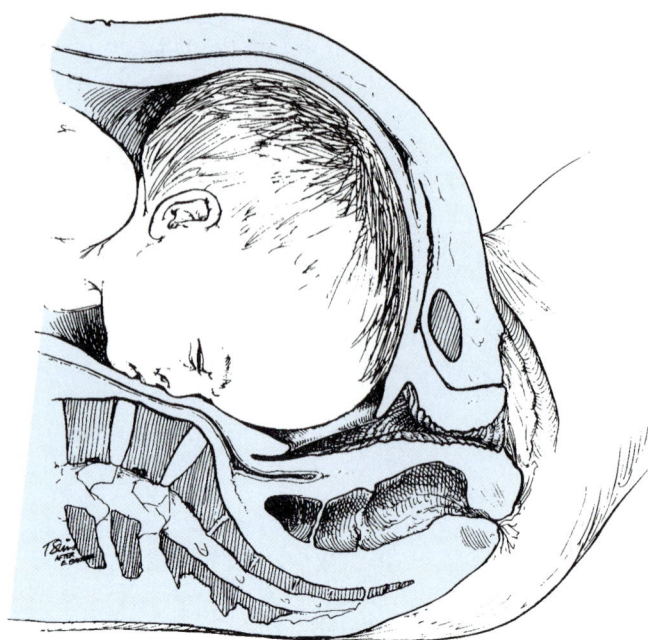

FIGURE 19–14. Severe dystocia from hydrocephalus, cephalic presentation. Note the disparity between the small size of the face and the rest of the cranium.

is found in at least a third of cases. Whatever the presentation, gross cephalopelvic disproportion is the rule, with serious dystocia the usual consequence (Figs. 19–14 and 19–15).

Hydrocephalus is somewhat more difficult to diag-

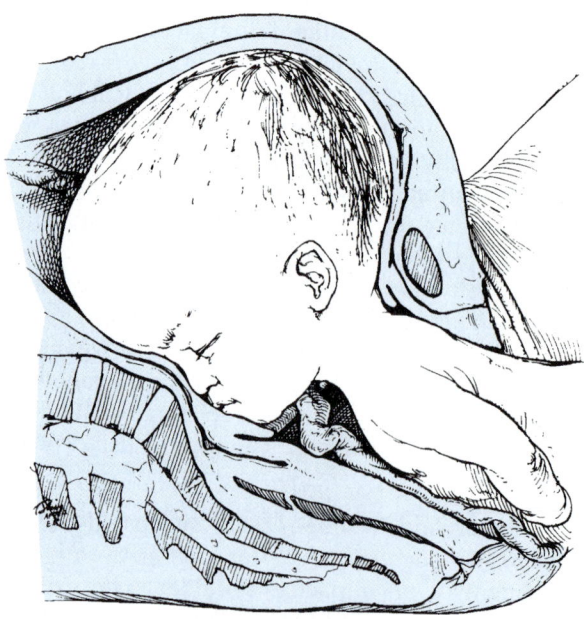

FIGURE 19–15. Severe dystocia from hydrocephalus, breech presentation. Note the distention of the lower uterine segment.

nose radiographically with a breech presentation, because the outline of a normal fetal head often appears enlarged to a degree suggestive of hydrocephalus. The difficulties inherent in radiological diagnosis are obviated by the use of sonography to compare the diameter of the lateral ventricles to the biparietal diameter of the head, and to evaluate the thickness of the cerebral cortex, as well as to compare the size of the head to that of the thorax and abdomen (Clark and associates, 1985).

MANAGEMENT. Most often, the size of the hydrocephalic head must be reduced if the head is to pass through the birth canal. Even with cesarean delivery, it may be desirable to remove cerebrospinal fluid just before incising the uterus in order to circumvent dangerous extensions of a low transverse or vertical incision and to avoid deliberately creating a very long vertical uterine incision. Removal of fluid by *cephalocentesis* was a mainstay in the historical management of fetal hydrocephalus with macrocephaly, but has come under considerable scrutiny in recent years. Chervenak and colleagues (1985) described results of cephalocentesis in 11 fetuses where the procedure was used to permit vaginal or cesarean delivery. Ten of these fetuses died either in utero or within 3 hours of delivery, and seven had intracranial bleeding at autopsy. Chervenak and McCullough (1986)

advocate that use of cephalocentesis be limited to fetuses with severe associated abnormalities. They recommended that all others be delivered abdominally. Such management requires precise knowledge of the extent of fetal malformations, which is not always possible.

TECHNIQUE OF CEPHALOCENTESIS. This varies depending on fetal presentation. With cephalic presentation, as soon as the cervix is dilated 3 to 4 cm, the ventricles may be tapped transvaginally with a needle. An 8-inch, 17-gauge needle is satisfactory for promptly removing appreciable volumes of cerebrospinal fluid. With a breech presentation, labor can be allowed to progress and the breech and trunk delivered. With the head over the inlet and the face toward the maternal back, the needle is inserted transvaginally just below the anterior vaginal wall and into the aftercoming head through the widened suture line. To protect the birth canal from the needle as it is passed toward the head, the more distal part of the needle, including the point, may be covered with a segment of sterile plastic tubing about 6 inches long cut from an intravenous infusion set. Alternatively, fluid may be withdrawn through a needle inserted via the maternal abdomen into the fetal head. After the bladder is emptied and the skin is cleansed, the needle is inserted in the midline somewhat

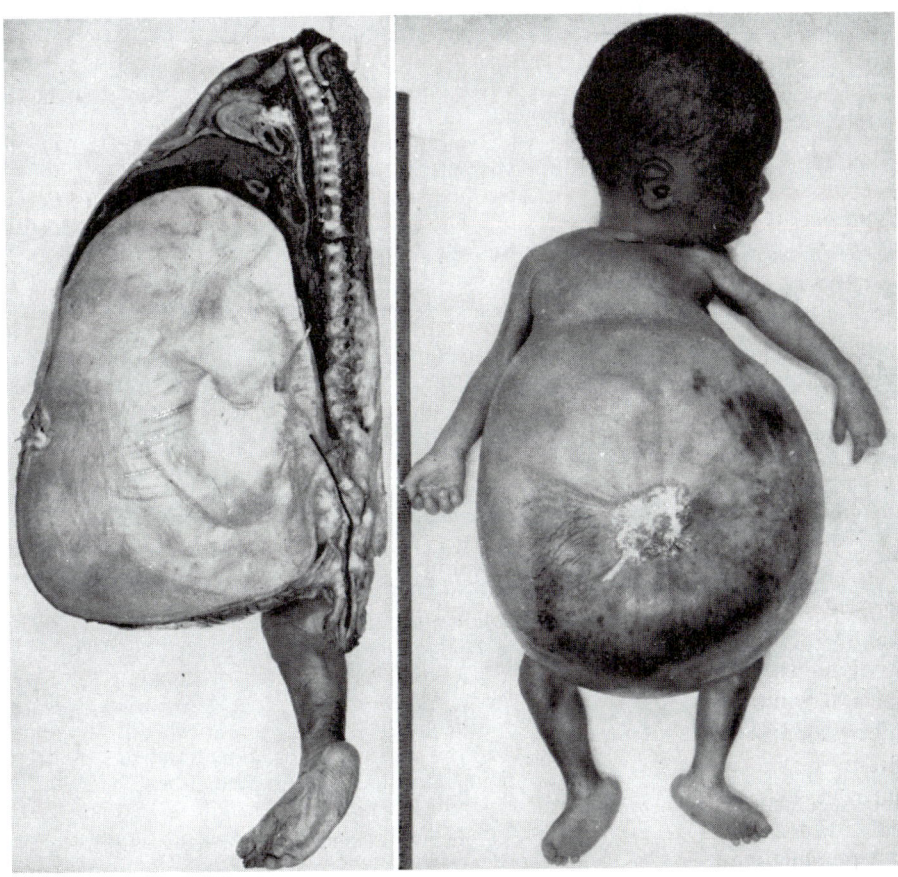

FIGURE 19–16. Fetal abdominal dystocia at 28 weeks caused by immensely distended bladder. Delivery was made possible by expression of fluid from bladder through perforation at umbilicus. Median sagittal section shows interior of bladder and compression of organs of abdominal and thoracic cavities. A black thread has been laid in the urethra. (From Savage, 1935.)

below the maternal umbilicus and inferior to the top of the fetal skull. The transabdominal approach to remove cerebrospinal fluid can also be used in the event of a cephalic presentation before trying to stimulate labor with oxytocin. The transabdominal approach has also been successfully applied in the breech fetus using ultrasound to guide the needle (Osathanondh and associates, 1980).

FETAL ABDOMEN AS A CAUSE OF DYSTOCIA

Enlargement of the fetal abdomen sufficient to cause dystocia is usually the result of a *greatly distended bladder* (Fig. 19–16), *ascites, or enlargement of the kidneys or liver.* Occasionally, the edematous fetal abdomen may attain such proportions that spontaneous delivery is impossible. Enlargement of the fetal abdomen may escape detection until fruitless attempts at delivery have demonstrated an obstruction. An enlarged abdomen and intra-abdominal accumulation of fluid can usually be diagnosed by ultrasound. If the diagnosis is made before delivery, the decision must be made whether or not to perform an abdominal delivery (Clark and associates, 1985). In general, prognosis is very poor, regardless of the method of delivery.

REFERENCES

American College of Obstetricians and Gynecologists: Fetal macrosomia. Practice Bulletin No. 22, November 2000

American College of Obstetricians and Gynecologists: Shoulder dystocia. Practice Pattern No. 7, October 1997

American College of Obstetricians and Gynecologists: Operative vaginal delivery. Technical Bulletin No. 152, February 1991

Baskett TF, Allen AC: Perinatal implications of shoulder dystocia. Obstet Gynecol 86:15, 1995

Beall MH, Spong C, McKay J, Ross MG: Objective definition of shoulder dystocia: A prospective evaluation. Am J Obstet Gynecol 179:934, 1998

Benedetti TJ, Gabbe SG: Shoulder dystocia. A complication of fetal macrosomia and prolonged second stage of labor with mid-pelvic delivery. Obstet Gynecol 52:526, 1978

Chervenak FA, Berkowitz RL, Tortona M, Hobbins JC: The management of fetal hydrocephalus. Am J Obstet Gynecol 151:933, 1985

Chervenak FA, McCullough LB: Ethical analysis of the intrapartum management of pregnancy complicated by fetal hydrocephalus with macrocephaly. Obstet Gynecol 68:720, 1986

Chez RA, Carlan S, Greenberg SL, Spellacy WN: Fractured clavicle is an unavoidable event. Am J Obstet Gynecol 171:797, 1994

Clark S, DeVore GR, Platt LD: The role of ultrasound in the aggressive management of obstructed labor secondary to fetal malformations. Am J Obstet Gynecol 152:1042, 1985

Cruikshank DP, White CA: Obstetric malpresentations: Twenty years' experience. Am J Obstet Gynecol 116:1097, 1973

Duff P: Diagnosis and management of face presentation. Obstet Gynecol 57:105, 1981

Fuchs K, Peretz BA, Marcovici R, Paldi E, Timor-Tritsch I: The grand multipara—is it a problem? Int J Gynaecol Obstet 73:321, 1985

Gardberg M, Laakkonen E, Salevaara M: Intrapartum sonography and persistent occiput posterior position: A study of 408 deliveries. Obstet Gynecol 91:746, 1998

Gardberg M, Tuppurainen M: Effects of the persistent occiput posterior presentation on the mode of delivery. Z Geburtshilfe Perinatol 198:117, 1994

Gherman RB, Ouzounian JG, Goodwin TM: Brachial plexus palsy: An in utero injury? Am J Obstet Gynecol 180:1303, 1999

Gherman RB, Ouzounian JG, Goodwin TM: Obstetric maneuvers for shoulder dystocia and associated fetal morbidity. Am J Obstet Gynecol 178:1126, 1998

Gherman RB, Tramont J, Muffley P, Goodwin TM: Analysis of McRoberts' maneuver by x-ray pelvimetry. Obstet Gynecol 95:43, 2000

Gonik B, Allen R, Sorab J: Objective evaluation of the shoulder dystocia phenomenon: Effect of maternal pelvic orientation on force reduction. Obstet Gynecol 74:44, 1989

Gonik B, Stringer CA, Held B: An alternate maneuver for management of shoulder dystocia. Am J Obstet Gynecol 145:882, 1983

Goodwin TM, Banks E, Millar LK, Phelan JP: Catastrophic shoulder dystocia and emergency symphysiotomy. Am J Obstet Gynecol 177:463, 1997

Goplerud J, Eastman NJ: Compound presentation: Survey of 65 cases. Obstet Gynecol 1:59, 1953

Gross SJ, Shime J, Farine D: Shoulder dystocia: Predictors and outcome: A five-year review. Am J Obstet Gynecol 156:334, 1987

Hardy AE: Birth injuries of the brachial plexus: Incidence and prognosis. J Bone Joint Surg 63:98, 1981

Hartfield VJ: Symphysiotomy for shoulder dystocia. Am J Obstet Gynecol 155:228, 1986

Hellman LM, Epperson JWW, Connally F: Face and brow presentation: The experience of the Johns Hopkins Hospital, 1896 to 1948. Am J Obstet Gynecol 59:831, 1950

Hernandez C, Wendel GD: Shoulder dystocia. In Pitkin RM (ed): Clinical Obstetrics and Gynecology, Vol XXXIII. Hagerstown, PA, Lippincott, 1990, p 526

Hibbard LT: Coping with shoulder dystocia. Contemp Ob/Gyn 20:229, 1982

Hopwood HG: Shoulder dystocia: Fifteen years' experience in a community hospital. Am J Obstet Gynecol 144:162, 1982

Jennett RJ, Tarby TJ, Kreinick CJ: Brachial plexus palsy: An old problem revisited. Am J Obstet Gynecol 166:1673, 1992

Johanson RB, Rice C, Doyle M, Arthur J, Anyanwu L, Ibrahim J, Warwick A, Redman CW, O'Brien PMS: A randomized prospective study comparing the new vacuum extractor policy with forceps delivery. Br J Obstet Gynaecol 100:524, 1993

Johnson CE: Transverse presentation of the fetus. JAMA 187:642, 1964

Keller JD, Lopez-Zeno JA, Dooley SL, Socol ML: Shoulder dystocia and birth trauma in gestational diabetes: A five-year experience. Am J Obstet Gynecol 165:928, 1991

McFarland M, Hod M, Piper JM, Xenakin EMJ, Langer D: Are labor abnormalities more common in shoulder dystocia? Am J Obstet Gynecol 173:1211, 1995

Menticoglou SM, Perlman M, Manning FA: High cervical spinal cord injury in neonates delivered with forceps: Report of 15 cases. Obstet Gynecol 86:589, 1995

Modanlou HD, Komatsu G, Dorchester W, Freeman RK, Bosu SK: Large-for-gestational-age neonates: Anthropometric reasons for shoulder dystocia. Obstet Gynecol 60:417, 1982

Neuman M, Beller U, Lavie O, Aboulafia Y, Rabinowitz R, Diamont Y: Intrapartum bimanual tocolytic-assisted reversal of face presentation: Preliminary report. Obstet Gynecol 84:146, 1994

Nocon JJ, McKenzie DK, Thomas LJ, Hansell RS: Shoulder dystocia: An analysis of risks and obstetric maneuvers. Am J Obstet Gynecol 168:1732, 1993

O'Leary JA: Shoulder Dystocia and Birth Injury. New York, McGraw-Hill, 1992, p 75

Osathanondh R, Birnholz JC, Altman AM, Driscoll SG: Ultrasonically guided transabdominal encephalocentesis. J Reprod Med 25:125, 1980

Parks DG, Ziel HK: Macrosomia: A proposed indication for primary cesarean section. Obstet Gynecol 52:407, 1978

Phelan JP, Boucher M, Mueller E, McCart D, Horenstein J, Clark SL: The nonlaboring transverse lie: A management dilemma. J Reprod Med 31:184, 1986

Phillips RD, Freeman M: The management of the persistent occiput posterior position: A review of 552 consecutive cases. Obstet Gynecol 43:171, 1974

Roberts SW, Hernandez C, Maberry MC, Adams MD, Leveno KJ, Wendel GD: Obstetric clavicular fracture: The enigma of normal birth. Obstet Gynecol 86:978, 1995

Rouse DJ, Owen J: Prophylactic cesarean delivery for fetal macrosomia diagnosed by means of ultrasonography—A Faustian bargain? Am J Obstet Gynecol 181:332, 1999

Rubin A: Management of shoulder dystocia. JAMA 189:835, 1964

Sandberg EC: The Zavanelli maneuver: A potentially revolutionary method for the resolution of shoulder dystocia. Am J Obstet Gynecol 152:479, 1985

Sandberg EC: The Zavanelli maneuver: 12 years of recorded experience. Obstet Gynecol 93:312, 1999

Savage JE: Dystocia due to dilation of the fetal urinary bladder. Am J Obstet Gynecol 29:267, 1935

Schramm M: Impacted shoulders—A personal experience. Aust NZ J Obstet Gynaecol 23:28, 1983

Smith RB, Lane C, Pearson JF: Shoulder dystocia: What happens at the next delivery? Br J Obstet Gynaecol 101:713, 1994

Spong CY, Beall M, Rodrigues D, Ross MG: An objective definition of shoulder dystocia: Prolonged head-to-body delivery intervals and/or the use of ancillary obstetric maneuvers. Obstet Gynecol 86:433, 1995

Tebes CC, Mehta P, Calhoun DA, Richards DS: Congenital ischemic forearm necrosis associated with a compound presentation. J Matern-Fetal Med 8:281, 1999

Woods CE: A principle of physics is applicable to shoulder delivery. Am J Obstet Gynecol 45:796, 1943

20

Induction and Augmentation of Labor

According to the National Center for Death Statistics, of the 3.9 million deliveries in the United States in 1995, 34 percent involved labor induction or augmentation (Ventura and colleagues, 1997). At Parkland Hospital, approximately 30 percent of labors are induced or augmented using oxytocin. At the University of Alabama at Birmingham Hospital, from 1996 through 1999, in over 17,000 deliveries, 20 percent of women were given oxytocin for labor induction and 35 percent for augmentation. Common indications for induction include membrane rupture without spontaneous onset of labor, maternal hypertension, nonreassuring fetal status, and postterm gestation. The purpose of this chapter is to describe techniques available in the United States to effect cervical ripening and for the induction or augmentation of labor.

GENERAL CONCEPTS

The concept of elective induction for either convenience of the practitioner and/or the patient is not recommended by us, or by the American College of Obstetricians and Gynecologists (1999a). This practice is associated with an increase in cesarean births, especially in nulliparas (Bland and colleagues, 2000; Maslow and Sweeny, 2000; Prysak and Castronova, 1998; Yeast and associates, 1999). Induction is indicated when the benefits to either the mother or fetus outweigh those of continuing the pregnancy. The spectrum of valid indications for induction includes emergent conditions such as ruptured membranes with chorioamnionitis or severe preeclampsia. There also are several relative indications that may approximate an elective induction. Some examples include women at term with a history of rapid labor and/or who reside an appreciable distance from the obstetrical facility. Such situations may be further aggravated by geographical (mountainous) and/or climatological (winter conditions) circumstances. Although less urgent, these situations present valid indications for induction at term.

Another general concept is the recognition that induction is associated with increased complications as compared with spontaneous labor. Complications include an increased incidence of chorioamnionitis and increased cesarean delivery. The latter may simply be due to the uterus being poorly prepared for labor; examples include an "unripe cervix" or a myometrium unable to achieve effective synchronous contractions. It is also likely that the increase in cesarean deliveries associated with labor induction is influenced by individual physician preferences regarding the duration of attempt at induction, especially in the circumstance of an "unripe cervix." For example, attempted labor induction with intravenous oxytocin for only 4 to 6 hours in a postterm nulliparous woman with an unripe cervix would not be expected to be successful (Rouse and colleagues, 2000).

Thus, the duration for either induction or augmentation, with the expectation of a successful progression of labor, has received too little attention. More precise data are needed considering the wide range of individual practitioner management.

CONTRAINDICATIONS

A number of uterine, fetal, or maternal conditions present contraindications to labor induction. Most of these are similar to those that would preclude spontaneous labor and delivery. **Uterine contraindications** primarily relate to a prior disruption such as a classical incision or uterine surgery. Placenta previa would also preclude labor. Fetal contraindications include appreciable macrosomia, some fetal anomalies such as hydrocephalus, malpresentations, or nonreassuring fetal status. **Maternal contraindications** are related to maternal size, pelvic anatomy, and selected medical conditions such as active genital herpes.

PREINDUCTION CERVICAL RIPENING

The condition or "favorability" of the cervix is important to labor induction. In many cases, the induction technique chosen depends upon the perceived ease of its anticipated success. Physical characteristics of the cervix and lower uterine segment are most important. The level of the presenting part, or station, is also important. One quantifiable method that is predictive of a successful labor induction is that described by Bishop (1964). Elements of the **Bishop score** include dilatation, effacement, station, consistence, and position of the cervix (Table 20–1). Induction to active labor is usually successful with a score of 9 or greater and is less successful with lower scores. Most practitioners would consider a woman whose cervix is 2 cm dilated, 80 percent effaced, soft and midposition, and with the fetal occiput at −1 station as likely to have a successful labor induction. In these circumstances, initiation of labor with a dilute intravenous oxytocin solution is usually successful.

Unfortunately, women too frequently have an indication for induction of labor but with various degrees of an unripe cervix. As the Bishop score decreases, there is an increasingly unsuccessful induction rate. Thus, considerable research has been directed toward various techniques to "ripen" the cervix prior to the stimulation of uterine contractions.

TABLE 20–1. Bishop Scoring System Used for Assessment of Inducibility

Score	Factor				
	Dilatation (cm)	Effacement (%)	Station[a]	Cervical Consistency	Cervical Position
0	Closed	0–30	−3	Firm	Posterior
1	1–2	40–50	−2	Medium	Midposition
2	3–4	60–70	−1.0	Soft	Anterior
3	≥5	≥80	+1, +2	—	—

[a] Station reflects a −3 to +3 scale.
From Bishop (1964), with permission.

PHARMACOLOGICAL TECHNIQUES

PROSTAGLANDIN E_2. Local application of prostaglandin E_2 gel (dinoprostone) is widely used for cervical ripening (American College of Obstetricians and Gynecologists, 1999a, 1999b). Histological changes include a dissolution of collagen bundles and an increase in submucosal water content (Rayburn and colleagues, 1994). These changes in cervical connective tissue at term are similar to those observed in early labor.

Rayburn (1989) reviewed cumulative experiences with intracervical or intravaginal prostaglandin E_2 preparations in over 5000 pregnancies comprising over 70 prospective clinical trials. He concluded that prostaglandin E_2 was superior to placebo in enhancing cervical effacement and dilation. The prostaglandin-induced cervical ripening process often included initiation of labor. Moreover, with the latter, labor is similar to that of normal spontaneous labor. Use of low-dose prostaglandin E_2 increases the chances of successful induction, decreases the incidence of prolonged labor, and reduces total and maximal oxytocin doses (Brindley and Sokol, 1988). Approximately half of treated women enter labor and deliver within 24 hours (Rayburn, 1989). The reported effects of prostaglandin on overall cesarean delivery rates, however, have been inconsistent. While some studies have shown a reduction, most have not shown a significant decrease (Bernstein, 1991; Brindley and Sokol, 1988; Keirse, 1993).

Early trials included various dosages of intracervical (0.3 to 0.5 mg) or intravaginal (3 to 5 mg) prostaglandin E_2, which were compared with untreated controls. In a meta-analysis of 18 such studies encompassing 1811 women, Owen and co-workers (1991) found that prostaglandin E_2 significantly improved Bishop scores and induction-to-delivery times. They found no benefit regarding the cesarean delivery rate.

In 1992, the Food and Drug Administration approved prostaglandin E_2 gel (Prepidil) for cervical ripening in women at or near term who have an indication for induction. The gel is available in a 2.5-mL syringe that contains 0.5 mg of dinoprostone. The intracervical route offers the advantages of prompting less uterine activity and greater efficacy in women with a very unripe cervix (Ekman and co-workers, 1983).

A 10-mg dinoprostone vaginal insert (Cervidil) also was approved in 1995 for cervical ripening. The insert provides slower release of medication (0.3 mg/hr) than the gel. Most trials with the insert have compared this formulation with intracervical gel (Chyu and Strassner, 1997; Rayburn and colleagues, 1992). Similar to results with dinoprostone gel, clinical trials demonstrate that these vaginal inserts shorten the interval from induction-to-delivery. One advantage is that the insert can be removed should hyperstimulation occur.

PATIENT SELECTION. A Bishop score of 4 or less (Table 20–1) is considered as identifying an unfavorable cervix and thus an indication for prostaglandin E_2 cervical ripening.

ADMINISTRATION. It is recommended that these preparations be administered either at or near the delivery suite, where continuous uterine activity and fetal heart rate monitoring can be performed (American College of Obstetricians and Gynecologists, 1995b). The woman remains recumbent for at least 30 minutes following application. An observation period ranging from 30 minutes to 2 hours may be prudent. If there is no change in uterine activity or fetal heart rate after this period, she then may be transferred or discharged. When contractions occur, they are usually apparent in the first hour and show peak activity in the first 4 hours (Bernstein, 1991; Miller and colleagues, 1991). If regular contractions persist, fetal heart rate monitoring should be continued and vital signs recorded.

A minimum safe time interval between prostaglandin E_2 administration and the initiation of oxytocin has not been established. According to manufacturer guidelines, oxytocin induction should be delayed for 6 to 12 hours.

SIDE EFFECTS. Reported rates of uterine hyperstimulation—defined as six or more contractions in 10 minutes for a total of 20 minutes—are 1 percent for intracervical gel (0.5-mg dose) and 5 percent for intravaginal gel (2- to 5-mg dose) (Brindley and Sokol, 1988; Rayburn, 1989). Because serious hyperstimulation or further fetal compromise can occur when prostaglandin is used with preexisting labor, such use is not generally accepted. When hyperstimulation occurs, it usually begins within 1 hour after the gel or insert is applied. Removing the insert by pulling on the tail of the net surrounding it will usually reverse this effect. Irrigation of the cervix and vagina to remove the gel has not been found to be helpful.

Systemic effects, including fever, vomiting, and diarrhea from low-dose prostaglandin E_2, are negligible. The manufacturers recommend caution when using any prostaglandin E_2 product in patients with glaucoma, severe hepatic or renal impairment, or asthma. This is despite that prostaglandin E_2 is a bronchodilator, and that neither bronchoconstriction nor significant blood pressure changes have been reported with low-dose gel.

Neonatal outcomes compare favorably with those achieved by oxytocin induction. The likelihood of a low Apgar score, need for resuscitation, admission to an intensive care nursery, or perinatal death is not increased with prostaglandin E_2 (Keirse, 1993).

PROSTAGLANDIN E_1. Misoprostol (Cytotec) is a synthetic prostaglandin E_1, and currently available as a 100-μg tablet for prevention of peptic ulcers. It has been used "off label" for preinduction cervical ripening and labor induction. Misoprostol is inexpensive with a cost less than $1 per 100-$\mu$g tablet compared with $75 for 0.5 mg of dinoprostone gel. It is stable at room temperature and easily administered orally or placed into the vagina, but not the cervix. In October, 2000, G. D. Searle & Company has notified physicians that misoprostol is not approved for labor induction or abortion. The American College of Obstetricians and Gynecologists (1999b, 2000) states that intravaginal administration of 25 μg not more frequently than every 3 to 6 h is effective in women with an unfavorable cervix.

VAGINAL MISOPROSTOL. Initial studies suggested that misoprostol tablets placed into the vagina were either superior to or equivalent in efficacy compared with intracervical prostaglandin E_2 gel (Chuck and Huffaker, 1995; Varaklis and colleagues, 1995; Wing and co-workers, 1995a, 1995b). The American College of Obstetricians and Gynecologists (1999b) reviewed 19 prospective randomized trials in which more than 1900 women were given misoprostol in intravaginal dosages ranging from 25 to 200 μg. The committee recommends

the use of intravaginal misoprostol in an approximate 25-μg dose (a quarter of a 100-μg tablet). Such usage is considered to decrease the need for oxytocin, achieve higher rates of vaginal delivery within 24 hours of induction, and significantly reduce induction-to-delivery intervals (Sanchez-Ramos and colleagues, 1997). Hofmeyr and associates (1999) reviewed data from the United Kingdom Cochrane Centre, and support these recommendations but cautioned that increased uterine hyperstimulation with fetal heart rate changes was of concern.

The 50-μg dose results in significantly increased tachysystole, meconium passage, and meconium aspiration compared with prostaglandin E_2 gel (Farah and colleagues, 1997; Wing and co-workers, 1995a, 1995b). There is also an increased incidence of cesarean delivery due to uterine hyperstimulation when compared with dinoprostone (Buser and collaborators, 1997). The 25-μg dose every 3 hours was associated with significantly fewer adverse effects than the 50-μg dose. Reports of uterine rupture in women with prior uterine surgery currently preclude the use of misoprostol in these women (Bennet, 1997; Sciscione and associates, 1998; Wing and colleagues, 1998). In one report, Plaut and associates (1999) described uterine rupture in 5 of 89 (6 percent) women with a previous cesarean delivery who were induced with misoprostol compared with only 1 of 423 such women not given misoprostol ($P = .0001$).

ORAL MISOPROSTOL. Windrim and associates (1997) reported that orally administered misoprostol was of similar efficacy for cervical ripening and labor induction as intravaginal administration. Bennett and colleagues (1998) and Toppozada and co-workers (1997) found a shorter interval-to-delivery with the vaginal application, but more frequent fetal heart rate abnormalities. Adair and colleagues (1998) concluded that oral and vaginal applications were of similar efficacy but that an oral dosage of 200 μg was associated with more frequent abnormal uterine contractility. Wing and collaborators (1999) reported that 50-μg oral misoprostol was less effective than 25 μg administered vaginally for cervical ripening and labor induction. These investigators (Wing and colleagues, 2000) subsequently reported that a 100-μg oral dose was as effective as the 25-μg intravaginal dose. Clearly, more information is needed regarding an optimum dosage and route of administration of misoprostol. Kinetics of oral absorption as well as vaginal absorption in regard to vaginal pH should also be studied (Karim and colleagues, 1989; Zieman and associates, 1997).

MECHANICAL TECHNIQUES. Cervical dilatation with a balloon catheter was first attributed to Barnes by Woodman (1863). Several variations of this method are

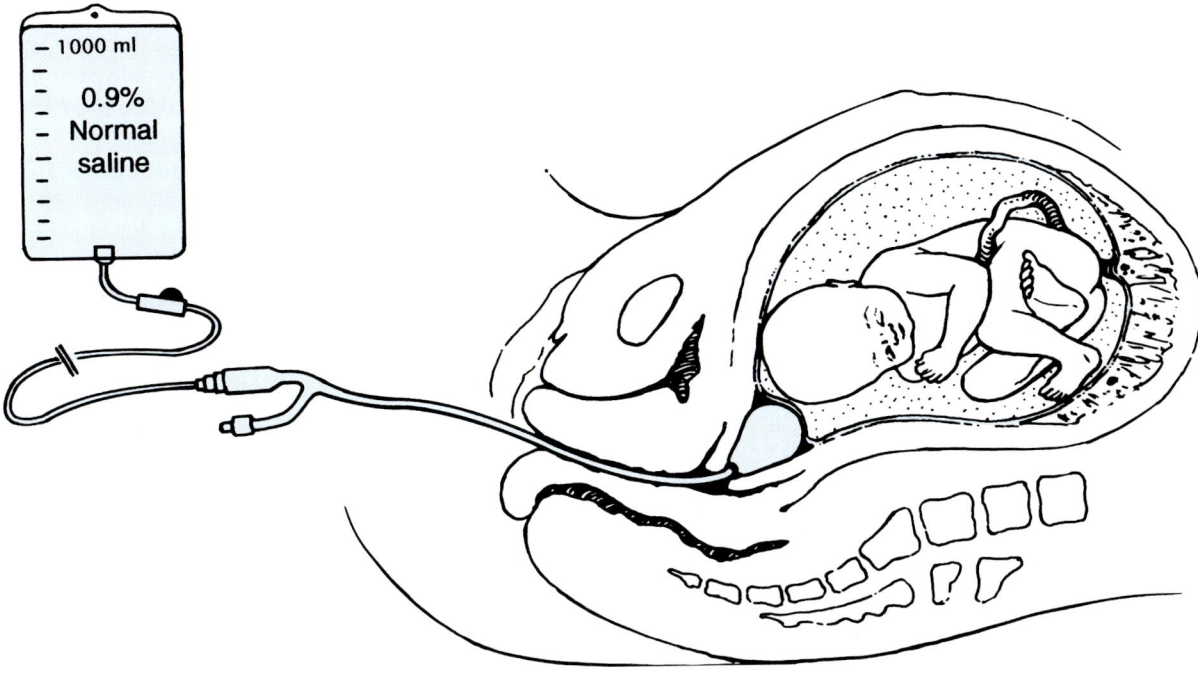

FIGURE 20–1. Extra-amnionic saline infusion (EASI) after Foley catheter placement and inflated 30 mL-balloon.

used currently. One method shown in Figure 20–1 includes the infusion of extra-amnionic normal saline and is referred to by some as **EASI.** Sherman and colleagues (1996) summarized the results of 13 trials with balloon catheters and concluded that, with or without saline infusion, the method resulted in rapid improvement in Bishop scores and shorter labors. In these 13 trials, the incidence of cesarean births ranged from 4 to 46 percent.

A number of comparative trials has been done. Schreyer and colleagues (1989) found that extra-amnionic saline infusion resulted in a greater increase in Bishop score in less time than vaginal prostaglandin E$_2$. Vengalil and colleagues (1998) reported similar outcomes with cesarean delivery rates and induction-to-delivery times with catheter infusion compared with 50-μg misoprostol administered vaginally every 4 hours. Studies by Hemlin and Möller (1998) and Sciscione and associates (1999) reported catheter infusion to be more efficacious for cervical ripening than 0.5 mg of intracervical prostaglandin E$_2$. Goldman and Wigton (1999) reported a significantly higher Bishop score at 6 and 12 hours with catheter infusion compared with intracervical dinoprostone. Abramovici and co-workers (1999) also found superior efficacy with catheter induction compared with 50-μg oral misoprostol every 4 hours in

nulliparas with a Bishop score of 5 or less. Almost 85 percent of those induced by catheter delivered within 24 hours compared with nearly 55 percent of these given misoprostol. Misoprostol and catheter/oxytocin had equivalent success rates.

Guinn and colleagues (2000) randomized women to intracervical prostaglandin E$_2$, laminaria plus intravenous oxytocin, or catheter infusion plus oxytocin. Cesarean delivery was similar with all three interventions. The randomization-to-delivery time of 18 hours with catheter infusion was significantly less than the 21.5 hours with laminaria plus oxytocin or 24.8 hours with prostaglandin E$_2$ gel. Buccellato and associates (2000) reported similar outcomes with 50-μg misoprostol compared with extra-amnionic saline.

HYGROSCOPIC CERVICAL DILATORS. Initiation of cervical dilatation with hygroscopic osmotic cervical dilators has long been accepted as efficacious prior to pregnancy termination (Hale and Pion, 1972; Chap. 33, p. 871). For labor induction with a viable pregnancy, less information is available regarding hygroscopic dilators to improve an "unripe cervix."

Krammer and colleagues (1995a, 1995b) and Gilson and associates (1996) reported that hygroscopic dilators resulted in rapid improvement of cervical status. Importantly, however, there was no beneficial effect on the cesarean delivery rate or randomization-to-delivery intervals. In the randomized study cited earlier, Guinn and co-workers (2000) reported that cervical ripening with cervical dilators plus oxytocin induction were similar in efficacy to either catheter infusion or prostaglandin E_2 cervical gel.

The attraction of these dilators is their low cost, ease of placement, and their ability to be quickly removed. Most recently, Guinn and colleagues (2000) at the University of Alabama compared cervical prostaglandin gel, cervical dilators, and EASI in women induced at term. Despite similar cesarean delivery rates, women randomized to cervical dilators had a significantly longer interval-to-delivery time compared with women assigned to EASI. The use of hygroscopic dilators appears to be safe, although anaphylaxis has followed laminaria insertion (Cole and Bruck, 2000; Nguyen and Hoffman, 1995). It is of some benefit for initiation of cervical dilation in women with an indication for induction of labor.

MEMBRANE STRIPPING. Induction of labor by membrane "stripping" or "sweeping" is a relatively common practice. In a randomized study of 180 women, McColgin and colleagues (1990a, 1990b) reported that membrane stripping was safe and associated with a decreased incidence of postterm gestation. These investigators observed significantly increased levels of plasma prostaglandins with membrane stripping (McColgin and co-authors, 1993). Allott and Palmer (1993) randomized 195 women with normal pregnancies beyond 40 weeks to digital cervical examination either with or without membrane stripping. Stripping was performed by inserting the index finger as far through the internal os as possible and rotating twice through 360 degrees to separate the membranes from the lower segment. Two thirds of those who underwent stripping entered spontaneous labor within 72 hours compared with a third of the other group. Ruptured membranes, infection, and bleeding were not increased, and induction for postterm pregnancy was significantly decreased with stripping.

Boulvain and colleagues (1999) reviewed 13 reports of sweeping of membranes to induce labor and prevent postterm pregnancy in almost 2000 women. Membrane stripping at term was considered to be safe in that maternal and neonatal infection and membrane rupture were similar in the intervention versus control groups. The cesarean delivery rate was also similar in both groups. Membrane stripping was considered beneficial because these women were significantly more likely to deliver within 48 hours, within 1 week, or before 41 weeks. Finally, significantly fewer women in the membrane-stripping group required labor induction.

SUMMARY OF PREINDUCTION CERVICAL RIPENING.
Induction of labor in the presence of an "unripe" cervix is frequently indicated. Initial pharmacological efforts to effect cervical ripening targeted cervical or vaginal prostaglandin E_2 preparations (dinoprostone). Subsequently developed pharmacological methods include either oral or vaginal prostaglandin E_1 (misoprostol). These pharmacological techniques have been compared in a few studies to mechanical techniques such as extra-amnionic saline infusion (EASI) through a transcervical 30-mL balloon Foley catheter or to insertion of hygroscopic cervical dilators. It is likely that all of the described techniques have some benefit when compared with no attempt at cervical ripening. Unfortunately, benefits are limited to either differences in an improved Bishop score and/or times to either active labor and/or delivery. There is little evidence and no consensus that any of these techniques have resulted in a significant reduction in cesarean births or in lower maternal or neonatal morbidity compared with untreated controls.

LABOR INDUCTION AND AUGMENTATION WITH OXYTOCIN

Synthetic oxytocin is one of the most commonly used medications in the United States. Oxytocin was the first polypeptide hormone synthesized, and the 1955 Nobel Prize in chemistry was awarded for this (DuVigneaud and co-workers, 1953). Virtually every parturient receives oxytocin following delivery and many also receive it to induce or augment labor. According to the National Center for Health Statistics, in 1995 more than 1.3 million American women were given oxytocin to stimulate labor (Ventura and colleagues, 1997).

In many cases, there is only a semantical difference between labor induction and augmentation. Induction of labor implies stimulation of contractions before the spontaneous onset of labor, with or without ruptured membranes. Augmentation refers to stimulation of spontaneous contractions that are considered inadequate because of failure of progressive dilatation and descent. Some practitioners consider augmentation to include stimulation of contractions following spontaneously ruptured membranes without labor. While some physicians use different oxytocin infusion regimens for each of these, we use the same technique that is described subsequently.

There are a myriad of obstetrical, medical, and fetal indications for labor induction. These are described throughout this book. The diagnosis of inadequate labor is discussed in detail in Chapter 18. The use of oxytocin given by intravenous infusion to augment inadequate labor—uterine dysfunction—is appropriate only after assessment to exclude fetopelvic disproportion. With oxytocin induction or augmentation, it is mandatory that the fetal heart rate and contraction pattern be observed closely. The American College of Obstetricians and Gynecologists (1999a) recommends fetal heart rate and uterine contraction monitoring similar to that for any high-risk pregnancy. This is done either by palpation of contraction frequency and relaxation or by electronic means of recording uterine activity (Chap. 14, p. 354). Uterine contraction pressures cannot be accurately quantified by palpation (Arrabal and Nagey, 1996).

TECHNIQUE FOR ADMINISTRATION OF INTRAVENOUS OXYTOCIN.

A variety of methods for stimulation of uterine contractions with oxytocin has been employed. The woman should have direct nursing supervision while oxytocin is being infused. The goal is to effect uterine activity that is sufficient to produce cervical change and fetal descent while avoiding uterine hyperstimulation and/or development of a nonreassuring fetal status. Contractions must be evaluated continually and oxytocin discontinued if they persist as greater than five in a 10-minute period or seven in a 15-minute period; if they last longer than 60 to 90 seconds; or if the fetal heart rate pattern becomes nonreassuring. With hyperstimulation, immediate discontinuation of oxytocin nearly always rapidly decreases the frequency of contractions. When oxytocin is stopped, its concentration in plasma rapidly falls because the mean half-life is approximately 5 minutes.

Seitchik and co-workers (1984) studied the pharmacokinetics of intravenously infused oxytocin and found that a uterine response occurs within 3 to 5 minutes of beginning infusion and that a plasma steady state is reached in 40 minutes. Response depends on preexisting uterine activity, sensitivity, and cervical status, which are related to pregnancy duration and to individual biological differences. Caldeyro-Barcia and Poseiro (1960) reported that uterine response to oxytocin increases from 20 to 30 weeks, but is unchanged from 34 weeks until term, at which time sensitivity rapidly increases (Chap. 14, p. 355). Satin and co-workers (1992b) studied factors affecting the oxytocin dosage required for adequate labor stimulation in 1773 pregnancies. Important predictors of oxytocin dosage included cervical dilatation, parity, and gestational age.

Synthetic oxytocin is usually diluted into 1000 mL of a balanced salt solution that is administered by infusion pump. Administration by any other route is not recommended for labor stimulation. To avoid bolus administration, the infusion should be inserted into the main intravenous line close to the venipuncture site. A typical oxytocin infusate consists of 10 to 20 units—equivalent to 10,000 to 20,000 mU—mixed into 1000 mL of lactated Ringer solution, resulting in an oxytocin concentration of 10 or 20 mU/mL, respectively.

At Parkland Hospital from 1996 through 1999, over 15,000 women were given oxytocin to induce or augment labor. Bedside attendance is provided by trained nursing personnel and continuous electronic monitoring of the fetal heart rate and uterine activity is conducted. Oxytocin is avoided generally in cases of abnormal fetal presentations and of marked uterine overdistention such as pathological hydramnios, an excessively large fetus, or multiple fetuses. Women of high parity (6 or more) are generally not given oxytocin because uterine rupture occurs more readily (Chap. 25, p. 646). At Parkland, oxytocin is usually withheld from women with a previous uterine scar and a live fetus (Chap. 25, p. 648). Conversely, a prior cesarean delivery is not a contraindication to induction or augmentation at the University of Alabama or the University of Texas at Houston. The fetal condition must be reassuring, as determined by heart rate and lack of thick meconium in amnionic fluid. A dead fetus is not a contraindication to oxytocin usage unless there is overt fetopelvic disproportion.

OXYTOCIN DOSAGE.

According to American College of Obstetricians and Gynecologists (1999a), any of a number of oxytocin regimens are appropriate for labor stimulation. Some are shown in Table 20–2. Until relatively recently, only variations of the low-dose protocol were used in the United States. In 1984, O'Driscoll and colleagues described a protocol for the active management of labor that called for oxytocin at a starting dose of 6 mU/min and advanced in 6-mU/min increments. Following this, various trials during the 1990s compared high-dose (4 to 6 mU/min) versus conventional low-dose (0.5 to 1.5 mU/min) regimens both for labor induction and augmentation.

At Parkland Hospital, Satin and colleagues (1992a) tested an oxytocin regimen of 1 mU/min compared with 6 mU/min. With the low-dose regimens, increases of 1 mU/min were given as needed at 20-minute intervals. With the high-dose protocol, increases of 6 mU/min were given as needed at 20-minute intervals to a maximum of 42 mU/min. The protocol allowed reduction of

TABLE 20–2. Oxytocin Regimens for Stimulation of Labor

Regimen	Starting Dose (mU/min)	Incremental Increase (mU/min)	Dosage Interval (min)	Maximum Dose (mU/min)
Low-dose	0.5–1	1	30–40	20
	1–2	2	15	40
High-dose	6	6[a], 3, 1	15–40	42

[a] The incremental increase is reduced to 3 mU/min in presence of recurrent hyperstimulation. Modified from the American College of Obstetricians and Gynecologists (1999a), with permission.

the dosage by 3 mU/min in the presence of uterine hyperstimulation. This flexible high-dose protocol was evaluated in nearly 5000 pregnancies and found to be more effective than the low-dose infusion. Specifically, of 1112 women with labor induction, the high-dose regimen had a significantly shorter mean admission-to-delivery time, fewer failed inductions, and there were no cases of neonatal sepsis. Of 1676 women who had labor augmentation, those who received the high-dose regimen had a significantly shorter duration-to-delivery time, fewer forceps deliveries, fewer cesarean deliveries for dystocia, less intrapartum chorioamnionitis, and less neonatal sepsis.

In this report by Satin and colleagues (1992a), hyperstimulation was identified in approximately half of women with the high-dose regimen. This was managed by oxytocin discontinuation followed by resumption when indicated but with only half the stopping dosage. Thereafter the dosage was increased at 3 mU/min when appropriate compared with 6 mU/min for women without hyperstimulation. Women who received the 6-mU/min regimen for labor augmentation underwent cesarean delivery for "fetal distress" in 6 compared with 3 percent of those in the low-dose group. No adverse neonatal effects were observed in either group.

Xenakis and colleagues (1995) reported benefits for a high-dose regimen starting at 4 mU/min with 4-mU/min incremental increases. Merrill and Zlatnik (1999) randomized 1307 women for labor induction (816) or augmentation (491) to either low-dose oxytocin given at 1.5 mU/min with incremental increases of 1.5 mU/min or to a higher-dose infusion begun at 4.5 mU/min and increased by 4.5-mU/min increments. Women randomized to the higher-dose regimen had a significantly decreased duration from induction-to-second-stage labor and from induction-to-delivery time. Nulliparas in the high-dose group had a trend toward a lower cesarean delivery rate for disproportion compared with those in the low-dose group (5.9 versus 11.9 percent, $P = .06$). In women whose labor was augmented, those randomized to the higher-dose regimen also had significantly shorter labors but a similar cesarean delivery rate.

The benefits favor the higher-dose regimens. In 1990, routine usage of the 6-mU/min oxytocin regimen was incorporated at Parkland Hospital. At the University of Alabama, the 2-mU/min oxytocin regimen is used. In both cases, these are used for either labor induction or augmentation, with graduated increased incremental dosages.

INCREASING DOSAGE INTERVALS. There are a number of suitable regimens with intervals to increase oxytocin dosage that vary from every 15 to 40 minutes (Table 20–2). Satin and colleagues (1994) compared a regimen beginning with 6 mU/min with incremental 6-

mU/min increases over 20- versus 40-minute intervals. Women given the 20-minute interval regimen for labor augmentation had a significant reduction in cesarean delivery for dystocia compared with the 40-minute interval regimen (8 versus 12 percent). In women with labor induction, uterine hyperstimulation was significantly more frequent with the 20-minute compared with the 40-minute regimen (40 versus 31 percent). This, however, was not observed in those undergoing labor augmentation (31 versus 28 percent). Because of the concern for hyperstimulation, the current Parkland protocol is to initiate oxytocin at 6 mU/min, with incremental increases every 40 minutes, but employing a flexible dosing schedule based on hyperstimulation.

Others report successful high-dose regimens escalated at more frequent intervals. Frigoletto and associates (1995) and Xenakis and co-workers (1995) began oxytocin at 4 mU/min with increases as needed every 15 minutes. Merrill and Zlatnik (1999) started with 4.5 mU/min with increases every 30 minutes. López-Zeno and colleagues (1992) began at 6 mU/min with increases every 15 minutes. Other variations are acceptable; for example, at the University of Alabama at Birmingham, intravenous oxytocin for labor induction or augmentation is begun at 2 mU/min and is increased as needed every 15 minutes to 4, 8, 12, 16, 20, 25, and 30 mU/min.

RISKS VERSUS BENEFITS. Oxytocin is a powerful drug, but previously described disasters of killed or maimed mothers and babies because of **uterine rupture** are uncommon today. This is because of several well-done studies to codify its administration and to quantify its efficacy and safety. As shown in Table 20–3, uterine rupture associated with oxytocin is rare even in parous women, unless the uterus is scarred.

Oxytocin has amino-acid homology similar to arginine vasopressin. Thus, when infused at high doses, it has significant antidiuretic action. Whenever 20 mU/min or more is infused, renal free water clearance decreases markedly. If aqueous fluids are infused in appreciable amounts along with oxytocin, **water intoxication** can lead to convulsions, coma, and even death.

UTERINE CONTRACTION PRESSURES WITH OXYTOCIN STIMULATION. Uterine contraction forces calculated in spontaneously laboring women range from 90 to 390 Montevideo units (Fig. 20–2). Caldeyro-Barcia and associates (1950) and Seitchik and colleagues (1984) found that the mean or median spontaneous uterine contraction pattern resulting in a progression to a vaginal delivery was between 140 and 150 Montevideo units (Chap. 14, p. 355).

In the management of arrest of active-phase labor, and with no contraindication to intravenous oxytocin, decisions are made knowing the safe upper range of

TABLE 20-3. Relationship of Overt Uterine Rupture to Parity, Prior
Cesarean Section, and Oxytocin Stimulation

Factor	Nulliparous	Parous	Prior Cesarean
Women delivered	27,829	48,718	2842
Overt uterine rupture	0	8	19
Uterine rupture with oxytocin	0	1	6

From Flannely and associates (1993), with permission.

uterine activity with spontaneous labor. Hauth and co-workers (1986) described an effective and safe protocol for labor augmentation with which over 90 percent of women achieved an average of 200 to 225 Montevideo units. Hauth and associates (1991) later reported that nearly all women whose arrest of labor persisted despite oxytocin were able to generate over 200 Montevideo units. Importantly, despite no labor progression, there were no adverse maternal or newborn effects following cesarean delivery.

The American College of Obstetricians and Gynecologists (1995a) recommends that prior to diagnosing an arrest of first-stage labor, the uterine contraction pattern should exceed 200 Montevideo units for 2 hours without cervical change. More data are needed regarding the precise safety and efficacy of contraction patterns in

subgroups of women with a prior cesarean delivery, with twins, with an overdistended uterus, and in those with chorioamnionitis.

DURATION OF OXYTOCIN ADMINISTRATION. In 1989 the American College of Obstetricians and Gynecologists defined arrest in first-stage labor as a completed latent phase along with a uterine contraction pattern of more than 200 Montevideo units that has been present for over 2 hours without cervical change. There are only sparse data to support a more accurate recommendation for the duration of augmentation for active phase arrest. Arulkumaran and associates (1987) extended the limits of the 2 hours to define failed augmentation. Using a 4-hour limit, they reported a cesarean rate of only 1.3 percent in those who continued to have adequate con-

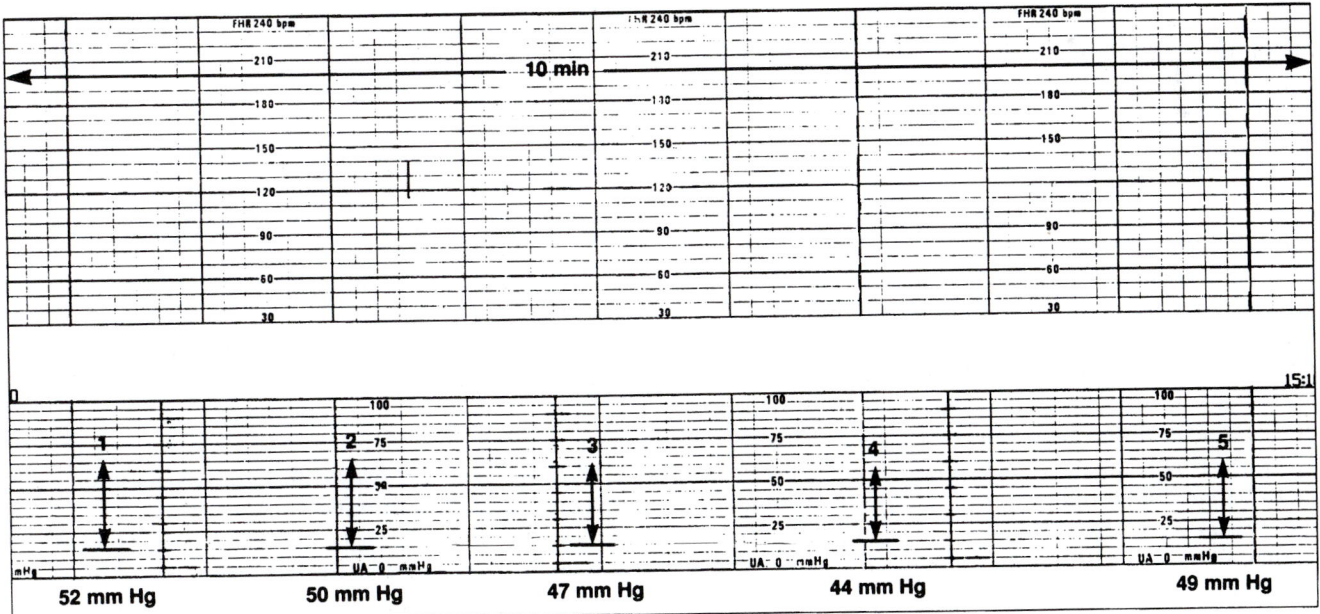

FIGURE 20-2. Montevideo units are calculated by subtracting the baseline uterine pressure from the peak contraction pressure for each contraction in a 10-minute window and adding the pressures generated by each contraction. In the example shown, there are five contractions in 10 minutes, producing pressure changes of 52, 50, 47, 44, and 49 mm Hg, respectively. The sum of these five contractions is 242 Montevideo units (From the American College of Obstetricians and Gynecologists, 1989, with permission).

tractions. For those without progress, another 4 hours were allowed, and a third of these were delivered vaginally.

Rouse and colleagues (1999) studied 542 women at term with active phase arrest who were managed within a prospective protocol. The protocol did not include the 2-hour rule, but rather included an intent to achieve a sustained pattern of over 200 Montevideo units for a minimum of 4 hours. This was increased up to 6 hours if activity of over 200 Montevideo units could not be sustained. Almost 92 percent of these women were delivered vaginally. Because women with a prior cesarean delivery, multifetal gestation, nonvertex presentations, or chorioamnionitis were excluded, these investigators recommended that further studies be performed.

These reports are suggestive that changes in management of labor may contribute to reducing the cesarean delivery rate. We anticipate increased attention to the duration of oxytocin augmentation in the active phase arrest disorders. If future studies confirm those of Arulkumaran and colleagues (1987) and Rouse and co-workers (1999) regarding the efficacy and safety of a longer duration of oxytocin augmentation, then this should be implemented.

AMNIOTOMY. Amniotomy or artificial rupture of the membranes, also referred to in Britain as surgical induction, is commonly used to induce or augment labor. The term amniorrhexis is used by some to signify either spontaneous or artificial membrane rupture, although this term and amniotomy erroneously imply rupture only of the amnion and not the chorion. Other common indications for amniotomy include internal electronic fetal heart rate monitoring when fetal jeopardy is anticipated and intrauterine assessment of contractions when labor has been unsatisfactory. Elective amniotomy to hasten spontaneous labor or detect meconium is also acceptable and commonly practiced.

Because amniotomy for these indications is so prevalent, it is difficult to find information on when during normal labor the fetal membranes would spontaneously rupture if left unperturbed. Fraser and co-workers (1991) studied elective amniotomy compared with no intervention in term pregnancies with spontaneous labor. Almost 60 percent of the nonintervention group reached 8 cm dilatation or more before the membranes ruptured spontaneously. It is likely that an even greater proportion of women would have entered second-stage labor with intact membranes because amniotomy for electronic internal monitoring or labor augmentation was performed in 38 percent.

Several precautions to minimize the risk of cord prolapse should be observed when membranes are ruptured artificially. Care should be taken to avoid dislodging the fetal head. An assistant applying fundal and suprapubic

pressure may reduce the risk of cord prolapse. Some prefer to rupture membranes during a contraction. The fetal heart rate should be assessed prior to and immediately after the procedure.

ELECTIVE AMNIOTOMY. Artificial membrane rupture with the intention of accelerating labor is among the most commonly performed procedures in obstetrics. Whether this procedure confers more benefit than harm has been the focus of controversy. There have been three investigations addressing this controversy recently, and these are summarized in Table 20–4. In all three studies, amniotomy at about 5 cm dilatation accelerated spontaneous labor 1 to 2 hours without increasing the overall rate of cesarean delivery or need for oxytocin stimulation. In the study by Garite and associates (1993), oxytocin use was decreased when early elective amniotomy was performed. Importantly, there were no adverse perinatal effects. These investigators, however, did identify increased mild and moderate umbilical cord compression patterns as a result of amniotomy. Despite this, severe decelerations were not increased and consequently cesarean delivery for fetal distress was unaffected.

AMNIOTOMY INDUCTION. Artifical rupture of the membranes can be used to induce labor, but it implies a firm commitment to delivery. The main disadvantage of amniotomy when used alone for labor induction is the unpredictable and occasionally long interval to the onset of contractions. Although this is widely practiced, there have been few investigations comparing amniotomy alone with other methods. In a randomized trial, Bakos and Bäckström (1987) found that amniotomy alone or combined with oxytocin was superior to oxytocin alone. Mercer and colleagues (1995) randomized 209 women undergoing oxytocin induction to amniotomy at 1 to 2 cm dilation (early amniotomy) or at 5 cm (late amniotomy). Early amniotomy was associated with significantly shorter labor (approximately 4 hours), but there was an increased incidence of chorioamnionitis (23 percent) and cord compression monitoring patterns (12 percent).

AMNIOTOMY FOR AUGMENTATION. It is common practice to perform amniotomy when spontaneous labor is abnormally slow. Given the evidence that is available from trials in established spontaneous labor and from labor induction, it is likely that amniotomy would enhance progress in dysfunctional labor. Rouse and co-workers (1994) performed a randomized study and found that the addition of amniotomy to oxytocin augmentation of arrest of labor in the active phase shortened labor by 44 minutes. It also significantly increased the incidence of chorioamnionitis. Amniotomy, as an

TABLE 20–4. Randomized Clinical Trials of Elective Amniotomy Early in Spontaneous Term Labor

Study	Number	Effects of Amniotomy					
		Mean Dilatation at Amniotomy	Mean Shortening of Labor	Need for Oxytocin	Cesarean Delivery Rate	Abnormal Tracing	Neonatal Effects
Fraser and co-workers (1993)	925	<5 cm	125 min	No effect	No effect[a]	No effect	None
Garite and associates (1993)	459	5.5 cm	81 min	Decreased	No effect	Increased[b]	None
UK Amniotomy Group (1994)	1463	5.1 cm	60 min	No effect	No effect	NA[c]	None

[a] No effect on overall rate; cesarean delivery for fetal distress significantly increased.
[b] Increased mild and moderate umbilical cord compression patterns.
[c] NA = not assessed.

adjunct to oxytocin infusion, did not affect the route of delivery compared with oxytocin alone.

ACTIVE MANAGEMENT OF LABOR

This term describes a codified approach to diagnosis and management of labor. It is discussed in detail in Chapter 18 (p. 446).

REFERENCES

Abramovici D, Goldwasser S, Mabie BC, Mercer BM, Goldwasser R, Sibai BM: A randomized comparison of oral misoprostol versus Foley catheter and oxytocin for induction of labor at term. Am J Obstet Gynecol 181:1108, 1999

Adair CD, Weeks JW, Barrilleaux S, Edwards M, Burlison K, Lewis DF: Oral or vaginal misoprostol administration for induction of labor: A randomized, double-blind trial. Obstet Gynecol 92:810, 1998

Allott HA, Palmer CR: Sweeping the membranes: A valid procedure in stimulating the onset of labour? Br J Obstet Gynaecol 100:898, 1993

American College of Obstetricians and Gynecologists: Response to Searle's drug warning on misoprostol. Committee on Obstetric Practice, 2000

American College of Obstetricians and Gynecologists: Induction of Labor. Practice Bulletin No. 10, November, 1999a

American College of Obstetricians and Gynecologists: Induction of Labor with Misoprostol. Committee Opinion No. 228, November, 1999b

American College of Obstetricians and Gynecologists: Dystocia and the Augmentation of Labor. Technical Bulletin No. 218, December, 1995a

American College of Obstetricians and Gynecologists: Induction of Labor. Technical Bulletin No. 217, December, 1995b

American College of Obstetricians and Gynecologists: Dystocia. Technical Bulletin No. 137, December, 1989

Arrabal PP, Nagey DA: Is manual palpation of uterine contractions accurate? Am J Obstet Gynecol 174:217, 1996

Arulkumaran S, Koh CH, Ingemarsson I, Ratnam SS: Augmentation of labour—mode of delivery related to cervimetric progress. Aust N Z J Obstet Gynaecol 27:304, 1987

Bakos, O, Bäckström T: Induction of labor: A prospective, randomized study into amniotomy and oxytocin as induction methods in a total unselected population. Acta Obstet Gynecol Scand 66:537, 1987

Bennet BB: Uterine rupture during induction of labor at term with intravaginal misoprostol. Obstet Gynecol 89:832, 1997

Bennett KA, Butt K, Crane JMG, Hutchens D, Young DC: A masked randomized comparison of oral and vaginal administration of misoprostol for labor induction. Obstet Gynecol 92:481, 1998

Bernstein P: Prostaglandin E_2 gel for cervical ripening and labour induction: A multi-centre placebo-controlled trial. Can Med Assoc J 145:1249, 1991

Bishop EH: Pelvic scoring for elective induction. Obstet Gynecol 24:266, 1964

Bland E, Oppenheimer L, Wen SW: The effect of a change in remuneration on obstetric intervention. Am J Obstet Gynecol 182:S20, 2000

Boulvain M, Irion O, Marcoux S, Fraser W: Sweeping of the membranes to prevent post-term pregnancy and to induce labour: A systematic review. Br J Obstet Gynaecol 106:481, 1999

Brindley BA, Sokol RJ: Induction and augmentation of labor. Basis and methods for current practice. Obstet Gynecol Surv 43:730, 1988

Buccellato CA, Stika CS, Frederiksen MC: A randomized trial of misoprostol versus extra-amniotic sodium chloride infusion with oxytocin for induction of labor. Am J Obstet Gynecol 182:1039, 2000

Buser D, Mora G, Arias F: A randomized comparison between misoprostol and dinoprostone for cervical ripening and labor induction in patients with unfavorable cervices. Obstet Gynecol 89:581, 1997

Caldeyro-Barcia R, Alvarez H, Reynolds SRM: A better understanding of uterine contractility through simultaneous recording with an internal and a seven channel external method. Surg Obstet Gynecol 91:641, 1950

Caldeyro-Barcia R, Poseiro JJ: Physiology of the uterine contraction. Clin Obstet Gynecol 3:386, 1960

Chuck FJ, Huffaker BJ: Labor induction with intravaginal misoprostol versus intracervical prostaglandin E_2 gel (Prepidel gel): Randomized comparison. Am J Obstet Gynecol 173:1137, 1995

Chyu JK, Strassner HT: Prostaglandin E_2 for cervical ripening: A randomized comparison of Cervidil versus Prepidil. Am J Obstet Gynecol 177:606, 1997

Cole DS and Bruck LR: Anaphylaxis after laminaria insertion. Obstet Gynecol 95:1025, 2000

DuVigneaud V, Ressler C, Swan JM, Roberts CW, Katsoyannis PG, Gordon S: The synthesis of oxytocin. J Am Chem Soc 75:4879, 1953

Ekman G, Forman A, Marsál K, Ulmsten U: Intravaginal versus intra-cervical application of prostaglandin E₂ in viscous gel for cervical priming and induction of labor at term in patients with an unfavorable cervical state. Am J Obstet Gynecol 147:657, 1983

Farah LA, Sanchez-Ramos L, Rosa C, Del Valle GO, Gaudier FL, Delke I, Kaunitz AM: Randomized trial of two doses of the prostaglandin E₁ analog misoprostol for labor induction. Am J Obstet Gynecol 177:364, 1997

Flannelly GM, Turner MJ, Rassmussen MJ, Strange JM: Rupture of the uterus in Dublin: An update. J Obstet Gynecol 13:440, 1993

Fraser W, Marcoux S, Moutquin JM, Christen A, and the Canadian Early Amniotomy Study Group: Effect of early amniotomy on the risk of dystocia in nulliparous women. N Engl J Med 328:1145, 1993

Fraser W, Sauve R, Parboosingh IJ, Fung T, Sokol R, Persaud D: A randomized trial of early amniotomy. Br J Obstet Gynaecol 98:84, 1991

Frigoletto FD, Lieberman E, Lang JM, Cohen A, Barrs V, Ringer S, Datta S: A clinical trial of active management of labor. N Engl J Med 333:745, 1995

Garite TJ, Porto M, Carlson NJ, Rumney PJ, Reinbold PA: The influence of elective amniotomy on fetal heart rate patterns and the course of labor in term patients: A randomized study. Am J Obstet Gynecol 168:1827, 1993

Gilson GJ, Russell DJ, Izquierdo LA, Qualls CR, Curet LB: A prospective randomized evaluation of a hygroscopic cervical dilator, Dilapan, in the preinduction ripening of patients undergoing induction of labor. Am J Obstet Gynecol 175:145, 1996

Goldman JB, Wigton TR: A randomized comparison of extraamniotic saline infusion and intracervical dinoprostone gel for cervical ripening. Obstet Gynecol 93:271, 1999

Guinn DA, Goepfert AR, Christine M, Owen J, Hauth JC: Extra-amniotic saline infusion, laminaria, or prostaglandin E₂ gel for labor induction with unfavorable cervix: A randomized trial. Obstet Gynecol 96:106, 2000

Hale RW, Pion RJ: Laminaria: An underutilized clinical adjunct. Clin Obstet Gynecol 15:829, 1972

Hauth JC, Hankins GD, Gilstrap LC III: Uterine contraction pressures achieved in parturients with active phase arrest. Obstet Gynecol 78:344, 1991

Hauth JC, Hankins GD, Gilstrap LC III, Strickland DM, Vance P: Uterine contraction pressures with oxytocin induction/augmentation. Obstet Gynecol 68:305, 1986

Hemlin J, Möller B: Extraamniotic saline infusion is promising in preparing the cervix for induction of labor. Acta Obstet Gynecol Scan 77:45, 1998

Hofmeyr GJ, Gülmezoglu AM, Alfirevic Z: Misoprostol for induction of labour: A systematic review. Br J Obstet Gynaecol 106:798, 1999

Karim A, Rozek LF, Smith ME, Kowalski KG: Effects of food and antacid on oral absorption of misoprostol, a synthetic prostaglandin E₂ analog. J Clin Pharmacol 29:439, 1989

Keirse MJNC: Prostaglandins in preinduction cervical ripening. Meta-analysis of worldwide clinical experience. J Reprod Med 38:89, 1993

Krammer J, O'Brien WF: Mechanical methods of cervical ripening. Clin Obstet Gynecol 38:280, 1995b

Krammer J, Williams MC, Sawai SK, O'Brien WF: Pre-induction cervical ripening: A randomized comparison of two methods. Obstet Gynecol 85:614, 1995a

López-Zeno JA, Peaceman AM, Adashek JA, Socol ML: A controlled trial of a program for the active management of labor. N Engl J Med 326:450, 1992

Maslow AS, Sweeny AL: Elective induction of labor as a risk factor for cesarean delivery among low-risk women at term. Obstet Gynecol 95:917, 2000

McColgin SW, Bennett WA, Roach H, Cowan BD, Martin JN, Morrison JC: Parturitional factors associated with membrane stripping. Am J Obstet Gynecol 169:71, 1993

McColgin SW, Hampton HL, McCaul JF, Howard PR, Andrew ME, Morrison JC: Stripping of membranes at term: Can it safely reduce the incidence of post-term pregnancy? Obstet Gynecol 76:678, 1990b

McColgin SW, Patrissi GA, Morrison JC: Stripping the fetal membranes at term: Is the procedure safe and efficacious? J Reprod Med 35:811, 1990a

Mercer BM, McNanley T, O'Brien JM, Randal L, Sibai BM: Early versus late amniotomy for labor induction: A randomized trial. Am J Obstet Gynecol 173:1371, 1995

Merrill DC, Zlatnik FJ: Randomized, double-masked comparison of oxytocin dosage in induction and augmentation of labor. Obstet Gynecol 94:455, 1999

Miller AM, Rayburn WF, Smith CV: Patterns of uterine activity after intravaginal prostaglandin E₂ during preinduction cervical ripening. Am J Obstet Gynecol 165:1006, 1991

Nguyen MT, Hoffman DR: Anaphylaxis to laminaria. J Allerg Clin Immunol 95:138, 1995

O'Driscoll K, Foley M, MacDonald D: Active management of labor as an alternative to cesarean section for dystocia. Obstet Gynecol 63:485, 1984

Owen J, Winkler CL, Harris BA, Hauth JC, Smith MC: A randomized, double-blind trial of prostaglandin E₂ gel for cervical ripening and meta-analysis. Am J Obstet Gynecol 165:991, 1991

Plaut MM, Schwartz ML, Lubarsky SL: Uterine rupture associated with the use of misoprostol in the gravid patient with a previous cesarean section. Am J Obstet Gynecol 180:1535, 1999

Prysak M, Castronova FC: Elective induction versus spontaneous labor: A case-control analysis of safety and efficacy. Obstet Gynecol 92:47, 1998

Rayburn WF: Prostaglandin E₂ gel for cervical ripening and induction of labor: A critical analysis. Am J Obstet Gynecol 160:529, 1989

Rayburn WF, Lightfoot SA, Newland JR, Smith CV, Christensen HD: A model for investigating microscopic changes induced by prostaglandin E₂ in the term cervix. J Mat Fet Invest 4:137, 1994

Rayburn WF, Wapner RJ, Barss VA, Spitzberg E, Molina RD, Mandsager N, Yonekura L: An intravaginal controlled-release prostaglandin E₂ pessary for cervical ripening and initiation of labor at term. Obstet Gynecol 79:374, 1992

Rouse D, Owen J, Hauth JC: Criteria for failed labor induction: Prospective evaluation of a standardized protocol. Am J Obstet Gynecol 182:S132, 2000

Rouse DJ, Owen J, Hauth JC: Active-phase labor arrest: Oxytocin augmentation for at least 4 hours. Obstet Gynecol 93:323, 1999

Rouse DJ, McCullough C, Wren AL, Owen J, Hauth JC: Active-phase labor arrest: A randomized trial of chorioamnion management. Obstet Gynecol 83:937, 1994

Sanchez-Ramos L, Kaunitz AM, Wears RL, Delke I, Gaudier FL: Misoprostol for cervical ripening and labor induction: A meta-analysis. Obstet Gynecol 89:633, 1997

Satin AJ, Leveno KJ, Sherman ML, Brewster DS, Cunningham FG: High- versus low-dose oxytocin for labor stimulation. Obstet Gynecol 80:111, 1992a

Satin AJ, Leveno KJ, Sherman ML, McIntire DD: High-dose oxytocin: 20- versus 40-minute dosage interval. Obstet Gynecol 83:234, 1994

Satin AJ, Leveno KJ, Sherman ML, McIntire DD: Factors affecting the dose response to oxytocin for labor stimulation. Am J Obstet Gynecol 166:1260, 1992b

Schreyer P, Sherman DJ, Ariely S, Herman A, Caspi E: Ripening the highly unfavorable cervix with extra-amniotic saline instillation or vaginal prostaglandin E_2 application. Obstet Gynecol 73:938, 1989

Sciscione AC, McCullough H, Manley JS, Shlossman PA, Pollock M, Colmorgen, GHC: A prospective, randomized comparison of Foley catheter insertion versus intracervical prostaglandin E_2 gel for preinduction cervical ripening. Am J Obstet Gynecol 180:55, 1999

Sciscione AC, Nguyen L, Manley JS, Shlossman PA, Colmorgen GHC: Uterine rupture during preinduction cervical ripening with misoprostol in a patient with a previous caesarean delivery. Aust N Z J Obstet Gynecol 38:96, 1998

Seitchik J, Amico J, Robinson AG, Castillo M: Oxytocin augmentation of dysfunctional labor, 4. Oxytocin pharmacokinetics. Am J Obstet Gynecol 150:225, 1984

Sherman DJ, Frenkel E, Tovbin J, Arieli S, Caspi E, Bukovsky I: Ripening of the unfavorable cervix with extraamniotic catheter balloon: Clinical experience and review. Obstet Gynecol Surv 51:621, 1996

Toppozada MK, Anwar MYM, Hassan HA, El-Gazaerly WS: Oral or vaginal misoprostol for induction of labor. Intl J Gyn Obstet 56:135, 1997

UK Amniotomy Group: A multicentre randomised trial of amniotomy in spontaneous first labour at term. Br J Obstet Gynaecol 101:307, 1994

Varaklis K, Gumina R, Stubblefield PG: Randomized controlled trial of vaginal misoprostol and intracervical prostaglandin E_2 gel for induction of labor at term. Obstet Gynecol 86:541, 1995

Vengalil SR, Guinn DA, Olabi NF, Burd LI, Owen J: A randomized trial of misoprostol and extra-amniotic saline infusion for cervical ripening and labor induction. Obstet Gynecol 91:774, 1998

Ventura SJ, Martin JA, Curtin SC, Mathews TJ, and the Division of Vital Statistics, National Center for Health Statistics, Centers for Disease Control and Prevention: Report of final mortality statistics. 1995 Mon Vital Stat Rep 45:1, 1997

Windrim R, Bennett K, Mundle W, Young DC: Oral administration of misoprostol for labor induction: A randomized controlled trial. Obstet Gynecol 89:392, 1997

Wing DA, Ham D, Paul RH: A comparison of orally administered misoprostol with vaginally administered misoprostol for cervical ripening and labor induction. Am J Obstet Gynecol 180:1155, 1999

Wing DA, Jones MM, Rahall A, Goodwin TM, Paul RH: A comparison of misoprostol and prostaglandin E_2 gel for preinduction cervical ripening and labor induction. Am J Obstet Gynecol 172:1804, 1995a

Wing DA, Lovett K, Paul RH: Disruption of prior uterine incision following misoprostol for labor induction in women with previous cesarean delivery. Obstet Gynecol 91:828, 1998

Wing DA, Park MR, Paul RH: A randomized comparison of oral and intravaginal misoprostol for labor induction. Obstet Gynecol 95:905, 2000

Wing DA, Rahall A, Jones MM, Goodwin TM, Paul RH: Misoprostol: An effective agent for cervical ripening and labor induction. Am J Obstet Gynecol 172:1811, 1995b

Woodman WB: Induction of labor at eight month, and delivery of a living child in less than four hours by Dr. Barnes's method. Lancet I:10, 1863

Xenakis EMJ, Langer O, Piper JM, Conway D, Berkus MD: Low-dose versus high-dose oxytocin augmentation of labor—a randomized trial. Am J Obstet Gynecol 173:1874, 1995

Yeast JD, Jones A, Poskin M: Induction of labor and the relationship to cesarean delivery: A review of 7001 consecutive inductions. Am J Obstet Gynecol 180:628, 1999

Zieman M, Fong SK, Benowitz NL, Banskter D, Darney PD: Absorption kinetics of misoprostol with oral or vaginal administration. Obstet Gynecol 90:88, 1997

VI

Operative Obstetrics

21

Forceps Delivery and Vacuum Extraction

Although there is periodic and vocal demand to delete assisted vaginal delivery, clinical experience provides recurring evidence that leaving all to natural forces or the scalpel will not accomplish this goal (American College of Obstetricians and Gynecologists, 2000; Robinson, 1994). When criteria for outlet forceps are met, and there is a nonreassuring fetal heart rate pattern, there is no question that assisted or operative vaginal delivery is indicated. The same heart rate pattern, but with the fetus at +1 station and as an occiput transverse, is an entirely different operation and a source of legitimate debate concerning optimal delivery route and risk for mother and fetus. Lack of skill and experience or emergency conditions do change the conditions of the debate and may seriously limit available options.

FORCEPS DELIVERY

Obstetrical forceps are designed for extraction of the fetus. True forceps were first devised in the late 16th or beginning of the 17th century. The reader is referred to the 19th and earlier editions of *Williams Obstetrics* for the history of their design and development.

DESIGN OF FORCEPS. Forceps vary considerably in size and shape, but basically consist of two crossing branches. Each branch has four components: the blade, shank, lock, and handle. Each blade has two curves, the cephalic and pelvic. The cephalic curve conforms to the shape of the fetal head, and the pelvic curve with that of the birth canal. Some varieties are fenestrated rather than solid to permit a more firm hold on the fetal head.

The cephalic curve (Fig. 21–1) should be large enough to grasp the fetal head firmly without compression. The pelvic curve (Fig. 21–1) corresponds more or

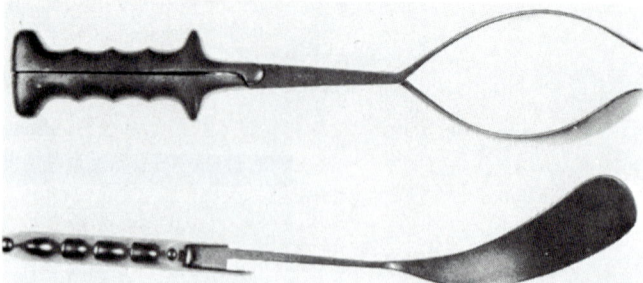

Figure 21–2. Tucker–McLane forceps. The blade is solid and the shank is narrow.

less to the axis of the birth canal, but varies considerably among different instruments. The blades are connected to the handles by the shanks, which give the requisite length to the instrument. The shanks are either parallel as in Simpson forceps or crossing as in Tucker–McLane forceps.

The kind of articulation, or forceps lock, varies among different instruments. The common method of articulation consists of a socket located on the shank at the junction with the handle, into which fits a socket similarly located on the opposite shank (Figs. 21–1 and 21–2). This form of articulation is commonly referred to as the English lock. A sliding lock is used in some forceps, such as Kielland forceps (Fig. 21–3) and allows the shanks to move forward and backward independently. In some cases, the operator chooses to use an axis-traction device to help maintain the appropriate vector for a necessary deliver (Fig. 21–4).

CLASSIFICATION OF FORCEPS DELIVERIES. The most appropriate and current classification for forceps operations is that proposed originally in 1988 and reaffirmed in 2000 by the American College of Obstetricians

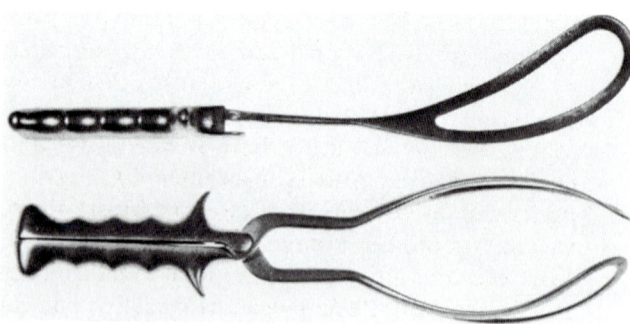

FIGURE 21–1. Simpson forceps. Note the ample pelvic curve in the single blade above and cephalic curve evident in the articulated blades below. The fenestrated blade and the wide shank in front of the English-style lock characterize the Simpson forceps.

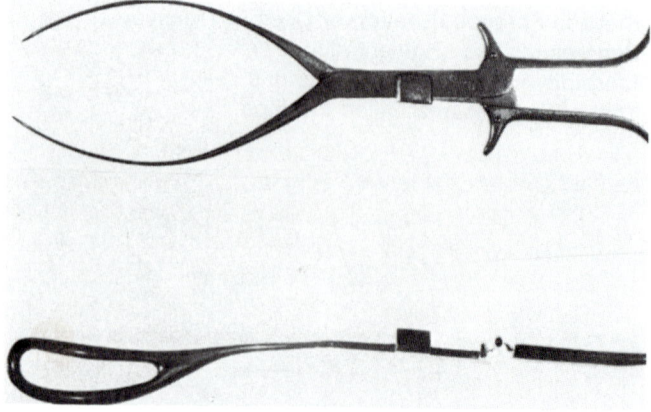

Figure 21–3. Kielland forceps. The characteristic features are the sliding lock, minimal pelvic curvature, and light weight.

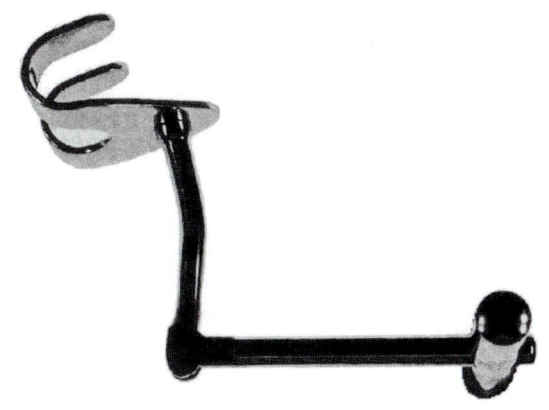

Figure 21–4. Bill axis-traction device which fits over handle of commonly used forceps. Proper use results in the hinge adjoining the handle at a 90-degree angle. (From Hankins and colleagues, 1995.)

and Gynecologists (Table 21–1). This same classification is utilized for vacuum deliveries. This classification emphasizes the two most important discriminators of risk for both mother and infant: station and rotation. It is emphasized that station contemporaneously is measured in centimeters (0 to +5), rather than by dividing the lower pelvis into thirds. Deliveries are categorized as outlet, low, and midforceps procedures. High forceps

TABLE 21–1. Classification of Forceps Delivery According to Station and Rotation

Procedure	Criteria
Outlet forceps	1. Scalp is visible at the introitus without separating the labia.
	2. Fetal skull has reached pelvic floor.
	3. Sagittal suture is in anteroposterior diameter or right or left occiput anterior or posterior position.
	4. Fetal head is at or on perineum.
	5. Rotation does not exceed 45 degrees.
Low forceps	Leading point of fetal skull is at station ≥ +2 cm, and not on the pelvic floor.
	• Rotation is 45 degrees or less (left or right occiput anterior to occiput anterior, or left or right occiput posterior to occiput posterior).
	• Rotation is greater than 45 degrees.
Midforceps	Station above +2 cm but head is engaged.
High	Not included in classification.

From American College of Obstetricians and Gynecologists (2000), with permission.

operations are those in which instruments are applied before engagement and have no place in modern obstetrics. Rotations of greater than 45 degrees are usually more difficult than lesser degrees (Hagadorn-Freathy and colleagues, 1991; Pearl and associates, 1993).

INCIDENCE OF FORCEPS DELIVERY. In any given institution, incidence will depend upon prevailing medical staff attitude, kinds of analgesia and anesthesia used for labor and delivery, and parity of the population. Zahniser and colleagues (1992) analyzed data from the National Hospital Discharge Survey to examine trends in the use of forceps, vacuum extraction, and cesarean section from 1980 to 1987. The rate of cesarean deliveries increased by 48 percent, while forceps procedures declined by 43 percent (Fig. 21–5). Learman (1998) reported data for the next 8 years, and as shown, operative vaginal delay remained at about 10 to 12 percent. By 1994, these were nearly evenly distributed between forceps and vacuum deliveries. Curtin and Park (1999) analyzed United States birth certificate data through 1997 and reported that forceps use was consistently declining as vacuum extraction deliveries consistently increased. More recently, DiMarco and associates (2000) have documented a decline in operative vaginal deliveries with parallel increase in cesarean deliveries.

The incidence varies geographically. Notzon and associates (1991) reported a decline in operative vaginal delivery rates in both the United States and Scotland, but a simultaneous increase in Norway. Ruderman and colleagues (1993) reported rates for Canadian family physicians and obstetricians, respectively, as follows: midforceps 10.1 and 13.5 percent; low forceps 5.3 and 10.5 percent; and vacuum 9.4 and 18.3 percent.

There is considerable regional difference in the United States on operative delivery (Table 21–2). The cesarean delivery rate declined but vacuum deliveries surpassed forceps deliveries in all but the southern United States. The frequency of operative delivery, including operative vaginal delivery, may also be related to maternal age. In a review of over 24,000 cases in women 40 years or older, Gilbert and colleagues (1999b) reported a higher rate of both cesarean delivery and operative vaginal delivery in women 40 or older compared with those aged 20 to 29 years. Most forceps and vacuum procedures are outlet or low pelvic procedures that pose very little risk to mother and fetus (Carmona and colleagues, 1995; Hagadorn-Freathy and associates, 1991).

TRAINING. Ramin and colleagues (1993) surveyed 295 residency training programs in the United States and Canada, of which 203 responded. These represented a

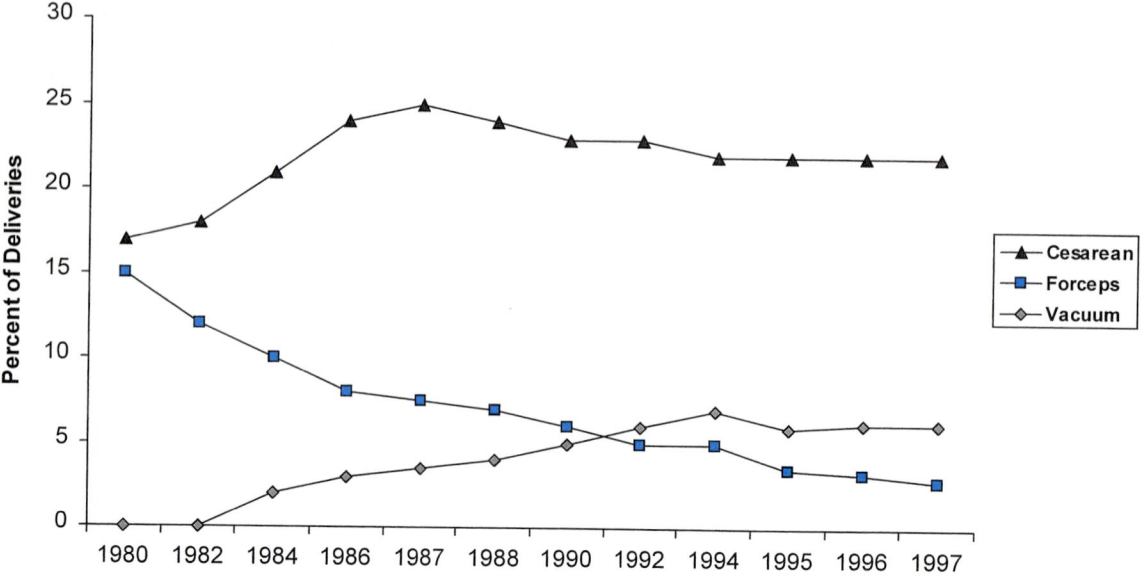

Figure 21–5. Rates of operative delivery in the United States from 1980 through 1997. (Data from 1980–1987 from Zahniser and associates, 1992; data from 1987–1994 from Learman, 1998; data from 1996–1997 from Curtin and Park, 1999.)

minimal total of 458,000 deliveries for 1990. Although two programs were not familiar with the revised 1998 classification of the American College of Obstetrics and Gynecologists, all but 20 percent of the remainder had incorporated these definitions. All responding programs utilized outlet and low forceps. Approximately half used outlet forceps for 5 percent or more of their deliveries, while about a third utilized low forceps for 5 percent or more of their deliveries. Midforceps operations were much less prevalent, and 15 percent of programs reported no use, while another 60 percent performed these operations for fewer than 1 percent of deliveries. Hospitals with high cesarean section rates did not perform fewer midforceps operations. With appropriate use and training, the "forceps cycle" described by Yeomans and Hankins (1992) can be avoided or broken.

EFFECTS OF REGIONAL ANALGESIA ON INSTRUMENTAL DELIVERY. Epidural analgesia is widely accepted as causative in failure of spontaneous rotation to occiput anterior position, as well as in slowing second-stage labor and decreasing maternal expulsive efforts. In some series its use has been associated with increases in forceps delivery from 4 percent to 31 percent and increased vacuum extraction rates of 0.7 to 3.5 percent (Ploeckinger and associates, 1995; Sizer and Nirmal, 2000).

In a randomized clinical trial conducted at Parkland Hospital, Ramin and colleagues (1995) compared segmental lumbar epidural analgesia with intermittent intravenous meperidine for pain relief during labor. As shown in Table 21–3, first- and second-stage labor were significantly prolonged, and this paralleled an increase in low-forceps and cesarean delivery, but not outlet forceps. In a follow-up study from the same institution, Sharma and colleagues (1997) found no increase in operative vaginal delivery in women receiving epidural analgesia compared with patient-controlled intravenous meperidine during labor. In a recent meta-analysis of epidural versus opioid analgesia, Halpern and colleagues (1998) reported that women receiving epidural analgesia were twice as likely to have an instrumental delivery, but not for dystocia.

Epidural blockade increases the frequency of malposition of the fetal head, especially the occiput posterior position, and this in turn may increase the frequency of instrumental delivery. Kaminski and associates (1987) documented occiput posterior positions in 27 percent of women given epidural analgesia compared with only 8 percent of those not given epidural analgesia.

In an attempt to decrease the incidence of forceps delivery associated with epidural analgesia, Saunders and colleagues (1989) compared routine second-stage oxytocin infusion with placebo in 225 nulliparous women who reached full dilatation without oxytocin stimulation. Oxytocin was associated with a significantly shorter second stage (134 versus 151 minutes), a reduction in the incidence of nonrotational forceps deliveries (33 versus 56 percent), and less perineal trauma. Routine oxytocin infusion, however, did not reduce the num-

TABLE 21–2. Operative Delivery Rates in the United States by Geographic Region, 1994

Mode by Region	Rate[a]	Operative Delivery Rates	
		Rate Ratio	95% CI
Cesarean delivery			
South	25.2	1.36	1.36, 1.37
Midwest	19.6	1.06	1.05, 1.06
Northeast	19.4	1.05	1.04, 1.05
West	18.5	1.0	Referent
Vacuum delivery			
South	5.4	1.0	Referent
Midwest	6.2	1.14	1.13, 1.15
Northeast	5.9	1.08	1.07, 1.09
West	9.8	1.81	1.79, 1.83
Forceps delivery			
South	7.5	3.22	3.17, 3.28
Midwest	3.4	1.46	1.43, 1.48
Northeast	2.3	1.0	Referent
West	2.4	1.03	1.01, 1.05

CI = confidence interval.
[a]Rates per 100 live births.
From Learman (1998), with permission.

rior positions of the occiput, forceps may be invaluable for rotation. In general, Simpson forceps are used to deliver the fetus with a molded head, as is common in nulliparous women. The Tucker–McLane instrument is often used for the fetus with a rounded head, which more characteristically is seen in multiparas. In most situations, however, either instrument is appropriate. In some circumstances, more specialized forceps such as the Kielland instrument may be preferable, as in some cases of deep transverse arrest with the fetal head in the transverse position well down in the pelvis with the occiput below the spines. If there is no apparent cephalopelvic disproportion and uterine contractions are inadequate, transverse arrest may sometimes be overcome with oxytocin stimulation.

FORCES EXERTED BY THE FORCEPS. From experiments conducted on women in labor more than a century ago, Joulin (1867) estimated that a pull in excess of 60 kg might damage the fetal skull. These crude studies and subsequent ones have furnished only a gross approximation, for the force produced by the forceps on the fetal skull is a complex function of pull and compression by the forceps and friction produced by the maternal tissues.

INDICATIONS FOR FORCEPS. The termination of labor by forceps, provided it can be accomplished safely, is indicated in any condition threatening the mother or fetus that is likely to be relieved by delivery. Maternal indications include heart disease, pulmonary injury or compromise, intrapartum infection, certain neurological conditions, exhaustion, or prolonged second-stage labor. The latter is defined by the American College of

ber of rotational forceps deliveries performed for malposition of the occiput.

FUNCTION OF FORCEPS. Forceps may be used as a tractor, rotator, or both. Its most important function is traction, although particularly in transverse and poste-

TABLE 21–3. Effects of Epidural Analgesia and Intermittent Intravenous Meperidine on Labor and Operative Deliveries

Factor	Labor Analgesia		Significance
	Epidural (n = 432)	Meperidine (n = 437)	
Admission to delivery			
Mean ± SD (hr)	7.2 ± 3.9	5.7 ± 3.3	P = .001
10 hr or greater	21%	39%	P < .001
Second-stage > 2 hr	7%	3%	P = .001
Delivery			
Spontaneous	82%	93%	P < .001
Outlet forceps	2%	2%	NS
Low forceps	8%	1%	P < .001
Cesarean	9%	4%	P = .002

NS = not stated.
From Ramin and colleagues (1995), with permission.

Obstetricians and Gynecologists (2000) as more than 3 hours with and more than 2 hours without regional analgesia in the nulliparous woman. In the parous woman, it is defined as more than 2 hours with and more than 1 hour without regional analgesia. Midforceps rarely are indicated for labor termination specifically for maternal reasons. Thus, shortening of second-stage labor for maternal reasons should generally be accomplished with either outlet or low forceps.

Fetal indications for operative vaginal delivery with either forceps or vacuum include prolapse of the umbilical cord, premature separation of the placenta, and a nonreassuring fetal heart rate pattern. In the case of a nonreassuring fetal heart rate pattern, it is prudent to describe the fetal heart rate pattern and the station of the planned forceps application in a precisely written note.

ELECTIVE AND OUTLET FORCEPS.
The vast majority of forceps operations performed in this country are elective. Some undoubtedly are related to the frequent use of epidural analgesia. Forceps generally should not be used electively until the criteria for outlet forceps have been met. The fetal head must be on the perineal floor with the sagittal suture no more than 45 degrees from the anteroposterior diameter. In these circumstances, forceps delivery is a simple and safe operation (Carmona and colleagues, 1995; Hagadorn-Freathy and associates, 1991). By allowing the woman in labor ample time, the criteria for outlet forceps can usually be met despite the effects of analgesia.

PROPHYLACTIC OUTLET FORCEPS.
DeLee (1920) recommended delivery by prophylactic outlet forceps, because it was held widely at the time that prolonged pressure of the fetal head against a rigid perineum might result in fetal brain damage. There is no evidence that use of prophylactic forceps is beneficial in the otherwise normal term labor and delivery. Likewise, such a practice has no immediate adverse effects on the newborn compared with spontaneous term vaginal delivery (Yancey and colleagues, 1991). Prophylactic outlet operations may be associated with increased perineal trauma in nulliparous women. Carmona and associates (1995), however, found no differences in maternal or infant outcomes with term pregnancies randomized to spontaneous or elective outlet forceps delivery.

PROPHYLACTIC OUTLET FORCEPS FOR SMALL FETUSES.
Bishop and associates (1965), after analyzing data from the Collaborative Perinatal Project, suggested that prophylactic outlet forceps delivery improved neonatal outcome in low-birthweight infants. Fairweather (1981) reported no significant differences in outcomes in neonates who weighed 500 to 1500 g and who were delivered spontaneously or by outlet forceps. Schwartz and colleagues (1983) reported similar findings. Anderson and associates (1988) presented findings consistent with the view that forceps delivery was protective against progression of periventricular hemorrhage in vaginally delivered neonates who weighed less than 1750 g. Currently, it would appear that there is no obvious advantage to routine outlet forceps delivery of a small fetus.

PREREQUISITES FOR FORCEPS APPLICATION.
There are at least six prerequisites for successful application of forceps:

1. The head must be engaged. Extensive caput succedaneum formation and molding might make determination of the station of the fetal head difficult at times. When difficulties of station assignment occur, it is important to realize that a "low-forceps" procedure may actually be a more difficult midforceps operation. Forceps should not be used until the station of the head is low enough to ensure a safe operative procedure. The same management principle applies to use of forceps for a nonreassuring fetal heart rate pattern when the head is not close to the pelvic floor.

2. The fetus must present as a vertex or by the face with the chin anterior.

3. The position of the fetal head must be precisely known so that cephalic placement of the forceps can be performed.

4. The cervix must be completely dilated before application of forceps. If prompt delivery becomes imperative before complete dilatation of the cervix, cesarean section is indicated.

5. Before forceps application, the membranes must be ruptured to permit a firm grasp of the fetal head by the forceps blades.

6. There should be no disproportion between the size of the head and that of the pelvic inlet or the midpelvis.

PREPARATION FOR FORCEPS DELIVERY.
Although pudendal block may prove adequate for outlet forceps operations, either regional analgesia or general anesthesia is usually preferred for low-forceps or midpelvic procedures. The bladder should be emptied by catheterization if a low- or midforceps delivery is planned. If spinal analgesia is to be used, the anesthetic agent is introduced before placing the woman in the lithotomy position for delivery. If general anesthesia is to be used, the woman is placed in the lithotomy position, the perineum is cleansed and draped, and the physician is ready to perform the delivery before anesthesia is induced.

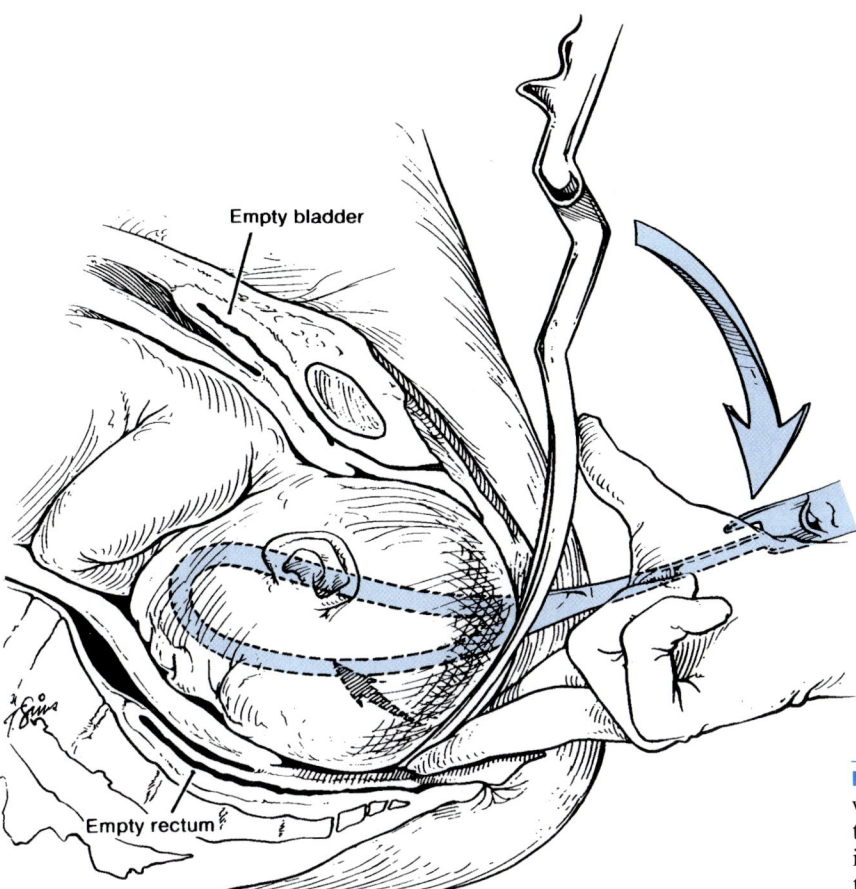

Figure 21-6. The fetus is presenting as vertex with occiput anterior crowning. The application of the left blade of the Simpson forceps is shown. Next, the right blade is applied and the blades are articulated.

Empty bladder

Empty rectum

FORCEPS APPLICATION. Forceps are constructed so that their cephalic curve is closely adapted to the sides of the fetal head (Fig. 21–6). The biparietal diameter of the fetal head corresponds to the greatest distance between the appropriately applied blades. Consequently, the head of the fetus is perfectly grasped only when the long axis of the blades corresponds to the occipitomental diameter, with the major portion of the blade lying over the face, while the concave margins of the blades are directed toward either the sagittal suture (occiput anterior position) or the face (occiput posterior position). Thus applied, the forceps should not slip, and traction may be applied most advantageously as illustrated in Figure 21–7. When forceps are applied obliquely, however (Fig. 21–8), with one blade over the brow and the other over the opposite mastoid region, the grasp is less secure, and the fetal head is exposed to injurious pressure. With most forceps, if one blade is applied over the brow and the other over the occiput, the instrument cannot be locked, or if locked, the blades slip off when traction is applied (Fig. 21–9). For these reasons, the forceps must be applied directly to the sides of the fetal head along the occipitomental diameter, in what is termed the biparietal or bimalar application.

IDENTIFICATION OF POSITION. Precise knowledge of the exact position of the fetal head is essential to a proper cephalic application. With the head low in the pelvis, determination of position is made by examination of the sagittal suture and the fontanels. When the head is at a higher station, an absolute determination can be made by locating the posterior ear.

OUTLET FORCEPS DELIVERY. Delivery by outlet forceps is illustrated in Figures 21–10 to 21–16. The obstacle to delivery is usually insufficient expulsive forces, appreciable resistance of the perineum, or both. In such circumstances, the sagittal suture occupies a principally anteroposterior diameter of the pelvic outlet, with the small (posterior) fontanel directed toward either the symphysis pubis or the concavity of the sacrum. In either event, the forceps, if applied to the sides of the pelvis, grasp the head ideally. The left blade is introduced by the left hand into the left side of the pelvis, and then the right blade is introduced by the right hand into the

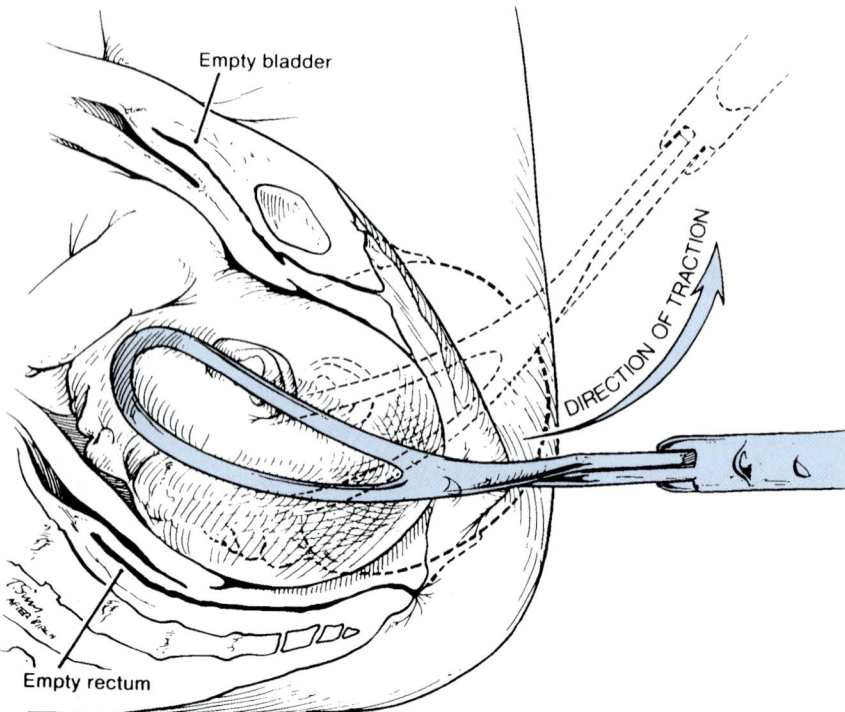

Figure 21–7. Occiput anterior. Delivery by outlet forceps (Simpson). The direction of gentle traction for delivery of the head is indicated.

right side of the pelvis, as follows: Two or more fingers of the right hand are introduced inside the left, posterior portion of the vulva and into the vagina beside the fetal head. The handle of the left branch is then grasped between the thumb and two fingers of the left hand, as in holding a pen, and the tip of the blade is gently passed into the vagina between the fetal head and the palmar surface of the fingers of the right hand, which serve as a guide (Fig. 21–10). The handle and branch are held

at first almost vertically; but as the blade adapts itself to the fetal head, they are depressed, eventually to a horizontal position.

Similarly, two or more fingers of the left hand are then introduced into the right, posterior portion of the vagina to serve as a guide for the right blade, which is held in the right hand and introduced into the vagina (Fig. 21–11). These guiding fingers are then withdrawn and the horizontally positioned branches are articulated.

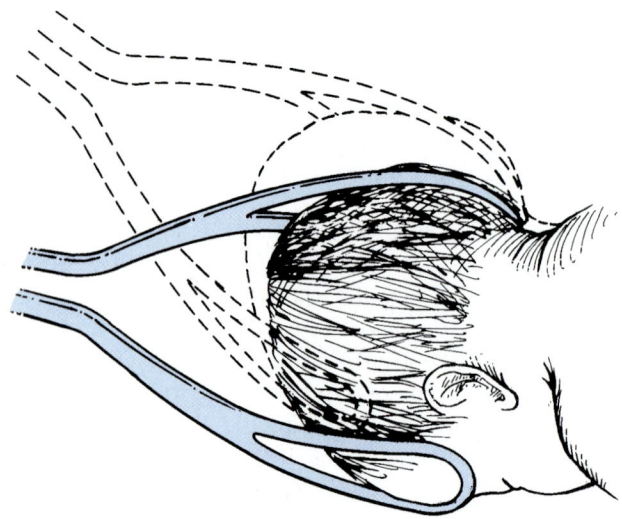

Figure 21–8. Incorrect application of forceps over brow and mastoid region.

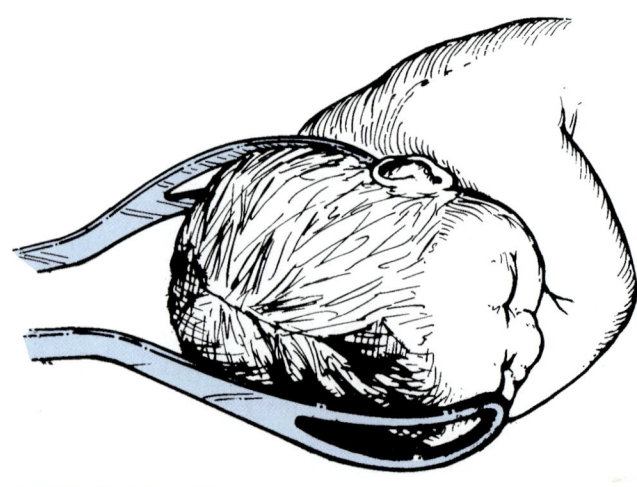

Figure 21–9. Incorrect application of forceps, one blade over the occiput and the other over the brow. Forceps cannot be locked and the head is extended with tendency of blades to slip off with traction.

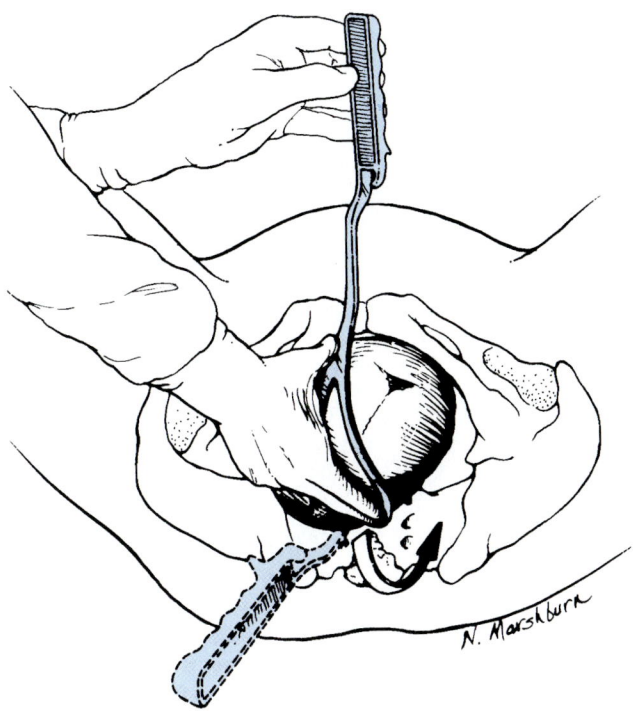

Figure 21–10. The left handle of the Simpson forceps is held in the left hand. The blade is introduced into the left side of the pelvis (*arrow*).

If necessary, one and then the other blade should be gently maneuvered until the handles are repositioned to effect easy articulation.

APPROPRIATENESS OF APPLICATION. The application now is checked before any traction is applied. For the occiput anterior position, appropriately applied blades are equidistant from the sagittal suture. In the occiput posterior position the blades are equidistant from the midline of the face and brow.

TRACTION. When it is certain that the blades are placed satisfactorily, gentle, intermittent, horizontal traction is exerted until the perineum begins to bulge. In some cases, rotation to occiput anterior (or occiput posterior) is performed before traction is applied (Fig. 21–12). Traction is always applied gently and never with excessive force. As the vulva is distended by the occiput, episiotomy may be performed if indicated (Fig. 21–13). More horizontal traction is applied (Fig. 21–14), and the handles are gradually elevated, eventually pointing almost directly upward as the parietal bones emerge (Fig. 21–15). With the fetal head in the occiput anterior position, this maneuver takes advantage of the smallest diameters of the fetal head and brings the suboccipital region beneath the symphysis. As the handles are raised, the head is extended. During upward traction, the four fingers should grasp the upper surface of the handles and shanks, while the thumb exerts the necessary force upon their lower surface.

During the birth of the head, spontaneous delivery should be simulated as closely as possible. Traction

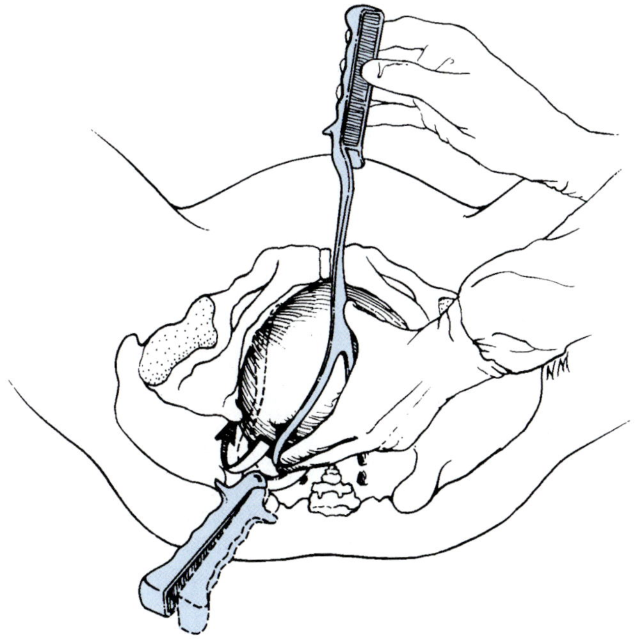

Figure 21–11. Left blade in place; introduction of right blade by right hand.

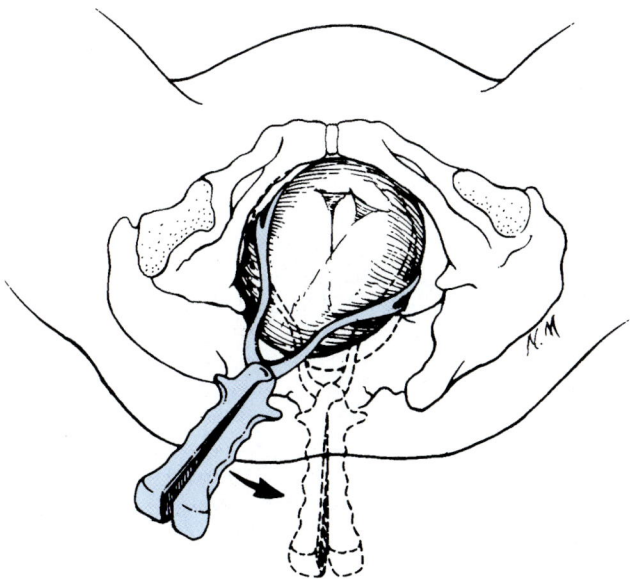

Figure 21–12. Forceps have been locked. Vertex is rotated from left occiput anterior to occiput anterior (*arrow*).

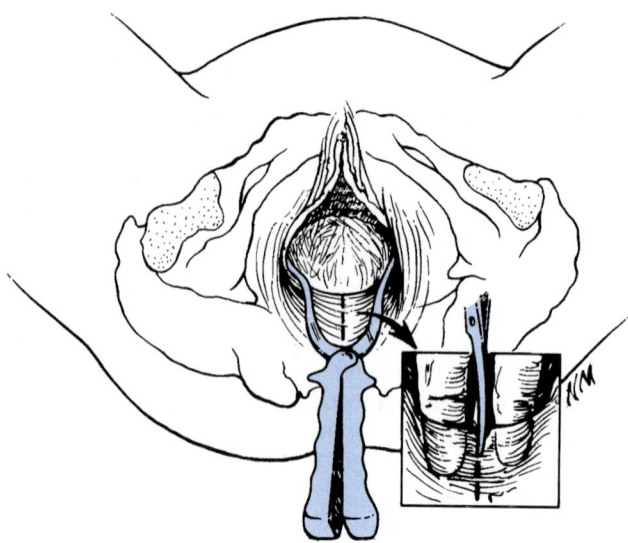

Figure 21–13. Forceps in place. Midline episiotomy is performed here.

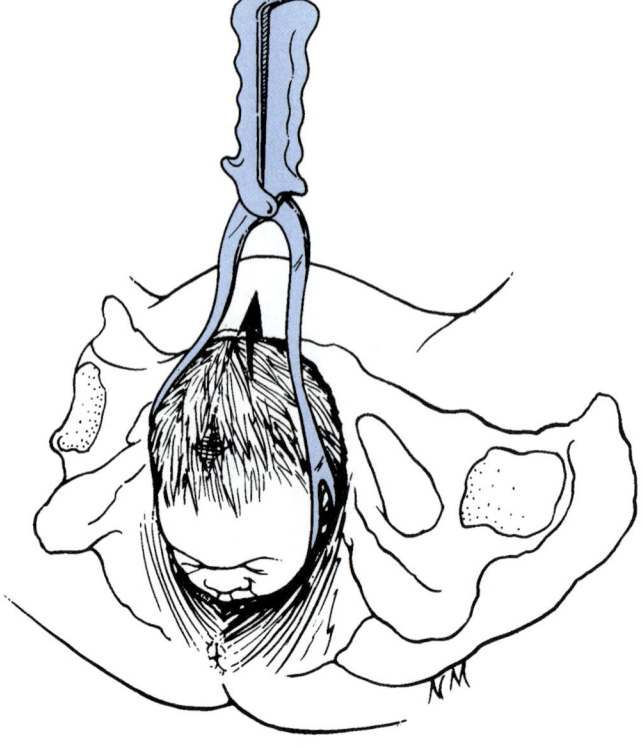

Figure 21–15. Upward traction (*arrow*) is applied as head is delivered. Forceps may be disarticulated after head is delivered.

should therefore be intermittent, and the head should be allowed to recede in intervals, as in spontaneous labor. Except when urgently indicated, as in severe fetal bradycardia, delivery should be sufficiently slow, deliberate, and gentle to prevent undue compression of the fetal head. It is preferable to apply traction with each uterine contraction.

After the vulva has been well distended by the head, and the brow can be felt through the perineum, the delivery may be completed in several ways. Some clinicians keep the forceps in place, in the belief that the greatest control of the advance of the head is thus maintained. The thickness of the blades many times add to

the distention of the vulva, however, thus increasing the likelihood of laceration or necessitating a large episiotomy. In such cases, the forceps may be removed and delivery completed by the modified Ritgen maneuver (Fig. 21–16), slowly extending the head by using upward

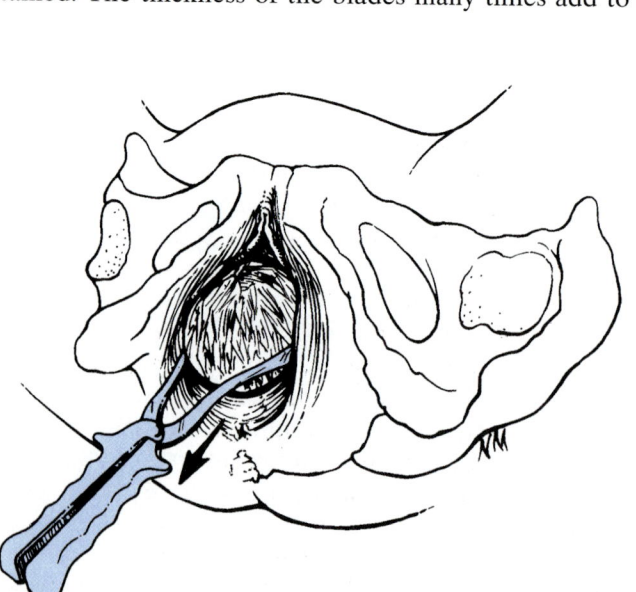

Figure 21–14. Horizontal traction; operator seated.

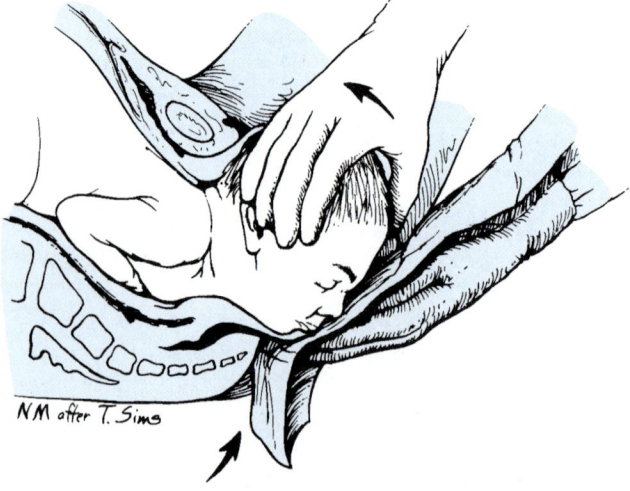

Figure 21–16. Forceps have been disarticulated and removed, and modified Ritgen maneuver (*arrow*) is used to complete delivery of the head.

pressure upon the chin through the posterior portion of the perineum, while covering the anus with a towel to minimize contamination from the bowel. If the forceps are removed prematurely, the modified Ritgen maneuver may prove to be a tedious and inelegant procedure.

LOW- AND MIDFORCEPS OPERATIONS. When the head lies above the perineum, the sagittal suture usually occupies an oblique or transverse diameter of the pelvis. In such cases, the forceps should always be applied to the sides of the head.

LEFT OCCIPUT ANTERIOR POSITION. In the left occiput anterior positions, the right hand, introduced into the left posterior segment of the vagina, should identify the posteriorly located left ear and at the same time serve as a guide for introduction of the left branch of the forceps, which is held in the left hand and applied over the left ear. The handle is held by an assistant or left unsupported, the blade usually retaining its position without difficulty. Two fingers of the left hand are then introduced into the right posterior portion of the pelvis. The right branch of the forceps, held in the right hand, is then introduced along the left hand as a guide. It must then be applied over the anterior ear of the fetus by gently sweeping the blade anteriorly until it lies directly opposite the blade that was introduced first. Of the two branches, when articulated, one occupies the posterior and the other the anterior extremity of the left oblique diameter.

RIGHT OCCIPUT ANTERIOR POSITION. In right positions, the blades are introduced similarly but in opposite directions, for in those cases the right ear of the fetus is the posterior ear, over which the first blade must be placed accordingly. After the blades have been applied to the sides of the head, the left handle and shank lie above the right. Consequently, the forceps do not immediately articulate. Locking of the branches is easily effected, however, by rotating the left around the right to bring the lock into proper position.

OCCIPUT TRANSVERSE POSITIONS. If the occiput is in a transverse position, the forceps are introduced similarly, with the first blade applied over the posterior ear and the second rotated anteriorly to a position opposite the first. In this case, one blade lies in front of the sacrum and the other behind the symphysis. The conventional Simpson or Tucker–McLane forceps (Figs. 21–1 and 21–2), or one of their modifications, or the specialized Kielland forceps (Fig. 21–3) may be used.

ROTATION FROM ANTERIOR AND TRANSVERSE POSITIONS. When the occiput is obliquely anterior, it gradu-

ally rotates spontaneously to the symphysis pubis as traction is exerted. When it is directly transverse, however, in order to bring it anteriorly a rotary motion of the forceps is required. The direction of rotation, of course, varies with the position of the occiput. Rotation counterclockwise from the left side toward the midline is required when the occiput is directed toward the left, and in the reverse direction when it is directed toward the right side of the pelvis.

Infrequently, when forceps are used in transverse positions in anteroposteriorly flattened (platypelloid) pelves, rotation should not be attempted until the fetal head has reached or approached the pelvic floor. Premature attempts at anterior rotation under such conditions may result in injury to the fetus and the mother. Regardless of the original position of the head, delivery is eventually effected by exerting traction downward until the occiput appears at the vulva; the rest of the operation is completed as previously described.

In exerting traction before the head appears at the vulva, one or both hands may be employed. The operator's body weight must not be used for traction.

OCCIPUT POSTERIOR POSITIONS. Prompt delivery may at times become necessary when the small (occipital) fontanel is directed toward one of the sacroiliac synchondroses, namely, in right occiput posterior and left occiput posterior positions. When delivery is required in either instance, the head is often imperfectly flexed. In some cases, when the hand is introduced into the vagina to locate the posterior ear, the occiput rotates spontaneously toward the anterior, indicating that manual rotation of the fetal head might easily be accomplished.

MANUAL ROTATION. A hand with the palm upward is inserted into the vagina and the fingers are brought in contact with the side of the fetal head that is to be pushed toward the anterior position, while the thumb is placed over the opposite side of the head (Fig. 21–17). With the occiput in a right posterior position, the left hand is used to rotate the occiput anteriorly in a clockwise direction; the right hand is used for the left occiput posterior position. At the beginning of the rotation, it may be helpful to dislodge the head slightly upward in the birth canal, but the head must not be disengaged. After the occiput has reached the anterior position, labor may be allowed to continue, or more commonly, forceps can be used to effect delivery. First one blade is applied to that side of the head that is held by the fingers to help maintain the occiput in the anterior position. The other blade is immediately applied and delivery accomplished.

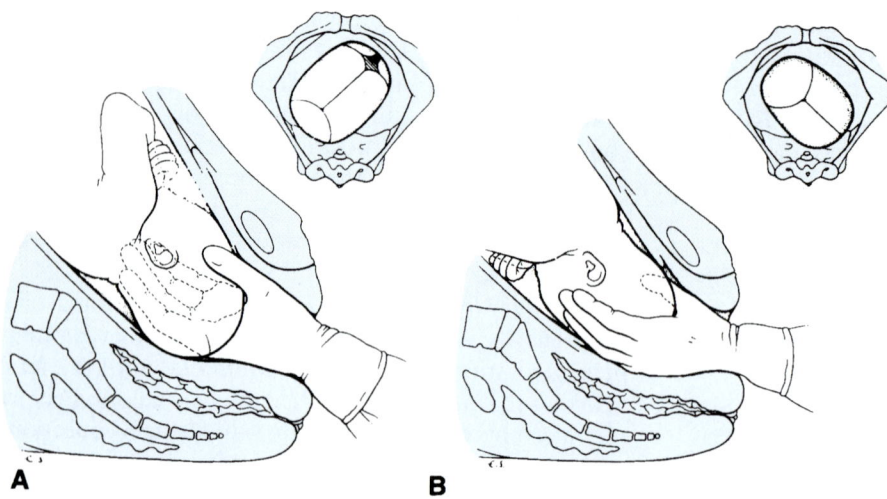

Figure 21–17. A. Manual rotation, left hand in position grasping the head (ROP). **B.** Manual rotation accomplished to right occiput anterior (ROA). Note that with rotation to the ROA position the fetal head may become more flexed. (From Douglas and Stromme, 1976.)

FORCEPS DELIVERY. If manual rotation cannot be easily accomplished, application of the blades to the head in the posterior position and delivery from the occiput posterior position may be the safest procedure (Fig. 21–18). In many cases, the cause of the persistent occiput posterior position and of the difficulty in accomplishing rotation is an anthropoid pelvis, the architecture of which predisposes to posterior delivery and opposes rotation. When the occiput is directly posterior, horizontal traction should be applied until the base of the nose is under the symphysis. The handles should then be slowly elevated until the occiput gradually emerges over the anterior margin of the perineum. Then, by imparting a downward motion to the instrument, the nose, face, and chin successively emerge from the vulva.

Occiput posterior extraction causes greater distention of the vulva, and a large episiotomy may be needed. Pearl and associates (1993) retrospectively reviewed 564 occiput posterior deliveries. These were compared with 1068 controls matched for race, parity, and delivery

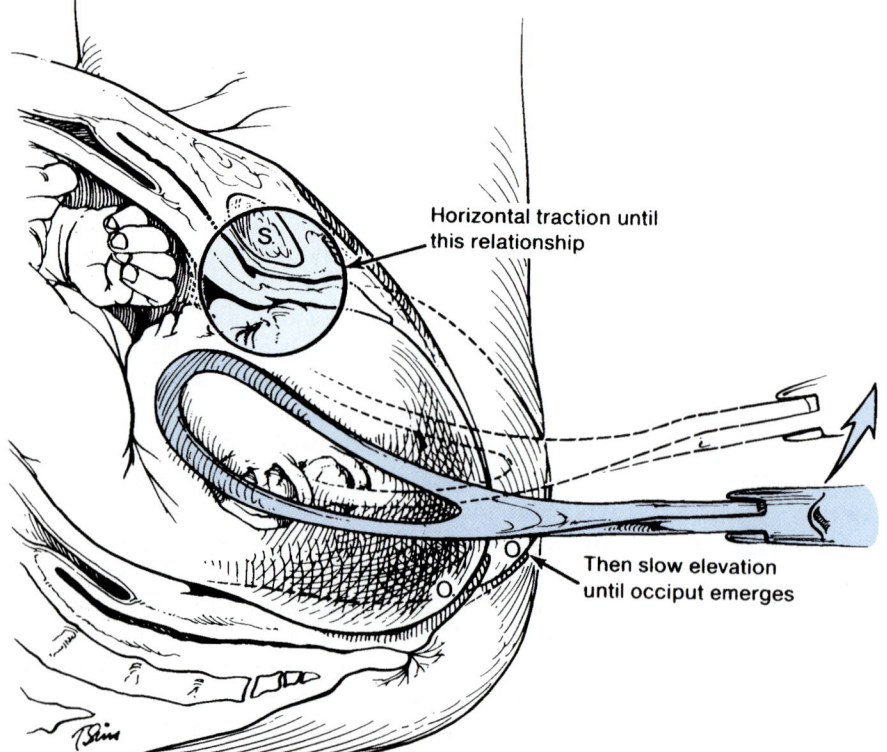

Horizontal traction until this relationship

Then slow elevation until occiput emerges

Figure 21–18. Occiput directly posterior. Low forceps (Simpson) delivery as an occiput posterior. (O = occiput, S = symphysis.) The *arrow* illustrates the point at which time the head should be flexed after the bregma passes under the symphysis. It is evident that to prevent serious perineal lacerations an extensive episiotomy is most often required.

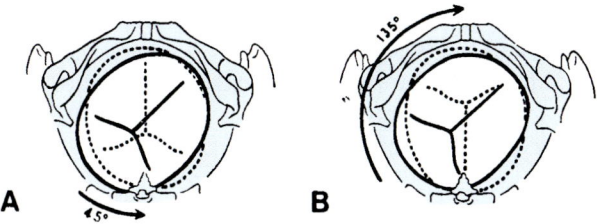

Figure 21–19. Rotation of obliquely posterior occiput to sacrum **(A)** and symphysis pubis **(B).**

method. The occiput posterior group had a higher incidence of severe perineal lacerations and extensive episiotomy compared with the occiput anterior group. Within the occiput posterior group, operative delivery was associated with a higher incidence of severe perineal lacerations (35 versus 16 percent), vaginal lacerations (18 versus 7 percent), and episiotomy (95 versus 74 percent) than was spontaneous delivery. The infants delivered from the occiput posterior position had a higher incidence of Erb (1 percent) and facial nerve (2 percent) palsy than did those delivered from the occiput anterior position.

FORCEPS ROTATIONS. Tucker–McLane, Simpson, or Kielland forceps may be used to rotate the fetal head. The oblique occiput may be rotated 45 degrees to the posterior position or 135 degrees to the anterior position (Fig. 21–19). If rotation is performed with Tucker–McLane or Simpson forceps, the head must be flexed, but this is not necessary with Kielland forceps because they have a more straightened pelvic curve. In rotating the occiput anteriorly with Tucker–McLane or Simpson forceps, the pelvic curvature, originally directed upward, at the completion of rotation is inverted and directed posteriorly. Attempted delivery with the instrument in that position is likely to cause serious maternal injury manifest as vaginal sulcus tears and sidewall lacerations. To avoid such trauma, it is essential to remove and reapply the instrument as described below.

KIELLAND FORCEPS ROTATION OF OCCIPUT TRANSVERSE. Kielland (1916) described forceps with narrow, somewhat bayonet-shaped blades that he claimed could be applied readily to the sides of the head in the occiput transverse position and surpassed all other models as a rotator (Fig. 21–3). Kielland forceps have a sliding lock and almost no pelvic curve. On each handle is a small knob that indicates the direction of the occiput.

The station of the fetal head must be accurately ascertained to be at, or preferably below, the level of the ischial spines. Often in these cases there has been extreme molding of the fetal head, and the caput succeda-

neum has descended to below the ischial spines, giving the erroneous impression that the head is engaged when actually the occiput is above the spines (Knight and colleagues, 1993). Forceps application under these circumstances is classified as high and is not to be attempted.

There are two methods of applying the anterior blade. In one, the anterior blade is introduced first with its cephalic curve directed upward; after it has entered sufficiently far into the uterine cavity, it is turned through 180 degrees to adapt the cephalic curvature to the head. Kielland also described a wandering or gliding method of application for the anterior blade when the uterus is tightly contracted about the head and the lower uterine segment is stretched and thin. In the wandering or gliding method, the anterior blade is introduced at the side of the pelvis over the brow or face to an anterior position, with the handle of the blade held close to the opposite maternal buttock throughout the maneuver. The second blade is introduced posteriorly and the branches are locked.

Because most cases amenable to Kielland forceps rotation are those in which there is deep transverse arrest—the fetal head is deep in the pelvis with the occiput well below the level of the ischial spines—rotation is usually accomplished by unwedging the fetal head from the pelvis by a small amount of upward pressure. From this slightly higher station, the rotation is accomplished. The head should not be pushed high enough to allow disengagement because the cord may prolapse.

In an early study, Rubin and Coopland (1970) summarized their experiences with 1000 consecutive cases of Kielland forceps rotation. Half were occiput posterior and half occiput transverse. Rotation was accomplished successfully in 970. There were eight perinatal deaths, including four with serious anomalies. Injuries to the infant were considered mostly minor for those contemporaneous times; however, there were 27 injuries that would not be considered minor today, including seven infants with a fractured skull!

Tan and associates (1992) reported more contemporaneous results with 137 midpelvic Kielland forceps deliveries. Common indications were prolonged second stage (73 percent), maternal distress (13 percent), or fetal distress (10 percent). Maternal complications included lacerations in 12 percent, and hemorrhage in 12 percent; 3 percent of the 137 women were given blood transfusions. Neonatal complications included cephalohematoma in 9 percent, and one infant each had a facial nerve or C_5 Erb palsy. In a later study by Krivak and colleagues (1999), 55 deliveries using Kielland rotation were compared with 213 nonrotational forceps. Jain and colleagues (1993) examined trends for delivery of deep transverse arrest from 1970 to 1990. Kielland forceps were used in 44 percent of cases in 1970, but by 1990 they were not used at all. Delivery in 1970 employed either or both manual rotation (63 percent), Kielland rotation (44 percent), or cesarean delivery (11 percent). By 1990, management involved cesarean delivery (42 percent), manual rotation (31 percent), or vacuum extraction (27 percent). Although the total number of women who had a deep transverse arrest is small—only 111—of the 25 infants delivered by Kielland forceps, eight required admission to the newborn intensive care unit. Two had facial nerve palsy and two had fractures of the right parietal bone. Importantly, if first manually rotated and then delivered by forceps, there were no injuries. In comparison, three delivered by cesarean had birth asphyxia.

For all of these reasons, in many centers forceps rotations of persistent occiput transverse positions are usually not done. Exceptions are cases associated with deep transverse arrest due to failure of rotation because of levator sling relaxation from epidural analgesia.

FORCEPS FOR FACE PRESENTATION.
In the face presentation, with the chin directed toward the symphysis (mentum anterior), the application of forceps is occasionally used to effect vaginal delivery. The blades are applied to the sides of the head along the occipitomental diameter, with the pelvic curve directed toward the neck. Downward traction is exerted until the chin appears under the symphysis. Then, by an upward movement, the face is slowly extracted, with the nose, eyes, brow, and occiput appearing in succession over the anterior margin of the perineum (Fig. 21–20). Forceps should not be applied to the mentum posterior presentation, because vaginal delivery is impossible as such.

MORBIDITY FROM FORCEPS OPERATIONS

MATERNAL MORBIDITY.
A valid and important question concerns the appropriate comparison group as regards forceps-related morbidity. Clearly it is not those women who deliver spontaneously, as forceps are usually not used absent a valid indication. Instead, the appropriate comparison group would be those women whose only options are either cesarean section or operative vaginal delivery by vacuum extractor.

Some generalizations can be made:

1. Elective outlet-forceps with rotations not exceeding 45 degrees may be used to shorten the second stage of labor with little, if any, increase in maternal morbidity (Carmona and colleagues, 1995).
2. Maternal injury increases significantly with rotations of greater than 45 degrees and at higher stations (Hagadorn-Freathy and associates, 1991; Hankins and Rowe, 1996).

3. Blood transfusions are increased with operative vaginal delivery (vacuum extraction 6.1 percent, forceps 4.2 percent) compared with uncomplicated cesarean (1.4 percent) or spontaneous vaginal delivery (0.4 percent) (Sherman and co-workers, 1993).

EPISIOTOMY AND LACERATIONS.
The very conditions that lead to the requirement for operative vaginal delivery would also be expected to increase the need for episiotomy. This is supported by the observation that women randomized to delivery with low forceps had no increase in perineal lacerations relative to those delivering spontaneously (Carmona and colleagues, 1995). Hagadorn-Freathy and co-workers (1991) reported rates for third- and fourth-degree episiotomies and vaginal lacerations of 13 percent for outlet, 22 percent for low-forceps with less than 45 degrees rotation, 44 percent for low-forceps with greater than 45 degrees rotation, and 37 percent for midforceps operations. Similarly, Bofill and colleagues (1996a, 1996b) found a significant association of moderate and severe perineal injuries with indicated operative deliveries, use of forceps versus vacuum extractor, need for episiotomy, and delivery other than outlet station.

Although Williams and associates (1991) did not stratify perineal injury by complexity of delivery, they reported an 18 percent vaginal laceration rate, 20 percent third-degree episiotomy rate, and 10 percent

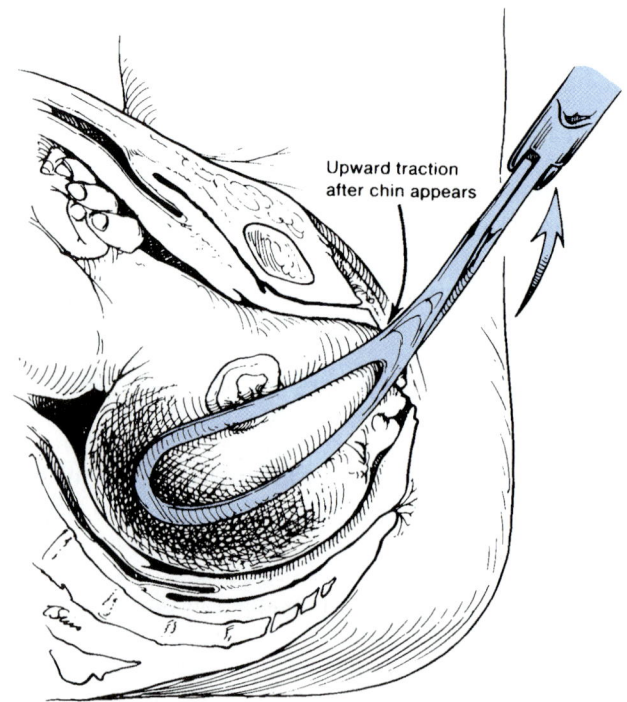

Upward traction after chin appears

Figure 21–20. Face presentation, mentum (chin) anterior. Delivery with outlet forceps (Simpson).

fourth-degree rate with forceps compared with 15 percent, 7 percent, and 22 percent respectively with vacuum extraction. Robinson and colleagues (1999) studied perineal trauma in 323 women delivered with forceps or vacuum extraction. Use of episiotomy with forceps delivery did not significantly increase perineal trauma which was already high (55 versus 46 percent, with and without episiotomy, respectively). Vacuum extraction, however, significantly increased such trauma (35 versus 9 percent, with and without episiotomy, respectively).

Others report less trauma with the vacuum extractor. Low and co-workers (1993) reported vaginal lacerations in 4.3 percent of women and fourth-degree episiotomy in 1.6 percent. Loghis and co-workers (1992) reported anal sphincter involvement in 3 percent of vacuum deliveries and vaginal vault extensions in 2.5 percent.

Ecker and colleagues (1997) reported a significant decrease in the rate of episiotomy use over a 10-year period from 1984 to 1994 for both forceps (96 versus 30 percent) and vacuum deliveries (89 versus 39 percent). During the same time period there was a decrease in fourth-degree and no change in third-degree lacerations. Eason and associates (2000) have recently reviewed this subject.

URINARY AND RECTAL INCONTINENCE. It appears that normal, spontaneous delivery may cause urinary and fecal incontinence in some women (Chap. 13, p. 325). For example, Dimpfl and colleagues (1992) suggest that as many as 6 percent of women who were continent before pregnancy develop permanent stress urinary incontinence after vaginal delivery. It is hypothesized that factors that increase trauma to the pelvic floor musculature and its innervation are causative, such as tears, no episiotomy, and forceps and vacuum delivery. This is unproven, however. Short-term effects of midcavity delivery and of rotations of greater than 45 degrees are associated with postpartum urinary retention and bladder dysfunction. Such complications also follow vacuum deliveries. Low and associates (1993) reported that 3 percent of women had voiding difficulties and required an indwelling catheter. Bladder rest by insertion of a Foley catheter, surveillance for urinary tract infection with early diagnosis and treatment, and bladder training usually result in restoration of normal function within a few days.

Anal sphincter trauma and resultant dysfunction may be associated with instrumental vaginal delivery. Sultan and colleagues (1993) described 43 nulliparas who had undergone forceps or vacuum vaginal delivery and compared them with women delivering spontaneously. A mediolateral episiotomy was performed in all 26 women undergoing forceps delivery and 13 of 17 in the vacuum group. In only one case was the rectal sphincter involved. The control group was composed of 47 randomly selected nulliparas delivered spontaneously who sustained a spontaneous second-degree tear or had a mediolateral episiotomy. Defecatory symptoms developed in 38 percent of women following forceps delivery, 12 percent following vacuum delivery, and 4 percent in the control group. Anal sphincter defects, diagnosed by anal endosonography, were present in 80 percent of forceps deliveries, 20 percent of vacuum deliveries, and 35 percent of controls.

In a subsequent study, Sultan and colleagues (1994) evaluated 50 women who had sustained third-degree tears. Anal incontinence or fecal urgency was present in half with tears compared with 13 percent without tears. Sonographic sphincter defects were identified in 85 percent of women who had a third-degree tear compared with 33 percent of controls. Every symptomatic woman had persistent combined internal and external sphincter defects that were associated with significantly lower anal pressures. Pudendal nerve conduction measurements were not different—suggesting that the injury is to the muscle and not the nerve.

In a 5-year follow-up study of women who had initially been randomized to either form of delivery, Sultan and colleagues (1998) reported that 32 percent of women delivered with forceps versus 16 percent of those delivered with vacuum had anal incontinence. Their study was small and the difference between the two groups was not significant. Tetzschner and colleagues (1998) reported that anal and urinary incontinence were associated with degree of sphincter rupture, use of vacuum extraction, and pudendal nerve terminal motor latencies of greater than 2.0 milliseconds.

Although the association of rectal incontinence and operative vaginal delivery, especially with forceps, is certainly disconcerting, the precise etiology of the lesion(s) or condition(s) producing the anal dysfunction is less than clear. Whether anal dysfunction associated with childbirth can even be prevented is also unclear. For example, factors other than operative vaginal delivery that have been associated with fecal incontinence include advanced parity, postmenopausal status, prior hysterectomy, and irritable bowel syndrome (Donnelly, 1998; Jackson, 1997; Nygaard, 1997, and their colleagues).

In a 30-year follow-up study, Nygaard and colleagues (1997) discovered flatus incontinence in 31, 43, and 36 percent of women in the disrupted anal sphincter, episiotomy, and cesarean groups respectively. These authors concluded that "regardless of the type of delivery, anal incontinence occurs in a surprisingly large number of middle-aged women." Moreover, Rieger and colleagues (1997) reported that normal vaginal delivery without evidence of sphincter injury was associated with significant effect on anal sphincter function.

Thus, not only do anal and urinary incontinence follow uncomplicated spontaneous delivery, they also may occur in women following cesarean delivery. Wilson and colleagues (1996) reported urinary incontinence in 5.2 percent of women delivered by cesarean and there was little difference between elective cesarean versus cesarean delivery following labor. MacArthur and colleagues (1997) reported fecal incontinence in six women who underwent emergency cesarean delivery. Fynes and colleagues (1998), in a cohort of 234 women, reported that cesarean delivery performed in late labor does not protect the anal sphincter mechanism.

At this time, the data do not support abandoning operative vaginal delivery techniques in favor of cesarean delivery in all women. Large randomized studies with controls are needed to address the effects of operative vaginal delivery and possible pelvic floor damage and incontinence. Current studies that address this are in progress in several institutions.

FEBRILE MORBIDITY. Postpartum metritis is far more frequent, and often more severe, in women following cesarean compared with operative vaginal delivery. Rates of metritis for vacuum delivery are about 8 percent, for forceps 16 percent, and for combined operations 40 percent (Williams and associates, 1991). Robertson and colleagues (1990), using the 1988 forceps classification, reported maternal morbidity in 60 to 70 percent of women undergoing cesarean delivery compared with 25 percent for those delivered by midforceps, and 33 percent by low forceps.

PERINATAL MORBIDITY. Operative vaginal delivery, especially if performed from the midpelvic level, may be associated with increased neonatal morbidity. Examples of such morbidity, as well as their frequencies, are shown in Table 21–4. This series consisted of 5 percent midpelvic operations and most low-forceps deliveries were done with less than 45-degree rotation.

Towner and colleagues (1999) studied 583,340 term nulliparous women delivered in California between 1992 and 1994. A third were delivered operatively—by cesarean, forceps, or vacuum. The incidence of intracranial hemorrhage, as shown in Table 21–5, was identified to be greatest in infants delivered by vacuum, forceps, or cesarean after labor. These investigators concluded that abnormal labor was the common risk factor.

White and associates (1996) found a significant association of facial nerve palsy with forceps delivery compared with spontaneous delivery or cesarean section. A seldom-reported complication of delivery is neonatal abducens nerve injury (Galbraith, 1994). This injury complicates virtually no cesarean deliveries, 0.1 percent of spontaneous vaginal deliveries, 2.4 percent of forceps deliveries (less common with outlet forceps), and 3.2 percent of vacuum extractions. Fortunately, almost all

resolve by 6 weeks. Gilbert and co-workers (1999a), using the California database cited above, found that either forceps (3.4-fold) or vacuum (2.7-fold) significantly increase the risk for brachial plexus injury compared with spontaneous delivery.

MIDFORCEPS DELIVERIES. The immediate consequences of midforceps rotations have been reviewed by several investigators whose reports included controlled

TABLE 21–4. Neonatal Complications with Vacuum and Forceps Delivery

Complications	Vacuum n = 41 (%)	Forceps n = 40 (%)
Apgar scores		
1 min < 7	4 (10)	4 (10)
5 min < 8	1 (2)	1 (2)
Cephalohematoma		
Mild	6 (15)	3 (7)
Moderate	1 (2)	2 (5)
Caput	14 (34)	7 (14)
Facial mark/injury	1 (2)	7 (18)[a]
Trauma		
Erb palsy (mild)	1 (2)	0
Fractured clavicle	1 (2)	0
Elevated bilirubin	8 (20)	4 (10)
Retinal hemorrhage		
Mild	6/37 (16)	3/36 (8)
Moderate or severe	8/37 (37)	3/36 (8)
Infant stay	3.4 days	3.1 days

[a]Significant difference between rates for vacuum and forceps deliveries.
From Williams and colleagues (1991), with permission.

TABLE 21–5. Effect of Method of Delivery on Incidence of Neonatal Intracranial Hemorrhage (ICH)

Delivery	Incidence of ICH
Vacuum and forceps	1:280
Forceps	1:664
Vacuum	1:860
Cesarean with labor	1:907
Spontaneous	1:1900
Cesarean without labor	1:2040

Data from Towner and colleagues (1999).

series. Chiswick and James (1979) reviewed neonatal morbidity and mortality with Kielland forceps deliveries compared with a matched group of babies born spontaneously. Birth trauma was evident in 15 percent of infants delivered with forceps. Neonatal mortality, most often from tentorial tears, occurred in 3 of 86 babies delivered with forceps, and two of these were in babies delivered by emergency cesarean section after attempts at instrumental delivery. More recent studies with Kielland forceps were discussed earlier (Jain and colleagues, 1993; Tan and associates, 1992).

Hughey and colleagues (1978) compared 458 midforceps operations with 17 cesarean deliveries. Women delivered by cesarean were selected when the cervix was completely dilated and the occiput failed to rotate to the anterior position from transverse or posterior. Using a perinatal morbidity index, an unfavorable result of 30 percent was reported for fetuses delivered by midforceps versus no morbidity with cesarean delivery. Bowes and Bowes (1980) compared fetal outcomes with midforceps deliveries with those delivered by cesarean delivery or vacuum extraction. Morbid events were identified in 14 of 71 midforceps deliveries (20 percent) compared with two morbid events in the 37 cesarean sections (5 percent) and three instances of fetal trauma in 15 vacuum extractions (20 percent).

Several factors must be taken into consideration when attempting to interpret the results of these studies. First and foremost, they were conducted prior to the redefined classification of forceps in 1988; thus, midforceps were not defined as clearly and included deliveries from relatively high stations (0 to +1), as well as difficult rotations. Second, spontaneous vaginal deliveries are not appropriate controls for midforceps as in the study by Chiswick and James (1979). Finally, there is no uniformity in the criteria utilized to define immediate fetal morbidity.

Gilstrap and colleagues (1984) retrospectively compared immediate maternal and neonatal outcomes of 234 women delivered by midforceps with those of women delivered spontaneously, by low forceps, or by cesarean. Importantly, forceps were not applied unless the fetal head was below zero station, or had descended to lower than +1 station (of 3 stations) in the case of transverse arrest. Almost 60 percent of women delivered by midforceps had epidural analgesia. These investigators found no difference in the incidence of neonatal acidosis between the groups when indications for delivery were matched. Likewise, they found no excessive trauma to fetuses delivered by midforceps.

Dierker and associates (1985) provided a retrospective review of 176 midforceps deliveries at Cleveland Metropolitan General Hospital from 1976 through 1982, and compared these with all other deliveries during the study period. Epidural analgesia was associated with

slightly more than half of the midforceps deliveries. Although cephalohematomas were identified more commonly in neonates delivered by midforceps (7 percent), they found no increased incidence of low Apgar scores, seizures, shoulder dystocia, and brachial or facial nerve palsy when these infants were compared with the general obstetrical population. Conversely, Falco and Eriksson (1990) described 92 cases of cranial VII nerve palsy in over 44,000 newborns delivered from 1982 to 1987 at Brigham and Women's Hospital. Of these, 74 (91 percent) were associated with forceps delivery.

Bashore and associates (1990) compared neonatal outcome in 358 midforceps deliveries with that of 486 cesarean deliveries. They found no increase in significant neonatal morbidity in the forceps group, although four newborns had transient facial palsy. Conversely, Robertson and associates (1990) used the 1988 classification of forceps and reported significantly higher neonatal morbidity in the midforceps group compared with infants delivered by cesarean.

In a prospective study of 357 forceps deliveries classified by both the old and new systems, Hagadorn-Freathy and colleagues (1991) reported that neonatal morbidity was effectively stratified using the 1988 classification. For example, facial nerve palsy developed in 1.3 percent of infants delivered by outlet forceps and 3.2 percent of those delivered by midforceps using the 1965 classification. This compared with 0.9 percent for outlet forceps, 1.7 percent for low forceps, and 9.2 percent for midforceps using the 1988 classification. Thus, the new classification of midforceps identifies a high-risk group for this complication. In the series of 99 women randomized to either forceps or vacuum by Williams and associates (1991), only five midpelvic deliveries were attempted. Of these, both vacuum deliveries were accomplished, but two of three forceps trials failed due to the inability to satisfactorily place the blades.

Because of the increased maternal and neonatal morbidity associated with midforceps deliveries compared with low forceps operations, they are seldom used contemporaneously. According to the American College of Obstetricians and Gynecologists (2000), midforceps procedures, including rotational delivery, are appropriate to teach and to use under the correct circumstances by an adequately trained individual.

LONG-TERM INFANT MORBIDITY. There has been significant controversy regarding possible associations of forceps delivery with long-term morbidity for the newborn. Although some earlier studies (Chefetz, 1965; Eastman and colleagues, 1962) reported an increased frequency of cerebral palsy with the use of midforceps, others did not find such an association (Amiel-Tison, 1969; Steer and Boney, 1962).

Of all the aspects of forceps use, none has engendered

more controversy than the possible association with decreased intelligence quotient (IQ). This issue is unsettled and is likely to remain so because of the multitude of variables affecting intelligence. Broman and co-workers (1975) used data from the Collaborative Perinatal Project and controlled for socioeconomic status, race, and gender, and reported that infants delivered by midforceps had slightly higher intelligence scores at 4 years of age than children delivered spontaneously. Friedman and associates (1977, 1984), using the same database, described intelligence assessments at least up to 7 years of age, and concluded that those children who had been delivered by midforceps had lower mean IQs compared with children delivered by outlet forceps. Dierker and colleagues (1986) assessed the long-term outcome of children delivered by midforceps, again from the same database, and compared them with children who had been delivered by cesarean section performed for dystocia. Clearly, this is the most appropriate control group. These children were assessed at a minimum of 2 years of age, and the investigators found no increased morbidity associated with delivery by midforceps.

Nilsen (1984) evaluated 18-year-old men drafted into the Norwegian Army and reported that those delivered by Kielland forceps had higher intelligence scores than those delivered spontaneously, by vacuum extraction, or by cesarean.

In a collaborative study of over 3000 school-age children, Wesley and colleagues (1992) found no significant difference in standardized intelligent scores according to the method of delivery. All were evaluated at age 5 for cognitive development. There were 1746 children who were delivered spontaneously compared with 1192 children who had been delivered by either low- or midforceps or vacuum operations; 114 were delivered by midforceps or vacuum extraction.

Seidman and colleagues (1991) studied over 52,000 persons who were examined by the Israeli Defense Forces draft board at age 17. They had been born between 1964 and 1972 in four West Jerusalem hospitals. Intelligence test scores were available through 1969, and data from these 32,425 deliveries are shown in Table 21–6. Data were adjusted by multiple regression for confounding effects of gender, birthweight, ethnic origin, birth order, maternal age, paternal and maternal education, and social class. Interestingly, prior to adjustment the mean intelligence scores at 17 years of age were significantly higher in the vacuum and forceps group than in the spontaneous delivery group. After adjustment for confounding factors, the IQ score of the cesarean delivery group was significantly lower than that of the spontaneous delivery group.

CONCLUSIONS REGARDING MORBIDITY FROM FORCEPS. When performed inappropriately, forceps deliv-

TABLE 21–6. Intelligence Test Scores at Age 17 for Subjects Born in Jerusalem between 1964 and 1970

Type of Delivery	Mean Intelligence Score (± SE)	
	Unadjusted	*Adjusted*[a]
Spontaneous (n = 29,136)	105.4 (0.1)	105.7 (0.1)
Forceps (n = 567)	108.2[b] (0.7)	104.6 (0.4)
Vacuum extraction (n = 1207)	109.6[b] (0.5)	105.9 (0.4)
Cesarean delivery (n = 1335)	105.4 (0.4)	103.7[b] (0.1)

SE = standard error.
[a]Adjusted by multiple regression for confounding effects of sex, birthweight, ethnic origin, birth order, maternal age, and paternal and maternal education and social class.
[b]$P < .0001$ compared with spontaneous delivery.
From Seidman and associates (1991), with permission.

ery can result in adverse maternal as well as fetal outcomes. It is clear that the greatest risk is incurred with true midforceps operations and when rotations of greater than 45 degrees are required. Most studies in which these morbid events were reported to be increased substantively were done when cesarean rates were still around 5 percent. Moreover, many of these earlier studies undoubtedly included forceps applications that would, in all likelihood, never be attempted today. In contrast, more contemporaneous studies appropriately emphasize that the majority of midforceps deliveries are done with the fetal vertex at +1 (of three stations) or lower station (Dierker and associates, 1986; Gilstrap and colleagues, 1984). It is unlikely that midforceps deliveries included in the Collaborative Perinatal Project during the 1960s were this conservative.

The impact of the popular use of epidural analgesia on the incidence of low- and midforceps deliveries cannot be discounted. The majority of such cases result from inadequate maternal expulsive forces against a relaxed pelvic sling, and thus they are not usually associated with either relative or absolute cephalopelvic disproportion. Although it is prudent in these cases to allow a longer second stage of labor, in some women and under some circumstances, delivery is indicated sooner. Low-forceps rotations for epidural-associated labor abnormalities are likely to be safer than the same operation performed in women with prolonged labors or midpelvic arrest unassociated with conduction analgesia.

It seems reasonable to conclude that outlet and low-forceps operations with rotation of 45 degrees or less, classified by the American College of Obstetricians and Gynecologists (2000) scheme, can be performed with safety for both mother and fetus if the basic guidelines set forth in this chapter are carefully observed.

TRIAL OF FORCEPS AND FAILED FORCEPS. In trial of forceps, the operator attempts delivery with the full knowledge that vaginal delivery may not be successful. With an operating room both equipped and staffed for immediate cesarean delivery, the trial may proceed. If a satisfactory application of the forceps cannot be achieved, then the procedure is abandoned and delivery accomplished by use of either vacuum extraction or cesarean. Once application has been achieved, gentle downward pulls are made on the instrument. If there is no descent, the procedure is abandoned. In some situations, vacuum extraction may be successful (Ezenagu and colleagues, 1999). If not deemed safe, or if it also fails to effect vaginal delivery, then cesarean delivery is performed.

In a study of 122 women who had a trial of midcavity forceps or vacuum extraction in a setting with full preparations to proceed to cesarean section, Lowe (1987) found no significant difference in immediate neonatal or maternal morbidity compared with 42 women delivered for similar indications by cesarean without such a trial of instrumentation. Conversely, neonatal morbidity was higher in 61 women who had "unexpected" forceps or vacuum failure in which there was no prior preparation for immediate cesarean delivery. Williams and colleagues (1991) reported good outcomes for both mother and infant by use of alternate or sequential forceps/vacuum delivery. They achieved an overall cesarean delivery rate of 3 percent in a group of 99 women, all 35 weeks or greater, and who had indications for assisted vaginal delivery.

Thus, as Lowe (1987) concluded, "a carefully conducted trial of instrumental delivery is an acceptable alternative to cesarean section for delay in the second stage due to a potentially difficult midcavity arrest." We agree with the American College of Obstetricians and Gynecologists (2000), which cautions that these are attempted only if the clinical assessment is highly suggestive of a successful outcome.

VACUUM EXTRACTION

Simpson introduced the idea of vacuum extraction in the 1840s, and there have been numerous attempts since to attach a traction device by suction to the fetal scalp. In the United States, the device is referred to as the vacuum extractor, while commonly in Europe it is referred to as a **ventouse** (from French, literally, *soft cup*). The theoretical advantages of the vacuum extractor over forceps include the avoidance of insertion of space-occupying steel blades within the vagina and their positioning precisely over the fetal head, as is required for forceps delivery; the ability to rotate the fetal head without impinging upon maternal soft tissues; and less intracranial pressure during traction. All previously described instruments were unsuccessful until Malmström (1954) applied a new principle, namely, traction on a metal cap so designed that the suction creates an artificial caput, or *chignon*, within the cup that holds firmly and allows adequate traction.

As with forceps choice, the decision to use a metal or a soft cup appears regional. In the United States, the metal cup generally has been replaced by newer soft cup vacuum extractors. As emphasized by Duchon and associates (1998), however, high-pressure vacuum generates large amounts of force regardless of the cup used. The silastic cup vacuum device is a reusable instrument with a soft, 65-mm diameter cup. The Mityvac instrument uses a disposable 60-mm diameter cup (Fig. 21–21), and the CMI Tender Touch uses a 62-mm cup (Fig. 21–22). Bofill and associates (1996b) reported good results with the Mityvac M-cup.

Loghis and colleagues (1992) compared results of 200 women delivered using a metal cup with 200 women in whom a pliable cup was used. No differences were found in the rate of birth canal trauma (11 versus 13 percent), major neonatal scalp trauma (6.5 percent versus 5.5 percent), neonatal jaundice (15.5 percent versus 13.5 percent), or Apgar scores. Kuit and co-workers (1993) found the only advantage of the soft cups to be a lower incidence of neonatal scalp injury. In this study, both rigid and pliable cups had an associated episiotomy extension rate of 14 percent. Vaginal lacerations were 16 percent with rigid cups and 10 percent with pliable cups.

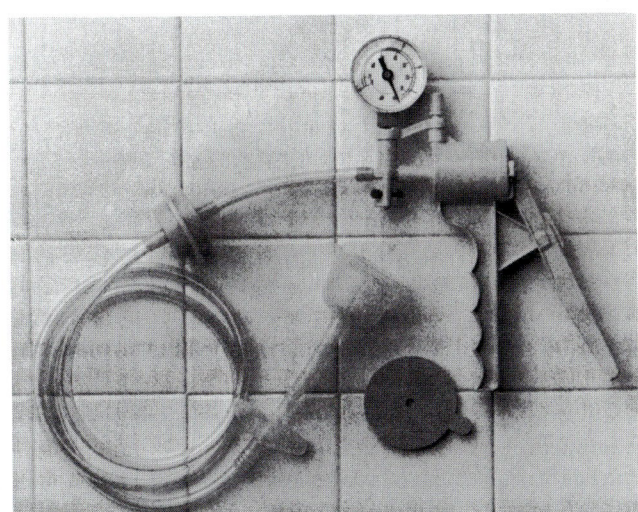

Figure 21–21. Mityvac obstetrical vacuum delivery system includes extractor cup and pump. (Photograph reproduced with permission of Prism Enterprises, Inc, Rancho Cucamonga, CA.)

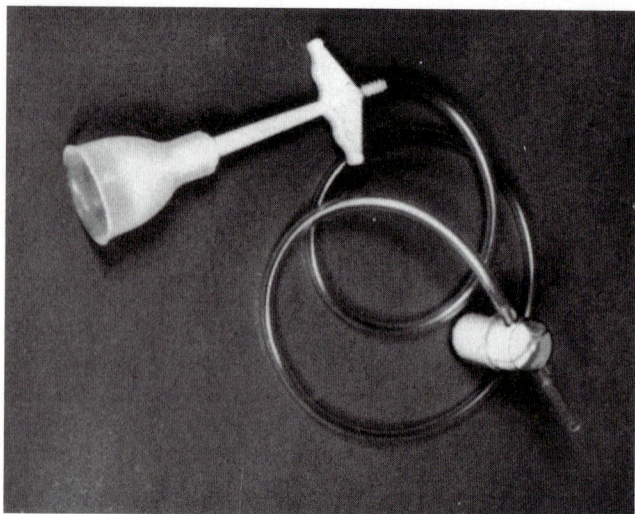

Figure 21–22. CMI Tender Touch extractor cup. (Photograph reproduced with permission of Utah Medical Products.)

Johanson and Menon (2000a) searched the Cochrane Pregnancy and Childbirth Group database and found nine randomized trials. They too found that soft cups had a higher failure rate (1.65 ×) but were associated with less scalp injury (0.45 ×) than rigid cups.

INDICATIONS AND PREREQUISITES. Generally, the indications and prerequisites for the use of the vacuum extractor for delivery are the same as for forceps delivery (American College of Obstetricians and Gynecologists, 2000). The tendency to attempt vacuum deliveries at stations higher than usually attempted with forceps is worrisome. Broekhuizen and colleagues (1987) reported that 3.5 percent of vacuum deliveries were performed with the vertex above zero station, and another 20 percent were at zero station. Relative contraindications for delivery using vacuum extraction include face or other nonvertex presentations, extreme prematurity, fetal coagulopathies, known macrosomia, and following recent scalp blood sampling.

TECHNIQUE. Proper cup placement is the most important determinant of success in vacuum extraction. The center of the cup should be over the sagittal suture and about 3 cm in front of the posterior fontanelle. Anterior placement on the fetal cranium—near the anterior fontanelle rather than over the occiput—will only aggravate the problem of cervical spine extension unless the fetus is small relative to the maternal pelvis. Similarly, asymmetrical placement relative to the sagittal suture may worsen asynclitism. The effects of asymmetrical or anterior misplacement of the cup are shown in Figure

21–23. Cup placement for elective use of the instrument in occiput anterior positions is seldom difficult. In contrast, when the indication for delivery is failure to descend caused by occipital malposition, with or without asynclitism or deflexion, cup placement can be very difficult (Lucas, 1994).

Entrapment of maternal soft tissue predisposes the mother to lacerations and hemorrhage and virtually assures cup "pop-off." The full circumference of the cup should be palpated both prior to as well as after the vacuum has been created, and prior to traction. When using rigid cups, it is recommended that the vacuum be created gradually by increasing the suction by 0.2 kg/cm² every 2 minutes until a negative pressure of 0.8 kg/cm² is reached. With soft cups, negative pressure can be increased to 0.8 kg/cm² over as little as 1 minute (Hankins and associates, 1995; Kuit and colleagues, 1993). Some authors suggest that 0.6 kg/cm² is optimal as higher amounts of pressure increase might potentially increase the risk of fetal scalp and/or cerebrocranial trauma without significantly increasing the rate of successful vaginal delivery (Lucas, 1994). Table 21–7 lists conversions of various units of pressures used by different instruments.

Traction should be intermittent and coordinated with maternal expulsive efforts. Traction may be initiated by using a two-handed technique; fingers of one hand are placed against the suction cup, while the other hand grasps the handle of the instrument. A theoretical advantage of the instrument is that it will usually detach prior to creating tractive forces sufficient to cause fetal injury. Vacuums offer no advantage for avoidance of shoulder dystocia. Manual torque to the cup should be avoided as it may cause cephalhematomas and lacerations—"cookie-cutter" type with metal cups—of the fetal scalp.

Vacuum extraction should be considered a trial, and without early and clear evidence of descent toward delivery, consideration for alternate delivery approach is given. As a general guideline, progress in descent should accompany each traction attempt. Neither data nor consensus are available regarding the number of pulls required to effect delivery, the maximum number of cup detachments that can be tolerated, or total duration of the procedure. A cup pop-off due to technical failure or because placement has been difficult to obtain, and thereby the amount of vacuum that can be developed or maintained is suboptimal, should not be equated with a pop-off under ideal conditions of exact cup placement and optimal vacuum maintenance. The former may merit several additional attempts at placement and delivery, or abandonment and use of forceps (Ezenagu and colleagues, 1999; Williams and co-workers, 1991). Conversely, the latter is highy suggestive of relative or absolute disproportion or asynclitism that is requiring

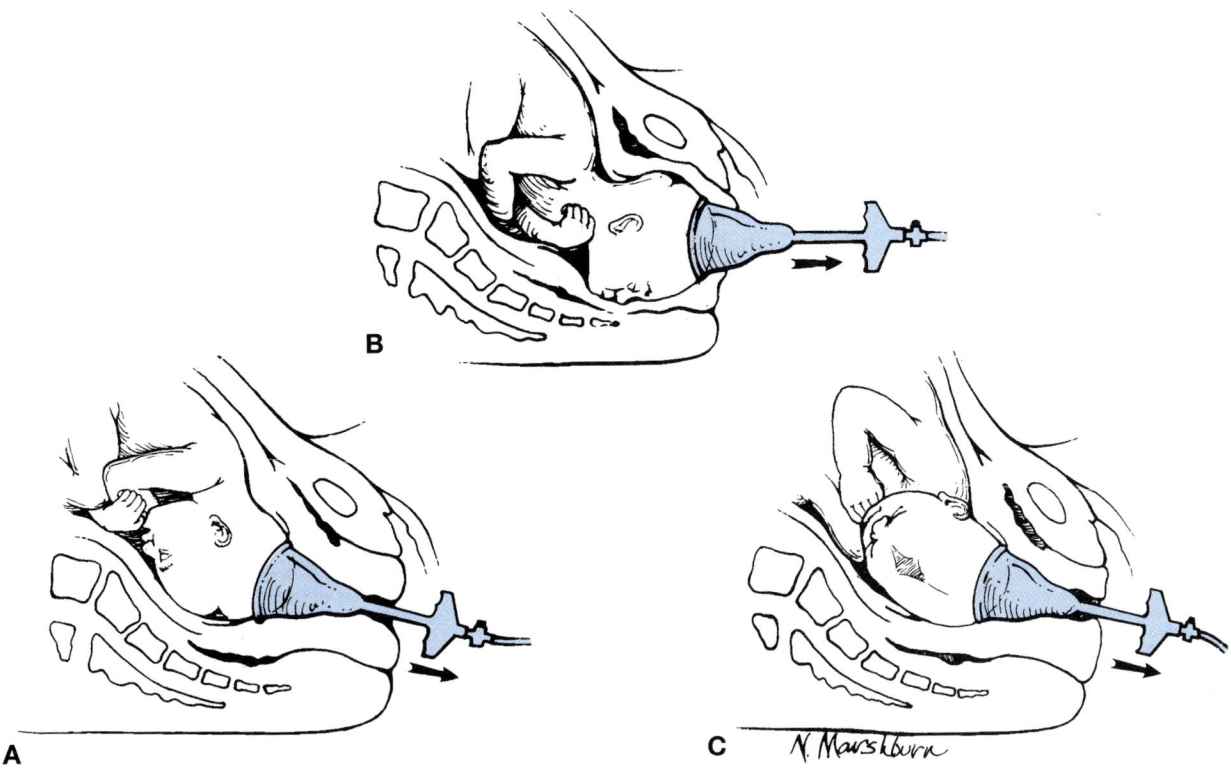

Figure 21–23. The effect of cup position on the attitude of the fetal head. **A.** The cup covers the posterior fontanelle. **B.** The anterior edge of the cup is on the posterior angle of the bregma. **C.** The cup is paramedian.

excessive tractive forces. As with forceps procedures, there should be a willingness to abandon attempts at vacuum extraction if satisfactory progress is not made (American College of Obstetricians and Gynecologists, 2000).

COMPLICATIONS. Complications include scalp lacerations and bruising, subgaleal hematoma, cephalohematomas, intracranial hemorrhage, neonatal jaundice, subconjunctival hemorrhage, clavicular fracture, shoulder dystocia, injury of sixth and seventh cranial nerves, Erb

TABLE 21–7. Table of Vacuum Pressure Conversions

mm Hg	in Hg	lb/in²	kg/cm²
100	3.9	1.9	0.13
200	7.9	3.9	0.27
300	11.8	5.8	0.41
400	15.7	7.7	0.54
500	19.7	9.7	0.68
600	23.6	11.6	0.82

From Lucas (1994), with permission.

palsy, retinal hemorrhage, and fetal death (Broekhuizen, 1987; Dell and associates, 1985; Galbraith, 1994; Govaert and colleagues, 1992). Significant scalp injuries, hematomas, and resulting hyperbilirubinemia are more common with the metal cup instruments compared with the soft cup devices (American College of Obstetricians and Gynecologists, 2000; Johanson and Menon, 2000a). In a review by Plauche (1979) of the Malmström vacuum extractor, scalp injury ranged from 0.8 to 33 percent, cephalohematomas from 1 to 26 percent, and subgaleal hemorrhage from 0 to 10 percent. Similar results have been reported by Benjamin and Kahn (1993) and Kuit and associates (1993). Berkus and associates (1985), on the other hand, found no increase in serious neonatal morbidity, including retinal hemorrhage, for the silastic vacuum extractor compared with spontaneous delivery.

The Food and Drug Administration issued a Public Health Advisory in 1998 regarding the possible association of vacuum-assisted delivery with serious or fetal complications, including death. During a 4-year period, the FDA received reports of nine serious fetal injuries and 12 newborn deaths, which was a significant increase over the preceding 11 years. In a response to this advisory, the American College of Obstetricians and Gynecologists (1998) issued a Committee Opinion recommending the continued use of vacuum-assisted delivery devices when appropriate. They estimated that there is approximately one adverse event per 45,455 vacuum extractions per year.

RECOMMENDATION REGARDING VACUUM DELIVERY. Considering the 1998 FDA Public Health Advisory, the following recommendations seem reasonable:

1. The classification of vacuum deliveries should be the same as that utilized for forceps deliveries (including station).
2. The same indications and contraindications utilized for forceps deliveries should be applied to vacuum-assisted deliveries.
3. The vacuum should not be applied to an unengaged vertex (i.e., above zero station).
4. The individual performing or assisting in the procedure should be an experienced operator.
5. The operator should be willing to abandon the procedure if it does not proceed easily or if the cup pops off more than three times.

COMPARISON OF VACUUM EXTRACTION WITH FORCEPS. There have been numerous studies comparing vacuum extraction with forceps deliveries. Vacca and associates (1983) conducted a randomized, prospective study comparing metal cup vacuum extraction with forceps delivery. They reported a higher frequency of maternal trauma and blood loss in the forceps group, but an increase in the incidence of neonatal jaundice in the vacuum group. Bofill and colleagues (1996b) randomized 637 women to forceps versus vacuum extraction with the Mityvac M-cup. There were significantly more third- and fourth-degree lacerations (29 versus 12 percent) in the forceps-delivered group. Conversely, the incidence of shoulder dystocia and cephalohematoma were doubled in the vacuum group. Others have found decreased maternal trauma and similar neonatal morbidity in babies delivered by vacuum compared with forceps (Berkus, 1985; Broekhuizen, 1987; Dell, 1985; Williams, 1991, and their colleagues). Although retinal hemorrhage is occasionally seen with vacuum usage, it has no apparent long-term effects. Johanson and Menon (2000b) searched the Cochrane Pregnancy and Childbirth Group database and analyzed 10 randomized trials. They confirmed that vacuum extraction was associated with less maternal trauma but increased cephalohematomas and retinal hemorrhages.

There are sparse data regarding long-term neurological outcome in newborns delivered by vacuum extraction. In the report of an 18-year follow-up by Nilsen (1984), the mean intelligence score of 38 male infants delivered by vacuum was not different from the national average. Seidman and associates (1991) reported a higher mean IQ score at age 17 in those delivered by vacuum or forceps compared with spontaneous delivery (Table 21–6).

Johanson and colleagues (1999) performed a 5-year follow-up of a randomized trial of forceps versus vacuum delivery in over 600 women. Almost half in each group reported urinary incontinence or fecal urgency. There was also no significant differences in child development.

REFERENCES

American College of Obstetricians and Gynecologists: Operative vaginal delivery. Practice Bulletin No. 17, June, 2000

American College of Obstetricians and Gynecologists: Delivery by vacuum extraction. Committee on Obstetric Practice, No. 208, 1998

American College of Obstetricians and Gynecologists, Committee on Obstetrics, Maternal and Fetal Medicine: Obstetric forceps. No. 59, February, 1998

Amiel-Tison C: Cerebral damage in full-term newborns, etiological factors, neonatal status and long-term follow-up. Biol Neonatorum 14:234, 1969

Anderson GD, Bada HS, Sibai BM, Korone SB: Obstetrical factors related to progression of periventricular hemorrhage in the preterm newborn. Abstract 401, presented at the 35th annual meeting of the Society for Gynecologic Investigation, Baltimore, March, 1988

Bashore RA, Phillips WH, Brankman CR III: A comparison of the morbidity of midforceps and cesarean delivery. Am J Obstet Gynecol 162:1428, 1990

Benjamin B, Khan MRH: Pattern of external birth trauma in southwestern Saudi Arabia. J Trauma 35:737, 1993

Berkus MD, Ramamurthy RS, O'Connor PS, Brown K, Hayashi RH: Cohort study of silastic obstetric vacuum cup deliveries, 1. Safety of the instrument. Obstet Gynecol 66:503, 1985

Bishop E, Israel L, Briscoe C: Obstetric influences on the premature infants' first year of development: A report from the Collaborative Study of Cerebral Palsy. Obstet Gynecol 26:628, 1965

Bofill JA, Rust OA, Devidas M, Martin RW, Morrison JC, Martin JN Jr: Prognostic factors for moderate and severe maternal genital tract laceration with operative vaginal delivery. Am J Obstet Gynecol 174:353, 1996a

Bofill JA, Rust OA, Schorr SJ, Brown RC, Martin RW, Martin JN Jr, Morrison JC: A randomized prospective trial of the obstetric forceps versus the M-cup. Am J Obstet Gynecol 174:354, 1996b

Bowes WS, Bowes C: Current role of midforceps operations. Clin Obstet Gynecol 23:549, 1980

Broekhuizen FF, Washington JM, Johnson F, Hamilton PR: Vacuum extraction versus forceps delivery: Indications and complications, 1979 to 1984. Obstet Gynecol 69:338, 1987

Broman SH, Nichols PL, Kennedy WA: Preschool IQ: Prenatal and Early Developmental Correlates. Hillside, NJ, Erlbaum, 1975

Carmona F, Martinez-Roman S, Manau D, Cararach V, Iglesias X: Immediate maternal and neonatal effects of lowforceps delivery according to the new criteria of The American College of Obstetricians and Gynecologists compared with spontaneous vaginal delivery in term pregnancies. Am J Obstet Gynecol 173:55, 1995

Chefetz MD: Etiology of cerebral palsy: Role of reproductive insufficiency and the multiplicity of factors. Obstet Gynecol 25:635, 1965

Chiswick ML, James DK: Kielland's forceps: Association with neonatal morbidity and mortality. BMJ 1:7, 1979

Curtin SC, Park MM: Trends in the attendant, place, and timing of births, and in the use of obstetric interventions: United States, 1989–97. Natl Vital Stat Rep 47:1, 1999

DeLee JB: The prophylactic forceps operation. Am J Obstet Gynecol 1:34, 1920

Dell DL, Sightler SE, Plauche WC: Soft cup vacuum extraction: A comparison of outlet delivery. Obstet Gynecol 66:624, 1985

Dierker LJ, Rosen MG, Thompson K, Debanne S, Linn P: The midforceps: Maternal and neonatal outcomes. Am J Obstet Gynecol 152:176, 1985

Dierker LJ, Rosen MG, Thompson K, Lynn P: Midforceps deliveries: Long-term outcome of infants. Am J Obstet Gynecol 154:764, 1986

DiMarco CS, Ramsey PS, Williams LH, Ramin KD: Temporal trends in operative obstetric delivery: 1992–1999. Obstet Gynecol 95:39S, 2000

Dimpfl T, Hesse U, Schussler B: Incidence and cause of postpartum urinary stress incontinence. Eur J Obstet Gynecol Reprod Biol 43:29, 1992

Donnelly VS, O'Herlihy C, Campbell DM, O'Connell PR: Postpartum fecal incontinence is more common in women with irritable bowel syndrome. Dis Colon Rectum 41:586, 1998

Douglas RB, Stormme WB: Operative Obstetrics, 3rd ed. New York, Appleton-Century-Crofts, 1976

Duchon MA, DeMund MA, Brown RH: Laboratory comparison of modern vacuum extractors. Obstet Gynecol 72:155, 1998

Eason E, Labrecque M, Wells G, Feldman P: Presenting perineal trauma during childbirth: A systematic review. Obstet Gynecol 95:464, 2000

Eastman NJ, Kohl SG, Maisel JE, Kaveler F: The obstetrical background of 753 cases of cerebral palsy. Obstet Gynecol Surv 17:459, 1962

Ecker JL, Tan WM, Bansal RK, Bishop JT, Kilpatrick SJ: Is there a benefit to episiotomy at operative vaginal delivery? Observations over ten years in a stable population. Am J Obstet Gynecol 176:411, 1997

Ezenagu LC, Kakaria R, Bofill JA: Sequential use of instruments at operative vaginal delivery: Is it safe? Am J Obstet Gynecol 180:1446, 1999

Fairweather D: Obstetric management and follow-up of the very low-birth-weight infant. J Reprod Med 26:387, 1981

Falco NA, Eriksson E: Facial nerve palsy in the newborn: Incidence and outcome. Plast Reconstr Surg 85:1, 1990

FDA Public Health Advisory: Need for CAUTION When Using Vacuum Assisted Delivery Devices. May 21, 1998

Friedman EA, Sachtleben MR, Bresky PA: Dysfunctional labor, 12. Long-term effects on the fetus. Am J Obstet Gynecol 127:779, 1977

Friedman EA, Sachtleben-Murray MR, Dahrouge D, Neff RK: Long-term effects of labor and delivery on offspring: A matched-pair analysis. Am J Obstet Gynecol 150:941, 1984

Fynes M, Donnelly VS, O'Connell PR, O'Herlihy C: Cesarean delivery and sphincter injury. Obstet Gynecol 92:496, 1998

Galbraith RS: Incidence of neonatal sixth nerve palsy in relation to mode of delivery. Am J Obstet Gynecol 170:1158, 1994

Gilbert WM, Nesbitt TS, Danielsen B: Associated factors in 1611 cases of brachial plexus injury. Obstet Gynecol 93:536, 1999a

Gilbert WM, Nesbitt TS, Danielsen B: Childbearing beyond age 40: Pregnancy outcome in 24,032 cases. Obstet Gynecol 93:9, 1999b

Gilstrap LC, Hauth JC, Schiano S, Connor KD: Neonatal acidosis and method of delivery. Obstet Gynecol 63:681, 1984

Govaert P, Vanhaesebrouck P, de Praeter C: Traumatic neonatal intracranial bleeding and stroke. Arch Dis Child 67:840, 1992

Hagadorn-Freathy AS, Yeomans ER, Hankins GDV: Validation of the 1988 ACOG forceps classification system. Obstet Gynecol 77:356, 1991

Halpern SH, Leighton BL, Ohisson A, Barrett JFR, Rice A: Effect of epidural vs parenteral opioid analgesia on the progress of labor. JAMA 280:2105, 1998

Hankins GDV, Clark SL, Cunningham FG, Gilstrap LC, III: Vacuum delivery. Operative Obstetrics, 9. Norwalk, CT, Appleton & Lange, 1995

Hankins GDV, Rowe TF: Operative vaginal delivery—Year 2000. Am J Obstet Gynecol 175:275, 1996

Hughey MJ, McElin JW, Lussky R: Forceps operation in perspective, 1. Midforceps rotation operations. J Reprod Med 20:253, 1978

Jackson SL, Weber AM, Hull TL, Mitchinson AR, Walters MD: Fecal incontinence in women with urinary incontinence and pelvic organ prolapse. Obstet Gynecol 89:423, 1997

Jain V, Guleria K, Gopalan S, Narang A: Mode of delivery in deep transverse arrest. Int J Gynaecol Obstet 43:129, 1993

Johanson RB, Heycock E, Carter J, Sultan AH, Walklate K, Jones PW: Maternal and child health after assisted vaginal delivery: Five-year follow up of a randomised controlled study comparing forceps and ventouse. Br J Obstet Gynaecol 106:544, 1999

Johanson R, Menon V: Soft versus rigid vacuum extractor cups for assisted vaginal delivery. Cochrane Database Syst Rev 2:CD000446, 2000a

Johanson RB, Menon BK: Vacuum extraction forceps for assisted vaginal delivery. Cochrane Database Syst Rev 2:CD000224, 2000b

Joulin M: Study on the use of force in obstetrics. Arch Gen Med, 6th series 9:149, 1867

Kaminski HM, Stafl A, Aiman J: The effect of epidural analgesia on the frequency of instrumental obstetric delivery. Obstet Gynecol 69:770, 1987

Kielland C: On the application of forceps to the unrotated head, with description of a new model of forceps. Monatsschrift fur Geburtshilfe und Gynkologie 43:48, 1916

Knight D, Newnham JP, McKenna M, Evans S: A comparison of abdominal and vaginal examinations for the diagnosis of engagement of the fetal head. Aust NZ J Obstet Gynaecol 33:154, 1993

Krivak TC, Drewes P, Horowitz GM: Kielland vs. nonrotational forceps for the second stage of labor. J Reprod Med 44:511, 1999

Kuit JA, Eppinga HG, Wallenburg HCS, Huikeshoven FJM: A randomized comparison of vacuum extraction delivery with a rigid and a pliable cup. Obstet Gynecol 82:280, 1993

Learman LA: Regional differences in operative obstetrics: A look to the south. Obstet Gynecol 92:514, 1998

Loghis C, Pyrgiotis E, Panayotopoulos N, Batalias L, Salamalekis E, Zourlas PA: Comparison between metal cup and silicon rubber cup vacuum extractor. Eur J Obstet Gynecol Reprod Biol 45:173, 1992

Low J, Ng TY, Chew SY: Clinical experience with the silicon-cup vacuum extractor. Singapore Med J 34:135, 1993

Lowe B: Fear of failure: A place for the trial of instrumental delivery. Br J Obstet Gynaecol 94:60, 1987

Lucas MJ: The role of vacuum extraction in modern obstetrics (review). Clin Obstet Gynecol 37:794, 1994

MacArthur C, Bick DE, Keighley MR: Faecal incontinence after childbirth. Br J Obstet Gynaecol 104:46, 1997

Malmström T: The vacuum extractor, an obstetrical instrument. Acta Obstet Gynecol Scand Suppl 4:33, 1954

Nilsen ST: Boys born by forceps and vacuum extraction examined at 18 years of age. Acta Obstet Gynecol Scand 63:549, 1984

Notzon FC, Bergsjo P, Cole S, Irgens LM, Daltveit AJ: International collaborative effort (ICE) on birth weight, plurality, perinatal, and infant mortality, 4. Differences in obstetrical delivery practice: Norway, Scotland and the United States. Acta Obstet Gynecol Scand 70:451, 1991

Nygaard IE, Rao SS, Dawson JD: Anal incontinence after anal sphincter disruption: A 30 year retrospective cohort study. Obstet Gynecol 89:896, 1997

Pearl ML, Roberts JM, Laros RK, Hurd WW: Vaginal delivery from the persistent occiput posterior position: Influence on maternal and neonatal morbidity. J Reprod Med 38:955, 1993

Plauche WC: Fetal cranial injuries related to delivery with the Malmström vacuum extractor. Obstet Gynecol 53:750, 1979

Ploeckinger B, Ulm MR, Chalubinski K, Gruber W: Epidural anaesthesia in labour: Influence on surgical delivery rates, intrapartum fever and blood loss. Gynecol Obstet Invest 39:24, 1995

Ramin S, Little B, Gilstrap L: Survey of operative vaginal delivery in North America in 1990. Obstet Gynecol 81:307, 1993

Ramin SM, Gambling DR, Lucas MJ, Sharma SK, Sidawi JE, Leveno KJ: Randomized trial of epidural versus intravenous analgesia during labor. Obstet Gynecol 86:783, 1995

Read AW, Prendiville WJ, Dawes VP, Stanley FJ: Cesarean section and operative vaginal delivery in low-risk primiparous women, western Australia. Am J Public Health 84:37, 1994

Rieger N, Schloithe A, Saccone G, Wattchow D: The effect of a normal vaginal delivery on anal function. Acta Obstet Gynecol Scand 76:769, 1997

Robertson PA, Laros RK, Zhao RL: Neonatal and maternal outcome in low-pelvic and mid-pelvic operative deliveries. Am J Obstet Gynecol 162:1436, 1990

Robinson JC: Forceps and vacuum extraction. Curr Opin Obstet Gynecol 6:414, 1994

Robinson JN, Norwitz ER, Cohen AP, McElrath TF, Lieberman ES: Episiotomy, operative vaginal delivery, and significant perinatal trauma in nulliparous women. Am J Obstet Gynecol 181:1180, 1999

Rubin L, Coopland AT: Kielland's forceps. Can Med Assoc J 103:505, 1970

Ruderman J, Carrol JC, Reid AJ, Murray MA: Are physicians changing the way they practice obstetrics? Can Med Assoc J 148:409, 1993

Saunders NJSG, Spiby H, Gilbert L, Fraser RB, Hall JM, Mutton PM, Jackson A, Edmonds DK: Oxytocin infusion during second stage of labour in primiparous women using epidural analgesia: A randomized double blind placebo controlled trial. BMJ 299:1423, 1989

Schwartz DB, Miodovnik M, Lavin JP Jr: Neonatal outcome among low birth weight infants delivered spontaneously or by low forceps. Obstet Gynecol 62:283, 1983

Seidman DS, Laor A, Gale R, Stevenson DK, Mashiach S, Danon YL: Long-term effects of vacuum and forceps deliveries. Lancet 2:1583, 1991

Sharma SK, Leveno KJ: Update: Epidural analgesia during labor does not increase cesarean births. Curr Anesth Rep 2:18, 2000

Sharma SK, Sidawi JE, Ramin SM, Lucas MJ, Leveno KJ, Cunningham FG: Cesarean delivery: A randomized trial of epidural versus patient-controlled meperidine analgesia during labor. Anesthesiology 87:487, 1997

Sherman SJ, Greenspoon JS, Nelson JM, Paul RH: Obstetric hemorrhage and blood utilization. J Reprod Med 38:929, 1993

Sizer AR, Nirmal DM: Occipitoposterior position: Associated factors and obstetric outcome in nulliparas. Obstet Gynecol 96:749, 2000

Steer CM, Boney W: Obstetric factors in cerebral palsy. Am J Obstet Gynecol 83:526, 1962

Sultan AH, Kamm MA, Bartram CI, Hudson CN: Anal sphincter trauma during instrumental delivery. Int J Gynaecol Obstet 43:263, 1993

Sultan AH, Kamm MA, Hudson CN, Bartram CI: Third degree obstetric anal sphincter tears: Risk factors and outcome of primary repair. BMJ 308:887, 1994

Sultan AH, Johanson RB, Carter JE: Occult anal sphincter trauma following randomized forceps and vacuum delivery. Int J Gynaecol Obstet 61:113, 1998

Tan KH, Sim R, Yam KL: Kielland's forceps delivery: Is it a dying art? Singapore Med J 33:380, 1992

Tetzschner T, Sorensen M, Lose G, Christiansen J: Anal and urinary incontinence after obstetric and sphincter rupture. Ugeskr Laeger 160:3218, 1998

Towner D, Castro MA, Eby-Wilkens E, Gilbert WM: Effect of mode of delivery in nulliparous women on neonatal intracranial injury. N Engl J Med 341:1709, 1999

Vacca A, Grant A, Wyatt G, Chalmers T: Portsmouth operative delivery trial: A comparison of vacuum extraction and forceps delivery. Br J Obstet Gynaecol 90:1107, 1983

Wesley B, Van den Berg B, Reece EA: The effect of operative vaginal delivery on cognitive development. Am J Obstet Gynecol 166:288, 1992

White DA, Pressman EK, Hanna GV, Odom MF, Callan NA, Blakemore K: Facial nerve palsy: Frequencies associated with spontaneous, forceps, and cesarean deliveries. Am J Obstet Gynecol 174:353, 1996

Williams MC, Knuppel RA, O'Brien WF, Weiss A, Kanarek KS: A randomized comparison of assisted vaginal delivery by obstetric forceps and polyethylene vacuum cup. Obstet Gynecol 78:789, 1991

Wilson PD, Herbison RM, Herbison GP: Obstetric practice and the prevalence of urinary incontinence three months after delivery. Br J Obstet Gynaecol 103:154, 1996

Yancey MK, Herpelsheimer A, Jordan GD, Benson WL, Brady K: Maternal and neonatal effects of outlet forceps delivery compared with spontaneous vaginal delivery in term pregnancies. Obstet Gynecol 78:646, 1991

Yeomans ER, Hankins GD: Operative vaginal delivery in the 1990s. Clin Obstet Gynecol 35:487, 1992

Zahniser SC, Kendrick JS, Franks AL, Saftlas AF: Trends in obstetric operative procedures, 1980 to 1987. Am J Public Health 82:1340, 1992

22

Breech Presentation and Delivery

Breech presentation is when the buttocks of the fetus enter the pelvis first. The term *breech* probably derives from the same word as *britches,* which described a cloth covering the loins and thighs. For a number of reasons, breech presentation is more common remote from term (Table 22–1). Most often, however, before the onset of labor the fetus turns spontaneously to a cephalic presentation so that breech presentation persists in only about 3 to 4 percent of singleton deliveries. For example, 3.5 percent of 136,256 singleton infants delivered from 1990 through 1999 at Parkland Hospital presented as breech.

ETIOLOGY

As term approaches, the uterine cavity most often accommodates the fetus in a longitudinal lie with the vertex presenting. Factors other than gestational age that appear to predispose to breech presentation include uterine relaxation associated with great parity, multiple fetuses, hydramnios, oligohydramnios, hydrocephalus, anencephalus, previous breech delivery, uterine anomalies, and pelvic tumors.

Fianu and Vaclavinkova (1978) provided sonographic evidence of a much higher prevalence of placental implantation in the cornual-fundal region for breech presentation (73 percent) than for vertex presentations (5 percent). The frequency of breech presentation is also increased with placenta previa, but only a small minority of breech presentations are associated with a previa. No strong correlation has been shown between breech presentation and a contracted pelvis.

A live fetus is *not* required for a fetus to change presentations spontaneously. One woman admitted to Parkland Hospital at term had a fetus known to be dead, confirmed by real-time sonography. The presentation was cephalic during the first oxytocin induction. Three days later, at the time of the second attempt at labor induction, the fetus was in a breech presentation. Three days later, at the time of a third and successful induction, the fetus was again in a cephalic presentation!

COMPLICATIONS

In the persistent breech presentation, an *increased* frequency of the following complications can be anticipated:

1. Perinatal morbidity and mortality from difficult delivery.
2. Low birthweight from preterm delivery, growth restriction, or both.
3. Prolapsed cord.
4. Placenta previa.
5. Fetal, neonatal, and infant anomalies.
6. Uterine anomalies and tumors.
7. Multiple fetuses.
8. Operative intervention, especially cesarean delivery.

DIAGNOSIS

The varying relations between the lower extremities and buttocks of breech presentations form the categories of frank, complete, and incomplete breech presentations (see Figs. 12–2 to 12–4). Chasen and D'Angelo (2000) reported a positive predictive value of 80 percent and a negative predictive value of 98.5 percent for abdominal and vaginal examination to diagnose breech presentation at 35 to 37 weeks. With a **frank breech** presentation, the lower extremities are flexed at the hips and extended at the knees, and thus the feet lie in close proximity to the head. A **complete breech** presentation differs in that one or both knees are flexed. With **incomplete breech** presentation, one or both hips are not flexed and one or both feet or knees lie below the breech, that is, a foot or knee is lowermost in the birth canal. The frank breech appears most commonly when the diagnosis is established radiologically near term.

ABDOMINAL EXAMINATION. Typically, with the first Leopold maneuver, the hard, round, readily ballotable fetal head is found to occupy the fundus (Fig. 22–1). The second maneuver indicates the back to be on one side of the abdomen and the small parts on the other. On the third maneuver, if engagement has not occurred—the intertrochanteric diameter of the fetal pelvis has not passed through the pelvic inlet—the breech is movable above the pelvic inlet. After engagement, the fourth maneuver shows the firm breech to be beneath the symphysis. Fetal heart sounds are usually heard loudest slightly above the umbilicus, whereas with engagement of the fetal head the heart sounds are loudest below the umbilicus.

TABLE 22–1. Fetal Presentation at Various Gestational Ages Determined Sonographically

Gestation (wks)	Total Number	Percent		
		Cephalic	Breech	Other
21–24	264	54.6	33.3	12.1
25–28	367	61.9	27.8	10.4
29–32	443	78.1	14.0	7.9
33–36	638	88.7	8.8	2.5
37–40	463	91.5	6.7	1.7

From Scheer and Nubar (1976).

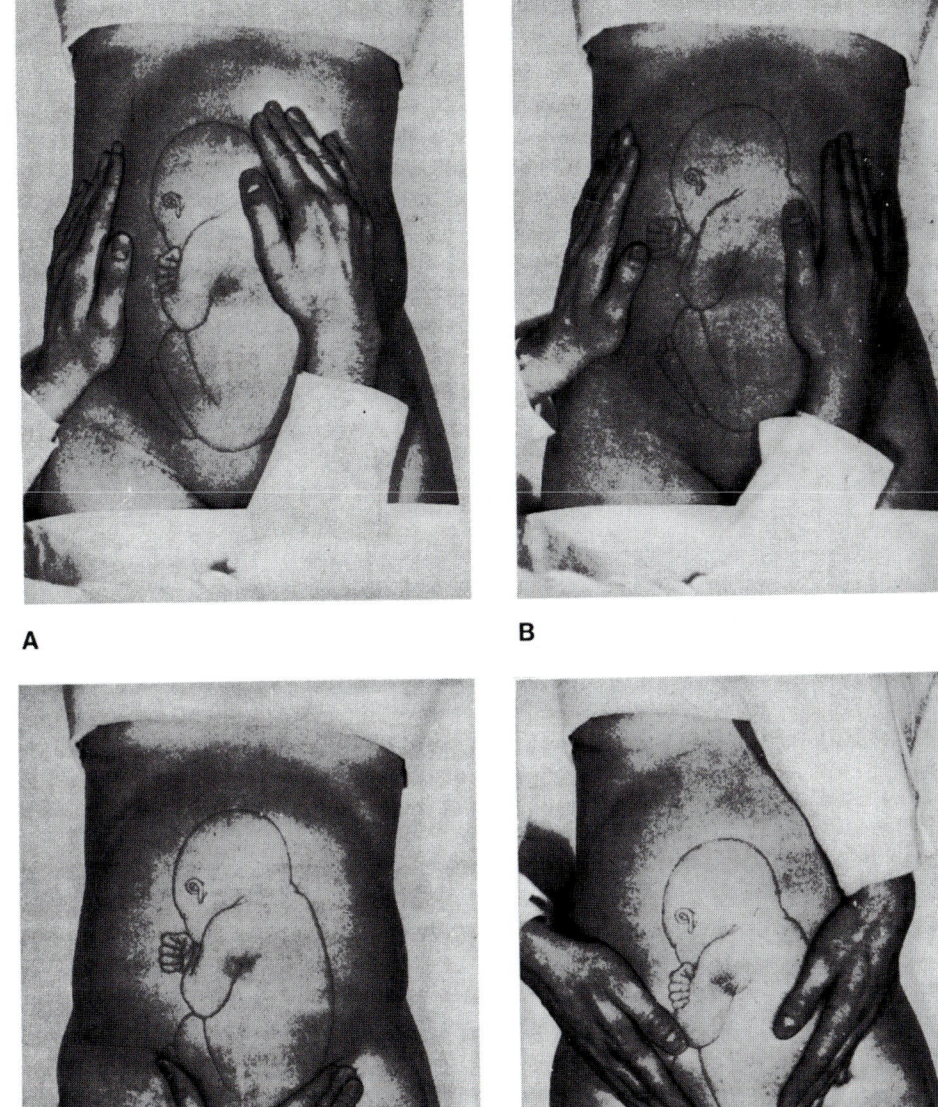

FIGURE 22–1. Palpation in left sacroanterior position. **A.** First Leopold maneuver. **B.** Second maneuver. **C.** Third maneuver. **D.** Fourth maneuver.

VAGINAL EXAMINATION. With the frank breech presentation, both ischial tuberosities, the sacrum, and the anus are usually palpable, and after further descent, the external genitalia may be distinguished. Especially when labor is prolonged, the buttocks may become markedly swollen, rendering differentiation of face and breech very difficult; the anus may be mistaken for the mouth, and the ischial tuberosities for the malar eminences. Careful examination, however, should prevent this error, because the finger encounters muscular resistance with the anus, whereas the firmer, less yielding jaws are felt through the mouth. Furthermore, the finger, upon removal from the anus, is sometimes stained with meconium. The mouth and malar eminences form a triangular shape, while the ischial tuberosities and anus are in a straight line. The most accurate information, however, is based on the location of the sacrum and its spinous processes, which establishes the diagnosis of position and variety.

In complete breech presentations, the feet may be

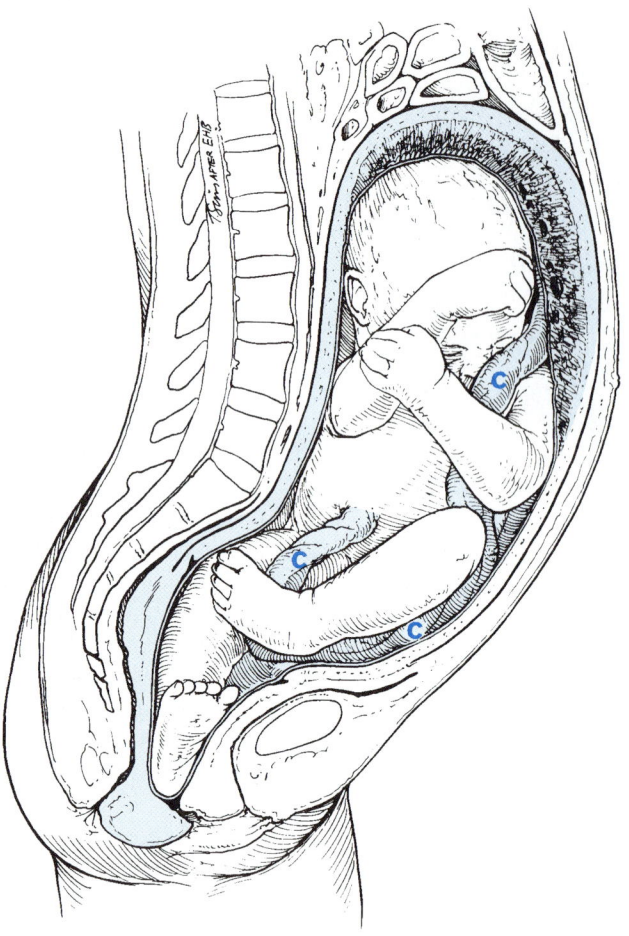

FIGURE 22–2. Double-footling breech presentation in labor with membranes intact. Note possibility of umbilical cord accident at any instant, especially after rupture of membranes.

felt alongside the buttocks, and in footling presentations, one or both feet are inferior to the buttocks (Fig. 22–2). In footling presentations, the foot can readily be identified as right or left on the basis of the relation to the great toe. When the breech has descended farther into the pelvic cavity, the genitalia may be felt.

IMAGING TECHNIQUES. Ultrasound ideally should be used to confirm a clinically suspected breech presentation and to identify, if possible, any fetal anomalies. Bruck and Sherer (1997) used intrapartum ultrasound to detect large lower uterine segment leiomyomas. If cesarean delivery is planned, x-rays are not indicated. If, however, vaginal delivery is considered, the type of breech presentation is of considerable importance. Radiation exposure may be reduced considerably by using computed tomographic pelvimetry (Kopelman and associates, 1986). These imaging techniques can be used to provide information regarding the type of breech

presentation, presence or absence of a flexed fetal head, and pelvic measurements (see Chap. 18, p. 438).

The role of x-ray pelvimetry in deciding mode of delivery for breech presentation is controversial (Morrison and co-authors, 1995). Cheng and Hannah (1993) comprehensively surveyed the literature on breech delivery at term and reviewed 15 studies in which x-ray pelvimetry was used and two studies in which CT pelvimetry was used as one of the criteria for allowing vaginal delivery. They concluded that the role of x-ray pelvimetry was complicated because pelvic dimensions for allowing labor varied among studies. Most authors, however, found no correlation between radiological pelvic measurements and the outcome of labor. Only one study demonstrated that the incidence of complicated labor rose with decreasing pelvic capacity (Ohlsén, 1975).

Magnetic resonance imaging for pelvimetry is considered more accurate than other methods. As emphasized by van Loon and colleagues (1997), this has no value if the results have no clinical benefits. They performed a randomized controlled trial in 235 women with breech presentation at term. The use of magnetic resonance pelvimetry did not decrease the overall cesarean delivery rate (42 percent) compared with controls not undergoing pelvimetry (50 percent).

PROGNOSIS

Both mother and fetus are at greater risk with breech compared with cephalic presentation, but to nowhere near the same degree. In an analysis of 57,819 pregnancies in the Netherlands, Schutte and colleagues (1985) reported that even after correction for gestational age, congenital defects, and birthweight, perinatal mortality was higher in breech infants. They concluded that it may be possible that breech presentation is not coincidental but is a consequence of poor fetal quality. Krebs and associates (1999) reported that cerebral palsy in breech-presenting fetuses was not related to the mode of delivery. Thus, it may be that medical intervention is unlikely to reduce perinatal mortality associated with breech presentation. This possibility had been suggested earlier by Hytten (1982) and by Susuki and Yamamuro (1985). This concept was strengthened by Nelson and Ellenberg (1986), who observed that a third of children with cerebral palsy who were in a breech presentation at birth had major noncerebral malformations.

MATERNAL MORBIDITY. Because of the greater frequency of operative delivery, including cesarean delivery, there is higher maternal morbidity and slightly higher mortality for pregnancies complicated by persistent breech presentation (Collea and co-authors, 1980).

This risk is likely increased even more with emergency operation instead of elective cesarean delivery (Bingham and Lilford, 1987). Labor is usually not prolonged and Hall and Kohl (1956) reported its median duration to be 9.2 hours for nulliparas and 6.1 hours for multiparas.

FETUS-INFANT MORBIDITY AND MORTALITY. The prognosis for the fetus in a breech presentation is considerably worse than when in a vertex presentation. The major contributors to perinatal loss are preterm delivery, congenital anomalies, and birth trauma. Almost 30 years ago, Brenner and associates (1974) reported the overall mortality rate for 1016 breech deliveries to be 25 percent compared with 2.6 percent for nonbreech deliveries. At every stage of gestation, they identified antepartum, intrapartum, and neonatal deaths to be significantly greater among breeches. Congenital abnormalities were identified in 6.3 percent of breech deliveries compared with 2.4 percent of nonbreech deliveries.

In a study of similar vintage, Tank and associates (1971) assessed outcomes of traumatic vaginal delivery. At autopsy, the organs most frequently found to be injured were, in order of frequency, the brain, spinal cord, liver, adrenal glands, and spleen. It is of interest that, in retrospective analysis of cases of "idiopathic" adrenal calcification, breech delivery was very common. Other injuries from vaginal delivery included the brachial plexus; the pharynx, in the form of tears or pseudodiverticula from the finger in the mouth as part of the Mauriceau maneuver (see p. 525); and the bladder, which might rupture if distended. Traction might injure the sternocleidomastoid muscle and, if not appropriately treated, lead to torticollis (Chap. 39, p. 1082).

These older reports are in contrast to more contemporaneous observations in which careful assessment is made before vaginal delivery is attempted, and cesarean delivery rates generally exceed 60 percent. Albrechtsen and colleagues (2000) have reported that perinatal mortality in 45,579 breeches decreased from 9 percent in 1967–1976 to 3 percent in 1987–1994.

COMPLICATIONS WITH VAGINAL DELIVERY

Delivery of the breech draws the umbilicus and attached cord into the pelvis, which compresses the cord. Therefore, once the breech has passed beyond the vaginal introitus, the abdomen, thorax, arms, and head must be delivered promptly. This involves delivery of successively less readily compressible parts. With a term fetus, some degree of head molding may be essential for it to negotiate the birth canal successfully. In this unfortunate circumstance, the alternatives with vaginal delivery are both unsatisfactory:

1. Delivery may be delayed many minutes while the aftercoming head accommodates to the maternal pelvis, but hypoxia and acidemia become severe; or
2. Delivery may be forced, causing trauma from compression, traction, or both.

With a preterm fetus, the disparity between the size of the head and buttocks is even greater than with a larger fetus. At times, the buttocks and lower extremities of the preterm fetus will pass through the cervix and be delivered, and yet the cervix will not be dilated adequately for the head to escape without trauma (Bodmer and associates, 1986). In this circumstance, *Dührssen incisions* of the cervix may be attempted. Even so, trauma to the fetus and mother may be appreciable, and fetal hypoxia may prove harmful. Robertson and colleagues (1995, 1996) observed no significant difference in the incidence of head entrapment by mode of delivery for breech infants at 28 to 36 weeks or from 24 to 27 weeks. They also found no association of adverse neonatal outcomes after head entrapment. Another mechanical problem with breech delivery is entrapment of the fetal arm behind the neck. A nuchal arm complicates up to 6 percent of vaginal breech deliveries and is associated with increased neonatal mortality (Cheng and Hannah, 1993).

The frequency of cord prolapse is increased when the fetus is small or when the breech is not frank. In the report by Collea and colleagues (1978), the incidence with frank breech presentation was about 0.5 percent, which is similar to 0.4 percent reported for cephalic presentations (Barrett, 1991). In contrast, the incidence of cord prolapse with footling presentation was 15 percent, and it was 5 percent with complete breech presentation.

Soernes and Bakke (1986) confirmed earlier observations that umbilical cord length is significantly shorter in breech compared with cephalic presentations. Moreover, multiple coils of cord entangling the fetus are more common with breech presentations (Spellacy and associates, 1966). These umbilical cord abnormalities likely play a role in the development of breech presentation as well as the relatively high incidence of a nonreassuring fetal heart rate pattern in labor. For example, Flanagan and co-workers (1987) selected 244 women with a variety of breech presentations (72 percent were frank breech) for a trial of labor, and there was a cord prolapse in 4 percent. Fetal distress not due to cord prolapse was diagnosed in another 5 percent of women selected for vaginal delivery. Overall, 10 percent of the women identified for vaginal birth underwent cesarean deliveries for fetal jeopardy in labor.

Apgar scores, especially at 1 minute, of vaginally delivered breech infants are generally lower than when elective cesarean delivery is performed (Flanagan and co-workers, 1987). Similarly, cord blood acid–base values are significantly different for vaginally delivered breech infants. Christian and Brady (1991) reported that umbilical artery blood pH was lower, P_{CO_2} higher, and HCO_3 lower compared with cephalic deliveries. Socol and colleagues (1988), however, concluded that cesarean delivery improved Apgar scores but not acid–base status. Flanagan and co-workers (1987) emphasized that ultimate infant outcome for breech birth was not worsened by these significant differences in Apgar scores or acid–base status at birth.

Albrechtsen and colleagues (1997) evaluated a protocol to select vaginal or cesarean delivery for breech presentation. In 1212 breech presentations, the vaginal delivery rate increased from 45 to 57 percent and cesarean delivery rate for a failed vaginal delivery declined from 21 to 6 percent. Birth asphyxia was diagnosed clinically among 2.5 percent of those with a vaginal delivery of a breech, but none delivered as vertex (P = .0001). Despite this, none of these infants died or had long-term sequelae. Daniel and co-workers (1998) reported similar success with a prospective protocol in 496 women at term with a singleton breech presentation. Conversely, Koo and associates (1998) observed increased perinatal morbidity and mortality in singleton term vaginal breech deliveries despite application of strict selection criteria.

UNFAVORABLE PELVIS. Because there is no time for molding of the aftercoming head, a moderately contracted pelvis that had not previously caused problems in delivery of an average-size cephalic fetus might prove dangerous with a breech. Rovinsky and colleagues (1973) urged not only accurate measurements of the pelvic dimensions but also precise evaluation of the pelvic architecture rather than reliance on pelvic indexes. Gynecoid (round) and anthropoid (elliptical) pelves are favorable configurations, but platypelloid (anteroposteriorly flat) and android (heart-shaped) pelves are not (Chap. 3, p. 57).

HYPEREXTENSION OF FETAL HEAD. In perhaps 5 percent of term breech presentations, the fetal head may be in extreme hyperextension (Fig. 22–3). These presentations have been referred to as "the stargazer fetus," and in Britain as "the flying foetus." With such hyperextension, vaginal delivery may result in injury to the cervical spinal cord. In general, marked hyperextension after labor has begun is considered an indication for cesarean delivery (Svenningsen and associates, 1985).

LABOR INDUCTION OR AUGMENTATION. Induction of labor in women with a breech presentation is defended by some and condemned by others. Brenner and associates (1974) found no significant differences

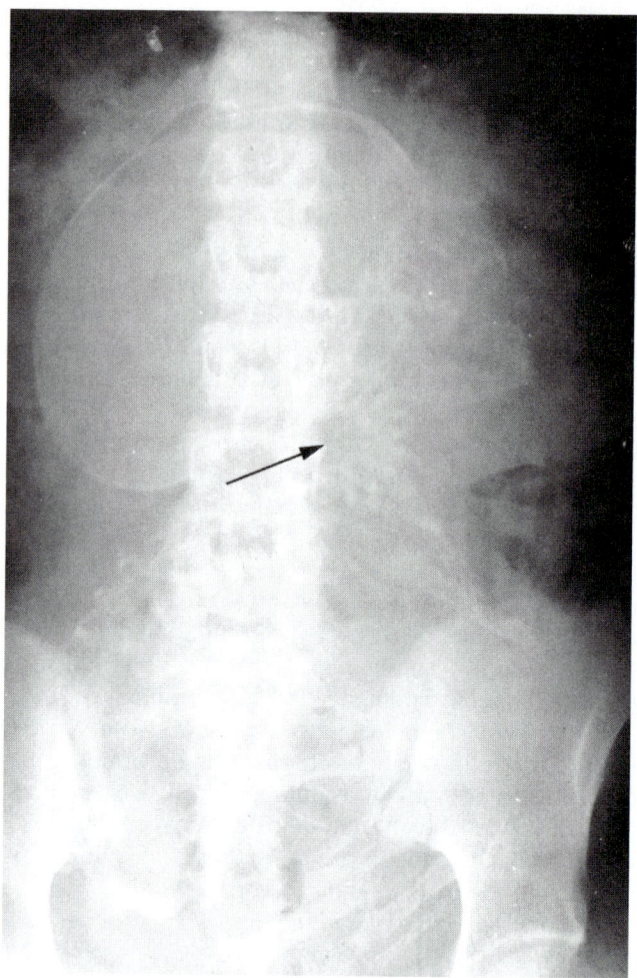

FIGURE 22–3. Radiograph of a complete breech presentation with a markedly hyperextended cervical spine (*arrow*) and head. Cesarean delivery resulted in a normal newborn infant.

in perinatal mortality and Apgar scores between infants with induced versus spontaneous labor. In oxytocin-augmented labor, however, infant mortality rates were higher, and Apgar scores were lower. Fait and colleagues (1998) reported that 12 of 23 women with a breech presentation and an unripe cervix who underwent induction had a successful vaginal delivery with no neonatal complications. At Jackson Memorial Hospital in Miami (Diro and associates, 1999), oxytocin is used in a manner similar to that for vertex presentations. By contrast, at Parkland Hospital, labor induction may be attempted by amniotomy, but cesarean delivery is preferred to oxytocin induction or augmentation of labor with a viable fetus.

FOOTLING BREECH PRESENTATIONS. The possibility of compression of a prolapsed cord or a cord entangled around the extremities as the breech fills the pelvis, if not before, is a threat to the fetus (see Fig. 12–2).

TERM FETUS. Cheng and Hannah (1993) conducted a systematic search of the world literature regarding term breech delivery and found 82 reports published in English between 1966 and 1992. A total of 24 studies were selected for analysis because these compared *planned* vaginal delivery with *planned* cesarean section for the term, singleton breech fetus. The effects of planned vaginal delivery on perinatal mortality, corrected for lethal congenital anomalies and antepartum fetal death, are shown in Table 22–2. The corrected perinatal mortality rate ranged from 0 to 48 per 1000 births and was higher among infants in the planned vaginal delivery groups.

All but two deaths were in the groups of women allowed to labor and deliver vaginally. The main causes of death were head entrapment, cerebral injury and hemorrhage, cord prolapse, and severe asphyxia. Cheng and Hannah (1993) observed that the overall neonatal mortality and morbidity resulting from trauma were increased significantly in the planned vaginal delivery groups, with a typical odds ratio of 3.86. They suggested that until a well-designed randomized trial with sufficient statistical power is performed, planned cesarean delivery should be strongly considered for persistent breech presentation at term. Similarly, Gifford and co-workers (1995b) performed a meta-analysis of outcomes after term breech delivery and observed that, given many methodological limitations of published studies, their analysis suggested an increased risk of injury or death after a trial of labor.

Only two of the 24 reports reviewed by Cheng and Hannah (1993) and Gifford and co-workers (1995b) were

TABLE 22–2. Causes of Neonatal Deaths in Term Breech Presentations in Relation to Planned Vaginal or Cesarean Delivery

Investigators	Neonatal Deaths/Deliveries		Odds Ratio	95% CI[a]	Cause of Death
	Vaginal	Cesarean			
Anderman et al (1984), Barlöv and Larsson (1986), Benson et al (1972), Bingham et al (1987), Bistoletti et al (1981), Christian et al (1990), Collea et al (1980), Crawford (1974), Flanagan et al (1987), Jaffa et al (1981), Mahomed (1988), Mecke et al (1989)	0/2287	0/1319	1.00	1.00–1.00	
El Gammal et al (1990)	1/21	0/30	11.34	0.21–99.99	Head entrapment
Fischer-Rasmussen and Trolle (1967)	8/365	0/55	3.22	0.41–25.58	Cerebral hemorrhage—1, cord prolapse—1, prolonged labor—2, head entrapment—2, unknown—2
Gimovsky et al (1983)	1/69	0/34	4.45	0.07–99.99	Inadequate resuscitation
Gimovsky and Petrie (1989)	2/204	1/463	5.50	0.47–64.35	Not specified
Kauppila (1975)	22/1383	0/287	3.40	1.11–10.36	Cerebral hemorrhage/injury ± head entrapment—7, cord prolapse—6, other cord complications, asphyxia—9
Mahomed et al (1989)	17/259	0/95	4.19	1.40–12.55	Not specified
Ohlsén (1975)	5/288	0/52	3.30	0.29–38.26	Tentorial rupture—2, asphyxia ± cord complication—3
Roumen and Luyben (1991)	2/234	0/13	2.89	0.01–99.99	Head entrapment—1, cord prolapse—1
Songane et al (1987)	6/602	0/255	4.19	0.72–24.22	Cerebral hemorrhage—1, tentorial tear—1, head entrapment—1, hypoxic cerebral damage—3
Svenningsen et al (1985)	1/284	0/46	3.20	0.01–99.99	Head entrapment, severe asphyxia, cerebral hemorrhage
Thorpe-Beeston et al (1992)	8/1990	1/1457	3.60	0.96–13.52	Not specified
Woodward and Callahan (1969)	2/95	0/5	2.90	0.00–99.99	Cerebral hemorrhage—1, unknown—1
Total	75/7695	2/4026			
Typical odds ratio			3.86	2.22–6.69	

[a]95% CI = confidence interval.
Modified after Cheng and Hannah (1993), with permission.

randomized trials, and both were from the same institution. Collea and colleagues (1980) reported the results of 208 women with frank breech fetuses at term. Almost half of these women were excluded from further consideration because of possible fetopelvic disproportion based on x-ray pelvimetry. A total of 60 infants were eventually delivered vaginally, and all survived, although two sustained brachial plexus injuries. There were no perinatal deaths, but half of the 148 women who had cesarean deliveries experienced significant morbidity compared with only 7 percent of 60 women who were delivered vaginally. Gimovsky and colleagues (1983) later evaluated 105 nonfrank breech fetuses and reported similar findings. Although these two trials concluded that vaginal breech delivery was relatively safe, only 110 fetuses were actually allowed a trial of labor. As emphasized by Eller and Van Dorsten (1995), this small number would not provide sufficient statistical power to demonstrate differences in uncommon adverse outcomes such as perinatal death and birth injury. Lindqvist and associates (1997), in a register-based nationwide study in Sweden from 1991 and 1992, found similar mortality with vaginal compared with cesarean delivery. The opposite conclusion was reached by Roman and colleagues (1998) in their study of almost 16,000 term breech births in Sweden between 1987 and 1993.

PRETERM FETUS. The aftercoming head of a preterm fetus may be trapped by a cervix that is sufficiently effaced and dilated to allow passage of the thorax but not the less compressible head. The consequences of vaginal delivery in this circumstance all too often have been both hypoxia and physical trauma, both of which are especially deleterious to the preterm infant.

There are no randomized studies regarding delivery of the preterm breech fetus. Penn and colleagues (1996) attempted such a study in 26 hospitals in England and discontinued the trial after 17 months because only 13 women could be recruited. Retrospective studies have yielded conflicting results. Bowes and colleagues (1979) and Main and co-workers (1983) found that infants undergoing cesarean delivery had a better prognosis. Others have concluded that vaginal delivery did not significantly increase perinatal mortality (Olshan and co-workers, 1984; Rosen and Chik, 1984; Westgren and co-workers, 1985a). More recently, Wolf and colleagues (1999) compared preterm breech fetuses delivered at two tertiary-care facilities in the Netherlands. At one center vaginal delivery was preferred and the cesarean delivery part was only 17 percent. At the other center, the cesarean delivery rate was 85 percent. These investigators found no difference in 2-year survival without disability or handicap.

The National Institute of Child Health and Human Development Neonatal Research Network (Malloy and co-workers, 1991) analyzed data from 437 very-low-birthweight breech infants admitted to seven neonatal intensive care centers. After adjusting for several variables, the risk of intraventricular hemorrhage and neonatal death was not significantly affected by the mode of delivery for fetuses weighing less than 1500 g. A similar analysis was reported from the Netherlands (Gravenhorst and co-workers, 1993). Perinatal follow-up data were collected on 899 singleton, nonanomalous infants of less than 32 weeks' gestation, whose birthweight was less than 1500 g. They could not conclusively resolve whether cesarean delivery was advantageous.

CURRENT STATUS OF VAGINAL BREECH DELIVERY. Eller and Van Dorsten (1995) surveyed the centers in the Maternal–Fetal Medicine Units Network to determine the feasibility of resolving the controversy regarding route of delivery by a randomized clinical trial. Virtually all participating obstetricians in the Network agreed that clear scientific evidence was needed to determine if mode of delivery of the breech affects outcome. They concluded, however, that the investigation was not feasible. This was because the number of skilled operators with the ability to safely deliver breech fetuses continues to dwindle and medicolegal concerns make it difficult to train residents to perform such deliveries. Indeed, at least two other groups of investigators who have attempted trials of breech delivery concluded that such studies were likely impossible (Penn and Steer, 1990; Zlatnik, 1993). Despite this, Hannah and colleagues (2000) reported results from a multinational randomized trial of vaginal versus cesarean delivery for term breeches. Almost 57 percent of 1042 women randomized to vaginal delivery were delivered as such. While they observed greater neonatal morbidity in the vaginally delivered group, the heterogeneity of the study populations makes their findings difficult to apply to contemporaneous obstetrical practices in developed countries.

What, then, is "standard of care" for delivery of term and preterm singleton breech fetuses in the United States? Despite the inadequacy of scientific evidence as discussed, most breech presentations are delivered by cesarean section. For example, in 1997, 85 percent of all malpresentations, including breeches, were delivered by cesarean (Ventura and associates, 1999). Still, as shown in Table 22–3, the number is variable throughout teaching centers. At Parkland Hospital and at the University of Alabama at Birmingham, the route of delivery is individualized depending upon clinical circumstances and with approval of the attending faculty.

Women with selected frank breech presentations estimated to be about 2000 g or more, but less than about 3500 g, are frequently offered planned vaginal delivery. Despite this, more than 80 percent of singleton breeches are delivered by cesarean. Thus, individualized cesarean

TABLE 22–3. **Method of Delivery for Breech-presenting Fetuses at Five University Hospitals**

Institution	Breech Fetuses		Delivery (*Percent*)	
	Size/Age	*Number*	*Vaginal*	*Cesarean*
Chicago Lying-In Hospital:				
Cibils et al (1994)	< 1500 g	262	60	40
Brown et al (1994)	> 1500 g	843	44	56
Jackson Memorial, Miami	Term	1021	14	86
Diro et al (1999)				
Parkland Hospital, Dallas	All	2364	19	81
University of Alabama, Birmingham	Preterm	376	36	64
	Term	263	14	86

or vaginal delivery are both reasonable and acceptable in current obstetrical practice.

RECOMMENDATIONS FOR DELIVERY. A diligent search for any other complication, actual or anticipated, that might justify cesarean delivery has become a feature of most philosophies for managing breech delivery. Cesarean delivery is commonly but not exclusively used in the following circumstances:

1. A large fetus.
2. Any degree of contraction or unfavorable shape of the pelvis.
3. A hyperextended head.
4. No labor, with maternal or fetal indications for delivery such as pregnancy-induced hypertension or ruptured membranes for 12 hours or more.
5. Uterine dysfunction.
6. Footling presentation.
7. An apparently healthy but preterm fetus of 25 to 26 weeks or more, with the mother in either active labor or in need of delivery.
8. Severe fetal growth restriction.
9. Previous perinatal death or children suffering from birth trauma.
10. A request for sterilization.

TECHNIQUES FOR BREECH DELIVERY

LABOR AND SPONTANEOUS DELIVERY. There are fundamental differences between labor and delivery in cephalic and breech presentations. With a cephalic presentation, once the head is delivered, typically the rest of the body follows without difficulty. With a breech, however, successively larger and very much less compressible parts of the fetus are born. Spontaneous complete expulsion of the fetus who presents as a breech, as described following, is seldom accomplished success-

fully. As a rule, either cesarean delivery or vaginal delivery requires skilled participation by the obstetrician for a favorable outcome.

Engagement and descent of the breech in response to labor usually takes place with the bitrochanteric diameter of the breech in one of the oblique diameters of the pelvis. The anterior hip usually descends more rapidly than the posterior hip, and when the resistance of the pelvic floor is met, internal rotation usually follows, bringing the anterior hip toward the pubic arch and allowing the bitrochanteric diameter to occupy the anteroposterior diameter of the pelvic outlet. Rotation usually takes place through an arc of 45 degrees. If the posterior extremity is prolapsed, however, it always rotates to the symphysis pubis, ordinarily through an arc of 135 degrees, but occasionally in the opposite direction past the sacrum and the opposite half of the pelvis through an arc of 225 degrees.

After rotation, descent continues until the perineum is distended by the advancing breech, while the anterior hip appears at the vulva. By lateral flexion of the body, the posterior hip then is forced over the anterior margin of the perineum, which retracts over the buttocks, thus allowing the infant to straighten out when the anterior hip is born. The legs and feet follow the breech and may be born spontaneously or with aid.

After the birth of the breech, there is slight external rotation, with the back turning anteriorly as the shoulders are brought into relation with one of the oblique diameters of the pelvis. The shoulders then descend rapidly and undergo internal rotation, with the bisacromial diameter occupying the anteroposterior diameter of the inferior strait. Immediately following the shoulders, the head, which is normally sharply flexed upon the thorax, enters the pelvis in one of the oblique diameters and then rotates in such a manner as to bring the posterior portion of the neck under the symphysis pubis. The head is then born in flexion.

The breech may engage in the transverse diameter

of the pelvis, with the sacrum directed anteriorly or posteriorly. The mechanism of labor in the transverse position differs only in that internal rotation occurs through an arc of 90 degrees.

Infrequently, rotation occurs in such a manner that the back of the infant is directed toward the vertebral column instead of toward the abdomen of the mother. Such rotation should be prevented if possible. Although the head may be delivered by allowing the chin and face to pass beneath the symphysis, the slightest traction on the body may cause extension of the head, which increases the diameter of the head that must pass through the pelvis.

METHODS OF VAGINAL DELIVERY. There are three general methods of breech delivery through the vagina:

- **Spontaneous breech delivery.** The infant is expelled entirely spontaneously without any traction or manipulation other than support of the infant.
- **Partial breech extraction.** The infant is delivered spontaneously as far as the umbilicus, but the remainder of the body is extracted/delivered with operator traction and assisted maneuvers with or without maternal expulsive efforts.
- **Total breech extraction.** The entire body of the infant is extracted by the obstetrician.

Because the technique of breech extraction differs in complete and incomplete breeches and frank breeches, it is necessary to consider these conditions in two separate sections later in the chapter. The varieties of breech presentation are illustrated in Chapter 12 (see Figs. 12–2 to 12–4).

MANAGEMENT OF LABOR. With a breech presentation, both mother and fetus are at considerably increased risk compared with a woman with a cephalic presentation (Kunzel, 1994). A rapid assessment should be made to establish the status of the fetal membranes, labor, and condition of the fetus. Close surveillance of fetal heart rate and uterine contractions should begin. An immediate recruitment of the necessary nursing and medical personnel to accomplish a vaginal or abdominal delivery should also be done. Included are nursery and anesthesia personnel.

An intravenous infusion through a venous catheter is begun as soon as the woman arrives in the labor suite. Possible emergency induction of anesthesia, or hemorrhage from lacerations or from uterine atony, are but two of many reasons that may require immediate intravenous access that can be used to administer medications or fluids, including blood.

STAGE OF LABOR. Assessment of cervical dilatation and effacement and the station of the presenting part are essential in planning the route of delivery. If labor is too far advanced, there may not be sufficient time to obtain pelvimetry. This alone should not force the decision for cesarean delivery. Biswas and Johnstone (1993) found that among 267 term breech presentations, fewer cesarean deliveries were done without adversely affecting neonatal outcome when x-ray pelvimetry was not used to select the mode of delivery. Satisfactory progress in labor was the best indicator of pelvic adequacy. Nwosu and colleagues (1993) reported similar findings.

FETAL CONDITION. The presence or absence of gross fetal abnormalities, such as hydrocephaly or anencephaly, can be rapidly ascertained with the use of sonography or x-ray. Such efforts will help to ensure that a cesarean delivery is not done under emergency conditions for an anomalous infant with no chance of survival. If vaginal delivery is planned, the fetal head should not be extended (Fig. 22–3). It is possible to ascertain head flexion and to exclude extension from sonography (Rojansky and co-workers, 1994). Most often, digital radiographs using computed tomographic pelvimetry will be adequate to document flexion or absence of extension of the fetal head (Berger and associates, 1994; Christian and colleagues, 1990). If not, a plain film of the abdomen may be necessary.

FETAL MONITORING. Guidelines for monitoring the high-risk fetus are applied as discussed in Chapter 13 (p. 313). Thus, the fetal heart rate is recorded at least every 15 minutes. Most authorities prefer continuous electronic monitoring of fetal heart rate and uterine contractions. The FIGO Committee on Perinatal Health has endorsed this (Kunzel, 1994). When membranes are ruptured, the risk of umbilical cord prolapse is appreciably increased. Therefore, a vaginal examination should be done following rupture of the membranes to check for cord prolapse. Special attention should be directed to the fetal heart rate for the first 5 to 10 minutes following membrane rupture, to ensure that there has not been an occult cord prolapse.

RECRUITMENT OF NURSING AND MEDICAL PERSONNEL. Additional help is required for managing labor and delivery of a breech. For labor, one-on-one nursing is ideal because of the risk of cord prolapse or occlusion, and all physicians must be readily available should there be an emergency.

ROUTE OF DELIVERY. Discussions of, and planning for, the route of delivery may have taken place before admission to labor and delivery. If not, they are accomplished as soon as possible after admission. The choice of abdominal or vaginal delivery is based upon the type of breech, flexion of the head, fetal size, quality of uterine contractions, and size of the maternal pelvis. The indications and contraindications for vaginal delivery of a breech have been discussed. The woman should be informed about all relevant facts and uncertainties before the breech delivery. The obstetrician should consider, and usually abide by, the preferences of the informed parents (Kunzel, 1994).

TIMING OF DELIVERY. In general, the ability to proceed with immediate breech extraction should exist when the buttocks or feet appear at the vulva. This is important because persistent fetal bradycardia is prone to develop from cord compression with further descent through the birth canal. It is essential that the delivery team include:

1. An obstetrician skilled in the art of breech extraction.
2. An associate to assist with the delivery.
3. An anesthesiologist who can assure adequate anesthesia when needed.
4. An individual trained to resuscitate the infant, including tracheal intubation.

Delivery is easier, and in turn, morbidity and mortality are probably lower, when the breech is allowed to deliver spontaneously to the umbilicus. If a nonreassuring fetal heart rate pattern develops before this time, however, a decision must be made whether to perform manual breech extraction or cesarean delivery. For a favorable outcome with any breech delivery, at the very minimum, the birth canal must be sufficiently large to allow passage of the fetus without trauma. The cervix must be fully dilated, and if not, then a cesarean delivery nearly always is the more appropriate method of delivery when suspected fetal compromise develops.

ASSISTED DELIVERY OF FRANK BREECH. The frank breech should ideally be allowed to deliver without assistance to at least the level of the umbilicus. Unless there is considerable relaxation of the perineum, an episiotomy should be made. The episiotomy is an important adjunct to any type of breech delivery. As the breech progressively distends the perineum, the posterior hip will deliver, usually from the 6 o'clock position, and often with sufficient pressure to evoke passage of thick meconium at this point (Fig. 22–4). The anterior hip then delivers followed by external rotation to the sacrum anterior position (Fig. 22–5). The mother should be encouraged to continue to push, as the cord is now drawn well down into the birth canal and is being compressed with resultant fetal bradycardia. Continued descent of the fetus will allow easy delivery of the legs by splinting the medial thighs of the fetus with the fingers positioned parallel to the femur and exertion of pressure laterally so as to sweep the legs away from the midline (Fig. 22–6).

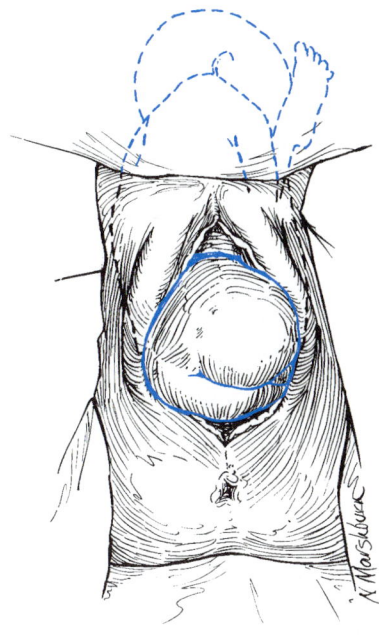

FIGURE 22–4. The posterior hip of the frank breech is delivering over the perineum. A generous midline episiotomy has been cut.

Following delivery of the legs, the fetal bony pelvis is grasped with both hands utilizing a cloth towel moistened with warm water. The fingers should rest on the anterior superior iliac crest and the thumbs on the sacrum, minimizing the chance of fetal abdominal soft tissue injury (Fig. 22–7). Maternal expulsive efforts are used in conjunction with continued gentle downward

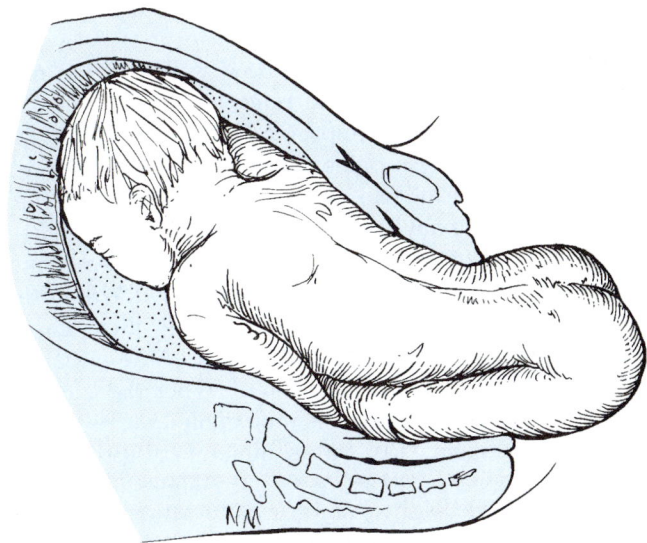

FIGURE 22–5. The anterior hip has now delivered and external rotation has occurred. The fetal thighs remain in flexion with extension at the knees.

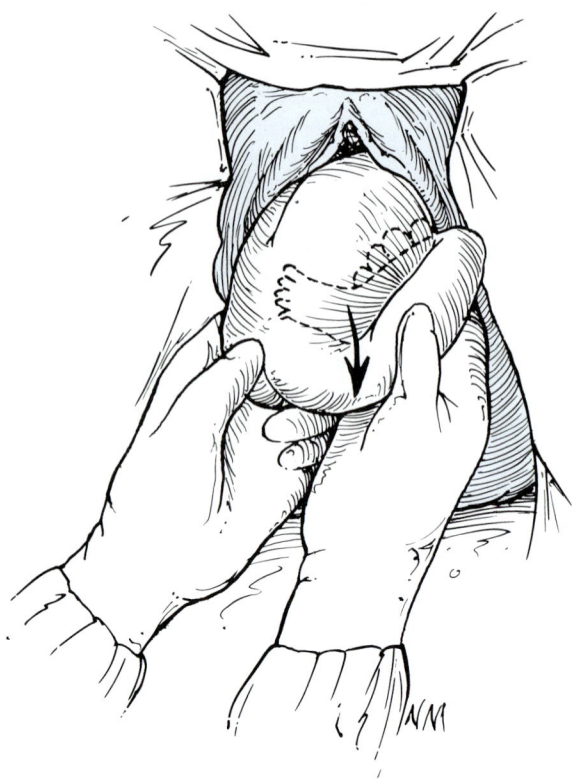

FIGURE 22–6. Spontaneous delivery has proceeded to beyond the level of the umbilicus. The operator now completes delivery of the legs by placing the fingers parallel with the medial aspect of the femur and displacing the femurs laterally and away from the midline.

operator rotational traction to effect delivery of the fetus. Gentle downward traction is combined with simultaneous 180 degree rotation of the fetal pelvis from either left to right sacrum transverse or from right to left (Figs. 22–8 and 22–9).

The depicted rotational and downward traction maneuver will decrease the occurrence of persistent nuchal arms. The latter may impact at the pelvic inlet and behind the symphysis pubis, thus preventing further descent. Nuchal arms can persist in term, preterm, and second twin vaginal breech deliveries. They are associated with increased fetal-newborn trauma and morbidity, and maneuvers to prevent this complication are warranted. These maneuvers are frequently most easily effected with the operator at the level of the maternal pelvis and with one knee on the floor. When the scapulas are clearly visible, delivery is then completed as subsequently described for the complete or incomplete breech.

FRANK BREECH EXTRACTION. At times, extraction of a frank breech may be required and can be accomplished by moderate traction exerted by a finger in each groin and facilitated by a generous episiotomy (Fig.

22–10). If moderate traction does not effect delivery of the breech, then vaginal delivery can be accomplished only by breech decomposition. This procedure involves intrauterine manipulation to convert the frank breech into a footling breech. The procedure is accomplished more readily if the membranes have ruptured recently, and it becomes extremely difficult if considerable time has elapsed since escape of amnionic fluid. In such cases, the uterus may have become tightly contracted over the fetus, and pharmacological relaxation by general anesthesia, intravenous magnesium sulfate, or small doses of nitroglycerin, (50 to 100 μg) or a β-mimetic such as terbutaline (250 μg) may be required.

Breech decomposition is accomplished by the maneuver attributed to Pinard (1889). It aids in bringing the fetal feet within reach of the operator. As shown in Figure 22–11, two fingers are carried up along one extremity to the knee to push it away from the midline. Spontaneous flexion usually follows, and the foot of the

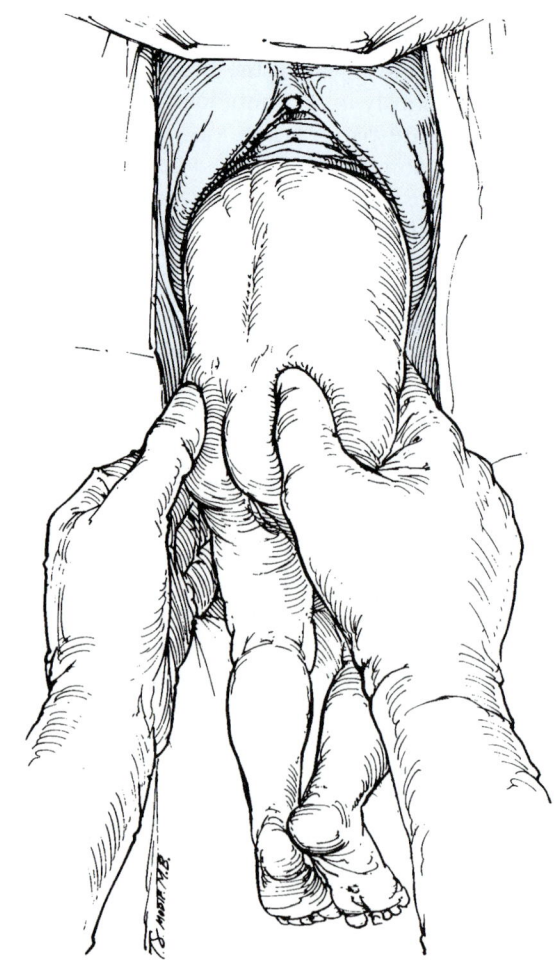

FIGURE 22–7. Delivery of the body. The hands are applied, but not above the pelvic girdle. Gentle downward rotational traction is accomplished until the scapulas clearly are visible.

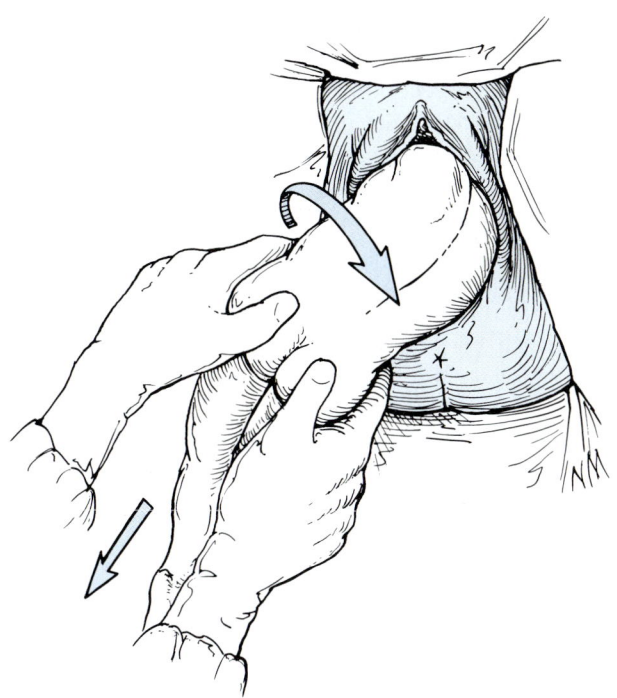

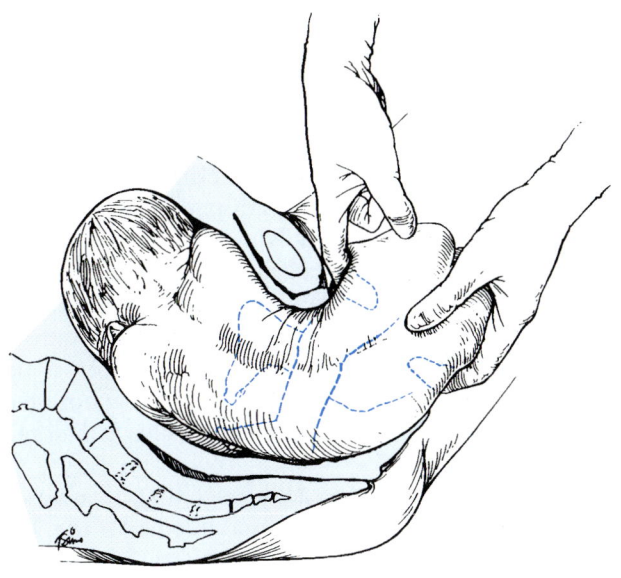

FIGURE 22–10. Extraction of a frank breech using fingers in groins.

FIGURE 22–8. Clockwise rotation of the fetal pelvis 180 degrees brings the sacrum from anterior to left sacrum transverse. Simultaneously, exerting gentle downward traction effects delivery to the scapula.

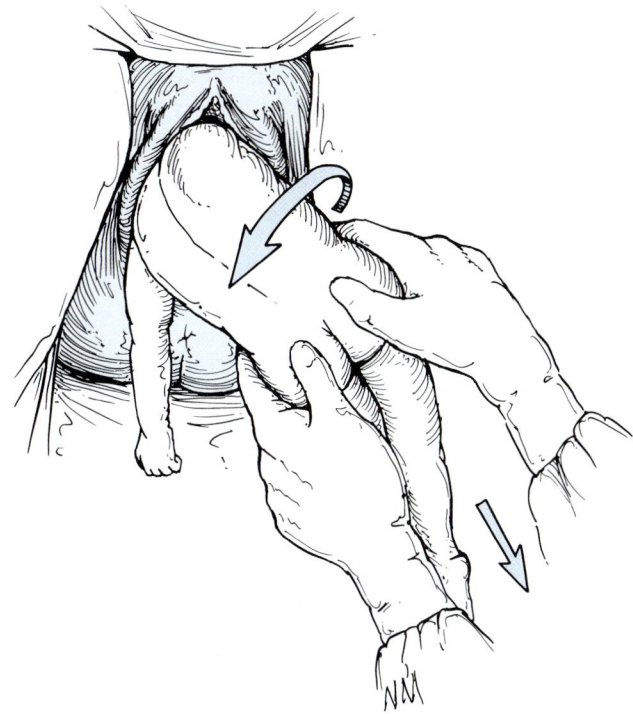

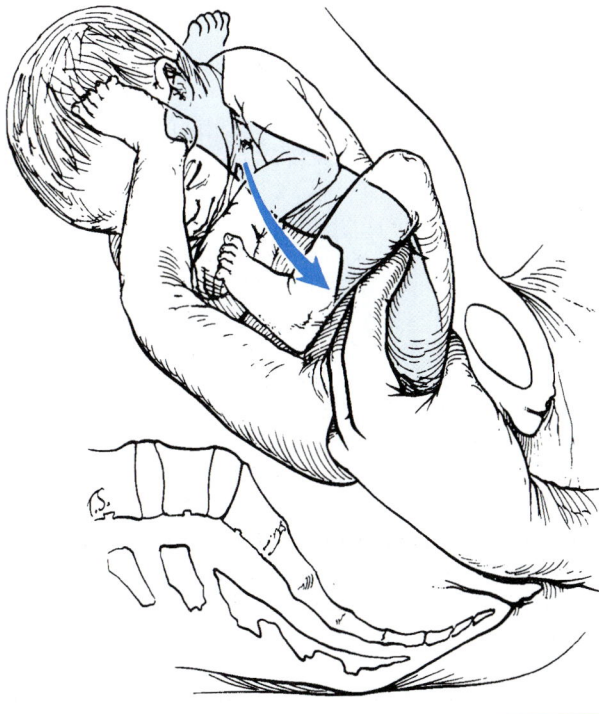

FIGURE 22–9. Counterclockwise rotation from sacrum anterior to right sacrum transverse along with gentle downward traction effects delivery to the right scapula.

FIGURE 22–11. Pinard maneuver, which is sometimes used in case of a frank breech presentation to deliver a foot into the vagina.

fetus is felt to impinge upon the back of the hand. The fetal foot then may be grasped and brought down.

COMPLETE OR INCOMPLETE BREECH EXTRACTION. During total extraction of a complete or incomplete breech, the hand is introduced through the vagina and both feet of the fetus are grasped. The ankles are held with the second finger lying between them and, with gentle traction, the feet are brought through the vulva. If difficulty is experienced in grasping both feet, first one foot should be drawn into the vagina but not through the introitus, and then the other foot is advanced in a similar fashion (Fig. 22–12). Now both feet are grasped and pulled through the vulva simultaneously.

As the legs begin to emerge through the vulva, downward gentle traction is then continued. As the legs emerge, successively higher portions are grasped, first the calves and then the thighs (Fig. 22–13). When the breech appears at the vulva, gentle traction is applied until the hips are delivered. As the buttocks emerge, the back of the infant usually rotates to the anterior. The thumbs are then placed over the sacrum and the fingers over the hips, and assisted breech delivery is effected as described previously (Fig. 22–7). As the scapulas become visible, the back of the infant tends to turn spontaneously toward the side of the mother to which it was originally directed (Fig. 22–13).

A cardinal rule in successful breech extraction is to employ steady, gentle, downward rotational traction un-

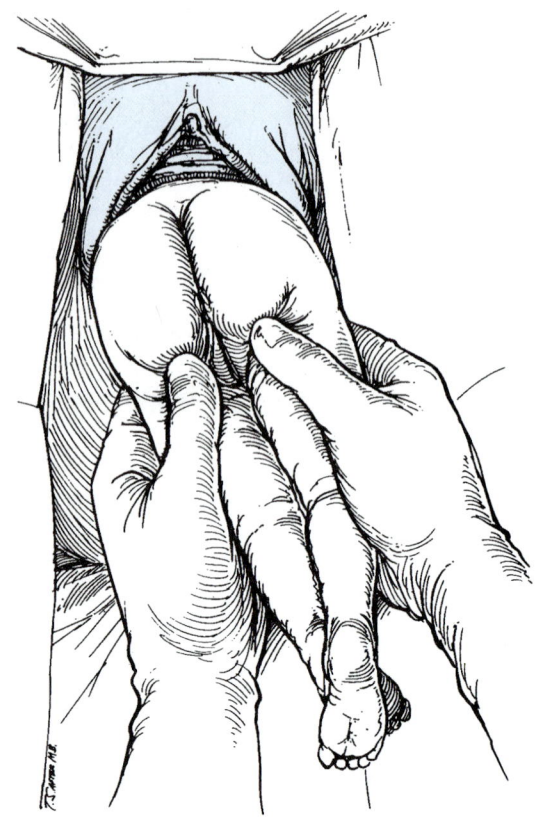

FIGURE 22–13. Breech extraction. Traction on the thighs. A warm, moist towel is most often applied over the fetal parts to reduce slippage from vernix as traction is applied.

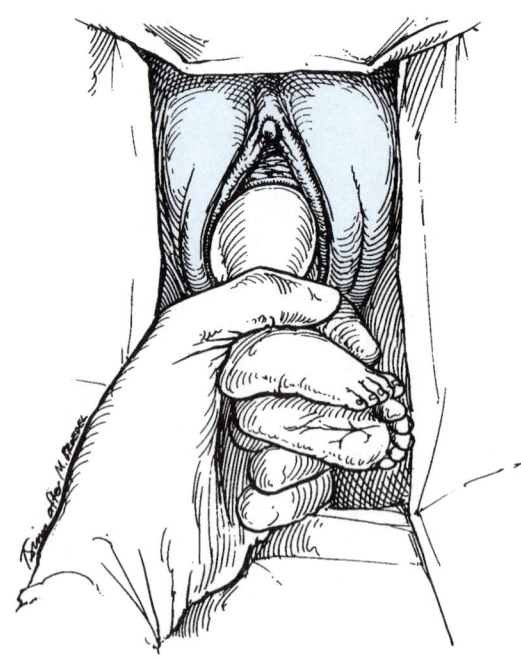

FIGURE 22–12. Breech extraction. Traction on the feet and ankles.

til the lower halves of the scapulas are delivered outside the vulva, making no attempt at delivery of the shoulders and arms until one axilla becomes visible. Failure to follow this rule frequently will make an otherwise easy procedure difficult. The appearance of one axilla indicates that the time has arrived for delivery of the shoulders. It makes little difference which shoulder is delivered first, and there are two methods for delivery of the shoulders, as follows.

In the first method, with the scapulas visible, the trunk is rotated in such a way that the anterior shoulder and arm appear at the vulva and can easily be released and delivered first. In Figure 22–14, the operator is shown rotating the trunk of the fetus counterclockwise to deliver the right shoulder and arm. The body of the fetus is then rotated in the reverse direction to deliver the other shoulder and arm.

In the second method, if trunk rotation is unsuccessful, the posterior shoulder must be delivered first. The feet are grasped in one hand and drawn upward over the inner thigh of the mother toward which the ventral surface of the fetus is directed. In this manner, leverage is exerted upon the posterior shoulder, which slides out over the perineal margin, usually followed by the arm

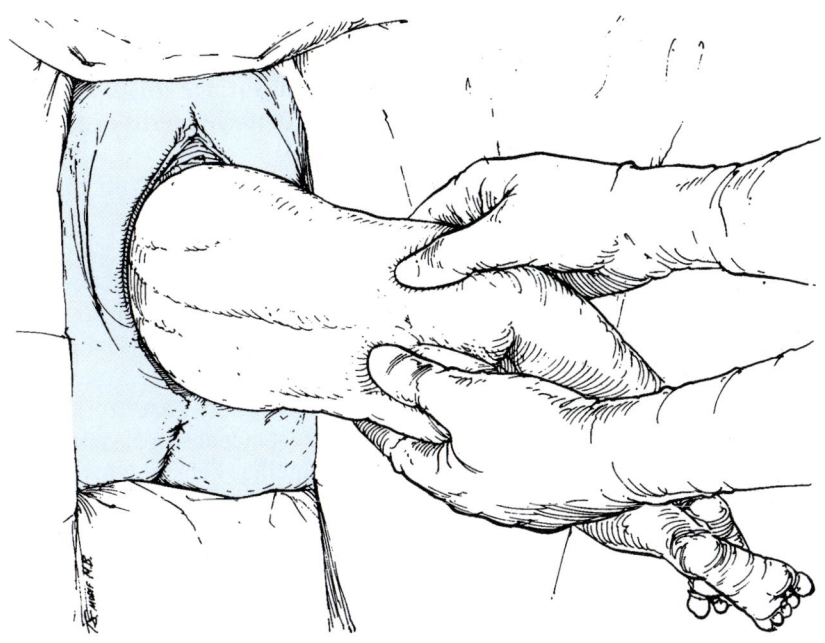

FIGURE 22–14. Breech extraction. The scapulas are visible and the body is rotating.

and hand (Fig. 22–15). Then, by depressing the body of the fetus, the anterior shoulder emerges beneath the pubic arch, and the arm and hand usually follow spontaneously (Fig. 22–16). Thereafter, the back tends to rotate spontaneously in the direction of the symphysis. If upward rotation fails to occur, it is effected by manual rotation of the body. Delivery of the head may then be accomplished.

Unfortunately, the process is not always so simple, and it is sometimes necessary first to free and deliver the arms. These maneuvers are much less frequently required today, presumably because of adherence to the principle of continuing rotational traction to prevent persistent nuchal arms and without attention to the shoulders until an axilla becomes visible. Attempts to free the arms immediately after the costal margins emerge should be avoided.

There is more space available in the posterior and lateral segments of the normal pelvis than elsewhere. Therefore, in difficult cases, the posterior arm should be freed first. Because the corresponding axilla already is visible, upward traction upon the feet is continued, and two fingers of the other hand are passed along the humerus until the elbow is reached (Fig. 22–15, inset). The fingers are placed parallel to the humerus and used to splint the arm, which is swept downward and delivered through the vulva. To deliver the anterior arm, depression of the body of the infant is sometimes all that is required to allow the anterior arm to slip out spontaneously. In other instances, the anterior arm can be swept down over the thorax using two fingers as a splint. Occasionally, however, the body must be held with the thumbs over the scapulas and rotated to bring

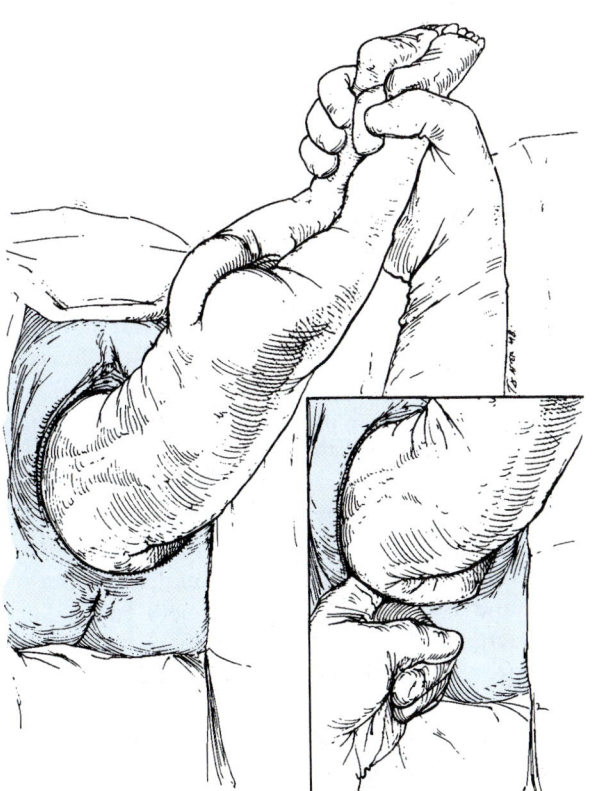

FIGURE 22–15. Breech extraction. Upward traction to effect delivery of the posterior shoulder, followed by freeing the posterior arm (inset).

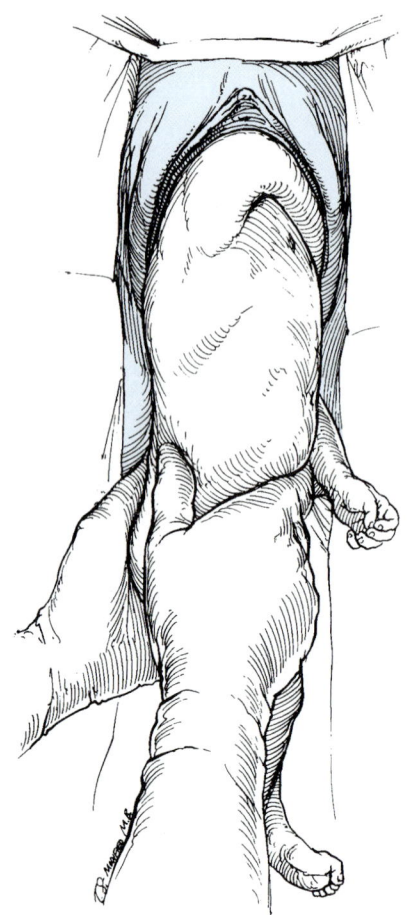

FIGURE 22–16. Breech extraction. Delivery of the anterior shoulder by downward traction. The anterior arm then may be freed the same way as the posterior arm in Figure 22–15.

the undelivered shoulder near the closest sacrosciatic notch. The legs then are carried upward to bring the ventral surface of the infant to the opposite inner thigh of the mother. Subsequently, the arm can be delivered as described previously. If the arms have become extended over the head, their delivery, although more difficult, can usually be accomplished by the maneuvers just described. In so doing, particular care must be taken to carry the fingers up to the elbow and to use the fingers as a splint to prevent fracture of the humerus.

As discussed earlier, one or both fetal arms occasionally is found around the back of the neck (nuchal arm) and impacted at the pelvic inlet. In this situation, delivery is more difficult. If the nuchal arm cannot be freed in the manner described, extraction may be facilitated, especially with a single nuchal arm, by rotating the fetus through half a circle in such a direction that the friction exerted by the birth canal will serve to draw the elbow toward the face. Should rotation of the fetus fail to free the nuchal arm(s), it may be necessary to push the fetus upward in an attempt to release it. If the rotation is

still unsuccessful, the nuchal arm is often extracted by hooking a finger(s) over it and forcing the arm over the shoulder, and down the ventral surface for delivery of the arm. In this event, fracture of the humerus or clavicle is very common.

The fetal head may then be extracted with forceps or by one of the following maneuvers.

MAURICEAU MANEUVER. This was first practiced by Mauriceau in 1721, but for some reason fell into disfavor. Much later Smellie (1876) described a similar procedure. Veit (1907) redirected attention to the Mauriceau maneuver, and in Germany the procedure frequently is named after Veit. The most accurate designation, however, is the Mauriceau-Smellie-Veit maneuver.

The index and middle finger of one hand are applied over the maxilla, to flex the head, while the fetal body rests upon the palm of the hand and forearm (Fig. 22–17). The forearm is straddled by the fetal legs. Two fingers of the other hand then are hooked over the fetal neck, and grasping the shoulders, downward traction is applied until the suboccipital region appears under the symphysis. Gentle suprapubic pressure simultaneously applied by an assistant helps keep the head flexed. The body of the fetus is then elevated toward the maternal abdomen, and the mouth, nose, brow, and eventually the occiput emerge successively over the perineum. It is emphasized that with this maneuver the operator uses both hands simultaneously and in tandem to exert continuous downward gentle traction bilaterally on the fetal neck and on the maxilla. At the same time, appropriate suprapubic pressure applied by an assistant is helpful in delivery of the head (Fig. 22–17).

PRAGUE MANEUVER. Rarely, the back of the fetus fails to rotate to the anterior. When this occurs, rotation of the back to the anterior may be achieved by using stronger traction on the fetal legs or bony pelvis. If the back still remains posteriorly, extraction may be accomplished using the Mauriceau maneuver and delivering the fetus back down. If this is impossible, the fetus still may be delivered using the modified Prague maneuver. This maneuver was recommended by Kiwisch (1846), who practiced in Prague. It had been described in London as early as 1754 by Pugh. The modified maneuver as practiced today consists of two fingers of one hand grasping the shoulders of the back-down fetus, from below, while the other hand draws the feet up over the maternal abdomen (Fig. 22–18).

BRACHT MANEUVER. With this maneuver, the breech is allowed to deliver spontaneously to the umbilicus. The fetal body then is held, but not pressed, against the maternal symphysis. This force is meant to be the equivalent of gravity (Bracht, 1936). The suspension of

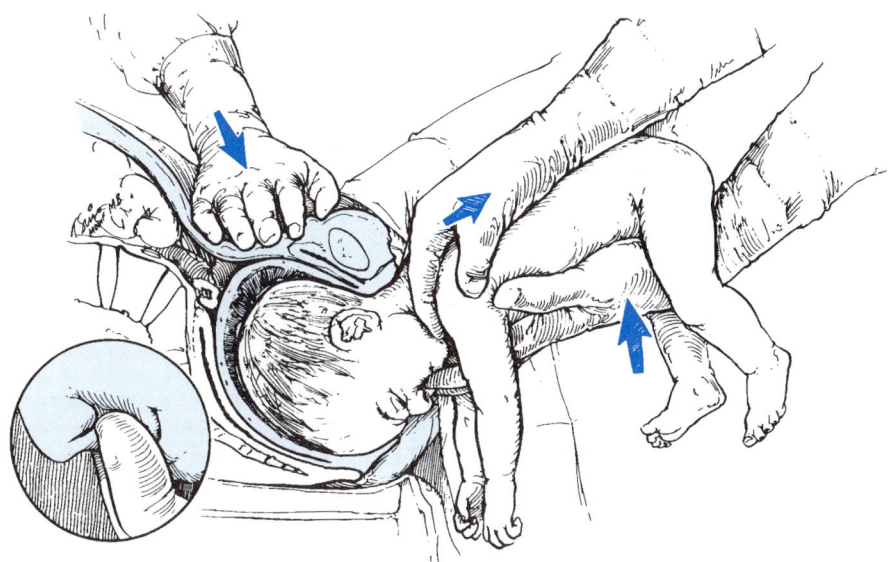

FIGURE 22–17. Delivery of the aftercoming head using the Mauriceau maneuver. Note that as the fetal head is being delivered, flexion of the head is maintained by suprapubic pressure provided by an assistant, and simultaneously by pressure on the maxilla (inset) by the operator as traction is applied.

the fetus in this position, coupled with the effects of uterine contractions and moderate suprapubic pressure by an assistant, often results in a spontaneous delivery. Despite its popularity in Europe, there is no proof that its use is associated with better long-term neurological outcomes (Krause and associates, 1991).

FORCEPS TO AFTERCOMING HEAD. Specialized forceps can be used to deliver the aftercoming head of the breech-presenting fetus. **Piper forceps,** shown in Figure 22–19, or divergent Laufe forceps may be applied electively or when the Mauriceau maneuver cannot be accomplished easily. The blades of the forceps should not be applied to the aftercoming head until it has been brought into the pelvis by gentle traction, combined

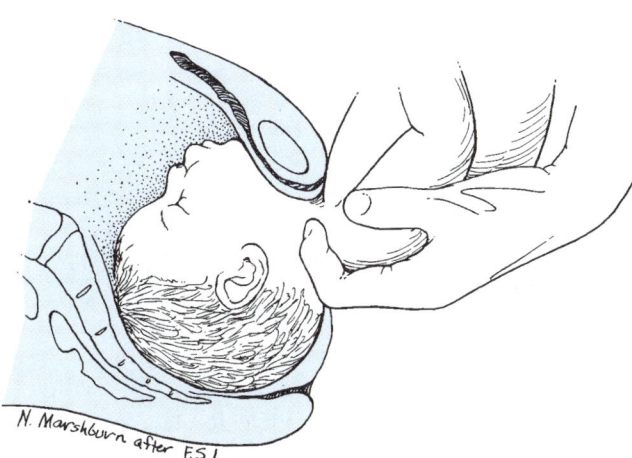

FIGURE 22–18. Delivery of the aftercoming head using the modified Prague maneuver necessitated by failure of the fetal trunk to rotate anteriorly.

with suprapubic pressure, and is engaged. Suspension of the body of the fetus in a towel helps keep the arms out of the way.

ENTRAPMENT OF THE AFTERCOMING HEAD. Occasionally, especially with small preterm fetuses, the incompletely dilated cervix will not allow delivery of the aftercoming head. With gentle traction on the fetal body, the cervix, at times, may be manually slipped over the occiput, or the Bracht maneuver may be tried. If these actions are not rapidly successful, *Dührssen incisions* can be made in the cervix.

Some advocate the use of intravenous nitroglycerin in doses of 50 to 100 μg to effect rapid uterine relaxation. Its use has been reported to be of benefit for intrapartum external version of a second twin, replacement of uterine inversion, and removal of a retained placenta (Abouleish and Corn, 1994; Altabef, 1992; DeSimone, 1990; Peng, 1989, and their colleagues). Its use for a "trapped" aftercoming fetal head with breech delivery has been suggested by Mayer and Weeks (1992) and Rolbin and associates (1991). Nitroglycerin, however, directly relaxes smooth muscle which constitutes only 15 percent of the cervix (Mercier and Benhamou, 1995). Its efficacy for fetal head entrapment has not been substantiated.

Replacement of the fetus higher into the vagina and uterus, followed by cesarean delivery, can be used successfully to rescue an entrapped breech that cannot be delivered vaginally. Iffy and colleagues (1986) described **abdominal rescue** by cesarean delivery for a 2050-g first twin whose fully deflexed head was entrapped after the arms had been delivered. The infant, delivered by emergency classical cesarean, had a small subarachnoid hemorrhage but remained neurologically normal. A similar maneuver to perform cesarean delivery for intractable

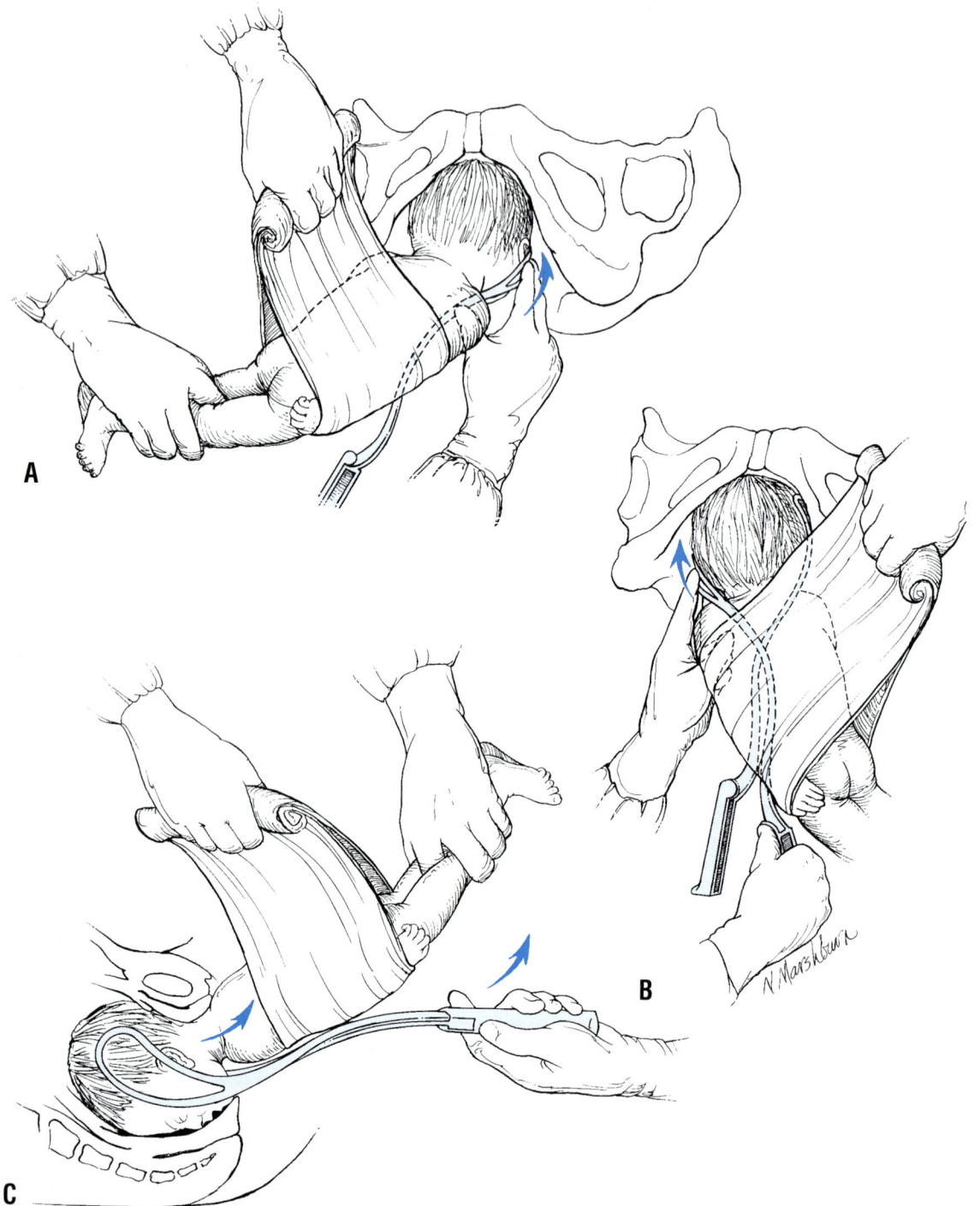

FIGURE 22–19. A. Left blade of Piper forceps applied to the aftercoming head. The fetal body is held elevated by using a warm towel. **B.** The right blade is applied. **C.** Forceps delivery of aftercoming head. Note the direction of movement (*arrow*).

shoulder dystocia is called the Zavanelli maneuver, but Sandberg (1999) found 11 published cases describing its use with a trapped aftercoming head.

ANALGESIA AND ANESTHESIA FOR LABOR AND DE-LIVERY. Continuous epidural analgesia (Chap. 15) has

been advocated by some as ideal for women in labor with a breech presentation (Kunzel, 1994; Mokriski, 1994). Confino and colleagues (1985) reviewed the outcomes of 371 nonanomalous singleton breech fetuses delivered vaginally. About 25 percent of these women had been given continuous epidural analgesia, and oxytocin augmentation was necessary to effect delivery in half of them. Although first-stage labor was not longer than in a control group not given epidural analgesia, the second stage was prolonged significantly in women whose fetuses weighed more than 2500 g. It was doubled if the fetus weighed more than 3500 g. Chadha and associates (1992) observed similar outcomes but also reported an increased incidence of cesarean delivery.

These potential disadvantages must be weighed against the advantage of better pelvic relaxation should extensive manipulation be required to effect delivery. Analgesia for episiotomy and intravaginal manipulations that are needed for breech extraction can usually be accomplished with pudendal block and local infiltration of the perineum. Nitrous oxide plus oxygen inhalation provides further relief from pain. If general anesthesia is required, it can be induced quickly with thiopental plus a muscle relaxant and maintained with nitrous oxide. Anesthesia for decomposition and extraction must provide sufficient relaxation to allow intrauterine manipulations. Although successful decomposition has been accomplished using epidural or spinal analgesia, increased uterine tone may render the operation more difficult. Under such conditions, one of the halogenated anesthetic agents may be required to relax the uterus as well as provide analgesia.

MORBIDITY AND MORTALITY

MATERNAL INJURIES. With complicated breech deliveries, there are increased maternal risks. Manual manipulations within the birth canal increase the risk of maternal infection. Intrauterine maneuvers, especially with a thinned-out lower uterine segment, or delivery of the aftercoming head through an incompletely dilated cervix, may cause rupture of the uterus, lacerations of the cervix, or both. Such manipulations also may lead to extensions of the episiotomy and deep perineal tears. Anesthesia sufficient to induce appreciable uterine relaxation may cause uterine atony and, in turn, postpartum hemorrhage. Even so, the prognosis in general for the mother whose fetus is delivered by breech extraction probably is somewhat better than with cesarean delivery.

FETAL INJURIES. For the fetus, the outlook is less favorable, and it is more serious the higher the presenting part is situated at the beginning of the breech extraction. In addition to the possibility of trauma, with incomplete breech presentations, cord prolapse is also much more common than with vertex presentations. Despite this, adverse outcomes for properly selected and managed vaginally delivered breeches are uncommon. Croughan-Minihane and associates (1990) reported that vaginally born infants were not at increased risk for adverse outcomes related to head trauma, neonatal seizures, cere-

bral palsy, mental retardation, or spasticity. Similarly, Roumen and Luyben (1991) described 247 consecutive women with term singleton breech fetuses, 95 percent of whom were allowed to labor. Excluded were cases of overt disproportion after previous cesarean delivery, abnormal presentation in combination with a congenital uterine anomaly, fetal distress, or a fetal biparietal diameter greater than 100 mm. Normal progression of labor during the first stage without secondary arrest or signs of fetal distress was used as the only factor to determine the feasibility of vaginal delivery. In this study, 196 of 234 (84 percent) delivered vaginally. One fetus died during breech extraction as a result of cephalopelvic disproportion.

Christian and colleagues (1990) reported no differences in Apgar scores, hospital stay, neonatal complications, and cord blood gases between vaginally delivered frank breeches and those delivered by cesarean section. All vaginal deliveries were in women with an adequate pelvis documented by CT pelvimetry, a frank breech presentation, and an estimated weight between 2000 and 4000 g. Christian and Brady (1991), but not Hommel and associates (1989), reported that breeches delivered vaginally had a lower mean cord blood pH and higher mean PCO_2 compared with cephalic-presenting infants delivered vaginally. In a long-term Scottish follow-up study, Danielian and colleagues (1996) found a similar incidence of neurological handicaps in infants born vaginally compared with cesarean delivery.

In a meta-analysis of 24 studies examining mode of planned delivery and perinatal outcome, Cheng and Hannah (1993) found a three- to fourfold significantly higher perinatal mortality rate and neonatal morbidity due to trauma in planned vaginally delivered infants, compared with those undergoing planned cesarean section. Gifford and associates (1995b) performed a similar analysis of nine studies. They concluded that the risk of any fetal injury, or any injury and death was tenfold increased after a trial of labor. Albrechtsen and colleagues (1998) Bartlett and colleagues (2000) studied early motor development of breech and control cephalic presenting infants. They concluded that the mode of delivery did not explain the excess neuromotor impairment detected in breech infants.

Fracture of the humerus and clavicle cannot always be avoided, and fracture of the femur may be sustained during difficult breech extractions (Fig. 22–20). Such fractures are associated with both vaginal and cesarean deliveries (Awwad and colleagues, 1993; Vasa and Kim, 1990). Neonatal perineal tears have been reported as a complication of spinal electrode use (Freud and associates, 1993). Hematomas of the sternocleidomastoid muscles occasionally develop after delivery, though they usually disappear spontaneously. More serious problems, however, may follow separation of the epiphyses of the scapula, humerus, or femur. There is no evidence that the incidence of congenital hip dislocations is in-

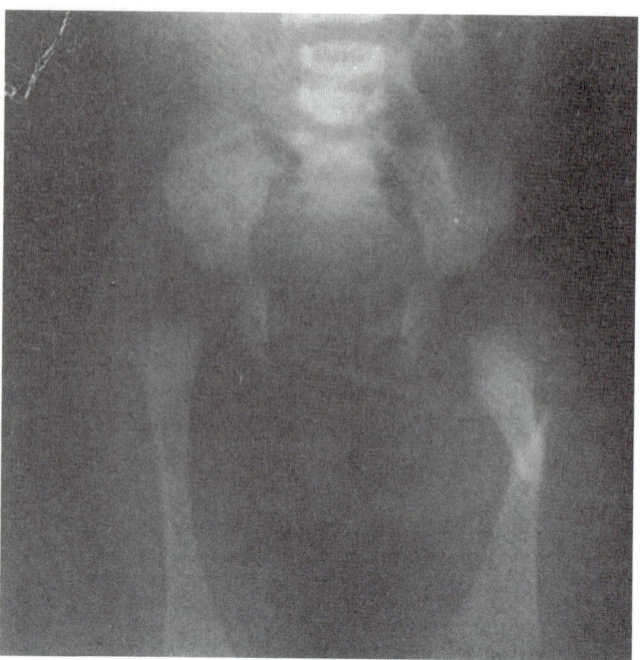

FIGURE 22–20. Midshaft right femoral fracture showing posterior displacement and lateral angulation. Injury occurred with extraction at cesarean delivery. (From Awwad and associates, 1993, with permission.)

creased by vaginal delivery of a breech (Clausen and Nielsen, 1988). Bartlett and colleagues (2000) studied early motor development of breech and control cephalic presenting infants. They concluded that the mode of delivery did not explain the excess neuromotor impairment detected in breech infants.

Paralysis of the arm may follow pressure upon the brachial plexus by the fingers in exerting traction, but more frequently it is caused by overstretching the neck while freeing the arms. Geutjens and colleagues (1996) observed a different pattern of brachial plexus injury in 36 newborns following vaginal breech delivery. In 80 percent, there was avulsion of the upper cervical spine roots. This injury cannot be treated by microsurgical nerve grafting and carries a worse prognosis for shoulder function. When the fetus is extracted forcibly through a contracted pelvis, spoon-shaped depressions or actual fractures of the skull may result. Occasionally, even the fetal neck may be broken when great force is employed. Testicular injury, in some cases severe enough to result in anorchia, may occur following vaginal breech delivery (Tiwary, 1989). Finally, vaginal breech delivery has also been reported to be associated with a sevenfold increased incidence of sudden infant death syndrome (Buck and co-workers, 1991).

Despite the potential fetal hazards of vaginal breech delivery, maternal morbidity associated with cesarean section must also be considered when planning delivery of the term frank or complete breech fetus (Gifford and colleagues, 1995a). In appropriately selected and managed cases, and with informed consent, both planned cesarean section and vaginal breech delivery remain appropriate and reasonable management options.

VERSION

Version is a procedure in which the presentation of the fetus is altered artificially, either substituting one pole of a longitudinal presentation for the other, or converting an oblique or transverse lie into a longitudinal presentation. According to whether the head or breech is made the presenting part, the operation is designated cephalic or podalic version, respectively. In *external version,* the manipulations are performed exclusively through the abdominal wall; whereas in *internal version,* the entire hand is introduced into the uterine cavity.

EXTERNAL CEPHALIC VERSION. The problems that have persisted until recently have not been whether external cephalic version could be accomplished and by what technique, but rather, whether the procedure was necessary, safe, and cost effective. With respect to necessity, it appears from the results of five randomized controlled studies totaling only 278 women, that if version is not performed, approximately 80 percent of noncephalic presentations diagnosed in the late third trimester will persist at delivery (Table 22–4). This is compared with only 30 percent of those who underwent a successful version. In their review, Laros and colleagues (1995) reported that external version was successful in 50 percent, however, even when the successful cesarean delivery rate was 30 percent.

External version was well known to our obstetrical predecessors, and it has received renewed interest in the past two decades coincidental with the availability of ultrasound, electronic fetal monitoring, and effective tocolytic agents. It is likely that these developments have improved the maternal and fetal safety of external version. Van Dorsten and co-workers (1981) rekindled interest in this procedure in the United States. In their first study, almost 70 percent of versions were successful, resulting in a 30 percent cesarean delivery rate compared with 75 percent when version was not attempted. The American College of Obstetricians and Gynecologists (2000) reviewed 20 studies and found a range from 35 to 85 percent success with an average of about 60.

Zhang and co-authors (1993) reviewed 25 selected reports on external cephalic version published between 1980 and 1991. Shown in Figure 22–21, and based on those data, are hypothetical results if all women with otherwise normal singleton breech presentations underwent attempted version at 35 to 37 weeks. Several points are noteworthy:

TABLE 22–4. Randomized Studies to Determine Effect of Cephalic Version on Noncephalic Births and Cesarean Deliveries

| | Noncephalic at Delivery | | | | Cesarean Delivery | | | |
| | Version | | Control | | Version | | Control | |
Investigators	No.	(%)	No.	(%)	No.	(%)	No.	(%)
Van Dorsten and colleagues (1981)	8/25	(32)	19/23	(83)	7/25	(28)	17/23	(74)
Hofmeyr (1983)	1/30	(3)	20/30	(67)	6/30	(20)	13/30	(43)
Brocks and associates (1984)	17/31	(55)	29/34	(85)	7/31	(23)	12/34	(35)
Van Veelen and co-workers (1989)	39/89	(44)	67/90	(74)	8/89	(9)	13/90	(14)
Mahomed and collaborators (1991)	18/103	(18)	87/105	(83)	13/103	(13)	35/105	(33)
Totals	83/278	(30)	222/282	(79)	41/278	(15)	90/282	(32)

Modified from Hofmeyr (1991).

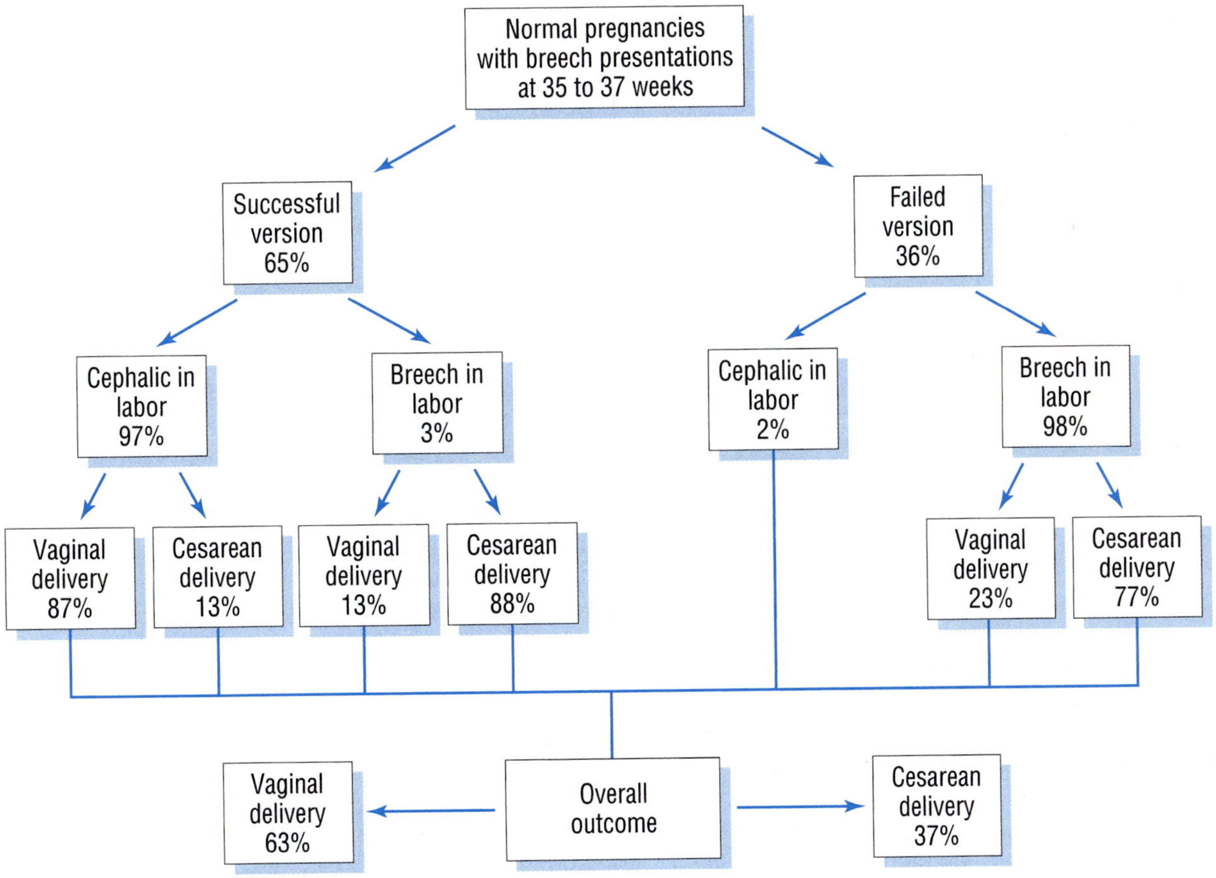

FIGURE 22–21. Hypothetical results of a trial of external cephalic version for breech presentation derived from reports totalling 1339 patients. (Modified from Zhang and co-workers, 1993, with permission.)

1. External cephalic version is successful in 65 percent of cases.
2. If version succeeds, almost all fetuses stay cephalic and vice versa.
3. Ultimately, and despite version attempts, 37 percent of women identified to have a late pregnancy breech will require cesarean delivery.

In a prospective study, Lau and associates (1997) observed that women who had a successful external version for breech presentation at term had an increased risk of a cesarean birth based on intrapartum events.

Zhang and co-workers (1993) estimated that universal application of external cephalic version could reduce the overall cesarean rate by no more than 2 percent. Morrison and co-workers (1986) attempted external cephalic version in 2.3 percent of pregnancies cared for at the University of Mississippi Medical Center between 1982 and 1984. Compared with the preceding 3 years at their institution, they decreased breech deliveries from 1.8 to 1.1 percent and cesarean deliveries performed for breeches from 2.8 to 1.6 percent. Ben-Arie and colleagues (1995) reported that introduction of an external version protocol at their institution decreased breech presentation at term from 3.9 to 2.4 percent. This was associated with a decrease of 5.5 percent in the cesarean section rate. Based on a decision analysis, Gifford and associates (1995a) concluded that routine use of external cephalic version would reduce cost and cesarean births. Adams and associates (2000) confirmed the independent cost benefit of attempting external cephalic version based on Medicaid billing. Conversely, Curet and co-workers (2000) reported that routine attempts at cephalic version resulted in *increased* costs per patient.

INDICATIONS. If a breech or shoulder presentation (transverse lie) is diagnosed in the last weeks of pregnancy, its conversion to a vertex may be attempted by external maneuvers, provided there is no marked disproportion between the size of the fetus and the pelvis, and provided there is no placenta previa. Chmait and colleagues (2000) reported good success in women who had undergone prior cesarean delivery.

FACTORS ASSOCIATED WITH SUCCESSFUL VERSION. The most consistent factor associated with the success of external cephalic version is parity (Zhang and colleagues, 1993). Hellstrom and co-workers (1990) identified only 3 of 16 variables to be associated with successful external version. The most important factor was parity, followed by fetal presentation, and then the amount of amnionic fluid. Version was more successful in a parous woman who has an unengaged fetus surrounded by a normal amount of amnionic fluid. Lau and associates (1997) also identified 3 of 19 studied variables to predict *failed* ver-

sion. These were engaged presenting part, difficulty in palpating the fetal head, and a uterus tense to palpation. With three of these present, there were no successes. With two, it was less than 20 percent. With none of these, success was 94 percent.

Gestational age is also important; the earlier external version is performed, the more likely it will be successful. Conversely, the more remote from term external version is performed, the higher the rate of spontaneous reversion (Westgren and colleagues, 1985b). Other reported, albeit controversial, determinants of unsuccessful version include diminished amnionic fluid volume, excessive maternal weight, anterior placental location, cervical dilatation, descent of the breech into the pelvis, and anterior or posterior positioning of the fetal spine (Newman and colleagues, 1993; Zhang and co-authors, 1993). Remarkably, Johnson and Elliott (1995) used fetal acoustic stimulation to startle breech fetuses to shift their spines laterally for successful Benifla and associates (1994) employed transabdominal amnioinfusion to facilitate successful external cephalic version in six women who had had previous unsuccessful version. According to Fortunato and colleagues (1988), external version using tocolysis is more likely to be successful if:

1. The presenting part has not descended into the pelvis.
2. There is a normal amount of amnionic fluid.
3. The fetal back is not positioned posteriorly.
4. The woman is not obese.

TRANSVERSE LIE. Women with a transverse lie are usually excluded from analyses of breech version because the overall success rate approaches 90 percent (Newman and colleagues, 1993).

TECHNIQUE. External cephalic version should be carried out in an area that has ready access to a facility equipped to perform emergency cesarean deliveries (American College of Obstetricians and Gynecologists, 2000). The labor and delivery unit is ideal for this, but Kornman and colleagues (1995) have performed selected versions in an office setting. Real-time ultrasonic examination is performed to confirm nonvertex term presentation, adequacy of amnionic fluid volume (vertical pocket of 2 cm or greater), and estimated fetal weight; to rule out obvious fetal anomalies; and to identify placental location. External monitoring is performed to assess fetal heart rate reactivity. A "forward roll" of the fetus is usually attempted first and the "back flip" technique is then tried if unsuccessful. Each hand grasps one of the fetal poles as shown in Figure 22–22. The fetal buttocks are elevated from the maternal pelvis, and displaced laterally. The buttocks are then gently guided toward the fundus, while the head is directed toward the pelvis. Version attempts are discontinued for excessive discomfort, per-

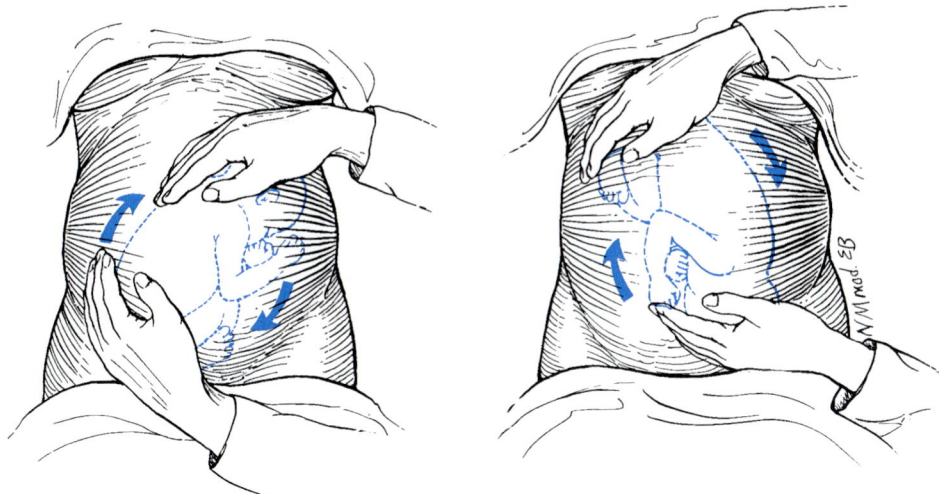

FIGURE 22–22. External cephalic version.

sistently abnormal fetal heart rate, or after multiple failed attempts. D-immune globulin is given to D-negative, unsensitized women. The nonstress test is repeated after version until a normal test result is obtained. This process takes about half a day and may cost as much as $1700 (Newman and colleagues, 1993).

Most authorities recommend uterine relaxation with a tocolytic agent, usually terbutaline 0.25 mg given subcutaneously. Some investigators have shown a benefit to tocolysis, while others have not. For example, Robertson and associates (1987) reported that ritodrine tocolysis did not improve their success. Similarly, Tan and colleagues (1989), in a prospective randomized trial, found that salbutamol did not improve their success rate. Conversely, in a randomized clinical trial, Fernandez and co-workers (1996) reported that terbutaline given subcutaneously significantly increased the success rate from 27 to 52 percent. Marquette and colleagues (1996) reported similar results with ritodrine infusion. Andarsio and Feng (2000) reported preliminary data in 35 women randomized to tocolysis with either nitroglycerin or terbutaline. With either agent, the success rate was about 50 percent. Yanny and associates (2000) found no advantages to glyceryl trinitrate over placebo.

Abdominal relaxation may also be helpful. Schorr and co-workers (1997), in a prospective randomized trial, found that epidural analgesia given with terbutaline tocolysis improved success (60 percent) with version, compared with the nonepidural group (30 percent). Mancuso and collaborators (2000) randomized 108 women and reported 59 versus 33 percent with epidural versus control groups. Neiger and associates (1998) used epidural analgesia with 56 percent success for failed versions. Conversely, Dugoff and colleagues (1999) randomized 102 women to terbutaline plus spinal analgesia versus terbutaline alone. The success rates were similar,

44 and 42 percent. According to the American College of Obstetricians and Gynecologists (2000), there is not enough consistent evidence to recommend conduction analgesia.

Lastly, to further emphasize our lack of understanding regarding the persistence of the breech presentation near term, several effective but unconventional interventions have been reported. Cardini and Weixen (1998) performed a randomized clinical trial to evaluate *moxibustion*—burning herbs to simulate acupuncture point BL67—to promote spontaneous breech version, possibly by increasing fetal activity. The intervention group experienced significantly increased fetal movements and cephalic presentations at birth. Mehl (1994) in a prospective matched series of 100 women with a breech presentation at 37 to 40 weeks, evaluated hypnosis with suggestions for relaxation. Significantly more fetuses in the intervention group (81 percent) converted to vertex than in the control group (48 percent).

COMPLICATIONS. Risks of external version include placental abruption, uterine rupture, amnionic fluid embolism, fetomaternal hemorrhage, isoimmunization, preterm labor, fetal distress, and fetal demise. According to Zhang and colleagues (1993), there have been no reported fetal deaths in the United States resulting directly from external version since 1980. Reported nonfatal complications include fetal heart rate decelerations in almost 40 percent of fetuses (Phelan and co-workers, 1984) and fetomaternal hemorrhage in 4 percent (Stine and colleagues, 1985). Petrikovsky and colleagues (1987) reported fetal brachial plexus injury after a successful external version. Stine and co-workers (1985) reported a death due to amnionic fluid embolus.

Because of the fear of uterine rupture, women who had undergone prior cesarean delivery were, in the past, excluded from most external cephalic version protocols. Flamm and co-workers (1991), however, reported no serious maternal or fetal complications associated with such attempts in 56 women with previous low transverse uterine incisions. They were successful in 82 percent. De Meeus and colleagues (1998) reported similar experiences in 38 women.

INTERNAL PODALIC VERSION. This maneuver consists of turning the fetus by inserting a hand into the uterine cavity, seizing one or both feet, and drawing them through the cervix while pushing transabdominally the upper portion of the fetal body in the opposite direction. The operation is followed by breech extraction. There are very few, if any, indications for internal podalic version other than for delivery of a second twin, which is discussed in detail in Chapter 30 (p. 800).

REFERENCES

Abouleish AE, Corn SB: Intravenous nitroglycerin for intrapartum external version of the second twin. Anesth Analg 78:808, 1994

Adams EK, Mauldin PD, Mauldin JG, Mayberry RM: Determining cost savings from attempted cephalic version in an inner city delivering population. Health Care Management Science 3:185, 2000

Albrechtsen S, Rasmussen S, Irgens LM: Secular trends in peri- and neonatal mortality in breech presentation, Norway 1967–1994. Acta Obstet Gynecol Scand 79:508, 2000

Albrechtsen S, Rasmussen S, Dalaker K, Irgens LM: Perinatal mortality in breech presentation sibships. Obstet Gynecol 92:775, 1998

Albrechtsen S, Rasmussen S, Reigstad H, Markestad T, Irgens LM, Dalaker K: Evaluation of a protocol for selecting fetuses in breech presentation for vaginal delivery or cesarean section. Am J Obstet Gynecol 177:586, 1997

Altabef KM, Spencer JT, Zinberg S: Intravenous nitroglycerin for uterine relaxation of an inverted uterus. Am J Obstet Gynecol 166:1237, 1992

American College of Obstetricians and Gynecologists: External cephalic version. ACOG Practice Bulletin No. 13, February 2000

Andarsio F, Feng TI: External cephalic version: Nitroglycerin versus terbutaline. (Abst.) Am J Obstet Gynecol 182:S161, 2000

Anderman S, Ellenbogen A, Jaschevatzky OE, Grunstein S: Is term breech presentation in primigravida an absolute indication for cesarean section? Eur J Obstet Gynecol Reprod Biol 18:11, 1984

Awwad JT, Nahhas DE, Karam KS: Femur fracture during cesarean breech delivery. Int J Gynaecol Obstet 43:324, 1993

Barlöv K, Larsson G: Results of a five-year prospective study using a feto-pelvic scoring system for term singleton breech delivery after uncomplicated pregnancy. Acta Obstet Gynecol Scand 65:315, 1986

Barrett JM: Funic reduction for the management of umbilical cord prolapse. Am J Obstet Gynecol 165:654, 1991

Bartlett DJ, Okun NB, Byrne PJ, Watt JM, Piper MC: Early

motor development of breech- and cephalic-presenting infants. Obstet Gynecol 95:425, 2000

Ben-Arie A, Kogan S, Schuachter M, Hagay ZJ, Insler V: The impact of external cephalic version on the rate of vaginal and cesarean breech deliveries: A 3-year cumulative experience. Eur J Obstet Gynecol Reprod Biol 63:125, 1995

Benifla JL, Goffinet F, Darai E, Madelenat P: Antepartum transabdominal amnioinfusion to facilitate external cephalic version after initial failure. Obstet Gynecol 84:1041, 1994

Benson WL, Boyce DC, Vaughn DL: Breech delivery in the primigravida. Obstet Gynecol 40:417, 1972

Berger R, Sawodny E, Bachmann G, Herrman S, Kunzel W: The prognostic value of magnetic resonance imaging for the management of breech delivery. Eur J Obstet Gynecol Reprod Biol 55:97, 1994

Bingham P, Lilford RJ: Management of the selected term breech presentation: Assessment of the risks of selected vaginal delivery versus cesarean section for all cases. Obstet Gynecol 69:965, 1987

Bistoletti P, Nisell H, Palme C, Lagercrantz H: Term breech delivery: Early and late complications. Acta Obstet Gynecol Scand 60:165, 1981

Biswas A, Johnstone MJ: Term breech delivery: Does x-ray pelvimetry help? Aust NZ J Obstet Gynaecol 33:150, 1993

Bodmer B, Benjamin A, McLean FH, Usher RH: Has use of cesarean section reduced the risks of delivery in the preterm breech presentation? Am J Obstet Gynecol 154:144, 1986

Bowes WA, Taylor VS, O'Brien M, Bowes C: Breech delivery: Evaluation of method of delivery on perinatal results and maternal morbidity. Am J Obstet Gynecol 135:965, 1979

Bracht E: Manual aid in breech presentation. Zeitschr Geburthshilfe Gynaekol 112:271, 1936

Brenner WE, Bruce RD, Hendricks CH: The characteristics and perils of breech presentation. Am J Obstet Gynecol 118:700, 1974

Brocks V, Philipsen T, Secher NJ: A randomized trial of external cephalic version with tocolysis in late pregnancy. Br J Obstet Gynaecol 91:653, 1984

Brown L, Karrison T, Cibils LA: Mode of delivery and perinatal results in breech presentation. Am J Obstet Gynecol 171:28, 1994

Bruck LR, Sherer DM: Intrapartum sonography of the lower uterine segment in patients with breech-presenting fetuses. Am J Perinatol 14:315, 1997

Buck GM, Michalek AM, Kramer AA, Batt RF: Labor and delivery events and risk of sudden infant death syndrome (SIDS). Am J Epidemiol 133:900, 1991

Cardini F, Weixin H: Moxibustion for correction of breech presentation: A randomized controlled trial. JAMA 280:1580, 1998

Chadha YC, Mahmood TA, Dick MJ, Smith NC, Campbell DM, Templeton A: Breech delivery and epidural analgesia. Br J Obstet Gynaecol 99:96, 1992

Chasen ST, D'Angelo M: Effectiveness of clinical assessment of fetal presentation at term. (Abst.) Am J Obstet Gynecol 182:S146, 2000

Cheng M, Hannah M: Breech delivery at term: A critical review of the literature. Obstet Gynecol 82:605, 1993

Chmait R, Fried M: Comparison of external cephalic version in multiparous women with and without prior history of cesarean section. (Abst.) Am J Obstet Gynecol 182:S152, 2000

Christian SS, Brady K: Cord blood acid–base values in breech-presenting infants born vaginally. Obstet Gynecol 78:778, 1991

Christian SS, Brady K, Read JA, Kopelman JN: Vaginal breech delivery: A five-year prospective evaluation of a protocol using computed tomographic pelvimetry. Am J Obstet Gynecol 163:848, 1990

Cibils LA, Karrison T, Brown L: Factors influencing neonatal outcomes in the very-low-birthweight fetus (1500 g) with a breech presentation. Am J Obstet Gynecol 171:35, 1994

Collea JV, Chein C, Quilligan EJ: The randomized management of term frank breech presentation: A study of 208 cases. Am J Obstet Gynecol 137:235, 1980

Collea JV, Rabin SC, Weghorst GR, Quilligan EJ: The randomized management of term frank breech presentation: Vaginal delivery vs cesarean section. Am J Obstet Gynecol 131:186, 1978

Clausen I, Nielsen KT: Breech position, delivery route and congenital hip dislocation. Acta Obstet Gynecol Scand 67:595, 1988

Confino E, Ismajovich B, Rudick V, David MP: Extradural analgesia in the management of singleton breech delivery. Br J Anaesth 57:892, 1985

Crawford JS: An appraisal of lumbar epidural blockade in patients with a singleton fetus presenting by the breech. J Obstet Gynaecol Br Commonw 81:867, 1974

Croughan-Minihane MS, Petitti DB, Gordis L, Golditch I: Morbidity among breech infants according to method of delivery. Obstet Gynecol 75:821, 1990

Curet LB, Gilson GJ, Christensen F: Cost effectiveness of routine external version for breech presentation. Am J Obstet Gynecol [abstract] 182:S156, 2000

Daniel Y, Fait G, Lessing JB, Jaffa A, David MP, Kupferminc MJ: Outcome of 496 term singleton breech deliveries in a tertiary center. Am J Perinatol 15:2, 1998

Danielian PJ, Wang J, Hall MH: Long term outcome by method of delivery of fetuses in breech presentation at term: Population based follow up. BMJ 312:1451, 1996

de Meeus JB, Ellia F, Magnin G: External cephalic version after previous cesarean section: A series of 38 cases. Eur J Obstet Gynecol Reprod Biol 81:65, 1998

DeSimone CA, Norris MC, Leighton BL: Intravenous nitroglycerin aids manual extraction of a retained placenta. Anesthesiology 73:787, 1990

Diro M, Puangsricharern A, Royer L, O'Sullivan MJ, Burkett G: Singleton term breech deliveries in nulliparous and multiparous women: A 5-year experience at the University of Miami-Jackson Memorial Hospital. Am J Obstet Gynecol 181:247, 1999

Dorn U: Hip screening in newborn infants. Clinical and ultrasound results. Wien Klin Wochenschr 181:3, 1990

Dugoff L, Stamm CA, Jones OW III, Mohling SI, Hawkins JL: The effect of spinal anesthesia on the success rate of external cephalic version: A randomized trial. Obstet Gynecol 93:345, 1999

El Gammal NA, Jallad KB, O'deh HMS: Breech vaginal delivery after one cesarean section: A retrospective study. Int J Gynaecol Obstet 33:99, 1990

Eller DP, Van Dorsten JP: Route of delivery for the breech presentation: A conundrum. Am J Obstet Gynecol 173:393, 1995

Fait G, Daniel Y, Lessing JB, Bar-Am A, Gull I, Shenhav M, Kupferminc MH: Can labor with breech presentation be induced? Gynecol Obstet Investig 469:181, 1998

Fernandez CO, Bloom S, Wendel G: A prospective, randomized, blinded comparison of terbutaline versus placebo for singleton, term external cephalic version. Am J Obstet Gynecol 174:326, 1996

Fianu S, Vaclavinkova V: The site of placental attachment as a factor in the aetiology of breech presentation. Acta Obstet Gynecol Scand 57:371, 1978

Fischer-Rasmussen W, Trolle D: Abdominal versus vaginal delivery in breech presentation: A retrospective study comparing 420 breech presentations and 9,291 cephalic presentations for infants weighing more than 2,500 g at birth. Acta Obstet Gynecol Scand Suppl 9:69, 1967

Flamm BL, Fried MW, Lonky NM, Giles WS: External cephalic version after previous cesarean section. Am J Obstet Gynecol 165:370, 1991

Flanagan TA, Mulchahey KM, Korenbrot CC, Green JR, Laros RK Jr: Management of term breech presentation. Am J Obstet Gynecol 156:1492, 1987

Fortunato SJ, Mercer LJ, Guzick DS: External cephalic version with tocolysis: Factors associated with success. Obstet Gynecol 72:59, 1988

Freud E, Orvieto R, Merlob P: Neonatal labioperineal tear from fetal scalp electrode insertion, a case report. J Reprod Med 36:647, 1993

Geutjens G, Gilbert A, Helsen K: Obstetric brachial plexus palsy associated with breech delivery. A different pattern of injury. J Bone Joint Surg [Br] 78:303, 1996

Gifford DS, Keeler E, Kahn KL: Reductions in cost and cesarean rate by routine use of external cephalic version: A decision analysis. Obstet Gynecol 85:930, 1995a

Gifford DS, Morton SC, Fiske M, Kahn K: A meta-analysis of infant outcomes after breech delivery. Obstet Gynecol 85:1047, 1995b

Gimovsky ML, Petrie RH: The intrapartum management of the breech presentation. Clin Perinatol 16:975, 1989

Gimovsky ML, Wallace RL, Schifrin BS, Paul RH: Randomized management of the nonfrank breech presentation at term: A preliminary report. Am J Obstet Gynecol 146:34, 1983

Gravenhorst JB, Schreuder AM, Veen S, Brand R. Verloove-Vanhorick SP, Verweij RA, van Zeben-van der Aa DM, Ens-Dokkum MH: Breech delivery in very preterm and very-low-birthweight infants in the Netherlands. Br J Obstet Gynaecol 100:411, 1993

Hall JE, Kohl SG: Breech presentation: A study of 1456 cases. Am J Obstet Gynecol 72:977, 1956

Hannah ME, Hannah WJ: Feasibility of a randomized controlled trial of planned cesarean section versus planned vaginal delivery for breech presentation at term. Am J Obstet Gynecol 174:1393, 1996

Hannah ME, Hannah WJ, Hewson SA, Hodnett ED, Saigal S, William AR, for the Term Breech Trial Collaborative Group: Planned caesarean section versus planned vaginal birth for breech presentation at term: A randomised multicentre trial. Lancet 356:1375, 2000

Hellstrom AC, Nilsson B, Stange L, Nylund L: When does external cephalic version succeed? Acta Obstet Gynecol Scand 69:281, 1990

Hofmeyr GJ: External cephalic version at term: How high are the stakes? Br J Obstet Gynaecol 98:1, 1991

Hofmeyr GJ: Effect of external cephalic version in late pregnancy on breech presentation and cesarean section rate: A controlled trial. Br J Obstet Gynaecol 90:392, 1983

Hommel U, Bellee H, Link M: The validity of parameters in neonatal diagnosis and fetal monitoring of breech deliveries, 1. Neonatal status after breech delivery. Zentralbl Gynakol 111:1293, 1989

Hytten FE: Breech presentation: Is it a bad omen? Br J Obstet Gynaecol 89:879, 1982

Iffy L, Apuzzio JJ, Cohen-Addad N, Zwolska-Demczuk B, Francis-Lane M, Olenczak J: Abdominal rescue after entrapment of the aftercoming head. Am J Obstet Gynecol 154:623, 1986

Irion O, Almagbaly PH, Morabia A: Planned vaginal delivery versus elective caesarean section: A study of 705 singleton term breech presentations. Br J Obstet Gynaecol 105:710, 1998

Jaffa AJ, Peyser MR, Ballas S, Toaff R: Management of term breech presentation in primigravidae. Br J Obstet Gynaecol 88:721, 1981

Johnson RL, Elliott JP: Fetal acoustic stimulation, an adjunct to external cephalic version: A blinded, randomized crossover study. Am J Obstet Gynecol 173:1369, 1995

Kauppila O: The perinatal mortality in breech deliveries and observations on affecting factors: A retrospective study on 2,227 cases. Acta Obstet Gynaecol Scand Suppl 39:1, 1975

Kiwisch FH: Beiträge zur Geburtskunde (Würzburg) 1:69, 1846

Koo MR, Dekker GA, van Geijn HP: Perinatal outcome of singleton term breech deliveries. Eur J Obstet Gynecol Reprod Biol 78:19, 1998

Kopelman JN, Duff P, Karl RT, Schipul AH, Read JA: Computed tomographic pelvimetry in the evaluation of breech presentation. Obstet Gynecol 68:455, 1986

Kornman MT, Kimball KT, Reeves KO: Preterm external cephalic version in an outpatient environment. Am J Obstet Gynecol 172:1743, 1995

Krause W, Voigt C, Donczik J, Michels W, Gstottner H: Assisted spontaneous delivery vs Bracht manual aid within the scope of vaginal delivery in breech presentation. Late morbidity in children 5–7 years of age. Z Geburtshilfe Perinatol 195:76, 1991

Krebs L, Topp M, Langhoff-Roos J: The relation of breech presentation at term to cerebral palsy. Br J Obstet Gynaecol 106:943, 1999

Kunzel W: Recommendations of the FIGO Committee on Perinatal Health on guidelines for the management of breech delivery. Int J Gynaecol Obstet 44:297, 1994

Laros RK Jr, Flanagan TA, Kilpatrick SJ: Management of term breech presentation: A protocol of external cephalic version and selective trial of labor. Am J Obstet Gynecol 172:1916, 1995

Lau TK, Lo KW, Rogers M: Pregnancy outcome after successful external cephalic version of breech presentation at term. Am J Obstet Gynecol 176:218, 1997

Lau TK, Lo KWK, Wan D, Rogers MS: Predictors of successful external cephalic version at term: A prospective study. Br J Obstet Gynaecol 104:798, 1997

Lindqvist A, Norden-Lindeberg S, Hanson U: Perinatal mortality and route of delivery in term breech presentations. Br J Obstet Gynaecol 104:1288, 1997

Mahomed K: Breech delivery: A critical evaluation of the mode of delivery and outcome of labor. Int J Gynaecol Obstet 27:17, 1988

Mahomed K, Seeras R, Coulson R: External cephalic version at term. A randomized controlled trial using tocolysis. Br J Obstet Gynaecol 98:8, 1991

Mahomed K, Seeras R, Coulson R: Outcome of term breech presentation. East Afr Med J 66:819, 1989

Main DM, Main BK, Maurer MM: Cesarean section versus vaginal delivery for the breech fetus weighing less than 1500 grams. Am J Obstet Gynecol 46:580, 1983

Malloy MH, Oustad L, Wright E: National Institute of Child Health and Human Development Neonatal Research Network: The effect of cesarean delivery on birth outcome in very-low-birthweight infants. Obstet Gynecol 77:498, 1991

Mancuso KM, Yancey MK, Murphy JA, Markenson GR: Epidural analgesia for cephalic version: A randomized trial. Obstet Gynecol 95:648, 2000

Marquette GP, Boucher M, Thériault D, Rinfret D: Does the use of a tocolytic affect the success rate of external cephalic version? Am J Obstet Gynecol 174:327, 1996

Mauriceau F: The method of delivering the woman when the infant presents one or two feet first. In: Traite des Maladies des Femmes Grosses, 6th ed. Paris, 1721, p 280

Mayer DC, Weeks SK: Antepartum uterine relaxation with nitroglycerin at caesarean delivery. Can J Anaesth 39:166, 1992

Mecke H, Weisner D, Freys I, Semm K: Delivery of breech presenting infants at term: An analysis of 304 breech deliveries. J Perinat Med 17:121, 1989

Mehl LE: Hypnosis and conversion of the breech to the vertex presentation. Arch Fam Med 81:654, 1994

Mercier FJ, Benhamou D: Nitroglycerin for fetal head entrapment during vaginal breech delivery? Anesth Analg 81:654, 1995

Mokriski B: Abnormal presentation and multiple gestation. In Chestnut, DH (ed): Obstetric Anesthesia. St Louis, Mosby, 1994, p 669

Morrison JC, Myatt RE, Martin JN, Meeks GR, Martin RW, Bucovarz ET, Wiser WL: External cephalic version of the breech presentation under tocolysis. Am J Obstet Gynecol 154:900, 1986

Morrison JJ, Sinnatamby R, Hackett GA, Tudor J: Obstetric pelvimetry in the UK: An appraisal of current practice. Br J Obstet Gynaecol 102:748, 1995

Neiger R, Hennessy MD, Patel M: Reattempting failed external cephalic version under epidural anesthesia. Am J Obstet Gynecol 179:1136, 1998

Nelson KB, Ellenberg JH: Antecedents of cerebral palsy: Multivariate analysis of risk. N Engl J Med 315:81, 1986

Newman RB, Peacock BS, Van Dorsten JP, Hunt HH: Predicting success of external cephalic version. Am J Obstet Gynecol 169:245, 1993

Nwosu EC, Walkinshaw S, Chia P, Manasse PR, Atlay RD: Undiagnosed breech. Br J Obstet Gynaecol 100:531, 1993

Ohlsén H: Outcome of term breech delivery in primigravidae. A feto-pelvic breech index. Acta Obstet Gynecol Scand 54:141, 1975

Olshan AF, Shy KK, Luthy DA, Hickok D, Weiss NS, Daling JR: Cesarean birth and neonatal mortality in very-low-birthweight infants. Obstet Gynecol 64:267, 1984

Peng AT, Gorman RS, Shulman SM, DeMarchis E, Nyunt K, Blancato L: Intravenous nitroglycerin for uterine relaxation in the postpartum patient with retained placenta. Anesthesiology 71:172, 1989

Penn ZJ, Steer PJ: Reasons for declining participation in a prospective randomized trial to determine the optimum mode of delivery of the preterm breech. Control Clin Trials 11:226, 1990

Penn ZJ, Steer PJ, Grant A: A multicentre randomised controlled trial comparing elective and selective caesarean section for the delivery of the preterm breech infant. Br J Obstet Gynaecol 103:684, 1996

Petrikovsky BM, DeSilva HN, Fumia FD: Erb's palsy and fetal bruising after external cephalic version: Case report. Am J Obstet Gynecol 157:258, 1987

Phelan JP, Stine LE, Mueller E, McCart D, Yeh S: Observations of fetal heart rate characteristics related to external cephalic version and tocolysis. Am J Obstet Gynecol 149:658, 1984

Pinard A: On version by external maneuvers. In: Traite de Palper Abdominal. Paris, 1889

Pugh A: Treatise on midwifery chiefly with regard to the operation. London, 1754

Robertson AW, Kopelman JN, Read JA, Duff P, Magelssen DJ, Dashow EE: External cephalic version at term: Is a tocolytic necesary? Obstet Gynecol 70:896, 1987

Robertson PA, Foran CM, Croughan-Minihane MS, Kilpatrick SJ: Head entrapment and neonatal outcome by mode of delivery in breech deliveries from 28 to 36 weeks of gestation. Am J Obstet Gynecol 174:1742, 1996

Robertson PA, Foran CM, Croughan-Minihane MS, Kilpatrick SJ: Head entrapment and neonatal outcome by mode of delivery in breech deliveries from twenty-four to twenty-seven weeks of gestation. Am J Obstet Gynecol 173:1171, 1995

Rojansky N, Tanos V, Lewin A, Weinstein D: Sonographic evaluation of fetal heart extension and maternal pelvis in cases of breech presentation. Acta Obstet Gynecol Scand 73:607, 1994

Rolbin SH, Hew EM, Bernstein A: Uterine relaxation can be life saving. Can J Anesth 38:939, 1991

Roman J, Bakos O, Cnattingius S: Pregnancy outcomes by mode of delivery among term breech births: Swedish experience 1987–1993. Obstet Gynecol 92:945, 1998

Rosen NG, Chik L: Effect of delivery route on outcome of breech presentation. Am J Obstet Gynecol 48:909, 1984

Roumen FJME, Luyben AG: Safety of term vaginal breech delivery. Eur J Obstet Gynecol Reprod Biol 40:171, 1991

Rovinsky JJ, Miller JA, Kaplan S: Management of breech presentation at term. Am J Obstet Gynecol 115:497, 1973

Sandberg EC: The Zavanelli maneuver: 12 years of recorded expeience. Obstet Gynecol 93:312, 1999

Scheer K, Nubar J: Variation of fetal presentation with gestational age. Am J Obstet Gynecol 125:269, 1976

Schorr SJ, Speights SE, Ross EL, Bofill Ja, Rust OA, Norman PF, Morrison JC: A randomized trial of epidural anesthesia to improve external cephalic version success. Am J Obstet Gynecol 177:1133, 1997

Schutte MF, van Hemel OJS, van de Berg C, van de Pol A: Perinatal mortality in breech presentations as compared to vertex presentations in singleton pregnancies: An analysis based upon 57,819 computer-registered pregnancies in the Netherlands. Eur J Obstet Gynecol Reprod Biol 19:391, 1985

Smellie W: Smellie's treatise on the theory and practice of midwifery. In McClintock AH (ed): Vol I. London, New Sydenham Society, 1876, p 305

Socol ML, Cohen L, Depp R, Dooley SL, Tamura RK: Apgar scores and umbilical cord arterial pH in the breech neonate. Int J Gynecol Obstet 27:37, 1988

Soernes T, Bakke T: The length of the umbilical cord in vertex and breech presentations. Am J Obstet Gynecol 154:1086, 1986

Songane FF, Thobani S, Malik H, Bingham P, Lilford RJ: Balancing the risks of planned elective cesarean section and trial of vaginal delivery for the mature, selected, singleton breech presentation. J Perinat Med 15:531, 1987

Spellacy WN, Gravem H, Fish RO: The umbilical cord complications of true knots, nuchal cords, and cord around the body. Am J Obstet Gynecol 94:1136, 1966

Stine LE, Phelan JP, Wallace R, Eglinton GS, Van Dorsten JP, Schifrin BS: Update on external cephalic version performed at term. Obstet Gynecol 65:642, 1985

Susuki S, Yamamuro T: Fetal movement and fetal presentation. Early Hum Dev 11:255, 1985

Svenningsen NW, Westgren M, Ingemarsson I: Modern strategy for the term breech delivery—A study with a 4-year follow-up of the infants. J Perinat Med 13:117, 1985

Tan GW, Jen SW, Tan SL, Salmon YM: A prospective randomised controlled trial of external cephalic version comparing two methods of uterine tocolysis with a non-tocolysis group. Singapore Med J 30:155, 1989

Tank ES, Davis R, Holt JF, Morley GW: Mechanism of trauma during breech delivery. Obstet Gynecol 38:761, 1971

Thorpe-Beeston JG, Banfield PJ, Saunders NJ: Outcome of breech delivery at term. BMJ 305:746, 1992

Tiwary CM: Testicular injury in breech delivery: Possible implications. Urology 34:210, 1989

Van Dorsten JP, Schifrin BS, Wallace RL: Randomized control trial of external cephalic version with tocolysis in late pregnancy. Am J Obstet Gynecol 141:417, 1981

Van Loon AJ, Mantingh A, Serlier EK, Kroon G, Mooyaart EL, Huisjes HJ: Randomised controlled trial of magnetic-resonance pelvimetry in breech presentation at term. Lancet 350:1799, 1997

Van Veelen AJ, Van Cappellen AW, Flu PK, Straub MJ, Wallenburg HC: Effect of external cephalic version in late pregnancy on presentation at delivery: A randomized controlled trial. Br J Obstet Gynaecol 96:916, 1989

Vasa R, Kim MR: Fracture of the femur at cesarean section: Case report and review of literature. Am J Perinatol 7:46, 1990

Veit G: On version by external manipulation. Hamburgisches Magazin für die Geburtshilfe, 1907

Ventura SJ, Martin JA, Curtin SC, Mathews TJ: Births: Final data for 1997. National Vital Statistics Reports 47:1, 1999

Yanny H, Johanson R, Baldwin KJ, Lucking L, Fitzpatrick R, Jones P. Double-blind randomised controlled trial of glyceryl trinitrate spray for external cephalic version. Br J Obstet Gynaecol 107:562, 2000

Walter RS, Donaldson JS, Davis CL, Shkolnick A, Binns HJ, Carroll NC, Brouillette RT: Ultrasound screening of high-risk infants: A method to increase early detection of congenital dysplasia of the hip. Am J Dis Child 146:230, 1992

Westgren LMR, Songster G, Paul RH: Preterm breech delivery: Another retrospective study. Obstet Gynecol 66:481, 1985a

Westgren M, Edvall H, Nordstrom L, Svalenius E, Ranstam J: Spontaneous cephalic version of breech presentation in the last trimester. Br J Obstet Gynaecol 92:19, 1985b

Wolf H, Schaap AHP, Bruinse HW, Smolders-de Haas H, van Ertbruggen I, Treffers PE: Vaginal delivery compared with caesarean section in early preterm breech delivery: A comparison of long term outcome. Br J Obstet Gynaecol 106:486, 1999

Woodward RW, Callahan WE: Breech labor and delivery in the primigravida. Obstet Gynecol 34:260, 1969

Yanny H, Johanson R, Baldwin KJ, Lucking L, Fitzpatrick R, Jones P: Double-blind randomised controlled trial of glyceryl trinitrate spray for external cephalic version. Br J Obstet Gynaecol 107:562, 2000

Zhang J, Bowes WA, Fortney JA: Efficacy of external cephalic version, including safety, cost-benefit analysis, and impact on the cesarean delivery rate. Obstet Gynecol 82:306, 1993

Zlatnick FJ: The Iowa premature breech trial. Am J Perinatol 10:60, 1993

23

Cesarean Delivery and Postpartum Hysterectomy

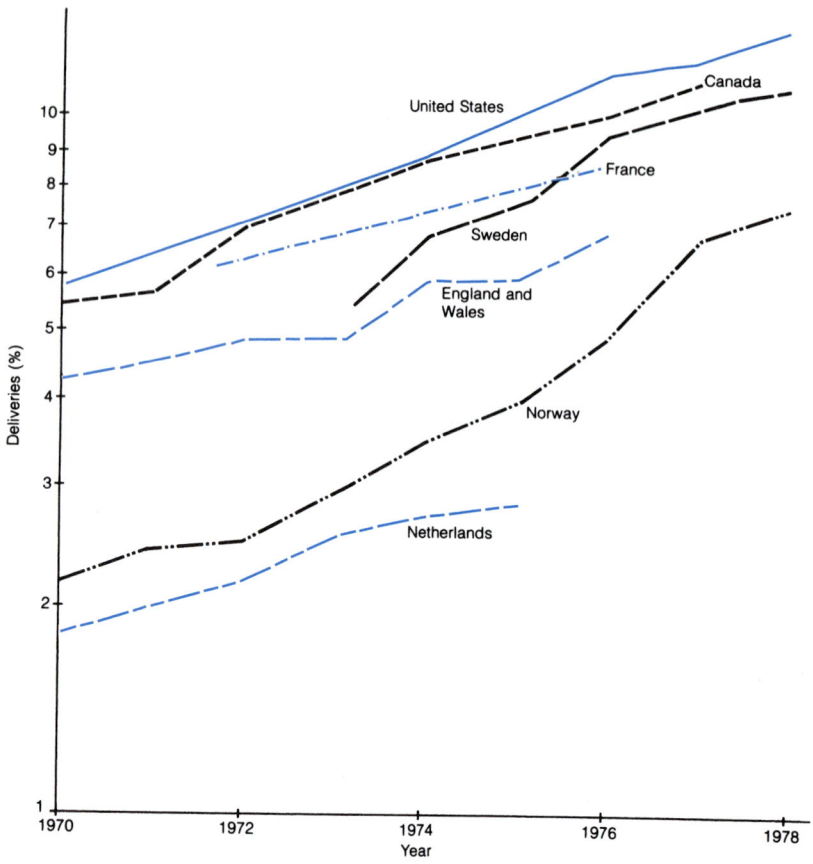

FIGURE 23-1. Percentage of deliveries by cesarean: Selected countries, 1970–1978. (From Smith, 1987.)

Cesarean delivery is defined as the birth of a fetus through incisions in the abdominal wall (laparotomy) and the uterine wall (hysterotomy). This definition does not include removal of the fetus from the abdominal cavity in the case of rupture of the uterus or in the case of an abdominal pregnancy.

CESAREAN DELIVERY

FREQUENCY. Currently, 1 out of every 10 American women delivered each year in the United States has had a previous cesarean delivery (Ventura and associates, 2000). This high prevalence represents the culmination of many years of escalating cesarean deliveries in the United States. Indeed, more than 825,000 women were delivered by cesarean in 1998, and 37 percent of these women had repeat procedures.

The overall cesarean delivery rate increased progressively in the United States each year between 1965 and 1988, rising from 4.5 percent of all deliveries to almost 25 percent (United States Public Health Service, 1991). Most of this increase took place in the 1970s and early 1980s and occurred throughout the western world (Fig. 23–1). According to Belizan and colleagues (1999), this

also occurred in Latin America. In one response to this increase, the United States Public Health Service (1991) set a goal of an overall 15 percent cesarean rate for the year 2000 (Fig. 23–2). An example of a unique response was the 1992 legislative mandate in Florida that stipulated dissemination of practice guidelines for obstetrical physicians (Studnicki and colleagues, 1997).

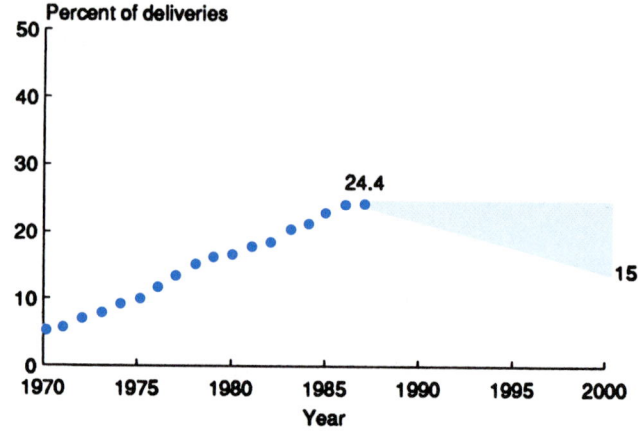

FIGURE 23-2. United States Public Health Service (1991) goal for the overall rate of cesarean delivery in the year 2000.

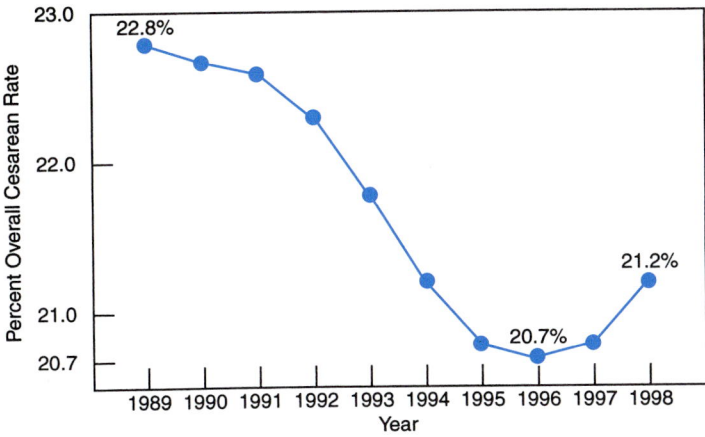

FIGURE 23–3. Percent overall cesarean delivery rate for the United State from 1989 to 1998. (From Ventura and associates, 2000.)

Between 1989 and 1996, and shown in Figure 23–3, the rate of cesarean delivery decreased in the United States. This was in large part due to increased vaginal birth after prior cesarean (VBAC) and to a lesser extent a small decrease in the primary cesarean rate (Table 23–1). As also shown in Figure 23–2 and Table 23–1, however, the rate of cesarean delivery has increased in the most recent years for which national data are available. Undoubtedly, one explanation for this change in direction of the national cesarean rate is increased concern about the fetal safety of labor in women with prior cesarean births (Sachs and colleagues, 1999).

It is now evident that the United States Public Health Service cesarean rate goal for the year 2000 was not achieved. The American College of Obstetricians and Gynecologists Task Force on Cesarean Delivery Rates (2000) has recommended two benchmarks for the United States for the year 2010:

1. A 15.5 percent cesarean rate in nulliparous women at 37 weeks or greater with singleton, cephalic presentations.
2. A 37 percent VBAC rate in women at 37 weeks or more with singleton cephalic presentations and one prior low-transverse cesarean delivery.

Reasons for quadrupling of the cesarean rate between 1965 and 1988 are not completely understood, but some explanations include the following.

1. There is **reduced parity,** and almost half of pregnant women are nulliparas. Therefore an increased number of cesarean births might be expected for conditions that are more common in nulliparous women.
2. Older women are having children. As shown in Figure 23–4 the frequency of cesarean deliveries increases with advancing age (see also Chap. 9, p. 208). In the past two decades, the rate of nulliparous births more than doubled for women aged 30 to 39 and increased by 50 percent in women 40 to 44 years old (Adashek and associates, 1993; Peipert and Bracken, 1993).
3. Since the early 1970s, **electronic fetal monitoring** has been used extensively. There is little question that this technique is associated with an increased cesarean rate compared with intermittent fetal heart rate auscultation. Although cesarean delivery performed primarily for "fetal distress" comprises only a minority of all such procedures, in many more cases concern for an abnormal fetal heart rate tracing prompts operative delivery with the listed indication being some form of labor arrest.
4. By 1990, 83 percent of all **breech presentations** were delivered abdominally (Notzon and associates, 1994).

TABLE 23–1. Total, Primary Cesarean and Vaginal Birth Rates After Previous Cesarean Delivery: United States, 1989–1998

Year	Cesarean Rate per 100 Deliveries		
	Total[a]	Primary[b]	VBAC Rate[c]
1989	22.8	16.1	18.9
1990	22.7	16.0	19.9
1991	22.6	15.9	21.3
1992	22.3	15.6	22.6
1993	21.8	15.3	24.3
1994	21.2	14.9	26.3
1995	20.8	14.7	27.5
1996	20.7	14.6	28.3
1997	20.8	14.6	27.4
1998	21.2	14.9	26.3

[a]Percent of all live births by cesarean delivery.
[b]Number of primary cesareans per 100 live births to women who have not had a previous cesarean.
[c]Number of vaginal births after previous cesarean (VBAC) delivery per 100 live births to women with a previous cesarean delivery.

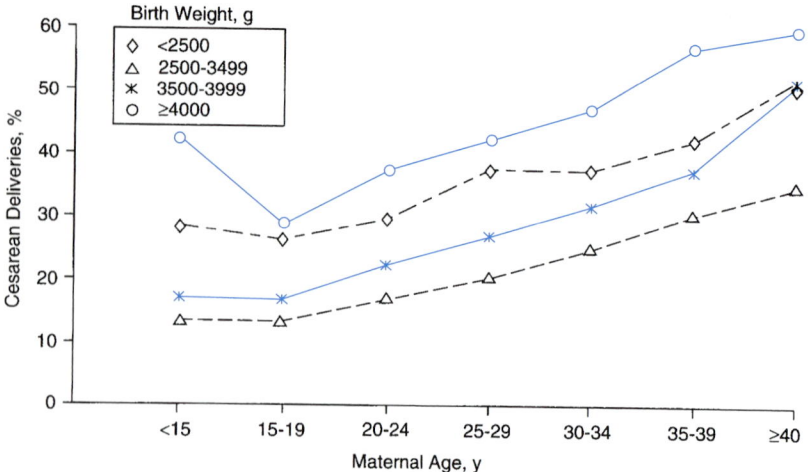

FIGURE 23–4. Primary cesarean deliveries by maternal age and birthweight among nulliparous women in Washington State, 1987–1990. (From Parrish and co-workers, 1994, with permission.)

5. The incidence of **midpelvic vaginal deliveries** has decreased. Indeed, according to the American College of Obstetricians and Gynecologists (1994), operative vaginal deliveries performed at stations higher than +2 should be performed only in rare emergencies and with simultaneous preparation for cesarean delivery.

6. Concern for **malpractice litigation** has contributed significantly to the present cesarean delivery rate. Failure to perform a cesarean and thus avoid adverse neonatal neurological outcome or cerebral palsy is the dominant claim in obstetrical malpractice litigation in the United States (Physicians Insurance Association of America, 1992). This trend is especially troubling in view of the well-documented lack of association between cesarean delivery and any reduction in childhood neurological problems, including both cerebral palsy and seizures (Lien and co-workers 1995; Scheller and Nelson, 1994).

7. Socioeconomic and demographic factors may play a role in cesarean birth rates. Gould and associates (1989) reported that the primary cesarean delivery rate in Los Angeles County was 23 percent for women from areas with a median family income of more than $30,000 compared with 13 percent for women with a median income less than $11,000. Similarly, Stafford (1990) reported significantly fewer vaginal births after a prior cesarean when comparing for-profit hospitals with university hospitals, those with private insurance with indigent patients, and low-volume to high-volume hospitals. Other factors implicated include unexplained variations in cesarean rates after risk adjustment, as shown in Figure 23–5.

According to the American College of Obstetricians and Gynecologists (2000), the highest variation occurs among nulliparous women with term singleton fetuses with cephalic presentation and without other complications. High-risk patients have much lower variations in cesarean delivery rates between practitioners and hospitals.

INDICATIONS. As shown in Table 23–2, repeat cesarean deliveries and those performed for labor dystocia have been the leading indications both in the United States and other western industrialized countries. Although it is not possible to catalog comprehensively all appropriate indications for cesarean delivery, over 85 percent are performed because of:

1. Prior cesareans.
2. Labor dystocia.
3. Fetal distress.
4. Breech presentation.

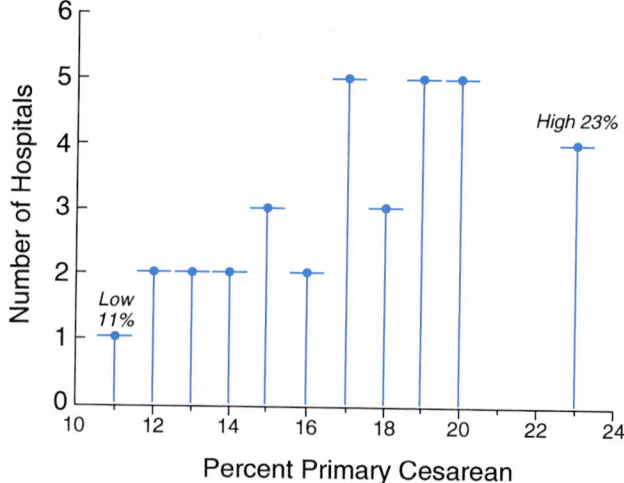

FIGURE 23–5. Risk-adjusted primary cesarean rates for 35 hospitals, representing 63,318 births, in the Dallas-Ft. Worth metroplex for 1995. (Data provided by Dallas-Ft. Worth Hospital Council Data Initiative.)

TABLE 23–2. Percent of Patients with Each Indication Delivered by Cesarean in Four Countries, 1990

Indication	Norway	Scotland	Sweden	United States
Previous section	94.3	86.7	47.1	80.5
Breech	60.8	79.6	66.3	83.1
Dystocia	31.6	34.6	22.8	59.7
Fetal distress	42.5	15.1	35.4	36.6
Other	4.7	4.0	3.1	4.6
Total	12.8	14.2	10.7	23.6

From Notzon and colleagues (1994), with permission.

PRIOR CESAREAN DELIVERY. For many years, the scarred uterus was believed to contraindicate labor out of fear of uterine rupture. In 1916, Cragin made his famous and now seemingly excessive pronouncement, "Once a cesarean, always a cesarean." It must be remembered, however, that when Cragin made this statement, obstetricians routinely used a "classical" vertical incision in the uterus. Indeed, the Kerr transverse incision was not recommended until 1921. It should also be pointed out that some of Cragin's contemporaries did not agree with his statement. Writing in the fourth edition of *Williams Obstetrics*, J. Whitridge Williams (1917) termed the statement "an exaggeration."

The year 1978 was an important year in the history of prior cesarean delivery. Merrill and Gibbs (1978) reported from the University of Texas at San Antonio that subsequent vaginal delivery was safely attempted in 83 percent of their patients with prior cesarean deliveries. This report served to rekindle interest in vaginal birth after prior cesarean (VBAC) at a time when only 2 percent of American women who had previously undergone cesarean birth were attempting vaginal delivery. Use of VBAC increased very significantly in the United States such that there was a 14-fold increase to 28 percent of women with prior cesareans delivering vaginally by 1996 (Table 23–1). Dr. Roy Pitkin, editor of *Obstetrics and Gynecology*, wrote in 1991 that ". . . without question, the most remarkable change in obstetric practice over the last decade was management of the woman with prior cesarean delivery."

Beginning in 1989, there have been several reports published from around the United States and Canada that suggest that VBAC may be riskier than anticipated (Leveno, 1999). For example, Scott (1991) suggested an "alternative viewpoint on mandatory trial of labor" based upon experiences with uterine rupture in Utah. He described 12 women who experienced uterine rupture during a trial of labor. Two women required hysterectomy, there were three perinatal deaths, and two infants suffered significant long-term neurological impairment. Porter and colleagues (1998) subsequently reported that there were 26 uterine ruptures in Salt Lake City between 1990 and 1996 and that 23 percent of the infants were dead or damaged as a result of intrapartum asphyxia.

Reports such as these raised serious concern about the safety of VBAC and have contributed to heightened controversy (Flamm, 1997). Indeed, the American College of Obstetricians and Gynecologists issued an updated Practice Bulletin in 1998 and 1999 urging a more cautious approach to attempting a trial of labor. In part, it reads: "Because uterine rupture may be catastrophic, VBAC should be attempted in institutions equipped to respond to emergencies with physicians immediately available to provide emergency care."

The American College of Obstetricians and Gynecologists (1999) observed that "It has become apparent that VBAC is associated with a small but significant risk of uterine rupture with poor outcomes for both mother and infant. . . . These developments, which have led to a more circumspect approach to trial of labor by even the most ardent supporters of VBAC, illustrate the need to reevaluate VBAC recommendations." In this section we will emphasize current VBAC recommendations (Table 23–3) by the American College of Obstetricians and Gynecologists (1998, 1999), which although urging caution, also strongly supports VBAC.

Recent reports from Northwestern Hospital in Chicago support the safety of VBAC as well as its cost-effectiveness in women with one or two prior low-transverse uterine incisions (Grobman and associates, 2000; Socol and Peaceman, 1999). Clark and colleagues (2000) concluded differently after comparing total medical costs of a trial of labor with those of elective repeat cesarean delivery. They found that "when costs as opposed to charges are considered and the cost of long-term care for neurologically injured infants is taken into account, trial of labor after previous cesarean is unlikely to be associated with a significant cost saving for the health care system."

TABLE 23–3. Recommendations of the American College of Obstetricians and Gynecologists (1999) for Selection of Candidates for Vaginal Birth after Cesarean Delivery (VBAC)

Selection Criteria
One or two prior low-transverse cesarean deliveries
Clinically adequate pelvis
No other uterine scars or previous rupture
Physician immediately available throughout active labor capable of monitoring labor and performing an emergency cesarean delivery
Availability of anesthesia and personnel for emergency cesarean delivery

From the American College of Obstetricians and Gynecologists (1999), with permission.

TYPE OF PRIOR UTERINE INCISION. Patients with transverse scars confined to the lower uterine segment have a small risk of symptomatic scar separation during a subsequent pregnancy. Shown in Table 23–4 are the rates of uterine rupture reported for various types of uterine incision at cesarean delivery. Generally, the lowest rates of rupture have been reported for low-transverse incisions and the highest for incisions extending into the fundus—the classical incision. Greene and colleagues (1997) reported a 7 percent uterine rupture rate before labor in 62 women with classical uterine incisions. The rates of uterine rupture have been reported to be similarly high (8 percent) in women with prior cesarean deliveries and unicornuate, bicornuate, didelphic, and septate uterine malformations (Ravasia and associates, 1999).

The rate of uterine rupture in women with prior vertical incisions not extending into the fundus is controversial. Given the indications today for vertical incisions, however, few do not extend into the active segment. Martin and co-authors (1997) and Shipp and colleagues

TABLE 23–4. Rates of Uterine Rupture According to the Type and Location of the Previous Uterine Incision

Type of Uterine Incision	Estimated Rupture (%)
Classical	4–9
T-shaped	4–9
Low-vertical	1–7
Low-transverse	0.2–1.5

From the American College of Obstetricians and Gynecologists (1999), with permission.

(1999) reported that women with prior low-vertical uterine incisions were not at increased risk for uterine rupture compared with women with transverse incisions. The American College of Obstetricians and Gynecologists (1999) concluded that although there is limited or inconsistent scientific evidence, women with a vertical incision within the lower uterine segment that does not extend into the fundus may be candidates for VBAC. In contrast, prior classical or T-shaped uterine incisions were considered contraindications to VBAC.

Women who have previously sustained a uterine rupture are at increased risk for recurrence. Those with a rupture confined to the lower segment were reported to have a 6 percent recurrence risk in subsequent labor, whereas those whose prior rupture included the upper uterus had a 32 percent recurrence risk (Reyes-Ceja and associates, 1969; Ritchie, 1971).

We are of the view that ideally women with prior uterine ruptures or classical or T-shaped incisions are delivered by cesarean upon achievement of fetal pulmonary maturity prior to the onset of labor, and that such women should be warned of the hazards of unattended labor and signs of possible uterine rupture. In preparing an operative report following any vertical uterine incision, it is essential to document the exact extent of the scar in a manner that cannot be misunderstood by subsequent surgeons.

NUMBER OF PRIOR CESAREANS. The risk of uterine rupture increases with the number of previous incisions. Miller and colleagues (1994) in a study of 12,707 women undergoing a trial of labor after cesarean delivery, reported rates of 0.6 percent and 1.8 percent for those with one and two prior cesareans deliveries, respectively. Caughey and colleagues (1999) compared uterine rupture rates in 3757 women with one prior uterine scar with 134 women with two prior incisions. The type of prior uterine incision was not specified other than to mention that classical incisions were usually delivered by elective repeat cesarean. The rate of uterine rupture was significantly increased fivefold in women with two previous uterine scars compared with those with one scar (3.7 percent versus 0.8 percent). The American College of Obstetricians and Gynecologists (1999) has taken the position that women with two prior low-transverse cesarean deliveries may be considered for VBAC (Table 23–3).

INDICATION FOR PRIOR CESAREAN. The success rate for trial of labor depends to a small extent upon the indication for the previous cesarean. Generally, about 60 to 80 percent of trials of labor after prior cesarean birth result in vaginal delivery (American College of Obstetricians and Gynecologists, 1999). The success rates are somewhat improved when the original cesarean was performed for breech presentation or fetal distress compared with dystocia. For example, in one large series, the VBAC success rate for women whose first cesarean was for breech presentation was 91 percent and the success rate was 84 percent when fetal distress was the original indication (Wing and Paul, 1998). In contrast, the success rate dropped to 77 percent in those with dystocia as the indication for cesarean delivery.

Impey and O'Herlihy (1998) reported that even when the strictest criteria are used to diagnose dystocia, a VBAC rate of 68 percent can be achieved. Hoskins and Gomez (1997) analyzed VBAC success rates in 1917 women in relation to the cervical dilation they achieved before the original cesarean delivery was performed for dystocia. The VBAC success rate was 67 percent for those whose cesarean was done at cervical dilatation of 5 cm or less, and it was 73 percent when the cervix was 6 to 9 cm dilated. The VBAC success rate fell to 13 percent when dystocia had been diagnosed in the second stage of labor. In contrast, Jongen and colleagues (1998) reported an 80 percent VBAC success rate in women delivered after prior cesarean performed during the second stage.

Previous vaginal delivery, either before or after a cesarean birth, significantly improves the prognosis for successful VBAC (Caughey and colleagues, 1998; Flamm and Geiger, 1997). Indeed, the most favorable prognostic factor is prior vaginal delivery.

According to the American College of Obstetricians and Gynecologists (1999), there has been a tendency to expand the indications for which VBAC may be appropriate. These include multiple previous cesarean deliveries, unknown uterine scar, breech presentation, twin gestation, postterm pregnancy, and suspected macrosomia. It has recommended, and we agree, that continuing study be done of the risk of adverse outcome before VBAC is routinely accepted in these circumstances.

ELECTIVE STERILIZATION. Desire for permanent sterilization in a woman with prior cesarean is not an indication for a repeat operation because the morbidity of vaginal birth and postpartum tubal ligation is considerably less than that of a repeat cesarean.

OXYTOCIN AND EPIDURAL ANALGESIA. Use of oxytocin to induce or augment labor has been implicated in uterine ruptures in women with prior cesarean deliveries. Turner (1997) observed that 13 of the 15 women with uterine ruptures encountered at the Coombe Hospital in Dublin between 1982 and 1991 occurred in women with prior cesareans and who had received an oxytoxic agent, usually for induction of labor.

In contrast, cautious use of intravenous oxytocin to *augment* labor in women with prior cesarean at this hospital was rarely associated with uterine rupture. Zelop and associates (1999) analyzed uterine ruptures at Brigham and Women's Hospital after induced or augmented labor in women with one prior cesarean delivery. Uterine rupture occurred in 2.3 percent of those induced compared with 1 and 0.4 percent of those whose labor was augmented or spontaneous, respectively. They urged caution when using oxytocin for labor stimulation in women with prior cesarean delivery. The American College of Obstetricians and Gynecologists (1999) has recommended close patient monitoring when oxytocin or prostaglandin gel are used in women with prior cesareans and undergoing a trial of labor.

The use of epidural analgesia has been debated in the past out of fear that such a technique might mask the pain of uterine rupture. In actuality, however, less than 10 percent of women with scar separation experience pain and bleeding, and fetal heart rate decelerations are the most likely sign of such an event (Flamm and associates, 1990). Several studies attest to the safety of properly conducted epidural analgesia (Farmer and colleagues, 1991; Flamm and associates, 1994).

EXAMINING THE SCAR. Although some obstetricians routinely document the integrity of the old scar by palpation following successful vaginal delivery, such uterine exploration is felt to be unnecessary by others. Currently it is not known what effect documentation of an asymptomatic scar has on subsequent reproduction or route of delivery. There is general agreement, however, that surgical correction of a scar dehiscence is necessary only if significant bleeding is encountered. Asymptomatic separations do not generally require exploratory laparotomy and repair.

ELECTIVE REPEAT CESAREAN DELIVERY. If repeat cesarean is elected, it is essential that fetal maturity be achieved prior to elective delivery. The American College of Obstetricians and Gynecologists (1991/1995) has established guidelines for timing an elective operation. According to these criteria, elective delivery may be considered at or beyond 39 weeks if at least one of the criteria outlined in Table 23–5 are met. In all other instances, fetal pulmonary maturity must be documented by amnionic fluid analysis before elective repeat cesarean is undertaken (Chap. 39, p. 1042). Alternately, the onset of spontaneous labor is awaited.

LABOR DYSTOCIA. This is the most frequent indication for primary cesarean delivery in the United States. An analysis of labor dystocia as a contributing factor to the cesarean rate is difficult, however, because of the heterogeneity inherent in the condition (Chap. 18). According to Notzon and associates (1994), there are 15 different ICD-9 codes describing cesarean delivery for

TABLE 23–5. Criteria for Timing of Elective Repeat Cesarean Delivery

At least one of these criteria must be met in a woman with normal menstrual cycles and no immediate antecedent use of oral contraceptives:

1. Fetal heart sounds have been documented for 20 weeks by nonelectronic fetoscope or for 30 weeks by Doppler.
2. It has been 36 weeks since a positive serum or urine chorionic gonadotropin pregnancy test was performed by a reliable laboratory.
3. An ultrasound measurement of the crown-rump length, obtained at 6–11 weeks, supports a gestational age of at least 39 weeks.
4. An ultrasound obtained at 12–20 weeks confirms the gestational age of at least 39 weeks determined by clinical history and physical examination.

labor dystocia! Descriptive terms vary from more precise definitions promulgated by Friedman (1978)—secondary arrest of dilatation, arrest of descent—to more ambiguous and commonly used terms such as *cephalopelvic disproportion* and *failure to progress*. It is meaningless to classify cesarean delivery performed after 8 hours of contractions at 3 cm dilatation for "failure to progress" in the same category as a woman undergoing cesarean delivery for arrest of descent after 3 hours of second-stage pushing with uterine contractions demonstrating 300 Montevideo units.

FETAL DISTRESS. The 1970s witnessed the development of electronic fetal heart rate monitoring as well as elegant descriptions of various fetal heart rate patterns and their association with fetal oxygenation and acid–base status. Such observations raised hopes that widespread recognition of various subtle parameters of "uteroplacental insufficiency" and timely cesarean delivery would allow the obstetrician to avoid childhood neurological abnormalities including cerebral palsy. Despite relatively poor specificity in the prediction of an abnormal newborn, a lack of scientific foundation for defining "normal" and "abnormal" newborn acid–base status, and widespread disagreement among experts regarding fetal heart rate interpretation, prompt recognition of various subtle patterns was often seen as the key to diagnosing "fetal distress" and preventing neurological damage (Chap. 14, p. 349).

Subsequently, it has become well established that management based upon electronic monitoring neither reduces the risk of cerebral palsy, nor improves any measurable indices of newborn outcome compared with intermittent heart rate auscultation (American College of Obstetricians and Gynecologists, 1992, 1995b; Free-

man, 1992; Nelson and co-workers, 1996). Scheller and Nelson (1994), in a report from the National Institutes of Health, and Lien and associates (1995) presented data specifically refuting any association between cesarean delivery and either cerebral palsy or seizures.

The American College of Obstetricians and Gynecologists (1992) recommends that facilities giving obstetrical care have the capability of initiating a cesarean delivery within 30 minutes of the decision for operation. This recommendation addresses facilities and does not govern clinical decision making. Misinterpretations of this guideline are common. There is no nationally recognized standard of care that codifies an acceptable time interval for performance of cesarean delivery. In most instances, operative delivery is **not** necessary within this 30-minute time frame. Indeed, Chauhan and co-workers (1997) reported that failure to achieve a cesarean decision-to-incision time of less than 30 minutes was not associated with a negative impact on neonatal outcome. In many cases of cesarean for indications such as labor arrest, a timely cesarean often will involve an interval considerably in excess of 30 minutes. On the other hand, when faced with an acute, catastrophic deterioration in fetal condition, cesarean may be indicated as rapidly as possible, and purposeful delays of any time period would be inappropriate.

BREECH PRESENTATION. Fetuses presenting as a breech are at increased risk of cord prolapse and head entrapment if delivered vaginally compared with those presenting cephalic. Nevertheless, prospective controlled trials are suggestive that with proper selection, certain fetuses may be delivered vaginally in breech presentations with minimal risk. The indications for cesarean versus vaginal delivery are discussed in Chapter 22. Suffice it to say, concern for fetal injury, as well as the infrequency with which a breech fetus meets criteria for a trial of labor, make it unlikely that significant reduction in the cesarean birth rate will come from a more liberal approach to vaginal breech delivery.

METHODS TO DECREASE CESAREAN DELIVERY RATES. Several investigators have documented the feasibility of achieving significant reductions in institutional cesarean rates without increased perinatal morbidity or mortality (DeMott, 1990; DeMuylder, 1990; Porreco, 1990; Pridijian, 1991; Sanchez-Ramos, 1990, and their co-workers). Programs aimed at reducing unnecessary cesarean deliveries are generally focused upon educational efforts and peer review, encouraging a trial of labor after prior transverse cesareans, and restricting cesareans for labor dystocia to women who meet strictly defined criteria.

TABLE 23–6. Maternal Mortality According to Delivery Method in Israel, 1984 to 1992

Delivery Method	Number	Maternal Mortality (per 100,000 births)
Vaginal	797,489	3.6
Cesarean		
Total	119,165	21.8
Emergency	83,416	30
Elective	35,749	2.8

From Yoles and Maschiach (1998).

MATERNAL MORTALITY AND MORBIDITY. In the United States, maternal death associated with cesarean delivery is rare. In 1980, Frigoletto and colleagues reported a series of 10,000 consecutive cesareans with no maternal deaths. In 1988, Sachs and associates observed only seven deaths as a direct result of cesarean births in over 121,000 cesareans performed between 1976 and 1984. In 1990, Lilford and co-workers, while documenting a sevenfold relative risk for maternal mortality associated with cesarean delivery, observed that most deaths were associated with complicated nonelective procedures. Indeed, the relative risk of death for elective cesareans under epidural analgesia was actually *lower* than that associated with all vaginal births. Yoles and Maschiach (1998) reviewed all deliveries in Israel between 1984 and 1992, and as shown in Table 23–6, the excess maternal mortality associated with cesarean delivery was attributable to emergency procedures rather than elective operations.

There is no doubt that maternal morbidity is increased dramatically in cesarean compared with vaginal delivery. Principle sources are endomyometritis, hemorrhage, urinary tract infection, and thromboembolism. As discussed in Chapter 48 (p. 1298), morbidity associated with cesarean delivery is increased dramatically in obese women (Isaacs and associates, 1994; Perlow and Morgan, 1994). These factors, as well as the increased recovery time associated with cesareans, result in a twofold increase in costs for cesarean compared with vaginal delivery (Book of Health Insurance Data, 1993).

BIRTH TRAUMA. Although cesarean delivery is sometimes performed in cases of malpresentation or with known excessive fetal size in an effort to avoid birth trauma, it is incorrect to assume that a cesarean delivery provides a guarantee against such injury. Numerous reports attest to the occurrence of Erb palsy, skull fractures, and fractures of other long bones in infants delivered by cesarean (Kaplan and colleagues, 1987; Skajaa and associates, 1987; Vasa and Kim, 1990).

TECHNIQUE FOR CESAREAN DELIVERY

ABDOMINAL INCISIONS

VERTICAL INCISION. An infraumbilical midline vertical incision is quickest to make. The incision should be of sufficient length to allow delivery of the infant without difficulty. Therefore, its length should correspond with the estimated fetal size. Sharp dissection is performed to the level of the anterior rectus sheath, which is freed of subcutaneous fat to expose a strip of fascia in the midline about 2 cm wide. Some surgeons prefer to incise the rectus sheath with the scalpel throughout the length of the fascial incision. Others prefer to make a small opening and then incise the fascial layer with scissors. The rectus and the pyramidalis muscles are separated in the midline by sharp and blunt dissection to expose transversalis fascia and peritoneum.

The transversalis fascia and preperitoneal fat are dissected carefully to reach the underlying peritoneum. The peritoneum near the upper end of the incision is opened carefully. Some surgeons elevate the peritoneum with two hemostats placed about 2 cm apart. The tented fold of peritoneum between the clamps is then visualized and palpated to be sure that omentum, bowel, or bladder are not adjacent. In women who have had previous intra-abdominal surgery, including cesareans, omentum or bowel may be adherent to the undersurface of the peritoneum. The peritoneum is incised superiorly to the upper pole of the incision and downward to just above the peritoneal reflection over the bladder.

TRANSVERSE INCISIONS. With the modified **Pfannenstiel incision,** the skin and subcutaneous tissue are incised using a lower transverse, slightly curvilinear incision. The incision is made at the level of the pubic hairline and is extended somewhat beyond the lateral borders of the rectus muscles. After the subcutaneous tissue has been separated from the underlying fascia for 1 cm or so on each side, the fascia is incised transversely the full length of the incision. The superior and inferior edges of the fascia are grasped with suitable clamps and then elevated by the assistant as the operator separates the fascial sheath from the underlying rectus muscles by blunt dissection with the scalpel handle. Blood vessels coursing between the muscles and fascia are clamped, cut, and ligated. Meticulous hemostasis is imperative. The fascial separation is carried near enough to the umbilicus to permit an adequate midline longitudinal incision of the peritoneum. The rectus muscles are then separated in the midline to expose the underlying peritoneum. The peritoneum is opened as discussed earlier. Closure in layers is carried out the same as with a vertical skin incision.

The cosmetic advantage of the transverse skin incision is apparent. While most believe the incision is stronger and less likely to undergo dehiscence, Hendrix and co-workers (2000) provided evidence that this is not the case. There are some disadvantages in its use. Exposure of the pregnant uterus and appendages in some women is not as good as with a vertical incision. Whenever more room is needed, the vertical incision can be rapidly extended around and above the umbilicus, whereas the Pfannenstiel incision cannot. If the woman is obese, the operative field may be even more restricted. In terms of morbidity it is not appropriate to compare the vertical incision, often performed under adverse conditions, with the transverse incision carried out under much more favorable circumstances. Importantly, at the time of repeat cesarean, reentry through a Pfannenstiel incision is likely to be more time consuming because of scarring.

When a transverse incision is desired and more room is needed, the **Maylard incision** provides a safe option. In this incision, the rectus muscles are divided with scissors or a scalpel. The incision may also be especially useful in women with significant scarring resulting from previous Pfannenstiel incisions. In the study by Ayers and Morley (1987), the mean incision length was 18.3 cm with the Maylard incision compared with 14.0 cm for the Pfannenstiel incision.

UTERINE INCISIONS. The so-called **classical cesarean incision,** a vertical incision into the body of the uterus above the lower uterine segment and reaching the uterine fundus, is seldom used today. Most always the incision is made in the lower uterine segment transversely (Kerr, 1926) or, less often, vertically (Krönig, 1912). The lower-segment transverse incision has the advantage of requiring only modest dissection of the bladder from the underlying myometrium. If the incision extends laterally, a laceration may involve one or both of the uterine vessels. The low-vertical incision may be extended upward so that in those circumstances where more room is needed, the incision can be carried into the body of the uterus. More extensive dissection of the bladder is necessary to keep the vertical incision within the lower uterine segment. Moreover, if the vertical incision extends downward, it may tear through the cervix into the vagina and possibly involve the bladder. Importantly, during the next pregnancy a vertical incision that extends into the upper myometrium is more likely to rupture than a transverse incision, especially during labor.

For a cephalic presentation, a transverse incision through the lower uterine segment is most often the operation of choice. Generally, the transverse incision:

1. Is easier to repair.
2. Is located at a site least likely to rupture with extrusion of the fetus into the abdominal cavity during a subsequent pregnancy.
3. Does not promote adherence of bowel or omentum to the incisional line.

TECHNIQUE FOR TRANSVERSE CESAREAN INCISION. Commonly, the uterus is found to be dextrorotated so that the left round ligament is more anterior and closer to the midline than the right. With thick meconium or infected amnionic fluid, some operators prefer to lay a moistened laparotomy pack in each lateral peritoneal gutter to absorb fluid and blood that escape from the opened uterus.

Typically the rather loose reflection of peritoneum above the upper margin of the bladder and overlying the anterior lower uterine segment is grasped in the midline with forceps and incised with a scalpel or scissors (Fig. 23–6). Scissors are inserted between the serosa and myometrium of the lower uterine segment and are pushed laterally from the midline, while partially opening the blades intermittently, to separate a 2-cm-wide strip of serosa, which is then incised. As the lateral margin on each side is approached, the scissors are aimed somewhat more cephalad (Fig. 23–7). The lower flap of peritoneum is elevated and the bladder is gently separated by blunt or sharp dissection from the underlying myometrium (Fig. 23–8). In general, the separation of bladder should not exceed 5 cm in depth and usually less. It is

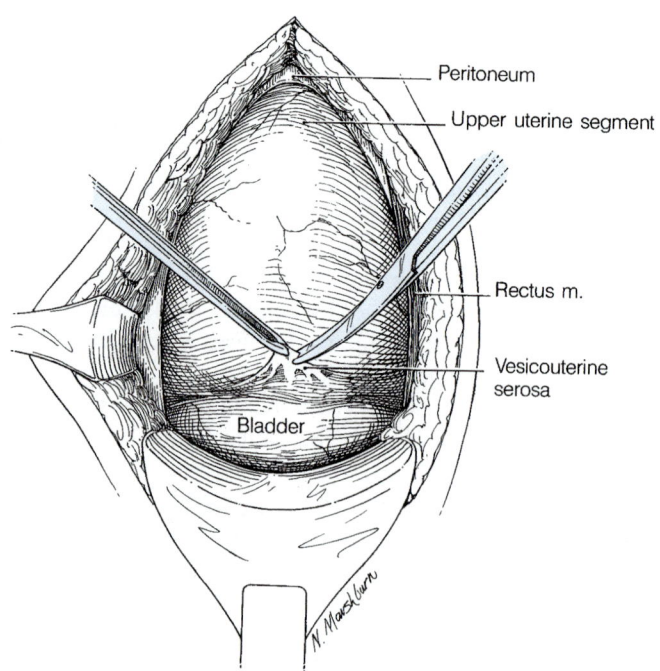

FIGURE 23–6. The loose vesicouterine serosa is grasped with the forceps. The hemostat tip points to the upper margin of the bladder. The retractor is firm against the symphysis.

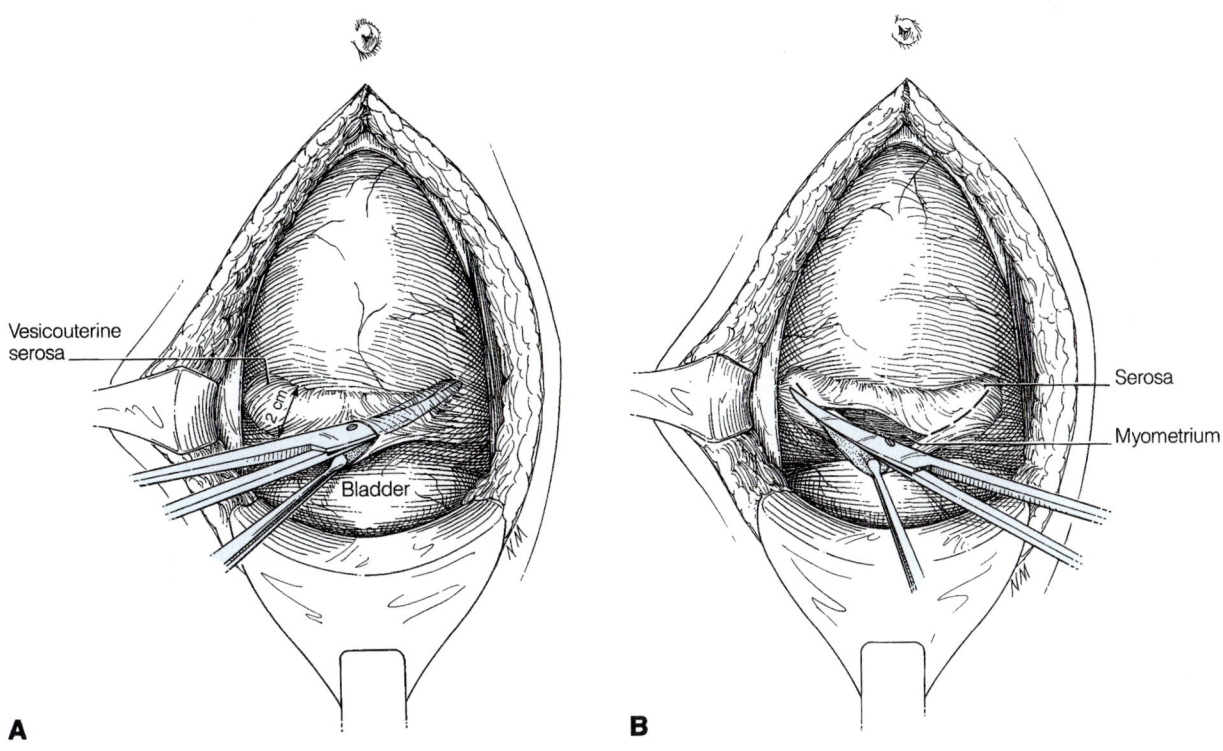

FIGURE 23–7. The loose serosa above the upper margin of the bladder is elevated and incised laterally.

possible, especially with an effaced, dilated cervix, to dissect downward so deeply as inadvertently to expose and then enter the underlying vagina rather than the lower uterine segment.

The uterus is opened through the lower uterine segment about 1 cm below the upper margin of the peritoneal reflection. It is important to place the uterine inci-

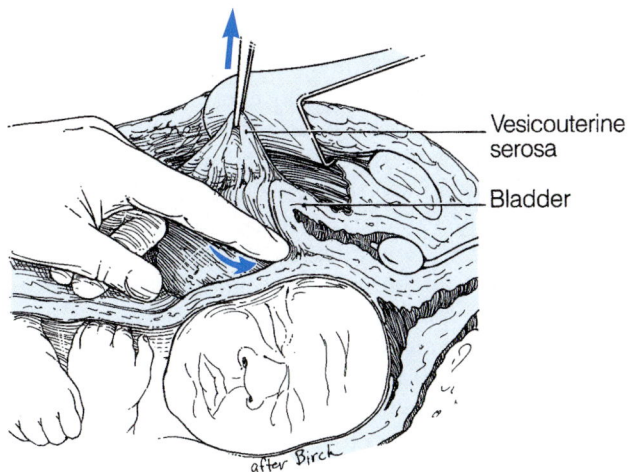

FIGURE 23–8. Low-segment cesarean. Cross-section showing dissection of bladder off uterus to expose lower uterine segment.

sion relatively higher in women with advanced or complete cervical dilatation in order to minimize lateral extension of the incision into the uterine arteries. The uterine incision can be made by a variety of techniques. Each is initiated by incising with a scalpel the exposed lower uterine segment transversely for 1 to 2 cm or so halfway between the latter margins. This must be done carefully so as to cut completely through the uterine wall but not deeply enough to wound the underlying fetus (Fig. 23–9). Careful blunt entry using hemostats to split the muscle may be helpful. Once the uterus is opened, the incision can be extended by cutting laterally and then slightly upward with bandage scissors. Alternatively, when the lower uterine segment is thin, the entry incision can be extended by simply spreading the incision, using lateral and upward pressure applied with each index finger (Fig. 23–10). Rodriguez and associates (1994) demonstrated that blunt and sharp extensions of the initial uterine incision are equivalent in terms of safely and postoperative complications. **It is very important to make the uterine incision large enough to allow delivery of the head and trunk of the fetus without either tearing into or having to cut into the uterine arteries and veins that course through the lateral margins of the uterus.** If the placenta is encountered in the line of incision, it must either be detached or incised. When the placenta is incised, fetal hemorrhage may be

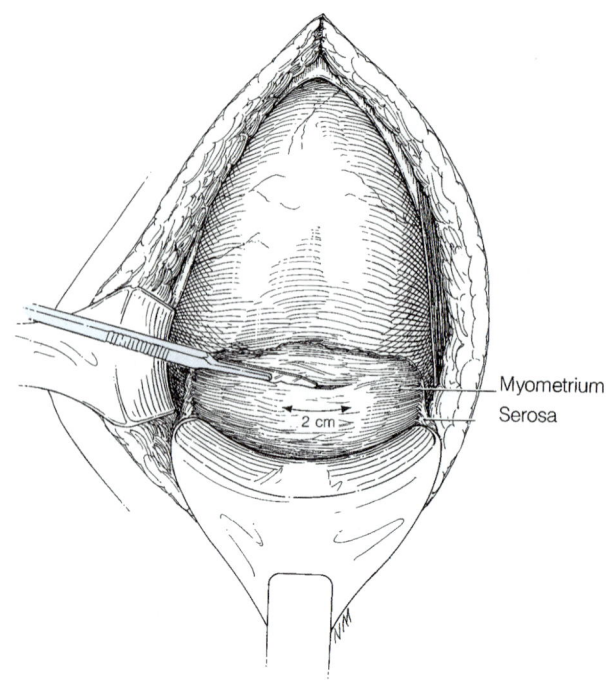

FIGURE 23–9. The myometrium is being incised carefully to avoid cutting the fetal head.

severe, and thus, the cord should be clamped as soon as possible in such cases.

DELIVERY OF THE INFANT. In cephalic presentation, a hand is slipped into the uterine cavity between the symphysis and fetal head, and the head is elevated gently

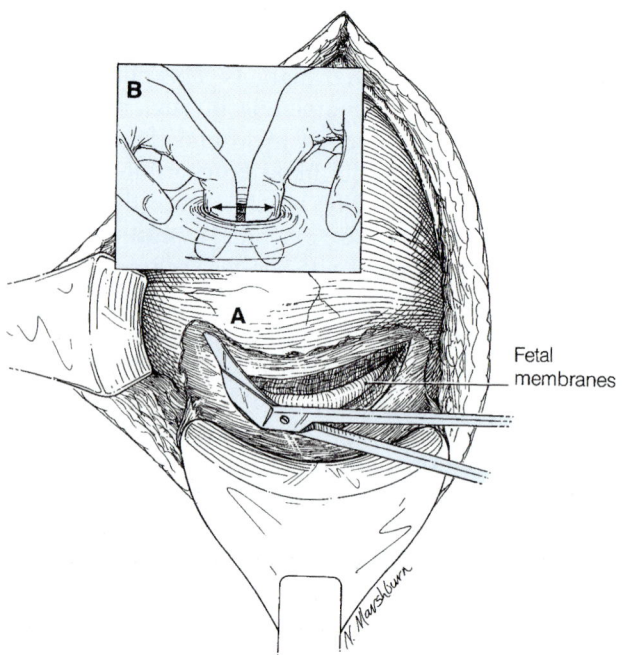

FIGURE 23–10. After entering the uterine cavity, the incision is extended laterally with either fingers or bandage scissors.

with the fingers and palm through the incision aided by modest transabdominal fundal pressure (Fig. 23–11). After a long labor with cephalopelvic disproportion, the fetal head may be rather tightly wedged in the birth canal. Upward pressure exerted through the vagina by an assistant will help to dislodge the head and allow its delivery above the symphysis. To minimize aspiration by the fetus of amnionic fluid and its contents, the exposed nares and mouth are aspirated with a bulb syringe before the thorax is delivered. The shoulders then are delivered using gentle traction plus fundal pressure. The rest of the body readily follows.

As soon as the shoulders are delivered (Fig. 23–12), an intravenous infusion containing about 20 units of oxytocin per liter is allowed to flow at a brisk rate of 10 mL/min until the uterus contracts satisfactorily, after which the rate can be reduced. Bolus doses of 5 to 10 units are avoided due to associated hypotension. The cord is clamped with the infant held at the level of the abdominal wall, and the infant is given to the member of the team who will conduct resuscitative efforts as they are needed.

If the fetus is not presenting cephalic, of if there are multiple fetuses or a very immature fetus in a woman who has had no labor, a vertical incision through the lower segment may, at times, prove to be advantageous. The fetal legs must be carefully distinguished from the arms to avoid premature extraction of an arm and a difficult delivery of the rest of the fetus.

The uterine incision is observed for any vigorously bleeding sites. These should be promptly clamped with Pennington or ring forceps, or similar instruments. Most surgeons recommend that the placenta be removed promptly manually, unless it is separating spontaneously (Fig. 23–13). Fundal massage, begun as soon as the fetus is delivered, reduces bleeding and hastens delivery of the placenta. In a randomized trial, Lasley and colleagues (1997) found a significant twofold postoperative infection rate with manual removal compared with spontaneous delivery. Some obstetricians prefer manual expression of the placenta using external uterine manipulation, but this has not been shown to be superior to manual removal (Cernadas and co-workers, 1998).

Recommendations from the *Guidelines for Perinatal Care* (American College of Obstetricians and Gynecologist, 1992) suggest that all births require the attendance of personnel capable of resuscitating the newborn. There are no specific recommendations for cesarean deliveries (Jacob and Pfenninger, 1997). In many institutions the standard of care mandates that pediatricians attend all cesarean deliveries regardless of fetal risk, whereas nurses attend to the newborn infant in low-risk vaginal deliveries. Jacob and Phenninger (1997) compared 834 cesarean deliveries with 834 low-risk vaginal deliveries. They concluded that repeat cesarean deliveries, and cesareans for dystocia without fetal heart

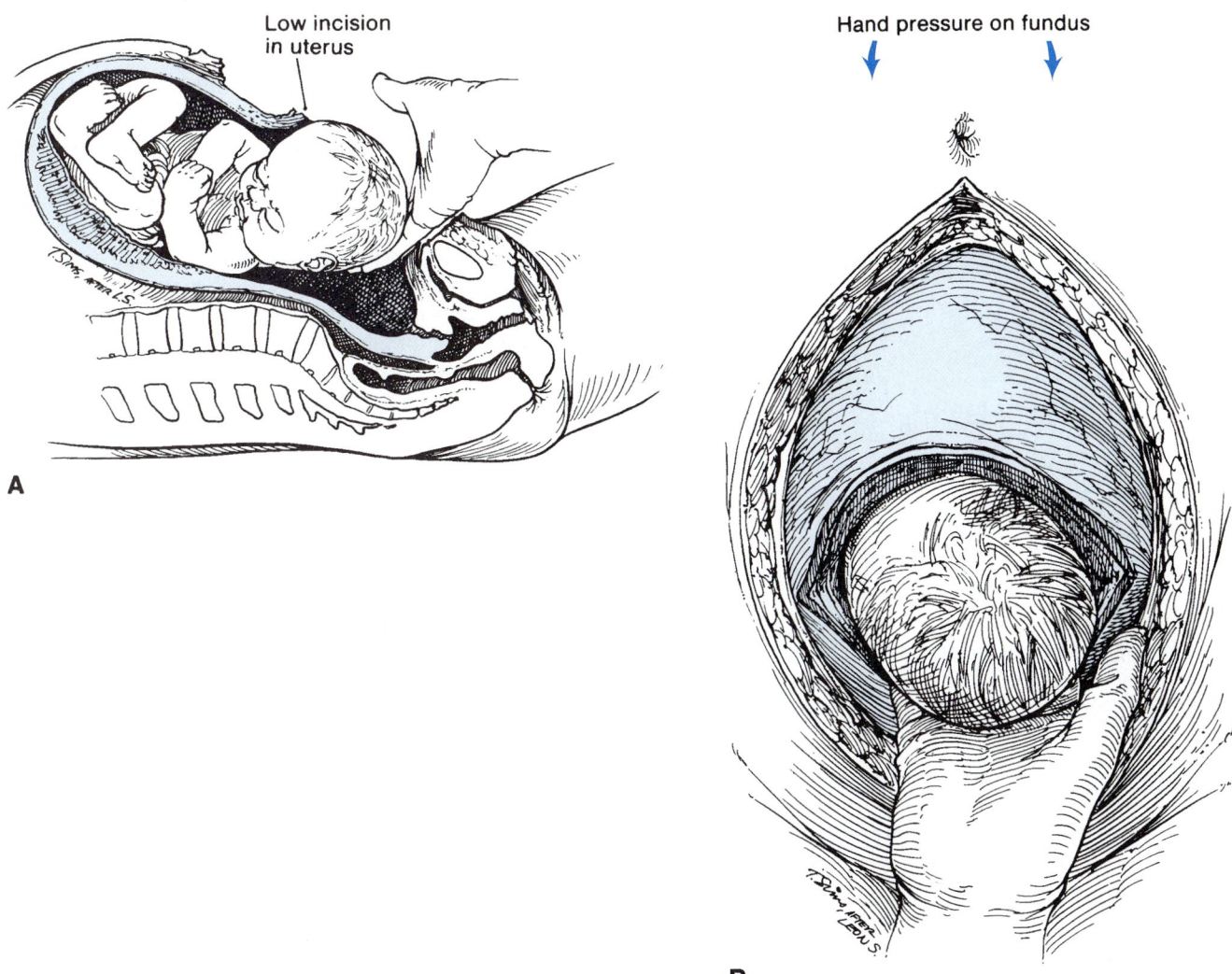

FIGURE 23–11. A. Immediately after incising the uterus and fetal membranes, the operator's fingers are insinuated between the symphysis pubis and the fetal head until the posterior surface is reached. The head is lifted carefully anteriorly and, as necessary, superiorly to bring it from beneath the symphysis forward through the uterine and abdominal incisions. **B.** As the fetal head is lifted through the incision, pressure usually is applied to the uterine fundus through the abdominal wall to help expel the fetus.

rate abnormalities and performed under regional anesthesia, do not need a pediatrician in attendance because of rare need for infant resuscitation. At Parkland Hospital, pediatric nurse practitioners attend uncomplicated, scheduled cesarean deliveries.

REPAIR OF THE UTERUS. After delivery of the placenta, the uterus may be lifted through the incision onto the draped abdominal wall and the fundus covered with a moistened laparotomy pack. Although some clinicians prefer to avoid this latter step, uterine exteriorization often has advantages that outweigh any disadvantages. The relaxed, atonic uterus can be recognized quickly and massage applied. The incision and bleeding points are visualized more easily and repaired, especially if

there have been extensions laterally. Adnexal exposure is superior and thus tubal sterilization is easier. The principal disadvantage is from discomfort and vomiting caused by traction in the woman given spinal or epidural analgesia. Neither febrile morbidity nor blood loss appears to be increased in women undergoing uterine exteriorization prior to repair (Magann and associates, 1993a; Wahab and co-workers, 1999).

Immediately after delivery and inspection of the placenta, the uterine cavity is inspected and wiped out with a gauze pack to remove avulsed membranes, vernix, clots, or other debris. The upper and lower cut edges and each angle of the uterine incision are examined carefully for bleeding vessels. The lower margin of an incision made through a thinned-out lower uterine seg-

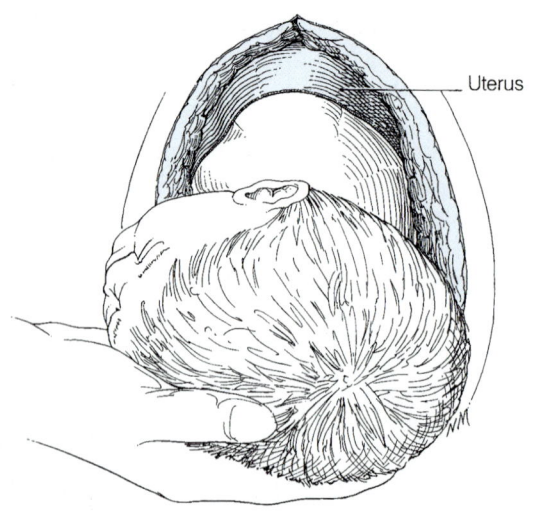

FIGURE 23–12. Just as shoulders are delivered, intravenous oxytocin is infused.

ment may be so thin as to be inadvertently ignored. At the same time, the posterior wall of the lower uterine segment may occasionally buckle anteriorly in such a way as to suggest that it is the lower margin of the incision.

The uterine incision is closed with one or two layers of continuous 0 or #1 absorbable suture. Traditionally, chromic suture is used, but some prefer synthetic nonabsorbable sutures. Zuidema and colleagues (1996) reviewed subsequent outcomes in 537 women in whom 237 had uterine chromic closure and 302 had closure with Vicryl. Subsequent scar separation was increased almost fourfold in the Vicryl group (4.6 versus 1.2 percent). From their review, Bivins and Gallup (2000) recommend one-layer uterine closure. Hauth and colleagues (1992) randomized 906 women to either one- or two-larger closure using 1-0 chromic gut. A continuous locking one-layer closure required less operative time and fewer uterine hemostatic sutures. In a follow-up report of 164 women delivered subsequently, the type of uterine closure did not significantly affect the next pregnancy (Chapman and associates, 1997).

Individually clamped large vessels are best ligated with a suture ligature. Concern has been expressed by some clinicians that sutures through the decidua may lead to endometriosis in the scar, but this is a rare complication. The initial suture is placed just beyond one angle of the incision. A running-lock suture is then carried out, with each suture penetrating the full thickness of the myometrium (Fig. 23–14). It is important to select carefully the site of each stitch and to avoid withdrawing the needle once it penetrates the myometrium. This minimizes the perforation of unligated vessels and subsequent bleeding. The running-lock suture is continued just beyond the opposite incision angle. Especially when the lower segment is thin, satisfactory approximation of the cut edges usually can be obtained with one layer of suture. If approximation is not satisfactory after a single-layer continuous closure, or if bleeding sites persist, either another layer of sutures may be placed so as to achieve approximation and hemostasis, or individual

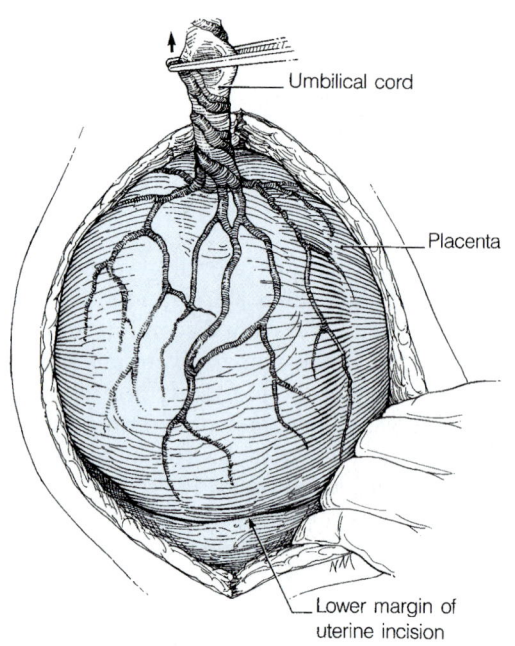

FIGURE 23–13. Placenta bulging through the uterine incision as uterus contracts.

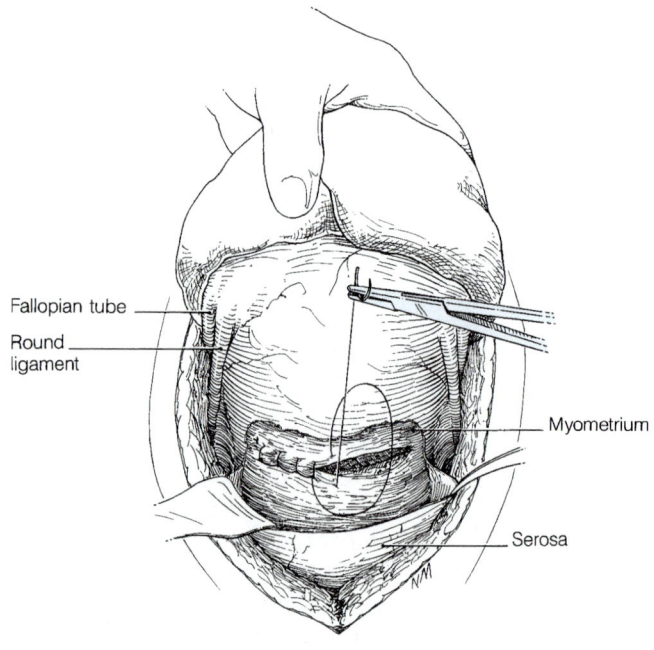

FIGURE 23–14. The cut edges of the uterine incision are closed with a running-lock suture.

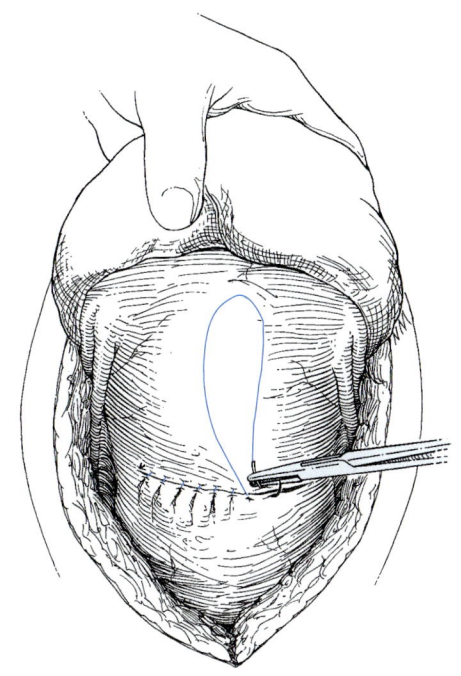

FIGURE 23–15. The serosal margins are approximated to reperitonealize the uterus.

bleeding sites can be secured with figure-of-eight or mattress sutures.

After hemostasis is obtained from uterine closure, serosal edges overlying the uterus and bladder in the past have been approximated with a continuous 2-0 chromic catgut suture (Fig. 23–15). After their review, Bivins and Gallup (2000) favor nonclosure of the peritoneum. Studies have demonstrated reduced need for postoperative analgesia and a quicker return of bowel function when both visceral and parietal peritoneum were left open (Hull and Varner, 1991; Pietrantoni and associates, 1991). It does not increase adhesion formation (Tulandi and co-workers, 1988).

If tubal sterilization is to be performed, it is now done. A partial midsegment salpingectomy, described in Chapter 59 (p. 1557), has a low failure rate.

ABDOMINAL CLOSURE. All packs are removed, and the gutters and cul-de-sac are emptied of blood and amnionic fluid by gentle suction. If general anesthesia is used, the upper abdominal organs may be palpated systematically. With conduction analgesia, however, this may produce considerable discomfort. After the sponge and instrument counts are found to be correct, the abdominal incision is closed (Fig. 23–16). Many omit peritoneal edge approximation. As each layer is closed, bleeding sites are located, clamped, and ligated. The rectus muscles are allowed to fall into place, and the subfascial space is meticulously checked for hemostasis. The overlying rectus fascia is closed either with inter-

rupted 0 nonabsorbable sutures that are placed lateral to the fascial edges and no more than 1 cm apart, or by continuous, nonlocking suture of a long-lasting absorbable or permanent type.

The subcutaneous tissue usually need not be closed separately if it is 2 cm or less in thickness, and the skin is closed with vertical mattress sutures of 3-0 or 4-0 silk or equivalent suture or skin clips. If there is more adipose tissue than this, or if clips or subcuticular closure are to be used, a few interrupted 3-0 plain catgut sutures will obliterate dead space and reduce tension on the skin edges. In a randomized prospective study of more than 1400 women undergoing cesarean delivery, Bohman and colleagues (1992) reported a significantly decreased frequency of superficial wound disruption when the subcutaneous layer was approximated. This was confirmed in a similar study by Naumann and co-workers (1995).

TECHNIQUE FOR CLASSICAL CESAREAN INCISION.
Occasionally it is necessary to use a classical incision for delivery. Some indications are:

1. If the lower uterine segment cannot be exposed or entered safely because the bladder is adherent densely from previous surgery, or if a myoma occupies the lower uterine segment, or if there is invasive carcinoma of the cervix.

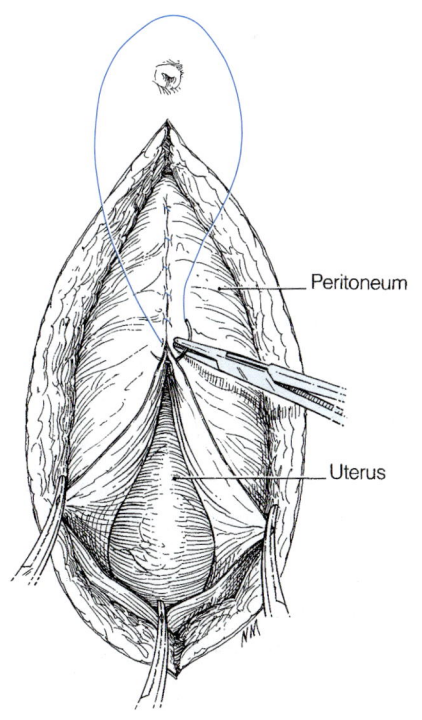

FIGURE 23–16. The cut margins of the parietal peritoneum are elevated, and closure has been initiated. Many choose to omit this step.

2. When there is a transverse lie of a large fetus, especially if the membranes are ruptured and the shoulder is impacted in the birth canal.

3. In some cases of placenta previa with anterior implantation.

4. In some cases of very small fetuses, especially presenting as breech, in which the lower uterine segment is not thinned out.

5. In some cases of massive maternal obesity where only the upper uterus is easily accessible.

UTERINE INCISION. Vertical uterine incision is initiated with a scalpel beginning as low as possible, but above the level of the attached bladder. Once sufficient room is made with the scalpel, the incision is extended cephaled with bandage scissors until it is sufficiently long to permit delivery of the fetus. Numerous large vessels that bleed profusely are commonly encountered within the myometrium. As soon as the fetus has been removed, these vessels may best be clamped and eventually ligated with chromic catgut sutures. Following birth of the infant, care is as described earlier.

UTERINE REPAIR. One method employs a layer of continuous 0- or 1-chromic catgut to approximate the inner halves of the incision. The outer half of the uterine incision is then closed with similar suture, using either a continuos stitch or figure-of-eight sutures. No unnecessary needle tracts should be made lest myometrial vessels be perforated with subsequent hemorrhage or hematomas. To achieve good approximation and to prevent the suture from tearing through the myometrium, it is helpful to have an assistant compress the myometrium on each side of the wound medially as each suture is placed and tied. The edges of the uterine serosa, if not already so, are approximated with continuous 2-0 chromic catgut. The operation is completed as described earlier.

EXTRAPERITONEAL CESAREAN DELIVERY. Early in the 20th century, Frank (1907) and Latzko (1909) recommended extraperitoneal cesarean rather than cesarean hysterectomy as a method of managing pregnancies with infected uterine contents. The goal of the operation was to open the uterus extraperitoneally by dissecting through the space of Retzius and then along one side and beneath the bladder to reach the lower uterine segment. Enthusiasm for the procedure has been transient, probably in large part because of the availability of a variety of effective antimicrobial agents (Wallace and associates, 1984).

POSTMORTEM CESAREAN DELIVERY. At times, cesarean delivery is performed on a woman who has just died, or who is expected to do so momentarily. A satis-factory infant outcome in such a situation is dependent upon:

1. Anticipation, if possible, of the death of the mother.
2. Gestational age of fetus.
3. Availability of personnel and appropriate equipment.
4. Availability of perimortem ventilation and cardiac massage for the mother.
5. Prompt delivery and effective neonatal resuscitation.

Although a few infants have survived with no apparent physical or intellectual compromise, most are not so fortunate. Both Katz and associates (1986) and Clark and colleagues (1995) stress the need for immediate cesarean delivery upon diagnosis of maternal cardiac arrest if neonatal outcome is to be optimized. In such cases, cesarean delivery is unlikely to adversely affect maternal outcome; indeed, only about 10 percent of patients suffering in-hospital cardiac arrest will survive to hospital discharge (Blackhall and associates, 1992; Niemann, 1992). Unfortunately, even with ideal management, maternal cardiac arrest often leads to survival of a neurologically impaired infant. Field and co-workers (1988) reported the successful delivery by cesarean of an infant whose mother, although brain dead, was maintained for 10 weeks on life-support systems in order for fetal maturation to occur. The issue of cesarean delivery to aid in cardiopulmonary resuscitation of the mother is further discussed in Chapter 43 (p. 1176).

POSTOPERATIVE COMPLICATIONS. Morbidity following cesarean delivery is influenced by the circumstances in which the procedure is performed. McMahon and colleagues (1996), in their analysis of women with prior cesarean delivery, reported the incidence of complications in women delivered by this method electively compared with after labor had failed in effecting vaginal delivery (Table 23–7). Potential complications included hysterectomy, operative injury to pelvic structures, as

TABLE 23–7. Morbidity after Elective Cesarean Delivery Compared with Cesarean Delivery after Labor in Women with Prior Cesarean Births

Morbidity	Elective Cesarean (%)	Cesarean after Labor (%)
Hysterectomy	0.2	0.3
Operative injury[a]	0.6	3
Puerperal fever	6.4	8
Transfusion	1.3	1.4
Wound infection	2.2	3.3

[a]Includes laceration of uterine artery, bladder, ureter, or bowel.
Modified from McMahon and colleagues (1996), with permission.

well as infection and need for transfusion. The incidence of some of these morbidities may be magnified by uterine rupture because the study included only those women with prior cesarean deliveries. Rajasekar and Hall (1997) specifically studied bladder and ureteral injuries. The incidence of bladder laceration at the time of cesarean operation was 1.4 per 1000 procedures, and that for ureteral injury was 0.3 per 1000. While bladder injury was immediate, diagnosis of ureteric injury was often delayed.

Lyndon-Rochelle and colleagues (2000) studied rehospitalizations within 60 days following cesarean deliveries in 54,074 women in Washington State. They compared these with 142,768 women delivered vaginally, and as shown in Table 23–8, rehospitalization was significantly increased in women with cesarean births. They calculated the risk of rehospitalization for women with cesarean births and discharged before 3 days, 3 to 5 days, and 6 days or longer after the operation. The risk of rehospitalization was significantly decreased for women discharged between 3 and 5 days following cesarean delivery compared with earlier discharge, suggesting that this interval may be optimal.

The diagnosis and treatment of pelvic and wound infections following cesarean delivery is discussed in Chapter 26. A rare but serious complication of cesarean delivery is necrotizing fasciitis. Goepfert and co-workers (1997) identified nine such women based on identification of necrotic fascia in febrile women undergoing postcesarean wound debridement. The incidence was approximately 2 per 1000 cesarean deliveries. Fasciitis was diagnosed an average of 10 days following cesarean delivery and these infections were polymicrobial. One woman died from sepsis.

POSTPARTUM HYSTERECTOMY

In some cases, and usually in those complicated by severe obstetrical hemorrhage, postpartum hysterectomy may be lifesaving. It is done primarily at laparotomy following vaginal delivery, or it may be done after cesarean delivery.

INDICATIONS. The majority of procedures are done to arrest hemorrhage either from intractable uterine atony, lower-segment bleeding associated with the uterine incision or placental implantation, a laceration of major uterine vessels, large myomas, severe cervical dysplasia, and carcinoma in situ. Placental implantation disorders, to include placenta previa and variations of placenta accreta, often in association with repeat cesarean delivery, are now the most common indications for cesarean hysterectomy (Miller and colleagues, 1997). These are discussed in Chapter 25 (p. 632).

Major deterrents to cesarean hysterectomy are concern for increased blood loss and the possibility of urinary tract damage. A major factor in the complication rate appears to be whether the operation is performed as an elective procedure or as an emergency. As shown in Table 23–9, morbidity associated with emergency hysterectomy is substantively increased. Recently, Seago and associates (1999) also reported increased blood loss, operative time, infection morbidity, and transfusion rates in women undergoing emergency compared with elective postpartum hysterectomy.

OPERATIVE TECHNIQUE. If done following vaginal delivery, the transverse bladder flap is deflected downward as for a cesarean incision, but extended farther down

TABLE 23–8. Incidence and Relative Risk of Rehospitalization in 54,074 Women with Cesarean Births Compared with 142,768 Women with Spontaneous Vaginal Deliveries in Washington State

Rehospitalization Diagnosis	Incidence per 1000 Women		Relative Risk (95% CI)
	Spontaneous Vaginal Delivery	Cesarean Delivery	
All diagnoses	10	17	1.8 (1.6–1.9)
Uterine infection	2.9	5.2	2.0 (1.7–2.4)
Surgical wounds	0.1	3.9	30.2 (19–47)
Postpartum hemorrhage	2.4	2.9	1.2 (1.0–1.5)
Gallbladder	2.2	2.8	1.5 (1.3–1.9)
Genitourinary	1.3	1.7	1.5 (1.2–2.0)
Cardiopulmonary	0.6	1.3	2.4 (1.8–3.4)
Thromboembolism	0.3	0.9	2.5 (1.5–3.5)
Appendicitis	0.3	0.5	1.8 (1.3–3.0)

Modified from Lyndon-Rochelle and colleagues (2000), with permission.

TABLE 23–9. Comparison of Morbidity with Elective versus Emergency Postpartum Hysterectomy

	Postpartum Hysterectomy	
Complications	Elective[a] (n = 189)	Emergency[b] (n = 184)
Blood transfusions	18%	91%
Bladder injury	3	9
Ureteral injury	None	3
Surgical infection	22%	29%
Death	0	3

[a]Data from Plauche (1995).
[b]Data from Zelop and colleagues (1993) and Zorlu and associates (1998).

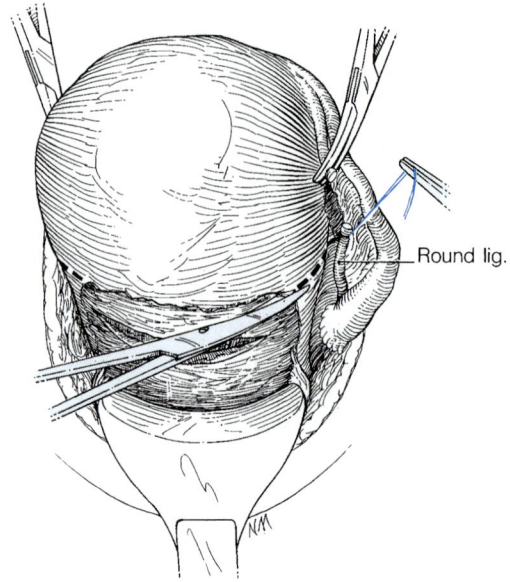

FIGURE 23–17. The incision in the vesicouterine serosa is extended laterally and upward through the anterior leaf of the broad ligament to reach the incised round ligaments.

to the level of the cervix is possible. If done after delivery of the infant by cesarean, the bladder flap is also deflected farther down. Supracervical or preferably total hysterectomy can be accomplished by standard operative techniques. Although all vessels are appreciably larger than those of the nonpregnant uterus, hysterectomy is usually facilitated by the ease of development of tissue planes in pregnant women. Blood loss is commonly appreciable because of the indications for the operation. When performed for hemorrhage, blood loss almost always is torrential. Indeed, as shown in Table 23–9, over 90 percent of women undergoing emergency postpartum hysterectomy required transfusions.

Following delivery, the major bleeding vessels are clamped and ligated quickly. The placenta is removed, and the uterine incision can be approximated with either a continuous suture or a few interrupted sutures. Alternatively, Pennington or sponge forceps can be applied, and if the incision is not bleeding appreciably, neither is necessary.

Next the round ligaments close to the uterus are divided between Heaney or Kocher clamps and doubly ligated. Either 0 or #1 sutures can be used. The incision in the vesicouterine serosa, made to mobilize the bladder for cesarean delivery, is extended laterally and upward through the anterior leaf of the broad ligament to reach the incised round ligaments (Fig. 23–17). The posterior leaf of the broad ligament adjacent to the uterus is perforated just beneath the fallopian tubes, utero-ovarian ligaments, and ovarian vessels (Fig. 23–18A). These then are doubly clamped close to the uterus (Fig. 23–18B), divided, and the lateral pedicle doubly suture ligated. The posterior leaf of the broad ligament is divided inferiorly toward the uterosacral ligaments (Fig. 23–19). Next, the bladder and attached peritoneal flap are again deflected and dissected from the lower uterine segment and retracted out of the operative field (Fig. 23–20). If the bladder flap is unusually

adherent, as it may be after previous cesarean incisions, careful sharp dissection may be necessary.

Special care is necessary from this point on to avoid injury to the ureters, which pass beneath the uterine arteries. The ascending uterine artery and veins on ei-

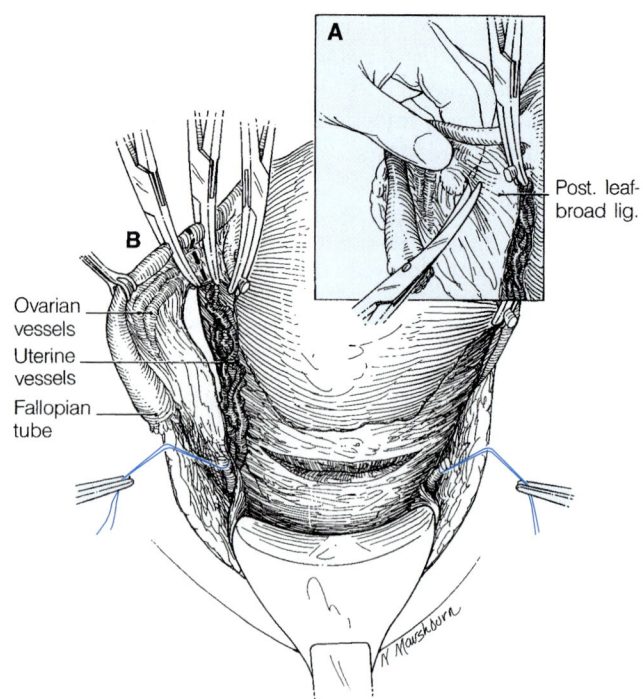

FIGURE 23–18. A. The posterior leaf of the broad ligament adjacent to the uterus is perforated just beneath the fallopian tube, utero-ovarian ligaments, and ovarian vessels. **B.** These then are doubly clamped close to the uterus and divided.

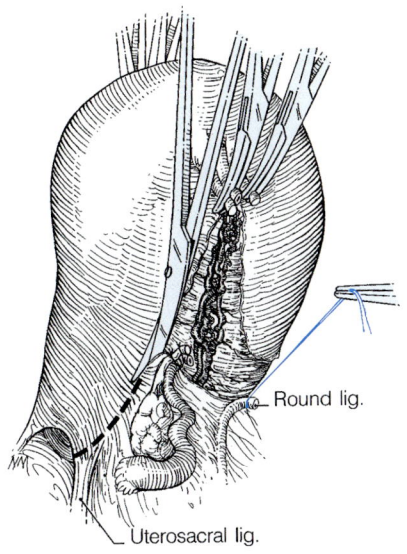

FIGURE 23–19. The posterior leaf of the broad ligament is divided inferiorly toward the uterosacral ligament.

ther side are identified and near their origin are doubly clamped immediately adjacent to the uterus, divided, and doubly suture ligated (Fig. 23–21).

In cases of profuse hemorrhage, it may be more advantageous to rapidly clamp all of the vascular pedicles and remove the uterus before suture ligating the pedicles.

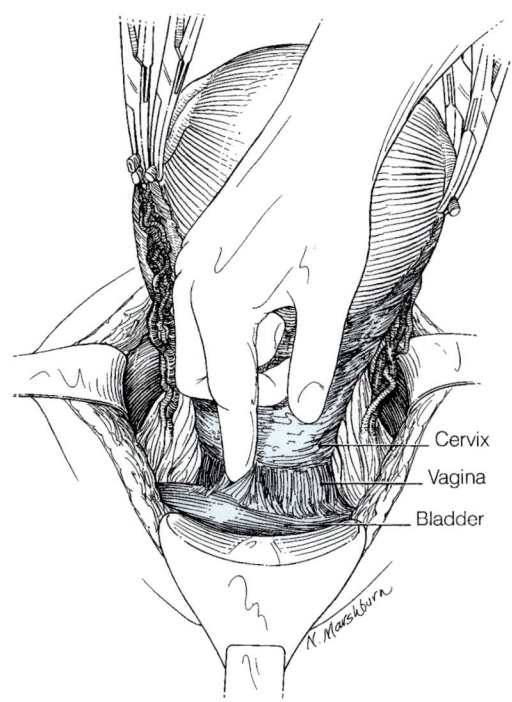

FIGURE 23–20. The bladder is further dissected from the lower uterine segment by blunt dissection with pressure directed toward the lower segment and not bladder. Sharp dissection may be necessary.

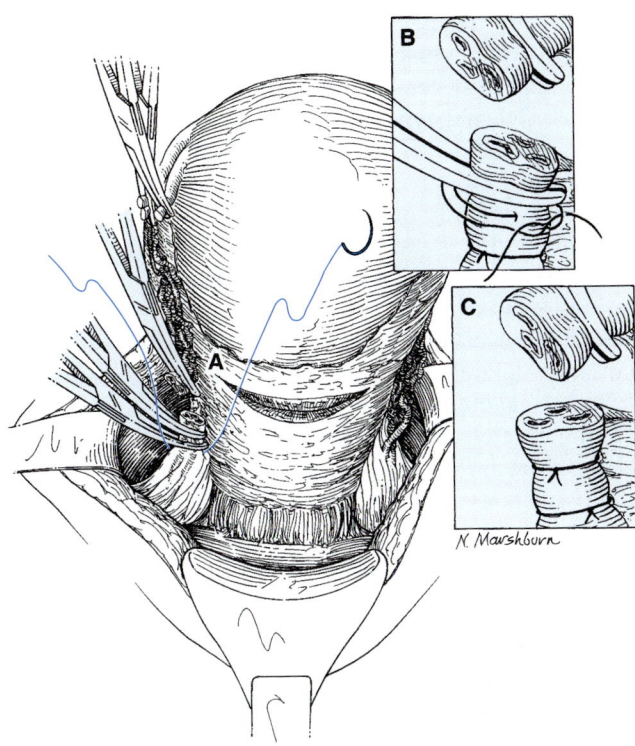

FIGURE 23–21. A. The uterine artery and veins on either side are doubly clamped immediately adjacent to the uterus and divided. **B, C.** The vascular pedicle is doubly suture ligated.

SUPRACERVICAL HYSTERECTOMY. To perform a subtotal hysterectomy, it is necessary only to amputate the body of the uterus at this level. The cervical stump may be closed with continuous or interrupted chromic sutures.

TOTAL HYSTERECTOMY. To perform a total hysterectomy, it is necessary to mobilize the bladder much more extensively in the midline and laterally. This will help carry the ureters caudad as the bladder is retracted beneath the symphysis and will also prevent laceration or suturing of the bladder during cervical excision and vaginal cuff closure. The bladder is dissected free for about 2 cm below the lowest margin of the cervix to expose the uppermost part of the vagina. If the cervix is effaced and dilated appreciably, the uterine cavity may be entered anteriorly in the midline either through the lower hysterotomy incision or through a stab would made at the level of the ligated uterine vessels. A finger is directed inferiorly through the incision to identify the free margin of the dilated, effaced cervix and the anterior vaginal fornix. The contaminated glove is removed and the hand regloved. Another useful method to identify the cervical margins is to place transvaginally four metal skin clips or brightly colored sutures at 12, 3, 6, and 9 o'clock positions on the cervical edges prior to planned hysterectomy.

The cardinal ligaments, uterosacral ligaments, and the many large vessels these ligaments contain are doubly clamped systematically with Heaney-type curved clamps, Ochsner-type straight clamps, or similar instruments (Fig. 23–22). The clamps are placed as close to the cervix as possible, and it is imperative not to include excessive tissue in each clamp. The tissue between the pair of clamps is incised, and suture ligated appropriately. These steps are repeated until the level of the lateral vaginal fornix is reached. In this way, the descending branches of the uterine vessels are clamped, cut, and ligated as the cervix is dissected from the cardinal ligaments posteriorly.

Immediately below the level of the cervix, a curved clamp is swung in across the lateral vaginal fornix, and the tissue is incised medially to the clamp (Fig. 23–23). The excised lateral vaginal fornix can be simultaneously doubly ligated and sutured to the stump of the cardinal ligament. The entire cervix is then excised from the vagina.

The cervix is inspected to insure that it has been completely excised, and the vagina is repaired. Each of the angles of the lateral vaginal fornix are secured to the cardinal and uterosacral ligaments (Fig. 23–24). Following this, some surgeons prefer to close the vagina using figure-of-eight chromic catgut sutures. Others achieve hemostasis by using a running-lock stitch of chromic catgut suture placed through the mucosa and

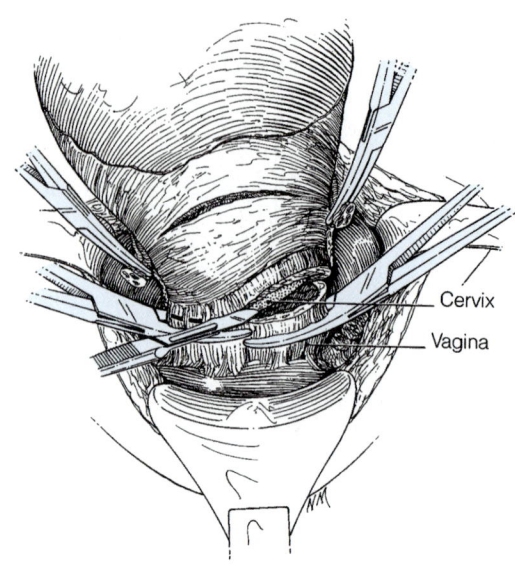

FIGURE 23–23. A curved clamp is swung in across the lateral vaginal fornix below the level of the cervix and the tissue incised medially to the point of the clamp.

adjacent endopelvic fascia around the circumference of the vagina (Fig. 23–25). The open vagina may promote drainage of fluids that would otherwise accumulate and contribute to hematoma formation and infection.

All sites of incision from the upper fallopian tube and ovarian ligament pedicles to the vaginal vault and bladder flap are examined carefully for bleeding. Bleeding sites are ligated with care to avoid the ureters.

Some clinicians choose to reperitonealize the pelvis (Fig. 23–26). One method employs a continuous chromic suture starting with the tip of the ligated pedicle of fallopian tube and ovarian ligament, which is inverted retroperitoneally. Sutures are then placed continuously so as to:

1. Approximate the leaves of the broad ligament.
2. Bury the stump of the round ligament.

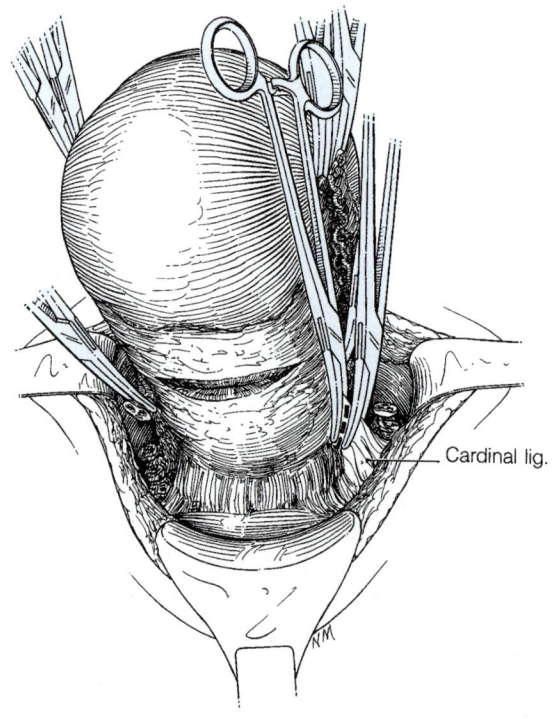

FIGURE 23–22. The cardinal ligaments are clamped, incised, and ligated.

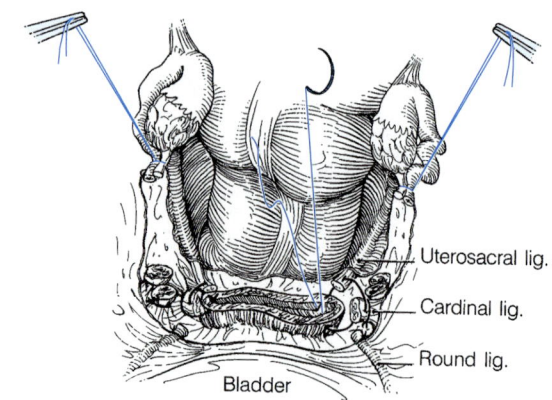

FIGURE 23–24. The lateral angles are secured to the cardinal and uterosacral ligaments.

3. Approximate the cut edge of the vesicouterine peritoneum over the vaginal vault posteriorly to the cut edge of peritoneum above the cul-de-sac.
4. Approximate the leaves of the broad ligament on the opposite side.
5. Bury the stump of the round ligament and pedicle of fallopian tube on the opposite side.

The abdominal wall normally is closed in layers, as previously described.

APPENDECTOMY AND OOPHORECTOMY. The benefits compared with the risks from incidental appendectomy at the time of cesarean or hysterectomy continue to be argued (Gilstrap, 1991). In one prospective study of 40 women undergoing elective appendectomy, Parsons and associates (1986) reported no significant morbidity and found that 20 percent of the removed appendices were abnormal. However, the procedure added 15 minutes to the operative time and a half-day to the hospital stay. Lydon-Rochelle and colleagues (2000) found an 80 percent increased risk of rehospitalization for appendicitis among women with cesarean delivery, an association not previously observed (Table 23–8). A plausible explanation is that the manipulation of abdominal contents during cesarean delivery may exacerbate or stimulate subclinical infection (Andersson and associates, 1995). Lacking, however, are results that demonstrate clearly that puerperal morbidity and mortality are not increased by appendectomy, especially with emergency cesarean delivery.

Most studies indicate that in 5 percent of postpartum hysterectomies, one adnexa will have to be removed to stop bleeding (Plauche, 1995). That said, during any hysterectomy, a decision as to the fate of the ovaries must be made. For women who are approaching menopause, the decision is not difficult, but few women who undergo cesarean hysterectomy are of this age. Thus,

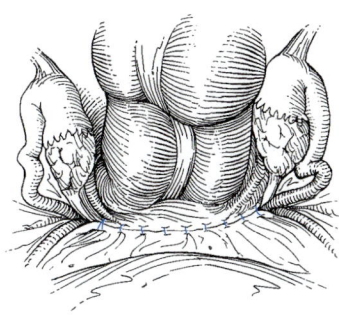

FIGURE 23–26. Reperitonealization of the pelvis. Many omit this step.

ovarian preservation is favored unless the ovaries are diseased. Even if oophorectomy is required, it rarely is necessary or desirable to remove both ovaries.

PERIPARTUM MANAGEMENT

PREOPERATIVE CARE. The woman scheduled for repeat cesarean delivery is typically admitted the day of surgery and evaluated by the obstetrician who will perform surgery and the anesthesiologist who will provide anesthesia. The hematocrit is rechecked, and if the indirect Coombs test is positive, then availability of compatible blood must be assured. A sedative, such as secobarbital 100 mg, may be given at bedtime the night before the operation. In general, no other sedatives, narcotics, or tranquilizers are administered until after the infant is born. Oral intake is stopped at least 8 hours before surgery. An antacid, such as Bicitra 30 mL, given shortly before the induction of a general anesthesia, minimizes the risk of lung injury from gastric acid should aspiration occur (Chap. 15, p. 366). This should be done routinely, even when conduction analgesia will be used, because at times it is necessary to switch to, or at least supplement, the regional analgesia with inhalation anesthesia.

INTRAVENOUS FLUIDS. Requirements for intravenous fluids, including blood during and after cesarean delivery, can vary considerably. The woman of average size with a hematocrit of 30 or more and a normally expanded blood volume and extracellular fluid volume most often will tolerate blood loss up to 2000 mL without difficulty. Unappreciated bleeding through the vagina during the procedure, bleeding concealed in the uterus after its closure, or both, commonly lead to underestimation. While blood loss averages about 1500 mL with elective cesarean hysterectomy, it is quite variable (Pritchard, 1965).

Intravenously administered fluids consist of either

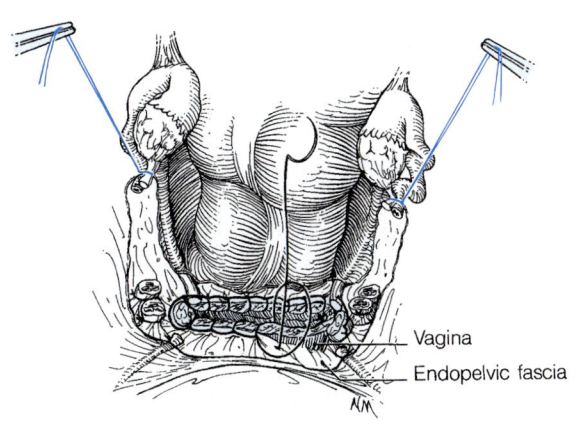

FIGURE 23–25. A running-lock stitch is placed through the edge of the vaginal mucosa.

Vagina
Endopelvic fascia

lactated Ringer solution or a similar crystalloid solution with 5 percent dextrose. Typically, 1 to 2 liters that contain electrolytes are infused during and immediately after the operation. Throughout the procedure, and subsequently while in the recovery area, the blood pressure and urine flow are monitored closely to ensure that perfusion of vital organs is satisfactory.

RECOVERY SUITE. In the recovery suite, the amount of bleeding from the vagina must be monitored closely, and the uterine fundus must be identified frequently by palpation to assure that the uterus is remaining firmly contracted. Unfortunately, as the woman awakens from general anesthesia or the conduction analgesia fades, palpation of the abdomen is likely to produce considerable discomfort. This can be made much more tolerable by giving an effective analgesic intravenously, such as meperidine, 75 to 100 mg, or morphine, 10 to 15 mg. A thick dressing with an abundance of adhesive tape over the abdomen interferes with fundal palpation and massage and later causes discomfort as the tape and perhaps skin are removed. Deep breathing and coughing are encouraged.

Once the mother is fully awake, bleeding is minimal, the blood pressure is satisfactory, and urine flow is at least 30 mL/hr, she may be returned to her room.

SUBSEQUENT CARE

ANALGESIA. For the woman of average size, meperidine, 75 to 100 mg, is given intramuscularly as often as every 3 hours as needed for discomfort, or morphine sulfate, 10 to 15 mg, is similarly administered. An antiemetic, such as promethazine, 25 mg, is usually given along with the narcotic. Intravenous meperidine or morphine via a patient-controlled pump is an even more effective alternative to bolus therapy in the immediate postoperative period.

VITAL SIGNS. After transfer, the woman is now evaluated at least hourly for 4 hours at the minimum, and blood pressure, pulse, urine flow, amount of bleeding, and status of the uterine fundus are checked at intervals of 4 hours, along with the temperature.

FLUID THERAPY AND DIET. Unless there has been pathological constriction of the extracellular fluid compartment from diuretics, sodium restriction, vomiting, fever, or prolonged labor without adequate fluid intake, the puerperium is characterized by excretion of fluid that was retained during pregnancy. Moreover, with the typical cesarean delivery, significant extracellular fluid sequestration in bowel wall and lumen does not occur, unless it was necessary to pack the bowel away from the operative field or peritonitis develops. Thus, the

woman who undergoes cesarean delivery rarely develops fluid sequestration in the so-called third space. Quite the contrary, she normally begins surgery with a physiologically enlarged third space that she acquired during pregnancy and that she now mobilizes and excretes after delivery. Therefore, large volumes of intravenous fluids during and subsequent to surgery are not needed to replace sequestered extracellular fluid. As a generalization, 3 L of fluid should prove adequate during the first 24 hours after surgery. If urine output falls below 30 mL/hr, however, then the woman should be reevaluated promptly. The cause of the oliguria may range from unrecognized blood loss to an antidiuretic effect from infused oxytocin.

BLADDER AND BOWEL FUNCTION. The bladder catheter most often can be removed by 12 hours after operation or, more conveniently, the morning after surgery. Subsequent ability to empty the bladder before overdistention develops must be monitored as with vaginal delivery. In uncomplicated cases, solid food may be offered within 8 hours of surgery (Burrows and associates, 1995; Kramer and colleagues, 1996). Although some degree of adynamic ileus follows virtually every abdominal operation, in most cases of cesarean delivery, it is negligible. Symptoms include abdominal distention and gas pains, and an inability to pass flatus or stool. The pathophysiology of postoperative ileus is complex, and involves hormonal, neural, and local factors that are incompletely understood (Livingston and Passaro, 1990). Treatment has changed little over the past several decades, and involves nasogastric decompression and intravenous fluid and electrolyte supplementation. Frequently, a 10-mg bisacodyl rectal suppository provides appreciable relief.

AMBULATION. In most instances, by at least the day after surgery the woman should get out of bed briefly at least twice with assistance. Ambulation can be timed so that a recently administered analgesic will minimize the discomfort. By the second day she may walk with assistance. With early ambulation, venous thrombosis and pulmonary embolism are uncommon.

WOUND CARE. The incision is inspected each day, and the skin sutures (or clips) are removed on the fourth day after surgery. By the third postpartum day, bathing by shower is not harmful to the incision. Thick subcutaneous tissue (greater than 3 cm) is a risk factor for wound infection (Vermillion and associates, 2000).

LABORATORY. The hematocrit is routinely measured the morning after surgery. It is checked sooner when there was unusual blood loss or when there is oliguria or other evidence to suggest hypovolemia. If the hematocrit is decreased significantly from the preoperative level, it is repeated, and a search is instituted to identify the cause of the decrease. If the lower hematocrit is stable, the mother can ambulate without any difficulty, and if there is little likelihood of further blood loss, hematological repair in response to iron therapy is preferred to transfusion.

BREAST CARE. Breast feeding can be initiated the day of surgery. If the mother elects not to breast feed, a binder that supports the breasts without marked compression will usually minimize discomfort (Chap. 17, p. 411).

HOSPITAL DISCHARGE. Unless there are complications during the puerperium, the mother is generally discharged on the third postpartum day (Chap. 17, p. 417). Strong and associates (1993) have presented data suggesting that discharge on day 2 may be appropriate for properly selected women. The woman's activities during the following week should be restricted to self-care and care of her baby with assistance. Brooten and colleagues (1994) successfully combined early discharge with nurse specialist transitional home care. In many cases, it may be advantageous to perform an initial postpartum evaluation during the first to third week after delivery for the reasons presented in Chapters 17 and 58.

PREVENTION OF POSTOPERATIVE INFECTION. Febrile morbidity is rather frequent after cesarean deliveries and appears to be more common among indigent than affluent women. A number of randomized clinical trials have demonstrated that a single-dose of an antimicrobial agent given at the time of cesarean delivery will serve to decrease infection morbidity appreciably. For women in labor or with ruptured membranes, most clinicians recommend a single 2-g dose of ampicillin, a cephalosporin, or an extended-spectrum penicillin after delivery of the infant. Postoperative pelvic infection is the most frequent cause of febrile morbidity and occurs despite peripartum prophylactic antimicrobials in approximately 20 percent of women (Brumfield and colleagues, 2000). Treatment of uterine infection and its complications are discussed in Chapter 26.

HISTORICAL BACKGROUND

The origin of the term cesarean is obscure. Three principal explanations have been suggested:

1. According to legend, Julius Caesar was born in this manner, with the result that the procedure became known as the Caesarean operation. Several circumstances weaken this explanation. First, the mother of Julius Caesar lived for many years after his birth in 100 BC, and as late as the 17th century, the operation was almost invariably fatal. Second, the operation, whether performed on the living or dead, is not mentioned by any medical writer before the Middle Ages. Historical details of the origin of the family name Caesar are found in Pickrell's monograph (1935).

2. It has been widely believed that the name of the operation is derived from a Roman law, supposedly created by Numa Pompilius (8th century BC), ordering that the procedure be performed upon women dying in the last few weeks of pregnancy in the hope of saving the child. This explanation then holds that this *lex regia,* as it was called at first, became the *lex caesarea* under the emperors, and the operation itself became known as the caesarean operation. The German term *Kaiserschnitt* ("Kaiser cut") reflects this derivation.

3. The word *caesarean* was derived sometime in the Middle Age from the Latin verb *caedere,* "to cut." An obvious cognate is the word caesura, a cutting, or pause, in a line of verse. This explanation of the term *caesarean* seems most logical, but exactly when it was first applied to the operation is uncertain. Because "section" is derived from the Latin verb *seco,* which also means "cut," the term *caesarean section* seems tautological.

It is customary in the United States to replace the "ae" in the first syllable of *caesarean* with the letter "e"; in Great Britain and Australia, however, the "ae" is still retained.

From the time of Virgil's Aeneas to Shakespeare's Macduff, poets repeatedly have referred to persons "untimely ripped" from their mother's womb. Ancient historians, such as Pliny, moreover, say that Scipio Africianus (the conqueror of Hannibal), Martius, and Julius Caesar were all born by cesarean. In regard to Julius Caesar, Pliny adds that it was from this circumstance that the surname arose by which the Roman emperors were known. Birth in this extraordinary manner, as described in ancient mythology and legend, was believed to confer supernatural powers and elevated the heroes so born above ordinary mortals.

In evaluating these references to abdominal delivery in antiquity, it is pertinent that no such operation is even mentioned by Hippocrates, Galen, Celsus, Paulus, Soranus, or any other medical writer of those periods. If a cesarean was actually employed, it is particularly surprising that Soranus, whose extensive work written in the second century AD covers all aspects of obstetrics, does not refer to cesarean delivery.

Several references to abdominal delivery appear in the Talmud, compiled between the second and sixth centuries AD, but whether they had any background in terms of clinical usage is conjectural. There can be no doubt, however, that cesareans in the dead were first practiced soon after the Christian Church gained dominance, as a measure directed at baptism of the child. Faith in the validity of some of these early reports is rudely shaken, however, when they glibly state that a living, robust child was obtained 8 to 24 *hours* after the death of the mother.

Cesarean deliveries in the living were first recommended, and the current name of the operation used, in the celebrated work of Francois Rousset (1581) entitled *Traité Nouveau de l'Hystérotomotokie ou l'Enfantement Césaerien.* Rousset had never performed or witnessed the operation; his information was based chiefly on letters from friends. He reported 14 successful cesarean deliveries, a fact in itself difficult to accept. When it is further stated that 6 of the 14 operations were performed on the same woman, the credulity of the most gullible is exhausted!

The apocryphal nature of most early reports on cesareans has been stressed because many of them have been accepted without question. Authoritative statements by dependable obstetricians about early use of the operation, however, did not appear in the literature until the mid-17th century, as for instance in the classical work of the French obstetrician, Francois Mauriceau, first published in 1668. These statements show without doubt that the operation was employed on the living in rare and desperate cases, and it was usually fatal. Details of the history of cesarean deliveries are to be found in Fasbender's classical text (1906).

The appalling maternal mortality rate of cesareans continued until the beginning of the 20th century. In Great Britain and Ireland, the maternal death rate from the operation in 1865 was 85 percent. In Paris, during the 90 years ending in 1876, not a single successful cesarean had been performed. Harris (1879) noted that as late as 1879, cesareans actually were more successful when performed by the patient herself or when the abdomen was ripped open by the horns of a bull! He collected from the literature nine such cases with five recoveries, and contrasted them with 12 cesareans performed in New York City during the same period, with only one recovery.

The turning point in the evolution of cesareans came in 1882, when Max Sänger, then a 28-year-old assistant of Credé in the University Clinic at Leipzig, introduced suturing of the uterine wall. The long neglect of so simple an expedient as uterine suture was not the result of oversight but stemmed from a deeply rooted belief that sutures in the uterus were superfluous as well as harmful by virtue of serving as the site for severe infection. In meeting these objections, Sänger, who had himself used sutures in only one case, documented their value not from the sophisticated medical centers of Europe but from frontier America. There, in outposts from Ohio to Louisiana, 17 cesarean deliveries had been reported in which silver wire sutures had been used, with the survival of eight mothers—an extraordinary record in those days. In a table included in his monograph, Sänger gives full credit to these frontier surgeons for providing the supporting data for his hypothesis. The problem of hemorrhage was the first and most serious problem to be solved. Details are found in Eastman's review (1932).

Although the introduction of uterine sutures reduced the mortality rate of the operation from hemorrhage, generalized peritonitis remained the dominant cause of death. Hence, various types of operations were devised to combat this scourge. The earliest was the Porro procedure (1876), which combined subtotal cesarean hysterectomy with marsupialization of the cervical stump. The first extraperitoneal operation was described by Frank in 1907 and, with various modifications, as introduced by Latzko (1909) and Waters (1940), was employed until recent years.

In 1912, Krönig contended that the main advantage of the extraperitoneal technique consisted not so much in avoiding the peritoneal cavity as in opening the uterus through its thin lower segment and then covering the incision with peritoneum. To accomplish this end, he cut through the vesical reflection of the peritoneum from one round ligament to the other and separated it and the bladder from the lower uterine segment and cervix. The lower portion of the uterus was then opened through a vertical median incision, and the child was extracted by forceps. The uterine incision was then closed and buried under the vesical peritoneum. With minor modifications, this low-segment technique was introduced into the United States by Beck (1919) and popularized by DeLee (1922) and others. A particularly important modification was recommended by Kerr in 1926, who preferred a transverse rather than a longitudinal uterine incision. The Kerr technique is the most commonly employed type of cesarean used today.

Two reviews of the history of cesarean delivery are recommended (Boley, 1991; Sewell, 1993).

REFERENCES

Adashek JA, Peaceman AM, Lopez-Zeno JA, Minogue JP, Socol ML: Factors contributing to the increased cesarean birth rate in older parturient women. Am J Obstet Gynecol 169:936, 1993

American College of Obstetricians and Gynecologists: Task Force on Cesarean Delivery Rates: Evaluation of cesarean delivery. June, 2000

American College of Obstetricians and Gynecologists: Vaginal birth after previous cesarean delivery. Practice Bulletin No. 5, July, 1999

American College of Obstetricians and Gynecologists: Vaginal birth after previous cesarean delivery. Practice Bulletin No. 2, October, 1998

American College of Obstetricians and Gynecologists: Fetal heart rate patterns: Monitoring, interpretation and management. Technical Bulletin No. 207, July, 1995a

American College of Obstetricians and Gynecologists: Vaginal delivery after previous cesarean birth. Practice Patterns No. 1, August, 1995b

American College of Obstetricians and Gynecologists: Operative vaginal delivery. Technical Bulletin No. 196, August, 1994

American College of Obstetricians and Gynecologists: Guidelines for Perinatal Care. Washington, DC, ACOG, 1992

American College of Obstetricians and Gynecologists. Committee on Obstetrics, Maternal and Fetal Medicine: Assessment of fetal maturity prior to repeat cesarean delivery or elective induction of labor. No. 98, September, 1991; reaffirmed 1995

American College of Obstetricians and Gynecologists: Management of Breech Presentations. Technical Bulletin No. 95, 1986

Andersson R, Hugander A, Thulin A, Nystrom P, Oliason G: Clusters of acute appendicitis: Further evidence for infectious aetiology. Int J Epidemiol 24:829, 1995

Ayers JWT, Morley GW: Surgical incision for cesarean section. Obstet Gynecol 70:706, 1987

Beck AC: Observations on a series of cases of cesarean section done at the Long Island College Hospital during the past six years. Am J Obstet Gynecol 79:197, 1919

Belizan JM, Althabe F, Barros FC, Alexander S: Rates and implication of cesarean sections in Latin America: Ecological study. BMJ 319:1397, 1999

Bivins Jr HA, Gallup DG: C/S closure techniques: Which work best? OBG Management 4:98, 2000

Blackhall LJ, Ziogas A, Azen SP: Low survival rate after cardiopulmonary resuscitation in a county hospital. Arch Intern Med 152:2045, 1992

Bohman VR, Gilstrap L, Leveno K, Ramin S, Santos-Ramos R, Goldaber K, Little B: Subcutaneous tissue: To close or not to close at cesarean section. Am J Obstet Gynecol 166:407, 1992

Boley JP: The history of cesarean section. Can Med Assoc J 145:319, 1991

Brooten D, Roncoli M, Finkler S, Arnold L, Cohen A, Mennuti M: A randomized trial of early hospital discharge and home follow-up of women having cesarean birth. Obstet Gynecol 84:832, 1994

Brumfield CG, Hauth JC, Andrews WW: Puerperal infection after cesarean delivery: Evaluation of a standardized protocol. Am J Obstet Gynecol 182:1147, 2000

Burrows WR, Gingo AJ Jr, Rose SM, Zwick SI, Kosty DL, Dierker LJ, Mann LI: Safety and efficacy of early postoperative solid food consumption after cesarean section. J Reprod Med 40:463, 1995

Caughey AB, Shipp TD, Repke JT, Zelop CM, Cohen A, Lieberman E: Rate of uterine rupture during a trial of labor in women with one or two prior cesarean deliveries. Am J Obstet Gynecol 181:872, 1999

Caughey AB, Shipp TD, Repke JT, Zelop CM, Cohen A, Lieberman E: Trial of labor after cesarean delivery: The effect of previous vaginal delivery. Am J Obstet Gynecol 179:938, 1998

Cernada M, Smulian JC, Giannina G, Ananth CV: Effects of placental delivery method and intraoperative glove changing on post cesarean febrile morbidity. J Matern-Fetal Med 7:100, 1998

Chapman SJ, Owen J, Hauth JC: One-versus two-layer closure

of a low transverse cesarean: The next pregnancy. Obstet Gynecol 89:16, 1997

Chauhan SP, Roach H, Naef RW, Magann EF, Morrison JC, Martin JN: Cesarean section for suspected fetal distress: Does the decision-incision time make a difference? J Reprod Med 42:347, 1997

Clark SL, Hankins GDV, Dudley DA, Dildy GA, Porter TF: Amniotic fluid embolism: Analysis of the National Registry. Am J Obstet Gynecol 172:1158, 1995

Clark SL, Scott JR, Porter TF, Schlappy DA, McClellan V, Burton DA: Is vaginal birth after cesarean less expensive than repeat cesarean delivery? Am J Obstet Gynecol 182:599, 2000

Cragin E: Conservatism in obstetrics. N Y Med J 104:1, 1916

DeLee JB, Cornell EL: Low cervical cesarean section (laparotrachelotomy). JAMA 79:109, 1922

DeMott RK, Sandmire HF: The Green Bay cesarean section study, 1. The physician factor as a determination of cesarean birth rates. Am J Obstet Gynecol 162:1593, 1990

DeMuylder X, Thiery M: The cesarean delivery rate can be safely reduced in a developing country. Obstet Gynecol 75:60, 1990

Eastman NJ: The role of frontier America in the development of cesarean section. Am J Obstet Gynecol 24:919, 1932

Farmer RM, Kirschbaun T, Potter D, Strong TH, Medearis AL: Uterine rupture during trial of labor after previous cesarean section. Am J Obstet Gynecol 165:996, 1991

Fasbender H: Geschichte der Geburtshilfe. Jena, 1906, p 979

Field DR, Gates EA, Creasy RK, Jonsen AR, Laros RK Jr: Maternal brain death during pregnancy. Medical and ethical issues. JAMA 260:816, 1988

Flamm BL: Once a cesarean, always a controversy. Obstet Gynecol 90:312, 1997

Flamm BL, Geiger AM: Vaginal birth after cesarean delivery: An admission scoring system. Obstet Gynecol 90:907, 1997

Flamm BL, Goings JR, Liu Y, Wolde-Tsadik G: Elective repeat cesarean delivery versus trial of labor: A prospective multicenter study. Obstet Gynecol 83:927, 1994

Flamm BL, Newman LA, Thomas SJ, Fallon D, Yoshida MM: Vaginal birth after cesarean delivery: Results of a 5-year multicenter collaborative study. Obstet Gynecol 76:750, 1990

Frank F: Suprasymphysial delivery and its relation to other operations in the presence of contracted pelvis. Arch Gynaekol 81:46, 1907

Freeman R: Intrapartum fetal monitoring—a disappointing story. N Engl J Med 322:624, 1992

Friedman EA: Labor, Clinical Evaluation and Management. New York, Appleton, 1978

Frigoletto FD Jr, Ryan KJ, Phillippe M: Maternal mortality rate associated with cesarean section: An appraisal. Am J Obstet Gynecol 136:969, 1980

Gilstrap LC III: Elective appendectomy during abdominal surgery. JAMA 265:1736 1991

Goepfert AR, Guinn DA, Andrews WA, Hauth JC: Necrotizing fasciitis after cesarean delivery. Obstet Gynecol 89:409, 1997

Gould JB, Davey B, Stafford RS: Socioeconomic differences in rates of cesarean section. N Engl J Med 321:233, 1989

Greene R, Gardeil F, Turner MJ: Long-term implications of cesarean delivery. Letter to the Editors. Am J Obstet Gynecol 176:254, 1997

Harris RP: Lessons from a study of the cesarean operation in the city and state of New York. Am J Obstet Gynecol 12:82, 1879

Hauth JC, Owen J, Davis RO, Lincoln T, Piazza J: Transverse

uterine incision closure: One versus two layers. Am J Obstet Gynecol 167:1108, 1992

Hendrix SL, Schimp V, Martin J, Singh A, Kruger M, McNeeley SG: The legendary superior strength of the Pfannenstiel incision: A myth? Am J Obstet Gynecol 182:1446, 2000

Hoskins IA, Gomez JL: Correlation between maximum cervical dilatation at cesarean delivery and subsequent vaginal birth after cesarean delivery. Obstet Gynecol 89:591, 1997

Hull DB, Varner MW: A randomized study of closure of the peritoneum at cesarean delivery. Obstet Gynecol 77:818, 1991

Impey L, O'Herlihy C: First delivery after cesarean delivery for strictly defined cephalopelvic disproportion. Obstet Gynecol 92:799, 1998

Isaacs JD, Magann EF, Martin RW, Chauhan SP, Morrison JC: Obstetric challenges of massive obesity complicating pregnancy. J Perinatol 14:10, 1994

Jacob J, Phenninger J: Cesarean deliveries: When is a pediatrician necessary? Obstet Gynecol 89:717, 1997

Jongen VHWM, Halfwek MGC, Brouwer WK: Vaginal delivery after previous cesarean section for failure of second stage of labour. Br J Obstet Gynaecol 105:1079, 1998

Kaplan M, Dollberg M, Wajntraub G, Itzchaki M: Fractured long bones in a term infant delivered by cesarean section. Pediatr Radiol 17:256, 1987

Katz VL, Dotters DJ, Droegemuller W: Perimortem cesarean delivery. Obstet Gynecol 68:571, 1986

Kerr JMM: The technic of cesarean section with special reference to the lower uterine segment incision. Am J Obstet Gynecol 12:729, 1926

Kerr JMM: Indications for cesarean section. J Obstet Gynaecol Br Emp 28:349, 1921

Kramer R, Van Someren J, Qualls C, Curet L: Postoperative management of cesarean section patients: The effect of immediate feeding on the incidence of ileus. Obstet Gynecol 88:29, 1996

Krönig B: Transperitonealer cervikaler Kaiserschnitt. In Doderlein A, Krönig B (eds): Operative Gynakologie. 1912, p 879

Lasley DS, Eblen A, Yancey MK, Duff P: The effect of placental removal method on the incidence of post cesarean infections. Am J Obstet Gynecol 176:1250, 1997

Latzko W: Ueber den extraperitonealen Kaiserschnitt. Zentralbl Gynaekol 33:275, 1909

Leveno KJ: Controversies in OB-Gyn: Should we rethink the criteria for VBAC? Contemporary OB-Gyn, January, 1999

Lien JM, Towers CV, Quilligan EJ, deVeciana M, Toohey JS, Morgan MA: Term early-onset neonatal seizures: Obstetric characteristics, etiologic classifications, and perinatal care. Obstet Gynecol 85:163, 1995

Lilford RJ, Van Coeverden de Groot HA, Moore PJ, Bingham P: The relative risks of caesarean section (intrapartum and elective) and vaginal delivery: A detailed analysis to exclude the effects of medical disorders and other acute pre-existing physiological disturbances. Br J Obstet Gynaecol 97:883, 1990

Livingston EH, Passaro EP: Postoperative ileus. Dig Dis Sci 35:21, 1990

Lyndon-Rochelle M, Holt VL, Martin DP, Easterling TR: Association between method of delivery and maternal rehospitalization. JAMA 283:2411, 2000

Magann EF, Dodson MK, Allbert JR, McCurdy CM Jr, Martin RW, Morrison JC: Blood loss at time of cesarean section by method of placental removal and exteriorization versus in situ repair of the uterine incision. Surg Gynecol Obstet 177:389, 1993

Martin JN, Perry KG, Roberts WE, Meydrech EF: The care for trial of labor in the patients with a prior low-segment vertical cesarean incision. Am J Obstet Gynecol 177:144, 1997

McMahon MJ, Luther ER, Bowes WA, Olshan AF: Comparison of a trial of labor with an elective second cesarean section. N Engl J Med 335:689, 1996

Merrill BS, Gibbs CE: Planned vaginal delivery following cesarean section. Obstet Gynecol 52:50, 1978

Miller DA, Chollet JA, Goodwin TM: Clinical risk factors for placenta previa-placenta accreta. Am J Obstet Gynecol 177:210, 1997

Miller DA, Diaz FG, Paul RH: Vaginal birth after cesarean: A 10-year experience. Obstet Gynecol 84:255, 1994

Naumann RW, Hauth JC, Owen J, Hodgkins PM, Lincoln T: Subcutaneous tissue approximation in relation to wound disruption after cesarean delivery in obese women. Obstet Gynecol 85:412, 1995

Nelson KB, Dambrosia JM, Ting TY, Grether JK: Uncertain value of electronic fetal monitoring in predicting cerebral palsy. N Engl J Med 334:613, 1996

Niemann JT: Cardiopulmonary resuscitation. N Engl J Med 327:1085, 1992

Notzon FC, Cnattingius S, Bergsjo P, Cole S, Taffel S, Irgens L, Daltveit AK: Cesarean section delivery in the 1980s: International comparison by indication. Am J Obstet Gynecol 170:495, 1994

Parrish K, Holt VL, Easterling TR, Connell FA, LoGerfo JP: Effect of changes in maternal age, parity and birth weight distribution on primary cesarean delivery rates. JAMA 271:443, 1994

Parsons AK, Sauer MY, Parsons MT, Tunca J, Spellacy WN: Appendectomy at cesarean section: A prospective study. Obstet Gynecol 68:479, 1986

Peipert JF, Bracken MB: Maternal age: An independent risk factor for cesarean delivery. Obstet Gynecol 81:200, 1993

Perlow JH, Morgan MA: Massive maternal obesity and perioperative cesarean morbidity. Am J Obstet Gynecol 170:560, 1994

Physicians Insurance Association of America: Data Sharing System, Report No. 4. Pennington, NJ, 1992

Pickrell K: An inquiry into the history of cesarean section. Bull Soc Med Hist (Chicago) 4:414, 1935

Pietrantoni M, Parsons MT, O'Brien WF, Collins E, Knuppel RA, Spellacy WN: Peritoneal closure or non-closure at cesarean. Obstet Gynecol 77:293, 1991

Pitkin RM: Once a cesarean? Obstet Gynecol 77:939, 1991

Plauche WC: Obstetric hysterectomy. In Hankins GDV, Clark SL, Cunningham FG, Gilstrap LC (eds): Operative Obstetrics. Norwalk, Appleton & Lange, 1995, p 333

Pliny the Elder: Natural History. Cambridge, Harvard University Press, 1942, book VII, chap IX. Translated by H. Rackham

Porreco RP: Meeting the challenge of the rising cesarean birth rate. Obstet Gynecol 75:133, 1990

Porro E: Della Amputazione Utero-ovarica. Milan, 1876

Porter TF, Clark SL, Esplin MS: Timing of delivery and neonatal outcomes in patients with clinically overt uterine rupture during VBAC. Abstract No. 73. Am J Obstet Gynecol 178:Part 2, 1998

Pridijian G, Hibbard JU, Moawad AH: Cesarean: Changing the trends. Obstet Gynecol 77:195, 1991

Pritchard JA: Changes in the blood volume during pregnancy and delivery. Anesthesiology 26:393, 1965

Rajasekar D, Hall M: Urinary tract injuries during obstetric intervention. Br J Obstet Gynaecol 104:731, 1997

Ravasia DJ, Brain PH, Pollard JK: Incidence of uterine rupture among women with mullerian duct anomalies who attempt vaginal birth after cesarean delivery. Am J Obstet Gynecol 181:877, 1999

Reyes-Ceja L, Cabrera R, Insfran E, Herrera-Lasso F: Pregnancy following previous uterine rupture: Study of 19 patients. Obstet Gynecol 34:387, 1969

Ritchie EH: Pregnancy after rupture of the pregnant uterus: A report of 36 pregnancies and a study of cases reported since 1932. J Obstet Gynaecol Br Commonw 78:642, 1971

Rodriguez AI, Porter KB, O'Brien WF: Blunt versus sharp expansion of the uterine incision in low-segment transverse cesarean section. Am J Obstet Gynecol 171:1022, 1994

Rousset F: Traité Nouveau de l'Hystérotomotokie ou l'Enfantement Césaerien. Paris, Denys deVal, 1581

Sachs BP, Kobelin C, Castro MA, Frigoletto F: The risks of lowering the cesarean-delivery rate. N Engl J Med 340:54, 1999

Sachs BP, Yeh J, Acker D, Driscoll S, Brown DAJ, Jewett JF: Cesarean section-related maternal mortality in Massachusetts, 1954–1985. Obstet Gynecol 71:385, 1988

Sanchez-Ramos L, Kaunitz AM, Peterson HB, Martinez-Schnell B, Thompson RJ: Reducing cesarean sections at a teaching hospital. Am J Obstet Gynecol 163:1081, 1990

Sänger M: Der Kaiserschnitt bei Uterusfibromen. Leipzig, 1882

Scheller JM, Nelson KB: Does cesarean delivery prevent cerebral palsy or other neurologic problems of childhood? Obstet Gynecol 83:624, 1994

Scott JR: Mandatory trial of labor after cesarean delivery: An alternative viewpoint. Obstet Gynecol 77:811, 1991

Seago DP, Roberts WE, Johnson VK, Martin RW, Morrison JC, Martin JN: Planned cesarean hysterectomy: A preferred alternative to separate operations. Am J Obstet Gynecol 180:1385, 1999

Sewell JE: Cesarean section—a brief history. Washington, DC, American College of Obstetricians and Gynecologists. 1993

Shipp TD, Zelop CM, Repke JT, Cohen A, Caughey AB, Lieberman E: Intrapartum uterine rupture and dehiscence in patients with prior lower uterine segment vertical and transverse incisions. Obstet Gynecol 94:735, 1999

Skajaa K, Hansen ES, Bendix J: Depressed fracture of the skull in a child born by cesarean section. Acta Obstet Gynecol Scand 66:275, 1987

Smith W: A profile of health and disease in America: Obstetrics Gynecology, and infant mortality. Facts on File Publications, New York, 1987, p 82

Socol ML, Peaceman AM: Vaginal birth after cesarean: An appraisal of fetal risk. Obstet Gynecol 93:674, 1999

Source Book of Health Insurance Data, Health Insurance Association of America. Orodell, NJ, Medical Economics, 1993

Stafford RS: Alternative strategies for controlling rising cesarean section rates. JAMA 263:683, 1990

Strong TH, Brown WL Jr, Brown WL, Curry CM: Experience with early postcesarean hospital dismissal. Am J Obstet Gynecol 169:116, 1993

Studnicki J, Remmel R, Campbell R, Werner DC: The impact of legislatively imposed practice guidelines as cesarean section rates: The Florida experience. Am J Med Quality 12:62, 1997

Tulandi T, Hum HS, Gelfand MM: Closure of laparotomy incisions with or without peritoneal suturing and second-look laparoscopy. Am J Obstet Gynecol 158:536, 1988

Turner MJ: Delivery after one previous cesarean section. Am J Obstet Gynecol 176:741, 1997

United States Department of Health and Human Services: Public Health Service. Health Resources and Services Administration: Maternal and Child Health Bureau. DHHS Publication No. HRSA-M-CH 91-2, 1991

Vasa R, Kim MR: Fracture of the femur at cesarean section: Case report and review of literature. Am J Perinatol 7:46, 1990

Ventura SJ, Martin JA, Curtin SC, Mathews TJ, Park MM: Births: Final data for 1998. National Vital Statistics Reports; Vol 48, No. 3. Hyattsville, MD: National Center for Health Statistics, 2000

Vermillion ST, Lamoutte C, Soper DE, Verdeja A: Wound infection after cesarean: Effect of subcutaneous tissue thickness. Obstet Gynecol 95:923, 2000

Wahab MA, Karantziz P, Eccersley PS, Russell IF, Thompson JW, Lindow SW: A randomized, controlled study of uterine exteriorization and repair at cesarean section. Br J Obstet Gynaecol 106:913, 1999

Wallace RC, Eglinton GS, Yonekura ML, Wallace TM: Extraperitoneal cesarean section: A surgical form of infection prophylaxis? Am J Obstet Gynecol 148:172, 1984

Waters EG: Supravesical extraperitoneal cesarean section: Presentation of a new technique. Am J Obstet Gynecol 39:423, 1940

Wing DA, Paul RH: Vaginal birth after cesarean section: Selection and management. Clin Obstet Gynecol 42:835, 1999

Yoles L, Maschiach S: Increased maternal mortality in cesarean section as compared to vaginal delivery? Time for reevaluation. Am J Obstet Gynecol 178:1, 1998

Zelop CM, Harlow BL, Frigoletto FD Jr, Safon LE, Saltzman DH: Emergency peripartum hysterectomy. Am J Obstet Gynecol 168:1443, 1993

Zelop CM, Shipp TD, Repke JT, Cohen A, Caughey AB, Lieberman E: Uterine rupture during induced or augmented labor in gravid women with one prior cesarean delivery. Am J Obstet Gynecol 181:882, 1999

Zorlu CG, Turan C, Isik AZ, Danisman N, Mungan T, Gokmen O: Emergency hysterectomy in modern obsteric practice. Changing clinical perspective in time. Acta Obstet Gynecol Scand 77:186, 1998

Zuidema L, Elderkin R, Cook C, Jelsema R: Is Vicryl suture closure of uterine wounds associated with more dehiscence? Am J Obstet Gynecol 174:357, 1996

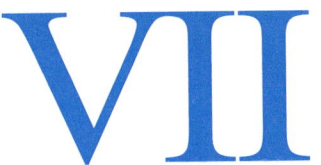

VII

SECTION

Common Complications of Pregnancy

24

Hypertensive Disorders in Pregnancy

Hypertensive disorders complicating pregnancy are common and form one of the deadly triad, along with hemorrhage and infection, that results in much of the maternal morbidity and mortality related to pregnancy. According to the National Center for Health Statistics in 1998, hypertension associated with pregnancy was the most common medical risk factor (Ventura and colleagues, 2000). It was identified in 146,320 women, or 3.7 percent of all pregnancies that ended in live births. In 12,345 of these women eclampsia was diagnosed, and maternal deaths from this complication still remain a threat. Berg and colleagues (1996) reported that almost 18 percent of 1450 maternal deaths in the United States from 1987 to 1990 were from complications of pregnancy-related hypertension.

How pregnancy incites or aggravates hypertension remains unsolved despite decades of intensive research, and hypertensive disorders remain among the most significant unsolved problems in obstetrics. Important ongoing research currently is sponsored by the National Institutes of Child Health and Human Development (NICHD) and its Maternal–Fetal Medicine Units Network. Another important stimulus for research is the International Society for the Study of Hypertension in Pregnancy (ISSHP). Also, the National Heart, Lung, and Breast Institute (NHLBI) encourages ongoing research and coordination through the National High Blood Pressure Education Program (NHBPEP) and its Working Group Report on High Blood Pressure in Pregnancy.

TERMINOLOGY

In former editions of this textbook, the authors preferred to use the term *pregnancy-induced hypertension* to describe any new-onset pregnancy-related hypertension. This designation was chosen because it served to emphasize the cause-and-effect connection between pregnancy and a unique form of hypertension manifest in women only during reproduction. It was also intended that *pregnancy-induced hypertension* would include the development of hypertension without proteinuria, including in nulliparous women. In this latter circumstance, *pregnancy-induced hypertension* was also a potential precursor to preeclampsia or eclampsia, which require proteinuria for diagnosis. Our purpose was to communicate that the development of hypertension in a previously normotensive pregnant woman should and must be considered potentially dangerous to both her and her fetus. The designation *pregnancy-induced hypertension* also had the advantage of signifying that most hypertensive nulliparous women had only *transient* uncomplicated hypertension that subsided promptly after delivery. Recently, the working group of the National

High Blood Pressure Education Program (2000) has proposed a classification system that accomplishes all the foregoing goals of the authors and thus will be adopted in this edition of *Williams Obstetrics*. The authors have taken this approach in an effort to deal with the nonuniform and confusing terminology that has long plagued the diagnosis of hypertension in pregnancy (American College of Obstetricians and Gynecologists, 1996).

DIAGNOSIS

The diagnosis of hypertensive disorders complicating pregnancy, as outlined by the Working Group (2000), is shown in Table 24–1. There are five types of hypertensive disease that include:

1. Gestational hypertension (formerly pregnancy-induced hypertension or transient hypertension).
2. Preeclampsia.
3. Eclampsia.
4. Preeclampsia superimposed on chronic hypertension.
5. Chronic hypertension.

An important consideration in this classification is differentiating hypertensive disorders that precede pregnancy from preeclampsia, which is a potentially more ominous disease.

Hypertension is diagnosed when *blood pressure* is 140/90 mm Hg or greater, using Korotkoff phase V to define diastolic pressure. Edema has been abandoned as a diagnostic criteria because it occurs in too many normal pregnant women to be discriminant. In the past, it had been recommended that an increment of 30 mm Hg systolic or 15 mm Hg diastolic blood pressure be used as a diagnostic criterion, even when absolute values were below 140/90 mm Hg. This criterion is no longer recommended because evidence shows that women in this group are not likely to suffer increased adverse pregnancy outcomes (Levine, 2000; North and colleagues, 1999). That said, women who have a rise of 30 mm Hg systolic or 15 mm Hg diastolic warrant close observation.

GESTATIONAL HYPERTENSION. As shown in Table 24–1, the diagnosis of gestational hypertension is made in women whose blood pressure reaches 140/90 mm Hg or greater for the first time during pregnancy, but in whom *proteinuria has not developed*. Gestational hypertension is termed *transient hypertension* if preeclampsia does not develop and the blood pressure has returned to normal by 12 weeks' postpartum. In this classification the final diagnosis that the woman does not have preeclampsia is made only postpartum. Thus, gestational

TABLE 24–1. Diagnosis of Hypertensive Disorders Complicating Pregnancy

Gestational Hypertension

BP ≥ 140/90 mm Hg for first time during pregnancy

No proteinuria

BP return to normal < 12 weeks' postpartum

Final diagnosis made only postpartum

May have other signs of preeclampsia, for example, epigastric discomfort or thrombocytopenia

Preeclampsia

Minimum criteria:

   BP ≥ 140/90 mm Hg after 20 weeks' gestation

   Proteinuria ≥ 300 mg/24 hours or ≥ 1+ dipstick

Increased certainty of preeclampsia:

   BP ≥ 160/110 mg Hg

   Proteinuria 2.0 g/24 hours or ≥ 2+ dipstick

   Serum creatinine > 1.2 mg/dL unless known to be previously elevated

   Platelets < 100,000/mm^3

   Microangiopathic hemolysis (increased LDH)

   Elevated ALT or AST

   Persistent headache or other cerebral or visual disturbance

   Persistent epigastric pain

Eclampsia

Seizures that cannot be attributed to other causes in a woman with preeclampsia

Superimposed Preeclampsia (on chronic hypertension)

New-onset proteinuria ≥ 300 mg/24 hours in hypertensive women but no proteinuria before 20 weeks' gestation

A sudden increase in proteinuria or blood pressure or platelet count < 100,000/mm^3 in women with hypertension and proteinuria before 20 weeks' gestation

Chronic Hypertension

BP ≥ 140/90 mm Hg before pregnancy or diagnosed before 20 weeks' gestation

or

Hypertension first diagnosed after 20 weeks' gestation and persistent after 12 weeks' postpartum

ALT = alanine aminotransferase; AST = aspartate aminotransferase; BP = blood pressure; LDH = lactate dehydrogenase.
Adapted from National High Blood Pressure Education Program Working Group Report on High Blood Pressure in Pregnancy (2000).

hypertension is a diagnosis of exclusion. Importantly, however, women with gestational hypertension may develop other signs associated with preeclampsia, for example, headaches, epigastric pain, or thrombocytopenia, which influence management.

When blood pressure rises appreciably during the latter half of pregnancy, it is dangerous—especially to the fetus—not to take action simply because proteinuria has not yet developed. As Chesley (1985) emphasized, 10 percent of eclamptic seizures develop before overt proteinuria. Thus, it is clear that when blood pressure begins to rise, both mother and fetus are at increased risk. Proteinuria is a sign of worsening hypertensive disease, specifically preeclampsia; and when it is overt and persistent, maternal and fetal risks are increased even more.

PREECLAMPSIA. Preeclampsia is a pregnancy-specific syndrome of reduced organ perfusion secondary to vasospasm and endothelial activation. *Proteinuria* is an important sign of preeclampsia, and Chesley (1985) rightfully concluded that the diagnosis is questionable in its absence. Proteinuria is described as 300 mg or more of urinary protein per 24 hours or persistent 30 mg/dL (1+ dipstick) in random urine samples. The degree of proteinuria may fluctuate widely over any 24-hour period, even in severe cases. Therefore, a single random sample may fail to demonstrate significant proteinuria.

McCartney and co-workers (1971), in their extensive study of renal biopsy specimens obtained from hypertensive pregnant women, invariably found that proteinuria was present when the glomerular lesion considered

TABLE 24–2. Hypertensive Disorders During Pregnancy: Indications of Severity

Abnormality	Mild	Severe
Diastolic blood pressure	< 100 mg Hg	110 mm Hg or higher
Proteinuria	Trace to 1+	Persistent 2+ or more
Headache	Absent	Present
Visual disturbances	Absent	Present
Upper abdominal pain	Absent	Present
Oliguria	Absent	Present
Convulsion	Absent	Present (eclampsia)
Serum creatinine	Normal	Elevated
Thrombocytopenia	Absent	Present
Liver enzyme elevation	Minimal	Marked
Fetal growth restriction	Absent	Obvious
Pulmonary edema	Absent	Present

to be characteristic of preeclampsia was evident. Importantly, both proteinuria and alterations of glomerular histology develop late in the course of hypertensive disorders due to pregnancy. In fact, preeclampsia becomes evident clinically only near the end of a covert pathophysiological process that may begin 3 to 4 months before hypertension develops (Gant and associates, 1973). As shown in Table 24–1, the minimum criteria for the diagnosis of preeclampsia are hypertension plus minimal proteinuria. The more severe the hypertension or proteinuria, the more certain is the diagnosis of preeclampsia (Table 24–2). Similarly, abnormal laboratory findings in tests of renal, hepatic, and hematological function increase the certainty of preeclampsia. Persistent premonitory symptoms of eclampsia such as headache and epigastric pain also increase the certainty of preeclampsia.

The combination of proteinuria and hypertension during pregnancy markedly increases the risk of perinatal mortality and morbidity (Ferrazzani and associates, 1990). Results from a 13-year prospective study reported by Friedman and Neff (1976) in over 38,000 pregnancies are shown in Table 24–3. Hypertension alone, defined by a diastolic blood pressure of 95 mm Hg or greater, was associated with a threefold increase in the fetal death rate. Worsening hypertension, especially if accompanied by proteinuria, was more ominous. Conversely, proteinuria without hypertension had little overall effect on the fetal death rate. Naeye and Friedman (1979) concluded that 70 percent of the excess fetal deaths in these same women were due to large placental infarcts, markedly small placental size, and abruptio placentae. They concluded that these causes usually develop late in the course of the disease. Certainly, persistent proteinuria of 2+ or more, or 24-hour urinary excre-

tion of 2 g or more, is severe preeclampsia. With severe renal involvement, glomerular filtration may be impaired, and plasma creatinine may rise.

Epigastric or right upper quadrant pain likely results from hepatocellular necrosis, ischemia, and edema that stretches Glisson's capsule. This characteristic pain is frequently accompanied by elevated serum liver enzymes, and usually is a sign to terminate the pregnancy. The pain presages hepatic infarction and hemorrhage as well as catastrophic rupture of a subcapsular hematoma. Fortunately, hepatic rupture is rare and most often associated with hypertension in older and multiparous women.

Thrombocytopenia is characteristic of worsening preeclampsia, and probably is caused by platelet activation and aggregation and microangiopathic hemolysis induced by severe vasospasm. Evidence for gross hemolysis such as hemoglobinemia, hemoglobinuria, or hyperbilirubinemia is indicative of severe disease.

Other factors indicative of severe hypertension include cardiac dysfunction with pulmonary edema as well as obvious fetal growth restriction.

SEVERITY OF PREECLAMPSIA. The severity of preeclampsia is assessed by the frequency and intensity of the abnormalities listed in Table 24–2. The more profound these aberrations, the more likely is the need for pregnancy termination. **Importantly, the differentiation between mild and severe preeclampsia can be misleading because apparently mild disease may progress rapidly to severe disease.**

Although hypertension is a requisite to diagnosing preeclampsia, blood pressure alone is not always a dependable indicator of its severity. For example, a thin adolescent woman may have 3+ proteinuria and convul-

TABLE 24–3. Fetal Death Rate per 1000 Births Analyzed According to Diastolic Pressure and Proteinuria

Diastolic Blood Pressure (mm Hg)	Degree of Proteinuria						
	None	Trace	1+	2+	3+	4+	Total
< 65	15.5[a]	13.6	6.2	—	—	—	13.6
65–74	9.3	8.1	5.6	32.9[a]	41.5	—	8.8
75–84	6.2	7.4	6.2	19.2[a]	—	—	6.8
85–94	8.7	9.3	23.6[a]	—	22.3	—	10.2
95–104	19.2[a]	17.4[a]	26.7[a]	55.8[a]	115.3[a]	143[a]	25.2
105+	20.5[a]	27.9[a]	62.6[a]	68.8[a]	125.2[a]	111[a]	41.5[a]
Total	8.6	9.5	12.9	23.2[a]	42.0[a]	57[a]	

[a]$P < .01$.
Modified from Friedman and Neff (1976).

sions while her blood pressure is 140/85 mm Hg, whereas most women with blood pressures as high as 180/120 mm Hg do not have seizures. Convulsions are usually preceded by an unrelenting severe headache or visual disturbances; thus, these symptoms are considered ominous.

ECLAMPSIA. Eclampsia is the occurrence of seizures in a woman with preeclampsia that cannot be attributed to other causes. The seizures are grand mal and may appear before, during, or after labor. Seizures that develop more than 48 hours postpartum, however, especially in nulliparas, may be encountered up to 10 days postpartum (Brown and colleagues, 1987; Lubarsky and associates, 1994).

PREECLAMPSIA SUPERIMPOSED UPON CHRONIC HYPERTENSION. All *chronic hypertensive disorders*, regardless of their cause, predispose to development of superimposed preeclampsia or eclampsia. These disorders can create difficult problems with diagnosis and management in women who are not seen until after midpregnancy. The diagnosis of chronic underlying hypertension is suggested by:

1. Hypertension (140/90 mm Hg or greater) antecedent to pregnancy.
2. Hypertension (140/90 mm Hg or greater) detected before 20 weeks (unless there is gestational trophoblastic disease).
3. Persistent hypertension long after delivery (Table 24–1).

Additional historical factors that help support the diagnosis are multiparity and hypertension complicating a previous pregnancy other than the first. There is also usually a strong family history of essential hypertension.

The diagnosis of chronic hypertension may be difficult to make if the woman is not seen until the latter half of pregnancy. This is because blood pressure decreases during the second and early third trimesters in both normotensive and chronically hypertensive women (Chap. 45, p. 1211). Thus, a woman with chronic vascular disease, who is seen for the first time at 20 weeks, will frequently have a normal blood pressure. During the third trimester, however, blood pressure may return to its former hypertensive level, thus presenting a diagnostic problem as to whether the hypertension is chronic or induced by pregnancy.

Some of the many causes of underlying hypertension that are encountered during pregnancy are listed in Table 24–4. Essential hypertension is the cause of underlying vascular disease in more than 90 percent of pregnant women. McCartney (1964) studied renal biopsies from women with "clinical preeclampsia," and found chronic glomerulonephritis in 20 percent of nulliparas and in nearly 70 percent of multiparas. Fisher and co-workers (1969), however, did not confirm this high prevalence of chronic glomerulonephritis.

Chronic hypertension causes morbidity whether or not a woman is pregnant. Specifically, as discussed in Chapter 45, it may lead to ventricular hypertrophy and cardiac decompensation, cerebrovascular accidents, or intrinsic renal damage. In some young women, hypertension develops as a consequence of underlying renal parenchymal disease. Dangers specific to pregnancy complicated by chronic hypertension include the risk of superimposed preeclampsia, which may develop in up to 25 percent of these women (Sibai and colleagues, 1998). Additionally, the risk of abruptio placentae is increased substantively especially in those women who develop superimposed preeclampsia (Chap. 25, p. 623). Moreover, the fetus of the woman with chronic hypertension is at increased risk for growth restriction and death.

Preexisting chronic hypertension worsens in some women, typically after 24 weeks. If accompanied by

TABLE 24–4. Underlying Chronic Hypertensive Disorders

Essential familial hypertension (hypertensive vascular disease)
Arterial abnormalities
　Renovascular hypertension
　Coarctation of the aorta
Endocrine disorders
　Diabetes
　Cushing syndrome
　Primary aldosteronism
　Pheochromocytoma
　Thyrotoxicosis
Glomerulonephritis (acute and chronic)
Renoprival hypertension
　Chronic glomerulonephritis
　Chronic renal insufficiency
　Diabetic nephropathy
Connective-tissue diseases
　Lupus erythematosus
　Scleroderma
　Periarteritis nodosa
Polycystic kidney disease
Acute renal failure
Obesity

proteinuria, superimposed preeclampsia is diagnosed. Often, superimposed preeclampsia develops earlier in pregnancy than "pure" preeclampsia, and it tends to be quite severe and accompanied in many cases by fetal growth restriction.

The diagnosis requires documentation of chronic underlying hypertension. Superimposed gestational hypertension is characterized by worsening hypertension, keeping in mind that both systolic and diastolic pressures normally rise after 26 to 28 weeks. Preeclampsia is accompanied by proteinuria. Indicators of severity shown in Table 24–2 are also used to further characterize these disorders.

INCIDENCE AND RISK FACTORS. Gestational hypertension more often affects nulliparous women. Older women, who accrue an increasing incidence of chronic hypertension with advancing age, are at greater risk for superimposed preeclampsia. Thus, women at either end of reproductive age are considered to be more susceptible (Chap. 9, p. 207).

The incidence of preeclampsia is commonly cited to be about 5 percent, although remarkable variations are reported. The incidence is markedly influenced by parity; it is related to race and ethnicity—and thus to

genetic predisposition; and environmental factors may also have a role. For example, Palmer and colleagues (1999) reported that high altitude in Colorado increased the incidence of preeclampsia. Some investigators have concluded that socioeconomically advantaged women have a lesser incidence of preeclampsia, even after racial factors are controlled. Conversely, in carefully controlled epidemiological studies in Scottish women, Baird and colleagues (1969) found that the incidence of preeclampsia was not different among five social classes.

The incidence of hypertensive disorders due to pregnancy in healthy nulliparous women has been carefully studied in a recent randomized trial of daily maternal dietary calcium supplementation (Hauth and colleagues, 2000). Of 4302 nulliparous women delivered at or beyond 20 weeks' gestation, a fourth developed a pregnancy-related hypertensive disorder. Of all nulliparas, preeclampsia was diagnosed in 7.6 percent and severe disease as defined in Table 24–2 developed in 3.3 percent.

Other risk factors associated with preeclampsia include multiple pregnancy, history of chronic hypertension, maternal age over 35 years, obesity, and African-American ethnicity (Conde-Agudelao and Belizan, 2000; Sibai and colleagues, 1997; Walker, 2000). The relationship between maternal weight and risk of preeclampsia is progressive, increasing from 4.3 percent for women with a body mass index less than 19.8 kg/m^2 to 13.3 percent for those greater than or equal to 35 kg/m^2. In women with twin gestations compared with those with singletons, the incidence of gestational hypertension (13 versus 6 percent) and preeclampsia (13 versus 5 percent) are both significantly increased (Sibai and co-authors, 2000). Moreover, women with twins and hypertensive disorders due to pregnancy experience higher rates of adverse neonatal outcomes than do those with singletons. Although maternal smoking causes a variety of adverse pregnancy outcomes, ironically, smoking during pregnancy has consistently been associated with a reduced risk of hypertension during pregnancy (Zhang and colleagues, 1999). Placenta previa has also been claimed to reduce the risk of hypertensive disorders due to pregnancy (Ananth and colleagues, 1997).

ECLAMPSIA. In general, eclampsia is preventable, and it has become less common in the United States because most women now receive adequate prenatal care. For example, in the 15th edition of *Williams Obstetrics* (1976), the incidence of eclampsia at Parkland Hospital was cited to be 1 in 700 deliveries for the prior 25-year period. For the 4-year period 1983 to 1986, the incidence was 1 in 1150 deliveries, and for 1990 to 2000 the incidence was approximately 1 in 2300 deliveries. Using figures from the National Vital Statistics Report, Ventura and colleagues (2000) estimated an incidence of about 1 in 3250 for the United States in 1998. Douglas and Redman (1994) cite an incidence of 1 in 2000 for the United Kingdom in 1992.

Mattar and Sibai (2000) have chronicled the hazards in 399 consecutive eclamptic women delivered between 1977 and 1998 at their center in Memphis. Major complications included abruptio placentae (10 percent), neurological deficits (7 percent), aspiration pneumonia (7 percent), pulmonary edema (5 percent), cardiopulmonary arrest (4 percent), acute renal failure (4 percent), and maternal death (1 percent).

PATHOLOGY

Pathological deterioration of function in a number of organs and systems, presumably as a consequence of vasospasm and ischemia, has been identified in severe preeclampsia and eclampsia. For descriptive purposes, these effects are separated into maternal and fetal consequences; however, these aberrations often occur simultaneously. Although there are many possible maternal consequences of hypertensive disorders due to pregnancy, for simplicity these effects are considered by analysis of cardiovascular, hematological, endocrine and metabolic, and regional blood flow changes with subsequent end-organ derangements. The major cause of fetal compromise occurs as a consequence of reduced uteroplacental perfusion.

CARDIOVASCULAR CHANGES. Severe disturbance(s) of normal cardiovascular function is common with preeclampsia or eclampsia. These basically are related to increased cardiac afterload caused by hypertension, cardiac preload which is substantively affected by pathologically diminished hypervolemia of pregnancy or iatrogenically increased by intravenous crystalloid or oncotic solutions, and endothelial activation with extravasation into the extracellular space, especially the lung. These interactions are discussed further in Chapter 43 (p. 1164).

HEMODYNAMIC CHANGES. The cardiovascular changes due to preeclampsia have been studied using invasive hemodynamic monitoring. Once preeclampsia has become clinically evident, however, such invasive hemodynamic studies are unlikely to provide meaningful information about the nature of the disease in earlier pregnancy. Bosio and colleagues (1999) used noninvasive Doppler hemodynamic monitoring in a longitudinal study commencing early in pregnancy in 400 nulliparous women. Gestational hypertension developed in 24 women, and 20 developed preeclampsia. Compared with normotensive women, those who developed pre-

eclampsia had significantly elevated cardiac outputs before clinical diagnosis, but total peripheral resistance was not significantly different during this preclinical phase. With clinical preeclampsia, there was a marked reduction in cardiac output and increased peripheral resistance. By contrast, women with gestational hypertension had significantly elevated cardiac outputs before and during the development of clinical hypertension.

Much of the data based upon invasive hemodynamic studies (Table 24–5) are confounded because (1) women with preeclampsia often have different severity and duration of disease, (2) underlying disease may modify the clinical presentation, or (3) therapeutic interventions may significantly alter these findings. Variables that define cardiovascular status range from high cardiac output with low vascular resistance to low cardiac output with high vascular resistance. Similarly, left ventricular filling pressures, estimated by pulmonary capillary wedge pressure determination, range from low to pathologically high. At least three factors may explain these differences:

1. Women with preeclampsia might present with a spectrum of cardiovascular findings dependent upon both severity and duration.
2. Chronic underlying disease may modify the clinical presentation.
3. Therapeutic interventions may significantly alter these findings.

It is likely that more than one of these is operative.

The studies listed in Table 24–5 are separated into three groups based on clinical management prior to initial hemodynamic observations:

1. No therapy for preeclampsia.
2. Magnesium sulfate and hydralazine without large volumes of intravenous fluid.
3. Magnesium sulfate and hydralazine plus intravenous volume loading.

Ventricular function from the studies listed in Table 24–5 is plotted in Figure 24–1. Cardiac function was hyperdynamic in all women, but filling pressures varied markedly.

Hemodynamic data obtained prior to active treatment of preeclampsia (Table 24–5) identified normal left ventricular filling pressures, high systemic vascular resistances, and hyperdynamic ventricular function. Benedetti (1980a), Hankins (1984), and their associates reported similar findings in women with severe preeclampsia or eclampsia who were being treated with magnesium sulfate, hydralazine, and intravenous crystalloid given at 75 to 100 mL/hour. Cardiac function in these women was appropriate, and the lower systemic vascular resistance was most likely due to hydralazine treatment.

TABLE 24–5. Severe Preeclampsia and Eclampsia: Associated Hemodynamic Measurements[a]

Therapy	No.	Cardiac Output (L/min)	Pulmonary Capillary Wedge Pressure (mm Hg)	Left Ventricular Stroke Work Index (g · m · m⁻²)	Systemic Vascular Resistance (dyne/sec) per cm⁻⁵)
Before Therapy					
Groenendijk et al (1984)	10	4.66	3.3	44	1943
Visser and Wallenberg (1995)	87	(3.3)[b]	7	NA	3003
Magnesium, Hydalazine, and Fluid Restriction					
Benedetti et al (1980a)	10	7.4	6.0	82	1322
Hankins et al (1984)	8	6.7	3.9	66	1357
Magnesium, Hydralazine, and Volume Expansion					
Rafferty and Berkowitz (1980)	3	11.0	7.0	89	780
Phelan and Yurth (1982)	10	9.3	16.0	89	1042

NA = not available.
[a]Values are those reported soon after pulmonary artery catheterization was performed, and are the means for each study.
[b]Reported as cardiac index (CI = L/min/m⁻²).

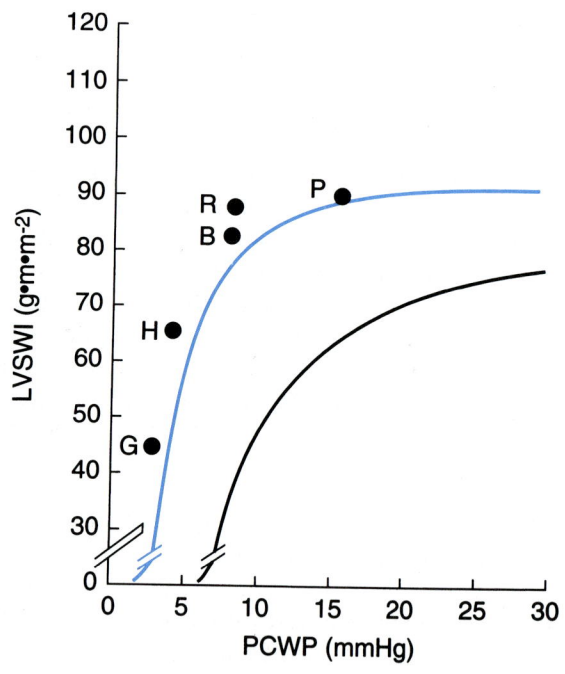

FIGURE 24–1. Ventricular function in severe preeclampsia–eclampsia. Data plotted represent mean values obtained in five of six studies cited in Table 24–5. Left ventricular stroke work index (LVSWI) and pulmonary artery capillary wedge pressure (PCWP) are plotted on a standard ventricular function curve. Points falling within the two solid lines represent normal function, while those below represent depressed function. Points above the solid lines represent hyperdynamic ventricular function. Each letter adjacent to the data points is the first initial of the last name of the investigator who reported this value. (From Hauth and Cunningham, 1999).

Women similarly treated with magnesium sulfate and hydralazine plus aggressive intravenous therapy or volume expansion had the lowest systemic vascular resistances and highest cardiac outputs. A comparison of volume restriction with aggressive hydration shows hyperdynamic ventricular function in most women in both groups, and two responses with respect to left ventricular stroke work index and pulmonary capillary wedge pressure (Fig. 24–2). Fluid restriction resulted in wedge pressures of less than 10 mm Hg, and most were less than 5 mm Hg. Thus, hyperdynamic ventricular function was largely a result of low wedge pressures and not a result of augmented left ventricular stroke work index, which more directly measures myocardial contractility. By comparison, women given appreciably larger volumes of fluid commonly had pulmonary capillary wedge pressures that exceeded normal; however, ventricular function remained hyperdynamic because of increased cardiac output. Subsequently, Visser and Wallenburg (1995) reported findings from 87 women with severe preeclampsia or eclampsia and described high systemic vascular resistance and hyperdynamic ventricular function in most.

From these studies, it is reasonable to conclude that aggressive fluid administration given to women with severe preeclampsia causes normal left-sided filling pressures to become substantively elevated, while increasing an already normal cardiac output to supranormal levels.

BLOOD VOLUME. It has been known for over 75 years that *hemoconcentration* is a hallmark of eclampsia. Pritchard and co-workers (1984) reported that in eclamp-

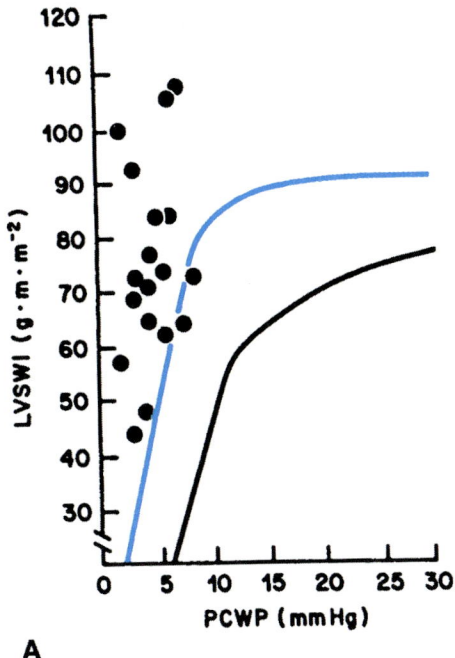

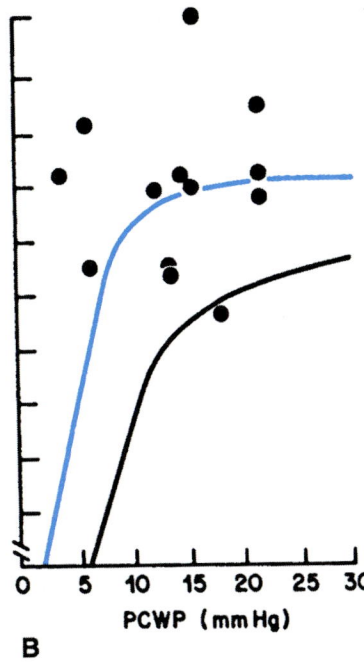

FIGURE 24-2. Ventricular function in women with severe preeclampsia–eclampsia. Left ventricular stroke work index (LVSWI) and pulmonary capillary wedge pressure (PCWP) are plotted. **A.** Restricted intravenous fluids. **B.** Aggressive fluid therapy. (From Hankins and colleagues, 1984.)

tic women the normally expected hypervolemia is usually absent (Table 24–6). Women of average size should have a blood volume of nearly 5000 mL during the last several weeks of a normal pregnancy, compared with about 3500 mL when nonpregnant. With eclampsia, however, much or all of the anticipated 1500 mL of blood normally present late in pregnancy is absent. The virtual absence of an expanded blood volume is likely the consequence of generalized vasoconstriction made worse by increased vascular permeability. In women with preeclampsia, these differences are not as marked, and women with gestational hypertension usually have a normal blood volume (Silver and Seebeck, 1996; Silver and colleagues, 1998). Silver and associates (2001) presented preliminary data that blood volume is decreased in women homozygous for the T235 angiotensinogen genotype associated with preeclampsia. An acute fall in

hematocrit is more likely the consequence of blood loss at delivery in the absence of normal pregnancy hypervolemia; or occasionally it is the result of intense erythrocyte destruction, as described next.

In the absence of hemorrhage, the intravascular compartment in eclamptic women is usually not underfilled. Vasospasm has contracted the space to be filled and the reduction persists until after delivery when the vascular system typically dilates, blood volume increases, and hematocrit falls. **The woman with eclampsia, therefore, is unduly sensitive to vigorous fluid therapy administered in an attempt to expand the contracted blood volume to normal pregnancy levels. She is sensitive as well to even normal blood loss at delivery.** Management of blood loss in these circumstances is considered in Chapter 25.

HEMATOLOGICAL CHANGES. Hematological abnormalities develop in some, but certainly not all, women who develop hypertensive disorders due to pregnancy. Among these are thrombocytopenia, which at times may become so severe as to be life threatening; the level of some plasma clotting factors may be decreased; and erythrocytes may be so traumatized that they display bizarre shapes and undergo rapid hemolysis.

COAGULATION. Subtle changes consistent with intravascular coagulation, and less often erythrocyte destruction, commonly are found with preeclampsia and especially eclampsia (Baker and Cunningham, 1999). Since the early description by Pritchard and co-workers (1954) of an eclamptic coagulopathy, we have found little evi-

TABLE 24–6. Blood Volumes in Five Women Measured with ^{51}Cr-tagged Erythrocytes During Antepartum Eclampsia, Again When Nonpregnant, and Finally at a Comparable Time in a Second Normotensive Pregnancy

	Eclampsia	Nonpregnant	Normal Pregnant
Blood volume (mL)	3530	3035	4425
Change (%)	+16		+47
Hematocrit	40.5	38.2	34.7

From Pritchard and colleagues (1984).

TABLE 24–7. Changes in Coagulation Factors that Imply Disseminated Intravascular Coagulation

	Normal Intrapartum Nulliparas	Most Abnormal Value for Each Case of Eclampsia
Platelets[a]		
Mean (per μL)	278,000	206,000
−2 standard deviations	150,000	—
< 150,000	0/20	24/91
< 100,000	0/20	14/91
< 50,000	0/20	3/91
Fibrin Degradation Products[b]		
8 μg/mL or less	17/20	51/59
16 μg/mL	3/20	6/59
> 16 μg/mL	0/20	2/59
Plasma Fibrinogen[a]		
Mean (mg/dL)	415	413
−2 standard deviations	285	—
< 285 mg per dL	0/20	7/89
Fibrin Monomer		
Positive	1/20	1/14

[a]Lowest value identified for each case of eclampsia.
[b]Highest value identified for each case of eclampsia.
From Pritchard and colleagues (1984).

dence that it is clinically significant. As presented in Table 24–7, thrombocytopenia, infrequently severe, was the most common finding. Unless some degree of placental abruption develops, plasma fibrinogen does not differ remarkably from levels found late in normal pregnancy and fibrin degradation products were elevated only occasionally. Barron and colleagues (1999) found routine laboratory evaluation of coagulation, including prothrombin time, activated partial thromboplastin time, and plasma fibrinogen level, to be unnecessary in the management of pregnancy-associated hypertensive disorders.

The *thrombin time* is somewhat prolonged in a third of the cases of eclampsia even when elevated levels of fibrin degradation products are not identified. The reason for this elevation is not known, but it has been attributed to hepatic derangements discussed subsequently (Leduc and associates, 1992). The coagulation changes just described are also identified in women with severe preeclampsia, but are certainly no more common. These observations in eclampsia are most consistent with the concept that coagulation changes are the consequence of preeclampsia–eclampsia, rather than the cause.

THROMBOCYTOPENIA. Maternal thrombocytopenia can be induced acutely by preeclampsia–eclampsia.

After delivery, the platelet count begins to increase progressively to reach a normal level within 3 to 5 days. The frequency and intensity of maternal thrombocytopenia vary in different studies, apparently dependent upon the intensity of the disease process, the length of delay between the onset of preeclampsia and delivery, and the frequency with which platelet counts are performed. Overt thrombocytopenia, defined by a platelet count less than 100,000/μL, indicates severe disease. In most cases, delivery is indicated because the platelet count continues to decrease.

The cause of thrombocytopenia likely results from platelet activation and consumption at the same time that platelet production is increased. Thrombopoietin, a cytokine that promotes proliferation of platelets from existing megakaryocytes, is increased in preeclamptic women with thrombocytopenia (Frolich and associates, 1998). In most studies, platelet aggregation is decreased compared with the normal increase seen in pregnancy (Baker and Cunningham, 1999). This likely is due to platelet "exhaustion" following in vivo activation. While the cause(s) is unknown, immunological processes or simply platelet deposition at sites of endothelial damage may be implicated (Pritchard and colleagues, 1976). Samuels and colleagues (1987) performed direct and indirect antiglobulin tests and found that platelet-bound and circulating platelet–bindable immunoglobulin were increased in preeclamptic women and their neonates. They interpreted these findings to suggest platelet surface alterations.

The clinical significance of thrombocytopenia, in addition to the obvious impairment in coagulation, is that it reflects the severity of the pathological process. In general, the lower the platelet count, the greater are maternal and fetal morbidity and mortality (Leduc and co-workers, 1992). The addition of elevated liver enzymes to this clinical picture is even more ominous. Weinstein (1982) referred to this combination of events as the *HELLP syndrome*—that is, hemolysis (H), elevated liver enzymes (EL), and low platelets (LP) (see "Fragmentation Hemolysis" below and "HELLP Syndrome" on p. 579).

NEONATAL THROMBOCYTOPENIA. Thiagarajah and co-workers (1984) and Weinstein (1985) reported thrombocytopenia in neonates whose mothers had preeclampsia. Conversely, Pritchard and colleagues (1987), in a large clinical study, did *not* observe severe thrombocytopenia in the fetus or infant at or very soon after delivery. In fact, no cases of fetal or neonatal thrombocytopenia were identified, despite severe maternal thrombocytopenia. Thrombocytopenia did develop later in some of these infants after hypoxia, acidosis, and sepsis developed. **Hence, maternal thrombocytopenia in hypertensive women is not a fetal indication for cesarean delivery.**

FRAGMENTATION HEMOLYSIS. Thrombocytopenia that accompanies severe preeclampsia and eclampsia may be accompanied by evidence of erythrocyte destruction characterized by hemolysis, schizocytosis, spherocytosis, reticulocytosis, hemoglobinuria, and occasionally hemoglobinemia (Pritchard and colleagues, 1954, 1976). These derangements result in part from microangiopathic hemolysis, and human and animal studies are suggestive that intense vasospasm causes endothelial disruption, with platelet adherence and fibrin deposition. Cunningham and associates (1985) described erythrocyte morphological characteristics using scanning electron microscopy. Women with eclampsia, and to a lesser degree those with severe preeclampsia, demonstrated schizocytosis and echinocytosis but not spherocytosis when compared with normally pregnant women. Sanchez-Ramos and colleagues (1994a) described increased erythrocyte membrane fluidity in women with HELLP syndrome and postulated that these changes predispose to hemolysis. Grisaru and associates (1997) have shown that erythrocytic membrane changes may facilitate the hypercoagulable state.

OTHER CLOTTING FACTORS. A severe deficiency of any of the soluble coagulation factors is very uncommon in severe preeclampsia–eclampsia unless another event coexists that predisposes to consumptive coagulopathy, such as placental abruption or profound hemorrhage due to hepatic infarction.

Antithrombin III has been reported to be lower in women with preeclampsia compared with normally pregnant women and those with chronic hypertension (Chang and co-workers, 1992). Unfortunately, early hope that antithrombin III levels could be used to predict the future development of preeclampsia and separate chronic hypertensive women from those with preeclampsia has not proven to be true (Sen and colleagues, 1994). *Fibronectin*, a glycoprotein associated with vascular endothelial cell basement membrane, is elevated in women with preeclampsia (Brubaker and colleagues, 1992). This observation is consistent with the view that preeclampsia causes vascular endothelial injury with subsequent hematological aberrations.

A number of clotting factor deficiencies or mutations lead to hypercoagulability that may be associated with early-onset preeclampsia. These are termed *thrombophilias* and are discussed in Chapter 49 (p. 1330).

ENDOCRINE AND METABOLIC CHANGES

ENDOCRINE CHANGES. Plasma levels of *renin, angiotensin II*, and *aldosterone* are increased during normal pregnancy. Hypertensive disorders due to pregnancy result in a decrease of these values toward the normal nonpregnant range (Weir and colleagues, 1973). With sodium retention, hypertension, or both, renin secretion by the juxtaglomerular apparatus decreases. Because renin catalyzes the conversion of angiotensinogen to angiotensin I (which is then transformed into angiotensin II by converting enzyme), angiotensin II levels decline, resulting in a decrease in aldosterone secretion. Despite this, women with preeclampsia avidly retain infused sodium (Brown and colleagues, 1988b).

Another potent mineralocorticoid, deoxycorticosterone (DOC), is increased strikingly in third-trimester plasma (Chap. 8, p. 194). This does not result from increased maternal adrenal secretion, but from conversion from plasma progesterone. Thus, it is not reduced by sodium retention or hypertension, and it may serve to explain why women with preeclampsia retain sodium.

Vasopressin levels are normal despite decreased plasma osmolality (Dürr and Lindheimer, 1999). As discussed in Chapter 8 (p. 177), *atrial natriuretic peptide* increases slightly during normal pregnancy. This peptide is released upon atrial wall stretching that results from blood volume expansion. It is vasoactive and promotes sodium and water excretion likely by inhibiting aldosterone, renin activity, angiotensin II, and vasopressin.

Atrial natriuretic peptide is further increased in women with preeclampsia (Gallery and Lindheimer, 1999). Increases in atrial natriuretic peptide following volume expansion result in comparable increases in cardiac output and decreases in peripheral vascular resistance in both normotensive and preeclamptic women (Nisell and associates, 1992). This observation may in part explain observations of a fall in peripheral vascular resistance following volume expansion in preeclamptic women.

FLUID AND ELECTROLYTE CHANGES. Commonly, the volume of *extracellular fluid*, manifest as edema, in women with severe preeclampsia–eclampsia has expanded beyond the normally increased volume that characterizes pregnancy. The mechanism responsible for the pathological expansion is not clear. Women with endothelial injury—manifest by significant proteinuria—have reduced plasma oncotic pressure which creates a filtration imbalance, displacing intravascular fluid into the surrounding interstitium.

Electrolyte concentrations do not differ appreciably in women with preeclampsia compared with those of normal pregnancy unless there has been vigorous diuretic therapy, sodium restriction, or administration of water with sufficient oxytocin to produce antidiuresis. Edema does not ensure a poor prognosis, and absence of edema does not ensure a favorable outcome.

Following an eclamptic convulsion, the *bicarbonate* concentration is lowered due to lactic acid acidosis and compensatory respiratory loss of carbon dioxide. The intensity of acidosis relates to the amount of lactic acid produced and its metabolic rate, as well as the rate at which carbon dioxide is exhaled.

KIDNEY. During normal pregnancy, renal blood flow and glomerular filtration rate are increased appreciably (Chap. 8, p. 186). With development of preeclampsia, renal perfusion and glomerular filtration are reduced. Levels that are much below normal nonpregnant values are the consequence of severe disease. Plasma uric acid concentration is typically elevated, especially in women with more severe disease. The elevation exceeds the reduction in glomerular filtration rate and creatinine clearance that accompanies preeclampsia (Chesley and Williams, 1945).

In the majority of preeclamptic women, mild to moderately diminished glomerular filtration appears to result from a reduced plasma volume resulting in plasma creatinine values approximately twice those expected for normal pregnancy of about 0.5 mg/dL. In some cases of severe preeclampsia, however, renal involvement is profound, and plasma creatinine may be elevated several times over nonpregnant normal values or up to 2 to 3 mg/dL. This is likely due to intrinsic renal changes caused by severe vasospasm (Pritchard and colleagues,

1984). Lee and associates (1987) reported normal ventricular filling pressures in seven severely preeclamptic women with oliguria, and concluded that this was consistent with intrarenal vasospasm. In most, urine sodium concentration was elevated abnormally, also suggesting an intrinsic renal etiology. Urine osmolality, urine:plasma creatinine ratio, and fractional excretion of sodium were also indicative that a prerenal mechanism was involved. *Importantly, intensive intravenous fluid therapy was not indicated for these women with oliguria.* When dopamine was infused into oliguric preeclamptic women, this renal vasodilator caused increased urine output, fractional sodium excretion, and free water clearance (Kirshon and co-workers, 1988).

Taufield and associates (1987) reported that preeclampsia is associated with diminished urinary excretion of calcium because of increased tubular reabsorption. This mechanism would explain the decreased calcium excretion in hypertensive pregnant women.

After delivery, in the absence of underlying chronic renovascular disease, complete recovery of renal function usually can be anticipated. This would not be the case, of course, if *renal cortical necrosis*, an irreversible but rare lesion, develops (Sibai and associates, 1990; also see Chap. 47, p. 1266).

PROTEINURIA. There should be some degree of proteinuria to establish the diagnosis of preeclampsia–eclampsia. Because proteinuria develops late, however, some women may be delivered before it appears. Meyer and colleagues (1994) emphasized that 24-hour urine excretion should be measured. They found that a urinary dipstick of 1+ proteinuria or greater was predictive of at least 300 mg per 24 hours in 92 percent of cases. Conversely, trace or negative proteinuria had a negative predictive value of only 34 percent in hypertensive women. Urine dipstick values of 3+ to 4+ were positively predictive of severe preeclampsia in only 36 percent of cases.

Albuminuria is an incorrect term to describe proteinuria of preeclampsia. As with any other glomerulopathy, there is increased permeability to most large-molecular-weight proteins; thus, abnormal albumin excretion is accompanied by other proteins, such as hemoglobin, globulins, and transferrin. Normally, these large protein molecules are not filtered by the glomerulus, and their appearance in urine signifies a glomerulopathic process. Some of the smaller proteins that usually are filtered but reabsorbed are also detected in urine.

ANATOMICAL CHANGES. Changes identifiable by light and electron microscopy are commonly found in the kidney. Sheehan (1950) observed that the glomeruli were enlarged by about 20 percent. The capillary loops variably are dilated and contracted. The endothelial cells are swollen, and deposited within and beneath them are fibrils that have been mistaken for thickening of the basement membrane.

Most electron microscopy studies of renal biopsies are consistent with glomerular capillary endothelial swelling. These changes, accompanied by subendothelial deposits of protein material, were called *glomerular capillary endotheliosis* by Spargo and associates (1959). The endothelial cells are often so swollen that they block or partially block the capillary lumens. Homogeneous deposits of an electron-dense substance are found between basal lamina and endothelial cells and within the cells themselves. On the basis of immunofluorescent staining, Lichtig and co-workers (1975) identified deposited fibrinogen or its derivatives in 13 of 30 renal biopsy specimens from women with preeclampsia. Kincaid-Smith (1991) found that these deposits disappear progressively in the first week postpartum.

Renal tubular lesions are common in women with eclampsia, but what has been interpreted as degenerative changes may represent only an accumulation within cells of protein reabsorbed from the glomerular filtrate. The collecting tubules may appear obstructed by casts from derivatives of protein, including, at times, hemoglobin.

Acute renal failure from *tubular* necrosis may develop. Such kidney failure is characterized by oliguria or anuria and rapidly developing azotemia (approximately 1 mg/dL increase in serum creatinine per day). Although this is more common in neglected cases, it is invariably induced by hypovolemic shock, usually associated with hemorrhage at delivery, for which adequate blood replacement is not given (Chap. 47, p. 1266). Haddad and colleagues (2000) reported that 5 percent of 183 women with hemolysis, elevated liver enzymes, and thrombocytopenia—*HELLP syndrome*—developed acute renal failure. Moreover, half of these also had a placental abruption, and most had postpartum hemorrhage. Rarely, *renal cortical necrosis* develops when the major portion of the cortex of both kidneys undergoes necrosis. Renal cortical necrosis is irreversible, and although it develops in nonpregnant women and in men, the lesion has most often been associated with pregnancy.

LIVER. With severe preeclampsia, at times there are alterations in tests of hepatic function and integrity, including delayed excretion of bromosulfophthalein and elevation of serum aspartate amniotransferase levels (Combes and Adams, 1972). Severe hyperbilirubinemia is uncommon even with severe preeclampsia (Pritchard and colleagues, 1976). Much of the increase in serum alkaline phosphatase is due to heat-stable alkaline phosphatase of placental origin. Oosterhof and co-workers (1994) described increased hepatic artery resistance

using Doppler sonography in 37 women with preeclampsia.

Periportal hemorrhagic necrosis in the periphery of the liver lobule is the most likely reason for increased serum liver enzymes (Fig. 24–3). Such extensive lesions are seldom identified in nonfatal cases with liver biopsy (Barton and colleagues, 1992). Bleeding from these lesions may cause *hepatic rupture*, or they may extend beneath the hepatic capsule and form a *subcapsular hematoma.* Such hemorrhages without rupture may be more common than previously suspected. Using computed tomography, Manas and colleagues (1985) showed that five of seven women with preeclampsia and upper abdominal pain had hepatic hemorrhage (Fig. 24–4). Prompt surgical intervention may be life saving. Rinehart and co-workers (1999) reviewed 121 cases of spontaneous hepatic rupture associated with preeclampsia, and the mortality rate was 30 percent. One woman at Parkland Hospital survived hepatic rupture after receiving blood and blood products from more than 200 donors. Hunter and co-workers (1995) described a similar women in whom liver transplant was considered life saving.

HELLP SYNDROME. Liver involvement in preeclampsia–eclampsia is serious and is frequently accompanied by evidence of other organ involvement, especially the kidney and brain, along with hemolysis and thrombocytopenia (De Boer and co-workers, 1991; Pritchard and associates, 1954; Weinstein, 1985). This is commonly referred to as *HELLP syndrome—He*molysis, *EL*evated liver enzymes, and *Low P*latelets. The Memphis group identified this constellation in almost 20 percent of women with severe preeclampsia or eclampsia (Sibai and co-workers, 1993b). Five of the 437 women died. In 13 of 33 women (40 percent) with laboratory evidence of HELLP syndrome and severe right upper quadrant pain, they found evidence of a subcapsular hematoma using imaging studies (Barton and Sibai, 1996). From the same group, Audibert and associates (1996) cited other complications, including placental abruption (7 percent), acute renal failure (2 percent), pulmonary edema (6 percent), and subcapsular liver hematoma (1 percent). Isler and co-authors (1999) have identified factors contributing to the death of 54 women with the HELLP syndrome, and these are shown in Figure 24–5.

Adverse outcomes in subsequent pregnancies are increased in women with HELLP syndrome. Sibai and colleagues (1995) observed a 3 percent incidence of recurrence of HELLP syndrome in 192 subsequent pregnancies, and Sullivan and associates (1994) found this to be 27 percent. Both groups confirmed a high incidence of recurrent preeclampsia, preterm delivery, fetal growth restriction, placental abruption, and cesarean delivery.

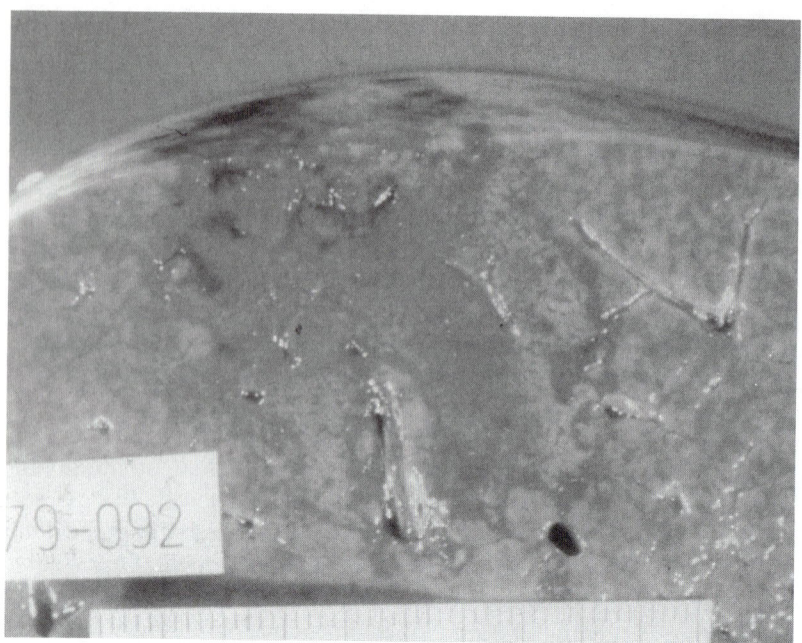

79-092

FIGURE 24–3. Gross liver specimen from a woman with preeclampsia who died from severe acidosis and liver failure. Periportal hemorrhagic necrosis was seen microscopically. (From Cunningham, 1993.)

BRAIN. Central nervous system manifestations of preeclampsia, and especially the convulsions of eclampsia, have been long known. In particular, visual symptoms have received much attention. The earliest description of brain involvement came from gross and histological examination, but with modern noninvasive techniques, imaging and Doppler studies have added new insight into cerebrovascular involvement.

ANATOMICAL PATHOLOGY. Two distinct but related types of cerebral pathology include gross hemorrhages due to ruptured arteries caused by severe hypertension. These can be seen in any woman with gestational hyper-

tension, and preeclampsia is not necessary for their development. These complications are more common with underlying chronic hypertension (Chap. 45).

The other lesions, variably demonstrated with preeclampsia, but likely universal with eclampsia, are more widespread and seldom fatal. The principal postmortem cerebral lesions are edema, hyperemia, focal anemia, thrombosis, and hemorrhage. Sheehan (1950) examined the brains of 48 eclamptic women very soon after death, and hemorrhages, ranging from petechiae to gross bleeding, were found in 56 percent. According to Sheehan, if the brain is examined within an hour after death, most often it is as firm as normal, and there is no obvious

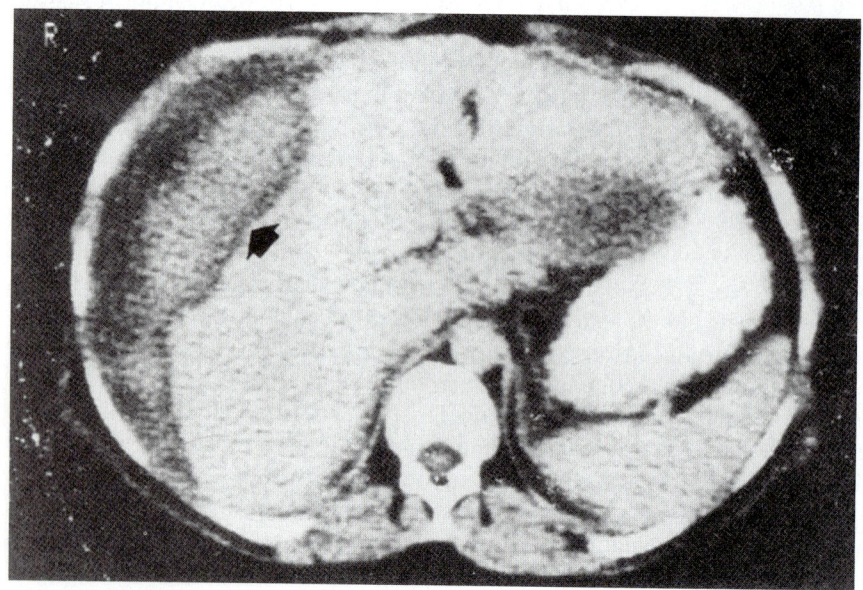

FIGURE 24–4. Computed tomographic scan of liver showing a subcapsular hematoma (*arrow*) along the right margin of the liver. (From Manas and colleagues, 1985, with permission.)

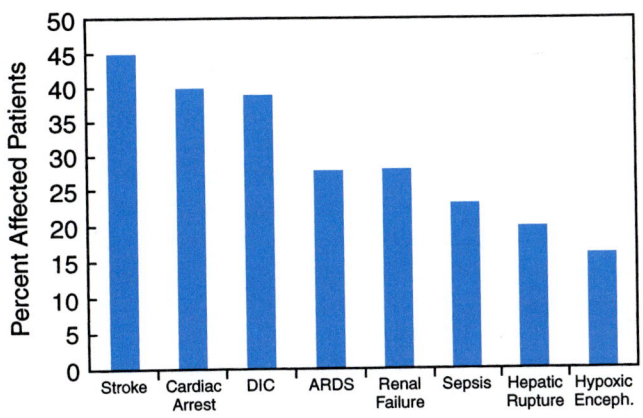

FIGURE 24–5. Contributing factors to deaths in 54 women with HELLP syndrome. (ARDS = acute respiratory distress syndrome; DIC = disseminated intravascular coagulopathy; Enceph. = encephalopathy.) (From Isler and co-authors, 1999, with permission.)

edema. This correlates with our findings that only 10 of 175 eclamptic women had evidence for cerebral edema (Cunningham and Twickler, 2000).

In another anatomical study, Govan (1961) concluded that cerebral hemorrhage was the cause of death in 39 of 110 fatal cases of eclampsia. In 40 of 47 women who died of cardiorespiratory failure, small cerebral hemorrhagic lesions were also found. A regular finding was fibrinoid changes in the walls of cerebral vessels. The lesions sometimes appeared to have been present for some time, as judged from the surrounding leukocytic response and hemosiderin-pigmented macrophages. These findings are consistent with the view that prodromal neurological symptoms and convulsions may be related to these lesions.

NEUROIMAGING STUDIES. The earliest abnormal imaging studies emerged with the use of computed tomographic scanning. In the earliest report from Parkland Hospital, Brown and colleagues (1988a) found that nearly half of eclamptic women studied had abnormal radiological findings. The most common were hypodense areas in the cerebral cortex, which corresponded to the petechial hemorrhages and infarction sites described at autopsy by Sheehan and Lynch (1973). While providing valuable insight to their number and locations, these studies did not answer the question concerning the cause of these localized areas of edema. It was still unknown if they were due to ischemic necrosis or hyperperfusion. The advent of magnetic resonance imaging allowed better resolution, but again the basic cause was not elucidated. For example, in another study from Parkland Hospital, Morriss and colleagues (1997) confirmed remarkable changes, especially in the area of the posterior cerebral artery.

These findings help to provide an explanation of why some women with preeclampsia convulse but others do not. The brain, like the liver and kidney, appears to be more involved in some women than in others. The extent and location of ischemic and petechial subcortical lesions likely influences the incidence of eclampsia. Their extent also explains more worrisome neurological complications such as blindness or coma. Recent findings indicate that these symptoms represent a continuum of involvement.

BLINDNESS. Although visual disturbances are common with severe preeclampsia, blindness, either alone or accompanying convulsions, is not. Most women with varying degrees of *amaurosis* are found to have radiographic evidence of extensive occipital lobe hypodensities. An example is shown in Figure 24–6 and is likely an exaggeration of the lesions described earlier. Over a 14-year period, we described 15 women with severe preeclampsia or eclampsia who also had blindness (Cunningham and associates, 1995). This persisted for 4 hours to 8 days, but in all it resolved completely.

Retinal artery vasospasm may also be associated with visual disturbances (Ohno and colleagues, 1999). Fortuitously, Belfort and associates (1992) showed that a 6-g bolus of magnesium sulfate caused retinal artery

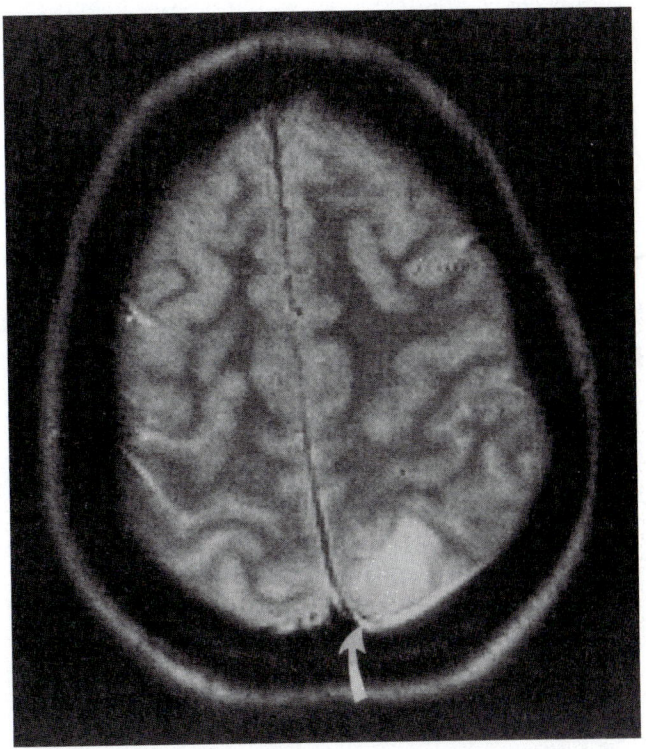

FIGURE 24–6. Magnetic resonance imaging in a 22-year-old eclamptic woman who had cortical blindness for 96 hours. A high-signal lesion (*arrow*) is apparent in the left occipital lobe. (From Cunningham and associates, 1995, with permission.)

vasodilation. *Retinal detachment* may also cause altered vision, although it is usually one sided and seldom causes total visual loss as in some women with cortical blindness. Surgical treatment is seldom indicated; prognosis is good, and vision usually returns to normal within a week.

CEREBRAL EDEMA.

Central nervous system manifestations from more widespread cerebral edema are worrisome. In some cases, obtundation and confusion are major features, and symptoms wax and wane. In a few cases, overt coma develops. Prognosis for these latter women is guarded and brainstem herniation is a serious complication.

During a 13-year period, we identified 10 of 175 eclamptic women at Parkland Hospital who had symptomatic cerebral edema (Cunningham and Twickler, 2000). Their symptoms ranged from lethargy, confusion, and blurred vision to obtundation and coma. Mental status changes correlated with the degree of involvement seen with computed tomographic and magnetic resonance imaging studies (Fig. 24–7). Three women with generalized cerebral edema were comatose and had impending transtentorial herniation on imaging studies and one of these died from herniation. It seems reasonable that this degree of involvement is related to both ischemic (cytotoxic) as well as hyperperfusion (vasogenic) edema. Conversely, Apollon and co-workers (2000) used single-photon-emission computed tomography and provided evidence for hyperperfusion and vasogenic (hydrostatic) edema.

CEREBRAL BLOOD FLOW.

As discussed, it is not known precisely what effects preeclampsia or eclampsia have on cerebral blood flow. Williams and Wilson (1999) used transcranial Doppler ultrasonography to study cerebral blood flow in six women with severe preeclampsia and in three women with eclampsia. Preeclampsia was associated with increased cerebral perfusion pressure counterbalanced by increased cerebrovascular resistance with no net change in cerebral blood flow. In eclampsia, and presumably due to loss of autoregulation of cerebral blood flow manifest as decreased vascular resistance, there was cerebral hyperperfusion similar to that seen in hypertensive encephalopathy unrelated to pregnancy. Belfort and colleagues (1999) also used transcranial Doppler ultrasound to estimate cerebral perfusion pressure in the middle cerebral artery in 79 preeclamptic women with and without headache. Women with headaches were more likely to have abnormal cerebral perfusion (either increased or decreased) than those without headaches. Those women with severe headaches tended to have high cerebral perfusion. Another important finding was that cerebral perfusion pressure may be normal in one hemisphere and very disordered in the other.

This evidence suggests that women with preeclampsia have cerebral vasospasm characterized by high or low cerebral perfusion pressure which varies from one hemisphere to the other. Women who develop eclampsia, however, ostensibly have suffered a transient loss of cerebral vascular autoregulation. This conclusion is also supported by evidence of widespread low-density areas confirmed by computed tomographic and magnetic resonance imaging (Cunningham and Twickler, 2000). According to Apollon and co-workers (2000), hyperperfusion likely causes vasogenic edema. Brackley and colleagues (2000) attributed cerebral vasospasm in preeclamptic women to increased cerebral arterial wall stiffness and vasoconstriction.

ELECTROENCEPHALOGRAPHY.

Nonspecific *electroencephalographic abnormalities* can usually be demonstrated for some time after eclamptic convulsions. Sibai and colleagues (1985a) observed that 75 percent of 65 eclamptic women had abnormal electroencephalograms within 48 hours of seizures. Half of these abnormalities persisted past 1 week, but most were normal by 3 months. An increased incidence of electroencephalographic abnormalities has been described in family members of eclamptic women, a finding suggestive that some eclamptic women have an inherited predisposition to convulse (Rosenbaum and Maltby, 1943).

UTEROPLACENTAL PERFUSION.

Compromised placental perfusion from vasospasm is almost certainly a major culprit in the genesis of increased perinatal morbidity and mortality associated with preeclampsia. For example, Brosens and associates (1972) reported that the mean diameter of myometrial spiral arterioles of 50 normal pregnant women was 500 μm. The same measurement in 36 women with preeclampsia was 200 μm. Attempts to measure human maternal and placental blood flow have been hampered by several obstacles, including inaccessibility of the placenta, the complexity of its venous effluent, and the unsuitability of certain investigative techniques for humans.

INDIRECT METHODS.

Everett and colleagues (1980) presented evidence that the clearance rate of dehydroisoandrosterone sulfate through placental conversion to estradiol-17β was an accurate reflection of maternal placental perfusion. Fritz and colleagues (1985) reported that the technique paralleled uteroplacental perfusion in primates. Normally, as pregnancy advances, this measurement increases greatly. The placental clearance rate decreases before the onset of overt hypertension (Worley and associates, 1975). Finally, placental

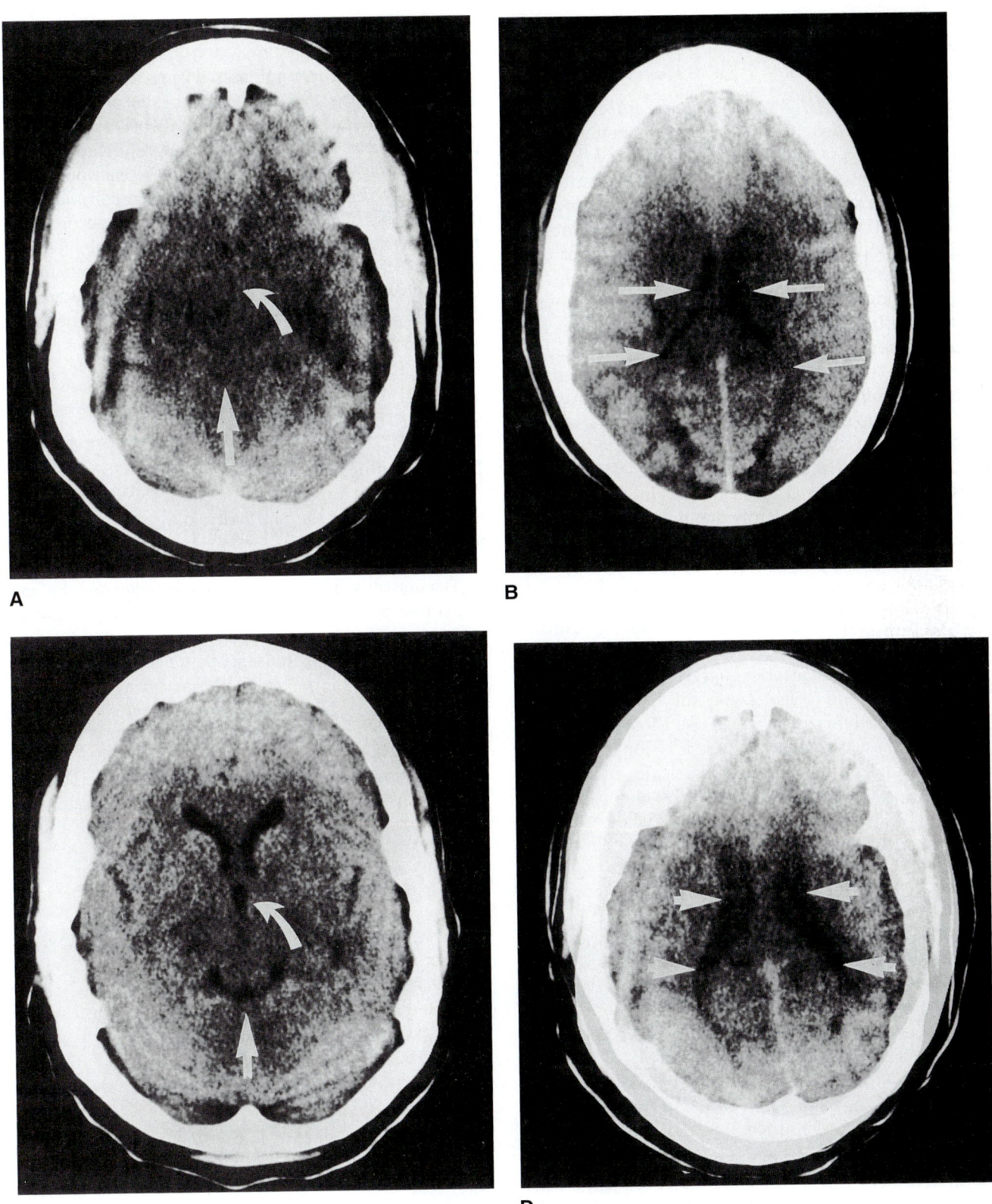

FIGURE 24–7. Patient with severe preeclampsia (BP 210/94 mm Hg; 3+ proteinuria) became disoriented intrapartum, and obtunded 5 hours postpartum: **A.** Base of skull axial computed tomographic image on day 1 with complete effacement of quadrigeminal plate cistern (*large arrow*) and third ventricle (*curved arrow*). **B.** More cephalad image on day 1 shows effacement of lateral ventricles (*white arrows*) and sulci and severe cerebral edema most obvious in occipital regions as low-density areas. **C.** Improved visualization on day 4 of quadrigemina plate cistern (*large arrow*) and third ventricle (*curved arrow*). **D.** Lateral ventricles (*arrows*) are larger on day 4, and low-density areas of occipital regions are less conspicuous. (From Cunningham and Twickler, 2000, with permission.)

clearance is decreased in women given diuretics or hydralazine (Gant and co-workers, 1976).

DOPPLER VELOCIMETRY. Doppler measurement of blood velocity through uterine arteries has been used to estimate uteroplacental blood flow (Chap. 41, p. 1133). Vascular resistance is estimated by comparing arterial systolic and diastolic velocity waveforms. Ducey and associates (1987) described systolic–diastolic velocity ratios from both uterine and umbilical arteries in 136 pregnancies complicated by hypertension. Among 51 women considered to have preeclampsia, 20 percent had normal umbilical artery velocity ratios; 15 percent had normal umbilical but abnormal uterine artery ratios; and in 40 percent both ratios were abnormal. Fleischer and colleagues (1986) and Trudinger and associates (1990) have also reported increased systolic–diastolic ratios in uterine arteries of women with preeclampsia. Others have not confirmed this (Hanretty and colleagues, 1988). These studies, in the aggregate, can be interpreted to imply that only a few women with preeclampsia have compromised uteroplacental circulations.

HISTOLOGICAL CHANGES IN THE PLACENTAL BED. Hertig (1945) identified in preeclamptic pregnancies a lesion of uteroplacental arteries characterized by prominent lipid-rich foam cells. Zeek and Assali (1950) termed this *acute atherosis* (Fig. 24–8). Most investigators are now in accord that there is a lesion, but they do not agree on its precise nature. Classically, in normal pregnancy, spiral arteries are invaded by endovascular trophoblast (Fig. 24–9). It seems that, in preeclampsia, decidual vessels, but not myometrial vessels, are invaded by endovascular trophoblasts. Using electron microscopy studies of arteries taken from the uteroplacental implantation site, De Wolf and co-workers (1980) reported that early preeclamptic changes included endothelial damage, insudation of plasma constituents into vessel walls, proliferation of myointimal cells, and medial necrosis. They also found that lipid accumulates first in myointimal cells and then in macrophages. Madazli and colleagues (2000) showed that the magnitude of defective trophoblastic invasion of the spiral arteries correlated with the severity of the hypertensive disorder.

PATHOPHYSIOLOGY

In 1903, and in some ways remarkably prescient as will be surmised in reading this section, J. Whitridge Williams reported on the pathophysiology of preeclampsia as follows:

> The present status of the question may therefore be summarized as follows: The clinical history and anatomical findings afford presumptive evidence that the disease is due to the circulation of some poisonous substance in the blood which gives rise to thrombosis in many of the smaller vessels, with consequent degenerative necrosis in the various organs.

Any satisfactory theory on the pathophysiology of preeclampsia must account for the observation that hy-

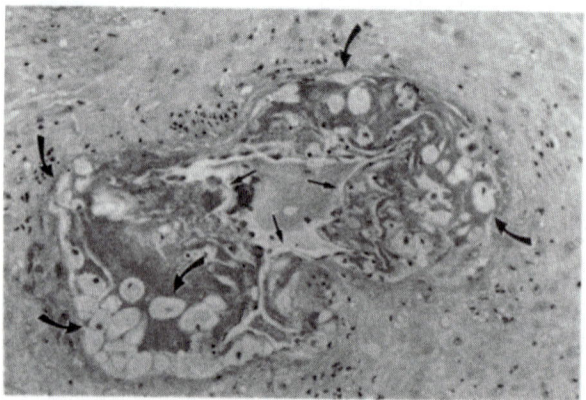
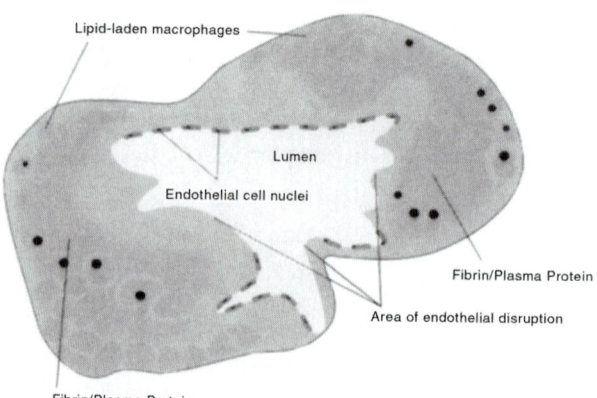

FIGURE 24–8. Atherosis is demonstrated in this blood vessel from the placental bed (left, photomicrograph; right schematic diagram of vessel). Disruption of the endothelium results in a narrowed lumen because of accumulation of plasma proteins and foamy macrophages beneath the endothelium. Some of the foamy macrophages are shown by *curved arrows* in the left photograph and *straight arrows* highlight areas of endothelial disruption. (From Rogers and colleagues, 1999, with permission.)

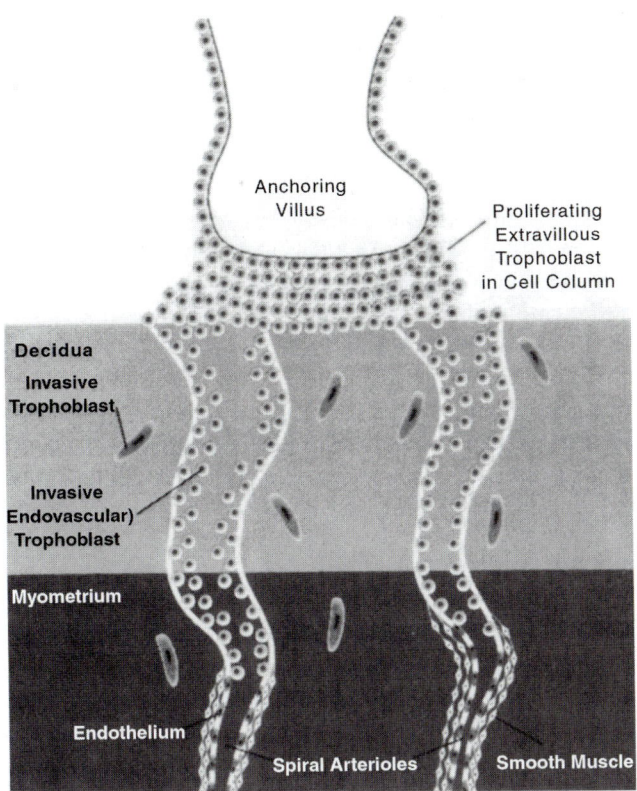

FIGURE 24–9. Normal placental implantation shows proliferation of extravillous trophoblasts, forming a cell column beneath the anchoring villus. The extravillous trophoblasts invade the decidua and extend down the inside of the spiral arteriole. This results in replacement of the endothelium and muscular wall of the vessel with subsequent enlargement of the blood vessel. (From Rogers and co-authors, 1999, with permission.)

pertensive disorders due to pregnancy are very much more likely to develop in the woman who:

1. Is exposed to chorionic villi for the first time.
2. Is exposed to a superabundance of chorionic villi, as with twins or hydatidiform mole.
3. Has preexisting vascular disease.
4. Is genetically predisposed to hypertension developing during pregnancy.

Although chorionic villi are essential, they need not support a fetus or be located within the uterus. An overview of the pathophysiology to be considered in this section is shown in Figure 24–10.

Vasospasm is basic to the pathophysiology of preeclampsia–eclampsia. This concept, first advanced by Volhard (1918), is based upon direct observations of small blood vessels in the nail beds, ocular fundi, and bulbar conjunctivae, and it has been surmised from histological changes seen in various affected organs (Hinselmann, 1924; Landesman and co-workers, 1954). Vascular constriction causes resistance to blood flow

and accounts for the development of arterial hypertension. It is likely that vasospasm itself also exerts a damaging effect on vessels. Moreover, angiotensin II causes endothelial cells to contract. These changes likely lead to endothelial cell damage and interendothelial cell leaks through which blood constituents, including platelets and fibrinogen, are deposited subendothelially (Brunner and Gavras, 1975). These vascular changes, together with local hypoxia of the surrounding tissues, presumably lead to hemorrhage, necrosis, and other end-organ disturbances that have been observed at times with severe preeclampsia. With this scheme, fibrin deposition is then likely to be prominent, as seen in fatal cases (McKay, 1965).

INCREASED PRESSOR RESPONSES. Normally pregnant women develop refractoriness to infused vasopressors (Abdul-Karim and Assali, 1961). Increased vascular reactivity to pressors in women with early preeclampsia has been identified by Raab and co-workers (1956) and Talledo and associates (1968) using either norepinephrine or angiotensin II, and by Dieckmann and Michel (1937) and Browne (1946) using vasopressin.

Gant and co-workers (1973) demonstrated that increased vascular sensitivity to angiotensin II clearly preceded the onset of pregnancy-induced hypertension. As

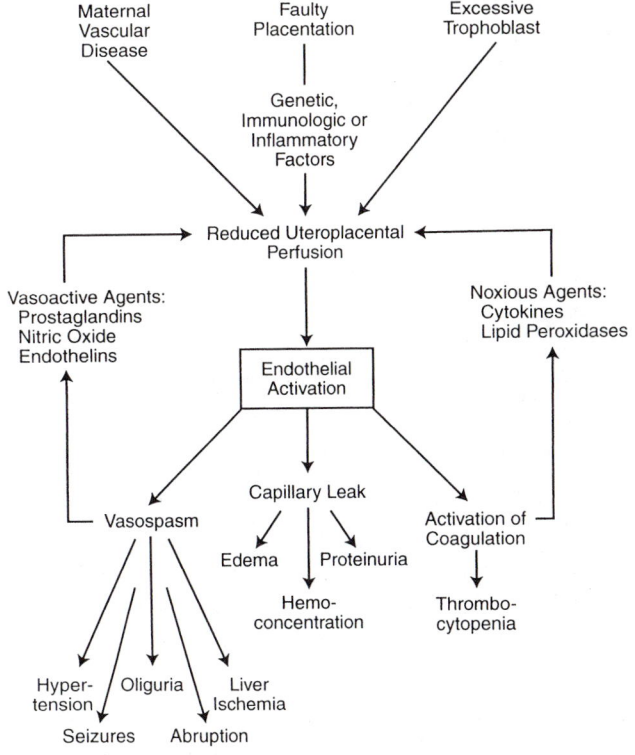

FIGURE 24–10. Pathophysiological considerations in the development of hypertensive disorders due to pregnancy. (Adapted from Friedman and Lindheimer, 1999.)

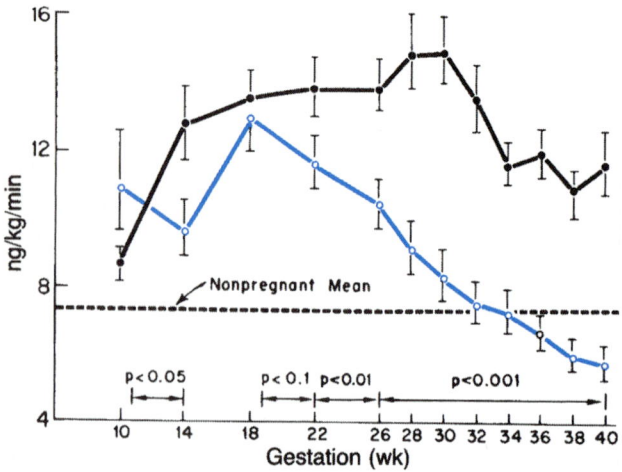

FIGURE 24–11. Comparison of the mean angiotensin II infusion doses required to evoke a pressor response in 120 nulliparous women who remained normotensive (solid circles) and 72 who subsequently developed pregnancy-induced hypertension (open circles). (From Gant and co-workers, 1973, with permission.)

shown in Figure 24–11, nulliparas who remained normotensive were refractory to the pressor effect of infused angiotensin II, while women who subsequently became hypertensive lost this refractoriness weeks before the onset of hypertension. Of women who required more than 8 ng/kg/min of angiotensin II to provoke a standardized pressor response between 28 and 32 weeks, 90 percent remained normotensive throughout pregnancy. Conversely, among normotensive nulliparas who required less than 8 ng/kg/min at 28 to 32 weeks, 90 percent subsequently developed overt hypertension. Women with underlying chronic hypertension have almost identical responses (Gant and colleagues, 1977).

PROSTAGLANDINS. Based on the findings of a number of studies, it has been concluded that the blunted pressor response described earlier is due principally to decreased vascular responsiveness mediated in part by vascular endothelial synthesis of prostaglandins or prostaglandin-like substances (Cunningham and associates, 1975; Gant and co-workers, 1974a). For example, refractoriness to angiotensin II in pregnant women is abolished by large doses of the prostaglandin synthase inhibitors (Everett and colleagues, 1978).

The exact mechanism by which prostaglandin(s) or related substances mediate vascular reactivity during pregnancy is unknown. From a number of observations, there is evidence that compared with normal pregnancy, prostacyclin production is decreased significantly and thromboxane A_2 significantly increased in preeclampsia (Walsh, 1985). Thus, in preeclamptic women, thromboxane is increased and prostacyclin and prostaglandin E_2

are decreased, resulting in vasoconstriction and sensitivity to infused angiotensin II.

Spitz and colleagues (1988) reported that 81 mg of aspirin given daily to future hypertensive women restored angiotensin II refractoriness by suppressing synthesis of thromboxane A_2 by about 75 percent; however, prostacyclin synthesis was decreased by only 20 percent and prostaglandin E_2 by 30 percent. These observations indicate that vessel reactivity may be mediated through a delicate balance of production and metabolism of these vasoactive prostaglandins. In this scheme, preeclampsia may follow inappropriately increased production or destruction of one prostaglandin, diminished synthesis or release of the other, or perhaps both. Unfortunately, these observations were not beneficial in clinical studies discussed subsequently.

NITRIC OXIDE. Previously termed *endothelium-derived relaxing factor* (*EDRF*), nitric oxide is synthesized by endothelial cells from L-arginine (Palmer and associates, 1988). It is a potent vasodilator whose absence or decreased concentration might play a role in the etiology of hypertensive disorders due to pregnancy. Its production appears to be increased in severe preeclampsia (Benedetto and associates, 2000). Withdrawal of nitric oxide from some pregnant animals results in the development of a clinical picture similar to preeclampsia (Conrad and Vernier, 1989; Weiner and associates, 1989). Inhibition of nitric oxide has been shown to increase mean arterial pressure, decrease heart rate, and reverse the pregnancy-induced refractoriness to vasopressors in some animals. Equally important, it appears to maintain the normal low-pressure vasodilated state characteristic of fetoplacental perfusion in the human (Chang and colleagues, 1992; Myatt and co-workers, 1992; Weiner and associates, 1992). Decreased nitric oxide release or production *has not been shown to develop prior to the onset of hypertension* (Anumba and colleagues, 1999). Thus, the changes in nitric oxide concentrations in women with hypertensive disorders due to pregnancy appear to be the consequence of hypertension and not the inciting event (Morris and colleagues, 1996).

ENDOTHELINS. These polypeptides are potent vasoconstrictors, and endothelin-1 is the only species produced by human endothelium (Mastrogiannis and co-workers, 1991). Plasma endothelin-1 is increased in normotensive laboring and nonlaboring women, and even higher levels have been reported in preeclamptic women (Clark, 1992; Nova, 1991; Schiff, 1992, and their associates). Otani and colleagues (1991), however, did not observe increased plasma endothelin levels, and Barton and associates (1993) did not find increased urinary endothelin-1 levels in preeclamptic women.

VASCULAR ENDOTHELIAL GROWTH FACTOR. This is a glycosalated glycoprotein that is selectively mitogenic for endothelial cells. Vascular endothelial growth factor (VEGF) is important in vasculogenesis and control of microvascular permeability and has been identified in the human placenta. Serum levels of VEGF increase in the first half of pregnancy concurrent with trophoblast and uterine vascular events characteristic of pregnancy. VEGF has been reported to be increased in serum from women with preeclampsia (Baker and associates, 1995). Simmons and co-workers (2000) studied uteroplacental vascular resistance, measured with Doppler ultrasound, and placental VEGF in pregnant women with and without preeclampsia. They found an increase in VEGF parallel to increased uteroplacental vessel resistance in women with preeclampsia. They concluded that increased placental VEGF may represent a compensatory mechanism attempting to restore uteroplacental blood flow toward normal.

GENETIC PREDISPOSITION. The tendency for preeclampsia–eclampsia is inherited. Chesley and Cooper (1986) studied the sisters, daughters, granddaughters, and daughters-in-law of eclamptic women delivered at the Margaret Hague Maternity Hospital from 1935 to 1984. They concluded that preeclampsia–eclampsia is highly heritable, and that the single-gene model, with a frequency of 0.25, best explained their observations. A multifactorial inheritance was also considered possible. Kilpatrick and associates (1989), but not Hayward and co-workers (1992), reported an association between the histocompatibility antigen HLA-DR4 and proteinuric hypertension. Hoff and associates (1992) concluded that a maternal humoral response directed against fetal anti-HLA-DR immunoglobulin antibody might influence the development of gestational hypertension.

Cooper and Liston (1979) examined the possibility that susceptibility to preeclampsia is dependent upon a single recessive gene. They calculated the expected first-pregnancy frequencies of daughters of women with eclampsia; daughters-in-law served as controls. The frequencies calculated by them and those actually observed by Chesley and co-workers (1968) in daughters and daughters-in-law of women with eclampsia are remarkably close. Ward and associates (1993) reported that women carrying the angiotensinogen gene variant T235 had a higher incidence of hypertensive disorders due to pregnancy. Morgan and colleagues (1995), however, could not confirm these findings. Morgan and colleagues (1999) subsequently showed that spiral arteries obtained at 8 weeks' gestation in women homozygous for the angiotensinogen gene failed to undergo the remodeling characteristic of normal implantation. They hypothesized that the failure to undergo such normal remodeling of the spiral arteries may predispose these women to

preeclampsia. Inherited thrombophilias, discussed in Chapter 49, predispose some women—either heterozygotes or homozygotes depending on the factor—to these syndromes.

IMMUNOLOGICAL FACTORS. The risk of hypertensive disorders due to pregnancy is appreciably enhanced in circumstances where formation of blocking antibodies to antigenic sites on the placenta *might* be impaired. This may arise where effective immunization by a previous pregnancy is lacking, as in first pregnancies; or where the number of antigenic sites provided by the placenta is unusually great compared with the amount of antibody, as with multiple fetuses (Beer, 1978). Strickland and associates (1986), however, provided data that do not support "immunization" by a previous pregnancy. They analyzed the outcomes of over 29,000 pregnancies at Parkland Hospital and reported that hypertensive disorders were decreased only slightly (22 versus 25 percent) in women who previously had miscarried (and thus were "immunized") and were now having their first baby. The immunization concept is supported by the observation that preeclampsia develops more frequently in multiparous women impregnated by a new consort (Trupin and colleagues, 1996).

Dekker and Sibai (1998) have reviewed the possible role of immune maladaptation in the pathophysiology of preeclampsia. Beginning in the early second trimester, women destined to develop preeclampsia have a significantly lower proportion of T-helper cells compared with women who remain normotensive (Bardeguez and associates, 1991). Antibodies against endothelial cells have been found in 50 percent of women with preeclampsia versus 15 percent of normotensive controls (Rappaport and colleagues, 1990). Immunological pathogenesis of acute atherosis shown in Figure 24–8 has also been suggested because of the morphological similarities to lesions seen in allograft rejection (Labarrere, 1988).

INFLAMMATORY FACTORS. Redman and colleagues (1999) have proposed that the endothelial cell dysfunction associated with preeclampsia can result from a "generalized perturbation of the normal, generalized maternal intravascular inflammatory adaptation to pregnancy" (Fig. 24–10). In this hypothesis, preeclampsia is considered a disease due to an extreme state of activated leukocytes in the maternal circulation (Faas and colleagues, 2000; Gervasi and co-workers, 2001).

The decidua contains an abundance of cells that, when activated, can release noxious agents (Staff and colleagues, 1999). These then serve as mediators to provoke endothelial cell injury (Fig. 24–10). Dekker and Sibai (1998) have reviewed this aspect of the pathophysiology of hypertensive disorders due to pregnancy.

Briefly, cytokines, to include tumor necrosis factor-alpha (TNF-α) and the interleukins, may contribute to the oxidative stress associated with preeclampsia. In this scheme, oxygen-free radicals lead to the formation of self-propagating lipid peroxides that in turn propagate highly toxic radicals which, in turn, injure endothelial cells. Such injury modifies endothelial cell production of nitric oxide, as well as interfering with prostaglandin balance. Other consequences of oxidative stress include production of the lipid-laden macrophage foam cells characteristics of atherosis (Fig. 24–8), activation of microvascular coagulation (thrombocytopenia), and increased capillary permeability (edema and proteinuria). These observations on the effects of oxidative stress in preeclampsia have given rise to increased interest in the potential benefit of antioxidant therapy given for the prevention of hypertensive disorders due to pregnancy. Antioxidants are a diverse family of components that function to prevent overproduction of and damage caused by noxious free radicals. Examples of antioxidants include vitamins E (α-tocopherol) and C (ascorbic acid) and β-carotene. Dietary supplementation with these antioxidants is discussed on page 590.

ENDOTHELIAL CELL ACTIVATION. Prevailing evidence is that endothelial cell activation is the centerpiece in the contemporary understanding of the pathogenesis of preeclampsia (Fig. 24–10). In this scheme, preeclampsia is an immunologically mediated deficiency in trophoblastic invasion of spiral arteries that leads to fetoplacental hypoperfusion. This results in the release of a factor(s) into the maternal circulation. These changes in turn provoke "activation" of the vascular endothelium, with the clinical syndrome of preeclampsia resulting from widespread changes in endothelial cell function (Hayman and associates, 2000; Ness and Roberts, 1996; Roberts, 2000; Walker, 2000). Intact endothelium has anticoagulant properties and blunts the response of vascular smooth muscle to agonists. Damaged endothelium, on the other hand, activates endothelial cells to promote coagulation, and increases sensitivity to vasopressor agents.

Further evidence of endothelial activation in preeclampsia includes the characteristic changes in glomerular capillary endothelial morphology, increased capillary permeability, and elevated blood levels of substances associated with such activation (see preceding section). Serum from preeclamptic women stimulates cultured endothelial cells to produce greater amounts of prostacyclin than serum from normotensive controls. Hyperhomocysteinemia is of interest in preeclampsia because elevated levels in men and nonpregnant women are an independent risk factor for atherosclerosis, which is very similar to implantation-site atherosis (Rogers and colleagues, 1999). Cotter and colleagues (2001) have presented preliminary data that

elevated serum homocysteine levels in early pregnancy increase preeclampsia risk threefold. Conversely, Laivuori and associates (2000) found no increased risk in carriers of the T677 allele for methylenetetrahydrofolate reductase.

PREDICTION AND PREVENTION

PREDICTION. A variety of biochemical and biophysical markers, based primarily on rationales implicated in the pathology and pathophysiology of hypertensive disorders due to pregnancy, have been proposed for the purpose of predicting the development of preeclampsia later in pregnancy. Investigators have attempted to identify early markers of faulty placentation, reduced placental perfusion, endothelial cell dysfunction, and activation of coagulation. Virtually all these attempts have resulted in testing strategies with low sensitivity for the prediction of preeclampsia. Friedman and Lindheimer (1999) concluded in their review that, at the present time, there are no screening tests for preeclampsia that are reliable, valid, and economical. Stamilio and colleagues (2000) reached a similar conclusion. Selected tests for prediction of preeclampsia are discussed in the following section.

ANGIOTENSIN II INFUSION. In this test, angiotensin II is infused in a stepwise fashion until there is a 20 mm Hg rise in diastolic blood pressure. Women requiring less than 8 ng/kg/min of angiotensin II had a positive-predictive value (true positive) of developing preeclampsia of 20 to 40 percent (Friedman and Lindheimer, 1999). While quite good when compared with other tests for prediction, angiotensin II infusion is difficult to perform and is therefore not used clinically.

ROLL-OVER TEST. A hypertensive response induced by having the woman assume the supine position after lying laterally recumbent was demonstrated in some pregnant women by Gant and colleagues (1974b). The majority of nulliparous women at 28 to 32 weeks who had increased diastolic pressure of at least 20 mm Hg when the maneuver ("roll-over test") was performed, later developed hypertension due to pregnancy. Conversely, most women whose blood pressure did not become elevated when this was done remained normotensive. Women who demonstrated a positive roll-over test were also abnormally sensitive to infused angiotensin II. It is hypothesized that a positive test result is a manifestation of increased vascular responsivity or sympathetic overactivity in women who will develop hypertension later in pregnancy. Using preeclampsia, rather than gestational hypertension as the end point, the positive-predictive value (true positive) was 33 percent, which is similar to that of the angiotensin infusion test (Dekker and colleagues, 1990).

URIC ACID. Elevated uric acid levels in maternal blood, presumably due to decreased renal urate excretion, are frequently found in women with preeclampsia. Jacobson and colleagues (1990) studied 135 pregnant women to determine if plasma uric acid levels, determined at 24 weeks' gestation, might predict the subsequent development of preeclampsia. Values exceeding 5.9 mg/dL were considered predictive. The positive-predictive value (true positive) for this test was 33 percent. It is unlikely that uric acid levels will prove very useful in predicting development of preeclampsia later in pregnancy given the observation that such levels have not even proven to be useful in differentiating established gestational hypertension from preeclampsia (Lim and co-authors, 1998).

CALCIUM METABOLISM. Alterations in calcium metabolism as well as deficiencies in dietary intake of calcium have been implicated in the pathophysiology of preeclampsia. Hypocalciuria has been identified with preeclampsia (Taufield and co-authors, 1987). Several investigators have thus performed studies to determine if midpregnancy urinary calcium levels might predict the development of preeclampsia. Sanchez-Ramos and colleagues (1991) measured 24-hour urinary calcium excretion in 103 nulliparous women between 10 and 24 weeks. The sensitivity in predicting preeclampsia was 88 percent and the positive-predictive value was 32 percent.

URINARY KALLIKREIN EXCRETION. Kallikrein is an important regulator of blood pressure, and it has been hypothesized its diminished excretion might precede the development of preeclampsia. Although Millar and colleagues (1996) found the predictive value of this test to be very good (sensitivity 83 percent, 91 percent positive-predictive value), others have not confirmed these findings (Kyle and associates, 1996).

FIBRONECTIN. There are many reports describing plasma fibronectin levels in women with impending or established preeclampsia. Endothelial cell injury, a centerpiece in the hypothesized pathophysiology of preeclampsia discussed previously, is the presumed source of elevated cellular fibronectin levels found in women with established hypertensive disease (Brubaker and associates, 1992). For example, Halligan and colleagues (1994) reported that fibronectin levels were elevated in the first trimester in women destined to develop preeclampsia. Paarlberg and colleagues (1998) measured plasma fibronectin levels during the second trimester in 347 healthy nulliparous women to predict hypertensive

disorders due to pregnancy. The sensitivity of this test was low (69 percent) as was the positive-predictive value (12 percent).

COAGULATION ACTIVATION. Thrombocytopenia and abnormalities of platelet function (aggregation) appear to be an integral feature of preeclampsia. Excessive platelet activation has been linked to maternal vasoconstriction, endothelial cell injury, placental infarction (atherosis and fetal growth restriction), and transient renal dysfunction. Platelet activation also leads to thromboxane A_2 release, which promotes vasospasm, further platelet aggregation, and endothelial cell injury. Thromboxane from platelets increases the thromboxane/prostacyclin ratio in women with preeclampsia (Fitzgerald and colleagues, 1987). This finding formed the basis for the concept that prophylactic administration of low-dose aspirin might prevent preeclampsia (see later discussion).

Clearly, the platelet count can be substantially decreased in women with severe preeclampsia. Platelet volume increases due to platelet consumption and resultant production of relatively younger (and therefore larger) platelets. Ahmed and associates (1993) found that high platelet volumes may be a marker of impending preeclampsia. Similarly, fibrinolytic activity is normally decreased in pregnancy due to increased plasminogen activator inhibitors (PAI) 1 and 2. In preeclampsia, PAI-1 is increased relative to PAI-2, and it may be a marker of endothelial cell dysfunction (Caron and colleagues, 1991).

MARKERS OF OXIDATIVE STRESS. Increased levels of lipid peroxides coupled with decreased activity of antioxidants in women with preeclampsia has raised the possibility that markers of oxidative stress might prove useful in the prediction of preeclampsia (Walsh, 1994). Possible markers include malondialdehyde lipid peroxidation (Hubel and co-authors, 1989); a variety of pro-oxidants or potentiators of pro-oxidants such as iron (Herbert and colleagues, 1994); homocysteine (Cotter and associates, 2001; Powers and colleagues, 2000); blood lipids to include triglycerides, free fatty acids, and lipoproteins (Hubel and colleagues, 1996); and antioxidants to include ascorbic acid and vitamin E (Mikhail and colleagues, 1994).

The decrease in prostaglandin synthesis described earlier has been reported to be detectable as early as the first trimester in women destined to develop preeclampsia. However, measuring prostacyclin metabolites in urine presents significant technical problems. Other prostaglandin isomers, for example, 8-isoprostane, a potent vasoconstrictor and a result of lipid peroxidation, has been also studied as a potential marker of impending preeclampsia (Regan and Fitzgerald, 1997).

IMMUNOLOGICAL FACTORS. Cytokines are protein messengers released by immune cells that serve to regulate the function of other immune cells and are produced by macrophages and lymphocytes at the interface of trophoblast and decidua. There are at least 50 cytokines, to include interleukins, interferons, growth factors, and tumor necrosis factors. Several of these cytokines have been found to be elevated in women with preeclampsia and are of interest as possible markers for the development of preeclampsia (Benyo, 2000; Dudley, 1996; Greer, 1994; Kupferminc, 1994, and all their colleagues).

PLACENTAL PEPTIDES. A variety of peptides produced by the placenta are of interest as possible markers for the prediction of preeclampsia. Examples include corticotropin-releasing hormone (Petraglia and colleagues, 1996), chorionic gonadotropin (Ashour and colleagues, 1997), and activin A and inhibin A (Aquilina and coauthors, 1999; Cuckle and associates, 1998; Muttukrishna and colleagues, 1997). Inhibin A and activin A appear to be particularly promising in the search for early pregnancy markers for the development of preeclampsia (Lindheimer and Woodruff, 1997).

DOPPLER VELOCIMETRY OF THE UTERINE ARTERIES. Uteroplacental vascular resistance can be assessed by Doppler ultrasound (Chap. 41, p. 1133). This has prompted studies to use Doppler measurements of uterine artery impedance in the second trimester as an early screening test for preeclampsia (Bewley and colleagues, 1991; Chappell and Bewley, 1998). The rationale for this is based upon the presumption that the pathophysiology of preeclampsia includes impaired trophoblastic invasion of the spiral arteries leading to obstruction in uteroplacental blood flow. Bower and colleagues (1993) screened 2026 pregnant women at 18 to 22 weeks using continuous-wave Doppler. Those women with increased uterine artery resistance (13 percent) underwent repeat testing using color Doppler at 24 weeks. The sensitivity of this two-stage test for prediction of preeclampsia was 78 percent, but the positive-predictive value was only 28 percent (Friedman and Lindheimer, 1999). Irion and associates (1998) found uterine artery Doppler velocimetry to be an unreliable screening test for preeclampsia in low-risk pregnancies. Clearly, none of the tests for prediction of preeclampsia described in this section are ideal.

PREVENTION. A variety of strategies have been used in attempts to prevent preeclampsia. Usually these strategies involve manipulation of diet and pharmacological attempts to modify the pathophysiological mechanisms thought to play a role in the development of preeclampsia. The latter includes use of low-dose aspirin and antioxidants.

DIETARY MANIPULATION. One of the earliest efforts aimed at preventing preeclampsia was salt restriction during pregnancy (De Snoo, 1937). The first randomized trial, however, was not published until 1998 (Knuist and colleagues). In this study of 361 women, prescribing a sodium-restricted diet was proven to be ineffective in preventing hypertensive disorders due to pregnancy.

Based primarily upon studies outside the United States, women with low dietary calcium were found to be at significantly increased risk for developing hypertension due to pregnancy (Belizan and Villar, 1980; López-Jaramillo and associates, 1989; Marya and colleagues, 1987). This has led to at least 14 randomized trials and resultant meta-analysis that showed calcium supplementation during pregnancy resulted in a significant reduction in blood pressure as well as prevention of preeclampsia (Bucher and colleagues, 1996). The apparently definitive study, however, was completed by Levine and co-workers (1997). This was a randomized trial sponsored by the National Institute of Child Health and Human Development. In this trial, using double-masking, 4589 healthy nulliparous women were randomly administered either 2 g per day of supplemental calcium or placebo. Supplemental calcium did not prevent any of the hypertensive disorders due to pregnancy, including gestational hypertension or preeclampsia.

Other dietary manipulations that have been tested for the purpose of preventing preeclampsia include administering four to nine capsules containing fish oil each day (Olsen and colleagues, 2000). This dietary supplement was chosen in an effort to modify the prostaglandin balance implicated in the pathophysiology of preeclampsia. Fish oil was ineffective in this study of 1474 pregnancies conducted at 19 hospitals in Europe.

LOW-DOSE ASPIRIN. In 1986, Wallenburg and co-workers reported their experiences with either 60 mg of aspirin or placebo given to angiotensin-sensitive primigravid women at 28 weeks' gestation. The reduced incidence of preeclampsia in the treated group was attributed to selective suppression of thromboxane synthesis by platelets and sparing of endothelial prostacyclin production. As a result of this report and others with similar results, multicenter randomized trials have been completed in both low-risk and high-risk women in the United States as well as in other countries (Caritis, 1998; CLASP Collaborative Group, 1994; Hauth, 1993; Sibai, 1993a, and their many colleagues). These trials have consistently shown that low-dose aspirin was ineffective in preventing preeclampsia. Hauth and colleagues (1998) in a secondary analysis of the high-risk intervention trial by Caritis and co-workers (1998), showed that administration of low-dose aspirin significantly reduced maternal thromboxane B_2 levels, but that this was without benefit because the incidence of preeclampsia was not decreased compared with placebo.

ANTIOXIDANTS. Sera of normal pregnant women contain antioxidant mechanisms that function to control lipid peroxidation which have been implicated in endothelial cell dysfunction associated with preeclampsia. Davidge and co-authors (1992) have shown that sera of women with preeclampsia have markedly reduced antioxidant activity. Schiff and colleagues (1996) tested the hypothesis that diminished antioxidant activity is involved in preeclampsia by studying dietary consumption as well as plasma concentration of vitamin E in 42 pregnancies complicated by preeclampsia compared with 90 controls. They found high plasma vitamin E levels in women with preeclampsia, but that the dietary vitamin E consumption was unrelated to preeclampsia. They speculated that the high vitamin E levels they observed were a response to the oxidative stress of preeclampsia.

Chappell and associates (1999) performed the first systematic study designed to test the hypothesis that treatment of pregnant women with antioxidants would alter endothelial cell injury linked to preeclampsia. A total of 283 women at risk for preeclampsia were randomized at 18 to 22 weeks' gestation to treatment with antioxidants or placebo. Antioxidant therapy significantly reduced endothelial cell activation, suggesting that such therapy might indeed be beneficial in the prevention of preeclampsia. There was also a significant reduction in the incidence of preeclampsia in those women given vitamins C and E compared with the control group (17 versus 11 percent, $P < .02$). A larger trial must be performed before concluding that such antioxidant therapy prevents preeclampsia.

MANAGEMENT

Basic management objectives for any pregnancy complicated by preeclampsia are:

1. Termination of pregnancy with the least possible trauma to mother and fetus.
2. Birth of an infant who subsequently thrives.
3. Complete restoration of health to the mother.

In certain cases of preeclampsia, especially in women at or near term, all three objectives are served equally well by induction of labor. **Therefore, the most important information that the obstetrician has for successful management of pregnancy, and especially a pregnancy that becomes complicated by hypertension, is precise knowledge of the age of the fetus.**

EARLY PRENATAL DETECTION. Traditionally, the timing of prenatal examinations has been scheduled at intervals of 4 weeks until 28 weeks, and then every 2 weeks until 36 weeks, and weekly thereafter. Increased prenatal visits during the third trimester facilitates early detection of preeclampsia. Women with overt hypertension ($\geq$ 140/90 mm Hg) are frequently admitted to the hospital for 2 to 3 days to evaluate the severity of new-onset pregnancy hypertension. Those with persistent severe disease are observed closely and many are delivered. Conversely, women with mild disease are often managed as outpatients.

Management of women without overt hypertension, but in whom early preeclampsia is suspected during routine prenatal visits, is primarily based upon increased surveillance. The protocol used successfully for many years at Parkland Hospital in women during the third trimester and with new-onset diastolic blood pressure readings between 81 and 89 mm Hg or sudden abnormal weight gain (more than 2 pounds per week) includes return visits at 3 to 4 day intervals. Such outpatient surveillance is continued unless overt hypertension, proteinuria, visual disturbances, or epigastric discomfort supervene.

HOSPITAL MANAGEMENT. Hospitalization is considered at least initially for women with new-onset hypertension if there is persistent or worsening hypertension or development of proteinuria. A systematic evaluation is instituted to include the following:

1. Detailed examination followed by daily scrutiny for clinical findings such as headache, visual disturbances, epigastric pain, and rapid weight gain.
2. Weight on admittance and every day thereafter.
3. Analysis for proteinuria on admittance and at least every 2 days thereafter.
4. Blood pressure readings in sitting position with an appropriate-size cuff every 4 hours, except between midnight and morning.
5. Measurements of plasma or serum creatinine, hematocrit, platelets, and serum liver enzymes, the frequency to be determined by the severity of hypertension.
6. Frequent evaluation of fetal size and amnionic fluid volume either clinically or with sonography.

If these observations lead to a diagnosis of severe preeclampsia (Table 24–2), further management is the same as described subsequently for eclampsia.

Reduced physical activity throughout much of the day is beneficial. Absolute bed rest is not necessary, and sedatives and tranquilizers are not prescribed. Ample, but not excessive, protein and calories should be included in the diet. Sodium and fluid intakes should not be limited or forced. Further management depends upon:

1. Severity of preeclampsia, determined by presence or absence of conditions cited.
2. Duration of gestation.
3. Condition of the cervix.

Fortunately, many cases prove to be sufficiently mild and near enough to term that they can be managed conservatively until labor commences spontaneously or until the cervix becomes favorable for labor induction. Complete abatement of all signs and symptoms, however, is uncommon until after delivery. *Almost certainly, the underlying disease persists until after delivery!*

TERMINATION OF PREGNANCY. Delivery is the cure for preeclampsia. Headache, visual disturbances, or epigastric pain are indicative that convulsions are imminent, and oliguria is another ominous sign. Severe preeclampsia demands anticonvulsant and usually antihypertensive therapy followed by delivery. Treatment is identical to that described subsequently for eclampsia. The prime objectives are to forestall convulsions, to prevent intracranial hemorrhage and serious damage to other vital organs, and to deliver a healthy infant.

When the fetus is known or suspected to be preterm, however, the tendency is to temporize in the hope that a few more weeks in utero will reduce the risk of neonatal death or serious morbidity. As discussed, such a policy certainly is justified in milder cases. Assessments of fetal well-being and placental function have been attempted, especially when there is hesitation to deliver the fetus because of prematurity. Most investigators recommend frequent performance of various tests currently used to assess fetal well-being as described by the American College of Obstetricians and Gynecologists (1999). These include the nonstress test or the *biophysical profile,* which are discussed in Chapter 40 (p. 1104). Measurement of the lecithin-sphingomyelin ratio in amnionic fluid may provide evidence of lung maturity. Even when this ratio is less than 2.0, however, respiratory distress may not develop; and if it does, it is usually not fatal (Chap. 39, p. 1006).

With moderate or severe preeclampsia that does not improve after hospitalization, delivery is usually advisable for the welfare of both mother and fetus. Labor should be induced by intravenous oxytocin. Many clinicians favor preinduction cervical ripening with a prostaglandin or osmotic dilator (see Chap. 20). Whenever it appears that labor induction almost certainly will not succeed, or attempts at induction of labor have failed, cesarean delivery is indicated for more severe cases.

For a woman near term, with a soft, partially effaced cervix, even milder degrees of preeclampsia probably carry more risk to the mother and her fetus-infant than does induction of labor by carefully monitored oxytocin induction. This is not likely to be the case, however, if the preeclampsia is mild but the cervix is firm and closed, indicating that abdominal delivery might be necessary if pregnancy is to be terminated. The hazard of cesarean delivery may be greater than that of allowing the pregnancy to continue *under close observation* until the cervix is more suitable for induction.

ELECTIVE CESAREAN DELIVERY. Once severe preeclampsia is diagnosed, the obstetrical propensity is for prompt delivery. Induced labor to effect vaginal delivery has traditionally been considered to be in the best interest of the mother. Several concerns, including an unfavorable cervix precluding successful induction of labor, a perceived sense of urgency because of the severity of preeclampsia, and the need to coordinate neonatal intensive care have led some practitioners to advocate cesarean delivery. Alexander and colleagues (1999) reviewed 278 singleton liveborn infants weighing 750 to 1500 g delivered of women with severe preeclampsia at Parkland Hospital. Half of the women had labor induced and the remainder were delivered by cesarean without labor. Induction of labor was not successful in 35 percent of the women in the induced group, but was not harmful to their very low-birthweight infants. Similar results were reported by Nassar and colleagues (1998).

ANTIHYPERTENSIVE DRUG THERAPY. The use of antihypertensive drugs in attempts to prolong pregnancy or modify perinatal outcomes in pregnancies complicated by various types and severities of hypertensive disorders has been of considerable interest.

Drug treatment for early mild preeclampsia has been disappointing (Table 24–8). Sibai and associates (1987a) performed a well-designed randomized study to evaluate the effectiveness of labetalol and hospitalization compared with hospitalization alone. They evaluated 200 nulliparous women with preeclampsia diagnosed between 26 and 35 weeks. Although women given labetalol had significantly lower mean blood pressure, there were no differences between the groups for mean pregnancy prolongation, gestational age at delivery, or birthweight. The cesarean delivery rates were similar, as were the number of infants admitted to special-care nurseries. **Growth-restricted infants were twice as frequent in women given labetalol compared with those treated by hospitalization alone (19 versus 9 percent).**

At least three other studies have been done to compare either the β-blocking agent, labetalol, or calcium-channel blockers, nifedipine and isradipine, with placebo, and the results are shown in Table 24–8. In none of these studies were any benefits of antihypertensive

TABLE 24–8. Summary of Randomized Placebo-controlled Clinical Trials of Antihypertensive Therapy for Early Mild Hypertension Due to Pregnancy

Study	Study Drug (no.)	Prolongation Pregnancy (days)	Severe Hypertension[a]	Cesarean Delivery (%)	Abruptio Placentae	Mean Birth-weight (g)	Growth Restriction (g)	Neonatal Deaths
Sibai et al (1987a)	Labetalol (100)	21.3	15[b]	32	0	2260	9[a]	0
200 inpatients	Placebo (100)	20.1	5	36	2	2205	19	1
Sibai et al (1992)	Nifedipine (100)	22.3	18[b]	35	2	2510	4	0
200 outpatients	Placebo (100)	22.5	9	43	3	2405	8	0
Pickles et al (1992)	Labetalol (70)	26.6	9	24	NS[c]	NS	NS	NS
144 outpatients	Placebo (74)	23.1	10	26	NS	NS	NS	NS
Wide-Swensson et al (1995)	Isradipine (54)	23.1	22	26	NS	NS	NS	0
111 outpatients	Placebo (57)	29.8	29	19	NS	NS	NS	0

[a]Includes postpartum hypertension.
[b]Significant ($P < .05$) when study drug compared with placebo.
[c]NS = not stated.

treatment shown. Von Dadelszen and associates (2000) performed a meta-analysis that included the aforementioned trials for the purpose of determining the relation between fetal growth and antihypertensive therapy. These investigators concluded that treatment-induced decreases in maternal blood pressure may adversely affect fetal growth.

In a somewhat unusual study, Easterling and colleagues (1999) identified 58 women at risk for preeclampsia because they had a high cardiac output at 24 weeks. Cardiac output was measured by Doppler technique and the women were randomized to either prophylactic atenolol or placebo. The incidence of preeclampsia was 18 percent in the control group compared with 4 percent in the atenolol group ($P = .04$).

The use of angiotensin-converting-enzyme (ACE) inhibitors during the second and third trimesters of pregnancy should be avoided (Chap. 38, p. 1014). Reported complications include oligohydramnios, fetal growth restriction, bony malformations, limb contractures, persistent patent ductus arteriosus, pulmonary hypoplasia, respiratory distress syndrome, prolonged neonatal hypotension, and neonatal death (Nightingale, 1992). Lip and colleagues (1997) reported that ACE inhibitors taken during early pregnancy do not carry an adverse outlook as long as these drugs are discontinued as soon as possible.

DELAYED DELIVERY WITH SEVERE PREECLAMPSIA.
Women with severe preeclampsia are usually delivered without delay. In recent years, a different approach in the treatment of women with severe preeclampsia remote from term has been advocated by several investigators worldwide (Many and colleagues, 1999). This approach advocates conservative or "expectant" man-

agement in a selected group of women with the aim of improving infant outcome without compromising the safety of the mother. Aspects of such conservative management always include careful daily and more frequent, monitoring of the pregnancy in the hospital with or without use of drugs to control hypertension.

Theoretically, antihypertensive therapy has potential usefulness when preeclampsia severe enough to warrant termination of pregnancy develops before neonatal survival is likely. Such management is controversial, and it may be catastrophic. Sibai and colleagues (1985b) from the University of Tennessee attempted to prolong pregnancy because of fetal immaturity in 60 women with severe preeclampsia diagnosed between 18 and 27 weeks. **The total perinatal mortality rate was 87 percent, and although no mothers died, 13 suffered placental abruption, 10 eclampsia, five consumptive coagulopathy, three renal failure, two hypertensive encephalopathy, one intracerebral hemorrhage, and one a ruptured hepatic hematoma.**

Sibai and associates (1994) subsequently performed a randomized controlled trial of expectant versus aggressive management of severe preeclampsia in 95 women at more advanced gestations of 28 to 32 weeks. Women with HELLP syndrome were specifically excluded from this trial. Aggressive management included glucocorticoid administration for fetal lung maturation followed by delivery in 48 hours. Expectantly managed women were treated with bed rest and either labetalol or nifedipine given orally. Pregnancy was prolonged for a mean of 15.4 days in the expectant management group with an improvement in neonatal outcome. Importantly, 4 percent in each group sustained placental abruption.

In a follow-up nonrandomized study from Memphis,

Abramovici and colleagues (1999) compared infant outcomes for deliveries between 24 and 36 weeks in 133 women with HELLP syndrome to 136 women with severe preeclampsia. Women with HELLP syndrome were subdivided into those with hemolysis plus elevated liver enzymes plus low platelets and those with partial HELLP syndrome defined as either one or two, but not three, of these laboratory findings. It was concluded that women with partial HELLP syndrome, as well as those with severe preeclampsia, could be managed expectantly. They also concluded that infant outcomes were related to gestational age rather than the hypertensive disorder per se. As shown in Table 24–9, these women were indeed severely hypertensive and had mean diastolic blood pressures of 110 mm Hg. The distinguishing feature between those with HELLP syndrome appears to be the platelet count: the mean value was 52,000/μL in women with complete HELLP syndrome compared with 113,000/μL in those with partial HELLP syndrome. Gestational age was about 2 weeks more advanced in women with severe preeclampsia compared with those with some degree of HELLP syndrome. Accordingly, neonatal outcomes, in terms of need for mechanical ventilation and neonatal death, were better in women with severe preeclampsia. Fetal growth restriction was not related to the severity of maternal disease and was prevalent in all three groups. Maternal morbidity was not described. However, Witlin and associates (2000) later reported that growth restriction adversely affected infant survival in such infants delivered in Memphis. Most importantly, the median elapsed time from admission to delivery was 0, 1 day, and 2 days for women with HELLP syndrome, partial HELLP syndrome, or severe preeclampsia, respectively.

Taken in toto, these three studies require comment about repeated claims that expectant management of severe preeclampsia and partial HELLP syndrome is beneficial. First, with expectant management, the interval from admission to delivery is very short at their center, particularly in pregnancies managed subsequent to their report claiming efficacy and safety. Second, it seems possible, even likely, that the gestational age difference between severe preeclampsia and HELLP syndrome is related to the timing of onset of the disease itself. That is, HELLP syndrome may develop earlier in pregnancy than severe preeclampsia. Third, fetal growth restriction is prevalent in women with severe disease and it adversely affects infant survival, *which* is not improved by the severity of maternal disease. Lastly, and most importantly, the authors overlook that the overriding reason to terminate pregnancies with severe preeclampsia is maternal safety. Results in Table 24–9 clearly confirm that severe preeclampsia is deleterious for fetal outcome. Conversely, these data in Table 24–9 do not prove that expectant management is beneficial for the mother.

Visser and Wallenburg (1995) compared clinical outcomes of expectant management in 256 women with severe preeclampsia prior to 34 weeks. Half of these women had *HELLP syndrome* and the other half had severe preeclampsia. They were able to prolong pregnancy in both groups for 10 to 14 days, but 5 percent had a placental abruption and three women developed eclampsia.

Hall and colleagues (2000b) managed 360 severely preeclamptic women with early-onset preeclampsia—before 34 weeks—by careful observation and blood pressure control. While these women gained a mean duration of 11 days, a fourth had major complications—20 percent had placental abruption, 2 percent pulmonary edema, and 1.2 percent had eclampsia. Reports such as these just cited serve to emphasize that it is prudent for clinicians to be concerned about maternal safety in women with severe hypertensive disorders due

TABLE 24–9. Results of Expectant Management of Severe Preeclampsia or HELLP Syndrome Before Term

Outcome	HELLP Syndrome (n = 68)	Partial HELLP Syndrome[a] (n = 65)	Severe Preeclampsia (n = 136)
Diastolic BP, mm Hg (mean ± SD)	109 ± 16	110 ± 15	110 ± 15
Platelet count (cells/μL ± SD)	52 ± 21	113 ± 56	199 ± 61
Gestational age at delivery (weeks, mean ± SD)	31 ± 3.2	31 ± 3.3	33 ± 3
Mechanical ventilation of infant	50%	40%	28%
Neonatal death	7%	8%	4%
Fetal growth restriction	28%	31%	22%
Diagnosis-to-delivery (median days)	0	1	2

BP = blood pressure; HELLP = hemolysis, elevated liver enzymes, and low platelet count; SD = standard deviation.
[a]See text for explanation.
From Abramovici and colleagues (1999), with permission.

to pregnancy before term. We are reluctant to advise clinicians that it is safe to expectantly manage women with persistent severe hypertension or significant hematological, cerebral, or liver abnormalities due to preeclampsia. Such women are not managed expectantly at Parkland Hospital.

GLUCOCORTICOIDS. In attempts to enhance fetal lung maturation, glucocorticoids have been administered to severely hypertensive pregnant women remote from term. Treatment does not seem to worsen maternal hypertension, and a decrease in the incidence of respiratory distress and improved fetal survival has been cited (Chap. 39, p. 1006). Thiagarajah and co-authors (1984) were the first to suggest that glucocorticoids might also have a role in treatment of the laboratory abnormalities associated with the HELLP syndrome. Tompkins and Thiagarajah (1999) more recently reported that glucocorticoids produced significant but transient improvement in the hematological abnormalities associated with the HELLP syndrome diagnosed upon admission in 52 women between 24 and 34 weeks. While platelet counts increased by an average of 23,000/μL, this salutary effect was short lived, and counts decreased by an average of 46,000/μL within 48 hours after completion of the glucocorticoid regimen. Importantly, few of the women studied had platelet counts less than 100,000/μL before glucocorticoid therapy, and hence, the efficacy of such treatment was not extensively tested in women with more severe hematological abnormalities.

One interpretation of these reports is that such use of glucocorticoids specifically administered as a therapy for the hematological abnormalities due to severe preeclampsia will not significantly delay the need for delivery. Most certainly, these reports should not be taken to imply that it is advisable to administer glucocorticoids to significantly delay delivery in women with severe laboratory abnormalities.

HIGH-RISK PREGNANCY UNIT. An inpatient High-Risk Pregnancy Unit was established at Parkland Hospital in 1973 in large part to provide care for women with hypertensive disorders. Initial results from this Unit were reported by Hauth (1976) and Gilstrap (1978) and their colleagues. The majority of women hospitalized have a salutary response characterized by disappearance or improvement of hypertension. **Importantly, these women are not "cured," because nearly 90 percent have recurrent hypertension before or during labor.** Through 2000, almost 8000 nulliparous women with mild to moderate early-onset hypertension during pregnancy have been successfully managed in the High-Risk Pregnancy Unit. The provider costs (as opposed to charges) for the relatively simple physical facility, modest nursing care, no drugs other than iron and folate supplements,

and the very few laboratory tests that are essential, are slight compared with the cost of neonatal intensive care for a preterm infant.

HOME HEALTH CARE. Many clinicians feel that further hospitalization is not warranted if hypertension abates within a few days, and this has legitimized third-party payors in the United States to refuse hospital reimbursement. Thus, many women with mild to moderate hypertension, and without proteinuria, are consequently managed at home. Such management may continue as long as the disease does not worsen and if fetal jeopardy is not suspected. Sedentary activity throughout the greater part of the day is recommended. These women should be instructed in detail about reporting symptoms. Home blood pressure and urine protein monitoring or frequent evaluations by a visiting nurse may be necessary.

Barton and colleagues (1994) managed 592 predominately nulliparous women with mild hypertension in such a manner. They were 24 to 36 weeks at enrollment and a fourth had proteinuria. Gestation was prolonged for a mean of 4 weeks and 60 percent were delivered after 37 weeks. Importantly, half developed severe hypertension and 10 percent had fetal jeopardy. These investigators concluded that in highly motivated women such management produced results similar to inpatient care. Helewa and associates (1993) reached similar conclusions with a home-care program.

In a study from Parkland Hospital, Horsager and associates (1995) randomized 72 nulliparas with new-onset hypertension from 27 to 37 weeks to continued hospitalization or outpatient care. In all of these women, proteinuria had receded to less than 500 mg per day when randomized. Outpatient management included daily blood pressure monitoring by the patient or her family and weight and spot urine protein were determined three times weekly. A home health nurse visited twice weekly and the women were seen weekly in the clinic. Although perinatal outcomes were similar, recurrence of severe preeclampsia was significantly more common in the home group than in hospitalized women (40 versus 25 percent, respectively).

Another approach that has been evaluated on a limited basis is day-care. Tuffnell and colleagues (1992) randomized 54 women with gestational hypertension after 26 weeks to either day-care or routine management by their individual physicians. Hospitalizations, the development of preeclampsia, and labor inductions were significantly increased in the routine management group.

ECLAMPSIA. Preeclampsia that is complicated by generalized tonic–clonic convulsions is termed eclampsia. Fatal coma without convulsions has also been called eclampsia; however, it is better to limit the diagnosis to women with convulsions and to regard deaths in nonconvulsive cases as due to severe preeclampsia. Once eclampsia has ensued, the risk to both mother and fetus is appreciable.

Almost without exception, preeclampsia precedes the onset of eclamptic convulsions. Depending on whether convulsions appear before, during, or after labor, eclampsia is designated as antepartum, intrapartum, or postpartum. Eclampsia is most common in the last trimester and becomes increasingly more frequent as term approaches. In 254 eclamptic women cared for at the University of Mississippi Medical Center, about 3 percent first developed seizures more than 48 hours postpartum (Miles and colleagues, 1990). Other diagnoses should be considered in women with the onset of convulsions more than 48 hours postpartum.

The convulsive movements usually begin about the mouth in the form of facial twitchings. After a few seconds, the entire body becomes rigid in a generalized muscular contraction. This phase may persist for 15 to 20 seconds. Suddenly the jaws begin to open and close violently, and soon after, the eyelids as well. The other facial muscles and then all muscles alternately contract and relax in rapid succession. So forceful are the muscular movements that the woman may throw herself out of her bed, and, if not protected, her tongue is bitten by the violent action of the jaws (Fig. 24–12). This phase, in which the muscles alternately contract and relax, may

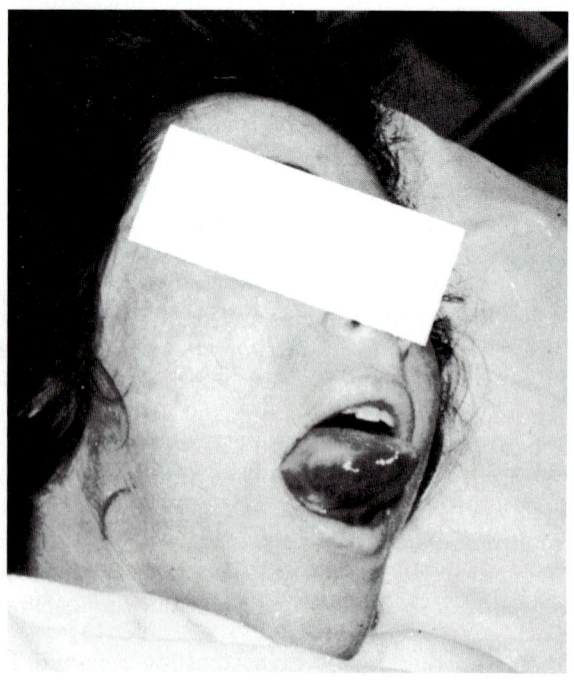

FIGURE 24–12. Hematoma of tongue from laceration during an eclamptic convulsion. Thrombocytopenia may have contributed to the bleeding.

last about a minute. Gradually, the muscular movements become smaller and less frequent, and finally the woman lies motionless. Throughout the seizure the diaphragm has been fixed, with respiration halted. For a few seconds the woman appears to be dying from respiratory arrest, but then she takes a long, deep, stertorous inhalation, and breathing is resumed. Coma then ensues. She will not remember the convulsion or, in all probability, events immediately before and afterward. Over time, these memories return.

The first convulsion is usually the forerunner of others, which may vary in number from one or two in mild cases to even 100 or more in untreated severe cases. In rare instances, convulsions follow one another so rapidly that the woman appears to be in a prolonged, almost continuous convulsion.

The duration of coma after a convulsion is variable. When the convulsions are infrequent, the woman usually recovers some degree of consciousness after each attack. As the woman arouses, a semiconscious combative state may ensue. In very severe cases, the coma persists from one convulsion to another, and death may result before she awakens. In rare instances, a single convulsion may be followed by coma from which the woman may never emerge, although, as a rule, death does not occur until after frequent convulsions.

Respirations after an eclamptic convulsion are usually increased in rate and may reach 50 or more per minute, in response presumably to hypercarbia from lactic acidemia, as well as to varying intensities of hypoxia. Cyanosis may be observed in severe cases. Fever of 39°C or more is a very grave sign, because it is probably the consequence of a central nervous system hemorrhage.

Proteinuria is almost always present and frequently pronounced. Urine output is likely diminished appreciably, and occasionally anuria develops. Hemoglobinuria is common, but hemoglobinemia is observed only rarely. Often, as shown in Figure 24–13, the edema is pronounced—at times, massive—but it may also be absent.

As with severe preeclampsia, after delivery an increase in urinary output is usually an early sign of improvement. Proteinuria and edema ordinarily disappear within a week (Fig. 24–13). In most cases, blood pressure returns to normal within a few days to 2 weeks after delivery. The longer hypertension persists postpartum, the more likely that it is the consequence of chronic vascular or renal disease (Table 24–1).

In antepartum eclampsia, labor may begin spontaneously shortly after convulsions ensue and progress rapidly, sometimes before the attendants are aware that the unconscious or stuporous woman is having effective uterine contractions. If the convulsion occurs during labor, contractions may increase in frequency and intensity, and the duration of labor may be shortened. Be-

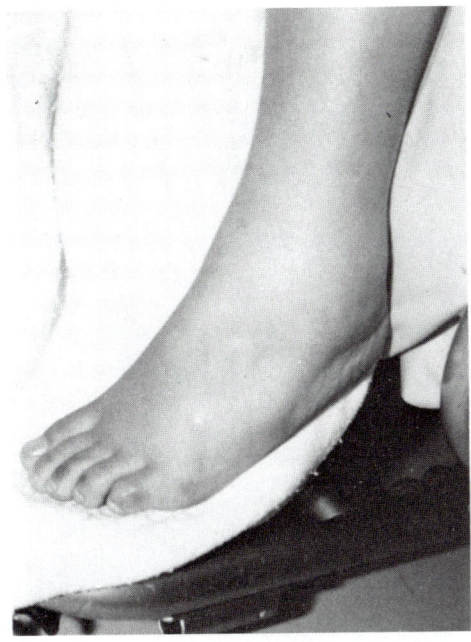

A

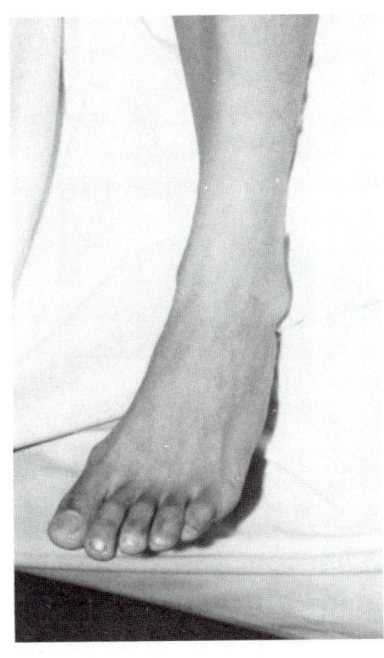

B

FIGURE 24–13. A. Severe edema in a young primigravida with antepartum eclampsia and a markedly reduced blood volume compared with normal pregnancy. **B.** The same woman 3 days after delivery. The remarkable clearance of pedal edema, accompanied by diuresis and a 28-pound weight loss, was spontaneous and unprovoked by any diuretic therapy. (From Cunningham and Pritchard, 1984.)

cause of maternal hypoxemia and lactic acidemia caused by convulsions, it is not unusual for fetal bradycardia to follow a seizure (Fig. 24–14). This usually recovers within 3 to 5 minutes; if it persists more than about 10 minutes, another cause must be considered, such as placental abruption or imminent delivery.

Pulmonary edema may follow eclamptic convulsions. There are at least two sources:

1. Aspiration pneumonitis may follow inhalation of gastric contents if simultaneous vomiting accompanies convulsions.
2. Cardiac failure may be the result of a combination of severe hypertension and vigorous intravenous fluid administration.

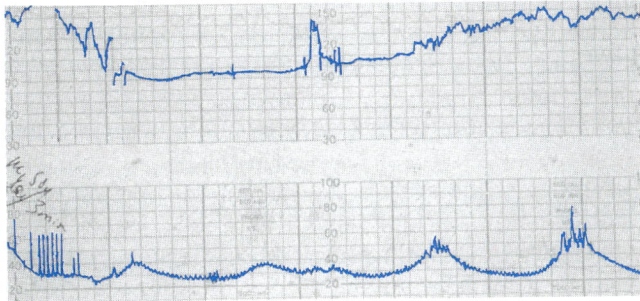

FIGURE 24–14. Fetal bradycardia developing in a woman with an intrapartum eclamptic convulsion. Bradycardia resolved and beat-to-beat variability returned about 5 minutes following the seizure. (From Cantrell and Cunningham, 1994.)

In some women with eclampsia, sudden death occurs synchronously with a convulsion or follows shortly thereafter, as the result of a massive cerebral hemorrhage (Fig. 24–15). Hemiplegia may result from sublethal hemorrhage. Cerebral hemorrhages are more likely in older women with underlying chronic hypertension. Rarely they may be due to a ruptured berry aneurysm or arteriovenous malformation (Witlin and co-workers, 1997a).

In about 10 percent of women, some degree of blindness will follow a seizure. Blindness may also develop spontaneously with preeclampsia. There are at least two causes:

1. Varying degrees of retinal detachment.
2. Occipital lobe ischemia, infarction, or edema.

Whether due to cerebral or retinal pathology, the prognosis for return of normal vision is good and usually complete within a week (Cunningham and associates, 1995). About 5 percent of women will have substantively altered consciousness, including persistent coma, following a seizure. This is due to extensive cerebral edema, and transtentorial uncal herniation may cause death (Cunningham and Twickler, 2000).

Rarely, eclampsia is followed by psychosis, and the woman becomes violent. This usually lasts for several days to 2 weeks, but the prognosis for return to normal is good, provided there was no preexisting mental illness. Chlorpromazine in carefully titrated doses has proved effective in the few cases of posteclampsia psychosis treated at Parkland Hospital.

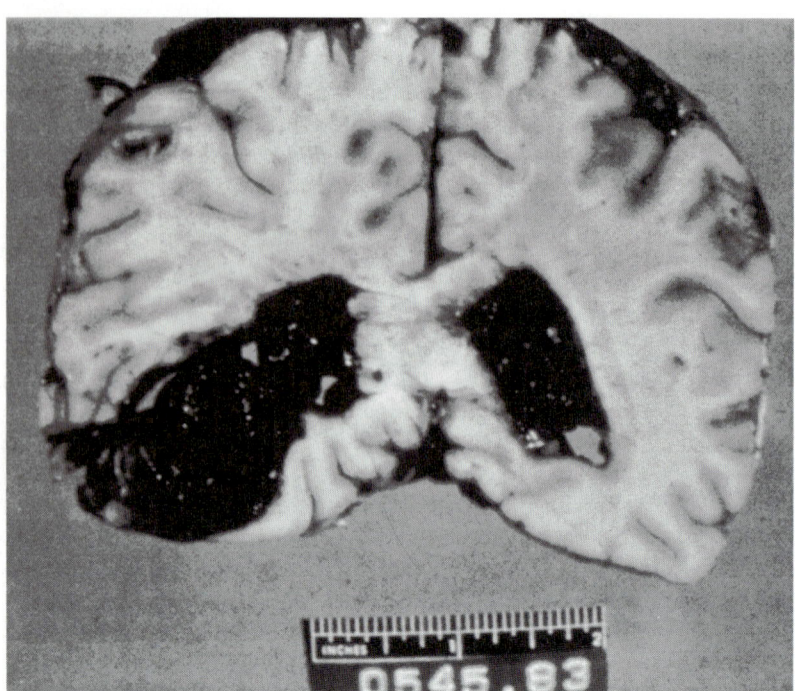

FIGURE 24–15. Hypertensive hemorrhage with eclampsia.

DIFFERENTIAL DIAGNOSIS. Generally, eclampsia is more likely to be diagnosed too frequently rather than overlooked, because epilepsy, encephalitis, meningitis, cerebral tumor, cysticercosis, and ruptured cerebral aneurysm during late pregnancy and the puerperium may simulate eclampsia. **Until other such causes are excluded, however, all pregnant women with convulsions should be considered to have eclampsia.**

PROGNOSIS. The prognosis for eclampsia is always serious; this is one of the most dangerous conditions that can afflict a pregnant woman and her fetus. Fortunately, maternal mortality due to eclampsia has decreased in the past three decades from 5 to 10 percent to less than 3 percent of cases (Eclampsia Trial Collaborative Group, 1995; Mattar and Sibai, 2000; Pritchard and associates, 1984). These experiences clearly underscore that eclampsia, as well as severe preeclampsia, are to be considered overt threats to maternal life. Indeed, 23 percent of maternal deaths recorded in the United States during 1997 were related to pregnancy hypertension and accounted for at least 64 deaths (Hoyert and colleagues, 1999).

TREATMENT. In 1955 Pritchard initiated a standardized treatment regimen at Parkland Hospital, and this was used through 1999 to manage over 400 women with eclampsia. The carefully analyzed results of treatment of 245 cases of eclampsia were reported by Pritchard and associates (1984). Most eclampsia regimens used in the United States adhere to a similar philosophy, the tenets of which include:

1. Control of convulsions using an intravenously administered loading dose of magnesium sulfate. This is followed by either a continuous infusion of magnesium sulfate or by an intramuscular loading dose and periodic intramuscular injections.
2. Intermittent intravenous or oral administration of an antihypertensive medication to lower blood pressure whenever the diastolic pressure is considered dangerously high. Some clinicians treat at 100 mm Hg, some at 105 mm Hg, and some at 110 mm Hg.
3. Avoidance of diuretics and limitation of intravenous fluid administration unless fluid loss is excessive. Hyperosmotic agents are avoided.
4. Delivery.

MAGNESIUM SULFATE TO CONTROL CONVULSIONS. In more severe cases of preeclampsia, as well eclampsia, magnesium sulfate administered parenterally is the effective anticonvulsant agent without producing central nervous system depression in either the mother or the infant. It may be given intravenously by continuous infusion or intramuscularly by intermittent injection (Table 24–10). The dosage schedule for severe preeclampsia is the same as for eclampsia. Because labor and delivery is a more likely time for convulsions to develop, women with preeclampsia–eclampsia usually are given magnesium sulfate during labor and for 24 hours postpartum. **Magnesium sulfate is not given to treat hypertension.**

Based on a number of studies cited subsequently, as well as extensive clinical observations, magnesium most likely exerts a specific anticonvulsant action on the cere-

TABLE 24–10. Magnesium Sulfate Dosage Schedule for Severe Preeclampsia and Eclampsia

Continuous Intravenous Infusion

1. Give 4- to 6-g loading dose of magnesium sulfate diluted in 100 mL of IV fluid administered over 15–20 min.

2. Begin 2 g/h in 100 mL of IV maintenance infusion.

3. Measure serum magnesium level at 4–6 h and adjust infusion to maintain levels between 4 and 7 mEq/L (4.8–8.4 mg/dL).

4. Magnesium sulfate is discontinued 24 h after delivery.

Intermittent Intramuscular Injections

1. Give 4 g of magnesium sulfate ($MgSO_4 \cdot 7H_2O$ USP) as a 20% solution intravenously at a rate not to exceed 1 g/min.

2. Follow promptly with 10 g of 50% magnesium sulfate solution, one-half (5 g) injected deeply in the upper outer quadrant of both buttocks through a 3-inch-long, 20-gauge needle. (Addition of 1.0 mL of 2% lidocaine minimizes discomfort.) If convulsions persist after 15 min, give up to 2 g more intravenously as a 20% solution at a rate not to exceed 1 g/min. If the woman is large, up to 4 g may be given slowly.

3. Every 4 h thereafter give 5 g of a 50% solution of magnesium sulfate injected deeply in the upper outer quadrant of alternate buttocks, but only after assuring that:

   a. the patellar reflex is present

   b. respirations are not depressed

   c. urine output during the previous 4 h exceeded 100 mL

4. Magnesium sulfate is discontinued 24 h after delivery.

---

bral cortex. Typically, the mother stops convulsing after the initial administration of magnesium sulfate, and within an hour or two regains consciousness sufficiently to be oriented as to place and time.

The magnesium sulfate dosage schedules presented in Table 24–10 usually result in plasma magnesium levels illustrated in Figures 24–16 and 24–17. When magnesium sulfate is given to arrest and prevent recurrent eclamptic seizures, about 10 to 15 percent of women will have a subsequent convulsion. An additional 2-g dose of magnesium sulfate in a 20 percent solution is administered slowly intravenously. In a small woman, an additional 2-g dose may be used once, and twice if needed in a larger woman. In only 5 of 245 women with eclampsia at Parkland Hospital was it necessary to use supplementary medication to control convulsions (Pritchard and associates, 1984). Sodium amobarbital is given slowly intravenously in doses up to 250 mg in women who are excessively agitated in the postconvulsion phase. Thiopental is suitable also. Maintenance magnesium sulfate therapy for eclampsia is continued for 24 hours after delivery. For eclampsia that develops postpartum, magnesium sulfate is administered for 24 hours after the onset of convulsions.

PHARMACOLOGY AND TOXICOLOGY OF MAGNESIUM SULFATE. Magnesium sulfate USP is $MgSO_4 \cdot 7H_2O$ and not $MgSO_4$. Parenterally administered magnesium is cleared almost totally by renal excretion, and magnesium intoxication is avoided by ensuring that urine output is adequate, the patellar or biceps reflex is present, and there is no respiratory depression. Eclamptic convulsions are almost always prevented by plasma magnesium levels maintained at 4 to 7 mEq/L (4.8 to 8.4 mg/dL or 2.0 to 3.5 mmol/L).

When administered as described in Table 24–10, the drug will practically always arrest eclamptic convulsions and prevent their recurrence. The initial intravenous infusion of 4 to 6 g is used to establish a prompt therapeutic level that is maintained by the nearly simultaneous intramuscular injection of 10 g of the compound, followed by 5 g intramuscularly every 4 hours, or by continuous infusion at 2 to 3 g per hour. With these dosage schedules, therapeutically effective plasma levels of 4 to 7 mEq/L are achieved compared with pretreatment plasma levels of less than 2.0 mEq/L.

Sibai and co-workers (1984) performed a prospective study in which they compared continuous intravenous magnesium sulfate and intramuscular magnesium sulfate. There was no significant difference between mean magnesium levels observed after intramuscular magnesium sulfate and those observed following a maintenance intravenous infusion of 2 g per hour (Fig. 24–17). In our experience many women will require 3-g-per-hour infusions to maintain effective plasma levels of magnesium.

Patellar reflexes disappear when the plasma magnesium level reaches 10 mEq per L (about 12 mg/dL), presumably because of a curariform action. This sign serves to warn of impending magnesium toxicity, because a further increase will lead to respiratory depression.

When plasma levels rise above 10 mEq/L, respiratory depression develops, and at 12 mEq/L or more, respiratory paralysis and arrest follow. Somjen and co-workers (1966) induced in themselves, by intravenous infusion, marked hypermagnesemia, achieving plasma levels up to 15 mEq/L. **Predictably, at such high plasma levels, respiratory depression developed that necessitated mechanical ventilation, but depression of the sensorium was not dramatic as long as hypoxia was prevented.** Treatment with calcium gluconate, 1 g intravenously, along with the withholding of magnesium sulfate usually reverses mild to moderate respiratory depression. Unfortunately, the effects of intravenously administered calcium may be short lived. For severe respiratory depression and arrest, prompt tracheal intubation and mechanical ventilation are life saving. Direct toxic effects on the myocardium from high levels of magnesium are uncommon. It appears that the cardiac dysfunction asso-

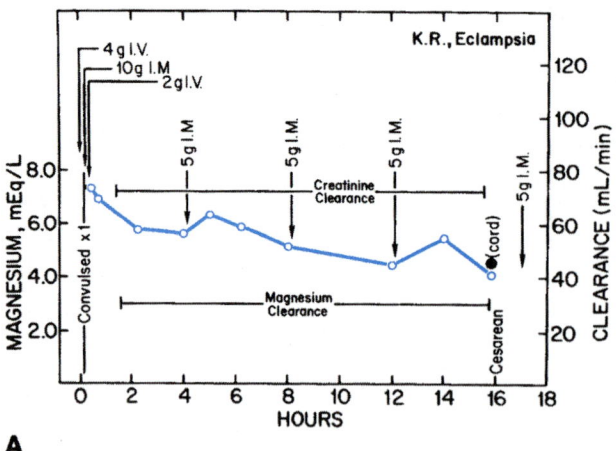

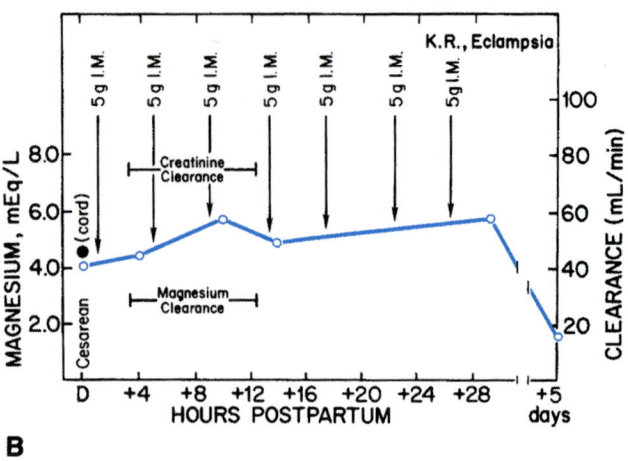

FIGURE 24–16. A. Plasma magnesium levels are plotted for a woman with antepartum eclampsia in whom 4 g of magnesium sulfate intravenously and 10 g intramuscularly were administered at the outset. When she soon convulsed again, 2 g more were injected slowly followed by 5 g intramuscularly every 4 hours, as described in Table 24–10. She did not convulse again. **B.** The same woman as in **A.** Maternal magnesium levels during the first 28 hours postpartum and 4 days after magnesium sulfate was discontinued are plotted. Before and the day after delivery the renal clearance of magnesium remained relatively constant at about 35 percent of the somewhat depressed creatinine clearance. The mother recovered fully and the baby thrived. (From Pritchard and associates, 1984.)

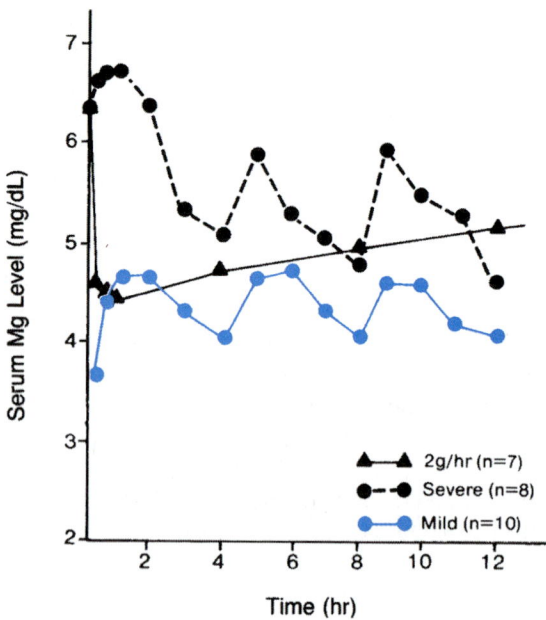

FIGURE 24–17. Comparison of serum magnesium levels following (1) mild preeclampsia—10-g intramuscular loading dose of magnesium sulfate and a 5-g maintenance dose every 4 hours (●–●); (2) severe preeclampsia—4-g intravenous loading dose followed by the same regimen as in (1) (●--●); compared with (3) 4-g intravenous loading dose followed by a continuous infusion of 2 g/hr (▲-▲). (From Sibai and co-workers, 1984, with permission.)

ciated with magnesium is due to respiratory arrest and hypoxia. With appropriate ventilation, cardiac action is satisfactory even when plasma levels are exceedingly high (McCubbin and colleagues, 1981).

IMPAIRED RENAL FUNCTION. Because magnesium is cleared almost exclusively by renal excretion, plasma magnesium concentration, using the doses described previously, will be excessive if glomerular filtration is decreased substantively. The initial standard dose of magnesium sulfate can be safely administered without knowledge of renal function. Renal function is thereafter estimated by measuring plasma creatinine, and whenever it is 1.3 mg/dL or higher, we give only half of the maintenance intramuscular magnesium sulfate dose outlined in Table 24–10. With this renal impairment dosage, plasma magnesium levels are usually within the desired range of 4 to 7 mEq/L. Whether magnesium sulfate is being given intravenously by continuous infusion, serum magnesium levels are used to adjust the infusion rate. **With either method, when there is renal insufficiency, plasma magnesium levels must be checked periodically.**

Acute cardiovascular effects of parenteral magnesium ion in women with severe preeclampsia have been studied by Cotton and associates (1986b), who obtained data using pulmonary and radial artery catheterization. Following a 4-g intravenous dose given over 15 minutes, mean arterial blood pressure fell slightly, and this was accompanied by a 13 percent increase in cardiac index. Thus, magnesium decreased systemic vascular resistance and mean arterial pressure, and at the same time increased cardiac output, without evidence of myocardial depression. These findings were coincidental with transient nausea and flushing, and the cardiovascular effects persisted for only 15 minutes despite continued infusion of magnesium sulfate at 1.5 g per hour.

Thurnau and colleagues (1987) showed that there was a small but highly significant increase in cerebrospinal fluid magnesium concentration after magnesium therapy for preeclampsia. The magnitude of the increase was directly proportional to the corresponding serum concentration. This increase cannot be due to the disease itself, because cerebrospinal fluid magnesium levels are unchanged in untreated severely preeclamptic women when compared with normotensive controls (Fong and associates, 1995).

Lipton and Rosenberg (1994) attribute anticonvulsant effects to blocked neuronal calcium influx through the glutamate channel. Cotton and associates (1992) induced seizure activity in the hippocampus region of rats because it is a region with a low seizure threshold and a high density of N-methyl-D-aspartate receptors. These receptors are linked to various models of epilepsy. Because hippocampal seizures can be blocked by magnesium, it is believed that this implicated the N-methyl-D-aspartate receptor in eclamptic convulsions (Hallak and colleagues, 1998). Importantly, results such as these suggest that magnesium has a central nervous system effect in blocking seizures.

UTERINE EFFECTS. Magnesium ions in relatively high concentration will depress myometrial contractility both in vivo and in vitro. With the regimen described earlier and the plasma levels that have resulted, no evidence of myometrial depression has been observed beyond a transient decrease in activity during and immediately after the initial intravenous loading dose. Indeed, Leveno and colleagues (1998) compared labor and delivery outcomes in 480 nulliparous women given phenytoin for preeclampsia with outcomes in 425 similar women given magnesium sulfate. Magnesium sulfate did not significantly alter oxytocin stimulation of labor, admission-to-delivery intervals, or route of delivery. Similar results have been reported by others (Atkinson and associates, 1995; Szal and co-workers, 1999; Witlin and colleagues, 1997b).

The mechanisms by which magnesium might inhibit uterine contractility is not established, but is generally assumed to depend on its effect on intracellular calcium (Watt-Morse and associates, 1995). The regulatory pathway leading to uterine contraction begins with an increase in the intracellular free Ca^{2+} concentration, which activates myosin light chain kinase (Mizuki and associates, 1993). High concentrations of extracellular magnesium have been reported not only to inhibit calcium entry into myometrial cells but to also lead to high intracellular magnesium levels.

This latter effect has been reported to inhibit calcium entry into the cell—presumably by blocking calcium channels (Mizuki and associates, 1993). These mechanisms for inhibition of uterine contractility appear to be dose dependent because serum magnesium levels of at least 8 to 10 mEq/L are necessary to inhibit uterine contractions (Watt-Morse and associates, 1995). This likely explains why there is no uterine effect clinically when magnesium sulfate is given for eclampsia treatment or prophylaxis. Specifically, magnesium sulfate when given either intravenously or intramuscularly for preeclampsia or eclampsia, consistently results in serum magnesium levels less than the 8 to 10 mEq/L necessary to inhibit uterine contractility (Fig. 24–16).

FETAL EFFECTS. Magnesium administered parenterally to the mother promptly crosses the placenta to achieve equilibrium in fetal serum and less so in amnionic fluid (Hallak and colleagues, 1993). The neonate may be depressed only if there is *severe* hypermagnesemia at delivery. We have not observed neonatal compromise after therapy with magnesium sulfate (Cunningham and Pritchard, 1984), nor have Green and associates (1983). Whether magnesium sulfate affects the fetal heat rate pattern, specifically beat-to-beat variability (Chap. 14, p. 336), is controversial. Hallak and colleagues (1999b), in a randomized investigation comparing an infusion of magnesium sulfate to saline, found that magnesium sulfate was associated with a small but clinically insignificant decrease in variability of the fetal heart rate.

There is a suggestion of a possible protective effect of magnesium against cerebral palsy in very-low-birthweight infants (Nelson and Grether, 1995; Schendel and colleagues, 1996). Murphy and colleagues (1995) found that preeclampsia, rather than magnesium sulfate, was protective against cerebral palsy in these infants. Kimberlin and colleagues (1996), however, found no advantage of maternal magnesium sulfate tocolysis in infants born weighing less than 1000 g.

CLINICAL EFFICACY OF MAGNESIUM SULFATE THERAPY. In 1995, results were reported from the multinational clinical trial of eclampsia therapy. The Eclampsia Trial Collaborative Group (1995) study was funded in part by the World Health Organization and coordination was provided by the National Perinatal Epidemiology Unit in Oxford, England. This study included 1687 women with eclampsia who were randomly allocated to different anticonvulsant regimens. The primary out-

Magnesium sulphate versus diazepam

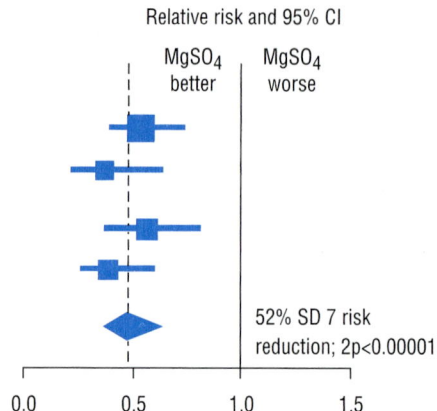

Entry characteristic	Recurrent convulsion/women MgSO₄	Recurrent convulsion/women Diazepam
Before delivery	46/325	83/308
After delivery	14/128	43/144
No prior anticonvulsant	33/198	64/218
Prior anticonvulsant	25/244	60/227
All women	60/453 (13.2%)	126/452 (27.9%)

52% SD 7 risk reduction; 2p<0.00001

Magnesium sulphate versus phenytoin

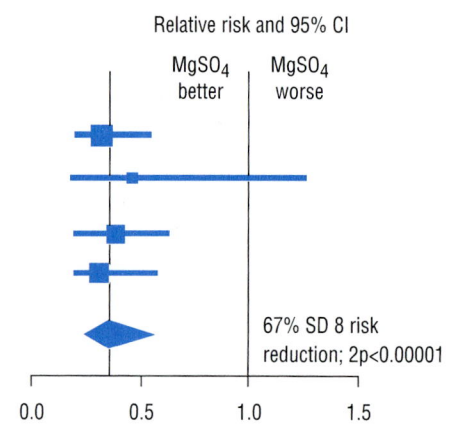

Entry characteristic	Recurrent convulsion/women MgSO₄	Recurrent convulsion/women Phenytoin
Before delivery	17/309	56/319
After delivery	5/79	10/68
No prior anticonvulsant	10/91	23/73
Prior anticonvulsant	12/294	43/308
All women	22/388 (5.7%)	66/387 (17.1%)

67% SD 8 risk reduction; 2p<0.00001

FIGURE 24–18. Effects of magnesium sulfate versus diazepam and phenytoin on recurrent convulsions. (From the Eclampsia Trial Collaborative Group, 1995, with permission.)

come measures were recurrence of convulsions and maternal deaths. In one study, 453 women were randomized to be given magnesium sulfate and compared with 452 given diazepam. Another 388 eclamptic women were randomized to be given magnesium sulfate and compared with 387 women given phenytoin.

As shown in Figure 24–18, women allocated to magnesium sulfate therapy had a 50 percent reduction in incidence of recurrent seizures compared with those given diazepam. Importantly, as shown in Table 24–11, maternal deaths were reduced in women given magnesium sulfate, and although these differences are clinically impressive, they are not statistically significant. Specifically, there were 3.8 percent deaths in 453 women randomized to magnesium sulfate compared with 5.1 percent of 452 given diazepam. Maternal and perinatal morbidity were not different between these two groups, and there was no difference in the number of labor inductions or cesarean deliveries.

In a second comparison, also shown in Figure 24–18,

women randomized to receive magnesium sulfate compared with phenytoin had a 67 percent reduction in recurrent convulsions. As shown in Table 24–11, maternal mortality was lower in the magnesium compared with the phenytoin group (2.6 versus 5.2 percent). This

TABLE 24–11. Maternal Mortality in Eclampsia Trial Collaborative Group

Regimen	No.	Mortality Maternal (%)	Mortality Perinatal (per 1000)
Magnesium sulfate	453	3.8	25
Diazepam	452	5.1	22
Magnesium sulfate	388	2.6	22
Pheytoin	387	5.2	31

From the Eclampsia Trial Collaborative Group (1995).

clinically impressive decreased maternal mortality of 50 percent again was not significant statistically.

In other comparisons, women allocated to magnesium sulfate therapy were less likely to be artificially ventilated, to develop pneumonia, and to be admitted to intensive care units than those given phenytoin. Neonates of women given magnesium sulfate were significantly less likely to require intubation at delivery and to be admitted to the neonatal intensive care unit compared with infants whose mothers received phenytoin.

The Collaborative Group concluded: "There is now compelling evidence in favour of magnesium sulfate, rather than diazepam or phenytoin, for the treatment of eclampsia." These results are even more impressive when it is emphasized that women in this study who received intravenous magnesium sulfate received only 1 g per hour!

ANTIHYPERTENSIVE TREATMENT ALONE TO CONTROL SEIZURES. There continues to be a question of whether antihypertensive medications alone can be used to prevent recurrent seizures (Duley and Johanson, 1994; Ramsay and colleagues, 1994). It is difficult and unwise to recommend withholding magnesium sulfate because even with the excellent results reported using both anticonvulsants and antihypertensive agents in the Collaborative Eclampsia Trial (1995), maternal mortality was still 4.1 percent of 1690 women.

PREVENTION OF ECLAMPSIA. Magnesium sulfate therapy also is superior to phenytoin in preventing eclamptic seizures. Lucas and colleagues (1995) reported results of a prospective study from Parkland Hospital in which women with gestational hypertension were randomized to receive magnesium sulfate or phenytoin during labor. The magnesium sulfate therapy consisted of the intramuscular regimen presented in Table 24–10. The phenytoin regimen consisted of a 1000-mg loading dose infused over a 1-hour period, followed by a 500-mg oral dose 10 hours later. Anticonvulsant therapy in both groups was continued for 24 hours postpartum. Ten of the 1089 women randomly assigned to the phenytoin regimen had eclamptic convulsions. There were no convulsions in the 1049 women given magnesium sulfate ($P = .004$). There were no significant differences in any risk factors for eclampsia between the two groups of women studied. Maternal and neonatal outcomes were similar in the two study groups. Women given phenytoin, and who developed eclampsia, did so despite "therapeutic" serum levels (10 to 25 μg/mL).

Debate still ensues—mostly outside the United States—over whether magnesium sulfate prophylaxis should be given routinely to all women in labor who have hypertension (Nelson and Grether, 1995; Robson, 1996). Burrows and Burrows (1995) described 467

women with preeclampsia in whom seizure prophylaxis was not given. A total of 3.9 percent developed eclamptic seizures. Hall and colleagues (2000a) reported this to be 1.5 percent in 318 preeclamptic women. This is in contrast to a failure rate of prophylaxis of 1 in 750 women treated with the regimen shown in Table 24–10 and reported by Cunningham and Leveno (1988). The debate hinges primarily on the position of some clinicians that a convulsion due to eclampsia does no immediate great harm to most mothers and fetuses. Presumably, those who embrace this view would reserve magnesium sulfate therapy for only those women who develop eclampsia. There may be, however, other previously unmeasured fetal effects of maternal eclampsia that could justify attempts to prevent as well as treat eclampsia. For example, Hallak and associates (1999a) have reported in experimental animals that maternal seizures were associated with fetal brain injury due to maternal hypoxia during the convulsion. Magnesium sulfate prevented this fetal damage.

The debate currently centers around which preeclamptic women should be given prophylaxis. To assess this, Coetzee and colleagues (1998) randomized 699 South African women with severe preeclampsia to intravenous magnesium sulfate or to saline placebo. Eclampsia developed in 1 of 30 of the women given saline, and although the maternal and fetal outcomes were good, the study was stopped. Benefits of prophylactic magnesium sulfate for women with mild preeclampsia is disputable because the estimated risk of eclampsia is 1 in 100 or less (Lucas and colleagues, 1995). Witlin and Sibai (1998) recently reviewed the evidence for the efficacy of magnesium sulfate for treatment and prevention of convulsions resulting from hypertensive disorders due to pregnancy. They concluded that although there is little question about the benefits of magnesium sulfate in women with severe preeclampsia and eclampsia, the need for its prophylactic administration to women with mild disease is unclear. We certainly agree that it is prudent to prevent eclampsia in women at high risk for convulsions.

HYDRALAZINE TO CONTROL SEVERE HYPERTENSION. At Parkland Hospital, hydralazine is given intravenously whenever the diastolic blood pressure is 110 mm Hg or higher. Some recommend treatment of diastolic pressures higher than 100 mm Hg and some use 105 mm Hg as a limit (Cunningham and Lindheimer, 1992; Sibai, 1996). Because precise data are lacking, the Working Group (National High Blood Pressure Education Program, 2000) recommended the compromise value of persistent systolic pressure greater than or equal to 160 mm Hg and/or diastolic pressure greater than 105 mm Hg.

A number of regimens have been used. Hydralazine

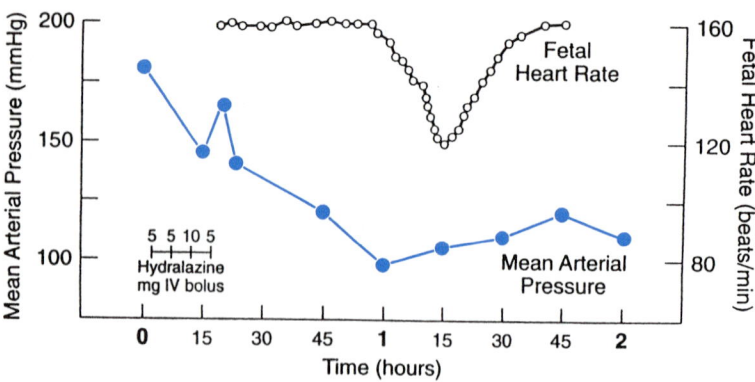

FIGURE 24–19. Effects of acute blood pressure decrease on fetal status. Hydralazine was given at 5-minute intervals instead of 15-minute intervals, and mean arterial pressure decreased from 180 to 90 mm Hg within 1 hour; this change was associated with fetal bradycardia.

is administered in 5- to 10-mg doses at 15- to 20-minute intervals until a satisfactory response is achieved. A satisfactory response antepartum or intrapartum is defined as a decrease in diastolic blood pressure to 90 to 100 mm Hg, but not lower lest placental perfusion be compromised. Hydralazine so administered has proven remarkably effective in the prevention of cerebral hemorrhage. At Parkland Hospital, approximately 8 percent of all women with hypertensive disorders are given hydralazine as described, and we estimate that more than 4000 women have been treated. Seldom was another antihypertensive agent needed because of poor response to hydralazine. In many European centers, hydralazine is also favored (Redman and Roberts, 1993).

The tendency to give a larger initial dose of hydralazine when the blood pressure is higher must be avoided. The response to even 5- to 10-mg doses cannot be predicted by the level of hypertension; thus we always give 5 mg as the initial dose. An example of very severe hypertension in a woman with chronic hypertension complicated by superimposed eclampsia that responded to repeated intravenous injections of hydralazine is shown in Figure 24–19. Hydralazine was injected more frequently than recommended in the protocol, and blood pressure decreased in less than 1 hour from 240–270/130–150 mm Hg to 110/80 mm Hg. Uteroplacental insufficiency fetal heart rate decelerations were evident when the pressure fell to 110/80 mm Hg, and persisted until maternal blood pressure increased.

LABETALOL. Intravenous labetalol is also used to treat acute hypertension of pregnancy. In 1994, hydralazine was not always available in the United States and more experience was gained with this α_1- and non-selective β-blocker. Mabie and associates (1987) compared intravenous hydralazine with labetalol for blood pressure control in 60 peripartum women. Labetalol lowered blood pressure more rapidly, and associated tachycardia was minimal, but hydralazine lowered mean arterial pressure to safe levels more effectively. We have evaluated labetalol given intravenously for women with

severe preeclampsia and our results are very similar. Our protocol calls for 10 mg intravenously initially. If the blood pressure has not decreased to the desirable level in 10 minutes, then 20 mg is given. The next 10-minute incremental dose is 40 mg followed by another 40 mg, and then 80 mg if a salutary response is not yet achieved.

The Working Group (2000) recommends starting with a 20-mg intravenous bolus. If not effective within 10 minutes, this is followed by 40 mg, then 80 mg every 10 minutes but not to exceed a 220-mg total dose.

OTHER ANTIHYPERTENSIVE AGENTS. The Working Group recommends **nifedipine** in a 10-mg oral dose to be repeated in 30 minutes if necessary. Scardo and colleagues (1996) gave 10-mg nifedipine orally to 10 women with preeclamptic hypertensive emergencies and reported no hypotension or fetal compromise. Mabie and colleagues (1988) administered nifedipine sublingually to 34 women with peripartum hypertension. Its antihypertensive effects were potent and rapid, and two women developed worrisome hypotension. Similar effects in nonpregnant patients have caused cerebrovascular ischemia, myocardial infarction, conduction disturbances, and death, leading Grossman and colleagues (1996) to call for a moratorium on its use in hypertensive emergencies. Vermillion and colleagues (1999) and Scardo and co-workers (1999) compared nifedipine with labetalol in randomized trials and found neither definitively superior to the other. Belfort and associates (1990) administered the calcium antagonist, **verapamil**, by intravenous infusion at 5 to 10 mg per hour. Mean arterial pressure was lowered by 20 percent. Belfort and co-workers (1996) reported that **nimodipine** given by continuous infusion as well as orally (1998) was effective to lower blood pressure in women with severe preeclampsia. Bolte and colleagues (1998) reported good results in 169 preeclamptic women treated with intravenous **ketanserin**, a selective serotonin$_2$ receptor blocker.

Nitroprusside is not recommended by the Working Group of the National High Blood Pressure Education

Program (2000) unless there is no response to hydralazine, labetalol, or nifedipine. A continuous infusion is begun with a dose of 0.25 μg/kg/min increased as necessary to 5 μg/kg/min. Fetal cyanide toxicity may occur after 4 hours.

PERSISTENT IMMEDIATE SEVERE POSTPARTUM HYPERTENSION. The potential problem of antihypertensive agents causing serious compromise of placental perfusion and fetal well-being is obviated by delivery. If there is a problem after delivery in controlling severe hypertension and intravenous hydralazine or another agent is being used repeatedly early in the puerperium to control persistent severe hypertension, then other regimens can be used. We have had success with intramuscular hydralazine, usually in 10- to 25-mg doses at 4- to 6-hour intervals. Once repeated blood pressure readings remain near normal, hydralazine is stopped.

If hypertension of appreciable intensity persists or recurs *in these postpartum women*, oral labetalol or a thiazide diuretic are given for as long as necessary. A variety of other antihypertensive agents have been utilized for this purpose, including other β-blockers and calcium-channel antagonists. The persistence or refractoriness of hypertension is likely due to at least two mechanisms:

1. Underlying chronic hypertension.
2. Mobilization of edema fluid with redistribution into the intravenous compartment.

Labetalol and a diuretic are effective treatment for both mechanisms.

PLASMA EXCHANGE. Over the years, the group at the University of Mississippi Medical Center has described an atypical syndrome in which severe preeclampsia–eclampsia persists despite delivery. Martin and associates (1995) described 18 such women over a 10-year period during which time they delivered nearly 43,000 patients. They advocate single or multiple plasma exchange for these women and in some cases, 3 L of plasma (representing 12 to 15 donors) were exchanged three times before a response was forthcoming. In our experiences of over 50,000 hypertensive women in nearly 350,000 pregnancies, we have not encountered this syndrome. In a very few women, persistent hypertension, thrombocytopenia, and renal dysfunction was found to be due to thrombotic microangiopathy (Dashe and colleagues, 1998).

DIURETICS AND HYPEROSMOTIC AGENTS. Potent diuretics further compromise placental perfusion, because their immediate effects include intravascular volume depletion, which most often is already reduced compared with normal pregnancy. Therefore, diuretics are not used to lower blood pressure lest they enhance the intensity of the maternal hemoconcentration and its adverse effects on the mother and the fetus (Zondervan and co-authors, 1988).

Once delivery is accomplished, in almost all cases of severe preeclampsia and eclampsia there is a spontaneous diuresis that usually begins within 24 hours and results in the disappearance of excessive extravascular fluid over the next 3 to 4 days, as demonstrated in Figure 24–13.

With infusion of hyperosmotic agents, the potential exists for an appreciable intravascular influx of fluid and, in turn, subsequent escape of intravascular fluid in the form of edema into vital organs, especially the lungs and brain. Moreover, an osmotically active agent that leaks through capillaries into lungs and brain promotes accumulation of edema at these sites. Most importantly, a sustained beneficial effect from their use has not been demonstrated. For all of these reasons, hyperosmotic agents have not been administered, and use of furosemide or similar drugs has been limited to the rare instances in which pulmonary edema was identified or strongly suspected.

FLUID THERAPY. Lactated Ringer solution is administered routinely at the rate of 60 mL to no more than 125 mL per hour unless there was unusual fluid loss from vomiting, diarrhea, or diaphoresis, or more likely, excessive blood loss at delivery. Oliguria, common in cases of severe preeclampsia and eclampsia, coupled with the knowledge that maternal blood volume is very likely constricted compared with normal pregnancy, makes it tempting to administer intravenous fluids more vigorously. The rationale for controlled, conservative fluid administration is that the typical eclamptic woman already has excessive extracellular fluid that is inappropriately distributed between the intravascular and extravascular spaces. Infusion of large fluid volumes could and does enhance the maldistribution of extravascular fluid and thereby appreciably increases the risk of pulmonary and cerebral edema (Sibai and colleagues, 1987b).

PULMONARY EDEMA. Women with severe preeclampsia–eclampsia who develop pulmonary edema most often do so postpartum (Cunningham and colleagues, 1986). Aspiration of gastric contents, the result of convulsions or perhaps from anesthesia, or oversedation, should be excluded; however, the majority of these women have cardiac failure. Some normal pregnancy changes, magnified by preeclampsia–eclampsia, predispose to pulmonary edema. Importantly, plasma oncotic pressure decreases appreciably in normal term pregnancy because of decreases in serum albumin, and oncotic pressure falls even more with preeclampsia (Zinaman and associates, 1985). Moreover, Øian and colleagues (1986) described increased extravascular fluid oncotic pressure in preeclamptic women, and this favors capillary fluid extravasation. Brown and associates (1989) verified increased capillary permeability in preeclamptic women. Bhatia and associates (1987) found a correlation between plasma colloid osmotic pressure and fibronectin concentration; this suggested to them that vascular protein loss was the result of increased vascular permeability caused by vessel injury.

The frequent findings of hemoconcentration, as well as the identification of reduced central venous and pulmonary capillary wedge pressures in women with severe preeclampsia, have tempted some investigators to infuse various fluids, starch polymers, or albumin concentrates, or all three, in attempts to expand blood volume and thereby somehow to relieve vasospasm and reverse organ deterioration. Thus far, clear-cut evidence of benefits from this approach is lacking; however, serious complications, especially pulmonary edema, have been reported. López-Llera (1982) reported that vigorous volume expansion was associated with a high incidence of pulmonary edema in more than 700 eclamptic women. Benedetti and colleagues (1985) described pulmonary edema in 7 of 10 severely preeclamptic women who were given colloid therapy. Sibai and colleagues (1987b) cited excessive colloid and crystalloid infusions as causing most of their 37 cases of pulmonary edema associated with severe preeclampsia–eclampsia. Finally, Lehmann and co-workers (1987) reported that pulmonary edema caused nearly a third of maternal deaths due to hypertensive disorders at Charity Hospital in New Orleans.

For these reasons, until it is understood how to contain more fluid within the intravascular compartment and, at the same time, less fluid outside the intravascular compartment, we remain convinced that, in the absence of marked fluid loss, fluids can be administered safely only in moderation. To date, no serious adverse effects have been observed from such a policy. Importantly, dialysis for renal failure was not required for any of the more than 400 cases of eclampsia so managed.

INVASIVE HEMODYNAMIC MONITORING. Much of what has been learned within the past decade about cardiovascular and hemodynamic pathophysiological alterations associated with severe preeclampsia–eclampsia has been made possible by invasive hemodynamic monitoring using a flow-directed pulmonary artery catheter. The need for clinical implementation of such technology for the woman with preeclampsia–eclampsia, however, has not been established. Gilbert and colleagues (2000) recently described a retrospective review of pulmonary artery catheterization in 17 women with eclampsia. Although they found this procedure subjectively "helpful" in clinical management, all of these women had undergone "multiple interventions," including volume expansion, prior to catheterization.

Use of pulmonary-artery catheterization has been reviewed by Nolan and colleagues (1992), Hankins and Cunningham (1991), and Clark and Cotton (1988). Two conditions frequently cited as indications for such monitoring are preeclampsia associated with oliguria and preeclampsia associated with pulmonary edema. Perhaps somewhat paradoxically, it is usually vigorous treatment of the former that results in most cases of the latter.

Because vigorous intravenous hydration and osmotically active agents are avoided at Parkland Hospital in women with severe preeclampsia and eclampsia, hemodynamic monitoring has not been used for the vast majority of these women. Such measures are usually reserved for women with accompanying severe cardiac disease and/or renal disease or in cases of refractory hypertension, oliguria, and pulmonary edema. Similar indications are used by Clark and associates (1997), Clark and Cotton (1988), Cowles (1994), and Easterling and co-workers (1989), as well as recommended by the American College of Obstetricians and Gynecologists (1988, 1996). The routine use of such monitoring even if pulmonary edema develops is questionable. Most of these women respond quickly to furosemide given intravenously. Afterload reduction with intermittent doses of intravenous hydralazine to lower blood pressure, as described earlier, may also be necessary, because women with chronic hypertension and severe superimposed preeclampsia are more likely to develop heart failure (Cunningham and colleagues, 1986). Obese women in these circumstances are even more likely to develop heart failure (Mabie and associates, 1988).

Invasive monitoring should be considered for those women with multiple clinical factors such as intrinsic heart disease and/or advanced renal disease that might cause pulmonary edema by more than one mechanism. This is particularly relevant if pulmonary edema is inexplicable or refractory to treatment. Still, in most of these cases it is not necessary to perform pulmonary artery catheterization for clinical management.

DELIVERY. To avoid maternal risks from cesarean delivery, steps to effect vaginal delivery are employed initially in women with eclampsia. After an eclamptic seizure, labor often ensues spontaneously or can be induced successfully even in women remote from term. An immediate cure does not immediately follow delivery by any route, but serious morbidity is less common during the puerperium in women delivered vaginally.

BLOOD LOSS AT DELIVERY. Hemoconcentration, or lack of normal pregnancy-induced hypervolemia, is an almost predictable feature of severe preeclampsia–eclampsia. **These women, who consequently lack normal pregnancy hypervolemia, are much less tolerant of blood loss than are normotensive pregnant woman.** It is of great importance to recognize that an appreciable fall in blood pressure very soon after delivery most often means excessive blood loss and not sudden dissolution of vasospasm. When oliguria follows delivery, the hematocrit should be evaluated frequently to help detect excessive blood loss that, if identified, should be treated appropriately by careful blood transfusion.

ANALGESIA AND ANESTHESIA. In the past, both spinal and epidural analgesia were avoided in women with severe preeclampsia and eclampsia. Physiological changes leading to these concerns centered on the hypotension induced by sympathetic blockade and, in turn, on dangers from pressor agents or large volumes of intravenous fluid used to correct iatrogenically induced hypotension. For example, rapid infusion of large volumes of crystalloid or colloid, given to counteract maternal hypovolemia caused by a variety of causes, including epidural analgesia, has been implicated as a cause of pulmonary edema (Sibai and colleagues, 1987b). There have also been concerns about fetal safety because sympathetic blockade–induced hypotension can dangerously lower uteroplacental perfusion (Montan and Ingemorsson, 1989). Another concern is that attempts to restore blood pressure pharmacologically with vasopressors may be hazardous because women with preeclampsia are extremely sensitive to such agents.

As regional analgesia techniques were improved during the past decade, epidural analgesia was promoted by some proponents for women with severe preeclampsia to ameliorate vasospasm and lower blood pressure (Gutsche and Creek, 1993). Moreover, many who favored epidural blockade believed that general anesthesia was inadvisable because stimulation caused by tracheal intubation may result in sudden hypertension, which may cause pulmonary edema, cerebral edema, or intracranial hemorrhage (Lavies and colleagues, 1989). Others have also cited that tracheal intubation may be particularly hazardous in women with airway edema due to preeclampsia (Chadwick and Easterling, 1991).

These differing perspectives on the advantages, disadvantages, and safety of the anesthetic method used in the cesarean delivery of women with severe preeclampsia have evolved so that most authorities believe that epidural analgesia is the preferred method. Wallace and colleagues (1995) evaluated these important issues by conducting a randomized investigation in women with severe preeclampsia cared for at Parkland Hospital.

There were 80 women with severe preeclampsia who were to be delivered by cesarean and who were randomized to general anesthesia or epidural or combined spinal–epidural analgesia. Their mean preoperative blood pressure was approximately 170/110 mm Hg, and all had proteinuria. Anesthetic and obstetrical management included antihypertensive drug therapy and limited intravenous fluids and other drug therapy. The infants, whose mean gestational age at delivery was 34.8 weeks, all were born in good condition as assessed by Apgar scores and umbilical arterial blood gas determinations. Maternal hypotension resulting from regional analgesia was managed without excessive intravenous fluid administration. Similarly, maternal blood pressure was managed without severe hypertensive effects in women undergoing general anesthesia (Fig. 24–20). There were no serious maternal or fetal complications attributable to any of the three anesthetic methods. It was concluded that general as well as regional anesthetic methods are equally acceptable for cesarean delivery in pregnancies complicated by severe preeclampsia if steps are taken to ensure a careful approach to either method.

The immense popularity and increasing availability of epidural analgesia for labor has led many anesthesiologists as well as obstetricians to develop the viewpoint that epidural analgesia is an important factor in the intrapartum *treatment* of women with preeclampsia (Chadwick and Easterling, 1991; Ramanathan, 1991). Although epidural analgesia is widely used during labor in women with preeclampsia, the effects of such analgesia on the mother and fetus have not been extensively investigated. In a study by Lucas and associates (2001) from Parkland Hospital, 738 laboring women at 36 weeks or more who had gestational hypertension of varying severity were randomized to epidural analgesia or patient-controlled intravenous meperidine analgesia. Maternal and infant outcomes were similar in the two study groups. As shown in Table 24–12, although epidural analgesia significantly lowered the maternal blood pressure compared with the meperidine-treated group, this provided no significant benefit in terms of preventing severe hypertension later in labor. It was concluded that epidural analgesia during labor was safe for women with pregnancy-associated hypertensive disorders; it should not be misconstrued to be a therapy for hypertension.

These results were similar to those published by the Maternal–Fetal Medicine Units Network of the National Institute of Child Health and Human Development. Hogg and colleagues (1999) performed a retrospective comparison of 327 women with severe hypertension, of whom 209 (65 percent) were given epidural analgesia during labor. There were no significant differences in the cesarean delivery rate or in neonatal

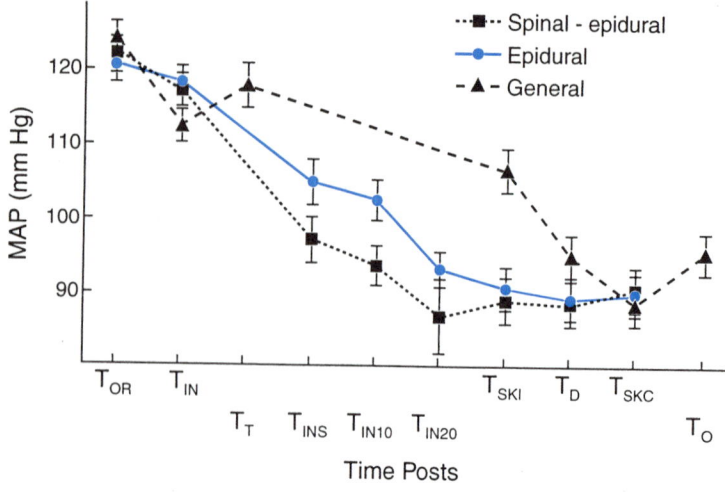

FIGURE 24–20. Blood pressure effects of general anesthesia versus epidural or spinal–epidural analgesia for cesarean delivery in 80 women with severe preeclampsia. (From Wallace and associates 1995, with permission.)

outcomes in those given epidural analgesia compared with those not receiving such analgesia. Importantly, 4.3 percent of the women given epidural analgesia developed pulmonary edema, presumably due in part to the intravenous crystalloid required to alleviate epidural-induced hypotension.

Newsome and colleagues (1986) studied the lowered mean arterial pressure that follows epidural blockade in a group of women with severe preeclampsia. Despite decreased blood pressure, the cardiac index did not fall and intravenous fluid loading caused elevation of pulmonary capillary wedge pressures as compared with women in whom fluids were restricted. It is clear that aggressive volume replacement in these women increases their risk for pulmonary edema, especially in the first 72 hours postpartum (Clark and colleagues, 1985; Cotton and associates, 1986a). When pulmonary edema develops there is also concern for development of cerebral edema. Finally, Heller and co-workers

(1983) demonstrated that the majority of cases of pharyngolaryngeal edema seen in women with severe preeclampsia were related to aggressive volume therapy.

LONG-TERM CONSEQUENCES

Women who develop hypertension during pregnancy should be evaluated during the immediate postpartum months and counseled about future pregnancies and also their cardiovascular risk later in life (Working Group of the National High Blood Pressure Education Program, 2000). As mentioned earlier, the longer hypertension diagnosed during pregnancy persists postpartum, the greater the likelihood that the cause is underlying chronic hypertension. Indeed, the Working Group has taken the position that hypertension attributable to pregnancy must resolve within 12 weeks of delivery.

TABLE 24–12. Effects of Epidural Analgesia During Labor on Maternal Blood Pressure in Women with Hypertensive Disorders Due to Pregnancy

	Type of Analgesia		
Outcome	Epidural (n = 372)	Meperidine (n = 366)	P Value
Mean maternal BP, change	−25 mm Hg	−13 mm Hg	< .001
Ephedrine for hypotension	11%	0	< .001
BP ≥ 160/110 mm Hg developed after analgesia	<1%	1%	NS

BP = blood pressure; NS = not significant.
From Lucas and colleagues (2001).

TABLE 24–13. Long-Term Consequences of Eclampsia in 270 Women Followed up to 43 Years After Diagnosis

	Long-Term Consequences	
Outcome	*Nulliparas with Eclampsia*	*Multiparas with Eclampsia*
Chronic hypertension[a]	Expected incidence	Increased incidence
Death[b]	Expected incidence	Increased 3-fold
Death related to hypertension	29%	80%

[a]Follow-up an average of 33 years after eclampsia diagnosed.
[b]Follow-up an average of 42 years after eclampsia diagnosed.
Adapted from Chesley and colleagues (1976).

Persistence of hypertension beyond this time is considered evidence of chronic hypertension (Chap. 45).

Although hypertension during pregnancy is common in occurrence, there are few reports concerning the long-term maternal consequences of hypertensive disorders during pregnancy. Most reports are focused on the risk of recurrence of hypertension during a subsequent pregnancy in women typically ascertained during the first months of such a pregnancy.

COUNSELING FOR FUTURE PREGNANCIES. Women who had preeclampsia are more prone to hypertensive complications in future pregnancies (Working Group of the National High Blood Pressure Education Program, 2000). Generally the earlier preeclampsia is diagnosed during the index pregnancy, the greater the likelihood of recurrence. For example, Sibai and colleagues (1986, 1991) found that nulliparous women diagnosed to have preeclampsia before 30 weeks have a recurrence risk as high as 40 percent during a subsequent pregnancy. The recurrence rate for women with one episode of HELLP syndrome is approximately 5 percent (Sibai and colleagues, 1995). Multiparous women who develop preeclampsia are at increased risk for recurrence of preeclampsia in subsequent pregnancy compared with nulliparas who develop preeclampsia (Trupin and associates, 1996).

Women with early-onset severe preeclampsia may be at risk for underlying thrombophilias such as factor V Leiden, protein S and C deficiency, and antiphospholipid antibodies, (Dekker and colleagues, 1995; Kupferminc and associates, 1999; Sibai, 1999; van Pampus and co-workers, 1999). These disorders, discussed in Chapter 49 (p. 1330), not only complicate subsequent pregnancies but also have an impact overall long-term health.

LONG-TERM PROGNOSIS. There is one truly remarkable and unparalleled effort to measure long-term maternal consequences of hypertension due to pregnancy.

Chesley and co-workers (1976) identified 270 women with eclampsia delivered at the Margaret Hague Maternity Hospital between 1931 and 1951 and meticulously followed these women through 1974—entailing a follow-up period of up to 43 years in some of the women. As shown in Table 24–13, the long-term cardiovascular prognosis depends on whether eclampsia occurred in nulliparous, compared with multiparous women. Chesley and co-workers (1976) also analyzed the long-term outcome in 54 nulliparous women with eclampsia in their index pregnancy and hypertension again during a subsequent pregnancy compared with 100 eclamptic nulliparous who were normotensive during all subsequent pregnancies. Those with recurrent pregnancy hypertension were at increased risk for chronic hypertension whereas those who remained normotensive during subsequent pregnancies were at decreased risk. Thus, normal blood pressure during subsequent pregnancies serves to define women not at risk for future chronic hypertension. According to the Working Group of the National High Blood Pressure Education Program (2000), women experiencing normotensive births have a reduced risk for remote hypertension. Thus, in some respects, repeated pregnancy serves as a screening test for future hypertension. Finally, and importantly, preeclampsia does not cause chronic hypertension (Fisher and colleagues, 1981).

REFERENCES

Abdul-Karim R, Assali NS: Pressor response to angiotonin in pregnant and nonpregnant women. Am J Obstet Gynecol 82:246, 1961

Abramovici D, Friedman SA, Mercer BM, Audibert F, Kao L, Sibai BM: Neonatal outcome in severe preeclampsia at 24 to 36 weeks' gestation: Does the HELLP (hemolysis, elevated liver enzyme, and low platelet count) syndrome matter? Am J Obstet Gynecol 180:221, 1999

Ahmed Y, van Iddekinge B, Paul C, Sullivan MHF, Elder MG: Retrospective analysis of platelet members and volumes in normal pregnancy and in preeclampsia. Br J Obstet Gynaecol 100:216, 1993

Alexander JM, Bloom SL, McIntire DD, Leveno KJ: Severe preeclampsia and the very low-birthweight infant: Is induction of labor harmful? Obstet Gynecol 93:485, 1999

American College of Obstetricians and Gynecologists: Antepartum Fetal Surveillance. Practice Bulletin No. 9, October 1999

American College of Obstetricians and Gynecologists: Hypertension in Pregnancy. Technical Bulletin No. 219, January 1996

American College of Obstetricians and Gynecologists: Invasive Hemodynamic Monitoring in Obstetrics and Gynecology. Technical Bulletin No. 121, October 1988

Ananth CV, Bowes WA, Savitz DA, Luther ER: Relationship between pregnancy-induced hypertension and placenta previa: A population-based study. Am J Obstet Gynecol 177:997, 1997

Anumba DOC, Ford GA, Boys RJ, Robson SC: Stimulated nitric oxide release and nitric oxide sensitivity in forearm arterial vasculature during normotensive and preeclamptic pregnancy. Am J Obstet Gynecol 181:1479, 1999

Apollon KM, Robinson JN, Schwartz RB, Norwitz ER: Cortical blindness in severe preeclampsia: Computed tomography, magnetic resonance imaging, and single-photon-emission computed tomography findings. Obstet Gynecol 95:1017, 2000

Aquilina J, Barnett A, Thompson O, Harrington K: Second-trimester maternal serum inhibin A concentrations as an early marker for preeclampsia. Am J Obstet Gynecol 181:131, 1999

Ashour AMN, Lieberman ES, Wilkins Haug LE, Repke JT: The value of elevated second trimester β-human chorionic gonadotropin in predicting development of preeclampsia. Am J Obstet Gynecol 176:438, 1997

Atkinson MW, Guinn D, Owen J, Hauth JC: Does magnesium sulfate affect the length of labor induction in women with pregnancy-associated hypertension. Am J Obstet Gynecol 173:1219, 1995

Audibert F, Friedman SA, Frangieh AY, Sibai BM: Diagnostic criteria for HELLP syndrome: Tedious or "HELLPFUL"? Am J Obstet Gynecol 174:454, 1996

Baird D: Combined Textbook of Obstetrics and Gynaecology for Students and Practitioners. Edinburgh, Livingston, 1969, p 631

Baker PN, Cunningham FG: Platelet and coagulation abnormalities. In Lindheimer MD, Roberts JM, Cunningham FG (eds): Chesley's Hypertensive Disorders in Pregnancy, 2nd ed. Stamford CT, Appleton & Lange, 1999, p 349

Baker PN, Krasnow J, Roberts JM, Yeo K: Elevated serum levels of vascular endothelial growth factor in patients with preeclampsia. Obstet Gynecol 86:815, 1995

Banias BB, Devoe LD, Nolan TE: Severe preeclampsia in preterm pregnancy between 26 and 32 weeks' gestation. Am J Perinatal 9:357, 1992

Bardeguez AD, McNerney R, Frieri M, Verma UL, Tejani N: Cellular immunity in preeclampsia: Alterations in T-lymphocyte subpopulations during early pregnancy. Obstet Gynecol 77:859, 1991

Barron WM, Heckerling P, Hibbard JU, Fister S: Reducing unnecessary coagulation testing in hypertensive disorders of pregnancy. Obstet Gynecol 94:364, 1999

Barton JR, Riely CA, Adamec TA, Shanklin DR, Khoury AD, Sibai BM: Hepatic histopathologic condition does not correlate with laboratory abnormalities in HELLP syndrome (hemolysis, elevated liver enzymes, and low platelet count). Am J Obstet Gynecol 167:1538, 1992

Barton JR, Sibai BM: Hepatic imaging in HELLP syndrome (hemolysis, elevated liver enzymes, and low platelet count). Am J Obstet Gynecol 174:1820, 1996

Barton JR, Sibai BM, Whybrew WD, Mercer BM: Urinary endothelin-1: Not a useful marker for preeclampsia. Am J Obstet Gynecol 168:599, 1993

Barton JR, Stanziano G, Sibai BM: Monitored outpatient management of mild gestational hypertension remote from term. Am J Obstet Gynecol 170:765, 1994

Beer AE: Possible immunologic bases of preeclampsia/eclampsia. Semin Perinatol 2:39, 1978

Belfort M, Anthony J, Saade G, the Nimodipine Study Group: Interim report of the nimodipine vs. magnesium sulfate for seizure prophylaxis in severe preeclampsia study: An international, randomized, controlled trial. Am J Obstet Gynecol 178:S7, 1998

Belfort MA, Anthony J, Buccimazza A, Davey DA: Hemodynamic changes associated with intravenous infusion of the calcium antagonist verapamil in the treatment of severe gestational proteinuric hypertension. Obstet Gynecol 75:970, 1990

Belfort MA, Saade GR, Grunewald C, Dildy GA, Abedejos P, Herd JA, Nisell H: Associates of cerebral perfusion pressure with headache in women with preeclampsia. Br J Obstet Gynaecol 106:814, 1999

Belfort MA, Saade GR, Moise KJ Jr: The effect of magnesium sulfate on maternal retinal blood flow in preeclampsia: A randomized placebo-controlled study. Am J Obstet Gynecol 167:1548, 1992

Belfort MA, Taskin O, Buhur A, Saade G, Yalcinoglu A: Intravenous nimodipine in the management of severe preeclampsia; Double blind, randomized, controlled clinical trial. Am J Obstet Gynecol 174:451, 1996

Belizan JM, Villar J: The relationship between calcium intake and edema-, proteinuria-, and hypertension-getosis: An hypothesis. Am J Clin Nutr 33:2202, 1980

Benedetti TJ, Cotton DB, Read JC, Miller FC: Hemodynamic observations in severe preeclampsia with a flow-directed pulmonary artery catheter. Am J Obstet Gynecol 136:465, 1980a

Benedetti TJ, Kates R, Williams V: Hemodynamic observations in severe preeclampsia complicated by pulmonary edema. Am J Obstet Gynecol 152:330, 1985

Benedetto C, Marozio L, Neri I, Giarola M, Volpe A, Facchinetti F: Increased L-citrulline/L-arginine plasma ratio in severe preeclampsia. Obstet Gynecol 96:395, 2000

Benyo DF, Adatisa P, Conrad KP: Levels of inflammatory cytokines in normal term and preeclamptic placentas and their regulation by oxygen. J Soc Gynecol Investig (Abstr 894), 7(1) (Suppl), 2000

Berg CJ, Atrash HK, Koonin LM, Tucker M: Pregnancy-related mortality in the United States, 1987–1990. Obstet Gynecol 88:161, 1996

Bewley S, Cooper D, Campbell S: Doppler investigation of uteroplacental blood flow resistance in the second trimester: A screening study for preeclampsia and intrauterine growth retardation. Br J Obstet Gynaecol 98:871, 1991

Bhatia RK, Bottoms SF, Saleh AA, Norman GS, Mammen EF, Sokol RJ: Mechanisms for reduced colloid osmotic pressure in preeclampsia. Am J Obstet Gynecol 157:106, 1987

Bolte AC, Gafar S, van Eyck J, van Geijn HP, Dekker GA: Ketanserin, a better option in the treatment of preeclampsia? Am J Obstet Gynecol 178:S118, 1998

Bosio PM, McKenna PJ, Conroy R, O'Herlihy C: Maternal central hemodynamics in hypertensive disorders of pregnancy. Obstet Gynecol 94:978, 1999

Bower S, Bewley S, Campbell S: Improved prediction of preeclampsia by two-stage screening of uterine arteries using the early diastolic notch and the cola Doppler imaging. Obstet Gynecol 82:78, 1993

Brackley KJ, Ramsay MM, Pipkin FB, Rubin PC: The maternal cerebral circulation in preeclampsia: Investigations using Laplace transform analysis of Doppler waveforms. Br J Obstet Gynaecol 107:492, 2000

Brosens IA, Robertson WB, Dixon HG: The role of the spiral arteries in the pathogenesis of preeclampsia. Obstet Gynecol Ann 1:177, 1972

Brown CEL, Cunningham FG, Pritchard JA: Convulsions in hypertensive, proteinura primiparas more than 24 hours after delivery: Eclampsia or some other cause? J Reprod Med 32:499, 1987

Brown CEL, Purdy PD, Cunningham FG: Head computed tomographic scans in women with eclampsia. Am J Obstet Gynecol 159:915, 1988a

Brown MA, Gallery EDM, Ross MR, Esber RP: Sodium excretion in normal and hypertensive pregnancy: A prospective study. Am J Obstet Gynecol 159:297, 1988b

Brown MA, Zammit VC, Lowe SA: Capillary permeability and extracellular fluid volumes in pregnancy-induced hypertension. Clin Sci 77:599, 1989

Browne FJ: Sensitization of the vascular system in preeclamptic toxaemia and eclampsia. Br J Obstet Gynaecol 53:510, 1946

Brubaker DB, Ross MG, Marinoff D: The function of elevated plasma fibronectin in preeclampsia. Am J Obstet Gynecol 166:526, 1992

Brunner HR, Gavras H: Vascular damage in hypertension. Hosp Pract 10:97, 1975

Bucher HC, Guyatt GH, Cook RJ, Hatala R, Cook DJ, Lang JD, Hunt D: Effect of calcium supplementation on pregnancy-induced hypertension and preeclampsia. JAMA 275:1113, 1996

Burrows RF, Burrows EA: The feasibility of a control population for a randomized control trial of seizure prophylaxis in the hypertensive disorders of pregnancy. Am J Obstet Gynecol 173:929, 1995

Cantrell DC, Cunningham FG: Epilepsy complicating pregnancy. Williams Obstetrics, 19th ed (Suppl 8). Norwalk, CT, Appleton & Lange, 1994

Caritis S, Sibai B, Hauth J, Lindheimer MD, Dkebanoff M, Thom E, Van Dorsten P, Landon M, Paul R, Miodovnik M, Meis P, Thurnau G: Low-dose aspirin to prevent preeclampsia in women at high risk. National Institute of Child Health and Human Development Network of Maternal–Fetal Medicine Units. N Engl J Med 338:701, 1998

Caron C, Goudemaud J, Marey A, Beague D, Ducroux G, Drouvin F: Are haemostatic and fibrinolytic parameters predictors of preeclampsia in pregnancy-associated hypertension? Thromb Haemost 66:410, 1991

Chadwick HS, Easterling T: Anesthetic concerns in the patient with preeclampsia. Semin Perinatol 15:397, 1991

Chang JK, Roman C, Heymann MA: Effect of endothelium-derived relaxing factor inhibition on the umbilical-placental circulation in fetal lambs in utero. Am J Obstet Gynecol 166:727, 1992

Chappell L, Bewley S: Preeclamptic toxaemia: The role of uterine artery Doppler. Br J Obstet Gynaecol 105:379, 1998

Chappell LC, Seed PT, Briley AL, Kelly FJ, Lee R, Hunt RJ, Parmar K, Bewley SJ, Shennan AH, Steer PJ, Poston L: Effect of antioxidants on the occurrence of preeclampsia in women at increased risk: A randomized trial. Lancet 354:810, 1999

Chesley LC: Diagnosis of preeclampsia. Obstet Gynecol 65:423, 1985

Chesley LC, Annitto JE, Cosgrove RA: The remote prognosis

of eclamptic women. Sixth periodic report. Am J Obstet Gynecol 124:446, 1976

Chesley LC, Annitto JE, Cosgrove RA: The familial factor in toxemia of pregnancy. Obstet Gynecol 32:303, 1968

Chesley LC, Cooper DW: Genetics of hypertension in pregnancy: Possible single gene control of preeclampsia and eclampsia in the descendants of eclamptic women. Br J Obstet Gynaecol 93:898, 1986

Chesley LC, Williams LO: Renal glomerular and tubular function in relation to the hyperuricemia of preeclampsia and eclampsia. Am J Obstet Gynecol 50:367, 1945

Clark SL, Cotton DB: Clinical indications for pulmonary artery catheterization in the patient with severe preeclampsia. Am J Obstet Gynecol 158:453, 1988

Clark BA, Halvorson L, Sachs B, Epstein FH: Plasma endothelin levels in preeclampsia: Elevation and correlation with uric acid levels and renal impairment. Am J Obstet Gynecol 166:962, 1992

Clark SL, Cotton DB, Hankin GDV, Phelan JP: Critical Care Obstetrics 3rd ed. Malden, MA, Blackwell Science, 1997

Clark SL, Divon MY, Phelan JP: Preeclampsia/eclampsia: Hemodynamic and neurologic correlations. Obstet Gynecol 66:337, 1985

CLASP Collaborative Group: A randomized trial of low-dose aspirin for the prevention and treatment of preeclampsia among 9364 pregnant women. Lancet 343:619, 1994

Coetzee EJ, Dommisse J, Anthony J: A randomized controlled trial of intravenous magnesium sulfate versus placebo in the management women with severe preeclampsia. Br J Obstet Gynecol 105:300, 1998

Combes B, Adams RH: Disorders of the liver in pregnancy. In Assali NS (ed): Pathophysiology of Gestation, Vol I. New York, Academic Press, 1972

Conde-Agudelo A, Belizan JM: Risk factors for preeclampsia in a large cohort of Latin American and Carribean women. Br J Obstet Gynaecol 107:75, 2000

Conrad KP, Vernier KA: Plasma level, urinary excretion and metabolic production of cGMP during gestation in rats. Am J Physiol 257:R847, 1989

Cooper DW, Liston WA: Genetic control of severe preeclampsia. J Med Gent 16:409, 1979

Cotter A, Molloy A, Scott JM, Daly SF: Elevated plasma homocysteine in early pregnancy: A risk factor for the development of severe preeclampsia. Presented at the 21st Annual Meeting of the Society of Maternal–Fetal Medicine, February 5–10, 2001 held in Reno, Nevada

Cotton DB, Janusz CA, Berman RF: Anticonvulsant effects of magnesium sulfate on hippocampal seizures: Therapeutic implications in preeclampsia–eclampsia. Am J Obstet Gynecol 166:1127, 1992

Cotton DB, Jones MM, Longmire S, Dorman KF, Tessen J, Joyce TH: Role of intravenous nitroglycerine in the treatment of severe pregnancy-induced hypertension complicated by pulmonary edema. Am J Obstet Gynecol 154:91, 1986a

Cotton DB, Longmire S, Jones MM, Dorman KP, Tessen J, Joyce TH III: Cardiovascular alterations in severe pregnancy-induced hypertension: Effects of intravenous nitroglycerin coupled with blood volume expansion. Am J Obstet Gynecol 154:1053, 1986b

Cowles T, Saleh A, Cotton DB: Hypertensive disorders in pregnancy. In James DK, Steer PJ, Weiner CP, Gonik B (eds): High Risk Pregnancy: Management Options. London, Saunders, 1994 p 253

Cuckle H, Sehmi I, Jones R: Maternal serum inhibin A can predict preeclampsia. Br J Obstet Gynaecol 105:1101, 1998

Cunningham FG: Liver disease complicating pregnancy. Williams Obstetrics, 19th ed (Suppl 1). Norwalk, CT, Appleton & Lange, 1993

Cunningham FG, Cox K, Gant NF: Further observations on the nature of pressor responsivity to angiotensin II in human pregnancy. Obstet Gynecol 146:581, 1975

Cunningham FG, Fernandez CO, Hernandez C: Blindness associated with preeclampsia and eclampsia. Am J Obstet Gynecol 172:1291, 1995

Cunningham FG, Leveno KJ: Management of pregnancy-induced hypertension. In Rubin PC (ed): Handbook of Hypertension. Vol X: Hypertension in Pregnancy. Amsterdam, Elsevier Science, 1988, p 290

Cunningham FG, Lindheimer MD: Hypertension in pregnancy. Current concepts. N Engl J Med 326:927, 1992

Cunningham FG, Lowe T, Guss S, Mason R: Erythrocyte morphology in women with severe preeclampsia and eclampsia. Am J Obstet Gynecol 153:358, 1985

Cunningham FG, Pritchard JA: How should hypertension during pregnancy be managed? Experience at Parkland Memorial Hospital. Med Clin North Am 68:505, 1984

Cunningham FG, Pritchard JA, Hankins GDV, Anderson PL, Lucas MJ, Armstrong KF: Peripartum heart failure: Idiopathic cardiomyopathy or compounding cardiovascular events? Obstet Gynecol 67:157, 1986

Cunningham FG, Twickler D: Cerebral edema complicating eclampsia. Am J Obstet Gynecol 182:94, 2000

Dashe JS, Ramin SM, Cunningham FG: The long-term consequences of thrombotic microangiopathy (thrombotic thrombocytopenic purpura and hemolytic uremic syndrome) in pregnancy. Obstet Gynecol 91:662, 1998

Davidge ST, Hubel CA, Braden RD, Capeless EC, McLaughlin MK: Sera antioxidant activity in uncomplicated and preeclamptic pregnancies. Obstet Gynecol 79:897, 1992

De Boer K, Büller HR, Ten Cate JW, Treffers PE: Coagulation studies in the syndrome of haemolysis, elevated liver enzymes and low platelets. Br J Obstet Gynaecol 98:42, 1991

De Snoo K: The prevention of eclampsia. Am J Obstet Gynecol 34:911, 1937

De Wolf F, De Wolf-Peeters C, Brosens I, Robertson WB: The human placental bed: Electron microscopic study of trophoblastic invasion of spiral arteries. Am J Obstet Gynecol 137:58, 1980

Dekker GA, de Vries JI, Doelitzsch PM, Huijgens PC, von Blomberg BME, Jakobs C, van Geijn HP: Underlying disorders associated with severe early-onset preeclampsia. Am J Obstet Gynecol 173:1042, 1995

Dekker GA, Makovitz JW, Wallenburg HCS: Prediction of pregnancy-induced hypertensive disorders by angiotensin II sensitivity and supine pressor test. Br J Obstet Gynaecol 97:817, 1990

Dekker GA, Sibai BM: Etiology and pathogenesis of preeclampsia: Current concepts. Am J Obstet Gynecol 179:1359, 1998

Dieckmann WJ: The Toxemias of Pregnancy, 2nd ed. St. Louis, Mosby, 1952

Dieckmann WJ, Michel HL: Vascular–renal effects of posterior pituitary extracts in pregnant women. Am J Obstet Gynecol 33:131, 1937

Douglas KA, Redman CWG: Eclampsia in the United Kingdom. BMJ 309:1395, 1994

Ducey J, Schulman H, Farmakides G, Rochelson B, Bracero L, Fleischer A, Guzman E, Winter D, Penny B: A classification of hypertension in pregnancy based on Doppler velocimetry. Am J Obstet Gynecol 157:680, 1987

Dudley DJ, Hunter C, Mitchell MD, Varner MW, Gately M: Elevations of serum interleukin-12 concentrations in women with severe preeclampsia and HELLP syndrome. J Reprod Immunol 31:97, 1996

Duley L, Johanson R: Magnesium sulfate for preeclampsia and eclampsia: The evidence so far. Br J Obstet Gynaecol 101, 565, 1994

Dürr JA, Lindheimer MD: Control of volume and body tonicity. In Lindheimer MD, Roberts JM, Cunningham FG (eds): Chesley's Hypertensive Disorders in Pregnancy, 2nd ed. Stanford, CT, Appleton & Lange, 1999, p 103

Easterling TR, Benedeti TJ, Schmucker BC, Carlson KL: Antihypertensive therapy in pregnancy directed by noninvasive hemodynamic monitoring. Am J Perinatol 6:86, 1989

Easterling TR, Brateng D, Schmucker B, Brown Z, Millard SP: Prevention of preeclampsia: A randomized trial of atenolol in hyperdynamic patients before onset of hypertension. Obstet Gynecol 93:725, 1999

Eclampsia Trial Collaborative Group: Which anticonvulsant for women with eclampsia? Evidence from the collaborative eclampsia trial. Lancet 345:1455, 1995

Everett RB, Porter JC, MacDonald PC, Gant NF: Relationship of maternal placental blood flow to the placental clearance of maternal plasma dehydroisoandrosterone sulfate through placental estriol formation. Am J Obstet Gynecol 136:435, 1980

Everett RB, Worley RJ, MacDonald PC, Gant NF: Effect of prostaglandin synthetase inhibitors on pressor response to angiotensin II in human pregnancy. J Clin Endocrinol Metab 46:1007, 1978

Faas MM, Schuiling GA, Linton EA, Sargent IL, Redman CWG: Activation of peripheral leukocytes in rate pregnancy and experimental preeclampsia. Am J Obstet Gynecol 182:351, 2000

Ferrazzani S, Caruso A, De Carolis S, Martino IV, Mancuso S: Proteinuria and outcome of 444 pregnancies complicated by hypertension. Am J Obstet Gynecol 162:366, 1990

Fisher ER, Pardo V, Paul R, Hayashi TT: Ultrastructural studies in hypertension, 4. Toxemia of pregnancy. Am J Pathol 55: 901, 1969

Fisher KA, Luger A, Spargo BH, Lindheimer MD: Hypertension in pregnancy: Clinical–pathological correlations and remote prognosis. Medicine 60:267, 1981

Fitzgerald DJ, Eutman SS, Mulloy K, Fitzgerald GA: Decreased prostacyclin biosynthesis preceding the clinical manifestation of pregnancy-induced hypertension. Circulation 75:956, 1987

Fleischer A, Schulman H, Farmakides G, Bracero L, Grunfeld L, Rochelson B, Koenigsberg M: Uterine artery Doppler velocimetry in pregnant women with hypertension. Am J Obstet Gynecol 154:806, 1986

Fong J, Gurewitsch ED, Vipe L, Wagner WE, Gomillion MC, August P: Baseline serum and cerebrospinal fluid magnesium levels in normal pregnancy and preeclampsia. Obstet Gynecol 85:444, 1995

Friedman SA, Lindheimer MD: Prediction and Differential Diagnosis. In Lindheimer MD, Roberts JM, Cunningham FG (eds): Chesley's Hypertensive Disorders in Pregnancy, 2nd ed. Stanford, CT, Appleton & Lange, 1999, p 201

Friedman EA, Neff RK: Pregnancy outcome as related to hypertension, edema, and proteinuria. In Lindheimer MD, Katz AI, Zuspan FP (eds): Hypertension in Pregnancy. New York, Wiley, 1976, p 13

Fritz MA, Stanczyk FZ, Novy MJ: Relationship of uteroplacental blood flow to the placental clearance of maternal dehydroepiandrosterone through estradiol formation in the pregnant baboon. J Clin Endocrinol Metab 61:1023, 1985

Frolich MA, Datta S, Corn SB: Thrombopoietin in normal pregnancy and preeclampsia. Am J Obstet Gynecol 179:100, 1998

Gallery EDM, Lindheimer MD: Alterations in volume homeostasis. In Lindhemier MD, Roberts JM, Cunningham FG (eds): Chesley's Hypertensive Disorders in Pregnancy, 2nd ed. Stamford, CT, Appleton & Lange, 1999, p 327

Gant NF, Chand S, Whalley PJ, MacDonald PC: The nature of pressor responsiveness to angiotensin II in human pregnancy. Obstet Gynecol 43:854, 1974a

Gant NF, Chand S, Worley RJ, Whalley PJ, Crosby UD, MacDonald PC: A clinical test useful for predicting the development of acute hypertension in pregnancy. Am J Obstet Gynecol 120:1, 1974b

Gant NF, Daley GL, Chand S, Whalley PJ, MacDonald PC: A study of angiotensin II pressor response throughout primigravid pregnancy. J Clin Invest 52:2682, 1973

Gant NF, Jimenez JM, Whalley PJ, Chand S, MacDonald PC: A prospective study of angiotensin II pressor responsiveness in pregnancies complicated by chronic essential hypertension. Am J Obstet Gynecol 127:369, 1977

Gant NF, Madden JD, Siiteri PK, MacDonald PC: The metabolic clearance rate of dehydroisoandrosterone sulfate, 4. Acute effect of induced hypertension, hypotension, and naturesis in normal and hypertensive pregnancies. Am J Obstet Gynecol 124:143, 1976

Garvasi M-T, Chaiworapongsa T, Pacora P, Naccasha N, Yoon BH, Maymon E, Romero R: Maternal systemic inflammation: A mechanism of disease in pre-eclampsia. Presented at the 21st Annual Meeting of the Society of Maternal–Fetal Medicine, February 5–10, 2001 held in Reno, Nevada

Gilbert WM, Towner DR, Field NT, Anthony J: The safety and utility of pulmonary artery catheterization in severe preeclampsia and eclampsia. Am J Obstet Gynecol 182:1397, 2000

Gilstrap LC, Cunningham FG, Whalley PJ: Management of pregnancy-induced hypertenson in the nulliparous patient remote from term. Semin Perinatol 2:73, 1978

Govan ADT: The pathogenesis of eclamptic lesions. Pathol Microbiol 24:561, 1961

Green KW, Key TC, Coen R, Resnik R: The effects of maternally administered magnesium sulfate on the neonate. Am J Obstet Gynecol 146:29, 1983

Greer IA, Lyall F, Perera T, Boswell F, Macaa LM: Increased concentrations of cytokines interleukin-6 and interleukin-1 receptor antagonist in plasma of women with preeclampsia: A mechanism for endothelial dysfunction? Obstet Gynecol 84:937, 1994

Grisaru D, Zwang E, Peyser MR, Lessing JB, Eldor A: The procoagulant activity of red blood cells from patients with severe preeclampsia. Am J Obstet Gynecol 177:1513, 1997

Groenendijk R, Trimbros JBM, Wallenburg HCS: Hemodynamic measurements in preeclampsia: Preliminary observations. Am J Obstet Gynecol 150:232, 1984

Grossman E, Messerli FH, Grodzicki T, Kowey P: Should a moratorium be placed on sublingual nifedipine capsules given for hypertensive emergencies and pseudoemergencies? JAMA 276:1328, 1996

Gutsche BB, Cheek TG: Anesthesia considerations in pre-eclampsia-eclampsia. In Shnider SM, Levinson G (eds): Anesthesia for obstetrics, 3rd ed. Baltimore, Williams & Wilkins, 1993, p 321

Haddad B, Barton JR, Livingston JC, Chahine R, Sibai BM: Risk factors for adverse maternal outcomes among women with HELLP (hemolysis, elevated liver enzymes, and low platelet count) syndrome. Am J Obstet Gynecol 183:444, 2000

Hall DR, Odendaal HJ, Smith M: Is the prophylactic administration of magnesium sulphate in women with pre-eclampsia indicated prior to labour? Br J Obstet Gynaecol 107:903, 2000a

Hall DR, Odendaal HJ, Steyn DW, Grové D: Expectant management of early onset, severe pre-eclampsia: Maternal outcome. Br J Obstet Gynaecol 107:1252, 2000b

Hallak M, Berry SM, Madincea F, Romero R, Evans MI, Cotton DB: Fetal serum and amniotic fluid magnesium concentrations with maternal treatment. Obstet Gynecol 81:185, 1993

Hallak M, Hotca JW, Evans JB: Magnesium sulfate affects the N-methyl-D-aspartate receptor binding in maternal rat brain. Am J Obstet Gynecol 178:S112, 1998

Hallak M, Kupsky WJ, Hotra JW, Evans JB: Fetal rat brain damage caused by maternal seizure activity: Prevention by magnesium sulfate. Am J Obstet Gynecol 181:828, 1999a

Hallak M, Martinez-Poyer J, Kruger ML, Hassan S, Blackwell SC, Sorokin Y: The effect of magnesium sulfate on fetal heart rate parameters: A randomized, placebo-controlled trial. Am J Obstet Gynecol 181:1122, 1999b

Halligan A, Bonnar J, Sheppard B, Darling M, Walshe J: Haemestatic, fibrinolytic and endothelial variables in normal pregnancies and preeclampsia. Br J Obstet Gynaecol 101:488, 1994

Hankins GDV, Cunningham FG: Severe preeclampsia and eclampsia: Controversies in management. Williams Obstetrics, 18th ed (Suppl 12). Norwalk, CT, Appleton & Lange, 1991

Hankins GDV, Wendel GW Jr, Cunningham FG, Leveno KJ: Longitudinal evaluation of hemodynamic changes in eclampsia. Am J Obstet Gynecol 150:506, 1984

Hanretty KP, Whittle MJ, Rubin PC: Doppler uteroplacental waveforms in pregnancy-induced hypertension: A re-appraisal. Lancet 1:850, 1988

Hauth JC, Cunningham FG: Pre-eclampsia–eclampsia. In Lindheimer MD, Roberts JM, Cunningham FG (eds): Chesley's Hypertensive Disorders in Pregnancy, 2nd ed. Stamford, CT, Appleton & Lange, 1999, p 169

Hauth JC, Cunningham FG, Whalley PJ: Management of pregnancy-induced hypertension in the nullipara. Obstet Gynecol 48:253, 1976

Hauth JC, Ewell MG, Levine RJ, Esterlitz JR, Sibai B, Curet LB, Catalano PM, Morris CD: Pregnancy outcomes in healthy nulliparas who developed hypertension. Obstet Gynecol 95:24, 2000

Hauth JC, Goldenberg RL, Parker CR Jr, Philips JB 3d, Copper RL, DuBard MB, Cutter GR: Low-dose aspirin therapy to prevent preeclampsia. Am J Obstet Gynecol 168:1083, 1993

Hauth J, Sibai B, Caritis S, VanDorsten P, Lindheimer M, Klebanoff M, MacPherson C, Landon M, Paul R, Miodovnik M, Meis P, Dombrowski M, Thurnau G, Walsh S, McNellis D, Robert JM, and the National Institute of Child Health and Human Development Network of Maternal-Fetal Medicine Units: Maternal serum thromboxane B_2 concentrations do not predict improved outcomes in high-risk pregnancies in a low-dose aspirin trial. Am J Obstet Gynecol 179:1193, 1998

Hayman R, Warren A, Brockelsby J, Johnson I, Baker P: Plasma from women with pre-eclampsia induces an in vitro alteration in the endothelium-dependent behaviors of myometrial resistant arteries. Brit J Obstet Gynaecol 107:108, 2000

Hayward C, Livingstone J, Holloway S, Liston WA, Brock DJH: An exclusion map for preeclampsia: Assuming autosomal recessive inheritance. Am J Hum Genet 50:749, 1992

Helewa M, Heaman M, Robinson M-A, Thompson L: Community-based home-care program for the management of preeclampsia: An alternative. Can Med Assoc J 149:829, 1993

Heller PJ, Scheider EP, Marx GF: Pharyngo-laryngeal edema

as a presenting symptom in preeclampsia. Obstet Gynecol 62:523, 1983

Herbert V, Shaw S, Jayatilleke E, Stopler-Kasdan T: Most free-radical injury is iron-related: It is promoted by iron, hemin, holoferritin and vitamin C, and inhibited by desferoxamine and apoferritin. Stern Cells 12:289, 1994

Hertig AT: Vascular pathology in the hypertensive albuminuric toxemias of pregnancy. Clinics 4:602, 1945

Hinselmann H: Die Eklampsie. Bonn, F Cohen, 1924

Hoff C, Peevy K, Giattina K, Spinnato JA, Peterson RDA: Maternal–fetal HLA-DR relationships and pregnancy-induced hypertension. Obstet Gynecol 80:1007, 1992

Hogg B, Hauth JC, Caritis SN, Sibai BM, Lindheimer M, VanDorsten JP, Klebanoff M, MacPherson C, Landon M, Paul R, Miodovnik M, Meis PJ, Thurnau GR, Dombrowski MP, McNellis D, Roberts JM, for the National Institute of Child Health and Human Development Maternal–Fetal Medicine Units Network: Safety of labor epidural anesthesia for women with severe hypertensive disease. Am J Obstet Gynecol 181:1096, 1999

Horsager R, Adams M, Richey S, Leveno KJ, Cunningham FG: Outpatient management of mild pregnancy-induced hypertension. Am J Obstet Gynecol 172:383, 1995

Hoyert DL, Kochanek KD, Murphy SL: Deaths: Final data for 1997. National Vital Statistics Reports; Vol 47, No. 19. Hyattsville, MD, National Center for Health Statistics, 1999

Hubel CA, McLaughlin MK, Evans RW, Hauth JA, Sims CJ, Roberts JM: Fasting serum triglycerides, free fatty acids, and malondialdehyde are increased in preeclampsia, are positively correlated, and decrease within 48 hours postpartum. Am J Obstet Gynecol 174:975, 1996

Hubel CA, Roberts JM, Taylor RN, Musci TJ, Rodgers GM, McLaughlin MK: Lipid peroxidation in pregnancy: New perspectives on preeclampsia. Am J Obstet Gynecol 161:1025, 1989

Hunter SK, Martin M, Benda JA, Zlatnik FJ: Liver transplant after massive spontaneous hepatic rupture in pregnancy complicated by preeclampsia. Obstet Gynecol 85:819, 1995

Irion O, Masse J, Forest JC, Moutquin JM: Prediction of preeclampsia; low birthweight for gestation and prematurity by uterine artery blood flow velocity waveform analysis in low risk nulliparous women. Br J Obstet Gynaecol 105:422, 1998

Isler CM, Rinehart BK, Terrone DA, Martin RW, Magann EF, Martin JN: Maternal mortality associated with HELLP (hemolysis, elevated liver enzymes, and low platelets) syndrome. Am J Obstet Gynecol 181:924, 1999

Jacobson SL, Imhof R, Manning N, Mannion V, Little D, Rey E, Redman C: The value of Doppler assessment of the uteroplacental circulation in predicting preeclampsia or intrauterine growth retardation. Am J Obstet Gynecol 162:110, 1990

Kilpatrick DC, Liston WA, Gibson F, Livingstone J: Association between susceptibility to preeclampsia within families and HLA-DR4. Lancet 2:1063, 1989

Kimberlin DF, Hauth JC, Goldenberg RL, MacPherson C, Thom E, Bottoms SF, McNellis D: The effect of maternal $MgSO_4$ treatment on neonatal morbidity in ≤ 1000 g neonates. Am J Obstet Gynecol 174:469, 1996

Kincaid-Smith P: The renal lesion of preeclampsia revisited. Am J Kidney Dis 17:144, 1991

Kirshon B, Lee W, Mauer MB, Cotton DB: Effects of low-dose dopamine therapy in the oliguric patient with preeclampsia. Am J Obstet Gynecol 159:604, 1988

Knuist M, Bonsel GJ, Zondervan HA, Treffers PE: Low sodium diet and pregnancy-induced hypertension: A multicentre randomized controlled trial. Br J Obstet Gynaecol 105:430, 1998

Kupferminc MJ, Eldor A, Steinman N, Many A, Bar-Am A, Jaffa A, Fait G, Lessing JB: Increased frequency of genetic thrombophilia in women with complications of pregnancy. N Engl J Med 340:9, 1999

Kupferminc MJ, Peaceman AM, Wigton TR, Rehnberg KA, Socol ML: Tumor necrosis factor-α is elevated in plasma and amniotic fluid of patients with severe preeclampsia. Am J Obstet Gynecol 170:1752, 1994

Kyle PM, Campbell S, Buckley D, Kissane J, de Swiet M, Albano J, Millar JG, Redman CW: A comparison of the inactive urinary kallikrein: creatinine ratio and the angiotension sensitivity test for prediction of pre-eclampsia. Br J Obstet Gynaecol 103:981, 1996

Labarrere C: Acute atherosis. A histopathological hallmark of immune aggression? Placenta 9:108, 1988

Laivuori H, Kaaja R, Turpeinen U, Stenman UH, Ylikorkala O: Serum activin A and inhibin A elevated in preeclampsia: No relation to insulin sensitivity. Br J Obstet Gynaecol 106:1298, 1999

Laivuori H, Kaaja R, Ylikorkala O, Hiltunen T, Kontula K: 677 C→T polymorphism of the methylenetetrahydrofolate reductase gene and preeclampsia. Obstet Gynecol 96:277, 2000

Landesman R, Douglas RG, Holze E: The bulbar conjunctival vascular bed in the toxemias of pregnancy. Am J Obstet Gynecol 68:170, 1954

Lavies NG, Meiklejohn BH, May AE, Achola KJ, Fell D: Hypertensive and catecholamine response to trachael intubation in patients with pregnancy-induced hypertension. Br J Anaesth 63:429, 1989

Leduc L, Wheeler JM, Kirshon B, Mitchell P, Cotton DB: Coagulation profile in severe preeclampsia. Obstet Gynecol 79:14, 1992

Lee W, Gonik B, Cotton DB: Urinary diagnostic indices in preeclampsia-associated oliguria: Correlation with invasive hemodynamic monitoring. Am J Obstet Gynecol 156:100, 1987

Lehmann DK, Mabie WC, Miller JM Jr, Pernoll ML: The epidemiology and pathology of maternal mortality: Charity Hospital of Louisiana in New Orleans, 1965–1984. Obstet Gynecol 69:833, 1987

Leveno KJ, Alexander JM, McIntire DD, Lucas MJ: Does magnesium sulfate given for prevention of eclampsia affect the outcome of labor? Am J Obstet Gynecol 178:707, 1998

Levine RJ: Should the definition of preeclampsia include a rise in diastolic blood pressure ≥ 15 mm Hg? Am J Obstet Gynecol 182:225, 2000

Levine RJ, Hauth JC, Curet LB, Sibai BM, Catalano PM, Morris CD, Der Simonian R, Esterlitz JR, Raymond EG, Bild DE, Clemens JD, Cutler JA: Trial of calcium to prevent preeclampsia. N Engl J Med 337:69, 1997

Lichtig C, Luger AM, Spargo BH, Lindheimer MD: Renal immunofluorescence and ultrastructural findings in preeclampsia. Clin Res 23:368A, 1975

Lim KH, Friedman SA, Ecker JL, Kao L, Kilpatrick SJ: The clinical utility of serum uric acid measurements in hypertensive disease of pregnancy. Am J Obstet Gynecol 178:1067, 1998

Lindheimer M, Woodruff TK: Activin A, inhibin A, and preeclampsia. Lancet 349:1266, 1997

Lip GYH, Churchill D, Beevers M, Auckett A, Beevers DG: Angiotensin-converting enzyme inhibitors in early pregnancy. Lancet 350:1446, 1997

Lipton SA, Rosenberg PA: Excitatory amino acids as a final common pathway for neurologic disorders. N Engl J Med 330:613, 1994

López-Llera M: Complicated eclampsia: Fifteen years' experience in a referral medical center. Am J Obstet Gynecol 142:28, 1982

López-Jaramillo P, Narváez M, Weigel RM, Yépez R: Calcium supplementation reduces the risk of pregnancy-induced hypertension in an Andes population. Br J Obstet Gynaecol 96:648, 1989

Lubarsky SL, Barto JR, Friedman SA, Nasreddine S, Ramadan MK, Sibai BM: Late postpartum eclampsia revisited. Obstet Gynecol 83:502, 1994

Lucas MJ, Leveno KJ, Cunningham FG: A comparison of magnesium sulfate with phenytoin for the prevention of eclampsia. N Engl J Med 333:201, 1995

Lucas MJ, Sharma S, McIntire DD, Sidawi JE, Ramin SM, Leveno KJ, Cunningham FG: A randomized trial of the effects of epidural analgesia on pregnancy-induced hypertension. Am J Obstet Gynecol 180:518, 2001

Mabie WC, Gonzalez AR, Sibai BM, Amon E: A comparative trial of labetalol and hydralazine in the acute management of severe hypertension complicating pregnancy. Obstet Gynecol 70:328, 1987

Mabie WC, Ratts TE, Ramanathan KB, Sibai BM: Circulatory congestion in obese hypertensive women: A subset of pulmonary edema in pregnancy. Obstet Gynecol 72:553, 1988

Mabie WC, Sibai BM, Anderson GD, Gonzalez-Ruiz AR, Moretti ML, Harvey CJ: Nifedipine in the treatment of severe peripartum hypertension. Soc Perinat Obstet (Abstr 87), February 1988.

Madazli R, Budak E, Calay Z, Aksu MF: Correlation between placental bed biopsy findings, vascular cell adhesion molecule and fibronectin levels in preeclampsia. Br J Obstet Gynaecol 107:514, 2000

Manas KJ, Welsh JD, Rankin RA, Miller DD: Hepatic hemorrhage without rupture in preeclampsia. N Engl J Med 312:426, 1985

Many A, Kuperminc MJ, Pausner D, Lessing JB: Treatment of severe preeclampsia remote from term: A clinical dilemia. Obstet Gynecol Surv 54:723, 1999

Martin JN Jr, Files JC, Blake PG, Perry KG Jr, Morrison JC, Norman PH: Postpartum plasma exchange for atypical preeclampsia–eclampsia as HELLP (hemolysis, elevated liver enzymes, and low platelets) syndrome. Am J Obstet Gynecol 172:1107, 1995

Marya RK, Rathee S, Manrow M: Effect of calcium and vitamin D supplementation on toxaemia of pregnancy. Gynecol Obstet Invest 24:38, 1987

Mastrogiannis DS, O'Brien WF, Krammer J, Benoit R: Potential role of endothelin-1 in normal and hypertensive pregnancies. Am J Obstet Gynecol 165:1711, 1991

Mattar F, Sibai BM: Eclampsia: VIII. Risk factors for maternal morbidity. Am J Obstet Gynecol 182:307, 2000

McCartney CP: Pathological anatomy of acute hypertension of pregnancy. Circulation (Suppl 2) 30:37, 1964

McCartney CP, Schumacher GFB, Spargo BH: Serum proteins in patients with toxemic glomerular lesion. Am J Obstet Gynecol 111:580, 1971

McCubbin JH, Sibai BM, Abdella TN, Anderson GD: Cardiopulmonary arrest due to acute maternal hypermagnesemia. Lancet 1:1058, 1981

McKay DG: Disseminated Intravascular Coagulation. New York, Harper & Row, 1965

Meyer NL, Mercer BM, Friedman SA, Bibai BM: Urinary dipstick protein: A poor predictor of absent or severe proteinuria. Am J Obstet Gynecol 170:137, 1994

Mikhail MS, Anyaegbunam A, Garfinkel D, Palan PR, Basu J, Romney SL: Preeclampsia and antioxidant nutrients: Decreased plasma levels of reduced ascorbic acid, α-tocopherol, and beta carotene in women with preeclampsia. Am J Obstet Gynecol 171:150, 1994

Miles JF, Martin JN Jr, Blake PG, Perry KG Jr, Martin RW, Meeds RG: Postpartum eclampsia: A recurring perinatal dilemma. Obstet Gynecol 76:328, 1990

Millar JGB, Campbell SK, Albano JDM, Higgins BR, Clark AD: Early prediction of pre-eclampsia by measurement of kallikrein and creatinine on a random urine sample. Br J Obstet Gynaecol 103:421, 1996

Mizuki J, Tasaka K, Masumoio N, Kasahara K, Miyake A, Tanizawa D: Magnesium sulfate inhibits oxytocin induced calcium mobilization in human puerperal myometrial cells: Possible involvement of intracellular free magnesium concentration. Am J Obstet Gynecol 109:134, 1993

Montan S, Ingemarsson I: Intrapartum fetal heart rate patterns in pregnancies complicated by hypertension. Am J Obstet Gynecol 160:283, 1989

Morgan L, Baker P, Broughton Pipkin F, Kalsheker N: Preeclampsia and the angiotensinogen gene. Br J Obstet Gynaecol 102:489, 1995

Morgan T, Craven C, Lalouel JM, Ward K: Angiotensinogen Thr[235] variant is associated with abnormal physiologic change of the uterine spiral arteries in first-trimester decidua. Am J Obstet Gynecol 180:95, 1999

Morris NH, Eaton BM, Dekker G: Nitric oxide, the endothelium, pregnancy and pre-eclampsia. Br J Obstet Gynaecol 103:4, 1996

Morriss MC, Twickler DM, Hatab MR, Clarke GD, Peshok RM, Cunningham FG: Cerebral blood flow and cranial magnetic resonance imaging in eclampsia and severe preeclampsia. Obstet Gynecol 89:561, 1997

Murphy DJ, Sellers S, Mackenzie IZ, Yudkin PK, Johnson AM: Case-control study of antenatal and intrapartum risk factors for cerebral palsy in very preterm singleton babies. Lancet 346:449, 1995

Muttukrishna S, Knight PG, Groome NP, Redman CW, Ledger WL: Activin-A and inhibin-A as possible endocrine markers for preeclampsia. Lancet 349:1285, 1997

Myatt L, Brewer AS, Langdon G, Brockman DE: Attenuation of the vasoconstrictor effects of thromboxane and endothelin by nitric oxide in the human fetal–placental circulation. Am J Obstet Gynecol 166:224, 1992

Naeye RL, Friedman EA: Causes of perinatal death associated with gestational hypertension and proteinuria. Am J Obstet Gynecol 133:8, 1979

Nassar AH, Adra AM, Chakhtoura N, Gomez-Marin O, Beydoun S: Severe preeclampsia remote from term: Labor induction or elective cesarean delivery? Am J Obstet Gynecol 179:1210, 1998

National High Blood Pressure Education Program: Working Group Report on High Blood Pressure in Pregnancy. Am J Obstet Gynecol 183:51, 2000

Nelson KB, Grether JK: Can magnesium sulfate reduce the risk of cerebral palsy in very low birthweight infants? Pediatrics 95:263, 1995

Ness RB, Roberts JM: Heterogeneous causes constituting the single syndrome of preeclampsia: A hypothesis and its implications. Am J Obstet Gynecol 175:1365, 1996

Newsome LR, Bramwell RS, Curling PE: Severe preeclampsia: Hemodynamic effects of lumbar epidural anesthesia. Anesth Analg 65:31, 1986

Nightingale FL: Warnings in the use of ACE inhibitors in the second and third trimester of pregnancy. JAMA 267:244, 1992

Nisell H, Carlström K, Cizinsky S, Grunewald C, Nylund L, Randmaa I: Atrial natriuretic peptide concentrations and hemodynamic effects of acute plasma volume expansion in normal pregnancy and preeclampsia. Obstet Gynecol 79:902, 1992

Nolan TE, Wakefield ML, Devoe LD: Invasive hemodynamic

monitoring in obstetrics. A critical review of its indications, benefits, complications, and alternatives. Chest 101:1429, 1992

North RA, Taylor RS, Schellenberg J-C: Evaluation of a definition of preeclampsia. Br J Obstet Gynaecol 106:767, 1999

Nova A, Sibai BM, Barton JR, Mercer BM, Mitchell MD: Maternal plasma level of endothelin is increased in preeclampsia. Am J Obstet Gynecol 165:724, 1991

Ohno Y, Kawai M, Wakahara Y, Kitagawa T, Kakihara M, Arii Y: Ophthalmic artery velocimetry in normotensive and preeclamptic women with or without photophobia. Obstet Gynecol 94:361, 1999

Øian P, Maltau JM, Noddleland H, Fadne HO: Transcapillary fluid balance in preeclampsia. Br J Obstet Gynaecol 93:235, 1986

Oláh KS, Redman CWG, Gee H: Management of severe, early preeclampsia: Is conservative management justified? Eur J Obstet Gynaecol Reprod Biol 51:175, 1993

Olsen SF, Secher NJ, Tabor A, Weber T, Walker JJ, Gluud C: Randomized clinical trials of fish oil supplementation in high risk pregnancies. Br J Obstet Gynaecol 107:382, 2000

Oosterhof H, Voorhoeve PG, Aarnoudse JG: Enhancement of hepatic artery resistance to blood flow in preeclampsia in presence or absence of HELLP syndrome (hemolysis, elevated liver enzymes, and low platelets). Am J Obstet Gynecol 171:526, 1994

Otani S, Usuki S, Saitoh T, Yanagisawa M, Iwasaki H, Tanaka J, Suzuki N, Fujino M, Goto K, Masaki T: Comparison of endothelin-1 concentrations in normal and complicated pregnancies. J Cardiovasc Pharmacol 17:S308, 1991

Paarlberg KM, DeJong CLD, Van Geijn HP, van Kamp GJ, Heinen AG, Dekker GA: Total plasma fibronectin as a marker of pregnancy-induced hypertensive disorders: A longitudinal study. Obstet Gynecol 91:383, 1998

Palmer RMJ, Ashton DS, Moncada S: Vascular endothelial cells synthesize nitric oxide from L-arginine. Nature 333:664, 1988

Palmer SK, Moore LG, Young DA, Cregger B, Berman JC, Zamudio S: Altered blood pressure and increased preeclampsia at high altitude (3100 meters) in Colorado. Am J Obstet Gynecol 180:1161, 1999

Petraglia F, Florio P, Benedetto C, Gallo C, Woods RJ, Genazzani AR, Lowry PJ: High levels of corticotropin-releasing factor (CRF) are inversely correlated with low levels of maternal CRF-binding protein in pregnant women with pregnancy-induced hypertension. J Clin Endocrinol Metab 81:852, 1996

Phelan JP, Yurth DA: Severe preeclampsia, 1. Peripartum hemodynamic observations. Am J Obstet Gynecol 144:17, 1982

Pickles CJ, Broughton Pipkin F, Symonds EM: A randomised placebo controlled trial of labetalol in the treatment of mild to moderate pregnancy induced hypertension. Br J Obstet Gynaecol 99:964, 1992

Powers RW, Evans RW, Ness RB, Crombleholme WR, Roberts JM: Homocysteine is increased in preeclampsia but not in gestational hypertension. J Sur Gynecol Investig (Abstr 375), 7(1) (Suppl), 2000

Pritchard JA, Cunningham FG, Mason RA: Coagulation changes in eclampsia: Their frequency and pathogenesis. Am J Obstet Gynecol 124:855, 1976

Pritchard JA, Cunningham FG, Pritchard SA: The Parkland Memorial Hospital protocol for treatment of eclampsia: Evaluation of 245 cases. Am J Obstet Gynecol 148:951, 1984

Pritchard JA, Cunningham FG, Pritchard SA, Mason RA: How often does maternal preeclampsia–eclampsia incite

thrombocytopenia in the fetus? Obstet Gynecol 69:292, 1987

Pritchard JA, Weisman R Jr, Ratnoff OD, Vosburgh G: Intravascular hemolysis, thrombocytopenia and other hematologic abnormalities associated with severe toxemia of pregnancy. N Engl J Med 250:87, 1954

Raab W, Schroeder G, Wagner R, Gigee W: Vascular reactivity and electrolytes in normal and toxemic pregnancy. J Clin Endocrinol 16:1196, 1956

Rafferty TD, Berkowitz RL: Hemodynamics in patients with severe toxemia during labor and delivery. Am J Obstet Gynecol 138:263, 1980

Ramanatham J: Anesthetic considerations in preeclampsia. Clin Perinatol 18:875, 1991

Ramsay MM, Rimoy GH, Rubin PC: Are anticonvulsants necessary to prevent eclampsia? Lancet 343:540, 1994

Rappaport VJ, Hirata G, Kim Yap H, Jordan SC: Anti-vascular endothelial cell antibodies in severe preeclampsia. Am J Obstet Gynecol 162::138, 1990

Redman CWG, Roberts JM: Management of pre-eclampsia. Lancet 341:1451, 1993

Redman CWG, Sacks GP, Sargent IL: Preeclampsia: An excessive maternal inflammatory response to pregnancy. Am J Obstet Gynecol 180:499, 1999

Regan CL, Fitzgerald DJ: Altered isoprostane to prostocyclin ratio in preeclampsia. Am J Obstet Gynecol 176:510, 1997

Rinehart BK, Terrone DA, Magann EF, Martin RW, May WL, Martin JN: Preeclampsia-associated hepatic hemorrhage and rupture: Mode of management related to maternal and perinatal outcome. Obstet Gynecol Surv 54:3, 1999

Roberts JM: Preeclampsia: What we know and what we do not know. Semin Perinatol 24:24, 2000

Roberts JM, Taylor RN, Musci TJ, Rodgers GM, Hubel CA, McLaughlin MK: Preeclampsia: An endothelial cell disorder. Am J Obstet Gynecol 161:1200, 1989

Robson SC: Magnesium sulphate: The timing of reckoning. Br J Obstet Gynaecol 103:99, 1996

Rogers BB, Bloom SL, Leveno KJ: Atherosis revisited: Current concepts on the pathophysiology of implantation site disorders. Obstet Gynecol Surv 54:189, 1999

Rosenbaum M, Maltby G: Cerebral dysrhythmia in relation to eclampsia. Arch Neurol Psychiatr 49:204, 1943

Samuels P, Main EK, Tomaski A, Mennuti MT, Gabbe SG, Cines DB: Abnormalities in platelet antiglobulin tests in preeclamptic mothers and their neonates. Am J Obstet Gynecol 157:109, 1987

Sanchez-Ramos L, Adair CD, Todd JC, Mollitt DL, Briones DK: Erythrocyte membrane fluidity in patients with preeclampsia and the HELLP syndrome: A preliminary study. J Mat Fet Invest 4:237, 1994a

Sanchez-Ramos L, Jones DC, Cullen MT: Urinary calcium as an early marker for preeclampsia. Obstet Gynecol 77:685, 1991

Scardo JA, Vermillion ST, Hogg BB, Newman RB: Hemodynamic effects of oral nifedipine in preeclampsia hypertensive emergencies. Am J Obstet Gynecol 175:336, 1996

Scardo JA, Vermillion ST, Newman RB, Chauhan SP, Hogg BB: A randomized, double-blind, hemodynamic evaluation of nifedipine and labetalol in preeclamptic hypertensive emergencies. Am J Obstet Gynecol 181:862, 1999

Schendel DE, Berg CJ, Yeargin-Allsopp M, Bogle CA, Decoufle P: Prenatal magnesium sulfate exposure and the risk for cerebral palsy or mental retardation among very low birthweight children aged 3 to 5 years. JAMA 276:1805, 1996

Schiff E, Ben-Baruch G, Peleg E, Rosenthal T, Alcalay M, Devir M, Mashiach S: Immunoreactive circulating endothelin-1 in normal and hypertensive pregnancies. Am J Obstet Gynecol 166:624, 1992

Schiff E, Friedman SA, Stampfer M, Kao L, Barrett PH, Sibai BM: Dietary consumption and plasma concentrations of vitamin E in pregnancies complicated by preeclampsia. Am J Obstet Gynecol 175:1024, 1996

Sen C, Madazh R, Kavuzlu L, Ocak V, Tolun N: The value of antithrombin-III and fibronectin in hypertensive disorders of pregnancy. J Perinat Med 22:29, 1994

Sheehan HL: Pathological lesions in the hypertensive toxaemias of pregnancy. In Hammond J, Browne FJ, Wolstenholme GEW (eds): Toxaemias of Pregnancy, Human and Veterinary. Philadelphia, Blakiston, 1950

Sheehan HL, Lynch JB (eds): Cerebral lesions. In: Pathology of Toxaemia of Pregnancy. Baltimore, Williams & Wilkins, 1973

Sibai BM: Thrombophilias and adverse outcomes of pregnancy—what should a clinician do? (editorial) N Engl J Med 340:50, 1999

Sibai BM: Treatment of hypertension in pregnant women. N Engl J Med 335:257, 1996

Sibai BM, Barton JR, Akl S, Sarinoglu C, Mercer BM: A randomized prospective comparison of nifedipine and bed rest alone in the management of preeclampsia remote from term. Am J Obstet Gynecol 167:879, 1992

Sibai BM, Caritis SN, Thom E, Klebanoff M, McNellis D, Rocco L, Paul RH, Romero R, Witter F, Rosen M, Depp R, National Institute of Child Health and Human Development Network of Maternal–Fetal Medicine Units: Prevention of preeclampsia with low-dose aspirin in healthy, nulliparous pregnant women. N Engl J Med 329:1213, 1993a

Sibai BM, El-Nazer A, Gonzalez-Ruiz A: Severe preeclampsia–eclampsia in young primigravid women: Subsequent pregnancy outcome and remote prognosis. Am J Obstet Gynecol 155:1011, 1986

Sibai BM, Ewell M, Levine RJ, Klebanoff MA, Estechitz J, Catalano PM, Goldenberg RL, Joffe G: Risk factors associated with preeclampsia in healthy nulliparous women. Am J Obstet Gynecol 177:1003, 1997

Sibai BM, Gonzalez AR, Mabie WC, Moretti M: A comparison of labetalol plus hospitalization versus hospitalization alone in the management of preeclampsia remote from term. Obstet Gynecol 70:323, 1987a

Sibai BM, Graham JM, McCubbin JH: A comparison of intravenous and intramuscular magnesium sulfate regimens in preeclampsia. Am J Obstet Gynecol 150:728, 1984

Sibai BM, Hauth J, Caritis S, Lindheimer MD, MacPherson C, Klebanoff M, VanDorsten JP, Landon M, Miodovnik M, Paul R, Meis P, Thurnau G, Dombrowski M, Roberts J, McNellis D, for the National Institute of Child Health and Human Development Network of Maternal–Fetal Medicine Units: Hypertensive disorders in twin versus singleton gestations. Am J Obstet Gynecol 182:938, 2000

Sibai BM, Lindheimer M, Hauth J, Caritis S, VanDorston P, Klebanoff M, MacPherson C, Landon M, Miodovnik M, Paul R, Meis P, Dombrowski M: Risk factors for preeclampsia, abruptio placentae, and adverse neonatal outcome among women with chronic hypertension. N Engl J Med 339:667, 1998

Sibai BM, Mabie BC, Harvey CJ, Gonzalez AR: Pulmonary edema in severe preeclampsia–eclampsia: Analysis of thirty-seven consecutive cases. Am J Obstet Gynecol 156:1174, 1987b

Sibai BM, Mercer B, Sarinoglu C: Severe preeclampsia in the second trimester: Recurrence risk and long-term prognosis. Am J Obstet Gynecol 165:1408, 1991

Sibai BM, Mercer BM, Schiff E, Friedman SA: Aggressive

versus expectant management of severe preeclampsia at 28 to 32 weeks' gestation: A randomized controlled trial. Am J Obstet Gynecol 171:818, 1994

Sibai BM, Ramadan MK, Chari RS, Friedman S: Pregnancies complicated by HELLP syndrome (hemolysis, elevated liver enzymes, and low platelets): Subsequent pregnancy outcome and long-term prognosis. Am J Obstet Gynecol 172:125, 1995

Sibai BM, Ramadan MK, Usta I, Salama M, Mercer BM, Friedman SA: Maternal morbidity and mortality in 442 pregnancies with hemolysis, elevated liver enzymes, and low platelets (HELLP syndrome). Am J Obstet Gynecol 169:1000, 1993b

Sibai BM, Spinnato JA, Watson DL, Lewis JA, Anderson GA: Eclampsia, 4. Neurological findings and future outcome. Am J Obstet Gynecol 152:184, 1985a

Sibai BM, Taslimi M, Abdella TN, Brooks TF, Spinnato JA, Anderson GD: Maternal and perinatal outcome of conservative management of severe preeclampsia in midtrimester. Am J Obstet Gynecol 152:32, 1985b

Sibai BM, Villar MA, Mabie BC: Acute renal failure in hypertensive disorders of pregnancy. Pregnancy outcome and remote prognosis in thirty-one consecutive cases. Am J Obstet Gynecol 162:777, 1990

Silver H, Morgan T, Ward K: Blood volume stratified by angiotensinogen genotypes in normal and hypertensive pregnancies. Presented at the 21st Annual Meeting of the Society of Maternal–Fetal Medicine, February 5–10, 2001 held in Reno, Nevada

Silver H, Seebeck M: Comparison of methods of blood volume measurement in normotensive and preeclamptic pregnancies. Am J Obstet Gynecol 174:452, 1996

Silver HM, Seebeck M, Carlson R: Comparison of total blood volume in normal, preeclamptic, and non-proteinuria gestational hypertensive pregnancy by simultaneous measurement of red blood cell and plasma volumes. Am J Obstet Gynecol 179:87, 1998

Simmons LA, Hennessy A, Gillin AG, Jeremy RW: Uteroplacental blood flow and placental vascular endothelial growth factor in normotensive and preeclamptic pregnancy. Br J Obstet Gynaecol 107:678, 2000

Somjen G, Hilmy M, Stephen CR: Failure to anesthetize human subjects by intravenous administration of magnesium sulfate. J Pharmacol Exp Ther 154:652, 1966

Spargo B, McCartney CP, Winemiller R: Glomerular capillary endotheliosis in toxemia of pregnancy. Arch Pathol 68:593, 1959

Spitz B, Magness RR, Cox SM, Brown CEL, Rosenfeld CR, Gant NF: Low-dose aspirin, 1. Effect on angiotensin II pressor responses and blood prostaglandin concentrations in pregnant women sensitive to angiotensin II. Am J Obstet Gynecol 159:1035, 1988

Staff AC, Ranheim T, Khoury J, Henriksen T: Increased contents of phospholipids, cholesterol, and lipid peroxides in decidua basalis in women with preeclampsia. Am J Obstet Gynecol 180:587, 1999

Stamilio DM, Sehder HM, Morgan MA, Propert K, Macones GA: Can antenatal clinical and biochemical markers predict the development of severe preeclampsia? Am J Obstet Gynecol 182:589, 2000

Strickland DM, Guzick DS, Cox K, Gant NF, Rosenfeld CR: The relationship between abortion in the first pregnancy and the development of pregnancy-induced hypertension in the subsequent pregnancy. Am J Obstet Gynecol 154:146, 1986

Sullivan CA, Magann EF, Perry KG Jr, Roberts WE, Blake PG, Martin JN Jr: The recurrence risk of the syndrome of hemolysis, elevated liver enzymes, and low platelets (HELLP) in subsequent gestations. Am J Obstet Gynecol 171:940, 1994

Szal SE, Croughan-Minibane MS, Kilpatrick SJ: Effect of magnesium prophylaxis and preeclampsia on the duration of labor. Am J Obstet Gynecol 180:1475, 1999

Talledo OE, Chesley LC, Zuspan FP: Renin-angiotensin system in normal and toxemic pregnancies, 3. Differential sensitivity to angiotensin II and norepinephrine in toxemia of pregnancy. Am J Obstet Gynecol 100:218, 1968

Taufield PA, Ales KL, Resnick LM, Druzin ML, Gertner JM, Laragh JH: Hypocalciuria in preeclampsia. N Engl J Med 316:715, 1987

Thiagarajah S, Bourgeois FJ, Harbert GM, Caudle MR: Thrombocytopenia in preeclampsia: Associated abnormalities and management principles. Am J Obstet Gynecol 150:1, 1984

Thurnau GR, Kemp DB, Jarvis A: Cerebrospinal fluid levels of magnesium in patients with preeclampsia after treatment with intravenous magnesium sulfate: A preliminary report. Am J Obstet Gynecol 157:1435, 1987

Tompkins MJ, Thiagarajah S: HELLP (hemalysis, elevated liver enzymes, and low platelet count) syndrome: The benefit of corticosteroids. Am J Obstet Gynecol 181:304, 1999

Trudinger BJ, Cook CM: Doppler umbilical and uterine flow waveforms in severe pregnancy hypertension. Br J Obstet Gynaecol 97:142, 1990

Trupin LS, Simon LP, Eskenazi B: Change in paternity: A risk factor for preeclampsia in multiparas. Epidemiology 7:240, 1996

Tuffnell DJ, Lilford RJ, Buchan PC, Prediville VM, Tuffnell AJ, Holgate MP, Jones MDG: Randomized controlled trial of day care for hypertension in pregnancy. Lancet 339:224, 1992

Van Pampus MG, Dekker GA, Wolf H, Huijgens PC, Koopman MMW, von Blomberg BME, Büller HR: High prevalence of hemostatic abnormalities in women with a history of severe preeclampsia. Am J Obstet Gynecol 180:1146, 1999

Ventura SJ, Martin JA, Curtin SC, Mathews TJ, Park MM: Births: Final data for 1998. National Vital Statistics Reports; Vol 48, No. 3. Hyattsville, MD, National Center Health Statistics, 2000

Vermillion ST, Scardo JA, Newman RB, Chauhan SP: A randomized, double-blind trial of oral nifedipine and intravenous labetalol in hypertensive emergencies of pregnancy. Am J Obstet Gynecol 181:858, 1999

Visser W, Wallenberg HCS: Temporizing management of severe preeclampsia with and without the HELLP syndrome. Br J Obstet Gynaecol 102:111, 1995

Volhard F: Die doppelseitigen haematogenen Nierenerkrankungen. Berlin, Springer, 1918

Von Dadelszen P, Ornstein MP, Bull SB, Logan AG, Koren G, Magee LA: Fall in mean arterial pressure and fetal growth restriction in pregnancy hypertension: A meta-analysis. Lancet 355:87, 2000

Walker JJ: Pre-eclampsia. Lancet 356:1260, 2000

Wallace DH, Leveno KJ, Cunningham FG, Giesecke AH, Shearer VE, Sidawi JE: Randomized comparison of general and regional anesthesia for cesarean delivery in pregnancies complicated by severe preeclampsia. Obstet Gynecol 86:193, 1995

Wallenburg HCS, Dekker GA, Makovitz JW, Rotmans P: Low-dose aspirin prevents pregnancy-induced hypertension and preeclampsia in angiotensin-sensitive primigravidae. Lancet 1:1, 1986

Walsh SC: Lipid peroxidation in pregnancy. Hypertens Peg 13:1, 1994

Walsh SW: Preeclampsia: An imbalance in placental prostacyclin and thromboxane production. Am J Obstet Gynecol 152:335, 1985

Ward K, Hata A, Jeunemaitre X, Helin C, Nelson L, Namikawa C, Farrington PF, Ogasawara M, Suzumori K, Tomoda S, Berrebi S, Sasaki M, Corvol P, Lifton RP, Lalouel JM: A molecular variant of angiotensinogen associated with preeclampsia (comment). Nat Genet 4:59, 1993

Watt-Morse ML, Caritis SN, Kridgen PL: Magnesium sulfate is a poor inhibitor of oxytocin-induced contractility in pregnant sheep. J Matern Fetal Med 4:139, 1995

Weiner C, Martinez E, Zhu LK, Ghodsi A, Chestnut D: In vitro release of endothelium-derived relaxing factor by acetylcholine is increased during the guinea pig pregnancy. Am J Obstet Gynecol 161:1599, 1989

Weiner CP, Thompson LP, Liu KZ, Herrig JE: Endothelium-derived relaxing factor and indomethacin-sensitive contracting factor alter arterial contractile responses to thromboxane during pregnancy. Am J Obstet Gynecol 166:1171, 1992

Weinstein L: Preeclampsia-eclampsia with hemolysis, elevated liver enzymes, and thrombocytopenia. Obstet Gynecol 66:657, 1985

Weinstein L: Syndrome of hemolysis, elevated liver enzymes and low platelet count: A severe consequence of hypertension in pregnancy. Am J Obstet Gynecol 142:159, 1982

Weir RJ, Fraser R, Lever AF, Morton JJ, Brown JJ, Kraszewski A, McIlevine GM, Robertson JIS, Tree M: Plasma renin, renin substrate, angiotensin II, and aldosterone in hypertensive disease of pregnancy. Lancet 1:291, 1973

Wide-Swensson DH, Ingemarsson I, Lunnell NO, Forman A, Skajaa K, Lindberg B, Lindeberg S, Marsál K, Andersson KE: Calcium channel blockade (isradipine) in treatment of hypertension in pregnancy: A randomized placebo-controlled study. Am J Obstet Gynecol 173:872, 1995

Williams Obstetrics, 15th ed. Pritchard JA, MacDonald PC (eds). Appleton-Century-Croft, New York, 1976, p 413

Williams JW: Obstetrics: A Text-Book for Students and Practitioners, 1st ed. New York, Appleton, 1903

Williams KP, Wilson S: Persistence of cerebral hemodynamic changes in patients with eclampsia: A report of 3 cases. Am J Obstet Gynecol 181:1162, 1999

Witlin AG, Friedman SA, Egerman RS, Frangieh AY, Sibai BM: Cerebrovascular disorders complicating pregnancy—Beyond eclampsia. Am J Obstet Gynecol 176:1139, 1997a

Witlin AG, Friedman SA, Sibai BA: The effect of magnesium sulfate therapy on the duration of labor in women with mild preeclampsia at term: A randomized, double-blind, placebo-controlled trial. Am J Obstet Gynecol 176:623, 1997b

Witlin AG, Saade GR, Mattar F, Sibai BM: Predictors of neonatal outcome in women with severe preclampsia or eclampsia between 24 and 33 weeks' gestation. Am J Obstet Gynecol 182:607, 2000

Witlin AG, Sibai BM: Magnesium sulfate therapy in preeclampsia and eclampsia. Obstet Gynecol 92:883, 1998

Worley RJ, Everett RB, MacDonald PC, Gant NF: Placental clearance of dehydroisoandrosterone sulfate and pregnancy outcome in three categories of hospitalized patients with pregnancy-induced hypertension. Gynecol Obstet Invest 6:28, 1975

Zeek PM, Assali NS: Vascular changes in decidua associated with eclamptogenic toxemia of pregnancy. Am J Clin Pathol 20:1099, 1950

Zhang J, Klebanoff MA, Levine RJ, Puri M, Moyer P: The puzzling association between smoking and hypertension during pregnancy. Am J Obstet Gynecol 181:1407, 1999

Zinaman M, Rubin J, Lindheimer MD: Serial plasma oncotic pressure levels and echoencephalography during and after delivery in severe preeclampsia. Lancet 1:1245, 1985

Zondervan HA, Oosting J, Smorenberg-Schoorl ME, Treffers PE: Maternal whole blood viscosity in pregnancy hypertension. Gynecol Obstet Invest 25:83, 1988

25

Obstetrical Hemorrhage

ANTEPARTUM HEMORRHAGE

Placental Abruption
Placenta Previa

POSTPARTUM HEMORRHAGE

Uterine Atony
Hemorrhage from Retained Placental Fragments
Placenta Accreta, Increta, and Percreta
Inversion of the Uterus
Genital Tract Lacerations
Puerperal Hematomas
Rupture of the Uterus
Rupture of the Unscarred Uterus

HYPOVOLEMIC SHOCK

Estimation of Blood Loss
Resuscitation and Acute Management

CONSUMPTIVE COAGULOPATHY

Abruptio Placentae
Fetal Death and Delayed Delivery
Amnionic Fluid Embolism
Septicemia
Abortion

Obstetrics is "bloody business." Even though the maternal mortality rate has been reduced dramatically by hospitalization for delivery and the availability of blood for transfusion, death from hemorrhage remains prominent in the majority of mortality reports in advanced countries. In the United States from 1979 through 1992, the Centers for Disease Control and Prevention analyzed 4915 nonabortion-related maternal deaths from the Pregnancy Mortality Surveillance System (Chichakli and colleagues, 1999). They found that hemorrhage was a direct cause in about 30 percent of these deaths. According to Bonnar (2000), hemorrhage was the major factor in maternal deaths in the United Kingdom between 1985 and 1996. There undoubtedly has been great improvement in mortality from hemorrhage with modernization of American obstetrics. For example, Sachs and associates (1987) reported that maternal deaths from obstetrical hemorrhage in Massachusetts decreased tenfold from the mid-1950s to the mid-1980s.

Unfortunately, despite improved outcomes, poor and minority women continue to die from hemorrhage and its complications at a disparately high rate. In the report from the Centers for Disease Control cited above, there was threefold increased mortality from hemorrhage in African-American compared with Caucasian women. In a similar analysis of 3777 pregnancy-related deaths from states that include Hispanic origin on death certificates, Hopkins and co-workers (1999) reported that hemorrhage caused 20 percent of maternal deaths. They showed disparate mortality in African-American and Hispanic women compared with Caucasians.

Causes of maternal death from hemorrhage are shown in Table 25–1. Obstetrical hemorrhage is most likely to be fatal in circumstances in which blood or components are not available immediately. The establishment and maintenance of facilities that allow prompt administration of blood are absolute requirements for acceptable obstetrical care. Hemorrhage may be **antepartum**—such as with placenta previa or placental abruption, or it more likely develops **postpartum**—from uterine atony or genital tract lacerations.

INCIDENCE AND PREDISPOSING CONDITIONS. Because of inexact definitions used, the incidence of obstetrical hemorrhage cannot be determined precisely. In one study of women delivered vaginally, Combs and colleagues (1991b) defined hemorrhage by a postpartum hematocrit drop of 10 volume percent or by need for transfusion. Using these criteria, the incidence was 3.9 percent. In women undergoing cesarean delivery it was 6 to 8 percent (Combs and associates, 1991a; Naef and co-workers, 1994).

Dickason and Dinsmoor (1992) reported transfusions in 6.8 percent of women undergoing cesarean delivery. Klapholz (1990) reviewed over 30,000 deliveries at the Beth Israel Hospital from 1976 to 1986. As expected, the incidence of transfusion has decreased over the years; in 1976 it was 4.6 percent, but by 1986 it was 1.9 percent.

Table 25–2 lists the many clinical circumstances in which risk of hemorrhage is appreciably increased. It is apparent that serious hemorrhage may occur at any time throughout pregnancy and the puerperium. The time of bleeding in pregnancy is widely used to classify obstetrical hemorrhage; however, the term *third-trimester* bleeding is imprecise and its use not recommended. One factor not generally considered as "predisposing" to hemorrhagic death is the lack of availability of obstetrical and anesthetic services. According to Bonnar (2000), the majority of deaths from hemorrhage in the United Kingdom cited earlier were associated with substandard care. Similarly, Nagaya and associates (2000) reviewed 197 maternal deaths in Japan in the 2-year period spanning 1991 and 1992. Hemorrhage caused 40 percent of these deaths, and they concluded that many of these were preventable because they were associated with inadequate obstetrical facilities. In Japan, 40 percent of deliveries take place in clinics with less than 20 beds, and frequently the physician functions both as obstetrician and anesthesiologist.

ANTEPARTUM HEMORRHAGE

Slight vaginal bleeding is common during active labor. This "bloody show" is the consequence of effacement and dilatation of the cervix, with tearing of small veins. Uterine bleeding from a site above the cervix before delivery is cause for concern. The bleeding may be the consequence of some separation of a placenta implanted in the immediate vicinity of the cervical canal—**placenta previa.** It may come from separation of a placenta located elsewhere in the uterine cavity—**abruptio placentae.** Rarely, the bleeding may be the consequence of

TABLE 25–1. Causes of 763 Pregnancy-related Deaths Due to Hemorrhage

Causes of Hemorrhage	Number (%)
Abruptio placentae	141 (19)
Laceration/uterine rupture	125 (16)
Uterine atony	115 (15)
Coagulopathies	108 (14)
Placenta previa	50 (7)
Placenta accreta/increta/percreta	44 (6)
Uterine bleeding	47 (6)
Retained placenta	32 (4)

From Chichakli and colleagues (1999).

TABLE 25–2. Conditions That Predispose to or Worsen Obstetrical Hemorrhage

Abnormal Placentation

Placenta previa

Placental abruption

Placenta accreta/increta/percreta

Ectopic pregnancy

Hydatidiform mole

Trauma During Labor and Delivery

Episiotomy

Complicated vaginal delivery

Low- or mid-forceps delivery

Cesarean delivery or hysterectomy

Uterine rupture—risk increased by

   Previously scarred uterus

   High parity

   Hyperstimulation

   Obstructed labor

   Intrauterine manipulation

   Midforceps rotation

Small Maternal Blood Volume

Small women

Pregnancy hypervolemia not yet maximal

Pregnancy hypervolemia constricted

   Severe preeclampsia

   Eclampsia

Other Factors

Obesity

Native American ethnicity

Previous postpartum hemorrhage

Uterine Atony

Overdistended uterus

   Large fetus

   Multiple fetuses

   Hydramnios

   Distention with clots

Anesthesia or analgesia

   Halogenated agents

   Conduction analgesia with hypotension

Exhausted myometrium

   Rapid labor

   Prolonged labor

   Oxytocin or prostaglandin stimulation

   Chorioamnionitis

Previous uterine atony

Coagulation Defects—Intensify Other Causes

Placental abruption

Prolonged retention of dead fetus

Amnionic fluid embolism

Saline-induced abortion

Sepsis with endotoxemia

Severe intravascular hemolysis

Massive transfusions

Severe preeclampsia and eclampsia

Congenital coagulopathies

Anticoagulant treatment

---

velamentous insertion of the umbilical cord with rupture and hemorrhage from a fetal blood vessel at the time of rupture of the membranes—**vasa previa.**

The source of uterine bleeding that originates above the level of the cervix is not always identified. In that circumstance, the bleeding typically begins with little or no other symptomatology, and then stops, and at delivery no anatomical cause is identified. Almost always the bleeding must have been the consequence of slight marginal separation of the placenta that did not expand. **The pregnancy in which such bleeding occurs remains at increased risk for a poor outcome even though the bleeding soon stops and placenta previa appears to have been excluded by sonography.** Lipitz and colleagues (1991) studied 65 consecutive women—almost 1 percent of their patients—who had uterine bleeding between 14 and 26 weeks. Almost a fourth had placental abruption or previa. Total fetal loss including abortions and perinatal deaths was 32 percent. Even in pregnancies with hemorrhage after 26 weeks that are not explained by placental abruption or previa, Ajayi and colleagues (1992) reported adverse outcomes in a third. For this reason, delivery should be considered in any woman at term with unexplained vaginal bleeding.

PLACENTAL ABRUPTION. The separation of the placenta from its site of implantation before the delivery of the fetus has been variously called placental abruption, abruptio placentae, and in Great Britain, accidental hemorrhage. The term *premature separation of the normally implanted placenta* is most descriptive because it differentiates the placenta that separates prematurely but is implanted some distance beyond the cervical internal os, from one that is implanted over the cervical internal os—that is, placenta previa. It is cumbersome, however, and hence the shorter term **abruptio placentae,** or **placental abruption,** has been employed. The Latin *abruptio placentae*, which means "rending asunder of the placenta," denotes a sudden accident, a clinical characteristic of most cases of this complication.

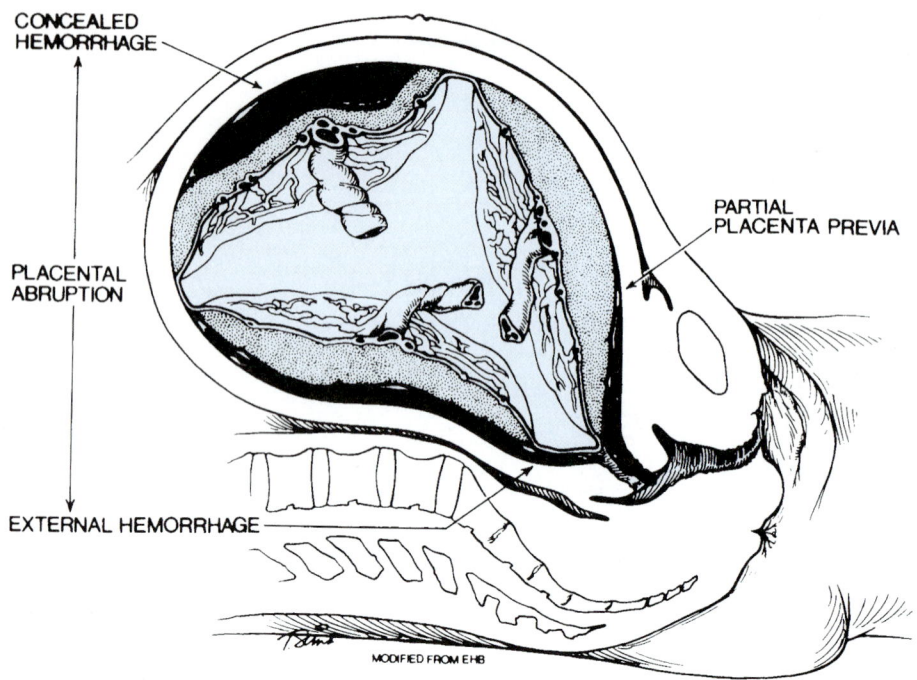

FIGURE 25–1. Hemorrhage from premature placental separation. Upper left: Extensive placental abruption but with the periphery of the placenta and the membranes still adherent, resulting in completely concealed hemorrhage. Lower: Placental abruption with the placenta detached peripherally and with the membranes between the placenta and cervical canal stripped from underlying decidua, allowing external hemorrhage. Right: Partial placenta previa with placental separation and external hemorrhage.

Some of the bleeding of placental abruption usually insinuates itself between the membranes and uterus, and then escapes through the cervix, causing *external hemorrhage* (Fig. 25–1). Less often, the blood does not escape externally but is retained between the detached placenta and the uterus, leading to *concealed hemorrhage* (Figs. 25–1 and 25–2). Placental abruption may be *total* (Figs. 25–1 and 25–2) or *partial* (Fig. 25–3). Placental abruption with concealed hemorrhage carries with it much greater maternal hazards, not only because of the possibility of consumptive coagulopathy, but also because the extent of the hemorrhage is not appreciated.

FREQUENCY, INTENSITY, AND SIGNIFICANCE. The frequency with which abruptio placentae is diagnosed will vary because criteria employed for diagnosis differ. The intensity of the abruption will often vary depending on how quickly the woman seeks and receives care following the onset of symptoms. With delay, the likelihood of extensive separation causing death of the fetus is increased remarkably.

The reported frequency for placental abruption averages about 1 in 200 deliveries. Käregärd and Gennser (1986) surveyed 849,619 births in Sweden and reported that 1 in 225 were complicated by abruptio placentae. Ananth and colleagues (1999a) reviewed 13 studies with nearly 1.6 million pregnancies and reported an incidence of 1 in 155.

At Parkland Hospital from 1988 through 1999, the incidence of abruption in over 169,000 deliveries has

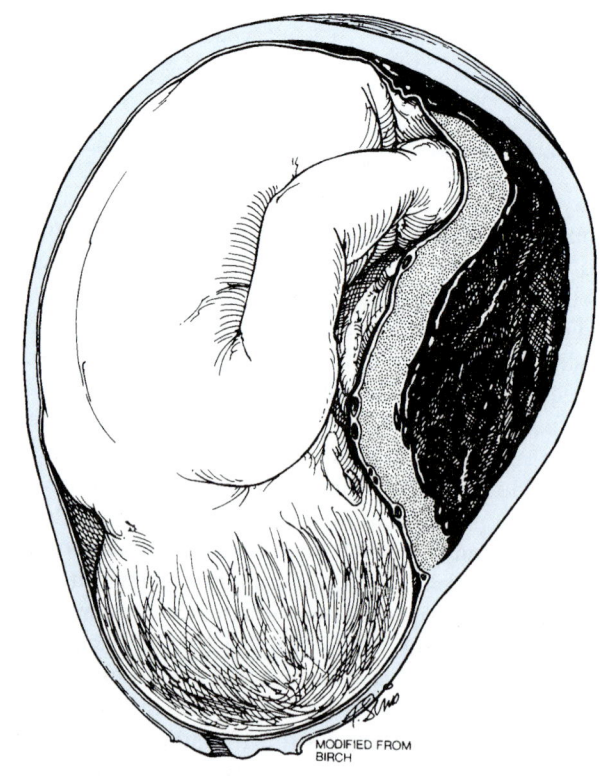

FIGURE 25–2. Total placental abruption with concealed hemorrhage. The fetus is now dead.

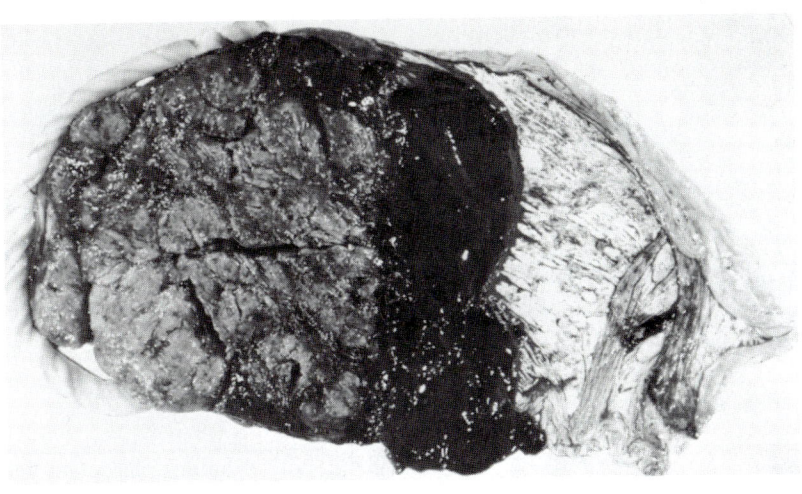

FIGURE 25–3. Partial placental abruption with adherent clot.

been 1 in 290. The incidence as well as severity have decreased over time. Applying the criterion of placental separation so extensive as to kill the fetus, the incidence was 1 in 420 deliveries from 1956 through 1967 (Pritchard and Brekken, 1967). As the number of high-parity women cared for decreased, and community-wide availability of prenatal care as well as emergency transportation improved, the frequency of abruption causing fetal death has dropped to about 1 in 830 deliveries from 1974 through 1989 (Pritchard and colleagues, 1991). From 1988 through 1999, it decreased to 1 in 1550.

PERINATAL MORBIDITY AND MORTALITY. In most reports, perinatal mortality with placental abruption is about 25 percent. In the large Swedish study by Käregärd and Gennser (1986) cited earlier, it was 20 percent. Krohn and associates (1987) reported that perinatal mortality was 20 percent in 884 pregnancies complicated by placental abruption in Washington State. Ananth and co-workers (1999b) studied 530 women with placental abruption at Mt. Sinai Hospital in New York and reported that 40 percent were delivered preterm.

As stillbirths from other causes have decreased appreciably, those from abruptio placentae have become especially prominent. For example, of all third-trimester stillbirths in over 40,000 deliveries at Parkland Hospital during 1992 and 1994, 12 percent were the consequence of placental abruption (Cunningham and Hollier, 1997). This frequency is similar to that described by Fretts and Usher (1997), who studied almost 62,000 births at the Royal Victoria Hospital in Montreal between 1978 and 1995. Abruptio placentae had become the leading known cause and accounted for 15 percent of stillborns.

Importantly, even if the infant survives, there may be adverse sequelae. Of the 182 survivors in the study by Abdella and associates (1984), 25 (14 percent) were identified to have significant neurological deficits within the first year of life.

ETIOLOGY. The primary cause of placental abruption is unknown, but there are several associated conditions. Some of these are listed in Table 25–3. As shown in Figure 25–4, the incidence increases with **maternal age.** While Pritchard and colleagues (1991) have also shown it to be higher in women of **great parity,** Toohey and associates (1995) did not find this in women para 5 or greater. Race or ethnicity appears to be important. In the 169,000-plus deliveries at Parkland Hospital, abruption was more common in African-American and Caucasian women (1 in 200) than in Asian (1 in 300) or Latin-American women (1 in 450).

By far the most commonly associated condition is

TABLE 25–3. Risk Factors for Abruptio Placentae

Risk Factor	Relative Risk (%)
Increased age and parity	NA
Preeclampsia	2.1–4.0
Chronic hypertension	1.8–3.0
Preterm ruptured membranes	2.4–3.0
Cigarette smoking	1.4–1.9
Thrombophilias	NA
Cocaine use	NA
Prior abruption	10–25
Uterine leiomyoma	NA

NA = not available.
Adapted from Cunningham and Hollier (1997); risk data from Ananth and colleagues (1999a, 1999b) and Kramer and associates (1997).

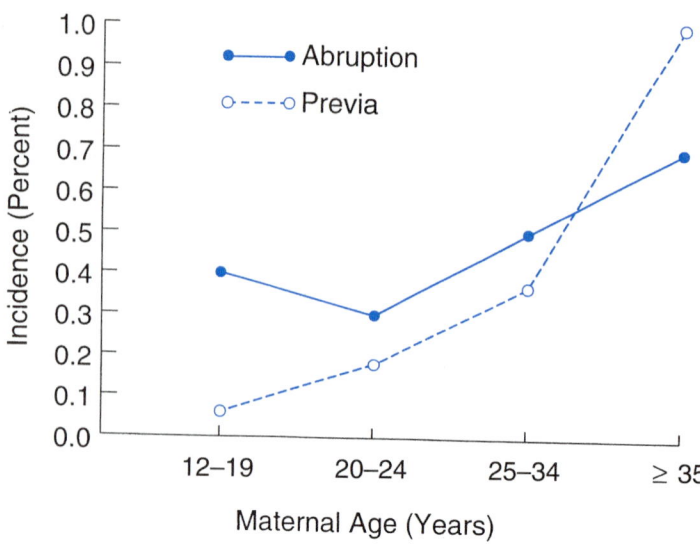

FIGURE 25-4. Incidence of abruptio placentae and placenta previa by maternal age in 169,108 deliveries at Parkland Hospital 1988 through 1999. (Data courtesy of Dr. Don McIntire.)

some type of **hypertension.** This includes preeclampsia, gestational hypertension, or chronic hypertension. In the earlier Parkland Hospital study of 408 cases of placental abruption so severe as to kill the fetus, maternal hypertension was apparent in about half of the women once the depleted intravascular compartment was adequately refilled (Pritchard and co-workers, 1991). Half of these women had chronic hypertension and the remainder had either gestational hypertension or preeclampsia. Morgan and colleagues (1994) found that hypertensive women were more likely to suffer a more severe abruption. According to Witlin and colleagues (1999), however, the severity of preeclampsia did not correlate with the incidence of abruption in 445 women. From the Maternal–Fetal Medicine Network, Sibai and co-workers (1998) reported that 1.5 percent of women with chronic hypertension suffered placental abruption. Ananth and associates (1999b) reported a threefold increased incidence of abruption with chronic hypertension and fourfold with severe preeclampsia.

There is an increased incidence of abruption with **preterm prematurely ruptured membranes.** Gonen and associates (1989) reported an incidence of 5.6 percent in 143 pregnancies of less than 34 weeks in which the membranes were ruptured for more than 24 hours. Major and colleagues (1995) described an incidence of 5 percent in 756 women with ruptured membranes between 20 and 36 weeks. Kramer and co-workers (1997) found an incidence of 3.1 percent in all patients if membranes were ruptured for longer than 24 hours. In a meta-analysis of 54 studies, Ananth and colleagues (1996) found a threefold risk of abruption with prematurely ruptured membranes.

In the earliest studies, from the Collaborative Perinatal Project, **cigarette smoking** was linked to an increased risk for abruption (Misra and Ananth, 1999; Naeye,

1980). In their meta-analysis of 1.6 million pregnancies, Ananth and colleagues (1999a, 1999b) found a twofold risk for abruption in smokers. This was increased to five- to eightfold if smokers had chronic hypertension and/or severe preeclampsia.

Cocaine abuse has been associated with an alarming frequency of placental abruption. In one report of 50 women who abused cocaine during pregnancy, there were eight stillbirths caused by placental abruption (Bingol and associates, 1987). Hoskins and collaborators (1991) reported a 13-percent rate of placental abruption in 112 women who were followed prospectively for cocaine abuse during pregnancy. Slutsker (1992) reviewed 10 studies of cocaine-using women and all showed that placental abruption was more common than in controls.

Over the past decade, a number of inherited or acquired **thrombophilias** have been described that are associated with thromboembolic disorders during pregnancy (Chap. 46, p. 1234). These clotting disorders also are associated with placental abruption and infarction (Gherman and Goodwin, 2000). Most of these are single-gene mutations that include genes for factor V Leiden, prothrombin, methylenetetrahydrofolate reductase, proteins S and C, and antithrombin III (Chap. 49, p. 1330). In addition, acquired antiphospholipid autoantibodies, including the lupus anticoagulant, are associated with placental abruption. For example, Kupferminc and colleagues (1999) found a sevenfold risk of abruption in women with a factor V, folate reductase, or prothrombin mutation.

As discussed in Chapter 43 (p. 1173), **external trauma** was implicated in only 3 of 207 cases of placental abruption causing fetal death at Parkland Hospital. Our experiences are similar to those of Kettel (1988) and Stafford (1988) and their co-workers, who stressed that abruption caused by relatively minor trauma may cause fetal jeopardy that is not always associated with immediate evidence for placental separation. In such cases, a period of monitoring for at least 4 hours is often necessary to exclude a subclinical abruption.

Uterine leiomyoma, especially if located behind the placental implantation site, predisposes to abruption (Chap. 35, p. 926). Rice and associates (1989) reported that 8 of 14 women with retroplacental myomas developed placental abruption; in four, fetal death ensued. By contrast, abruption developed in only 2 of 79 women whose myoma was not retroplacental.

RECURRENT ABRUPTION. Pritchard and co-workers (1970) identified a recurrence rate of severe abruption in 1 in 8 pregnancies. Importantly, of the 14 recurrent placental abruptions, eight caused fetal death for a second time. Käregärd and Gennser (1986) reported that the recurrent placental abruption risk was increased tenfold, from 0.4 to 4 percent. Management of the subsequent pregnancy is made difficult in that the placental separation may suddenly occur at any time, even remote from term. In the majority of cases, fetal well-being was normal beforehand, and thus currently available methods of fetal evaluation are usually not predictive. In an extreme example, Seski and Compton (1976) documented both a normal nonstress test and a normal contraction stress test done 4 hours before the onset of placental abruption that promptly killed the fetus.

PATHOLOGY. Placental abruption is initiated by hemorrhage into the decidua basalis. The decidua then splits, leaving a thin layer adherent to the myometrium. Consequently, the process in its earliest stages consists of the development of a decidual hematoma that leads to separation, compression, and the ultimate destruction of the placenta adjacent to it. In its early stage, there may be no clinical symptoms. The condition is discovered only upon examination of the freshly delivered organ, which will present on its maternal surface a circumscribed depression measuring a few centimeters in diameter, and covered by dark, clotted blood. Undoubtedly, it takes at least several minutes for these anatomical changes to materialize. Thus, a very recently separated placenta may appear no different from a normal placenta at delivery. According to Benirschke and Kaufmann (2000), the "age" of the retroplacental clot cannot be determined exactly.

In some instances, a decidual spiral artery ruptures to cause a retroplacental hematoma, which as it expands disrupts more vessels to separate more placenta. The area of separation rapidly becomes more extensive and reaches the margin of the placenta. Because the uterus is still distended by the products of conception, it is unable to sufficiently contract to compress the torn vessels that supply the placental site. The escaping blood may dissect the membranes from the uterine wall and eventually appear externally, or may be completely retained within the uterus (Figs. 25–1 and 25–2).

CONCEALED HEMORRHAGE. Retained or concealed hemorrhage is likely when:

1. There is an effusion of blood behind the placenta but its margins still remain adherent.
2. The placenta is completely separated yet the membranes retain their attachment to the uterine wall.
3. Blood gains access to the amnionic cavity after breaking through the membranes.
4. The fetal head is so closely applied to the lower uterine segment that the blood cannot make its way past it.

In most cases, however, the membranes are gradually dissected off the uterine wall, and blood sooner or later escapes.

CHRONIC PLACENTAL ABRUPTION. In some women, hemorrhage with retroplacental hematoma formation is somehow arrested completely without delivery. We have been able to document this phenomenon by labeling maternal red cells with ^{51}chromium. This technique served to demonstrate that red blood cells concealed as clot within the uterus at delivery 3 weeks later contained no chromium and therefore were shed before.

FETAL-TO-MATERNAL HEMORRHAGE. Bleeding with placental abruption is almost always maternal. In nontraumatic placental abruption, evidence for fetomaternal hemorrhage was found in 20 percent of 78 cases; however, in all instances it was less than 10 mL (Stettler and colleagues, 1992). Significant fetal bleeding is more likely to be seen with traumatic abruption (Chap. 43, p. 1173). Pearlman and associates (1990) found fetal bleeding that averaged 12 mL in a third of women with a traumatic abruption. Stettler and colleagues (1992) reported that there was fetomaternal hemorrhage of 80 to 100 mL in 3 of 8 cases of traumatic placental abruption.

CLINICAL DIAGNOSIS. It is emphasized that the signs and symptoms with abruptio placentae can vary considerably. For example, external bleeding can be profuse, yet placental separation may not be so extensive as to compromise the fetus directly. Rarely, there may be no external bleeding but the placenta may be completely sheared off and the fetus dead as the direct consequence. In one very unusual case, a multiparous woman near term presented to the Parkland Hospital obstetrical emergency room because of nosebleed. There was no abdominal or uterine pain or tenderness and no vaginal bleeding but her fetus was dead. Her blood did not clot

TABLE 25–4. Signs and Symptoms Determined Prospectively in 59 Women with Abruptio Placentae

Sign or Symptom	Frequency (%)
Vaginal bleeding	78
Uterine tenderness or back pain	66
Fetal distress	60
High frequency contractions	17
Hypertonus	17
Idiopathic preterm labor[a]	22
Dead fetus	15

[a]All treated with tocolytic agents.
From Hurd and associates (1983), with permission.

and the plasma fibrinogen level was 25 mg/dL. Labor was induced, and at delivery a total abruption with fresh clots was found.

Hurd and co-workers (1983), in a relatively small prospective study of abruptio placentae, identified the frequency of a variety of pertinent signs and symptoms (Table 25–4). Bleeding and abdominal pain are the most frequent findings. **In 22 percent of cases, idiopathic preterm labor was considered to be the diagnosis until subsequent fetal death or distress developed.** Other findings that developed were serious bleeding, back pain, uterine tenderness, frequent uterine contractions, or persistent uterine hypertonus. In older studies, ultrasound infrequently confirmed the diagnosis of abruption. For example, Sholl (1987) confirmed the clinical diagnosis sonographically in only 25 percent of women. Preliminary data from Yeo and colleagues (1999) indicated a 100-percent positive-predictive value and an 88-percent negative-predictive value in 25 women with preterm prematurely ruptured membranes and vaginal bleeding. In 48 women with vaginal bleeding and intact membranes, these corresponding numbers were 92 and 63 percent. **Importantly, negative findings with ultrasound examination do not exclude placental abruption.**

SHOCK. It was once held that the shock sometimes seen with placental abruption was out of proportion to the amount of hemorrhage. Supposedly, thromboplastin from decidua and placenta entered the maternal circulation and incited intravascular coagulation and other features of the amnionic fluid embolism syndrome, including hypotension. This sequence is rare, and the intensity of shock is seldom out of proportion to maternal blood loss. Pritchard and Brekken (1967) studied blood loss in 141 women with placental abruption so severe as to kill the fetus and found that it often amounted to at

least half of the pregnant blood volume. Neither hypotension nor anemia is obligatory in cases of concealed hemorrhage, even when the acute hemorrhage has achieved considerable magnitude. Oliguria caused by inadequate renal perfusion but responsive to vigorous treatment of hypovolemia may also be observed in these circumstances.

DIFFERENTIAL DIAGNOSIS. In severe cases of placental abruption, the diagnosis is generally obvious. Milder and more common forms of abruption are difficult to recognize with certainty, and the diagnosis is often made by exclusion. Therefore, with vaginal bleeding complicating a viable pregnancy, it often becomes necessary to rule out placenta previa and other causes of bleeding by clinical inspection and ultrasound evaluation. It has long been taught, perhaps with some justification, that painful uterine bleeding means abruptio placentae, while painless uterine bleeding is indicative of placenta previa. Unfortunately, the differential diagnosis is not that simple. Labor accompanying placenta previa may cause pain suggestive of abruptio placentae. On the other hand, abruptio placentae may mimic normal labor, or it may cause no pain at all. The latter is more likely with a posteriorly implanted placenta.

There are neither laboratory tests nor diagnostic methods that accurately detect lesser degrees of placental separation. The cause of the vaginal bleeding at times remains obscure even after delivery. Magriples and colleagues (1999) found that **thrombomodulin**—an endothelial cell marker—was significantly elevated in eight women with placental abruption compared with 17 women without an abruption.

CONSUMPTIVE COAGULOPATHY. One of the most common causes of clinically significant consumptive coagulopathy in obstetrics is placental abruption. Overt *hypofibrinogenemia*—less than 150 mg/dL of plasma—along with elevated levels of fibrinogen–fibrin degradation products, D-dimer, and variable decreases in other coagulation factors is found in about 30 percent of women with placental abruption severe enough to kill the fetus. Such severe coagulation defects are seen less commonly in those cases in which the fetus survives. Our experience has been that serious coagulopathy, when it develops, is usually evident by the time the symptomatic woman seeks care.

The major mechanism is almost certainly the induction of coagulation intravascularly and, to a lesser degree, retroplacentally. Although an appreciable amount of fibrin is commonly deposited within the uterine cavity in cases of severe placental abruption and hypofibrinogenemia, the amounts are insufficient to account for all of the fibrinogen missing from the circulation (Pritchard and Brekken, 1967). Moreover, Bonnar and co-workers

(1969) have observed, and we have confirmed, that the levels of fibrin degradation products are higher in serum from peripheral blood than in serum from blood contained in the uterine cavity. The reverse would be anticipated in the absence of significant intravascular coagulation.

An important consequence of intravascular coagulation is the activation of plasminogen to plasmin, which lyses fibrin microemboli, thereby maintaining patency of the microcirculation. In every instance of placental abruption severe enough to kill the fetus, we have identified clearly pathological levels—greater than 100 μg/mL—of fibrinogen-fibrin degradation products in maternal serum. At the outset, severe hypofibrinogenemia may or may not be accompanied by overt thrombocytopenia. After repeated blood transfusions, however, thrombocytopenia is common.

RENAL FAILURE. Acute renal failure that persists for any length of time is seen in severe forms of placental abruption. This includes those in which treatment of hypovolemia is delayed or incomplete (Chap. 47, p. 1266). Of 57 cases of acute renal failure in pregnant women described by Grünfeld and Pertuiset (1987), 23 percent were associated with placental abruption. Fortunately, reversible acute tubular necrosis accounts for three fourths of cases of renal failure (Turney and colleagues, 1989). According to Lindheimer and associates (2000), acute cortical necrosis in pregnancy is usually caused by abruptio placentae, and 7 of 19 women with this lesion indeed had a placental abruption in the report by Grünfeld and Pertuiset (1987).

Seriously impaired renal perfusion is the consequence of massive hemorrhage. Because preeclampsia frequently coexists with placental abruption, renal vasospasm is likely intensified (Hauth and Cunningham, 1999). Even when placental abruption is complicated by severe intravascular coagulation, prompt and vigorous treatment of hemorrhage with blood and crystalloid solution will often prevent clinically significant renal dysfunction. During nearly 45 years at Parkland Hospital, more than 500 cases of placental abruption so severe as to kill the fetus have received fluid replacement therapy consisting of blood and lactated Ringer solution. In only one instance has dialysis for renal failure been necessary.

For unknown reasons, *proteinuria* is common, especially with more severe forms of placental abruption. It usually clears soon after delivery.

COUVELAIRE UTERUS. There may be widespread extravasation of blood into the uterine musculature and beneath the uterine serosa (Fig. 25–5). This so-called *uteroplacental apoplexy*, first described by Couvelaire in the early 1900s, is now frequently called *Couvelaire uterus*. Such effusions of blood are also occasionally

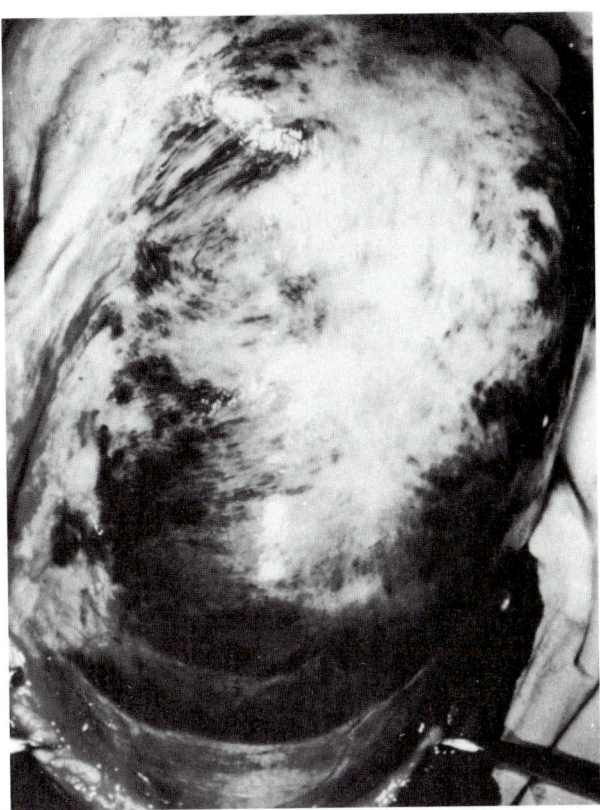

FIGURE 25–5. Couvelaire uterus with total placental abruption before cesarean section. Blood had markedly infiltrated much of the myometrium to reach the serosa. After the infant was delivered and the uterus closed, the uterus remained well contracted despite extensive extravasation of blood into the uterine wall.

seen beneath the tubal serosa, in the connective tissue of the broad ligaments, and in the substance of the ovaries, as well as free in the peritoneal cavity. Its precise incidence is unknown because it can only be demonstrated conclusively at laparotomy. These myometrial hemorrhages seldom interfere with uterine contractions sufficiently to produce severe postpartum hemorrhage and are not an indication for hysterectomy.

MANAGEMENT. Treatment for placental abruption will vary depending upon gestational age and the status of the mother and fetus. With a live and mature fetus, and if vaginal delivery is not imminent, then emergent cesarean delivery is chosen by most. As discussed later in the section Hypovolemic Shock (p. 652), with massive external bleeding, intensive resuscitation with blood plus crystalloid and prompt delivery to control the hemorrhage are life saving for the mother and, it is hoped, for the fetus. If the diagnosis is uncertain and the fetus is alive but without evidence of fetal compromise, very close observation, with facilities for immediate intervention, can be practiced.

EXPECTANT MANAGEMENT IN PRETERM PREGNANCY. Delaying delivery may prove beneficial when the fetus is immature. Sholl (1987) described 72 women with pregnancies between 26 and 37 weeks who had clinically diagnosed placental abruption. About half were delivered within 3 days of admission because of progression to serious hemorrhage, fetal distress, or both. Interestingly, the cesarean rate was about 50 percent for those delivered soon after admission, as well as those in whom delivery was postponed for at least 3 days. In another study, Bond and associates (1989) expectantly managed 43 women with abruptio placentae before 35 weeks; 31 of these were given tocolytic therapy. The mean time to delivery in all 43 was about 12 days and there were no stillborns. Cesarean delivery was performed in 75 percent.

Women with evidence for very early abruption frequently develop oligohydramnios, either with or without premature membrane rupture. Elliott and associates (1998) described 24 women with abruptions who had a mean gestation of 20 weeks and who also developed oligohydraminos. They were delivered at a mean of 28 weeks.

Lack of ominous decelerations does not guarantee the safety of the intrauterine environment for any period of time. The placenta may further separate at any instant and seriously compromise or kill the fetus unless delivery is performed immediately. Some of the immediate causes of fetal distress from abruptio placentae are shown in Figure 25–6. It is important for the welfare of the distressed fetus that steps be initiated immediately to correct maternal hypovolemia, anemia, and hypoxia so as to restore and maintain the function of any placenta that is still implanted. Little can be done to favorably modify the other causes that contribute to fetal distress except to deliver the fetus.

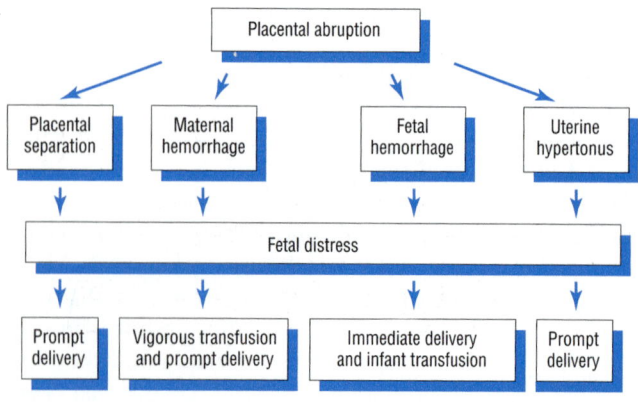

FIGURE 25–6. Various causes of fetal distress from placental abruption and their treatment.

TOCOLYSIS. Some have advocated tocolysis for preterm pregnancy complicated by suspected abruption. Hurd and associates (1983) found that abruption went unrecognized for dangerously long periods if tocolysis was initiated. Conversely, Sholl (1987) as well as Combs and co-workers (1992), provided data that tocolysis improved outcome in a highly selected group of preterm pregnancies complicated by partial abruption. Towers and co-workers (1999) administered magnesium sulfate, terbutaline, or both to 95 of 131 women with abruptio placentae diagnosed before 36 weeks. The perinatal mortality was 5 percent and did not differ from the nontreated group. They concluded that a randomized clinical trial could be safely conducted. Until then, we are of the view that clinically evident placental abruption should be considered a contraindication to tocolytic therapy.

CESAREAN DELIVERY. Rapid delivery of the fetus who is alive but in distress practically always means cesarean delivery. An electrode applied directly to the fetus may rarely provide misleading information, as in the case illustrated in Figure 25–7. At first impression at least, fetal bradycardia of 80 to 90 beats/min, with a degree of beat-to-beat variability, seemed evident. The fetus, however, was dead. There were no audible fetal heart sounds, and the maternal pulse rate was identical to that recorded through the fetal scalp electrode. Cesarean section at this time would likely have proved dangerous for the mother because she was profoundly hypovolemic and had severe consumptive coagulopathy.

VAGINAL DELIVERY. If placental separation is so severe that the fetus is dead, vaginal delivery is preferred unless hemorrhage is so brisk that it cannot be successfully managed even by vigorous blood replacement, or there are other obstetrical complications that prevent vaginal delivery. Serious coagulation defects are likely to prove especially troublesome with cesarean delivery. The abdominal and uterine incisions are prone to bleed excessively when coagulation is impaired. Hemostasis at the placental implantation site depends primarily upon myometrial contraction. Therefore, with vaginal delivery, stimulation of the myometrium pharmacologically and by uterine massage will cause these vessels to be constricted so that serious hemorrhage is avoided even though coagulation defects persist. Moreover, bleeding that does occur is shed through the vagina. An example of an indication for abdominal delivery despite documented fetal demise is now illustrated:

> Although placental abruption was suspected, because rupture of a prior cesarean incision could not be excluded, repeat cesarean section was performed for a 26-week stillborn fetus. The patient had profound hypofibrinogenemia

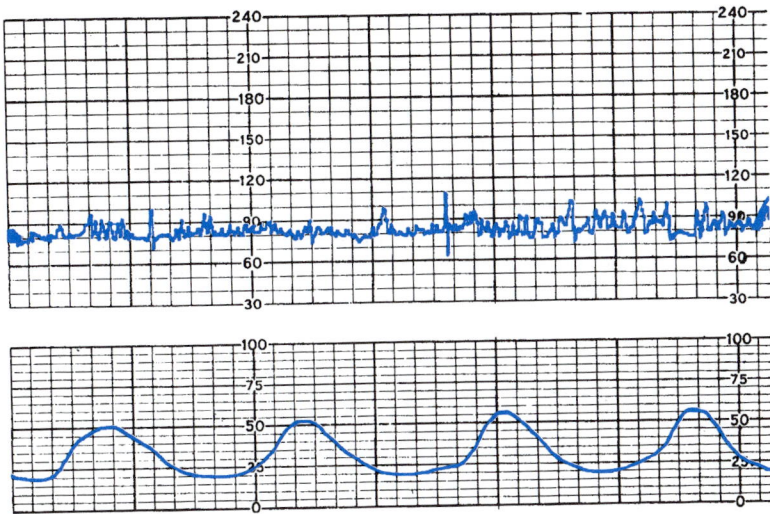

FIGURE 25-7. A recording of uterine pressures and presumed fetal heart rate in a case of placental abruption so severe as to have killed the fetus. The scalp electrode conducted the maternal ECG signal. Note the increased uterine basal tone.

and serious bleeding was encountered from all surgical incisions. Persistent bleeding necessitated hysterectomy followed by internal iliac artery ligation. Lactated Ringer solution was given along with 17 units of blood, 8 units of plasma, and 10 units of platelets to maintain perfusion and treat the coagulopathy, which finally resolved intraoperatively.

AMNIOTOMY. Rupture of the membranes as early as possible has long been championed in the management of placental abruption. The rationale for amniotomy is that the escape of amnionic fluid might both decrease bleeding from the implantation site and reduce the entry into the maternal circulation of thromboplastin and perhaps activated coagulation factors from the retroplacental clot. There is no evidence, however, that either is accomplished by amniotomy. If the fetus is reasonably

mature, rupture of the membranes may hasten delivery. If the fetus is immature, the intact sac may be more efficient in promoting cervical dilatation than will a small fetal part poorly applied to the cervix.

LABOR. With extensive placental abruption, the uterus will likely be persistently hypertonic. The baseline intra-amnionic pressure may be 50 mm Hg or higher, with rhythmic increases up to 75 to 100 mm Hg. Because of persistent hypertonus, it may be difficult at times to determine by palpation if the uterus is contracting and relaxing to any degree (Fig. 25-8).

OXYTOCIN. Although hypertonicity characterizes myometrial function in most cases of severe placental abruption, if no rhythmic uterine contractions are superimposed, then oxytocin is given in standard doses. Uter-

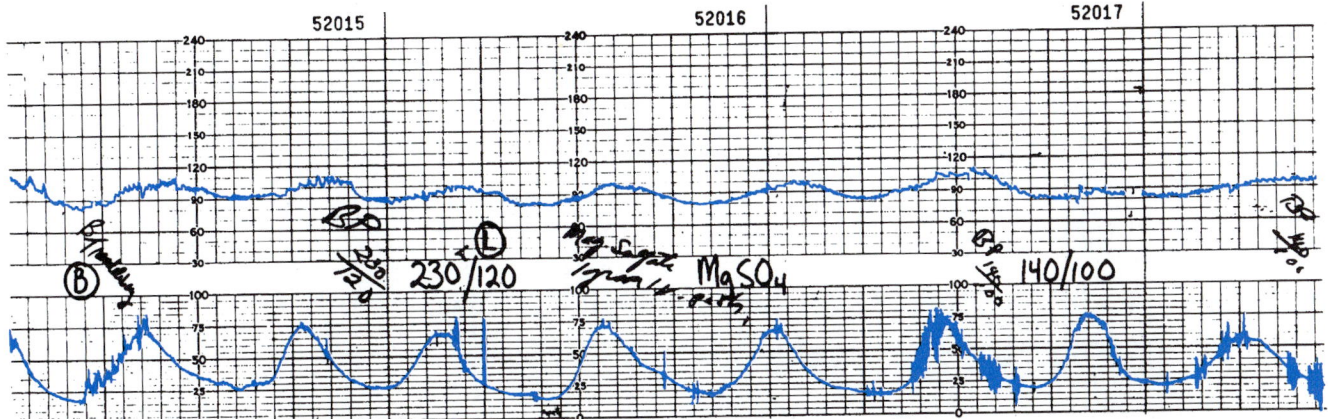

FIGURE 25-8. Placental abruption in a woman with severe preeclampsia. Persistent uterine hypertonus is demonstrated by an elevated baseline pressure of 20 to 25 mm Hg and frequent contractions. The fetal heart rate demonstrates baseline bradycardia with repetitive late decelerations.

ine stimulation to effect vaginal delivery provides benefits that override the risks. The use of oxytocin has been challenged on the basis that it might enhance the escape of thromboplastin into the maternal circulation and thereby initiate or enhance consumptive coagulopathy or amnionic fluid embolism syndrome. There is no evidence to support this fear (Clark and colleagues, 1995; Pritchard and Brekken, 1967).

TIMING OF DELIVERY AFTER SEVERE PLACENTAL ABRUPTION.

When the fetus is dead or previable, there is no evidence that establishing an arbitrary time limit for delivery is necessary. Experiences at both the University of Virginia and Parkland Hospitals indicate that the maternal outcome depends upon the diligence with which adequate fluid and blood replacement therapy is pursued, rather than upon the interval to delivery (Brame and associates, 1968; Pritchard and Brekken, 1967). At the University of Virginia Hospital, women with severe placental abruption who were transfused for 18 hours or more before delivery, experienced complications that were neither more numerous nor greater in severity than did the group in which delivery was accomplished sooner. Our observations are similar; Figure 25–9 summarizes serial findings from one of the most severe cases in terms of the prolonged interval between the onset of symptoms and delivery and the necessity of transfusing a large volume of blood.

PLACENTA PREVIA

DEFINITION.

In placenta previa, the placenta is located over or very near the internal os. Four degrees of this abnormality have been recognized:

1. **Total placenta previa.** The internal cervical os is covered completely by placenta (Fig. 25–10).
2. **Partial placenta previa.** The internal os is partially covered by placenta (Figs. 25–1 and 25–10).
3. **Marginal placenta previa.** The edge of the placenta is at the margin of the internal os.
4. **Low-lying placenta.** The placenta is implanted in the lower uterine segment such that the placenta edge actually does not reach the internal os but is in close proximity to it.

Another condition, termed **vasa previa,** is where the fetal vessels course through membranes and present at the cervical os. This is an uncommon cause of antepartum hemorrhage and is associated with a high rate of fetal death. Prenatal diagnosis by ultrasonography improves perinatal salvage (Lee and colleagues, 2000). It is discussed in detail in Chapter 32.

The degree of placenta previa will depend in large measure on the cervical dilatation at the time of examination. For example, a low-lying placenta at 2 cm dilatation may become a partial placenta previa at

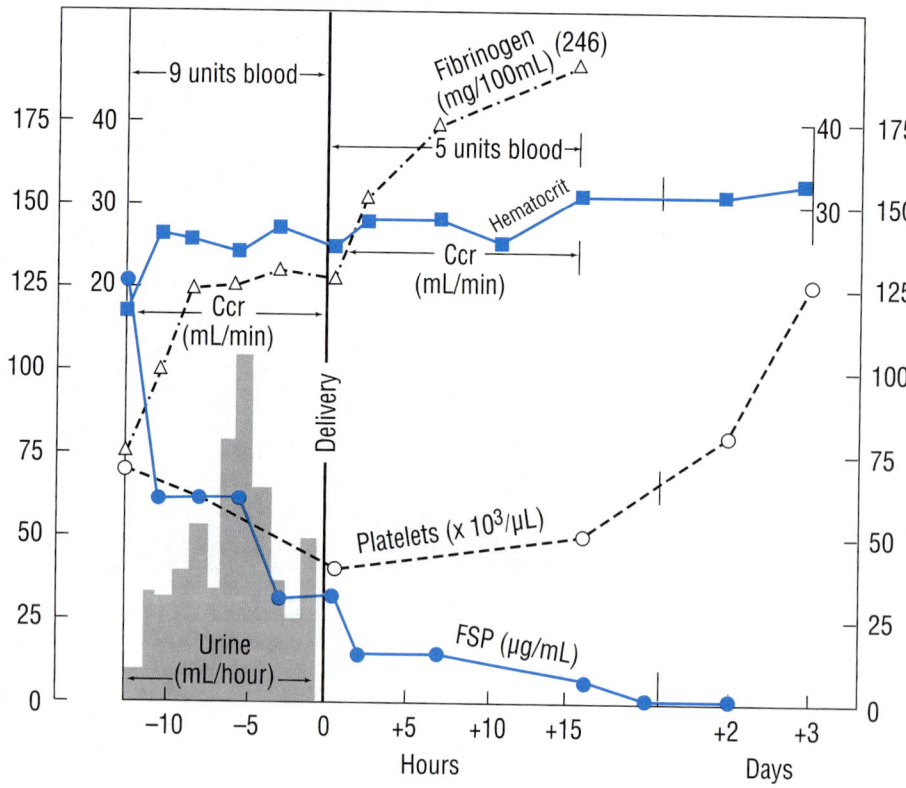

FIGURE 25–9. Serial data from a case of placental abruption so extensive as to kill the fetus and induce serious consumptive coagulopathy. Symptoms of abruption began 2 hours before hospitalization and 14 hours before delivery. Note the normal creatinine clearances (Ccr). The patient left the hospital on the third postpartum day.

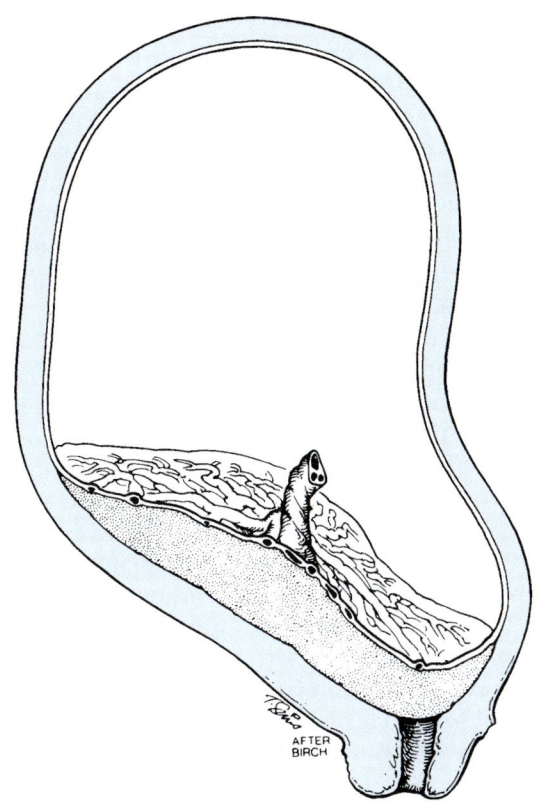

FIGURE 25–10. Total placenta previa. Even with the modest cervical dilatation illustrated, copious hemorrhage would be anticipated.

8 cm dilatation because the dilating cervix has uncovered placenta. Conversely, a placenta previa that appears to be total before cervical dilatation may become partial at 4 cm dilatation because the cervix dilates beyond the edge of the placenta (Fig. 25–11). **Digital palpation to try to ascertain these changing relations between the edge of the placenta and the internal os as the cervix dilates can incite severe hemorrhage!**

In both the total and partial placenta previa, a certain degree of spontaneous placental separation is an inevitable consequence of the formation of the lower uterine segment and cervical dilatation. Such separation is associated with hemorrhage from blood vessels so disrupted.

INCIDENCE. Iyasu and co-workers (1993), in an analysis of the National Hospital Discharge Survey from 1979 to 1987, found that placenta previa complicated 0.5 percent (1 in 200) deliveries. At Prentice Women's Hospital, Frederiksen and colleagues (1999) reported that 0.55 percent (1 in 180) of nearly 93,500 deliveries were complicated by previa. Crane and associates (1999) found the incidence to be 0.33 percent (1 in 300) in almost 93,000 deliveries in the province of Nova Scotia. At Parkland Hospital, the incidence was 0.26 percent (1 in 390) for more than 169,000 deliveries over 12 years.

These statistics are remarkably similar considering the lack of precision in definition and identification for reasons already discussed. A question difficult to answer is whether painless bleeding from focal separation of a placenta implanted in the lower uterine segment but away from a partially dilated cervical os should be classified as placenta previa or placental abruption. Obviously, it is both.

ETIOLOGY. Advancing **maternal age** increases the risk of placenta previa. As shown in Figure 25–4, in over 169,000 deliveries at Parkland Hospital from 1988 through 1999, the incidence of previa increased significantly with each age group. At the extremes, it is 1 in 1500 for women 19 or less and for women over 35 it is 1 in 100. Frederisken and colleagues (1999) reported that the incidence of previa increased from 0.3 percent in 1976 to 0.7 percent in 1997. They attributed this to a shift to an older obstetrical population.

Multiparity is associated with previa. In a study of

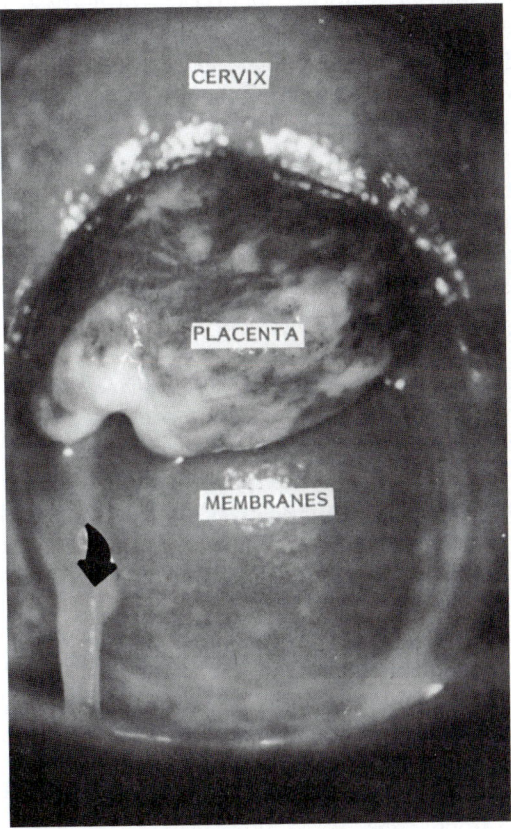

FIGURE 25–11. Partial placenta previa seen through a cervix 3- to 4-cm dilated at 22 weeks' gestation. The arrow points to mucus dripping from the cervix. Uterine cramping was evident, but earlier intermittent bleeding had stopped 1 month before. The fetus weighed 410 g when delivered vaginally the next day. Blood loss was not massive. (Photograph courtesy of Dr. Rigoberto Santos.)

314 women who were para 5 or greater, Babinszki and collaborators (1999) reported that the incidence of previa of 2.2 percent was increased significantly compared with women of lower parity. In the 169,000-plus women at Parkland Hospital the incidence was 1 in 175 in women para 3 or greater.

Prior cesarean delivery increases the likelihood of placenta previa. Nielsen and colleagues (1989) found a fivefold increased incidence of placenta previa in Swedish women with a prior cesarean delivery. At Parkland, the incidence was increased twofold from 1 in 400 to 1 in 200 with at least one prior cesarean section. Miller and associates (1996) cited a threefold increase of previa in women with prior cesarean delivery in over 150,000 deliveries at Los Angeles County Women's Hospital. The incidence increased with the number of previous cesarean deliveries—it was 1.9 percent with two prior cesareans and 4.1 percent with three or more. Certainly, a prior cesarean incision with a previa increases the incidence of hysterectomy. Frederiksen and co-workers (1999) reported a 25-percent hysterectomy rate in women with repeat cesarean for a previa compared with only 6 percent of those undergoing primary cesarean for placenta previa.

Williams and colleagues (1991b) found the relative risk of placenta previa to be increased twofold related to **smoking.** They theorized that carbon monoxide hypoxemia caused compensatory placental hypertrophy. These findings were confirmed by Handler and colleagues (1994). Perhaps related, defective decidual vascularization, the possible result of inflammatory or atrophic changes, has been implicated in the development of previa.

PLACENTA ACCRETA, INCRETA, AND PERCRETA.

Placenta previa may be associated with *placenta accreta* or one of its more advanced forms, *placenta increta* or *percreta.* Such abnormally firm attachment of the placenta might be anticipated because of poorly developed decidua in the lower uterine segment. Almost 7 percent of 514 cases of previa reported by Frederiksen and collaborators (1999) had an associated abnormal placental attachment. Biswas and co-workers (1999) performed placental bed biopsies at cesarean delivery in 50 women with previas and 50 control women. While about half of specimens from previas showed myometrial spiral arterioles with trophoblastic giant-cell infiltration, only 20 percent from those normally implanted had these changes.

CLINICAL FINDINGS.

The most characteristic event in placenta previa is painless hemorrhage, which usually does not appear until near the end of the second trimester or after. Some abortions, however, may result from such an abnormal location of the developing placenta.

Frequently, bleeding from placenta previa has its onset without warning, presenting without pain in a woman who has had an uneventful prenatal course. Fortunately, the initial bleeding is rarely so profuse as to prove fatal. Usually it ceases spontaneously, only to recur. In some cases, particularly those with a placenta implanted near but not over the cervical os, bleeding does not appear until the onset of labor, when it may vary from slight to profuse hemorrhage and may clinically mimic placental abruption.

The cause of hemorrhage is reemphasized. When the placenta is located over the internal os, the formation of the lower uterine segment and the dilatation of the internal os result inevitably in tearing of placental attachments. The bleeding is augmented by the inability of the myometrial fibers of the lower uterine segment to contract and thereby constrict the torn vessels.

Hemorrhage from the placental implantation site in the lower uterine segment may continue after delivery of the placenta, because the lower uterine segment is more prone to contract poorly than is the uterine body. Bleeding may also result from lacerations in the friable cervix and lower uterine segment, especially following manual removal of a somewhat adherent placenta.

COAGULATION DEFECTS.

In our experiences, coagulopathy is rare with placenta previa, even when extensive separation from the implantation site has occurred. Wing and colleagues (1996b) studied 87 women with antepartum bleeding from placenta previa and found no evidence for coagulopathy. Presumably thromboplastin that incites intravascular coagulation that commonly characterizes abruptio placentae readily escapes through the cervical canal rather than being forced into the maternal circulation.

DIAGNOSIS.

In women with uterine bleeding during the latter half of pregnancy, placenta previa or abruptio placentae should always be suspected. The possibility of placenta previa should not be dismissed until appropriate evaluation, including sonography, has clearly proved its absence. The diagnosis of placenta previa can seldom be established firmly by clinical examination unless a finger is passed through the cervix and the placenta is palpated. **Such examination of the cervix is never permissible unless the woman is in an operating room with all the preparations for immediate cesarean delivery, because even the gentlest examination of this sort can cause torrential hemorrhage.** Furthermore, such an examination should not be made unless delivery is planned, for it may cause bleeding of such a degree that immediate delivery becomes necessary even though the fetus is immature. Such a "double set-up" examination is rarely necessary as placental location can almost always be obtained by sonography.

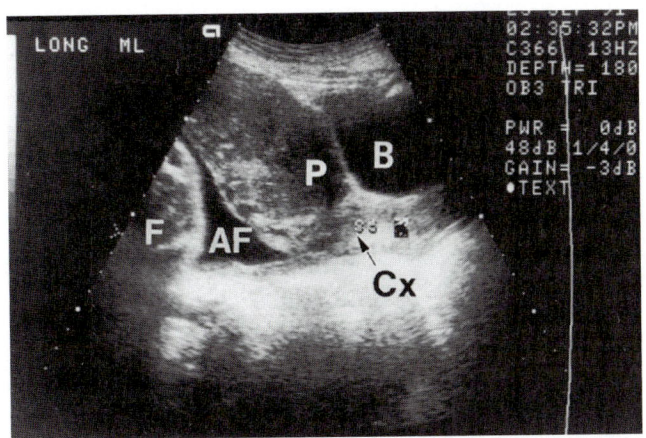

FIGURE 25–12. Partial anterior placenta previa at 36 weeks' gestation. Placenta (P) extends anteriorly and downward toward cervix (Cx). Fetus (F), amnionic fluid (AF), and bladder (B) are seen. (Courtesy of Dr. Rigoberto Santos.)

LOCALIZATION BY SONOGRAPHY. The simplest, most precise, and safest method of placental localization is provided by *transabdominal sonography,* which is used to locate the placenta with considerable accuracy (Figs. 25–12 and 25–13). According to Laing (1996), the average accuracy is about 96 percent, and rates as high as 98 percent have been obtained. **False-positive results are often a result of bladder distention. Therefore, ultrasonic scans in apparently positive cases should be repeated after emptying the bladder.** An uncommon source of error has been identification of abundant placenta implanted in the uterine fundus but failure to appreciate that the placenta was large and extended downward all the way to the internal os of the cervix.

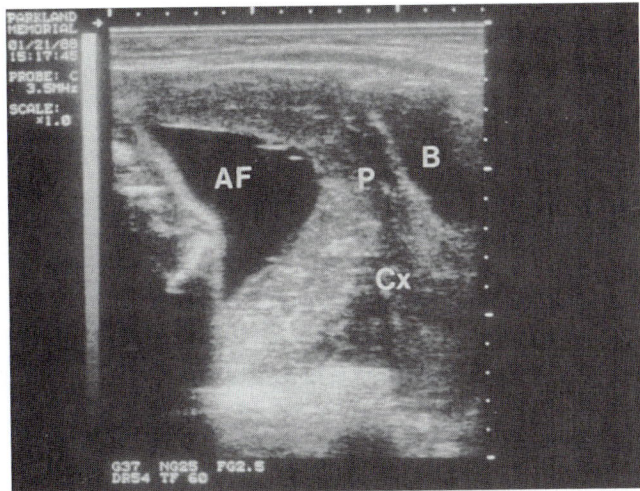

FIGURE 25–13. Total placenta previa at 34 weeks' gestation. Placenta (P) completely overlies cervix (Cx). Bladder (B) and amnionic fluid (AF) are also visualized clearly. (Courtesy of Dr. Rigoberto Santos.)

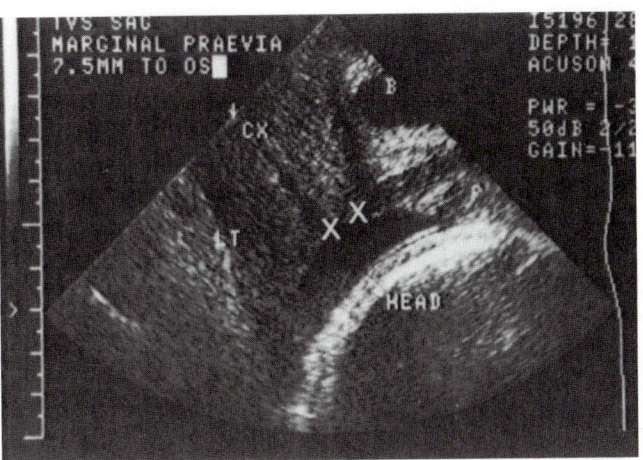

FIGURE 25–14. Transvaginal ultrasonic scan at 34 weeks' gestation. Cervical canal is clearly visible (CX) and distance from internal os to placental edge, measured between calipers (X) is 0.75 cm. The patient was delivered by cesarean section 4 weeks later because of vaginal bleeding. (B = bladder; P = placenta.) (From Oppenheimer and colleagues, 1991, with permission.)

The use of *transvaginal ultrasonography* has substantively improved diagnostic accuracy of placenta previa. Farine and associates (1988) were able to visualize the internal cervical os in all cases with the transvaginal technique, in contrast to only 70 percent using transabdominal equipment. An example is shown in Figure 25–14. Leerentveld and colleagues (1990) studied 100 women suspected of having placenta previa. They reported a 93-percent positive-predictive value and 98-percent negative-predictive value for transvaginal ultrasonography. Tan and co-workers (1995) reported less accuracy with the technique. In studies comparing abdominal ultrasound with transvaginal imaging, Smith (1997) and Taipale (1998) and their colleagues found the transvaginal technique to be superior. Most now agree that confirmatory transvaginal imaging is indicated if the placenta is low lying or appears to be covering the cervical os by transabdominal sonography.

Hertzberg and associates (1992) demonstrated that *transperineal sonography* allowed visualization of the internal os in all 164 cases examined because transabdominal sonography disclosed a previa or was inconclusive. Placenta previa was correctly excluded in 154 women, and in 10 in whom it was diagnosed sonographically, nine had a previa confirmed at delivery. The positive-predictive value was 90 percent and the negative-predictive value was 100 percent.

MAGNETIC RESONANCE IMAGING. A number of investigators have used magnetic resonance imaging to visualize placental abnormalities, including placenta previa. Kay and Spritzer (1991) discussed the many posi-

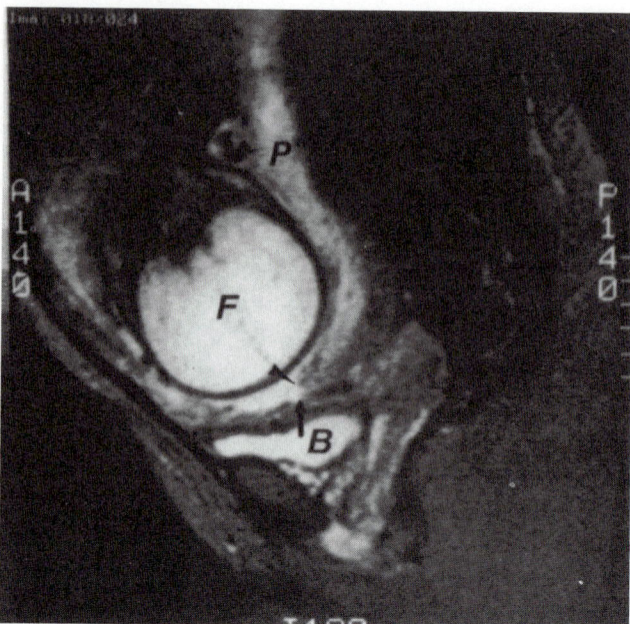

FIGURE 25–15. A sagittal T2-weighted (2000/80 ms) image of a patient with a posterior marginal placenta previa. The arrowhead points to the placental edge and the arrow indicates the internal os. (B = maternal bladder; F = fetal head; P = placenta.) (From Kay and Spritzer, 1991, with permission.)

TABLE 25–5. **Ultrasonic Identification of Placenta Previa and Subsequent Clinical Outcome**

Gestational Age at Sonography (wk)	Previa or Hemorrhage at Delivery (%)
< 20	2.3
20–25	3.2
25–30	5.2
30–25	24

Adapted from Comeau and associates (1983).

tive attributes of such technology (Fig. 25–15). It is unlikely that this will replace ultrasonic scanning for routine evaluation in the near future.

PLACENTAL "MIGRATION." Since the report by King (1973), the apparent peripatetic nature of the placenta has been well established. In earlier studies, "low-lying placentas" were evaluated and McClure and Dornal (1990) found these in 25 percent of 1490 routine scans at 18 weeks. At delivery, only seven of these 385 low-lying placentas persisted. Sanderson and Milton (1991) found that only 12 percent of placentas were "low lying" in 4300 women at 18 to 20 weeks. Of those not covering the internal os, previa did not persist and hemorrhage was not encountered. Conversely, of those covering the os at midpregnancy, about 40 percent persisted as a previa.

Thus, placentas that lie close to the internal os, but not over it, during the second trimester, or even early in the third trimester, are very unlikely to persist as previas by term. These data were amplified by Taipale and co-workers (1998), who found that 57 of 3696 (1.5 percent) unselected women had a placenta previa at 18 to 23 weeks. Only 20 percent of those with the placental edge extending less than 15 mm from the os had a previa at delivery. If the placental edge extended to 25 mm or more, however, 40 percent had a previa.

The low frequency with which placenta previa per-

sists when it has been identified sonographically before 30 weeks is shown in Table 25–5. It is apparent from these data that in the absence of any other abnormality, sonography need not be frequently repeated simply to follow placental position, and restriction of activity need not be practiced unless the previa persists beyond 30 weeks, or becomes clinically apparent before that time.

The mechanism of apparent placental movement is not completely understood. The term *migration* is clearly a misnomer, however, as invasion of chorionic villi into the decidua on either side of the cervical os will persist. The apparent movement of the low-lying placenta relative to the internal os probably results from inability to precisely define this relationship in a three-dimensional manner using two-dimensional sonography in early pregnancy. This difficulty is coupled with differential growth of lower and upper myometrial segments as pregnancy progresses. Thus, those placentas that "migrate" most likely never had actual circumferential villus invasion that reached the internal cervical os in the first place.

MANAGEMENT. Women with a placenta previa may be considered as follows:

1. Those in whom the fetus is preterm but there is no indication for delivery.
2. Those in whom the fetus is reasonably mature.
3. Those in labor.
4. Those in whom hemorrhage is so severe as to mandate delivery despite fetal immaturity.

Management with a preterm fetus, but with no active bleeding, consists of close observation. In some cases prolonged hospitalization may be ideal; however, the woman is usually discharged after bleeding has ceased and the fetus is judged to be healthy. The women and her family must fully appreciate the problems of placenta previa and be prepared to transport her to the hospital immediately. In properly selected patients, there appears to be no benefit to inpatient versus outpatient management of placenta previa (Mouer, 1994). Drost and Keil (1994) demonstrated a 50 percent reduction in hospital days, a 50 percent reduction in maternal cost, and a 40 percent reduction in cost for mother–infant pairs, with no differences in maternal or fetal morbidity with outpatient compared with inpatient management. Wing and colleagues (1996a) reported preliminary results from their randomized clinical trial of inpatient versus home management of 53 women with bleeding from a previa at 24 to 36 weeks. Maternal and perinatal morbidity was similar in each group, but home management saved $15,000 per case. Importantly, 33 (62 percent) of these 53 women had recurrent bleeding and in 28 it required expeditious cesarean delivery.

DELIVERY. Cesarean delivery is necessary in practically all cases of placenta previa. In most cases a transverse uterine incision is made. Because fetal bleeding may result from an incision into an anterior placenta, a vertical incision is sometimes recommended in these circumstances. Even when the incision extends through the placenta, however, maternal or fetal outcome is rarely compromised.

Because of the poorly contractile nature of the lower uterine segment, there may be uncontrollable hemorrhage following placental removal. This can occur even without histological confirmation of placenta accreta. Under these circumstances, management appropriate for placenta accreta is indicated (see p. 632). When placenta previa is complicated by degrees of placenta accreta that render control of bleeding from the placental bed difficult by conservative means, other methods of hemostasis are necessary. Oversewing the implantation site with 0-chromic sutures may provide hemostasis. In some cases, bilateral uterine artery ligation is helpful, and in others, bleeding ceases with internal iliac artery ligation. Cho and colleagues (1991) have described placing circular interrupted 0-chromic sutures around the lower segment, above and below the transverse incision, which controlled hemorrhage in all eight women in whom this was employed. Druzin (1989) described four cases in which the lower uterine segment was tightly packed with gauze that successfully arrested hemorrhage. The pack was removed transvaginally 12 hours later.

If these conservative methods fail, and bleeding is brisk, then hysterectomy is necessary. In some cases, uterine or internal iliac artery ligation as described on page 652 may provide hemostasis. Pelvic artery embolization has gained acceptance also (Hansch and colleagues, 1999; Pelage and associates, 1999). For women whose placenta previa is implanted anteriorly in the site of a prior cesarean section incision, there is an increased likelihood of associated placenta accreta and need for hysterectomy (see p. 632).

PROGNOSIS. A marked reduction in maternal mortality from placenta previa has been achieved, a trend that began in 1927 when Bill advocated adequate transfusion and cesarean delivery. Since 1945, when Macafee and Johnson independently suggested expectant therapy for patients remote from term, a similar trend has been evident in perinatal loss. Although half of women are near term when bleeding first develops, preterm delivery still poses a formidable problem for the remainder, because not all women with placenta previa and a preterm fetus can be treated expectantly.

PERINATAL MORBIDITY AND MORTALITY. Preterm delivery is a major cause of perinatal death even though expectant management of placenta previa is practiced. In their study of almost 93,000 deliveries, Crane and co-investigators (1999) reported a preterm delivery rate of 47 percent. Mortality from complications of preterm birth, however, was not increased when compared with infants of similar gestational age born to women without a previa. Although suggested earlier by some investigators that congenital malformations are increased with a previa, Crane and co-workers (1999) were the first to confirm this and to control for maternal age. For reasons that are unclear, fetal anomalies were increased 2.5-fold.

It is unclear if there is associated fetal growth restriction with a previa. Brar and colleagues (1988) reported that the incidence was nearly 20 percent. Conversely, Crane and co-workers (1999) found no increased incidence after controlling for gestational age. Wolf and associates (1991), in a case-control study of 179 women with placenta previa, found the incidence of growth restriction to be 5 percent for both groups.

POSTPARTUM HEMORRHAGE

Hemorrhage following delivery is the consequence of excessive bleeding from the placental implantation site, trauma to the genital tract and adjacent structures, or both (Table 25–6). Thus, postpartum hemorrhage is a description of an event, and not a diagnosis. In the United Kingdom, half of maternal deaths from hemorrhage are due to postpartum events (Bonnar, 2000). When excess bleeding is encountered, a specific etiology should be sought. Uterine atony, degrees of retained placenta—including placenta accreta and its variants, and genital tract lacerations account for most cases of postpartum hemorrhage. In the past 20 years, placenta accreta has overtaken uterine atony as the most common cause of postpartum hemorrhage of sufficient severity to mandate hysterectomy (Chestnut and colleagues, 1985; Clark and associates, 1984; Zelop and co-workers, 1993).

TABLE 25–6. Predisposing Factors and Causes of Immediate Postpartum Hemorrhage

Bleeding from Placental Implantation Site

Hypotonic myometrium—uterine atony

    Some general anesthetics—halogenated hydrocarbons

    Poorly perfused myometrium—hypotension

        Hemorrhage

        Conduction analgesia

    Overdistended uterus—large fetus, twins, hydramnios

    Following prolonged labor

    Following very rapid labor

    Following oxytocin-induced or augmented labor

    High parity

    Uterine atony in previous pregnancy

    Chorioamnionitis

Retained placental tissue

    Avulsed cotyledon, succenturiate lobe

    Abnormally adherent—accreta, increta, percreta

Trauma to the Genital Tract

Large episiotomy, including extensions

Lacerations of perineum, vagina, or cervix

Ruptured uterus

Coagulation Defects

Intensify all of the above

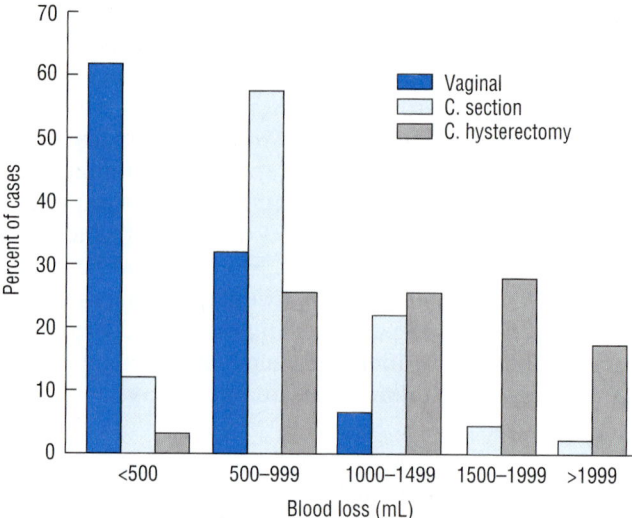

FIGURE 25–16. Blood loss associated with vaginal delivery, repeat cesarean section, and repeat cesarean section plus hysterectomy. (From Pritchard and associates, 1962, with permission.)

DEFINITION. Traditionally postpartum hemorrhage has been defined as the loss of 500 mL or more of blood after completion of the third stage of labor. Nonetheless, nearly a half of all women who are delivered vaginally shed that amount of blood or more, when measured quantitatively (Fig. 25–16). This compares with 1000 mL blood loss for cesarean section, 1400 mL for elective cesarean hysterectomy, and 3000 to 3500 mL for emergency cesarean hysterectomy (Chestnut and associates, 1985; Clark and colleagues, 1984). The woman with normal pregnancy-induced hypervolemia usually increases her blood volume by 30 to 60 percent, which for an average-sized woman amounts to 1 to 2 L (Pritchard, 1965). Consequently, she will tolerate, without any remarkable decrease in postpartum hematocrit, blood loss at delivery that approaches the volume of blood she added during pregnancy. In one study, the mean postpartum hematocrit decline ranged from 2.6 to 4.3 volume percent; a third of women had no decline or had an actual increase (Combs and colleagues, 1991b). Women undergoing cesarean delivery had a mean drop in hematocrit of 4.2 volume percent, but 20 percent had no decline (Combs and co-workers, 1991a).

Therefore, blood loss somewhat in excess of 500 mL by accurate measurement is not necessarily an abnormal event for vaginal delivery. Pritchard and associates (1962) found that about 5 percent of women delivering vaginally lost more than 1000 mL of blood. **They also observed that estimated blood loss is commonly only about half the actual loss.** Based on an estimated blood loss greater than 500 mL, postpartum hemorrhage has been found in about 5 percent of deliveries. An estimated blood loss in excess of 500 mL in many institutions, therefore, should call attention to mothers who are bleeding excessively and warn the physician that dangerous hemorrhage is imminent. Hemorrhage after the first 24 hours is designated *late postpartum hemorrhage* and is discussed in Chapter 17 (p. 406).

HEMOSTASIS AT THE PLACENTAL SITE. Near term, it is estimated that approximately 600 mL/min of blood flows through the intervillous space. With separation of the placenta, the many uterine arteries and veins that carry blood to and from the placenta are severed abruptly. Elsewhere in the body, hemostasis in the absence of surgical ligation depends upon intrinsic vasospasm and formation of blood clot locally. At the placental implantation site, most important for achieving hemostasis are contraction and retraction of the myometrium to compress the vessels and obliterate their lumens. Adherent pieces of placenta or large blood clots will prevent effective contraction and retraction of the myometrium and thereby impair hemostasis at the implantation site. Fatal postpartum hemorrhage can occur from a hypotonic uterus while the maternal blood coagulation mechanism is quite normal. Conversely, if the myometrium at and adjacent to the denuded implantation site contracts and retracts vigorously, fatal hemorrhage *from the placental implantation site* is unlikely even though the coagulation mechanism is severely impaired.

PROLONGED THIRD STAGE.

Occasionally, the placenta does not separate promptly. A question to which there is still no definite answer concerns the length of time that should elapse in the absence of bleeding before the placenta is removed manually. Management is discussed in Chapter 13 (p. 321). Obstetrical tradition has set somewhat arbitrary limits on third-stage duration in attempts to define *abnormally retained placenta,* and thus reduce blood loss due to excessively prolonged placental separation. Combs and Laros (1991) studied 12,275 singleton vaginal deliveries and reported the median third-stage duration to be 6 minutes, and 3.3 percent were more than 30 minutes. Several measures of hemorrhage, including curettage or transfusion, increased with third stages nearing 30 minutes or longer.

UTERINE ATONY.

Failure of the uterus to contract properly following delivery is a common cause of obstetrical hemorrhage. In many cases, postpartum hemorrhage can be predicted well in advance of delivery (Table 25–6). Examples in which trauma may lead to postpartum hemorrhage include delivery of a large infant, midforceps delivery, forceps rotation, any intrauterine manipulation, and perhaps vaginal delivery after cesarean section or other uterine incisions. Uterine atony causing hemorrhage can be anticipated whenever excessive concentrations of halogenated anesthetic agents are used that will relax the uterus (Gilstrap and colleagues, 1987). The overdistended uterus is very likely to be hypotonic after delivery. Thus, the woman with a large fetus, multiple fetuses, or hydramnios is prone to hemorrhage from uterine atony. Blood loss with delivery of twins, for example, averages nearly 1000 mL and may be much greater (Pritchard, 1965). The woman whose labor is characterized by uterine activity that is either remarkably vigorous or barely effective is also likely to bleed excessively from uterine atony after delivery.

Similarly, labor either initiated or augmented with oxytocin is more likely to be followed by postdelivery uterine atony and hemorrhage. The woman of high parity may be at increased risk for uterine atony. Fuchs and colleagues (1985) described the outcomes of nearly 5800 women para 7 or greater. They reported that the 2.7 percent incidence of postpartum hemorrhage in these women was increased fourfold compared with the general obstetrical population. Babinszki and colleagues (1999) reported the incidence of postpartum hemorrhage to be 0.3 percent in women of low parity, but it was 1.9 percent in those para 4 or greater.

Another risk is if the woman has previously suffered postpartum hemorrhage. Finally, mismanagement of the third stage of labor involves an attempt to hasten delivery of the placenta short of manual removal. **Constant kneading and squeezing of the uterus that already is contracted likely will impede the physiological mechanism of placental detachment, causing incomplete placental separation and increased blood loss.**

CLINICAL CHARACTERISTICS.

Postpartum hemorrhage before placental delivery is called **third-stage hemorrhage.** Contrary to general opinion, whether bleeding begins before or after placental delivery, or at both times, there may be no sudden massive hemorrhage but rather steady bleeding that at any given instant appears to be moderate, but persists until serious hypovolemia develops. Especially with hemorrhage after placental delivery, the constant seepage may lead to enormous blood loss.

The effects of hemorrhage depend to a considerable degree upon the nonpregnant blood volume, magnitude of pregnancy-induced hypervolemia, and degree of anemia at the time of delivery. A treacherous feature of postpartum hemorrhage is the failure of the pulse and blood pressure to undergo more than moderate alterations until large amounts of blood have been lost. The normotensive woman may actually become somewhat hypertensive in response to hemorrhage, at least initially. Moreover, the already hypertensive woman may be interpreted to be normotensive although remarkably hypovolemic. Tragically, the hypovolemia may not be recognized until very late.

As emphasized in Chapter 24, the woman with severe preeclampsia has usually lost her pregnancy-induced hypervolemia. Thus, she frequently is very sensitive or even intolerant of what may be considered normal blood loss. **Therefore, when excessive hemorrhage is even suspected in the woman with severe pregnancy-induced hypertension, efforts should be made immediately to identify those clinical and laboratory findings that would prompt vigorous crystalloid and blood replacement.**

In instances in which the fundus has not been adequately monitored after delivery, the blood may not escape vaginally but instead may collect within the uterus. The uterine cavity may thus become distended by 1000 mL or more of blood while an inattentive attendant fails to identify the large uterus or, having done so, erroneously massages a roll of abdominal fat. The care of the postpartum uterus, therefore, must not be left to an inexperienced person.

DIAGNOSIS.

Except possibly when intrauterine and intravaginal accumulation of blood are not recognized, or in some instances of uterine rupture with intraperitoneal bleeding, the diagnosis of postpartum hemorrhage should be obvious. The differentiation between bleeding from uterine atony and from lacerations is tentatively made on the condition of the uterus. If bleeding persists despite a firm, well-contracted uterus, the cause of the hemorrhage most probably is from lacerations. Bright red blood also suggests lacerations. **To ascertain the role of lacerations as a cause of bleeding, careful inspection of the vagina, cervix, and uterus is essential.**

Sometimes bleeding may be caused by both atony and trauma, especially after major operative delivery. In general, inspection of the cervix and vagina should be performed after every delivery to identify hemorrhage from lacerations. Anesthesia should be adequate to prevent discomfort during such an examination. Examination of the uterine cavity, the cervix, and all of the vagina is essential after breech extraction, after internal podalic version, and following vaginal delivery in a woman who previously underwent cesarean section. The same is true when unusual bleeding is identified during the second stage of labor.

SHEEHAN SYNDROME. Severe intrapartum or early postpartum hemorrhage is on rare occasions followed by pituitary failure. In the classical case of Sheehan syndrome, this is characterized by failure of lactation, amenorrhea, breast atrophy, loss of pubic and axillary hair, hypothyroidism, and adrenal cortical insufficiency (Chap. 50, p. 1354). The exact pathogenesis is not well understood, because such endocrine abnormalities do not develop in most women who hemorrhage severely. In some but not all instances of Sheehan syndrome, varying degrees of anterior pituitary necrosis with impaired secretion of one or more trophic hormones account for endocrine abnormalities. The anterior pituitary of some women who develop hypopituitarism after puerperal hemorrhage does respond to various releasing hormones, which at the least implies impaired hypothalamic function. Moreover, Whitehead (1963) identified specific atrophic changes in hypothalamic nuclei histologically in some cases. Lactation after delivery usually, but not always, excludes extensive pituitary necrosis. In some women, failure to lactate may not be followed until many years later by other symptoms of pituitary insufficiency. In the series reported by Ammini and Mathur (1994), the average duration of onset of symptoms was 5 years.

The incidence of Sheehan syndrome was originally estimated to be 1 per 10,000 deliveries (Sheehan and Murdoch, 1938). It appears to be even more rare today in the United States. Application of tests of hypothalamic and pituitary function now available should identify milder forms of the syndrome and define their prevalence (Grimes and Brooks, 1980). Bakiri and colleagues (1991) used computed tomography to study 54 women

with documented Sheehan syndrome. In all of these, the appearance of the pituitary was abnormal; the sella turcica was either totally or partially empty.

MANAGEMENT OF THIRD-STAGE BLEEDING. Some bleeding is inevitable during the third stage as the result of transient partial separation of the placenta. As the placenta separates, the blood from the implantation site may escape into the vagina immediately (*Duncan mechanism*) or it may be concealed behind the placenta and membranes (*Schultze mechanism*) until the placenta is delivered.

In the presence of any external hemorrhage during the third stage, the uterus should be massaged if it is not contracted firmly. If the signs of placental separation have appeared, expression of the placenta should be attempted by manual fundal pressure as described in Chapter 13 (p. 321). Descent of the placenta is indicated by the cord becoming slack. If bleeding continues, manual removal of the placenta is mandatory.

TECHNIQUE OF MANUAL REMOVAL. Adequate analgesia or anesthesia is mandatory. Aseptic surgical technique should be employed. After grasping the fundus through the abdominal wall with one hand, the other hand is introduced into the vagina and passed into the uterus, along the umbilical cord. As soon as the placenta is reached, its margin is located and the ulnar border of the hand insinuated between it and the uterine wall (Fig. 25–17). Then with the back of the hand in contact

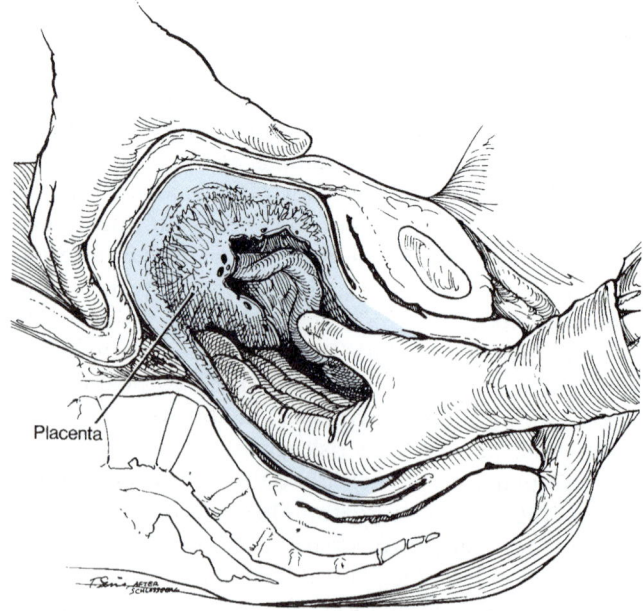

Placenta

FIGURE 25–17. Manual removal of placenta. The fingers are alternately abducted, adducted, and advanced until the placenta is completely detached.

with the uterus, the placenta is peeled off its uterine attachment by a motion similar to that employed in separating the leaves of a book. After its complete separation, the placenta should be grasped with the entire hand, which is then gradually withdrawn. Membranes are removed at the same time by carefully teasing them from the decidua, using ring forceps to grasp them as necessary. Some clinicians prefer to wipe out the uterine cavity with a sponge. If this is done, it is imperative that a sponge not be left in the uterus or vagina.

MANAGEMENT AFTER DELIVERY OF PLACENTA. The fundus should always be palpated following placental delivery to make certain that the uterus is well contracted. If it is not firm, vigorous fundal massage is indicated. Most often, 20 U of oxytocin in 1000 mL of lactated Ringer or normal saline proves effective when administered intravenously at approximately 10 mL/min (200 mU of oxytocin per minute) simultaneously with effective uterine massage. Oxytocin should never be given as an undiluted bolus dose as serious hypotension or cardiac arrhythmias may follow (Chap. 13, p. 323).

ERGOT DERIVATIVES. If oxytocin given by rapid infusion does not prove effective, some administer methylergonovine, 0.2 mg intramuscularly or intravenously. This may stimulate the uterus to contract sufficiently to control hemorrhage. Any superior therapeutic effects of ergot derivatives over oxytocin are speculative, and if intravenously administered they may cause dangerous hypertension, especially in the woman with preeclampsia.

PROSTAGLANDINS. The 15-methyl derivative of prostaglandin $F_{2\alpha}$ (carboprost tromethamine) was approved in the mid-1980s by the Food and Drug Administration for treatment of uterine atony. The initial recommended dose is 250 μg (0.25 mg) given intramuscularly, and this is repeated if necessary at 15- to 90-minute intervals up to a maximum of eight doses. Oleen and Mariano (1990) studied use of carboprost for postpartum hemorrhage at 12 cooperating obstetrical units. Arrest of bleeding was considered successful in 208 of 237 (88 percent) women treated. An additional 17 women required other oxytocics for control of hemorrhage. The remaining 12 women in whom drug treatment failed required surgical intervention.

Carboprost is associated with side effects in about 20 percent of women (Oleen and Mariano, 1990). In descending order of frequency, these include diarrhea, hypertension, vomiting, fever, flushing, and tachycardia. We have encountered serious hypertension in a few women so treated. In addition, Hankins and colleagues (1988) observed that intramuscular carboprost was followed by arterial oxygen desaturation that averaged 10

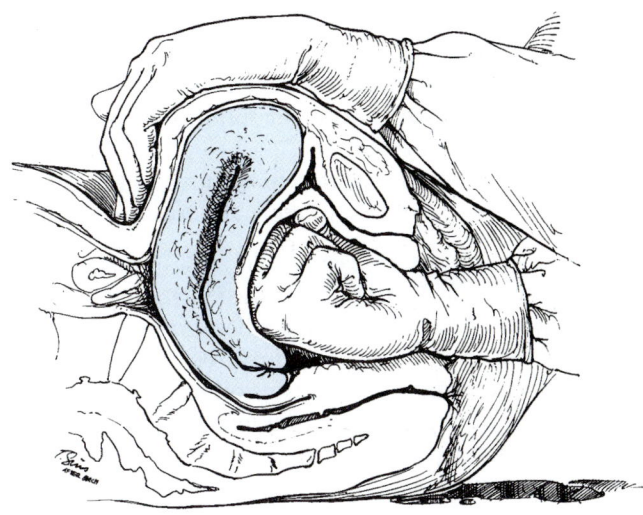

FIGURE 25–18. Bimanual compression of the uterus and massage with the abdominal hand usually will effectively control hemorrhage from uterine atony.

percent and developed within 15 minutes. They concluded that this was due to pulmonary airway and vascular constriction.

Rectally administered prostaglandin E_2 20-mg suppositories have been used for uterine atony, but not studied in clinical trials. O'Brien and colleagues (1998) reported that misoprostol, 1000 μg given rectally, was effective in 14 women unresponsive to usual oxytocics.

BLEEDING UNRESPONSIVE TO OXYTOCICS. Continued bleeding after multiple oxytocic administrations may be from unrecognized genital tract lacerations, including in some cases uterine rupture. Thus, if bleeding persists, no time should be lost in haphazard efforts to control hemorrhage, but the following management should be initiated immediately:

1. Employ bimanual uterine compression (Fig. 25–18). The technique of consists simply of massage of the posterior aspect of the uterus with the abdominal hand and massage through the vagina of the anterior uterine aspect with the other fist. This procedure will control most hemorrhage.
2. Obtain help!
3. Begin blood transfusions. The blood group of every obstetrical patient should be known, if possible, before labor, and an indirect Coombs test done to detect erythrocyte antibodies. If the latter is negative, then cross-matching of blood is not necessary (see p. 655). In an extreme emergency, type O D-negative "universal donor" blood is given.
4. Explore the uterine cavity manually for retained placental fragments or lacerations.

5. Thoroughly inspect the cervix and vagina after adequate exposure.
6. Add a second large-bore intravenous catheter so that crystalloid with oxytocin is continued at the same time as blood is given.
7. A Foley catheter is inserted to monitor urine output, which is a good measure of renal perfusion.

Resuscitation is then carried out as described subsequently (see p. 652). Blood transfusion should be considered in any case of postpartum hemorrhage in which abdominal uterine massage and oxytocic agents fail to control the bleeding. With transfusion and simultaneous manual uterine compression and intravenous oxytocin, additional measures are rarely required. Intractable atony may mandate hysterectomy as a lifesaving measure (Chap. 23, p. 553). Alternatively, uterine artery ligation, internal iliac artery ligation, or angiographic embolization as described on page 647 may prove successful.

HEMORRHAGE FROM RETAINED PLACENTAL FRAGMENTS. Immediate postpartum hemorrhage is seldom caused by retained small placental fragments, but a remaining piece of placenta is a common cause of bleeding late in the puerperium. Inspection of the placenta after delivery must be routine. If a portion of placenta is missing, the uterus should be explored and the fragment removed, particularly with continuing postpartum bleeding. Retention of a succenturiate lobe (see Fig. 5–15) is an occasional cause of postpartum hemorrhage. The late bleeding that may result from a placental polyp is discussed in Chapter 17 (p. 406).

PLACENTA ACCRETA, INCRETA, AND PERCRETA. In most instances, the placenta separates spontaneously from its implantation site during the first few minutes after delivery of the infant. The precise reason for delay in detachment beyond this time is not always obvious, but quite often it seems to be due to inadequate uterine contraction. Very infrequently, the placenta is unusually adherent to the implantation site, with scanty or absent decidua, so that the physiological line of cleavage through the decidual spongy layer is lacking. As a consequence, one or more cotyledons are firmly bound to the defective decidua basalis or even to the myometrium. When the placenta is densely anchored in this fashion, the condition is called placenta accreta.

DEFINITIONS. The term *placenta accreta* is used to describe any placental implantation in which there is abnormally firm adherence to the uterine wall. As the consequence of partial or total absence of the decidua basalis and imperfect development of the fibrinoid layer (*Nitabuch layer*), placental villi are attached to the myo-

metrium in **placenta accreta,** actually invade the myometrium in **placenta increta,** or penetrate through the myometrium in **placenta percreta** (Figs. 25–19 and 25–20). The abnormal adherence may involve all of the cotyledons (total placenta accreta), a few to several cotyledons (partial placenta accreta), or a single cotyledon (focal placenta accreta). According to Benirschke and Kaufmann (2000), histological diagnosis of accreta cannot be made from the placenta alone and the entire uterus or curettings with myometrium are necessary.

SIGNIFICANCE. An abnormally adherent placenta, although an uncommon condition, assumes considerable significance clinically because of morbidity and, at times, mortality from severe hemorrhage, uterine perforation, and infection. The incidence of placenta accreta, increta, and percreta have increased because of the increased cesarean delivery rate. In earlier reports, Breen and associates (1977) reviewed studies published since 1891 and found an average incidence of about 1 in 7000. Read and co-workers (1980) reported an incidence of about 1 per 2500 deliveries. Zelop and colleagues (1993) reported that abnormally adherent placentation caused 65 percent of cases of intractable postpartum hemorrhage requiring emergency peripartum hysterectomy at Brigham and Women's Hospital. Zaki and associates (1998) found an incidence of 1 in 1900 from 1990 to 1996 during which time there were over 23,000 deliveries at their hospital.

ETIOLOGICAL FACTORS. Abnormal placental adherence is found when decidual formation is defective. Associated conditions include implantation in the lower uterine segment; over a previous cesarean section scar or other previous uterine incisions; or after uterine curettage. In his review of 622 cases collected between 1945 and 1969, Fox (1972) noted the following characteristics:

1. Placenta previa was identified in a third of affected pregnancies.
2. A fourth of the women had been previously delivered by cesarean section.
3. Nearly a fourth had previously undergone curettage.
4. A fourth were gravida 6 or more.

Zaki and associates (1998) found that 10 percent of 112 consecutive cases of placenta previa had associated accreta. Hardardottir and colleagues (1996) observed that almost half of placentas in women with a prior cesarean delivery had adherent myometrial fibers detected microscopically.

Other risk factors for placenta accreta were analyzed by Hung and co-workers (1999) in their study of over 9300 women screened for Down syndrome at 14 to 22 weeks. Compared with the normal population, they

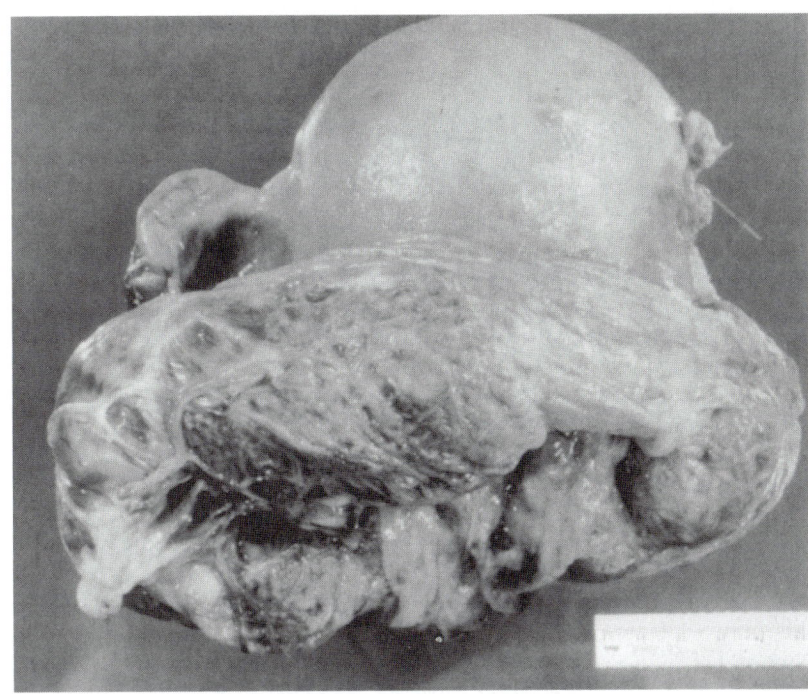

FIGURE 25–19. Placenta percreta in a woman at term with a known placenta previa. The placenta had grown into the entire lower uterine segment. (Photograph courtesy of Dr. Tom Dowd.)

found a 54-fold increased risk for accreta with placenta previa; an 8.3-fold risk when maternal serum alpha-fetoprotein levels exceeded 2.5 multiples of the median (MOM); or a 3.9-fold risk when maternal free β-hCG levels were greater than 2.5 MOM; and a 3.2-fold risk with maternal age of 35 or older.

CLINICAL COURSE AND DIAGNOSIS. Early in pregnancy, the maternal serum alpha-fetoprotein level may be increased (Chap. 37, p. 983). Antepartum hemorrhage is common, but in the great majority of cases, bleeding before delivery is the consequence of coexisting placenta previa. Myometrial invasion by placental villi at the site of a previous cesarean section scar may lead to uterine rupture before labor (Berchuck and Sokol, 1983). We have seen this as early as 12 weeks in a woman explored for an ectopic pregnancy. Archer and Furlong (1987) described massive hemoperitoneum caused by placenta percreta at 21 weeks. In women whose pregnancies go to term, however, labor will most likely be normal in the absence of an associated placenta previa or an involved uterine scar.

The possibility exists that placenta increta might be diagnosed antepartum. Cox and associates (1988) described a case of placenta previa in which they also were able to identify placenta increta ultrasonically from *the lack of the usual subplacental sonolucent space.* They hypothesize that the presence of this normal subplacental sonolucent area represents the decidua basalis and the underlying myometrial tissue. The absence of this sonolucent area is consistent with the presence of a

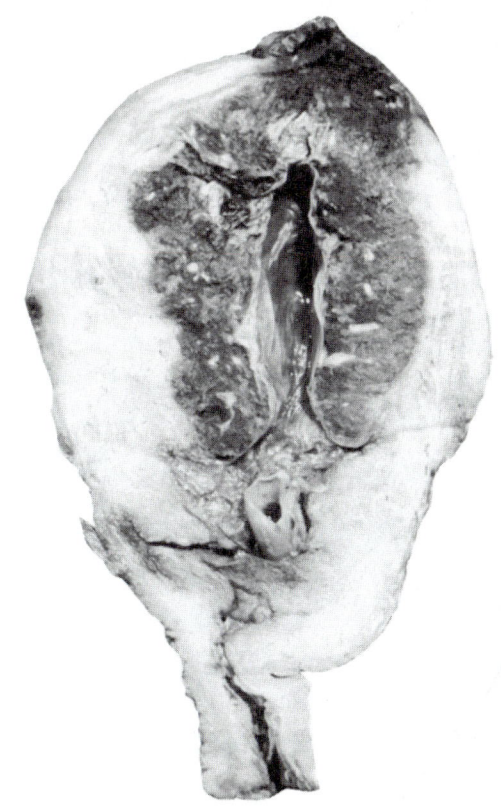

FIGURE 25–20. Placenta percreta. The placenta is fungating through the fundus above the old classical cesarean scar. The variable penetration of the fundus by the placenta is evident. (From Morison, 1978.)

placenta increta. Pasto and associates (1983) confirmed that the *absence* of a subplacental sonolucent or "hypo-echoic retroplacental zone" is consistent with placenta increta.

More recently, magnetic resonance imaging has been used to diagnose placenta accreta (Maldjian and co-workers, 1999).

MANAGEMENT. The problems associated with delivery of the placenta and subsequent developments vary appreciably, depending upon the site of implantation, depth of myometrial penetration, and number of cotyledons involved. It is likely that focal placenta accreta with implantation in the upper uterine segment develops much more often than is recognized. The involved cotyledon is either pulled off the myometrium with perhaps somewhat excessive bleeding, or the cotyledon is torn from the placenta and adheres to the implantation site with increased bleeding, immediately or later. According to Benirschke and Kaufmann (2000), this may be one mechanism for formation of so-called placental polyps (Chap. 17, p. 406).

With more extensive involvement, hemorrhage becomes profuse as delivery of the placenta is attempted. In some cases, the placenta invades the broad ligament and entire cervix (Lin and co-workers, 1998). Such a case is shown in Figure 25–19. Successful treatment depends upon immediate blood replacement therapy as described on page 652 and nearly always prompt hysterectomy. Alternative measures are discussed subsequently (p. 647), and include uterine or internal iliac artery ligation or angiographic embolization. Scarantino and associates (1999) described use of argon beam coagulation for hemostasis in the lower uterine segment.

With total placenta accreta, there may be very little or no bleeding, at least until manual placental removal is attempted. At times, traction on the umbilical cord will invert the uterus, as described in the next section. Moreover, usual attempts at manual removal will not succeed because a cleavage plane between the maternal placental surface and the uterine wall cannot be developed. In the past, the most common form of "conservative" management was manual removal of as much placenta as possible and then packing of the uterus. In the review by Fox (1972), 25 percent of women managed conservatively died. Thus, the safest treatment in this circumstance is prompt hysterectomy.

INVERSION OF THE UTERUS. Complete uterine inversion after delivery of the infant is almost always the consequence of strong traction on an umbilical cord attached to a placenta implanted in the fundus (Fig. 25–21). Incomplete uterine inversion may also occur (Fig. 25–22). Contributing to uterine inversion is a tough cord that does not readily break away from the placenta,

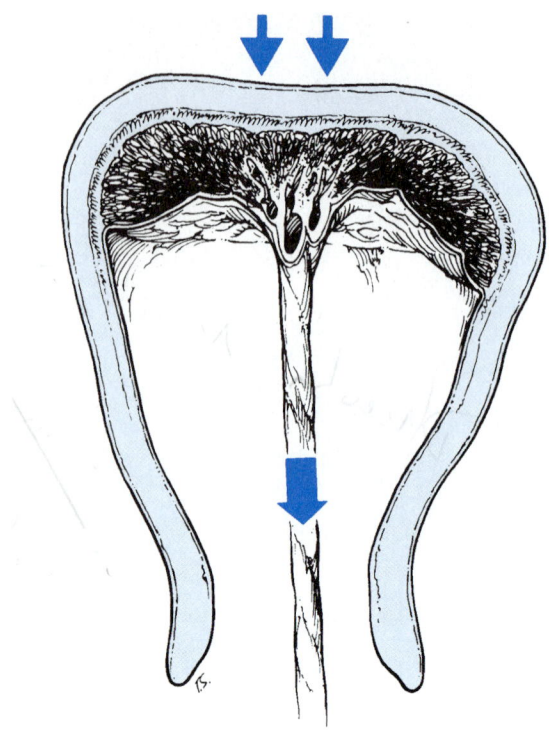

FIGURE 25–21. Most likely site of placental implantation in cases of uterine inversion. With traction on the cord and the placenta still attached, the likelihood of inversion is obvious.

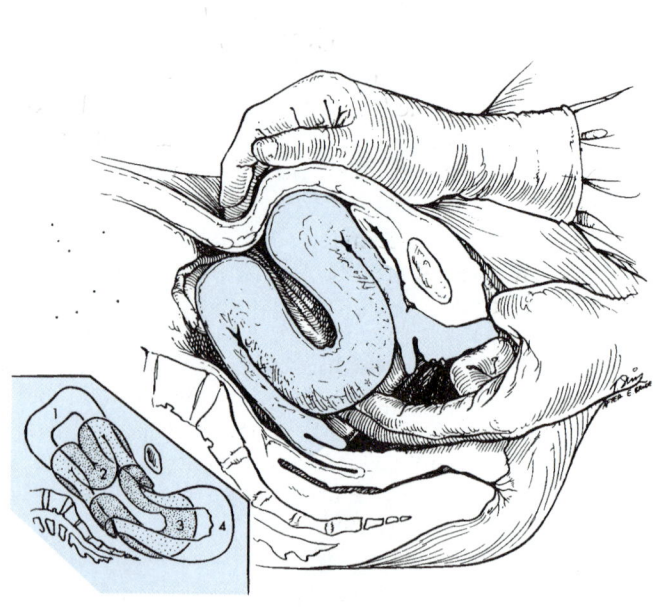

FIGURE 25–22. Incomplete uterine inversion. The diagnosis is made by abdominal palpation of the craterlike depression and vaginal palpation of the fundal wall in the lower segment and cervix. Progressive degrees of inversion are shown in the inset.

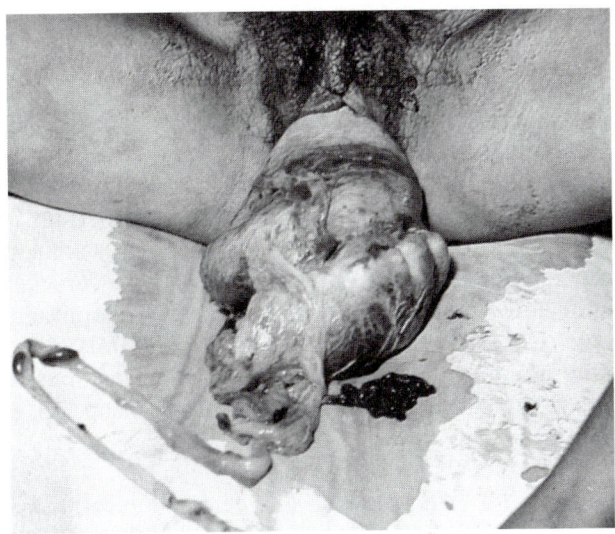

FIGURE 25–23. A fatal case of inverted uterus associated with placenta accreta following delivery at home.

combined with fundal pressure and a relaxed uterus, including the lower segment and cervix. Placenta accreta may be implicated, although uterine inversion can occur without the placenta being so firmly adherent.

Shah-Hosseini and Evrard (1989) reported an incidence of about 1 in 6400 deliveries at the Women and Infants Hospital of Rhode Island. Of the 11 inversions identified, most were in primiparous women; immediate vaginal replacement of the inverted uterus was successful in nine instances. Platt and Druzin (1981) reported 28 cases in over 60,000 deliveries, for an incidence of about 1 in 2100. On the busy obstetrical service at Parkland Hospital, we encounter several cases annually and the vast majority are in "low-risk" deliveries.

CLINICAL COURSE. Uterine inversion is most often associated with immediate life-threatening hemorrhage, and without prompt treatment it may be fatal (Fig. 25–23). In the past it was stated that shock tends to be disproportionate to blood loss. Careful evaluation of the effects from transfusion of large volumes of blood in such cases does not support this concept, but instead makes it very apparent that blood loss in such circumstances was often massive but greatly underestimated (Watson and associates, 1980).

TREATMENT. Delay in treatment increases the mortality rate appreciably. It is imperative that a number of steps be taken immediately and simultaneously:

1. Assistance, including an anesthesiologist, is summoned immediately.

2. The freshly inverted uterus with placenta already separated from it may often be replaced simply by immediately pushing up on the fundus with the palm of the hand and fingers in the direction of the long axis of the vagina.

3. Preferably two intravenous infusion systems are made operational, and lactated Ringer solution and blood are given to treat hypovolemia.

4. If attached, the placenta is not removed until the infusion systems are operational, fluids are being given, and anesthesia, preferably halothane or enflurane, has been administered. Tocolytic drugs such as terbutaline, ritodrine, or magnesium sulfate have been used successfully for uterine relaxation and repositioning (Catanzarite and associates, 1986; Kovacs and DeVore, 1984; Thiery and Delbeke, 1985). In the meantime, the inverted uterus, if prolapsed beyond the vagina, is replaced within the vagina.

5. After removing the placenta, the palm of the hand is placed on the center of the fundus with the fingers extended to identify the margins of the cervix. Pressure is then applied with the hand so as to push the fundus upward through the cervix.

6. As soon as the uterus is restored to its normal configuration, the agent used to provide relaxation is stopped and simultaneously oxytocin is started to contract the uterus while the operator maintains the fundus in normal relationship.

Initially, bimanual compression (Fig. 25–18) will aid in control of further hemorrhage until uterine tone is recovered. After the uterus is well contracted, the operator continues to monitor the uterus transvaginally for any evidence of subsequent inversion.

SURGICAL INTERVENTION. Most often, the inverted uterus can be restored to its normal position by the techniques described. If the uterus cannot be reinverted by vaginal manipulation because of a dense constriction ring (Fig. 25–24), laparotomy is imperative. The fundus then may be simultaneously pushed upward from below and pulled from above. A traction suture well placed in the inverted fundus may be of aid. If the constriction ring still prohibits reposition, it is carefully incised posteriorly to expose the fundus. This surgical technique was described by Van Vugt and associates (1981). After replacement of the fundus, the anesthetic agent used to relax the myometrium is stopped, oxytocin infusion is begun, and the uterine incision repaired.

GENITAL TRACT LACERATIONS

PERINEAL LACERATIONS. All except the most superficial perineal lacerations are accompanied by varying degrees of injury to the lower portion of the vagina.

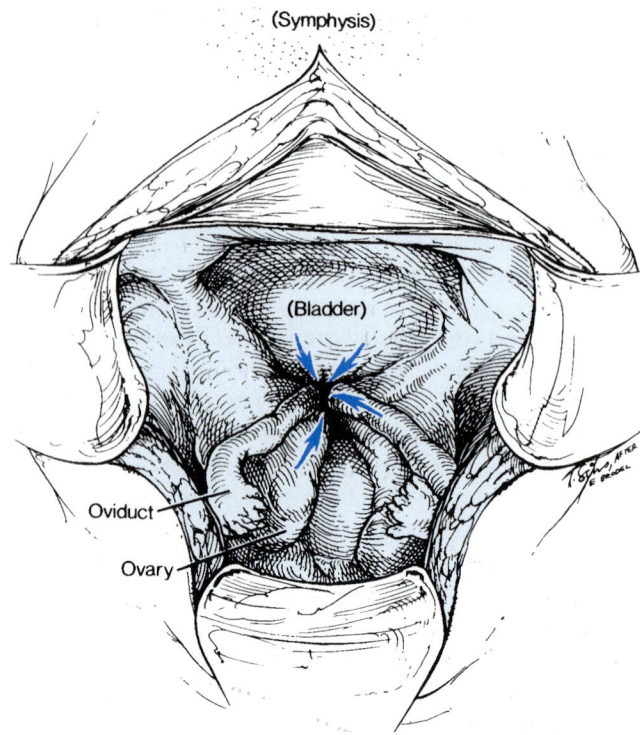

(Symphysis)

(Bladder)

Oviduct

Ovary

FIGURE 25-24. Completely inverted uterus viewed from above.

Such tears may reach sufficient depth to involve the anal sphincter and may extend to varying depths through the walls of the vagina. Bilateral lacerations into the vagina are usually unequal in length and separated by a tongue-shaped portion of vaginal mucosa (see Fig. 13–17). Their repair should form part of every operation for the restoration of a lacerated perineum. If the underlying perineal and vaginal fascia and muscle are not sutured, this may lead to relaxation of the vaginal outlet and may contribute to rectocele and cystocele formation.

VAGINAL LACERATIONS. Isolated lacerations involving the middle or upper third of the vagina but unassociated with lacerations of the perineum or cervix are observed less commonly. These are usually longitudinal and frequently result from injuries sustained during a forceps or vacuum operation, but they may even develop with spontaneous delivery. Such lacerations frequently extend deep into the underlying tissues and may give rise to significant hemorrhage, which usually is controlled by appropriate suturing. They may be overlooked unless thorough inspection of the upper vagina is performed. **Bleeding while the uterus is firmly contracted is strong evidence of genital tract laceration, retained placental fragments, or both.**

Lacerations of the anterior vaginal wall in close prox-

imity to the urethra are relatively common. They are often superficial with little to no bleeding, and repair is usually not indicated. If such lacerations are large enough to require extensive repair, difficulty in voiding can be anticipated and an indwelling catheter placed.

INJURIES TO LEVATOR ANI. These are the result of overdistention of the birth canal. Muscle fibers are separated and diminution in their tonicity may be sufficient to interfere with the function of the pelvic diaphragm. In such cases, the woman may develop pelvic relaxation. If these injuries involve the pubococcygeus muscle, urinary incontinence also may develop (Chap. 13, p. 325).

INJURIES TO THE CERVIX. The cervix is lacerated in over half of vaginal deliveries (Fahmy and associates, 1991). Most of these are less than 0.5 cm. Deep cervical tears may extend to the upper third of the vagina. In rare instances, however, the cervix may be entirely or partially avulsed from the vagina, with colporrhexis in the anterior, posterior, or lateral fornices. Such injuries sometimes follow difficult forceps rotations or deliveries performed through an incompletely dilated cervix with the forceps blades applied over the cervix. Rarely, cervical tears may extend to involve the lower uterine segment and uterine artery and its major branches, and even through the peritoneum. They may be totally unsuspected, but much more often they become manifest by excessive external hemorrhage or by hematoma formation. Extensive tears of the vaginal vault should be explored carefully. If there is question of peritoneal perforation, or of retroperitoneal or intraperitoneal hemorrhage, laparotomy should be considered. With damage of this severity, intrauterine exploration for possible rupture is also mandatory. Surgical repair is usually required, and effective anesthesia, vigorous blood replacement, and capable assistance are mandatory.

Cervical lacerations up to 2 cm must be regarded as inevitable in childbirth. Such tears heal rapidly and are rarely the source of any difficulty. In healing, they cause a significant change in the round shape of the external os before cervical effacement and dilatation to that of appreciable lateral elongation after delivery. As the consequence of such tears, there may be eversion of the cervix with exposure of the delicate mucus-producing endocervical glands.

Occasionally, during labor the edematous anterior lip of the cervix may be caught and compressed between the head and the symphysis pubis. If ischemia is severe, the cervical lip may undergo necrosis and separation. More rarely, the entire vaginal portion may be avulsed from the rest of the cervix. Such *annular or circular detachment of the cervix* is uncommon in modern obstetrics.

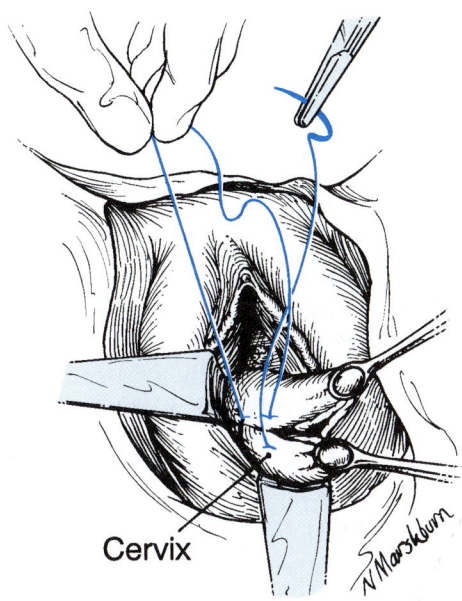

FIGURE 25–25. Cervical laceration exposed for repair.

DIAGNOSIS. A deep cervical tear should always be suspected in cases of profuse hemorrhage during and after third-stage labor, particularly if the uterus is firmly contracted. Thorough examination is necessary, and the flabby cervix often makes digital examination alone unsatisfactory. Thus, the extent of the injury can be fully appreciated only after adequate exposure and visual inspection of the cervix. The best exposure is gained by the use of right-angle vaginal retractors by an assistant while the operator grasps the patulous cervix with a ring forceps (Fig. 25–25).

In view of the frequency with which deep tears follow major operative procedures, the cervix should be inspected routinely at the conclusion of the third stage after all difficult deliveries, even if there is no bleeding.

TREATMENT. Deep cervical tears require surgical repair. When the laceration is limited to the cervix, or even when it extends somewhat into the vaginal fornix, satisfactory results are obtained by suturing the cervix after bringing it into view at the vulva. Visualization is best accomplished when an *assistant* makes firm downward pressure on the uterus while the operator exerts traction on the lips of the cervix with fenestrated ovum or sponge forceps. Right-angle vaginal wall retractors are often helpful (Fig. 25–25). Because the hemorrhage usually comes from the upper angle of the wound, the first suture is applied just above the angle and sutured outward toward the operator. Associated vaginal lacerations may be tamponaded with gauze packs to retard hemorrhage while cervical lacerations are repaired. Either interrupted or running absorbable sutures are suitable. Overzealous suturing in an attempt to restore the normal cervical appearance may lead to subsequent stenosis during uterine involution.

PUERPERAL HEMATOMAS. From a review of six series, the incidence of puerperal hematomas was found to vary from 1 in 300 to 1 in 1000 deliveries (Gilstrap and colleagues, 2001). Nulliparity, episiotomy, and forceps delivery are the most commonly associated risk factors (Propst and Thorp, 1998; Ridgway, 1995). In many other cases, however, hematomas develop following injury to a blood vessel without laceration of the superficial tissues. These may develop with spontaneous or operative delivery. Occasionally, the hemorrhage is delayed.

Puerperal hematomas may be classified as vulvar, vulvovaginal, paravaginal, or retroperitoneal. Vulvar hematomas most often involve branches of the pudendal artery, including the posterior rectal, transverse perineal, or posterior labial artery, whereas paravaginal hematomas may involve the descending branch of the uterine artery (Zahn and Yeomans, 1990). Infrequently, the torn vessel lies above the pelvic fascia. In that event, the hematoma develops above it. In its early stages, the hematoma forms a rounded swelling that projects into the upper portion of the vaginal canal and may almost occlude its lumen. If the bleeding continues, it dissects retroperitoneally, and thus may form a tumor palpable above the Poupart ligament, or it may dissect upward, eventually reaching the lower margin of the diaphragm. Branches of the uterine artery may be involved with these types of hematomas.

VULVAR HEMATOMAS. These hematomas, such as the one shown in Figure 25–26, particularly those that develop rapidly, may cause excruciating pain, which often is the first symptom noticed. Hematomas of moderate

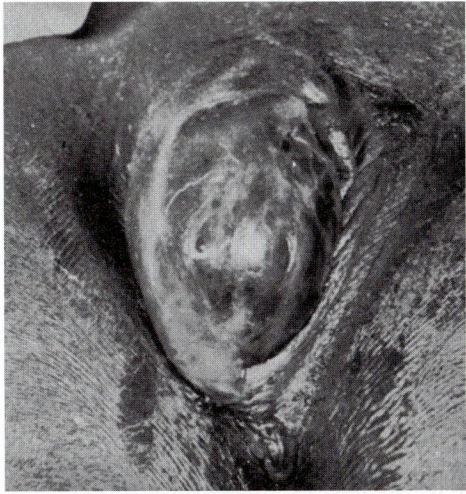

FIGURE 25–26. Vulvar hematoma bulging into the right vaginal wall.

size may be absorbed spontaneously. The tissues overlying the hematoma may give way as a result of necrosis caused by pressure, and profuse hemorrhage may follow. In other cases, the contents of the hematoma may be discharged in the form of large clots. In the subperitoneal variety, extravasation of blood beneath the peritoneum may be massive and occasionally fatal.

DIAGNOSIS. A vulvar hematoma is readily diagnosed by severe perineal pain and the sudden appearance of a tense, fluctuant, and sensitive tumor of varying size covered by discolored skin. When the mass develops adjacent to the vagina, it may escape detection temporarily; but symptoms of pressure, if not pain, or inability to void should prompt a vaginal examination with discovery of a round, fluctuant tumor encroaching on the lumen. When the hematoma extends upward between the folds of the broad ligament, it may escape detection unless a portion of the tumor can be felt on abdominal palpation or unless hypovolemia develops. These are worrisome because large hematomas have led to death.

TREATMENT. Smaller vulvar hematomas identified after leaving the delivery room may be treated expectantly (Propst and Thorp, 1998). If, however, the pain is severe, or if the hematoma continues to enlarge, the best treatment is prompt incision. This is done at the point of maximal distention along with evacuation of blood and clots and ligation of bleeding points. The cavity may then be obliterated with mattress sutures. Often, no sites of bleeding are identified after the hematoma has been drained. In such cases, the vagina—and not the hematoma cavity—is packed for 12 to 24 hours. **With hematomas of the genital tract, blood loss is nearly always considerably more than the clinical estimate.** Hypovolemia and severe anemia should be prevented by adequate blood replacement. In about half of women with hematomas requiring surgical repair, transfusions are necessary (Zahn and Yeomans, 1990).

Subperitoneal and supravaginal hematomas are more difficult to treat. They can be evacuated by incision of the perineum; but unless there is complete hemostasis, which is difficult to achieve by this route, laparotomy is advisable.

ANGIOGRAPHIC EMBOLIZATION. This technique has become popular for management of intractable puerperal hematomas. In can be used primarily, or usually when hemostasis is not obtained by surgical methods. A case in which embolization was carried out with occlusion of the internal pudendal artery and its vaginal branch as well as the uterine artery is shown in Figure 25–27. Alvarez and co-workers (1992) and Hsu and Wan (1998) have reviewed indications for angiographic embolization and described cases in which it was employed.

RUPTURE OF THE UTERUS. The incidence of uterine rupture may vary appreciably among institutions. According to the Centers for Disease Control and Prevention (2000), use of hospital discharge data is inaccurate for surveillance purposes. Although the frequency of uterine rupture from all causes has probably not decreased remarkably during the past several decades, the etiology of rupture has changed appreciably and the outcome has improved significantly. Still, maternal mortality is reported (Ripley, 1999). Indeed, 20 percent of maternal deaths from hemorrhage were due to ruptured uterus (Nagaya and colleagues, 2000).

Eden and associates (1986) reviewed experiences with uterine rupture over a 53-year period at Duke University. From 1931 to 1950 the incidence was 1 in 1280 deliveries compared with 1 in 2250 from 1973 to 1983. Rachagan and colleagues (1991) reported a similar incidence of about 1 in 3000 over a 21-year period. Miller and Paul (1996) reported an incidence of about 1 in 1235 in nearly 190,000 deliveries from Los Angeles County–University of Southern California Women's Hospital. More than 90 percent of these were associated with a prior cesarean delivery. In our experiences, true uterine rupture, as will be defined, has become exceedingly rare. For the 5-year period from 1990 through 1994, during which time nearly 74,000 women were delivered at Parkland Hospital, there were only four uterine ruptures for an incidence of 1 in 18,500 deliveries. This low rate is related to our policy of not inducing or augmenting labor with oxytocin in women with a prior cesarean delivery (Chap. 23, p. 540).

ETIOLOGY. Uterine rupture may develop as a result of preexisting injury or anomaly, it may be associated with trauma, or it may complicate labor in a previously unscarred uterus. A classification of the etiology of uterine rupture is presented in Table 25–7.

The most common cause of uterine rupture is separation of a previous cesarean section scar. As discussed in Chapter 23 (p. 542), this is increasing with the developing trend of allowing a trial of labor following prior transverse cesarean section(s). Farmer and colleagues (1991) reported that two thirds of over 11,000 women with a prior cesarean delivery underwent a trial of labor with an incidence of overt uterine rupture of 0.8 percent. In the study cited above by Miller and Paul (1996), only 11 of 153 cases of uterine rupture were not associated with prior cesarean section. Midtrimester uterine rupture is rare (Levrant and Wingate, 1996). However, women undergoing midpregnancy termina-

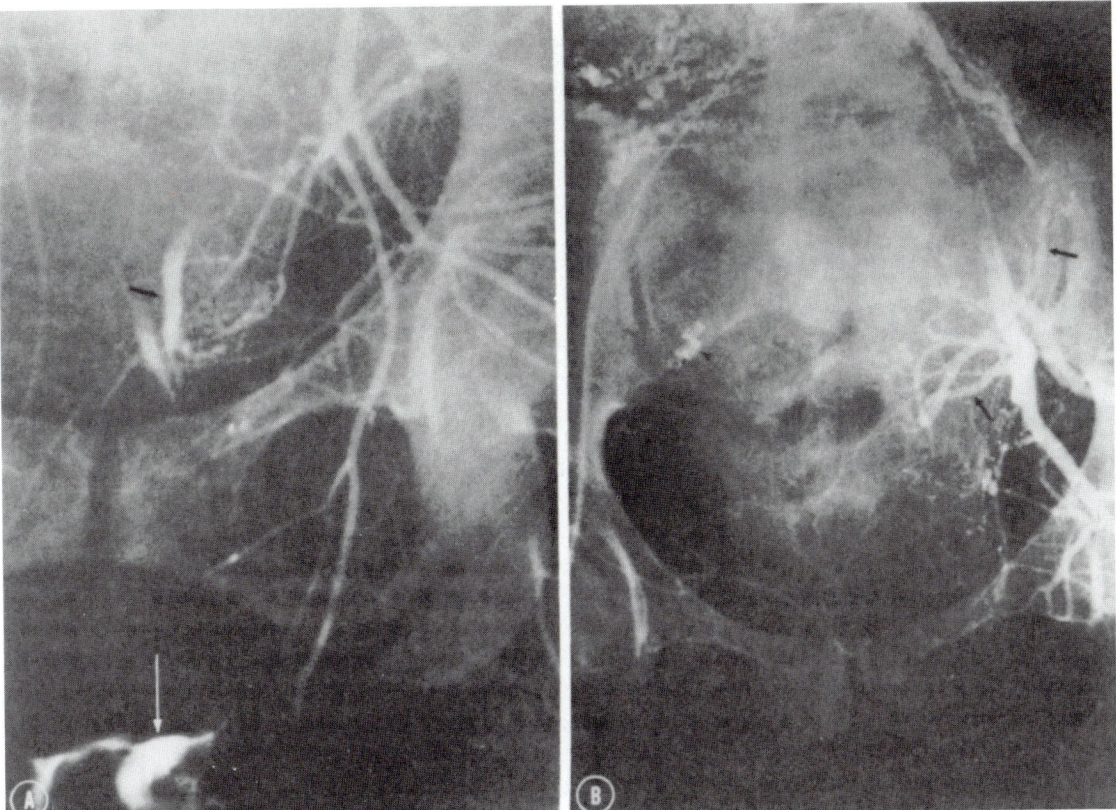

FIGURE 25–27. **A.** Selective left internal iliac arteriogram before embolization. Note marked extravasation from vaginal (*black arrow*) and vulvar branches (*white arrow*) of left internal pudendal artery. **B.** After embolization the branches of the left internal pudendal artery are occluded. Patency of the left uterine artery (*arrows*) and coils in the right internal iliac artery (*arrowhead*) are noted. (From Chin and colleagues, 1989, with permission.)

tions following a prior cesarean were found to have a 3.8 percent risk of rupture (Chapman and associates, 1996).

Other common predisposing factors to uterine rupture are previous traumatizing operations or manipulations such as curettage, perforation, or myomectomy (Fedorkow and colleagues, 1987; Pelosi and Pelosi, 1997). Excessive or inappropriate uterine stimulation with oxytocin, a previously common cause, has become very uncommon. Mishra and colleagues (1995) described a 43-year-old woman who suffered a ruptured vertical cesarean incision associated with inhaled crack cocaine.

DEFINITIONS. Rupture of the uterus may communicate directly with the peritoneal cavity (*complete*) or may be separated from it by the visceral peritoneum over the uterus or that of the broad ligament (*incomplete*).

It is important to differentiate between *rupture versus dehiscence of a cesarean section scar.* Rupture refers to separation of the old uterine incision throughout most of its length, with rupture of the fetal membranes so that the uterine cavity and the peritoneal cavity commu-

nicate. In these circumstances, all or part of the fetus is usually extruded into the peritoneal cavity. In addition, there is usually significant bleeding from the edges of the scar or from an extension of the rent into previously uninvolved uterus. By contrast, with dehiscence of a cesarean section scar, the fetal membranes are not ruptured and the fetus is not extruded into the peritoneal cavity. Typically, with dehiscence, the separation does not involve all of the previous uterine scar, the peritoneum overlying the defect is intact, and bleeding is absent or minimal.

CLASSICAL VERSUS LOWER-SEGMENT CESAREAN SECTION SCARS. With prior cesarean delivery, the American College of Obstetricians and Gynecologists (1999) cite the following figures for a trial of labor and uterine rupture: 1 to 7 percent with a prior low-vertical cesarean incision, 4 to 9 percent with a T-shaped incision, and 4 to 9 percent with a classical scar. Importantly, in about a third of cases the classical scar ruptures before labor, and not infrequently, it takes place several weeks before term. We recently encountered a term abdominal pregnancy in a woman whose prior classical incision had

TABLE 25–7. Classification of Causes of Uterine Rupture

Uterine Injury or Anomaly Sustained Before Current Pregnancy	Uterine Injury or Abnormality During Current Pregnancy
1. Surgery involving the myometrium	1. Before delivery
Cesarean delivery or hysterotomy	Persistent, intense, spontaneous contractions
Previously repaired uterine rupture	Labor stimulation—oxytocin or prostaglandins
Myomectomy incision through or to the endometrium	Intra-amnionic instillation—saline or prostaglandins
Deep cornual resection of interstitial oviduct	Perforation by internal uterine pressure catheter
Metroplasty	External trauma—sharp or blunt
	External version
	Uterine overdistention—hydramnios, multiple pregnancy
2. Coincidental uterine trauma	2. During delivery
Abortion with instrumentation—curette, sounds	Internal version
Sharp or blunt trauma—accidents, bullets, knives	Difficult forceps delivery
Silent rupture in previous pregnancy	Breech extraction
	Fetal anomaly distending lower segment
	Vigorous uterine pressure during delivery
	Difficult manual removal of placenta
3. Congenital anomaly	3. Acquired
Pregnancy in undeveloped uterine horn	Placenta increta or percreta
	Gestational trophoblastic neoplasia
	Adenomyosis
	Sacculation of entrapped retroverted uterus

separated weeks to months before she was delivered by repeat cesarean.

RUPTURE OF A CESAREAN SECTION SCAR. As discussed in detail in Chapter 23 (p. 540), the current trend is to offer and even encourage a trial of labor for women who had one previous transverse cesarean delivery (American College of Obstetricians and Gynecologists, 1999). The main drawback is that separation of the previous scar complicates about 1 in 200 trials of labor. This is higher in women with two or more prior operations who have a trial of labor, either spontaneous or with oxytocin stimulation.

The experience at Parkland Hospital has been that separation of the transverse uterine incision that develops antepartum or during early labor usually is limited to dehiscence without an appreciable increase in maternal or perinatal morbidity. From 1986 through 1990, there were a total of 7049 women at Parkland Hospital with prior cesarean sections, and 2044, or almost 30 percent, were allowed a trial of labor. Of the women undergoing such a trial, 1482 (73 percent) delivered vaginally. Uterine rupture with part of the fetus extruded outside of the uterus developed in three women, for a rate of 1.5 per 1000. In the entire group, there were two stillbirths (1 per 1000) and four women required hysterectomy (2 per 1000). In another 307 women un-

dergoing a trial of labor who were given oxytocin, there were three uterine ruptures (10 per 1000). **Since 1990, when we discontinued the use of oxytocin for labor induction or augmentation for women with prior cesarean deliveries, there have been no uterine ruptures in these women.**

Separation of a vertical (classical) scar is more likely to result in severe hemorrhage with increased perinatal morbidity and mortality. It also more likely will require hysterectomy (Fig 25–28).

MORBIDITY AND MORTALITY. Maternal risks are related to whether there is rupture of an intact uterus versus a prior cesarean scar. Scar separation following a trial of labor in a woman with a prior transverse incision has not been associated with maternal deaths (Flamm and colleagues, 1988; Rachagan and associates, 1991). Conversely, in the 24 cases of uterine rupture principally unassociated with prior incisions, Eden and associates (1986) reported one maternal death and a 46 percent perinatal loss. Likewise, Rachagan and colleagues (1991) reported fetal mortality to be almost 70 percent with either spontaneous or traumatic uterine rupture. As discussed in Chapter 23 (p. 542), perinatal morbidity and mortality can be substantive with rupture during labor of a prior uterine incision.

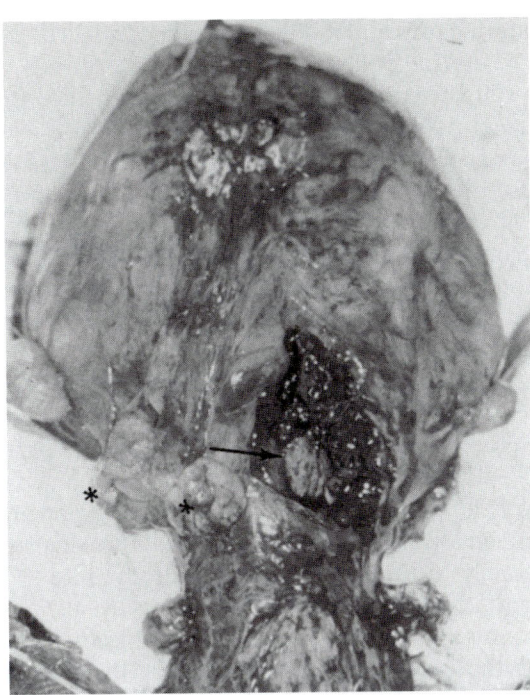

FIGURE 25–28. Ruptured vertical cesarean section scar (*arrow*) identified at time of repeat cesarean section early in labor; asterisks indicate some of the sites of densely adherent omentum.

HEALING OF THE CESAREAN SECTION SCAR. There is little information that deals with healing of cesarean section scars. Williams (1921) believed that the uterus heals by regeneration of the muscular fibers and not by scar tissue formation. For example, upon inspection of the unopened uterus at repeat cesarean delivery, there is usually no trace of the former incision, or at most, an almost invisible linear scar. Also, when the uterus is removed and fixed in formalin, often no scar is visible, or only a shallow vertical furrow in the external and internal surfaces of the anterior uterine wall is seen, with no trace of scar tissue between them.

Schwarz and co-workers (1938) concluded that healing occurs mainly by fibroblast proliferation. They studied the uterine incision site some days after cesarean incision and observed that as the scar shrinks, connective tissue proliferation becomes less obvious. If the cut surfaces of the uterus are closely apposed, the proliferation of connective tissue is minimal, and the normal relation of smooth muscle to connective tissue is gradually reestablished. Even when the healing is so poor that marked thinning has resulted, the remaining tissue often is entirely muscular.

RUPTURE OF THE UNSCARRED UTERUS

TRAUMATIC RUPTURE. Although the uterus is surprisingly resistant to blunt trauma, pregnant women sus-

taining blunt trauma to the abdomen should be watched carefully for signs of a ruptured uterus (Chap. 43, p. 1173). Miller and Paul (1996) described only three cases due to trauma in over 150 women with a ruptured uterus. The likelihood of placental abruption with blunt trauma is greater. Conversely, penetrating abdominal wounds are much more likely to involve the large pregnant uterus.

In the past, traumatic rupture during delivery often was caused by internal podalic version and extraction. Other causes of traumatic rupture include difficult forceps delivery, breech extraction (Fig. 25–29), and unusual fetal enlargement, such as hydrocephaly.

SPONTANEOUS RUPTURE. In the study cited earlier by Miller and Paul (1996), the incidence of spontaneous uterine rupture was only about 1 in 15,000 deliveries. They also found that rupture is more likely in women of high parity (Miller and colleagues, 1997). Oxytocin stimulation of labor has been rather commonly associated with uterine rupture, especially in women of high parity (Fuchs and co-workers, 1985; Rachagan and associates, 1991). Maymon and associates (1991) as well as Bennett (1997) have reported uterine rupture with labor induction using prostaglandin E_2 gel or E_1 vaginal tab-

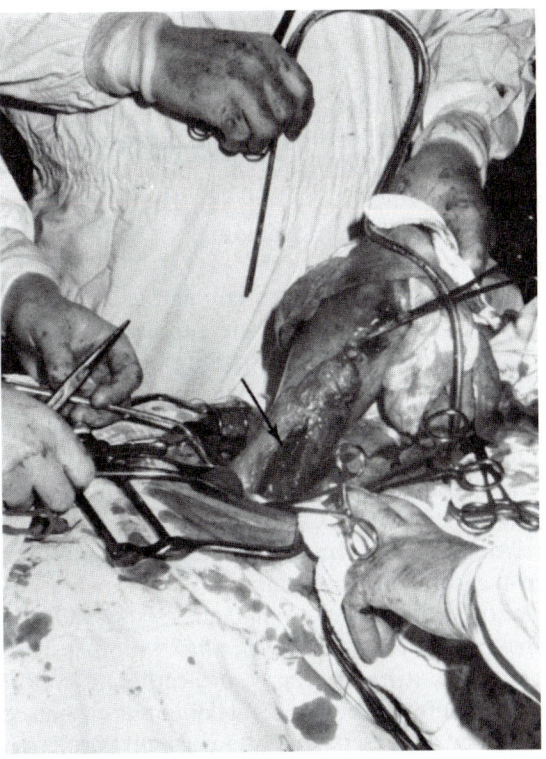

FIGURE 25–29. Ruptured uterus with vaginal breech delivery. At laparotomy, there was extensive bleeding beneath the uterine serosa, bladder, and left broad ligament. The extent of rupture is shown by the *arrow*.

lets. For these reasons, oxytocin should be given with great caution to stimulate labor in women of high parity. Similarly, in women of high parity, a trial of labor in the presence of suspected cephalopelvic disproportion, or abnormal presentation such as a brow, must be undertaken with caution.

PATHOLOGICAL ANATOMY. The role in uterine rupture of excessive stretching of the lower uterine segment with the development of a pathological retraction ring is described in Chapter 18. Rupture of the previously intact uterus at the time of labor most often involves the thinned-out lower uterine segment. The rent, when it is in the immediate vicinity of the cervix, frequently extends transversely or obliquely. Usually the tear is longitudinal when it occurs in the portion of the uterus adjacent to the broad ligament (Fig. 25–29). Although developing primarily in the lower uterine segment, it is not unusual for the laceration to extend further upward into the body of the uterus or downward through the cervix into the vagina. At times, the bladder may also be lacerated (Rachagan and colleagues, 1991). After complete rupture, the uterine contents escape into the peritoneal cavity, unless the presenting part is firmly engaged, when only a portion of the fetus may be extruded from the uterus.

With uterine rupture in which the peritoneum remains intact, hemorrhage frequently extends into the broad ligament. In such circumstances, hemorrhage tends to be less severe than with intraperitoneal rupture. Such bleeding results in a large retroperitoneal hematoma that may involve sufficient blood loss to cause death. Fatal exsanguination may also supervene after rupture of the hematoma relieves the tamponading effect of the intact broad ligament.

CLINICAL COURSE. Prior to circulatory collapse from hemorrhage, the symptoms and physical findings may appear bizarre unless the possibility of uterine rupture is kept in mind. For example, hemoperitoneum from a ruptured uterus may result in irritation of the diaphragm and pain referred to the chest—leading one to a diagnosis of pulmonary or amnionic fluid embolus instead of uterine rupture.

Although once taught, it appears that few women experience cessation of contractions following uterine rupture. Rodriguez and colleagues (1989) described data from 39 of 76 women with uterine rupture in whom there was an intrauterine pressure catheter. In none of these was there a loss of intrauterine pressure or cessation of labor. Four women had increased baseline pressure associated with severe variable decelerations (Fig. 25–30). The most common finding in all of these 76 cases was sudden, severe fetal heart rate decelerations, seen in almost 80 percent of cases. They concluded that intrauterine pressure monitoring added little to the diagnosis of uterine rupture.

In other women, the appearance is identical to that of placental abruption. In still others, rupture is unaccompanied by appreciable pain and tenderness. Also, because most women in labor are given something for discomfort (either narcotics or lumbar epidural analgesia), pain and tenderness may not be readily apparent and the condition becomes evident because of signs of fetal distress, maternal hypovolemia from concealed hemorrhage, or both.

In some cases in which the fetal presenting part had entered the pelvis with labor, there is *loss of station* detected by pelvic examination. If the fetus is partly or totally extruded, abdominal palpation or vaginal examination is helpful to identify the presenting part, which has moved away from the pelvic inlet. A firm contracted uterus may at times be felt alongside the fetus. Often fetal parts are more easily palpated than usual. On vaginal examination, it is sometimes possible to palpate a tear in the uterine wall through which the fingers can be passed into the peritoneal cavity. **Failure to detect the tear by no means proves its absence.** In suspected cases, it is imperative that thorough examination be performed by an experienced examiner before the suspicion is abandoned. Sonography, performed on site, may be useful.

PROGNOSIS. With rupture and expulsion of the fetus into the peritoneal cavity, the chances for intact fetal survival are dismal, and mortality rates reported in various studies range from 50 to 75 percent. If the fetus is alive at the time of the rupture, the only chance of continued survival is afforded by immediate delivery, most often by laparotomy. Otherwise, hypoxia from both placental separation and maternal hypovolemia is inevitable. If untreated, most of the women die from hemorrhage or, less often, later from infection. Prompt diagnosis, immediate operation, the availability of large amounts of blood, and antimicrobial therapy have greatly improved the prognosis. Conversely, Nkata (1996) reported 44 percent maternal deaths in 32 women with a ruptured uterus in Zambia.

HYSTERECTOMY VERSUS REPAIR. In cases of scar separation without bleeding following vaginal birth after cesarean section, exploratory laparotomy is not indicated. With spontaneous uterine rupture, or frank rupture during a trial of labor after cesarean delivery, hysterectomy is frequently required. In two recent reports by McMahon (1996) and Miller (1997) and their colleagues, 10 to 20 percent of these women required hysterectomy for hemostasis. In selected cases, suture of the wound with uterine preservation may be performed. Sheth (1968) described outcomes

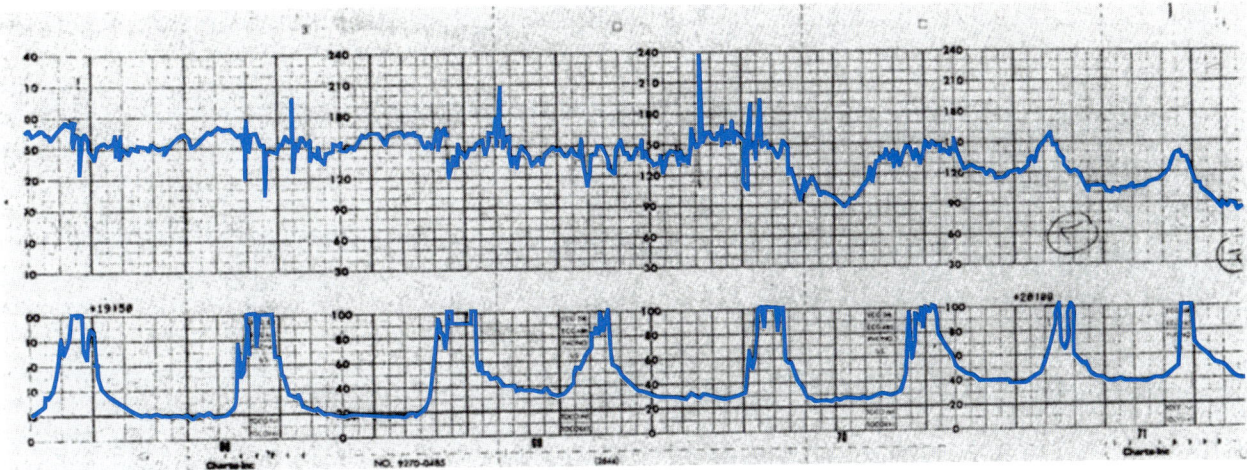

FIGURE 25–30. Internal monitor tracing demonstrates fetal heart rate decelerations, increase in uterine tone, and continuation of uterine contractions in a woman with uterine rupture. (From Rodriguez and colleagues, 1989, with permission.)

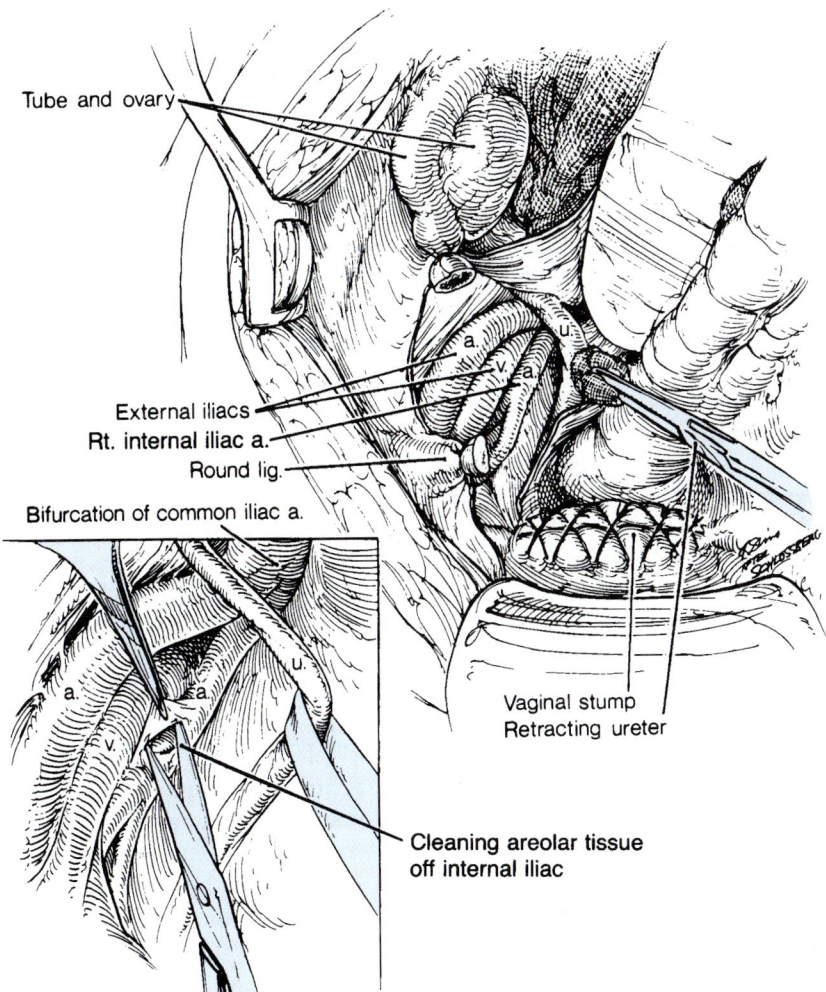

Tube and ovary

External iliacs
Rt. internal iliac a.
Round lig.

Bifurcation of common iliac a.

Vaginal stump
Retracting ureter

Cleaning areolar tissue
off internal iliac

FIGURE 25–31. Ligation of the right internal iliac artery. In the lower left insert, the areolar sheath covering the artery is being opened. (a. = artery; lig. = ligament; rt. = right; u. = ureter; v. = vein.)

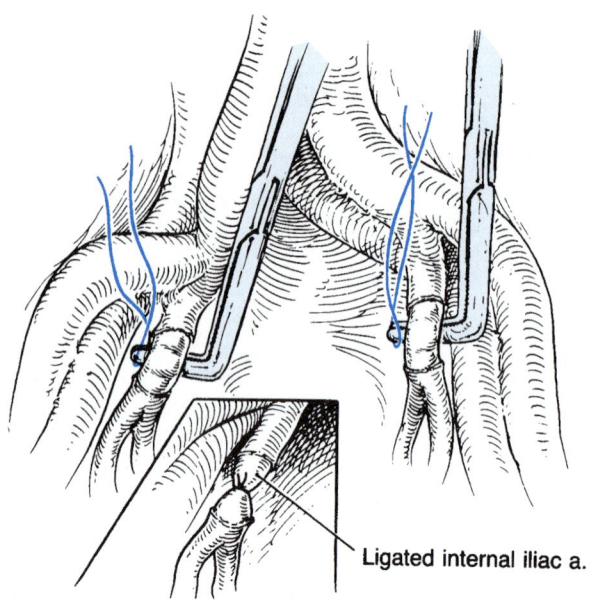

Ligated internal iliac a.

FIGURE 25–32. Ligation of both internal iliac arteries. After the covering sheath has been opened and the artery has been carefully freed from the immediately adjacent veins, a ligature is carried beneath the artery with a right angle clamp and firmly tied. (a. = artery.)

from a series of 66 cases in which repair of a uterine rupture was elected rather than hysterectomy. In 25 instances, the repair was accompanied by tubal sterilization. Thirteen of the 41 mothers who did not have tubal sterilization had a total of 21 subsequent pregnancies, but uterine rupture recurred in four instances. Martin and colleagues (1990) described a woman in whom recurrent uterine lateral fundal separation at 19 weeks was repaired using a Gore-Tex soft tissue patch. When delivered by cesarean section at 33 weeks, the patch was intact and epithelialized.

In the presence of a large hematoma in the broad ligament, identification and ligation of the uterine vessels can be extremely difficult. In general, efforts to control hemorrhage by clamping indiscriminately at the site of rupture involving the lower segment should be avoided. To do otherwise often leads to clamping and ligation of the ureter, bladder, or both. With uterine ruptures involving the lower uterine segment, bleeding vessels must be visualized free of surrounding tissue before clamping, or the ureter and bladder must be demonstrated to be remote from the tissue that is clamped. In some cases, the transected uterine artery has retracted laterally and is displaced to the pelvic sidewall by the hematoma that resulted. Placement of clamps to control bleeding carries little risk when rupture involves the body of the uterus remote from the ureters and bladder. The broad ligament may be entered and the ascending uterine artery and veins safely

clamped. Usually, the ovarian vessels should be promptly clamped adjacent to the uterus.

INTERNAL ILIAC ARTERY LIGATION. Ligation of the internal iliac arteries at times reduces the hemorrhage appreciably (Allahbadia, 1993; Clark and colleagues, 1985). This operation is more easily performed if the midline abdominal incision is extended upward above the umbilicus. With adequate exposure, ligation is accomplished by opening the peritoneum over the common iliac artery and dissecting down to the bifurcation of the external and internal iliac arteries. The areolar sheath covering the internal iliac artery is incised longitudinally, and a right-angle clamp is carefully passed just beneath the artery. Care must be taken not to perforate contiguous large veins, especially the internal iliac vein. Suture, usually nonabsorbable, is then inserted into the open clamp, the jaws are locked, the suture is carried around the vessel, and the vessel is securely ligated (Figs. 25–31 and 25–32). Pulsations in the external iliac artery, if present before tying the ligature, should be present afterward as well. If not, pulsations must be identified after arterial hypotension has been successfully treated, in order to assure that the blood flow through the external iliac vessel has not been compromised by the ligature. The most important mechanism of action with internal iliac artery ligation is an 85 percent reduction in pulse pressure in those arteries distal to the ligation (Burchell, 1968), thus turning an arterial pressure system into one with pressures approaching those in the venous circulation and more amenable to hemostasis via simple clot formation. Bilateral ligation of these arteries does not appear to interfere seriously with subsequent reproduction. Mengert and associates (1969) documented successful pregnancies in five women after bilateral internal iliac artery ligation. In three, the ovarian arteries were also ligated.

In some women, pelvic vessel bleeding may continue even after internal iliac artery ligation. Angiographically directed arterial embolization has been reported to successfully arrest hemorrhage. This was described on page 647 and in Figure 25–27.

HYPOVOLEMIC SHOCK

Shock from hemorrhage evolves through several stages. Early in the course of massive bleeding, there are decreases in mean arterial pressure, stroke volume, cardiac output, central venous pressure, and pulmonary capillary wedge pressure. Increases in arteriovenous oxygen content difference reflect a relative increase in tissue oxygen extraction, although overall oxygen consumption falls (Bland and colleagues, 1985).

Blood flow to capillary beds in various organs is controlled by arterioles, which are resistance vessels that in turn are controlled by the central nervous system. At least 70 percent of total blood volume is contained in venules, which are passive resistance vessels controlled by humoral factors. Catecholamine release during hemorrhage causes a generalized increase in venular tone, resulting in an autotransfusion from this capacitance reservoir (Barber and colleagues, 1999). These changes are accompanied by compensatory increases in heart rate, systemic and pulmonary vascular resistance, and myocardial contractility. In addition, there is redistribution of cardiac output and blood volume by selective centrally mediated arteriolar constriction. This results in diminished perfusion to the kidneys, splanchnic beds, skin, and uterus with relative maintenance of blood flow to the heart, brain, and adrenal glands, organs that autoregulate their own flow (Barber and associates, 1999).

As blood volume deficit exceeds 25 percent, compensatory mechanisms usually are inadequate to maintain cardiac output and blood pressure. At this point, additional small losses of blood result in rapid clinical deterioration. Despite an initial increase in *total oxygen extraction* by maternal tissue, maldistribution of blood flow results in *local* tissue hypoxia and metabolic acidosis, producing a vicious cycle of vasoconstriction, organ ischemia, and cellular death. Hemorrhage also activates the CD-18 locus of lymphocytes and monocytes, which mediates leukocyte–endothelial cell interactions. These events lead to loss of capillary membrane integrity and additional loss of intravascular volume. A number of these adverse effects appear to be mediated by peptide leukotrienes and cytokines and may be experimentally improved by their pharmacological antagonism mediators (Bitterman and colleagues, 1988). There is also increased platelet aggregation in hypovolemic shock, resulting in the release of a number of vasoactive mediators that cause small vessel occlusion and further impairment of microcirculatory perfusion.

Often overlooked is the importance of extracellular fluid and electrolyte shifts in both pathophysiology and successful treatment of hypovolemic shock. This involves changes in the cellular transport of various ions, in which sodium and water enter skeletal muscles and cellular potassium is lost to the extracellular fluid (Chiao and colleagues, 1990). Replacement of extracellular fluid is thus an important component of therapy in hypovolemic shock. Indeed, survival appears to be reduced in acute hemorrhagic shock when blood alone—compared with blood and lactated Ringer solution—is administered (Barber and co-workers, 1999).

ESTIMATION OF BLOOD LOSS. Visual inspection is most often used but is notoriously inaccurate. In some reports, the amount of blood estimated to have been lost by inspection was on average about half the measured loss. Importantly, in obstetrics, part or all of the hemorrhage may be concealed. It is important to realize that in a situation of acute hemorrhage, the immediate hematocrit may not reflect actual blood loss. After the loss of 1000 mL, the hematocrit typically falls only 3 volumes percent in the first hour. However, rapid infusion of intravenous crystalloids will allow for more rapid equilibration.

Urine output is one of the most important parameters to follow in the bleeding patient. **When carefully measured, the rate of urine formation, in the absence of diuretics, reflects the adequacy of renal perfusion and, in turn, perfusion of other vital organs, because renal blood flow is especially sensitive to blood volume changes.** Urine flow of at least 30 mL and preferably 60 mL per hour should be maintained. With potentially serious hemorrhage, an indwelling catheter should be inserted promptly to measure urine flow. Potent diuretics such as furosemide invalidate the relationship between urine flow and renal perfusion. This need not be a problem in the management of the woman who is hemorrhaging, however, because the use of diuretics is contraindicated. Further intravascular volume reduction with diuretics is harmful in a hypovolemic patient. Another effect of furosemide is venodilation, which further reduces cardiac venous return, thereby further compromising cardiac output.

RESUSCITATION AND ACUTE MANAGEMENT. Whenever there is any suggestion of excessive blood loss, it is essential that steps be immediately taken to identify the presence of uterine atony, retained placental fragments, or genital tract lacerations. It is imperative that at least one or two intravenous infusion systems of large caliber be established immediately to allow rapid administration of crystalloid solutions and blood. An operating room, surgical team, and anesthesiologist should always be immediately available. The management of specific causes of postpartum hemorrhage were discussed earlier in this chapter.

FLUID AND BLOOD REPLACEMENT. Treatment of serious hemorrhage demands prompt and adequate refilling of the intravascular compartment. Crystalloid solutions typically are used for initial volume resuscitation. Such solutions rapidly equilibrate into the extravascular space and only 20 percent of crystalloid remains in the circulation of critically ill patients after 1 hour (Shoemaker and co-workers, 1991). Because of such equilibration, initial fluid infusion should involve about three times as much crystalloid as the estimated blood loss.

There is debate concerning fluid resuscitation of hypovolemic shock with colloid versus crystalloid solutions. According to their review, Schierhout and Roberts (1998) found a 4-percent excessive mortality in nonpregnant patients resuscitated with colloid compared with crystalloid. The Cochrane Injuries Group Albumin Reviewers (1998) found a 6-percent excess mortality in albumin-treated nonpregnant patients with shock. We concur with Bonnar (2000) that fluid resuscitation preferably should be with crystalloid and blood.

Considerable debate also surrounds the hematocrit level or hemoglobin concentration that mandates blood transfusion. According to deliberations of a Consensus Development Conference (1988), cardiac output does not substantively increase until the hemoglobin concentration falls to about 7 g/dL. Although the committee reported that otherwise healthy anesthetized animals survived isovolemic anemia with hematocrit decreases down to 5 volume percent, they further cited that there was significant functional deterioration well before that point. It is difficult to define a universal hematocrit or hemoglobin value below or above which transfusion is either mandatory or contraindicated. However, the recommendations of the Consensus Development Conference should be considered in clinical decision making. According to these guidelines, red blood cells are not infused for moderate anemia in stable women.

For the woman acutely bleeding, we recommend rapid blood infusion if the hematocrit is less than 25 volume percent. Similarly, Morrison and colleagues (1993) recommend transfusion if the hematocrit is less than 24 volume percent or if hemoglobin is less than 8 g/dL if there is imminent surgery, acute operative blood loss, acute hypoxia, vascular collapse, or other factors present. Further support for these recommendations was provided by Czer and Shoemaker (1978). In 94 critically ill postoperative patients, mortality rates were lowest when hematocrit values were maintained between 27 and 33 volume percent.

Hebert and associates (1999) reported results from the Canadian Critical Care Trials Group. A total of 838 critically ill nonpregnant patients were randomized to restrictive red cell transfusions to maintain hemoglobin concentration over 7 g/dL, or to liberal transfusions to maintain the hemoglobin 10 to 12 g/dL. The 30-day mortality rate was similar (19 versus 23 percent, restrictive versus liberal), however, in the less ill patients (APACHE score 20 or less) the 30-day mortality was significantly lower in the restrictive group (9 versus 26 percent). Morrison and colleagues (1991) reported no benefits of red cell transfusions given to women who had suffered postpartum hemorrhage and who were *isovolemic but anemic* with a hematocrit between 18 and 25 volume percent. **Clearly, the level to which a woman is transfused depends not only on the present red cell mass, but also on the likelihood of additional blood loss.**

BLOOD AND COMPONENT REPLACEMENT. Contents and effects of transfusion of various blood components are shown in Table 25–8. **Compatible whole blood is ideal for treatment of hypovolemia from catastrophic acute hemorrhage.** It has a shelf life of 40 days, and 70 percent of the transfused red cells remain viable for at least 24 hours following transfusion. It replaces many coagulation factors, and especially fibrinogen, and its plasma expands the hypovolemia from hemorrhage. Overall, the bleeding patient is resuscitated with fewer blood donor exposures with whole blood. One unit of whole blood will raise the hematocrit by 3 to 4 volume percent. For two decades, in most cases of obstetrical hemorrhage, as well as most every other field of medicine, red cell replacement has been used and usually proves to be sufficient. The exception is the woman with torrential bleeding.

Autotransfusion has been used for many years in surgical procedures and is becoming more popular (Schwartz, 1999). The safety of intraoperative autologous blood salvage and autotransfusion was evaluated in a multicenter historical cohort study by Rebarber and colleagues (1998). When 139 women undergoing cesarean delivery and given autotransfusion were compared with 87 control women, there were no differences in adverse outcomes. Specifically, there was no evidence for respiratory distress or amnionic fluid embolism.

Fractionation of whole blood makes available specific components—clotting factors and platelets—that otherwise would be scarce and thus unavailable for specific deficiencies. According to the National Institutes of Health (1993), component therapy provides better treatment because only the specific component needed is given. It also conserves blood resources because components from one unit of blood can be used for several patients. For these reasons, the infusion of whole banked blood is usually not necessary and rarely, available (Barber and colleagues, 1999; Bonnar, 2000; Klein, 1994).

DILUTIONAL COAGULOPATHY. When blood loss is massive, replacement with crystalloid solutions and packed red blood cells usually results in a depletion of platelets and soluble clotting factors, leading to a functional coagulopathy that clinically is indistinguishable from disseminated intravascular coagulopathy (p. 657). This impairs hemostasis and further contributes to blood loss. The most frequent coagulation defect found in women with blood loss and multiple transfusions is thrombocytopenia (Counts and associates, 1979; Wilson and associates, 1971). Because stored whole blood is deficient in factors V, VIII, XI, and platelets, and all soluble clotting factors are absent from packed red blood cells, severe hemorrhage without factor replacement may also cause hypofibrinogenemia and

TABLE 25–8. Blood Components Commonly Transfused in Obstetrics

Product	Indication	Contents	Effect
Whole blood (450 mL)	Symptomatic anemia with large volume deficits	All components	Increases hematocrit 3–4 vol% per unit
Packed red cells (250 mL)	Symptomatic anemia	Erythrocytes	Increases hematocrit 3–4 vol% per unit
Fresh-frozen plasma (250 mL)	Deficit of labile and stable coagulation factors	All clotting factors	Supplies fibrinogen 150 mg per unit and other factors
Cryoprecipitate (50 mL)	Hypofibrinogenemia	Factors VIII, vWF, XIII, fibronectin, fibrinogen	Supplies select clotting factors
Platelets (50 mL/U)	Bleeding from thrombocyto-penia	Platelets	Increases platelet count 5000–8000/μL per unit

Modified from the American Association of Blood Banks (1994).

prolongation of the prothrombin and partial thromboplastin times. In some cases, frank consumptive coagulopathy may accompany shock and confuse the distinction between dilutional and consumptive coagulopathy. Fortunately, in most situations encountered in obstetrics, treatment of both is the same.

Although various algorithms have been proposed to guide the replacement of platelets and clotting factors according to the volume of blood loss, there is great patient variability. Thus, component replacement is rarely necessary with acute replacement of 5 to 10 units of packed red blood cells or less. However, when blood loss exceeds this amount, consideration should be given to laboratory evaluation of platelet count, clotting studies, and fibrinogen levels. Fortunately, in practice the level of various clotting factors required for adequate hemostasis is quite minimal.

In the bleeding woman, the platelet count should be maintained above 50,000/μL with the infusion of platelet concentrates. A fibrinogen level of less than 100 mg/dL or sufficiently prolonged prothrombin or partial thromboplastin times in a patient with surgical bleeding is an indication for fresh-frozen plasma administration in doses of 10 to 15 mL/kg. If fibrinogen is severely depleted and the woman is bleeding, 15 units of cryoprecipitate given rapidly will result in plasma levels above 100 mg/dL.

TYPE AND SCREEN VERSUS CROSS-MATCH. Blood transfusion is usually not needed in most women delivered vaginally, and even with cesarean section, only 2 to 5 percent will require transfusion (Dickason and Dinsmoor, 1992; Klapholtz, 1990). In any women at significant risk for hemorrhage, typing and screening or cross-matching is essential. The screening procedure involves mixing the maternal serum with standard reagent red cells that contain the antigens with which most of the common clinically significant antibodies will react.

A cross-match, on the other hand, involves the use of actual donor erythrocytes rather than standard red cells. Only 0.03 to 0.07 percent of patients who are determined not to have antibodies in a type and screen procedure subsequently will have antibodies as determined by cross-match (Boral and colleagues, 1979). Thus, in an emergency, administration of screened blood very rarely results in adverse clinical sequela. Not testing for a cross-match also decreases blood bank costs. Further, blood that is cross-matched is held exclusively for a single potential recipient, whereas with screening, blood is available for more than one potential recipient and wastage of banked blood is reduced. For these reasons, type and screen is preferred in most obstetrical situations.

PACKED RED BLOOD CELLS. Cells packed from a unit of whole blood have a hematocrit of 60 to 70 volumes percent, depending upon the method used for preparation and storage. A unit of packed red blood cells contains the same volume of erythrocytes as whole blood, and will also raise the hematocrit by 3 to 4 volume percent. Packed red blood cell and crystalloid infusion are the mainstays of transfusion therapy for most cases of obstetrical hemorrhage.

PLATELETS. When transfusion is needed, it is preferable to give platelets obtained by apheresis from one donor. In this scheme, the equivalent of platelets from six individual donors is given as a one-unit one-donor transfusion. Such units generally cannot be stored more than 5 days. The donor plasma must be compatible with recipient erythrocytes. Further, because some red blood cells are invariably transfused along with the platelets, only platelets from D-negative donors should be given to D-negative recipients. Platelet transfusion is considered in a bleeding patient with a platelet count below 50,000/μL. In the **nonsurgical patient,** bleeding is rarely encountered if the platelet count exceeds 5000 to 10,000/μL (Sachs, 1991).

If single-donor platelets are not available, random donor platelet packs are used. These are prepared from individual units of whole blood by centrifugation, then resuspended in 50 to 70 mL of plasma. One unit of random donor platelets contains about 5.5×10^{10} platelets; 6 to 10 such units are generally transfused. Each unit transfused should raise the platelet count by 5000/μL (National Institutes of Health, 1993).

FRESH-FROZEN PLASMA. This component is prepared by separating plasma from whole blood and then freezing it. It is a source of all stable and labile clotting factors, including fibrinogen. It is often used in the acute treatment of women with consumptive or dilutional coagulopathy. Fresh-frozen plasma is not appropriate for use as a volume expander in the absence of specific clotting factor deficiency. It should be considered in a bleeding woman with a fibrinogen level below 100 mg/dL and abnormal prothrombin and partial thromboplastin times.

CRYOPRECIPITATE. This component is prepared from fresh-frozen plasma. It contains factor VIII: C, factor VIII: von Willebrand factor, fibrinogen (at least 150 mg), factor XIII, and fibronectin in less than 15 mL of plasma from which it was derived (American Association of Blood Banks, 1994). There is no advantage to the use of cryoprecipitate for general clotting factor replacement in the bleeding woman instead of fresh-frozen plasma. Cryoprecipitate is only indicated in states of general factor deficiency where potential volume overload is a problem, and in a few conditions involving deficiency of specific factors. A major indication for this fraction is with severe hypofibrinogenemia caused by placental abruption in a woman with surgical incisions.

AUTOLOGOUS TRANSFUSIONS. Under some circumstances, autologous blood storage for transfusion may be considered. McVay and colleagues (1989) reported observations from 273 pregnant women in whom blood was drawn in the third trimester. Minimal requirements were a hemoglobin concentration 11 g/dL or a hematocrit of 34 volume percent. However, almost three fourths of these women donated only one unit, a volume of questionable value. They reported no complications. Further, the need for transfusion generally cannot be predicted. Sherman and colleagues (1992) studied 27 women given two or more transfusions in over 16,000 deliveries. In only 40 percent was an antepartum risk factor identified. Andres and co-workers (1990) and Etchason and associates (1995) concluded that autologous transfusions were not cost effective.

TRANSFUSION-RELATED INFECTIONS. With each unit of blood or any component thereof, the recipient is exposed to the risk of blood-borne infections. In a multihospital prospective follow-up done in London, Regan and colleagues (2000) tested almost 5600 recipients of nearly 22,000 units of blood. All were seronegative when tested 9 months after transfusion for hepatitis B and C, human immunodeficiency virus (HIV) infection, and human T-cell leukemia/lymphoma virus (HTLV) types I and II.

Fortunately, the most feared infection—**human immunodeficiency virus (HIV)**—is the least common. Earlier estimates with donor screening for viral antibody placed the risk of infection at 1 in 40,000 to 1 in 310,000 (National Institutes of Health, 1993). Unfortunately, more than 60 percent of recipients of HIV-positive blood become seropositive, and half develop acquired immunodeficiency syndrome (AIDS) within 7 years (Ward and associates, 1988). Because of improved sensitivity of enzyme immunosorbent assays, the risk of HIV transmission in screened blood is currently computed to be 1 in 500,000 to 1 million donations (Cohn, 2000; Lackritz and associates, 1995; Schreiber and co-workers, 1996).

The likelihood of **HIV-2** infection is even less. After implementation of a combined HIV-1/HIV-2 screening of blood donors in 1992, only three units of 74 million tested through 1995 were positive for HIV-2 (Centers for Disease Control and Prevention, 1995).

Until relatively recently, the transmission of **non-A, non-B hepatitis virus** was much more likely to complicate transfusions. The prevalence of hepatitis C is 1 to 2 percent of donors. In the past, most cases were undetected because they caused anicteric infection, although chronic hepatitis was common (Chap. 48, p. 1289). Serological testing for hepatitis C antibody became available in 1990 and the American Association of Blood Banks mandated hepatitis C testing for all donors. With current testing techniques, the risk of hepatitis C transmission is approximately 1 in 3300 to 1 in 103,000 (Schreiber and associates, 1996; Sloand and colleagues, 1995). The risk of transmitting other infectious disease with transfusion, such as malaria and cytomegalovirus, is estimated to be less than 1 in 1 million (National Institutes of Health, 1993).

RED-CELL SUBSTITUTES. These are of three varieties: perfluorochemicals, liposome-encapsulated hemoglobin, and hemoglobin-based oxygen carriers. Their history and development was recently reviewed by Cohn (2000). Fluoridated hydrocarbons are biologically inert liquids with relatively high oxygen solubility. The use of such emulsions allows oxygen to be transported and delivered to tissues by simple diffusion. The most commonly used emulsion, Fluosol, must be stored frozen and thawed within 24 hours of use. Clinical benefits of these emulsions are not well established, but they may decrease the need for blood with extensive hemorrhage (Klein, 2000). Liposome-encapsulated hemoglobin has not proved promising. One formulation of a hemoglobin-based oxygen carrier, diaspirin cross-linked hemoglobin (DCLHb), proved to be dangerous (Sloan and colleagues, 1999). More recently, Mullon and co-workers (2000) have described successful use of polymerized bovine hemoglobin, HBOC-201, as a blood substitute for a nonpregnant women with severe autoimmune hemolytic anemia.

CONSUMPTIVE COAGULOPATHY

In 1901, DeLee reported that "temporary hemophilia" developed in a woman with a placental abruption and another with a long-dead macerated fetus. Observations that extensive placental abruption, as well as other accidents of pregnancy, were frequently associated with hypofibrinogenemia, stimulated interest in causes of intense intravascular coagulation. Although these observations were initially almost totally confined to obstetrical cases, subsequently they were made for almost all areas of medicine (Baglin, 1996). These syndromes are commonly termed **consumptive coagulopathy or disseminated intravascular coagulation.**

PREGNANCY HYPERCOAGULABILITY. Pregnancy normally induces appreciable increases in the concentrations of coagulation factors I (fibrinogen), VII, VIII, IX, and X. Other plasma factors and platelets do not change so remarkably. Plasminogen levels are increased considerably, yet plasmin activity antepartum is normally decreased compared with the nonpregnant state. Various stimuli act to incite the conversion of plasminogen to plasmin, and one of the most potent is activation of coagulation.

PATHOLOGICAL ACTIVATION OF COAGULATION. In normal circumstances, there is no appreciable continuous physiological intravascular coagulation. During pregnancy, there does appear to be increased activation of platelet, clotting, and fibrinolytic mechanisms in vivo. Gerbasi and colleagues (1990) found significant increases in fibrinopeptide A, β-thromboglobulin, platelet factor 4, and fibrinogen–fibrin degradation products. They concluded that this compensated, accelerated intravascular coagulation may serve for maintenance of the uteroplacental interface.

In pathological states, coagulation may be activated via the extrinsic pathway by thromboplastin from tissue destruction and perhaps via the intrinsic pathway by collagen and other tissue components when there is loss of endothelial integrity (Fig. 25–33). Tissue factor is released and complexes with factor VII. This is turn activates tenase (factor IX) and prothrombinase (factor X) complexes (Fig. 25–34). Common inciting factors in obstetrics include thromboplastin from placental abruption as well as endotoxin and exotoxins. Another mechanism is by direct activation of factor X by proteases, for example, as present in mucin or produced by neoplasms. Amnionic fluid contains abundant mucin from fetal squames, and this likely causes rapid defibrination with amnionic fluid embolism.

Consumptive coagulopathy is almost always seen as a complication of an identifiable, underlying pathological process against which treatment must be directed to reverse defibrination. Thus identification and prompt elimination of the source of the coagulopathy is the first priority in dealing with it. With pathological activation of procoagulants that triggers disseminated intravascular coagulation, there is consumption of platelets and coagulation factors in variable quantities. As a consequence, fibrin may be deposited in small vessels of virtually every organ system. Fortunately, this seldom causes organ failure. Small vessels are protected because coagulation releases fibrin monomers that combine with tissue plasminogen activator (t-PA) and plasminogen, which releases plasmin. In turn, plasmin lyses fibrinogen, fibrin monomer, and fibrin polymers to form a series of fibrinogen–fibrin derivatives. These share immunological determinants known as fibrin degradation products or split products.

SIGNIFICANCE. In addition to bleeding and circulatory obstruction, which may cause ischemia from hypoperfusion, consumptive coagulopathy may be associated with microangiopathic hemolysis. This is caused by mechanical disruption of the erythrocyte membrane within small vessels in which fibrin has been deposited. Varying degrees of hemolysis with anemia, hemoglobinemia, hemoglobinuria, and erythrocyte morphological changes are produced. This process likely causes or contributes to the hemolysis encountered with the so-called *HELLP syndrome* (Pritchard and colleagues, 1976).

In obstetrical syndromes involving consumptive coagulopathy, the importance of vigorous restoration and maintenance of the circulation to treat hypovolemia and persistent intravascular coagulation cannot be overemphasized. With adequate perfusion of vital organs, activated coagulation factors and circulating fibrin and fibrin degradation products are promptly removed by the reticuloendothelial system. At the same time, hepatic and endothelial synthesis of procoagulants is promoted.

The likelihood of life-threatening hemorrhage in obstetrical situations complicated by defective coagulation will depend not only on the extent of the coagulation defects but—of great importance—on whether or

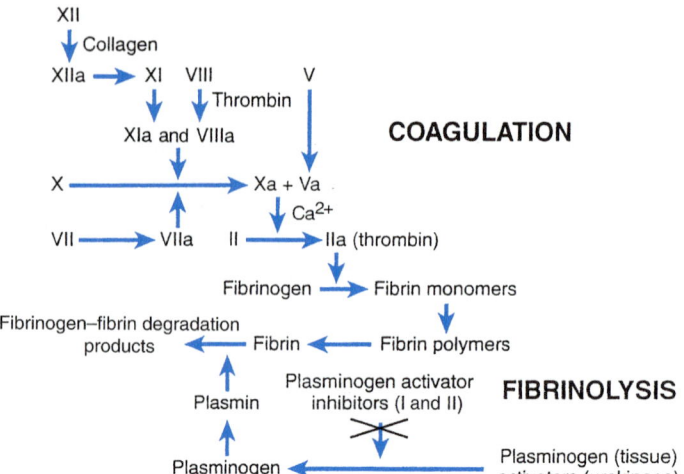

FIGURE 25–33. The coagulation and fibrinolysis cascades. (From Baker and Cunningham, 1999.)

not the vasculature is intact or disrupted. With gross derangement of blood coagulation, there may be fatal hemorrhage when vascular integrity is disrupted, yet no hemorrhage as long as all blood vessels remain intact.

**CLINICAL AND LABORATORY EVIDENCE OF DEFEC-
TIVE HEMOSTASIS.** *Bioassay* is an excellent method to clinically detect or suspect significant coagulopathy. **Excessive bleeding at sites of modest trauma characterizes defective hemostasis.** Persistent bleeding from venipuncture sites, nicks from shaving the perineum or abdomen, trauma from insertion of a catheter, and spontaneous bleeding from the gums or nose are signs of possible coagulation defects. Purpuric areas at pressure sites may indicate incoagulable blood, or more com-

monly, clinically significant thrombocytopenia. A surgical procedure provides the ultimate bioassay for coagulation. Continuous generalized oozing from the skin, subcutaneous and fascial tissues, and vascular retroperitoneal space, should at least suggest coagulopathy. Such evidence also may be gained by observing continuous oozing from episiotomy incisions or perineal lacerations.

HYPOFIBRINOGENEMIA. In late pregnancy, plasma fibrinogen levels typically are 300 to 600 mg/dL. With activation of coagulation, these high levels may sometimes serve to protect against clinically significant hypofibrinogenemia. To promote clinical coagulation, fibrinogen levels must be around 150 mg/dL. If serious *hypofibrinogenemia* is present, the clot formed from whole blood in a glass tube may initially be soft but not necessarily remarkably reduced in volume. Then, over the next half hour or so, it becomes quite small, so that many of the erythrocytes are extruded and the volume of liquid clearly exceeds that of the clot.

FIBRIN AND FIBRINOGEN DERIVATIVES. Fibrin degradation products in serum may be detected by a number of sensitive test systems. Monoclonal antibodies to detect the D-dimer are commonly used. With clinically significant consumption coagulopathy, these measurements are always abnormally high.

THROMBOCYTOPENIA. Serious thrombocytopenia is likely if petechiae are abundant, clotted blood fails to retract over a period of an hour or so, or if platelets are rare in a stained blood smear. Confirmation is provided by platelet count.

**PROTHROMBIN AND PARTIAL THROMBOPLASTIN
TIMES.** Prolongation of these coagulation tests may be the consequence of appreciable reductions in those co-

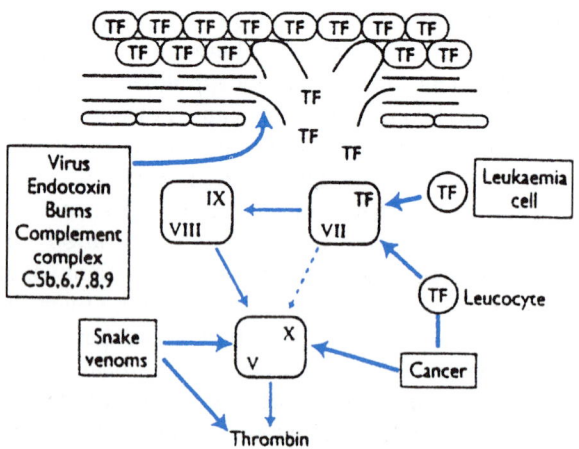

FIGURE 25–34. Pathological thrombin generation can be triggered at almost any point in the coagulation pathway. Thrombin generation driven by uncontrolled tissue factor (TF) is a major component in most forms of consumptive coagulopathy. (From Baglin, 1996, with permission.)

agulants essential for generating thrombin, a fibrinogen concentration below a critical level of about 100 mg/dL, or appreciable amounts of circulating fibrinogen–fibrin degradation products. Prolongation of the prothrombin time and partial thromboplastin time need not be the consequence of disseminated intravascular coagulation.

HEPARIN. **The infusion of heparin to try to block disseminated intravascular coagulation associated with placental abruption or other situations in which the integrity of the vascular system is compromised is mentioned only to condemn its use.**

EPSILON-AMINOCAPROIC ACID. Epsilon-aminocaproic acid has been administered to try to control fibrinolysis by inhibiting the conversion of plasminogen to plasmin and the proteolytic action of plasmin on fibrinogen, fibrin monomer, and fibrin polymer (clot). Failure to clear fibrin polymer from the microcirculation could result in organ ischemia and infarction, such as renal cortical necrosis. Its use in most types of obstetrical coagulopathy is **not** recommended.

ABRUPTIO PLACENTAE. Abruptio placentae is the most common cause of severe consumptive coagulopathy in obstetrics. It is discussed on page 621.

FETAL DEATH AND DELAYED DELIVERY. Although in most women with fetal death, spontaneous labor eventually ensues—most often within 2 weeks—the psychological stress imposed by carrying a dead fetus usually prompts induction of labor at the time of discovery. This also obviates the dangers of coagulation defects that may develop. Undoubtedly, the advent of more effective methods of labor induction have enhanced the desirability of early delivery (Chap. 20).

COAGULATION CHANGES. Weiner and associates reported in 1950 that some isoimmunized D-negative women who carried a dead fetus developed coagulation defects. Prospective studies indicated that gross disruption of the maternal coagulation mechanism rarely developed before less than 1 month after fetal death (Pritchard, 1959, 1973). If the fetus was retained longer, however, about 25 percent of the women developed a coagulopathy.

Typically the fibrinogen concentration falls to levels that are normal for the nonpregnant state, and in some cases it falls to potentially dangerous concentrations of 100 mg/dL or less (Pritchard, 1973). The rate of decrease commonly found is demonstrated in Figure 25–35. Simultaneously, fibrin degradation products are elevated in serum. The platelet count tends to decrease in these instances, but severe thrombocytopenia is uncommon even if the fibrinogen level is quite low. Although coagu-

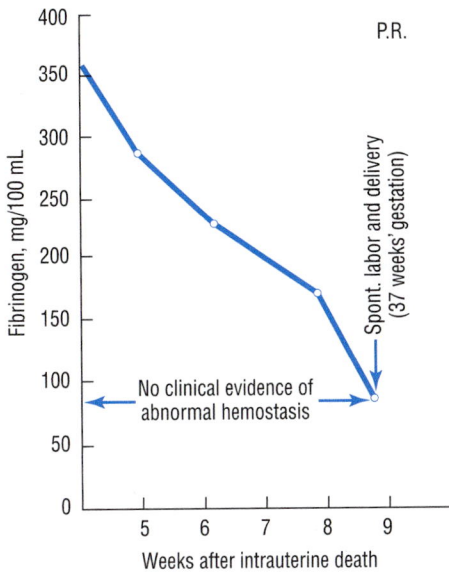

FIGURE 25–35. Slow development of maternal hypofibrinogenemia following fetal death and delayed delivery. (From Pritchard, 1959, with permission.)

lation defects may correct spontaneously before evacuation, this is unusual and happens quite slowly (Pritchard, 1959).

PATHOGENESIS. It was clearly established that consumptive coagulopathy, presumably mediated by thromboplastin from the dead products of conception, is operational in these cases (Jimenez and Pritchard, 1968; Lerner and associates, 1967). Heparin infused alone over a few days corrected the coagulation defects, but ε-aminocaproic acid did not.

HEPARIN. Correction of coagulation defects has been accomplished using low doses of heparin—5000 U two to three times daily—under carefully controlled conditions *in women with an intact circulation* (Weiner, 1991). Heparin appropriately administered can block further pathological consumption of fibrinogen and other clotting factors, thereby slowing or temporarily reversing the cycle of consumption and fibrinolysis. Such correction should be undertaken only if the patient is not actively bleeding, and with simultaneous steps to effect delivery.

FETAL DEATH IN MULTIFETAL PREGNANCY. It is uncommon that an obvious coagulation derangement develops in multifetal pregnancy complicated by death of at least one fetus and survival of another (Landy and Weingold, 1989). Carlson and Towers (1989) described 642 multifetal gestations of which 3 percent were complicated by death of only one fetus. Fusi and Gordon (1990) reported 11 of 485 twin pairs in which one fetus

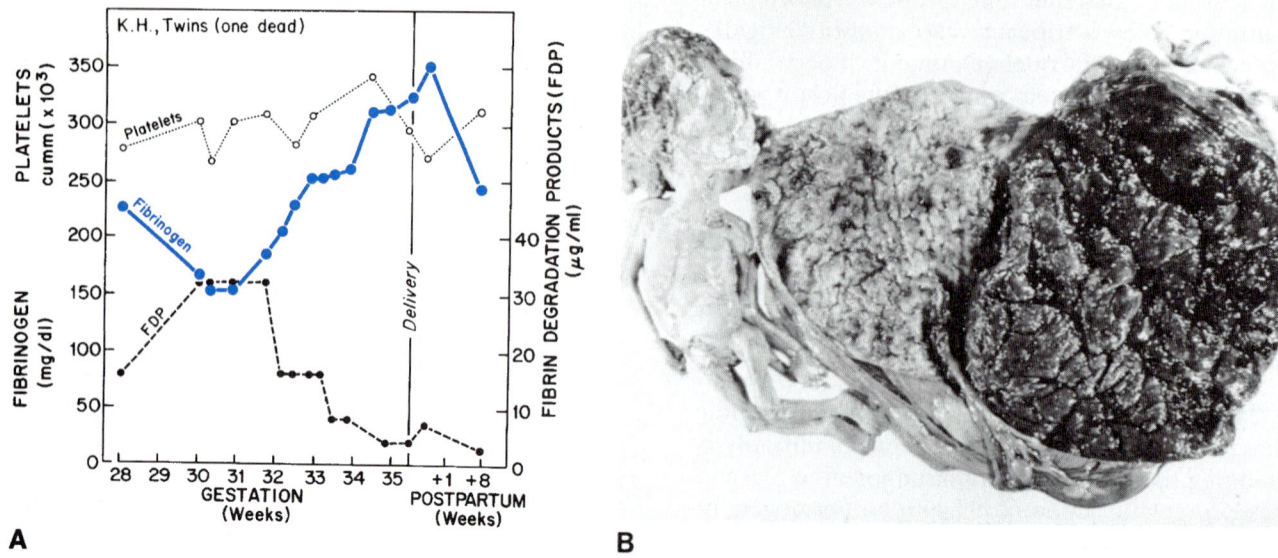

A   **B**

FIGURE 25–36. **A.** Death of one twin was confirmed sonographically at 28 weeks' gestation. Coagulation studies then demonstrated a somewhat low plasma fibrinogen concentration and abnormal amounts of fibrin degradation products (FDP). These abnormalities became more intense 2 weeks later. Then, spontaneously, the fibrinogen concentration rose, and the fibrin degradation products fell in mirror fashion. The live-born infant was healthy, and coagulation studies on cord plasma and serum were normal. **B.** The fibrin-filled placenta of the long-dead fetus is apparent. Presumably, the fibrin curtailed the escape of thromboplastin from the dead products into the maternal circulation.

died. Santema and associates (1995) followed 29 consecutive pregnancies in which one twin died after 20 weeks. Chitkara and colleagues (1989) performed selective termination in 17 twin pairs between 20 and 24 weeks. Petersen and Nyholm (1999) followed 22 multifetal pregnancies with one fetal death after the first trimester. In none of these almost 100 cases was a coagulopathy detected.

Chescheir and Seeds (1988) reported a woman in whom, following death of one of twin fetuses, there was progressive but transient fall in plasma fibrinogen concentration and rise in fibrin split products. We have encountered only a few such cases at Parkland Hospital, and one is shown in Figure 25–36. Coagulation changes ceased spontaneously, and the surviving fetus, when delivered near term, was healthy. The placenta of the long-dead fetus was filled with fibrin. Most cases are in monochorionic twins with vascular anastomoses (Chap. 30, p. 784). The survivor-twin has an extremely high risk of cerebral palsy and other cerebral impairment (Pharoah and Adi, 2000). Although perfusion abnormalities seem the likely cause of these problems, some investigators attribute cerebral hemorrhage to disseminated intravascular coagulation and have recommended heparin administration for women with one dead twin (Romero and colleagues, 1984).

AMNIONIC FLUID EMBOLISM. This is a complex disorder classically characterized by the abrupt onset of hypotension, hypoxia, and consumptive coagulopathy. There is great individual variation in its clinical manifestation and women will be encountered in whom one of these three clinical hallmarks dominates, or is entirely absent. The syndrome is uncommon in an absolute sense; however, it is a common cause of maternal death (Berg and associates, 1996; Koonin and colleagues, 1997). Using data from 1.1 million deliveries in California, Gilbert and Danielsen (1999) estimated a frequency of about 1 case per 20,000 deliveries.

In obvious cases, the clinical picture frequently is dramatic. Classically, a woman in the late stages of labor or immediately postpartum begins gasping for air, and then rapidly suffers seizure or cardiorespiratory arrest complicated by disseminated intravascular coagulation, massive hemorrhage, and death. There appears to be great variation in clinical presentations of this condition. We have managed a number of women in whom otherwise uncomplicated vaginal delivery was followed by severe acute disseminated intravascular coagulation without cardiorespiratory symptoms. Thus, in some women, consumptive coagulopathy appears to be the *forme fruste* of amnionic fluid embolism (Davies, 1999; Porter and colleagues, 1996).

PATHOGENESIS. Amnionic fluid embolism was originally described in 1941 by Steiner and Luschbaugh, who found evidence of fetal debris in the pulmonary circulation of a group of women dying during labor. Subsequent studies by Adamsons and associates (1971) and Stolte and co-workers (1967), however, clearly demonstrated that amnionic fluid itself is innocuous, even when infused in large amounts. Cumulative data from the National Amniotic Fluid Embolism Registry suggested a clinical picture similar to that seen in human anaphylaxis and unlike an embolic phenomenon as commonly understood (Clark and co-workers, 1995).

Amnionic fluid enters the circulation as a result of a breach in the physiological barrier that normally exists between maternal and fetal compartments. Such events appear to be common, if not universal, with both squames of presumed fetal origin and trophoblasts being commonly found in the maternal circulation (Clark and colleagues, 1986; Lee and co-workers, 1986). There may be maternal exposure to various fetal elements during pregnancy termination, following amniocentesis or trauma, or more commonly during labor or delivery as small lacerations develop in the lower uterine segment or cervix. Alternately, cesarean section affords ample opportunity for mixture of maternal blood and fetal tissue.

In most cases, these events are innocuous. In certain women, however, such exposure initiates a complex series of physiological reactions mimicking those seen in human anaphylaxis and sepsis (Table 25–9). A similar process has been shown for traumatic fat embolism, a process once felt to involve simple vascular obstruction following trauma (Peltier, 1984). The pathophysiological cascade likely is caused by a number of chemokines and cytokines. For example, Khong (1998) found intense expression of endothelin-1 in fetal squames recovered from the lungs of two fatal cases.

PATHOPHYSIOLOGY. Studies in primates using homologous amnionic fluid injection, as well as a carefully performed study in the goat model, have provided important insights into central hemodynamic aberrations (Adamsons and co-workers, 1971; Hankins and colleagues, 1993; Stolte and colleagues, 1967). After a brief initial phase of pulmonary and systemic hypertension, there is decreased systemic vascular resistance and left ventricular stroke work index (Clark and colleagues, 1988). Transient but profound oxygen desaturation is often seen in the initial phase, resulting in neurological injury in most survivors (Harvey and associates, 1996). In women who live beyond the initial cardiovascular collapse, a secondary phase of lung injury and coagulopathy often ensues.

The association of uterine hypertonus with cardiovascular collapse appears to be the effect of amnionic fluid embolism rather than the cause (Clark and co-workers, 1995). Indeed, uterine blood flow ceases completely when intrauterine pressures exceed 35 to 40 mm Hg (Towell, 1976), thus, a hypertonic contraction is the *least* likely time for fetal–maternal exchange to take place. Similarly, there is no causal association between oxytocin use and amnionic fluid embolism, and the frequency of oxytocin use is not increased in these women (American College of Obstetricians and Gynecologists, 1993).

DIAGNOSIS. In the past, the detection of squamous cells or other debris of fetal origin in the central pulmonary circulation was felt to be pathognomonic for amnionic fluid embolism. Indeed, in fatal cases, histopathological findings may be dramatic, especially in those involving meconium-stained amnionic fluid (Fig. 25–37). The detection of such debris, however, may require extensive special staining and even then it is often not seen. In the National Registry, fetal elements were detected in 75 percent of autopsies and 50 percent of specimens

TABLE 25–9. Clinical Findings in 84 Women with Amnionic Fluid Embolism

Clinical Findings	Clark et al (1995) (n = 46)	Weiwen (2000) (n = 38)
Hypotension	43	38
Fetal distress	30/30	NS
Pulmonary edema or ARDS	28/30	11
Cardiopulmonary arrest	40	38
Cyanosis	38	38
Coagulopathy	38	12/16
Dyspnea	22/45	38
Seizure	22	6

ARDS = acute respiratory distress syndrome; NS = not stated.

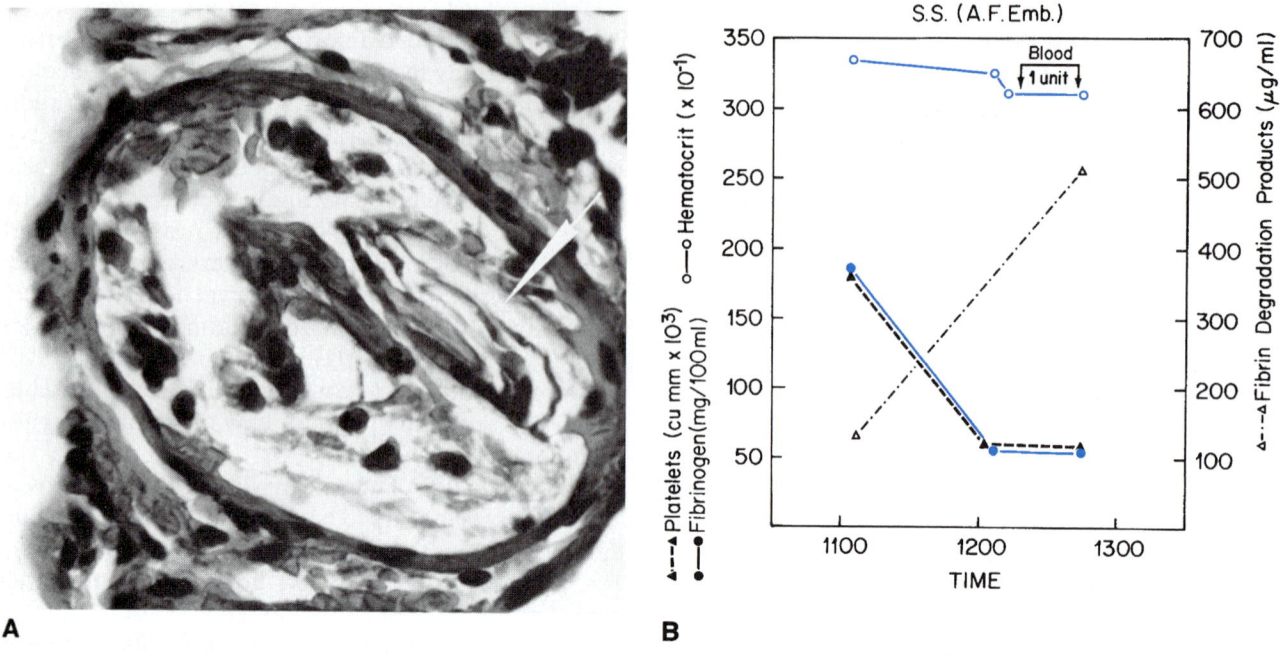

FIGURE 25–37. A. Fetal squames (*arrow*) packed into a small pulmonary artery from a fatal case of amnionic fluid embolism. Most of the empty spaces within the vessel were demonstrated by appropriate staining for lipid to have been filled with vernix caseosa. **B.** Levels of fibrinogen, fibrinogen–fibrin degradation products, and platelets during fatal amnionic fluid embolism.

prepared from concentrated buffy coat aspirates from a pulmonary artery catheter before death. Further, several studies have demonstrated that squamous cells, trophoblasts, and other debris of fetal origin may commonly be found in the central circulation of women with conditions other than amnionic fluid embolism. Thus, this finding is neither sensitive nor specific, and the diagnosis is generally made by identifying clinically characteristic signs and symptoms. In less typical cases, diagnosis is contingent upon careful exclusion of other causes.

MANAGEMENT. Although an initial period of systemic and pulmonary hypertension appears to be involved in amnionic fluid embolism, this phase is transient. Women who survive long enough to receive any treatment other than cardiopulmonary resuscitation should receive therapy directed at oxygenation and support of the failing myocardium. Circulatory support and blood and component replacement are paramount. **There are no data that any type of intervention improves maternal prognosis with amnionic fluid embolism.** In undelivered women suffering cardiac arrest, consideration should be given to emergency perimortem cesarean delivery in an effort to improve newborn outcome. However, for the mother who is hemodynamically unstable, but who has not suffered arrest, such decision making becomes more complex.

PROGNOSIS. The dismal outcomes with amnionic fluid embolism are undoubtedly related to reporting biases. Also, the syndrome likely is underdiagnosed in all but the most severe cases. In the National Registry series, there was a 60 percent maternal mortality rate. In the California database of 1.1 million deliveries by Gilbert and Danielson (1999), only a fourth of reported cases were fatal. Weiwen (2000) has provided preliminary data from 38 cases in the Suzhou region of China. Almost 90 percent of these women died. Death can be amazingly rapid, and of the 34 women who died in the series from China, 12 died with 30 minutes.

Profound neurological impairment is common in survivors. Of women reported to the National Registry who had cardiac arrest in conjunction with initial symptoms, only 8 percent survived neurologically intact. Outcome is also poor for fetuses of these latter women and is related to arrest-to-delivery interval. Overall neonatal survival is 70 percent, but almost half suffer residual neurological impairment.

SEPTICEMIA. Infections that lead to bacteremia and septic shock in obstetrics are most commonly due to septic abortion, antepartum pyelonephritis, or puerperal sepsis. Other aspects of septic shock are discussed in Chapter 43 (p. 1167).

COAGULOPATHY. The lethal properties of bacterial toxins, and especially endotoxins, are undoubtedly mediated largely by disruption of vascular endothelium. It is unclear, however, whether this is the major mechanism that initiates consumptive coagulopathy. For example, in experimental animals, endothelial damage is greatest 24 hours after endotoxin is given, but intravascular coagulation can usually be identified during the first few hours. More likely, as shown in Figure 25–34, endotoxin activates the extrinsic clotting mechanism through cytokine-induced tissue factor expression on the surface of activated monocytes (Levi and colleagues, 1993). The intrinsic route seems unimportant in this role.

MANAGEMENT. Therapy for women with septicemia from any cause is outlined in Chapter 43 (p. 1167). In general, treatment of the inciting cause will be followed by reversal of the coagulopathy. In some cases, especially if surgical procedures are performed before sepsis is controlled and the coagulopathy is reversed, treatment with fresh-frozen plasma and platelet packs usually will arrest such bleeding. **Heparin therapy is dangerous and should not be given.**

ABORTION. Remarkable blood loss may occur as the consequence of abortion. Hemorrhage during early pregnancy is less likely to be severe unless abortion was induced and the procedure was traumatic. When pregnancy is more advanced, the mechanisms responsible for hemorrhage are most often the same as those described for placental abruption and placenta previa— that is, the disruption of a large number of maternal blood vessels at the site of placental implantation.

COAGULATION DEFECTS. Serious disruption of the coagulation mechanism as the consequence of abortion may develop in the following circumstances:

1. Prolonged retention of a dead fetus, as already described.
2. Sepsis, a notorious cause.
3. Intrauterine instillation of hypertonic saline or urea solutions.
4. Medical induction with a prostaglandin.
5. During instrumental termination of the pregnancy.

The kinds of changes in coagulation that have been identified with abortion induced with *hypertonic solutions* imply at least that thromboplastin is released from placenta, fetus, decidua, or all three by the necrobiotic effect of the hypertonic solutions, which then initiates coagulation within the maternal circulation (Burkman and associates, 1977). Coagulation defects have been observed to develop rarely during induction of abortion with prostaglandin. Saraiya and colleagues (1999) reported 62 spontaneous-abortion related deaths reported

to the Pregnancy Mortality Surveillance System. Almost 60 percent of deaths were caused by infection and half of these women had consumptive coagulopathy.

Consumptive coagulopathy has been an uncommon but serious complication among women with **septic abortion.** The incidence of coagulation defects in the past at Parkland Hospital was highest in those with *Clostridium perfringens* sepsis and intense intravascular hemolysis (Pritchard and Whalley, 1971). Management consists of prompt restoration and maintenance of the circulation, and appropriate steps to control the infection, including evacuation of the infected products (Chap. 33, p. 877).

REFERENCES

Abdella TN, Sibai BM, Hays JM Jr, Anderson GD: Perinatal outcome in abruptio placentae. Obstet Gynecol 63:365, 1984

Adamsons K, Mueller-Heubach E, Myer RE: The innocuousness of amniotic fluid infusion in the pregnant rhesus monkey. Am J Obstet Gynecol 109:997, 1971

Ajayi RA, Soothill PW, Campbell S, Nicolaides KH: Antenatal testing to predict outcome in pregnancies with unexplained antepartum haemorrhage. Br J Obstet Gynaecol 99:122, 1992

Allahbadia G: Hypogastric artery ligation: A new perspective. J Gynecol Surg 9:35, 1993

Alvarez M, Lockwood CJ, Ghidini A, Dottino P, Mitty HA, Berkowitz RL: Prophylactic and emergent arterial catheterization for selective embolization in obstetric hemorrhage. Am J Perinatol 9:441, 1992

American Association of Blood Banks: Circular of information for the use of human blood and blood components. American Red Cross 1751, March 1994

American College of Obstetricians and Gynecologists: Vaginal birth after previous cesarean delivery. ACOG Practice Bulletin No. 5, July 1999

American College of Obstetricians and Gynecologists: Prologue—Obstetrics, 3rd ed. 1993, p 65

Ammini AC, Mathur SK: Sheehan syndrome: An analysis of possible aetiological factors. Aust NZ J Obstet Gynecol 34:534, 1994

Ananth CV, Berkowitz GS, Savitz DA, Lapinski RH: Placental abruption and adverse perinatal outcomes. JAMA 282:1646, 1999b

Ananth CV, Savitz DA, Williams MA: Placental abruption and its association with hypertension and prolonged rupture of membranes: A methodologic review and meta-analysis. Obstet Gynecol 88:309, 1996

Ananth CV, Smulian JC, Vintzileos AM: Incidence of placental abruption in relation to cigarette smoking and hypertensive disorders during pregnancy: A meta-analysis of observational studies. Obstet Gynecol 93:622, 1999a

Andres RL, Piacquadio KM, Resnik R: A reappraisal of the need for autologous blood donation in the obstetric patient. Am J Obstet Gynecol 163:1551, 1990

Archer GE, Furlong LA: Acute abdomen caused by placenta percreta in the second trimester. Am J Obstet Gynecol 157:146, 1987

Babinszki A, Kerenyi T, Torok O, Grazi V, Lapinski RH,

Berkowitz RL: Perinatal outcome in grand and great-grand multiparity: Effects of parity on obstetric risk factors. Am J Obstet Gynecol 181:669, 1999

Baglin T: Disseminated intravascular coagulation: Diagnosis and treatment. BMJ 312:683, 1996

Baker PN, Cunningham FG: Platelet and coagulation abnormalities. In Lindheimer ML, Roberts JM, Cunningham FG (eds): Chesley's Hypertensive Disorders in Pregnancy, 2nd ed. Stamford, CT, Appleton & Lange, 1999, p 349

Bakiri F, Bendib SE, Maoui R, Bendib A, Benmiloud M: The sella turcica in Sheehan's syndrome: Computerized tomographic study in 54 patients. J Endocrinol Invest 14:193, 1991

Barber A, Shires GT III, Shires GT: Shock. In Schwartz SI, Shires GT, Spencer FC, Daly JM, Fischer JE, Galloway AC (eds): Principles of Surgery, 7th ed. New York, McGraw-Hill, 1999, p 101

Benirschke K, Kaufmann P (eds): Pathology of the Human Placenta. 4th ed. New York, Springer, 2000, p 554

Bennett BB: Uterine rupture during induction of labor at term with intravaginal misoprostol. Obstet Gynecol 89:832, 1997

Berchuck A, Sokol RJ: Previous cesarean section, placenta increta, and uterine rupture in second-trimester abortion. Am J Obstet Gynecol 145:766, 1983

Berg CJ, Atrash HK, Koonin LM, Tucker M: Pregnancy-related mortality in the United States, 1987–1990. Obstet Gynecol 88:161, 1996

Bill AH: The treatment of placenta previa by prophylactic blood transfusion and cesarean section. Am J Obstet Gynecol 14:523, 1927

Bingol N, Fuchs M, Diaz V, Stone RK, Gromish DS: Teratogenicity of cocaine in humans. J Pediatr 110:93, 1987

Biswas R, Sawhney H, Dass R, Saran RK, Vasishta K: Histopathological study of placental bed biopsy in placenta previa. Acta Obstet Gynecol Scan 78:173, 1999

Bitterman H, Smith BA, Lefer AM: Beneficial actions of antagonism of peptide leukotrienes in hemorrhagic shock. Circ Shock 24:159, 1988

Bland RD, Shoemaker WC, Abraham E, Cobo JC: Hemodynamic and oxygen transport patterns in surviving and nonsurviving postoperative patients. Crit Care Med 13:85, 1985

Bond AL, Edersheim TG, Curry L, Druzin ML, Hutson JM: Expectant management of abruptio placentae before 35 weeks gestation. Am J Perinatol 6:121, 1989

Bonnar J: Massive obstetric hemorrhage. Baillieres Clin Obstet Gynaecol 14:1, 2000

Bonnar J, McNicol GP, Douglas AS: The behavior of the coagulation and fibrinolytic mechanism in abruptio placentae. J Obstet Gynaecol Br Commonw 76:799, 1969

Boral LI, Hill SS, Apollon CJ, Folland A: The type and antibody screen, revisited. Am J Clin Pathol 71:578, 1979

Brame RG, Harbert GM Jr, McGaughey HS Jr, Thornton WN Jr: Maternal risk in abruption. Obstet Gynecol 31:224, 1968

Brar HS, Platt DL, DeVore GR, Horenstein J: Fetal umbilical velocimetry for the surveillance of pregnancies complicated by placenta previa. J Reprod Med 33:741, 1988

Breen JL, Neubecker R, Gregori CA, Franklin JE Jr: Placenta accreta, increta, and percreta: A survey of 40 cases. Obstet Gynecol 49:43, 1977

Burchell RC: Physiology of internal iliac artery ligation. J Obstet Gynaecol Br Commonw 75:642, 1968

Burkman RT, Bell WR, Atienza MF, King TM: Coagulopathy with midtrimester induced abortion: Association with hyperosmolar urea administration. Am J Obstet Gynecol 127:533, 1977

Carlson NJ, Towers CV: Multiple gestation complicated by the death of one fetus. Obstet Gynecol 73:685, 1989

Catanzarite VA, Moffitt KD, Baker ML, Awadalla SG, Argubright KF, Perkins RP: New approaches to the management of acute puerperal uterine invasion. Obstet Gynecol 68:7S, 1986

Centers for Disease Control and Prevention: Use of hospital discharge data to monitor uterine rupture—Massachusetts, 1990–1997. MMWR 49:245, 2000

Centers for Disease Control and Prevention: Update: HIV-2 infection among blood and plasma donors–United States, June 1992–June 1995. MMWR 44:603, 1995

Chapman S, Crispens MA, Owen J, Savage K: Complications of mid-trimester pregnancy terminations: The effect of prior cesarean delivery. Am J Obstet Gynecol 174:356, 1996

Chescheir NC, Seeds JW: Spontaneous resolution of hypofibrinogenemia associated with death of a twin in utero: A case report. Am J Obstet Gynecol 159:1183, 1988

Chestnut DH, Eden SD, Gall SA, Parker RT: Peripartum hysterectomy: A review of cesarean and postpartum hysterectomy. Obstet Gynecol 65:365, 1985

Chiao J, Minei JP, Shires GT: In vivo myocyte sodium activity and concentration during hemorrhagic shock. Am J Physiol 258:R864, 1990

Chichakli LO, Atrash HK, Mackay AP, Musani AS, Berg BJ: Pregnancy-related mortality in the United States due to hemorrhage: 1979–1992. Obstet Gynecol 94:721, 1999

Chin HG, Scott DR, Resnik R, Davis GB, Lurie AL: Angiographic embolization of intractable puerperal hematomas. Am J Obstet Gynecol 160:434, 1989

Chitkara U, Berkowitz RL, Wilkins IA, Lynch L, Mehalek KE, Alvarez M: Selective second-trimester termination of the anomalous fetus in twin pregnancies. Obstet Gynecol 75:690, 1989

Cho JY, Kim SJ, Cha KY, Kay CW, Kim MI, Cha KS: Interrupted circular suture: Bleeding control during cesarean delivery in placenta previa accreta. Obstet Gynecol 78:876, 1991

Clark SL, Cotton DB, Gonik B, Greenspoon J, Phelan JP: Central hemodynamic alterations in amniotic fluid embolism. Am J Obstet Gynecol 158:1124, 1988

Clark SL, Hankins GDV, Dudley DA, Dildy GA, Porter TF: Amniotic fluid embolism: Analysis of the National Registry. Am J Obstet Gynecol 172:1159, 1995

Clark SL, Pavlova Z, Greenspoon J, Horenstein J, Phelan JP: Squamous cells in the maternal pulmonary circulation. Am J Obstet Gynecol 154:104, 1986

Clark SL, Phelan JP, Yeh SY: Hypogastric artery ligation for obstetric hemorrhage. Obstet Gynecol 66:353, 1985

Clark SL, Yeh SY, Phelan JP, Paul RH: Emergency hysterectomy for obstetric hemorrhage. Obstet Gynecol 64:376, 1984

Cochrane Injuries Group Albumin Reviewers: Human albumin administration in critically ill patients: Systematic review of randomised control trials. BMJ 317:235, 1998

Cohn SM: Blood substitutes in surgery. Surgery 127:599, 2000

Combs CA, Laros RK: Prolonged third stage of labor: Morbidity and risk factors. Obstet Gynecol 77:863, 1991

Combs CA, Murphy EL, Laros RKL Jr: Factors associated with hemorrhage in cesarean deliveries. Obstet Gynecol 77:77, 1991a

Combs CA, Murphy EL, Laros RKL Jr: Factors associated with postpartum hemorrhage with vaginal birth. Obstet Gynecol 77:69, 1991b

Combs CA, Nyberg DA, Mack LA, Smith JR, Benedetti TJ:

Expectant management after sonographic diagnosis of placental abruption. Am J Perinatol 9:170, 1992

Comeau J, Shaw L, Marcell CC, Lavery JP: Early placenta previa and delivery outcome. Obstet Gynecol 61:577, 1983

Consensus Development Conference: Perioperative red cell transfusion. Bethesda, National Institutes of Health, June 27–29, 1988, Vol 7, No. 4

Counts RB, Haisch C, Simon TL, Maxwell NG, Heimbach DM, Carrico CJ: Hemostasis in massively transfused trauma patients. Ann Surg 190:91, 1979

Cox SM, Carpenter RJ, Cotton DB: Placenta percreta: Ultrasound diagnosis and conservative surgical management. Obstet Gynecol 72:452, 1988

Crane JMG, Van Den Hof MC, Dodds L, Armson A, Liston R: Neonatal outcomes with placenta previa. Obstet Gynecol 93:541, 1999

Cunningham FG, Hollier LM: Fetal death. In: Williams Obstetrics, 20th ed (Suppl 4). Norwalk, CT, Appleton & Lange, August/September, 1997

Czer LSC, Shoemaker WC: Optimal hematocrit value in critically ill postoperative patients. Surg Gynecol Obstet 147:363, 1978

Davies S: Amniotic fluid embolism and isolated disseminated intravascular coagulation. Can J Anaesth 46:456, 1999

DeLee JB: A case of fatal hemorrhagic diathesis, with premature detachment of the placenta. Am J Obstet Gynecol 44:785, 1901

Dickason LA, Dinsmoor MJ: Red blood cell transfusion and cesarean section. Am J Obstet Gynecol 167:327, 1992

Drost S, Keil K: Expectant management of placenta previa: Cost-benefit analysis of outpatient treatment. Am J Obstet Gynecol 170:1254, 1994

Druzin ML: Packing of lower uterine segment for control of postcesarean bleeding in instances of placenta previa. Surg Gynecol Obstet 169:543, 1989

Eden RD, Parker RT, Gall SA: Rupture of the pregnant uterus: A 53-year review. Obstet Gynecol 68:671, 1986

Elliott JP, Gilpin B, Strong TH Jr, Finberg HJ: Chronic abruption–oligohydramnios sequence. J Reprod Med 43:418, 1998

Etchason J, Petz L, Keeler E, Calhoun L, Kleinman S, Snider C, Fink A, Brook R: The cost effectiveness of preoperative autologous blood donations. N Engl J Med 332:719, 1995

Fahmy K, el-Gazar A, Sammour M, Nosair M, Salem A: Postpartum colposcopy of the cervix: Injury and healing. Int J Gynaecol Obstet 34:133, 1991

Farine D, Fox HE, Jakobson S, Timor-Tritsch IE: Vaginal ultrasound for diagnosis of placenta previa. Am J Obstet Gynecol 159:566, 1988

Farmer RM, Kirschbaum T, Potter D, Strong TH, Medearis AL: Uterine rupture during trial of labor after previous cesarean section. Am J Obstet Gynecol 165:996, 1991

Fedorkow DM, Nimrod CA, Taylor PJ: Ruptured uterus in pregnancy: A Canadian hospital's experience. Can Med Assoc J 137:27, 1987

Flamm BL, Lim OW, Jones C, Fallon D, Newman LA, Mantis JK: Vaginal birth after cesarean section: Results of a multicenter study. Am J Obstet Gynecol 158:1079, 1988

Fox H: Placenta accreta, 1945–1969. Obstet Gynecol Surv 27:475, 1972

Frederiksen MC, Glassenberg R, Stika CS: Placenta previa: A 22-year analysis. Am J Obstet Gynecol 180:1432, 1999

Fretts RC, Usher RH: Causes of fetal death in women of advanced maternal age. Obstet Gynecol 89:40, 1997

Fuchs K, Peretz B-A, Marcovici R, Paldi E, Timor-Tritsch I:

The "grand multipara"—Is it a problem? A review of 5785 cases. Int J Gynaecol Obstet 23:321, 1985

Fusi L, Gordon H: Twin pregnancy complicated by single intrauterine death: Problems and outcome with conservative management. Br J Obstet Gynaecol 97:511, 1990

Gerbasi FR, Bottoms S, Farag A, Mammen E: Increased intravascular coagulation associated with pregnancy. Obstet Gynecol 75:385, 1990

Gherman RB, Goodwin TM: Obstetric implications of activated protein C resistance and factor V Leiden mutation. Obstet Gynecol Surv 55:117, 2000

Gilbert WM, Danielsen B: Amniotic fluid embolism: Decreased mortality in a population-based study. Obstet Gynecol 93:973, 1999

Gilstrap LC, Hauth JC, Hankins GDV, Patterson AR: Effect of type of anesthesia on blood loss at cesarean section. Obstet Gynecol 69:328, 1987

Gilstrap LC, Van Dorsten PV, Cunningham FG: Puerperal hematomas and genital tract lacerations. In: Operative Obstetrics, 2nd ed. New York, McGraw-Hill, 2001, in press

Gonen R, Hannah ME, Milligan JE: Does prolonged preterm premature rupture of the membranes predispose to abruptio placenta? Obstet Gynecol 74:347, 1989

Grimes HG, Brooks MH: Pregnancy in Sheehan's syndrome. Report of a case and review. Obstet Gynecol Surv 35:481, 1980

Grünfeld JP, Pertuiset N: Acute renal failure in pregnancy: 1987. Am J Kid Dis 9:359, 1987

Handler AS, Mason ED, Rosenberg DL, Davis FG: The relationship between exposure during pregnancy to cigarette smoking and cocaine use and placenta previa. Am J Obstet Gynecol 170:884, 1994

Hankins GDV, Berry GK, Scott RT Jr, Hood D: Maternal arterial desaturation with 15-methyl prostaglandin F_2 alpha for uterine atony. Obstet Gynecol 65:605, 1988

Hankins GDV, Snyder RR, Clark SL, Schwartz L, Patterson WR, Butzin CA: Acute hemodynamic and respiratory effects of amniotic fluid embolism in the pregnant goat model. Am J Obstet Gynecol 168:1113, 1993

Hansch E, Chitkara U, McAlpine J, El-Sayed Y, Dake MD, Razavi MK: Pelvic arterial embolization for control of obstetric hemorrhage: A five-year experience. Am J Obstet Gynecol 180:1454, 1999

Hardardottir H, Borgida AF, Sanders MM, Ernst L, Campbell WA: Histologic myometrial fibers adherent to the placenta: Impact of method of placental removal. Am J Obstet Gynecol 174:358, 1996

Harvey C, Hankins G, Clark S: Amniotic fluid embolism and oxygen transport patterns. Am J Obstet Gynecol 174:304, 1996

Hauth JC, Cunningham: Preeclampsia-eclampsia. In: Lindheimer ML, Roberts JM, Cunningham FG, (eds): Chesley's Hypertensive Disorders in Pregnancy, 2nd ed. Stamford CT, Appleton & Lange, 1999, p 179

Hebert PC, Wells G, Blajchman MA, Marshall J, Martin C, Pagliarello G, Tweeddale M, Schweitzer I, Yetisir: A multicenter, randomized, controlled clinical trial of transfusion requirements in critical care. Transfusion Requirements in Critical Care Investigators, Canadian Critical Care Trials Group. N Engl J Med 340:1056, 1999

Hertzberg BS, Bowie JD, Carroll BA, Kliewer MA, Weber TM: Diagnosis of placenta previa during the third trimester: Role of transperineal sonography. AJR 159:83, 1992

Hopkins FW, Mackay AP, Koonin LM, Berg CJ, Irwin M, Atrash HK: Pregnancy-related mortality in Hispanic women in the United States. Obstet Gynecol 94:747, 1999

Hoskins IA, Friedman DM, Frieden FJ, Ordorica SA, Young BK: Relationship between antepartum cocaine abuse, abnormal umbilical artery Doppler velocimetry, and placental abruption. Obstet Gynecol 78:279, 1991

Hsu YR, Wan YL: Successful management of intractable puerperal hematoma and severe postpartum hemorrhage with DIC through transcatheter arterial embolization—two cases. Acta Obstet Gynecol Scand 77:129, 1998

Hung TH, Shau WY, Hsieh CC, Chiu TH, Hsu JJ, Hsieh TT: Risk factors for placenta accreta. Obstet Gynecol 93:545, 1999

Hurd WW, Miodovnik M, Hertzberg V, Lavin JP: Selective management of abruptio placentae: A prospective study. Obstet Gynecol 61:467, 1983

Iyasu S, Saftlas AK, Rowley DL, Koonin LM, Lawson HW, Atrash HK: The epidemiology of placenta previa in the United States, 1979 through 1987. Am J Obstet Gynecol 168:1424, 1993

Jandl JH: Secondary defects of red cell membrane defects. In: Blood: Textbook of Hematology, 2nd ed. Boston: Little, Brown, 1996, p 404

Jimenez JM, Pritchard JA: Pathogenesis and treatment of coagulation defects resulting from fetal death. Obstet Gynecol 32:449, 1968

Johnson HW: The conservative management of some varieties of placenta previa. Am J Obstet Gynecol 50:248, 1945

Käregärd M, Gennser G: Incidence and recurrence rate of abruptio placentae in Sweden. Obstet Gynecol 67:523, 1986

Kay HH, Spritzer CE: Preliminary experience with magnetic resonance imaging in patients with third-trimester bleeding. Obstet Gynecol 78:424, 1991

Kettel LM, Branch DW, Scott JR: Occult placental abruption after maternal trauma. Obstet Gynecol 71:449, 1988

Khong TY: Expression of endothelin-1 amniotic fluid embolism and possible pathophysiological mechanism. Br J Obstet Gynecol 105:802, 1998

King DL: Placental migration demonstrated by ultrasonography. Radiology 109:163, 1973

Klapholz H: Blood transfusion in contemporary obstetric practice. Obstet Gynecol 75:940, 1990

Klein HG: The prospects for red-cell substitutes. N Engl J Med 342:1666, 2000

Klein HG: Blood groups and blood transfusion. In Isselbacher KJ, Braunwald E, Wilson JD, Martin JB, Fauci AS, Kasper DL (eds): Harrison's Principles of Internal Medicine, 13th ed. New York, McGraw-Hill, New York, 1994, p 1788

Koonin LM, MacKay AP, Berg CJ, Atrash HK, Smith JC: Pregnancy-related mortality surveillance—United States, 1987–1990. MMWR 46:17, 1997

Kovacs BW, DeVore GR: Management of acute and subacute puerperal uterine inversion with terbutaline sulfate. Am J Obstet Gynecol 150:784, 1984

Kramer MS, Usher RH, Pollack R, Boyd M, Usher S: Etiologic determinants of abruptio placentae. Obstet Gynecol 89:221, 1997

Krohn M, Voigt L, McKnight B, Daling JR, Starzyk P, Benedetti TJ: Correlates of placental abruption. Br J Obstet Gynaecol 94:333, 1987

Kupferminc MJ, Eldor A, Steinman N, Many A, Bar-Am A, Jaffa A, Fait G, Lessing JB: Increased frequency of genetic thrombophilia in women with complications of pregnancy. N Engl J Med 340:9, 1999

Lackritz EV, Satten GA, Aberle-Grasse J, Dodd RY, Raimondi VP, Janssen RS, Lewis WF, Notari EP, Petersen LR: Estimated risk of transmission of the human immunodeficiency virus by screened blood in the United States. N Engl J Med 333:1721, 1995

Laing FC: Ultrasound evaluation of obstetric problems relating to the lower uterine segment and cervix. In Fleischer AC, Manning FA, Jeanty P, Romero R (eds): Sonography in Obstetrics and Gynecology: Principles and Practice, 5th ed. Appleton & Lange, Stamford CT, 1996, p 720

Landy HJ, Weingold AB: Management of a multiple gestation complicated by an antepartum fetal demise. Obstet Gynecol Surv 44:171, 1989

Lee W, Ginsburg KA, Cotton DB, Kauffman RH: Squamous and trophoblastic cells in the maternal pulmonary circulation identified by invasive hemodynamic monitoring during the peripartum period. Am J Obstet Gynecol 155:999, 1986

Lee W, Lee VA, Kirk JS, Sloan CT, Smith RS, Comstock CH: Vasa previa: Prenatal diagnosis, natural evolution, and clinical outcome. Obstet Gynecol 95:572, 2000

Leerentveld RA, Gilberts ECAM, Aronld MJCWJ, Wladimiroff JW: Accuracy and safety of transvaginal sonographic placental localization. Obstet Gynecol 76:759, 1990

Lerner R, Margolin M, Slate WG: Heparin in the treatment of hypofibrinogenemia complicating fetal death in utero. Am J Obstet Gynecol 97:373, 1967

Levi M, ten Cate H, van der Poll T, van Deventer SJH: Pathogenesis of disseminated intravascular coagulation in sepsis. JAMA 270:975, 1993

Levrant SG, Wingate M: Midtrimester uterine rupture. J Reprod Med 41:186, 1996

Lin CC, Adamszyk CJ, Montag AG, Zelop CM, Snow JC: Placenta previa percreta involving the left broad ligament and cervix. A case report. J Reprod Med 43:839, 1998

Lindheimer MD, Grünfeld JP, Davison JM: Renal disorders. In Barron WM, Lindheimer MD (eds): Medical Disorders During Pregnancy. St Louis, Mosby, 2000, p 39

Lipitz S, Admon D, Menczer J, Ben-Baruch G, Oelsner G: Midtrimester bleeding: Variables which affect the outcome of pregnancy. Gynecol Obstet Invest 32:24, 1991

Macafee CHG: Placenta previa: A study of 174 cases. J Obstet Gynaecol Br Emp 52:313, 1945

Magriples U, Chan DW, Bruzek D, Copel JA, Hsu CD: Thrombomodulin: A new marker for placental abruption. Thromb Haemost 81:32, 1999

Major CA, deVeciana M, Lewis DF, Morgan MA: Preterm premature rupture of membranes and abruptio placentae: Is there an association between these pregnancy complications? Am J Obstet Gynecol 172:672, 1995

Maldjian C, Adam R, Pelosi M, Pelosi M III, Rudelli RD, Maldjian J: MRI appearance of placenta percreta and placenta accreta. Magn Reson Imaging 17:965, 1999

Martin JN Jr, Brewer DW, Rush LV Jr, Martin RW, Hess LW, Morrison JC: Successful pregnancy outcome following mid-gestational uterine rupture and repair using Gore-Tex soft tissue patch. Obstet Gynecol 75:518, 1990

Maymon R, Shulman A, Pomeranz M, Holtzinger M, Haimovich L, Bahary C: Uterine rupture at term pregnancy with the use of intracervical prostaglandin E₂ gel for induction of labor. Am J Obstet Gynecol 165:368, 1991

McClure N, Dornal JC: Early identification of placenta praevia. Br J Obstet Gynaecol 97:959, 1990

McMahon MJ, Luther ER, Bowes WA Jr, Olshan AF: Comparison of a trial of labor with an elective second cesarean section. N Engl J Med 335:689, 1996

McVay PA, Hoag RA, Hoag S, Toy PTCY: Safety and use of autologous blood donation during the third trimester of pregnancy. Am J Obstet Gynecol 160:1479, 1989

Mengert WJ, Burchell RC, Blumstein RW, Daskal JL: Pregnancy after bilateral ligation of the internal iliac and ovarian arteries. Obstet Gynecol 34:664, 1969

Miller DA, Diaz FG, Paul RH: Incidence of placenta previa with previous cesarean. Am J Obstet Gynecol 174:345, 1996

Miller DA, Goodwin TM, Gherman RB, Paul RH: Intrapartum rupture of the unscarred uterus. Obstet Gynecol 89:671, 1997

Miller DA, Paul RH: Rupture of the unscarred uterus. Am J Obstet Gynecol 174:345, 1996

Mishra A, Landzberg BR, Parente JT: Uterine rupture in association with alkaloidal ("crack") cocaine abuse. Am J Obstet Gynecol 243, 1995

Misra DP, Ananth CV: Risk factor profiles of placental abruption in first and second pregnancies: Heterogeneous etiologies. J Clin Epidemiol 52:453, 1999

Morgan MA, Berkowitz KM, Thomas SJ, Reimbold P, Quilligan EJ: Abruptio placentae: Perinatal outcome in normotensive and hypertensive patients. Am J Obstet Gynecol 170:1595, 1994

Morison JE: Obstetrics and Gynecology Annual. New York, Appleton-Century-Crofts, 1978, p 113

Morrison JC, Martin RW, Dodson MK, Roberts WE, Morrison FS: Blood transfusions after postpartum hemorrhage due to uterine atony. J Mat Fetal Invest 1:209, 1991

Morrison JC, Sumrall DD, Chavalier SP, Robinson SV, Morrison FS, Wiser WL: The effect of provider education on blood utilization practices. Am J Obstet Gynecol 169:1240, 1993

Mouer JR: Placenta previa: Antepartum conservative management, inpatient versus outpatient. Am J Obstet Gynecol 170:1683, 1994

Mullon J, Giacoppe G, Clagett C, McCune D, Dillard T: Transfusions of polymerized bovine hemoglobin in a patient with severe autoimmune hemolytic anemia. N Engl J Med 342:1638, 2000

Naef RW, Chauhan SP, Chevalier SP, Roberts WE, Meydrech EF, Morrison JC: Prediction of hemorrhage at cesarean delivery. Obstet Gynecol 83:923, 1994

Naeye RL: Abruptio placentae and placenta previa: Frequency, perinatal mortality, and cigarette smoking. Obstet Gynecol 55:701, 1980

Nagaya K, Fetters MD, Ishikawa M, Kubo T, Koyanagi T, Saito Y, Sameshima H, Sugimoto M, Takagi K, Chiba Y, Honda H, Mukubo M, Kawamura M, Satoh S, Neki R: Causes of maternal mortality in Japan. JAMA 283:2661, 2000

National Institutes of Health: Indications for the use of red blood cells, platelets and fresh frozen plasma. Washington, DC, US Department of Health and Human Services, Pub. No. 89-2974A, August, 1993

Nielsen TF, Hagberg H, Ljungblad U: Placenta previa and antepartum hemorrhage after previous cesarean section. Gynecol Obstet Invest 27:88, 1989

Nkata M: Rupture of the uterus: A review of 32 cases in a general hospital in Zambia. Br Med J 312:1204, 1996

O'Brien P, El-Rafaey H, Gordon A, Geary M, Rodeck CH: Rectally administered misoprostol for the treatment of postpartum hemorrhage unresponsive to oxytocin and ergometrine: A descriptive study. Obstet Gynecol 92:212, 1998

Oleen MA, Mariano JP: Controlling refractory atonic postpartum hemorrhage with Hemabate sterile solution. Am J Obstet Gynecol 162:205, 1990

Oppenheimer LW, Farine D, Ritchie JWK, Lewinsky RM, Telford J, Fairbanks LA: What is a low-lying placenta? Am J Obstet Gynecol 165:1035, 1991

Pasto ME, Kurtz AB, Rifkin MD, Cole-Beuglet C, Wapner RJ, Goldberg BB: Ultrasonographic findings in placenta increta. J Ultrasound Med 2:155, 1983

Pearlman MD, Tintinalli JE, Lorenz RP: A prospective controlled study of outcome after trauma during pregnancy. Am J Obstet Gynecol 162:1502, 1990

Pelage JP, Le Dref O, Jacob D, Soyer P, Herbreteau D, Rymer R: Selective arterial embolization of the uterine arteries in the management of intractable post-partum hemorrhage. Acta Obstet Gynecol Scand 78:698, 1999

Pelosi MA III, Pelosi MA: Spontaneous uterine rupture at thirty-three weeks subsequent to previous superficial laparoscopic myomectomy. Am J Obstet Gynecol 177:1547, 1997

Peltier LF: Fat embolism: A reappraisal of the problem. Clin Orthop 187:3, 1984

Petersen IR, Nyholm HC: Multiple pregnancies with single intrauterine demise. Description of twenty-eight pregnancies. Acta Obstet Gynecol Scand 78:22, 1999

Pharoah POD, Adi Y: Consequences of in-utero death in a twin pregnancy. Lancet 355:1597, 2000

Platt LD, Druzin ML: Acute puerperal inversion of the uterus. Am J Obstet Gynecol 141:187, 1981

Porter TF, Clark SL, Dildy GA, Hankins GDV: Isolated disseminated intravascular coagulation and amniotic fluid embolism. Am J Obstet Gynecol 174:486, 1996

Pritchard JA: Haematological problems associated with delivery, placental abruption, retained dead fetus, and amniotic fluid embolism. Clin Haematol 2:563, 1973

Pritchard JA: Changes in the blood volume during pregnancy and delivery. Anesthesiology 26:393, 1965

Pritchard JA: Fetal death in utero. Obstet Gynecol 14:573, 1959

Pritchard JA, Baldwin RM, Dickey JC, Wiggins KM: Blood volume changes in pregnancy and the puerperium, 2. Red blood cell loss and changes in apparent blood volume during and following vaginal delivery, cesarean section, and cesarean section plus total hysterectomy. Am J Obstet Gynecol 84:1271, 1962

Pritchard JA, Brekken AL: Clinical and laboratory studies on severe abruptio placentae. Am J Obstet Gynecol 97:681, 1967

Pritchard JA, Cunningham FG, Mason RA: Coagulation changes in eclampsia: Their frequency and pathogenesis. Am J Obstet Gynecol 124:855, 1976

Pritchard JA, Cunningham FG, Pritchard SA, Mason RA: On reducing the frequency of severe abruptio placentae. Am J Obstet Gynecol 165:1345, 1991

Pritchard JA, Mason R, Corley M, Pritchard S: Genesis of severe placental abruption. Am J Obstet Gynecol 108:22, 1970

Pritchard JA, Whalley PJ: Abortion complicated by Clostridium perfringens infection. Am J Obstet Gynecol 11:484, 1971

Propst AM, Thorp JM Jr: Traumatic vulvar hematomas: Conservative versus surgical management. South Med J 91:144, 1998

Rachagan SP, Raman S, Balasundram G, Balakrishnan S: Rupture of the pregnant uterus—A 21-year review. Aust NZ J Obstet Gynaecol 31:37, 1991

Read JA, Cotton DB, Miller FC: Placenta accreta: Changing clinical aspects and outcome. Obstet Gynecol 56:31, 1980

Rebarber A, Lonser R, Jackson S, Copel JA, Sipes S: The safety of intraoperative autologous blood collection and autotransfusion during cesarean section. Am J Obstet Gynecol 179:715, 1998

Regan FAM, Hewitt P, Barbara JAJ, Contreras M: Prospective investigation of transfusion transmitted infection in recipients of over 20,000 units of blood. BMJ 320:403, 2000

Rice JP, Kay HH, Mahony BS: The clinical significance of uterine leiomyomas in pregnancy. Am J Obstet Gynecol 160:1212, 1989

Ridgway LE: Puerperal emergency: Vaginal and vulvar hematomas. Obstet Gynecol Clin North Am 22:275, 1995

Ripley DL: Uterine emergencies: Atony, inversion, and rupture. Obstet Gynecol Clin 26:419, 1999

Rodriguez MH, Masaki DI, Phelan JP, Diaz FG: Uterine rupture: Are intrauterine pressure catheters useful in the diagnosis? Am J Obstet Gynecol 161:666, 1989

Romero R, Duffy TP, Berkowitz RL, Chang E, Hobbins JC: Prolongation of a preterm pregnancy complicated by death of a single twin in utero and disseminated intravascular coagulation: Effects of treatment with heparin. N Engl J Med 310:772, 1984

Sachs DA: Blood and component therapy in obstetrics. In Clark SL, Cotton DB, Hankins GDV, Phelan JP (eds): Critical Care Obstetrics, 2nd ed. Boston, Blackwell, 1991, p 599

Sachs BP, Brown DAJ, Driscoll SG, Schulman E, Acker D, Ransil BJ, Jewett JF: Maternal mortality in Massachusetts: Trends and prevention. N Engl J Med 316:667, 1987

Sanderson DA, Milton PJD: The effectiveness of ultrasound screening at 18–20 weeks gestational age for predication of placenta previa. J Obstet Gynaecol 11:320, 1991

Santema JG, Swaak AM, Wallenburg HCS: Expectant management of twin pregnancy with single fetal death. Br J Obstet Gynaecol 102:26, 1995

Saraiya M, Green CA, Berg CJ, Hopkins FW, Koonin LM, Atrash HK: Spontaneous abortion-related deaths among women in the United States—1981–1991. Obstet Gynecol 94:172, 1999

Scarantino SE, Reilly JG, Moretti ML, Pillari VT: Argon beam coagulation in the management of placenta accreta. Obstet Gynecol 94:825, 1999

Schierhout G, Roberts I: Fluid resuscitation with colloid or crystalloid solutions in critically ill patients: A systemic review of randomised trials. BMJ 315:961, 1998

Schreiber GB, Busch MP, Kleinman SH, Korelitz JJ for the Retrovirus Epidemiology Donor Study: The risk of transfusion-transmitted viral infections. N Engl J Med 334:1685, 1996

Schwartz SI: Hemostasis, surgical bleeding, and transfusion. In Schwarz SI, Shires GT, Spencer FC, Daly JM, Fisher JE, Galloway AC (eds): Principles of Surgery, 7th ed. New York, McGraw-Hill, 1999, p 77

Schwarz O, Paddock R, Bortnick AR: The cesarean scar: An experimental study. Am J Obstet Gynecol 36:962, 1938

Seski JC, Compton AA: Abruptio placentae following a negative oxytocin challenge test. Am J Obstet Gynecol 125:276, 1976

Shah-Hosseini R, Evrard JR: Puerperal uterine inversion. Obstet Gynecol 73:567, 1989

Sheehan HL, Murdoch R: Postpartum necrosis of the anterior pituitary: Pathological and clinical aspects. Br J Obstet Gynaecol 45:456, 1938

Sherman SJ, Greenspoon JS, Nelson JM, Paul RH: Identifying the obstetric patient at high risk of multiple-unit blood transfusions. J Reprod Med 37:649, 1992

Sheth SS: Results of treatment of rupture of the uterus by suturing. J Obstet Gynaecol Br Commonw 75:55, 1968

Shoemaker WC, Kram HB: Comparison of the effects of crystalloids and colloids on hemodynamic oxygen transport, mortality and morbidity. In Simmons RS, Udeko AJ (eds): Debates in General Surgery. Chicago, Year Book, 1991

Sholl JS: Abruptio placentae: Clinical management in nonacute cases. Am J Obstet Gynecol 156:40, 1987

Sibai BM, Lindheimer M, Hauth J, Caritis S, Van Dorsten P, Klebanoff M, MacPherson C, Landon M, Miodovnik M, Paul R, Meis P, Dombrowski M: Risk factors for preeclampsia, abruptio placentae, and adverse neonatal outcomes among women with chronic hypertension. N Engl J Med 339:667, 1998

Sloan EP, Koenigsberg M, Gens D, Cipolle M, Runge J, Mallory MN, Rodman G Jr: Diaspirin cross-linked hemoglobin (DCLHb) in the treatment of severe traumatic hemorrhagic shock: A randomized controlled efficacy trial. JAMA 282:1857, 1999

Sloand EM, Pitt E, Klein HG: Safety of the blood supply. JAMA 274:1368, 1995

Slutsker L: Risks associated with cocaine use during pregnancy. Obstet Gynecol 79:778, 1992

Smith RS, Lauria MR, Comstock CH, Treadwell MC, Kirk JS, Lee W, Bottoms SF: Transvaginal ultrasonography for all placentas that appear to be low-lying or over the internal cervical os. Ultrasound Obstet Gynecol 9:22, 1997

Stafford PA, Biddinger PW, Zumwalt RE: Lethal intrauterine fetal trauma. Am J Obstet Gynecol 159:485, 1988

Steiner PE, Luschbaugh CC: Maternal pulmonary embolism by amniotic fluid. JAMA 117:1245, 1941

Stettler RW, Lutich A, Pritchard JA, Cunningham FG: Traumatic placental abruption: A separation from traditional thought. Presented at the American College of Obstetricians and Gynecologists Annual Clinical Meeting, Las Vegas, April 27, 1992

Stolte L, van Kessel H, Seelen J, Eskes T, Wagatsuma T: Failure to produce the syndrome of amniotic fluid embolism by infusion of amniotic fluid and meconium into monkeys. Am J Obstet Gynecol 98:694, 1967

Taipale P, Hiilesmaa V, Ylostalo P: Transvaginal ultrasonography at 18–23 weeks in predicting placenta previa at delivery. Ultrasound Obstet Gynecol 12:422, 1998

Tan NH, Abu M, Woo JL, Tahir HM: The role of transvaginal sonography in the diagnosis of placenta praevia. Aust NZ J Obstet Gynaecol 35:42, 1995

Thiery M, Delbeke L: Acute puerperal uterine inversion: Two-step management with a β-mimetic and a prostaglandin. Am J Obstet Gynecol 153:891, 1985

Toohey JS, Keegan KA Jr, Morgan MA, Francis J, Task S, deVeciana M: The "dangerous multipara": Fact or fiction? Am J Obstet Gynecol 172:683, 1995

Towell ME: Fetal acid–base physiology and intrauterine asphyxia. In Goodwin JW, Godden JO, Chance GW (eds): Perinatal Medicine. Baltimore, Williams & Wilkins, 1976, p 200

Towers CV, Pircon RA, Heppard M: Is tocolysis safe in the management of third-trimester bleeding? Am J Obstet Gynecol 180:1572, 1999

Turney TH, Ellis CM, Parsons FM: Obstetric acute renal failure 1956–1987. Br J Obstet Gynaecol 96:679, 1989

Van Vugt PJH, Baudoin P, Blom VM, van Duersen TBM: Inversio uteri puerperalis. Acta Obstet Gynecol Scand 60:353, 1981

Ward JW, Bush TJ, Perkins HA, Lieb LE, Allen JR, Goldfinger D, Samson SM: Transfusion of human immunodeficiency virus (HIV) by blood transfusions screened as negative for HIV antibody. N Engl J Med 318:473, 1988

Watson P, Besch N, Bowes WA Jr: Management of acute and subacute puerperal inversion of the uterus. Obstet Gynecol 55:12, 1980

Weiner CP: Disseminated intravascular coagulopathy associated with pregnancy. In Clark SL, Hankins GDV, Cotton DB, Phelan JP (eds): Critical Care Obstetrics, 2nd ed. Boston, Blackwell, 1991

Weiwen Y: Study of the diagnosis and management of amniotic fluid embolism: 38 cases of analysis. Obstet Gynecol 95:385, 2000

Whitehead R: The hypothalamus in post-partum hypopituitarism. J Pathol Bacteriol 86:55, 1963

Williams JW: A critical analysis of 21 years' experience with cesarean section. Bull Johns Hopkins Hosp 32:173, 1921

Williams MA, Mittendorf R, Lieberman E, Monson RR, Schoenbaum SC, Genest DR: Cigarette smoking during pregnancy in relation to placenta previa. Am J Obstet Gynecol 165:28, 1991b

Wilson RF, Mammem E, Walt AJ: Eight years of experience with massive blood transfusions. Trauma 11:275, 1971

Wing DA, Paul RH, Millar LK: Management of symptomatic placenta previa: A randomized, controlled trial of in-patient versus out-patient expectant management. Am J Obstet Gynecol 174:305, 1996a

Wing DA, Paul RH, Millar LK: The usefulness of coagulation studies and blood banking in the symptomatic placenta previa. Am J Obstet Gynecol 174:346, 1996b

Witlin AG, Saade GR, Mattar F, Sibai BM: Risk factors for abruptio placentae and eclampsia: Analysis of 445 consecutively managed women with severe preeclampsia and eclampsia. Am J Obstet Gynecol 180:1322, 1999

Wolf EJ, Mallozzi A, Rodis JF, Egan JFX, Vintzileos AM, Campbell WA: Placenta previa is not an independent risk factor for small for gestational age infant. Obstet Gynecol 77:707, 1991

Yeo L, Vintzileos AM, Guzman ER, Shen-Shwartz S, Ananth CV, Smulian JC: The sonographic diagnostic accuracy of abruptio placenta in patients with premature rupture of the membranes vs. intact membranes. Am J Obstet Gynecol 180:S166, 1999

Zahn CM, Yeomans ER: Postpartum hemorrhage: Placenta accreta, uterine inversion and puerperal hematomas. Clin Obstet Gynecol 33:422, 1990

Zaki AMS, Bahar AM, Ali ME, Albar HAM, Gerais MA: Risk factors and morbidity in patients with placenta previa accreta compared to placenta previa non-accreta. Acta Obstet Gynecol Scand 77:391, 1998

Zelop CM, Harlow BL, Frigeletto FD, Safon LE, Saltzman DH: Emergency peripartum hysterectomy. Am J Obstet Gynecol 168:1443, 1993

26

Puerperal Infection

Puerperal infection is a general term used to describe any bacterial infection of the genital tract after delivery. Pelvic infections are the most common serious complications of the puerperium, and along with preeclampsia and obstetrical hemorrhage, for many decades of this century formed the lethal triad of causes of maternal deaths. Fortunately, maternal deaths from infection have become uncommon. Koonin and associates (1997) reported results from the National Pregnancy Mortality Surveillance System representing almost 1500 maternal deaths in the United States from 1987 through 1990. Infection comprised 13 percent of pregnancy-related deaths and was the fourth leading cause. In an earlier review of 2644 maternal deaths in the United States from 1979 to 1986, infection was associated with 8 percent of the total (Atrash and colleagues, 1990). Jacob and co-workers (1998) reported a similar rate of 10 percent for pregnancy-related deaths in Utah from 1982 through 1994.

PUERPERAL FEVER

Because most temperature elevations in the puerperium are caused by pelvic infection, the incidence of fever after childbirth is a reasonably reliable index of their incidence. The Joint Committee on Maternal Welfare was convened in 1919 (Mussey and colleagues, 1935). Several years later it modified European standards and defined puerperal morbidity as follows: *Temperature 38.0°C (100.4°F) or higher, the temperature to occur on any 2 of the first 10 days postpartum, exclusive of the first 24 hours, and to be taken by mouth by a standard technique at least four times daily.* This is still a commonly employed definition in the United States, and although it suggests that all puerperal fevers are the consequence of pelvic infection, temperature elevations may be the result of other causes.

DIFFERENTIAL DIAGNOSIS OF FEVER. When temperature persists at 38°C or more postpartum, the woman should be evaluated for extrapelvic causes of fever as well as for puerperal infection. **Most persistent fevers after childbirth are caused by genital tract infection.** Filker and Monif (1979) reported that only about 20 percent of febrile women (first 24 hours) delivered vaginally were subsequently diagnosed with pelvic infection, in contrast to 70 percent of those delivered by cesarean section. It must be emphasized that a high-spiking fever—39°C or higher—developing within the first 24 hours after birth may be associated with very virulent pelvic infection caused by either group A or group B streptococcus. The extragenital causes of puerperal fever described next need to be emphasized because they are more common.

BREAST ENGORGEMENT. This condition commonly causes a brief temperature elevation. About 15 percent of all postpartum women develop fever from breast engorgement, which rarely exceeds 39°C in the first few postpartum days. The fever characteristically lasts no longer than 24 hours (Chap. 17, p. 413). By contrast, the fever of **bacterial mastitis** develops later and usually is sustained. It is associated with other signs and symptoms of breast infection that become overt within 24 hours.

RESPIRATORY COMPLICATIONS. These problems are most often seen within the first 24 hours following delivery, and almost invariably are in women delivered by cesarean section. They are much less common if conduction analgesia is used. Complications include **atelectasis, aspiration pneumonia,** or occasionally, **bacterial pneumonia.** Atelectasis is best prevented with the use of routine coughing and deep breathing on a fixed schedule, usually every 4 hours for at least 24 hours following operative delivery. Hypoventilation causes alveolar collapse. Airway obstruction from thick secretions and diminished cough reflex increase this possibility. Fever associated with atelectasis is thought to be due to infection with normal flora that proliferate distal to the obstruction. Engoren (1995) found no association with fever and radiographic findings of atelectasis. With worsening symptoms, and because of severe sequelae, the possibility of aspiration must be suspected. These latter women most often will develop a high-spiking fever, varying degrees of respiratory wheezing, and in most instances, obvious signs of hypoxemia.

PYELONEPHRITIS. Acute renal infection may be difficult to distinguish from pelvic infection. In the typical case, bacteriuria, pyuria, costovertebral angle tenderness, and spiking temperature clearly indicate renal infection; however, the clinical picture varies. For example, in the puerperal woman the first sign of renal infection may be a temperature elevation, with costovertebral angle tenderness, nausea, and vomiting developing later. Actually, these infections are not as common as might be expected from their antenatal prevalence (Chap. 47, p. 1255). This likely is due to the brisk diuresis that normally begins early in the puerperium.

THROMBOPHLEBITIS. Superficial or deep venous thrombosis of the legs may cause minor temperature elevations in the puerperal woman. The diagnosis is made by the observation of a painful, swollen leg, usually accompanied by calf tenderness, or occasionally femoral triangle area tenderness. Diagnosis and treatment are discussed in Chapter 46 (p. 1235).

UTERINE INFECTION

Postpartum uterine infection has been called variously *endometritis, endomyometritis,* and *endoparametritis.* Because infection actually involves not only the decidua but also the myometrium and parametrial tissues, we prefer the term **metritis with pelvic cellulitis.** Uterine infections are relatively uncommon following uncomplicated vaginal delivery, but they continue to be a major problem in women delivered by cesarean section. **The route of delivery is the single most significant risk factor for the development of postpartum uterine infection.**

PREDISPOSING FACTORS

VAGINAL DELIVERY. Compared with cesarean section, metritis following vaginal delivery is relatively uncommon. Sweet and Ledger (1973) reported that the incidence of postpartum uterine infections after vaginal delivery was 2.6 percent. A 6-month survey during 1987 of nearly 5000 women delivered vaginally at Parkland Hospital showed that only 1.3 percent were given treatment for metritis. However, when women at high risk—defined by prolonged membrane rupture and labor, multiple cervical examinations, and internal fetal monitoring—were analyzed separately, the incidence of metritis after vaginal delivery was nearly 6 percent. If there is intrapartum chorioamnionitis, the risk of infection increases to 13 percent (Maberry and colleagues, 1991). Libombo and colleagues (1994) reported that metritis following vaginal delivery developed more frequently in women who had pregnancies associated with adverse fetal outcomes, including stillbirth, low birthweight, preterm delivery, and serious neonatal morbidity. Interestingly, women readmitted to the hospital with postpartum metritis are more likely to have been delivered vaginally (Atterbury and colleagues, 1998).

CESAREAN DELIVERY. The incidence of metritis following surgical delivery varies with socioeconomic factors, and over the years this has been altered substantively by the almost universal use of perioperative antimicrobials (Chap. 23, p. 559). Prior to use of antimicrobial prophylaxis, Sweet and Ledger (1973) reported an overall incidence of uterine infection of 13 percent among affluent women undergoing cesarean section at the University of Michigan Hospital; however, they reported the incidence to be 27 percent in indigent women delivered at Wayne County Hospital. Cunningham and associates (1978) found an overall incidence of about 50 percent in women delivered by cesarean section at Parkland Hospital. Important risk factors for infection included duration of labor and membrane rupture, multiple cervical examinations, and internal fetal monitoring. Women with all of these factors delivered for cephalopelvic disproportion, who were not given perioperative prophylaxis, had an incidence of serious pelvic infection that was nearly 90 percent (DePalma and colleagues, 1982; Gilstrap and Cunningham, 1979).

OTHER RISK FACTORS. It is generally accepted—albeit unknown why—that pelvic infection is more common in women of lower socioeconomic status compared with middle- or upper-class patients. Goldenberg and associates (1996) have shown significant racial differences in vaginal colonization during pregnancy with potential pathogens. Precise reasons for these differences are unclear, but they could not be attributed to differences in health behavior.

The evidence that **anemia** increases the likelihood of infection is not conclusive (Cook and Lynch, 1986). The results obtained from both animal and in vitro experiments are consistent with the view that iron-deficiency anemia does not predispose to infection, and some believe it may actually prevent infection. For example, transferrin, which is increased in iron-deficiency anemia, appears to have significant antibacterial action. Moreover, growth of a variety of pathogenic bacteria in vitro is inhibited by lack of iron. Finally, there is no impairment of wound healing in animals previously made iron deficient.

The role of **nutrition** in the genesis of infection is also unclear, although cell-mediated immunity is impaired in malnourished laboratory animals. An increased incidence of puerperal infection resulting from recent **sexual intercourse** has not been clearly demonstrated.

Bacterial colonization of the lower genital tract with certain microorganisms—for example, group B streptococcus, *Chlamydia trachomatis, Mycoplasma hominis,* and *Gardnerella vaginalis*—has been associated with an increased risk of postpartum infection (Berenson and colleagues, 1990; Berman and associates, 1987). In a study of almost 8000 women, Krohn and colleagues (1999) reported an increased risk of intrapartum but not postpartum infection in women with heavy versus light group B streptococcal colonization. Of 345 cases of group B bacteremia identified by an active surveillance program, Schrag and co-workers (2000) reported one maternal death. While Watts and associates (1990) reported an increased risk of puerperal metritis with bacterial vaginosis, Carey and collaborators (2000) reported that its treatment antepartum did not affect the postpartum infection rate. Andrews and colleagues (1995) reported that colonization with *Ureaplasma urealyticum* of intact membranes was a significant risk factor for infection following cesarean delivery.

Some other factors include cesarean delivery for **multifetal gestation** (Suonio and Huttunen, 1994). **Young maternal age and nulliparity** are associated with a higher incidence of metritis following cesarean delivery (Magee and associates, 1994; Suonio and Huttunen, 1994; Tran and co-workers, 2000). Bahn and associates (1998), as well as many others before, reported an increased risk of maternal infectious morbidity associated with **prolonged labor induction.** Tran and colleagues (2000) found a twofold increase in cesarean infections for every 5-unit increase in body mass index. Finally, Rotmensch and associates (1999) reported an increase in infection-related maternal morbidity with three or more courses of **betamethasone** given to women at risk for preterm delivery.

BACTERIOLOGY. Organisms that invade the placental implantation site, incisions, or lacerations as a consequence of delivery typically are those that normally colonize the cervix, vagina, and perineum. Most of these bacteria are of relatively low virulence and seldom initiate infection in healthy tissues. Although an occasional epidemic caused by group A β-hemolytic streptococcus has been reported, these are usually endemic (Anteby and associates, 1999).

Over the past decade, there have been reports of this organism causing toxic shock-like syndrome (Dotters and Katz, 1991; Nathan and Leveno, 1994; Whitted and colleagues, 1990). Udagawa and associates (1999) recently reviewed 30 cases of group A infections in women either peripartum or postpartum. Of 17 women in whom infection manifest before or during labor, or within 12 hours of delivery, maternal mortality was 88 percent and fetal mortality was 60 percent. In 13 women who deteriorated more than 12 hours postpartum, the maternal death rate was 55 percent and there were no fetal deaths. Anteby and associates (1999) reviewed their experiences with 47 women who had group A streptococcal infections intrapartum or in the puerperium. A prominent risk factor was prematurely ruptured membranes. Three women had septic shock.

COMMON PATHOGENS. In the great majority of instances, bacteria responsible for pelvic infection are those that normally reside in the bowel and also colonize the perineum, vagina, and cervix. Bacteria commonly responsible for female genital tract infections are listed in Table 26–1. Usually, multiple species of bacteria are isolated, and although typically considered to be of relatively low virulence, they may become pathogenic as a result of hematomas and devitalized tissue.

Although the cervix and lower genital tract routinely harbor such bacteria, the uterine cavity is usually sterile before rupture of the amnionic sac. As the consequence of labor and delivery and associated manipulations, the amnionic fluid and perhaps the uterus commonly become contaminated with anaerobic and aerobic bacteria (Fig. 26–1). Gilstrap and Cunningham (1979), from cul-

TABLE 26–1. Bacteria Commonly Responsible for Female Genital Infections

Aerobes
Group A, B, and D streptococci
Enterococcus
Gram-negative bacteria—*Escherichia coli, Klebsiella,* and *Proteus* species
Staphylococcus aureus
Gardnerella vaginalis

Anaerobes
Peptococcus species
Peptostreptococcus species
Bacteroides fragilis group
Clostridium species
Fusobacterium species
Mobiluncus species

Other
Mycoplasma species
Chlamydia trachomatis
Neisseria gonorrhoeae

Data from the American College of Obstetricians and Gynecologists (1998).

tures of amnionic fluid obtained at cesarean delivery in women in labor with membranes ruptured more than 6 hours, identified anaerobic and aerobic organisms in 63 percent, anaerobes alone in 30 percent, and aerobes alone in 7 percent. Predominant anaerobic organisms were gram-positive cocci (*Peptostreptococcus* and *Peptococcus* species), 45 percent; *Bacteroides* species, 9 percent; and *Clostridium* species, 3 percent. Gram-positive aerobic cocci also were common (*Enterococcus,* 14 percent, and group B streptococcus, 8 percent). *Escherichia coli* comprised 9 percent of isolates. An average of 2.5 organisms was identified from each specimen. Walmer and colleagues (1988) provided evidence for *Enterococcus* species in the pathogenesis of these infections. Sherman and co-workers (1999) showed that bacterial isolates from the lower uterine segment at cesarean delivery correlated with isolates taken at 3 days postpartum when metritis had developed.

Chlamydia trachomatis has been implicated as a cause of late-onset, indolent metritis that may develop in a third of women who had antepartum chlamydial cervical infection (Ismail and co-workers, 1985). Berenson and colleagues (1990) reported that *C. trachomatis* was isolated significantly more often from adolescents with postcesarean metritis compared with adults. Of interest, *Gardnerella vaginalis* also was isolated more often in the younger women. Whether these organisms are truly pathogenic or simply "markers" of risk factors for infection is unclear. Gibbs and colleagues (1987)

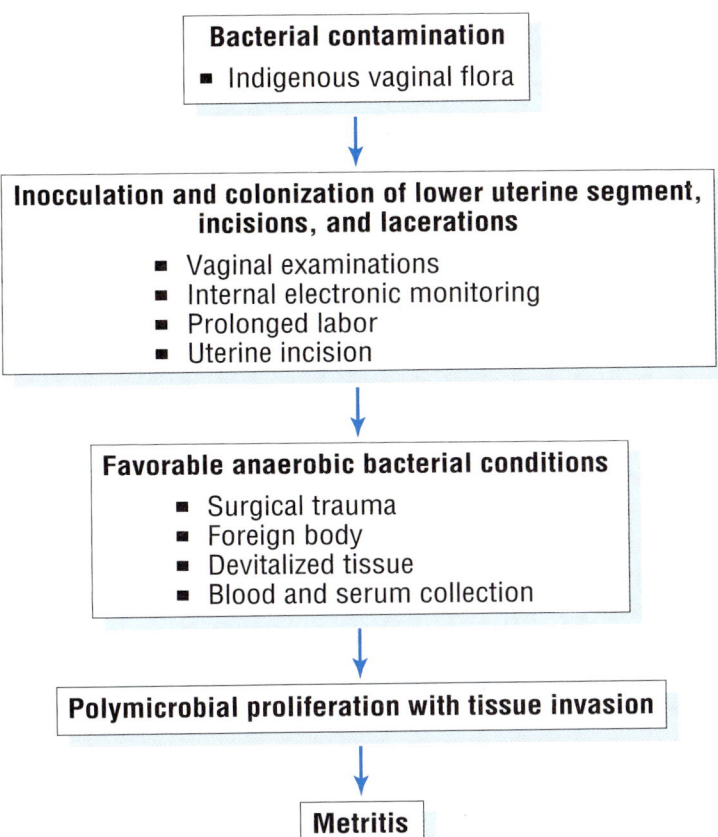

FIGURE 26–1. Pathogenesis of metritis following cesarean section. (From Gilstrap and Cunningham, 1979.)

reported that *Gardnerella* lacked a pathogenic role in puerperal infections. The role of genital mycoplasmas and ureaplasma is less clear, but some researchers have implicated these organisms in the etiology of puerperal metritis (Andrews and co-workers, 1995; Blanco and colleagues, 1983).

BACTERIAL CULTURES. Precise identification of bacteria specifically responsible for any puerperal infection is quite difficult. For example, using double-lumen catheters, Gibbs and associates (1975) cultured one or more pathogens from the uterine cavity in 70 percent of clinically healthy puerperal women. For these reasons, routine pretreatment genital tract cultures are of little clinical utility, and they add significantly to hospitalization costs. Similarly, the utility of routine blood cultures obtained before antimicrobials are given is questionable. In two earlier studies, blood cultures were positive in 13 percent of women at Parkland Hospital and 24 percent at Los Angeles County Hospital who had postcesarean pelvic infections (Cunningham and colleagues, 1978; DiZerega and co-workers, 1979).

PATHOGENESIS. Puerperal infection following vaginal delivery primarily involves the placental implantation site and the decidua and adjacent myometrium. In some cases, the discharge is foul, profuse, bloody, and sometimes frothy. In others, the discharge is scant. Uterine involution may be retarded. Microscopical sections may show a superficial layer of necrotic material containing bacteria and a thick zone of leukocytic infiltration.

As shown in Figure 26–1, the pathogenesis of uterine infection following cesarean delivery is that of an infected surgical incision. Bacteria that colonized the cervix and vagina gain access to amnionic fluid during labor, and postpartum they invade devitalized uterine tissue at the hysterotomy site. Parametrial cellulitis next follows with infection of the pelvic retroperitoneal fibroareolar connective tissue (Fig. 26–2). It may be caused by the lymphatic spread of organisms from an infected cervical laceration or uterine incision or laceration. The process is usually limited to the paravaginal tissue and rarely extends deeply into the pelvis.

CLINICAL COURSE. Whenever fever develops postpartum, uterine infection should be suspected. Fever is probably proportional to the extent of infection, and when confined to the endometrium (decidua) and superficial myometrium, cases are mild and associated with minimal fever. More commonly, temperature exceeds 38 to 39°C. Chills may accompany fever and suggest

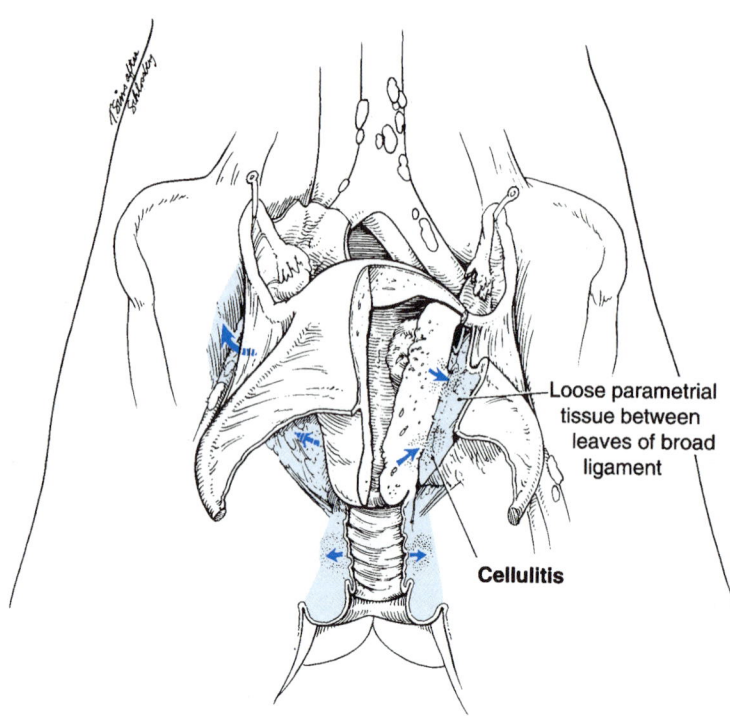

Loose parametrial
tissue between
leaves of broad
ligament

Cellulitis

FIGURE 26–2. Pelvic cellulitis (parametritis) associated with puerperal infection. Bacteria may enter the parametrial tissue between the leaves of the broad ligament by direct extension or by lymphatic transmission from cervical lacerations or foci of trauma within the uterus, including the placental implantation site or cesarean incision. Bacterial spread may also develop across the wall of an infected vein. Lacerations of the perineum or vagina usually cause only localized cellulitis, but may extend to pelvic lymphatics.

bacteremia, which is documented in 10 to 20 percent of women with pelvic infection following cesarean delivery. The pulse rate typically follows the temperature curve.

The woman usually complains of abdominal pain, and parametrial tenderness is elicited upon abdominal and bimanual examination. Because of incisional pain, abdominal and uterine fundal tenderness may be more helpful in establishing the diagnosis of metritis in women following vaginal than cesarean delivery. Even in the early stages, an offensive odor may develop; however, in many women foul-smelling lochia without other evidence for infection is found. Some infections, and notably those due to group A β-hemolytic streptococci, are frequently associated with scanty, odorless lochia. Leukocytosis may range from 15,000 to 30,000 cells/μL. The average increase in the leukocyte count postpartum is 22 percent (Hartmann and co-workers, 2000). **Thus, fever after exclusion of other causes remains the most important criterion for the diagnosis of postpartum metritis.** If the process is localized to the uterus, the temperature may return to normal without antimicrobial treatment. Indeed, localized metritis may be misdiagnosed as a urinary infection, breast engorgement, or pulmonary atelectasis. Without treatment, uterine and pelvic cellulitis worsen; however, resolution usually is prompt with appropriate antimicrobial therapy.

TREATMENT. For mild cases of metritis following vaginal delivery diagnosed after discharge, an oral agent may suffice. For moderately to severely infected women, however, including those delivered by cesarean, parenteral therapy with a broad-spectrum antimicrobial regimen is indicated. Improvement will follow in 48 to 72 hours in nearly 90 percent of women treated with one of the regimens discussed next. Persistence of fever after this interval mandates a careful search for causes of refractory pelvic infection, although nonpelvic sources are occasionally found. Complications of metritis that cause persistent fever despite appropriate therapy include parametrial phlegmons or intense cellulitis, surgical incisional and pelvic abscesses, infected hematomas, and septic pelvic thrombophlebitis. Bacteria resistant to initial therapy occasionally may be a cause of persistent fever, but this is rare in our experiences. Drug fever also is very uncommon.

In the usual contemporaneous practice, the woman is discharged without further therapy after she has been afebrile for at least 24 hours. Dinsmoor and colleagues (1991) found no differences in infection-related complications when oral antimicrobials were compared with placebo for afebrile women discharged following intravenous therapy.

PRINCIPLES OF ANTIMICROBIAL TREATMENT. Few, if any, antimicrobial regimens are effective against all putative pathogens that cause pelvic infection and initial antibiotic therapy is empirical. Despite this, initial treatment following cesarean delivery is directed against at least most of the polymicrobial and mixed flora that typically cause puerperal infections (Table 26-1). Fortunately, selection of an agent(s) effective against the most common ones usually proves suitable. Such broad-spectrum coverage is often not necessary to treat infection following vaginal delivery, and up to 90 percent of such women will respond to regimens such as ampicillin plus gentamicin. In contrast, the importance of including anaerobic coverage for those with infections following cesarean delivery is exemplified in that only 60 to 70 percent have a satisfactory response to ampicillin plus gentamicin. A number of effective regimens is shown in Table 26-2.

In 1979, DiZerega and colleagues compared the effectiveness of clindamycin plus gentamicin with penicillin G plus gentamicin given for treatment of pelvic infections following cesarean section. Women given the **clindamycin-gentamicin** regimen had a favorable response 95 percent of the time, and this regimen now is considered by most to be the standard by which others are measured. Walmer and colleagues (1988) later provided evidence that enterococcal infections may be associated with its clinical failure; thus, many add ampicillin to the clindamycin-gentamicin regimen, either initially or if there is no response by 48 to 72 hours. Most recently, vancomycin-resistant enterococcal infections have been problematic in nonobstetrical units (Murray, 2000).

Brumfield and colleagues (2000) at the University of Alabama at Birmingham reaffirmed the efficacy of this regimen given to 322 women with postcesarean metritis and pelvic cellulitis. Over half (54 percent) were cured with the original two-drug regimen and another 40

percent in whom ampicillin was added at 48 hours responded. Of the 19 women (6 percent) who did not respond to "triple therapy," 7 had a wound infection that required drainage.

Although many authorities recommend that serum gentamicin levels be periodically monitored, we do not feel it necessary to measure peak and trough serum concentrations in most women. Liu and associates (1999) compared multiple- versus single-daily dosing with gentamicin and found that both provided adequate serum levels which avoided the need for routine measurement. Because of the potential for nephrotoxicity and ototoxicity with gentamicin in the event of diminished glomerular filtration, some have recommended a combination of clindamycin and a second-generation cephalosporin to treat such women. Others have recommended a combination of clindamycin and aztreonam, a monobactam compound with activity against gram-negative aerobic pathogens similar to aminoglycosides (American College of Obstetricians and Gynecologists, 1998).

The spectra of **β-lactam antimicrobials** include activity against many anaerobic pathogens, and these antimicrobials have been used successfully for decades to treat such infections. Some examples include cephalosporins—cefoxitin, cefotetan, cefotaxime, and others—as well as extended-spectrum penicillins such as piperacillin, ticarcillin, and mezlocillin. Beta-lactam antimicrobials are inherently safe, and except for allergic reactions, are free of major toxicity. Another advantage is the cost-effectiveness of administering only one drug. The **β-lactamase inhibitors,** clavulanic acid, sulbactam, and tazobactam, have been combined with ampicillin, amoxicillin, ticarcillin, and piperacillin to extend their spectra, and these also have been proven effective.

Metronidazole has superior in vitro activity against most anaerobes, and it is recommended by some to be given intravenously in combination with gentamicin. The use of metronidazole plus ampicillin and an aminoglycoside provides coverage against most organisms encountered in serious pelvic infections.

Imipenem is a carbapenem that has broad-spectrum coverage against the majority of organisms associated with metritis. It is used in combination with **cilastatin,** which inhibits renal metabolism of imipenem. Although this combination will most certainly be effective in most cases of metritis, it seems reasonable from both a medical and economic standpoint to reserve it for more serious infections.

TABLE 26-2. Antimicrobial Regimens for Pelvic Infection Following Cesarean Delivery

Regimen	Comments
Clindamycin 900 mg + gentamicin 1.5 mg/kg, q8h intravenously	Most widely studied regimen, 90–97% efficacy, once-daily gentamicin dosing acceptable
plus ampicillin	Added to regimen with sepsis syndrome or suspected enterococcal infection
plus aztreonam	Gentamicin substitute with renal insufficiency
Extended-spectrum penicillins	Piperacillin, ampicillin/sulbactam
Extended-spectrum cephalosporins	Cefotetan, cefoxitin, cefotaxime
Imipenem + cilastatin	Reserved for special indications

Data from the American College of Obstetricians and Gynecologists (1998).

COMPLICATIONS OF PELVIC INFECTIONS

In over 90 percent of women, metritis responds within 48 to 72 hours to treatment with one of the aforementioned regimens. In the others, any of a number of complications may arise.

WOUND INFECTIONS. The incidence of abdominal incisional infections following cesarean delivery ranges from 3 to 15 percent, with an average of about 6 percent (Faro, 1990; Owen and Andrews, 1994). When prophylactic antibiotics are given, the incidence is probably 2 percent or less. According to Soper and co-workers (1992), wound infection is the most common cause of antimicrobial failure in women treated for metritis. Risk factors for wound infections include obesity, diabetes, corticosteroid therapy, immunosuppression, anemia, and poor hemostasis with hematoma formation.

Incisional abscesses that develop following cesarean section usually cause fever beginning on about the fourth postoperative day. In many cases, these are preceded by uterine infection, and there is persistent fever despite adequate antimicrobial therapy. Erythema and drainage may also be present. Wound cultures are almost always positive (Owen and Andrews, 1994; Roberts and colleagues, 1993). Organisms causing these infections are usually the same as those isolated from amnionic fluid at cesarean delivery, but hospital-acquired pathogens must be suspected (Emmons and colleagues, 1988; Owen and Andrews, 1994). Treatment is with antimicrobials and surgical drainage, with careful inspection to ensure that the fascia is intact; if not, secondary closure must be performed.

WOUND DEHISCENCE. Wound disruption, dehiscence, or "burst abdomen" refers to separation of the wound involving the fascial layer. McNeely and colleagues (1998) studied 8590 women undergoing cesarean delivery at Hutzel Hospital in Detroit. They reported that 27 of these women developed fascial dehiscence—about 1 in 300 operations. Most disruptions do not manifest until about the fifth postoperative day, at which time there is a serosanguinous discharge. Most instances of wound dehiscence develop following treatment for post-cesarean metritis. Two thirds of the 27 fascial dehiscences identified by McNeely and associates (1998) were associated with infection and tissue necrosis.

Fascial dehiscence is a serious complication. Treatment includes secondary closure of the incision in the operating room with adequate anesthesia. Surgical debridement is carried out first, followed by fascial or myofascial closure.

NECROTIZING FASCIITIS. Fortunately, this most serious of wound infections is rare, but it is associated with very high mortality. It may involve abdominal incisions following cesarean delivery or it may complicate episiotomy or perineal lacerations (see p. 682). As the name implies, these infections are associated with significant tissue necrosis. Of the risk factors for fasciitis summarized by Owen and Andrews (1994), three of these—diabetes, obesity, and hypertension—are relatively common in pregnant women. Infections are either monobacterial, as with group A β-hemolytic streptococcus, but more commonly they are polymicrobial. Bacterial isolates are those shown in Table 26–1. Occasionally, these infections are caused by rarely encountered pathogens (Barber and Swygert, 2000).

At the University of Alabama, Goepfert and colleagues (1997) reviewed their experiences with incisional necrotizing fasciitis following cesarean delivery. From 1987 through 1994, there were nine cases in 5048 cesarean deliveries—1.8 per 1000 cesareans. In two women, including one with metastatic breast cancer, the infection was fatal.

Adequate antimicrobial therapy is continued as discussed previously. Zimbleman and co-workers (1999) reported preliminary observations that clindamycin given along with a β-lactam agent may be the most effective regimen. Additional treatment includes prompt and aggressive wide debridement in the operating room. With extensive resection, fascial closure may require synthetic mesh to eventually effect closure (McNeely and associates, 1998).

PERITONITIS. This complication is rarely seen with prompt therapy, but may be encountered with infections following cesarean delivery when there is uterine incisional necrosis and dehiscence. It also is occasionally seen in women who have undergone vaginal delivery following prior cesarean section. Also rare, late in the course of pelvic cellulitis, a parametrial or adnexal abscess may rupture and produce catastrophic generalized peritonitis.

Clinically, puerperal peritonitis resembles surgical peritonitis, except that abdominal rigidity usually is less prominent because of the abdominal stretching associated with pregnancy. Pain may be severe. Marked bowel distention is a consequence of paralytic ileus. It is important to identify the cause of the generalized peritonitis. If the infection began in the uterus and extended into the peritoneum, the treatment is usually medical. Conversely, peritonitis as the consequence of a bowel lesion or uterine incisional necrosis is usually best treated surgically. Antimicrobial therapy is continued, but septicemic shock may supervene (Chap. 43, p. 1167).

ADNEXAL INFECTIONS. Most often with puerperal infections the fallopian tubes are involved only with perisalpingitis without subsequent tubal occlusion and sterility. An *ovarian abscess* rarely develops as a complication of puerperal infection, presumably from bacterial invasion through a rent in the ovarian capsule (Wetchler and Dunn, 1985). The abscess is usually unilateral and women typically present 1 to 2 weeks after delivery. In many cases, rupture causes peritonitis, which prompts surgical exploration.

PARAMETRIAL PHLEGMON. In some women in whom metritis develops following cesarean delivery, parametrial cellulitis is intensive and forms an area of induration, termed a *phlegmon,* within the leaves of the broad ligament (Fig. 26–3). These infections should be considered when fever persists after 72 hours despite adequate treatment of pelvic infections that complicate cesarean delivery (DePalma and colleagues, 1982). In some cases, infection may not manifest before discharge. Kindig and colleagues (1998) described a woman with uterine dehiscence at 6 weeks postpartum.

Areas of parametrial cellulitis are more often unilateral, and although they frequently may remain limited to the base of the broad ligament, if the inflammatory reaction is more intense, cellulitis extends along natural lines of cleavage. The most common form of extension is directly laterally, along the base of the broad ligament, with a tendency to extend to the lateral pelvic wall. Posterior extension may involve the rectovaginal septum, producing a firm mass posterior to the cervix.

Intensive cellulitis of the uterine incision may cause necrosis and separation with extrusion of purulent material into the peritoneal cavity. Clinical findings then are as described earlier for peritonitis. Frequently, the first symptoms of peritonitis are those of *adynamic ileus,* which usually is absent or mild following uncomplicated cesarean delivery. Because puerperal metritis with cellulitis is typically a retroperitoneal infection, evidence for peritonitis suggests the possibility of uterine incisional necrosis, or less commonly a bowel injury or other lesion.

In the majority of women with a phlegmon, clinical response follows continued treatment with one of the intravenous antimicrobial regimens previously discussed. These women usually remain febrile for 5 to 7 days, and in some cases even longer. Absorption of the induration follows, but it may take several days to weeks to dissipate completely. Surgery is reserved for women in whom uterine incisional necrosis is suspected. Hysterectomy and surgical debridement are usually difficult, and there is often appreciable blood loss. Frequently, the cervix and lower uterine segment are involved with an intensive inflammatory process that extends to the pelvic sidewall to encompass one or both ureters, and

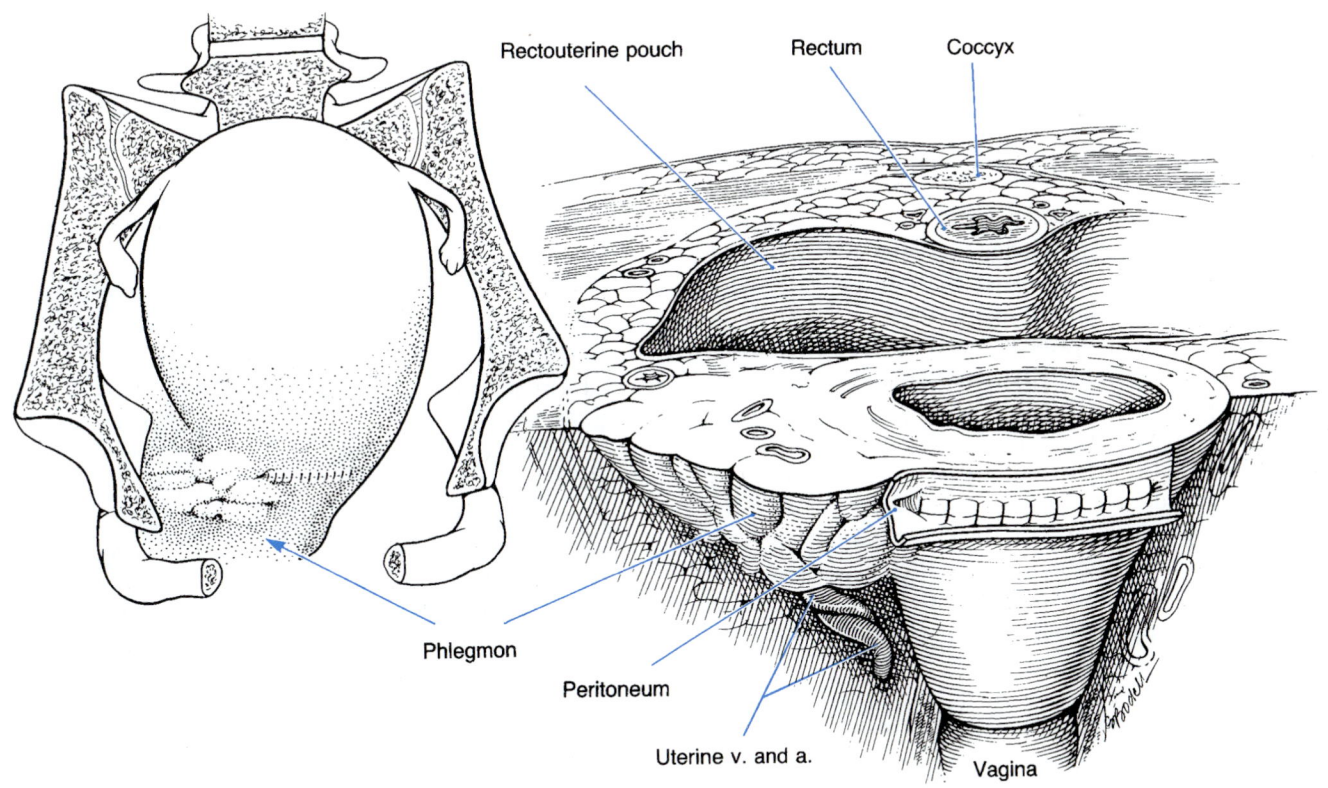

FIGURE 26–3. Parametrial phlegmon. Cellulitis in the right parametrium begins adjacent to the cesarean incision and extends to the pelvic sidewall. On pelvic examination, the phlegmon is palpable as a firm, three-dimensional mass.

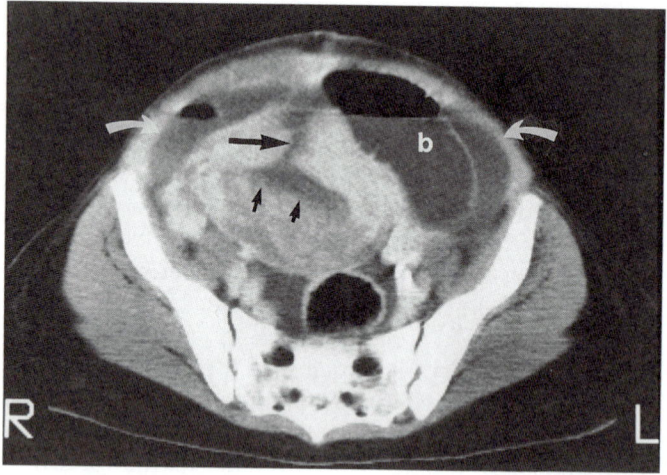

FIGURE 26–4. Pelvic computed tomography of dehiscence from infection of a vertical cesarean incision. Endometrial fluid (*small black arrows*) communicates with parametrial fluid (*curved white arrow*) through the uterine dehiscence (*black arrow*). A dilated bowel loop (b) is adjacent to the uterus on the left. (Courtesy of Dr. Diane Twickler.)

supracervical hysterectomy should be considered. The adnexae are seldom involved, and depending on their appearance, one or both ovaries may be conserved.

IMAGING STUDIES. Evaluation of persistent pelvic infections using sonography has been less than satisfactory because these areas of cellulitis usually have ultrasonic characteristics suggesting an abscess. As discussed, surgical drainage of a phlegmon is inadvisable. Brown and colleagues (1991) described the use of computed tomography in 74 women to assess refractory pelvic infections, and there was at least one abnormal radiological finding in three fourths of these women. Lev-Toaff and colleagues (1991) reported similar findings in 31 women using ultrasound along with computed tomography or magnetic resonance imaging. Only two of these women had negative findings. Utilizing magnetic resonance imaging, Maldjian and associates (1999) studied 50 women with persistent low-grade fever following cesarean delivery. Bladder flap hematomas were found in two thirds, three had parametrial edema, and two had pelvic hematomas.

Sometimes evidence for uterine incisional dehiscence can be detected using computed tomographic scanning (Figs. 26–4 and 26–5). It is important that these x-ray findings be interpreted along with the clinical course, because apparent uterine incisional defects can be visualized after cesarean section with no other evidence for infection or other complications (Twickler and colleagues, 1991).

PELVIC ABSCESS. Rarely, despite prompt and appropriate antimicrobial treatment for metritis, a parametrial phlegmon will suppurate, forming a fluctuant broad ligament mass that may point above the Poupart ligament. Should the abscess rupture into the peritoneal cavity, life-threatening peritonitis may develop as pre-

viously described. More likely, these abscesses will dissect anteriorly, and may be amenable to needle drainage directed by computed tomography (Fig. 26–5). Occasionally they dissect posteriorly to the rectovaginal septum, where surgical drainage is easily effected by colpotomy incision. Segal and colleagues (1996) have described two cases of **psoas abscess** following normal delivery.

Sometimes following cesarean section, collections of blood develop under the bladder flap (Maldjian and associates, 1999). Hematomas may also form in the broad ligament near the uterine incision. These may become infected and require drainage. They usually can be aspirated using computed tomography guidance.

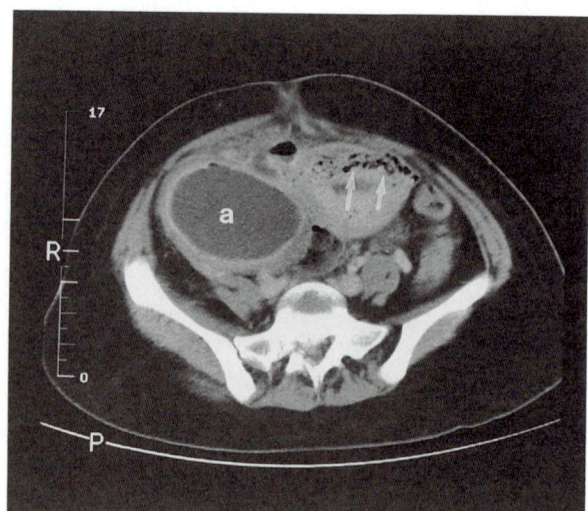

FIGURE 26–5. Pelvic computed tomograph showing necrosis of the uterus with gas in the myometrium (*arrows*) and a large right-sided parametrial abscess (a). (Courtesy of Dr. Diane Twickler.)

SEPTIC PELVIC THROMBOPHLEBITIS. The first reports of surgical excision for pelvic thrombophlebitis appeared at the turn of the last century in the German literature. In 1909, Williams reported a 50 percent mortality rate among 56 women undergoing excision of thrombosed pelvic veins complicating "puerperal pyemia." In 1919, Halban and Köhler performed autopsies in 163 women who died from puerperal infection and reported that half of these had pelvic thrombophlebitis. In 1951, Collins and colleagues described the pathogenesis of suppurative pelvic thrombophlebitis in 70 women cared for from 1937 through 1946 at Charity Hospital at New Orleans. Septic embolization was common in these women and caused a third of maternal deaths during those times. With the advent of antimicrobial therapy, the mortality from these infections diminished as did the need for surgical therapy.

PATHOGENESIS. Bacterial infection begins as usual in the placental implantation site, or more commonly, the uterine incision. These infections are associated with myometrial venous thromboses. As shown in Figures 26–2 and 26–6, puerperal infection may extend along venous routes. There often is coexisting lymphangitis. As shown in Figure 26–7, the ovarian veins may then become involved because they drain the upper uterus, which most often includes veins draining the placental site. The experiences of Witlin and Sibai (1995) and Brown and colleagues (1999) suggest that puerperal septic thrombophlebitis is likely to involve one or both ovarian venous plexuses. In a fourth of women with pelvic thrombosis, clot extends into the inferior vena cava (Fig. 26–8). Septic phlebitis of the left ovarian vein may extend to the renal vein (Bahnson and colleagues, 1985).

INCIDENCE. During a 5-year survey of 45,000 women delivered at Parkland Hospital, Brown and associates (1999) found an incidence of septic thrombophlebitis of 1 : 9000 for vaginal and 1:800 for cesarean delivery. The overall incidence of 1:3000 deliveries was very similar to 1 : 2000 reported by Dunnihoo and colleagues (1991), who used modern imaging techniques to study women with prolonged fever in a population of over 60,000 deliveries.

CLINICAL FINDINGS. Women with septic thrombophlebitis usually experience most aspects of clinical improvement of pelvic infection following antimicrobial treatment; however, they continue to have hectic fever spikes. They usually do not appear clinically ill, and may be asymptomatic except for chills. This clinical picture was aptly termed *enigmatic fever* by Dunn and Van Voorhis (1967). In some women, the cardinal symptom of ovarian vein thrombophlebitis is pain typically manifest on the second or third postpartum day (Munsick and Gillanders, 1981). In some cases, a tender mass is palpable just beyond the uterine cornu on either side. In many cases, pelvic findings are inconclusive by clinical examination. Thus, diagnosis is by either pelvic computed tomography or magnetic resonance imaging. Us-

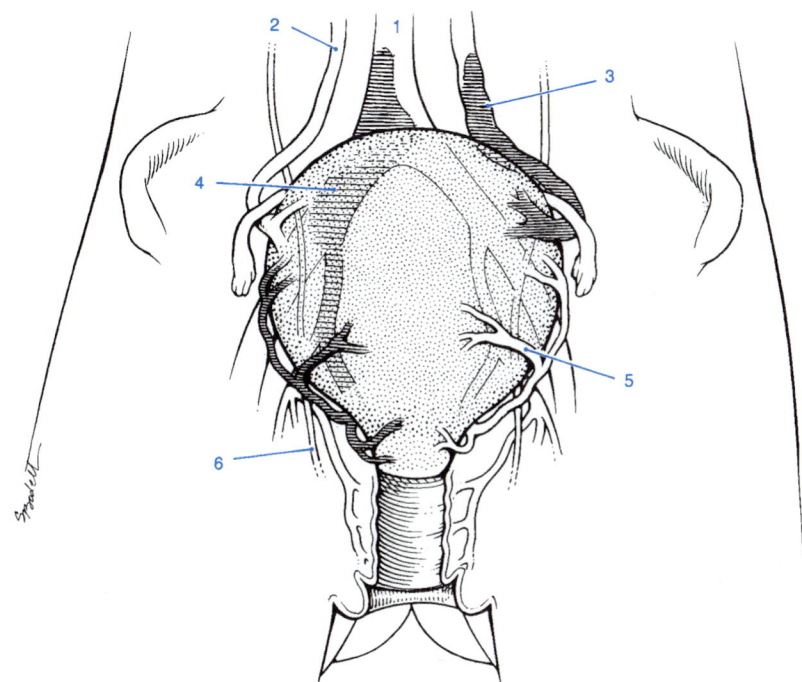

FIGURE 26–6. Routes of extension of septic pelvic thrombophlebitis. Any pelvic vessels and the inferior vena cava may be involved: (1) inferior vena cava; (2) right ovarian vein; (3) left ovarian vein; (4) clot in right common iliac vein which extends from the uterine and internal iliac veins and into the inferior vena cava; (5) left uterine vein; and (6) right ureter.

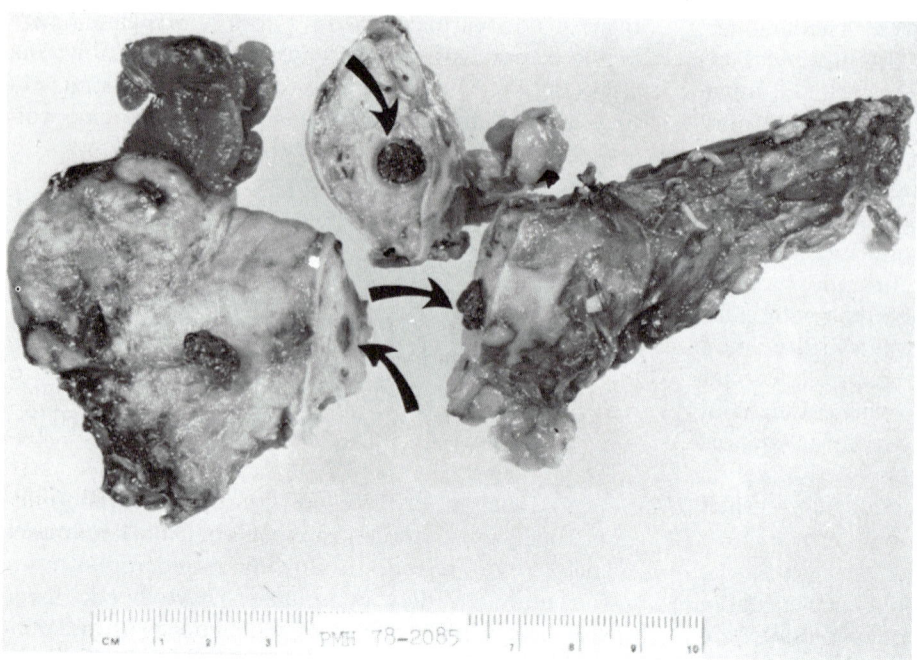

FIGURE 26–7. Ovarian vein thrombophlebitis: resected thrombosed right ovarian vein plus right oviduct.

ing these, Brown and co-workers (1999) found that 20 percent of 69 women who had fever despite 5 days of appropriate antimicrobial therapy for metritis had confirmed septic phlebitis.

Because variable degrees of pelvic thrombophlebitis accompany most cases of metritis and parametrial cellulitis, initial treatment is directed at both. Before imaging methods were available to confirm clinical suspicions

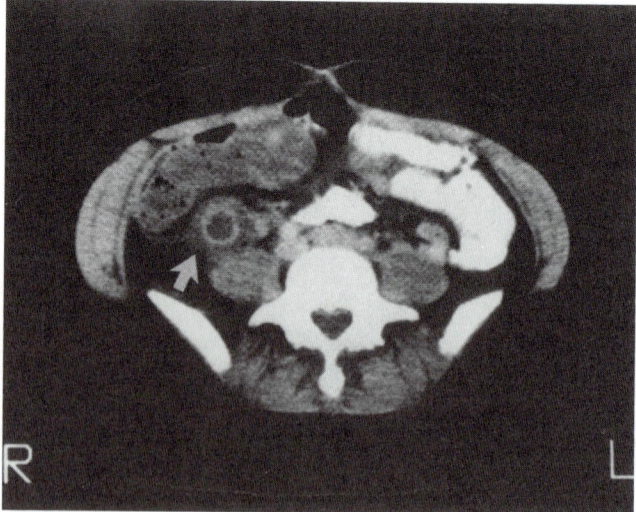

FIGURE 26–8. Computed tomograph after administration of intravenous and oral contrast shows enlargement of right ovarian vein, low density of lumen, and vessel-wall enhancement consistent with thrombosis (*arrow*). Associated low-density area surrounding vein represents perivascular edema. (From Brown and colleagues, 1999, with permission.)

of venous involvement, the *heparin challenge test* was advocated. Supposedly, after intravenous heparin was given, there was lysis of fever; this was taken as diagnostic of pelvic phlebitis and heparin treatment continued (Duff and Gibbs, 1983; Josey and Staggers, 1974). This was subsequently disproven by Brown and colleagues (1986) who showed that despite withholding heparin from 6 of 11 women with computed tomography–proven pelvic thrombophlebitis, continued antimicrobial therapy resulted in clinical resolution. Conversely, in five women given heparin along with antimicrobial drugs, the prolonged febrile course was not appreciably abbreviated. Witlin and Sibai (1995) reported similar observations in 11 women with ovarian vein thrombophlebitis. In a follow-up randomized study of 14 women by Brown and associates (1999), the addition of heparin to antimicrobial therapy for septic thrombophlebitis did not improve outcome nor did it hasten the time to defervescence or hospital discharge.

INFECTIONS OF THE PERINEUM, VAGINA, AND CERVIX

Surprisingly, infections of perineal wounds, including episiotomy incisions and repaired lacerations, are relatively uncommon considering the degree of bacterial contamination that accompanies normal delivery. Sweet and Ledger (1973) reported only 21 infected episiotomies (0.35 percent) among nearly 6000 women delivered vaginally at the University of Michigan and Wayne County Hospitals. Owen and Hauth (1990) described only 10 (0.05 percent) episiotomy infections with over 20,000 deliveries at the University of Alabama at Birmingham. Ramin and colleagues (1992) reported a 0.5 percent incidence of episiotomy breakdown at Parkland Hospital, and 80 percent of these were due to infection. Perhaps not surprisingly, serious infection is more likely in women who sustain a fourth-degree laceration. Goldaber and colleagues (1993) described the clinical courses of 390 such women of whom 5.4 percent had morbidity: dehiscence developed in 1.8 percent, infection and dehiscence in 2.8 percent, and infection only in 0.8 percent. Although rare, life-threatening septic shock may still occur as a result of an infected episiotomy wound (Soltesz and colleagues, 1999).

PATHOGENESIS AND CLINICAL COURSE. The apposing wound edges become red, brawny, and swollen. The sutures then often tear through the edematous tissues, allowing the necrotic wound edges to gape, with the result that serous, serosanguineous, or frankly purulent material exudes. Episiotomy breakdown or dehiscence is most commonly associated with infection. Other reported predisposing factors include coagulation disorders, cigarette smoking, and human papillomavirus (Ramin and Gilstrap, 1994). Local pain and dysuria, with or without urinary retention, are common symptoms. Ramin and colleagues (1992), in a series of 34 women with episiotomy dehiscence, reported that the most common signs and symptoms were pain (65 percent), purulent discharge (65 percent), and fever (44 percent). In extreme cases, the entire vulva may become edematous, ulcerated, and covered with exudate. Fortunately, provided drainage is good, superficial infections are seldom severe.

Vaginal lacerations may become infected directly or by extension from the perineum. The mucosa becomes edematous and hyperemic and may then become necrotic and slough. Parametrial extension may result in lymphangitis.

Cervical infection is probably more common than appreciated because lacerations are common and the cervix normally harbors potentially pathogenic organisms. Moreover, because deep cervical lacerations often extend directly into the tissue at the base of the broad ligament, infections may cause lymphangitis, parametritis, and bacteremia.

TREATMENT. Infected perineal wounds, like other infected surgical wounds, should be treated by establishing drainage. In most cases, sutures are removed and the infected wound opened. In some women with obvious cellulitis but no purulence, broad-spectrum antimicrobial therapy with close observation is appropriate. In others, drainage is necessary. Classically, it has been recommended with episiotomy dehiscence—especially if associated with infection—that a repair not be attempted for at least 3 to 4 months. It was postulated that such a delay would allow for adequate vascularization of the involved tissue and resolution of infection and cellulitis. This approach was challenged by Hauth and colleagues (1986), who advocated early repair after evidence of infection subsided. Subsequently, two large studies have attested to the efficacy of such practices. Hankins and co-workers (1990) described their experiences with early repair of episiotomy breakdown in 31 women. The average duration from breakdown to episiotomy repair was 6 days. All but two women had a successful repair; both developed a pinpoint rectovaginal fistula soon after repair and both were treated successfully with a small rectal flap. Ramin and colleagues (1992) reported successful early repair of episiotomy breakdown associated with infection in 32 of 34 women (94 percent).

TECHNIQUE FOR EARLY REPAIR. A preoperative protocol for early repair is summarized in Table 26–3. **Prior to attempting early repair of episiotomy dehiscence, the surgical wound must be properly cleaned and free of infection.** As shown in Figure 26–9, once the surface of the episiotomy wound is free of infection and exudate and covered by pink granulation tissue, secondary repair can be accomplished in the operating suite. Good tissue mobility must be accomplished, including identification and mobilization of the sphincter ani muscle. Secondary closure of the episiotomy is accomplished in layers as described for primary episiotomy closure in Chapter 13 (p. 326). Postoperative care includes local care, low-residue diet, stool softeners that avoid diarrhea, and nothing per vagina or rectum until healed.

TABLE 26–3. Preoperative Protocol for Early Repair of Episiotomy Dehiscence

1. Intravenous antimicrobial therapy
2. Remove sutures and open wound entirely
3. Wound care
   Meperidine as indicated
   1% lidocaine jelly applied to wound
   Debridement of all necrotic tissue
   Scrub wound twice daily with a Betadine-impregnated scrub brush
   Sitz bath several times daily
4. Mechanical bowel preparation evening before surgery[a]
5. NPO evening before surgery

[a] For fourth-degree repairs.
From Ramin and Gilstrap (1994), with permission.

NECROTIZING FASCIITIS. A rare but frequently fatal complication of perineal and vaginal wound infections is deep soft tissue infection involving muscle and fascia. These may also complicate vulvar infections in diabetic and immunocompromised women, and they rarely develop in otherwise healthy women. The microbiology of these serious perineal infections appears to be similar to those that cause other pelvic infections, as well as necrotizing fasciitis of the abdominal incision described previously. Although uncommon today, Shy and Eschenbach (1979) reported that necrotizing fasciitis was responsible for 20 percent of 15 maternal deaths in King County, Washington in the 1970s.

Necrotizing fasciitis of the episiotomy site may involve any of the several superficial or deep perineal fascial layers, and thus it may extend to the thighs, buttocks, and abdominal wall (Fig. 26–10). Although some infections may develop within a day of delivery, they more commonly do not cause symptoms until 3 to 5 days afterward. Clinical symptoms vary, and it is frequently difficult to differentiate superficial perineal infections from deep fascial ones. A high index of suspicion, with surgical exploration if the diagnosis is uncertain, may be lifesaving. Stamenkovic and Lew (1984) recommend biopsy of the fascial edges with frozen section microscopical examination when the diagnosis is uncertain. We have not found this advantageous, but aggressively pursue early exploration. Certainly, if myofasciitis progresses, the woman becomes very ill from septicemia, there is profound hemoconcentration from

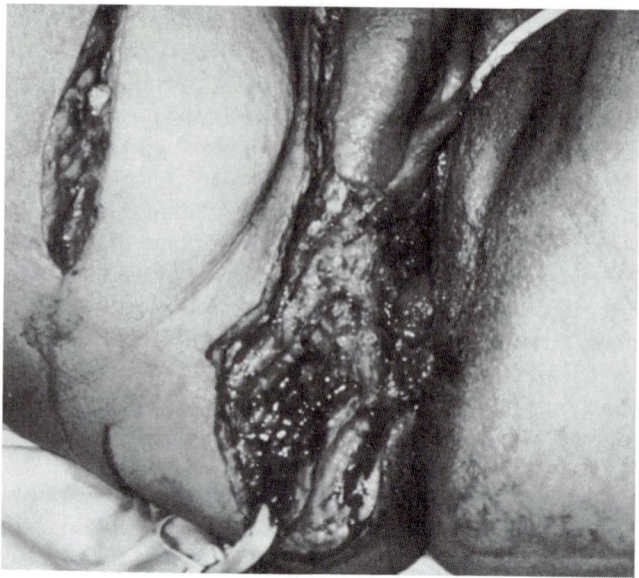

FIGURE 26–10. Necrotizing fasciitis complicating episiotomy infection. Three days postpartum this woman had severe perineal pain and edema of the episiotomy site. Prompt extensive debridement was carried out. Bacteria cultured from the infected episiotomy included *Escherichia coli*, *Streptococcus viridans*, group D streptococcus, *Corynebacterium* species, *Bacteroides fragilis*, and *Clostridium* species. Blood cultures were positive for *Bacteroides fragilis*.

capillary leakage with circulatory failure, and death soon follows. Early diagnosis, surgical debridement, antibiotics, and intensive care are of paramount importance in the successful treatment of necrotizing soft tissue infections (Urschel, 1999).

Aggressive surgical treatment is indicated and includes wide debridement of all infected tissue. As shown in Figure 26–10, this may include extensive vulvar debridement with unroofing and excision of abdominal, thigh, or buttock fascia. Split-thickness skin grafts later are used to repair the defects. **Mortality is virtually universal without surgical treatment, and it approaches 50 percent even if aggressive excision is performed.**

TOXIC SHOCK SYNDROME

Although not typically a puerperal infection, toxic shock syndrome is considered here because it has been reported in the puerperium. This is an acute febrile illness with severe multisystem derangement and a case-fatality rate of 10 to 15 percent. The illness is usually characterized by fever, headache, mental confusion, diffuse macular erythematous rash, subcutaneous edema, nausea, vomiting, watery diarrhea, and marked hemoconcentration. Renal failure followed by hepatic failure, disseminated intravascular coagulation, and circulatory

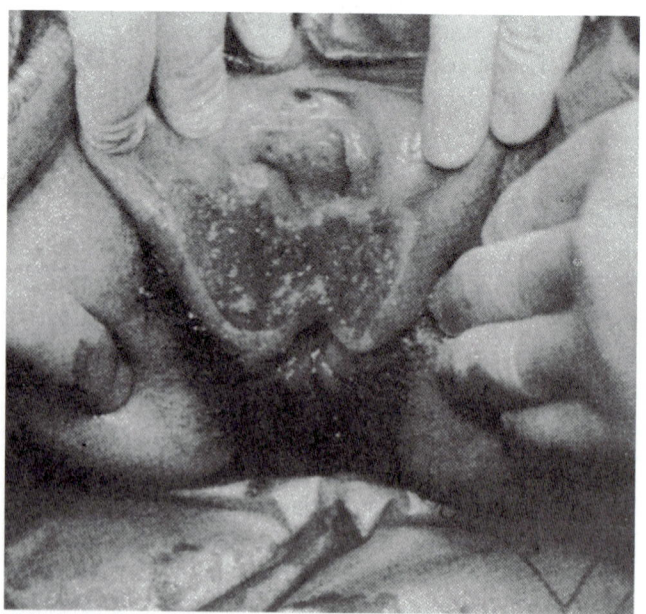

FIGURE 26–9. Dehiscence of fourth-degree episiotomy. Secondary repair is done when the wound surface is free of exudate and covered by pink granulation tissue. (From Ramin and Gilstrap, 1994, with permission.)

collapse may follow in rapid sequence. During recovery, the rash-covered areas undergo desquamation. *Staphylococcus aureus* has been recovered from almost all of afflicted persons, and a staphylococcal exotoxin, termed *toxic shock syndrome toxin-1,* and formerly called both *enterotoxin F* and *pyrogenic exotoxin C,* causes the syndrome by provoking profound endothelial injury.

In many cases, infection is not documented and colonization alone is found. McGregor and colleagues (1988) have described almost identical findings in women with infection complicated by *Clostridium sordelli* colonization.

When first described, toxic shock syndrome was associated with young menstruating women who used tampons. Because of educational efforts, as well as changes in tampon manufacture, it is much less prevalent. It has, however, been reported in a variety of other clinical situations. Nearly 10 percent of pregnant women have vaginal colonization with *S. aureus;* thus it is not surprising that the disease develops in postpartum women (Guerinot and co-workers, 1982). It has also been described in a mother-and-newborn pair (Green and La-Peter, 1982).

There have been several reports of a **toxic shock-like syndrome** associated with group A β-hemolytic streptococcal infection. Whitted and colleagues (1990) described this in a woman 2 weeks postpartum. Dotters and Katz (1991) reported a similar case in a 40-year-old woman following spontaneous abortion. As previously discussed, we have experienced similar cases of severe group A streptococcal infection in postpartum women (Nathan and colleagues, 1994). The toxin is quite potent, and the mortality rate correspondingly high.

Principal therapy for toxic shock is supportive, while allowing reversal of capillary endothelial injury. Treatment is similar to that for septic shock, discussed in Chapter 43 (p. 1169). In severe cases, it requires massive fluid replacement, mechanical ventilation with positive end-expiratory pressure, and renal dialysis. Antimicrobial therapy with specific antistaphylococcal drugs is given, although their value is questioned in cases without infection. With evidence for infection, for example wound cellulitis, antimicrobial therapy must include agents used for all puerperal infections.

HISTORY OF PUERPERAL INFECTION

The earliest reference to puerperal infection is found in the 5th century BC works of Hippocrates. In his discussion of women, *De Muliebrum Morbis,* he described the condition and attributed it to retention of bowel contents. By AD 200, Celsus and Galen had written in support of the theories of Hippocrates, and they recommended purgation. It was not until the late 1500s that lochial putrefaction or uterine inflammation were suspected as the cause of childbed fever, which had been linked to difficult labor. William Harvey (1651) aptly described the placental implantation site as a "vast internal ulcer" that may lead to gangrene. In 1659, Willis wrote on the subject of *febris puerperarum,* although the English term *puerperal fever* was probably first employed by Strother in 1716.

The theory of *milk metastasis* of Puzos (1686) followed next and predominated for 100 years, but in the 1700s, uterine inflammation was again thought to cause febrile morbidity. John Leake (1772) first suggested the contagious nature of puerperal infection, and Alexander Hamilton embraced this in 1781. Alexander Gordon of Aberdeen, in a treatise on epidemic puerperal fever in 1795, discussed its infectious and contagious nature, antedating Holmes (1855) and Semmelweis (1861) by half a century. Charles White (1773) of Manchester postulated that puerperal fever was dependent on lochial stagnation, and advised complete isolation of infected women.

It was not until the mid-1800s that such views were becoming acceptable. In 1843, Oliver Wendell Holmes presented *Contagiousness of Puerperal Fever* before the Boston Society for Medical Improvement. He showed clearly that at least the epidemic forms of the infection could always be traced to the lack of proper precautions on the part of the physician or nurse. Four years later, Semmelweis, then an assistant at the Vienna Lying-In Hospital, began a careful inquiry into the causes of the frightful mortality rate following delivery in that institution, as compared with the relatively small number of women who died as a result of infection following home delivery. He concluded that the morbid process was essentially a wound infection caused by the introduction of septic material by the examining finger. He issued stringent orders that physicians, students, and midwives disinfect their hands with chlorine water, the forerunner of Dakin solution, before examining parturient women. Despite immediate and surprising results in which the mortality rate fell from over 10 percent to 1 percent, both his work and that of Holmes were ridiculed by many prominent physicians of the time. His discovery remained unappreciated until Lister's teachings in 1867 regarding antisepsis, and the development of bacteriology by Pasteur.

The history of puerperal infection is discussed in greater detail in prior editions of *Williams Obstetrics.* The reader is also referred to the monographs of Eisenmann (1837), Burtenshaw (1904), and Peckham (1935). Willson (1988) provided a review of cesarean section infections, and Raju (1999) presented the theories of Simmelweis regarding neonatal infections transmitted at delivery in the woman with puerperal fever.

REFERENCES

American College of Obstetricians and Gynecologists: Antimicrobial therapy for obstetric patients. ACOG Educational Bulletin No. 245, March, 1998

Andrews WW, Shah SR, Goldenberg RL, Cliver SP, Hauth JC, Cassell GH: Association of post-cesarean delivery endometritis with colonization of the chorioamnion by *Ureaplasma urealyticum.* Obstet Gynecol 85:509, 1995

Anteby EY, Yagel S, Hanoch J, Shapiro M, Moses AE: Puerperal and intrapartum group A streptococcal infection. Infect Dis Obstet Gynecol 7:276, 1999

Atrash HK, Koonin LM, Lawson HW, Franks AL, Smith JC: Maternal mortality in the United States, 1979–1986. Obstet Gynecol 76:1055, 1990

Atterbury JL, Groome LJ, Baker SL, Ross EL, Hoff C: Hospital readmission for postpartum endometritis. J Matern Fetal Med 7:250, 1998

Bahn SA, Jacobson J, Petersen F: Maternal and neonatal outcome following prolonged labor induction. Obstet Gynecol 92:403, 1998

Bahnson RR, Wendel EF, Vogelzang RL: Renal vein thrombosis following puerperal ovarian vein thrombophlebitis. Am J Obstet Gynecol 152:290, 1985

Barber GR, Swygert JS: Necrotizing fasciitis due to *Photobacterium damsela* in a man lashed by a stingray. N Engl J Med 342:824, 2000

Berenson AB, Hammill HA, Martens MG, Faro S: Bacteriologic findings of post-cesarean endometritis in adolescents. Obstet Gynecol 75:627, 1990

Berman SM, Harrison HR, Boyce WT, Haffner WJJ, Lewis M, Arthur JB: Low birth weight, prematurity, and postpartum endometritis. JAMA 257:1189, 1987

Blanco JD, Gibbs RS, Malherbe H, Strickland-Cholmley M, St Clair PJ, Castaneda YS: A controlled study of genital mycoplasmas in amniotic fluid from patients with intra-amniotic infection. J Infect Dis 147:650, 1983

Brown CEL, Dunn DH, Harrell R, Setiawan H, Cunningham FG: Computed tomography for evaluation of puerperal infection. Surg Gynecol Obstet 172:2, 1991

Brown CEL, Lowe TW, Cunningham FG, Weinreb JC: Puerperal pelvic thrombophlebitis: Impact on diagnosis and treatment using x-ray computed tomography and magnetic resonance imaging. Obstet Gynecol 68:789, 1986

Brown CEL, Stettler RW, Twickler D, Cunningham FG: Puerperal septic pelvic thrombophlebitis: Incidence and response to heparin therapy. Am J Obstet Gynecol 181:143, 1999

Brumfield CG, Hauth JC, Andrews WW: Puerperal infections following cesarean delivery: Evaluation of a standardized protocol. Am J Obstet Gynecol 182:1147, 2000

Burtenshaw JH: The fever of the puerperium. NY and Philadelphia Med J, June/July 1904

Carey JC, Klebanoff MA, Hauth JC, Hillier SL, Thom EA, Ernest JM, Heine RP, Nugent RP, Fischer ML, Leveno KL, Wapner R, Varner M, and the National Institute of Child Health and Human Development Network of Maternal-Fetal Medicine Units: Metronidazole to prevent preterm delivery in pregnant women with asymptomatic bacterial vaginosis. N Engl J Med 342:534, 2000

Collins CG, McCallum EA, Nelson EW, Weinstein BB, Collins JH: Suppurative pelvic thrombophlebitis: 1. Incidence, pathology, etiology; 2. Symptomatology and diagnosis; 3. Surgical techniques: A study of 70 patients treated by ligation of the inferior vena cava and ovarian veins. Surgery 30:298, 1951

Cook JD, Lynch SR: The liabilities of iron deficiency. Blood 68:803, 1986

Cunningham FG, Hauth JC, Strong JD, Kappus SS: Infectious morbidity following cesarean: Comparison of two treatment regimens. Obstet Gynecol 52:656, 1978

DePalma RT, Cunningham FG, Leveno KJ, Roark ML: Continuing investigation of women at high risk for infection following cesarean delivery. Obstet Gynecol 60:53, 1982

Dinsmoor MJ, Newton ER, Gibbs RS: A randomized, double-blind placebo-controlled trial of oral antibiotic therapy following intravenous antibiotic therapy for postpartum endometritis. Obstet Gynecol 77:60, 1991

DiZerega G, Yonekura L, Roy S, Nakamura RM, Ledger WJ: A comparison of clindamycin-gentamicin and penicillin-gentamicin in the treatment of post-cesarean section endomyometritis. Am J Obstet Gynecol 134:238, 1979

Dotters DJ, Katz VL: Streptococcal toxic shock associated with septic abortion. Obstet Gynecol 78:549, 1991

Duff P, Gibbs RS: Pelvic vein thrombophlebitis: Diagnostic dilemma and therapeutic challenge. Obstet Gynecol Surv 38:365, 1983

Dunn LJ, Van Voorhis LW: Enigmatic fever and pelvic thrombophlebitis. N Engl J Med 276:265, 1967

Dunnihoo DR, Gallaspy JW, Wise RB, Otterson WN. Postpartum ovarian vein thrombophlebitis: A review. Obstet Gynecol Surv 46:415, 1991

Eisenmann GE: Die Wundfieber und die Kindbettfieber. Erlangen, 1837

Emmons SL, Krohn M, Jackson M, Eschenbach DA: Development of wound infections among women undergoing cesarean section. Obstet Gynecol 72:559, 1988

Engoren M: Lack of association between atelectasis and fever. Chest 107:81, 1995

Faro S: Soft tissue infections. In Gilstrap LC, Faro S (eds): Infections in Pregnancy. New York, Wiley-Liss, 1990, p 75

Filker R, Monif GRG: The significance of temperature during the first 24 hours postpartum. Obstet Gynecol 53:359, 1979

Gibbs RS, O'Dell TN, MacGregor RR, Schwarz RH, Morton H: Puerperal endometritis: A prospective microbiologic study. Am J Obstet Gynecol 121:919, 1975

Gibbs RS, Weiner MH, Walmer K, St. Clair PJ: Microbiologic and serologic studies of *Gardnerella vaginalis* in intra-amniotic infection. Obstet Gynecol 70:187, 1987

Gilstrap LC III, Cunningham FG: The bacterial pathogenesis of infection following cesarean section. Obstet Gynecol 53:545, 1979

Goepfert AR, Guinn DA, Andrews WW, Hauth JC: Necrotizing fasciitis after cesarean section. Obstet Gynecol 89:409, 1997

Goldaber KG, Wendel PJ, McIntire DD, Wendel GD Jr: Postpartum perineal morbidity after fourth degree perineal repair. Am J Obstet Gynecol 168:489, 1993

Goldenberg RL, Klebanoff MA, Nugent R, Krohn MA, Hillier S, Andrews WW: Bacterial colonization of the vagina during pregnancy in four ethnic groups. Am J Obstet Gynecol 174:1618, 1996

Gordon A: A Treatise on Epidemic Puerperal Fever of Aberdeen. London, CG & J Robinson, 1795

Green SL, LaPeter KS: Evidence for postpartum toxic-shock syndrome in a mother–infant pair. Am J Med 72:169, 1982

Guerinot GT, Gitomer SD, Sanko SR: Postpartum patient with toxic shock syndrome. Obstet Gynecol 59:43S, 1982

Halban J, Köhler R: Die pathologische Anatomie des Puerperalprozesses. Vienna, 1919

Hamilton A: A Treatise on Midwifery. London, 1781

Hankins GDV, Hauth JC, Gilstrap LC, Hammond TL, Yeomans ER, Snyder RR: Early repair of episiotomy dehiscence. Obstet Gynecol 75:48, 1990

Hauth JC, Gilstrap LC III, Ward SC, Hankins GDV: Early repair of an external sphincter ani muscle and rectal mucosal dehiscence. Obstet Gynecol 67:806, 1986

Hippocrates: Liber Prior de Muliebrum Morbis

Holmes OW: Puerperal Fever as a Private Pestilence. Boston, Ticknor & Fields, 1855

Ismail MA, Chandler AE, Beem ME: Chlamydial colonization of the cervix in pregnant adolescents. J Reprod Med 30:549, 1985

Jacob S, Bloebaum L, Shah G, Varner MW: Maternal mortality in Utah. Obstet Gynecol 91:187, 1998

Josey WE, Staggers SR Jr: Heparin therapy in septic pelvic thrombophlebitis: A study of 46 cases. Am J Obstet Gynecol 120:228, 1974

Kindig M, Cardwell M, Lee T: Delayed postpartum uterine dehiscence. Case report. J Reprod Med 43:591, 1998

Koonin LM, Mackay AP, Berg CJ, Atrash HK, Smith JC: Pregnancy-related mortality surveillance—United States, 1987–1990. MMWR 46:17, 1997

Krohn MA, Hillier SL, Baker CJ: Maternal peripartum complications associated with vaginal group B streptococci colonization. J Infect Dis 179:1410, 1999

Leake J: Practical Observations on the Child-bed Fever; Also on the Nature and Treatment of Uterine Haemorrhages, Convulsions, and Such Other Acute Disease as Are Most Fatal to Women During the State of Pregnancy. London, J Walter, 1772

Lev-Toaff AS, Baka JJ, Toaff ME, Friedman AC, Radecki PD, Caroline DF: Diagnostic imaging in puerperal febrile morbidity. Obstet Gynecol 78:50, 1991

Libombo A, Folgosa E, Bergstrom S: Risk factors in puerperal endometritis-myometritis. An incident case-referent study. Gynecol Obstet Invest 38:198, 1994

Lister J: On the antiseptic principle in the practice of surgery. Br Med J 2:246, 1867

Liu C, Abate B, Reyes M, Gonik B: Single daily dosing of gentamicin: Pharmacokinetic comparison of two dosing methodologies for postpartum endometritis. Infect Dis Obstet Gynecol 7:133, 1999

Maberry MC, Gilstrap LC, Bawdon RE, Little BB, Dax JS: Anaerobic coverage for intra-amnionic infection: Maternal and perinatal impact. Am J Perinatol 8:338, 1991

Magee KP, Blanco JD, Graham JM, Rayburn C, Prien S: Endometritis after cesarean: The effect of age. Am J Perinatol 11:24, 1994

Maldjian C, Adam R, Maldjian J, Smith R: MRI appearance of the pelvis in the post cesarean-section patient. Magn Reson Imaging 17:223, 1999

McGregor JA, Soper D, Lovell G: A toxic shock-like syndrome caused by Clostridia sordelli affecting postpartum women. Abstract 30 presented at meeting of Infectious Disease Society in Obstetrics and Gynecology, Aspen, CO, August 1988

McNeeley SG Jr, Hendrix SL, Bennett SM, Singh A, Ransom SB, Kmak DC, Morley GW: Synthetic graft placement in the treatment of fascial dehiscence with necrosis and infection. Am J Obstet Gynecol 179:1430, 1998

Munsick RA, Gillanders LA: A review of the syndrome of puerperal ovarian vein thrombophlebitis. Obstet Gynecol Surv 36:57, 1981

Murray BE: Vancomycin-resistant enterococcal infections. N Engl J Med 342:710, 2000

Mussey RD, DeNormandie RL, Adair FL: The American Committee on Maternal Welfare, Inc: Its organization, purposes and activities. Am J Obstet Gynecol 28:754, 1935

Nathan L, Leveno KJ: Group A streptococcal puerperal sepsis: Historical review and 1990s resurgence. Infect Dis Obstet Gynecol 1:252, 1994

Owen J, Andrews WW: Wound complications after cesarean section. Clin Obstet Gynecol 27:842, 1994

Owen J, Hauth JC: Episiotomy infection and dehiscence. In Gilstrap LC III, Faro S (eds): Infections in Pregnancy. New York, Liss, 1990, p 61

Peckham CH: A brief history of puerperal infection. Bull Hist Med 3:187, 1935

Puzos N: Première mémoire sur les depots laiteux. In: Traités des Accouchements. Paris, 1686, p 341

Raju TN: Ignac Semmelweis and the etiology of fetal and neonatal sepsis. J Perinatol 19:307, 1999

Ramin SM, Gilstrap LC: Episiotomy and early repair of dehiscence. Clin Obstet Gynecol 37:816, 1994

Ramin SM, Ramus R, Little B, Gilstrap LC: Early repair of episiotomy dehiscence associated with infection. Am J Obstet Gynecol 167:1104, 1992

Roberts S, Maccato M, Faro S, Pinell P: The microbiology of post-cesarean section wound morbidity. Obstet Gynecol 81:383, 1993

Rotmensch S, Vishne TH, Celentano C, Dan M, Ben-Rafael Z: Maternal infectious morbidity following multiple courses of betamethasone. J Infect 39:49, 1999

Schrag SJ, Zywicki S, Farley MM, Reingold A, Harrison LH, Lefkowitz LB, Hadler JL, Danila R, Cieslak PR, Schuchat A: Group B streptococcal disease in the era of intrapartum antibiotic prophylaxis. N Engl J Med 342:15, 2000

Segal S, Gemer O, Sestopal-Epelman M, London D, Velkes S, Jakim I: Retroperitoneal abscess after normal delivery. A report of two cases. J Reprod Med 41:276, 1996

Semmelweis IP: Die Aetiologie, der Begriff und die Prophylaxis des Kindbettfiebers. Pest, 1861

Sherman D, Lurie S, Betzer M, Pinhasi Y, Arieli S, Boldur I: Uterine flora at cesarean and its relationship to postpartum endometritis. Obstet Gynecol 94:787, 1999

Shy KK, Eschenbach DA: Fatal perineal cellulitis from an episiotomy site. Obstet Gynecol 52:293, 1979

Soltesz S, Biedler A, Ohlmann P, Molter G: Puerperal sepsis due to infected episiotomy wound. Zentralbl Gynakol 121:441, 1999

Soper DE, Brockwell WJ, Dalton HP: The importance of wound infection in antibiotic failures in the therapy of postpartum endometritis. Surg Gynecol Obstet 174:265, 1992

Stamenkovic I, Lew PD: Early recognition of potentially fatal necrotizing fasciitis: The use of frozen-section biopsy. N Engl J Med 310:1689, 1984

Strother E: Critical Essay on Fevers. London, 1716

Suonio S, Huttunen M: Puerperal endometritis after abdominal twin delivery. Acta Obstet Gynecol Scand 73:313, 1994

Sweet RL, Ledger WJ: Puerperal infectious morbidity. A two-year review. Am J Obstet Gynecol 117:1093, 1973

Tran TS, Jamulitrat S, Chongsuvivatwong V, Geater A: Risk factors for postcesarean surgical site infection. Obstet Gynecol 95:367, 2000

Twickler DM, Setiawan AT, Harrell RS, Brown CEL: CT appearance of the pelvis after cesarean section. Am J Radiol 156:523, 1991

Udagawa H, Oshio Y, Shimizu Y: Serious group A streptococcal infection around delivery. Obstet Gynecol 94:153, 1999

Urschel JD: Necrotizing soft tissue infections. Postgrad Med J 75:645, 1999

Walmer D, Walmer KR, Gibbs RS: Enterococci in post-cesarean endometritis. Obstet Gynecol 71:159, 1988

Watts DH, Krohn MA, Hillier SL, Eschenbach DA: Bacterial vaginosis as a risk factor for post-cesarean endometritis. Obstet Gynecol 75:52, 1990

Wetchler SJ, Dunn LJ: Ovarian abscess. Report of a case and a review of the literature. Obstet Gynecol Surv 40:476, 1985

White C: Treatise on the Management of Pregnancy and Lying-in Women and the Means of Curing But More Especially of Preventing the Principal Disorders to Which They Are Liable. London, EC Dilly, 1773

Whitted RW, Yeomans ER, Hankins GDV: Group A β-hemolytic streptococcus as a cause of toxic shock. A case report. J Reprod Med 35:558, 1990

Williams JW. Ligation or excision of thrombosed veins in the treatment of puerperal pyemia. Am J Obstet Gynecol 59:758, 1909

Willis T: Diatribae duae medico-philosophical . . . de febribus. London, T Raycroft, 1659

Willson JR: The conquest of cesarean section related infections: A progress report. Obstet Gynecol 72:519, 1988

Witlin AG, Sibai BM: Postpartum ovarian vein thrombosis after vaginal delivery: A report of 11 cases. Obstet Gynecol 85:775, 1995

Zimbelman J, Palmer A, Todd J: Improved outcome of clindamycin compared with beta-lactam antibiotic treatment for invasive *Streptococcus pyogenes* infections. Pediatr Infect Dis J 18:1096, 1999

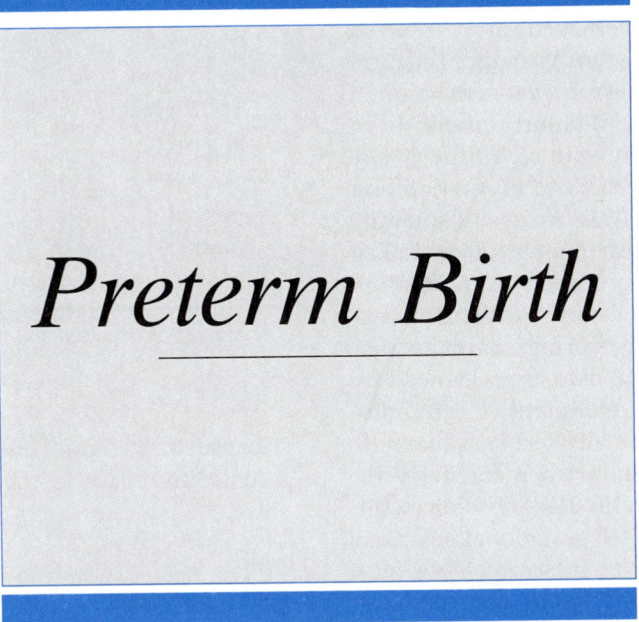

27

Preterm Birth

Low birthweight is the term used to define infants who are born too small, and *preterm* or *premature birth* are the terms used to define infants who are born too soon. Prior to the last century, when the expression premature birth was first used, infants delivered before term were usually referred to as "weaklings" or "congenitally debilitated babies" (Cone, 1985). Indeed, prior to 1872, infants were not even weighed at birth whether full term or premature. In 1900, Ransom wrote that in the United States "of the thousands of premature infants born . . . most are quietly laid away with . . . little if any effort being made for their rescue." In his first edition of this textbook, Williams (1903) wrote: "Generally speaking, premature children weighing less than 1500 g (3 lbs 3 oz) have practically no chance of life, though exceptional cases have been reported." As the 20th century progressed, there was an increasing awareness that preterm infants required special care, as evidenced by the development of incubators and intensive care nurseries. Prematurity became nationally visible as the most frequent cause of death in infancy when country-wide statistics became available with the 1949 revision of the birth certificate, which specified gestational age and birthweights.

More recently, infant mortality has become a benchmark for international comparisons of health-care systems. In this regard, the United States has ranked poorly. For example, in 1995 the United States ranked 25th in the world, well behind Japan, Singapore, Germany, and most of the Scandinavian countries (National Center for Health Statistics, 1999). Those countries with higher rates of preterm delivery have higher rates of infant mortality. Moreover, within the United States, African-Americans are disproportionately affected by preterm delivery and infant mortality. As shown in Table 27–1, more than 28,000 infants died during infancy in 1998 in the United States, and 66 percent of these were within 4 weeks of birth. Moreover, preterm birth is implicated in at least two thirds of these early infant deaths.

Sachs and associates (1995) have legitimately challenged international comparisons of infant mortality,

TABLE 27–2. Live Births in the United States in 1998 According to Gestational Age at Delivery

Gestational Age	Live Births	Percent
Total	3,941,553	100
36 weeks or less	452,275	11
< 28 weeks	29,037	0.7
28–31 weeks	47,486	1.2
32–35 weeks	212,210	5
36 weeks	163,542	4
37–39 weeks	1,859,198	47
40 weeks	853,416	22
41 weeks	443,502	11
42 weeks or greater	292,766	7

Adapted from Ventura and colleagues (2000).

because they found enormous regional and international differences in the way preterm births are classified.

DEFINITIONS

In 1935, the American Academy of Pediatrics defined prematurity as a live-born infant weighing 2500 g or less (Cone, 1985). These criteria were used widely until it became apparent that there were discrepancies between gestational age and birthweight because of restricted fetal growth. The World Health Organization in 1961 added gestational age as a criterion for premature infants, defined as those born at 37 weeks or less. A distinction was made between low birthweight (2500 g or less) and prematurity (37 weeks or less). Others have suggested that preterm birth be defined as those infants delivered prior to the completion of 37 weeks (American College of Obstetricians and Gynecologists, 1995).

With continued improved care of the preterm infant, other definitions have been developed. For example, the Collaborative Group on Antenatal Steroid Therapy (1981) reported that the great preponderance of mortality and serious morbidity from preterm birth is prior to 34 weeks. Moreover, low birthweight, defined as less than 2500 g, has been modified now to describe very-low birthweight, infants weighing 1500 g or less; and extremely-low birthweight, those who weigh 1000 g or less. As shown in Table 27–2, almost 90 percent of live births in the United States occur at 37 weeks or later in gestation, and progressively fewer births are recorded with decreasing gestational weeks at delivery. The disproportionate contribution of multiple gestations to preterm births is discussed in Chapter 30 (p. 780).

In many industrialized countries including the United

TABLE 27–1. Infant Mortality in the United States for 1998

	Infants	Rate per 100,000 Live Births
Total live births	3,944,046	—
Infant deaths	28,486 (100%)	722
0–27 days	18,832 (66%)	477
28 days–1 year	9,654 (34%)	245

Adapted from Martin and colleagues (1999).

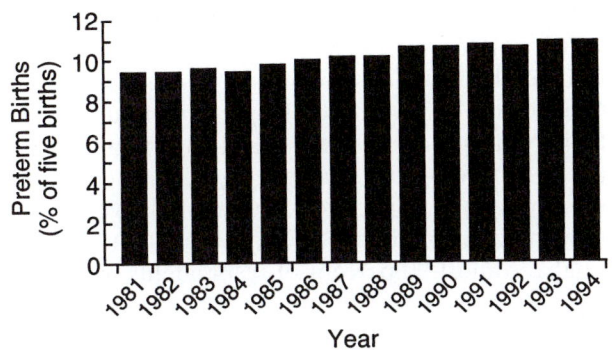

FIGURE 27-1. Preterm births in the United States, 1981 through 1994. (Data are from the National Center for Health Statistics, 1996.)

increased use of ultrasound for estimating gestational age (Joseph and associates, 1998). Similar factors are undoubtedly operative in the rise in preterm births that has occurred in the United States.

The importance of low birthweight, which is approximately equivalent to birth before 37 weeks, as a predictor of infant death within 28 days of birth (neonatal death), is shown in Figure 27–2. Neonatal mortality rates by state are directly proportional to the delivery of low-birthweight infants. Those states with large urban populations, or where poverty is common, have the highest incidence. In response, the United States greatly expanded the Medicaid program in 1986 with the aim of increasing prenatal and other health services for pregnant women (Dubay and colleagues, 1995). Similarly, the federal government also initiated the Healthy Start Program in 1991 for the 15 urban areas with the worst infant mortality rates.

States (Fig. 27–1), the proportion of infants born before term has increased in the past 20 years (Joseph and associates, 1998). In Canada, for instance, births at 36 weeks' gestation or less increased from 6.3 percent in 1981 to 6.8 percent in 1992. This increase in preterm births has been attributed to changes in the frequency of multiple births, increases in obstetrical intervention, improved ascertainment of early preterm births, and

With respect to gestational age, a fetus or infant may be preterm, term, or postterm. With respect to size, the fetus or infant may be normally grown or appropriate for gestational age, small in size or small for gestational age, or overgrown and consequently large for gestational age. In recent years, the term *small for gestational age* has been widely used to categorize an infant whose

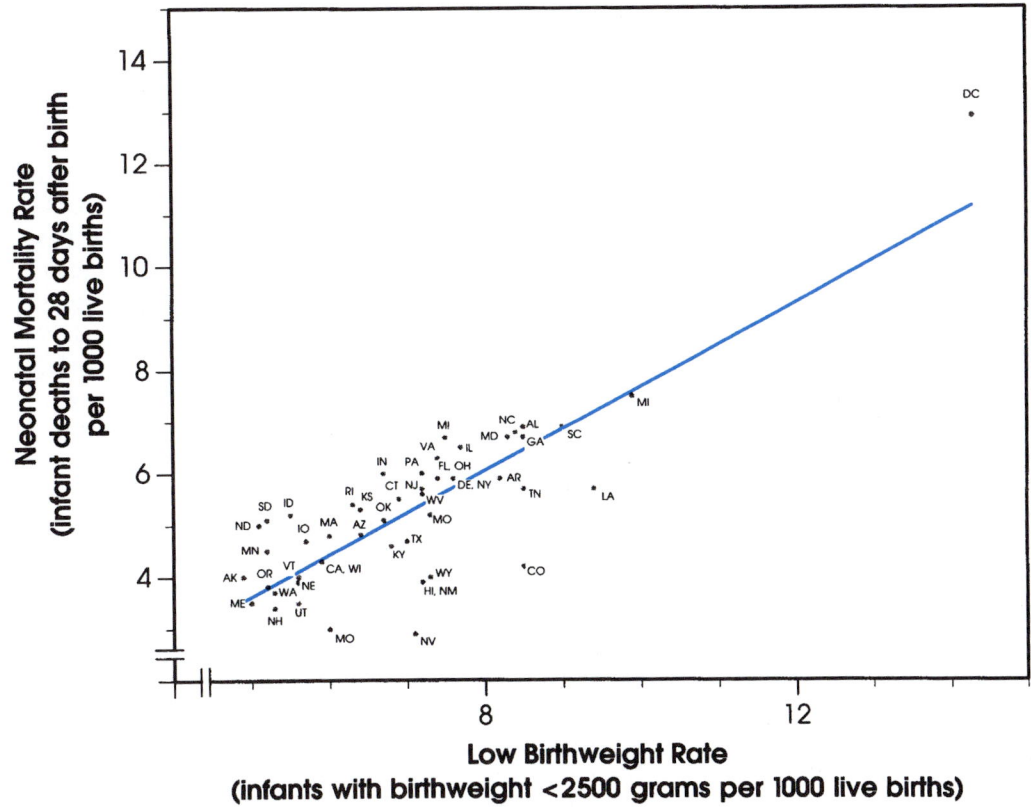

FIGURE 27–2. Neonatal mortality rate in relation to low birthweight in the 50 states and Washington, DC. (From Paneth, 1995, with permission.)

birthweight is usually below the 10th percentile for its gestational age. Other often-used terms have included *fetal growth retardation* or *intrauterine growth retardation*. Within the past 5 years the term *restriction* has largely replaced *retardation*, because the latter may erroneously convey mental delay rather than only the intended suboptimal fetal growth (Chap. 29, p. 745). The infant whose birthweight is above the 90th percentile has been categorized as *large for gestational age*, and the infant whose weight is between the 10th and 90th percentiles is designated *appropriate for gestational age*. Thus, an infant born before term can be small or large for gestational age and still be preterm according to chronological gestational age. Moreover, some preterm infants have also suffered growth restriction in utero. It is important to recognize that preterm birth also frequently includes infants who have suffered subnormal in utero growth. Fetal growth restriction is discussed in Chapter 29, and this chapter will focus on preterm births where the only perceived problem is delivery before full maturation. Shown in Table 29–1 are birthweight percentiles for each gestational week between 20 and 44 weeks, which may be helpful in estimating when a preterm infant's birthweight is subnormal or excessive.

IMPACT OF PRETERM BIRTH

Obstetrical approaches to preterm labor and delivery are guided in large part by expectations that the obstetrician has for survival of the premature neonate as well as the therapeutic alternatives available for management of preterm labor (Bottoms and colleagues, 1997). That some very small infants do survive when provided with prolonged, very expensive intensive care has created serious problems in decision making. The obstetrician faces the challenge of effecting delivery in such a way as to optimize the status of the fetus-infant at birth, in the event that intensive care will be applied. The neonatologist in turn must make a judgment as how best to dispense the finite resources for medical care provided by the insurance carrier, the family, governmental agencies, the hospital, and the health-care team.

Aside from survival, another important issue is the quality of life achieved by quite immature, extremely-low-birthweight infants. It is apparent that appreciable compromise, both physical and intellectual, afflicts many such children. Given these concerns, at what time in gestation should obstetrical interventions be practiced? Although it is impossible to precisely set the earliest limit for neonatal survival, certain factors inevitably have an impact on the clinical decision-making process.

Obstetrical perception of viability probably influences survival of extremely-low-birthweight infants.

Amon and co-workers (1992) and Bottoms and co-workers (1997) surveyed American obstetricians to determine their clinical opinions regarding intrapartum management of the severely preterm fetus requiring delivery. Intrapartum fetal heart rate monitoring was initiated at 23, 24, and 25 weeks by 10, 45, and 65 percent of respondents, respectively. Cesarean delivery was not performed at less than 24 weeks or less than 500 g fetal weight. Almost 90 percent of respondents were willing to perform cesarean delivery for fetal distress or breech presentation at 26 weeks or 750 g fetal weight. Delivery management prior to 26 weeks, or for fetuses smaller than 750 g, was variable and individualized. Haywood and associates (1994) found that physicians significantly underestimated survival and handicap-free survival rates, particularly in those infants delivered between 23 and 29 weeks. Doron and co-workers (1998) analyzed delivery room decisions by neonatologists to provide or withhold resuscitation for 41 infants born between 23 and 26 weeks' gestation. They concluded that the delivery room is not the best place to decide on withholding life support and that this decision is best made later in the neonatal course.

It is important to emphasize that the obstetrical decision not to perform cesarean delivery or use intrapartum monitoring does not necessarily imply that the fetus is "nonviable" or "written off." For example, Kitchen and co-workers (1992) analyzed the outcomes of live-born infants weighing 500 to 999 g and found that although 50 percent of the infants survived and only 7 percent were severely disabled, these outcomes were unrelated to the use of cesarean delivery or electronic monitoring.

Perceptions of the potential for survival are inevitably confused by difficulties incurred by imprecisely known gestational age. Most survival data are based upon birthweight, which may vary appreciably between 24 and 26 weeks. For example, infants born between 24 and 26 weeks can vary in weight from 435 g to 1640 g (Alexander and associates, 1996). Perinatal mortality and morbidity decreases markedly from 24 to 26 weeks' gestation. Indeed, survival increases from approximately 20 percent at 24 weeks' gestation up to 50 percent at 25 weeks, or an increase of almost 4 percent each day. Similarly, serious perinatal morbidity also markedly decreases each day from 24 to 26 weeks' gestation. Clinically, this daily marked association with improved outcomes is of immense importance when determining obstetrical management at the lowest end of gestational ages.

The birthweight-linked survival rates for live births during 1999 at Parkland Hospital are shown in Table 27–3. Survival data for infants 500 to 1500 g are remarkably similar to rates reported by Fanaroff and colleagues (1995) for the National Institutes of Health (NIH)-sponsored Neonatal Research Network. Chances for

TABLE 27–3. Survival Rates by Birthweight for 14,733 Infants Born at Parkland Hospital in 1999

Birthweight (g)	Live Births (no.)	Neonatal Deaths[a] (no.)	Survival (%)
500–750	34	20	41
751–1000	52	6	85
1001–1250	54	6	89
1251–1500	52	3	94
1501–1750	82	3	96
1751–2000	138	3	98
2001–2500	667	11	98
2501–3000	2,488	3	99.9
3001–3500	5,695	3	99.9
3501–4000	4,071	1	100
> 4000	1,400	2	100
Total	14,733	61	99.6

[a] Approximately 85% of all neonatal deaths were in live-born infants weighing less than 2500 g and 57% in those less than 1500 g.

survival increase appreciably at or above 1000-g birthweight. These data indicate that survival is possible for infants weighing 500 to 750 g. Many of these extremely-low-birthweight infants, however, were growth restricted and therefore of more advanced maturity. For example, survival of a 380-g infant has been reported, but the gestational age was confirmed to be $25^{3/7}$ weeks (Ginsberg and associates, 1990). Clearly, expectations for neonatal survival are primarily influenced by gestational age and maturity rather than simply by birthweight.

LOWER LIMIT OF SURVIVAL. The frontier for infant survival has been progressively pushed earlier into gesta-

tion primarily as a result of continued innovations in neonatal intensive care. Copper and associates (1993) compiled gestational age–specific neonatal mortality rates for 3386 live-born infants prospectively enrolled between 1982 and 1986 in the March of Dimes Multicenter Preterm Birth Prevention Project. As shown in Figure 27–3, neonatal mortality decreased from 100 percent at 23 weeks to about 10 percent at 29 weeks, with little additional improvement through 34 weeks. Virtually identical mortality rates for 2678 live-born infants delivered in England between 1990 and 1993 were reported by Rutter (1995). The period of gestation from 23 to 25 weeks poses the greatest dilemma for both the obstetrician and pediatrician. As shown in Figure 27–3, the probability of neonatal death before 26 weeks exceeds 75 percent. Stevenson and colleagues (1998) reported very similar low-birthweight outcomes from an inborn cohort of the NICHD Neonatal Research Network in 1993 and 1994. Based on the "best obstetrical assignment of gestational age," death, severe infant morbidities, or both were great before 26 weeks' gestation and almost universal before 24 weeks' gestation. Bottoms and co-workers (1999), for the NICHD Maternal–Fetal Medicine Units Network, concluded that in newborns weighing less than 1000 g, ultrasound assessment of either fetal femur length or gestational age were most predictive of neonatal mortality.

LONG-TERM OUTCOMES. Whereas few infants with birthweights below 750 g were actively treated during the 1970s, beginning in the 1980s, treatment was often practiced for infants with birthweights of at least 500 g and those born at 24 weeks or more (Hack and colleagues, 1994). The high rate of significant neonatal morbidity in these tiny infants, and the likelihood of a normal life, must be weighed against the apparent tri-

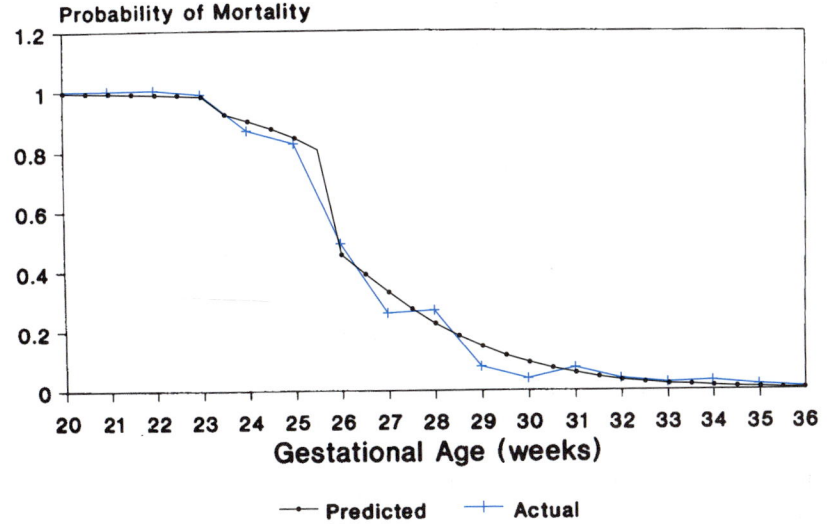

FIGURE 27–3. Probability of neonatal mortality before hospital discharge in 3386 births between 20 and 37 weeks. The predicted mortality curves serve to smooth the data points. (From Copper and colleagues, 1993, with permission.)

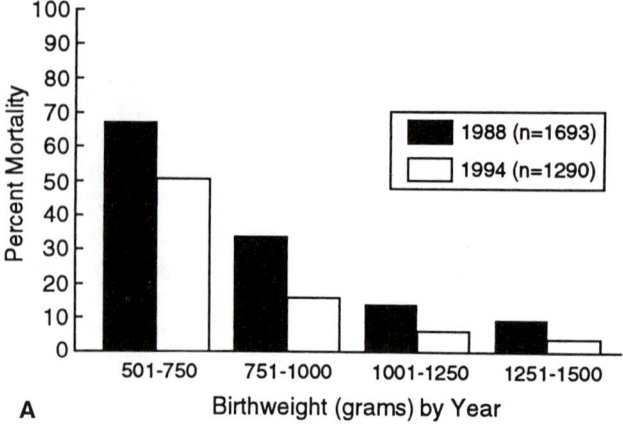

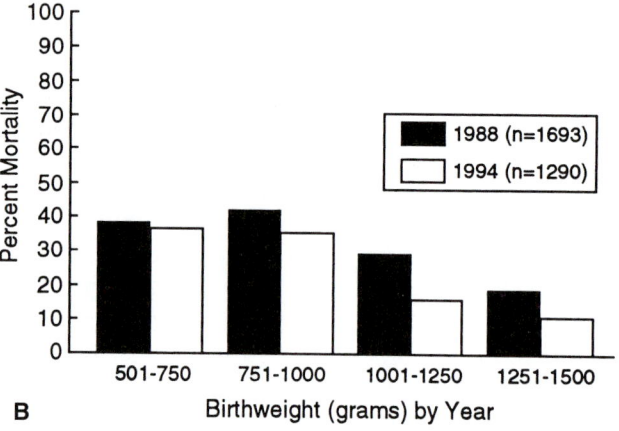

FIGURE 27–4. Mortality (**A**) and morbidity (**B**) rates for very low birthweight infants cared for in the NICHD Neonatal Research Network Centers from 1988 to 1994. (From Stevenson and colleagues, 1998, with permission.)

umph of survival. As shown in Figure 27–4, among 501- to 1500-g newborns in the National Institute of Child Health and Human Development (NICHD) Neonatal Research Network Centers, mortality and major morbidity among survivors decreased from 1988 to 1994, but both occurred in half of newborns at 501- to 750-g birthweight. Allen and co-workers (1993) described outcomes to 6 months of life for infants delivered at 22 to 25 weeks, and who were aggressively supported with intensive care. No infants survived at 22 weeks, and virtually all survivors at 23 and 24 weeks had significant brain abnormalities (Table 27–4). They concluded that whether the occasional child who is born at 23 or 24 weeks and does well justifies the considerable mortality and morbidity of the majority is a question that should be discussed by parents, health-care providers, and society. More recently, Wood and colleagues (2000) con-

firmed these data in a similar study from the United Kingdom.

Several groups of investigators have attempted to measure long-term outcomes in infants delivered at the very frontier of survival during the 1980s. Whyte and co-workers (1993) prospectively followed for a minimum of 2 years 321 infants born at their hospital between 23 and 26 weeks. There were no survivors among infants delivered at 23 weeks, and only 6 percent of the survivors at 24 weeks did not sustain major long-term morbidity. Approximately half of infants delivered at 25 and 26 weeks were intact at a minimum of 2 years of age. Doyle and colleagues (1994) followed infants born at 24 to 26 weeks for 5 years or longer. Even fewer infants (approximately 20 percent) were totally free of impairment with longer intervals of survival. Hack and colleagues (1994) studied the health and developmental outcomes at early school age of 68 children with birthweights below 750 g who were born from 1982 through 1986. They concluded from their unique study that children with birthweights below 750 g who survived are at "serious disadvantage in every skill required for adequate performance." Specifically, 45 percent of the survivors needed special education facilities, 21 percent had subnormal intelligence quotient (IQ) (less than 70), and many had subnormal growth and visual ability. Rutter (1995) concluded in his review of outcomes in extremely preterm infants that full resuscitation and intensive care should definitely be given at 26 weeks, probably be given at 25 weeks, possibly be given at 24 weeks, but not at 23 weeks or earlier.

Vohr and co-workers (2000) assessed neurodevelopmental and functional outcomes at 18 to 22 months corrected age of 1151 (401 to 1000 g) survivors cared for in the 12 participating centers of the NICHD Neonatal Research Network and who were born in 1993 and 1994. Only half of the 1151 survivors had a normal neurodevelopmental and sensory assessment, and those at the

TABLE 27–4. Outcomes of Live-born Infants Delivered Between 22 and 25 Weeks and Given Intensive Care

Weeks of Gestation	Live Births	Alive at 6 Months (%)	Infants without Severe Brain Abnormalities[a] (%)
22	29	0	—
23	40	6 (15)	1 (3)
24	34	19 (56)	7 (21)
25	39	31 (79)	28 (72)

[a] Grade III or IV intraventricular hemorrhage or periventricular leukomalacia.
From Allen and colleagues (1993), with permission.

lower birthweights had markedly worse outcomes as predicted by chronic lung disease, grades 3 and 4 intraventricular hemorrhage, and periventricular leukomalacia.

Wood and associates (2000) reported results from the EPI Cure Study Group of the United Kingdom. They performed careful mental and psychomotor evaluations at a median of 30 months in 283 surviving infants born at 25 completed weeks or less. Infant neurological survival without disability was reported in 1 of 138 infants born during the 22nd week; 11 of 241 (5 percent) during the 23rd week; 45 of 382 (12 percent) during the 24th week; and 98 of 424 (23 percent) born during the 25th week.

UPPER LIMIT OF SIGNIFICANT PREMATURITY. Not only has the frontier for neonatal survival been pushed earlier into pregnancy, but survival of larger preterm infants has become as good as that for term infants. Is there a birthweight or gestational age threshold after which attempts to delay delivery are unwarranted? In an effort to address this question, Robertson and colleagues (1992) analyzed neonatal outcomes between 1983 and 1986 from five tertiary care centers in the United States. A total of 20,680 carefully dated pregnancies without complications such as diabetes or hypertension were identified. Most thresholds—defined as the gestational week at which the incidence of complications attributable to preterm delivery became indistinguishable from term infants—were between 32 and 34 weeks. Respiratory distress syndrome, although decreasing precipitously between 33 and 34 weeks (31 to 13 percent), still developed in about 6 percent of births between 35 and 38 weeks. DePalma and co-workers (1992) found that the birthweight threshold for neonatal mortality at Parkland Hospital was 1600 g, and the threshold for neonatal morbidity due to complications of preterm delivery was approximately 1900 g. They concluded that aggressive obstetrical attempts to prevent preterm births for infants whose weights exceed 1900 g offer few apparent benefits.

ECONOMIC IMPACT OF PRETERM BIRTH. The dollar cost of the resources used to care for low-birthweight infants is one measure of the national burden of preterm birth. These dollar costs are shown in Table 27–5. A proportionately small number of births in the United States (approximately 7 percent) consume more than a third of health-care expenditures during the first year of life. On an individual basis, it is not uncommon for the smallest surviving infants to incur special care nursery costs exceeding several hundred thousand dollars (Walker and associates, 1984). Costs exceeding $1 million are possible in those hospitalized for up to a year or longer. Moreover, because of the long-term outcomes already described, additional expenditures for developmental handicaps are necessary during the remainder of childhood for many infants.

Recently, St. John and associates (2000) used a cost-analysis model to determine that 12 percent of initial neonatal care dollars in the United States were spent on infants born between 24 and 26 weeks' gestation for 1989 through 1992, and that 43 percent was spent on those born at 37 weeks' gestation or later.

CAUSES OF PRETERM BIRTH

A wide spectrum of causes and demographic factors have been implicated in the birth of preterm infants (Table 27–6).

MEDICAL AND OBSTETRICAL COMPLICATIONS. Meis and colleagues (1995b, 1998) analyzed the causes of delivery before 37 weeks in a population-based study of singleton pregnancies performed in the NICHD Maternal–Fetal Medicine Units Network. Approximately 28 percent of preterm births were indicated due to preeclampsia (43 percent), fetal distress (27 percent), fetal growth restriction (10 percent), abruptio placentae (7 percent), and fetal death (7 percent). The remaining 72 percent were due to spontaneous preterm labor with or without ruptured membranes. Women with placenta

TABLE 27–5. Health-care Costs During the First Year of Life by Birthweight, United States, 1988

Birthweight Group	Births No. (%)	Cost per Birth	Total Costs for Group	Percentage of Infant Health-care Costs
≥ 2500 g	3,600,000 (93)	$ 1,900	$7.4 billion	65
< 2500 g	271,000 (7)	$15,000	$4 billion	35
< 1500 g	57,000 (1.4)	$32,000	$1.8 billion	16

From Lewit and co-workers (1995), with permission.

TABLE 27–6. Causes of Preterm Birth at 23 to 36 Weeks in 50 Consecutive Pregnancies

Cause	Percent[a]
Placenta previa or abruption	50
Amnionic fluid infection	38
Immunological—e.g., antiphospholipid antibody syndrome	30
Cervical incompetence	16
Uterine—anomaly, hydramnios, fibroids	14
Maternal—preeclampsia, drug intoxication	10
Trauma or surgery	8
Fetal anomalies	6
No cause	4

[a] Some women had more than one cause identified.
From Lettieri and associates (1993), with permission.

previa and multiple gestations, both common associations of preterm birth, were excluded from this analysis.

LIFESTYLE FACTORS. Behaviors such as cigarette smoking, poor nutrition and poor weight gain during pregnancy, and use of drugs such as cocaine or alcohol have been reported to play important roles in the incidence and outcome of low-birthweight infants. Some of this effect is undoubtedly due to restricted fetal growth (Chap. 29, p. 745) as well as preterm birth. Hickey and colleagues (1995), however, have shown that low maternal prenatal weight gain is associated specifically with an increased risk for preterm birth.

Alcohol abuse has been linked not only to preterm birth but also to substantially increased risk of brain injury in premature infants (Holzman and co-workers, 1995). DiFronza and Lew (1995) reviewed smoking during pregnancy and reported that tobacco use was responsible for 32,000 to 61,000 low-birthweight infants each year in the United States.

Other maternal factors implicated include young maternal age (Satin and co-workers, 1994), poverty (Meis and colleagues, 1995b), short stature (Kramer and colleagues, 1995), and occupational factors (Henriksen and co-workers, 1995; Luke and associates, 1995).

Another lifestyle factor that seems intuitively important, yet has seldom been formally studied, is psychological stress in the mother. Hedegaard and associates (1993) performed a prospective follow-up study of measures of psychological stress, using questionnaires in 5872 women with singleton pregnancies. A direct association was found between psychological stress in the 30th week of pregnancy and delivery before 37 weeks' gestation. Peacock and co-workers (1995) also found an association between psychological stress and preterm birth.

Copper and colleagues (1996), from the NICHD Maternal–Fetal Medicine Units Network Preterm Prediction Study, reported that maternal stress was associated with spontaneous preterm birth at less than 35 weeks' gestation and after adjustment for maternal demographic and behavioral characteristics.

GENETIC FACTORS. It has been observed for many years that preterm delivery is a condition that runs in families. This observation plus the recurrent nature of preterm birth and its differing prevalence between races has led to the suggestion of a genetic cause for preterm labor. Hoffman and Ward (1999) have reviewed the possible genetic factors implicated in preterm delivery.

AMNIONIC FLUID AND CHORIOAMNIONIC INFECTION. Chorioamnionic infection caused by a variety of microorganisms has emerged as a possible explanation for many heretofore unexplained cases of ruptured membranes and/or preterm labor. Although female reproductive tract infection was associated with prematurity more than 45 years ago (Knox and Hoerner, 1995), there was renewed interest when Bobbitt and Ledger (1977) implicated subclinical amnionic fluid infection as a cause of preterm labor. For example, pathogenic bacteria have typically been recovered at transabdominal amniocentesis from approximately 20 percent of women in preterm labor without evidence of overt clinical infection and with intact fetal membranes (Cox and associates, 1996a; Watts and co-workers, 1992). Hillier and colleagues (1995) and Hauth and co-workers (1998) have reported that an appreciable number of women with spontaneous preterm birth have pathogenic organisms recovered from the chorioamnion. Indeed, the frequency of recovery of these organisms is increased in women with spontaneous onset of preterm labor with and without amnion rupture, but not increased in women delivered preterm for a medical or obstetrical complication such as maternal hypertension or hemorrhage (Hauth and co-workers, 1998). The recovery of upper genital tract pathogens is, therefore, increased in women with spontaneous labor and delivery and is inversely associated with gestational age (Fig. 27–5) and birthweight (Fig. 27–6).

PATHOGENESIS. Schwarz and co-workers (1976) suggested that term labor is initiated by activation of phospholipase A_2, which cleaves arachidonic acid from within fetal membranes, thereby making free arachidonic acid available for prostaglandin synthesis. Subsequently, Bejar and colleagues (1981) reported that many microorganisms produce phospholipase A_2, and thus potentially may initiate preterm labor. Bennett and Elder (1992) have shown that common genital tract bacteria do not themselves produce the prostaglandins. Cox and

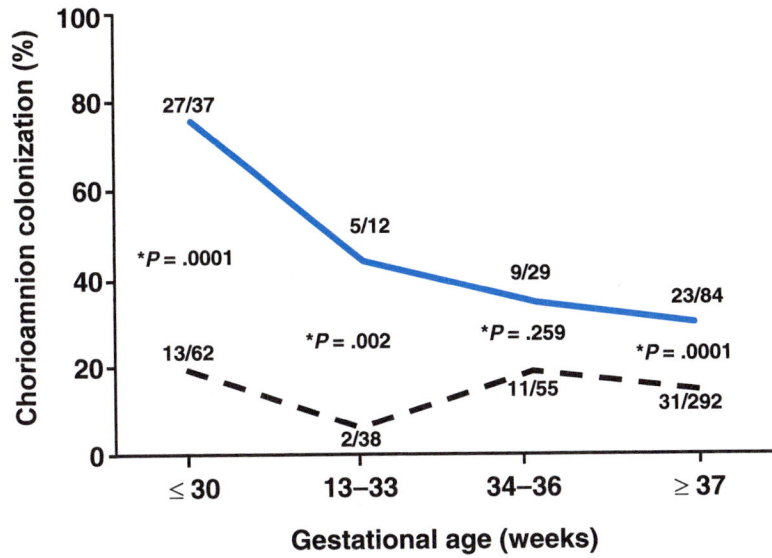

FIGURE 27–5. Chorioamnion colonization as a function of gestational age in women with spontaneous labor (solid line) and in those whose delivery was indicated for maternal medical or obstetrical complications (dashed line). (From Hauth and colleagues, 1998, with permission.)

associates (1989) provided data that bacterial endotoxin (lipopolysaccharide) introduced into the amnionic fluid stimulates decidual cells to produce cytokines and prostaglandins that may initiate labor. Romero and co-workers (1987, 1988) and Cox and associates (1988a) reported that endotoxin was present in the amnionic fluid. Andrews and colleagues (1995) found a markedly higher mean amnionic fluid interleukin-6 concentration versus gestational age in women with the spontaneous onset of labor compared with women with indicated deliveries (Fig. 27–7).

It has now been established that endogenous host products secreted in response to infection are responsible for many of the effects of infection. In endotoxin shock, for example, bacterial endotoxins exert their deleterious effect through the release of endogenous cell mediators (cytokines) of the inflammatory response. Similarly, preterm parturition due to infection is thought to be initiated by secretory products resulting from monocyte (macrophage) activation (Fig. 27–8). Cytokines, including interleukin-1, tumor necrosis factor, and interleukin-6, are such secretory products implicated in preterm labor. Narahara and Johnston (1993) have suggested that platelet-activating factor, which is found in the amnionic fluid, is synergistically involved in activating the cytokine network (Fig. 27–8). Platelet-activating factor is thought to be produced in the fetal lungs and kidneys. Thus, the fetus appears to play a synergistic

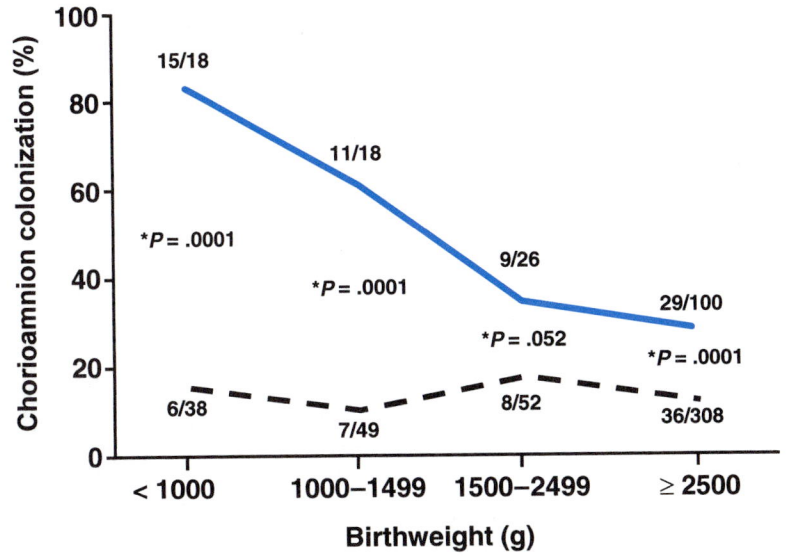

FIGURE 27–6. Chorioamnion colonization as a function of birthweight in women with spontaneous labor (solid line) and in those who delivery was indicated for maternal medical or obstetrical complications (dashed line). (From Hauth and colleagues, 1998, with permission.)

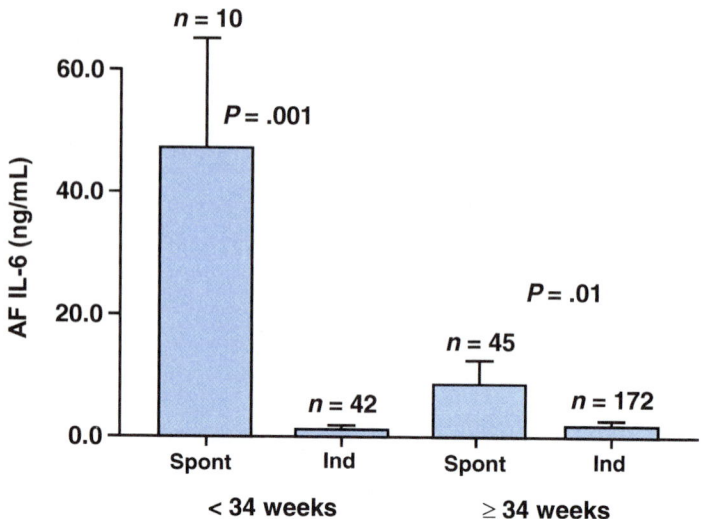

FIGURE 27-7. Mean amnionic fluid interleukin-6 (IL-6) concentration and gestational age at birth in women with the spontaneous onset of labor (Spont) compared with women with indicated deliveries (Ind). (From Andrews and colleagues, 1995, with permission.)

role in the initiation of preterm birth due to bacterial infection. Teleologically, this could be advantageous to the fetus interested in extricating itself from an infected environment.

Gravett and colleagues (1994), in a remarkable experiment with rhesus monkeys, have provided the first direct evidence that infection incites preterm labor. Group B streptococci were injected into the amnionic fluid in preterm rhesus monkeys, and concentrations of cytokines and prostaglandins shown in Figure 27–8 were serially measured. Amnionic fluid cytokine concentrations increased about 9 hours after introduction of the bacteria, followed sequentially by production of the prostaglandins E_2 and $F_{2\alpha}$ and finally, uterine contractions. As observed in humans with preterm labor due to amnionic fluid infection, there was no clinical evi-

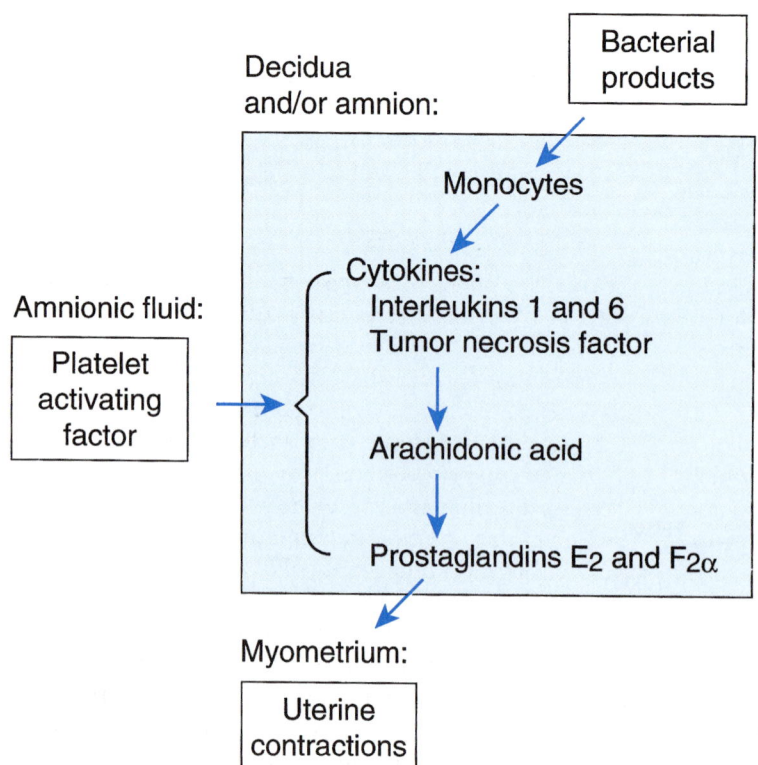

FIGURE 27-8. Proposed schematic mechanism of action for bacteria to incite preterm labor. Examples of bacterial products include cell wall lipopolysaccharide (endotoxin). (Compiled from Berry, 1995; Gravett, 1994; Molnar, 1993; Narahara and Johnston, 1993, and their colleagues.)

dence of chorioamnionitis in these rhesus monkeys until after preterm labor ensued.

Although the pathway for bacteria to enter the amnionic fluid is obvious after membrane rupture, the route of access with intact membranes is unclear. Gyr and colleagues (1994) found that *Escherichia coli* can permeate living chorioamnionic membranes. Thus, intact fetal membranes at the cervix are not necessarily a barrier to ascending bacterial invasion of the amnionic fluid. Alternatively, the pathway for bacterial initiation of preterm labor described in Figure 27–8 may not require colonization of the amnionic fluid. For example, Cox and co-workers (1993) found that the cytokine network of cell-mediated immunity can be activated locally in decidual tissue that lines the forebag fetal membranes.

DIAGNOSIS. The interest in a possible microbial pathogenesis of preterm labor has prompted many investigators to evaluate amniocentesis for management. Garite and colleagues (1979) successfully performed sonar-directed amniocentesis in 30 of 59 women with ruptured membranes between 28 and 35 weeks. As none had clinical infection, their purpose was to establish fetal lung maturity while evaluating Gram stain and culture of amnionic fluid. Surprisingly, the fluids from nine women (30 percent) contained bacteria; six of these women developed chorioamnionitis and two neonates developed infection. Despite these reports, it has not been shown that amniocentesis used to diagnose infection is associated with improved pregnancy outcome. Feinstein and colleagues (1986) compared 73 cases of preterm ruptured membranes managed with the aid of amniocentesis with 73 matched historical controls. There were no differences in fetal condition at delivery, incidence of neonatal infection, or perinatal mortality.

In centers using amniocentesis in the management of preterm labor, several laboratory methods have been reported helpful for the rapid detection of intra-amnionic infection. Romero and colleagues (1993) evaluated the diagnostic value of amnionic fluid white blood cell count, low glucose and high interleukin-6 concentration, and Gram-stained positive bacteria in 120 women with preterm labor and intact fetal membranes. Those women with positive amnionic fluid cultures were considered infected. A negative Gram stain was the most reliable test to exclude amnionic fluid bacteria (specificity 99 percent), and a high interleukin-6 was the most sensitive test (sensitivity 82 percent) in detecting amnionic fluids containing bacteria. Andrews and colleagues (1995) also found good correlation between amnionic fluid interleukin-6 and chorioamnionic microbial colonization. Yoon and associates (1996) compared the accuracy of C-reactive protein levels or white blood cell counts in maternal blood with amnionic fluid white blood cell counts and found the latter to be superior in the confirmation of amnionic fluid infection.

Gonik and colleagues (1985) reported that oligohydramnios identified by ultrasound was linked to antepartum clinical chorioamnionitis. Vintzileos and colleagues (1986) found a similar association between oligohydramnios and bacterial colonization of amnionic fluid collected by amniocentesis. Vintzileos and associates (1985) observed that fetal infection could be predicted reliably using daily biophysical profiles; however, this was not confirmed by others (Carroll and colleagues, 1995b; DeVoe and colleagues, 1994; Gauthier and co-workers, 1992; Miller and associates, 1990).

PRETERM RUPTURED MEMBRANES. An intense inflammatory reaction at the site of prematurely ruptured membranes was noted as early as 1950, and this suggested infection. McGregor and colleagues (1987) demonstrated that in vitro exposure to bacterial proteases reduced the bursting load of fetal membranes. Thus, microorganisms given access to fetal membranes may be capable of causing membrane rupture, preterm labor, or both.

BACTERIAL VAGINOSIS. Bacterial vaginosis is a condition in which the normal, hydrogen peroxide–producing lactobacillus-predominant vaginal flora is replaced with anaerobic bacteria, *Gardnerella vaginalis*, *Mobiluncus* species, and *Mycoplasma hominis* (Hillier and colleagues, 1995; Nugent and co-workers, 1991). Clinical diagnostic features described by Amsel and associates (1983) include:

1. Vaginal pH greater than 4.5.
2. An amine odor when vaginal secretions are mixed with potassium hydroxide.
3. Vaginal epithelial cells heavily coated with bacilli—"clue cells."
4. A homogeneous vaginal discharge.

Bacterial vaginosis can also be diagnosed with Gram staining of vaginal secretions as reported by Nugent and co-workers (1991). Typically a Gram stain of vaginal secretion in women with bacterial vaginosis shows few white cells along with a mixed flora as compared with the normal predominance of lactobacilli.

Bacterial vaginosis has been associated with spontaneous preterm birth, preterm ruptured membranes, infection of the chorion and amnion, as well as amnionic fluid infection (Hillier and colleagues, 1995; Kurki and co-authors, 1992). Platz-Christensen and colleagues (1993) have provided some evidence that bacterial vaginosis may precipitate preterm labor by a mechanism similar to the cytokine network pathway proposed for amnionic fluid bacteria (Fig. 27–8). In contrast, Thorsen and associates (1996), in a prospective study of 3600

Danish women, found that bacterial vaginosis diagnosed before 24 weeks was not related to ruptured membranes before 37 weeks or to low birthweight. The contrasting reports may relate to the diagnosis of the clinical syndrome of bacterial vaginosis. Because of its imprecise diagnosis, it is difficult to correlate each level of Gram stain score with adverse outcomes, and specifically with spontaneous preterm birth or membrane rupture. Hauth and colleagues (2000) presented data from the large prospective NICHD Maternal–Fetal Medicine Units Network observational trial that confirmed a significant increase in spontaneous preterm birth when the vaginal pH is greater than 5.0 compared with 4.7 or less, and when the Gram stain score is 9 or 10 compared with 7 or 8 or less.

TRICHOMONAS AND CANDIDA VAGINITIS. Cotch and associates (1997), after adjusting for multiple confounding factors, including bacterial vaginosis, found that women with *Trichomonas vaginalis* were at 30 percent increased risk of having low-birthweight infants, 30 percent increased risk of preterm birth, and a nearly doubled risk of perinatal death. Meis and co-workers (1995a) examined 2929 women at 24 and 28 weeks using 10-percent potassium hydroxide wet mount preparations and found that detection of *Trichomonas* or *Candida* had no significant association with preterm birth. Most recently, Carey and colleagues (2000a) for the NICHD Maternal–Fetal Medicine Units Network reported that of 617 women with asymptomatic vaginal trichomonas, 19 percent assigned to metronidazole treatment, compared with 11 percent assigned to placebo treatment, had a preterm birth ($P = .004$). These authors concluded that routine screening and treatment for this condition cannot be recommended.

CHLAMYDIAL INFECTION. Although *Chlamydia trachomatis* is the most common sexually transmitted bacterial pathogen in the United States (Webster and colleagues, 1993), the possible influence of cervical infection with this organism on preterm birth is unclear (McGregor and French, 1991). Ryan and associates (1990) used erythromycin to treat 1323 pregnant women with positive cervical cultures for *Chlamydia* at enrollment for prenatal care. Pregnancy outcomes in these women were compared with 1110 similar, but untreated women. Low birthweight and ruptured membranes more than 1 hour before labor were significantly decreased with erythromycin therapy. The effects on preterm birth, however, were not specified. Andrews and colleagues (2000) from the NICHD Maternal–Fetal Medicine Units Network Preterm Prediction Study reported that genitourinary chlamydial infection at 24 weeks' gestation—but not at 28 weeks—detected via a ligase chain reaction assay was associated with a twofold

increase in subsequent spontaneous preterm birth. The Centers for Disease Control and Prevention guidelines for screening (1993) and treatment (1998) of chlamydial infection during pregnancy are based on the prevalence of the infection in various populations, for example, teenagers, and on the likely benefit of third-trimester screening and treatment to reduce newborn ophthalmia neonatorum or pneumonitis, rather than reduce the incidence of preterm birth (Chap. 57, p. 1493).

IDENTIFICATION OF WOMEN AT RISK FOR PRETERM BIRTH

Obstetrical approaches to preterm birth have traditionally been focused primarily on treatment interventions rather than prevention of preterm labor. The first step in prevention is early identification of women at risk for preterm birth.

RISK-SCORING SYSTEMS. A risk-scoring system devised by Papiernik and modified by Creasy and colleagues (1980) has been tested in several regions of the United States. In this system, scores of 1 through 10 are given to a variety of pregnancy factors, including socioeconomic status, reproductive history, daily habits, and current pregnancy complications. Women with scores of 10 or more are considered to be at high risk for preterm delivery.

Although Creasy and associates (1980) and Covington and co-workers (1988) reported salutary results with this risk scoring coupled with an educational prevention program, the experiences of Main and colleagues (1989) in Philadelphia using this scoring system with indigent women was less satisfactory. Similar disappointing results in indigent women were obtained by Mueller-Heubach and Guzick (1989) and Owen and associates (1990b). The Creasy program also was not successful to reduce preterm birth in the multicenter randomized trial of 2395 pregnancies managed at five centers by the Collaborative Group on Preterm Birth Prevention (1993). Hueston and colleagues (1995) reviewed all published studies and found no benefits. Subsequently, the NIH-sponsored Maternal–Fetal Medicine Network Units study showed that risk assessment failed to identify most women who have preterm delivery (Mercer and colleagues, 1996).

Although these scoring systems have been unsuccessful in identifying pregnancies at risk for preterm labor, certain features may be more useful than others in predicting the risk of preterm delivery. Complex combinations of risk scoring systems and other screening tests have been reported to increase the prediction of spontaneous preterm birth (Crane and associates, 1999; Goldenberg and co-workers, 1998).

TABLE 27–7. Recurrent Spontaneous Preterm Births According to Prior Outcome in 6072 Scottish Women

First Birth	Second Birth	Next Birth Preterm (%)
Term	—	5
Preterm	—	15
Term	Preterm	24
Preterm	Preterm	32

From Carr-Hill and Hall (1985), with permission.

PRIOR PRETERM BIRTH. A history of prior preterm delivery strongly correlates with subsequent preterm labor. Table 27–7 gives the incidence of recurrent spontaneous preterm birth in over 6000 Scottish women. The risk of recurrent preterm delivery for those whose first delivery was preterm increased threefold compared with women whose first infant reached term. Strikingly, almost a third of women whose first two infants were preterm subsequently delivered preterm infants during their third pregnancies. Almost identical results were obtained in an analysis of 13,967 pregnancies in Danish women (Kristensen and co-workers, 1995). Iams and colleagues (1998a) used the NICHD Maternal–Fetal Medicine Units Network Preterm Prediction Study to detail the increased risk of spontaneous preterm birth before 36 weeks' gestation in women who had had a prior preterm birth. This increased risk was substantially further increased in association with a positive (≥ 50 μg/dL) midtrimester vaginal fetal fibronectin test or in relation to cervical shortening measured with ultrasound, especially in women with a cervix measurement at or below the 10th percentile (≤ 25 mm) at 24 weeks' gestation.

Not only are women who deliver preterm at risk themselves for recurrence, but recent evidence suggests that this risk is also transmitted to their children. Wang and associates (1995) and Porter and colleagues (1996) have found familial aggregation of preterm birth.

CERVICAL DILATATION. Asymptomatic cervical dilatation after midpregnancy has gained attention as a risk factor for preterm delivery. Some authorities have considered such dilatation to be a normal anatomical variant, particularly in parous women. Recent studies have suggested that parity alone is not sufficient to explain cervical dilatation discovered early in the third trimester. Cook and Ellwood (1996) longitudinally studied the cervix between 18 and 30 weeks using transvaginal ultrasound in both nulliparous and parous women. Cervical length and diameter were identical in both groups of women throughout these critical weeks.

Table 27–8 gives the results of routine cervical examinations performed between 26 and 30 weeks in 185 women cared for at Parkland Hospital. Approximately a fourth of the women whose cervices were dilated 2 or 3 cm delivered prior to 34 weeks. Many of these women had experienced the same complication in earlier pregnancies. Similarly, Papiernik and colleagues (1986), in a study of cervical status before 37 weeks in 4430 women, found that precocious cervical dilatation increased the risk of preterm birth. Stubbs and colleagues (1986) performed cervical examinations in 191 women between 28 and 34 weeks and found that those with dilatation of 1 cm or more, or effacement of more than 30 percent, were at increased risk for preterm delivery. Copper and associates (1995) examined 570 women at risk for preterm birth at about 28 weeks and found that cervical condition predicted delivery before 37 weeks.

ULTRASONIC MEASUREMENT OF CERVICAL LENGTH. Iams and co-workers (1996) used transvaginal sonography to measure the length of the cervix in 2915 women at approximately 24 weeks and again at 28 weeks. As shown in Figure 27–9, the mean cervical length at 24 weeks was about 35 mm, and those women with progressively shorter cervices experienced increased rates of preterm birth. These findings were supported by investigations of Hartmann and colleagues (1999). In another study performed in the NICHD Maternal–Fetal Medicine Units Network, Owen and co-workers (2000) corre-

TABLE 27–8. Cervical Dilatation Between 26 and 30 Weeks and Risk of Delivery Before 34 Weeks

	Cervical Status at 26–30 Weeks			
	Total (n = 185)	< 1 cm (n = 170)	2–3 cm (n = 15)	
	no. (%)	no. (%)	no. (%)	Comparison
Prior low birthweight[a]	9 (5)	6 (4)	3 (20)	$P < .001$
Current pregnancy low birthweight	7 (4)	3 (2)	4 (27)	$P < .002$

[a] Less than 2200 g (50th percentile for 34 weeks).
From Leveno and associates (1986a), with permission.

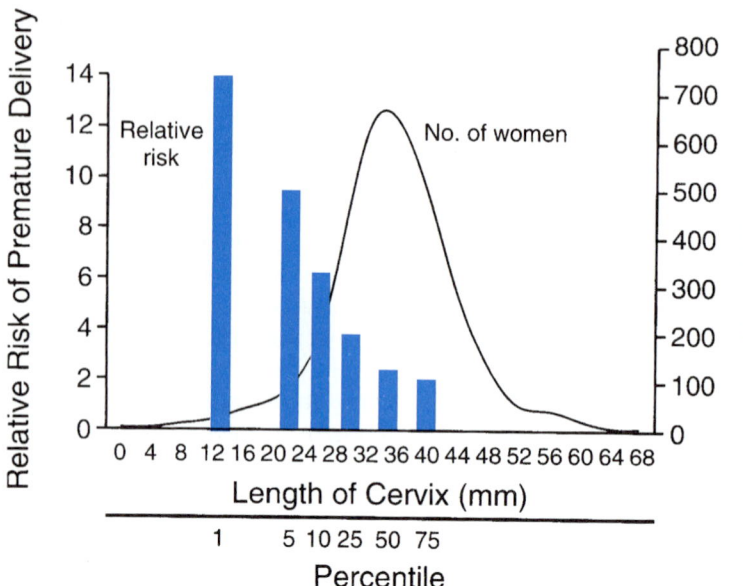

FIGURE 27-9. Percentile distribution of pregnancies based upon cervical length measured with transvaginal sonography at 24 weeks (solid line) and the relative risk of spontaneous preterm delivery before 35 weeks. (From Iams and co-workers, 1996, with permission.)

lated cervical length at 16 to 24 weeks' gestation with subsequent preterm birth before 35 weeks. Guzman and colleagues (2001) longitudinally evaluated 237 at-risk women with singletons between 15 and 24 weeks' gestation. At all testing periods the sensitivity and negative predictive value of cervical length to predict spontaneous preterm birth prior to 30 weeks' gestation were excellent.

Transvaginal ultrasound cervical assessment requires special expertise. Yost and colleagues (1999) caution those who perform these examinations to be wary of falsely reassuring findings due to potential anatomical and technical pitfalls. In recent small randomized trials, cervical cerclage has not been found to be beneficial in preventing delivery before 35 weeks (Althuisius and co-workers, 2000; Rust and colleagues, 2000). Rust and colleagues (2001) used ultrasonic cervical measurement criteria for cervical dilatation obtained between 16 and 24 weeks to identify and randomize 55 women to cerclage and 58 to a no cerclage intervention. The survival curve, generated with respect to gestational age at delivery, showed no significant difference between groups. However, Althuisius and colleagues (2001) randomized 35 women at high risk for cervical incompetence to either therapeutic cerclage or to bed rest. Women randomized to cerclage had significantly fewer births prior to 34 weeks and less neonatal morbidity.

Although it seems clear that pregnant women with cervical dilatation and effacement diagnosed early in the third trimester by direct cervical digital examination are at increased risk for preterm birth, it has not been established that detection appreciably improves pregnancy outcome. Buekens and colleagues (1994) random-ized 2719 European women to routine cervical examinations at each prenatal visit compared with 2721 women in whom cervical examinations were not performed. Knowledge of antenatal cervical dilatation did not affect any pregnancy outcome related to preterm birth or the frequency of interventions practiced in the management of preterm labor. Importantly, cervical examinations were not related to preterm ruptured membranes. Thus, prenatal cervical examinations were neither beneficial nor harmful.

SIGNS AND SYMPTOMS. In addition to painful or painless uterine contractions, symptoms such as pelvic pressure, menstrual-like cramps, watery or bloody vaginal discharge, and pain in the low back have been empirically associated with impending preterm birth. Such symptoms are thought by some to be common in normal pregnancy, and are therefore often dismissed by patients, physicians, and nurses. The importance of these signs and symptoms has been emphasized by some investigators (Iams and associates, 1990; Kragt and Keirse, 1990). Conversely, Copper and colleagues (1990) did not find these to be meaningful in the prediction of preterm birth. Iams and colleagues (1994), in a follow-up investigation to their 1990 study, found that the signs and symptoms signaling preterm labor, including uterine contractions, only appeared within 24 hours of preterm labor. Thus, these are a late warning sign of preterm birth.

FETAL FIBRONECTIN. Fibronectin is a glycoprotein produced in 20 different molecular forms by a variety of cell types, including hepatocytes, malignant cells, fibroblasts, endothelial cells, and fetal amnion. It is present in high concentrations in maternal blood and in amnionic fluid, and is thought to have a role in intercellular adhesion in relation to implantation as well as in the maintenance of adhesion of the placenta to the decidua (Leeson and colleagues, 1996). Fetal fibronectin can be detected in cervicovaginal secretions in normal pregnancies with intact membranes at term, and appears to reflect stromal remodeling of the cervix prior to labor. Lockwood and co-workers (1991) reported that detection of fetal fibronectin in cervicovaginal secretions prior to membrane rupture may be a marker for impending preterm labor. This report has stimulated considerable interest in the use of fibronectin assays for the prediction of preterm birth. Fetal fibronectin is measured using an enzyme-linked immunosorbent assay and values exceeding 50 ng/mL are considered a positive result. Contamination of the sample by amnionic fluid and maternal blood should be avoided.

Leeson and associates (1996) and Peaceman and co-workers (1996) have found that although fibronectin-positive tests are associated with preterm birth, negative results are more consistently meaningful in predicting that preterm labor will not ensue. Cox and co-workers (1996b) found cervical dilatation to be superior to detection of fibronectin to predict preterm birth. Goldenberg and colleagues (1996a) using the NICHD Network Preterm Prediction Study reported that a positive cervical or vaginal fetal fibronectin at 24 weeks' gestation was a powerful predictor of subsequent spontaneous preterm birth. Most recently, Goldenberg and co-authors (2000) reported that detection of fetal fibronectin in cervical/vaginal secretions as early as 18 to 22 weeks' gestation was predictive of preterm delivery. In a meta-analysis of 27 studies, Leitich and associates (1999) also found it to be an effective predictor of preterm delivery.

Importantly, other factors such as cervical manipulation and peripartum infection can stimulate fetal fibronectin release (Goldenberg and colleagues, 1996b; Thorp and Lukes, 1996). Similarly, Jackson and colleagues (1996) have shown that human amnion cells in vitro produce fetal fibronectin when stimulated by inflammatory products implicated in the initiation of preterm labor due to infection (Fig. 27–8).

AMBULATORY UTERINE CONTRACTION TESTING.

The diagnosis of preterm labor, before it is irreversibly established, is a goal of management. To this end, uterine activity monitoring, using tocodynamometry, has received considerable interest. In 1957, Smyth described an external tocodynamometer with an innovative sensor that employed the so-called guard-ring principle. The abdominal wall is flattened by an outer ring, thus permitting the inner contraction–sensing transducer to be applied more directly to the underlying uterine wall. Several preterm birth–prevention programs incorporating such a device have been commercially available since 1985 for ambulatory uterine monitoring. The contraction sensor is belted around the abdomen and connected to a small electronic recorder worn at the waist. This recorder is used to transmit uterine activity via phone on a daily basis. Patients are educated concerning signs and symptoms of preterm labor, and their attending physicians are kept apprised of their progress. The program is expensive; for example, in Dallas in 1996 the list price was $55 to $154 per day, depending on the patient's risk status.

As shown in Figure 27–10, Katz and associates (1986) found that women who subsequently had a preterm delivery experienced increased uterine activity beginning at about 30 weeks. Subsequent widespread clinical application of home uterine contraction monitoring for the purpose of preventing preterm birth has provoked considerable controversy in the United States. Currently, the American College of Obstetricians and Gynecologists (1995) continues to take the following position: "It is not clearly demonstrated that this expensive and burdensome system can be used to actually affect the rate of preterm delivery."

Recent studies continue to show that home uterine activity monitoring is ineffective in the prevention of preterm birth. In the Collaborative Home Uterine Monitoring Study (1995), sham transducers were used in 655 women and outcomes compared with 637 women with functioning monitors. Home monitoring was ineffective in the prevention of preterm birth. Iams and colleagues (1998b) longitudinally assessed uterine activity with daily home monitoring and reported on 34,908 hours of uterine contraction data

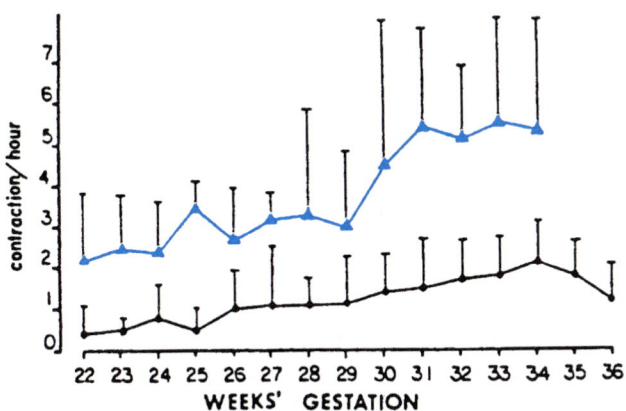

FIGURE 27–10. Mean frequency (±SD) of contractions during pregnancy in women having preterm labor (▲) compared with those with term labor (●). (From Katz and colleagues, 1986, with permission.)

from 306 women. Contraction frequency increased with advancing gestational age but did not efficiently predict preterm birth.

Dyson and colleagues (1998), in a multicenter trial conducted at Kaiser Permanente Hospital in California, also found no benefits for home uterine activity monitoring. They randomzed 2422 women at risk for preterm birth (including 844 women with twins) to weekly contact with a nurse or to contraction monitoring at home. There were no differences in delivery before 35 weeks' gestation nor in birthweight less than 1500 g or less than 2500 g. Undesirable outcomes included a significant increase in unscheduled visits to obstetricians and significantly increased prophylactic tocolytic drug therapy in women with twins.

SALIVARY ESTRIOL. Several investigators have reported an association between increased maternal salivary estriol concentration and subsequent preterm birth (Goodwin, 1996; Heine, 1999; McGregor, 1995; and their co-workers). Goodwin (1999) reviewed the potential value of maternal salivary estriol and concluded that this test requires further evaluation. We are also of the view that use of salivary estriol to predict preterm delivery is investigational.

MANAGEMENT OF PRETERM LABOR

There are a number of factors important in directing management of the woman with possible preterm labor. Foremost is its correct identification, along with whether there is accompanying membrane rupture.

DIAGNOSIS. Early differentiation between true and false labor is difficult before there is demonstrable cervical effacement and dilatation. Uterine contractions alone can be misleading because of *Braxton Hicks contractions* (Chap. 14, p. 355). These contractions, described as irregular, nonrhythmical, and either painful or painless, can cause considerable confusion in the diagnosis of preterm labor. Not infrequently, women who deliver before term have uterine activity that is attributed to Braxton Hicks contractions, prompting an incorrect diagnosis of false labor.

Because uterine contractions alone may be misleading, the American Academy of Pediatrics and the American College of Obstetricians and Gynecologists (1997) has proposed the following criteria to document preterm labor between 20 and 37 weeks' gestation:

1. Contractions occurring at a frequency of four in 20 minutes or eight in 60 minutes plus progressive change in the cervix.
2. Cervical dilatation greater than 1 cm.
3. Cervical effacement of 80 percent or greater.

ANTEPARTUM MANAGEMENT. It is not apparent that making prenatal care available to more women or making more visits available has reduced preterm births (Buescher and associates, 1988; Donaldson and colleagues, 1984; Fink and co-workers, 1992; Fiscella, 1995). Despite this, women with pregnancies identified to be at risk for preterm birth, and also those who present with signs and symptoms of impending preterm delivery, have become candidates for a large number of interventions intended to improve infant outcomes. In the absence of maternal or fetal indications that warrant intentional delivery, most interventions are expected to forestall preterm birth or enhance the infants' ability to cope with the extrauterine environment. In many instances, the interventions described in the following section should be considered and not necessarily recommended for clinical practice.

PRETERM PREMATURELY RUPTURED MEMBRANES. Attempts to avoid delivery when there is preterm ruptured membranes are of two primary forms:

1. Nonintervention or expectant management, in which spontaneous labor is simply awaited.
2. Intervention that may include corticosteroids, given with or without tocolytic agents to arrest preterm labor in order that the corticosteroids have sufficient time to induce fetal maturation.

The American College of Obstetricians and Gynecologists (1998a) has recently reviewed preterm ruptured membranes.

Known risk factors for preterm rupture of the membranes include preceding preterm birth (Guinn and co-workers, 1995), occult amnionic fluid infection (see p. 696), multiple fetuses (Chap. 30, p. 778), and abruptio placentae (Major and colleagues, 1995).

NATURAL HISTORY OF PRETERM MEMBRANE RUPTURE. Cox and associates (1988b) described the pregnancy outcomes of 298 consecutive women delivered following spontaneously ruptured membranes between 24 and 34 weeks. Although this complication was identified in only 1.7 percent of pregnancies, it contributed to 20 percent of all perinatal deaths during that time period. Preterm membrane rupture was found to be associated with other obstetrical complications that affect perinatal outcome, including multifetal gestation, breech presentation, chorioamnionitis, and intrapartum fetal distress. As a consequence of these complications, cesarean delivery was done in nearly 40 percent of women. At admission, 75 percent of the women were already in labor, 5 percent were delivered for other complications, and another 10 percent were delivered following spontaneous labor within 48 hours. In only 7 percent was delivery delayed 48 hours or more after membrane rupture. This latter subgroup, however, appeared to benefit from delayed delivery, because no neonatal deaths occurred. This was in contrast to a neonatal death rate of 80 per 1000 in infants delivered within 48 hours of membrane rupture. Nelson and colleagues (1994) reported similar results. In women already in labor upon admission, about half were undelivered at 48 hours after membrane rupture but only 13 percent were undelivered at 7 days. Both of these studies attest to the inevitability of preterm labor and birth after preterm membrane rupture.

The time period from preterm ruptured membranes to delivery is inversely proportional to the gestational age when the membranes ruptured (Carroll and associates, 1995a). As shown in Figure 27–11, very few days were gained when membranes ruptured during the third compared with the second trimester.

EXPECTANT MANAGEMENT. Despite an extensive literature concerning expectant management of preterm ruptured membranes, few randomized studies have been performed. An exception is the report by Garite and colleagues (1981), who studied 160 pregnancies with preterm ruptured membranes between 28 and 34 weeks. The women were divided into two groups that included expectant management only or corticosteroids plus tocolysis with either intravenous ethanol or magnesium sulfate. The authors concluded that active interventions did not improve perinatal outcomes and may have aggravated infection-related complications. Subsequent randomized studies by Garite and associates (1987) and Nelson and colleagues (1985) failed to show benefits for tocolysis, either with or without steroid therapy. Morales and co-workers (1989) studied 165 pregnancies with preterm ruptured membranes and lecithin:sphingomyelin ratios less than two. These were randomized to four treatment groups that included (1) expectant management only, (2) corticosteroids for fetal lung maturation, (3) ampicillin only, and (4) ampicillin plus corticosteroids. They concluded that ampicillin plus corticosteroids were beneficial because of less respiratory disease. Unfortunately, neonatal survival was not ultimately affected by any intervention, nor was the length of gestation.

Alexander and colleagues (2000), in a study performed in the NICHD Maternal–Fetal Medicine Units Network, found that one or two digital cervical examinations performed with expectant management of ruptured membranes between 24 and 32 weeks' gestation were associated with a significantly shorter rupture-to-delivery interval (3 days) compared with avoidance of such examinations (5 days). Importantly, however, this difference in latency from rupture-to-delivery interval did not worsen maternal or neonatal outcomes.

SECOND-TRIMESTER RUPTURED MEMBRANES. There are both maternal and infant risks to be considered when contemplating expectant management of ruptured membranes before 25 to 26 weeks. Maternal risks include the consequences of uterine infection and

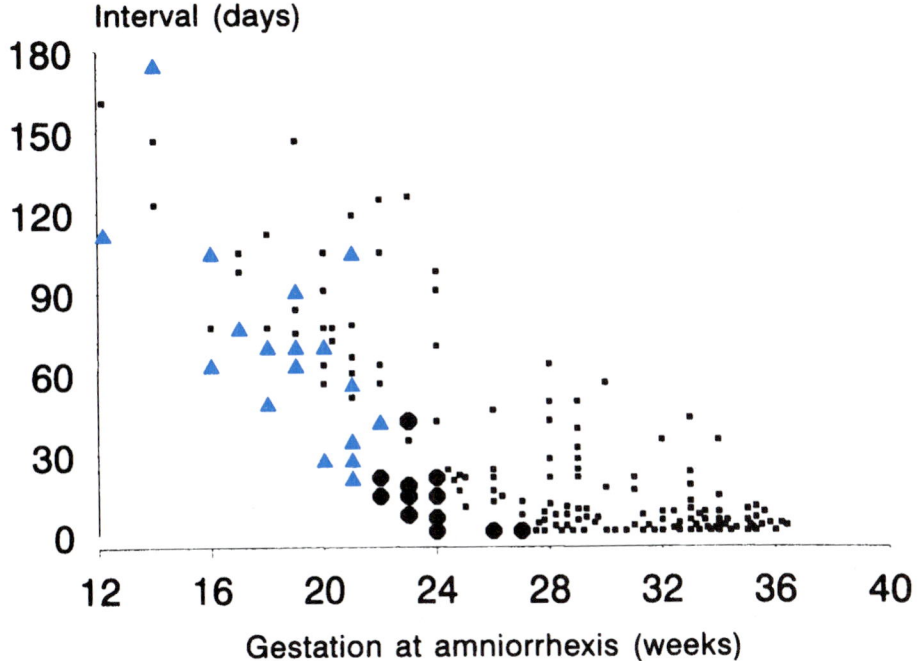

FIGURE 27–11. Relationship of time interval between preterm membrane rupture and delivery in 172 singleton pregnancies. (Squares = survivors; circles = deaths due to prematurity; triangles = deaths due to pulmonary hypoplasia.) (From Carroll and co-workers, 1995a, with permission.)

sepsis. Fetal risks include pulmonary hypoplasia and limb compression deformities, which have been associated with prolonged periods of oligohydramnios due to ruptured membranes (Chap. 31, p. 822). Morales and Talley (1993) expectantly managed 94 women with singleton pregnancies and ruptured membranes prior to 25 weeks and found that 41 percent ultimately survived to 1 year of age and 27 percent were neurologically normal. The average time gained during expectant management was 11 days. Similar results were reported by Farooqi and colleagues (1998) and Winn and associates (2000). In contrast, Hibbard and colleagues (1993) analyzed neonatal mortality, morbidity, and health-care costs in 44 pregnancies expectantly managed after membrane rupture at 25 weeks or less. They concluded that immediate delivery of the fetus less than 24 weeks may be the most cost-effective plan. In this report, 77 percent of the women expectantly managed developed chorioamnionitis.

The volume of amnionic fluid and fetal age at membrane rupture appears to have prognostic importance in pregnancies before 26 weeks. Hadi and associates (1994) analyzed 178 pregnancies with ruptured membranes between 20 and 25 weeks' gestation and 40 percent had oligohydramnios defined as no sonographic pockets of 2 cm or greater. Virtually all those with oligohydramnios delivered before 25 weeks, whereas 85 percent of those with adequate amnionic fluid volume delivered in the third trimester. Carroll and colleagues (1995a) observed no cases of pulmonary hypoplasia in fetuses born after membrane rupture at 24 weeks or beyond, suggesting 23 weeks or less is the threshold for lung hypoplasia.

HOSPITALIZATION. Most obstetricians hospitalize women with pregnancies complicated by preterm ruptured membranes. Concerns about the costs of lengthy hospitalizations are usually moot, because most women enter labor within a week or less of membrane rupture. Carlan and co-workers (1993) randomized 67 carefully selected pregnancies with ruptured membranes to home versus hospital management. All women were hospitalized until 72 hours after rupture; 20 women were ultimately sent home and 25 others randomized to hospitalization. No benefits were found for hospitalization and maternal hospital stay was reduced by 50 percent in those sent home (14 to 7 days). Three women sent home delivered at outside hospitals because their labor was too advanced to return to the research hospital. Importantly, these investigators emphasize that this study was too small to conclude that home management was safe.

Unfortunately, perinatal outcome in surviving infants in whom labor is delayed is not always satisfactory. In a previous study from Parkland Hospital, Hankins and associates (1984) reported that 30 percent of 176 such infants required ventilator therapy. Overall, 13 percent died in the neonatal period and another 3 percent died before age 1. Care of these infants born preterm required over 5100 newborn hospital days (almost 14 years) and cost $2.3 million (in 1984 dollars) just for bed space. Importantly, follow-up to 4 years was carried out for 105 of these infants, and neurological abnormalities of varying degrees were found in 16 percent. Similarly, Spinillo and colleagues (1995) found that preterm infants delivered 48 hours or more after ruptured membranes were at high risk for subsequent moderate to severe neurodevelopmental impairment compared with infants born after spontaneous preterm labor with intact membranes.

INTENTIONAL DELIVERY. The prospect of deliberately delivering a pregnancy preterm seems imprudent, although intentional delivery was widely practiced prior to the 1970s due to fear of infection (Reid and Christian, 1974). Another more recent rationale for intentional delivery is to avoid the uncommon fetal death that occurs in pregnancies managed expectantly after preterm rupture. The typically very short interval from membrane rupture to onset of spontaneous labor also lends support to the rationale for intentional delivery, because so little time is gained from expectant management, especially later in the third trimester (Fig. 27–11).

There have been two randomized trials of intentional delivery of pregnancies complicated by preterm ruptured membranes. Mercer and colleagues (1993) randomized 93 pregnancies with ruptured membranes between 32 and 36 weeks to delivery compared with expectant management. All had documented fetal lung maturity. Intentional delivery reduced the length of maternal hospitalization and also reduced infection rates in both mothers and neonates. Cox and Leveno (1995) similarly randomized 129 women with ruptured membranes between 30 and 34 weeks. There was one fetal death (due to sepsis) in those pregnancies managed expectantly and three neonatal deaths (two of which were due to sepsis and one due to pulmonary hypoplasia) among those intentionally delivered. Neither management approach was felt to be satisfactory.

OVERT CHORIOAMNIONITIS. Assuming that no untoward perinatal outcome occurs due to an entangled or prolapsed cord or from placental abruption, the greatest concern with prolonged membrane rupture is the risk of maternal or fetal infection. If chorioamnionitis is diagnosed, prompt efforts to effect delivery, preferably vaginally, are initiated. Unfortunately, fever is the only reliable indicator for making this diagnosis; a temperature of 38°C (100.4°F) or higher accompanying ruptured membranes implies infection. Maternal leukocytosis by itself has been found to be unreliable by most investigators, and this has also been our experience.

With chorioamnionitis, fetal and neonatal morbidity are substantively increased. In a prospective study of nearly 700 women between 26 and 34 weeks with preterm ruptured membranes, Morales (1987) reported that 13 percent developed chorioamnionitis diagnosed by oral temperatures of 38°C and no other cause for fever. Infants born to women with chorioamnionitis had a fourfold increased neonatal mortality and a threefold increase in the incidence of respiratory distress, neonatal sepsis, and intraventricular hemorrhage. Alexander and colleagues (1998) studied the effects of clinical chorioamnionitis in 1367 very-low-birthweight infants delivered at Parkland Hospital. Approximately 7 percent of the infants were exposed to chorioamnionitis and the outcomes of these infants were compared with those without overt infection. Neonatal sepsis, respiratory distress syndrome, seizures in the first 24 hours of life, intraventricular hemorrhage, and periventricular leukomalacia were all increased with chorioamnionitis. It was concluded that very-low-birthweight infants were vulnerable to neurological injury attributable to chorioamnionitis. Similarly, Yoon and colleagues (2000) found that intra-amnionic infection in preterm infants was related to cerebral palsy at 3 years of age.

ACCELERATED MATURATION OF PULMONARY FUNCTION. A variety of clinical events—some well defined and others not—have been proposed to accelerate surfactant production sufficient to protect against respiratory distress. Gluck (1979) emphasized that surfactant production is likely to be accelerated remote from term in pregnancies complicated by a number of maternal or fetal conditions or stresses. Examples included chronic renal or cardiovascular disease, long-standing hypertensive disorders due to pregnancy, heroin addiction, fetal growth restriction, placental infarction, chorioamnionitis, or preterm ruptured membranes. This view is widely held, although more recent data refute this association. For example, Owen and associates (1990a) concluded that a ''stressed'' pregnancy (primarily pregnancy-associated hypertension) conferred a negligible fetal survival advantage. Similarly, Hallak and Bottoms (1993) reviewed 1395 pregnancies delivered between 24 and 35 weeks and found that prematurely ruptured membranes was not associated with accelerated pulmonary maturation.

ANTIMICROBIAL THERAPY. The microbial pathogenesis for preterm ruptured membranes (Fig. 27–8) has prompted investigations of various antimicrobials to forestall delivery. Mercer and Arheart (1995) reviewed 13 randomized studies concerning the efficacy of antimicrobials compared with placebo treatment for ruptured membranes before 35 weeks. There was a combined total of 1594 pregnancies reported between 1974 and 1993. A total of 10 outcomes were subjected to meta-analysis and only three showed a possible beneficial effect of antimicrobials: fewer women developed chorioamnionitis, fewer infants developed sepsis, and pregnancy was more often prolonged 7 days in those given antimicrobials. Neonatal survival was unaffected, as was the incidence of necrotizing enterocolitis, respiratory distress, or intracranial hemorrhage.

To further address this issue, the NICHD Maternal–Fetal Medicine Units Network conducted a prospective randomized trial of ampicillin or amoxicillin plus erythromycin in women with preterm rupture between 24 and 32 weeks' gestation (Mercer and colleagues, 1997). Tocolysis, corticosteroid treatment, or both were not given in this trial. There were significantly fewer newborns with respiratory distress syndrome, necrotizing enterocolitis, or a composite adverse outcome in pregnancies in which antimicrobials were given. Latency from membrane rupture to delivery was significantly longer at 7, 14, and 21 days in women given antibiotics compared with placebo. At 7 days, 50 percent of these women remained undelivered compared with only 25 percent of those assigned to placebo. These benefits were apparent whether or not the patient had a positive test for cervicovaginal group B streptococcus at the time of amnion rupture.

Prolonged antimicrobial therapy in such pregnancies may have unwanted consequences. Kyle and Turner (1996) reported superinfection with *Pseudomonas aeruginosa* as a result of prolonged antibiotic therapy for preterm ruptured membranes. Carroll and colleagues (1996) and Mercer and associates (1999) have also voiced concern that such therapy potentially increases the risk for selection of resistant pathogens.

DIAGNOSIS AND MANAGEMENT OF PRETERM MEMBRANE RUPTURE AT PARKLAND HOSPITAL. Pregnancy complicated by preterm rupture of the membranes is managed as follows:

1. In women with possible amnion rupture one sterile speculum examination is performed to identify fluid coming from the cervix or pooled in the vagina. Demonstration of visible fluid is indicative of ruptured membranes and is usually accompanied by ultrasound examination to confirm oligohydramnios, to identify the presenting part, and to estimate gestational age. Nitrazine paper testing of vaginal pH has an appreciable false-positive rate associated with blood contamination, semen, or bacterial vaginosis. The microscopic inspection of cervicovaginal dried secretions for NaCl crystallization (ferning) also has

an appreciable false-positive rate. Infrequently, a compelling maternal history of amnion rupture is not supported by either gross visualization or vaginal pooling of amnionic fluid or ultrasound confirmation of decreased amnionic fluid. In these instances, instillation of indigo carmine dye (one ampule) into the amnionic fluid and assessing leakage of blue fluid into the vagina can be helpful in ascertaining the integrity of the membranes.

Attempts are made to visualize the extent of cervical effacement and dilatation, but a digital examination is not performed.

2. If the gestational age is less than 34 weeks and there are no other maternal or fetal indications for delivery, the woman is observed closely in Labor and Delivery. Continuous fetal heart rate monitoring is employed to look for evidence of cord compression, especially if labor supervenes.

3. If the fetal heart rate is reassuring, and if labor does not follow, the woman is transferred to the High Risk Pregnancy Unit for close observation for signs of labor, infection, or fetal jeopardy.

4. If the gestational age is greater than 34 completed weeks and if labor has not begun following adequate evaluation, labor is induced with intravenous oxytocin unless contraindicated. If induction fails, cesarean delivery is performed.

5. Dexamethasone, 5 mg intramuscularly every 12 hours for 4 doses, is given for enhancement of fetal maturation.

6. When labor is diagnosed, ampicillin, 2 g, is given intravenously every 6 hours prior to delivery for prevention of group B streptococcal infection in the neonate.

PRETERM LABOR WITH INTACT FETAL MEMBRANES.
Antepartum management of women with signs and symptoms of preterm labor and intact mambranes is much the same as already described for pregnancies with preterm ruptured membranes. That is, the cornerstone of treatment is to avoid delivery prior to 34 weeks' gestation if possible. Drugs intended to abate or suppress uterine contractions are commonly employed, and these will be discussed later. As in pregnancies with preterm ruptured membranes, antimicrobials, for the purpose of delaying delivery in women with preterm labor, have been studied specifically in women with intact membranes. Results with a variety of antimicrobial agents have been disappointing (Cox, 1996a; Gordon, 1995; Klebanoff, 1995, Romero, 1993, and their co-workers). Two smaller trials of metronidazole and ampicillin in women with suspected spontaneous preterm labor have shown a modest benefit (Norman and associates, 1994; Svare and colleagues, 1997). It is likely that administration of antimicrobials after preterm labor has begun

is too late to interfere with propagation of the biochemical cascade that modulates uterine activity (Fig. 27–8).

GLUCOCORTICOID THERAPY.
On the basis of previous observations that corticosteroids administered to the ewe accelerated lung maturation in the preterm fetus, Liggins and Howie (1972) performed a randomized study to evaluate the effects of maternally administered betamethasone (12 mg intramuscularly in two doses, 24 hours apart) to prevent respiratory distress in the subsequently delivered preterm infant. Infants born before 34 weeks had a significantly lowered incidence of respiratory distress and neonatal mortality from hyaline membrane disease if birth was delayed for at least 24 hours after completion of 24 hours of betamethasone given to the mother and for up to 7 days after completion of steroid therapy. This study served to stimulate more than 20 years of research on fetal maturation, which culminated in 1995 with a position statement on usage of corticosteroids for fetal therapy by the National Institutes of Health (NIH Consensus Development Panel, 1995).

The mechanism by which betamethasone or other corticosteroids are currently thought to reduce the frequency of respiratory distress involves induction of proteins that regulate biochemical systems within type II cells in the fetal lung that produce surfactant (Ballard and Ballard, 1995). The reported physiological effects of glucocorticoids on the developing lungs include increased alveolar surfactant, compliance, and maximal lung volume.

COLLABORATIVE STUDY ON ANTENATAL STEROID THERAPY.
The NIH-sponsored trial by the Collaborative Group on Antenatal Steroid Therapy (1981) was designed to study the effects of corticosteroid therapy on preterm fetuses. This double-blind collaborative trial was conducted at five centers, and of nearly 8000 women identified to be in preterm labor, 696 women at risk for preterm birth were enrolled. Women randomized to therapy were given intramuscular dexamethasone, 5 mg every 12 hours for a total of up to 4 doses. Including twins, a total of 720 infants was available for analysis. A significantly fewer number of infants whose mothers were given dexamethasone developed respiratory distress (13 versus 18 percent). Importantly, more than 80 percent in each study group did not develop respiratory distress. Neonatal mortality was not reduced by treatment. Similar results were obtained from a multicenter randomized trial of betamethasone performed in the United Kingdom between 1975 and 1978 (Gamsu and colleagues, 1989).

In 1985, a workshop reviewed the results of the Collaborative Study (Avery and colleagues, 1986). The group agreed that no differences in terms of cognitive, motor, or neurological function were found when 406 of the study infants were followed to 36 months of age, suggesting that steroid treatment did not adversely affect subsequent short-term neurological development (Collaborative Group, 1984). They further concluded that dexamethasone appeared beneficial only to a female fetus of older than 30 weeks and when the treatment-to-delivery interval exceeded 24 hours. Such therapy was not helpful in multiple gestations. These many caveats concerning the benefits (or lack thereof) of corticosteroids undoubtedly limited widespread use of this fetal therapy (Jobe and colleagues, 1993).

NATIONAL INSTITUTE OF HEALTH CONSENSUS DEVELOPMENT CONFERENCE ON CORTICOSTEROIDS FOR FETAL MATURATION. The proceedings of this conference were described in detail in the *American Journal of Obstetrics and Gynecology* (NIH Consensus Development Conference Statement, 1995). The resulting consensus on prescribing corticosteroids to accomplish fetal maturation was hailed by some as the most important development in perinatal care during 1995 (Hayward and Diaz-Rossello, 1995). Grimes (1995) took the position that because of the delay between 1972 and 1995 in adopting corticosteroids for fetal maturation, "tens of thousands of neonates died needlessly . . . and our nation squandered millions of health care dollars treating preventable complications of prematurity."

The centerpiece used by the National Institutes of Health panel on corticosteroids to establish the efficacy of this therapy was a meta-analysis of randomized controlled trials (Crowley, 1995). Such analyses pool individual randomized controlled trials together to arrive at an overall estimate of the effect of an intervention, in this case, corticosteroids. This analytical approach assumes that the pooled studies are identical or nearly so in experimental design, definitions of disease endpoints, patient populations, and treatment regimens. It is likely that most current meta-analyses have several sources of between-trial heterogeneity that could skew interpretation of pooled results (Moher and Olkin, 1995). For example, some trials included could use correctly concealed treatment allocation to randomize subjects whereas others may not be this rigorous in design. This is crucial, because trials with inadequate concealment generally produce results indicating that a particular treatment or intervention is beneficial (Martyn, 1996). An example of this type of heterogeneity can be found in the corticosteroid meta-analysis. Morales and colleagues (1986), in their randomized trial of corticosteroids for fetal maturation in 245 pregnancies with preterm ruptured membranes, used hospital medical record numbers in an unspecified design to randomize patients. This method of allocation to treatment or nontreatment

with corticosteroids was thus not concealed from the clinicians. Despite this, the study by Morales and colleagues (1986) was pooled in the meta-analysis with other trials with more rigorous experimental design.

The next three figures include examples of meta-analysis on the fetal effects of corticosteroids using respiratory distress syndrome (Fig. 27–12), neonatal death (Fig. 27–13), and the summary of multiple effects on infant outcome (Fig. 27–14). A total of 15 randomized trials were chosen by Crowley (1995) to be included in the meta-analysis. Each horizontal line represents the results of one trial and the shorter the line, the more certain the result. If a horizontal line (study trial) touches the solid vertical line it means that that particular trial found no significant benefit. The total at the bottom of each figure is the result when all 15 trials are pooled together.

In the case of respiratory distress syndrome, nine trials found no benefit for corticosteroids and three others found only marginal benefits (Fig. 27–12). The total effect, however, when all the trials are pooled indicates that corticosteroids reduce respiratory distress by 50 percent. This beneficial effect is heavily dependent on the largest and original trial by Liggins and Howie (1972). An alternative interpretation could also be that no group of investigators has ever been able to reproduce that original trial. For neonatal deaths, 10 of the 15 trials analyzed showed no benefit (Fig. 27–13). Pooling of the data, however, indicates that corticosteroids reduced neonatal mortality by 50 percent. Meta-analysis for multiple infant outcomes related to corticosteroid therapy is shown in Figure 27–14.

Table 27–9 summarizes recommendations for use of corticosteroids for fetal maturation by the NIH Consensus Development Panel (1995). Data were deemed insufficient to assess effectiveness of corticosteroids in pregnancies complicated by hypertension, diabetes, multiple gestation, fetal growth restriction, and fetal hydrops. The Consensus Panel concluded, however, that in the absence of evidence of adverse effects, it is reasonable to use corticosteroids with these complications. It was also concluded, however, that there were insufficient data to comment on the benefits or risks of repeating maternal corticosteroid treatment weekly to enhance fetal maturation. The national response to dissemination of the NIH Consensus Panel recommendations was dramatic, and the use of corticosteroids to enhance fetal maturation doubled within 12 months (Leviton and colleagues, 1999).

The American College of Obstetricians and Gynecologists Committee on Obstetric Practice (1994) supported the conclusions of the NIH Consensus Panel with the exception of the recommendation for treatment of women with preterm ruptured membranes. They recommended further research. Indeed, Chapman and col-

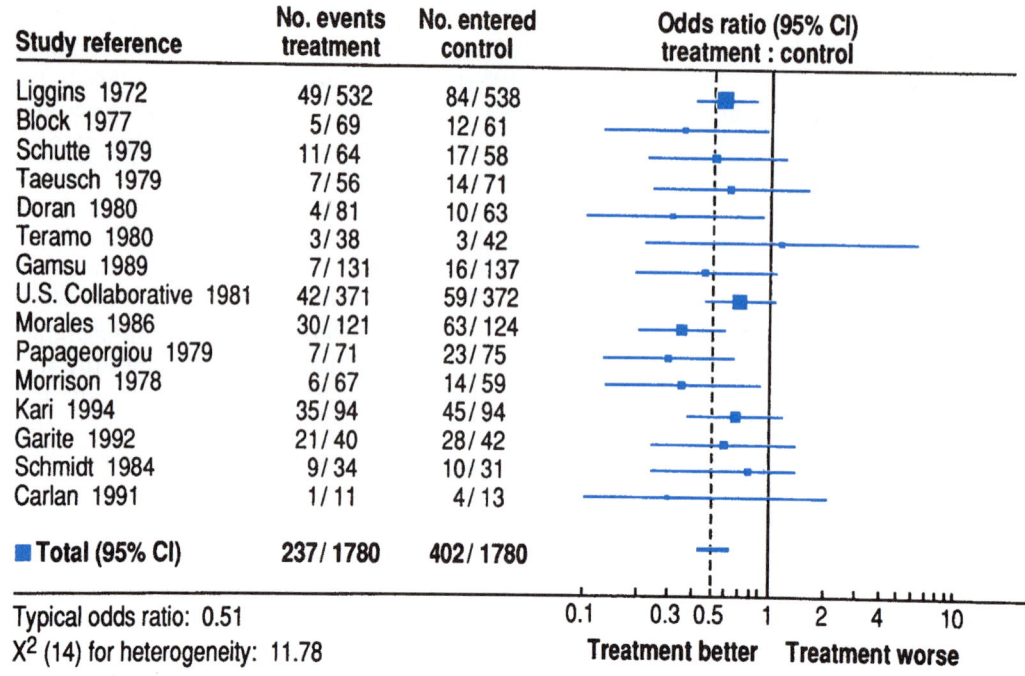

Study reference	No. events treatment	No. entered control	Odds ratio (95% CI) treatment : control
Liggins 1972	49/ 532	84/ 538	
Block 1977	5/ 69	12/ 61	
Schutte 1979	11/ 64	17/ 58	
Taeusch 1979	7/ 56	14/ 71	
Doran 1980	4/ 81	10/ 63	
Teramo 1980	3/ 38	3/ 42	
Gamsu 1989	7/ 131	16/ 137	
U.S. Collaborative 1981	42/ 371	59/ 372	
Morales 1986	30/ 121	63/ 124	
Papageorgiou 1979	7/ 71	23/ 75	
Morrison 1978	6/ 67	14/ 59	
Kari 1994	35/ 94	45/ 94	
Garite 1992	21/ 40	28/ 42	
Schmidt 1984	9/ 34	10/ 31	
Carlan 1991	1/ 11	4/ 13	
■ Total (95% CI)	237/ 1780	402/ 1780	

Typical odds ratio: 0.51
χ^2 (14) for heterogeneity: 11.78

Treatment better   Treatment worse

FIGURE 27–12. Meta-analysis of the effects of maternal corticosteroid therapy to prevent neonatal respiratory distress syndrome. (From Crowley, 1995, with permission.)

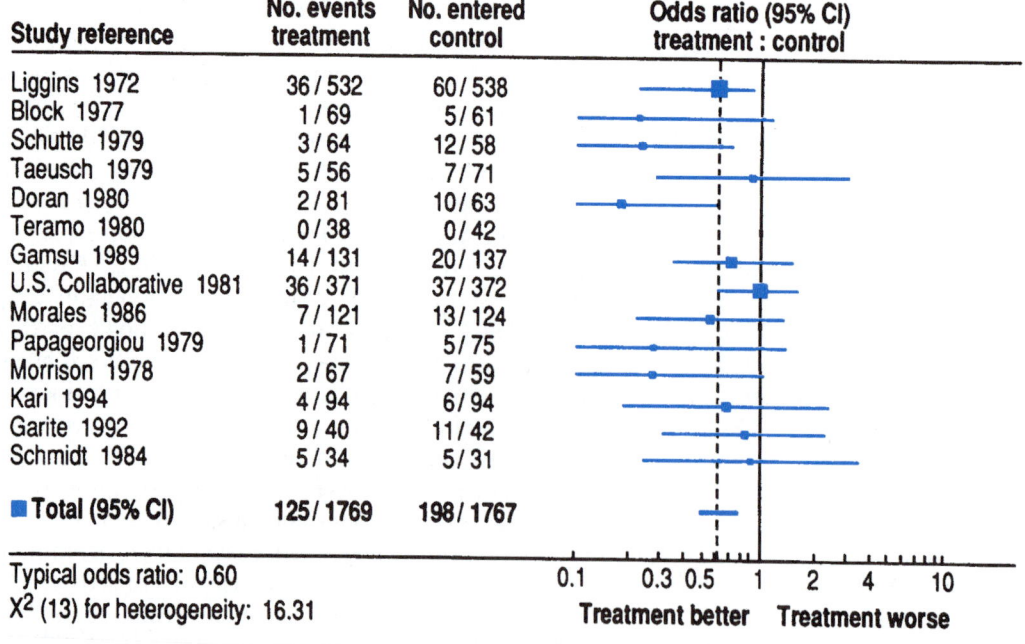

Study reference	No. events treatment	No. entered control	Odds ratio (95% CI) treatment : control
Liggins 1972	36/ 532	60/ 538	
Block 1977	1/ 69	5/ 61	
Schutte 1979	3/ 64	12/ 58	
Taeusch 1979	5/ 56	7/ 71	
Doran 1980	2/ 81	10/ 63	
Teramo 1980	0/ 38	0/ 42	
Gamsu 1989	14/ 131	20/ 137	
U.S. Collaborative 1981	36/ 371	37/ 372	
Morales 1986	7/ 121	13/ 124	
Papageorgiou 1979	1/ 71	5/ 75	
Morrison 1978	2/ 67	7/ 59	
Kari 1994	4/ 94	6/ 94	
Garite 1992	9/ 40	11/ 42	
Schmidt 1984	5/ 34	5/ 31	
■ Total (95% CI)	125/ 1769	198/ 1767	

Typical odds ratio: 0.60
χ^2 (13) for heterogeneity: 16.31

Treatment better   Treatment worse

FIGURE 27–13. Meta-analysis of the effects of maternal corticosteroid therapy to prevent neonatal death. (From Crowley, 1995, with permission.)

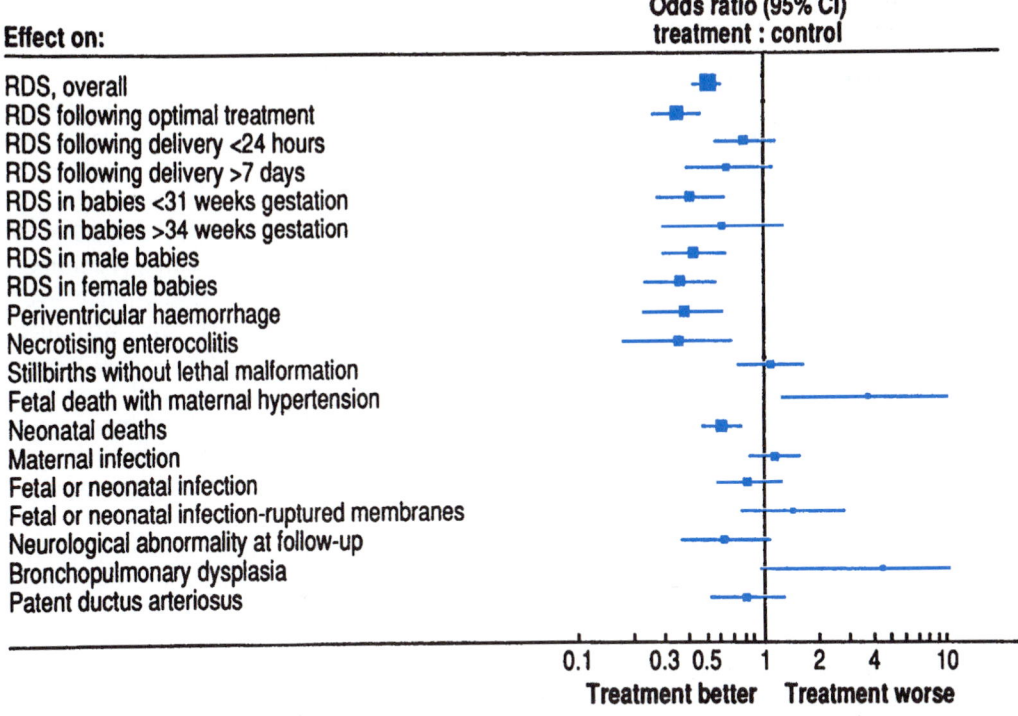

Odds ratio (95% CI)
treatment : control

Effect on:

RDS, overall
RDS following optimal treatment
RDS following delivery <24 hours
RDS following delivery >7 days
RDS in babies <31 weeks gestation
RDS in babies >34 weeks gestation
RDS in male babies
RDS in female babies
Periventricular haemorrhage
Necrotising enterocolitis
Stillbirths without lethal malformation
Fetal death with maternal hypertension
Neonatal deaths
Maternal infection
Fetal or neonatal infection
Fetal or neonatal infection-ruptured membranes
Neurological abnormality at follow-up
Bronchopulmonary dysplasia
Patent ductus arteriosus

0.1   0.3 0.5   1   2   4   10
Treatment better   Treatment worse

FIGURE 27–14. Summary of maternal and infant effects of maternal corticosteroid therapy given before preterm delivery (15 trials). (RDS = respiratory distress syndrome.) (From Crowley, 1995, with permission.)

leagues (1996) concluded that corticosteroid treatment for women with preterm ruptured membranes who were delivered of infants weighing less than 1000 g was not beneficial. More recently, the American College of Obstetricians and Gynecologists Committee on Obstetric

TABLE 27–9. Quality of Evidence to Support Use of Corticosteroids to Promote Fetal Maturation

	Evidence
Neonatal mortality	Good
Repiratory distress syndrome	Good
Intraventricular hemorrhage	Good
Preterm ruptured membranes	Fair
Delivery at 24–28 weeks	Good
Delivery at 29–34 weeks	Good
Delivery at > 34 weeks	Inadequate for or against
Treatment-to-delivery interval	
< 24 hr	Fair
24 hr–7 days	Good
> 7 days	Inadequate for or against

From NIH Consensus Development Panel on the Effect of Corticosteroids for Fetal Maturation on Perinatal Outcome (1995), with permission.

Practice (1998) expressed concern about adverse fetal effects and possible effects on maternal immune status of repeated weekly courses of steroids. The College recommended that following the initial course of corticosteroids, repeated doses should be given only on an as-needed basis (i.e., a "rescue" dose given when the threat of preterm delivery recurred).

In the previous edition of this textbook, we predicted that "It is likely that some of the many benefits attributed to corticosteroid therapy by the Consensus Panel will be reassessed in the future." **Indeed, the Consensus Panel was reconvened on August 17–18, 2000 to reconsider the safety and efficacy of repeated courses of corticosteroids given for fetal maturation.** The conclusions of the panel are shown in Table 27–10. To summarize, it is now recommended that repeated courses of antenatal corticosteroids be used only in clinical trials.

ADVERSE EFFECTS OF CORTICOSTEROIDS. Studies initiated in the 1970s, which followed the development of children treated antenatally with corticosteroids up to the age of 12 years, showed no adverse outcomes in the areas of long-term neurodevelopment. These were measured by learning, behavioral, and motor or sensory disturbances (NIH Consensus Development Panel, 1995). There are, however, short-term maternal effects to include pulmonary edema, infection, and more difficult glucose control in diabetic women. No long-term adverse maternal effects have been reported.

Liggins and Howie (1972) based their use of corticosteroids to promote fetal lung maturation on experiments in sheep that indicated that such therapy not only affected lung maturation but also stimulated labor. Corticosteroids were reported to induce labor in humans more than 20 years ago (Jenssen and Wright, 1977; Mati and colleagues, 1973). Elliott and Radin (1995) confirmed that corticosteroids induce uterine contractions and preterm labor in humans.

Adverse fetal-newborn and long-term effects have been reported in regard to repeated versus single courses of maternal corticosteroid treatment to enhance pulmonary maturation. Esplin and colleagues (2000) compared mental and psychomotor development of 429 low-birthweight infants exposed to two courses or more of antenatal corticosteroids with infants exposed to a single course or to no exposure. The authors found no benefits for repeated doses, and exposure to multiple courses of corticosteroids was independently and significantly associated with abnormal psychomotor development. Vermillion and colleagues (2000), in an analysis of 453 infants, determined that early-onset neonatal sepsis, chorioamnionitis, and neonatal death were significantly associated with multiple maternal dosing with betamethasone. Thorp (2000) and Guinn (2001) and their associates conducted large prospective trials and found no benefits of multiple steroid courses. Importantly, in a secondary analysis, Thorp and co-workers (2001) reported a significant reduction in head circumference in infants exposed to steroids. Likewise, Mercer and associates (2001) reported a dose-dependent decrease in birth weight and length in neonates exposed to antenatal steroid therapy. Some of these results were available and they played a prominent role in the conclusions reached by the reconvened Consensus Panel (Table 27–10).

USE OF CORTICOSTEROIDS AT PARKLAND HOSPITAL. As a result of the original Consensus Panel recommendations, dexamethasone, 5 mg intramuscularly every 12 hours for four doses every 7 days, was introduced at Parkland Hospital in May 1994 for selected women at risk for preterm birth between 24 and 34 weeks. Corticosteroids were not used for fetal maturation prior to this date. Outcomes of 370 singleton pregnancies ending between 24 and 34 weeks during 12 months before dexamethasone therapy was begun were compared with outcomes of 370 similar pregnancies in which dexamethasone therapy was subsequently given. We were unable to demonstrate much benefit, if any, in this before–after population based study. Publication of this experience has not been possible.

THYROTROPIN-RELEASING HORMONE FOR FETAL MATURATION. Knight and colleagues (1994) from New Zealand reported that administration of thyrotropin-releasing hormone (400 mg intravenously) in addition to betamethasone augmented fetal lung maturation compared with betamethasone used alone. This effect is based on experimental observations that tri-iodothyronine enhances surfactant synthesis. Crowther and co-workers (1995) and the Australian Collaborative Study Group randomized 1234 women to receive thyrotropin-releasing hormone in addition to corticosteroids or to corticosteroids alone and were unable to reproduce these beneficial results. Indeed, the incidence of respiratory disease was increased in the thyrotropin-treated group! In this ACTOBAT study, the investigators also observed that 7 percent of the mothers became overtly hypertensive as a result of thyrotropin therapy. They concluded that thyrotropin-releasing hormone given to augment fetal maturation "is associated with maternal and perinatal risks and cannot be recommended." Ballard and associates (1998) enrolled 996 women before 30 weeks' gestation in a multicenter randomized double-blind, placebo-controlled trial of maternal thyrotropin-releasing hormone treatment to decrease neonatal pulmonary morbidity. All women also received betamethasone treatment. The primary outcome was chronic lung disease or infant death before 28 days. Primary and secondary outcomes were almost identical in both groups. They concluded that antenatal administration of thyrotropin-releasing hormone was not beneficial.

ANTENATAL PHENOBARBITAL AND VITAMIN K THERAPY. As reviewed by Thorp and colleagues (1995), several studies have suggested that antenatal phenobarbital and vitamin K given to the mother may reduce the incidence of intracranial hemorrhage. They randomized 272 women at risk for preterm birth to placebo or treatment with phenobarbital and vitamin K and found that such therapy did not reduce the frequency or severity of neonatal intracranial hemorrhage.

CERCLAGE. Prophylactic cervical cerclage, which is typically recommended in the United States for women with a supporting history and recurrent midtrimester losses, has also been used in Europe to prevent preterm birth. Two randomized trials of cerclage included more than 700 women at risk for preterm delivery, and neither study showed a benefit (Lazar and colleagues, 1984; Rush and associates, 1984). Prophylactic cerclage in twin pregnancies has also been shown to be of no benefit in a randomized trial (Dor and associates, 1982). The Medical Research Council of the Royal College of Obstetricians and Gynaecologists (1993) studied 1292 women from 12 countries with heterogenous and often unclear indications for cerclage to assess if this procedure prolonged pregnancy. Approximately 75 percent of women enrolled in this randomized study had previously delivered preterm infants. In 647 women, cervical sutures were placed at about 16 weeks and their outcomes compared with 645 women randomized to no cerclage. A small—from 17 to 13 percent—but significant decrease in births before 33 weeks was observed in women undergoing cerclage. Importantly, there was no difference in neonatal death between the two groups. The use of cerclage, however, was linked to increased interventions such as tocolysis and hospital admission. The investigators concluded that cervical sutures should be offered to women with a history of three or more pregnancies ending before 37 weeks.

Althuisius and co-workers (2000) randomized 73 women who had had a prior preterm birth before 34 weeks' gestation either to cerclage or observation. These latter women were followed with transvaginal measurement of cervical length until 27 weeks, and cerclage was placed if the cervical length shortened to less than 25 mm. Delivery before 34 weeks and neonatal survival were similar in the two study groups. In a subgroup analysis, however, preterm birth was significantly reduced in women who received cerclage after developing ultrasound evidence of cervical shortening. Rust and colleagues (2000) randomized 61 women to cerclage or to expectant management based on ultrasound evidence of cervical funneling between 16 to 24 weeks' gestation. No benefits were apparent in the women randomized to cervical cerclage.

BACTERIAL VAGINOSIS. Hillier and colleagues (1995) detected bacterial vaginosis in 16 percent of 10,397 pregnant women without risk factors for preterm birth who were screened between 23 and 26 weeks. Bacterial vaginosis was linked to poverty and to significantly increased preterm birth at 32 weeks or less but not to premature membrane rupture. Microbes most strongly associated with bacterial vaginosis included *Gardnerella vaginalis, Bacteroides species,* and *Mycoplasma hominis.*

Hauth and co-workers (1995) studied 624 women at risk for preterm birth either because they had previously delivered preterm infants or because they weighed less than 50 kg before pregnancy. In this double-blind study, women were randomized to treatment with metronidazole, 250 mg three times a day for 7 days; erythromycin, 333 mg three times a day for 14 days; or placebo. About 40 percent of women in each arm had bacterial vaginosis at 22 to 24 weeks. Delivery before 37 weeks in women with bacterial vaginosis was significantly decreased from 40 to 25 percent when metronidazole or erythromycin was given. Morales and co-workers (1994) reported a similar benefit in 80 women at increased risk for preterm birth and with bacterial vaginosis and who were treated with metronidazole.

Carey and colleagues (2000), in a multicenter NICHD Maternal–Fetal Medicine Units Network trial, found that metronidazole treatment of asymptomatic pregnant women with bacterial vaginosis did not improve pregnancy outcomes despite that bacterial vaginosis resolved in 78 percent of women assigned to metronidazole treatment compared with 37 percent assigned to a placebo. Specifically, the incidence of preterm birth was similar in the 953 women treated with metronidazole compared with the 966 in the placebo group. Finally, treatment with metronidazole did not reduce clinical intra-amnionic or postpartum infections, neonatal sepsis, or admission to the neonatal intensive care unit.

Intravaginal topical treatment of bacterial vaginosis using clindamycin cream has not been shown to be effective to prevent preterm birth (Joesoef and colleagues, 1995; McGregor and associates, 1994).

METHODS USED TO INHIBIT PRETERM LABOR. A great number of drugs and other interventions have been used to inhibit preterm labor, but unfortunately, none has been completely effective (American College of Obstetricians and Gynecologists, 1995). Potential maternal complications of tocolytic drugs are shown in Table 27–11. Their importance cannot be underestimated. For example, tocolysis was the third most common cause of acute respiratory distress syndrome and death in pregnant women during a 14-year period in Jackson, Mississippi (Perry and associates, 1996). The American College of Obstetricians and Gynecologists

TABLE 27–11. Potential Complications of Tocolytic Agents

Beta-adrenergic Agents
  Hyperglycemia
  Hypokalemia
  Hypotension
  Pulmonary edema
  Cardiac insufficiency
  Arrhythmias
  Myocardial ischemia
  Maternal death

Magnesium Sulfate
  Pulmonary edema
  Respiratory depression[a]
  Cardiac arrest[a]
  Maternal tetany[a]
  Profound muscular paralysis[a]
  Profound hypotension[a]

Indomethacin
  Hepatitis[b]
  Renal failure[b]
  Gastrointestinal bleeding[b]

Nifedipine
  Transient hypotension

[a] Effect is rare; seen with toxic levels.
[b] Effect is rare; associated with chronic use.
From the American College of Obstetricians and Gynecologists (1995), with permission.

(1998) has recommended that tocolysis be used in the presence of regular uterine contractions plus documented cervical change or appreciable cervical dilatation and effacement.

BED REST. The treatment regimen that has been used most often is bed rest either in the hospital or at home. Goldenberg and colleagues (1994) have reviewed bed rest used to treat a variety of pregnancy complications and found no conclusive evidence that bed rest was helpful in preventing preterm birth. Kovacevich and associates (2000) reported that enforced bed rest (except for bathroom privileges) for 3 days or more increased the risk of thromboembolic complications from 1 per 1000 women without bed rest to 16 per 1000 in those with bed rest for threatened preterm delivery.

HYDRATION AND SEDATION. Helfgott and associates (1994) performed the first randomized trial of hydration and sedation compared with bed rest alone in the treat-ment of 119 women in preterm labor. Women randomized to treatment received 500 mL of lactated Ringer solution intravenously over 30 minutes and 8 to 12 mg of intramuscular morphine sulfate. Such therapy was not found to be more beneficial than bed rest.

BETA-ADRENERGIC RECEPTOR AGONISTS. Earlier in this century, epinephrine in low doses was demonstrated to exert a depressant effect on pregnant myometrium. Its tocolytic effects, however, proved to be rather weak, quite transient, and likely to be accompanied by troublesome cardiovascular effects. Several compounds capable of reacting predominantly with β-adrenergic receptors have subsequently been investigated. Some of these now are used in obstetrics, but only ritodrine hydrochloride has been approved (1980) by the Food and Drug Administration to treat preterm labor.

The adrenergic receptors are located on the outer surface of the smooth muscle cell membrane, where specific agonists can couple with them. Adenyl cyclase in the cell membrane is activated by the receptor stimulation. Adenyl cyclase enhances the conversion of ATP to cyclic AMP, which in turn initiates a number of reactions that reduce the intracellular concentration of ionized calcium and thereby prevent activation of contractile proteins (also see Chap. 11, p. 271). Flier and Underhill (1996) have comprehensively reviewed adrenergic receptors.

There are two classes of β-adrenergic receptors: β_1-receptors, dominant in the heart and intestines; and β_2-receptors, dominant in the myometrium, blood vessels, and bronchioles. A number of compounds generally similar in structure to epinephrine have been evaluated in the search for one that ideally would provide optimal stimulation of myometrial β_2-receptors and thus inhibit uterine contractions while simultaneously causing few adverse effects from stimulation of receptors elsewhere. Thus far, no compound has exhibited these utopian properties. In the United States, β-agonist compounds employed to arrest preterm labor include ritodrine and terbutaline.

RITODRINE. In a multicenter United States study, infants whose mothers were treated with ritodrine for presumed preterm labor had a lower mortality rate, developed respiratory distress less often, and achieved a gestational age of 36 weeks or a birthweight of 2500 g more often than did infants whose mothers were not so treated (Merkatz and colleagues, 1980). Hesseldahl (1979), however, in a multicenter controlled study in Denmark, did not find any of several ritodrine regimens tested to be more efficacious than treatment with bed rest, glucose infusion, and placebo tablets.

Because of contemporaneous concerns for the efficacy and safety of ritodrine, we evaluated the drug on the obstetrical service at Parkland Hospital (Leveno and associates, 1986b). Preterm labor was carefully defined to include cervical dilatation plus regular uterine contractions, and 106 women between 24 and 33 weeks were randomly allocated to receive either intravenous ritodrine or no tocolysis. Although ritodrine treatment significantly delayed delivery for 24 hours or less, it did not significantly modify ultimate perinatal outcomes. A significant delay in delivery at 48 hours was found in a randomized study involving 708 pregnancies reported by the Canadian Preterm Labor Investigators Group (1992). A likely explanation for the transient uterine tocolytic effects of ritodrine and ultimate failure of such therapy may be the phenomenon of β-adrenergic receptor desensitization (Hausdorff and colleagues, 1990).

The infusion of ritodrine, as well as the other β-adrenergic agonists, has resulted in frequent and at times serious side effects (Table 27–11). Maternal tachycardia, hypotension, apprehension, chest tightness or pain, electrocardiographic S-T segment depression, pulmonary edema, and death have all been observed. Maternal metabolic effects include hyperglycemia, hyperinsulinemia (unless diabetic), hypokalemia, and lactic and ketoacidosis. Less serious but nonetheless troublesome side effects include emesis, headaches, tremulousness, fever, and hallucinations.

A single mechanism has not been identified to explain the development of pulmonary edema, but maternal infection appears to increase the risk (Hatjis and Swain, 1988). The cause of the pulmonary edema appears to be multifactorial. Beta-adrenergic agonists cause retention of sodium and water, and thus with time—usually 24 to 48 hours—may lead to volume overload (Hankins and colleagues, 1988). The drugs have also been implicated as a cause of increased capillary permeability, disturbances of cardiac rhythm, and myocardial ischemia. Simultaneous administration of glucocorticoids to try to hasten fetal maturation may also contribute, although pulmonary edema has developed in their absence.

Only parenteral ritodrine is now available in the United States since the manufacturer discontinued distribution of tablets in 1995. The efficacy of oral ritodrine had been challenged on pharmacokinetic grounds (Schiff and colleagues, 1993).

TERBUTALINE. This β-agonist is commonly used to forestall preterm labor although, like ritodrine, toxicity—especially maternal pulmonary edema and glucose intolerance—have been evident with its use (Angel and associates, 1988).

Lam and colleagues (1988) described long-term subcutaneous administration of low-dose terbutaline using a portable pump in nine pregnancies. It was claimed that the lower dose of terbutaline used likely prevented β-adrenergic desensitization, resulting in less "breakthrough tocolysis." The Tokos Corporation promptly marketed this approach, and between 1987 and 1993 had used these pumps in nearly 25,000 women with preterm labor (Perry and colleagues, 1995). The list price for terbutaline pump therapy in Dallas in 1996 was $484 per day. The only other reports concerning terbutaline pumps include a sudden maternal death (Hudgens and Conradi, 1993) and a description of newborn myocardial necrosis after the mother used the pump for 12 weeks (Fletcher and colleagues, 1991).

Two prospective randomized trials have not found any benefit for terbutaline pump therapy. Wenstrom and colleagues (1997) randomized 42 women to therapy with a terbutaline pump, a saline pump, or to oral terbutaline. These three groups had similar gestational ages at entry and at delivery. Guinn and associates (1998) in a double-blind trial, randomized 52 women to terbutaline pump or to saline pump therapy. A sample size of 48 women was required to detect a 2-week intergroup difference in mean time to delivery. Terbutaline pump therapy did not significantly prolong pregnancy, prevent preterm delivery, or improve neonatal outcomes.

Oral terbutaline therapy has been reported ineffective by several groups (How and associates, 1995; Parilla and co-workers, 1993). In a double-blind trial, Lewis and colleagues (1996) randomized 203 women with preterm labor following successful intravenous tocolysis at 24 to 34 weeks' gestation, to 5 mg oral terbutaline every 4 hours or placebo. Delivery at one week was similar in both groups as was median latency, mean gestational age at delivery, and the incidence of recurrent preterm labor. Post hoc analysis, however, of 96 women enrolled before 32 weeks' gestation suggested significant pregnancy prolongation with maintenance oral terbutaline.

OVERVIEW OF BETA-ADRENERGIC DRUGS TO INHIBIT PRETERM LABOR. Several meta-analyses of parenteral β-agonists given to prevent preterm birth have consistently confirmed that these agents delay delivery for no more than 48 hours (Canadian Preterm Labor Group, 1992). Moreover, this delay has not proven to be beneficial despite repeated attempts to revisit the data (Lamont, 1993). Finally, Macones and colleagues (1995) used meta-analysis to assess the available data on the efficacy of oral β-agonist therapy and found no benefits.

Thus, oral β-agonist therapy has convincingly been shown to be ineffective, and parenteral therapy can only delay delivery for a short time that has not been shown to be beneficial. Keirse (1995b) suggests that the brief delay in delivery afforded may be useful to facilitate maternal transport to tertiary care centers, and also delay delivery sufficiently to effect fetal maturation with glucocorticoids. Unfortunately, there are no data to support this viewpoint.

MAGNESIUM SULFATE. It has been recognized for some time that ionic magnesium in a sufficiently high concentration can alter myometrial contractility in vivo as well as in vitro. Its role is presumably that of a calcium antagonist.

Steer and Petrie (1977) concluded that intravenously administered magnesium sulfate, 4 g given as a loading dose followed by a continuous infusion of 2 g/hr, will usually arrest labor. Elliott (1983), in a retrospective study, found tocolysis with magnesium sulfate to be successful, inexpensive, and relatively nontoxic. He reported 87 percent success when the cervix was dilated 2 cm or less, but the period of inhibited labor was as short as 48 hours. Spisso and co-workers (1982) were also favorably impressed by the efficacy of magnesium sulfate when given intravenously in relatively large doses to women in the early latent phase of labor.

Watt-Morse and associates (1995) studied the inhibitory effects of magnesium concentrations up to 8.3 mEq/L in preterm sheep with oxytocin-induced contractions. They concluded that magnesium sulfate in tolerable, nontoxic doses has no direct effect on uterine contractility.

There have been only two randomized controlled studies of the tocolytic properties of magnesium sulfate in humans. Cotton and associates (1984) compared magnesium sulfate with ritodrine as well as with a placebo, and they identified little difference in outcomes. Cox and associates (1990) randomized 156 women in preterm labor with intact membranes to infusions of magnesium sulfate or normal saline. Magnesium sulfate (20 percent solution) was begun using a 4-g loading dose followed by 2 g/hr intravenously. If contractions persisted after 1 hour, the infusion was increased to 3 g/hr. Treated women had a mean plasma magnesium concentration of 5.5 mEq/L. No benefits for such therapy were found, and this method of tocolysis was abandoned at Parkland Hospital. Similar results were subsequently reported in an evaluation of nonrandomized women in preterm labor who were delivered of infants weighing less than 1000 g (Kimberlin and associates, 1996a).

Hollander and colleagues (1987) used an unprecedented infusion dose of magnesium sulfate that averaged 4.5 g/hr. They reported that such therapy was equivalent to ritodrine. Conversely, Semchyshyn and associates (1983) failed to stop labor in a woman who inadvertently was given 17.3 g of magnesium sulfate in 45 minutes! Women given high-dosage magnesium sulfate must be monitored very closely for evidence of hypermagnesemia that might prove toxic to them and their fetus-infants. The pharmacology and toxicology of parenterally administered magnesium are considered in more detail in Chapter 24 (p. 599).

PROSTAGLANDIN INHIBITORS. Compounds that inhibit prostaglandins have been the subject of considerable interest since it was appreciated that prostaglandins are intimately involved in myometrial contractions of normal labor (Chap. 11, p. 274). Antiprostaglandin agents may act by inhibiting the synthesis of prostaglandins or by blocking the action of prostaglandins on target organs. A group of enzymes collectively called prostaglandin synthase is responsible for the conversion of free arachidonic acid to prostaglandins. Several drugs are known to block this system, including aspirin and other salicylates, indomethacin, naproxen, and sulindac.

Unfortunately, prostaglandin synthase inhibitors may adversely affect the fetus, and this has prevented widespread use of these agents for tocolysis. Complications include closure of the ductus arteriosus, necrotizing enterocolitis, and intracranial hemorrhage (Norton and co-workers, 1993). Parilla and colleagues (2000) have challenged the association of indomethacin with necrotizing enterocolitis. Van der Heijden and colleagues (1994) linked long-term perinatal indomethacin to anemia, neonatal death, and cystic renal damage. The mother can be adversely affected by indomethacin therapy, and Lunt and associates (1994) reported that indomethacin tocolysis caused profound prolongation of maternal bleeding time.

Sulindac, closely related to indomethacin in structure, has been reported to have fewer side effects when used for tocolysis (Rasanen and Jouppila, 1995). Preliminary trials, however, indicate that oral sulindac therapy may not be very useful in the prevention of preterm birth (Carlan and associates, 1995). Kramer and colleagues (1996) measured the effects of sulindac on fetal urine production and amnionic fluid volume and compared them with terbutaline in a randomized, double-blind study. Sulindac administration decreased fetal urine flow and amnionic fluid volume. Two fetuses also developed severe ductal constriction. Thus, sulindac shares many of the fetal side effects associated with indomethacin.

Panter and colleagues (1996) reviewed all randomized trials that have compared indomethacin with β-agonists for tocolysis. Indomethacin was found to be more effective in delaying delivery by 48 hours, and there were fewer maternal side effects compared with ritodrine. Indomethacin was, however, associated with increased neonatal morbidity. These investigators concluded that indomethacin needs to be further evaluated before it is used routinely for tocolysis.

CALCIUM-CHANNEL-BLOCKING DRUGS. Smooth muscle activity, including myometrium, is directly related to free calcium within the cytoplasm, and a reduction in calcium concentration inhibits contraction. Calcium ions reach the cytoplasm through specific membrane portals or channels, and calcium-channel blockers act to inhibit, by a variety of different mechanisms, the entry of calcium through the cell membrane channels. Calcium-entry blockers, because of their smooth muscle arteriolar relaxation effects, are currently being used for the treatment of coronary artery disease and hypertension.

The possibility that calcium-channel–blocking drugs might have applications in the treatment of preterm labor has been the subject of research in both animals and humans since the late 1970s. Saade and colleagues (1994), using in vitro human myometrial strips, showed that nifedipine caused relaxation similar to ritodrine and more effectively than magnesium. The first clinical trial in which nifedipine was given for preterm labor was from Denmark by Ulmsten and colleagues (1980). Nifedipine treatment postponed delivery at least 3 days in 10 women with preterm labor at 33 weeks or less. No serious maternal or fetal side effects were noted. There have been several subsequent studies of nifedipine tocolysis, and these have been reviewed comprehensively by Childress and Katz (1994). In all the studies, nifedipine was as successful or better than ritodrine in stopping preterm contractions without adverse fetal effects. Maternal side effects were much worse with ritodrine.

As promising as calcium-channel blockers may appear for treatment of preterm labor, some investigators caution that more research is needed to clarify their potential maternal or fetal dangers. This is because smooth muscle relaxation by nifedipine is not limited to uterine muscle, but also includes the systemic and uterine vasculature. Nifedipine-induced decreased vascular resistance can lead to maternal hypotension and thus decreased uteroplacental perfusion. Parisi and colleagues (1986) reported that hypercapnia, acidosis, and possibly hypoxemia developed in fetuses of hypertensive ewes given nicardipine. Similarly, Lirette and colleagues (1987) observed a fall in uteroplacental blood flow in pregnant rabbits. Other investigators, however, have not found these adverse fetal effects (Childress and Katz, 1994).

The efficacy of calcium-channel blockers, such as nifedipine, in suppressing preterm contractions or labor has not been adequately studied. Small trials have arrived at inconclusive results (Kupferminc and colleagues, 1993; Papatsonis and co-workers, 1997; Read and associates, 1986; Smith and Woodland, 1993). In a review from the Cochrane Database comparing nifedipine and β-sympathomimetics, Keirse (1995a) concluded that nifedipine treatment reduced births less than 2500 g, but more infants were admitted to neonatal intensive care. Results such as these mandate further study of their safety and efficacy.

The combination of nifedipine and magnesium for tocolysis is potentially dangerous. Ben-Ami and colleagues (1994) and Kurtzman and associates (1993) have reported that nifedipine enhances the toxicity of magnesium to produce neuromuscular blockade that can interfere with both pulmonary and cardiac function. Carr and colleagues (1999) found that maintenance therapy with oral nifedipine did not significantly prolong pregnancy in women initially treated with intravenous magnesium sulfate for preterm labor.

ATOSIBAN. A nonapeptide oxytocin analog, atosiban has been shown to be a competitive oxytocin-vasopressin antagonist capable of inhibiting oxytocin-induced uterine contractions. Goodwin and colleagues (1995) reviewed atosiban and described its pharmacokinetics in pregnant women. Results of a multicenter, double-blind, placebo-controlled trial in 501 women assigned to intravenous atosiban or placebo were recently published (Romero and colleagues, 2000). Atosiban therapy did not significantly improve any clinically relevant infant outcome. Safety considerations were of great concern with more fetal-infant deaths in the atosiban group. Food and Drug Administration approval for the use of atosiban to arrest preterm labor has been denied due to concerns regarding efficacy and fetal-newborn safety (FDA, personal communication).

NITRIC OXIDE DONOR DRUGS. Nitric oxide is a potent endogenous smooth-muscle relaxant in the vasculature, the gut, and the uterus. Nitroglycerin is an example of a nitric oxide donor drug. Clavin and colleagues (1996) randomized 34 women in preterm labor to tocolysis with intravenous nitroglycerin or magnesium sulfate. There was no difference in the tocolytic efficacy of these two drugs, but 3 of 15 women given nitroglycerin had severe hypotension. Lees and colleagues (1999) randomized 245 women in preterm labor to transdermal glycerl trinitrate or intravenous ritodrine. There was no overall superiority of glyceryl trinitrate in the inhibition of preterm labor.

COMBINED THERAPY. The use of multiple drugs to inhibit preterm labor suggests that no single drug is completely satisfactory. Unfortunately, there are no studies in which tocolytic combinations were compared with placebo. Kosasa and colleagues (1994) used long-term tocolysis with combined intravenous terbutaline and magnesium sulfate in 1000 pregnancies. The mean duration of intravenous therapy was 61 days in women with intact membranes, and one woman received this therapy for 123 days. This approach was claimed to be effective and safe because only 2 to 4 percent of the women developed pulmonary edema.

INTRAPARTUM MANAGEMENT. In general, the more immature the fetus, the greater the risks from labor and delivery.

LABOR. Whether labor is induced or spontaneous, abnormalities of fetal heart rate and uterine contractions should be sought, preferably by continuous electronic monitoring. Fetal tachycardia, especially in the presence of ruptured membranes, is suggestive of sepsis. There is some emerging evidence that intrapartum acidemia may intensify some of the neonatal complications usually attributed solely to prematurity. For example, Low and colleagues (1995) observed that intrapartum acidosis—umbilical artery blood pH less than 7.0—had an important role in neonatal complications. Similarly, Kimberlin and colleagues (1996b) found that increasing umbilical artery blood acidemia was related to more severe respiratory disease in preterm neonates, although no effects were found in short-term neurological outcomes that included intracranial hemorrhages.

Importantly, just as the markedly preterm infant is to be afforded special care in the neonatal intensive care unit, the mother and fetus should be observed very closely in the labor and delivery unit. Especially skilled physicians should monitor the labor and delivery of the markedly preterm fetus.

PREVENTION OF NEONATAL GROUP B STREPTOCOCCAL INFECTIONS. As discussed in Chapter 56 (p. 1471), group B streptococcal infections are common and dangerous in the preterm neonate. Since 1996 the Centers for Disease Control and Prevention, along with the American College of Obstetricians and Gynecologists, recommend either penicillin G or ampicillin intravenously every 6 hours until delivery for women in labor prior to 37 weeks and whose culture status is unknown or positive for group B streptococcus.

DELIVERY. In the absence of a relaxed vaginal outlet, an episiotomy for delivery may be advantageous once the fetal head reaches the perineum. Argument persists as to the merits of spontaneous delivery versus forceps delivery to protect the fragile preterm fetal head (Chap. 21, p. 490). It is doubtful whether use of forceps in most instances produces less trauma. Indeed, to compress and pull on the head of a grossly preterm infant might be more traumatic than natural expulsion. The use of outlet forceps of appropriate size may be of assistance when conduction analgesia is used and voluntary expulsion efforts are obtunded.

A physician and staff proficient in resuscitative techniques and fully oriented to the specific problems of the case should be present at delivery. Principles of resuscitation described in Chapter 16 are applicable, including prompt tracheal intubation and ventilation.

The importance of the availability of specialized personnel and facilities in the case of preterm infants is underscored by the improved survival of these infants when they are delivered in tertiary care centers (Powell and colleagues, 1995).

PREVENTION OF NEONATAL INTRACRANIAL HEMORRHAGE. Preterm infants frequently have germinal matrix bleeding that can extend to more serious intraventricular hemorrhage (Bejar and colleagues, 1980). It was hypothesized that cesarean delivery to obviate trauma from labor and vaginal delivery might prevent these complications. These initial observations have not been validated by most subsequent studies. In the largest study, Malloy and colleagues (1991) analyzed 1765 infants with birthweights less than 1500 g and found that cesarean delivery did not lower the risk of mortality or intracranial hemorrhage. Anderson and colleagues (1988), however, made an interesting observation regarding the role of cesarean delivery in the prevention of neonatal intracranial hemorrhages. These hemorrhages were related to whether or not the fetus had been subjected to the active phase of labor, defined as the interval before 5 cm cervical dilatation. As emphasized by Anderson and colleagues (1988), avoidance of active-phase labor is impossible in most preterm births because the route of delivery cannot be decided until labor is firmly established.

Nelson and Grether (1995) reported that magnesium sulfate given to women delivered preterm for either tocolysis or preeclampsia was associated with a significantly reduced incidence of cerebral palsy when surviving infants with birthweights less than 1500 g were followed to 3 years of age. It was suggested that magnesium given to the fetus via the mother perhaps played a role in regulation of the vasculature supplying the germinal matrix of the preterm fetal brain that is especially vulnerable to hemorrhage. Murphy and colleagues (1995), however, found that severe preeclampsia and delivery without labor were protective against cerebral palsy. They concluded that magnesium could not be the protective agent because this drug is not used for preeclampsia in England.

REFERENCES

Alexander GR, Himes JH, Kaufman RB, Mor J, Kogan M: A United States national reference for fetal growth. Obstet Gynecol 87:163, 1996

Alexander JM, Gilstrap LC, Cox SM, McIntire DM, Leveno KJ: Clinical chorioamnionitis and the prognosis for very low birthweight infants. Obstet Gynecol 91:725, 1998

Alexander JM, Merer BM, Miodovnik M, Thurnau GR, Goldenberg RL, Das AF, Meis PJ, Moawad AH, Iams JD, Van Dorsten JP, Paul RH, Dombrowski MP, Roberts JM, McNellis D, the NICHD/MFMU Network: The impact of digital cervical examination on expectantly managed preterm ruptured membranes. Am J Obstet Gynecol 183:1003, 2000

Allen MC, Donohue PK, Dusman AE: The limit of viability—neonatal outcome of infants born at 22 to 25 weeks' gestation. N Engl J Med 329:1597, 1993

Althuisius SM, Dekker GA, van Geijn HP, Bekedam DJ, Hummel P: Cervical incompetence prevention randomized cerclage trial, preliminary results. Am J Obstet Gynecol 182:S20, 2000

Althuisiua S, Dekker G, Hummel P, Bekedam D, van Geijn H: Cervical incompetence prevention randomized cerclage trial: Therapeutic cerclage with bed rest versus bed rest, final results. Am J Obstet Gynecol 184:S2, 2001

American Academy of Pediatrics: Guidelines for prevention of Group B streptococcal (GBS) infection by chemoprophylaxis. Committee on Infectious Diseases and Committee on Fetus and Newborn. Pediatrics 90:775, 1992

American Academy of Pediatrics and the American College of Obstetricians and Gynecologists: Guidelines for Perinatal Care, 4th ed. 1997, p 100

American College of Obstetricians and Gynecologists: Premature Rupture of Membranes. ACOG Practice Bulletin No. 1, June 1998a

American College of Obstetricians and Gynecologists: Procedure: Tocolysis. Criteria Set No. 34, June 1998b

American College of Obstetricians and Gynecologists: Preterm Labor. Technical Bulletin No. 206, June 1995

American College of Obstetricians and Gynecologists Committee on Obstetric Practice: Antenatal Corticosteroid Therapy for Fetal Maturation. Committee Opinion No. 210, October 1998

American College of Obstetricians and Gynecologists Committee on Obstetric Practice: Prevention of Early Onset Group B Streptococcal Disease in Newborns. Committee Opinion No. 173, June 1996

American College of Obstetricians and Gynecologists Committee on Obstetric Practice: Antenatal Corticosteroid Therapy for Fetal Maturation. Committee Opinion No. 147, December 1994

Amon E, Shyken JM, Sibai BM: How small is too small and how early is too early? A survey of American obstetricians specializing in high-risk pregnancies. Am J Perinatol 9:17, 1992

Amsel R, Totten PA, Spiegel CA, Chen KC, Eschenbach D, Holmes KK: Nonspecific vaginitis: Diagnostic criteria and microbial and epidemiologic associations. Am J Med 74:14, 1983

Anderson GD, Bada HS, Sibai BM, Harvey C, Korones SB, Magill HL, Wong SP, Tullis K: The relationship between labor and route of delivery in the preterm infant. Am J Obstet Gynecol 158:1382, 1988

Andrews WW, Goldenberg RL, Mercer B, et al: The Preterm Prediction Study: Association of mid-trimester genitourinary chlamydia infection with subsequent spontaneous preterm birth. Am J Obstet Gynecol 183:662, 2000

Andrews WW, Hauth JC, Goldenberg RL, Gomez R, Romero R, Cassell GH: Amniotic fluid interleukin-6: Correlation with upper genital tract microbial colonization and gestational age in women delivered after spontaneous labor versus indicated delivery. Am J Obstet Gynecol 173:606, 1995

Angel JL, O'Brien WF, Knuppel RA, Morales WJ, Sims CJ: Carbohydrate intolerance in patients receiving oral tocolytics. Am J Obstet Gynecol 159:762, 1988

Avery ME, Aylward G, Creasy R, Little AB, Stripp B: Update on prenatal steroid for prevention of respiratory distress: Report of a conference—September 26–28, 1985. Am J Obstet Gynecol 155:2, 1986

Ballard PL, Ballard RA: Scientific basis and therapeutic regimens for use of antenatal glucocorticoids. Am J Obstet Gynecol 173:254, 1995

Ballard RA, Ballard PL, Cnaan A, Pinto-Martin J, Davis DJ, Padbury JF, Phibbs RH, Parer JT, Hart MC, Mannino FL, Sawai SK: Antenatal thyrotropin-releasing hormone to prevent lung disease in preterm infants. N Engl J Med 338:493, 1998

Bejar R, Curbelo V, Coen RW, Leopold G, James H, Gluck L: Diagnosis and follow-up of intraventricular and intracerebral hemorrhages by ultrasound studies of infant's brain through the fontanelles and sutures. Pediatrics 66:661, 1980

Bejar R, Curbelo V, Davis C, Davis C, Gluck L: Premature labor, II. Bacterial sources of phospholipase. Obstet Gynecol 57:479, 1981

Ben-Ami M, Giladi Y, Shalev E: The combination of magnesium sulphate and nifedipine: A cause of neuromuscular blockade. Br J Obstet Gynaecol 101:262, 1994

Bennett PR, Elder MG: The mechanisms of preterm labor: Common genital tract pathogens do not metabolize arachidonic acid to prostaglandins or to other eicosanoids. Am J Obstet Gynecol 166:1541, 1992

Berry SM, Romero R, Gomez R, Puder KS, Ghezzi F, Cotton DB, Bianchi DW: Premature parturition is characterized by in utero activation of the fetal immune system. Am J Obstet Gynecol 173:1315, 1995

Bobbitt JR, Ledger WJ: Unrecognized amnionitis and prematurity: A preliminary report. J Reprod Med 19:8, 1977

Bottoms SF, Paul RH, Iams JD, Mercer BM, Thom EA, Roberts JM, Caritis SN, Moawad AH, Van Dorsten JP, Hauth JC, Thurnau GR, Miodovnik M, Meis PM, McNellis D: Obstetric determinants of neonatal survival: Influence of willingness to perform cesarean delivery on survival of extremely low-birth-weight infants. National Institute of Child Health and Human Development Network of Maternal–Fetal Medicine Units. Am J Obstet Gynecol 176:960, 1997

Bottoms SF, Paul RH, Mercer BM, MacPherson CA, Caritis SN, Moawad AH, Van Dorsten JP, Hauth JC, Thurnau GR, Miodovnik M, Meis PM, Roberts JM, McNellis D, Iams JD: Obstetric determinants of neonatal survival: Antenatal predictors of neonatal survival and morbidity in extremely low birth weight infants. Am J Obstet Gynecol 180:665, 1999

Buekens P, Alexander S, Boutsen M, Blondel B, Kaminski M, Reid M: Randomised controlled trial of routine cervical examinations in pregnancy. Lancet 344:841, 1994

Buescher PA, Meis PJ, Ernest JM, Moore ML, Michielutte R, Sharp P: A comparison of women in and out of a prematurity prevention project in a North Carolina perinatal care region. Am J Public Health 78:264, 1988

Canadian Preterm Labor Investigators Group: Treatment of preterm labor with the beta-adrenergic agonist ritodrine. N Engl J Med 327:308, 1992

Carey JC, Klebanoff M, for the NICHD MFMU Network: Metronidazole treatment increased the risk of preterm birth in asymptomatic women with trichomonas. Am J Obstet Gynecol 182:S17, 2000a

Carey JC, Klebanoff MA, Hauth JC, Hillier SL, Thom EA, Ernest JM, Heine RP, Nugent RP, Fischer ML, Leveno KJ, Wapner R, Varner M: Metronidazole to prevent preterm delivery in pregnant women with asymptomatic bacterial vaginosis. N Engl J Med 342:534, 2000b

Carlan SJ, O'Brien WF, Jones MH, O'Leary TD, Roth L: Outpatient oral sulindac to prevent recurrence of preterm labor. Obstet Gynecol 85:769, 1995

Carlan SJ, O'Brien WF, Parsons MT, Lense JJ: Preterm premature rupture of membranes: A randomized study of home versus hospital management. Obstet Gynecol 81:61, 1993

Carr DB, Clark AL, Kernek K, Spinnato JA: Maintenance oral nifedipine for preterm labor: A randomized clinical trial. Am J Obstet Gynecol 181:822, 1999

Carr-Hill RA, Hall MH: The repetition of spontaneous preterm labour. Br J Obstet Gynaecol 92:921, 1985

Carroll SG, Blott M, Nicolaides KH: Preterm prelabor amniorrhexis: Outcome of live births. Obstet Gynecol 86:18, 1995a

Carroll SG, Papaionnou S, Nicolaides KH: Assessment of fetal activity and amniotic fluid volume in the prediction of intrauterine infection in preterm labor amniorrhexis. Am J Obstet Gynecol 172:1427, 1995b

Carroll SG, Papaionnou S, Ntumazah IL, Philpott-Howard J, Nicolaides KH: Lower genital tract swabs in the prediction of intrauterine infection in preterm prelabour rupture of the membranes. Br J Obstet Gynaecol 103:54, 1996

Centers for Disease Control and Prevention: 1998 Guidelines for treatment of sexually transmitted diseases. MMWR 47 (RR-1), 1998

Centers for Disease Control and Prevention: Prevention of perinatal group B streptococcal disease: A public health perspective. MMWR 45 (RR-7):1, 1996

Centers for Disease Control and Prevention: Recommendations for the prevention and management of Chlamydia trachomatis infections. MMWR 42 (RR-12):1, 1993

Chapman S, Hauth JC, Goldenberg RL, Owen J, Bottoms SF, McNellis D, MacPherson C, Thom E: Lack of apparent corticosteroid benefits in 1000 g infants born after preterm amnion rupture. Am J Obstet Gynecol 174:316, 1996

Childress CH, Katz VL: Nifedipine and its indications in obstetrics and gynecology. Obstet Gynecol 83:616, 1994

Clavin DK, Bayhi DA, Nolan TE, Rigby FB, Cork RC, Miller JM: Comparison of intravenous magnesium sulfate and nitroglycerin for preterm labor: Preliminary data. Am J Obstet Gynecol 174:307, 1996

Collaborative Group on Antenatal Steroid Therapy: Effects of antenatal dexamethasone administration in the infant: Long-term follow-up. J Pediatr 104:259, 1984

Collaborative Group on Antenatal Steroid Therapy: Effect of antenatal dexamethasone administration on the prevention of respiratory distress syndrome. Am J Obstet Gynecol 141:276, 1981

Collaborative Group on Preterm Birth Prevention: Multicenter randomized, controlled trial of preterm birth prevention program. Am J Obstet Gynecol 169:352, 1993

Collaborative Home Uterine Monitoring Study Group: A multicenter randomized controlled trial of home uterine monitoring: Active versus sham device. Am J Obstet Gynecol 173:1170, 1995

Cone TE Jr: History of the Care and Feeding of the Premature Infant. Boston, Little, Brown, 1985, pp 1, 180

Cook CM, Ellwood DA: A longitudinal study of the cervix in pregnancy using transvaginal ultrasound. Br J Obstet Gynaecol 103:16, 1996

Copper RL, Goldenberg RL, Creasy RK, DuBard MB, Davis RO, Entman SS, Iams JD, Cliver SP: A multicenter study of preterm birthweight and gestational age-specific neonatal mortality. Am J Obstet Gynecol 168:78, 1993

Copper RL, Goldenberg RL, Das A, Elder N, Swain M, Norman G, Ramsey R, Cotroneo P, Collins BA, Johnson F, Jones P, Meier AM: The preterm prediction study: Maternal stress is associated with spontaneous preterm birth at less than thirty-five weeks' gestation. National Institute of Child Health and Human Development Maternal–Fetal Medicine Units Network. Am J Obstet Gynecol 175:1286, 1996

Copper RL, Goldenberg RL, Davis RO, Cutter GR, DuBard MB, Corliss DK, Andrews JB: Warning symptoms, uterine contractions, and cervical examination findings in women at risk of preterm delivery. Am J Obstet Gynecol 162:748, 1990

Copper RL, Goldenberg RL, Dubard MB, Hauth JC, Cutter GR: Cervical examination and tocodynamometry at 28 weeks' gestation: Prediction of spontaneous preterm birth. Am J Obstet Gynecol 172:666, 1995

Cotch MF, Pastorek JG 2nd, Nugent RP, Hillier SL, Gibbs RS, Martin DH, Eschenbach DA, Edelman R, Carey JC, Regan JA, Krohn MA, Klebanoff MA, Rao AV, Rhoads GG: Trichomonas vaginalis associated with low birth weight and preterm delivery. The Vaginal Infections and Prematurity Study Group. Sex Transm Dis 24:353, 1997

Cotton DB, Strassner HT, Hill LM, Schifrin BS, Paul RH: Comparison between magnesium sulfate, terbutaline and a placebo for inhibition of preterm labor: A randomized study. J Reprod Med 29:92, 1984

Covington DL, Carl J, Daley JG, Cushing D, Churchill MP: Effects of the North Carolina Prematurity Program among public patients delivering at New Hanover Memorial Hospital. Am J Public Health 78:1493, 1988

Cox SM, Bohman VR, Sherman ML, Leveno KJ: Randomized investigation of antimicrobials for the prevention of preterm birth. Am J Obstet Gynecol 174:206, 1996a

Cox SM, King MR, Casey ML, MacDonald PC: Interleukin-1 beta, -1 alpha, and -6 and postaglandins in vaginal/cervical fluids of pregnant women before and during labor. J Clin Endocrinol Metab 77:805, 1993

Cox SM, Leveno KJ: Intentional delivery versus expectant management with preterm ruptured membranes at 30–34 weeks' gestation. Obstet Gynecol 86:875, 1995

Cox SM, Little B, Dax J, Leveno K: Fetal fibronectin and preterm delivery. Am J Obstet Gynecol 174:306, 1996b

Cox SM, MacDonald PC, Casey ML: Cytokines and prostaglandins in amniotic fluid of preterm labor pregnancies: Decidual origin in response to bacterial toxins (lipopolysaccharide [LPS] and lipotechnoic acid [LTA]). Abstract presented at the 36th annual meeting of the Society of Gynecologic Investigation, San Diego, March 1989

Cox SM, MacDonald PC, Casey ML: Assay of bacterial endotoxin (lipopolysaccharide) in human amniotic fluid: Potential usefulness in diagnosis and management of preterm labor. Am J Obstet Gynecol 159:99, 1988a

Cox SM, Sherman ML, Leveno KJ: Randomized investigation of magnesium sulfate for prevention of preterm birth. Am J Obstet Gynecol 163:767, 1990

Cox SM, Williams ML, Leveno KJ: The natural history of preterm ruptured membranes: What to expect of expectant management. Obstet Gynecol 71:558, 1988b

Crane JM, Armson BA, Dodds L, Feinberg RF, Kennedy W, Kirkland SA: Risk scoring, fetal fibronectin, and bacterial vaginosis to predict preterm delivery. Obstet Gynecol 93:517, 1999

Creasy RK, Gummer BA, Liggins GC: System for predicting spontaneous preterm birth. Obstet Gynecol 55:692, 1980

Crowley PA: Antenatal corticosteroid therapy: A meta-analysis of randomized trials, 1972 to 1994. Am J Obstet Gynecol 173:322, 1995

Crowther CA, Hiller JE, Haslam RR, Robinson JS: Australian collaborative trial of antenatal thyrotropin-releasing hormone (ACTOBAT) for prevention of neonatal respiratory disease. Lancet 345:877, 1995

DePalma RT, Leveno KJ, Kelly MA, Sherman ML, Carmody TJ: Birth weight threshold for postponing preterm birth. Am J Obstet Gynecol 167:1145, 1992

DeVoe LD, Youssef AE, Croom CS, Watson J: Can fetal biophysical observations anticipate outcome in preterm labor or preterm rupture of membranes? Obstet Gynecol 84:432, 1994

DiFronza JR, Lew RA: Effect of maternal cigarette smoking on pregnancy complications and sudden infant death syndrome. J Fam Pract 40:385, 1995

Donaldson PJ, Billy JO: The impact of prenatal care on birth weight: Evidence from an international data set. Med Care 22:177, 1984

Dor J, Shalev J, Mashiach S, Blankstein J, Serr DM: Elective cervical suture of twin pregnancies diagnosed ultrasonically in the first trimester following induced ovulation. Gynecol Obstet Invest 13:55, 1982

Doron MW, Veness-Meehan KA, Margolis LH, Holoman EM, Stiles AD: Delivery room resuscitation decisions for extremely premature infants. Pediatrics 102:574, 1998

Doyle LW, Permezel M, Ford GW, Knoches AM, Rickards AL, Kelly EA, Callanan C: The obstetrician and the extremely immature fetus (24–26 weeks): Outcome to 5 years of age. Aust N Z J Obstet Gynaecol 34:421, 1994

Dubay LC, Kenney GM, Norton SA, Cohen BC: Local responses to expanded Medicaid coverage for pregnant women. Milbank Q 73:535, 1995

Dyson DC, Danbe KH, Bamber JA, Crites YM, Field DR, Maier JA, Newman LA, Ray DA, Walton DL, Armstrong MA: Monitoring women at risk for preterm labor. N Engl J Med 338:15, 1998

Elliott JP: Magnesium sulfate as a tocolytic agent. Am J Obstet Gynecol 147:277, 1983

Elliott JP, Radin TG: The effect of corticosteroid administration on uterine activity and preterm labor in high-order multiple gestations. Obstet Gynecol 85:250, 1995

Esplin MS, Fausett MB, Smith S, Oshiro BT, Porter TF, Branch DW, Varner MW: Multiple courses of antenatal steroids are associated with a delay in long-term psychomotor development in children with birth weights ≤ 1500 grams. Am J Obstet Gynecol (Abstr 27) 182:S24, 2000

Fanaroff AA, Wright LL, Stevenson DK, Shankaran S, Donovan EF, Ehrenkranz RA, Younes N, Korones SB, Stoll BJ, Tyson JE, Bauer CR, Oh W, Lenors JA, Papile LA, Verter J: Very-low-birthweight outcomes of the National Institute of Child Health and Human Development Neonatal Research Network, May 1991 through December 1992. Am J Obstet Gynecol 173:1423, 1995

Farooqi A, Holmgren PA, Engberg S, Serenius F: Survival and 2-year outcome with expectant management of second-trimester rupture of membranes. Obstet Gynecol 92:895, 1998

Feinstein SJ, Vintzileos AM, Lodeiro JG, Campbell WA, Weinbaum PJ, Nochimson DJ: Amniocentesis with premature rupture of membranes. Obstet Gynecol 68:147, 1986

Fink A, Yano EM, Goya D: Prenatal programs: What the literature reveals. Obstet Gynecol 80:867, 1992

Fiscella K: Does prenatal care improve birth outcomes? A critical review. Obstet Gynecol 85:468, 1995

Fletcher SE, Fyfe DA, Case CL, Wiles HB, Upshur JK, Newman RB: Myocardial necrosis in a newborn after long-term maternal subcutaneous terbutaline infusion for suppression of preterm labor. Am J Obstet Gynecol 165:1401, 1991

Flier JS, Underhill LH: Adrenergic receptors-evolving concepts and clinical implications. N Engl J Med 334:580, 1996

Gamsu HR, Mullinger BM, Donnai P, Dash CH: Antenatal administration of betamethasone to prevent respiratory distress syndrome in preterm infants: Report of a UK multicentre trial. Br J Obstet Gynaecol 96:401, 1989

Garite TJ, Freeman RK, Linzey EM, Braly PS, Dorchester WL: Prospective randomized study of corticosteroids in the management of premature rupture of the membranes and the premature gestation. Am J Obstet Gynecol 141:508, 1981

Garite TJ, Freeman RK, Linzey EM, Braly PS: The use of amniocentesis in patients with premature rupture of membranes. Obstet Gynecol 54:226, 1979

Garite TJ, Keegan KA, Freeman RK, Nageotte MP: A randomized trial of ritodrine tocolysis versus expectant management in patients with premature rupture of membranes at 25 to 30 weeks of gestation. Am J Obstet Gynecol 157:388, 1987

Gauthier DW, Meyer WJ, Bieniarz A: Biophysical profile as a predictor of amniotic fluid culture results. Obstet Gynecol 80:102, 1992

Ginsberg HG, Goldsmith JP, Stedman CM: Survival of a 380-g infant. N Engl J Med 322:1753, 1990

Gluck L: Fetal lung maturity. Paper presented at the 78th Ross Conference on Pediatric Research, San Diego, May 1979

Goldenberg RL: Vaginal fetal fibronectin (V-fFN) levels at 8-22 weeks and subsequent spontaneous preterm birth. Am J Obstet Gynecol (Abstr 44) 183:S32, 2000

Goldenberg RL, Cliver SP, Bronstein J, Cutter GR, Andrews WW, Mennemeyer ST: Bed rest in pregnancy. Obstet Gynecol 84:131, 1994

Goldenberg RL, Mercer BM, Meis PJ, Cooper RL, Das A, McNellis D: The preterm prediction study: Fetal fibronectin testing and spontaneous preterm birth. NICHD Maternal Fetal Medicine Units Network. Obstet Gynecol 87:643, 1996a

Goldenberg RL, Thom E, Moawad AH, Johnson F, Roberts J, Caritis SN: The preterm prediction study: Fetal fibronectin, bacterial vaginosis, and peripartum infection. NICHD Maternal Fetal Medicine Units Network. Obstet Gynecol 87:656, 1996b

Goldenberg RL, Iams JD, Mercer BM, Meis PJ, Moawad AH, Cooper RL, Das A, Thom E, Johnson F, McNellis D, Miodovnik M, Van Dorsten JP, Caritis SN, Thurnau GR, Bottoms SF: The preterm prediction study: The value of new vs standard risk factors in predicting early and all spontaneous preterm births. NICHD MFMU Network. Am J Public Health 88:233, 1998

Gonik B, Bottoms SF, Cotton DB: Amniotic fluid volume as a risk factor in preterm premature rupture of the membranes. Obstet Gynecol 65:456, 1985

Goodwin TM: A role of estriol in human labor, term and preterm. Am J Obstet Gynecol 180:S208, 1999

Goodwin TM, Jackson GM, McGregor JA, Lachelin GC, Artal R, Dullien V: Increased incidence of preterm labor and preterm delivery associated with increased salivary estriol level. Am J Obstet Gynecol (Abstr 59) 174:326, 1996

Goodwin TM, Millar L, North L, Abrams LS, Weglein RC, Holland ML: The pharmacokinetics of the oxytocin antagonist atosiban in pregnant women with preterm uterine contractions. Am J Obstet Gynecol 173:913, 1995

Gordon M, Samuels P, Shubert P, Johnson F, Gebauer C, Iams J: A randomized, prospective study of adjunctive ceftizoxime in preterm labor. Am J Obstet Gynecol 172:1546, 1995

Gravett MG, Witkin SS, Haluska GJ, Edwards JL, Cook MJ, Novy MJ: An experimental model of intraamniotic infection and preterm labor in rhesus monkeys. Am J Obstet Gynecol 171:1660, 1994

Grimes DA: Introducing evidence-based medicine into a department of obstetrics and gynecology. Obstet Gynecol 86:451, 1995

Guinn DA and BMZ Study Group: Multicenter randomized trial of single versus weekly courses of antenatal corticosteroids (ACS). Am J Obstet Gynecol 184:S6, 2001

Guinn DA, Goepfert AR, Owen J, Wenstrom KD, Hauth JC: Terbutaline pump maintenance therapy for prevention of preterm delivery: A double-blind trial. Am J Obstet Gynecol 179:874, 1998

Guinn DA, Goldenberg RL, Hauth JC, Andrews WW, Thom E, Romero R: Risk factors for the development of preterm premature rupture of the membranes after arrest of preterm labor. Am J Obstet Gynecol 173:1310, 1995

Guzman E, Walters C, Benito C, Yeo L, Sharma S, Vintzileos A: Cervical sonography in predicting spontaneous preterm birth at-risk singleton gestations. Am J Obstet Gynecol 184:S27, 2001

Gyr TN, Malek A, Mathez-Loic F, Altermatt HJ, Bodmer T, Nicolaides K, Schneider H: Permeation of human chorio-amniotic membranes by *Escherichia coli* in vitro. Am J Obstet Gynecol 170:223, 1994

Hack M, Taylor HG, Klein V, Eiben R, Schatschneider C, Mercuri-Minich N: School-age outcomes in children with birth weights under 750 g. N Engl J Med 331:753, 1994

Hadi HA, Hodson CA, Strickland D: Premature rupture of the membranes between 20 and 25 weeks' gestation: Role of amniotic fluid volume in perinatal outcome. Am J Obstet Gynecol 170:1139, 1994

Hallak M, Bottoms SF: Accelerated pulmonary maturation from preterm premature rupture of membranes: A myth. Am J Obstet Gynecol 169:1045, 1993

Hankins GD, Hauth JC, Cissik JH, Kuehl TJ: Effects of ritodrine hydrochloride on arteriovenous blood gas and shunt in healthy pregnant yellow baboons. Am J Obstet Gynecol 158:658, 1988

Hankins GDV, Leveno KJ, Whalley PJ, DePalma RT, Williams ML, Nelson S: Maternal, fetal, neonatal, and infant outcomes with expectant management for preterm rupture of the membranes. Paper presented at the Society of Perinatal Obstetricians, San Antonio, February 1984

Hartmann K, Thorp JM Jr, McDonald TL, Savitz DA, Granados JL: Cervical dimensions and risk of preterm birth: A prospective cohort study. Obstet Gynecol 93:504, 1999

Hatjis CG, Swain M: Systemic tocolysis for premature labor is associated with an increased incidence of pulmonary edema in the presence of maternal infection. Am J Obstet Gynecol 159:723, 1988

Hausdorff WP, Caron MG, Lefkowitz RJ: Turning off the signal: Desensitization of beta-adrenergic receptor function. FASEB J 4:2881, 1990

Hauth JC, for the NICHD MFMU Network: Mid-trimester threshold vaginal pH and gram stain scores predictive of subsequent preterm birth. Am J Obstet Gynecol (Abstr 45) 182:S32, 2000

Hauth JC, Andrews WW, Goldenberg RL: Infection-related risk factors predictive of spontaneous preterm labor and birth. Prenat Neonat Med 3:86, 1998

Hauth JC, Goldenberg RL, Andrews WW, DuBard MB, Copper RL: Reduced incidence of preterm delivery with metro-nidazole and erythromycin in women with bacterial vaginosis. N Engl J Med 333:1732, 1995

Hayward PE, Diaz-Rossello JL: New evidence for preventive perinatal care. Lancet 346:S17, 1995

Haywood JL, Goldenberg RL, Bronstein J, Nelson KG, Carlos WA: Comparison of perceived and actual rates of survival and freedom from handicap in premature infants. Am J Obstet Gynecol 171:432, 1994

Hedegaard M, Henriksen TB, Sabroe S, Secher NJ: Psychological distress in pregnancy and preterm delivery. BMJ 307:234, 1993

Heine RP, McGregor JA, Dullien VK: Accuracy of salivary estriol testing compared to traditional risk factor assessment in predicting preterm birth. Am J Obstet Gynecol 180:S214, 1999

Helfgott AW, Willis DC, Blanco JD: Is hydration and sedation beneficial in the treatment of threatened preterm labor? A preliminary report. J Matern Fetal Med 3:37, 42, 1994

Henriksen TB, Hedegaard M, Secher NJ, Wilcox AJ: Standing at work and preterm delivery. Br J Obstet Gynaecol 102:198, 1995

Hesseldahl H: A Danish multicenter study of ritodrine in the treatment of pre-term labour. Dan Med Bull 26:116, 1979

Hibbard JU, Hibbard MC, Ismail M, Arendt E: Pregnancy outcome after expectant management of premature rupture of the membranes in the second trimester. J Reprod Med 38:945, 1993

Hickey CA, Cliver SP, McNeal SF, Hoffman HJ, Goldenberg RL: Prenatal weight gain patterns and spontaneous preterm birth among nonobese black and white women. Obstet Gynecol 85:909, 1995

Hillier SL, Nugent RP, Eschenbach DA, Krohn MA, Gibbs RS, Martin DH, Cotch MF, Edelman R, Pastorek JG 2nd, Rao AV, McNellis D, Regan JA, Carey JC, Klebanoff MA: Association between bacterial vaginosis and preterm delivery of a low-birthweight infant. N Engl J Med 333:1737, 1995

Hoffman JD, Ward K: Genetic factors in preterm delivery. Obstet Gynecol Surv 54:203, 1999

Hollander DI, Nagey DA, Pupkin MJ: Magnesium sulfate and ritodrine hydrochloride: A randomized comparison. Am J Obstet Gynecol 156:631, 1987

Holzman C, Paneth N, Little R, Pinto-Martin J: Perinatal brain injury in premature infants born to mothers using alcohol in pregnancy. Pediatrics 95:66, 1995

How HY, Hughes SA, Vogel RL, Gall SA, Spinnato JA: Oral terbutaline in the outpatient management of preterm labor. Am J Obstet Gynecol 173:1518, 1995

Hudgens DR, Conradi SE: Sudden death associated with terbutaline sulfate administration. Am J Obstet Gynecol 169:120, 1993

Hueston WJ, Knox MA, Eilers G, Pauwels J, Lonsdorf D: The effectiveness of preterm-birth prevention educational program for high-risk women: A meta-analysis. Obstet Gynecol 86:705, 1995

Iams JD, for the NICHD MFMU Network: Prediction of preterm birth with ambulatory measurement of uterine contraction frequency. Am J Obstet Gynecol (Abstr 2) 178:S2, 1998b

Iams JD, Goldenberg RL, Meis PJ, Mercer BM, Moawad A, Das A, Thom E, McNellis D, Copper RL, Johnson F, Roberts JM: The length of the cervix and the risk of spontaneous premature delivery. National Institute of Child Health and Human Development Maternal–Fetal Medicine Unit Network. N Engl J Med 334:567, 1996

Iams JD, Goldenberg RL, Mercer BM, Moawad A, Thom E,

Meis PJ, McNellis D, Caritis SN, Miodovnik M, Menard MK, Thurnau GR, Bottoms SE, Roberts JM: The Preterm Prediction Study: Recurrence risk of spontaneous preterm birth. National Institute of Child Health and Human Development Maternal–Fetal Medicine Units Network. Am J Obstet Gynecol 178:1035, 1998a

Iams JD, Johnson FF, Parker M: A prospective evaluation of the signs and symptoms of preterm labor. Obstet Gynecol 84:227, 1994

Iams JD, Stilson R, Johnson FF, Williams RA, Rice R: Symptoms that precede preterm labor and preterm premature rupture of the membranes. Am J Obstet Gynecol 162:486, 1990

Jackson GM, Edwin SS, Varner MW, Casal D, Mitchell MD: Regulation of fetal fibronectin production in human amnion cells. J Soc Gynecol Investig 3:85, 1996

Jenssen H, Wright PB: The effect of dexamethasone therapy in prolonged pregnancy. Acta Obstet Gynecol Scand 56:467, 1977

Jobe AH, Mitchell BR, Gunkel JH: Beneficial effects of the combined use of prenatal corticosteroids and postnatal surfactant on preterm infants. Am J Obstet Gynecol 168:508, 1993

Joesoef MR, Hillier SL, Wiknjosastro G, Sumampouw H, Linnan M, Norojono W, Idajadi A, Utomo B: Intravaginal clindamycin treatment for bacterial vaginosis: Effects on preterm delivery and low birth weight. Am J Obstet Gynecol 173:1527, 1995

Joseph KS, Kramer MS, Marcoux S, Ohlsson A, Wen SW, Allen A, Platt R: Determinants of preterm birth rates in Canada from 1981 through 1983 and from 1992 through 1994. N Engl J Med 339:1434, 1998

Katz M, Newman RB, Gill PJ: Assessment of uterine activity in ambulatory patients at high risk of preterm labor and delivery. Am J Obstet Gynecol 154:44, 1986

Keirse MJNC. Calcium antagonists vs. betamimetics in preterm labour. In Neilson JP, Crowther C, Hodnett ED, et al (eds): Pregnancy and Childbirth Module. Cochrane Database of Systematic Reviews, Issue 2, Oxford, Update Software, 1995a

Keirse MJNC: New perspectives for the effective treatment of preterm labor. Am J Obstet Gynecol 173:618, 1995b

Kimberlin DF, Hauth JC, Goldenberg RL, MacPherson C, Thom E, Bottoms SF, McNellis D: The effect of maternal MgSO4 treatment on neonatal morbidity in < 1000 g neonates. Am J Obstet Gynecol 174:469, 1996a

Kimberlin DF, Hauth JC, Goldenberg RL, MacPherson C, Thom E, Bottoms SF, McNellis D: Relationship of acid–base status and neonatal morbidity in 1000 g infants. Am J Obstet Gynecol 174:382, 1996b

Kitchen WH, Permezel MJ, Doyle LW, Ford GW, Rickards AL, Kelly EA: Changing obstetric practice and 2-year outcome of the fetus of birthweight under 1000 g. Obstet Gynecol 79:268, 1992

Klebanoff MA, Regan JA, Rao AV, Nugent RP, Blackwelder WC, Eschenbach DA, Pastorek JG 2nd, Williams S, Gibbs RS, Carey JC: Outcome of the Vaginal Infections and Prematurity Study: Results of a clinical trial of erythromycin among pregnant women colonized with group B streptococci. Am J Obstet Gynecol 172:1540, 1995

Knight DB, Liggins GC, Wealthall SR: A randomized, controlled trial of antepartum thyrotropin-releasing hormone and betamethasone in the prevention of respiratory disease in preterm infants. Am J Obstet Gynecol 171:11, 1994

Knox IC Jr, Hoerner JK: The role of infection in premature

rupture of the membranes: 1950. Am J Obstet Gynecol 173:951, 1995

Kosasa TS, Busse R, Wahl N, Hirata G, Nakayama RT, Hale RW: Long-term tocolysis with combined intravenous terbutaline and magnesium sulfate: A 10-year study of 1000 patients. Obstet Gynecol 84:369, 1994

Kovacevich GJ, Gaich SA, Lavin JP, Hopkins MP, Crane SS, Stewart J, Nelson D, Lavin LM: The prevalence of thromboembolic events among women with extended bed rest prescribed as part of the treatment for premature labor or preterm premature rupture of membranes. Am J Obstet Gynecol 182:1089, 2000

Kragt H, Keirse MJ: How accurate is a woman's diagnosis of threatened preterm delivery? Br J Obstet Gynaecol 97:317, 1990

Kramer MS, Coates AL, Michoud MC, Dagenais S, Hamilton EF, Papageorgiou A: Maternal anthropometry and idiopathic preterm labor. Obstet Gynecol 86:744, 1995

Kramer W, Saade G, Belfort M, Dorman K, Mayes M, Moise K: Randomized, double-blind study comparing sulindac to terbutaline: Fetal renal and amniotic fluid effects. Am J Obstet Gynecol 174:244, 1996

Kristensen J, Langhoff-Ross J, Kristensen FB: Implications of idiopathic preterm delivery for previous and subsequent pregnancies. Obstet Gynecol 86:800, 1995

Kupferminc M, Lessing JB, Yaron Y, Peyser MR: Nifedipine versus ritodrine for suppression of preterm labour. Br J Obstet Gynaecol 100:1090, 1993

Kurki T, Sivonen A, Renkonen OV, Savia E, Ylikorkala O: Bacterial vaginosis in early pregnancy and pregnancy outcome. Obstet Gynecol 80:173, 1992

Kurtzman JL, Thorp JM Jr, Spielman FJ, Mueller RC, Cefalo RC: Do nifedipine and verapamil potentiate the cardiac toxicity of magnesium sulfate? Am J Perinatol 10:450, 1993

Kyle P, Turner DP: Chorioamnionitis due to pseudomonas aeruginosa: A complication of prolonged antibiotic therapy for premature rupture of membranes. Br J Obstet Gynaecol 103:181, 1996

Lam F, Gill P, Smith M, Kitzmiller JL, Katz M: Use of the subcutaneous terbutaline pump for long-term tocolysis. Obstet Gynecol 72:810, 1988

Lamont RF: The contemporary use of beta-agonists. Br J Obstet Gynaecol 100:890, 1993

Lazar P, Gueguen S, Dreyfus J, Renaud R, Pontonnier G, Papiernik E: Multicentred controlled trial of cervical cerclage in women at moderate risk of preterm delivery. Br J Obstet Gynaecol 91:731, 1984

Lees CC, Lojacono A, Thompson C, Danti L, Black RS, Tanzi P, White IR, Campbell S: Glyceryl trinitrate and ritodrine in tocolysis: An international multicenter randomized study. Obstet Gynecol 94:403, 1999

Leeson SC, Maresh MJA, Martindale EA, Mahmood T, Muotune A, Hawkes N, Baldwin KJ: Detection of fetal fibronectin as a predictor of preterm delivery in high risk symptomatic pregnancies. Br J Obstet Gynaecol 103:48, 1996

Leitich H, Egarter C, Kaider A, Hohlagschwandtner M, Berghammer P, Husslein P: Cervicovaginal fetal fibronectin as a marker for preterm delivery: A meta-analysis. Am J Obstet Gynecol 180:1169, 1999

Lettieri L, Vintzileos AM, Rodis JF, Albini SM, Salafia CM: Does "idiopathic" preterm labor resulting in preterm birth exist? Am J Obstet Gynecol 168:1480, 1993

Leveno KJ, Cox K, Roark ML: Cervical dilatation and prematurity revisited. Obstet Gynecol 68:434, 1986a

Leveno KJ, Klein VR, Guzick DS, Young DR, Hankins DV,

Williams ML: Single-centre randomised trial of ritodrine hydrochloride for preterm labour. Lancet 1:1293, 1986b

Leviton LC, Goldenberg RL, Baker CS, Schwartz RM, Freda MC, Fish LJ, Cliver SP, Rouse DJ, Chazotte C, Merkatz IR, Raczynski JM: Methods to encourage the use of antenatal corticosteroid therapy for fetal maturation: A randomized controlled trial. JAMA 281:46, 1999

Lewis R, Mercer BM, Salama M, Walsh MA, Sibai BM: Oral terbutaline after parenteral tocolysis: A randomized, double-blind, placebo-controlled trial. Am J Obstet Gynecol 175:834, 1996

Lewit EM, Baker LS, Corman H, Shiono PH: The direct cost of low birth weight. Future Child 5:35, 1995

Liggins GC, Howie RN: A controlled trial of antepartum glucocorticoid treatment for prevention of the respiratory distress syndrome in premature infants. Pediatrics 50:515, 1972

Lirette M, Holbrook RH, Katz M: Cardiovascular and uterine blood flow changes during nicardipine HCl tocolysis in the rabbit. Obstet Gynecol 69:79, 1987

Lockwood CJ, Senyei AE, Dische MR, Casal D, Shah KD, Thung SN, Jones L, Deligdisch L, Garite TJ: Fetal fibronectin in cervical and vaginal secretions as a predictor of preterm delivery. N Engl J Med 325:669, 1991

Low JA, Panagiotopoulos C, Derrick EJ: Newborn complication after intrapartum asphyxia with metabolic acidosis in the preterm fetus. Am J Obstet Gynecol 172:805, 1995

Luke B, Mamelle N, Keith L, Munoz F, Minogue J, Papiernik E, Johnson TR: The association between occupational factors and preterm birth: A United States nurses study. Am J Obstet Gynecol 173:849, 1995

Lunt CC, Satin AJ, Barth WH Jr, Hankins GD: The effect of indomethacin tocolysis on maternal coagulation status. Obstet Gynecol 84:820, 1994

Macones GA, Berlin M, Berlin JA: Efficacy of oral beta-agonist maintenance therapy in preterm labor: A meta-analysis. Obstet Gynecol 85:313, 1995

Main DM, Richardson DK, Hadley CB, Gabbe SG: Controlled trial of a preterm labor detection program: Efficacy and costs. Obstet Gynecol 74:873, 1989

Major CA, de Veciana M, Lewis DF, Morgan MA: Preterm premature rupture of membranes and abruptio placentae: Is there an association between these pregnancy complications? Am J Obstet Gynecol 172:672, 1995

Malloy MH, Onstad L, Wright E: The effect of cesarean delivery on birth outcome in very low birth weight infants. Obstet Gynecol 77:498, 1991

Martin JA, Smith BL, Mathews TJ, Ventura SJ: Births and deaths: Preliminary data for 1998. Natl Vital Stat Rep 47:1, 1999

Martyn C: Not quite as random as I pretended. Lancet 347:70, 1996

Mati JK, Horrobin DF, Bramley PS: Induction of labour in sheep and in humans by single doses of corticosteroids. BMJ 2:149, 1973

McGregor JA, French JI: *Chlamydia trachomatis* infection during pregnancy. Am J Obstet Gynecol 164:1782, 1991

McGregor JA, French JI, Lawellin D, Franco-Buff A, Smith C, Todd JK: Bacterial protease–induced reduction of chorioamniotic membrane strength and elasticity. Obstet Gynecol 69:167, 1987

McGregor JA, Jackson GM, Lachelin GC, Goodwin TM, Artal R, Hastings C, Dullein V: Salivary estriol as risk assessment for preterm labor: A prospective trial. Am J Obstet Gynecol 173:1337, 1995

McGregor JA, French JI, Jones W, Milligan K, McKinney PJ, Patterson E, Parker R: Bacterial vaginosis is associated with prematurity and vaginal fluid mucinase and sialidase: Results of a controlled trial of topical clindamycin cream. Am J Obstet Gynecol 170:1048, 1994

Medical Research Council/Royal College of Obstetricians and Gynaecologists Working Party on Cervical Cerclage: Final reporting of the Medical Research Council/Royal College of Obstetricians and Gynaecologists Multicenter Randomized Trial of Cervical Cerclage. Br J Obstet Gynaecol 100:516, 1993

Meis PJ, Goldenberg RL, Mercer BM, Iams JD, Moawad AH, Miodovnik M, Menard MK, Caritis SN, Thurnau GR, Bottoms SF, Das A, Roberts JM, McNellis D: The preterm prediction study: Risk factors for indicated preterm births. Maternal–Fetal Medicine Units Network of the National Institute of Child Health and Human Development. Am J Obstet Gynecol 178:562, 1998

Meis PJ, Goldenberg RL, Mercer B, Moawad A, Das A, McNellis D, Johnson F, Iams JD, Thom E, Andrews WW: The preterm prediction study: Significance of vaginal infections. National Institute of Child Health and Human Development Maternal–Fetal Medicine Units Network. Am J Obstet Gynecol 173:1231, 1995a

Meis PJ, Michielutte R, Peters TJ, Wells HB, Sands RE, Coles EC, Johns KA: Factors associated with preterm birth in Cardiff, Wales, I. Univariable and multivariable analysis. Am J Obstet Gynecol 173:590, 1995b

Mercer BM, Arheart KL: Antimicrobial therapy in expectant management of preterm premature rupture of the membranes. Lancet 346:1271, 1995

Mercer BM, Carr TL, Beazley DD, Crouse DT, Sibai BM: Antibiotic use in pregnancy and drug-resistant infant sepsis. Am J Obstet Gynecol 181:816, 1999

Mercer BM, Crocker LG, Boe NM, Sibai BM: Induction versus expectant management in premature rupture of the membranes with mature amniotic fluid at 32 to 36 weeks: A randomized trial. Am J Obstet Gynecol 169:775, 1993

Mercer B, Egerman R, Beazley D, Sibai B, Carr T, Sepesi J: Steroids reduce fetal growth: Analysis of a retrospective trial. Am J Obstet Gynecol 186:S7, 2001

Mercer BM, Goldenberg RL, Das A, Moawad AH, Iams JD, Meis PJ, Copper RL, Johnson F, Thom E, McNellis D, Miodovnik M, Menard MK, Caritis SN, Thurnau GR, Bottoms SF, Roberts J: The preterm prediction study: A clinical risk assessment system. Am J Obstet Gynecol 174:1885, 1996

Mercer BM, Miodovnik M, Thurnau GR, Goldenberg RL, Das AF, Ramsey RD, Rabello YA, Meis PJ, Moawad AH, Iams JD, Van Dorsten JP, Paul RH, Bottoms SF, Merenstein G, Thom EA, Roberts JM, McNellis D: Antibiotic therapy for reduction of infant morbidity after preterm premature rupture of the membranes. JAMA 278:989, 1997

Merkatz IR, Peter JB, Barden TP: Ritodrine hydrochloride: A betamimetic agent for use in preterm labor, II. Evidence of efficacy. Obstet Gynecol 56:7, 1980

Miller JM Jr, Kho MS, Brown HL, Gabert HA: Clinical chorioamnionitis is not predicted by an ultrasonic biophysical profile in patients with premature rupture of membranes. Obstet Gynecol 76:1051, 1990

Moher D, Olkin I: Meta-analysis of randomized controlled trials: A concern for standards. JAMA 274:1962, 1995

Molnar M, Romero R, Hertelendy F: Interleukin-1 and tumor necrosis factor stimulate arachidonic acid release and physiolipid metabolism in human myometrial cells. Am J Obstet Gynecol 169:825, 1993

Morales WJ: The effect of chorioamnionitis on the developmental outcome of preterm infants at one year. Obstet Gynecol 70:183, 1987

Morales WJ, Angel JL, O'Brien WF, Knuppel RA: Use of ampicillin and corticosteroids in premature rupture of membranes: A randomized study. Obstet Gynecol 73:721, 1989

Morales WJ, Diebel ND, Lazar AJ, Zadrozny D: The effect of antenatal dexamethasone administration on the prevention of respiratory distress syndrome in preterm gestations with premature rupture of the membranes. Am J Obstet Gynecol 154:591, 1986

Morales WJ, Schorr S, Albritton J: Effect of metronidazole in patients with preterm birth in preceding pregnancy and bacterial vaginosis: A placebo-controlled, double-blind study. Am J Obstet Gynecol 171:345, 1994

Morales WJ, Talley T: Premature rupture of membranes < 25 weeks: A management dilemma. Am J Obstet Gynecol 168:503, 1993

Mueller-Heubach E, Guzick DS: Evaluation of risk scoring in a preterm birth prevention study of indigent patients. Am J Obstet Gynecol 160:829, 1989

Murphy DJ, Sellers S, MacKenzie IZ, Yudkin PL, Johnson AM: Case-control study of antenatal and intrapartum risk factors for cerebral palsy in very preterm singleton babies. Lancet 346:1449, 1995

Narahara H, Johnston JM: Effects of endotoxins and cytokines on the secretion of platelet-activating factor acetylhydrolase by human decidual macrophages. Am J Obstet Gynecol 169:531, 1993

National Center for Health Statistics: Health, United States, 1996. Hyattsville, MD, US Department of Health and Human Services, 1996

National Center for Health Statistics. Health, United States 1999. Hyattsville, MD, US Department of Health and Human Services, 1999

National Institutes of Health Consensus Development Conference: Statement on Repeat Courses of Antenatal Corticosteroids. Bethesda, MD. August 17–18, 2000. http://consensus.nih.gov

Nelson KB, Grether JK: Can magnesium sulfate reduce the risk of cerebral palsy in very-low-birthweight infants? Pediatrics 95:263, 1995

Nelson LH, Anderson RL, O'Shea M, Swain M: Expectant management of preterm premature rupture of the membranes. Am J Obstet Gynecol 171:350, 1994

Nelson LH, Meis PJ, Hatjis CG, Ernest JM, Dillard R, Schey HM: Premature rupture of membranes: A prospective, randomized evaluation of steroids, latent phase, and expectant management. Obstet Gynecol 66:55, 1985

NIH Consensus Development Conference Statement: Effect of corticosteroids for fetal maturation on perinatal outcomes. Am J Obstet Gynecol 173:246, 1995

NIH Consensus Development Panel: Effect of Corticosteroids for Fetal Maturation on Perinatal Outcomes. JAMA 173:413, 1995

Norman K, Pattinson RC, de Souza J, de Jong P, Moller G, Kirsten G: Ampicillin and metronidazole treatment in preterm labour: A multicentre, randomised controlled trial. Br J Obstet Gynaecol 101:404, 1994

Norton ME, Merrill J, Cooper BA, Kuller JA, Clyman RI: Neonatal complications after the administration of indomethacin for preterm labor. N Engl J Med 329:1602, 1993

Nugent RP, Krohn MA, Hillier SL: Reliability of diagnosing bacterial vaginosis by a standardized method of gram stain interpretation. J Clin Microbiol 29:297, 1991

Owen J: Endovaginal sonography at 16-18 weeks of gestation predicts subsequent spontaneous preterm delivery in high-risk women. J Soc Gynecol Investig (Abstr 520) 7:189A, 2000

Owen J, Baker SL, Hauth JC, Goldenberg RL, Davis RO, Copper RL: Is indicated or spontaneous preterm delivery more advantageous for the fetus? Am J Obstet Gynecol 163:868, 1990a

Owen J, Goldenberg RL, Davis RO, Kirk KA, Copper RL: Evaluation of a risk scoring system as a predictor of preterm birth in an indigent population. Am J Obstet Gynecol 163:873, 1990b

Paneth NS: The problem of low birth weight. Future Child 5:19, 1995

Panter K, Tan B, Hannah M: Indomethacin vs mimetics for the tocolysis of preterm labor: A meta-analysis of RCTs. Am J Obstet Gynecol 174:466, 1996

Papatsonis DN, Van Geijn HP, Ader HJ, Lange FM, Bleker OP, Dekker GA: Nifedipine and ritodrine in the management of preterm labor: A randomized multicenter trial. Obstet Gynecol 90:230, 1997

Papiernik E, Bouyer J, Collin D, Winisdoerffer G, Dreyfus J: Precocious cervical ripening and preterm labor. Obstet Gynecol 67:238, 1986

Parilla BV, Dooley SL, Minogue JP, Socol ML: The efficacy of oral terbutaline after intravenous tocolysis. Am J Obstet Gynecol 169:965, 1993

Parilla BV, Grobman WA, Holtzman RB, Thomas HA, Dooley SL: Indomethacin tocolysis and risk of necrotizing enterocolitis. Obstet Gynecol 96:120, 2000

Parisi V, Salina J, Stockman E: Fetal cardiorespiratory responses to maternal administration of nicardipine in the hypertensive ewe. Abstract presented at meeting of the Society of Perinatal Obstetricians, San Antonio, January 30–February 1, 1986

Peaceman AM, Andrews WW, Thorp JM, Cliver SP, Lukes A: Fetal fibronectin as a predictor of preterm birth in symptomatic patients—a multicenter trial. Am J Obstet Gynecol 174:303, 1996

Peacock JL, Bland JM, Anderson HR: Preterm delivery: Effects of socioeconomic factors, psychological stress, smoking, alcohol, and caffeine. BMJ 311:531, 1995

Perry KG, Martin RW, Blake PC, Roberts WE, Martin JN: Maternal outcome associated with adult respiratory distress syndrome. Am J Obstet Gynecol 174:391, 1996

Perry KG Jr, Morrison JC, Rust OA, Sullivan CA, Martin RW, Naef RW 3rd: Incidence of adverse cardiopulmonary effects with low-dose continuous terbutaline infusion. Am J Obstet Gynecol 173:1273, 1995

Platz-Christensen JJ, Mattsby-Baltzer I, Thomsen P, Wiqvist N: Endotoxin and interleukin-1 alpha in the cervical mucus and vaginal fluid of pregnant women with bacterial vaginosis. Am J Obstet Gynecol 169:1161, 1993

Porter TF, Varner MW, Fraser AM, Ward RH: The familial aggregation of prematurity. J Soc Gynecol Invest 3 (Suppl):353, 1996

Powell SL, Holt VL, Hickok DE, Easterling T, Connell FA: Recent changes in delivery site of low-birthweight infants in Washington: Impact on birth weight-specific mortality. Am J Obstet Gynecol 173:1585, 1995

Ransom SW: The care of premature and foeble infants. Pediatrics (NY) 9:321, 1900

Rasanen J, Jouppila P: Fetal cardiac function and ductus arteriosus during indomethacin and sulindac therapy for threatened preterm labor: A randomized study. Am J Obstet Gynecol 173:20, 1995

Read MD, Wellby DE: The use of a calcium antagonist (nifedipine) to suppress preterm labour. Br J Obstet Gynaecol 93:933, 1986

Reid DE, Christian CD: Controversy in Obstetrics and Gynecology, 2nd ed. Philadelphia, Saunders, 1974, p 33

Richey SD, Ramin KD, Roberts SW, Ramin SM, Cox SM, Twickler DM: The correlation between transperineal sonography and digital examination in the evaluation of the third-trimester cervix. Obstet Gynecol 85:745, 1995

Robertson PA, Sniderman SH, Laros RK Jr, Cowan R, Heilbron D, Goldenberg RL, Iams JD, Creasy RK: Neonatal morbidity according to gestational age and birth weight from five tertiary care centers in the United States, 1983 through 1986. Am J Obstet Gynecol 166:1629, 1992

Romero R, Kadar N, Hobbins JC, Duff GW: Infection and labor: The detection of endotoxin in amniotic fluid. Am J Obstet Gynecol 157:815, 1987

Romero R, Roslansky P, Oyarzun E, Wan M, Emamian M, Novitsky TJ, Gould MJ, Hobbins JC: Labor and infection, II: Bacterial endotoxin in amniotic fluid and its relationship to the onset of preterm labor. Am J Obstet Gynecol 158:1044, 1988

Romero R, Sibai BM, Sanchez-Ramos L, Valenzuela GJ, Veille JC, Tabor B, Perry KG, Varner M, Goodwin TM, Lane R, Smith J, Shangold G, Creasy GW: An oxytocin receptor antagonist (atosiban) in the treatment of preterm labor: A randomized, double-blind, placebo-controlled trial with tocolytic rescue. Am J Obstet Gynecol 182:1173, 2000

Romero R, Yoon BH, Mazor M, Gomez R, Diamond MP, Kenney JS, Ramirez M, Fidel PL, Sorokin Y, Cotton D, Sehgal P: The diagnostic and prognostic value of amniotic fluid white blood cell count, glucose, interleukin-6 and gram stain in patients with preterm labor and intact membranes. Am J Obstet Gynecol 169:805, 1993

Rush RW, Isaacs S, McPherson K, Jones L, Chalmers I, Grant A: A randomized controlled trial of cervical cerclage in women at high risk of spontaneous preterm delivery. Br J Obstet Gynaecol 91:724, 1984

Rust O, Atlas R, Jones K, Benham B, Balducci J: A randomized trial of cerclage vs. no cerclage in patients with sonographically detected 2nd trimester premature dilation of the internal os. Am J Obstet Gynecol (Abstr 8) 182:S13, 2000

Rust O, Atlas R, Reed J, Van Gaalen J, Balducci J: Revisiting the clinical efficacy of cerclage in the treatment of second-trimester sonographically detected premature dilation of the internal os. Am J Obstet Gynecol 184:S3, 2001

Rutter N: The extremely preterm infant. Br J Obstet Gynaecol 102:682, 1995

Ryan GM Jr, Abdella TN, McNeeley SG, Baselski VS, Drummond DE: Chlamydia trachomatis infection in pregnancy and effect of treatment on outcome. Am J Obstet Gynecol 162:34, 1990

Saade GR, Taskin O, Belfort MA, Erturan B, Moise KJ Jr: In vitro comparison of four tocolytic agents, alone and in combination. Obstet Gynecol 84:374, 1994

Sachs BP, Fretts RC, Gardner R, Hellerstein S, Wampler NS, Wise PH: The impact of extreme prematurity and congenital anomalies on the interpretation of international comparisons of infant mortality. Obstet Gynecol 85:941, 1995

Satin AJ, Leveno KJ, Sherman ML, Reedy NJ, Lowe TW, McIntire DD: Maternal youth and pregnancy outcomes: Middle school versus high school age groups compared to women beyond the teen years. Am J Obstet Gynecol 171:184, 1994

Schiff E, Sivan E, Terry S, Dulitzky M, Friedman SA, Mashiach S, Sibai BM: Currently recommended oral regimen for ritodrine tocolysis result in extremely low plasma levels. Am J Obstet Gynecol 169:1059, 1993

Schwarz BE, Schultz FM, MacDonald PC, Johnston JM: Initiation of human parturition, IV. Demonstration of phospholipase A2 in the lysosomes of human fetal membranes. Am J Obstet Gynecol 125:1089, 1976

Semchyshyn S, Zuspan FP, O'Shaughnessy R: Pulmonary edema associated with the use of hydrocortisone and a tocolytic agent for the management of premature labor. J Reprod Med 28:47, 1983

Smith CS, Woodland MB: Clinical comparison of oral nifedipine and subcutaneous terbutaline for initial tocolysis. Am J Perinatol 10:280, 1993

Smyth CN: The guard-ring tocodynamometer: Absolute measurement of intra-amniotic pressure by a new instrument. J Obstet Gynaecol Br Commonw 64:59, 1957

Spinillo A, Capuzzo E, Stronati M, Ometto A, Orcesi S, Fazzi E: Effect of preterm premature rupture of membranes in neurodevelopmental outcome: Follow up at two years of age. Br J Obstet Gynaecol 102:882, 1995

Spisso KR, Harbert GM Jr, Thiagarajah S: The use of magnesium sulfate as the primary tocolytic agent to prevent premature delivery. Am J Obstet Gynecol 142:840, 1982

St. John EB, Nelson KG, Cliver SP, Bishnoi RR, Goldenberg RL: Cost of neonatal care according to gestational age at birth and survival status. Am J Obstet Gynecol 182:170, 2000

Steer CM, Petrie RH: A comparison of magnesium sulfate and alcohol for the prevention of premature labor. Am J Obstet Gynecol 129:1, 1977

Stevenson DK, Wright LL, Lemons JA, Oh W, Korones SB, Papile LA, Bauer CR, Stoll BJ, Tyson JE, Shankaran S, Fanaroff AA, Donovan EF, Ehrenkranz RA, Verter J: Very low birth weight outcomes of the National Institute of Child Health and Human Development Neonatal Research Network, January 1993 through December 1994. Am J Obstet Gynecol 179:1632, 1998

Stubbs TM, Van Dorsten P, Miller MC 3d: The preterm cervix and preterm labor: Relative risks, predictive values, and change over time. Am J Obstet Gynecol 155:829, 1986

Svare J, Langhoff-Roos J, Andersen LF, Kryger-Baggesen N, Borch-Christensen H, Heisterberg L, Kristensen J: Ampicillin-metronidazole treatment in idiopathic preterm labour: A randomised controlled multicentre trial. Br J Obstet Gynaecol 104:892, 1997

Thorp JA, Clark R, Jones PG, D'Angelo L: The effect of antenatal steroids on head circumference at birth. Am J Obstet Gynecol 186:S2, 2001

Thorp JA, Ferrette-Smith D, Gaston LA, Johnson J, Yeast JD, Meyer B: Combined antenatal vitamin K and phenobarbital therapy for preventing of intracranial hemorrhage of newborns less than 34 weeks gestation. Obstet Gynecol 86:1, 1995

Thorp JM, Lukes AG: Predictors of positivity for cervico-fetal fibronectin in patients with symptoms of preterm labor. J Soc Gynecol Invest 3 (Suppl):247, 1996

Thorp JA, Yeast JD, Cohen GR, et al. Repeated antenatal betamethasone and perinatal outcome. Am J Obstet Gynecol (Abstr 23) 182:S21, 2000

Thorsen P, Molsted K, Jensen IP, Arpi M, Bremmelgaard A, Jeune B, Møller BR: Bacterial vaginosis in a population of 3600 pregnant women and relationship to preterm birth. Am J Obstet Gynecol 174:331, 1996

Ulmsten U, Andersson KE, Wingerup L: Treatment of premature labor with the calcium antagonist nifedipine. Arch Gynecol 229:1, 1980

Van der Heijden BJ, Carlus C, Narcy F, Bavoux F, Delezoide AL, Gubler MC: Persistent anuria, neonatal death, and renal microcystic lesions after prenatal exposure to indomethacin. Am J Obstet Gynecol 171:617, 1994

Ventura SJ, Martin JA, Curtin SC, Mathews TJ, Park MM: Births: Final data for 1998. Natl Vital Stat Rep 48:1, 2000

Vermillion S, Soper D, Newman R: Neonatal sepsis and death after multiple doses of antenatal betamethasone. Am J Obstet Gynecol (Abstr 28) 182:S24, 2000

Vintzileos AM, Campbell WA, Nochimson DJ, Connolly ME, Fuenfer MM, Hoehn GJ: The fetal biophysical profile in patients with premature rupture of the membranes—an early predictor of fetal infection. Am J Obstet Gynecol 152:510, 1985

Vintzileos AM, Campbell WA, Nochimson DJ, Weinbaum PJ, Escoto DT, Mirochnick MH: Qualitative amniotic fluid volume versus amniocentesis in predicting infection in preterm premature rupture of the membranes. Obstet Gynecol 67:579, 1986

Vohr BR, Wright LL, Dusick AM, Mele L, Verter J, Steichen JJ, Simon NP, Wilson DC, Broyles S, Bauer CR, Delaney-Black V, Yolton KA, Fleisher BE, Papile LA, Kaplan MD: Neurodevelopmental and functional outcomes of extremely low birth weight infants in the National Institute of Child Health and Human Development Neonatal Research Network, 1993–1994. Pediatrics 105:1216, 2000

Walker DJ, Feldman A, Vohr BR, Oh W: Cost-benefit analysis of neonatal intensive care for infants weighing less than 1,000 grams at birth. Pediatrics 74:20, 1984

Wang X, Zuckerman B, Coffman GA, Corwin MJ: Familial aggregation of low birth weight among whites and blacks in the United States. N Engl J Med 333:1744, 1995

Watt-Morse ML, Caritis SN, Kridgen PL: Magnesium sulfate is a poor inhibitor of oxytocin-induced contractility in pregnant sheep. J Matern Fetal Med 4:139, 1995

Watts DH, Krohn MA, Hillier SL, Eschenbach DA: The association of occult amniotic fluid infection with gestational age and neonatal outcome among women in preterm labor. Obstet Gynecol 79:351, 1992

Webster LA, Greenspan JR, Nakashima AK, Johnson RE: An evaluation of surveillance for *Chlamydia trachomatis* infections in the United States, 1987 to 1991. MMWR 43 (Suppl 5–3):21, 1993

Wenstrom K, Weiner CP, Merrill D, Niebyl J: A placebo-controlled randomized trial of the terbutaline pump for prevention of preterm delivery. Am J Perinatol 14:87, 1997

Whyte HE, Fitzhardinge PM, Shennan AT, Lennox K, Smith L, Lacy J: Extreme immaturity: Outcome of 568 pregnancies of 23–26 weeks' gestation. Obstet Gynecol 82:1, 1993

Williams JW: Obstetrics: A Text-Book for Students and Practitioners, 1st ed. New York, Appleton, 1903, p 133

Winn HN, Chen M, Amon E, Leet TL, Shumway JB, Mostello D: Neonatal pulmonary hypoplasia and perinatal mortality in patients with mid-trimester rupture of amniotic membranes—a critical analysis. Am J Obstet Gynecol 182:1638, 2000

Wood NS, Marlow N, Costeloe K, Gibson AT, Wilkinson AR for the EPICure Study Group: Neurologic and development disability after extremely preterm birth. N Engl J Med 343:378, 2000

Yoon BH, Romero R, Park JS, Kim CJ, Kim SH, Choi JH, Han TR: Fetal exposure to an intra-amniotic inflammation and the development of cerebral palsy at the age of three years. Am J Obstet Gynecol 182:675, 2000

Yoon BH, Yang SH, Jun JK, Park KH, Kim CJ, Romero R: Maternal blood C-reactive protein, white blood cell count, and temperature in preterm labor: A comparison with amniotic fluid white blood cell count. Obstet Gynecol 87:231, 1996

Yost NP, Bloom SL, Twickler DM, Leveno KJ: Pitfalls in ultrasonic cervical length measurement for predicting preterm birth. Obstet Gynecol 93:510, 1999

28

Postterm Pregnancy

For almost three quarters of the 20th century, prolonged pregnancy was considered a nonproblem except that such pregnancies were sometimes associated with macrosomia and difficult delivery. Labor induction was recommended only when the intention was to circumvent continued fetal growth to prevent dystocia. In the 1950s, the possibility of increased perinatal mortality in pregnancies at or beyond 42 weeks was considered insufficient to warrant intervention. Induction, especially with an unfavorable cervix, was considered a greater hazard. By the 1970s, however, it was accepted that perinatal mortality increased appreciably in these pregnancies, and this led to interventions such as delivery or scrutiny of fetal health.

DEFINITIONS

The terms *postterm, prolonged, postdates,* and *postmature* are often loosely used interchangeably to signify pregnancies that have exceeded a duration considered to be the upper limit of normal. Imprecision in their use, along with varying definitions of the upper limit of normal pregnancy, make a search of the literature on postterm pregnancy bewildering.

Postmature should be used to describe the infant with recognizable clinical features indicating a pathologically prolonged pregnancy. **Postdates** probably should be abandoned, because the real issue in many postterm pregnancies is "post-*what* dates?" Therefore, **postterm** or **prolonged pregnancy** are the preferred expressions for extended pregnancies, and "postmature" is reserved for a specific clinical syndrome. Importantly, few infants from prolonged pregnancies are postmature, and indiscriminate use of this term can falsely imply a pathologically prolonged pregnancy.

The standard internationally recommended definition of prolonged pregnancy, endorsed by the American College of Obstetricians and Gynecologists (1997), is 42 completed weeks (294 days) or more from the first day of the last menstrual period.

It is important to emphasize the phrase "42 completed weeks." Pregnancies between 41 weeks 1 day and 41 weeks 6 days, although in the 42nd week, do not complete 42 weeks until the seventh day has elapsed. Thus, technically speaking, prolonged pregnancy could begin either on day 294 or on day 295 following the onset of the last menses. Which is it? Day 294 or 295? We cannot solve this question, and emphasize this dilemma only to ensure that litigators and others understand that some imprecision is inevitable when attempting to define prolonged pregnancy. Amersi and Grimes (1998) have cautioned against use of ordinal numbers such as "42nd week" because of their imprecision. For example, "42nd week" refers to 41 weeks and 1 through

6 days whereas the cardinal number "42 weeks" refers precisely 42 completed weeks.

MENSTRUAL DATES. The definition of postterm pregnancy as one that persists for 42 weeks or more from the onset of a menstrual period assumes that the last menses was followed by ovulation 2 weeks later. Although this may include perhaps 10 percent of pregnancies, some may not be actually postterm but rather the result of an error in estimation of gestational age. It is likely that there are two categories of pregnancies that reach 42 completed weeks:

1. Those truly 42 weeks past conception.
2. Those with less advanced gestations due to variations in timing of ovulation.

Munster and associates (1992) described a high incidence of large variations in menstrual cycles in normal women. Boyce and associates (1976) studied 317 French women with conceptional basal body temperature profiles and found that 70 percent who completed 42 postmenstrual weeks had less advanced gestations based on their ovulation dates. Reuss and co-workers (1995) found similar results when early pregnancy ultrasound dating was prospectively studied in 764 women. Postterm pregnancies decreased from 10 percent using menstrual history to 3 percent when ultrasound criteria were used. Finally, a small number of women ovulate sooner than expected, giving rise to the possibility that 40 completed postconceptional weeks could be achieved by 41 weeks of amenorrhea.

Thus, most pregnancies reliably 42 completed weeks beyond the last menses probably are not biologically prolonged, and a few not yet 42 weeks might be postterm. These variations in menstrual cycle likely explain, at least partially, why approximately 10 percent of human pregnancies reach 42 completed weeks, yet a relatively small proportion of fetuses have evidence of *postmaturity.* Because there is no method to identify pregnancies that are truly prolonged, all pregnancies judged to be 42 completed weeks should be managed as if abnormally prolonged.

INCIDENCE

Postterm pregnancy varies greatly depending on the criteria used for diagnosis, and reported frequencies range from 4 to 14 percent with an average of about 10 percent (Bakketeig and Bergsjø, 1991). As shown in Figure 28–1 approximately 8 percent of 4 million infants born in the United States during 1997 were estimated to have been delivered at 42 weeks or more. In comparison, 11 percent of live births were preterm, defined as 36 weeks or less.

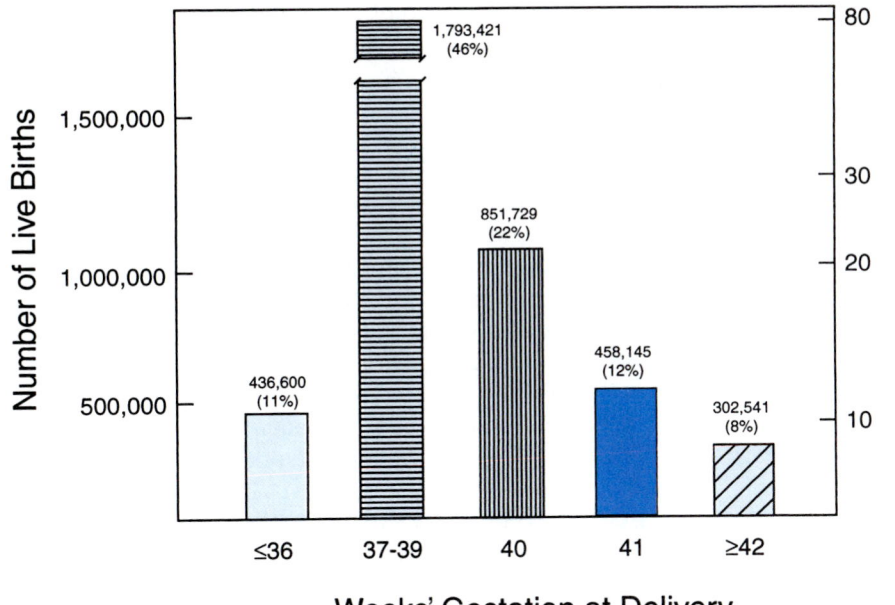

FIGURE 28-1. Gestational age at delivery of 4 million live births in the United States during 1997. (Adapted from Ventura and colleagues, 1999).

Contradictory results have been found concerning the significance of a variety of maternal demographic factors such as parity, prior postterm birth, socioeconomic class, and age. One interesting feature, the tendency for some mothers to repeat postterm births, suggests that some prolonged pregnancies are biologically determined. In an analysis of 27,677 births to Norwegian women, the incidence of a subsequent postterm birth increased from 10 to 27 percent if the first birth was postterm and to 39 percent if there had been two previous successive postterm deliveries (Bakketeig and Bergsjø, 1991). Mogren and colleagues (1999) reported that prolonged pregnancy also recurred across generations in Swedish women. When the mother had had a prolonged pregnancy in delivering her daughter, the risk for postterm pregnancy in the daughter's pregnancy was increased two- to threefold.

PERINATAL MORTALITY

The historical basis for the concept of an upper limit of human pregnancy duration was the observation that perinatal mortality increased after the expected due date was passed. This is best seen when perinatal mortality is analyzed from times before widespread use of interventions for pregnancies exceeding 42 weeks. As shown in Figure 28–2, after reaching a nadir at 39 to 40 weeks, perinatal mortality increased in Sweden as pregnancy exceeded 41 weeks. The most recent data from Sweden (Table 28–1) indicate that this late-pregnancy trend has persisted for almost 50 years despite

dramatic improvement in gestational age-specific mortality rates.

Lucas and co-workers (1965) compared perinatal outcomes in 6624 postterm pregnancies with almost 60,000 singleton pregnancies delivered between 38 and 41 weeks. The study was done before intentional delivery at 42 weeks was practiced. All components of perinatal mortality—antepartum, intrapartum, and neonatal

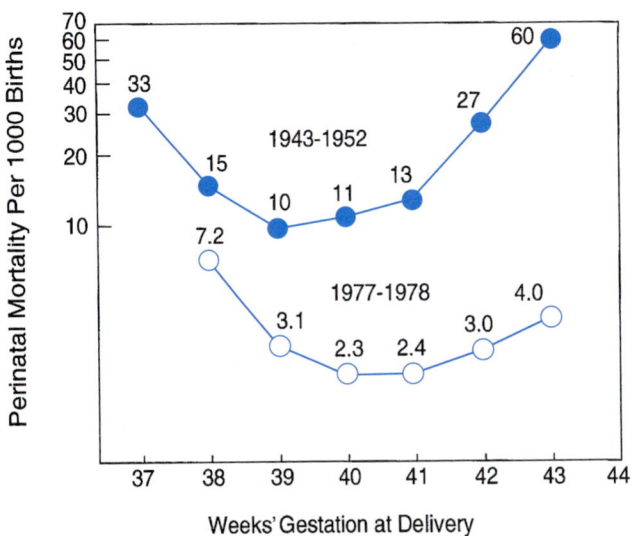

FIGURE 28-2. Perinatal mortality in late pregnancy according to gestational age in Sweden 1943–1952 compared with 1977–1978. Logarithm scale is used for convenience in depiction. (Adapted from Bakketeig and Bergsjø, 1991, and Lindell, 1956.)

TABLE 28–1. Adjusted[a] Odds Ratios for Perinatal Mortality As a Function of Gestational Age for 181,524 Births in Sweden (1987–1992)

Gestational Age (wk)	Fetal Death Odds Ratio (95% CI)	Neonatal Mortality Odds Ratio (95% CI)
40	1.0 (ref)	1.0 (ref)
41	1.48 (1.13–1.95)[b]	1.24 (0.90–1.70)
42	1.77 (1.22–2.56)[b]	1.44 (0.92–2.24)
≥43	2.90 (1.27–6.61)[b]	1.89 (0.60–5.99)

CI = Confidence interval.
[a]Adjusted for maternal age, parity, smoking, and fetal sex.
[b]$P < .05$ (over referent group).
From Divon and co-authors (1998).

deaths—were increased at 42 weeks and beyond. The most significant increases occurred intrapartum. The major causes included pregnancy hypertension, prolonged labor with cephalopelvic disproportion, "unexplained anoxia," and malformations. Using data from the Collaborative Perinatal Project comprising 53,158 pregnancies delivered in the 1960s, Naeye (1978) also reported that malformations in postterm stillborns was common. As discussed in Chapter 39 (p. 1074), most malformed fetuses are detected earlier in pregnancy, and thus the incidence of malformations is not currently increased compared with the general obstetrical population (Clausson and co-workers, 1999).

In 62,804 births at the National Maternity Hospital in Dublin between 1979 and 1986, excess perinatal mortality attributable to postterm pregnancy occurred only in the intrapartum and neonatal periods (Crowley, 1991). Intrapartum asphyxia and meconium aspiration were implicated in almost three fourths of these deaths. Moreover, early neonatal seizures, often used as an index of intrapartum events, occurred in 5.4 per 1000 postterm infants compared with 0.9 per 1000 infants born at term.

Thus, intrapartum perinatal risk is increased in prolonged pregnancies, particularly when meconium is present (Chap. 14, p. 351). Meconium is found in more than a fourth of postterm pregnancies and, as shown in Table 28–2, meconium aspiration syndrome is significantly increased. Labor induction, cesarean delivery, macrosomia, and shoulder dystocia are also significantly increased (Eden and associates, 1987).

The specific congenital malformations—anencephaly and adrenal hypoplasia—associated with prolonged pregnancy share a common feature of pituitary insufficiency and lack of the usually high estrogen levels that characterize normal pregnancy (Chap. 6, p. 120). In these cases, the precursor hormone, dehydroisoandrosterone sulfate, is secreted in insufficient amounts for

conversion to estradiol and indirectly to estriol in the placenta (MacDonald and Siiteri, 1965).

PATHOPHYSIOLOGY

Clifford (1954) described a recognizable clinical syndrome in some infants delivered after term that did much to dispel the prevailing obstetrical opinion that prolonged human pregnancy did not exist (Calkins, 1948). Infants, either live or stillborn, and demonstrating these clinical characteristics, are now diagnosed to be pathologically *postmature*. Actually, the postmature infant Clifford described had been reported more than 50 years earlier by Ballantyne (1902).

POSTMATURITY SYNDROME Clifford's 1954 description of the postmature infant was based on 37 births that typically occurred 300 or more days after the last menstruation. He divided postmaturity into three stages: in stage 1 the amnionic fluid was clear, in stage 2 the skin was stained green, and in stage 3 the skin discoloration was yellow-green.

The postmature infant presents a unique and characteristic appearance (Fig. 28–3). This includes wrinkled, patchy peeling skin, a long, thin body suggesting wasting, and advanced maturity because the infant is open-eyed, unusually alert, old, and worried-looking. Skin wrinkling can be particularly prominent on the palms and soles. The nails are typically quite long. Most such postmature infants are not growth restricted, because their birthweight seldom falls below the 10th percentile for gestational age. Severe growth restriction, however, which logically must have preceded completion of 42 weeks, can occur. Many of Clifford's postmature infants died, and many were seriously ill due to birth asphyxia and meconium aspiration. Several survivors were brain damaged.

TABLE 28–2. Outcomes in Postterm Pregnancies (42 Weeks or Greater) Compared with Pregnancies Delivered at 40 Weeks

Outcome[a]	40 Weeks (n = 8135) %	Postterm (n = 3457) %
Meconium	19	27
Oxytocin induction	3	14
Shoulder dystocia	8	18
Cesarean delivery	0.7	1.3
Macrosomia (>4500 g)	0.8	2.8
Meconium aspiration	0.6	1.6

[a]For all comparisons between 40- and 42-week groups, $P < .05$. From Eden and associates (1987), with permission.

The incidence of postmaturity syndrome in infants at 41, 42, or 43 weeks, respectively, has not been conclusively determined. Shime and colleagues (1984), in one of the rare contemporary reports to chronicle postmaturity, found that this syndrome occurred in about 10 percent of pregnancies between 41 and 43 weeks and increased to 33 percent at 44 weeks. Associated oligohydramnios substantially increases the likelihood of postmaturity. Trimmer and colleagues (1990) diagnosed oligohydramnios when the ultrasonic maximum vertical amnionic fluid pocket measured 1 cm or less at 42 weeks and 88 percent of the infants were postmature.

PLACENTAL DYSFUNCTION. Clifford (1954) proposed that the skin changes of postmaturity were due to loss of the protective effects of vernix caseosa. His second hypothesis that continues to influence contemporary concepts attributes postmaturity syndrome to placental senescence. Clifford could not, however, demonstrate placental degeneration histologically. Indeed, in the ensuing 40 years, no morphological or significant quantitative changes have been found (Larsen and co-workers, 1995; Rushton, 1991). Of interest, Smith and Barker (1999) recently reported that placental apoptosis—programmed cell death—was significantly increased at 41 to 42 completed weeks compared with 36 to 39 weeks. The clinical significance of such apoptosis is unclear at this time.

Jazayeri and co-workers (1998) investigated umbilical cord plasma erythropoietin levels in 124 appropriately grown newborns delivered from 37 to 43 weeks. They sought to assess whether fetal oxygenation may be compromised, presumably due to placental aging, in

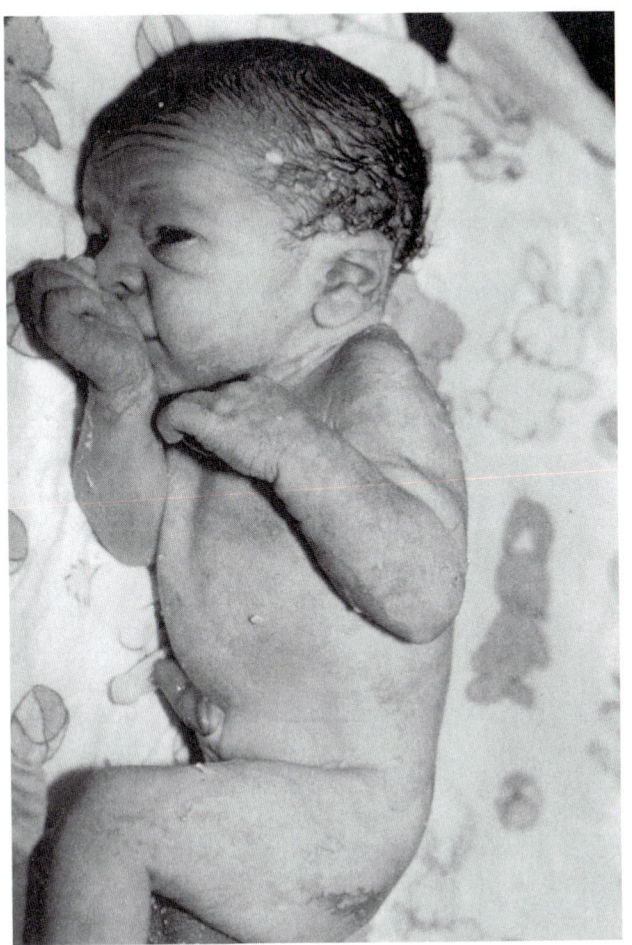

FIGURE 28–3. Postmature infant delivered at 43 weeks' gestation. Thick, viscous meconium coated the desquamating skin. Note the long, thin appearance and wrinkling of the palms of the hands.

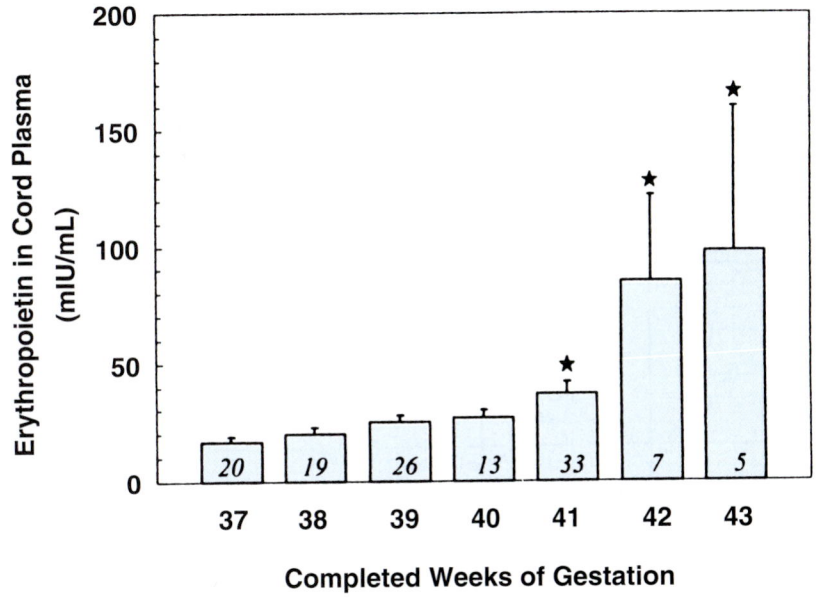

FIGURE 28–4. Umbilical cord plasma erythropoietin levels (mean ± S.E.M) at 37 to 43 weeks' gestation. Analysis of variance showed a significant difference between the groups ($P < .001$). Numbers inside the bars indicate the number of infants tested. (Adapted from Hendricks, 1964, with permission.)

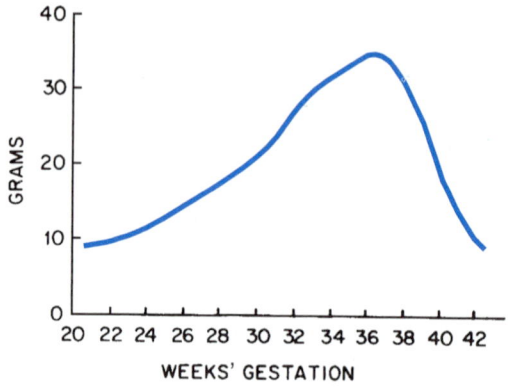

FIGURE 28–5. Mean daily fetal growth during previous week of gestation. (From Jazayeri and co-workers, 1998, with permission.)

pregnancies proceeding beyond their due data. Decreased partial oxygen pressure is the only known stimulator of erythropoietin. Each woman studied had an uncomplicated labor and delivery course without evidence of fetal stress or meconium passage. Cord plasma erythropoietin levels were significantly increased in pregnancies reaching 41 weeks or more (Fig. 28–4), and although Apgar scores and umbilical cord blood gases were not abnormal in these infants, the authors concluded that there was decreased fetal oxygenation in some postterm gestations.

The postterm fetus may continue to gain weight and thus be an unusually large infant at birth. That the fetus continues to grow serves to suggest that placental function is not compromised. Indeed, continued fetal growth, although at a slower rate, is characteristic between 38 and 42 weeks (Fig. 28–5). Nahum and colleagues (1995) more recently confirmed that fetal growth continues at least up until 42 weeks.

FETAL DISTRESS AND OLIGOHYDRAMNIOS. The principal reasons for increased risks to postterm fetuses were described by Leveno and associates (1984). They reported that both antepartum fetal jeopardy and intrapartum fetal distress were the consequence of cord compression associated with oligohydramnios. In their analysis of 727 postterm pregnancies, intrapartum fetal distress detected with electronic monitoring was not associated with late decelerations characteristic of uteroplacental insufficiency. Instead, one or more prolonged decelerations (Fig. 28–6) preceded three fourths of emergency cesarean deliveries for fetal jeopardy. In all but two cases, there were also variable decelerations (Fig. 28–7). Another common fetal heart rate pattern, although not ominous by itself, was the saltatory baseline shown in Figure 28–8. These findings are consistent with cord occlusion as the proximate cause of fetal distress. Other correlates found were oligohydramnios and viscous meconium. These observations on the pathophysiology of postterm pregnancy were confirmed by Phelan and co-workers (1985) and Bochner and associ-

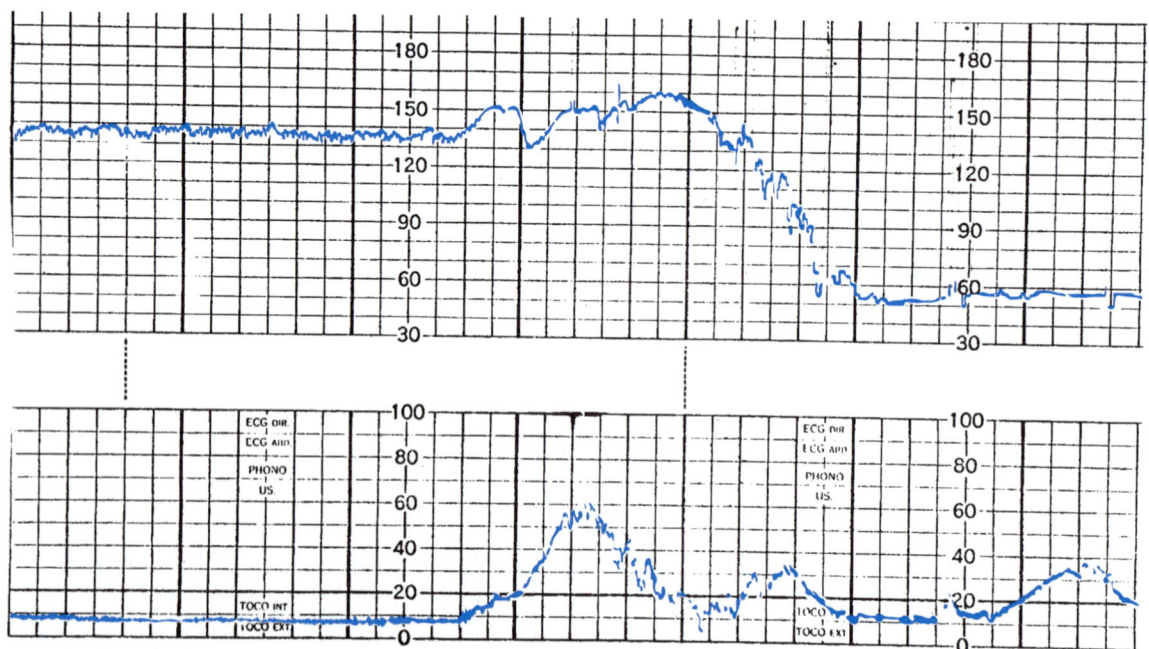

FIGURE 28–6. Prolonged fetal heart rate deceleration prior to emergency cesarean delivery in postterm pregnancy with oligohydramnios. (From Leveno and co-workers, 1984, with permission.)

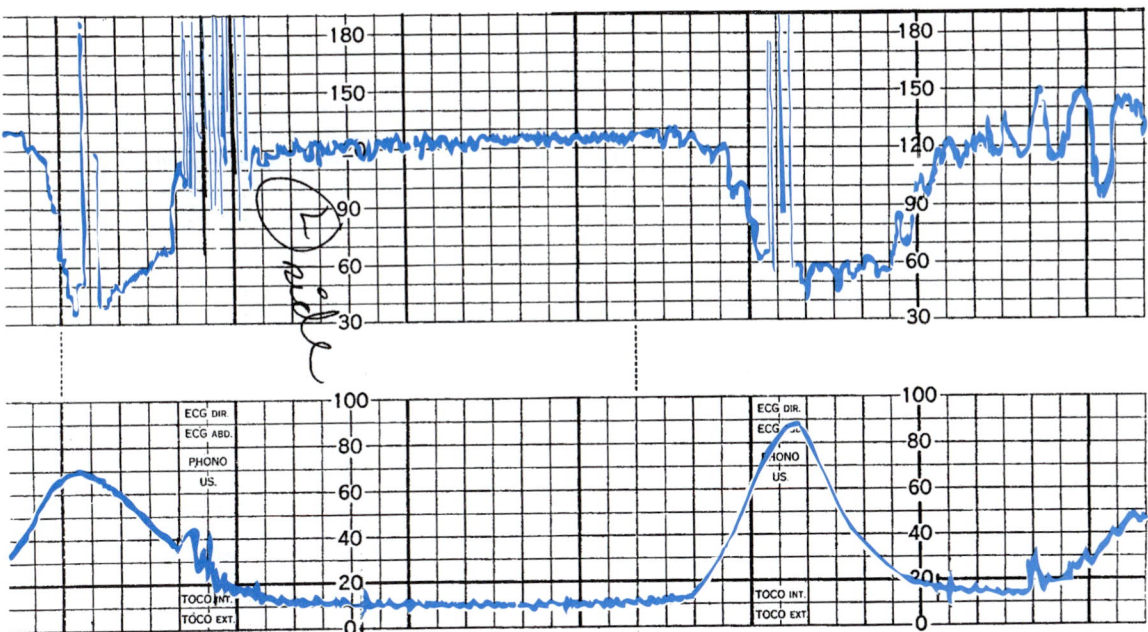

FIGURE 28-7. Severe—less than 70 bpm for 60 seconds or longer—variable decelerations in postterm pregnancy with oligohydramnios and cesarean delivery for fetal jeopardy. (From Leveno and co-workers, 1984, with permission.)

ates (1987). Silver and colleagues (1987) also reported that decreased umbilical cord diameter, measured ultrasonically, was predictive of intrapartum fetal distress, especially if associated with oligohydramnios.

Decreased amnionic fluid volume commonly devel-

ops as pregnancy advances beyond 42 weeks (Fig. 28-9). It is also likely that fetal release of meconium (Chap. 14, p. 351) into an already reduced amnionic fluid volume is the reason for the thick, viscous meconium implicated in meconium aspiration syndrome.

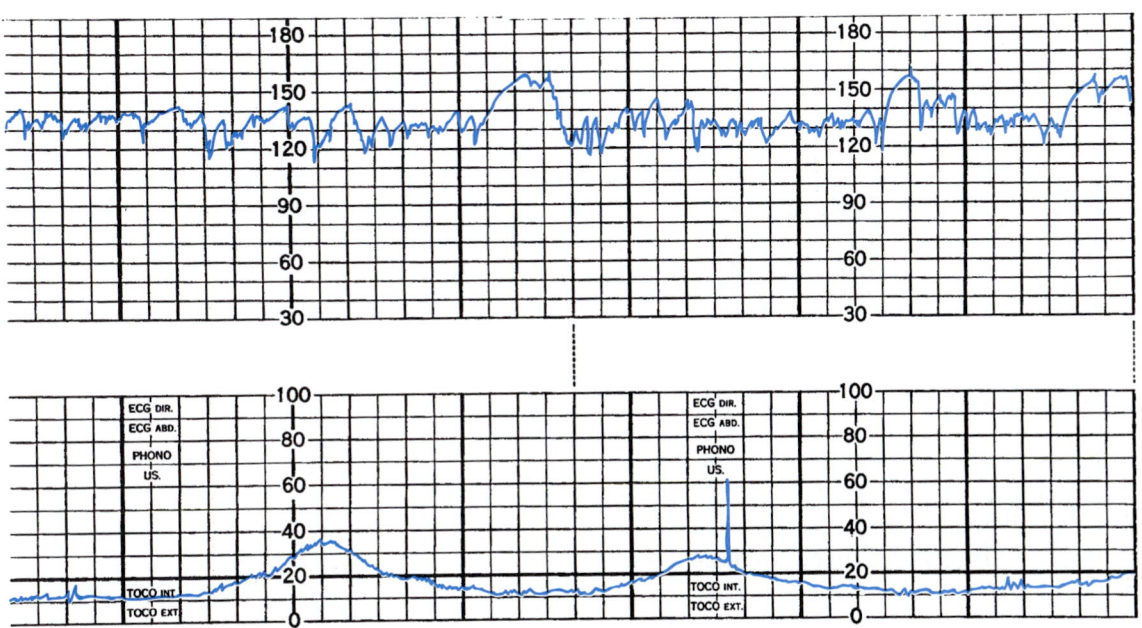

FIGURE 28-8. Saltatory baseline fetal heart rate showing oscillations exceeding 20 bpm and associated with oligohydramnios in postterm pregnancy. (From Leveno and co-workers, 1984, with permission.)

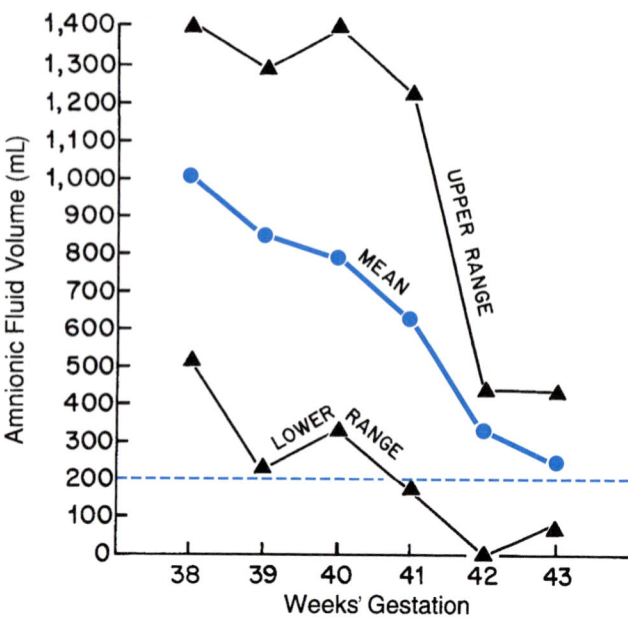

FIGURE 28–9. Volume of amnionic fluid during the last weeks of pregnancy. (Adapted from Elliott and Inman, 1961, with permission.)

TABLE 28–3. Effects of Fetal Growth Restriction[a] on Stillbirth Rates in Pregnancies Reaching 42 Weeks or More Compared with 37 to 41 Weeks in Sweden (1991–1995)

Outcome	Pregnancy Duration	
	37–41 Weeks	≥42 Weeks
Births	469,056	40,973
Fetal growth restriction (%)[a]	10,312 (2)	1558 (4)
Stillbirths (per 1000)		
Appropriate growth	650 (1.4)	69 (1.8)
Fetal growth restriction	116 (11)	23 (15)

[a]Fetal growth restriction was defined as birthweight below two standard deviations from the mean birthweight for fetal gender and gestational age.
From Clausson and colleagues, 1999, with permission.

Trimmer and co-workers (1990) measured hourly fetal urine production using sequential ultrasonic bladder volume measurements in 38 pregnancies of 42 weeks or more. Diminished urine production was found to be associated with oligohydramnios. It was hypothesized, however, that decreased fetal urine flow was likely the result of preexisting oligohydramnios that limited fetal swallowing of amnionic fluid. Veille and co-workers (1993), using pulsed Doppler waveforms, reported that fetal renal blood flow is reduced in postterm pregnancies with oligohydramnios.

FETAL GROWTH RESTRICTION. Until quite recently, the clinical significance of fetal growth restriction in the otherwise uncomplicated pregnancy has received little attention. Divon and co-authors (1998) and Clausson and co-workers (1999) have analyzed births of almost 700,000 women between 1987 and 1995 using the National Swedish Medical Birth registry. As shown in Table 28–3, fetal growth restriction was implicated in stillbirths at 42 weeks or beyond as well as for term infants. Indeed, a third of the postterm stillbirths were growth restricted. At the time of these births in Sweden, induction of labor and antenatal fetal testing was usually commenced at 42 weeks. Alexander and colleagues (2000b) compared infant outcomes for 355 postterm infants (≥42 weeks) with birthweights less than or equal to the third percentile for gestational age with the remaining 14,520 infants in higher percentiles delivered at Parkland Hospital. Morbidity and mortality were sig-

nificantly increased in the growth-restricted infants. Indeed, a fourth of all stillbirths associated with prolonged pregnancy were in this comparatively small number of growth-restricted infants.

MANAGEMENT

It is generally accepted that antepartum interventions are indicated in management of prolonged pregnancies. The type(s) of interventions and when to employ them are somewhat controversial. One major issue is whether to intervene at 41 or 42 weeks. Another is whether labor induction is warranted compared with expectant management using antepartum fetal testing. Roussis and colleagues (1993) surveyed members of the Society for Maternal–Fetal Medicine in 1990 and found that approximately two thirds induced labor at 41 weeks if the cervix was favorable. Antepartum fetal testing was advocated at 41 weeks when the cervix was unfavorable. At 42 weeks, virtually all respondents induced labor when the cervix was favorable, and 58 percent would do this even when the cervix was unfavorable. Others (42 percent) recommended antepartum testing when the cervix was unfavorable at 42 weeks. Clearly, the inducibility of the cervix has considerable impact on management.

UNFAVORABLE CERVIX. It is difficult to precisely define the "unfavorable cervix" in prolonged pregnancies because investigators have used different criteria. For example, Harris and colleagues (1983) reported that 92 percent of women at 42 weeks had an unfavorable cervix defined by Bishop scores less than 7. Hannah and colleagues (1992), however, found that 40 percent of 3407 women with 41-week pregnancies had undilated cervices. Importantly, women with dilatation of 3 cm or more were excluded from their study. Cervical dilatation is an important prognostic indicator for induction success. Alexander and associates (2000c) evaluated 800 women induced for postterm pregnancy at Parkland Hospital. They reported that women with no cervical dilatation had a twofold increased cesarean delivery rate for dystocia.

In the past 10 years, a number of investigations to evaluate management for prolonged pregnancies have included use of prostaglandin E_2 for cervical ripening. The Maternal–Fetal Medicine Units Network of the National Institute of Child Health and Human Development (1994) evaluated prostaglandin E_2 gel and found that it was not more effective than placebo. Sawai and colleagues (1994) used 2-mg prostaglandin E_2 vaginal suppositories daily for an average of 4 days in 42 women with a 41-week gestation and an unfavorable cervix (Bishop score less than 9). Although such treatment improved the Bishop score in an average of 4 days, it had no significant effect on any subsequent intrapartum outcomes. Alexander and associates (2000d) studied 393 women with postterm pregnancy who were given prostaglandin E_2 for cervical ripening. These women were treated even if the cervix was "favorable." They reported that almost half of the 84 women with cervical dilatation of 2 to 4 cm entered labor with prostaglandin E_2 alone. The American College of Obstetricians and Gynecologists (1997) has concluded that prostaglandin gel can be used safely in postterm pregnancies. Use of prostaglandin for cervical ripening is discussed in Chapter 20 (p. 471).

Fassett and colleagues (2000) presented preliminary data to indicate that mifepristone (RU486) did not stimulate sufficient uterine activity to effect cervical favorability in 97 women with postterm pregnancy.

Sweeping, or stripping of the membranes to induce labor and prevent postterm pregnancy has been studied in 15 randomized trials during the 1990s (Chap. 20, p. 474). Boulvain and co-authors (1999) performed a meta-analysis of these and found that membrane stripping at 38 to 40 weeks decreased the frequency of postterm pregnancy. Membrane stripping, however, did not modify the risk of cesarean delivery nor were maternal or neonatal infections increased. The authors emphasized that membrane stripping could be painful and might provoke vaginal bleeding and irregular contractions.

INDUCTION VERSUS FETAL TESTING.
A logical plan for reducing perinatal mortality and morbidity associated with prolonged pregnancy is to terminate pregnancy before such events occur. There have been doubts about the value of labor induction, mainly because it was feared that this would result in more operative

intervention without preventing perinatal death. As a result, many clinicians prefer to employ fetal testing to avoid inductions. Major studies designed to resolve these questions have been done in both Canada and the United States.

Hannah and colleagues (1992) randomized 3407 Canadian women with pregnancies at 41 or more weeks to labor induction or fetal testing. Women assigned to fetal testing were asked to count the number of times they felt the fetus move over a 2-hour period each day, and they also underwent nonstress testing three times weekly. Amnionic fluid volume was assessed two to three times each week, and pockets less than 3 cm were considered abnormal. Labor induction resulted in a significantly lower cesarean rate (21 percent) compared with pregnancies managed with antepartum testing (24 percent). There were two stillbirths in the fetal testing group and none in the induction group. The lower cesarean rate in the induction group was due to fewer procedures for fetal distress. A cost-effectiveness analysis of the Canadian data was later reported by Goeree and colleagues (1995). The mean cost per patient managed with fetal testing was $3132 compared with $2939 in those who underwent labor induction. Thus, managing postterm pregnancy with labor induction resulted in more favorable outcomes than fetal testing and at a lower cost. A similar analysis, however, of the Maternal–Fetal Medicine Network study, showed no cost advantages for either scheme (Gardner and associates, 1996).

In the Maternal–Fetal Medicine Network randomized trial of induction versus fetal testing, nonstress tests and ultrasonic estimations of amnionic fluid volume were done twice weekly in 175 women whose pregnancies had reached 41 weeks or more. Their outcomes were compared with 265 women randomized to oxytocin induction with or without cervical ripening with prostaglandin E_2 gel. Oligohydramnios was diagnosed in the fetal testing group when the largest pocket of amnionic fluid was less than 2 cm. There were no perinatal deaths in any study subgroup, and the rate of cesarean delivery was not significantly different when labor induction was compared with expectant management. Thus, this study supported the validity of either management scheme.

Crowley (1997) used the Oxford Database of Perinatal Trials to perform a meta-analysis of 18 studies that assessed management of postterm pregnancy. Routine induction after 41 weeks resulted in reduced perinatal mortality without increased risk of cesarean or instrumental delivery. Roberts and colleagues (1999), in a study of 540,116 births, concluded that this meta-analysis prompted routine induction after 41 weeks to be widely adopted in New South Wales, Australia. Specifically, from 1990 to 1996 there was a significant decrease in births at 42 completed weeks or more—4.6 compared with 2.8 percent, respectively. This also was associated with an increased induction rate at 41 weeks. Importantly, the cesarean delivery rate also increased. Because infant outcomes were not described in this report, any beneficial neonatal effects are undetermined.

Because macrosomia is more prevalent, O'Reilly-Green (1996) tested the predictive value of sonographic estimates of fetal weight greater than 4500 g in 202 consecutive postterm pregnancies. They concluded that using 4500-g fetal weight estimates as an indication for cesarean delivery would be imprudent because two thirds of these were incorrect. Importantly, almost a fourth of these infants weighed more than 4000 g, thus attesting to the association of large infants with prolonged pregnancies.

INTERVENTION AT 41 VERSUS 42 WEEKS. Evidence to substantiate intervention—whether induction or fetal testing—commencing at 41 versus 42 weeks is limited. Most evidence used to justify intervention at 41 weeks is from the randomized Canadian and American investigations cited earlier. No randomized studies have specifically assessed intervention at 41 weeks versus an identical intervention employed at 42 weeks. Importantly, a national policy of intervention for prolonged pregnancy at 41 versus 42 weeks would mean that approximately 500,000 additional women would be subjected to interventions that are not conclusively proven necessary nor harmful.

Three randomized studies published between 1978 and 1986 compared induction at 40 weeks versus 42 weeks. The only benefit was reported by Martin and associates (1978), and this was limited to less frequent meconium-stained amnionic fluid. Tylleskar and colleagues (1979) found no benefits. In the study by Husslein and co-workers (1986), fetal testing was used be-

tween 40 and 42 weeks, but still no benefits were found. In subsequent observational studies, Bochner and colleagues (1988) and Guidetti and associates (1989) have advocated antepartum fetal testing beginning at 41 weeks. In none of these reports is there convincing evidence that starting fetal testing at 41 weeks significantly changed any outcome. Indeed, the reverse interpretation, that beginning fetal testing at 41 weeks offered no benefit, could have been easily made.

As previously seen in Figure 28–2, perinatal mortality does not appreciably increase at 41 weeks, but does so at 42 weeks. Usher and colleagues (1988) analyzed several outcomes in 7663 pregnancies with gestational ages determined to be 40, 41, or 42 weeks confirmed by early ultrasound examinations. Perinatal death rates, corrected for malformations, were 1.5, 0.7, and 3.0 per 1000 for 40, 41, and 42 weeks, respectively. These results could be used to challenge the concept of routine intervention at 41 instead of 42 weeks. Interestingly, Divon and colleagues (1996) found that, although adverse fetal outcomes increased at 41 compared with 40 weeks, these were associated with growth restriction. They suggested that management strategies should be focused on fetal growth rather than simply gestational age in pregnancies reaching 41 weeks.

Based on results summarized in Table 28–4, 41-week pregnancies without other complications such as hypertension are considered normal pregnancies at Parkland Hospital. No interventions are practiced solely on the basis of fetal age until 42 completed weeks. It is our view that large, randomized studies should be performed before 41-week gestations are routinely considered pathologically prolonged.

OLIGOHYDRAMNIOS. Several authors have suggested that the identification of diminished amnionic fluid de-

TABLE 28–4. Perinatal Deaths, Excluding Infants with Malformations, and Labor Complications in Singleton Births at 40, 41, and 42 Weeks at Parkland Hospital (1988–1997)

Outcome	Gestational Age		
	40 Weeks	41 Weeks	42 Weeks
Pregnancies	31,034	17,122	11,441
Inductions (%)	667 (2)	990 (6)	3,519 (31)
Meconium (%)	6,438 (21)	4,339 (25)	2,626 (23)
Cesarean (%)			
Total	1813 (6)	1524 (9)	1444 (13)
Dystocia	1012 (3)	852 (5)	888 (8)
Fetal distress	629 (2)	532 (3)	450 (4)
Perinatal deaths (per 1000)	1.7	1.8	2.2

From Alexander and co-workers (2000a), with permission.

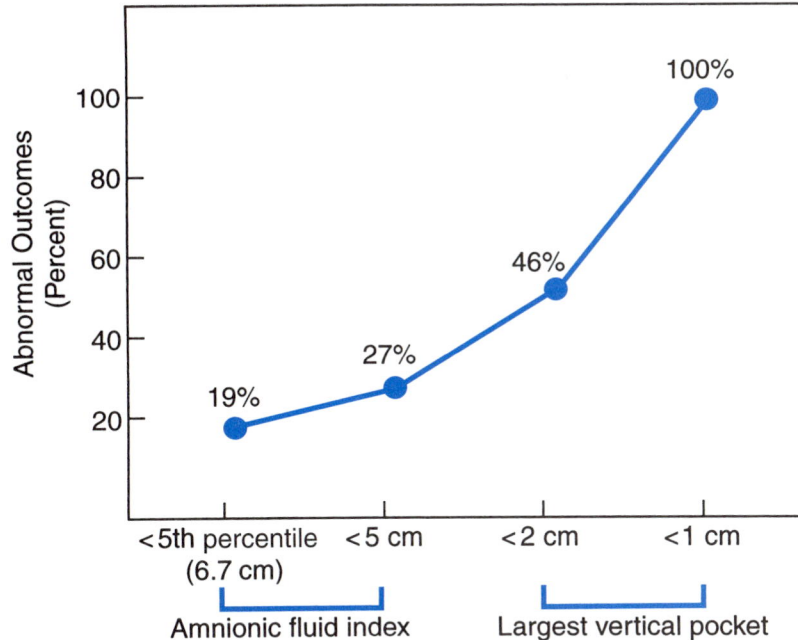

FIGURE 28–10. Comparison of diagnostic value of various ultrasonic estimates of amnionic fluid in prolonged pregnancies. Abnormal outcomes include cesarean or operative vaginal delivery for fetal jeopardy, 5-minute Apgar score of 6 or less, umbilical arterial blood pH less than 7.1, or admission to the neonatal intensive care unit. (Adapted from Fischer and associates, 1993.)

termined by various ultrasonic methods may be helpful to identify a postterm fetus in jeopardy. There is no doubt that when amnionic fluid is decreased in a postterm pregnancy—or for that matter in any pregnancy—the fetus is at increased risk. Many different criteria for ultrasonic diagnosis of oligohydramnios have been proposed. Fischer and colleagues (1993) attempted to determine which criteria were most predictive of normal versus abnormal outcomes in postterm pregnancies. As shown in Figure 28–10, the smaller the amnionic fluid pocket, the greater the likelihood that there was clinically significant oligohydramnios. Normal amnionic fluid volume, however, did not preclude abnormal outcomes. Alfirevic and co-authors (1997) randomized 500 women with postterm pregnancies—defined as 290 days or longer gestation—to assessment of amnionic fluid volume using either the amnionic fluid index or deepest vertical pocket. They concluded that the amnionic fluid index overestimated the number of abnormal outcomes in postterm pregnancies.

Regardless of criteria used to diagnose oligohydramnios in postterm pregnancies, most investigators have found an increased incidence of "fetal distress" during labor. Thus, oligohydramnios by most definitions is a clinically meaningful finding. Conversely, reassurance of continued fetal well-being in the presence of "normal" amnionic fluid volume is tenuous because it is unknown how quickly pathological oligohydramnios develops. Clement and co-workers (1987) reported six postterm pregnancies in which amnionic fluid volume diminished abruptly over 24 hours and one fetus died. Wing and colleagues (1996) recommended that amnionic fluid vol-

ume be assessed twice weekly in all pregnancies beginning at 41 weeks.

AMERICAN COLLEGE OF OBSTETRICIANS AND GYNECOLOGISTS RECOMMENDATIONS FOR 1997 AND 1999. Management recommendations for pregnancies at 42 weeks or more are summarized in Table 28–5.

TABLE 28–5. Recommendations by the American College of Obstetricians and Gynecologists (1997) for Evaluation and Management of Prolonged Pregnancies

1. Antenatal surveillance of postterm pregnancies should be initiated by 42 weeks despite a lack of evidence that monitoring improves outcomes.

2. There is insufficient evidence that initiating antenatal surveillance between 40 and 42 completed weeks improves outcomes.

3. No single antenatal surveillance protocol for monitoring fetal well-being in a postterm pregnancy appears superior to another.

4. It is unknown whether induction or expectant management (antenatal surveillance) is preferable in the postterm patient with a *favorable cervix*.

5. There is good evidence that either induction or expectant management will result in good outcomes in postterm patients with *unfavorable cervices*.

6. Prostaglandin gel can be used safely in postterm pregnancies to promote cervical changes and induce labor.

Used with permission, from the American College of Obstetricians and Gynecologists (1997).

The recommendations, although providing flexibility in the evaluation and management of pregnancies completing 42 weeks, indicate that either antenatal testing or labor induction should be commenced at 42 weeks. There was insufficient evidence to recommend a management strategy between 40 and 42 completed weeks.

Postterm pregnancy has been identified by the American College of Obstetricians and Gynecologists (1999) as a high-risk condition where twice weekly antepartum fetal testing may be indicated. Doppler velocimetry was not recommended. Oligohydramnios detected using ultrasound, defined as no vertical pocket of amnionic fluid greater than 2 cm or an amnionic fluid index (AFI) 5 cm or less, is considered an indication for either delivery or close fetal surveillance.

MANAGEMENT OF POSTTERM PREGNANCY AT PARKLAND HOSPITAL. In women with a *certain* gestational age, labor is induced at the completion of 42 weeks (Fig. 28–11). Almost 90 percent of such women are induced successfully, or enter labor within 2 days of induction. For those who do not deliver with the first induction, a second induction is performed within 3 days. Almost all women will be delivered by this plan of management, but in the unusual few who are not delivered, management decisions are a third (or more) induction versus cesarean delivery.

Women classified as having *uncertain* postterm pregnancies are followed on a weekly basis and without intervention unless fetal jeopardy is suspected. The latter is based upon clinical or sonographic perception of decreased amnionic fluid volume. Equally worrisome is

diminished fetal movement reported by the mother. If fetal jeopardy is suspected by either method, labor induction is carried out as described previously for the woman with certain postterm gestation. Other details of management are summarized in Figure 28–11. This protocol has been used successfully for almost 20 years with very few adverse fetal or neonatal outcomes.

MEDICAL OR OBSTETRICAL COMPLICATIONS. In the event of a medical or another obstetrical complication, it is generally unwise to allow a pregnancy to continue past 42 weeks. Indeed, in many such instances *early* delivery is indicated. Timing of delivery will depend on the individual complication. Common examples include pregnancy-induced hypertension, prior cesarean delivery, and diabetes.

INTRAPARTUM MANAGEMENT. Labor is a particularly dangerous time for the postterm fetus. Therefore, it is important that women whose pregnancies are known or suspected to be postterm come to the hospital as soon as they suspect they are in labor. Upon arrival, while being observed for possible labor, we recommend that fetal heart rate and uterine contractions be monitored electronically for variations consistent with fetal distress (American College of Obstetricians and Gynecologists, 1995).

When to perform amniotomy is problematic. Further reduction in fluid volume following amniotomy can certainly enhance the possibility of cord compression. Conversely, amniotomy will aid diagnosis of thick meconium, which may be dangerous to the fetus if aspirated.

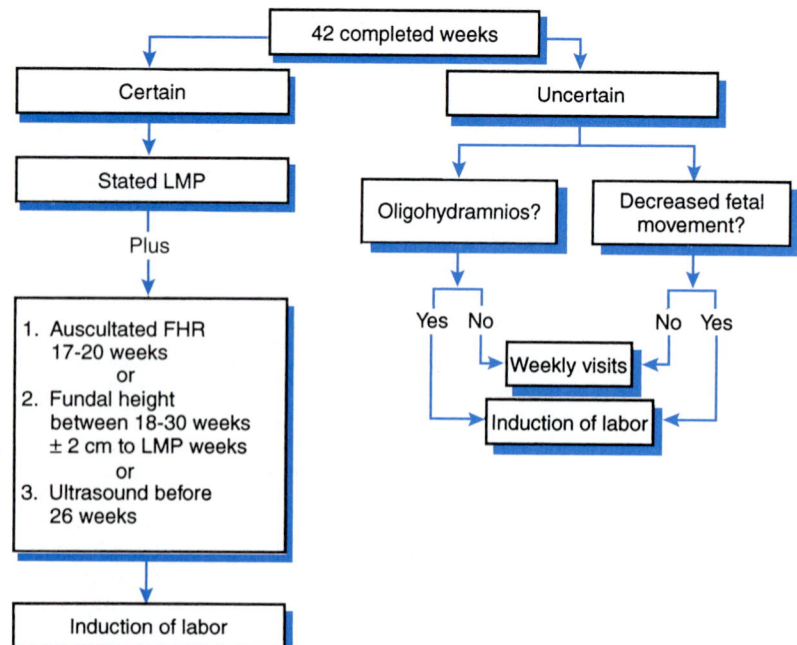

FIGURE 28–11. Parkland Hospital protocol for management of prolonged pregnancies. (FHR = fetal heart rate; LMP = last menstrual period.)

Moreover, once the membranes are ruptured, a scalp electrode and intrauterine pressure catheter can be placed, which usually provide more precise data concerning fetal heart rate and uterine contractions.

Identification of *thick meconium* in the amnionic fluid is particularly worrisome. The viscosity probably signifies the lack of liquid and thus oligohydramnios. Aspiration of thick meconium may cause severe pulmonary dysfunction and neonatal death (Chap. 39, p. 1044). This may be minimized but not eliminated by effective suctioning of the pharynx as soon as the head is delivered but before the thorax is delivered. If meconium is identified, the trachea should be aspirated as soon as possible after delivery. Immediately thereafter, the infant should be ventilated as needed. The likelihood of successful vaginal delivery is reduced appreciably for the nulliparous woman who is in early labor with thick, meconium-stained amnionic fluid. Therefore, when the woman is remote from delivery, strong consideration should be given to prompt cesarean section, especially when cephalopelvic disproportion is suspected or either hypotonic or hypertonic dysfunctional labor is evident. Some practitioners choose to avoid oxytocin use in these cases.

At times, the continued growth of the fetus postterm will result in a *large-for-gestational-age* infant, and shoulder dystocia may develop. Therefore, an obstetrician experienced in managing this complication should be available to effect delivery (Chap. 19, p. 459).

REFERENCES

Alexander JM, McIntire DD, Leveno KJ: Forty weeks and beyond: Pregnancy outcomes by week of gestation. Obstet Gynecol 96:291, 2000a

Alexander JM, McIntire DD, Leveno KJ: The effect of fetal growth restriction on neonatal outcome in postterm pregnancy. Abstract No. 463. Am J Obstet Gynecol 182: S148, 2000b

Alexander JM, McIntire DD, Leveno KJ: Postterm pregnancy: Does induction increase cesarean rates? J Soc Gynecol Invest 7: 79A, 2000c

Alexander JM, McIntire DD, Leveno KJ: Postterm pregnancy: Is cervical "ripening" being used in the right patients? J Soc Gynecol Invest 7:247A, 2000d

Alfirevic Z, Luckas M, Walkinshaw SA, McFarlane M, Curran R: A randomized comparison between amniotic fluid index and maximum pool depth in the monitoring of postterm pregnancy. Br J Obstet Gynaecol 104:207, 1997

American College of Obstetricians and Gynecologists: Antepartum fetal surveillance. Technical Bulletin No. 9, October 1999

American College of Obstetricians and Gynecologists: Management of postterm pregnancy. Practice Pattern No. 6, October 1997

American College of Obstetrics and Gynecologists: Fetal heart rate patterns: Monitoring, interpretation, and management. Technical Bulletin No. 207, July 1995

Amersi S, Grimes DA: The case against using ordinal numbers for gestational age. Obstet Gynecol 91:623, 1998

Bakketeig LS, Bergsjø P: Post-term pregnancy: Magnitude of the problem. In Chalmers I, Enkin M, Keirse M (eds): Effective Care in Pregnancy and Childbirth. Oxford, Oxford University Press, 1991, p 765

Ballantyne JW: The problem of the postmature infant. J Obstet Gynaecol Br Emp 2:522, 1902

Bochner CJ, Medearis AL, Davis J, Oakes GK, Hobel CJ, Wade ME: Antepartum predictors of fetal distress in postterm pregnancy. Am J Obstet Gynecol 157:353, 1987

Bochner CJ, Williams J III, Castro L, Medearis A, Hobel CJ, Wade M: The efficacy of starting postterm antenatal testing at 41 weeks as compared with 42 weeks of gestational age. Am J Obstet Gynecol 159:550, 1988

Boulvain M, Irion O, Marcoux S, Fraser W: Sweeping of the membranes to prevent post-term pregnancy and to induce labour: A systematic review. Br J Obstet Gynaecol 106: 481, 1999

Boyce A, Magaux MJ, Schwartz D: Classical and "true" gestational post maturity. Am J Obstet Gynecol 125:911, 1976

Calkins LA: Postmaturity. Am J Obstet Gynecol 56:167, 1948

Clausson B, Cnattingus S, Axelsson O: Outcomes of postterm births: The role of fetal growth restriction and malformations. Obstet Gynecol 94:758, 1999

Clement D, Schifrin BS, Kates RB: Acute oligohydramnios in post date pregnancy. Am J Obstet Gynecol 157:884, 1987

Clifford SH: Postmaturity with placental dysfunction. Clinical syndromes and pathologic findings. J Pediatr 44:1, 1954

Crowley P: Interventions to prevent or improve outcome for deliveries at or beyond term. In Neilson JP, Crowther CA, Hodnett ED, Hofmeyr GJ (eds): Pregnancy and Childbirth Module of the Cochrane Database of Systematic Reviews [updated September 1997]. The Cochrane Library. The Cochrane Collaboration; Issue 4, Oxford: Update Software, 1997

Crowley P: Post-term pregnancy: Induction of surveillance? In Chalmers I, Enkin M, Keirse M (eds): Effective Care in Pregnancy and Childbirth. Oxford, Oxford University Press, 1991, p 776

Divon MY, Haglund B, Nisell H, Otterblad PO, Westgren M: Fetal and neonatal mortality in the postterm pregnancy: The impact of gestational age and fetal growth restriction. Am J Obstet Gynecol 178:726, 1998

Divon MY, Haglund B, Nisell H, Otterblad PO, Westgren M: Perinatal outcome in a large cohort of postdates pregnancies. Am J Obstet Gynecol 174:351, 1996

Eden RD, Seifert LS, Winegar A, Spellacy WN: Perinatal characteristics of uncomplicated postdate pregnancies. Obstet Gynecol 69:296, 1987

Elliott PM, Inman WH: Volume of liquor amnii in normal and abnormal pregnancy. Lancet 2:835, 1961

Fassett MJ, Wing DA: Uterine activity after oral mifepristone administration in the postterm pregnancy. J Soc Gynecol Invest 7:191A, 2000

Fischer RL, McDonnell M, Bianculli KW, Perry RL, Hediger ML, Scholl TO: Amniotic fluid volume estimation in the postdate pregnancy: A comparison of techniques. Obstet Gynecol 81:698, 1993

Gardner M, Rouse D, Goldenberg R, Lanning J, Thom E, Zachary J, NIH Maternal-Fetal Medicine Unit Network: Cost comparison of induction of labor at 41 weeks versus expectant management in the postterm pregnancy. Am J Obstet Gynecol 174:351, 1996

Goeree R, Hannah M, Hewson S: Cost-effectiveness of induction of labour versus serial antenatal monitoring in the Canadian Multicentre Postterm Pregnancy Trial. Can Med Assoc J 152:1445, 1995

Guidetti DA, Divon MY, Langer O: Postdate fetal surveillance: Is 41 weeks too early? Am J Obstet Gynecol 161:91, 1989

Hannah ME, Hannah WJ, Hellman J, Hewson S, Milner R, Willan A, Canadian Multicenter Post-Term Pregnancy Trial Group: Induction of labor as compared with serial antenatal monitoring in post-term pregnancy. N Engl J Med 326:1587, 1992

Harris BA Jr, Huddleston JF, Sutliff G, Perlis HW: The unfavorable cervix in prolonged pregnancy. Obstet Gynecol 62:171, 1983

Hendricks CH: Patterns of fetal and placental growth: The second half of normal pregnancy. Obstet Gynecol 24:357, 1964

Husslein P, Egarter C, Sevelda P, Genger H, Salzer H, Kofler E: Induction of labour with prostaglandin E_2 vaginal tablets: A revival of elective induction. Results of a randomized trial. Geburtshilfe Frauenheilkd 46:83, 1986

Jazayeri A, Tsibris JC, Spellacy WN: Elevated umbilical cord plasma erythropoietin levels in prolonged pregnancies. Obstet Gynecol 92:61, 1998

Larsen LG, Clausen HV, Andersen B, Graem N: A stereologic study of postmature placentas fixed by dual perfusion. Am J Obstet Gynecol 172:500, 1995

Leveno KJ, Quirk JG, Cunningham FG, Nelson SD, Santos-Ramos R, Toofanian A, DePalma RT: Prolonged pregnancy, 1. Observations concerning the causes of fetal distress. Am J Obstet Gynecol 150:465, 1984

Lindell A: Prolonged pregnancy. Acta Obstet Gynecol Scand 35:136, 1956

Lucas WE, Anefil AO, Callagan DA: The problem of postterm pregnancy. Am J Obstet Gynecol 91:241, 1965

MacDonald PC, Siiteri PK: Origin of estrogen in women pregnant with an anencephalic fetus. J Clin Invest 44:465, 1965

Martin DH, Thompson W, Pinkerton JHM, Watson JD: A randomized controlled trial of selective planned delivery. Br J Obstet Gynaecol 85:109, 1978

Mogren I, Stenlund H, Högberg U: Recurrence of prolonged pregnancy. Int J Epidemiol 28:253, 1999

Munster K, Schmidt L, Helm P: Length and variation in the menstrual cycle—a cross-sectional study from a Danish county. Br J Obstet Gynaecol 99:422, 1992

Naeye RL: Causes of perinatal excess in prolonged gestations. Am J Epidemiol 108:429, 1978

Nahum GG, Stanislaw H, Huffaker BJ: Fetal weight gain at term: Linear with minimal dependence on maternal obesity. Am J Obstet Gynecol 172:1387, 1995

National Institute of Child Health and Human Development Network of Maternal–Fetal Medicine Units: A clinical trial of induction of labor versus expectant management in postterm pregnancy. Am J Obstet Gynecol 170:716, 1994

O'Reilly-Green C: Positive and negative predictive values of estimated fetal weight for macrosomia in postdate patients. Am J Obstet Gynecol 174:350, 1996

Phelan JP, Platt LD, Yeh SY, Boussard P, Paul RH: The role of ultrasound assessment of amniotic fluid volume in the management of the postdate pregnancy. Am J Obstet Gynecol 151:304, 1985

Reuss ML, Hatch MC, Susser M: Early ultrasound dating of pregnancy: Selection and measurement biases. J Clin Epidemiol 48:667, 1995

Roberts CL, Taylor L, Henderson-Smart D: Trends in births at and beyond term: Evidence of a change? Br J Obstet Gynaecol 106:937, 1999

Roussis P, Cox SM, Campbell BA, Miller FC: Survey on the management of postdate pregnancy. J Mat Fetal Med 2:155, 1993

Rushton DI: Pathology of placenta. In Wigglesworth JS, Singer DB (eds): Textbook of Fetal and Perinatal Pathology. Boston, Blackwell, 1991, p 171

Sawai SK, O'Brien WF, Mastrogiannis DS, Krammer J, Mastry MG, Porter GW: Patient-administered outpatient intravaginal prostaglandin E_2 suppositories in postdate pregnancies: A double-blind, randomized placebo-controlled study. Obstet Gynecol 84:807, 1994

Shime J, Gare DJ, Andrews J, Bertrand M, Salgado J, Whilliams G: Prolonged pregnancy: Surveillance of the fetus and the neonate and the course of labor and delivery. Am J Obstet Gynecol 148:547, 1984

Silver RK, Dooley SL, Tamura RK, Depp R: Umbilical cord size and amniotic fluid volume in prolonged pregnancy. Am J Obstet Gynecol 157:716, 1987

Smith SC, Baker PN: Placental apoptosis is increased in postterm pregnancies. Br J Obstet Gynaecol 106:861, 1999

Trimmer KJ, Leveno KJ, Peters MT, Kelly MA: Observation on the cause of oligohydramnios in prolonged pregnancy. Am J Obstet Gynecol 163:1900, 1990

Tylleskar J, Finnstrom O, Leijon I, Hedenskop S, Ryden G: Spontaneous labour and elective induction—a prospective randomized study, 1: Effect on mother and fetus. Acta Obstet Gynecol Scand 59:513, 1979

Usher RH, Boyd ME, McLean FH, Kramer MS: Assessment of fetal risk in postdate pregnancies. Am J Obstet Gynecol 158:259, 1988

Veille JC, Penry M, Mueller-Heubach E: Fetal renal pulsed Doppler waveform in prolonged pregnancies. Am J Obstet Gynecol 169:882, 1993

Ventura SJ, Martin JA, Curtin SC, Mathews TJ: Births: Final Data for 1997. National Vital Statistics Reports, Vol 47, No. 18. Hyattsville, MD, National Center for Health Statistics, 1999

Wing DA, Fishman A, Gonzalez C, Paul RH: How frequently should the amniotic fluid index be performed during the course of antepartum testing? Am J Obstet Gynecol 174:33, 1996

29

Fetal Growth Disorders

Each year, about a fifth of the almost 4 million infants in the United States are born at the low and high extremes of fetal growth (Fig. 29–1). Low birthweight, defined as less than 2500 g, constitutes just less than half of these 700,000 births and includes preterm infants as well as those whose growth has been impaired in utero. Although the majority of these infants are preterm, the National Institutes of Health estimated that approximately 40,000 are at term, having suffered abnormal intrauterine growth (Frigoletto, 1986). Macrosomia, defined as birthweight of 4000 g or greater, occurred in 1 out of every 10 births in the United States in 1997. The incidence of macrosomic infants, however, has been declining since 1991 after peaking at about 11 percent in the 1980s (Ventura and co-authors, 1999).

NORMAL FETAL GROWTH

Human fetal growth is characterized by sequential patterns of tissue and organ growth, differentiation, and maturation that are determined by maternal provision of substrate, placental transfer of these substrates, and fetal growth potential governed by the genome. Steer (1998) has summarized the potential effects of evolutionary pressures on human fetal growth:

> Over the last 3.5 million years the human species has become adapted to the upright posture, and the pelvis has maneuvered to facilitate walking. During the last 500,000 years human brain volume has increased from about 750 mL (*Homo erectus*) to about 1000 to 1800 mL (*Homo sapiens*); this compares with only 300–400 mL in chimpanzees. Because the head has to pass through the pelvis during parturition, there has developed an increasing conflict between the need to walk (requiring a narrow pelvis) and the need to think (requiring a large brain and therefore a large head), which leads to difficulty in labor (dystocia). This has to some extent been resolved by an evolutionary

modification, known as neoteny, whereby humans are born increasingly early. If humans were born with the same level of functional maturity as the chimpanzee, human gestation would last 17 months. Another way the human fetus may be resolving this dilemma is by acquiring the ability to restrict its growth late in pregnancy. This characteristic "tail off" of fetal growth rates from 38 weeks onward as seen in human pregnancies is not evident in other mammals. Thus, the ability to "growth restrict" may be an adaptation which in the majority of cases is not pathological. . . .

Fetal growth has been divided into three consecutive cell growth phases (Lin and Santolaya-Forgas, 1998). The initial phase of hyperplasia occurs during the first 16 weeks and is characterized by a rapid increase in cell number. The second phase, which extends up to 32 weeks, includes both cellular hyperplasia and hypertrophy. After 32 weeks, fetal growth occurs via cellular hypertrophy and it is during this phase that most fetal fat and glycogen deposition takes place. The corresponding fetal growth rates during these three cell growth phases are from 5 g/day at 15 weeks, 15 to 20 g/day at 24 weeks, and 30 to 35 g/day at 34 weeks (Williams and co-authors, 1982). Owen and colleagues (1996) measured the rate of human fetal growth using ultrasound in 274 normal pregnancies, and as shown in Figure 29–2, there was considerable biological variation in the velocity of fetal growth in the last half of gestation.

Although many factors have been implicated in the process of fetal growth, the precise cellular and molecular mechanisms by which normal fetal growth occurs are not well understood. In early fetal life the major determinant of growth is the fetal genome, but later in pregnancy environmental, nutritional, and hormonal influences become increasingly important (Holmes and colleagues, 1998).

There is considerable evidence that insulin and insulin-like growth factors-I (IGF-I) and -II (IGF-II) have a role in the regulation of fetal growth and weight gain (Verhaeghe and colleagues, 1993). Insulin is secreted by fetal pancreatic β-cells primarily during the second half of gestation and is believed to stimulate somatic growth and adiposity. The insulin-like growth factors, structurally proinsulin-like polypeptides, are produced by virtually all fetal organs from early development onward and are potent stimulators of cell division and differentiation. Verhaeghe and colleagues (1993) have found that IGF-I and IGF-II and fetal insulin in the umbilical circulation are all related to fetal growth and weight gain, but that IGF-I correlates best with birthweight. Insulin is mainly related to fetal overgrowth (macrosomia), whereas IGF-binding protein may be a growth inhibitor. Holmes and colleagues (1998) found maternal levels of IGF-I to be low in women with

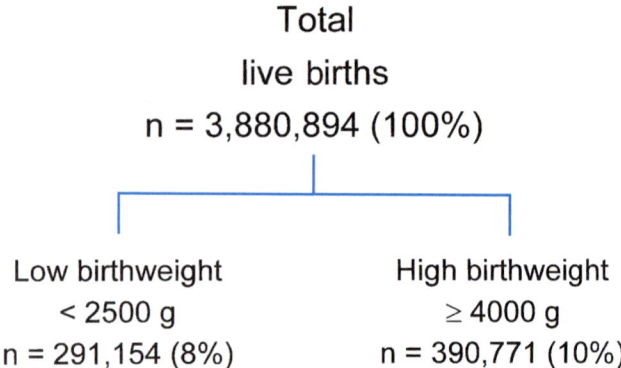

FIGURE 29–1. Births in the United States in 1997 at the extremes of fetal growth. (Ventura and co-authors, 1999.)

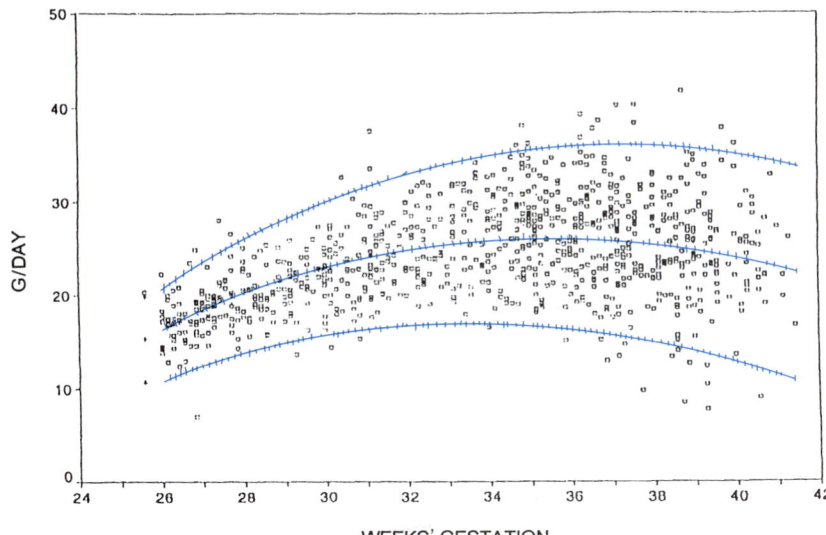

FIGURE 29–2. Increments in fetal weight in grams per day from 24 to 42 weeks' gestation. The lines represent the mean and ± 2 standard deviations. (Adapted from Owen and colleagues, 1996.)

growth-restricted fetuses and attributed this to compromised placental transfer.

Since the discovery of the "obesity gene" and its protein product, leptin, which is synthesized in adipose tissue, there has been interest in leptin levels in maternal and umbilical circulations. Fetal levels increase during the first two trimesters, and they correlate with birthweight (Sivan and colleagues, 1998; Tamura and colleagues, 1998).

Fetal growth is also dependent on an adequate supply of nutrients. Indeed, Williams (1903) in the first edition of this text aptly commented, "the increase in size of the foetus affords conclusive evidence that materials in solution must, pass from the maternal to the foetal circulation. . . ." Glucose transfer has been extensively studied during pregnancy as a result of interest in diabetes mellitus (Chap. 51). Both excessive and diminished maternal glucose availability to the fetus have been shown to affect fetal growth. In this scheme, excessive glycemia produces macrosomia whereas diminished glucose levels have been associated with fetal growth restriction. Indeed, the macrosomic infant of the mildly diabetic mother is the prototypical example of the effects of excessive maternal glucose supply. Characteristics of these infants include fetal hyperinsulinism and elevated umbilical cord levels of IGF-I and IGF-II (Roth and colleagues, 1996).

There is relatively less information concerning the physiology of maternal–fetal transfer of other nutrients such as amino acids and lipids. Ronzoni and colleagues (1999) studied maternal–fetal concentrations of amino acids in 26 normal pregnancies at the time of cesarean delivery. An increase in maternal amino acid levels lead to an increase in levels of most amino acids in the fetus. In growth-restricted fetuses, amino acid disturbance similar to the biochemical changes seen in postnatal protein-starvation states have been detected (Economides and colleagues, 1989a).

Although specific changes in lipid metabolism are associated with pregnancy—plasma triglycerides, low-density lipoprotein cholesterol, and total cholesterol all normally increase throughout gestation—studies of their fetal effects are limited. Jones and colleagues (1999) studied 38 growth-restricted infants and found impaired utilization of circulating triglycerides consistent with peripheral adipose depletion.

FETAL GROWTH RESTRICTION

In the past, low-birthweight infants who were small-for-gestational age were designated as suffering from *intrauterine growth retardation.* To avoid undue alarm in parents, to whom the term "retardation" implies abnormal mental function, the term *fetal growth restriction* is now preferred. It is estimated that from 3 to 10 percent of infants are growth restricted (Divon and Hsu, 1992).

It was not until about 30 years ago that physicians first recognized that *runting*—fetal growth restriction—was a human as well as an animal phenomenon. In 1961, Warkany and co-workers reported normal values for infant weights, lengths, and head circumferences which served to define fetal growth restriction. Gruenwald (1963) reported that approximately a third of low-birthweight infants were mature and that their small size could be explained by *chronic placental insufficiency.* These as well as observations by many others generated the concept that birthweight was governed not only by gestational length but also by fetal growth rate. It has been suggested that fetal size is largely determined in the first trimester or second half of pregnancy (Dickey and Gasser, 1993; Gluckman and Liggins, 1984). Smith and colleagues (1998) examined the relation between the outcome of 4229 pregnancies and the difference between the measured and expected ultrasound crown-rump length in the first trimester. Suboptimal first-trimester growth was associated with fetal growth restriction as well as preterm delivery between 24 and 32 weeks. It may be that suboptimal environment in the first weeks of gestation limits fetal growth for the remainder of pregnancy and that such an environment may precipitate extremely preterm delivery.

DEFINITION. In 1963 Lubchenco and co-workers from Denver published detailed comparisons of gestational ages to birthweights in an effort to derive norms for expected fetal size, and therefore growth, at a given gestational week. Battaglia and Lubchenco (1967) then classified *small-for-gestational-age* (SGA) infants as those whose weights were below the 10th percentile for their gestational age. Such infants were shown to be at increased risk for neonatal death. For example, the neonatal mortality rate of a small-for-gestational-age infant born at 38 weeks was 1 percent compared with 0.2 percent in those with appropriate birthweights. Seeds and Peng (1998) concluded that the threshold for impaired growth, based upon the risk of fetal death, should be set even higher, at the 15th birthweight percentile.

Not all infants with birthweights less than the 10th percentile are pathologically growth restricted; some are small simply because of constitutional factors. Indeed, Manning and Hohler (1991) and Gardosi and colleagues (1992) concluded that 25 to 60 percent of infants conventionally diagnosed to be small-for-gestational age were in fact appropriately grown when determinants of birthweight such as maternal ethnic group, parity, weight, and height were considered.

A definition based upon birthweight below the fifth percentile has also been proposed (Seeds, 1984). In addition, Usher and McLean (1969) proposed that fetal growth standards should be based on mean values with normal limits defined by ±2 standard deviations because this definition would limit small-for-gestational-age infants to 3 percent of births instead of 10 percent with use of the 10th percentile. From a clinical standpoint, the definition proposed by Usher and McLean (1969) appears to be most meaningful. This is because, as shown in Figure 29–3, most poor outcomes are in those infants with birthweights below the third percentile. In a study of 122,754 pregnancies delivered at Parkland Hospital, McIntire and colleagues (1999) found that mortality and morbidity were significantly increased among infants born at term only when their birthweights

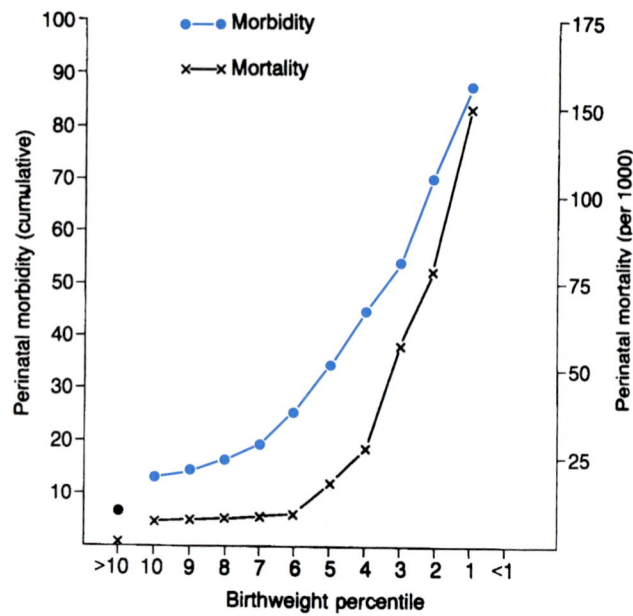

FIGURE 29–3. Relationship between birthweight percentile and perinatal mortality and morbidity observed in 1560 small-for-gestational-age fetuses. A progressive increase in both mortality and morbidity is observed as birthweight percentile falls. (From Manning, 1995, with permission.)

were at or below the third percentile for their gestational age.

NORMAL INFANT BIRTHWEIGHT. Normative data for fetal growth based upon birthweight have evolved considerably in the aftermath of the pioneering work done in Denver by Lubchenco and co-workers (1963). Their data were derived exclusively from births to white and Hispanic women who resided at high altitudes, and such infants are smaller than those born at sea level. For example, term infants average 3400 g at sea level, 3200 g at 5000 feet, and 2900 g at 10,000 feet altitude. Several fetal growth curves have been developed from various populations and geographic locations throughout the United States in the more than 30 years since Lubchenko and colleagues first described gestational age-specific birthweights. Brenner and colleagues (1976) used white and black infants delivered in Cleveland and aborted fetuses from North Carolina. Williams (1975) used live births in California to examine fetal growth curves in four ethnic groups. Ott (1993) used postnatal assessments of infants born in St. Louis. Overpeck and colleagues (1999) described birthweight standards specific to Mexican-American women. Because each of these curves was based on specific ethnic or regional groups, they were not considered to be necessarily representative of the entire population. For these reasons, fetal growth data have been derived on a nationwide

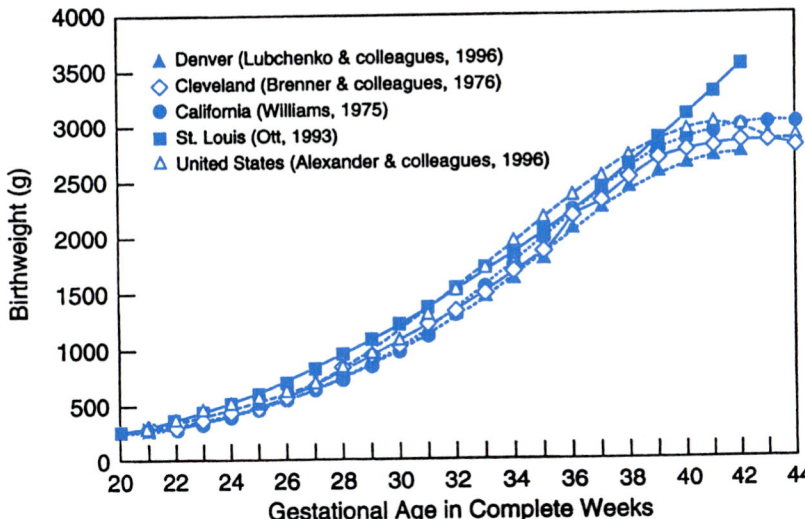

FIGURE 29–4. Comparison of fetal growth curves for infants born in different regions of the United States compared with the nation at large. (Modified from Alexander and colleagues, 1996, with permission.)

basis in both the United States and Canada (Alexander and colleagues, 1996; Arbuckle and colleagues, 1993).

Single live births to over 3.1 million mothers in the United States during 1991 were used to derive the growth curve shown in Figure 29–4. Also shown in Figure 29–4 is a comparison of the U.S. curve to those previously reported from different regions. In general, the previously published fetal growth curves underestimated the 1991 U.S. curve when used as a reference. This underestimation was most apparent between 33 and 38 weeks. Table 29–1 shows the percentiles of birthweight for each week of gestation between 20 and 44 weeks.

BIRTHWEIGHT VERSUS GROWTH. Most of what is known about normal and abnormal human fetal growth is actually based on birthweight standards, which is the endpoint of fetal growth. These standards do not reveal the *rate* of fetal growth. Indeed, such birthweight curves only reveal compromised growth at the extreme of impaired growth. Importantly, these curves cannot currently be used to identify the fetus who fails to achieve an expected or potential size, but whose birthweight exceeds the 10th percentile. Thus, birthweight percentile is an incomplete measure of growth failure. Infants of apparently appropriate birthweight, but who "cross centiles," may be exhibiting signs of malnutrition because they have not achieved their full genetic potential (Owen and colleagues, 1996). Interest in the rate or velocity of human fetal growth is very recent and depends on serial ultrasonic fetal anthropometry. Early reports suggest that a diminished growth velocity is related to cesarean delivery for fetal distress and significant fetal growth restriction (Owen and colleagues, 1997; Owen and Khan, 1998).

TABLE 29–1. Smoothed Percentiles of Birthweight (g) for Gestational Age in the United States Based on 3,134,879 Single Live Births

| Age (wk) | Percentile | | | | |
	5th	10th	50th	90th	95th
20	249	275	412	772	912
21	280	314	433	790	957
22	330	376	496	826	1023
23	385	440	582	882	1107
24	435	498	674	977	1223
25	480	558	779	1138	1397
26	529	625	899	1362	1640
27	591	702	1035	1635	1927
28	670	798	1196	1977	2237
29	772	925	1394	2361	2553
30	910	1085	1637	2710	2847
31	1088	1278	1918	2986	3108
32	1294	1495	2203	3200	3338
33	1513	1725	2458	3370	3536
34	1735	1950	2667	3502	3697
35	1950	2159	2831	3596	3812
36	2156	2354	2974	3668	3888
37	2357	2541	3117	3755	3956
38	2543	2714	3263	3867	4027
39	2685	2852	3400	3980	4107
40	2761	2929	3495	4060	4185
41	2777	2948	3527	4094	4217
42	2764	2935	3522	4098	4213
43	2741	2907	3505	4096	4178
44	2724	2885	3491	4096	4122

From Alexander and associates (1996), with permission.

METABOLIC ABNORMALITIES. Fetal blood sampling from the umbilical vein done for karyotyping of severely growth-impaired fetuses has permitted remarkable insights into pathophysiology of fetal growth (Chap. 37, p. 991). Soothill and colleagues (1987) at Kings College Hospital in London measured umbilical venous P_{O_2}, P_{CO_2}, pH, lactate and glucose concentrations, nucleated red cell count, and hemoglobin concentrations in 38 growth-restricted fetuses. The severity of fetal hypoxia correlated significantly with fetal hypercapnia, acidosis, lactic acidemia, hypoglycemia, and erythroblastosis. Subsequently, Economides and Nicolaides (1989b) found that the major cause of hypoglycemia in small-for-gestational-age fetuses was reduced supply rather than increased fetal consumption or decreased endogenous glucose production. Economides and co-workers (1989c) later found that these fetuses also had hypoinsulinemia, which they attributed to pancreatic dysfunction, as well as hypoglycemia. The degree of fetal growth restriction, however, did not correlate with plasma insulin, suggesting that it is not the primary determinant of poor fetal growth.

In children with *kwashiorkor,* the ratio of nonessential to essential amino acids is increased, presumably because of decreased intake of essential amino acids. Economides and colleagues (1989a) measured the glycine/valine ratio in umbilical vessel blood from growth-restricted fetuses and found ratios similar to those observed in children with protein deprivation and kwashiorkor. Moreover, protein deprivation correlated with fetal hypoxemia.

Economides and associates (1990) also measured plasma triglyceride concentrations in small but appropriate-for-gestational-age fetuses as well as growth-restricted fetuses. Growth-restricted fetuses demonstrated hypertriglyceridemia that was correlated with the degree of fetal hypoxemia. They hypothesized that hypoglycemic, growth-restricted fetuses mobilize adipose tissue, and that the hypertriglyceridemia is the result of lipolysis of fetal fat stores. Other findings include observations that growth-restricted fetuses may be thrombocytopenic, and that the degree of platelet abnormality is correlated with the degree of growth restriction, hypoxemia, and acidemia (Van den Hof and Nicolaides, 1990).

In fetuses with growth restriction, plasma adenosine concentrations are elevated. Yoneyama and associates (1994) postulate that this represents an adaptive response to chronic asphyxia. Elevations in interleukin-10, placental atrial natriuretic peptide, and plasma endothelin-1 concentrations, as well as a defect in epidermal growth factor function, have also been described in growth-restricted fetuses (Varner and colleagues, 1996). These findings suggest a possible role for abnormal immune activation and abnormal placentation in the gene-

sis of this condition (Gabriel, 1994; Heyborne, 1994; Kingdom, 1994; McQueen, 1993; Neerhof, 1995, and all their associates). In animals, chronic reduction in nitric oxide, an endothelium-derived, locally acting vasorelaxant, has also been shown to result in diminished fetal growth (Diket and associates, 1994).

Fetal heart rate monitoring for 30 to 60 minutes was performed immediately before cordocentesis and results compared with fetal blood gases (Visser and colleagues, 1990). Repetitive fetal heart rate decelerations best identified hypoxemic growth-restricted fetuses. Several small infants with low normal P_{O_2} values still demonstrated heart rate acceleration. Such accelerations, however, indicated the absence of potentially damaging degrees of hypoxemia or acidosis.

MORTALITY AND MORBIDITY. As shown in Figure 29–3, fetal growth restriction is associated with substantive perinatal morbidity and mortality. Fetal demise, birth asphyxia, meconium aspiration, and neonatal hypoglycemia and hypothermia are all increased, as is the prevalence of abnormal neurological development (Paz and associates, 1995; Piper and colleagues, 1996). This is true for both term and preterm infants (Minior and Divon, 1998). Kok and colleagues (1998) analyzed the outcome up to 9 years of age of growth-restricted infants less than 32 weeks at birth. They found the mortality risk for growth-restricted infants was significantly increased compared with appropriately grown preterm infants. Growth-restricted preterm infants also more often required special education.

Postnatal growth and development of the growth-restricted fetus depends on the cause of restriction, nutrition in infancy, and the social environment (Kliegman, 1997). Infants with growth restriction due to congenital viral, chromosomal, or maternal constitutional factors remain small throughout life. Those infants with in utero growth restriction due to placental insufficiency will often have catch-up growth after birth and approach their inherited growth potential when provided with an optimal environment. Similarly, neurodevelopmental outcome of the growth-restricted fetus is influenced by postnatal environment. Such infants born to families of higher socioeconomic status demonstrate few developmental problems during follow-up, whereas those born to poorer families have significant developmental handicaps.

ACCELERATED MATURATION. There have been numerous reports describing accelerated fetal pulmonary maturation in complicated pregnancies associated with growth restriction (Perelman and colleagues, 1985). One explanation for this phenomenon is that the fetus responds to a stressed environment by increasing adrenal glucocorticoid production, which leads to earlier or accelerated fetal lung maturation (Laatikainen and associates, 1988). Although this concept pervades modern perinatal thinking, there is little clinical information to substantiate that pregnancy complications convey a fetal advantage.

Owen and associates (1990) analyzed perinatal outcomes in 178 pregnancies delivered primarily because of hypertension. They compared these with 159 pregnancies delivered because of spontaneous preterm labor or ruptured membranes. They concluded that a "stressed" pregnancy, which often resulted in small-for-gestational-age infants, did not confer an appreciable survival advantage. Similar findings were reported by Friedman and colleagues (1995) in women with fetal growth restriction due to severe preeclampsia. Two studies from Parkland Hospital substantiate that fetal growth restriction confers no apparent advantage to the preterm infant (McIntire and colleagues, 1999; Tyson and colleagues, 1995). Smulian and colleagues (2000) analyzed U.S. national linked birth–infant death data for 1995 and 1996 to determine deaths during the first 12 months of life for infants with birthweights less than the 10th percentile. Compared with uncomplicated pregnancies, growth-restricted infants had higher death rates during infancy.

SYMMETRICAL VERSUS ASYMMETRICAL FETAL GROWTH RESTRICTION. Campbell and Thoms (1977) described the use of the sonographic *head-to-abdomen circumference ratio* (*HC/AC*) to differentiate fetuses into the subtypes "symmetrical," meaning proportionately small, and "asymmetrical," referring to those with disproportionately lagging abdominal growth. These authors constructed an HC/AC ratio nomogram from approximately 500 normal fetuses and evaluated its use in 31 fetuses at risk for uteroplacental insufficiency. The 70 percent of fetuses with an HC/AC ratio above the 95th percentile were termed asymmetrical. They found that although asymmetrical fetuses had relatively larger brains and were "preferentially protected from the full effects of the growth-retarding stimulus," they were at significantly greater risk for severe preeclampsia, fetal distress, operative intervention, and lower Apgar scores than their symmetrical counterparts.

It is compelling to relate the type of growth restriction to the onset or etiology of a particular insult. An early insult due to chemical exposure, viral infection, or inherent cellular development abnormality caused by aneuploidy could theoretically result in a relative decrease in cell number as well as cell size. The resultant proportionate reduction in both head and body size has been termed *symmetrical growth restriction.* Conversely, a late pregnancy insult such as placental insufficiency associated with hypertension would theoretically affect primarily cell size. Because placental insufficiency may

result in diminished glucose transfer and hepatic storage, fetal abdominal circumference—which reflects liver size—would be reduced. This concept, however, has been challenged (Roberts and co-authors, 1999). Simultaneously, it is proposed that there is preferential shunting of oxygen and nutrients to the brain, which allows normal brain and head growth. This sequence of events can theoretically result in *asymmetrical growth restriction* with an abnormally increased relative brain size compared with the small liver. Because the fetal brain is normally relatively large and the liver relatively small, the ratio of brain weight to liver weight—usually about 3 to 1—over the last 12 weeks is increased to 5 to 1 or more in many severely growth-restricted infants (Fig. 29–5).

Although these generalizations about the potential pathophysiology of symmetrical versus asymmetrical growth restriction are interesting from a conceptual standpoint, there is considerable evidence that fetal growth patterns are more complex. For example, Nicolaides and co-authors (1991) compared the ratios of fetal head-to-abdominal circumference in 376 growth-restricted fetuses with and without normal karyotypes. Those with aneuploidy typically had disproportionately large head sizes and were therefore *asymmetrically* growth restricted rather than the hypothetically expected symmetrical pattern. Similarly, most preterm infants with growth restriction due to preeclampsia and associated uteroplacental insufficiency demonstrate a

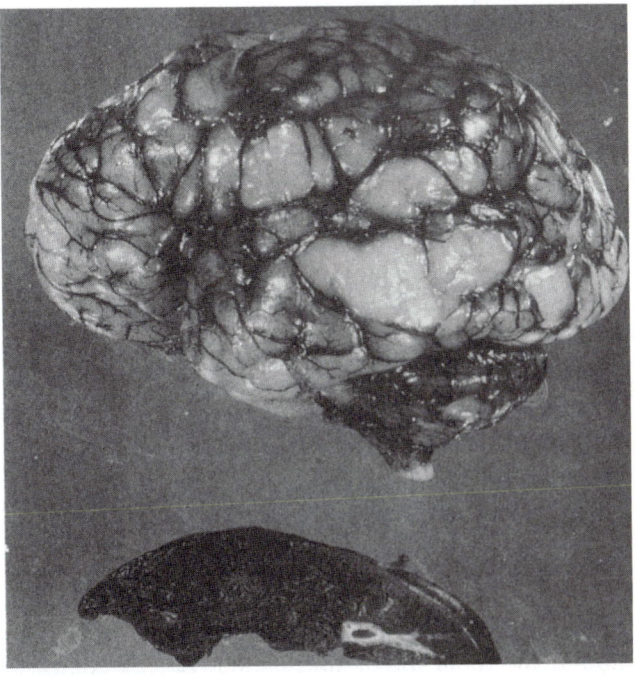

FIGURE 29–5. Brain and coronal liver slice from an infant of 1100 g in weight at 34 weeks. Brain-to-liver weight ratio is 6:1. (From Wigglesworth and Singer, 1991, with permission.)

symmetrical pattern of growth impairment rather than the hypothesized asymmetrical pattern (Salafia and co-authors, 1995).

Recognition of symmetrical and asymmetrical patterns of impaired fetal growth has prompted considerable interest in the antepartum diagnosis of these two forms because the pattern may potentially reveal the cause. This has been particularly true with ultrasonic evaluation of fetal growth restriction, where several fetal dimensions are now measured and can be related to each other. Crane and Kopta (1980) analyzed several anthropometric measurements in growth-restricted newborns and concluded that the concept of brain sparing was erroneous and could not be used to diagnose the cause of individual fetal growth restriction. Dashe and colleagues (2000) analyzed head-to-abdominal circumference ratios in 8722 consecutive liveborn singletons delivered at Parkland Hospital and who underwent ultrasound examinations within 4 weeks of delivery. Only 20 percent of growth-restricted fetuses demonstrated head-to-abdomen asymmetry, but importantly, these fetuses were at increased risk for intrapartum and neonatal complications. Symmetrically growth-restricted fetuses with birthweights less than the 10th percentile, when compared with those appropriately grown, were not at increased risk for adverse outcomes. It was concluded that asymmetrical fetal growth restriction represented significantly disordered fetal growth, whereas symmetrical growth restriction more likely represented normal, genetically determined small stature.

RISK FACTORS

CONSTITUTIONALLY SMALL MOTHERS. Small women typically have smaller babies. If a woman begins pregnancy weighing less than 100 pounds, the risk of delivering a small-for-gestational-age infant is increased at least twofold (Simpson and colleagues, 1975). Data from a longitudinal study of all births during one week in 1958 in England, Wales, and Scotland indicate that there are intergenerational effects on birthweight that are transmitted through the maternal line (Emanuel and associates, 1992). Klebanoff and co-authors (1997) also reported that reduced intrauterine growth of the mother is a risk factor for reduced intrauterine growth of her children. Whether or not the phenomenon of a small mother giving birth to a small infant is nature or nurture is unclear. Brooks and co-authors (1995) analyzed 62 births after ovum donation to examine the relative influence of the donor versus the recipient on birthweight. They concluded that the environment provided by the mother was more important than her genetic contribution to birthweight. Cryopreservation of embryos does not adversely affect fetal or postnatal growth (Wennerholm and colleagues, 1998).

POOR MATERNAL WEIGHT GAIN AND NUTRITION. In the woman of average or low weight, lack of weight gain throughout pregnancy may be associated with fetal growth restriction (Simpson and colleagues, 1975). Lack of weight gain in the second trimester is strongly correlated with decreased birthweight (Abrams and Selvin, 1995). If the mother is large and otherwise healthy, however, below-average maternal weight gain without maternal disease is unlikely to be associated with appreciable fetal growth restriction.

As discussed in Chapter 10 (p. 231), marked restriction of weight gain during the last half of pregnancy should not be encouraged. Even so, it appears that caloric restriction to less than 1500 kcal/day adversely affects fetal growth only minimally (Lechtig and co-workers, 1975). The best documented effect of famine on fetal growth was in the winter of 1944 in Holland, when the German Army restricted dietary intake to 600 kcal/day for all citizens, including pregnant women. The famine persisted for 28 weeks and there was an average birthweight decrease of 250 g (Stein and colleagues, 1975). Although there was only a small mean decrease in birthweight, fetal mortality rates increased significantly.

SOCIAL DEPRIVATION. The effect of social deprivation on birthweight is interconnected to the effects of associated lifestyle factors such as smoking, alcohol or other substance abuse, and poor nutrition. Wilcox and associates (1995), in a study of 7493 British women, found that the most socially deprived mothers had the smallest babies. Similarly, Dejin-Karlsson and colleagues (2000) prospectively studied a cohort of Swedish women and found that lack of psychosocial resources influenced the risk of growth-restricted infants. Almost 100 years ago, Williams, commenting in the first edition of this text (1903), wrote: "The social condition of the mother and the comforts by which she is surrounded also exert a marked influence upon the child's weight, heavier children being more common in the upper walks of life."

FETAL INFECTIONS. Viral, bacterial, protozoan, and spirochetal infections have been implicated in up to 5 percent of cases of fetal growth restriction (Klein and Remington, 1995). The best known of these are infections caused by rubella and cytomegalovirus (Lin and Evans, 1984; Stagno and associates, 1977). Mechanisms affecting fetal growth appear to be different with these two viral infections. *Cytomegalovirus* is associated with direct cytolysis and loss of functional cells. *Rubella* infection causes vascular insufficiency by damaging the endothelium of small vessels. Cell division rate is also reduced in congenital rubella infections (Pollack and Divon, 1992). *Hepatitis A and B* are associated with preterm delivery but may also adversely affect fetal growth (Waterson, 1979). *Listeriosis, tuberculosis,* and *syphilis* have been reported to cause fetal growth restriction. Paradoxically, in cases of syphilis, the placenta is almost always increased in weight and size due to edema and perivascular inflammation (Varner and Galask, 1984). *Toxoplasmosis* is the protozoan infection most often associated with compromised fetal growth, but *congenital malaria* may produce the same result (Varner and Galask, 1984).

CONGENITAL MALFORMATIONS. In a study of over 13,000 infants with major structural anomalies, 22 percent had accompanying growth restriction (Khoury and associates, 1988). In general, the more severe the malformation, the more likely the fetus is to be small-for-gestational age. This is especially evident in fetuses with chromosomal abnormalities or those with serious cardiovascular malformations.

CHROMOSOMAL ABNORMALITIES. Placentas of fetuses with autosomal trisomies have a reduced number of small muscular arteries in the tertiary stem villi (Rochelson and associates, 1990). Thus, both placental insufficiency and primary abnormal cellular growth and differentiation may contribute to the significant degree of fetal growth restriction often associated with karyotype abnormalities. In a series of 458 fetuses with no sonographically visible structural anomalies, Snijders and co-workers (1993) found karyotype abnormalities in 20 percent. In the presence of growth restriction and fetal anomalies, the prevalence of chromosome abnormalities was even greater.

Although postnatal growth failure is prominent in children with *trisomy 21,* fetal growth restriction is generally mild (Thelander and Pryor, 1966). In fact, their mean birthweight was 2900 g. A significant first-trimester lag in crown-rump length among fetuses with trisomy 21 has been observed by some investigators, but not others (Golbus 1978; Stephens and Shepard, 1980). After the first trimester, the length of all long bones in fetuses with trisomy 21 lags behind those of normal fetuses (Fitzsimmons and colleagues, 1990). Both shortened femur length and hypoplasia of the middle phalanx have been documented with increased frequency with trisomy 21.

In contrast to the mild and variable growth restriction that accompanies trisomy 21, fetuses with *trisomy 18* are virtually always significantly affected. In one series of trisomy 18 newborns, 10 of 11 weighed less than 2500 g at birth (Moerman and associates, 1982). Growth failure has been documented as early as the first trimester. By the second trimester, long bone measurements typically fall below the third percentile for age, and the upper extremity is more severely affected than the lower

(Droste and co-workers, 1990). Visceral organ growth is also abnormal in this condition (Droste, 1992). Some degree of growth restriction is also commonly present in fetuses with trisomy 13, but it is generally not as severe as in trisomy 18.

Significant fetal growth restriction is not seen with *Turner syndrome* (45,X or gonadal dysgenesis) or *Klinefelter syndrome* (47,XXY) (Droste, 1992).

TRISOMY 16. Trisomy 16 is the most common trisomy in spontaneous abortions and is usually, if not always, lethal to the fetus in the nonmosaic state (Lindor and associates, 1993). As discussed in Chapter 36 (p. 949), patches of trisomy 16 in the placenta—called *confined placental mosaicism*—lead to placental insufficiency that may account for many cases of previously unexplained fetal growth restriction (Kalousek and colleagues, 1993). In these pregnancies, the chromosome abnormality is confined to the placenta. Wolstenholme (1995) has reviewed the significance of trisomy 16 placental mosaicism from gametogenesis to term and onwards.

PRIMARY DISORDERS OF CARTILAGE AND BONE. Numerous inherited syndromes such as *osteogenesis imperfecta* and various chondrodystrophies are associated with fetal growth restriction (Chap. 39, p. 1068).

CHEMICAL TERATOGENS. Any teratogen is capable of adversely affecting fetal growth. These are considered in detail in Chapter 38. Some *anticonvulsants,* such as phenytoin and trimethadione, may produce specific and characteristic syndromes that include fetal growth restriction (Hanson and co-workers, 1976). *Cigarette smoking* causes growth restriction as well as preterm delivery in a direct relationship with the number of cigarettes smoked (Cliver and associates, 1995; Shah and Bracken, 2000). *Narcotics* and related drugs act by decreasing maternal food intake and fetal cell number. *Alcohol* is a potent teratogen that acts in a linear dose-related fashion. *Cocaine* use is also associated with poor fetal weight gain (LeBlanc and co-workers, 1987). Miller and associates (1995) have suggested that this may be a result of frequent cigarette use and poor prenatal care, rather than a direct effect of cocaine.

VASCULAR DISEASE. Chronic vascular disease, especially when further complicated by superimposed preeclampsia, commonly causes growth restriction. Preeclampsia itself may cause fetal growth failure, especially when the onset is before 37 weeks (Xiong and colleagues, 1999). As discussed in Chapter 24 (p. 570), fetal growth restriction with preeclampsia is a marker of severity.

CHRONIC RENAL DISEASE. Renal disease may be accompanied by restricted fetal growth (Cunningham and colleagues, 1990; Stettler and Cunningham, 1992).

CHRONIC HYPOXIA. When exposed to a chronically hypoxic environment, some fetuses have significant reduction in birthweight. As discussed earlier, fetuses of women who reside at high altitude usually weigh less than those born to women who live at a lower altitude. Lichty and colleagues (1957), reported a mean difference of 250 g among infants born to Peruvian women at altitudes above 10,000 feet compared with those at sea level. As discussed in Chapter 44 (p. 1193), fetuses of women with cyanotic heart disease are frequently severely growth-restricted (Patton and co-worker, 1990).

MATERNAL ANEMIA. In most cases, anemia does not cause growth restriction. Exceptions include sickle cell disease or other inherited anemias associated with serious maternal disease. Conversely, deficient total maternal blood volume early in pregnancy has been linked to fetal growth restriction (Duvekot and colleagues, 1995).

PLACENTAL AND CORD ABNORMALITIES. Chronic partial placental separation, extensive infarction, or chorioangioma are likely to cause restricted fetal growth. A circumvallate placenta or a placenta previa may impair growth, but usually the fetus is not markedly smaller than normal. Marginal insertion of the cord and especially velamentous insertions are more likely to be accompanied by a growth-restricted fetus (Chap. 32, p. 833).

Many cases of fetal growth restriction occur in pregnancies with apparently normal fetuses with grossly normal placentas. Growth failure in these cases is often presumed to be due to *uteroplacental insufficiency.* Women with otherwise unexplained fetal growth restriction demonstrated a fourfold reduction in uteroplacental blood flow compared with normally grown fetuses (Lunell and Nylund, 1992). Similar reductions were also seen in growth-restricted fetuses with congenital malformations, suggesting that maternal blood flow may in part be regulated by the fetus (Howard, 1987; Rankin and McLaughlin, 1979). Uteroplacental blood flow is also reduced in women with preeclampsia compared with normotensive women. Interestingly, macrosomic infants do not have increased uteroplacental blood flow (Lunell and Nylund, 1992).

MULTIPLE FETUSES. As shown in Figure 29–6, pregnancy with two or more fetuses is more likely to be complicated by diminished growth of one or both fetuses compared with normal singletons (Chap. 30, p. 778). Growth restriction has been reported in 10 to 50 percent of twins (Hill and associates, 1994).

ANTIPHOSPHOLIPID ANTIBODY SYNDROME. Two classes of antiphospholipid antibodies have been associated with fetal growth restriction—*anticardiolipin antibodies* and *lupus anticoagulant* (Lockwood and Rand, 1994). These syndromes are considered in detail in Chapters 33 (p. 860) and 52 (p. 1384). Pregnancy outcome in women with these antibodies is often poor, and may also involve early-onset preeclampsia and second or third trimester fetal demise (Branch and associates, 1992). Maternal morbidity due to vascular thrombotic events is not uncommon. Pathophysiological mechanisms in the fetus appear to be caused by maternal platelet aggregation and placental thrombosis. These

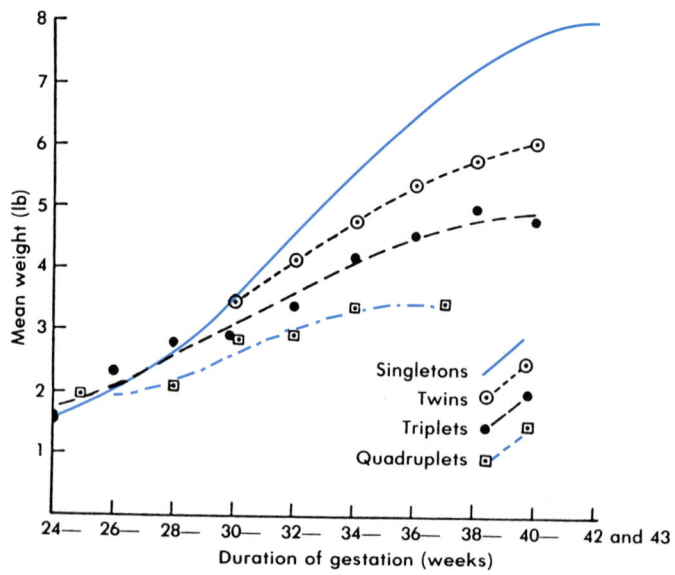

FIGURE 29–6. Birthweight and gestational age relationships in multifetal gestations. (From McKeown and Record, 1952, with permission.)

antibodies may also be suspected in women demonstrating repetitive second-trimester fetal loss or early-onset fetal growth restriction, especially when accompanied by early, severe hypertensive disease.

EXTRAUTERINE PREGNANCY. The fetus gestated outside the uterus is usually growth-restricted (Chap. 34, p. 887). Also, some maternal uterine malformations have been linked to impaired fetal growth (Chap. 35, p. 915).

SCREENING AND IDENTIFICATION OF FETAL GROWTH RESTRICTION. Early establishment of gestational age, attention to maternal weight gain, and careful measurement of uterine fundal growth throughout pregnancy will serve to identify many cases of abnormal fetal growth in women without risk factors. Identification of risk factors, including a *previously growth-restricted fetus,* should raise the possibility of recurrence during the current pregnancy. In women with significant risk factors, consideration should be given to serial sonography. Although their frequency will vary depending upon clinical circumstances, an initial dating examination, followed by a second examination at 32 to 34 weeks, should serve to identify many cases of growth restriction. If clinical findings suggest inadequate fetal growth prior to this time, earlier sonography is done. *Definitive diagnosis,* however, usually cannot be made until delivery.

Identification of the inappropriately growing fetus remains a challenge. This is underscored by the fact that such identification is not always possible even in the nursery. Regardless, there are both simple clinical techniques and more complex technologies that may prove useful in helping to exclude and diagnose fetal growth restriction. Some of the widely used techniques, as well as those of potential use, are described next.

UTERINE FUNDAL HEIGHT. Carefully performed serial fundal height measurements throughout gestation are a simple, safe, inexpensive, and reasonably accurate *screening* method to detect many small-for-gestational-age fetuses (Gardosi and Francis, 1999). Its principal drawback is imprecision. Jensen and Larsen (1991) and Walraven and colleagues (1995) found that symphysis-to-fundus measurements helped to correctly identify only 40 percent of such infants. Thus, small-for-age infants were both overlooked and overdiagnosed. Despite this, these results do not diminish the importance of carefully performed fundal measurements as a simple screening method.

The method used in most clinics in the United States was reported by Jimenez and colleagues (1983). Briefly this consists of a tape calibrated in centimeters being applied over the abdominal curvature from the upper edge of the symphysis to the upper edge of the uterine fundus, which is identified by palpation or percussion. The tape is applied with the markings away from the examiner to avoid bias. Between 18 and 30 weeks, the uterine fundal height in centimeters coincides with weeks of gestation. If the measurement is more than 2 to 3 cm from the expected height, inappropriate fetal growth may be suspected.

ULTRASONIC MEASUREMENTS. Central to the debate over whether all pregnancies should routinely receive ultrasonic evaluations is the potential for diagnosis of fetal growth restriction (Ewigman and colleagues, 1993) (Chap. 41, p. 1113). Typically, such routine screening incorporates an ultrasound examination at 16 to 20 weeks to establish gestational age and rule out visible anomalies, and then follow-up imaging at 32 to 34 weeks to evaluate fetal growth.

The optimal ultrasonographic method of estimating fetal size, and therefore fetal growth restriction, was reviewed by Manning (1995). Combining head, abdomen, and femur dimensions should in theory enhance the accuracy of predictions of fetal size. Unfortunately, any potential improvement is apparently lost by the cumulative error inherent in measurement of each individual fetal dimension. As a result, abdominal circumference measurements have been accepted by most experts as the most reliable index of fetal size (Manning, 1995; Smith and colleagues, 1997; Snijders and Nicolaides, 1994). In these studies, the estimated fetal weight calculated with abdominal circumference measurements was almost always within 10 percent of the actual birthweight (Fig. 29–7).

Interestingly, abdominal circumference measured directly in the newborn was also shown to be an important anatomical marker of growth restriction (Deter and colleagues, 1995). The elegant observations on the metabolic effects of fetal growth restriction, performed at Kings College Hospital and described earlier, were all obtained in fetuses diagnosed to have growth restriction because their ultrasonic abdominal circumference was less than the fifth percentile for age (Snijders and Nicolaides, 1994). As shown in Figure 29–8, such small abdominal circumferences are linked to decreased P_{O_2} and pH. These observations emphasize that sonographic measurements of the abdominal circumference can meaningfully signify pathological fetal growth restriction.

Use of ultrasound for detection of fetal growth restriction does not preclude missed diagnoses. Dashe and colleagues (2001) studied 8400 live births at Parkland Hospital who had antepartum ultrasound within 4 weeks of delivery. They found that although 70 percent of growth-restricted fetuses were detected, 30 percent were missed.

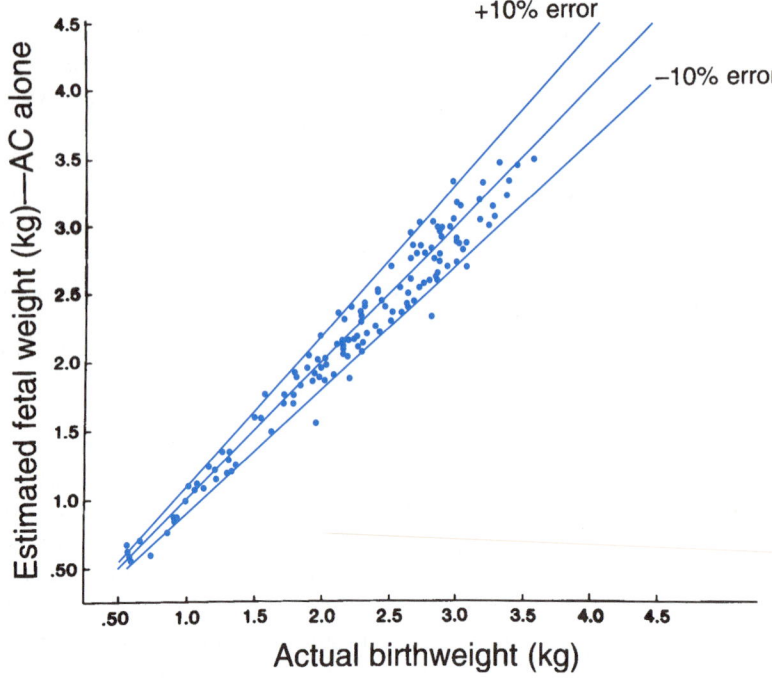

FIGURE 29–7. Correlation of fetal weight estimation using abdominal circumference (AC) with actual birthweight in 175 fetuses with birthweights ranging from 400 to 3600 g. Within this weight range, the range of error was ± 10 percent in all but eight perinates. (From Manning, 1995, with permission.)

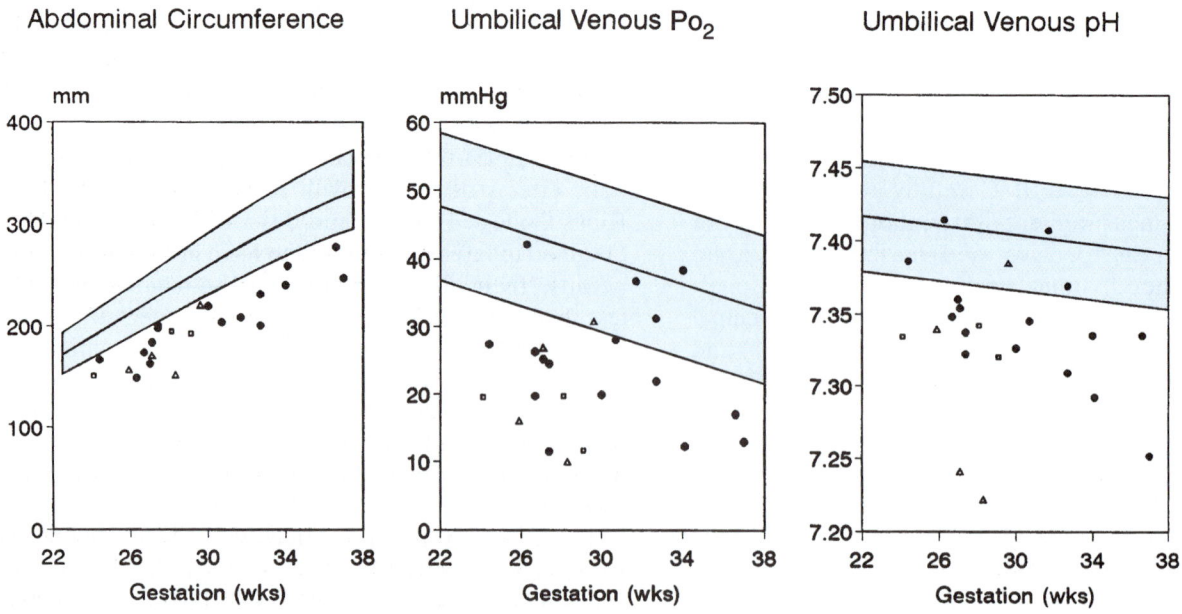

FIGURE 29–8. Abdominal circumference and umbilical venous blood Po_2 and pH in growth-restricted fetuses (▲ = fetal deaths; ● = neonatal deaths). The lines within and bordering the shaded areas are the mean, 5th, and 95th percentiles for gestational age. (From Hecher and colleagues, 1995, with permission.)

Larsen and colleagues (1992) performed ultrasound beginning at 28 weeks and every 3 weeks thereafter in 1000 pregnancies at risk for fetal growth restriction. They randomly withheld the results from clinicians. Revealing the results of ultrasonic estimates of growth during the third trimester significantly increased diagnosis of small-for-gestational-age fetuses. In this same group, elective deliveries also increased, but without overall improvement in neonatal mortality or morbidity. Thus, while this method of screening improved the diagnosis, it did not improve fetal outcome. Goldenberg and colleagues (1989) found that as the percentage of pregnancies undergoing ultrasound increased, fetal growth restriction decreased. This was attributed to accurate gestational age information obtained using ultrasound.

An association between oligohydramnios and pathological fetal growth restriction has long been recognized (Chap. 31, p. 821). As shown in Figure 29–9, the smaller the vertical dimension of a sonographically measured pocket of amnionic fluid, the greater the perinatal mortality. The likely explanation for oligohydramnios (Nicolaides and associates, 1990) is diminished fetal urine production caused by hypoxia and diminished renal blood flow.

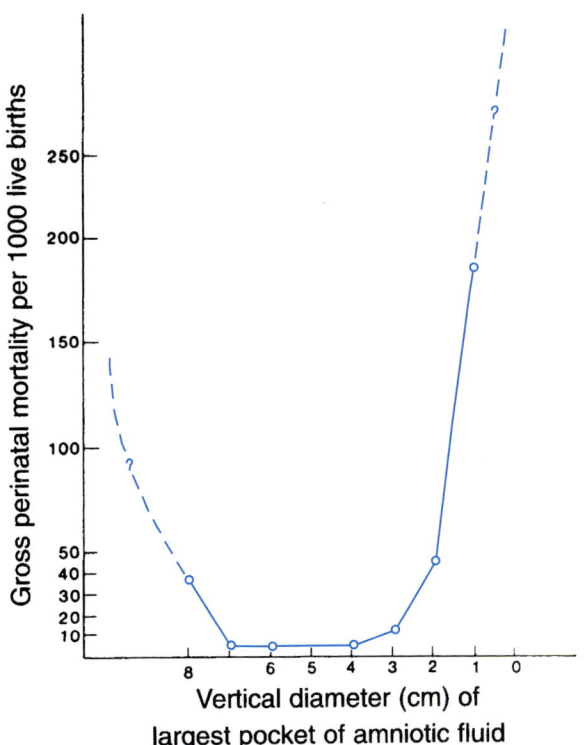

FIGURE 29–9. Relationship of amnionic fluid volume, as determined by the largest vertical pocket method, to perinatal mortality. Mortality rises significantly when the largest pocket of fluid falls below 2 cm. (From Manning, 1995, with permission.)

DOPPLER VELOCIMETRY. Abnormal umbilical artery Doppler velocimetry—characterized by absent or reversed end-diastolic flow signifying increased impedance—has been uniquely associated with fetal growth restriction (American College of Obstetricians and Gynecologists, 2000). An example of this is shown in Figure 29–10. The use of Doppler velocimetry in the management of fetal growth restriction has been recommended as a possible adjunct to other fetal evaluation techniques such as nonstress tests or biophysical profiles (American College of Obstetricians and Gynecologists, 2000a). Doppler velocimetry is more extensively reviewed in Chapter 41 (p. 1132).

MANAGEMENT. Once a growth-restricted fetus is suspected, efforts should be made to confirm the diagnosis, and if so, to determine if the fetus has anomalies or is in poor physiological condition. Some practitioners have performed cordocentesis for rapid karyotyping because detection of lethal aneuploidy may obviate cesarean delivery. Conversely, the American College of Obstetricians and Gynecologists (2000a) has concluded that there are not enough data to warrant cordocentesis for management of fetal growth restriction. The timing of delivery is crucial and the clinician must often weigh the risks of fetal death against the hazards of preterm delivery.

GROWTH RESTRICTION NEAR TERM. Prompt delivery is likely to afford the best outcome for the fetus who is considered growth restricted at or near term. In the presence of significant oligohydramnios, most fetuses will be delivered if gestational age has reached 34 weeks or beyond. Assuming that the fetal heart rate pattern is reassuring, vaginal delivery may be attempted. Unfortunately, such fetuses often tolerate labor less well than their appropriately grown counterparts, and cesarean delivery is necessary for intrapartum fetal compromise. Importantly, uncertainty about the diagnosis of fetal growth restriction should preclude intervention until fetal lung maturity is assured. Expectant management can be guided using antepartum fetal surveillance techniques described in Chapter 40.

GROWTH RESTRICTION REMOTE FROM TERM. When a growth-restricted fetus is diagnosed prior to 34 weeks, and amnionic fluid volume and antepartum fetal surveillance are normal, observation is recommended. A sonographic search is made for fetal anomalies. Sonography is repeated at intervals of 2 to 3 weeks. As long as there is continued growth and fetal evaluation remains normal, pregnancy is allowed to continue until fetal maturity is achieved; otherwise, delivery is effected. At times, amniocentesis for assessment of pulmonary maturity may be helpful in clinical decision making.

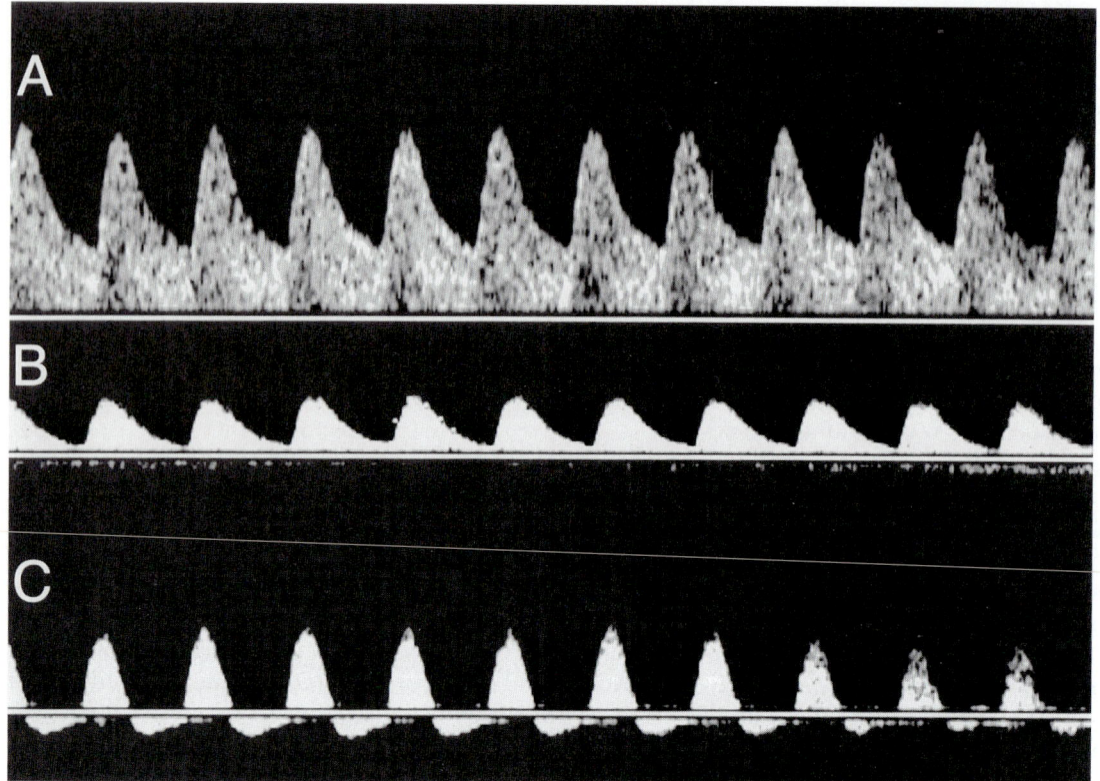

FIGURE 29–10. Fetal umbilical arterial Doppler velocimetry studies, ranging from normal to markedly abnormal. **A.** Normal velocimetry pattern with an S/D ratio of <30. **B.** The diastolic velocity of zero reflects increased placental vascular resistance. **C.** During diastole, arterial velocity is reversed (negative S/D ratio). This is an ominous sign that may precede fetal demise. (Courtesy of Dr. Diane Twickler.)

Oligohydramnios is highly suggestive of fetal growth failure although a normal amnionic fluid volume does not preclude fetal growth restriction. Screening for toxoplasmosis, rubella, cytomegalovirus, herpes, and other viral agents is recommended by some clinicians, but we have not generally found this to be productive in most cases.

With growth restriction remote from term, there is no specific treatment that will ameliorate the condition. There is no evidence that bed rest actually results in accelerated fetal growth or improved outcome in growth-restricted fetuses. Despite this, many clinicians advise a program of modified rest in the lateral recumbent position in which maternal cardiac output—and presumably placental perfusion—is maximized. Nutrient supplementation, plasma volume expansion, oxygen therapy, antihypertensive drugs, heparin, and aspirin have not been shown to be effective (American College of Obstetricians and Gynecologists, 2000a).

In most cases of growth restriction diagnosed prior to term, neither a precise etiology nor a specific therapy is apparent. Management decisions in such cases hinge upon an assessment of the relative risks of fetal death with continued antepartum evaluation versus risks from preterm delivery. Although reassuring tests of fetal well-being will in many cases allow safe observation and continued maturation of preterm significantly growth-restricted fetuses, there is concern for their long-term neurological outcome (Blair and Stanley, 1992). Indeed, although it is generally believed various tests of fetal well-being appear to be effective in reducing risks for fetal death, some challenge this belief. Weiner and colleagues (1996) performed nonstress tests, biophysical profiles, and umbilical artery velocimetry within 3 days of delivery in 135 fetuses who, at birth, were confirmed to have growth restriction. Other than metabolic acidosis at birth, which was predicted by absent or reversed end-diastolic umbilical artery velocimetry, morbidity and mortality in the growth-restricted fetuses were determined primarily by gestational age and birthweight and not by abnormal fetal testing. Moreover, there is no convincing evidence that any such testing scheme reduces the risk of survival with long-term neurological deficit (American College of Obstetricians and Gynecologists, 2000a). Thus, the optimal management of the preterm growth-restricted fetus remains problematic.

LABOR AND DELIVERY. Throughout labor, spontaneous or induced, those fetuses suspected of being growth restricted should be monitored for evidence of compromise, most commonly manifested by fetal heart rate abnormalities. Fetal growth restriction is commonly the result of insufficient placental function as a consequence of faulty maternal perfusion, ablation of functional placenta, or both. These conditions are likely aggravated by labor. Importantly, diminished amnionic fluid volume also predisposes to cord compression and its dangers. Cesarean delivery is also increased in fetal growth restriction because breech presentation occurs more commonly (Sherer and colleagues, 1996).

It can be anticipated that the infant may need expert assistance in making a successful transition to air breathing. The fetus is at risk of being born hypoxic and of having aspirated meconium. It is essential that care for the newborn be provided immediately by someone who can skillfully clear the airway below the vocal cords, especially of meconium, and ventilate the infant as needed. The severely growth-restricted newborn is particularly susceptible to hypothermia and may also develop other metabolic derangements such as hypoglycemia, polycythemia, and hyperviscosity.

RECURRENT FETAL GROWTH RESTRICTION. The risk of fetal growth restriction is increased in subsequent pregnancies (Bakketeig and colleagues, 1986). This is particularly true in women with both a history of growth restriction and a continuing medical complication (Patterson and colleagues, 1986).

BARKER HYPOTHESIS. Barker and colleagues at the United Kingdom Medical Research Unit have over the past 12 years been responsible for a series of remarkable publications in which causes of adult mortality and morbidity have been related to fetal and infant life (Fraser and Cresswell, 1997). Most interesting, in the context of fetal growth restriction, is the suggestion that there is a relationship between suboptimal fetal nutrition and an increased risk for hypertension and atherosclerosis later in life. Although fascinating, it is important to emphasize the investigational nature of this hypothesis.

MACROSOMIA

Macrosomia is a term used rather imprecisely to describe a very large fetus-neonate. There is general agreement among obstetricians that newborns weighing less than 4000 g are not excessively large; but a similar consensus has not been reached that permits a precise definition of macrosomia. Indeed, the term macrosomia does not appear in the *New Shorter Oxford English Dictionary* (1993) although *Stedman's Medical Dictionary* (1995) offers the definition of "abnormally large size of the body." The key word is "abnormal." What is the threshold for the upper limit of normal human fetal growth above which birthweight is abnormal? What criteria should be used to define "abnormal"? For example, should the threshold for abnormal high birthweight be simply mathematically derived or should it include features of adverse pregnancy outcome? Given that the major hazard of excessive fetal growth is birth injury due to shoulder dystocia, should the threshold for excessive growth be defined in terms of the risk of brachial plexus injury? But this approach cannot entirely suffice to diagnose excessive and abnormal fetal growth because shoulder dystocia would not be expected in an overgrown but preterm and thus physically small infant.

Newborn weight rarely exceeds 11 pounds (5000 g) and excessively large infants are still a curiosity. The birth of a 16-pound (7300 g) infant in the United States in 1979 was widely publicized. Two of the largest newborn weights ever recorded were those of a nearly 24-pound (10,800 g) infant described by Beach in 1879 (Barnes, 1957), and a 25-pound stillborn cited in Chapter 7 (p. 134). Among almost 170,000 infants who were delivered at Parkland Hospital between 1988 and 1999, only one weighed 6000 g or more for an incidence less than 1 in 200,000 births. This infant weighed 6025 g (13 lbs 4 oz) and was delivered by repeat cesarean incision to a 329-lb diabetic woman. The incidence of excessively large infants seems to have increased during the 20th century. For example, the incidence of birthweight 5000 g or greater was approximately 1 to 2 per 10,000 births at the beginning of the 20th century (Williams, 1903) compared with 15 per 10,000 at Parkland Hospital in 1999.

DEFINITIONS. As discussed, there is no precise definition of macrosomia. Several definitions are in general clinical use. In one scheme, macrosomia is viewed as those weights that exceed certain percentiles for populations. Another common scheme includes use of empirical birthweights.

BIRTHWEIGHT DISTRIBUTION. Commonly used definitions of macrosomia are based upon mathematical distributions of birthweight such as shown in Figure 29–11. Birthweights exceeding the 90th percentile for a given gestational week are usually used as the threshold for macrosomia. For example, the 90th percentile at 39 weeks is 4000 g whereas the corresponding birthweight at 42 weeks is 4400 g. If, on the other hand, birthweights two standard deviations above the mean were used to define excessive fetal growth, the percentile threshold would be between the 97th and 99th percentile, or substantially larger infants when compared with

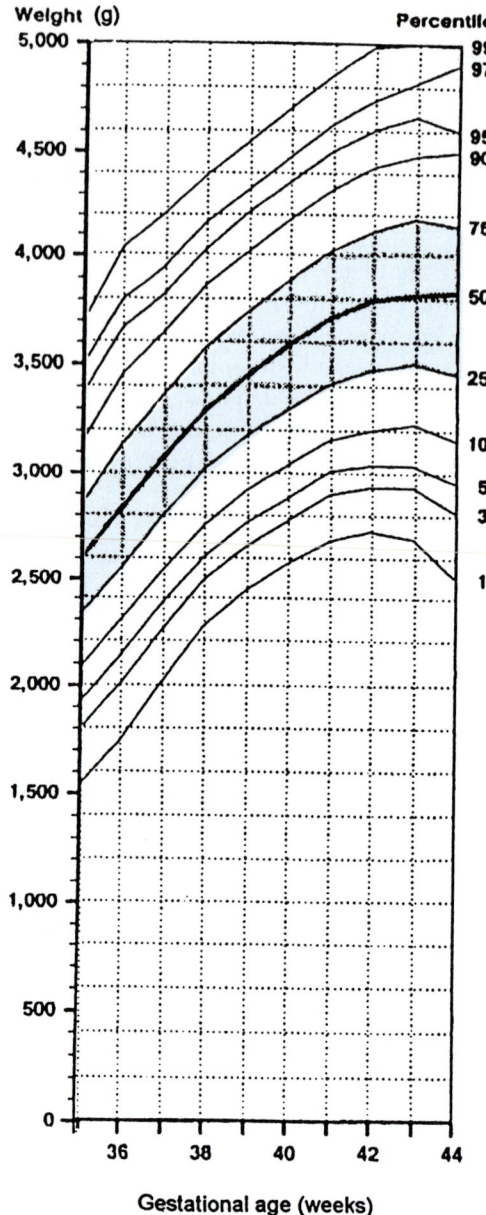

Weight (g)

Percentile

Gestational age (weeks)

FIGURE 29-11. Birthweight percentiles for male singleton live births, Canada. (Adapted from Arbuckle and colleagues, 1993.)

TABLE 29–2. Birthweight Distribution of 169,886 Infants Born at Parkland Hospital Between 1988 and 1999[a]

Birthweight (g)	Births		Percent Maternal Diabetes
	No.	Percent	
500–3999	156,079	91.9	2
4000–4249	8,254	4.9	4
4250–4499	3,470	2.0	7
4500–4649	1,329	0.8	9
4700–4999	500	0.3	12
5000–5249	164	0.1	18
5250–5499	59	—	29
5500–5749	19	—	32
5750–5999	11	—	18
6000–6249	1[b]	—	100
Total	169,886	—	2.4

[a] Also shown is the association of birthweight with maternal diabetes.
[b] 6025-g infant (13 lb 4 oz) delivered by repeat cesarean at 38 weeks to a 329-lb diabetic woman.

Table 29–2, birthweights of 4500 g or more are rare. Over a 12-year period at Parkland Hospital, during which time there were almost 170,000 singleton births, only about 1 percent weighed 4500 g or more. We are of the view that the upper limit of fetal growth, above which growth can be deemed abnormal, is likely two standard deviations above the mean, representing perhaps 3 percent of births. At 40 weeks such a threshold would correspond to approximately 4500 g. This definition of excessive growth is clearly more restrictive than using the upper 10 percent to define macrosomia. The American College of Obstetricians and Gynecologists (2000b) concluded that the term "macrosomia" was an appropriate designation for fetuses who, at birth, weigh 4500 g or more.

RISK FACTORS. Maternal diabetes is an important risk factor for development of fetal macrosomia (Chap. 51, p. 1364). As shown in Table 29–2, the incidence of maternal diabetes increases as birthweight above 4000 g increases. It should be emphasized, however, that maternal diabetes is associated with but a small percentage of such large infants. For example, of the 13,805 infants shown in Table 29–2 who weighed 4000 g or more, only 823 or 6 percent were born to diabetic mothers. Among macrosomic fetuses of diabetic women, there is a greater shoulder circumference and a greater shoulder circumference-to-head circumference ratio. Consequent to this is a greater risk of shoulder dystocia compared with

the 90th percentile. For example, the birthweight threshold at 39 weeks would be approximately 4500 g (97th percentile) rather than 4000 g (90th percentile).

EMPIRICAL BIRTHWEIGHT. Absolute birthweight exceeding a specific threshold is also commonly used to define macrosomia. Newborn weight exceeding 4000 g (8 lbs 13½ oz) is a frequently used threshold. Others use 4250 g or even 4500 g (almost 10 lb). As shown in similar bodyweight fetuses of nondiabetic women (Modenlau and colleagues, 1982; Neiger, 1992; Sachs, 1993).

Among macrosomic fetuses of similar bodyweight, the presence of a relatively greater proportion of body fat is associated independently with an increased risk of labor dystocia and cesarean delivery (Bernstein and Catalano, 1994). For these reasons, and in the absence of a commonly agreed-upon definition of macrosomia, a generally accepted obstetrical management plan optimal for this pregnancy complication has not evolved.

There are several other factors that also favor the likelihood of a large fetus:

1. Large size of the parents, especially obesity of the mother.
2. Multiparity.
3. Prolonged gestation.
4. Maternal age.
5. Male fetus.
6. Previous infant weighing more than 4000 g.
7. Race and ethnicity (Benito and co-workers, 1996; Chervenak, 1992; Johnson and co-workers, 1992; Perlow and associates, 1992; Sachs, 1993).

When the pregnant woman weighs more than 300 pounds, her fetus has a 30 percent risk of macrosomia. Among women who are simultaneously diabetic, obese, and postterm, the incidence of fetal macrosomia can range from 5 to 15 percent (Arias, 1987; Chervenak, 1992). Known maternal risk factors, however, are identified in only 40 percent of women who deliver macrosomic infants (Boyd and associates, 1983).

DIAGNOSIS. Currently, an accurate estimate of excessive fetal size is not possible; consequently, the diagnosis of macrosomia most commonly is not made until after delivery. Inaccuracy in clinical estimates of fetal weight by physical examination is often attributable, at least in part, to maternal obesity.

Numerous attempts have been made to improve the accuracy of fetal weight estimations by analysis of various measurements obtained by ultrasonography. A number of formulas have been proposed to estimate fetal weight using ultrasonic measurements of head, femur, and abdomen. The estimates provided by these computations, although reasonably accurate for predicting the weight of small, preterm fetuses are less valid in predicting the weight of very large fetuses. For example, and as shown in Figure 29–12, an infant predicted to weigh 4000 g can actually weigh considerably more or less than predicted. Similar results were described by Jazayeri and colleagues (1999). Rouse and co-authors (1996) reviewed 13 studies from 1985 to 1995 which reported sensitivity (true positive) and specificity (true negative) for ultrasonic prediction of macrosomic fetuses. The methods were found to have only fair sensi-

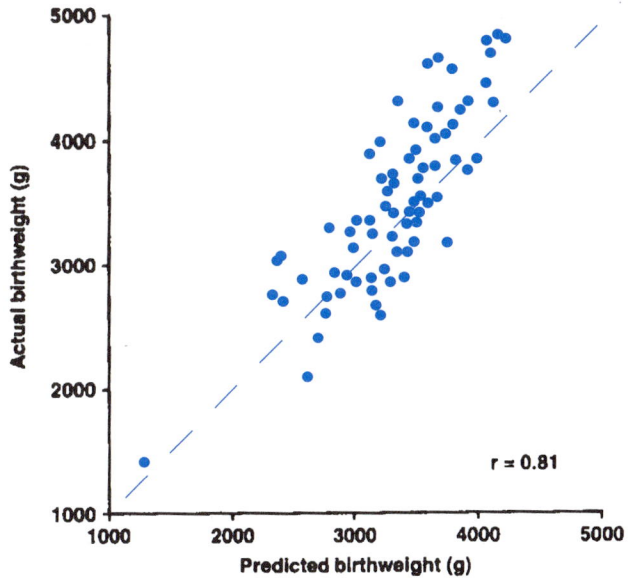

FIGURE 29–12. Relation between predicted birthweight from ultrasound measurement of abdominal circumference within 7 days and actual birthweight. (From Johnstone and colleagues, 1996.)

tivity (60 percent) in the accurate diagnosis of macrosomia but higher specificity (90 percent) in excluding excessive fetal size.

Unfortunately, a formula that gives estimates of fetal macrosomia with sufficiently accurate predictive value to be useful in constructing clinical management decisions has not been derived (American College of Obstetricians and Gynecologists, 2000b). In a comprehensive review of estimates of fetal weight from ultrasonic measurements to identify macrosomia, Sandmire (1993) argued that the use of such data in clinical decision making may cause more harm than good. He suggested that a moratorium be placed on the reporting and clinical use of sonographic data in estimates of excess fetal weight. Indeed, Adashek and colleagues (1996) found that women who had ultrasonography in the last 4 weeks of pregnancy were at significantly increased risk for cesarean delivery if estimated fetal size exceeded 4000 g, regardless of actual newborn weight.

We conclude that the estimation of fetal weight from ultrasonic measurements is not proven to be reliable. Nonetheless, sonographic measurements to evaluate excess fetal weight to assist in clinical management decisions may be warranted in rare circumstances. Routine use of these estimates to identify macrosomia is not recommended; indeed, the findings of several studies are indicative that estimates of fetal weight by physician-conducted physical examination of the pregnant woman are as reliable as, or even superior to, those made from ultrasonic fetal measurements (Sherman and colleagues, 1998).

CONTROVERSIES. Precise knowledge of fetal weight might permit the avoidance of vaginal delivery for women with pregnancies in which labor most likely would be arrested because of true fetopelvic disproportion or delivery complicated by shoulder dystocia. Avoidance of such complications has given rise to the controversies now described.

"PROPHYLACTIC" LABOR INDUCTION. Some have proposed induction of labor upon diagnosis of macrosomia in nondiabetic women as a way to avoid further fetal growth and thereby reduce potential delivery complications. Theoretically, induction should reduce the risk of cesarean delivery and shoulder dystocia by preempting further fetal growth. Gonen and colleagues (1997) randomized 273 nondiabetic women with ultrasonic fetal weight estimates 4000 to 4500 g to either induction or expectant management. Labor induction did not decrease the rate of cesarean delivery or shoulder dystocia. Similar results were reported by Leaphart and colleagues (1997) with the added finding that induction unnecessarily increased the rate of cesarean delivery. According to the American College of Obstetricians and Gynecologists (2000b), current evidence does not support a policy for early induction with suspected macrosomia.

ELECTIVE CESAREAN DELIVERY. Rouse and colleagues (1996, 1999) analyzed the potential effects of a policy of elective cesarean delivery for ultrasonically diagnosed fetal macrosomia compared with standard obstetrical management. They concluded that for women who are not diabetic, a policy of elective cesarean delivery was medically and economically unsound. They did, however, conclude that a policy of elective cesarean delivery in *diabetic* women with macrosomic fetuses was a tenable approach. Conway and Langer (1998) reported that introduction of a protocol of routine cesarean delivery for ultrasonic estimates of 4250 g or greater in diabetic women significantly reduced the rate of shoulder dystocia from 2.4 to 1.1 percent.

PREVENTION OF SHOULDER DYSTOCIA. A major concern for delivery of macrosomic infants is shoulder dystocia and attendant risks of permanent brachial plexus palsy. Shoulder dystocia occurs when the maternal pelvis is of sufficient size to permit delivery of the fetal head, but not large enough to allow delivery of the very large-diameter fetal shoulders. In this circumstance, the anterior shoulder becomes impacted against the maternal symphysis pubis (Chap. 19, p. 459). Even with expert obstetrical assistance at delivery, stretching and injury of the brachial plexus of the affected shoulder may be inevitable (Chap. 39, p. 1080). Fortunately, fewer than 10 percent of all shoulder dystocia cases result in a persistent brachial plexus injury (American College of Obstetricians and Gynecologists, 1997a). Ecker and colleagues (1997) analyzed 80 cases of brachial plexus injury in 77,616 consecutive deliveries at Brigham and Women's Hospital in Boston and concluded that an excessive number of otherwise unnecessary cesarean deliveries would be needed to prevent a single brachial plexus injury in infants born to women without diabetes. As previously cited, however, elective cesarean delivery in diabetic women may be helpful in preempting shoulder dystocia (Conway and Langer, 1998).

The American College of Obstetricians and Gynecologists (1997b, 2000) has concluded that most cases of shoulder dystocia cannot be predicted or prevented. Planned cesarean delivery on the basis of suspected macrosomia in the *general population* was deemed an unreasonable strategy because of the number and cost of additional cesarean deliveries. Again, it was concluded that planned cesarean delivery may be a reasonable strategy for diabetic women with estimated fetal weights exceeding 4250 to 4500 g.

REFERENCES

Abrams B, Selvin S: Maternal weight gain pattern and birth weight. Obstet Gynecol 86:163, 1995

Adashek JA, Lagrew DC, Iriye BK, Carr MH, Porto M, Freeman RK: The influence of ultrasound examination at term on the rate of cesarean section. Am J Obstet Gynecol 174:327, 1996

Alexander GR, Himes JH, Kaufman RB, Mor J, Kogan M: A United States national reference for fetal growth. Obstet Gynecol 87:163, 1996

American College of Obstetricians and Gynecologists. Intrauterine growth restriction. Practice Bulletin No. 12, January, 2000a

American College of Obstetricians and Gynecologists. Fetal macrosomia. Practice Bulletin No. 22, November 2000b

American College of Obstetricians and Gynecologists. Shoulder dystocia. Practice Pattern No. 7, October, 1997a

American College of Obstetricians and Gynecologists. Utility of antepartum umbilical artery Doppler velocimetry in intrauterine growth restriction. Committee Opinion No. 18, October, 1997b.

Arbuckle TE, Wilkins R, Sherman GJ: Birth weight percentiles by gestational age in Canada. Obstet Gynecol 81:39, 1993

Arias F: Predictability of complications associated with prolongation of pregnancy. Obstet Gynecol 70:101, 1987

Bakketeig LS, Bjerkedal T, Hoffman HJ: Small-for-gestational age births in successive pregnancy outcomes: Results from a longitudinal study of births in Norway. Early Hum Dev 14:187, 1986

Barnes AC: An obstetric record from the Medical Record. Obstet Gynecol 9:237, 1957

Battaglia FC, Lubchenco LO: A practical classification of newborn infants by weight and gestational age. J Pediatr 71:159, 1967

Benito CW, Thayer CF, Lake MF, Knuppel RA, Vintzileos

AM: Predictors of fetal macrosomia. Am J Obstet Gynecol 174:350, 1996

Bernstein IM, Catalano PM: Examination of factors contributing to the risk of cesarean delivery in women with gestational diabetes. Obstet Gynecol 83:462, 1994

Blair E, Stanley F: Intrauterine growth and spastic cerebral palsy, 2. The association with morphology at birth. Early Hum Dev 28:91, 1992

Boyd ME, Usher PH, McLean FH: Fetal macrosomia: Prediction, risks and proposed management. Obstet Gynecol 61:715, 1983

Branch DW, Silver RM, Blackwell JL, Reading JC, Scott JR: Outcome of treated pregnancies in women with antiphospholipid syndrome: An update of the Utah experience. Obstet Gynecol 80:614, 1992

Brenner WE, Edelman DA, Hendricks CH: A standard of fetal growth for the United States of America. Am J Obstet Gynecol 126:555, 1976

Brooks AA, Johnson MR, Steer PJ, Pawson ME, Abdalla HI: Birthweight: Nature or nurture? Early Hum Dev 2:29, 1995

Campbell S, Thoms A: Ultrasound measurement of the fetal head to abdomen circumference ratio in the assessment of growth retardation. Br J Obstet Gynaecol 84:165, 1977

Chervenak JL: Macrosomia in the postdates pregnancy. Clin Obstet Gynecol 35:161, 1992

Cliver SP, Goldenberg RL, Cutter GR, Hoffman JH, Davis RO, Nelson KG: The effect of cigarette smoking on neonatal anthropmetric measurements. Obstet Gynecol 85:625, 1995

Conway DL, Langer O: Elective delivery of infants with macrosomia in diabetic women: Reduced shoulder dystocia versus increased cesarean deliveries. Am J Obstet Gynecol 178:922, 1998

Crane JP, Kopta MM: Comparative newborn anthropometric data in symmetric versus asymmetric intrauterine growth retardation. Am J Obstet Gynecol 138:518, 1980

Cunningham FG, Cox SM, Harstad TW, Mason RA, Pritchard JA: Chronic renal disease and pregnancy outcome. Am J Obstet Gynecol 163:453, 1990

Dashe JS, Lo JY, McIntire DD, Bloom, SL, Leveno KJ: Antepartum ultrasound for the detection of fetal growth restriction. Presented at the Society for Gynecologic Investigation, Toronto, Canada, March 14–17, 2001

Dashe JS, McIntire DD, Lucas MJ, Leveno KJ: Impact of asymmetric versus symmetric fetal growth restriction on pregnancy outcomes. SGI abstract 96:321, 2000

Dejin-Karlsson E, Hanson BS, Ostergren P-O, Lindgren A, Sjoberg N-O, Marsal K: Association of a lack of psychosocial resources and the risk of giving birth to small for gestational age infants: A stress hypothesis. Br J Obstet Gynaecol 107:89, 2000

Deter RL, Nazar R, Milner LL: Modified neonatal growth assessment score: A multivariate approach to the detection of intrauterine growth retardation in the neonate. Ultrasound Obstet Gynecol 6:400, 1995

Dickey RP, Gasser RF: Ultrasound evidence of variability in the size and development of normal human embryos before the tenth post-insemination week after assisted reproductive technologies. Hum Reprod 8:331, 1993

Diket AL, Pierce MR, Munshi UK, Voelker CA, Eloby-Childress S, Greenberg SS, Zhang XJ, Clark DA, Miller MJ: Nitric oxide inhibition causes intrauterine growth retardation and hind-limb disruptions in rats. Am J Obstet Gynecol 171:1243, 1994

Divon MY, Hsu HW: Maternal and fetal blood flow velocity waveforms in intrauterine growth retardation. Clin Obstet Gynecol 35:156, 1992

Droste S: Fetal growth in aneuploid conditions. Clin Obstet Gynecol 35:119, 1992

Droste S, Fitzsimmons J, Pascoe-Mason J, Shepard T: Growth of linear parameters in trisomy 18 fetuses. Am J Obstet Gynecol 163:158, 1990

Duvekot JJ, Cheriex EC, Pieters FAA, Menheere PPCA, Schouten HJA, Peeters LLH: Maternal volume homeostasis in early pregnancy in relation to fetal growth restriction. Obstet Gynecol 85:361, 1995

Ecker JL, Greenberg JA, Norwitz ER, Nadel AS, Repke JT: Birthweight as a predictor of brachial plexus injury. Obstet Gynecol 89:643, 1997

Economides DL, Crook D, Nicolaides KH: Hypertriglyceridemia and hypoxemia in small-for-gestational-age fetuses. Am J Obstet Gynecol 162:387, 1990

Economides DL, Nicolaides KH, Gahl WA, Bernardini I, Bottoms S, Evans M: Cordocentesis in the diagnosis of intrauterine starvation. Am J Obstet Gynecol 161:1004, 1989a

Economides DL, Nicolaides KH: Blood glucose and oxygen tension levels in small-for-gestational-age fetuses. Am J Obstet Gynecol 160:385, 1989b

Economides DL, Proudler A, Nicolaides KH: Plasma insulin in appropriate- and small-for-gestational-age fetuses. Am J Obstet Gynecol 160:1091, 1989c

Emanuel I, Alberman HFE, Evans SJ: Intergenerational studies of human birthweight from the 1958 birth cohort, 1. Evidence for a multi-generational effect. Br J Obstet Gynaecol 99:67, 1992

Ewigman BG, Crane JP, Frigoletto FD, LeFevre ML, Bain RP, McNellis D: Effect of prenatal ultrasonic screening on perinatal outcome. N Engl J Med 329:821, 1993

Fitzsimmons J, Droste S, Shepard T, Pascoe-Mason J, Fantel A: Growth failure in second trimester fetuses with trisomy 21. Teratology 42:337, 1990

Fraser R, Cresswell J: What should obstetricians be doing about the Barker hypothesis? Br J Obstet Gynaecol 104:645, 1997

Friedman SA, Schiff E, Kao L, Sibai BM: Neonatal outcome after preterm delivery for preeclampsia. Am J Obstet Gynecol 172:1785, 1995

Frigoletto F: Diagnostic Ultrasound Imaging in Pregnancy. Pub. No. 84667. Washington, DC, US Department of Health and Human Services, Public Health Service, National Institutes of Health, 1986

Gabriel R, Alsat E, Evion-Brion D: Alteration of epidermal growth factor receptor in placental membranes of smokers: Relationship with intrauterine growth retardation. Am J Obstet Gynecol 170:1238, 1994

Gardosi J, Chang A, Kalyan B, Sahota D, Symonds EM: Customized antenatal growth charts. Lancet 339:283, 1992

Gardosi J, Francis A: Controlled trial of fundal height measurement plotted on customized antenatal growth charts. Br J Obstet Gynaecol 106:309, 1999

Gluckman PD, Liggins GC: Regulation of fetal growth. In Beard RW, Nathanielsz PW (eds): Fetal Physiology and Medicine: The Basis of Perinatology, 2nd ed. Rev. Vol 6 of Reproductive Medicine. New York, Marcel Dekker, 1984, p 511

Golbus MS: Development in the first half of gestation of genetically abnormal fetuses. Teratology 18:333, 1978

Goldenberg RL, Cutter GR, Hoffman HJ, Foster JM, Nelson KG, Hauth JC: Intrauterine growth retardation: Standards for diagnosis. Am J Obstet Gynecol 161:271, 1989

Gonen O, Rosen DJD, Dolfin Z, Tepper R, Markov S, Fejgin MD: Induction of labor versus expectant management in macrosomia: A randomized study. Obstet Gynecol 89:913, 1997

Gruenwald P: Chronic fetal distress and placental insufficiency. Biol Neonate 5:215, 1963

Hanson JW, Myrianthopoulas NC, Harvey MAS, Smith DW: Risks to the offspring of women treated with hydantoin anticonvulsants, with emphasis on the fetal hydantoin syndrome. J Pediatr 89:662, 1976

Hecher K, Snijder R, Campbell S, Nicolaides K: Fetal venous, intracardiac, and arterial blood flow measurements in intrauterine growth retardation: Relationship with fetal blood gases. Am J Obstet Gynecol 173:10, 1995

Heyborne KD, McGregor JA, Henry G, Witkin SS, Abrams JS: Interleukin-10 in amniotic fluid at midtrimester: Immune activation and suppression in relation to fetal growth. Am J Obstet Gynecol 171:55, 1994

Hill LM, Guzick D, Chevenvey P, Boyles D, Nedzesky P: The sonographic assessment of twin growth discordancy. Obstet Gynecol 84:501, 1994

Holmes RP, Holly JMP, Soothill PW: A prospective study of maternal serum insulin-like growth factor-I in pregnancies with appropriately grown or growth restricted fetuses. Br J Obstet Gynaecol 105:1273, 1998

Howard RB: Control of human placental blood flow. Med Hypotheses 23:51, 1987

Jazayeri A, Heffron JA, Phillips R, Spellacy WN: Macrosomia prediction using ultrasound fetal abdominal circumference of 35 centimeters or more. Obstet Gynecol 93:523, 1999

Jensen OH, Larsen S: Evaluation of symphysis fundus measurements and weighing during pregnancy. Acta Obstet Gynecol Scand 70:13, 1991

Jimenez JM, Tyson JE, Reisch J: Clinical measurements of gestational age in normal pregnancies. Obstet Gynecol 61:438, 1983

Johnson JWC, Longmate JA, Frentzen B: Excessive maternal weight and pregnancy outcome. Am J Obstet Gynecol 167:353, 1992

Johnstone FD, Prescott RJ, Steel JM, Mao JH, Chamber S, Muir N: Clinical and ultrasound prediction of macrosomia in diabetic pregnancy. Br J Obstet Gynaecol 103:747, 1996

Jones JW, Gercel-Taylor C, Taylor DD: Altered cord serum lipid levels associated with small for gestational age infants. Obstet Gynecol 93:527, 1999

Kalousek DK, Langlois S, Barrett I, Yam I, Wilson DR, Howard-Peebles PN, Johnson MD, Giorgiutti E: Uniparental disomy for chromosome 16 in humans. Am J Hum Genet 52:8, 1993

Khoury MJ, Erickson JD, Cordero JF, McCarthy BJ: Congenital malformations and intrauterine growth retardation: A population study. Pediatrics 82:83, 1988

Kingdom JCP, McQueen J, Ryan G, Connell JMC, Whittle MJ: Fetal vascular atrial natriuretic peptide receptors in human placenta: Alteration in intrauterine growth retardation and preeclampsia. Am J Obtet Gynecol 170:142, 1994

Klebanoff MA, Schulsinger C, Mednick BR, Secher NJ: Preterm and small-for-gestational-age birth across generations. Am J Obstet Gynecol 176:521, 1997

Klein JO, Remington JS: Current concepts of infections of the fetus and newborn infant. In Remington JS, Klein JO, (eds): Infectious Diseases of the Fetus and Newborn Infant, 4th ed. Philadelphia, Saunders, 1995, p 1

Kliegman RM: Intrauterine growth retardation. In Fanuroff AA, Martin RJ (eds): Neonatal-Perinatal Medicine, 6th ed. New York, Mosby, 1997, p 203

Kok JH, den Ouden AL, Verloove-Vanhorick SP, Brand R: Outcome of very preterm small for gestational age infant: The first nine years of life. Br J Obstet Gynaecol 105:162, 1998

Laatikainen TJ, Raisanen IJ, Salminen KR: Corticotrophin-releasing hormone in amnionic fluid during gestation and labor and in relation to fetal lung maturation. Am J Obstet Gynecol 59:891, 1988

Larsen T, Larsen JF, Petersen S, Greisen G: Detection of small-for-gestation-age fetuses by ultrasound screening in a high risk population: A randomized controlled study. Br J Obstet Gynaecol 99:469, 1992

Leaphart WL, Meyer MC, Capeless EL: Labor induction with a prenatal diagnosis of fetal macrosomia. J Matern Fetal Med 6:99, 1997

LeBlanc PE, Parekh AJ, Naso B, Glass L: Effects of interuterine exposure to alkaloidal cocaine ("crack"). Am J Dis Child 141:937, 1987

Lechtig A, Delgado H, Lasky RE, Yarbrough C, Klein RE, Habicht JP, Behar M: Maternal nutrition and fetal growth in developing societies. Am J Dis Child 129:434, 1975

Lichty JA, Ting RY, Bruns PD, Dyar E: Studies of babies born at high altitude, 1. Relation of altitude to birth weight. Am J Dis Child 93:666, 1957

Lin CC, Evans MI: Introduction. In Lin CC, Evans MI (eds): Intrauterine Growth Retardation. New York, McGraw-Hill, 1984

Lin CC, Santolaya-Forgas J: Current concepts of fetal growth restriction: Part I. Causes, classification, and pathophysiology. Obstet Gynecol 92:1044, 1998

Lindor NM, Jalal SM, Thibedeau SM, Bonde D, Sauser KL, Karnes PS: Mosaic trisomy 16 in a thriving infant: Maternal heterodisomy for chromosome 16. Clin Genet 44:185, 1993

Lockwood CJ, Rand JH: The immunobiology and obstetrical consequences of antiphospholipid antibodies. Obstet Gynecol Surv 49:432, 1994

Lubchenco LO, Hansman C, Dressler M, Boyd E: Intrauterine growth as estimated from liveborn birth-weight data at 24 to 42 weeks of gestation. Pediatrics 32:793, 1963

Lunell NO, Nylund L: Uteroplacental blood flow. Clin Obstet Gynecol 35:108, 1992

Manning FA: Intrauterine growth retardation. In: Fetal Medicine. Principles and Practice. Norwalk, CT, Appleton & Lange, 1995, p 317

Manning FA, Hohler C: Intrauterine growth retardation: Diagnosis, prognostication, and management based on ultrasound methods. In Fleischer AC, Romero R, Manning FA, Jeanty P, James AE (eds): The Principles and Practices of Ultrasonography in Obstetrics and Gynecology, 4th ed. Norwalk, CT, Appleton & Lange, 1991, p 331

McIntire DD, Bloom SL, Casey BM, Leveno KJ: Birthweight in relation to morbidity and mortality among newborn infants. N Engl J Med 340:1234, 1999

McKeown T, Record RG: Observations on foetal growth in multiple pregnancy in man. Endocrinology 8:386, 1952

McQueen J, Kingdom JCP, Connell JMC, Whittle MJ: Fetal endothelin levels and placental vascular endothelin receptors in intrauterine growth retardation. Obstet Gynecol 82:992, 1993

Miller JM, Boudreaux MC, Regan FA: A case-control study of cocaine use in pregnancy. Am J Obstet Gynecol 172:180, 1995

Minior VK, Divon MY: Fetal growth restriction at term: Myth or reality? Obstet Gynecol 92:57, 1998

Modenlau HD, Komatsu G, Dorchester W, Freeman RK,

Bosu SK: Large for gestational age neonates: Anthropomorphic reasons for shoulder dystocia. Obstet Gynecol 60:417, 1982

Moerman P, Fryns JP, Goodeeris P, Lauweryns JM: Spectrum of clinical and autopsy findings in trisomy 18 syndrome. J Hum Genet 30:17, 1982

Neerhof MG: Causes of intrauterine growth restriction. Clin Perinatol 22:375, 1995

Neiger R: Fetal macrosomia in the diabetic patient. Clin Obstet Gynecol 35:138, 1992

New Shorter Oxford English Dictionary. Brown L (ed). Oxford, Clarendon Press, 1993

Nicolaides KH, Peters MT, Vyas S, Rabinowitz R, Rosen DJ, Campbell S: Relation of rate of urine production to oxygen tension in small-for-gestational-age infants. Am J Obstet Gynecol 162:387, 1990

Nicolaides KH, Snijders RJM, Noble P: Cordocentesis in the study of growth-retarded fetuses. In Divon MY (ed): Abnormal Fetal Growth. New York, Elsevier, 1991

Ott W: Intrauterine growth retardation and preterm delivery. Am J Obstet Gynecol 168:710, 1993

Overpeck MD, Hediger ML, Zhang J, Turnbule AC, Klebanoff MA: Birthweight for gestational age of Mexican American infants born in the United States. Obstet Gynecol 93:943, 1999

Owen J, Baker SL, Hauth JC, Goldenberg RL, Davis RO, Copper RL: Is indicated or spontaneous preterm delivery more advantageous for the fetus? Am J Obstet Gynecol 163:868, 1990

Owen P, Donnet ML, Ogston SA, Christie AD, Howie PW, Patel NB: Standards for ultrasound fetal growth velocity. Br J Obstet Gynaecol 103:60, 1996

Owen P, Harrold AJ, Farrell T: Fetal size and growth velocity in the prediction of intrapartum cesarean section for fetal distress. Br J Obstet Gynaecol 104:445, 1997

Owen P, Khan KS: Fetal growth velocity in the prediction of intrauterine growth restriction in a low risk population. Br J Obstet Gynaecol 105:536, 1998

Patterson RM, Gibb CE, Wood RC: Birthweight percentile and perinatal outcome: Recurrence of intrauterine growth retardation. Obstet Gynecol 68:464, 1986

Patton DE, Lee W, Cotton DB, Miller J, Carpenter RJ Jr, Hahta J, Hankins G: Cyanotic maternal heart disease in pregnancy. Obstet Gynecol Surv 45:594, 1990

Paz I, Gale R, Laor A, Danon YL, Stevenson DK, Seidman DS: The cognitive outcome of full-term small-for-gestational age infants at late adolescence. Obstet Gynecol 85:452, 1995

Perelman RH, Farrell PM, Engle MJ, Kemnitz JW: Development aspects of lung lipids. Ann Rev Physiol 47:803, 1985

Perlow JH, Morgan MA, Montgomery D, Towers CV, Porto M: Perinatal outcome in pregnancy complicated by massive obesity. Am J Obstet Gynecol 167:958, 1992

Piper JM, Xenakis EMJ, McFarland M, Elliot BD, Berkens MD, Langer O: Do growth-retarded premature infants have different rates of perinatal morbidity and mortality than appropriate-grown premature infants? Obstet Gynecol 87:169, 1996

Pollack RN, Divon MY: Intrauterine growth retardation: Definition, classification and etiology. Clin Obstet Gynecol 35:99, 1992

Rankin JHG, McLaughlin MK: The regulation of the placental blood flows. J Dev Physiol 1:3, 1979

Roberts AB, Mitchele J, McCowan LM, Barker S: Ultrasonographic measurement of liver length in the small-for-gestational-age fetus. Am J Obstet Gynecol 180:634, 1999

Rochelson B, Kaplan C, Guzman E, Arato M, Hansen K, Trunca C: A quantitative analysis of placental vasculature in the third trimester fetus with autosomal trisomy. Obstet Gynecol 75:59, 1990

Ronzoni S, Marconi AM, Cetin I, Paolini CL, Teng C, Pardi G, Battaglia FC: Umbilical amino acid uptake at increasing maternal amino acid concentrations: Effect of a maternal amino acid infusate. Am J Obstet Gynecol 181:477, 1999

Roth S, Abernathy MP, Lee WH, Pratt L, Denne S, Golichowski A, Pescovitz OH: Insulin-like growth factors I and II peptide and messenger RNA levels in macrosomic infants of diabetic pregnancies. J Soc Gynecol Investig 3:78, 1996

Rouse DJ, Owen J: Prophylactic cesarean delivery for fetal macrosomia diagnosed by means of ultrasonography—A Faustian bargain? Am J Obstet Gynecol 181:332, 1999

Rouse DJ, Owen J, Goldenberg RL, Cliver SP: The effectiveness and costs of elective cesarean delivery for fetal macrosomia diagnosed by ultrasound. JAMA 276:1480, 1996

Sachs DA: Fetal macrosomia and gestational diabetes: What's the problem? Obstet Gynecol 81:775, 1993

Salafia CM, Minior VK, Pezzullo JC, Pipek EJ, Rosenkrantz TS, Vintzileos AM: Intrauterine growth restriction in infants of less than 32 weeks' gestation: Associated placental pathologic features. Am J Obstet Gynecol 173:1049, 1995

Sandmire HF: Whither ultrasonic prediction of fetal macrosomia? Obstet Gynecol 82:860, 1993

Seeds JW: Impaired fetal growth: Definition and clinical diagnosis. Obstet Gynecol 64:303, 1984

Seeds JW, Peng T: Impaired growth and risk of fetal death: Is the tenth percentile the appropriate standard? Am J Obstet Gynecol 178:658, 1998

Shah NR, Bracken MB: A systematic review and meta-analysis of prospective studies on the association between maternal cigarette smoking and preterm delivery. Am J Obstet Gynecol 182:465, 2000

Sherer DM, Salafia CM, Spong CY, Minior VK: In deliveries < 32 weeks, breech presentation is associated with an increased incidence of intrauterine growth retardation. Am J Obstet Gynecol 174:344, 1996

Sherman DJ, Arieli S, Tovbin J, Siegel G, Caspi E, Bukovsky I: A comparison of clinical and ultrasonic estimations of fetal weight. Obstet Gynecol 91:212, 1998

Simpson JW, Lawless RW, Mitchell AC: Responsibility of the obstetrician to the fetus, 2. Influence of prepregnancy weight and pregnancy weight gain on birth weight. Obstet Gynecol 45:481, 1975

Sivan E, Whittaker PG, Sinha D, Homko CJ, Lin M, Reece EA, Boden G: Leptin in human pregnancy: The relationship with gestation hormones. Am J Obstet Gynecol 179:1128, 1998

Smith GCS, Smith MFS, McNay MB, Fleming JEE: First-trimester growth and the risk of low birthweight. N Engl J Med 339:1817, 1998

Smith GCS, Smith MFS, McNay MB, Fleming JEE: The relation between fetal abdominal circumference and birthweight: Findings in 3512 pregnancies. Br J Obstet Gynaecol 104:186, 1997

Smulian JC, Anauth CV, Martins ME, Vintzileos AM, Knuppel RA: Timing of infant death by gestational age at delivery in pregnancies complicated by intrauterine growth-restriction: A population based study. Am J Obstet Gynecol Abstract 166, 182:S68, 2000

Snijders RJM, Nicolaides KJ: Fetal biometry at 14 to 40 weeks' gestation. Ultrasound Obstet Gynecol 4:34, 1994

Snijders RJM, Sherrod C, Gosden CM, Nicolaides KH: Fetal growth retardation: Associated malformations and chromosomal abnormalities. Am J Obstet Gynecol 168:547, 1993

Soothill PW, Nicolaides KH, Campbell S: Prenatal asphyxia, hyperlacticaemia, hypoglycaemia and erythroblastosis in growth retarded fetuses. BMJ 294:1046, 1987

Stagno S, Reynolds DW, Hwang ES: Congenital cytomegalovirus infection. N Engl J Med 296:1254, 1977

Stedmans Medical Dictionary, 26th ed. Spraycar M (ed). Baltimore, Williams & Wilkins, 1995, p 1052

Steer P: Fetal growth. Br J Obstet Gynaecol 105:1133, 1998

Stein Z, Susser M, Saenger G, Marolla F: In: Famine and Human Development: The Dutch Hunger Winter of 1944–1945. New York, Oxford University Press, 1975

Stephens TD, Shepard TH: The Down syndrome in the fetus. Teratology 22:37, 1980

Stettler RW, Cunningham FG: Natural history of chronic proteinura complicating pregnancy. Am J Obstet Gynecol 167:1219, 1992

Tamura T, Goldenberg RL, Johnston KE, Cliver SP: Serum leptin concentrations during pregnancy and their relationship to fetal growth. Obstet Gynecol 91:389, 1998

Thelander HE, Pryor HB: Abnormal patterns of growth and development in mongolism. Clin Pediatr 5:493, 1966

Tyson JE, Kennedy K, Broyles S, Rosenfeld CR: The small for gestational age infant: Accelerated or delayed pulmonary maturation? Increased or decreased survival? Pediatrics 95:534, 1995

Usher R, McLean F: Intrauterine growth of live-born caucasian infants at sea level: Standards obtained from measurements in 7 dimensions of infants born between 25 and 44 weeks' gestation. J Pediatr 74:901, 1969

Van den Hof MC, Nicolaides KH: Platelet count in normal, small, and anemic fetuses. Am J Obstet Gynecol 162:730, 1990

Varner MW, Dildy GA, Hunter BS, Dudley DJ, Clark SL, Mitchell MD: Amniotic fluid epidermal growth factor levels in normal and abnormal pregnancies. J Soc Gynecol Invest 3:17, 1996

Varner MW, Galask RP: Infectious causes. In Linc CC, Evans MI (eds): Intrauterine Growth Retardation. New York, McGraw-Hill, 1984

Ventura SJ, Martin JA, Curtin SC, Mathews TJ: Births: Final Data for 1997. National Vital Statistics Reports, Vol 47, No. 18. Hyattsville, MD, National Center for Health Statistics, 1999

Verhaeghe J, VanBree R, VanHerck E, Laureys J, Bouillon R, Van Assche FA: C-peptide, insulin-like growth factors I & II, and insulin-like growth factor binding protein-1 in umbilical cord serum: Correlations with birthweight. Am J Obstet Gynecol 169:89, 1993

Visser GH, Sadovsky G, Nicolaides KH: Antepartum heart rate patterns in small-for-gestational-age third-trimester fetuses: Correlations with blood gas values obtained at cordocentesis. Am J Obstet Gynecol 162:698, 1990

Walraven GEL, Mkanje RJB, van Roosmalen J, van Dongen PWJ, van Asten HAGH, Domans WMV: Single pre-delivery symphysis-fundal height measurement as a predictor of birthweight and multiple pregnancy. Br J Obstet Gynaecol 102:525, 1995

Warkany JB, Monroe B, Sutherland BSS: Intrauterine growth retardation. Am J Dis Child 102:24, 1961

Waterson AP: Viral infections (other than rubella) during pregnancy. BMJ 2:564, 1979

Weiner Z, Divon MY, Katz VK, Minior VK, Nasseri A, Girz B: Multivariant analysis of antepartum fetal tests in predicting neonatal outcome of growth retarded fetus. Am J Obstet Gynecol 174:339, 1996

Wennerholm UB, Albertsson-Wikland K, Bergh C, Hamberger L, Niklasson A, Nilsson L, Thiringer K, Wennergren M, Wikland M, Borres MP: Postnatal growth and health in children born after cryo preservation of embryos. Lancet 351:1085, 1998

Wigglesworth JS, Singer DB: Fetal growth and maturation: Standards for body and region development. In: Textbook of Fetal and Perinatal Pathology. Cambridge, Blackwell, 1991, p 28

Wilcox MA, Smith SJ, Johnson IR, Maynard PV, Clivers CED: The effect of social deprivation on birthweight, excluding physiological and pathological effects. Br J Obstet Gynaecol 102:918, 1995

Williams JW: Obstetrics: A Text-Book for Students and Practitioners, 1st ed. New York, Appleton, 1903, 133

Williams RL: Intrauterine growth curves. Intra- and international comparisons with different ethnic groups in California. Present Med 4:163, 1975

Williams RL, Creasy RK, Cunningham GC, Hawes WE, Norris FD, Tashiro M: Fetal growth and perinatal viability in California. Obstet Gynecol 59:624, 1982

Wolstenholme J: An audit of trisomy 16 in man. Prenat Diagn 15:109, 1995

Xiong X, Mayes D, Demianczuk N, Olson DM, Davidge ST, Newburn-Cook C, Saunders LD: Impact of pregnancy-induced hypertension on fetal growth. Am J Obstet Gynecol 180:207, 1999

Yoneyama Y, Wakatsuki M, Sawa R, Kamoi S, Takahashi H, Shin S, Kawamura T, Power GG, Araki T: Plasma adenosine concentration in appropriate- and small-for-gestational-age fetuses. Am J Obstet Gynecol 170:684, 1994

30

Multifetal Pregnancy

The number and rate of twin and triplet and other higher order multiple births have increased in the United States at an unprecedented pace over the past two decades (Kogan and colleagues, 2000; Martin and Park, 1999). As shown in Figure 30–1, between 1980 and 1997, the number of twin deliveries rose 52 percent and the number of triplets and other higher order multiple births soared 404 percent. Singleton births, in contrast, rose only 6 percent. This extraordinary increase in multiple births is a public health concern because these infants are less likely to survive and more likely to suffer life-long disability due to preterm delivery. Jewell and Yip (1995) profiled women delivering plural births in the United States during the 1980s and observed that the increase in multiple births was due to use of fertility-stimulating therapy by older, typically white women with high-education status. Multiple gestation currently accounts for 3 percent of all pregnancies (American College of Obstetricians and Gynecologists, 1998).

Powers and Kiely (1994) used United States linked birth/infant death certificates for 7.4 million singleton births and 156,690 twin births in 1985 and 1986 to measure the impact of twins on national infant morbidity and mortality. Although twins were relatively infrequent in the United States—approximately 1 in 94 pregnancies—they accounted for a disproportionately large share of adverse pregnancy outcomes, primarily as a consequence of preterm delivery. Similarly, at Parkland Hospital, twin infants represent only 1 in 45 births and yet account for 1 in 11 perinatal deaths (Table 30–1). In addition to the perinatal mortality and morbidity attributable to preterm delivery, fetuses in multiple gestations are vulnerable to a variety of unique complications such as structural malformations and twin-to-twin transfusion syndrome, so that stillbirth rates are also appreciably increased. As Powers and Kiely (1994) emphasized, postponing preterm delivery in twin pregnancy should become a national health priority because of its disproportionate adverse pregnancy outcomes. As also shown in Table 30–1, maternal complications are increased with multiple gestations. Conde-Agudelo and co-workers (2000) studied over 15,000 twin pregnancies and found a twofold significant risk for preeclampsia, postpartum hemorrhage, and maternal death.

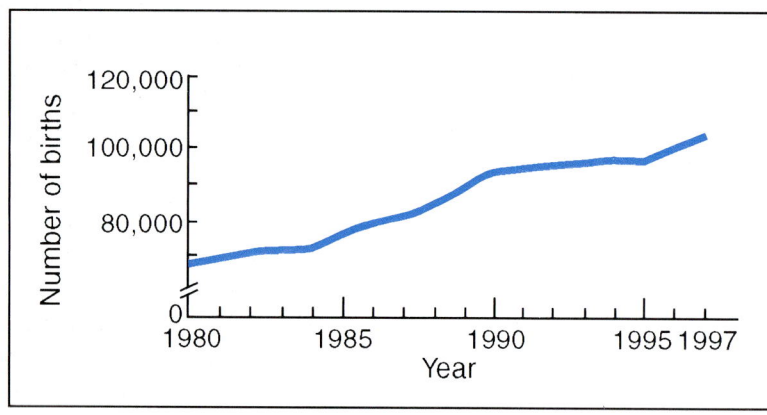

A

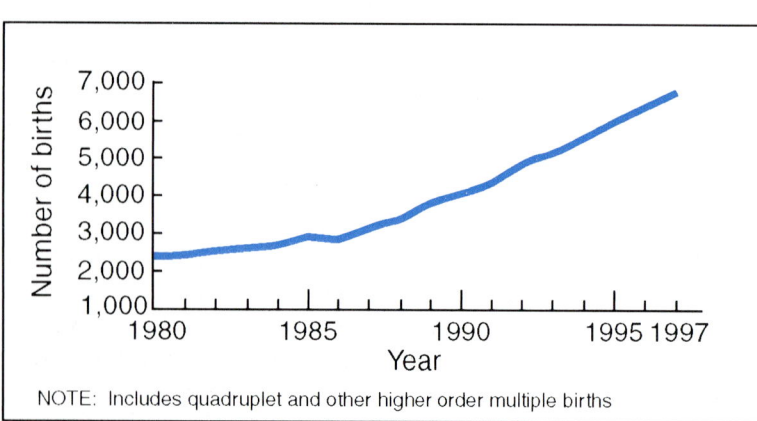

NOTE: Includes quadruplet and other higher order multiple births

B

FIGURE 30–1. Number of twin **(A)** and triplet or higher multiple births **(B),** United States, 1980–1997. (From Martin and Park, 1999, with permission.)

TABLE 30–1. Selected Outcomes in Twin Pregnancies Compared with Singletons Delivered at Parkland Hospital in 1999

Outcome	Singletons	Twins[a]
Women delivered	14,503	162
Births	14,503	324
Stillbirths (per 1000)	85 (6)	8 (25)
Neonatal deaths (per 1000)	57 (4)	6 (18)
Perinatal deaths (per 1000)	142 (10)	14 (43)
Very-low birthweight (< 1500 g)	1.4%	12%
Pregnancy hypertension	12%	20%
Cesarean delivery	19%	60%

[a]Represented 1 in 44 births and 1 in 8 perinatal deaths.

ETIOLOGY OF MULTIPLE FETUSES

Twin fetuses commonly result from fertilization of two separate ova, that is, double-ovum, dizygotic, or fraternal twins. About a third as often, twins arise from a single fertilized ovum that subsequently divides into two similar structures, each with the potential for developing into a separate individual, that is, single-ovum, monozygotic, or identical twins. Either or both processes may be involved in the formation of higher numbers of fetuses. Quadruplets, for example, may arise from one to four ova.

FRATERNAL VERSUS IDENTICAL TWINS. Dizygotic twins are not in a strict sense true twins because they result from the maturation and fertilization of two ova during a single ovulatory cycle (Fig. 30–2). Also, monozygotic or identical twins are usually not identical. As discussed subsequently, the process of division of one fertilized zygote into two does not necessarily result in equal sharing of protoplasmic materials. Furthermore, the process of monozygotic twinning is in a sense a teratogenic event, and monozygotic twins have an increased incidence of (often discordant) structural malformations. In fact, dizygotic or fraternal twins of the same sex may appear more nearly identical at birth than do monozygotic twins, while growth of monozygotic twin fetuses may be discordant and at times dramatically so.

GENESIS OF MONOZYGOTIC TWINS. The physiological basis of monozygotic twinning is slowly coming to light. Evidence now suggests that the division of the fertilized ovum may occur as the result of a delay in the timing of normal developmental events. In humans, evidence suggests that delayed transport through the tube increases the risk of twinning. Because progestational agents and combination contraceptives decrease tubal motility, delayed tubal transport and implantation are believed to increase the risk of twinning in pregnancies conceived in close proximity to contraceptive use (Bressers and colleagues, 1987). It is also possible that minor trauma to the blastocyst during assisted reproduction techniques is responsible for the increased incidence of monozygotic twinning observed in pregnancies conceived in this manner (Wenstrom and co-workers, 1993).

The outcome of the twinning process depends on when the division occurs:

- If division occurs before the inner cell mass (morula) is formed and the outer layer of blastocyst is not yet committed to become chorion, that is, within the first 72 hours after fertilization, two embryos, two amnions, and two chorions will develop (Fig. 30–3). There will evolve a diamonionic, dichorionic, and monozygotic twin pregnancy. There may be two distinct placentas or a single fused placenta (Fig. 30–4).
- If division occurs between the fourth and eighth day, after the inner cell mass is formed and cells destined to become chorion have already differentiated but those of the amnion have not, two embryos will develop, each in separate amnionic sacs (Fig. 30–3). The two amnionic sacs will eventually be covered by a common chorion, thus giving rise to diamnionic, monochorionic, monozygotic twin pregnancy (Fig. 30–4C).
- If, however, the amnion has already become established, which occurs about 8 days after fertilization, division will result in two embryos within a common amnionic sac, or a monoamnionic, monochorionic, monozygotic twin pregnancy.
- If division is initiated even later, that is after the embryonic disk is formed, cleavage is incomplete and conjoined twins are formed.

CHIMERISM. A chimera is an individual whose cells originated from more than one fertilized ovum. Chimerism is to be distinguished from mosaicism, in which two or more cell lines of different chromosomal composition arise from the same zygote as the consequence of nondisjunction during meiotic division (Chap. 36). One possible mechanism for chimerism is the transfer of genetic

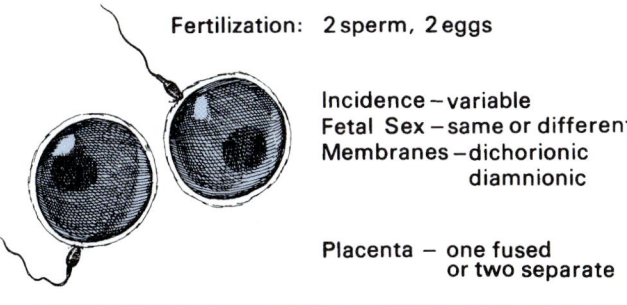

Fertilization: 2 sperm, 2 eggs

Incidence – variable
Fetal Sex – same or different
Membranes – dichorionic
                       diamnionic

Placenta – one fused
                   or two separate

FIGURE 30–2. Mechanism of dizygotic twinning.

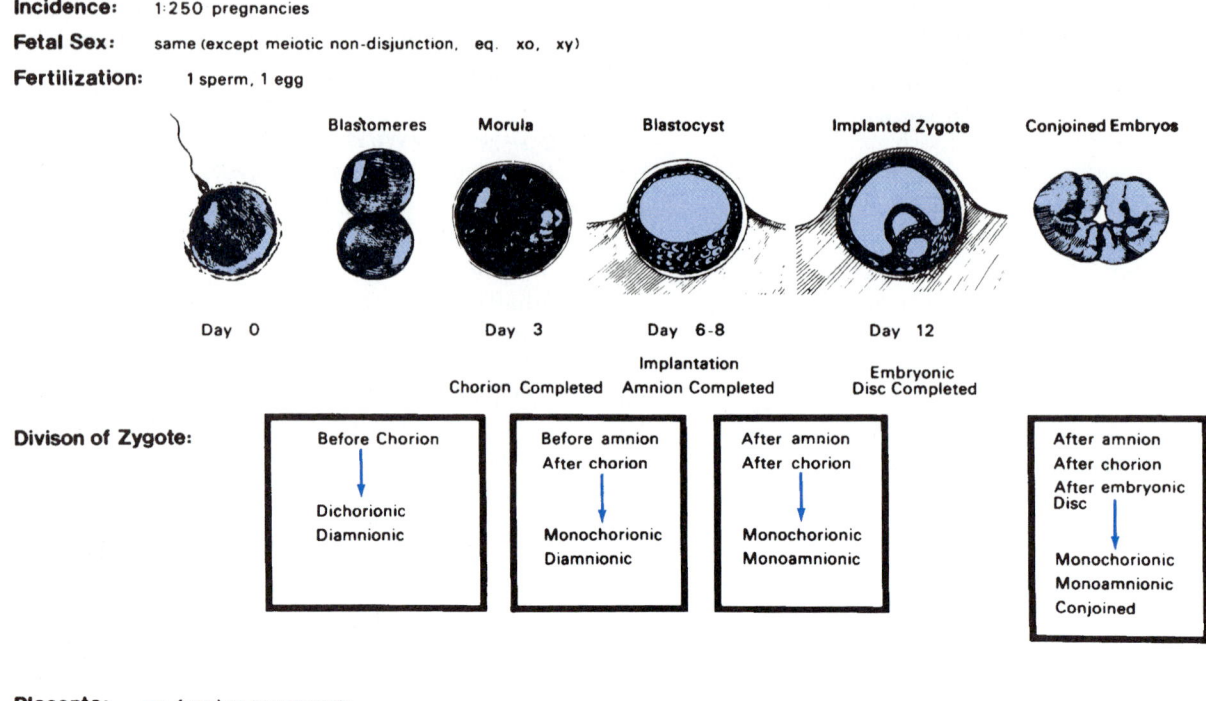

Incidence: 1:250 pregnancies

Fetal Sex: same (except meiotic non-disjunction, eq. xo, xy)

Fertilization: 1 sperm, 1 egg

Placenta: one fused or two separate
(two separate ⟶ dichorionic)

FIGURE 30–3. Mechanism of monozygous twinning.

material from one nonidentical twin fetus to the other across chorionic vascular anastomoses. The transposed cells are not destroyed, because the transfer occurs before the maturation of the fetal immune system and the recipient fetus becomes tolerant to the dissimilar antigens on the donor tissues. Blood chimerism is most commonly discovered at the time of blood typing when cells with two different blood types are found in one individual (Benirschke, 1974).

SUPERFETATION AND SUPERFECUNDATION. In superfetation, an interval as long as or longer than an ovulatory cycle intervenes between fertilizations. Superfetation requires ovulation during the course of an established pregnancy, which would theoretically be possible until the uterine cavity is obliterated by the fusion of the decidua capsularis to the decidua vera. Although known to occur in mares, superfetation is as yet unproven in humans. Most authorities believe that the alleged cases of human superfetation result from marked inequality in growth and development of twin fetuses of the same gestational age.

Superfecundation refers to the fertilization of two ova within a short period of time but not at the same

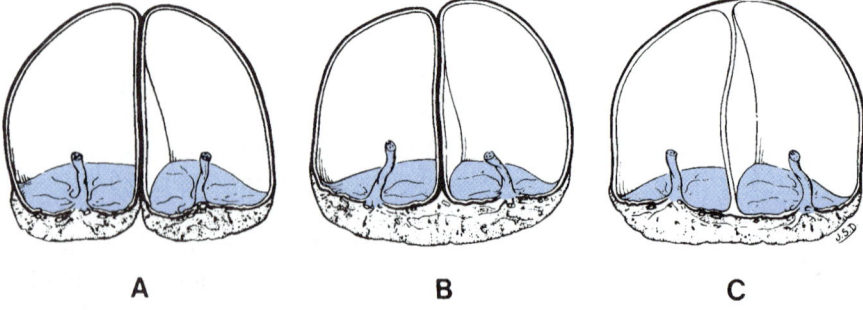

    A   **B**   **C**

FIGURE 30–4. Placenta and membranes in twin pregnancies. **A.** Two placentas, two amnions, two chorions (from either dizygotic twins or monozygotic twins with cleavage of zygote during first 3 days after fertilization). **B.** Single placenta, two amnions, and two chorions (from either dizygotic twins or monozygotic twins with cleavage of zygote during first 3 days). **C.** One placenta, one chorion, two amnions (monozygotic twins with cleavage of zygote from the fourth to the eighth day after fertilization).

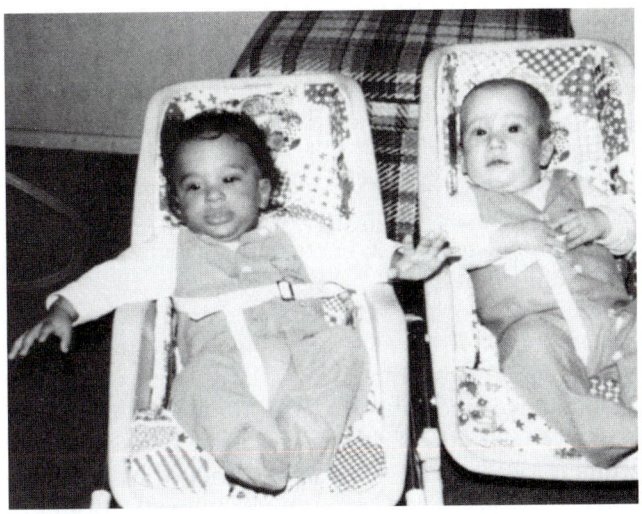

FIGURE 30–5. An example of dizygotic twin boys as the consequence of superfecundation. (Courtesy of Dr. David Harris.)

coitus, nor necessarily by sperm from the same male. It may be that twin ova are not fertilized by sperm from the same ejaculate, but that fact can be demonstrated only in exceptional circumstances.

An instance of superfecundation, documented by Harris (1982), is demonstrated in Figure 30–5. The mother was raped on the 10th day of her menstrual cycle and had intercourse 1 week later with her husband. She went into labor very near term and was delivered of a black infant whose blood type was A and a white infant whose blood type was O. The blood type of both the mother and her husband was O. HLA typing was not done. Terasaki and co-workers (1978) described the use of HLA typing to establish that dizygotic twins were sired by different fathers.

FREQUENCY OF TWINS. The frequency of monozygotic twin births is relatively constant worldwide, at approximately one set per 250 births, and is largely independent of race, heredity, age, and parity. The frequency was once thought to be independent of therapy for infertility; however, there is now evidence that the incidence of zygotic splitting is increased following assisted reproductive technologies. The incidence of dizygotic twinning is influenced remarkably by race, heredity, maternal age, parity, and especially, fertility drugs.

THE "VANISHING TWIN." Improved ultrasound technology has facilitated sonographic studies of early gestations which show that the first trimester incidence of twins is much greater than the incidence of twins at birth. Multiple gestations are now estimated to occur in 12 percent of all spontaneous conceptions, but only

14 percent of these survive to term (Boklage, 1990). Monochorionic twins have a significantly greater risk of abortion than dichorionic twins (Sebire and colleagues, 1997). In some cases the entire pregnancy is lost, but in many cases, only one fetus is lost and the pregnancy delivers as a singleton. Studies in which pregnancies were evaluated with ultrasound in the first trimester have shown that one twin is lost or "vanishes" before the second trimester in 21 to 63 percent of spontaneous twin conceptions (Kol and associates, 1993; Landy and colleagues, 1986; Parisi and co-workers, 1983). Undoubtedly, some threatened abortions have resulted in actual abortion of one embryo from an unrecognized twin gestation while the other embryo continued its growth and development (Jauniaux and co-workers, 1988).

This event can be upsetting to patients who worry about the fate of the remaining fetus. Usually, there is no evidence of the lost fetus at birth, and patients can be reassured that losing a fetus in this manner does not increase the risk of pregnancy complications. It is important to establish the diagnosis, however, because it may complicate maternal serum screening for Down syndrome or neural-tube defects, and can result in abnormal genetic testing. The vanishing twin can cause a discrepancy between the karyotype established by chorionic villous sampling and the fetal karyotype when tissue from the vanished twin is inadvertently sampled. For these reasons, amniocentesis for karyotype may be preferable (Reddy and associates, 1991). It can also cause an elevated maternal serum alpha-fetoprotein level as well as an elevated amnionic fluid alpha-fetoprotein level and a positive acetylcholinesterase assay (Winsor and associates, 1987).

Multiple embryos and fetuses may develop ectopically, that is, outside the uterus. Such multiple ectopic pregnancies, as well as combined pregnancies in which there are one or more extrauterine embryos or fetuses as well as one or more intrauterine, are considered in Chapter 34.

RACE. The frequency of multiple fetal births varies significantly among different races and ethnic groups (Table 30–2). Myrianthopoulos (1970) identified the birth of twins in 1 of every 100 pregnancies among white women, compared with 1 of 80 pregnancies for black women. In some areas of Africa the frequency of twinning is very high. Knox and Morley (1960), in a survey of one rural community in Nigeria, found that twinning occurred once in every 20 births! Twinning in Asia is less common. In Japan, for example, among more than 10 million pregnancies analyzed, twinning was identified in only 1 of 155 births. These marked differences in twinning frequency may be the consequence of racial variations in follicle-stimulating hormone levels which

TABLE 30–2. Twinning Rates per 1000 Births by Zygosity

Country	Monozygotic	Dizygotic	Total
Nigeria	5.0	49	54
United States			
Black	4.7	11.1	15.8
White	4.2	7.1	11.3
England and Wales	3.5	8.8	12.3
India (Calcutta)	3.3	8.1	11.4
Japan	3.0	1.3	4.3

From MacGillivray (1986), with permission.

can lead to multiple ovulation. In the Nigerian population, mean follicle-stimulating hormone levels are higher at the peak and for four days before and after the peak in women who have had one set of twins than in women who have had only singletons. Women who have had more than one set of twins have even higher follicle-stimulating hormone levels (Nylander, 1973).

HEREDITY. As a determinant of twinning, the family history of the mother is much more important than that of the father. White and Wyshak (1964), in a study of 4000 records of the General Society of the Church of Jesus Christ of Latter-day Saints, found that women who themselves were a dizygotic twin gave birth to twins at the rate of 1 set per 58 births. Women not a twin, but whose husbands were a dizygotic twin, gave birth to twins at the rate of 1 set per 116 pregnancies. One explanation is that it is the tendency to multiple ovulation which is inherited. A Belgian–Dutch group has reported that dizygotic twinning may be influenced by an autosomal dominant gene carried by approximately 15 percent of the population (Meulemans and colleagues, 1996). If true, this gene may exert its effects only in women.

MATERNAL AGE AND PARITY. The rate of twinning rises from 0 at puberty, a time of minimal ovarian activity, to a peak at age 37, when maximal hormonal stimulation increases the rate of double ovulation (Bulmer, 1959). This is in accordance with the first consistently observed sign of reproductive aging, an isolated rise in serum follicle-stimulating hormone (Klein and co-workers, 1996). The fall in incidence after age 37 probably reflects exhaustion of the Graafian follicles. Fertility, as reflected by any increase in parity up to 7, also increases the twinning rate independent of maternal age. Increasing maternal age and parity have been shown to increase the incidence of twinning in all populations studied. Waterhouse demonstrated that twin pregnancies were a third as common in women under 20 with no previous children, as in women 35 to 40 years old

with four or more previous children (1950). In Sweden, Pettersson and associates (1976) determined that the frequency of multiple fetuses in first pregnancies was 1.3 percent, compared with 2.7 percent in the fourth pregnancy. In Nigeria, Azubuike (1982) showed that the frequency of twinning increased from 1 in 50 (2 percent) pregnancies among women pregnant for the first time to 1 in 15 (6.6 percent) for women pregnant six or more times!

NUTRITIONAL FACTORS. In animals the litter size increases with the nutritional level. Evidence from a variety of sources indicates that this occurs in humans as well. Nylander (1971) showed a definite gradient in the twinning rate related to nutritional status as reflected by maternal size. Taller, heavier women had a twinning rate 25 to 30 percent higher than short, nutritionally deprived women. MacGillivray (1986) also found that dizygotic twinning is more common in large and tall women than in small women. Evidence that the twinning rate is related more to nutrition than to body size alone was acquired during and after World War II. Widespread undernourishment in Europe during those years was associated with a marked fall in the dizygotic twinning rate (Bulmer, 1959). More recently, Czeizel and colleagues (1994), in a randomized trial of periconceptional folic acid supplementation, found that women who received folic acid supplementation had an increased incidence of multiple gestations.

PITUITARY GONADOTROPIN. The common factor linking race, age, weight, and fertility to multiple gestation may be follicle-stimulating hormone levels. Benirschke and Kim (1973) presented intriguing reasons for implicating elevated levels of endogenous follicle-stimulating hormone in the genesis of spontaneous dizygous twinning. In addition to the data cited earlier, this theory is supported by the fact that increased fecundity and a higher rate of dizygous twinning have been reported in women who conceive within 1 month after stopping oral contraceptives, but not during subsequent months (Rothman, 1977). This may be due to the sudden release of pituitary gonadotropin in amounts greater than usual during the first spontaneous cycle after stopping contraception.

INFERTILITY THERAPY. The induction of ovulation by use of gonadotropins (follicle-stimulating hormone plus chorionic gonadotropin) or clomiphene remarkably enhances the likelihood of multiple ovulations. The incidence of multiple gestation following conventional gonadotropin therapy is 16 to 40 percent, with 75 percent being twins (Schenker and co-workers, 1981). Tuppin and colleagues (1993) reported that in France the incidence of twin and triplet deliveries and the sale of human menopausal gonadotropin rose in parallel between 1972 and 1989, so that by 1989, half of triplet pregnancies resulted from ovulation induction. Superovulation therapy, which increases the chance of pregnancy by recruiting multiple follicles, results in multiple gestation rates of 25 to 30 percent (Bailey-Pridham and associates, 1990). Therapy with pulsatile gonadotrophin-releasing hormone is associated with a 10 percent incidence of multiple gestation, of which the majority are twins (Blunt and Butt, 1988; Homburg and co-authors, 1989).

Risk factors for multiple fetuses after ovarian stimulation with human menopausal gonadotropin include increased estradiol levels on the day of chorionic gonadotropin injection and sperm characteristics such as increased concentration and motility (Dickey and associates, 1992; Pasqualotto and colleagues, 1999). Recognition of these factors plus the ability to sonographically monitor follicle growth and size and cancel cycles likely to lead to a multiple gestation have led to a reduction in the incidence of multiple births. Although clomiphene therapy was previously associated with a lower incidence of multiple gestation than human menopausal gonodotropin, the majority of multiple gestations resulting from ovulation induction are currently caused by clomiphene (Rein and colleagues, 1990).

Ovulation induction increases both dizygotic and monozygotic twinning. Derom and colleagues (1987) studied the incidence of monozygotic twinning in almost 1000 twin-pairs delivered in East Flanders, Belgium, and reported that the incidence of zygotic splitting was doubled after induced ovulation. Multiple gestation resulting from ovulation induction has also been associated with an increased risk of mendelian, chromosomal, and multifactorial fetal anomalies (Brambati and associates, 1995; Shoham and colleagues, 1991). This risk is related to the age and family history of the women undergoing therapy, however, and not to the treatment itself.

ASSISTED REPRODUCTION TECHNOLOGIES (ART). Techniques designed to increase the probability of pregnancy increase the probability of multiple gestation as well. Typically, patients undergo superovulation, and in vitro fertilization is attempted in all retrieved ova. Because the likelihood of a successful pregnancy increases according to the number of blastocysts transferred, as many as five blastocysts may be replaced (Bradshaw and colleagues, 1992). This practice not only increases multiple gestation, it increases the incidence of high-order multiples, that is, pregnancies with four or more fetuses.

High-order multiple gestation entails significant risk to both mother and fetuses (discussed later) and reduces the chances of both a live birth or the birth of a child without significant handicap. The only remedy is a selective reduction procedure, which also increases risk. Ad-

ditionally, it is expensive. Goldfarb and colleagues (1996) estimated the combined costs of in vitro fertilization plus prenatal care and delivery was $39,249 for singletons or twins, and this increased to $342,788 for triplets or higher-order multiple gestations. Most of the costs for singletons or twins were attributed to in vitro fertilization, whereas most of the costs with triplets or more were due to intensive care. Gleicher and co-workers (1995) found that most couples considered the possibility of twins desirable, but higher-order multiple births were typically rejected because of the risks and costs.

The high morbidity and mortality associated with high-order multiples has motivated a concerted effort by the reproductive endocrinology community to reduce the incidence of this outcome, with favorable results. It has been shown that the chances of a live birth increase along with the number of eggs successfully fertilized, presumably because it improves the selection of embryos for transfer (Templeton and Morris, 1998). Selection is further improved by culturing the embryos for 5 days to the blastocyst stage, because it allows identification of the most viable blastocysts and an acceptable chance of pregnancy with the transfer of fewer embryos (Scholtes and Zeilmaker, 1996). This and similar data have led to a protocol in which many eggs are retrieved, fertilized, and grown to the blastocyst stage, but then only one to three of the healthiest are transferred. Two-embryo transfer for women with a good prognosis has been advocated as a way to maintain the successful pregnancy rate while decreasing the number of high-order multiples (Meldrum and Gardner, 1998). This has been promoted by the American Society for Reproductive Medicine (1999). Less intensive gonadotropin stimulation, another strategy to reduce high-order multiple pregnancy, has proved of limited value (Gleicher and colleagues, 2000).

SEX RATIOS WITH MULTIPLE FETUSES. The percentage of male conceptuses in the human species decreases as the number of fetuses per pregnancy increases. Strandskov and co-workers (1946) found the sex ratio, or percentage of males, for 31 million singleton births in the United States to be 51.6 percent. For twins it was 50.9 percent; for triplets, 49.5 percent; and for quadruplets, 46.5 percent. There is an even greater excess of females in twins resulting from late twinning events. Seventy percent of monochorionic–monoamnionic twins and 75 percent of conjoined twins are female (Machin, 1996). Two explanations have been offered. First, there is a well-known differential fetal mortality between the sexes, which persists for the newborn infant, child, and adult. Survival is always in favor of the female and against the male. The population pressure with multiple fetuses in utero may exaggerate the biological tendency noted in singleton pregnancies. A sec-

TABLE 30–3. Overview of the Incidence of Twin Pregnancy Zygosity and Corresponding Twin-specific Complications

Type of Twinning	Twins	Twin-specific Complication (%)			
		Fetal Growth Restriction	Preterm Delivery[a]	Placental Vascular Anastomosis	Perinatal Mortality
Dizygous	80	25	40	0	10–12
Monozygous	20	40	50		15–18
Diamnionic/dichorionic	6–7	30	40	0	18–20
Diamnionic/monochorionic	13–14	50	60	100	30–40
Monoamnionic/monochorionic	<1	40	60–70	80–90	58–60
Conjoined	0.002 to 0.008	—	70–80	100	70–90

[a]Delivery before 37 weeks.
Modified from Manning (1995), with permission.

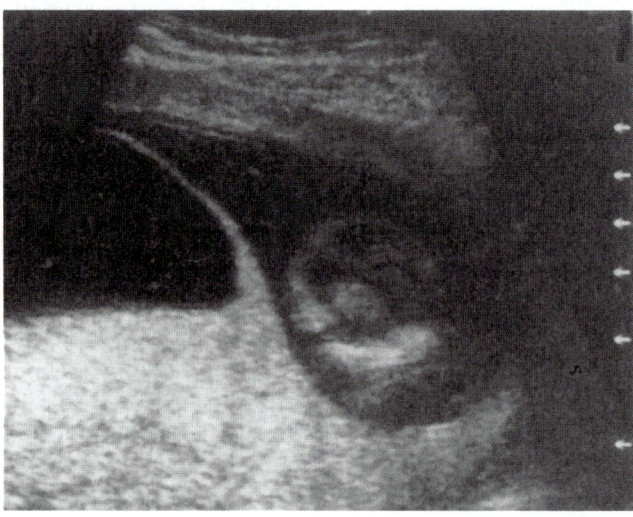

A

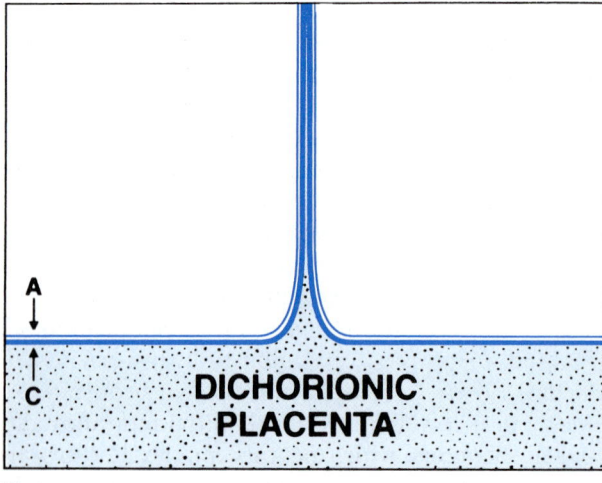

B

FIGURE 30–6. A. Ultrasound image of "twin peak" sign showing an extension of placental tissue into the intertwin membrane, confirming dichorionic twinning. **B.** Schematic diagram of the twin peak sign. (From Finberg, 1992, with permission.)

ond explanation is that the female-producing zygote has a greater tendency to divide into twins, triplets, and quadruplets.

DETERMINATION OF ZYGOSITY. The main reason to determine zygosity antenatally is that it is beneficial in assessing obstetrical risks as well as guiding management of multiple gestations (Fisk and Bryan, 1993). Twin-specific complications in relation to zygosity are summarized in Table 30–3. Clearly, monochorial twin gestations are at increased risk for a variety of pregnancy complications, some of which may be minimized by early antepartum diagnosis and treatment. Of particular importance are those monozygotic twins with shared circulation (twin-to-twin transfusion syndrome), shared amnionic sac (cord entanglement), and shared organs (conjoined twins).

Another important reason to encourage determination of zygosity is that this knowledge may facilitate inter-twin organ transplantation later in life. Determination of zygosity frequently requires sophisticated genetic tests because dizygotic twins can look alike, while monozygotic twins are not always identical. Monozygotic twins may actually be discordant for genetic mutations as the result of a postzygotic mutation, or may have the same genetic disease but with marked variability in expression. In female fetuses, skewed lyonization can produce differential expression of X-linked traits or diseases. Most interestingly, monozygotic twins may be discordant for malformations which involve asymmetrical organs. For example, a fetus who is the mirror image of his twin may have a heart defect caused by reversed looping or laterality (Machin, 1996).

SONOGRAPHIC EVALUATION. Zygosity can be determined prenatally only if the fetuses are monoamnionic or monochorionic. Dichorionic, diamnionic twins may be either dizygotic or monozygotic. A third of monozygotic twins have dichorionic placentas, separate or fused (Machin, 1996). For obstetrical reasons, it is more important to determine the number of chorions. Chorionicity can be determined as early as the first trimester using multiple sonographic signs. The presence of two separate placental sites and a thick dividing membrane that generally is 2 mm or greater (Fig. 30–6A) supports dichorionicity. Fetuses of opposite gender are almost always dizygotic as well (Mahony and co-workers, 1985).

In pregnancies in which there is a single placental mass, it may be difficult to distinguish one large placenta from two placentas lying side by side or "fused." In this situation it is important to examine the point of origin of the dividing membrane on the placental surface. If there is a triangular projection of placental tissue extending beyond the chorionic surface between the layers of the dividing membrane—termed the "twin peak"

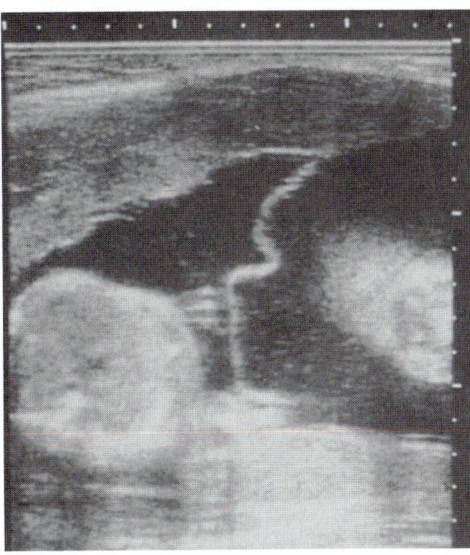

FIGURE 30–7. Sonogram of twins at 18 weeks' gestational age. Two fetal poles are separated by intervening membranes that divide the amnionic sacs. (Courtesy of Dr. R. Santos.)

sign—there are actually two fused placentas present (Fig. 30–6B).

Monochorionic pregnancies have a dividing membrane that is so thin it may not be visualized at all until the second trimester. The membrane is generally less than 2 mm in thickness, and magnification reveals only two layers (Scardo and associates, 1995). As shown in Figure 30–7, ultrasonic evaluation of the dividing membrane is easiest and most accurate in the first half of pregnancy when the fetuses are smaller (Stagiannis and colleagues, 1995). A monochorionic pregnancy with discordant amnionic fluid volume, discordant fetal size, and little or no change in the position of one twin, should raise suspicion of twin-twin transfusion syndrome (discussed later). Scardo and colleagues (1995) used the combination of placental location, dividing membrane thickness, presence or absence of the twin peak sign, and fetal gender to determine the chorionicity, amnionicity, and zygosity in 110 consecutive twins at midgestation. Compared to the pathological diagnosis made by examining the placenta after delivery, the ultrasound determination had 91 percent sensitivity and specificity. In 35 percent of cases, however, zygosity could not be determined even by placental pathology, emphasizing that determination of zygosity often requires sophisticated genetic testing.

PLACENTAL EXAMINATION. A knowledgeably performed examination of the placenta and membranes serves to establish zygosity promptly in about two thirds of cases. The following system for examination is recommended: As the first infant is delivered, one clamp is placed on the portion of the cord coming from the pla-

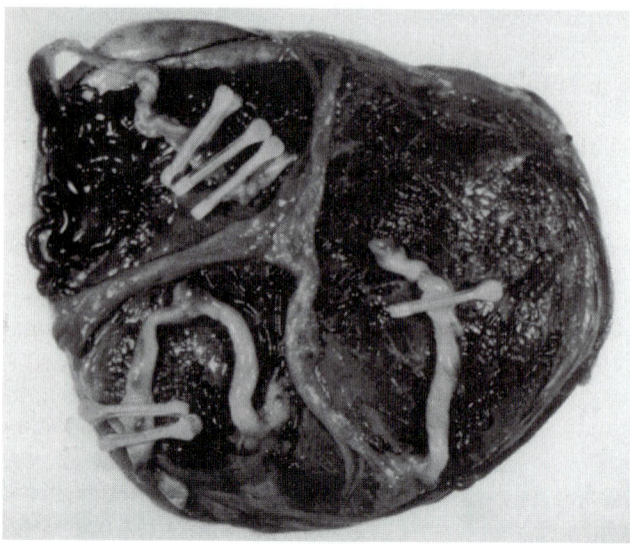

FIGURE 30–8. Placenta from a triplet gestation showing umbilical cord clamps placed in order of delivery of the infants. This identification system aids determination of zygosity.

centa (Fig. 30–8). Cord blood is not collected until after delivery of the co-twin, unless it has been clearly shown that there are two placentas. As the second infant is delivered, two clamps are placed on that cord. Three clamps are used to mark the cord of a third infant, and so on as necessary. Until the delivery of the last fetus is completed, it is important that each cord segment remain clamped to prevent hemorrhage through anastomoses in the placenta.

Delivery of the placenta should be accomplished with care to preserve the attachment of the amnion and chorion to the placenta, because identification of the relationship of the membranes to each other is critical. With one common amnionic sac, or with juxtaposed amnions not separated by chorion arising between the fetuses, the infants are monozygotic. If adjacent amnions are separated by chorion, the fetuses could be either dizygotic or monozygotic, but dizygosity is more common (Figs. 30–4, 30–9, and 30–10). If the infants are of the same sex, blood typing of cord blood samples might be helpful. Different blood types confirms dizygosity, although demonstrating the same blood type in each fetus is not enough to confirm monozygosity. For definitive diagnosis, more complicated techniques such as DNA fingerprinting can be used, but these tests are generally not performed at birth unless there is a pressing medical indication (Azuma and associates, 1989).

INFANT SEX AND ZYGOSITY. Twins of opposite sex are almost always dizygotic. Very rarely, monozygotic twins may be discordant for phenotypic sex. This occurs when one twin is phenotypically female due to Turner syndrome (45,X) and its sibling is 46,XY.

DIAGNOSIS OF MULTIPLE FETUSES

Widespread use of prenatal ultrasound imaging has greatly decreased the incidence of overlooked twin gestations prior to delivery.

ULTRASOUND. By careful ultrasonic examination, separate gestational sacs can be identified very early in twin pregnancy (Fig. 30–11). Subsequently, the identification of each fetal head should be made in two perpendicular planes so as not to mistake a cross-section of the fetal trunk for a second fetal head. Ideally, two fetal heads or two abdomens should be seen in the same plane, to avoid scanning the same fetus twice and interpreting it as twins. Sonographic scanning should detect practically all sets of twins. Indeed, one argument in favor of routine ultrasound screening is earlier detection of multiple fetuses (Chap. 41, p. 1113). In the Routine Antenatal Diagnostic Imaging and Ultrasound Study (RADIUS), LeFevre and co-workers (1993) randomized 7617 women to undergo ultrasound examinations at 18 to 20 weeks and again at 31 to 35 weeks. Another 7534 women were randomized to undergo ultrasound scanning only when clinically indicated. Virtually all multiple gestations (99 percent) were diagnosed before 26 weeks when routine ultrasound was used compared with 62 percent in women scanned only for specific indications. A total of 87 percent of multiple gestations were ultimately diagnosed sonographically before labor in these latter women. Higher-order multiple gestations are harder to evaluate. Even in the first trimester it can be difficult to determine the correct number of fetuses and their position, which is important for nonselective pregnancy reduction and essential for selective termination (discussed later).

HISTORY AND CLINICAL EXAMINATION. A maternal family history of twins, older maternal age, high parity, large maternal size, and a previous history of twins provide weak clues, but knowledge of recent administration of either clomiphene or gonadotropins or pregnancy accomplished by assisted reproductive technology provide strong ones.

Clinical examination with accurate measurement of fundal height, as described in Chapter 10 (p. 228), is essential. During the second trimester, the uterine size is larger than expected for gestational age determined from menstrual data. Rouse and co-workers (1993) measured fundal heights in 336 well-dated twin pregnancies. Between 20 and 30 weeks, fundal heights were on average about 5 cm greater than expected for singletons of the same fetal age.

In the case of a woman with a uterus that appears large for gestational age, the following possibilities are considered:

1. Multiple fetuses.
2. Elevation of the uterus by a distended bladder.
3. Inaccurate menstrual history.
4. Hydramnios.
5. Hydatidiform mole.
6. Uterine myomas.
7. A closely attached adnexal mass.
8. Fetal macrosomia late in pregnancy.

OTHER DIAGNOSTIC AIDS. A variety of techniques may be used to clinically suspect or diagnose multifetal gestation.

FETAL PARTS. When uterine palpation leads to diagnosis of twins, it is most often because two fetal heads have been detected, often in different uterine quadrants. In general, however, it is difficult to diagnose twins by palpation of fetal parts before the third trimester. Even late in pregnancy it may be very difficult to identify twins by transabdominal palpation, especially if one twin overlies the other, if the woman is obese, or if hydramnios is present.

FETAL HEART SOUNDS. Late in the first trimester, fetal heart action may be detected with generally available Doppler ultrasonic equipment. Sometime thereafter it becomes possible to identify two fetal hearts if their rates are clearly distinct from each other as well as from

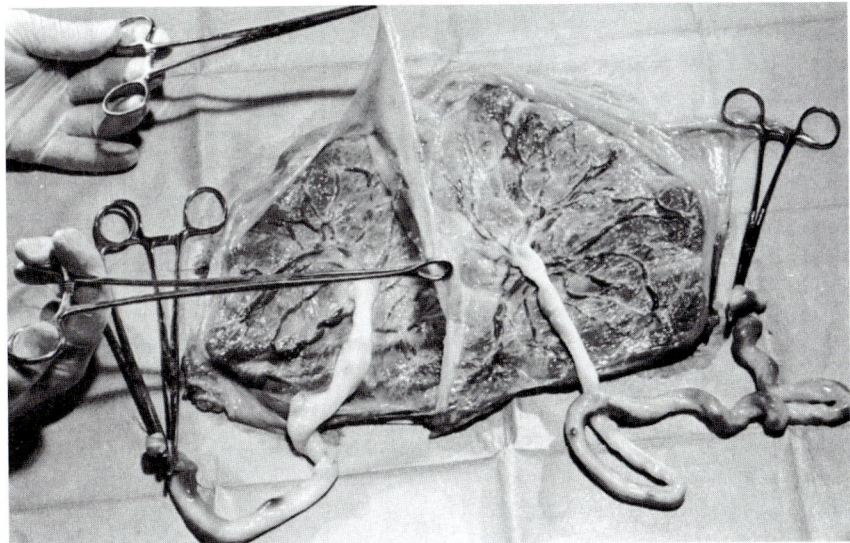

A

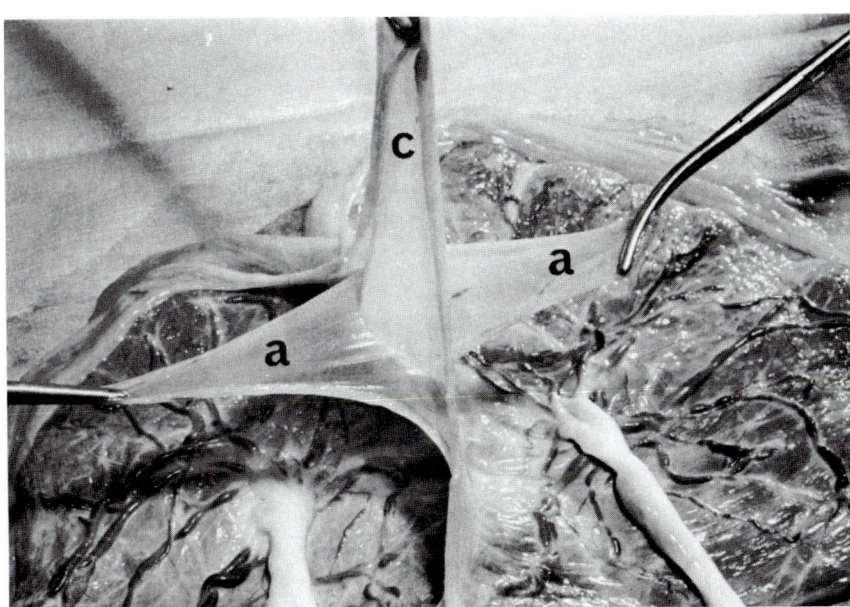

B

FIGURE 30–9. A. The membrane partition that separated twin fetuses is elevated. **B.** The membrane partition consists of chorion (c) between two amnions (a).

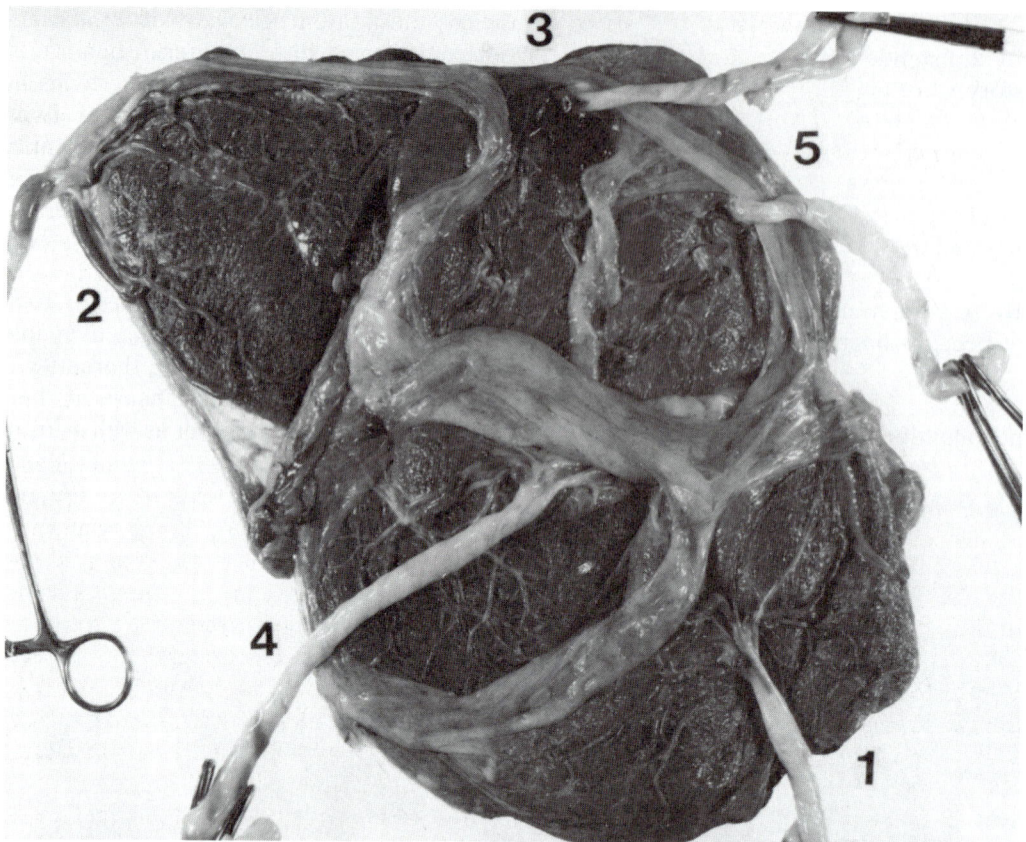

FIGURE 30–10. Quintuplet placenta with five separate amnionic sacs delivered at 32 weeks. Amnionic sacs of numbers 3 and 5 were not separated by chorion and therefore those infants are monozygous. Infant birthweights ranged from a high of 1530 g (no. 1) to 860 g (no. 5). All of the infants survived.

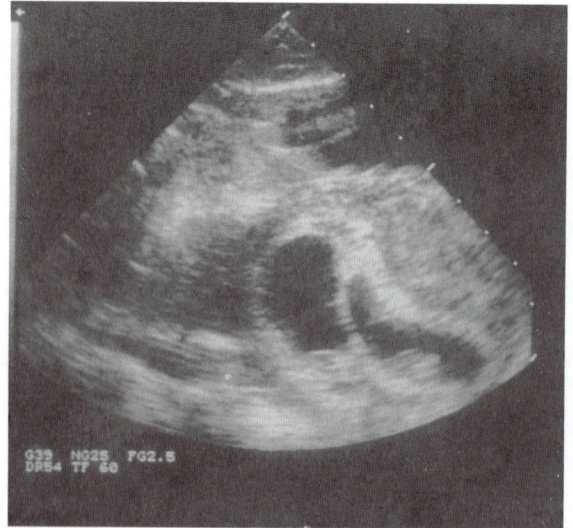

FIGURE 30–11. Longitudinal sonogram demonstrating two gestational sacs, each containing a fetus, at 7 weeks menstrual age. (Courtesy of J. and J. Ackerman and Dr. R. Santos.)

that of the mother. It is possible by careful examination to identify fetal heart sounds in twins with the usual aural fetal stethoscopes at 18 to 20 weeks.

RADIOLOGICAL EXAMINATION. A radiograph of the maternal abdomen to try to demonstrate multiple fetuses can be helpful in rare circumstances, usually when there is a high-order multiple gestation and it is unclear how many fetuses are present. Even more rarely, one of the fetuses may be suspected of having a bone dysplasia best visualized radiologically. Radiographs are otherwise frequently not useful and may be responsible for an incorrect diagnosis for the following reasons:

1. The film is taken before 18 weeks when the fetal skeletons are insufficiently radiopaque.
2. The film is of poor quality from inappropriate exposure time or from malposition of the mother so that her upper abdomen and the fetus beneath are excluded from the x-ray.
3. The mother is obese.
4. There is hydramnios.
5. One or more fetuses moves during the exposure.

BIOCHEMICAL TESTS. The amounts of chorionic gonadotropin in plasma and in urine, on average, are higher than those found with a singleton pregnancy, but not so high as to allow a definite diagnosis of multiple fetuses. Twins are frequently diagnosed during an evaluation for an elevated maternal serum alpha-fetoprotein level, although this alone is not diagnostic (Chap. 37, p. 980). Currently, there is no biochemical test that in any individual case will reliably differentiate between the presence of one and more than one fetus.

MATERNAL ADAPTATION

In general, the degree of maternal physiological change is greater with multiple fetuses than with a single fetus. Beginning in the first trimester, women with multiple gestation often have nausea and vomiting in excess of that characterizing singleton pregnancies, for reasons that are not clear. The normal maternal blood volume expansion is greater in twin pregnancies (Pritchard, 1965). Whereas the average increase in late pregnancy is about 40 to 50 percent with a single fetus, it is about 50 to 60 percent with twins, which amounts to a maternal blood volume about 500 mL greater. The red cell mass increases as well, but proportionately less in twin pregnancies than in singletons, resulting in a more pronounced "physiological anemia." Women with twins have an average hemoglobin concentration of 10 g/dL from 20 weeks onward (Campbell, 1986). The average blood loss with vaginal delivery of twins is 935 mL, or nearly 500 mL more than with delivery of a single fetus. Both the remarkable increase in maternal blood volume and the increased iron and folate requirements imposed by a second fetus predispose to a greater prevalence of maternal anemia.

Veille and associates (1985) used M-mode echocardiography to assess cardiac function in women with twin pregnancies. As expected, cardiac output was increased compared with singleton pregnancy, but end-diastolic ventricular dimensions were the same. During the third trimester, cardiac output was increased as a result of both increased heart rate and increased stroke volume. Stroke volume was higher by virtue of increased fractional shortening, which suggests increased contractility. Women carrying twins also have a typical pattern of arterial blood pressure change. Compared with mothers of singletons, their diastolic blood pressure is lower at 20 weeks, and 74 percent have a diastolic pressure less than 80 mm Hg compared with 66 percent of singletons. This is followed by a greater rise in diastolic pressure between midpregnancy and delivery, and 95 percent of women with twins have a 15 mm Hg or greater increase compared with only 54 percent of singleton pregnancies (Campbell, 1986).

The larger size of the uterus with multiple fetuses intensifies the anatomical changes that occur during pregnancy. The uterus and its contents may achieve a volume of 10 L or more and weigh in excess of 20 pounds! Especially with monozygotic twins, rapid accumulation of grossly excessive amounts of amnionic fluid, that is, acute hydramnios, may develop. In these circumstances it is easy to envision appreciable compression and displacement of many of the abdominal viscera as well as the lungs by the elevated diaphragm. The size and weight of the very large uterus may preclude more than a very sedentary existence for the woman.

In multiple gestation complicated by hydramnios, maternal renal function may become seriously impaired, most likely as the consequence of obstructive uropathy. Quigley and Cruikshank (1977) described two pregnancies with twin fetuses plus acute and severe hydramnios in which oliguria and azotemia developed. Maternal urine output and plasma creatinine levels promptly returned to normal after delivery. In the case of severe hydramnios, therapeutic amniocentesis may be employed to provide relief for the mother and, it is hoped, to allow the pregnancy to continue (Chap. 31, p. 820). Unfortunately, the hydramnios is often characterized by acute onset remote from term and by rapid reaccumulation following amniocentesis.

The various stresses of pregnancy and the likelihood of serious maternal complications will almost invariably be greater with multiple fetuses than with a singleton. This should be taken into account, especially when counseling the woman whose health is compromised and whose multiple gestation is recognized early. The same is true for a woman who is not pregnant but is considering infertility treatment by ovulation induction or assisted reproductive technology.

PREGNANCY OUTCOME

ABORTION. Spontaneous abortion is more likely with multiple fetuses. Detailed reviews have identified three times more twins among aborted pregnancies when compared with the ratios at term (Livingston and Poland, 1980; Uchida and co-authors, 1983). Monochorial twins greatly outnumber dichorial twins by 18 to 1, implicating monozygosity as a risk factor for spontaneous abortion. Anomalies and chromosomal errors, as in singletons, are also often found in twin abortuses.

MALFORMATIONS. The incidence of congenital malformations is appreciably increased in twin and higher-order multiple gestations compared with singletons. Major malformations occur in 2 percent and minor malformations in 4 percent of twins. (Cameron and colleagues, 1983; Kohl and Casey, 1975). This increase is almost entirely due to the high incidence of structural defects in monozygotic twins. According to Schinzel and associates (1979), anomalies in monozygotic twins generally fall into one of three categories:

1. Defects resulting from twinning itself, which some consider to be a teratogenic event. This category includes conjoined twins, amorphous twins, sirenomelia, neural-tube defects, and holoprosencephaly.
2. Defects resulting from vascular interchange between monochorionic twins. Vascular connections can give rise to reverse flow with acardia in one twin, or if one twin dies, intravascular coagulation with embolization to the living twin can cause defects such as microcephaly, hydranencephaly, intestinal atresia, aplasia cutis, or limb amputation.
3. Defects that occur as the result of crowding. Examples include talipes or congenital hip dislocation.

Dizygotic twins can have malformations of the type that occur in singletons as well as defects due to crowding. Baldwin (1991) has comprehensively reviewed anomalies occurring in twins.

Persistent or chronic hydramnios is more likely to be associated with fetal anomalies of one or both twins. Hashimoto and colleagues (1986) subjectively identified increased amnionic fluid in a fourth of twin pregnancies. In half, hydramnios at midpregnancy was transient, and all of these fetuses were normal. In the 10 pregnancies in which hydramnios persisted, nine fetuses had anomalies.

BIRTHWEIGHT. Multifetal gestations are more likely to be characterized by low birthweight than singletons, due mostly to restricted fetal growth and preterm delivery (Buekens and Wilcox, 1993). In general, the larger the number of fetuses, the greater the degree of growth restriction. Two thirds of twin and even more triplet pregnancies are complicated by fetal growth restriction. However, this assessment of growth is based on growth curves established for singletons. Several authorities have made the argument that fetal growth in multiple gestation is different from that of singletons, and that abnormal growth should be diagnosed only when fetal size is less than expected for *multiple gestation*. Triplet growth curves have been created for this purpose (Rodis and associates, 1999). In dizygotic pregnancies, marked size discordance usually results from unequal placentation, with one placental site receiving a better blood supply than the other, but can also reflect different genetic growth potentials. In the third trimester, the larger fetal mass leads to advanced placental maturation and relative placental insufficiency. Size discordance can also be caused by umbilical cord abnormalities such as velamentous or marginal insertion or vasa previa, or discordance for malformations, genetic syndromes, or infection. Figure 30–12 shows dizygotic twins, one

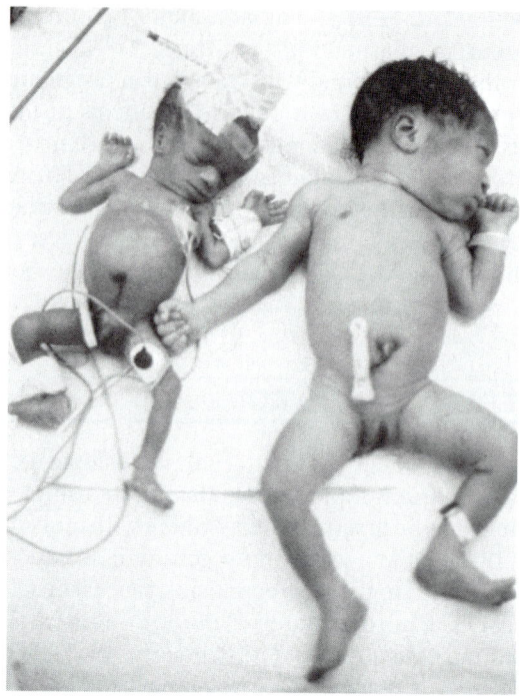

FIGURE 30–12. Marked discordance in dizygotic twins. The larger infant weighted 2300 g, appropriate for gestational age. The markedly growth-restricted smaller infant weighed only 785 g. Both thrived.

of whom weighed 2300 and the other 785 g, delivered at Parkland Hospital. Both survived, but one remains appreciably smaller than the other.

The degree of growth restriction in monozygotic twins is likely to be greater than in dizygotic pairs. For example, the quintuplets shown in Figure 30–13 represent three dizygotic and two monozygotic fetuses. When delivered at 31 weeks, the three infants from separate ova weighed 1420, 1530, and 1440 g, whereas the two derived from the same ovum weighed 990 and 860 g. Monozygotic twins are also more likely to be discordant in size. At the time of the split, the allocation of blastomeres may not be equal between the two embryos, vascular communications within a monochorionic placenta may cause unequal distribution of nutrients and oxygen, and discordant structural anomalies resulting from the twinning event itself may affect growth.

Twin fetuses have been of particular interest to investigators seeking clues on the relative roles of nature versus nurture in human fetal growth. Excluding anomalies, fetal gender influences, and birthweight disparity due to placental insufficiency or vascular communications, restricted fetal growth of twins appears to be primarily a result of diminished nurture during the third trimester. Figure 30–14 compares birthweights in more than 500,000 male singleton infants with more than 10,000 male twin infants. Twin birthweights closely parallel singletons until about 28 to 30 weeks, when twins

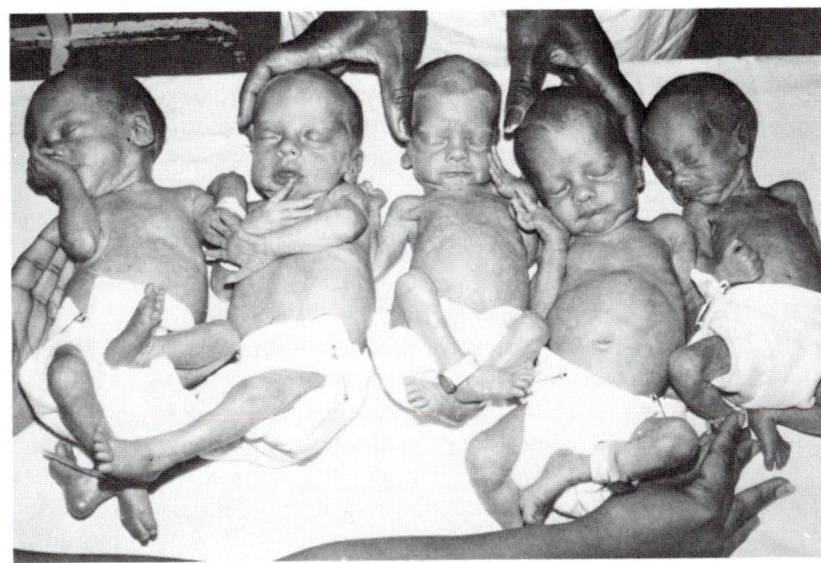

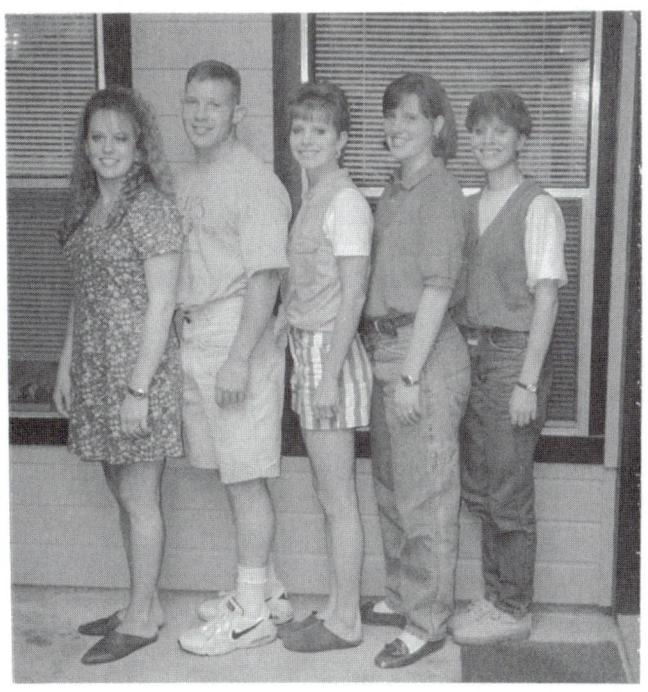

FIGURE 30–13. A. Davis quintuplets at 3 weeks of age. The first, second, and fourth infants from the left each arose from separate ova, whereas the third and fifth infants are from the same ovum. **B.** Davis quintuplets at 20 years of age.

begin to become progressively smaller than singletons. At approximately 34 to 35 weeks and thereafter, twin birthweights clearly diverge from singletons. Interestingly, it is also at this stage of gestation when the combined weight of twin fetuses reaches 4000 to 5000 g, the latter weight being quite rare in singletons. For example, only 2 per 1000 births at Parkland Hospital in 1999 weighed more than 5000 g.

Thus, the empirical upper fetal growth limit for sin-gletons, and presumably upper limit of maternal support capacity, occurs at about 34 or 35 weeks in twin gestation. Moreover, twin growth restriction intensifies as the third trimester continues, such that at 38 weeks or later, the incidence of overt growth restriction quadruples to include almost half of twin births.

There is other circumstantial evidence that in utero crowding by multiple fetuses affects nurture, presumably by overtaxing the capacity of the mother, the uterus, or

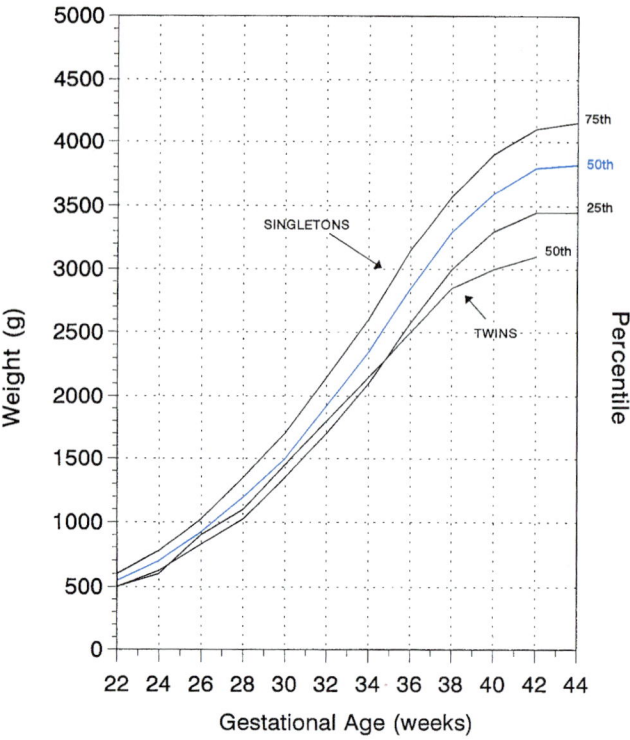

FIGURE 30–14. Birthweight percentiles (25 to 75) for singleton male infants compared with the 50th birthweight percentile for twin males, Canada, 1986–1988. (Modified from Arbuckle and colleagues, 1993, with permission.)

both to provide nutrients. For example, both Lipitz and co-workers (1996) and Smith-Levitin and colleagues (1996) have reported that selective reduction of triplets to twins before 12 weeks results in a growth pattern typical of twins rather than triplets, which are typically growth restricted compared with twins. Thus, the number of fetuses residing in the uterus later in pregnancy, and not their embryonic potential, seems to govern growth. Another example that the maternal supply line is affected by the number of fetuses is provided by Casele and co-authors (1996) in their studies of maternal metabolic responses to eating and extended overnight fasting. Women with twins were more vulnerable to starvation ketosis after fasting compared with women with singleton pregnancies. This finding suggests that more maternal metabolic resources are funneled to twin fetuses.

DURATION OF GESTATION. As the number of fetuses increases, the duration of gestation decreases (Fig. 30–15). Approximately half of twins deliver at 36 weeks or less. The mean age at delivery of triplets is 33.5 weeks, with 90 percent, 24 percent, and 8 percent delivered before 37, 32, and 28 weeks, respectively (Berkowitz and colleagues, 1996). The average age at delivery was 31 weeks in 37 quadruplet pregnancies (Barton and colleagues, 1996).

PRETERM BIRTH. Delivery before term is the major reason for the increased risk of neonatal death and morbidity in twins. Gardner and associates (1995) found that the causes of preterm birth differed between twins and singletons. Spontaneous preterm labor accounted for a larger proportion of twins delivered before 37 weeks compared with singletons, whereas the reverse was true for preterm ruptured membranes. Indicated preterm delivery accounted for equal proportions of prematurely delivered twins and singletons. Maternal hypertension, fetal growth restriction, and placental abruption were the main indications for preterm delivery of twins.

Although the causes of preterm delivery in twins and singletons may be different, once delivered the neonatal outcome is generally the same at similar gestational ages. Gardner and colleagues (1995) compared neonatal outcomes of preterm twin infants with preterm singletons delivered at the same gestational ages and found that preterm twins did not have significantly more respiratory distress syndrome, intraventricular hemorrhage, or necrotizing enterocolitis than same-gestational-age singletons. Similar findings were reported by Kilpatrick and colleagues (1996). Thus, the primary neonatal problem with twin gestation is simply more frequent preterm delivery, not increased vulnerability to the morbidity of preterm delivery.

The previous statements apply to twins who are essentially concordant. As one would expect, the neonatal outcome for preterm twins who are markedly discordant may not be comparable to that of singletons because whatever caused the discordance may have long-lasting effects. Sonntag and co-workers (1996) compared 27 weight-discordant twin pairs to 72 concordant twins. They found that the discordant twins had a significantly higher neonatal mortality (19 versus 2 percent), and

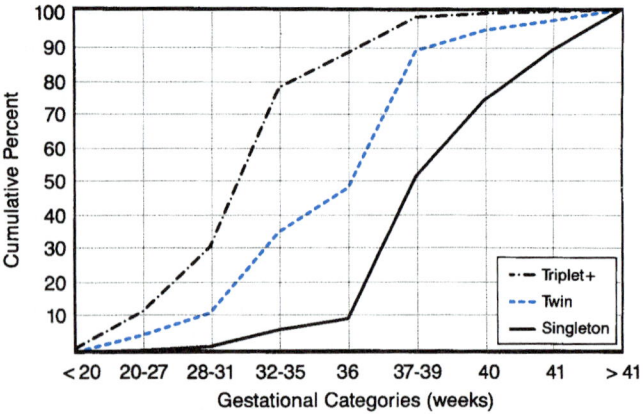

FIGURE 30–15. Cumulative percent of singleton, twin, triplet, or higher-order multiple births according to gestational age at delivery in the United States during 1990. (From Luke, 1994, with permission.)

were more likely to have severe intracranial hemorrhage and persistent ductus arteriosus. Most of the increase in morbidity and mortality was due to the sequelae of chronic twin-twin transfusion, and nearly half of the discordant pairs fulfilled the criteria for this disorder.

PROLONGED PREGNANCY. Is there a safe upper limit of twin gestation? More than 30 years ago Bennett and Dunn (1969) suggested that a twin pregnancy of 40 weeks or more should be considered postterm. This was based on the observation that twin stillborn infants delivered at 40 weeks or beyond had features similar to postmature singletons (Chap. 28, p. 738). Kiely (1990) later reported that twins born at 40 weeks or more were actually lighter than those born at 38 to 39 weeks, suggesting that intrauterine growth for twins stops after 39 weeks. Similarly, Luke and colleagues (1993) as well as Minakami and Sato (1996) concluded that twins were postterm after 38 weeks. They arrived at this conclusion because the incidence of fetal growth restriction and associated morbidity increased significantly in twins delivered between 39 and 41 weeks compared with delivery at 38 weeks or less. At Parkland Hospital, twin gestations have empirically been considered for many years to be prolonged at about 40 weeks gestation.

SUBSEQUENT DEVELOPMENT. In Norway, Nilsen and associates (1984) evaluated the physical and intellectual development of male twins at 18 years of age. Compared with singletons, twice as many twins were found to be physically unfit for military service. They attributed this to sequelae of preterm delivery such as visual impairment rather than twinning. General intelligence did not appear to differ.

At least one study has suggested that long-term physical development might be different for twins. Silva and colleagues (1982, 1985) carefully monitored 24 twins up to 11 years of age, and compared their outcomes to 1013 singletons who had similar gestational ages and weights at birth and who experienced similar antenatal and neonatal complications. Twins had delays in achieving developmental milestones, and at age 11 years lagged behind singletons in intelligence quotient (IQ) scores. At each age twins were similar in height to singletons 3 months younger, and similar in weight to singletons 6 months younger.

The pattern of subsequent development of discordant twins varies. For example, Babson and Phillips (1973) reported that in monozygotic twins whose birthweights differed on the average by 35 percent, the twin who was smaller at birth remained so into adulthood. Height, weight, head circumference, and intelligence often remained superior in the twin who weighed more at birth. Fujikura and Froelich (1974), however,

failed to confirm a significant difference in mental and motor scores.

Baigts and co-workers (1982) studied 17-year-old monozygotic twins who had body frames that were similar, but who were remarkably dissimilar in weight, as they were at birth. The investigators documented hyperplasia of adipocytes in the heavier twin compared with her lighter sister. They suggested that intrauterine nutritional status helps to determine adipocyte numbers and the way the body evolves. Others have concluded that genetic heritage in twins is more important than environment in determining body mass (Bouchard and co-workers, 1990; Stunkard and co-workers, 1990).

UNIQUE COMPLICATIONS

There are a number of unique complications that occur in multiple fetuses. While these have been best described in twins, they also occur in higher-order multiple gestations.

MONOAMNIONIC TWINS. There is an extremely high fetal death rate with the relatively rare variety of monozygous twinning in which both fetuses occupy the same amnionic sac. A common cause of death is intertwining of their umbilical cords, which has been estimated to complicate at least half of cases. An example is provided in Figure 30–16. Approximately 1 percent of monozygotic twins are monoamnionic. Diamnionic twins can become monoamnionic, and have all the associated morbidity and mortality, if the dividing membrane ruptures (Gilbert and colleagues, 1991).

Once diagnosed, management of monoamnionic twins is somewhat problematic due to the unpredictability of fetal death resulting from cord entanglement and the lack of an effective means of monitoring for it. There are some data that suggest that morbid cord entanglement is likely to occur early, and that monoamnionic pregnancies that have successfully reached 30 to 32 weeks are at greatly reduced risk. Carr and co-authors (1990) reviewed 24 sets of monoamnionic twins where all the fetuses were known to be alive before 18 weeks. At 30 weeks, 70 percent of the fetuses were alive and there were no additional deaths prior to delivery at an average of 36 weeks. They concluded that the risks due to early delivery to prevent cord accidents outweighed the risks of fetal death from cord entanglement, especially after 30 weeks. A similar experience was reported by Tessin and Zlatnik (1991) in their description of 20 monoamnionic twin pregnancies at the University of Iowa Hospital. There were no fetal deaths after 32 weeks, again suggesting that prophylactic preterm delivery may not be indicated in all cases.

Umbilical cord entanglement occurs frequently, but

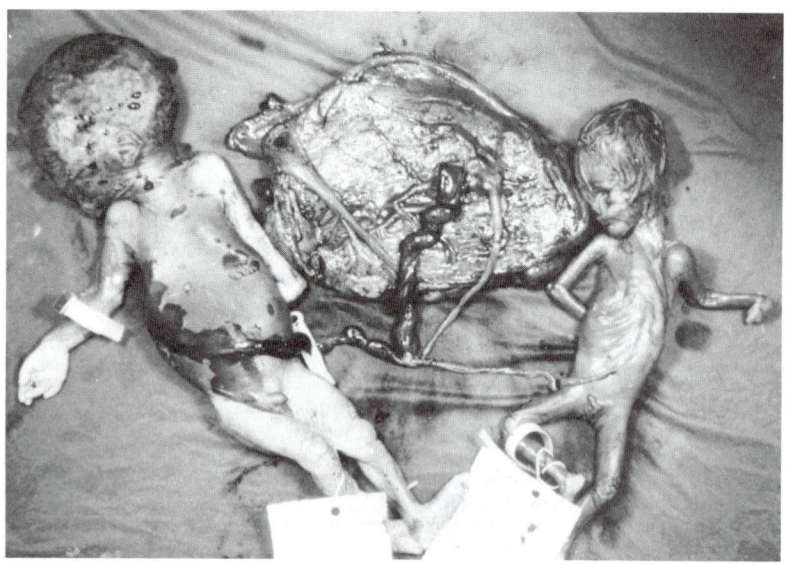

FIGURE 30–16. Monozygotic twins in a single amnionic sac. The smaller fetus apparently died first and the second subsequently succumbed when the umbilical cords entwined.

the factors that lead to pathological umbilical vessel constriction during entanglement are unknown. Belfort and colleagues (1993) and Aisenbrey and co-workers (1995) used color-flow Doppler ultrasonography to diagnose umbilical cord entanglement in 10 monoamnionic twin pregnancies. The recognition of cord entanglement in seven of these pregnancies prompted hospital admission, increased fetal surveillance, or both. Interestingly, only one set of entangled twins required immediate delivery. In fact, the pregnancies continued for an average of 6 weeks after the diagnosis, and one pregnancy continued for 12 weeks!

CONJOINED TWINS. In the United States, united or conjoined twins are commonly referred to as Siamese twins, after Chang and Eng Bunker of Siam (Thailand), who were displayed worldwide by P. T. Barnum. If twinning is initiated after the embryonic disc and the rudimentary amnionic sac have formed, and if division of the embryonic disc is incomplete, conjoined twins result (see Fig. 30–2). When each of the joined twins is nearly complete, the commonly shared body site may be:

1. Anterior (thoracopagus).
2. Posterior (pyopagus).
3. Cephalic (craniopagus).
4. Caudal (ischiopagus).

The majority are of the thoracopagus variety (Figs. 30–17 and 30–18).

When the bodies are duplicated only partly, the attachment is usually lateral. The incomplete division of the embryonic disc may begin at either or both poles and produce two heads; two, three, or four arms; two, three, or four legs; or some combination thereof. The frequency of conjoined twins is not well established. At Kandang Kerbau Hospital in Singapore, Tan and co-workers (1971) identified seven cases of conjoined twins among somewhat more than 400,000 deliveries (1 in 60,000).

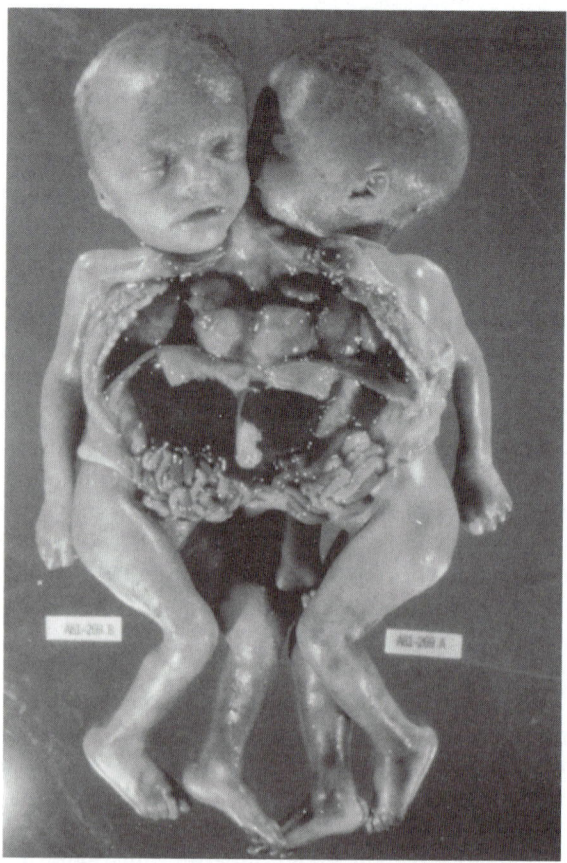

FIGURE 30–17. Conjoined twins delivered at 22 weeks and showing a shared liver.

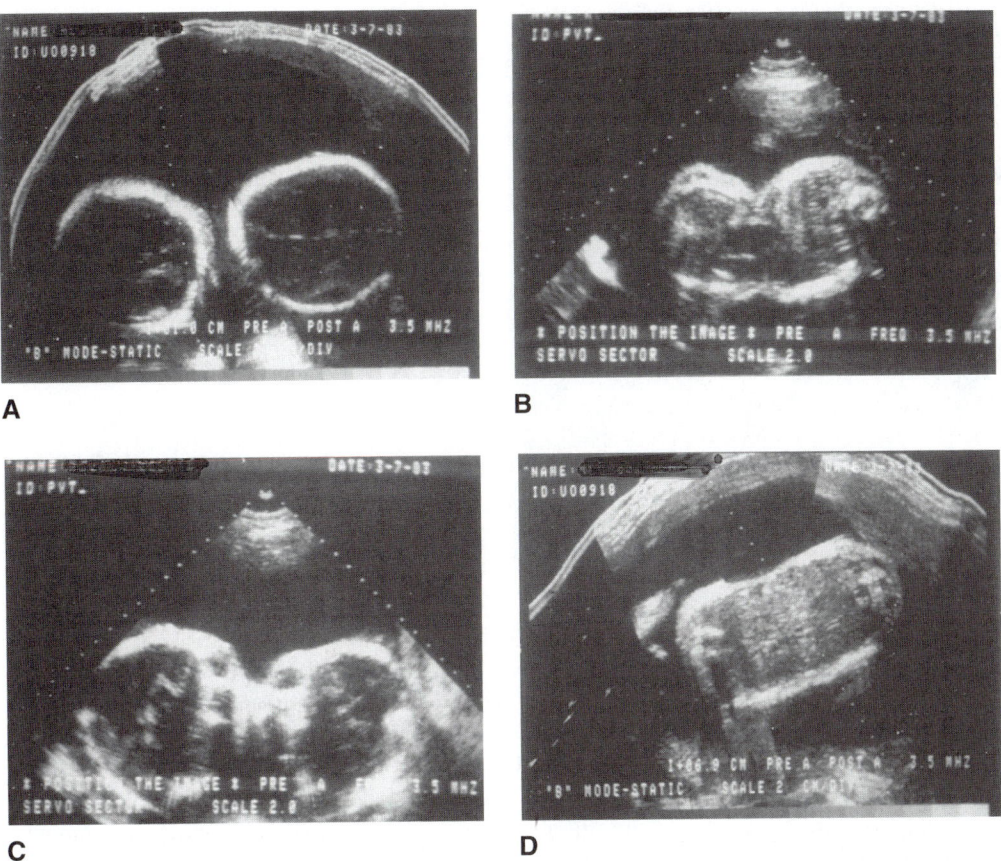

FIGURE 30–18. Transverse sonograms of thoracopagus twins at about 28 weeks' gestation. **A.** Axial view of fetal heads. **B.** Fused thorax with conjoined hearts. **C.** Oblique view of the heads showing the proximity of the two faces. **D.** Fusion of the abdomen with a common liver. (Courtesy of Dr. R. Santos.)

As reviewed by van den Brand and associates (1994), the diagnosis of conjoined twins can frequently be made at midpregnancy using sonography, which allows the parents to decide whether or not to continue the pregnancy. A thorough targeted ultrasound examination, including a careful evaluation of the point of connection and the organs involved, is essential before counseling is provided. Surgical separation of nearly complete conjoined twins may be successful when organs essential for life are not shared. Chang and Eng Bunker, for example, were reportedly connected only by a thin bridge of tissue containing abdominal wall structures and possibly some liver. Consultation with a pediatric surgeon often facilitates parental decision making. It must also be remembered that monozygotic twins are at increased risk to be discordant for structural malformations, most likely because the process of twinning is a teratogenic event which disturbs the timing of normal developmental processes. As a result, conjoined twins may have discordant structural anomalies that further complicate decisions about whether or not to continue the pregnancy. For example, one of the conjoined twins

shown in Figure 30–19 was anencephalic. Vaginal delivery of conjoined twins for the purpose of pregnancy termination is possible because the union is most often pliable, although dystocia is common. If the fetuses are mature, vaginal delivery may be traumatic.

ACARDIAC TWIN. Twin reversed-arterial-perfusion (TRAP) sequence is a rare (1 in 35,000 births), but serious complication of monochorionic, monozygotic multiple gestation. In the TRAP sequence, there is usually a normally formed donor twin who has features of heart failure, and a recipient twin without a normal heart (acardius) and missing various other structures (van Allen and colleagues, 1983). It has been hypothesized that the TRAP sequence is caused in the embryo by a sizable artery-to-artery placental shunt, often accompanied by a vein-to-vein shunt. The perfusion pressure of one twin overpowers the other who then has reverse blood flow from the co-twin (Jones, 1997). The "used" arterial blood reaching the recipient twin preferentially goes to the iliac vessels and thus perfuses only the lower part of the body, leading to disruption or deteriora-

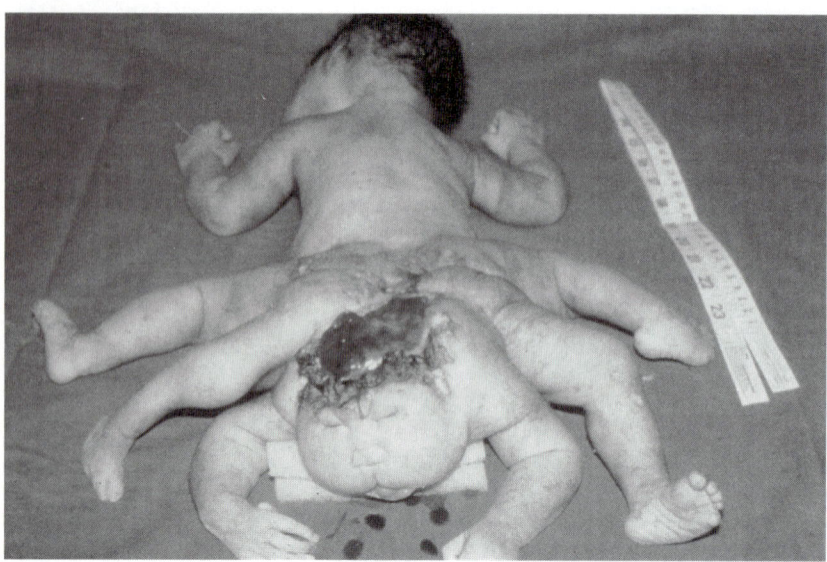

FIGURE 30–19. Conjoined twins in which one was anencephalic. (Courtesy of Dr. Craig Syrop, University of Iowa.)

tion of growth and development of the upper body. Failure or disrupted growth of the head is called *acardius acephalus;* a partially developed head with identifiable limbs is called *acardius myelacephalus;* and failure of any recognizable structure to form is *acardius amorphous*

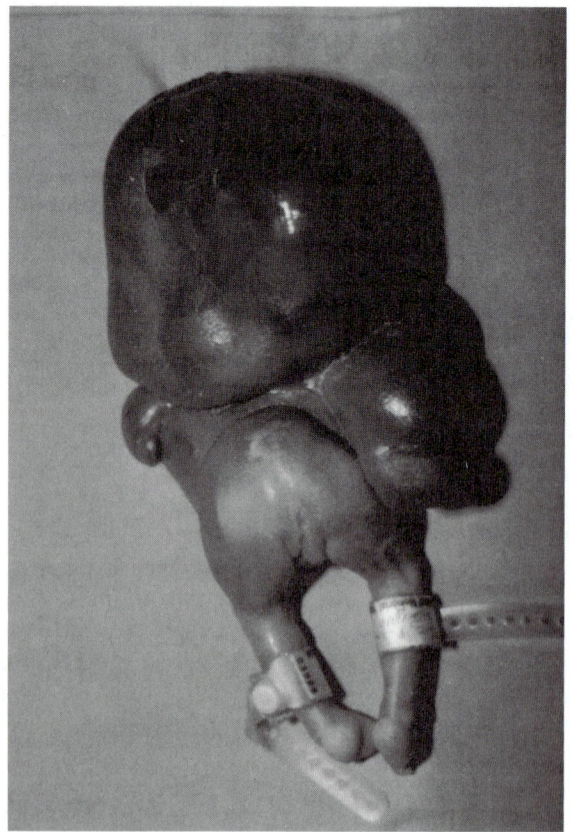

FIGURE 30–20. Acardiac twin photographed from the rear and showing acephalus with total deformity of the upper torso. (Photo courtesy of Dr. Paul Wendel.)

(Robie and colleagues, 1989). An example of an acardiac twin is shown in Figure 30–20. It demonstrates acephalus as well as complete malformation of the upper torso. Without treatment the pump twin dies in 50 to 75 percent of cases (Moore and colleagues, 1990). Recently, Norwitz and associates (2000) described prenatal planning for neonatal surgery using three-dimensional modeling with magnetic resonance imaging.

Quintero and colleagues (1994) have reviewed methods of in utero treatment of acardiac twinning where the goal is interruption of the vascular communication between the pump and recipient twins. They also have described successful use of transabdominal fetoscopy to ligate the umbilical cord of 11 acardiac twins at approximately 21 weeks (Quintero and co-authors, 1996).

VASCULAR COMMUNICATIONS BETWEEN FETUSES. With rare exceptions, vascular communications between twins are present only in monochorial placentas (Baldwin, 1991; Robertson and Neer, 1983). Nearly 100 percent of monochorial placentas have vascular anastomoses, but there is marked variation in the number, size, and direction of these seemingly haphazardly formed connections. Artery-to-artery anastomoses on the chorionic surface of the placenta have been identified in up to 75 percent of monochorial placentas and are the commonest pattern (Fig. 30–21). Vein-to-vein and artery-to-vein communications are each found in approximately 50 percent of similar placentas. One vessel may have several connections, sometimes to both arteries and veins. In contrast to these vascular connections on the surface of the chorion, there are artery-to-vein communications through the capillary bed of the villous tissue of the placenta. These deep arteriovenous anastomoses create a common villous district or third circula-

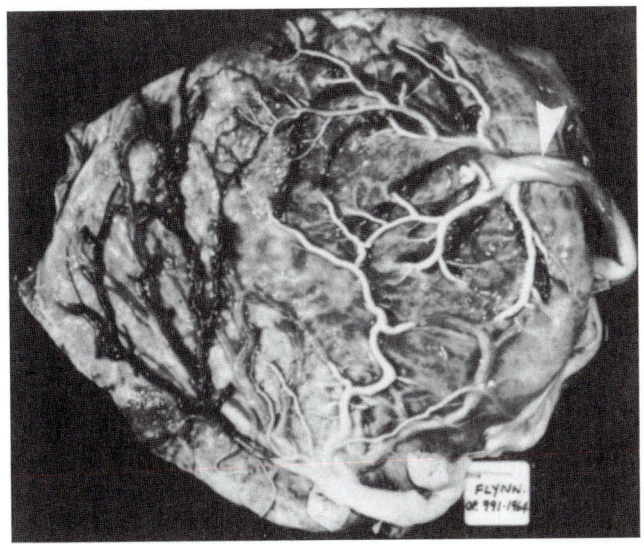

FIGURE 30–21. Monochorionic twin placenta from which the amnion has been stripped. The arteries of cord 1 (*arrow*) have been injected with barium solution and a direct communication with an artery from cord 2 (*label*) is apparent. A major artery of cord 2 was injected with India ink and a communication with veins in placenta 1 is evident, indicating a deep vascular communication. (From Fox, 1978, with permission.)

tion that has been identified in approximately half of monochorial placentas (Fig. 30–22).

Most of these vascular communications are hemodynamically balanced and of little fetal consequence. Rarely, however, they can cause hemodynamically significant shunts between fetuses. There are two patterns of hemodynamically significant anastomotic circulations: acardiac twining (see preceding description) and the twin-to-twin transfusion syndrome. The incidence of the latter syndrome is unclear, but up to approximately a fourth of monochorial twins have some clinical features of this syndrome (Galea and co-workers, 1982).

TWIN-TO-TWIN TRANSFUSION SYNDROME. Blood is transfused from the donor twin to its recipient sibling such that the donor becomes anemic and its growth may be restricted, while the recipient becomes polycythemic and may develop circulatory overload manifest as hydrops. As shown in Figure 30–23, the donor twin is pale and its recipient sibling is plethoric. Similarly, one portion of the placenta often appears quite pale compared with the rest of the placenta.

The neonatal period may be complicated by dangerous circulatory overload with heart failure if severe hypervolemia and hyperviscosity are not identified promptly and treated. Occlusive thrombosis is also much

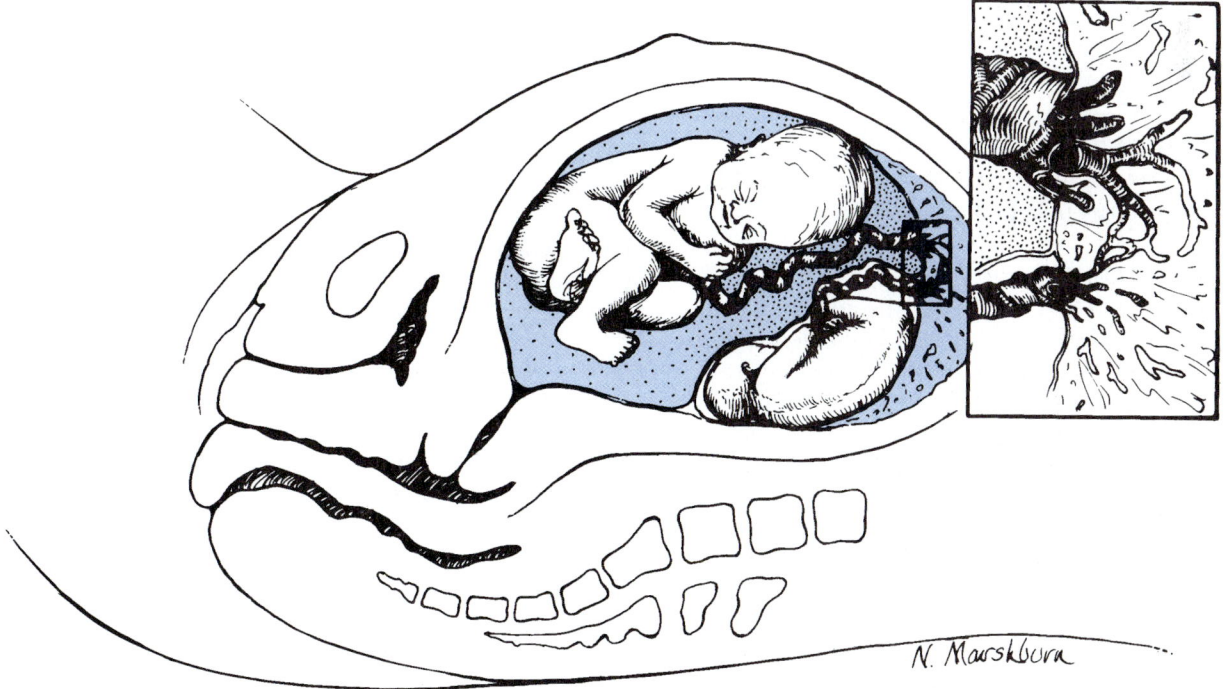

FIGURE 30–22. Schematic representation of arteriovenous anastomosis deep with the villous tissue forming a "common villous district" or "third circulation" that has been identified in monochorial placentas. Also shown is a growth-restricted discordant twin fetus with markedly reduced amnionic fluid, causing it to be "stuck."

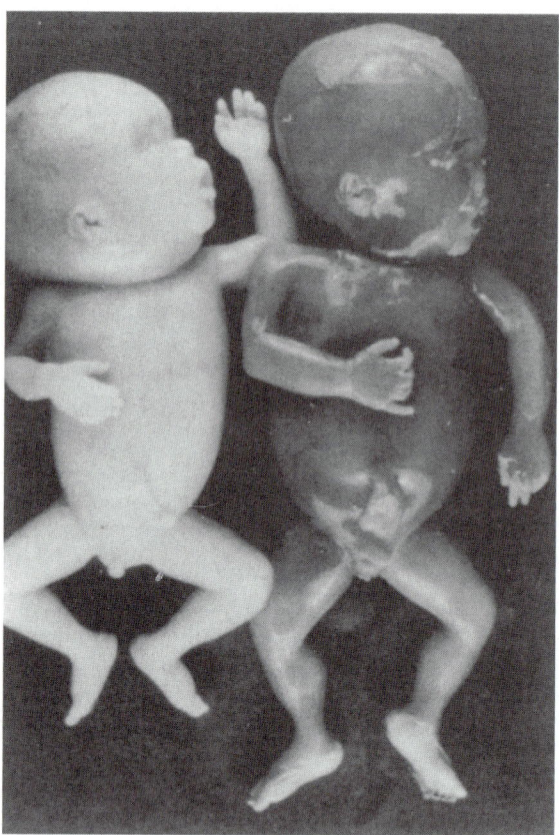

FIGURE 30–23. Twin-to-twin transfusion syndrome at 23 weeks. Pale donor twin (690 g) is shown on the left. The plethoric recipient twin (730 g) on the right also had hydramnios. The donor twin had oligohydramnios. (From Mahone and co-authors, 1993, with permission.)

more likely to develop in this setting. Polycythemia may lead during the neonatal period to severe hyperbilirubinemia and kernicterus (Chap. 39, p. 1067).

PATHOPHYSIOLOGY. Bajoria and colleagues (1995) perfused 30 monochorial placentas with anticoagulant solution immediately after delivery and then delineated anastomoses by dye-contrast injection. Ten were from pregnancies with evidence of midtrimester twin-to-twin transfusion syndrome and 10 were from monochorial twin pregnancies without this complication. The vascular communications found in these two groups were remarkably different. Those without twin-to-twin transfusion syndrome had multiple superficial anastomoses. In contrast, those with the twin-to-twin transfusion syndrome had solitary, deep arteriovenous capillary channels within the villous tissue. Bajoria and colleagues (1995) hypothesized that multiple superficial vascular communications were protective against the transfusion syndrome because this arrangement permitted bi-directional, and thus, balanced, blood flow. Conversely, the single deep arteriovenous villous anastomoses without

multiple superficial connections were one-way arteriovenous shunts from a donor fetus to its recipient sibling, and thereby hemodynamically imbalanced.

There are other data to suggest that placental pathophysiology may be more complex. Bendon (1995) injected 21 monochorionic placentas from live-born twins, scored surface vessel anastomoses and venous return areas, and correlated them with neonatal birthweight and hematocrit. Birthweight and hematocrit did not correlate with each other or with vessel anastomoses, and only the placental area allotted to each twin correlated with neonatal size.

This pathophysiological scenario does not explain all instances of twin-to-twin transfusion. Hecher and colleagues (1994) described two monochorial twin pregnancies with features of twin-to-twin transfusion syndrome in which Doppler was used to demonstrate artery-to-artery anastomoses and opposing pulsatile blood flows. Although there were intermittent episodes of flow reversal, there was no net forward flow from one fetus to the other that could account for a shift of blood from one fetus to its sibling. They postulated that the intermittent blood flow reversal or sudden hypotension in one twin could cause cerebral damage in the donor twin.

Another hemodynamic explanation for twin-to-twin transfusion syndrome was offered by Fries and co-workers (1993). They postulated that velamentous umbilical cord insertions may contribute to the development of unequal fetal blood volumes because the membranously inserted cord can be easily compressed, restricting blood flow to one twin. Talbert and colleagues (1996) used a computerized model to study the hemodynamics of unidirectional and bi-directional intertwin transfusion via placental anastomoses. They determined that the net direction of blood flow is determined by the donor arterial pressure and not the number of anastomoses, and that the fetal physiological response to the unequal blood volume, primarily relating to changes in urine production and colloid osmotic pressure, determines whether or not blood flow will be equilibrated.

FETAL BRAIN DAMAGE. Cerebral palsy, microcephaly, porencephaly, and multicystic encephalomalacia are serious complications associated with vascular communications in twin gestations. It is most likely that such neurological damage is caused by ischemic necrosis leading to cavitary brain lesions. In the donor twin, ischemia results from hypotension and/or anemia. In the recipient, ischemia is from blood pressure instability and episodes of severe hypotension (Larroche and colleagues, 1990). Denbow and colleagues (1998) reviewed 17 sets of live-born, monochorionic twins who had twin-to-twin transfusion syndrome and found that one had a cerebral infarction and 10 had other antenatally acquired cerebral lesions; both donors and recipients were affected.

Cerebral pathology may occur after the death of one twin. In this case, damage may be due to emboli of thromboplastic material originating in the dead fetus, but more likely results from acute hypotension at the time of death (Benirschke, 1993). Fusi and co-workers (1990, 1991) observed that at the time of death of one twin fetus, acute twin-to-twin anastomotic transfusion from the high-pressure vessels of the living twin to the very low resistance vessels of the dead twin leads to rapid hemodynamic changes and ischemic antenatal brain damage in the survivor. This group described eight monochorial twin pregnancies in which one twin died but the pregnancy continued. Careful follow-up showed that none developed disseminated intravascular coagulopathy, and yet there was a high frequency of neurological damage. Pharoah and Adi (2000) surveyed 348 survivors whose co-twin had died in utero. The prevalence of cerebral palsy was 83 per 1000 live births—a 40-fold risk. Okamura and colleagues (1994) performed cordocentesis on seven surviving twin fetuses within 24 hours of sibling death. They found acute anemia in the surviving twin, and hypothesized that cerebral abnormalities in survivors were produced by hypotensive cerebral ischemia due to acute hemorrhage through placental vascular channels. Such sibling brain damage has been reported following death of one fetus as early as 16 weeks (Anderson and co-workers, 1990).

The pathological importance of hemodynamic fluctuation and fetal response, reflected by urine output, in causing brain damage was shown by Bejar and co-workers (1990). They reviewed neonatal echoencephalographic studies in 89 twins and 12 triplets and diagnosed antenatal necrosis of cerebral white matter in 15 percent of the infants (Fig. 30–24). The neurological damage was linked to hydramnios, co-twin fetal death, hydrops, and multiple vascular connections. The most important factor in this study appeared to be vein-to-vein anastomosis within the placenta, because 90 percent of such infants had brain damage. Denbow and colleagues (2000) confirmed this and reported that arterioarterial anastomoses are usually harmless.

The acute nature of the twin-to-twin transfusion and hypotension following the death of one twin makes successful intervention after the death nearly impossible. Even with delivery immediately after the demise is recognized, the hypotension that occurs at the moment of death has likely already caused irreversible damage (Langer and associates, 1997; Wada and co-authors, 1998).

DIAGNOSIS. The diagnosis of twin-to-twin transfusion syndrome, whether made antenatally or postnatally, is problematic. The postnatal diagnosis was classically made based on an intertwin weight discordance of 15 or 20 percent and a hemoglobin difference of 5 g/dL or greater, with the smaller twin being anemic. It is now recognized, however, that significant intertwin weight differences can have a variety of etiologies such as discordance for anomalies, infection, or placental support. Also, hemoglobin discordance can occur acutely at the time of delivery. Wenstrom and colleagues (1992) illustrated this by reviewing the birthweights and hemoglobin concentrations in 97 monochorionic twin pregnancies. They found that 37 percent of weight concordant twins and 50 percent of discordant twins had a significant hemoglobin discordance. Twin B had the higher value in 63 percent, including a third of the discordant twins in which twin B was the smaller, suggesting that the hemoglobin discordance was due to acute transfusion after the delivery of twin A and before the delivery of twin B. Although this pattern met the criteria for twin-to-twin transfusion, it was not clinically important because it was an acute phenomena. Classical features of twin-to-twin transfusion, namely weight discordance with the smaller twin being anemic, occurred in only 11 of these 97 twin pairs. Danskin and Neilson (1989) also concluded that this syndrome cannot be established definitively if based solely upon birthweight or newborn hemoglobin differences.

Clinically important twin-to-twin transfusion syndrome is chronic, and results from significant antenatal vascular volume discrepancies between the twins. The syndrome typically presents in the midtrimester when the donor fetus becomes oliguric due to decreased renal perfusion (Mari and co-authors, 1993). This fetus develops oligohydramios, while the recipient fetus develops severe polyhydramnios, presumably due to increased urine production. Virtual absence of amnionic fluid in the donor sac prevents fetal motion, giving rise to the description of **stuck fetus** (Berry and co-workers, 1995). This polyhydramnios–oligohydramnios combination can lead to growth restriction, contractures, and pulmonary hypoplasia in one twin, and premature rupture of the membranes and heart failure in the other.

The goal of antenatal diagnosis is to prevent fetal morbidity and mortality by selecting candidates for prenatal therapy or delivery. Antenatal criteria recommended for defining the twin-to-twin transfusion syndrome include the following: same sex fetuses, monochorionicity with placental vascular connections, intertwin weight difference greater than 20 percent, hydramnios in the large twin, oligohydramnios or stuck twin in the smaller twin, and hemoglobin difference greater than 5 g/dL (Bruner and Rosemond, 1993). All of these criteria except hemoglobin levels can be determined sonographically. Cordocentesis is required to measure hemoglobin concentration in each twin antenatally. Berry and co-workers (1995) performed cordocentesis on 38 twin pairs, and found when the intertwin hemoglobin difference was 2.5 g/dL or greater that all cases had stuck twin syndrome.

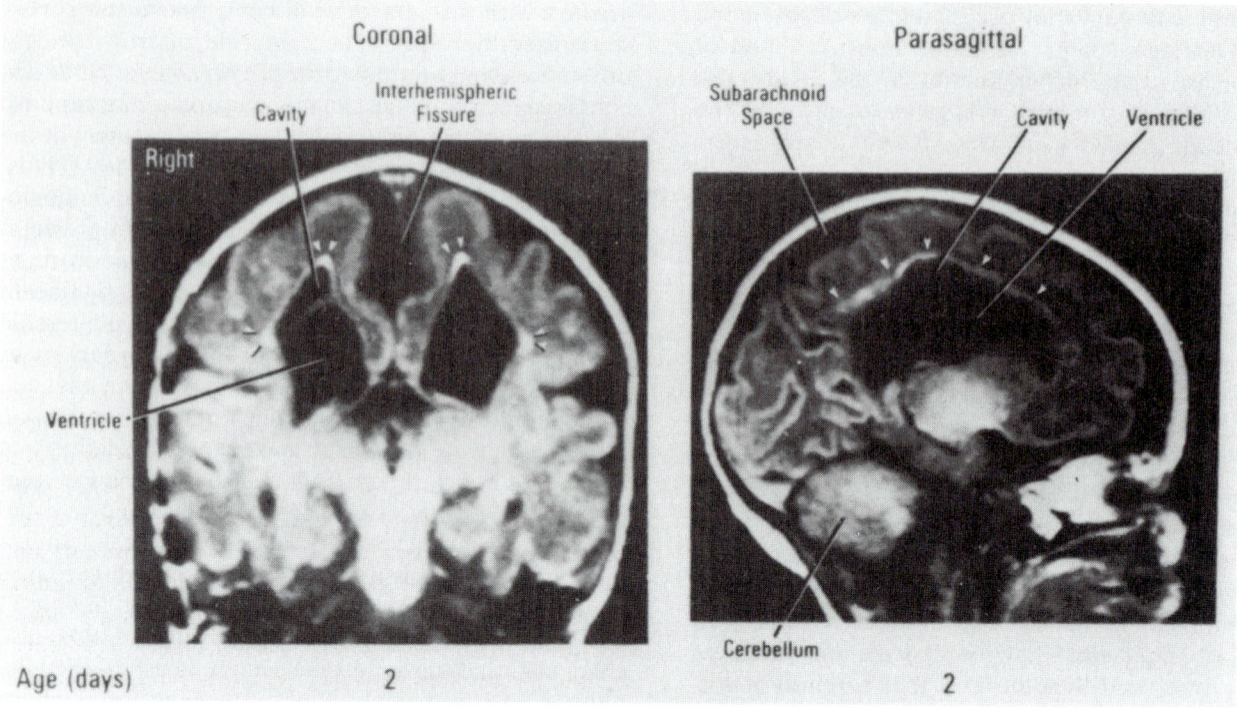

FIGURE 30–24. Cranial magnetic resonance imaging study of diamnionic–monochorionic twin performed on day 2 of life. The subarachnoid space and lateral ventricles are markedly enlarged. There are large cavitary lesions in the white matter adjacent to the ventricles. The bright signals (*arrowheads*) in the periphery of the cavitary lesions most probably correspond to gliosis. (From Bejar and colleagues, 1990, with permission.)

Shared circulation can also be confirmed in twin-to-twin transfusion syndrome by another invasive technique. Both Bruner and Rosemond (1993) and Weiner and Ludomirski (1994) have used adult red blood cells as a marker injected into the donor twin's umbilical vein, and then performed cordocentesis in the recipient twin to verify the presence of the adult cells.

In situations in which the diagnosis must be confirmed, for example before consideration of a high-risk therapy (see later discussion), such invasive testing is required because the sonographic diagnosis is sometimes incorrect. Saunders and co-workers (1991) used cordocentesis to show that none of four sets of monochorionic twins with all the sonographic features of twin-to-twin transfusion actually had discordant hemoglobin concentrations. Bruner and Rosemond (1993) used cordocentesis and adult red blood cell infusion to show that only four of nine monochorionic twin pregnancies with sonographic features of twin-to-twin transfusion actually had the syndrome. The cause of the discordant amnionic fluid volumes in these cases is unknown. When fetal hemoglobin concentrations have not been determined antenatally, it may be more accurate to refer to this situation as the "stuck twin" syndrome or the "polyhydramnios–oligohydramnios syndrome," to acknowledge that twin-to-twin transfusion has not been confirmed as the cause of the sonographic findings.

THERAPY AND OUTCOME. The prognosis for multiple gestations complicated by twin-to-twin transfusion syndrome is extremely guarded. Not only is brain damage a possibility, but antenatal death of one twin as well as neonatal death due to preterm delivery are other hazards. Generally, the earlier in gestation that twin-to-twin transfusion is diagnosed, the worse the prognosis (Bebbington and Wittmann, 1989). Unfortunately, the most serious form of twin-to-twin transfusion syndrome, with acute hydramnios in one sac and a stuck twin with anhydramnios in the other sac, usually presents between 18 and 26 weeks. The survival rate for those diagnosed before 28 weeks has been reported to be between 20 and 45 percent (Gonsoulin and co-workers, 1990; Shah and Chaffin, 1989).

Several therapies for twin-to-twin transfusion have been reported. Serial amnioreduction to decompress the hydramnios has the least risk. It is reported to be beneficial for at least two reasons. First, it relieves uterine overdistention and thus forestalls preterm labor

(Mahony and co-workers, 1990; Pinette and colleagues, 1993). Second, there is evidence that it may correct the hemodynamic inequalities by reducing intra-amnionic fluid pressure and placental compression, thus improving perfusion. Bower and colleagues (1995) used color flow Doppler imaging to evaluate uterine artery blood flow before and after amnioreduction in eight twin-to-twin transfusion pregnancies, seven singletons with acute hydramnios, and six controls. They found that quantitative blood flow increased by 75 percent after the procedure. Garry and associates (1996) have reported that use of repetitive decompression amniocentesis significantly reduced amnionic fluid pressure, and Mari and co-workers (1996) concluded, based on their experience in 24 twin pregnancies, that therapeutic amniocentesis was beneficial.

In contrast, Bruner and Anderson (1996) found decompression amniocentesis in eight pregnancies to be of no benefit to donor twins. Gonsoulin and co-workers (1990) also observed that amniocentesis for decompression failed to decrease perinatal mortality. There may be a pathological explanation for these therapeutic failures. For example, Bajoria (1998) correlated placental vascular anatomy with pregnancy outcome in 26 monochorial pregnancies treated by serial amnioreduction. He found that when the placenta had no superficial anastomoses, more procedures were required and were associated with a higher risk of fetal and neonatal death. It may be that amnioreduction improves pressure and blood flow primarily in superficial vessels, and is ineffective in pregnancies in which polyhydramnios–oligohydramnios is due to deeper vascular anastomoses.

Other more invasive therapies have been attempted. De Lia and associates (1990) reported the use of fetoscopic laser occlusion of placental vessels in severe twin-to-twin transfusion syndrome. The theoretical advantage is hemodynamic and hematological isolation of the living fetus, which could obviate embolic and hypotensive injury. The procedure is controversial in part because it results in occlusion of surface vessels only, and thus may not improve hemodynamics in placentas in which the offending anastomoses are deeper (as previously described). Branisteanu-Demitrascu and co-workers (1999), however, used a sheep model to show that laser coagulation of the superficial chorionic vessels leads to complete infarction of all treated cotyledons, and thus does eventually impact the deep vessels.

Laser occlusion entails more risk than amniocentesis and it is technically difficult. Placental vessel perforation was reported by De Lia and colleagues (1990). Their later report of 100 treated cases excluded outcome data from the first 33 procedures which were performed early on the "learning curve" (De Lia and associates, 1999). Fetal limb necrosis and skin loss have been reported

(Lundvall and co-workers, 1999; Stone and colleagues, 1998).

Despite these early concerns, accumulated data indicate that in experienced hands the procedure may be safe and beneficial. Ville and colleagues (1998) reported the results of a multicenter trial of laser coagulation in 132 pregnancies with severe, early twin-to-twin transfusion syndrome. There was at least one surviving fetus in 73 percent of cases, and at 1 year of age only six survivors were suspected of having a neurological handicap. A descriptive study of severe twin-to-twin transfusion syndrome by Hecher and co-workers (1999) compared 73 women treated with laser coagulation at one center with 43 similar patients treated with serial amnioreduction at another center. Although the overall fetal survival rate was not different, there was a higher proportion of pregnancies with at least one survivor in the laser group. This group also had fewer fetal deaths and abnormal sonographic findings in the brains of survivors. They also had higher birthweights, longer intervals-to-delivery, and longer gestational ages at delivery. Zikulnig and co-workers (1999) evaluated 121 cases treated with laser and found improved outcome with less severe stigmata of twin-to-twin transfusion before the procedure, and Doppler evidence of successful vessel ablation after the procedure. Ryan (2000) cited over 300 cases worldwide in his recent review. Serial amnioreduction is associated with 60 percent average survival, with 20 percent neurological disability in surviving infants. Laser ablation has a 75 to 80 percent survival of at least one twin, 5 to 60 percent for both, and a 5 percent neurological disability at 1 year of age.

Selective fetocide of one twin has also been reported. This has been considered when severe amnionic fluid and growth disturbances occur very early, generally before 20 weeks, and it is likely that both fetuses would die without intervention. Selection of the twin to be sacrificed has been based on evidence of fetal damage and comparison of each twin's prognosis. Because any substance injected into one twin may affect the co-twin, techniques have included saline cardiac tamponade followed by intracardiac potassium chloride, injection of an occlusive substance into the umbilical vein, or fetoscopic ligation, laser coagulation, or monopolar coagulation and bipolar cautery of the umbilical cord (Challis and co-workers, 1999; Donner and associates, 1997; Weiner, 1987; Wittmann and colleagues, 1986). The complication rate after these procedures is high.

DISCORDANT TWINS. Unequal size of twin fetuses may be a sign of pathological growth restriction in one fetus, and is defined using the larger twin as the index. Generally, as the weight difference within a twin pair increases, perinatal mortality increases proportionately. Restricted growth of one twin fetus usually develops late in the second and early third trimester, and is often asymmetrical (Leveno and co-workers, 1979). Earlier discordancy is usually symmetrical and indicates higher risk; generally, the earlier in pregnancy discordancy is recognized, the more serious the sequelae. Weissman and colleagues (1994) diagnosed discordancy between 6 and 11 weeks in five twin gestations, and all of the smaller twins had major malformations.

PATHOLOGY. The cause of birthweight inequality in twin fetuses is often unclear, but evidence indicates that the etiology of discordance is different in monochorionic and dichorionic twins. In monochorionic twins, discordancy is usually attributed to placental vascular communications causing hemodynamic imbalance between the twins. Reduced pressure and perfusion of the donor twin may then cause its placental portion to fail to grow (Benirschke, 1993). Rarely, monochorionic twins are discordant in size because they are discordant for structural anomalies occurring during twinning.

Different etiologies are believed to cause discordance in dichorionic twins. One source of discordance is that dizygous fetuses have different genetic growth potential, especially if they are of opposite genders. It is also possible that, because the placentas are separate and require more implantation space, one of the placentas is likely to have a suboptimal implantation site. The observation that the incidence of discordance doubles in triplets compared with twins lends additional credence to the view that in utero crowding plays a role in fetal growth restriction (Mordel and colleagues, 1993).

Eberle and co-workers (1993) performed an evaluation of placental pathology in 147 twin gestations that provides important insight into the etiology of discordant twins. They quantified placental lesions usually associated with singleton growth restriction. Placentas from the smaller fetus in discordant dichorionic twin pairs demonstrated the lesions typical of singleton fetal growth restriction, whereas these lesions were not found in discordant monochorionic twin pairs.

Additional evidence supports that discordancy in dichorionic twins is due to placental insufficiency whereas that seen in discordant monochorionic twins is due to hemodynamic imbalance. Rizzo and colleagues (1994) used serial Doppler recordings to evaluate the fetal circulation in 15 women with discordant dichorionic twins compared with 10 discordant monochorionic twin pairs. Discordant dichorionic twins showed Doppler results similar to those described for singleton growth restriction due to placental insufficiency, whereas the smaller of discordant monochorionic twin fetuses had Doppler findings consistent with anemia.

DIAGNOSIS. There are two areas of uncertainty in detection of discordant twins. First, which ultrasonic anatomi-

cal measurements most reliably predict discordance? Second, what fetal weight difference is clinically significant?

Size discordancy between twins can be determined in several ways. One common method is to use all fetal measurements to compute the estimated weight of each twin, and then to compare the weight of the smaller twin to that of the larger twin (weight of larger twin minus weight of smaller twin, divided by weight of larger twin). Considering that growth restriction is the primary concern and the abdominal circumference reflects fetal nutrition, some authors diagnose discordance when there is more than 20 mm difference in abdominal circumferences. Hill and colleagues (1994) evaluated the sonographic assessment of twin discordancy and found that abdominal circumference was superior to head circumference, femur length, or transverse cerebellar diameter as the most useful index of unequal size fetuses.

Several different intertwin weight differences have been used to define discordance. Accumulated data suggest that a greater than 25 to 30 percent weight discordance, usually with growth restriction in one or both twins, most accurately predicts an adverse perinatal outcome. Hollier and co-workers (1999) retrospectively evaluated 1370 twin pairs delivered at Parkland Hospital and stratified twin discordance in 5 percent increments from 15 to 40 percent. They found that the incidence of respiratory distress, intraventricular hemorrhage, seizures, periventricular leukomalacia, sepsis, and necrotizing enterocolitis increased directly with the degree of discordance, with a large risk increase beginning at 25 percent discordance. The relative risk of fetal death increased significantly only when there was over 30 percent discordance, which was associated with a relative risk of 5.6 and increased to 18.9 at over 41 percent discordance.

MANAGEMENT. Sonographic monitoring of growth within a twin pair, which provides a means to detect growth disturbance and discordance, has become a mainstay in the management of twin gestations. Other sonographic findings, such as oligohydramnios in the smaller twin, may be helpful in gauging fetal risk. Additionally, discordance with growth restriction should prompt fetal heart rate testing or a biophysical profile to evaluate fetal well being. Delivery is not performed for size discordance alone, but is indicated if there is fetal stress unlikely to respond to intervention and the gestational age is such that survival is expected. Many authorities advise determination of fetal lung maturity before delivery of discordant twin fetuses where the only finding is difference in the ultrasonic estimates of fetal size.

DEATH OF ONE FETUS. On occasion, one fetus succumbs remote from term, but the pregnancy continues with one living fetus. Factors influencing pregnancy loss in twins have been described by Rydhström (1994), who used the Medical Birth Registry in Stockholm to review fetal death in 15,066 twin pairs weighing 500 g or more. Same sex twins were at highest risk. Loss of one or both twins occurred in 1.1 percent of opposite sex twins and 2.6 percent of same sex twins. Size discordancy also increased the risk of loss. However, in opposite sex twins the risk of loss remained constant at 1.2 percent or higher until the discordance exceeded 40 to 50 percent or 1000 grams, while anything greater than a 20 percent or 250 g discordance increased the risk in same sex twins. After loss of one twin, the risk of subsequently losing the surviving twin was sixfold greater in same sex twins. Although chorionicity was not known in all cases, the authors estimated that the loss rate for same sex dizygotic twins was the same as for opposite sex twins (0.8 percent), and that monochorionic twins had the greatest risk of loss (3 percent). Saito and co-workers (1999) reviewed 481 twin pregnancies and reported that the risk of single fetal death in a twin pregnancy was 6.2 percent.

At delivery, the dead fetus with placenta and membranes may be identifiable but may be compressed appreciably (fetus compressus) or may be flattened remarkably through loss of fluid and most of the soft tissue (fetus papyraceous). The papyraceous fetus shown in Figure 30–25 died at midpregnancy while the other fetus and placenta thrived. The dead fetus shown in Figure 30–26 has become almost a shadow of itself compressed onto its placenta, which was separate from the placenta of the surviving twin.

Both the maternal risk and the prognosis for the surviving twin depend on the gestational age at the time of the demise, the chorionicity, and the length of time between the demise and delivery of the surviving twin.

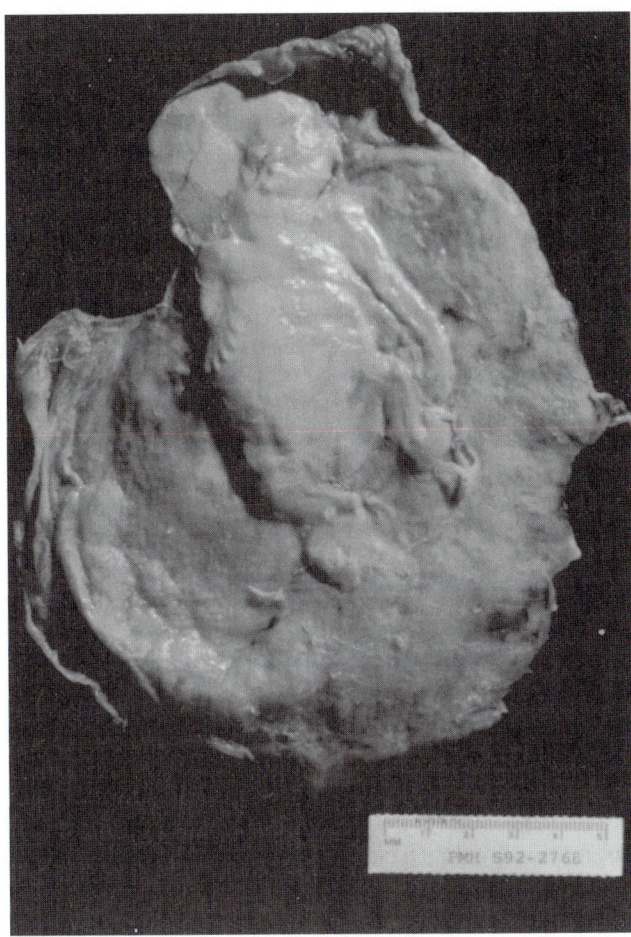

FIGURE 30–26. A long-dead twin fetus compressed onto its placenta. A separate placenta supported the surviving twin fetus.

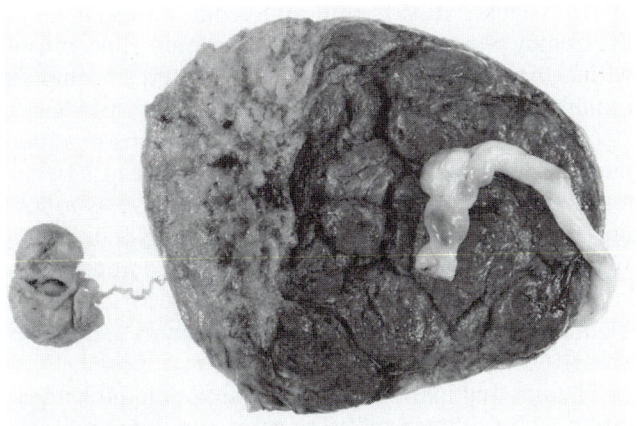

FIGURE 30–25. To the left is a fetus papyraceous that died at midpregnancy, its cord, and its pale placenta. To the right are the normal placenta and cord of the healthy 3200-g twin.

Early loss such as a "vanishing twin" does not appear to increase the risk of losing the surviving fetus after the first trimester. Selective reduction of a high-order multiple pregnancy (discussed later) increases the risk of losing the entire pregnancy but does not appear to increase the risk of other maternal or fetal complications.

Later in gestation, the death of one of multiple fetuses could theoretically trigger coagulation defects in the mother. Only a few cases of maternal coagulopathy after a single fetal death in a twin pregnancy have been reported, probably because the co-twin is usually delivered within a few weeks of the demise (Chap. 25, p. 659).

We have observed transient, spontaneously corrected consumptive coagulopathy when one fetus died and was retained in utero along with the other who was alive. The fibrinogen concentration initially dropped but then rose spontaneously and the level of serum fibrinogen–fibrin degradation products fell to normal. At delivery the portions of the placenta that supplied the living fetus appeared quite normal, whereas the part that had once provided for the dead fetus was the site of massive fibrin deposition. This may have accounted directly for the fall in maternal fibrinogen and in turn an increase in fibrin degradation products, or it may have served to block the escape of thromboplastin from fetus and placenta into the maternal circulation and thereby prevented disseminated intravascular coagulation. Both mechanisms may also have been operational until extensive fibrosis was achieved. The surviving fetus continued to thrive in utero and had normal plasma fibrinogen levels, serum fibrinogen–fibrin degradation products, and platelet counts at birth.

Management decisions should be based on the cause of death and the risk to the surviving fetus. The majority of cases of a single fetal death in twin pregnancy involve monochorionic placentation. Evidence indicates that morbidity in the monochorionic survivor is almost always due to vascular anastomoses, which first cause the demise of one twin and then produce sudden hypotension in the other. Benirschke (1993) has concluded that it is implausible that degenerating material from a dead fetus could be transported back to a living sibling. Considering that coagulopathy takes at least 5 weeks to develop, it is unlikely that there would still be shared circulation at that time. Bajoria and colleagues (1999) compared 50 monochorionic and 42 dichorionic twin pregnancies complicated by death of one fetus. The risk of fetal demise was more than 10 times greater in monochorionic twins, and the monochorionic survivors were significantly more likely to be anemic (51 versus 0 percent) and to have intracranial lesions at birth (46 versus 0 percent). The risk was highest if there was twin-to-twin transfusion and the recipient was the one who died. In monochorionic twins without twin-to-twin transfusion, those with superficial artery-to-artery or vein-to-vein anastomoses were at greater risk than those with bi-directional anastomoses. Yoshida and Matayoshi (1990) described 33 pairs of monochorionic twin pregnancies complicated by death of one fetus, in which 8 of 33 survivors had porencephaly, cerebral palsy, or other abnormalities. These complications generally occurred only when the death was in the latter half of pregnancy. As discussed earlier, in this situation delivery does not necessarily prevent morbidity in the survivor.

Less frequently, death results from a maternal complication such as diabetic ketoacidosis or severe preeclampsia with abruption, and pregnancy management is based on the diagnosis and the status of both mother and the surviving fetus. When the death of one dichorionic twin is due to a discordant congenital anomaly, its cause of death should not affect its co-twin. Santema and co-workers (1995b) assessed the cause and outcome of 29 consecutive twin pregnancies where one of the fetuses died after 20 weeks. The causes of fetal death were not clear in all cases; the most common associations were monochorionic placentation and severe preeclampsia. These investigators concluded that in most cases the benefit derived from continuation of multiple pregnancy exceeded the risks of preterm delivery after diagnosis of fetal death, and recommended conservative management of the living fetuses.

IMPENDING DEATH OF ONE FETUS. Abnormal antepartum tests of fetal health in one twin fetus but not the other pose a particular dilemma because delivery may be the best option for the compromised fetus, yet may result in death from immaturity of the second (Fig. 30–27). When fetal lung maturity is confirmed, salvage of both the healthy fetus and its jeopardized sibling is possible. Unfortunately, ideal management when the healthy fetus is very immature is problematic, but should be based on an estimate of the chances of intact survival in both fetuses. Often the compromised fetus is severely growth restricted or anomalous. An advantage of performing genetic amniocentesis for advanced maternal age in twin pregnancies, even when the mother will continue the pregnancy regardless of the diagnosis, is that the detection of aneuploidy in one fetus allows rational decisions about intervention to be made. In the case of twin-to-twin transfusion syndrome, the stuck twin often decompensates first and in addition to growth restriction has a high risk of pulmonary hypoplasia.

DEATH OF BOTH TWIN FETUSES. Rarely, both twin fetuses will die during the antepartum period. Rydhström (1996) reported that both fetuses died in 0.5 percent of twin pregnancies. Causes implicated in these deaths were monochorionic placentation and discordant fetal growth.

COMPLETE HYDATIDIFORM MOLE AND COEXISTING FETUS. This entity is different from a partial molar pregnancy because there are two separate conceptuses, with a normal placenta in one twin and a complete molar gestation in the other. As discussed in Chapter 32 (p. 836), the distinction between partial and complete mole has important clinical implications because persistent trophoblastic tumor occurs more commonly following complete mole (Berkowitz and Goldstein, 1992). Approximately 60 percent of women with complete molar twinning will require chemotherapy for persistent gestational trophoblastic tumors (Fishman and associates, 1998; Steller and colleagues, 1994).

The optimal management of complete mole with coexisting fetus is uncertain. These frequently require preterm delivery because of bleeding complications or severe preeclampsia. Bristow and colleagues (1996) reviewed 26 well-documented cases and found that 73

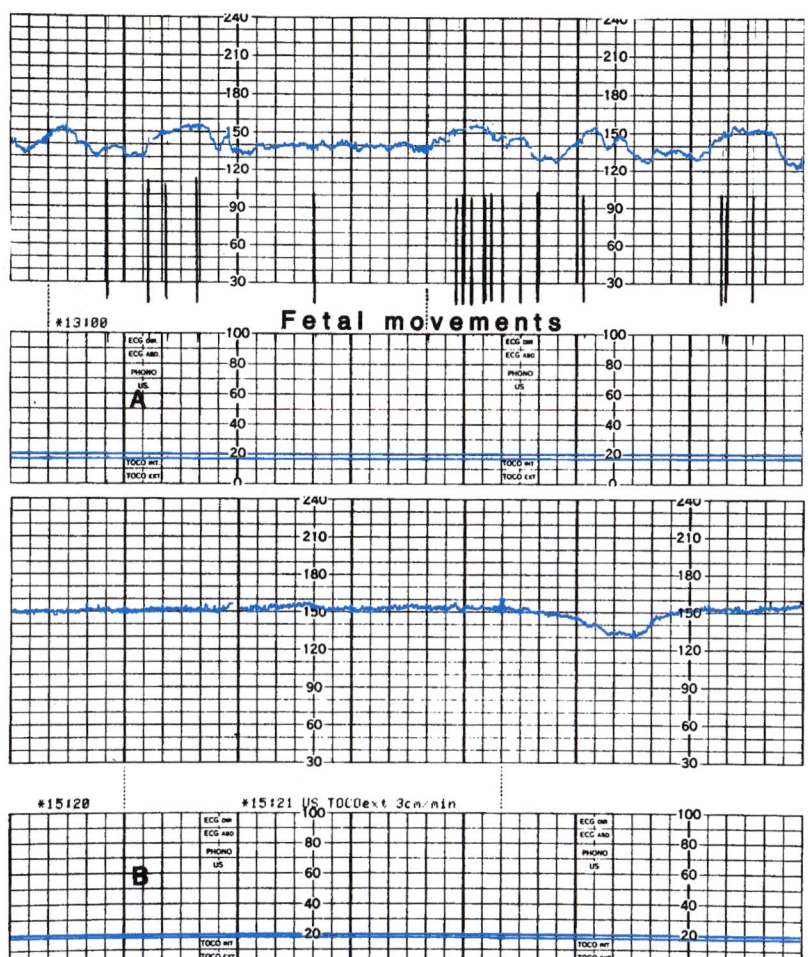

FIGURE 30–27. Antepartum fetal heart rate recordings in discordant twin fetuses at 31 weeks. Shown in panel A are accelerations in response to movements for twin A (birthweight 1200 g). Spontaneous uteroplacental insufficiency-type decelerations were observed in twin B (birthweight 700 g). This fetus also failed to move or accelerate its heart rate. Because of these findings, cesarean section was performed. Both twins died 3 days after delivery: twin A died of hyaline membrane disease and twin B died due to anoxic encephalopathy.

percent required evacuation before fetal viability, but the remainder continued until fetal viability without serious complications. The pregnancies resulting in liveborn infants had evidence of less exuberant tumor growth and their uterine size was only 1 week greater than expected, compared with 8 weeks greater in those requiring evacuation. The mean hCG levels were significantly lower (168,000 mIU/mL) compared with those evacuated early (1,000,000 mIU/mL).

ANTEPARTUM MANAGEMENT OF TWIN PREGNANCY

To reduce perinatal mortality and morbidity in pregnancies complicated by twins, it is imperative that:

1. Delivery of markedly preterm infants be prevented.
2. Failure of one or both fetuses to thrive be identified and fetuses so afflicted be delivered before they become moribund.
3. Fetal trauma during labor and delivery be eliminated.
4. Expert neonatal care be provided.

DIET. The requirements for calories, protein, minerals, vitamins, and essential fatty acids are further increased in women with multiple fetuses. The Recommended Dietary Allowances made by the Food and Nutrition Board of the National Research Council for uncomplicated pregnancy should not only be met but in most instances exceeded (Chap. 10). Consumption of energy sources should be increased by another 300 kcal/day. Brown and Carlson (2000) have recommended that weight gain be based in part on prepregnancy weight, but that women with triplet pregnancies should gain 50 pounds. Iron supplementation of 60 to 100 mg/day is recommended. Folic acid, 1 mg/day, is also given.

MATERNAL HYPERTENSION. Hypertensive disorders due to pregnancy are much more likely to develop with multiple fetuses. The exact incidence attributable to twin gestation is difficult to determine because twin pregnancies are more likely to deliver preterm before preeclampsia can develop, and because women with twin pregnancies are often older and multiparous. Santema and co-workers (1995a) performed a case control study in which 187 twin and 187 singleton pregnancies were matched for maternal age, parity, and gestational age at delivery. They found that the incidence of hypertension was significantly higher in the twin pregnancies (15 versus 6 percent). Coonrad and colleagues (1995) reviewed the outcomes of 3407 twin and 8287 singleton pregnancies to determine the contribution of other independent risk factors for preeclampsia. They found that twin pregnancy carries an overall fourfold increased risk of preeclampsia independent of race and parity, and that nulliparous twin pregnancies have a 14-fold increased risk compared with parous singleton pregnancies. Mastrobattista and colleagues (1997) compared 53 triplet with 53 twin pregnancies and observed that the rate of severe preeclampsia was significantly higher in triplets (23 versus 5.7 percent).

These data suggest that fetal number and placental mass are involved in the pathogenesis of preeclampsia (Chap. 24). Hypertension not only develops more often but also tends to develop earlier and to be more severe. Interestingly, Hardardottir and colleagues (1996) have reported that women with preeclampsia due to high-order multifetal gestations more often develop epigastric pain, hemolysis, and thrombocytopenia as a result of their disease. As shown in Table 30–1, the incidence of pregnancy hypertension in women with twins is 20 percent at Parkland Hospital.

ANTEPARTUM SURVEILLANCE. As discussed earlier, fetal growth is slower in multiple pregnancies than in singleton gestations, and it also may be unequal within a twin pair. For these reasons serial sonography is usually employed throughout the third trimester. Appropriate interval growth is reassuring, and size discordance is a concern primarily when one fetus is growth restricted. Assessment of amnionic fluid volume is also important, as associated oligohydramnios may indicate uteroplacental pathology, and should prompt further evaluation of fetal well being.

Magann and colleagues (1995b), using dye-dilution technique, measured amnionic fluid volumes in each sac in 47 uncomplicated twin gestations between 27 and 38 weeks. The average amnionic fluid volume per twin sac was 877 mL, which is similar to that reported for singletons. The normal range for one fetus was 215 to 2500 mL. These results suggest that in the aggregate, a diamnionic twin gestation has twice the amnionic fluid volume of a singleton.

Quantifying amnionic fluid volume in multiple gestation can be difficult. Some clinicians measure the deepest vertical pocket is each sac, or assess the fluid subjectively. If the sacs are side by side—as opposed to one on top of the other—measurement of the amnionic fluid index (AFI) may be helpful. Using data from 405 normal twin pregnancies, Porter and associates (1996) described

a protocol for measuring the AFI in twins and provided normal values. As in singletons, the deepest vertical pocket in each quadrant was measured, regardless of the location of the dividing membrane. An AFI of less than 8 cm (below the 5th percentile) and over 24 cm (above the 95th percentile) were abnormal at all gestational ages from 28 to 40 weeks. If the overall AFI is abnormal, the sonologist must determine which sac is responsible and attempt to quantify the degree of abnormality. Subjective assessment is often required, and is not always accurate. Magann and co-workers (1995a) reported that oligohydramnios, defined as less than 500 mL, is poorly identified by any sonographic method in twin gestations.

TESTS OF FETAL HEALTH. As described in Chapter 40, there are several methods of assessing fetal health in singleton pregnancies. Use of the nonstress test or biophysical profile is common in management of twin or higher-order multiple gestations. The complexity of complications associated with multiple gestations as well as the potential technical difficulties in separating fetuses during antepartum testing appears to limit the usefulness of these methods. For example, Saacks and co-workers (1995) observed that the antepartum death rate of twin fetuses did not change between 1952 to 1962 and 1983 to 1993 despite the availability of fetal testing during the latter decade. Devoe and Ware (1995) evaluated a fetal monitoring protocol for twins that included ultrasound assessment of fetal growth and amnionic fluid, Doppler velocimetry of the umbilical artery, and nonstress and biophysical profile testing. Nonstress testing and Doppler velocimetry were more predictive of fetal well-being than amnionic fluid volume or biophysical profile. In either case, both could be inaccurate because amnionic fluid measurement was difficult. Elliot and Finberg (1995) evaluated the biophysical profile with nonstress testing as a backup for monitoring of high-order multiple gestations. They reported that 4 of 24 monitored pregnancies had a poor outcome despite reassuring biophysical profile scores.

Whatever method is used, care must be taken to evaluate each fetus separately. Gallagher and colleagues (1992) analyzed fetal heart rate accelerations, fetal movement, and other behavioral states in 15 twin pairs. If one twin of a pair was awake or asleep so was its sibling; however, accelerations and movements were usually not coincidental. An example of such asynchrony of accelerations is shown in Figure 30–28.

DOPPLER VELOCIMETRY. As discussed in Chapters 40 and 41, Doppler evaluation of vascular resistance may provide a measure of fetal well-being. Increased resistance with diminished diastolic flow velocity often accompanies restricted fetal growth. Doppler values

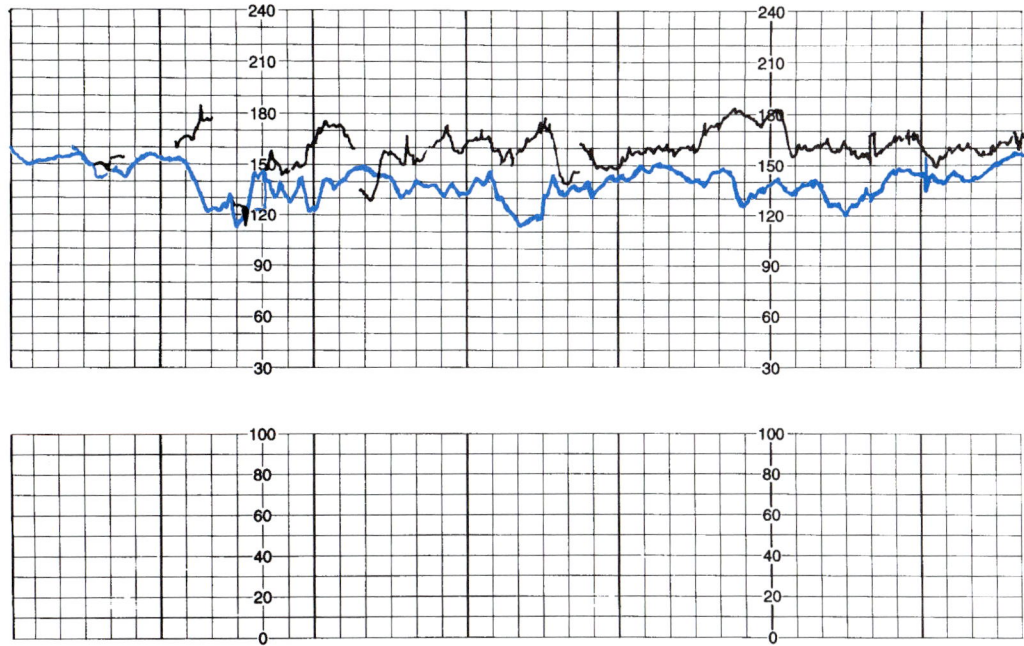

FIGURE 30–28. Simultaneous antepartum fetal heart rate recordings from twin fetuses showing that accelerations are not necessarily synchronous.

in twins and triplets are the same as in singletons, and can thus be used in a similar manner. Akiyama and co-workers (1999) performed Doppler studies of the descending aorta and the middle cerebral, umbilical, splenic, renal, and femoral arteries of 35 singleton, 52 twin, and 12 triplet fetuses every 2 weeks from 15 weeks to term. They found no differences in absolute values or in the patterns of change in regional arterial vascular resistance between singleton and multiple gestations. As in singletons, however, the clinical utility of these findings is controversial.

Gerson and co-workers (1987) used duplex Doppler ultrasound to measure umbilical venous blood flow and arterial systolic–diastolic velocity ratios in twins. Normal studies correctly predicted 44 of 45 concordant twin pairs, while abnormal values, especially of the umbilical artery, correctly predicted 9 of 11 sets of discordant twins. Conversely, DiVou and co-workers (1989) reported that velocimetry alone was not uniformly successful in identifying twin discordance. Ezra and colleagues (1999) found that in triplets and quadruplets, as in singletons, only absent end-diastolic blood flow in the umbilical artery was associated with low birthweight and perinatal mortality.

PREVENTION OF PRETERM DELIVERY. Several techniques have been applied in attempts to prolong multifetal gestations. These include bed rest, especially through hospitalization, prophylactic administration of beta-mimetic drugs, and prophylactic cervical cerclage.

BED REST. Most evidence suggests that routine hospitalization is not beneficial in prolonging multifetal pregnancy. For example, Crowther and co-workers (1990) randomized hospitalization in 139 Zimbabwean women with twin pregnancies and found that hospitalized bed rest did not prolong pregnancy or improve infant survival, although it did improve fetal growth. Arabin and colleagues (1997) demonstrated sonographically that in multiple gestation the cervix shortens several millimeters and often shows funneling when the woman is in the erect position. In this study, however, bed rest did not improve pregnancy outcome.

At Parkland Hospital, elective hospitalization at 26 weeks was compared longitudinally with outpatient management and no advantages were found for routine hospitalization (Andrews and colleagues, 1991). Importantly, almost half of the twin pregnancies studied required admission for specific indications such as hypertension or threatened preterm delivery. Similarly, Adams and colleagues (1998) compared 32 triplet pregnancies managed with outpatient bed rest to a historical cohort of 34 triplets managed with routine hospitalization in the third trimester. The outpatient group delivered one week earlier (32.5 versus 33.5 weeks), but neonatal hospitalization was similar between the groups. The outpatient group had a significantly higher rate of preeclampsia (31 versus 9 percent) and significantly more of their neonates had intraventricular hemorrhages (10 versus 1 percent).

Special prenatal clinic sessions, limited physical activity, early work leave, and structured maternal education on the risks of preterm delivery have been advocated to be effective in reducing preterm births in women with multiple fetuses. Unfortunately, there is little evidence that these measures substantially change outcome. For example, Pons and co-workers (1998) found virtually no difference in outcomes of 70 triplet pregnancies managed intensively from 1987 to 1993 and compared with 21 triplet pregnancies managed routinely between 1975 and 1986. The only major difference between these two periods was that neonates in the later group had significantly less hyaline membrane disease (13 versus 31 percent), which these investigators attributed to the use of corticosteroids.

TOCOLYTIC THERAPY. As in singleton pregnancies, most randomized trials of beta-mimetics in twin pregnancies have not shown significant reductions in preterm delivery rates. Garite and colleagues (1990) monitored the contraction patterns of 39 twin, 20 triplet, and 10 quadruplet pregnancies daily and thus diagnosed preterm labor before advanced cervical dilatation had occurred. Despite this, they found that tocolytic therapy was not effective in diminishing the crescendo of uterine activity that preceded preterm labor. Ashworth and associates (1990) were also unable to substantiate any benefits for prophylactic beta-mimetic therapy with salbutamol in twin gestations. As described in Chapter 27 (p. 714), most randomized studies of other tocolytic drugs compared with untreated controls exclude multiple gestation, and few specifically focus on multiple gestation.

Tocolytic therapy in women with multiple gestation entails a higher risk than in singletons, in part because the increased plasma volume and cardiovascular demands make such patients especially susceptible to pulmonary edema after receiving hydration and beta-mimetic therapy. Gabriel and colleagues (1994) compared the outcomes of 26 twin and 6 triplet pregnancies with 51 singletons treated with a beta-mimetic for preterm labor without ruptured membranes. They found that women with multiple gestation had significantly more cardiovascular complications (43 versus 4 percent), including three cases of pulmonary edema. Magnesium sulfate can also increase risk, especially when used with prolonged bed rest as is commonly prescribed for multiple gestation. Levav and co-authors (1998) reported a case of osteoporosis and bilateral stress fractures of the calcanei in a woman with triplets treated with magnesium sulfate and prolonged bed rest.

CORTICOSTEROIDS FOR FETAL LUNG MATURATION. There is no satisfactory evidence that corticosteroids benefit multiple fetuses. For example, Turrentine and colleagues (1996) found no difference in neonatal

outcome between 21 twin pairs who received optimal corticosteroid treatment and 63 pairs who received no treatment. Although acknowledging the preceding, the Consensus Development Conference on the Effect of Corticosteroids for Fetal Maturation (1994) sponsored by the National Institutes of Health essentially recommended treatment for women with multiple gestations and impending delivery.

CERCLAGE. No significant reduction in preterm delivery or perinatal deaths has been demonstrated from prophylactic cervical cerclage in multiple pregnancies. For example, Elimian and colleagues (1999) compared the outcomes of 20 triplet pregnancies managed with prophylactic cerclage and 39 triplet pregnancies managed expectantly. The incidence of low-birthweight infants was higher in the no cerclage group because this group had an increased proportion of deliveries before 31 weeks. Despite this, there was no difference in mean age at delivery (32.8 weeks in the cerclage group versus 31.5 weeks in the control group) or in the incidence of antenatal, perinatal, or neonatal complications.

PRETERM LABOR PREDICTION. Goldenberg and colleagues (1996) prospectively screened 147 twin pregnancies for more than 50 potential risk factors for preterm birth and found that only cervical length and fetal fibronectin predicted preterm birth. At 24 weeks, a cervical length over 25 mm was the best predictor of birth before 32 weeks, and at 28 weeks, a positive fetal fibronectin was the best predictor. Similarly, Souka and co-workers (1999) sonographically measured the cervices of 215 women with twin pregnancies at 23 weeks and found that a length of 25 mm or less had a 100 percent, 80 percent, 47 percent, and 35 percent sensitivity in predicting birth before 28, 30, 32, and 34 weeks, respectively. Conversely, Imseis and colleagues (1997) measured cervical length at 24 to 26 weeks' gestation in 85 twin pregnancies. They found that a cervix measuring 35 mm or less had 49 percent sensitivity, 94 percent specificity, and 97 and 31 percent positive and negative predictive values in identifying women at *low* risk for delivery before 34 weeks.

PULMONARY MATURATION. As measured by determination of the lecithin-sphingomyelin ratio, pulmonary maturation is usually synchronous in twins (Leveno and associates, 1984). Moreover, although this ratio usually exceeds 2 by 36 weeks in singleton pregnancies, it often does so by about 32 weeks in multifetal pregnancy. In some cases, however, there may be marked disparity of pulmonary function, with the smallest, most stressed fetus being more mature. We observed the lecithin–sphingomyelin ratio with quintuplets to vary from less than 2 for the largest infant, who weighed 1530 g at 32 weeks and was of appropriate size, to greater than 5 for the severely growth-restricted smallest infant, who weighed 860 g. The largest infant developed appreciable respiratory distress, whereas the smallest infant did not.

Friedman and co-workers (1997) studied 224 twins from 112 otherwise uncomplicated twin pregnancies delivered before 35 weeks because of refractory preterm labor. When compared to 224 normal singleton fetuses from similarly uncomplicated pregnancies who were matched for gestational age at birth, gender, and mode of delivery, there was no difference in the incidence of respiratory distress syndrome, grades 3 and 4 intraventricular hemorrhage, grades 2 and 3 necrotizing enterocolitis, or neonatal death. However, significantly more twins required admission to the neonatal intensive care unit (88 versus 72 percent).

EXPECTANT MANAGEMENT OF RUPTURED MEMBRANES. Twin gestations with preterm ruptured membranes are managed expectantly much like singleton pregnancies (Chap. 27, p. 704). Mercer and colleagues (1993) compared outcomes of twin and singleton pregnancies with prematurely ruptured membranes at 19 to 36 weeks and found that labor ensued earlier in twins. Specifically, the median time from rupture to delivery was 1.1 days in twins compared with 1.7 days in singletons. Over 90 percent in both groups delivered within 7 days of ruptured membranes. Similarly, Hsieh and colleagues (1999) studied 131 twins and 48 singletons with preterm premature rupture and found that the latency in twins was 1.2 days shorter when rupture was at 30 weeks or sooner. Regardless of the gestational age at rupture, 50 percent of twins compared with 27 percent of singletons delivered within 48 hours, and 92 percent of twins and 86 percent of singletons delivered within 7 days.

DELAYED DELIVERY OF SECOND TWIN. Cases have been reported in which one or more of multiple fetuses was expelled very preterm, and because uterine activity then ceased the pregnancy was allowed to continue with delivery of another fetus days to even many weeks later. Trivedi and Gillett (1998) reviewed the English literature and found 45 case reports of asynchronous birth in multiple gestation. Most often, the first birth resulted from preterm rupture of the membranes, and the survival rate for these infants was very poor. However, the pregnancies with a surviving twin or triplet continued for an average of 49 days. Management with tocolytics, prophylactic antibiotics, and cerclage, appeared to make no difference. If asynchronous birth is attempted, there must be careful evaluation for infection, abruption, and congenital anomalies, and the woman is counseled thoroughly about these risks.

DELIVERY OF TWIN FETUSES

LABOR. Many complications of labor and delivery, including preterm labor, uterine dysfunction, abnormal presentations, prolapse of the umbilical cord, premature separation of the placenta, and immediate postpartum hemorrhage, are encountered much more often with multiple fetuses. For these reasons, certain precautions and special arrangements are prudent when delivery of two or more fetuses is expected. Recommendations for intrapartum management follow.

1. An appropriately trained obstetrical attendant should remain with the mother throughout labor. Continuous external electronic monitoring or, if the membranes are ruptured and the cervix dilated, evaluation of both fetuses by simultaneous internal and external electronic monitoring, is typically employed.
2. Blood transfusion products should be readily available.
3. An intravenous infusion system capable of delivering fluid rapidly should be established. In the absence of hemorrhage or metabolic disturbance during labor, lactated Ringer with aqueous dextrose solution is infused at a rate of 60 to 120 mL/hr.
4. Ampicillin, 2 g intravenously, is administered every 6 hours for prevention of group B *Streptococcus* neonatal infection when preterm labor is diagnosed.
5. An obstetrician skilled in intrauterine identification of fetal parts and intrauterine manipulation of the fetus should be present.
6. If possible, an ultrasound machine should be available in the delivery room to facilitate evaluation of position and status of the second twin after delivery of the first.
7. An experienced anesthesiologist should be immediately available in the event that intrauterine manipulation or cesarean delivery is necessary.
8. For each fetus, two people, one of whom is skilled in resuscitation and care of newborns, are appropriately informed of the case and remain immediately available.
9. The delivery area should provide adequate space for all members of the team to work effectively. Moreover, the site should be appropriately equipped to take care of all possible maternal problems plus resuscitation and maintenance of each infant.

PRESENTATION AND POSITION. With twins, all possible combinations of fetal positions may be encountered. Either or both fetuses may present cephalic, breech, or shoulder. As shown in Figure 30–29, the most common presentations at admission for delivery are cephalic–cephalic, cephalic–breech, and cephalic–transverse. Importantly, these presentations, especially those other

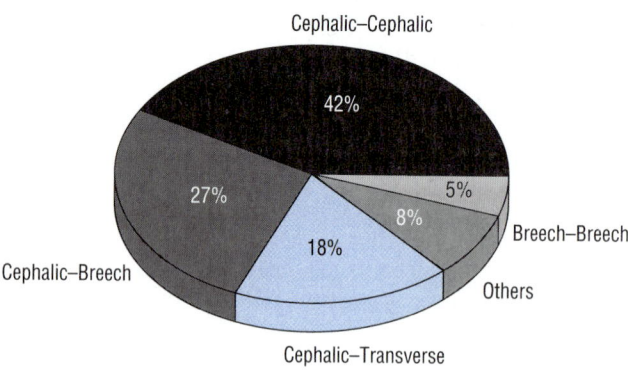

Cephalic–Cephalic
42%
5%
8%
Breech–Breech
27%
18%
Cephalic–Breech
Others
Cephalic–Transverse

FIGURE 30–29. Presentations of twin fetuses on admission for delivery. (From Divon and colleagues, 1993, with permission.)

than cephalic–cephalic, are unstable before and during labor or delivery. Compound, face, brow, and footling breech presentations are relatively common, especially when the fetuses are quite small, there is excess amnionic fluid, or maternal parity is high. Prolapse of the cord is fairly common in these circumstances.

The presentation can often be ascertained by sonography. If any confusion about the relationship of the twins to each other or to the maternal pelvis persists, a single anteroposterior x-ray of the abdomen may be helpful.

INDUCTION OR STIMULATION OF LABOR. Labor is generally shorter with twins (Schiff and associates, 1998), but rupture of the membranes without effective labor, and prolonged inefficient labor with or without previous rupture of the membranes, do develop. These problems are often handled better by cesarean delivery unless there is little hope of salvaging the infants because of their gross immaturity. Termination of pregnancy is occasionally desirable before the spontaneous onset of labor, as with severe pregnancy-induced hypertension. In these circumstances, if the presenting part is well fixed in the pelvis and the cervix dilated somewhat, amniotomy will often initiate labor and effect delivery. If the woman meets all criteria for administration of oxytocin for labor initiation (Chap. 20, p. 477), the American College of Obstetricians and Gynecologists (1995) has stated that multifetal gestation is not a contraindication to labor induction, but is a condition that warrants special attention. There is no reluctance by some obstetricians to give oxytocin by dilute intravenous infusion to initiate or to stimulate labor in pregnancies complicated by multiple fetuses. Satin and co-workers (1996) compared outcomes in 55 women with twins who were given oxytocin for augmentation or induction for labor with 55 matched singleton pregnancies.

Women with twin pregnancies responded similarly to women with singletons.

ANALGESIA AND ANESTHESIA. During labor and delivery of multiple fetuses, deciding what to use for analgesia and for anesthesia is unusually difficult because of the frequency of and problems imposed by:

1. Prematurity.
2. Maternal hypertension.
3. Desultory labor.
4. Need for intrauterine manipulation.
5. Uterine atony and hemorrhage after delivery.

Epidural analgesia is recommended by some clinicians because it provides: (1) pain relief, (2) skeletal muscle relaxation that would be required for internal podalic version, and (3) it can be rapidly extended cephalad if cesarean delivery is required (Koffel, 1999). Special care must be taken in hypertensive women or those who have hemorrhaged because epidural analgesia may cause hypotension with inadequate perfusion of vital organs, especially the placenta.

Therefore, placement and maintenance of continuous epidural analgesia should be by someone knowledgeable in obstetrics and preceded by adequate hydration, and the block should be allowed to come up slowly to avoid a hypotensive episode. Because the woman pregnant with multiple fetuses is even more vulnerable to supine hypotension during labor and delivery, she should be placed in full lateral position during and after induction of epidural analgesia, and left uterine displacement should be maintained for cesarean delivery.

It is likely that the effects of epidural analgesia on the progress of labor seen in singleton pregnancy would also be found in twins, but few studies include multiple gestations. These effects are discussed in Chapter 15 (p. 374). Crawford (1987) described 105 women with twins delivered vaginally who were given epidural analgesia. It prolonged the interval from complete dilatation until delivery by approximately 60 minutes. Interestingly, the mean delivery intervals between delivery of the first and second twins were not altered by epidural analgesia.

Either balanced general anesthesia or regional epidural or subarachnoid analgesia has proved satisfactory at Parkland Hospital for cesarean delivery of twins. When general anesthesia is used, the increased oxygen demand and decreased functional residual capacity associated with multiple gestation increase the risk of hypoxemia, thus making adequate preoxygenation essential. Pudendal block skillfully administered along with nitrous oxide plus oxygen can provide relief of pain for spontaneous delivery. When intrauterine manipulation is necessary, as with internal podalic version, uterine relaxation can also be accomplished rapidly with isoflurane. Although these agents provide effective relaxation for intrauterine manipulation, they also cause an increase in blood loss during the third stage. Some use intravenous or sublingual nitroglycerine for relaxation (Vinatier and associates, 1996).

VAGINAL DELIVERY. The presenting twin typically bears the major brunt of dilating the cervix and the remaining soft tissues of the birth canal. When the first twin is cephalic, delivery is usually uncomplicated, and can be accomplished spontaneously or with outlet forceps. As in singletons, when the first fetus presents as a breech, major problems are most likely to develop if:

1. The fetus is unusually large and the aftercoming head taxes the capacity of the birth canal.
2. The fetus is quite small so that the extremities and trunk are delivered through a cervix inadequately effaced and dilated for the head to escape easily.
3. The umbilical cord prolapses.

When these problems are anticipated or identified, cesarean delivery will often be the better way to effect delivery, except in those instances in which the fetuses are so immature that they will not survive. Otherwise, breech delivery may be accomplished as described in Chapter 22.

The phenomenon of locked twins is rare, and according to Cohen and co-workers (1965) occurred only once in 817 twin gestations. For locking to occur, the first fetus must present by the breech and the second as cephalic. With descent of the breech through the birth canal, the chin of the first fetus locks in the neck and chin of the second cephalic fetus. Cesarean delivery is recommended when the potential for locking is identified.

Many obstetricians plan vaginal delivery for cephalic–cephalic presenting twins if satisfactory labor has been established. The optimal delivery route for cephalic–noncephalic twins is controversial, particularly when very-low-birthweight is a concern (American College of Obstetricians and Gynecologists, 1998). Many of the issues involved in vaginal delivery of breech second twins are similar to those for singletons, with the added concern that second-born twins have historically fared worse than their first-born siblings. Kurzel and colleagues (1997) reviewed the delivery events of 541 twin pregnancies at the University of California in Los Angeles from 1987 to 1995. The overall cesarean delivery rate was 35 percent, including 5 percent solely for twin B. Cesareans were performed in 14 percent of twins in which twin A was cephalic, compared with 67 percent when twin A was breech and 100 percent when twin A was transverse. The proportion of primary cesarean deliveries when twin B was breech or transverse was similar. Of the twins who were cephalic–cephalic, cesar-

ean delivery of the second twin was performed in 26 percent, primarily for cord prolapse. Of the cephalic–noncephalic twins, cesarean delivery of twin B was done in 52 percent, primarily for failed internal podalic version and extraction when twin B was transverse.

There are several reports attesting to the safety of vaginal delivery of second noncephalic twins who are larger than 1500 g (Blickstein, 1987; Chervanak, 1985; Gocke, 1989, and their associates) as well as those weighing less than 1500 g (Davidson and co-workers, 1992; Rydhström, 1990). More recently, Mauldin and colleagues (1998) retrospectively reviewed the delivery courses of 84 cephalic–noncephalic twins, and found that vaginal delivery of twin A with breech extraction of twin B resulted in significantly shorter maternal and neonatal hospital stays and lowered hospital charges than either vaginal delivery of A with external version of B or cesarean delivery. Hospital stays were shorter for both mother and infant in part because vaginally extracted breech twins had less respiratory disease and infections. Unfortunately, and as emphasized by Chauhan and colleagues (1995), there are no large randomized trials to help resolve the uncertainty about vaginal or cesarean delivery for noncephalic second twins.

When the first twin is breech, most clinicians plan a cesarean delivery. The American College of Obstetricians and Gynecologists (1998) has concluded that, in general, cesarean delivery is the method of choice when the first twin is noncephalic, such as breech or transverse presentation. More recently, however, Blickstein and colleagues (2000) reported the collective experience from 1990 to 1997 of 13 European centers that allowed vaginal delivery in 239 of 613 twin pairs when twin A was breech. Although twin A breech infants weighing less than 1500 g were more likely to suffer neonatal death (45 versus 8 percent), the death rates were not significantly different in those weighing more than 1500 g (0.3 versus 0.2 percent).

VAGINAL DELIVERY OF THE SECOND TWIN. As soon as the first twin has been delivered, the presenting part of the second twin, its size, and its relationship to the birth canal are quickly ascertained by careful combined abdominal, vaginal, and at times intrauterine examination. Sonography also has proven quite valuable in some cases.

If the fetal head or the breech is fixed in the birth canal, moderate fundal pressure is applied and membranes are ruptured. Immediately afterward, the examination is repeated to identify prolapse of the cord. Labor is allowed to resume while the fetal heart rate is monitored. With re-establishment of labor there is no need to hasten delivery unless there is a nonreassuring fetal heart rate or bleeding. Hemorrhage indicates placental separation, which can be deleterious to both the fetus

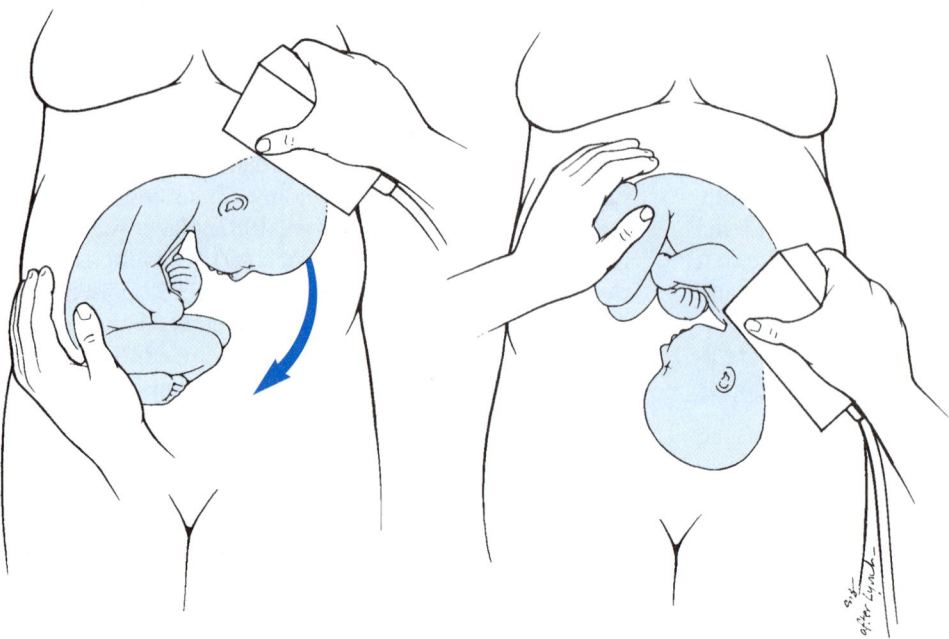

FIGURE 30–30. External version of second breech twin fetus. Ultrasound transducer is being used to help guide vertex into pelvis. (Redrawn from Chervenak and colleagues, 1983, with permission.)

and the mother. If contractions do not resume within approximately 10 minutes, dilute oxytocin may be used to stimulate appropriate myometrial activity, leading to spontaneous delivery or delivery assisted by outlet forceps.

If the occiput or the breech presents immediately over the pelvic inlet but is not fixed in the birth canal, the presenting part can often be guided into the pelvis with a vaginal hand while a hand on the uterine fundus exerts moderate pressure. Alternatively, an assistant can direct the presenting part into the pelvis using ultrasound for guidance and to monitor heart rate. Intrapartum external version of the noncephalic second twin has also been described (Chervanak and co-workers, 1983). Using the method shown in Figure 30–30, the fetus who presents as breech or shoulder may be gently converted into a cephalic presentation. Once the presenting part is fixed in the pelvic inlet, membranes are ruptured and delivery is carried out as described earlier.

If the occiput or the breech is not over the pelvic inlet and cannot be so positioned by gentle pressure on the presenting part, or if appreciable uterine bleeding develops, delivery of the second twin can be problematic. So as to take maximum advantage of the dilated cervix before the uterus contracts and the cervix retracts, procrastination must be avoided. An obstetrician skilled in intrauterine fetal manipulation and an anesthesiologist skilled in providing anesthesia to effectively relax the uterus are essential for vaginal delivery with a favorable outcome. Prompt delivery of the second fetus by

cesarean delivery is the better choice if no one present is skilled in the performance of internal podalic version (described in the following section) or if anesthesia that will provide effective uterine relaxation is not immediately available.

INTERNAL PODALIC VERSION. In internal podalic version, the fetus is turned so as to deliver the feet first, which then enables the obstetrician to effect delivery by breech extraction. Chauhan and colleagues (1995) compared outcomes of 23 second twins delivered by podalic version and breech extraction with 21 who underwent external cephalic version. Breech extraction was considered superior to external version because there was less fetal distress.

Through careful abdominal, vaginal, and intrauterine examinations, the various parts of the fetus can be identified. A hand is used to rupture the membranes and both feet are identified and grasped, and only then are they gently pulled toward the birth canal (Fig. 30–31). With the other hand applied to the abdomen, or with the help of an assistant, the head simultaneously is elevated gently (Fig. 30–32). An episiotomy is made or extended whenever more room is needed for uterine and vaginal manipulation. The legs are drawn slowly through the birth canal until the buttocks are visible anteriorly just beyond the maternal symphysis. A moist, warm towel is applied to the buttocks, and gentle traction is continued until the lower thirds of both scapulas are visible. Next,

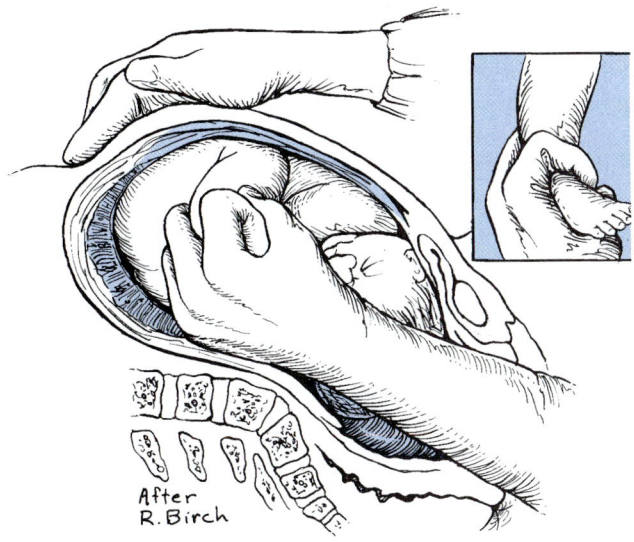

FIGURE 30–31. Internal podalic version.

the trunk is slowly rotated with gentle traction until the shoulder and arm on one side of the fetus are delivered. Rotation of the fetal trunk now is gently reversed to deliver the other arm and shoulder into the vagina. Care must be taken to avoid or at least recognize the presence of a nuchal arm (Chap. 22, p. 524). A nuchal arm can be reduced by rotating the trunk 90 degrees or more in the direction of the trapped arm (for example, if the left arm is trapped, rotate the trunk to the patient's left), bringing the arm into extension in front of the trunk where it can be grasped and gently pulled down. The aftercoming head may then be delivered either by simultaneous suprapubic external pressure to flex the

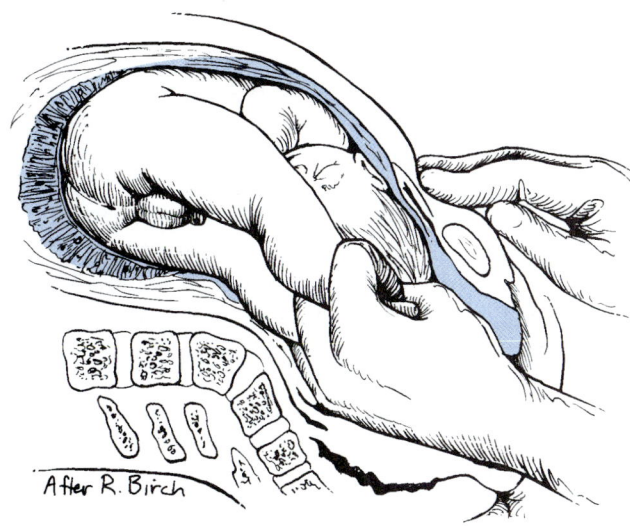

FIGURE 30–32. Internal podalic version. Upward pressure on head is applied as downward traction is exerted on feet.

head and gentle traction applied to the trunk, or by use of Piper forceps (Chap. 22, p. 524).

The cord is clamped promptly with two clamps on the placental side to identify it as the cord of the second infant. The placenta or placentas are delivered immediately by manual removal, if necessary. The uterus is promptly explored for defects and for retained pregnancy products. As these steps are being carried out, the uterine-relaxing anesthetic agent is discontinued, and as soon as uterine exploration has been completed, oxytocin is administered through an intravenous infusion system. Fundal massage or, preferably, manual compression of the uterus with one hand in the vagina against the lower uterine segment and the other transabdominally over the uterine fundus is applied to hasten and enhance myometrial contraction.

The cervix, vagina, periurethral region, vulva, and perineum are inspected carefully. Lacerations likely to bleed are repaired along with the episiotomy.

INTERVAL BETWEEN FIRST AND SECOND TWINS. In the past, the interval between delivery of the first and second twins was commonly cited to be safest if less than 30 minutes. Subsequently, as shown by Rayburn and colleagues (1984) as well as others, if continuous fetal monitoring is employed, there is a good outcome even if this interval is longer. Of 115 twin pairs at 34 weeks or more, the mean interval between delivery of twins was 21 minutes, but it ranged from 1 to 134 minutes. In 60 percent, the interval was 15 minutes or less. Importantly, there was no excess trauma or evidence for fetal depression in those born after the 15-minute interval. As expected, the cesarean delivery rate was much higher if the interval was more than 15 minutes (18 percent) than if the interval was less than 15 minutes (3 percent). Saacks and co-workers (1995) found that the time interval between delivery of twin A and twin B increased significantly between 1952 and 1993. The median interval was 11 minutes in the most recent years they studied, however, probably indicating that the spontaneous delivery interval between twins is typically quite brief. The American College of Obstetricians and Gynecologists (1998) has determined that the interval between delivery of twins is not critical in determining the outcome of twin B.

CESAREAN DELIVERY. Twin fetuses create unusual intraoperative problems. The mother is likely to be even less tolerant of the supine position, and therefore it is important to rotate her position so as to deflect the uterus off the aorta (Chap. 8, p. 182). Hypotension can be detected with simultaneous monitoring of brachial and popliteal blood pressures. The incision should be large enough to allow atraumatic delivery of both fetuses. In some cases, a vertical incision in the lower uterine segment may be advantageous. For example, if a fetus is in transverse position, with the back down, and the arms are inadvertently delivered first, it is much easier and safer to extend a vertical uterine incision upward than to extend a transverse incision. If twin B is breech and delivery of the head is obstructed, Piper forceps can be used just as for a vaginal delivery.

It is important that the uterus be well contracted during completion of the cesarean delivery and thereafter. Remarkable blood loss may be concealed within the uterus and vagina and beneath the drapes during the time taken to close the incisions.

At times, attempts to deliver the second twin vaginally after delivery of the first twin are not only unwise but also impossible, and prompt cesarean delivery is required. Cesarean delivery of twin B may be necessary, for example, when the second fetus is much larger than the first, and is in a breech position or in a transverse lie. Even more perplexing, cesarean delivery may be required because the cervix promptly contracts and thickens after delivery of the first infant and does not dilate subsequently.

TRIPLETS OR MORE

All of the problems of twin gestation are remarkably intensified by the presence of additional fetuses. Improved neonatal care has lead to the expectation of 95 percent infant survival, but triplets still suffer morbidity. Kaufman and colleagues (1998) compared the outcomes of 55 triplet pregnancies with 357 twin and 959 singleton pregnancies delivered from 1992 to 1996. They reported that the survival rates were similar at 95, 95, and 97 percent, respectively. Compared with singletons, however, triplets were at significantly higher risk to have mild intraventricular hemorrhage (RR 6.2), mild retinopathy of prematurity (RR 20.0), and severe retinopathy (RR 46.7). The mortality rate for triplets was 121 per 1000, regardless of birth order.

Labor and delivery entails increased risk as well. Fetal heart rate monitoring during labor is challenging. A scalp electrode can be attached to the presenting fetus, but it is difficult to assure that the other two triplets are each being monitored separately. With vaginal delivery, the first infant is usually born spontaneously or with little manipulation. However, subsequent infants are delivered according to the presenting part, which often requires complicated obstetrical maneuvers such as total breech extraction with or without internal podalic version, or may even necessitate cesarean delivery. Associated with malposition of the fetuses is an increased incidence of cord prolapse and fetal collision. Moreover, reduced placental perfusion and hemorrhage from separating placentas are more likely during delivery.

For all these reasons, many clinicians believe that delivery of pregnancies complicated by three or more fetuses is best accomplished by cesarean section. Vaginal delivery is reserved for those circumstances in which survival is not expected because the fetuses are markedly immature, or maternal complications make cesarean delivery hazardous to the mother. There are other clinicians who believe that vaginal delivery is safe under certain circumstances. For example, Alamia and colleagues (1998) evaluated a protocol for vaginal delivery of triplet pregnancies in which the presenting fetus was cephalic, and all three fetuses could be continuously monitored. A total of 23 sets of triplets were analyzed and a third were delivered vaginally. Neonatal outcomes were the same in the vaginal and cesarean groups, with no morbidity and 100 percent survival. As in any obstetrical procedure, the safety of vaginal triplet delivery depends on the skill and experience of the operator.

SELECTIVE REDUCTION OR TERMINATION

In some cases of higher-order multifetal gestations, reduction in the number of fetuses to two or three will improve survival for the remaining fetuses. Selective reduction implies early pregnancy intervention whereas selective termination is done later.

SELECTIVE REDUCTION. Reduction of a selected fetus or fetuses in a multiple gestation may be chosen as a therapeutic intervention to enhance survivability of the co-fetuses. Multifetal pregnancy reduction was developed at Mount Sinai Medical Center in New York in an effort to improve the poor prognosis of pregnancies with three or more fetuses that typically resulted from assisted reproduction technologies (Berkowitz and associates, 1988). Pregnancy reduction can be performed transcervically, transvaginally, or transabdominally, but the transabdominal route is easiest. Transabdominal reductions are typically performed between 10 and 13 weeks. This time was chosen because any spontaneous fetal losses have already occurred, the remaining fetuses are big enough to be evaluated sonographically, the amount of devitalized fetal tissue remaining after the procedure is small, and the risk of losing the entire pregnancy as a result of the procedure is low. The smallest fetuses and any anomalous fetuses are targeted for reduction and potassium chloride is then injected into the heart or thorax of each selected fetus under ultrasound guidance, taking care not to enter or traverse the sacs of the fetuses selected for retention. In most cases, pregnancies are reduced to twins in order to increase the chances of delivering at least one viable fetus.

Berkowitz and co-workers (1996), in describing their experience with 400 reductions performed by very expe-

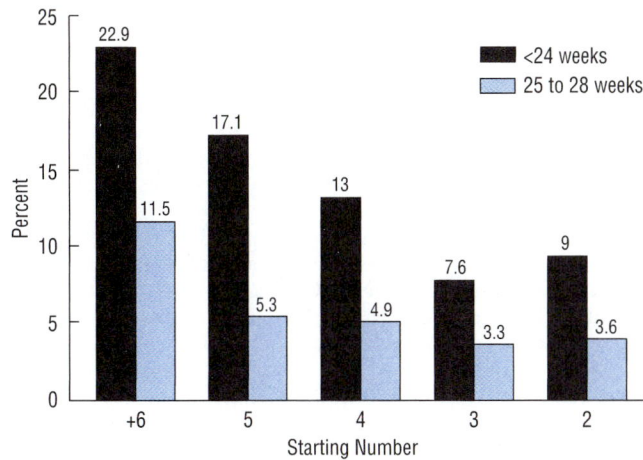

FIGURE 30–33. Histogram showing the rate of pregnancy losses (less than 24 weeks) and preterm birth (25 to 28 weeks) as a function of higher starting number of multiple fetuses in 1789 pregnancies undergoing selective reduction. (Modified from Evans and associates, 1996, with permission.)

rienced operators, reported a pregnancy loss rate of 8 percent. The remaining 92 percent delivered one or more viable fetus after 24 weeks. Evans and associates (1996) described a multicenter collaborative experience with this procedure in 1789 patients. They reported an overall pregnancy loss rate of 12 percent, which varied from a low of 8 percent for triplets reduced to twins, and increased with each additional starting fetus to 23 percent for sextuplets or higher. The loss rate early on was higher than for the last two years, attesting to the importance of operator skill and experience. Early preterm deliveries were more likely in pregnancies starting as higher-order gestations, reinforcing the concept that higher-order multiple gestations are hazardous to both the fetuses and the mothers (Fig. 30–33).

SELECTIVE TERMINATION. With the identification of multiple fetuses discordant for structural or genetic abnormalities, three options are available:

1. Abortion of all fetuses.
2. Selective termination of the abnormal fetus.
3. Continuation of the pregnancy.

Because anomalies are typically not discovered until the second trimester, selective termination is performed later in gestation than selective reduction and entails more risk. This procedure is therefore usually not performed unless the anomaly is severe but not lethal, meaning that the anomalous fetus would survive and require lifetime care, or the estimated risk of continuing the pregnancy is greater than the risk of the procedure. For example, a triplet pregnancy in which one fetus has Down syndrome might be a candidate for selective

termination, while a twin pregnancy in which one has trisomy 18 might not. In some cases, termination is considered because the abnormal fetus may jeopardize the normal one. For example, pathological hydramnios developing in a twin with esophageal atresia could lead to preterm birth of its sibling. Prerequisites to selective termination include a precise diagnosis for the anomalous fetus and absolute certainty as to its location. In the case of an aneuploidy detected after genetic amniocentesis for advanced maternal age, for example, a map of the uterus with the locations of all the fetuses clearly labeled should be made at the time of the diagnostic procedure.

Evans and co-workers (1999) have provided the most comprehensive results to date on second-trimester selective termination for fetal abnormalities. A total of 402 cases from the eight most experienced centers worldwide were analyzed. Included were 345 twins, 39 triplets, and 18 quadruplets. Selective termination using potassium chloride resulted in the delivery of a viable infant in more than 90 percent of cases, with a mean age at delivery of 35.7 weeks. The loss rate was 7.1 percent in pregnancies reduced to singletons and was 13 percent in those reduced to twins, again attesting to the increased risk of higher-order multiples. The gestational age at the time of the procedure did not appear to affect the outcome—the rate was 5.4 percent when the procedure was performed at 9 to 12 weeks; 8.7 percent at 13 to 18 weeks; 6.8 percent at 19 to 24 weeks; and 9.1 percent at 25 weeks. Several losses occurred because the pregnancy was actually monochorionic and potassium chloride killed the normal fetus through placental vascular shunts. Lynch and colleagues (1996) reported that termination of the presenting fetus or selective termination after 20 weeks significantly increased the risk of preterm prematurely membrane rupture and delivery.

ETHICS. The ethical issues associated with these techniques are almost limitless. The interested reader is referred to the excellent reviews by Evans and co-workers (1988) and Simpson and Carson (1996).

INFORMED CONSENT. Prior to initiation of infertility therapy or any attempt to perform selective termination or reduction, the couple should be counseled about the risks and benefits and informed consent obtained. Counseling should include a discussion of the morbidity and mortality expected if the pregnancy is continued, according to the number of fetuses; the morbidity and mortality expected with twins or triplets, whichever the couple would reduce to; and the risks of the procedure itself. Specific risks that are common to selective termination or reduction include:

1. Abortion of the remaining fetuses.
2. Abortion of the wrong (normal) fetus in twins.
3. Retention of genetic or structurally abnormal fetuses after a reduction in number.
4. Damage without death to a fetus.
5. Preterm labor complicating pregnancies with the remaining fetuses.
6. Development of discordant twins or growth restricted fetuses.
7. Maternal infection, hemorrhage, or possible disseminated intravascular coagulopathy owing to retained products of conception.

The procedure should be performed by an operator skilled and experienced in ultrasound-guided procedures. Because selective reduction will increase the maternal serum alpha-fetoprotein level, the couple should be informed that this screening test will not be helpful to them after the procedure (Lynch and Berkowitz, 1993). Instead, they are offered a second-trimester targeted ultrasound evaluation.

PSYCHOLOGICAL REACTIONS. Women and their spouses who elect to undergo selective termination or reduction find this decision highly stressful. Schreiner-Engel and associates (1995) retrospectively studied the emotional reactions of 100 women following selective reduction. Although 70 percent of the women mourned for their lost fetus(es), most grieved only for 1 month. Persistent depressive symptoms were mild, although moderately severe sadness and guilt continued for many. Fortunately, the large majority were reconciled to the termination of some fetuses to preserve the lives of a remaining few. Indeed, 93 percent of the women would have made the same decision again.

REFERENCES

Adams DM, Sholl JS, Haney EI, Russell TL, Silver RK: Perinatal outcome associated with outpatient management of triplet pregnancy. Am J Obstet Gynecol 178:843, 1998

Aisenbrey GA, Catanzarite VA, Hurley TJ, Spiegel JH, Schrimmer DB, Mendoza A: Monoamniotic and pseudomonoamniotic twins: Sonographic diagnosis, detection of cord entanglement, and obstetric management. Obstet Gynecol 86:218, 1995

Akiyama M, Kuno A, Tanaka Y, Tanaka H, Hayashi K, Yanagihara T, Hata T: Comparison of alterations in fetal regional arterial vascular resistance in appropriate-for-gestational-age singleton, twin and triplet pregnancies. Hum Reprod 14:2635, 1999

Alamia V Jr, Royek AB, Jaekle RK, Meyer BA: Preliminary experience with a prospective protocol for planned vaginal delivery of triplet gestations. Am J Obstet Gynecol 179:1133, 1998

American College of Obstetricians and Gynecologists: Special problems of multiple gestation. Education Bulletin No. 253, 1998

American College of Obstetricians and Gynecologists: Induction of labor. Technical Bulletin No. 217, 1995

American Society for Reproductive Medicine. A Practice Committee Report: Guidelines on number of embryos transferred. Birmingham, Alabama, November 1999

Anderson RL, Golbus MS, Curry CJ, Callen PW, Hastrup WH: Central nervous system damage and other anomalies in surviving fetus following second trimester antenatal death of co-twin. Prenat Diagn 10:513, 1990

Andrews WW, Leveno KJ, Sherman ML, Mutz J, Gilstrap LC III, Whalley PJ: Elective hospitalization in the management of twin pregnancies. Obstet Gynecol 77:826, 1991

Arabin B, Aardenburg R, van Eyck J: Maternal position and ultrasonic cervical assessment in multiple pregnancy. Preliminary observations. J Reprod Med 42:719, 1997

Arbuckle TE, Wilkins R, Sherman GJ: Birthweight percentiles by gestational age in Canada. Obstet Gynecol 81:39, 1993

Ashworth MF, Spooner SF, Verkuyl DA, Waterman R, Ashurst HM: Failure to prevent preterm labour and delivery in twin pregnancy using prophylactic oral salbutamol. Br J Obstet Gynaecol 97:878, 1990

Azubuike JC: Multiple births in Igbo women. Br J Obstet Gynaecol 89:77, 1982

Azuma C, Kamiura S, Nobunaga T, Negoro T, Saji F, Tanizawa O: Zygosity determination of multiple pregnancy by deoxyribonucleic acid finger prints. Am J Obstet Gynecol 160:734, 1989

Babson SG, Phillips DS: Growth and development of twins dissimilar in size at birth. N Engl J Med 289:937, 1973

Baigts F, Dunica S, Fumeron F, Apfelbaum M: Birthweight difference in monozygous twins followed by differences in development of body weight. Lancet 2:274, 1982

Bailey-Pridham DD, Reshef E, Drury K, Cook CL, Hurst HE, Yussman MA: Follicular fluid lidocaine levels during transvaginal oocyte retrieval. Fertil Steril 53:171, 1990

Bajoria R: Chorionic plate vascular anatomy determines the efficacy of amnioreduction therapy for twin-twin transfusion syndrome. Hum Reprod 13:1709, 1998

Bajoria R, Wee LY, Anwar S, Ward S: Outcome of twin pregnancies complicated by single intrauterine death in relation to vascular anatomy of the monochorionic placenta. Hum Reprod 14:2124, 1999

Bajoria R, Wigglesworth J, Fisk NM: Angioarchitecture of monochorionic placentas in relation to the twin-twin transfusion syndrome. Am J Obstet Gynecol 172:856, 1995

Baldwin VJ: Pathology of multiple pregnancy. In Wigglesworth JS, Singer J (eds): Textbook of Fetal and Perinatal Pathology. Boston, Blackwell, 1991, p 238

Barton JR, O'Brien JM, Jacques DL, Bergauer NK, Stanziano GJ, Sibai BM: Perinatal outcome in quadruplet gestations. Am J Obstet Gynecol 174:478, 1996

Bebbington MW, Wittmann BK: Fetal transfusion syndrome: Antenatal factors predicting outcome. Am J Obstet Gynecol 160:913, 1989

Bejar R, Vigliocco G, Gramajo H, Solana C, Benirschke K, Berry C, Coen R, Resnik R: Antenatal origin of neurological damage in newborn infants, 2. Multiple gestations. Am J Obstet Gynecol 162:1230, 1990

Belfort MA, Moise KJ, Kirshon B, Saade G: The use of color flow Doppler ultrasonography to diagnose umbilical cord entanglement in monoamniotic twin gestations. Am J Obstet Gynecol 168:601, 1993

Bendon RW: Twin transfusion: Pathological studies of the monochorionic placenta in liveborn twins and of the perinatal autopsy in monochorionic twin pairs. Pediatric Pathology & Laboratory Medicine 15:363, 1995

Benirschke K: Intrauterine death of a twin: Mechanisms, implications for surviving twin, and placental pathology. Semin Diagn Pathol 10:222, 1993

Benirschke K: Chimerism and mosaicism. Two different entities. In Wynn RM (ed): Obstetrics and Gynecology Annual. New York, Appleton, 1974, p 33

Benirschke K, Kim CK: Multiple pregnancy. N Engl J Med 288:1276, 1973

Bennett D, Dunn LC: Genetical and embryological comparisons of semilethal t-alleles from wild mouse populations. Genetics 61:411, 1969

Berkowitz RL, Lynch L, Chitkara U, Wilkins I, Mehalek KE, Alvarez M: Selective reduction of multifetal pregnancies in the first trimester. N Engl J Med 318:1043, 1988

Berkowitz RL, Lynch L, Stone J, Alvarez M: The current status of multifetal pregnancy reduction. Am J Obstet Gynecol 174:1265, 1996

Berkowitz RS, Goldstein DP: Management of molar pregnancy and gestational trophoblastic tumors. In Knapp RC, Berkowitz RS (eds): Gynecologic Oncology, 2nd ed. New York, McGraw-Hill, 1992, p 328

Berry SM, Puder KS, Bottoms SF, Uckele JE, Romero R, Cotton DB: Comparison of intrauterine hematologic and biochemcial values between twin pairs with and without stuck twin syndrome. Am J Obstet Gynecol 172:1403, 1995

Blickstein I, Goldman RD, Kupferminc M: Delivery of breech first twins: A multicenter retrospective study. Obstet Gynecol 95:37, 2000

Blickstein I, Schwartz-Shoham Z, Lancet M, Borenstein R: Vaginal delivery of the second twin in breech presentation. Obstet Gynecol 68:774, 1987

Blunt SM, Butt WR: Pulsatile GnRH therapy for the induction of ovulation in hypogonadotropic hypogonadism. Acta Endocrinol (Copenh) 288:58, 1988

Boklage CE: Survival probability of human conceptions from fertilization to term. Int J Fertil 35:75, 1990

Bouchard C, Trembley A, Despres JP, Nadeau A, Lupien PJ, Teriault G, Dussault J, Moorjani S, Pinalt S, Fournier G: The response to long-term over feeding in identical twins. N Engl J Med 322:1477, 1990

Bower, SJ, Flack NJ, Sepulveda W, Talbert DG, Fisk NM: Uterine artery blood flow response to correction of amniotic fluid volume. Am J Obstet Gynecol 173:502, 1995

Bradshaw KD, Marshburn PB, Cunningham FG: Assisted reproductive technology. Williams Obstetrics, 18th ed (Suppl 17). Norwalk, CT, Appleton & Lange, April/May 1992

Brambati B, Tului-Baldi M, Guercilena S: Genetic analysis prior to selective fetal reduction in multiple pregnancy: Technical aspects and clinical outcome. Hum Reprod 10:818, 1995

Branisteanu-Dumitrascu I, Deprest JA, Evrard VA, Van Ballaer PP, Van Schoubroeck D, Gratacos E, Pijnenborg R: Time-related cotyledonary effects of laser coagulation of superficial chorionic vessels in an ovine model. Prenatal Diagnosis 19:205, 1999

Bressers WM, Eriksson AW, Kostense PJ, Parisi P: Increasing trend in the monozygotic twinning rate. Acta Genet Med Gemellol (Roma) 36:397, 1987

Bristow RE, Shumway JB, Khouzami AN, Witter FR: Complete hydatidiform mole and surviving coexistent twin. Obstet Gynecol Surv 51:705, 1996

Brown JE, Carlson M: Nutrition and multifetal pregnancy. J Am Diet Assoc 100:343, 2000

Bruner J, Anderson T: Management of the twin oligohydramnios–polyhydramnios sequence and twin-to-twin transfusion. Am J Obstet Gynecol 174:379, 1996

Bruner JP, Rosemond RL: Twin-to-twin transfusion syndrome: A subset of the twin oligohydramnios–polyhydramnios sequence. Am J Obstet Gynecol 169:925, 1993

Buekens P, Wilcox A: Why do small twins have a lower mortality rate than small singletons? Am J Obstet Gynecol 168:937, 1993

Bulmer MG: The effect of parental age, parity, and duration of marriage on the twinning rate. Hum Genet 23:454, 1959

Cameron AH, Edwards JH, Derom R, Theiry M, Boelaert R: The value of twin surveys in the study of malformation. Eur J Obstet Gynecol Reprod Biol 14:347, 1983

Campbell DM: Maternal adaptation in twin pregnancy. Semin Perinatol 10:14, 1986

Carr SR, Aronson MP, Coustan DR: Survival rates of monoamnionic twins do not decrease after 30 weeks gestation. Am J Obstet Gynecol 163:719, 1990

Casele H, Daley S, Metzger B: Metabolic response to meal eating and extended overnight fasting in twin gestation. Am J Obstet Gynecol 174:375, 1996

Challis D, Gratacos E, Deprest JA: Cord occlusion techniques for selective termination in monochorionic twins. J Perinat Med 27:327, 1999

Chauhan SP, Roberts WE, McLaren RA, Roach H, Morrison JC, Martin JN: Delivery of the nonvertex second twin: Breech extraction versus external cephalic version. Am J Obstet Gynecol 173:1015, 1995

Chervanak FA, Johnson RE, Berkowitz RL, Hobbins JC: Intrapartum external version of the second twin. Obstet Gynecol 62:160, 1983

Chervanak FA, Johnson RE, Youcha S, Hobbins JC, Berkowitz RL: Intrapartum management of twin gestation. Obstet Gynecol 65:119, 1985

Cohen M, Kohl SG, Rosenthal AH: Fetal interlocking complicating twin gestation. Am J Obstet Gynecol 91:407, 1965

Conde-Agudelo A, Belizán JM, Lindmark G: Maternal morbidity and mortality associated with multiple gestations. Obstet Gynecol 95:899, 2000

Consensus Development Conference on the Effect of Corticosteroids for Fetal Maturation on Perinatal Outcomes, February 28–March 2, 1994 Report. Bethesda, US Department of Health and Human Services, Public Health Service and National Institutes of Child Health and Human Development. NIH Publ. No. 95-3784, November 1994

Coonrad DV, Hickok DE, Zhu K, Easterling TR, Daling JR: Risk factors for preeclampsia in twin pregnancies: A population-based cohort study. Obstet Gynecol 85:645, 1995

Crawford JS: A prospective study of 200 consecutive twin deliveries. Anaesthesia 42:33, 1987

Crowther CA, Neilson JP, Ashurst HM, Verkuyl DA, Bannerman C: The effects of hospitalization for rest on fetal growth, neonatal morbidity and length of gestation in twin pregnancy. Br J Obstet Gynaecol 97:872, 1990

Czeizel AE, Metneki J, Dudas I: The higher rate of multiple births after periconceptional multivitamin supplementation: An analysis of causes. Acta Genet Med Gemellol (Roma) 43:175, 1994

Danskin FH, Neilson JP: Twin-to-twin transfusion syndrome: What are appropriate diagnostic criteria? Am J Obstet Gynecol 161:365, 1989

Davidson L, Easterling TR, Jackson JC, Benedetti TJ: Breech extraction of low-birth-weight second twins. Am J Obstet Gynecol 166:497, 1992

De Lia JE, Cruikshank DP, Keye WR: Fetoscopic neodymium: Yag laser occlusion of placental vessels in severe twin-twin transfusion syndrome. Obstet Gynecol 75:1046, 1990

De Lia JE, Kuhlmann RS, Lopez KP: Treating previable twin-twin transfusion syndrome with fetoscopic laser surgery: Outcomes following the learning curve. J Perinat Med 27:61, 1999

Denbow ML, Battin MR, Cowan F, Azzopardi D, Edwards AD, Fisk NM: Neonatal cranial ultrasonographic findings in preterm twins complicated by severe fetofetal transfusion. Am J Obstet Gynecol 178:479, 1998

Denbow ML, Cox P, Taylor M, Hammal DM, Fisk NM: Placental angioarchitecture in monochorionic twin pregnancies: Relationship to fetal growth, fetofetal transfusion syndrome, and pregnancy outcome. Am J Obstet Gynecol 182:417, 2000

Derom C, Derom R, Vlietinck R, Van den Berghe H, Thiery M: Increased monozygotic twinning rate after ovulation induction. Lancet 1:1237, 1987

Devoe LD, Ware DJ: Antenatal assessment of twin gestation. Semin Perinatol 19:413, 1995

Dickey RP, Olar TT, Taylor SN, Curole DN, Rye PH: Relationship of follicle number and other factors to fecundability and multiple pregnancy in clomiphene citrate–induced intrauterine insemination cycles. Fert Steril 57:613, 1992

Divon MY, Marin MJ, Pollack RN, Katz NT, Henderson C, Aboulafia Y, Merkatz IR: Twin gestation: Fetal presentation as a function of gestational age. Am J Obstet Gynecol 168:1500, 1993

DiVou MY, Girz BA, Sklar A, Guidetti DA, Langer O: Discordant twins—a prospective study of the diagnostic value of real time ultrasonography combined with umbilical artery velocimetry. Am J Obstet Gynecol 161:757, 1989

Donner C, Shahabi S, Thomas D, Noel JC, Kirkpatrick C, Rysselberghe MV, Hubinon C, Vermeylen D, Masters L, Rodesch F: Selective feticide by embolization in twin-twin transfusion syndrome. A report of two cases. J Reprod Med 42:747, 1997

Eberle AM, Levesque D, Vintzileos AM, Egan JFX, Tsapanos V, Salafia CM: Placental pathology in discordant twins. Am J Obstet Gynecol 169:931, 1993

Elimian A, Figueroa R, Nigam S, Verma U, Tejani N, Kirshenbaum N: Perinatal outcome of triplet gestation: Does prophylactic cerclage make a difference? J Matern Fetal Med 8:119, 1999

Elliott JP, Finberg HJ: Biophysical profile testing as an indicator of fetal well-being in high-order multiple gestations. Am J Obstet Gynecol 172:508, 1995

Evans MI, Dommergues M, Wapner RJ, Goldberg JD, Lynch L, Zador IE, et al: International collaborative experience in 1798 patients having multifetal pregnancy reduction: A plateauing of risks and outcomes. J Soc Gynecol Invest 3:23, 1996

Evans MI, Fletcher JC, Zador IE, Newton BW, Quigg MH, Struyk CD: Selective first-trimester termination in octuplet and quadruplet pregnancies: Clinical and ethical issues. Obstet Gynecol 71:289, 1988

Evans MI, Goldberg JD, Horenstein J, Wapner RJ, Ayoub MA, Stone J, et al: Selective termination for structural, chromosomal, and mendelian anomalies: International experience. Am J Obstet Gynecol 181:893, 1999

Ezra Y, Jones J, Farine D: Umbilical artery waveforms in triplet and quadruplet pregnancies. Gynecol Obstet Invest 47:239, 1999

Finberg HJ: The "twin peak" sign: Reliable evidence of dichorionic twinning. J Ultrasound Med 11:571, 1992

Fishman DA, Padilla LA, Keh P, Cohen L, Frederiksen M, Lurain JR: Management of twin pregnancies consisting of a complete hydatidiform mole and normal fetus. Obstet Gynecol 91:546, 1998

Fisk NM, Bryan E: Routine prenatal determination of chorionicity in multiple gestations: A plea to the obstetrician. Br J Obstet Gynaecol 100:975, 1993

Fox H: Pathology of the Placenta. London, Saunders, 1978, p 77

Friedman SA, Schiff E, Kao L, Kuint J, Sibai BM: Do twins mature earlier than singletons? Results from a matched cohort study. Am J Obstet Gynecol 176:1193, 1997

Fries MH, Goldstein RB, Kilpatrick SJ, Golbus MS, Callen PW, Filly RA: The role of velamentous cord insertion in the etiology of twin-twin transfusion syndrome. Obstet Gynecol 81:569, 1993

Fujikura T, Froelich LA: Mental and motor development in monozygotic co-twins with dissimilar birth weights. Pediatrics 53:884, 1974

Fusi L, Gordon H: Twin pregnancy complicated by single intrauterine death. Problems and outcome with conservative management. Br J Obstet Gynaecol 97:511, 1990

Fusi L, McParland P, Fisk N, Nicolini U, Wigglesworth J: Acute twin-twin transfusion: A possible mechanism for brain-damaged survivors after intrauterine death of a monochorionic twin. Obstet Gynecol 78:517, 1991

Gabriel R, Harika G, Saniez D, Durot S, Quereux C, Wahl P: Prolonged intravenous ritodrine therapy: A comparison between multiple and singleton pregnancies. Eur J Obstet Gynecol Reprod Biol 57:65, 1994

Galea P, Scott JM, Goel KM: Feto-fetal transfusion syndrome. Arch Dis Child 57:781, 1982

Gallagher MW, Costigan K, Johnson TRB: Fetal heart rate accelerations, fetal movement, and fetal behavior patterns in twin gestations. Am J Obstet Gynecol 167:1140, 1992

Gardner MO, Goldenberg RL, Cliver SP, Tucker JM, Nelson KJ, Copper RL: The origin and outcome of preterm twin pregnancies. Obstet Gynecol 85:553, 1995

Garite TJ, Bentley DL, Hamer CA, Porto ML: Uterine activity characteristics in multiple gestations. Obstet Gynecol 76:56S, 1990

Garry D, Lysikiewicz A, Mays J, Tejani N: Intra-amnionic pressure reduction in twin-to-twin transfusion syndrome. Am J Obstet Gynecol 174:311, 1996

Gerson AG, Wallace DM, Bridgens NK, Ashmead GG, Weiner S, Bolognese RJ: Duplex Doppler ultrasound in the evaluation of growth in twin pregnancies. Obstet Gynecol 70:419, 1987

Gilbert WM, Davis SE, Kaplan C, Pretorius D, Merritt TA, Benirschke K: Morbidity associated with prenatal disruption of the dividing membrane in twin gestations. Obstet Gynecol 78:623, 1991

Gleicher N, Campbell DP, Chan CL, Karande V, Rao R, Balin M, Pratt D: The desire for multiple births in couples with infertility problems contradicts present practice patterns. Hum Reprod 10:1079, 1995

Gleicher N, Oleske DM, Tur-Kaspa I, Vidali A, Karande V: Reducing the risk of high-order multiple pregnancy after ovarian stimulation with gonadotropins. N Engl J Med 343:2, 2000

Gocke SE, Nageotte MP, Garite T, Towers CV, Dorcester W: Management of the non-vertex second twin: Primary cesarean section, external version, or primary breech extraction. Am J Obstet Gynecol 161:111, 1989

Goldenberg RL, Iams JD, Miodovnik M, Van Dorsten JP, Thurnau G, Bottoms S, et al, and the National Institute of

Child Health and Human Development Maternal–Fetal Medicine Units Network: The preterm prediction study: Risk factors in twin gestations. Am J Obstet Gynecol 175:1047–53, 1996

Goldfarb JM, Austin C, Lisbona H, Peskin B, Clapp M: Cost-effectiveness of in vitro fertilization. Obstet Gynecol 87: 18, 1996

Gonsoulin W, Moise KJ, Kirshon B, Cotton DB, Wheeler JM, Carpenter RJ: Outcome of twin–twin transfusion diagnosed before 28 weeks of gestation. Obstet Gynecol 75: 214, 1990

Hardardottir H, Kelly K, Bork MD, Cusick W, Campbell WA, Rodis JF: Atypical presentation of preeclampsia in high-order multifetal gestations. Obstet Gynecol 87:370, 1996

Harris DW: Letter to the editors. J Reprod Med 27:39, 1982

Hashimoto B, Callen PW, Filly RA, Laros RK: Ultrasound evaluation of polyhydramnios and twin pregnancy. Am J Obstet Gynecol 154:1069, 1986

Hecher K, Jauniaux E, Campbell S, Deane C, Nicolaides K: Artery-to-artery anastomosis in monochorionic twins. Am J Obstet Gynecol 171:570, 1994

Hecher K, Plath H, Bregenzer R, Hansmann M, Hackeloer BJ: Endoscopic laser surgery versus serial amniocenteses in the treatment of severe twin-twin transfusion syndrome. Am J Obstet Gynecol 180:717, 1999

Hill LM, Guzick D, Chenevey P, Boyles D, Nedzesky P: The sonographic assessment of twin discordancy. Obstet Gynecol 84:501, 1994

Hollier LM, McIntire DD, Leveno KJ: Outcome of twin pregnancies according to intrapair birth weight differences. Obstet Gynecol 94:1006, 1999

Homburg R, Eshel A, Armar NA, Tucker M, Mason PW, Adams J, Kilborn J, Sutherland IA, Jacobs HS: One hundred pregnancies after treatment with pulsatile luteinizing hormone releasing hormone to induce ovulation. Br Med J 298:809, 1989

Hsieh YY, Chang CC, Tsai HD, Yang TC, Lee CC, Tsai CH: Twin vs. singleton pregnancy. Clinical characteristics and latency periods in preterm premature rupture of membranes. J Reprod Med 44:616, 1999

Imseis HM, Albert TA, Iams JD: Identifying twin gestations at low risk for preterm birth with a transvaginal ultrasonographic cervical measurement at 24 to 26 weeks' gestation. Am J Obstet Gynecol 177:1149, 1997

Jauniaux E, Elkazen N, Leroy F, Wilkin P, Rodesch F, Hustin J: Clinical and morphologic aspects of the vanishing twin phenomenon. Obstet Gynecol 72:577, 1988

Jewell SE, Yip R: Increasing trends in plural births in the United States. Obstet Gynecol 85:229, 1995

Jones KL: Smith's Recognizable Patterns of Human Malformation, 5th ed. Philadelphia, Saunders, 1997, p 658

Kaufman GE, Malone FD, Harvey-Wilkes KB, Chelmow D, Penzias AS, D'Alton ME: Neonatal morbidity and mortality associated with triplet pregnancy. Obstet Gynecol 91:342, 1998

Kiely JL: The epidemiology of perinatal mortality in multiple births. Bull NY Acad Med 66:618, 1990

Kilpatrick SJ, Jackson R, Croughan-Minihane MS: Perinatal mortality in twins and singletons matched for gestational age at delivery at 30 weeks. Am J Obstet Gynecol 174: 66, 1996

Klein NA, Battaglia DE, Clifton DK, Bremner WJ, Soules MR: The gonadotropin secretion pattern in normal women of advanced reproductive age in relation to the monotropic FHS rise. J Soc Gynecol Invest 3:27, 1996

Knox G, Morley D: Twinning in Yoruba women. J Obstet Gynaecol Br Emp 67:981, 1960

Koffel B: Abnormal presentation and multiple gestation. In Chestnut DH (ed). Obstetrical Anesthesia, Mosby, St Louis, Missouri, 2nd ed. 1999, p 694

Kogan MD, Alexander GR, Kotelchuck M, MacDorman MF, Buekens P, Martin JA, Papiernik E: Trends in twin birth outcomes and prenatal care utilization in the United States, 1981–1997. JAMA 283:335, 2000

Kohl SG, Casey G: Twin gestation. Mt Sinai J Med 42:523, 1975

Kol S, Levron J, Lewit N, Drugan A, Itskovitz-Eldor J: The natural history of multiple pregnancies after assisted reproduction: Is spontaneous fetal demise a clinically significant phenomenon. Fertil Steril 60:127, 1993

Kurzel RB, Claridad L, Lampley EC: Cesarean section for the second twin. J Reprod Med 42:767, 1997

Landy HJ, Weiner S, Corson SL, Batzer FR, Bolognese RJ: The "vanishing twin" Ultrasonographic assessment of fetal disappearance in the first trimester. Am J Obstet Gynecol 150:14, 1986

Langer B, Boudier E, Gasser B, Christmann D, Messer J, Schlaeder G: Antenatal diagnosis of brain damage in the survivor after the second trimester death of a monochorionic monoamniotic co-twin: Case report and literature review. Fetal Diagn Ther 12:286, 1997

Larroche JC, Droulle P, Delezoide AL, Narcy F, Nessmann C: Brain damage in monozygous twins. Biol Neonate 57:261, 1990

LeFevre ML, Bain RP, Ewigman BG, Frigoletto FD, Crane JP, McNellis D: A randomized trial of prenatal ultrasonographic screening: Impact on maternal management and outcome. RADIUS (Routine Antenatal Diagnostic Imaging with Ultrasound) study group. Am J Obstet Gynecol 169:483, 1993

Levav AL, Chan L, Wapner RJ: Long-term magnesium sulfate tocolysis and maternal osteoporosis in a triplet pregnancy: A case report. Am J Perinatology 15:43, 1998

Leveno KJ, Quirk JG, Whalley PJ, Herbert WNP, Trubey R: Fetal lung maturation in twin gestation. Am J Obstet Gynecol 148:405, 1984

Leveno KJ, Santos-Ramos R, Duenhoelter JH, Reisch JS, Whalley PJ: Sonar cephalometry in twins: A table of biparietal diameters for normal twin fetuses and a comparison with singletons. Am J Obstet Gynecol 135:727, 1979

Lipitz S, Uval J, Achiron R, Schiff E, Lusky A, Reichman B: Outcome of twin pregnancies reduced from triplets compared with nonreduced twin gestations. Obstet Gynecol 87:511, 1996

Livingston JE, Poland BJ: A study of spontaneously aborted twins. Teratology 21:139, 1980

Luke B: The changing patterns of multiple births in the United States: Maternal and infant characteristics, 1973 and 1990. Obstet Gynecol 84:101, 1994

Luke B, Minogue J, Witter FR, Keith LG, Johnson TRB: The ideal twin pregnancy: Patterns of weight gain, discordancy, and length of gestation. Am J Obstet Gynecol 169:588, 1993

Lundvall L, Skibsted L, Graem N: Limb necrosis associated with twin-twin transfusion syndrome treated with YAG-laser coagulation. Acta Obstet Gynecol Scand 78:349, 1999

Lynch L, Berkowitz RL: Maternal serum alpha-fetoprotein and coagulation profiles after multifetal pregnancy reduction. Am J Obstet Gynecol 169:987, 1993

Lynch L, Berkowitz RL, Stone J, Alvarez M, Lapinski R: Preterm delivery after selective termination in twin pregnancies. Obstet Gynecol 87336, 1996

MacGillivray I: Epidemiology of twin pregnancy. Semin Perinatol 10:4, 1986

Machin GA: Some causes of genotypic and phenotypic discordance in monozygotic twin pairs. Am J Med Genet 61:216, 1996

Magann EF, Chauhan SP, Martin JN, Whitworth NS, Morrison JC: Ultrasound assessment of the amniotic fluid volume in diamniotic twins. J Soc Gynecol Invest 2:609, 1995a

Magann EF, Whitworth NS, Bass JD, Chauhan SP, Martin JN, Morrison JC: Amniotic fluid volumes of third-trimester diamniotic twin pregnancies. Obstet Gynecol 85:957, 1995b

Mahone PR, Sherer DM, Abramowicz JS, Woods JR: Twin-twin transfusion syndrome: Rapid development of severe hydrops of the donor following selective feticide of the hydropic recipient. Am J Obstet Gynecol 169:166, 1993

Mahony BS, Filly RA, Callen PW: Amnionicity and chorionicity in twin pregnancies. Radiology 155:205, 1985

Mahony BS, Petty CN, Nyberg DA, Luthy DA, Hickok DE, Hirsch JH: The stuck twin phenomenon: Ultrasonographic findings, pregnancy outcome, and management with serial amniocentesis. Am J Obstet Gynecol 163:1513, 1990

Manning FA: Fetal biophysical profile scoring. In: Fetal Medicine: Principles and Practices. Norwalk, CT, Appleton & Lange, 1995, p 288

Mari G, Abuhamad A, Verpairojkit B, Jones D, Gomez K, Bohado-Singh R, Soper R, Copel JA: Treatment of twin-to-twin transfusion syndrome: Is the therapeutic amniocentesis still a good management option? Am J Obstet Gynecol 174:487, 1996

Mari G, Kirshon B, Abuhamad A: Fetal renal artery flow velocity waveforms in normal pregnancies and pregnancies complicated by polyhydramnios and oligohydramnios. Obstet Gynecol 81:560, 1993

Martin JA, Park MM: Trends in twin and triplet births; 1980–97. National Vital Statistics Reports; Vol 47, No. 24. Hyattsville, MD, National Center for Health Statistics, 1999

Mastrobattista JM, Skupski DW, Monga M, Blanco JD, August P: The rate of severe preeclampsia is increased in triplet as compared to twin gestations. Am J Perinatol 14:263, 1997

Mauldin JG, Newman RB, Mauldin PD: Cost-effective delivery management of the vertex and nonvertex twin gestation. Am J Obstet Gynecol 179:864, 1998

Meldrum DR, Gardner DK: Two-embryo transfer—the future looks bright (editorial). N Eng J Med 339:624, 1998

Mercer B, Crocker LG, Pierce WF, Sibai BM: Clinical characteristics and outcome of twin gestation complicated by preterm premature rupture of the membranes. Am J Obstet Gynecol 168:467, 1993

Meulemans WJ, Lewis CM, Boomsma DI, Derom CA, Van den Berghe H, Orlebeke JF, Vlietinck RF, Derom RM: Genetic modelling of dizygotic twinning in pedigrees of spontaneous dizygotic twins. Am J Med Genet 61:258, 1996

Minakami H, Sato I: Reestimated date of delivery in multifetal pregnancies. JAMA 275:1996

Moore TR, Gale S, Bernirschke K: Perinatal outcome of forty-nine pregnancies complicated by acardiac twinning. Am Obstet Gynecol 163:907, 1990

Mordel N, Benshushan A, Zajicek G, Laufer N, Schenker JC, Sadovsky E: Discordancy in triplets. Am J Perinatol 10:224, 1993

Myrianthopoulos NC: An epidemiologic survey of twins in a large prospectively studied population. Am J Hum Genet 22:611, 1970

Nilsen ST, Bergsjo P, Nome S: Male twins at birth and 18 years later. Br J Obstet Gynaecol 91:122, 1984

Norwitz ER, Hoyte LPJ, Jenkins KJ, Van Der Velde ME, Ratiu P, Rodriguez-Thompson D, Wilkins-Haug L, Tempany CMC, Fishman SJ: Separation of conjoined twins with the twin reversed-arterial-perfusion sequence after prenatal planning with three-dimensional modeling. N Engl J Med 343:399, 2000

Nylander PPS: Serum levels of gonadotropins in relation to multiple pregnancy in Nigeria. Br J Obstet Gynaecol 80:651, 1973

Nylander PPS: Biosocial aspects of multiple births. J Biosoc Sci 3:29, 1971

Okamura K, Murotsuki J, Tanigawara S, Uehara S, Yajima A: Funipuncture for evaluation indices in the surviving twin following co-twin's death. Obstet Gynecol 83:975, 1994

Parisi P, Gatti M, Prinzi G, Caperna G: Familial incidence of twinning. Nature 304:626, 1983

Pasqualotto EB, Falcone T, Goldberg JM, Petrauskis C, Nelson DR, Agarwal A: Risk factors for multiple gestation in women undergoing intrauterine insemination with ovarian stimulation. Fertil Steril 72:613, 1999

Pettersson F, Smedby B, Lindmark G: Outcome of twin birth: Review of 1636 children born in twin birth. Acta Paediatr Scand 64:473, 1976

Pharoah PO, Adi Y: Consequences of in-utero death in twin pregnancy. Lancet 355:1597, 2000

Pinette MG, Pan Y, Pinette SG, Stubblefield PG: Treatment of twin-twin transfusion syndrome. Obstet Gynecol 82:841, 1993

Pons JC, Charlemaine C, Dubreuil E, Papiernik E, Frydman R: Management and outcome of triplet pregnancy. Eur J Obstet Gynecol Reprod Biol 76:131, 1998

Porter TF, Dildy GA, Blanchard JR, Kochenour NK, Clark SL: Normal values for amnionic fluid index during uncomplicated twin pregnancy. Obstet Gynecol 87:699, 1996

Powers WF, Kiely JL: The risks confronting twins: A national perspective. Am J Obstet Gynecol 170:456, 1994

Pritchard JA: Changes in blood volume during pregnancy. Anesthesiology 26:393, 1965

Quigley MM, Cruikshank DP: Polyhydramnios and acute renal failure. J Reprod Med 19:92, 1977

Quintero RA, Goncalves L, Johnson MP, Reich H, Romero R, Carreno C, Evans MI: Percutaneous umbilical-cord ligation in complicated monochorionic multiple gestations. Am J Obstet Gynecol 174:326, 1996

Quintero RA, Reich H, Puder KS, Bardicef M, Evans MI, Cotton DB, Romero R: Brief report: Umbilical-cord ligation in an acardiac twin by fetoscopy at 19 weeks gestation. N Engl J Med 330:469, 1994

Rayburn WF, Lavin JP Jr, Miodovnik M, Varner MW: Multiple gestation: Time interval between delivery of the first and second twins. Obstet Gynecol 63:502, 1984

Reddy KS, Petersen MB, Antonarakis SE, Blakemore KJ: The vanishing twin: An explanation for discordance between chorionic villus karyotype and fetal phenotype. Prenat Diagn 11:679, 1991

Rein MS, Barbieri RL, Greene MF: The causes of high-order multiple gestation. Inter J Fert 35:154, 1990

Rizzo G, Arduini D, Romanini C: Cardiac and extracardiac flows in discordant twins. Am J Obstet Gynecol 170:1371, 1994

Robertson EG, Neer KJ: Placental injection studies in twin gestation. Am J Obstet Gynecol 147:170, 1983

Robie GF, Payne GG, Morgan MA: Selective delivery of an acardiac, acephalic twin. N Engl J Med 320:512, 1989

Rodis JF, Lawrence A, Egan JFX, Borgida AF, Leo MV, Campbell WA: Comprehensive fetal ultrasonographic growth measurements in triplet gestations. Am J Obstet Gynecol 181:1128, 1999

Rothman KJ: Fetal loss, twinning and birthweight after oral-contraceptive use. N Engl J Med 297:468, 1977

Rouse DJ, Skopec GS, Zlatnik FJ: Fundal height as a predictor of preterm twin delivery. Obstet Gynecol 81:211, 1993

Ryan G: Laser as alternative to amnioreduction. Presented at the Society for Obstetricians and Gynecologists of Canada. Ob Gyn News 35:1, 2000

Rydhström H: Pregnancy with stillbirth of both twins. Br J Obstet Gynaecol 103:25, 1996

Rydhström H: Discordant birthweight and late fetal death in like-sexed and unlike-sexed twin pairs: A population-based study. Br J Obstet Gynecol 101:765, 1994

Rydhström H: Prognosis for twins with birthweight < 1,500 g: The impact of cesarean section in relation to fetal presentation. Am J Obstet Gynecol 163:528, 1990

Saacks CB, Thorp JM, Hendricks CH: Cohort study of twinning in an academic health center: Changes in management and outcome over forty years. Am J Obstet Gynecol 172:432, 1995

Saito K, Ohtsu Y, Amano K, Nishijima M: Perinatal outcome and management of single fetal death in twin pregnancy: A case series and review. J Perinat Med 27:473, 1999

Santema JG, Koppelaar I, Wallenburg HC: Hypertensive disorders in twin pregnancy. Eur J Obstet Gynecol Reprod Biol 58:9, 1995a

Santema JG, Swaak AM, Wallenburg HCS: Expectant management of twin pregnancy with single fetal death. Br J Obstet Gynaecol 102:26, 1995b

Satin AJ, Fausett MB, Gordon MC, Barth WH: Oxytocin labor stimulation of twin gestations: Effective and efficient. Am J Obstet Gynecol 174:483, 1996

Saunders NJ, Snijders RJ, Nicolaides KH: Twin-twin transfusion syndrome during the 2nd trimester is associated with small intertwin hemoglobin differences. Fetal Diagn Ther 6:34, 1991

Scardo JA, Ellings JM, Newman RB: Prospective determination of chorionicity, amnionicity, and zygosity in twin gestations. Am J Obstet Gynecol 173:1376, 1995

Schenker JG, Yarkoni S, Granat M: Multiple pregnancies following induction of ovulation. Fertil Steril 35:105, 1981

Schiff E, Cohen SB, Dulitzky M, Novikov I, Friedman SA, Mashiach S, Lipitz S: Progression of labor in twins versus singleton gestations. Am J Obstet Gynecol 179:1181, 1998

Schinzel AA, Smith DW, Miller JR: Monozygotic twinning and structural defects. J Pediatr 95:951, 1979

Scholtes MCW, Zeilmaker GH: A prospective, randomized study of embryo transfer results after 3 or 5 days of embryo culture in vitro fertilization. Fertil Steril 65:1245, 1996

Schreiner-Engel P, Walther VN, Mindes J, Lynch L, Berkowitz RL: First-trimester multifetal pregnancy reduction: Acute and persistent psychologic reactions. Am J Obstet Gynecol 172:544, 1995

Sebire NJ, Snijders RJ, Hughes K, Sepulveda W, Nicolaides KH: The hidden mortality of monochorionic twin pregnancies. Br J Obstet Gynaecol 104:1203, 1997

Shah DM, Chaffin D: Perinatal outcome in very preterm births with twin–twin transfusion syndrome. Am J Obstet Gynecol 161:1111, 1989

Shoham Z, Zosmer A, Insler V: Early miscarriage and fetal malformations after induction of ovulation (by clomiphene citrate and/or human menotropins), in vitro fertilization, and gamete intrafallopian transfer. Fert Steril 55:1, 1991

Silva PA, Crosado B: The growth and development of twins compared with singletons at ages 9 and 11. Aust Paediatr J 21:265, 1985

Silva PA, McGee RO, Powell J: Growth and development of twins compared with singletons at ages five and seven: A follow-up report from the Dunedin Multidisciplinary Child Development Study. Aust Paediatr J 18:35, 1982

Simpson JL, Carson SA: Multifetal reduction in high-order gestations: A nonelective procedure? J Soc Gynecol Invest 3:1, 1996

Smith-Levitin M, Kowalik A, Birnholz J, Hutson M, Skupski D, Rosenwaks Z, Chervenak F: Comparison of birthweight of twin gestations resulting from embryo reduction of higher order gestations to birthweights of twin and triplet gestations using a novel way to correct for gestational age at delivery. Am J Obstet Gynecol 174:346, 1996

Sonntag J, Waltz S, Schollmeyer T, Schuppler U, Schroder H, Weisner D: Morbidity and mortality of discordant twins up to 34 weeks of gestational age. Eur J Pediatr 155:224, 1996

Souka AP, Heath V, Flint S, Sevastopoulou I, Nicolaides KH: Cervical length at 23 weeks in twins in predicting spontaneous preterm delivery. Obstet Gynecol 94:450, 1999

Stagiannis KD, Sepulveda W, Southwell D, Price DA, Fisk NM: Ultrasonic measurement of the dividing membrane in twin pregnancy during the second and third trimesters: A reproducibility study. Am J Obstet Gynecol 173:1546, 1995

Steller MA, Genest DR, Bernstein MR, Lage JM, Goldstein DP, Berkowitz RS: Natural history of twin pregnancy with complete hydatidiform mole and coexisting fetus. Obstet Gynecol 83:35, 1994

Stone CA, Quinn MW, Saxby PJ: Congenital skin loss following Nd:YAG placental photocoagulation. Burns 25:192, 1998

Strandskov HH, Edelen EW, Siemens GJ: Analysis of the sex ratios among single and plural births in the total white and colored U.S. populations. Am J Phys Anthropol 4:491, 1946

Stunkard AJ, Harris JR, Pedersen NL, McClearn GE: The body-mass index of twins who have been reared apart. N Engl J Med 322:1483, 1990

Talbert DG, Bajoria R, Sepulveda W, Bower S, Fisk N: Hydrostatic and osmotic pressure gradients produce manifestations of fetofetal transfusion syndrome in a computerized model of monochorial twin pregnancy. Am J Obstet Gynecol 174:598, 1996

Tan KL, Goon SM, Salmon Y, Wee JH: Conjoined twins. Acta Obstet Gynecol Scand 50:373, 1971

Templeton A, Morris JK: Reducing the risk of multiple births by transfer of two embryos after in vitro fertilization. N Eng J Med 339:573, 1998

Terasaki PI, Gjertson D, Bernoco D, Perdue S, Mickey MR, Bond J: Twins with two different fathers identified by HLA. N Engl J Med 299:590, 1978

Tessen JA, Zlatnick FJ: Monoamnionic twins: A retrospective controlled study. Obstet Gynecol 77:832, 1991

Trivedi AN, Gillett WR: The retained twin/triplet following a preterm delivery—an analysis of the literature. Aust NZ J Obstet Gynaecol 38:461, 1998

Tuppin P, Blondel B, Kaminski M: Trends in multiple deliveries and infertility treatments in France. Br J Obstet Gynaecol 100:383, 1993

Turrentine MA, Wilson PD, Wilkins IA: A retrospective analysis of the effect of antenatal steroid administration on the incidence of respiratory distress syndrome in preterm twin pregnancies. Am J Perinatol 13:351, 1996

Uchida IA, Freeman VCP, Gedeon M, Goldmaker J: Twinning rate in spontaneous abortions. Am J Hum Genet 35:987, 1983

Van Allen MI, Smith DW, Shepard TH: Twin reversed atrial perfusion (TRAP) sequence: A study of 14 twin pregnancies with acardius. Semin Perinatol 7:285, 1983

Van den Brand SF, Nijhuis JG, van Dongen PW: Prenatal ultrasound diagnosis of conjoined twins. Obstet Gynecol Surv 49:656, 1994

Veille JC, Morton MJ, Burry KJ: Maternal cardiovascular adaptations to twin pregnancy. Am J Obstet Gynecol 153:261, 1985

Ville Y, Hecher K, Gagnon A, Sebire N, Hyett J, Nicolaides K: Endoscopic laser coagulation in the management of severe twin-to-twin transfusion syndrome. Br J Obstet Gynaecol 105:446, 1998

Vinatier D, Defour P, Beard J: Utilization of intravenous nitroglycerin for obstetrical emergencies. Int J Gynecol Obstet 55:129, 1996

Wada H, Nunogami K, Wada T, Niida Y, Yachie A, Koizumi S: Diffuse brain damage caused by acute twin-twin transfusion during late pregnancy. Acta Paediatr Jpn 40:370, 1998

Waterhouse JAH: Twinning in twin pedigrees. Br J Soc Med 4:197, 1950

Weiner CP: Diagnosis and treatment of twin to twin transfusion in the mid-second trimester of pregnancy. Fetal Ther 2:71, 1987

Weiner CP, Ludomirski A: Diagnosis, pathophysiology, and treatment of chronic twin-to-twin transfusion syndrome. Fetal Diagn Ther 9:283, 1994

Weissman A, Achiron R, Lipitz S, Blickstein I, Mashiach S: The first-trimester growth-discordant twin: An ominous prenatal finding. Obstet Gynecol 84:110, 1994

Wenstrom KD, Syrop CH, Hammitt DG, VanVoorhis BJ: Increased risk of monochorionic twinning associated with assisted reproduction. Fertil Steril 60:510, 1993

Wenstrom KD, Tessen JA, Zlatnik FJ, Sipes SL: Frequency, distribution, and theoretical mechanisms of hematologic and weight discordance in monochorionic twins. Obstet Gynecol 80:257, 1992

White C, Wyshak G: Inheritance in human dizygotic twinning. N Engl J Med 271:1003, 1964

Winsor EJ, Brown BS, Luther ER, Heifetz SA, Welch JP: Deceased co-twin as a cause of false positive amniotic fluid AFP and AChE. Prenat Diagn 7:485, 1987

Wittmann BK, Farquharson DF, Thomas WD, Baldwin VJ, Wadsworth LD: The role of feticide in the management of severe twin transfusion syndrome. Am J Obstet Gynecol 155:1023, 1986

Yoshida K, Matayoshi K: A study of prognosis of surviving co-twin. Acta Genet Med Gemellol 39:383, 1990

Zikulnig L, Hecher K, Bregenzer T, Baz E, Hackeloer BJ: Prognostic factors in severe twin-twin transfusion syndrome treated by endoscopic laser surgery. Ultrasound Obstet Gynecol 14:380, 1999

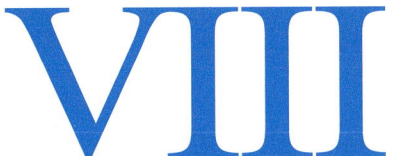

VIII

SECTION

Placental Disorders

31

Abnormalities of the Fetal Membranes and Amnionic Fluid

ABNORMALITIES OF THE CHORIOAMNION

Meconium Staining
Chorioamnionitis
Other Abnormalities

DISORDERS OF AMNIONIC FLUID VOLUME

Hydramnios
Oligohydramnios

Fetal membranes include the amnion and chorion. Their development, physiology, and histology are detailed in Chapter 5 (p. 86). A number of physiological and pathological events cause perceptible anatomical changes in the amnion, chorion, or both.

ABNORMALITIES OF THE CHORIOAMNION

MECONIUM STAINING. The presence of meconium is relatively common. In a summary of 17 series, Katz and Bowes (1992) reported that the incidence of meconium passage ranged from 7 to 22 percent. Wiswell and associates (1990) identified it in 12 percent of more than 175,000 live-born infants. Benirschke and Kaufmann (2000) identified visible meconium staining in 18 percent of nearly 13,000 consecutive placentas. It has been remarkably constant over the past 16 years at Parkland Hospital. Of almost 200,000 women delivered during this period, about 20 percent had amnionic fluid that contained some meconium identified during labor or at delivery.

Meconium passage is seldom seen in preterm fetuses, and it may be confused with pigments arising from fetal hemolysis. It is uncommon prior to 38 weeks, and it increases after 40 weeks (Table 31–1). Staining of the amnionic membranes is obvious within 1 to 3 hours after meconium passage (Miller and colleagues, 1985). Although more prolonged exposure results in staining of the chorion, umbilical cord, and decidua, according

to Benirschke and Kaufmann (2000), it cannot be dated accurately.

In a global sense, meconium passage is associated with increased perinatal morbidity and mortality. Fujikura and Klionsky (1975) identified meconium-stained membranes or fetuses in about 10 percent of 43,000 live-born infants in the Collaborative Study of Cerebral Palsy. The neonatal mortality rate was 3.3 percent in the group with meconium-stained membranes compared with 1.7 percent in those without such staining. Nathan and co-workers (1994) retrospectively compared perinatal outcomes in over 8000 women delivered at Parkland Hospital in whom meconium was identified intrapartum. The control group consisted of over 34,500 similar pregnancies with clear amnionic fluid. Perinatal mortality was increased significantly in the meconium group (1.5 versus 0.3 per 1000). Likewise, severe fetal acidemia—cord arterial pH less than 7.0—was significantly more common with meconium-stained births (7 versus 3 per 1000). Finally, cesarean delivery was doubled in the meconium group (14 versus 7 percent). These global findings are not applicable in individual cases. Despite this, according to Benirschke and Kaufmann (2000), meconium has assumed great importance in many medicolegal pursuits.

Neonatal mortality associated with meconium is primarily the result of aspiration of thick, tenacious meconium (Chap. 39, p. 1044). Houlihan and Knuppel (1994) and Cleary and Wiswell (1998) have reviewed this subject.

CHORIOAMNIONITIS. Inflammation of the fetal membranes is a manifestation of an intrauterine infection, and it is frequently associated with prolonged membrane rupture and long labors (Fox, 1978). When mononuclear and polymorphonuclear leukocytes infiltrate the chorion, the resulting microscopical finding is designated chorioamnionitis (Fig. 31–1). If they are found in amnionic fluid, it is termed *amnionitis.* Inflammation of the umbilical cord is *funisitis* and placental infection is manifest by *villitis* (Goldenberg and co-workers, 2000). According to some investigators, these findings may be nonspecific and are not always associated with other evidence for fetal or maternal infection. For example, Yamada and colleagues (2000) found that meconium-stained fluid is a chemoattractant for leukocytes. Conversely, Benirschke and Kaufmann (2000) believe that microscopic chorioamnionitis is always due to infection. Before 20 weeks, almost all polymorphonuclear leukocytes are maternal in origin, but later the inflammatory response is primarily fetal (Sampson and colleagues, 1997).

Management of clinical chorioamnionitis is antimicrobial administration and expedient delivery (Chap. 27, p. 707). Occult chorioamnionitis, caused by a wide

TABLE 31–1. Meconium Passage as a Function of Gestational Age

Study	Meconium Passage (%)
Eden et al (1987)	
39 weeks	14
40 weeks	19
42 weeks	26
> 42 weeks	29
Usher et al (1988)	
39–40 weeks	15
41 weeks	27
42 weeks or greater	32
Steer et al (1989)	
< 36 weeks	3
36–39 weeks	13
40–41 weeks	19
42 weeks or greater	23

From Katz and Bowes (1992), with permission.

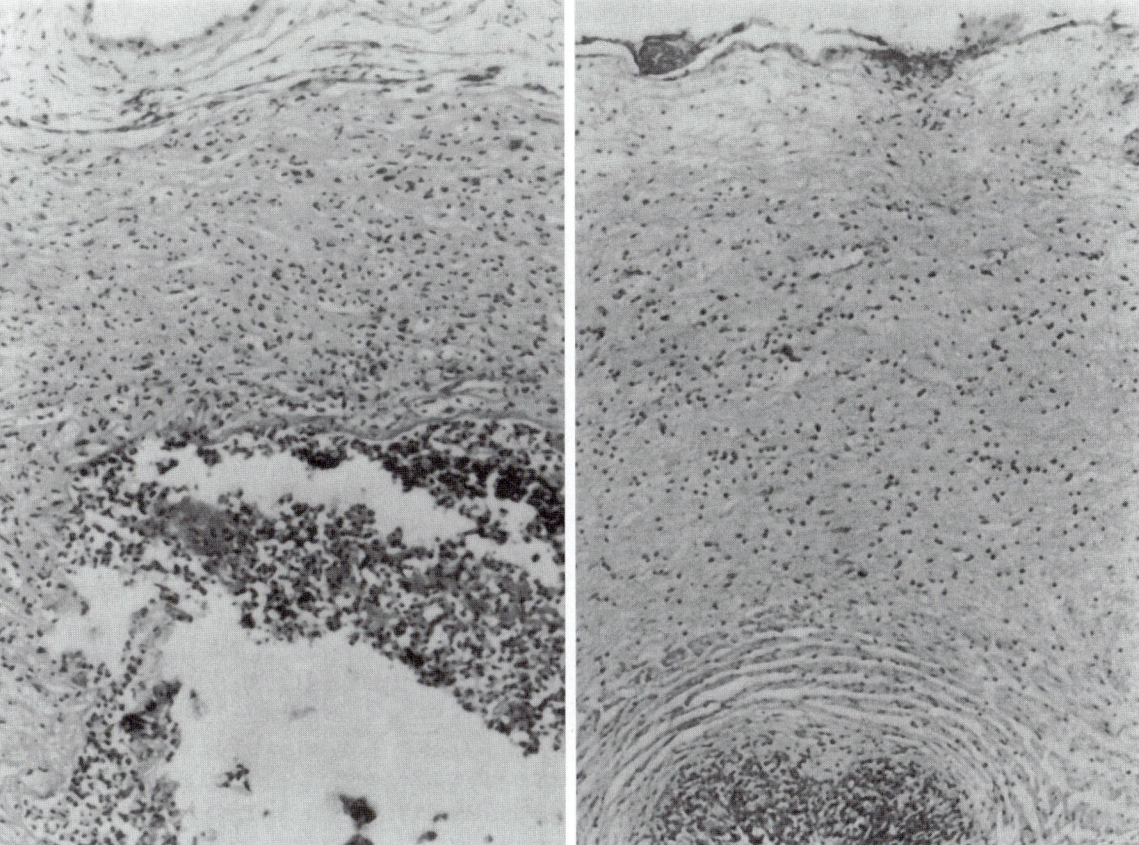

FIGURE 31–1. Placental surface from a woman delivered at 30 weeks. The membranes had been ruptured for 40 hours and the 1200-g neonate had congenital pneumonia. Note exudation of leukocytes from the intervillous space on the left. Minimal vascular necrosis along with amnion necrosis is seen on the right. (From Benirschke and Kaufmann, 2000, with permission.)

variety of microorganisms, has recently emerged as a possible explanation for many heretofore unexplained cases of ruptured membranes, preterm labor, or both (Chaps. 11, p. 282 and 27, p. 696).

OTHER ABNORMALITIES. Small **amnionic cysts** lined by typical amnionic epithelium are occasionally formed. The common variety results from fusion of amnionic folds, with subsequent retention of fluid.

Amnion nodosum are nodules in the amnion that are sometimes called squamous amnionic metaplasia or amnionic caruncles. They are most commonly seen in the amnion in contact with the chorionic plate, but they may also be found elsewhere. They usually appear near the insertion of the cord as shiny grayish-yellow opaque elevations that are multiple, rounded, or oval, and they vary from 1 mm to 5 mm in diameter. The nodules are made up of fetal ectodermal debris, including vernix caseosa with hair, squames, and sebum. They are associated with oligohydramnios and are most commonly found in fetuses with renal agenesis or prolonged prema-

turely ruptured membranes or in the placenta of the donor fetus with twin–twin transfusion syndrome (Benirschke and Kaufmann, 2000).

Amnionic bands are caused when disruption of the amnion leads to formation of bands or strings that adhere to the fetus and impair growth and development of the involved structure. Some conditions that appear to be the consequence of this phenomenon, including intrauterine amputations, are considered in Chapter 39 (p. 1082).

DISORDERS OF AMNIONIC FLUID VOLUME

Normally, amnionic fluid volume increases to about 1 L, or somewhat more by 36 weeks, but decreases thereafter (Table 31–2). Postterm, there may be only 100 to 200 mL or less. Diminished fluid volume is termed *oligohydramnios*. Somewhat arbitrarily, more than 2000 mL of amnionic fluid is considered excessive and is termed *hydramnios* and sometimes called *polyhydramnios*. In

TABLE 31-2. Typical Amnionic Fluid Volume

Weeks' Gestation	Fetus (g)	Placenta (g)	Amnionic Fluid (mL)	Percent Fluid
16	100	100	200	50
28	1000	200	1000	45
36	2500	400	900	24
40	3300	500	800	17

From Queenan (1991), with permission.

TABLE 31-3. Amnionic Fluid Index Values (mm) for Normal Pregnancies

	Amnionic Fluid Index Percentile Values					
Week	2.5th	5th	50th	95th	97.5th	Number
16	73	79	121	185	201	32
17	77	83	127	194	211	26
18	80	87	133	202	220	17
19	83	90	137	207	225	14
20	86	93	141	212	230	25
21	88	95	143	214	233	14
22	89	97	144	216	235	14
23	90	98	146	218	237	14
24	90	98	147	219	238	23
25	89	97	147	221	240	12
26	89	97	147	223	242	11
27	85	95	146	226	245	17
28	86	94	146	228	249	25
29	84	92	145	231	254	12
30	82	90	145	234	258	17
31	79	88	145	238	263	26
32	77	86	144	242	269	25
33	74	83	143	245	274	30
34	72	81	142	248	278	31
35	70	79	140	249	279	27
36	68	77	138	249	279	39
37	66	75	135	244	275	36
38	65	73	132	239	269	27
39	64	72	127	226	255	12
40	63	71	123	214	240	64
41	63	70	116	194	216	162
42	63	69	110	175	192	30

From Moore and Cayle (1990), with permission.

rare instances, the uterus may contain an enormous quantity of fluid, with reports of as much as 15 L. In most instances, chronic hydramnios develops, which is the gradual increase of excessive fluid. In acute hydramnios, the uterus may become markedly distended within a few days.

MEASUREMENT OF AMNIONIC FLUID. Over the past two decades, a number of ultrasonic methods have been used to measure the amount of amnionic fluid. Limitations of using a single pocket of amnionic fluid to determine accurate quantification of fluid were obvious. Accordingly, Phelan and colleagues (1987) described the clinical utility of quantification using the **amnionic fluid index.** This is calculated by adding the vertical depths of the largest pocket in each of four equal uterine quadrants. According to their calculations, significant hydramnios is defined by an index greater than 24 cm. Moore and Cayle (1990) reported normal values for 791 normal pregnancies from 16 to 42 weeks (Table 31-3). Hallak and colleagues (1993) studied 892 normal pregnancies and reported similar trends, but lower absolute numbers (Fig. 31-2). Porter and associates (1996) and Hill and co-workers (2000) have provided normal values for twin pregnancies (Chap. 30, p. 794).

The group from the University of Mississippi has performed several investigations to correlate ultrasonic accuracy of predicting abnormal amnionic fluid volume with actual measurement by dye dilution. Magann and associates (1992) used the dye-dilution technique to measure amnionic fluid in 40 women undergoing amniocentesis in late pregnancy. They found that the amnionic fluid index was reasonably reliable in determining normal or increased amnionic fluid, but was inaccurate in diagnosing oligohydramnios. In a later study, Chauhan and co-workers (1997) evaluated 144 women and found a poor correlation of fluid volume with both the amnionic fluid index and the 2-diameter fluid pocket method.

Williams (1993) reviewed techniques and concluded that there is good inter- and intra-observer variability. In a preliminary study, Bootstaylor and associates (1996)

found that assessment of the index with the woman in the lateral decubitus position correlated well with supine values. Peedicayil and colleagues (1994) emphasized that borderline values should be repeated before interventions are undertaken.

Importantly, several factors may modulate the amnionic fluid index. Yancey and Richards (1994) reported that high altitude (6000 ft) was associated with an increased index. Bush and associates (1996) and Kilpatrick and Safford (1993), but not Kerr and associates (1996), showed that maternal hydration increased the index. Conversely, fluid restriction or dehydration may lower the index. Ross and colleagues (1996) administered 1-deamino-[8-D-arginine] vasopressin to women with oligohydramnios. The resulting maternal serum hypoosmolality (285 to 265 mOsm/kg) was associated with

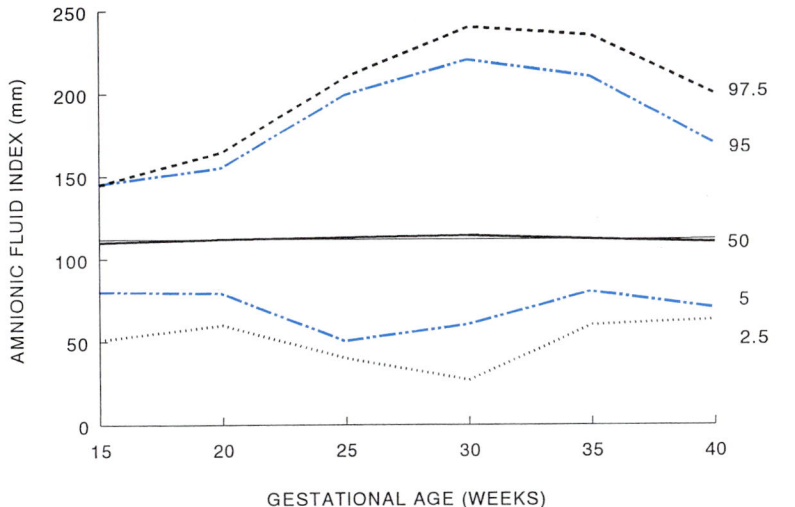

FIGURE 31–2. Normal percentiles for the amnionic fluid index. (Redrawn from Hallak and colleagues, 1993.)

an increased amnionic fluid index from 4 to 8 cm within 8 hours.

HYDRAMNIOS. Minor to moderate degrees of hydramnios—2 to 3 L—are rather common. Because of the difficulty of complete collection and measurement of fluid, the diagnosis is usually clinical (Fig. 31–3) and

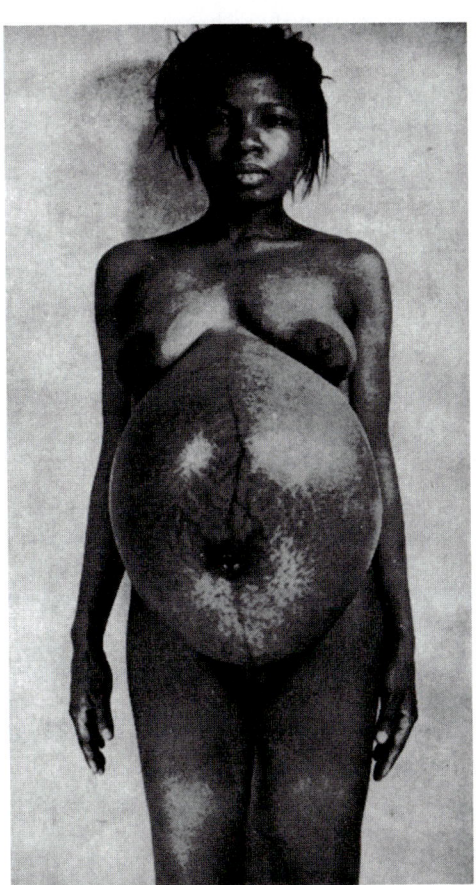

FIGURE 31–3. Advanced degree of hydramnios—5500 mL of amnionic fluid was measured at delivery.

confirmed by sonographic estimation. The frequency of the diagnosis varies appreciably with different observers.

INCIDENCE. Hydramnios is identified in around 1 percent of all pregnancies. Most clinical studies define hydramnios as an amnionic fluid index of greater than 24 to 25 cm—corresponding to greater than either the 95th or 97.5th percentiles. Using an index of 25 cm or greater, Biggio and colleagues (1999) at the University of Alabama reported a 1 percent incidence in nearly 36,450 women examined.

In an earlier study by Hill and associates (1987) from the Mayo Clinic, more than 9000 prenatal patients underwent routine ultrasonic evaluation near the beginning of the third trimester. The incidence of hydramnios was 0.9 percent. Mild hydramnios—defined as pockets measuring 8 to 11 cm in vertical dimension—was present in 80 percent of cases with excessive fluid. Moderate hydramnios—defined as a pocket containing only small parts and measured 12 to 15 cm deep—was found in 15 percent. Only 5 percent had severe hydramnios defined by a free-floating fetus found in pockets of fluid of 16 cm or greater. Although two thirds of all cases were idiopathic, the other third were associated with fetal anomalies, maternal diabetes, or multifetal gestation. Golan and co-workers (1993) reported remarkably similar findings in nearly 14,000 women.

CAUSES OF HYDRAMNIOS. The degree of hydramnios, as well as its prognosis, is related to the cause. Many reports are significantly biased because they consist of observations from women referred for targeted ultrasonic evaluation. Others are population based, but still may not reflect an accurate incidence unless universal ultrasonic screening is done. In either case, obvious pathological hydramnios is frequently associated with

TABLE 31–4. Outcomes in 370 Women with Hydramnios after 20 Weeks Compared with 36,426 Women with a Normal Amnionic Fluid Index

	AFI			Hydramnios (n = 370)		
Factor Studied	*Hydramnios* *(n = 370)*	*Normal* *(n = 36,426)*	P	*Diabetic* *(n = 71)*	*Nondiabetic* *(n = 299)*	P
Perinatal outcomes						
Anomalies	8.4%	0.3%	< .001	0	10.4	.005
Growth restriction	3.8%	6.7%	0.3	0	4.7%	NS
Aneuploidy	1/370	1/3643	.10	0/71	1/299	NS
Mortality	49/1000	14/1000	< .001	0/1000	60/1000	.03
Maternal						
Cesarean delivery	47%	16.4%	< .001	70%	42%	< .001
Diabetes	19.5%	3.2%	< .001			

AFI = amnionic fluid index; NS = not stated.
From Biggio and colleagues (1999).

fetal malformations, especially of the central nervous system or gastrointestinal tract. For example, hydramnios accompanies about half of cases of anencephaly and esophageal atresia. In the study cited earlier by Hill and associates (1987) of nonreferred Mayo Clinic prenatal patients, the cause of mild hydramnios was identified in only about 15 percent of cases. Conversely, with moderately or severely increased amnionic fluid, the cause was identified in more than 90 percent of cases. Specifically, in almost half of cases with moderate and severe hydramnios, a fetal anomaly was identified. The opposite is not true, however, and in the Spanish Collaborative Study of Congenital Malformations (ECEMC) with over 27,000 anomalous fetuses, only 3.7 percent had hydramnios (Martinez-Frias and colleagues, 1999). Another 3 percent had oligohydramnios.

In another population-based study, Biggio and coworkers (1999) reviewed sonographic examinations in over 40,000 women at the University of Alabama at Birmingham. They identified 370 women with hydramnios defined as an index of 25 cm or greater, largest vertical pocket of 8 cm or more, or subjective impression by an experienced sonographer. Using over 36,000 women with a normal index as controls, hydramnios was found to portend a significantly increased risk for a number of adverse outcomes as shown in Table 31–4. One quite interesting finding was that most perinatal adverse outcomes were in nondiabetic women with hydramnios.

Damato and colleagues (1993) reported results from 105 women referred for evaluation of excessive fluid. Using definitions similar to those described by Hill and associates (1987), these investigators observed that almost 65 percent of the 105 pregnancies were abnormal

(Table 31–5). There were 47 singletons with one or more anomalies: gastrointestinal (15), nonimmune hydrops (12), central nervous system (12), thoracic (9), skeletal (8), chromosomal (7), and cardiac (4). Among 19 twin pregnancies, only two were normal. Twelve of the remaining 17 had twin–twin transfusion.

Using an amnionic fluid index of greater than 24 or 25 cm to define hydramnios, most studies indicate that perinatal mortality is increased substantively. In a report by Carlson and associates (1990) of 49 women with an index of 24 cm or more, 22 (44 percent) had fetal malformations and six of these also had aneuploidy. There were 14 perinatal deaths among these 49 women. Brady and colleagues (1992) used an index of 25 cm or greater in 5000 nonreferred women and found unexplained or idiopathic hydramnios in 125 cases. They identified two fetuses with trisomy 18 and two with trisomy 21. Panting-Kemp and co-workers (1999) found

TABLE 31–5. Pregnancy Outcomes in 105 Women Referred for Hydramnios

Largest Pocket (cm)	Abnormal Outcome No. (%)
8.0–9.5	19 (50)
10–11.5	16 (62)
12–13.5	14 (67)
14–15.5	10 (83)
>16	7 (88)
Total	66/105 (63)

From Damato and colleagues (1993), with permission.

that idiopathic hydramnios was not associated with increased adverse outcomes except for cesarean delivery.

PATHOGENESIS. Early in pregnancy, the amnionic cavity is filled with fluid very similar in composition to extracellular fluid. During the first half of pregnancy, transfer of water and other small molecules takes place not only across the amnion but through the fetal skin. During the second trimester, the fetus begins to urinate, swallow, and inspire amnionic fluid (Abramovich and colleagues, 1979; Duenhoelter and Pritchard, 1976). These processes almost certainly have a significant modulating role in the control of fluid volume. Although the major source of amnionic fluid in hydramnios has most often been assumed to be the amnionic epithelium, no histological changes in amnion or chemical changes in amnionic fluid have been found.

Because the fetus normally swallows amnionic fluid, it has been assumed that this mechanism is one of the ways by which the volume is controlled. The theory gains validity by the nearly constant presence of hydramnios when swallowing is inhibited, as in cases of esophageal atresia. Fetal swallowing is by no means the only mechanism for preventing hydramnios. Both Pritchard (1966) and Abramovich (1970) quantified this and found in some instances of gross hydramnios that appreciable volumes of fluid were swallowed.

In cases of anencephaly and spina bifida, increased transudation of fluid from the exposed meninges into the amnionic cavity may be an etiological factor. Another possible explanation in anencephaly, when swallowing is not impaired, is excessive urination caused either by stimulation of cerebrospinal centers deprived of their protective coverings, or lack of antidiuretic effect because of impaired arginine vasopressin secretion. The converse is well established—that fetal defects that cause anuria are nearly always associated with oligohydramnios.

In hydramnios associated with monozygotic twin pregnancy, the hypothesis has been advanced that one fetus usurps the greater part of the circulation common to both twins and develops cardiac hypertrophy, which in turn results in increased urine output (Chap. 30, p. 777). Naeye and Blanc (1972) identified dilated renal tubules, enlarged bladder, and an increased urinary output in the early neonatal period, suggesting that increased fetal urine production is responsible for hydramnios. Conversely, donor members of parabiotic transplacental transfusion pairs had contracted renal tubules with oligohydramnios.

Hydramnios that rather commonly develops with maternal diabetes during the third trimester remains unexplained. One explanation is that maternal hyperglycemia causes fetal hyperglycemia that results in osmotic diuresis. Bar-Hava and associates (1994) have provided

evidence that third-trimester amnionic fluid volume in 399 gestational diabetes reflected recent glycemic status. Yasuhi and co-workers (1994) reported increased fetal urine production in fasted diabetic women compared with nondiabetic controls. Of interest, fetal urine production increased in nondiabetic women after eating, but this was not observed in diabetic women.

SYMPTOMS. Major symptoms accompanying hydramnios arise from purely mechanical causes and result principally from pressure exerted within and around the overdistended uterus upon adjacent organs. When distention is excessive, the mother may suffer from severe dyspnea and, in extreme cases, she may be able to breathe only when upright. Edema, the consequence of compression of major venous systems by the very large uterus, is common, especially in the lower extremities, the vulva, and the abdominal wall. Rarely, severe oliguria may result from ureteral obstruction by the very large uterus (Chap. 47, p. 1252).

With chronic hydramnios, the accumulation of fluid takes place gradually and the woman may tolerate the excessive abdominal distention with relatively little discomfort. In acute hydramnios, however, distention may lead to disturbances sufficiently serious to be threatening. Acute hydramnios tends to develop earlier in pregnancy than does the chronic form—often as early as 16 to 20 weeks—and it may rapidly expand the hypertonic uterus to enormous size. As a rule, acute hydramnios leads to labor before 28 weeks, or the symptoms become so severe that intervention is mandatory. In the majority of cases of chronic hydramnios, and thus differing from acute hydramnios, the amnionic fluid pressure is not appreciably higher than in normal pregnancy.

DIAGNOSIS. The primary clinical finding with hydramnios is uterine enlargement in association with difficulty in palpating fetal small parts and in hearing fetal heart tones. In severe cases, the uterine wall may be so tense that it is impossible to palpate any fetal parts (Fig. 31–3).

The differentiation between hydramnios, ascites, or a large ovarian cyst can usually be made without difficulty by ultrasonic evaluation. Large amounts of amnionic fluid can nearly always be readily demonstrated as an abnormally large, echo-free space between the fetus and the uterine wall or placenta (Fig. 31–4). At times, a fetal abnormality such as anencephaly or other neural-tube defects, or a gastrointestinal tract anomaly, may be seen.

PREGNANCY OUTCOME. In general, the more severe the degree of hydramnios, the higher the perinatal mortality rate. The outlook for the infant in pregnancies with marked hydramnios is poor. Even when sonography and x-ray show an apparently normal fetus, the prognosis is

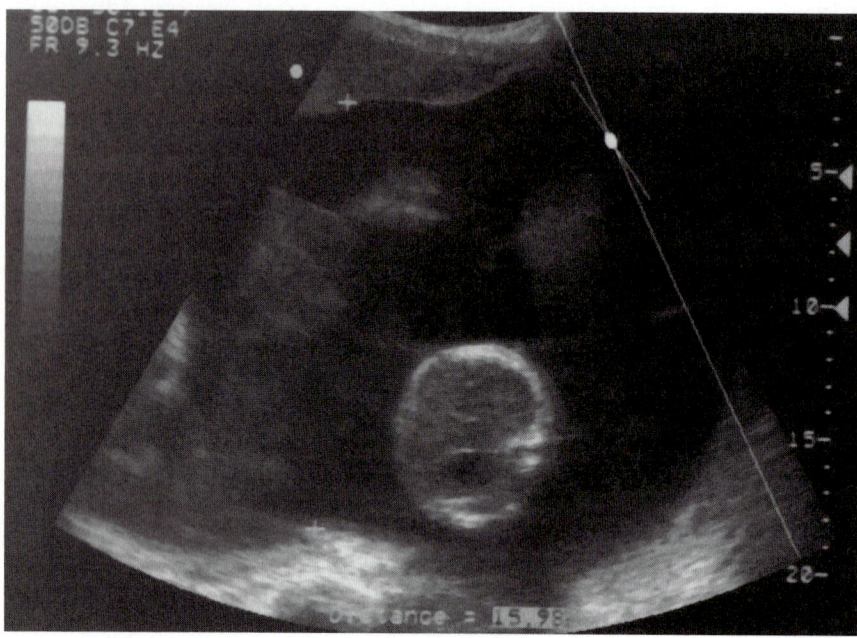

FIGURE 31–4. Marked hydramnios in a 24-week twin gestation with twin–twin transfusion syndrome. (Courtesy of Dr. Diane Twickler.)

still guarded, because fetal malformations and chromosomal abnormalities are common. Furman and co-workers (2000) described substantively increased adverse perinatal outcomes if fetal growth restriction accompanies hydramnios. Perinatal mortality is increased further by preterm delivery, even with a normal fetus. Many and colleagues (1995) reported that 20 percent of 275 women with an amnionic fluid index of at least 25 cm delivered preterm. Moreover, preterm delivery was more common in women with an anomalous fetus (40 percent). Erythroblastosis, difficulties encountered by infants of diabetic mothers, prolapse of the umbilical cord when the membranes rupture, and placental abruption as the uterus rapidly decreases in size, add still further to bad outcomes.

The most frequent maternal complications associated with hydramnios are placental abruption, uterine dysfunction, and postpartum hemorrhage. Extensive premature separation of the placenta sometimes follows escape of massive quantities of amnionic fluid because of the decrease in the area of the emptying uterus beneath the placenta (Chap. 25 p. 621). Uterine dysfunction and postpartum hemorrhage result from uterine atony consequent to overdistention. Abnormal fetal presentations and operative intervention are also more common.

MIDTRIMESTER HYDRAMNIOS. The prognosis of midtrimester hydramnios depends on the severity. Mild hydramnios has a reasonably good outcome. Glantz and co-workers (1994) studied 47 consecutive singleton pregnancies with a single deepest pocket of 6 to 10 cm that was identified at 14 to 27 weeks. Excessive fluid

resolved spontaneously in three fourths and perinatal outcomes were similar to matched controls without hydramnios. In the group in which hydramnios persisted, 2 of 10 had fetal aneuploidy.

MANAGEMENT. Minor degrees of hydramnios rarely require treatment. Even moderate degrees with some discomfort can usually be managed without intervention until labor ensues or until the membranes rupture spontaneously. If there is dyspnea or abdominal pain, or if ambulation is difficult, hospitalization becomes necessary. Bed rest rarely has any effect, and diuretics and water and salt restriction are likewise ineffective. Recently, indomethacin therapy has been used for symptomatic hydramnios.

AMNIOCENTESIS. The principal purpose of amniocentesis is to relieve maternal distress, and to that end it is transiently successful. Amnionic fluid can also be tested to predict fetal lung maturity as described in Chapter 39 (p. 1042). Piazze and co-workers (1998) showed that dilution may cause false-negative results. Therapeutic amniocentesis appears at times to initiate labor even though only a part of the fluid is removed. Elliott and associates (1994) reported results from 200 therapeutic amniocenteses in 94 women with hydramnios. Common causes included twin–twin transfusion (38 percent), idiopathic (26 percent), fetal or chromosomal anomalies (17 percent), and diabetes (12 percent). They removed a mean of 1650 mL of fluid at each procedure and gained an average duration of 7 weeks to delivery. Only three procedures were complicated: one woman had ruptured membranes, one developed chorioamnionitis, and another suffered placental abruption after 10 L of fluid was removed.

TECHNIQUE

To remove amnionic fluid, a commercially available plastic catheter that tightly covers an 18-gauge needle is inserted through the locally anesthetized abdominal wall into the amnionic sac, the needle is withdrawn, and an intravaneous infusion set is connected to the catheter hub. The opposite end of the tubing is dropped into a graduated cylinder placed at floor level, and the rate of flow of amnionic fluid is controlled with the screw clamp so that about 500 mL/ h is withdrawn. After about 1500 to 2000 mL have been collected, the uterus has usually decreased in size sufficiently so that the catheter may be withdrawn from the amnionic sac. At the same time, maternal relief is dramatic and the danger of placental separation from decompression is very slight. Using strict aseptic technique, this procedure can be repeated as necessary to make the woman comfortable. Elliott and colleagues (1994) used wall suction and removed 1000 mL over 20 minutes (50 mL/min); however, we prefer more gradual removal.

AMNIOTOMY. The disadvantages inherent in rupture of the membranes through the cervix is the possibility of cord prolapse and especially of placental abruption. Slow removal of the fluid by amniocentesis helps to obviate these dangers.

INDOMETHACIN THERAPY. In their review of several studies, Kramer and colleagues (1994) concluded that indomethacin impairs lung liquid production or enhances absorption, decreases fetal urine production, and increases fluid movement across fetal membranes. Doses employed by most investigators range from 1.5 to 3 mg/kg per day.

Cabrol and associates (1987) treated eight women with idiopathic hydramnios from 24 to 35 weeks with indomethacin for 2 to 11 weeks. Hydramnios, defined by at least one 8-cm fluid pocket, improved in all cases. There were no serious adverse effects and the outcome was good in all cases. Kirshon and associates (1990) treated eight women (three sets of twins) with hydramnios from 21 to 35 weeks. In all of these, two therapeutic amniocenteses had been done before indomethacin was given. Of 11 fetuses, three were stillborn associated with twin–twin transfusion syndrome and one newborn died at 3 months of age. The remaining seven infants did well. Mamopoulos and colleagues (1990) treated 15 women—11 were diabetic—who had hydramnios at 25 to 32 weeks. Indomethacin was given and amnionic fluid volume decreased in all women, from a mean of 10.7 cm at 27 weeks to 5.9 cm after therapy. The outcome was good in all 15 newborns.

A major concern for the use of indomethacin is the potential for closure of the fetal ductus arteriosus (Chap. 38, p. 1027). Moise and colleagues (1988) reported that 50 percent of 14 fetuses whose mothers received indomethacin had ductal constriction detected by Doppler ultrasound. Persistent constriction was not demonstrated in the studies described earlier, nor has it been described in studies in which indomethacin was given for tocolysis (Kramer and colleagues, 1994).

OLIGOHYDRAMNIOS. In rare instances, the volume of amnionic fluid may fall far below the normal limits and occasionally be reduced to only a few mL of viscid fluid. The cause of this condition is not completely understood. In general, oligohydramnios developing early in pregnancy is less common and frequently has a bad prognosis. By contrast, diminished fluid volume may be found relatively often with pregnancies that continue beyond term. Marks and Divon (1992) found oligohydramnios—defined as an amnionic fluid index of 5 cm or less—in 12 percent of 511 pregnancies of 41 weeks' duration or greater. In 121 women studied longitudinally, there was a mean decrease in the amnionic fluid index of 25 percent per week beyond 41 weeks. The risk of cord compression, and in turn fetal distress, is increased as the consequence of diminished fluid in all labors, but especially in postterm pregnancy (Grubb and Paul, 1992; Leveno and colleagues, 1984).

EARLY-ONSET OLIGOHYDRAMNIOS. A number of conditions have been associated with diminished amnionic fluid (Table 31–6). Oligohydramnios is almost always evident when there is either obstruction of the fetal urinary tract or renal agenesis. Therefore, anuria almost certainly has an etiological role in such cases. A chronic leak from a defect in the membranes may reduce the volume of fluid appreciably, but most often labor soon

TABLE 31–6. Conditions Associated with Oligohydramnios

Fetal	Maternal
Chromosomal abnormalities	Uteroplacental insufficiency
Congenital anomalies	Hypertension
Growth restriction	Preeclampsia
Demise	Diabetes
Postterm pregnancy	**Drugs**
Ruptured membranes	Prostaglandin synthase inhibitors
Placenta	Angiotensin-converting enzyme inhibitors
Abruption	
Twin–twin transfusion	**Idiopathic**

From Peipert and Donnenfeld (1991), with permission.

TABLE 31-7. Congenital Anomalies Associated with Oligohydramnios

Amnionic band syndrome

Cardiac: Tetralogy of Fallot, septal defects

Central nervous system: holoprosencephaly, meningocoele, encephalocoele, microcephaly

Chromosomal abnormalities: triploidy, trisomy 18, Turner syndrome

Cloacal dysgenesis

Cystic hygroma

Diaphragmatic hernia

Genitourinary: renal agenesis, renal dysplasia, urethral obstruction, bladder exstrophy, Meckel–Gruber syndrome, ureteropelvic junction obstruction, prune-belly syndrome

Hypothyroidism

Skeletal: sirenomelia, sacral agenesis, absent radius, facial clefting

TRAP (twin reverse arterial perfusion) sequence

Twin–twin transfusion

VACTERL (vertebral, anal, cardiac, tracheo-esophageal, renal, limb) association

Adapted from McCurdy and Seeds (1993) and Peipert and Donnenfeld (1991).

ated with oligohydramnios prior to 37 weeks had a significant threefold increase in preterm birth, but not growth restriction or fetal death.

Newbould and colleagues (1994) described autopsy findings in 89 infants with the oligohydramnios sequence. Only 3 percent had a normal renal tract; 34 percent had bilateral renal agenesis; 34 percent bilateral cystic dysplasia, 9 percent unilateral agenesis with dysplasia, and 10 percent minor urinary abnormalities.

Otherwise normal infants may suffer the consequences of early-onset severely diminished amnionic fluid. Adhesions between the amnion and fetal parts may cause serious deformities including amputation. Moreover, subjected to pressure from all sides, the fetus assumes a peculiar appearance, and musculoskeletal deformities such as clubfoot are observed frequently.

PULMONARY HYPOPLASIA. The incidence of pulmonary hypoplasia at birth has been unchanged and ranges from 1.1 to 1.4 per 1000 infants (Moessinger and colleagues, 1989). When amnionic fluid is scant, pulmonary hypoplasia, such as that shown in Figure 31–5, is common. Winn and associates (2000) performed a prospective cohort study in 163 cases of oligohydramnios that

ensues. Exposure to angiotensin-converting enzyme inhibitors has been associated with oligohydramnios (Chap. 38, p. 1014). Anywhere from 15 to 25 percent of cases are associated with the fetal anomalies shown in Table 31–7. Pryde and co-workers (2000) were able to visualize fetal structures in only half of women referred for ultrasonic evaluation of midtrimester oligohydramnios. They performed amnioinfusion and were then able to visualize 77 percent of routinely imaged structures. Identification of associated anomalies increased from 12 to 31 percent.

PROGNOSIS. Fetal outcome is poor with early-onset oligohydramnios. Shenker and colleagues (1991) described 80 such pregnancies and only half of these fetuses survived. Mercer and Brown (1986) described 34 midtrimester pregnancies complicated by oligohydramnios diagnosed ultrasonically by the absence of amnionic fluid pockets greater than 1 cm in any vertical plane. Nine of these fetuses (26 percent) had anomalies, and 10 of the 25 who were phenotypically normal either aborted spontaneously or were stillborn because of severe maternal hypertension, restricted fetal growth, or placental abruption. Of the 14 live-born infants, eight were preterm and seven died. The six infants who were delivered at term did well. Garmel and co-workers (1997) observed that appropriately grown fetuses associ-

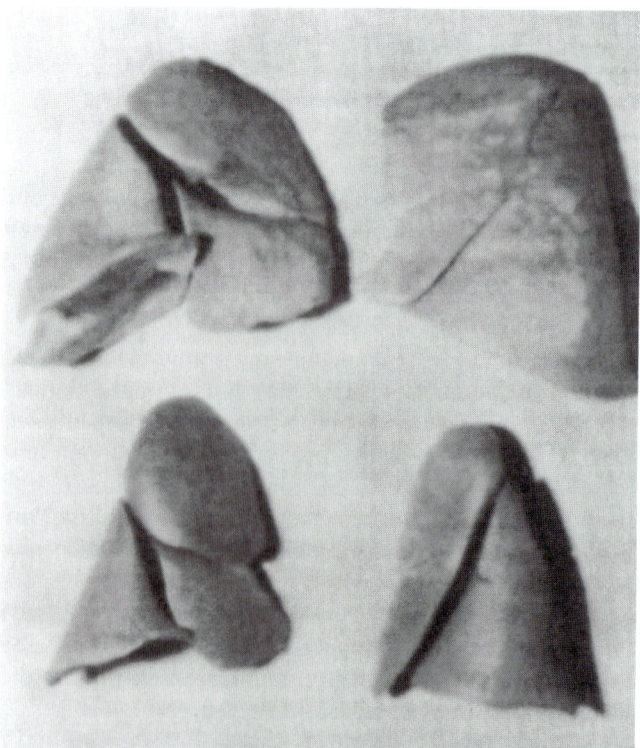

FIGURE 31–5. Normal-sized lungs (above) are shown in comparison with hypoplastic lungs (below) of fetuses at the same gestational age. (From Newbould and colleagues, 1994, with permission.)

followed prematurely ruptured membranes at 15 to 28 weeks. Almost 13 percent of fetuses developed pulmonary hypoplasia. This was more common as gestational age decreased. Kilbride and co-workers (1996) studied 115 women with prematurely ruptured membranes before 29 weeks. There ultimately were seven stillbirths and 40 neonatal deaths for a perinatal mortality of 409 per 1000. The risk of lethal pulmonary hypoplasia was 20 percent. Adverse outcomes were more likely with earlier rupture as well as duration exceeding 14 days.

According to Fox and Badalian (1994) and Lauria and colleagues (1995), there are three possibilities that account for pulmonary hypoplasia. First, thoracic compression may prevent chest wall excursion and lung expansion. Second, lack of fetal breathing movements decreases lung inflow. The third and most widely accepted model involves a failure to retain amnionic fluid or increased outflow with impaired lung growth and development.

The appreciable volume of amnionic fluid demonstrated by Duenhoelter and Pritchard (1976) to be inhaled by the normal fetus is suggestive of a role for the inspired fluid in expansion, and in turn growth, of the lung. Fisk and colleagues (1992), however, concluded that fetal breathing impairment does not cause pulmonary hypoplasia with oligohydramnios. In a unique experiment, McNamara and associates (1995) described findings from two sets of monoamnionic twins with discordant renal anomalies. They provided evidence that normal amnionic fluid volume in the presence of fetal renal obstruction allows normal lung development.

OLIGOHYDRAMNIOS IN LATE PREGNANCY. As shown in Table 31–3 and Figure 31–2, amnionic fluid volume diminishes normally after 35 weeks. Using an amnionic fluid index of less that 5 cm, Casey and co-workers (2000) found an incidence of oligohydramnios of 2.3 percent in over 6400 pregnancies undergoing sonography after 34 weeks at Parkland Hospital. They confirmed previous observations that this is associated with an increased risk of adverse perinatal outcomes (Table 31–8). In pregnancies selected because of "high risk," Magann and co-workers (1999) did not find that associated oligohydramnios (amnionic fluid index of less than 5 cm) increased risks for intrapartum complications such as thick meconium, variable heart-rate decelerations, cesarean delivery for fetal distress, or neonatal acidemia.

Chauhan and associates (1999) performed meta-analysis of 18 studies with over 10,500 pregnancies in which the intrapartum amnionic fluid index was less than 5 cm. Compared with controls whose index was over 5 cm, women with oligohydramnios had significantly increased risks for cesarean delivery for fetal dis-

TABLE 31–8. Pregnancy Outcomes in 147 Women with Oligodydramnios at 34 Weeks

Factor Studied	Oligo-hydramnios (n = 147)	Normal AFI (n = 6276)	P
Labor induction	42%	18%	< .001
Nonreassuring FHR	48%	39%	< .03
Cesarean for FHR	5%	3%	.18
Stillbirth	14/1000	3/1000	< .03
Neonatal ICU	7%	2%	< .001
Meconium aspiration	1%	0.1%	< .001
Neonatal death	5%	0.3%	< .001
Growth restriction	24%	9%	< .001
Malformation	10%	2.5%	< .001

AFI = amnionic fluid index; FHR = fetal heart rate pattern; ICU = intensive care unit.
From Casey and co-workers (2000).

tress risk ratio [RR] 2.2) and 5-minute Apgar of less than 7 (RR 5.2).

Cord compression during labor is common with oligohydramnios. Sarno and co-workers (1989, 1990) reported that an index of 5 cm or less was associated with a fivefold increased cesarean delivery rate. Baron and colleagues (1995) reported a 50 percent increase in variable decelerations during labor and a sevenfold increased cesarean delivery rate in these women. By contrast, Casey and co-workers (1999) showed a 25 percent increase in nonreassuring fetal heart rate patterns when women with oligohydramnios were compared with normal controls; however, the cesarean rate for this increased only from 3 to 5 percent (Table 31–8).

Divon and associates (1995) studied 638 postterm pregnancies in labor and observed that only women whose amnionic fluid index was 5 cm or less had fetal heart rate decelerations and meconium. Interestingly, Chauhan and collaborators (1995) showed that diminished amnionic fluid index increased the cesarean delivery rate only in women whose labor attendants were made aware of the findings!

AMNIOINFUSION. Infusion of crystalloid to replace pathologically diminished amnionic fluid has most often been used during labor to prevent umbilical cord compression (Chap. 14, p. 345). Results with intrapartum amnioinfusion to prevent fetal morbidity from meconium-stained fluid—often associated with oligohydramnios—are mixed. Pierce and colleagues (2000) performed meta-analysis of 13 studies with 1924 such women randomized to amnioinfusion or no treatment. They found significantly decreased adverse outcomes: meconium beneath the cords (OR 0.18), meconium aspiration syndrome (OR 0.30), neonatal acidemia (OR 0.42), and cesarean delivery rate (0.74). Wenstrom and associates (1995) surveyed academic obstetrical departments and reported that amnioinfusion is widely performed with relatively few complications. It is discussed in greater detail in Chapter 39 (p. 1045) and the technique is described in Chapter 14 (p. 345).

REFERENCES

Abramovich DR: Fetal factors influencing the volume and composition of liquor amnii. J Obstet Gynaecol Br Commonw 77:865, 1970

Abramovich DR, Garden A, Jandial L, Page KR: Fetal swallowing and voiding in relation to hydramnios. Obstet Gynecol 54:15, 1979

Bar-Hava I, Scarpelli SA, Barnhard Y, Divon MY: Amniotic fluid volume reflects recent glycemic status in gestational diabetes mellitus. Am J Obstet Gynecol 171:952, 1994

Baron C, Morgan MA, Garite TJ: The impact of amniotic fluid volume assessed intrapartum on perinatal outcome. Am J Obstet Gynecol 173:167, 1995

Benirschke K, Kaufmann P: Pathology of the Human Placenta. New York, Springer-Verlag, 2000

Biggio JR Jr, Wenstrom KD, Dubard MB, Cliver SP: Hydramnios prediction of adverse perinatal outcome. Obstet Gynecol 94:773, 1999

Bootstaylor B, Rigaud-Echols S, Barry J, Ohana S, Saltzman D: Influence of the lateral decubitus position on the amniotic fluid index. Am J Obstet Gynecol 174:338, 1996

Brady K, Polzin WJ, Kopelman JN, Read JA: Risk of chromosomal abnormalities in patients with idiopathic polyhydramnios. Obstet Gynecol 79:234, 1992

Bush J, Minkoff H, McCalla S, Moy S, Chung H: The effect of intravenous fluid load on amniotic fluid index in patients with oligohydramnios. Am J Obstet Gynecol 174:379, 1996

Cabrol D, Landesman R, Muller J, Uzan M, Sureau C, Saxena BB: Treatment of polyhydramnios with prostaglandin synthetase inhibitor (indomethacin). Am J Obstet Gynecol 157:422, 1987

Carlson DE, Platt LD, Medearis AL, Hornestein J: Quantifiable polyhydramnios: Diagnosis and management. Obstet Gynecol 75:989, 1990

Casey BM, McIntire DD, Bloom SL, Lucas MJ, Santos R, Twickler DM, Ramus RM, Leveno KJ: Pregnancy outcomes after antepartum diagnosis of oligohydramnios at or beyond 34 weeks' gestation. Am J Obstet Gynecol 182:909, 2000

Chauhan SP, Magan EF, Morrison JC, Whitworth NS, Hendrix NW, Devoe LD: Ultrasonographic assessment of amniotic fluid does not reflect actual amnioic fluid volume. Am J Obstet Gynecol 177:291, 1997

Chauhan SP, Sanderson M, Hendrix NW, Magann EF, Devoe LD: Perinatal outcome and amniotic fluid index in the antepartum and intrapartum periods: A meta-analysis. Am J Obstet Gynecol 181:1473, 1999

Chauhan SP, Washburne JF, Magann EF, Perry KG Jr, Martin JN Jr, Morrison JC: A randomized study to assess the efficacy of the amniotic fluid index as a fetal admission test. Obstet Gynecol 86:9, 1995

Leary GM, Wiswell TE: Meconium-stained amniotic fluid and the meconium aspiration syndrome. An update. Pediatr Clin North Am 45:511, 1998

Damato N, Filly RA, Goldstein RB, Callen PW, Goldberg J, Golbus M: Frequency of fetal anomalies in sonographically detected polyhydramnios. J Ultrasound Med 12:11, 1993

Divon MY, Marks AD, Henderson CE: Longitudinal measurement of amniotic fluid index in postterm pregnancies and its association with fetal outcome. Am J Obstet Gynecol 172:142, 1995

Duenhoelter JH, Pritchard JA: Fetal respiration: Quantitative measurements of amnionic fluid inspired near term by human rhesus fetuses. Am J Obstet Gynecol 125:306, 1976

Eden RD, Seifert LS, Winegar A, Spellacy W: Perinatal characteristics of uncomplicated postdate pregnancies. Obstet Gynecol 69:296, 1987

Elliott JP, Sawyer AT, Radin TG, Strong RE: Large-volume therapeutic amniocentesis in the treatment of hydramnios. Obstet Gynecol 84:1025, 1994

Fisk NM, Talbert DG, Nicolini U, Vaughan J, Rodeck CH: Fetal breathing movements in oligohydramnios are not increased by amnioinfusion. Br J Obstet Gynaecol 99:464, 1992

Fox HE: Pathology of the placenta. Monograph, Vol VII. Philadelphia, Saunders, 1978

Fox HE, Badalian SS: Ultrasound prediction of fetal pulmonary hypoplasia in pregnancies complicated by oligohydramnios and in cases of congenital diaphragmatic hernia: A review. Am J Perinatol 11:104, 1994

Fujikura T, Klionsky B: The significance of meconium staining. Am J Obstet Gynecol 121:45, 1975

Furman B, Erez O, Senior L, Shoham-Vardi I, Bar-David J, Maymon E, Mazor M: Hydramnios and small for gestational age: Prevalence and clinical significance. Acta Obstet Gynecol Scand 79:31, 2000

Garmel SH, Chelmow D, Sha SJ, Roan JT, D'Alton ME: Oligohydramnios and the appropriately grown fetus. Am J Perinatol 14:359, 1997

Glantz JC, Abramowicz JS, Sherer DM: Significance of idiopathic midtrimester polyhydramnios. Am J Perinatol 11:305, 1994

Golan A, Wolman I, Saller Y, David MP: Hydramnios in singleton pregnancy: Sonographic prevalence and etiology. Gynecol Obstet Invest 35:91, 1993

Goldenberg, RL, Hauth JC, Andrews WW: Intrauterine infection and preterm delivery. N Engl J Med 342:1500, 2000

Grubb DK, Paul RH: Amniotic fluid index and prolonged antepartum fetal heart rate decelerations. Obstet Gynecol 79:588, 1992

Hallak M, Kirshon B, Smith EO, Cotton DB: Amniotic fluid index. Gestational age-specific values for normal human pregnancy. J Reprod Med 38:853, 1993

Hill LM, Breckle R, Thomas ML, Fries JK: Polyhydramnios: Ultrasonically detected prevalence and neonatal outcome. Obstet Gynecol 69:21, 1987

Hill LM, Krohn M, Lazebnik N, Tush B, Boyles D, Ursiny JJ: The amniotic fluid index in normal twin pregnancies. Am J Obstet Gynecol 182:950, 2000

Houlihan CM, Knuppel RA: Meconium-stained amniotic fluid: Current controversies. J Reprod Med 39:888, 1994

Katz VL, Bowes WA: Meconium aspiration: Reflections on a murky subject. Am J Obstet Gynecol 166:171, 1992

Kerr J, Borgida AF, Hardardottir H, Calhoun S, Galetta J, Egan JFX: Maternal hydration and its effect on the amniotic fluid index. Am J Obstet Gynecol 174:416, 1996

Kilbride HW, Yeast J, Thibeault DW: Defining limits of survival: Lethal pulmonary hypoplasia after midtrimester premature rupture of membranes. Am J Obstet Gynecol 175:675, 1996

Kilpatrick SJ, Safford KL: Maternal hydration increases amniotic fluid index in women with normal amniotic fluid. Obstet Gynecol 81:49, 1993

Kirshon B, Mari G, Moise KJ: Indomethacin therapy in the treatment of symptomatic polyhydramnios. Obstet Gynecol 75:202, 1990

Kramer WB, Van den Veyver IB, Kirshon B: Treatment of polyhydramnios with indomethacin. Clin Perinatol 21:615, 1994

Lauria MR, Gonik B, Romero R: Pulmonary hypoplasia: Pathogenesis, diagnosis, and antenatal prediction. Obstet Gynecol 86:466, 1995

Leveno KJ, Quirk JG Jr, Cunningham FG, Nelson SD, Santos-Ramos R, Toofanian A, DePalma RT: Prolonged pregnancy, 1. Observations concerning the causes of fetal distress. Am J Obstet Gynecol 150:465, 1984

Magann EF, Kinsella MJ, Chauhan SP, McNamara MF, Gehring BW, Morrison JC: Does an amniotic fluid index of ≤5 cm necessitate delivery in high-risk pregnancies? A case-control study. Obstet Gynecol 180:1354, 1999

Magann EF, Nolan TE, Hess LW, Martin RW, Whitworth NS, Morrison JC: Measurement of amniotic fluid volume: Accuracy of ultrasonography techniques. Am J Obstet Gynecol 167:1533, 1992

Mamopoulos M, Assimakopoulos E, Reece EA, Andreou A, Zheng XZ, Mantalenakis S: Maternal indomethacin therapy in the treatment of polyhydramnios. Am J Obstet Gynecol 162:1225, 1990

Many A, Hill LM, Lazebnik N, Martin JG: The association between polyhydramnios and preterm delivery. Obstet Gynecol 86:389, 1995

Marks AD, Divon MY: Longitudinal study of the amniotic fluid index in postdated pregnancy. Obstet Gynecol 79:229, 1992

Martinez-Frias ML, Bermejo E, Rodriguez-Pinilla E, Frias JL: Maternal and fetal factors related to abnormal amniotic fluid. J Perinatol 19:514, 1999

McCurdy CM, Seeds JW: Oligohydramnios: Problems and treatment. Semin Perinatol 17:183, 1993

McNamara MF, McCurty CM, Reed KL, Phillips AF, Seeds JW: The relation between pulmonary hypoplasia and amniotic fluid volume: Lessons learned from discordant urinary tract anomalies in monoamniotic twins. Obstet Gynecol 85:867, 1995

Mercer LJ, Brown LB: Fetal outcome with oligohydramnios in the second trimester. Obstet Gynecol 67:840, 1986

Miller PW, Coen RW, Benirschke K: Dating the time interval from meconium passage to birth. Obstet Gynecol 66:459, 1985

Moessinger AC, Santiago A, Paneth NS, Rey HR; Blanc WA, Driscoll JM Jr: Time-trends in necropsy prevalence and birth prevalence of lung hypoplasia. Paediatr Perinatal Epidemiol 3:421, 1989

Moise KJ Jr, Huhta JC, Sharif DS, Ou CN, Kirshon B, Wasserstrum N, Cano L: Indomethacin in the treatment of premature labor: Effects on the fetal ductus arteriosus. N Engl J Med 319:327, 1988

Moore TR, Cayle JE: The amniotic fluid index in normal human pregnancy. Am J Obstet Gynecol 162:1168, 1990

Naeye RL, Blanc WA: Fetal renal structure and the genesis of amniotic fluid disorders. Am J Pathol 67:95, 1972

Nathan L, Leveno KJ, Carmody TJ III, Kelly MA, Sherman

ML: Meconium: A 1990s perspective on an old obstetric hazard. Obstet Gynecol 83:329, 1994

Newbould MJ, Lendon M, Barson AJ: Oligohydramnios sequence: The spectrum of renal malformation. Br J Obstet Gynaecol 101:598, 1994

Panting-Kemp A, Nguyen T, Chang E, Quillen E, Castro L: Idiopathic polyhydramnios and perinatal outcome. Am J Obstet Gynecol 181:1079, 1999

Peedicayil A, Mathai M, Regi AN, Aseelan LJ, Rekha K, Jasper P: Inter- and intra-observer variation in the amniotic fluid index. Obstet Gynecol 84:848, 1994

Peipert JF, Donnenfeld AE: Oligohydramnios: A review. Obstet Gynecol Surv 46:325, 1991

Phelan JP, Smith CV, Broussard P, Small M: Amniotic fluid volume assessment with the four-quadrant technique at 36–42 weeks' gestation. J Reprod Med 32:540, 1987

Piazze JJ, Maranghi L, Cosmi EV, Anceschi MM: The effect of polyhydramnios and oligohydramnios on fetal lung maturity indexes. Am J Perinatol 15:249, 1998

Pierce J, Gaudier FL, Sanchez-Ramos L: Intrapartum amnioinfusion for meconium-stained fluid: Meta-analysis of prospective clinical trials. Obstet Gynecol 95:1051, 2000

Porter TF, Dildy GA, Blanchard JR, Kochenour NK, Clark SL: Normal values for amniotic fluid index during uncomplicated twin pregnancy. Obstet Gynecol 87:699, 1996

Pritchard JA: Fetal swallowing and amniotic fluid volume. Obstet Gynecol 28:606, 1966

Pryde PG, Hallak M, Lauria MR, Littman L, Bottoms SF, Johnson MP, Evans MI: Severe oligohydramnios with intact membranes: An indication for diagnostic amnioinfusion. Fetal Diagn Ther 15:46, 2000

Queenan JT: Polyhydramnios and oligohydramnios. Contemp Obstet Gynecol 36:60, 1991

Ross MG, Cedars L, Nijland MJM, Agundipe A: Treatment of oligohydramnios with maternal 1-deamino-[8-D-arginine] vasopressin–induced plasma hypoosmolality

Sampson JE, Theve RP, Blatman RN, Shipp TD, Bianchi DW, Ward BE, Jack RM: Fetal origin of amniotic fluid polymorphonuclear leukocytes. Am J Obstet Gynecol 176:77, 1997

Sarno AP, Ahn MO, Brar HS, Phelan JP, Platt LD: Intrapartum Doppler velocimetry, amniotic fluid volume, and fetal heart rate as predictors of subsequent fetal distress, 1. An initial report. Am J Obstet Gynecol 161:1508, 1989

Sarno AP, Anh MO, Phelan JP: Intrapartum anionic fluid volume at term: Association of ruptured membranes, oligohydramnios, and increased fetal risk. J Reprod Med 35:719, 1990

Shenker L, Reed KL, Anderson CF, Borjon JA: Significance of oligohydramnios complicating pregnancy. Am J Obstet Gynecol 164:1597, 1991

Steer PJ, Eigbe F, Lissauer TJ, Beard RW: Interrelationships among abnormal cardiocograms in labor, meconium staining of the amniotic fluid, arterial cord blood pH and Apgar scores. Obstet Gynecol 74:715, 1989

Usher RH, Boyd ME, McLean FH, Kramer MS: Assessment of fetal risk in postdate pregnancies. Am J Obstet Gynecol 158:259, 1988

Wenstrom K, Andrews WW, Maher JE: Amnioinfusion survey: Prevalence, protocols, and complications. Obstet Gynecol 86:572, 1995

Williams K: Amniotic fluid assessment. Obstet Gynecol Surv 48:795, 1993

Winn HN, Chen M, Amon E, Leet TL, Shumway JB, Mostello D: Neonatal pulmonary hypoplasia and perinatal mortality in patients with midtrimester rupture of amniotic membranes—a critical analysis. Am J Obstet Gynecol 182:1638, 2000

Wiswell TE, Tuggle JM, Turner BS: Meconium aspiration syndrome: Have we made a difference? Pediatrics 85:715, 1990

Yamada T, Minakami H, Matsubara S, Yatsuda T, Kohmura Y, Sato I: Meconium-stained amniotic fluid exhibits chemotactic activity for polymorphonuclear leukocytes in vitro. J Reprod Immunol 46:21, 2000

Yancey MK, Richards DS: Effect of altitude on the amniotic fluid index. J Reprod Med 39:101, 1994

Yasuhi I, Ishimaru T, Hirai M, Yamabe T: Hourly fetal urine production rate in the fasting and the postprandial state of normal and diabetic pregnant women. Obstet Gynecol 84:64, 1994

32

Diseases and Abnormalities of the Placenta

With the basic understanding of the process of implantation and placental development presented in Chapter 5 (p. 87), it is much easier to visualize the development of abnormal placental types. In addition to these, there are a number of tumors that involve the placenta. These include trophoblastic tumors such as hydatidiform mole, stromal tissue tumors such as chorioangiomas, and tumors metastatic to the placenta.

ABNORMALITIES OF PLACENTATION

ABNORMAL SHAPES. There are a number of normal placental shape variations.

MULTIPLE PLACENTAS WITH A SINGLE FETUS. Occasionally, the placenta may be separated into lobes. When the division is incomplete and the vessels of fetal origin extend from one lobe to the other before uniting to form the umbilical cord, the condition is termed *placenta bipartita* or *bilobata* (Fig. 32–1). Its reported incidence varies widely, and Fox (1978) cited it at about 1 of 350 deliveries. If the two lobes are separated entirely and the vessels remain distinct, the condition is designated *placenta duplex*. Occasionally, there is *placenta triplex,* with three distinct lobes.

SUCCENTURIATE PLACENTA. This variation results when one or more small accessory lobes are developed in the membranes at a distance from the periphery of the main placenta, to which they usually have vascular connections of fetal origin (see Fig. 5–15). It is a smaller version of the bilobed placenta and its incidence is about 5 percent (Benirschke and Kaufmann, 2000). The accessory lobe may sometimes be retained in the uterus after expulsion of the main placenta, and may subsequently give rise to serious hemorrhage. If, on placental examination, defects are seen in the membranes a short distance from the placental margin, retention of a succenturiate lobe should be suspected. The suspicion is confirmed if vessels extend from the placenta to the margins of the tear.

RING-SHAPED PLACENTA. This is a rare anomaly seen in fewer than 1 in 6000 deliveries. The placenta is annular in shape and sometimes a complete ring of placental tissue is present, but because of atrophy of a portion of the tissue of the ring, a horseshoe shape is more common. These abnormalities appear to be associated with a greater likelihood of antepartum and postpartum bleeding and fetal growth restriction. This anomaly may be a variant of membranaceous placenta (Fox, 1978).

MEMBRANACEOUS PLACENTA. In rare circumstances, all of the fetal membranes are covered by functioning villi, and the placenta develops as a thin membranous structure occupying the entire periphery of the chorion. *Placenta membranacea* (Fig. 32–2) is also referred to as *placenta diffusa*. It may occasionally give rise to serious hemorrhage because of associated placenta previa, and diagnosis can often be made using sonography. After delivery, the placenta may not separate readily. Bleeding resembles that seen in central placenta previa, and it may be necessary to perform a hysterectomy to control bleeding from the large area of implantation.

FENESTRATED PLACENTA. This is a rare anomaly in which the central portion of a discoidal placenta is missing. In some instances, there is an actual hole in the

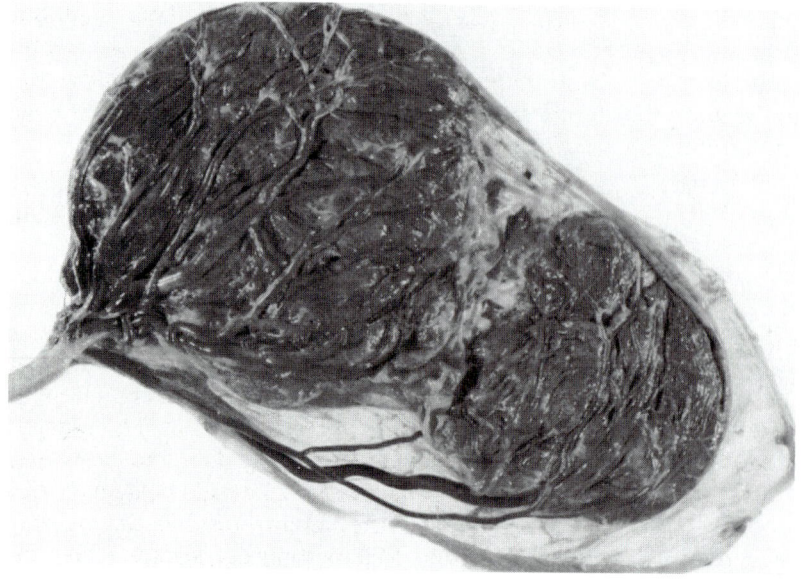

FIGURE 32–1. Placenta demonstrating bilobed structure, marginal insertion of umbilical cord, and partial velamentous insertion of cord (fetal vessels traversing membranes to reach smaller placental lobe on right).

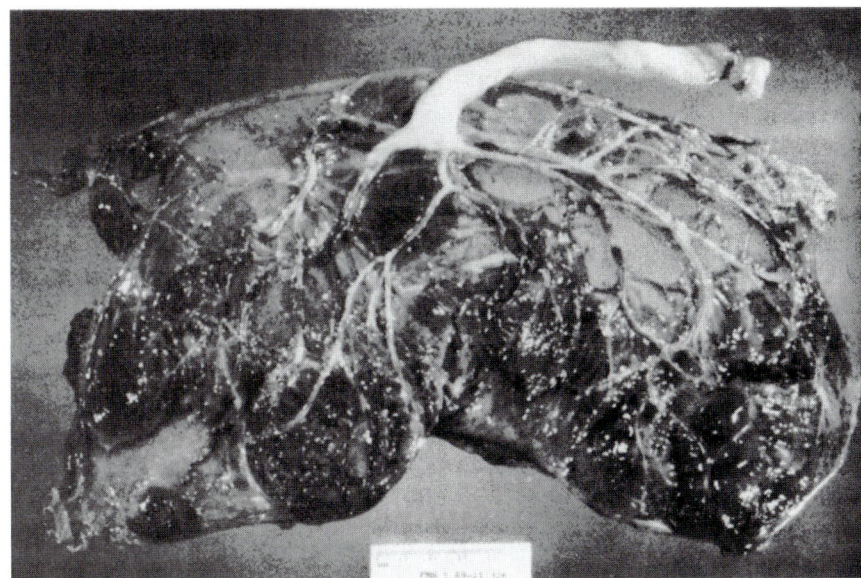

FIGURE 32–2. Placenta membranacea. (From Ramin and Gilstrap, 1992, with permission.)

placenta, but more often the defect involves villous tissue only, and the chorionic plate is intact. The clinical significance of this anomaly is that it may be mistakenly considered to represent a missing portion that has been retained in the uterus.

EXTRACHORIAL PLACENTA. This is a common variation and Benirschke and Kaufmann (2000) found it in 5.3 percent of over 13,500 consecutive placentas. It forms when the chorionic plate, which is on the fetal side of the placenta, is smaller than the basal plate, which is located on the maternal side. If the fetal surface of such a placenta presents a central depression surrounded by a thickened, grayish-white ring, it is called a *circumvallate placenta.* When the ring coincides with the placental margin, the condition is sometimes described as a *circummarginate placenta.* Within the ring, the fetal surface presents the usual appearance, gives attachment to the umbilical cord, and shows the usual large vessels, which terminate abruptly at the margin of the ring. In a circumvallate placenta, the ring is composed of a double fold of amnion and chorion, with degenerated decidua and fibrin in between. In a marginate placenta, the chorion and amnion are raised at the margin by interposed decidua and fibrin, without folding of the membranes (Fig. 32–3). The cause of circumvallate and circummarginate placentation is not completely understood. Antepartum hemorrhage—both from placental abruption and fetal hemorrhage, preterm delivery, perinatal deaths, and fetal malformations are reported to be increased with circumvallate placentas (Benirschke, 1974; Lademacher and co-workers, 1981).

PLACENTA ACCRETA, INCRETA, AND PERCRETA. In these cases, trophoblastic tissues invade the myometrial

tissues. Because of their importance clinically, these are discussed in Chapter 25 (p. 632).

CIRCULATORY DISTURBANCES

PLACENTAL INFARCTS. The most common placental lesions, though of diverse origin, are referred to collectively as placental infarcts. Fox (1978) found that about a fourth of placentas from uncomplicated term pregnancies have infarcts, while pregnancies complicated by severe hypertensive disease are infarcted in about two thirds of cases. They result from occlusion of the maternal vascular supply, that is, the intervillous circulation (Benirschke and Kaufmann, 2000). The principal histopathological features include fibrinoid degeneration of the trophoblast, calcification, and ischemic infarction from occlusion of spiral arteries. Overclassification of these infarcts has led to unnecessary confusion. Small subchorionic and marginal foci of degeneration are present in almost every term placenta. In simplest terms, degenerative lesions of the placenta have two etiological factors in common:

1. Changes associated with aging of the trophoblast.
2. Impairment of the uteroplacental circulation causing infarction.

Although the placenta is by no means a dying organ at term, there are morphological indications of aging. During the latter half of pregnancy, syncytial degeneration begins and *syncytial knots* are formed. The villous stroma usually undergoes hyalinization. The syncytium may then break away, exposing the connective tissue directly to maternal blood. Clotting occurs as a result, and propagation of the clot may result in the incorporation of other villi. Macroscopically, such a focus closely

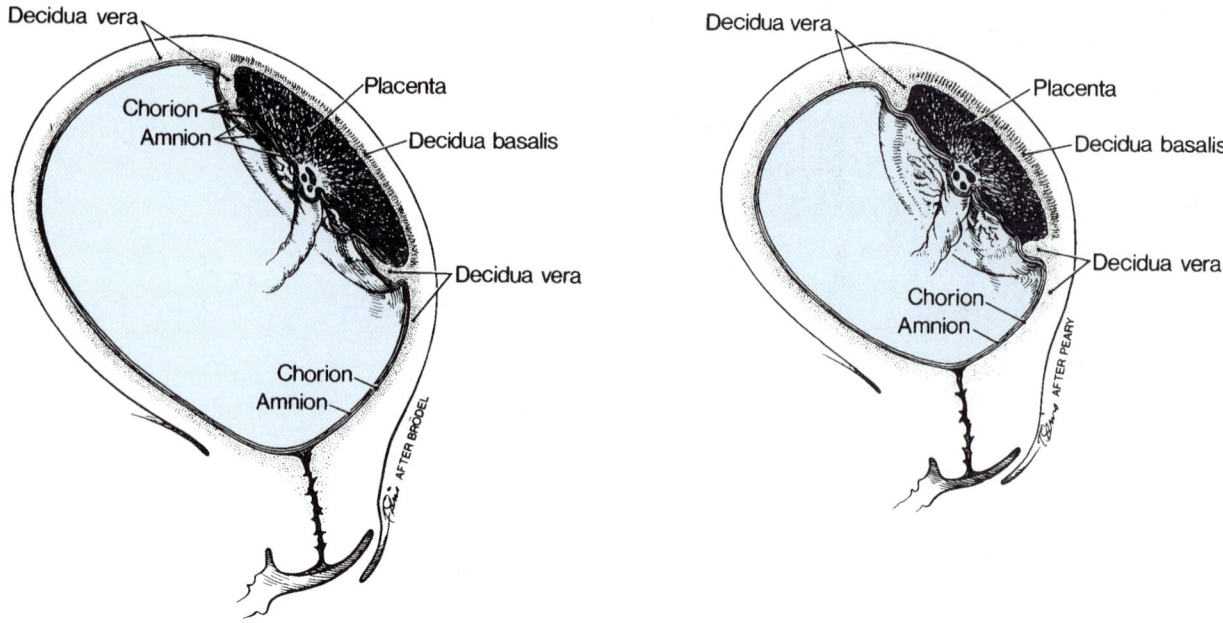

FIGURE 32–3. Circumvallate (*left*) and marginate (*right*) varieties of extrachorial placentas.

resembles an ordinary blood clot, but if not observed until it has become thoroughly organized, on section a firm, white island of tissue is seen.

Around the edge of nearly every term placenta there is a dense yellowish-white fibrous ring representing a zone of degeneration and necrosis, which usually is termed a *marginal infarct.* Underneath the chorionic plate, there are nearly always similar lesions, most often pyramidal shaped, ranging from 2 mm to 3 cm across the base, and extending downward with their apices in the intervillous space (*subchorionic infarcts*). Similar lesions may be noted about the intercotyledonary septa. Occasionally, these lesions meet and form a column of cartilage-like material extending from the maternal surface to the fetal surface. Less frequently, round or oval islands of similar tissue occupy the central portions of the placenta (Fig. 32–4).

PLACENTAL CALCIFICATION. Small calcareous nodules or plaques are frequently observed on the maternal surface of the placenta. An extensive deposition of calcium is shown in Figure 32–5. Placental calcification may be visualized using sonography, and Spirit and colleagues (1982) reported that by 33 weeks more than half of placentas have some degree of calcification, which increases substantively until term. Placental calcification graded ultrasonically has been correlated with fetal lung maturity (Grannum and co-workers, 1979); however, this correlation is not of sufficient strength to justify elective delivery.

VILLOUS (FETAL) ARTERY THROMBOSIS. Thrombosis of a stem artery produces a sharply demarcated area of avascularity. Fox (1978) found single-artery thrombosis in 4.5 percent of placentas from normal pregnancies and in 10 percent of those involving diabetic women. He estimated that thrombosis of a single fetal stem artery will deprive only 5 percent of the villi of their blood supply. However, he also observed a few placentas from recent stillbirths in which 40 to 50 percent of the villi were so deprived. According to Benirschke and Kaufmann (2000), these lesions indicate a pathological prenatal environment.

CLINICAL SIGNIFICANCE. In general, placental infarcts, caused either by local deposition of fibrin or by the more acute process of intervillous thrombosis, have little clinical significance. Nonetheless, in certain maternal diseases, notably severe hypertension, the reduction in functioning placenta through infarction, coupled with reduced blood flow to the uterus, may be sufficient to cause fetal growth restriction or death.

Villous (fetal) vessels may show endarteritic thickening and obliteration in association with fetal death. This is termed *hemorrhagic endovasculitis* (*HEV*). When the placental villi are excluded from their supply of maternal blood by fibrin deposits, hematomas, or direct blockage of the decidual circulation, they become infarcted and die. Histologically, the compromised villi are characterized by fibrosis, obliteration of fetal vessels, and gradual disappearance of the syncytium. Shen-

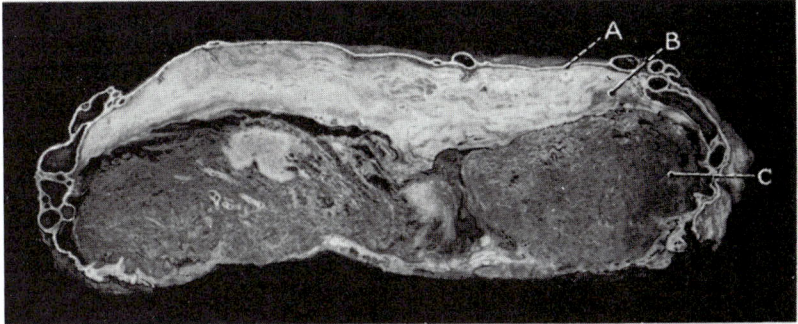

A

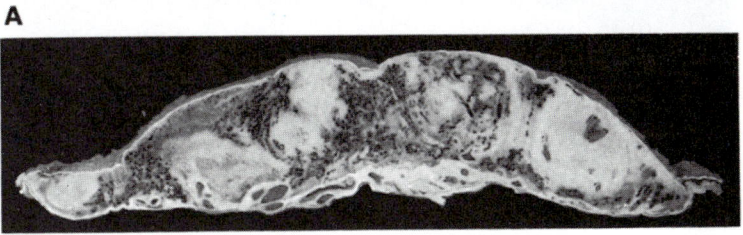

B

FIGURE 32–4. **A.** Placental infarcts. (A = chorio-amnionic membrane; B = fibrin deposited locally beneath the chorion; C = normal placental tissue.) In this instance, the infarct was unusually extensive, most likely contributing to the death of the fetus. **B.** Generalized fibrin deposition with little normal tissue remaining.

Schwarz and associates (1988) described hemorrhagic endovasculitis in less than 1 percent of placentas.

HYPERTROPHIC LESIONS OF THE CHORIONIC VILLI. Striking enlargement of the chorionic villi is commonly seen in association with severe erythroblastosis and fetal hydrops. It has also been described in diabetes and occasionally in severe fetal congestive heart failure.

MICROSCOPIC PLACENTAL ABNORMALITIES. Beginning after 32 weeks, clumps of syncytial nuclei are found to project into the intervillous space, and these are called *syncytial knots.* By term, up to 30 percent of villi may be involved; however, formation of knots by more than one third of villi is considered abnormal (Fox, 1978). In prolonged pregnancies there are marked increases in syncytial knots and avascular villi as the consequence of fetal artery thrombosis. Generally, increased numbers of syncytial knots are found in placentas in which there may have been reduced uteroplacental blood flow, as with preeclampsia.

It is well recognized that the number of *cytotrophoblastic* cells becomes progressively reduced as pregnancy advances. In a normal mature placenta, cytotrophoblastic cells are found in about 20 percent of the villi (Fox, 1978). Most often, at this stage of pregnancy such cells are few and inconspicuous. However, numerous cytotrophoblastic cells are found in placentas of pregnant women with diabetes mellitus, erythroblastosis fetalis, and pregnancy-induced hypertension.

PLACENTAL INFLAMMATION. Changes that are now recognized as various forms of degeneration and necro-

sis were formerly described under the term *placentitis.* For example, small placental cysts with grumous contents were formerly thought to be abscesses. Nonetheless, especially in cases of prolonged rupture of the membranes, pyogenic bacteria do invade the fetal surface of the placenta, and after gaining access to the chorionic vessels, give rise to fetal infection.

ABNORMALITIES OF THE UMBILICAL CORD (FUNIS). The cord develops in close association with the amnion (Chap. 5, p. 105).

LENGTH. Umbilical cord length varies appreciably, with the mean length at term being about 55 to 60 cm (Benirschke and Kaufmann, 2000). Extremes in cord length in abnormal instances range from apparently no cord (achordia) to lengths up to 300 cm. Vascular occlusion by thrombi and true knots are more common in excessively long cords, and they are more likely to prolapse through the cervix. Rarely, excessively short umbilical cords may be instrumental in abruptio placentae and uterine inversion.

Determinants of cord length are intriguing. Studies performed on animals and experiments of nature in human pregnancy support the concept that cord length is positively influenced by the volume of amnionic fluid and by fetal mobility. Miller and associates (1981) identified the human umbilical cord to be shortened appreciably when there had been either chronic fetal constraint from oligohydramnios or decreased fetal movement because of limb dysfunction. Excessive cord length may be the consequence of entanglement of cord and fetus with stretching during fetal movement. Soernes and

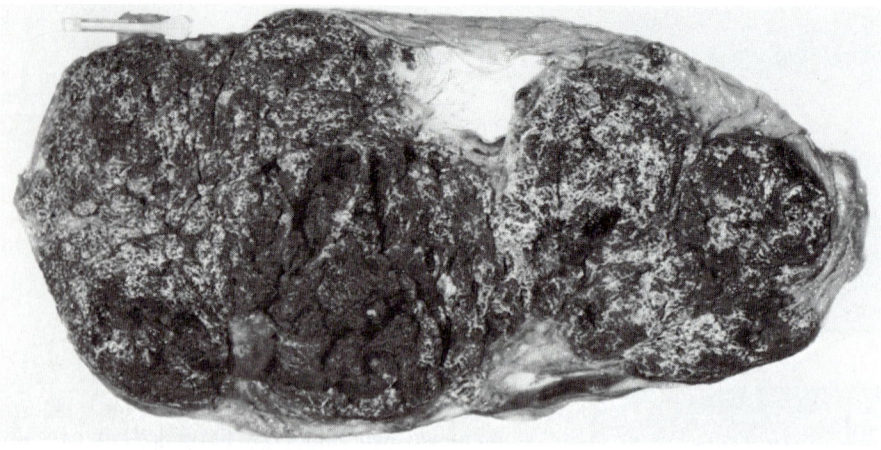

A

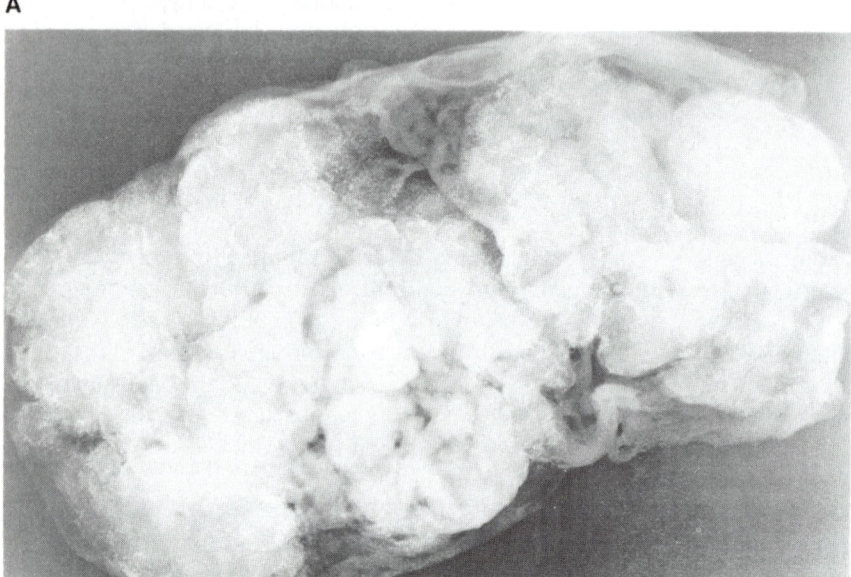

B

FIGURE 32–5. A. Placental calcification is evident as gray plaques on the maternal surface of the placenta, a common finding at term. **B.** A radiograph of the same placenta emphasizes the extensive calcification.

Bakke (1986) reported that the mean cord length in fetuses with breech presentations was about 5 cm shorter than those with vertex presentations.

SINGLE UMBILICAL ARTERY. The absence of one umbilical artery, according to Benirschke and Dodds (1967), characterized 0.85 percent of all cords in singletons and 5 percent of the cords of at least one twin. **About 30 percent of all infants with only one umbilical artery had associated congenital anomalies.** The incidence ranged from 18 to 68 percent (Herrmann and Sidiropoulos, 1988; Leung and Robson, 1989). Bryan and Kohler (1975) identified single-artery umbilical cords of 143 infants out of nearly 20,000 examined (0.72 percent). Infants with a single-artery cord had an 18 percent incidence of major malformations, 34 percent were growth-restricted, and 17 percent delivered preterm. The authors followed 90 infants and found previously unrecognized malformations in another 10.

The incidence of a single umbilical artery is increased considerably in newborns of women with diabetes, epilepsy, preeclampsia, antepartum hemorrhage, oligohydramnios, and hydramnios (Leung and Robson, 1989). Most of these conditions are associated with a threefold increase in anomalous fetuses.

Two-vessel cords are more frequently identified in fetuses aborted spontaneously. For example, Byrne and Blanc (1985) studied 879 consecutively aborted fetuses and identified a single umbilical artery in 1.5 percent. Eight of these 13 fetuses had serious malformations, most associated with chromosomal abnormalities.

Parilla and colleagues (1995) reviewed 50 neonates with a two-vessel umbilical cord as an isolated finding on prenatal ultrasound. They reported that as an isolated finding, a single umbilical artery was not associated with adverse outcomes. All 17 women who underwent amniocentesis had a fetus with a normal karyotype. Catanzarite (1995), however, cautioned that an isolated single umbilical artery may be associated with adverse outcomes. Two fetuses were reported with lethal chromosomal abnormalities and one fetus with a tracheoesophageal fistula out of 46 infants with a single umbilical artery.

Pavlopoulos and colleagues (1998) found an increase in renal aplasia, limb-reduction defects, and atresia of hollow organs in such fetuses, suggesting a vascular etiology. In a Doppler velocimetry study of 45 fetuses with single umbilical arteries compared with 124 normal controls, Goldkrand and colleagues (1999) found indices in the normal range but lower than in normal cords beginning at 26 weeks. Congenital anomalies were present in approximately 10 percent of fetuses with a single umbilical artery and fetal growth restriction was present in 20 percent of such fetuses. Raio and colleagues (1999) reported an association between single umbilical artery and a reduction of Wharton jelly. They postulated that such reduction may be responsible, at least in part, for the increased morbidity and mortality in these fetuses.

CORD COILING. In most cases, the umbilical vessels course through the umbilical cord in a spiraled manner. Several authors have observed a significant increase in various indices of adverse perinatal outcome in fetuses with hypocoiled cords, including meconium staining, preterm birth, and operative delivery for fetal distress (Strong and colleagues, 1993, 1994). Shen-Schwarz and associates (1996) reported an association between "absent" cord twist and marginal and velamentous cord insertion. Rana and associates (1995) also demonstrated a higher incidence of preterm delivery and cocaine abuse in women with hypercoiled cords.

FOUR-VESSEL CORD. Additional umbilical vessels are rarely apparent on casual inspection; however, careful inspection may disclose a venous remnant in 5 percent of cases (Fox, 1978). Its significance is unknown.

CORD INSERTION. The umbilical cord usually, but not always, is inserted at or near the center of the fetal surface of the placenta.

MARGINAL INSERTION. Cord insertion at the placental margin is sometimes referred to as a *Battledore placenta.* It is found in about 7 percent of term placentas (Benirschke and Kaufmann, 2000). With the exception of the cord being pulled off during delivery of the placenta, it is of little clinical significance.

VELAMENTOUS INSERTION. This type of cord insertion is of considerable practical importance because the umbilical vessels separate in the membranes at a distance from the placental margin, which they reach surrounded only by a fold of amnion (Figs. 32–1 and 32–6).

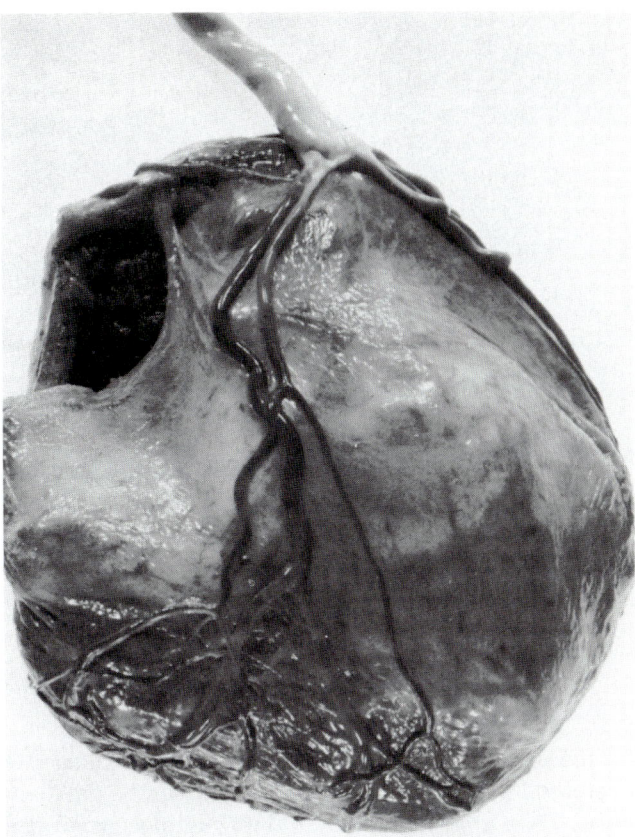

Figure 32–6. Velamentous insertion of the cord. The placenta (*bottom*) and membranes have been inverted to expose the amnion. Note the large fetal vessels within membranes (*top*) and their proximity to the site of rupture of the membranes.

In a review of the literature totaling almost 195,000 cases, Benirschke and Kaufmann (2000) found an average of 1.1 percent of singleton deliveries to have velamentous insertion. It occurs much more frequently with twins, and it is almost the rule with triplets.

VASA PREVIA. This is associated with velamentous insertion when some of the fetal vessels in the membranes cross the region of the internal os and occupy a position ahead of the presenting part. At times, the careful examiner will be able to palpate a tubular fetal vessel in the membranes overlying the presenting part. Compression of the vessels between the examining finger and the presenting part is likely to induce changes in the fetal heart rate. At times, the vessels may be visualized directly, or they may be seen on ultrasonic examination (Fig. 32–7). With vasa previa, there is considerable potential danger to the fetus, for rupture of the membranes may be accompanied by rupture of a fetal vessel, causing exsanguination.

Fung and Lau (1998) described three cases of vasa previa and reviewed the literature of other cases re-

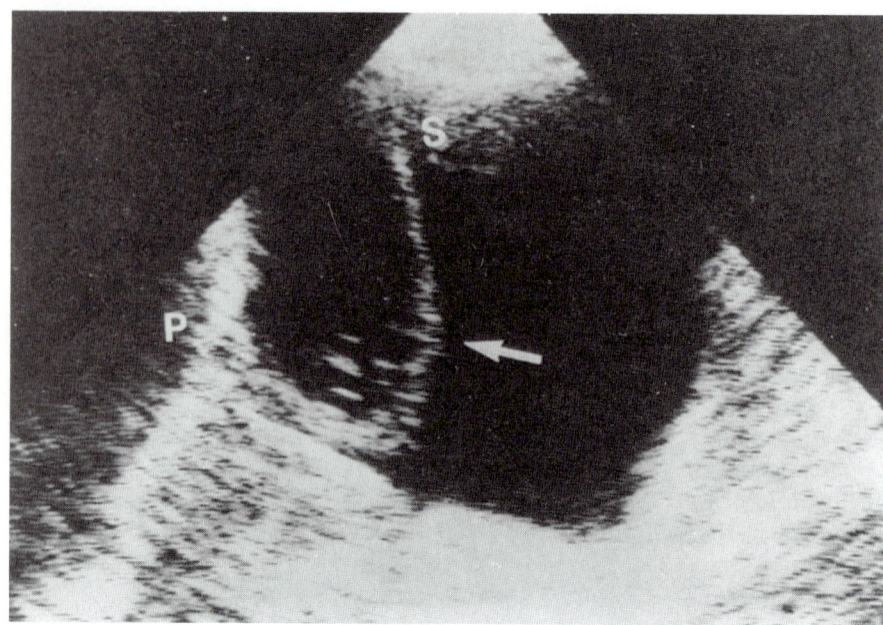

FIGURE 32–7. Sonogram showing placenta (P), succenturiate lobe (S), and leading fetal vessels in *vasa previa* (*arrow*). (From Gianopoulos and colleagues, 1987, with permission.)

ported since 1980. These authors reported a significantly decreased fetal mortality associated with antenatal diagnosis. They also found that a low-lying placenta was a risk factor in 80 percent of cases. In another review by Oyelese and colleagues (1999), transvaginal ultrasound with color Doppler was recommended for antenatal diagnosis in women with risk factors such as a bilobed or succenturiate placenta, low-lying placenta, multiple pregnancy, or pregnancy resulting from in vitro fertilization. In a prospective study of 45 women with placenta previa in the third trimester, Megier and colleagues (1999) found 20 previas over the internal cervical os and three of these had vasa previa.

In an 8-year survey of over 90,000 women who had gray-scale ultrasonography, Lee and colleagues (2000) utilized endovaginal and Doppler studies to confirm vasa previa in women whose initial ultrasound demonstrated an "echogenic parallel or circular line near the cervix." These authors were able to detect vasa previa in asymptomatic women as early as the midtrimester. Likewise, Nomiyama and colleagues (1998) were able to diagnose two cases of vasa previa at 18 weeks with transvaginal color Doppler imaging.

Whenever there is hemorrhage antepartum or intrapartum, the possibility of vasa previa and a ruptured fetal vessel exists. Unfortunately, the amount of fetal blood that can be shed without killing the fetus is relatively small. A quick, readily available approach to detecting fetal blood is to smear the blood on glass slides, stain the smears with Wright stain, and examine for nucleated red cells, which normally are present in cord blood but not maternal blood.

CORD ABNORMALITIES CAPABLE OF IMPEDING BLOOD FLOW. Several mechanical and vascular abnormalities of the umbilical cord are capable of impairing fetal–placental blood flow.

KNOTS. *False knots,* which result from kinking of the vessels to accommodate to the length of the cord, should be distinguished from *true knots,* which result from active fetal movements. In nearly 17,000 deliveries in the Collaborative Study on Cerebral Palsy, Spellacy and coworkers (1966) found an incidence of true knots of 1.1 percent. Perinatal loss was 6 percent in the presence of true knots. The incidence of true knots is especially high in monoamnionic twins.

LOOPS. The cord frequently becomes coiled around portions of the fetus, usually the neck. In 1000 consecutive deliveries studied by Kan and Eastman (1957), the incidence of the umbilical cord around the neck ranged from one loop in 21 percent to three loops in 0.2 percent. Fortunately, coiling of the cord around the neck is an uncommon cause of fetal death. Typically, as labor progresses and the fetus descends the birth canal, contractions compress the cord vessels, which cause fetal heart rate deceleration that persists until the contraction ceases. Hankins and colleagues (1987a) reported 110 pregnancies in which labor at term was complicated by a nuchal cord. Compared with control infants, those with a nuchal cord had more moderate or severe variable fetal heart rate decelerations (20 versus 5 percent). They also were more likely to have a lower umbilical artery pH. Interestingly, none of the newborns had pathological fetal acidemia (pH less than 7.00).

TORSION. As a result of fetal movements, the cord normally becomes twisted. Occasionally, the torsion is so marked that fetal circulation is compromised. Extreme degrees may occur after the death of the fetus by a mechanism that is not understood. In monoamnionic twinning, a significant fraction of the high perinatal mortality rate is attributed to entwining of the umbilical cords before labor.

STRICTURE. Most, but not all, infants with cord stricture are stillborns; the stricture probably has a role in fetal death. Cord stricture, for unknown reasons, is associated with an extreme focal deficiency in Wharton jelly. Stricture is commonly and causally associated with torsion.

HEMATOMA. These occasionally result from the rupture of a varix, usually of the umbilical vein, with effusion of blood into the cord (Fig. 32–8). Cord hematomas have also been described as resulting from ultrasound-directed umbilical vessel venipuncture.

CYSTS. Occasionally found along the course of the cord, cysts are designated true and false, according to their origin. True cysts are quite small and may be derived from remnants of the umbilical vesicle or of the allantois. False cysts, which may attain considerable size, result from liquefaction of Wharton jelly. Such cysts may be detected by sonography but are difficult to identify precisely. For example, the cyst demonstrated in Figure

32–9 was thought to possibly be a meningocele when detected by sonography, because the cyst maintained a close and constant relationship over time with the lower spine of the fetus.

EDEMA. Placental and cord edema are rarely seen alone, but are frequently associated with edema of the fetus. They are very common with macerated fetuses.

PATHOLOGICAL EXAMINATION. The College of American Pathologists (1991) recommends routine pathological examination of the placenta with certain obstetrical and neonatal conditions. Conversely, the American College of Obstetricians and Gynecologists (1993a) feels that there are insufficient data to support this recommendation, which is costly and time consuming. Certainly, the placenta and cord—including the number of vessels—should be grossly examined following all deliveries. Although pathological examination may be useful in the diagnosis of some unusual conditions, such as microabscesses seen with listeriosis, the possible correlation of specific placental findings with both short- and long-term neonatal outcome is still unclear. Currently, routine placental examination in all births does not appear to be justified on either a scientific or cost-effective basis. Pathological placental examination, however, as well as fetal autopsy, frequently prove useful in determining the cause of stillbirth (Chap. 39, p. 1074).

GESTATIONAL TROPHOBLASTIC DISEASE

There is a spectrum of pregnancy-related trophoblastic proliferative abnormalities, the classification of which for many years was based principally on histological criteria and included hydatidiform mole, invasive mole, and choriocarcinoma. Subsequently, a classification was proposed based principally upon clinical findings and serial determinations of serum levels of chorionic gonadotropin which is secreted by the abnormal tissue (Hammond and colleagues, 1973). Although these two classifications have caused some confusion, the clinical approach is now accepted.

In 1983, the World Health Organization Scientific Group on Gestational Trophoblastic Diseases published specific recommendations regarding terminology for the definition, classification, and staging of trophoblastic disease. Basically, gestational trophoblastic disease can be divided into **hydatidiform mole** and **gestational trophoblastic tumors** (Table 32–1). The term *gestational trophoblastic neoplasia* is no longer employed because invasive moles are not true neoplasms (Miller and Lurain, 1988). As shown in Table 32–1, gestational trophoblastic tumors can be classified clinically as nonmeta-

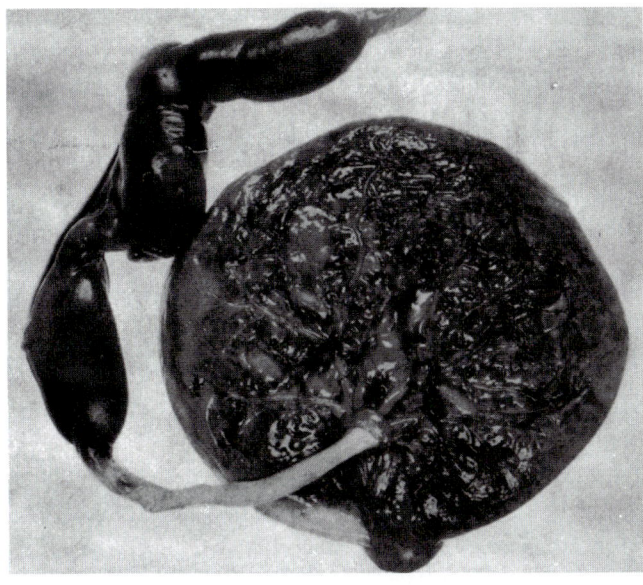

FIGURE 32–8. Hematoma of the umbilical cord.

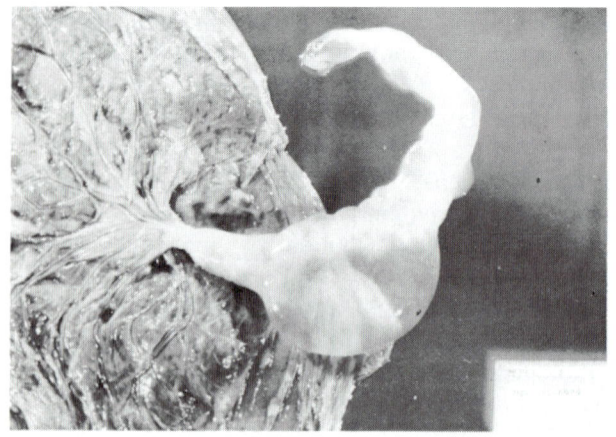

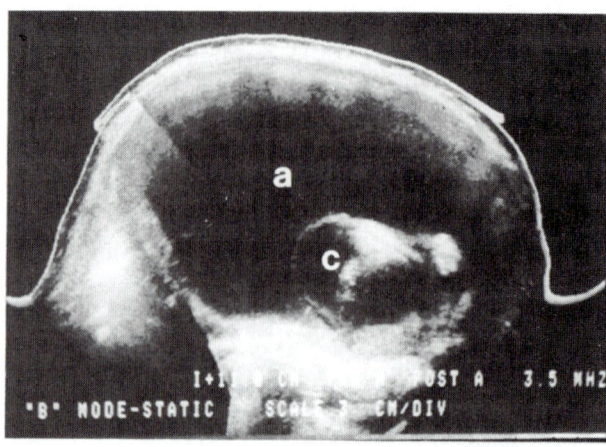

A   **B**

FIGURE 32–9. A. Cyst of umbilical cord at 27 weeks' gestation in a monoamnionic twin pregnancy, further complicated by symptomatic acute hydramnios and marked discordance in the size of the fetuses. **B.** Sonogram from the same case demonstrating the cyst of the cord (c) and marked hydramnios (a). The possibility that the cyst was a meningocele was considered originally. (Courtesy of Dr. R. Santos.)

static and metastatic, and the latter are subdivided into low risk and high risk.

HYDATIDIFORM MOLE (MOLAR PREGNANCY). Molar pregnancy is characterized histologically by abnormalities of the chorionic villi consisting of varying degrees of trophoblastic proliferation and edema of villous stroma. Moles usually occupy the uterine cavity; however, they may occasionally be located in the oviduct and even the ovary (Stanhope and associates, 1983). The absence or presence of a fetus or embryonic elements has been used to classify them into *complete* and *partial* moles (Table 32–2). As emphasized by Benirschke and Kaufmann (2000), in many cases this is difficult.

COMPLETE HYDATIDIFORM MOLE. The chorionic villi are converted into a mass of clear vesicles (Fig. 32–10). The vesicles vary in size from barely visible to a few centimeters in diameter and often hang in clusters from thin pedicles. The histological structure demonstrated in Figure 32–11 is characterized by:

1. Hydropic degeneration and swelling of the villous stroma.
2. Absence of blood vessels in the swollen villi.
3. Proliferation of the trophoblastic epithelium to a varying degree.
4. Absence of fetus and amnion.

Hydropic or molar degeneration, which may be confused with a true mole, is not classified as trophoblastic disease (Berkowitz and associates, 1991).

Cytogenetic studies of complete molar pregnancies have identified the chromosomal composition most of-

ten (85 percent or more) to be 46, XX, with the chromosomes completely of paternal origin (Wolf and Lage, 1995). This phenomenon is referred to as *androgenesis.* Typically, the ovum has been fertilized by a haploid sperm, which then duplicates its own chromosomes after meiosis, and thus the chromosomes are homozygous. The chromosomes of the ovum are either absent or inactivated. Occasionally, the chromosomal pattern in a complete mole may be 46,XY, that is, heterozygous due to dispermic fertilization (Bagshawe and Lawler, 1982; Lawler and colleagues, 1991).

TABLE 32–1. Classification of Gestational Trophoblastic Disease

Hydatidiform Mole
Complete
Partial
Gestational trophoblastic tumors
Nonmetastatic
Metastatic
Low risk—no risk factors
High risk—any risk factor
Pretherapy hCG level > 40,000 mIU/mL
Duration > 4 months
Brain or liver metastases
Prior chemotherapy failure
Antecedent term pregnancy

hCG = human chorionic gonadotropin.
From the American College of Obstetricians and Gynecologists (1993b), with permission.

TABLE 32–2. Features of Partial and Complete Hydatidiform Moles

Feature	Partial Mole	Complete Mole
Karyotype	Most commonly 69,XXX or 69,XXY	46,XX or 46,XY
Pathology		
Fetus	Often present	Absent
Amnion, fetal red blood cells	Often present	Absent
Villous edema	Variable, focal	Diffuse
Trophoblastic proliferation	Variable, focal, slight to moderate	Variable, slight to severe
Clinical presentation		
Diagnosis	Missed abortion	Molar gestation
Uterine size	Small for dates	50% large for dates
Theca-lutein cysts	Rare	25–30%
Medical complications	Rare	Frequent
Postmolar disease	Less than 5–10%	20%

From the American College of Obstetricians and Gynecologists (1993b), with permission.

Lawler and colleagues (1991) described 202 hydatidiform moles; 151 were complete and 49 partial moles. The genetic ploidy of these moles is summarized in Table 32–3. The majority (85 percent) of complete moles are diploid whereas most partial moles (86 percent) are triploid. Other variations have been described, such as 45,X. Thus, a morphologically complete mole can result from a variety of chromosomal patterns (Wolfe and Lage, 1995). The risk of trophoblastic tumors developing from a complete mole is approximately 20 percent (Table 32–2).

PARTIAL HYDATIDIFORM MOLE. When the hydatidiform changes are focal and less advanced, and maybe some fetal tissues, usually at least an amnionic sac, is seen, the condition is classified as a partial hydatidiform mole. There is slowly progressing hydatidiform swelling of some usually avascular villi, while other vascular villi with a functioning fetal–placental circulation are spared. Trophoblastic hyperplasia is focal rather than generalized.

As shown in Table 32–3, the karyotype typically is triploid—69,XXX, 69,XXY, or 69,XYY—with one maternal but usually two paternal haploid complements (Berkowitz and colleagues, 1986, 1991; Wolfe and Lage, 1995). The fetus of a partial mole typically has stigmata of triploidy, which includes multiple congenital malformations and growth restriction, and it is nonviable. In the report by Lawler and colleagues (1991), 86 percent of partial moles were triploid and 2 percent were diploid.

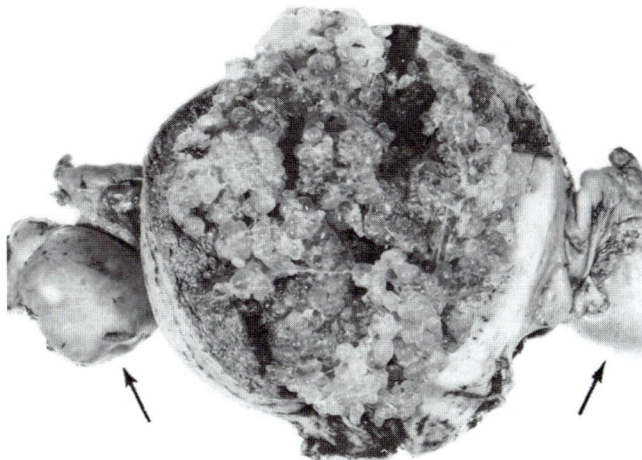

FIGURE 32–10. A complete (classic) hydatidiform mole characterized grossly by abundance of edematous enlarged chorionic villi but no fetus or fetal membranes. Note theca-lutein cysts in each ovary (*arrows*).

TABLE 32–3. Chromosomal Composition of 200 Hydatidiform Moles

Chromosomes	Complete (n = 151) No. (%)	Partial (n = 49) No. (%)
Haploid	1 (0.7)	—
Diploid	128 (85)	1 (2)
Triploid	3 (2)	42 (86)
Tetraploid	—	2 (4)
Unknown	19 (13)	4 (8)

Adapted from Lawler and colleagues (1991), with permission.

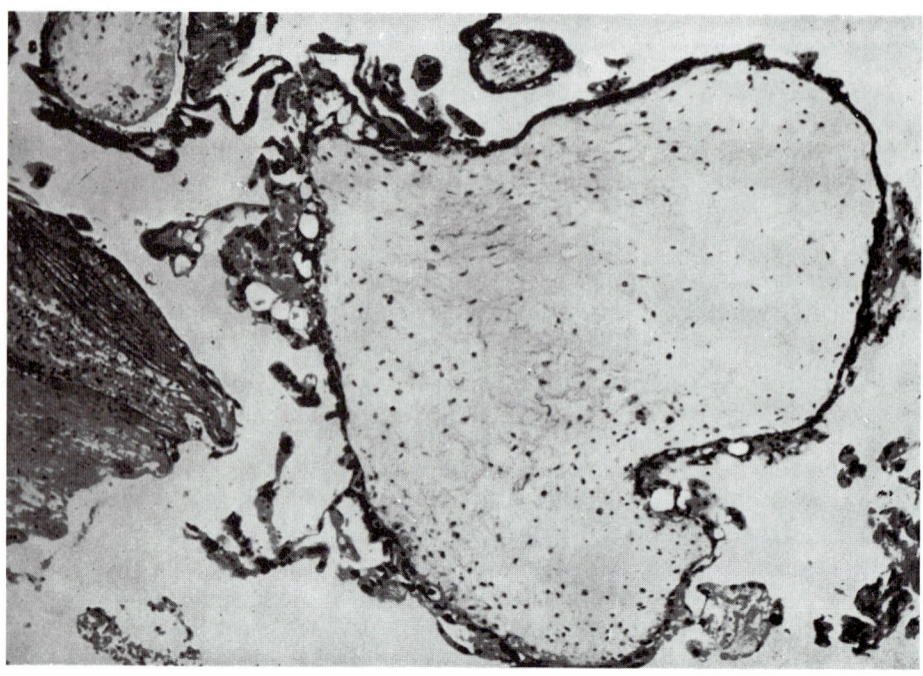

FIGURE 32–11. Photomicrograph of a hydatidiform mole with slight to moderate trophoblastic hyperplasia, confined to the syncytium and considered as probably benign. (From Smalbraak, 1957.)

Jauniaux (1999), in a review of partial moles, reported that 82 percent of fetuses with triploid karyotypes had symmetrical growth restriction. Jauniaux and colleagues (1998) also reported a case of partial mole with trisomy 13. Lembet and colleagues (2000) recently reported a case of partial hydatidiform mole with a diploid karyotype and a live fetus.

A twin gestation of a complete mole and a normal fetus and placenta is sometimes misdiagnosed as a diploid partial mole (Fig. 32–12). It is important to attempt to distinguish between the two, because twin pregnancies consisting of a normal fetus and a complete mole have a 50 percent chance of subsequent persistent trophoblastic disease compared with a much lower rate with triploid partial moles (Bruchim and associates, 2000). Van de Kaa and colleagues (1995) described the use of interphase cytogenetics and DNA cytometric analysis to help distinguish between these two entities.

Nonmetastatic trophoblastic tumors may follow hydatidiform mole in 4 to 8 percent of cases (Berkowitz

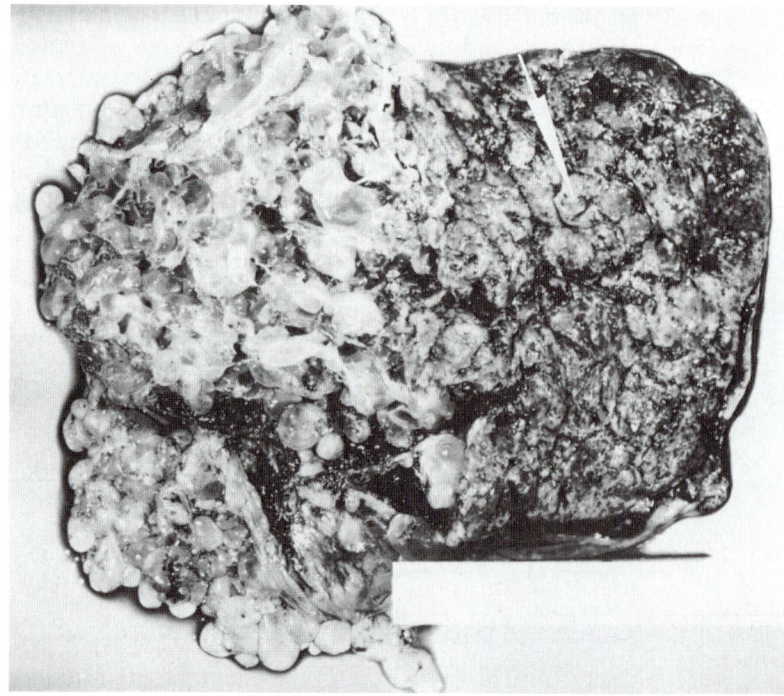

FIGURE 32–12. Molar placenta on the left and normal placenta (*white arrow*) on the right. The molar placenta was identified by sonography late in pregnancy when the mother developed preeclampsia. A healthy fetus was delivered near term by cesarean section. Most likely, these were twins consisting of a placenta with a fetus from one ovum and a complete mole developing from the other ovum.

and colleagues, 1986; Szulman and Surti, 1982). The risk of choriocarcinoma arising from a partial mole is very low. Seckl and associates (2000) described 3000 cases of partial mole and documented only three cases of choriocarcinoma.

Vejerslev (1991) reviewed the outcomes of pregnancies reported with a hydatidiform mole coexistent with a normal fetus. Of 113 pregnancies, 52 (45 percent) of fetuses progressed to 28 weeks, and survival was 70 percent. Thus, when providing counseling for women with a coexistent mole and a fetus, both cytogenetic and high-resolution ultrasound studies are of paramount importance.

HISTOLOGICAL DIAGNOSIS. Attempts to relate the histological structure of individual complete hydatidiform moles to their subsequent malignant tendencies have generally been disappointing. Novak and Seah (1954), for example, were unable to precisely establish such a relation in 120 cases of hydatidiform mole or in the molar tissue in 26 cases of choriocarcinoma following hydatidiform mole.

THECA-LUTEIN CYSTS. In many cases of hydatidiform mole, the ovaries contain multiple theca-lutein cysts (Fig. 35–10). These may vary from microscopic size to 10 cm or more in diameter. The surfaces of the cysts are smooth, often yellowish, and lined with lutein cells. The incidence of obvious cysts in association with a mole is reported to be from 25 to 60 percent. These cysts are thought to result from overstimulation of lutein elements by large amounts of chorionic gonadotropin secreted by proliferating trophoblast. In general, extensive cystic change is usually associated with larger hydatidiform moles and a long period of stimulation. Montz and colleagues (1988) reported that persistent trophoblastic disease was more likely in women with theca-lutein cysts, especially if bilateral. Cysts are not limited to cases of hydatidiform mole, and are associated with placental hypertrophy with fetal hydrops or multifetal pregnancy. Some of these, especially very large cysts, may undergo torsion, infarction, and hemorrhage. Because the cysts regress after delivery, oophorectomy should not be performed unless the ovary is extensively infarcted.

INCIDENCE. Hydatidiform mole develops in approximately 1 in 1000 pregnancies in the United States and Europe. Although it has been reported to be more frequent in other countries, especially in parts of Asia, much of this information was based on hospital studies (Schorge and associates, 2000). Based on population studies, the incidence in most of the world is probably similar to that in the United States (Miller and colleagues, 1989; Semer and Macfee, 1995).

AGE. There is a relatively high frequency of hydatidiform mole among pregnancies at the beginning or end of the childbearing period (Semer and Macfee, 1995). The most pronounced effect is seen in women over 45, when the relative frequency of the lesion is more than 10 times greater than at ages 20 to 40 (Schorge and colleagues, 2000). There are numerous authenticated cases of hydatidiform mole in women 50 years old and older.

PREVIOUS MOLE. Recurrence of hydatidiform mole is seen in about 1 to 2 percent of cases (Miller and co-workers, 1989). In a review of 12 series totaling almost 5000 deliveries, the frequency of recurrent moles was 1.3 percent (Loret de Mola and Goldfarb, 1995). Kim and associates (1998) found a 4.3 percent recurrence rate in 115 women followed in Seoul, Korea. In a review of repetitive hydatidiform moles with different partners, Tuncer and colleagues (1999) concluded that there may be "a primary oocyte problem."

OTHER FACTORS. The role of gravidity, parity, other reproductive factors, estrogen status, oral contraceptives, and dietary factors in the risk of gestational trophoblastic disease is unclear (Semer and Macfee, 1995).

CLINICAL COURSE. The clinical presentation of most molar pregnancies has changed appreciably over 20 years because use of transvaginal ultrasound and quantitive serum hCG have led to earlier diagnosis (Coukos and colleagues, 1999). Later in the first trimester and during the second trimester, a number of changes are often evident. Symptoms are more likely to be dramatic with a complete mole. Schlaerth and colleagues (1988) reported complications in two thirds of 381 women with molar pregnancies.

BLEEDING. Uterine bleeding is almost universal, and may vary from spotting to profuse hemorrhage (Rose, 1995). It may begin just before abortion or, more often, it may occur intermittently for weeks or even months. A dilutional effect from appreciable hypervolemia has been demonstrated in some women with larger moles. At times there may be considerable hemorrhage concealed within the uterus. Iron-deficiency anemia is a common finding and infrequently megaloblastic erythropoiesis is evident, presumably as a result of poor dietary intake because of nausea and vomiting coupled with increased folate requirement imposed by rapidly proliferating trophoblast.

UTERINE SIZE. The growing uterus often enlarges more rapidly than usual. It is the most common finding, and in about half of cases, uterine size clearly exceeds that expected from the duration of gestation. The uterus may be difficult to identify precisely by palpation, particularly in the nulliparous woman, because of its soft consistency beneath a firm abdominal wall. At times ovaries appreciably enlarged by multiple theca-lutein cysts may be difficult to distinguish from the enlarged uterus.

FETAL ACTIVITY. Even though the uterus is enlarged sufficiently to reach well above the symphysis, typically no fetal heart action is detected. Rarely, there may be twin placentas with a complete molar pregnancy developing in one, while the other placenta and its fetus appear normal (Fig. 32–12). Also, very infrequently there may be extensive but incomplete molar change in the placenta accompanied by a living fetus.

PREGNANCY-INDUCED HYPERTENSION. Of special importance is the possible association of preeclampsia with molar pregnancies that persist into the second trimester. Because pregnancy-induced hypertension is rarely seen before 24 weeks, preeclampsia that develops before this time should at least suggest hydatidiform mole or extensive molar change.

HYPEREMESIS. Significant nausea and vomiting may occur. Of interest, none of the 24 complete moles reported by Coukos and colleagues (1999) had preeclampsia, hyperemesis, or clinical hyperthyroidism.

THYROTOXICOSIS. Plasma thyroxine levels in women with molar pregnancy are often elevated, but clinically apparent hyperthyroidism is unusual. Amir and colleagues (1984) and Curry and associates (1975) identified hyperthyroidism in about 2 percent of cases. Plasma thyroxine elevation may be the effect primarily of estrogen, as in normal pregnancy, in which case free thyroxine levels are not elevated. As discussed in Chapter 6 (p. 113), serum free thyroxine is elevated as the consequence of either the thyrotropin-like effect of chorionic gonadotropin or its variants (Amir and co-workers, 1984; Mann and colleagues, 1986). Miller and Seifer (1990) reviewed the endocrinological aspects of gestational trophoblastic diseases.

EMBOLIZATION. Variable amounts of trophoblast with or without villous stroma escape from the uterus in the venous outflow at evacuation. The volume may be such as to produce signs and symptoms of acute pulmonary embolism and even a fatal outcome (Fig. 32–13). Such fatalities are rare. Hankins and colleagues (1987b) obtained hemodynamic measurements using a pulmonary artery catheter in six women with large molar pregnancies. They also searched for evidence of **trophoblastic deportation** before and during molar evacuation. Only small numbers of multinucleated giant cells and mononuclear cells, presumably trophoblasts, were identified. They found no evidence for acute cardiore-

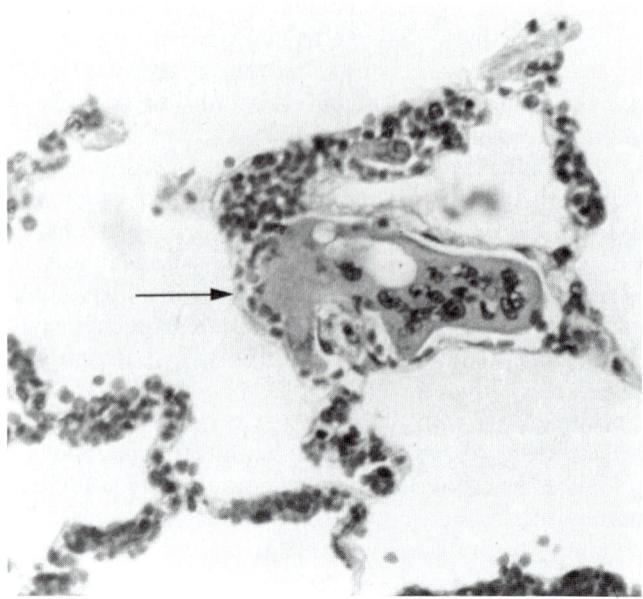

FIGURE 32–13. An embolus of trophoblast within a small pulmonary vein (*arrow*). The woman died from trophoblastic embolization further complicated by massive hemorrhage soon after hysterotomy to evacuate a large hydatidiform mole.

spiratory changes, and concluded that massive trophoblastic embolization with molar evacuation was probably infrequent.

Some, but not most, practitioners believe that medical induction prior to evacuation of a hydatidiform mole may increase the risk of trophoblast embolization or persistent trophoblastic disease. Schlaerth and co-workers (1988) identified respiratory complications in 15 percent of women with a mole larger than 20 weeks' size. In many of these, pregnancy was terminated by hysterotomy or labor induction.

Even though trophoblast, with or without villous stroma, embolizes to the lungs in volumes too small to produce overt blockade of the pulmonary vasculature, these can subsequently invade the pulmonary parenchyma to establish metastases that are evident radiographically. The lesions may consist of trophoblast alone (metastatic choriocarcinoma) or trophoblast with villous stroma (metastatic hydatidiform mole). The subsequent course of such lesions is unpredictable, and some have been observed to disappear spontaneously either soon after uterine evacuation or even weeks to months later, while others proliferate and cause death without treatment.

DIAGNOSTIC FEATURES. In some cases, hydatid vesicles that resemble grapes are passed before the mole is aborted spontaneously or removed by operation (Rose, 1995). Spontaneous expulsion is most likely around 16 weeks and is rarely delayed beyond 28 weeks. Clinical

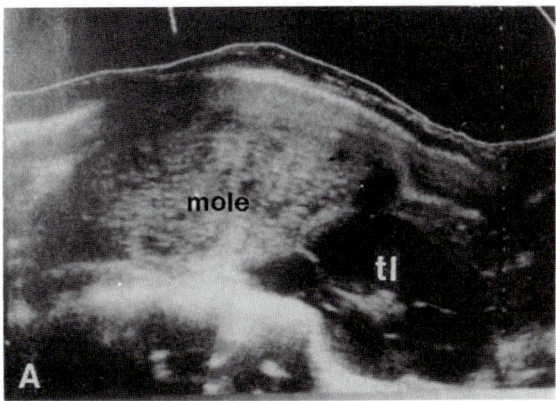
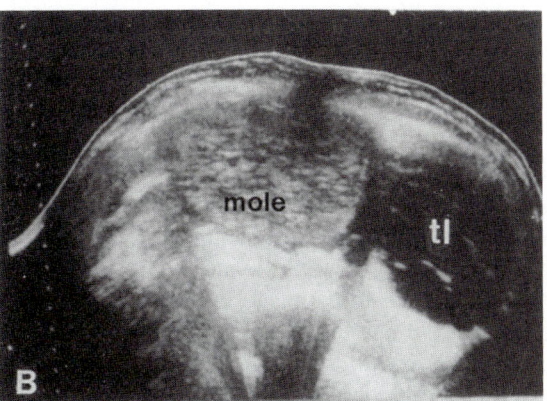

FIGURE 32–14. A. Longitudinal sonogram demonstrating a complete hydatidiform mole that fills a uterus enlarged to well above the umbilicus. A large theca-lutein cyst (tl) is seen above the uterus. **B.** Transverse sonogram of the same woman. (Courtesy of Dr. R. Santos.)

findings of persistent bleeding and a uterus larger than the expected size arouse suspicion for a molar pregnancy. Consideration must be given to an error in menstrual data or a pregnant uterus further enlarged by myomas, hydramnios, or especially multiple fetuses. The greatest diagnostic accuracy is obtained from the characteristic ultrasonic appearance of hydatidiform mole (Fig. 32–14). Occasionally, other structures may have an appearance similar to that of a mole, including uterine myoma and pregnancies with multiple fetuses.

In summary, the clinical and diagnostic features of a complete hydatidiform mole are the following:

- Continuous or intermittent bloody discharge evident by about 12 weeks, usually not profuse, and often more nearly brown rather than red.
- Uterine enlargement out of proportion to the duration of pregnancy in about half of the cases.
- Absence of fetal parts and fetal heart sounds even though the uterus may be enlarged to the level of the umbilicus or higher.
- Characteristic ultrasonic appearance.
- Serum chorionic gonadotropin level higher than expected for the stage of gestation.
- Preeclampsia–eclampsia developing before 24 weeks.
- Hyperemesis gravidarum.

PROGNOSIS. Current mortality from moles has been practically reduced to zero by more prompt diagnosis and appropriate therapy. With advanced molar pregnancies, these women are usually anemic and bleeding acutely. Infection and sepsis in these cases may cause serious morbidity (Schlaerth and colleagues, 1988).

Earlier evacuation unfortunately has not diminished the development of persistent tumors (Schorge and co-workers, 2000).

Nearly 20 percent of complete moles progress to gestational trophoblastic tumor. Lurain and colleagues

(1983) reported follow-up results of 738 patients from 1962 to 1978 following evacuation of a hydatidiform mole. Spontaneous regression occurred in 596 women (81 percent), while gestational trophoblastic tumors developed in 142 (19 percent). Of this latter group, 125 (17 percent) had an invasive mole and 17 (2 percent) had choriocarcinoma. All 142 women with trophoblastic tumors were cured and all 738 patients were free of disease at 4 to 18 years follow-up.

TREATMENT. Hydatidiform mole treatment consists of two phases: immediate evacuation of the mole, and subsequent follow-up for detection of persistent trophoblastic proliferation or malignant change. Initial evaluation prior to evacuation or hysterectomy includes at least a cursory search for metastatic disease. A chest radiograph should be done to look for pulmonary lesions. Although Mutch and colleagues (1986) showed that using computed tomography increased the likelihood of detecting metastatic disease, its routine use has not been evaluated and did not affect prognosis. Unless there is other evidence of extrauterine disease, computed tomography or magnetic resonance imaging to evaluate the liver or brain is not done routinely.

The rare circumstance of twinning with a complete hydatidiform mole plus a fetus and placenta presents an unusual therapeutic dilemma, especially in the absence of karyotypic aberrations or gross fetal anomalies. Neither the risks to the mother nor the likelihood of a healthy offspring have been established. Suzuki and associates (1980) and Vejerslev (1991) reviewed cases in which the outcome was good for both infant and mother.

TERMINATION OF MOLAR PREGNANCY. Because of greater awareness, and certainly because of better technique for diagnosis, moles now are terminated more often when they are still small, and under controlled circumstances rather than the chaos common when they abort spontaneously. Thus, there is time for adequate evaluation of the woman who may be anemic, hypertensive, or fluid depleted.

PROPHYLACTIC CHEMOTHERAPY. The role of prophylactic chemotherapy for women with a hydatidiform mole is controversial (Bloss and Miller, 1995; Goldstein and Berkowitz, 1995). There is no evidence, however, that such therapy improves the long-term prognosis. Not only will the majority of women experience a spontaneous regression of disease following evacuation, but the follow-up of all patients, including those receiving chemotherapy, is essentially the same. Moreover, the toxicity from prophylactic chemotherapy may be significant, including death (Bloss and Miller, 1995).

VACUUM ASPIRATION. Suction evacuation is the treatment of choice for hydatidiform mole, regardless of uterine size (Bloss and Miller, 1995; Miller and colleagues, 1989). For large moles, compatible blood is made ready and an intravenous system is established for its rapid infusion, if needed. Cervical dilating agents described in Chapter 20 (p. 470) are used if the cervix is long, very firm, and closed. Further dilatation can be safely accomplished under anesthesia to a diameter sufficient to allow insertion of a plastic suction curet.

After the great bulk of the mole has been removed by aspiration and oxytocin is given, and the myometrium has contracted, *thorough but gentle* curettage with a large sharp curet is usually performed. Evacuation of all the contents of a large mole is not always easily accomplished, and intraoperative ultrasonic examination may be helpful to establish that the uterine cavity is empty. Facilities and personnel for immediate laparotomy are mandatory in case there is uncontrollable hemorrhage or serious trauma to the uterus.

OXYTOCIN, PROSTAGLANDINS, AND HYSTEROTOMY. Labor induction rarely is used in this country for evacuation of hydatidiform moles, and there are many who feel that medical termination and hysterotomy have no role in the management (Miller and co-workers, 1989; Stone and Bagshawe, 1979).

HYSTERECTOMY. If age and parity are such that no further pregnancies are desired, then hysterectomy may be preferred to suction curettage. Hysterectomy is a logical procedure in women of 40 or over, because of the frequency with which malignant trophoblastic disease ensues in this age group. Tow (1966) reported that 37 percent of women over age 40 with a complete mole went on to develop gestational trophoblastic tumor. Although hysterectomy does not eliminate trophoblastic tumor, it does appreciable reduce the likelihood of recurrent disease.

FOLLOW-UP PROCEDURES. The prime objective of follow-up is prompt detection of any change suggestive of malignancy. A general method of follow-up is the following:

- Prevent pregnancy during the follow-up period—at a minimum, for 1 year.
- Measure serum chorionic gonadotropin (hCG) levels every 2 weeks. Although weekly assays are recommended by some, no distinct benefit has been demonstrated.
- Withhold therapy as long as these serum levels continue to regress. A rise or persistent plateau in the level demands evaluation and usually treatment.
- Once the level is normal—that is, once it has reached the lower limit of measurement—then test monthly for 6 months, and then every 2 months for a total of 1 year.
- Follow-up may be discontinued and pregnancy allowed after 1 year.

Thus current follow-up and management centers on serial measurement of serum hCG values to detect persistent trophoblastic tumor. As shown in Figure 32–15, chorionic gonadotropin levels should progressively fall to undetectable levels, otherwise trophoblast persists. An increase signifies trophoblastic proliferation that is most likely malignant unless the woman is again preg-

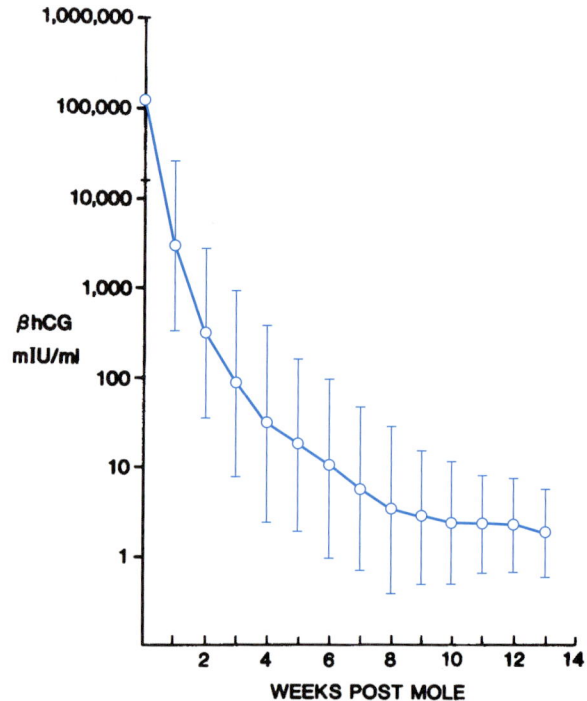

FIGURE 32–15. The mean value and 95 percent confidence limits describing the normal postmolar β-subunit chorionic gonadotropin regression curve. (From Schlaerth and associates, 1981, with permission.)

nant. Treatment of suspected persistent trophoblastic tumor is discussed subsequently.

Estrogen–progestin contraceptives have often been used to prevent a subsequent pregnancy and to suppress pituitary luteinizing hormone that cross-reacts with some tests for chorionic gonadotropin. Yuen and Burch (1983) reported that neither the duration that chorionic gonadotropin persisted nor the frequency of invasive complications was increased in women who used oral contraceptives after molar evacuation. Deicas and associates (1991) studied the effect of contraception on subsequent development of postmolar tumor in 162 women with hydatidiform mole and 137 with trophoblastic tumor. Of the women using oral contraceptives, 33 percent developed tumors compared with 57 percent who did not.

TREATMENT OF PERSISTENT TROPHOBLASTIC TUMOR. Following evacuation of a hydatidiform mole, about 20 percent of women will subsequently undergo further treatment for suspected persistent gestational trophoblastic tumor (Lurain and co-workers, 1983). If serum chorionic gonadotropin values have plateaued or are rising, if there is no evidence for disease beyond the uterus, and if the uterus is not important for future reproduction, hysterectomy will effect a cure in most cases. Often chorionic gonadotropin will disappear and the woman remains well. However, if the uterus is to be preserved, if there is radiographic evidence of lung lesions, or if there are vaginal metastases, chemotherapy is started. Most often, such treatment has been successful. Very small amounts of viable trophoblastic tumor can be detected by hCG assay. Once gonadotropin activity has decreased to the limit of measurement, therapy can be stopped safely without likelihood of recurrence.

GESTATIONAL TROPHOBLASTIC TUMOR. This term refers to the pathological entities of invasive mole, choriocarcinoma, and placental site trophoblastic tumor. It may follow molar pregnancy or normal pregnancy, or develop after abortive outcomes, including ectopic pregnancy. As shown in Table 32–1, malignant gestational trophoblastic disease is divided into two clinical categories, nonmetastatic and metastatic. The latter is further divided into those women who are at high risk and low risk with regard to prognosis.

ETIOLOGY. Gestational trophoblastic tumor most always develops with or follows some form of pregnancy. Very rarely, choriocarcinoma may arise from a teratoma. Approximately half of cases follow a hydatidiform mole, 25 percent follow an abortion, and 25 percent develop after an apparently normal pregnancy. Of 48 fatal cases from the Brewer Trophoblastic Disease Center, only 14 (30 percent) developed in association with

a hydatidiform mole (Lurain and co-workers, 1982). The remainder were associated with term or near-term pregnancies, abortions, or ectopic pregnancies. Tanos and associates (1994) described a woman who developed recurrence of gestational trophoblastic disease after two attempts at in vitro fertilization.

Malignancy has rarely been identified in the placenta of a seemingly normal pregnancy. In a case described by Brewer and Mazur (1981), widespread malignant trophoblast was evident at 18 weeks, and a primary choriocarcinoma of the placenta was detected. A case in which malignant trophoblast metastasized to the fetus has also been described (Kruseman and colleagues, 1977). Others have reported intraplacental choriocarcinoma associated with a live fetus (Aonahata and co-workers, 1998; Jacques and associates, 1998). Lele and colleagues (1999) presented another case and a review of the literature.

PATHOLOGY. In most cases of gestational trophoblastic tumor, the diagnosis is made primarily by persistent serum chorionic gonadotropin. **Clinical management is no longer dictated by histological findings.** In fact, in most cases, no tissue is submitted for pathological study. In those cases with tissue submitted, either choriocarcinoma or invasive mole are most often found.

CHORIOCARCINOMA. This extremely malignant form of trophoblastic tumor may be considered a carcinoma of the chorionic epithelium, although in its growth and metastasis it often behaves like a sarcoma. Factors involved in malignant transformation of the chorion are unknown. In choriocarcinoma, the predisposition of normal trophoblast to invasive growth and erosion of blood vessels is greatly exaggerated. The characteristic gross picture is that of a rapidly growing mass invading both uterine muscle and blood vessels, causing hemorrhage and necrosis (Fig. 32–16A). The tumor is dark red or purple and ragged or friable. If it involves the endometrium, then bleeding, sloughing, and infection of the surface usually occur early. Masses of tissue buried in the myometrium may extend outward, appearing on the uterus as dark, irregular nodules that eventually penetrate the peritoneum.

Microscopically, columns and sheets of trophoblast penetrate the muscle and blood vessels, sometimes in plexiform arrangement and at other times in complete disorganization, interspersed with clotted blood (Fig. 32–16B). An important diagnostic feature of choriocarcinoma, in contrast to hydatidiform mole or invasive mole, is absence of a villous pattern. Both cytotrophoblast and syncytial elements are involved, although one or the other may predominate. Cellular anaplasia exists, often in marked degrees, but is less valuable as a criterion of trophoblastic malignancy than in other tumors.

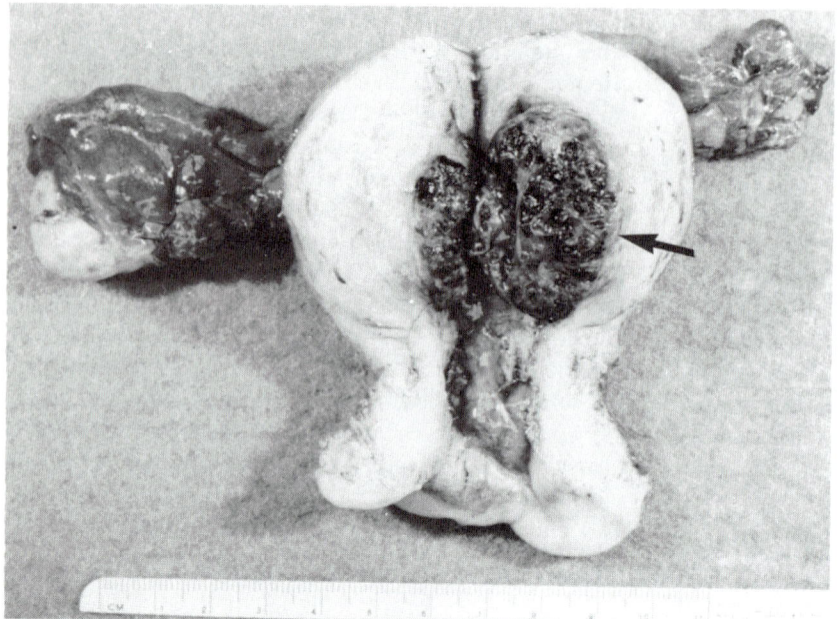

A

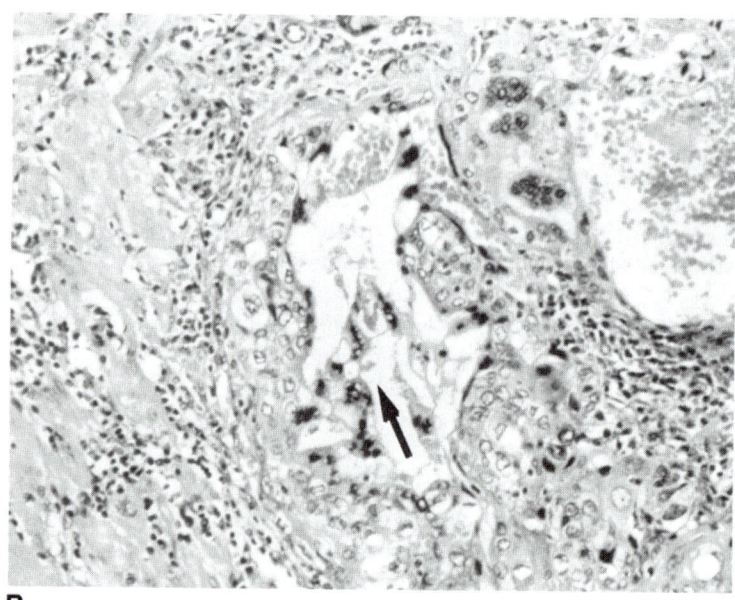

B

FIGURE 32–16. A. Choriocarcinoma (*arrow*) invading the uterus. Persistent trophoblastic disease was demonstrated by curettage subsequent to the expulsion of a hydatidiform mole. Chemotherapy was given, consisting of repeated courses of actinomycin D, then methotrexate, and finally triple therapy with actinomycin D, 5-fluorouracil, and cyclophosphamide. When these failed to destroy the malignancy, hysterectomy and bilateral salpingo-oophorectomy were performed. The woman was known to be alive without detectable chorionic gonatodropin 10 years later. **B.** Histological characteristics of the choriocarcinoma demonstrated in **A.** Malignant syncytio- and cytotrophoblast without villous stroma invade the myometrium and vascular spaces (*arrow*) accompanied by necrosis and hemorrhage.

The difficulty of cytological evaluation is one of the factors leading to error in the diagnosis of choriocarcinoma from examination of uterine curettings. Cells of normal trophoblast at the placental site have been erroneously diagnosed as choriocarcinoma.

Metastases often develop early and are generally blood-borne because of the affinity of trophoblast for blood vessels. The most common sites of metastasis are the lungs (over 75 percent) and the vagina (about 50 percent). The vulva, kidneys, liver, ovaries, brain, and bowel also contain metastases in many cases (Fig.

32–17). Ovarian theca-lutein cysts are identified in over a third of cases.

INVASIVE MOLE. The distinguishing features of invasive mole are excessive trophoblastic overgrowth and extensive penetration by the trophoblastic elements, including whole villi, into the depths of the myometrium, sometimes to involve the peritoneum or the adjacent parametrium or vaginal vault. Such moles are locally invasive, but generally lack the pronounced

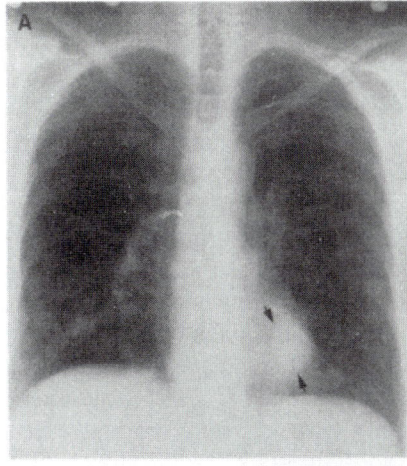
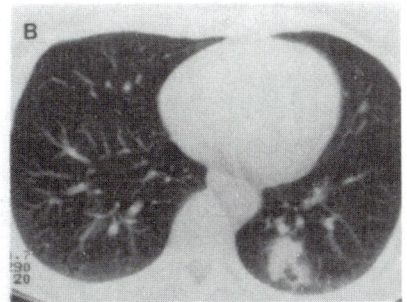
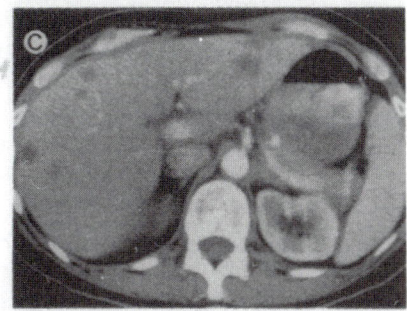
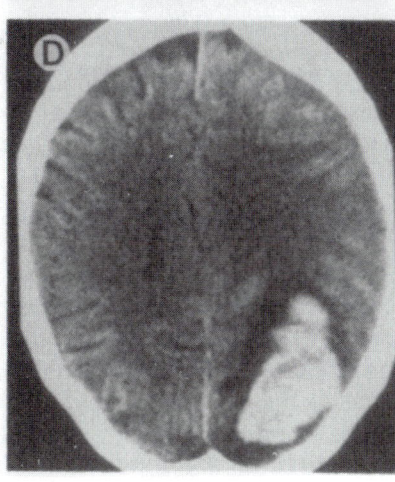

FIGURE 32-17. Metastatic choriocarcinoma. A chest radiograph **(A)** and a computed tomographic scan **(B)** demonstrate a left lower lobe metastatic lesion having poorly defined, irregular borders ("alveolar type") thought to be secondary to peripheral hemorrhage. **C.** Tomographic scan of the abdomen at the level of the liver shows multiple low-density hepatic metastasis. **D.** Tomographic scan of the brain performed without contrast shows a large hemorrhagic metastasis in the left parietal lobe. (From DeBaz and Lewis, 1995, with permission.)

tendency to widespread metastasis characteristic of choriocarcinoma.

PLACENTAL SITE TROPHOBLASTIC TUMOR. Very rarely, a trophoblastic tumor arises from the placental implantation site following either a normal term pregnancy or abortion. This tumor is characterized histologically by predominantly cytotrophoblastic cells, and immunohistochemical staining reveals many prolactin-producing cells and few gonadotropin-producing ones (Miller and associates, 1989). Thus, gonadotropin levels may be normal to elevated. Bleeding is the main presenting symptom. Brewer and colleagues (1992) described erythrocytosis associated with a placental-site trophoblastic tumor. Polycythemia resolved after hysterectomy. Disease confined to the uterus can usually be cured by hysterectomy, although women with metastatic disease have a much worse progress. Randall and col-

leagues (2000) described a woman with prolonged remission following recurrent metastatic placental site tumor and chemotherapy. Gillespie and colleagues (2000) reviewed their experience with seven women with placental site tumor. Three were treated successfully with hysterectomy for tumor confined to the uterus, two are doing well following chemotherapy for pulmonary metastases, and two have died from metastatic disease despite therapy.

CLINICAL COURSE. Gestational trophoblastic tumor may follow hydatidiform mole, abortion, ectopic pregnancy, or normal pregnancy. The most common, though not constant sign, is irregular bleeding after the immediate puerperium in association with uterine subinvolution. The bleeding may be continuous or intermittent, with sudden and sometimes massive hemorrhages. Uterine perforation by the growth may cause intraperitoneal hemorrhage.

In many cases, the first indication may be a metastatic lesion. Vaginal or vulvar tumors may be found. The woman may complain of cough and have bloody sputum from pulmonary metastases. In a few cases it has been impossible to find choriocarcinoma in the uterus or pelvis, the original lesion having disappeared, leaving only distant metastases growing actively. If untreated, choriocarcinoma is rapidly progressive, and death usually follows within a few months in the majority of cases. The most common cause of death is hemorrhage in various locations.

DIAGNOSIS. All women with a hydatidiform mole are at risk and need to be followed as described. **Recognition of the possibility of the lesion is the most important factor in diagnosis.** Any case of unusual bleeding after term pregnancy or abortion should be investigated by curettage, but especially by measurements of chorionic gonadotropin, because absolute reliance cannot be placed on histological findings. Solitary or multiple nodules present in the chest radiograph (Fig. 32–17) that cannot be otherwise explained are suggestive of the possibility of choriocarcinoma. Persistent or rising gonadotropin levels in the absence of pregnancy are indicative of trophoblastic tumor. Occasionally, some nontrophoblastic tumors secrete small amounts of chorionic gonadotropin (Shane and Naftolin, 1975).

Other evaluation before treatment is given includes computed tomography to evaluate the brain, lungs, liver, and pelvis. Hricak and colleagues (1986) reported the use of magnetic resonance imaging in nine women with trophoblastic tumor and concluded that this method was superior to sonography and computed tomography to evaluate the degree of uterine involvement. Yamashita and co-workers (1995) recently reported that contrast-enhanced magnetic resonance imaging was superior to conventional spin-echo imaging for demonstrating myometrial involvement of postmolar trophoblastic tumor.

TREATMENT. Single-agent chemotherapy is given for nonmetastatic or low-risk metastatic disease (Table 32–1). Methotrexate and other agents effective against malignant tumors, especially actinomycin D, have been widely used with considerable success. In some cases, such as with brain metastases, chemotherapy is given along with radiotherapy (Evans and associates, 1995).

The pharmacology and clinical use of methotrexate have been reviewed extensively by Jolivet and colleagues (1983). The overall cure rate in past years for persistent gestational trophoblastic tumor of all severities has been about 90 percent (American College of Obstetricians and Gynecologists, 1993b). Patients classi-

fied as having nonmetastatic tumors or good-prognosis gestational trophoblastic tumors have been cured virtually 100 percent of the time. (Schorge and colleagues, 2000). Cure has usually been achieved for these low-risk women following single-agent chemotherapy. Such treatment reduces serious toxicity.

A number of regimens have been used with success. Barter and associates (1987) reported success with methotrexate given orally. Homesley and associates (1988) reported similar results with weekly intramuscular methotrexate. Petrilli and colleagues (1987) found that single-dose actinomycin D given every 2 weeks was highly effective in women with nonmetastatic disease. Lurain and Elfstrand (1995) reported similar results from the Brewer Trophoblastic Disease Center at Northwestern Medical School. A total of 253 women with nonmetastatic disease were treated with 5-day intravenous methotrexate repeated every 14 days. Additional therapy was required in about 10 percent and all eventually were cured.

HIGH-RISK TROPHOBLASTIC TUMOR. Patients are classified as high risk because they have metastatic trophoblastic tumor that is unlikely to be cured with single-agent chemotherapy based on the following risk factors: disease for more than 4 months, serum gonadotropin levels greater than 40,000 mIU/mL, liver or brain metastases, tumor following term pregnancy, or previous chemotherapy without success. In these women, combination chemotherapy, in spite of increased toxicity, has produced the highest cure rate. According to Schorage and colleagues (2000), the EMA-CO regimen results in response rates of about 90 percent and survival rates of 80 to 100 percent. This combination employs etoposide, methotrexate, actinomycin, cyclophosphamide, and vincristine.

PLACENTAL SITE TUMORS. The most efficacious treatment for placental site trophoblastic tumor is unknown, although Miller and colleagues (1989) recommend that most women are best treated by hysterectomy. Although chemotherapy is recommended for metastatic disease, it does not appear to be as effective as for other gestational trophoblastic tumors (Gillespie and colleagues, 2000; Randall and associates, 2000).

PROGNOSIS. Women with nonmetastatic malignant trophoblastic disease have an extremely good prognosis if single-agent chemotheraphy is started as soon as persistent disease is identified. Previously cited were the remarkable results of Lurain and colleagues (1983) of women with molar pregnancies from the Brewer Trophoblastic Disease Center of Northwestern University. From 1962 to 1978, 738 women with molar pregnancy were managed as generally outlined above. Che-

TABLE 32–4. Brewer Score for Gestational Trophoblastic Tumors

Factor	Score
Lung and/or vaginal metastasis	0
One to four metastases	1
Metastasis other than lung and/or vaginal metastases, and prior chemotherapy	
Five to eight metastases	2
More than eight metastases	3

Adapted from Lurain and associates (1991), with permission.

motherapy was given for persistent disease in 19 percent, and all were living and disease-free 4 to 18 years later.

Women with low-risk malignant metastatic gestational disease who are treated aggressively with single- or multiagent chemotherapy in general do almost as well as those with nonmetastatic disease (DuBeshter and associates, 1987; Hammond and colleagues, 1980; Jones, 1987). Women with high-risk metastatic disease have appreciable mortality that depends on which factors were considered "high risk" (Soper and associates, 1988). Remission rates have been reported to vary from about 45 to 65 percent. Lurain (1987) analyzed 53 deaths from the Brewer Trophoblastic Center and concluded that the three factors primarily responsible were:

1. Extensive choriocarcinoma at initial diagnosis.
2. Lack of appropriately aggressive initial treatment.
3. Failure of currently used chemotherapy.

There have been several prognostic scoring systems and an anatomical staging system reported (Bagshawe, 1976; Pettersson and colleagues, 1985; World Health Organization, 1983). Lurain and associates (1991) presented a simplified prognostic scoring system based on multivariate analysis of almost 400 women treated for gestational trophoblastic tumor. This system, known as the Brewer Score, is summarized in Table 32–4. This score is derived by adding the component scores for the three significant variables from the multivariate analysis. In the 168 women with metastatic trophoblastic tumors, survival was 100 percent with a score of 1, 88 percent for a score of 2, 63 percent for a score of 3, and only 30 percent for a score of 4.

PREGNANCY AFTER TROPHOBLASTIC DISEASE.
There is no difficulty with fertility or normal pregnancy outcome following trophoblastic disease, even if standard chemotherapy was given (Schorge and associates, 2000; Woolas and co-workers, 1998). Women who had trophoblastic disease are at increased risk for developing trophoblastic disease in a subsequent pregnancy.

Berkowitz and colleagues (1987) reported that 1.3 percent of 1048 women treated at the New England Trophoblastic Disease Center for gestational trophoblastic disease had a recurrent molar pregnancy. Kim and associates (1998) reported a 4.3 percent recurrence in 115 Korean women. Importantly, women who have been given chemotherapy do not have an increased risk for anomalous fetuses in subsequent pregnancies (Rustin and colleagues, 1984; Song and associates, 1988).

OTHER TUMORS OF THE PLACENTA

CHORIOANGIOMA (HEMANGIOMA). Various angiomatous tumors of the placenta ranging widely in size have been described. Because of the resemblance of their components to the blood vessels and stroma of the chorionic villus, the term *chorioangioma,* or *chorangioma,* has been considered the most appropriate designation. These are the only benign tumors of the placenta (Benirschke and Kaufmann, 2000). The tumors are most likely hamartomas of primitive chorionic mesenchyme. Their incidence has been reported to be about 1 percent. Larger chorioangiomas may be strongly suspected on the basis of sonographic changes within the placenta. A dramatic example is provided in Figure 32–18.

Small growths are essentially asymptomatic, but large tumors may be associated with hydramnios or antepartum hemorrhage. Fetal death and malformations are uncommon complications, although there may be a positive correlation with low birthweight. Stiller and Skafish

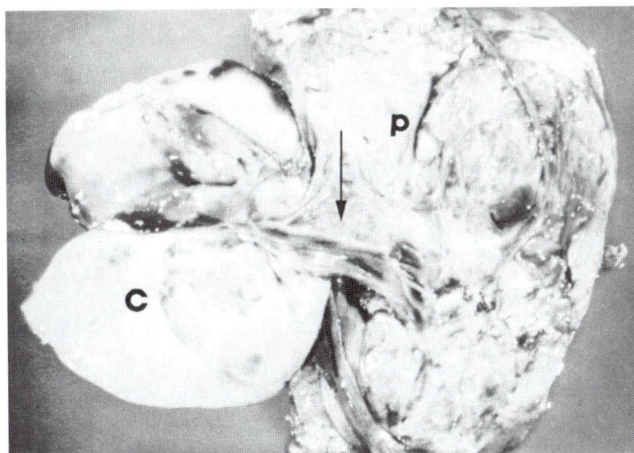

FIGURE 32–18. Placenta (p) and discrete 450-g chorioangioma (c) connected to the placenta by vascular stalk (*arrow*). The 34-week fetus was identified by sonography to have marked hydrothorax. Demonstrated in cord blood were severe hypofibrinogenemia, thrombocytopenia, hypoprothrombinemia, and microangiopathic hemolysis. The infant had cardiomegaly, heart failure, pleural effusion, and hepatomegaly. After several cardiac arrests the infant succumbed 3 days after birth.

TABLE 32–5. Maternal Cancer Metastatic to the Products of Conception (1966–1987)

Tumor Type	Cases to POC	Cases to Placenta	Cases to Fetus	Cases with Fetal Involvement
Malignant melanoma	16	12	7	3
Leukemia and lymphoma	8	5	4	2
Breast carcinoma	7	7	0	0
Lung carcinoma	6	6	0	0
Sarcoma	5	5	0	0
Gastric carcinoma	2	2	0	0
Other carcinoma—lung, liver, ethmoid, cervical, adrenal, ovarian, rectal, pancreas, neck				
Total	53	45	12	6

POC = products of conception.
From Dildy and associates (1989), with permission.

(1986) described a case with multiple placental chorio-angiomas in which a blood group A fetus bled acutely into her O group mother. The mother showed evidence of acute hemolysis without anemia, and the fetus developed a sinusoidal heart rate pattern frequently seen in severe anemia. We have identified severe iron-deficiency anemia in the neonate as the consequence of chronic fetal to maternal hemorrhage associated with multiple small chorioangiomas. Large chorioangiomas provide an arteriovenous shunt in the fetal circulation that can lead to heart failure with all of its complications. Chorioangiomas may result in fetal anemia even without hydrops fetalis. Haak and colleagues (1999) described a case of severe anemia requiring intrauterine transfusion in a fetus with a placental chorioangioma but without hydrops fetalis. With a large chorioangioma, consumptive coagulopathy and microangiopathic hemolytic anemia have also been observed in the fetus-infant. Figure 32–18 shows a placenta and a very large, discrete chorioangioma that led to heart failure, consumptive coagulopathy, and microangiopathic hemolysis in the fetus.

TUMORS METASTATIC TO THE PLACENTA. Metastases of malignant tumors are rare. This was reviewed by Read and Platzer (1981) and Dildy and associates

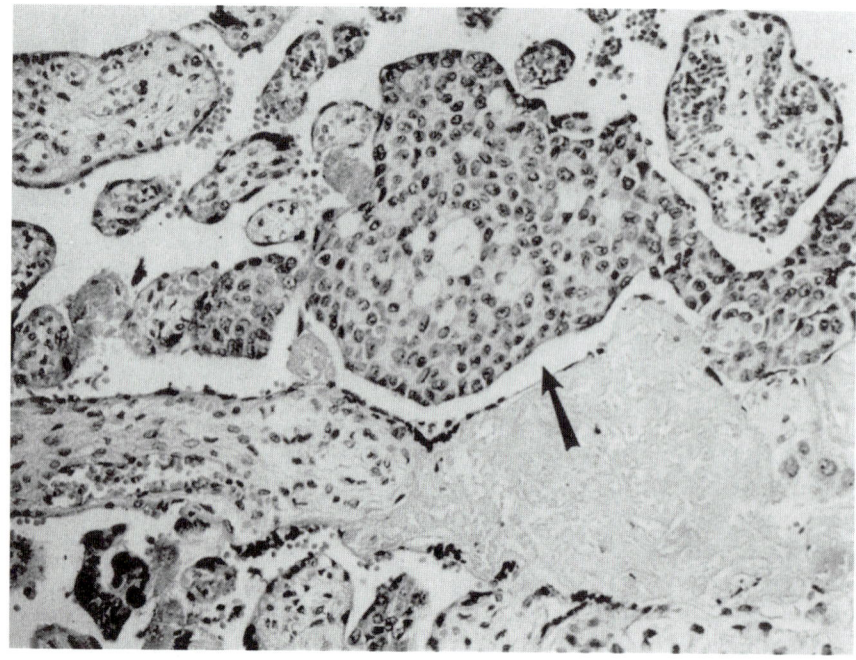

FIGURE 32–19. Adenocarcinoma of the breast metastatic to the intervillous space (*arrow*). (From Benirschke and Kaufmann, 2000, with permission.)

(1989), who reported that malignant melanoma is the most common malignancy metastatic to the placenta; it makes up nearly a third of reported cases. Leukemias and lymphomas comprise another third. In most cases, tumor cells are in the intervillous space; however, as shown in Table 32–5, the fetus is involved with malignant tumor in about a fourth of cases. Despite this, malignant cells seldom proliferate in the fetus to cause clinical disease (Baergen and colleagues, 1997). Any tumor with hematogenous spread is a potential source of placental metastases, as evidenced by the case of large-cell undifferentiated lung carcinoma metastatic to the placenta (Fig. 32–19). The mother succumbed but the child remained healthy by 16 months. Eltorky and colleagues (1995) reported two breast cancers and one pancreatic cancer with placental metastasis.

REFERENCES

American College of Obstetricians and Gynecologists: Committee on Obstetrics: Maternal-Fetal Medicine. Placental Pathology, No. 125, July, 1993a

American College of Obstetricians and Gynecologists: Management of Gestational Trophoblastic Disease. Technical bulletin No. 178, March, 1993b

Amir SM, Osathanondh R, Berkowitz RS, Goldstein DP: Human chorionic gonadotropin and thyroid function in patients with hydatidiform mole. Am J Obstet Gynecol 150:723, 1984

Aonahata M, Masuzawa Y, Tsutsui Y: A case of intraplacental choriocarcinoma associated with placental hemangioma. Pathol Int 48:897, 1998

Baergen RN, Johnson D, Moore T, Benirschke K: Maternal melanoma metastatic to the placenta. A case report and review of the literature. Arch Pathol Lab Med 121:508, 1997

Bagshawe KD: Risk and prognostic factors in trophoblastic neoplasia. Cancer 38:1373, 1976

Bagshawe KD, Lawler SD: Commentary: Unmasking moles. Br J Obstet Gynaecol 89:255, 1982

Barter JF, Soong SJ, Hatch KD, Orr JW Jr, Partridge EC, Austin JM Jr, Shingleton HM: Treatment of nonmetastatic gestational trophoblastic disease with oral methotrexate. Am J Obstet Gynecol 157:1166, 1987

Benirschke K: Disease of the placenta. In Gluck L (ed): Modern Perinatal Medicine. Chicago, Year Book, 1974, p 99

Benirschke K, Dodds JP: Angiomyxoma of the umbilical cord with atrophy of an umbilical artery. Obstet Gynecol 30:99, 1967

Benirschke K, Kaufmann P: Pathology of the Human Placenta, 4th ed. New York, Springer-Verlag, 2000

Berkowitz RS, Goldstein DP, Bernstein MR: Advances in management of partial molar pregnancy. Contemp Ob/Gyn 36:33, 1991

Berkowitz RS, Goldstein DP, Bernstein MR: Management of partial molar pregnancy. Contemp Obstet Gynecol 27:77, 1986

Berkowitz RS, Goldstein DP, Bernstein MR, Sablinska B: Subsequent pregnancy outcome in patients with molar pregnancy and gestational trophoblastic tumors. J Reprod Med 32:680, 1987

Bloss J, Miller D: Gestational trophoblastic disease. In Hankins GDV, Clark SL, Cunningham FG, Gilstrap LC (eds): Operative Obstetrics. Norwalk, CT, Appleton & Lange, 1995, p 695

Brewer CA, Adelson MD, Elder RC: Erythrocytosis associated with a placental-site trophoblastic tumor. Obstet Gynecol 79:846, 1992

Brewer JI, Mazur MT: Gestational choriocarcinoma: Its origin in the placenta during a seemingly normal pregnancy. Am J Surg Pathol 5:267, 1981

Bruchim I, Kidron D, Amiel A, Altaras M, Fejgin MD: Complete hydatidiform mole and a coexistent viable fetus: Report of two cases and review of the literature. Gynecol Oncol 77:197, 2000

Bryan EM, Kohler HG: The missing umbilical artery, 2. Paediatric follow-up. Arch Dis Child 50:714, 1975

Byrne J, Blanc WA: Malformations and chromosome anomalies in spontaneously aborted fetuses with single umbilical artery. Am J Obstet Gynecol 151:340, 1985

Catanzarite VA: The clinical significance of a single umbilical artery as an isolated finding on prenatal ultrasound. Obstet Gynecol 86:155, 1995

College of American Pathologists: Conference XIX, the examination of the placenta: Patient care and risk management. Arch Pathol Lab Med 115:641, 1991

Coukos G, Makrigiannakis A, Chung J, Randall TC, Rubin SC, Benjamin I: Complete hydatidiform mole. A disease with a changing profile. J Reprod Med 44:698, 1999

Curry SL, Hammond CB, Tyrey L, Creasman WT, Parker RT: Hydatidiform mole: Diagnosis, management, and long-time follow-up of 347 patients. Obstet Gynecol 45:1, 1975

DeBaz BP, Lewis TJ: Imaging of gestational trophoblastic disease. Semin Oncol 22:130, 1995

Deicas RE, Miller DS, Rademaker AW, Lurain JR: The role of contraception in the development of postmolar gestational trophoblastic tumor. Obstet Gynecol 78:221, 1991

Dildy GA III, Moise KJ Jr, Carpenter RJ, Klima T: Maternal malignancy metastatic to the products of conception: A review. Obstet Gynecol Surv 44:535, 1989

DuBeshter B, Berkowitz RS, Goldstein DP, Cramer DW, Bernstein MR: Metastatic gestational trophoblastic disease: Experience at the New England Trophoblastic Disease Center, 1965 to 1985. Obstet Gynecol 69:390, 1987

Eltorky M, Khare VK, Osborne P, Shanklin DR: Placental metastasis from maternal carcinoma: A report of three cases. J Reprod Med 40:399, 1995

Evans AC, Soper JT, Clarke-Pearson DL, Berchuck A, Rodriguez GC, Hammond CB: Gestational trophoblastic disease metastatic to the central nervous system. Gynecol Oncol 59:226, 1995

Fox H: Pathology of the placenta. Monograph, Vol VII. Philadelphia, Saunders, 1978

Fung TY, Lau TK: Poor perinatal outcome associated with vasa previa: Is it preventable? A report of three cases and review of the literature. Ultrasound Obstet Gynecol 12:430, 1998

Gianopoulas J, Carver T, Tomich PG, Karlman R, Gadwood K: Diagnosis of vasa previa with ultrasonography. Obstet Gynecol 69:488, 1987

Gillespie AM, Liyim D, Goepel JR, Coleman RE, Hancock BW: Placental site trophoblastic tumour: A rare but potentially curable cancer. Br J Cancer 82:1186, 2000

Goldkrand JW, Lentz SU, Turner AD, Clements S, Sefter H, Bryant J: Doppler velocimetry in the fetus with a single umbilical artery. J Reprod Med 44:346, 1999

Goldstein DP, Berkowitz RS: Prophylactic chemotherapy of complete molar pregnancy. Semin Oncol 22:157, 1995

Grannum PAT, Berkowitz RL, Hobbins JC: The ultrasonic changes in the maturing placenta and their relation to fetal pulmonic maturity. Am J Obstet Gynecol 133:915, 1979

Haak MC, Oosterhof H, Mouw RJ, Oepkes D, Vandenbussche FP: Pathophysiology and treatment of fetal anemia due to placental chorioangioma. Ultrasound Obstet Gynecol 14:68, 1999

Hammond CB, Borchert I, Tyrey I, Creasman WT, Parker RT: Treatment of metastatic trophoblastic disease: Good and poor prognosis. Am J Obstet Gynecol 115:451, 1973

Hammond CB, Weed JC, Currie JL: The role of operation in the current therapy of gestational trophoblastic disease. Am J Obstet Gynecol 136:844, 1980

Hankins GDV, Snyder RR, Hauth JC, Gilstrap LC III, Hammond T: Nuchal cords and neonatal outcome. Obstet Gynecol 70:687, 1987a

Hankins GDV, Wendel GW, Snyder RR, Cunningham FG: Trophoblastic embolization during molar evacuation: Central hemodynamic observations. Obstet Gynecol 69:368, 1987b

Herrmann UJ Jr, Sidiropoulos D: Single umbilical artery: Prenatal findings. Prenat Diagn 8:275, 1988

Homesley HD, Blessing JA, Rettenmaier M, Capizzi RL, Major FJ, Twiggs LB: Weekly intramuscular methotrexate for nonmetastatic gestational trophoblastic disease. Obstet Gynecol 72:413, 1988

Hricak H, Demas BE, Braga CA, Fisher MR, Winkler ML: Gestational trophoblastic neoplasm of the uterus: MR assessment. Radiology 161:11, 1986

Jacques SM, Qureshi F, Doss BJ, Munkarah A: Intraplacental choriocarcinoma associated with viable pregnancy: Pathologic features and implications for the mother and infant. Pediatr Dev Pathol 1:380, 1998

Jauniaux E: Partial moles: From postnatal to prenatal diagnosis. Placenta 20:379, 1999

Jauniaux E, Halder A, Partington C: A case of partial mole associated with trisomy 13. Ultrasound Obstet Gynecol 11:62, 1998

Jolivet J, Cowan KH, Curt GA, Clendeninn NH, Chaber BA: The pharmacology and clinical use of methotrexate. N Engl J Med 309:1094, 1983

Jones WB: Current management of low-risk metastatic gestational trophoblastic disease. J Reprod Med 32:655, 1987

Kan PS, Eastman NJ: Coiling of the umbilical cord around the foetal neck. Br J Obstet Gynaecol 64:227, 1957

Kim JH, Park DC, Bae SN, Namkoong SE, Kim SJ: Subsequent reproductive experience after treatment for gestational trophoblastic disease. Gynecol Oncol 71:108, 1998

Kruseman AC, Lent MV, Blom AH, Lauw GP: Choriocarcinoma in mother and child, identified by immunoenzyme histochemistry. Am J Clin Pathol 67:279, 1977

Lademacher DS, Vermeulen RCW, Harten JJVD, Arts NFT: Circumvallate placenta and congenital malformation. Lancet 1:732, 1981

Lawler SD, Fisher RA, Dent J: A prospective genetic study of complete and partial hydatidiform moles. Am J Obstet Gynecol 164:1270, 1991

Lee W, Lee VL, Kirk JS, Sloan CT, Smith RS, Comstock CH: Vasa previa: Prenatal diagnosis, natural evolution and clinical outcome. Obstet Gynecol 95:572, 2000

Lele SM, Crowder SE, Grafe MR: Asymptomatic intraplacental choriocarcinoma diagnosed on routine placental examination. J Perinatol 19:244, 1999

Lembet A, Zorlu CG, Yalcin HR, Seckin B, Ekici E: Partial hydatidiform mole with diploid karyotype in a live fetus. Int J Gynaecol Obstet 69:149, 2000

Leung A, Robson W: Single umbilical artery: A report of 159 cases. Am J Dis Child 143:108, 1989

Loret de Mola JR, Goldfarb JM: Reproductive performance of patients after gestational trophoblastic disease. Semin Oncol 22:193, 1995

Lurain JR: High-risk metastatic gestational trophoblastic tumors. Current management. J Reprod Med 39:217, 1994

Lurain JR: Causes of treatment failure in gestational trophoblastic disease. J Reprod Med 32:677, 1987

Lurain JR, Brewer JI, Mazur MT, Torok EE: Fatal gestational trophoblastic disease: An analysis of treatment failures. Am J Obstet Gynecol 144:391, 1982

Lurain JR, Brewer JI, Torek EE, Halpern B: Natural history of hydatidiform mole after primary evacuation. Am J Obstet Gynecol 145:591, 1983

Lurain JR, Casanova LA, Miller DS, Rademaker AW: Prognostic factors in gestational trophoblastic tumors: A proposed new scoring system based on multivariate analysis. Am J Obstet Gynecol 164:611, 1991

Lurain JR, Elfstrand EP: Single-agent methotrexate chemotherapy for the treatment of nonmetastatic gestational trophoblastic tumors. Am J Obstet Gynecol 172:574, 1995

Mann K, Schneider N, Hoermann R: Thyrotropic activity of acidic isoelectric variants of human chorionic gonadotropin and trophoblastic tumors. Endocrinology 118:1558, 1986

Megier P, Gorin V, Desroches A: Ultrasonography of placenta previa at the third trimester of pregnancy: Research for signs of placenta accreta/percreta and vasa previa. Prospective color and pulsed Doppler ultrasonography study of 45 cases. J Gynecol Obstet Biol Reprod (Paris) 28:239, 1999

Miller DS, Ballon SC, Teng NNH: Gestational trophoblastic diseases. In Brody SA, Ueland K (eds): Endocrine Disorders in Pregnancy. Norwalk, CT, Appleton & Lange, 1989, p 451

Miller DS, Lurain JR: Classification and staging of gestational trophoblastic tumors. Obstet Gynecol Clin North Am 15:477, 1988

Miller DS, Seifer DB: Endocrinologic aspects of gestational trophoblastic diseases. Int J Fertil 35:137, 1990

Miller ME, Higginbottom M, Smith DW: Short umbilical cord: Its origin and relevance. Pediatrics 67:618, 1981

Montz FJ, Schlaerth JB, Morrow CP: The natural history of theca lutein cysts. Obstet Gynecol 72:247, 1988

Mutch DG, Soper JT, Baker ME, Bandy LC, Cox EB, Clarke-Pearson DL, Hammond CB: Role of computed axial tomography of the chest in staging patients with nonmetastatic gestational trophoblastic disease. Obstet Gynecol 68:348, 1986

Nomiyama M, Toyota Y, Kawano H: Antenatal diagnosis of velamentous umbilical cord insertion and vasa previa with color Doppler imaging. Ultrasound Obstet Gynecol 12:426, 1998

Novak E, Seah CS: Choriocarcinoma of the uterus. Am J Obstet Gynecol 67:933, 1954

Oyelese KO, Turner M, Lees C, Campbell S: Vasa previa: An avoidable obstetric tragedy. Obstet Gynecol 54:138, 1999

Parilla BV, Tamura RK, MacGregor SN, Geibel LJ, Sabbagha RE: The clinical significance of a single umbilical artery as an isolated finding on prenatal ultrasound. Obstet Gynecol 85:570, 1995

Pavlopoulos PM, Konstantinidou AE, Agapitos E, Christodoulou CN, Davaris P: Association of single umbilical artery with congenital malformations of vascular etiology. Pediatr Dev Pathol 1:487, 1998

Petrilli ES, Twiggs LB, Blessing JA, Teng NNH, Curry S: Single-dose actinomycin-D treatment for nonmetastatic gestational trophoblastic disease: A prospective phase II trial of the Gynecologic Oncology Group. Cancer 60:2173, 1987

Pettersson F, Kolstad P, Ludwig H: Annual report on the results of treatment in gynecologic cancer. Stockholm, International Federation of Gynecology and Obstetrics, 1985

Raio L, Ghezzi F, Di Naro E, Franchi M, Bruhwiler H, Luscher KP: Prenatal assessment of Wharton's jelly in umbilical cords with single artery. Ultrasound Obstet Gynecol 14:42, 1999

Ramin SM, Gilstrap LC III: Placental abnormalities: Previa, abruption and accreta. In Plauche W, Morrison JC, O'Sullivan MJ (eds): Surgical Obstetrics. Philadelphia, Saunders, 1992, p 203

Rana J, Ebert GA, Kappy KA: Adverse perinatal outcome in patients with an abnormal umbilical coiling index. Obstet Gynecol 85:573, 1995

Randall TC, Coukos G, Wheeler JE, Rubin SC: Prolonged remission of recurrent, metastatic placental site trophoblastic tumor after chemotherapy. Gynecol Oncol 76:115, 2000

Read EJ, Platzer PB: Placental metastasis from maternal carcinoma of the lung. Obstet Gynecol 58:387, 1981

Rose P: Hydatidiform mole: Diagnosis and management. Semin Oncol 22:149, 1995

Rustin GJ, Booth M, Dent J, Salt S, Rustin F, Bagshawe KD: Pregnancy after cytotoxic chemotherapy for gestational trophoblastic tumours. BMJ 288:103, 1984

Schlaerth JB, Morrow CP, Kletzky OA, Nalick RH, D'Ablaing GA: Prognostic characteristics of serum human chorionic gonadotropin titer regression following molar pregnancy. Obstet Gynecol 58:478, 1981

Schlaerth JB, Morrow CP, Montz F, d'Ablaing G: Initial management of hydatidiform mole. Am J Obstet Gynecol 158:1299, 1988

Schorge JO, Goldstein DP, Bernstein MR, Berkowitz RS: Recent advances in gestational trophoblastic disease. J Reprod Med 45:692, 2000

Seckl MJ, Fisher RA, Salerno G, Rees H, Paradinas FJ, Foskett M, Newlands ES: Choriocarcinoma and partial hydatidiform moles. Lancet 356:36, 2000

Semer DA, Macfee MS: Gestational trophoblastic disease: Epidemiology. Semin Oncol 22:109, 1995

Shane JM, Naftolin F: Aberrant hormone activity by tumors of gynecologic importance. Am J Obstet Gynecol 121:133, 1975

Shen-Schwarz S, King E, Benito C, Guzman E, Simullian J, Vintzileos A: Umbilical cord twist: Relationship with placental gross morphology. Am J Obstet Gynecol 174:361, 1996

Shen-Schwarz S, Macpherson TA, Mueller-Heubach E: The clinical significance of hemorrhagic endovasculitis of the placenta. Am J Obstet Gynecol 159:48, 1988

Smalbraak J: Trophoblastic Growths. Haarlem, Netherlands, Elsevier, 1957

Soernes T, Bakke T: The length of the human umbilical cord in vertex and breech presentations. Am J Obstet Gynecol 154:1086, 1986

Song HZ, Wu PC, Wang YE, Yang XE, Dong SY: Pregnancy outcomes after successful chemotherapy for choriocarcinoma and invasive mole: Long-term follow-up. Am J Obstet Gynecol 158:538, 1988

Soper JT, Clarke-Pearson D, Hammond CB: Metastatic gestational trophoblastic disease: Prognostic factors in previously untreated patients. Obstet Gynecol 71:338, 1988

Spellacy WN, Gravem H, Fisch RO: The umbilical cord complications of true knots, nuchal coils and cords around the body. Am J Obstet Gynecol 94:1136, 1966

Spirit BA, Cohen WN, Weinstein HM: The incidence of placental calcification in normal pregnancies. Radiology 142:707, 1982

Stanhope CR, Stuart GCE, Curtis KL: Primary ovarian hydatidiform mole: Review of the literature and report of a case. Am J Obstet Gynecol 145:886, 1983

Stiller AG, Skafish PR: Placental chorioangioma: A rare cause of fetomaternal transfusion with maternal hemolysis and fetal distress. Obstet Gynecol 67:296, 1986

Stone M, Bagshawe KD: An analysis of the influence of maternal age, gestational age, contraceptive method, and the mode of primary treatment of patients with hydatidiform moles on the incidence of subsequent chemotherapy. Br J Obstet Gynaecol 86:782, 1979

Strong TH, Elliot JP, Radin TG: Noncoiled umbilical blood vessels: A new marker for the fetus at risk. Obstet Gynecol 81:409, 1993

Strong TH, Jarles DL, Vega JS, Feldman DB: The umbilical coiling index. Am J Obstet Gynecol 170:29, 1994

Suzuki M, Matsunobu A, Wakita K, Nishijima M, Osanai K: Hydatidiform mole with a surviving coexisting fetus. Obstet Gynecol 56:384, 1980

Szulman AE, Surti U: The clinicopathologic profile of the partial hydatidiform mole. Obstet Gynecol 59:597, 1982

Tanos V, Meirow D, Reubenoff BE, Anteby SO: Recurrent gestational trophoblastic disease following in vitro fertilization. Human Reprod 9:2010, 1994

Tow WSH: The classification of malignant growths of the chorion. Br J Obstet Gynaecol 73:1000, 1966

Tuncer ZS, Bernstein MR, Wang J, Goldstein DP, Berkowitz RS: Repetitive hydatidiform mole with different male partners. Gynecol Oncol 75:224, 1999

Van de Kaa CA, Robben JC, Hopman AH, Hanselaar AG, Vooijs GP: Complete hydatidiform mole in twin pregnancy: Differentiation from partial mole with interphase cytogenetic and DNA cytometric analyses on paraffin embedded tissues. Histopathology 26:123, 1995

Vejerslev LO: Clinical management and diagnostic possibilities in hydatidiform mole with coexistent fetus. Obstet Gynecol Surv 46:577, 1991

Wolf NG, Lage JM: Genetic analysis of gestational trophoblastic disease: A review. Semin Oncol 22:113, 1995

Woolas RP, Bower M, Newlands ES, Seckl M, Short D, Holden L: Influence of chemotherapy for gestational trophoblastic disease on subsequent pregnancy outcome. B J Obstet Gynaecol 105:1032, 1998

World Health Organization Scientific Group on Gestational Trophoblastic Diseases: Gestational Trophoblastic Diseases. Technical Report Series No. 692. Geneva, World Health Organization, 1983

Yamashita Y, Torashima M, Takahashi M, Mizutani H, Miyazaki K, Matsuura K, Okamura H: Contrast-enhanced dynamic MR imaging of postmolar gestational trophoblastic disease. Acta Radiologica 36:188, 1995

Yuen BH, Burch P: Relationship of oral contraceptives and the intrauterine contraceptive devices to the regression of concentrations of the beta subunits of human chorionic gonadotropin and invasive complications after molar pregnancy. Am J Obstet Gynecol 145:214, 1983

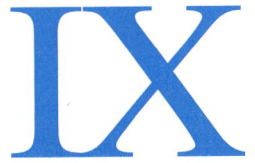

SECTION

Reproductive Success and Failure

33

Abortion

The definition of *abortion* is the termination of pregnancy by any means before the fetus is sufficiently developed to survive. In the United States this definition is confined to the termination of pregnancy before 20 weeks based upon the date of the first day of the last normal menses. Another commonly used definition is the delivery of a fetus-neonate that weighs less than 500 g.

SPONTANEOUS ABORTION

When abortion occurs without medical or mechanical means to empty the uterus, it is referred to as spontaneous. Another widely used term is *miscarriage*.

PATHOLOGY. Hemorrhage into the decidua basalis and necrotic changes in the tissues adjacent to the bleeding usually accompany abortion. The ovum becomes detached, and this stimulates uterine contractions that result in expulsion. When the sac is opened, fluid is commonly found surrounding a small macerated fetus, or alternatively there may be no visible fetus in the sac, the so-called *blighted ovum.*

Blood or *carneous mole* is an ovum that is surrounded by a capsule of clotted blood. The capsule is of varying thickness, with degenerated chorionic villi scattered through it. The small, fluid-containing cavity within appears compressed and distorted by thick walls of old blood clot.

In later abortions, several outcomes are possible. The retained fetus may undergo *maceration*. The bones of the skull collapse and the abdomen becomes distended with blood-stained fluid. The skin softens and peels off in utero or at the slightest touch, leaving behind the corium. Internal organs degenerate and undergo necrosis. Amnionic fluid may be absorbed when the fetus becomes compressed upon itself and desiccated to form a *fetus compressus*. Occasionally, the fetus eventually becomes so dry and compressed that it resembles parchment, so-called *fetus papyraceous.*

RESUMPTION OF OVULATION. Ovulation may resume as early as 2 weeks after an abortion. Lähteenmäki and Luukkainen (1978) detected a surge of luteinizing hormone (LH) 16 to 22 days after abortion in 15 of 18 women studied. Moreover, plasma progesterone level, which had plummeted after the abortion, increased soon after the LH surge. These hormonal events are in temporal agreement with histological changes observed in endometrial biopsies as described by Boyd and Holmstrom (1972). **Therefore, it is important that effective contraception be initiated soon after abortion.**

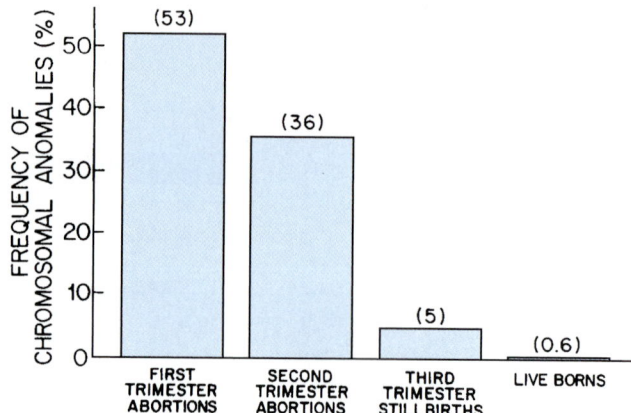

FIGURE 33-1. Frequency of chromosomal anomalies in abortuses and stillbirths for each trimester compared with the frequency of chromosomal anomalies in live-born infants. The percentage for each group is shown in parentheses. (Data adapted from Warburton, 1980, and Fantel, 1980, and their associates.)

ETIOLOGY. More than 80 percent of abortions occur in the first 12 weeks, and the rate decreases rapidly thereafter (Harlap and Shiono, 1980). Chromosomal anomalies cause at least half of these early abortions, and their incidence likewise decreases thereafter (Fig. 33-1). The risk of spontaneous abortion increases with parity as well as with maternal and paternal age (Warburton and Fraser, 1964; Wilson and associates, 1986). The frequency of clinically recognized abortion increases from 12 percent in women less than 20 years old to 26 percent in those over age 40. The effect of advancing maternal age is illustrated in Figure 33-2. For the same paternal ages, the increase is from 12 to 20 percent. Finally, the incidence of abortion is increased if a woman conceives within 3 months of a term birth (Harlap and Shiono, 1980).

The exact mechanisms responsible for abortion are not always apparent, but in the very early months of pregnancy, spontaneous expulsion of the ovum is nearly always preceded by death of the embryo or fetus. For this reason, etiological considerations of early abortion involve ascertaining whenever possible the cause of fetal death. In the subsequent months, the fetus frequently does not die in utero before expulsion, and other explanations for its expulsion must be invoked.

FETAL FACTORS

ABNORMAL ZYGOTE DEVELOPMENT. The most common morphological finding in early spontaneous abortions is an abnormality of development of the zygote, embryo, early fetus, or at times the placenta. In an analysis of 1000 spontaneous abortions, Hertig and Sheldon (1943) observed pathological ("blighted") ova

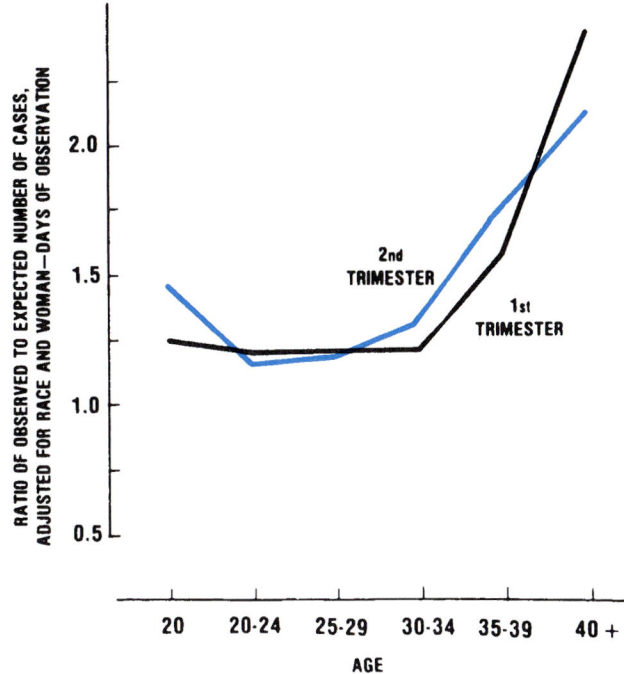

FIGURE 33-2. First- and second-trimester spontaneous abortions by maternal age. (From Harlap and colleagues, 1980, with permission.)

in which the embryo was degenerated or absent in half. Such an abnormal ovum can be seen in Figure 33–3.

Poland and co-workers (1981) identified morphological disorganization of growth in 40 percent of abortuses that were expelled spontaneously before 20 weeks.

Among embryos of less than 30 mm crown–rump length, the frequency of abnormal morphological development was 70 percent. Of the embryos on which tissue culture and chromosomal analyses were performed, 60 percent had chromosomal abnormalities. For fetuses of 30 to 180 mm crown–rump length, the frequency of chromosomal abnormalities was 25 percent.

ANEUPLOID ABORTION. Chromosomal abnormalities are common among embryos and early fetuses that are aborted spontaneously, and account for much or most of early pregnancy wastage. Approximately 50 to 60 percent of early spontaneous abortions are associated with a chromosomal anomaly of the conceptus (Table 33–1). Jacobs and Hassold (1980) reported that approximately one fourth of chromosomal abnormalities were due to maternal gametogenesis errors and 5 percent to paternal errors. In a study of fetuses and newborns with trisomy 13, Robinson and colleagues (1996) reported that in 21 of 23 cases, the extra chromosome was of maternal origin.

Autosomal trisomy is the most frequently identified chromosomal anomaly associated with first-trimester abortions (Table 33–1). As discussed in Chapter 36, trisomies can be the result of an **isolated nondisjunction,** maternal or paternal **balanced translocation,** or **balanced chromosomal inversion.** Balanced structural chromosomal rearrangements are present in 2 to 3 percent of couples with a history of recurrent abortions (American College of Obstetricians and Gynecologists, 1995). Translocations may be identified in either parent.

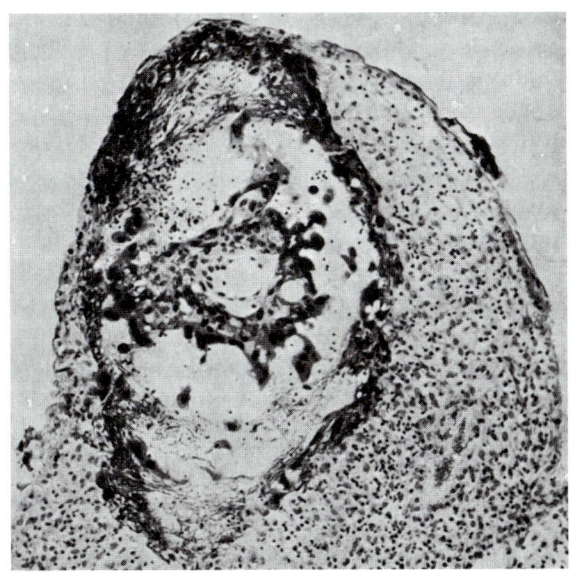

FIGURE 33-3. Abnormal ovum. A cross-section of a defective ovum showing an empty chorionic sac embedded within a polypoid mass of endometrium. (From Hertig and Rock, 1944.)

TABLE 33–1. Chromosomal Findings in Human Abortuses

Chromosomal Studies	Kajii et al (1980) (%)	Simpson (1980) (%)
Normal (euploid), 46XY and 46XX	46	54
Abnormal (aneuploid)		
Autosomal trisomy	31	22
Monosomy X (45,X)	10	9
Triploidy	7	8
Tetraploidy	2	3
Structural anomaly	3	2
Double trisomy	2	0.7
Triple trisomy	0.4	NL
Others—XXY, monosomy 21	0.8	NL
Autosomal monosomy G	NL	0.1
Mosaic trisomy	NL	1.3
Sex chromosome polysomy	NL	0.2
Abnormality not specified	NL	0.9

NL = not listed.

Balanced chromosomal inversions may also be identified in couples with recurrent abortions. Trisomies for all autosomes except chromosome number 1 have been identified in abortuses, but autosomes 13, 16, 18, 21, and 22 are most common.

Monosomy X (45,X) is the next most common chromosomal abnormality and is compatible with live-born females (Turner syndrome). **Triploidy** is often associated with hydropic placental degeneration. Incomplete hydatidiform moles may have fetal development that is triploid or trisomic for chromosome number 16. Fetuses associated with these frequently abort early, and the few carried longer are all grossly malformed. Advanced maternal and paternal age are not associated with this abnormality. **Tetraploid abortuses** are rarely live born and are most often aborted very early in gestation.

Chromosomal structural abnormalities are unusual causes of abortion and have been identified only since the development of banding techniques. Some of these infants are live born with balanced translocations and can be normal. **Autosomal monosomy** is extremely rare and is incompatible with life. **Sex chromosomal polysomy (47,XXX or 47,XXY)** is unusual in abortus material but is commonly seen in live births.

EUPLOID ABORTION. Kajii and co-workers (1980) reported that three fourths of aneuploid abortions were before 8 weeks, while euploid abortions peaked at about 13 weeks. Stein and associates (1980) presented evidence that the incidence of euploid abortions increases dramatically after the maternal age of 35 years. The reasons for euploid abortions are generally unknown, but the following are possibilities:

1. A genetic abnormality such as an isolated mutation or polygenic factors.
2. Various maternal factors.
3. Possibly some paternal factors.

Simpson (1980) observed that approximately 0.5 percent of live births have chromosomal abnormalities, while at least 2 percent of live births have diseases associated with a single-gene mutation or a polygenic mechanism of inheritance.

MATERNAL FACTORS. A variety of medical disorders, environmental conditions, and developmental abnormalities have been implicated in euploidic abortion.

INFECTIONS. Some chronic infections have been implicated in causing abortion. *Brucella abortus* and *Campylobacter fetus* are well-known causes of chronic abortion in cattle, but they are not a significant cause in humans (Sauerwein and associates, 1993). Evidence that *Toxoplasma gondii* causes abortion in humans is inconclusive. There is no evidence in humans that either *Listeria*

monocytogenes or *Chlamydia trachomatis* produce abortions (Feist and associates, 1999; Osser and Persson, 1996; Paukku and associates, 1999). Herpes simplex, however, has been associated with an increased incidence of abortion following genital infection in early pregnancy. Temmerman and colleagues (1992) reported that spontaneous abortion was independently associated with maternal human immunodeficiency virus-1 (HIV-1) antibody, with maternal syphilis seroreactivity, and with vaginal colonization with group B streptococci. Serological evidence supportive of a role for *Mycoplasma hominis* and *Ureaplasma urealyticum* in abortion was provided by Quinn and co-workers (1983). Conversely, Temmerman and associates (1992) found no association between genital mycoplasma and spontaneous abortion. Interestingly, Berg and associates (1999) reported that erythromycin treatment for women with mycoplasma culture-positive amnionic fluid undergoing genetic amniocentesis resulted in a significant decrease in midtrimester losses (11 versus 44 percent).

CHRONIC DEBILITATING DISEASES. In early pregnancy, chronic wasting diseases such as tuberculosis or carcinomatosis have seldom caused abortion. Hypertension is seldom associated with abortion before 20 weeks, but rather may lead to fetal death and preterm delivery. Celiac sprue has been reported to cause both male and female infertility and recurrent abortions (Sher and colleagues, 1994).

ENDOCRINE ABNORMALITIES

HYPOTHYROIDISM. There does not appear to be an increased incidence of abortion associated with clinical hypothyroidism (Montoro and associates, 1981). Thyroid autoantibodies were associated with an increased incidence of abortion despite the lack of overt hypothyroidism (Dayan and Daniels, 1996; Stagnaro-Green and associates, 1990). Conversely, others have found no increase in the incidence of antithyroid antibodies in women who have recurrent abortions when compared with normal controls (Esplin and colleagues, 1998; Pratt and associates, 1994).

DIABETES MELLITUS. As reviewed recently by Greene (1999), spontaneous abortion and major congenital malformations are both increased in women with insulin-dependent diabetes. The risk is related to the degree of metabolic control in the first trimester. In a prospective study, Mills and associates (1988) reported that early glucose control (within 21 days of conception) resulted in a similar spontaneous abortion rate compared with nondiabetic controls. Lack of glucose control, however, resulted in a marked increase in the abortion rate. In a study from the Children's Hospital of Pittsburgh, Dorman and associates (1999) reported a significantly higher rate of spontaneous abortion (27 versus 8 percent) for diabetic women compared with nondiabetic partners of type I diabetic men. There was a temporal decline in the spontaneous abortion rate in these diabetic women from 26 percent before 1969 to 5.7 percent from 1980 to 1989. These authors postulated that this decrease may be secondary to changes in medical care such as glucose self-monitoring.

PROGESTERONE DEFICIENCY. Insufficient progesterone secretion by the corpus luteum or placenta has been associated with an increased incidence of abortion. It has been suggested that abnormal levels of one or more hormones might help to forecast abortion. Unfortunately, reduced levels of these hormones are usually the consequence rather than the cause (Salem and co-workers, 1984). There are well-documented cases of luteal phase defects, but they are uncommon.

NUTRITION. There is no conclusive evidence that dietary deficiency of any one nutrient or moderate deficiency of all nutrients is an important cause of abortion. The nausea and vomiting that develop rather commonly during early pregnancy, and any inanition so induced, are rarely followed by spontaneous abortion.

DRUG USE AND ENVIRONMENTAL FACTORS. A variety of different agents has been reported, but not confirmed, to be associated with an increased incidence of abortion.

TOBACCO. Smoking has been associated with an increased risk for euploidic abortion (Harlap and Shiono, 1980). For women who smoked more than 14 cigarettes a day, the risk was approximately twofold compared with controls (Kline and associates, 1980). Armstrong and associates (1992) calculated that the abortion risk increased in a linear fashion by a factor of 1.2 for each 10 cigarettes smoked per day.

ALCOHOL. Both spontaneous abortion and fetal anomalies may result from frequent alcohol use during the first 8 weeks of pregnancy (Floyd and associates, 1999). Spontaneous abortion was increased even when alcohol was consumed "in moderation." Kline and co-workers (1980) reported that the abortion rate was doubled in women drinking twice weekly and trebled in women who consumed alcohol daily compared with nondrinkers. Armstrong and colleagues (1992) computed that abortion risk increased by an average of 1.3 for each drink per day. In contrast, Cavallo and associates (1995), in a prospective study of 546 women, reported that a low level of alcohol consumption during pregnancy was not associated with a significant risk for abortion. Some-

what worrisome is the fact that in one cross-sectional study from the Centers for Disease Control and Prevention, Floyd and associates (1999) found that half of all pregnant women in the study drank alcohol during the 3 months preceding pregnancy recognition and 5 percent drank moderate to heavy levels!

CAFFEINE. Coffee consumption at greater than four cups per day appears to slightly increase the risk of abortion (Armstrong and associates, 1992). The risk appears to increase with increasing amounts. In a study by Klebanoff and associates (1999), maternal paraxanthine (a caffeine metabolite) levels were associated with a significant twofold risk of spontaneous abortion only if extremely high. These authors concluded that moderate consumption of caffeine was unlikely to be associated with spontaneous abortion.

RADIATION. In sufficient doses, radiation is a recognized abortifacient. As discussed in Chapter 42, the human dose is not precisely known.

CONTRACEPTIVES. There is no evidence to support that oral contraceptives or spermicidal agents used in contraceptive creams and jellies are associated with an increased incidence of abortion. Intrauterine devices, however, are associated with an increased incidence of septic abortion after contraceptive failure (Chap. 58, p. 1538).

ENVIRONMENTAL TOXINS. In some studies abortion rates in exposed women were not increased (Axelsson and Rylander, 1982). Rowland and associates (1995) reported an increased risk for spontaneous abortion among dental assistants exposed to 3 or more hours of nitrous oxide in offices without scavenging equipment, but not in offices using such equipment. In a meta-analysis, Boivin (1997) concluded that there was an increased risk of spontaneous abortion for women occupationally exposed to anesthetic gases based on data from the prescavenging era.

In most instances, there is little information to indict any specific environmental agent; however, there is evidence that arsenic, lead, formaldehyde, benzene, and ethylene oxide may cause abortion (Barlow and Sullivan, 1982). Video display terminals and exposure to the accompanying electromagnetic fields do not increase the risk of abortion (Schnorr and co-workers, 1991). Short-waves and ultrasound also do not increase the risk (Taskinen and colleagues, 1990).

IMMUNOLOGICAL FACTORS. Much attention has focused on the immune system as important in recurrent pregnancy loss. Two primary pathophysiological models that have evolved are the autoimmune theory (immunity against self) and the alloimmune theory (immunity against another person).

AUTOIMMUNE FACTORS. It has been determined from compiled studies that approximately 15 percent of over 1000 recurrent pregnancy loss patients have recognized autoimmune factors (Kutteh and Pasquarette, 1995). The most significant antibodies have specificity against negatively charged phospholipids and are most commonly detected by testing for lupus anticoagulant (LAC) and anticardiolipin antibody (ACA). Women with both a history of early fetal loss and high levels of antibodies may suffer a 70 percent miscarriage recurrence (Dudley and Branch, 1991). Pooling studies totaling 1500 women with recurrent loss yields an average incidence of 17 percent for anticardiolipin antibody and 7 percent for the lupus anticoagulant. In contrast, only 1 to 3 percent of normal obstetrical patients are found to have either of these (Harris and Spinnato, 1991; Lockwood and colleagues, 1989). In a prospective study of 860 women screened for anticardiolipin antibody in the first trimester, Yasuda and colleagues (1995) reported that 7 percent were positive. Spontaneous abortion occurred in 25 percent of the antibody-positive group compared with 10 percent of the negative group. In another recent study, however, Simpson and associates (1998) found no association between early pregnancy loss and the presence of either anticardiolipin antibody or lupus anticoagulant. Despite these controversies with early abortion, there is a consensus regarding increased midtrimester pregnancy losses and the antiphospholipid antibody syndrome (Blumenfeld and Brenner, 1999; Cowchock, 1997; Simpson and associates, 1998).

The lupus anticoagulant is an immunoglobulin (IgG, IgM, or both) that interferes with one or more of the phospholipid-dependent tests of in vitro coagulation. The term is a misnomer because it is associated with clinically important increases in thromboembolic events. Importantly, the lupus anticoagulant is most often diagnosed in patients who do not meet the diagnostic criteria for lupus.

Antiphospholipid antibodies are acquired antibodies targeted against a phospholipid. They can be of the IgG, IgA, or IgM isotype. The mechanism of pregnancy loss in these women is thought to involve placental thrombosis and infarction. One mechanism may involve the inhibition of prostacyclin release (Fig. 33–4). This product of endothelial cells is a potent vasodilator and inhibitor of platelet aggregation. On the other hand, platelets produce thromboxane A_2, a vasoconstrictor and platelet aggregator. These antibodies therefore may reduce prostacyclin production, facilitating a thromboxane dominant milieu that leads to thrombosis. In addition, they have been shown to inhibit protein C activation. Investigators have proposed various treatments for

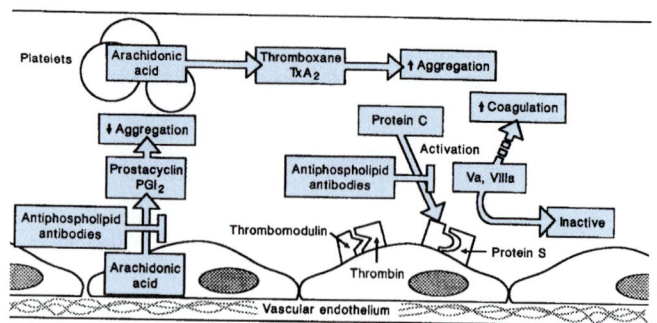

FIGURE 33–4. Possible mechanisms of antiphospholipid antibody–induced thrombosis. Three potential mechanisms are shown: (1) Endothelial cells normally convert plasma membrane arachidonic acid into prostacyclin, which is released into the circulation and prevents platelet aggregation. Antiphospholipid antibodies may predispose to thrombosis by inhibiting endothelial cells from producing prostacyclin. (2) Platelets normally convert plasma membrane arachidonic acid into thromboxane, which is released and induces platelet aggregation. Antiphospholipid antibodies may increase thrombosis by enhancing thromboxane release. (3) During clotting, thrombin forms a complex on the surface of endothelial cells with its receptor, thrombomodulin. The thrombin/thrombomodulin complex is enzymatically active and can activate circulating protein C. The activated protein C binds with protein S on the surface of endothelial cells (and platelets). The protein C/protein S complex degrades circulating activated components of the clotting cascade, factors Va and VIIIa. If factors Va and VIIIa were allowed to remain in the circulation, they would increase coagulation activity of the blood. (From Rote, 1989, with permission.)

the antiphospholipid antibody syndrome, including low-dose aspirin, prednisone, heparin, and intravenous immunoglobulin (Coulam, 1995). These treatments are thought to counteract the adverse action of antibodies by affecting both the immune and coagulation systems. Cowchock and colleagues (1992) performed a randomized trial comparing prednisone to low-dose heparin therapy in 20 women with antibodies and recurrent pregnancy loss. Live-birth rates were equal (75 percent) for both groups. However, those women receiving a glucocorticoid demonstrated a significantly greater incidence of maternal and fetal morbidity. Kutteh (1996) described 50 such women who were treated with either heparin and low-dose aspirin or aspirin alone. Heparin was initiated at 5000 units subcutaneously twice daily with a positive pregnancy test and titrated according to the partial thromboplastin time and platelet count. Although 76 percent of women in the heparin plus aspirin group delivered viable infants, only 44 percent of those treated with aspirin alone had a live birth. Maternal and obstetrical complications were low in both groups. Recent data indicate that antibodies bind directly to heparin in vitro and function in a similar way in vivo, thereby decreasing the adverse effects of the antibodies (Ermel and associates, 1995).

Branch and associates (2000) conducted a placebo-controlled pilot study of immune globulin for the treatment of the antiphospholipid antibody syndrome during pregnancy and found that intravenous immune globulin did not improve pregnancy outcomes above that achieved with heparin and low-dose aspirin.

ALLOIMMUNE FACTORS. A number of women with recurrent pregnancy loss have been diagnosed as having an alloimmune cause. They have received a variety of therapies targeted at stimulating maternal immune tolerance of fetal material. Diagnosis of an alloimmune factor has centered on several tests:

1. Maternal and paternal HLA comparison.
2. Assessment of maternal serum for the presence of cytotoxic antibodies to paternal leukocytes.
3. Maternal serum testing for blocking factors for maternal–paternal mixed lymphocyte reactions.

In essence, those couples determined to have significant HLA-type homology, or in which the women were found to have minimal antipaternal antibodies, were judged to represent an alloimmune disorder.

The validity of this model remains doubtful. For example, human HLA sharing clearly does not preclude successful pregnancies (Ober and co-workers, 1983). Most importantly, other studies have compared HLA sharing frequency in couples with recurrent losses with those with reproductive success and observed no differences (Bellingard, 1995; Houwert-de Jong, 1989; Sargent, 1988; and their associates). Although some investigators have found the presence of lymphocytotoxic antibodies and mixed lymphocyte culture inhibitors to be associated with women with successful pregnancies, Coulam (1992) has conclusively shown these to be a function of the duration and number of pregnancies rather than a reason for pregnancy loss. Furthermore, the results of these three tests were found to have no predictive value in assessing risks for subsequent pregnancy outcome in a population of women with recurrent losses (Cowchock and Smith, 1992).

Notwithstanding the uncertainties surrounding the most prevalent hypotheses of alloimmune causes of recurrent pregnancy loss, a number of studies have described outcomes following therapy to improve the maternal immune milieu. The majority of these women received either paternal leukocytes or pooled human immunoglobulin. Fraser and associates (1993) performed meta-analysis of 19 case series and concluded that immunotherapy does not significantly improve pregnancy outcome. A retrospective worldwide observational study and meta-analysis on allogenic leukocyte immunization therapy for recurrent pregnancy loss in

over 400 cases demonstrated marginal improvement for immunized women (Coulam and colleagues, 1994). The considerable expense and potential morbidity associated with immunization therapy make full disclosure of relevant information and informed consent important (Bux and co-workers, 1992; Katz and associates, 1992).

Some physicians have infused pooled human immunoglobulin as an alternative to paternal lymphocyte therapy. A prospective, double-blind, placebo-controlled trial using intravenous gamma globulin to treat women with recurrent loss demonstrated an improvement in women receiving this treatment versus placebo (Coulam, 1995). In another prospective study of 47 women with a history of three or more unexplained pregnancy losses, Stricker and associates (2000) reported that low-dose intravenous immunoglobulin (IVIG) was beneficial in improving pregnancy outcome. Of the 24 women receiving IVIG therapy who subsequently became pregnant, 22 had a term pregnancy. There were 11 women who refused IVIG therapy and seven subsequently became pregnant but all had first-trimester spontaneous abortions.

INHERITED THROMBOPHILIA. There have been numerous reports of an association of spontaneous abortions and inherited thrombophilias (Blumenfeld, 1999; Girling, 1998; Nelen, 1997; Ridker; 1998; Souza, 1999; Younis, 2000 and all their associates). As discussed in Chapter 49 (p. 1330), other pregnancy complications have also been associated with these thrombophilias (Table 33–2). In a study of 78 consecutive women with two or more first- or second-trimester losses, Younis and associates (2000) reported that 38 percent versus 8 percent of controls had activated protein C resistance and 19 percent versus 6 percent of controls had factor V Leiden mutation. Nelen and colleagues (2000) reported that elevated serum homocysteine levels were also a risk factor. Blumenfeld and Brenner (1999) recently reviewed thrombophilia-associated pregnancy wastage.

The optimal treatment for the various thrombophilias during pregnancy is unclear, but heparin (including low molecular weight heparin) appears to be efficacious for the treatment of antithrombin III deficiency as well as protein C and S deficiency. Aspirin plus heparin seems to be efficacious for treatment of factor V Leiden mutation and antiphospholipid syndrome (Blumenfeld and Brenner, 1999).

AGING GAMETES. Guerrero and Rojas (1975) found an increased incidence of abortion relative to successful pregnancies when insemination occurred 4 days before or 3 days after the time of shift in basal body temperature. They concluded, therefore, that aging of the gametes within the female genital tract before fertilization increased the chance of abortion. Dickey and colleagues

TABLE 33–2. **Maternal and Fetal Complications Associated with Thrombophilia**

Thrombophilia	Abortion	Fetal Demise	Preeclampsia
Antithrombin III deficiency	Possible	Definite	Possible
Protein C deficiency	Possible	Definite	Possible
Protein S deficiency	Possible	Definite	Possible
Factor V Leiden mutation	Definite	Definite	Definite
Hyperhomocysteinemia	Possible	Possible	Possible

Adapted from Blumenfeld and Brenner (1999), with permission.

(1992) reported that infertility patients over 35 had a higher incidence of *small amnionic sac syndrome* and an increased incidence of euploidic abortion. Whether ovulation induction or in vitro fertilization result in aging of gametes prior to implantation is not known.

LAPAROTOMY. There is no evidence that surgery performed during early pregnancy causes increased abortions (Chap. 42, p. 1144). For example, ovarian tumors and pedunculated myomas are generally removed without interfering with pregnancy. Peritonitis increases the likelihood of abortion.

PHYSICAL TRAUMA. Trauma that failed to interrupt the pregnancy is often forgotten. Only the particular event apparently related temporally to abortion is remembered. Most spontaneous abortions, however, occur some time after death of the embryo or fetus.

UTERINE DEFECTS

ACQUIRED UTERINE DEFECTS. Even large and multiple uterine leiomyomas usually do not cause abortion. When associated with abortion, their location is apparently more important than their size (Chap. 35, p. 927). Uterine synechiae (Asherman syndrome) are caused by destruction of large areas of endometrium by curettage. This in turn results in amenorrhea and recurrent abortions believed to be due to insufficient endometrium to support implantation. The diagnosis can be made by a hysterosalpingogram that shows characteristic multiple filling defects, but the most accurate and direct diagnosis is made by hysteroscopy (Raziel and colleagues, 1994). Romer (1994) reported that the incidence of intrauterine adhesions diagnosed by hysteroscopy was about the same after the first incomplete or missed abortion (20 percent), but was significantly higher in women with recurrent abortions (approximately 50 percent). Recommended treatment is lysis of the adhesions via hysteroscopy and placement of an intrauterine contraceptive device to prevent recurrence. Continous high-dose es-

trogen therapy is also recommended by some practitioners for 60 to 90 days. March and Israel (1981) reported that abortions decreased from 80 to 15 percent with such therapy.

DEVELOPMENTAL UTERINE DEFECTS. These defects are the consequence of abnormal müllerian duct formation or fusion; or they may occur spontaneously or be induced by in utero exposure to diethylstilbestrol (Chap. 35). Some types, such as uterine septa, may be associated with abortions. Porcu and associates (2000) described pregnancy outcomes in 63 women with a septate uterus. They all underwent hysteroscopic resection of the septa because of repeat pregnancy loss or abnormal fetal presentation. There were 26 term live births following this procedure. In a recent review, Homer and associates (2000) reported that hysteroscopic septoplasty resulted in improved pregnancy outcome in women with repeated pregnancy loss.

INCOMPETENT CERVIX. The term *incompetent cervix* is applied to a discrete obstetrical entity. It is characterized by painless cervical dilatation in the second trimester or perhaps early in the third trimester, with prolapse and ballooning of membranes into the vagina, followed by rupture of membranes and expulsion of an immature fetus. Unless effectively treated, this sequence tends to repeat in each pregnancy.

Numerous methods have been described in nonpregnant women to make the diagnosis, usually by documenting a more widely dilated internal cervical os than is normal. Methods have included hysterography, pull-through techniques of inflated catheter balloons, and acceptance without resistance at the internal os of specifically sized cervical dilators (Ansari and Reynolds, 1987). During pregnancy, attempts have been made with moderate success to predict premature cervical dilation using ultrasonic techniques (Michaels and associates, 1989). Iams and co-workers (1995) performed a cross-sectional study of cervical length measured by transvaginal ultrasonography in women with a prior preterm delivery, those with cervical incompetence, and normal controls delivered at term. Gestational age at the first preterm delivery was significantly correlated with cervical length in the pregnancy evaluated at each gestational age between 20 and 30 weeks. Andrews and associates (2000), in a study of 53 women with ultrasound evaluation prior to 20 weeks, reported an association of short cervical lengths or funneling of the internal cervical os and early spontaneous preterm births. Several authors have reported on the use of transfundal pressure during transvaginal ultrasound evaluation of the cervix as an aid in the detection of asymptomatic incompetent cervix (Guzman and colleagues, 1997a, 1997b, 1998; Rocco and Garrone, 1999).

Kurup and Goldkrand (1999), in a study comparing elective, emergent, or urgent cerclage, concluded that ultrasound was useful in identifying women with subtle changes in the cervix who would benefit from urgent cerclage. Ultrasound has also been utilized to demonstrate an increase in cervical length after prophylactic or therapeutic cerclage (Althuisius and co-workers, 1999; Funai and colleagues, 1999). The use of magnetic resonance imaging in the diagnosis of incompetent cervix was recently reported by Maldjian and associates (1999).

There is little doubt that ultrasound, especially transvaginal, is a useful adjunct for the diagnosis of cervical shortening or funneling of the internal os and in the early detection of cervical incompetence. The diagnosis, however, remains difficult in most women and is still often based on clinical examination and history.

ETIOLOGY. Although the cause of cervical incompetence is obscure, previous trauma to the cervix—especially in the course of dilatation and curettage, conization, cauterization, or amputation—appears to be a factor in many cases. In other instances, abnormal cervical development, including that following exposure to diethylstilbestrol in utero, plays a role (Chap. 35, p. 918).

TREATMENT. The treatment of cervical incompetence is surgical, consisting of reinforcement of the weak cervix by some type of purse-string suture. Bleeding, uterine contractions, or ruptured membranes are usually contraindications to surgery.

PREOPERATIVE EVALUATION. Cerclage should generally be delayed until after 14 weeks so that early abortions due to other factors will be completed. There is no consensus as to how late in pregnancy the procedure should be performed. The more advanced the pregnancy, the more likely surgical intervention will stimulate preterm labor or membrane rupture. For these reasons, some clinicians prefer bed rest rather than cerclage some time after midpregnancy. We usually do not perform cerclage after 24 to 26 weeks.

Aarts and associates (1995) provided a review of late second-trimester cerclage, commonly known as an *emergency cerclage*. They concluded that emergency cerclage can be of benefit in some women, but that the incidence of complications, especially infection, is high. According to Schorr and Morales (1996), bulging membranes are associated with significantly increased failure rates. Caruso and associates (2000) reported their experience with emergency cerclage in 23 women with a dilated cervix and protruding membranes (gestational age 17 to 27 weeks). There were 11 live-born infants and they concluded that the success of the procedure was unpredictable. In a 10-year review of 75 emergency cerclages, Chasen and Silverman (1998) reported that 65 percent of the women delivered at 28 weeks or later, and half delivered at 37 weeks or greater. Only 44 percent of those with bulging membranes at the time of cerclage reached 28 weeks. Amnioreduction at the time of emergency cerclage may improve pregnancy prolongation (Locatelli and associates, 1999).

Sonography to confirm a living fetus and to exclude major fetal anomalies is done prior to cerclage. Obvious cervical infection should be treated, and cultures for gonorrhea, chlamydia, and group B streptococci are recommended. For at least a week before and after surgery, there should be no sexual intercourse.

If there is a question as to whether cerclage should be performed, the woman is placed at decreased physical activity. Proscription of intercourse is essential, and frequent cervical examinations should be conducted to assess cervical effacement and dilatation. Weekly ultrasonic surveillance of the lower uterine segment between 14 and 27 weeks may prove useful in some women (Guzman and associates, 1998; Michaels and colleagues, 1989). Unfortunately, rapid effacement and dilatation develop even with such precautions (Witter, 1984).

CERCLAGE PROCEDURES. Three types of operations are commonly used during pregnancy. One is a simple procedure recommended by McDonald (1963) and illustrated in Figure 33–5. The second is the more complicated Shirodkar operation (1955). The third is the modified Shirodkar procedure shown in Figure 33–6. There is less trauma and blood loss with both the McDonald and modified Shirodkar procedures than with the original Shirodkar procedure.

In many cases, filling the bladder with 600 mL of saline through an indwelling Foley catheter will serve to push the fetus and membranes upward from the ballooning lower segment. Some clinicians recommended placement of a 30-mL balloon Foley catheter through the cervix and inflating the balloon with saline to deflect the amnionic sac cephalad.

Success rates approaching 85 to 90 percent are achieved with both McDonald and modified Shirodkar techniques (Caspi and associates, 1990; Kuhn and Pep-

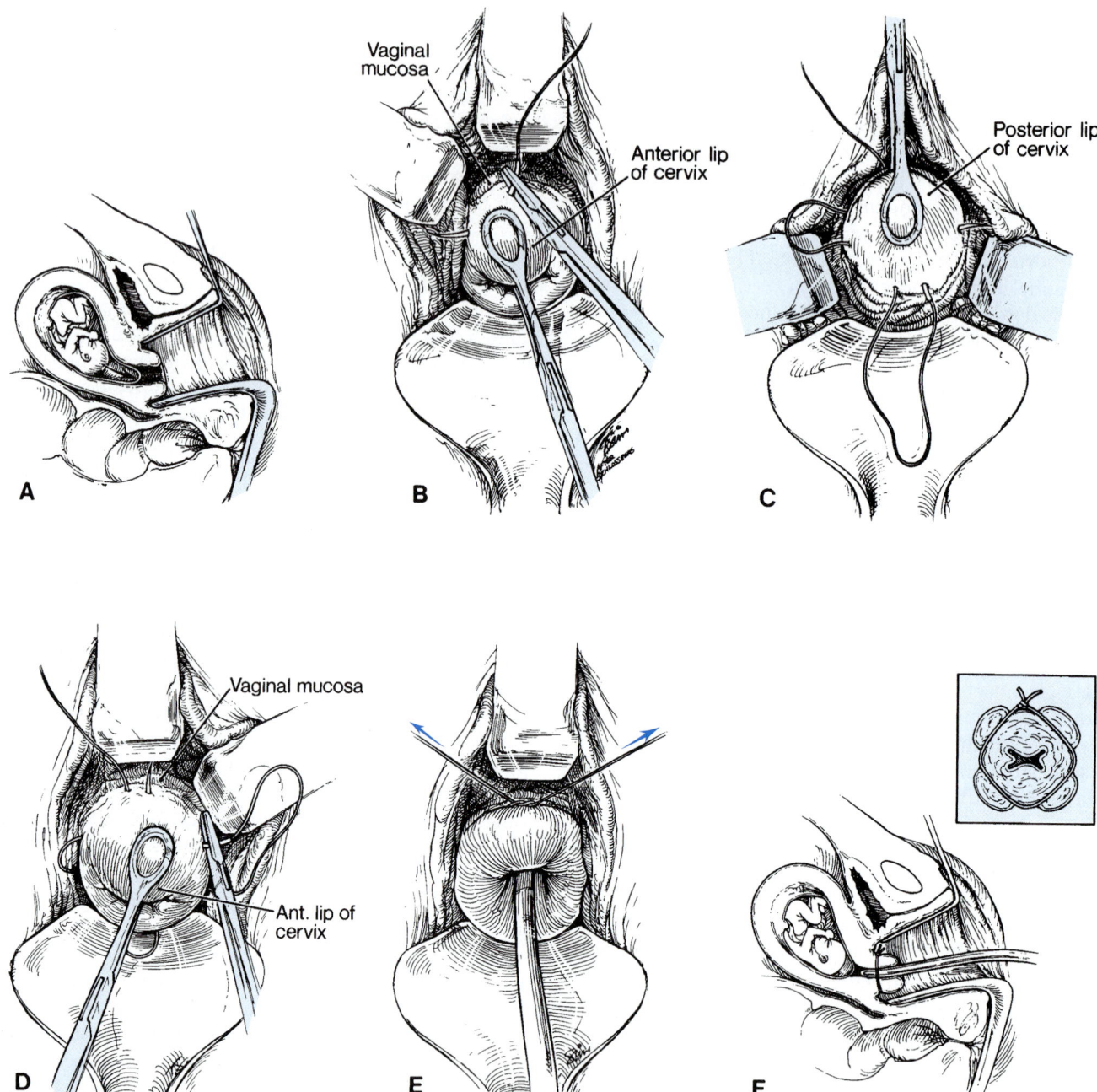

FIGURE 33–5. Incompetent cervix treated with McDonald cerclage procedure. **A.** Somewhat dilated cervical canal and beginning prolapse of membranes (*arrow*). **B.** Start of the cerclage procedure with a suture of #2 monofilament being placed superiorly in the body of the cervix very near the level of the internal os. **C.** Continuation of suture placement in the body of the cervix so as to encircle the os. **D.** Completion of encirclement. **E.** The suture is tightened around the cervical canal sufficiently to reduce the diameter of the canal to 5 to 10 mm. In the illustration the *small* dilator has been placed just through the level of ligation to maintain patency of the canal when the suture is tied. A second suture similarly placed but somewhat higher may be of value, especially if the first is not in close proximity to the internal os. **F.** The effect of the suture placement on the cervical canal is apparent.

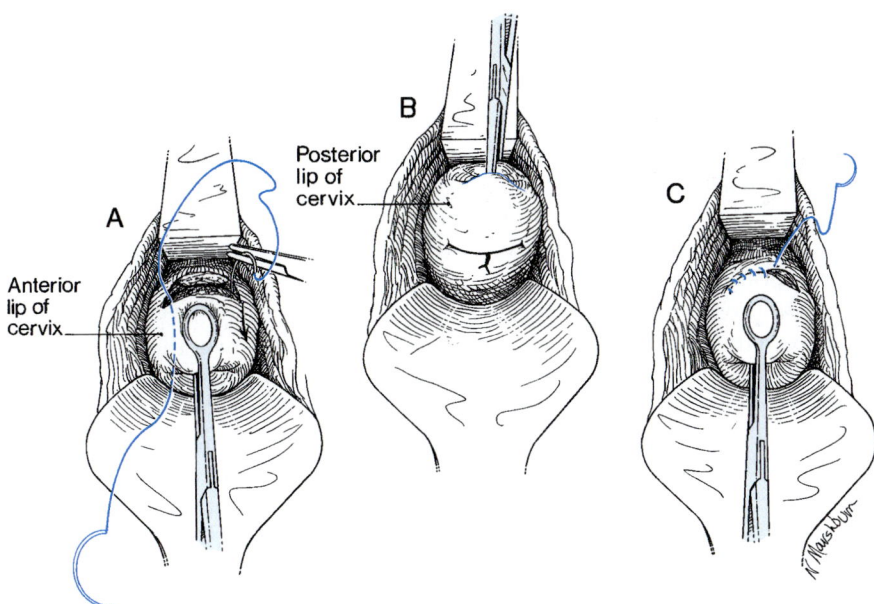

FIGURE 33-6. Modified Shirodkar cerclage. **A.** After transverse cervical incision, the bladder has been pushed cephalad. Double-needled ligature is passed anteriorly to posteriorly on each side of cervix. **B.** Ligature is tied posteriorly, usually around a 10-mm dilator. **C.** Cervical mucosa is run with chromic suture to bury the anterior purse-string suture.

perell, 1977). Thus, there appears to be little reason for performing the more complicated original Shirodkar procedure. The modified Shirodkar procedure is often reserved for previous McDonald cerclage failures and structural cervical abnormalities. Success rates are higher when cervical dilatation was minimal and membrane prolapse was absent.

Transabdominal cerclage placed at the level of the uterine isthmus has been recommended in some instances, especially in cases of anatomical defects of the cervix or failed transvaginal cerclage (Cammarano and colleagues, 1995; Gibb and Salaria, 1995; Herron and Parer, 1988). The procedure requires laparotomy for placement of the suture and another laparotomy for its removal, for delivery of the fetus, or both. The potential for trauma and other complications initially and subsequently is much greater with this procedure than with the vaginal procedures. Turnquest and colleagues (1999) recently described fetal salvage in 9 of 11 women with abdominal cerclage.

COMPLICATIONS. Charles and Edward (1981) identified complications, especially infection, to be much less frequent when cerclage was performed by 18 weeks. When performed much after 20 weeks, there was a high incidence of membrane rupture, chorioamnionitis, and intrauterine infection. With clinical infection, the suture should be cut, and labor induced.

There is no evidence that prophylactic antibiotics prevent infection, or that progestational agents or β-mimetic drugs are of any adjunctive value (Thomason and co-workers, 1982). In the event that the operation fails and signs of imminent abortion or delivery develop, it is urgent that the suture be released at once; failure

to do so may result in grave sequelae. Rupture of the uterus or cervix may be the consequence of vigorous uterine contractions with the ligature in place. Membrane rupture during suture placement or within the first 48 hours of surgery is considered by some to be an indication to remove the cerclage. Kuhn and Pepperell (1977) reported that when the membranes rupture in the absence of labor, the likelihood of serious fetal or maternal infection is increased appreciably if the suture is left in situ and delivery is delayed. Still, the range of management options spans from observation, to removal of the cerclage with observation, to removal of the cerclage and labor induction (Barth, 1995). There are insufficient data upon which to base any firm recommendation, and the optimal management of such patients remains controversial (O'Connor and associates, 1999).

Following the Shirodkar operation, the suture can be left in place if it remains covered by mucosa, and cesarean delivery performed near term. Conversely, the Shirodkar suture may be removed and vaginal delivery permitted.

PATERNAL FACTORS. Little is known about paternal factors in the genesis of spontaneous abortion. Certainly, chromosomal translocations in sperm can lead to abortion. Kulcsar and associates (1991) found adenovirus or herpes simplex virus in nearly 40 percent of semen samples obtained from sterile men. The viruses were detected in latent form in 60 percent of the cells, and the same viruses were found in abortuses.

CATEGORIES AND TREATMENT OF SPONTANEOUS ABORTION. It is convenient to consider the clinical aspects of spontaneous abortion under five subgroups: threatened, inevitable, incomplete, missed, and recurrent abortion.

THREATENED ABORTION. The clinical diagnosis of threatened abortion is presumed when any bloody vaginal discharge or bleeding appears during the first half of pregnancy. It is an extremely commonplace occurrence, and one out of four or five women has vaginal spotting or heavier bleeding during early gestation. Of those women who bleed in early pregnancy, approximately half will abort. The bleeding of threatened abortion frequently is slight, but it may persist for days or weeks. Unfortunately, an increased risk of suboptimal pregnancy outcome in the form of preterm delivery, low birthweight, and perinatal death persists (Batzofin and associates, 1984; Funderburk and colleagues, 1980). Importantly, the risk of a malformed infant does not appear to be increased.

Some bleeding about the time of expected menses may be physiological. Cervical lesions are likely to bleed in early pregnancy, especially after intercourse. Polyps presenting at the external cervical os as well as decidual reaction in the cervix tend to bleed in early gestation. A significant clinical point is that lower abdominal pain and persistent low backache do not accompany bleeding from these benign causes.

Because most physicians consider any bleeding in early pregnancy to be a sign of threatened abortion, any treatment of so-called threatened abortion has a considerable likelihood of success. Most women who actually are threatening to abort will ultimately do so no matter what is done. If, however, bleeding is attributable to one of the unrelated causes mentioned previously, it is likely to disappear, regardless of treatment.

If an intrauterine device is still present and the "string" is visible, the device should be removed for reasons cited in Chapter 58 (p. 1539).

Bleeding usually begins first, and cramping abdominal pain follows a few hours to several days later. The pain of abortion may be anterior and clearly rhythmic; it may be a persistent low backache, associated with a feeling of pelvic pressure; or it may be a dull, midline, suprapubic discomfort. Whichever form the pain takes, prognosis for pregnancy continuation in the presence of bleeding and pain is poor. Higher perinatal mortality rates are observed in women whose pregnancies were complicated early by threatened abortion.

Each woman should be examined for there is always the possibility that the cervix already is dilated and abortion is inevitable, or there is a serious complication such as extrauterine pregnancy or torsion of an unsuspected ovarian cyst. She may be kept at home in bed with analgesia given to help relieve the pain. If the bleeding persists, she should be reexamined and the hematocrit rechecked. If blood loss is sufficient to cause anemia or hypovolemia, evacuation of the pregnancy is generally indicated.

Women with threatened abortion have been treated with progesterone intramuscularly or with a wide variety of synthetic progestational agents orally or intramuscularly. Unfortunately, there evidence of effectiveness is lacking. "Success" from the use of these agents often results in no more than a missed abortion.

Occasionally, slight bleeding may persist for weeks. It then becomes essential to decide whether there is any possibility of continuation of the pregnancy. Vaginal sonography, serial serum quantitative chorionic gonadotropin (hCG) levels, and serum progesterone values, measured alone or in various combinations, have proven helpful in ascertaining if a live intrauterine pregnancy is present. Fossum and associates (1988) reported that a fetal sac can usually be seen using vaginal sonography between 33 and 35 days from the last menstrual period (Table 33–3). This was associated with a chorionic gonadotropin level of about 1000 mIU/mL. Thus, if a gestational sac can be seen and serum hCG is less than 1000 mIU/mL, the gestation is not likely to survive. If any doubt exists, however, serial gonadotropin levels should be measured.

Al-Sebai and associates (1995) reported that a single progesterone measurement had an 88 percent sensitivity and specificity in predicting a live versus dead intrauterine fetus or a tubal pregnancy. Stovall and associates (1992) reported that only about 1 percent of abnormal pregnancies (spontaneous incomplete abortions and ectopic pregnancies) have a serum progesterone level of 25 ng/mL or greater. A serum progesterone value of less than 5 ng/mL was associated with a dead conceptus, but this did not localize the pregnancy as uterine or extrauterine. Hahlin and colleagues (1990) reported that no live intrauterine pregnancy had a progesterone level less than 10 ng/mL; and 88 percent of ectopic pregnancies and 83 percent of spontaneous abortions had lower values. Therefore, with a fetal sac clearly visible, a

TABLE 33–3. Temporal Values for Gestational Age, Serum β-hCG Levels, and Vaginal Ultrasound Findings in Normal Pregnancy

Days from Last Menses	β-hCG (mIU/mL)	Vaginal Ultrasonography
34.8 ± 2.2[a]	914 ± 106	Fetal sac
40.3 ± 3.4[b]	3783 ± 683	Fetal pole
46.9 ± 6.0[b]	13,178 ± 2898[b]	Fetal heart activity

[a] ± Standard error of the mean.
[b] $P < .05$ when compared with fetal sac.
Modified from Fossum and colleagues (1988).

gonadotropin level of less than 1000 mIU/mL, and a serum progesterone value of less than 5 ng/mL, there almost certainly is not an intrauterine pregnancy.

Sonographic demonstration of a distinct, well-formed gestational ring with central echoes from the embryo implies that the products of conception are reasonably healthy (Table 33–3). A gestational sac with no central echoes from an embryo or fetus implies strongly, but does not prove, death of the conceptus. When abortion is inevitable, mean gestational sac diameter is frequently smaller than appropriate for gestational age. All viable intrauterine pregnancies are visible by transvaginal ultrasonography by 41 days' gestation (Lipscomb and colleagues, 2000). Moreover, by approximately 45 days after the last menses and thereafter, fetal heart action should be discernible using real-time ultrasound. Emerson and associates (1992) and Pellerito and colleagues (1992) reported excellent results in identifying live intrauterine gestations using vaginal color and pulsed Doppler flow imaging techniques.

After death of the conceptus, the uterus should be emptied. All tissue passed should be examined to determine whether the abortion is complete. Unless all of the fetus and placenta can be positively identified, curettage may be required. Vaginal probe or abdominal ultrasound may assist in this decision-making process. If significant amounts of material are retained within the uterine cavity, curettage is recommended by most clinicians. Ectopic pregnancy should always be considered in the differential diagnosis of threatened abortion. This is especially so if the gestational sac or fetus are not identified. Frozen section of the curettings may further assist with diagnosis.

Women who are D negative with a threatened abortion probably should receive anti-D immunoglobulin (Chap. 39, p. 1067). Von Stein and associates (1992) reported that more than 10 percent of such women had significant fetomaternal hemorrhage.

INEVITABLE ABORTION. Inevitability of abortion is signaled by gross rupture of the membranes in the presence of cervical dilatation. Under these conditions, abortion is almost certain. Rarely, a gush of fluid from the uterus during the first half of pregnancy is without serious consequence. The fluid may have collected previously between the amnion and chorion. Most often, however, either uterine contractions begin promptly, resulting in expulsion of the pregnancy, or infection develops.

With obvious membrane rupture during the first half of pregnancy, the possibility of salvaging the pregnancy is very unlikely. If in early pregnancy the sudden discharge of fluid, suggesting ruptured membranes, occurs before any pain or bleeding, the woman may be put to bed and observed for further leakage of fluid, bleeding, cramping, or fever. If after 48 hours there has been no further escape of amnionic fluid, no bleeding or pain, and no fever, she may get up and, except for any form of vaginal penetration, continue her usual activities. If, however, the gush of fluid is accompanied or followed by bleeding and pain, or if fever ensues, abortion should be considered inevitable and the uterus emptied.

INCOMPLETE ABORTION. The fetus and placenta are likely to be expelled together in abortions occurring before 10 weeks, but separately thereafter. When the placenta, in whole or in part, is retained in the uterus, bleeding ensues sooner or later, to produce the main sign of incomplete abortion. With abortions that are more advanced, bleeding occasionally may be massive to the point of producing profound hypovolemia.

In instances of incomplete abortion, it is often unnecessary to dilate the cervix before curettage. In many cases, the retained placental tissue simply lies loose in the cervical canal and can be lifted from an exposed external os with ovum or ring forceps. Suction curettage, as described later, is effective for evacuating the uterus. A woman with a more advanced pregnancy, or a woman who is bleeding heavily, should be hospitalized and the retained tissue removed without delay. Hemorrhage from incomplete abortion is occasionally severe but rarely fatal. Fever is not a contraindication to curettage once appropriate antibiotic treatment has been started (p. 877).

Nielsen and Hahlin (1995) performed a randomized study comparing expectant management with curettage for spontaneous abortions less than 13 weeks. Spontaneous resolution of pregnancy occurred within 3 days in 80 percent of women treated conservatively, although vaginal bleeding lasted on the average one day longer. Complications were similar between the groups.

MISSED ABORTION. This is defined as retention of dead products of conception in utero for several weeks. The rationale for an exact time period is not clear, and it serves no useful clinical purpose. In the typical instance, early pregnancy appears to be normal, with amenorrhea, nausea and vomiting, breast changes, and growth of the uterus. After fetal death, there may or may not be vaginal bleeding or other symptoms denoting a threatened abortion. For a time, the uterus seems to remain stationary in size, but mammary changes usually regress. The woman is likely to lose a few pounds. Thereafter, it becomes apparent that the uterus not only has ceased to enlarge but also has become smaller. Many women have no symptoms during this period except persistent amenorrhea. If the missed abortion terminates spontaneously, and most do, the process of expulsion is the same as in any abortion. If retained several weeks after death, it becomes a shriveled sac containing a macerated

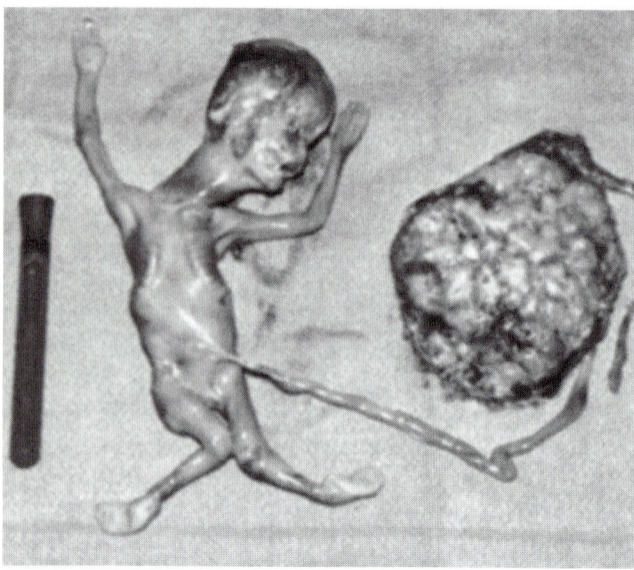

FIGURE 33–7. Dead immature fetus retained in utero with placenta for many weeks. Characteristic thick, opaque amnionic fluid is contained in the stoppered tube.

fetus (Fig. 33–7). Egarter and associates (1995) reported that gemeprost vaginal suppositories (prostaglandin E_1) were effective in the termination of first-trimester missed abortions in 77 percent of women.

Occasionally, after prolonged retention of the dead fetus, serious coagulation defects develop. This is more likely when the gestation reached the second trimester before fetal death. The woman may note troublesome bleeding from the nose or gums and especially from sites of slight trauma. The pathogenesis and treatment of coagulation defects and any attendant hemorrhage in instances of prolonged retention of a dead fetus are considered in Chapter 25 (p. 659).

The reason some abortions do not terminate after fetal death is not clear. The use of potent progestational compounds to treat threatened abortion, however, may contribute to this. Smith and co-workers (1978) observed that 73 percent of women with threatened abortion given hormonal treatment did abort, but on the average 20 days later. In women who received no hormonal support, 67 percent aborted at a mean of 5 days.

RECURRENT ABORTION. This has been defined by various criteria of number and sequence, but probably the most generally accepted definition refers to three or more consecutive spontaneous abortions. Repeated spontaneous abortions are likely to be chance phenomena in the majority of cases. Accepting an independent risk of miscarriage occurrence to be 15 percent, a second loss could be calculated to occur at a rate of 2.3 percent and a third loss in 0.34 percent of women. In a study of women doctors, the occurrences of one, two, and

three miscarriages were reported to be 10.4, 2.3, and 0.34 percent, respectively (Alberman, 1988). Approximately 1 to 2 percent of women of reproductive age will experience three or more spontaneous, consecutive abortions, and as many as 5 percent will have two or more recurrent abortions (Blumenfeld and Brenner, 1999).

Epidemiologically, there is some uniformity in the proportion of recurrent pregnancy loss with chromosomal anomalies. Despite this, however, there are significant discrepancies when compared with the relative prevalence of other categories. There are several reasons to explain this: First, differences in definition make direct comparisons between various studies questionable. For example, some authors included women with only two losses into their analysis. Second, methods used to assign women to various diagnostic categories differ. Complicating this issue is that many diagnoses under consideration are debatable, both as to the criteria used and to their actual contribution to pregnancy loss. Third, the intensity of evaluation applied prior to categorizing a woman as "unexplained" varied among these studies. In general, the majority of studies have observed that women with three or more miscarriages more commonly are determined to have a chromosomal anomaly, endocrinological disorder, or an altered immune system (Table 33–4).

PROGNOSIS. With the exception of antiphospholipid antibodies and an incompetent cervix, the apparent "cure rate" after as many as three consecutive spontaneous abortions will range between 70 and 85 percent regardless of treatment. That is, the loss rate will be higher, but not a great deal higher, than that anticipated for pregnancies in general. In fact, Warburton and Fraser (1964) reported that the likelihood of recurrent abortion was 25 to 30 percent regardless of the number of previous abortions. Poland and associates (1977) noted that if a woman had previously delivered a live-born

TABLE 33–4. Diagnosis in Normal Women and in Women with Recurrent Pregnancy Loss[a]

Diagnosis	Normal (%)	Recurrent Loss (%)
Genetic (parental)	0.2	2–5
Endocrinological	3–8	5–29
Anatomical	5–15	1–28
Immunological	1–3	6–65
Idiopathic	—	15–50

[a] Percentages refer to estimated frequencies of diagnosis that can be made in normal women and in women with recurrent pregnancy loss.
Data from Coulam (1995), Harger (1983), Makino (1992), Stray-Pedersen (1984), Tho (1979), and all their colleagues.

infant, the risk for each recurrent abortion was approximately 30 percent. If, however, the woman had no live-born infants and had experienced at least one spontaneous fetal loss, the risk of abortion was 46 percent. Women with three or more spontaneous abortions are at increased risk in a subsequent pregnancy for preterm delivery, placenta previa, breech presentation, and fetal malformation (Thom and colleagues, 1992).

INDUCED ABORTION

Induced abortion is the *medical or surgical termination of pregnancy before the time of fetal viability*. In 1996, a total of 1,221,585 legal abortions were reported to the Centers for Disease Control and Prevention (1999). Approximately 20 percent of these women were 19 years of age or less and the majority were less than 25 years of age, white, and unmarried (Centers for Disease Control and Prevention, 2000). About 88 percent of abortions were performed before 13 weeks, 55 percent before 8 weeks, and 16 percent at 6 weeks or less.

LEGAL ASPECTS. Until the United States Supreme Court decision of 1973, only therapeutic abortions could be performed legally in most states. The most common legal definition of therapeutic abortion until then was termination of pregnancy before the period of fetal viability for the purpose of saving the life of the mother. A few states extended their laws to read "to prevent serious or permanent bodily injury to the mother" or "to preserve the life or health of the woman." Some states allowed abortion if pregnancy was likely to result in the birth of an infant with grave malformations.

The stringent abortion laws in effect until 1973 were of fairly recent origin. Abortion before quickening—the first definite perception of fetal movement, which most often occurs between 16 and 20 weeks' gestation—was either lawful or widely tolerated in both the United States and Great Britain until 1803. In that year, as part of a general restructuring of British criminal law, a statute was enacted that made abortion before quickening illegal. The Roman Catholic Church's traditional condemnation of abortion did not receive the ultimate sanction of universal law (excommunication) until 1869 (Pilpel and Norwich, 1969).

It was not until 1821 that Connecticut enacted the nation's first abortion law. Subsequently, throughout the United States, abortion became illegal except to save the life of the mother. Because therapeutic abortion to save the life of the woman is rarely necessary or definable, it follows that the great majority of such operations previously performed in this country went beyond the letter of the law. Borgmann and Jones (2000) have extensively reviewed legal issues in providing abortions.

INDICATIONS. Some indications for therapeutic abortion are discussed with the diseases that commonly lead to the operation. Well-documented indications are persistent heart disease after previous cardiac decompensation and advanced hypertensive vascular disease. Another is invasive carcinoma of the cervix. The American College of Obstetricians and Gynecologists (1987) established guidelines for therapeutic abortion:

- When continuation of pregnancy may threaten the life of the woman or seriously impair her health. In determining whether or not there is such a risk to health, account may be taken of her total environment, actual or reasonably foreseeable.
- When pregnancy has resulted from rape or incest. In this case, the same medical criteria should be employed in evaluation of the woman.
- When continuation of pregnancy is likely to result in the birth of a child with severe physical deformities or mental retardation. Issues such as maternal HIV-1 infection are less clear-cut but problematic (Araneta and colleagues, 1992).

ELECTIVE (VOLUNTARY) ABORTION. Elective or voluntary abortion is the interruption of pregnancy before viability at the request of the woman but not for reasons of impaired maternal health or fetal disease. Most abortions done today fall into this category; in fact, there is approximately one elective abortion for every three live births in the United States.

LEGALITY. It was only about 25 years ago when elective abortion was again legalized in the United States. Several Supreme Court decisions are noteworthy in the history of abortion.

ROE VERSUS WADE. The legality of elective abortion was established by the United States Supreme Court in its 1973 decision in *Roe v Wade*. It defined the extent to which states might regulate abortion:

(a) For the stage prior to approximately the end of the first trimester, the abortion decision and its effectuation must be left to the medical judgment of the attending physician.

(b) For the stage subsequent to approximately the end of the first trimester, the State, in promoting its interest in the health of the mother, may, if it chooses, regulate the abortion procedures in ways that are reasonably related to maternal health.

(c) For the stage subsequent to viability, the State, in promoting its interest in the potential of human life, may, if it chooses, regulate, and even proscribe, abortion, except where necessary, in appropriate medical judgment, for the preservation of the life or health of the mother.

WEBSTER VERSUS REPRODUCTIVE HEALTH SERVICES. Since the *Roe v Wade* decision, many different pieces of legislation, both state and national, have been introduced, and some enacted, to regulate or even dismantle its three provisions. All such attempts were unsuccessful until the United States Supreme Court ruled in the 1989 *Webster v Reproductive Health Services* that states could place restrictions interfering with provision of abortion services on such items as waiting periods, specific informed consent requirements, parental/spousal notification, and hospital requirements. Based upon this decision, numerous challenges have arisen to limit a woman's choice and access to abortion services.

PLANNED PARENTHOOD OF SOUTHEASTERN PENNSYLVANIA VERSUS ROBERT P. CASEY. In 1992, the United States Supreme Court considered whether a state could require, prior to an abortion, a woman's informed consent, a 24-hour waiting period, spousal consent, parental consent in the case of a minor, and a physician's description of the fetus and the abortion technique to be employed. In a 5 to 4 decision, the court upheld a state's right to require all these except spousal consent. The court also reconsidered and reaffirmed the *Roe v Wade* decision by a 5 to 4 vote.

STENBERG VERSUS CARHART. The United States Supreme Court in 2000 considered whether the state of Nebraska, as represented by Attorney General Don Stenberg, could by state law prevent the performance of so-called "partial birth abortions," and specifically those performed by Dr. Leroy Carhart. The court, in a 5 to 4 decision, struck down the Nebraska law. The court ruled that the Nebraska law was too broad, and that such a prohibition could jeopardize abortions that involve more common surgical procedures. The court also noted that the Nebraska law "would place some women at unnecessary risk" because it did not include a health exception.

HILL VERSUS COLORADO. In this 6 to 4 decision rendered also in 2000, the United States Supreme Court upheld the 1993 Colorado statute that is used to regulate speech-related conduct within 100 feet of the entrance to any health-care facility. The specific portion of the statute that was challenged by Leila J. Hill and others dealt with the provision that made it unlawful to "knowingly approach" within 8 feet of another person without that person's consent "for the purpose of passing a leaflet or handbill to, displaying a sign to, or engaging in oral protest, education, or counseling with such other person. . . ."

The Colorado law had been enacted to prevent the disruption of normal functions at medical facilities by protests conducted for any reason. The Supreme Court's decision to uphold the Colorado law does not prevent protests against abortion facilities, but it certainly reduces the likelihood of confrontations between patients and demonstrators. That is, the court noted that the Colorado law insured "the right to be left alone" and did not violate the First Amendment because the law is "content neutral."

COUNSELING BEFORE ELECTIVE ABORTION. There are only three choices available to the woman considering an abortion. These are continued pregnancy with its risks and responsibilities; continued pregnancy with its risks and arranged adoption; or the choice of abortion with its risks. In any event, knowledgeable and compassionate counselors are invaluable. For instance, women who delay abortion decisions to later gestational ages have been shown to exhibit greater disturbances in the basic sense of self as noted in indications of gender/sexual conflict and lower achievement or striving orientation (Cancelmo and associates, 1992).

ABORTION TECHNIQUES. Abortion can be performed either medically or surgically. In a randomized comparison of the efficacy and acceptability of these techniques, Creinin (2000) reported that medical abortion seemed to be slightly less costly than surgical techniques. Paul and colleagues (1999) have provided detailed summaries for each method shown in Table 33–5.

Prior to an elective abortion, if bacterial vaginosis is found, the woman should be treated with metronidazole to reduce the postoperative infection rate (Larsson and colleagues, 1992). Vaginal application of 2 percent clindamycin cream for 3 days reduces postabortion pelvic infection fourfold compared with placebo (Larsson and co-workers, 2000). Treatment of D-negative women after abortion with anti-D immunoglobulin is recommended, because about 5 percent of D-negative women become sensitized after an abortion (Chap. 39, p. 1066).

Goldstein and associates (1994) emphasized the utility of both ultrasound and immediate tissue examination in 674 women undergoing elective first-trimester abortion. Each woman was scanned with an empty bladder using the transabdominal technique. If no gestational sac was seen, endovaginal sonography was performed. All specimens underwent modified gross examination at 33 times magnification and tissue was sent for histopathological analysis. Transabdominal sonogram demonstrated uterine gestational tissue in 612 women (91 percent) and 595 of these were less than 12 weeks. There were 17 women (2.5 percent) who were 13 weeks or greater. In 62 women (9 percent) with no sac seen transabdominally, endovaginal ultrasound showed 34 uterine and two unruptured ectopic pregnancies. Of the remaining women, chorionic villi (17) and decidua without villi (4) were seen on tissue examination. Of the latter

TABLE 33–5. Abortion Techniques

Surgical Techniques

Cervical dilatation followed by uterine evacuation

    Curettage

    Vacuum aspiration (suction curettage)

    Dilatation and evacuation (D & E)

    Dilatation and extraction (D & X)

Menstrual aspiration

Laparotomy

    Hysterotomy

    Hysterectomy

Medical Techniques

Oxytocin intravenously

Intra-amnionic hyperosomotic fluid

    20% saline

    30% urea

Prostaglandins E_2, $F_{2\alpha}$, and analogues

    Intra-amnionic injection

    Extraovular injection

    Vaginal insertion

    Parenteral injection

    Oral ingestion

Antiprogesterones—RU 486 (mifepristone) and epostane

Various combinations of the above

four, two had rising serum hCG levels and were diagnosed with ectopic pregnancy, and two with falling levels were managed expectantly.

SURGICAL TECHNIQUES FOR ABORTION. The pregnancy may be removed surgically through an appropriately dilated cervix or transabdominally by either hysterotomy or hysterectomy.

DILATATION AND CURETTAGE. Surgical abortion is performed by first dilating the cervix and then evacuating the pregnancy by mechanically scraping out the contents (sharp curettage), by vacuum aspiration (suction curettage), or both. The technique for early manual vacuum has been recently reviewed by MacIsaac and Jones (2000). The likelihood of complications—including uterine perforation, cervical laceration, hemorrhage, incomplete removal of the fetus and placenta, and infection—increases after the first trimester. For this reason, curettage or vacuum aspiration should be performed before 14 weeks.

After 16 weeks, dilatation and evacuation (D & E) is performed. This consists of wide cervical dilatation followed by mechanical destruction and evacuation of fetal parts. With complete removal of the fetus, a large-bore vacuum curette is used to remove the placenta and remaining tissue. A dilatation and extraction (D & X) is similar to a D & E except that with a D & X, part of the fetus is first extracted through the dilated cervix to facilitate the procedure.

In the absence of maternal systemic disease, pregnancies are usually terminated by curettage or by evacuation or extraction without hospitalization. When abortion is not performed in a hospital setting, it is imperative that capabilities for effective cardiopulmonary resuscitation be available, and that immediate access to hospitalization be possible.

HYGROSCOPIC DILATORS. Trauma from mechanical dilatation can be minimized by using a device to slowly dilate the cervix. These devices draw water from cervical tissues and also are used for preinduction cervical ripening (Chap. 20, p. 473). Laminaria tents are commonly used to help dilate the cervix (Fig. 33–8). They are

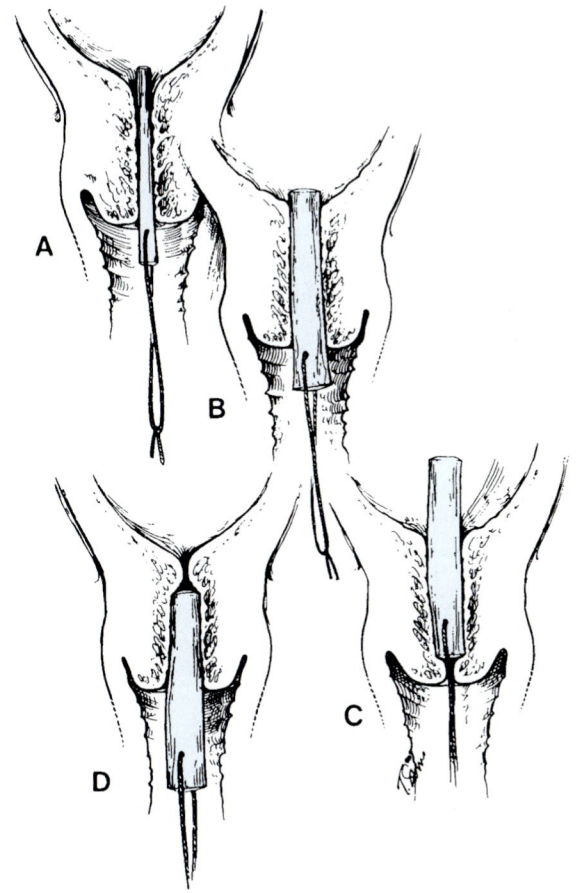

FIGURE 33–8. Insertion of laminaria prior to dilatation and curettage. **A.** Laminaria immediately after being appropriately placed with its upper end just through the internal os. **B.** The swollen laminaria and dilated, softened cervix several hours later. **C.** Laminaria inserted too far through the internal os; the laminaria may rupture the membranes. **D.** Laminaria not inserted far enough to dilate the internal os.

made from the stems of *Laminaria digitata* or *Laminaria japonica,* a brown seaweed. The stems are cut, peeled, shaped, dried, sterilized, and packaged according to size (small, 3 to 5 mm diameter; medium, 6 to 8 mm; and large, 8 to 10 mm). The strongly hygroscopic laminaria are thought to act by drawing water from proteoglycan complexes, causing them to dissociate and thereby allowing the cervix to soften and dilate.

Synthetic hygroscopic dilators have also been used. *Lamicel* is a polyvinyl alcohol polymer sponge impregnated with anhydrous magnesium sulfate (Nicolaides and co-workers, 1983). Stornes and Rasmussen (1991) reported that although both lamicel tents and gemeprost pessaries were effective for cervical dilatation preparatory to first-trimester abortions, further dilatation was significantly easier after gemeprost.

Dilapan is made of hydrogel polymer, and while it was used for some time, it is not available now in the United States. It has been claimed that it dilates the cervix more rapidly than dilators made of traditional seaweed (Blumenthal, 1988; Chvapil and co-workers, 1982). Patsner (1996) found same-day Dilapan insertion successful in preparing the cervix for dilatation and evacuation for second-trimester abortion. Hern (1994) compared Dilapan with laminaria in 1001 women as overnight dilators. Although both were equally effective dilators, women receiving the Dilapan were at least twice as likely to experience problems in cervical dilatation or problems resulting from poor dilatation or disintegration of the device than women who used the seaweed preparation.

An interesting dilemma is presented by the woman who has an osmotic dilator placed overnight preparatory to elective abortion, but who then changes her mind. Among seven first-trimester and 14 second-trimester pregnancies in which this occurred, the dilator was removed and 14 had term deliveries, two had preterm deliveries, and one had a spontaneous abortion 2 weeks later (Schneider and associates, 1991). None suffered infectious morbidity, including three untreated women with cervical cultures positive for chlamydia.

TECHNIQUE FOR INSERTION. The cleansed cervix is grasped anteriorly with a tenaculum. The cervical canal is carefully sounded, without rupturing the membranes, to identify its length. A laminaria of appropriate size is then inserted so that the tip rests just at the level of the internal os using a uterine packing forceps or a radium capsule forceps (Fig. 33–8). Later, usually after 4 to 6 hours, the laminaria will have swollen and thereby dilated the cervix sufficiently to allow easier mechanical dilatation and curettage. The laminaria may cause cramping.

PROSTAGLANDINS. Rather than using a hygroscopic dilator to effect cervical softening, prostaglandin pessaries (suppositories) have been inserted into the vagina against the cervix 3 hours or so before attempting dilatation. Chen and Edler (1983) reported good results from applying 1 mg of prostaglandin E_1 methyl ester. Several newer prostaglandin products have been used to induce labor or to efface the cervix prior to labor induction. Many of these same products have also been used to prepare the cervix prior to mechanical dilatation for induction of abortion. These prostaglandins are also discussed in Chapter 20 (p. 471).

TECHNIQUE FOR DILATATION AND CURETTAGE. The anterior cervical lip is grasped with a toothed tenaculum. A local anesthetic such as 5 mL of 1 or 2 percent lidocaine is injected bilaterally into the cervix. Alternatively, a paracervical block may be used.

The uterus is sounded carefully to identify the status of the internal os and to confirm uterine size and position. The cervix is further dilated with Hegar or Pratt dilators until a vacuum aspirator suction curet of appropriate diameter can be inserted. As shown in Figure 33–9, the fourth and fifth fingers of the hand introducing the dilator should rest on the perineum and buttocks as the dilator is pushed through the internal os. This provides a further safeguard against uterine perforation.

Suction curettage then is used to aspirate pregnancy products. The vacuum aspirator is moved over the surface systematically in order eventually to cover all the uterine cavity. Once this is done and no more tissue is aspirated, then gentle sharp curettage is done if it is thought that any placenta or fetal fragments remain. A sharp curet is more efficacious, and its dangers need not be greater than those of the dull instrument. Uterine perforations rarely occur on the downstroke of the curet, but they may occur when any instrument is introduced into the uterus. As shown in Figure 33–10, manipulations should be carried out with the thumb and forefingers only.

In cases advanced past 16 weeks, the fetus is extracted, usually in parts, using Sopher or similar forceps and other destructive instruments. These late abortions are unpleasant for medical and nursing personnel and more dangerous for the woman undergoing the procedure. The risks of uterine perforation and laceration are increased due to the larger fetus and the thinner uterine walls.

It is reemphasized that morbidity, immediate and remote, will be kept to a minimum if:

1. The cervix is adequately dilated without trauma before attempting to remove the fetus and gestational tissues.

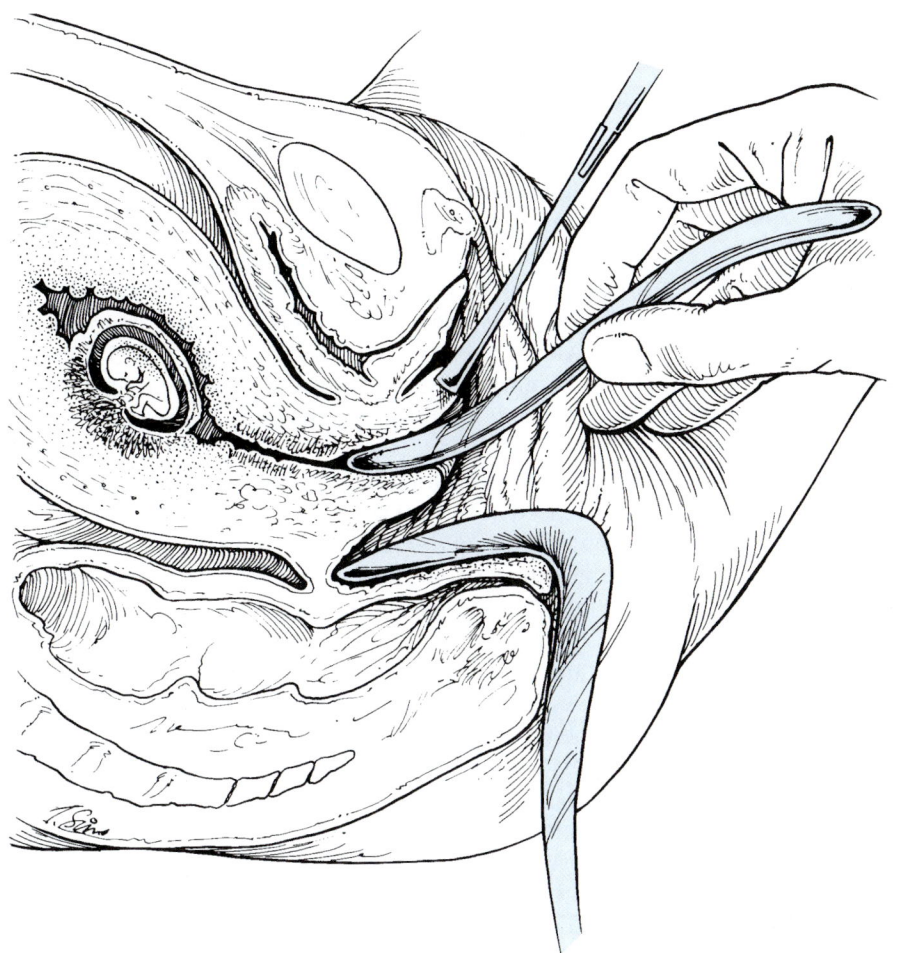

FIGURE 33–9. Dilatation of cervix with a Hegar dilator. Note that the fourth and fifth fingers rest against the perineum and buttocks, lateral to the vagina. This maneuver is a most important safety measure because if the cervix relaxes abruptly, these fingers prevent a sudden and uncontrolled thrust of the dilator, a common cause of uterine perforation.

2. Removal of the pregnancy is accomplished without perforating the uterus.
3. All pregnancy tissue is removed.

UTERINE PERFORATION. Accidental uterine perforation may occur during sounding of the uterus, dilatation, or curettage. The incidence of uterine perforation associated with elective abortion varies. Two important determinants of this complication are the skill of the physician and the position of the uterus, with a much greater likelihood of perforation if the uterus is retroverted. Accidental uterine perforation is recognized easily, as the instrument passes without hindrance further than it should have. Observation may be sufficient therapy if the uterine perforation is small, as when produced by a uterine sound or narrow dilator.

Considerable intra-abdominal damage can be caused by instruments passed through a uterine defect into the peritoneal cavity. This is especially true for suction and sharp curets. In this circumstance, laparotomy to examine the abdominal contents, especially the bowel, is the safest course of action. Unrecognized bowel injury causes severe peritonitis and sepsis (Kambiss and associ-

ates, 2000). We have also cared for a woman transferred to us after much of her right ureter had been removed at the time of attempted abortion using suction curettage! Similar cases have been observed by others (Keegan and Forkowitz, 1982).

Some women may develop cervical incompetence or uterine synechiae following dilatation and curettage. The possibility of these complications should be explained to those contemplating abortion. In general, their risk is very slight. Unfortunately, more advanced abortion performed by curettage may induce sudden, severe consumptive coagulopathy, which can prove fatal.

MENSTRUAL ASPIRATION. Aspiration of the endometrial cavity using a flexible 5- or 6-mm Karman cannula and syringe within 1 to 3 weeks after a missed menstrual period has been referred to as menstrual extraction, menstrual induction, instant period, traumatic abortion, and mini-abortion. Problems include the woman not being pregnant, the implanted zygote being missed by the curet, failure to recognize an ectopic pregnancy, and rarely, uterine perforation.

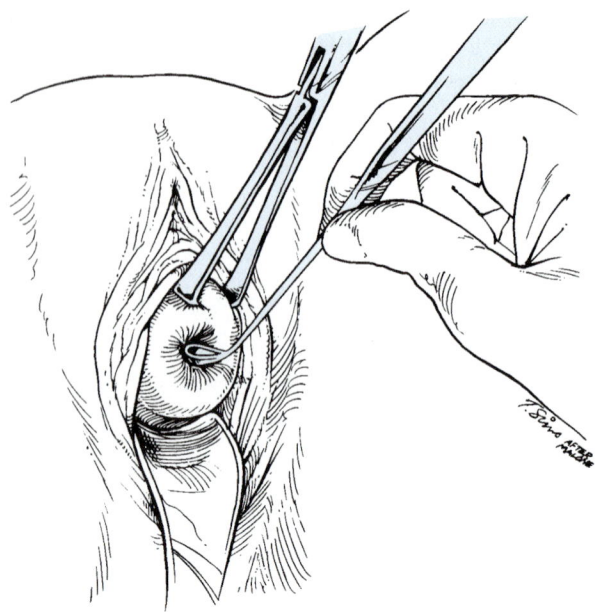

FIGURE 33–10. Introduction of a sharp curet. Note that the instrument is held with the thumb and forefinger; in the upward movement of the curet, only the strength of these two fingers should be used.

A positive pregnancy test will eliminate a needless procedure on a nonpregnant woman whose period has been delayed for other reasons. MacIsaac and Jones (2000) recommend the following technique for identifying placenta in the aspirate. First, the syringe contents are placed in a clear plastic container and examined with back lighting. Tap water is used to wash the tissue held in a strainer. The tissue is immersed in clear water. Placenta is macroscopically soft, fluffy, feathery, and villous. A magnifying lens or culposcope provides visualization. If there is doubt as to whether the tissue is placenta or decidua, microscopic examination of a small piece under a cover glass with high-light contrast will allow differentiation. Placental villi are obvious.

LAPAROTOMY. In a few circumstances, abdominal hysterotomy or hysterectomy for abortion is preferable to either curettage or medical induction. If significant uterine disease is present, hysterectomy may provide ideal treatment. If sterilization is to be performed, either hysterotomy with tubal ligation or hysterectomy on occasion may indicated. At times, hysterotomy or hysterectomy becomes necessary because of failure of a medical induction during the second trimester.

MEDICAL INDUCTION OF ABORTION. Throughout history, many naturally occurring substances have been tried as abortifacients by women desperate not to be pregnant. Most often, serious systemic illness or even death has been the result rather than abortion. Even today, there are only a few effective, safe abortifacient drugs.

OXYTOCIN. Successful induction of second-trimester abortion is possible with high doses of oxytocin administered in small volumes of intravenous fluids. One regimen we have found effective is to add 10 1-mL ampules of oxytocin (10 IU/mL) to 1000 mL of lactated Ringer solution. This solution contains 100 mU oxytocin per mL. An intravenous infusion is started at 0.5 mL/min (50 mU/min). The rate of infusion is increased at 15- to 30-minute intervals up to a maximum rate of 2 mL/min (200 mU/min). If effective contractions are not established at this infusion rate, the concentration of oxytocin is increased in the infused solution. It is safest to discard all but 500 mL of the remaining solution, which contains a concentration of 100 mU oxytocin per mL. To this 500 mL is added an additional five ampules of oxytocin. The resulting solution now contains 200 mU/mL, and the rate of infusion is reduced to 1 mL/min (200 mU/min). A resumption of a progressive rate increase is commenced up to a rate of 2 mL/min (400 mU/min) and left at this rate for an additional 4 to 5 hours, or until the fetus is expelled.

Similar regimens have been shown to be highly effective by Winkler (1991) and Owen (1992) and their associates. In a retrospective comparison of prostaglandin E_2 (PGE_2) vaginal suppositories and high-dose oxytocin, Winkler and colleagues (1991) reported successes of 93 percent and 91 percent, respectively. The mean duration of labor was 13.1 hours with PGE_2 and 8.2 hours with oxytocin. The mean dose of PGE_2 was 65 mg and of oxytocin was 200 units. Side effects were limited to the PGE_2 group, with nausea (46 percent), vomiting (37 percent), fever (64 percent), and diarrhea (20 percent).

In a subsequent randomized trial, Owen and co-workers (1992) concluded that concentrated oxytocin is a satisfactory alternative to prostaglandin E_2 for midtrimester abortion. The same group also compared concentrated oxytocin plus low-dose prostaglandin with prostaglandin E_2 vaginal suppositories for second trimester terminations (Owen and Hauth, 1996). The women in the prostaglandin-only group received a 20-mg PGE_2 vaginal suppository every 4 hours, and those in the combined group received a 10-mg PGE_2 suppository every 6 hours. The success rate was 81 versus 89 percent, but the side effects were significantly higher for the vaginal PGE_2-only group. In a more recent trial, the Alabama group compared vaginal misoprostol (200 μg vaginally every 12 hours) with a regimen of concentrated oxytocin plus 10-mg PGE_2 suppositories every 6 hours (Owen and Hauth, 1999). They concluded that misoprostol vaginal tablets in this dose were not satisfactory for second-trimester pregnancy termination.

With concentrated oxytocin, careful attention must be directed to the frequency and intensity of uterine contractions, because each increase in infusion rate markedly increases the amount of oxytocin infused. If the initial induction is unsuccessful, serial inductions on a daily basis for 2 to 3 days are almost always successful. The chance of a successful induction with high-dose oxytocin is enhanced greatly by the use of hygroscopic dilators such as laminaria tents inserted the night before.

INTRA-AMNIONIC HYPEROSMOTIC SOLUTIONS. In order to effect abortion during the second trimester, 20 to 25 percent saline or 30 to 40 percent urea have been injected into the amnionic sac to stimulate uterine contractions and cervical dilatation. These techniques are used infrequently in the United States, and according to the American College of Obstetricians and Gynecologists (1987), they have been replaced by dilatation and evacuation. Benefits of the latter cited included speed, lower cost, and less pain and emotional trauma.

In a study from Thailand, among 125 pregnancies undergoing midtrimester termination using hypertonic saline, the mean induction-to-delivery time was 31.7 hours (Herabutya and O-Prasertsawat, 1994). Retained placenta developed in 63 percent and pyrexia in 39 percent. In a study from India, Allahbadia (1992) reported success rates of 96 percent in pregnancies ranging from 14 to 20 weeks when 200 mL of 20 percent saline was instilled. This compared favorably with a success rate of 90 percent with intramuscular $PGF_{2\alpha}$, and 100 percent with extra-amnionic instillation of 5 percent povidone-iodine mixed with normal saline.

Hypertonic saline may result in serious complications, including death (Jasnosz and colleagues, 1993). Other complications include:

1. Hyperosmolar crisis following entry of hypertonic saline into the maternal circulation.
2. Cardiac failure.
3. Septic shock.
4. Peritonitis.
5. Hemorrhage.
6. Disseminated intravascular coagulation.
7. Water intoxication.

HYPEROSMOTIC UREA. Urea, 30 to 40 percent, dissolved in 5 percent dextrose solution, has been injected into the amnionic sac, followed by intravenous oxytocin at about 400 mU/min. Urea plus oxytocin is as efficacious an abortifacient as hypertonic saline, but is less likely to be toxic. Urea plus prostaglandin $F_{2\alpha}$ injected into the amnionic sac is similarly effective.

PROSTAGLANDINS. Because of shortcomings of other medical methods of inducing abortion, prostaglandins and their analogues are used extensively to terminate pregnancies, especially in the second trimester. Compounds commonly used are prostaglandin E_2, prostaglandin $F_{2\alpha}$, and certain analogues, especially 15-methyl-prostaglandin $F_{2\alpha}$ methyl ester, PGE_1-methyl ester (gemeprost), and misoprostol. Mechanisms of action of the prostaglandins are considered in detail in Chapter 20 (p. 471).

TECHNIQUE. Prostaglandins can act effectively on the cervix and uterus when:

1. Placed in the vagina as a suppository or pessary immediately adjacent to the cervix.
2. Administered as a gel through a catheter into the cervical canal and lowermost uterus extraovularly.
3. Injected intramuscularly.
4. Injected into the amnionic sac by amniocentesis.
5. Taken orally.

Various treatment regimens are outlined in Table 33–6.

Christin-Maitre and colleagues (2000) provided a recent update on the medical termination of pregnancy. They reviewed numerous studies regarding the efficacy and side effects of prostaglandins and methotrexate utilized alone or in various combinations. They also reviewed the efficacy and side effects of mifepristone utilized with a prostaglandin. Kahn and associates (2000) provided a meta-analysis regarding medical abortion with mifepristone and misoprostol, mifepristone with other prostaglandins, and methotrexate with misoprostol. They concluded that these regimens had high levels of success for early gestations. Parenteral approaches reduce appreciably, but do not eliminate, the unpleasant systemic effects, especially gastrointestinal, that accompany oral administration. Repeated doses of prostaglandin are often required and hygroscopic cervical dilators are often used concurrently.

Effectiveness of the various treatment regimens has ranged from 86 to 95 percent. Induction-to-delivery intervals ranged from 4 hours to more than 48 hours. In one study of 932 second-trimester terminations using gemeprost, the median induction-to-abortion interval was 18 hours in nulliparas and 15 hours in parous women (Thong and associates, 1992).

Prostaglandin vaginal suppositories applied to the cervix are also used in a lower dose during the first and early second trimesters to ripen or soften and dilate the cervix before curettage or as an adjunct for mifepristone termination (Healy and Evans, 1994). The safety of late induced abortion after a previous cesarean delivery using prostaglandins or mifepristone was reported by Boulot and associates (1993). At a mean gestational age of almost 24 weeks, vaginal evacuation was achieved in 20 of 23 women. At hysterotomy in the three treatment failures, one uterine rupture was found and successfully

TABLE 33–6. Prostaglandin Analogue Regimes Used for Midtrimester Abortion

Investigators	Prostaglandin	Route	Dose and Interval
Allahbadia (1992)	$F_{2\alpha}$	Intramuscular	Unspecified dose at regular intervals
el-Refaey et al (1995)	E_1 (misoprostol)	Oral	800 μg once
		Vaginal	800 μg once
Ferguson et al (1993)	15 methyl-$PGF_{2\alpha}$	Intra-amnionic	2.0 mg once
Herabutya and O-Prasertsawat (1994)	E_2	Intracervical	3 mg q 6 h × 2
Jaschevatzky et al (1992, 1994)	$F_{2\alpha}$	Extra-amnionic	20 mg per 500 mL NS once
Owen et al (1992, 1996)	E_2	Vaginal	20 mg q 4 h
Papageorgiou et al (1991)	$PGF_{2\alpha}$	Intra-amnionic	40 mg once
Thong and Baird (1992), Thong et al (1992)	E_1 (gemeprost)	Vaginal pessary	5 × 1 mg q 3 h
Winkler et al (1991)	E_2	Vaginal	20 mg q 4 h

repaired. Chapman and colleagues (1996) reported a uterine rupture rate of 3.8 percent in 79 women undergoing termination by induction at a mean age of 21 weeks.

MIFEPRISTONE (RU 486). This oral antiprogesterone has been used to effect abortions in early gestation, either alone or in combination with oral prostaglandins (Baird and colleagues, 1992; el-Refaey and associates, 1995; Newhall and Winikoff, 2000; World Health Organization Task Force, 1994). The effectiveness of the drug as an abortifacient is based upon its high receptor affinity for progesterone-binding sites (Healy and colleagues, 1983). A single 600-mg dose of RU 486 administered prior to 6 weeks results in an 85 percent abortion rate. In first trimester nondeveloping pregnancies, a single dose of 600-mg of mifepristone induced expulsion in 82 percent of women (Lelaidier and co-workers, 1993).

Ulmann and associates (1992) reported their results from over 16,000 women in whom RU 486 was given followed by a prostaglandin analogue for medical termination. Overall success rate was 95 percent, with no difference regarding the nature or dose of prostaglandin used. Median duration of bleeding was 8 days and it was 12 days or less in 90 percent of women. Bleeding necessitated vacuum aspiration or curettage in 0.8 percent of cases. Transfusion was required in 1 per 1000 women.

As discussed in Chapter 58 (p. 1548), RU 486 is also highly effective for emergency postcoital contraception if given within 72 hours (Glasier and associates, 1993). After 72 hours, the agent is progressively less effective. The addition of various oral, vaginal, or injected prostaglandins to this regimen results in abortion rates over 95 percent.

Side effects of RU 486 include nausea, vomiting, and gastrointestinal cramping. The major associated risk is hemorrhage due to partial expulsion of the pregnancy and due to intra-abdominal hemorrhage from an early unsuspected ectopic pregnancy. The duration of vaginal bleeding is approximately 2 weeks after RU 486 alone and approximately 1 to 2 weeks after RU 486 is given with a prostaglandin.

EPOSTANE. This 3β-hydroxysteroid dehydrogenase inhibitor block the synthesis of endogenous progesterone. If administered within 4 weeks of the last menstrual period, the drug will induce an abortion in approximately 85 percent of women (Crooij and associates, 1988). Clinical responses are likely related to circulating endogenous progesterone levels. Nausea is a frequent side effect, and hemorrhage is a risk if the abortion is incomplete. Other antiprogestins such as ZK 98,734 are under study, and appear to be promising for induction of early abortion (Swahn and colleagues, 1994).

CONSEQUENCES OF ELECTIVE ABORTION

MATERNAL MORTALITY. Legally induced abortion is a relatively safe surgical procedure, especially when performed during the first 2 months of pregnancy. The risk of death from abortion performed during the first 2 months is about 0.6 per 100,000 procedures (Berg and co-workers, 1996; Centers for Disease Control, 1986; Grimes, 1994). The relative risk of dying as the consequence of abortion is approximately doubled for each 2 weeks of delay after 8 weeks' gestation. Atrash and colleagues (1988) reported that the proportion of abortion-related deaths caused by general anesthesia had increased from 8 percent in 1975 to 29 percent in 1985. This likely reflects an absolute decrease in deaths from nonanesthetic complications. LeBolt and co-workers (1982) estimated that during the 1970s, overall risk of death from legal abortion was 15 percent of the risk from childbirth. Indeed, in 1987 six maternal deaths were reported among 1.3 million legal abortions

(Grimes, 1994). In his recent review, de Swiet (2000) emphasized that prior to the United Kingdom Abortion Act in 1968, 40 percent of maternal deaths were due to criminal abortion. In 1994 through 1996, only 4 percent of deaths were related to abortion, and none were illegal.

IMPACT ON FUTURE PREGNANCIES. Hogue (1986), in a scholarly review of the impact of elective abortion upon subsequent pregnancy outcome, summarized data from more than 200 publications. She emphasized that consideration must be given for the method of inducing abortion, and that women chosen as controls should be nulliparous because parous women had a reduced risk of complications in subsequent pregnancies.

Fertility is not altered by an elective abortion. A possible exception is the small risk from pelvic infection. Vacuum aspiration results in no increased incidence of midtrimester spontaneous abortions, preterm deliveries, or low-birthweight infants in subsequent pregnancies. Dilatation and curettage, however, in primigravidas results in an increased risk for subsequent ectopic pregnancy, midtrimester abortion, and low-birthweight infants.

Subsequent ectopic pregnancies are not increased if the first termination is done by vacuum aspiration. Possible exceptions are in women with preexisting chlamydial infection or those who develop postabortion infection. Multiple elective abortions do not increase the incidence of preterm delivery and low-birthweight infants (Mandelson and associates, 1992). Placenta previa was reported to be increased following elective abortion (Barrett and associates, 1981). Hogue (1986) discounted this study because of failure to control for maternal age.

Induced midtrimester abortions apparently carry little risk to subsequent pregnancies if injection techniques are used. There are not enough procedure-specific data available to permit valid conclusions regarding the risks to future pregnancies following any midtrimester abortion.

SEPTIC ABORTION. Serious complications of abortion have most often been associated with criminal abortion. Severe hemorrhage, sepsis, bacterial shock, and acute renal failure have all developed in association with legal abortion but at a very much lower frequency. Metritis is the usual outcome, but parametritis, peritonitis, endocarditis, and septicemia may all occur (Vartian and Septimus, 1991). In 300 septic abortions at Parkland Hospital, a positive blood culture was found in a fourth. Almost two thirds were anaerobic bacteria and coliforms were also common. Other organisms reported as causative of septic abortion include *Haemophilus influenzae, Campylobacter jejuni,* and group A streptococcus (Denton and Clarke, 1992; Dotters and Katz, 1991; Pinhas-Hamiel and associates, 1991). Treatment of infection includes prompt evacuation of the products of conception along with broad-spectrum antimicrobials given intravenously. If sepsis and shock supervenes, then supportive care is essential as discussed in Chapter 43 (p. 1167). Septic abortion has also been associated with disseminated intravascular coagulopathy (Chap. 25, p. 657).

REFERENCES

Aarts JM, Brons JT, Bruinse HW: Emergency cerclage: A review. Obstet Gynecol Surv 50:459, 1995

Alberman E: The epidemiology of repeated abortion. In Beard RW, Sharp F (eds): Early Pregnancy Loss: Mechanisms and Treatment. London, RCOG, 1988, p 9

Allahbadia G: Comparative study of midtrimester termination of pregnancy using hypertonic saline, ethacridine lactate, prostaglandin analogue and iodine-saline. J Indian Med Assoc 90:237, 1992

Al-Sebai MA, Kingsland CR, Diver M, Hipkin L, McFadyen IR: The role of a single progesterone measurement in the diagnosis of early pregnancy failure and the prognosis of fetal viability. Br J Obstet Gynaecol 102:364, 1995

Althuisius SM, Dekker GA, van Geijn HP, Hummel P: The effect of therapeutic McDonald cerclage on cervical length as assessed by transvaginal ultrasonography. Am J Obstet Gynecol 180:366, 1999

American College of Obstetricians and Gynecologists: Early pregnancy loss. Technical Bulletin No. 212, September, 1995

American College of Obstetricians and Gynecologists: Methods of midtrimester abortion. Technical Bulletin No. 109, October, 1987

Andrews WW, Copper R, Hauth JC, Goldenberg RL, Neely C, Dubard M: Second-trimester cervical ultrasound: Association with increased risk for recurrent early spontaneous delivery. Obstet Gynecol 95:222, 2000

Ansari AH, Reynolds RA: Cervical incompetence: A review. J Reprod Med 32:161, 1987

Araneta MR, Weisfuse IB, Greenberg B, Schultz S, Thomas PA: Abortions and HIV-1 infection in New York City, 1987–1989. AIDS 6:1195, 1992

Armstrong BG, McDonald AD, Sloan M: Cigarette, alcohol, and coffee consumption and spontaneous abortion. Am J Public Health 82:85, 1992

Atrash HK, Cheek TG, Hogue CJR: Legal abortion mortality and general anesthesia. Am J Obstet Gynecol 158:420, 1988

Axelsson G, Rylander R: Exposure to anesthetic gases and spontaneous abortion: Response bias in a postal questionnaire study. Int J Epidemiol 11:250, 1982

Baird DT, Norman JE, Thong KJ, Glasier AF: Misoprostol, mifepristone, and abortion. Lancet 339:313, 1992

Barlow S, Sullivan FM: Reproductive Hazards of Industrial Chemicals: An Evaluation of Animal and Human Data. New York, Academic Press, 1982

Barrett JM, Boehm FH, Killam AP: Induced abortion: A risk factor for placenta previa. Am J Obstet Gynecol 141:769, 1981

Barth WH: Operative procedures of the cervix. In Hankins GDV, Clark SL, Cunningham FG, Gilstrap LC (eds): Operative Obstetrics. Norwalk, CT, Appleton & Lange, 1995, p 753

Batzofin JH, Fielding WL, Friedman EA: Effect of vaginal

bleeding in early pregnancy on outcome. Obstet Gynecol 63:515, 1984

Bellingard V, Hedon B, Eliaou JF, Seignalet J, Clot J, Viala JL: Immunogenetic study of couples with recurrent spontaneous abortions. Eur J Obstet Gynecol Reprod Biol 60:53, 1995

Berg CJ, Atrash HK, Koonin LM, Tucker M: Pregnancy-related mortality in the United States, 1987–1990. Obstet Gynecol 88:161, 1996

Berg TG, Philpot KL, Welsh MS, Sanger WG, Smith CV: *Ureaplasma/Mycoplasma*-infected amniotic fluid: Pregnancy outcome in treated and nontreated patients. J Perinatol 19:275, 1999

Blumenthal PD: Prospective comparison of dilapan and laminaria for pretreatment of the cervix in second-trimester induction abortion. Obstet Gynecol 72:243, 1988

Blumenfeld Z, Brenner B: Thrombophilia—associated pregnancy wastage. Fertil Steril 72:765, 1999

Boivin JF: Risk of spontaneous abortion in women occupationally exposed to anaesthetic gases: A meta-analysis. Occup Environ Med 54:541, 1997

Borgmann CE, Jones BS: Legal issues in the provision of medical abortion. Am J Obstet Gynecol 183:S84, 2000

Boulot P, Hoffet M, Bachelard B, Lefort G, Hedon B, Laffargue F, Viala JL: Late vaginal induced abortion after a previous cesarean birth: Potential for uterine rupture. Gynecol Obstet Invest 36:87, 1993

Boyd EF Jr, Holmstrom EG: Ovulation following therapeutic abortion. Am J Obstet Gynecol 113:469, 1972

Branch DW, Peaceman AM, Druzin M, Silver RK, El-Sayed Y, Silver RM, Esplin MS, Spinnato J, Harger J: A multicenter, placebo-controlled pilot study of intravenous immune globulin treatment and antiphospholipid syndrome during pregnancy. The Pregnancy Loss Study Group. Am J Obstet Gynecol 182:122, 2000

Bux J, Westphal E, de Sousa F, Mueller-Eckhardt G, Mueller-Eckhardt C: Alloimmune neonatal neutropenia is a potential side effect of immunization with leukocytes in women with recurrent spontaneous abortions. J Reprod Immunol 22:299, 1992

Cammarano CL, Herron MA, Parer JT: Validity of indications for transabdominal cervicoisthmic cerclage for cervical incompetence. Am J Obstet Gynecol 172:1871, 1995

Cancelmo JA, Hart B, Herman JL, Rashbaum WK, Stein JL: Psychodynamic aspects of delayed abortion decisions. Br J Med Psych 65:333, 1992

Caruso A, Trivellini C, De Carolis S, Paradisi G, Mancuso S, Ferrazzani S: Emergency cerclage in the presence of protruding membranes: Is pregnancy outcome predictable? Acta Obstet Gynecol Scand 79:265, 2000

Caspi E, Schneider DF, Mor Z, Langer R, Weinraub Z, Bukovsky I: Cervical internal os cerclage: Description of a new technique and comparison with Shirodkar operation. Am J Perinatol 7:347, 1990

Cavallo F, Russo R, Zotti C, Camerlengo A, Ruggeni AM: Moderate alcohol consumption and spontaneous abortion. Alcohol 30:195, 1995

Centers for Disease Control: Abortion surveillance: Preliminary analysis—United States, 1982–1983. MMWR 35:7SS, 1986

Centers for Disease Control and Prevention: Abortion surveillance: Preliminary analysis—United States, 1997. MMWR 48:1171, 2000

Centers for Disease Control and Prevention: Abortion surveillance: United States, 1996. MMWR 48:1, 1999

Chapman S, Crispens MA, Owen J, Savage J: Complications

of midtrimester pregnancy terminations: The effect of prior cesarean delivery. Am J Obstet Gynecol 174:356, 1996

Charles D, Edward WR: Infectious complications of cervical cerclage. Am J Obstet Gynecol 141:1065, 1981

Chasen ST, Silverman NS: Mid-trimester emergent cerclage: A ten year single institution review. J Perinatol 18:338, 1998

Chen JK, Edler MG: Preoperative cervical dilatation by vaginal pessaries containing prostaglandin F_1 analogue. Obstet Gynecol 62:339, 1983

Christin-Maitre S, Bouchard P, Spitz IM: Drug therapy: Medical termination of pregnancy. N Engl J Med 342:946, 2000

Chvapil M, Droegemueller W, Meyer T, Mascalka R, Stoy V, Suciu T: New synthetic laminaria. Obstet Gynecol 60:729, 1982

Coulam CB: Immunotherapy for recurrent spontaneous abortion: Early pregnancy. Bio Med 1:13, 1995

Coulam CB: Immunologic tests in the evaluation of reproductive disorders: A critical review. Am J Obstet Gynecol 167:1844, 1992

Coulam CB, Clark DA, Collins J, Scott JR Schlesselman JS: Recurrent Miscarriage Immunotherapy Trialists Group: World wide collaborative and observational study and meta-analysis on allogenic leukocyte immunotherapy for recurrent spontaneous abortion. Am J Reprod Immunol 32:55, 1994

Cowchock S: Autoantibodies and pregnancy loss. N Engl J Med 337:197, 1997

Cowchock FS, Reece EA, Balaban D, Branch DW, Plouffe L: Repeated fetal losses associated with antiphospholipid antibodies: A collaborative randomized trial comparing prednisone with low-dose heparin treatment. Am J Obstet Gynecol 166:1318, 1992

Cowchock FS, Smith JB: Predictors for live birth after unexplained spontaneous abortions: Correlations between immunologic test results, obstetric histories, and outcome of next pregnancy without treatment. Am J Obstet Gynecol 167:1208, 1992

Creinin MD: Randomized comparison of efficacy and acceptability of medical versus surgical abortion. Obstet Gynecol 95:S83, 2000

Crooij MJ, Coenraad CA, deNoyyer CCA, Rao BR, Berends GT, Gooren LJG, Janssens J: Termination of early pregnancy by the 3β-hydroxy-steroid dehydrogenase inhibitor epostane. N Engl J Med 319:813, 1988

Dayan CM, Daniels GH: Chronic autoimmune thyroiditis. N Engl J Med 335:99, 1996

de Swiet, M: Maternal mortality: Confidential inquiries into maternal deaths in the United Kingdom. Am J Obstet Gynecol 182:760, 2000

Denton KJ, Clarke T: Role of *Campylobacter jejuni* as a placental pathogen. J Clin Pathol 45:171, 1992

Dickey RP, Olar TT, Taylor SN, Curole DN, Matulich EM: Relationship of small gestational sac–crown-rump length differences to abortion and abortus karyotypes. Obstet Gynecol 79:554, 1992

Dorman JS, Burke JP, McCarthy BJ, Norris JM, Steeinkiste AR, Aarons JH, Schmeltz R, Cruickshanks KJ: Temporal trends in spontaneous abortion associated with Type 1 diabetes. Diabetes Res Clin Pract 43:41, 1999

Dotters DJ, Katz VL: Streptococcal toxic shock associated with septic abortion. Obstet Gynecol 78:549, 1991

Dudley DJ, Branch W: Antiphospholipid syndrome: A model for autoimmune pregnancy loss. Infert Reprod Med Clin North Am 2:149, 1991

Egarter C, Lederhilger J, Kurz C, Karas H, Reisenberger

K: Gemeprost for first trimester missed abortion. Arch Gynecol Obstet 256:29, 1995

el-Refaey H, Rajasekar D, Abdalla M, Calder L, Templeton A: Induction of abortion with mifepristone (RU 486) and oral or vaginal misoprostol. N Engl J Med 332:983, 1995

Emerson DS, Cartier MS, Altieri LA, Felker RE, Smith WC, Stoval TG, Gray LA: Diagnostic efficacy of endovaginal color Doppler flow imaging in an ectopic pregnancy screening program. Radiology 183:413, 1992

Ermel LD, Marshburn PB, Kutteh WH: Interaction of heparin with antiphospholipid antibodies (APA) from the sera of women with recurrent pregnancy loss (RPL). Am J Reprod Immunol 33:14,1995

Esplin MS, Branch DW, Silver R, Stagnaro-Green A: Thyroid autoantibodies are not associated with recurrent pregnancy loss. Am J Obstet Gynecol 179:1583, 1998

Fantel AG, Shepard TH, Vadheim-Roth C, Stephens TD, Coleman C: Embryonic and fetal phenotypes: Prevalence and other associated factors in a large study of spontaneous abortion. In Porter IH, Hook EM (eds): Human Embryonic and Fetal Death. New York, Academic Press, 1980, p 71

Feist A, Sydler T, Gebbers JJ, Pospischil A, Guscetti F: No association of *Chlamydia* with abortion. J R Soc Med 92:237, 1999

Ferguson JE 2d, Burkett BJ, Pinkerton JV, Thiagarajah S, Flather MM, Martel MM, Hogge WA: Intraamniotic 15(s)-15-methyl prostaglandin F2 alpha and termination of middle and late second-trimester pregnancy for genetic indications: A contemporary approach. Am J Obstet Gynecol 169:332,1993

Floyd RL, Decoufle P, Hungerford DW: Alcohol use prior to pregnancy recognition. Am J Prev Med 17:101, 1999

Fossum GT, Davajan V, Kletzky OA: Early detection of pregnancy with transvaginal ultrasound. Fertil Steril 49:788, 1988

Fraser EJ, Grimes DA, Schulz KF: Immunization as therapy for recurrent spontaneous abortion: A review and meta-analysis. Obstet Gynecol 82:854, 1993

Funai EF, Paidas MJ, Rebarber A, O'Neill L, Rosen TJ, Young BK: Change in cervical length after prophylactic cerclage. Obstet Gynecol 94:117, 1999

Funderburk SJ, Guthrie D, Meldrum D: Outcome of pregnancies complicated by early vaginal bleeding. Br J Obstet Gynaecol 87:100, 1980

Gibb DM, Salaria DA: Transabdominal cervicoisthmic cerclage in the management of recurrent second trimester miscarriage and preterm delivery. Br J Obstet Gynaecol 102:802, 1995

Girling J, de Swiet M: Inherited thrombophilia and pregnancy. Curr Opin Obstet Gynecol 10:135, 1998

Glasier A, Thong KJ, Dewar M, Mackie M, Baird DT: Mifepristone (RU 486) compared with high-dose estrogen and progestogen for emergency postcoital contraception. N Engl J Med 328:354, 1993

Goldstein SR, Danon M, Watson C: An updated protocol for abortion surveillance with ultrasound and immediate pathology. Obstet Gynecol 83:55, 1994

Greene MF: Spontaneous abortions and major malformations in women with diabetes mellitus. Semin Reprod Endocrinol 17:127, 1999

Grimes DA: The morbidity and mortality of pregnancy: Still risky business. Am J Obstet Gynecol 170:1489-94, 1994

Guerrero R, Rojas OI: Spontaneous abortion and aging of human ova and spermatozoa. N Engl J Med 293:573, 1975

Guzman ER, Mellon C, Vintzileos AM, Ananth CV, Walters C, Gipson K: Longitudinal assessment of endocervical ca-nal length between 15 and 24 weeks' gestation in women at risk for pregnancy loss or preterm birth. Obstet Gynecol 92:31, 1998

Guzman ER, Pisatowski DM, Vintzileos AM, Benito CW, Hanley ML, Ananth CV: A comparison of ultrasonographically detected cervical changes in response to transfundal pressure, coughing, and standing in predicting cervical incompetence. Am J Obstet Gynecol 177:660, 1997a

Guzman ER, Vintzileos AM, McLean DA, Martins ME, Benito CW, Hanley ML: The natural history of a positive response to transfundal pressure in women at risk for cervical incompetence. Am J Obstet Gynecol 176:634, 1997b

Hahlin M, Wallin A, Sjoblom P, Lindblom B: Single progesterone assay for early recognition of abnormal pregnancy. Hum Reprod 5:662, 1990

Harger JH, Archer DF, Marchese SG, Muracca-Clemens M, Garver KL: Etiology of recurrent pregnancy losses and outcome of subsequent pregnancies. Obstet Gynecol 62:574, 1983

Harlap S, Shiono PH: Alcohol, smoking, and incidence of spontaneous abortions in the first and second trimester. Lancet 2:173, 1980

Harlap S, Shiono PH, Ramcharan S: A life table of spontaneous abortions and the effects of age, parity and other variables. In Porter IH, Hook EB (eds): Human Embryonic and Fetal Death. New York, Academic Press, 1980, p 145

Harris EN, Spinnato JA: Should anticardiolipin tests be performed in otherwise healthy pregnant women? Am J Obstet Gynecol 165:1272, 1991

Healy DL, Baulieu EE, Hodgen GD: Induction of menstruation by an antiprogesterone steroid (RU 486) in primates: Site of action, dose–response relationships, and hormonal effects. Fertil Steril 40:253, 1983

Healy DL, Evans AJ: Mifepristone (RU486) and emergency contraception. Med J Aust 161:403, 1994

Herabutya Y, O-Prasertsawat P: Mid-trimester abortion using hypertonic saline or prostaglandin E2 gel: An analysis of efficacy and complications. J Med Assoc Thailand 77:148, 1994

Hern WM: Laminaria versus Dilapan osmotic cervical dilators for outpatient dilation and evacuation abortion: Randomized cohort comparison of 1001 patients. Am J Obstet Gynecol 171:1324, 1994

Herron MA, Parer JT: Transabdominal cerclage for fetal wastage due to cervical incompetence. Obstet Gynecol 71:865, 1988

Hertig AT, Rock J: On the development of the early human ovum, with special reference to the trophoblast of the previllous stage: A description of 7 normal and 5 pathologic human ova. Am J Obstet Gynecol 47:149, 1944

Hertig AT, Sheldon WH: Minimal criteria required to prove prima facie case of traumatic abortion or miscarriage: An analysis of 1,000 spontaneous abortions. Ann Surg 117:596, 1943

Hogue CJR: Impact of abortion on subsequent fecundity. Clin Obstet Gynaecol 13:95, 1986

Homer HA, Li TC, Cooke ID: The septate uterus: A review of management and reproductive outcome. Fertil Steril 73:1, 2000

Houwert-de Jong MH, Termijtelen A, Eskes TKAB, Mantingh A, Bruinse HW: The natural course of habitual abortion. Eur J Obstet Gynecol Reprod Biol 33:221, 1989

Iams JD, Johnson FF, Sonek J, Sachs L, Gebauer C, Samuels P: Cervical competence as a continuum: A study of ultrasonographic cervical length and obstetric performance. Am J Obstet Gynecol 172:1097, 1995

Jacobs PA, Hassold TJ: The origin of chromosomal abnormalities in spontaneous abortion. In Porter IH, Hook EB (eds): Human Embryonic and Fetal Death. New York, Academic Press, 1980, p 289

Jaschevatzky OE, Dascalu S, Noy Y, Rosenberg RP, Anderman S, Ballas S: Intrauterine PGF2 alpha infusion for termination of pregnancies with second-trimester rupture of membranes. Obstet Gynecol 79:32, 1992

Jaschevatzky OE, Rosenberg RP, Noy Y, Dascalu S, Anderman S, Ballas S: Comparative study of extra-amniotic prostaglandin F2 alpha infusion and increasing intravenous oxytocin for termination of second trimester missed abortion. J Am Coll Surg 178:435, 1994

Jasnosz KM, Shakir AM, Perper JA: Fatal *Clostridium perfringens* and *Escherichia coli* sepsis following urea-instillation abortion. Am J Forensic Med Path 14:151, 1993

Kahn JG, Becker BJ, MacIsaa L, Amory JK, Neuhaus J, Olkin I, Creinin MD: The efficiacy of medical abortion: A meta-analysis. Contraception 61:29, 2000

Kajii T, Ferrier A, Niikawa N, Takahara H, Ohama K, Avirachan S: Anatomic and chromosomal anomalies in 639 spontaneous abortions. Hum Genet 55:87, 1980

Kambiss SM, Hibbert ML, Macedonia C, Potter ME: Uterine perforation resulting in bowel infarction: Sharp traumatic bowel and mesentery injury at the time of pregnancy termination. Mil Med 165:81, 2000

Katz I, Fisch B, Amit S, Ovadia J, Tadir Y: Cutaneous graft-versus-host-like reaction after paternal lymphocyte immunization for prevention of recurrent abortion. Fertil Steril 57:927, 1992

Keegan GT, Forkowitz MJ: A case report: Uretero-uterine fistula as a complication of elective abortion. J Urol 128:137, 1982

Klebanoff MA, Levine RJ, DerSimonian R, Clemens JD, Wilkins DG: Maternal serum paraxanthine, a caffeine metabolite, and the risk of spontaneous abortion. N Engl J Med 341:1639, 1999

Kline J, Stein ZA, Shrout P, Susser M: Drinking during pregnancy and spontaneous abortion. Lancet 2:176, 1980

Kuhn RPJ, Pepperell RJ: Cervical ligation: A review of 242 pregnancies. Aust NZ J Obstet Gynaecol 17:79, 1977

Kulcsar G, Csata S, Nasz I: Investigations into virus carriership in human semen and mouse testicular cells. Acta Microb Hungarica 38:127, 1991

Kurup M, Goldkrand JW: Cervical incompetence: Elective, emergent, or urgent cerclage. Am J Obstet Gynecol 181:240, 1999

Kutteh WH: Antiphospholipid antibody–associated recurrent pregnancy loss: Treatment with heparin and low-dose aspirin is superior to low-dose aspirin alone. Am J Obstet Gynecol 174:1584, 1996

Kutteh WH, Pasquarette MM: Recurrent pregnancy loss. Adv Obstet Gynecol 2:147, 1995

Lähteenmäki P, Luukkainen T: Return of ovarian function after abortion. Clin Endocrinol 8:123, 1978

Larsson PG, Platz-Christensen JJ, Dalaker K, Eriksson K, Fahraeus L, Irminger K, Jerve F, Stray-Pedersen B, Wolner-Hanssen P: Treatment with 2% clindamycin vaginal prior to first trimester surgical abortion to reduce signs of postoperative infection: A prospective, double-blinded, placebo-controlled, multicenter study. Acta Obstet Gynecol Scand 79:390, 2000

Larsson PG, Platz-Christensen JJ, Thejls H, Forsum U, Påhlson C: Incidence of pelvic inflammatory disease after

first-trimester legal abortion in women with bacterial vaginosis after treatment with metronidazole: A double-blind, randomized study. Am J Obstet Gynecol 166:100, 1992

LeBolt SA, Grimes DA, Cates W Jr: Mortality from abortion: Are the populations comparable? JAMA 248:188, 1982

Lelaidier C, Baton-Saint-Mleux C, Fernandez H, Bourget P, Frydman R: Mifepristone (RU 486) induces embryo expulsion in first trimester non-developing pregnancies: A prospective randomized trial. Hum Reprod 8:492, 1993

Lipscomb GH, Stovall TG, Ling TW: Nonsurgical treatment of ectopic pregnancy. N Engl J Med 343:1325, 2000

Locatelli A, Vergani P, Bellini P, Strobelt N, Arreghini A, Ghidini A: Amnioreduction in emergency cerclage with prolapsed membranes: Comparison of two methods for reducing the membranes. Am J Perinatol 16:73, 1999

Lockwood CJ, Romero R, Feinberg RF, Clyne LP, Coster B, Hobbins JC: The prevalence and biologic significance of lupus anticoagulant and anticardiolipin antibodies in a general obstetric population. Am J Obstet Gynecol 161:369, 1989

MacIsaac L, Darney P: Early surgical abortion: An alternative to and backup for medical abortion. Am J Obstet Gynecol 183:S76, 2000

Makino T, Hara T, Oka C, Toyoshima K, Sugi T, Iwasaki K, Umeuchi M, Iizuka R: Survey of 1120 Japanese women with a history of recurrent spontaneous abortions. Eur J Obstet Gynecol Reprod Biol 44:123, 1992

Maldjian C, Adam R, Pelosi M, Pelosi M 3rd: MRI appearance of cervical incompetence in a pregnant patient. Magn Reson Imaging 17:1399, 1999

Mandelson MT, Maden CB, Daling JR: Low birth weight in relation to multiple induced abortions. Am J Public Health 82:391, 1992

March CM, Israel R: Gestational outcome following hysteroscopic lysis of adhesions. Fertil Steril 36:455, 1981

McDonald IA: Incompetent cervix as a cause of recurrent abortion. J Obstet Gynaecol Br Commonw 70:105, 1963

Michaels WH, Thompson HO, Schreiber FR, Berman JM, Ager J, Olson K: Ultrasound surveillance of the cervix during pregnancy in diethylstilbestrol-exposed offspring. Obstet Gynecol 73:230, 1989

Mills JL, Simpson JL, Driscoll SG, Jovanovic-Peterson L, Van Allen M, Aarons JH, Metzger B, Bieber FR, Knopp RH, Holmes LB: Incidence of spontaneous abortion among normal women and insulin-dependent diabetic women whose pregnancies were identified within 21 days of conception. N Engl J Med 319:1618, 1988

Montoro M, Collea JV, Frasier D, Mestman J: Successful outcome of pregnancy in women with hypothyroidism. Ann Intern Med 94:31, 1981

Munsick RA: Clinical test for placenta in 300 consecutive menstrual aspirations. Obstet Gynecol 60:738, 1982

Nelen WL, Blom HJ, Steegers EA, Heijer MD, Thomas CM, Eskes TK: Homocysteine and folate levels as risk factors for recurrent early pregnancy loss. Obstet Gynecol 95:519, 2000

Nelen WLDM, Steegers EAP, Eskes TKAB, Blom JH: Genetic risk factor for unexplained recurrent early pregnancy loss. Lancet 350:861, 1997

Newhall EP, Winikoff B: Abortion with mifepristone and misoprostol: Regimens, efficacy, acceptability and future directions. Am J Obstet Gynecol 183:S44, 2000

Nicolaides KH, Welch CC, Koullapis EN, Filshie GM: Cervical dilatation by Lamicel—studies on the mechanism of action. Br J Obstet Gynaecol 90:1060, 1983

Nielsen S, Hahlin M: Expectant management of first-trimester spontaneous abortion. Lancet 345:84, 1995

Ober CL, Martin AO, Simpson JL, Hauck WW, Amos DB, Kostyu DD, Fotino M, Allen FH Jr: Shared HLA antigens and reproductive performance among Hutterites. Am J Hum Genet 35:994, 1983

O'Connor S, Kuller JA, McMahon MJ: Management of cervical cerclage after preterm premature rupture of membranes. Obstet Gynecol Surv 54:391, 1999

Osser S, Persson K: Chlamydial antibodies in women who suffer miscarriage. Br J Obstet Gynaecol 103:137, 1996

Owen J, Hauth JC: Vaginal misoprostol vs. concentrated oxytocin plus low-dose prostaglandin E2 for second trimester pregnancy termination. J Matern Fetal Med 8:48, 1999

Owen J, Hauth JC: Concentrated oxytocin plus low-dose prostaglandin E_2 compared with prostaglandin E_2 vaginal suppositories for second-trimester pregnancy termination. Obstet Gynecol 88:110, 1996

Owen J, Hauth JC, Winkler CL, Gray SE: Midtrimester pregnancy termination: A randomized trial of prostaglandin E2 versus concentrated oxytocin. Am J Obstet Gynecol 167:1112, 1992

Papageorgiou I, Minaretzis D, Tsionou C, Michalas S: Late midtrimester medical pregnancy terminations: Three different procedures with prostaglandin F2 alpha and laminaria tents. Prostaglandins 41:487, 1991

Patsner B: Same-day Dilapan insertion before second-trimester dilatation and evacuation for a fetal anomaly or death. J Reprod Med 41:71, 1996

Paukku M, Tulppala M, Puolakkainen M, Anttila T, Paavonen J: Lack of association between serum antibodies to Chlamydia trachomatis and a history of recurrent pregnancy loss. Fertil Steril 72:427, 1999

Paul M, Lichtenberg S, Borgatta L, Grimes DA, Stubblefield PG (eds): A Clinician's Guide to Medical and Surgical Abortion. New York, Churchill Livingstone, 1999

Pellerito JS, Taylor KJW, Quedens-Case C, Hammers LW, Scoutt LM, Ramos IM, Meyer WR: Ectopic pregnancy: Evaluation with endovaginal color flow imaging. Radiology 183:407, 1992

Pilpel HF, Norwich KP: When should abortion be legal? New York, Public Affairs Committee, No. 429, 1969

Pinhas-Hamiel O, Schiff E, Ben-Baruch G, Mashiach S, Reichman B: A life-threatening sexually transmitted Haemophilus influenzae in septic abortion: A case report. Am J Obstet Gynecol 165:66, 1991

Poland BJ, Miller JR, Harris M, Livingston J: Spontaneous abortion: A study of 1961 women and their abortuses. Acta Obstet Gynecol Scand 102:1, 1981

Poland BJ, Miller JR, Jones DC, Trimble BK: Reproductive counseling in patients who have had a spontaneous abortion. Am J Obstet Gynecol 127:685, 1977

Porcu G, Cravello L, D'Ercole C, Cohen D, Roger V, de Montgolfier R, Blanc B: Hysteroscopic metroplasty for septate uterus and repetitive abortions: Reproductive outcome. Eur J Obstet Gynecol Reprod Biol 88:81, 2000

Pratt D, Novotny M, Kaberlein G, Dudkiewicz A, Gleicher N: Antithyroid antibodies and the association with non-organ-specific antibodies in recurrent pregnancy loss. Am J Obstet Gynecol 170:956, 1994

Quinn PA, Shewchuck AB, Shuber J, Lie KI, Ryan E, Sheu M, Chipman ML: Serologic evidence of Ureaplasma urealyticum infection in women with spontaneous pregnancy loss. Am J Obstet Gynecol 145:245, 1983

Raziel A, Arieli S, Bukovsky I, Caspi E, Golan A: Investigation of the uterine cavity in recurrent aborters. Fertil Steril 62:1080, 1994

Ridker PM, Miletich JP, Buring JE, Ariyo AA, Price DT, Manson JE, Hill JA: Factor V Leiden mutation as a risk factor for recurrent pregnancy loss. Ann Intern Med 128:1000, 1998

Robinson WP, Bernasconi F, Dutly F, Lefort G, Romain DR, Binkert F, Schinzel AA: Molecular studies of translocations and trisomy involving chromosome 13. Am J Med Gen 61:158, 1996

Rocco BP, Garrone C: Can examination of the cervix provide useful information for prediction of cervical incompetence and following preterm labour? Aust N Z J Obstet Gynecol 39:296, 1999

Romer T: Post-abortion-hysteroscopy—a method for early diagnosis of congenital and acquired intrauterine causes of abortions. Eur J Obstet Gynecol Reprod Biol 57:171, 1994

Rote NS: Pregnancy-associated immunological disorders. Curr Opin Immunol 1:1165, 1989

Rowland AS, Baird DD, Shore DL, Weinberg CR, Savitz DA, Wilcox AJ: Nitrous oxide and spontaneous abortion in female dental assistants. Am J Epidemiol 141:531, 1995

Salem HT, Ghaneimah SA, Shaaban MM, Chard T: Prognostic value of biochemical tests in the assessment of fetal outcome in threatened abortion. Br J Obstet Gynaecol 91:382, 1984

Sargent IL, Wilkins T, Redman CW: Maternal immune responses to the fetus in early pregnancy and recurrent miscarriage. Lancet 2:1099, 1988

Sauerwein RW, Bisseling J, Horrevorts AM: Septic abortion associated with Campylobacter fetus subspecies fetus infection: Case report and review of the literature. Infection 21:33, 1993

Schneider D, Golan A, Langer R, Caspi E, Bukovsky I: Outcome of continued pregnancies after first- and second-trimester cervical dilatation by laminaria tents. Obstet Gynecol 78:1121, 1991

Schnorr TM, Grajewski BA, Hornung RW, Thun MJ, Egeland GM, Murray WE, Conover DL, Halperin WE: Video display terminals and the risk of spontaneous abortion. N Engl J Med 324:727, 1991

Schorr SJ, Morales WJ: Obstetric management of incompetent cervix and bulging fetal membranes. J Reprod med 41:235, 1996

Sher KS, Jayanthi V, Probert CS, Stewart CR, Mayberry JF: Infertility, obstetric and gynaecological problems in coeliac sprue. Digest Dis 12:186, 1994

Shirodkar VN: A new method of operative treatment for habitual abortions in the second trimester of pregnancy. Antiseptic 52:299, 1955

Simpson JL: Genes, chromosomes, and reproductive failure. Fertil Steril 33:107, 1980

Simpson JL, Carson SA, Chesney C, Conley MR, Metzger B, Aarons J, Holmes LB, Jovanovic-Peterson L, Knopp R, Mills JL: Lack of association between antiphospholipid antibodies and first trimester spontaneous abortion: Prospective study of pregnancies detected within 21 days of conception. Fertil Steril 69:814, 1998

Smith C, Gregori CA, Breen JL: Ultrasonography in threatened abortion. Obstet Gynecol 51:173, 1978

Souza SS, Ferriani RA, Pontes AG, Zago MA, Franco RF: Factor V leiden and factor II G20210A mutations in patients with recurrent abortion. Hum Reprod 14:2448, 1999

Stagnaro-Green A, Roman SH, Cobin RH, el-Harazy E, Alvarez-Marfany M, Davies TF: Detection of at-risk pregnancy by means of highly sensitive assays for thyroid autoantibodies. JAMA 264:1422, 1990

Stein Z, Kline J, Susser E, Shrout P, Warburton D, Susser

M: Maternal age and spontaneous abortion. In Porter IH, Hook EB (eds): Human Embryonic and Fetal Death. New York, Academic Press, 1980, p 107

Stornes I, Rasmussen KL: A comparison of Lamicel tents and gemeprost (Cervagem) pessaries prior to first trimester abortion. Arch Gynecol Obstet 249:67, 1991

Stovall TG, Ling FW, Carson SA, Burke JE: Serum progesterone and uterine curettage in differential diagnosis of ectopic pregnancy. Fertil Steril 57:456, 1992

Stray-Pedersen B, Stray-Pedersen S: Etiologic factors and subsequent reproductive performance in 195 couples with a prior history of habitual abortion. Am J Obstet Gynecol 148:140, 1984

Stricker RB, Steinleitner A, Bookoff CN, Weckstein LN, Winger EE: Successful treatment of immunologic abortion with low-dose intravenous immunoglobulin. Fertil Steril 73:536, 2000

Supreme Court of the United States: Don Stenberg et al v Leroy Carhart. Opinion No. 99-830, June 28, 2000

Supreme Court of the United States: Leila Jeanne Hill et al v Colorado et al. Opinion No. 98-1856, June 28, 2000

Supreme Court of the United States: Planned Parenthood of Southeastern Pennsylvania v Robert P. Casey. Opinion No. 91-744 and 91-902, June 29, 1992

Supreme Court of the United States: William Webster v Reproductive Health Services. Opinion No. 88-605, July 3, 1989

Supreme Court of the United States: Jane Roe et al v Henry Wade, District Attorney of Dallas County. Opinion No. 70-18, January 22, 1973

Swahn ML, Kovacs L, Cekan SZ, Aedo AR, Westlund P: Termination of early pregnancy with ZK 98, 734: Pharmacokinetic behaviour and clinical effect. Hum Reprod 9:57, 1994

Taskinen H, Kyyrönen P, Hemminki K: Effects of ultrasound, shortwaves, and physical exertion on pregnancy outcome in physiotherapists. J Epidemiol Community Health 44:196, 1990

Temmerman M, Lopita MI, Sanghvi HC, Sinei SK, Plummer FA, Piot P: The role of maternal syphilis, gonorrhoea and HIV-1 infections in spontaneous abortion. Int J STD AIDS 3:418, 1992

Tho PT, Byrd JR, McDonough PG: Etiologies and subsequent reproductive performance of 100 couples with recurrent abortion. Fertil Steril 32:389, 1979

Thom DH, Nelson LM, Vaughan TL: Spontaneous abortion and subsequent adverse birth outcomes. Am J Obstet Gynecol 166:111, 1992

Thomason JL, Sampson MB, Beckman CR, Spellacy WN: The incompetent cervix: A 1982 update. J Reprod Med 27:187, 1982

Thong KJ, Baird DT: A study of gemeprost alone, dilapan or

mifepristone in combination with gemeprost for the termination of second trimester pregnancy. Contraception 46:11, 1992

Thong KJ, Robertson AJ, Baird DT: A retrospective study of 932 second trimester terminations using gemeprost (16, 16 dimethyl-trans delta 2 PGE1 methyl ester). Prostaglandins 44:65, 1992

Turnquest MA, Britton KA, Brown HL: Outcome of patients undergoing transabdominal cerclage: A descriptive study. J Matern Fetal Med 8:225, 1999

Ulmann A, Silvestre L, Chemama L, Rezvani Y, Renault M, Aguillaume CJ, Baulieu EE: Medical termination of early pregnancy with mifepristone (RU 486) followed by a prostaglandin analogue. Study in 16,369 women. Acta Obstet Gynecol Scand 71:278, 1992

Vartian CV, Septimus EJ: Tricuspid valve group B streptococcal endocarditis following elective abortion. Review Infect Dis 13:997, 1991

Von Stein GA, Munsick RA, Stiver K, Ryder K: Fetomaternal hemorrhage in threatened abortion. Obstet Gynecol 79:383, 1992

Warburton D, Fraser FC: Spontaneous abortion risks in man: Data from reproductive histories collected in a medical genetics unit. Am J Hum Genet 16:1, 1964

Warburton D, Stein Z, Kline J, Susser M: Chromosome abnormalities in spontaneous abortion: Data from the New York City study. In Porter IH, Hook EB (eds): Human Embryonic and Fetal Death. New York, Academic Press, 1980, p 261

Wilson RD, Kendrick V, Wittmann BK, McGillivray B: Spontaneous abortion and pregnancy outcome after normal first-trimester ultrasound examination. Obstet Gynecol 67:352, 1986

Winkler CL, Gray SE, Hauth JC, Owen J, Tucker JM: Mid-second-trimester labor induction: Concentrated oxytocin compared with prostaglandin E2 vaginal suppositories. Obstet Gynecol 77:297, 1991

Witter FR: Negative sonographic findings followed by rapid cervical dilatation due to cervical incompetence. Obstet Gynecol 64:136, 1984

World Health Organization: Task Force on Postovulatory Methods of Fertility Regulation: Cervical ripening with mifepristone (RU 486) in late first trimester abortion. Contraception 50:461, 1994

Yasuda M, Takakuwa K, Tokunaga A, Tanaka K: Prospective studies of the association between anticardiolipin antibody and outcome of pregnancy. Obstet Gynecol 86:555, 1995

Younis JS, Brenner B, Ohel G, Tal J, Lanir N, Ben-Ami M: Activated protein C resistance and factor V Leiden mutation can be associated with first- as well as second-trimester recurrent pregnancy loss. Am J Reprod Immunol 43:31, 2000

34

Ectopic Pregnancy

The blastocyst normally implants in the endometrial lining of the uterine cavity. Implantation anywhere else is an ectopic pregnancy. More than 1 in every 100 pregnancies in the United States is ectopic and over 95 percent of ectopic pregnancies involve the oviduct. The risk of death from an extrauterine pregnancy is greater than that for a vaginal delivery or an induced abortion. Moreover, prognosis for a successful subsequent pregnancy is reduced in these women. With earlier diagnosis, both maternal survival and conservation of reproductive capacity are enhanced.

GENERAL CONSIDERATIONS

ETIOLOGY AND PATHOGENESIS. There are a number of risk factors that lead to tubal damage and dysfunction. While there is overlap, these can be generalized as mechanical and functional factors (Table 34–1).

MECHANICAL FACTORS. These factors prevent or retard passage of the fertilized ovum into the uterine cavity. Prior tubal surgery, either to restore patency or to perform sterilization, confers the highest risk (Ankum, 1996; Hendrix, 1998; Mol, 1995, and their colleagues). After one previous ectopic pregnancy, the chance of another is 7 to 15 percent (Ankum and colleagues, 1996;

TABLE 34–1. Risk Factors for Ectopic Pregnancy

Risk Factor	Risk[a]
High Risk	
Tubal corrective surgery	21.0
Tubal sterilization	9.3
Previous ectopic pregnancy	8.3
In utero DES exposure	5.6
Intrauterine device	4.5–45
Documented tubal pathology	3.8–21
Moderate Risk	
Infertility	2.5–21
Previous genital infection	2.5–3.7
Multiple partners	2.1
Slight Risk	
Previous pelvic/abdominal surgery	0.93–3.8
Smoking	2.3–2.5
Douching	1.1–3.1
Intercourse < 18 yr	1.6

DES = diethylstilbestrol.
[a]Single values are common odds ratio from homogeneous studies; double values are range of values from heterogenous studies.
Modified from Pisarska and Carson (1999), with permission.

Coste and associates, 1991). The increased risk likely is due to previous salpingitis which causes agglutination of the mucosal arborescent folds with luminal narrowing or formation of blind pockets (Sherman and co-workers, 1990). Reduced ciliation due to infection also may contribute to tubal implantation. According to the American College of Obstetricians and Gynecologists (1998), prior pelvic inflammatory disease, especially that caused by *Chlamydia trachomatis,* is the most common risk factor. Bjartling and colleagues (2000) showed that peak salpingitis rates in Malmo, Sweden, mirrored the peak ectopic pregnancy rates. Peritubal adhesions subsequent to postabortal or puerperal infection, appendicitis, or endometriosis may cause tubal kinking and narrowing of the lumen (Coste and associates, 1991). These may be associated with the slightly increased risk of ectopic pregnancy following previous induced abortion (Tharaux-Deneux and co-workers, 1998). In utero exposure to diethylstilbestrol predisposes to developmental tubal abnormalities, especially diverticula, accessory ostia, and hypoplasia. Finally, previous cesarean delivery has been linked to a small increase in ectopic pregnancy risk (Hemminki and Meriläinen, 1996).

FUNCTIONAL FACTORS. Some tubal factors delay passage of the fertilized ovum into the uterine cavity. Altered tubal motility may follow changes in serum levels of estrogens and progesterone, likely from upregulation of adrenergic receptors in smooth muscle (Jacobson and associates, 1987). An increased incidence of ectopic pregnancies has been reported with use of progestin-only oral contraceptives (Ory, 1981); with use of intrauterine devices—with and without progesterone (Sivin, 1991); after use of postovulatory high-dose estrogens to prevent pregnancy—the "morning after pill" (Chap. 58, p. 1546; Morris and Van Wagenen, 1973); and after ovulation induction. The rate of tubal ectopic pregnancy has also been reported to be significantly increased in women with luteal phase defects (Guillaume and colleagues, 1995), with cigarette smoking (Phillips and colleagues, 1992; Saraiya and associates, 1998), and with vaginal douching (Kendrick and co-workers, 1997).

ASSISTED REPRODUCTION. The increase in ectopic pregnancies with assisted reproduction is likely related to tubal factors that cause infertility. Tubal pregnancy is increased following gamete intrafallopian transfer (GIFT) and in vitro fertilization (IVF) (Coste and associates, 1991; Guirgis and Craft, 1991). The Society for Assisted Reproductive Technology and the American Society of Reproductive Medicine (1998) cited the 1995 incidence to be 2.8 percent for these pregnancies.

"Atypical" implantations are more common following assisted reproductive techniques. Chen and associates (1998) reported 11 ectopic gestations following 1014

IVF cycles, and 3 of 11 were cornual implantations. Similarly, extratubal as well as heterotypic tubal pregnancies are also increased after these procedures (Botta and co-workers, 1995; Glassner and colleagues, 1990; Marcus and associates, 1995; Pisarska and Carson, 1999). Berliner and associates (1998) described a triplet heterotypic pregnancy following ovulation induction and intrauterine insemination. Heterotypic cervical and ovarian pregnancy also have been reported (Bayati and associates, 1989; DeMuylder and co-workers, 1994).

Abdominal pregnancy has been reported following gamete intrafallopian transfer and in vitro fertilization (Balmaceda and associates, 1993; Ferland and associates, 1991; Vignali and co-workers, 1990). Cervical pregnancy may be increased after in vitro fertilization (Bennett, 1993; Ginsberg, 1994; Pattinson, 1994; Peleg, 1994, and their colleagues). Finally, ovarian pregnancy also may be increased after in vitro fertilization (Marcus and Brinsden, 1995).

FAILED CONTRACEPTION. With any form of contraceptive, the actual number of ectopic pregnancies is decreased because pregnancy occurs less often. In some contraceptive failures, however, there is an increased incidence of ectopic compared with uterine pregnancies. Examples include some forms of tubal sterilization and in women using intrauterine devices or taking progestin-only minipills (Sivin, 1991).

As shown in Table 34–1, pregnancy following tubal sterilization has an ectopic pregnancy rate that is increased ninefold. The highest rates follow laparoscopic fulguration. Yamada and Kasamatsu (2000) recently described a woman who developed a tubal pregnancy in each tube at different times following puerperal tubal sterilization. Tubal pregnancy may occasionally follow hysterectomy. Isaacs and colleagues (1996) reviewed 36 such cases, and in 24 instances, a recently fertilized ovum was trapped in the oviduct at the time of hysterectomy. In the 12 cases remote from hysterectomy (1 to 11 years), sperm migrated from a fistulous communication in the vaginal vault.

EPIDEMIOLOGY. There has been a marked increase in both the absolute number and rate of ectopic pregnancies in the United States in the past two decades. The actual number has increased out of proportion to population growth.

The incidence of ectopic pregnancy for nonwhite women is higher in every age category than for whites, and this disparity increases with age (Fig. 34–1). Overall, in 1989 a nonwhite woman had a 1.4 times increased risk for ectopic pregnancy compared with a white woman (Goldner and associates, 1993). The combined factors of race and increasing age are at least additive. For example, nonwhite women 35 to 44 years of age were five times more likely to have an ectopic pregnancy than white women aged 15 to 24 years.

As shown in Table 34–2, the rate of ectopic pregnancy per 1000 reported pregnancies increased fourfold from 1970 to 1992. This increase was greater for nonwhite than white women, and for both, the incidence increased with age. Put another way, in 1992, almost 2 percent of all pregnancies were ectopic. Importantly, ectopic pregnancy accounted for 10 percent of all pregnancy-related deaths (Centers for Disease Control and Prevention, 1995; Koonin and colleagues, 1997).

The apparent fall in the number of ectopic pregnancies after 1989 as shown in Table 34–2 unfortunately is not real. For example, the number in 1992 was 108,800 rather than 55,200. This difference is because of contem-

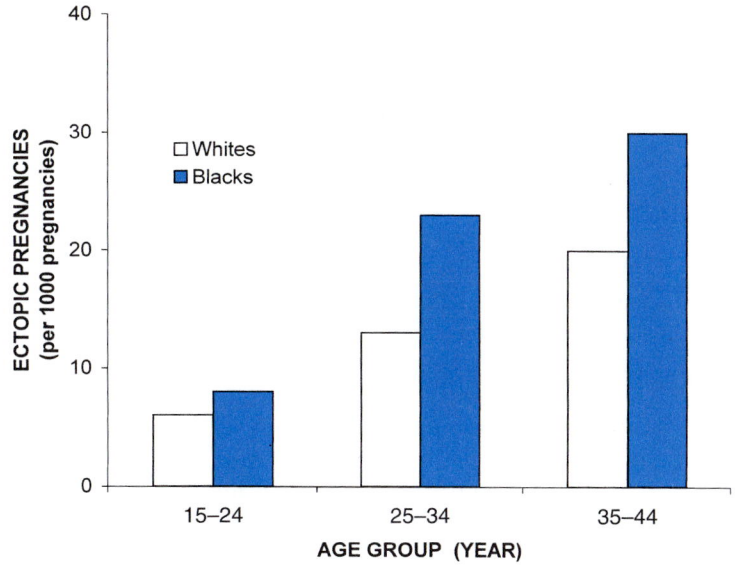

FIGURE 34–1. Ectopic pregnancy rates for white and black women—United States, 1970 through 1990. (Data from Goldner and colleagues, 1993.)

TABLE 34–2. **Numbers and Rate of Reported Ectopic Pregnancies in the United States, 1970–1992**

Year	Number[a]	Rates		
		Females 15 to 44 years[b]	Live Births[c]	Reported[d] Pregnancies
1970	17,800	—	—	4.5
1975	30,500	6.5	9.8	7.6
1980	52,200	9.9	14.5	10.5
1985	78,400	14.0	20.9	15.2
1989	88,400	—	—	16.0
1990	60,400	—	—	11.4
1992[e]	55,200	—	—	10.6
1992[f]	108,800	—	—	19.7
1993[g]	53,000	—	—	—
1995[g]	40,000	—	—	—
1996[g]	37,000	—	—	—
1997[g]	25,000	—	—	—

[a]Rounded to nearest hundred.
[b]Rate per 10,000 females.
[c]Rate per 1000 live births.
[d]Rate per 1000 reported pregnancies (live births, legal abortions, and ectopic).
[e]Number and rate based upon conventional data reported from hospitals.
[f]Number and rate based upon hospitalizations and ambulatory management of ectopic pregnancies.
[g]Number based on National Hospital Discharge Survey.
From Centers for Disease Control and Prevention (1988, 1995, 1999); Goldner and colleagues (1993); and Nederlof and associates (1990).

poraneous ambulatory management of very early ectopic pregnancies. Medical therapy usually does not require hospitalization. Therefore, accurate figures are currently obtained through the National Hospital Ambulatory Medical Care Survey (NHAMCS), along with inpatient statistics from the National Hospital Discharge Survey (NHDS).

CAUSES FOR INCREASED ECTOPIC PREGNANCY RATES. The reasons for increased ectopic pregnancies in the United States are not entirely clear. Similar increases have been reported from Eastern Europe, Scandinavia, and Great Britain. Some likely causes include:

1. Increased prevalence of sexually transmitted tubal infection (Brunham and associates, 1992; Maccato and colleagues, 1992).
2. Earlier diagnosis with sensitive assays for chorionic gonadotropin and transvaginal ultrasound—in some, resorption would occur before diagnosis in the past.
3. Popularity of contraception that prevents intrauterine but not extrauterine pregnancies.
4. Unsuccessful tubal sterilizations.
5. Induced abortion followed by infection.
6. Increased use of assisted reproductive techniques.
7. Tubal surgery, including prior salpingotomy for tubal pregnancy as well as tuboplasty.

MORTALITY. Deaths from ectopic pregnancy in the United States decreased from 63 in 1970, to 46 in 1980, and to 30 in 1987. Unfortunately, the proportion of all maternal deaths attributed to ectopic pregnancy increased from 8 percent in 1970 to 11 percent in the 3-year period ending 1990 (Koonin and associates, 1997). As shown in Figure 34–2, the death rate has plateaued for white women and for black women since 1986. The case-fatality rate, however, decreased 10-fold, from 35.5 per 10,000 ectopic pregnancies in 1970 to 3.8 per 10,000 in 1989. Ectopic pregnancy remains a leading cause of maternal mortality in the United States, and is the most common cause of maternal mortality in the first trimester (Centers for Disease Control and Prevention, 1995).

The dramatic decrease in deaths from ectopic pregnancies is probably due to improved diagnosis and management. For example, massive hemorrhage causing death was often the result of abdominal and interstitial tubal pregnancies, which were likely to become symptomatic later in gestation. An important consideration for improvement is the markedly high mortality rate in 15- to 19-year-old nonwhite women (Nederlof and colleagues, 1990). This almost certainly is due in part to lack of early care.

ANATOMICAL CONSIDERATIONS. The fertilized ovum may develop in any portion of the oviduct, giving rise to ampullary, isthmic, and interstitial tubal pregnancies (see Fig. 3–16, p. 47). In rare instances, the fertilized ovum may be implanted in the fimbriated extremity. The ampulla is the most frequent site, and the isthmus the next most. Interstitial pregnancy accounts for only about 3 percent of all tubal gestations. From these primary types, certain secondary forms of tubo-abdominal, tubo-ovarian, and broad ligament pregnancies occasionally develop.

ZYGOTE IMPLANTATION. The fertilized ovum promptly burrows through the epithelium and the zygote comes to lie in the muscular wall because the tube lacks a submucosa. At the periphery of the zygote is a capsule of rapidly proliferating trophoblast, which invades and erodes the subjacent muscularis. At the same time, maternal blood vessels are opened, and blood pours into the spaces lying within the trophoblast or between it and the adjacent tissue.

Although decidual cells usually can be recognized,

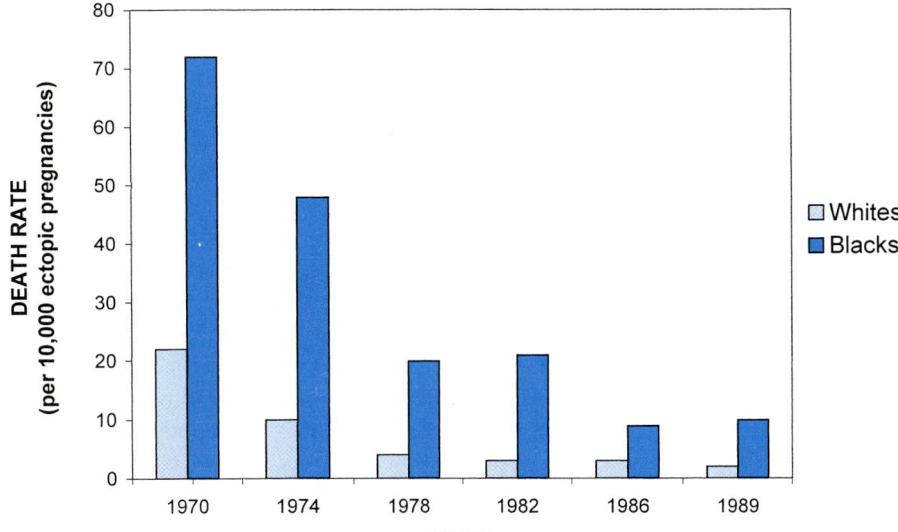

FIGURE 34–2. Death rate from ectopic pregnancy for white and black women—United States, 1970 through 1989. (From Goldner and co-workers, 1993.)

the tube normally does not form an extensive decidua. Tubal wall in contact with the zygote offers only slight resistance to invasion by the trophoblast, which soon burrows through it, opening maternal vessels (Fig. 34–3). The embryo or fetus in an ectopic pregnancy is often absent or stunted.

UTERINE CHANGES. The uterus undergoes some of the changes associated with early normal pregnancy, including softening of the cervix and isthmus and an increase in size. Even so, of 1125 women with a proven ectopic pregnancy, 75 percent had a normal-sized uterus (Stabile and Grudzinskas, 1990). Thus, lack of uterine changes do not exclude an ectopic pregnancy.

The degree to which the endometrium is converted to decidua is variable. The finding of uterine decidua without trophoblast suggests ectopic pregnancy but is not absolute. In 1954, Arias-Stella described, as had others before him, these changes. Enlarged epithelial cells with nuclei that are hypertrophic, hyperchromatic, lobular, and irregularly shaped. Cytoplasm may be vacuolated and foamy, and occasional mitoses are found. These endometrial changes—the *Arias-Stella reaction*—are not specific for ectopic and may occur with a normal implantation.

External bleeding—seldom severe—is seen commonly in cases of tubal pregnancy and is uterine in origin from degeneration and sloughing of the uterine decidua.

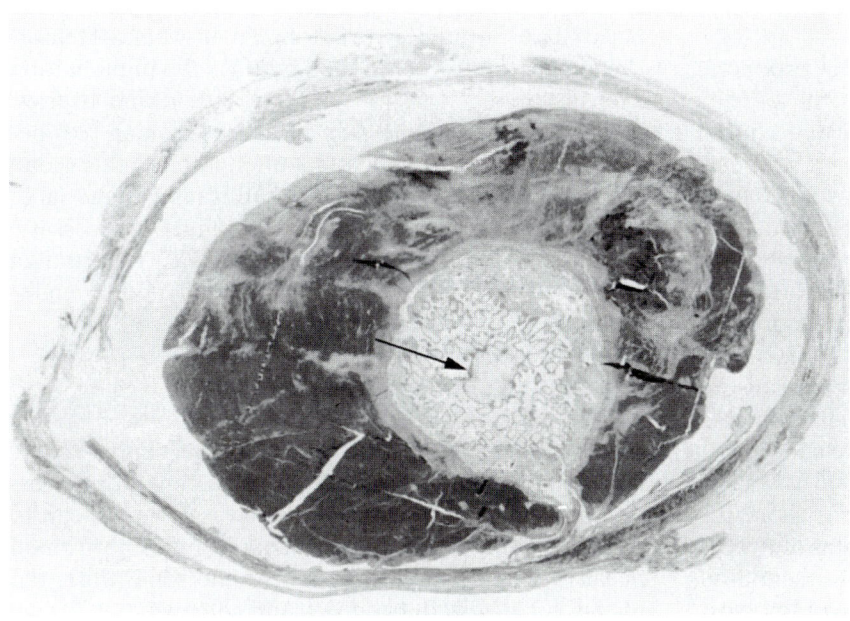

FIGURE 34–3. Early tubal pregnancy. Amnionic sac (*arrow*) is surrounded by chorionic villi, which in turn are encased in blood clot. (Courtesy of Dr. Richard Voet.)

Soon after embryonic death, the decidua degenerates and is usually shed in small pieces. Occasionally it is cast off intact, as a decidual cast of the uterine cavity. Absence of decidual tissue, however, does not exclude an ectopic pregnancy. Romney and co-workers (1950) identified secretory endometrium in 40 percent of cases of ectopic pregnancy, proliferative in 30 percent, and menstrual in 6 percent, while decidua was present in only 20 percent.

NATURAL HISTORY OF TUBAL PREGNANCY

TUBAL ABORTION. The frequency of tubal abortion depends in part upon the implantation site. Tubal abortion is common in ampullary tubal pregnancy, whereas rupture is the usual outcome with isthmic pregnancy. The immediate consequence of tubal hemorrhage is further disruption of the connection between the placenta and membranes and the tubal wall. If placental separation is complete, all of the products of conception may be extruded through the fimbriated end into the peritoneal cavity. At this point, hemorrhage may cease and symptoms eventually disappear.

Some bleeding usually persists as long as products remain in the oviduct. Blood slowly trickles from the tubal fimbria into the peritoneal cavity and typically pools in the rectouterine cul-de-sac. If the fimbriated extremity is occluded, the fallopian tube may gradually become distended by blood, forming a hematosalpinx.

After incomplete tubal abortion, pieces of the placenta or membranes may remain attached to the tubal wall and, after becoming surrounded by fibrin, give rise to a placental polyp. The process is similar to that in the uterus after an incomplete abortion.

TUBAL RUPTURE. The invading, expanding products of conception may rupture the oviduct at any of several sites. Before sophisticated methods to measure chorionic gonadotropin were available, many cases of tubal pregnancy ended during the first trimester by intraperitoneal rupture. As a rule, whenever there is tubal rupture in the first few weeks, the pregnancy is situated in the isthmic portion of the tube. When the fertilized ovum is implanted well within the interstitial portion, rupture usually occurs later.

Rupture is usually spontaneous, but it may be caused by trauma associated with coitus or a bimanual examination. With intraperitoneal rupture, the entire conceptus may be extruded from the tube, or if the rent is small, profuse hemorrhage may occur without extrusion. In either event, the woman commonly shows signs of hypovolemia. If an early conceptus is expelled essentially undamaged into the peritoneal cavity, it may reimplant almost anywhere, establish adequate circulation, survive, and grow. This outcome is most unlikely, however, because of damage during the transition. The conceptus, if small, may be resorbed or, if larger, may remain in the cul-de-sac for years as an encapsulated mass or even become calcified to form a *lithopedion*.

ABDOMINAL PREGNANCY. If only the fetus is extruded at the time of rupture, the effect upon the pregnancy will vary depending on the extent of injury sustained by the placenta. The fetus dies if the placenta is damaged appreciably, but if the greater portion of the placenta retains its tubal attachment, further development is possible. The fetus may then survive for some time, giving rise to an abdominal pregnancy. Typically, in such cases, a portion of the placenta remains attached to the tubal wall and the periphery grows beyond the tube and implants on surrounding structures.

BROAD-LIGAMENT PREGNANCY. When original zygote implantation is toward the mesosalpinx, rupture may occur at the portion of the tube not immediately covered by peritoneum, and the gestational contents may be extruded into a space formed between the folds of the broad ligament. This is designated an intraligamentous or broad-ligament pregnancy.

INTERSTITIAL PREGNANCY. Implantation within the tubal segment that penetrates the uterine wall results in an interstitial or cornual pregnancy (Fig. 34–4). These account for about 3 percent of all tubal gestations. There is variable asymmetry of the uterus that is often difficult to distinguish from a uterine pregnancy. Hence, early diagnosis is more frequently overlooked than in other types of tubal implantation. Because of the greater distensibility of the myometrium covering the tube, rupture occurs later, usually between 8 and 16 weeks. Hemorrhage may rapidly prove fatal because the implantation site is located between the ovarian and uterine arteries. In fact, tubal pregnancies in which the woman dies before she can reach the hospital often fall into this group (Dorfman and associates, 1984). Because of the large uterine defect, hysterectomy is commonly necessary. Despite this, Moon and colleagues (2000) reported 24 women with an interstitial pregnancy treated by endoscopic surgery.

MULTIFETAL ECTOPIC PREGNANCY

HETEROTYPIC ECTOPIC PREGNANCY. Tubal pregnancy may be accompanied by a coexisting uterine gestation. Such a heterotypic pregnancy is quite difficult to diagnose clinically. Typically, laparotomy is performed because of a tubal pregnancy. At the same time, the uterus is congested, softened, and somewhat enlarged.

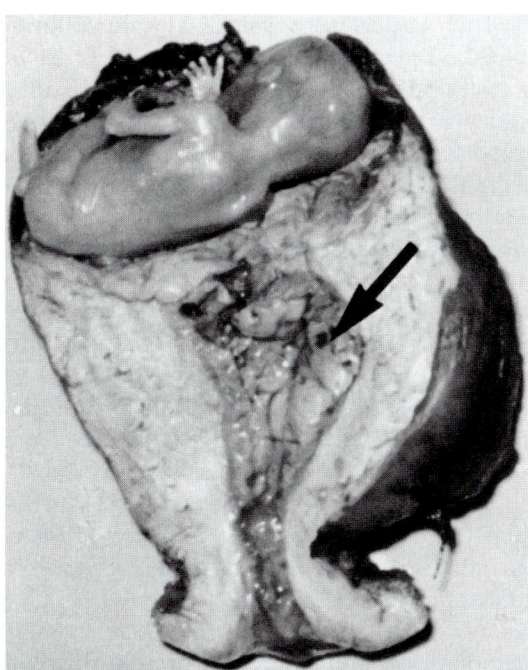

FIGURE 34–4. Right interstitial tubal pregnancy. Fetus weighed 55 g and measured 90 mm crown to rump (14 to 15 weeks' gestational age). Note abundant decidua (*arrow*) filling the uterine cavity. The patient sought medical help because of sudden severe abdominal pain with syncope following intercourse. Hysterectomy and 2000 mL blood transfusion were necessary.

Although these features are suggestive of uterine pregnancy, they are commonly induced by tubal pregnancy. Using ultrasound, gestational products are demonstrable within the uterine cavity in practically all instances of heterotypic pregnancy.

Until recently, heterotypic pregnancies were rare with an incidence of 1 per 30,000 pregnancies (Glassner and associates, 1990). Currently, because of assisted reproduction, the incidence is likely 1 in 7000 overall, and following ovulation induction it may be as high as 1 in 900 (Glassner and associates, 1990). In vitro fertilization and embryo transfer also increases the incidence (Dimitry and colleagues, 1990; Marcus and associates, 1995). According to Pisarska and Carson (1999), almost 12 percent of pregnancies following assisted reproduction are heterotypic.

A heterotypic pregnancy is more likely, and should be considered:

1. After assisted reproduction techniques.
2. With persistent or rising chorionic gonadotropin levels after dilatation and curettage for an induced or spontaneous abortion.
3. When the uterine fundus is larger than menstrual dates.
4. With more than one corpus luteum.
5. With absence of vaginal bleeding in the presence of signs and symptoms of an ectopic pregnancy.
6. When there is ultrasound evidence of uterine and extrauterine pregnancy (Kouyoumdjian and Kirkpatrick, 1990; Nugent, 1992).

Sherer and associates (1995) reported a heterotypic quadruplet pregnancy after in vitro fertilization and embryo transfer complicated by a ruptured interstitial pregnancy at 8 weeks. Cases of cervical and ovarian heterotypic pregnancy have been described (Bayati and associates, 1989; Hirose and associates, 1994; Peleg and colleagues, 1994).

MULTIFETAL TUBAL PREGNANCY. Twin tubal pregnancy has been reported with both embryos in the same tube, as well as with one in each tube. Simultaneous pregnancy in both fallopian tubes is the rarest form of double-ovum twinning. Quadruplet tubal pregnancy in the same oviduct was described by Fujii and associates (1981).

TUBO-UTERINE, TUBO-ABDOMINAL, AND TUBO-OVARIAN PREGNANCIES. A tubo-uterine pregnancy results from the gradual extension into the uterine cavity of products of conception that originally implanted in the interstitial portion of the tube. Tubo-abdominal pregnancy is derived from a tubal pregnancy in which the zygote, originally implanted near the fimbriated end of the tube, gradually extends into the peritoneal cavity. In such circumstances, the portion of the fetal sac projecting into the peritoneal cavity may form troublesome adhesions to surrounding organs. Both of these conditions are very uncommon.

A tubo-ovarian pregnancy occurs when the fetal sac is adherent partly to tubal and partly to ovarian tissue. Such cases arise from zygote development in a tubo-ovarian cyst or in a tube, the fimbriated extremity of which was adherent to the ovary or soon after fertilization. Rarely, the fetus and placenta may achieve appreciable size before rupture.

CLINICAL AND LABORATORY FEATURES OF TUBAL PREGNANCY

Clinical manifestations of a tubal pregnancy are diverse and depend on whether rupture has occurred. Earlier presentation and more precise diagnostic technology have enabled identification before there is rupture in most cases. Usually, the woman does not suspect pregnancy, or thinks that she is normally pregnant, or that she is aborting a uterine pregnancy.

In what used to be considered "classical" cases, normal menstruation is replaced by variably delayed slight vaginal bleeding, or "spotting." Suddenly, the woman is stricken with severe lower abdominal pain, frequently described as sharp, stabbing, or tearing in character. Vasomotor disturbances develop, ranging from vertigo to syncope. There is tenderness on abdominal palpation, and vaginal examination, especially cervical motion, causes exquisite pain. The posterior vaginal fornix may bulge because of blood in the cul-de-sac, or a tender, boggy mass may be felt to one side of the uterus. Symptoms of diaphragmatic irritation, characterized by pain in the neck or shoulder, especially on inspiration, develop in perhaps 50 percent of women with sizable intraperitoneal hemorrhage.

The diagnosis of such cases with rupture is not difficult to make. Even though symptoms and signs of ectopic pregnancy often range from indefinite to bizarre, most women are now seeking care before this classical clinical picture develops. Every reasonable effort is made to diagnose the condition before catastrophic events occur.

SYMPTOMS AND SIGNS

PAIN. Symptoms are related to whether the ectopic pregnancy has ruptured. According to Pisarska and colleagues (1998), women at high risk should be screened early and before they become symptomatic. For others, the most frequently experienced symptoms of ectopic pregnancy are pelvic and abdominal pain (95 percent) and amenorrhea with some degree of vaginal spotting or bleeding (60 to 80 percent). With more advanced gestation, Dorfman and associates (1984) reported that gastrointestinal symptoms (80 percent) and dizziness or light-headedness (58 percent) were common. With rupture, pain may be anywhere in the abdomen. Pleuritic chest pain may occur from diaphragmatic irritation caused by the hemorrhage.

ABNORMAL MENSTRUATION. About a fourth of women do not report amenorrhea; they mistake uterine bleeding that frequently occurs with tubal pregnancy for true menstruation. When endocrine support for the endometrium declines, bleeding is usually scanty, dark brown, and may be intermittent or continuous. Although profuse vaginal bleeding is suggestive of an incomplete abortion rather than an ectopic gestation, such bleeding is occasionally seen with tubal gestations.

ABDOMINAL AND PELVIC TENDERNESS. Exquisite tenderness on abdominal and vaginal examination, especially on motion of the cervix, is demonstrable in over three fourths of women with ruptured or rupturing tubal pregnancies. Such tenderness, however, may be absent prior to rupture.

UTERINE CHANGES. Because of placental hormones, in about 25 percent of cases, the uterus grows during the first 3 months of a tubal gestation to nearly the same size as it would with a normal pregnancy (Stabile and Grudzinskas, 1990). Its consistency may be similar as long as the fetus is alive. The uterus may be pushed to one side by an ectopic mass, or if the broad ligament is filled with blood, the uterus may be greatly displaced. Uterine decidual casts are passed by only 5 to 10 percent of women. Their passage may be accompanied by cramps similar to those with a spontaneous abortion.

BLOOD PRESSURE AND PULSE. Before rupture, vital signs generally are normal. Early responses to moderate hemorrhage may range from no change in vital signs to a slight rise in blood pressure, or a vasovagal response with bradycardia and hypotension. Blood pressure will fall and pulse rise only if bleeding continues and hypovolemia becomes significant.

Even with modern diagnostic methods, women with a ruptured ectopic pregnancy may present with hypovolemia and shock. Stabile and Grudzinskas (1990) reviewed several reports totaling almost 2400 women with surgically confirmed ectopic pregnancy. Almost a fourth presented in shock, but this proportion ranged from 1 to 50 percent in various series.

TEMPERATURE. After acute hemorrhage, the temperature may be normal or even low. Temperatures up to 38°C may develop, but higher temperatures are rare in the absence of infection. Fever is important in distinguishing a ruptured tubal pregnancy from some cases of acute salpingitis.

PELVIC MASS. On bimanual examination, a pelvic mass is palpable in about 20 percent of women. Its size ranges between 5 and 15 cm, and such masses are often soft and elastic. With extensive infiltration of blood into the tubal wall, the mass may be firm. It is almost always either posterior or lateral to the uterus. Pain and tenderness often preclude identification of the mass by palpation.

In some cases, there is gradual disintegration of the tubal wall followed by slow leakage of blood into the lumen, peritoneal cavity, or both. Signs of active hemorrhage are absent, and even mild symptoms may subside. Gradually, however, trickling blood collects in the pelvis, more or less walled off by adhesions, and a pelvic hematocele results. In some cases, this is eventually absorbed, and the patient recovers without operation. In others, it may rupture into the peritoneal cavity, or it may become infected and form an abscess.

CULDOCENTESIS. This is a simple technique for identifying hemoperitoneum. The cervix is pulled toward the symphysis with a tenaculum, and a long 16- or 18-gauge needle is inserted through the posterior fornix into the cul-de-sac. If present, fluid can be aspirated; however, failure to do so is interpreted only as unsatisfactory entry into the cul-de-sac and does not exclude an ectopic pregnancy, either ruptured or unruptured. Fluid-containing fragments of old clots, or bloody fluid that does not clot, are compatible with the diagnosis of hemoperitoneum resulting from an ectopic pregnancy. If the blood subsequently clots, it may have been obtained from an adjacent perforated blood vessel rather than from a bleeding ectopic pregnancy.

LABORATORY TESTS. Measurement of hemoglobin, hematocrit, and leukocyte count, as well as serum levels of chorionic gonadotropin and progesterone, are useful in certain cases if their limitations are understood.

HEMOGLOBIN, HEMATOCRIT, AND LEUKOCYTE COUNT. After hemorrhage, depleted blood volume is restored toward normal by hemodilution over the course of a day or longer. Even after substantive hemorrhage, therefore, hemoglobin or hematocrit readings may at first show only a slight reduction. For the first few hours after an acute hemorrhage, a decrease in hemoglobin or hematocrit level while the woman is under observation is a more valuable index of blood loss than is the initial reading.

The degree of leukocytosis varies considerably in ruptured ectopic pregnancy. In about half of women, it is normal, but in the remainder, varying degrees of leukocytosis up to $30,000/\mu L$ may be documented.

CHORIONIC GONADOTROPIN ASSAYS. Ectopic pregnancy cannot be diagnosed by a positive pregnancy test alone. The key issue, however, is whether the woman is pregnant. In virtually all cases of ectopic gestation, human chorionic gonadotropin (β-hCG) can be detected in serum, but usually at markedly reduced concentrations compared with normal pregnancy.

URINARY PREGNANCY TESTS. Urine tests are most often latex agglutination inhibition slide tests with sensitivities for chorionic gonadotropin in the range of 500 to 800 mIU/mL. Their simplicity is offset by only a 50 to 60 percent chance of being positive with an ectopic pregnancy. Even when tube-type tests are used, detection of chorionic gonadotropin is within 150 to 250 mIU/mL, and the test is positive only in 80 to 85 percent of ectopic pregnancies. Tests using enzyme-linked immunosorbent assays (ELISA) are sensitive to 10 to 50 mIU/mL, and are positive in 95 percent of ectopic pregnancies.

SERUM β-hCG ASSAYS. Radioimmunoassay is the most precise method, and virtually any pregnancy can be detected. In fact, because of the sensitivity of this assay, a pregnancy may be confirmed before there are grossly visible changes in the fallopian tube. Absence of pregnancy can be established only when there is a negative assay for serum gonadotropin that has a sensitivity of 5 to 10 mIU/mL. Because a single positive serum assay does not exclude an ectopic pregnancy, several different methods have been devised to use serial quantitative serum values to establish the diagnosis. These may be used alone, but more commonly are used in conjunction with sonography.

SERUM PROGESTERONE. A single progesterone measurement can often be used to establish that there is a normally developing pregnancy. A value exceeding 25 ng/mL excludes ectopic pregnancy with 97.5 percent sensitivity (Lipscomb and co-workers, 1999a; Pisarska and colleagues, 1998; Stoval and associates, 1992). Values less than 5 ng/mL suggest that the fetus-embryo is dead, but not its location. Progesterone levels between 5 and 25 ng/mL—unfortunately common—are inconclusive (McCord and colleagues, 1996).

According to DeCherney (1996), 10 percent of women with a normal pregnancy have serum progesterone values less than 25 ng/mL. Hahlin and co-workers (1990) reported that no woman with a uterine pregnancy had progesterone levels less than 10 ng/mL, while 88 percent of those with ectopic pregnancies and 83 percent of those with spontaneous abortions had lower values.

ULTRASOUND IMAGING

ABDOMINAL SONOGRAPHY. Identification of pregnancy products in the fallopian tube is difficult using abdominal sonography. If a gestational sac is clearly identified within the uterine cavity, it is unlikely an ectopic pregnancy coexists. Moreover, with sonographic absence of a uterine pregnancy, a positive pregnancy test, fluid in the cul-de-sac, and an abnormal pelvic mass, ectopic pregnancy is almost certain (Romero and associates, 1988). Unfortunately, ultrasonic findings suggestive of early uterine pregnancy may be apparent in some cases of ectopic pregnancy. The sonographic appearance of a small sac (very early pregnancy) or a collapsed sac (dead fetus) may actually be a blood clot or decidual cast (Coleman and colleagues, 1985). A uterine pregnancy is usually not recognized using abdominal ultrasound until 5 to 6 menstrual weeks or 28 days after timed ovulation (Batzer and co-workers, 1983). Conversely, demonstration of an adnexal or cul-de-sac mass by sonography is not necessarily helpful. Corpus luteum cysts and matted bowel sometimes look like tubal pregnancies sonographically. Identification with sonography of fetal heart

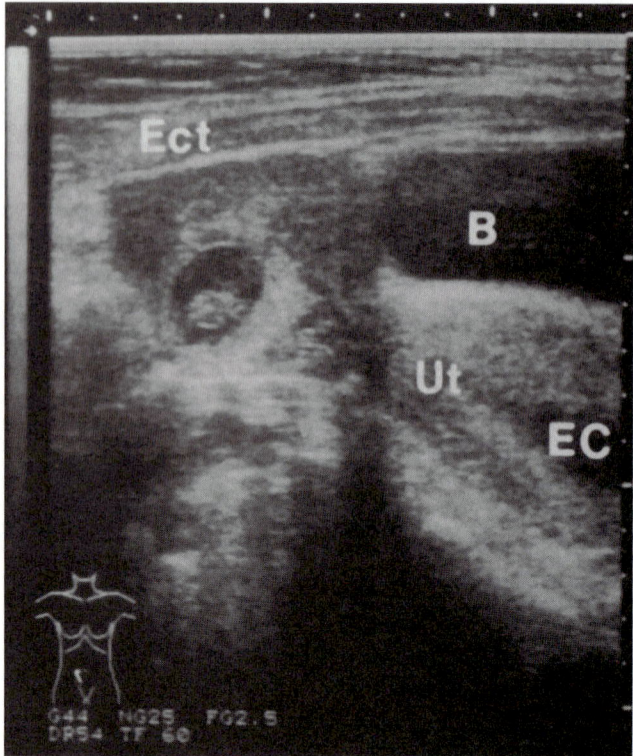

FIGURE 34–5. Longitudinal midline abdominal sonogram showing a well-defined ectopic pregnancy (Ect) overlying the uterus (Ut). (B = bladder; EC = endometrial cavity.) (Courtesy of Dr. Rigoberto Santos.)

action clearly outside the uterine cavity, however, provides firm evidence of an ectopic pregnancy (Fig. 34–5).

VAGINAL SONOGRAPHY. Sonography with a vaginal transducer can be used to detect uterine gestation as early as 1 week after missed menses when the serum β-hCG level is greater than 1500 mIU/mL. In a study by Barnhart and colleagues (1994), an empty uterus with a serum β-hCG concentration of 1500 mIU/mL or higher was 100 percent accurate in identifying an ectopic pregnancy.

Vaginal sonography is also used to detect adnexal masses. This, however, can be misleading, and ectopic pregnancies may be missed when a tubal mass is small or obscured by bowel (Cacciatore and colleagues, 1990). Sadek and Schiatz (1995) reported that the sensitivity and specificity of vaginal ultrasound for ectopic pregnancy was 96 and 99 percent, respectively, when free peritoneal fluid was identified. With visualization of a tubal mass, these were 81 and 99 percent, respectively.

Vaginal sonography results in earlier and more specific diagnoses of uterine pregnancy. With a serum β-hCG level of 1000 mIU/mL, 50 percent of gestational sacs are seen (DeCherney, 1996). Criteria include identification of a 1- to 3-mm or larger gestational sac, ec-

centrically placed in the uterus, and surrounded by a decidual-chorionic reaction. A fetal pole within the sac is diagnostic, especially when accompanied by fetal heart action.

Vaginal sonography, such as shown in Figures 34–6 and 34–7, can be used alone to diagnose ectopic pregnancy in more than 90 percent of cases (Cacciatore and co-workers, 1990). Accurate clinical diagnosis is based upon two possibilities:

1. Uterine pregnancy is identified as described.
2. Or, an empty uterus and an ectopic pregnancy are seen based upon visualization of an adnexal mass separate from two clearly identified ovaries.

The mass must be complex, or contain a gestational saclike adnexal ring with or without a fetal pole (fetal echoes or yolk sac).

Without these criteria, the study may be nondiagnostic. A heterotypic pregnancy is an exception (Hirsch and associates, 1992). In the event of a nondiagnostic study, most clinicians favor serial sonography along with serial β-hCG measurements because the change in concentration is important (Tay and colleagues, 2000). In some cases, laparoscopy or laparotomy may be necessary.

VAGINAL COLOR AND PULSED DOPPLER ULTRASOUND. This technique consists of identifying a uterine or extrauterine site of vascular color in a characteristic placental shape, the so-called *ring-of-fire* pattern, and a high-velocity low-impedance flow pattern that is compatible with placental perfusion. If this pattern is seen outside the uterine cavity, which is also "cold" with respect to blood flow, the diagnosis of ectopic pregnancy is apparent.

The technique significantly improves the correct diagnosis of a live uterine pregnancy as well as an ectopic pregnancy or incomplete abortion (Emerson and colleagues, 1992; Pellerito and co-workers, 1992). It has been used successfully to diagnose cervical pregnancy and to monitor its regression following methotrexate therapy (Chao and colleagues, 1993; Roussis and co-workers, 1992). Unfortunately, the equipment is expensive and interpretation is complex.

DIAGNOSIS OF ECTOPIC PREGNANCY

During the past decade, as modern refinements for identification of ectopic pregnancy have evolved, the majority—perhaps 80 percent—are diagnosed before rupture. Coincidentally, the death rate has decreased appreciably (Fig. 34–2). A number of diagnostic algorithms have been proposed and are described next.

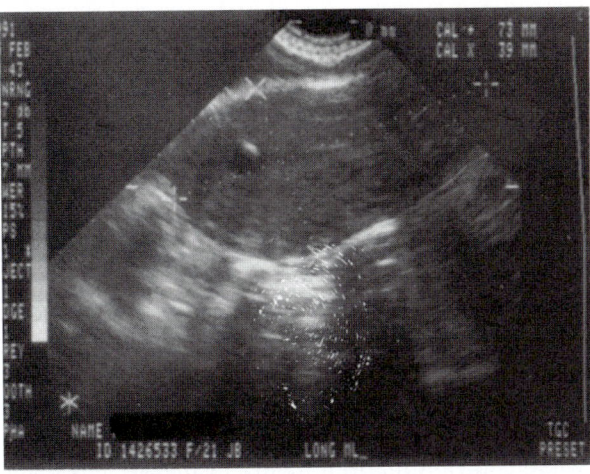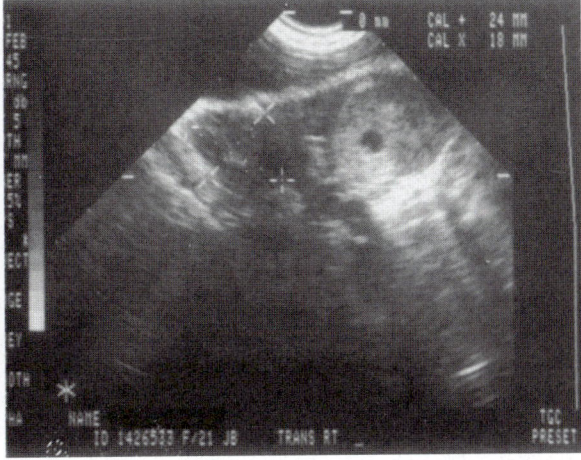

FIGURE 34-6. Vaginal sonogram of an ectopic pregnancy.

QUANTITATIVE SERUM β-hCG PLUS SONOGRAPHY.
When pregnancy is diagnosed in a hemodynamically stable woman suspected of having an ectopic pregnancy, subsequent management is based upon serial serum β-hCG values and sonography. When the β-hCG value is less than 1500 mIU/mL and there is an empty uterus with vaginal sonography, no definitive diagnosis can be made. While a positive assay for serum β-hCG can confirm a pregnancy as early as 8 days after fertilization, a uterine gestational sac cannot be reliably identified with vaginal ultrasound until 28 days after conception, or about 6 weeks of amenorrhea. This time between 8 and 28 days is called the *20-day window* (Daus and colleagues, 1989). During this time, the woman may abort, she may continue her pregnancy and develop a normal gestational sac, or she may develop evidence of an ectopic pregnancy.

Kadar and Romero (1987) confirmed earlier work demonstrating that in women with normal pregnancies, mean doubling time for β-hCG in serum was approximately 48 hours, and the lowest normal value for this increase was 66 percent (Table 34–3). They calculated this number by subtracting the initial value for β-hCG from the 48-hour value and dividing the result by the initial value, which is multiplied by 100 to obtain a percentage. They found that more reliable values could be obtained at 48-hour intervals. They concluded that failure to maintain this rate of increased β-hCG production, along with an empty uterus, was suggestive for an ectopic pregnancy. This plan delays surgery at least 48

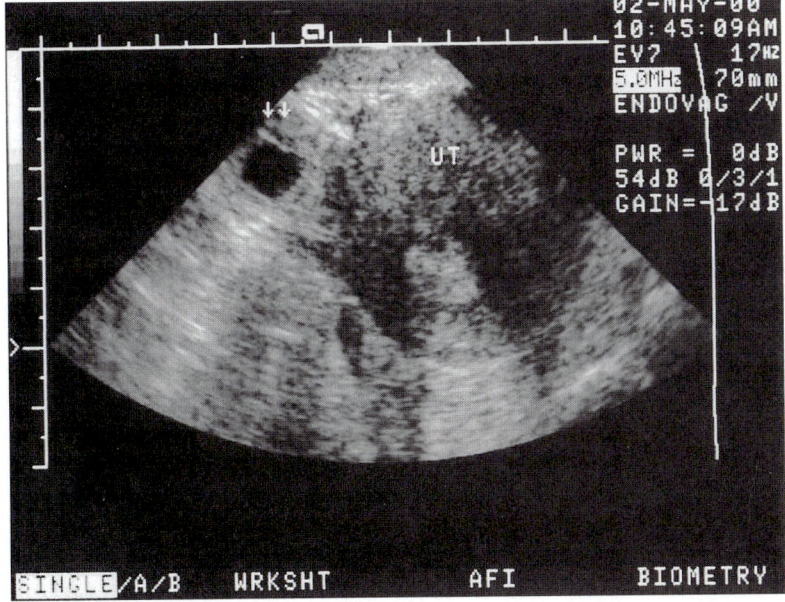

FIGURE 34-7. Vaginal sonogram showing right tubal ectopic pregnancy with the echogenic ring of trophoblastic tissue with the tube (*arrows*) adjacent to the uterus (UT). (Courtesy of Dr. Diane Twickler.)

TABLE 34–3. Lower Normal Limits for Percentage Increase of Serum β-hCG During Early Uterine Pregnancy

Sampling Interval (days)	Increase from Initial Value (%)
1	29
2	66
3	114
4	175
5	255

Modified from Kadar and co-workers (1981) with permission.

hours. Moreover, the test would still falsely identify 15 percent of normal women as likely to have an ectopic pregnancy and falsely identify 13 percent of women with an ectopic pregnancy as normal.

SURGICAL DIAGNOSIS

CURETTAGE. Differentiation between threatened or incomplete abortion and a tubal pregnancy may be accomplished in many instances by office curettage. Stovall and colleagues (1992) recommend curettage in suspected cases of incomplete abortion versus ectopic pregnancy when serum progesterone is less than 5 ng/mL, β-hCG levels are rising abnormally (less than 2000 mU/mL), and a uterine pregnancy is not seen using transvaginal sonography. If an embryo, fetus, or placenta is identified, the diagnosis is apparent. When none of these is identified, tubal pregnancy is a probability and further follow-up is done using serial β-hCG levels and sonography.

LAPAROSCOPY. Advantages of diagnostic laparoscopy include:

1. A definitive diagnosis in most cases.
2. A concurrent route to remove the ectopic mass using operative laparoscopy.
3. A direct route to inject chemotherapeutic agents into the ectopic mass.

Complete visualization of the pelvis may be impossible if there is pelvic inflammation or active bleeding. At times, identification of an early unruptured tubal pregnancy may be difficult, even if the tube is fully visualized.

LAPAROTOMY. This is preferred when the woman is hemodynamically unstable, or if laparoscopy is not feasible. Laparotomy should not be delayed while laparoscopy is performed in a woman with obvious abdominal hemorrhage that requires immediate defin-

itive treatment. Laparoscopy is more cost-effective, and there is a shorter postoperative recovery (Gray and colleagues, 1995).

TREATMENT AND PROGNOSIS OF TUBAL PREGNANCY

In the past, salpingectomy was usually done to remove a damaged, bleeding oviduct. Over the past two decades, technical advances with earlier diagnosis and treatment of high-risk women have allowed definitive management of an unruptured ectopic pregnancy even before there are clinical symptoms. Importantly, early diagnosis, while contributing to a higher incidence, has made many cases of ectopic pregnancy amenable to medical therapy. Indeed, according to Pisarska and colleagues (1998), ectopic pregnancy is evolving into a medical disorder. Mol and associates (1999) evaluated costs for 100 women in a randomized study to compare salpingostomy with methotrexate therapy. They reported that medical therapy costs were lower if confirmatory laparoscopy was not performed. Lecuru and colleagues (2000) analyzed costs in a nonrandomized prospective evaluation of 59 women treated by methotrexate or laparoscopic salpingectomy. The cost for surgical therapy was more than twice than for methotrexate. Morlock and colleagues (2000) used decision-analysis of published data and calculated cost savings of $3000 in 1998 for methotrexate therapy for each resolved ectopic pregnancy.

SURGICAL MANAGEMENT. Subsequent pregnancy and lower recurrent ectopic pregnancy rates are observed in women in whom surgery is performed prior to rupture. Laparoscopy is preferred over laparotomy unless the woman is unstable (Tulandi and Saleh, 1999). Even though reproductive outcome—including rates of uterine and recurrent ectopic pregnancies—is similar, laparoscopy is more cost effective and has a shorter recovery time—1.3 versus 3.1 days (Tay and colleagues, 2000).

Tubal surgery for ectopic pregnancy is considered *conservative* when there is tubal salvage. Examples include salpingostomy, salpingotomy, and fimbrial expression of the ectopic. *Radical surgery* is defined by salpingectomy. Shown in Table 34–4 are four retrospective studies of fertility subsequent to surgical treatment. The rates of uterine and recurrent ectopic pregnancies are not different when conservative procedures were compared with salpingectomy.

SALPINGOSTOMY. This procedure is used to remove a small pregnancy that is usually less than 2 cm in length and located in the distal third of the fallopian tube (Fig.

TABLE 34–4. Reproductive Performance After Conservative versus Radical Surgery for Ectopic Pregnancy

Series	Total	Conservative[a] No.	Conservative[a] Uterine (%)	Conservative[a] Ectopic (%)	Radical[b] No.	Radical[b] Uterine (%)	Radical[b] Ectopic (%)
Ory et al (1993)	188	38	50	21	50	58	8
Silva et al (1993)	143	60	60	18	26	54	8
Tuomivaara and Kauppila (1988)	523	86	69	12	237	71	11
Sherman et al (1982)	250	47	83	6	104	72	6
Total	1104	231	66	14	417	69	9

[a]Includes salpingostomy, fimbrial expression, and ovarian and tubo-uterine implantation.
[b]Salpingectomy performed.
Modified after Tulandi and Seleh (1999).

34–8). A linear incision, 10 to 15 mm in length or less, is made on the antimesenteric border immediately over the ectopic pregnancy. The products usually will extrude from the incision and can be carefully removed or flushed out. Small bleeding sites are controlled with needlepoint electrocautery or laser, and the incision is left unsutured to heal by secondary intention. This procedure is readily performed through a laparoscope and currently is the "gold standard" of surgical methods used for an unruptured ectopic pregnancy (Tulandi and Saleh, 1999).

SALPINGOTOMY. The procedure is the same as for salpingostomy except that the incision is closed with 7-0 Vicryl or similar suture. According to Tulandi and Saleh (1999), there is no difference in prognosis with or without suturing.

SALPINGECTOMY. Tubal resection can be performed through an operative laparoscope and may be used for both ruptured and unruptured ectopic pregnancies. It is performed if the fallopian tube is extensively diseased or damaged (Tay and associates, 2000). When removing

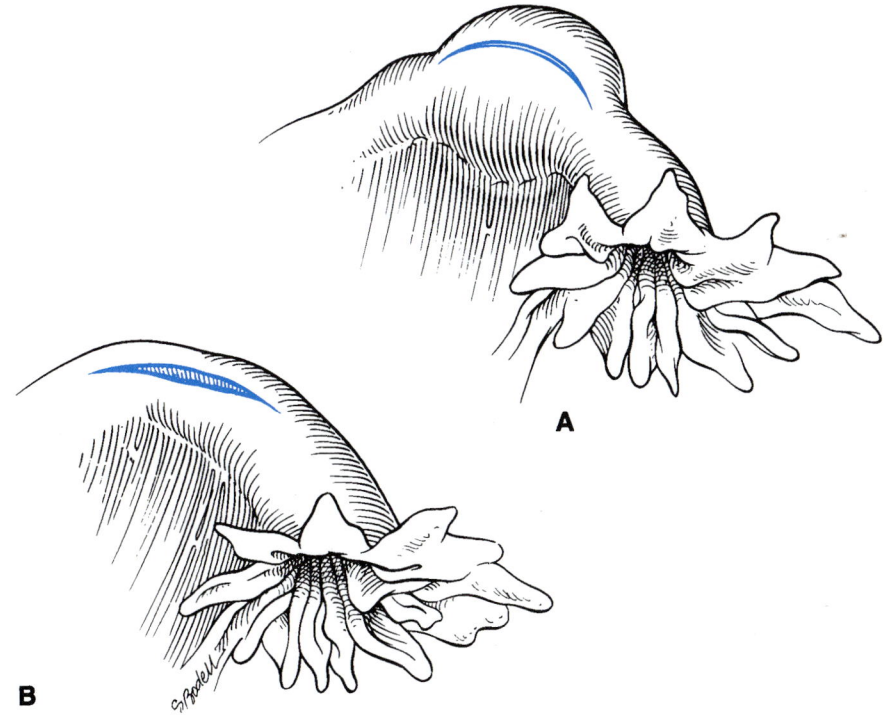

FIGURE 34–8. A. Linear salpingostomy for removal of a small tubal pregnancy in distal third of fallopian tube. **B.** The incision is not sutured.

the oviduct, it is advisable to excise a wedge no more than the outer third of the interstitial portion of the tube. This so-called *cornual resection* is done in an effort to minimize the rare recurrence of pregnancy in the tubal stump. Even with cornual resection, a subsequent interstitial pregnancy may not be prevented (Kalchman and Meltzer, 1966).

In some women with an interstitial pregnancy, hysterectomy is necessary to stop life-threatening hemorrhage. Conversely, Moon and co-workers (2000) described 24 women with an interstitial pregnancy who were successfully treated by endoscopic surgery. In 15 of these, the endoloop technique was used.

SEGMENTAL RESECTION AND ANASTOMOSIS.
Resection of the mass and tubal anastomosis is sometimes used for an unruptured isthmic pregnancy. This procedure is used because salpingostomy may cause scarring and subsequent narrowing of the small lumen (Stangel and associates, 1976). After the tubal segment is exposed, the mesosalpinx beneath the tube is incised, and the tubal isthmus containing the ectopic mass is resected. The mesosalpinx is sutured, thus reapproximating the tubal stumps. The segments of the tube are then apposed to one another in layers with interrupted 7-0 Vicryl sutures, preferably using magnification. Three sutures are used in the muscularis and three in the serosa, with strict attention to avoid the tubal lumen.

PERSISTENT TROPHOBLAST.
Following salpingostomy or salpingectomy, serum β-hCG levels usually fall quickly and are at about 10 percent of preoperative values by day 12 (Hajenius and colleagues, 1995; Vermesh and associates, 1988). Persistent ectopic pregnancy is the result of incomplete removal of trophoblast. It is the most common complication of salpingostomy, with a frequency of 5 to 20 percent (Graczykowski and Mishell, 1997). Yao and Tulandi (1997) summarized almost 700 tubal pregnancies removed at laparoscopy, and persistent pregnancy was identified in 8 percent. The number was 4 percent in 230 women undergoing laparotomy. Because of these high rates, Spandorfer and co-workers (1997) studied the predictive value of a day 1 serum hCG value. If the level at this time had decreased to less than 50 percent of that done preoperatively, then persistent ectopic trophoblast was rare.

According to Seifer (1997), factors that increase the risk of persistent ectopic include:

1. Small pregnancies, viz, less than 2 cm.
2. Early therapy, viz, before 42 menstrual days.
3. β-hCG serum levels exceeding 3000 mIU/mL.
4. Implantation medial to the salpingostomy site.

To avoid persistent ectopic pregnancy, some clinicians choose to give single-dose prophylactic methotrexate

(1 mg/kg) to women in these high-risk categories. In either case, with persistent or increasing values, the choice of reexploration or methotrexate chemotherapy must be made.

MEDICAL MANAGEMENT

METHOTREXATE.
Tanaka and associates (1982) were first to recommend use of methotrexate for interstitial pregnancy. Subsequently, Miyazaki (1983) and Ory and colleagues (1986) reported its use as first-line therapy for ectopic pregnancies. Since these initial reports, there have been numerous reports describing successful treatment of all varieties of ectopic pregnancies using a number of methotrexate regimens. Indeed, as experience was gained, medical treatment became comparable with the "gold standard" of salpingostomy (Buster and Pisarska, 1999). Despite this, there still may be reluctance to use medical therapy for fear of subsequent tubal rupture (Kucera and associates, 2000; Lipscomb and colleagues, 2000).

In the largest single-center series, Lipscomb and colleagues (1999a) reported a 91 percent success rate in 350 women given methotrexate therapy. Of these, 283 women were given a single dose of methotrexate, 60 women two doses, six women three doses, and one woman four doses. In a randomized trial from the Netherlands by Hajenius and colleagues (1997), comparable results were described with systemic methotrexate and laparoscopic salpingostomy.

Active intra-abdominal hemorrhage is a contraindication to chemotherapy. The size of the ectopic mass is also important, and Pisarska and colleagues (1998) recommend that methotrexate not be used if the pregnancy is more than 4 cm. Success is greatest if the gestation is less than 6 weeks, the tubal mass is not more than 3.5 cm in diameter, the fetus is dead, and the β-hCG is less than 15,000 mIU (Lipscomb and colleagues, 1999a; Stovall, 1995). According to the American College of Obstetricians and Gynecologists (1998), other contraindications include breast feeding, immunodeficiency, alcoholism, liver or kidney disease, blood dyscrasias, active pulmonary disease, and peptic ulcer.

PATIENT SELECTION.
Candidates for methotrexate therapy must be hemodynamically stable with a normal hemogram and normal liver and renal function. They are instructed that:

1. Medical therapy fails in 5 to 10 percent of cases, and this rate is higher in pregnancies past 6 weeks gestation or with a tubal mass greater than 4 cm in diameter.
2. Failure of medical therapy results in re-treatment, either medically or with elective surgery, or if tubal

TABLE 34-5. Methotrexate Therapy for Primary Treatment of Ectopic Pregnancy

Regimen	Follow-up

Single Dose[a]
  Methotrexate, 50 mg/m^2 IM
	Measure β-hCG days 4 and 7:
	  If difference is ≥15%, repeat weekly until <15 mIU/mL
	  If difference <15%, repeat methotrexate dose and begin new day 1
	  If fetal cardiac activity present day 7, repeat methotrexate dose, begin new day 1
	  Surgical treatment if β-hCG levels not decreasing or fetal cardiac activity persist after three doses methotrexate

Variable Dose
  Methotrexate, 1 mg/kg IM, days 1, 3, 5, 7
  plus
  Leukovorin, 0.1 mg/kg IM, days 2, 4, 6, 8
	Continue alternate-day injections until β-hCG levels decrease >15% in 48 h, or four doses methotrexate given
	  Then, weekly β-hCG until <5.0 mIU/mL

IM = intramuscularly.
[a]Preferred by editors.
Regimens from Buster and Pisarska (1999), Lipscomb and co-workers (1999b), and Pisarska and colleagues (1998, 1999).

rupture occurs—a 5 percent chance—emergency surgery.

3. If treated as an outpatient, rapid transportation must be available.
4. Signs and symptoms of tubal rupture such as vaginal bleeding, abdominal and pleuritic pain, weakness, dizziness, or syncope must be reported promptly.
5. Sexual intercourse is prohibited until after serum β-hCG is undetectable.
6. No alcohol is consumed.
7. Multivitamins with folic acid should not be taken.

DOSE AND ADMINISTRATION. Methotrexate is an antineoplastic drug that acts as a folic acid antagonist and is highly effective against rapidly proliferating trophoblast. Its use is discussed in greater detail in Chapter 32 (p. 846). The two general schemes used for methotrexate administration for ectopic pregnancy are shown in Table 34–5. While single-dose treatment is easier to administer and monitor than variable-dose methotrexate therapy, it is associated with a higher failure rate, defined as persistent ectopic pregnancy (Table 34–6). This likely

is related to the pharmokinetics of methotrexate. Creinin and Krohn (1997) reported that with 50 or 60 mg/m^2 given intramuscularly, serum levels peaked within 2 hours and were undetectable by 72 hours.

Most methotrexate regimens studied include a dose of 50 mg/m^2. Recently, Yalcinkaya and colleagues (2000) compared 50 mg/m^2 with 25 mg/m^2 in a randomized study of clinically stable patients. Their preliminary results show that either dose resulted in similar outcomes. Importantly, the need for a second injection was about the same (25 to 30 percent) for each group.

MONITORING METHOTREXATE TOXICITY. Although toxicity may be severe, fortunately, most regimens have been associated with minimal laboratory changes and symptoms. Kooi and Kock (1992) reviewed 16 studies that reported side effects that all resolved in 3 to 4 days after methotrexate was discontinued. The most common were liver dysfunction (12 percent), stomatitis (6 percent), and gastroenteritis (1 percent); however, one woman had bone marrow depression. Case reports also describe life-threatening neutropenia and

TABLE 34-6. Success Rates and Subsequent Pregnancy Following Primary Treatment for Ectopic Pregnancy

Treatment	Studies	Patients	Treatment Success (%)[a]	Tubal Patency (%)[b]	Subsequent Pregnancy Uterine (%)	Subsequent Pregnancy Ectopic (%)
Conservative laaparoscopic surgery	32	1626	93	76	57	13
Variable-dose	12	338	93	75	58	7
Single-dose methotrexate	7	393	87	81	61	8

[a]Success defined as resolution of ectopic pregnancy with initial treatment scheme.
[b]Only 12 to 55% of all women tested for patency.

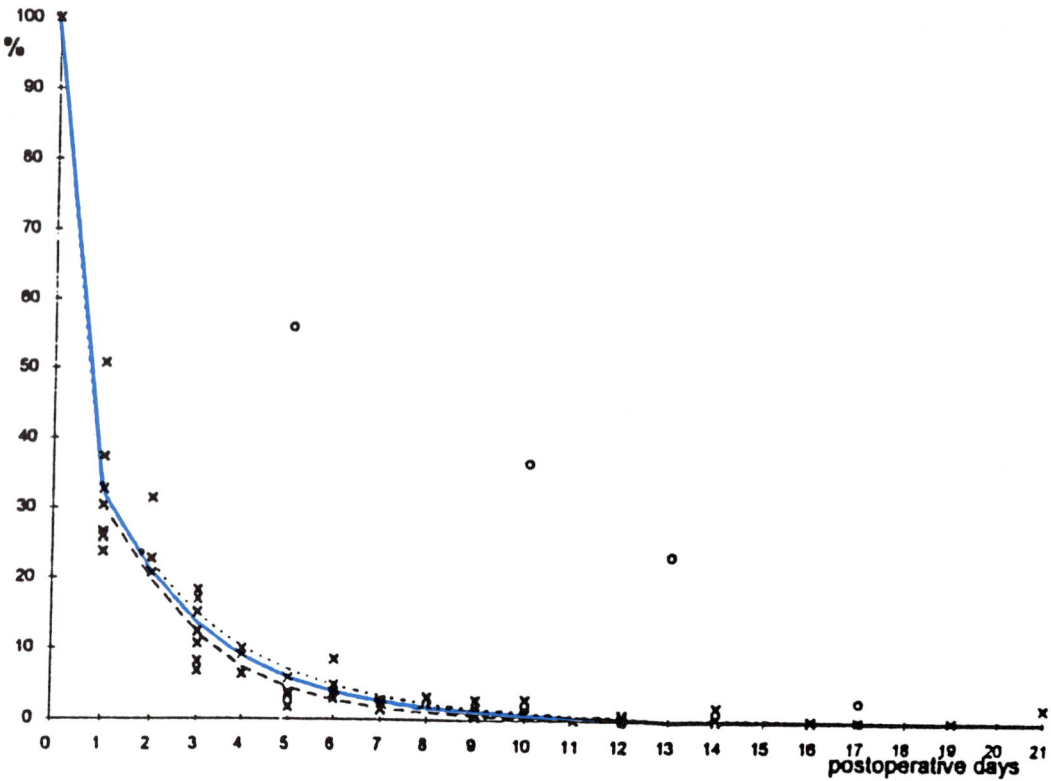

FIGURE 34–9. Serum chorionic gonadotropin (β-hCG) clearance curve in percentage of the initial serum β-hCG concentration on the day of surgery in patients successfully treated by salpingostomy via laparoscopy (n = 19). (Dashed and dotted lines indicate 95 percent confidence limits; ○ = patient with a slow but steady decline.) (From Hajenius and associates, 1995.)

fever, transient drug-induced pneumonitis, and alopecia (Buster and Pisarska, 1999).

MONITORING EFFICACY OF THERAPY. Various placental protein and steroid hormones have been used to monitor trophoblastic function (and mass) following medical and surgical therapy for ectopic pregnancies. The most widely used is serial serum β-hCG determinations, but values frequently continue to rise until day 4 after methotrexate therapy (Lipscomb and colleagues, 2000).

After methotrexate administration, β-hCG usually disappears from plasma between 14 and 21 days (Fig. 34–9). Lipscomb and colleagues (1998) treated 287 women successfully and found the average time to resolution (< 15 mIU/mL) was 34 days. The longest time was 109 days. As shown in Table 34–5, monitoring single-dose therapy calls for repeat serum β-hCG determinations at 4 and 7 days. With variable-dose methotrexate, serum concentrations are measured at 48-hour intervals until they fall more than 15 percent. After successful treatment, weekly serum β-hCG determinations are measured until less than 5 mIU/mL. Outpatient surveillance is preferred, but if there is any ques-

tion of safety, the woman is hospitalized. Failure is judged when there is no decline in β-hCG level, there is persistence of the ectopic mass, or there is any intraperitoneal bleeding.

PERSISTENT ECTOPIC PREGNANCY. Failure of initial medical or surgical therapy usually can be resolved with methotrexate therapy. About 20 percent of women given single-dose methotrexate will need a second dose (Lipscomb and associates, 2000). Aggregate studies shown in Table 34–6 suggest comparable efficacy—93 percent—of conservative surgery and variable-dose methotrexate. In the only randomized trial, however, Hajenius and colleagues (1997) observed persistent trophoblast in only 4 percent of women given variable-dose methotrexate compared with 20 percent of women undergoing salpingostomy.

Persistent pregnancy is suspected in women with abdominal pain. This is problematic because 65 to 75 percent of women given methotrexate will have increasing pain beginning several days after therapy. This **separation pain** generally is mild and relieved by nonnarcotic analgesics. For 20 percent of 258 patients with pain severe enough to require evaluation in the clinic or emergency room, Lipscomb and colleagues (1999b) reported that 10 of 53 ultimately underwent surgical exploration. Careful clinical observation, along with vaginal sonography and serum β-hCG determinations, is warranted.

Rupture of persistent ectopic pregnancy is the most catastrophic form of primary therapy failure. Its incidence is not known for certain, but Graczykowski and Seifer (1999) estimate it to be about 25 percent. Lipscomb and associates (1998) described a 14-day mean time to rupture, but one woman had tubal rupture 32 days after single-dose methotrexate therapy.

Reproductive outcomes after treatment for persistent ectopic pregnancy were reviewed by Seifer and colleagues (1994). At 36-month follow-up, 60 percent of 32 women trying had a successful uterine pregnancy. There were no recurrent ectopic pregnancies reported. These data are comparable to those shown in Table 34–6 for successes following primary medical or surgical therapy.

OTHER TREATMENTS

ACTINOMYCIN. Neary and Rose (1995) reported that a 5-day course of intravenous *actinomycin* resulted in complete resolution of an ectopic pregnancy in a woman who had failed methotrexate therapy. Fishman and associates (1998) reported successful treatment of a diaphragmatic pregnancy with thorascopic excision and actinomycin chemotherapy.

DIRECT INJECTION. A number of cytotoxic drugs have been injected directly into the ectopic mass, either by laparoscopy or transvaginally by culdocentesis. Treatment with methotrexate by salpingocentesis usually is a single 50-mg injection, but as little as 5 mg has been used successfully (Fernandez and colleagues, 1995). Natofsky and associates (1999) reviewed 406 ectopic pregnancies treated by salpingocentesis. In the majority, methotrexate was injected and the success rate was 81 percent. This is much lower than the 93 percent success rate with either conservative surgery or variable-dose methotrexate as determined by Pisarska and colleagues (1998).

Paulsson and colleagues (1995) reported their results of laparoscopic injection of **prostaglandin F$_{2\alpha}$** into 127 ectopic pregnancies. While 85 to 90 percent effective, prostaglandin therapy caused cardiac arrhythmias, transient hypertension, pulmonary edema, and atrioventricular block.

Tubal pregnancy injection with **hyperosmolar glucose** has also been reported to be successful for unruptured ectopic pregnancies (Yeko and associates, 1995).

Because of the much lower success rate and side effects with direct injection, coupled with the need for laparoscopic guidance, these techniques are not used widely.

EXPECTANT MANAGEMENT. Some practitioners choose to observe very early tubal pregnancies that are associated with stable or falling serum β-hCG levels. As many as a third of women with ectopic pregnancies will present with declining β-hCG levels (Shalev and colleagues, 1995). Stovall and Ling (1992) restrict this to women with these criteria:

1. Decreasing serial β-hCG levels.
2. Tubal pregnancies only.
3. No evidence of intraabdominal bleeding or rupture using vaginal sonography.
4. Diameter of the ectopic mass not greater than 3.5 cm.

Trio and colleagues (1995) reported spontaneous resolution of ectopic pregnancy in 49 of 67 women (73 percent) treated expectantly. This was more likely if the initial serum β-hCG level was less than 1000 mIU/mL. In a study of 60 women observed initially with expectant management, Shalev and associates (1995) reported spontaneous resolution in 28 women (48 percent).

ANTI-D IMMUNE GLOBULIN. If the woman is D-negative but not yet sensitized to D-antigen, then anti-D immunoglobulin should be administered.

ABDOMINAL PREGNANCY

Almost all cases of abdominal pregnancy follow early rupture or abortion of a tubal pregnancy into the peritoneal cavity. Primary peritoneal implantation of the fertilized ovum is very rare, and six well-documented cases have been reported (Thomas and co-workers, 1991a). The Centers for Disease Control estimated that the incidence of abdominal pregnancy is 1 in 10,000 live births (Atrash and co-workers, 1987). At Parkland Hospital, where ectopic pregnancy is common, advanced abdominal pregnancy is rare and encountered in perhaps 1 in 25,000 births.

Typically, the growing placenta, after penetrating the oviduct wall, maintains its tubal attachment but gradually encroaches upon and implants in the neighboring serosa. Meanwhile, the fetus continues to grow within the peritoneal cavity. Occasionally, the placenta is found in the general region of the oviduct and over the posterior aspect of the broad ligament and uterus (Fig. 34–10). In other cases, after tubal rupture, the conceptus reimplants elsewhere in the peritoneal cavity. In some cases a prior cesarean incision will rupture early in pregnancy to give rise to a pregnancy under the vesicouterine peritoneal fold (Marcus and colleagues, 1999). We recently encountered a woman whose pregnancy

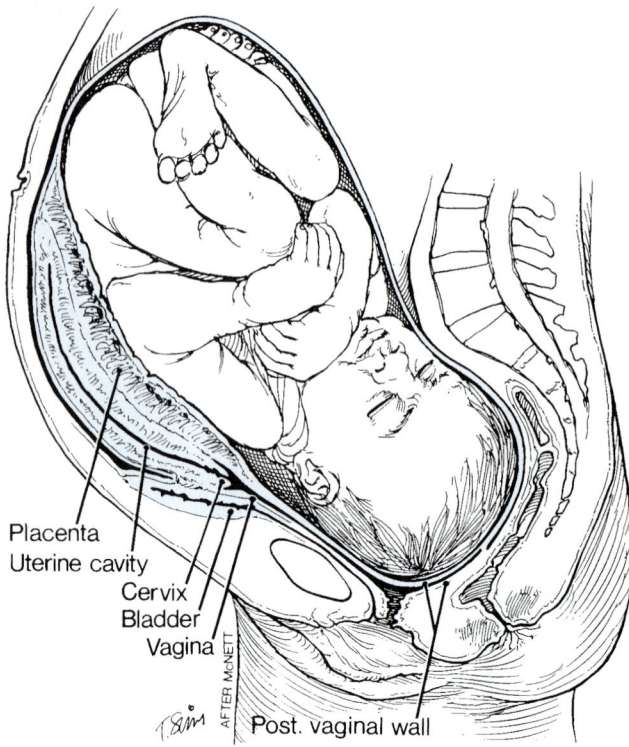

Placenta
Uterine cavity
Cervix
Bladder
Vagina
AFTER McNETT
Post. vaginal wall

FIGURE 34–10. Abdominal pregnancy at term. Placenta is implanted on posterior wall of uterus and broad ligament. The enlarged, flattened uterus is located just beneath the anterior abdominal wall. Cervix and vagina are dislodged anteriorly and superiorly by the large fetal head in the cul-de-sac.

had ruptured through a prior vertical cesarean incision at some point remote from delivery. The placenta remained implanted in the lower uterine segment and repeat cesarean delivery near term disclosed the abdominal pregnancy with the healthy fetus outside of the uterus.

The incidence of abdominal pregnancy is increased after gamete intrafallopian transfer, in vitro fertilization, and induced abortion (Ferland and associates, 1991; Pisarska and Carson, 1999). Endometriosis, tuberculosis, and intrauterine devices may also contribute to an increased incidence (Børlum and Blom, 1988; Durukan and co-workers, 1990).

FETAL OUTCOME. Fetal salvage in an abdominal pregnancy is exceedingly precarious, and the great majority succumb. In a world literature review, Ware (1948) cited a perinatal loss of 75 percent, but this figure may have been falsely low because of the tendency to report cases with good outcomes. Some authors report an incidence of a malformed fetus as high as 50 percent. In his extensive review of abdominal pregnancies since the year 1809, Stevens (1993) found that survival of infants born after 30 weeks was 63 percent. Moreover, fetal malfor-

mations and deformations were only 20 percent. The most common deformations were facial and/or cranial asymmetry and various joint abnormalities. The most common malformations were limb deficiency and central nervous system malformations. Even the lack of amnionic fluid surrounding the fetus is not always associated with fetal lung hypoplasia (Dubinsky and colleagues, 1994).

Some clinicians await fetal viability with in-hospital expectant management if pregnancy is diagnosed after 24 weeks, (Cartwright and associates, 1986; Hage and colleagues, 1988). Such management carries a risk for sudden, life-threatening, intraabdominal bleeding. Because of this risk, termination of pregnacy is generally indicated when abdominal pregnancy is diagnosed. In cases where amnionic fluid volume is minimal or absent, and in cases less than 24 weeks, conservative treatment is rarely justified because fetal survival is extremely poor.

If the fetus dies after reaching a size too large to be resorbed, it may undergo suppuration, mummification, or calcification. Bacteria may gain access to the gestational products, particularly when they are adherent to intestine, resulting in suppuration. Eventually, the abscess ruptures, and if the woman does not die of peritonitis and septicemia, fetal parts may be extruded through the abdominal wall or more commonly into the intestine or bladder (Emembolu, 1989). Mummification and formation of a lithopedion occasionally ensue, and calcified products of conception may be carried for years. There are instances in which a period of 20 to 50 years elapsed before removal of a lithopedion at operation or autopsy. Much more rarely, the fetus is converted into a yellowish, greasy mass to which the term adipocere is applied. The various bizarre terminations of abdominal pregnancy have been discussed, with illustrative cases graphically described by King (1954).

DIAGNOSIS. Because early rupture or abortion of a tubal pregnancy is the usual antecedent of an abdominal pregnancy, in retrospect, a suggestive history can usually be obtained. Abnormalities likely to be recalled include spotting or irregular bleeding along with abdominal pain that usually was most prominent in one or both lower quadrants. Costa and associates (1991) presented an excellent and extensive review of this subject.

Women with an abdominal pregnancy are likely to be uncomfortable but not sufficiently so to warrant thorough evaluation. Nausea, vomiting, flatulence, constipation, diarrhea, and abdominal pain may each be present in varying degrees. Multiparas may state that the pregnancy does not "feel right." Late in pregnancy, fetal movements may cause pain.

Abnormal fetal positions can frequently be palpated, but the ease of palpating fetal parts is not a reliable sign. Fetal parts sometimes feel exceedingly close to the examining fingers even in normal pregnancies, especially in thin, multiparous women. Abdominal massage over the pregnancy does not stimulate the mass to contract as it almost always does with advanced intrauterine pregnancy. As depicted in Figure 34–10, the cervix is usually displaced, depending in part on the fetal position, and it may dilate but appreciable effacement is unusual. The uterus may be outlined over the lower part of the pregnancy mass. Small parts or the fetal head may occasionally be palpated through the fornices and identified as clearly outside the uterus.

LABORATORY TESTS. An unexplained transient anemia early in pregnancy may accompany the initial tubal rupture or abortion. Almost all other laboratory values, including those reflecting fetal well-being, are normal until fetal demise occurs. An otherwise unexplained increase in serum alpha-fetoprotein value suggests the possibility of abdominal pregnancy (Bombard, 1994; Costa, 1991; el Kareh, 1993; Jackson, 1993, and their associates). Interestingly, despite two elevated maternal serum alpha-fetoprotein values, amnionic fluid alpha-fetoprotein was normal in the abdominal pregnancy reported by Jackson and colleagues (1993). Doppler waveform analyses also have been reported to be normal in abdominal gestations (Hage and co-workers, 1988; Kirkinen and colleagues, 1988).

OXYTOCIN STIMULATION. Cross and co-workers (1951) emphasized that oxytocin stimulation could be a valuable aid to diagnose abdominal pregnancy. If no uterine activity is detected using a sensitive strain gauge applied over the products of conception while oxytocin is infused, the diagnosis of extrauterine pregnancy may be suspected. Hertz and co-workers (1977) could detect no uterine activity while infusing oxytocin in excess of 50 mU/min because the empty uterus was posterior to the fetus. If the uterus were anterior, as in Figure 34–10, it might contract in response to oxytocin and possibly lead to the false diagnosis of intrauterine pregnancy.

Orr and associates (1979) reported that before the diagnosis of an abdominal pregnancy was made, the uterus contracted in response to oxytocin, and an oxytocin challenge test was interpreted as negative on two occasions. Nonstress testing has been normal in most series, and as noted earlier, contraction stress testing may lead to varying results depending upon placental location (Costa and associates, 1991).

SONOGRAPHY. Ultrasonic findings with an abdominal pregnancy most often do not allow an unequivocal diagnosis to be made. In some suspected cases, however, these findings may be diagnostic. For example, if the fetal head is seen to lie immediately adjacent to the maternal bladder with no interposed uterine tissue, a specific diagnosis can be made (Kurtz and associates, 1982). Even with ideal conditions, however, a sonographic diagnosis of abdominal pregnancy is missed in half of cases (Costa and associates, 1991).

Akhan and colleagues (1990) reported the following sonographic criteria to be suggestive of abdominal pregnancy:

1. Visualization of the fetus separate from the uterus.
2. Failure to visualize uterine wall between the fetus and urinary bladder.
3. Close approximation of fetal parts to the maternal abdominal wall.
4. Eccentric position (relation of fetus to uterus) or abnormal fetal attitude (relation of fetal parts to one another) and visualization of extrauterine placental tissue.

The consensus is that sonography is not a definitive diagnostic procedure for abdominal pregnancy (Angtuaco and colleagues, 1994; Sherer and associates, 1994).

MAGNETIC RESONANCE IMAGING. This technique has been used to confirm abdominal pregnancy following a suspicious sonographic examination. The technique appears to be very accurate and specific (Harris and associates, 1988; Wagner and Burchardt, 1995). Even so, in our institutions, abdominal pregnancy has been incorrectly diagnosed as a placenta previa, and an intrauterine pregnancy with degenerating fibroids has been misdiagnosed as an abdominal pregnancy.

COMPUTED TOMOGRAPHY. Costa and associates (1991) maintain that computed tomography is superior to magnetic resonance imaging, but its use is limited because of the concern for fetal radiation. In cases of fetal demise, computed tomography may be diagnostic and should be considered (Glew and Sivanesaratnam, 1989).

TREATMENT. Surgery for abdominal pregnancy may precipitate torrential hemorrhage, and it is essential to have adequate blood immediately available. Preoperatively, two intravenous infusion systems, each capable of delivering large volumes of fluid at a rapid rate, should be functioning. Techniques for monitoring the adequacy of the circulation should be employed, as described in Chapter 25 (p. 652). Whenever time allows, a mechanical bowel preparation should be done.

The massive hemorrhage that often ensues with surgery for abdominal pregnancy is related to the lack of constriction of hypertrophied opened blood vessels after placental separation. Partial placental separation occasionally occurs spontaneously and mandates laparotomy. Even if the fetus has been dead for several weeks, bleeding may still be torrential.

MANAGEMENT OF THE PLACENTA. Because placental removal always carries the risk of hemorrhage, blood vessels supplying the placenta should be ligated before its removal. Partial separation can develop spontaneously or, more likely, in the course of the operation while attempting to locate the exact site of placental attachment. Therefore, it is best to avoid unnecessary exploration of surrounding organs. In general, the infant should be delivered, the cord severed close to the placenta, and the abdomen closed.

Unfortunately, if left in the abdominal cavity, the placenta commonly causes infection, abscesses, adhesions, intestinal obstruction, and wound dehiscence (Bergstrom and colleagues, 1998; Martin and associates, 1988). Reversible maternal hydronephrosis may also develop (Weiss and Stone, 1994). Piering and colleagues (1993) described persistent preeclampsia for 99 postpartum days until the placenta was removed! The woman was normotensive before pregnancy and again after placental removal. Although the complications of leaving the placenta are troublesome and usually lead to subsequent laparotomy, they may be less grave than the hemorrhage that sometimes results from placental removal during initial surgery.

If the placenta is left, its involution may be monitored using ultrasound and a variety of placental hormones. Serum β-hCG levels have been shown to be accurate (France and Jackson, 1980; Martin and associates, 1990). In many cases, placental function rapidly declines, and the placenta is resorbed. In a case described by Belfar and associates (1986), placental resorption took over 5 years! Methotrexate use is controversial. It has been recommended to hasten involution but may cause accelerated placental destruction with accumulation of necrotic tissue and infection with abscess formation (Rahman and associates, 1982).

ARTERIAL EMBOLIZATION. Percutaneous femoral artery catheterization and pelvic angiography, followed by embolization of specific bleeding sites is discussed in Chapter 25 (p. 646). This technique has been lifesaving in instances of massive pelvic hemorrhage (Kivikoski and associates, 1988; Martin and colleagues, 1990). Kerr and associates (1993) advocate preoperative transcatheter embolization followed by surgical intervention.

MATERNAL PROGNOSIS. Maternal mortality is increased substantively compared with normal pregnancy. With appropriate preoperative planning, however, maternal mortality has been reduced from approximately 20 percent to less than 5 percent in the past 20 years (Stevens, 1993). Morbidity in surviving women is excessive in many cases (Costa and colleagues, 1991; Martin and associates, 1988; Martin and McCall, 1990).

OVARIAN PREGNANCY

Ectopic pregnancy implanted in the ovary is rare. In 1878, Spiegelberg formulated criteria for diagnosis of ovarian pregnancy:

1. The tube on the affected side must be intact.
2. The fetal sac must occupy the position of the ovary.
3. The ovary must be connected to the uterus by the ovarian ligament.
4. Definite ovarian tissue must be found in the sac wall.

Bobrow and Winkelstein (1956) reviewed 154 cases that satisfied these criteria. Hallatt (1982) described 25 cases of primary ovarian pregnancy, and Grimes and co-workers (1983) reported 24 more.

Traditional risk factors for tubal pregnancy are similar for ovarian ectopic pregnancy. Concurrent use of an intrauterine contraceptive device seems to be inordinately associated with ovarian pregnancy (Golan and associates, 1991; Pisarska and Carson, 1999). Gray and Ruffolo (1978) described four instances of ovarian pregnancy in which the women conceived with a copper-7 device in situ.

Although the ovary can accommodate itself more readily than the tube to the expanding pregnancy, rupture at an early period is the usual consequence. Nonetheless, there are recorded cases in which ovarian pregnancy went to term, and a few infants survived. Williams and associates (1982), while attempting a cesarean delivery because of a fetal transverse lie at 41 weeks, found an ovarian pregnancy. The infant, who weighed about 3500 g, survived. The ovary, placenta, and membranes were resected, and the severed right ureter was reimplanted in the bladder. Belfar and colleagues (1991) reported ultrasound diagnosis in a case where the infant survived.

DIAGNOSIS. Findings are likely to mimic those of a tubal pregnancy or a bleeding corpus luteum. Serious bleeding is seen in about a third of cases. At surgery, early ovarian pregnancies are likely to be considered corpus luteum cysts or a bleeding corpus luteum. The increased use of vaginal ultrasound has resulted in the more frequent diagnosis of unruptured ovarian pregnancies (Marcus and Brinsden, 1993; Sidek and colleagues, 1994). Early diagnosis of an intact ovarian pregnancy allows for a medical approach.

MANAGEMENT. The classical management for ovarian pregnancies has been surgical. Early bleeding for small lesions has been managed by ovarian wedge resection or cystectomy (Schwartz and colleagues, 1993). In the presence of larger lesions, ovariectomy is most often performed. Recently, laparoscopy has been used to resect or to perform laser ablation of ovarian pregnancies (Carter and colleagues, 1993; Goldenberg and associates, 1994). Finally, methotrexate has been used successfully to treat unruptured ovarian pregnancies (Chelmow, 1994; Raziel, 1993; Shamma, 1992, and their associates).

CERVICAL PREGNANCY

In the past, cervical pregnancy was a rare form of ectopic gestation. Dees (1966) estimated the incidence to be 1 in 18,000 pregnancies. In our experience, it is even less common. The incidence is increasing, again in part due to assisted reproduction, but especially after in vitro fertilization and embryo transfer (Ginsburg, 1994; Pattinson, 1994; Peleg, 1994, and their associates). According to Pisarska and Carson (1999), prior dilatation and curettage precedes 70 percent of cases.

In a typical case, the endocervix is eroded by trophoblast, and the pregnancy proceeds to develop in the fibrous cervical wall (Fig. 34–11). The duration of preg-

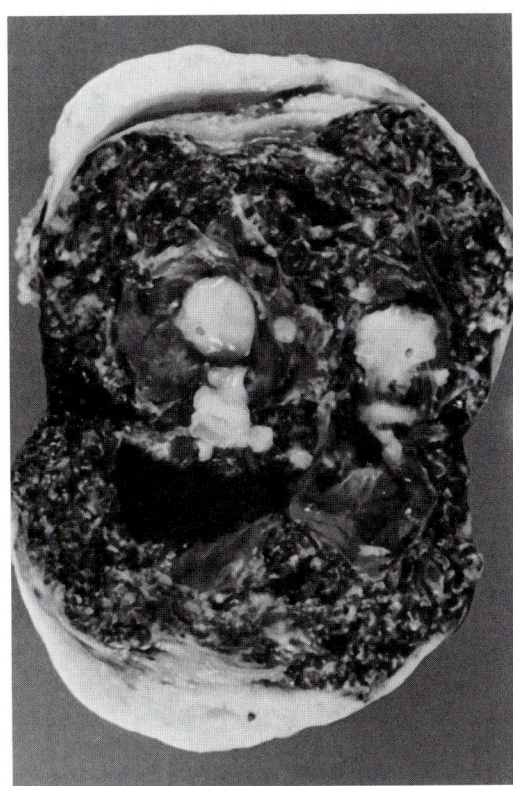

FIGURE 34–11. Cervical pregnancy in situ removed by hysterectomy nearly 3 months after last normal menstrual period and 1 month after onset of vaginal bleeding. (Courtesy of Drs. D. Rubell and A. Brekken.)

nancy is dependent upon the site of embryo implantation. The higher it is implanted in the cervical canal, the greater is its capacity to grow and cause hemorrhage.

Painless vaginal bleeding is present in 90 percent of cervical pregnancies, and a third of these have massive hemorrhage (Ushakov and colleagues, 1996). Only a fourth had abdominal pain with bleeding. As pregnancy progresses, a distended, thin-walled cervix with the external os partially dilated may be evident. Above the cervical mass, a slightly enlarged uterine fundus may be palpated. Gabbe and co-workers (1975) reported two women with high fever that initially was attributed to septic abortion. Cervical pregnancy rarely goes beyond 20 weeks, and usually is surgically terminated because of bleeding. A case of cervical-isthmic pregnancy has been reported to advance to term (Jelsema and Zuidema, 1992).

Thus, identification of cervical pregnancy is based upon a high degree of clinical suspicion confirmed with sonography (Frates and colleagues, 1994; Kligman and associates, 1995). Sonographic findings include an empty uterus and a gestation filling the cervical canal (Fig. 34–12). If any doubt remains, magnetic resonance imaging most often confirms the diagnosis, as shown in Figure 34–13 (Bader-Armstrong and associates, 1989; Rafal and co-workers, 1990). We have used color Doppler to determine extent of the implantation.

Rubin and co-workers (1983) have described pathological criteria that establish the diagnosis of cervical pregnancy:

1. Cervical glands must be present opposite placental attachment.
2. Attachment of placenta to cervix must be intimate.
3. The placenta must be below the entrance of uterine vessels or below the peritoneal reflection on the anteroposterior uterine surfaces.
4. Fetal elements must not be present in the uterine corpus.

SURGICAL MANAGEMENT. In the past, hysterectomy was often the only choice available because of profuse hemorrhage that accompanied attempts at removal of the cervical pregnancy. Even with hysterectomy, hemorrhage was excessive, and urinary tract injury frequent due to the enlarged barrel-shaped cervix.

CERCLAGE. Bernstein and associates (1981) and Bachus and colleagues (1990) successfully managed cervical pregnancy by placing a heavy silk ligature around the cervix similar to a McDonald cerclage (see Chap. 27, p. 713). We do not recommend this.

FOLEY CATHETER. Nolan and associates (1989) and Thomas and co-workers (1991b) recommend placement

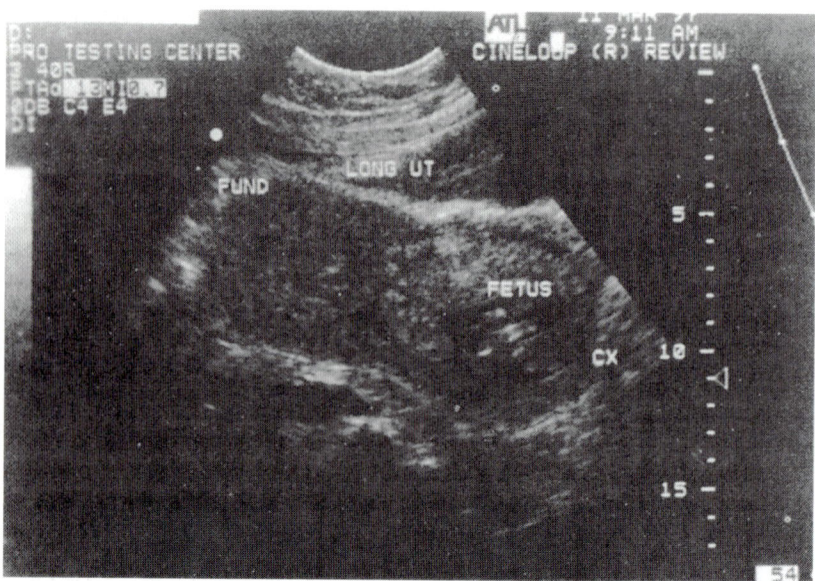

FIGURE 34–12. Sonogram showing longitudinal view of 11-week cervical pregnancy. (From Eblen and colleagues, 1999, with permission.)

of hemostatic cervical sutures at 3 and 9 o'clock. Suction curettage is then performed, followed immediately by insertion of a Foley catheter into the cervical canal. The 30-mL catheter bulb is inflated, and the vagina is packed tightly with gauze to further tamponade bleeding. A suction catheter tip may be left above the vaginal packing to ensure adequate drainage and to monitor blood loss.

ARTERIAL EMBOLIZATION. Lobel and colleagues (1990), Saliken and co-workers (1994), and others have

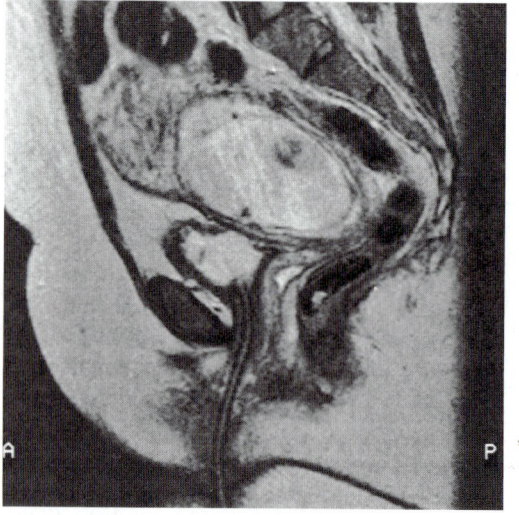

FIGURE 34–13. Magnetic resonance imaging showing a cervical ectopic pregnancy of 12 weeks' gestation. The uterus is above the pregnancy, which is ovoid in shape. The placenta and fetus are seen with amnionic fluid. There is a Foley catheter in the bladder. (Courtesy of Dr. Diane Twickler.)

reported success with selective preoperative uterine artery embolization using Gelfoam (see Chap. 25, p. 646).

MEDICAL MANAGEMENT. To avoid the risks of uncontrolled hemorrhage, methotrexate and other drug treatments have been successfully used. Currently, surgical techniques are generally used only when chemotherapy fails or in emergency situations when a woman, usually undiagnosed, presents with life-threatening acute hemorrhage (Wolcott and associates, 1988).

The general rules for methotrexate use were described earlier in the chapter (p. 897). The drug has been injected directly into the gestational sac with or without potassium chloride to induce fetal death; it has been given systemically in single high-dose therapy with folinic acid rescue; it has been given in lower-dose prolonged courses; it has been given as a single low-dose regimen; and finally, it has been given in various combinations, usually intra-amnionically after failure of systemic therapy (Dotters, 1995; Kaplan, 1990; Marcovici, 1994; Roussis, 1992; Timor-Tritsch, 1994, and their colleagues). Pregnancies of greater than 6 weeks' duration generally require induction of fetal death (usually with potassium chloride) or high-dose and prolonged methotrexate therapy. Kung and Chang (1999) reviewed 62 cases treated with methotrexate. Women in whom the fetus was alive (35 cases) had a higher failure rate with single-dose methotrexate. Almost 45 percent of these needed a surgical procedure compared with 4 percent in the group without a live fetus.

Brand and associates (1993) reported the successful treatment of a cervical pregnancy using actinomycin D. This is a logical approach, but confirmation is necessary before recommending this agent. Segna and colleagues (1990) reported successful treatment of a 6-week cervical pregnancy with etoposide, which is a semisynthetic derivative of podophyllotoxin.

OTHER SITES OF ECTOPIC PREGNANCY

Primary **splenic pregnancy** was reported by Mankodi and associates (1977). Findings that led to laparotomy included epigastric and left shoulder pain, hypotension, tachycardia, syncope, and pelvic tenderness. A rent in the hilar surface of the spleen prompted splenectomy and chorionic villi were identified microscopically. A similar case was reported by Yackel and associates (1988). A few cases of primary **hepatic pregnancy** have been described, including one with lithopedion formation (Børlum and Blom, 1988; De Almeida Barbosa and associates, 1991; Schlatter and colleagues, 1988). An upper **retroperitoneal pregnancy** was reported by Ferland and associates (1991) after in vitro fertilization and embryo transfer. Finally, Fishman and co-workers (1998) described implantation of a 6-week **diaphragmatic pregnancy** in a women with abdominal and shoulder pain, dyspnea, and a hemothorax.

REFERENCES

Akhan O, Cekirge S, Senaati S, Besim A: Sonographic diagnosis of an abdominal ectopic pregnancy. Am J Radiol 155:197, 1990

American College of Obstetricians and Gynecologists: Medical management of tubal pregnancy. ACOG Practice Bulletin No. 3, December, 1998

Angtuaco TL, Shah HR, Neal MR, Quirk JG: Ultrasound evaluation of abdominal pregnancy (review). Crit Rev Diagn Imaging 35:1, 1994

Ankum WW, Mol BWJ, Van der Veen F, Bossuyt PMM: Risk factors for ectopic pregnancy: A meta-analysis. Fertil Steril 65:1093, 1996

Arias-Stella J: Atypical endometrial changes associated with the presence of chorionic tissue. Arch Pathol 58:112, 1954

Atrash HK, Friede A, Hogue CJR: Abdominal pregnancy in the United States: Frequency and maternal mortality. Obstet Gynecol 69:333, 1987

Bachus KE, Stone D, Suh B, Thickman D: Conservative management of cervical pregnancy with subsequent fertility. Am J Obstet Gynecol 162:450, 1990

Bader-Armstrong B, Shah Y, Rubens D: Use of ultrasound and magnetic resonance imaging in the diagnosis of cervical pregnancy. J Clin Ultrasound 17:283, 1989

Balmaceda JP, Bernardini L, Asch RH, Stone SC: Early primary abdominal pregnancy after in vitro fertilization and embryo transfer. J Assist Reprod Genet 10:317, 1993

Barnhart K, Mennuti MT, Benjamin I, Jacobson S, Goodman D, Coutifaris C: Prompt diagnosis of ectopic pregnancy in an emergency department setting. Obstet Gynecol 84:1010, 1994

Batzer FR, Weiner S, Corson SL, Schlaff S, Otis C: Landmarks during the first forty-two days of gestation demonstrated by the β-subunit of human chorionic gonadotropin and ultrasound. Am J Obstet Gynecol 146:973, 1983

Bayati J, Garcia JE, Dorsey JH, Padilla SL: Combined intrauterine and cervical pregnancy from in vitro fertilization and embryo transfer. Fertil Steril 51:725, 1989

Belfar H, Heller K, Edelston DI, Hill LM, Martin JG: Ovarian pregnancy resulting in a surviving neonate. Ultrasound findings. J Ultrasound Med 10:465, 1991

Belfar HL, Kurtz AB, Wapner RJ: Long-term follow-up after removal of an abdominal pregnancy: Ultrasound evaluation of the involuting placenta. J Ultrasound Med 5:521, 1986

Bennett S, Waterstone J, Parsons J, Creighton S: Two cases of cervical pregnancy following in vitro fertilization and embryo transfer to the lower uterine cavity. J Assist Repord Genet 10:100, 1993

Bergstrom R, Mueller G, Yankowitz J: A case illustrating the continued dilemmas in treating abdominal pregnancy and a potential explanation for the high rate of postsurgical febrile morbidity. Gynecol Obstet Invest 46:268, 1998

Berliner I, Mesbah M, Zalud I, Maulik D: Heterotopic triplet pregnancy. Report of a case with successful twin intrauterine gestation. J Reprod Med 43:237, 1998

Bernstein D, Holzinger M, Ovadia J, Frishman B: Conservative treatment of cervical pregnancy. Obstet Gynecol 58:741, 1981

Bjartling C, Osser S, Persson K: The frequency of salpingitis and ectopic pregnancy as epidemiologic markers of *Chlamydia trachomatis*. Acta Obstet Gynecol Scand 79:123, 2000

Bobrow ML, Winkelstein LB: Intrafollicular ovarian pregnancy. Am J Surg 91:991, 1956

Bombard AT, Nakagawa S, Runowicz CD, Cohen BL, Mikhail MS, Nitowsky HM: Early detection of abdominal pregnancy by maternal serum AFP+ screening. Prenat Diagn 14:1155, 1994

Børlum KG, Blom R: Primary hepatic pregnancy. Int J Gynecol Obstet 27:427, 1988

Botta G, Fortunato N, Merlino G: Heterotopic pregnancy following administration of human menopausal gonadotropin and following in vitro fertilization and embryo transfer: Two case reports and review of the literature. Eur J Obstet Gynecol Reprod Biol 59:211, 1995

Brand E, Gibbs RS, Davidson SA: Advanced cervical pregnancy treated with actinomycin-D. Br J Obstet Gynaecol 100:491, 1993

Brunham RC, Pelling R, Maclean I, Kosseim ML, Paraskevas M: *Chlamydia trachomatis*–associated ectopic pregnancy: Serologic and histologic correlates. J Infect Dis 165:1076, 1992

Buster JE, Pisarska MD: Medical management of ectopic pregnancy. Clin Obstet Gynecol 42:23, 1999

Cacciatore B, Stenman UH, Ylöstalo P: Diagnosis of ectopic pregnancy by vaginal ultrasonography in combination with a discriminatory serum hCG level of 1000 IU/1 (IRP). Br J Obstet Gynaecol 97:904, 1990

Carter JE, Ekuan J, Kallins GJ: Laparoscopic diagnosis and excision of an intact ovarian pregnancy. A case report. J Reprod Med 38:962, 1993

Cartwright PS, Brown JE, Davis RJ, Thieme GA, Boehm FH: Advanced abdominal pregnancy associated with fetal pulmonary hypoplasia: Report of a case. Am J Obstet Gynecol 155:396, 1986

Centers for Disease Control: Ectopic-pregnancy—United States, 1984 and 1985. MMWR 37:637, 1988

Centers for Disease Control and Prevention: Ectopic pregnancy—United States, 1990–1992. MMWR 1:46, 1995

Centers for Disease Control and Prevention: Sexually transmitted disease surveillance, 1998. Atlanta, GA, September, 1999

Chao KH, Shyu MK, Juang GT, Hsieh FJ, Chen HY: Methotrexate treatment for cervical pregnancy: Experience of four cases. J Formos Med Assoc 92:426, 1993

Chelmow D, Gates E, Penzias AS: Laparoscopic diagnosis and methotrexate treatment of an ovarian pregnancy: A case report. Fertil Steril 62:879, 1994

Chen CD, Chen SU, Chao KH, Wu MY, Ho HN, Yang YS: Cornual pregnancy after IVF-ET. A report of three cases. J Reprod Med 43:393, 1998

Coleman BG, Baron RL, Arger PH, Arenson RL, Axel L, Mayer DP, Costello P: Ectopic embryo detection using real-time sonography. J Clin Ultrasound 13:545, 1985

Costa SD, Presley J, Bastert G: Advanced abdominal pregnancy. Obstet Gynecol Surv 46:515, 1991

Coste J, Job-Spira N, Fernandez H, Papiernik E, Spira A: Risk factors for ectopic pregnancy: A case-control study in France, with special focus on infectious factors. Am J Epidemiol 133:839, 1991

Creinin MD, Krohn MA: Methotrexate pharmacokinetics and effects in women receiving methotrexate 50 mg and 60 mg per square meter for early abortion. Am J Obstet Gynecol 177:1444, 1997

Cross JB, Lester WM, McCain J: The diagnosis and management of abdominal pregnancy with a review of 19 cases. Am J Obstet Gynecol 63:303, 1951

Daus K, Mundy D, Graves W, Slade BA: Ectopic pregnancy. What to do during the 20-day window. J Reprod Med 34:162, 1989

De Almeida Barbosa A, Rodrigues de Freitas LA, Andrade Mota M: Primary pregnancy in the liver: A case report. Path Res Pract 187:329, 1991

DeCherney AH: Case records of the Massachusetts General Hospital. Case 3-1996. N Engl J Med 334:255, 1996

Dees HC: Cervical pregnancy associated with uterine leiomyomas. South Med J 59:900, 1966

DeMuylder X, DeLoecker P, Campo R: Heterotopic ovarian pregnancy after clomiphene ovulation induction. Eur J Obstet Gynecol Reprod Biol 53:65, 1994

Dimitry ES, Subak-Sharpe R, Mills M, Margara R, Winston R: Nine cases of heterotopic pregnancies in 4 years of in vitro fertilization. Fertil Steril 53:107, 1990

Dorfman SF, Grimes DA, Cates W Jr, Binkin NJ, Kafrissen ME, O'Reilly KR: Ectopic pregnancy mortality, United States, 1979 to 1980: Clinical aspects. Obstet Gynecol 64:386, 1984

Dotters DJ, Katz VL, Kuller JA, McCoy MC: Successful treatment of a cervical pregnancy with a single low dose methotrexate regimen. Eur J Obstet Gynecol Reprod Biol 60:187, 1995

Dubinsky TJ, Guella F, Ivankovic M, Robert A, Gonzalez P, Espinoza R, Gormaz G: Normal pulmonary development in two anhydramniotic abdominal pregnancies. J Ultrasound Med 13:412, 1994

Durukan T, Urman B, Yarali H, Arikan Õ, Beykal Ö: An abdominal pregnancy 10 years after treatment for pelvic tuberculosis. Am J Obstet Gynecol 163:594, 1990

Eblen AC, Pridham DD, Tatum CM: Conservative management of an 11-week cervical pregnancy. J Reprod Med 44:61, 1999

El Kareh A, Beddoe AM, Brown BL: Advanced abdominal pregnancy complicated by bilateral ureteral obstruction. A case report. J Reprod Med 38:900, 1993

Emembolu JO: Celo-intestinal fistulae complicating advanced extra-uterine pregnancy. Int J Gynecol Obstet 28:177, 1989

Emerson DS, Cartier MS, Altieri LA, Felker RE, Smith WC, Stovall TG, Gray LA: Diagnostic efficacy of endovaginal color doppler flow imaging in an ectopic pregnancy screening program. Radiology 183:413, 1992

Ferland RJ, Chadwick DA, O'Brien JA, Granai CO III: An ectopic pregnancy in the upper retroperitoneum following in vitro fertilization and embryo transfer. Obstet Gynecol 78:544, 1991

Fernandez H, Pauthier S, Doumerc S, Lelaidier C, Olivennes F, Ville Y, Frydman R: Ultrasound-guided injection of methotrexate versus laparoscopic salpingotomy in ectopic pregnancy. Fertil Steril 63:25, 1995

Fishman DA, Padilla LA, Joob A, Lurain JR: Ectopic pregnancy causing hemothorax managed by thoracoscopy and actinomycin D. Obstet Gynecol 91:837, 1998

France JT, Jackson P: Maternal plasma and urinary hormone levels during and after a successful abdominal pregnancy. Br J Obstet Gynaecol 87:356, 1980

Frates MC, Benson CB, Doubilet PM, DiSalvo DN, Brown DL, Laing FC, Rein MS, Osathanondh R: Cervical ectopic pregnancy: Results of conservative treatment. Radiology 191:773, 1994

Fujii S, Ban C, Okamura H, Nishimura T: Unilateral tubal quadruplet pregnancy. Am J Obstet Gynecol 141:840, 1981

Gabbe SG, Kitzmiller JL, Kosasa TS, Driscoll SG: Cervical pregnancy presenting as septic abortion. Am J Obstet Gynecol 123:212, 1975

Ginsburg ES, Frates MC, Rein MS, Fox JH, Hornstein MD, Friedman AJ: Early diagnosis and treatment of cervical pregnancy in an in vitro fertilization program. Fertil Steril 61:966, 1994

Glassner MJ, Aron E, Eskin BA: Ovulation induction with clomiphene and the rise in heterotopic pregnancies cases. J Reprod Med 35:175, 1990

Glew SS, Sivanesaratnam V: Advanced extrauterine pregnancy mimicking intrauterine fetal death: Case reports. Aust NZ J Obstet Gynecol 29:450, 1989

Golan A, Raziel A, Neuman M, Schneider D, Bukovsky I, Caspi E: Fertility before and after surgery for primary ovarian pregnancy. Fertil Steril 55:200, 1991

Goldenberg M, Bider D, Mashiach S, Raminovici J, Dulitzky M, Oelsner G: Laparoscopic laser surgery of primary ovarian pregnancy. Hum Reprod 9:1337, 1994

Goldner TE, Lawson HW, Xia Z, Atrash HK: Surveillance for ectopic pregnancy—United States, 1970–1989. MMWR 42:73, 1993

Graczykowski JW, Mishell DR Jr: Methotrexate prophylaxis for persistent ectopic pregnancy after conservative treatment by salpingostomy. Obstet Gynecol 89:118, 1997

Graczykowski JW, Seifer DB: Diagnosis of acute and persistent ectopic pregnancy. Clin Obstet Gynecol 42:9, 1999

Gray CL, Ruffolo EH: Ovarian pregnancy associated with intrauterine contraceptive devices. Am J Obstet Gynecol 132:134, 1978

Gray DT, Thorburn J, Lundorff P, Strandell A, Lindblom B: A cost-effectiveness study of a randomized trial of laparoscopy versus laparotomy for ectopic pregnancy. Lancet 345:1139, 1995

Grimes HG, Nosal RA, Gallagher JC: Ovarian pregnancy: A series of 24 cases. Obstet Gynecol 61:174, 1983

Guillaume AJ, Benjamin F, Sicuranza B, Deutsch S, Spitzer M: Luteal phase defects and ectopic pregnancy. Fertil Steril 3:30, 1995

Guirgis RR, Craft IL: Ectopic pregnancy resulting from gamete intrafallopian transfer and in vitro fertilization. Role of ultrasonography in diagnosis and treatment. J Reprod Med 36:793, 1991

Hage ML, Wall LL, Killam A: Expectant management of abdominal pregnancy. A report of two cases. J Reprod Med 33:407, 1988

Hahlin M, Wallin A, Sjoblom P, Lindblom B: Single progesterone assay for early recognition of abnormal pregnancy. Hum Reprod 5:662, 1990

Hajenius PG, Engelsbel B, Mol WJ, Van der Veen F, Ankum WM, Bossuy PMM, Hemrika DJ, Lammes FB: Randomized trial of systemic methotrexate versus laparoscopic salpingostomy in tubal pregnancy. Lancet 350:774, 1997

Hajenius PJ, Mol BWJ, Ankum WM, van der Veen F, Bossuyt PMM, Lammes FB: Clearance curves of serum human chorionic gonadotropin for the diagnosis of persistent trophoblast. Hum Reprod 10:682, 1995

Hallatt JG: Primary ovarian pregnancy: A report of 25 cases. Am J Obstet Gynecol 143:55, 1982

Harris MB, Angtuaco T, Frazier CN, Mattison DR: Diagnosis of a viable abdominal pregnancy by magnetic resonance imaging. Am J Obstet Gynecol 159:150, 1988

Hemminki E, Meriläinen J: Long-term effects of cesarean sections: Ectopic pregnancies and placental problems. Am J Obstet Gynecol 174:1569, 1996

Hendrix NW, Chauhan SP, Maier RC: Ectopic pregnancy in sterilized and non-sterilized women. A comparison. J Reprod Med 43:515, 1998

Hertz RH, Timor-Tritsch I, Sokol RJ, Zador I: Diagnostic studies and fetal assessment in advanced extrauterine pregnancy. Obstet Gynecol 50 (suppl):63, 1977

Hirose M, Nomura T, Wakuda K, Ishiguro T, Yoshida Y: Combined intrauterine and ovarian pregnancy: A case report. Asia Oceania J Obstet Gynaecol 20:25, 1994

Hirsch E, Cohen L, Hecht BR: Heterotopic pregnancy with discordant ultrasonic appearance of fetal cardiac activity. Obstet Gynecol 79:824, 1992

Isaacs JD, Cesare CD Sr, Cowan BD: Ectopic pregnancy following hysterectomy: An update for the 1990s. Obstet Gynecol 88:732, 1996

Jackson S, Hollingworth T, Macpherson M: Elevated serum alpha fetoprotein and normal liquor alpha fetoprotein values in association with an abdominal pregnancy. Aust NZ J Obstet Gynaecol 33:214, 1993

Jacobson L, Riemer RK, Goldfien AC, Lykins D, Siiteri PK, Roberts JM: Rabbit myometrial oxytocin and alpha 2-adrenergic receptors are increased by estrogen but are differentially regulated by progesterone. Endocrinology 120:184, 1987

Jelsema RD, Zuidema L: First-trimester diagnosed cervicoisthmic pregnancy resulting in term delivery. Obstet Gynecol 80:517, 1992

Kadar N, DeVore G, Romero R: The discriminatory hCG zone: Its use in the sonographic evaluation for ectopic pregnancy. Obstet Gynecol 58:156, 1981

Kadar N, Romero R: Observations on the log human chorionic gonadotropin-time relationship in early pregnancy and its practical implications. Am J Obstet Gynecol 157:73, 1987

Kalchman GG, Meltzer RM: Interstitial pregnancy following homolateral salpingectomy: Report of 2 cases and a review of the literature. Am J Obstet Gynecol 96:1139, 1966

Kaplan BR, Brandt T, Javaheri G, Scommegna A: Nonsurgical treatment of a viable cervical pregnancy with intra-amniotic methotrexate. Fertil Steril 53:941, 1990

Kendrick JS, Atrash HK, Strauss LT, Gargiullo PM, Ahn YW: Vaginal douching and the risk of ectopic pregnancy among black women. Am J Obstet Gynecol 176:991, 1997

Kerr A, Trambert J, Mikhail M, Hodges L, Runowicz C: Preoperative transcatheter embolization of abdominal pregnancy: Report of three cases. J Vasc Interv Radiol 4:733, 1993

King G: Advanced extrauterine pregnancy. Am J Obstet Gynecol 67:712, 1954

Kirkinen P, Lauper U, Huch R, Huch A: Case report. Normal placental function and fetoplacental blood circulation in advanced abdominal pregnancy. Acta Obstet Gynecol Scand 67:283, 1988

Kivikoski AI, Martin C, Weyman P, Picus D, Giudice L: Angiographic arterial embolization to control hemorrhage in abdominal pregnancy: A case report. Obstet Gynecol 71:456, 1988

Kligman I, Adachi TJ, Katz E, McClamrock HD, Jockle GA, Barakat B: Conserving fertility with early management of cervical pregnancy: A case report. J Reprod Med 40:743, 1995

Kooi S, Kock HC: A review of the literature on nonsurgical treatment in tubal pregnancy. Obstet Gynecol Surv 47:739, 1992

Koonin LM, Mackay AP, Berg CJ, Atrash HK, Smith JC: Pregnancy-related morality surveillance—United States, 1987–1990. MMWR 46:17, 1997

Kouyoumdjian A, Kirkpatrick J: Coexistence of an intrauterine pregnancy with both an ectopic pregnancy and salpingitis in the right fallopian tube: A case report. J Reprod Med 35:824, 1990

Kucera E, Schindl M, Klem I, Sam C, Hanzal E, Kölbl H, Leodolter S, Sliutz G: Could we treat more unruptured ectopic pregnancies with intramuscular methotrexate? Gynecol Obstet Invest 49:6, 2000

Kung FT, Chang SY: Efficacy of methotrexate treatment in viable and nonviable cervical pregnancies. Am J Obstet Gynecol 181:1438, 1999

Kurtz AB, Dubbins PA, Wapner RJ, Goldberg BB: Problem of abnormal fetal position. JAMA 247:3251, 1982

Lecuru F, Robin F, Chasset S, Leonard F, Guitti S, Taurelle R: Direct cost of single dose methotrexate for unruptured ectopic pregnancy. Prospective comparison with laparoscopy. Eur J Obstet Gynecol Reprod Biol 88:1, 2000

Lipscomb GH, Bran D, McCord ML, Portera C, Ling FW: Analysis of three hundred fifteen ectopic pregnancies treated with single-dose methotrexate. Am J Obstet Gynecol 178:1354, 1998

Lipscomb GH, McCord ML, Stovall TG, Huff, G, Portera SG, Ling FW: Predictors of success of methotrexate treatment in women with tubal ectopic pregnancies. N Engl J Med 341:1974, 1999a

Lipscomb GH, Puckett KJ, Bran D, Ling FW: Management of separation pain after single-dose methotrexate therapy for ectopic pregnancy. Obstet Gynecol 93:590, 1999b

Lipscomb GH, Stovall TG, Ling FW: Nonsurgical treatment of ectopic pregnancy. N Engl J Med 343:1325, 2000

Lobel SM, Meyerovitz MF, Benson CC, Goff B, Bengtson JM: Preoperative angiographic uterine artery embolization in the management of cervical pregnancy. Obstet Gynecol 76:938, 1990

Maccato M, Estrada R, Hammill H, Faro S: Prevalence of

active *Chlamydia trachomatis* infection at the time of exploratory laparotomy for ectopic pregnancy. Obstet Gynecol 79:211, 1992

Mankodi RC, Sankari K, Bhatt SM: Primary splenic pregnancy. Br J Obstet Gynaecol 84:634, 1977

Marcovici I, Rosenzweig BA, Brill AI, Khan M, Scommegna A: Cervical pregnancy: Case reports and a current literature review. Obstet Gynecol Surv 49:49, 1994

Marcus SF, Brinsden PR. Analysis of the incidence and risk factors associated with ectopic pregnancy following in vitro fertilization and embryo transfer. Hum Repro 10:199, 1995

Marcus SF, Brinsden PR: Primary ovarian pregnancy after in vitro fertilization and embryo transfer: Report of seven cases. Fertil Steril 60:167, 1993

Marcus S, Cheng E, Goff B: Extrauterine pregnancy resulting from early uterine rupture. Obstet Gynecol 94:804, 1999

Marcus SF, Macnamee M, Brinsden P: Heterotopic pregnancies after in-vitro fertilization and embryo transfer. Human Reprod 10:1232, 1995

Martin JN Jr, McCaul JF IV: Emergent management of abdominal pregnancy. Clin Obstet Gynecol 33:438, 1990

Martin JN Jr, Ridgway LE III, Connors JJ, Sessums JK, Martin RW, Morrison JC: Angiographic arterial embolization and computed tomography-directed drainage for the management of hemorrhage and infection with abdominal pregnancy. Obstet Gynecol 76:941, 1990

Martin JN Jr, Sessums JK, Martin RW, Pryor JA, Morrison JC: Abdominal pregnancy: Current concepts of management. Obstet Gynecol 71:549, 1988

McCord M, Muram D, Buster JE, Arheart KL, Stoval TG, Carson SA: Single serum progesterone as a screen for ectopic pregnancy: Exchanging specificity and sensitivity to obtain optimal test performance. Fertil Steril 66:513, 1996

Miyazaki Y: Nonsurgical therapy of ectopic pregnancy. Hokkaido Igaku Zasshi 58:132, 1983

Mol BWJ, Ankum WM, Bossuyt PMM, Van Der Veen F: Contraception and the risk of ectopic pregnancy: A meta-analysis. Contraception 52:337, 1995

Mol BWJ, Hajenius PJ, Engelsbel S, Ankum WM, Hemrika DJ, Van der Veen F, Bossuyt PMM: Treatment of tubal pregnancy in the Netherlands: an economic comparison of systemic methotrexate administration and laparoscopic salpingostomy. Am J Obstet Gynecol 181:945, 1999

Moon HS, Choi YJ, Park YH, Kim SG: New simple endoscopic operations for interstitial pregnancies. Am J Obstet Gynecol 182:114, 2000

Morlock RJ, Lafata JE, Eisenstein D: Cost-effectiveness of single-dose methotrexate compared with laparoscopic treatment of ectopic pregnancy. Obstet Gynecol 95:407, 2000

Morris JM, Van Wagenen G: Interception: The use of postovulatory estrogens to prevent implantation. Am J Obstet Gynecol 115:101, 1973

Natofsky JG, Lense J, Mayer JC, Yeko TR: Ultrasound-guided injection of ectopic pregnancy. Clin Obstet Gynecol 42:39, 1999

Neary BA, Rose PG: Complete response of a persistent ectopic pregnancy to dactinomycin after methotrexate failure: A case report. J Reprod Med 40:160, 1995

Nederlof KP, Lawson HW, Saftlas AF, Atrash HK, Finch EL: Ectopic pregnancy surveillance, United States, 1970–1987. MMWR 39 (suppl 4):9, 1990

Nolan TE, Chandler PE, Hess LW, Morrison JC: Cervical

pregnancy managed without hysterectomy. A case report. J Reprod Med 34:241, 1989

Nugent PJ: Ruptured ectopic pregnancy in a patient with a recent intrauterine abortion. Ann Emerg Med 21:5, 1992

Orr JW Jr, Huddleston JF, Knox GE, Goldenberg RL, Davis RO: False negative oxytocin challenge test associated with abdominal pregnancy. Am J Obstet Gynecol 133:108, 1979

Ory HW: The woman's health study: Ectopic pregnancy and intrauterine contraceptive devices: New perspectives. Obstet Gynecol 57:137, 1981

Ory SJ, Nnadi E, Herrmann R, O'Brien PS, Melton LJ 3rd: Fertility after ectopic pregnancy. Fertil Steril 60:231, 1993

Ory SJ, Villaneuva AL, Sand PK, Tamura RK: Conservative treatment of ectopic pregnancy with methotrexate. Am J Obstet Gynecol 154:1299, 1986

Pattinson HA, Dunphy BC, Wood S, Saliken J: Cervical pregnancy following in vitro fertilization: Evacuation after uterine artery embolization with subsequent successful intrauterine pregnancy. Aust NZ J Obstet Gynaecol 34:492, 1994

Paulsson G, Kvint S, Labecker BM, Lofstrand T, Lindblom B: Laparoscopic prostaglandin injection in ectopic pregnancy: Success rates according to endocrine activity. Fertil Steril 63:473, 1995

Peleg D, Bar-Hava I, Neuman-Levin M, Ashkenazi J, Ben-Rafael Z: Early diagnosis and successful nonsurgical treatment of viable combined intrauterine and cervical pregnancy. Fertil Steril 62:405, 1994

Pellerito JS, Taylor KJW, Quedens-Case C, Hammers LW, Scoutt LM, Ramos IM, Meyer WR: Ectopic pregnancy: Evaluation with endovaginal color flow imaging. Radiology 183:407, 1992

Phillips RS, Tuomala RE, Feldblum PJ, Schachter J, Rosenberg MJ, Aronson MD: The effect of cigarette smoking, *Chlamydia trachomatis* infection, and vaginal douching on ectopic pregnancy. Obstet Gynecol 79:85, 1992

Piering WF, Garancis JG, Becker CG, Beres JA, Lemann J Jr: Preeclampsia related to a functioning extrauterine placenta: Report of a case and 25-year follow-up. Am J Kidney Dis 21:310, 1993

Pisarska MD, Carson SA: Incidence and risk factors for ectopic pregnancy. Clin Obstet Gynecol 42:2, 1999

Pisarska MD, Carson SA, Buster JE: Ectopic pregnancy. Lancet 351:1115, 1998

Rafal RB, Kosovsky PA, Markisz JA: Case Report. MR appearance of cervical pregnancy. J Comput Assist Tomogr 14:482, 1990

Rahman MS, Al-Suleiman SA, Rahman J, Al-Sibai MH: Advanced abdominal pregnancy—observations in 10 cases. Obstet Gynecol 59:366, 1982

Raziel A, Golan A: Primary ovarian pregnancy successfully treated with methotrexate. Am J Obstet Gynecol 169:1362, 1993

Romero R, Kadar N, Castro D, Jeanty P, Hobbins JC, DeCherney AH: The value of adnexal sonographic findings in the diagnosis of ectopic pregnancy. Am J Obstet Gynecol 158:52, 1988

Romney SL, Hertig AT, Reid DE: The endometria associated with ectopic pregnancy. Surg Gynecol Obstet 91:605, 1950

Roussis P, Ball RH, Fleischer AC, Herbert CM III: Cervical pregnancy. A case report. J Reprod Med 37:479, 1992

Rubin GL, Peterson HB, Dorfman SF, Layde PM, Maze JM, Ory HW, Cates W Jr: Ectopic pregnancy in the United States: 1970 through 1978. JAMA 249:1725, 1983

Sadek AL, Schiotz HA: Transvaginal sonography in the management of ectopic pregnancy. Acta Obstet Gynecol Scand 74:293, 1995

Saliken JC, Normore WJ, Pattinson HA, Wood S: Embolization of the uterine arteries before termination of a 15-week cervical pregnancy. Can Assoc Radiol J 45:399, 1994

Saraiya M, Berg CJ, Kendrick JS, Strauss LT, Atrash HK, Ahn YW: Cigarette smoking as a risk factor for ectopic pregnancy. Am J Obstet Gynecol 178:493, 1998

Schlatter MC, DePree B, Vanderkolk KJ: Hepatic abdominal pregnancy: A case report. J Reprod Med 33:921, 1988

Schwartz LB, Carcangiu ML, DeCherney AH: Primary ovarian pregnancy. A case report. J Reprod Med 38:155, 1993

Segna RA, Mitchell DR, Misas JE: Successful treatment of cervical pregnancy with oral etoposide. Obstet Gynecol 76:945, 1990

Seifer DB: Persistent ectopic pregnancy: An argument for heightened vigilance and patient compliance. Fertil Steril 68:402, 1997

Seifer DB, Silva PD, Grainger DA, Barber SR, Grant WD, Gutmann JN: Reproductive potential after treatment for persistent ectopic pregnancy. Fertil Steril 62:194, 1994

Shalev E, Peleg D, Tsabari A, Romano S, Bustan M: Spontaneous resolution of ectopic tubal pregnancy: Natural history. Fertil Steril 63:15, 1995

Shamma FN, Schwartz LB: Primary ovarian pregnancy successfully treated with methotrexate. Am J Obstet Gynecol 167:1307, 1992

Sherer DM, Scibetta JJ, Sanko SR: Heterotopic quadruplet gestation with laparoscopic resection of ruptured interstitial pregnancy and subsequent successful outcome of triplets. Am J Obstet Gynecol 172:216, 1995

Sherer DM, Smith SA, Sanko SR: Uterine sacculation sonographically mimicking an abdominal pregnancy at 20 weeks' gestation. Am J Perinatol 11:350, 1994

Sherman D, Langer R, Sadovsky G, Bukovsky I, Caspi E: Improved fertility following ectopic pregnancy. Fertil Steril 37:497, 1982

Sherman KJ, Daling JR, Stergachis A, Weiss NS, Foy HM, Wang SP, Grayston JT: Sexually transmitted diseases and tubal pregnancy. Sex Transm Dis 17:115, 1990

Sidek S, Lai SF, Lim-Tan SK: Primary ovarian pregnancy: Current diagnosis and management. Singapore Med J 35:71, 1994

Silva PD, Schaper AM, Rooney B: Reproductive outcome after 143 laparoscopic procedures for ectopic pregnancy. Obstet Gynecol 81:710, 1993

Sivin I: Alternative estimates of ectopic pregnancy risks during contraception. Am J Obstet Gynecol 165:1900, 1991

Society for Assisted Reproductive Technology and the American Society of Reproductive Medicine: Assisted reproductive technology in the United States and Canada: 1995 results generated from the American Society for Reproductive Medicine/Society for Assisted Technology registry. Fertil Steril 69:389, 1998

Spandorfer SD, Sawin SW, Benjamin I, Barnhart KT: Postoperative day 1 serum human chorionic gonadotropin level as a predictor of persistent ectopic pregnancy after conservative surgical management. Fertil Steril 68:430, 1997

Spiegelberg O: Casuistry in ovarian pregnancy. Arch Gynaekol 13:73, 1878

Stabile I, Grudzinskas JG: Ectopic pregnancy: A review of incidence, etiology and diagnostic aspects. Obstet Gynecol Surv 45:335, 1990

Stangel JJ, Reyniak V, Stone ML: Conservative surgical management of tubal pregnancy. Obstet Gynecol 48:241, 1976

Stevens CA: Malformations and deformations in abdominal pregnancy Am J Med Genet 47:1189, 1993

Stovall TG: Medical management should be routinely used as primary therapy for ectopic pregnancy. Clin Obstet Gynecol 38:3436, 1995

Stovall TG, Ling FW: Some new approaches to ectopic pregnancy management. Contemp Obstet Gynecol 37:35, 1992

Stovall TG, Ling FW, Carson SA, Buster JE: Serum progesterone and uterine curettage in differential diagnosis of ectopic pregnancy. Fertil Steril 57:456, 1992

Tanaka T, Hayashi H, Kutsuzawa T, Fujimoto S, Ichinoe K: Treatment of interstitial ectopic pregnancy with methotrexate: Report of a successful case. Fertil Steril 37:851, 1982

Tay JI, Moore J, Walker JJ: Ectopic pregnancy. BMJ 320:916, 2000

Tharaux-Deneux C, Bouyer J, Job-Spira N, Coste J, Spira A: Risk of ectopic pregnancy and previous induced abortion. Am J Public Health 88:401, 1998

Thomas JS Jr, Willie JO, Clark JFJ: Primary peritoneal pregnancy: A case report. J Natl Med Assoc 83:635, 1991a

Thomas RL, Gingold BR, Gallagher MW: Cervical pregnancy. A report of two cases. J Reprod Med 36:459, 1991b

Timor-Tritsch IE, Monteagudo A, Mandeville EO, Pisner DB, Anaya GP, Pirrone EC: Successful management of viable cervical pregnancy by local injection of methotrexate guided by transvaginal ultrasonography. Am J Obstet Gynecol 170:737, 1994

Trio D, Strobelt N, Picciolo C, Lapinski RH, Ghidini A: Prognostic factors for successful expectant management of ectopic pregnancy. Fertil Steril 6:469, 1995

Tulandi T, Saleh A: Surgical management of ectopic pregnancy. Clinical Obstet Gynecol 42:31, 1999

Tuomivaara L, Kauppila A: Radical or conservative surgery for ectopic pregnancy? A follow-up study patients. Fertil Steril 50:580, 1988

Ushakov FB, Elchalal U, Aceman PJ, Schenker JG: Cervical pregnancy: Past and future. Obstet Gynecol 52:45, 1996

Vermesh M, Silva PD, Sauer MV, Vargyas JM, Lobo RA: Persistent tubal ectopic gestation: Patterns of circulating β-human chorionic gonadotropin and progesterone and management options. Fertil Steril 50:584, 1988

Vignali M, Busacca M, Brigante C, Doldi N, Spagnolo D, Belloni C: Abdominal pregnancy as a result of gamete intrafallopian transfer (GIFT) and subsequent treatment with methotrexate: Case report. Int J Fertil 35:280, 1990

Wagner A, Burchardt AJ: MR imaging in advanced abdominal pregnancy. A case report of fetal death. Acta Radiol 36:193, 1995

Ware HH: Observations on thirteen cases of late extrauterine pregnancy. Am J Obstet Gynecol 55:561, 1948

Weiss RE, Stone NN: Persistent maternal hydronephrosis after intra-abdominal pregnancy. J Urol 152:1196, 1994

Williams PC, Malvar TC, Kraft JR: Term ovarian pregnancy with delivery of a live female infant. Am J Obstet Gynecol 142:589, 1982

Wolcott HD, Kaunitz AM, Nuss RC, Benrubi GE: Successful pregnancy after previous conservative treatment of an advanced cervical pregnancy. Obstet Gynecol 71:1023, 1988

Yackel DB, Panton ONM, Martin DJ, Lee D: Splenic pregnancy-case report. Obstet Gynecol 71:471, 1988

Yalcinkaya TM, Brown SE, Mertz HL, Thomas DW, DePond RT, Heywood ER: A comparison of 25 mg/m^2 vs 50 mg/m^2

dose of methotrexate (MTX) for the treatment of ectopic pregnancy. J Soc Gynecol Investig 7:179A, 2000

Yamada T, Kasamatsu H: Bilateral tubal pregnancy after puerperal tubal ligation. J Am Assoc Gynecol Laparosc 7:161, 2000

Yao M, Tulandi T: Current status of surgical and nonsurgical management of ectopic pregnancy. Fertil Steril 67:421, 1997

Yeko TR, Mayer JC, Parsons AK, Maroulis GB: A prospective series of unruptured ectopic pregnancies treated by tubal injection with hyperosmolar glucose. Obstet Gynecol 85:265, 1995

35

Abnormalities of the Reproductive Tract

In some cases, pregnancy is complicated by abnormalities of the reproductive tract. In general, these are considered as developmental anomalies incurred during embryogenesis or they may be acquired and caused by events that usually occur during adulthood.

DEVELOPMENTAL REPRODUCTIVE TRACT ABNORMALITIES

A number of genitourinary defects from abnormal embryogenesis occur sporadically. Serious defects often result in significant fetal and maternal hazards. In some, even minor defects may result in an increased incidence of threatened abortion and abnormal fetal lie.

EMBRYOGENESIS OF THE REPRODUCTIVE TRACT. In order to understand the etiology of developmental abnormalities of the vagina, cervix, and uterus, it is important to first understand how the structures are formed. Briefly, development begins when the metanephric ducts emerge and connect with the cloaca between the third and fifth gestational weeks. Between the fourth and fifth weeks, two ureteric buds develop distally from the mesonephric ducts and begin to grow cephalad toward the mesonephros. Müllerian (paramesonephric) ducts form bilaterally between the developing gonad and the mesonephros. The müllerian ducts extend downward and laterally to the mesonephric ducts, and finally turn medially to meet and fuse together in the midline. The fused müllerian duct descends to the urogenital sinus to join the müllerian tubercle. **The close association between the müllerian and mesonephric ducts has clinical relevance, because damage to either duct system will most often be associated with damage to both—uterine horn, kidney, and ureter.**

The uterus is formed by the union of the two müllerian ducts at about the 10th week. Fusion begins in the middle and then extends caudally and cephalad. The characteristic uterine shape is now formed, with cellular proliferation at the upper portion and a simultaneous dissolution of cells at the lower pole, thus establishing the first uterine cavity. This cavity is at the lower pole with a thick wedge of tissue above. The upper thick wedge of tissue (septum) is dissolved slowly, creating the uterine cavity. This process is usually completed by the 20th week. Any failure to fuse the two müllerian ducts or failure to resorb the cavity between them results in separate uterine horns or some degree of persistent uterine septum.

The vagina forms between the urogenital sinus and the müllerian tubercle by a dissolution of the cell cord between the two structures. It is believed that this dissolution starts at the hymen and moves upward toward the cervix. Failure of this process will be associated with persistence of the cell cord, and vaginal agenesis or lesser abnormalities of this process will result in varying degrees of septum formation.

GENESIS AND CLASSIFICATION OF MÜLLERIAN ABNORMALITIES. Because fusion of the two müllerian ducts forms the vagina, cervix, and uterine body, the principal groups of deformities arising from three types of embryological defects can be classified as follows:

1. Defective canalization of the vagina results in a transverse vaginal septum, or in the most extreme form, absence of the vagina.
2. Unilateral maturation of the müllerian duct with incomplete or absent development of the opposite duct results in defects associated with upper urinary tract abnormalities.
3. The most common abnormality is absent or faulty midline fusion of the müllerian ducts. Complete lack of fusion results in two entirely separate uteri, cervices, and vaginas. Incomplete tissue resorption between the two fused müllerian ducts results in a uterine septum.

Various classifications of these anomalies have been proposed, but none is completely satisfactory. One for müllerian duct abnormalities suggested by Buttram and Gibbons (1979) is based upon the failure of normal development. The classification separates a diversity of anomalies into groups with similar clinical characteristics, prognosis for pregnancy, and treatment (Table 35–1). The classification includes a category for abnormalities associated with fetal exposure to diethylstilbestrol (DES). Vaginal anomalies were not classified because they were not associated with fetal loss. Vaginal anomalies using their scheme were most often associated with uterine didelphys and bicornuate anomalies.

VULVAR ABNORMALITIES. Complete *atresia of the vulva*, or the lower portion of the vagina, unless corrected, precludes conception. More frequently, vulvar atresia is incomplete, resulting from adhesions or scars following injury or infection. The defect may present a considerable obstacle to delivery, but the resistance usually is overcome eventually by continued pressure exerted by the fetal head. This may result in deep perineal tears unless prevented by an adequate episiotomy.

VAGINAL ABNORMALITIES. Several developmental abnormalities of the vagina are possible:

1. *Single.* The normal vagina.
2. *Longitudinally septate.* More or less complete longitudinal septum.
3. *Double.* It is often difficult to distinguish the double from the completely septate vagina. The true double

TABLE 35–1. Classification of Müllerian Anomalies

I. Segmental müllerian agenesis or hypoplasia
    A. Vaginal
    B. Cervical
    C. Fundal
    D. Combined anomalies
II. Unicornuate uterus
    A. With rudimentary horn
        1. With endometrial cavity
            a. Communicating
            b. Noncommunicating
        2. Without endometrial cavity
    B. Without rudimentary horn
III. Uterine didelphys
IV. Bicornuate uterus
    A. Complete (division down to internal os)
    B. Partial
    C. Arcuate
V. Septate uterus
    A. Complete (septum to internal os)
    B. Partial
VI. Diethylstilbestrol

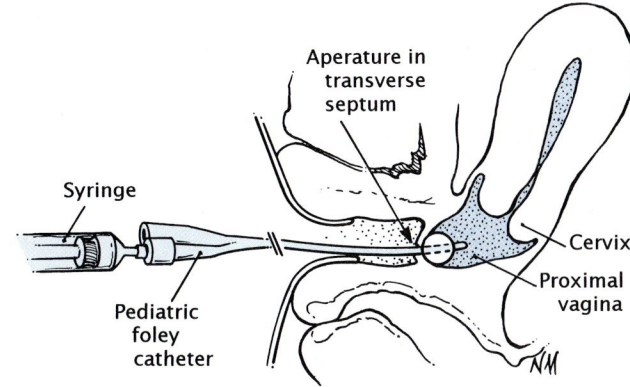

FIGURE 35–1. Sagittal view of a transverse vaginal septum with communication through a small opening into the distal vagina.

vagina includes a double introitus and resembles a double-barreled shotgun, with each passage terminating in a distinct, separate cervix. At times with double vaginas, one may end blindly.

4. *Transversely septate.* These result from faulty canalization of the united müllerian anlage rather than faulty longitudinal fusion. The septate vagina is usually discovered during routine pelvic examinations or by the woman who notices that vaginal tampons are not always effective in absorbing menses.

OBSTETRICAL SIGNIFICANCE OF VAGINAL ABNORMALITIES. In most cases, vaginal anomalies present few problems, but if so, they are usually obstruction to delivery.

SEPTAE AND STRICTURES. A complete longitudinal septum usually does not cause dystocia because the half of the vagina through which the fetus descends gradually dilates satisfactorily. An incomplete septum, however, occasionally interferes with descent. In these cases, the septum may become stretched around the presenting part as a band of varying thickness. Occasionally such septae are sufficiently resistant that either they must be divided or cesarean delivery must be performed.

Infrequently, the vagina may be obstructed by a congenital *annular stricture* or band. These strictures are unlikely to interfere seriously with delivery because they

usually soften during pregnancy and yield before the oncoming head. An incision rarely is required.

Sometimes the upper vagina is separated from the rest of the canal by a *transverse septum* with a small opening, as shown in Figure 35–1 Some of these are associated with in utero exposure to diethylstilbestrol (p. 918). Such a stricture is occasionally mistaken for the upper limit of the vaginal vault, and at the time of labor, the opening in the septum is erroneously considered to be an undilated external os. After the external os has dilated completely, the head impinges upon the septum and causes it to bulge downward. If the septum does not yield, slight pressure upon its opening usually will lead to further dilatation, but occasionally cruciate incisions may be required to permit delivery.

A communicating transverse vaginal septum as illustrated in Figure 35–1 is better corrected prior to pregnancy. Such a lesion in pregnancy may lead to significant vaginal lacerations or to a cesarean delivery. The surgical correction should follow an attempt to identify the extent of the lesion. As illustrated in Figure 35–1, a Foley catheter is inserted through the communicating tract. Normal saline is used to flush the area before filling the distal vagina. With saline filling the distal vagina, a vaginal probe sonogram is used to map the distal vaginal area and outline any additional cervical abnormalities. Following this mapping procedure and under the same anesthetic, a Z-plasty removal of the septum should be performed. Patency of the distal vagina must be maintained using a vaginal stent for several months, even in sexually active women.

ATRESIA. Complete congenital *vaginal atresia*, unless corrected operatively, forms an effective bar to pregnancy (Chakravarty and colleagues, 2000). Incomplete atresia can be a manifestation of faulty development as shown in Figure 35–2A, C, and D, or it results from

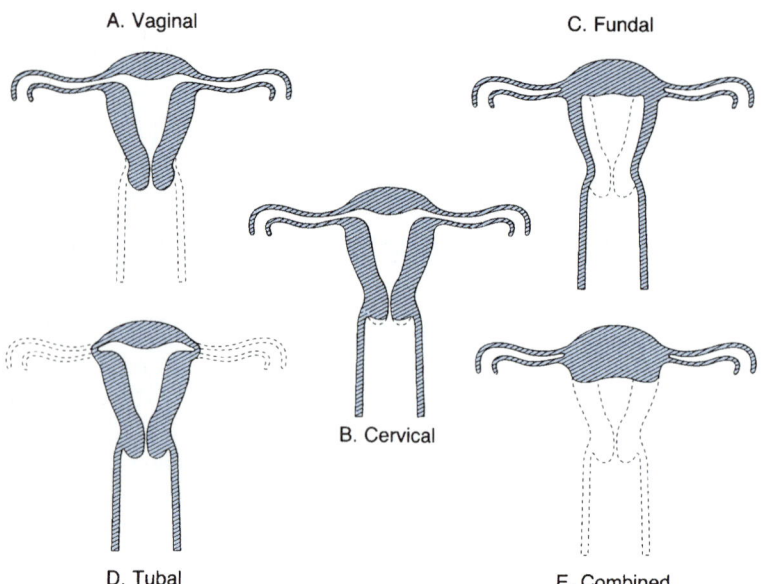

FIGURE 35–2. Class I: Segmental müllerian agenesis or hypoplasia with subdivisions.

accidents such as scarring from injury or inflammation (p. 923). In most cases of partial atresia, because of pregnancy-induced tissue softening, obstructions are gradually overcome by pressure exerted by the presenting part. Less often, manual or hydrostatic dilatation or incisions or even cesarean delivery are necessary.

CERVICAL AND UTERINE ABNORMALITIES

TYPES OF CERVICES. As with development there are a number of cervical anomalies that are encountered.

1. *Single.* The normal cervix.
2. *Septate.* Cervix consisting of a single muscular ring partitioned by a septum. The septum may be confined to the cervix, or more often, it may be the downward continuation of a uterine septum or the upward extension of a vaginal septum.
3. *Double.* Two distinct cervices, each resulting from separate müllerian duct maturation. Both septate and true double cervices are frequently associated with a longitudinal vaginal septum. Unfortunately, many septate cervices are erroneously classified as double.
4. *Single hemicervix.* This arises from a unilateral müllerian maturation.

DIAGNOSIS OF CERVICAL AND UTERINE MALFORMATIONS.
Some of these are discovered by simple inspection or during bimanual examination. Frequently they are discovered at cesarean delivery or during manual exploration of the uterine cavity after delivery. Fundal notching, palpated abdominally, is most often indicative of a malformed uterus. Ultrasonic screening for uterine anomalies, although 98 percent specific, has only a 43 percent sensitivity (Nicolini and associates, 1987). It is

difficult to distinguish a septate from bicornuate uterus without radiological examination, high-resolution sonography, direct visualization of the uterine cavity, and often laparoscopic examination. *Hysteroscopic examination* and *hysterography* are of value in ascertaining the configuration of the uterine cavity. When combined with a laparoscopic confirmation of the absence or presence of an external division of the uterus and the presence or absence of a rudimentary uterine horn, virtually all uterine abnormalities can be described and classified accurately as subsequently described.

INCIDENCE. Accurate figures are not available for these anomalies. Green and Harris (1976) identified 80 uterine developmental anomalies during the course of 31,836 deliveries (1 in 400). They emphasized that detection was greatest during a period when one especially interested staff member espoused uterine exploration at delivery, and when an anomaly was suspected, hysterosalpingography was performed 6 to 8 weeks postpartum.

Sonography may be used to identify abnormal uterine development, although it lacks the precision of diagnosis provided by hysteroscopy and hysterosalpingography. During actual or suspected pregnancy, however, ultrasonic evaluation can be quite informative (Raga and co-workers, 1996; Salle and associates, 1998). *Magnetic resonance imaging* may be more specific (Kelley and associates, 1990).

UROLOGICAL EVALUATION. When asymmetrical development of the reproductive tract is found, urological evaluation is indicated because of the frequent association of urinary tract anomalies. When there is uterine atresia on one side or when one side of a double vagina terminates blindly, an ipsilateral urological anomaly is common (Fedele and associates, 1987; Heinonen, 1983, 1984; Wiersma and colleagues, 1976).

AUDITORY EVALUATION. Up to a third of women with müllerian defects have been reported to have auditory defects (Letterie and Vauss, 1991). These are characterized as mild to severe sensorineural hearing defects in the high-frequency range.

UTERINE ANOMALIES IN WILMS TUMOR SURVIVORS. Survivors of this rare malignancy appear to have an increased incidence of urinary and reproductive tract anomalies (Nicholson and colleagues, 1996). The authors suggest that this observation might partially explain infertility noted in female survivors.

OBSTETRICAL SIGNIFICANCE OF CERVICAL ABNORMALITIES. Complete atresia of the cervix is incompatible with conception (Chakravarty and associates, 2000). Cicatrical *cervical stenosis* may follow various forms of cervical trauma (p. 924). Because there usually is tissue softening during pregnancy, cervical stenosis gradually yields during labor. In rare instances, stenosis may be so pronounced that dilatation appears improbable and cesarean delivery is necessary.

OBSTETRICAL SIGNIFICANCE OF UTERINE HYPOPLASIA OR AGENESIS

BUTTRAM AND GIBBONS CLASS I. The range of anomalies seen with müllerian agenesis is shown in Figure 35–2. As discussed, vaginal hypoplasia or agenesis renders pregnancy virtually impossible, and even in rare cases in which a uterus is reattached surgically to a neovagina, successful pregnancy is unusual. The various types of vaginal septa can be dilated, displaced, or surgically divided. The septate cervix functions remarkably well, but during labor there is possible danger of rupture and hemorrhage.

BUTTRAM AND GIBBONS CLASSES II THROUGH V. Major obstetrical difficulties arise from uterine anomalies (Raga and co-workers, 1997). Uterine defects that result from development of only one müllerian duct, or from lack of fusion, often give rise to a hemiuterus that fails to dilate and hypertrophy appropriately. This may result in a number of possible difficulties, including miscarriage, ectopic pregnancy, rudimentary horn pregnancy, preterm delivery, fetal growth restriction, abnormal fetal lie, uterine dysfunction, and uterine rupture (Ben-Rafael and associates, 1991; Michalas, 1991). Surprisingly, even in conditions where only a uterine septum is present, miscarriage is increased (Buttram and

Gibbons, 1979; Buttram, 1983). Because of these obstetrical problems, each uterine defect is discussed within the classification outlined in Table 35–1.

REPRODUCTIVE PERFORMANCE OF WOMEN WITH UNICORNUATE UTERUS (BUTTRAM AND GIBBONS CLASS II). Developmental anomalies that result in a unicornuate uterus are shown in Figure 35–3. Its incidence in a series of 1160 uterine anomalies was 14 percent (Zanetti and associates, 1978). This was likely an underestimate, because the major diagnostic technique used was hysterosalpingography, which cannot identify noncommunicating rudimentary horns. O'Leary and O'Leary (1963) estimated that in 90 percent of unicornuate uteri with rudimentary horns there was no communication between the horns. The increased incidence of infertility, endometriosis, and dysmenorrhea in such cases is certainly more easily understood (Fedele and associates, 1987, 1995; Heinonen, 1983).

As shown in Table 35–2, pregnancy outcome is poor, and fetal wastage is over 40 percent. This likely is due to anatomical defects, and increased pregnancy loss may be partially explained by smaller uterine size or implantation of the zygote in a communicating rudimentary horn. The smaller hemiuterine size is almost certainly an explanation for the increased rates of preterm delivery, fetal growth restriction, breech presentation, dysfunctional labor, and increased cesarean delivery (Andrews

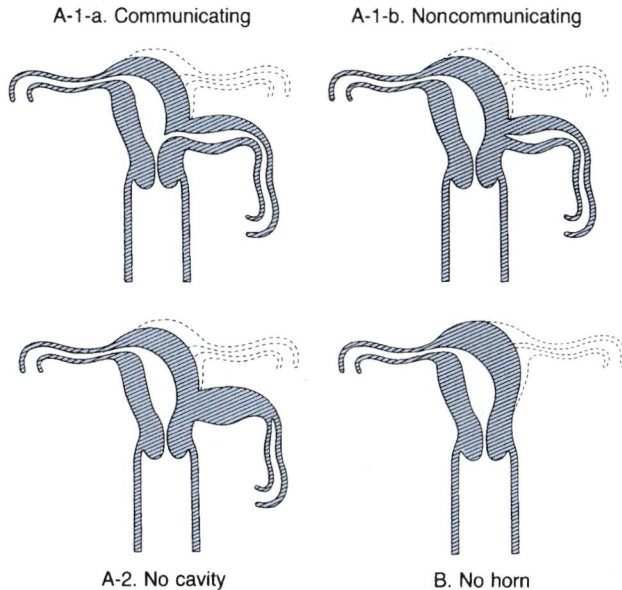

A-1-a. Communicating   A-1-b. Noncommunicating

A-2. No cavity   B. No horn

FIGURE 35–3. Class II: Unicornuate uterus with either rudimentary horn (A) or without rudimentary horn (B). Those with a rudimentary horn are divided into groups with an endometrial cavity (A-1) or without an endometrial cavity (A-2). Those with an endometrial cavity either have a communication with the opposite uterine horn (A-1-a) or do not have a communication with the opposite horn (A-1-b).

TABLE 35–2. Pregnancy Outcomes in Women with a Unicornuate Uterus

Outcome	Heinonen (1983)	Moutos et al. (1992)	Acien (1993)	Fedele et al. (1995)	Total
Patients	15	20	24	26	85
Pregnancies	35	36[a]	55	57	183
Spontaneous abortions (%)[b]	4 (11)	13 (36)	12 (22)	33 (58)	62 (34)
Ectopic pregnancies (%)[b]	4 (11)	1 (2.8)	1 (1.8)	3 (5.2)[c]	9 (5)
Deliveries (%)[b]	27 (77)	22 (61)	42 (76)	21 (37)	112 (61)
Breech presentations[d]	9 (33)	—	13 (31)	—	—
Cesarean deliveries[d]	8 (30)	8 (36)	—	—	—
Preterm deliveries[d]	4 (15)	3 (14)	9 (21)[e]	5 (24)	21 (19)
Term deliveries[d]	23 (85)	19 (86)	33 (79)	16 (76)	91 (21)
Fetal survival[b]	25 (71)	21 (58)	39 (71)	20 (35)	105 (57)

[a] This number excludes four elective abortions.
[b] Of all pregnancies.
[c] This number includes one blind horn pregnancy.
[d] Of deliveries, this number excludes abortions and ectopic pregnancies.
[e] This number includes one preterm infant who did not survive.

and Jones, 1982; Fedele and associates, 1995; Heinonen, 1983, 1997).

Tubal pregnancies and pregnancies in the noncommunicating rudimentary horn are special problems. Rolen and associates (1966) reported that in 70 pregnancies with implantation in rudimentary horns, uterine rupture usually occurred prior to 20 weeks. Intraperitoneal hemorrhage in such cases may be massive and life-threatening, but rare cases of fetal survival have been reported (Akhtar, 1988; Heinonen and Aro, 1988). In one case, surviving twins were delivered 8 days apart (Nahum, 1997). In another, pregnancy in a rudimentary noncommunicating horn was mistaken for uterine incarceration with sacculation (Nwosu and Thatcher, 1993). The more liberal use of magnetic resonance imaging may result in an earlier diagnosis of such problems in pregnancy (Lawhon and associates, 1998).

Pregnancy in a rudimentary uterine horn at 15 weeks is shown in Figure 35–4. There was no connection between the rudimentary horn and the opposite horn or the vagina. Sperm had to migrate out the oviduct of the patent horn and cross transperitoneally to enter the oviduct attached to the rudimentary horn. At 15 weeks, the woman complained of sudden, severe, cramping lower abdominal pain. A tender mass was felt to the left of a somewhat enlarged uterus. Fetal heart motion was identified in this mass. At laparotomy, about 200 mL of blood was found free in the peritoneal cavity. A total hysterectomy and left salpingo-oophorectomy were performed. Her three previous pregnancies, all breech presentations, resulted in infants who weighed 750 g (expired), 1220 g (lived), and 2815 g (lived).

REPRODUCTIVE PERFORMANCE IN WOMEN WITH UTERINE DIDELPHYS (BUTTRAM AND GIBBONS CLASS III). Uterine didelphys is distinguished from bicornuate and septate uteri by the presence of complete reduplication of cervices and hemiuterine cavities (Fig. 35–5. In a series of 26 such women, Heinonen (1984) reported that all had a longitudinal vaginal septum as well. Except for ectopic and rudimentary horn pregnancies, problems associated with uterine didelphys are similar to those seen with a unicornuate uterus. Heinonen (1984) reported an overall successful pregnancy outcome of 70 percent. In addition to 30 percent miscarriages, there was preterm delivery in 20 percent, fetal growth restriction in 10 percent, breech presentation in 43 percent, and the cesarean delivery rate was 82 percent. Subsequent trial of labor results in a higher uterine rupture rate (Ravasia and colleagues, 1999). The case shown in Figure 35–6 is illustrative of these complications.

Multifetal gestation is unusual but not rare in women with uterine didelphys (Heinonen, 1984; Hochner-Celnikier and colleagues, 1983). Mashiach and associates (1981) reported a case of triplets with a delivery interval of 72 days!

REPRODUCTIVE PERFORMANCE IN WOMEN WITH BICORNUATE AND SEPTATE UTERI (BUTTRAM AND GIBBONS CLASSES IV AND V). In both classes IV and V (Figs. 35–7 and 35–8), there is a marked increase in spontaneous miscarriage. This is likely due to the abundant muscular tissue in the septum (Dabirashrafi and colleagues, 1995). The exception is for the

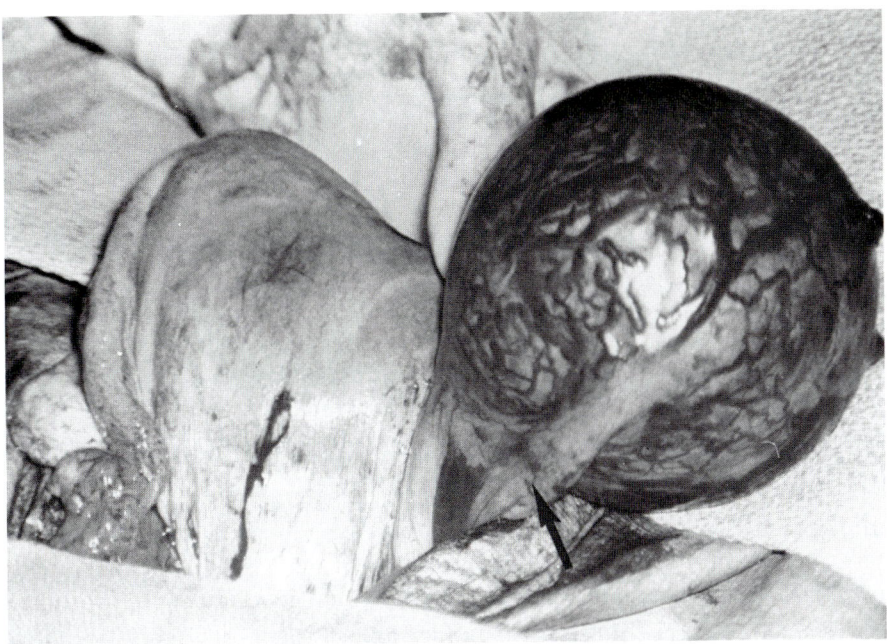

A

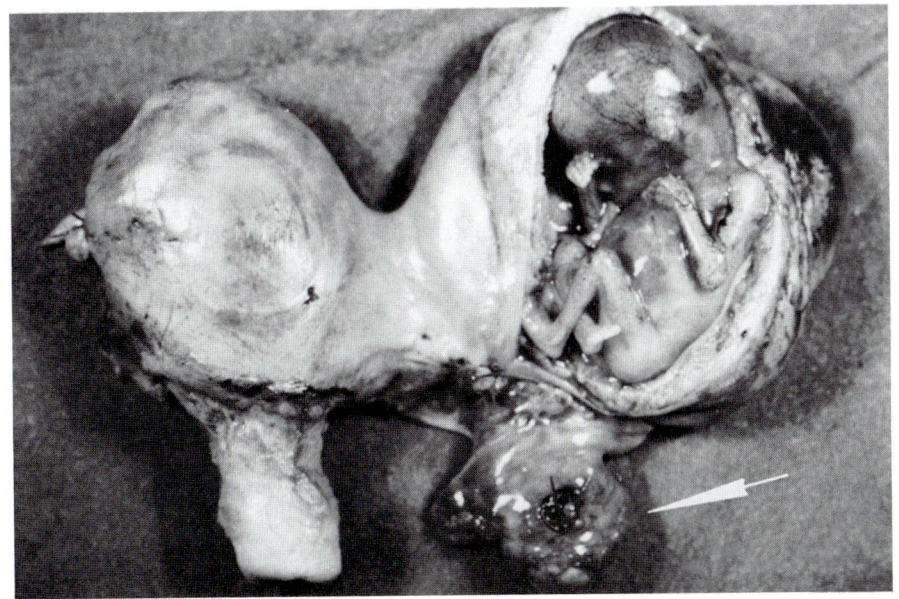

B

FIGURE 35–4. A. Pregnancy of 15 weeks in a left rudimentary hemiuterus as seen at laparotomy. The tense, vascular rudimentary uterus was bleeding from veins over its extremely vascular surface. The attached oviduct (*arrow*) was patent and the adjacent left ovary contained the corpus luteum of pregnancy. **B.** Hysterectomy specimen from **A,** now with left hemiuterus opened to display the fetus and placenta. The intact mass (*arrow*) consists of left tube and ovary. There is no cervix on the left and no communication with the right hemiuterus, which does have a cervix that communicated with the vagina.

arcuate uterus, which is merely a slight deviation from normal. Pregnancy losses in the first 20 weeks were observed by Buttram and Gibbons (1979) to be 70 percent for bicornuate and 88 percent for septate uteri. This extraordinarily high pregnancy wastage likely is due to partial or complete implantation on the largely avascular septum (Fedele and co-workers, 1989; Gast and Martin, 1992). In 255 women with uterine malformations, three with a septate uterus had newborns with limb reduction defects (Heinonen, 1999). Leible and

associates (1998) showed that two-thirds of women with lateral placental müllerian anomalies had implantation and that the nonplacental uterine artery in these cases had an abnormally high systolic/diastolic ratio. Once pregnancy is well established, overall outcome is associated with an increased incidence of preterm delivery, abnormal fetal lie, and cesarean delivery. Subsequent trials of labor have a high uterine rupture rate (Ravasia and associates, 1999).

A hysterosalpingogram usually cannot be used alone

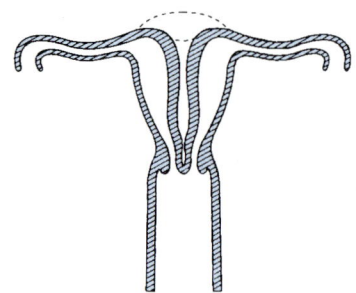

FIGURE 35-5. Class III: Uterine didelphys.

to differentiate the septate and bicornuate uterus, but transvaginal hysterosonography markedly improves the diagnostic accuracy (Salle and associates, 1998). Three-dimensional ultrasound also has been reported to improve diagnostic accuracy, but like hysterosonography, is not 100 percent accurate (Raga and co-workers, 1996). Buttram and Gibbons (1979) stressed the necessity of laparoscopy to establish the presence of an external uterine division. This diagnosis now can be established in a noninvasive manner using magnetic resonance imaging techniques (Kelley and associates, 1990). Subsequent trials of labor have a high uterine rupture rate (Ravasia and associates, 1999).

MANAGEMENT OF UTERINE ANOMALIES. Abnormal fetal presentations are commonly seen with an abnormal uterus. Attempts at external podalic version are less likely to be successful and may prove dangerous. If uterine dysfunction develops, it seems unwise to stimulate these defective uteri with oxytocin. Cesarean delivery is safer, but unfortunately the diagnosis is often unexpected.

CERCLAGE. Therapeutic and prophylactic cervical cerclages may be indicated in women with uterine didelphys and unicornuate or bicornuate uteri (Golan and Caspi, 1992; Golan and associates, 1990b, 1992; Maneschi and colleagues, 1988; Seidman and co-workers, 1991). Transabdominal cerclage offers the best hope of successful pregnancy outcome in women with partial cervical atresia or cervical hypoplasia (Hampton and colleagues, 1990; Welker and associates, 1988). Caspi and associates (1990) have described a modified Shirodkar cerclage that closes the internal os without resorting to an abdominal procedure. This technique is performed by making a small transverse incision at the anterior vaginal–bladder junction and advancing the bladder up to the level of the internal os. A large round needle is used to insert a monofilament suture around either side of the cervix under the vaginal mucosa. The suture is brought out from under the vaginal mucosa in the cul-de-sac and ligated. This procedure was performed in

women with short or lacerated cervices and in women with previous McDonald cerclage failures. The results obtained were similar to those achieved with a Shirodkar cerclage, but operative time and blood loss were less. Transvaginal cervical cerclage has been successfully in DES-exposed women with cervical hypoplasia (Ludmir and co-workers, 1991). The question of whether to place a suture in both cervices of a uterine didelphys is unresolved (Heinonen, 1984). There appears to be no reason for cerclage with an arcuate uterus. Cerclage should not be needed after successful resection of a uterine septum, but probably should still be used following abdominal metroplasties for uterine didelphys and bicornuate uteri. If active labor supervenes, procrastination in severing a cerclage ligature must be avoided because of the increased risk of uterine rupture.

METROPLASTY. Women with septate or bicornuate anomalies and poor reproductive outcomes are likely to benefit from uterine repair (Ayhan, 1992; Khalifa, 1993; Musich, 1978; Teti, 1991; Zorlu, 1996, and all their co-workers).

Repair of a bicornuate uterus (classes IV-A and IV-B, Fig. 35–7) is by transabdominal metroplasty involving septal resection and recombination of the fundi (Candiani and associates, 1990; Gitsch and colleagues, 1990; Kessler and co-workers, 1986). Following repair, uterine activity is normal if anatomically symmetrical uterine horns have been conjoined (Oliva and associates, 1992).

Repair of a septate uterus (class V, Fig. 35–8) is best done by hysteroscopic resection of the septum (Daly, 1989; Grigoris, 1998; Hassiakos, 1990; Israel, 1984; Jourdain, 1998, and all their co-workers). Excessive infusion of dextran during these hysteroscopic procedures can result in life-threatening pulmonary edema and induce a severe coagulopathy (Vercellini and colleagues, 1992). Laser septal resection apparently only adds time and expense to the procedure (Candiani and associates, 1991). Postoperative intrauterine device insertion and hormonal therapy are not necessary to prevent septal fusion (Vercellini and associates, 1989).

Fedele and associates (1988) reported improved pregnancy outcomes following abdominal metroplasty to correct uterine didelphys (class III, Fig. 35–5). Cerclage was used only once following uterine repair.

DIETHYLSTILBESTROL-INDUCED REPRODUCTIVE TRACT ABNORMALITIES. For nearly a quarter of a century, until the early 1970s, diethylstilbestrol (DES), a synthetic, nonsteroidal estrogen, was prescribed for an estimated 3 million pregnant women in the United States. Early uncontrolled reports claimed the drug was useful in treating abortion, preeclampsia, diabetes, and preterm labor. Other than its lack of effectiveness, the first serious problem to be linked to its use was identifi-

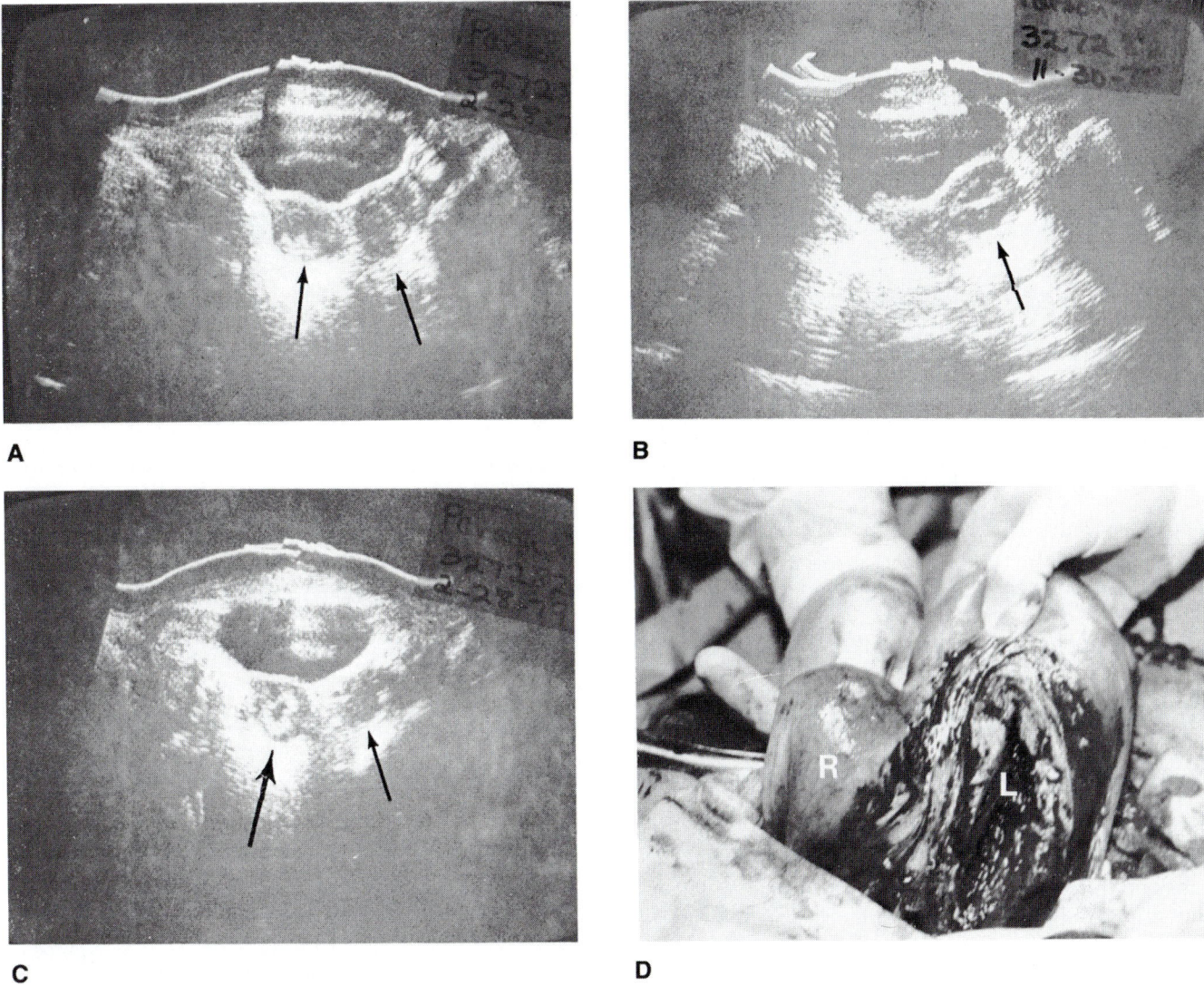

FIGURE 35–6. Woman with uterine didelphys who had experienced seven consecutive abortions. In this eighth pregnancy, as illustrated in transverse sonogram **A**, two uterine cavities are apparent above the arrows. In sonogram **B**, a pregnancy ring, probably abnormal, is seen in the left uterine cavity above the arrow. In sonogram **C**, 90 days later, a normal pregnancy ring is seen in the right uterine cavity above the larger arrow but not in the left uterine cavity above the smaller arrow. A 2900-g healthy infant was delivered from the right uterus as a double footling breech by cesarean at 38 weeks' gestation. The left kidney was absent. Necrotic placental villi from the missed abortion were expelled from the left uterus 2 days postpartum. **D.** The same woman in **C** conceived again 3 years later in the left uterus (L). A growth-restricted fetus who thrived after cesarean birth was delivered at 37 weeks through a vertical uterine incision. The small right uterus (R) is larger than when nonpregnant.

cation of vaginal clear-cell adenocarcinoma in some daughters who were exposed in utero (Herbst and co-workers, 1971). It has been established that the risk of malignancy is from 0.14 to 1.4 per 1000 exposed daughters observed through the age of 24 years. Subsequently, it was established that these women also had an increased risk of developing small-cell cervical carcinoma (Herbst, 2000). Cervical intraepithelial neoplasia may also be more common (Fowler and associates, 1981).

Several non-neoplastic abnormalities of the vagina and cervix have been reported. The most frequent of these are vaginal adenosis and cervical ectropion. Major structural abnormalities of the vagina, cervix, uterus, and fallopian tubes have also been reported, and these are associated with an increased incidence of poor reproductive outcome (Goldberg and Falcone, 1999; Kaufman and colleagues, 2000; Managan and associates, 1982; Senekjian and co-workers, 1988).

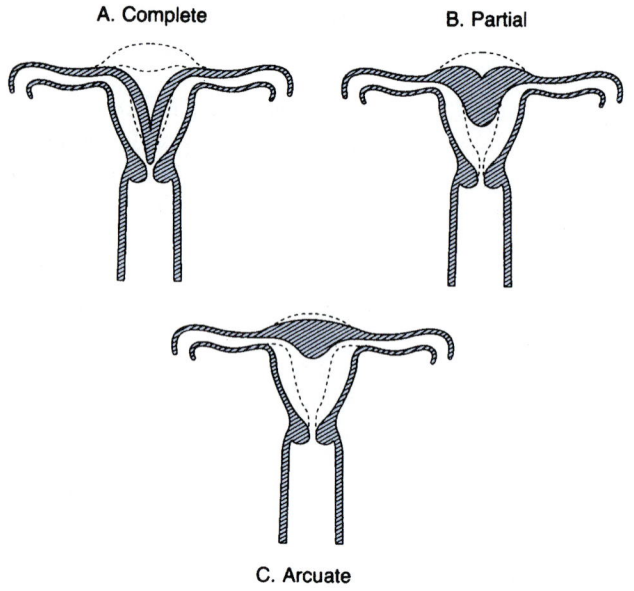

FIGURE 35–7. Class IV: Bicornuate uterus in which the septum is complete down to the internal os (**A**), partial (**B**), or arcuate (**C**).

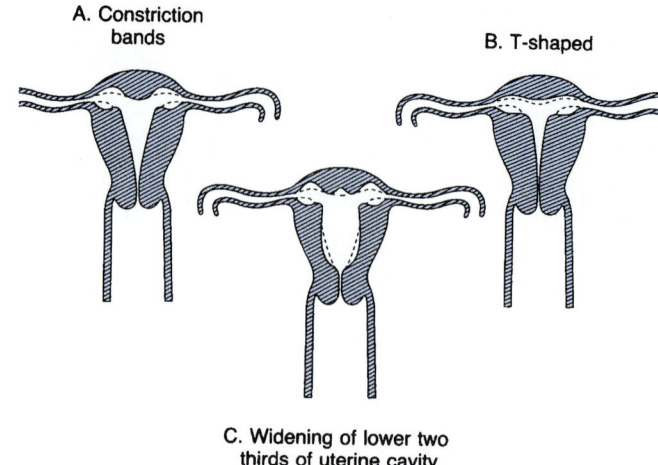

FIGURE 35–9. Class VI: DES anomalies, including uteri with luminal changes, such as constriction bands in the uterine cavity with lateral internal uterine wall spurs and internal fundal arcuate abnormalities (**A**), T-shaped cavity (**B**), and widening of the lower two thirds of the uterine cavity (**C**). (Modified from Buttram and Gibbons, 1979.)

STRUCTURAL ABNORMALITIES. From a fourth to a half of women exposed to DES in utero have identifiable structural variations in the cervix and vagina. These include transverse septa, circumferential ridges involving the vagina and cervix, and cervical collars. Uterine cavity anomalies are evident on hysterography in perhaps two thirds of exposed women (Kaufman and associates, 1980). Significantly smaller uterine cavities, shortened upper uterine segments, and T-shaped cavities have also been described (Figs. 35–9 and 35–10). About half of women with uterine defects also have cervical defects, especially a hypoplastic cervix. Finally, a variety of abnormalities of the oviduct have been described, including shortening, narrowing, and absence of fimbriae. Kipersztok and colleagues (1996) believe that hysterosalpingography remains the procedure of choice when compared with magnetic resonance imaging and

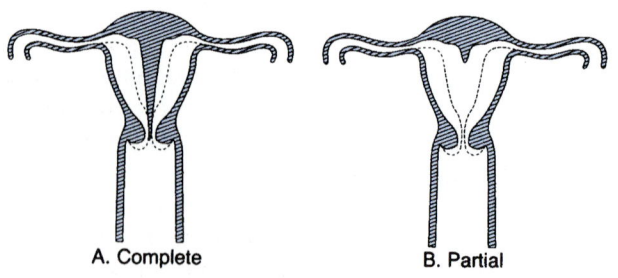

FIGURE 35–8. Class V: Septate uterus with complete septum to the internal or external os (**A**) or partial septum (**B**).

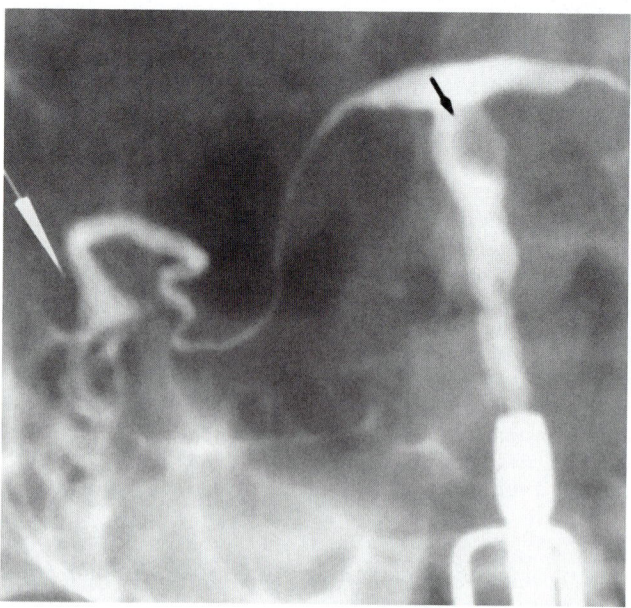

FIGURE 35–10. Hysterosalpingogram from a woman who was exposed in utero to DES. Note the T-shaped uterine cavity filled with contrast material that also has spilled from the end of the right oviduct (*white arrow*), demonstrating tubal patency. The filling defect within the uterine cavity (*black arrow*) is probably hyperplastic myometrium, the consequence of the DES exposure. She has since been pregnant successfully. (Courtesy of Dr. Bruce R. Carr.)

transvaginal ultrasonography in identifying these anomalies.

REPRODUCTIVE PERFORMANCE. Lower conception rates are reported for women exposed to DES in utero (Goldberg and Falcone, 1999; Senekjian and co-workers, 1988). Of those who conceive, spontaneous miscarriage, ectopic pregnancies, and preterm births are increased (Herbst and co-workers, 1981, 1989; Kaufman and associates, 1984, 2000). The risk is greatest for women with demonstrated structural abnormalities.

ECTOPIC PREGNANCY. The incidence of ectopic pregnancy was reported to be 7 percent compared with none for controls (Herbst and colleagues, 1989, 2000). The etiology is likely due to tubal anomalies, but decreased uterine size may also be a factor (Kaufman and associates, 1980, 1984).

MISCARRIAGE AND PRETERM LABOR. The incidence of preterm labor is increased, likely due to uterine and cervical anomalies (de Haas and associates, 1991). Spontaneous abortion is increased, but the mechanism responsible for early abortion is not well understood. Cervical incompetence appears to be responsible for the increased incidence of midpregnancy losses and preterm labor (Ayers and associates, 1988; Ludmir and colleagues, 1987). This was shown graphically by Michaels and co-workers (1989) in their serial prospective ultrasonic study of DES-exposed women. In 5 of 21 pregnancies, preterm cervical effacement and dilatation were identified using serial sonographic evaluation of the lower uterine segment, cervix, and vagina. A cerclage was applied in each of the five cases, and all continued to at least 36 weeks.

Michaels and co-workers (1989) advise these women that they are at risk for preterm labor. They are followed weekly with serial ultrasound surveillance of the lower uterine–cervicovaginal area, beginning at 14 weeks and continuing through 27 weeks. If there is progressive cervical effacement and dilatation, cerclage is performed. Ayers and associates (1988) and Ludmir and co-workers (1987, 1991) recommend cervical cerclage in most of these women, but especially those with cervical hypoplasia. Hampton and colleagues (1990) recommend abdominal cerclage for women with partial atresia or hypoplasia of the cervix.

INFERTILITY. Reduced fertility in these women is poorly understood but is associated with cervical hypoplasia and atresia. Surgical correction with vaginal and cervical reanastomosis has been accomplished (Welker and co-workers, 1988). Successful pregnancies have been achieved using a variety of different zygote intra-fallopian transfer techniques (Thijssen and associates, 1990).

TREATMENT. Treatment of DES-exposed women consists of continued surveillance for development of clear-cell carcinoma of the vagina and cervix (American College of Obstetricians and Gynecologists, 1996). Annual examinations are adequate for most women, but they should be done twice yearly in women with extensive vaginal adenosis. Women with cervical or vaginal atypia should be examined as often as indicated. No specific therapy is recommended for adenosis in the absence of cellular atypia. The treatment of clear-cell carcinoma of the vagina involves irradiation or radical extirpation.

Surgical management of structural anomalies has been reported to improve reproductive performance. Garbin and associates (1998) recommend hysteroscopic metroplasty using a monopolar hook to resect the lateral spurs of the upper interior uterine walls of a T-shaped uterus. They also resect the arcuate fundus of the uterine cavity to further increase uterine volume. They reported a decrease in abortions from 88 to 13 percent and an increase in term deliveries from 3 to 88 percent. Nagel and Malo (1993) and Katz and colleagues (1996) reported improved pregnancy outcomes with hysteroscopic uterine resection using scissors, electrocoagulation, and a cutting electrode.

ACQUIRED REPRODUCTIVE TRACT ABNORMALITIES

VULVAR ABNORMALITIES

EDEMA. In women with the nephrotic syndrome and hypoproteinemia, troublesome vulvar edema may be problematic even by midpregnancy. Sometimes in normal women and especially those with severe preeclampsia, the vulva may become edematous during labor. Venous thromboses and hematomas may also cause edema and significant pain and make an episiotomy difficult to perform.

INFLAMMATORY LESIONS. Extensive perineal inflammation and scarring from *hidradenitis suppurativa, lymphogranuloma venereum*, or Crohn disease may create difficulty with vaginal delivery, episiotomy, and repair. A mediolateral episiotomy may prevent some of these difficulties and rectal lacerations.

BARTHOLIN ABSCESS. Drainage must be established whenever an abscess develops during pregnancy. In some cases, local analgesia will suffice but with large abscesses with cellulitis, drainage is best performed in the operating room. After incision and drainage, the cut edges of the abscess cavity, if actively bleeding, are sutured with fine chromic catgut. A gauze drain should be inserted to keep the ostium open until granulation is complete. Both aerobic and anaerobic bacteria can be identified in pus from such abscesses, but *Neisseria gonorrhoeae* has been identified in less than 10 percent. A broad-spectrum antibiotic should be administered until cellulitis resolves.

BARTHOLIN CYSTS. Because of pregnancy-induced hyperemia, treatment of asymptomatic cysts is best postponed until after delivery. Rarely is a labial cyst of sufficient size to cause difficulty at delivery. If so, needle aspiration will suffice as a temporary measure.

URETHRAL AND BLADDER LESIONS. Trauma to the urethra or infection of its glands may result in periurethral abscesses, cysts, and diverticulae. Abscesses usually resolve spontaneously, with asymptomatic cyst formation as a sequela. A urethral diverticulum may fill with debris that intermittently empties through the urethra to give rise to proteinuria of obscure etiology. In general, surgical excision of cysts or diverticulae should not be done during pregnancy.

Obstruction of labor by bladder stones resulting in cesarean delivery has been reported by Rai and Ramesh (1998) and by Penning and associates (1997). Hendry (1997) reviewed the literature concerning bladder tumors and concluded that cesarean delivery was required in some cases of bladder cancer.

CONDYLOMA ACUMINATA. Genital infection with the human papillomavirus results in condyloma acuminata, often called *venereal warts.* Treatment of these sexually transmitted lesions is discussed in Chapter 57 (p. 1505). In some cases, genital condyloma may be so extensive that vaginal delivery is undesirable.

FEMALE GENITAL MUTILATION. Inaccurately called female circumcision, female genital mutilation refers to medically unnecessary modification. Currently, such female mutilation is practiced in countries throughout Africa and the Middle East and in Muslim populations of Indonesia and Malaysia. It affects 80 to 110 million women worldwide. According to the World Health Organization (1992), female circumcision is significantly associated with poverty, illiteracy, and low status of women. Increasing numbers of such patients are seen by physicians in the United States. Jones and colleagues (1997) estimated that nearly 170,000 such women live in this country.

There are different kinds of surgical modifications to female genitalia. The World Health Organization (1997) classifies female genital mutilation into four types as listed in Table 35–3. Others have described three forms. *Sunna* is the only type of female genital procedure that could properly be called circumcision. It is the least extreme form and consists of a subtotal clitoridectomy, the degree of which varies. When performed under sterile conditions—which is often not the case—long-term adverse physical consequences are rare (Toubia, 1994). The second type is known as *excision.* It consists of clitoridectomy and sometimes the removal of part or all of the labia minora. More severe medical consequences of this procedure can ensue.

The third and most extreme form is known as *infibulation* or *pharaonic circumcision* (Fig. 35–11). It consists of the removal of the entire clitoris, the whole labia minora, and at least two thirds of the labia majora. The two sides of the vulva are then stitched together by silk or catgut or are held together by thorns. A small opening is left—usually made by the insertion of a matchstick—for the passage of menstrual blood and urine. The legs of the girl are then bound from hip to ankle for up to 40 days so that scar tissue will form. Infibulation has the most severe medical consequences. Knight and co-workers (1999) reported that almost 80 percent of "circumcised" women who presented to the Royal Women's Hospital in Melbourne had undergone infibulation.

The procedure is typically performed at the age of 7 years, though it is known to be practiced on girls any time between infancy and puberty. The surgery is usually performed without anesthesia by a midwife or village woman. The instruments most commonly used to perform female genital mutilation are razor blades, kitchen knives, scissors, glass, and in some regions, the teeth of the midwife.

The most immediate danger of female genital mutilation is exsanguination. Severe infections may develop within a few days. A common problem with infibulated women is urinary retention due to wound pain and a narrowly sewn introitus. Long-term complications include chronic vaginal and uterine infections, which can lead to sterility, urinary infections and increasingly dif-

TABLE 35–3. World Health Organization Classification of Female Genital Mutilation

Type 1. Excision of the prepuce with or without excision of the clitoris.

Type 2. Excision of the clitoris and partial or total excision of the labia minora.

Type 3. Excision of part or all of the external genitalia and infibulation.

Type 4. Unclassified; includes pricking, piercing, incision, stretching, and introduction of corrosive substances into the vagina.

Adapted from the World Health Organization (1997).

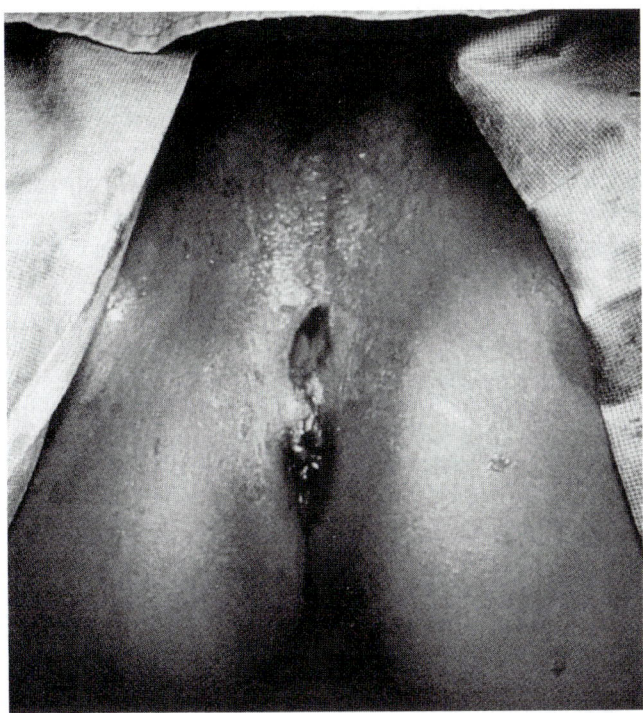

FIGURE 35–11. Infibulation: mutilation procedure done for female circumcision included clitoridectomy, excision of labia minora, incision of labia majora. Remnant labia majora have been approximated, leaving a small neo-introitus. (From Nour, 2000, with permission.)

ficult urination, dysmenorrhea, dyspareunia, and apareunia (Knight and colleagues, 1999; Nour, 2000). It may predispose to human immunodeficiency virus infection (Kun, 1997).

These women experience a number of obstetrical complications due to birth canal obstruction by scar tissue. For many reasons, they do not desire deinfibulation until pregnant. Nour (2000) recommends that this be done at midpregnancy under spinal anesthesia. If not, the scar must usually be cut open at delivery by anterior episiotomy. Failure to do so will result in severe vaginal tearing and can obstruct labor. If the circumcision scar is cut early enough, a conventional episiotomy may not be needed (Baker and colleagues, 1993). These women also suffer the consequences of anterior episiotomy such as vesicovaginal and rectovaginal fistulas.

The American College of Obstetricians and Gynecologists (1995) has long been opposed to female genital mutilation. In 1999, the College made available to its fellows a slide lecture kit containing materials that include photographs, illustrations, and case studies which address the following issues:

1. How to care for these women including during pregnancy.
2. How to discuss this procedure with such women in a culturally sensitive manner.

3. How to manage complication(s) due to these procedures.
4. How and when to refer these women for emotional and social needs.

Copies of this kit are available by calling the ACOG Distribution Center at 800-762-2264. Additional information about the ACOG Task Force on Female Circumcisions/Female Genital Mutilation can be obtained at 800-673-8444.

The Council on Scientific Affairs of the American Medical Association (1995) recommends support of legislation to eliminate the performance of female genital mutilation in the United States and to protect girls and women at risk of undergoing the procedure. The American Academy of Pediatrics (1998) similarly opposes all forms of female genital mutilation and encourages development of community educational programs for immigrant populations. We agree with Barstow (1999) that female genital mutilation is the penultimate form of gender abuse. Fortunately, albeit slowly, even in countries where this procedure has been routinely performed, laws are being enacted to prohibit such mutilation (Ciment, 1999; Eke and Nkanginieme, 1999).

VAGINAL ABNORMALITIES

PARTIAL ATRESIA. Incomplete atresia may result from scarring from injury or inflammation. Following an infection in which much of the lining of the vagina sloughs, the vaginal lumen may be obliterated almost entirely during the healing process. Injuries that lead to extensive scarring, such as trauma during rape of a child, also may cause vaginal atresia.

During labor, partial atresias are usually overcome by pressure exerted by the presenting part. Less often, manual or hydrostatic dilatation or incisions are necessary. If the structure is so resistant that spontaneous dilatation appears improbable, cesarean delivery is performed early in labor.

GARTNER DUCT CYST. These cysts may protrude into the vagina and even through the introitus to such a degree that they may be confused with a *cystocele*. During labor, cystocele may be managed successfully by bladder catheterization and upward manual pressure on the prolapsed anterior vaginal wall. A Gartner duct cyst may slip above the presenting part; if it does not, the cyst may be aspirated.

GENITAL TRACT FISTULAS FROM PARTURITION. In obstructed labor, the tissues of various parts of the genital tract may be compressed between the fetal head and the bony pelvis. If the pressure is brief, it is without significance; but if it is prolonged, necrosis results and is followed in a few days by sloughing and perforation. In most cases, the perforation develops between the vagina and the bladder, giving rise to a *vesicovaginal fistula*. Miklos and colleagues (1995) described a *vesicouterine fistula* that developed following vaginal delivery after a prior low-transverse cesarean delivery. In other rare cases, the anterior cervical lip is compressed against the symphysis pubis, and an abnormal communication eventually is established between the cervical canal and the bladder, a *vesicocervical fistula*. If the woman has no infection, the fistula may heal spontaneously. More often it persists, requiring subsequent repair.

CERVICAL ABNORMALITIES

STENOSIS. Cicatrical *cervical stenosis* may follow extensive cauterization or difficult labor associated with infection and considerable tissue destruction (Cardwell, 1988; Melody, 1957). Of the 10 cases of severe cervical dystocia following cervical treatment reported by Gibbs and Moore (1968), previous conization was responsible in six. Cryotherapy and laser therapy are less likely to produce stenosis (Spitzer and colleagues, 1995). Likewise, large-loop excision of the transformation zone (LLETZ) with diathermy loop does not seem to impair subsequent pregnancy outcome (Cruickshank and associates, 1995). Amputation of the cervix, with suturing to effect hemostasis and promote reepithelialization, may lead to stenosis, although cervical incompetence is much more likely.

Due to cervical effacement with labor, a *conglutinated cervix* may undergo complete obliteration, but the cervical os may not dilate. Thus, the presenting part is often separated from the vagina by only a thin layer of cervical tissue. Ordinarily, complete dilatation promptly follows pressure with a fingertip, although in rare instances manual dilatation or cruciate incisions may be required. Cervical stenosis almost always yields during labor.

CARCINOMA OF THE CERVIX.

Dystocia may be caused by extensive cervical infiltration by carcinoma because dilatation is inadequate even with uterine contractions. Carcinoma of the cervix complicating pregnancy is discussed in Chapter 55 (p. 1450).

UTERINE DISPLACEMENT

ANTEFLEXION. Exaggerated degrees of anteflexion frequently observed in early pregnancy are without significance. In later months, particularly when the abdominal wall is very lax, the uterus may fall forward. The sagging occasionally is so exaggerated that the fundus lies considerably below the lower margin of the symphysis pu-

bis. Marked anteflexion of the enlarging pregnant uterus usually is associated with *diastasis recti* and a pendulous abdomen. When the abnormal uterine position prevents the proper transmission of uterine contractions to the cervix, cervical dilatation, as well as engagement of the presenting part, is impeded. Marked improvement may follow maintenance of the uterus in an approximately normal position by means of a properly fitting abdominal binder.

RETROFLEXION. The retroflexed uterus is not a pathological finding in itself. Treatment is seldom needed during pregnancy, and an exception is in the rare circumstance in which the growing retroflexed uterus remains incarcerated in the hollow of the sacrum (Fig. 35–12). Women with a retroflexed uterus should be evaluated frequently early in the second trimester to ensure that the uterus is not incarcerated.

Symptoms from an incarcerated uterus usually include abdominal discomfort and inability to void. Acute urinary retention may also occur (Myers and Scotti, 1995). As pressure from the full bladder increases, small amounts of urine are passed involuntarily, but the bladder never empties entirely—*paradoxical incontinence*. Urinary obstruction can be so severe as to cause azotemia. With relief of obstruction, there may be a marked diuresis. After bladder catheterization, the uterus can usually be pushed out of the pelvis when the woman is placed in the knee-chest position. Occasionally spinal analgesia or general anesthesia will be necessary to effect repositioning. Seubert and associates (1999) used colonoscopy to dislodge an incarcerated uterus in five women. When passed above the level of the fundus, the endoscope causes anterior pressure to dislodge the uterus. A catheter is left in place until bladder tone returns. Insertion of a soft pessary usually will prevent reincarceration. Lettieri and colleagues (1994) described seven cases of uterine incarceration of which three were not relieved by these simple procedures. In two women, laparoscopy was used at 13 to 14 weeks to displace the uterus out of the pelvis using the round ligaments for traction.

SACCULATION OF THE UTERUS. Persistent entrapment of the pregnant uterus in the pelvis may result in an anterior uterine sacculation. Friedman and associates (1986) reported a posterior uterine sacculation following aggressive treatment for intrauterine adhesions (Asherman syndrome).

Rarely, the persistently entrapped uterus produces few symptoms, and yet extensive dilatation of the lower portion of the body of the uterus takes place to accommodate the fetus (Jackson and associates, 1988; Lettieri and co-workers, 1994). In one case at Parkland Hospital, at the time of cesarean delivery, the Foley catheter bulb

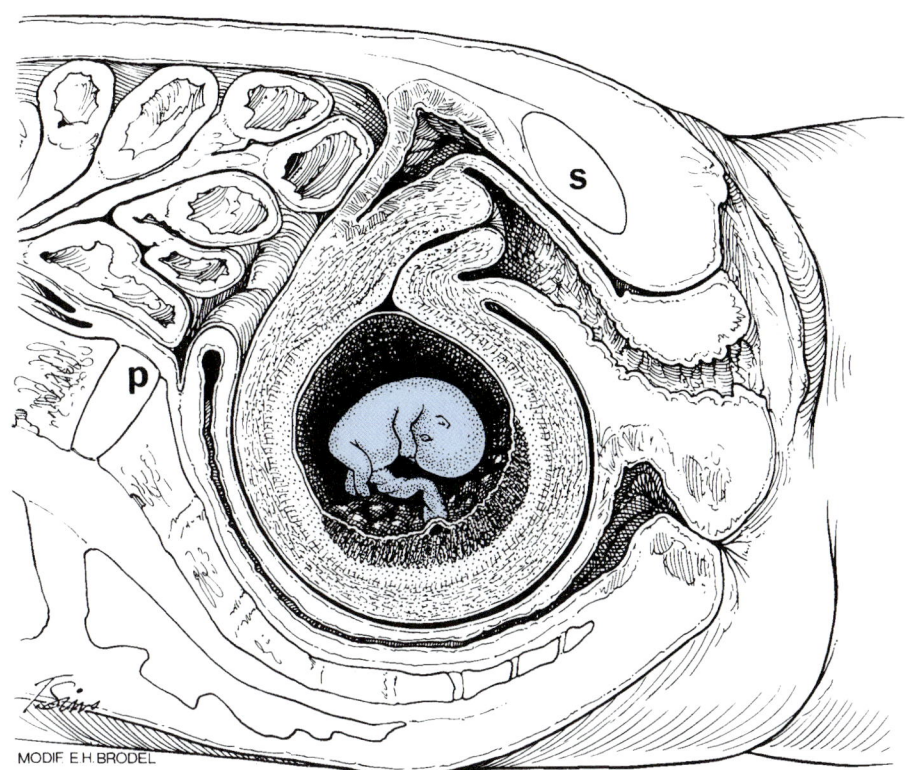

FIGURE 35-12. Incarcerated, retroflexed uterus. (p = sacral promontory, s = symphysis.)

MODIF E.H. BRODEL

lay just above the urethra in the bladder at the level of the umbilicus. The cervix was at an equally high level. Most of the 2500-g living fetus, amnionic fluid, and fetal membranes were contained in a remarkably thin sacculation of the anterior wall of the lower segment. The fetal head was entrapped in the most superior part of the sacculation, along with three loops of cord, by a constricting ring of myometrium. The fundus of the uterus and the placenta were contained in the true pelvis beneath a sharp sacral promontory. After delivery, the uterus soon contracted and retracted to assume a more normal shape.

Spearing (1978) stressed the importance of describing the distorted anatomy. He suggested that the finding of an elongated vagina passing above the level of a fetal head deeply placed into the pelvis is suggestive of a sacculation or an abdominal pregnancy. He also recommended extension of the abdominal incision to above the umbilicus and delivery of the entire gravid uterus from the abdomen before an attempt was made to incise it. **This simple procedure will restore anatomy to the correct relationships and prevent inadvertent incisions into and through the vagina and bladder.**

Engel and Rushovich (1984) reported a true uterine diverticulum confused with sacculation. Finally, uterine retroversion can be mistaken for uterine sacculations (Hill and associates, 1993).

PROLAPSE OF THE PREGNANT UTERUS. The cervix, and occasionally a portion of the body of the uterus, may protrude to a variable extent from the vulva during the early months of pregnancy. As pregnancy progresses, however, the body of the uterus usually rises above the pelvis, and may draw the cervix up with it. If the uterus persists in its prolapsed position, symptoms of incarceration may develop during the third or fourth month.

Early in pregnancy, the uterus should be replaced and held in position with a suitable pessary. If, however, the pelvic floor is too relaxed to permit retention of the pessary, the woman should be kept recumbent as long as possible until after the fourth month. If much of the cervix persists outside the vulva and cannot be replaced, the pregnancy should be terminated. Successful pregnancies and even vaginal deliveries have been reported following sacrospinous uterosacral fixation of the uterus to correct severe uterine prolapse (Kovac and Cruikshank, 1993).

CYSTOCELE AND RECTOCELE. Attenuation of fascial support that normally is interposed between the vagina and the bladder leads to prolapse of the bladder into the vagina, or cystocele. Attenuation of fascia between the vagina and the rectum results in a rectocele. Urinary stasis associated with a large cystocele predisposes to infection. A large rectocele may fill with feces that, at times, can only be evacuated manually. During labor, both lesions can block normal fetal descent unless they are emptied and pushed out of the way. A cystocele often is associated with *urinary stress incontinence* due to loss of the posterior urethrovesical angle. This may be made worse during pregnancy by the enlarging uterus and increased intra-abdominal pressure. These women have low urethral closing pressures that do not increase sufficiently to compensate for the progressive increase in bladder pressure induced by the enlarging uterus (Iosif and Ulmsten, 1981).

ENTEROCELE. In rare instances, an enterocele of considerable size filled with loops of intestine may complicate pregnancy. If symptomatic, the protrusion should be replaced and the woman kept in a recumbent position. If the mass interferes with delivery, it should be pushed up or held out of the way.

Surgical repair of uterine prolapse, cystocele, rectocele, and enterocele should not be attempted during the antepartum or intrapartum periods. Definitive repair, often with vaginal hysterectomy for associated uterine prolapse and sterilization, should be carried out after pregnancy-induced pelvic hyperemia has subsided completely.

TORSION OF THE PREGNANT UTERUS. Rotation of the pregnant uterus, most often to the right, is common during pregnancy. Torsion of sufficient degree to arrest uterine circulation and produce an acute abdominal catastrophe, however, is rare. Bakos and Axelsson (1987) reported a case of severe levotorsion associated with repeated fetal heart rate decelerations that prompted cesarean delivery. As a consequence of the extreme uterine torsion, the incision inadvertently was made in the posterior side of the uterus! As emphasized by Spearing (1978), the uterus should be removed from the abdomen prior to making the uterine incision. Sherer and colleagues (1994) stress the fact that this condition can be confused with an abdominal pregnancy (Chap. 34, p. 900). The accuracy of an antepartum diagnosis may be improved with magnetic resonance imaging and the identification of the "X" sign (Dietz and co-workers, 1998; Nicholson and associates, 1995). This sign is based upon the fact that the vagina is normally seen on magnetic resonance imaging as an H-shaped structure; but with torsion of the uterus and upper vagina, the vagina appears as an X-shaped structure. An extensive review of this subject has been provided by Jensen (1992).

UTERINE LEIOMYOMAS. Uterine leiomyomas or myomas, which are also erroneously called "fibroids," commonly are found during pregnancy. Rice and colleagues

(1989) found that 1.4 percent of over 6700 pregnancies were complicated by myomas. Katz and associates (1989) reported that 1 in 500 pregnant women were admitted for a complication related to a myoma.

Uterine myomas may be located immediately beneath the endometrial or decidual surface of the uterine cavity (*submucous*), immediately beneath the uterine serosa (*subserous*), or may be confined to the myometrium (*intramural*). An intramural myoma, as it grows, may develop a significant subserous or submucous component, or both. Submucous and subserous myomas may at times be attached to the uterus by only a stalk (*pedunculated*). These may undergo torsion with necrosis to the extent that the myoma is detached from the uterus. At times, a subserous myoma may become *parasitic*, and much or all of its blood is supplied through a highly vascularized omentum.

Myomas during pregnancy or the puerperium occasionally undergo "red" or "carneous" degeneration that is caused by *hemorrhagic infarction.* The symptoms and signs are focal pain, with tenderness on palpation and sometimes low-grade fever. Moderate leukocytosis is common. On occasion, the parietal peritoneum overlying the infarcted myoma becomes inflamed and a peritoneal friction rub develops. Red degeneration is difficult to differentiate at times from appendicitis, placental abruption, ureteral stone, or pyelonephritis, but the imaging techniques discussed later will likely prove helpful (Kawakami and associates, 1994). Treatment consists of analgesia such as codeine. Most often, signs and symptoms abate within a few days, but inflammation may stimulate labor.

Myomas may become infected during the course of puerperal metritis or septic abortion. They are especially likely to do so if the myoma is located immediately adjacent to the placental implantation site or if an instrument, such as a sound or curette, perforates the myoma. If the myoma is infarcted, the risk of infection is increased, and the likelihood of cure of the infection, except by hysterectomy, is reduced.

EFFECTS OF PREGNANCY. The stimulatory effects of pregnancy on uterine myoma growth have been noted clinically for many years. These actions were later assumed to be via estrogen and progesterone receptors that have been identified in normal uterine tissue and myomas (Soules and McCarty, 1982). Actually, the normal rapid uterine expansion that occurs during pregnancy is likely a more complex mechanism mediated in part by estrogen, progesterone, and some growth factors, especially *platelet-derived growth factor* (Mendoza and co-workers, 1990).

Estrogen receptors are reduced in number in normal myometrium during the secretory phase of the menstrual cycle and during pregnancy (Benassayag and colleagues, 1999). In myomas, estrogen receptors are present throughout the menstrual cycle, but they are suppressed during pregnancy. Progesterone receptors are present in both myometrium and myomas throughout the menstrual cycle and pregnancy. The Ki-67 cell proliferation-associated antigen is more abundant in myometrial cells during pregnancy, but it is even higher in myomas throughout the menstrual cycle and pregnancy (Kawaguchi and associates, 1991). Thus, factors that stimulate normal uterine growth during pregnancy appear to be estrogen, progesterone, various growth factors, and an increase in cells with Ki-67 antigen.

Stimulatory effects of uterine myomas in the nonpregnant woman appear to be from increased estrogen and estrogen receptors, progesterone and progesterone receptors, Ki-67 cells, and *epidermal growth factor* (EGF) (Ichimura and co-workers, 1998; Lumsden and associates, 1988). It is likely that EGF is stimulated by estrogen.

These observations support the concept that the same or similar hormonal and growth factors that normally cause uterine growth during pregnancy, also stimulate growth of leiomyomas early in pregnancy. This may serve to explain the paradoxical observations that large myomas remain unchanged or decrease in size late in pregnancy. It is likely that during pregnancy, myoma estrogen receptors are downregulated due to massive amounts of estrogen. Without effective estrogen receptors, and thus estrogen action in the myomas, epidermal growth factor binding is also decreased.

Lev-Toaff and co-workers (1987), using serial ultrasonic monitoring, observed that only half of myomas changed significantly in size during pregnancy (Table 35–4). Specifically, during the first trimester, myomas of all sizes either remained unchanged or increased in size (early response due to increased estrogen). During the second trimester, smaller myomas (2 to 6 cm) usually remained unchanged or *increased* in size, whereas larger myomas become smaller (start of downregulation of estrogen receptors). Regardless of *initial* myoma size,

during the third trimester, myomas usually remained unchanged or decreased in size (estrogen receptors downregulated). The importance of these observations is that an accurate prediction of myoma growth in pregnancy cannot be made.

EFFECTS OF MYOMA SIZE, LOCATION, AND NUMBER ON PREGNANCY. Several investigators have attempted to assess the effects on pregnancy of myoma size, location, and number (Tables 35–5 and 35–6). With respect to size alone, Rice and associates (1989) concluded that women with myomas greater than 3 cm had significantly increased rates of preterm labor, placental abruption, pelvic pain, and cesarean delivery. Tumors less than 3 cm were not clinically significant. Lev-Toaff and colleagues (1987) noted that as both size and number of myomas increased, there was a significantly higher frequency of retained placenta, fetal malpresentation, and preterm contractions. Hasan and co-workers (1990) found no association with respect to myoma size except for an increased likelihood of obstructed labor when myoma size was more than 6 cm. Davis and associates (1990) as well as Roberts and co-workers (1999) observed no relationship of complications with myoma size, location, or number.

Coronado and co-workers (2000) reviewed pregnancy outcomes in 2065 women with leiomyoma who were ascertained from Washington state birth certificates. Placental abruption and breech presentation were increased fourfold, first-trimester bleeding and dysfunctional labor twofold, and cesarean delivery sixfold. The likelihood of placental abruption appears to be increased if the placenta is in contact with or covers a uterine myoma (Table 35–6). Abortion and postpartum hemorrhage were not increased unless the placenta was adjacent to or implanted over a myoma. Although the *incidence* of postpartum hemorrhage was not increased, if hemorrhage did occur, it was massive, unrelenting, and often corrected only by hysterectomy (Hasan and associates, 1990). Lev-Toaff and colleagues (1987)

TABLE 35–4. Ultrasonically Measured Changes in Myomas During Pregnancy

	Small Myomas[a] (n = 111)			Large Myomas[b] (n = 51)		
	No Change	Increase	Decrease	No Change	Increase	Decrease
Trimester	No. (%)	No. (%)	No. (%)	No. (%)	No. (%)	No. (%)
First	7 (58)	5 (42)	0 (0)	1 (20)	4 (80)	0 (0)
Second	42 (55)	23 (30)	11 (15)	11 (38)	4 (14)	14 (48)
Third	14 (61)	1 (4)	8 (35)	5 (29)	2 (12)	10 (59)

[a] Small myomas = 2.0–5.9 cm.
[b] Large myomas = 6.0–11.9 cm.
Modified from Lev-Toaff and co-workers (1987).

TABLE 35-5. Pregnancy Complications Associated with Uterine Myomas

Study	Antepartum Pain and/or Bleeding	Placental Abruption	Preterm Ruptured Membranes	Preterm Labor	Complications (%) Abortion	Fetal Malpresentation	Postpartum Hemorrhage	Obstructed Labor	Cesarean Delivery Indicated	Elective
Winer-Muram et al (1984)	Table 35–6[a]	NS	NS	5/79 (6)	10/89 (11)	NS	Table 35–6[a]	NS	11/79 (14)	—
Lev-Toaff et al (1987)										
Uterine corpus	NS	NS	0/68	NS	6/68 (9)	NS	NS	1/68 (2)	11/68 (16)	10/68 (15)
Lower uterine segment	NS	NS	0/68	NS	0/68	NS	NS	8/45 (18)	15/45 (33)	9/45 (20)
Rice et al (1989)[a]	Table 35–6[a]	10/93 (11)	NS	20/93 (22)	NS	11/93 (12)	NS	NS	26/39 (38)	—
Katz et al (1989)	Increased	0/28	6/24 (25)	2/24 (8)	2/24 (8)	4/24 (17)	NS	NS	9/24 (38)	—
Hasan et al (1990)	NS	NS	NS	16/60 (27)	NS	22/60 (37)	10/60 (17)	9/60 (21)	24/60 (40)	20/60 (33)
Davis et al (1990)	NS	NS	6/85 (7)	15/85 (18)	NS	NS	NS	NS	NS	NS

NS = not stated.
[a] Additional data presented in Table 35–6.

928

TABLE 35–6. **Pregnancy Complications and Relationships of Myoma to Placenta**

Study	Complication	Myoma (%)	
		No Contact with Placenta	Contact with Placenta
Winer-Muram et al (1984)	Bleeding and pain	5/54 (9)	8/35 (23)
	Major complications		
	Abortion	1/54 (2)	9/35 (26)
	Preterm labor	0	5/35 (14)
	Postpartum hemorrhage	0	4/35 (11)
Rice et al (1989)	Major complications		
	Preterm labor	19/79 (24)	1/14 (7)
	Abruption	2/79 (3)	8/14 (57)
Total		48/133 (36)	35/49 (71)

found an increased incidence of retained placenta in cases with lower uterine segment myomas.

Several conclusions can be derived from these reports:

1. Growth of myomas during pregnancy cannot be predicted.
2. Placental implantation over or in contact with a myoma increases the likelihood of placental abruption, abortion, preterm labor, and postpartum hemorrhage.
3. Multiple myomas are associated with an increased incidence of fetal malposition and preterm labor.
4. Degeneration of myomas may be associated with a characteristic sonographic pattern.
5. The incidence of cesarean delivery is increased (Vergani and colleagues, 1994).

Serial ultrasonic examinations should be considered throughout pregnancy in women with uterine myomas.

CERVICAL MYOMAS. Myomas in the cervix or lower uterine segment may obstruct labor and may be confused with the fetal head. Sonograms from such a case early in pregnancy are shown in Figure 35–13. At term, cesarean hysterectomy was necessary (Fig. 35–14). Myomas that lie within or contiguous to the birth canal earlier in pregnancy may be carried upward as the uterus enlarges, with relief of obstruction to vaginal delivery. A decision regarding the method of delivery should usually not be made before the onset of labor.

IMAGING OF MYOMAS. The critical issue to be resolved after the detection of an abdominopelvic mass is its etiology. Ultrasound has helped tremendously not only in correctly identifying such masses but also in following the progression, regression, and response to therapy. Limitations of sonography in evaluating pelvic masses have been established (Exacoustos and Rosati,

1993; Kier and co-workers, 1990; Strobelt and associates, 1994). Ovarian masses (both benign and malignant), molar pregnancies, ectopic pregnancies, missed abortions, bowel abnormalities, and even fetal heads have all been confused with uterine myomas. In some cases the use of color Doppler imaging has been recommended (Kessler and colleagues, 1993; Locci and associates, 1993).

To improve accuracy, some clinicians recommend that magnetic resonance imaging supersede, or at least serve as an adjunct to ultrasound (Hricak and associates, 1992; Karasick and colleagues, 1992; Kier and co-workers, 1990). Comparisons of ultrasound with magnetic resonance imaging have been made in the same women,

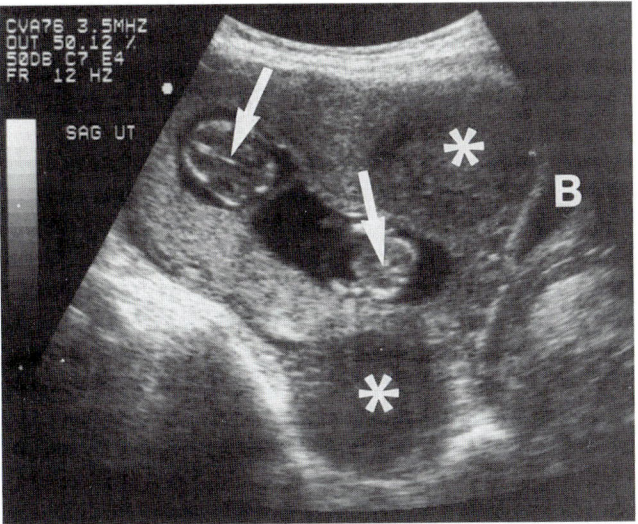

FIGURE 35–13. Two uterine myomas (*), one posterior and one anterior, are seen in this 13-week pregnancy. Arrows point to fetal head and body. (B = bladder.) (Photo courtesy of Dr. R. Santos.)

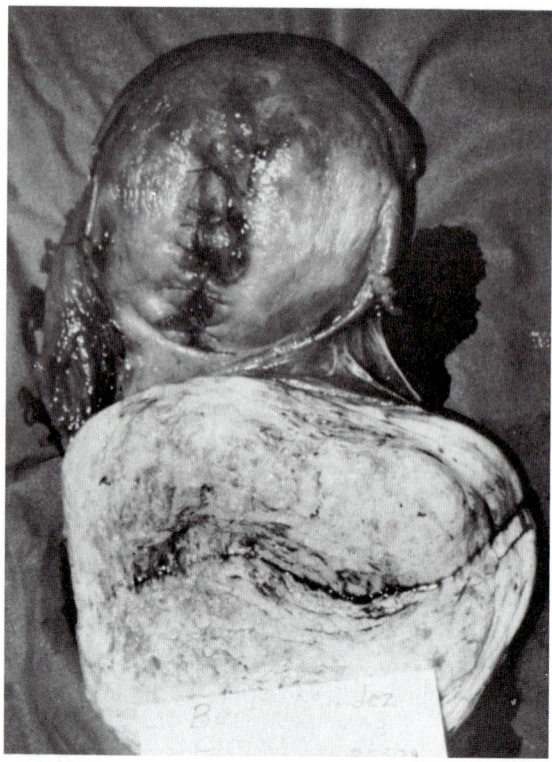

FIGURE 35-14. Same case as shown in Figure 35-13. Cesarean hysterectomy specimen. The upper mass is the body of the uterus that was just emptied by cesarean delivery. The lower mass is a huge myoma arising low in the uterus and now incised. The infant weighed 3250 g, and the uterus with myoma weighed 2900 g. Red degeneration was not found.

and magnetic resonance imaging was found superior to ultrasound, especially in correctly identifying uterine myomas (Weinreb and associates, 1990; Zawin and colleagues, 1990). Even with magnetic resonance imaging, however, errors are made in diagnosing uterine myomas (Brown and associates, 1990). This emphasizes again the importance and the difficulty in establishing a noninvasive diagnosis for an abdominopelvic mass during pregnancy. Several investigators have described techniques using magnetic resonance imaging which markedly improve the reliability of identifying uterine myomas when compared with other pelvic structures (Mayer and Shipilov, 1995; Schwartz and associates, 1998; Torashima and colleagues, 1998).

MYOMECTOMY DURING PREGNANCY. Myomectomy during pregnancy should be limited to myomas with a discrete pedicle that can be clamped and easily ligated (Burton and associates, 1989). Myomas should not be dissected from the uterus during pregnancy or at the time of delivery, because bleeding may be profuse and, at times, hysterectomy may be required. Although Glavind and associates (1990) maintain that a more

aggressive approach will not increase pregnancy losses compared with nonsurgical controls; this remains to be confirmed. Typically, myomas will undergo remarkable involution after delivery; therefore, myomectomy should be deferred until involution has occurred.

MYOMECTOMY BEFORE PREGNANCY. Removal of an intramural leiomyoma is especially hazardous for subsequent pregnancy. **After myomectomy there is a significant risk of uterine rupture during a subsequent pregnancy.** Furthermore, rupture may occur early in gestation at a time remote from labor (Golan and associates, 1990a). When a myomectomy results in a defect through or immediately adjacent to the endometrium, subsequent pregnancies should be delivered before active labor begins. Arterial embolization of uterine myomas recently has been performed in nonpregnant women (Katsumori and colleagues, 1999). The outcome and complications in pregnancies following this procedure is unknown.

ENDOMETRIOSIS. Severe, active endometriosis is an uncommon complication of pregnancy. Bizarre and vexing clinical symptoms may be caused by rupture of an endometrial cyst. There may be clinical features suggestive of pyelonephritis, acute appendicitis, or tubal pregnancy (Rossman and associates, 1983). Rarely, an enlarging pelvic endometrioma may cause dystocia; but most women with endometriosis go through pregnancy and labor without complications.

ADENOMYOSIS. Azziz (1986) reviewed the literature from the prior 80 years and reported that adenomyosis and pregnancy coexisted in 17 percent of women over age 35. Fortunately, it was rarely associated with obstetrical or surgical problems. When complications occurred, however, they were serious and included uterine rupture, ectopic pregnancy, uterine atony, and placenta previa. Live births may follow treatment of adenomyosis with gonadotropin-releasing hormone agonists (Hirata and co-workers, 1993; Silva and colleagues, 1994). The accurate, noninvasive diagnosis of adenomyosis is now possible using magnetic resonance imaging techniques (Kataoka and co-workers, 1998; Lipson and Hricak, 1996; Troiano and colleagues, 1998).

OVARIAN MASSES. Any type of ovarian mass may complicate pregnancy. The incidence of tumors and cysts varies with age groups studied, as well as the use of routine sonography during pregnancy. From their review, Katz and colleagues (1993) found an average incidence of adnexal masses of 1 in 200 pregnancies. Whitecar and associates (1999) reported an incidence of 1 in 1300 pregnancies of masses that required laparotomy. Koonings and co-workers (1988) reported finding one adnexal neoplasm for every 197 cesarean deliveries.

The most common ovarian tumors are cystic (Fig. 35–15). Whitecar and associates (1999) described 130 adnexal masses diagnosed during pregnancy; 30 percent were cystic teratomas, 28 percent were serous or mucinous cystadenomas, 13 percent were corpus luteal cysts, and 7 percent other benign cysts. Of the 130 masses, 5 percent were malignant. Half of malignancies were serous carcinomas of low-malignant potential. Similar observations were reported by Sunoo and colleagues (1990). Hopkins and Duchon (1986) found that benign cystic teratomas and corpus luteum cysts each accounted for about a third of adnexal masses. In a report by Comerci and associates (1994), half of 27 mature cystic teratomas in pregnancy were found at cesarean delivery.

The most frequent and most serious complication of benign ovarian cysts during pregnancy is torsion. This complicated 5 percent of the 130 adnexal masses reported by Whitecar and colleagues (1999). Torsion is most common in the first trimester, and may result in cyst rupture into the peritoneal cavity. Cyst rupture may also occur during labor or during surgical removal. When a tumor blocks the pelvis, it may lead to uterine rupture.

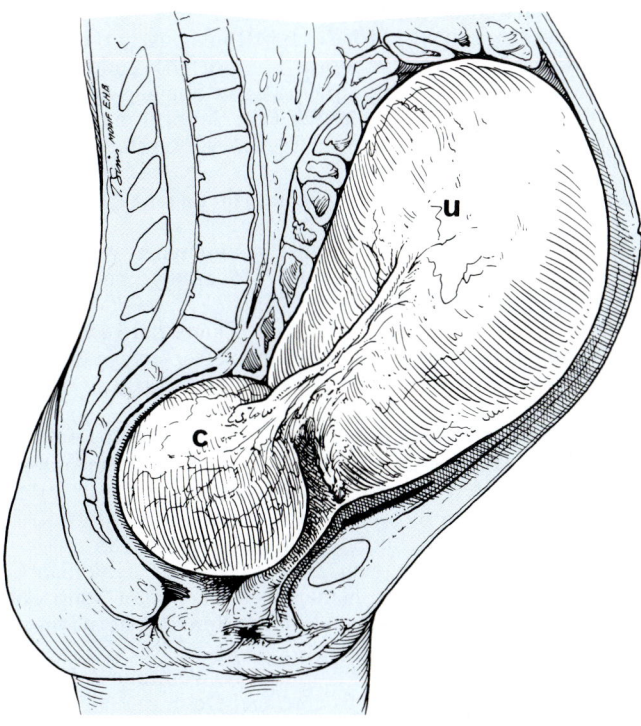

FIGURE 35–15. Ovarian cyst filling most of true pelvis and causing dystocia. (c = ovarian cyst; u = pregnant uterus.)

MANAGEMENT. Early in pregnancy, an ovary may be enlarged, creating a suspicion of neoplasm. Ovaries less than 6 cm in diameter usually are the consequence of corpus luteum formation. Thornton and Wells (1987) reported that with the advent of high-resolution sonography, a conservative approach to management of ovarian cysts might be adopted based upon their sonographic characteristics. They recommend resection of all cysts suspected of rupture, torsion, or obstruction of labor, and those over 10 cm in diameter because of the increased risk of cancer in large cysts. Cysts 5 cm or less could be left alone. Cysts between 5 and 10 cm in diameter also could be managed expectantly if they had a simple cystic appearance. Whitecar and co-workers (1999) caution against this approach because half of 41 women with a simple cyst on sonography had a neoplasm. Of these 20, there were two who had a serous tumor of low malignant potential. Most agree that if the 5- to 10-cm cysts contain septae or nodules, or if there are solid components, then the cysts should be resected.

Fleischer and associates (1990) recommend observation in asymptomatic women with masses less than 5 cm. If a mass increases in size, become symptomatic, or has sonographic characteristics that are suspicious, then malignancy should be strongly considered. Some of these changes include irregular septae, papillary excrescences, or large solid areas. Caspi and co-workers (2000) provided support for these recommendations. They described 49 women with ultrasonically diagnosed ovarian cystic teratomas that were less than 6 cm. Excluding abortions, there were 63 pregnancies during which no torsion, rupture, or labor obstruction developed.

Hess and colleagues (1988) recommend elective resection of any ovarian mass 6 cm or larger that persists after 16 weeks. They reported better perinatal outcome in such women compared with those in whom an emergency procedure was required for resection of a ruptured, twisted, or infarcted cyst. Platek and colleagues (1995) described such management of *persistent* adnexal masses that were 6 cm or greater—including those that were simple or complex. They cited an incidence of this complication as 1 in 1400 in over 43,000 women after 16 weeks. The study was retrospective and multi-institutional; thus management varied. Of 31 women with a persistent mass, 60 percent had operative intervention. Most of these (13 of 19) were benign cysts, and 6 of 19 were benign cystic teratomas. Of 12 women managed conservatively, five became symptomatic and benign ovarian cysts were drained percutaneously and had negative cytological findings. In another retrospective study, Parker and co-workers (1996) described laparoscopy between 9 and 17 weeks to remove a benign cystic teratoma in 12 women. Although 10 of 12 of these tumors—5 to 13 cm—ruptured intraoperatively, there was no evidence of peritonitis.

The major questions to be answered once a pelvic mass is discovered include the following:

1. What is the mass and is it malignant?
2. Is there a good likelihood that the mass will regress?
3. Will the mass result in dystocia and/or torsion and possible rupture?

Only time, serial ultrasonic surveillance, and labor will provide answers to the last two questions. As for the first question, Kier and associates (1990) reported that magnetic resonance imaging correctly identified the origin of unknown pelvic masses in 17 of 17 cases versus 12 of 17 cases (70 percent) using sonography. They concluded that magnetic resonance imaging was a valuable complement to sonography for preoperative evaluation. Kurjak and Zalud (1990) claim that transvaginal color Doppler assessment of tumor vascularity can be used for better characterization of adnexal tumors and may potentially be useful as a screening test for ovarian malignancy. Most clinicians recommend exploratory laparotomy if a reasonable doubt exists as to the possibility of malignancy.

TUMOR MARKERS. Measurement of serum ovarian tumor markers are rarely helpful during pregnancy. Frederiksen and associates (1991) and Montz and co-workers (1989) reported that elevated serum alpha-fetoprotein values obtained during routine screening for neural-tube defects led to the diagnosis of an immature ovarian teratoma in two women. A similar discovery of an ovarian endodermal sinus tumor was reported (van der Zee and associates, 1991). The role of tumor markers CA54/61, CASA, CA15-3, inhibin, macrophage colony-stimulating factor, and CA125 remains unproven even for management of nonpregnant women with ovarian malignancies. Thus, use of these markers during pregnancy is even more problematical (Devine and associates, 1994; Spitzer and colleagues, 1998).

CARCINOMA OF THE OVARY. Malignant ovarian neoplasms are unusual during pregnancy, but their incidence is probably increasing due to the recognition of borderline tumors of low malignant potential and the widespread use of ultrasound. The diagnosis and treatment of ovarian malignancies are discussed in Chapter 55 (p. 1452).

REFERENCES

Acien P: Reproductive performance of women with uterine malformations. Hum Reprod 8:122, 1993

Akhtar AZ: Term pregnancy in a rudimentary horn of a bicornuate uterus with foetal salvage: A case report. Asia Oceania J Obstet Gynaecol 14:143, 1988

American Academy of Pediatrics, Committee on Bioethics: Female genital mutilation. Pediatrics 102:153, 1998

American College of Obstetricians and Gynecologists: Committee opinion: Diethylstilbestrol. Committee on Gynecologic Practice, No. 131, December 1993; reaffirmed, 1996

American College of Obstetricians and Gynecologists: Committee opinion: Female genital mutilation. Committee on Gynecologic Practice, No. 151, January 1995

Andrews MC, Jones HW Jr: Impaired reproductive performance of unicornuate uterus: Intrauterine growth retardation, infertility and recurrent abortion in five cases. Am J Obstet Gynecol 144:173, 1982

Ayers JWT, DeGrood RM, Compton AA, Barclay M, Ansbacher R: Sonographic evaluation of cervical length in pregnancy: Diagnosis and management of preterm cervical effacement in patients at risk for premature delivery. Obstet Gynecol 71:939, 1988

Ayhan A, Yucel I, Tuncer ZS, Kisnisci HA: Reproductive performance after conventional metroplasty: An evaluation of 102 cases. Fertil Steril 57:1194, 1992

Azziz R: Adenomyosis in pregnancy: A review. J Reprod Med 31:223, 1986

Baker CA, Gilson GJ, Vill MD, Curet LB: Female circumcision: Obstetric issues. Am J Obstet Gynecol 169:1616, 1993

Bakos O, Axelsson O: Pathologic torsion of the pregnant uterus. Acta Obstet Gynecol Scand 66:85, 1987

Barstow DG: Female genital mutilation: The penultimate gender abuse. Child Abuse Negl 23:501, 1999

Benassayag C, Leroy MJ, Rigourd V, Robert B, Honore JC, Mignot T, Vacher-Lavenu MC, Chapron C, Ferre F: Estrogen receptors (ERalpha/ERbeta) in normal and pathologic growth of the human myometrium: Pregnancy and leiomyoma. Am J Physiol 276:E1112, 1999

Ben-Rafael Z, Seidman DS, Recabi K, Bider D, Mashiach S: Uterine anomalies. A retrospective, matched-control study. J Reprod Med 36:723, 1991

Brown JJ, Thurnher S, Hricak H: MR imaging of the uterus: Low-signal-intensity abnormalities of the endometrium and endometrial cavity. Magn Reson Imaging 8:309, 1990

Burton CA, Grimes DA, March CM: Surgical management of leiomyomata during pregnancy. Obstet Gynecol 74:707, 1989

Buttram VC: Müllerian anomalies and their management. Fertil Steril 57:416, 1983

Buttram VC, Gibbons WE: Müllerian anomalies: A proposed classification (an analysis of 144 cases). Fertil Steril 32:40, 1979

Candiani GB, Fedele L, Parazzini F, Zamberletti D: Reproductive prognosis after abdominal metroplasty in bicornuate or septate uterus: A life table analysis. Br J Obstet Gynaecol 97:613, 1990

Candiani GB, Vercellini P, Fedele L, Garsia S, Brioschi D, Villa L: Argon laser versus microscissors for hysteroscopic incision of uterine septa. Am J Obstet Gynecol 164:87, 1991

Cardwell MS: Severe cervical stenosis with the twin-to-twin transfusion syndrome. South Med J 81:940, 1988

Caspi B, Levi R, Appelman Z, Rabinerson D, Goldman G, Hagay Z: Conservative management of ovarian cystic teratoma during pregnancy and labor. Am J Obstet Gynecol 182:503, 2000

Caspi E, Schneider DF, Mor Z, Langer R, Weinraub Z, Bukovsky I: Cervical internal os cerclage: Description of a new technique and comparison with Shirodkar operation. Am J Perinatol 7:347, 1990

Chakravarty B, Konar H, Chowdhury NN: Pregnancies after

reconstructive surgery for congenital cervicovaginal atresia. Am J Obstet Gynecol 183:421, 2000

Ciment J: Senegal outlaws female genital mutilation. BMJ 318:318, 1999

Comerci JT Jr, Licciardi F, Bergh PA, Gregori C, Breen JL: Mature cystic teratoma: A clinicopathologic evaluation of 517 cases and review of the literature. Obstet Gynecol 84:22, 1994

Coronado GD, Marshall LM, Schwartz SM: Complications in pregnancy, labor, and delivery with uterine leiomyomas: A population-based study. Obstet Gynecol 95:764, 2000

Council on Scientific Affairs, American Medical Association: Female genital mutilation. JAMA 274:1714, 1995

Cruickshank ME, Flannelly G, Campbell DM, Kitchener HC: Fertility and pregnancy outcome following large loop excision of the cervical transformation zone. Br J Obstet Gynaecol 102:467, 1995

Dabirashrafi H, Bahadori M, Mohammad K, Alavi M, Moghadami-Tabrizi N, Zandinejad K, Ghafari V: Septate uterus: New idea on the histologic features of the septum in this abnormal uterus. Am J Obstet Gynecol 172:105, 1995

Daly DC, Maier D, Soto-Albors C: Hysteroscopic metroplasty: Six years' experience. Obstet Gynecol 73:201, 1989

Davis JL, Ray-Mazumder S, Hobel CJ, Baley K, Sassoon D: Uterine leiomyomas in pregnancy: A prospective study. Obstet Gynecol 75:41, 1990

de Haas I, Harlow BL, Cramer DW, Frigoletto FD Jr: Spontaneous preterm birth: A case-control study. Am J Obstet Gynecol 165:1290, 1991

Devine PL, McGuckin MA, Quin RJ, Ward BG: Serum markers CASA and CA 15-3 in ovarian cancer: All MUC1 assays are not the same. Tumour Biol 15:337, 1994

Dietz HP, Teare AJ, Wilson PD: Sacculation and retroversion of the gravid uterus in the third trimester. Aust NZ J Obstet Gynaecol 38:343, 1998

Eke N, Nkanginieme KE: Female genital mutilation: A global bug that should not cross the millenium bridge. World J Surg 23:1082, 1999

Engel G, Rushovich AM: True uterine diverticulum: A partial Müllerian duct duplication? Arch Pathol Lab Med 108:734, 1984

Exacoustos C, Rosati P: Ultrasound diagnosis of uterine myomas and complications in pregnancy. Obstet Gynecol 82:97, 1993

Fedele L, Bianchi S, Tozzi L, Marchini M, Busacca M: Fertility in women with unicornuate uterus. Br J Obstet Gynaecol 102:1007, 1995

Fedele L, Dorta M, Brioschi D, Giudici MN, Candiani GB: Pregnancies in septate uteri: Outcome in relation to site of uterine implantation as determined by sonography. Am J Roentgenol 152:781, 1989

Fedele L, Zamberletti D, D'Alberton A, Vercellini P, Candiani GB: Gestational aspects of uterus didelphys. J Reprod Med 33:353, 1988

Fedele L, Zamberletti D, Vercellini P, Dorta M, Candiani GB: Reproductive performance of women with unicornuate uterus. Fertil Steril 47:416, 1987

Fleischer AC, Dinesh MS, Entman SS: Sonographic evaluation of maternal disorders during pregnancy. Radiol Clin North Am 28:51, 1990

Fowler WC Jr, Schmidt G, Edelman DA, Kaugman DG, Fenoglio CM: Risks of cervical intraepithelial neoplasia among DES exposed women. Obstet Gynecol 58:720, 1981

Frederiksen MC, Casanova L, Schink JC: An elevated maternal serum alphafetoprotein leading to the diagnosis of an immature teratoma. Int J Gynaecol Obstet 35:343, 1991

Friedman A, DeFazio J, DeCherney A: Severe obstetric complications after aggressive treatment of Asherman syndrome. Obstet Gynecol 67:864, 1986

Garbin O, Ohl J, Bettahar-Lebugle K, Dellenbach P: Hysteroscopic metroplasty in diethylstilboestrol-exposed and hypoplastic uterus: A report on 24 cases. Human Reprod 13:2751, 1998

Gast MJ, Martin CM: Pregnancy in a woman with a uterine septum. J Reprod Med 37:85, 1992

Gibbs CE, Moore SF: The scarred cervix in pregnancy and labor. Gen Pract 37:85, 1968

Gitsch G, Riss P, Janisch H: Surgical correction of uterus abnormalities: Experiences with the Tompkins method. Geburtshilfe Frauenheilkd 50:467, 1990

Glavind K, Palvio DHB, Lauritsen JG: Uterine myoma in pregnancy. Acta Obstet Gynecol Scand 69:617, 1990

Golan D, Aharoni A, Gonen R, Boss Y, Sharf M: Early spontaneous rupture of the post myomectomy gravid uterus. Int J Gynecol Obstet 31:167, 1990a

Golan A, Caspi E: Congenital anomalies of the müllerian tract. Contemp Obstet Gynecol 37:39, 1992

Golan A, Langer R, Neuman M, Wexler S, Segev E, David MP: Obstetric outcome in women with congenital uterine malformations. J Reprod Med 37:233, 1992

Golan A, Langer R, Wexler S, Segev E, Niv D, David MP: Cervical cerclage—its role in the pregnant anomalous uterus. Int J Fertil 35:164, 1990b

Goldberg JM, Falcone T: Effect of diethylstilbestrol on reproductive function. Fertil Steril 72:1, 1999

Green LK, Harris RE: Uterine anomalies: Frequency of diagnosis and associated obstetric complications. Obstet Gynecol 47:427, 1976

Grigoris G, Camus M, Clasen K, Tournaye H, De Munck L, Devroey P: Hysteroscopic septum resection in patients with recurrent abortions or infertility. Human Reprod 13:1188, 1998

Hampton HL, Meeks GR, Bates GW, Wiser WL: Pregnancy after successful vaginoplasty and cervical stenting for partial atresia of the cervix. Obstet Gynecol 76:900, 1990

Hasan F, Arumugam K, Sivanesaratnam V: Uterine leiomyomata in pregnancy. Int J Gynaecol Obstet 34:45, 1990

Hassiakos DK, Zourlas PA: Transcervical division of uterine septa. Obstet Gynecol Surv 45:165, 1990

Heinonen PK: Limb anomalies among offspring of women with a septate uterus: Report of three cases. Early Hum Dev 56:179, 1999

Heinonen PK: Unicornuate uterus and rudimentary horn. Fertil Steril 68:224, 1997

Heinonen PK: Uterus didelphys: A report of 26 cases. Eur J Obstet Gynecol Reprod Biol 17:345, 1984

Heinonen PK: Clinical implications of the unicornuate uterus with rudimentary horn. Int J Gynaecol Obstet 21:145, 1983

Heinonen PK, Aro P: Rupture of pregnant noncommunicating uterine horn with fetal salvage. Eur J Obstet Gynecol Reprod Biol 27:261, 1988

Hendry WF: Management of urological tumours in pregnancy. Br J Urol 1:24, 1997

Herbst AL: Behavior of estrogen-associated female genital tract cancer and relation to neoplasia following intrauterine exposure to diethylstilbestrol (DES). Gynecol Oncol 76:147, 2000

Herbst AL, Hubby MM, Azizi F, Makii MM: Reproductive and gynecologic surgical experiences in diethylstilbestrol-exposed daughters. Am J Obstet Gynecol 141:1019, 1981

Herbst AL, Senekjian EK, Frey KW: Abortion and pregnancy loss among diethylstilbestrol-exposed women. Semin Reprod Endocrinol 7:124, 1989

Herbst AL, Ulfelder H, Poskanzer DC: Adenocarcinoma of the vagina. N Engl J Med 284:878, 1971

Hess LW, Peaceman A, O'Brien WF, Winkel CA, Cruikshank DW, Morrison JC: Adnexal mass occurring with intrauterine pregnancy: Report of fifty-four patients requiring laparotomy for definitive management. Am J Obstet Gynecol 158:1029, 1988

Hill LM, Chenevey P, DiNofrio D: Sonographic documentation of uterine retroversion mimicking uterine sacculation. Am J Perinatol 10:398, 1993

Hirata JD, Moghissi KS, Ginsburg KA: Pregnancy after medical therapy of adenomyosis with a gonadotropin-releasing hormone agonist. Fertil Steril 59:444, 1993

Hochner-Celnikier D, Yagel S, Beller U, Milwidsky A: Simultaneous pregnancy in each cavity of a double uterus: A case report. Int J Gynaecol Obstet 21:51, 1983

Hopkins MP, Duchon MA: Adnexal surgery in pregnancy. J Reprod Med 31:1035, 1986

Hricak H, Finck S, Honda G, Göranson H: MR imaging in the evaluation of benign uterine masses: Value of gadopentetate dimeglumine-enhanced T$_1$-weighted images. AJR 158:1043, 1992

Ichimura T, Kawamura N, Ito F, Shibata S, Minakuchi K, Tsujimura A, Umesaki N, Ogita S: Correlation between the growth of uterine leiomyomata and estrogen and progesterone receptor content in needle biopsy specimens. Fertil Steril 70:967, 1998

Iosif S, Ulmsten U: Comparative urodynamic studies of continent and stress incontinent women in pregnancy and in the puerperium. Am J Obstet Gynecol 140:645, 1981

Israel R, March CM: Hysteroscopic incision of the septate uterus. Am J Obstet Gynecol 149:66, 1984

Jackson D, Elliott JP, Pearson M: Asymptomatic uterine retroversion at 36 weeks' gestation. Obstet Gynecol 71:466, 1988

Jensen JG: Uterine torsion in pregnancy. Acta Obstet Gynecol Scand 71:260, 1992

Jones W, Smith J, Kieke B, Wilcox L: Female genital mutilation/female circumcision. Who is at risk in the U.S.? Public Health Rep 112:368, 1997

Jourdain O, Dabysing F, Harle T, Lajus C, Roux D, Dallay D: Management of septate uterus by flexible hysteroscopy and Nd:YAG laser. Inter J Gynecol Obstet 63:159, 1998

Karasick S, Lev-Toaff AS, Toaff ME: Imaging of uterine leiomyomas. AJR 158:799, 1992

Kataoka ML, Togashi K, Konishi I, Hatabu H, Morikawa K, Kojima N, Kuroda H, Fujimoto R, Kataoka N, Konishi J: MRI of adenomyotic cyst of the uterus. J Comp Assis Tomogr 22:555, 1998

Katsumori T, Nakajima K, Hanada Y: MR Imaging of a uterine myoma after embolization. AJR 172:248, 1999

Katz VL, Dotters DJ, Droegemueller W: Complications of uterine leiomyomas in pregnancy. Obstet Gynecol 73:593, 1989

Katz VL, Watson WJ, Hansen WF, Washington JL: Massive ovarian tumor complicating pregnancy. A case report. J Reprod Med 38:907, 1993

Katz Z, Ben-Arie A, Lurie S, Manor M, Insler V: Beneficial effect of hysteroscopic metroplasty on the reproductive outcome in a "T-shaped" uterus. Gynecol Obstet Invest 41:41, 1996

Kaufman RH, Adam E, Hatch EE, Noller K, Herbst AL, Palmer JR, Hoover RN: Continued follow-up of pregnancy outcomes in diethylstilbestrol-exposed offspring. Obstet Gynecol 96:483, 2000

Kaufman RH, Noller K, Adam E, Irvine J, Gray M, Jeffries JJ,

Hilton J: Upper genital tract abnormalities and pregnancy outcome in DES-exposed progeny. Am J Obstet Gynecol 148:973, 1984

Kaufman RH, Adam E, Binder GL, Gerthoffer E: Upper genital tract changes and pregnancy outcome in offspring exposed in utero to diethylstilbestrol. Am J Obstet Gynecol 137:299, 1980

Kawaguchi K, Fujii S, Konishi I, Iwai T, Nanbu Y, Nonogaki H, Ishikawa Y, Mori T: Immunohistochemical analysis of oestrogen receptors, progesterone receptors and Ki-67 in leiomyoma and myometrium during the menstrual cycle and pregnancy. Virchows Arch 419:309, 1991

Kawakami S, Togashi K, Konishi I, Kimura I, Fukuoka M, Mori T, Konishi J: Red degeneration of uterine leiomyoma: MR appearance. J Comp Assis Tomogr 18:925, 1994

Kelley JL III, Edwards RP, Wozney P, Vaccarello L, Laifer SA: Magnetic resonance imaging to diagnose a müllerian anomaly during pregnancy. Obstet Gynecol 75:521, 1990

Kessler A, Mitchell DG, Kuhlman K, Goldberg BB: Myoma vs. contraction in pregnancy: Differentiation with color Doppler imaging. J Clin Ultrasound 21:241, 1993

Kessler I, Lancet M, Appelman Z, Borenstein R: Indications and results of metroplasty in uterine malformations. Int J Gynaecol Obstet 24:137, 1986

Khalifa E, Toner JP, Jones HW Jr: The role of abdominal metroplasty in the era of operative hysteroscopy. Surg Gynecol Obstet 176:208, 1993

Kier R, McCarthy SM, Scoutt LM, Viscarello RR, Schwartz PE: Pelvic masses in pregnancy: MR imaging. Radiology 176:709, 1990

Kipersztok S, Javitt M, Hill MC, Stillman RJ: Comparison of magnetic resonance imaging and transvaginal ultrasonography with hysterosalpingography in the evaluation of women exposed to diethylstilbestrol. J Reprod Med 41:347, 1996

Knight R, Hotchin A, Bayly C, Grover S: Female genital multilation—Experience of The Royal Women's Hospital, Melbourne. Aust NZ J Obstet Gynaecol 39:50, 1999

Koonings PP, Platt LD, Wallace R: Incidental adnexal neoplasms at cesarean section. Obstet Gynecol 72:767, 1988

Kovac SR, Cruikshank SH: Successful pregnancies and vaginal deliveries after sacrospinous uterosacral fixation in five of nineteen patients. Am J Obstet Gynecol 168:1778, 1993

Kun KE: Female genital mutilation: The potential for increased risk of HIV infection. Int J Gynecol Obstet 59:153, 1997

Kurjak A, Zalud I: Transvaginal color Doppler for evaluating gynecologic pathology of the pelvis. Ultraschall Med 11:164, 1990

Lawhon BP, Wax JR, Dufort RT: Rudimentary uterine horn pregnancy diagnosed with magnetic resonance imaging. Obstet Gynecol 91:869, 1998

Leible S, Munoz H, Walton R, Sabaj V, Cumsille F, Sepulveda W: Uterine artery blood flow velocity waveforms in pregnant women with müllerian duct anomaly: A biologic model for uteroplacental insufficiency. Am J Obstet Gynecol 178:1048, 1998

Letterie GS, Vauss N: Müllerian tract abnormalities and associated auditory defects. J Reprod Med 36:765, 1991

Lettieri L, Rodis JF, McLean DA, Campbell WA, Vintzileos AM: Incarceration of the gravid uterus. Obstet Gynecol Surv 49:642, 1994

Lev-Toaff AS, Coleman BG, Arger PH, Mintz MC, Arenson RL, Toaff ME: Leiomyomas in pregnancy: Sonographic study. Radiology 164:375, 1987

Lipson SA, Hricak H: MR Imaging of the female pelvis. Radiol Clin N Amer 34:1157, 1996

Locci M, Nazzaro G, DePlacido G, Nazzaro A, DiRenzo GC: Angiogenesis: A new diagnostic aspect of obstetric and gynecologic echography. J Perinatol Med 21:453, 1993

Ludmir J, Jackson GM, Samuels P: Transvaginal cerclage under ultrasound guidance in cases of severe cervical hypoplasia. Obstet Gynecol 78:1067, 1991

Ludmir J, Landon MB, Gabbe SG, Samuels P, Mannuti MT: Management of the diethylstilbestrol-exposed pregnant patient: A prospective study. Am J Obstet Gynecol 157:665, 1987

Lumsden MA, West CP, Bramley T, Rumgay L, Baird DT: The binding of epidermal growth factor to the human uterus and leiomyomata in women rendered hypo-oestrogenic by continuous administration of an LHRH agonist. Br J Obstet Gynaecol 95:1299, 1988

Managan CE, Borow L, Burtnett-Rubin MM, Egan V, Giuntoli RL, Mikuta JJ: Pregnancy outcome in 98 women exposed to diethylstilbestrol in utero, their mothers, and unexposed siblings. Obstet Gynecol 59:315, 1982

Maneschi M, Maneschi F, Fuc'a G: Reproductive impairment of women with unicornuate uterus. Acta Eur Fertil 19:273, 1988

Mashiach S, Ben-Rafael Z, Dor J, Serr DM: Triplet pregnancy in uterus didelphys with delivery interval of 72 days. Obstet Gynecol 58:519, 1981

Mayer DP, Shipilov V: Ultrasonography and magnetic resonance imaging of uterine fibroids. Obstet Gynecol Clin N Amer 22:667, 1995

Melody GF: Obstructed cervix: A study of 100 patients. Obstet Gynecol 10:190, 1957

Mendoza AE, Young R, Orkin SH, Collins T: Increased platelet-derived growth factor A-chain expression in human uterine smooth muscle cells during the physiologic hypertrophy of pregnancy. Proc Natl Acad Sci USA 87:2177, 1990

Michaels WH, Thompson HO, Schreiber FR, Berman JM, Ager J, Olson K: Ultrasound surveillance of the cervix during pregnancy in diethylstilbestrol-exposed offspring. Obstet Gynecol 73:230, 1989

Michalas SP: Outcome of pregnancy in women with uterine malformation: Evaluation of 62 cases. Int J Gynaecol Obstet 35:215, 1991

Miklos JR, Sze E, Parobeck D, Karram MM: Vesicouterine fistula: A rare complication of vaginal birth after cesarean. Obstet Gynecol 86:638, 1995

Montz FJ, Horenstein J, Platt LD, d'Ablaing G, Schlaerth JB, Cunningham G: The diagnosis of immature teratoma by maternal serum alpha-fetoprotein screening. Obstet Gynecol 73:522, 1989

Moutos DM, Damewood MD, Schlaff WD, Rock JA: A comparison of the reproductive outcome between women with a unicornuate uterus and women with a didelphic uterus. Fertil Steril 58:88, 1992

Musich J Jr, Behrman SJ: Obstetric outcomes before and after metroplasty in women with uterine anomalies. Obstet Gynecol 52:63, 1978

Myers DL, Scotti RJ: Acute urinary retention and the incarcerated, retroverted, gravid uterus. A case report. J Reprod Med 40:487, 1995

Nagel TC, Malo JW: Hysteroscopic metroplasty in the diethylstilbestrol-exposed uterus and similar non-fusion anomalies: Effects of subsequent reproductive performance; a preliminary report. Fertil Steril 59:502, 1993

Nahum GG: Rudimentary uterine horn pregnancy: A case report on surviving twins delivered eight days apart. J Reprod Med 42:525, 1997

Nicholson HS, Blask AN, Markle BM, Reaman GH, Byrne J: Uterine anomalies in Wilms' tumor survivors. Cancer 78:887, 1996

Nicholson WK, Coulson CC, McCoy MC, Semelka RC: Pelvic magnetic resonance imaging in the evaluation of uterine torsion. Obstet Gynecol 85:888, 1995

Nicolini V, Bellotti M, Bannazzi B, Zamberletti D, Candiani GB: Can ultrasound be used to screen uterine malformations? Fertil Steril 47:89, 1987

Nour NM: Female circumcision and genital mutilation: A practical and sensitive approach. Contemp Ob/Gyn 45:50, 2000

Nwosu UC, Thatcher S: Pregnancy in a non-communicating uterine horn mimicking incarceration with sacculation of a retroflexed uterus. Acta Obstet Gynecol Scand 72:580, 1993

O'Leary JL, O'Leary JA: Rudimentary horn pregnancy. Obstet Gynecol 22:371, 1963

Oliva GC, Fratoni A, Genova M, Romanini C: Uterine motility in patients with bicornuate uterus. Int J Gynaecol Obstet 37:7, 1992

Parker WH, Childers JM, Canis M, Philips DR, Topel H: Laparoscopic management of benign cystic teratomas during pregnancy. Am J Obstet Gynecol 174:1499, 1996

Penning SR, Cohen B, Tewari D, Curran M, Weber P: Pregnancy complicated by vesical calculus and vesicocutaneous fistula. Obstet Gynecol 176:728, 1997

Platek DN, Henderson CE, Goldberg GL: The management of a persistent adnexal mass in pregnancy. Am J Obstet Gynecol 173:1236, 1995

Raga F, Bauset C, Remohi J, Bonilla-Musoles F, Simón C, Pellicer AN: Reproductive impact of congenital Müllerian anomalies. Human Reprod 12:2277, 1997

Raga F, Bonilla-Musoles F, Blanes J, Osborne NG: Congenital Müllerian anomalies: Diagnostic accuracy of three-dimensional ultrasound. Fertil Steril 65:523, 1996

Rai L, Ramesh K: Obstructed labour due to a vesical calculus. Aust NZ J Obstet Gynaecol 38:474, 1998

Ravasia DJ, Brain PH, Pollard JK: Incidence of uterine rupture among women with mullerian duct anomalies who attempt vaginal birth after cesarean delivery. Am J Obstet Gynecol 181:877, 1999

Rice JP, Kay HH, Mahony BS: The clinical significance of uterine leiomyomas in pregnancy. Am J Obstet Gynecol 160:1212, 1989

Roberts WE, Fulp KS, Morrison JC, Martin JN Jr: The impact of leiomyomas on pregnancy. Aust NZ J Obstet Gynecol 39:43, 1999

Rolen AC, Choquette AJ, Semmens JP: Rudimentary uterine horn: Obstetric and gynecologic implications. Obstet Gynecol 27:806, 1966

Rossman F, D'Ablaing G III, Marrs RP: Pregnancy complicated by ruptured endometrioma. Obstet Gynecol 62:519, 1983

Salle B, Sergeant P, Gaucherand P, Guimont I, de Saint Hilaire P, Rudigoz RC: Transvaginal hysterosonographic evaluation of septate uteri: A preliminary report. Hum Reprod 11:1004, 1996

Schwartz LB, Zawin M, Carcangiu ML, Lange R, McCarthy S: Does pelvic magnetic resonance imaging differentiate among the histologic subtypes of uterine leiomyomata? Fertil Steril 70:580, 1998

Seidman DS, Ben-Rafael Z, Bider D, Recabi K, Mashiach S: The role of cervical cerclage in the management of uterine anomalies. Surg Gynecol Obstet 173:384, 1991

Senekjian EK, Potkul RK, Frey K, Herbst AL: Infertility

among daughters either exposed or not exposed to diethylstilbestrol. Am J Obstet Gynecol 158:493, 1988

Seubert DE, Puder KS, Goldmeier P, Gonik B: Colonoscopic release of the incarcerated gravid uterus. Obstet Gynecol 94:792, 1999

Sherer DM, Smith SA, Sanko SR: Uterine sacculation sonographically mimicking an abdominal pregnancy at 20 weeks' gestation. Am J Perinatol 11:350, 1994

Silva PD, Perkins HE, Schauberger CW: Live birth after treatment of severe adenomyosis with a gonadotropin-releasing hormone agonist. Fertil Steril 61:171, 1994

Soules MR, McCarty KS Jr: Leiomyomas: Steroid receptor content. Am J Obstet Gynecol 143:6, 1982

Spearing GJ: Uterine sacculation. Obstet Gynecol 51:11S, 1978

Spitzer M, Herman J, Krumholz BA, Lesser M: The fertility of women after cervical laser surgery. Obstet Gynecol 86:504, 1995

Spitzer M, Kaushal N, Benjamin F: Maternal CA-125 levels in pregnancy and the puerperium. J Reprod Med 43:387, 1998

Strobelt N, Ghidini A, Cavallone M, Pensabene I, Ceruti P, Vergani P: Natural history of uterine leiomyomas in pregnancy. J Ultrasound Med 13:399, 1994

Sunoo CS, Terada KY, Kamemoto LE, Hale RW: Adnexal masses in pregnancy: Occurrence by ethnic group. Obstet Gynecol 75:38, 1990

Teti G, Maffei S, Pippi E, Fioretti P: Reproductive capacity and outcome of pregnancy after metroplasty following the technique of Bret-Palmer partially modified in the pathological symmetric malformations of müllerian ducts. Clin Exp Obstet Gynecol 18:65, 1991

Thijssen RF, Hollanders JM, Willemsen WN, van der Heyden PM, van Dongen PW, Rolland R: Successful pregnancy after ZIFT in a patient with congenital cervical atresia. Obstet Gynecol 76:902, 1990

Thornton JG, Wells M: Ovarian cysts in pregnancy: Does ultrasound make traditional management inappropriate? Obstet Gynecol 69:717, 1987

Torashima M, Yamashita Y, Matsuno Y, Takahashi M, Nakahara K, Onitsuka Y, Ohtake H, Tanaka N, Okamura H: The value of detection of flow voids between the uterus and the leiomyoma with MRI. JMRI 8:427, 1998

Toubia N: Female circumcision as a public health issue. N Engl J Med 331:712, 1994

Troiano RN, Flynn SD, McCarthy S: Cystic adenomyosis of the uterus: MRI. J Magn Reson Imaging 8:1198, 1998

Van der Zee AG, de Bruijn HW, Bouma J, Aalders JG, Oosterhuis JW, de Vries EG: Endodermal sinus tumor of the ovary during pregnancy: A case report. Am J Obstet Gynecol 164:504, 1991

Vercellini P, Fedele L, Arcaini L, Rognoni MT, Candiani GB: Value of intrauterine device insertion and estrogen administration after hysteroscopic metroplasty. J Reprod Med 34:447, 1989

Vercellini P, Rossi R, Pagnoni B, Fedele L: Hypervolemic pulmonary edema and severe coagulopathy after intrauterine dextran instillation. Obstet Gynecol 79:838, 1992

Vergani P, Ghidini A, Strobelt N, Roncaglia N, Locatelli A, Lapinski RH, Mangioni C: Do uterine leiomyomas influence pregnancy outcome? Am J Perinatol 11:356, 1994

Weinreb JC, Barkoff ND, Megibow A, Demopoulos R: The value of MR imaging in distinguishing leiomyomas from other solid pelvic masses when sonography is indeterminate. Am J Roentgenol 154:295, 1990

Welker B, Krebs D, Lang N: Pregnancy following repair of a congenital atresia of the uterine cervix and upper vagina. Arch Gynecol Obstet 243:51, 1988

Whitecar P, Turner S, Higby K: Adnexal masses in pregnancy: A review of 130 cases undergoing surgical management. Am J Obstet Gynecol 181:19, 1999

Wiersma AF, Peterson LF, Justema EJ: Uterine anomalies associated with renal agenesis. Obstet Gynecol 47:654, 1976

Winer-Muram HT, Muram D, Gillieson MS: Uterine myomas in pregnancy. J Assoc Can Radiol 35:168, 1984

World Health Organization: Female genital mutilation: A joint WHO/UNICEF/UNFPA statement. Geneva: World Health Organization, 1997

World Health Organization, International Federation of Gynecology and Obstetrics: Female circumcision. Eur J Obstet Gynecol Reprod Biol 45:153, 1992

Zanetti E, Ferrari LR, Rossi G: Classification and radiographic features of uterine malformations: Hysterosalpingographic study. Br J Radiol 51:161, 1978

Zawin M, McCarthy S, Scoutt LM, Comite F: High-field MRI and US evaluation of the pelvis in women with leiomyomas. Magn Reson Imaging 8:371, 1990

Zorlu CG, Yalçin H, Ugur M, Özden S, Kara-Soysal S, Gökmen O: Reproductive outcome after metroplasty. Int J Gynecol Obstet 55:45, 1996

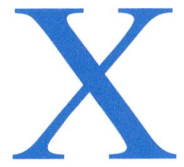

SECTION

X

Fetal Abnormalities

INHERITED AND ACQUIRED DISORDERS

36

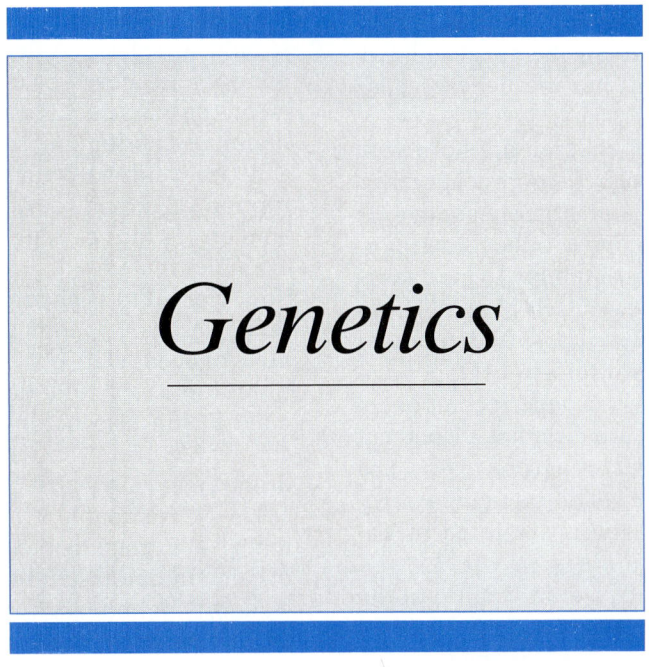

Genetics

Simply put, genetics is the study of biological variation. Medical genetics is the investigation of individual variation in the incidence of and susceptibility to disease, as well as disease mechanisms, response to therapy, and results of genetic tests. The genetic basis of normal biological variation as well as that of many common diseases is rapidly being elucidated, and soon will be incorporated into the daily practice of medicine.

Between 2 and 3 percent of children are born with a congenital birth defect. By age 18, approximately 8 percent are discovered to have one or more anomalies. While correct, these figures comprise only a small portion of genetic disease. Both susceptibility to most common diseases as well as the disease itself have a genetic basis. Finally, most cancers develop as the result of cumulative mutations. Thus, two thirds of the population will experience a disease with a genetic component in their lifetime, and if cancers are included, 91 percent will be affected (Rimoin and colleagues, 1997). The types and estimated frequencies of all categories of genetic conditions by age at diagnosis are listed in Table 36–1.

The **Human Genome Project,** a joint venture of the United States Department of Energy and the National Institutes of Health, has as its goal the mapping of the complete human genome. As the result of unprecedented worldwide cooperation from both the private and public sectors, this enterprise was completed in 2000, and nearly 3 years ahead of schedule (Collins, 1999). It is hoped that mapping the approximately 80,000 genes that comprise the haploid human genome will facilitate further studies of normal and abnormal gene function, and will provide the basis for future diagnosis and therapy. Within a decade or so, consideration of genetic background and specific traits and susceptibilities may thus become part of routine patient care. If true, then knowledge of genetic principles will be essential for all practitioners.

ETIOLOGY OF BIRTH DEFECTS

Birth defects can arise in at least three ways (Fig. 36–1). In a **malformation** the fetus or structure is genetically abnormal and thus "programmed" to develop abnormally. An example is limb contractures resulting from diastrophic dysplasia. A **deformation** is when a genetically normal fetus develops in an abnormal uterine environment, causing structural changes. An example is oligohydramnios causing limb contractures. In a **disruption,** a genetically normal fetus suffers an insult resulting in disruption of normal development. An example is early amnion rupture causing limb deformities. These three examples illustrate that identical-appearing abnormalities, referred to as **phenocopies,** can have widely varying etiologies. It is apparent that phenocopies make the diagnosis of even relatively simple defects difficult.

Multiple structural defects or developmental abnormalities can also occur together in one individual. A cluster of several anomalies or defects can be a **syndrome,** meaning that all the abnormalities have the same cause—for example, trisomy 18; a **sequence,** meaning that all abnormalities occurred sequentially as the result of one initial insult—for example, oligohydramnios leading to pulmonary hypoplasia, limb contractures, and facial deformities; or an **association,** meaning that these particular anomalies occur together frequently, but do not seem to be linked etiologically—for example, *CHARGE association,* which is combination of *colo*boma, *h*eart defects, *a*tresia choanae, mental *r*etardation, *g*rowth deficiency, and *e*ar anomalies. Classification of anomalies can thus be challenging, and reclassification may be required as more is learned.

In this chapter the various known genetic causes of disease are considered, starting with the most obvious defects such as chromosomal abnormalities, and proceeding to the most obscure, illustrated by genetic imprinting. Descriptions of certain genetic diseases are provided for illustrative purposes only, with the caveat that these descriptions may be rendered incomplete or

TABLE 36–1. Types and Frequency of Genetic Disease by Age

Type	Frequency by Age 25 (per 1000 live births)	Lifetime Frequency (per 1000 live births)
Chromosome disorders	1.8	4
Single-gene disorders	3.6	20
Multifactorial disease	46.4	646
Somatic cell (cancer) disease	—	240
Total	52	910

Adapted from Baird and colleagues (1988).

Types of Problems in
MORPHOGENESIS

Poor Formation
of Tissue

Unusual Forces
on Normal Tissue

Breakdown
of Normal Tissue

MALFORMATION
or
Malformation Sequence

DEFORMATION
or
Deformation Sequence

DISRUPTION
or
Disruption Sequence

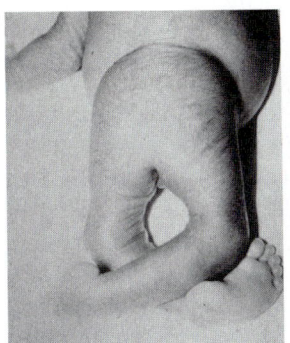 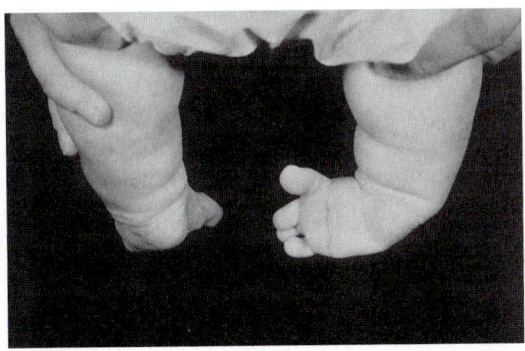 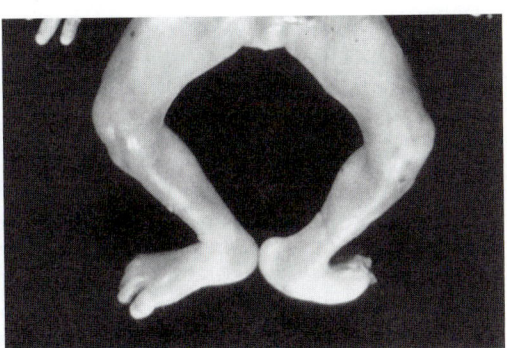

FIGURE 36–1. The three major types of problems in morphogenesis. **Malformation Sequence** (left): infant with diastrophic dysplasia which results in multiple joint contractures due to abnormal connective tissue. **Deformation Sequence** (center): infant experienced prolonged oligohydramnios from 17 weeks until birth. **Disruption Sequence** (right): infant has limb and body wall defects that resulted from disruption after early amnion rupture and localized hemorrhages. (Adapted from Graham, 1988, with permission.)

even inaccurate as understanding of the genetic basis of disease advances.

CHROMOSOMAL ABNORMALITIES

STANDARD NOMENCLATURE. By convention, karyotypes are reported using nomenclature agreed upon by the genetics community and codified in 1985 by the International System for Human Cytogenetic Nomenclature (ISCN). The total number of chromosomes is listed first, and corresponds to the number of *centromeres* present. This is followed by the sex chromosomes (XX or XY), and then by a description of any variation or abnormality detected. Specific abnormalities are indi-

cated by standard abbreviations, such as *dup* (*duplicated*), *der* (*derivative*), *t* (*translocated*), and many more. The standard nomenclature for writing a karyotype is shown in Table 36–2.

Chromosome abnormalities figure prominently in assessments of the impact of genetic disease, viz, 50 percent of embryonic deaths, 5 to 7 percent of fetal losses, 6 to 11 percent of stillbirths and neonatal deaths, and 0.9 percent of live-born children (Hook, 1992; Tolmie, 1995).

ANEUPLOIDY. There are a total of 44 autosomes, arranged in pairs numbered from 1 to 22, and one pair of sex chromosomes. The most obvious or easily recognized chromosomal abnormalities are numerical. In

TABLE 36–2. Standard Nomenclature for Chromosome Karyotypes

Karyotype	Description
46,XY	Normal male chromosome constitution
47,XX,+21	Female with trisomy 21 Down syndrome
47,XY,+21/46,XY	Male who is a mosaic of trisomy 21 cells and normal cells
46,XY,del(4)(p14)	Male with distal deletion of the short arm of chromosome 4 band designated 14
46,XX,dup(5p)	Female with duplication of the short arm of chromosome 5
45,XY,−13,−15,t(13q;14q)	A male with a balance Robertsonian translocation of chromosome 13 and karyotype shows that one normal 13 and one normal 14 are missing
46,XY,t(11;22)(q23;q22)	A male with a balanced reciprocal translocation between chromosomes 11 and 22; breakpoints are at 11q23 and 22q22
46,XX,inv(3)(p21;q13)	An inversion of chromosome 3 that extends from p21 to q13; because it includes the centromere, this is a pericentric inversion
46,X,r(X)	A female with one normal X chromosome and one ring X chromosome
46,X,l(xq)	A female with one normal X chromosome and an isochromosome of the long arm of the X chromosome

From Jorde and colleagues (1995), with permission.

TABLE 36–3. Estimates of Frequency of Chromosomal Abnormalities in a Population of Unselected Newborns

	Incidence	
	Per 1000 Births	Per Birth
Sex chromosomes		
Male	1.15	1/870
Female	0.75	1/1333
Autosomal trisomy	1.42	1/700
Structural abnormality		
Unbalanced	0.61	1/1600
Balanced	5.22	1/200
Triploidy	0.02	1/50,000
Total	9.17	1/109

Adapted from Jacobs and colleagues (1992), with permission.

these, the affected individual inherits an extra chromosome—**trisomy;** is missing a chromosome—**monosomy;** or has an abnormal number of haploid chromosome complements—**polyploidy.** The estimated incidence of aneuploidy and other chromosomal abnormalities among unselected newborns is shown in Table 36–3. The incidence of chromosome abnormalities of 9 per 1000 is derived from data using high-resolution banding (350 to 550 bands), which allows accurate identification of deletions and rearrangements. While the pathophysiological basis of all aneuploidy is not completely understood, most trisomies and nonmosaic monosomies result from an abnormality in meiosis.

TRISOMY. Numerical abnormalities most often result from nondisjunction, in which the chromosomes pair up properly but then fail to separate. They can also occur after premature separation of the paired chromosomes,

or from failure to pair up in the first place (Gardner and Sutherland, 1996; Sherman and colleagues, 1991). The risk of nondisjunction increases with maternal age (Table 36–4). Oocytes are held suspended in midprophase of meiosis I from birth until ovulation, in some cases for 50 years! Aging is thought to break down chiasmata that keep paired chromosomes aligned. When meiosis is completed at the time of ovulation, nondisjunction leads to one daughter gamete receiving two copies of the chromosome in question, resulting in trisomy. The other gamete receives no copies, leading to monosomy if fertilized.

Although 3 to 4 percent of sperm and 10 to 20 percent of oocytes are aneuploid as the result of meiotic errors, these abnormal gametes are less likely to result in conception than normal gametes. If fertilization does occur, selection results in early loss of most aneuploid conceptions. Each of the 23 chromosome pairs is equally likely to be involved in a segregation error (Kamiguchi and associates, 1993). Despite this, only a few trisomies are typically identified because those causing the most severe abnormalities result in preimplantation or early loss. For example, trisomy 1 has never been reported even in the earliest abortus tissue. Trisomy 16 accounts for 16 percent of all first-trimester loss, but it is never seen later in pregnancy. Of the autosomal aneuploidies associated with survival past the first trimester, trisomies 13, 18, and 21 can result in term viable pregnancies in 57, 14, and 70 percent cases respectively (Table 36–5). In their review, McIntosh and colleagues (1995) confirmed that 32 percent of Down syndrome fetuses in women 35 years and older are lost in the interval between chorionic villus sampling at 10 weeks and amniocentesis at 16 weeks; half are lost by term.

TABLE 36–4. Regression-derived Estimated Rates (per 1000 Births) of Cytogenetic Abnormalities by Maternal Age at the Time of Amniocentesis

Maternal Age (years)	47,+21	47,+18	47,+13	47,XXX	47,XXY	Other Clinically Significant	All Abnormalities
33	2.4	0.3	0.4	0.4	0.4	1.1	4.6–5.4
35	4.0	1.0	0.5	0.6	0.6	1.3	7.4–8.0
37	6.7	1.8	0.8	0.8	1.0	1.4	12.1–12.2
40	14.5	3.3	1.0	1.4	1.9	1.7	25.0–23.8
43	31.1	8.8	1.5	2.4	3.8	2.0	51.9–47.5
45	51.8	10.8	2.0	3.4	5.9	2.3	84.3–78.0
47	88.2	18.9	2.7	4.9	9.3	2.6	137.1–122.8
49	143.5	26.9	3.8	7.0	14.8	2.9	222.9–198.6

From Hook and colleagues (1983), with permission.

MONOSOMY. Although non-dysfunction leads to both nullisomic and disomic gametes, there is no clinically recognized association between maternal age and monosomy. Most likely, monosomy is almost universally incompatible with life, and monosomic conceptuses are lost prior to implantation (Garber and co-workers, 1996). As a rule, missing a portion of chromosomal material is much more devastating to the organism than having extra chromosome material. One exception is *monosomy X*, or *Turner syndrome*. Although it accounts for about 20 percent of first-trimester loss, a small proportion survive.

POLYPLOIDY. Abnormalities of ploidy account for about 20 percent of early losses and are rarely seen in late pregnancies. Two thirds of **triploidy** cases result from fertilization of one egg by two sperm. The remainder are caused by failure of one of the meiotic divisions, resulting in a diploid chromosome complement in the egg or more frequently, the sperm. If the extra set of chromosomes is paternal, the result is usually a partial hydatidiform mole, and no fetal structures are detected (Chap. 32, p. 836). Rarely, a fetus develops. In this situation, the origin of the extra chromosomes determines the phenotype. With an extra maternal haplotype (digynic), the fetus and placenta will be severely growth restricted. If the extra haplotype is paternal (diandric), the fetus may be relatively normal in size but the placenta will be abnormally large and cystic. Triploides of either kind can be dysmorphic. If a woman has a triploid pregnancy involving a fetus that survived past the first trimester, the recurrence risk is 1 to 1.5 percent, which justifies offering prenatal diagnosis in subsequent pregnancy (Gardner and Sutherland, 1996).

Tetraploids are always 96,XXXX or 92,XXYY, indicating that they result from postzygotic failure to com-

TABLE 36–5. Incidences of Common Aneuploids According to Gestational Age

Chromosomal Defect	Loss Rate (%)		Observed
	Estimated		
	10 Weeks–Birth	16 Weeks–Birth	16 Weeks–Birth
Trisomy 21	47	31	30
Trisomy 18	86	74	86
Trisomy 13	83	71	43
Turner syndrome	76	52	75
47,XXX	~5	~3	0
47,XXY	~5	~3	1
47,XYY	~5	~3	3
Triploidy	> 99	> 99	100

From Snijders and colleagues (1995), with permission.

plete an early cleavage division (Thompson and colleagues, 1991). The recurrence risk for tetraploidy is minimal.

PATERNAL EFFECTS. Unlike advanced maternal age, there is no association between aneuploidy and paternal age. This likely is because aneuploid sperm cannot fertilize an egg. Advanced paternal age does, however, logarithmically increase the risk of new mutations causing autosomal dominant diseases (Friedman, 1981). These new mutations may also be a factor in early pregnancy loss. The absolute frequency of new autosomal dominant mutations among newborns whose fathers are 40 years old is at least 0.3 percent. In one example, Orioli and colleagues (1995) compared nonfamilial cases of three diseases caused relatively frequently by new mutations—achondroplasia, thanatophoric dysplasia, and osteogenesis imperfecta—with matched controls. Half of neonates with achondroplasia and thanatophoric dwarfism, and a third of those with osteogenesis imperfecta, were born to fathers above age 35. Marfan syndrome is another example.

There is some evidence that paternal age may affect the incidence of isolated structural abnormalities (McIntosh and colleagues, 1995). Finally, paternal chromosome abnormalities are increased when conception is induced by **intracytoplasmic sperm injection (ICSI).** These fetuses are at increased risk to have Y chromosome deletions (In't Velt and colleagues, 1997). They do not appear to be at risk for other chromosome abnormalities (ESHRE Task Force, 1998; Loft and associates, 1999).

AUTOSOMAL TRISOMIES

TRISOMY 21. This is also called **Down syndrome** after J.L.H. Down who described it in 1866. A trisomy 21 karyotype is shown in Figure 36–2. Its incidence is 1 in 800 to 1000 newborns. Because it is the most common nonlethal trisomy, this condition is the focus of most genetic screening and testing protocols. Almost 95 percent of Down syndrome is due to maternal nondisjunction of chromosome 21—75 percent during meiosis I and 25 percent in meiosis II. The remaining cases result from mosaicism or translocation. Affected children have marked hypotonia, tongue protrusion, and a small head, flattened occiput, flat nasal bridge, and epicanthal folds with up-slanting palpebral fissures (Fig. 36–3). There is frequently loose skin at the nape of the neck, short and stubby fingers, and a single palmar crease, and the fifth fingers are curved inward (clinodactyly) due to absence or hypoplasia of the middle phalanx. Associated major abnormalities include heart defects (particularly endocardial cushion defects) in 30 to 40 percent, gastrointestinal atresias, neonatal or childhood leukemia, and thyroid disease. The intelligence quotient (IQ) ranges from 25 to 50, with a few individuals testing higher, and most affected children have social skills averaging 3 to 4 years ahead of their mental age. The chromosome region responsible for the mental deficit is located at 22q 22.13 to 22.2.

RECURRENCE RISK. Once a woman has had a child with trisomy 21 resulting from nondisjunction, her risk to have another with any trisomy is 1 percent until her age-related risk exceeds this; then her age-related risk predominates. This justifies offering invasive prenatal diagnosis. Parental chromosome studies are not necessary unless the trisomy was due to a translocation (approximately 3 percent).

Females with Down syndrome are fertile, and approximately a third of their offspring will have Down syndrome (Scharrer and colleagues, 1975). Males are almost always sterile, and only one case of reproduction has been reported (Simpson and associates, 1982).

TRISOMY 18. This is known as **Edward syndrome** and occurs in 1 in 8000 newborns. The incidence is much higher in the first trimester, but 85 percent of fetuses with this syndrome are lost between 10 weeks and term (Snijders and colleagues, 1995).

Trisomy 18 fetuses and neonates are usually growth restricted with a mean birthweight of 2340 g. Striking facial features include prominent occiput, rotated and malformed auricles, short palpebral fissures, and a small mouth (Jones, 1997). Virtually every organ system can be affected by trisomy 18. Almost 95 percent have cardiac defects, most commonly ventricular or atrial septal defect or patent ductus arteriosus. Horseshoe kidney, radial aplasia, hemivertebrae, clinched hands with overlapping fingers, and syndactyly may be present. Hernias, diastasis, or imperforate anus may be evident. These infants are usually feeble, have frequent apneic spells, and half die in the first week. Another 45 percent die before one year and those who survive past 12 months are profoundly retarded. There are rare reports of individuals with trisomy 18 surviving to age 10 or more.

In view of the extremely poor outcome, prenatal diagnosis should prompt discussion of pregnancy termination. If not chosen, the mode of delivery must be discussed. Because it is extremely unlikely that cesarean delivery will change the outcome, it is reasonable to plan vaginal delivery regardless of whether the fetus tolerates labor, recognizing that intrapartum fetal demise may occur. Fetuses with trisomy 18 commonly have fetal heart rate abnormalities during labor. Schneider and colleagues (1989) reported that the primary cesarean delivery rate was 56 percent in 48 pregnancies—85 percent of these were performed for "fetal distress."

TRISOMY 13. Known as **Patau syndrome,** trisomy 13 occurs in approximately 1 in 20,000 births. Common

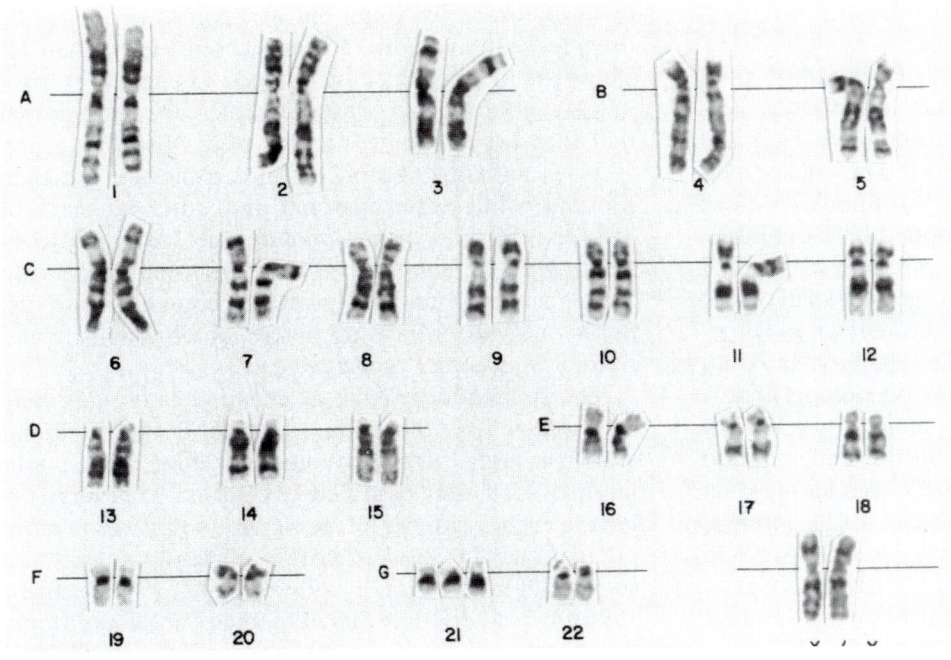

FIGURE 36-2. Abnormal female karyotype with trisomy 21, consistent with Down syndrome; 47,XXX +21. (Courtesy of Dr. Nancy R. Schneider.)

abnormalities include cardiac defects in 80 to 90 percent and holoprosencephaly in 70 percent. Other abnormalities are moderate microcephaly, microphthalmia, cleft lip and/or cleft palate, abnormal ears, omphalocele, polycystic kidneys, and radial aplasia. The occurrence of *cutis aplasia* (localized punched-out appearing scalp defects) and *polydactyly* together strongly suggests either trisomy 13 or the usually lethal deletion 4p. The median survival for infants is about 3 days, and 90 percent die within the first month. The few surviving trisomy 13 individuals are profoundly retarded. Counseling is approached as previously described with trisomy 18.

OTHER TRISOMIES. It is rare to see live-born infants with other autosomal trisomies, although mosaicism involving a few other autosomal chromosomes has been reported. Information concerning characteristic malformation patterns and genetic counseling for these aneuploidies can be provided by a genetic counselor.

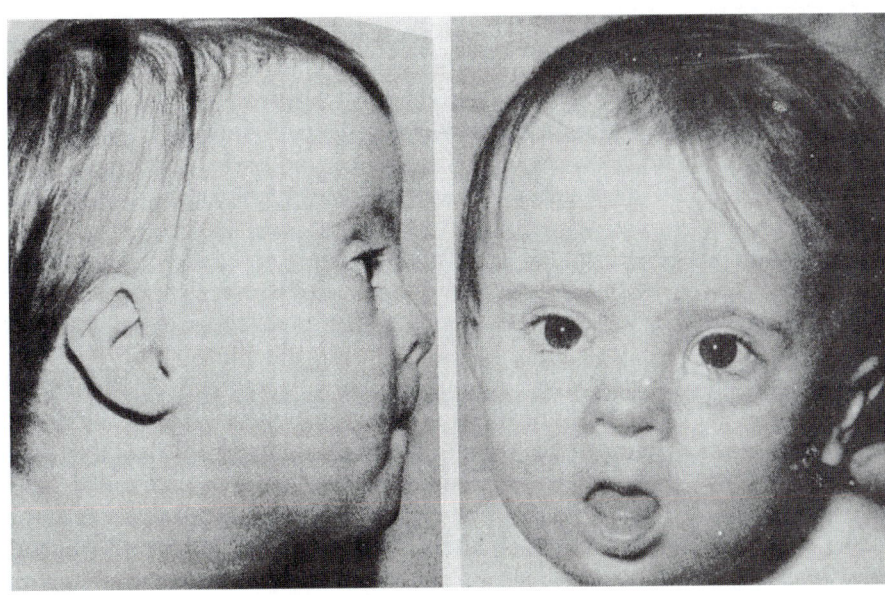

FIGURE 36-3. Young infant with Down syndrome, trisomy 21. (From Jones, 1997, with permission.)

SEX CHROMOSOME ABNORMALITIES

XXX AND XXY. Robinson and colleagues (1991) used Barr-body analysis to screen 40,000 infants consecutively born at two Denver hospitals between 1964 and 1974. Karyotypes were performed on those who screened positive, and 43 (1 in 930) infants with sex chromosome aneuploidy were identified. These children were then followed prospectively with annual physical and psychometric evaluations until age 24. Females with 47,XXX and males with 46,XXY (also known as Klinefelter syndrome) had very similar phenotypes. Both tended to be tall, but had no striking phenotypic abnormalities. Pubertal development in females was usually normal, but XXY males did not virilize and required testosterone therapy. While XXX females had normal fertility, XXY males were more likely to be infertile from gonadal dysgenesis and to have gynecomastia and small testicles. Neither XXX or XXY was strongly associated with mental retardation, but there was a great deal of variability in intellectual function. The IQ range was 71 to 122 and the mean IQ of XXY males was 95 while that of XXX females was 87—both within normal limits, but lower than controls. Most XXX and XXY study subjects have developmental problems, speech disabilities, and neuromotor and learning disabilities.

Females with more than three X chromosomes (48,XXXX; 49,XXXXX) are likely to have physical abnormalities that are apparent at birth, and to exhibit varying degrees of mental retardation. For both males and females, a drop in IQ occurs with each additional X chromosome.

47,XYY. These males are tall but phenotypically normal. They generally have normal intelligence, although their IQs may be lower than those of their siblings. They often have learning disabilities. The syndrome was once associated with criminal or violent behavior, and the XYY karyotype has even been used as a defense in several sensational murder trials (Brogger, 1985). Most early reports were biased, however, because prisoners or men with serious psychological dysfunction were tested preferentially. In their prospective study, Robinson and colleagues (1997) found only an increased risk of emotional difficulties, including mild depression, and increased hyperactivity and aggressiveness in XYY men.

Males with more than two extra Y chromosomes (48,XYYY) or with both additional X and Y chromosomes (48,XXYY; 49,XXXYY) have obvious physical abnormalities and significant mental retardation.

45,X. This is called **Turner syndrome** and it is the only monosomy compatible with life. It is the most common aneuploidy in abortuses and accounts for 20 percent of chromosomally abnormal first-trimester losses. Its prevalence in live-born infants is about 1 in 5000 births. There are three distinct phenotypes. The first comprises 98 percent of 45,X conceptuses which are so abnormal that they are spontaneously aborted. A second group survives until the second or third trimester, but then presents with cystic hygroma and other stigmata of Turner syndrome, or as a fetal demise. Incredibly, considering the outcomes for the majority, the third group has a phenotype mild enough to be compatible with life. Survivors usually have relatively minor problems and normal intellectual capacity.

The tremendous range of phenotypes of 45,X may be explained by the finding that 45,X abortuses and stillbirths are generally nonmosaic with only one population of 45,X cells identified. In contrast, 45,X survivors have a high incidence of mosaicism with two or more populations of cells identified; for example, some 45,X; some 46,XX or XY (Held and colleagues, 1992; Saenger, 1996). It is likely that this nonlethal Turner syndrome does not occur as the result of maternal age-related meiotic nondisjunction, but rather as the result of a postzygotic mitotic error. This causes one population of cells in a zygote to lose an X chromosome during mitotic cleavage. The missing X chromosome does not appear to be lost randomly, as the maternal X is retained in 80 percent of all surviving 45,X cases (Cockwell and colleagues, 1991; Hassold and associates, 1991). If ultimately the majority of cells are 45,X, that individual will have the Turner phenotype, but modified by the presence of the other cell populations (Koeberl and co-workers, 1995). Several large studies have shown that up to half of surviving women with Turner syndrome are mosaics; the remainder may have mosaicism expressed only in tissues that are not routinely tested (Fernandez, 1996; Kim, 1999; Nazarenko, 1999, and their colleagues).

Women with a 45,X or 45,X mosaic karyotype usually have a fairly specific phenotype. This includes short stature, broad chest with widely spaced nipples, congenital lymphedema with puffy fingers and toes, low hairline with webbed posterior neck, and minor bone and cartilage abnormalities. Ovarian dysgenesis and infertility are found in over 90 percent, who will require life-long hormone therapy beginning just before adolescence. Mosaicism can modify this phenotype, for example, a 46,XY cell line usually results in increased height. Some mosaic individuals with a normal 46,XX cell line may reproduce, although as a rule they have premature ovarian failure (Saenger, 1996). Between 30 and 50 percent have a major cardiac malformation, and most of these have aortic coarctation or bicuspid aortic valves and may develop subsequent aortic dissection. Intelligence is generally in the normal range, however, 45,X females have visual–spatial organization deficits and difficulty with nonverbal problem solving and interpretation of subtle social cues (Jones, 1997).

Deletions of portions of the X chromosome can also produce features of Turner syndrome. Deletion or complete absence of the short arm of the X chromosome results in short stature, while loss of the long arm results in streak ovaries and amenorrhea. As discussed later, the same phenotypes are found with isochromosomes consisting of either the long or short arms of X.

CHROMOSOMAL DELETIONS. A deletion refers to a portion of a chromosome that is missing. These are usually described by the location of the two chromosomal break points or, if the deletion is common, by an eponym—for example, **del 5p** is also called **cri du chat syndrome.** Most deletions occur during meiosis and result from malalignment or mismatching during pairing of homologous chromosomes. If the two chromosomes are not aligned properly, the unaligned loop may be deleted (Fig. 36–4). If the mismatch remains and the two chromosomes recombine, the result may be a deletion in one and a duplication in the other. If a deletion is identified, the parents should be tested to find if it is associated with a familial translocation that would have a recurrence risk.

CHROMOSOMAL BANDING. Recognition of a deletion during cytogenetic analysis is facilitated by various staining methods used to create light and dark chromosome bands. These banding patterns are unique and allow identification of each chromosome as well as recognition of missing segments. Recently, several genetic conditions have been identified that are caused by **microdeletions**—deletions too small to be detected by older methods. These may be recognized with high-resolution banding and molecular techniques, or by fluorescence in situ hybridization using a probe for the deleted region (Driscoll and colleagues, 1993; Korf, 2000).

The genes in a deleted chromosome segment often control individual traits. **Contiguous gene deletion syndromes** usually involve serious but unrelated phenotypic and functional abnormalities. Although deletions can occur in any area of any chromosome, some now discussed are found more frequently than expected by chance alone. This is probably because certain regions are predisposed to breakage.

DELETION 4p. Known as **Wolf-Hirschhorn syndrome,** this is deletion of material from the short arm of chromosome number 4. There is marked fetal growth restriction, hypotonia, characteristic facial appearance, severe mental deficiency, and posterior midline scalp defects (cutis aplasia). Children often have severe seizures and seldom survive childhood. Approximately 85 percent of deletions occur de novo, and in 80 percent the deleted chromosome is paternal.

DELETION 5p. The partial deletion of the short arm of chromosome 5 causes the **cri du chat syndrome.** Affected infants are growth restricted, hypotonic, and severely retarded. They are sometimes identified by their mewling, high-pitched, catlike cry, attributed to abnormal laryngeal development.

SHPRINTZEN SYNDROME AND DIGEORGE SEQUENCE. These both result from the same 22q11.2 microdeletion (Driscoll and colleagues, 1993). Shprintzen syndrome is also called **velo-cardio-facial syndrome.** Individuals with this deletion have cleft palate, velopharyngeal incompetence, prominent nose, a long face with retruded mandible, cardiac defects, learning difficulties, and short stature. By contrast, the DiGeorge sequence is characterized by thymus hypo- or aplasia, parathyroid hypo- or aplasia, and aortic arch malformations. Typical facies includes short palpebral fissures, micrognathia with a short philtrum, and ear anomalies. Mental development and heights are usually normal.

It has been hypothesized that DiGeorge and Shprintzen syndromes represent two extremes of a spectrum of abnormalities associated with the identical deletion. It is also possible that each condition represents a separate contiguous gene deletion syndrome of genes located at 22q11.2, but that current cytogenetic methods cannot distinguish differences between the two.

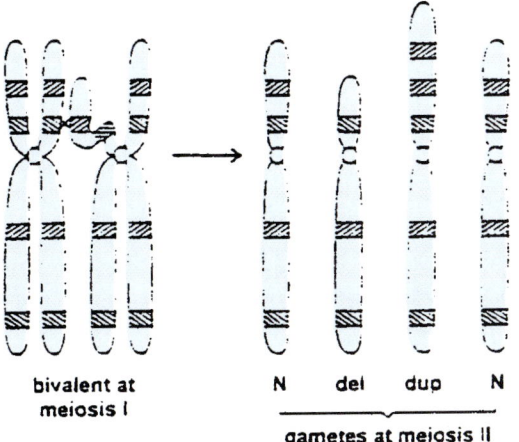

bivalent at meiosis I

N   del   dup   N

gametes at meiosis II

FIGURE 36–4. One mechanism to produce a duplication and a deletion. Similar sequences (crosshatched segments) exist at numerous places along the chromosome. Misalignment of two nonhomologous sequences, followed by illegitimate recombination within these two sequences (X), produces recombinant products that are reciprocally imbalanced: one with a duplication of the chromatin between the two sequences, and the other with a deficiency. (From Gardner and Sutherland, 1996, with permission.)

CHROMOSOMAL TRANSLOCATIONS

RECIPROCAL TRANSLOCATIONS. A reciprocal or double-segment translocation is a rearrangement of chromosomal material in which breaks occur in two different chromosomes. The fragments are exchanged before the breaks are repaired. The rearranged chromosome is called a **derivative (der) chromosome.** If no chromosomal material is gained or lost in this process, it is a *balanced translocation.* Although the transposition of chromosome segments can cause abnormalities due to repositioning of specific genes, in most cases genetic function in the balanced carrier is not affected. Offspring who inherit either the two normal chromosomes or the two translocated chromosomes are also usually normal. Despite this, Fryns and associates (1992) reported a 6.4 percent total risk (including background) for anomalies with a balanced translocation.

Carriers of a balanced translocation can produce unbalanced gametes that result in abnormal offspring. As shown in Figure 36–5, if one of the translocated chromosomes and one of the normal co-chromosomes are included in the oocyte or sperm, the result is monosomy for part of one chromosome and trisomy for part of another. The observed risk for each translocation can be provided by a genetic counselor, but in general, translocation carriers identified after the birth of an abnormal child have a 5 to 30 percent risk of having unbalanced

offspring. Carriers identified for other reasons, for example, during an infertility workup, have up to 5 percent risk, probably because their conceptions with unbalanced chromosome segments are nonviable.

ROBERTSONIAN TRANSLOCATIONS. These result from the centric fusion of two acrocentric chromosomes, which are 13, 14, 15, 21, and 22 (Fig. 36–2). Robertsonian translocations are common. Their incidence in newborns is approximately 1 in 1000, which is equal to all other translocations combined. Almost all translocations involve chromosome 14, with material translocated to 13, 14, or 15 most commonly (Levitan, 1988). Fusion at the centromeres results in the loss of one centromere and the *satellite regions* on the short arms. These regions contain only genes coding for ribosomal RNA, which are also present in multiple copies on other acrocentric chromosomes. As long as the fused q arms are intact, the translocation carrier is usually phenotypically normal. The normal carrier of a robertsonian translocation will have only 45 chromosomes because the number of centromeres determines the chromosome count.

Robertsonian carriers have reproductive difficulties. If the fused chromosomes are homologous, for example, made up of both copies of chromosome 21, the carrier makes only unbalanced gametes. Each egg or sperm contains either two copies of the translocated chromo-

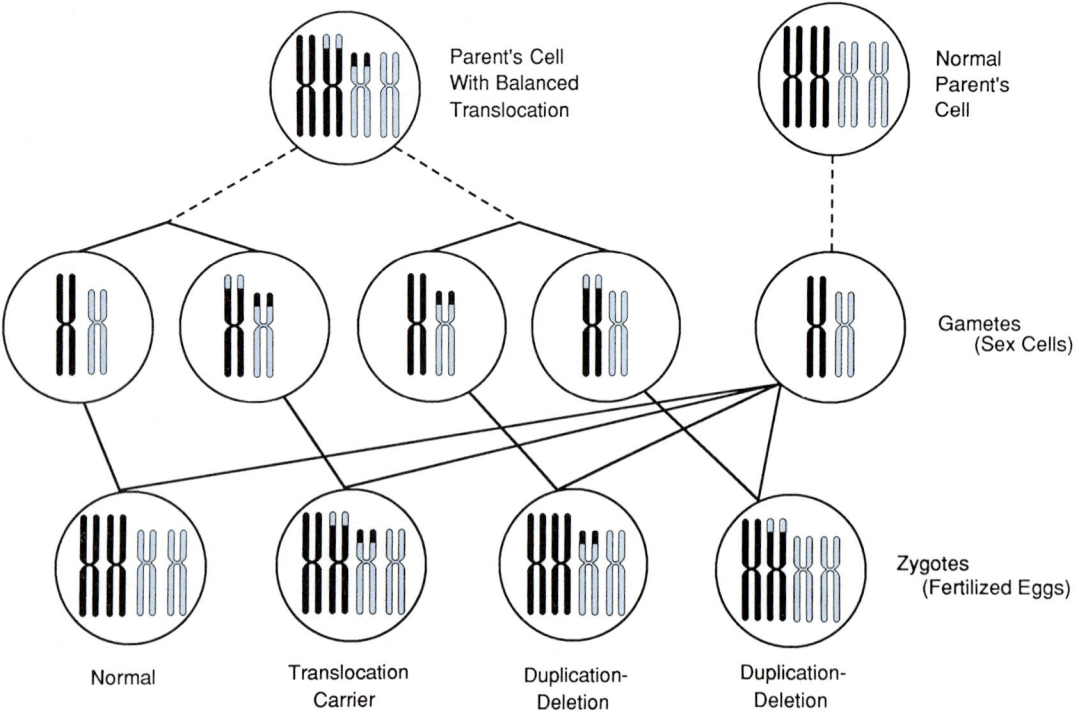

Parent's Cell With Balanced Translocation

Normal Parent's Cell

Gametes (Sex Cells)

Zygotes (Fertilized Eggs)

Normal   Translocation Carrier   Duplication-Deletion   Duplication-Deletion

FIGURE 36–5. Gametes produced by a balanced translocation carrier. (From Greenwood Genetics Center, 1995, with permission.)

some which would result in trisomy if fertilized, or no copy, which results in monosomy.

The fused chromosomes may be nonhomologous. While the most common translocation involves 14 and 21, any acrocentric chromosomes can be involved. Gametes produced in this situation could have any of six potential chromosome combinations, of which four would result in abnormal offspring. In general, the recurrence risk is 15 percent if carried by the mother, and 2 percent if carried by the father because several possible gametes would be nonviable. Robertsonian translocations are not a major cause of miscarriage and occur in less that 5 percent of couples with recurrent pregnancy loss (Smith and Gaha, 1990). Still, identification of these translocations has tremendous impact on reproductive plans, and may have implications for other family members. Chromosome studies should be obtained on both parents if their offspring is found to have a translocation trisomy. When robertsonian translocations occur spontaneously, neither parent is a carrier and the recurrence risk is low.

ISOCHROMOSOMES. These are composed of either two q (long) arms or two p (short) arms of one chromosome fused together. Isochromosomes are thought to arise when the centromere breaks transversely instead of longitudinally during meiosis II or mitosis. They also may result from a meiotic error in a chromosome with a robertsonian translocation. Robertsonian 21/21 translocation is a kind of isochromosome. An isochromosome made up of an acrocentric chromosome (q arms only) behaves like a homologous robertsonian translocation in that no important genetic material is lost. In these cases, the carrier is usually phenotypically normal but produces only abnormal gametes. Conversely, when an isochromosome involves nonacrocentric chromosomes that have p arms containing functional genetic material, the carrier is usually phenotypically abnormal and produces abnormal gametes. One of these isochromosomes is frequently lost during cell division. Thus, all the genes located on the lost chromosome will be deleted, and phenotypic abnormalities specific to that gene deletion result. An example is *isochromosome X*. The carrier has an isochromosome with two q arms but is missing all the genes from the p arm. This causes the full Turner syndrome phenotype including streak gonads. An individual with an X isochromosome composed of only the two p arms has streak gonads, but not the short stature or any other characteristic features of the 45,X phenotype.

CHROMOSOMAL INVERSIONS. These inversions result when two breaks occur in the same chromosome, and the intervening genetic material is inverted before the breaks are repaired. Although no genetic material is lost or duplicated, the rearrangement may alter gene function. **Paracentric inversions** are those in which the inverted material is from only one arm, and the centromere is not within the inverted segment (Fig. 36–6). The carrier has either normal (balanced) gametes, or gametes that are so abnormal as to preclude fertilization. Thus, although infertility may be a problem, the risk of abnormal offspring is extremely low.

Pericentric inversions occur when the breaks are in each arm, and the inversion includes the centromere. Because of problems in alignment during meiosis, the carrier is at high risk to produce abnormal offspring. The risk can be calculated individually for each unique inversion. In general, however, the observed risk is 5 to 10 percent if ascertainment occurred after the birth of an abnormal child, and 1 to 3 percent if ascertainment occurred by some other means (Gardner and Sutherland, 1996).

RING CHROMOSOMES. When there are deletions from both ends of a chromosome, the ends may unite, forming a ring chromosome. If the deletions are substantial, the carrier is phenotypically abnormal. If only the telomeres are lost, all important genetic material is retained and the carrier is essentially balanced. However, the ring disrupts cell division during meiosis. This causes abnormal growth of many tissues with small stature, borderline to moderate mental deficiency, and minor dysmorphisms (Gardner and Sutherland, 1996).

A ring chromosome may occur de novo or may be inherited from a carrier. In all cases of parent-to-child transmission, the mother is the carrier. This may be because a ring chromosome somehow compromises spermatogenesis. The clinical significance of a ring chromosome depends on the amount and function of the lost genetic material. *Ring X chromosome* is associated with Turner syndrome. The ring configuration may interfere with normal chromosomal segregation and production of abnormal gametes and pregnancy loss.

CHROMOSOMAL MOSAICISM. This is defined as two or more cytogenetically distinct cell lines in the same individual. In many cases, mosaicism is a cell-culture artifact that must be differentiated from true mosaicism (Claussen and co-workers, 1984). While true mosaicism is rarely encountered either in a fetus or in amniocytes, *placental mosaicism* is relatively common. Chorionic villus sampling has shown that 2 percent of placentas are mosaic, although the associated fetus is usually normal (Henderson and associates, 1996). Such *confined placental mosaicism* likely results from nondisjunction during early mitotic divisions in one or more cells destined to become the placenta. Another mechanism is that the conceptus was trisomic, but "correction" occurred and the extra chromosome was lost in all fetal

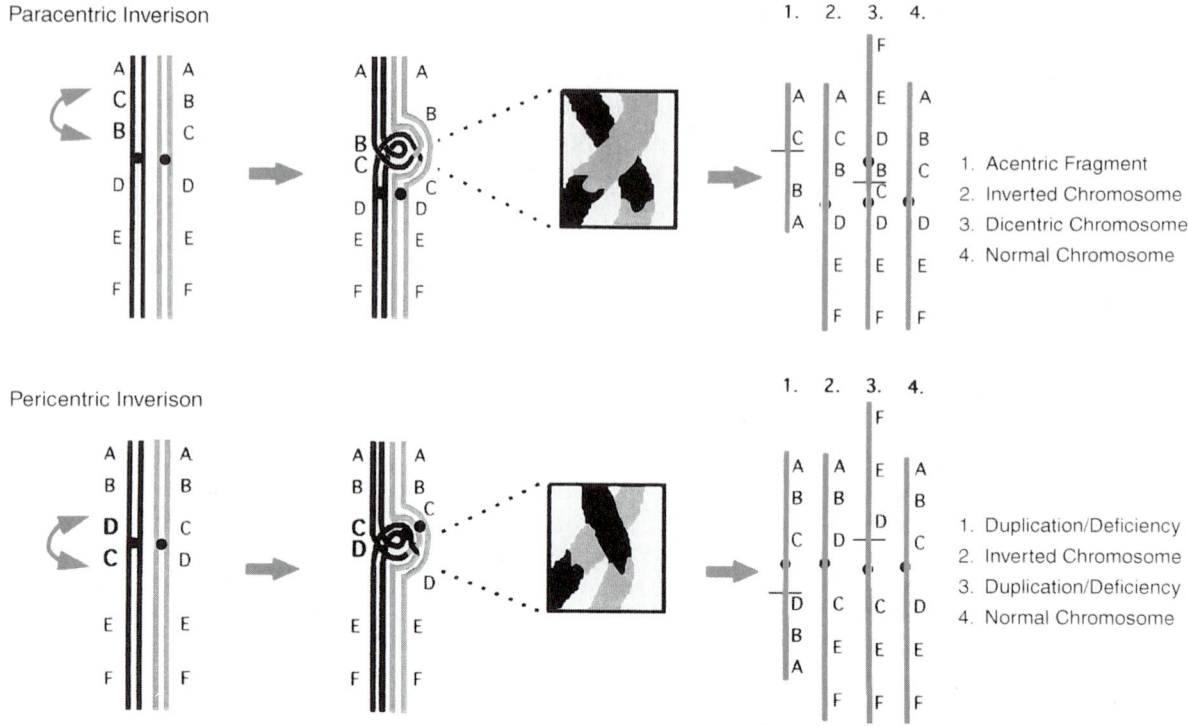

FIGURE 36–6. Meiosis in chromosomes with pericentric and paracentric inversions. (Adapted from Greenwood Genetics Center, 1995, with permission.)

cells but only in some placental cells. Mosaicism likely is chromosome specific, and with chromosomes 2, 7, 8, 10, and 12, it is usually caused by mitotic error. Alternatively, mosaicism for chromosomes 9, 16, and 22 tends to result from partial correction of a meiotic error (Robinson and colleagues, 1997).

Phenotypic expression of mosaicism depends on many factors, including whether the cytogenetically abnormal cells involve the placenta, the fetus, parts of the fetus, or some combination. If an individual with somatic mosaicism has a high percentage of abnormal cells, the phenotype may be abnormal. Conversely, the phenotype of an aneuploid fetus may be ameliorated by a co-population of normal cells. Suspected but unproven mosaicism may accout for the phenotype of surviving fetuses with Turner syndrome as discussed earlier. This may also explain phenotypic variation in some trisomic individuals who have high function.

Confined placental mosaicism may also have either positive or negative effects. It may play a role in survival of some cytogenetically abnormal fetuses. For example, trisomy 18 and 13 fetuses that survive to term may do so only because of early "correction" of the trisomy in some cells destined to become trophoblasts (Kalousek and co-workers, 1989). Conversely, some cytogeneti-

cally normal but severely growth-restricted fetuses may have placental chromosomal abnormalities that presumably impair placental and thus fetal growth (Kalousek and Dill, 1983). In these cases, the trisomic cells destined to become the fetus lost the extra chromosome (corrected), while some cells that became the placenta remained trisomic. Growth restriction is also influenced by which chromosome was lost during the "correction." If the fetus has two normal copies of the chromosome in question, but both copies came from the same parent, growth may also be impaired. This is referred to as *uniparental disomy* and is discussed later.

Gonadal mosaicism is confined to the gonads and may arise as the result of a mitotic error in the zygote. If the error occurs in cells destined to become the gonad, a portion of the germ cells may be abnormal. Because spermatogonia and oogonia continue to divide throughout fetal life, gonadal mosaicism could also occur as the result of a meiotic error in previously normal dividing germ cells. Gonadal mosaicism may explain de novo autosomal dominant mutations in the offspring of normal parents, causing such diseases as achondroplasia or osteogenesis imperfecta, or X-linked diseases such as Duchenne muscular dystrophy. It also explains the recurrence of such diseases in more than one offspring in a previously unaffected family. Because of the potential for gonadal mosaicism, the recurrence risk after the birth of a child with a disease due to a "new" mutation is approximately 6 percent.

SINGLE-GENE (MENDELIAN) DISORDERS

A mendelian disorder is caused by a mutation or alteration in a single locus or gene, in one or both members of a gene pair. Approximately 0.4 percent of the population has a genetic abnormality caused by a single-gene mutation discovered by age 25, and 2 percent will have single-gene disorder diagnosed during their lifetime (Table 36–1). As of December 2000, 12,126 monogenic disorders had been identified. While they are classified according to their mode of inheritance—11,357 autosomal, 632 X-linked, 37 Y-linked, and 60 mitochondrial—it must be emphasized that it is the *phenotype* that is dominant or recessive, not the genes. In some dominant diseases, for example, the normal gene may still be directing the production of normal protein, but the phenotype is determined by protein produced by the abnormal gene. Likewise, the heterozygous carrier of some recessive diseases may produce detectable levels of the abnormal gene product, but does not display features of the disease because the phenotype is directed by the product of the normal co-gene.

The expression of many so-called single gene disorders is strongly influenced by modifying genes, or by alterations in a combination of additional genes, often with environmental influences. Some common "single-gene disorders" affecting adults are listed in Table 36–6. Although transmission patterns of these diseases are consistent with mendelian inheritance, their phenotypes are strongly influenced by modifying genes and environmental factors. Ironically, although single-gene (mendelian) disorders were the first genetic conditions identified, diseases caused solely by single genes are actually relatively rare.

AUTOSOMAL DOMINANT. If only one member of a gene pair determines the phenotype, that gene is considered to be dominant. Likewise, a gene with a dominant mutation specifies the phenotype in preference to the normal gene. The carrier of a gene causing an autosomal dominant disease has a 50 percent chance of passing on the affected gene with each conception. Importantly, several factors influence the ultimate phenotype of the affected individual.

PENETRANCE. This term describes whether or not the mutant gene is expressed at all. A dominant gene with some kind of recognizable phenotypic expression in all individuals who carry the gene has 100 percent pene-

TABLE 36–6. Some Relatively Frequent Mendelian Disorders Affecting Adults

Autosomal Dominant

Achondroplasia

Acute intermittent porphyria

Adult polycystic kidney disease

BRCA1 and BRCA2 breast cancer

Familial hypercholesterolemia

Familial hypertrophic cardiomyopathy

Hereditary hemorrhagic telangiectasia

Hereditary spherocytosis

Huntington chorea

Marfan syndrome

Myotonic dystrophy

Neurofibromatosis

Osteogenesis imperfecta tarda

Polyposis of the colon

Tuberous sclerosis

von Willebrand disease

Autosomal Recessive

Albinism

Cystic fibrosis

Deafness

Friedrich ataxia

Hemochromatosis

Hereditary emphysema

Homocystinuria

Phenylketonuria

Sickle-cell anemia

β-Thalassemia

Wilson disease

X Linked

Chronic granulomatous disease

Color blindness

Fabry disease

Fragile X syndrome

Glucose-6-phosphate deficiency

Hemophilia A and B

Hypophosphatemic rickets

Muscular dystrophy

Ocular albinism

Testicular feminization

From Goldstein and Brown (1994).

trance. If the carrier of the abnormal gene displays *no* features of the associated disease, the gene is not penetrant. Penetrance is thus described by only two options, yes or no. The degree of penetrance of a specific gene is usually quantitatively expressed as the ratio of gene carriers who have any phenotypic characteristics associated with the altered gene to the total number of gene carriers. A gene that is 80 percent penetrant is expressed in some way in 80 percent of individuals who have that gene. Incomplete or reduced penetrance explains why some autosomal dominant diseases appear to "skip" generations.

Some mechanisms responsible for reduced penetrance have been elucidated in various disorders. For example, in retinoblastoma, reduced penetrance is explained by the fact that an individual carrying the gene must also acquire a somatic mutation affecting the normal retinoblastoma allele in order to develop the disease. If the normal allele is not mutated, the disease is not penetrant. Reduced penetrance does not explain all skipped generations. In some disorders, there is delayed onset of disease. Symptoms of Huntington disease, for example, may not become apparent until age 40. If the parent of an affected individual died before the abnormal gene had been expressed, the gene would appear to have skipped that generation.

EXPRESSIVITY. This refers to the *degree* to which the phenotypic features are expressed. If all individuals carrying the affected gene do not have identical phenotypes, the gene has *variable expressivity.* Expressivity of a gene can range from complete or severe manifestations to only mild features of the disease. An example of a disease with variable expressivity is neurofibromatosis.

ANTICIPATION. This term describes a phenomenon observed in certain autosomal dominant diseases in which the disease symptoms seem to be more severe and to occur at an earlier age in each successive generation. Important examples are fragile X syndrome and myotonic dystrophy. Bias of ascertainment does account for many cases of apparent anticipation. When an individual with a severe phenotype is identified, the search for other affected family members often reveals milder cases in previous generations. The reverse rarely occurs, however, in that an individual with a very mild phenotype may not even be recognized, and family members in previous generations would not be evaluated. One explanation for anticipation is expansion of triplet repeat regions discussed later.

AUTOSOMAL RECESSIVE. These traits often are expressed only when both copies of the gene function identically. Thus, autosomal recessive diseases require that both gene copies be abnormal. Heterozygotes or carriers who have only one abnormal gene may have some phenotypic alteration, but only individuals who have two copies of the affected gene (homozygotes) have the disease. Phenotypic alterations in gene carriers are usually clinically undetectable, but may be recognized at the biochemical or cellular level. For example, many enzyme deficiency diseases are autosomal recessive. The enzyme level in the carrier will be about half of normal, but because enzymes are made in great excess this reduction usually does not cause disease. It does, however, represent a phenotypic alteration, and can be used for screening purposes (Chap. 37, p. 978). Other recessive conditions do not produce any phenotypic changes in the carrier, and can be identified only by molecular methods.

Besides screening programs, carriers are usually recognized only after the birth of an affected child or diagnosis of an affected family member. Because the disease is often present in only one generation, this type of inheritance is sometimes referred to as *horizontal transmission.* A couple whose child has an autosomal recessive disease has a 25 percent recurrence risk with each conception. The likelihood that a normal sibling of an affected child is a carrier of the gene is two out of three—¼ of offspring will be homozygous normal, ¾ will be heterozygote carriers, and ¼ will be homozygous abnormal—thus, three of four children will be phenotypically normal and two of these three will be carriers. The carrier child will not have affected children, unless his or her partner is also a carrier or is affected. Because genes leading to rare autosomal recessive conditions have a low prevalence in the general population, the chance that a partner will be a gene carrier is low unless the couple is related or consanguineous (see below).

INBORN ERRORS OF METABOLISM. Most of these autosomal recessive diseases result from the absence of a crucial enzyme leading to incomplete metabolism of proteins, sugars, or fats. The metabolic intermediates that build up are toxic to a variety of tissues, resulting in mental retardation and other abnormalities.

PHENYLKETONURIA (PKU). This classical example of an autosomal recessive defect results from diminished or absent phenylalanine hydroxylase activity. Homozygotes are unable to metabolize phenylalanine to tyrosine. If the diet is unrestricted, incomplete protein metabolism leads to abnormally high phenylalanine levels that cause neurological damage, mental retardation, and hypopigmented hair, eyes, and skin. (Phenylalanine competitively inhibits tyrosine hydrolase which is essential for melanin production.) The disease is rare and affects 1 in 10,000 to 15,000 white infants. There is tremendous geographic and ethnic variation, with incidences ranging from 5 to 190 cases per million.

PKU is notable for two reasons. First, it is one of the few metabolic disorders for which treatment exists. Homozygotes who ingest a phenylalanine-free diet can avoid many of the clinical consequences of the disease. Thus, early diagnosis is important because limitation of dietary phenylalanine beginning in infancy is essential to prevent neurological damage. The special diet should be continued indefinitely; it is now believed that patients who abandon the phenylalanine-free diet may have some decline in IQ. All states and many countries now mandate newborn screening for phenylketonuria, and about 100 cases per million births are identified worldwide.

The second reason is that phenylalanine readily crosses the placenta and high maternal serum levels can result in pregnancy loss. It can also induce birth defects such as microcephaly with mental retardation and cardiac defects in the heterozygote fetus who otherwise would not be affected. Importantly, these defects can be prevented with dietary treatment (Williamson and associates, 1981). Women with PKU who plan to conceive and are not already on a phenylalanine-restricted diet are counseled to adhere to the diet before conception and throughout pregnancy. The Maternal Phenylketonuria Collaborative Study enrolled nearly 600 women in a 12-year study (Platt and colleagues, 2000). They reported that maintenance of serum phenylalanine levels in the 160 to 360 μmol/L (2 to 6 mg/dL) range significantly reduces the risk of fetal abnormalities.

CONSANGUINITY. Two individuals are considered consanguineous if they have at least one ancestor in common. The term usually refers to mating between third-degree relatives such as first cousins who share $\frac{1}{16}$ of genes, half uncle/aunt and niece/nephew, or more distantly related individuals. First cousin marriage is legal in 30 states and is actually preferred in some countries, for example, some parts of the Middle East (Bennett, 1987; Shami and colleagues, 1991). Incest is defined as a sexual relationship between first-degree relatives such as parent/child or brother/sister, and is universally illegal.

Consanguineous unions are at increased risk to produce children with genetic abnormalities, specifically autosomal recessive or multifactorial diseases. This is because consanguineous partners are more likely to share the same deleterious genes. Individuals from very isolated or restricted religious or ethnic groups may also share many genes. Consanguinity or being a member of a restricted group often prompts a request for preconceptional counseling. First cousin marriages, the most frequent consanguineous mating, carry a twofold risk of abnormal offspring if there is no family history of genetic disease. If there is a family history of genetic disease, the risk increases appreciably.

First-degree relatives share half their genes, second-degree relatives share $\frac{1}{8}$, and third-degree relatives (cousins) share $\frac{1}{16}$. If first cousins marry and one of the partners has a sibling with a rare autosomal recessive disease, the risk of affected offspring is many times higher than if he or she had chosen an unrelated partner. Incest carries a much higher risk of abnormal outcome, because the partners have half their genes in common. Up to 30 to 40 percent of offspring of an incestuous union will be abnormal as a result of both recessive and multifactorial disorders (Friere-Maia, 1984, Nadiri, 1979).

CO-DOMINANT GENES. If alleles in a gene pair are different from each other, but both are expressed in the phenotype, they are considered to be co-dominant. An example is the genes responsible for hemoglobinopathies. The individual with one gene directing production of sickle hemoglobin gene and the other directing production of hemoglobin C produces both S and C hemoglobins. Genes determining human blood type are also co-dominant, as individuals are capable of expressing simultaneously both A and B red-cell antigens.

X-LINKED AND Y-LINKED GENES. X-linked diseases are usually recessive. The best known X-linked recessive diseases are color blindness, hemophilia A, and Duchenne muscular dystrophy. Women carrying an X-linked recessive gene are generally unaffected, unless unfavorable lyonization—inactivation of one X chromosome in every cell—results in the majority of cells expressing the abnormal gene. When a woman carries a gene causing an X-linked recessive condition, there is a 50–50 chance of passing on the gene with each conception; thus, each son has a 50 percent risk of being affected and each daughter has a 50 percent chance of being a carrier.

Men carrying an X-linked recessive gene are usually affected because they lack a second X chromosome to express the normal dominant gene. When a man has an X-linked disease, all his sons will be unaffected because they cannot receive the affected X chromosome from him. In the rare situation in which the female partner of a man with an X-linked recessive disease is a carrier for the same disease, both their daughters and sons have a 50 percent chance of being affected. For complex reasons, fragile X syndrome does not conform to these rules of X-linked inheritance (see later discussion).

X-linked dominant disorders affect females predominantly because they tend to be lethal in male offspring. Examples include focal dermal hypoplasia, vitamin D–resistant rickets, and incontinentia pigmenti.

The Y chromosome carries genes important for sex

determination and a variety of cellular functions such as spermatogenesis and bone development. Deletion of genes on the long arm of the Y chromosome results in severe spermatogenic defects, while genes at the tip of the short arm are critical for chromosome pairing during meiosis and fertility.

NONMENDELIAN PATTERNS OF INHERITANCE

HEREDITARY UNSTABLE DNA. Mendel's first law states that genes are passed unchanged from parent to progeny. Barring the occurrence of new mutations, that law still applies to many genes or traits. Certain genes, however, are unstable, and their size and consequently their function may be altered as they are transmitted from parent to child.

FRAGILE X SYNDROME (MARTIN–BELL SYNDROME). This syndrome is the most common form of familial mental retardation. It accounts for 4 to 8 percent of all retardation in males and females in all ethnic and racial groups. Affected individuals have mild to severe mental retardation, autistic behavior, attention deficit-hyperactivity disorder, speech and language problems, narrow face with large jaw, long prominent ears, and macroorchidism in postpubertal males. The carrier rate for clinically important fragile X mutations is variable between populations, ranging from about 1 in 165 to 1 in 1540 (Rousseau and colleagues, 1995). The incidence of the full fragile X syndrome is generally cited as 1 in 1000 males and 1 in 2000 females (Rousseau and co-workers, 1995; Turner and colleagues, 1996).

The fragile X mutation is a region of unstable DNA on the X chromosome (Kremer, 1991; Oberle, 1991; Yu, 1991, and all of their colleagues). The region is best described as a series of CGG (cytosine–guanine–guanine) repeats at Xq27. If the number of repeats and thus the region reaches a critical size, it can be methylated and thus inactivated (Migeon, 1993). The number of repeats and the degree of methylation determines whether or not an individual is affected (Cutillo, 1994). Individuals carrying 2 to 49 repeats are phenotypically normal. Those carrying 50 to 199 repeats have a *premutation,* and although they are also phenotypically normal, they may have affected children. Those with more than 200 repeats have the *full* mutation and, if methylation occurs, are affected. The number of repeats usually remains stable when the gene is transmitted by a male. In the female, however, the gene can expand during meiosis. The risk of expansion with maternal transmission generally correlates with the number of repeats in the mother's premutation, and mutations with 100 repeats or more expand 100 percent of the time. Thus, if a woman carries a premutation that increases in size as she transmits it to her offspring, it is possible for her child to manifest fragile X syndrome (Cutillo, 1994).

Approximately 80 percent of males and 50 to 70 percent of females carrying the full mutation are retarded (deVries and co-workers, 1996; Jones, 1997; Sutherland and colleagues, 1991). Males are moderately to severely affected, with an IQ of 35 to 45, while the IQ in females is generally higher (Nelson, 1995). Surprisingly, 20 percent of males and 10 percent of females carrying the expanded gene are either unaffected or have the mildest phenotype. This phenotypic variability is caused by lyonization (in females) and mosaicism in both for the size of the expansion, the degree of methylation, or both (Cutillo, 1994). Both types of mosaicism can occur during mitosis in the zygote, and thus cannot be predicted by analysis of parental genes or fetal cells (Maddalena and colleagues, 1996; Mingroni-Netto and associates, 1996). The best example of this is provided by Kruyer and colleagues (1994), who described two sets of monozygotic carrier twins in which each twin had a very different phenotype due to discordant mosaicism.

Until recently, the diagnosis of fragile X syndrome was made using cytogenetic techniques, which were unreliable. With the use of restriction endonuclease digestion and Southern blot analysis, the number of CGG repeats and the methylation status of the gene can now be accurately determined (see discussion that follows). Amniocentesis may be preferred for prenatal diagnosis because methylation status is difficult to determine in chorionic villus cells. Women with a confirmed family or personal history of fragile X syndrome should be offered prenatal diagnosis. It is reasonable to refer individuals with a nonspecific history of mental retardation, developmental delay of unknown etiology, or autism for genetic evaluation. From 2 to 6 percent of individuals with these characteristics will be determined to have fragile X (Curry and colleagues, 1997; Wenstrom and associates, 1999). Universal screening (screening of low-risk women), however, is controversial. It currently is not recommended by either the American College of Medical Genetics (1994) or the American College of Obstetricians and Gynecologists (1995), primarily because screening for fetal disease should not be considered unless accurate prenatal diagnosis is available.

MYOTONIC DYSTROPHY. This is the most common form of adult myopathy with an age of onset from birth to 70 years (Jones, 1997). Affected family members tend to have successively earlier and more severe symptoms with each generation. The affected gene on the long arm of chromosome 9 contains a region of unstable trinucleotide (CTG) repeats (Buxton and co-workers, 1992). Normal individuals have 3 to 30 repeats, and although they can expand up to 3000, an increase to as few as 40 has been associated with myotonic dystrophy. In contrast to fragile X, there are three distinct phenotypes, depending on the number of repeats. With around 100 repeats there is mild disease; with around 1300 there is a 90 percent chance of having the full syndrome; and individuals with an intermediate number from 200 to 800 have an intermediate phenotype (Gennarelli and colleagues, 1996). In contrast to fragile X, the number of repeats can increase from transmission from either parent. Increased repeats cause successively more severe symptoms, i.e., "anticipation."

HUNTINGTON DISEASE. This disorder is characterized by progressive chorea, bradykinesia, and rigidity with an insidious deterioration of intellectual function. The mean age at diagnosis is about 40 years. The gene on chromosome 4 contains a region of CAG triplet repeats. Normal individuals have 10 to 35 CAG repeats, while those with the disease have 36 to 121 repeats. Like myotonic dystrophy, there is a significant correlation between the number of repeats and the age of onset (Andrew and colleagues, 1993). Interestingly, there is also a correlation between *paternal* inheritance and early disease (Clarke, 1990). Thus, the gene appears to be most unstable when transmitted by the father.

OTHER DNA-TRIPLET REPEAT DISEASES. These include Friedrich ataxia, X-linked spinal and bulbar muscular atrophy (Kennedy disease), spinocerebellar ataxia types 1 and 2, dentato-rubro-pallido-luysian atrophy, and Machado–Joseph disease.

IMPRINTING. This term describes the process by which certain genes are inherited in an inactivated or *transcriptionally silent* state (Hall, 1990). This type of gene inactivation correlates directly with the gender of the transmitting parent and is reversible in the next generation. Imprinting affects gene expression by *epigenetic control;* that is, it is a factor that changes the phenotype without permanently altering the genotype. When a gene is inherited in an imprinted state, gene function is necessarily directed entirely by the co-gene inherited from the other parent. Thus, imprinting exerts an effect in part by controlling the "dosage" of specific genes. Certain important genes appear to be *monoallelic;* that is, under normal circumstances only one member of the gene pair is functioning—as opposed to most genes in the genome, which are bi-allelic.

Teleological reasons for imprinting are incompletely understood. The fetus carries the imprinting pattern inherited from its parents in all of its somatic cells but not in its germ cells. In the immediate post-zygote period, the inherited methylation pattern in germ cells is erased and a new imprinting pattern corresponding to

the sex of the fetus is imposed. Thus, during reproduction, the subsequent adult will pass on the imprinting pattern unique to its own gender. One interesting example of imprinting concerns chromosomal deletion at 15q11–13 which causes two very different diseases. *Prader–Willi syndrome* is characterized by obesity and hyperphagia; short stature; small hands, feet, and external genitalia; and mild mental retardation. The other disorder is *Angelman syndrome,* which includes normal stature and weight, severe mental retardation, absent speech, and seizure disorder; ataxia and jerky arm movements; and paroxysms of inappropriate laughter. While both diseases are associated with the same deletion, if the maternally derived chromosome 15 region is missing the result is Angelman syndrome, and if the paternally derived chromosome 15 region is missing Prader–Willi syndrome results.

There are a number of other examples of imprinting important to obstetrician-gynecologists. *Complete hydatidiform mole,* which has a paternally derived, diploid chromosome complement, is characterized by the abundant growth of placental tissue, but no fetal structures (Chap. 32, p. 836). Conversely, *ovarian teratoma,* which has a maternally derived diploid chromosome complement, is characterized by the growth of various fetal tissues but no placental structures (Porter and Gilks, 1993). It thus appears that paternal genes are vital for placental development and maternal genes are essential for fetal development, but both must be present in every cell in order for normal fetal growth and development. This concept is also illustrated by triploidy, discussed earlier. Imprinting also is operative in some malignancies.

UNIPARENTAL DISOMY. This term describes the situation in which both members of one pair of chromosomes are inherited from the same parent (Fig. 36–7). This appears to occur as the result of "correction" of a trisomic zygote by loss of a chromosome. The chromosome transmitted by one parent is lost, and the two chromosomes transmitted by the other parent are retained. **Isodisomy** is the unique situation in which an individual receives two identical copies of one chromosome in a pair from one parent. This mechanism explains some cases of cystic fibrosis, in which only one parent was a carrier but the fetus inherited two copies of the same abnormal chromosome (Spence and co-workers, 1988; Spotila and colleagues, 1992). It has also been implicated in abnormal growth related to placental mosaicism (Robinson and colleagues, 1997).

MITOCHONDRIAL INHERITANCE. Each human cell contains hundreds of mitochondria, each containing its own genome and associated replication systems. In a sense, mitochondria behave autonomously. Interest-

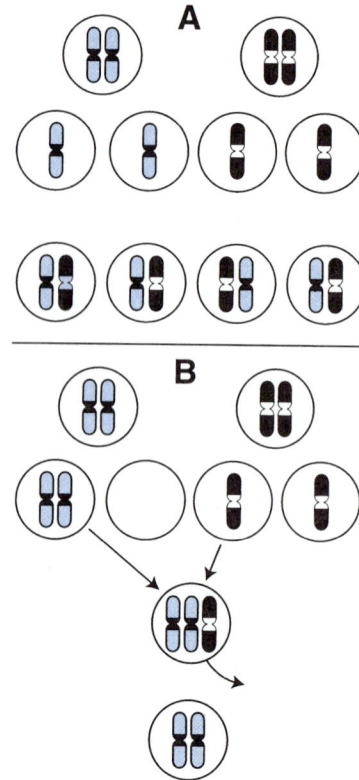

FIGURE 36–7. Diagrammatic representation of how uniparental disomy may arise.

ingly, these organelles are derived exclusively from the mother. While human oocytes contain approximately 100,000 mitochondria and mitochondrial DNAs, sperm contains only 100, and these are selectively eliminated after fertilization. Each mitochondrian contains multiple copies of a 16.5-kb circular DNA molecule. This DNA encodes 13 peptides that are subunits of proteins. These are required for oxidative phosphorylation, as well as ribosomal and transfer RNAs.

Because mitochondria contain genetic information, mitochondrial inheritance allows the transmission of genes from mother to offspring without the possibility of recombination. If a mitochondrial mutation occurs, it may segregate into a daughter cell during cell division and thus be propagated. Over time, the percentage of mutant mitochondrial DNAs in different cell lines can drift toward either normal or pure mutant (Wallace, 1995). If an oocyte containing largely mutant mitochondrial DNAs is fertilized, the offspring might have a mitochondrial disease.

Mitochondrial diseases have a characteristic transmission pattern—individuals of both sexes can be affected, but transmission is only through females. Mitochondrial genetic diseases include myoclonic epilepsy with ragged red fibers (MERRF), Leber hereditary optic neuropathy, Leigh syndrome, and pigmentary retinopathy.

POLYGENIC AND MULTIFACTORIAL INHERITANCE.
Polygenic traits are determined by the combined effects of many genes. **Multifactorial traits** are determined by multiple genes and environmental factors. It is now believed that the majority of inherited traits are multifactorial or polygenic. Birth defects caused by such inheritance are recognized by their tendency to recur in families, but not according to a mendelian inheritance pattern. The empirical recurrence risk for first-degree relatives is usually quoted as 2 to 3 percent (Thompson and colleagues, 1991). Multifactorial traits can be classified in several ways, but the most logical is to categorize them as:

1. Continuously variable.
2. Threshold.
3. Complex adult disorders.

CONTINUOUSLY VARIABLE TRAITS.
These traits have a normal distribution in the general population. By convention, abnormality is defined as a trait or measurement greater than two standard deviations above or below the population mean. These are typically measurable or quantitative traits such as height or head size, and are believed to result from the individually small effects of many genes combined with environmental factors. Such traits tend to be less extreme in the offspring of affected individuals, because of the statistical principle of regression to the mean.

THRESHOLD TRAITS.
These traits do not appear until a certain threshold of liability is exceeded (Fig. 36–8). Factors creating liability to the malformation are assumed to be continuously distributed, and only individ-

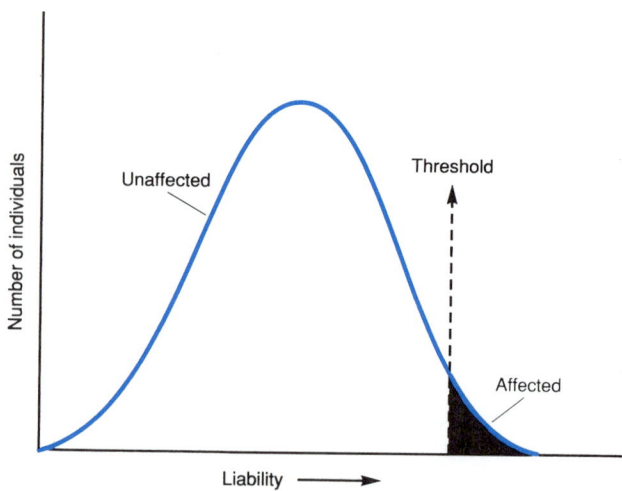

FIGURE 36–8. Example of a threshold trait. Liability to a trait is distributed normally, with a threshold dividing the population into unaffected and affected segments. (From Thompson and colleagues, 1991, with permission.)

uals at the extreme of this distribution exceed the threshold and have the trait or defect. The phenotypic abnormality is thus an all-or-none phenomenon. Individuals in high-risk families have enough abnormal genes or environmental influences that their liability is close to the threshold. Usually for unknown reasons, some factor(s) increases the liability for certain family members still further, and the threshold is crossed. Cleft lip and palate and pyloric stenosis are some examples of threshold traits.

Certain threshold traits have a predilection for one gender, indicating that males and females have a different liability threshold. Thus, when a family includes an affected member who is the less frequently affected gender, it indicates that even more abnormal genes or environmental influences are present. Their first-degree relatives (siblings) thus have an even higher liability for that particular trait. An example is pyloric stenosis, which is more common in males. If a female has pyloric stenosis, she or her parents have even more abnormal genes or predisposing factors than usually necessary to produce pyloric stenosis. The recurrence risk for her siblings or for her future children is thus higher than the expected 2 to 3 percent. Male siblings or offspring would have the highest liability, because they are the most susceptible sex *and* they will inherit more than the usual number of predisposing genes.

Finally, the recurrence risk for threshold traits is also higher if the defect is severe, again suggesting the presence of more abnormal genes or influences. For example, the recurrence risk after the birth of a child with bilateral cleft lip and palate is 8 percent, compared with only 4 percent after unilateral cleft lip without cleft palate (Melnick and associates, 1980).

COMPLEX DISORDERS OF ADULT LIFE. These are traits in which many genes determine the susceptibility to environmental factors, with disease resulting from the most unfavorable combination of both. Examples include common diseases such as heart disease or hypertension. These disorders are usually familial and behave as threshold traits but with a very strong environmental influence. The genetic mechanisms of many common adult diseases have not yet been elucidated, although several associated genes have been identified. In some cases, the identity of the associated gene provides a clue to pathogenesis, while in others the related gene may simply be used as a disease marker. For example, premature cardiovascular disease is associated with the gene for apolipoprotein E, which likely influences pathology of the disease. By way of contrast, the association of type I diabetes with HLA-DR3/4 is less clear. Some multifactorial adult-onset diseases and associated genes are listed in Table 36–7.

TABLE 36–7. Multifactorial Adult-Onset Disease and Their Associated Genes

Approach	Disease	Major Gene
Working from the phenotype down, using physiological abnormalities	Coronary artery disease	Hypercholesterolemia; combined hyperlipidemia
	Hypertension	Ion transport abnormalities
	Pernicious anemia	Atrophic gastritis
	Peptic ulcer	Hyperpepsinogenemia I
	Lactose intolerance	Lactase deficiency
	Hemochromatosis	Increased iron absorption
	Diabetes mellitus	Glucose intolerance; pancreatic autoimmunity
	Colon cancer	Single adenomatous polyp
Working from the genotype up, using genetic markers	Celiac disease	Associated with HLA-DR3
	Hemochromatosis	Associated with HLA-A3, linked to HLA region (chromosome 6)
	Insulin-dependent diabetes	Associated with HLA-DR3 and HLA-DR4
	Rheumatoid arthritis	Associated with HLA-DR4
	Ankylosing spondylitis	Associated with HLA-B27
	Alzheimer disease	Linked to amyloid β-protein RFLP (chromosome 21)

From King and associates (1992), with permission.

EXAMPLES OF MULTIFACTORIAL OR POLYGENIC DEFECTS. A variety of isolated structural birth defects and a number of common diseases in the population are associated with multifactorial or polygenic inheritance. All of these traits have certain characteristics that help to distinguish them from disorders with other modes of inheritance, and which can be cited in patient counseling (Table 36–8). When counseling regarding risks for a familial multifactorial trait, it is important to consider the affected relative's degree of relatedness to the *fetus,* not the parents. An affected first-degree relative (the fetus's parents or siblings) results in a substantial risk increase. After this, risk declines exponentially with successively more distant relationships. Two examples are given next to illustrate principles of these disorders.

NEURAL TUBE DEFECTS (NTDs). The neural folds in the brain and spinal cord regions fuse in the midline, converting the neural plate into the neural tube by days 26 to 28 of embryonic life (Fig. 36–9). Recent data indicate that closure occurs in separate regions that then fuse (Golden and Chernoff, 1995). Clinical data suggest five possible closure sites. Neural-tube defects likely result from either failure of closure in one or more sites, or failure of two sites to meet.

After cardiac defects, isolated (nonsyndromic) neural-tube defects are the most common congenital structural defects with a worldwide incidence of 1.4 to 2 per 1000 live births. They can also occur as part of a genetic syndrome or constellation of abnormalities. They are a major cause of stillbirth, neonatal and infant death, and lifelong severe handicap. With treatment, 80 to 90 percent of infants with isolated spina bifida survive with

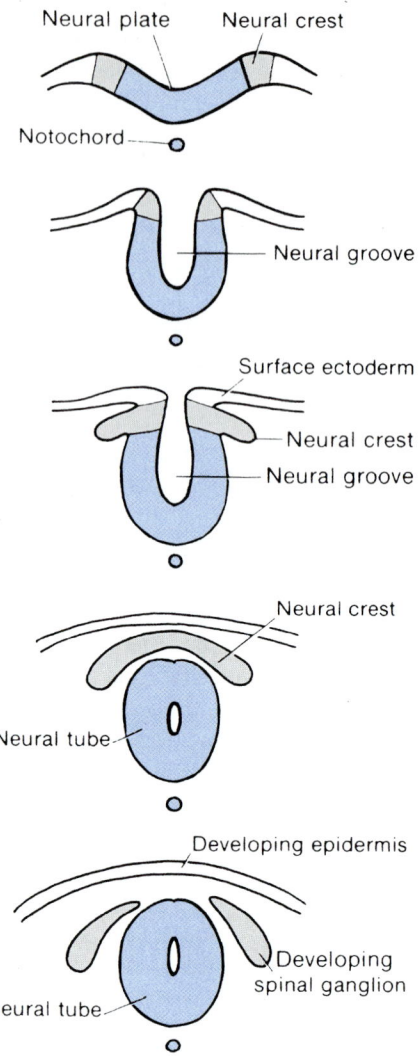

FIGURE 36–9. Schematic representation of neural tube closure before 28 days. (From Moore, 1977, with permission.)

varying degrees of handicap. Factors that influence eventual neurological function include the size and location of the defect, trauma to exposed neural tissue, timing of surgical closure, degree of associated ventriculomegaly, and occurrence of complications such as infection.

The most common neural-tube anomalies are listed in Table 36–9. **Anencephaly** is the most severe defect, in which the forebrain, meninges, vault of the skull, and scalp all fail to form (Fig. 36–10). It is lethal, resulting in stillbirth or early neonatal demise. Other cranial defects include:

1. **Exencephaly**—failure of scalp and skull formation with exteriorization of an abnormally formed brain.
2. **Encephalocele**—extrusion of brain tissue through a defect in the skull.

TABLE 36–8. Characteristics of Multifactorial Traits

1. Multiple family members are affected, but there is no specific inheritance pattern.
2. The risk to first-degree relatives is approximately the square root of the population risk.
3. The risk is sharply lower for second-degree relatives, and declines rapidly for more distant relatives.
4. The recurrence risk is higher if more than one family member is affected.
5. The recurrence risk is higher if the defect is severe.
6. If the trait is more frequent in one gender, the risk for relatives is higher if the person with the defect is of the less frequently affected gender.
7. The concordance rate in dizygotic twins is less than a quarter of the rate in monozygotic twins.
8. The recurrence risk is higher if the parents are consanguineous.

Adapted from Thompson and colleagues (1991).

3. **Iniencephaly**—a defect of the cervical and upper thoracic vertebrae and base of the skull with abnormally formed brain tissue and extreme retroflexion of the upper spine.

Spina bifida involves failure of fusion of the vertebral arches, so that meninges **(meningocele)** or neural tissue plus meninges **(meningomyelocele)** are exposed to the amniotic fluid and eventually to the environment (Fig. 36–11). Neural tissue is damaged by such exposure, causing the structures supplied by the damaged nerves to be dysfunctional. Lesions in the lumbosacral area can lead to paraplegia and lack of bowel or bladder control. Higher lesions result in even greater handicap. Open defects are often associated with *ventriculomegaly* (en-

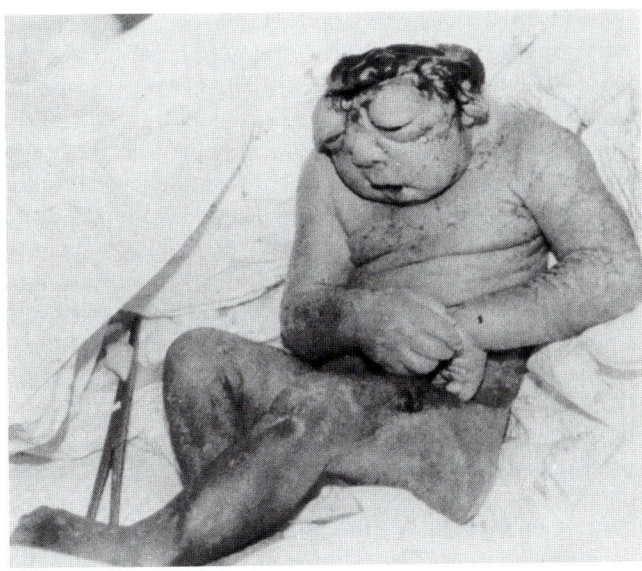

FIGURE 36–10. Anencephalic infant.

largement of the ventricles) or *hydrocephalus* (enlargement of the cranium due to ventriculomegaly) as a result of a block to cerebrospinal fluid circulation. The increased intracranial pressure may cause pressure atrophy of the developing brain, although neurological dysfunction cannot be reliably estimated from the thickness of the compressed cortical mantle. **Rachischisis** describes the situation in which none of the vertebral arches fuse, and the entire spine is open. This condition is generally incompatible with life.

Neural-tube defects are classical examples of multifactorial inheritance. Their occurrence is influenced by environment, diet, physiological abnormalities such as hyperthermia or hyperglycemia, teratogen exposure, family history, ethnic origin, fetal gender, amnionic fluid nutrients, and various genes. The variety of defects associated with these risk factors suggest that many genes are likely to be involved in neural-tube development. For example, insulin-dependent diabetes is preferentially associated with cranial or cervical-thoracic defects; hyperthermia is usually associated with anencephaly, and valproic acid exposure almost always causes lumbosacral defects (Becerra and colleagues, 1990; Hunter, 1984; Lindhout and associates, 1992). Moreover, each defect type appears to have a unique recurrence risk. Hall and colleagues (1988) reported a 7.8 percent recurrence risk with high spina bifida, 0.7 percent with low spina bifida, 2.2 percent with anencephaly, and no increased risk for craniorachischisis, encephalocele, or multiple defects. Because of this, it is not surprising that familial neural-tube defects usually involve the same location (Cowchock and collaborators, 1980; Toriello and Higgins, 1985). Thus far, only one clearly associated

TABLE 36–9. Basic Types of Neural-Tube Defects (Myelodysplasia)

Defect	Definition
Spina bifida occulta	Vertebral defect characterized by failure of closure of the posterior elements of the vertebral arch without a sac containing neural tissue visible on the back. The defect may or may not be associated with an abnormality of the spinal cord.
Spina bifida cystica	Vertebral defect with cystic protrusion of the meninges or of the spinal cord and meninges.
Meningocele	Protrusion of the meninges and cerebrospinal fluid into a sac covered by epithelium. Clinical symptoms vary according to underlying spinal cord anomalies.
Myelomeningocele	Most common and serious defect that includes the spinal cord, nerve roots, meninges, and cerebrospinal fluid. Commonly occurs in the lumbar area. The level of the lesion is usually reflected in severity of the clinical deficit, with higher lesions having more pronounced deficits.
Lipomeningocele	Vertebral defect associated with a superficial fatty mass that merges with lower levels of the spinal cord. Neurological deficits vary. There is no associated hydrocephalus.
Encephalocele	A protrusion of scarred brain, cerebrospinal fluid, and meninges through a bony skull defect. It is usually occipital, but can be frontal or through the skull base.
Anencephaly	Failure of fusion of the cranial end of the neural tube, resulting in exposure of a malformed brain.

From Ryan and colleagues (1991), with permission.

gene has been identified, and its teratogenic effects are strongly influenced by diet.

Although Hibbard and Smithells (1965) postulated more than 30 years ago that abnormal folate metabolism was responsible for many neural-tube malformations, a specific gene defect associated with folic acid metabolism has only recently been implicated. A thermolabile variant of 5,10-methylenetetrahydrofolate reductase (MTHFR) has the mutation 677C→T, which results in a substitution of valine for alanine. This variant enzyme has reduced activity leading to altered homocysteine metabolism. The culpability of this particular enzyme defect makes biological sense. Folic acid supplementation reduces neural-tube defect recurrences by 70 percent and significantly reduces first occurrences (Czeizel and Dudas, 1992; MRC Vitamin Study Research Group, 1991). Folic acid likely works by overcoming this relative enzyme deficiency. Because some defects occur in fetuses with normal 677C→T alleles, and because folic acid supplementation does not prevent all cases, other unknown genes or factors are presumed to cause some cases. Without folic acid supplementation, the empirical recurrence risk after one affected child is 3 to 4 percent, and after two affected children it is 10 percent. With supplementation, the risk after one affected child is less than 1 percent.

CONGENITAL HEART DISEASE. Cardiac anomalies are the most common birth defects with a worldwide incidence of 7 per 1000 births. They outnumber all other isolated structural defects combined (Burn and Goodship, 1996). Cardiac anomalies may occur as the result of aneuploidy or other chromosomal abnormality,

or be part of a recognized single-gene disorder or another genetic syndrome. The majority of isolated malformations have traditionally been considered multifactorial, with environmental factors playing a major role. More recently, however, the reproductive experiences of adult survivors with congenital heart disease have challenged this view. Specifically, the recurrence of the same or similar defect in the offspring of women with congenital cardiac defects, despite different environmental exposures, suggests that genetic factors are more important, and this supports polygenic inheritance.

Many genes involved in normal and abnormal cardiac development have not yet been identified. Defects associated with gene deletion syndromes provide clues to the function and location of some cardiac genes. For example, association of the DiGeorge deletion with conotruncal cardiac defects has prompted a search for the causative genes within a small region of chromosome 22q11.2.

More than 50 genes believed to be involved in cardiovascular morphogenesis have been identified. These include those directing production of various transcription factors, secreted proteins, extracellular proteins, and protein receptors (Chin, 1998). Although these gene products seem to be involved in the structural development of the defect, their mechanism(s) remains unknown. For example, reduced elastin production is clearly related to supravalvular aortic stenosis, but the pathophysiological basis is unclear (Keating, 1994).

Epidemiological studies have contributed to the understanding of environmental influences on heart development. Ferencz and colleagues (1997) described results from the Baltimore–Washington Infant Study. This

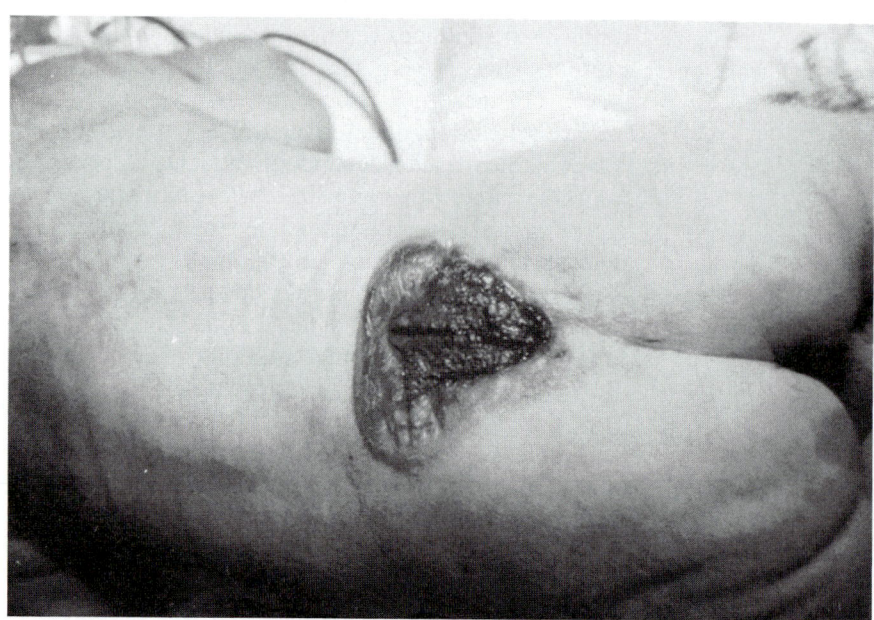

FIGURE 36–11. Large lumbar meningomyelocele. (Courtesy of Dr. Victor Klein.)

TABLE 36–10. Recurrence Risk (Percent) for Congenital Heart Defects if Siblings or Parents are Affected

	Father	Mother	1 Sibling	2 Siblings
Ventricular septal defects	2	6–10	3	10
Atrial septal defects	1.5	4–4.5	2.5	8
Fallot tetralogy	1.5	2.5	2.5	8
Pulmonary stenosis	2	4–6.5	2	6
Aortic stenosis	3	13–18	2	6
Coarctation	2	4	2	6

Adapted from Nora and Nora (1988), with permission.

large, comprehensive case-control study included all live-born infants in a specific geographic region with congenital cardiac disease over an 8-year period. Maternal diabetes, influenza or fever, previous poor obstetrical outcomes, cigarette smoking, exposure to pesticides and solvents, marijuana use, and exposure to certain medications all increased the risk threefold for fetal cardiac anomalies.

The recurrence risk for cardiac malformations is difficult to determine because of multiple potential biases. For example, until relatively recently, patients with severe heart defects often did not reproduce, and many parents with a child with a serious heart defect choose not to have more children. One method used to approximate risk for first-degree relatives is to examine the relatives of children with congenital heart disease to determine *recurrence risk*. Lin and Garver (1988) and Nora and Nora (1988) summarized several studies in which the various cardiac defects were categorized according to the abnormal developmental mechanism. There are two situations in which their data can be used to approximate recurrence risk, as follows.

1. Risk after birth of an affected child. Obstructive defects related to abnormal blood flow of the left side of the heart have a familial recurrence rate four- to sixfold higher than other cardiac defects. Some of these defects include hypoplastic left heart (15 percent risk), bicuspid aortic valve (11 percent risk), and aortic coarctation (8 percent risk). Defects categorized as involving abnormal cell migration (conotruncal defects), cell death (Ebstein anomaly), growth of the extracellular matrix (AV canal), or targeted growth (anomalous pulmonary venous return) had relatively low recurrence rates.

2. Risk if parent or sibling has a cardiac defect. Recurrence risks for some congenital heart defects are shown in Table 36–10. For counseling, if the exact nature of the defect is known, the most specific risk should be quoted. Otherwise, couples can be informed of the empirical risk of having a child with a cardiac defect. This

is 5 to 6 percent if the mother has the defect, and 2 to 3 percent if the father has the defect (Burn and associates, 1998).

MOLECULAR GENETICS

Significant advances in DNA technology in the last decade now allow isolation and sophisticated analysis of human genes. The Human Genome Project, a cooperative international project whose goal was mapping the entire human genome, was completed in 2000. Watson (1991), however, cautions that "Our descendants will be working for hundreds if not thousands of years to fully understand all the information contained in the 3 billion DNA base pairs that constitute the human genome." These 3 billion base pairs make up approximately 80,000 genes in each human nucleus (Table 36–11). Of these, several thousand have been assigned to a particular chromosome and hundreds have been cloned. The following is a cursory review of molecular

TABLE 36–11. Relative Size of Genomes, Chromosomes, and Cloned DNA

	Size (base pairs)
Size	
Human genome	3,000,000,000
Human chromosome (average)	130,000,000
Yeast genome	15,000,000
Escherichia coli genome	5,000,000
Cloning Capacity	
YAC (yeast artificial chromosome)	1,000,000
Cosmid	45,000
Bacteriophage	25,000

Adapted from Green and Waterston (1991), with permission.

genetics as related to obstetrics as well as to prenatal diagnosis, which is discussed in Chapter 37.

ORGANIZATION OF THE GENOME. The 2 meters of DNA in every cell must be packaged according to a very elaborate system in order to be maintained and transmitted without interruption. The DNA is wrapped very compactly around basic proteins called histones to form nucleosomes. These are then organized into solenoid structures and looped around a nonhistone protein scaffold to form chromatin (Fig. 36–12). As the cell enters prophase, the chromatin begins to condense until it assumes the familiar structure of metaphase chromosomes. Each chromosome is composed of densely packed nontranscribed DNA near the centromeres, called heterochromatin, and less densely packed transcribed DNA called euchromatin.

About 75 percent of the genome is unique, single copy DNA, and the rest consists of various classes of repetitive DNA. Surprisingly, virtually all of the repetitive DNA and a large portion of the single copy DNA has no apparent or recognized function. Less than 10 percent of the genome encodes genes! Single copy DNA is intensely studied because it contains all the genes necessary to make and sustain the organism, and repetitive DNA is of interest because it contains unique markers that identify each individual and can be used to study genetic variation.

CODING DNA

GENES. A gene is a unique series of four purine and pyrimidine bases that specifies the amino acid sequence for a single polypeptide chain of a protein molecule. A gene is not one continuous segment of DNA, but is typically composed of multiple coding sequences called *exons,* interrupted by nontranscribed regions called *introns* that must be excised prior to translation. Each gene also has a regulatory region called a *promoter,* a 5′ untranslated region that has regulatory functions, and a 3′ untranslated region containing the signal for messenger RNA maturation and function. In the nucleus, genetic information is transcribed from DNA into a single-stranded RNA identical in sequence with one of the strands of the DNA helix. The RNA is processed (the introns are excised) and transported into the cytoplasm where it is translated into the amino acid sequence that constitutes a protein. Post-translational processing of the protein follows in the cytoplasm. The polypeptide chain is folded into a unique three-dimensional structure, and two or more polypeptide chains may combine or the structure may be chemically modified by the addition of carbohydrate or other moieties.

Many genes exist in several alternate but normal forms called **alleles.** For example, CDE and major blood group genes all have several normal alleles. A **mutation** is an alteration of DNA sequencing that occurs in a coding region (gene), results in a change in protein structure or function, and is passed on to future progeny. Mutations can be visible chromosome alterations, such as deletions or insertions, or they may involve a change in one or more of the purine or pyrimidine bases of a single gene. Single nucleotide substitutions that result in the wrong amino acid being selected are called **missense mutations;** those that cause a premature stop codon to be inserted are **nonsense mutations.** Some mutations cause an error in RNA splicing at the intron/exon splice sites. The distinction between an allele and a mutation can be blurred; many normal alleles probably result from ancient mutations that either did not affect survival or conferred some selective advantage. In current usage, the DNA changes characterized as mutations generally have adverse effects on protein structure or function, and occur infrequently in the population.

The vast majority—99.8 percent—of DNA is identical in all humans. There are however, minor differences that distinguish one person from another. These differ-

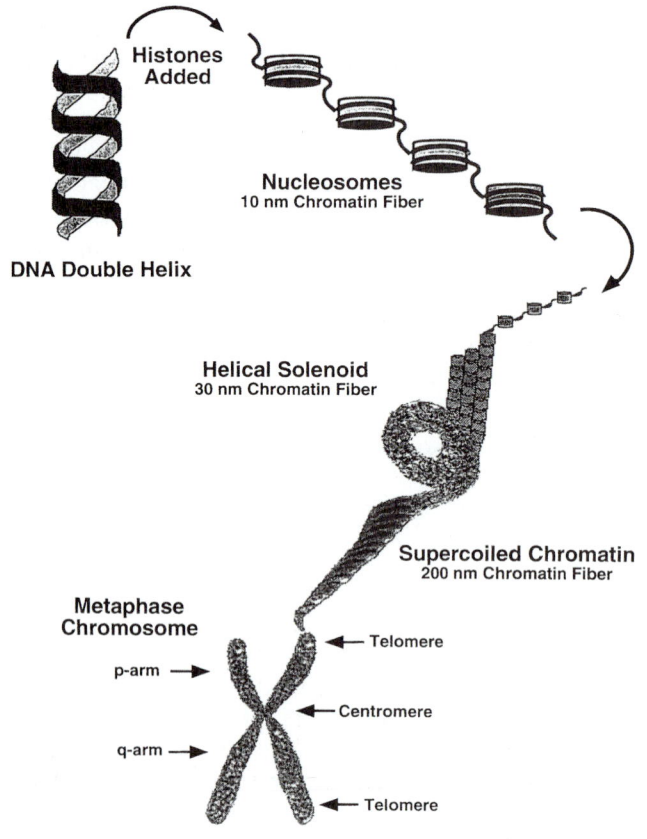

FIGURE 36–12. Schematic representation of the structural organization of DNA. (Adapted from Elsa and Patel, 1998, with permission.)

ences, called **polymorphisms,** generally consist of a single nucleotide change about every 200 to 500 base pairs. These changes are primarily in noncoding regions of the genome, but can also be found in introns and in gene coding regions. They are silent, meaning that they do not affect gene structure or function. They can, however, be used for identification and to determine the origin of inherited DNA sequences.

Diseases caused by a single mutation, such as sickle cell disease, are rare. Physiological processes and pathways are highly redundant, and a single mutation located in the coding region of a gene may be clinically silent. Most frequently, pathological phenotypic changes occur only when multiple genes are affected or when specific environmental influences are present. The genetic mutations and other conditions necessary for phenotypic alteration are in general poorly understood. When newly discovered genes are being analyzed, it can thus be difficult to distinguish a normal allele from a polymorphism or a mutation. For example, over 100 variations of the BRCA1 gene, one of the major genes associated with familial breast and ovarian cancers, have been identified. It is not currently known whether all of these variations are actually mutations associated with disease, or if some could be polymorphisms or allelic variants (Collins, 1996). The ability to distinguish alleles from mutations is obviously essential to any molecular screening program.

CONTROL OF GENE EXPRESSION

METHYLATION. Genomic DNA methylation is believed to be the major form of DNA modification that permits control of many aspects of gene expression (Thompson and McInnes, 1991). It occurs only at one specific nucleotide in the human genome: the cytosine of a CpG dinucleotide repeat. Most CpG dinucleotides are located in gene regulatory regions, where methylation would prevent transcription and thus effectively turn off that gene.

Methylation is very common as about half of all CpG sequences are methylated (Barsh and Epstein, 1996). Methylation is believed to be the mechanism for imprinting and plays a role in producing the fragile X phenotype discussed earlier. Its most important function, however, is to control the tissue-specific activation of certain genes. Every cell in the body contains the entire genome, but the body contains many pathophysiologically different cells because the expression of genes that are not essential for each specific tissue type is prevented by methylation. For example, the globin genes are methylated in all nonerythroid tissues, ensuring that only erythrocytes produce hemoglobin (Barsh and Epstein, 1996).

NEW MUTATIONS AND GENE REGULATION. New mutations are also linked to DNA methylation. As previously stated, most CpG dinucleotides appear to be located primarily in gene regulatory regions. They are also found within certain gene coding regions. The function of the CpGs within gene coding regions is not completely understood, and cytosine methylation here does not prevent gene transcription. However, if a methylated cytosine residue is deaminated to thymidine, the methylcytosine on the opposite strand is likely to be changed to thymidine. This mutation can lead to premature termination of translation or production of an abnormal protein. This specific mutation is extremely common. Methylated CpGs are the single most mutated dinucleotides in the genome and cause a third of all germline point mutations leading to genetic disease (Mancini and associates, 1997; Ollila and colleagues, 1996; Tornaletti and Pfeifer, 1995). Certain *hot spots* of the human genome have an abundance of CpGs and are especially vulnerable. Mutations at sites with multiple CpG dinucleotides occur at a frequency 10- to 40-fold higher than at any other sites and account for more than a third of nucleotide substitutions in inherited diseases (Cooper and Krawczak, 1990; Youssoufian and co-workers, 1986).

CpG dinucleotides have been associated with mutations in a variety of genes. The most mutable nucleotide in the entire genome is a CpG dinucleotide in the fibroblast growth receptor 3 gene (FGFR3 1138 guanosine), which accounts for more than 97 percent of all cases of achondroplasia (Bellus and colleagues, 1995). The majority of new mutations causing hemophilia A, half of point mutations causing mucopolysaccharidosis type II, and 10 to 15 percent of mutations causing retinoblastoma are in CpG doublets (Mancini and collaborators, 1997; Rathmann and associates, 1996). Other genes with high mutation rates are those causing neurofibromatosis, polycystic kidney disease, and aniridia. Certain lethal autosomal dominant diseases such as osteogenesis imperfecta or thanatophoric dwarfism *always* result from new mutations. These affected individuals have "reduced reproductive fitness"; that is, they die before they can reproduce.

OTHER FORMS OF GENE REGULATION. In a small number of genes, the mRNA sequence is modified ("mRNA editing") before it is transcribed, so that it is no longer complementary to the DNA template (Barsh and Epstein, 1996). The initiation of mRNA translation can also be regulated, controlling the quantity of gene product produced. Finally, DNA can actually be rearranged to produce a unique protein such as immunoglobulin (Harriman and colleagues, 1993).

NONCODING DNA. Approximately 1 percent of all the nucleotides in the noncoding regions are polymorphic.

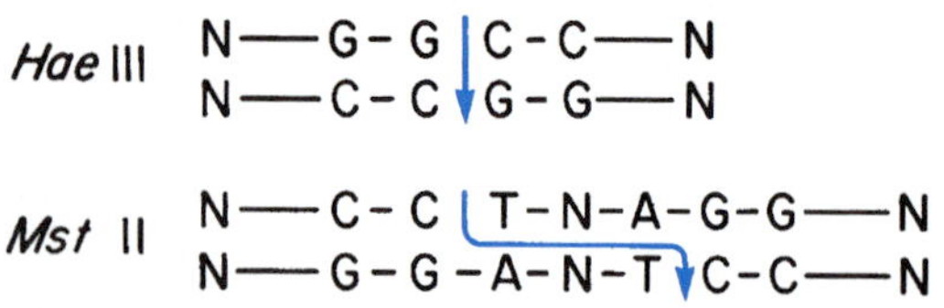

Hae III
N——G- G | C - C——N
N——C - C ↓ G - G——N

Mst II
N——C - C | T- N- A- G- G——N
N——G- G - A- N- T ↓ C- C——N

FIGURE 36–13. Restriction endonucleases. *Hae* III (*H influenzae* III) cleaves a four-base sequence. *Mst* II (*Microcoleus*) cleaves a seven-base sequence, the center of which is a nonspecific nucleotide, shown here as N.

These sites can be identified by *restriction endonuclease* digestion, or they may be areas of repeated sequences with variable length.

RESTRICTION FRAGMENT LENGTH POLYMORPHISMS (RFLPs).

The entire human genome, composed of 3 billion base pairs of DNA, is so large that searching for a specific gene within it is a monumental task. The first step is to break the genomic DNA into manageable fragments. This is accomplished by bacterial enzymes termed **restriction endonucleases.** Each endonuclease locates and cleaves a specific sequence of base pairs, wherever it occurs along the genome. As shown in Figure 36–13, some enzymes recognize sequences of four nucleotides, some six, and others seven. More than 200 different restriction enzymes have been identified. The number and size of fragments produced by enzyme digestion are determined by the frequency or location of the particular sequences recognized by the enzyme. Each enzyme thus produces its own unique pattern of DNA fragments.

Certain restriction endonuclease sites are the same in all humans. Others, however, are unique to each individual. These unique endonuclease sites, leading to unique DNA fragment lengths, are called restriction fragment length polymorphisms, or RFLPs. RFLPs are not mutations or abnormalities, but are merely individual differences in nucleotide sequences that are present roughly once in every 250 base pairs throughout the genome (Marian, 1995). Each RFLP generally has two alleles and is inherited in mendelian fashion. Because of this, they can be used for identification purposes, for diagnostic testing, or to confirm or rule out transmission of a specific DNA segment from parent to child. The different cleavage locations and fragment lengths obtained with different endonucleases can also be used as *markers* to help locate a particular gene or to facilitate analysis of the inheritance pattern of a trait.

REPETITIVE DNA.

These segments are characterized by short nucleotide sequences that are repeated many times throughout the genome. A large part of the noncoding genome consists of repetitive DNA. They are of interest because they include polymorphisms that can be used as markers. They can also be very useful for following alleles through a family and have been used to analyze certain genes. **Clustered repetitive DNA** makes up 10 to 15 percent of the genome (Elsa and Patel, 1998). These segments are called *simple sequence DNA* or *satellite DNA* because of their physical properties. This class of DNA includes several distinct types of repeated sequences. One class is characterized by a *variable number of tandem repeats* **(VNTRs),** consisting of multiple copies of short DNA sequences. VNTRs are more *polymorphic* than RFLPs because they usually have up to several dozen alleles compared with only two alleles at each RFLP site. **Short tandem repeats (STRs),** also called CA dinucleotides or GT repeats, are areas of dinucleotide or trinucleotide repeats scattered throughout the genome. STRs are also highly polymorphic, with 4 to 10 alleles typically identified at each site. VNTRs and STRs are considered more *informative* than RFLPs because their allelic variation makes them more useful for identification and other purposes. **Interspersed repetitive DNA** accounts for 15 percent of the total DNA, and occurs randomly throughout the genome. These sequences include **SINES (short interspersed sequences)** and **LINES (long interspersed sequences).**

All these repetitive sequences and other types of polymorphic markers can be used to determine the relative locations of markers to each other and to gene(s) of interest. Thus, they can be used to generate a DNA map. Such a linkage map of the whole genome, containing almost 6000 markers located less than 1 million base-pairs apart, has already been accomplished by the Human Genome Project (Murray and co-workers, 1994).

GENETIC TESTS

CYTOGENETIC ANALYSIS.

Any tissue containing dividing cells or cells that can be stimulated to divide is suitable for cytogenetic analysis. The dividing cells are blocked in metaphase and the chromosomes are stained to reveal light and dark bands. The banding pattern of each chromosome facilitates its identification and detection of any deleted, duplicated, or rearranged segments. The accuracy of band analysis increases along with the number of bands produced. Most laboratories now routinely perform high-resolution metaphase banding, which yields 350 to 550 visible bands per haploid chromosome set. Banding of prophase chromosomes generally yields 850 bands.

Because only dividing cells can be evaluated, cells must be cultured for analysis. The rapidity with which results are obtained thus correlates with the rapidity of cell growth in culture. Bone marrow cell results are usually available in less than a day. Adult blood yields results in 3 to 4 days. Fetal blood often produces results in 24 to 48 hours. Amniocytes, which are fetal fibroblasts, sloughed gastrointestinal mucosal cells, and amnion cells, require 7 to 14 days. Fibroblasts usually require 3 to 6 weeks, but this is often because the skin sample is obtained postmortem and stimulation of growth is difficult.

FLUORESCENCE IN SITU HYBRIDIZATION (FISH). This is a rapid method for determining ploidy for a few specific chromosomes, or confirming the presence or absence of a gene or large DNA sequence (Fig. 36–14). It is not comparable to cytogenetic evaluation because the chromosomes appear squat and the banding patterns are much less distinctive. Chromosome duplications, deletions, and rearrangements often cannot be detected by FISH. Cells are fixed on a glass slide, and fluorescently labeled chromosome or gene probes are allowed to hybridize to the fixed chromosomes. Each probe is complementary to a unique area of the chromosome or gene, thus preventing cross reaction with other chromosomes. If the chromosome or gene of interest is present, hybridization is detected as a bright signal visible by micros-

copy. The number of signals indicates the number of chromosomes or genes of that type in the cell being analyzed. FISH is usually used when ploidy status would change clinical management, and time constraints prevent waiting for a cytogenetic analysis.

SPECTRAL KARYOTYPE ANALYSIS. This is a FISH procedure in which a labeled probe for *every* chromosome is used simultaneously. Chromosomes can be distinguished from each other because each probe emits a unique, defined spectrum of a different color. The results are analyzed by computer, making it a rapid and accurate test. It is currently available for research only.

LINKAGE ANALYSIS. RFLPs, STRs, and other markers can be used to locate a specific gene for research or diagnostic purposes if certain criteria are met (Beaudet and Ballabio, 1994). First, a large family with multiple members affected by the disease in question must be identified. Next, specific markers scattered throughout the genome are selected for study or, if the gene is believed to be located on a specific chromosome, markers on that chromosome are chosen. DNA from each

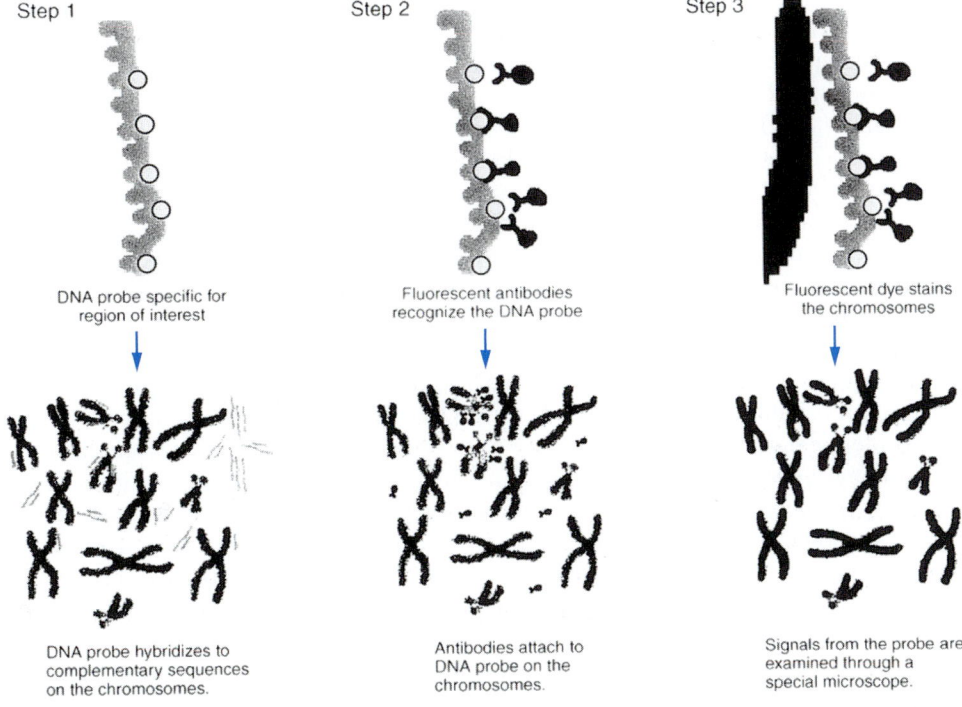

Step 1

DNA probe specific for
region of interest

DNA probe hybridizes to
complementary sequences
on the chromosomes.

Step 2

Fluorescent antibodies
recognize the DNA probe

Antibodies attach to
DNA probe on the
chromosomes.

Step 3

Fluorescent dye stains
the chromosomes

Signals from the probe are
examined through a
special microscope.

FIGURE 36–14. Steps in fluorescence in situ hybridization (FISH). (Adapted from Greenwood Genetics Center, 1995, with permission.)

family member is then analyzed to determine whether any of the selected markers are transmitted together (segregate) with the disease. If individuals with the disease have the marker, and individuals without the disease do not, the gene causing the disease and the marker are said to be *linked,* or close to each other on the same chromosome.

Linkage analysis allows determination of locations of different genes and their approximate distances from each other. The approximate distance between genes or markers is estimated using the crossover frequency, a measure of how often a crossover moves the gene away from the marker to the other chromosome in the pair. The farther apart the genes or markers are, the more likely they are to crossover. This then provides the basis for more detailed molecular study. It can also be used for diagnosis if members of the affected family have informative markers with multiple alleles. Thus, they are helpful if the marker associated with the disease-causing gene represents one allele, and the marker associated with that normal gene is a different allele.

In cases in which the specific gene has not been identified, linkage analysis can be used to estimate the likelihood that an individual, for example, a fetus, has inherited the abnormal gene. Linkage analysis is imprecise, and dependent on family size, availability of family members for testing, presence of informative markers near the gene, and frequency of crossover events. In informative cases it provides some information about the likelihood of inheritance.

COMPLEMENTARY DNA (cDNA). When the nucleic acid sequence of a gene or DNA region of interest is known, it can be studied directly using complementary DNA. This cDNA is a laboratory-made copy of a DNA segment or gene. It is synthesized utilizing *reverse transcriptase,* an enzyme isolated from tumor viruses which can synthesize a DNA copy from nuclear messenger RNA. cDNA is usually single stranded and, because messenger RNA is the template, it does not contain the introns which are removed during processing of mRNA. Radioactive bases are inserted into the sequence to label cDNA so that the resulting probe can be visualized if it bonds with a matching sequence or identical gene.

Many isolated genes or DNA fragments have been collected in cDNA *libraries.* The source of the copied genes is usually a single tissue or chromosome, which substantially aids the search for specific genes. For example, to study the β-globin gene, it would be much easier to isolate the gene from a cDNA library prepared from red blood cells, where β-globin represents the major mRNA transcript, than from a library representing the whole genome, where it is present at only one part per million. Likewise, a search for a gene thought to be

on chromosome 9 would be easier if the chromosome 9 library was used to focus the search.

FLUORESCENCE-ACTIVATED CHROMOSOME SORTING. Large quantities of a specific chromosome can be obtained by fluorescence-activated chromosome sorting. Chromosomes are stained with fluorescent dyes, and are distinguished from each other by intensity of fluorescence. Stained metaphase chromosomes are passed through a laser beam which deflects each chromosome according to its unique intensity.

GEL SEPARATION. Once the desired chromosome has been isolated, it can be fragmented with endonuclease. The fragments are screened for the gene or DNA sequence of interest. This process is greatly facilitated by separating the fragments with electrophoresis. Smaller fragments move faster and farther than larger fragments. The DNA fragments can be visualized directly or by fluorescent staining to facilitate removal for further study.

POLYMERASE CHAIN REACTION (PCR). This is a rapid technique for synthesizing large amounts of a specific DNA sequence or gene (Beaudet and Ballabio, 1994). Using PCR, a million copies of the original gene or DNA segment can be made in a few hours using very minute quantities of DNA. However, either the entire gene sequence or the sequences at the beginning and end of the gene must be known. PCR involves three steps that are repeated many times. First, double-stranded DNA is denatured by heating. Oligonucleotide primers anneal to the target sequence on each strand of separated DNA. A mixture of nucleotides and heat-stable DNA polymerase is added, and new complementary strands of DNA are synthesized. In just a few minutes, the original DNA has been duplicated. The procedure is repeated over and over with exponential amplification of the DNA segment. PCR is used to generate large quantities of DNA for testing or it is used to amplify a particular gene or mutation to identify it.

SOUTHERN BLOTTING. Named for its inventor, Edward Southern, this technique allows identification of one or several DNA fragments of interest from among the million or so typically obtained by enzyme digestion of the human genome. It applies the principles of gel separation and nucleic acid hybridization illustrated in Figure 36–15, but on a much larger scale. The cDNA probe may be a normal gene, in which case hybridization confirms the presence of a normal copy while lack of hybridization indicates a mutation. Because hybridization can occur even with incomplete sequence homology, only relatively large mutations or changes such as deletions can be detected by cDNA probes.

The probe can also be a fragment of DNA produced

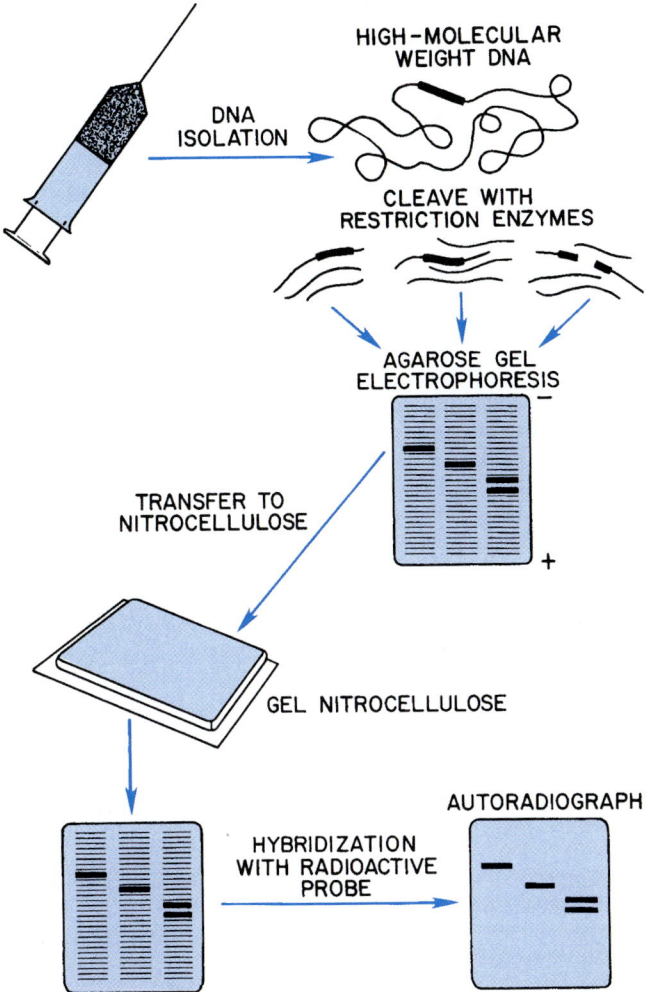

HIGH-MOLECULAR WEIGHT DNA

DNA ISOLATION

CLEAVE WITH RESTRICTION ENZYMES

AGAROSE GEL ELECTROPHORESIS

TRANSFER TO NITROCELLULOSE

GEL NITROCELLULOSE

AUTORADIOGRAPH

HYBRIDIZATION WITH RADIOACTIVE PROBE

FIGURE 36–15. Southern blotting analysis. Genomic DNA is isolated from leukocytes or amniocytes and digested with a restriction enzyme. This yields a series of reproducible fragments that are separated by agarose gel electrophoresis. The separated DNA fragments are then transferred ("blotted") to a nitrocellulose membrane that binds DNA. The membrane is treated with a solution containing a radioactive single-stranded nucleic acid probe, which forms a double-stranded nucleic acid complex at membrane sites when homologous DNA is present. These regions are then detected by autoradiography using x-ray film.

by endonuclease digestion. In this case, individuals with a normal gene would have fragments of a different size than individuals carrying the abnormal gene. Before the sickle cell gene was identified, this method was used for prenatal diagnosis by Chang and Kan in 1982. They developed an assay using the restriction enzyme Mst II. The sickle cell mutation results in loss of the Mst II recognition site, yielding one large fragment instead of two smaller ones after endonuclease digestions.

Basic principles of the Southern blot technique can also be applied to RNA, in which case it is called **Northern blotting,** and to proteins, as **Western blotting.**

ALLELE SPECIFIC OLIGONUCLEOTIDE (ASO) PROBES.
If a mutation of interest consists of a change in only one or two base pairs, a cDNA probe will not detect it. A few mismatches will not prevent the cDNA probe from hybridizing to the gene. For single nucleotide mutations, an allele specific oligonucleotide probe must be used instead. An ASO is a short DNA probe, 15 to 25 bases in length, which is synthesized by sequential addition of each nucleotide and is homologous to a specific DNA sequence (Layman, 1992). ASOs can be used instead of cDNA in the Southern blotting technique shown in Figure 36–15. They are useful for testing family members at risk for a small, well-characterized familial mutation.

MULTIPLEX POLYMERASE CHAIN REACTION.
If primers spanning the DNA region of interest are available, PCR can be used to amplify any DNA segment, including genes with deletions or mutations. If a variety of mutations in one gene have been identified in association with a certain disorder, they can all be amplified simultaneously using multiplex PCR.

OLIGONUCLEOTIDE LIGATION ASSAY (OLA).
This technique provides great sensitivity in detecting single-base insertions, deletions, or substitutions. Two probes, each corresponding to an adjacent region of the gene in question, are allowed to hybridize to contiguous regions of the DNA region of interest. They are then ligated using DNA ligase. The label attached to one probe is released by the ligation, indicating that the DNA sequence of interest corresponds exactly to the sequences of the two probes. This procedure provides a higher degree of accuracy than can be achieved with single-probe assays (Winn-Deen, 1996).

LIGATION CHAIN REACTION (LCR).
LCR is the amplification counterpart of OLA, and may be used to screen for many different small or single-gene mutations simultaneously. In a single tube, the specimen is submitted to multiplex PCR, and then evaluated with simultaneous OLA analysis for multiple different mutations. LCR it is used by many laboratories for cystic fibrosis screening for 30 of the most common mutations.

CLONING.
A clone is a large number of molecules or cells all identical to one ancestral molecule or cell (Lewin, 1997). Cloning refers to the replication of genetic material, although a new definition has been created by the popular media that includes replication of whole animals. Technically, cloning includes several laboratory techniques that enable pieces of DNA to be copied in large quantities by lower organisms. These techniques utilize various vectors, which are DNA molecules that replicate autonomously in its host cell. Re-

striction enzymes are used to cleave both the DNA sequence of interest and the vector DNA at appropriate sites, and DNA ligase is used to insert the DNA segment into the vector. The inserted DNA will then be replicated along with vector DNA, and large quantities of the DNA insert can then be retrieved for study.

The first vectors used for cloning were bacterial plasmids which are circular double-stranded DNA molecules that replicate separately from bacterial chromosomes. Plasmids are used for small DNA inserts, usually less than 5 to 10 kb in size. DNA fragments were later cloned in bacteriophages with inserts up to 20 kb; or modified plasmids called cosmids with inserts up to 50 kb. Burke and colleagues (1987) then developed a method to insert 100 to 1000 kb of DNA into a *yeast artificial chromosome* or *YAC*. These chromosomes have their own centromeres and telomeres and replicate like normal yeast chromosomes. YAC libraries, with each YAC containing a different fragment of the genome, have been established to greatly simplify gene isolation.

POSITIONAL CLONING. This is sometimes referred to as "reverse genetics" because it involves attempting to clone the gene responsible for a specific disease based on its location, without knowing the nature of the gene product. This is only possible once the gene has been localized to a specific part of a given chromosome (Gelehrter and Collins, 1990). Localization or mapping of the abnormal gene to a specific chromosome region usually involves narrowing the search to a sequence of over a million base pairs. This is easier if the affected individual also has a cytogenetic abnormality such as a chromosomal deletion to mark the most likely location. Examples of genes that have been cloned using this technique include cystic fibrosis, Duchenne muscular dystrophy, retinoblastoma, colonic polyposis, neurofibromatosis, and Huntington disease (Beaudet and Ballabio, 1994).

DNA CHIPS. These take advantage of the principles of PCR and nucleic acid hybridization to screen DNA for many genes or mutations simultaneously. Many cDNA probes or ASOs, each representing a different gene mutation, are tagged with different colored fluorescent dyes and arrayed on a tiny chip. DNA from the test individual is amplified by PCR and exposed to the probes fixed on the chip. Hybridization to any of the probes is recognized by the color pattern, and indicates that the individual carries the mutation represented by that particular cDNA. It is anticipated that this technology will revolutionize genetic screening. For example, although over 800 mutations causing cystic fibrosis have been identified, most laboratories currently test patient samples only for a panel of 16 to 32 of the most common mutations. Using a DNA chip, the patient could be screened for all 750 mutations simultaneously.

REFERENCES

American College of Medical Genetics: Fragile X syndrome: Diagnostic and carrier testing. Working group of the genetic screening subcommittee of the clinical practice committee. Am J Med Gen 53:380, 1994

American College of Obstetricians and Gynecologists: Committee on Genetics: Fragile X syndrome. ACOG Committee Opinion No. 161, October 1995

Andrew SE, Goldberg YP, Kremer B: The relationship between trinucleotide repeat length (CAG) and clinical features of Huntington disease. Nat Genet 4:398, 1993

Barsh GS, Epstein CJ: Gene structures and function. In Rimoin DL, Connor JM, Pyeritz RE (eds): Emery and Rimoin's Principles and Practice of Medical Genetics, 3rd ed. New York, Churchill Livingstone, 1996, p 35

Beaudet AL, Ballabio A: Molecular genetics and medicine. In Isselbacher KJ, Braunwald E, Wilson JD, Martin JB, Fauci AS, Kasper DL (eds): Harrison's Principles of Internal Medicine, 13th ed. New York, McGraw-Hill, 1994, p 349

Becerra JE, Khoury MJ, Cordero JF, Erickson JD: Diabetes mellitus during pregnancy and the risks for specific birth defects: A population-based case-control study. Pediatrics 85:1, 1990

Bellus G, Hefferon TW, Ortiz de Luna RI, Hecht JT, Horton WA, Machado M: Achondroplasia is defined by recurrent G380R mutations of FGFR-3. Am J Hum Genet 56:368, 1995

Bennett RL: The genetic risks of incest and consanguinity. Genet Northwest 2:2, 1987

Brogger A: XYY and its relation to criminality. In: The Y Chromosome, Part B: Clinical Aspects of Y Chromosome Abnormalities. New York, Liss, 1985, p 345

Burke DT, Carle CF, Olson MV: Cloning of large segments of exogenous DNA into yeast by means of artificial chromosome vectors. Science 236:806, 1987

Burn J, Brennan P, Little J, Holloway S, Coffey R, Somerville J: Recurrence risks in offspring of adults with major heart defects: Results from first cohort of British collaborative study. Lancet 351:311, 1998

Burn J, Goodship J: Developmental genetics of the heart. Curr Opin Genet Dev 6:322, 1996

Buxton J, Shelbourne P, Davies J: Detection of an unstable fragment of DNA specific to individuals with myotonic dystrophy. Nature 355:547, 1992

Chang JC, Kan YW: A sensitive new prenatal test for sickle-cell anemia. N Engl J Med 307:30, 1982

Chin AJ: Congenital heart disease. In Jameson JL (ed): Principles of Molecular Medicine. Totowa, NJ, Humana Press, 1998, p 117

Clarke A: Genetic imprinting in clinical genetics. Dev Suppl, p 131, 1990

Claussen U, Schafer H, Trampisch HJ: Exclusion of chromosomal mosaicism in prenatal diagnosis. Hum Genet 67:23, 1984

Cockwell A, MacKenzie M, Youings S, Jacobs P: A cytogenetic and molecular study of a series of 45 X fetuses and their parents. J Med Genet 28:151, 1991

Collins FS: Shattuck lecture—Medical and societal consequences of the human genome project. N Engl J Med 341:28, 1999

Collins FS: BRA1—Lots of mutations, lots of dilemmas. N Engl J Med 334:186, 1996

Cooper DN, Krawczak M: The mutational spectrum of single base pair subscriptions causing human genetic disease: Patterns and predictions. Hum Genet 85:55, 1990

Cowchock S, Ainbender E, Prescott G, Crandall B, Lau L, Heller R: The recurrence risk for neural tube defects in the United States: A collaborative study. Am J Med Genet 5:309, 1980

Curry CJ, Stevenson RE, Aughton D, Byrne J, Carey JC, Cassidy S, Cunniff C Jr, Graham JM, Jones MC, Kaback MM, Moeschler J, Schaefer GB, Schwartz S, Tarleton J, Opitz J: Evaluation of mental retardation: Recommendations of a consensus conference. Am J Med Genet 72:468, 1997

Cutiollo DM: Fragile X syndrome. Genet Teratol 2:1, 1994

Czeizel AE, Dudas I: Prevention of the first occurrence of neural-tube defects by periconceptional vitamin supplementation. N Engl J Med 327:1832, 1992

DeVries BB, Weigers AM, Smits APT, Mohkamsing S, Diuvenvoovden HJ, Fryns J-P, Curfs LMG: Mental status of females with an FMR1 gene full mutation. Am J Hum Genet 58:1025, 1996

Driscoll DA, Salvin J, Sellinger B, Budarf ML, McDonald-McGinn DM, Zackai EH, Emanuel BS: Prevalence of 22q11 microdeletions in DiGeorge and velocardiofacial syndromes: Implications for genetic counseling and prenatal diagnosis. J Med Genet 30:813, 1993

Elsa SH, Patel PI: Organization of the human genome, chromosomes, and genes. In Jameson JL (ed): Principles of Molecular Medicine. Totowa, NJ, Humana Press, 1998, p 4

ESHRE Task Force on Intracytoplasmic Sperm Injection: Assisted reproduction by intracytoplasmic sperm injection: A survey on the clinical experience in 1994 and the children born after ICSI, carried out until 31 December 1993. Hum Reprod 13:1737, 1998

Ferencz C, Correa-Villasenor A, Loffredo CA, Wilson PD: Perspectives in Pediatric Cardiology. Vol 5: Genetic and Environmental Risk Factors of Major Cardiovascular Malformations: The Baltimore-Washington Infant Study: 1981–1989. New York, Futura, 1997

Fernandez R, Mendez J, Pasaro E: Turner syndrome: A study of chromosomal mosaicism. Hum Genet 98:29, 1996

Friedman JM: Genetic disease in the offspring of older fathers. Obstet Gynecol 57:745, 1981

Friere-Maia N: Effects of consanguineous marriages on morbidity and precocious mortality: Genetic counseling. Am J Med Genet 18:401, 1984

Fryns JP, Kleczkowski A, Kubien E, Van der Bergehe H: On the excess of mental retardation and/or congenital malformations in apparently balanced reciprocal translocations. A critical review of the Leuven data. Genet Counsel 2:185, 1992

Garber AP, Schreck R, Carlson DE: Fetal loss. In Rimoin DL, Connor JM, Pyeritz RE (eds): Emery and Rimoin's Principles and Practice of Medical Genetics, 3rd ed. New York, Churchill Livingstone, 1996

Gardner RJM, Sutherland GR: Chromosome abnormalities and genetic counseling, 2nd ed. Oxford Monographs on Medical Genetics No. 29. Oxford, Oxford University Press, 1996

Gelehrter TD, Collins FS: Anatomy of the human genome: Gene mapping and linkage. In Gelehrter TD, Collins FS (eds): Principles of Medical Genetics. Baltimore, Williams & Wilkins, 1990, p 193

Gennarelli M, Novelli G, Bassi FA, Martorell L, Cornet M,

Menegazzo E, Mostacciuolo ML, Martinez JM, Angelini C, Pizzuti A, Baiget M, Dallapiccola B: Prediction of myotonic dystrophy clinical severity based on the number of intragenic [CTG]n trinucleotide repeats. Am J Med Genet 65:342, 1996

Golden JA, Chernoff GF: Multiple sites of anterior neural tube closure in humans: Evidence from anterior neural tube defects (anencephaly). Pediatrics 4:506, 1995

Goldstein JC, Brown MS: Genetic aspects of disease. In Isselbacher KJ, Braunwald E, Wilson JD, Martin JB, Fauci AS, Kasper DL (eds): Harrison's Principles of Internal Medicine, 13th ed. New York, McGraw-Hill, 1994, p 339

Graham JM Jr: Smith's Recognizable Patterns of Human Deformation, 2nd ed. Philadelphia, Saunders, 1988

Green ED, Waterston RH: The human genome project: Prospects and implications for clinical medicine. JAMA 266:1966, 1991

Greenwood Genetics Center: Fluorescence In situ hybridization (FISH). In: Counseling Aids for Geneticists, 3rd ed. Greenville, SC, Keys Printing, 1995, p 23

Hall JG: Genomic imprinting: Review and relevance to human diseases. Am J Hum Genet 46:857, 1990

Hall JG, Friedman JM, Kenna BA, Popkin J, Jawanda M, Arnold W: Clinical, genetic, and epidemiological factors in neural tube defects. Am J Hum Genet 43:827, 1988

Harriman W, Volk H, Defranoux N, Wabl M: Immunoglobulin class switch recombination. Ann Rev Immunol 11:361, 1993

Hassold T, Arnovitz K, Jacobs PA, May K, Robinson D: The parental origin of the missing or additional chromosome in 45,X and 47,XXX females. Birth Defects: Original Article Series 26:297, 1991

Held KR, Kerber S, Kaminsky E: Mosaicism in 45X Turner syndrome: Does survival in early pregnancy depend on the presence of two sex chromosomes? Hum Genet 88:288, 1992

Henderson KG, Shaw TE, Barrett IJ, Telenius AHP, Wilson RD, Kalousek DK: Distribution of mosaicism in human placentae. Hum Genet 97:650, 1996

Hibbard ED, Smithells RW: Folic acid metabolism and human embryopathy. Lancet, 1:1254, 1965

Hodges, P, Scott J: Spolipoprotein β μ RNA editing: A new tier for the control of gene expression. Trends Biochem Sci 17:77, 1992

Hook EB: Prevalence, risks, and recurrence. In Brock DJH, Rodeck CH, Ferguson-Smith MA (eds): Prenatal Diagnosis and Screening. Edinburgh, Churchill Livingstone, 1992, p 351

Hook EB, Cross PK, Schreinemachers DM: Chromosomal abnormality rates at amniocentesis and in live-born infants. JAMA 249:2034, 1983

Hunter AGW: Neural tube defects in Eastern Ontario and Western Quebec: Demography and family data. Am J Med Genet 19:45, 1984

In't Velt P, Halley DJJ, Van Hemel JO, Niermeijer MF, Dohle G, Weber RFA: Genetic counseling before intracytoplasmic sperm injection. Lancet 350:490, 1997

Jacobs PA, Browne C, Gregson N, Joyde C, White H: Estimates of the frequency of chromosome abnormalities detectable in unselected newborns using moderate levels of banding. J Med Genet 29:103, 1992

Jones KL: Smith's Recognizable Patterns of Human Malformation. 5th ed. Philadelphia, Saunders, 1997

Jorde LB, Carey JC, White RL: Clinical cytogenetics: The chromosome basis of human disease. In: Medical Genetics. St Louis, Mosby, 1995, p 102

Kalousek DK, Barrett IJ, McGillivray BC: Placental mosaicism and intrauterine survival of trisomies 13 and 18. Am J Hum Genet 44:338, 1989

Kalousek DK, Dill FJ: Chromosomal mosaicism confined to the placenta in human conceptions. Science 221:665, 1983

Kalousek DK, Langlois S, Barrett I, Yam I, Wilson DR, Howard-Peebles PN, Johnson MP, Giorgiutti E: Uniparental disomy for chromosome 16 in humans. Am J Hum Genet 52:8, 1993

Kamiguchi Y, Rosenbusch B, Sterzik K, Mikamo K: Chromosomal analysis of unfertilized human oocytes prepared by a gradual fixation-air drying method. Hum Genet 90:533, 1993

Keating M: Elastin and vascular disease. Trends Cardiovasc Med 4:165, 1994

Kim SS, Jung SC, Kim JH, Moon HR, Lee JS: Chromosome abnormalities in a referred population for suspected chromosomal aberrations: A report of 4117 cases. J Korean Med Sci 14:373, 1999

King RA, Rotter JI, Motulsky AG: The approach to genetic bases of common diseases. In King RA, Rotter JI, Motulsky AG (eds): The Genetic Basis of Common Disease. New York, Oxford University Press, 1992, p 3

Koeberl DD, McGillivray B, Sybert VP: Prenatal diagnosis of 45,X/46,XX mosaicism and 45,X: Implications for postnatal outcome. Am J Hum Genet 57:661, 1995

Korf BR: New genetics of hearing loss. Teratology 61:163, 2000

Kremer EJ, Pritchard M, Lynch M, Yu S, Holman K, Baker E, Warren ST, Schlessinger D, Sutherland GR, Richards RI: Mapping of DNA instability at the fragile X to a trinucleotide repeat sequence p(CCG)n. Science 252:1711, 1991

Kruyer H, Mila M, Glover G, Carbonell P, Ballesta F, Estivill X: Fragile X syndrome and the (CGG)n mutation: Two families with discordant MZ twins. Am J Hum Genet 54:437, 1994

Layman LC: Basic concepts of molecular biology as applied to pediatric and adolescent gynecology. Obstet Gynecol Clin North Am 19:1, 1992

Levitan M: Textbook of Human Genetics, 3rd ed. New York, Oxford University Press, 1988

Lewin B: DNA biotechnology. In: Genes VI. Oxford, Oxford University Press, 1997, p 623

Lin AE, Garver KL: Genetic counseling for congenital heart defects. J Pediatr 113:1105, 1988

Lindhout D, Omtzigt JGC, Cornel MC: Spectrum of neural tube defects in 34 infants prenatally exposed to antiepileptic drugs. Neurology 42 (Suppl 5):111, 1992

Loft A, Petersen K, Erb K, Mikkelsen AL, Grinsted J, Hald F: A Danish national cohort of 730 infants born after intracytoplasmic sperm injection (ICSI). Hum Reprod 14:2143, 1999

Maddalena A, Yadvish KN, Spence WC, Howard-Peebles PN: A fragile X mosaic male with a cryptic full mutation detected in epithelium but not in blood. Am J Med Genet 64:309, 1996

Mancini D, Singh S, Ainsworth P, Rodenhiser D: Constitutively methylated CpG dinucleotides as mutation hot spots in the retinoblastoma gene (RB1). Am J Hum Genet 61:80, 1997

Marian AJ: Molecular approaches for screening of genetic diseases. Chest 108:255, 1995

McIntosh GC, Olshan AF, Baird PA: Paternal age and the risk of birth defects in offspring. Epidemiology 6:282, 1995

Melnick M, Bixler D, Fogh-Anderson P: Cleft lip and +/− cleft palate: An overview of the literature and an analysis of Danish cases born between 1941 and 1968. Am J Med Genet 6:83, 1980

Migeon BR: Role of DNA methylation in X inactivation and the fragile X syndrome. Am J Med Genet 47:685, 1993

Mingroni-Netto RC, Haddad LA, Vianna-Morgante AM: The number of CGG repeats of the FMR1 locus in premutated and fully mutated heterozygotes and their offspring: Implications for the origin of mosaicism. Am J Med Genet 64:270, 1996

Moore KL: Before We Are Born. Philadelphia, Saunders, 1977, p 46

MRC Vitamin Study Research Group: Prevention of neural tube defects: Results of the Medical Research Council Vitamin Study. Lancet 338:131, 1991

Murray JC, Buetow KH, Weber JL: A comprehensive human linkage map with centimorgan density. Science 265:2049, 1994

Nadiri S: Congenital abnormalities in newborns of consanguineous and non-consanguineous parents. Obstet Gynecol 53:195, 1979

Nazarenko SA, Timoshevsky VA, Sukhanova NN: High frequency of tissue-specific mosaicism in Turner syndrome patients. Clin Genet 56:59, 1999

Nelson DL: The fragile X syndromes. Sem Cell Biol 6:5, 1995

Nora JJ, Nora AH: Updates on counseling the family with a first-degree relative with a congenital heart defect. Am J Med Genet 29:137, 1988

Oberle I, Rosseau F, Heitz D, Kretz C, Devys D, Hanauer A, Boue J, Bertheas MF, Mandel JL: Instability of a 550-base pair DNA segment and abnormal methylation in fragile X syndrome. Science 252:1097, 1991

Ollila J, Lappalainen I, Vihinen M: Sequence specificity in CpG mutation hotspots. FEBS Lett 396:119, 1996

Orioli IM, Castilla EE, Scarano G, Mastroiacovo P: Effect of paternal age in achondroplasia, thanatophoric dysplasia, and osteogenesis imperfecta. Am J Med Genet 59:209, 1995

Platt LD, Koch R, Hanley WB, Levy HL, Matalon R, Rouse B, Trefz F, de la Cruz F, Guttler F, Azen C, Friedman EG: The international study of pregnancy outcome in women with maternal phenylketonuria: Report of a 12-year study. Am J Obstet Gynecol 182:326, 2000

Porter S, Gilks CB: Genomic imprinting: A proposed explanation for the different behaviors of testicular and ovarian germ cell tumors. Med Hypotheses 41:37, 1993

Rathmann M, Bunge S, Beck M, Kresse H, Tylki-Szymanska A, Gal A: Mucopolysaccharidosis type II (Hunter syndrome): Mutation "hotspots" in the iduronate-2-sulfatase gene. Am J Hum Genet 59:1202, 1996

Rimoin DL, Connor JM, Pyeritz RE (eds): Emery and Rimoin's Principles and Practice of Medical Genetics, 3rd ed. New York: Churchill Livingstone, 1997, pp 31, 277, 767

Robinson A, Bender BG, Linden MG, Salbenblatt JA: Sex chromosome aneuploidy: The Denver prospective study. Birth Defects: Original Article Series 26:59, 1991

Robinson WP, Barrett IJ, Bernard L, Telenius A, Bernasconi F, Wilson RD, Best RG, Howard-Peebles PN, Langlois S, Kalousek DK: Meiotic origin of trisomy in confined placental mosaicism is correlated with presence of fetal uniparental disomy, high levels of trisomy in trophoblast, and increased risk of fetal intrauterine growth restriction. Am J Hum Genet 60:917, 1997

Rosenberg RN: DNA-triplet repeats and neurologic disease. N Engl J Med 335:1222, 1996

Rousseau F, Rouillard P, Morel M-L, Khandjian EW, Morgan K: Prevalence of carriers of premutation-size alleles of the

FMRI gene—and implications for the population genetics of the fragile X syndrome. Am J Hum Genet 57:1006, 1995

Ryan KD, Ploski C, Emans JB: Myelodysplasia—The musculoskeletal problem: Habilitation from infancy to adulthood. Phys Ther 71:935, 1991

Saenger P: Turner's syndrome. N Engl J Med 335:1749, 1996

Scharrer S, Stengel-Rutkowski S, Rodewald-Rudescu A, Erdlen E, Zang KD: Reproduction in a female patient with Down's syndrome. Case report of a 46,XY child showing slight phenotypical anomalies born to a 47,XX,+21 mother. Hummangenetik 26:207, 1975

Schneider AS, Mennuti MT, Zackai EH: High cesarean section rate in trisomy 18 births: A potential indication for late prenatal diagnosis. Am J Obstet Gynecol 140:367, 1981

Shami SA, Qaisar R, Bittles AH: Consanguinity and adult morbidity in Pakistan. Lancet 338:954, 1991

Sherman SL, Takaesu N, Freeman SB, Grantham M, Phillips C, Blackston RD, Jacobs PA: Trisomy 21: Association between reduced recombination and nondisjunction. Am J Hum Genet 46:608, 1991

Simpson JL, Golbus MS, Martin AO, Sarto GE (eds): Genetics in Obstetrics and Gynecology. New York, Grune & Stratton, 1982

Smith A, Gaha TJ: Data on families of chromosome translocation carriers ascertained because of habitual spontaneous abortion. Aust NZ J Obstet Gynaecol 30:57, 1990

Snijders RJM, Sebire NJ, Nicolaides KH: Maternal age and gestational age-specific risk for chromosomal defects. Fetal Diagn Ther 10:356, 1995

Spence JE, Perciaccante RG, Greig FM, Willard HF, Ledbetter DH, Hejtmancik JF, Pollack MS: Uniparental disomy as a mechanism for human genetic disease. Am J Hum Genet 42:217, 1988

Spotila LD, Sereda L, Prockop DJ: Partial isodisomy for maternal chromosome 7 and short stature in an individual with a mutation at the COLIA2 locus. Am J Hum Genet 51:1396, 1996

Sutherland GR, Haan EA, Kremer E, Lynch M, Pritchard M, Yu S, Richards RI: Hereditary unstable DNA: A new explanation for some old genetic questions? Lancet 338:289, 1991

Thompson MW, McInnes RR, Huntington FW: Thompson & Thompson—Genetics in Medicine, 5th ed. Philadelphia, Saunders, 1991

Tolmie JL: Chromosome disorders. In Whittle MJ, Connor JM (eds): Prenatal Diagnosis in Obstetric Practice. Oxford, Blackwell Scientific, 1995, p 34

Toriello HV, Higgins JV: Possible causal heterogeneity in spina bifida cystica. Am J Med Genet 21:13, 1985

Tornaletti S, Pfiefer GP: Complete and tissue-independent methylation of CpG sites in the p53 gene: Implications for mutations in human cancers. Oncogene 10:1493, 1995

Turner G, Webb T, Wake S, Robinson H: The prevalence of the fragile X syndrome. Am J Med Genet 64:196, 1996

Wallace DC: 1994 William Allan Award Address. Mitochondrial DNA variation in human evolution, degenerative disease, and aging. Am J Hum Genet 57:201, 1995

Watson JD: The human genome initiative: A statement of need. Hosp Pract October 15, 1991

Wenstrom KD, Descartes M, Franklin J, Cliver SP: A five year experience with fragile X screening of high risk gravidas. Am J Obstet Gynecol 181:789, 1999

Williamson ML, Koch R, Azen C, Chang C: Correlates of intelligence test results in treated phenylketonuric children. Pediatrics 68:161, 1981

Winn-Deen ES: Multi-mutation screening using PCR and ligation—Principles and applications. TIBTECH 14:113, 1996

Youssoufian H, Kazazian HH, Philips DG: Recurrent mutations in hemophilia A: Evidence for CpG dinucleotides as mutation hotspots. Nature 324:380, 1986

Yu S, Pritchard M, Kremer E, Lynch M, Nancarrow J, Baker E, Holman K, Mulley JC, Warren ST, Schlessinger D, Sutherland GR, Richards RI: Fragile X genotype characterized by an unstable region of DNA. Science 252:1179, 1991

37

Prenatal Diagnosis and Fetal Therapy

Prenatal diagnosis is the art and science of identifying structural or functional abnormalities in the developing fetus. As discussed in Chapter 36, 2 to 3 percent of all neonates have a major abnormality discovered at birth. Congenital abnormalities have a major impact on the health of the pediatric population and have emerged as a major cause of neonatal death; indeed, more than a fourth of all pediatric hospital admissions result from genetic disorders (Ling, 1992). Prenatal diagnosis is thus an important bridge between obstetrics and pediatrics, and concerns a unique group of patients with specific medical, social, and psychiatric needs. Many fetal anomalies can be identified prenatally, and technology has provided an ever-expanding number of prenatal treatment options. In other cases, prenatal diagnosis allows optimization of delivery or consideration of pregnancy termination, but in either event, it offers an opportunity to influence the incidence and severity of genetic disease.

Prenatal diagnosis typically involves the evaluation of three major categories of patients:

1. Fetuses at high risk for a genetic or congenital disorder.
2. Those at unknown risk for common congenital abnormalities.
3. Fetuses discovered sonographically to have structural or developmental abnormalities.

Current prenatal (fetal) therapy includes optimization of the intrauterine environment and delivery conditions, blood transfusion, administration of medication, amnioreduction, placement of shunts, and surgery. The near future will likely include hematopoietic stem cell transplantation and other methods for gene transfer.

FETUSES AT HIGH RISK FOR GENETIC OR CONGENITAL DISORDERS

FETAL ANEUPLOIDY. At least 8 percent of conceptuses are aneuploid, accounting for 50 percent of first-trimester abortions and 5 to 7 percent of all stillbirths and neonatal deaths (Hook, 1992; Rimoin and colleagues, 1997). Chromosome defects compatible with life but causing significant morbidity occur in 0.65 percent of newborns, and another 0.2 percent have structural chromosomal rearrangements that will eventually affect reproduction (Milunsky, 1992).

Women aged 35 and older have traditionally, if somewhat arbitrarily, been offered genetic amniocentesis because at age 35 the incidence of trisomy starts to rapidly increase (Fig. 37–1). Also at this time, the term risk of any aneuploidy roughly equals the oft-quoted risk of amniocentesis-related pregnancy loss of 1 in 200, thus justifying the test (Table 37–1). Because only 8 to 12

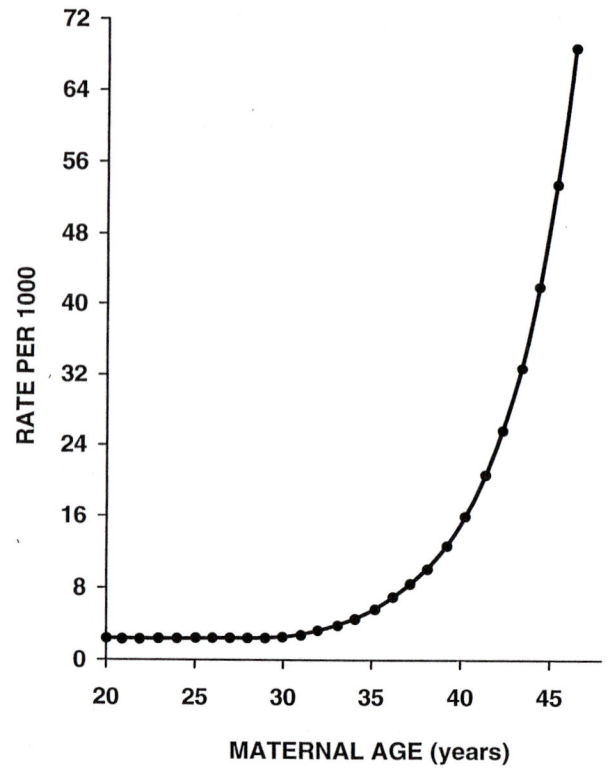

FIGURE 37–1. Maternal age-related incidence of fetal trisomy. (Data from Ferguson-Smith MA and Colleagues, 1984.)

percent of all children are born to these older women, at most only 20 percent of all Down syndrome pregnancies would be identified by this policy. Put another way, because younger women have the majority of pregnancies, younger women give birth to the majority (80 percent) of all children with Down syndrome (Shreinemachers and co-workers, 1982).

Several safe, accurate, and well-established procedures to obtain fetal cells for definitive fetal diagnosis are currently available. The challenge comes in determining which women are at high risk for fetal aneuploidy and should be offered these tests. "High risk" can be defined in many ways. Most commonly, it means a risk greater than fetal loss associated with the diagnostic procedure being considered. Thus, if the risk of postamniocentesis pregnancy loss is approximately 1 in 200, a genetic amniocentesis would not typically be offered unless the risk of fetal aneuploidy was estimated to be greater than 1 in 200. As listed in Table 37–2, women with a risk of fetal aneuploidy high enough to justify an invasive diagnostic procedure include the following:

1. Women with a singleton pregnancy who will be at least age 35 at delivery. The midtrimester risk of a 35-year-old woman to be carrying a fetus with Down syn-

TABLE 37-1. Maternal Age-Related Midtrimester Risk of Down Syndrome and All Aneuploidies

Weeks' Gestation	Midtrimester Incidence		Term Live-born Incidence	
	Down Syndrome	**All Aneuploidies**	**Down Syndrome**	**All Aneuploidies**
33	1/417	1/208	1/625	1/345
34	1/333	1/152	1/500	1/278
35	1/250	1/132	1/384	1/204
36	1/192	1/105	1/303	1/167
37	1/149	1/83	1/227	1/130
38	1/115	1/65	1/175	1/103
39	1/89	1/53	1/137	1/81
40	1/69	1/40	1/106	1/63
41	1/53	1/31	1/81	1/50
42	1/41	1/25	1/64	1/39
43	1/31	1/19	1/50	1/30
44	1/25	1/15	1/38	1/24
45	1/19	1/12	1/30	1/19

From Hook and colleagues (1983), with permission.

drome is 1 in 250 and the risk of any numerical aneuploidy is 1 in 132 (Table 37–1). These numbers are higher than the term risks because a large proportion of aneuploid pregnancies is lost spontaneously before term delivery. The risks at term are 1 in 384 for Down syndrome and 1 in 204 for all numeric aneuploidies.

2. Women with a dizygotic twin gestation who will be at least age 31 at delivery. With two fetuses, the laws of probability dictate that the chance that one or both will have Down syndrome is greater than if there was only one fetus. The risk of trisomy 21 in a twin pregnancy must be calculated after considering the maternal age-related Down syndrome risk, the maternal race- and age-related incidence of dizygotic twinning, and the

TABLE 37-2. Women with Risk of Fetal Aneuploidy High Enough to Justify Risk of Amniocentesis

Singleton pregnancy with age ≥ 35 at delivery
Dizygotic twin pregnancy with age ≥ 31 at delivery
Previous autosomal trisomy birth
Previous 47,XXX or 47,XXY birth
Patient or partner is carrier of chromosome translocation
Patient or partner is carrier of chromosomal inversion
History of triploidy
Some cases with repetitive early pregnancy losses
Patient or partner has aneuploidy
Major fetal structural defect by ultrasound

probability that either or both fetuses could be affected. The analysis by Meyers and colleagues (1997) shown in Table 37–3 indicates that, for both white and African American women, the midtrimester risk of fetal Down syndrome in a dizygotic twin pregnancy at age 31 is approximately 1 in 190, thus justifying the risk of an amniocentesis. Counseling in this situation should also include a discussion of options for pregnancy management if only one fetus is affected. These options include terminating both twins, selective second-trimester termination of the affected fetus only, continuing the pregnancy with monitoring of the normal fetus only, or continued monitoring of both fetuses.

3. Women who have previously had a pregnancy complicated by autosomal trisomy. Women who have had at least one trisomic pregnancy have approximately a 1 percent occurrence with the same or different autosomal trisomy. This is so until their age-related risk exceeds 1 percent at which time the higher risk predominates (Warburton, 1987).

4. Women who have previously had a pregnancy complicated by triple X (47, XXX) or Klinefelter syndrome (47, XXY). The extra X may be maternal or paternal in origin. As with autosomal trisomies, the recurrence risk is 1 percent until the maternal age-related risk exceeds 1 percent, at which time this risk predominates (Gardner and Sutherland, 1996). Women whose previous child was 47,XYY are *not* at high risk for recurrence, as the extra chromosome in this situation is paternal in origin, and paternal errors have minimal chance of recurring. Likewise, 45, X has a very low recurrence risk.

TABLE 37–3. Maternal Age-Related Midtrimester Risk of Down Syndrome in One or Both Fetuses of a Dizygotic Twin Pregnancy

Weeks' Gestation	Down Syndrome		All Aneuploidies	
	Midtrimester	*Term*	*Midtrimester*	*Term*
25	1/481	1/679	1/833	1/259
26	1/447	1/636	1/650	1/258
27	1/415	1/599	1/509	1/245
28	1/387	1/566	1/398	1/234
29	1/364	1/535	1/310	1/223
30	1/342	1/508	1/243	1/206
31	1/324	1/483	1/190	1/205
32	1/256	1/409	1/149	1/171
33	1/206	1/319	1/116	1/151
34	1/160	1/257	1/91	1/126
35	1/125	1/199	1/71	1/101
36	1/98	1/153	1/56	1/82
37	1/77	1/118	1/44	1/67
38	1/60	1/92	1/35	1/54
39	1/47	1/72	1/27	1/44
40	1/37	1/56	1/21	1/35
41	1/29	1/44	1/17	1/28
42	1/23	1/33	1/13	1/22
43	1/18	1/27	1/10	1/18
44	1/14	1/20	1/8	1/14
45	1/11	1/16	1/6	1/11

From Meyers and colleagues (1997), with permission.

5. Women or their partners who are chromosome translocation carriers. The risk of having abnormal offspring must be estimated individually, taking into account the chromosomes involved, the sex of the transmitting parent, and the method of ascertainment. For most translocations, the observed risk of abnormal liveborn children is less than the theoretical risk, because a portion of gametes produces nonviable conceptions. The observed risk specific to the translocation can be provided by a geneticist or genetic counselor. In general, however, translocation carriers identified after the birth of an abnormal child have a 5 to 30 percent risk of having unbalanced offspring, while those identified for other reasons, for example during an infertility workup, have a 0 to 5 percent risk (Gardner and Sutherland, 1996).

6. Women or their partners who are carriers of chromosome inversions. Each carrier's risk is determined by the method of ascertainment, the chromosome involved, and the size of the inversion, and thus should be determined individually. In general, the observed risk is approximately 5 to 10 percent if ascertainment occurred after the birth of an abnormal child, and 1 to 3 percent if ascertainment occurred by some other means (Gardner and Sutherland, 1996).

7. History of triploidy. Over 99 percent of triploid conceptions are lost in the first or early second trimesters (Chap. 32, p. 837). Rarely, a fetus will develop. If the triploidy involved a fetus surviving past the first trimester, the recurrence risk is 1 to 1.5 percent, sufficient to justify prenatal diagnosis (Gardner and Sutherland, 1996).

8. Repetitive spontaneous first-trimester pregnancy losses. If an abortus is karyotyped, it is unclear as to how to use the data. A history of one early loss caused by a fetal trisomy does not increase the maternal age-related risk for recurrent trisomic pregnancy. The majority of *repetitive* early losses are euploid (Boue and co-workers, 1976; Morton and associates, 1987; Stray-Pedersen and Stray-Pedersen, 1984; Warburton and colleagues, 1987). The few repetitive early pregnancy losses associated with an aneuploidy tend to be caused by maternal or paternal inversions or translocations. These nontrisomic aneuploidies do increase the risk of having another pregnancy with the same karyotypic abnormality. This justifies prenatal diagnosis in subsequent pregnancies if there is not early loss. Considering these facts, karyotyping the *parents,* but not the aborted tissue, after repetitive early losses yields the most useful information about recurrence risks (Warburton and associates, 1987).

9. Parental aneuploidy. Trisomic individuals are often sterile. However, women with trisomy 21 or with 47, XXX, as well as men with 47, XYY are usually fertile and have a 30-percent risk to have trisomic offspring. Men with trisomy 21 or those with 47, XXY are usually sterile.

10. A fetus with a major structural defect identified by ultrasound. This increases the risk of aneuploidy sufficiently to warrant genetic testing of the fetus, regardless of maternal age or parental karyotypes (Marchese and colleagues, 1985; Waldimiroff and co-workers 1998; Williamson and Pringle, 1987).

ISOLATED STRUCTURAL ANOMALIES. Certain structural malformations are multifactorial or polygenic in origin, and thus have a recurrence risk for first-degree relatives of at least 2 to 3 percent. This warrants prenatal counseling and diagnosis. Any woman whose fetus has an affected first-degree relative—sibling, mother, or father—should be offered evaluation. The risk conferred by an affected second-degree relative—aunt, uncle, grandparents, half-siblings—is much lower, but many such patients will still request evaluation. For most multifactorial disorders, the risk resulting from affected third-degree relatives—cousins—is not substantively different than background risk (Thompson and col-

TABLE 37–4. High-Resolution Ultrasonography for Detection of Fetal Anomalies

Head	Gastrointestinal
Anencephaly	Duodenal atresia
Ventriculomegaly/hydrocephaly	Omphalocele
Encephalocele	Gastroschisis
Intracranial lesions	**Urinary Tract**
Neck	Bilateral renal agenesis
Cystic hygroma	Polycystic kidneys
Branchial cleft cysts	Multicystic kidneys
Teratomas	**Skeletal**
Spinal	Achondroplasia
Myelomeningocele	Agenesis or hypoplasia of bones
Sacrococcygeal teratomas	
Chest	Osteogenesis imperfecta
Diaphragmatic hernia	Camptomelic dysplasia
Pleural effusion	**Cardiac**[a]

[a]Frequently requires echocardiography.
Adapted from Vintzileos and colleagues (1987), with permission.

leagues, 1991). For life-threatening or otherwise severe malformations, efforts should be made to complete the evaluation as early in the pregnancy as possible, allowing time for pregnancy termination to be considered. If the parents have decided that they will continue the pregnancy regardless, and the method and location of the delivery will not be altered by the presence of the defect, for example with familial cleft lip, an ultrasound is done for patient reassurance. Table 37–4 lists the kinds of structural defects that can be identified by an ultrasound examination performed by an experienced sonologist using high-resolution equipment.

CONGENITAL HEART DEFECTS. These are the most common isolated structural defects. They have an incidence of 7 per 1000 and a recurrence rate as high as 11 to 13 percent for obstructive left-sided lesions (Burn and colleagues, 1998). Prenatal diagnosis typically involves a careful sonographic evaluation of the heart, usually including an echocardiogram, at approximately 20 to 22 weeks (Chap. 41, p. 1123). This gestational age is optimal because it is advanced enough to allow visualization of all cardiac structures, but still early enough to allow time for a complete workup and consideration of pregnancy termination if an anomaly is found. If the previous lesion was related to abnormal blood flow—for example, hypoplastic left heart, coarctation of the aorta, or pulmonary or aortic stenosis—then a follow-up examination should be scheduled at 24 to 26 weeks. Flow-related defects are believed to result from a change in blood flow through the still-developing cardiac chambers, and

have been reported to develop as late as the third trimester (Hornberger and associates, 1996).

NEURAL-TUBE DEFECTS. Women at increased risk of having a child with a neural-tube defect are offered alpha-fetoprotein *testing* as part of the diagnostic workup. The patient should be counseled and offered prenatal diagnosis with targeted ultrasound and amniocentesis if indicated. As shown in Table 37–5, factors indicating increased risk include the following:

1. Family history of neural-tube defects. This is the most important risk factor for neural-tube defects. Because they are multifactorial in inheritance, the risk to a first-degree relative is approximately 2 to 3 percent. While this is lower than the risk of an autosomal dominant or recessive disorder it is 20 to 30 times higher than the risk of neural-tube defects in the general population. The level of risk is directly related to the number of affected relatives and their degree of relatedness to the *fetus,* and should be estimated individually for each family (Bonaiti-Pellie and Smith, 1974).

2. Exposure to certain environmental agents. A few of these have been implicated in neural-tube defect formation. Exposure must occur during the first 28 days of gestation when the neural tube is developing. **Hyperglycemia,** usually from insulin-dependent diabetes, increases the risk for neural-tube defects (Becerra and colleagues, 1990). The exact mechanism is unknown, but may involve inhibition of fetal glycolysis, a functional deficiency of arachidonic acid or myoinositol in the developing embryo, or alterations in the yolk sac (Reece and Hobbins, 1986). **Hyperthermia** during neural-tube formation has also been implicated to cause defects. Maternal fever and sauna baths have both been reported to increase the relative risk up to sixfold. The duration and intensity of temperature elevation necessary to produce an effect, as well as the embryological mechanism are unknown (Milunsky, 1992). Women concerned about exposing their fetus to acetaminophen should be counseled that exposure to a high fever is more dangerous than exposure to the medication. Certain **drugs** are thought to be causative. *Anticonvulsants,* most notably

TABLE 37–5. Risk Factors for Neural-Tube Defects

Family history of neural-tube defects
Exposure to certain environmental agents
Diabetes (hyperglycemia)
Hyperthermia
Drugs and medications
Genetic syndrome with known recurrence risk
Some racial or ethnic groups and/or living in high-risk geographic regions

valproic acid and *carbamazepine,* impart a significantly increased malformation risk (Chap. 38, p. 1013). *Aminopterin* and *isotretinoin* have been associated with a constellation of abnormalities that can include anencephaly or encephalocele.

3. Neural-tube defects occurring as part of a genetic syndrome with a known recurrence risk. Some inherited syndromes known to include neural-tube defects include Meckel–Gruber, Roberts–SC phocomelia, Jarco–Levin, and HARDE syndromes. These are all autosomal recessive with 25 percent recurrence risk. Trisomies 13 and 18 and triploidy all have a 1 percent recurrence risk (Jones, 1997). Cloacal exstrophy and sacrococcygeal teratoma may be associated with spina bifida. Amnionic bands may cause spina bifida or anencephaly, but these are believed to occur sporadically and have minimal recurrence risk.

4. Individuals belonging to high-risk racial or ethnic groups and/or living in high-risk geographic regions. The United Kingdom has the highest frequency of neural-tube defects, with an incidence of almost 1 percent compared with 0.2 percent in the United States. China, Egypt, and India also have a very high incidence. The frequency of defects in these areas is probably related to both the ethnic (genetic) background of the inhabitants and environmental influences such as diet. This is illustrated by Indian Sikhs living in British Columbia, Canada, who experience less than half the neural-tube defect rate of Sikhs living in India (Thompson and co-workers, 1991). Likewise, individuals of Celtic origin living in the United States and ingesting a fortified American diet are at lower risk than those living in the United Kingdom (Main and Mennuti, 1986; Thompson and co-workers, 1991). These interactions are discussed in greater detail in Chapter 36 (p. 958).

FAMILIAL GENETIC DISEASE. Couples with a personal or family history of a heritable genetic disorder should be offered genetic counseling. Using various laboratory methods discussed in Chapter 36, potential parents can often be offered prenatal diagnosis or at least be provided with a more precise risk of having an affected child. Specific molecular tests for some common genetic diseases are available. The risk of diseases for which the responsible gene has not been identified can sometimes be estimated by comparing fetal DNA with that of affected and unaffected family members (RFLP analysis). The risk of diseases for which no laboratory test has been developed may, in some cases, be refined by ultrasound examination—if the disease is associated with fetal structural abnormalities, or by determination of fetal sex—if the disease is X-linked.

Although ongoing research will undoubtedly result in the development of genetic tests for a great number of diseases, a major issue that remains unresolved for many disorders is phenotype prediction. Because of variable penetrance and expressivity, identification of a specific disease gene is often not enough to predict the phenotype of the affected fetus, even when there have been other affected siblings or family members. The phenotypes of cystic fibrosis, for example, can vary widely within a family (Chap. 36, p. 956). Phenotype prediction is especially difficult when there are no other living affected family members, as would be the case if prenatal diagnosis was offered because of a remote family history or after screening parents at unknown risk.

ETHNIC GROUPS AT HIGH RISK. Although single-gene disorders are generally rare, some ethnic groups are at higher risk than the general population to have certain diseases, and should be counseled and offered genetic testing accordingly. Most of these diseases are caused by otherwise rare autosomal recessive genes that have increased in frequency in certain racial or ethnic groups after generations of mating only within those groups. Individuals from specific geographic regions can also be at increased risk because of genetic isolation, or a phenomenon called the *founder effect.* Autosomal recessive diseases found with increased frequency in ethnic groups living in the United States are listed in Table 37–6 and discussed next.

AFRICAN, MEDITERRANEAN, CARIBBEAN, LATIN AMERICAN, OR MIDDLE EASTERN DESCENT. A number of clinically significant hemoglobin mutations are more prevalent in patients from these areas. Their clinical impact is considered in Chapter 49 (p. 1314). African Americans are at increased risk of having sickle

TABLE 37–6. Autosomal Recessive Diseases Found with Increased Frequency in Certain Ethnic Groups

Disease	Heritage of Groups at Increased Risk
Hemoglobinopathies	African, Mediterranean, Caribbean, Latin American, Middle Eastern
Thalassemia	Mediterranean, Asian
Inborn errors of metabolism: Tay–Sachs, Canavan, Gaucher, Niemann–Pick, Fanconi anemia (type C), Bloom syndrome	Ashkenazi Jewish
Cystic fibrosis	Caucasians of Northern European descent, Ashkenazi Jewish, Native American (Zuni, Pueblo)
Tyrosinemia, fragile X	French Canadian

cell anemia, a severe hemolytic disorder and the most common hemoglobinopathy in the United States. Southeast Asians are at increased risk to carry hemoglobin E, the second most common abnormal hemoglobin in the world.

MEDITERRANEAN OR ASIAN ORIGIN. These individuals are at increased risk of having α- or β-thalassemia (Chap. 49, p. 1320).

JEWISH ANCESTRY. These individuals are at increased risk for Tay–Sachs, Canavan, and Gaucher disease, each of which is caused by a different enzyme deficiency (hexosaminidase A, aspartoacyclase, and glucocerebrosidase, respectively). The carrier rate among individuals of Ashkenazi Jewish heritage is 1 in 30 for Tay–Sachs disease, 1 in 40 for Canavan disease, and 1 in 12 to 25 for Gaucher disease. The American College of Obstetricians and Gynecologists (1995b) recommends that counseling and carrier screening for Tay–Sachs and Canavan disease be offered to all patients of Jewish heritage. Prenatal diagnosis is possible for both diseases. Gaucher disease is more complex because diagnosis requires molecular analysis, and there are three phenotypes that range from mild to severe. Prenatal screening for Gaucher disease, as well as Niemann-Pick, Bloom syndrome, and Fanconi anemia are controversial (Zauri and associates, 1998).

CAUCASIANS OF NORTHERN EUROPEAN DESCENT. Cystic fibrosis is the most common monogenic disorder in this population. It is transmitted in autosomal recessive fashion and has a carrier frequency of about 1 in 25 in Caucasian Americans, 1 in 30 in Native Americans, 1 in 50 in Hispanics, and it ranges from 1 in 90 to 1 in 25 in individuals of Jewish heritage (National Institutes of Health, 1997). More than 800 different gene mutations are known to cause cystic fibrosis. The most common cystic fibrosis mutation in Caucasians is $\Delta F508$ (75 percent) and in the Jewish population are 5T and W12828 (50 percent). If a specific gene mutation or mutations have been identified in an affected family, individuals at risk can be screened for those particular mutations. If both members of the couple carry a cystic fibrosis mutation, prenatal diagnosis is possible.

SCREENING FOR COMMON CONGENITAL ABNORMALITIES

The majority of neural-tube defects, Down syndrome, and many other fetal abnormalities occur in families with no prior history of birth defects. Prenatal evaluation of only high-risk women would thus fail to identify most affected pregnancies. Women with no family history of genetic abnormalities can now be offered screening tests for certain fetal disorders. The screening test does not provide a diagnosis, but identifies individuals whose risk is high enough that they would benefit from further evaluation. A positive screening test must be followed by a definitive test. Screening tests by design have a high false-positive and false-negative rate.

Genetic screening tests should meet the criteria generally accepted for other types of screening tests. These include that the disorder is well defined and serious; treatment or prevention is available, but not possible without the screening test; the test is cost effective and reliable; and there is a reliable diagnostic test (Wald and associates, 1997).

NEURAL-TUBE DEFECTS (NTDs). The pathogenesis of neural-tube defects (NTDs) is discussed in Chapter 36 (p. 958). These defects are the second most common serious fetal malformation in the United States (Centers for Disease Control and Prevention, 1995b). Because only 5 percent of children with NTDs are born into families with other affected members, the majority occur in families with no prior history. Prior to the late 1970s, there was no way to identify these (unexpectedly) affected pregnancies, but then it was discovered that amnionic fluid and maternal serum alpha-fetoprotein was a marker for affected pregnancies.

ALPHA-FETOPROTEIN (AFP). This glycoprotein is synthesized by the fetal yolk sac early in gestation and later by the gastrointestinal tract and liver (Chap. 7). It circulates in fetal serum and passes into fetal urine and amnionic fluid. Although its function is unknown, it is the major serum protein in the embryo-fetus, analogous to albumin. Its concentration increases steadily in both fetal serum and amnionic fluid until 13 weeks, after which these levels rapidly decrease (Burton, 1988). AFP passes into the maternal circulation by diffusion across the placental membranes and may also be transported via the placental circulation (Brumfield and colleagues, 1990). It is found in steadily increasing quantities in maternal serum after 12 weeks (Fig. 37–2). When there is a fetal abnormality such as an opening uncovered by integument somewhere in the body or a number of other problems, then maternal AFP serum levels are increased.

Brock and Sutcliffe (1972) showed that amnionic fluid AFP levels were much higher in pregnancies complicated by fetal anencephaly. Subsequently, Brock and colleagues (1973) demonstrated that maternal serum AFP levels were also elevated in affected pregnancies. The first large prospective trial for maternal serum AFP screening was the UK Collaborative Study on Alphafetoprotein in Relation to Neural-tube Defects (1977). Screening for neural-tube defects was subsequently confirmed by others and adopted in the United States and Europe (Burton and associates, 1983; Haddow and colleagues, 1983; Milunsky and co-workers, 1980).

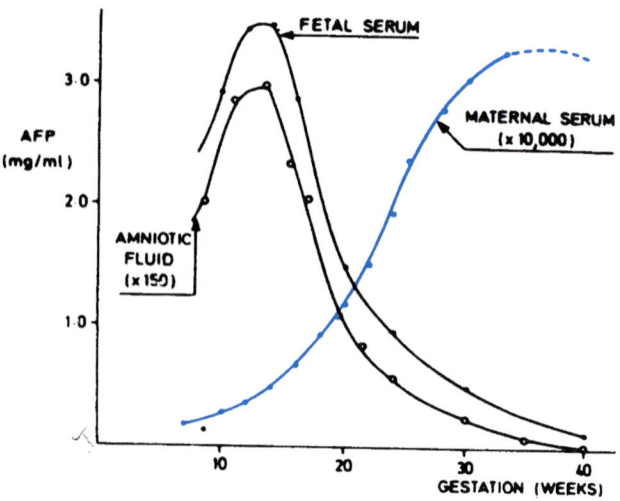

FIGURE 37–2. Maternal and fetal serum and amnionic fluid alpha-fetoprotein levels corresponding with gestational age. (From Roberts and colleagues, 1983, with permission.)

MATERNAL SERUM AFP SCREENING. This is usually done between 15 and 22 weeks, although it has the greatest sensitivity at 16 to 18 weeks. Factors that influence the result include maternal age, weight, race, diabetic status, and number of fetuses as well as gestational age determined by accurate menstrual history or sonography. Maternal serum AFP is measured in ng/mL and reported as a multiple of median (MOM) of the unaffected population. The latter is used because AFP levels do not follow a Gaussian distribution, and because it aids comparison of results from different laboratories and populations (Fig. 37–3). A confirmed increase in

maternal serum AFP to greater than or equal to 2.0 to 2.5 MOM (for most laboratories) indicates increased risk for a fetal NTD or other structural anomaly and warrants further evaluation.

Evaluation for elevated maternal serum AFP begins with a basic ultrasound examination to determine fetal age and the number of fetuses, and to exclude fetal death (Fig. 37–4). Incorrect gestational age assessment accounts for a large proportion of abnormal test results. In some cases, a repeat serum AFP measurement may be helpful. As can be seen in Figure 37–3, the distributions of serum AFP levels overlap in affected and unaffected pregnancies. If the level is within the range of the overlap—the indiscriminate zone of 2.5 to 3.5 MOM—then repeating the measurement may determine to which distribution the sample belongs, that is, affected or unaffected. Because repeated sample values tend to regress toward the mean of population to which they belong, a truly elevated serum AFP level will still be elevated in the repeat sample, while a level corresponding to an unaffected pregnancy may normalize.

Maternal serum AFP levels greater than 3.5 MOM need not be repeated, as levels this high are outside the AFP distribution of unaffected pregnancies and clearly indicate increased fetal risk. In general, the likelihood that the fetus is affected increases along with the AFP level. In a study of 773 women with elevated serum AFP levels, Reichler and colleagues (1994) reported that there was a progressive increase in the frequency of neural-tube defects, ventral wall defects, and total anomalies as a direct function of maternal serum levels (Fig. 37–5). Approximately 40 percent of pregnancies were abnormal when the AFP level was greater than 7 MOM.

The majority of women with an abnormally elevated maternal serum AFP level do not have a fetus with a neural-tube defect. In some, other fetal anomalies or pregnancy abnormalities are the cause of increased levels (Table 37–7). The American College of Obstetricians and Gynecologists (1996c) recommends that all pregnant women be offered second-trimester maternal serum AFP screening. This is done only within a coordinated system that includes quality control, counseling, follow-up, and high-resolution sonographic facilities. Using an MSAFP level of 2.0 or 2.5 MOM as the upper limit of normal, most laboratories report a screen-positive rate of 3 to 5 percent, a sensitivity of at least 90 percent, and a positive-predictive value of 2 to 6 percent (Milunsky and associates, 1989). Because only 1 in 16 to 33 women with an elevated serum AFP level actually has an affected fetus, women should be counseled regarding the high false-positive rates, risks with amniocentesis, and the rationale for the screening program.

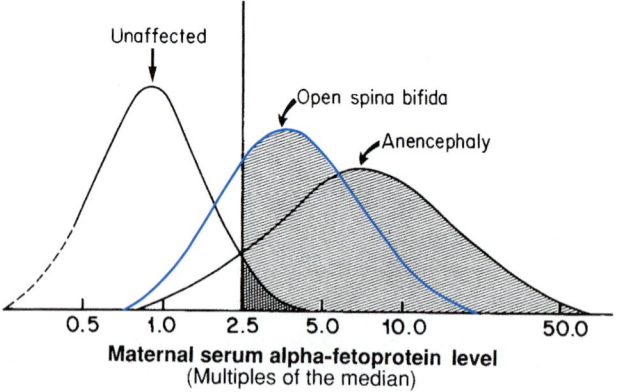

FIGURE 37–3. Maternal serum alpha-fetoprotein levels in singleton gestations 16 to 18 weeks. The cutoff value of 2.5 multiples of the median results in both false-positive and false-negative diagnosis. Any cutoff point chosen, however, would result in false-positive (cross-hatched area) and false-negative rates. (Redrawn from American College of Obstetricians and Gynecologists, 1986, with permission.)

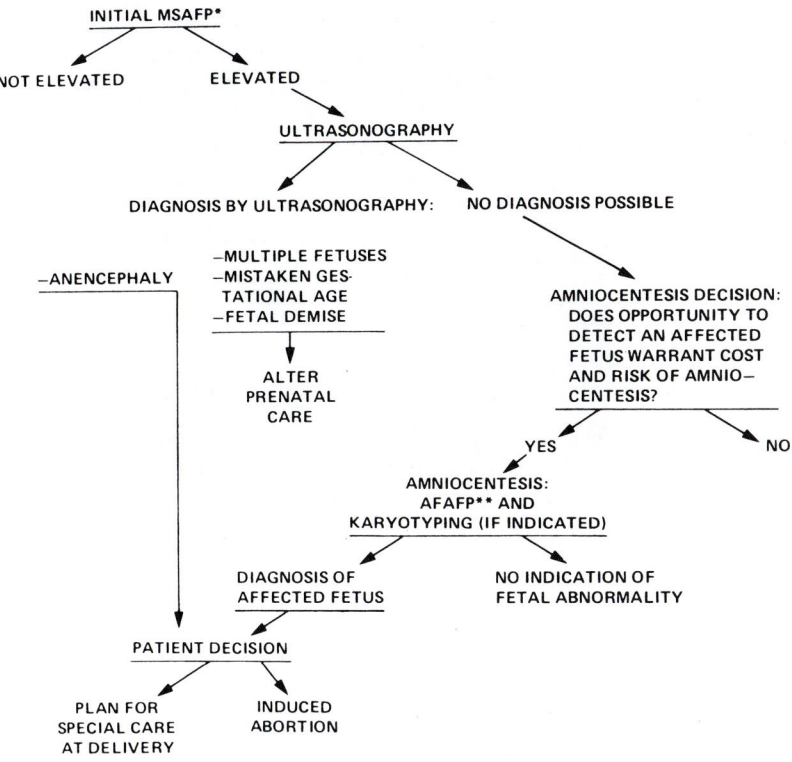

FIGURE 37–4. Algorithm for evaluating an elevated maternal serum alpha-fetoprotein (MSAFP) level. (From Adams and colleagues, 1984, with permission.)

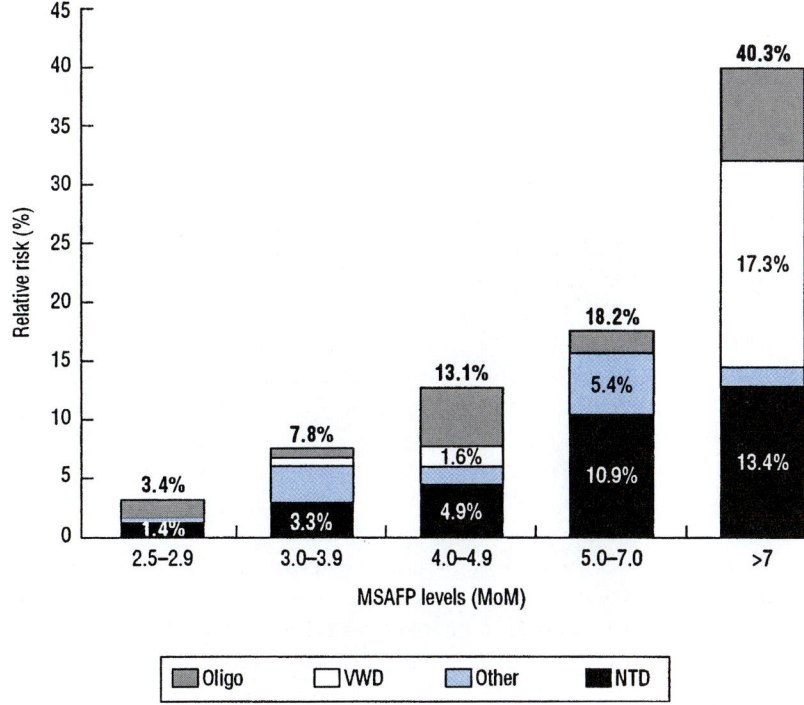

FIGURE 37–5. Anomalies and oligohydramnios distribution as function of elevated maternal serum alpha-fetoprotein levels (MSAFP). (MoM = multiples of median; NTD = neural-tube defect; Oligo = oligohydramnios; Other = subchorionic bleeding, intraabdominal echogenicity, hydronephrosis, echogenic bowel, dilated kidney, heart defect; VWD = ventral wall defect.) (From Reichler and colleagues, 1994, with permission.)

TABLE 37–7. Some Conditions Associated with Abnormal Maternal Serum Alphafetoprotein Concentrations

Elevated Levels
Neural-tube defects
Pilonidal cysts
Esophageal or intestinal obstruction
Liver necrosis
Cystic hygroma
Sacrococcygeal teratoma
Abdominal wall defects—omphalocele, gastroschisis
Urinary obstruction
Renal anomalies—polycystic or absent kidneys
Congenital nephrosis
Osteogenesis imperfecta
Congenital skin defects
Cloacal exstrophy
Chorioangioma of placenta
Low birthweight
Oligohydramnios
Multifetal gestation
Decreased maternal weight
Underestimated gestational age
Maternal hepatoma or teratoma
Low Levels
Chromosomal trisomies
Gestational trophoblastic disease
Fetal death
Increased maternal weight
Overestimated gestational age

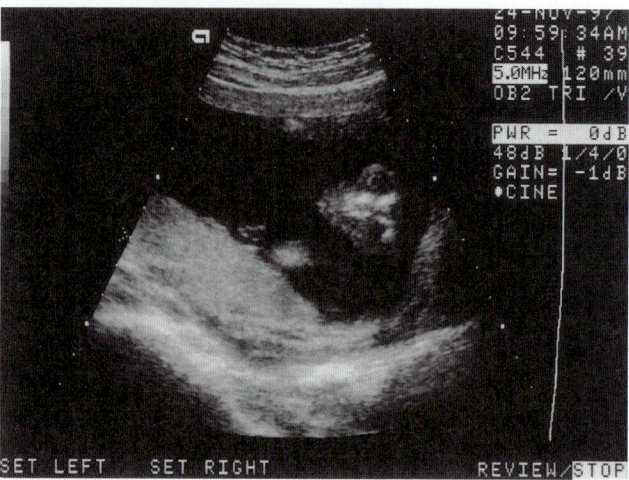

FIGURE 37–6. Anencephalic fetus with the face visualized by sonography. (Courtesy of Dr. Jodi Dashe.)

authors recommend that a woman with an elevated serum AFP level could be counseled that the risk of a neural-tube defect is reduced by 95 percent if no spine defects or cranial findings are seen (Hogge, 1989; Morrow, 1991; Van den Hof, 1990, and their colleagues). In fact, nearly 100 percent accuracy of detection of neural-tube defects with ultrasound has been reported (Nadel and colleagues, 1990; Sepulveda and associates, 1995).

Ultrasound is also helpful in identifying other causes of elevated AFP levels such as fetal death or multiple gestation; structural abnormalities such as gastroschisis, omphalocele, bladder exstrophy, sacrococcygeal teratoma, cystic hygroma, hydrops, esophageal or intestinal obstruction, and renal abnormalities; and placental ab-

ULTRASOUND EXAMINATION. When elevated serum AFP levels are confirmed, the fetus is evaluated by targeted ultrasound. As shown in Figure 37–6, anencephaly and other major cranial defects are usually readily visualized. Most spine defects can be detected as well (Limb and Holmes, 1994). They may be diagnosed by visualization of the open spinal lesion itself (Fig. 37–7). In some cases, the lesions are suspected following identification of certain associated cranial abnormalities (Chap. 41, p. 1120). In a review of 234 fetuses with spina bifida from nine different studies, Watson and associates (1991) reported that 99 percent had at least one of five specific cranial anomalies detected by ultrasound. These include frontal notching, also called the *lemon sign* (Fig. 37–8); ventriculomegaly with the lateral ventricle width greater than 10 mm; obliteration of the cisterna magna; small biparietal diameter; and elongated cerebellum referred to as the *banana sign* (Fig. 37–8). These cranial anomalies are most clearly visible in the second trimester, and some (lemon sign) may resolve later in pregnancy. Some

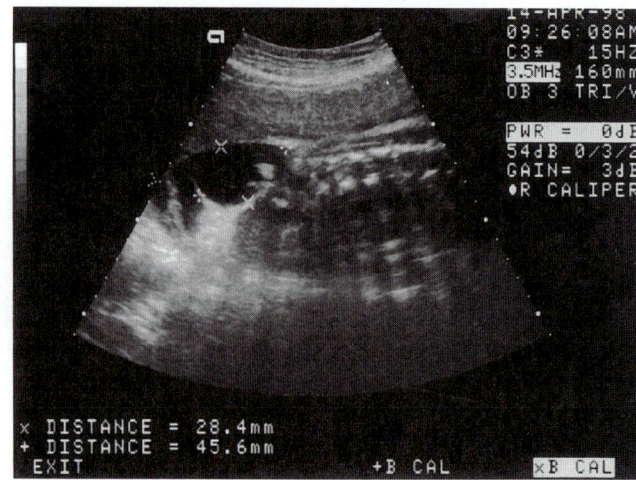

FIGURE 37–7. Lumbosacral view of meningomyelocele. (Courtesy of Dr. Jodi Dashe.)

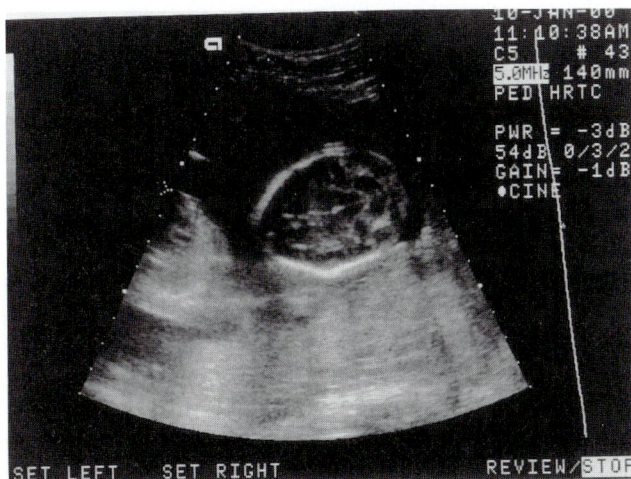

FIGURE 37-8. Cranial ultrasound in fetus with Arnold–Chiari malformation showing frontal scalloping (lemon sign) on the left and effacement of the cisterna magna (banana sign) on the right. (Courtesy of Dr. Jodi Dashe.)

normalities such as chorioangioma or oligohydramnios (Table 37–7).

Although during the first decade of AFP screening, all women with elevated serum levels were offered amniocentesis routinely, current ultrasound resolution has made the need to measure amnionic fluid AFP controversial. Although some investigators have reported nearly 100 percent diagnostic accuracy with ultrasound without amniocentesis, others have not. Perhaps more realistic "real world" findings were described by Platt and co-workers (1992) from a statewide screening program that included ultrasound performed by a variety of practitioners. They reported that 6 of 161 open spina bifida cases were not recognized. Alternatively, amnionic fluid AFP analysis identifies all open neural-tube defects but misses the 3 to 5 percent of fetuses whose spinal defect is covered by skin (Crandall and Matsumoto, 1984). The decision for amniocentesis thus is individualized, and considers both ultrasound quality and patient desires.

AMNIOCENTESIS. Amnionic fluid AFP levels are measured if an NTD is suspected or if the ultrasound is nondiagnostic in the presence of elevated maternal serum AFP. If elevated, the presence or absence of acetylcholinesterase is determined in amnionic fluid. The presence of this enzyme verifies that there is exposed neural tissue or another open fetal defect. Elevation of the amnionic fluid AFP level without acetylcholinesterase suggests another etiology or from fetal blood contamination. Importantly, it frequently is prognostic of other adverse outcomes (American College of Obstetricians and Gynecologists, 1996c).

There is another reason for amniocentesis with sono-

graphic diagnosis of an isolated neural-tube defect. Because of a small associated risk of aneuploidy, which would affect the prognosis considerably, fetal karyotyping may be indicated. Hume and associates (1996), in a review of over 17,000 prenatal diagnosis cases, observed a 2 percent rate of aneuploidy in the 106 fetuses with isolated neural-tube defects. Harmon and colleagues (1995) found that 7 of 43 fetuses with isolated neural-tube defects were aneuploid.

If the targeted ultrasound survey is normal when the maternal serum AFP level is clearly outside the indiscriminate zone—that is, greater than 3.5 MOM—then amniocentesis for fetal karyotype is controversial. Thiagarajah and colleagues (1995) studied 658 women with elevated maternal serum AFP levels and concluded that there was no justification for routine fetal karyotyping with a normal targeted ultrasonography. In contrast, Feuchtbaum and associates (1995) reported results from 8097 women who underwent amniocentesis and fetal karyotyping under these circumstances and they found a twofold increased rate of chromosomal anomalies compared with the general population. Watson and colleagues (1991) reported an aneuploidy rate of 1 in 164 composed of sex chromosome abnormalities, translocations, or triploidies.

Some clinicians evaluate the fetal karyotype only if both the maternal serum and amnionic fluid AFP are elevated. Gonzalez and associates (1996) reported that routine karyotyping was not necessary in women with elevated serum AFP but with normal amnionic fluid levels. If the amnionic fluid AFP was abnormal, however, the incidence of chromosomal abnormalities was elevated fivefold over background risk.

INCIDENTAL AMNIONIC FLUID AFP MEASUREMENT. When amniocentesis is done primarily for fetal cytogenetic analysis such as advanced maternal age, amnionic fluid AFP is often routinely measured. It is not known if this practice is cost-effective. In a retrospective analysis of 1737 such amnionic fluid specimens, Sepulveda and associates (1995) reported that ultrasonography correctly identified all fetuses with abnormal amnionic fluid AFP levels, and that routine measurement was probably unnecessary if targeted ultrasonography was normal. Shields and colleagues (1996), in a review of almost 7000 women who underwent second-trimester genetic amniocentesis, reported that measurement of amnionic fluid AFP did not increase the detection of fetal anomalies.

OTHER CAUSES OF ELEVATED SERUM AFP LEVELS. Maternal serum screening as described has a sensitivity of about 90 percent, but unfortunately has a positive-predictive value of only 2 to 6 percent (Milunsky and colleagues, 1989). Thus, the majority of women with elevated levels do not have a fetus with a neural-tube defect; however, some may be at increased risk for other conditions shown in Table 37–7.

UNEXPLAINED ELEVATED ABNORMAL AFP LEVELS.
Even if there are no obvious fetal abnormalities, unexplained high serum levels may forecast a poor pregnancy outcome. Several large studies have documented increased perinatal morbidity and mortality, including low birthweight, oligohydramnios, placental abruption, and fetal death in these women (Katz, 1990; Simpson, 1991; Waller, 1991, and their associates). Wenstrom and co-workers (1992) showed that the first serum determination is most predictive and that serial measurements are not helpful. Simpson and colleagues (1991) did a cohort study and reported that there was a significant association between second-trimester but not third-trimester elevation of maternal serum AFP levels and preterm prematurely ruptured membranes, preterm birth, and low-birthweight infants. Ramus and associates (1996), in a study of 241 women with unexplained serum AFP elevations, reported a higher incidence of preterm delivery compared with women who had normal levels (22 versus 11 percent). The incidence of preterm delivery was highest (47 percent) in the 38 women who had both an otherwise unexplained elevated serum level along with placental sonolucencies on ultrasound.

Unfortunately, neither the etiology of the majority of elevated serum values, nor the most appropriate management for these women is clear. There is no evidence that such outcomes are favorably affected by any specific program of maternal or fetal surveillance (American College of Obstetricians and Gynecologists, 1996c; Cunningham and Gilstrap, 1991).

MANAGEMENT OF THE FETUS WITH A NEURAL-TUBE DEFECT. Other than termination of pregnancy, options are limited. Anencephaly, exencephaly, and iniencephaly are lethal disorders, but some women with these diagnoses elect to continue their pregnancy and should receive routine prenatal care. Antenatal fetal testing, intrapartum fetal heart rate monitoring, and cesarean delivery for fetal indications are not recommended.

A woman whose fetus has another type of neural-tube defect may benefit from counseling by a pediatric neurosurgeon, neurologist, or other specialists in pediatric development. The fully informed couple is more likely to make the best decision and to be prepared for pregnancy outcomes.

If pregnancy is continued, serial sonographic examinations are done. Generally, delivery at term is optimal. Rapidly increasing ventriculomegaly, however, may prompt delivery before term so that a shunting procedure can be performed. The optimal timing and method of delivery remain controversial. All studies of vaginal versus cesarean delivery are retrospective, and all suffer from various biases (Bensen and co-workers, 1988; Luthy and colleagues, 1991; Sakala and Andree, 1990). Theoretically, cesarean delivery possibly avoids mechanical trauma and infection of the fetal spine. It also allows precise timing of the delivery so that the appropriate consultants can be available.

DOWN SYNDROME. The vast majority—97 percent—of Down syndrome pregnancies occur de novo in families with no previous history of this or other aneuploidy. Moreover, 80 percent are born to women who are younger than age 35 (Chap. 36, p. 942). Prior to the mid-1980s, diagnosis was limited to women 35 and older by genetic amniocentesis. In 1984, Merkatz and colleagues reported that Down syndrome screening was possible because these pregnancies were associated with unusually low maternal serum AFP levels. Cuckle and colleagues (1984) and Haddow and associates (1983) confirmed this, and neural-tube defect screening programs began to include Down syndrome screening. Because maternal age-related risk is still the most powerful predictor of fetal aneuploidy, screening programs eventually calculated risk by converting the serum AFP level to a likelihood ratio. The maternal age-related risk was multiplied by this ratio (New England Regional Genetics Group, 1989). Women with a calculated Down syndrome risk greater than a predetermined cutoff—usually either the midtrimester or term risk of a 36-year-old—were offered amniocentesis for definitive diagnosis.

MULTIPLE MARKER SCREENING. Serum analytes other than AFP were also found to be altered by fetal aneuploidy. These include elevated serum levels of chorionic gonadotropin and decreased unconjugated estriol with Down syndrome (Bogart and colleagues, 1987; Wald and associates, 1988a, 1988b). Although both hCG and estriol can individually distinguish Down syndrome from euploid pregnancies, when used together with AFP, they are more predictive. Thus, the three relative risks are combined and multiplied by the age-related risk. This combination is termed the *expanded AFP test, AFP plus, triple screen,* or *multiple marker screening test.* The test has been validated and has become the preferred Down syndrome screening test in most centers (Burton, 1993; Cheng, 1993; Haddow, 1992; Wenstrom, 1993, and their colleagues). At a cutoff associated with about a 5 percent screen-positive rate, the multiple marker screening test identifies approximately 60 percent of all Down syndrome pregnancies in women under age 35 (Table 37–8). In women over 35, it detects over 75 percent of Down syndrome and a portion of other aneuploidies (Haddow and co-workers, 1994).

Many permutations of these analytes are in current use. Estriol measurement is a subject of debate, and

TABLE 37–8. Maternal Age-Related Down Syndrome Detection and Screen-Positive Rates Using the Multiple Marker Screening Test[a]

Maternal Age	False-Positive Rate (%)	Detection Rate (%)
20	2.4	41
25	2.9	44
30	5	52
35	14	71
40	40	91

[a]Employs levels of maternal serum alpha-fetoprotein, unconjugated estriol, and chorionic gonadotropin, which are then correlated with the age-adjusted risk.
From Haddow and colleagues (1994), with permission.

some centers offer AFP and hCG alone. Some prefer free β-hCG measurement to the intact hCG molecule. A variety of other multiple-marker screening tests has been reported (Bahado-Singh, 2001; Morris, 2001; Wenstrom, 1999, and their colleagues).

The multiple-marker test has a high false-positive rate, and only 6 percent of all screen-positive samples are associated with an affected fetus. Likewise, it has a false-negative rate. A negative multiple-marker screening test indicates "no increased risk," but does not mean that the fetus is normal. If gestational age is confirmed by sonography, these women with a positive screen are offered amniocentesis for karyotyping (American College of Obstetricians and Gynecologists, 1996c).

FIRST-TRIMESTER DOWN SYNDROME SCREENING. Identification of fetal aneuploidy earlier than is currently possible with traditional amniocentesis is desirable for many reasons, including that more options for pregnancy termination would be available. First-trimester screening protocols under study include maternal serum analyte screening, ultrasound evaluation, a combination of both, or urinary screening. The most discriminatory analytes at this gestational age appear to be free β-hCG and pregnancy-associated plasma protein A (PAPP-A) (Haddow and associates, 1998; Wald and colleagues, 1998). The median free β-hCG level in affected pregnancies is approximately 1.79 MOM, while the median PAPP-A level is approximately 0.43 MOM.

Dimeric inhibin A and AFP levels are too similar in affected and unaffected pregnancies to be of value in first-trimester screening (Wald and associates, 1988b). Some problems include that free β-hCG is not markedly elevated in Down syndrome pregnancies until 12 weeks, while PAPP-A loses discrimination after 13 weeks. Accurate assessment of gestational age and careful timing of the screening test are thus essential (Wald and co-workers, 1998). Several investigative protocols combine

maternal serum analytes, ultrasound assessment of the nuchal fold, long bone measurements, and other parameters as discussed later.

SERUM SCREENING IN WOMEN OVER AGE 35. If serum screening were totally accurate, empirical amniocentesis could be avoided. There is, however, no currently available screening test capable of determining with 100 percent accuracy which women over 35 have an aneuploid fetus. For some older women, serum screening facilitates the decision to undergo invasive testing.

ELECTIVE GENETIC AMNIOCENTESIS IN WOMEN UNDER AGE 35. Maternal age 35 was chosen somewhat arbitrarily as the age cutoff above which genetic amniocentesis should be routinely offered to all women. As discussed, this cutoff was chosen in part because, at age 35, the midtrimester risk of any aneuploidy roughly equals the risk of amniocentesis-associated pregnancy loss. With development of more sophisticated sonographic guidance, there now is a lower procedure-associated loss rate in many centers. Also, the relative weights of the two risks being considered—risk of aneuploidy versus the risk of pregnancy loss—may not be considered equal by all women. Thus, these must be determined individually according to each couple's own values and belief (Pauker and Pauker, 1994).

Because of the foregoing, some women under 35 may request amniocentesis despite reassuring maternal serum screening and ultrasound findings. Druzin and co-workers (1993) offered elective amniocentesis to 592 women younger than 35, and 161 (22 percent) accepted. There were no procedure-related losses. They concluded that they did not invoke any psychological issues to compel young women to accept invasive testing, and that the women were able to resist the "technological imperative." Each diagnostic center must develop its own protocol to handle such requests. Some consider requests by women at least 30 years old, who have a midtrimester risk for all aneuploidies of 1 in 384, to be reasonable, but they discourage younger women.

URINARY ANALYTES. Screening for fetal Down syndrome by urine testing is appealing because of ease and simplicity. Maternal urinary total estriol and the various forms of degraded hCG (intact and nicked hCG, free α- and β-subunits, and β-core fragment) seem to have the most potential for Down syndrome screening (Canick and co-workers, 1995; Cuckle and colleagues, 1994). In a large multicenter international trial to investigate first trimester urinary β-core hCG fragment screening, Cuckle and associates (1999) reported a low discriminatory power. They analyzed 6730 samples from 16 centers, and only a fourth of all aneuploidies screened positive. Further research in this area is ongoing.

SCREENING FOR HERITABLE GENETIC DISEASES

The development of molecular tests for various genetic diseases has raised the possibility of population screening. Current debate centers on screening for fragile X and cystic fibrosis, but will no doubt extend to other conditions as more disease-specific genes are identified. The issues complicating fragile X and cystic fibrosis screening illustrate problems likely to be faced with other genetic screening tests. The wide range of phenotypes and the difficulty in predicting phenotypes make it unclear that the diseases in question are always well-defined and serious; there is often no treatment available other than pregnancy termination; the tests are usually expensive; and a reliable diagnostic test does not always exist.

FRAGILE X SYNDROME. This is the most common cause of familial mental retardation, and is discussed in detail in Chapter 36 (p. 954). Although it is an X-chromosome linked anomaly, inheritance of fragile X does not conform to the usual rules governing X-linked traits. This is because the fragile X mutation is an unstable region of repeated CGG trinucleotides that can expand only when transmitted by a female. When the expansion reaches a critical size (more than 230 repeats), it is methylated and thus inactivated. Female carriers of a "premutation" who have 56 to 229 CGG repeats are at risk to pass on an expanded gene, and the individual inheriting the gene is at high risk to exhibit fragile X phenotype (Fisch and colleagues, 1995).

CARRIER SCREENING. Based on current knowledge, fragile X does not meet criteria established for a good screening test. The prevalence of the premutation in the general population is unknown, so it is not clear who should be offered testing. It is estimated to be approximately 1 in 700, an incidence that is much lower than that of other genetic diseases for which screening is usually considered (Hagerman and co-workers, 1991). Currently, it is not possible to predict whether a female carrier will pass on an expanded gene. Scandinavian studies have demonstrated that even large premutations can be passed unchanged through several generations (Holmgren and co-workers, 1988). Finally, phenotype prediction in a fetus carrying the full mutation is also imprecise. Because of lyonization, as many as half of females inheriting the full fragile X mutation will be intellectually normal (deVries and colleagues, 1996). There also is wide phenotypic variation due to mosaicism in males inheriting the gene.

TESTING. Given the preceding concerns, it is currently recommended that any individual with unexplained mental retardation be tested for fragile X, especially if there are clinical findings consistent with the syndrome, or a family history (Cutillo, 1994). In this setting, approximately 2 to 6 percent of males and 2 to 4 percent of females will be determined to have the full mutation (Curry and associates, 1997). Family members of patients with documented fragile X syndrome should also be offered fragile X testing. The goal is to identify premutation carriers and allow them to make informed reproductive choices. Based on available data, it seems unlikely that it will be cost effective to test relatives of patients with unexplained mental retardation *not* known to be due to fragile X (Curry and co-workers, 1997; Wenstrom and collaborators, 1999a). Testing of women without a family history of neurodevelopmental disorders is not recommended by the American College of Obstetricians and Gynecologists (1995c).

CYSTIC FIBROSIS. This autosomal recessive disorder is caused by a gene with a frequency of about 1 in 25 in Caucasians of Northern European heritage. As discussed in Chapter 46 (p. 1243), in its classical form it is marked by abnormal sweat chloride levels, chronic pulmonary disease, pancreatic insufficiency, liver disease, and obstructive azoospermia (Rosenstein and Zeitlin, 1998). The tremendous range of clinical expression likely reflects both the degree to which protein function is changed by the mutation, and variation in susceptibility to environmental factors associated with the altered protein. Although there have been improvements in care, there is no advantage to diagnosing cystic fibrosis prenatally other than to consider pregnancy termination.

CARRIER SCREENING. The CF gene on the long arm of chromosome 7 encodes the protein that is the *cystic fibrosis conductance transmembrane regulator (CFTR)*. Over 800 mutations in this large gene have been described thus far. Because it is not possible to screen for all known mutations during carrier testing, unless there is a family history, most laboratories screen for the 16 to 32 mutations causing most CF cases. The ΔF508 mutation is always included as it accounts for 75 percent of cases in Caucasians, and the 5T and W1282X mutations are included if the patient is Jewish. It is obvious that a negative test does not preclude possibilities of carrying another of the over 800 known mutations. Negative screening for 32 mutations does, however, reduce the risk substantively from the background rate.

Because CF is a recessive disorder, a fetus must inherit an affected gene from each parent to have the disease. If only one partner undergoes CF screening, the couple's risk to have a child with CF can be calculated assuming that the other partner has a 1 in 25 background risk. Some patients will be reassured by this analysis if the only goal is to determine the risk to the fetus. The key to CF screening is knowing which mutations to test for, which requires knowledge of the CF mutations common to different heritages. Currently, CF screening is most accurate for Caucasians of Northern European descent and for those of Ashkenazi Jewish heritage.

FETAL TESTING. If both parents are carriers, the fetus can be tested for homozygosity for the same mutation. Phenotype prediction is fairly accurate if the mutations are Δ508 or W1282X. Other mutations are less closely associated with disease symptoms, making phenotype prediction and decisions about the fate of the pregnancy difficult. Importantly, there is poor genotype–phenotype correlation of these other mutations with pulmonary disease, which is the most severe aspect of CF. For all of these reasons, individuals who have an affected first- or second-degree relative should be offered counseling and possible cystic fibrosis screening. Although some authors have recommended that screening be offered to all pregnant women, the American College of Obstetricians and Gynecologists (1991, 1995a) recommends against widespread screening until the standard screening battery includes more mutations and thus reduces the risk further.

ULTRASOUND SCREENING

INCIDENTAL FINDING OF A MAJOR STRUCTURAL DEFECT. Major structural fetal anomalies or minor dysmorphic features are often discovered in otherwise low-risk pregnancies during ultrasonography performed for other indications. In addition to concerns about the anomaly itself, the *etiology* of the anomaly is important. For example, if the defect is part of a genetic syndrome, the fetus may have other abnormalities that are undetectable by ultrasound but which affect the prognosis— for example, mental retardation. Fetal aneuploidy is usually at the top of the differential diagnosis list, because such fetuses often have major anatomical malformations and minor dysmorphic features. The specific risk associated with several relatively common major anomalies is listed in Table 37–9.

Fetal aneuploidy can only be diagnosed by evaluating the karyotype. The nature of the structural abnormality is used to estimate the risk of aneuploidy and to facilitate decisions regarding invasive testing. In general, any abnormality involving a major organ or structure, or the finding of multiple minor structural abnormalities in the same fetus, indicate a sufficiently significant risk of aneuploidy to justify amniocentesis (Wladimiroff and associates, 1998; Williamson and colleagues, 1987). Although some combinations of anomalies may indicate a genetic syndrome not resulting from aneuploidy, fetal karyotype analysis is still warranted because aneuploidy-associated abnormalities can mimic other syndromes.

SONOGRAPHIC SCREENING FOR MAJOR STRUCTURAL ANOMALIES. Routine early second-trimester ultrasonography specifically to look for structural fetal abnormalities in low-risk women is controversial. Before this issue can be resolved, the detection and false-negative rates for such screening examinations need to be determined. The largest study to date addressing these issues is the RADIUS trial reported by Ewigman and colleagues (1993) and discussed in Chapter 41 (p. 1114). Almost 16,000 low-risk women were examined sonographically and one important finding was that only 17 percent of all major congenital anomalies were detected before 24 weeks. Although tertiary centers have higher detection rates, it appears that even under ideal circumstances, the detection rate for major anomalies may not be high enough to warrant routine screening with ultrasound in low-risk women.

SONOGRAPHIC SCREENING FOR MINOR ABNORMALITIES. By themselves, minor abnormalities or dysmorphisms usually do not affect the fetal prognosis in any substantive way, but they are of extreme interest because they can be associated with fetal aneuploidy. To date, dysmorphisms have been studied mostly in high-risk women. It is controversial whether ultrasound evaluation for fetal dysmorphisms should be offered as a Down syndrome screening test in low-risk women— instead of or as a supplement to maternal serum screening. Down syndrome risks resulting from ultrasonically detected dysmorphisms such as thickened nuchal fold, mild hydronephrosis, echogenic bowel, slightly shortened long bones, choroid plexus cysts, and others derived from high-risk women are listed in Table 37–10. Nuchal fold thickness appears to be the best discriminator of affected and unaffected pregnancies in the first trimester.

NUCHAL FOLD. This fold is seen as a sonolucency at the back of the fetal neck in the midsagittal plane. Although its precise etiology and significance are unknown, it may represent one end of the spectrum of lymphatic obstruction sequence. Most data regarding the utility of nuchal fold measurements have been obtained in the first trimester. Several investigators have reported that, even under optimal circumstances, first-trimester nuchal fold measurements typically identify less than half of all Down syndrome cases (Brambati and colleagues, 1995; Haddow and Palomaki, 1996).

The nuchal fold is difficult to measure accurately and reproducibly at this early age (Roberts and co-workers, 1995). Normal measurements are between 0 and 5 mm,

TABLE 37-9. Aneuploidy Risk Associated with Major Structural Fetal Malformations

Defect	Population Incidence	Aneuploidy Risk	Most Common Aneuploidy (Trisomy)
Cystic hygroma	1/120 EU–1/6000 B	60–75%	45 X (80%), 21, 18, 13, XXY
Hydrops	1/1500–4000 B	30–80%[a]	13, 21, 18, 45, X
Hydrocephalus	3–8/10,000 LB	3–8%	13, 18, triploidy
Hydranencephaly	2/1000 IA	Minimal	
Holoprosencephaly	1/16,000 LB	40–60%	13, 18, 18p-
Cardiac defects	7–9/1000 LB	5–30%	21, 18, 13, 22, 8, 9
Diaphragmatic hernia	1/3500–4000 LB	20–25%	13, 18, 21, 45, X
Omphalocele	1/5800 LB	30–40%	13, 18
Gastroschisis	1/10,000–15,000 LB	Minimal	
Duodenal atresia	1/10,000 LB	20–30%	21
Bowel obstruction	1/2500–5000 LB	Minimal	
Bladder outlet obstruction	1–2/1000 B	20–25%	13, 18
Facial cleft	1/700 LB	1%	13, 18, deletions
Limb reduction	4–6/10,000 LB	8%	18
Club foot	1.2/1000 LB	20–30%	18, 13, 4p-, 18q-
Single umbilical artery	1/100 LB	Minimal	

B = birth; EU = early ultrasound; IA = infant autopsy; LB = live birth.
[a]30% if diagnosed ≥24 weeks; 80% if diagnosed ≤17 weeks.
Data from Marchese (1985); Nyberg (1990); Wald (1998); Wladimiroff (1998); Williamson (1987), and all their colleagues.

TABLE 37-10. Down Syndrome Risk Associated with Minor Fetal Abnormalities and Dysmorphic Features

Ultrasound Marker	Risk (%)	False-Positives (%)
Nuchal fold ≥ 6 mm	38	1.3
Femur length (O/E)	34	5.9
Femur length (BPD/FL)	22	5.9
Humerus length (O/E)	37	5.3
Femur plus humerus (O/E)	36	3.7
Pyelectasis	19	2.4
Hyperechogenic bowel	11	0.7
Ventricular dilatation	6	0
Choroid plexus cyst	0	1.8
Ear length	78	8.0
Fifth midphalanx hypoplasia	75	18
Increased iliac length	50	2
Short frontal lobe	21	4.8

BPD = biparietal diameter; FL = fetal length; O/E = observed compared with expected.
Adapted from Wald and colleagues (1998), with permission.

with an overlap of 2 to 3 mm in affected and unaffected populations. Flexion or extension of the head can change measurements by as much as 0.62 mm, while an unfavorable fetal position or maternal obesity may prevent measurement. Roberts and colleagues (1995) and Haddow and Palomaki (1996) have reported that first-trimester measurement is technically impossible in up to 20 percent of women. Finally, most prevalence data is from high-risk pregnancy, and it is unclear whether these can or should be extrapolated to younger, low-risk women (Wald and colleagues, 1998).

MATERNAL AGE. If one of a number of minor dysmorphisms is identified, then a better risk estimate can sometimes be calculated for Down syndrome using maternal age (Vintzileos and associates, 1995; Wald and colleagues, 1998). This has been done for both nuchal fold thickening and choroid plexus cysts (Fig. 41–6, p. 1121). Gupta and colleagues (1997) used data from 200,000 ultrasound examinations and concluded that isolated choroid plexus cysts in women over age 32 carried a significant enough risk of trisomy 18 to justify fetal karyotyping.

Another technique undergoing testing is revision of risk estimate of biochemical analytes by ultrasound findings. For example, it may be possible that combining dysmorphisms with AFP screening may provide a more accurate risk assessment for Down syndrome.

DIAGNOSTIC TECHNIQUES

SECOND-TRIMESTER AMNIOCENTESIS. Amniocentesis for genetic diagnosis is usually performed between 15 and 20 weeks. A number of multicenter studies have confirmed its safety as well as its more than 99 percent diagnostic accuracy (Canadian Early and Mid-Trimester Amniocentesis Trial Group, 1998; NICHD National Registry for Amniocentesis Study Group, 1976). Typically, ultrasound guidance is used to pass a 20- to 22-gauge spinal needle into the amnionic sac while avoiding the placenta, umbilical cord, and fetus. The initial aspirate of 1 or 2 mL of fluid is discarded to decrease the chance of maternal cell contamination, and then after approximately 20 mL of fluid is collected, the needle is removed. The puncture site is observed for bleeding, and the patient is shown the beating fetal heart and remaining amnionic fluid at the conclusion of the procedure. Several studies have confirmed that the incidence of bloody taps, amnionic fluid leakage, and multiple punctures are inversely related to the operator experience (Leschot and co-workers, 1985; Romero and colleagues, 1985).

Minor complications are infrequent and include transient vaginal spotting or amnionic fluid leakage in 1 to 2 percent and chorioamnionitis in fewer than 1 in 1000. Needle injuries to the fetus are rare when ultrasound guidance is used. Cell culture failure is also rare, but is more likely if the fetus is abnormal (Persutte and Lenke, 1995). The fetal loss rate is 0.5 percent or less (1 in 200), and it does not appear possible to reduce this further (Simpson, 1990; Wilson and colleagues, 1984). It may be that some losses result from preexisting abnormalities and were destined to occur whether or not amniocentesis was performed. These might include placental abruption, abnormal placental implantation, uterine anomalies, and infection. Wenstrom and colleagues (1996) analyzed 66 postamniocentesis losses following nearly 12,000 second-trimester procedures, and found that 12 percent were caused by preexisting intrauterine infection.

EARLY AMNIOCENTESIS. This is performed between 11 and 14 weeks and has been widely studied (Johnson, 1994; Nicolaides, 1994; Shulman, 1994; Sundberg, 1997, and all of their associates). The technique is the same as for traditional amniocentesis, although lack of membrane fusion to the uterine wall makes puncture of the sac difficult, and less fluid is withdrawn (usually 1 mL for each week of gestation). For reasons that are not yet

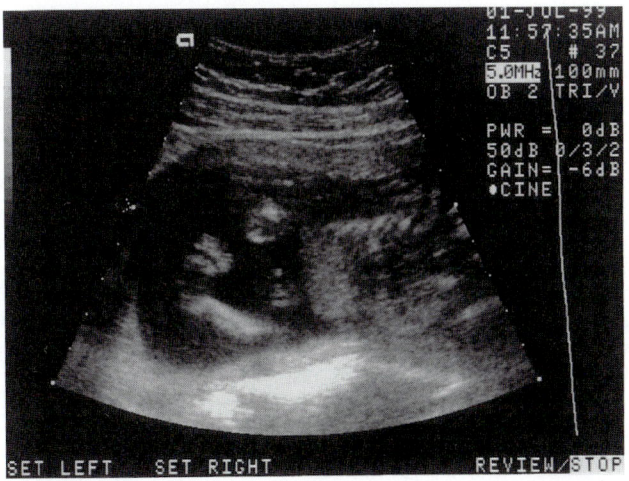

FIGURE 37–9. Clubfoot or talipes equinus varus. (Courtesy of Dr. Jodi Dashe.)

clear, early amniocentesis results in significantly higher pregnancy loss and complication rates than traditional amniocentesis. In a recent multicenter randomized trial, in which all procedures were performed by skilled operators, the spontaneous pregnancy loss rate following early amniocentesis was 2.5 percent compared with 0.7 percent with traditional amniocentesis (Canadian Early and Mid-Trimester Amniocentesis Trial Group, 1998). These rates are consistent with those of many other studies.

Early amniocentesis has also been associated with significantly more positional foot deformities than traditional amniocentesis (Fig. 37–9). Most large studies report an incidence of talipes of 1 to 1.4 percent after the early procedure compared with 0.1 percent (the same as the background rate) after traditional amniocentesis. The Canadian study also found that membrane rupture was more likely after the early procedure, and the incidence of talipes was 15 percent in cases with early postprocedure fluid leak. Because oligohydramnios was transitory, it is likely that the foot deformities resulted from a disruption caused by damage to the vascular supply of the developing leg and foot, rather than a deformation caused by oligohydramnios forcing the foot into one position for a prolonged period. Finally, significantly more cell culture failures occurred after the early procedure, necessitating an additional invasive procedure. For all these reasons, many centers no longer offer amniocentesis before 14 weeks.

CHORIONIC VILLOUS SAMPLING (CVS). The indications for biopsy of chorionic villi are essentially the same as for amniocentesis, except for a few analyses that require amnionic fluid rather than cells or tissue. The primary advantage of CVS is that results are available

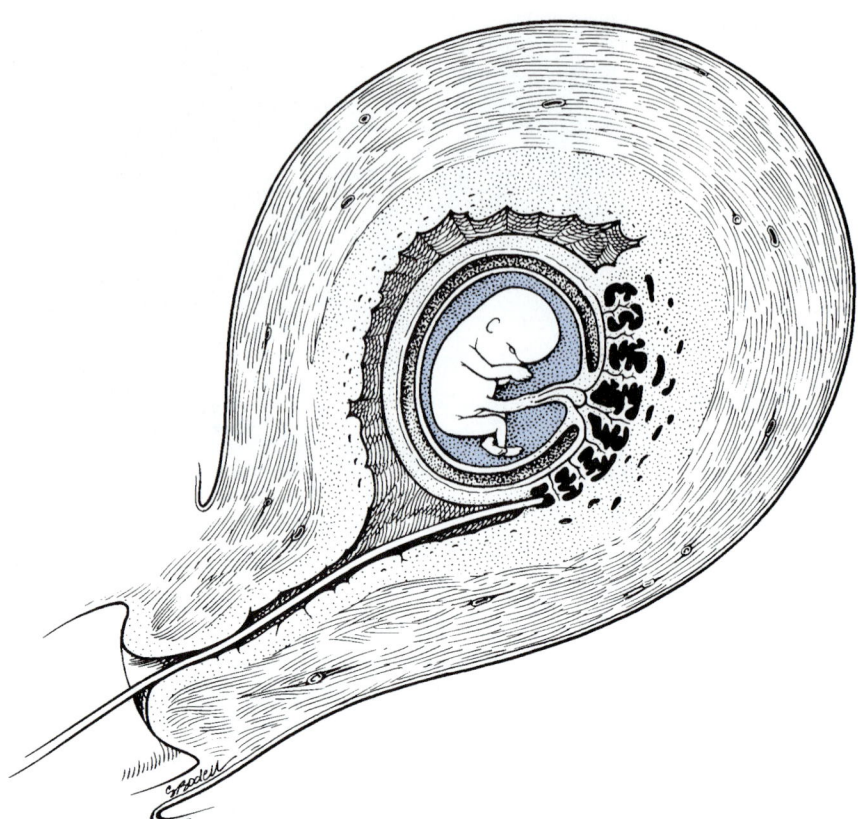

FIGURE 37–10. Transcervical chorionic villus sampling.

earlier in pregnancy, which decreases parental anxiety when results are normal and, allows earlier and safer methods of pregnancy termination when they are abnormal. Chorionic villus sampling is generally performed at 10 to 13 weeks. Placental villi may be obtained through transcervical, transabdominal, or transvaginal access to the placenta (Fig. 37–10). Later in pregnancy, when a fetal abnormality is associated with severe oligohydramnios, transabdominal CVS may be preferred. Skill in ultrasound-guided procedures and specialized training are required before attempting CVS, and maintenance of skills is essential. Relative contraindications include vaginal bleeding or spotting, extreme ante- or retroversion of the uterus, and patient body habitus precluding easy access to the uterus or clear visualization of its contents with ultrasound. Active infection is a contraindication. Complications of CVS are similar to those of amniocentesis.

A number of randomized and case-control trials have compared the safety of CVS with amniocentesis, and of transabdominal CVS with the transcervical procedure. Wald and colleagues (1998) summarized eight randomized trials and found that transcervical CVS has an excess fetal loss rate of 3.7 percent compared with transabdominal CVS or traditional amniocentesis. This rate is similar to that for early amniocentesis.

There have been small series or case reports that suggest an association between CVS and limb-reduction defects, oromandibular defects, and cavernous hemangiomas (Burton, 1992; Firth, 1991, 1994; Hsieh, 1995, and their colleagues). The accumulated experience, however, of nearly 139,000 CVS cases reported to an International Registry of the World Health Organization refutes this. Kuliev and colleagues (1996) showed that the global 10-year experience with CVS done after 9 weeks had an incidence of limb-reduction defects of 6 per 10,000, which is the same as background. A National Institute of Child Health and Human Development workshop of CVS and limb-reduction defects concluded that the frequency of oromandibular-limb hypogenesis appeared to be more common after CVS only when the procedure was performed before 9 weeks (Bianchi and associates, 1993; Kalousek and Dill, 1983). Transabdominal CVS performed after 9 weeks appears to be as safe as second-trimester amniocentesis.

LABORATORY RESULTS. Midtrimester amniocentesis is associated with the lowest number of uninformative results (up to 0.8 percent), compared with transcervical CVS (0.8 to 1.5 percent) or transabdominal CVS (1 percent) (Canadian Collaborative CVS–Amniocentesis Clinical Trial Group, 1989; Rhoads and colleagues, 1989). Uninformative results are primarily due to a failure to obtain a sample or the detection of apparent mosaicism. The latter is the finding of more than one distinct cell line obtained from a single chorionic villus sample. Mosaicism may (rarely) represent true fetal mosaicism, but usually indicates *confined placental mosaicism,* or *pseudomosaicism* (Chap. 36, p. 949).

PERCUTANEOUS UMBILICAL CORD BLOOD SAMPLING (PUBS). Umbilical cord blood was first obtained under direct visualization by Valenti in 1973 who used a surgical endoamnioscope and general anesthesia. Fetal blood sampling in the second trimester by placental aspiration using fetoscopy was subsequently described, but was not ideal (Cao and associates, 1982; Rodeck and Campbell, 1978). Daffos and colleagues (1983) then described the technique now known as percutaneous umbilical cord blood sampling (PUBS) or cordocentesis. After evaluation by Hobbins (1985), Daffos (1985), Nicolaides (1986b), Hogge (1988), Weiner (1988), and others, cordocentesis became a routine procedure for specific fetal indications. Some of these include evaluation of fetal abnormalities, severe growth restriction, congenital infection, thrombocytopenia, hydrops, twin-to-twin transfusion syndrome, and certain genetic diseases.

The umbilical vein is punctured under direct ultrasound guidance, usually at or near its placental origin, and blood is withdrawn (Fig. 37–11). Currently, and as discussed in Chapter 39, it is performed primarily for assessment and treatment of confirmed red cell or platelet alloimmunization, and for the analysis of nonimmune hydrops (Fisk and Bower, 1993). It can also be used to obtain fetal blood cells for genetic analysis when CVS or amniocentesis results are confusing or when rapid diagnosis is necessary. For example, cord blood sampling can be performed when a fetal malformation or severe growth restriction is detected late in pregnancy, and when fetal diagnosis might change management of labor and delivery. Karyotype analysis of fetal blood can usually be accomplished within 24 to 48 hours. The fetal blood sample can also be sent as necessary for metabolic and hematological studies, acid–base analysis, viral cultures, and immunological studies.

COMPLICATIONS. Many complications are similar to those for amniocentesis. Ghidini and colleagues (1993) reviewed unique complications and the most common were umbilical cord vessel bleeding (50 percent), hematoma (17 percent), fetal–maternal hemorrhage (66 percent with an anterior placenta and 17 percent with a posterior placenta), and fetal bradycardia (3 to 12 percent). Most complications were transitory, with complete fetal recovery; however, fetal death does occur. Ghidini and associates (1993) estimated that the procedure-related loss rate was 2.7 percent. This rate appears to be strongly related to the indication for the procedure.

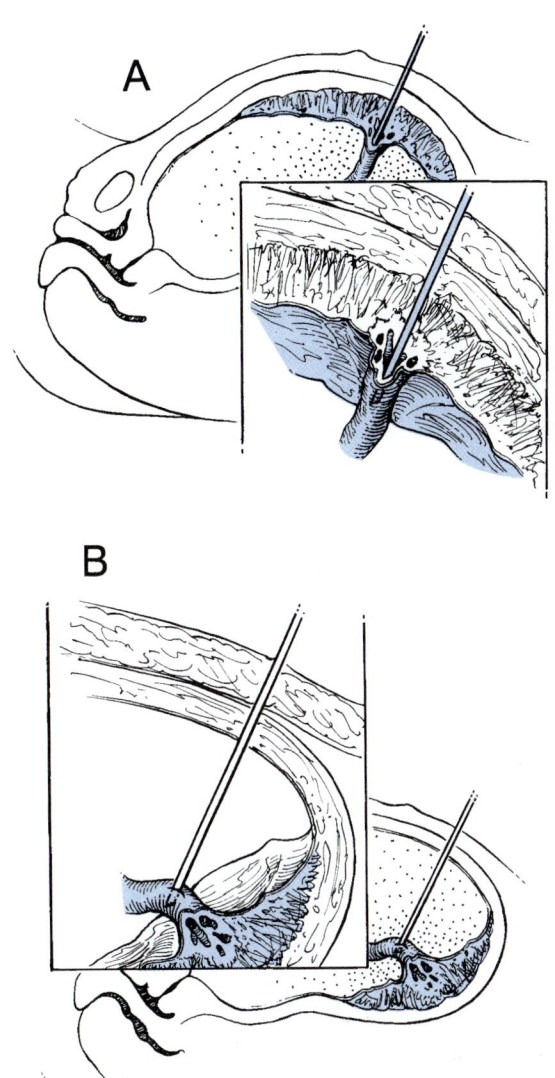

FIGURE 37–11. Umbilical cord blood sampling. Access to the umbilical artery or vein varies, depending upon both the placental location and the position of cord insertion into the placenta. **A.** With an anterior placenta, the needle may traverse the placenta. **B.** With posterior implantation, the needle usually passes through the amnionic fluid before penetrating an umbilical vessel.

It was lower with evaluation of possible isoimmunization in a healthy fetus and higher for evaluation of a severely compromised growth-restricted fetus or a fetus with an anomaly (Maxwell and colleagues, 1991).

FETAL TISSUE BIOPSY. Some genetic conditions affecting the fetus cannot be diagnosed by molecular genetic techniques. Linkage analysis has been used for diagnosis, but is helpful only if there are other living, informative, affected family members (Chap. 36, p. 965).

In some of these conditions, prenatal diagnosis can sometimes be performed by direct analysis of fetal tissue obtained by sonographically guided skin or muscle biopsy. As with other invasive procedures, biopsy requires specific training, and the outcome appears to be directly related to operator skill and experience.

The technique has been used by Evans and colleagues (1994) for muscle biopsy to diagnose muscular dystrophy and mitochondrial myopathy in 12 high-risk fetuses. Elias and co-workers (1994) used skin biopsy in 17 fetuses at high-risk for epidermolysis bullosa.

PREIMPLANTATION DIAGNOSIS. The identification of genes responsible for certain severe hereditary diseases and the development of techniques for in vitro fertilization have provided access to the early embryo and the means to perform preimplantation diagnosis. It is hoped that preimplantation diagnosis will allow selection of only healthy embryos to avoid pregnancy termination. Applications include diagnosis of single-gene disorders such as cystic fibrosis or sickle cell disease, sex determination in X-linked diseases, and identification of aneuploidy with advanced maternal age or parental chromosome rearrangements.

Several variations in technique have been reported. Some clinicians favor *polar body analysis,* reasoning that the first polar body is expelled anyway and its removal should not affect fetal development. A second technique utilizes the 3-day embryo (6- to 10-cell stage), and involves *blastomere biopsy* through a hole made in the zone pellucida. Loss of one totipotent cell at this stage supposedly has little or no effect on the developing embryo, although too few children have been followed to be certain of this. Genetic testing of the removed cell is performed and unaffected embryos are transferred. This technique is still under development. Prenatal diagnosis using only one isolated cell can be very difficult and fraught with errors (Simpson and Carson, 1992; Viville and associates, 1996).

FETAL CELLS IN THE MATERNAL CIRCULATION. Since the 1950s, various types of fetal cells have been identified in the maternal circulation (Douglas and colleagues, 1959; Kleihauer and associates, 1957). It is now known that virtually all women have at least a small number of fetal cells in their bloodstream (Goldberg, 1997). If these fetal cells could be analyzed for prenatal diagnosis, it would obviate the need for invasive procedures. Walnowska and co-workers (1969) used cumbersome cytogenetic techniques to correctly determine fetal sex in 19 of 22 women carrying a male fetus. Fetal cell isolation was advanced by the development of cell-sorting techniques in the late 1970s (Steele and associates, 1996). These take advantage of unique cell surface proteins and other characteristics that distinguish fetal from maternal cells. These can be separated by density-gradient or protein separation techniques, fluorescence-activated cell sorting, or magnetic-activated cell sorting. Nucleated red blood cells are most easily isolated.

Isolated fetal cells have been evaluated for autosomal recessive diseases such as β-thalassemia (Camaschella and associates, 1990). It has also been used for fetal red cell D antigen typing (Geifman-Holtzman and colleagues, 1996). Fetal cells can be karyotyped using fluorescence in situ hybridization (FISH) (Poon and co-workers, 2000; Price and colleagues, 1991). Bianchi and colleagues (1997) have reported a sixfold increase in fetal cells in the maternal blood if the fetus is aneuploid.

A number of problems must be resolved before these techniques can be used clinically for fetal diagnosis. Currently, an ongoing multicenter trial sponsored by the National Institutes of Health promises to perfect the technique for widespread application (Simpson and Elias, 1998). Even if all limitations are not overcome, fetal cell isolation may be useful as a screening test for aneuploidy.

FETAL THERAPY

PREGNANCY TERMINATION. Unfortunately, there is no antenatal therapy available for most congenital anomalies. Despite this, the patient and her family still benefit from prenatal diagnosis because it allows an informed decision about pregnancy continuation and psychological preparation. In addition to maternal–fetal medicine or genetics referral, consultation with a pediatric neurosurgeon, gastrointestinal surgeon, cardiologist, or urologist may be helpful. In some cases, only one of twin fetuses is involved. In cases of high-order multiple fetuses, selective reduction results in better outcomes (Chap. 30, p. 777). A complete summary of the counseling session is placed in the medical record. Techniques for pregnancy termination are discussed in Chapter 33 (p. 870).

TWIN-TO-TWIN TRANSFUSION SYNDROME. This is a unique complication of monochorionic twin pregnancies that is discussed in detail in Chapter 30 (p. 785). All monochorionic twins share a placenta which contains vascular anastomoses potentially connecting the two circulations. Schatz recognized as early as 1875 that a small proportion of such twins have unequal blood flow as the result of unbalanced anastomoses, and they have varying degrees of discordancy of weight, intravascular volume, hemoglobin concentration, and amnionic fluid volume. In the extreme case, one twin is severely growth restricted with no amnionic fluid—giving it the sonographic appearance of being "stuck" to one spot in the uterus—while the co-twin is larger, often plethoric, and has hydramnios (Mahony and associates, 1985). Approximately 15 percent of monozygotic twin pregnancies develop some degree of this complication (Nicolaides and Petterson, 1994).

Therapeutic options for twin-to-twin transfusion are limited. It has been shown that removal of fluid from the sac with hydramnios somehow improves the pressure differential between the two fetal circulations and occasionally may even reverse the unequal fluid balance between the twins (Elliott and co-workers, 1991; Mahony and colleagues, 1990; Pinette and associates, 1993). Others have reported intentional creation of an opening in the amnion separating the fetuses, allowing fluid to interchange and supposedly equalizing pressure differences (Vetter and Schneider, 1988). A more invasive therapy is endoscopic laser ablation of placental vascular anastomoses, literally separating the surface of the placenta into two halves (De Lia and collaborators, 1995). Because many offending anastomoses are deep in the placenta, this procedure is not always successful and has a high complication rate (Fisk and associates, 1990). The most aggressive therapy is selective feticide of the donor twin, usually considered for early severe cases that would otherwise result in the death of both twins (Arabin and associates, 1998; Weiner, 1987). When severe twin-to-twin transfusion occurs before 24 weeks, the prognosis is poor regardless of therapy (Bebbington and Wittmann, 1989).

FETAL TRANSFUSION

ISOIMMUNIZATION. Intraperitoneal red blood cell transfusion for treatment of fetal anemia from red cell isoimmunization was the first invasive fetal therapy accepted into routine practice (Berkowitz and Hobbins, 1981; Bowman, 1976; Frigoletto and colleagues, 1981). Using fluoroscopic guidance and a large-bore trocar and needle, blood placed into the fetal abdominal cavity is gradually absorbed by the subdiaphragmatic lymphatics. Severely affected fetuses, especially those with ascites or hydrops, often were not able to absorb enough blood to survive. In addition, the procedure entailed significant risk. Subsequently, Rodeck and colleagues (1981, 1984) described fetoscopically guided intraumbilical blood transfusion, using a 2.4- to 3.0-mm cannula. This was followed by accounts of ultrasonically guided transfusion directly into the hepatic portion of the umbilical vein or the fetal heart (Bang and associates, 1982; deCrespigny and colleagues, 1985; Westgren and co-workers, 1988).

Grannum and colleagues (1986) described the currently used technique of sonographically directed transfusion into the umbilical cord vein using a 22-gauge needle. With a few modifications, this technique has proved efficacious and safe (Berkowitz, 1986; Nicolaides, 1986a; Weiner, 1991, and their colleagues). The large fetal–placental volume allows infusion of a relatively large quantity of blood over a short period, and direct sonographic guidance allows direct fetal monitoring. Furosemide can also be administered directly along with the blood, to relax the capacitance vessels and facilitate the clearance of excess plasma. In Table 37–11, the outcomes of 44 isoimmunized women managed with intraumbilical transfusion are compared with the outcomes of 44 women managed by intraperitoneal transfusion. These groups were matched for severity of disease, gestational age, and placental site. The results highlight the greater efficacy and lower morbidity of the intraumbilical procedure.

PARVOVIRUS INFECTION. A small number of fetuses affected by parvovirus B19 infection will develop severe transient aplastic anemia (Chap. 56, p. 1466). Fetuses infected before 20 weeks are most likely to develop severe anemia with heart failure and subsequent hydrops. While an unknown number spontaneously recover and survive, others that are severely compromised will die. Some of these moribund fetuses can be rescued with blood transfusion (Peters and Nicolaides, 1990; Sahakian and colleagues, 1991). In a fetus with nonimmune hydrops, cord blood sampling can be performed to confirm anemia. Fetal and maternal blood is used to identify parvovirus DNA by polymerase chain reaction (Dieck and associates, 1999). Transfusions are not always lifesaving, probably because some infections include lethal viral myocarditis which cannot be diagnosed antenatally.

OTHER INDICATIONS. Transfusion may also be considered after a severe, but not ongoing fetal–maternal hemorrhage. It has also been described in a case of fetal hemoglobin Bart disease (Chap. 49, p. 1319). Copel and co-workers (1991) have administered platelet transfusion for severe alloimmune thrombocytopenia using the same technique (Chap. 39, p. 1072).

FETAL MEDICAL THERAPY. In a unique number of instances, fetal therapy is accomplished by maternal treatment with the desired medication. In other cases, medication is administered directly to the fetus by intramuscular injection or intravenous infusion through the umbilical vein. There are many examples of fetal treatment with maternally administered medications. The obvious example is that treatment of many infections is directed at both patients, for example, syphilis. In other cases, only the fetus is affected, such as the woman with Graves disease who has been rendered euthyroid by radioiodine ablation. The IgG thyroid-stimulating antibody crosses the placenta and causes fetal thyrotoxicosis with up to 25 per-

TABLE 37–11. Comparison of Outcomes with Intraperitoneal versus Intravascular Fetal Transfusion for Isoimmunization

Factor	Method of Transfusion		P value
	Intraperitoneal (n = 44)	Intravascular (n = 44)	
Attempts per successful transfusion	1.8 ± 0.9	1.2 ± 0.3	.02
Procedural complication	31/104 (30%)	17/173 (9.8%)	.003
Traumatic death	8/44 (18%)	1/44 (2.2%)	< .001
Completed planned treatment	17/44 (39%)	37/44 (84%)	< .0001
Gestational age at delivery (wk)	30.7 ± 5.5	34.1 ± 3.7	.01
Apgar score < 7 at 5 min	13/34 (38%)	6/42 (14%)	< .02
Neonatal exchange transfusions	1.8 ± 2.0	0.8 ± 1.2	.007
Neonatal ICU (days)	8.2 ± 16.2	6.1 ± 13.9	.04

Adapted from Harman and colleagues (1990).

cent mortality (Bruinse and colleagues, 1988). In fetuses with suspected compromise, thyroid status can be assessed by cordocentesis, and maternal treatment given with propylthiouracil that crosses the placenta to suppress the fetal thyroid (Wenstrom and associates, 1990). Also, David and Forest (1984) reported that maternally administered corticosteroids resulted in fetal adrenal suppression and thus prevented fetal masculinization in congenital adrenal hyperplasia.

Up to 1 percent of fetuses have a cardiac arrhythmia, however, only a small number are hemodynamically significant (Copel and associates, 2000). Most arrhythmias are tolerated without compromise or the arrhythmia resolves spontaneously (Simpson and colleagues, 1997). When there is sustained tachyarrhythmia, the fetus may begin to show cardiac decompensation, which can progress to hydrops. Maternally administered antiarrhythmic agents cross the placenta in therapeutic doses. Digoxin, verapamil, propranolol, procainamide, quinidine, flecainide, sotalol, and amiodarone have all been given for fetal arrhythmias with reasonable results in nonhydropic fetuses (Edwards and colleagues, 1999; Sonesson and associates, 1998). With fetal hydrops, however, these drugs do not enter the fetal circulation as well (Younis and Granat, 1987). In these cases, medication is administered directly to the fetus through the umbilical cord or by intramuscular injection in the buttock (Mangione and co-workers, 1999; Parilla and colleagues, 1996).

CONGENITAL INFECTION. Several infectious agents can cross the placenta and cause fetal infection with serious consequences. Because effective antenatal treatment can ameliorate some or all of the most severe associated fetal morbidity, treatment of maternal infections constitutes fetal therapy. Diagnosis and treatment of syphilis, gonorrhea, toxoplasmosis, and a number of sexually

transmitted or other infectious diseases are discussed in Chapters 56 and 57.

FETAL SURGERY. With only a few exceptions, fetal surgery is still in the pioneering stages. There are a few in utero surgical procedures that are commonplace, but most are considered experimental. Fetal surgery is performed in only a few centers by teams trained in multidisciplinary techniques required for complete care of both mother and fetus. Some of these procedures are discussed in greater detail in the second edition of *Operative Obstetrics* (Gilstrap and colleagues, 2001).

Recent technical advances, especially in ultrasound and laparoscopic surgical techniques, make it possible to consider surgical correction of structural fetal malformation. There are a number of requisites that are necessary before surgical intervention is considered. Importantly, the natural history of the condition, both with and without therapy, must be known. Because intervention entails substantial fetal and maternal risks, as well as risk to subsequent pregnancies, it should not be considered unless withholding such intervention is absolutely certain to be catastrophic. There must be certainty that the surgical treatment, barring unforeseen complications, will improve outcome. The importance of this criterion is underscored by early experiences with antenatal ventriculoamnionic shunt placement to correct fetal obstructive hydrocephalus. The results of the first 44 procedures reported to the International Fetal Surgery Registry were discouraging (Manning and colleagues, 1986). The procedure-related fetal death rate was 10 percent, and 18 of the 34 survivors had serious neurological handicaps. It eventually became clear that the natural history of the condition without (and with) shunting was unknown, and appropriate selection criteria for the procedure could not be determined. A third criteria is that the procedure has been perfected and tested successfully in experimental animals, preferably a primate (Harrison and colleagues, 1980; Moise and associates, 1995). The surgery, usually considered experimental, must be performed by an experienced operator. Rigorous evaluation of the efficacy of these techniques should be expected prior to their widespread use.

While early enthusiasm for fetal surgery has waned somewhat, there is progress concerning the complex influences on fetal development and the unique features of various defects. Along with this understanding, there are a few fetal lesions for which antenatal surgical intervention is considered.

URINARY SHUNTS. As discussed, in many cases the presence of a major urinary tract malformation indicates aneuploidy or another genetic syndrome usually associated with a poor prognosis. An isolated malformation, however, may have the potential for a good prognosis with correction. This is not possible with malformations such as cystic dysplasia or renal agenesis in which associated oligohydramnios has prevented development of the fetal lungs. This mechanism is considered in Chapter 31 (p. 822).

Because fetal urine is the major source of amnionic fluid after 16 weeks, any urinary obstruction can be lethal (Fig. 37–12). Such lesions include posterior urethral

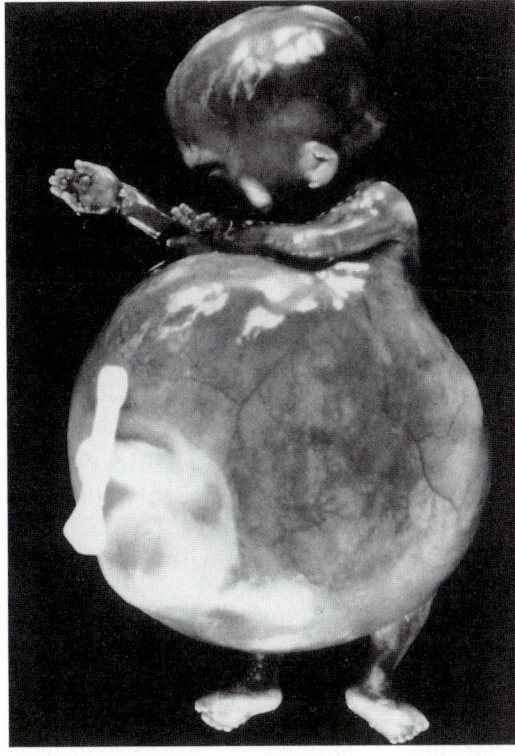

FIGURE 37–12. Fetus with megacystis as the result of urethral atresia.

valves, urethral atresia, and ureteropelvic junction obstruction. Outflow obstruction increases intrarenal pressure and produces dysplastic renal changes (Adzick and Harrison, 1994). Almost 20 years ago, it was theorized that, if fetal urine could somehow be shunted into the uterine cavity, then pulmonary hypoplasia and related problems could be avoided. In the early 1980s, a double-pigtail catheter was placed to reduce pressure and restore amnionic fluid volume (Berkowitz and colleagues, 1982; Harrison and associates, 1982). It was positioned under ultrasound guidance as shown in Figure 37–13. In experienced hands, fetal survival after such surgery was 70 percent (Holzgreve and Evans, 1993).

Because most of the poor outcomes are related to serious renal pathology in survivors, the biggest problem is selecting appropriate fetuses for treatment. It has become clear that many fetuses with bladder outlet obstruction already have significant renal dysfunction (Johnson and associates, 1995). Because correct determination of the cause of the obstruction is important for prognosis, Quintero and associates (1995) have investigated the use of percutaneous fetal cystoscopy.

THORACIC SHUNTS. Accumulation of thoracic fluid can also cause pulmonary hypoplasia by compressing developing lung structures. Some causes include chylothorax, infection, and chest tumors. While successful outcomes after thoracic shunt placement for isolated fetal hydrothorax have been reported, a review by Hagay and colleagues (1993) suggested that the procedure may not significantly change perinatal outcomes. Of 82 cases, 54 were managed conservatively and 24 were treated either with a thoracic shunt or serial thoracentesis. About a third of fetuses died in each group.

Intrathoracic masses leading to pulmonary hypoplasia include pulmonary sequestration, congenital cystic adenomatoid malformation, and nonspecific cysts (Harrison and co-workers, 1998). Their diagnosis is considered in Chapter 41 (p. 1123). Fetal goiter or tracheal atresia also may prevent egress of pulmonary fluid. Thoracic shunt placement has been described for all these entities, with variable success. Although fluid drainage immediately following the procedure is usually good, obstruction or displacement of the shunt leads to rapid reaccumulation. Shunt placement in the presence of hydrops is generally not curative, probably because the fetus has already suffered damage, is moribund at the time of the procedure, or because the hydrops itself indicates a more serious abnormality with a poor prognosis (Adzick and co-workers, 1993; Weiner and colleagues, 1986).

CONGENITAL DIAPHRAGMATIC HERNIA. This is one of the first malformations for which ex utero fetal surgery was performed. The incidence of this defect in the general population is about 1 in 3700 (Wenstrom and col-

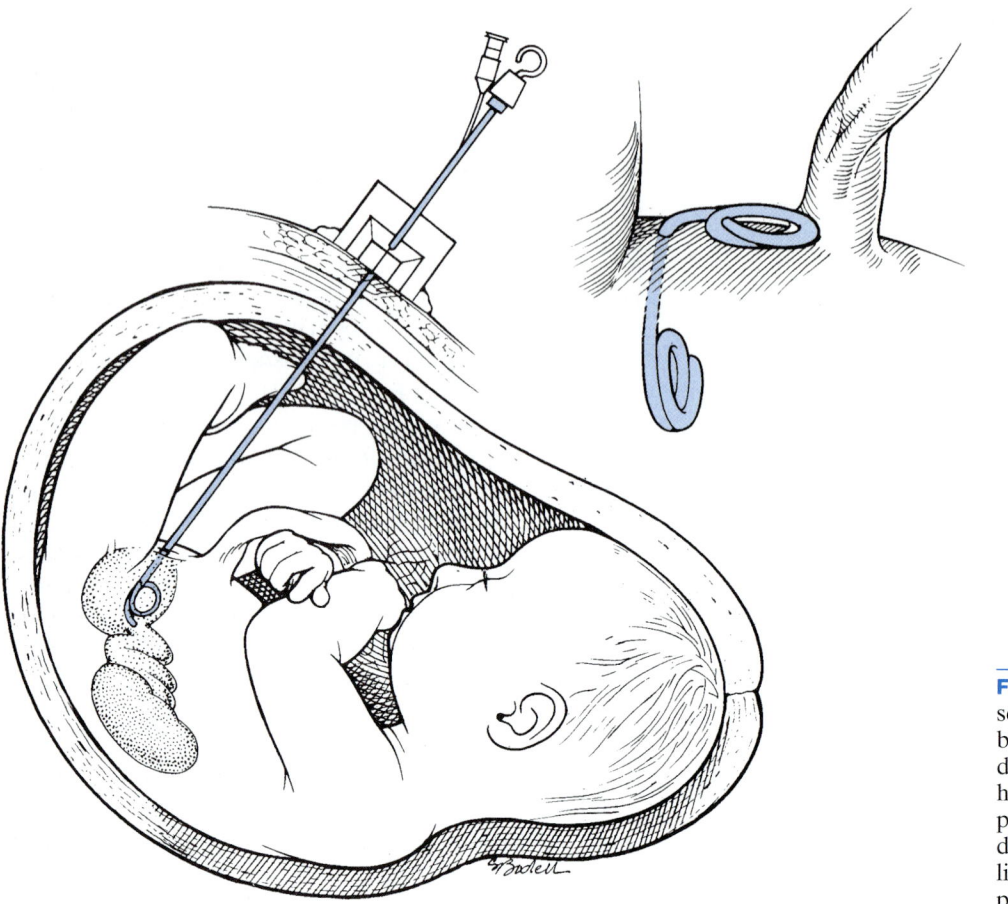

FIGURE 37–13. Schematic representation of placement of fetal bladder shunt through a specially designed cannula. The catheter has pigtail curls at each end, which prevent the catheter from being dislodged. (Redrawn from Williamson and Pringle, 1987, with permission.)

leagues, 1991). Up to half of these fetuses have genetic syndromes or other associated defects that may be lethal (Powers and Phillips, 1990). In those with isolated malformations, some survive intact. Harrison and associates (1990b) postulated that antenatal surgical correction of the diaphragmatic defect might restore normal intrathoracic anatomy to allow pulmonary development and prevent pulmonary hypoplasia (Fig. 37–14). Fetal surgery was justified by data suggesting perinatal mortality of up to 80 percent (Adzick and co-workers, 1985), however, this rate was challenged (Wenstrom and colleagues, 1991). Early attempts had survival rates of 25 percent with antenatal intervention. Unfortunately, complication rates, including prematurely ruptured membranes and preterm labor were common. It now seems clear that fetuses with late or intermittent left-sided herniation do well after neonatal surgery, while fetuses with early herniation, mediastinal shift, and dilated intrathoracic stomach or liver do poorly despite repair (Harrison, 1996).

Another approach to prevent pulmonary hypoplasia has been evaluated by Harrison and colleagues (1998). They reasoned that if normal pulmonary efflux could be prevented, the lungs would inflate with fluid and fill the thorax. This would mechanically keep bowel out of the chest, and thus pulmonary growth would continue. They also took advantage of fetal endoscopic surgical techniques, collectively called *Fetendo* (Deprest and colleagues, 1997; Vanderwall and co-workers, 1996). They used these techniques to band or plug the trachea in fetuses with congenital diaphragmatic hernia—this protocol is called *Plug the Lung Until it Grows,* or *PLUG.* This procedure was offered only to women whose fetus had a poor prognosis due to liver herniation diagnosed before 25 weeks. In 34 fetuses with poor prognoses, parents chose postnatal treatment with extracorporeal membrane oxygenation in 13, open fetal surgery for tracheal occlusion in 13, or fetoscopic tracheal occlusion in eight (Harrison and colleagues, 1998). The survival rate in the fetoscopic surgery group was 75 percent compared with only 15 percent in the open surgery group and 40 percent in the neonatal therapy group.

SACROCOCCYGEAL TERATOMA. This is a congenital germ cell tumor composed of tissues representing all three germ layers. It arises from totipotent cells in Hensen node or from ectopic primordial germ cells in

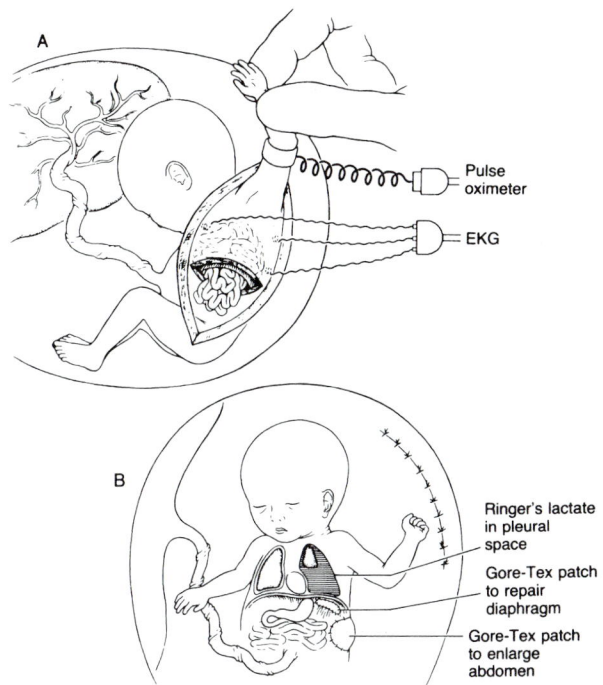

FIGURE 37–14. Techniques used to repair a fetal diaphragmatic hernia at 24 weeks' gestation. **A** shows the hysterotomy, made on the posterior side of the uterus to avoid an anterior placenta. The fetus was continuously monitored by pulse oximetry, Electrocardiography (EKG), and sonography while the intestines, dilated stomach, spleen, and some of the liver were removed from the chest. **B** shows the closure of the diaphragmatic defect with a patch. The left hemithorax was filled with warm Ringer lactate, and the fetal abdomen was enlarged with a patch to accommodate the viscera. (From Harrison and colleagues, 1990b, with permission.)

the sacral area. In addition to a malignant potential of 10 to 20 percent, perinatal morbidity is high because teratomas are very vascular with numerous arteriovenous shunts. Vascular steal syndromes or hemorrhage result in fetal anemia, heart failure, and hydrops (Altman and colleagues, 1974). Early detection usually indicates an aggressive tumor. Survival is less than 10 percent in fetuses whose tumors are identified before 30 weeks, compared with 75 percent in those discovered later (Malone and co-workers, 1990).

In view of the very poor prognosis for early aggressive lesions, prenatal surgical excision has been attempted, but largely without success (Langer and colleagues, 1989). An alternative approach is to attempt palliative surgery (debulking) in order to prevent hydrops, and to reserve the definitive repair until after birth. Graf and colleagues (1998) reported good results with debulking in four of five fetuses. Harrison (1996) has suggested the possibility to debulk or reduce the blood supply to the tumor endoscopically.

CONGENITAL CYSTIC ADENOMATOID MALFORMATION AND PULMONARY SEQUESTRATION. These two pulmonary lesions may be amenable to fetal surgical therapy. Congenital cystic adenomatoid malformations (CCAMs) are pulmonary hamartomas consisting of overgrown terminal bronchioles. Type I has large cysts, type II has multiple small cysts less than 1.2 cm, and type III is essentially solid. Type III lesions have the worst prognosis. Pulmonary sequestration is a tissue mass that becomes completely separated from normal lung, which receives its blood supply from the systemic circulation. The intralobar variety is located inside the pleura adjacent to normal lung, while the extralobar variety has its own separate pleura, like an accessory lobe.

Both of these may enlarge, eventually leading to mediastinal shift, pleural effusions, hydramnios, and perinatal death from hydrops or pulmonary hypoplasia. Alternatively either may regress spontaneously. Adzick and colleagues (1993) found that 28 of 39 (72 percent) sequestrations regressed before delivery compared with only 15 of 120 (13 percent) of CCAMs. While half of the latter continued to grow, they did not cause hydrops, and fetuses without hydrops did well after neonatal surgery.

There is a subgroup of fetuses with either lesion who are good candidates for fetal surgery because the natural history of the lesions are known, and those with a poor prognosis can be readily identified. Those whose lesions rapidly enlarge leading to early hydropic changes usually do not survive, even with aggressive neonatal therapy. Thus, early or fully hydropic fetuses are candidates for serial cyst drainage or antenatal surgical resection. Adzick and colleagues (1993) offered fetal surgery only to fetuses with a poor prognosis. All 25 fetuses with large cystic CCAMs and hydrops died with expectant management. Conversely, there were eight survivors of 13 hydropic fetuses managed with open fetal lobectomy. There were 5 of 6 survivors with thoracoamnionic shunting. Fetuses with a large cyst do well with such shunting (Adzick and Nance, 2000).

NEURAL-TUBE DEFECTS. Isolated open spine defects that are not part of a genetic syndrome or associated with other anomalies, often result in permanent neurological damage (Chap. 36, p. 958). Observations are consistent with a *two-hit hypothesis* in these fetuses. The first "hit" is the defect itself, and the second comes from continued exposure to amnionic fluid (Heffez and colleagues, 1990). Several investigators have theorized that antenatal closure or coverage of the spine defect might avert some of the neurological damage. Currently, both open surgical closure and laparoscopic techniques are being evaluated.

With the fetal sheep model, Harrison's group has shown that repair of induced fetal spine defects prevents tissue damage and "rescues" neurological function (Meuli and co-workers, 1995, 1996). Bruner and colleagues (1999a) described four human fetuses whose open lower-spine defects were covered endoscopically with a maternal skin graft at 22 to 24 weeks. It was hoped that this would prevent herniation of the hindbrain into the foramen magnum with obstruction and ventriculomegaly—the *Arnold–Chiari malformation.* The two survivors were delivered at 28 and 35 weeks had only mild somatosensory deficit. Bruner and co-workers (1999b) also compared 10 fetuses who underwent open surgical repair at 26 to 30 weeks with 20 fetuses without antenatal repair. The surgically treated fetuses had a significantly decreased need for ventriculoperitoneal shunt placement after delivery. Unfortunately, the open surgical procedure was associated with serious complications, including preterm delivery and even extrusion of fetal small parts through the uterine incision. Because only very preliminary observations of these procedures have thus far been reported, and most of the children are still too young to assess mobility or control of bodily functions, the procedure remains experimental (Adzick and Nance, 2000). It also remains controversial because spina bifida is not a lethal defect.

STEM CELL TRANSPLANTATION

This is a therapeutic option for several hematological diseases. Because immunocompetence in the human fetus does not develop until 18 weeks, it would appear possible that the fetus would be tolerant to foreign antigens before that time. Hematopoietic stem cells might also serve as a delivery vehicle for gene transfer. A number of animal models have been developed to study fetal bone marrow transplantation. Crombleholme (1989), Harrison (1989), and others have identified the optimal time interval for transplantation in primate models, and have investigated sources of hematopoietic stem cells including fetal liver, umbilical cord blood, and adult bone marrow. Therapeutic fetal bone marrow transplantation has been attempted in the human fetus for such diseases as bare lymphocyte syndrome, severe combined immunodeficiency syndrome, thalassemia, metachromatic leukodystrophy, and group D isoimmunization. Unfortunately, there has been very limited success; however, research efforts are ongoing (Crombleholme and Bianchi, 1994; Westgren and co-workers, 1996).

GENE TRANSFER

With advances in genetic technologies and progress in the identification of genes responsible for inherited disease, the possibility of gene transfer for definitive ther-

apy is being explored. Fetal gene transfer is appealing for several reasons, which are summarized in an excellent review by Pergament and Fiddler (1995). First, certain inherited metabolic conditions are particularly devastating because tissue damage begins shortly after or even before birth. In Tay–Sachs disease, for example, central nervous system cells exhibit the characteristic pathology as early as 9 weeks after conception (Grabowski and colleagues, 1984). Second, early therapy holds out the prospect of being administered only one time, definitive, and having a lifetime impact. Third, parents could be assured of healthy children without having to choose termination of affected pregnancies.

A number of criteria are considered requisite for the development of therapeutic gene transfer. These criteria, which have not been met, include:

1. That the normal gene can be inserted into the target cells and remain there long enough to have the desired effect.
2. That the level of gene expression in the new gene will be appropriate.
3. That the new gene will not harm the cell or the individual (Anderson, 1984).

Other unresolved issues include the timing of the procedure, viz., preconceptional, at the time of fertilization, prior to implantation, or during embryogenesis or fetal development; the best DNA vectors to use; the ideal recipient or target cells; and the safest methods. Efficient techniques for in vivo gene targeting have yet to be developed, and the possibility of ex vivo gene transfer raises ethical considerations. Ethical questions remaining to be resolved include whether or not to target fetal gonadal tissues—which would affect future generations—and how to prevent gene transfer from being used for enhancement of phenotype rather than disease prevention (eugenics). Gene transfer is still in its earliest experimental stages, and it must be thoroughly investigated in animals and adult humans before it can be extended to fetuses.

REFERENCES

Adams MJ, Windham GC, Greenberg F, Clayton-Hopkins JA, Reimer CB, Oakley GP: Clinical interpretation of maternal serum α-fetoprotein concentrations. Am J Obstet Gynecol 148:241, 1984

Adzick NS, Harrison MR: Fetal surgical therapy. Lancet 343:897, 1994

Adzick NS, Harrison MR, Flake AW, Howell LJ, Golbus MS, Filly RA, UCSF Fetal Treatment Center: Fetal surgery for cystic adenomatoid malformation of the lung. J Pediatr Surg 28:806, 1993

Adzick NS, Harrison MR, Glick PL, Golbus MS, Anderson RL, Mahony BS, Callen PW, Hirsch JH, Luthy DA, Filly RA, deLorimier AA: Fetal cystic adenomatoid malformation: Prenatal diagnosis and natural history. J Pediatr Surg 20:483, 1985

Adzick NS, Nance ML: Pediatric surgery: Second of two parts. N Engl J Med 342:1726, 2000

Altman RP, Randolph JG, Lilly JR: Sacrococcygeal teratoma. American Academy of Pediatric Surgical Section Survey. J Ped Surg 9:389, 1974

American College of Obstetricians and Gynecologists: Maternal serum screening. Educational Bulletin No. 228, September 1996c

American College of Obstetricians and Gynecologists: Preconceptional care. Technical Bulletin No. 205, May 1995a

American College of Obstetricians and Gynecologists: Screening for Tay Sachs disease. Committee on Genetics. Committee Opinion No. 162, November 1995b

American College of Obstetricians and Gynecologists: Fragile X syndrome. Comittee Opinion No. 161, October 1995c

American College of Obstetricians and Gynecologists: Current status of cystic fibrosis carrier screening. Committee Opinion No. 101, November 1991

American College of Obstetricians and Gynecologists: Prenatal detection of neural tube defects. Technical Bulletin No. 99, 1986

Anderson WF: Prospects for human gene therapy. Science 226:401, 1984

Arabin B, Laurini RN, van Eyck J, Nicolaides KH: Treatment of twin–twin transfusion syndrome by laser and digoxin: Biophysical and angiographic evaluation. Fetal Diagn Ther 13:141, 1998

Bahado-Singh R, Oz UA, Baumgarten A, Shahabi S, Cermik D, Cole L, Mahoney M, Karaca M: The comprehensive mid-trimester test (CMT): Highly-sensitive for Down syndrome detection (Abstract 0055). Presented at the Society for Maternal-Fetal Medicine, Reno, Nevada, February 5-10, 2001

Bang J, Bock JE, Trolle D: Ultrasound-guided fetal intravenous transfusion for severe Rhesus hemolytic disease. Br Med J 284:373, 1982

Bebbington MW, Wittmann BK: Fetal transfusion syndrome: Antenatal factors predicting outcome. Am J Obstet Gynecol 160:913, 1989

Becerra JE, Khoury MJ, Cordero JF, Erickson JD: Diabetes mellitus during pregnancy and the risks for specific birth defects: A population based study. Pediatrics 85:1, 1990

Bensen JT, Dillard RG, Burton BK: Open spina bifida: Does cesarean section delivery improve prognosis? Obstet Gynecol 71:532, 1988

Berkowitz RA, Chitkara U, Goldberg JD, Wilkins I, Chervensk FA, Lynch L: Intrauterine intravascular transfusions for severe red blood cell isoimmunization: Ultrasound-guided percutaneous approach. Am J Obstet Gynecol 155:574, 1986

Berkowitz RL, Glickman MG, Smith GJ, Siegel NJ, Weiss RM, Mahoney MJ, Hobbins JC: Fetal urinary tract obstruction: What is the role of surgical intervention in utero? Am J Obstet Gynecol 144:367, 1982

Berkowitz RL, Hobbins JC: Intrauterine transfusing utilizing ultrasound. Obstet Gynecol 57:33, 1981

Bianchi DW, Demaria M, Vadnars TI, Zickwolf GK, Weil GJ: Trials in recovering fetal cells from maternal blood. In Zakut II (ed): Seventh International Conference on Early Prenatal Diagnosis. Bologna, Monduzzi Editore, 1994, p 7

Bianchi DW, Wilkins-Haug LE, Enders AC, Hay ED: Origin of extraembryonic mesoderm in experimental animals: Relevance to chorionic mosaicism in humans. Am J Med Genet 46:542, 1993

Bianchi DW, Williams JM, Sullivan LM, Hanson FW, Klinger KW, Shuber AP: PCR quantification of fetal cells in maternal blood in normal and aneuploid pregnancies. Am J Hum Genet 61:822, 1997

Bogart MH, Pandian MR, Jones OW: Abnormal maternal serum chorionic gonadotropin levels in pregnancies with fetal chromosome abnormalities. Prenat Diagn 7:623, 1987

Bonaiti-Pellie C, Smith C: Risks tables for genetic counseling in some common congenital malformations. J Med Genet 11:374, 1974

Boue J, Boue H, Lazar P: Retrospective and prospective epidemiological studies of 1500 karyotyped spontaneous human abortuses. Teratology 14:3, 1976

Bowman JM: The management of Rh-isoimmunization. Obstet Gynecol 52:1, 1976

Brambati B, Cislaghi C, Tului L, Alberti E, Amidani M, Columbo U, Zuliani G: First trimester Down's syndrome screening using nuchal translucency: A prospective study in patients undergoing chorionic villus sampling. Ultrasound Obstet Gynecol 5:9, 1995

Brock DJH, Bolton AE, Monaghan JM: Prenatal diagnosis of anencephaly through maternal serum-alphafetoprotein measurement. Lancet ii:923, 1973

Brock DJH, Sutcliffe RG: Alphafetoprotein in the antenatal diagnosis of anencephaly and spina bifida. Lancet ii:197, 1972

Bruinse HW, Vermeulen-Meiners C, Wit JM: Fetal treatment for thyrotoxicosis in non-thyrotoxic pregnant women. Fetal Ther 3:152, 1988

Brumfield CG, Cloud GA, Davis RO, Finley SC, Hauth JC, Boots L: The relationship between maternal serum and amniotic fluid α-fetoprotein in women undergoing early amniocentesis. Am J Obstet Gynecol 163:903, 1990

Bruner JP, Richards WO, Tulipan NB, Arney TL: Endoscopic coverage of fetal myelomeningocele in utero. Am J Obstet Gynecol 180:153, 1999a

Bruner JP, Walsh WF, Boehm FH, Paschall RL, Reed GW, Silva SR, Vrabcak EK, Tulipan N: Open fetal repair of myelomeningocele improves neurologic outcome in the neonate. Am J Obstet Gynecol 19th Annual Meeting of the Society for Maternal–Fetal Medicine 180:S31, 1999b

Burn J, Brennan P, Little J, Holloway S, Coffey R, Somerville J, Dennis NR, Allan L, Arnold R, Deanfield JE, Godman M, Houston A, Keeton B, Oakley C, Scott O, Silove E, Wilkinson J, Pembrey M, Hunter AS: Recurrence risks in offspring of adults with major heart defects: Results from first cohort of British collaborative study. Lancet 351:311, 1998

Burton BK: Elevated maternal serum alpha-fetoprotein (MSAFP): Interpretation and follow-up. Clin Obstet Gynecol 31:293, 1988

Burton BK, Sowers SG, Nelson LH: Maternal serum α-fetoprotein screening in North Carolina: Experience with more than twelve thousand pregnancies. Am J Obstet Gynecol 146:439, 1983

Burton BK, Schulz CJ, Burd LI: Limb anomalies associated with chorionic villus sampling. Obstet Gynecol 79:726, 1992

Burton BK, Prins GS, Verp MS: A prospective trial of prenatal screening for Down syndrome by means of maternal serum α-fetoprotein, human chorionic gonadotropin, and unconjugated estriol. Am J Obstet Gynecol 169:526, 1993

Camaschella C, Alfarno A, Gattardi E, Travis M: Prenatal diagnosis of fetal haemoglobin Lepore-Boston disease on maternal peripheral blood. Blood 75:2101, 1990

Canadian Collaborative CVS–Amniocentesis Clinical Trial

Group: Multicentre randomised clinical trial of chorion villus sampling and amniocentesis. Lancet 7:1, 1989

Canadian Early and Mid-Trimester Amniocentesis Trial (CEMAT) Group: Randomised trial to assess safety and fetal outcome of early and midtrimester amniocentesis. Lancet 351:242, 1998

Canick JA, Kellner LH, Saller DN, Palomaki GE, Walker RP, Osathanondh R: Second-trimester levels of maternal urinary gonadotropin peptide in Down syndrome pregnancy. Prenat Diagn 15:739, 1995

Cao A, Furbetta M, Angius A, Ximenes A, Rosatelli C, Tuveri T, Scalas MT, Falchi AM, Angioni G, Caminiti F: Haematological and obstetric aspects of antenatal diagnosis of β-thalassaemia: Experience with 200 cases. J Med Genet 19:81, 1982

Centers for Disease Control and Prevention: Economic costs of birth defects and cerebral palsy—United States, 1992. MMWR 44:694, 1995b

Cheng EY, Luthy DA, Zebelman AM, Williams MA, Luppman RE, Hickok DE: A prospective evaluation of a second trimester screening test for fetal Down syndrome using maternal serum fetoprotein, hCG, and unconjugated estriol. Obstet Gynecol 81:72, 1993

Copel JA, Liang RI, Demasio K, Ozeren S, Kleinman CS: The clinical significance of the irregular fetal heart rhythm. Am J Obstet Gynecol 182:813, 2000

Copel JA, Gollin YG, Grannum PA: Alloimmune disorders and pregnancy. Semin Perinatol 15:251, 1991

Crandall BF, Matsumoto M: Routine amniotic fluid α-fetoprotein measurement in 34,000 pregnancies. Am J Obstet Gynecol 149:744, 1984

Crombleholme TM, Bianchi DW: In utero hematopoietic stem cell transplantation and gene therapy. Semin Perinatol 18:376, 1994

Crombleholme TM, Longaker MG, Langer JC: In utero transplantation of fetal liver hematopoietic stem cells in monkeys. Lancet 2:1425, 1989

Cuckle HS, Iles RK, Chard T: Urinary B-Core human chorionic gonadotrophin: A new approach to Down syndrome screening. Prenat Diagn 14:953, 1994

Cuckle HS, Shahabi S, Semni IK, Jones R, Cole LA: Maternal urine hyperglycosylated in hCG in pregnancies with Down syndrome. Prenat Diagn 19:918, 1999

Cuckle HS, Wald NJ, Lindenbaum RH: Maternal serum alpha-fetoprotein measurement: A screening test for Down syndrome. Lancet 1:926, 1984

Cunningham FG, Gilstrap LC: Maternal serum alpha-fetoprotein screening. N Engl J Med 325:55, 1991

Curry CJ, Stevenson RE, Aughton D, Byrne J, Carey JC, Cassidy S, Cunniff C, Graham JM Jr, Jones MC, Kaback MM, Moeschler J, Schaefer GB, Schwartz S, Tarleton J, Opitz J: Evaluation of mental retardation: Recommendations of a consensus conference. Am J Med Genet 72:468, 1997

Cutillo DM: Fragile X syndrome. Genet Teratol 2:1, 1994

Daffos F, Capella-Pavlovsky M, Forestier F: Fetal blood sampling during pregnancy with use of a needle guided by ultrasound: A study of 606 consecutive cases. Am J Obstet Gynecol 153:655, 1985

Daffos F, Capella-Pavlovsky M, Forestier F: A new procedure for fetal blood sampling in utero: Preliminary results of fifty-three cases. Am J Obstet Gynecol 146:985, 1983

David M, Forest MG: Prenatal treatment of congenital adrenal hyperplasia resulting from 21-hydroxylase deficiency. J Pediatr 105:799, 1984

De Lia JE, Kuhlmann RS, Harstad TW, Cruikshank DP: Fetoscopic laser ablation of placental vessels in severe previa-

ble twin–twin transfusion syndrome. Am J Obstet Gynecol 172:1202, 1995

deCrespigny LC, Robinson HP, Quinn M, Doyle L, Ross A, Cauchi M: Ultrasound-guided fetal blood transfusion for severe Rhesus isoimmunization. Obstet Gynecol 66:529, 1985

Deprest JA, Lerut TE, Vandenberghe K: Operative fetoscopy: New perspective in fetal therapy? Prenat Diagn 17:1247, 1997

deVries BBA, Wiegers AM, Smits APT, Mohkamsing S, Duivenvoorden HJ, Fryns J-P, Curfs LMG, Halley DJJ, Oostra BA, van den Ouweland AMW, Niermeijer MF: Mental status of females with an FMR1 gene full mutation. Am J Hum Genet 58:1025, 1996

Dieck D, Schild RL, Hansmann M, Eis-Hubinger AM: Prenatal diagnosis of congenital parvovirus B19 infection: Value of serological and PCR techniques in maternal and fetal serum. Prenat Diagn 19:1119, 1999

Douglas GW, Thomas L, Carr M, Cullen NM, Morris R: Trophoblasts in the circulating blood during pregnancy. Am J Obstet Gynecol 58:960, 1959

Druzin ML, Chervenak F, McCullough LB, Blatman RN, Neidich JA: Should all pregnant patients be offered prenatal diagnosis regardless of age? Obstet Gynecol 81:615, 1993

Edwards A, Peek MJ, Curren J: Transplacental flecainide therapy for fetal supraventricular tachycardia in a twin pregnancy. Aust NZ J Obstet Gynaecol 39:110, 1999

Elias S, Emerson DS, Simpson JL, Shulman LP, Holbrook KA: Ultrasound-guided fetal skin sampling for prenatal diagnosis of genodermatoses. Obstet Gynecol 83:337, 1994

Elliott JP, Urig MA, Clewell WH: Aggressive therapeutic amniocentesis in the treatment of acute twin–twin transfusion syndrome. Obstet Gynecol 77:337, 1991

Evans MI, Hoffman EP, Cadrin C, Johnson MP, Quintero RA, Golbus MS: Fetal muscle biopsy: Collaborative experience with varied indications. Obstet Gynecol 84:913, 1994

Ewigman BG, Crane JP, Frigoletto FD, LeFevre ML, Bain RP, McNellis D: Effect of prenatal ultrasound screening on perinatal outcome. N Engl J Med 329:821, 1993

Ferguson-Smith MA, Yates JRW: Maternal age specific rates for chromosome aberrations and factors influencing them: A report of a collaborative European study on 52,965 amniocenteses. Prenat Diagn 4:5, 1984

Feuchtbaum LB, Cunningham G, Waller DK, Lustig LS, Tompkinson DG, Hook EB: Fetal karyotyping for chromosome abnormalities after an unexplained elevated maternal serum alpha-fetoprotein screening. Obstet Gynecol 86:248, 1995

Firth HV, Boyd PA, Chamberlain P, MacKenzie IZ, Lindenbaum RH, Huson SM: Severe limb abnormalities after chorion villus sampling at 56–66 days' gestation. Lancet 337:762, 1991

Firth HV, Boyd PA, Chamberlain PF, MacKenzie IZ, Morriss-Kay GM, Huson SM: Analysis of limb reduction defects in babies exposed to chorionic villus sampling. Lancet 343:1069, 1994

Fisch GS, Snow K, Thibodeau SN, Chalifaux M, Holden JJ, Nelson DL, Howard-Peebles PN, Maddalena A: The fragile X premutation in carriers and its effect on mutation size in offspring. Am J Hum Genet 56:1147, 1995

Fisk NM, Borrell A, Hubinont C, Tannirandorn Y, Nicolini U, Rodeck CH: Fetofetal transfusion syndrome: Do the neonatal criteria apply in utero? Arch Dis Child 65:657, 1990

Fisk NM, Bower S: Fetal blood sampling in retreat: A casualty of advances in molecular genetics, cytogenetics, and Doppler imaging. BMJ 307:143, 1993

Frigoletto FD Jr, Umansky I, Birnholz J, Acker D, Easterday CL, Harris GB, Griscom NT: Intrauterine fetal transfusion in 365 fetuses during fifteen years. Am J Obstet Gynecol 139:781, 1981

Gardner RJM, Sutherland GR: Chromosome Abnormalities and Genetic Counseling, 2nd ed. Oxford Monographs on Medical Genetics No. 29. Oxford, Oxford University Press, 1996

Geifman-Holtzman O, Bernstein IM, Berry SM, Holtzman EJ, Vadnais TJ, DeMaria MA, Bianchi DW: Fetal RhD genotyping in fetal cells flow sorted from maternal blood. Am J Obstet Gynecol 174:818, 1996

Ghidini A, Sepulveda W, Lockwood CJ, Romero R: Complications of fetal blood sampling. Am J Obstet Gynecol 168:1339, 1993

Gilstrap LC, Van Dorsten P, Cunningham FG: Fetal surgery. In Operative Obstetrics, 2nd ed. New York, McGraw-Hill, 2001

Goldberg JD: Fetal cells in maternal circulation: Progress in analysis of a rare event. Am J Hum Genet 61:806, 1997

Gonzalez D, Barret T, Apuzzio J: Utility of routine fetal karyotyping for patients undergoing amniocentesis for elevated maternal serum alpha-fetoprotein. Am J Obstet Gynecol 174:436, 1996

Grabowski GA, Kruse JR, Goldberg JD, Chockkalingam K, Gordon RE, Blakemore KJ, Mahoney MJ, Desnick RJ: First trimester prenatal diagnosis of Tay–Sachs disease. Am J Hum Genet 36:1369, 1984

Graf JL, Housely HT, Albanese CT, Adzick NS, Harrison MR: A surprising histological evolution of preterm sacrococcygeal teratoma. J Pediatr Surg 33:177, 1998

Grannum PA, Copel JA, Plaxe SC, Scioscia AL, Hobbins JC: In utero exchange transfusion by direct intravascular injection in severe erythroblastosis fetalis. N Engl J Med 314:1431, 1986

Gupta JK, Khan KS, Thornton JG, Lilford RJ: Management of fetal choroid plexus cysts. Br J Obstet Gynaecol 104:881, 1997

Haddow JE, Kloza EM, Smith DE, Knight GJ: Data from an alphafetoprotein pilot screening program in Maine. Obstet Gynecol 62:556, 1983

Haddow JE, Palomaki GE: Down's syndrome screening. Lancet 347:1625, 1996

Haddow JE, Palomaki GE, Knight GJ, Cunningham GC, Lustig LS, Boyd PA: Reducing the need for amniocentesis in women 35 years of age or older with serum markers for screening. N Engl J Med 330:1114, 1994

Haddow JE, Palomaki GE, Knight GJ, Williams J, Miller WA, Johnson A: Screening of maternal serum for fetal Down syndrome in the first trimester. N Engl J Med 338:955, 1998

Haddow JE, Palomaki GE, Knight GJ, Williams J, Pulkkinen A, Canick JA, Saller DN Jr, Bowers GB: Prenatal screening for Down syndrome with use of maternal serum markers. N Engl J Med 327:588, 1992

Hagay Z, Reece EA, Roberts A, Hobbins JC: Isolated fetal pleural effusion: A prenatal management dilemma. Obstet Gynecol 81:147, 1993

Hagerman RJ, Amiri K, Cronister A: Fragile X checklist. Am Med Genet 38:283, 1991

Harman CR, Bowman JM, Manning FA, Menticoglou SM: Intrauterine transfusion—Intraperitoneal versus intravascular approach: A case-control comparison. Am J Obstet Gynecol 162:1053, 1990

Harmon JP, Hiett AK, Palmer CG, Golichowski AM: Prenatal ultrasound detection of isolated neural tube defects: Is cytogenetic evaluation warranted? Obstet Gynecol 86:595, 1995

Harrison ME, Crombleholme TM, Slotnick NR: In utero transplantation of fetal liver hematopoietic stem cells in monkeys. Lancet 2:1425, 1989

Harrison MR: Fetal surgery. Am J Obstet Gynecol 174:1255, 1996

Harrison MR, Adzick NS, Jennings RW: Antenatal intervention for congenital cystic adenomatoid malformation. Lancet 336:96507, 1990a

Harrison MR, Adzick NS, Longaker MT, Goldberg JD, Rosen MA, Filly RA, Evans MI, Golbus MS: Successful repair in utero of a fetal diaphragmatic hernia after removal of herniated viscera from the left thorax. N Engl J Med 322:1582, 1990b

Harrison MR, Golbus MS, Filly RA, Nakayama DK, Callen PW, deLorimier AA, Hricak H: Management of the fetus with congenital hydronephrosis. J Pediatr Surg 17:728, 1982

Harrison MR, Jester JA, Ross NA: Correction of congenital diaphragmatic hernia in utero. I. The model: Intrathoracic balloon produces fatal pulmonary hypoplasia. Surgery 88:174, 1980

Harrison MR, Mychaliska GB, Albanese CT, Jennings RW, Farrell JA, Hawgood S, Sandberg P, Levine AH, Lobo E, Filly RA: Correction of congenital diaphragmatic hernia in utero IX: Fetuses with poor prognosis (liver herniation and low lung-to-head ratio) can be saved by fetoscopic temporary tracheal occlusion. J Pediatr Surg 33:1017, 1998

Heffez DS, Aryaupur J, Hutchins GM, Freeman JM: The paralysis associated with myelomeningocele: Clinical and experimental data implicating a preventable spinal cord injury. Neurosurgery 26:987, 1990

Hobbins JC, Grannum PA, Romero R, Reece EA, Mahoney MJ: Percutaneous umbilical blood sampling. Am J Obstet Gynecol 152:1, 1985

Hogge WA, Thiagarajah S, Brenbridge AN, Harbert GM: Fetal evaluation by percutaneous blood sampling. Am J Obstet Gynecol 158:132, 1988

Hogge WA, Thiagarajah S, Ferguson JE, Schnatterly PT, Harbert GM: The role of ultrasonography and amniocentesis in the evaluation of pregnancies at risk for neural tube defects. Am J Obstet Gynecol 161:520, 1989

Holmgren G, Blomiquist K, Son H, Drugge U, Gustavson KH: Fragile X families in a northern Swedish county: A geneological study of possible affected individuals in the nineteenth century. Am J Med Genet 30:673, 1988

Holzgreve W, Evans MI: Nonvasular needles and shunt placements for fetal therapy. West J Med 159:333, 1993

Hook EB: Prevalence, risks, and recurrence. In Brock DJH, Rodeck CH, Ferguson-Smith MA (eds): Prenatal Diagnosis and Screening. Edinburgh, Churchill-Livingstone, 1992, p 351

Hook EB, Cross PK, Schreinemachers DM: Chromosomal abnormality rates of amniocentesis and in live-born infants. JAMA 249:2034, 1983

Hornberger LK, Need L, Benacerraf BR: Development of significant left and right ventricular hypoplasia in the second and third trimester fetus. J Ultrasound Med 15:655, 1996

Hsieh FJ, Shyu MK, Sheu BC, Lin SP, Chen CP, Huang FY: Limb defects after chorionic villus sampling. Obstet Gynecol 85:84, 1995

Hume RF Jr, Drugan A, Reichler A, Lampinen J, Martin LS, Johnson MP, Evans MI: Aneuploidy among prenatally detected neural tube defects. Am J Med Genet 61:171, 1996

Johnson JM, Wilson RD, Winor RD, Winsor EJ, Singer J, Dansereau J, Kalousek DK: The early amniocentesis versus mid-trimester amniocentesis for fetal karyotyping at 10–13 weeks' gestation. Lancet 344:435, 1994

Johnson MP, Corsi P, Bradfield W, Hume RF, Smith C, Flake AW, Qureshi F, Evans MI: Sequential urinalysis improves evaluation of fetal renal function in obstructive uropathy. Am J Obstet Gynecol 173:59, 1995

Jones KL: Smith's Recognizable Patterns of Human Malformation, 5th ed. Philadelphia, Saunders, 1997

Kalousek DJ, Dill FJ: Chromosomal mosaicism confined to the placenta in human conceptions. Science 221:665, 1983

Katz VL, Chescheir NC, Cefalo RC: Unexplained elevations of maternal serum alpha-fetoprotein. Obstet Gynecol Surg 45:719, 1990

Kleihauer E, Braun H, Betke K: Demonstration von fetalem hemaglobin in den erythrocyten eines Blutausstrines. Klinische Wochenschrif 35:637, 1957

Kuliev A, Jackson L, Froster U, Brambati B, Simpson JL, Verlinsky Y, Ginsberg N, Smidt-Jensen S, Zakut H: Chorionic villus sampling safety. Report of World Health Organization/EURO meeting in association with the Seventh International Conference on Early Prenatal Diagnosis of Genetic Diseases, Tel-Aviv, Israel, May 21, 1994. Am J Obstet Gynecol 174:807, 1996

Lammer EJ, Sever LE, Oakley GP: Teratogen update: Valproic acid. Teratology 35:465, 1987

Langer JC, Harrison MR, Schmidt KG, Silverman NH, Anderson RL, Goldberg JD, Filly RA, Crombleholme TM, Longaker MT, Golbus MS: Fetal hydrops and death from sacrococcygeal teratoma: Rationale for fetal surgery. Am J Obstet Gynecol 160:1145, 1989

Leschot NJ, Verjaal M, Treffers PE: Risks of midtrimester amniocentesis; assessment in 3000 pregnancies. Br J Obstet Gynaecol 92:804, 1985

Limb CJ, Holmes LB: Anencephaly: Changes in prenatal detection and birth status, through 1990. Am J Obstet Gynecol 170:1333, 1994

Ling EWY: Frequency and load of congenital anomalies in a neonatal intensive care unit, prenatal diagnosis, and perinatal management. Semin Perinatol 16:352, 1992

Luthy DA, Wardinsky T, Shurtleff DB, Hollenbach KA, Hickok DE, Nyberg DA, Beneditti TJ: Cesarean section before the onset of labor and subsequent motor function in infants with meningomyelocele diagnosed antenatally. N Engl J Med 324:662, 1991

Mahony BS, Filly RA, Callen PW: Amnionicity and chorionicity in twin pregnancies: Prediction using ultrasound. Radiology 155:205, 1985

Mahony BS, Petty CN, Nyberg DA, Luthy DA, Hickok DE, Hirsch JH: The "stuck twin" phenomenon: Ultrasonographic findings, pregnancy outcome, and management with serial amniocenteses. Am J Obstet Gynecol 163:1513, 1990

Main DM, Mennuti MT: Neural tube defects: Issues in prenatal diagnosis and counseling. Obstet Gynecol 67:1, 1986

Malone PS, Spitz L, Kiely EM, Brereton RJ, Duffy PG, Ransley PG: The functional sequelae of sacrococcygeal teratomas. J Pediatr Surg 25:679, 1990

Mangione R, Guyon F, Vergnaud A, Jimenez M, Saura R, Horovitz J: Successful treatment of refractory supraventricular tachycardia by repeat intravascular injection of amiodarone in a fetus with hydrops. Eur J Obstet Gynecol Reprod Biol 86:105, 1999

Manning FA, Harrison MR, Rodeck C: Catheter shunts for fetal hydronephrosis and hydrocephalus. Report of the International Fetal Surgery Registry. N Engl J Med 315:336, 1986

Marchese CA, Carozzi F, Mosso R, et al: Fetal karyotype in malformations detected by ultrasound. Am J Hum Genet 37:A223, 1985

Maxwell DJ, Johnson P, Hurley P, Neales K, Allan L, Knott P: Fetal blood sampling and pregnancy loss in relation to indication. Br J Obstet Gynaecol 98:892, 1991

Merkatz IR, Nitowsky HM, Macri JN, Johnson WE: An association between low maternal serum α-fetoprotein and fetal chromosomal abnormalities. Am J Obstet Gynecol 148:886, 1984

Meuli M, Meuli-Simmen C, Hutchins GM, Yingling CD, Hoffman KM, Harrison MR, Adzick NS: In utero surgery rescues neurological function at birth in sheep with spina bifida. Nat Med 1:342, 1995

Meuli M, Meuli-Simmen C, Yingling CD, Hutchins GM, Timmel GB, Harrison MR, Adzick NS: In utero repair of experimental myelomeningocele saves neurological function at birth. J Pediatr Surg 31:397, 1996

Meyers C, Adam R, Dungan J, Prenger V: Aneuploidy in twin gestations: When is maternal age advanced? Obstet Gynecol 89:248, 1997

Milunsky A: Genetic Disorders and the Fetus: Diagnosis, Prevention, and Treatment, 3rd ed. Baltimore, Johns Hopkins University Press, 1992, p 1

Milunsky A, Alpert E, Neff RK, Frigoletto FD Jr: Prenatal diagnosis of neural tube defects. IV. Maternal serum alpha-fetoprotein screening. Obstet Gynecol 55:60, 1980

Milunsky A, Jick SS, Bruell CL, MacLaughlin DS, Tsung YK, Jick H, Rothman KJ, Willett W: Predictive values, relative risks, and overall benefits of high and low maternal serum α-fetoprotein screening in singleton pregnancies: New epidemiologic data. Am J Obstet Gynecol 161:291, 1989

Moise KJ Jr, Belfort M, Saade G: Iatrogenic gastroschisis in the treatment of diaphragmatic hernia. Am J Obstet Gynecol 172:715, 1995

Morris C, Stringer J, Biggio J, Owen J: Prenatal screening strategies for Down Syndrome (Abstract 0057). Presented at the Society for Maternal–Fetal Medicine, Reno, Nevada, February 5-10, 2001

Morrow RJ, McNay MB, Whittle MJ: Ultrasound detection of neural tube defects in patients with elevated maternal serum alpha-fetoprotein. Obstet Gynecol 78:1055, 1991

Morton NE, Chiu D, Holland C, Jacobs PA, Pettay D: Chromosome anomalies as predictors of recurrence risk for spontaneous abortion. Am J Med Genet 28:353, 1987

Nadel AS, Green JK, Holmes LB, Frigoletto FD Jr, Benacerraf BR: Absence of need for amniocentesis in patients with elevated levels of maternal serum alpha-fetoprotein and normal ultrasonographic examinations. N Engl J Med 323:557, 1990

National Institutes of Health: Genetic testing for cystic fibrosis. NIH Consensus Conference. Washington, DC, 1997

New England Regional Genetics Group Prenatal Collaborative Study of Down Syndrome Screening: Combining maternal serum α-fetoprotein measurements and age to screen for Down syndrome in pregnant women under age 35. Am J Obstet Gynecol 160:575, 1989

NICHD National Registry for Amniocentesis Study Group: Midtrimester amniocentesis for prenatal diagnosis. JAMA 236:1471, 1976

Nicolaides K, Brizot M de L, Patel F, Snijders R: Comparison of chorionic villus sampling and amniocentesis for fetal karyotyping at 10–13 weeks' gestation. Lancet 344:435, 1994

Nicolaides K, Pettersen H: Fetal therapy. Curr Opin Obstet Gynecol 6:468, 1994

Nicolaides K, Soothill PW, Rodeck CH, Campbell S: Ultrasound-guided sampling of umbilical cord and placental blood to assess fetal well being. Lancet 1:1065, 1986a

Nicolaides KH, Soothill PW, Rodeck CH, Clewell W: Rh disease: Intravascular fetal blood transfusion by cordocentesis. Fetal Ther 1:185, 1986b

Nyberg DA, Mahony BS, Pretorius DH: Diagnostic ultrasound of fetal anomalies: Text and atlas. Mosby Year Book, St. Louis, MO, 1990 p 481

Parilla BV, Strasburger JF, Socol ML: Fetal supraventricular tachycardia complicated by hydrops fetalis: A role for direct fetal intramuscular therapy. Am J Perinatol 13:483, 1996

Pauker SP, Pauker SG: Prenatal diagnosis—Why is 35 a magic number? N Engl J Med 330:1151, 1994

Pergament E, Fiddler M: Prenatal gene therapy: Prospects and issues. Prenat Diagn 15:1303, 1995

Persutte WH, Lenke RR: Failure of amniotic-fluid-cell growth: Is it related to fetal aneuploidy? Lancet 345:96, 1995

Peters MT, Nicolaides KH: Cordocentesis for the diagnosis and treatment of human fetal parvovirus infection. Obstet Gynecol 75:501, 1990

Pinette MC, Pay Y, Pinette SG, Stubblefield PG: Treatment of twin–twin transfusion syndrome. Obstet Gynecol 82:841, 1993

Platt LD, Feuchtbaum L, Filly R, Lustig L, Simon M, Cunningham GC: The California Maternal Serum α-Fetoprotein Screening Program: The role of ultrasonography in the detection of spina bifida. Am J Obstet Gynecol 166:1328, 1992

Poon LL, Leung TN, Lau TK, Dennis YM: Prenatal detection of fetal Down's syndrome from maternal plasma. Lancet 356:1819, 2000

Powers RJ, Phillips BL: Repair in utero of a fetal diaphragmatic hernia. N Engl J Med 323:1279, 1990

Price JO, Elias S, Wachtel SS, Klinger K, Dockter M, Tharapel A, Shulman LP, Phillips OP, Meyers CM, Shook D: Prenatal diagnosis using fetal cells isolated from maternal blood by multiparameter flow cytometry. Am J Obstet Gynecol 165:1731, 1991

Quintero RA, Johnson MP, Romero R, Smith C, Arias F, Guevara-Zuloaga F, Cotton DB, Evans MI: In utero percutaneous cystoscopy in the management of fetal lower obstructive uropathy. Lancet 346:537, 1995

Ramus R, Martin L, Dowd T, Lucas M, Santos-Ramos R, Twickler D: Elevated maternal serum alpha-fetoprotein and placental sonolucencies. Am J Obstet Gynecol 174:423, 1996

Reece EA, Hobbins JC: Diabetic embryopathy: Pathogenesis, prenatal diagnosis and prevention. Obstet Gynecol Surv 41:325, 1986

Reed KL: Fetal arrhythmias: Etiology, diagnosis, pathophysiology, and treatment. Semin Perinatol 13:294, 1989

Reichler A, Hume RF Jr, Drugan A, Bardicef M, Isada NB, Johnson MP, Evans MI: Risk of anomalies as a function of level of elevated maternal serum α-fetoprotein. Am J Obstet Gynecol 171:1052, 1994

Rhoads GG, Jackson LG, Schlesselman SE, de la Cruz FF, Desnick RJ, Golbus MS, Ledbetter DH, Lubs HA, Mahoney MJ, Pergament E: The safety and efficacy of chorionic villus sampling for early prenatal diagnosis of cytogenetic abnormalities. N Engl J Med 320:609, 1989

Rimoin DL, Conner JM, Pyeritz RE: Nature and frequency of genetic disease. In Rimoin DL, Conner JM, Pyeritz RE (eds): Emery and Rimoin's Principles and Practices of Medical Genetics, 3rd ed. New York, Churchill-Livingstone, 1997, p 31

Roberts LJ, Bewley S, MacKinson AM, Rodeck CH: First trimester fetal nuchal translucency: Problems with screening the general population 1. Br J Obstet Gynaecol 102:381, 1995

Roberts NS, Dunn LK, Weiner S, Godmilow L, Miller R: Midtrimester amniocentesis: Indications, technique, risk and potential for prenatal diagnosis. J Reprod Med 28:167, 1983

Rodeck CH, Campbell S: Sampling pure fetal blood by fetoscopy in second trimester of pregnancy. BMJ 2:728, 1978

Rodeck CH, Kemp JR, Holman CA, Whitmore DN, Karnicki J, Austin MA: Direct intravascular fetal blood transfusion by fetoscopy in severe rhesus isoimmunization. Lancet 1:625, 1981

Rodeck CH, Nicolaides KH, Warsof SL, Fysh WJ, Gamsu HR, Kemp JR: The management of severe rhesus isoimmunization by fetoscopic intravascular transfusions. Am J Obstet Gynecol 150:769, 1984

Romero R, Jeanty P, Reece EA, Grannum P, Bracken M, Berkowitz R, Hobbins JC: Sonographically monitored amniocentesis to decrease intraoperative complications. Obstet Gynecol 65:426, 1985

Rosenstein BJ, Zeitlin PL. Cystic fibrosis. Lancet 351:277, 1998

Sahakian V, Weiner CP, Naides SJ, Williamson RA, Scharosch LL: Intrauterine transfusion treatment of nonimmune hydrops fetalis secondary to human parvovirus B19 infection. Am J Obstet Gynecol 164:1090, 1991

Sakala EP, Andree I: Optimal route of delivery for meningomyelocele. Obstet Gynecol Surv 45:209, 1990

Schatz F: Arch Gynsekol 7:336, 1875

Sepulveda W, Donaldson A, Johnson RD, Davies G, Fisk NM: Are routine alpha-fetoprotein and acetylcholinesterase determinations still necessary at second-trimester amniocentesis? Impact of high-resolution ultrasonography. Obstet Gynecol 85:107, 1995

Shields LE, Ultrich SB, Komarniski CA, Werner MH, Winter TC: Amniotic fluid alpha-fetoprotein determination at the time of genetic amniocentesis: Has it outlived its usefulness? J Ultrasound Med 15:735, 1996

Shreinemachers DM, Cross PK, Hook EB: Rates of trisomies 21, 18, 13, and other chromosomal abnormalities in about 20,000 prenatal studies compared with estimated rates in live births. Hum Genet 61:318, 1982

Shulman LP, Elias S, Phillips OP, Grevengood C, Dungan JS, Simpson JL: Amniocentesis performed at 14 weeks' gestation or earlier: Comparison with first-trimester transabdominal chorionic villus sampling. Obstet Gynecol 83:543, 1994

Simpson JL: Incidence and timing of pregnancy losses: Relevance to evaluating safety of early prenatal diagnosis. Am J Med Genet 35:165, 1990

Simpson JL, Carson SA: Preimplantation genetic diagnosis. N Engl J Med 327:951, 1992

Simpson JL, Elias S: Isolating fetal cells in the maternal circulation. Hum Reprod 1:409, 1998

Simpson JL, Elias S, Morgan LD, Anderson RN, Shulman LP, Sibai BM, Mercer BH, Skoll A: Does unexplained second trimester (15 to 20 weeks' gestation) maternal serum alpha-fetoprotein elevation presage adverse perinatal outcome? Pitfalls and preliminary studies with late second and third trimester maternal serum alphafetoprotein. Am J Obstet Gynecol 164:829, 1991

Simpson LL, Marx GR, D'Alton ME: Supraventricular tachycardia in the fetus: Conservative management in the absence of hemodynamic compromise. J Ultrasound Med 16:459, 1997

Sonesson SE, Fouron JC, Wesslen-Eriksson E, Jaeggi E, Winberg P: Foetal supraventricular tachycardia treated with sotalol. Acta Paediatr 87:584, 1998

Steele CD, Wapner RJ, Smith JB, Haynes MK, Jackson LG: Prenatal diagnosis using fetal cells isolated from maternal peripheral blood: A review. Clin Obstet Gynecol 39:801, 1996

Stray-Pedersen B, Stray-Pedersen S: Etiologic factors and subsequent reproductive performance in 195 couples with a prior history of habitual abortion. Am J Obstet Gynecol 148:140, 1984

Sundberg K, Bang J, Smidt-Jensen S, Brocks V, Lundsteen C, Parner J, Keiding N, Philip J: Randomised study of risk of fetal loss related to early amniocentesis versus chorionic villus sampling. Lancet 350:697, 1997

Thiagarajah S, Stroud CB, Vavelidis F, Schnorr JA, Schnatterly PT, Ferguson JE II: Elevated maternal serum α-fetoprotein levels: What is the risk of fetal aneuploidy? Am J Obstet Gynecol 173:388, 1995

Thompson MW, McInnes RR, Huntington WF: Genetics of disorders with multifactorial inheritance. In: Genetics in Medicine, 5th ed. Philadelphia, Saunders, 1991, p 349

UK Collaborative Study on Alphafetoprotein in Relation to Neural-tube Defects: Maternal serum-alphafetoprotein measurement in antenatal screening for anencephaly and spina bifida in early pregnancy. Lancet 11:1323, 1977

Valenti C: Antenatal detection of hemoglobinopathies: A preliminary report. Am J Obstet Gynecol 115:851, 1973

Van den Hof MC, Nicolaides KH, Campbell J, Campbell S: Evaluation of the lemon and banana signs in one hundred thirty fetuses with open spina bifida. Am J Obstet Gynecol 162:322, 1990

VanderWall KJ, Bruch SW, Meuli M, Kohl T, Szabo Z, Adzick NS, Harrison MR: Fetal endoscopic ("Fetendo") tracheal clip. J Pediatr Surg 31:1101, 1996

Vetter K, Schnieder KTM: Iatrogenous remission of twin transfusion syndrome. Am J Obstet Gynecol 158:221, 1988

Vintzileos AM, Campbell WA, Nochimson DJ, Weinbaum PJ: Antenatal evaluation and management of ultrasonically detected fetal anomalies. Obstet Gynecol 69:640, 1987

Vintzileos AM, Egan JFX: Adjusting the risk for trisomy 21 on the basis of second-trimester ultrasonography. Am J Obstet Gynecol 172:837, 1995

Viville S, Ray P, Viville B, Handyside A, Gerlinger P: Diagnostic genetique preimplantatoire: Techniques et resultats. Med Sci 12:1378, 1996

Wald NJ, Cuckle HS, Densem JW, Nanchahal K, Canick JA, Haddow JE, Knight GJ, Palomaki GE: Maternal serum unconjugated oestriol as an antenatal screening test for Down's syndrome. Br J Obstet Gynaecol 95:334, 1988a

Wald NJ, Cuckle HS, Densem JW, Nanchahal K, Royston P, Chard T, Haddow JE, Knight GJ, Palomaki GE, Canick JA: Maternal serum screening for Down syndrome in early pregnancy. BMJ 297:883, 1988b

Wald NJ, Densem JW, George L, Muttukrishna S, Knight PG: Prenatal screening for Down's syndrome using inhibin-A as a serum marker. Prenat Diagn 16:143, 1996a

Wald NJ, George L, Smith D, Densem JW, Petterson K: Serum screening for Down syndrome between 8 and 14 weeks of pregnancy. Br J Obstet Gynaecol 103:407, 1996b

Wald NJ, Kennard A, Hackshaw A, McGuire A: Antenatal screening for Down syndrome. Health Technol Assess 2:i, 1, 1998

Wald NJ, Kennard A, Hackshaw A, McGuire A: Antenatal screening for Down's syndrome. J Med Screen 4:181, 1997

Waller DK, Lustig LS, Cunningham GC, Golbus MS, Hook EB: Second-trimester maternal serum alpha-fetoprotein levels and the risk of subsequent fetal death. N Engl J Med 325:6, 1991

Walnowska J, Conte FA, Grumback MM: Practical and theoretical implications of fetal/maternal lymphocyte transfer. Lancet 1:1119, 1969

Warburton D, Kline J, Stein Z, Hutzler M, Chin A, Hassold T: Does the karyotype of a spontaneous abortion predict the karyotype of a subsequent abortion? Evidence from 273 women with two karyotyped spontaneous abortions. Am J Hum Genet 41:465, 1987

Watson WJ, Chescheir NC, Katz VL, Seeds JW: The role of ultrasound in evaluation of patients with elevated maternal serum alpha-fetoprotein: A review. Obstet Gynecol 78:123, 1991

Weiner C, Varner M, Pringle K, Hein H, Williamson R, Smith WL: Case reports: Antenatal diagnosis and palliative treatment of nonimmune hydrops fetalis secondary to pulmonary extralobar sequestration. Obstet Gynecol 68:275, 1986

Weiner CP: The role of cordocentesis in fetal diagnosis. Clin Obstet Gynecol 31:285, 1988

Weiner CP: Diagnosis and treatment of twin to twin transfusion in the mid-second trimester of pregnancy. Fet Ther 2:71, 1987

Weiner CP, Williamson RA, Wenstrom KD, Sipes SL, Widness JA, Grant SS, Estle L: Management of fetal hemolytic disease by cordocentesis. II. Outcome of treatment. Am J Obstet Gynecol 165:1302, 1991

Wenstrom KD, Andrews WW, Tamura T, DuBard MB, Johnston KE, Hemstreet P: Elevated amniotic fluid interleukin-6 levels at genetic amniocentesis predict subsequent pregnancy loss. Am J Obstet Gynecol 174:830, 1996

Wenstrom KD, Descartes M, Franklin J, Cliver SP: A five-year experience with fragile X screening of high-risk gravid women. Am J Obstet Gynecol 181:789, 1999a

Wenstrom KD, Owen J, Chu DC, Boots L: Prospective evaluation of free βhCG and dimeric inhibin A for aneuploidy detection. Am J Obstet Gynecol 181:887, 1999b

Wenstrom KD, Sipes SL, Williamson RA, Grant SS, Trawick DC, Estle LC: Prediction of pregnancy outcome with single versus serial maternal serum α-fetoprotein tests. Am J Obstet Gynecol 167:1529, 1992

Wenstrom KD, Weiner CP, Hanson JW: A five-year statewide experience with congenital diaphragmatic hernia. Am J Obstet Gynecol 165:838, 1991

Wenstrom KD, Weiner CP, Williamson RA, Grant SS: Prenatal diagnosis of fetal hyperthyroidism using funipuncture. Obstet Gynecol 76:513, 1990

Wenstrom KD, Williamson RA, Grant SS, Hudson JD, Getchell JP: Evaluation of multiple-marker screening for Down syndrome in a state-wide population. Am J Obstet Gynecol 169:793, 1993

Westgren M, Ringden O, Eik-Nes S, Ek S, Anvret M, Brubakk AM, Bui TH, Giambona A, Kiserud T, Kjaeldgaard A, Maggio A, Markling L, Seiger A, Orlandi F: Lack of evidence of permanent engraftment after in utero fetal stem cell transplantation in congenital hemoglobinopathies. Transplantation 61:1176, 1996

Westgren M, Selbing A, Stangenberg M: Fetal intracardiac transfusions in patients with severe rhesus isoimmunisation. BMJ 296:885, 1988

Williamson RA, Pringle KC: Correcting hydrocephalus and fetal uropathy: How good are the prospects? Contemp Obstet Gynecol 30:77, 1987

Williamson RA, Weiner CP, Patil S, Benda J, Varner MW, Abu-Yousef MM: Abnormal pregnancy sonogram: Selective indication for fetal karyotype. Obstet Gynecol 69:15, 1987

Wilson RD, Kendrick V, Witman BK, McGillivray BC: Risk of spontaneous abortion in ultrasonographically normal pregnancies. Lancet 2:290, 1984

Wladimiroff JW, Sachs ES, Reuss A, Stewart PA, Pijpers L, Niermeijer MF: Prenatal diagnosis of chromosome abnormalities in the presence of fetal structural defects. Am J Med Genet 28:289, 1998

Younis JS, Granat M: Insufficient transplacental digoxin transfer in severe hydrops fetalis. Am J Obstet Gynecol 157:1268, 1987

Zauri J, Elstein D, Lahad A, Abrahamov A, Hadas-Halpern I, Zimran A: Asymptomatic Gaucher disease—implications for large-scale screening. Genet Test 2:4, 1998

38

Teratology, Drugs, and Medications

A birth defect is defined as a major deviation from normal morphology or function that is congenital in origin. Birth defects are common, and 3 percent of all children born in the United States have a major structural malformation detectable at birth. In addition, by 1 year of age, 7 percent have developmental disorders identified, 12 to 14 percent by the time they enter school, and 17 percent before age 18 (Boyle and associates, 1994; Kimmel and colleagues, 1993). Less than a third of all patients seeking genetic counseling for birth defects have a primarily genetic condition (Hanson, 1996). The majority of congenital abnormalities are due to nonheritable factors. Only about 10 percent of malformations identified at birth are caused by teratogens (Shepard, 1998). Only a small number of the latter have been positively identified.

TERATOLOGY

A teratogen is any agent that acts during embryonic or fetal development to produce a permanent alteration of form or function (Shepard, 1998). Teratology is the study of all environmental contributions to abnormal development. Currently recognized teratogens include chemicals, viruses, environmental agents, physical factors, and drugs. Women commonly ingest medications or drugs while pregnant. In a study of almost 9000 Medicaid prenatal patients in Michigan, Piper and colleagues (1987) reported that each woman received an average of 3.1 prescriptions for drugs other than vitamins. Commonly used drugs include antiemetics, antacids, antihistamines, analgesics, antimicrobials, antihypertensives, tranquilizers, hypnotics, and diuretics. A substantial number of pregnant women also abuse recreational drugs during pregnancy. A study by Vega and colleagues (1993) found that 5.2 percent of 29,494 women presenting for delivery in 202 California hospitals were using one or more illicit drugs, including amphetamines, barbiturates, benzodiazepines, cannabinoid, cocaine, methadone, opiates, or phencyclidine. Another 6.7 percent were using alcohol, and 8.8 percent smoked cigarettes prior to delivery.

The word *teratogen* is derived from the Greek *teratos*, meaning monster. Because this derivation implies obvious, visible defects, a teratogen is most properly defined as an agent that produces structural abnormalities. Since recognition of a structural anomaly at birth is often straightforward, its association with a specific agent is more likely to be suspected. Some congenital abnormalities, however, do not become apparent until later. A *hadegen*—after Hades, the god who possessed a helmet conferring invisibility—is an agent that interferes with normal maturation and function of an organ. A *trophogen* is an agent that alters growth. Hadegens and trophogens generally affect processes occurring after organogenesis or even after birth. Chemical or physical exposures that act as hadegens or trophogens are much harder to document. For simplification, most authors use the word teratogen to refer to all three types of agents.

EVALUATION OF POTENTIAL TERATOGENS. A birth defect in a child exposed prenatally to a certain drug, chemical, or environmental agent naturally arouses concern that the agent was a teratogen. Before such culpability is established, and as shown in Table 38–1 and described next, certain criteria must be met.

THE DEFECT MUST BE COMPLETELY CHARACTERIZED. This should be done preferably by a geneticist or dysmorphologist. A wide variety of genetic and environmental factors can often produce the same anomaly. For example, although cleft lip and palate are associated with antenatal hydantoin exposure, there are also more than 300 known genetic causes (Murray, 1995). Identical defects with different etiologies are called *phenocopies* (Chap. 36, p. 940). In general, it is easiest to prove causation when a rare drug exposure produces a rare defect, when at least three cases have been identified, and when the defect is relatively severe. For example, it has not been difficult to show that isotretinoin is a teratogen because relatively few pregnant women have

TABLE 38–1. Criteria for Proof of Human Teratogenicity

1. Proven exposure to agent at critical time(s) in prenatal development—prescriptions, office records, dates.

2. Consistent findings by two or more epidemiological studies of high quality:
   a. Control of confounding factors
   b. Sufficient numbers
   c. Exclusion of positive and negative bias factors
   d. Prospective studies, if possible
   e. Relative risk of six or more (?).

3. Careful delineation of clinical cases—specific defect or syndrome, if present, is very helpful.

4. Rare environmental exposure associated with rare defect. Probably three or more cases—examples: oral anticoagulants and nasal hypoplasia, methimazole and scalp defects (?), and heart block and maternal rheumatism.

5. Teratogenicity in experimental animals important but not essential.

6. The association should make biological sense.

7. Proof in an experimental system that the agent acts in an unaltered state. Important information for prevention.

Note: Items 1, 2, and 3 or 1, 3, and 4 are essential criteria. Items 5, 6, and 7 are helpful but not essential.

From Shepard (1998), with permission.

taken it during pregnancy, and one associated defect—agenesis of the ears—is an otherwise rare and severe abnormality.

THE AGENT MUST CROSS THE PLACENTA. The drug or chemical must cross in sufficient doses to directly influence fetal development, or alter maternal or placental metabolism to exert an indirect fetal effect. Placental transfer depends on maternal metabolism, protein binding and storage, molecular size, electrical charge, and lipid solubility. Additionally, placental tissue contains an array of enzymes including cytochrome P-450, which may metabolize offending substances, and in the first trimester has a relatively thick membrane which slows diffusion (Leppik and Rask, 1988). These requirements are illustrated by the vitamin A analogs. *Isotretinoin* given for cystic acne readily crosses the placenta and produces severe fetal defects, while its topical form, *tretinoin,* is not absorbed in appreciable amounts and thus has no apparent fetal effects (Shepard, 1998).

EXPOSURE MUST OCCUR DURING A CRITICAL DEVELOPMENTAL PERIOD. Gestation is divided into the following periods:

1. Preimplantation period, the 2 weeks from fertilization to implantation.
2. Embryonic period, from the second through the eighth week.
3. Fetal period, from 9 weeks until term.

Syndromes from drug exposure are named accordingly—major effects occurring within the first 8 weeks result in an *embryopathy;* after 8 weeks, a *fetopathy.*

The **preimplantation period** has been called the "all or none" period. The zygote undergoes cleavage and cells divide into an outer and inner cell mass. An insult damaging a large number of cells usually causes death of the embryo. If only a few cells are injured, compensation is usually possible with continued normal development (Clayton-Smith and Donnai, 1996). Some animal research studies have challenged this concept by showing that an insult that diminishes the number of cells in the inner cell mass can produce a dose-dependent diminution in body length or size (Iahnaccone and co-workers, 1987).

The **embryonic period** is the most crucial with regard to structural malformations because it encompasses organogenesis. Figure 38–1 illustrates the critical structural development period for each organ system. For example, the heart undergoes major structural development between 3.5 and 6 weeks, and is completely formed by the eighth week. Drugs associated with cardiac malformations can only exert an effect if ingested during this time. It follows that if pregnancy is diagnosed at 10 weeks in a woman ingesting a known cardiac teratogen, there is no advantage to discontinuing the drug.

Throughout the **fetal period** maturation that is important for functional development continues but the fetus remains vulnerable. For example, the brain remains susceptible throughout pregnancy to environmental influences such as alcohol exposure. Alteration in cardiac blood flow during the fetal period can result in deformations such as hypoplastic left heart or aortic coarctation (Clark, 1984). Any agent that reduces amnionic fluid volume between 20 to 25 weeks can cause pulmonary hypoplasia.

CAUSE AND EFFECT MUST BE BIOLOGICALLY PLAUSIBLE. After consideration of the pharmacology of the drug and maternal and fetal metabolism, is it biologically plausible that the suspected agent caused the defect? Because both birth defects and drug or environmental exposures are common, it is always possible that an exposure and a defect are temporally but not causally related. For example, pregnant women often express concern over ingesting food or drinks containing aspartame (Nutrasweet). However, aspartame is metabolized to aspartic acid, which does not cross the placenta; phenylalanine, which is normally metabolized; and methanol, which is produced in levels lower than are found in an equivalent amount of fruit juice.

EPIDEMIOLOGICAL STUDIES MUST BE CONSISTENT. Recurrent findings of characteristic abnormalities in association with a possible environmental exposure should prompt suspicion. Abnormalities include fetal wastage, fetal growth restriction, structural abnormalities, and altered neurological function (Hanson, 1996). The initial evaluation of teratogen exposure is usually retrospective, and is likely to be hampered by recall bias, inadequate reporting, and incomplete assessment of the exposed population. This is further confounded by a variety of doses, concomitant drug therapy, and maternal disease(s). Familial and environmental factors can also influence development of birth defects. Thus, an important criterion for proving teratogenicity is that two or more high-quality epidemiological studies report similar findings.

Epidemiological studies can be **descriptive,** monitoring the change in frequency of a certain birth defect in a specified population over time; **analytic,** looking for an association between certain exposures and specific outcomes; or **experimental,** in which the exposure occurs as the result of the study. Optimally, epidemiological studies are controlled for confounding factors, exclude positive and negative biases, include a sufficient number of cases, and are carried out prospectively. Additionally, a relative risk greater than three is generally necessary to support the hypothesis; a lesser risk should

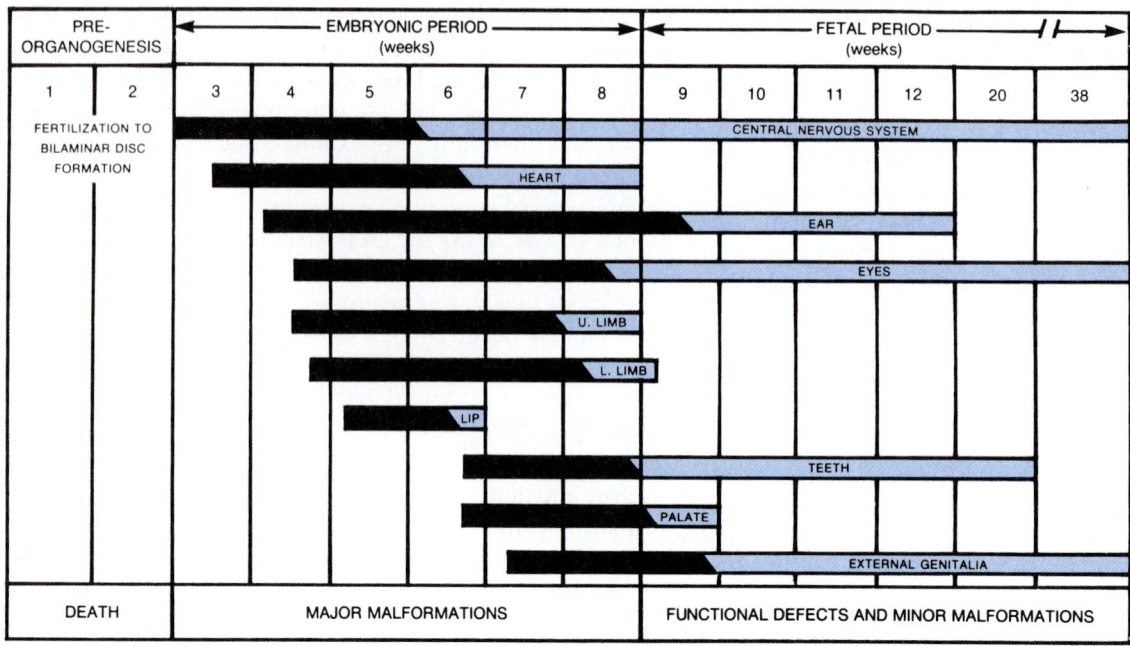

FIGURE 38–1. Timing of organogenesis during the embryonic period. (From Sadler, 1990, with permission.)

be interpreted with caution (Khouri and colleagues, 1992).

An illustration of the advantages of prospective evaluation is the Canadian multicenter study of lithium exposure during pregnancy (Jacobson and colleagues, 1992). Case reports had linked lithium to the rare cardiac malformation, *Ebstein anomaly.* In the study, 138 women taking lithium were monitored prospectively, with confounding factors carefully detailed. A control group was monitored identically, and children born to both groups were evaluated by echocardiography. There was no difference in the incidence of birth defects between the two groups, nor was there an association between lithium and any cardiac malformation.

Suspected teratogens are rarely evaluated epidemiologically, and as a result drug safety information is derived from case reports and small series. Nonscientific and biased reporting has contributed to subsequently proved false assertions that such widely used drugs as benzodiazepines and spermicides were teratogenic. In many cases this prompted litigation and cessation of manufacture of some very useful drugs. An example is Bendectin, a drug that was safe and effective for the treatment of nausea and vomiting in early pregnancy. More than 30 million women used this drug worldwide and the 3 percent congenital anomaly rate among exposed fetuses was not different from the background rate (McKeague and associates, 1994). Despite scientific evidence that Bendectin did not cause birth defects, it was the subject of numerous lawsuits. The financial burden of defending these suits forced its withdrawal, after which hospitalizations for hyperemesis gravidarum increased (Koren and co-workers, 1998). Brent (1985), concluded that although a drug may not be a teratogen, it may be a *litogen!*

THE SUSPECTED TERATOGEN CAUSES A DEFECT IN AN ANIMAL. If a suspected teratogen causes birth defects in experimental animals, the agent may be harmful to the human fetus (Jelovsek and colleagues, 1989). The more species in which a drug produces an effect, especially if testing includes subhuman primates, the more likely it is to have an effect on humans. However, drugs under development are often tested in animals at the equivalent of toxic human doses, making fetal outcomes difficult to interpret. Additionally, different species of animals often have different responses to the same drug. Reliance solely on animal data is imperfect as illustrated by thalidomide. This drug is one of the most potent teratogens ever prescribed, but this was not immediately recognized because it produced no defects in mice and rats (Shepard, 1998). Conversely, corticosteroids have been withheld in pregnancy because they cause cleft lip in rodents, although, there is no evidence that they cause human structural malformations (Czeizel and Rockenbauer, 1997).

FOOD AND DRUG ADMINISTRATION CLASSIFICATIONS. The rating system developed to provide therapeutic guidance based on potential benefits and mater-

TABLE 38–2. **Food and Drug Administration Categories for Drugs and Medications**

Category A

Controlled studies in humans have demonstrated no fetal risks. There are a few category A drugs, and examples include multivitamins or prenatal vitamins, but not "megavitamins."

Category B

Animal studies indicate no fetal risks, but there are no human studies; or adverse effects have been demonstrated in animals, but not in well-controlled human studies. Several classes of commonly used drugs, for example, penicillins, are in this category.

Category C

There are either no adequate studies, either animal or human, or there are adverse fetal effects in animal studies but no available human data. Many drugs or medications commonly taken during pregnancy are in this category.

Category D

There is evidence of fetal risk, but benefits are thought to outweigh these risks. Carbamazepine and phenytoin are examples.

Category X

Proven fetal risks clearly outweigh any benefits. An example is the acne medication isotretinoin, which may cause multiple central nervous system, facial, and cardiovascular anomalies.

From Food and Drug Administration Drug Bulletin (1980).

nal and fetal risks is shown in Table 38–2. However, it may be based on case reports or limited animal data, and updates of these ratings are sometimes slow—for example, oral contraceptives were listed as category X for many years after their teratogenicity was disproved. Friedman and colleagues (1990) concluded that these categories have no correlation with teratogenic risk. The Teratology Society Public Affairs Committee (1994) has proposed that the current rating system be abandoned in favor of an evidence-based rating system which is currently under development. The most current information can be obtained from a drug information service (offered by many academic centers) or an on-line reproductive toxicity service such as reprotox.

GENETIC AND PHYSIOLOGICAL MECHANISMS OF TERATOGENICITY

Teratogens likely act by disturbing specific pathogenetic processes, leading to cell death, altered tissue growth, abnormal cellular differentiation, or disruption of normal development. The mechanism by which most teratogens disturb these processes is unknown. Presumed mechanisms of several agents have been inferred from clinical observations and animal research. Some teratogens disrupt one or more of these processes, and combinations of drugs may be additive. Two established mechanisms of teratogenesis are disruption of folic acid metabolism and production of oxidative intermediates.

DISRUPTION OF FOLIC ACID METABOLISM. Several congenital anomalies, including neural-tube defects, cardiac defects, and cleft lip and palate are thought to arise from disturbance of folic acid metabolic pathways. Folic acid is essential for the production of methionine, which is a co-factor in RNA and DNA synthesis, and is required for methylation of proteins, lipids, and myelin (Scott and associates, 1994). Hydantoin, carbamazepine, valproic acid, and phenobarbital all impair folate absorption or act as antagonists (Donaldson, 1989). There may be a relationship between decreased preconceptional folate levels in epileptic women and fetal malformations (Dansky and colleagues, 1987; Hiilesmaa and co-workers, 1983). Periconceptional folate supplementation decreases malformations in offspring exposed to maternal anticonvulsant therapy (Biale and Lewenthal, 1984; Zhu and Zhou, 1989).

OXIDATIVE INTERMEDIATES. Hydantoin, carbamazepine, and phenobarbital are metabolized by microsomes to arene oxides or epoxides. These oxidative intermediates are detoxified by cytoplasmic *epoxide hydrolase*. The fetus produces arene oxides from anticonvulsants, but because fetal epoxide hydrolase activity is weak, oxidative intermediates accumulate in fetal tissue (Horning and colleagues, 1974). These free oxide radicals have carcinogenic, mutagenic, and other toxic affects (Buehler and associates, 1990). These effects are dose related and increase with multidrug therapy (Lindhout and co-workers, 1984). Damage resulting from toxic intermediates may be common to other teratogens.

Because abnormal physiological processes are induced in many different cells or tissues, teratogen exposure commonly results in multiple effects. Conversely, different drugs that disturb similar pathophysiological processes can produce similar phenotypes. The **fetal hydantoin syndrome** illustrates these concepts (p. 1013). Exposure may cause any combination of growth deficiency, borderline mental deficiency, craniofacial abnormalities, hypoplasia of the distal phalanges, and widely spaced nipples. This phenotype also results from prenatal exposure to carbamazepine, and it is similar to fetal alcohol syndrome (Vorhees and associates, 1988).

EFFECTS OF MATERNAL DISEASES. The interaction of maternal disease and maternal and fetal genetic makeup will determine some drug effects. For example, alcoholic women often have poor nutrition and abuse other drugs. Fetuses exposed to these combined adverse influences are at higher risk for malformation than those exposed to alcohol alone. Heredity and socioeconomic factors appear to influence the development of birth defects in offspring of epileptic women. Even untreated epileptic women have an increased risk of fetal anomalies (American Academy of Neurology, 1998).

FETAL GENETIC COMPOSITION. It is likely that many anomalies now categorized as multifactorial are caused by the interaction of environment and certain altered genes. For example, fetuses exposed to hydantoin are most likely to develop anomalies if they are homozygous for a gene mutation resulting in abnormally low levels of epoxide hydrolase (Buehler and associates, 1990). Another example is a reported association between cigarette smoking and isolated cleft palate, but observed only in individuals with an uncommon polymorphism in the gene for transforming growth factor α-1. The risk of clefts in individuals with this allele is increased two- to sevenfold (Hwang and colleagues, 1995; Shaw and co-workers, 1996).

HOMEOBOX GENES. Certain genes are found in all humans and confer equal susceptibility to specific agents. For example, all vertebrates carry groups of highly conserved genes which share a region of homology and are called **homeobox genes.** These regulatory genes encode nuclear proteins that act as transcription factors to control the expression of other developmentally important genes (Boncinelli, 1997). They are essential for establishing positional identity of various structures along the body axis from the branchial area to the coccyx. The arrangement of the genes along the chromosome corresponds to the arrangement of the body areas they control, and the order in which they are activated. Genes at the 3′ end control the cranial region and are expressed before those at the 5′ end, which control the caudal region (Faiella and collaborators, 1994). During normal embryogenesis, retinoids such as vitamin A activate some of these genes essential for normal growth and tissue differentiation. The potent teratogen, retinoic acid, can activate these genes prematurely, resulting in chaotic gene expression at sensitive stages of development (Soprano and Soprano, 1995). This mechanism has been linked to abnormalities in the hindbrain and limb buds. Valproic acid may preferentially activate a homeobox gene near the 5′ end that regulates axial skeletal patterning. This corresponds with clinical observations that most neural-tube defects caused be valproic acid are in the lumbosacral area.

PATERNAL EXPOSURES. It is possible that paternal exposures to drugs or environmental influences may increase the risk of adverse fetal outcome (Robaire and Hales, 1993). Several mechanisms have been postulated.

One is the induction of a gene mutation or chromosome abnormality in sperm. Because the process by which germ cells mature into functional spermatogonia takes 64 days, drug exposure at any time during the 2 months prior to conception could result in a mutation. A second possibility is that a drug in seminal fluid could gain exposure to the fetus during intercourse. Third, male germ cell exposure to drugs or environmental agents may alter genomic imprinting or cause other changes in gene expression (Trasler and Doerksen, 1999).

Some studies support these hypotheses. Ethyl alcohol, cyclophosphamide, lead, and certain opiates have been associated with an increased risk of behavioral defects in the offspring of exposed male rodents (Nelson and colleagues, 1996). In humans, paternal environmental exposure to mercury, lead, solvents, pesticides, anesthetic gases, or hydrocarbons has been associated with early pregnancy loss although the data is of varying quality (Savitz and associates, 1994). Offspring of men employed in the art or textile industries have been reported to be at increased risk for stillbirth, preterm delivery, and growth restriction. Others who may have an increased risk of congenital fetal anomalies include janitors, woodworkers, firemen, printers, and painters (Olshan and co-workers, 1991; Schnitzer and associates, 1995). There have been no adverse outcomes associated with paternal therapeutic or recreational drug exposure, atomic radiation exposure, or Agent Orange (Centers for Disease Control, 1998, Trasler and Doerksen, 1999).

COUNSELING FOR TERATOGEN EXPOSURE

Women who request genetic counseling for drug exposure during pregnancy often have misconceptions regarding their risk. Koren and colleagues (1989) reported that a fourth of pregnant women seeking counseling because of exposure to nonteratogenic drugs thought they had a 25 percent risk of fetal anomalies, equivalent to thalidomide exposure. These women may also underestimate the background risk of birth defects in the general population. Such misconceptions can be amplified by the referral source, who may exaggerate risk—and even offer pregnancy termination—or by inaccurate articles in the lay press. Counseling should include discussion of possible teratogenic risks of the condition for which the drug was prescribed as well as its genetic implications, in addition to any fetal risks from drug exposure. Ideally, women should be counseled preconceptionally (Chap. 9). In reality, however, patients often report such exposure after conception.

With a few notable exceptions, most commonly prescribed drugs and medications can be used with relative safety during pregnancy. For the few believed to be teratogenic, counseling should emphasize *relative risk.*

All women have about a 3 percent chance of having a child with a birth defect, and although exposure to a confirmed teratogen may increase this risk, it is usually increased by only 1 or 2 percent or at most doubled or tripled. The concept of *risk versus benefit* should also be introduced. Some untreated diseases pose a more serious threat to both mother and fetus than any theoretical risks from medication exposure.

KNOWN TERATOGENS

The number of drugs or medications strongly suspected or proven to be human teratogens is small (Table 38–3). New or infrequently used drugs should be considered to have possible teratogenic potential, and given in pregnancy only if benefits outweigh any theoretical risks.

ALCOHOL. Ethyl alcohol is one of the most potent teratogens. As many as 70 percent of Americans imbibe alcohol socially. During pregnancy, alcohol use varies by population, but its prevalence has been reported to be 1 to 2 percent (Chasnoff and associates, 1990; Little and colleagues, 1989a). The fetal effects of alcohol abuse have been recognized at least since the 1800s, and the consequences of antenatal exposure were first described in a medical journal in 1900 by Sullivan. In 1968, Lemoine and associates reported the wide spectrum of alcohol-related fetal defects culminating in what is now called *fetal alcohol syndrome* (Table 38–4). According to data from the Birth Defects Monitoring Program, the reported rate of the syndrome has increased from 1 per 10,000 births in 1979 to more than 6 per 10,000 births in 1993 (Centers for Disease Control and Prevention,

TABLE 38–4. Features of Fetal Alcohol Syndrome

Growth restriction
Behavioral disturbances
Brain defects
Cardiac defects
Spinal defects
Craniofacial anomalies
    Absent to hypoplastic philtrum
    Broad upper lip
    Flattened nasal bridge
    Hypoplastic upper lip vermilion
    Micrognathia
    Microphthalmia
    Short nose
    Short palpebral tissues

1995). It is one of the most frequent recognizable causes of mental retardation in the United States, a tragedy that could be avoided (Hanson, 1996). The affected child typically has hyperactivity and persistent irritability in the early years. This is followed by developmental delay, growth deficiency, a variable degree of mental retardation, hyperactivity, poor coordination, and distinctive facial features listed in Table 38–4 and shown in Figure 38–2. Congenital heart and joint defects are common. The affected child is typically recognized because of failure to thrive and persistent irritability in early years.

EXPOSURE DOSE. A safe threshold dose for alcohol use during pregnancy has never been established. Women at highest risk to have affected children are those who chronically ingest large quantities and those who engage in binge drinking. Although some studies indicate that fetal injury can result from consuming as little as 1 to 2 drinks per day, the effects of binge drinking may have been obscured by computing a daily average alcohol consumption. For example, Jacobson and co-workers (1993) reported that the threshold below which no alcohol-related effects occurred was 0.5 oz of absolute alcohol per day, however, also stated that most women with affected children actually drank 4 to 6 drinks per occasion, which averaged out to lower daily doses. Subsequently, Jacobson and associates (1998) found that 80 percent of functionally impaired infants were born to women who drank more than five drinks per occasion, on several occasions weekly.

The effects of alcohol thus appear to be biphasic, with a linear dose-response observed only once a threshold of six drinks per occasion is met (Abel, 1999). Alcoholic women ingesting eight or more drinks daily throughout

TABLE 38–3. Drugs or Substances Suspected or Proven to Be Human Teratogens

ACE inhibitors	Etretinate
Alcohol	Isotretinoin
Aminopterin	Lithium
Androgens	Methimazole
Busulfan	Methotrexate
Carbamazepine	Penicillamine
Chlorbiphenyls	Phenytoin
Coumarins	Radioactive iodine
Cyclophosphamide	Tetracycline
Danazol	Trimethadione
Diethylstilbestrol (DES)	Valproic acid

ACE = angiotensin-converting enzyme.
Adapted from Shepard (1986, 1989).

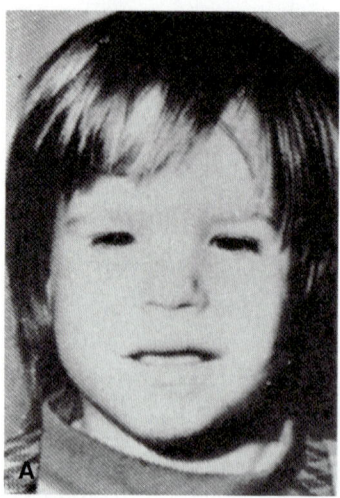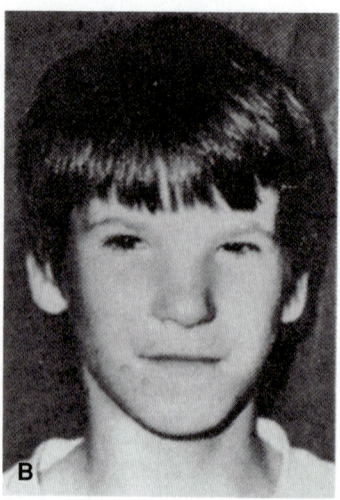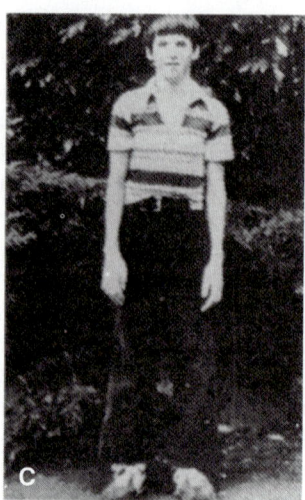

FIGURE 38–2. Fetal alcohol syndrome. **A.** At 2 years 6 months. **B, C.** At 12 years. Note persistence of short palpebral fissures, epicanthal folds, flat midface, hyoplastic philtrum, and thin upper vermilion border. He also has the short, lean prepubertal stature characteristic of young males with fetal alcohol syndrome. (From Streissguth and colleagues, 1985, with permission.)

pregnancy have a 30 to 50 percent risk of having a child with all features of the alcohol syndrome.

Early cessation of alcohol consumption may result in amelioration of some effects. In a prospective study of 60 fetuses exposed to heavy alcohol consumption, Autti-Rämö and colleagues (1992) did not identify any abnormalities of language or mental development in children exposed to heavy drinking only in the first trimester. Those exposed to heavy drinking throughout pregnancy, however, had significantly lower scores in these two areas. Prenatal alcohol exposure also increases the risk of pregnancy complications such as intraventricular hemorrhage and white-matter brain damage in preterm neonates (Holzman and colleagues 1995). Maternal age may contribute independently to increased fetal risk. Jacobson and co-workers (1998) have speculated that susceptibility may be the result of age-related increases in the body fat-to-water ratio and a faster rate of alcohol metabolism in older women.

Fetal alcohol syndrome cannot be diagnosed prenatally. Persutte and associates (1996) reported no correlation between alcohol use and ultrasonically detectable facial and intracranial biometrical measurements in 167 high-risk women compared with controls. While cardiac defects or cleft lip can be diagnosed sonographically, failure to identify major organ defects does not preclude other alcohol effects.

Despite the preceding data, even low levels of alcohol consumption cannot be recommended during pregnancy. Besides individual variation of "threshold dose," there are confounding effects of maternal age, other drug and environmental exposures, and pregnancy com-

plications. However, the data can be used to reassure women who have inadvertently exposed their fetuses to low levels of alcohol.

ANTICONVULSANT MEDICATIONS. It is well established that women with epilepsy have an increased risk of fetal malformations even without exposure to anticonvulsant medication (Yerby, 1997, 1993). In a review of over 750,000 pregnancies from 13 cohort studies, Kelly (1984) calculated a malformation rate of 70 per 1000 for infants of epileptic mothers compared with 30 per 1000 for controls. The most frequently reported defects, whether or not the mother takes medication, include orofacial clefts and congenital heart disease (Table 38–5). Clefts occur almost 10 times more frequently than in the general population (Yerby, 1997, 1993).

The association of minor facial anomalies with drug exposure was first reported by Meadow (1968). Most studies since then have supported that anticonvulsant

TABLE 38–5. Some Malformations Associated with Epilepsy and Anticonvulsant Drugs

Major Malformations	Minor Anomalies
Congenital heart defects	Mental subnormality
Oral–facial clefts	Hypertelorism
Neural-tube defects	Palmar creases
Microcephaly	Digital hypoplasia

From Cantrell and Cunningham (1994).

use is directly related to adverse fetal outcome, with risk increasing directly with the number of drugs. Malformations are more prevalent with high serum anticonvulsant concentrations, and polytherapy imposes a higher risk than monotherapy (Dansky and associates, 1980; Omtzigt and colleagues, 1992). A Japanese collaborative study reported that the rate of fetal malformations was 1.9 percent if the epileptic mother took no anticonvulsants during pregnancy, 5.5 percent if two drugs were taken, 11 percent if three were taken, and 23 percent if four were taken (Nakane and colleagues, 1980; Okuma and associates, 1980). Because the need for drug therapy, high serum levels, and multiple medications also reflect severity of maternal disease, it is possible that at least part of the increased risk is related to epilepsy itself.

PHENYTOIN. Hanson and Smith (1975) were the first to report that this commonly prescribed anticonvulsant caused craniofacial defects, limb abnormalities, and mental deficiency (Table 38–6 and Fig. 38–3). Hanson and colleagues (1976) estimated that 7 to 10 percent of exposed infants have sufficient features of this **fetal hydantoin syndrome** to be recognizable in infancy, while a third display minor craniofacial and digital anomalies. Kelly (1984) confirmed these estimates, and Scolnik and colleagues (1994) also described lower global intelligence quotient (IQ) scores in phenytoin-exposed children compared with controls. Teratogenicity is strongly influenced by the fetal genetic makeup, with inability to produce normal levels of epoxide hydrolase increasing risk as discussed earlier. This in part explains observations by Van Dyke and co-workers (1988) that some families include many exposed but normal offspring while other families include multiple affected children.

CARBAMAZEPINE. This commonly prescribed anticonvulsant was considered for years to be the drug of choice in pregnancy. Jones and co-workers (1989), however, subsequently described a significant excess of carbamazepine-exposed children with three or more of the minor malformations shown in Table 38–6, similar to the fetal hydantoin syndrome. These were primarily craniofacial defects (11 percent), fingernail hypoplasia (26 percent), and developmental delay (20 percent). This study was subsequently criticized because of methodological flaws, including the fact that a large proportion of the subjects were taking multiple medications and the proportion of children with developmental delay was not different than that expected based on the normal distribution of test scores (Bortnichak and Wetter, 1989; Keller, 1989; Scialli and Lione, 1989). Thus, the teratogenic potential of carbamazepine is unclear. Because it is metabolized through the arene oxide pathway, there is potential for accumulation of toxic intermediates and alteration of the phenotype in susceptible individuals with some enzyme deficiencies.

TRIMETHADIONE AND PARAMETHADIONE. These are used infrequently to treat petit mal seizures. A characteristic pattern of severe malformations including those in Table 38–6 was found to be associated with their use (German and associates, 1970; Zackai and co-workers, 1975). Because of their high potential for teratogenicity, they are avoided.

VALPROIC ACID. Fetuses exposed to this drug in the first trimester have a 1 to 2 percent—20 times background—risk of spina bifida (Robert and colleagues, 1983). Because these defects are located almost exclusively in the lumbosacral region, it is likely that this agent acts directly on a homeobox gene governing the development of caudal structures (see earlier discussion). Valproic acid has also been associated with several minor facial features (Clayton-Smith and Donnai, 1995).

TABLE 38–6. Some Aspects of Anticonvulsant Embryopathies

Hydantoin Syndrome	Carbamazepine Syndrome
Craniofacial abnormalities	Craniofacial abnormalities
Cleft lip/palate	Upslanting palpebral fissures
Broad nasal bridge	Short nose
Hypertelorism	Epicanthal folds
Epicanthal folds	Limb defects
Limb defects	Hypoplasia of distal phalanges, nails
Hypoplasia of distal phalanges, nails	Growth deficiency
Growth deficiency	Mental deficiency
Mental deficiency	

From Hanson and Smith (1975) and Jones and colleagues (1989).

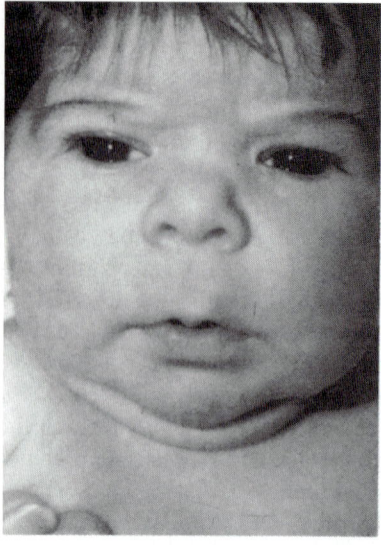
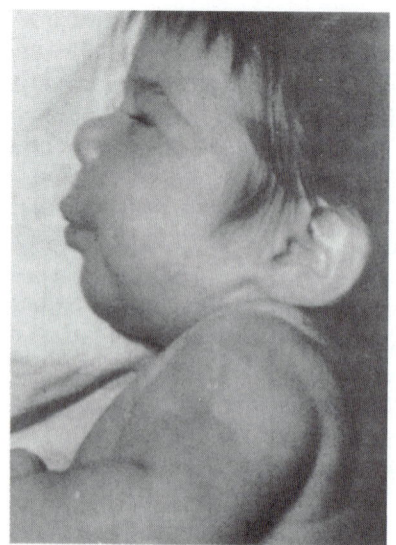
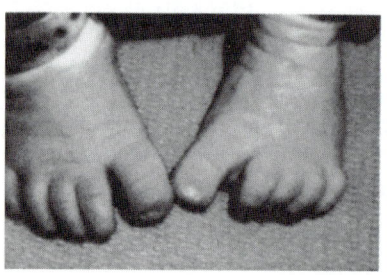
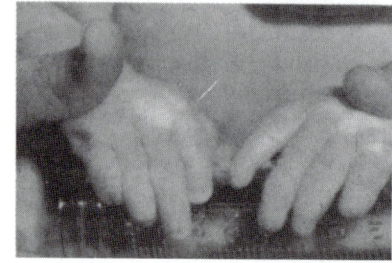

FIGURE 38–3. Fetal hydantoin syndrome. Upper facial features including upturned nose, mild midfacial hypoplasia, and long upper lip with thin vermilion border. Lower distal digital hypoplasia. (From Buehler and colleagues, 1990, with permission).

Reported cardiac malformations and oral clefts probably are related to the epilepsy itself (Lammer and colleagues, 1987).

WARFARIN COMPOUNDS. These drugs have a low molecular weight, readily cross the placenta, and can cause significant adverse teratogenic and fetal effects. Hall and co-workers (1980) estimated that a sixth of exposed pregnancies result in an abnormal live-born infant, and a sixth will result in abortion or stillbirth. Ginsberg and Hirsh (1989) reviewed 186 studies including 1325 exposed pregnancies and reported that 9 percent of exposed fetuses suffered permanent deformity or disability, and 17 percent of these died.

Distinct defects with two different etiologies result from exposure during two different developmental periods. If exposure occurs between the sixth and ninth week, the fetus is at increased risk for **warfarin embryopathy** characterized by nasal hypoplasia (Fig. 38–4) and stippled vertebral and femoral epiphyses. It is doubtful that this embryopathy results from fetal hemorrhage because vitamin K clotting factors are not demonstrable in the embryo at this age. Instead, these derivatives are thought to exert their teratogenic effect by inhibiting post-translational carboxylation of coagulation proteins (Hall and associates, 1980). These pro-

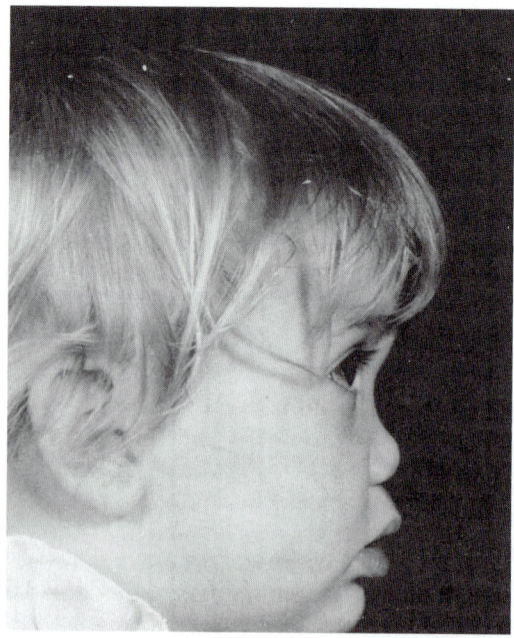

FIGURE 38–4. Warfarin embryopathy or fetal warfarin syndrome: nasal hypoplasia and depressed nasal bridge. (Photograph courtesy of Dr. Mary Jo Harrod.)

teins are called *osteocalcins* because of their role in embryonic control of calcification, and their deficiency could result in many features of warfarin embryopathy. The syndrome is a phenocopy of *chondrodysplasia punctata,* a group of genetic diseases thought to be caused by inherited defects in osteocalcin.

During the second and third trimester, the defects associated with fetal exposure to warfarin likely result from hemorrhage leading to subsequent dysharmonic growth and deformation from scarring in any of several organs (Warkany, 1976). Defects may be regionally extensive and include dorsal midline central nervous system dysplasia such as agenesis of the corpus callosum, Dandy–Walker malformation, and midline cerebellar atrophy; ventral midline dysplasia such as microphthalmia, optic atrophy, and blindness; and developmental delay and mental retardation (Hall and colleagues, 1980).

ANGIOTENSIN-CONVERTING ENZYME (ACE) INHIBITORS.

These antihypertensive agents have been associated with many reports of fetal damage. The most frequently associated agent is *enalapril,* although *captopril* and *lisinopril* have been implicated. No structural malformations from first-trimester exposure have been documented, although animals given doses comparable to those used in humans have an increased incidence of fetal wastage (fetotoxicity). Most commonly, there is late-onset growth restriction and oligohydramnios, followed by prolonged and profound neonatal hypotension and anuria. The most severe consequence is renal tubular dysgenesis, which causes early-onset oligohydramnios, pulmonary hypoplasia and limb contractures, and perinatal death (Table 38–7). Hypocalvaria—hypoplasia of the membranous skull bones—is strongly linked to ACE inhibitor exposure (Barr and Cohen, 1991). Relative limb shortening has also been described (Pryde and co-workers, 1993).

All of these abnormalities are believed to result from prolonged fetal hypotension and hypoperfusion that causes renal ischemia, renal tubular dysgenesis, and then anuria (Pryde and colleagues, 1993; Schubiger and associates, 1988). The resulting oligohydramnios prevents normal lung development and causes limb contractures. Reduced perfusion also causes growth restriction. Hypotension also explains maldevelopment of the calvar-

ium because it is formed from membranous bone which requires extensive vascularity and high oxygen tension for growth. Because these changes occur during the fetal period they are termed **ACE inhibitor fetopathy.** This is not a syndrome, but instead is a classical example of a *sequence* in which one initial insult leads to a cascade of other problems (Chap. 36, p. 940).

Not all fetuses are affected, and the lack of epidemiological data prevents estimation of risk. However, the variable fetal response may be due to genetic variation in the ACE gene. Individuals homozygous for a 50-bp deletion in this gene have high serum ACE activity, while those homozygous for an insertion of the same fragment have low activity (Lee, 1994; Rigat and associates, 1990). The relationship between ACE exposure and the fetal ACE gene has yet to be explored.

RETINOIDS. Retinoids, especially vitamin A, are essential for normal growth, tissue differentiation, reproduction, and vision (Gudas, 1994). As discussed earlier, retinoids are believed to activate four clusters of homeobox genes during embryogenesis (Soprano and Soprano, 1995). While vitamin A deficiency is a health problem worldwide, it is rare in the United States.

VITAMIN A. There are two forms of vitamin A in nature. **Beta-carotene** is a precursor of provitamin A. It is found in fruits and vegetables and has never been shown to cause birth defects (Oakley and Erickson, 1995). **Retinol** is preformed vitamin A. Many foods contain vitamin A, but only livers from animals raised in Europe and polar bear liver contain toxic doses. Levels found in animal liver available in markets in the United States are not dangerous (American College of Obstetricians and Gynecologists, 1998). Likewise, the 5000-IU dose of vitamin A contained in common prenatal vitamins is not harmful.

It is uncertain whether high doses of vitamin A are teratogenic. Several case reports and small series have associated high doses with congenital anomalies. These reports concern vitamin A supplements, and in general have been hampered by small numbers, unknown daily dose, and absence of any recognizable pattern in the small number of observed defects. Two cohort studies have also been inconclusive. Conway (1958) gave 12,500 IU of vitamin A daily prior to and through 3 months' gestation as an experimental therapy to prevent recurrence in 59 women who had a child with cleft lip or palate. They observed no defects. Rothman and co-workers (1995) evaluated outcomes of 317 women ingesting at least 10,000 IU of vitamin A daily during the first 12 weeks of pregnancy. Only 1 in 57 of these, the same incidence as in the general population, had a child with a congenital anomaly.

The largest prospective series evaluated a cohort of

TABLE 38–7. Adverse Fetal Effects Associated with Angiotensin-converting Enzyme Inhibitors

Oligohydramnios	Hypocalvaria
Renal anomalies	Growth restriction
Neonatal renal failure	Death
Pulmonary hypoplasia	

423 women who ingested from 10,000 to 300,000 IU of vitamin A daily during the first 9 weeks and who contacted one of 13 European Teratology Services (Mastroiacovo and associates, 1999). Only three children had birth defects, and there was no relationship between vitamin dose and outcome. Their conclusion supports the opinion that in developed countries there is no scientific basis for vitamin A supplementation and doses higher than the daily allowance should be avoided (American College of Obstetricians and Gynecologists, 1995).

ISOTRETINOIN. Some isomers display the biological activity of vitamin A, and because they stimulate epithelial cell differentiation, are used chiefly for dermatological disorders (Chap. 54, p. 1435). Isotretinoin is 13-*cis*-retinoic acid and is highly effective for treatment of cystic acne. It is also considered one of the most potent teratogens in common use. First-trimester exposure is associated with a high rate of fetal loss and malformations in survivors at a rate similar to that for thalidomide (Lammer and co-workers, 1985). Abnormalities have been described only with first-trimester use. Its mean serum half-life is 12 hours, and anomalies are not increased in women who discontinue therapy before conception (Dai and colleagues, 1989).

Malformations typically involve the cranium and face, heart, central nervous system, and thymus. The craniofacial malformation most strongly associated with isotretinoin is bilateral but often asymmetrical microtia or anotia, frequently with agenesis or stenoses of the external ear canal (Fig. 38–5). Other defects include maldevelopment of the facial bones and cranium, and

cleft palate. The most frequent cardiac defects are conotruncal, and hydrocephalus is the most common central nervous system defect. Thymic abnormalities include aplasia, hypoplasia, or malposition.

Dai and colleagues (1992) summarized 433 exposed pregnancies reported to the manufacturer. Elective abortion was chosen in half. Of the others exposed before 12 weeks, a third spontaneously aborted and a third had an infant with at least one major malformation. There did not appear to be any safe first-trimester exposure period or dose. The incidence was unaffected by the length of exposure, and a third of women who used the drug for less than 1 week had malformed infants.

Despite that isotretinoin has been listed as a category X drug since its introduction, and there have been at least three packaging changes to highlight reproductive risks, exposures continue to be reported. In the aforementioned report, almost 30 percent of women were pregnant when they started the drug, and 65 percent conceived while taking the drug because of improper contraceptive use. A pregnancy test before initiating the drug and a mistake-proof method of birth control such as Norplant are now required by many clinics prior to beginning therapy.

ETRETINATE. This orally administered retinoid is used to treat psoriasis. It is associated with severe anomalies similar to those with isotretinoin. In contrast to isotretinoin, however, anomalies are observed even when conception is after discontinuation of therapy. Etretinate is lipophilic and has a half-life of 120 days. It has been detected in serum almost 3 years after cessation of ther-

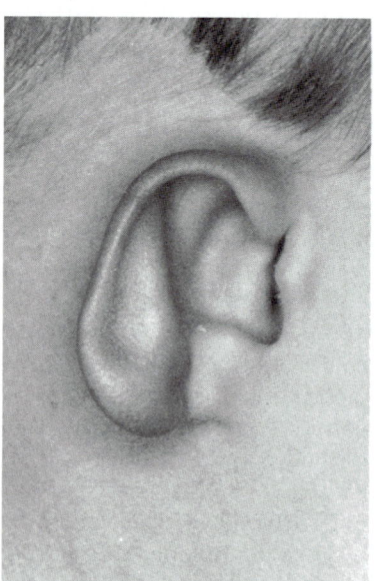
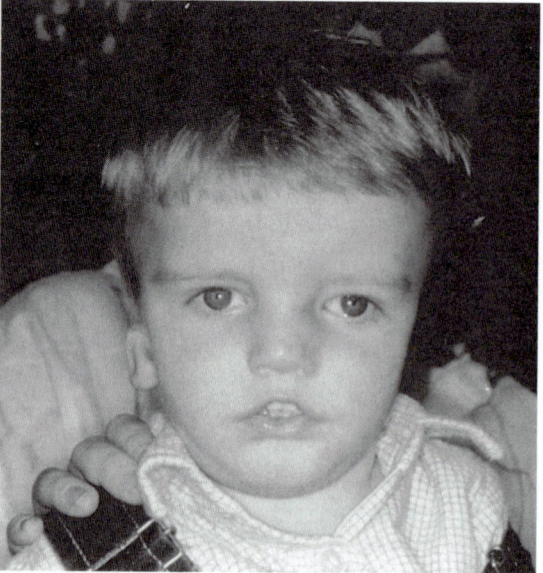

FIGURE 38–5. Isotretinoin embryopathy. Left: bilateral microtia or anotia with stenosis of external ear canal. Right: flat depressed nasal bridge and ocular hypertelorism. (Photograph courtesy of Dr. Edward Lammer.)

apy (DiGiovanna and colleagues, 1984; Thomson and Cordero, 1989). It is unknown how long the teratogenic effects persist, but malformations have been described up to 51 weeks after its discontinuation (Lammer, 1988). If possible, women who have not completed their child bearing should not use this drug. If etretinate use cannot be avoided, Geiger and associates (1994) suggest that the woman wait at least 2 years after treatment before conceiving.

TRETINOIN. This is all-*trans*-retinoic acid and is prescribed for treatment of acne vulgaris. It is available only as a topical gel. The skin metabolizes most of the drug without apparent absorption. Jick and colleagues (1993) found no increase in congenital anomalies in 212 infants born to women who used tretinoin during early pregnancy.

HORMONES. The primordial structures that will become the external genitalia are bipotential for the first 9 weeks (Chap. 7, p. 157). Between 9 and 14 weeks, the testis secretes androgen and the male fetus develops a male perineal phenotype. Because the ovaries do not secrete androgens, the female fetus continues to develop a female phenotype which is completed by 20 weeks (Speroff and colleagues, 1994). Exposure to exogenous sex hormones before 7 completed weeks generally has no effect on external structures. Between 7 and 12 weeks, however, female genital tissue is very responsive to exogenous androgens and exposure can result in full masculinization. The tissue continues to exhibit some response until 20 weeks, and up to then partial masculinization or genital ambiguity can develop.

Those areas of the brain with high concentrations of estrogen and androgen receptors are also influenced by hormone exposure, which programs the central nervous system for gender identity, sexual behavior, levels of aggression and gender-specific play behaviors. The critical period for hormonal influence on behavior is much later that that for the external genitalia, with the degree of behavioral alteration proportional to dose and length of exposure.

ANDROGENS. An example of the effects of early androgen exposure is autosomal recessive *congenital adrenal hyperplasia.* Fetal adrenal glands ordinarily begin functioning by 12 weeks, but because of certain enzyme deficiencies, the glands are unable to hydroxylate cortisol precursors. Androgenic intermediates accumulate, masculinizing female external genitalia and producing abnormal male genital growth (Chrousos and associates, 1985). Early androgen exposure may also result in a more masculine orientation with stronger homosexual and/or weaker heterosexual interests, as well as increased male gender identity (Dittman and co-workers,

1990, 1992; Meyer-Bahlburg and collaborators, 1996; Zucker and associates, 1996). Maternal exposure to androgens can induce similar fetal effects; however, in contrast to congenital adrenal hyperplasia, masculinization does not progress after birth (Stevenson, 1993b).

TESTOSTERONE AND ANABOLIC STEROIDS. Androgen exposure in reproductive-age women occurs primarily as the result of anabolic steroid use by athletes wishing to increase lean body mass and muscular strength. The most effective agents are synthetic testosterones, which are taken in doses 10 to 40 times higher than those used therapeutically. These cause extreme and irreversible virilization, liver dysfunction, and mood and libido disorders in women. Exposure of a female fetus results in varying degrees of virilization, including labioscrotal fusion after first-trimester exposure and phallic enlargement later (Grumbach and Ducharme, 1960; Schardein, 1985). Normal female maturation can be anticipated at puberty, although surgical correction may be necessary for genital defects.

ANDROGENIC PROGESTINS. These agents are currently used as contraceptives. Antenatal exposure to *medroxyprogesterone acetate,* an intramuscular depot contraceptive, has been associated with virilization of the female fetus and a small increase in heart defects (Barlow and Knight, 1983; Prahalada and associates, 1985). *Norethindrone,* a progesterone-only contraceptive, is estimated to cause female fetus masculinization in 1 percent of exposures (Schardein, 1985).

DANOCRINE. This ethinyltestosterone derivative has weak androgenic activity that inhibits the pituitary–ovarian axis. It is primarily prescribed for endometriosis but is also used to treat immune thrombocytopenic purpura, migraine headaches, premenstrual syndrome, and some breast diseases. In a review of its inadvertant use during early pregnancy, Brunskill (1992) reported that 40 percent of 57 exposed female fetuses were virilized. There was a dose-related pattern of clitoromegaly, fused labia, and urogenital sinus malformation, most of which required surgical correction.

ESTROGENS. Of many compounds, most estrogenic substances do not affect fetal development. Oral contraceptives are discussed on page 1029.

DIETHYLSTILBESTROL (DES). From 1940 to 1971, between 2 and 10 million pregnant women took DES to "support" high-risk pregnancies (Giusti and co-workers, 1995; Smith, 1948). The drug later was shown to have no salutary effects, and its use for this purpose was abandoned. Herbst and colleagues (1971) subsequently presented their classical study showing that vaginal adenocarcinoma developed between ages 15 and 22 in eight prenatally exposed women. These observations were subsequently confirmed. Moreover, when ingested before 18 weeks, the drug affects normal development of both female and male reproductive structures. DES is thus a carcinogen and teratogen.

The most striking associated malignancy is clear-cell adenocarcinoma of the cervix and/or vagina (Herbst and Anderson, 1990). The absolute risk is substantially increased to about 1 per 1000 DES-exposed daughters. The Registry for Research on Hormonal Transplacental Carcinogenesis reported that half of 384 cancer patients were exposed before 12 weeks and 70 percent before 17 weeks (Melnick and colleagues, 1987). Malignancy was not dose related and there was no relationship between location of the tumor and timing of exposure. For these reasons and because its absolute risk is low, some categorize DES as an *incomplete carcinogen*.

DES produces both structural and functional abnormalities (Salle and colleagues, 1996). One is interruption of normal vaginal development. By 18 weeks, the müllerian-derived cuboidal-columnar epithelium lining the vagina should be replaced by squamous epithelium originating from the urogenital sinus. DES interrupts this transition in up to half of exposed female fetuses, resulting in excess cervical eversion (ectropion) and ectopic vaginal glandular epithelium (adenosis). The Diethylstilbestrol Adenosis (DESAD) Project showed that these lesions have malignant potential, as DES-exposed women have a twofold increase in vaginal and cervical intraepithelial neoplasia (Vessey, 1989).

There are structural abnormalities of the cervix or vagina in a fourth of exposed females (Robboy and associates, 1984). As many as two thirds have uterine abnormalities and their embryological mechanism is unknown (Kaufman and co-workers, 1980). The most commonly reported abnormalities include hypoplastic T-shaped uterine cavity; cervical collars, hoods, septa, and coxcombs; and "withered" fallopian tubes (Falcone, 1999). As discussed in Chapter 35 (p. 918), these exposed women are at increased risk for poor pregnancy outcomes related to the uterine malformation, decreased endometrial thickness, and reduced uterine perfusion (Kaufman and colleagues, 2000). Exposed men have normal sexual function and fertility, but are at increased risk for epididymal cysts, microphallus, cryptorchidism, and testicular hypoplasia (Stillman, 1982).

ANTINEOPLASTIC DRUGS. By their mechanisms of action, many anticancer drugs intuitively would be thought to be teratogenic or carcinogenic. Fortunately, this is not the case for most, as discussed in Chapter 55. There are notable exceptions, as follows.

CYCLOPHOSPHAMIDE. This alkylating agent inflicts a chemical insult on developing fetal tissues, resulting in cell death and heritable DNA alterations in surviving cells. Fetal anomalies have been described after exposure during early pregnancy. The most commonly reported are missing and hypoplastic digits on hands and feet. These defects are believed to be caused by necrosis of limb buds and DNA damage in surviving cells (Manson and associates, 1982). Other defects include cleft palate, single coronary artery, imperforate anus, and fetal growth restriction with microcephaly (Kirshon and colleagues, 1988). It has been reported that nurses who administer cyclophosphamide may be at increased risk for fetal loss, but the data are hard to interpret and there are no adequate epidemiological studies (Glantz, 1994). Alkylating agents should be avoided during early pregnancy if possible, but can be given during the second and third trimester.

METHOTREXATE/AMINOPTERIN. Closely related, both are associated with a rare but strikingly similar pattern of anomalies. Teratogenic potential is from alteration of folic acid metabolism essential for cell replication (Sutton and co-workers, 1998). Methotrexate is commonly prescribed as an abortifacient, for ectopic pregnancy, and for psoriasis and some connective-tissue diseases. Principal features of fetal methotrexate/aminopterin syndrome are growth restriction, failure of calvarial ossification, craniosynostosis, hypoplastic supraorbital ridges, small posteriorly rotated ears, micrognathia, and severe limb abnormalities (Del Campo and associates, 1999). Feldcamp and Carey (1993) reviewed 20 first-trimester exposures and calculated that a dose of 10 mg per week is necessary to produce abnormalities. This dose is exceeded during standard therapy for ectopic pregnancy or elective abortion. Ongoing pregnancies after methotrexate treatment require immediate follow-up (Creinin and Vittinghoff, 1994).

ANTIMICROBIALS

TETRACYCLINES. These drugs, including doxycycline and minocycline, may cause yellow-brown discoloration of deciduous teeth or be deposited in fetal long bones (Kutscher and associates, 1966). Tetracycline causes acute fatty liver changes in pregnant women with renal insufficiency (Whalley and colleagues, 1964). One acceptable use is treatment of maternal syphilis in penicillin-allergic women for whom desensitization is impractical (Chap. 57, p. 1489).

AMINOGLYCOSIDES. Maternal administration results in significant fetal blood levels (Gilstrap and co-workers, 1988). *Streptomycin* is associated with fetal cranial nerve VIII damage when given for protracted periods (Conway and Birt, 1965). The risk of ototoxicity with any aminoglycoside is approximately 1 to 2 percent.

SULFONAMIDES. While these agents readily cross the placenta, fetal blood levels are lower than maternal levels. These drugs compete for bilirubin-binding sites, and may be associated with hyperbilirubinemia if used near delivery in the preterm infant (Landers and colleagues, 1983). There have been no studies exploring a possible association of sulfa drugs with congenital anomalies. *Trimethoprim* is used in conjunction with a sulfonamide, and because it is a folate antagonist, some authors caution against its use; however, congenital anomalies are not reportedly increased (Brumfitt and Pursell, 1973).

GRISEOFULVIN. This oral fungicide is used for treatment of mycotic infections of the skin, nails, and scalp. There is one report of possible association with conjoined twins (Rosa and associates, 1987a, 1987b). Animal studies indicate increased anomalies of the central nervous system and skeleton.

RIBAVIRIN. This antiviral is given by aerosol inhalation to treat respiratory syncytial virus infections in infants and young children. Pregnant women may be exposed to the drug while working in intensive care nurseries. Based on animal studies, the drug has significant teratogenic potential. It consistently produces hydrocephalus and limb abnormalities in rodent models.

TOBACCO. Cigarette smoke contains a number of potential teratogens, including nicotine, continine, cyanide, thiocyanate, carbon monoxide, cadmium, lead, and a variety of hydrocarbons. In addition to being fetotoxic, many of these substances have vasoactive effects or reduce oxygen levels. The best documented reproductive outcome related to smoking is fetal growth restriction. Smoking has a direct dose-response effect on fetal growth. Infants of mothers who smoke are on average 200 g lighter than those of nonsmokers, and heavy smoking results in more severe weight reduction (D'Souza and associates, 1981). The risk of low birthweight is doubled, and that of a small-for-gestational age infant is increased 2.5-fold (Werler, 1997). Women who stop smoking early in pregnancy generally have infants with normal birthweights (Cliver and co-workers, 1995). Smoking also may cause slightly increased incidence of subfertility, spontaneous abortion, placenta previa and abruption, and preterm delivery (Werler, 1997).

While it is plausible that vasoactive properties of smoking would produce defects related to vascular disturbances, most studies indicate no increased risk of congenital malformations involving the cardiac or central nervous systems, or of gastroschisis. A twofold increased risk of Poland sequence—caused by an interruption in the vascular supply to the chest and arm—was reported by Martinez-Frias and colleagues (1999). Smoking has been associated with cleft lip and palate, but only in individuals heterozygous or homozygous for an uncommon polymorphism in the gene for transforming growth factor-α (Shaw and colleagues, 1996). In individuals carrying this allele, the risk of cleft lip and palate is doubled and the risk of cleft palate is increased four- to sevenfold (Hwang and associates, 1995; Shaw and co-workers, 1996).

COCAINE. This alkaloid is derived from the leaves of the South American tree, *Erythroxylon coca.* It is a highly effective topical anesthetic and local vasoconstrictor, and through sympathomimetic action via dopamine, it is also a central nervous system stimulant. Cocaine is currently one of the most widely abused drugs in the United States. In a 1994 Georgia study, the Centers for Disease Control and Prevention (1996) determined that 1 in 20 pregnancies was associated with cocaine use. A population-based study of over 29,000 racially and socioeconomically diverse obstetrical patients from 202 California hospitals found that 1.1 percent had a positive urine test for cocaine (Vega and colleagues, 1993).

Many adverse outcomes associated with cocaine are from its vasoconstrictive and hypertensive effects. Although an impressive number of adverse sequelae have been reported, placental abruption is the most frequently cited (Chasnoff and colleagues, 1985). In their review, Shiono and colleagues (1995) found that cocaine use was associated with a fourfold increase in placental abruption. Cocaine use has been associated with myocardial infarction, arrhythmias, aortic rupture, strokes, seizures, bowel ischemia, hyperthermia, and sudden death.

Risk of vascular disruption within the embryo, fetus, or placenta is highest after the first trimester, and likely accounts for the increased incidence of stillbirth (Hoyme and associates, 1990). A number of cocaine-related congenital anomalies due to vascular-based disruptions have been described. They include skull defects, cutis aplasia, porencephaly, ileal atresia, cardiac anomalies, and visceral infarcts (Little and colleagues, 1989b; Stevenson, 1993a). Cohen and associates (1994b) have identified subependymal and periventricular cysts in term infants. One mechanism by which brain defects may develop after cocaine exposure is shown in Figure 38–6.

Reports of increased limb-reduction defects are disputed (Hume and co-workers, 1997). However, cocaine is especially likely to disrupt urinary tract development separate from genital organ development. Chavez and colleagues (1988) utilized the population-based Atlanta Birth Defects Case-Control Study and concluded that

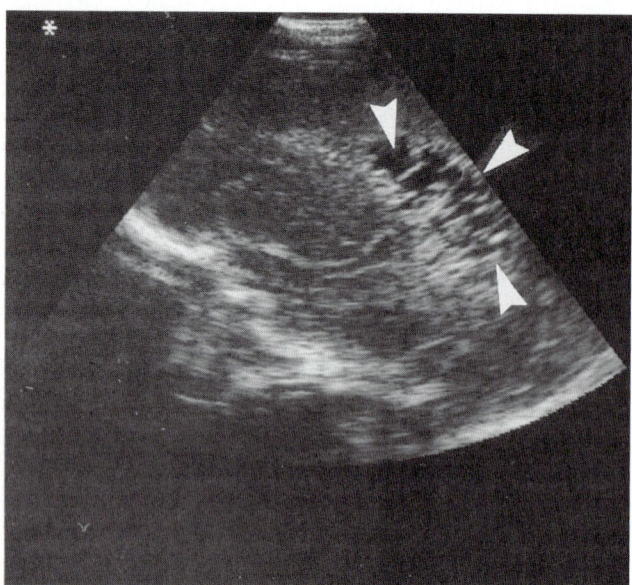

FIGURE 38–6. Cocaine-induced brain infarction causing periventricular leukomalacia. Arrows indicate large area of multilocular cavitation that was posterior and lateral to lateral ventricles. (Sonogram courtesy of Dr. Jeff Perlman.)

cocaine use increased the risk of urinary tract defects by 4.39. Finally, prune-belly anomaly has been reported (Bingol and co-workers, 1986; Chasnoff and colleagues, 1985, 1988).

THALIDOMIDE. This is an anxiolytic and sedative drug that is a notorious human teratogen. It produces malformations in approximately 20 percent of exposed pregnancies, primarily limited to structures derived from the mesodermal layer such as limbs, ears, cardiovascular system, and bowel musculature. A wide variety of limb-reduction defects have been associated with thalidomide, with upper limbs usually more severely affected. Bone defects range from abnormal shape or size to total absence of a bone or limb segment.

Thalidomide was available from 1956 to 1960 before its teratogenicity, along with several teratological principles, were forcefully demonstrated. Prior to this, the placenta was believed to be a perfect barrier that was impervious to toxic substances unless given in such high doses that the mother was killed (Dally, 1998). The extreme variability in species susceptibility to drugs and chemicals also was not appreciated. Thalidomide produced no defects in experimental mice and rats and thus was assumed safe in humans. The thalidomide experience also demonstrated the very close relationship between time of exposure and the presence and type of defect produced (Knapp and co-workers, 1962). For example, upper limb phocomelia occurred after ingestion during days 27 to 30, coincidental with appearance of the upper limb buds at 27 days. Lower limb phocome-

lia was associated with treatment during days 30 to 33 at the time of lower limb bud development.

Recently, thalidomide has again become available in the United States. It is used for refractory cutaneous lupus erythematosus, chronic graft-versus-host disease with bone marrow transplantation, and for treatment of leprosy (Cole and colleagues, 1994; Duna and Cash, 1995). Reproductive-age women taking thalidomide need excellent birth control, as thalidomide-affected children continue to be born in countries where the drug is available, and despite ample warnings (Castilla and co-investigators, 1996).

DRUGS COMMONLY USED IN PREGNANCY

INFECTIONS. A number of bacterial, viral, fungal, and parasitic infections are commonly encountered during pregnancy. Some of the agents used to treat them are listed in Table 38–8. Virtually all antimicrobial and chemotherapeutic medications readily cross the placenta.

ANTIBACTERIAL AGENTS. As a group, **penicillins** are probably the safest antimicrobial to use during pregnancy. They include agents with broad-spectrum activity such as piperacillin and mezlocillin, as well as those combined with the β-lactamase inhibitors, clavulanic acid, sulbactam, and tazobactam.

Erythromycin is a macrolide often given to penicillin-allergic patients, especially for community-acquired pneumonia (Chap. 46, p. 1225). The fetus is not always treated effectively when erythromycin is given for maternal syphilis because only small amounts of the drug gain fetal access (Chap. 57, p. 1489). **Azithromycin** has proven efficacy for treatment of community-acquired pneumonias and for treatment of chlamydial cervicitis. It is listed as a category B drug.

There are numerous oral and parenteral **cephalosporins.** When given during pregnancy, all cross the placenta, although their half-life is likely shorter during pregnancy because of increased renal clearance (Gilstrap and colleagues, 1988). Limited data suggest no adverse embryo-fetal effects and as a group they are listed in category B.

Aztreonam is a monobactam used primarily as an aminoglycoside alternative. It is not associated with either renal or ototoxicity, and although there are no well-controlled human studies, it is not teratogenic for rodents.

Imipenem is a carbapenem that is effective against aerobic and anaerobic organisms commonly isolated from intra-abdominal and female pelvic infections. Although there are no available human data regarding its safety during pregnancy, there are few specific indications for its use.

TABLE 38–8. Classification of Some Antimicrobial Agents Commonly Used in Pregnancy

Agent	FDA Category[a]
Antibacterials	
Aminoglycosides	C/D
Azithromycin	B
Aztreonam	C
Cephalosporins	B
Chloroquine	C
Erythromycin	B
Fluoroquinolones	C
Imipenem	C
Metronidazole	B
Nitrofurantoin	B
Penicillins	B
Quinolones	C
Rifabutin	B
Sulfonamides	B
Tetracyclines	D
Trimethoprim	C
Vancomycin	C
Antivirals	
Acyclovir	C
Didanosine (ddl)	B
Ganciclovir	C
Stavudine (d4T)	C
Zalcitabine (ddC)	C
Zidovudine	C
Antiprotozoals	
Lindane	B
Mebendazole	C
Pyrantel	C
Quinine	D
Antifungals	
Amphotericin	B
Fluconazole	C
Itraconazole	C
Miconazole	C
Nystatin	B

[a] Classification from manufacturers' guidelines.

Clindamycin readily crosses the placenta and may result in significant fetal blood levels (Gilstrap and associates, 1988). There have been no studies of potential adverse embryo-fetal effects from its use during pregnancy, although clinical experience suggests that this drug is relatively safe.

Chloramphenicol readily crosses the placenta and results in significant fetal blood levels. In almost 100 infants exposed to this antimicrobial in early pregnancy, congenital anomalies were not increased (Heinonen and associates, 1977). The *gray baby syndrome,* manifested by cyanosis, vascular collapse, and death, has been reported with large doses of chloramphenicol given to the preterm neonate. It seems unlikely that fetal levels obtained from maternal administration would cause this syndrome.

Nitrofurantoin is commonly used for urinary infections during pregnancy. In a prospective study of 100 women treated with this drug, congenital anomalies were not increased (Lenke and colleagues, 1983). Nitrofurantoin has been associated with hemolytic anemia in women with glucose-6-phosphate dehydrogenase deficiency. In our experiences with more than 20,000 pregnant women given this drug for asymptomatic bacteriuria, hemolytic anemia has not been observed in either the mother or the fetus.

Vancomycin is used primarily for bacterial endocarditis prophylaxis in penicillin-allergic patients or as the drug of choice for *Clostridium difficile* pseudomembranous colitis. While there are no available human reproductive studies, vancomycin is associated with maternal nephrotoxicity and ototoxicity, and theoretically could cause these in the embryo or fetus (Hermans and Wilhelm, 1987).

Quinolones—ciprofloxacin, norfloxacin, ofloxacin, and enoxacin—are especially useful for treatment of urinary infections. Although there are no well-controlled studies in pregnant women, Berkovitch and colleagues (1994) observed no congenital anomalies among 10 fetuses exposed to ciprofloxacin. No teratogenic effects have been demonstrated in animal studies. Fluoroquinolones are reported by their manufacturer to be associated with irreversible arthropathy in immature dogs and are not recommended during pregnancy except for resistant infections.

Commonly used tuberculostatic drugs include **rifampicin, isoniazid,** and **ethambutol** (Chap. 46, p. 1241). Snyder and co-workers (1980) reviewed studies of several hundred pregnant women given these drugs, and reported no increase in congenital anomalies. **Rifabutin,** a category C drug, is used to treat *Mycobacterium avium complex* (*MAC*) disease in patients with human immunodeficiency infection.

ANTIFUNGAL AGENTS. Vaginal candidiasis is common during pregnancy. Three commonly used agents for its treatment are **clotrimazole, miconazole,** and **nystatin.** In one report there was no increase in congenital malformations reported with their use (Rosa and associates, 1987b). **Fluconazole** and **itraconazole** are category C antifungal agents commonly used in immunocompromised patients. There are no human studies of **butoconazole** use during early pregnancy; however, it is not teratogenic in rodents.

Amphotericin B is used primarily to treat systemic histoplasmosis, coccidioidomycosis, cryptococcosis, and candidiasis. In more than 30 fetuses exposed to this agent, there was no evidence for congenital anomalies (Dean and associates, 1994).

ANTIVIRAL AGENTS. Experience with use of antiviral medications during pregnancy is limited. There is ample reason for concern because they inhibit host–intracellular viral replication through their action on RNA or DNA substrates. A great deal of emphasis has been placed on these agents in light of the epidemic of human immunodeficiency virus (HIV) infection that began in the 1980s.

Zidovudine, previously called azidothymidine or AZT, is a thymidine analog that decreases DNA synthesis by reverse transcriptase inhibition. It is used specifically to treat HIV infections. It has been given to delay the onset of clinical disease in asymptomatic seropositive persons and prophylactically following accidental HIV exposure. Transplacental passage of the drug has been documented (Pons and colleagues, 1991). In 1994, the Centers for Disease Control reported data from the Zidovudine in Pregnancy Registry which was established in 1989 by the Glaxo Wellcome Company as discussed in Chapter 57 (p. 1501), and later renamed the Antiretroviral Pregnancy Registry (1996). Both registers indicate that birth defects are not increased with first-trimester zidovudine exposure (Briggs and colleagues, 1998).

Zalcitabine (ddC), **didanosine** (ddI), **stavudine** (d4T), and **lamivudine** (3TC) are similar to zidovudine. They are nucleoside analogs that inhibit reverse transcriptase. These nucleoside analogs are combined with protease inhibitors and given along with zidovudine because combination therapy dramatically lowers viral titers and reverses HIV-related complications. Although currently recommended for use in pregnant women, their efficacy in preventing vertical transmission is unknown (Public Health Service Task Force, 2000). While there is limited information of use during pregnancy, reports from the manufacturers indicate that these agents do not cause malformations in animals, and there are no reports of associated defects in human fetuses (Antiretroviral Pregnancy Registry, 1996; Briggs and colleagues, 1998).

Acyclovir and **ganciclovir** are purine nucleoside analogs that are effective for treating primary herpes and possibly varicella infections. Both drugs are category B. The Acyclovir Pregnancy Registry (1998) reported the outcome of 739 pregnancies in which this agent was given during the first trimester. There were nine infants

with anomalies but with no distinctive pattern. Topical administration of acyclovir results in minimal systemic absorption. There is limited information on ganciclovir, with only 25 first-trimester exposures reported by the Valacyclovir Pregnancy Registry (1998).

Amantadine is used to prevent or modify influenza infections (Chap. 46, p. 1227). This drug has not been studied in human pregnancy, but it is embryotoxic and teratogenic in animals in high doses. Experience with 51 pregnancies in which amantadine was given during the first trimester resulted in five major anomalies (Briggs and colleagues, 1998).

Oseltamivir, a viral neuraminidase inhibitor, is used to treat influenza (Chap. 56, p. 1464). No data on safety in humans is available. In animals, doses producing blood levels 50 to 100 times higher than achieved therapeutically caused maternal toxicity and minor skeletal malformations (Reprotox, 2000e).

Interferons are a family of proteins and glycoproteins with antiviral, antineoplastic, and immunomodulating actions. Interferon-α is approved for treating hairy cell leukemia, and it is effective for some viral infections. Interferons β1b and γ1b are also used therapeutically. Animal studies indicate that interferons have a very low potential for toxicity. Experience in pregnant women is very limited but it appears safe (Briggs and associates, 1998).

Idoxuridine is effective against adenovirus, cytomegalovirus, varicella, and vaccinia viral infections. **Trifluridine** is effective in treating herpes virus infections, and **vidarabine** is effective against herpesvirus and poxvirus infections. **Idoxuridine** has not been investigated in human pregnancy, and may have the same potential for damage as other cytotoxic drugs such as trifluridine and vidarabine, which were developed originally as antineoplastics.

ANTIPARASITIC AGENTS. Parasitic infections during pregnancy are quite common, are usually asymptomatic, and in general do not need to be treated until after delivery. **Metronidazole** is a nitroimidazole that is effective for treatment of vaginal trichomoniasis and bacterial vaginosis. Although carcinogenic in rodents and mutagenic in certain bacteria, there was no increase in congenital anomalies in over 1700 fetuses exposed to metronidazole during the first trimester (Piper and associates, 1993; Rosa and colleagues, 1987a). In a meta-analysis of seven studies, Burtin and colleagues (1995) found no association with increased teratogenic risk. It is classified as category B and is recommended by the Centers for Disease Control and Prevention (1998) for treatment of trichomoniasis in pregnancy (Chap. 57, p. 1506).

Lindane, used topically for the treatment of pediculosis pubis and scabies, was not teratogenic for a variety of animals. In adults, a significant amount of lindane is absorbed systemically, but rarely it causes central nervous system toxicity (Orkin and Maibach, 1983). Because of this, some recommend a combination of **pyrethrins** and **piperonyl butoxide** as initial treatment of pediculosis pubis during pregnancy, with lindane reserved for resistant infections. Crotamiton in 10 percent lotion or cream or 6 percent sulfur in petrolatum can also be used as first-line treatment for scabies during pregnancy.

Chloroquine is a valuable first-line antimalarial. There was no increase in congenital anomalies in over 150 offspring of mothers who received this drug during pregnancy (Wolfe and Cordero, 1985). It is also used at much lower doses for chemoprophylaxis against malaria in pregnant women who must travel to or live in countries in which malaria is endemic. **Mefloquine** has been used more recently for chloroquine-resistant falciparum malaria. Accumulated evidence supports its safety (Briggs and colleagues, 1998). **Quinine** and **quinidine** are reserved for severely ill women with chloroquine-resistant malaria. Malformations primarily involving the central nervous system, hearing, limb, and urogenital structures were reported during the 1930s when large doses of quinine were used to induce abortion. Defects have not been reported at therapeutic doses. It should be avoided if possible during pregnancy, but should not be withheld from severely ill women because of fetal concerns.

Pyrimethamine is an antiparasitic folic acid antagonist used to treat malaria and toxoplasmosis. Hengst (1972) reported no increased frequency of malformations in 64 newborns exposed in early pregnancy. **Spiramycin** has been used to treat toxoplasmosis; there is no evidence of adverse embryo-fetal effects. Sulfadiazine plus pyrimethamine also has been used for toxoplasmosis. The efficacy of all of these agents for either the prevention or amelioration of embryo-fetal effects of toxoplasmosis is uncertain. Despite therapy, newborns may have chorioretinitis, hydrocephalus, and intracranial calcifications (Chap. 56, p. 1476).

Mebendazole is effective for treatment of a variety of helminths, including enterobiasis (pinworm), trichuriasis (whipworm), ascariasis (roundworm), and uncinariasis (hookworm). It is teratogenic for animals given several times the human adult dose. In a number of studies, there did not appear to be increased teratogenic risks (Briggs and co-workers, 1998). **Thiabendazole** is a similar antihelmintic used primarily to treat strongyloidiasis, trichinosis, and cutaneous larval migrans. It is also used as second-line therapy to treat pinworm, whipworm, roundworm, and hookworm infections. It has not been reported to be teratogenic for animals, but there are no adequate human studies. **Pyrantel pomoate** is primarily used for the treatment of ascariasis and en-

TABLE 38–9. Classification of Some Cardiovascular Drugs Commonly Used in Pregnancy

	FDA Category[a]
ACE inhibitors	C/D
Adenosine	C
Amiodarone	D
β-blockers	C
Calcium antagonists	C
Coumarins	D
Digoxin	C
Furosemide	C
Heparin (conventional)	C
Heparin (low molecular weight)	B
Local anesthetic antiarrhythmics	B/C
Methyldopa	C
Quinidine	C
Streptokinase	C
Thiazides	D
Urokinase	B

ACE = angiotensin-converting enzyme.
[a] Classification from manufacturers' guidelines.

terobiasis. It has not been reported as teratogenic for animals, and there are no human studies.

CARDIOVASCULAR DISEASES. Almost 1 percent of pregnant women have some form of heart disease. They are often given a myriad of drugs and medications, the majority of which are safe during pregnancy (Table 38–9).

HEART FAILURE AND ARRHYTHMIAS. Cardiac glycosides are prescribed for heart failure, atrial fibrillation or flutter, and other supraventricular tachycardias. **Digoxin** is the most commonly used preparation, and although it rapidly crosses the placenta, there is no convincing evidence that it causes adverse fetal effects. Antiarrhythmic drugs have been administered both maternally and directly to the fetus in attempts to control fetal tachycardias (Harrigan and associates, 1981; Kerenyi and colleagues, 1980; Weiner and Thompson, 1988). This is discussed in Chapter 37 (p. 994).

Quinidine, discussed earlier for malaria treatment, is commonly used to treat supraventricular tachycardias and some ventricular arrhythmias. The drug readily crosses the placenta, and has been given to the mother to treat fetal supraventricular tachycardias (Killeen and Bowers, 1987). There are no epidemiological studies of congenital anomalies following its use during the first trimester, but it is relatively safe during later pregnancy (Rotmensch and colleagues, 1987).

A number of β-**adrenergic blocking** drugs are used to treat supraventricular and ventricular tachycardias, as well as chronic hypertension and hyperthyroidism. Propranolol has been used widely in pregnancy now for several decades and is not teratogenic (Briggs and associates, 1998). Earlier it was associated with fetal growth restriction; however, in a review of five prospective studies, such complications were identified in only 4 percent of pregnancies (Rotmensch and colleagues, 1983). Other β-blockers may be associated with fetal growth restriction (Chap. 45, p. 1216).

Some **antiarrhythmic drugs** include disopyramide, amiodarone, adenosine, bretylium, diltiazem, local anesthetics (procainamide, lidocaine, and tocainide), and calcium antagonists (nifedipine and verapamil). All cross the placenta, and many have been used to treat fetal arrhythmias without adverse effects (Dumesic and colleagues, 1982; Rey and associates, 1985). Amiodarone is structurally similar to thyroxine but readily crosses the placenta at levels 10 to 30 percent of maternal serum levels. Fetal and neonatal hypothyroidism after exposure has been reported (De Catte and co-workers, 1994; Grosso and colleagues, 1998). Although most exposed fetuses have no drug-related abnormalities, amiodarone use in pregnancy should be avoided.

ANTIHYPERTENSIVE DRUGS. Undoubtedly **methyldopa** is the most widely used of these agents during pregnancy for the treatment of chronic hypertension (Chap. 45, p. 1217). There are no large epidemiological studies in early pregnancy, but its many years of use attest to its safety. **Hydralazine** is commonly utilized to treat hypertension in women in the latter half of pregnancy without apparent adverse fetal effects. There are no human reproduction studies of **sodium nitroprusside;** however, this drug readily crosses the placenta (Lewis and colleagues, 1977). Theoretically its use may result in the accumulation of cyanide in fetal liver. **Clonidine** is an α-adrenergic blocker that has been used to treat hypertension in pregnant women without apparent adverse fetal effects (Horvath and co-workers, 1985).

A number of β-**adrenergic blocking agents** are used primarily for the treatment of chronic hypertension. These include propranolol, labetalol, atenolol, metoprolol, nadolol, and timolol. Several are also useful for the chronic treatment of angina pectoris, certain cardiac arrhythmias, and for treatment of hyperthyroidism. There is little information regarding their use in early gestation; however, increasing numbers of reports indicate no apparent adverse effects in pregnant women in the United Kingdom. In two studies, Sibai and associates (1987, 1990) reported that infants of women given labetalol were more likely to be growth restricted than those born to chronically hypertensive women not given the drug (Chap. 45, p. 1218). There are now a number of studies that have not found an association with growth restriction, bradycardia, or neonatal hypoglycemia, and some have reported a beneficial effect of labetalol on birthweight (Reprotox, 2000c).

Calcium-channel antagonists are also commonly used to treat chronic hypertension. **Verapamil** is used to treat hypertension, angina, and supraventricular tachycardias. Although it is commonly employed to treat hypertension in pregnant women without apparent adverse effects, it may cause decreased uterine blood flow (Murad and colleagues, 1985). First-trimester use has been associated with limb defects (Magee and associates, 1996). Although cause and effect have not been proven, many embryogenic processes are calcium dependent and could theoretically be blocked by calcium-channel blockers (Bilozur and colleagues, 1982; Lee and Nagel, 1986). Verapamil has also been associated with fetal cardiac depression and arrest when used transplacentally in combination with digoxin for treatment of fetal supraventricular tachycardias (Owen and associates, 1988). Whether **nifedipine** is associated with similar adverse effects is unclear at this time. Sibai and associates (1992) used nifedipine to treat women with preeclampsia remote from term. Although no adverse fetal effects were noted, there was also no improvement in perinatal outcome. Other calcium antagonists include **diltiazem** and **nicardipine.**

DIURETICS. These drugs are prescribed during pregnancy for some women with chronic hypertension, and are also given acutely or chronically to treat pulmonary edema. Congenital anomalies were not increased among over 60 women who took **chlorothiazide** in the first trimester, or among over 5000 who took it later (Heinonen and co-workers, 1977). Similarly, **hydrochlorothiazide** use during early pregnancy was not associated with increased congenital anomalies (Jick and colleagues, 1981). Thiazides have been associated with neonatal thrombocytopenia, bleeding, and electrolyte disturbances when given near the time of delivery.

Acetazolamide is a carbonic anhydrase inhibitor used as a diuretic and to treat glaucoma and epilepsy. Although the drug has been consistently reported to be associated with an unusual type of limb abnormality in rodents, similar defects could not be induced in primates and have not been observed in humans (Heinonen and co-workers, 1977; Hirsch and colleagues, 1983). **Spironolactone** is a commonly used potassium-sparing diuretic that has not been widely studied in human pregnancy. It causes feminization of male rat fetuses and delayed sexual maturation of female rat fetuses, but these effects have not been observed in humans (Messina and colleagues, 1979).

Ethacrynic acid and **furosemide** are loop diuretics that are usually not used chronically during pregnancy.

Furosemide crosses the placenta and increases fetal urine production. There is some evidence that it stimulates the renal synthesis of prostaglandin E_2, which increases the incidence of patent ductus arteriosus in preterm infants (Green and colleagues, 1983). No adverse fetal effects have been associated with its acute administration. Ethacrynic acid has ototoxic effects in vitro, but only one report has been made of associated ototoxicity in vivo (Jones, 1973).

ANTICOAGULANTS. Deep vein thrombosis or pulmonary embolus is estimated to complicate about 1 in 2500 pregnancies (Chap. 46, p. 1237). **Coumarin** derivatives cause embryo-fetal defects and should not be used in pregnancy (p. 1014). **Heparin** is the anticoagulant of choice. Unfractionated heparin is a group of large (m.w. 4000 to 30,000) highly polar molecules that do not cross the placenta and are not associated with congenital anomalies. It may be given intravenously, either continuously or intermittently, or by subcutaneous injection. Its protracted use may cause maternal osteopenia, osteoporosis, and thrombocytopenia (Chap. 46, p. 1239). The newer low-molecular weight (4000 to 6000) heparins such as **enoxaparin** have been used for anticoagulation. In a review by Fejgin and Lourwood (1994), low-molecular weight heparin was not found to cross the placenta. Although Nelson-Piercy and co-workers (1997) reported five miscarriages, four midtrimester losses, and seven preterm deliveries in 69 pregnancies treated with enoxaparin, they attributed the poor outcomes to the antiphospholipid antibody syndrome. In another study of 108 pregnant women, Schneider and colleagues (1997) found no adverse fetal effects associated with either preparation.

Thrombolytic agents have been used during pregnancy. Examples of these agents include **streptokinase, urokinase,** and **tissue plasminogen activator (t-PA).** Urokinase is normally produced by the ovary and cytotrophoblast, and case reports suggest it can be used safely in pregnancy (Kramer, 1995; La Valleur, 1996; Turrentine, 1995, and their associates). In two reports of 166 pregnancies, streptokinase was not associated with adverse fetal effects (Ludwig, 1973). The few reports of use of tissue plasminogen activator during pregnancy do not support a teratogenic risk (Briggs and colleagues, 1998).

ASTHMA. Most medications for treatment of asthma can be used with apparent safety during pregnancy (Chap. 46, p. 1230). For acute asthma, **epinephrine** and **terbutaline** may be given subcutaneously as there is little evidence that these agents cause adverse fetal effects. In one long-term study of exposed fetuses, Wallace and colleagues (1978) reported no increase in complications. **Metaproterenol** and **albuterol** are self-administered by

inhalation. There is little information regarding their possible teratogenicity following first-trimester use.

Theophylline salts are commonly used bronchodilators. **Aminopylline** is the only salt available for parenteral use, but there are numerous oral forms of which many contain other bronchodilators such as **ephedrine.**

Cromolyn inhibits mast cell histamine release and is given chronically for asthma prophylaxis. There are no large studies in pregnant women, nor are there reports of congenital anomalies after first-trimester use.

Inhaled corticosteroids, including beclomethasone and triamcinolone acetonide, are now used commonly for asthma. Oral prednisone may be given as a dose pack or methylprednisolone given intravenously. Similar to other corticosteroids, beclomethasone has been associated with fetal resorption and cleft lip and palate in mice and rabbits (Esaki and associates, 1976; Oguro and co-workers, 1970). However, two clinical studies including 101 pregnant women treated with beclomethasone and/or prednisone for severe asthma showed no increase in congenital malformation (Fitzsimons and colleagues, 1986; Greenberger and Patterson, 1983). Triamcinolone is a more potent teratogen in animals than either hydrocortisone or cortisone, but has not been associated with adverse fetal effects in humans (Dombrowski and co-investigators, 1996).

SEIZURE DISORDERS. The most commonly used anticonvulsants are teratogenic, as discussed earlier (p. 1012). **Phenobarbital** has been used frequently in combination with these other anticonvulsants. Over 1000 mother–infant pairs with first-trimester exposure to phenobarbital were included in the Collaborative Perinatal Project database, and no increased frequency of either minor or major birth defects was observed compared with unexposed controls (Heinonen and associates, 1977). The effects of phenobarbital on fetal development have been obscured by the co-administration of hydantoin and the increased risk of anomalies due to epilepsy itself (Briggs and associates, 1998). Reinisch and colleagues (1995) studied over 9000 offspring in the Danish perinatal cohort, and reported that 114 phenobarbital-exposed men tested at age 22 or older had decreased cognitive performance compared with nonexposed controls.

Ethosuximide and **methsuximide** are succinimide anticonvulsants used for petit mal seizures. There are no human reproduction studies available or reports of malformations attributed solely to either of these agents. They are classified as category C drugs.

Newer anticonvulsants include **felbamate, gabapentin, lamotrigine, oxcarbazepine, tiagabine, topiramate,** and **vigabatrin.** Information about the safety of these agents in pregnancy is limited, as relatively few exposed pregnancies have been reported (Briggs and associates,

1998). Based on what is known about the likely mechanisms of teratogenesis in the more traditional anticonvulsants, several of these new drugs may actually be safer for the fetus. For example, none of these agents has antifolate effects; none except tiagabine results in the production of arene oxide metabolites; and most have minimal or no effect on the cytochrome p450 system (Morrell, 1996). Whether they are as efficacious as older drugs for management of epilepsy in pregnancy remains to be seen.

PSYCHIATRIC CONDITIONS. Medications used to treat psychiatric illness include sedatives, hypnotics, tranquilizers, antidepressants, and antipsychotics (Table 38–10). Some of these treatments are discussed in Chapter 53.

BENZODIAZEPINES. These minor tranquilizers may be required for women who have severe and debilitating anxiety disorders or who are psychotic and assaultive or agitated. **Diazepam** is the most widely used and it has been associated with an increased risk of cleft palate and limb malformations in rodents. Although some studies have associated high doses of benzodiazepines with multiple defects, determination of cause and effect has been complicated by frequent concomitant alcohol and substance abuse (Bergman and associates, 1992; Laegrid and colleagues, 1989). More recent studies have not found an association between diazepam alone and fetal anomalies (Czeizel, 1987/88). Likewise, lorazepam and midazolam have not been linked to adverse fetal outcomes other than transient sedation at birth. Alprazolam is commonly used for panic disorder. It has been available for less time than other benzodiazepines and thus the data are not conclusive. There have been few reports associating alprazolam with congenital abnormalities, although one study found that the rate of malformations following over 400 first-trimester exposures was 4.7 percent (St. Clair and Schirmer, 1992). Exposed neonates should be watched for signs of hypotonia.

ANTIDEPRESSANT DRUGS. Commonly used antidepressants are listed in Table 38–10. The most commonly used antidepressants are the **selective serotonin reuptake inhibitors (SSRIs).** The older compounds, **fluoxetine** and **sertraline,** have not been reported to cause birth defects in animals or humans. A summary of 796 fluoxetine-exposed pregnancies reported to the manufacturer described rates of early pregnancy loss and congenital abnormalities not different from those in historical controls (3.5 percent). This report and others also failed to identify a specific pattern of defects or a predilection for any particular organ system in the small number of affected offspring (Goldstein and associates, 1993, 1997). In a study comparing first-trimester treat-

TABLE 38–10. Commonly Used Medications for Psychiatric Disorders and Their Classification Regarding Use During Pregnancy

	FDA Category[a]
Tricyclic Antidepressants	
Amitriptyline	D
Amoxapine	C
Clomipramine	C
Desipramine	C
Doxepin	C
Imipramine	D
Nortriptyline	D
Selective Serotonin Reuptake Inhibitors	
Fluoxetine	B
Paroxetine	B
Sertraline	B
Monoamine Oxidase Inhibitors	
Isocarboxazid	C
Phenelzine	C
Tranylcypromine	C
Other	
Bupropion	B
Trazodone	C
Antipsychotics	
Chlorpromazine	C
Clozapine	B
Fluphenazine	C
Haloperidol	C
Loxapine	C
Perphenazine	C
Thioridazine	C
Trifluporazine	C
Benzodiazepines	
Alprazolam	D
Chlordiazepoxide	D
Clonazepam	C
Diazepam	D
Lorazepam	C
Midazolam	D
Oxazepam	C

Classification according to manufacturer or Briggs and colleagues (1998).

ment with fluoxetine, standard tricyclic antidepressants, or another nonteratogen, there were no differences in malformations or fetal losses (Pastuszak and colleagues, 1993). Because these agents have few side effects compared with other antidepressants, they are a good therapeutic choice for pregnant women requiring treatment.

Some malformations, particularly those affecting limbs, have been reported in conjunction with first-trimester use of **tricyclic antidepressants** (Elia and colleagues, 1987). In the largest study investigating the rate of malformations in over 1 million women exposed to these antidepressants during pregnancy, however, no increase in fetal malformations was found (Rowe, 1973). These agents are unlikely to be potent teratogens (Briggs and colleagues, 1998).

Lithium salts, especially lithium carbonate, are used for treatment of affective mental illness. In an early study, Weinstein (1980) reported that 8 percent of 225 lithium-exposed infants in an international registry had serious congenital cardiovascular abnormalities. Six of these affected infants—2.7 percent of those exposed—had the otherwise rare defect *Ebstein anomaly*. Because of this, lithium was presumed to be a teratogen. However, methodological problems with this study clouded interpretation. In a subsequent prospective study, Jacobson and colleagues (1992) followed 148 women given lithium in the first trimester and reported a 2.8 percent major congenital malformation rate (one fetus had Ebstein anomaly), similar to the 2.4 percent observed in controls. They concluded that lithium is not a major teratogen. Epidemiological data would indicate that the risk of Ebstein anomaly from first-trimester lithium exposure is much lower than previously estimated (Cohen and associates, 1994a). Considering these data, lithium can be taken throughout pregnancy if necessary, or it may be discontinued at least until 6 to 8 weeks, when cardiac structures have formed (Briggs and colleagues, 1998).

Monoamine oxidase (MAO) inhibitors are used less frequently today because patients must follow a low tyramine diet and hypertensive crises can occur after dietary indiscretion. Administration of meperidine and some anesthetic agents coincident with MAO inhibitor use can stimulate a life-threatening hyperthermic crisis. Such severe adverse reactions are especially undesirable in pregnant women, and this class of medication is generally avoided (Mortola, 1989).

ANTIPSYCHOTIC MEDICATIONS. Many of these agents are **phenothiazines,** which have been used in pregnancy to treat both psychotic disorders and hyperemesis, although most safety information has been derived from their use as antiemetics. Most information concerns chlorpromazine, and the largest study of this and other phenothiazines from the Collaborative Perinatal Project reported no increased risk of fetal malformations after prenatal exposure (Slone and colleagues, 1977). When used for hyperemesis, these drugs are ingested intermittently at low doses, and their safety when taken at high continuous doses for antipsychotic therapy is generally difficult to assess. Infants born to mothers with certain psychiatric illnesses such as schizophrenia are independently at greater risk for malformations (Elia and colleagues, 1987). Also, affected women often take a number of other prescription medications as well as known teratogens such as alcohol. Because of widespread use without serious fetal effects, the teratogenic potential of most antipsychotic agents is considered to be minimal (Briggs and associates, 1998).

ANALGESICS

SALICYLATES AND ACETAMINOPHEN. In one review of over 1000 women, Streissguth and colleagues (1987) reported that almost half of pregnant women used salicylates and acetaminophen. Most investigators have found no association between maternal salicylate ingestion and fetal anomalies (Heinonen, 1977; Slone, 1976; Turner, 1975, and their associates). Because **aspirin** is a potent prostaglandin inhibitor, there is a theoretical concern that antenatal exposure could lead to premature closure of the ductus arterious and associated cardiac and pulmonary abnormalities. Although the fetal effects of chronic high-dose aspirin ingestion are not known, no adverse outcomes have been reported after low-dose exposure. DiSessa and colleagues (1994) performed echocardiograms from 15 to 40 weeks in 63 fetuses exposed to 60 mg aspirin given daily to prevent preeclampsia. They found consistently normal ductus flow velocity, and normal output from both ventricles. **Acetaminophen** was not found to be associated with an increased risk of anomalies in over 500 exposed offspring (Aselton and colleagues, 1985; Heinonen and associates, 1977). Liver toxicity may result from maternal overdose with acetaminophen (Chap. 48, p. 1294).

OTHER NONSTEROIDAL ANTI-INFLAMMATORY DRUGS (NSAIDs). There are a variety of nonsteroidal anti-inflammatory drugs with analgesic action, but **ibuprofen, naproxen,** and **ketoprofen** are used most often. **Indomethacin** has also been employed as a tocolytic agent (Niebyl and colleagues, 1980). These drugs are not considered to be teratogenic but may have reversible fetal effects when used in the third trimester. Indomethacin and other prostaglandin inhibitors have been associated with constriction of the fetal ductus arteriosus and subsequent persistent fetal circulation (pulmonary hypertension) in the neonate (Csaba and associates, 1978). It also causes decreased urine output and reduced amnionic fluid volume after prolonged usage (Hickok and colleagues, 1989). For these reasons, the drug is used to treat hydramnios (Chap. 31, p. 820). Most studies have shown that these effects are reversible as long as the drug is not given after 34 weeks (Dudley and Hardie, 1985; Niebyl, 1991). Case reports have associated indomethacin with other adverse fetal effects such as intraventricular hemorrhage, bronchopulmonary dysplasia, and necrotizing enterocolitis. Infants are at highest risk if delivery occurs within 48 hours of instituting therapy (Major and associates, 1994; Norton and co-workers, 1993). Doppler studies in neonates suggest that these problems may be related to hypotension and decreased blood flow in blood vessels supplying the bowel and brain (Van Bel and co-workers, 1990).

NARCOTIC ANALGESICS. Commonly used opioids include **meperidine** and **morphine.** Heinonen and colleagues (1977) found no association between either of these agents and congenital anomalies. As with all narcotics, chronic maternal ingestion may be associated with a neonatal withdrawal syndrome (Chap. 29, p. 751). **Codeine, propoxyphene, oxycodone,** and **hydrocodone** have not been found to be associated with congenital anomalies (Bracken and Holford, 1981; Heinonen and colleagues, 1977). **Butorphanol** has been associated with neonatal respiratory depression and withdrawal, and 20 percent of fetuses exposed to it exhibit a sinusoidal heart rate pattern (Hatjis and Meis, 1986; Welt, 1985).

LOCAL ANALGESIA AND ANESTHESIA

GENERAL ANESTHESIA. As discussed in Chapter 42 (p. 1144), nonobstetrical surgery is occasionally performed during pregnancy. All general anesthetic agents cross the placenta to some degree, and some local analgesics have the potential for systemic absorption. Although risk-benefit analysis during a surgical emergency in pregnancy usually clearly supports surgery, it is appropriate to counsel the woman about any potential fetal risks. None of the currently used anesthetic agents is a known teratogen, and the exposures during pregnancy are generally brief and not at toxic levels. However, data supporting this conclusion is imperfect. It is difficult to clearly differentiate any adverse fetal effects from anesthetic exposure from any harmful sequelae of the conditions leading to surgery. Other confounding factors include maternal hypotension, hypoxia, metabolic disturbances, and the interaction of multiple drugs. The Collaborative Perinatal Project did not identify any anesthesia-related teratogenic effects in the first 4 months of pregnancy, even though the analysis was not controlled for confounding factors (Heinonen and colleagues, 1977). Because halothane appears to interfere with normal fetal cardiovascular homeostasis in animals

(fetal lambs), it is not recommended for fetal surgery (Sabik and colleagues, 1993). A large Swedish study likewise failed to find an association between anesthesia exposure and adverse fetal outcome (Mazze and Kallen, 1989). This 8-year study included 720,000 pregnant women who underwent 5405 nonobstetrical operations. In a case-control study, Czeizel and associates (1998) also found no increased malformations from anesthesia exposure.

Of 152 women given **thiopental** in early pregnancy, the frequency of congenital malformations was not increased (Heinonen and colleagues, 1977). Thiopental also does not increase the rate of malformations in rodents at three times the usual dose (Tanimura and colleagues, 1967). Although none has been examined in a large study, **ketamine, methohexital, thiamylal, etomidate, alphaxalone, sodium oxylate,** and **thialbarbitone** have not been associated with fetal malformations when used in pregnant women. The two most commonly used muscle relaxants, **curare** and **succinylcholine,** have not been associated with teratogenic effects in humans.

A wide variety of inhalation agents are employed for general anesthesia, but the most commonly used is **nitrous oxide.** The frequency of malformations was not increased in offspring of mothers exposed to nitrous oxide during the first 4 months of pregnancy (Friedman, 1988; Heinonen and co-workers, 1977). **Halogenated agents** are commonly used to supplement nitrous oxide. **Halothane** has been reported to be teratogenic in some animal studies, but not in others (Friedman, 1988). It was not associated with increased malformations in the offspring of 25 women who were given this agent during the first 4 months of pregnancy (Heinonen and colleagues, 1977). There have been no epidemiological studies regarding the use of either **isoflurane, enflurane,** or **methoxyflurane** during pregnancy. Chronic exposure of mouse and rabbit embryos to isoflurane and enflurane at doses causing maternal toxicity has caused impaired development, but similar effects have not been seen in humans (Reprotox, 2000a, 2000b).

Older reports suggested that women with an occupational exposure to inhalation agents—anesthesiologists, surgeons, nurse anesthetists, operating room nurses, dental hygienists—had an increased risk of pregnancy loss or decreased fertility. In general, however, these studies are marred by their retrospective designs, recall bias among subjects, inadequate documentation of the dose or timing of exposure, and failure to show a dose-response relationship (Friedman, 1988; Shnider and Levinson, 1987). Most of these also concerned exposures which occurred before nitrous oxide scavenging equipment was routinely utilized (Rowland and associates, 1992). Epidemiological studies did not find significantly increased risk of either pregnancy loss or fetal malformations in women exposed when scavenging equipment is used. Current safety guidelines require stringent ventilation and scavenging equipment in areas where inhalation agents are used.

LOCAL ANESTHESIA. A variety of local anesthetic agents may be employed for spinal or epidural analgesia. **Lidocaine** is used frequently, and in one review of almost 300 children whose mothers were given lidocaine in early pregnancy, the frequency of congenital malformations was not increased (Heinonen and colleagues, 1977). The frequency of malformations in offspring exposed to the other "caine" anesthetics also was not greater than expected in the general population. The main concern with these agents is the possibility of associated fetal bradycardia or hyperthermia, both of which could be detrimental to the fetus, but would likely not produce structural anomalies (Macaulay and co-workers, 1992; Stavrous and colleagues, 1990).

ANTIEMETICS. **Bendectin,** a combination of doxylamine and pyridoxine, is no longer available in the United States because of the litigation it engendered as discussed earlier (p. 1008). It can essentially be reconstituted by ingesting **vitamin B$_6$** along with an over-the-counter sleep aid, **doxylamine,** neither of which is considered to have teratogenic potential (Niebyl, 2000). A variety of other antiemetics are used during pregnancy such as the piperazines (**meclizine, cyclizine**) and phenothiazines (**chlorpromazine, prochlorperazine, promethazine**). Teratogenic effects of **metoclopramide** have not been seen in a variety of experimental animals, and no adverse effects in humans have been reported (Berkovitch and associates, 2000; Reprotox, 2000d). There is no evidence that any antiemetics are associated with an increased risk of congenital anomalies (Farkas and Farkas, 1971; Heinonen and colleagues, 1977).

Ondansetron hydrochloride is used primarily for nausea associated with cancer chemotherapy. There are no large human studies with the drug. It is given by intravenous infusion and is especially helpful in pregnant women with hyperemesis refractory to other medications. This antiemetic is often reserved for use after 12 weeks.

IMMUNOSUPPRESSIVE DRUGS. Immunosuppressants are given primarily for the treatment of autoimmune disease and for organ transplantation maintenance. **Corticosteroids** such as prednisone and dexamethasone are most commonly used and are discussed on page 1025.

Azathioprine is primarily used to prevent organ transplant rejection or to treat inflammatory bowel disease. Although teratogenic for animals, most investigators have found the drug safe for use during human pregnancy (Briggs and colleagues, 1998). Neonatal hematological abnormalities, including fatal pancytopenia, have been described in association with maternal therapy (Davidson and co-workers, 1985; DeWitte and associates, 1984).

Cyclosporine is an antibiotic used as an immunosuppressant to prevent organ transplant rejection. It is widely used for liver and heart allografts, and has recently also been used for renal transplantation. The drug causes significant maternal toxicity, especially nephrotoxicity. There are no large epidemiological reports regarding its use in pregnancy, but it appears to be safe for the fetus (Briggs and co-workers, 1998). Moreover, the benefits appear to outweigh any theoretical risks.

Cyclophosphamide, often prescribed for immune suppression after organ transplant or for systemic lupus erythematosus, is a suspected teratogen (p. 1018).

HORMONES. Some hormones are teratogenic as discussed on page 1017. Initial findings from the Collaborative Perinatal Project indicated that high-dose **oral contraceptives** were associated with an increased risk for cardiovascular and limb-reduction defects. Subsequent analysis, however, has shown no difference when compared with control women (Wiseman and Dodds-Smith, 1984). In 1988, the Food and Drug Administration approved the removal of the package insert rejoinder that warned against birth defects. In a meta-analysis of first-trimester sex hormone exposure, including oral contraceptives, Raman-Wilms and colleagues (1995) found no association between exposure and fetal genital malformations.

Gonadotropin-releasing hormone agonists (GnRH) have been used to treat infertility as well as other gynecological conditions. There is little information regarding their use during pregnancy. In a review of five women who were exposed to GnRH agonists during the first trimester, Young and colleagues (1993) reported three term pregnancies without complications and two abortions.

NATURAL (HERBAL) REMEDIES. It is difficult to estimate the risk or safety of various herbal remedies because they are not regulated as prescription or over-the-counter drugs. Often, the identity and quantity of all ingredients are unknown. Virtually no human or animal studies of their teratogenic potential have been reported, and knowledge of complications is essentially limited to acute toxicity (Sheehan, 1998). Because it is not possible to assess the safety of various herbal remedies during pregnancy, pregnant women should be counseled to avoid these substances. Several remedies do contain substances with pharmaceutical properties that could theoretically have adverse fetal effects. **Echinaceae,** which is believed to have anti-inflammatory properties, causes fragmentation of hamster sperm at high concentrations (Ondrizek and associates, 1999). **Black cohosh,** used to speed labor and treat premenstrual symptoms, contains a chemical that acts like estrogen. **Garlic** and **willow barks** have anticoagulant properties that may intensify the effects of anticoagulant drugs. **Gingko,** touted as an aid to memory and mental clarity, can apparently interfere with the effects of MAO-inhibiting drugs and has anticoagulant properties. Real **licorice** contains **glycyrrhizin,** which has hypertensive and potassium wasting effects. **Valerian** intensifies the effects of prescription sleep aids. **Ginseng,** which is ingested to increase energy, interferes with MAO-inhibiting drugs. **Soy** products contain phytoestrogen.

Certain herbal remedies are used as abortifacients, for example, **blue** and **black cohosh** appear to directly stimulate uterine musculature. **Pennyroyal** has been used as an abortifacient, and appears to work by irritating the bladder and uterus and causing strong uterine contractions. The drug can also cause liver damage, renal failure, and disseminated intravascular coagulation, and has been associated with several maternal deaths (Black, 1985).

ILLICIT DRUGS. The American College of Obstetricians and Gynecologists (1994) estimates that 10 percent is a minimal prevalence for substance abuse in pregnant women. In one survey of 715 pregnant women screened for alcohol, opiates, cocaine, and cannabinoids, 15 percent had positive urine toxicological tests (Chasnoff and associates, 1990). It has been estimated that from 350,000 to over 700,000 infants may be exposed to illicit substances in utero each year (Chasnoff, 1991; Gomby and Shiono, 1991). While solid information is lacking for most drugs of abuse, **cocaine** and alcohol are potent and commonly used teratogenic substances (pp. 1019 and 1011).

POLYDRUG ABUSE. Illicit drug users seldom abuse only one drug. In a review of patterns of substance abuse during pregnancy, Little and colleagues (1990b) analyzed the use of methamphetamine, cocaine, heroin, and "t's and blues" in a primarily indigent population. Overall, 75 percent of these women reported that they abused more than one drug during pregnancy. Alcohol is a common co-factor, and appears to increase the risk of congenital anomalies and growth retardation. For example, infants born to women who abuse "t's and blues" are at a 3- to 14-fold risk of alcohol-induced embryo-fetal damage compared with infants born to abusers of other drugs (Little and co-workers, 1990b). Similarly, in a study of 104,000 pregnant women registered in the Swedish public health insurance system, 10 percent of offspring of women who abused benzodiazepines during pregnancy had birth defects thought to be caused by the additive effects of heavy alcohol use and

exposure to other substances (Bergman and colleagues, 1992).

IMPURITIES AND DILUTANTS. Most illegal substances contain impurities and contaminants. Examples include lead, cyanide, cellulose, herbicides, and pesticides. Many substances are used as dilutants, including fine glass beads, powdered sugar, finely ground sawdust, strychnine, arsenic, and antihistamines. Coumadin has been used to "cut" heroin. Some of these dilutants and impurities may have serious adverse effects on both the mother and her fetus.

SPECIFIC SUBSTANCES. There are not enough data concerning substance use during pregnancy to allow full assessment of risks, especially to the embryo-fetus. Available information is usually confounded by factors that include poor maternal health, malnutrition, infectious diseases, and especially the use of multiple drugs.

Marijuana or **hashish** is used by nearly 15 percent of pregnant women (Abel and Sokol, 1988; Chasnoff and colleagues, 1990). The active ingredient is **delta-9-tetrahydrocannabinol (THC)** which in high doses is teratogenic for animals; however, there is no evidence that marijuana is associated with human anomalies. In one study, birthweight was lower in exposed infants than controls, however, larger studies failed to corroborate this (Greenland, 1983; Linn, 1983; Shiono, 1995, and their colleagues).

Amphetamines are sympathomimetic agents used as central nervous system stimulants, anorectics, and to treat narcolepsy. Various amphetamines are teratogenic in mice and rabbits, producing cleft palate, exencephaly, and eye defects when given at very high doses (Reprotox, 2000g). Retrospective human studies and case reports have linked amphetamines to congenital heart disease, biliary atresia, and limb-reduction defects (Bays, 1991; Nora and colleagues, 1970). In four cohort studies of 818 women who took amphetamines during early pregnancy, however, the frequencies of major and minor congenital anomalies were no greater than controls (Heinonen and colleagues, 1983; Little and associates, 1988; Milkovich and van den Berg, 1977).

Methamphetamines are used medically to treat narcolepsy and hyperkinetic children, but are largely ineffective in the treatment of obesity. These drugs are often used to dilute other illicit drugs. In one cohort study of medically supervised methamphetamine use, the frequency of congenital anomalies was not increased compared with controls (Heinonen and co-workers, 1977). In two investigations, symmetrical fetal growth retardation was increased compared with control women, but the frequency of congenital anomalies was not different (Little and colleagues, 1988; Ramin and associates, 1992). Methylamphetamine, known as speed, ice, crank, and crystal meth, is a drug of abuse that produces defects in mice, rats, and rabbits, but has not been associated with defects in humans.

In most studies, the frequency of congenital anomalies is not higher among infants born to mothers addicted to **heroin** (Little and associates, 1990c). In one cohort study of 830 exposed infants, the frequency of anomalies of 2.4 percent was similar to background risk (Ostrea and Chavez, 1979). Other morbidity is common, and fetal growth restriction, perinatal death, and several perinatal complications were reported with high frequency in offspring of narcotic-addicted mothers (Lifschitz and colleagues, 1983; Little and co-workers, 1990c). It is not clear whether these effects are due to fetal heroin exposure or to generally poor maternal health. Postnatal growth of these children appears to be normal in most cases, although the average head circumference is smaller than that of unexposed children (Lifschitz and co-workers, 1983). In addition, Chasnoff and colleagues (1986), as well as others, have reported mild developmental delay or behavioral disturbances in the children of narcotic-addicted women. Withdrawal symptoms in exposed neonates are common. Tremors, irritability, sneezing, vomiting, fever, diarrhea, and occasionally seizures are observed in 40 to 80 percent of infants born to heroin-addicted women (Alroomi and colleagues, 1988). Although these symptoms can be of prolonged duration, they usually persist for less than 10 days. Abnormal respiratory function during sleep often persists after withdrawal is complete, and may be a factor in the increased incidence of sudden infant death syndrome seen in exposed infants (Kandall and associates, 1993).

Methadone is a synthetic opiate narcotic that structurally resembles propoxyphene. Its principal medical use is maintenance therapy for heroin addiction. In large doses, methadone causes exencephaly and central nervous system defects in rodents. However, congenital anomalies were not increased above background in cohort studies and clinical series of infants born to heroin-addicted women treated with methadone (Stimmel and Adamsons, 1976). Conversely, withdrawal symptoms frequently develop and birthweight is lower than in unexposed infants (Briggs and colleagues, 1998). Chasnoff and co-workers (1987) compared 52 cocaine-using pregnant women to 73 women who were former heroin addicts maintained on methadone, and found a significantly higher rate of preterm labor, rapid labor, abruptio placentae, and meconium staining among cocaine users. Withdrawal from methadone is more severe than from heroin and more protracted (up to 3 weeks), due to the much longer half-life of methadone.

Lysergic acid amides, classically known as **lysergic acid diethylamide (LSD),** are amine alkaloids obtained only through chemical synthesis. There is no evidence that this drug is a human teratogen. Some investigators have found increased frequencies of chromosomal breakage in somatic cells of mothers who used lysergic acid as well as their prenatally exposed infants. This also has been observed in human cells incubated in vitro with the drug (Long, 1972). Such breakage, however, does not appear to correlate with an increased risk for congenital anomalies.

Phencyclidine (PCP), known as angel dust, is no longer manufactured legally, although it is still used illegally. Wachsman and cohorts (1989) described 57 infants whose mothers used phencyclidine throughout pregnancy, including embryogenesis, and reported the frequency of congenital anomalies to be no greater than background. Neonatal withdrawal characterized by tremors, jitteriness, and irritability was observed in more than half of exposed infants. A study of 94 phencyclidine-exposed infants did not identify an increase in structural malformations, but did confirm an increased incidence of newborn behavioral and developmental abnormalities (Golden and colleagues, 1987).

"T's and blues" is a street mixture of the narcotic analgesic *pentazocine* (*Talwin*) and the over-the-counter antihistamine *tripelennamine* (*Pyribenzamine*). Since 1972 this mixture has gained popularity in urban centers among lower socioeconomic groups as a less costly substitute for heroin. Although its abuse by pregnant women has been reported to increase the risk of fetal growth restriction, an increased frequency of congenital anomalies was not found (Little and co-workers, 1990a; von Almen and Miller, 1984). Exposed infants often suffer from withdrawal symptoms.

REFERENCES

Abel EL: What really causes FAS? Teratology 59:4, 1999

Abel EL, Sokol RJ: Marijuana and cocaine use during pregnancy. In Niebyl J (ed): Drug Use in Pregnancy, 2nd ed. Philadelphia, Lea & Febiger, 1988, p 223

Acyclovir Pregnancy Registry: Interim report. Project office. Glaxo Wellcome, Research Triangle Park, NC, July 31, 1998

Alroomi LG, Davidson J, Evans TJ, Galea P, Howat R: Maternal narcotic abuse and the newborn. Arch Dis Child 63:81, 1988

American Academy of Neurology: Practice parameter: Management issues for women with epilepsy (summary statement). Epilepsia 39:1225, 1998

American College of Obstetricians and Gynecologists: Vitamin A supplementation during pregnancy. Committee Opinion No. 196, January 1998

American College of Obstetricians and Gynecologists: Vitamin A supplementation during pregnancy. Committee Opinion No. 157, September 1995

American College of Obstetricians and Gynecologists: Substance abuse in pregnancy. Technical Bulletin No. 195, July 1994

Antiretroviral Pregnancy Registry: Interim report. Project office. Glaxo Wellcome, Research Triangle Park, NC, December 31, 1996

Aselton P, Jick H, Milunsky A, Hunter JR, Stergachis A: First trimester drug use and congenital disorders. Obstet Gynecol 65:451, 1985

Autti-Rämö I, Korkman M, Hilakivi-Clark L, Lehtonen M, Halmesmäki E, Granström ML: Mental development of 2-year-old children exposed to alcohol in utero. J Pediatr 120:740, 1992

Barlow SM, Knight AF: Teratogenic effects of silastic intrauterine devices in the rat with or without added medroxyprogesterone acetate. Fertil Steril 39:224, 1983

Barr M, Cohen MM: ACE inhibitor fetopathy and hypocalvaria: The kidney skull connection. Teratology 44:485, 1991

Bays J: Fetal vascular disruption with prenatal exposure to cocaine or methamphetamine [letter]. Pediatrics 87:416, 1991

Bergman U, Rosa FZ, Baum C, Wiholm BE, Faich GA: Effects of exposure to benzodiazepine during fetal life. Lancet 340:694, 1992

Berkovitch M, Elbirt D, Addis A, Schuler-Faccini L, Ornoy A: Fetal effects of metochlopramide therapy for nausea and vomiting of pregnancy. N Engl J Med 343:445, 2000

Berkovitch M, Pastoszak A, Gazarian M, Lewis M, Koren G: Safety of quinolones in pregnancy. Pediatr Res 35:91A, 1994

Biale Y, Lewenthal H: Effect of folic acid supplementation on congenital malformations due to anticonvulsant drugs. Eur J Obstet Gynecol Reprod Biol 18:211, 1984

Bilozur M, Powers RD: Two sites for calcium action in compaction of the mouse embryo. Exp Cell Res 142:39, 1982

Bingol N, Fuchs M, Holipas N, Henriquez R, Pagan M, Diaz V: Prune belly syndrome associated with maternal cocaine abuse. Am J Hum Gen 39:A51, 1986

Black DR: Pregnancy unaffected by pennyroyal usage. J Am Osteopath Assoc 85:282, 1985

Boncinelli E: Homeobox genes and disease. Curr Opin Genet Dev 7:331, 1997

Bortnichak EA, Wetter MS: Teratogenic effects of carbamazepine. Correspondence to the editor. N Engl J Med 321:1480, 1989

Boyle CA, Deccoufle PK, Yeargig-Allsopp M: Prevalence and health impact of developmental disabilities in US children. Pediatrics 93:399, 1994

Bracken MB, Holford TR: Exposure to prescribed drugs in pregnancy and association with congenital malformations. Obstet Gynecol 58:336, 1981

Brent RL: Teratogen update: Bendectin. Teratology 31:429, 1985

Briggs GG, Freeman RK, Yaffe SJ: Drugs in Pregnancy and Lactation, 5th ed. Baltimore, Williams & Wilkins, 1998

Brumfitt W, Pursell R: Trimethoprim/sulfamethoxazole in the treatment of bacteriuria in women. J Infect Dis 128:657, 1973

Brunskill PJ: The effects of fetal exposure to danazol. Br J Obstet Gynaecol 99:212, 1992

Buehler BA, Delimont D, van Waes M, Finnell RH: Prenatal prediction of risk of the fetal hydantoin syndrome. N Engl J Med 322:1567, 1990

Burtin P, Taddio A, Ariburnu O, Einarson TR, Koren G: Safety of metronidazole in pregnancy: A meta-analysis. Am J Obstet Gynecol 172:525, 1995

Cantrell DC, Cunningham FG: Epilepsy complicating pregnancy. Supplement to Williams Obstetrics, 19th ed. Stamford, CT, Appleton & Lange, August/September 1994

Castilla EE, Ashton-Prolla O, Barreda-Mejia E, Brunoni D, Cavalcanti DP, Correa-Neto J, et al: Thalidomide, a current teratogen in South America. Teratology 54:273, 1996

Centers for Disease Control: Centers for Disease Control Vietnam Experience Study. Health status of Vietnam veterans III. Reproductive outcomes and child health. JAMA 259:2715, 1998

Centers for Disease Control and Prevention: Population-based prevalence of perinatal exposure to cocaine—Georgia, 1994. MMWR 45:887, 1996

Centers for Disease Control and Prevention: Update: Trends in fetal alcohol syndrome United States, 1979–1993. MMWR 44:249, 1995

Centers for Disease Control and Prevention: Birth outcomes following zidovudine therapy in pregnant women. MMWR 43:409, 1994

Chasnoff IJ: Drugs, alcohol, pregnancy, and the neonate: Pay now or pay later. JAMA 266:1567, 1991

Chasnoff IJ, Burns KA, Burns WJ, Schnoll SH: Prenatal drug exposure: Effects on neonatal and infant growth development. Neurotoxicol Teratol 8:357, 1986

Chasnoff IJ, Burns KA, Burns WJ: Cocaine use in pregnancy: Perinatal morbidity and mortality. Neurotoxicol Teratol 9:291, 1987

Chasnoff IJ, Burns WJ, Schnoll SH, Burns KA: Cocaine use in pregnancy. N Engl J Med 313:666, 1985

Chasnoff IJ, Chisum GM, Kaplan WE: Maternal cocaine use and genitourinary tract malformations. Teratology 37:201, 1988

Chasnoff IJ, Landress HJ, Barrett ME: The prevalence of illicit drug or alcohol use during pregnancy and the discrepancies in mandatory reporting in Pinellas County, Florida. N Engl J Med 322:1202, 1990

Chavez GF, Mulinare J, Cordero JF: Maternal cocaine use and the risk for genitourinary tract defects: An epidemiologic approach. Am J Hum Genet 43:A43, 1988

Chrousos GP, Evans MI, Loriaux DL, McCluskey J, Fletcher JC, Schulman JD: Prenatal therapy in congenital adrenal hyperplasia. Attempted prevention of abnormal external genital masculinization by pharmacologic suppression of the fetal adrenal gland in utero. Ann N Y Acad Sci 458:156, 1985

Clark EB: Neck web and congenital heart defects: A pathogenic association in 45 X-O Turner syndrome? Teratology 29:355, 1984

Clayton-Smith J, Donnai D: Human malformations. In Rimoin DL, Connor JM, Pyeritz RE (eds): Emery and Rimoin's Principles and Practice of Medical Genetics, 3rd ed. New York, Churchill Livingston, 1996, p 383

Clayton-Smith H, Donnai D: Fetal valproate syndrome. J Med Genet 32:724, 1995

Cliver SP, Goldenberg RL, Lutter R, Hoffman H, Dans RO, Nelson KG: The effect of cigarette smoking on neonatal anthropometric measurements. Obstet Gynecol 85:625, 1995

Cohen LS, Friedman JM, Jefferson JW, Johnson EM, Weiner ML: A reevaluation of risk of in utero exposure to lithium. JAMA 271:1485, 1994a

Cohen HL, Sloves JH, Laungani S, Glass L, DeMarinis P: Neurosonographic findings in full-term infants born to maternal cocaine abusers: Visualization of subependymal and periventricular cysts. J Clin Ultrasound 22:327, 1994b

Cole CH, Rogers PC, Pritchard S, Phillips G, Chan KW: Thalidomide in the management of chronic graft-versus-host disease in children following bone marrow transplantation. Bone Marrow Transplant 14:937, 1994

Conway H: Effect of supplemental vitamin therapy on the

limitation of incidence of cleft lip and cleft palate in humans. Plast Reconstr Surg 22:450, 1958

Conway N, Birt DN: Streptomycin in pregnancy: Effect on the fetal ear. BMJ 2:260, 1965

Creinin MD, Vittinghoff E: Methotrexate and misoprostol vs misoprostol alone for early abortion: A randomized controlled trial. JAMA 272:1190, 1994

Csaba I, Sulyok FE, Ertl T: Relationship of maternal treatment with indomethacin to persistence of fetal circulation syndrome. J Pediatr 92:484, 1978

Czeizel A: Lack of evidence of teratogenicity of benzodiazepine drugs in Hungary. Reprod Toxicol 1:183, 1987/88

Czeizel AE, Pataki T, Rockenbauer M: Reproductive outcome after exposure to surgery under anesthesia during pregnancy. Arch Gynecol Obstet 261:193, 1998

Czeizel AE, Rockenbauer M: Population-based case-control study of teratogenic potential of corticosteroids. Teratology 56:335, 1997

D'Souza SW, Black P, Richards B: Smoking in pregnancy: Associations with skinfold thickness, maternal weight gain, and fetal size at birth. BMJ 282:1661, 1981

Dai WS, Hsu MA, Itri LM: Safety of pregnancy after discontinuation of isotretinoin. Arch Dermatol 125:362, 1989

Dai WS, LaBraico JM, Stern RS: Epidemiology of isotretinoin exposure during pregnancy. J Am Acad Dermatol 26:599, 1992

Dally A: Thalidomide: Was the tragedy preventable? Lancet 351:1197, 1998

Dansky LV, Andermann E, Rosenblatt D, Sherwin AL, Andermann F: Anticonvulsants, folate levels, and pregnancy outcome: A prospective study. Ann Neurol 21:176, 1987

Dansky LV, Andermann E, Sherwin AL, Andermann F, Kinch RA: Maternal epilepsy and congenital malformations: A prospective study with monitoring of plasma anticonvulsant levels during pregnancy. Neurology 3:15, 1980

Davidson JM, Dallagrammatikas H, Parkin JM: Maternal azathioprine therapy and depressed hemopoiesis in the babies of renal allograft patients. Br J Obstet Gynaecol 92:233, 1985

De Catte L, De Wolf D, Smitz J, Bougatef A, De Schepper J, Foulon W: Fetal hypothyroidism as a complication of amiodarone treatment for persistent fetal supraventricular tachycardia. Prenat Diagn 14:762, 1994

Dean JL, Wolf JE, Ranzini AC, Laughlin MA: Use of amphotericin B during pregnancy: Case report and review. Clin Infect Dis 18:364, 1994

Del Campo M, Kosaki K, Bennett FC, Jones KL: Developmental delay in fetal aminopterin/methotrexate syndrome. Teratology 60:10, 1999

DeWitte DB, Buick MK, Cyran SE, Maisels MJ: Neonatal pancytopenia and severe combined immunodeficiency associated with antenatal administration of azathioprine and prednisone. J Pediatr 105:625, 1984

DiGiovanna JJ, Zezh LA, Ruddel ME, Gantt G, McClean SW, Gross EG, Peck GL: Etretinate: Persistent serum levels of a potent teratogen. Clin Res 32:579A, 1984

DiSessa TG, Moretti ML, Khouri A, Pulliam DA, Arheart RL, Sibar BM: Cardiac function in fetuses and newborns exposed to low dose aspirin during pregnancy. Am J Obstet Gynecol 171:892, 1994

Dittman RW, Kappes ME, Kappes MH: Sexual behavior in adolescent and adult females with congenital adrenal hyperplasia. Psychoneuroendocrinology 17:153, 1992

Dittman RW, Kappes MH, Kappes ME, Borger D, Stegner H, Willig RH, Wallis H: Congenital adrenal hyperplasia I: Gender-related behavior and attitudes in female patients and sisters. Psychoneuroendocrinology 15:401, 1990

Dombrowski MP, Brown CL, Berry SM: Preliminary experience with triamcinolone acetonide during pregnancy. J Matern Fetal Med 5:310, 1996

Donaldson J: Neurology of Pregnancy, 2nd ed. Philadelphia, Saunders, 1989, p 229

Dudley DKL, Hardie MJ: Fetal and neonatal effects of indomethacin used as a tocolytic agent. Am J Obstet Gynecol 151:181, 1985

Dumesic DA, Silverman NH, Tobias S, Golbus MS: Transplacental cardioversion of fetal supraventricular tachycardia with procainamide. N Engl J Med 307:1128, 1982

Duna GF, Cash JM: Treatment of refractory cutaneous lupus erythematosus. Rheum Dis Clin North Am 21:99, 1995

Elia J, Katz IR, Simpson GM: Teratogenicity of psychotherapeutic medications. Psychopharmacol Bull 23:531, 1987

Esaki K: Effects of inhalant administration of beclomethasone dipropionate on reproduction in mice. CIEA Preclin Rep 2:213, 1976

Faiella A, Zappavigna V, Mavilio F, Boncinelli E: Inhibition of retinoic acid-induced activation of 3′ human HOXB genes by antisense oligonucleotides affects sequential activation of genes located upstream in the four HOX clusters. Proc Natl Acad Sci USA 7:5335, 1994

Farkas VG, Farkas G: Teratogenic action of hyperemesis in pregnancy and of medication used to treat it. Zentralbl Gynaekol 93:325, 1971

Fejgin MD, Lourwood DL: Low molecular weight heparins and their use in obstetrics and gynecology. Obstet Gynecol Surv 49:424, 1994

Feldcamp M, Carey JC: Clinical teratology counseling and consultation case report: Low dose methotrexate exposure in the early weeks of pregnancy. Teratology 47:533, 1993

Fitzsimons R, Greenberger PA, Patterson R: Outcome of pregnancy in women requiring corticosteroids for severe asthma. J Allergy Clin Immunol 78:349, 1986

Food and Drug Administration: Drug bulletin. Fed Reg 44:37434, 1980

Friedman JM: Teratogen update: Anesthetic agents. Teratology 37:69, 1988

Friedman JM, Little BB, Brent RL, Cordero JF, Hanson JW, Shepard TH: Potential human teratogenicity of frequently prescribed drugs. Obstet Gynecol 75:594, 1990

Geiger JM, Baudin M, Saurat JH: Teratogenic risk with etretinate and acitretin treatment. Dermatology 189:109, 1994

German J, Kowal A, Ellers KH: Trimethadione and human teratogenesis. Teratology 3:349, 1970

Gilstrap LC, Bawdon RE, Burris JS: Antibiotic concentration in maternal blood, cord blood, and placental membranes in chorioamnionitis. Obstet Gynecol 72:124, 1988

Ginsberg JS, Hirsh J: Anticoagulants during pregnancy. Ann Rev Med 40:79, 1989

Giusti RM, Iwamoto K, Hatch EE: Diethylstilbestrol revisited: A review of the long-term health effects. Ann Intern Med 122:778, 1995

Glantz JC: Reproductive toxicology of alkylating agents. Obstet Gynecol Surv 49:709, 1994

Golden NL, Kuhnert BR, Sokol RJ, Martier S, Williams T: Neonatal manifestations of maternal phencyclidine exposure. J Perinat Med 15:185, 1987

Goldstein DJ, Corbin LA, Sundell KL: Effects of first-trimester fluoxetine exposure on the newborn. Obstet Gynecol 89:713, 1997

Goldstein DJ, Marvel DE, Lily E: Psychotropic medications during pregnancy: Risk to the fetus. JAMA 270:2177, 1993

Gomby DS, Shiono PH: Estimating the number of substance-exposed infants. Future Child 1:17, 1991

Green TP, Thompson TR, Johnson DE, Lock JE: Furosemide promotes patent ductus arteriosus in premature infants with the respiratory-distress syndrome. N Engl J Med 308:743, 1983

Greenberger PA, Patterson R: Beclomethasone dipropionate for severe asthma during pregnancy. Ann Intern Med 98:478, 1983

Greenland S, Richwald GA, Honda GD: The effects of marijuana use during pregnancy, 2. A study in a low-risk home-delivery population. Drug Alcohol Depend 11:359, 1983

Grosso S, Berardi R, Cioni M, Morgese G: Transient neonatal hypothyroidism after gestational exposure to amiodarone: A follow-up of two cases. J Endocrinol Invest 21:699, 1998

Grumbach MM, Ducharme JR: The effects of androgens on fetal sexual development. Androgen-induced female pseudohermaphrodism. Fertil Steril 11:157, 1960

Gudas LJ: Retinoids and vertebrate development [review]. J Biol Chem 269:15399, 1994

Hall JG, Pauli RM, Wilson K: Maternal and fetal sequelae of anticoagulation during pregnancy. Am J Med 68:122, 1980

Hanson JW: Human teratology. In Rimoin DL, Connor JM, Pyeritz RE (eds): Emery and Rimoin's Principles and Practice of Medical Genetics, 3rd ed. New York, Churchill Livingston, 1996, p 697

Hanson JW, Myrianthopoulos NC, Harvey MS, Smith DW: Risks to the offspring of women treated with hydantoin anticonvulsants, with emphasis on the fetal hydantoin syndrome. J Pediatr 89:662, 1976

Hanson JW, Smith DW: The fetal hydantoin syndrome. J Pediatr 87:285, 1975

Harrigan JT, Kangos JJ, Sikka KR, Spisso KR, Natarajan N, Rosenfeld D, Leiman S, Korn D: Successful treatment of fetal congestive failure secondary to tachycardia. N Engl J Med 304:1527, 1981

Hatjis CG, Meis PJ: Sinusoidal fetal heart rate pattern associated with butorphanol administration. Obstet Gynecol 67:377, 1986

Heinonen OP, Slone D, Shapiro S: Birth Defects and Drugs in Pregnancy. Littleton, MA, John Wright Publishing Sciences Group, 1983

Heinonen OP, Slone D, Shapiro S: Birth defects and drugs in pregnancy. Littleton, MA, Publishing Sciences Group, 1977, p 441

Hengst VP: Investigations of the teratogenicity of Daraprim (pyrimethamine) in humans. Zentralbl Gynakol 94:551, 1972

Herbst AL, Ulfelder H, Poskanzer DC: Adenocarcinoma of the vagina. Association of maternal stilbestrol therapy. N Engl J Med 284:878, 1971

Hermans PE, Wilhelm MP: Vancomycin. Mayo Clin Proc 62:901, 1987

Hickok DE, Hollenbach KA, Reilley SF, Nyberg DA: The association between decreased amniotic fluid volume and treatment with nonsteroidal anti-inflammatory agents for preterm labor. Am J Obstet Gynecol 160:1525, 1989

Hiilesmaa VK, Teramo K, Granstrom ML, Brady AH: Serum folate concentrations in women with epilepsy. BMJ 287:577, 1983

Hirsch KS, Wilson JG, Scott WJ, Oflaherty EJ: Acetazolamide teratology and its association with carbonic anhydrase inhibition in the mouse. Teratogenesis Carcinog Mutagen 3:133, 1983

Holzman C, Paneth N, Little R, Pinto-Martin J, and the Neonatal Brain Hemorrhage Study Team: Perinatal brain injury in premature infants born to mothers using alcohol in pregnancy. Pediatrics 94:66, 1995

Horning MG, Stratton C, Wilson A, Horning EC, Hill RM: Detection of 5-(3,4)-diphenylhydantoin in the newborn human. Anal Lett 4:537, 1974

Horvath JS, Phippard A, Korda A, Henderson-Smart DS, Child A, Tiller DJ: Clonidine hydrochloride: A safe and effective antihypertensive agent in pregnancy. Obstet Gynecol 66:634, 1985

Hoyme HE, Jones KL, Dixon SD, Jewett T, Hanson JW, Robinson LK, Msaii ME, Allanson JE: Prenatal cocaine exposure and fetal vascular disruption. Pediatrics 85:743, 1990

Hume RF Jr, Martin LS, Bottoms SF, Hassan SS, Banker-Collins K, Tomlinson M, Johnson MP, Evans MI: Vascular disruption birth defects and history of prenatal cocaine exposure: A case control study. Fetal Diagn Ther 12:292, 1997

Hwang SJ, Beaty TH, Panny SR, Street NA, Joseph JH, Gordon S, McIntosh I, Francomano CA: Association study of transforming growth factor alpha (TGFα) Tag 1 polymorphism and oral clefts. Am J Epidemiol 14:629, 1995

Iahnaccone PM, Bossert NL, Connelly CS: Disruption of embryonic and fetal development due to preimplantation chemical insults: A critical review. Am J Obstet Gynecol 157:476, 1987

Jacobson JL, Jacobson SW, Sokol RJ, Ager JW: Relation of maternal age and pattern of pregnancy drinking to functionally significant cognitive deficit in infancy. Alcohol Clin Exp Res 22:345, 1998

Jacobson JL, Jacobson SW, Sokol RJ, Martier SS, Ager JW, Kaplan-Estrin MG: Teratogenic effects of alcohol on infant development. Alcohol Clin Exp Res 17:174, 1993

Jacobson SJ, Jones K, Johnson K, Ceolin L, Kaur P, Sahn D, Donnenfeld AE, Rieder M, Santelli R, Smythe J, Pastuszak A, Einarson T, Koren G: Prospective multicentre study of pregnancy outcome after lithium exposure during first trimester. Lancet 339:530, 1992

Jelovsek FR, Mattison DR, Chen JJ: Prediction of risk for human developmental toxicity: How important are animal studies for hazard identification? Obstet Gynecol 74:624, 1989

Jick H, Holmes LB, Hunter JR, Madsen S, Stergachis A: First-trimester drug use and congenital disorders. JAMA 246:343, 1981

Jick SS, Terris BZ, Jick H: First trimester topical tretinoin and congenital disorders. Lancet 341:1664, 1993

Jones HC: Intrauterine ototoxicity: A case report and review of the literature. J Natl Med Assoc 65:201, 1973

Jones KL, Lacro RV, Johnson KA, Adams J: Patterns of malformations in the children of women treated with carbamazepine during pregnancy. N Engl J Med 320:1661, 1989

Kandall SR, Gaines J, Habel L, Davidson G, Jessop D: Relationship of maternal substance abuse to subsequent sudden infant death syndrome in offspring. J Pediatr 123:120, 1993

Kaufman RH, Adam E, Binder Gl, Gerthoffer E: Upper genital tract changes and pregnancy outcome in offspring exposed in utero to diethylstilbestrol. Am J Obstet Gynecol 137:299, 1980

Kaufman RH, Adam E, Hatch EE, Noller K, Herbst AL, Palmer JR, Hoover RN: Continued follow-up of pregnancy outcomes in diethylstilbestrol-exposed offspring. Obstet Gynecol 96:483, 2000

Keller DM: Teratogenic effects of carbamazepine. Correspondence to the editor. N Engl J Med 321:1480, 1989

Kelly TE: Teratogenicity of anticonvulsant drugs. 1. Review of the literature. Am J Med Gen 19:413, 1984

Kerenyi TD, Gleicher N, Meller J, Brown E, Steinfeld L, Chitkara U, Raucher H: Transplacental cardioversion of intrauterine supraventricular tachycardia with digitalis. Lancet 2:393, 1980

Khouri MI, James IM, Flanders WD, Erickson JD: Interpretation of recurring weak association obtained from epidemiologic studies of suspected human teratogens. Teratology, 46:69, 1992

Killeen AA, Bowers LD: Fetal supraventricular tachycardia treated with high-dose quinidine: Toxicity associated with marked elevation of the metabolite, 3(S)-3-hydroxyquinidine. Obstet Gynecol 70:445, 1987

Kimmel CA, Generoso WM, Thomas RD, Bakshi KS: A new frontier in understanding the mechanisms of developmental abnormalities. Toxicol Appl Pharmacol 119:159, 1993

Kirshon B, Wasserstrum N, Willis R, Herman GE, McCabe ERB: Teratogenic effects of first trimester cyclophosphamide therapy. Obstet Gynecol 72:462, 1988

Knapp K, Lenz W, Nowack E: Multiple congenital abnormalities. Lancet 2:725, 1962

Koren G, Bologa M, Long D, Feldman Y, Shear NH: Perception of teratogenic risk by pregnant women exposed to drugs and chemicals during the first trimester. Am J Obstet Gynecol 160:1190, 1989

Koren G, Pastuszak A, Ito S: Drugs in pregnancy. N Engl J Med 338:1128, 1998

Kramer WB, Belfort M, Saade GR, Surani S, Moise KJ: Successful urokinase treatment of massive pulmonary embolism in pregnancy. Obstet Gynecol 86:600, 1995

Kutscher AH, Zegarelli EV, Tovell HM, Hochberg B, Hauptman J: Discoloration of deciduous teeth induced by administration of tetracycline antepartum. Am J Obstet Gynecol 96:291, 1966

La Valleur J, Molina E, Williams PP, Rolnick SJ: Use of urokinase in pregnancy. Two success stories. Postgrad Med 99:269; 272, 1996

Laegrid L, Olegard R, Walstrom J, Conradi N: Teratogenic effects of benzodiazepine use during pregnancy. J Pediatr 114:126, 1989

Lammer EJ: Embryopathy in infant conceived one year after termination of maternal etretinate. Lancet 2:1080, 1988

Lammer EJ, Chen DT, Hoar RM, Agnish ND, Benke PJ, Braun JT, Curry CJ, Fernhoff PM, Griz AW Jr, Lott IT, Richard JM, Sun SC: Retinoic acid embryopathy. N Engl J Med 313:837, 1985

Lammer EJ, Hayes AM, Schunior A, Holmes LB: Risk for major malformation among human fetuses exposed to isotretinoin (13-cis-retinoic acid). Teratology 35:68A, 1987

Landers DV, Green JR, Sweet RL: Antibiotic use during pregnancy and the postpartum period. Clin Obstet Gynecol 26:391, 1983

Lee EJD: Population genetics of the angiotensin-converting enzyme in Chinese. Br J Clin Pharmacol 37:212, 1994

Lee H, Nagel RG: Toxic and teratologic effects of verapamil on early chick embryos: Evidence for the involvement of calcium in neural tube closure. Teratology 33:203, 1986

Lemoine P: Les enfants de parents alcooliques. Ovest Med 21:476, 1968

Lenke RR, VanDorsten JP, Schifrin BS: Pyelonephritis in pregnancy: A prospective randomized trial to prevent recurrent disease evaluating suppressive therapy with nitrofu-

rantoin and close surveillance. Am J Obstet Gynecol 146:953, 1983

Leppik IE, Rask CA: Pharmacokinetics of antiepileptic drugs during pregnancy. Semin Neurol 8:240, 1988

Lewis PE, Cefalo RC, Naulty JS, Rodkey FL: Placental transfer and fetal toxicity of sodium nitroprusside. Gynecol Invest 8:46, 1977

Lifschitz MH, Wilson GS, Smith EO, Desmond MM: Fetal and postnatal growth of children born to narcotic-dependent women. J Pediatr 102:686, 1983

Lindhout D, Rene JE, Hoppener A, Meinardi H: Teratogenicity of antiepileptic drug combinations with special emphasis on epioxidation of carbamazepine. Epilepsia 25:77, 1984

Linn S, Schoenbaum SC, Monson RR, Rosner R, Stubblefield PC, Ryan KJ: The association of marijuana use with outcome of pregnancy. Am J Public Health 73:1161, 1983

Little BB, Snell LM, Gilstrap LC: Methamphetamine abuse during pregnancy: Outcome and fetal effects. Obstet Gynecol 72:541, 1988

Little BB, Snell LM, Gilstrap LC, Breckenridge JD, Knoll KA: Effects of ts and blues abuse during pregnancy on maternal and infant health status. Am J Perinatol 7:359, 1990a

Little BB, Snell LM, Gilstrap LC, Gant NF, Rosenfeld CR: Alcohol abuse during pregnancy: Changes in frequency in a large urban hospital. Obstet Gynecol 74:547, 1989a

Little BB, Snell LM, Gilstrap LC, Johnston WL: A review of patterns of substance abuse during pregnancy: Implications for the mother and fetus. South Med J 83:507, 1990b

Little BB, Snell LM, Klein VR, Gilstrap LC: Cocaine abuse during pregnancy: Maternal and fetal implications. Obstet Gynecol 73:157, 1989b

Little BB, Snell LM, Klein VR, Gilstrap LC, Knoll KA, Breckenridge JD: Maternal and fetal effects of heroin addiction during pregnancy. J Reprod Med 35:159, 1990c

Long SY: Does LSD induce chromosomal damage and malformations? A review of the literature. Teratology 6:75, 1972

Ludwig H: Results of streptokinase therapy in deep venous thrombosis during pregnancy. Postgrad Med J 49:65, 1973

Macaulay JH, Bond K, Steer PJ: Epidural analgesia in labor and fetal hyperthermia. Obstet Gynecol 80:665, 1992

Magee LA, Schick B, Donnenfeld, Sage SR, Conover B, Cook L, McElhatton PR, Schmidt MA, Koren G: The safety of calcium channel blockers in human pregnancy: A prospective, multicenter cohort study. Am J Obstet Gynecol 174:823, 1996

Major CA, Lewis DF, Harding JA, Porto MA, Garite TJ: Tocolysis with indomethacin increases the incidence of necrotizing enterocolitis in the low-birth-weight neonate. Am J Obstet Gynecol 170:102, 1994

Manson JM, Papa L, Miller ML, Boyd C: Studies of DNA damage and cell death in embryonic limb buds induced by teratogenic exposure to cyclophosphamide. Teratog Carcinog Mutagen 2:47, 1982

Martinez-Frias ML, Czeizel AE, Rodriguez-Pinilla E, Bermejo E: Smoking during pregnancy and Poland sequence: Results of a population-based registry and a case-control registry. Teratology 59:35, 1999

Mastroiacovo P, Mazzone T, Addis A, Elephant E, Carlier P, Vial T, Garbis H, Robert E, Bonati M, Ornoy A, Finardi A, Schaffer C, Caramelli L, Rodriguez-Pinilla E, Clementi M: High vitamin A intake in early pregnancy and major malformations: A multicenter prospective controlled study. Teratology 59:7, 1999

Mazze RI, Kallen B: Reproductive outcome after anesthesia

and operation during pregnancy a registry study of 5405 cases. Am J Obstet Gynecol 161:1178, 1989

McKeague PM, Lamm SH, Linn S, Kutcher JS: Bendectin and birth defects: I. A metal analysis of the epidemiologic studies. Teratology 50:27, 1994

Meadow SR: Anticonvulsant drugs and congenital abnormalities. Lancet 2:1296, 1968

Melnick S, Cole P, Anderson D, Herbst A: Rates and risks of diethylstilbestrol-related clear-cell adenocarcinoma of the vagina and cervix. N Engl J Med 316:514, 1987

Messina M, Biffignandi P, Ghigo E, Jeantet MG, Molinatti GM: Possible contraindication of spironolactone during pregnancy. J Endocrinol Invest 2:222, 1979

Meyer-Bahlburg HFL, Gruen RS, New MI, Bell JJ, Morishima A, et al: Gender change from female to male in classical congenital adrenal hyperplasia. Horm Behav 3:319, 1996

Milkovich L, van den Berg BJ: Effects of antenatal exposure to anorectic drugs. Am J Obstet Gynecol 129:637, 1977

Morrell MJ: The new antiepileptic drugs and women: Efficacy reproductive health, pregnancy, and fetal outcome. Epilepsia 37:S34, 1996

Mortola JF: The use of psychotropic agents in pregnancy and lactation. Psychiatr Clin North Am 12:69, 1989

Murad SH, Tabsh KM, Shilyanski G, Kapur PA, Ma C, Lee C, Conklin KA: Effects of verapamil on uterine blood flow and maternal cardiovascular function in the awake pregnant ewe. Anesth Analg 64:7, 1985

Murray JC: Face facts: Genes, environment, and clefts. Am J Hum Genet 57:3227, 1995

Nakane Y, Okuma T, Takahashi R, Sato Y, Wada T, Sato T, et al: Multi-institutional study on the teratogenicity and fetal toxicity of antiepileptic drugs: A report of a collaborative study group in Japan. Epilepsia 21:663, 1980

Nelson BK, Moorman WJ, Schrader SM: Review of experimental male-mediated behavioral and neurochemical disorders. Neurotoxicol 18:611, 1996

Nelson-Piercy C, Letsky EA, de Swiet M: Low-molecular-weight heparin for obstetric thromboprophylaxis: experience of sixty-nine pregnancies in sixty-one women at high risk. Am J Obstet Gynecol 176:1062, 1997

Niebyl JR: Management of nausea and vomiting in pregnancy: traditional therapies. Contemp Ob/Gyn 45:130, 2000

Niebyl JR: Perinatal effects of indomethacin. Biweekly Rev Clin Obstet Gynecol 11:22, 1991

Niebyl JR, Blake D, White R, Kumor KM, Dubin NH, Robinson JC, Egnor PG: The inhibition of premature labor with indomethacin. Am J Obstet Gynecol 136:1014, 1980

Nora JJ, Vargo TA, Nora AH, Love KE, McNamara DG: Dexamphetamine: A possible environmental trigger in cardiovascular malformations. Lancet 1:1290, 1970

Norton ME, Merrill J, Cooper BA, Kuller JA, Clyman RI: Neonatal complications after the administration of indomethacin for preterm labor. N Engl J Med 329:1602, 1993

Oakley GP, Erickson JD: Vitamin A and birth defects. N Engl J Med 333:1414, 1995

Oguro Y: Pharmacological and toxicological studies on beclomethasone dipropionate. Yamaguch Igaku 19:65, 1970

Okuma T, Takahashi R, Wada T: A collaborative study of the teratogenicity and fetal toxicity of antiepileptic drugs in Japan. In Wada A, Penry JK (eds): Advances in Epileptology: The 10th Epilepsy International Symposium. New York, Raven, 1980, p 511

Olshan AF, Teschke K, Baird PA: Paternal occupation and congenital anomalies. Am J Ind Med 20:447, 1991

Omtzigt JGC, Los RJ, Grobbee DE, Pijpers L, Jahoda MGJ, Brandenburg H, et al: The risk of spina bifida aperta after first trimester valproate exposure in a prenatal cohort. Neurology 42(S5):119, 1992

Ondrizek RR, Chan PJ, Patton WC, King A: An alternative medicine study of herbal effects on the penetration of zona-free hamster oocytes and the integrity of sperm deoxyribonucleic acid. Fertil Steril 71:517, 1999

Orkin M, Maibach HI: Scabies and pediculosis pubis. Dermatol Clin 1:111, 1983

Ostrea EM, Chavez CJ: Perinatal problems (excluding neonatal withdrawal) in maternal drug addiction: A study of 830 cases. J Pediatr 94:292, 1979

Owen J, Clovin EV, Davis RO: Fetal death after successful conversion of fetal supraventricular tachycardia with digoxin and verapamil. Am J Obstet Gynecol 158:1169, 1988

Pastuszak A, Schick-Boschetto B, Ziber C, Feldkamp M, Pirelli M, Sihn S, et al: Pregnancy outcome following first-trimester exposure to fluoxetine. JAMA 269:2246, 1993

Persutte WH, Wass T, Hobbins J: Assessment of facial and intracranial biometry using prenatal ultrasound in identifying fetal alcohol syndrome/effects: A pilot study. Am J Obstet Gynecol 174:433, 1996

Piper JM, Baum C, Kennedy DL: Prescription drug use before and during pregnancy in a Medicaid population. Am J Obstet Gynecol 157:148, 1987

Piper JM, Mitchell EF, Ray WA: Prenatal use of metronidazole and birth defects: No association. Obstet Gynecol 82:348, 1993

Pons JC, Taburet AM, Singlas E, Delfraissy JF, Papiernik E: Placental passage of azathiothymidine (AZT) during the second trimester of pregnancy: study by direct fetal blood sampling under ultrasound. Eur J Obstet Gynecol Reprod Biol 40:229, 1991

Prahalada S, Carroad E, Hendrickx AG: Embryotoxicity and maternal serum concentrations of medroxyprogesterone acetate (MPA) in baboons (Papio cynocephalus). Contraception 32:497, 1985

Pryde PG, Sedman AB, Nugent CE, Barr M Jr: Angiotensin-converting enzyme inhibitor fetopathy. J Am Soc Nephrol 3:1575, 1993

Public Health Service Task Force: Recommendations for use of antiretroviral drugs in pregnant HIV-1 infected women for maternal health and interventions to reduce perinatal HIV-1 transmission in the United States. November, 2000

Raman-Wilms L, Lin-in Tseng A, Wighardt S, Einarson TR, Koren G: Fetal genital effects of first-trimester sex hormone exposure: A meta-analysis. Obstet Gynecol 85:141, 1995

Ramin SM, Little BB, Trimmer KJ, Standard DI, Blakeley CA, Snell LM: Methamphetamine use during pregnancy. Am J Obstet Gynecol 166:353, 1992

Reinisch JM, Sanders SA, Mortensen EL, Rubin DB: In utero exposure to phenobarbital and intelligence deficits in adult men. JAMA 274:1518, 1995

Reprotox: Reproductive Toxicology Center: Enflurane. 2000a, http://reprotox.org/data/2680.html

Reprotox: Reproductive Toxicology Center: Isoflurane. 2000b, http://reprotox.org/data/1252.html

Reprotox: Reproductive Toxicology Center: Labetalol. 2000c, http://reprotox.org/data/2175.html

Reprotox: Reproductive Toxicology Center: Metoclopramide. 2000d, http://reprotox.org/data/1135.html

Reprotox: Reproductive Toxicology Center: Oseltamivir. 2000e, http://reprotox.org/data/4141.html

Reprotox: Reproductive Toxicology Center: Thalidomide. 2000f, http://reprotox.org/data/2487.html

Reprotox: Reproductive Toxicology Center: Amphetamines, 2000g, http://reprotox.org/data

Rey E, Duperron L, Gautheir R, Lemay M, Grignon A, Le Lorier J: Transplacental treatment of tachycardia-induced fetal heart failure with verapamil and amiodarone: A case report. Am J Obstet Gynecol 153:311, 1985

Rigat B, Hubert C, Alhenc-Gelas F, Cambien F, Corvol P, Soubrier F: An insertion/deletion polymorphism in the angiotensin I-converting enzyme gene accounting for half the variance of serum enzyme levels. J Clinic Invest 86:1343, 1990

Robaire B, Hales BF: Paternal exposure to chemicals before conception. BMJ 307:341, 1993

Robboy SJ, Noller KL, OBrien P, Kaufman RH, Townsend D, Barnes AB, Gundersen J, Lawrence D, Bergstrahl E, McGorray S, Tilley BC, Anton J, Chazen G: Increased incidence of cervical and vaginal dysplasia in 3,980 diethylstilbestrol-exposed young women. Experience of the National Collaborative Diethylstilbestrol Adenosis Project. JAMA 252:2979, 1984

Robert E, Robert JM, Lapras C: Is valproic acid teratogenic? Rev Neurol 139:445, 1983

Rosa FW, Baum C, Shaw M: Pregnancy outcomes after first trimester vaginitis drug therapy. Obstet Gynecol 69:751, 1987b

Rosa FW, Hernandez C, Carlo WA: Griseofulvin teratology, including two thoracopagus conjoined twins. Lancet 1:171, 1987a

Rothman KJ, Moore LL, Singer MR, Nguyen UDT, Mannino S, Milunsky A: Teratogenicity of high vitamin A intake. N Engl J Med 333:1369, 1995

Rotmensch HH, Elkayam U, Frishman W: Antiarrhythmic drug therapy during pregnancy. Ann Intern Med 98:487, 1983

Rotmensch HH, Rotmensch S, Elkayam U: Management of cardiac arrhythmias during pregnancy: Current concepts. Drugs 33:623, 1987

Rowe I: Prescriptions of psychotropic drugs by general practitioners: Antidepressants. Med J Aust 1:642, 1973

Rowland AS, Baird DD, Weinberg CR, Shore DL, Shy CM, Wilcox AJ: Reduced fertility among women employed as dental assistants exposed to high levels of nitrous oxide. N Engl J Med 327:993, 1992

Sabik JF, Assad RS, Hanley FL: Halothane as an anesthetic for fetal surgery. J Pediatr Surg 28:542, 1993

Sadler TW: Langman's Medical Embryology, 6th ed. Baltimore, MD, Williams & Wilkins, 1990

Salle B, Sergeant P, Awada A, Bied-Damon V, Gaucherand P, Boisson C, Guibaud S, Benchaib M, Rudigoz RC: Transvaginal ultrasound studies of vascular and morphological changes in uteri exposed to diestilbestrol in utero. Hum Reprod 11:2531, 1996

Savitz DA, Sonnenfeld N, Olshan AF: Review of epidemiological studies of paternal occupational exposure and spontaneous abortion. Am J Ind Med 25:361, 1994

Schardein JL: Congenital abnormalities and hormones during pregnancy: A clinical review. Teratology 22:251, 1985

Schneider DM, von Tempelhoff G-F, Heilmann L: Retrospective evaluation on the safety and efficacy of low-molecular-weight heparin as thromboprophylaxi during pregnancy. Am J Obstet Gynecol 177:1567, 1997

Schnitzer PG, Olshan AF, Erickson JD: Paternal occupation and risk of birth defects in the offspring. Epidemiology 6:577, 1995

Schubiger G, Flury G, Nussberger J: Enalapril for pregnancy-induced hypertension: Acute renal failure in the neonate. Ann Int Med 108:215, 1988

Scialli AR, Lione A: Teratogenic effects of carbamazepine. Correspondence to the editor. N Engl J Med 321:1480, 1989

Scolnik D, Nulman I, Rovet J, Gladstone D, Czuchta D, Gardner A, Gladstone R, Ashby P, Weksberg R, Einarson T, Koren G: Neurodevelopment of children exposed in utero to phenytoin and carbamazepine monotherapy. JAMA 271:767, 1994

Scott JM, Weir DG, Molloy A, McPartlin J, Daly L, Kirke P: Folic acid metabolism and mechanisms of neural tube defects. Ciba Foundation Symposium. Manchester, England, John Wiley, 1994, p 181

Shaw GM, Velie EM, Schaffer D: Risk of neural tube defect-affected pregnancies among obese women. JAMA 275:1093, 1996

Sheehan DM: Herbal medicines, phytoestrogens and toxicity: Risk:benefit considerations. Proc Soc Exp Biol Med 217:379, 1998

Shepard TH: Catalog of Teratogenic Agents, 9th ed. Baltimore, John Hopkins University Press, 1998

Shepard TH: Catalog of Teratogenic Agents, 6th ed. Baltimore, Johns Hopkins University Press, 1989

Shepard TH: Human teratogenicity. Adv Pediatr 33:225, 1986

Shiono PH, Klebanoff MA, Nugent RP, Cotch MF, Wilkins DG, Rollins DE, Carey JC, Behrman RE: The impact of cocaine and marijuana use on low birth weight and preterm birth: A multicenter study. Am J Obstet Gynecol 172:19, 1995

Shnider SM, Levinson G: Anesthesia for surgery during pregnancy. In Shnider SM, Levinson G (eds): Anesthesia for Obstetrics, 2nd ed. Baltimore, Williams & Wilkins, 1987, p 188

Sibai BM, Barton JR, Sarinoglu C, Mercer BM: A randomized prospective comparison of nifedipine and bed rest alone in the management of preeclampsia remote from term. Am J Obstet Gynecol 166:280, 1992

Sibai BM, Gonzalez AR, Mabie WC, Moretti M: A comparison of labetalol plus hospitalization versus hospitalization alone in the management of preeclampsia remote from term. Obstet Gynecol 70:323, 1987

Sibai BM, Mabie WC, Shamsa F, Villar GD: A comparison of no medication versus methyldopa or labetalol in chronic hypertension during pregnancy. Am J Obstet Gynecol 162:960, 1990

Slone D, Sikskind V, Heinonen OP, Manson RR, Kaufman DW, Shapiro S: Antenatal exposure to the phorothiazines in relation to congenital malformations, perinatal mortality rate, birth weight, and intelligence quotient score. Am J Obstet Gynecol 128:486, 1977

Slone D, Siskind V, Heinonen OP, Manson RR, Kaufman DW, Shapiro S: Aspirin and congenital malformations. Lancet 1:1372, 1976

Smith OW: Diethylstilbestrol in the prevention and treatment of complications of pregnancy. Am J Obstet Gynecol 46:821, 1948

Snyder DE, Layde PM, Johnson MW, Lyle MA: Treatment of tuberculosis during pregnancy. Am Rev Respir Dis 122:65, 1980

Soprano DR, Soprano KJ: Retinoids as teratogens. Annu Rev Nutr 15:111, 1995

Speroff L, Glass RH, Kase NG: Normal and abnormal sexual development. In: Clinical Gynecologic Endocrinology and Infertility, 5th ed. Baltimore, Williams & Wilkins, 1994, 321

St. Clair SM, Schirmer RG: First trimester exposure to alprazolam. Obstet Gynecol 80:843, 1992

Stavrous C, Hofmeyer GJ, Boezaart AP: Prolonged fetal bradycardia during epidural analgesia. S Afr Med J 77: 66, 1990

Stevenson RE: Causes of human anomalies: An overview and historical perspective. Human malformations and related anomalies. In Stevenson RE, Hall JG, Goodman RM (eds): Human Malformations and Related Anomalies. New York, Oxford University Press, 1993a, p 3

Stevenson RE: The environmental basis of human anomalies. In Stevenson RE, Hall JG, Goodman RM (eds): Human malformations and Related Anomalies. New York, Oxford University Press, 1993b, p. 137

Stillman RJ: In utero exposure to diethylstilbestrol: Adverse effects on the reproductive tract and reproductive performance in male and female offspring. Am J Obstet Gynecol 142:905, 1982

Stimmel B, Adamsons K: Narcotic dependency in pregnancy. Methadone maintenance compared to use of street drugs. JAMA 235:1121, 1976

Streissguth AP, Clarren SK, Jones KL: Natural history of the fetal alcohol syndrome: A 10-year follow-up of eleven patients. Lancet 2:85, 1985

Streissguth AP, Treder RP, Barr HM, Shepard TH, Bleyer WA, Sampson PD, Martin DC: Aspirin and acetaminophen use by pregnant women and subsequent child IQ and attention decrements. Teratology 35:211, 1987

Sullivan WC: The children of the female drunkard. Med Temp Rev 1:72, 1900

Sutton C, McIvor RS, Vagt M, Doggett B, Kapur RP: Methotrexate-resistant form of dihydroreductase protests transgenic murine embryos from teratogenic effects of methotrexate. Pediatr Dev Pathol 1:503, 1998

Tanimura T, Owaki Y, Nishimura H: Effect of administration of thiopental sodium to pregnant mice upon the development of their offspring. Okaji-mas Folia Anat Jpn 43:219, 1967

Teratology Society Public Affairs Committee, Teratology Society, Reston, VA, 1994

Thomson EJ, Cordero JF: The new teratogens: Accutane and other vitamin-A analogs. MCN 14:244, 1989

Trasler JM, Doerksen T: Teratogen update: Paternal exposures—reproductive risks. Teratology 60:161, 1999

Turner G, Collins E: Fetal effects of regular salicylate ingestion in pregnancy. Lancet 2:338, 1975

Turrentine MA, Braems G, Ramirez MM: Use of thrombolytics for the treatment of thromboembolic disease during pregnancy. Obstet Gynecol Surv 50:534, 1995

Valacyclovir Pregnancy Registry: Interim report. Project office. Glaxo Wellcom, Research Triangle Park, NC, July 31, 1998

Van Bel F, Van Zoeren D, Schipper J, Guit GL, Baan J: Effect of indomethacin on superior mesenteric artery blood flow velocity in preterm infants. J Pediatrics 116:965, 1990

Van Dyke DC, Hodge SE, Heide F, Hill LR: Family studies in fetal phenytoin exposure. J Pediatr 113:301, 1988

Vega WA, Kolody B, Hwang J, Noble A: Prevalence and magnitude of perinatal substance exposures in California. N Engl J Med 329:850, 1993

Vessey MP: Epidemiological studies of the effects of diethylstilbestrol. IARC Sci Publ 335, 1989

Von Almen WF, Miller JM: Ts and blues in pregnancy. J Reprod Med 31:236, 1984

Vorhees CV, Minck Dr, Berry HK: Anticonvulsants and brain development. Prog Brain Res 73:229, 1988

Wachsman L, Schuetz S, Chan LS, Wingert WA: What happens to babies exposed to phencyclidine (PCP) in utero? Am J Drug Alcohol Abuse 15:31, 1989

Wallace R, Caldwell D, Ansbacher R, Otterson W: Inhibition of premature labor by terbutaline. Obstet Gynecol 51:387, 1978

Warkany J: Warfarin embryopathy. Teratology 14:205, 1976

Weiner CP, Thompson MIB: Direct treatment of fetal supraventricular tachycardia after failed transplacental therapy. Am J Obstet Gynecol 158:570, 1988

Weinstein MR: Lithium treatment of women during pregnancy and in the post-delivery period. In Johnson FN (ed): Handbook of Lithium Therapy. Baltimore, University Park Press, 1980, p 421

Welt SI: Sinusoidal fetal heart rate and butorphanol administration. Am J Obstet Gynecol 152:362–3, 1985

Werler MM: Teratogen update: Smoking and reproductive outcomes. Teratology 55:382, 1997

Whalley PJ, Adams RH, Combes B: Tetracycline toxicity in pregnancy: Liver and pancreatic dysfunction. JAMA 189:357, 1964

Wiseman RA, Dodds-Smith IC: Cardiovascular birth defects and antenatal exposure to female sex hormones: A reevaluation of some basic data. Teratology 30:359, 1984

Wolfe MS, Cordero JF: Safety of chloroquine in chemosuppression of malaria during pregnancy. BMJ 290:1466, 1985

Yerby MS: Epilepsy and pregnancy. New issues for an old disorder. Neurol Clin 11:777, 1993

Young DC, Snabes MC, Poindexter AN: GnRH agonist exposure during the first trimester of pregnancy. Obstet Gynecol 81:587, 1993

Zackai EH, Mellman WJ, Neiderer B, Hanson JW: The fetal trimethadione syndrome. J Pediatr 87:280, 1975

Zhu M, Zhou S: Reduction of the teratogenic effects of phenytoin by folic acid and a mixture of folic acid, vitamins, amino acids: A preliminary trial. Epilepsia 30:246, 1989

Zucker KJ, Bradley SJ, Oliver G, et al. Psychosexual development of women with congenital adrenal hyperplasia. Hormones and Behavior, 30:300, 1996

39

Diseases and Injuries of the Fetus and Newborn

The fetus and newborn are subject to a great variety of diseases. Those that are the direct consequence of maternal disease have been considered in other chapters along with specific maternal illnesses. This chapter provides an introduction to other fetal and neonatal diseases and injuries of major clinical importance.

DISEASES OF THE FETUS AND NEWBORN

HYALINE MEMBRANE DISEASE. To provide blood-gas exchange after birth, the infant's lungs must rapidly fill with air while being cleared of fluid, and the volume of blood that perfuses the lungs must increase remarkably. Some of the fluid is expressed as the chest is compressed during vaginal delivery, and the remainder is absorbed through the pulmonary lymphatics. The presence of sufficient surfactant synthesized by the type II pneumonocytes is essential to stabilize the air-expanded alveoli by lowering surface tension and thereby preventing lung collapse during expiration (Chap. 7, p. 151). If surfactant is inadequate, respiratory distress develops. This is characterized by the formation of hyaline membranes in the distal bronchioles and alveoli.

Hyaline membrane disease has decreased as a cause of neonatal death in the United States. According to most experts, surfactant therapy and administration of antenatal corticosteroids are responsible for much of this decrease (Avery, 1995; National Institutes of Health, 1994). Boys are more prone than girls to develop these problems, and white infants appear to be more often and more severely affected than are black infants (Hulsey and associates, 1993). Neither preeclampsia nor prematurely ruptured membranes appear to accelerate fetal lung maturation (Hallack and Bottoms, 1993; Schiff and colleagues, 1993).

CLINICAL COURSE. In the typical case, tachypnea develops and the chest wall retracts, while expiration is often accompanied by a whimper and grunt—a combination called "grunting and flaring." Grunting is common in the newborn whenever there is uneven expansion of the lungs or lower airway obstruction. Progressive shunting of blood through nonventilated lung areas contributes to hypoxemia and metabolic and respiratory acidosis. Poor peripheral circulation and systemic hypotension may be evident. The chest x-ray shows a diffuse reticulogranular infiltrate with an air-filled tracheobronchial tree (air bronchogram).

Respiratory insufficiency can also be caused by sepsis, pneumonia, meconium aspiration, pneumothorax, diaphragmatic hernia, persistent fetal circulation, and heart failure. Common causes of cardiac decompensation in the early newborn period are patent ductus arteriosus and congenital cardiac malformations.

PATHOLOGY. Hyaline membrane disease is the consequence of inadequate surfactant production. Without surfactant, the alveoli are not stable and low pressures cause collapse on end expiration. Nutrition of lung cells is compromised by hypoxia and systemic hypotension. There may be only partial maintenance of the fetal circulation (pulmonary hypertension) and a relative right-to-left shunt. Ischemic necrosis of the cells lining the airway eventually occurs. When oxygen therapy is initiated, the pulmonary vascular bed dilates and the shunt (if there is one) reverses. Protein filled fluid leaks into the alveolar ducts, and cells lining the alveolar ducts slough. Hyaline membranes of fibrin-rich protein and cellular debris line the dilated alveoli and terminal bronchioles, and the epithelium underlying the membrane becomes necrotic. In fatal cases, the atelectatic lungs on gross examination resemble liver. Histologically, many alveoli are collapsed while some are dilated widely, and the alveolar duct epithelium appears vacuolated.

TREATMENT. The most important factor influencing survival is admission to a neonatal intensive care unit. This has dramatically reduced the number of deaths from respiratory distress syndrome. An arterial P_{O_2} below 40 mm Hg is indicative of the need for oxygen therapy. Because excess oxygen can damage the pulmonary epithelium and retina, the oxygen concentration administered should be at the lowest level sufficient to relieve hypoxia and acidosis. Arterial oxygen tensions of 50 to 70 mm Hg are adequate.

Continuous positive airway pressure (*CPAP*) prevents the collapse of unstable alveoli and has brought about an appreciable reduction in the mortality rate. Successful ventilation usually allows high inspired oxygen concentrations to be reduced and thereby minimizes toxicity. Disadvantages are that venous return is impaired and there is always the possibility of barotrauma. Although positive pressure ventilation has undoubtedly improved survival, it is also an important factor in the genesis of bronchopulmonary dysplasia.

Mechanical ventilation results in repeated alveolar overstretching, which can disturb the integrity of the endothelium and epithelium and cause barotrauma (Verbrugge and Lachmann, 1999). To obviate this, *high-frequency oscillatory ventilation* is used to maintain an optimal lung volume and to clear CO_2 by using a constant low distending pressure and small variations or oscillations that promote alveolar recruitment. It can be used in combination with inhaled nitric oxide for severe cases of pulmonary hypertension (Biarent, 1999).

SURFACTANT TREATMENT. Because hyaline membrane disease is caused by lack of surfactant, important preventive therapy is the administration of exogenous surfactant. Following an initial report by Fujiwara and colleagues (1980) that aerosolized surfactant treatment appeared to ameliorate the severity of the respiratory distress syndrome, many clinical trials have confirmed its efficacy. Preparations included biological or animal surfactants such as human, bovine (Survanta), calf lung surfactant extract (CLSE), porcine (Curosurf), or synthetic surfactant (Exosurf).

The introduction of surfactant therapy has been credited by both the Centers for Disease Control and the Surgeon General for the largest drop in infant mortality observed in 20 years. It has been utilized for **prophylaxis** of preterm infants at risk for respiratory distress, as well as for **rescue** of those with established disease. Long and co-workers (1995) summarized the many published clinical trials of surfactant use, and found that it has reduced morbidity substantively with a net savings of over $8000 per added year of life. Moreover, both early and late follow-up of treated infants over a wide range of birthweights indicate that surfactant does not result in more survivors with impairments.

Jobe (1993) summarized the results of 35 randomized controlled studies of surfactant utilized either as prophylaxis or rescue therapy, and found that it substantially reduced the incidence of pneumothorax and death in the first 28 days (Table 39–1). There was also a greater reduction in overall death rate and deaths due to respiratory distress syndrome when antenatal corticosteroids and surfactant were given together. These findings were confirmed by Kari and associates (1994). In a report from a large multicenter trial conducted under the auspices of the National Institute of Child Health and Human Development Neonatal Research Network, Horbar and associates (1993) reported a decrease in

mortality from 28 to 20 percent from surfactant therapy alone.

Surfactant treatment is also beneficial for the very-low-birthweight infant. Hamvas and co-workers (1996) described a preferential improvement in neonatal mortality for white versus black very-low-birthweight infants. Ferrara and colleagues (1994) demonstrated improved intact survival in a group of infants born between 23 and 26 weeks. These findings were confirmed by a large multicenter trial of infants weighing 500 to 750 g (Smyth and associates, 1995). The superiority of prophylactic versus rescue surfactant for the very-low-birthweight infant was demonstrated in the large trial conducted by the OSRIS Collaborative Group (1992). For the older preterm infant, prophylactic versus rescue surfactant use continues to be debated (Dunn, 1993).

COMPLICATIONS. As previously described, persistent hyperoxia injures the lung, especially the alveoli and capillaries. High oxygen concentrations given at high pressures can cause *bronchopulmonary dysplasia*, or *oxygen toxicity lung disease*. This is a chronic condition in which alveolar and bronchiolar epithelial damage leads to hypoxia, hypercarbia, and oxygen dependence, followed by peribronchial and interstitial fibrosis. *Pulmonary hypertension* is another frequent complication. If hyperoxemia is sustained, the infant is also at risk of developing *retinopathy of prematurity*, formerly called *retrolental fibroplasia*. Thus, the oxygen concentration must be reduced appropriately as the arterial P_{O_2} rises.

PREVENTION. There is no method of diagnosis or treatment of preterm labor that has significantly reduced the incidence of preterm birth or improved any index of

TABLE 39–1. Effects of Surfactant Treatment in Infants with Respiratory Distress Syndrome or at High Risk for the Disease

Surfactant and Strategy	Percent Change in Incidence[a] (incidence in untreated infants)		
	Pneumothorax	Bronchopulmonary Dysplasia	Death by Day 28
Synthetic surfactant			
Delivery-room prophylaxis	−34 (15)	+ 7 (18)	−30 (24)
Treatment of disease	−33 (22)	−30 (8)	−34 (14)
Natural surfactant			
Delivery-room prophylaxis	−64 (23)	−6 (44)	−39 (18)
Treatment of disease	−58 (31)	0 (38)	−31 (29)

[a] Percentages were calculated from the total numbers of patients studied in the trials that served as the basis for each meta-analysis.
From Soll (1991a–d). Data compiled by Jobe (1993) and includes 35 randomized controlled trials. Used with permission.

neonatal outcome (American College of Obstetricians and Gynecologists, 1995c). Elective preterm birth, however, can be avoided. It is clearly inexcusable to electively deliver an infant without a certain knowledge of gestational age, or confirmation of pulmonary maturity (see Table 23–5, p. 544). When preterm delivery is indicated, for example in some cases of preeclampsia, it is also important to weigh the relative risks of immaturity and maternal disease (Wigton and co-workers, 1993).

AMNIOCENTESIS FOR FETAL LUNG MATURITY.

Certainly, there are times when the risks to the fetus from a hostile intrauterine environment are greater than the risk of respiratory distress. If the criteria for elective delivery at term are not met, however, then amniocentesis is often utilized to confirm fetal lung maturity. A number of methods are used to determine the relative concentration of surfactant-active phospholipids. The technique is similar to that described for second-trimester amniocentesis in Chapter 37 (p. 989).

LECITHIN-TO-SPHINGOMYELIN (L/S) RATIO.

Lecithin (dipalmitoyl phosphatidylcholine) plus phosphatidylinositol and especially phosphatidylglycerol are important in the formation and stabilization of the surface-active layer that prevents alveolar collapse and respiratory distress (Chap. 7, p. 152). Before 34 weeks, lecithin and sphingomyelin are present in amnionic fluid in similar concentrations. At about 34 weeks, the concentration of lecithin relative to sphingomyelin begins to rise (Fig. 39–1).

Gluck and co-workers (1971) reported that the risk

TABLE 39–2. Respiratory Support Requirements Compared with Lecithin–Sphingomyelin (L/S) Ratio

L/S Ratio	Mechanical Ventilation (%)	Any Support (%)
< 1.0	24	59
1.0–1.5	22	53
1.6–2.0	9	44
2.1–2.5	3	28

Modified from Harper and Lorenz (1993), with permission.

of neonatal respiratory distress is very slight whenever the concentration of lecithin is at least twice that of sphingomyelin (L/S ratio). Conversely, there is increased risk of respiratory distress when this ratio is below 2. Because lecithin and sphingomyelin are found in blood and meconium, contamination with these substances may confound the results. Blood has an L/S ratio of 1.3 to 1.5 and could thus either raise or lower the true value, whereas meconium usually lowers the L/S ratio (Buhi and Spellacy, 1975). Harper and Lorenz (1993) found an immature L/S ratio to be more predictive of the need for ventilatory support than gestational age or birthweight (Table 39–2).

Unfortunately, with some pregnancy complications, respiratory distress may develop despite a mature L/S ratio. This outcome has been reported most frequently with diabetes, but this concept is controversial. Kjos and co-workers (1990) presented data to suggest that standard methods of lung assessment are valid in infants of diabetic mothers, and that cases of respiratory distress in infants with "mature" studies are unrelated to surfactant deficiency. Low and colleagues (1994) opined that additional factors causing metabolic compromise, such as acidosis or sepsis, may also adversely impact the development of respiratory distress despite a mature L/S ratio. Berkowitz and associates (1996) reported that 96 percent of 585 diabetic women and 90 percent of 628 nondiabetic women had mature L/S ratios at 39 weeks. They concluded that lung maturation is not delayed. Piper and Langer (1996), however, in a study of 621 diabetic pregnancies, found that delayed pulmonary maturation is associated with poor glucose control.

Ethnic background may also affect the predictive value of the L/S ratio and the likelihood of respiratory distress (Hulsey and colleagues, 1993). Richardson and Torday (1994) studied 135 black infants and found no case of respiratory distress syndrome when the L/S ratio was greater than 1.5.

PHOSPHATIDYLGLYCEROL.

Because of uncertainty about the predictive value of the L/S ratio, some clini-

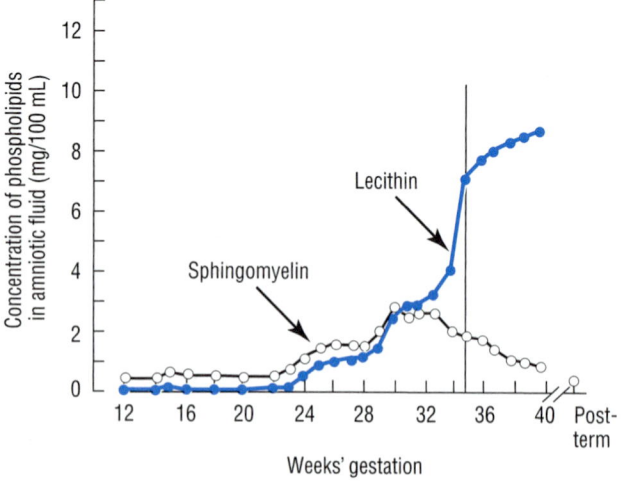

FIGURE 39–1. Changes in mean concentrations of lecithin and sphingomyelin in amnionic fluid during gestation in normal pregnancy. (From Gluck and Kulovich, 1973, with permission.)

cians consider the presence of phosphatidylglycerol to be mandatory prior to elective delivery of the diabetic mother (Ojomo and Coustan, 1990). Phosphatidylglycerol is believed to enhance the surface-active properties of lecithin and sphingomyelin (Chap. 7, p. 152). Its identification in amnionic fluid provides more assurance, but not necessarily an absolute guarantee, that respiratory distress will not develop. Because phosphatidylglycerol is not detected in blood, meconium, or vaginal secretions, these contaminants do not confuse the interpretation. While the presence of phosphatidylglycerol is reassuring, its absence is not necessarily a strong indicator that respiratory distress is likely to develop after delivery.

TDx-FLM. This automated assay measures the surfactant-albumin ratio in uncentrifuged amnionic fluid and gives results in approximately 30 minutes. In a study of 374 consecutive amnionic fluid specimens, Steinfeld and associates (1992) reported that a TDx value of 50 or greater predicted fetal lung maturity in 100 percent of cases. Subsequent investigations by Hagen and associates (1993) and Herbert and co-workers (1993) found the TDx-FLM to be equal or superior to the L/S ratio, foam stability index, or phosphatidylglycerol assessment in predicting both positive and negative tests. Eriksen and associates (1996) reported that the TDx-FLM test has a sensitivity, specificity, and negative-predictive value for evaluating fetal lung maturity in diabetic women comparable to the L/S ratio. Many hospitals use the TDx-FLM as their first-line test of pulmonary maturity, followed by the L/S ratio in indeterminant samples.

OTHER TESTS. The **foam stability** or **shake test** was introduced by Clements and associates (1972) to reduce the time and effort inherent in precise measurement of the L/S ratio. The test depends on the ability of surfactant in amnionic fluid, when mixed appropriately with ethanol, to generate stable foam at the air–liquid interface. There are two problems with the test:

1. Slight contamination of amnionic fluid, reagents, or glassware, as well as errors in measurement may alter the test results.
2. A false-negative test is rather common.

Some laboratories use this as a screening test, and if negative, use another test to better quantify the L/S ratio.

The **Lumadex-FSI test** is based on the principle of foam stability to identify surfactant activity in amnionic fluid. It has also been found to be reliable (Herbert and associates, 1993). **Fluorescent polarization (microviscometry)** is a test in which the microviscosity of lipid aggregates in amnionic fluid are assayed by mixing the

fluid with a specific fluorescent dye that incorporates into hydrocarbons of surfactant lipids. The intensity of the fluorescence induced by polarized light is then measured. The technique is rapid and simple to perform, but expensive (Barkai and associates, 1982). **Amnionic fluid absorbance at 650-nm** wavelength has been reported to correlate well with the L/S ratio (Sbarra and co-workers, 1977). Tsai and associates (1983) reported that the test is most informative at low and high absorbance. Between these extremes, however, false-positive and false-negative values proved troublesome. Kjos and colleagues (1990) found this test to be reliable even in infants of diabetic mothers.

Welsch and colleagues (1996) used the **lamellar body count** to study 849 amnionic fluid specimens. They reported that a count of at least 35,000/mL was a reliable predictor of fetal lung maturity and compared favorably with the L/S ratio. They concluded that this assay was rapid, simple, and an accurate method for assessing fetal lung maturity. Alvarez and Ludmir (1996) reported that measurement of the concentration of **dipalmitoylphosphatidylcholine (DPPC test)** in amnionic fluid had a sensitivity and specificity of 100 percent and 96 percent, respectively, for prediction of respiratory distress.

RETINOPATHY OF PREMATURITY. Formally known as retrolental fibroplasia, retinopathy of prematurity had become by 1950 the largest single cause of blindness in this country. After the discovery that the etiology of the disease was hyperoxemia, its frequency decreased remarkably.

PATHOLOGY. The retina vascularizes centrifugally from the optic nerve starting about the fourth month and continuing until shortly after birth. During the time of vascularization, retinal vessels are easily damaged by excessive oxygen. The temporal portion of the retina is most vulnerable. Oxygen induces severe vasoconstriction, endothelial damage, and vessel obliteration. When the oxygen level is reduced, there is neovascularization at the site of previous vascular damage. The new vessels penetrate the retina and extend intravitreally, where they are prone to leak proteinaceous material or burst with subsequent hemorrhage. Adhesions then form, which detach the retina.

PREVENTION. Precise levels of hyperoxemia that can be sustained without causing retinopathy are not known. Retinopathy is unlikely if inhaled air is enriched with oxygen to no more than 40 percent. Unfortunately, very immature infants who develop respiratory distress will most likely require ventilation with high oxygen concentrations to maintain life until respiratory distress clears. Administration of relatively large doses of vitamin E to prevent oxidation has produced conflicting results (Mino, 1992).

RESPIRATORY DISTRESS IN THE TERM INFANT.
Term infants can also have respiratory complications, although much less frequently than those born preterm. Common causes in term infants include sepsis and intrauterine-acquired pneumonia, persistent pulmonary hypertension of the newborn (PPHN), meconium aspiration syndrome, and pulmonary hemorrhage. Septicemia, especially from group B streptococcal disease, is a relatively common cause of respiratory distress in the term infant (Chap. 56, p. 1471). Persistent pulmonary hypertension is more common after elective cesarean delivery or premature closure of the ductus arteriosus. Meconium aspiration syndrome is frequently associated with oligohydramnios, uteroplacental insufficiency, and fetal stress. Frequently, most of these diagnoses are completely unexpected.

Treatment is similar to that for respiratory distress from surfactant deficiency in preterm neonates, described previously. Advances in neonatal care have improved the survival rate and decreased the morbidity of these conditions. One is high-frequency oscillatory ventilation, discussed earlier, and another is the use of nitric oxide as a pulmonary vasodilator that has no effect on systemic vasculature. Finer and Barrington (2000) performed a meta-analysis of 11 trials of nitric oxide use in term or near-term infants with respiratory failure. When compared with traditional therapy, nitric oxide significantly improved oxygenation and reduced the incidence of death or the need for extracorporeal membrane oxygenation (ECMO). Furthermore, its effects seem to be enhanced when used along with high-frequency oscillatory ventilation. Nitric oxide apparently does not have similar beneficial effects for infants born before 34 weeks (Kinsella and co-workers, 1999).

MECONIUM ASPIRATION.
This is a severe pulmonary disease characterized by chemical pneumonitis and mechanical obstruction of the airways. It results from peripartum inhalation of meconium-stained amnionic fluid, leading to inflammation of pulmonary tissues and hypoxia. There is also evidence that the free fatty acids in meconium strip away alveolar surfactant (Clark and colleagues, 1987). In severe cases, the pathological process progresses to persistent pulmonary hypertension, other morbidity, and death. Even with prompt and appropriate therapy, seriously affected infants frequently die or suffer long-term neurological sequelae.

RISK FACTORS.
In about 20 percent of pregnancies at term, amnionic fluid is contaminated by the passage of fetal meconium. In the past, this was considered a sign of "fetal distress" occurring only in response to hypoxia.

It is now recognized, however, that in the majority of cases meconium passage is a manifestation of a normally maturing gastrointestinal tract, or is the result of vagal stimulation from umbilical cord compression (Nathan and co-workers, 1994). In a global sense, however, it is still considered a marker for adverse perinatal outcomes (Chap. 31, p. 814).

Aspiration of meconium-stained amnionic fluid before labor is thus a relatively common occurrence. In healthy, well-oxygenated fetuses with normal amnionic fluid volume, meconium is diluted and is readily cleared from the lungs by normal physiological mechanisms. In some infants, however, the inhaled meconium is not cleared, and meconium aspiration syndrome results. The syndrome may occur after otherwise normal labor, but it is more often encountered in postterm pregnancy or in association with fetal growth restriction. Meconium varies in concentration, and the syndrome is more likely when meconium is thick. Putting these together, pregnancies at highest risk are those in which there is diminished amnionic fluid volume, along with cord compression or uteroplacental insufficiency that may cause meconium passage. In these, meconium remains thick and undiluted, and the compromised fetus cannot clear it. Leveno and colleagues (1984) reported that meconium aspiration syndrome may follow transient episodes of umbilical-cord compression, an event more likely if there is oligohydramnios. In a study by Davis and co-workers (1985), meconium aspiration syndrome was strongly associated with thick meconium and fetal heart rate abnormalities, which mostly were severe variable decelerations from cord compression.

Unfortunately, pathological meconium aspiration cannot be predicted. Dooley and co-workers (1985) studied 272 pregnancies with meconium-stained fluid, and found that the 20 percent of fetuses who had aspirated meconium did not have fetal heart decelerations during labor or any other predictive heart rate pattern. They reported that liberal cesarean delivery (60 percent) for meconium and fetal heart rate abnormalities did not alter the frequency of meconium found beneath the cords. Moreover, the single death was not prevented by aggressive peripartum airway management.

PREVENTION.
In 1976, Carson and colleagues reported that meconium aspiration syndrome could be prevented by **oropharyngeal suctioning** of the infant following delivery of the head, but before delivery of the chest. This maneuver was followed by laryngoscopic visualization of the cords and, when meconium was visualized, additional suctioning of the trachea. In this study, meconium aspiration syndrome was reduced but not eliminated, suggesting that delivery factors were not solely responsible. In the two decades since this report, this combined obstetric–pediatric delivery protocol became common.

In subsequent studies, Davis and colleagues (1985) found that strict adherence to this protocol in 1420 pregnancies failed to reduce the incidence of meconium aspiration syndrome below 2.1 percent. Wiswell and colleagues (1990) found no reduction in the risk of meconium aspiration syndrome with perinatal suctioning maneuvers in a study involving more than 175,000 neonates over a 14-year period. Linder and associates (1988) demonstrated that nondepressed infants with meconium-stained fluid who underwent routine tracheal suctioning actually had increased respiratory morbidity compared with those not suctioned.

During this time, Murphy and associates (1984) presented evidence that development of newborn pulmonary hypertension with this syndrome depended upon a chronic or recurring antenatal insult. This in turn would cause abnormal muscularization of the interacinar arteries beginning well before birth, and thus would be unaffected by maneuvers at delivery. Cornish and colleagues (1994) used a baboon model and found that meconium aspiration, either alone or combined with peripartum asphyxia, did not produce pathophysiological effects which led to long-term damage or death in the human neonate.

Katz and Bowes (1992) concluded from their review that the etiology of the meconium aspiration syndrome is primarily chronic fetal asphyxia rather than simply damage from meconium. They postulated that chronic antepartum asphyxia causes pathophysiological changes leading to pulmonary vascular damage, pulmonary hypertension, and persistent fetal circulation. Affected infants are unable to clear aspirated meconium. Thus, the 2 percent of infants who do not respond to suctioning at delivery are likely to be those who have sustained this type of antenatal damage. These findings agree with those provided by Richey and colleagues (1995) who found no correlation between markers of acute asphyxia—umbilical artery pH, lactate, or hypoxanthine—and meconium. One marker of chronic asphyxia, erythropoietin, was significantly elevated in newborns with meconium-stained fluid. This latter observation was confirmed by Bloom and associates (1996).

AMNIOINFUSION. Gabbe and co-workers (1976) demonstrated the utility of amnioinfusion for relief of variable decelerations in labor in a rhesus monkey model. Miyazaki and Taylor (1983) applied the technique to human fetuses experiencing variable heart rate decelerations in labor. It was then suggested that amnioinfusion might also prevent meconium aspiration because fetal gasping would be less likely with reduced variable decelerations from cord compression. To test this, Wenstrom and Parsons (1989) performed a randomized trial of amnioinfusion in pregnancies complicated by thick meconium. They showed that it significantly decreased the

incidence of meconium below the cords and operative delivery, and that no infants receiving amnioinfusion developed meconium aspiration syndrome. At the same time, Sadovsky and colleagues (1989) reported similar results. A number of studies since then have generally confirmed these findings, and in a meta-analysis of 13 studies, Pierce and co-workers (2000) found that amnioinfusion significantly lowered the incidence of meconium beneath the vocal cords (OR 0.18), meconium aspiration syndrome (OR 0.30), and neonatal acidemia (OR 0.42).

Amnioinfusion for meconium may be beneficial only when the meconium is thick and there are recurrent variable decelerations that could provoke aspiration (Spong and colleagues, 1994). While amnioinfusion appears to be beneficial only for some pregnancies, it probably poses little or no increased risk (Wenstrom and co-workers, 1995). Finally, it does not benefit fetuses in whom meconium aspiration has occurred well before the onset of labor (Byrne and Gau, 1987; Manning and colleagues, 1978).

MANAGEMENT. According to guidelines of the American Academy of Pediatrics and American Heart Association (1994), at delivery the infant's mouth and nares should be carefully suctioned before the shoulders are delivered. A suction bulb is usually adequate. The DeLee trap can also be used, but should be connected to wall suction and not suctioned by mouth. Locus and colleagues (1990) studied 80 women whose labors were complicated by moderate to thick meconium-stained amnionic fluid. Fetuses were randomly assigned to undergo suction at delivery of the head by either bulb or DeLee trap. Although both methods were equally efficacious, even with careful suctioning, 5 percent of these infants developed meconium aspiration syndrome.

For infants who are depressed, or those who have passed thick, particulate meconium, the infant is placed on the radiant warmer and residual meconium in the hypopharynx is removed by suctioning under direct visualization. The trachea is then intubated and meconium suctioned from the lower airway. The stomach is emptied to avoid the possibility of further meconium aspiration. It remains controversial whether a vigorous infant with thinly meconium-stained fluid requires tracheal suctioning. These guidelines are followed with the realization that their efficacy in preventing long-term neonatal morbidity or mortality is, as outlined, undocumented. Nevertheless, when skillfully and promptly performed, these procedures carry little risk of harm (Yoder, 1994).

INTRAVENTRICULAR HEMORRHAGE. There are four major categories of neonatal intracranial hemorrhage: **subdural hemorrhage** is usually due to trauma. **Subarachnoid** and **intracerebellar hemorrhage** usually result from trauma in term infants, but are commonly due to hypoxia in preterm infants. **Periventricular–intraventricular hemorrhage** results from either trauma or asphyxia in half of term infants, but has no discernible cause in 25 percent of cases (Volpe, 1995). In preterm neonates, the pathogenesis of periventricular hemorrhage is multifactorial and includes hypoxic-ischemic events, anatomical considerations, coagulopathy, and many others. The prognosis after hemorrhage depends on the location and extent of the bleeding. Subdural and subarachnoid hemorrhage, for example, often results in minimal if any neurological abnormalities. Bleeding into the parenchyma of the brain, however, can cause serious permanent damage.

PERIVENTRICULAR–INTRAVENTRICULAR HEMORRHAGE.
When the fragile capillaries in the germinal matrix rupture, this leads to bleeding into surrounding tissues which may extend into the ventricular system and brain parenchyma. Unfortunately, it is a common problem in preterm neonates. Although a variety of external perinatal and postnatal influences undoubtedly alter its incidence and severity, preterm birth before 32 weeks has the greatest impact. These lesions can develop at later gestational ages, and are occasionally seen in term neonates.

Most hemorrhages develop within 72 hours of birth, but they have been observed as late as 24 days (Perlman and Volpe, 1986). Almost half are clinically silent, and most small germinal matrix hemorrhages and those confined to the cerebral ventricles resolve without impairment (Weindling, 1995). Large lesions can result in hydrocephalus or *periventricular leukomalacia,* a correlate of cerebral palsy discussed later. Because intraventricular hemorrhages are usually recognized within 3 days of delivery, their genesis is often erroneously attributed to birth events. It is important to realize that prelabor intraventricular hemorrhage is well recognized (Achiron and associates, 1993; Asakura and co-workers, 1994; Nores and associates, 1996).

PATHOLOGY. The primary pathological process is damage to the germinal matrix capillary network, which predisposes to subsequent extravasation of blood into the surrounding tissue. This capillary network is especially fragile in preterm infants:

1. The subependymal germinal matrix provides poor support for the vessels coursing through it.
2. Venous anatomy in this region cause venous stasis and congestion susceptible to vessel bursting with increased intravascular pressure.
3. Vascular autoregulation is impaired before 32 weeks (Volpe and Hill, 1987).

If extensive hemorrhage or other complications of preterm birth do not cause death, survivors can have major neurodevelopmental handicaps (Papile and co-workers, 1983).

DeVries and colleagues (1985) attribute most long-term sequelae of intraventricular–periventricular hemorrhage to cystic areas called *periventricular leukomalacia.* These areas develop more commonly as a result of ischemia and less commonly in direct response to hemorrhage, and are discussed subsequently.

INCIDENCE AND SEVERITY. The incidence of ventricular hemorrhage undoubtedly depends on gestational age at birth (Fig. 39–2). About half of all neonates born before 34 weeks will have evidence of some hemorrhage, and this incidence decreases to 4 percent at term (Hayden and associates, 1985). Perlman and Volpe (1986) have shown that very-low-birthweight infants have the earliest onset of hemorrhage, the greatest likelihood for progression into parenchymal tissue, and thus the highest mortality rate.

The severity of intraventricular hemorrhage can be assessed by ultrasound and computed tomography, and various grading schemes are used to quantify the extent of the lesion. The scheme proposed by Papile and colleagues (1978) is commonly used:

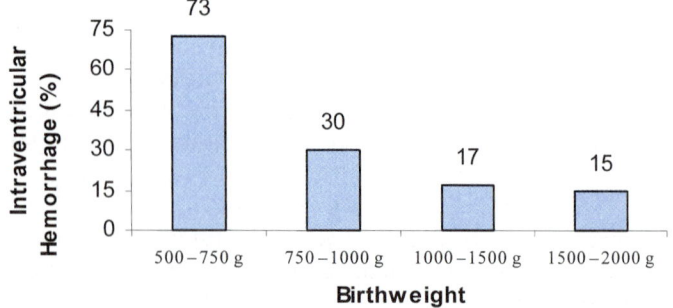

FIGURE 39–2. Incidence of intraventricular hemorrhage as a function of birthweight in 210 neonates admitted to the Parkland Hospital neonatal intensive care unit. The overall incidence was 30 percent. (Data courtesy of Dr. Jeffrey Perlman.)

- *Grade I*—Hemorrhage limited to the germinal matrix
- *Grade II*—Intraventricular hemorrhage
- *Grade III*—Hemorrhage with ventricular dilatation
- *Grade IV*—Parenchymal extension of hemorrhage

The severity of the hemorrhage strongly influences prognosis. Jakobi and colleagues (1992) showed that infants with grades I or II intraventricular hemorrhage had over 90 percent survival with 3.2 percent handicap. This was the same as for control infants of the same age but without hemorrhage. The survival rate for infants with grades III or IV hemorrhage, however, was only 50 percent. Vergani and co-workers (1996) also correlated the degree of hemorrhage with outcome. Very preterm infants are at increased risk of sustaining severe intracranial hemorrhage. In a report of 1765 very-low-birthweight infants studied by the National Institute of Child Health and Development (NICHD)-sponsored Neonatal Intensive Care Network, the incidence of intraventricular hemorrhage was 45 percent, and about 20 percent of these infants had grade III or IV hemorrhage (Hack and colleagues, 1991).

CONTRIBUTING FACTORS. Events that predispose to germinal matrix hemorrhage and subsequent periventricular leukomalacia are multifactorial and complex. Most recognized risk factors relate to immaturity characterized by fragile intracranial blood vessels. Associated complications of preterm birth, which for example is frequently associated with infection, predispose to tissue ischemia. Luthy and co-workers (1987) reported a threefold increased risk for grade III or IV hemorrhage when the cord arterial pH was less than 7.2. Respiratory distress syndrome and mechanical ventilation are commonly associated factors. Lesko and colleagues (1986) reported that heparin, often used to maintain vascular catheter patency in intensive care units, was associated with a fourfold increased risk of germinal matrix hemorrhage. In a review of 232 infants who weighed less than 1500 g, Wallin and co-workers (1990) reported that associated postnatal factors include respiratory distress, ventilator therapy, a P_{CO_2} of 60 mm Hg or greater, a P_{O_2} less than 40 mm Hg at 2 hours of life or greater, and pneumothorax.

PREVENTION AND TREATMENT. Administration of corticosteroids before delivery appears to prevent intraventricular hemorrhage. Based in part on the data of Garite and associates (1992) and the March of Dimes Multicenter Study Group (Maher and colleagues, 1994), a consensus statement was developed by a panel of the National Institutes of Health (1994). The advisory panel concluded that antenatal corticosteroid therapy reduced mortality, respiratory distress, and intraventricular hemorrhage in preterm infants born between 24 and 32 weeks' gestation. These benefits are additive with those from surfactant therapy. Even though the original Consensus Conference concluded that benefits of antenatal steroid therapy probably extended to preterm premature membrane rupture, the American College of Obstetricians and Gynecologists (1994) concluded that further research was needed in this area.

Silver and associates (1996) reported that antenatal dexamethasone administered to surfactant-treated infants born before 30 weeks' gestation resulted in fewer grade III and IV hemorrhages than placebo plus surfactant. Conversely, Cox and associates (1996) found no benefits of dexamethasone with regard to grade III or IV hemorrhage in preterm infants delivered at Parkland Hospital. The type of corticosteroid administered may be important. Baud and colleagues (1999) found that *betamethasone* decreased the incidence of periventricular leukomalacia but *dexamethasone* did not. Canterino and associates (1996), in a study of 716 consecutive newborns less than 34 weeks' gestation, reported that antenatal corticosteroid therapy decreased the risk of periventricular leukomalacia.

The efficacy of phenobarbital or vitamin K in diminishing the frequency and severity of intracranial hemorrhage, when administered either to the neonate or to the mother during labor, remains controversial (Thorp and colleagues, 1995). While vitamin E given to high-risk neonates reportedly decreases the incidence and severity of hemorrhage, it did not affect mortality (Chiswick and colleagues, 1991). Indomethacin given to neonates weighing less than 1000 g was associated with a similar incidence of hemorrhage, but a higher mortality rate than untreated controls (Hanigan and colleagues, 1988). Data from a variety of sources suggest that magnesium sulfate may prevent the sequelae of periventricular hemorrhage (see later discussion).

It is generally agreed that avoiding significant hypoxia both before and after preterm delivery is of paramount importance (Low and co-workers, 1995). There is presently no convincing evidence, however, that routine cesarean delivery for the preterm fetus presenting cephalic will decrease the incidence of periventricular hemorrhage (Tejani and co-workers, 1987; Welch and Bottoms, 1986). Strauss and colleagues (1985) found no association with presence of labor or its duration. In a study of 106 preterm infants weighing less than 1750 g, Anderson and associates (1992) found no significant difference in the overall frequency of hemorrhage in infants whose mothers were not in labor compared with those in latent or active labor. There was, however, an increased frequency of grade III or IV hemorrhage in infants of women in active labor. In contrast, data presented by Ment and associates (1995) suggested a reduction in early intracranial hemorrhage with cesarean delivery.

OUTCOME IN EXTREME PREMATURITY. All of the concerns described are amplified as the limits of viability are reached in the 22- to 25-week age group (Holtrop and co-workers, 1994; Wood and colleagues, 2000). Not only is the mortality rate in this age group high, but survivors frequently have devastating neurological, ophthalmological, or pulmonary injury due to immaturity. Allen and associates (1993) provided outcome data for 142 infants born at 22 to 25 weeks in whom surfactant therapy was routinely administered (Table 39–3). No infant born prior to 23 weeks survived. Although survival increased at or beyond 23 weeks, severe abnormalities seen on cranial ultrasonography, which usually lead to major neurological impairment, were inversely associated with age. In all, 98 percent of infants born at 23 weeks, 79 percent at 24 weeks, and 31 percent at 25 weeks either died or had severe neurological abnormalities. Wood and associates (2000) provided follow-up of 283 of 308 survivors born at 25 or fewer completed weeks. Formal assessment at a median of 30 months showed that half had neurological disability and half of these (25 percent of the total group) had severe disability.

BRAIN DISORDERS. The etiology of cerebral palsy has been debated since 1862 when a London orthopedist, William Little, described 47 children with spastic rigidity and concluded that abnormalities of birth could cause this clinical picture. Sigmund Freud questioned this over 100 years ago because abnormal birth processes frequently produced no effects. It is now recognized that cerebral palsy is caused by a combination of genetic, physiological, environmental, and obstetrical factors. Although it inarguably is a complex multifactorial disease, Paneth (1986) emphasized that the presumed birth-injury etiology for cerebral palsy has endured and has influenced the opinions and practices of countless obstetricians and pediatricians. This myth likely is one of the major reasons that at least one in four infants in the United States is currently born by cesarean delivery. Unfortunately, despite the substantive increase in cesarean delivery over 50 years, there has not been any significant decline in the rate of cerebral palsy.

In 1985, the National Institutes of Health convened a panel of experts to set some guidelines crucial to resolving issues that often surround cerebral palsy, mental retardation, learning disabilities, and seizures (Freeman, 1985). Progress has been made and understanding improved as to what antepartum, intrapartum, and neonatal factors are, and—possibly more important—are not associated with neurological abnormalities and cerebral palsy. Despite this, some obstetricians, pediatricians, and neurologists—and most if not all plaintiff attorneys—still erroneously attribute many cases of cerebral palsy to intrapartum or perinatal asphyxia.

Unfortunately, although "asphyxia" has been clearly defined, the term is still widely misused. According to the American College of Obstetricians and Gynecologists (1998), birth asphyxia is defined by (*1*) *profound metabolic or mixed acidemia (pH < 7.00) determined*

TABLE 39–3. Outcomes in 6-Month Survivors Born at 23 to 25 Weeks

Outcome	23 Weeks (n = 6)	24 Weeks (n = 19)	25 Weeks (n = 31)
	Mean ± SD		
Mechanical ventilation (days)	60 ± 29	51 ± 42	24 ± 19
Oxygen administration (days)	89 ± 40	81 ± 48	52 ± 33
Age oxygen discontinued (week)	36 ± 6	36 ± 7	32 ± 5
Length of stay (days)	120 ± 23	107 ± 37	76 ± 23
	Percent		
Retinopathy of prematurity	83	53	32
Intraventricular hemorrhage			
Any	83	74	32
Grade III	17	11	10
Grade IV	33	32	0
Periventricular leukomalacia	33	21	3
Severe abnormality on cranial ultrasonography	83	64	13

From Allen and co-workers (1993), with permission.

on an umbilical cord arterial blood sample, (2) persistent Apgar score of 0 to 3 for longer than 5 minutes; and (3) evidence of neonatal neurological sequelae such as seizures, coma, or hypotonia, or dysfunction of one or more of the following systems: cardiovascular, gastrointestinal, hematological, pulmonary, or renal. Despite this precise definition, the diagnosis is frequently based on low Apgar scores alone, which may be caused by other factors such as preterm birth, maternal sedation, anesthesia, vigorous suctioning or intubation, congenital malformations, and newborn musculoskeletal, neurological, or cardiorespiratory disease (Gilstrap and Crosby, 1994).

CEREBRAL PALSY. The National Institutes of Health defines cerebral palsy as a nonprogressive motor disorder of early infant onset involving one or more limbs, with resulting muscular spasticity or paralysis. Epilepsy and mental retardation may also be associated with cerebral palsy, but are usually not associated with perinatal asphyxia in the absence of cerebral palsy (American College of Obstetricians and Gynecologists, 1992; Freeman and Nelson, 1988). Cerebral palsy may be categorized by the type of neurological dysfunction (spastic, dyskinetic, or ataxic) and by the number and distribution of limbs involved (quadriplegia, diplegia, hemiplegia, or monoplegia).

The major types of cerebral palsy are:

1. *Spastic quadriplegia*—which has an increased association with mental retardation and seizure disorders.
2. *Diplegia*—which is common in preterm or low-birthweight infants.
3. *Hemiplegia.*
4. *Choreoathetoid types.*
5. *Mixed varieties* (Freeman and Nelson, 1988).

From their review, Rosen and Dickinson (1992) reported that approximately 35 percent of cases were of the diplegic type, 30 percent were hemiplegic, 20 percent quadriplegic, and 15 percent were of the extrapyramidal type. Significant mental retardation, defined as an intelligence quotient (IQ) less than 50, was associated with 25 percent of cerebral palsy cases.

INCIDENCE AND EPIDEMIOLOGICAL CORRELATES. The incidence of cerebral palsy is approximately 1 to 2 per 1000 livebirths (American College of Obstetricians and Gynecologists, 1992). Importantly, as emphasized by many groups, the incidence has remained essentially unchanged since the 1950s, and it may actually have increased in some countries (Freeman and Nelson, 1988; Torfs and colleagues, 1990). As perhaps expected, cerebral palsy has increased coincidentally with an increase in survival of low-birthweight babies (Stanley and Blair, 1991). Advances in the care of very preterm infants

has improved their survival, but not without significant handicaps, as discussed earlier. In their review of 11 studies published from 1985 through 1990, Rosen and Dickinson (1992) reported that the average cumulative rate for cerebral palsy at ages 5 to 7 years was 2.7 per 1000 livebirths. The rate for infants born weighing less than 2500 g was 15 per 1000, and for survivors weighing 500 to 1500 g at birth, the rate was 13 to 90 per 1000. In the study by Wood and co-workers (2000), half of all surviving infants born before 25 completed weeks had a neurological disability.

Nelson and Ellenberg (1984, 1985, 1986a, 1986b) have made important contributions to our understanding of cerebral palsy. They analyzed data from the Collaborative Perinatal Project, which followed offspring of 54,000 pregnancies regularly until age 7. They determined that important antecedents and most commonly associated risk factors of cerebral palsy were:

1. Evidence of genetic abnormalities such as maternal mental retardation, microcephaly, and congenital malformations.
2. Birthweight less than 2000 g.
3. Gestational age less than 32 weeks.
4. Infection.

They further found that obstetrical complications were not strongly predictive of cerebral palsy. Indeed, only about 20 percent of affected children had markers of perinatal asphyxia, whereas over half had associated congenital malformations, low birthweight, microcephaly, or another explanation for the brain disorder. They concluded that the causes of most cases of cerebral palsy are unknown and that no foreseeable single intervention is likely to prevent a large proportion of cases.

Torfs and associates (1990) presented data that confirm these observations. They reported an incidence of cerebral palsy of 0.3 percent among 19,044 live-born children from the California Child Health and Development Studies database. Of the 55 children with cerebral palsy, 14 (25 percent) had neural-tube defects or obvious postnatal causes, such as infection or injury. There were only nine infants (22 percent) with cerebral palsy who had "perinatal asphyxia"—defined erroneously as a time-to-cry interval longer than 5 minutes. Importantly, all nine had birth defects, gestational risk factors, or both. The strongest predictors for cerebral palsy were the presence of a major or minor congenital anomaly, low birthweight, low placental weight, or abnormal fetal position (which is often associated with neurological abnormality) such as face, breech, or transverse lie. These factors were similar to those identified in the Collaborative Perinatal Project (Table 39–4). Interestingly, instrumental delivery—including low, mid, or even high forceps—or cesarean delivery did not correlate with cerebral palsy. More recent observations from

TABLE 39–4. Prenatal and Perinatal Risk Factors in Children with Cerebral Palsy

Risk Factors	Risk Ratio	95% CI
Long menstrual cycle (> 36 days)[a]	9.0	2.2–37.1
Hydramnios[a]	6.9	1.0–49.3
Premature placental separation[a]	7.6	2.7–21.1
Intervals between pregnancies < 3 months or > 3 years	3.7	1.0–4.4
Birthweight < 2000 g[a]	4.2	1.8–10.2
Breech, face, or transverse lie[a]	3.8	1.6–9.1
Severe birth defect[a]	5.6	8.1–30.0
Nonsevere birth defect	6.1	3.1–11.8
Time-to-cry more than 5 min[a]	9.0	4.3–18.8
Low placental weight[a]	3.6	1.5–8.4

[a] Also associated with cerebral palsy in the Collaborative Perinatal Project (Nelson and Ellenberg, 1985, 1986a, 1986b).
Adapted from Torfs and associates (1990), with permission.

the Maternal Fetal Medicine Network of nearly 800 infants weighing less than 1000 g were that only low birthweight and early gestational age correlated with neonatal neurological morbidity (Goepfert and associates, 1996).

INTRAPARTUM EVENTS. Obstetricians and the legal system naturally want to know whether cerebral palsy is related to intrapartum events—the mismanagement of labor—which could be prevented or avoided. Data from several studies indicate that this usually is not the case. Stanley and Blair (1991) performed a case-control study of all cases of cerebral palsy in western Australia from 1975 to 1980. Antepartum, intrapartum, and neonatal events were carefully reviewed. They found that in 92 percent of cases, intrapartum injury as the cause of cerebral palsy was not likely; in 3.3 percent, intrapartum injury was possible; and in only 4.9 percent was it likely. Phelan and associates (1996) reviewed fetal monitor tracings of 209 neurologically impaired neonates and classified 75 percent as nonpreventable.

The role of continuous electronic fetal monitoring in predicting or allowing prevention of cerebral palsy has been studied. Data from a variety of sources indicate that such monitoring neither predicts nor reduces the risk of cerebral palsy when compared with intermittent auscultation (American College of Obstetricians and Gynecologists, 1992; Freeman, 1990; Thacker and colleagues, 1995). MacDonald and associates (1985) performed a randomized, prospective study of over 13,000 pregnancies comparing continuous electronic monitoring with intermittent auscultation. In a later analysis, Grant and associates (1989) found an equal number of cases of cerebral palsy (3) in each group. The American College of Obstetricians and Gynecologists (1995a) concluded that "a substantial body of evidence disproves the hypothesis that electronic fetal monitoring would reduce long-term neurological impairment and cerebral palsy in newborns so monitored."

Importantly, there does not appear to be any specific fetal heart rate pattern that predicts cerebral palsy. Furthermore, the recognition of abnormal patterns, usually leading to cesarean delivery, has not decreased the incidence of cerebral palsy. In fact, in cases that ultimately result in cerebral palsy, the abnormal heart rate pattern may reflect preexisting neurological abnormality and not ongoing, remedial injury (Phelan and Ahn, 1994). This in part accounts for the unchanged incidence of cerebral palsy in the United States, despite a fivefold increase in the cesarean delivery rate since 1965. A number of studies found no relationship between an appropriate response to abnormal fetal heart rate patterns and neurological outcome (Melone and associates, 1991; Nelson and co-workers, 1996; Niswander and colleagues, 1984). Indeed, Shy and co-workers (1990) found a significant increase in cerebral palsy among a group of preterm infants monitored electronically when compared with intermittent auscultation.

APGAR SCORES. Since their inception, Apgar scores have been used to predict neurological impairment in childhood. It is now clear that they are poor predictors except in certain circumstances. Nelson and Ellenberg (1984) studied the interaction between obstetrical complications and a low Apgar score as a predictor of poor neurological outcome. A variety of late pregnancy complications were identified in 62 percent of pregnancies, and when considered alone, they were not associated strongly with cerebral palsy. However, in infants with complicated births who also had 5-minute Apgar scores of 3 or less, the incidences of mortality and cerebral palsy were increased appreciably. In the absence of complications, low Apgar scores alone were not associated with a high level of risk. Dijxhoorn and colleagues (1986) reported similar findings and concluded that most neonatal neurological abnormalities were due to factors other than perinatal hypoxia. Luthy and associates (1987) reported that in low-birthweight infants with 1-minute Apgar scores of 3 or less, the incidence of death was increased fivefold and the incidence of cerebral palsy was increased threefold.

Because it is predictive of increased neonatal death, recent data suggest that a low 5-minute Apgar score might be predictive of future neurological impairment. Casey and colleagues (2001) studied over 150,000 live-born infants delivered at Parkland Hospital from 1988 through 1998. They found that a 5-minute Apgar score of 0 to 3 predicts an increased incidence of neonatal death in preterm, but especially term, infants (Table 39–5). For infants born before 37 completed weeks whose 5-minute Apgar score was 0 to 3, the risk for neonatal death was increased 75-fold. In infants born at 38 weeks or more, the 5-minute Apgar of 0 to 3 was associated with a 1460-fold increase in death within 28 days.

The American College of Obstetricians and Gynecologists (1996) has summarized the use and misuse of the Apgar score to assess asphyxia and to predict future neurological deficit (Chap. 16, p. 387). It was concluded that low scores at 1 and 5 minutes are excellent indicators for identification of those infants who need resuscitation. It was further concluded, however, that low Apgar scores alone are not evidence for hypoxia sufficient to result in neurological damage. In a child found to have cerebral palsy, low 1- or 5-minute Apgar scores provide insufficient evidence that the damage was due to hypoxia.

UMBILICAL CORD BLOOD GAS. As summarized in Chapter 16 (p. 389), an important criterion in the definition of asphyxia is metabolic acidosis. In its absence, significant intrapartum hypoxia or asphyxia is generally excluded. Although there has been significant enthusiasm for the clinical use of umbilical cord acid–base determinations, when used alone, they have proven no more helpful than the 1- and 5-minute Apgar scores in predicting long-term neurological sequelae. Dijxhoorn and associates (1986), in a study of 805 term newborns delivered vaginally, reported that the largest number of neurologically abnormal infants had a normal umbilical arterial pH but low Apgar scores. These authors concluded that intrapartum hypoxia was not a major cause of neurological morbidity. Others have reported that neither pH measurements nor acidemia correlated with long-term neurological outcome in term infants (American College of Obstetricians and Gynecologists, 1992; Fee and associates, 1990). Subsequently, it was reported that the pH cutoff for clinically significant acidemia most likely is less than 7.0 instead of the earlier arbitrarily chosen level of less than 7.2 (American College of Obstetricians and Gynecologists, 1995d; Gilstrap and associates, 1989; Goldaber and associates, 1991). Nagel and associates (1995) reported long-term follow-up in 30 infants whose umbilical artery pH was less than 7.0. Of the 28 survivors, only two had mild neurological sequelae. They concluded that infants with this degree of acidosis did well if they had no major neonatal problems.

In the previously cited study by Casey and co-workers (2001) of over 150,000 live-born infants, the umbilical artery pH was also used to assess predictability of neonatal death within 28 days. As the pH fell to 7.0 or less, the likelihood of neonatal death increased, and it was 1400-fold increased with a cord pH of less than or equal to 6.8 in term newborns. When cord pH was 7.0 or below and the 5-minute Apgar score was 0 to 3, the relative risk of neonatal death was 3204!

TABLE 39–5. Correlation of Low (0–3) 5-Minute Apgar Score with Neonatal Death within 28 Days of Birth

Infants	5-Minute Apgar Score and Neonatal Death		Umbilical Artery pH and Neonatal Death	
	Apgar Score (n)	Relative Risk (98% CI)	pH (n)	Relative Risk (95% CI)
Preterm infants (n)	0–3 (92)	59 (40, 87)	≤ 7.0 (125)	20 (11, 34)
	4–6 (556)	13 (9, 20)	≤ 6.9 (59)	22 (11, 46)
	7–10 (12,827)	1.0 (referent)	≤ 6.8 (26)	43 (21, 91)
Term infants	0–3 (86)	1460 (835, 2555)	≤ 7.0 (598)	180 (97, 334)
	4–4 (561)	53 (20, 140)	≤ 6.9 (135)	708 (381, 1320)
	7–10 (131, 581)	1.0 (referent)	≤ 6.8 (51)	1407 (736, 2689)

From Casey and colleagues (2001), with permission.

NUCLEATED RED BLOOD CELLS. Nucleated erythrocytes are immature cells that enter the circulation in response to hypoxia. Their measurement has been proposed as a means to quantify the degree of hypoxia and determine its duration. Some investigators have reported an association with cord blood nucleated red blood cells and fetal asphyxia (Korst and associates, 1996). Conversely, Salafia and colleagues, (1996), in a study of 465 preterm newborns, found no correlation with nucleated red cells and fetal hypoxia. Instead, these were found to be hematological markers associated with maternal and newborn infection, as well as placental histological evidence of infection.

Naeye and Localio (1995) provided data that serial lymphocyte and normoblast counts in the neonate helped to accurately identify the time before birth when hypoxic ischemic encephalopathy took place. They studied 16 newborns in whom intrapartum events allowed accurate assessment of the time of injury. Counts peaked 2 hours after injury and normalized in 24 to 36 hours. Further studies of both nucleated erythrocytes and lymphocytes are needed before these premises are accepted for clinical use.

PERIVENTRICULAR LEUKOMALACIA. This term refers to cystic areas deep in the white matter of the brain which develop after hemorrhagic infarction and ischemia. Tissue ischemia leads to regional necrosis, and because brain tissue does not regenerate, these irreversibly damaged areas appear as echolucent cysts on neuroimaging studies. They generally require at least 2 weeks to develop, and have been reported to develop up to 104 days after the initial insult (Goetz and colleagues, 1995). Accordingly, the presence of cystic areas at birth may determine the timing of the hemorrhagic event (Hayakawa and co-workers, 1999).

A variety of clinical and pathological data link severe intracranial hemorrhage and periventricular leukomalacia to cerebral palsy. Luthy and colleagues (1987) reported that more than 40 percent of low-birthweight infants with cerebral palsy had grade III or IV hemorrhages. They computed a 16-fold increased risk for cerebral palsy for these infants compared with those who had either no hemorrhage or grade I or II hemorrhage. DeVries and colleagues (1993) followed 504 infants born at 34 weeks or less and found that only 11 percent of those with transient cysts developed cerebral palsy. Conversely, 67 percent with localized cystic periventricular leukomalacia and 100 percent of those with extensive cystic areas developed cerebral palsy. Allan and co-workers (1997) evaluated multiple prenatal, perinatal, and postnatal variables in 505 infants with birthweights between 600 and 1250 g. They found that the highest rates of cerebral palsy were associated with periventricular leukomalacia (37 percent) and ventricu-

lomegaly (30 percent). Hsu and colleagues (1996) showed that the size of the cyst(s) correlated directly with the risk of cerebral palsy. Fujimoto and colleagues (1994) demonstrated that symmetrical cystic lesions portended the highest risk.

Although some of the same factors that appear to cause intraventricular hemorrhage are associated with periventricular leukomalacia, the latter condition seems to be more strongly linked to infection and inflammation, as discussed subsequently. Zupan and colleagues (1996) studied 753 infants born between 24 and 32 weeks. About 9 percent developed periventricular leukomalacia, and those born before 28 weeks, or who had inflammatory events during the last days to weeks before delivery, or both, were at highest risk. Perlman and co-workers (1996) found that periventricular leukomalacia was strongly associated with neonatal hypotension, prolonged rupture of the membranes, and chorioamnionitis. Spinillo and colleagues (1995, 1998) found a strong association of leukomalacia with first-trimester hemorrhage, maternal urinary infection in labor, low birthweight, smoking, preterm labor, neonatal acidosis, meconium staining, and more than 72 hours of ritodrine therapy.

PRETERM FETUS AND PERIVENTRICULAR LEUKOMALACIA. Consideration of brain development explains why very preterm infants are most susceptible to intraventricular hemorrhage and periventricular leukomalacia. Before 32 weeks, the blood supply to the brain is composed of two systems: one penetrates into the cortex—the *ventriculopedal system,* and the other reaches down to the ventricles, but then curves to flow outward—the *ventriculofugal system* (Weindling, 1995). The area between these two blood supplies corresponds to an area near the lateral cerebral ventricles through which the pyramidal tracts pass. It is called the *watershed area* because there are no vascular anastomoses where these two blood supplies meet, and thus it is very vulnerable to ischemia. Any intracranial vascular injury occurring before 32 weeks and leading to ischemia would affect the watershed area first, damaging the pyramidal tracts and resulting in spastic diplegia. After 32 weeks, the blood supply shifts away from the brainstem and basal ganglia toward the cortex. Hypoxic injury after this time primarily damages the cortical region.

PERINATAL INFECTION. Fetal infection may be a key element in the pathway between preterm birth, intracranial hemorrhage, periventricular leukomalacia, and cerebral palsy (Dammann and Leviton, 1997; Yoon and colleagues, 1997a, 2000, 2001). In the pathway proposed in Figure 39–3, antenatal reproductive tract infection is characterized by the production of cytokines such as interleukins-1, -6, and -8, and tumor necrosis factor.

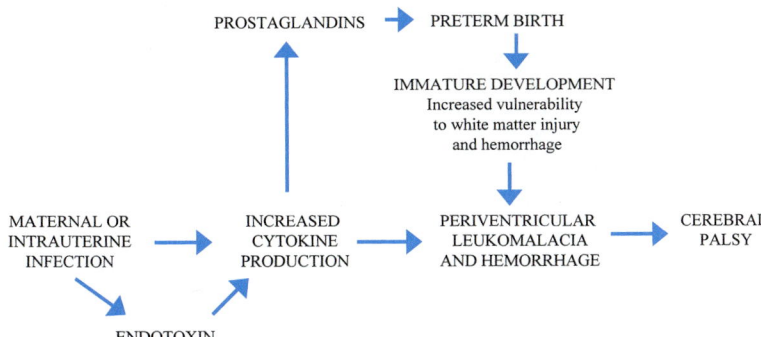

FIGURE 39-3. Schematic representation of hypothesized pathway between maternal or intrauterine infection, preterm birth, and cerebral palsy. (Courtesy of Dr. Robert Goldenberg.)

These stimulate prostaglandin production, which may cause preterm birth (Chap. 11, p. 274). Because of their incomplete development, discussed earlier, intracranial blood vessels are susceptible to rupture and damage. The cytokines that stimulate preterm labor also have direct toxic effects on oligodendrocytes and myelin. Thus, vessel rupture, tissue hypoxia, and cytokine-mediated damage results in massive cell death. Glutamate that is released may cause damage to cerebral white matter. Glutamate causes membrane receptor changes that allow excess calcium to enter the neurons, and the high intracellular calcium levels are toxic (Levene, 1992). Glutamate may also be directly toxic to oligodendroglia (Oka and associates, 1993).

Both animal and clinical data support the role of infection and cytokines. Yoon and colleagues (1997a) have shown that inoculation of rabbit embryos with *Escherichia coli* causes histological white matter damage. In another study, Yoon and associates (1997b) also showed that tumor necrosis factor and interleukin-6 were more frequently found in the brains of infants who died with periventricular leukomalacia. Cytokines have been strongly linked to white matter lesions even when infectious organisms cannot be demonstrated. In a study in which amnionic fluid cultures were performed and cytokines were measured in 123 preterm infants, Yoon and colleagues (2000) showed that, while only 45 percent of the infants with cerebral palsy had microorganisms in amnionic fluid, 85 percent had abnormally elevated interleukin-6 and -8 levels.

The importance of infection separate from preterm birth has also been demonstrated. Verma and colleagues (1997) compared 285 infants born after preterm labor and 279 infants born after preterm prematurely ruptured membranes with 149 infants who were delivered preterm for other reasons. The incidence and severity of intraventricular hemorrhage and periventricular leukomalacia was highest in those infants with spontaneous labor or membrane rupture. In both cases, cerebral damage was significantly increased if chorioamnionitis was diagnosed. Bejar and co-workers (1988) showed that the most significant clinical correlates of white matter

necrosis in preterm infants were funisitis, purulent amnionic fluid, and placental vascular anastomoses. Grether and Nelson (1997) performed a population-based case-control study of cerebral palsy in which they focused only on affected children whose birthweight was more than 2500 g and who had no congenital brain malformations or genetic abnormalities. They found a significant ninefold increased risk of cerebral palsy after either maternal fever in labor or chorioamnionitis, and a 19-fold risk after neonatal infection.

PREVENTION. The benefits of corticosteroid therapy were discussed earlier in reference to intraventricular hemorrhage (p. 1040). Discovery of the link between infection, cytokines, and cerebral palsy may allow another step toward prevention. Aggressive treatment of or prophylaxis against infection in the woman delivering preterm may be neuroprotective.

Magnesium sulfate has been shown to stabilize intracranial vascular tone, minimize fluctuations in cerebral blood flow, reduce reperfusion injury, and block calcium-mediated intracellular damage (Marret and associates, 1995). It also appears to reduce synthesis of cytokines and bacterial endotoxins, and thus may minimize the inflammatory effects of infection (Grether and Nelson, 1997). Epidemiological evidence suggests that prenatal exposure to maternal magnesium sulfate therapy has a neuroprotective effect (Schendel and co-workers, 1996). This may be limited to preeclamptic women (Grether and colleagues, 2000). This is currently being evaluated in the *BEAM study* sponsored by the National Institutes of Health—*Randomized Clinical Trial of the **B**eneficial **E**ffects of **A**ntenatal **M**agnesium Sulfate.*

NEURORADIOLOGICAL IMAGING. Computed tomography and magnetic resonance performed later in childhood have been used to define the neuropathology and timing of cerebral palsy (Perlman and Cunningham, 1993). Wiklund and colleagues (1991a, 1991b) used computed tomography to study 28 preterm infants and 83 term infants with hemiplegic cerebral palsy between 5 and 16 years of age. Only 25 percent of these children

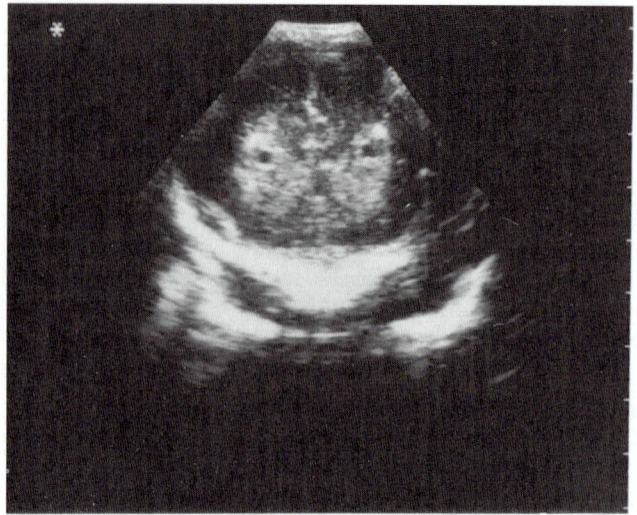
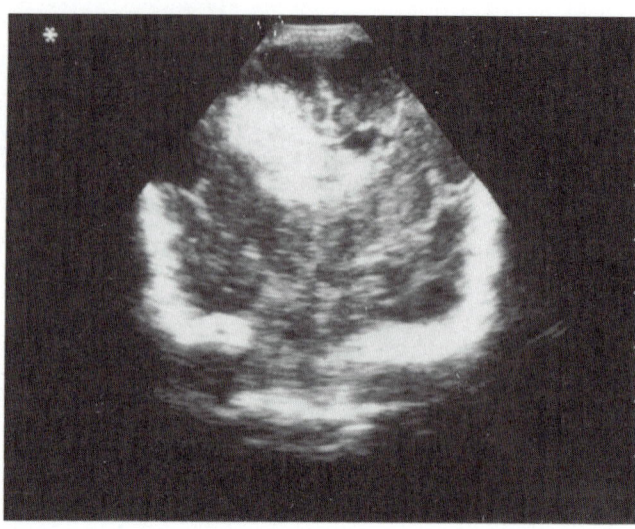

A   **B**

FIGURE 39–4. Preterm infant delivered at 27 weeks because of placental abruption. **A.** Head ultrasound performed on the first postnatal day shows small bilateral cysts in the periventricular white matter and bilateral germinal-matrix hemorrhages. These findings indicate a much older lesion than one caused by perinatal asphyxia. **B.** Repeat ultrasound of same infant on day 3 of life showed bilateral intraventricular hemorrhage and a large intraparenchymal echodensity on the right. (Courtesy of Dr. Jeffrey Perlman.)

had computed tomographic findings that were considered normal. Moreover, in 70 percent of preterm infants, findings confirmed an insult at early age. In term infants, computed tomographic findings suggested a prenatal injury in over half of cases—that is, periventricular atrophy in 37 percent and maldevelopment in 17 percent. Cortical and subcortical injury suggestive of a perinatal injury was found in 19 percent.

Truwit and colleagues (1992) used magnetic resonance imaging, and the predominant finding in 80 percent of preterm infants was evidence of periventricular white matter damage which is indicative of hypoxic ischemic brain injury. It was difficult to determine its exact chronology. In contrast, 50 percent of term infants had imaging findings consistent with antenatal brain damage. These included gyral abnormalities such as polymicrogyria, consistent with midpregnancy injury, and isolated periventricular leukomalacia. In 25 percent of these cases, magnetic resonance imaging findings, coupled with clinical events, were suggestive of hypoxic ischemic injury at birth.

Cranial ultrasound also provides useful information. The development of periventricular leukomalacia is shown in Figure 39–4. Because ultrasonic evolution of cysts takes days to weeks to develop, ultrasound performed on the first day was critical in diagnosing antenatal brain injury. Intraventricular hemorrhage was found to be a secondary insult that developed in the nursery. Sometimes head ultrasound reveals findings different

but complimentary to those with computed tomography. A grade III intraventricular hemorrhage diagnosed at birth by computed tomographic scan is shown in Figure 39–5A. A head ultrasound done the same day, however, also disclosed periventricular leukomalacia, which documents injury well before birth (Fig. 39–5B).

Magnetic resonance imaging in the neonate is also valuable to study intracranial lesions relevant to the development of cerebral palsy (Battin and associates, 1998; Okumura and colleagues, 1997). In a study of 30 children with cerebral palsy, Fedrizzi and colleagues (1996) found that magnetic resonance imaging between the ages of 1 and 2 years predicted the specific pattern of neuropsychological dysfunction, thus enabling early intervention. The severity of ventricular dilatation, the degree and extent of white matter loss, involvement of optic structures, and the degree of thinning of the corpus collosum correlated with the Wechsler full scale and performance IQ test. Jaw and co-workers (1998) have used magnetic resonance imaging to determine the most likely time of the brain insult in 86 pediatric patients with cerebral palsy.

NEONATAL ENCEPHALOPATHY. Term infants can also suffer neurological insults resulting in permanent compromise. Neonatal encephalopathy is used to describe a defined syndrome of disturbed neurological function in the earliest days of life in the term infant. It consists of difficulty in initiating and maintaining res-

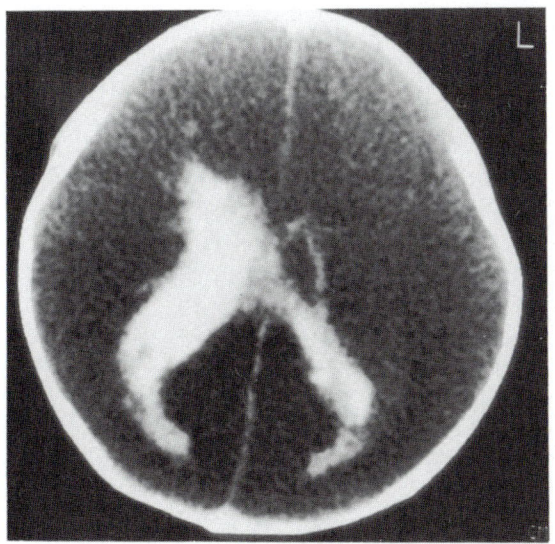
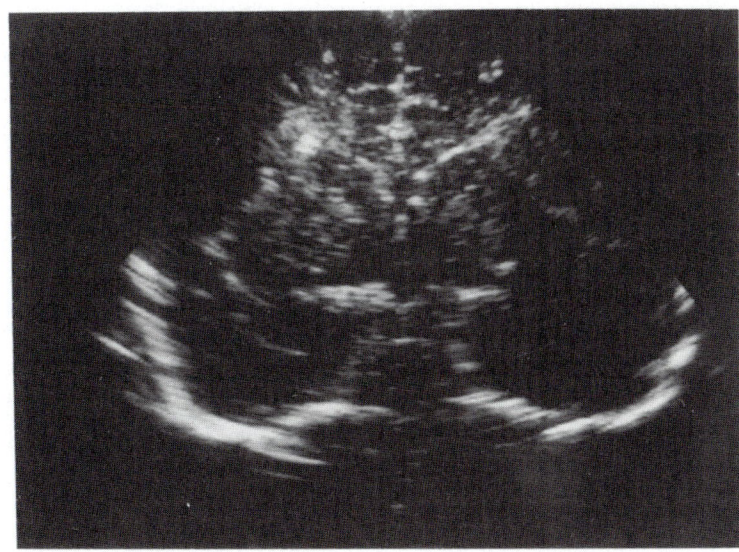

A   B

FIGURE 39–5. This term infant was born depressed. **A.** Computed tomographic scan demonstrates a grade III intraventricular hemorrhage. **B.** Ultrasound scan confirmed intraventricular hemorrhage and, in addition, bilateral cystic periventricular leukomalacia was seen, which was not observed on the computed tomographic scan. These findings documented a severe antenatal brain insult of 4 to 5 weeks' duration. (From Perlman and Cunningham, 1993.)

piration, depressed tone and reflexes, subnormal level of consciousness, and frequently seizures (Nelson and Leviton, 1991). It is generally believed to be the consequence of an hypoxic-ischemic insult, although the timing of the insult is not always known. Mild encephalopathy is generally defined as hyperalertness, irritability, jitteriness, and hypertonia and hypotonia. Moderate encephalopathy includes lethargy, severe hypertonia, and occasional seizures. Severe encephalopathy is defined by coma, multiple seizures, and recurrent apnea. Severe encephalopathy is an important predictor of cerebral palsy and future cognitive defects. In the report by Robertson and Finer (1985), none of the infants with severe encephalopathy had a normal neurological outcome. In contrast, normal outcomes were documented in 80 percent with moderate encephalopathy, and in all newborns with mild hypoxic encephalopathy. Low and colleagues (1985) studied 303 high-risk preterm and term neonates, 30 percent of whom had newborn encephalopathy. A total of 17 percent of infants developed cognitive and motor deficits; in a quarter of these there was mild or moderate encephalopathy, whereas half had severe encephalopathy. Respiratory complications were the most commonly identifiable risk factor, and perinatal hypoxia was associated with or contributed to 26 percent of cases of mild to moderate encephalopathy and 66 percent of these with severe encephalopathy. Cordes and colleagues (1994) performed serial head circumference measurements of 54 term infants with hypoxic-

ischemic encephalopathy. They found that a decrease in the head circumference of more than 3.1 percent relative to that expected for age in the first 4 months of life predicted microcephaly, and thus permanent impairment, with 90 percent specificity.

MENTAL RETARDATION. Etiological factors for severe mental retardation, which has a prevalence of 3 per 1000 children, are shown in Table 39–6. Some genetic causes

TABLE 39–6. Some Etiological Factors for Severe Mental Retardation

Factor	Percent
Prenatal	73
Chromosomal	36
Mutant genes	7
Multiple congenital anomalies	20
Acquired infections, diabetes, growth restriction	10
Prenatal	10
Asphyxia or hypoxia	5
Unidentified causes	5
Postnatal	11
Unknown	6

Modified from Rosen and Hobel (1986), with permission.

of mental retardation are discussed in Chapter 36. In the National Institutes of Health report, the panel ascertained that isolated mental retardation—that is, mental retardation without epilepsy or cerebral palsy—was associated with perinatal hypoxia in less than 5 percent of cases.

SEIZURE DISORDERS. Although seizure disorders may accompany cerebral palsy, isolated seizure disorders or epilepsy are not usually caused by perinatal hypoxia. Nelson and Ellenberg (1986b) determined that the major predictors of seizure disorders were fetal malformations (cerebral and noncerebral), family history of seizure disorders, and neonatal seizures.

ANEMIA. After 35 weeks, the mean cord hemoglobin concentration is about 17 g/dL and values below 14 g/dL are abnormal. During the first several hours of life, the hemoglobin value may rise by as much as 20 percent due to delayed cord clamping, resulting in an appreciable volume of blood being expressed from the placenta through the cord into the infant. Alternatively, if the placenta is cut or torn, a fetal vessel is perforated or lacerated, or the infant is held well above the level of the placenta for some time before cord clamping, the hemoglobin concentration may fall after delivery.

FETAL-TO-MATERNAL HEMORRHAGE. The presence of fetal red cells in the maternal circulation may be identified by use of the acid elution principle first described by Kleihauer, Brown, and Betke, or any of several modifications. This test is based on the fact that fetal erythrocytes contain hemoglobin F, which is more resistant to acid elution than hemoglobin A. After exposure to acid, only fetal hemoglobin remains. Fetal red cells can then be identified by uptake of a special stain and quantified on a peripheral smear (Fig. 39–6).

Very small volumes of blood cells commonly escape from the fetal intravascular compartment across the placental barrier into the maternal intervillous space. This routine fetal–maternal bleeding may someday serve as the basis of a screening test for fetal aneuploidy using maternal peripheral blood samples (Chap. 37, p. 985). Choavaratana and colleagues (1997) performed serial Kleihauer–Betke tests in 2000 pregnant women and found that, although the incidence of fetal–maternal hemorrhage in each trimester was high, the volume transfused from fetus to mother was very small (Table 39–7). Large hemorrhages are uncommon, and Bowman (1985) reported that only 21 of 9000 women had fetal hemorrhage at delivery exceeding 30 mL. A number of events may cause sufficient fetal–maternal hemorrhage to incite isoimmunization (Table 39–8).

The presence of D-positive fetal red blood cells in maternal blood can also be determined by the rosette

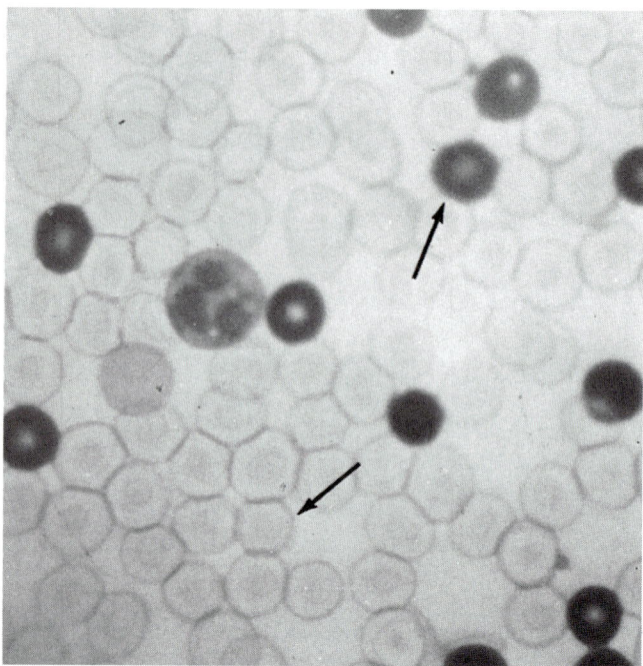

FIGURE 39–6. Massive fetal-to-maternal hemorrhage. After acid-elution treatment, fetal red cells rich in hemoglobin F stain darkly (*upper arrow*), whereas maternal red cells with only very small amounts of hemoglobin F stain lightly (*lower arrow*).

test. In this test, maternal red cells are mixed with anti-D antibodies, which coat any fetal D-positive cells in the sample. Indicator red cells bearing the D antigen are then added, and "rosettes" form around the fetal cells as the indicator cells are attached to them by the antibodies. The presence of rosettes indicates that fetal D-positive cells are present. Using the erythrocyte rosette test, Stedman and colleagues (1986) reported fetal hemorrhage exceeding 30 mL in only 6 of 1000 women. Because the Kleihauer–Betke test is based on the detection of fetal hemoglobin, the rosette test is probably more accurate in certain cases, such as when fetal cells

TABLE 39–7. Incidence and Volume of Fetal–Maternal Hemorrhage During Pregnancy

Stage of Pregnancy	Hemorrhage (%)	Volume (mL)
First trimester	54	0.07
Second trimester	63	0.08
Third trimester	71	0.13
Delivery	76	0.19

From Choavaratana and colleagues (1997), with permission.

TABLE 39–8. Pregnancy Events Causing Fetal–Maternal Hemorrhage

Event	Incidence (%)
Early pregnancy loss	3–5
Elective abortion	6–20
Ectopic pregnancy	5–8
Amniocentesis	4–11
Chorionic villous sampling	8–15
Cordocentesis	30–50
Antepartum trauma	Variable
Placental abruption	Low
Fetal demise	Variable
Manual placental extraction	Variable
External version	Variable

carry excess fetal hemoglobin as the result of a hemoglobinopathy (Goldman and associates, 1991).

The fetus who is severely anemic is more likely to demonstrate an ominous heart rate pattern. The sinusoidal pattern shown in Figure 39–7 is commonly caused by severe anemia, but is not pathognomonic. It should, however, prompt immediate evaluation. In general, anemia occurring gradually or chronically as in isoimmunization is better tolerated by the fetus than if it develops acutely. Chronic anemia may not produce fetal heart rate abnormalities until the fetus is moribund. Significant hemorrhage, either chronic or acute, often causes profound neurological fetal impairment. Acute hemorrhage causes fetal hypotension, diminished perfusion, ischemia, and cerebral infarction. Unfortunately, after an acute hemorrhage, subsequent obstetrical management usually will not change the outcome. For example, deAlemida and Bowman (1994) described 27 cases of

fetal–maternal hemorrhage exceeding 80 mL. Despite appropriate management, almost half of these infants suffered death or spastic diplegia. In some cases, and as discussed on page 1056, fetal-to-maternal hemorrhage may be so severe as to kill the fetus (Fig. 39–6). Samadi and colleagues (1996) found that such hemorrhage was responsible for fetal death in about 5 percent of 319 cases (see also p. 1075).

The cause of a large fetal-to-maternal hemorrhage is often undetermined. In some cases, a placental lesion—for example, a chorioangioma—may be the cause. Placental abruption does not commonly cause appreciable fetal-to-maternal hemorrhage, although if due to trauma, the likelihood is increased (Chap. 43, p. 1173).

In addition to recognizing fetal–maternal hemorrhage, it is important to try to quantify the volume of fetal blood lost. The volume may influence obstetrical management, and is essential to determining the appropriate dose of D-immune globulin when the women is D negative.

Using basic physiological principles, the amount of fetal hemorrhage may be calculated from the results of a Kleihauer–Betke (KB) stain using the formula:

$$\text{Fetal red cells} = \frac{\text{MBV} \times \text{maternal Hct} \times \% \text{ fetal cells in KB}}{\text{Newborn Hct}}$$

where MBV = maternal blood volume (about 5000 mL in normal-sized normotensive women at term) and Hct = hematocrit. Thus for 1.7 percent positive KB-stained cells in a woman of average size with a hematocrit of 35 percent giving birth to an infant weighing 3000 g:

$$\text{Fetal red cells} = \frac{5000 \times 0.35 \times 0.017}{0.5} = 60 \text{ mL}$$

The fetal–placental blood volume at term is 125 mL/kg and the hematocrit is 50 percent. Thus, this fetus has lost 60 mL of red cells over time into the maternal circulation. This is equivalent to 120 mL of whole blood or about a third of its blood volume of 375 mL.

ISOIMMUNIZATION. In 1892, Ballantyne established clinicopathological criteria for the diagnosis of hydrops fetalis. In 1932, Diamond, Blackfan, and Baty reported that fetal anemia characterized by numerous circulating erythroblasts was associated with this syndrome. Certainly ranking as a major contribution to medicine is the subsequent delineation of the pathogenesis of most cases of hemolytic disease in the fetus and newborn, including the related discovery of the Rhesus factor by Landsteiner and Weiner in 1940. In 1941, Levine and associates confirmed that erythroblastosis was due to maternal isoimmunization with paternally inherited fetal factors, and the subsequent development of effective maternal prophylaxis was attributed to Finn and associ-

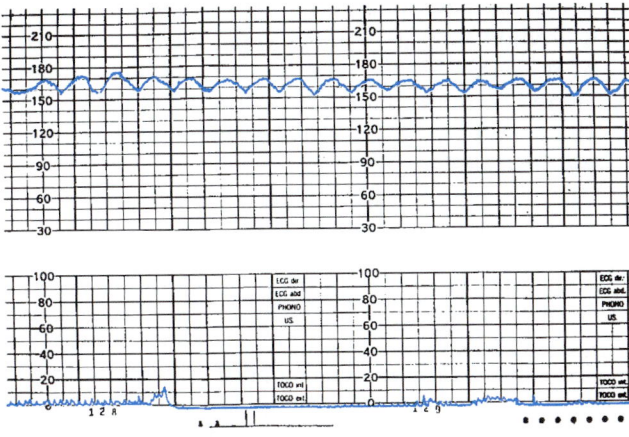

FIGURE 39–7. Sinusoidal fetal heart rate pattern in a fetus with significant fetal–maternal hemorrhage during labor.

ates (1961) in England, and Freda and co-workers (1963) in the United States.

Over 400 red cell antigens have been identified. Although some of them are immunologically and genetically important, fortunately many are so rare as to be of little clinical significance. Individuals who lack a specific red cell antigen may potentially produce an antibody when exposed to that antigen. The antibody could prove harmful to the individual in the case of a blood transfusion or to a fetus during pregnancy. The vast majority of humans have at least one antigen inherited from their father but lacking in their mother. Although the mother could be sensitized if enough erythrocytes from the fetus were to reach her circulation to elicit an immune response, isoimmunization occurs infrequently. Factors explaining its rarity include:

1. Varying rates of occurrence of red cell antigens.
2. Their variable antigenicity.
3. Insufficient transplacental passage of antigen or antibody.
4. Variability of the maternal immune response to the antigen.
5. Protection from isoimmunization by ABO incompatibility of fetus and mother.

The latter confers some protection against D-isoimmunization because fetal red cells entering the mother usually are rapidly destroyed before they can elicit an antigenic response, viz., there is only a 2 percent chance of D-isoimmunization in all women by 6 months postpartum. Another factor benefitting the fetus is that isoimmunization does not always lead to erythroblastosis fetalis.

The incidence of sensitization to red cell antigens at each stage of pregnancy has been studied most extensively in D-negative women. A D-negative woman delivered of a D-positive, ABO-compatible infant has a likelihood of isoimmunization of 16 percent (Bowman, 1985). About 2 percent of such women will be immunized by the time of delivery, another 7 percent will have anti-D antibody by 6 months postpartum, and the remaining 7 percent will be "sensibilized"; that is, they do not ordinarily produce anti-D antibodies but will demonstrate D-isoimmunization when challenged in a subsequent pregnancy by another D-positive fetus.

ABO BLOOD GROUP SYSTEM. Incompatibility for the major blood group antigens A and B is the most common cause of hemolytic disease in the newborn. About 20 percent of all infants have an ABO maternal blood group incompatibility, and 5 percent are clinically affected. Fortunately, ABO incompatibility invariably causes only mild disease, evident as neonatal jaundice or anemia but not erythroblastosis fetalis, and treatment is most often limited to phototherapy.

ABO incompatibility is different from CDE incompatibility for several reasons:

1. ABO disease is frequently seen in firstborn infants. This is because most group O women have anti-A and anti-B isoagglutinins antedating pregnancy, believed to result from exposure to bacterial antigens that are very similar to the A and B antigens. Anti-A or -B antibody production accelerates during the first pregnancy and is likely to recur in subsequent pregnancies.
2. Although the disease is common, it is invariably milder than D-isoimmunization and rarely results in significant anemia. Most species of A and B isoantibodies are immunoglobulin M, which cannot cross the placenta or gain access to fetal erythrocytes. Also, fetal red cells have fewer A and B antigenic sites than adult cells and are thus less immunogenic. Thus, while ABO isoimmunization can cause hemolytic disease of the newborn, it does not cause hydrops fetalis and is a disease of pediatric rather than obstetrical concern.
3. ABO incompatibility can affect future pregnancies but, unlike CDE disease, rarely gets progressively more severe. Katz and co-workers (1982) identified a recurrence rate of 87 percent of whom 62 percent required treatment, most often limited to phototherapy.
4. In contrast to D-isoimmunization, which preferentially affects Caucasians, African-American infants are more likely to develop ABO disease (Kirkman, 1977).

There is no need for antenatal detection as ABO incompatibility does not cause severe fetal anemia. Careful observation is essential in the neonatal period, however, because hyperbilirubinemia may require treatment. The usual criteria for diagnosis of neonatal hemolysis due to ABO incompatibility include the following:

1. The mother is blood group O, with anti-A and anti-B antibodies in her serum, while the fetus is group A, B, or AB.
2. There is onset of jaundice within the first 24 hours.
3. There are varying degrees of anemia, reticulocytosis, and erythroblastosis.
4. There has been careful exclusion of other causes of hemolysis.

Unlike CDE hemolytic disease, the Coombs test in ABO incompatibility may be negative although it is usually positive.

The principles of management of the newborn with ABO hemolytic disease are similar to those for the infant born with D-isoimmunization. For simple transfusion or exchange transfusion, group O blood is used. Because the incidence of stillbirths among ABO-incompatible pregnancies is not increased, there is no justification for early labor induction or for performing amniocentesis.

CDE (RHESUS) BLOOD GROUP SYSTEM.
These red cell antigens are of considerable clinical importance because the majority of individuals who lack its major antigenic determinant, the D or Rhesus antigen, become immunized after a single exposure. The CDE genes are inherited independent of other blood group genes and are located on the short arm of chromosome 1. Like most gene products, there is no difference in the distribution of the CDE antigens with regard to sex, but there are important racial differences. Native Americans, Inuits, and Chinese and other Asiatic peoples are almost all D-positive (99 percent). Approximately 92 to 93 percent of African Americans are D-positive, but only 87 percent of Caucasians carry the D antigen. Of all racial and ethnic groups studied thus far, the Basques show the highest incidence of D-negativity (34 percent).

The Rhesus blood group system includes five red cell proteins or antigens: c, C, D, e, and E. No "d" antigen has been identified, and D-negativity is defined as the absence of "D." The C, c, E, and e antigens have lower immunogenicity than the D antigen, but they can cause erythroblastosis fetalis. All pregnant women should be tested routinely for the presence or absence of D antigen on their erythrocytes and for other irregular antibodies in their serum. Barss and colleagues (1988) have argued convincingly that this need be done only once during pregnancy in D-positive women.

OTHER BLOOD GROUP INCOMPATIBILITIES.
Proportionately more cases of significant antenatal hemolytic disease are now caused by rarer red cell antigens because of prevention of anti-D isoimmunization. Such sensitization may be suspected from the results of the indirect Coombs test done to screen for abnormal antibodies in maternal serum (Table 39–9).

An idea of the frequency of some of these antibodies comes from the report of Bowell and colleagues (1986a), who screened 70,000 pregnant women over a 2-year period. They identified 677 pregnancies with atypical red cell antibodies, for an incidence of nearly 1 percent. One fourth of these were from the Lewis system, which do not cause fetal hemolysis because Lewis antigens do not develop on erythrocytes until a few weeks after birth. Of the remaining 544 antibodies, 72 percent were of the CDE group, and anti-D was most common (158), followed by anti-E (130), anti-c (49), and anti-C (19). Antibodies to the Kell system antigens also were common (76). More recently, Howard and colleagues (1998) evaluated all clinically important cases of isoimmunization occurring in Liverpool during a 12-month period. They also found that 1 percent of 22,264 pregnancies

were sensitized, and anti-D immunization accounted for 40 percent while non-D antibodies accounted for the majority.

KELL ANTIGEN.
This antigen is uncommon, and 91 percent of Caucasians are Kell negative. While 90 percent of cases of sensitization result from transfusion with Kell-positive blood, it can also occur as the result of maternal–fetal incompatibility (Mayne and associates, 1990). Maternal sensitization to Kell is different from D sensitization in that it results in a more rapid and more severe fetal anemia. Furthermore, severe anemia may not be predicted by either maternal serum antibody titer or amnionic fluid bilirubin studies. Sensitized pregnancies often have only mild or moderately increased amnionic fluid bilirubin levels as discussed below. Caine and colleagues (1986) described 13 Kell-sensitized pregnancies with a Kell-positive fetus in which five resulted in hydrops or perinatal death, despite favorable amnionic fluid studies one week prior to delivery. Bowman and colleagues (1992a) reviewed 20 Kell-sensitized pregnancies, and in four, exchange transfusions were required and four fetuses died.

According to Weiner and Widness (1996), anti-Kell antibodies attack fetal erythrocyte precursor cells directly in the bone marrow, which prevents the hematopoietic response to anemia. Because fewer erythrocytes are produced, there is less hemolysis, and less bilirubin despite severe anemia. Because of this disparate severity of Kell sensitization, some authorities recommend evaluation when the maternal anti-Kell titer is 1:8 or greater as discussed subsequently. Weiner and Widness (1996) further recommend that the initial evaluation be accomplished by cordocentesis instead of amniocentesis because of their observations indicating that Kell sensitization produces fetal anemia out of proportion to the amnionic fluid evidence of hemolysis.

OTHER ANTIGENS.
Kidd (Jk^a), Duffy (Fy^a), c, E, and to a lesser extent C can all cause erythroblastosis as severe as that associated with sensitization to D (Table 39–9). Two Duffy antigens have been identified, Fy^a and Fy^b, and among blacks there is a type that lacks both. Fy^a is the most immunogenic. The Kidd system also has two antigens, Jk^a and Jk^b, with a distribution in the population as follows: Jk (a+b−), 26 percent; Jk (a−b+), 24 percent; and jK (a+b+), 50 percent (Alper, 1977). Most cases of isoimmunization to these antigens occur after blood transfusions.

The clinical importance of anti-C isoimmunization has been emphasized by Wenk (1986) and Bowell (1986b) and their colleagues. This antibody was the next most common cause of clinically significant isoimmunization following anti-D. Although anti-C isoimmunization most commonly resulted from previous pregnan-

TABLE 39–9. Some Red Cell Antigens and Their Propensity to Cause Hemolytic Disease in the Fetus-Infant Whose Mother Is Isoimmunized

Blood Group System	Antigen	Severity of Hemolytic Disease	Proposed Management
CDE (Rh)	D	Mild to severe with hydrops fetalis	Amnionic fluid studies
	C	Mild to moderate	Amnionic fluid studies
	c	Mild to severe	Amnionic fluid studies
	E	Mild to severe	Amnionic fluid studies
	E	Mild to moderate	Amnionic fluid studies
I		Not a proven cause of hemolytic disease	
Lewis		Not a proven cause of hemolytic disease	
Kell	K	Mild to severe with hydrops fetalis	Amnionic fluid studies
	k	Mild to severe	Amnionic fluid studies
Duffy	Fy^a	Mild to severe with hydrops fetalis	Amnionic fluid studies
	Fy^b	Not a cause of hemolytic disease	
Kidd	Jk^a	Mild to severe	Amnionic fluid studies
	Jk^b	Mild to severe	Amnionic fluid studies
MNSs	M	Mild to severe	Amnionic fluid studies
	N	Mild	Expectant
	S	Mild to severe	Amnionic fluid studies
	s	Mild to severe	Amnionic fluid studies
	U	Mild to severe	Amnionic fluid studies
Lutheran	Lu^a	Mild	Expectant
	Lu^b	Mild	Expectant
Diego	Di^a	Mild to severe	Amnionic fluid studies
	Di^b	Mild to severe	Amnionic fluid studies
Xg	Xg^a	Mild	Expectant
P	$PP_{1Pk(Tja)}$	Mild to severe	Amnionic fluid studies
Public Antigens	Yt^a	Moderate to severe	Amnionic fluid studies
	Yt^b	Mild	Expectant
	Lan	Mild	Expectant
	En^a	Moderate	Amnionic fluid studies
	Ge	Mild	Expectant
	Jr^a	Mild	Expectant
	Co^a	Severe	Amnionic fluid studies
Private Antigens	Co^{a-b}	Mild	Expectant
	Batty	Mild	Expectant
	Becker	Mild	Expectant
	Berrens	Mild	Expectant
	Biles	Moderate	Amnionic fluid studies
	Evans	Mild	Expectant
	Gonzales	Mild	Expectant
	Good	Severe	Amnionic fluid studies
	Heibel	Moderate	Amnionic fluid studies
	Hunt	Mild	Expectant
	Jobbins	Mild	Expectant
	Radin	Moderate	Amnionic fluid studies
	Rm	Mild	Expectant
	Ven	Mild	Expectant
	$Wright^a$	Severe	Amnionic fluid studies
	$Wright^b$	Mild	Expectant
	Zd	Moderate	Amnionic fluid studies

Modified with permission from the American College of Obstetricians and Gynecologists (1990).

cies, those fetuses whose mothers had been transfused were more likely to have moderate to severe hemolysis. In a review by Bowman and colleagues (1992b) of 98 ongoing pregnancies with either anti-C or anti-Ce alloimmunization, there were 33 affected fetuses, of which eight required treatment after birth and none had severe diseases.

If an IgG red cell antibody is detected and there is any doubt as to its significance, the clinician should err on the side of caution and the pregnancy should be evaluated. As shown in Table 39–9, many rare or *private antigens* have been associated with severe isoimmunization (Rouse and Weiner, 1990).

IMMUNE HYDROPS. The pathological changes in the organs of the fetus and newborn infants vary with the severity of the process. Excessive and prolonged hemolysis serves to stimulate marked erythroid hyperplasia of the bone marrow as well as large areas of extramedullary hematopoiesis, particularly in the spleen and liver, which may in turn cause hepatic dysfunction (Nicolini and associates, 1991). Histological examination of the liver may also disclose fatty degenerative parenchymal changes as well as deposition of hemosiderin and engorgement of hepatic canaliculi with bile. There may be cardiac enlargement and pulmonary hemorrhages. When the severely affected fetus or infant shows considerable subcutaneous edema as well as effusion into the serous cavities, this is called *hydrops fetalis.* It is defined as the presence of abnormal fluid in two or more sites such as thorax, abdomen, or skin. The diagnosis is usually made easily using sonography (Fig. 39–8). The placenta is also markedly edematous, appreciably enlarged and boggy, with large, prominent cotyledons and edematous villi. Fetal ascites, hepatomegaly, and splenomegaly may be so massive as to lead to severe dystocia. Hydrothorax may be so severe as to affect lung development and compromise respirations after birth.

The precise pathophysiology of hydrops remains obscure. Theories of its causation include heart failure from profound anemia, capillary leakage caused by hypoxia from severe anemia, portal and umbilical venous hypertension from hepatic parenchymal disruption by extramedullary hematopoiesis, and decreased colloid oncotic pressure from hypoproteinemia caused by liver dysfunction. Nicolaides and colleagues (1985) performed percutaneous umbilical artery blood sampling in 17 severely D-isoimmunized fetuses at 18 to 25 weeks. All fetuses with hydrops had hemoglobin values of less than 3.8 g/dL as well as plasma protein concentrations less than 2 standard deviations from the mean for normal fetuses of the same age. The hydropic fetuses also had substantive protein concentrations in ascitic fluid. Conversely, all nonhydropic fetuses had hemoglobin values exceeding 4 g/dL; however, 6 of 10 had hypoproteinemia of the same magnitude as the hydropic fetuses. These investigators concluded that the degree and duration of anemia and resulting hypoxia most strongly influenced the severity of ascites, which is made worse by hypoproteinemia. They also hypothesized that the severe chronic anemia associated with tissue hypoxia actually causes capillary endothelial leakage with protein loss. Weiner and co-workers (1989) came to similar conclusions after their evaluation of umbilical venous pressure during 20 antenatal transfusions in isoimmunized pregnancies. They found that the fetuses with immune hydrops had significantly elevated pressures that normalized within 24 hours of the transfusion. This suggests that elevated pressure was due to hypoxic myocardial dysfunction and not to portal hypertension.

Fetuses with hydrops may die in utero from profound anemia and circulatory failure (Fig. 39–9). A sign of severe anemia and impending death is the sinusoidal fetal heart rate pattern shown in Figure 39–7. The liveborn hydropic infant appears pale, edematous, and limp at birth, often requiring resuscitation. The spleen and liver are enlarged, and there may be widespread ecchymosis or scattered petechiae. Dyspnea and circulatory collapse are common.

HYPERBILIRUBINEMIA. Less severely affected infants may appear well at birth, only to become jaundiced within a few hours. Marked hyperbilirubinemia, if untreated, may lead to *kernicterus,* a form of central nervous system damage that especially affects the basal ganglia. Anemia, in part resulting from impaired erythropoiesis, may persist for many weeks to months in the

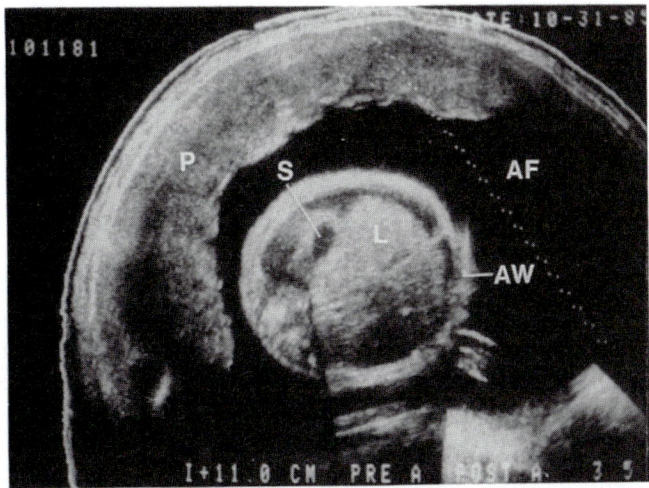

FIGURE 39–8. Transverse sonogram of a hydropic fetus. Illustrated are the edematous fetal abdominal wall (AW) and the fetal liver (L) and stomach (S). Increased amnionic fluid (AF) is apparent, and there is also a large placenta (P). (Courtesy of Dr. R. Santos.)

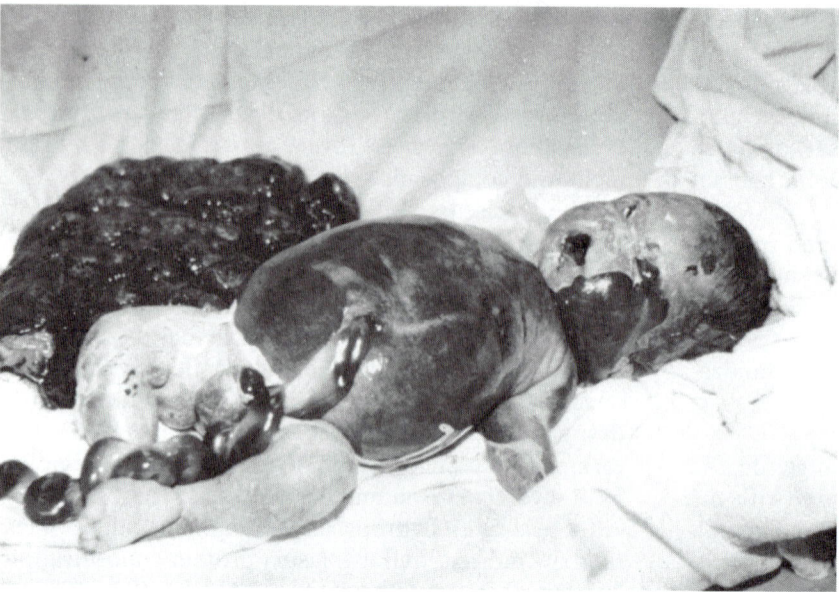

FIGURE 39–9. Severe erythroblastosis fetalis. Hydropic macerated stillborn infant and characteristically large placenta.

infant who had demonstrated hemolytic disease at birth. In the absence of hypoxia, erythrocyte production normally falls after birth, especially in the preterm infant.

MORTALITY. Perinatal deaths from hemolytic disease caused by D-isoimmunization have decreased dramatically because of administration of D-immune globulin to D-negative women during or immediately after pregnancy. Another reason is that the fetus who is most likely to be seriously affected can be treated by antenatal transfusions or be delivered preterm. In the province of Manitoba, the number of perinatal deaths from hemolytic disease decreased from 29 in 1964 to only 1 in 1975 (Bowman and colleagues, 1977). Similarly, Fretts and colleagues (1992) reviewed the changing patterns of fetal death in their tertiary care center from 1961 to 1988 and found that death from D-isoimmunization has also virtually disappeared.

IDENTIFICATION OF THE ISOIMMUNIZED PREGNANCY. With the exception of ABO incompatibility, which requires only neonatal treatment, the management of isoimmunization is the same regardless of the inciting antigen. The first step is identifying the woman at risk by performing a type and antibody screen at the first prenatal appointment during all pregnancies. Maternal serum antibodies are detected by the *indirect Coombs test,* because the anti-D antibodies are unbound and are absorbed to red cells only in the fetal circulation.

The fetus is evaluated by the *direct Coombs test,* as the anti-red cell antibodies produced by the mother are largely absorbed to the D-positive fetal erythrocytes.

The absorbed antibodies act as hemolysins, leading to an accelerated rate of red cell destruction. The neonate also is evaluated with the direct Coombs test. Maternal antibodies detectable at birth gradually disappear from over a period of 1 to 4 months. If the fetal blood type has not been determined antenatally by invasive methods discussed subsequently, then the blood type is determined at birth but may yield inaccurate results. This is because neonatal red cells may be so thoroughly coated with anti-D antibody that D antigens are not detectable and the neonate is reported incorrectly to be D-negative.

If maternal red cell antibodies are present, they are identified and determined to be either IgG or IgM. Only IgG antibodies are of concern because IgM antibodies do not usually cross the placenta in amounts that cause fetal hemolysis. The antibody titer is quantified. If the antibodies are IgG and are known to cause fetal hemolytic anemia (Table 39–9), and if the titer is above a critical level, further evaluation is indicated. For anti-D antibodies, the titer below which the fetus will not die from hemolytic disease is usually 1:16, although this varies between laboratories. A titer equal to or higher than this *critical titer* indicates the possibility of severe hemolytic disease. This critical titer of 1:16 is often extrapolated to other antibodies, but there are insufficient data to support this. An example is anti-Kell antibody discussed earlier. Conversely, for less immunogenic antigens like c or E, the critical titer may be 1:32 or higher.

The presence of maternal anti-D antibodies does not necessarily mean that the fetus will be affected or is even D-positive. For example, the titer in a previously sensitized woman may rise to high levels during a subsequent pregnancy even though her fetus is D-negative—the *amnestic response.* Because half of D-positive white males are heterozygous for the D antigen, a fourth of all fetuses of women at risk will be D-negative (Race, 1975). Similarly, many women sensitized to atypical red cell antigens become immunized after a blood transfusion and not by exposure to their antigen-negative husband.

ESTIMATING FETAL GENOTYPE. Along with paternal blood type, the most likely arrangement of his CDE genes can be estimated—the *presumed genotype.* This provides a basis for predicting whether or not the father is a heterozygote and thus whether the fetus could be D-negative. The CDE blood group gene locus is located on chromosome 1p34-p36. One gene encodes the C/c and E/e proteins and a second gene encodes D—there is no "d" gene or gene product. The laboratory first identifies all CDE antigens made by the father, and then estimates his presumed genotype based on the most common arrangement of genes for those particular antigens in men of his race. Predicting the most likely gene arrangement is improved somewhat in that cross-overs rarely occur within this gene group. For example, if the father has antigens C, c, D, and e, he could either be homozygous for D (D,D) or heterozygous (D, "d"). If he is white, there is a 94 percent chance that the arrangement of these alleles is Cde/cde; that is, he has a 94 percent chance of being heterozygous for D and thus a 47 percent (94 ÷ 2) chance of having a D-negative fetus.

If the women is sensitized to an atypical antigen, the paternal antigen type will determine whether the fetus is at risk. Before such testing is pursued, any possibility of nonpaternity must be disclosed, as testing the wrong father could be disastrous for the fetus.

MANAGEMENT OF ISOIMMUNIZATION. After identification of isoimmunization and the fetus potentially at risk, for optimal outcome, subsequent management is individualized. It is aided by the obstetrical history, with emphasis on fetal outcome(s). Fetal anemia from hemolytic disease tends to occur earlier and be more severe with every pregnancy. Accurate dating of pregnancy is essential. If below the critical titer, maternal antibody measurements are repeated at timely intervals. If these exceed the critical titer, then further evaluation is done by spectrophotometric analysis of amnionic fluid or analysis of fetal blood.

If the results of evaluation of all these factors is that the fetus is likely to be anemic, it must be tested and therapy provided as appropriate. Early studies showed that if no treatment is given for the sensitized D-negative women with a D-positive fetus, the perinatal mortality rate is about 30 percent (Freda, 1973). With aggressive management, including diagnostic amniocentesis or studies performed on fetal blood obtained by cordocentesis, repeated ultrasound examinations, and intrauterine transfusions in selected cases, the perinatal mortality rate is lowered remarkably (Harman and co-workers, 1983; Queenan and colleagues, 1993).

AMNIONIC FLUID EVALUATION. When fetal blood cells undergo hemolysis, breakdown pigments, mostly bilirubin, are present in the supernatant of amnionic fluid. The amount of amnionic fluid bilirubin correlates roughly with the degree of hemolysis and thus indirectly predicts the severity of the fetal anemia. Because these bilirubin concentrations are so low (compared with serum), its concentration is measured by a continuously recording spectrophotometer and is demonstrable as a change in absorbance at 450 nm, referred to as ΔOD_{450} (Fig. 39–10). The likelihood that the fetus is anemic is determined by plotting the ΔOD_{450} on a graph originated by Liley (1961), who compared ΔOD_{450} measurements with fetal outcome in 101 isoimmunized pregnancies (Fig. 39–11).

Subsequent studies have correlated the zones of the Liley graph with fetal hemoglobin concentration. Optical density values in zone 1 generally indicate a D-negative fetus or one who will only have mild disease. In zone 2, the fetus is at moderate to severe risk; in lower zone 2, the expected fetal hemoglobin concentration is between 11.0 and 13.9 g/dL, whereas in upper zone 2,

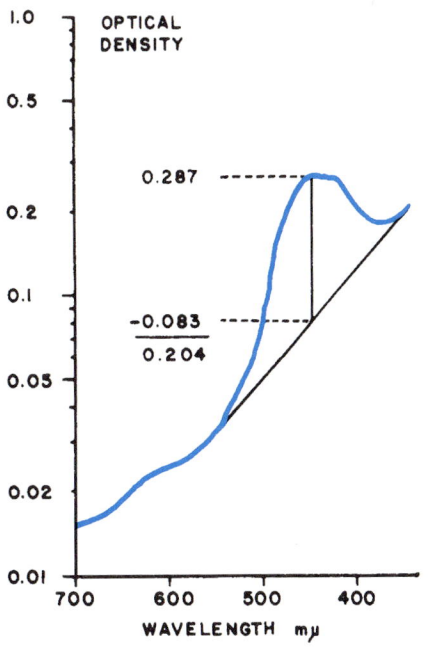

FIGURE 39–10. Spectral absorption curve of amnionic fluid in hemolytic disease.

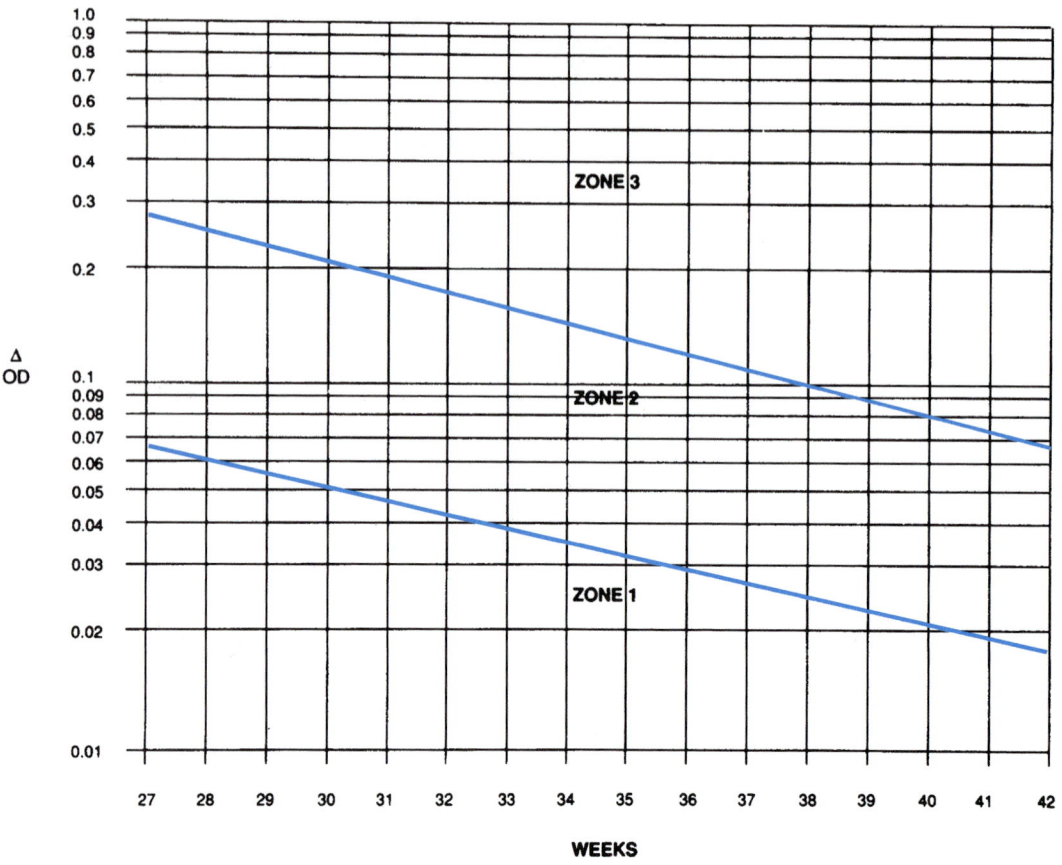

FIGURE 39–11. Liley graph used to depict severity of fetal hemolysis with red cell isoimmunization. (From Liley, 1961, with permission.)

the anticipated hemoglobin level ranges from 8.0 to 10.9 g/dL. Values in zone 3 indicate a severely affected fetus with a hemoglobin level less than 8.0 g/dL, and without therapy, death within 7 to 10 days may be expected.

Values in zone 3 demand immediate fetal red blood cell transfusion or delivery. Values in zones 1 or 2 should be followed by a repeat sampling in 1 to 2 weeks, and the trend of the two values used to estimate the severity of the hemolytic process. For pregnancies in which the trend of samples forms a line parallel to the lines on the graph or decreasing within the zone, thus indicating an unaffected fetus or a stable process, amniocentesis is repeated at 2- to 3-week intervals until either transfusion or delivery are required (American College of Obstetricians and Gynecologists, 1990). Pregnancies in which the process is unstable, that is, those in which the trend of ΔOD_{450} values is rising within zone 2 or has risen into zone 3, require immediate evaluation followed by transfusion or delivery as indicated. Vaginal delivery as close to term as possible, without subjecting the fetus to excess high-risk procedures, is always the goal.

EXPANDED LILEY GRAPH. Because of the age of viability contemporaneous to those times, the Liley graph

only included pregnancies from 27 to 41 weeks. As the age of viability decreased, and because isoimmunized fetuses are at risk of being severely anemic well before 27 weeks, management was originally planned by extrapolation of the Liley curve back to 18 to 20 weeks. This subsequently was found to be inaccurate, because prior to 25 weeks, bilirubin concentration is normally higher and amnionic fluid ΔOD_{450} results do not accurately predict the fetal hemoglobin level (Nicolaides and colleagues, 1986).

These findings led to development of modified Liley curves for pregnancies before 27 weeks. Queenan and colleagues (1993) examined 845 amnionic fluid samples from 75 D-immunized and 520 unaffected pregnancies and constructed a Liley-type curve that begins at 14 weeks. This is shown in Figure 39–12, and there is a large "indeterminate" zone in which values do not accurately predict fetal hemoglobin concentration. For these reasons, many clinicians forego amniocentesis in favor of fetal blood sampling when evaluation indicates there is likely to be severe fetal anemia or hydrops before 25 weeks.

FETAL BLOOD SAMPLING. Cordocentesis is used for obtaining fetal blood. The technique for this invasive

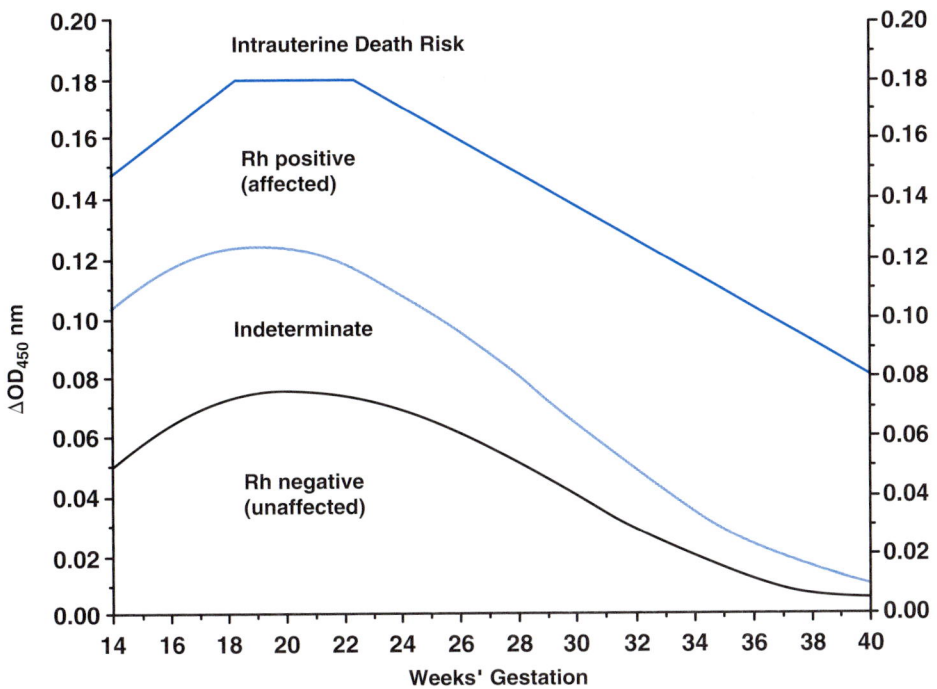

FIGURE 39–12. Proposed amnionic fluid ΔOD_{450} management zones in pregnancies from 14 to 40 weeks. (From Queenan and colleagues, 1993, with permission.)

procedure is discussed in Chapter 37 (p. 991). Its risks exceed those of amniocentesis. For a while, some clinicians used cordocentesis primarily to evaluate all isoimmunized pregnancies, regardless of gestational age. This was because fetal blood sampling had the added advantages of determination of blood type. Advances in molecular genetic techniques now allow the fetal D-antigen type to be determined from amniocytes in amnionic fluid (Bennett and associates, 1993). This is invaluable, especially for pregnancies in which the father is a presumed heterozygote, and thus the fetus could be D-negative. In these cases, a single amniocentesis for fetal D typing and ΔOD_{450} measurement may be the only invasive test needed. Van Den Veyver and colleagues (1996) reported 100 percent accuracy using this procedure in 112 of 114 amnionic fluid samples. Yankowitz and co-workers (1997) evaluated 765 adult blood samples and reported that this procedure had 99.7 percent sensitivity and 94 percent specificity. Several reference laboratories are now able to analyze amniocytes for the E, c, Kell, and Cellano antigens as well.

When the ΔOD_{450} measurement indicates the possibility of fetal anemia, ultrasonography reveals fetal hepatomegaly or hydrops, or fetal testing indicates physiological stress, either fetal transfusion or delivery must be performed. As discussed earlier, cordocentesis is also a consideration for fetuses likely to be affected before

27 weeks. Cordocentesis allows determination of the fetal hemoglobin and hematocrit, as well as the reticulocyte count and indirect Coombs titer (Weiner and associates, 1991a).

Nicolaides and co-workers (1988) recommend that transfusions be commenced when the hemoglobin is at least 2 g/dL below the mean for normal fetuses of corresponding gestational age (Fig. 39–13). Others perform transfusions when the fetal hematocrit is below 30 percent, which is 2 SD below the mean at all gestational ages (Weiner and co-workers, 1991b). Intraperitoneal and intraumbilical blood transfusions are discussed in Chapter 37 (p. 993).

SUBSEQUENT CHILD DEVELOPMENT. According to Bowman (1978), the great majority of fetal transfusion survivors developed normally. When 89 of these children were tested at 18 months of age or older, 74 were completely normal, four were abnormal, and development in the other 11 appeared somewhat delayed, perhaps because of preterm birth.

OTHER METHODS TO MINIMIZE FETAL HEMOLYSIS. In an attempt to prevent D-antibody formation, to remove antibody already formed, or to block antibody action on the red cell, a number of techniques have been tried without consistent success. Plasmapheresis

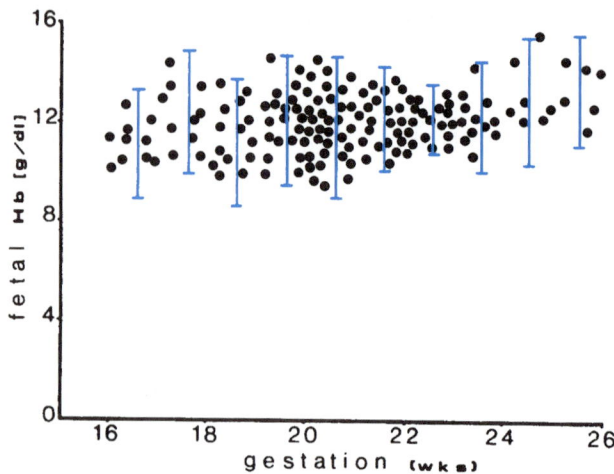

FIGURE 39–13. Reference range (mean + 2 SD) and distribution of individual values for fetal hemoglobin concentration from 153 pregnancies not complicated by fetal hemolysis. (From Nicolaides and colleagues, 1986, with permission.)

does not appear to provide benefits that outweigh the risks and the costs. Promethazine in large doses has been cited by some as being beneficial; however, this remains unproven (Charles and Blumenthal, 1982). D-positive erythrocyte membrane in enteric-coated capsules has been administered orally to sensitized women throughout pregnancy. It was hoped that such treatment might induce T-suppressor cell formation that would in turn reduce antibody response to challenges by the antigen. Unfortunately, this approach also does not appear to provide any benefit (Gold and co-workers, 1983). Attempts at immunosuppression with corticosteroids have also proven to be of no benefit.

DELIVERY. Vaginal delivery at or near term is the goal of management. Whether serial amnionic fluid ΔOD_{450} measurement or intrauterine transfusions are being performed, the pregnancy is usually closely monitored with tests of fetal well being described in Chapter 40. Their initiation is determined by history as well as severity in the current pregnancy. Gestational age is usually the most important consideration in choosing which treatment option to pursue. The very immature fetus may benefit from intrauterine resuscitation by transfusions, while the fetus near term should be delivered. Fortunately, with careful monitoring and transfusions when appropriate, very early preterm delivery can usually be avoided.

In carefully monitored cases, labor can be induced as soon as pulmonary maturity is documented. The severely compromised fetus, however, may benefit from cesarean delivery. The time of birth is set and the most experienced personnel can be assembled to provide for optimal treatment. Scheduling of labor induction could have similar advantages.

EXCHANGE TRANSFUSION IN THE NEWBORN. Cord blood analysis should be carried out immediately for any pregnancy in which the D-negative mother is known to be sensitized. Cord blood hemoglobin concentration and direct Coombs test are of considerable importance when the infant is D-positive. If the infant is overtly anemic, it is often best to carry out the initial exchange promptly to correct anemia. Type O, D-negative red cells, recently collected, are used. For infants who are not overtly anemic, the need for exchange transfusion is determined by the rate of increase in bilirubin concentration, the maturity of the infant, and the presence of other complications. Because close neonatal monitoring is required, delivery should be at a center familiar with management of this disease.

PREVENTION. Anti-D immunoglobulin is a 7S immune globulin G extracted by cold alcohol fractionation from plasma containing high-titer D-antibody. Each dose provides not less than 300 μg of D-antibody as determined by radioimmunoassay. It is given to the D-negative nonsensitized mother to prevent the hazards of sensitization described above.

Freda and co-workers (1975) summarized their 10 years of clinical experience with D-immune globulin, confirming their original observations that such globulin given to the previously unsensitized D-negative woman within 72 hours of delivery is highly protective. Any pregnancy-related events that could result in fetal–maternal hemorrhage require D-immune globulin prophylaxis (Table 39–8). Anti-D immune globulin should be provided to D-negative women after miscarriage, abortion, or evacuation of a molar or ectopic pregnancy. Up to 2 percent of women with a spontaneous abortion and 5 percent of those undergoing elective termination become isoimmunized without D-immune globulin. Blajchman and co-workers (1974) reported detectable fetal–maternal hemorrhage after 6 percent of amniocenteses. Boucher and associates (1996) documented hemorrhage following external cephalic version.

ROUTINE ANTEPARTUM ADMINISTRATION. In addition to the previously described situations, anti-D immune globulin is also given prophylactically to all D-negative women at about 28 weeks (American College of Obstetricians and Gynecologists, 1999b). It is again given after delivery if the infant is D-positive. Bowman and Pollock (1978) showed that without such prophylaxis, 1.8 percent of D-negative women will become isoimmunized during pregnancy as the consequence of spontaneous silent fetal–maternal hemorrhages remote from delivery. They administered 300 μg of antibody intramuscularly at 28 weeks, at 34 weeks, and if the infant was D-positive, again after delivery. This program was followed by a reduction in the incidence of D-isoimmunization during pregnancy from 1.8 percent to 0.07 percent. Subsequently, they showed that a single dose at about 28 weeks was almost as effective as were the two doses antepartum. Indeed, only 2 of 1799 D-negative women developed D-isoimmunization despite antenatal prophylaxis.

The half life of immune globulin is 24 days, and titers decrease with time. The initial dose of 300 μg will produce a weakly positive (1:1 to 1:4) indirect Coombs titer. If an amniocentesis is performed or uterine bleeding occurs more than 3 weeks after the 28-week prophylactic dose, but before delivery, a second dose of 300 μg will protect the mother against a hemorrhage of up to 15 mL of D-positive red cells, or 30 mL of fetal blood. The small amount of antibody that crosses the placenta results at times in a weakly positive direct Coombs test in cord and infant blood. If the positive Coombs test is due to D-immune globulin, there is no evidence of anemia or exaggerated hyperbilirubinemia.

Some patients express concern that the human immunodeficiency virus or other viruses may be transmitted by plasma-derived products such as anti-D immunoglobulin. The risk of this is very low because individuals who are antibody or antigen positive for various hepatitis viruses are excluded from blood donation, and the human immunodeficiency virus is inactivated by the manufacturing process (Centers for Disease Control, 1987; Misbah and Chapel, 1993).

D-negative women who receive blood or blood fractions are also at risk of becoming sensitized. Red cell and platelet transfusions and plasmapheresis can provide sufficient D-antigen to cause sensitization, which can be prevented by an injection of D-antiglobulin. **Freda (1973), as well as Bowman (1985), emphasize that when there is doubt about whether to give anti-D immune globulin, then it should be given.**

LARGE FETAL-TO-MATERNAL HEMORRHAGE. In the case of a large fetal–maternal hemorrhage, one dose of D-immune globulin may not be sufficient to neutralize the transfused fetal cells. Bowman (1985) estimated the incidence of excessive fetal–maternal bleeding sufficient so as not to be neutralized by one dose of immune globulin to be 1 in 1250 deliveries. Ness and colleagues (1987), however, provided different data regarding this incidence. Using the enzyme-linked antiglobulin test, they studied almost 800 D-negative mothers giving birth to D-positive infants, and found evidence in 1 percent of the mothers for fetal–maternal bleeding in excess of 30 mL. Another 5.6 percent of these pregnancies had fetal–maternal hemorrhage of between 11 and 30 mL. Thus, at least 1 percent, and perhaps more, of suscepti-

ble mothers would have been given insufficient immune globulin if not tested. Importantly, they determined that if extra D-immune globulin is only considered for women with risk factors such as abdominal trauma, placental abruption, placenta previa, intrauterine manipulation, multiple gestation, or manual removal of the placenta, that half of women requiring more than the 300 μg dose would be missed. They thus recommended that all women be tested at delivery with the Kleihauer–Betke or rosette test. Stedman and co-workers (1986), utilizing the erythrocyte rosette test, reported similar results. The dosage of anti-D immunoglobulin is calculated as described on page 1066. The fetal red cell volume is divided by 15, which is the volume that one 300-mg ampule will neutralize.

D^u ANTIGEN. The identification of the D^u antigen in a maternal blood type often causes confusion. Most laboratories designate this blood type as "weak D-positive." The D^u antigen is a variant of the D antigen. The woman confirmed to be D^u-positive does not need immune globulin (American College of Obstetricians and Gynecologists, 1999b). Maternally detected D^u antigen (rarely) indicates the transfer of D^u-positive fetal cells into a D-negative mother. Bowman (1985) cites only five instances in 750,000 pregnancies in which a D^u-positive mother produced anti-D antibody. Fortunately, in none of these was the fetus severely affected. If the maternal blood type is known to be D^u-positive before conception, most authorities would treat her as D-positive, and if a D-negative woman delivers a D^u-positive infant, she should be given D-immune globulin. As before, if there is any doubt about D-antigen status, then globulin should be given.

MATERNAL-TO-FETAL HEMORRHAGE. Rarely, the D-negative fetus is exposed in utero to D antigen from the mother and becomes sensitized as a result. When such a female fetus becomes an adult, she will produce anti-D antibodies indicating sensitization even before or early in her first pregnancy. This mechanism of isoimmunization is called the "grandmother theory" because the fetus in the current pregnancy is jeopardized by antibodies initially provoked by its grandmother's blood. This accounts for very few cases of D sensitization. Major blood group (ABO) incompatibility offers appreciable protection against D-sensitization. Furthermore, maternal–fetal hemorrhage is uncommon. Jennings and Clauss (1978) and Bowman (1985), on the basis of their extensive studies, do not recommend D-immune globulin prophylaxis for D-negative babies born to D-positive mothers.

HYPERBILIRUBINEMIA

DISPOSAL OF BILIRUBIN. Unconjugated or free bilirubin is readily transferred across the placenta from fetal to maternal circulation—and vice versa, if the maternal plasma level of unconjugated bilirubin is high. Bilirubin glucuronide is water soluble and normally excreted into the bile by the liver and into the urine by the kidney when the plasma level is elevated. Conversely, unconjugated bilirubin is not excreted in the urine or to any extent in the bile.

KERNICTERUS. The great concern over unconjugated hyperbilirubinemia in the newborn, especially the preterm neonate, is its association with kernicterus. Yellow staining of the basal ganglia and hippocampus by bilirubin is indicative of profound degeneration in these regions. Surviving infants show spasticity, muscular incoordination, and varying degrees of mental retardation. There is a positive correlation between kernicterus and unconjugated bilirubin levels above 18 to 20 mg/dL, although kernicterus may develop at much lower concentrations, especially in very preterm infants.

Factors other than the serum bilirubin concentration contribute to the development of kernicterus. Hypoxia and acidosis enhance bilirubin toxicity. Both hypothermia and hypoglycemia predispose the infant to kernicterus by raising the level of nonesterified fatty acids, which compete with bilirubin for binding sites on albumin and inhibit bilirubin conjugation. Sepsis contributes to kernicterus, although the mechanism is not clear. Although it is extremely unlikely that they lead to kernicterus, sulfonamides and salicylates may increase the level of bilirubin because they compete with unconjugated bilirubin for protein-binding sites. Sodium benzoate, in injectable diazepam, furosemide, and gentamicin, displaces bilirubin from albumin. Excessive doses of vitamin K analogs may be associated with hyperbilirubinemia. The importance of the serum albumin concentration and the binding sites so provided is obvious.

BREAST MILK JAUNDICE. Jaundice in breast-fed infants has been attributed to the excretion of pregnane-$3\alpha,20\beta$-diol into breast milk. This steroid was reported by Arias and colleagues (1964) to block bilirubin conjugation by inhibiting glucuronyl transferase activity. Breast milk samples from mothers of infants with hyperbilirubinemia have been described to have an unusually high lipolytic activity and to liberate large quantities of fatty acids that inhibit bilirubin conjugation (Foliot and co-workers, 1976). Another explanation is that bilirubin is broken down in the intestine to form free bilirubin, which can be reabsorbed. Usually, bovine and human milk appear to block the reabsorption of free bilirubin, whereas the milk of mothers with jaundiced offspring does not, and may even enhance its reabsorption. With breast milk jaundice, the serum bilirubin level rises from about the fourth day after birth to a maximum by 15 days. If breast feeding is continued, the high levels persist for another 10 to 14 days and slowly decline over the next several weeks. No cases of overt bilirubin encephalopathy have been reported as a result of this phenomenon (Maisels, 1979).

PHYSIOLOGICAL JAUNDICE. By far the most common form of unconjugated nonhemolytic jaundice is so-called physiological jaundice. In the mature infant, the serum bilirubin increases for 3 to 4 days to achieve serum levels up to 10 mg/dL or so and then falls rapidly. In preterm infants, the rise is more prolonged and may be more intense.

TREATMENT. Phototherapy is now widely used to treat hyperbilirubinemia. By some unknown mechanism, light seems to promote hepatic excretion of unconjugated bilirubin. In most instances, its use leads to oxidation of bilirubin resulting in a lower bilirubin level. Light that penetrates the skin also increases peripheral blood flow, which further enhances photo-oxidation. As much surface area as possible should be exposed, and the infant should be turned every 2 hours with close temperature monitoring to prevent dehydration. The fluorescent bulbs must be appropriate wavelength and the eyelids should be closed and completely shielded from light. Serum bilirubin should be monitored for at least 24 hours after discontinuance of phototherapy. Rarely, exchange transfusion is required.

NONIMMUNE HYDROPS FETALIS. Hydrops is defined by the presence of excess fluid in two or more body areas, such as thorax, abdomen, or skin, and is usually associated with hydramnios and placental thickening. Because ultrasound examination has become routine, hydrops is identified frequently and the etiology is often discovered. Santolaya and colleagues (1992) reviewed ultrasound studies performed in 12,572 pregnant women and identified hydrops in 0.6 percent. The etiology was determined in 77 percent of cases (Fig. 39–14). Similarly, Heinonen and colleagues (2000) reported a hydrops incidence of 1 in 1700, of which the etiology was discovered in 95 percent.

ETIOLOGY. A variety of pathogenic mechanisms can lead to hydrops. **Cardiac abnormalities,** either structural, rhythm related, or both are associated with 20 to 45 percent of cases of nonimmune hydrops (Allan, 1986; Castillo, 1986; Gough, 1986; Santolaya, 1992, and their co-workers). **Fetal heart failure** can also result from infection leading to myocarditis or hepatitis. Approximately 35 percent of cases of hydrops are due to **chromosomal anomalies** or other **malformations.** Shulman and colleagues (2000) have reported that chromosomal abnormalities are commonly associated with *space suit hydrops*—dramatic and extensive subcutaneous hy-

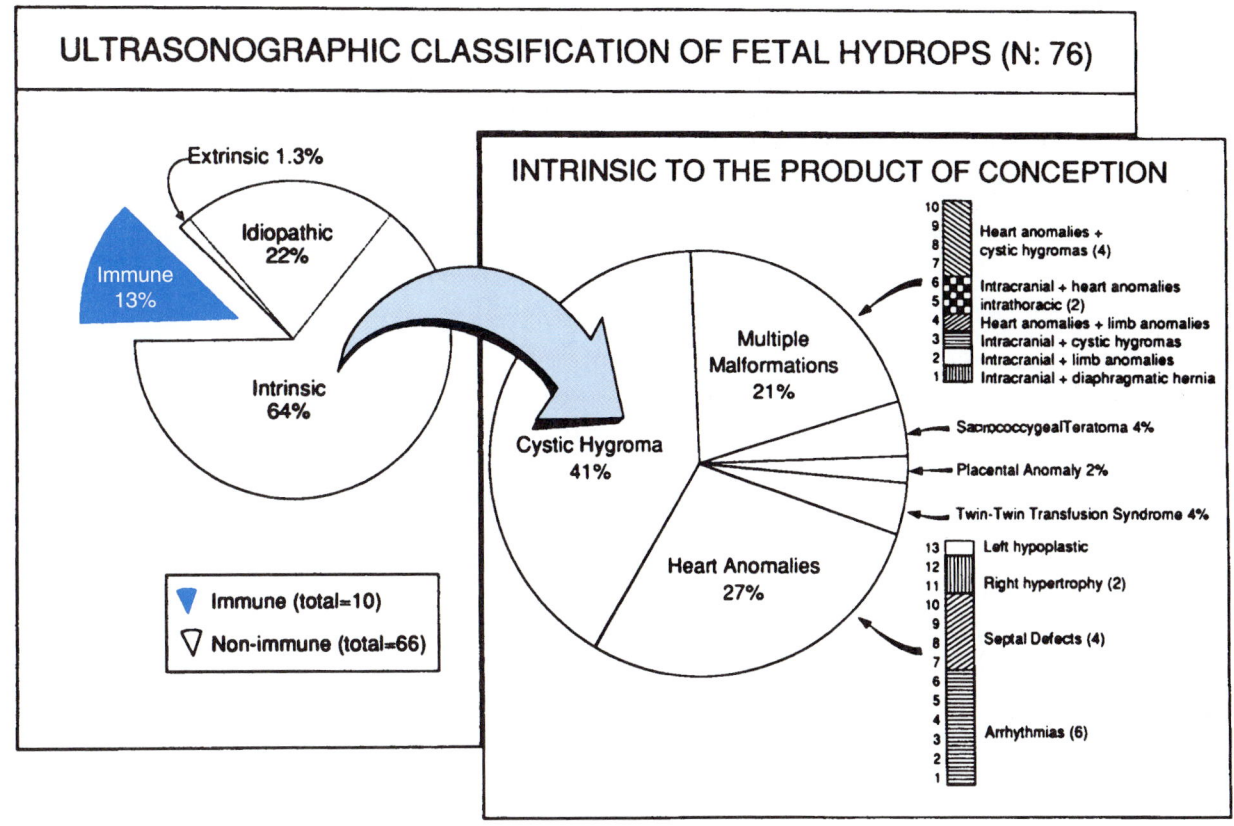

FIGURE 39-14. Classification and cause in 76 cases of fetal hydrops in which the etiology could be diagnosed by ultrasound. (From Santolaya and associates, 1992, with permission.)

drops recognized in the first trimester. Of 30 such fetuses less than 14 weeks, 87 percent had an aneuploidy, of which over half involved sex chromosomes. About 10 percent of hydrops cases are associated with **twin-to-twin transfusion syndrome** (Chap. 30, p. 785). Usually the recipient twin develops heart failure from volume overload, or the donor twin develops hydrops after the death of the recipient. Hydrops can also be caused by **severe anemia** such as might occur with parvovirus infection, acute fetal–maternal hemorrhage, or α-thalassemia (American College of Obstetricians and Gynecologists, 1999a). **Inborn errors of metabolism** such as Gaucher disease, GM 1 gangliosidosis, or sialidosis can cause recurrent hydrops (Lefebvre and colleagues, 1999). Rarely, an **anomalous lymph system** can result in lymph accumulating to cause chylothorax or chylous ascites.

The great variety of causes of hydrops were tabulated by Holzgreve and associates (1984) and are presented in Table 39–10. The precise incidence of these various causes of hydrops is unclear, and varies according to the sophistication of the evaluation and the population studied. For example, the San Francisco group, with a large Asian population, reported a 10 percent incidence of hydrops caused by α-thalassemia (Holzgreve and colleagues, 1984).

PROGNOSIS. The outcome for hydrops caused by any of these mechanisms is poor. McCoy and colleagues (1995) reviewed 82 cases of nonimmune hydrops attributed to cardiovascular abnormalities (23 percent), aneuploidy (16 percent), thoracic anomalies (13 percent), genetic syndromes (11 percent), anemia and infection (9 percent), twin-to-twin transfusion (6 percent), and idiopathic causes (22 percent). The mortality rate for hydrops before 24 weeks was 95 percent. Fetuses with hydrops who survived to at least 24 weeks, and who had no congenital heart defect and were euploid, had a survival rate of 20 percent.

DIAGNOSIS. Ultrasound evaluation may provide a diagnosis. Depending on circumstances, maternal blood analysis might include hemoglobin electrophoresis, Kleihauer–Betke smear, indirect Coombs, and serological tests for syphilis, toxoplasmosis, cytomegalovirus, rubella, and parvovirus B-19. Cordocentesis is considered for karyotyping, hemoglobin concentration and

TABLE 39–10. Causes of Nonimmune Hydrops Fetalis and Associated Clinical Conditions

Category	Condition	Category	Condition
Cardiovascular	Tachyarrhythmia	Urinary	Urethral stenosis or atresia
	Congenital heart block		Posterior neck obstruction
	Anatomical defects (atrial septal defect, ventricular defect, hypoplastic left heart, pulmonary valve insufficiency, Ebstein sub-aortic stenosis, dilated heart, atrioventricular canal defect, single ventricle, tetralogy of Fallot, premature closure of foramen ovale, subendocardial fibroelastosis, dextrocardia in combination with pulmonic stenosis)		Spontaneous bladder perforation
			Prune belly
			Neurogenic bladder with reflux
			Ureterocele
Chromosomal	Down syndrome (trisomy 21)	Gastrointestinal	Jejunal atresia
	Other trisomies		Midgut volvulus
	Turner syndrome		Malrotation of intestines
	Triploidy		Duplication of intestinal tract
			Meconium peritonitis
Malformation syndromes	Thanatophoric dwarfism	Medications	Antepartum indomethacin (taken to stop preterm labor, causing fetal ductus closure and secondary nonimmune hydrops fetalis)
	Arthrogryposis multiplex congenita		
	Asphyxiating thoracic dystrophy		
	Hypophosphatasia		
	Osteogenesis imperfecta		
	Achondroplasia		
	Achondrogenesis		
	Neu–Laxova syndrome		
	Recessive cystic hygroma		
	Saldino–Noonan syndrome		
	Penna–Shokeir type I syndrome		
Hematological	α-Thalassemia	Infections	Cytomegalovirus
	Arteriovenous shunts (vascular tumors)		Toxoplasmosis
	Chronic fetal–maternal transfusion		Syphilis
	Kasabach–Merritt syndrome		Congenital hepatitis
	In utero closed-space hemorrhage		Rubella
	Caval, portal, or femoral thrombosis		Parvovirus
			Leptospirosis
			Chaga disease
Twin pregnancy	Twin-to-twin transfusion syndrome		
	Parabiotic (acardiac) twin syndrome		
Respiratory	Diaphragmatic hernia	Miscellaneous	Amnionic band syndrome
	Cystic adenomatous malformation		Cystic hygroma
	Pulmonary hypoplasia		Congenital lymphedema
	Hamartoma of lung		Polysplenia syndrome
	Mediastinal teratoma		Congenital neuroblastoma
	Congenital chylothorax		Tuberous sclerosis
			Torsion of ovarian cyst
			Fetal trauma
			Sacrococcygeal teratoma

Modified from Holzgreve and co-workers (1984).

electrophoresis, liver transaminases, and serological testing for IgM-specific antibodies to infectious agents. In view of the data from McCoy and associates (1995) described previously, a fetal echocardiogram and karyotype analysis may be the most important elements of the evaluation in predicting prognosis for fetuses still alive after 24 weeks.

MANAGEMENT. In a few cases, depending on the cause of hydrops, treatment is available. Some cardiac arrhythmias can be treated pharmacologically, severe anemia due to fetal–maternal hemorrhage or parvovirus infection can be treated with blood transfusions, and hydrops of one fetus in twin-to-twin transfusion syndrome may resolve with therapeutic amniocentesis (Chap. 30, p. 788). Because most lesions associated with these syndromes ultimately prove fatal for the fetus or newborn, however, treatment is often not possible. In general, when hydrops persists, cardiac abnormalities and aneuploidy have been ruled out, and if the fetus is mature enough that survival is likely, then delivery should be accomplished. Very preterm fetuses usually are managed expectantly. Although hydrops usually persists or worsens with time, it occasionally resolves spontaneously (Mueller-Heubach and Mazer, 1983).

MATERNAL COMPLICATIONS. A unique complication of hydrops is the so-called maternal **mirror syndrome** (Midgley and Hardrug, 2000). Believed to be caused by vascular changes in the swollen hydropic placenta, it is called the mirror syndrome because the mother develops preeclampsia with severe edema similar to the fetus. This type of preeclampsia may develop early and (rarely) may be resolved with fetal treatment. Duthie and Walkinshaw (1995) described a woman with parvovirus-associated fetal hydrops and severe preeclampsia whose hypertension receded at 25 weeks when fetal transfusion reversed the fetal hydrops. In most cases, however, treatment is not possible and thus delivery is necessary. Preterm labor is common because of hydramnios. Postpartum hemorrhage sometimes occurs as the result of sudden decompression of an overdistended uterus, and retained placenta is common.

FETAL CARDIAC ARRHYTHMIAS. Recognition of fetal cardiac rhythm disturbances has become more common because of extensive use of real-time ultrasound technology. Whereas most of these arrhythmias are transient and benign, some tachyarrhythmias, if sustained, can result in congestive heart failure, nonimmune hydrops, and fetal death. Sustained bradycardia, although less often associated with hydrops, may signify underlying cardiac pathology that includes structural lesions or autoimmune myocarditis.

Kleinman and associates (1985) summarized their ex-

TABLE 39–11. Types of Arrhythmias in 198 Fetuses from Pregnancies Referred to Yale University

Arrhythmias	Number
Isolated extrasystoles	164
Atrial	145
Ventricular	19
Sustained arrhythmias	34
Supraventricular tachycardia	15
Complete heart block	8
Atrial flutter or fibrillation	5
Ventricular tachycardia	2
Second-degree heart block	2
Sinus bradycardia	2

From Kleinman and colleagues (1985).

perience with fetal arrhythmias (Table 39–11). Premature atrial contractions accounted for 63 percent of cases. Fortunately, this arrhythmia is benign, related to immaturity, and usually resolves with further fetal development. Rarely this rhythm converts to a sustained supraventricular tachycardia. If the rate is more than 200 beats/min, it may cause cardiac failure, and thus requires treatment as discussed in Chapter 37 (p. 994).

The prognosis for the fetus with bradycardia is less promising. Bradycardia typically results from a major structural abnormality such as complete atrial-ventricular canal, or from heart block. Taylor and colleagues (1986) demonstrated that half of the mothers of children with congenital heart block have antibodies to fetal myocardial tissue. Anti-SS-A (anti-Ro) antibody is one of the most common, and appears to bind to the conduction tissue. Unfortunately, tissue inflammation provoked by these antibodies leads to permanent damage, and survivors frequently require a pacemaker at birth.

Fetal cardiac antigens to which anti-SS-A affixes are not confined to the conduction system, and if there is extensive myocarditis, the prognosis is poor. Many of these women have, or subsequently develop, lupus erythematosus or another connective-tissue disease. Anti-SS-A actually causes fetal heart block in the minority, and only 1 in 20 fetuses born to women positive for this antibody have cardiac disease (Chap. 52, p. 1389). Of seven affected infants described by Ramsey-Goldman and colleagues (1986), three died within 9 months, two required permanent pacemakers, and two underwent cardiac surgery. Only one infant had no problems. Fetal therapy in the form of maternal corticosteroid ingestion has been reported (Chua and colleagues, 1991; Finkelstein and associates, 1997).

Cameron and associates (1988) and Shenker and colleagues (1987) reported that fetal cardiac anomalies are common with heart block in the absence of connective-tissue disease. They recommend fetal echocardiography and consideration for karyotyping.

HEMORRHAGIC DISEASE OF THE NEWBORN. This is a disorder of the newborn characterized by spontaneous internal or external bleeding accompanied by hypoprothrombinemia and very low levels of other vitamin K–dependent coagulation factors (V, VII, IX, and X). Bleeding may begin any time after birth but is typically delayed for a day or two. The infant may be mature and healthy in appearance, although there is a greater incidence of the disease in preterm infants.

The prothrombin and partial thromboplastin times are greatly prolonged. Causes other than vitamin K deficiency include hemophilia, congenital syphilis, sepsis, thrombocytopenia purpura, erythroblastosis, and intracranial hemorrhage.

Hypoprothrombinemia appears to be the consequence of poor placental transport of vitamin K_1 to the fetus. Plasma vitamin K_1 levels are somewhat lower in pregnant women than in nonpregnant adults, and it is not clear to what extent vitamin K crosses the placenta. Shearer and associates (1982) gave 1 mg of vitamin K_1 intravenously to mothers shortly before delivery and showed that maternal plasma levels were remarkably raised, but cord plasma levels still were very low. However, Pomerance and colleagues (1987) reported that prothrombin activity was improved in preterm neonates whose mothers were given intramuscular vitamin K_1 during labor.

The main cause of hemorrhagic disease of the newborn from vitamin K deficiency appears to be a dietary deficiency of vitamin K as the consequence of ingesting solely breast milk, which contains only very small amounts of the vitamin. Keenan and colleagues (1971) showed that the prothrombin time 24 hours after the start of feedings with cow milk is comparable to that found 24 hours after vitamin K administration, whereas in infants fed with human milk it remains prolonged.

Vitamin K–dependent clotting factors may also be reduced in infants of mothers taking anticonvulsant drugs (Mountain and associates, 1970). These drugs apparently have a mechanism similar to warfarin and act by depressing hepatic synthesis of several coagulation factors (VII, IX, and X). Like warfarin, anticonvulsant-induced vitamin K deficiency may produce a phenotype similar to that of *chondrodysplasia punctata* (Chap. 38, p. 1014). This is also called *Conradi–Hunermann syndrome* and is an inherited bony dystrophy resulting in typical facial abnormalities (Howe and colleagues, 1995).

PROPHYLAXIS. Hemorrhagic disease of the newborn can be avoided by the intramuscular injection of 1 mg

TABLE 39–12. Some Causes of Neonatal Thrombocytopenia

Immune disorders
Passive—Maternal immune thrombocytopenia, lupus, drugs
Active—Alloimmune, erythroblastosis fetalis
Infections
Drugs
Congenital
Thrombocytopenia absent radius (TAR) syndrome
Fanconi anemia
Chédiak–Higashi syndrome
Megakaryocytic hypoplasia
Leukemia
Histiocytosis
Osteopetrosis
Bone marrow disease
Disseminated intravascular coagulation
Inherited
Wiskott–Aldrich syndrome
May–Hegglin syndrome

of vitamin K_1 (phytonadione) at delivery. For treatment of active bleeding, it is injected intravenously.

THROMBOCYTOPENIA. The differential diagnosis of neonatal thrombocytopenia is provided in Table 39–12. Thrombocytopenia tends to be more severe in preterm fetuses, especially those with respiratory distress and hypoxia or sepsis.

IMMUNE THROMBOCYTOPENIA. Rarely, antiplatelet IgG is transferred from the mother to cause thrombocytopenia in the fetus-neonate. The most severe cases are usually due to alloimmune thrombocytopenia, discussed next, but this disorder can also be found in association with maternal autoimmune disease, especially immune thrombocytopenia. Maternal thrombocytopenia therapy consists of corticosteroids, which increase maternal platelet levels; however, such treatment generally does not affect fetal thrombocytopenia. A detailed discussion of management and perinatal outcomes is presented in Chapter 49 (p. 1324).

ALLOIMMUNE (ISOIMMUNE) THROMBOCYTOPENIA (ATP). This type of thrombocytopenia differs from immunological thrombocytopenia in several important ways. Because it is caused by maternal isoimmunization to fetal platelet antigens in a manner similar to D-antigen isoimmunization (see p. 1057), the maternal platelet count is always normal. Thus, alloimmunization is not suspected until after the birth of an affected child. Another important difference is that the fetal thrombocytopenia associated with ATP is frequently severe. It thus can cause fetal intracranial hemorrhage. The incidence of ATP is reported to be from 1 in 5000 to 1 in 10,000 live births (Nicolaides and Snijders, 1992; Silver and colleagues, 2000).

Fetal thrombocytopenia follows maternal isoimmunization usually against fetal platelet antigens HPA-1a, which is found in 98 percent of the population. Thus, the mother lacks the common platelet antigen and becomes immunized when exposed to the antigen by fetal platelets that enter the maternal circulation. Based on the incidence of HPA-1a negativity, 1 in 50 pregnancies is at risk. The rarity of the condition results from the fact that fetal–maternal hemorrhage significant enough to provoke an immune response must occur. The disease primarily affects offspring of women with HLA type DR-3 or B-8 (Reznikoff-Etievant and colleagues, 1983).

The diagnosis often can be made correctly on clinical grounds if the mother has a normal platelet count with no evidence of any immunological disorder, and her infant has thrombocytopenia without evidence of other disease. Fetal thrombocytopenia recurs in 70 to 90 percent of subsequent pregnancies (Silver and associates, 2000). It is often severe and occurs earlier with each successive pregnancy. Most clinicians document recurrent fetal thrombocytopenia by cordocentesis followed by maternally administered intravenous immunoglobulin in massive doses (Chap. 37, p. 991).

PREECLAMPSIA AND ECLAMPSIA. Neonatal thrombocytopenia has been suggested by some to result from preeclampsia–eclampsia. In a large number of infants born to women with pregnancy-induced hypertension at Parkland Hospital, however, Pritchard and colleagues (1987) identified no cases in which neonatal thrombocytopenia correlated with maternal thrombocytopenia (Chap. 24, p. 577).

POLYCYTHEMIA AND HYPERVISCOSITY. Several conditions predispose to neonatal polycythemia and blood hyperviscosity. These include chronic hypoxia in utero and placental transfusion from a twin or, much more rarely, from the mother. As the hematocrit rises above 65, blood viscosity markedly increases. Signs and symptoms include plethora, cyanosis, and neurological aberrations. Laboratory findings include hyperbilirubinemia, thrombocytopenia, fragmented erythrocytes, and hypoglycemia. Treatment consists of lowering the hematocrit by partial exchange transfusion with plasma.

NECROTIZING ENTEROCOLITIS. This bowel disorder commonly presents with clinical findings of abdominal distention, ileus, and bloody stools. There is usually radiological evidence of *pneumatosis intestinalis* caused by intestinal wall gas as the consequence of invasion by gas-forming bacteria and bowel perforation. Abdominal distention or blood in the stools may signal developing enterocolitis. At times it is so severe that bowel resection is necessary.

The disease is primarily seen in low-birthweight infants, but occasionally is encountered in mature neonates. Various causes have been suggested, including perinatal hypotension, hypoxia, or sepsis, as well as umbilical catheters, exchange transfusions, and the feeding of cow milk and hypertonic solutions (Kliegman and Fanaroff, 1984). The disease tends to occur in clusters, and coronaviruses have been suspected of having an etiological role. Kanto and colleagues (1987) reported that 5.7 percent of 2123 preterm infants developed necrotizing enterocolitis. The incidence of the disease was related to birthweight, but not to other perinatal factors. They concluded that gastrointestinal immaturity and not ischemia is the major causative factor for necrotizing enterocolitis. Orally administered immunoglobulin was shown to prevent enterocolitis when given to preterm infants (Eibl and associates, 1988).

FETAL DEATH

From the foregoing sections, it is apparent that a number of maternal and fetal conditions may result in fetal demise. With advances in obstetrics, clinical genetics, maternal–fetal and neonatal medicine, and perinatal pathology, a number of stillbirths which had previously been categorized as "unexplained" can now be attributed to specific causes. Because of this information, management of subsequent pregnancy is made easier. An advantage of the common use of ultrasound technology is the ease with which the suspicion of fetal death is confirmed. Conversely, because the diagnosis can be verified immediately, labor induction in a woman with an unfavorable cervix has become a problem (Chap. 20, p. 470).

DEFINITION OF FETAL MORTALITY. The National Center for Health Statistics and the American College of Obstetricians and Gynecologists (1995b) recommend that statistics of perinatal outcomes include only those dead fetuses and neonates born weighing 500 g or more. As shown in Figure 39–15, stillbirths are much more common with decreasing gestational age. According to Copper and colleagues (1994), almost 80 percent of all stillbirths occur before term, and more than half are before 28 weeks.

Along with the decline in stillbirth rate over the past five decades, the pattern of causes of stillbirths has changed appreciably. Fretts and colleagues (1992) re-

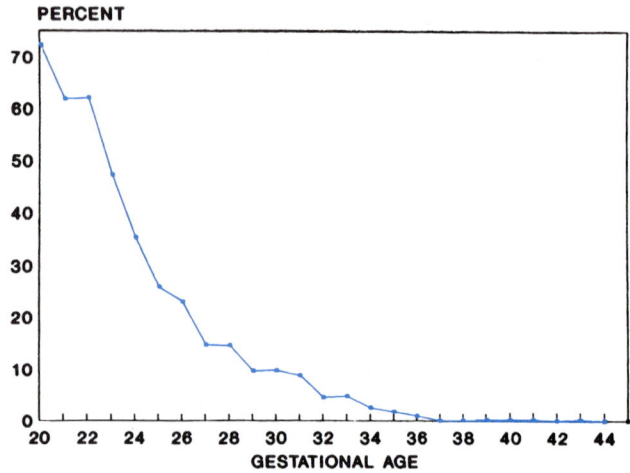

FIGURE 39–15. Relationship between gestational age and incidence of stillbirth. (From Copper and colleagues, 1994, with permission.)

viewed causes of 709 stillbirths among almost 89,000 deliveries at the Royal Victoria Hospital in Montreal. The fetal death rate per 1000 births decreased from 11.5 in the 1960s to 5.1 in the 1980s. The fetal death rate due to lethal anomalies declined by almost half between the 1970s and 1980s, from 10.8 to 5.4 per 10,000 births. This was because deaths of infants with anomalies were replaced by early pregnancy terminations. The more common recognized causes of fetal death through the 1980s included infection, malformations, fetal growth restriction, and abruptio placentae. More than a fourth of all fetal deaths during the 1980s were still unexplained, although in the previously cited Montreal study, this category diminished from 38.1 to 13.6 per 10,000 births.

CAUSES OF FETAL DEATH. There are many explanations for fetal death which generally can be categorized as fetal, placental, or maternal causes. In the past, a definable cause could not always be assigned and there was only mild enthusiasm for necropsy. Currently, however, it is recognized that a fetal autopsy performed by a pathologist with expertise in fetal and placental disorders, assisted by a team including maternal–fetal medicine, genetics, and pediatric specialists, often determines the cause of death (Craven and colleagues, 1990). Faye-Peterson and associates (1999) reviewed 139 fetal autopsies performed by such a team, and found that autopsy determined the cause of death in 94 percent. Some causes of fetal death or stillbirth determined by autopsy are shown in Table 39–13.

FETAL CAUSES. Up to 25 to 40 percent of stillbirths have fetal causes. In a carefully defined population of stillborn infants referred to the Wisconsin Stillbirth Ser-

vice Program, Pauli and Reiser (1994) found that 25 percent of 789 deaths could be ascribed to fetal problems, while Fretts and Usher (1997) attributed 35 to 40 percent of 278 fetal deaths to fetal causes. These included anomalies, infections, malnutrition, nonimmune hydrops, and anti-D isoimmunization.

The reported incidence of **major congenital malformations** in stillborns is highly variable, and depends on whether a necropsy was performed and, if so, the experience and training of the person performing it (Cartlidge and co-workers, 1995). Pauli and Reiser (1994) reported that the vast majority of 193 stillborns attributed to fetal causes had a major malformation to explain fetal death. Conversely, in a study of 403 stillbirths reported by Copper and colleagues (1994), without information from fetal autopsies, malformations were identified (prenatally) in only 5.6 percent. Faye-Peterson and colleagues (1999) found that a third of fetal deaths were caused by structural anomalies, of

TABLE 39–13. Some Causes of Fetal Death

Fetal (25–40%)
   Chromosomal anomalies
   Nonchromosomal birth defects
   Nonimmune hydrops
   Infections—viruses, bacteria, protozoa
Placental (25–35%)
   Abruption
   Fetal–maternal hemorrhage
   Cord accident
   Placental insufficiency
   Intrapartum asphyxia
   Previa
   Twin-to-twin transfusion
   Chorioamnionitis
Maternal (5–10%)
   Antiphospholipid antibodies
   Diabetes
   Hypertensive disorders
   Trauma
   Abnormal labor
   Sepsis
   Acidosis
   Hypoxia
   Uterine rupture
   Postterm pregnancy
   Drugs
Unexplained (25–35%)

From Cunningham and Hollier (1997).

which neural-tube defects, hydrops, isolated hydrocephalus, and complex congenital heart disease were the most common. Major structural anomalies, hydrops, and aneuploidy are particularly amenable to antenatal diagnosis.

The incidence of stillbirths caused by **fetal infection** appears to be remarkably consistent. From five studies totaling 2676 stillbirths, 5.6 percent were attributed to infection (Cartlidge, 1995; Copper, 1994; Fretts, 1992; Lammer, 1989, and all of their colleagues; Pauli and Reiser, 1994). Most were diagnosed as "chorioamnionitis," and some as "fetal or intrauterine sepsis." In indigent and inner-city women, congenital syphilis is another common cause of fetal death. For example, 6.3 percent of the stillbirths at Parkland Hospital from 1988 to 1995 were attributable to syphilis. Other potentially lethal infections include cytomegalovirus, parvovirus B-19, rubella, varicella, and listeriosis.

PLACENTAL CAUSES. The causes of fetal death due to placental abnormalities shown in Table 39–13 are somewhat arbitrary. For example, placental abruption is associated with pregnancy-induced hypertension in about half of cases; thus, such cases could be classified as "maternal causes." This is also true for placental insufficiency due to chronic hypertensive diseases and antiphospholipid antibodies. With these caveats in mind, approximately 15 to 25 percent of fetal deaths are attributed to problems of the placenta, membranes, or cord (Alessandri and colleagues, 1992; Fretts and Usher, 1997).

Placental abruption is the most common single identifiable cause of fetal death (also see Chap. 25, p. 621). Fretts and Usher (1997) determined this to be the cause of death in 14 percent of 278 stillborns. Our experiences are similar, and 12 percent of third-trimester stillbirths in over 40,000 deliveries at Parkland Hospital from 1992 through 1994 were the consequence of placental abruption.

Clinically significant **placental and membrane infection** rarely occurs in the absence of significant fetal infection. Some exceptions perhaps are tuberculosis and malaria. In some cases, microscopic examination of the placenta and membranes may help to identify an infectious cause. Chorioamnionitis is characterized by mononuclear and polymorphonuclear leukocytes infiltrating the chorion. While many consider these findings to be nonspecific and not always associated with fetal or maternal infection, Benirschke and Kaufmann (2000) believe that microscopic chorioamnionitis is always due to infection (Chap. 31, p. 814).

Placental infarcts show fibrinoid trophoblastic degeneration, calcification, and ischemic infarction from spiral artery occlusion (Chap. 32, p. 829). Other common lesions are marginal and subchorionic infarcts. Fox (1978) found that a fourth of placentas from uncomplicated term deliveries have infarcts. When there is severe hypertension, two thirds of placentas are so involved.

Fetal–maternal hemorrhage can be of such severity as to induce fetal death. Samadi and associates (1996) analyzed 319 fetal deaths at Los Angeles County Women's Hospital in which Kleihauer–Betke stains of maternal blood had been performed. Massive fetal–maternal hemorrhage was found in 4.7 percent. With severe maternal trauma, life-threatening fetal–maternal hemorrhage may be encountered (Chap. 43, p. 1173). Finally, twin-to-twin transfusion is a common cause of fetal death in monochorionic multifetal pregnancy (Chap. 30, p. 785).

MATERNAL CAUSES. Perhaps surprisingly, maternal disorders make only a small contribution to fetal deaths. This is true partially because placental abruption has been designated a "placental cause." Hypertensive disorders and diabetes are the two most commonly cited maternal diseases associated with 5 to 8 percent of stillborn infants (Alessandri and colleagues, 1992; Fretts and Usher, 1997).

Lupus anticoagulant and anticardiolipin antibodies are associated with decidual vasculopathy, placental infarction, fetal growth restriction, recurrent abortion, and fetal death (Chap. 52, p. 1412). While women with these autoantibodies clearly are at increased risk for adverse pregnancy outcomes, the contribution to otherwise unexplained stillbirths is minimal (Haddow and co-workers, 1991; Infante-Rivard and associates, 1991).

Recently, hereditary thrombophilias have been associated with placental abruption, fetal growth restriction, and stillbirths. These disorders are discussed in detail in Chapter 49 (p. 1330).

UNEXPLAINED STILLBIRTHS. With careful assessment of the clinical course, meticulous examination of the fresh stillborn, and appropriate laboratory investigations including necropsy, only about 10 percent of fetal deaths will remain unclassified. The difficulty of assessing the cause of fetal death appears to be greatest in preterm infants (Yudkin and colleagues, 1987).

EVALUATION OF THE STILLBORN INFANT. It is important to try to determine the cause of fetal death. First, the psychological adaptation to a significant loss may be eased by knowledge of a specific etiology. Second, it may help to assuage the guilt that is part of grieving. Most importantly, appropriate diagnosis makes counseling regarding recurrence more accurate and may allow therapy or some intervention to prevent a similar outcome in the next pregnancy. Identification of inherited syndromes also provides useful information for other family members.

CLINICAL EXAMINATION. A thorough examination of the infant, placenta, and membranes should be performed at delivery. This information may aid in subsequent determination of the etiology. The checklist used at Parkland Hospital to format the stillbirth note is outlined in Table 39–14.

GENETIC EVALUATION. If autopsy and chromosomal studies are performed when indicated, up to 35 percent of stillborn infants are discovered to have congenital structural anomalies (Faye-Peterson and associates, 1999; Mueller and colleagues, 1983). As many as 8 percent of stillbirths have chromosomal abnormalities, and about 20 percent have dysmorphic features or skeletal abnormalities (Pauli and Reiser, 1994; Saller and colleagues, 1995). It is probably not cost effective to perform cytogenetic analyses in all stillbirths. Instead, the American College of Obstetricians and Gynecologists (1996) recommends consideration of cytogenetic studies for infants with dysmorphic features, inconsistent growth measurements, anomalies, hydrops, or growth restriction. Such studies might also be considered in cases in which absolutely no other explanation for the loss is found. Another indication is a parent who is a carrier for a balanced translocation, a mosaic chromosomal pattern, or a history of recurrent losses or stillbirths in first-degree relatives.

Appropriate consent must be obtained to take skin and other tissue samples, including fluid obtained by needle postmortem. A total of 3 mL of fetal blood, obtained from the umbilical cord (preferably) or by cardiac puncture, is placed into a sterile, heparinized (green top) tube for cytogenetic studies. Skin samples with attached dermal tissue should measure 1 cm^2 and be washed with sterile saline prior to placement in saline or sterile cytogenetic medium. Placement in formalin or alcohol prohibits cytogenetic analysis because the cells must remain alive for study. If the skin is macerated, 1-cm^2 samples of fascia should be obtained from the thigh, inguinal region, or Achilles tendon. Because a traditional cytogenetic study requires that fetal cells be stimulated to divide, it may not be possible in cases with prolonged intrauterine retention. However, fluorescent in situ hybridization (FISH) might be used to rule out trisomies or to look for certain common deletions such as DiGeorge syndrome.

AUTOPSY. As autopsy rates for adults have decreased, so have those for stillborns. Patients should be counseled that, even if they do not allow a full autopsy to be performed, valuable information can still be obtained from limited studies. Mueller and colleagues (1983) demonstrated the importance of gross autopsy for stillbirths. This, along with photography, radiography, bacterial cultures, and selective use of more expensive procedures such as chromosomal and histopathological studies can often determine the cause of death.

Cartlidge and Stewart (1995) performed a cohort analysis of 400 consecutive fetal deaths in Wales and found that the clinicopathological classification was altered by necropsy in 13 percent. New information was obtained in another 26 percent. Thus, autopsy provided important information in almost 40 percent of stillborns. Faye-Peterson and colleagues (1999) reported that autopsy results changed the recurrence risk estimates and parental counseling in 26 percent of cases. Similar findings were reported by Saller and associates (1995).

If the family refuses autopsy because of personal or religious objections, valuable information can still be obtained noninvasively. With appropriate permission, x-rays are performed to evaluate the bony skeleton, and high-resolution magnetic resonance imaging can be considered to evaluate soft tissue, depending on the degree of maceration. The fetus should be photographed to facilitate evaluation by a dysmorphologist, and if indicated, bacterial cultures should be taken from the ear canal (Brookes and colleagues, 1996).

TABLE 39–14. Protocol for Examination of Stillborns

Infant Description
  Malformations
  Skin staining
  Degree of maceration
  Color—pale, plethoric
Umbilical Cord
  Prolapse
  Entanglement—neck, arms, legs
  Hematomas or strictures
  Number of vessels
  Length
Amnionic Fluid
  Color—meconium, blood
  Consistency
  Volume
Placenta
  Weight staining
  Adherent clots
  Structural abnormalities—circumvallate or accessory lobes, velamentous insertion
  Edema—hydropic changes
Membranes
  Stained
  Thickening

From Cunningham and Hollier (1997).

STILLBORN PROTOCOL. The protocol shown in Table 39–14 includes a systematic review of all stillbirths. A detailed note should be written regarding prenatal events, and the infant, placenta, and membranes should be carefully examined and pertinent positive and negative findings recorded. Autopsy, either complete (preferably) or limited, is encouraged. Samples are sent for cytogenetic analysis in case of fetal malformation, multiple pregnancy losses, or growth restriction, to name a few. Other laboratory evaluations include fetography and maternal blood for Kleihauer–Betke staining, testing for antiphospholipid antibodies and lupus anticoagulant if indicated, and serum glucose to exclude overt diabetes.

In many centers, maternal records and autopsy findings are reviewed on a monthly basis by a Stillbirth Committee composed of maternal–fetal medicine and neonatology fellows and faculty, clinical geneticists, and perinatal pathologists. If possible, the cause of death is assigned based on available evidence. Most importantly, parents should then be contacted and offered counseling regarding the cause of death, the recurrence risk, if any, and strategies to avoid recurrence in future pregnancies.

PSYCHOLOGICAL ASPECTS.

Fetal death is a psychologically traumatic event for the woman and her family. Radestad and colleagues (1996) found that an interval of more than 24 hours from the diagnosis of fetal death to the induction of labor was related to excessive anxiety. Other factors included when the woman did not see her infant for as long as she wished and when she had no tokens of remembrance. The woman experiencing a stillbirth is at increased risk for postpartum depression and should be closely monitored (Chap. 53, p. 1421).

Even early miscarriage may provoke depression in as many as a third of women (Neugebauer, 1992). Janssen and colleagues (1996) prospectively followed 227 women who had a pregnancy loss and 213 control women who had a live birth for 18 months. Up to 6 months after pregnancy loss, women with stillborns showed greater depression, anxiety, and somatization than control women. Fortunately, the mental health of these women improved over time and at one year was comparable with that of women who had live births. During the study period, only 3 percent of the women were given psychotherapy. Importantly, Hughes and associates (1999) showed vulnerability to depression and anxiety during the next pregnancy. This risk diminished with time, and they recommended an interval of 12 months before conception.

MANAGEMENT OF WOMEN WITH A PREVIOUS STILLBIRTH.

A woman with a prior stillbirth has long been accepted to be at increased risk for adverse outcomes in subsequent pregnancies. Fortunately, however, there are very few conditions associated with recurrent stillbirth. Other than hereditary disorders, only maternal conditions such as diabetes, chronic hypertension, or hereditary thrombophilia increase risk of recurrence.

RISKS. Several studies have cited rates of recurrent stillbirth to range from 0 to 8 percent, depending on the specific population studied (Freeman, 1985; Samueloff, 1993; Weeks, 1995, and their colleagues). Earlier pregnancy losses, although not technically all stillborns, are associated with subsequent adverse outcomes. Goldenberg and colleagues (1993) identified 95 women who had a pregnancy loss at 13 to 24 weeks. Almost 40 percent of these had a preterm delivery in their next pregnancy, 5 percent had a stillbirth, and 6 percent had a neonatal death. Knowledge of the cause of fetal death allows a more precise individual recurrence risk to be calculated. For example, aneuploidy generally has a 1 percent recurrence risk, familial DiGeorge syndrome has a 50 percent recurrence, while a cord accident would not be expected to recur.

PRENATAL EVALUATION. If the cause of the previous stillbirth can be ascertained, then risk for the current pregnancy may be quantified. In general, with proper treatment infectious causes would be unlikely to recur. If there was a previous stillbirth with an abnormal karyotype or polygenic cause, then chorionic villous sampling or amniocentesis could facilitate early detection and allow termination to be considered. Maternal medical disorders associated with prior stillborns will likely be easily identified. Although early studies demonstrated a reduction in fetal death in women with treated chronic hypertension, a randomized trial by Sibai and colleagues (1990) showed no reduction. Importantly, placental abruption is often associated with chronic hypertension, and Pritchard and colleagues (1991) demonstrated an abruption recurrence rate of 10 percent.

With diabetes, a significant portion of perinatal mortality is attributable to congenital anomalies. Intensive glycemic control in the periconceptional period has been shown to reduce the incidence of malformations and generally improve outcome (Chap. 51, p. 1369). Such control requires that the pregnancy be planned, and lack of planning may account for the fact that unexplained losses still account for half of stillborns of diabetic mothers (Hanson and Persson, 1993).

There is some evidence that recurrent fetal loss due to antiphospholipid antibodies can be decreased with treatment (Chap. 52, p. 1390). In women who have an unexplained fetal loss in the second trimester, we usually test for antiphospholipid antibodies. Conversely, such testing is not recommended for the woman with a normally grown, unexplained third-trimester stillborn.

MANAGEMENT. There are few studies that address management of the woman who has suffered a prior fetal death. In a report from the University of California at Irvine, Freeman (1985) and colleagues evaluated the significance of a prior stillbirth in women followed with fetal heart rate testing. In 5 percent of women referred for evaluation, prior stillbirth was the indication for testing. None of these women had a recurrent stillbirth. Those with a prior stillbirth, however, were more likely to have a positive contraction stress test than the other women. This difference was primarily accounted for by women with hypertension (12 percent) or those suspected of having fetal growth restriction (17 percent). Importantly, offspring of women with prior stillborns had an increased incidence of respiratory distress syndrome compared with those of women tested for other reasons. This suggests that early delivery was performed empirically in women with a prior stillbirth.

The Irvine group later conducted a nonconcurrent cohort study of women with a prior stillbirth as the only indication for antepartum testing (Weeks and colleagues, 1995). There was only one recurrent still-birth among 300 study patients. Interestingly, there was no relationship between the gestational age of the previous stillborn and the incidence or timing of abnormal tests or fetal distress in the subsequent pregnancy. Only three women had an abnormal antepartum test at less than 32 weeks, and they were subsequently delivered without incident at term. These investigators concluded that antepartum surveillance should begin at 32 weeks or later in the otherwise healthy woman with a history of stillbirth. This agrees with recommendations of the American College of Obstetricians and Gynecologists (1999a).

INJURIES OF THE FETUS AND NEWBORN

Considered here are several varieties of birth injuries. Others are described elsewhere in connection with specific obstetrical complications that led to or contributed to the injury.

INTRACRANIAL HEMORRHAGE. Hemorrhage within the head of the fetus-infant may be located at any of several sites: subdural, subarachnoid, cortical, white matter, cerebellar, intraventricular, and periventricular. A classification is shown in Table 39–15. Intraventricular hemorrhage into the germinal matrix is the most common type of intracranial hemorrhage encountered, and as discussed on page 1045, it usually is a result of immaturity or an antepartum cerebrovascular accident. Isolated intraventricular hemorrhage in the absence of subarachnoid or subdural bleeding is not a traumatic injury. Hayden and colleagues (1985) reported that nearly 4 percent of otherwise normal newborns at term have sonographic evidence for subependymal germinal matrix hemorrhages unrelated to obstetrical factors.

Birth trauma is no longer a common cause of intracranial hemorrhage. The head of the fetus has consider-

TABLE 39–15. **Major Types of Intracranial Hemorrhage in the Newborn**

Type	Gestational Age	Incidence and Severity	Cause(s) and Pathogenesis
Subdural	Term > Preterm	Uncommon Serious	Venous tears Trauma common
Primary subarachnoid	Preterm > term	Common Benign	Trauma—term "Hypoxia"—preterm
Intracerebellar	Preterm > term	Uncommon Serious	Multifactorial
Intraventricular	Preterm	Common Serious	Thin-walled vessels of germinal matrix Multifactorial causes
Miscellaneous	Term > preterm	Uncommon Variable	Trauma, hemorrhagic infarction, coagulopathy, vascular defect, ECMO

ECMO = extracorporeal membrane oxygenation.
Data from Volpe (1995).

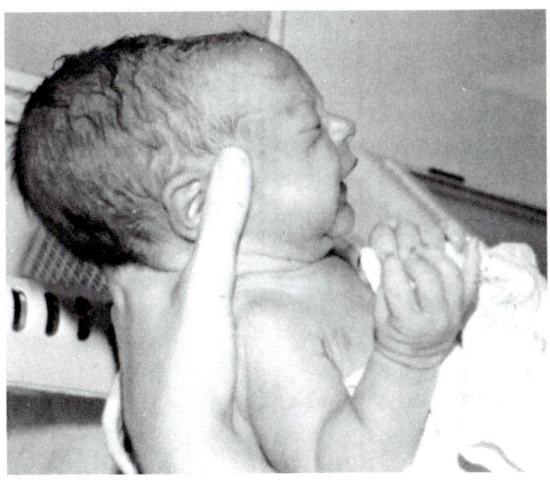

FIGURE 39–16. Molding of the head in normal newborn.

able plasticity and may undergo appreciable molding during passage through the birth canal. The skull bones, the dura mater, and the brain itself permit considerable alteration in the shape of the fetal head without untoward results. The dimensions of the head are changed, with lengthening especially of the occipitofrontal diameter of the skull (Fig. 39–16). With severe molding and marked overlap of the parietal bones, bridging veins from the cerebral cortex to the sagittal sinus may tear. Less common is rupture of the internal cerebral veins, the vein of Galen at its junctions with the straight sinus, or the tentorium itself. Compression of the skull can stretch the tentorium cerebelli and may tear the vein of Galen or its tributaries.

Illingworth (1979) observed that because of superficial thinking, obstetricians have been blamed unjustifiably for causing brain damage and other injuries, the genesis of which was not limited just to difficulties during labor and delivery, but actually involved prenatal factors, including those that were genetic and environmental in nature. Nonetheless, the elimination of difficult forceps operations and appropriate management of breech delivery have contributed significantly to a reduction in the incidence of all birth injuries, including intracranial hemorrhage. It must be emphasized that intracranial hemorrhage often occurs following an apparently uneventful vaginal delivery.

As discussed in detail in Chapter 21 (p. 501), it has been well documented that low or outlet forceps or vacuum delivery do not lead to an increased incidence of intracranial hemorrhage or other neonatal injury (American College of Obstetricians and Gynecologists, 2000; Hagadorn-Freathy and associates, 1991; Yancy and colleagues, 1991). In a series of predominantly low pelvic operative deliveries, Williams and associates

(1991) found no cases of intraventricular hemorrhage with forceps and vacuum delivery. The spectrum of subgaleal and bone injury encountered in 23 infants undergoing vacuum delivery had been described by Govaert and co-workers (1992). The use of pliable as opposed to rigid vacuum cups has been associated with less neonatal scalp trauma (Kuit and associates, 1993).

CLINICAL FINDINGS. According to Volpe (1995), there are few clinical neurological data available concerning infants suffering intracranial hemorrhage from mechanical injury. With subdural hemorrhage from tentorial tears and massive infratentorial hemorrhage, there is neurological disturbance from the time of birth. Severely affected infants—usually those weighing more than 4000 g—have stupor or coma, nuchal rigidity, and opisthotonus. Over minutes to hours, these problems worsen. Some infants are born depressed, but appear to improve until about 12 hours of age. Then drowsiness, apathy, feeble cry, pallor, failure to nurse, dyspnea, cyanosis, vomiting, and convulsions may become evident.

Subarachnoid hemorrhage most commonly is minor with no symptoms, but seizures with a normal interictal period may manifest. In some there is catastrophic deterioration. Head scanning using sonography, computed tomography, or magnetic resonance imaging not only had proven diagnostic value but has also contributed appreciably to an understanding of the etiology and frequency of some forms of intracranial hemorrhage (Perlman and Cunningham, 1993). For example, periventricular and intraventricular hemorrhages occur often in infants born quite preterm and these hemorrhages usually develop without birth trauma.

CEPHALOHEMATOMA. A cephalohematoma usually is caused by injury to the periosteum of the skull during labor and delivery, although it may also develop in the absence of birth trauma. The incidence is 2.5 percent, according to the 10-year review by Thacker and colleagues (1987). Hemorrhages may develop over one or both parietal bones. The periosteal limitations with definite palpable edges differentiate the cephalohematoma from caput succedaneum (Fig. 39–17). The caput, also shown in Figure 39–16, consists of a focal swelling of the scalp from edema that overlies the periosteum. Furthermore, a cephalohematoma may not appear for hours after delivery, often growing larger and disappearing only after weeks or even months. In contrast, caput succedaneum is maximal at birth, grows smaller, and usually disappears within a few hours if small, and within a few days if very large.

Increasing size of the hematoma and other evidence of extensive hemorrhage are indications for additional

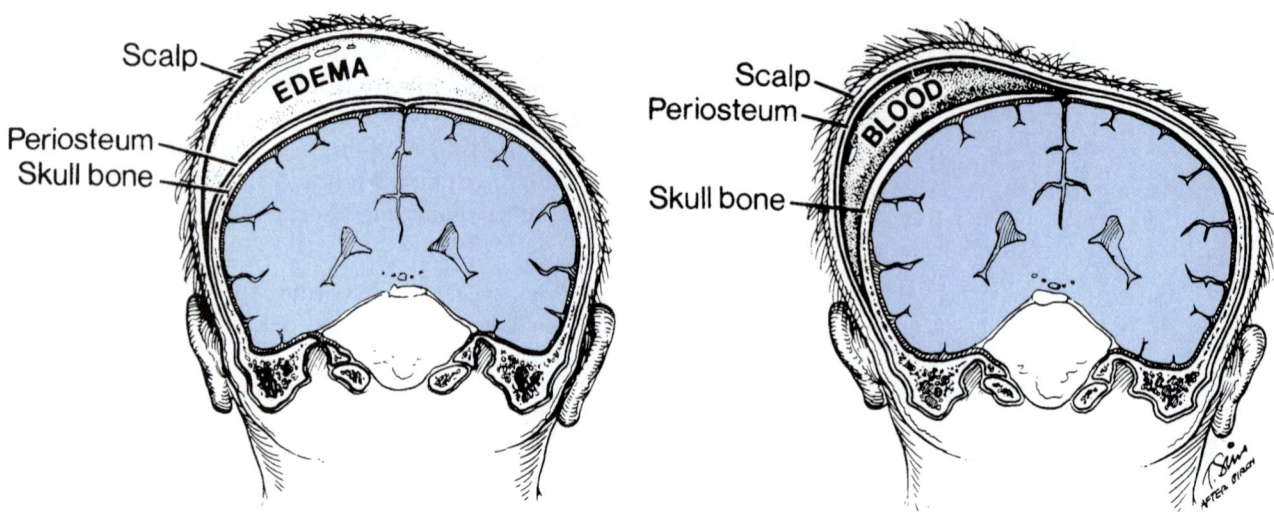

FIGURE 39–17. Difference between a large caput succedaneum (*left*) and cephalohematoma (*right*). In a caput succedaneum, the effusion overlies the periosteum and consists of edema fluid; in a cephalohematoma, it lies under periosteum and consists of blood.

investigation, including radiographic studies and assessment of coagulation factors.

NERVE INJURIES

SPINAL INJURY. Overstretching the spinal cord and associated hemorrhage may follow excessive traction during a breech delivery, and there may be actual fracture or dislocation of the vertebrae. Menticoglou and associates (1995) described 15 neonates with a high cervical spinal cord injury and found that all were associated with forceps rotations.

BRACHIAL PLEXUS INJURY. These injuries are relatively common and are encountered in between 1 in 500 to 1 in 1000 term births (Boo and colleagues, 1991; Salonen and Uüsitalo, 1990). In a review of over 21,500 live births, Oppenheim and colleagues (1990) reported 58 clavicular fractures (2.7 per 1000), three of which were associated with Erb palsy. Increasing birthweight and breech deliveries are significant risk factors and are discussed in detail in Chapter 29 (p. 760).

Duchenne, or *Erb paralysis* is incorrectly thought to occur only with large infants with shoulder dystocia. In reality, only 30 percent of brachial plexus injuries occur in macrosomic infants (Walle and Hartikainen-Sorri, 1993). These neurological lesions involve paralysis of the deltoid and infraspinatus muscles, as well as the flexor muscles of the forearm, causing the entire arm to fall limply close to the side of the body with the forearm extended and internally rotated. The function of the fingers usually is retained. The lesion likely results from stretching or tearing of the upper roots of the brachial plexus. Because lateral head traction is frequently employed to effect delivery of the shoulders in normal vertex presentations, Erb paralysis can result without the delivery appearing to be difficult. As emphasized by Sandmire and DeMott (2000), however, the propulsive efforts of delivery may actually cause nerve stretching with damage. Ubachs and colleagues (1995) described 130 infants who underwent surgical treatment for brachial plexus injuries. Most cases that involved C_{5-6} nerve roots were associated with breech delivery, whereas more extensive forms—involving C_{5-7} or C_5–T_1 roots—followed difficult cephalic deliveries.

Less frequently, trauma is limited to the lower nerves of the brachial plexus, which leads to paralysis of the hand, or *Klumpke paralysis.*

As discussed in Chapter 29, risk factors for shoulder dystocia are common and nonspecific. Nocon and associates (1993), after an analysis of over 12,000 vaginal deliveries, concluded:

> Most of the traditional risk factors for shoulder dystocia have no predictive value; shoulder dystocia itself is an unpredictable event and infants at risk for permanent injury are virtually impossible to predict. In addition, no delivery method in shoulder dystocia was superior to another with respect to injury.

FACIAL PARALYSIS. The incidence likely is influenced by the vigor with which it is sought. For example, Levine and colleagues (1984) reported facial nerve injury in 7.5 per 1000 term births. White and associates (1996)

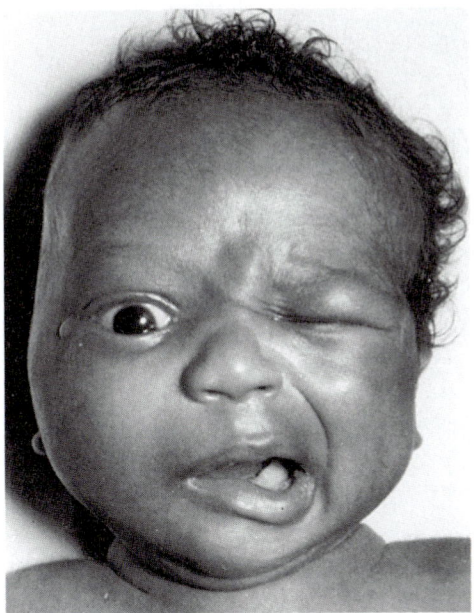
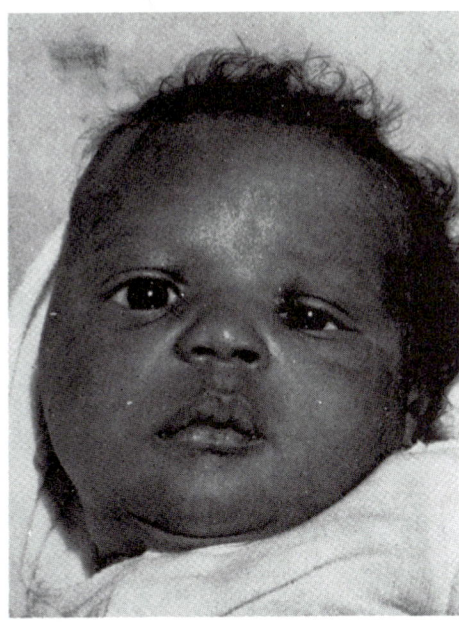

A   **B**

FIGURE 39–18. A. Paralysis of right side of face 15 minutes after forceps delivery. **B.** Same infant 24 hours later. Recovery was complete in another 24 hours.

reported 27 cases of facial nerve palsy in 18,500 deliveries for an incidence of 1.4 per 1000. Salonen and Uüsitalo (1990) observed only one case of facial nerve palsy in over 14,000 live births.

Facial paralysis may be apparent at delivery or it may develop shortly after birth (Fig. 39–18). It is seen with delivery of an infant in which the head has been seized obliquely with forceps. The injury is caused by pressure exerted by the posterior blade of the forceps on the stylomastoid foramen, through which the facial nerve emerges. Facial marks from the forceps may be obvious (Fig. 39–19). The condition is also encountered after spontaneous delivery. White and associates (1996) observed that only 18 percent of facial nerve palsies were associated with forceps delivery and that the majority followed spontaneous vaginal or cesarean delivery. Levine and co-workers (1984) reported that a third of cases followed spontaneous delivery. Spontaneous recovery within a few days is the rule (Fig. 39–17). Galbraith (1994) described an increase in injuries to the sixth cranial nerve with resultant lateral rectus paralysis following operative vaginal delivery.

SKELETAL AND MUSCLE INJURIES

FRACTURES. Clavicular fractures are surprisingly common if a careful search is made. They have been identified in up to 18 per 1000 live births (Oppenheim and colleagues, 1990; Salonen and Uüsitalo, 1990; Turpenny

and Nimmo, 1993). Chez and colleagues (1994) reported an incidence of 9 per 1000 vaginally delivered newborns and were unable to identify any specific factor that could be changed to avoid such fractures. Roberts and associates (1995) identified 215 clavicular fractures in infants born to nearly 65,000 women at Parkland Hospital for

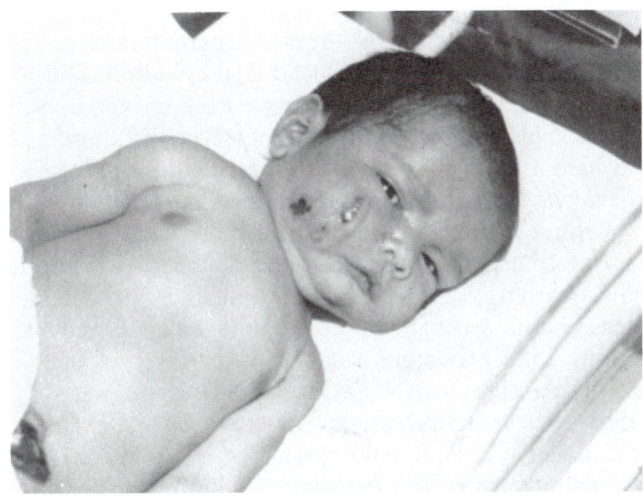

FIGURE 39–19. Healing abrasions and lacerations from a difficult forceps delivery. Palsy of the right facial nerve has nearly cleared.

an incidence of 3.3 per 1000 deliveries. Both of these latter investigators concluded that clavicular fracture was an unpredictable and unavoidable complication of normal birth.

Humeral fractures are less common. Difficulty encountered in the delivery of the shoulders in cephalic deliveries and extended arms in breech deliveries often produce such fractures. Up to 70 percent of cases, however, follow uneventful delivery (Turpenny and Nimmo, 1993). Upper extremity fractures associated with delivery are often of the greenstick type, although complete fracture with overriding of the bones may occur. Palpation of the clavicles and long bones should be performed on all newborns when a fracture is suspected, and any crepitation or unusual irregularity should prompt radiographic examination.

Femoral fractures are relatively uncommon and usually associated with breech delivery.

Skull fracture may follow forcible attempts at delivery, especially with forceps, spontaneous delivery, or even cesarean section (Saunders and colleagues, 1979; Skajaa and associates, 1987). In the radiograph shown in Figure 39–20, a focal, but marked, depressed skull fracture is apparent. Labor was characterized by vigorous contractions, full dilatation of the cervix, and arrest of descent of the head, which was tightly wedged in the pelvis. The fracture was the consequence of compression of the skull against the sacral promontory of the mother, or perhaps from pressure from an assistant's hand in the vagina or as the head was pushed upward out of the birth canal at cesarean delivery. Surgical decompression was successful.

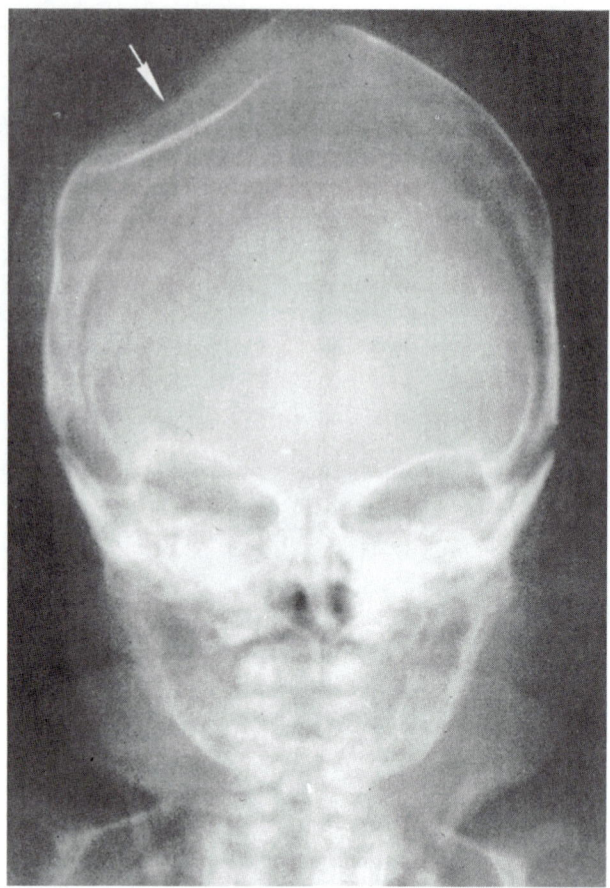

FIGURE 39–20. Depressed skull fracture evident immediately after birth. Delivery followed vigorous but obstructed labor and dislodgement upward of the fetal head from the birth canal by an assistant's hand in the vagina at the time of cesarean section.

MUSCULAR INJURIES. Injury to the sternocleidomastoid muscle may occur, particularly during a breech delivery. There may be a tear of the muscle or possibly of the fascial sheath, leading to a hematoma and gradual cicatricial contraction. As the neck lengthens in the process of normal growth, the head is gradually turned toward the side of the injury, because the damaged muscle is less elastic and does not elongate at the same rate as its normal contralateral counterpart, thus producing *torticollis.* Roemer (1954) reported that 27 of 44 infants showing this deformity had been delivered by breech or internal podalic version. He postulated that lateral hyperextension sufficient to rupture the sternocleidomastoid may occur as the aftercoming head passes over the sacral promontory.

CONGENITAL INJURIES

AMNIONIC BAND SYNDROME. Focal ring constrictions of the extremities and actual loss of a digit or a limb are rare complications. Their genesis is debated. Streeter (1930), and others since, maintain that localized failure of germ plasm usually is responsible for the abnormalities. Torpin (1968) and others contend that the lesions are the consequence of early rupture of the amnion, which then forms adherent tough bands that constrict and at times actually amputate an extremity of the fetus. Occasionally, the amputated part may be found within the uterus.

CONGENITAL POSTURAL DEFORMITIES. Mechanical factors arising from chronically low volumes of amnionic fluid and restrictions imposed by the small size and inappropriate shape of the uterine cavity may mold the growing fetus into distinct patterns of deformity, including talipes or clubfoot (Fig. 37–9, p. 989), scoliosis, and hip dislocation (Miller and co-workers, 1981). Hypoplastic lungs also can result from oligohydramnios (Chap. 31, p. 822).

REFERENCES

Achiron R, Pinchas OH, Reichman B, Heyman Z, Schimmel M, Eidelman A, Mashiach S: Fetal intracranial haemorrhage: Clinical significance of in-utero ultrasonic diagnosis. Br J Obstet Gynaecol 100:995, 1993

Alessandri LM, Stanley FJ, Garner JB, Newnham J, Walters BNJ: A case-control study of unexplained antepartum stillbirths. Br J Obstet Gynaecol 99:711, 1992

Allan LD, Crawford DC, Sheridan R, Chapman MG: Aetiology of non-immune hydrops: The value of echocardiography. Br J Obstet Gynaecol 93:223, 1986

Allan WC, Vohr B, Makuch RW, Katz KH, Ment LR: Antecedents of cerebral palsy in a multicenter trial on indomethacin for intraventricular hemorrhage. Arch Pediatr Adolesc Med 151:580, 1997

Allen MC, Donohue PK, Dusman AE: The limit of viability—neonatal outcome of infants born at 22 to 25 weeks gestation. N Engl J Med 329:1597, 1993

Alper CA: Blood groups I. Physiology. In Beck WS (ed): Hematology. Cambridge, MA, MIT Press, 1977, p 299

Alvarez JG, Ludmir J: Improved DPPC test for the assessment of fetal lung maturity by high-pressure liquid chromatography. Am J Obstet Gynecol 174:473, 1996

American Academy of Pediatrics/American Heart Association: Neonatal Resuscitation Manual. American Academy of Pediatrics, 1994

American College of Obstetricians and Gynecologist: Operative vaginal delivery. Educational Bulletin No. 17, June 2000

American College of Obstetricians and Gynecologists: Antepartum fetal surveillance. Practice bulletin No. 9, October 1999a

American College of Obstetricians and Gynecologists: Prevention of RhD alloimmunization. Clinical Management Guidelines No. 4, May 1999b

American College of Obstetricians and Gynecologists: Inappropriate use of the terms fetal distress and birth asphyxia. Committee Opinion No. 174, 1998

American College of Obstetricians and Gynecologist: Genetic evaluation of stillbirths and neonatal deaths. Committee Opinion No. 178, November 1996

American College of Obstetricians and Gynecologists: Fetal heart rate patterns: Monitoring, interpretation, and management. Technical Bulletin No. 207, July 1995a

American College of Obstetricians and Gynecologists: Perinatal and infant mortality statistics. Committee Opinion No. 167, December 1995b

American College of Obstetricians and Gynecologists: Preterm labor. Technical Bulletin No. 206, June 1995c

American College of Obstetricians and Gynecologists: Umbilical artery blood acid–base analysis. Technical Bulletin No. 216, November 1995d

American College of Obstetricians and Gynecologists: Antenatal corticosteroid therapy for fetal maturation. Committee on Obstetrics, Maternal and Fetal Medicine, and on the Fetus and Newborn, No. 147, December 1994

American College of Obstetricians and Gynecologists: Fetal and neonatal neurologic injury. Technical Bulletin No. 163, January 1992

American College of Obstetricians and Gynecologists: Management of isoimmunization in pregnancy. Technical Bulletin No. 148, October 1990

Anderson GD, Bada HS, Shaver DC, Harvey CJ, Korones SB, Wong SP, Arheart KL, Magill HL: The effect of cesarean section on intraventricular hemorrhage in the preterm infant. Am J Obstet Gynecol 166:1091, 1992

Arias IM, Gartner LM, Seifter S, Furman M: Prolonged neonatal unconjugated hyperbilirubinemia associated with breast feeding and steroid, pregnane-3a, 20b-diol in maternal milk that inhibits glucuronide formation in vitro. J Clin Invest 43:2037, 1964

Asakura H, Schifrin BS, Myers SA: Intrapartum, atraumatic, nonasphyxial intracranial hemorrhage in a full-term infant. Obstet Gynecol 84:680, 1994

Avery ME: Historical overview of antenatal steroid use. Pediatrics 126:133, 1995

Ballantyne JW: The diseases and deformities of the foetus. Oliver and Boyd, 1892–1895

Barkai G, Mashiach S, Lanzer D, Kayam Z, Brish M, Goldman B: Determination of fetal lung maturity from amniotic fluid microviscosity in high-risk pregnancy. Obstet Gynecol 59:615, 1982

Barss VA, Frigoletto FD, Konugres A: The cost of irregular antibody screening. Am J Obstet Gynecol 159:428, 1988

Battin MR, Maalouf EF, Counsell SJ, Herlihy AH, Rutherford MA, Azzopardi D: Magnetic resonance imaging of the brain in very preterm infants: Visualization of the germinal matrix, early myelination, and cortical folding. Pediatrics 101:957, 1998

Baud O, Foix-L'Helias L, Kaminski M, Audibert F, Jarreau PH, Papiernik E: Antenatal glucocorticoid treatment and cystic periventricular leukomalacia in very premature infants. N Engl J Med 341:1190, 1999

Bejar R, Wozniak P, Allard M, Benirschke K, Vaucher Y, Coen R: Antenatal origin of neurologic damage in newborn infants. I. Preterm infants. Am J Obstet Gynecol 159:357, 1988

Benirschke K, Kaufmann P (eds): Infectious diseases. In: Pathology of the Human Placenta, 4th ed. New York, Springer-Verlag, 2000, p 468

Bennett PR, Le Van Kim C, Colin Y, Warwich RM, Cherif-Zahar B, Fisk NM, Cartron JP: Prenatal determination of fetal RhD type by DNA amplification. N Engl J Med 329:607, 1993

Berkowitz K, Reyes C, Sadaat P, Kjos S: Comparison of fetal lung maturation in well dated diabetic and non-diabetic pregnancies. Am J Obstet Gynecol 174:373, 1996

Biarent D: New tools in ventilatory support: High frequency ventilation, nitric oxide, tracheal gas insufflation, non-invasive ventilation. Ped Pulmon 18:178, 1999

Blajchman MA, Maudsley RF, Uchida I, Zipursky A: Diagnostic amniocentesis and fetal–maternal bleeding. Lancet 1:993, 1974

Bloom S, Ramin S, Neyman S, Little B, Gilstrap: Meconium-stained amniotic fluid: Is it associated with elevated erythropoietin levels? Am J Obstet Gynecol 174:360, 1996

Boo NY, Lye MS, Kanchanamala M, Ching CL: Brachial plexus injuries in Malaysian neonates: Incidence and associated risk factors. J Trop Pediatr 37:327, 1991

Boucher M, Rinfret D, Varin J: Feto-maternal hemorrhage after external cephalic version: An overestimated risk. Am J Obstet Gynecol 174:3349, 1996

Bowell PJ, Allen DL, Entwistle CC: Blood group antibody screening tests during pregnancy. Br J Obstet Gynaecol 93:1038, 1986a

Bowell PJ, Brown SE, Dike AE, Inskip MJ: The significance of anti-c alloimmunization. Br J Obstet Gynaecol 93:1044, 1986b

Bowman JM: Controversies in Rh prophylaxis: Who needs Rh immune globulin and when should it be given? Am J Obstet Gynecol 151:289, 1985

Bowman JM: The management of Rh-isoimmunization. Obstet Gynecol 52:1, 1978

Bowman JM, Chown B, Lewis M, Pollock J: Rh isoimmunization, Manitoba, 1963–1975. Can Med Assoc J 116:282, 1977

Bowman JM, Pollock JM: Antenatal Rh prophylaxis: 28 week gestation service program. Can Med Assoc J 118:622, 1978

Bowman JM, Pollock JM, Manning FA, Harman CR, Menticoglou S: Maternal Kell blood group alloimmunization. Obstet Gynecol 79:239, 1992a

Bowman JM, Pollock JM, Manning FA, Harman CR: Severe anti-C hemolytic disease of the newborn. Am J Obstet Gynecol 166:1239, 1992b

Brookes JAS, Hall-Craggs MA, Sams VR, Lees WR: Noninvasive perinatal necropsy by magnetic resonance imaging. Lancet 348:1139, 1996

Buhi WC, Spellacy WN: Effects of blood or meconium on the determination of the amniotic fluid lecithin/sphingomyelin ration. Am J Obstet Gynecol 121:321, 1975

Byrne DL, Gau G: In utero meconium aspiration: An unpreventable cause of neonatal death. Br J Obstet Gynecol 94:813, 1987

Caine ME, Mueller-Heuback E: Kell sensitization in pregnancy. Am J Obstet Gynecol 154:85, 1986

Cameron A, Nicholson S, Nimrod C, Harder J, Davies D, Fritzler M: Evaluation of fetal cardiac dysrhythmias with two-dimensional, M-mode, and pulsed Doppler ultrasonography. Am J Obstet Gynecol 158:286, 1988

Canterino J, Roberts A, Carr A: Prenatal diagnosis and management of fetuses with intracranial hemorrhage. Am J Obstet Gynecol 174:475, 1996

Carson BS, Losey RW, Bowes WA Jr, Simmons MA: Combined obstetric and pediatric approach to prevent meconium aspiration syndrome. Am J Obstet Gynecol 126:712, 1976

Cartlidge PHT, Dawson AT, Stewart JH, Vujanic GM: Value and quality of perinatal and infant postmortem examination: Cohort analysis of 400 consecutive deaths. BMJ 310:155, 1995

Cartlidge PHT, Stewart JH: Effect of changing the stillbirth definition on evaluation of perinatal mortality rates. Lancet 346:486, 1995

Casey BM, McIntire DD, Leveno KJ: Continuous value of the Apgar score in assessing infant well-being. N Engl J Med 2001 (in press)

Castillo RA, Devoe LD, Hadi HA, Martin S, Giest D: Nonimmune hydrops fetalis: Clinical experience and factors related to a poor outcome. Am J Obstet Gynecol 155:812, 1986

Centers for Disease Control: Lack of transmission of human immunodeficiency virus through Rh$_o$ (D) immune globulin (human). MMWR 36:728, 1987

Charles AG, Blumenthal LS: Promethazine hydrochloride therapy in severe Rh-sensitized pregnancies. Obstet Gynecol 60:627, 1982

Chez RA, Carlan S, Greenberg SL, Spellacy WN: Fractured clavicle is an unavoidable event. Am J Obstet Gynecol 174:797, 1994

Chiswick M, Gladman G, Sinha S, Toner N, Davies J: Vitamin E supplementation and periventricular hemorrhage in the newborn. Am J Clin Nutr 53:370S, 1991

Chua S, Ostman-Smith I, Sellers S, Redman CW: Congenital heart block with hydrops fetalis treated with high-dose dexamethasone: A case report. Eur J Obstet Gynecol Reprod Biol 42:155, 1991

Choavaratana R, Uer-Areewong S, Makanantakocol S: Feto-

maternal transfusion in normal pregnancy and during delivery. J Med Assoc Thailand 80:96, 1997

Clark DA, Nieman GF, Thompson JE, Paskanik AM, Rokhar JE, Bredenberg CE: Surfactant displacement by meconium free fatty acids: An alternative explanation for atelectasis in meconium aspiration syndrome. J Pediatr 110:765, 1987

Clements JA, Platzker ACG, Tierney DF, Hobel CL, Creasy RK, Margolis AJ, Thibeault DW, Tooley WH, Oh W: Assessment of the risk of respiratory distress syndrome by a rapid test for surfactant in amniotic fluid. N Engl J Med 286:1077, 1972

Copper RL, Goldenberg RL, DuBard MB, Davis RO, and the Collaborative Group on Preterm Prevention: Risk factors for fetal death in white, black, and hispanic women. Obstet Gynecol 94:490, 1994

Cordes I, Roland EH, Lupton BA, Hill A: Early prediction of the development of microcephaly after hypoxic ischemic encephalopathy in the full-term newborn. Pediatrics 93:703, 1994

Cornish JD, Dreyer GL, Snyder GE, Kuehl TJ, Gerstmann DR, Null DM Jr, Coalson JJ, deLemos RA: Failure of acute perinatal asphyxia or meconium aspiration to produce persistent pulmonary hypertension in a neonatal baboon model. Am J Obstet Gynecol 171:43, 1994

Cox SM, Leveno KJ, Cunningham DFG, Engle W, Rosenfeld CR, Kelly MA, Sherman ML: Introduction of corticosteroids for fetal maturation in a large obstetric service: A 2-year before/after comparison. Am J Obstet Gynecol 174:467, 1996

Craven CM, Dempsey S, Carey JC, Kochenour NK: Evaluation of a perinatal autopsy protocol: Influence of the prenatal diagnosis conference team. Obstet Gynecol 76:684, 1990

Cunningham FG, Hollier LM: Fetal death. Williams Obstetrics, 20th ed (Suppl 4). Norwalk, CT, Appleton & Lange, August/September, 1997

Dammann O, Leviton A: Maternal intrauterine infection, cytokines, and brain damage in the preterm newborn. Pediatr Res 42:1, 1997

Davis RO, Phillips JB III, Harris BA Jr, Wilson ER, Huddleston JF: Fatal meconium aspiration syndrome occurring despite airway management considered appropriate. Am J Obstet Gynecol 141:731, 1985

DeAlemida V, Bowman JM: Massive fetomaternal hemorrhage: Manitoba experience. Obstet Gynecol 83:323, 1994

DeVries LS, Dubowitz V, Lary S, Whitelaw A, Dubowitz LMS, Kaiser A, Silverman M, Wigglesworth JS: Predictive value of cranial ultrasound in the newborn baby: A reappraisal. Lancet 2:137, 1985

DeVries LS, Eken P, Groenendaal F, van Haastert IC, Meiners LC: Correlation between the degree of periventricular leukomalacia diagnosed using cranial ultrasound and MRI later in infancy in children with cerebral palsy. Neuropediatrics 24:263, 1993

Diamond LK, Blackfan KP, Baty JM: Erythroblastosis fetalis and its association with universal edema of the fetus, icterus gravis neonatorum and anemia of the newborn. J Pediatr 1:269, 1932

Dijxhoorn MJ, Visser GHA, Fidler VJ, Touwen BCL, Huisjes HJ: Apgar score, meconium and acidaemia at birth in relation to neonatal neurological morbidity in term infants. Br J Obstet Gynaecol 86:217, 1986

Dooley SL, Pesavento DJ, Depp R, Socol ML, Tamura RK, Wiringa KS: Meconium below the vocal cords at delivery: Correlation with intrapartum events. Am J Obstet Gynecol 153:767, 1985

Dunn MS: Surfactant replacement therapy: Prophylaxis or treatment? Pediatrics 92:148, 1993

Duthie SJ, Walkinshaw SA: Parvovirus associated fetal hydrops: Reversal of pregnancy induced proteinuric hypertension by in utero fetal transfusion. Br J Obstet Gynaecol 102:1011, 1995

Eibl MM, Wolf HM, Fürnkranz H, Rosenkranz A: Prevention of necrotizing enterocolitis in low-birth-weight infants by IgA-IgG feeding. N Engl J Med 319:1, 1988

Eriksen N, Tey A, Prieto J, O'Sullivan E, Wong S, Blanco J: Fetal lung maturity in diabetic patients using the TDX-FLM assay. Am J Obstet Gynecol 174:348, 1996

Faye-Petersen OM, Guinn DA, Wenstrom KD: The value of perinatal autopsy. Obstet Gynecol 96:915, 1999

Fedrizzi E, Inverno M, Bruzzone MG, Botteon G, Saletti V, Farionotti M: MRI features of cerebral lesions and cognitive functions in preterm spastic diplegic children. Pediatr Neurol 15:207, 1996

Fee SC, Malee K, Deddish R, Minogue JP, Min D, Socol ML: Severe acidosis and subsequent neurologic status. Am J Obstet Gynecol 162:802, 1990

Ferrara TB, Hoekstra RE, Couser RJ, Gaziano EP, Calvin SE, Payne NR, Fangman JJ: Survival and follow-up of infants born at 23 to 26 weeks of gestational age: Effects of surfactant therapy. J Pediatr 124:119, 1994

Finer NN, Barrington KJ: Nitric oxide therapy for the newborn. Semin Perinatol 24:59, 2000

Finkelstein Y, Adler Y, Harel L, Nussinovitch M, Youinou P: Anti-Ro (SSA) and anti-La (SSB) antibodies and complete congenital heart block [Review]. Anales de Medicine Interna 148:205, 1997

Finn R, Clarke CA, Donohoe W, McConnell RB, Sheppard PM, Lehane D, Kulke W: Experimental studies on the prevention of Rh haemolytic disease. BMJ 1:1486, 1961

Foliot A, Ploussard JP, Housset E, Christoforov B: Breast milk jaundice: In vitro inhibition of rat liver bilirubin-uridine diphosphate glucuronosyltransferase activity and Z protein-bromosulfophthalein binding by human breast milk. Pediatr Res 10:594, 1976

Fox H: Pathology of the placenta. Monograph, Vol VI. Philadelphia, Saunders, 1978

Freda V: Hemolytic disease. Clin Obstet Gynecol 16:72, 1973

Freda VJ, Gorman JG, Pollack W: Successful prevention of sensitization to Rh with an experimental anti-Rh gamma$_2$ globulin antibody preparation. Fed Proc 22:374, 1963

Freda VJ, Gorman JG, Pollack W, Bowe E: Prevention of Rh hemolytic disease: Ten years' clinical experience with Rh immune globulin. N Engl J Med 292:1014, 1975

Freeman J (ed): Prenatal and perinatal factors associated with brain disorders. US Department of Health and Human Services, Public Health Service, National Institutes of Health, NIH Publication No. 85-1149, 1985

Freeman JM, Nelson KB: Intrapartum asphyxia and cerebral palsy. Pediatrics 82:240, 1988

Freeman R: Intrapartum fetal monitoring—a disappointing story. N Engl J Med 322:624, 1990

Freeman RK, Dorchester W, Anderson G, Garite TJ: The significance of a previous stillbirth. Am J Obstet Gynecol 151:7, 1985

Fretts RC, Boyd ME, Usher RH, Usher HA: The changing pattern of fetal death, 1961–1988. Obstet Gynecol 79:35, 1992

Fretts RC, Usher RH: Causes of fetal death in women of advanced maternal age. Obstet Gynecol 89:40, 1997

Freud S: Infantile Cerebrallahmung. Notnagel's Specielle Pathologie und Therapie 9, Vol XII. Vienna, A. Holder, 1897

Fujimoto S, Yamaguchi N, Togari H, Wada Y, Yokochi K: Cerebral palsy of the cystic periventricular leukomalacia in low-birth-weight infants. Acta Paediatr 83:397, 1994

Fujiwara T, Maeta H, Shida S, Morita T, Watabe Y, Abe T: Artificial surfactant therapy in hyaline-membrane disease. Lancet 1:55, 1980

Gabbe SG, Ettinger BB, Freeman RK, Martin CB: Umbilical cord compression associated with amniotomy: Laboratory observations. Am J Obstet Gynecol 126:353, 1976

Galbraith RS: Incidence of sixth nerve palsy in relation to mode of delivery. Am J Obstet Gynecol 170:1158, 1994

Garite TJ, Rumney PJ, Briggs GG, Harding JA, Nageotte MP, Towers CV, Freeman RK: A randomized placebo controlled trial of betamethasone for the prevention of respiratory distress syndrome at 24–28 weeks gestation. Am J Obstet Gynecol 166:646, 1992

Gilstrap LC III, Crosby UD: When is fetal asphyxia alarming? Contemp Ob/Gyn 39:34, 1994

Gilstrap LC III, Leveno KJ, Burris J, Williams ML, Little BB: Diagnosis of asphyxia on the basis of fetal pH, Apgar score, and newborn cerebral dysfunction. Am J Obstet Gynecol 161:825, 1989

Gluck L, Kulovich MV: Lecithin/sphingomyelin ratios in amniotic fluid in normal and abnormal pregnancy. Am J Obstet Gynecol 115:539, 1973

Gluck L, Kulovich MV, Borer RC Jr, Brenner PH, Anderson GG, Spellacy WN: Diagnosis of the respiratory distress syndrome by amniocentesis. Am J Obstet Gynecol 109:440, 1971

Goepfert AR, Goldenberg RL, Hauth JC, Owen J, MacPherson C, Thom E, Bottoms S, McNellis D: Obstetrical determinants of neonatal neurological morbidity. Am J Obstet Gynecol 174:470, 1996

Goetz MC, Gretebeck RJ, Oh KS, Shaffer D, Hermansen MC: Incidence, timing, and follow-up of periventricular leukomalacia. Am J Perinatol 12:325, 1995

Gold WR Jr, Queenan JT, Woody J, Sacher RA: Oral desensitization in Rh disease. Am J Obstet Gynecol 146:980, 1983

Goldaber KJ, Gilstrap LC, Leveno KJ, Dax JS, McIntire DD: Pathologic fetal acidemia. Obstet Gynecol 78:1103, 1991

Goldenberg RL, Mayberry SK, Cooper RL, Dubard MB, Hauth JC: Pregnancy outcome following a second-trimester loss. Obstet Gynecol 81:444, 1993

Goldman M, Blajchman MA, Ati MA: Overestimation of feto-maternal hemorrhage by the acid-elution technique in mothers with beta-thalassemia minor. Transfus Med 1:129, 1991

Gough JD, Keeling JW, Castle B, Iliff PJ: The obstetric management of non-immunological hydrops. Br J Obstet Gynaecol 93:226, 1986

Govaert P, Vanhaesebrouck P, De Praeter C, Moens K, Leroy J: Vacuum extraction, bone injury and neonatal subgaleal bleeding. Eur J Pediatr 151:532, 1992

Grant A, O'Brien N, Joy MT, Hennessy E, MacDonald D: Cerebral palsy among children born during the Dublin randomised trial of intrapartum monitoring. Lancet 2:1233, 1989

Grether JK, Nelson KB: Maternal infection and cerebral palsy in infants of normal birth weight. JAMA 278:207, 1997

Hack M, Horbar JD, Malloy MH, Tyson JE, Wright E, Wright L: Very low-birth-weight outcomes of the National Institute of Child Health and Human Development neonatal network. Pediatrics 87:587, 1991

Haddow JE, Rote NS, Dostal-Johnson D, Palomaki GE, Pulkinen AJ, Knight GJ: Lack of an association between late fetal death and antiphospholipid antibody measurements in the second trimester. Am J Obstet Gynecol 165:1308, 1991

Hagadorn-Freathy AS, Yeomans ER, Hankins GDV: Validation of the 1988 ACOG forceps classification system. Obstet Gynecol 77:356, 1991

Hagen E, Link JC, Arias F: A comparison of the accuracy of the TDx-FLM assay, lecithin–sphingomyelin ratio, and phosphatidyl glycerol in the prediction of neonatal respiratory distress syndrome. Obstet Gynecol 82:1004, 1993

Hallack M, Bottoms SF: Accelerated pulmonary maturation from preterm premature rupture of the membranes: A myth. Am J Obstet Gynecol 169:1045, 1993

Hamvas A, Wise PH, Yang RK, Wampler NS, Noguchi A, Maurer MM, Walentik CA, Schramm WF, Cole FS: The influence of the wider use of surfactant therapy on neonatal mortality among blacks and whites. N Engl J Med 334: 1635, 1996

Hanigan WC, Kennedy G, Roemisch F, Anderson R, Cusack T, Powers W: Administration of indomethacin for the prevention of periventricular–intraventricular hemorrhage in high-risk neonates. J Pediatr 112:941, 1988

Hanson J, Persson B: Outcome of pregnancies complicated by type 1 insulin-dependent diabetes in Sweden: Acute pregnancy complications, neonatal mortality and morbidity. Am J Perinatol 4:330, 1993

Harman CR, Manning FA, Bowman JM, Lange IR: Severe Rh disease—poor outcome is not inevitable. Am J Obstet Gynecol 145:823, 1983

Harper MA, Lorenz WB Jr: Immature lecithin/sphingomyelin ratios and respiratory course. Am J Obstet Gynecol 168: 495, 1993

Hayakawa F, Okumura A, Kato T, Kuno K, Watanabe K: Determination of timing of brain injury in preterm infants with periventricular leukomalacia with serial neonatal electroencephalography. Pediatrics 104:1077, 1999

Hayden CK, Shattuck KE, Richardson CJ, Ahrendt DK, House R, Swischuk LE: Subependymal germinal matrix hemorrhage in full-term neonates. Pediatrics 75:714, 1985

Heinonen S, Ruynamen M, Kirkinen P: Etiology and outcome of second trimester nonimmunological fetal hydrops. Scand J Obstet Gynecol 79:15, 2000

Herbert WNP, Chapman JE, Schnoor MM: Role of the TDx FLM assay in fetal lung maturity. Am J Obstet Gynecol 168:808, 1993

Holtrop PC, Ertzbischoff LM, Roberts CL, Batton DG, Lorenz RP: Survival and short-term outcome in newborns of 23–25 weeks gestation. Am J Obstet Gynecol 170:1266, 1994

Holzgreve W, Curry CJR, Golbus MS, Callen PW, Filly RA, Smith JC: Investigation of nonimmune hydrops fetalis. Am J Obstet Gynecol 150:805, 1984

Horbar JD, Wright EC, Onstad L: Decreasing mortality associated with the introduction of surfactant therapy: An observational study of neonates weighing 601 to 1300 grams at birth. Pediatrics 92:191, 1993

Howard H, Martlew V, McFadyen I, Clarke C, Duguid J, Bromilow I, Eggington J: Consequences for fetus and neonate of maternal red cell allo-immunization. Arch Dis Childhood Fetal Neonat Ed 78:F62, 1998

Howe AM, Lipson AH, Sheffield LJ, Haan EA, Halliday JL, Jenson F, David DJ, Webster WS: Prenatal exposure to phenytoin, facial development, and a possible role for vitamin K. Am J Med Gen 58:238, 1995

Hsu N, Hung KL, Tsai ML, Wu CH, Kua KE: The association of periventricular echodensity of cerebral palsy in preterm infants. Chung-Hua Min Kuo Hsiao Erh Koi Hsueh Hui Tsa Chih 37:433, 1996

Hughes PM, Turton P, Evans CDH: Stillbirth as risk factor for depression and anxiety in the subsequent pregnancy: Cohort study. BMJ 318:1721, 1999

Hulsey TC, Alexander GR, Robillard PY, Annibale DJ, Keenan A: Hyaline membrane disease: The role of ethnicity and maternal risk characteristics. Am J Obstet Gynecol 168:572, 1993

Illingworth RS: Why blame the obstetrician? A review. BMJ 1:797, 1979

Infante-Rivard C, David M, Gautheir R, Rivard GE: Lupus anticoagulants, anticardiolipin antibodies, and fetal loss: A case-control study. N Engl J Med 325:1063, 1991

Jakobi P, Weissman A, Zimmer EZ, Blazer S: Survival and long-term morbidity in preterm infants with and without a clinical diagnosis of periventricular, intraventricular hemorrhage. Eur J Obstet Gynecol Reprod Biol 46:73, 1992

Janssen HJ, Cuisinier MC, Hoogduin KA, de Graauw KP: Controlled prospective study on the mental health of women following pregnancy loss. Am J Psychiatry 153: 226, 1996

Jaw TS, Jong YJ, Sheu RS, Liu GC, Chou MS, Yang RC: Etiology, timing of insult, and neuropathology of cerebral palsy evaluated with magnetic resonance imaging. J Formos Med Assoc 97:239, 1998

Jennings ER, Clauss B: Maternal–fetal hemorrhage: Its incidence and sensitizing effects. Am J Obstet Gynecol 131:725, 1978

Jobe AH: Pulmonary surfactant therapy. N Engl J Med 328:861, 1993

Kanto WP Jr, Wilson R, Breart GL, Zierler S, Purohit DM, Peckham GJ, Ellison RC: Perinatal events and necrotizing enterocolitis in premature infants. Am J Dis Child 141:167, 1987

Kari MA, Hallman M, Eronen M, Teramo K, Virtanen M, Koivisto M, Ikonen RS: Prenatal dexamethasone treatment in conjunction with rescue therapy of human surfactant: A randomized placebo-controlled multicentered study. Pediatrics 93:730, 1994

Katz LV, Bowes WA: Meconium aspiration syndrome: Reflections on a murky subject. Am J Obstet Gynecol 166: 171, 1992

Katz MA, Kanto WP Jr, Korotkein JH: Recurrence rate of ABO hemolytic disease of the newborn. Obstet Gynecol 59:611, 1982

Keenan WJ, Jewitt T, Glueck HI: Role of feeding and vitamin K in hypoprothrombinemia of the newborn. Am J Dis Child 121:271, 1971

Kinsella JP, Walsh WF, Bose CL, Gerstmann DR, Labella JJ, Sardesai S: Inhaled nitric oxide in premature neonates with severe hypoxaemic respiratory failure: A randomised controlled trial. Lancet 354:2126, 1999

Kirkman HN Jr: Further evidence for a racial difference in the frequency of ABO hemolytic disease. J Pediatr 90:717, 1977

Kjos SL, Walther FJ, Montoro M, Paul RH, Diaz F, Stabler M: Prevalence and etiology of respiratory distress in infants of diabetic mothers: Predictive value of fetal lung maturation tests. Am J Obstet Gynecol 163:898, 1990

Kleinman CS, Copel JA, Weinstein EM, Santulli TV, Hobbins JC: In utero diagnosis and treatment of fetal supraventricular tachycardia. Semin Perinatol 9:113, 1985

Kliegman RM, Fanaroff AA: Necrotizing enterocolitis. N Engl J Med 310:1093, 1984

Korst LM, Ahn MO, Phelan JP: Nucleated red blood cells:

An update on the marker for fetal asphyxia. Am J Obstet Gynecol 174:318, 1996

Kuit JA, Eppinga HG, Wallenburg HCS, Huikeshoven FJM: A randomized comparison of vacuum extraction delivery with a rigid and a pliable cup. Obstet Gynecol 82:280, 1993

Lammer EJ, Brown LE, Anderka MT, Guyer B: Classification and analysis of fetal deaths in Massachusetts. JAMA 261:1757, 1989

Landsteiner K, Weiner AS: An agglutinable factor in human blood recognized by immune sera for rhesus blood. Proc Soc Exp Biol Med 43:223, 1940

Lefebvre G, Wehbe G, Heron D, VautgoerBrouzes D, Choukroun JB, Dubois Y: Recurrent nonimmune hydrops fetalis: A prepresentation of sciatic acid storage disease. Gen Coun 10:277, 1999

Lesko SM, Mitchell AA, Epstein MF, Louik C, Giacoia GP, Shapiro S: Heparin use as a risk factor for intraventricular hemorrhage in low-birth-weight infants. N Engl J Med 314:1156, 1986

Levene M: Role of excitatory amino acid antagonists in the management of birth asphyxia. 62:248, 1992

Leveno KJ, Quirk JG, Cunningham FG, Nelson SD, Santo-Ramos R, Toofanian A, DePalma RT: Prolonged pregnancy, 1. Observations concerning the causes of fetal distress. Am J Obstet Gynecol 150:465, 1984

Levine MG, Holroyde J, Woods JR, Siddiqi TA, Scott M, Miodovnik M: Birth trauma: Incidence and predisposing factors. Obstet Gynecol 63:792, 1984

Levine P, Katzin KM, Burnham L: Isoimmunization in pregnancy: Its possible bearing on the etiology of erythroblastosis fetalis. JAMA 116:825, 1941

Liley AW: Liquor amnii analysis in management of pregnancy complicated by rhesus sensitization. Am J Obstet Gynecol 82:1359, 1961

Linder N, Aranda JV, Tsur M, Matoth I, Yatsiv I, Mandelberg H, Rottem M, Feigenbaum D, Ezra Y, Tamir I: Need for endotracheal intubation and suction in meconium-stained neonates. J Pediatr 112:613, 1988

Locus P, Yeomans E, Crosby U: The efficacy of bulb versus DeLee suction at deliveries complicated by meconium-stained amniotic fluid. Perinatology 7:87, 1990

Long W, Zucker J, Kraybill E: Symposium on synthetic surfactant II: Perspective and commentary. J Pediatr 126:1, 1995

Low JA, Galbraith RS, Muir DW, Killen HL, Karchmar EJ: The relationship between perinatal hypoxia and newborn encephalography. Am J Obstet Gynecol 152:256, 1985

Low JA, Panagiotopoulos C, Derrick EJ: Newborn complications after intrapartum asphyxia with metabolic acidosis in the preterm fetus. Am J Obstet Gynecol 172:805, 1995

Low JA, Panagiotopoulos C, Derrick EJ: Newborn complications after intrapartum asphyxia with metabolic acidosis in the term fetus. Am J Obstet Gynecol 170:1081, 1994

Luthy DA, Shy KK, Strickland D, Wilson J, Bennett FC, Brown ZA, Benedetti TJ: Status of infants at birth and risk for adverse neonatal events and long-term sequelae: A study in low birthweight infants. Am J Obstet Gynecol 157:676, 1987

MacDonald D, Grant A, Sheridan-Pereira M, Boylan P, Chalmers I: The Dublin randomized control trial of intrapartum fetal heart rate monitoring. Am J Obstet Gynecol 152:524, 1985

Maher JE, Cliver SP, Goldenberg RL, Davis RO, Copper RL: The effect of corticosteroid therapy in the very premature infant. Am J Obstet Gynecol 170:869, 1994

Maisels MJ: Neonatal jaundice, 3. Breast feeding and jaundice. Perinatol Press 3:19, 1979

Manning FA, Schrieber J, Turkel SB: Fatal meconium aspiration "in utero": A case report. Am J Obstet Gynecol 132:111, 1978

Marret S, Gressens P, Gadisseux JF, Evrard P: Prevention by magnesium of excitotoxic neuronal death in the developing brain: An animal model for clinical intervention studies. Dev Med Child Neurol 34:473, 1995

Mayne KM, Bowell PJ, Pratt GA: The significance of anti-Kell sensitization in pregnancy. Clin Lab Hematol 12:379, 1990

McCoy MC, Katz VL, Could N, Kuller JA: Non-immune hydrops after 20 weeks' gestation: Review of 10 years' experience with suggestions for management. Obstet Gynecol 85:578, 1995

Melone PJ, Ernest JM, O'Shea MD Jr, Klinepeter KL: Appropriateness of intrapartum fetal heart rate management and risk of cerebral palsy. Am J Obstet Gynecol 165:272, 1991

Ment LR, Oh W, Ehrenkranz RA, Philip AGS, Duncan CC, Makuch RW: Antenatal steroids, delivery mode and intraventricular hemorrhage in preterm infants. Am J Obstet Gynecol 172:795, 1995

Menticoglou SM, Perlman M, Manning FA: High cervical spinal cord injury in neonates delivered with forceps: Report of 15 cases. Obstet Gynecol 86:589, 1995

Midgley DY, Hardrug K: The mirror syndrome. Euro J Obstet Gynecol and Reprod Biol 8:201, 2000

Miller ME, Graham JM Jr, Higginbotton MC, Smith DW: Compression-related defects from early amnion rupture: Evidence for mechanical teratogenesis. J Pediatr 98:292, 1981

Mino M: Clinical uses and abuses of vitamin E in children. Proc Soc Exp Biol Med 200:266, 1992

Misbah SA, Chapel HM: Adverse effects of intravenous immunoglobulin. Drug Saf 9:254, 1993

Miyazaki FS, Taylor NA: Saline amnioinfusion for relief of variable or prolonged decelerations. A preliminary report. Am J Obstet Gynecol 146:670, 1983

Mountain K, Hirsh J, Gallus AS: Neonatal coagulation defect and maternal anti-convulsant treatment. Lancet 1:265, 1970

Mueller RF, Sybert VP, Johnson J, Brown ZA, Chen W-J: Evaluation of a protocol for postmortem examination of stillbirths. N Engl J Med 309:586, 1983

Mueller-Heubach E, Mazer J: Sonographically documented disappearance of fetal ascites. Obstet Gynecol 61:253, 1983

Murphy JD, Vawter GF, Reid LM: Pulmonary vascular disease in fatal meconium aspiration. J Pediatr 194:758, 1984

Naeye RL, Localio AR: Determining the time before birth when ischemia and hypoxemia initiated cerebral palsy. Obstet Gynecol 86:713, 1995

Nagel HTC, Vandenbussche FPHA, Oepkes D, Jennekens-Schinkel A, Laan LAEM, Gravenhorst JB: Follow-up of children born with an umbilical arterial blood pH < 7. Am J Obstet Gynecol 173:1758, 1995

Nathan L, Leveno KJ, Carmody TJ, Kelly MA, Sherman ML: Meconium: A 1990s perspective on an old obstetric hazard. Obstet Gynecol 83:329, 1994

National Institutes of Health: Consensus Development Conference on the effects of corticosteroids for fetal maturation on perinatal outcomes. Consensus Development Conference statement. Bethesda, MD, 1994

Nelson KB, Dambrosia JM, Ting TY, Brether JC: Uncertain value of electronic fetal monitoring in predicting cerebral palsy. N Engl J Med 334:613, 1996

Nelson KB, Ellenberg JH: Antecedents of cerebral palsy: Multivariate analysis of risk. N Engl J Med 315:81, 1986a

Nelson KB, Ellenberg JH: Antecedents of seizure disorders in early childhood. Am J Dis Child 140:1053, 1986b

Nelson KB, Ellenberg JH: Antecedents of cerebral palsy: Univariate analysis of risks. Am J Dis Child 139:1031, 1985

Nelson KB, Ellenberg JH: Obstetric complications as risk factors for cerebral palsy or seizure disorders. JAMA 251:1843, 1984

Nelson KB, Leviton A: How much of neonatal encephalopathy is due to birth asphyxia? Am J Dis Child 145:1325, 1991

Ness PM, Baldwin ML, Niebyl JR: Clinical high-risk designation does not predict excess fetal–maternal hemorrhage. Am J Obstet Gynecol 156:154, 1987

Neugebauer R, Kline J, O'Connor P, Shrout P, Johnson J, Skodol A, Wicks J, Susser M: Determinants of depressive symptoms in the early weeks after miscarriage. Am J Public Health 82:1332, 1992

Nicolaides KH, Clewell WH, Mibashan RS, Soothill PW, Rodeck CH, Campbell S: Fetal haemoglobin measurement in the assessment of red cell isoimmunization. Lancet 1:1073, 1988

Nicolaides KH, Rodeck CH, Mibashan RS, Kemp JR: Have Liley charts outlived their usefulness? Am J Obstet Gynecol 155:90, 1986

Nicolaides KH, Snijders RJM: Cordocentesis. In Evans MI (ed): Reproductive Risks and Prenatal Diagnosis. Norwalk, CT, Appleton & Lange, 1992, p 201

Nicolaides KH, Warenski JC, Rodeck CH: The relationship of fetal plasma protein concentration and hemoglobin level to the development of hydrops in rhesus isoimmunization. Am J Obstet Gynecol 152:341, 1985

Nicolini U, Nicolaides P, Tannirandorn Y, Fisk N, Nasrat H, Rodeck CH: Fetal liver dysfunction in Rh alloimmunization. Br J Obstet Gynaecol 98:287, 1991

Niswander K, Henson G, Elbourne D, Chalmers I, Redman C, Macfarlane A, Tizard P: Adverse outcome of pregnancy and the quality of obstetric care. Lancet 2:827, 1984

Nocon JJ, McKenzie DK, Thomas LJ, Hansell RS: Shoulder dystocia: An analysis of risks and obstetric maneuvers. Am J Obstet Gynecol 168:1732, 1993

Nores J, Roberts A, Carr S: Prenatal diagnosis and management of fetuses with intracranial hemorrhage. Am J Obstet Gynecol 174:424, 1996

Ojomo EO, Coustan DR: Absence of evidence of pulmonary maturity at amniocentesis in term infants of diabetic mothers. Am J Obstet Gynecol 163:954, 1990

Oka A, Belliveau MJ, Rosenberg PA, Volpe JJ: Vulnerability of oligodendroglia to glutamate: Pharmacology, mechanisms, and prevention. J Neuroscience 13:1441, 1993

Okumura A, Kato T, Juno K, Hayakawa F, Watanabe K: MRI findings in patients with spastic cerebral palsy. II: Correlation with type of cerebral palsy. Dev Med Child Neurol 39:369, 1997

Oppenheim WL, Davis A, Growdon WA, Dorey FJ, Davlin LB: Clavicle fractures in the newborn. Clin Ortho 250:176, 1990

OSRIS Collaborative Group: Early versus delayed neonatal administration of synthetic surfactant: The judgment of OSRIS. Lancet 340:1363, 1992

Paneth N: Birth and the origins of cerebral palsy. N Engl J Med 315:124, 1986

Papile LA, Burstein J, Burstein R, Koffler H: Incidence and evolution of subependymal and intraventricular hemorrhage: A study of infants with birth weights less than 1500 gm. J Pediatr 92:529, 1978

Papile LA, Munsick-Bruno G, Schaefer A: Relationship of

cerebral intraventricular hemorrhage and early childhood neurologic handicaps. J Pediatr 103:273, 1983

Pauli RM, Reiser CA: Wisconsin Stillbirth Service Program: II. Analysis of diagnoses and diagnostic categories in the first 1,000 referrals. Am J Med Genet 50:135, 1994

Perlman JM, Cunningham FG: Fetal and neonatal hypoxic ischemic cerebral injury. Williams Obstetrics, 18th ed (Suppl 21). Norwalk, CT, Appleton & Lange, December/January 1993

Perlman JM, Risser R, Broyles RS: Bilateral cystic periventricular leukomalacia in the premature infant: Associated risk factors. Pediatrics 97:822, 1996

Perlman JM, Volpe JJ: Intraventricular hemorrhage in extremely small premature infants. Am J Dis Child 140:1122, 1986

Phelan JP, Ahn MO: Perinatal observations in forty-eight neurologically impaired term infants. Am J Obstet Gynecol 171, 424, 1994

Phelan JP, Ahn MO, Korst L, Martin GI: Is intrapartum fetal brain injury in the term fetus preventable? Am J Obstet Gynecol 174:318, 1996

Piper J, Langer O: Delayed pulmonary maturation is associated with poor glucose control in diabetic pregnancies. Am J Obstet Gynecol 174:396, 1996

Pomerance JJ, Jeal JG, Gogolok JF, Brown S, Stewart ME: Maternally administered antenatal vitamin K_1: Effect on neonatal prothrombin activity, partial thromboplastin time and intraventricular hemorrhage. Obstet Gynecol 70:235, 1987

Pritchard JA, Cunningham G, Pritchard SA, Mason RA: On reducing the frequency of severe abruptio placentae. Am J Obstet Gynecol 165:1345, 1991

Pritchard JA, Cunningham FG, Pritchard SA, Mason RA: How often does maternal preeclampsia–eclampsia incite thrombocytopenia in the fetus? Obstet Gynecol 69:292, 1987

Queenan JT, Thomas PT, Tomai TP, Ural SH, King JC: Deviation in amniotic fluid optical density at a wavelength of 450 nm in Rh isoimmunized pregnancies from 14 to 40 weeks gestation: A proposal for clinical management. Am J Obstet Gynecol 168:1370, 1993

Race RR, Sanger R: Blood Groups in Man, 6th Ed. Blackwell, Oxford, England, 1975

Radestad I, Steineck G, Nordin C, Sjögren B: Psychological complications after stillbirth—influence of memories and immediate management: population based study. BMJ 312:1505, 1996

Ramsey-Goldman R, Hom D, Deng J, Ziegler GC, Kahl LE, Steen VD, LaPorte RE, Medsger TA Jr: Anti-SS-A antibodies and fetal outcome in maternal systemic lupus erythematosus. Arthritis Rheum 29:1269, 1986

Reznikoff-Etievant MF, Muller JY, Julien F, Patereau C: An immune response gene liked to MHC in man. Tissue Antigens 22:312, 1983

Richardson DK, Torday JS: Racial differences in predictive value of the lecithin/sphingomyelin ratio. Am J Obstet Gynecol 170:1273, 1994

Richey S, Ramin SM, Bawdon RE, Roberts SW, Dax J, Roberts J, Gilstrap LC: Markers of acute and chronic asphyxia in infants with meconium-stained amniotic fluid. Am J Obstet Gynecol 172:1212, 1995

Roberts SW, Hernandez C, Maberry MC, Adams MD, Leveno KJ, Wendel GD Jr: Obstetric clavicular fracture: The enigma of normal birth. Obstet Gynecol 86:978, 1995

Robertson C, Finer N: Term infants with hypoxic-ischemic encephalopathy: Outcome at 3.5 years. Dev Med Child Neurol 27:473, 1985

Roemer RJ: Relation of torticollis to breech delivery. Am J Obstet Gynecol 67:1146, 1954

Rosen MG, Dickinson JC: The incidence of cerebral palsy. Am J Obstet Gynecol 167:417, 1992

Rosen MG, Hobel CJ: Prenatal and perinatal factors associated with brain disorders. Obstet Gynecol 68:416, 1986

Rouse D, Weiner C: Ongoing fetomaternal hemorrhage treated by serial fetal intravascular transfusions. Obstet Gynecol 76:974, 1990

Sadovsky Y, Amon E, Bade ME, Petrie RH: Prophylactic amnioinfusion during labor complicated by meconium: A preliminary report. Am J Obstet Gynecol 161:613, 1989

Salafia CM, Minior UK, Pezzullo JC, Ghidini A, Ernst LM, Sherer DM: Premature rupture of membranes and premature labor neonatal nucleated erythrocyte number (nRBCs) is related to histologic acute inflammation and not to placental markers of hypoxia. Am J Obstet Gynecol 174:318, 1996

Saller DN Jr, Lesser KB, Harrel U, Rogers BB, Oyer CE: The clinical utility of the perinatal autopsy. JAMA 273:663, 1995

Salonen IS, Uüsitalo R: Birth injuries: Incidence and predisposing factors. Zeitschr fur Kinderch 45:133, 1990

Samadi R, Miller D, Settlage R, Gviazda I, Paul R, Goodwin TM: Massive fetomaternal hemorrhage and fetal death: Is it predictable? Am J Obstet Gynecol 174:391, 1996

Samueloff A, Xenakis EMJ, Berkus MD, Huff RW, Langer O: Recurrent stillbirth: Significance and characteristics. J Reprod Med 88:883, 1993

Sandmire HF, DeMott RK: Erb's palsy: Concepts of causation. Obstet Gynecol 95:941, 2000

Santolaya J, Alley D, Jaffe R, Warsof SL: Antenatal classification of hydrops fetalis. Obstet Gynecol 79:256, 1992

Saunders BS, Lazoritz S, McArtor RD, Marshall P, Bason WM: Depressed skull fracture in the neonate. J Neurosurg 50:512, 1979

Sbarra AJ, Michlewitz H, Selvaraj RJ, Mitchell GW, Cetrulo CL, Kelley EC, Kennedy JL, Herschell MJ, Paul BB, Louis F: Relation between optical density at 650 nm and L/S ratio. Obstet Gynecol 50:273, 1977

Schendel DE, Berg CJ, Yeargin-Allsopp M, Boyle CA, Decoufle P: Prenatal magnesium sulfate exposure and the risk for cerebral palsy or mental retardation among very low-birth-weight children aged 3 to 5 years. JAMA 276:1805, 1996

Schiff E, Friedman SA, Mercer BM, Sibai BM: Fetal lung maturity is not accelerated in preeclamptic pregnancies. Am J Obstet Gynecol 169:1096, 1993

Shearer MJ, Barkhan P, Rahim S, Stimmler L: Plasma vitamin K_1 in mothers and their newborn babies. Lancet 2:460, 1982

Shenker L, Reed KL, Anderson CF, Marx GR, Sobonya RE, Graham AR: Congenital heart block and cardiac anomalies in the absence of maternal connective tissue disease. Am J Obstet Gynecol 157:248, 1987

Shulman LP, Phillips OP, Emerson DS, Felker RE, Tharapel AT: Fetal "space-suit" hydrops in the first trimester: Differentiating risk for chromosome abnormalities by delineating characteristics of nuchal translucency. Prenatal Diagn 20:30, 2000

Shy KK, Luthy DA, Bennett FC, Whitfield M, Larson EB, van Belle G, Hughes JP, Wilson JA, Stenchever MA: Effects of electronic fetal heart rate monitoring, as compared with periodic auscultation, on the neurologic development of premature infants. N Engl J Med 322:588, 1990

Sibai BM, Mabie WC, Shasma F, Villar MA, Anderson GD: A comparison of no medication versus methyldopa or labe-talol in chronic hypertension complicating pregnancy. Am J Obstet Gynecol 162:960, 1990

Silver RM, Porter TF, Branch DW, Esplin MS, Scot JR: Neonatal alloimmune thrombocytopenia: Antenatal management. Am J Obstet Gynecol 182:1233, 2000

Silver RK, Vyskocil C, Solomon SL, Ragin A, Neerhof MG, Farrell EE: Randomized trial of antenatal dexamethasone in surfactant-treated infants delivered before 30 weeks' gestation. Obstet Gynecol 87:683, 1996

Skajaa K, Hansen ES, Bendix J: Depressed fracture of the skull in a child born by cesarean section. Acta Obstet Gynecol Scand 66:275, 1987

Smyth J, Allen A, MacMurray B, Peliowski A, Sankaran K, Volberg F, Shukla A, Long W: Double-blind, randomized, placebo-controlled Canadian multicenter trial of two doses of synthetic surfactant or air placebo in 224 infants weighing 500 to 749 gm with respiratory distress syndrome. J Pediatr 126:S81, 1995

Soll RF: Natural surfactant extract treatment of RDS. In Chalmers I (ed): Oxford Database of Perinatal Trials. Version 1.2, disk issue 6, record 5206 1991a

Soll RF: Prophylactic administration of natural surfactant extract. In Chalmers I (ed): Oxford Database of Perinatal Trials. Version 1.2, disk issue 6, record 5207, 1991b

Soll RF: Prophylactic administration of synthetic surfactant treatment of RDS. In Chalmers I (ed): Oxford Database of Perinatal Trials. Version 1.2, disk issue 6, record 5253, 1991c

Soll RF: Synthetic surfactant treatment of RDS. In Chalmers I (ed): Oxford Database of Perinatal Trials. Version 1.2, disk issue 6, record 5252, 1991d

Spinillo A, Capuzzo E, Stronati M, Ometto A, DeSantolo A, Acciano S: Obstetric risk factors for periventricular leukomalacia among preterm infants. Br J Obstet Gynaecol 105:865, 1998

Spinillo A, Ometto A, Bottino R, Piazzi G, Iasci A, Rondini G: Antenatal risk factors for germinal matrix hemorrhage and intraventricular hemorrhage in preterm infants. Eur J Obstet Gynecol Reprod Biol 60:13, 1995

Spong CY, Ogundipe OA, Ross MG: Prophylactic amnioinfusion for meconium stained amniotic fluid. Am J Obstet Gynecol 171:931, 1994

Stanley FJ, Blair E: Why have we failed to reduce the frequency of cerebral palsy? Med J Aust 154:623, 1991

Stedman CM, Baudin JC, White CA, Cooper ES: Use of the erythrocyte rosette test to screen for excessive fetomaternal hemorrhage in Rh-negative women. Am J Obstet Gynecol 154:1363, 1986

Steinfeld JD, Samuels P, Bulley MA, Cohen AW, Goodman DBP, Senior MB: The utility of the TDx test in the assessment of fetal lung maturity. Obstet Gynecol 79:460, 1992

Strauss A, Kirz D, Modanlou HD, Freeman RK: Perinatal events and intraventricular/subependymal hemorrhage in the very low-birth-weight infant. Am J Obstet Gynecol 151:1022, 1985

Streeter GL: Contrib Embryol 22:1, 1930

Taylor PV, Scott JS, Gerlis LM, Esscher E, Scott O: Maternal antibodies against fetal cardiac antigens in congenital complete heart block. N Engl J Med 315:667, 1986

Tejani N, Verma U, Hameed C, Chayen B: Method and route of delivery in the low-birth-weight vertex presentation correlated with early periventricular/intraventricular hemorrhage. Obstet Gynecol 69:1, 1987

Thacker KE, Lim T, Drew JH: Cephalhaematoma: A 10-year review. Aust NZ J Obstet Gynaecol 27:210, 1987

Thacker SB, Stroup DF, Peterson HB: Efficacy and safety of

intrapartum electronic fetal monitoring: an update. Obstet Gynecol 86:613, 1995

Thorp JA, Ferette-Smith D, Gaston L, Johnson J, Caspers D, Yeast JD, Cohen Gr, Meyer BA: Antenatal vitamin K and phenobarbital for preventing intracranial hemorrhage in the premature newborn: A randomized double-blind placebo-controlled trial. Am J Obstet Gynecol 172:253, 1995

Torfs CP, van den Berg B, Oechsli FW, Cummins S: Prenatal and perinatal factors in the etiology of cerebral palsy. J Pediatr 116:615, 1990

Torpin R: Fetal malformations caused by amnion rupture during gestation. Springfield, IL, Thomas, 1968

Truwit CL, Barkovich AJ, Koch TK, Ferriero DM: Cerebral palsy: MR findings in 40 patients. AJNR 13:67, 1992

Tsai MY, Josephson MW, Knox GE: Absorbance of amniotic fluid at 650 nm as a fetal lung maturity test: A comparison with the lecithin/sphingomyelin ratio and tests for desaturated phosphatidylcholine and phosphatidylglycerol. Am J Obstet Gynecol 146:963, 1983

Turpenny PD, Nimmo A: Fractured clavicle of the newborn in a population with a high prevalence of grand-multiparity: Analysis of 78 consecutive cases. Br J Obstet Gynaecol 100:338, 1993

Ubachs JMH, Slooff ACJ, Peeters LLH: Obstetric antecedents of surgically treated obstetric brachial plexus injuries. Br J Obstet Gynaecol 102:813, 1995

Van Den Veyver IB, Subramanian SB, Hudson KM, Werch J, Moise KJ Jr, Hughes MR: Prenatal diagnosis of the RhD fetal blood type on amniotic fluid by polymerase chain reaction. Obstet Gynecol 87:419, 1996

Verbrugge SJ, Lachmann B: Mechanisms of ventilation-induced lung injury: Physiological rationale to prevent it. Monaldi Arch Chest Dis 54:22, 1999

Vergani P, Strobetl N, Locatelli A, Paterlini G, Tagliabue P, Parravicini E, Chidini A: Clinical significance of fetal intracranial hemorrhage. Am J Obstet Gynecol 175:536, 1996

Verma U, Tajani N, Klein S, Reale MR, Beneck D, Figueroa R, Visintainer P: Obstetric antecedents of intraventricular hemorrhage and periventricular leukomalacia in the low-birth-weight neonatal. Am J Obstet Gynecol 176:275, 1997

Volpe JJ: Neurology of the Newborn, 3rd ed. Philadelphia, Saunders, 1995, p 373

Volpe JJ, Hill A: Neurologic disorders. In Avery GB (ed): Neonatology, 3rd ed. Philadelphia, JB Lippincott, 1987, p 10723

Walle T, Hartikainen-Sorri AL: Obstetric shoulder dystocia: Associated risk factors, prediction and prognosis. Acta Obstet Gynecol Scand 72:450, 1993

Wallin LA, Rosenfeld CR, Laptook AR, Maravilla AM, Strand C, Campbell N, Dowling S, Lasky RE: Neonatal intracranial hemorrhage, 2. Risk factor analysis in an inborn population. Early Hum Dev 23:129, 1990

Weeks JW, Asrat T, Morgan MA, Nagoette M, Thomas SJ, Freeman RK: Antepartum surveillance for a history of stillbirth: When to begin? Am J Obstet Gynecol 172:486, 1995

Weindling M: Periventricular haemorrhage and periventricular leukomalacia. Br J Obstet Gynaecol 102:278, 1995

Weiner CP, Pelzer GD, Heilskov J, Wenstrom KD, Williamson RA: The effect of intravascular transfusion on umbilical venous pressure in anemic fetuses with and without drops. Am J Obstet Gynecol 161:1498, 1989

Weiner CP, Wenstrom KD, Sipes SL, Williamson RA: Risk factors for cordocentesis and fetal intravascular transfusion. Am J Obstet Gynecol 165:1020, 1991a

Weiner CP, Widness JA: Decreased fetal erythropoiesis and hemolysis in Kell hemolytic anemia. 174:547, 1996

Weiner CP, Williamson RA, Wenstrom KD, Sipes SL, Grant SS, Widness JA: Management of fetal hemolytic disease by cordocentesis: I. Prediction of fetal anemia. Am J Obstet Gynecol 165:546, 1991b

Weiner CP, Williamson RA, Wenstrom KD, Sipes SL, Widness JA, Grant SS, Estle L: Management of fetal hemolytic disease by cordocentesis, 2. Outcome of treatment. Am J Obstet Gynecol 165:1302, 1991c

Welch RA, Bottoms SF: Reconsideration of head compression and intraventricular hemorrhage in the vertex very low-birth-weight fetus. Obstet Gynecol 68:29, 1986

Welsch C, Woods J, Yancey M, Sarno A: The efficacy of a rapid lamellar body count assay in predicting fetal lung maturity. Am J Obstet Gynecol 174:335, 1996

Wenk RE, Goldstein P, Felix JK: Alloimmunization by hr' (c), hemolytic disease of newborns, and perinatal management. Obstet Gynecol 67:623, 1986

Wenstrom KD, Andrews WW, Maher JE: Amnioinfusion survey: Prevalence, protocols, and complications. ACOG 86:572, 1995

Wenstrom KD, Parsons MT: The prevention of meconium aspiration in labor using amnioinfusion. Obstet Gynecol 73:647, 1989

White DA, Pressman EK, Hanna GV, Odon MF, Callan NA, Blakemore K: Facial nerve palsy—frequencies associated with spontaneous, forceps and cesarean deliveries. Am J Obstet Gynecol 174:353, 1996

Wigton TR, Tamura RK, Wickstrom E, Atkins V, Deddish R, Socol ML: Neonatal morbidity after preterm delivery in the presence of documented lung maturity. Am J Obstet Gynecol 169:951, 1993

Wiklund LM, Uvebrant P, Flodmark O: Computed tomography as an adjunct in etiological analysis of hemiplegic cerebral palsy, 1. Children born preterm. Neuropediatrics 22:50, 1991a

Wiklund LM, Uvebrant P, Flodmark O: Computed tomography as an adjunct in etiological analysis of hemiplegic cerebral palsy, 2. Children born at term. Neuropediatrics 22:121, 1991b

Williams MC, Knuppel RA, O'Brien WF, Weiss A, Kanarek KS: A randomized comparison of assisted vaginal delivery by obstetric forceps and polyethylene vacuum cup. Obstet Gynecol 78:789, 1991

Wiswell TE, Tuggle JM, Turner BS: Meconium aspiration syndrome: Have we made a difference? Pediatrics 85:715, 1990

Wood NS, Marlow N, Costeloe K, Gibson AT, Wilkinson AR: Neurologic and developmental disability after extremely preterm birth. N Engl J Med 343:378, 2000

Yancy MK, Herpolsheimer A, Jordan GD, Benson WL, Brady K: Maternal and neonatal effects of outlet forceps delivery compared with spontaneous vaginal delivery in term pregnancies. Obstet Gynecol 78:646, 1991

Yankowitz J, Li S, Weiner CP: Polymerase chain reaction determination of RhC, Rhc, and RhE blood types: An evaluation of accuracy and clinical utility. Am J Obstet Gynecol 176:1107, 1997

Yoder BA: Meconium stained amniotic fluid and respiratory complications: Impact of selective tracheal suction. Obstet Gynecol 83:77, 1994

Yoon BH, Kim CJ, Romero R, Jun JK, Park KH, Choi ST: Experimentally induced intrauterine infection causes fetal brain white matter lesions in rabbits. Am J Obstet Gynecol 177:797, 1997a

Yoon BH, Romero R, Kim CJ, Koo JN, Choe G, Syn HC, Chi JG: High expression of tumor necrosis factor-alpha and interleukin-6 in periventricular leukomalacia. Am J Obstet Gynecol 177:406, 1997b

Yoon BH, Romero R, Park JS, Kim CJ, Kim SH, Choi JH, Han TR: Fetal exposure to an intra-amniotic inflammation and the development of cerebral palsy at the age of three years. Am J Obstet Gynecol 182:675, 2000

Yoon BH, Romero R, Kim M, Oh M, Kim JC, Lee J-S, Moon JB, Park JS: Elevated amniotic fluid matrix metalloproteinase-8 and the subsequent development of cerebral palsy. Am J Obstet Gynecol 186:S2, 2001

Yudkin PL, Wood L, Redman CWG: Risk of unexplained stillbirth at different gestational ages. Lancet 1:1192, 1987

Zupan V, Conzalez P, Lacaze-Masmonteil T, Boithias C, d'Allest AM, Dehan M, Gabilan JC: Periventricular leukomalacia: Risk factors revisited. Dev Med Child Neurol 38:1061, 1996

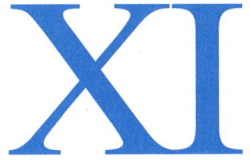

XI

Techniques Used to Assess Fetal Health

40

Antepartum Assessment

The rate of foetal heart is subject to considerable variations which afford us a fairly reliable means of judging as to the well-being of the child. As a general rule, its life should be considered in danger when the heart-beats fall below 100 or exceed 160.

J. Whitridge Williams

The preceding statement is the only comment on judging fetal well-being in the 1903 first edition of *Williams Obstetrics*. At that time, the mother was the patient for whom care was given, and the fetus was simply a transient maternal organ. During the past two decades, remarkably intimate knowledge of the fetus along with technological developments have prompted a new phenomenon in medicine: forecasts of fetal health. The fetus is now a second patient, who faces greater risks of serious morbidity and mortality than the mother. The technological boundary for fetal assessment has even been extended to the embryonic period—for example, Oasin and colleagues (1997) found that embryonic heart rates may be predictive of pregnancy outcome!

In this chapter, the evolution of several techniques employed to forecast fetal well-being is considered. Focus is on contemporary testing procedures that depend upon fetal physical activities, including movement, breathing, amnionic fluid production, and heart rate. According to the American College of Obstetricians and Gynecologists (1999), the goal of antepartum fetal surveillance is to prevent fetal death. In most cases, a normal test result is highly reassuring since fetal deaths within 1 week of a normal test result are rare. Indeed, the negative predictive values (true negative test) for most of the tests described in this chapter are 99.8 percent or higher. In contrast, estimates of the positive predictive values (true positive test) for abnormal test results are quite low and range between 10 percent and 40 percent (American College of Obstetricians and Gynecologists, 1999). Importantly, the widespread use of antepartum fetal surveillance is primarily based on circumstantial evidence because there have been no definitive randomized clinical trials.

FETAL MOVEMENTS

Passive unstimulated fetal activity commences as early as 7 weeks and becomes more sophisticated and coordinated by the end of pregnancy (Vindla and James, 1995). Indeed, beyond 8 menstrual weeks, fetal body movements are never absent for time periods exceeding 13 minutes (DeVries and co-workers, 1985). Between 20 and 30 weeks, general body movements become organized and the fetus starts to show rest–activity cycles (Soronkin and co-workers, 1982). In the third trimester, fetal movement maturation continues until about 36

weeks, when behavioral states are established in 80 percent of normal fetuses. Nijhuis and colleagues (1982) studied fetal heart rate patterns, general body movements, and eye movements and described four fetal behavioral states:

- **State 1F** is a quiescent state (quiet sleep), with narrow oscillatory bandwidth of the fetal heart rate.
- **State 2F** includes frequent gross body movements, continuous eye movements, and wider oscillation of the fetal heart rate. This state is analogous to rapid eye movement (REM) or active sleep in the neonate.
- **State 3F** includes continuous eye movements in the absence of body movements and no accelerations of the heart rate. The existence of this state is disputed (Pillai and James, 1990a).
- **State 4F** is one of vigorous body movement with continuous eye movements and fetal heart rate accelerations. This state corresponds to the awake state in infants.

Fetuses spend most of their time in states 1F and 2F. For example, at 38 weeks, 75 percent of their time is spent in states 1F and 2F (Nijuis and colleagues, 1982).

These behavioral states, particularly 1F and 2F, corresponding to quiet sleep and active sleep, have been used to develop an increasingly sophisticated understanding of fetal behavior. Oosterhof and co-workers (1993) studied fetal urine production in normal pregnancies in states 1F or 2F. As shown in Figure 40–1, bladder volumes increased during quiet sleep (state 1F). During state 2F, the fetal heart rate baseline bandwidth increased appreciably, and bladder volume was signifi-

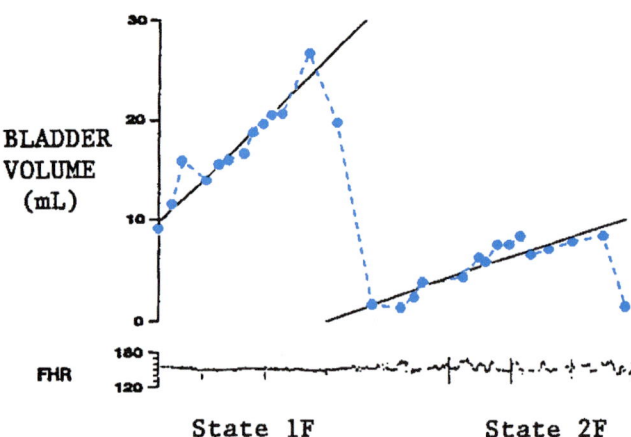

FIGURE 40–1. Fetal bladder volume measurements together with fetal heart rate variation record in relation to 1F or 2F behavior states. State 1F fetal heart rate has a narrow bandwidth consistent with quiet sleep. State 2F heart rate shows wide oscillation of the baseline consistent with active sleep. (Modified from Oosterhof and co-workers, 1993, with permission.)

cantly diminished. The latter occurred due to fetal voiding as well as decreased urine production. These phenomena were interpreted to represent reduced renal blood flow during active sleep.

An important determinant of fetal activity appears to be sleep–awake cycles, which are independent of the maternal sleep–awake state. "Sleep cyclicity" has been described to vary from about 20 minutes to as much as 75 minutes. Timor-Tritsch and associates (1978) reported that the mean length of the quiet or inactive state for term fetuses was about 23 minutes. Patrick and associates (1982) measured gross fetal body movements with real-time ultrasound for 24-hour periods in 31 normal pregnancies and found the longest period of inactivity to be 75 minutes. Amnionic fluid volume is another important determinant of fetal activity. Sherer and colleagues (1996) assessed the number of fetal movements in 465 pregnancies during biophysical profile testing (see p. 1104) in relation to amnionic fluid volume estimated using ultrasound. They observed decreased fetal activity with diminished amnionic volumes, and suggested that a restricted intrauterine space might physically limit fetal movements.

Sadovsky and colleagues (1979b) studied fetal movements in 120 normal pregnancies and classified the movements into three categories according to both maternal perceptions and independent recordings using piezoelectric sensors. Weak, strong, and rolling movements were described, and their relative contributions to total weekly movements throughout the last half of pregnancy were quantified. As pregnancy advances, weak movements decrease and are superseded by more vigorous movements, which increase for several weeks then subside at term. Presumably, declining amnionic fluid and intrauterine space account for diminishing activity at term. Figure 40–2 shows fetal movements during the last half of gestation in 127 pregnancies with normal outcomes. The mean number of weekly movements calculated from 12-hour daily recording periods increased from about 200 at 20 weeks to a maximum of 575 movements at 32 weeks. Fetal movements then declined to an average of 282 at 40 weeks. Normal weekly counts of fetal movements ranged between 50 and 950, with large daily variations that included counts as low as 4 to 10 per 12-hour day in normal pregnancies.

CLINICAL APPLICATION OF FETAL MOVEMENT ASSESSMENT. Since Sadovsky and Yaffe (1973) described seven case reports of pregnancies with decreased fetal activity that preceded fetal death, there have been various methods described to quantify fetal movement to prognosticate well-being. Methods include use of a tocodynamometer, visualization with real-time ultrasound, and maternal subjective perceptions. Most investigators have reported excellent correlation between maternally perceived fetal motion and movements documented by instrumentation. For example, Rayburn (1980) found that 80 percent of all movements seen during ultrasonic monitoring were perceived by the mother. In contrast, Johnson and colleagues (1992) reported that beyond 36 weeks, mothers perceived only 16 percent of fetal body movements recorded by a Doppler device. Fetal motions lasting more than 20 seconds were identified more accurately by the mother than shorter episodes.

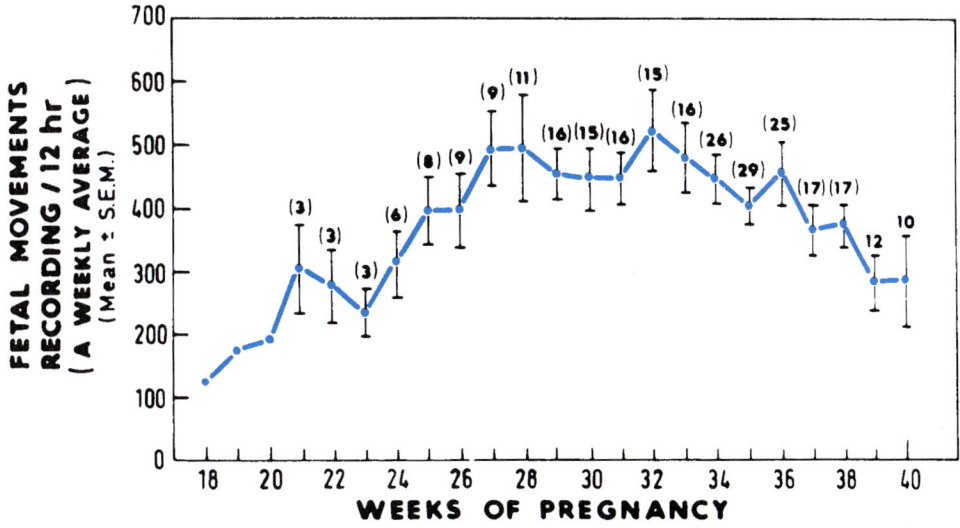

FIGURE 40–2. Weekly average fetal movements calculated from Daily Fetal Movement Records during normal pregnancy (means ± SEM). (From Sadovsky, 1979a, with permission.)

Although several fetal movement counting protocols have been used, neither the optimal number of movements nor the ideal duration for counting them has been defined. For example, in one method, perception of 10 fetal movements in up to 2 hours is considered normal (Moore and Piaquadio, 1989). In another, women are instructed to count fetal movements for 1 hour a day and the count is accepted as reassuring if it equals or exceeds a previously established baseline count (Neldam, 1983).

A particularly bothersome clinical situation occurs when women present in the third trimester with a chief complaint of subjectively reduced fetal movement. This is not uncommon, and Harrington and colleagues (1998) reported that 7 percent of 6793 women delivered at a London hospital presented with a complaint of decreased fetal movement. Fetal heart rate monitoring tests were employed if ultrasound scans for fetal growth or Doppler velocimetry were abnormal. The pregnancy outcomes for women who complained of decreased fetal movement were not significantly different than those of women without this complaint. Nonetheless, the authors recommended evaluation to reassure the mother.

Grant and co-workers (1989) performed an unparalleled investigation of maternally perceived fetal movements and pregnancy outcome. More than 68,000 pregnancies, regardless of risk category, were randomized between 28 and 32 weeks. Women in the fetal movement arm of the study were instructed by specially employed midwives to record the time needed to feel 10 movements each day. This required an average of 2.7 hours of counting time each day. Women in the control group were informally asked about movements during prenatal visits. Reports of decreased fetal motion were evaluated with tests of fetal well-being. Antepartum death rates for normally formed singletons were similar in the two study groups regardless of prior risk status. Despite the counting policy, most of the fetuses who died were dead by the time the mothers received medical attention. Importantly, these investigators did not conclude that maternal perceptions of fetal activity were meaningless. Conversely, they concluded that informal maternal perceptions were as good as formally counted and recorded fetal movement.

FETAL BREATHING

After decades of uncertainty as to whether the fetus normally breathes, Dawes and co-workers (1972) showed small inward and outward flows of tracheal fluid indicating fetal thoracic movement in sheep. These chest wall movements differed from those following birth in that they were discontinuous. Another interesting feature of fetal respiration was *paradoxical chest wall move-*

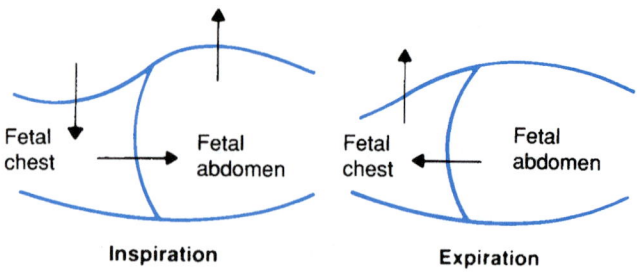

FIGURE 40–3. Paradoxical chest movement with fetal respiration. (From Johnson and co-workers, 1988, with permission.)

ment. As shown in Figure 40–3, during inspiration the chest wall paradoxically collapses and the abdomen protrudes (Johnson and co-authors, 1988). In the newborn or adult, the opposite occurs. One interpretation of the paradoxical respiratory motion might be coughing to clear amnionic fluid debris. Although the physiological basis for the breathing reflex is not completely understood, such exchange of amnionic fluid appears to be essential for normal lung development.

Two types of respiratory movements have been identified: (1) *gasps (or sighs)*, which occurred at a frequency of 1 to 4 per minute; and (2) *irregular bursts of breathing,* occurring at rates up to 240 cycles per minute (Dawes, 1974). The latter rapid respiratory movements were associated with REM. Badalian and co-workers (1993) studied the maturation of normal fetal breathing using color flow and spectral Doppler analysis of nasal fluid flow as an index of lung function. They suggested that fetal respiratory rate decreased in conjunction with increased respiratory volume at about 33 to 36 weeks, coincidental with lung maturation.

Many investigators have examined fetal breathing movements utilizing ultrasound to determine whether monitoring chest wall movements might be of benefit to evaluate fetal health. Several variables in addition to hypoxia were found to affect fetal respiratory movements. These included labor—during which it is normal for respiration to cease—hypoglycemia, sound stimuli, cigarette smoking, amniocentesis, impending preterm labor, gestational age, and the fetal heart rate itself.

Because fetal breathing movements are episodic, interpretation of fetal health when respirations are absent may be tenuous. Patrick and associates (1980) performed continuous 24-hour observation periods using real-time ultrasonography in an effort to characterize fetal breathing patterns during the last 10 weeks of pregnancy. A total of 1224 hours of fetal observation was completed in 51 pregnancies. Figure 40–4 shows the percentage of time spent breathing near term. Clearly, there is diurnal variation, because breathing substantively diminishes during the night. In addition, breathing activity increases somewhat following maternal meals.

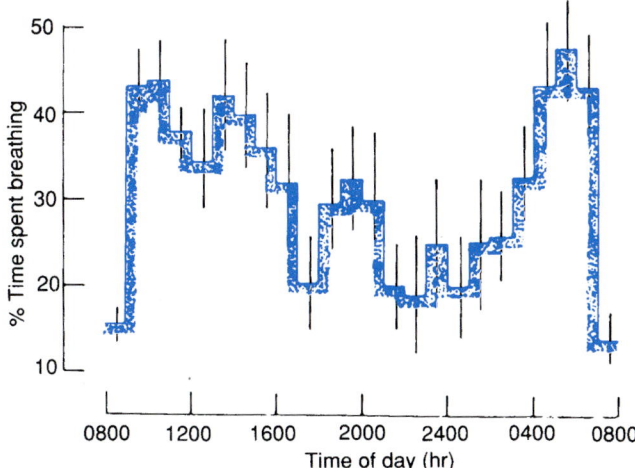

FIGURE 40–4. The percentage of time spent breathing (± SEM) by 11 fetuses at 38 to 39 weeks demonstrated significant increase in fetal breathing activity after breakfast. Breathing activity diminished over the day and reached its minimum between 1900 and 2400 hours. There was a significant increase in the percentage of time spent breathing between 0400 and 0700 hours when mothers were asleep. (From Patrick and co-workers, 1980, with permission.)

Total absence of breathing was observed in some of these normal fetuses for up to 122 minutes, indicating that fetal evaluation to diagnose absent respiratory motion may require long periods of observation.

The potential for breathing activity to be an important marker of fetal health is unfulfilled because of the multiplicity of factors that normally affect breathing. Most clinical applications have included assessment of other fetal biophysical indices, such as heart rate. More recently, as will be discussed, fetal breathing has become a component of the *biophysical profile.*

CONTRACTION STRESS TESTING

As amnionic fluid pressure increases with uterine contractions, myometrial pressure exceeds collapsing pressure for vessels coursing through uterine muscle, ultimately isolating the intervillous space. Brief periods of impaired oxygen exchange result, and if uteroplacental pathology is present, these elicit late fetal heart rate decelerations (Chap. 14). Uterine contractions may also produce a pattern of variable decelerations due to cord compression suggesting oligohydramnios, which is often a concomitant of placental insufficiency.

Ray and colleagues (1972) used this concept in 66 complicated pregnancies and developed what they termed the **oxytocin challenge test,** and later called the **contraction stress test.** Contractions were induced using intravenous oxytocin, and the fetal heart rate response

was recorded using standard monitoring. The criterion for a positive (abnormal) test was uniform repetitive fetal heart rate decelerations. These reflected the uterine contraction waveform and had an onset at or beyond the acme of a contraction. Such late decelerations could be due to uteroplacental insufficiency. The tests were generally repeated on a weekly basis, and the investigators concluded that negative (normal) contraction stress tests forecast fetal health. One disadvantage cited was that the average contraction stress test required 90 minutes to complete.

Fetal heart rate and uterine contractions are simultaneously recorded with an external monitor. If at least three spontaneous contractions of 40 seconds or longer are present in 10 minutes, no uterine stimulation is necessary (American College of Obstetricians and Gynecologists, 1999). Contractions are induced with either oxytocin or nipple stimulation (see discussion that follows) if there are fewer than three in 10 minutes. If oxytocin is preferred, a dilute intravenous infusion is initiated at a rate of 0.5 mU/min and doubled every 20 minutes until a satisfactory contraction pattern is established (Freeman, 1975). The results of the contraction stress test are interpreted according to the criteria shown in Table 40–1.

Nipple stimulation in lieu of oxytocin-induced uterine contractions has been reported to be usually successful for contraction stress testing (Huddleston and associates, 1984). One method recommended by the American College of Obstetricians and Gynecologists (1999) involves the woman rubbing one nipple through her clothing for 2 minutes or until a contraction begins. She is instructed to restart after 5 minutes if the first nipple stimulation did not induce three contractions in 10 minutes. Advantages include reduced cost and shortened testing times. Although Schellpfeffer and associates (1985) reported unpredictable uterine hyperstimu-

TABLE 40–1. Criteria for Interpretation of the Contraction Stress Test

Negative: no late or significant variable decelerations.

Positive: late decelerations following 50% or more of contractions (even if the contraction frequency is fewer than three in 10 min).

Equivocal-suspicious: intermittent late decelerations or significant variable decelerations.

Equivocal-hyperstimulatory: fetal heart rate decelerations that occur in the presence of contractions more frequent than every 2 min or lasting longer than 90 sec.

Unsatisfactory: fewer than three contractions in 10 min or an uninterpretable tracing.

From the American College of Obstetricians and Gynecologists (1999), with permission.

lation with fetal distress, others did not find excessive nipple-stimulated induced uterine activity to be harmful (Frager and Miyazaki, 1987).

NONSTRESS TESTING

Freeman (1975) and Lee and colleagues (1975) introduced the **nonstress test** to describe fetal heart rate acceleration in response to fetal movement as a sign of fetal health. This test involved the use of Doppler-detected fetal heart rate acceleration coincident with fetal movements perceived by the mother. By the end of the 1970s, the nonstress test had become the primary method of testing fetal health. The nonstress test was much easier to perform, and normal results were used to further discriminate false-positive contraction stress tests. Simplistically, the nonstress test is primarily a test of *fetal condition,* and it differs from the contraction stress test, which is a test of *uteroplacental function.* Currently, nonstress testing is the most widely used primary testing method for assessment of fetal well-being and has also been incorporated into the biophysical profile testing system (see later discussion).

PHYSIOLOGY OF FETAL HEART RATE ACCELERATION.
Fetal heart rate is normally increased or decreased on a beat-to-beat basis by autonomic influences mediated by sympathetic or parasympathetic impulses from brainstem centers. Thus, fetal heart rate acceleration is believed to be an indication of fetal autonomic function. Beat-to-beat variability is also under the control of the autonomic nervous system (Matsuura and colleagues, 1996). Consequently, pathological loss of acceleration may be seen in conjunction with significantly decreased beat-to-beat variability of the fetal heart rate (see p. 346). Loss of such reactivity, however, is most commonly associated with sleep cycles (discussed earlier), and may be due to central depression from medications.

The nonstress test is based on the hypothesis that the heart rate of a fetus who is not acidotic as a result of hypoxia or neurological depression, will temporarily accelerate in response to fetal movement. An example that supports this hypothesis is shown in Figure 40–5. Similarly, Smith and colleagues (1988) observed a decrease in the number of accelerations in preterm fetuses subsequently found to have lower umbilical artery blood PO_2 values compared with those who had normal heart rate characteristics. Thus, nonstress testing is considered to reflect fetal condition.

Gestational age influences acceleration or reactivity of fetal heart rate. Pillai and James (1990b) studied the development of fetal heart rate acceleration patterns during normal pregnancy. The percentage of body movements accompanied by acceleration and the amplitude of these accelerations increased with gestational

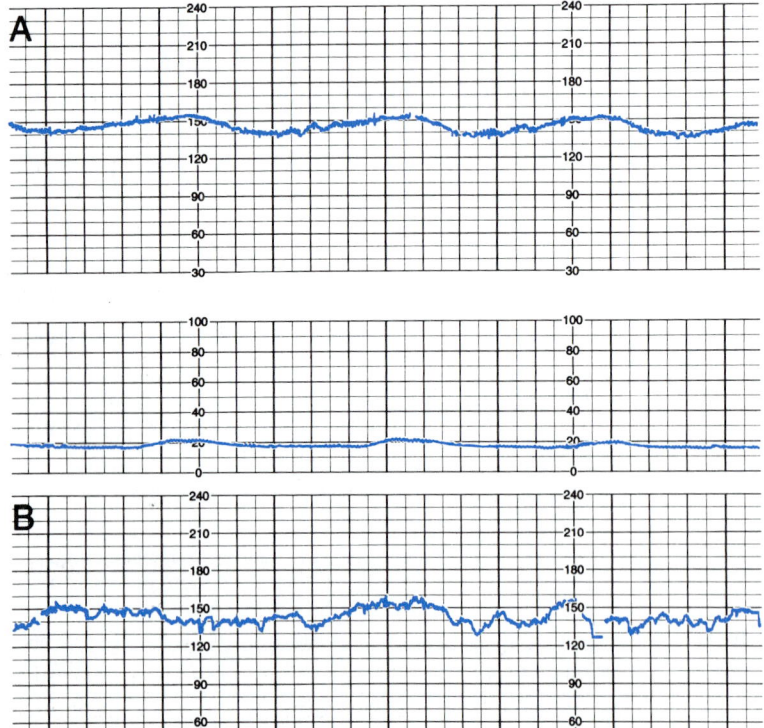

FIGURE 40–5. Antepartum fetal heart rate tracings at 28 weeks' gestation in a woman with diabetic ketoacidosis. Tracing **A,** obtained during maternal and fetal acidemia, shows absence of accelerations, diminished variability, and late decelerations with weak spontaneous contractions. Tracing **B** shows return of normal accelerations and variability of the fetal heart rate following correction of maternal acidemia.

age (Fig. 40–6). Guinn and colleagues (1998) studied nonstress test results between 25 and 28 weeks in 188 pregnancies that ultimately had normal outcomes. Only 70 percent of these normal fetuses demonstrated the required 15 bpm or more of heart rate acceleration (see next paragraph). Lesser degrees of acceleration, i.e., 10 bpm, occurred in 90 percent of the tested pregnancies.

The National Institute of Child Health and Human Development fetal monitoring workshop (1997) has defined acceleration based on gestational age. The acme of acceleration is 15 bpm or more above the baseline rate and the acceleration lasts 15 seconds or longer for less than 2 minutes in fetuses at or beyond 32 weeks. Before 32 weeks, accelerations are defined as having an acme 10 bpm or more for 10 seconds or longer.

DEFINITION OF NORMAL NONSTRESS TESTS. There have been many different definitions of normal nonstress test results. They vary as to the number, amplitude, and duration of accelerations, as well as the test duration. The definition currently recommended by the American College of Obstetricians and Gynecologists (1999) is two or more accelerations that peak at 15 bpm or more, each lasting 15 seconds or more, and all occurring within 20 minutes of beginning the test (Fig. 40–7). It was also recommended that accelerations with or without fetal movements be accepted, and that a 40-minute or longer tracing—to account for fetal sleep cycles—should be performed before concluding that there was insufficient fetal *reactivity*. Miller and colleagues (1996) reviewed fetal outcomes after nonstress tests considered as nonreactive because there was only one acceleration. They concluded that one acceleration was just as reliable in predicting healthy fetal status as were two.

Although a normal number and amplitude of accelerations seems to reflect fetal well-being, "insufficient acceleration" does not invariably predict fetal compromise. Indeed, some investigators have reported false-positive nonstress test rates in excess of 90 percent when acceleration was considered insufficient (Devoe and colleagues, 1986). Because healthy fetuses may not move for periods of up to 75 minutes, Brown and Patrick (1981) considered that a longer duration of nonstress testing might increase the positive predictive value of an abnormal, or nonreactive test. They concluded that either the test became reactive during a period of time up to 80 minutes, or that the test remained nonreactive for 120 minutes, indicating that the fetus was very ill.

Not only are there many different definitions of normal nonstress test results, but the reproducibility of interpretations is problematic. For example, Hage (1985) mailed five nonstress tests, blinded to specific patient clinical data, to a national sample of obstetricians for their interpretations. He concluded that although nonstress testing is very popular, the reliability of test interpretation needs improvement. Such problems with subjective interpretation have prompted efforts to computerize analysis of nonstress tests. Bracero and co-authors (1999) randomized 404 women to either human or computer interpretation of nonstress tests. They concluded that computerized analysis was a more cost-effective, reliable, and objective method of fetal surveillance.

ABNORMAL NONSTRESS TESTS. There are abnormal nonstress test patterns that reliably forecast severe fetal jeopardy. Hammacher and co-workers (1968) described not only acceleration in response to movement, but also antepartum fetal heart rate tracings with what they termed a *silent oscillatory pattern*. This pattern consisted of a fetal heart rate baseline that oscillated less than 5 bpm and presumably indicated absent acceleration as well as beat-to-beat variability. Hammacher considered this pattern ominous.

Visser and associates (1980) described a "terminal cardiotocogram," which included:

1. Baseline oscillation of less than 5 bpm.
2. Absent accelerations.
3. Late decelerations with spontaneous uterine contractions.

These results were very similar to experiences from Parkland Hospital in which absence of accelerations during an 80-minute recording period in 27 pregnancies was associated consistently with evidence of uteroplacental pathology (Leveno and associates, 1983). The

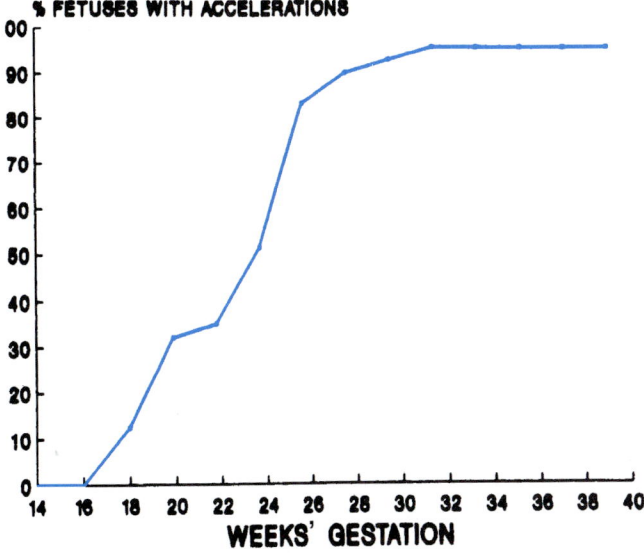

FIGURE 40–6. Percentage of fetuses with at least one acceleration (15 beats/min sustained for 15 sec) with movement. (From Pillai and James, 1990b, with permission.)

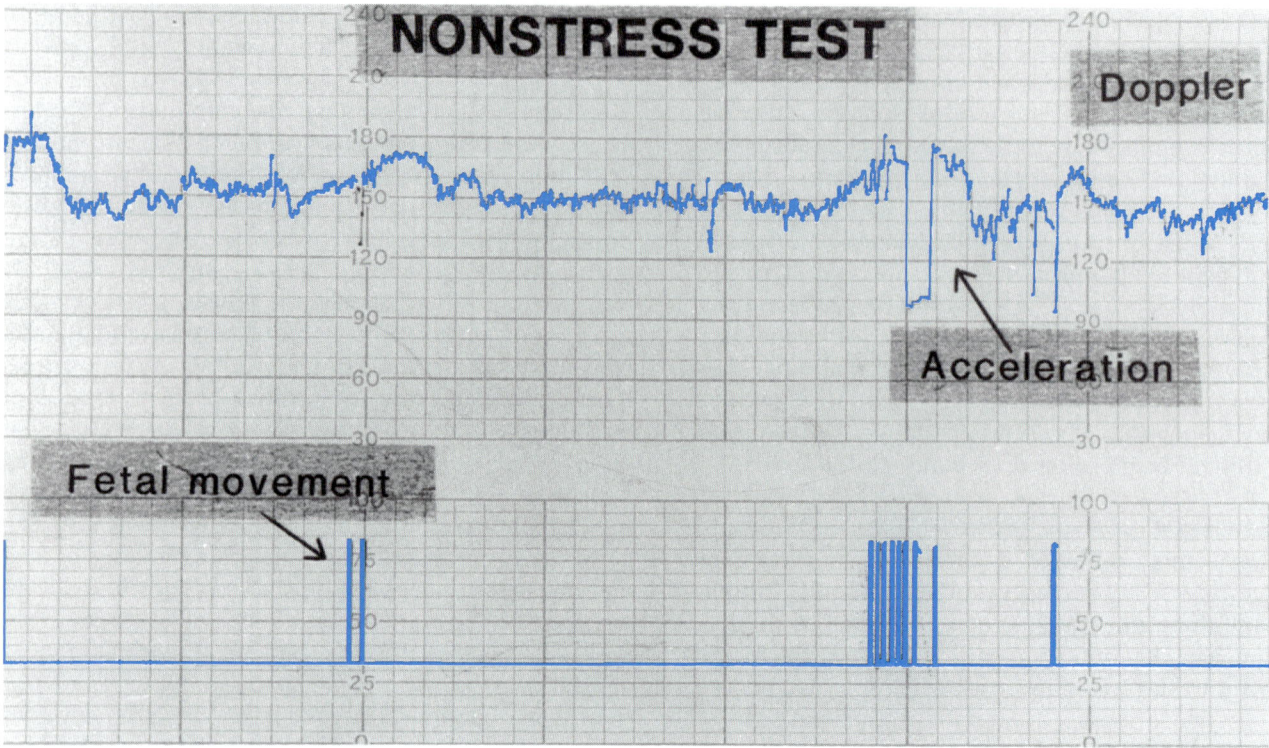

FIGURE 40–7. Reactive nonstress test. Notice increase of fetal heart rate to more than 15 beats/min for longer than 15 sec following fetal movements, indicated by the vertical marks on the lower part of the recording.

latter included fetal growth restriction (75 percent), oligohydramnios (80 percent), fetal acidosis (40 percent), meconium (30 percent), and placental infarction (93 percent). We concluded that inability of the fetus to accelerate its heart rate, when not due to maternal sedation, was an ominous finding (Fig. 40–8). Similarly, Devoe and co-workers (1985) concluded that nonstress tests that were nonreactive for 90 minutes were almost invariably (93 percent) associated with significant perinatal pathology.

INTERVAL BETWEEN TESTING. The interval between tests, originally rather arbitrarily set at 7 days, appears to have been shortened as experience evolved with nonstress testing. According to the American College of Obstetricians and Gynecologists (1999), more frequent testing is advocated by some investigators for women with postterm pregnancy, type 1 diabetes, fetal growth restriction, or pregnancy-induced hypertension. In these circumstances, some investigators perform twice-weekly tests with additional testing performed for maternal or fetal deterioration regardless of time elapsed since the last test. Some clinicians perform nonstress tests daily or even more frequently. For example, Chari and co-workers (1995) recommend daily fetal testing in women with severe preeclampsia remote from term.

DECELERATIONS DURING NONSTRESS TESTING. Fetal movements may produce heart rate decelerations. Timor-Tritsch and co-authors (1978) reported that decelerations may be observed during nonstress testing in half to two thirds of tracings, depending on the vigor of the fetal motion. Such a high incidence of decelerations inevitably makes interpretation of their significance problematic. Indeed, Meis and co-workers (1986) reported that variable fetal heart rate decelerations during nonstress tests were not a sign of fetal compromise. The American College of Obstetricians and Gynecologists (1999) has concluded that variable decelerations, if nonrepetitive and brief (less than 30 seconds), do not indicate fetal compromise nor the need for obstetrical intervention. In contrast, repetitive variable decelerations—at least three in 20 minutes—even if mild, have been associated with an increased risk of cesarean delivery for fetal distress. Decelerations lasting 1 minute or longer have been reported to have an even worse prognosis (Bouregeois and colleagues, 1984; Druzin and colleagues, 1981; Pazos and colleagues, 1982).

Hoskins and associates (1991) attempted to refine interpretation of testing that shows variable decelerations by adding ultrasonic estimation of amnionic fluid volume. The incidence of cesarean delivery for intrapar-

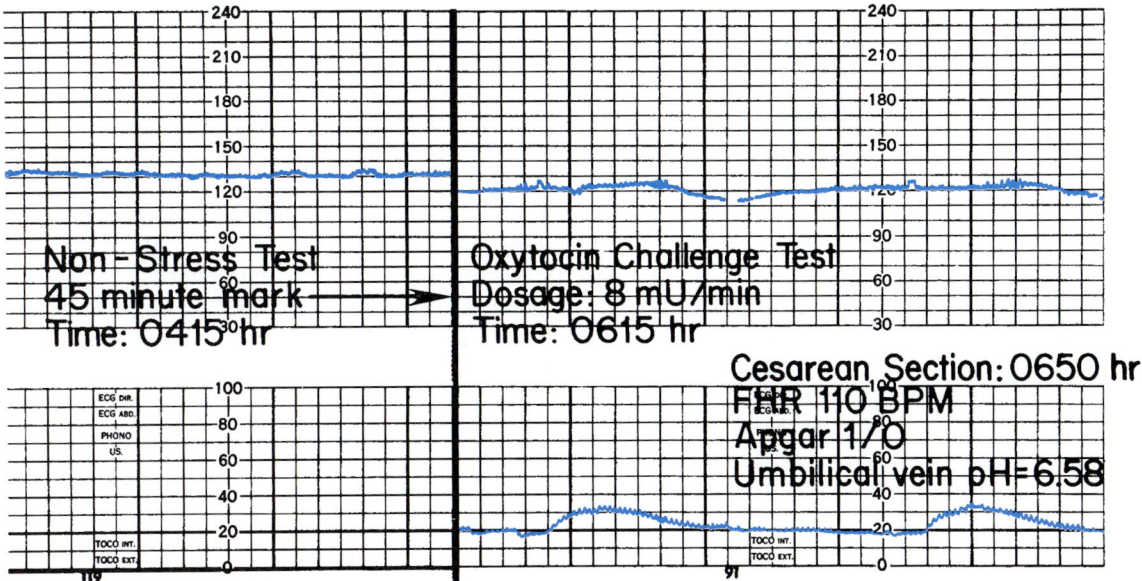

FIGURE 40–8. Nonreactive nonstress test followed by contraction stress test showing mild late decelerations. Cesarean delivery was performed and the severely acidemic fetus could not be resuscitated.

tum fetal distress progressively increased coincidentally with the severity of variable decelerations and diminished amnionic fluid volume. For example, severe variable decelerations during a nonstress test plus an amnionic fluid index of 5 cm or less resulted in a 75 percent cesarean rate. Fetal distress in labor, however, also frequently developed in those pregnancies with variable decelerations but with normal amounts of amnionic fluid. Similar results were reported by Grubb and Paul (1992).

FALSE-NORMAL NONSTRESS TESTS. Smith and associates (1987) performed a detailed analysis of the causes of fetal death within 7 days of normal nonstress tests. The most common indication for testing was postterm pregnancy. The mean interval between testing and death was 4 days, with a range of 1 to 7 days. The single most common autopsy finding was meconium aspiration, often associated with some type of umbilical cord abnormality. They concluded that an acute asphyxial insult had provoked fetal gasping. They also concluded that nonstress testing was inadequate to preclude such an acute asphyxial event and that other biophysical characteristics might be beneficial adjuncts. For example, assessment of amnionic fluid volume was considered likely of value. Other ascribed frequent causes of fetal death included intrauterine infection, abnormal cord position, malformations, and placental abruption.

ACOUSTIC STIMULATION TESTS

In 1935 Sontag and Wallace reported that the fetus responds to sound. Benzaquen (1990) and Richards (1992) and their colleagues used miniaturized hydrophones to study the intrauterine sound environment during labor. External low frequency sounds of less than 125 Hz are enhanced, but sounds of greater frequency are attenuated with maximum attenuation at 4000 Hz. Sound levels of the maternal voice were enhanced at an average of 5 dB whereas external male or female voices were attenuated by 2 to 3 dB. Maternal cardiovascular sounds as well as bowel sounds are also audible inside the uterus. Uterine contractions did not affect the fetal sound environment. The background noise level was about 60 dB and consisted primarily of low-frequency sounds; that is, less than 100 Hz. This investigation indicates that the intrauterine environment is relatively quiet. Hykin and colleagues (1999), using functional magnetic resonance imaging, detected fetal brain activity in response to music played over the woman's abdomen.

Loud external sounds have been used to startle the fetus, provoking acceleration of the heart rate. Acoustic devices used to stimulate the fetus during antepartum surveillance tests generate sound pressures considerably above those just described. Eller and associates (1995) used a commercially available acoustic stimulator (Corometrics model 146) to measure intrauterine sound levels. Satisfactory sound intensity between 100 and 105 dB (100 dB is generated by a jet plane at takeoff) was maintained until the stimulator was moved more than 20 cm from the maternal abdomen. To perform acoustic stimulation, an artificial larynx is positioned on the maternal abdomen and a stimulus of 1 to 2 seconds is applied. This may be repeated up to three times for up to 3 seconds (American College of Obstetricians and Gynecologists, 1999).

Read and Miller (1977) were the first to suggest that acoustic stimulation could be used to examine fetal health. Romero and co-authors (1988), in their review of acoustic stimulation for determination of fetal well-being, recommended vigorous clinical evaluation before such testing becomes a part of standard obstetrical care.

BIOPHYSICAL PROFILE

Manning and colleagues (1980) proposed the combined use of five fetal biophysical variables as a more accurate means of assessing fetal health than any one used alone. They hypothesized that consideration of five variables could significantly reduce both false-positive and false-negative tests. Required equipment includes a real-time ultrasound device and Doppler ultrasound to record fetal heart rate. Typically, these tests require 30 to 60 minutes of examiner time. Shown in Table 40–2 are the five biophysical components assessed, which include:

1. Fetal heart rate acceleration.
2. Fetal breathing.
3. Fetal movements.
4. Fetal tone.
5. Amnionic fluid volume.

Normal variables were assigned a score of two each and abnormal variables a score of zero. Thus, the highest score possible for a normal fetus is 10.

Manning and colleagues (1987) tested over 19,000 pregnancies using the biophysical profile interpretation and management shown in Table 40–3. They reported a false-normal test rate, defined as an antepartum death of a structurally normal fetus, of approximately 1 per 1000. Importantly, more than 97 percent of the pregnancies tested had normal test results. The most common identifiable causes of fetal death after normal biophysical profiles include fetal–maternal hemorrhage, umbilical cord accidents, and placental abruption (Dayal and colleagues, 1999). Identifiable causes could be found in almost two thirds of fetal deaths. Manning and co-authors (1993) published a remarkable description of 493 fetuses in which biophysical scores were performed immediately before measurement of umbilical venous blood pH values obtained via cordocentesis. Approximately 20 percent of tested fetuses had growth restriction and the remainder had alloimmune hemolytic anemia. As shown in Figure 40–9, a biophysical score of zero was invariably associated with significant fetal acidemia, whereas normal scores of 8 or 10 were associated with normal pH. An equivocal test result—a score of 6—was a poor predictor of abnormal outcome. A decrease from an abnormal result—a score of 2 or 4—to a very abnormal score (zero) was a progressively more accurate predictor of abnormal outcome. Similarly, Salvesen and colleagues (1993) correlated the biophysical profile with umbilical venous blood pH obtained at cordocentesis in 41 pregnancies complicated by diabetes. They also found that abnormal pH was significantly associated with abnormal biophysical profile scores. They concluded, however, that the biophysical profile

TABLE 40–2. Components and Their Scores for the Biophysical Profile

Component	Score 2	Score 0
Nonstress test[a]	≥ 2 accelerations of ≥ 15 beats/min for ≥ 15 sec in 20–40 min	0 or 1 acceleration in 20–40 min
Fetal breathing	≥ 1 episode of rhythmic breathing lasting ≥ 30 sec within 30 min	< 30 sec of breathing in 30 min
Fetal movement	≥ 3 discrete body or limb movements within 30 min	≤ 2 movements in 30 min
Fetal tone	≥ 1 episode of extension of a fetal extremity with return to flexion, or opening or closing of hand	No movements or no extension/flexion
Amnionic fluid volume[b]	Single vertical pocket > 2 cm	Largest single vertical pocket ≤ 2 cm

[a] May be omitted if all four ultrasound components are normal.
[b] Further evaluation warranted, regardless of biophysical composite score, if largest vertical amnionic fluid pocket ≤ 2 cm.
From the American College of Obstetricians and Gynecologists (1999), with permission.

TABLE 40–3. Modified Biophysical Profile Score, Interpretation, and Pregnancy Management

Biophysical Profile Score	Interpretation	Recommended Management
10	Normal nonasphyxiated fetus	No fetal indication for intervention; repeat test weekly except in diabetic patient and postterm pregnancy (twice weekly)
8/10 Normal fluid 8/8	Normal nonasphyxiated fetus	No fetal indication for intervention; repeat testing per protocol
8/10 Decreased	Chronic fetal asphyxia suspected	Deliver
6	Possible fetal asphyxia	If amnionic fluid volume abnormal, deliver
		If normal fluid at > 36 weeks with favorable cervix, deliver
		If repeat test ≤ 6 deliver
		If repeat test > 6, observe and repeat per protocol
4	Probable fetal asphyxia	Repeat testing same day; if biophysical profile score ≤ 6, deliver
0–2	Almost certain fetal asphyxia	Deliver

From Manning and colleagues (1987), with permission.

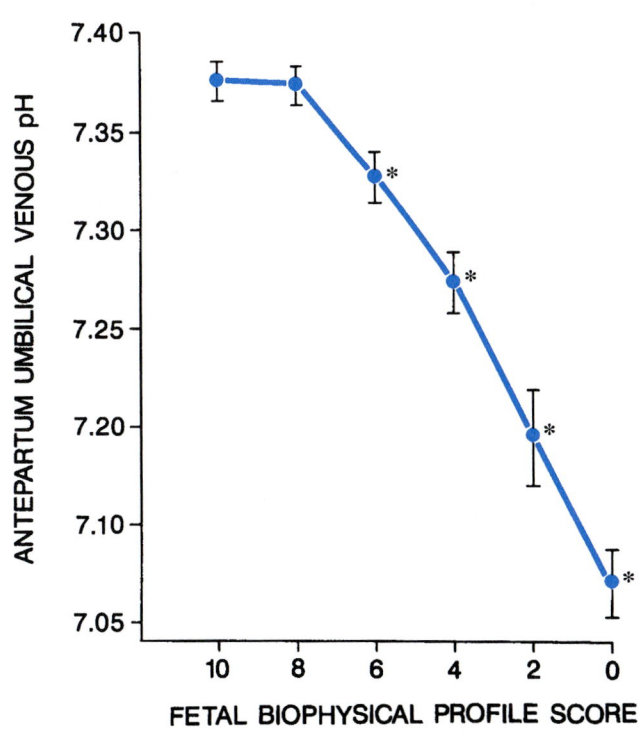

FIGURE 40–9. Mean umbilical vein pH ($\pm$ 2 SD) in relation to fetal biophysical profile score category. (From Manning and associates, 1993, with permission.)

was of limited value in the prediction of fetal pH, because nine mildly acidemic fetuses had normal antepartum tests. Weiner and colleagues (1996) assessed the meaning of antepartum fetal tests in 135 overtly growth-restricted fetuses and came to a similar conclusion. They found that morbidity and mortality in severe fetal growth restriction was primarily determined by gestational age and birthweight and not by abnormal fetal tests.

MODIFIED BIOPHYSICAL PROFILE. Because the biophysical profile is labor-intensive and requires a person trained in ultrasonic visualization of the fetus, Clark and co-workers (1989) used an abbreviated biophysical profile as their first-line antepartum screening test. Specifically, a vibroacoustic nonstress test and amnionic fluid index were performed twice weekly in 2628 singleton pregnancies. Amnionic fluid indices less than 5 cm were considered abnormal. The typical test required only 10 minutes to perform. These investigators concluded that this abbreviated biophysical profile was a superb method of antepartum surveillance because there were no unexpected fetal deaths.

Nageotte and colleagues (1994) also combined biweekly nonstress tests with ultrasonic assessment of amnionic fluid. An index of 5 cm or less was also considered abnormal in their study. They performed 17,429 modified biophysical profiles in 2774 women and concluded that such testing was an excellent method of fetal surveillance. They randomized women with abnormal test results to backup testing with either a complete biophysical profile or a contraction stress test. Contraction stress testing increased intervention for a false-abnormal test. Miller and associates (1996) reported results of over 54,000 modified biophysical profiles in 15,400 high-risk pregnancies at the University of Southern California. They described a false-negative rate of 0.8 per 1000 and a false-positive rate of 1.5 percent. The American College of Obstetricians and Gynecologists (1999) has concluded that the modified biophysical profile test is an acceptable means of antepartum fetal surveillance.

AMNIONIC FLUID VOLUME

Assessment of amnionic fluid has become an integral component in the antepartum assessment of pregnancies at risk for fetal death. This is based on the rationale that decreased uteroplacental perfusion may lead to diminished fetal renal blood flow, decreased micturition, and ultimately, oligohydramnios. The amnionic fluid index (Rutherford and colleagues, 1987), the largest vertical pocket (Chamberlain and co-authors, 1984), and the 2×2 cm pocket of the biophysical profile (Manning and colleagues, 1984) are some ultrasonic techniques used to estimate amnionic fluid volume. Chauhan and colleagues (1999) reviewed 42 reports on the amnionic fluid index published between 1987 and 1997 and concluded that an index of 5.0 cm or less significantly increased the risk of either cesarean delivery for fetal distress or a low 5-minute Apgar score. Similarly, Casey and colleagues (2000), in a retrospective analysis of 6423 pregnancies managed at Parkland Hospital, found that an amnionic fluid index of 5 cm or less was associated with significantly increased perinatal morbidity and mortality. In contrast, Magann and colleagues (1999) evaluated the utility of amnionic fluid indices of 5 cm or less in 1001 pregnancies receiving antepartum fetal testing. About 20 percent of pregnancies studied had amnionic fluid index values of less than 5 cm. They concluded that the index was a poor diagnostic test. A similar conclusion was reached by Schucker and colleagues (1996) in their analysis of 136 pregnancies complicated by severe preeclampsia. In the only randomized trial reported to date, Conway and colleagues (2000) concluded that nonintervention to permit spontaneous onset of labor was as effective as induction in term pregnancies with amnionic fluid index values of 5 cm or less.

UMBILICAL ARTERY DOPPLER VELOCIMETRY

Doppler ultrasonography is a noninvasive technique to assess blood flow by characterizing downstream imped-

ance. The umbilical artery systolic/diastolic ratio (S/D), the most commonly used index, is considered abnormal if it is elevated above the 95th percentile for gestational age or if diastolic flow is either absent or reversed. Absent or reversed end-diastolic flow signifies increased impedance (Fig. 40–10), and it is uniquely associated with fetal growth restriction (American College of Obstetricians and Gynecologists, 2000). Such increased impedance to umbilical artery blood flow is reported to result from poorly vascularized placental villi (Todros and co-authors, 1999). Absent, or reversal of end-diastolic flow is seen in the most extreme cases of fetal growth restriction and may suggest fetal compromise. For example, Zelop and colleagues (1996) reported that perinatal mortality for reversed end-diastolic flow was approximately 33 percent and that for absent end-diastolic flow was about 10 percent.

Doppler ultrasonography has been subjected to more rigorous and extensive assessment with randomized controlled trials than has any previous test of fetal health (Alfirevic and Neilson, 1995). Williams and colleagues (2000) randomized 1240 high-risk women to either non-stress tests or Doppler velocimetry and found these two fetal surveillance tests to be equivalent in their ability to predict pregnancy outcome. The utility of umbilical artery Doppler velocimetry has been reviewed by the American College of Obstetricians and Gynecologists (1999, 2000). It was concluded that no benefit has been demonstrated for umbilical artery velocimetry for conditions other than suspected fetal growth restriction (American College of Obstetricians and Gynecologists, 1999). The use of Doppler velocimetry in the management of fetal growth restriction, however, has been recommended as a possible adjunct to other fetal evaluation techniques such as nonstress testing or biophysical profile (American College of Obstetricians and Gynecologists, 2000). No benefit has been demonstrated for umbilical artery velocimetry for other conditions such as postterm pregnancy, diabetes, systemic lupus erythematosus, or antiphospholipid antibody syndrome. Similarly, velocimetry has not proved of value as a screening test for detecting fetal compromise in the general obstetrical population.

It is possible to evaluate blood flow in other fetal vessels in addition to the umbilical artery. The middle cerebral artery has received particular attention because of observations that the hypoxic fetus compensates by "brain sparing" via reduced impedance—increased blood flow—in cerebral vessels. Based upon this premise, it has been suggested that the ratio of the middle cerebral artery S/D value to umbilical artery S/D value might reflect fetal compromise (Mari and Deter, 1992). Studies to date of this premise have been inconclusive. For example, Ott and colleagues (1998) randomized 665 women undergoing modified biophysical profiles to either this test alone or combined with middle cerebral

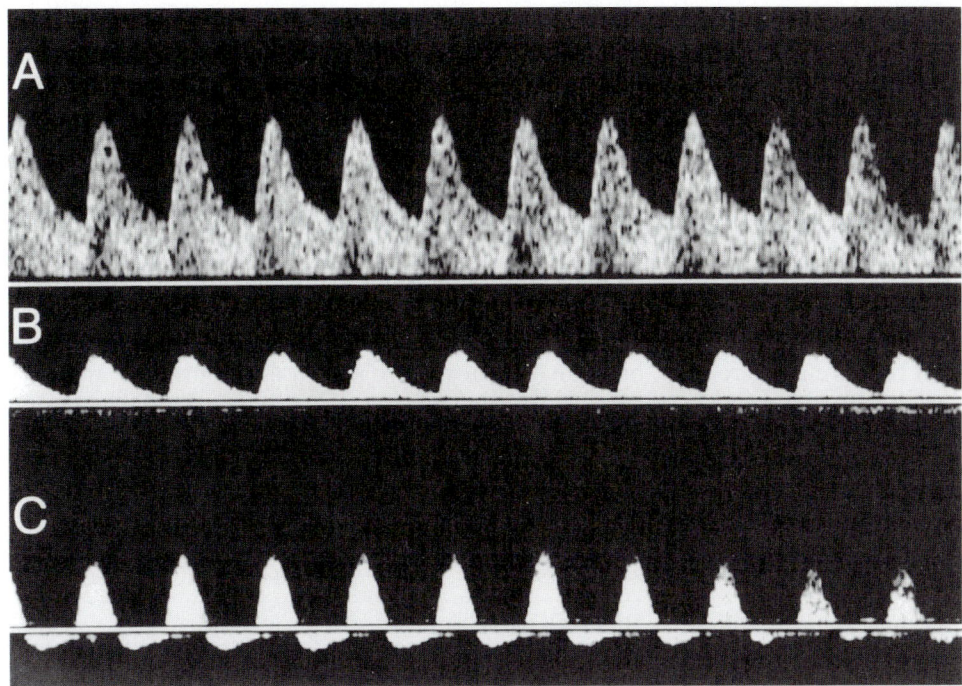

FIGURE 40–10. Three studies of fetal umbilical arterial velocimetry. The peaks represent systolic velocity and the troughs show the diastolic velocity. **A.** Normal velocimetry pattern. **B.** Velocity is zero during diastole (trough reaches the horizontal line). **C.** Arterial velocity is reversed during diastole (trough is below horizontal line). (Courtesy of Dr. Diane Twickler.)

artery to umbilical artery velocity flow ratios. There were no significant differences in pregnancy outcomes between these two study groups. This technique currently is considered investigational by the American College of Obstetricians and Gynecologists (1999).

CURRENT ANTENATAL TESTING RECOMMENDATIONS

According to the American College of Obstetricians and Gynecologists (1999), there is no overall agreement regarding the best test to evaluate fetal well-being. All three testing systems—contraction stress test, nonstress test, and biophysical profile—have different end points that are considered depending on the clinical situation.

The most important consideration in deciding when to begin antepartum testing is the prognosis for neonatal survival. The severity of maternal disease is another important consideration. In general, with the majority of high-risk pregnancies, most authorities recommend that testing begin by 32 to 34 weeks. Pregnancies with severe complications might require testing as early as 26 to 28 weeks. The frequency for repeating tests has been arbitrarily set at 7 days, but more frequent testing is often done.

At Parkland Hospital, antepartum fetal heart rate recordings have been limited to about 700 women ad-

mitted to the High-Risk Pregnancy Unit each year. Such recordings are often obtained several times throughout the week—for example, Monday, Wednesday, and Friday—in these pregnancies. The primary focus of fetal heart rate assessments is detection of decelerations, and delivery is not withheld simply because accelerations are witnessed. Clinical and ultrasonic estimations of amnionic fluid volume may also be used to assess fetal health. Outpatients do not undergo fetal heart rate testing. If there is concern about fetal movement or amnionic fluid volume, then the woman may be observed in the labor suite with fetal heart rate monitoring. Depending on results, she is either discharged, transferred to the High-Risk Unit, or labor is induced. Despite this limited use of antepartum testing, the fetal death rate in structurally normal infants is quite low in high-risk women. Indeed, most antepartum fetal deaths that we encounter are in low-risk pregnancies and are attributable to unpreventable placental abruptions and umbilical cord accidents.

SIGNIFICANCE OF FETAL TESTING

Does antenatal fetal forecasting really make a difference? Platt and co-workers (1987) reviewed the impact of fetal testing between 1971 and 1985 at Los Angeles County Hospital. During this 15-year period, more than

200,000 pregnancies were managed at their hospital and nearly 17,000 of these underwent antepartum testing of various types. Fetal surveillance increased from less than 1 percent of pregnancies in the early 1970s to 15 percent in the mid-1980s. They concluded that such testing was clearly beneficial because the fetal death rate was significantly less in the tested high-risk pregnancies compared with the rate in those not tested.

A contrasting opinion on the benefits of antenatal fetal testing was offered by Thacker and Berkelman (1986). It was their view that efficacy is best evaluated in randomized controlled trials. After reviewing 600 reports, they found only four such trials, all performed with the nonstress test and none with the contraction stress test. The numbers in these four trials were considered too small to detect important benefits. They projected that the costs of such testing exceeded $200 million per year in 1986 and that published studies did not support the use of either test.

Mohide and Keirse (1991), using the Oxford Database of Perinatal Trials, exhaustively reviewed evidence from controlled clinical trials concerning antepartum fetal surveillance. They found virtually no investigations where the antepartum test was compared with management without some other test of fetal well-being. The few suitable studies revealed no benefits. They concluded that use of these tests has not been demonstrated to confer benefits in the care of an individual woman. Indeed, antepartum tests were subsequently described as "forms of care likely to be ineffective or harmful" (Erkin and co-authors, 1995).

Another important and unanswered question is whether antepartum fetal surveillance identifies fetal asphyxia early enough to prevent brain damage. Todd and co-workers (1992) attempted to correlate cognitive development in infants up to 2 years following either abnormal Doppler velocimetry or nonstress tests. Abnormal nonstress tests were associated with marginally poorer cognitive outcomes, but not those associated with abnormal Doppler velocimetry. Importantly, these investigators concluded that by the time fetal compromise is diagnosed with antenatal testing, fetal damage has already been sustained.

Manning and co-authors (1998) studied the incidence of cerebral palsy in 26,290 high-risk pregnancies managed with serial biophysical profile testing compared with 58,657 low-risk pregnancies that did not receive antepartum testing. The rate of cerebral palsy was 1.3 per 1000 in tested pregnancies compared with 4.7 per 1000 in untested women. In a prior report, however, Manning and colleagues (1996) also found that cerebral palsy was significantly associated with low biophysical profile scores suggesting that identification of the truly compromised fetus may be too late.

Antenatal forecasts of fetal health have clearly been

the focus of intense interest for more than two decades. When such testing is reviewed, several themes emerge. First, the methods of fetal forecasting have evolved continually, a phenomenon that itself suggests dissatisfaction with the efficacy of any given method. Second, the biophysical performance of the human fetus is characterized by wide ranges of normal variation, resulting in difficulty determining when such performance should be considered abnormal. *How many movements, respirations, or accelerations? In what time period?* Unable to easily quantify normal fetal biophysical performance, most investigators have resorted to somewhat arbitrary answers for such questions. Third, despite the invention of increasingly complex testing methods, abnormal results are seldom reliable, prompting many clinicians to use antenatal testing to forecast fetal *wellness* rather than *illness*.

REFERENCES

Alfirevic Z, Neilson JP: Doppler ultrasonography in high-risk pregnancies: Systematic review with meta-analysis. Am J Obstet Gynecol 172:1379, 1995

American College of Obstetricians and Gynecologists. Intrauterine growth restriction. Practice Bulletin No. 12, January 2000

American College of Obstetricians and Gynecologists: Antepartum fetal surveillance. Practice Bulletin No. 9, October 1999

Badalian SS, Chao CR, Fox HE, Timor-Tritsch IE: Fetal breathing-related nasal fluid flow velocity in uncomplicated pregnancies. Am J Obstet Gynecol 169:563, 1993

Benzaquen S, Gagnon R, Hunse C, Foreman J: The intrauterine sound environment of the human fetus during labor. Am J Obstet Gynecol 163:484, 1990

Bourgeois FJ, Thiagarajah S, Harbert GN: The significance of fetal heart rate decelerations during nonstress testing. Am J Obstet Gynecol 150:213, 1984

Bracero LA, Morgan S, Byrne DW: Comparison of visual and computerized interpretation of nonstress test results in a randomized controlled trial. Am J Obstet Gynecol 181:1254, 1999

Brown R, Patrick J: The nonstress test: How long is enough? Am J Obstet Gynecol 141:646, 1981

Casey BM, McIntire DD, Bloom SL, Lucas MJ, Santos R, Twickler DM, Ramus RM, Leveno KJ: Pregnancy outcomes after antepartum diagnosis of oligohydramnios at or beyond 34 weeks gestation. Am J Obstet Gynecol 182:909, 2000

Chamberlain PF, Manning FA, Morrison I, Harman CR, Lange IR: Ultrasound evaluation of amniotic fluid volume. II. The relationship of increased amniotic fluid volume to perinatal outcome. Am J Obstet Gynecol 150:250, 1984

Chari RS, Friedman SA, O'Brien JM, Sibai BM: Daily antenatal testing in women with severe preeclampsia. Am J Obstet Gynecol 173:1207, 1995

Chauhan SP, Sanderson M, Hendrix NW, Magann EF, Devoe LD: Perinatal outcomes and amniotic fluid index in the antepartum and intrapartum periods: A meta-analysis. Am J Obstet Gynecol 181:1473, 1999

Clark SL, Sabey P, Jolley K: Nonstress testing with acoustic stimulation and amnionic fluid volume assessment: 5973 tests without unexpected fetal death. Am J Obstet Gynecol 160:694, 1989

Conway DL, Groth S, Adkins WB, Langer O: Management of isolated oligohydramnios in the term pregnancy: A randomized clinical trial. Am J Obstet Gynecol 182:S21, 2000

Dawes GS: Breathing before birth in animals and man. An essay in medicine. Physiol Med 290:557, 1974

Dawes GS, Fox HE, Leduc BM, Liggins GC, Richards RT: Respiratory movements and rapid eye movement sleep in the foetal lamb. J Physiol 220:119, 1972

Dayal AK, Manning FA, Berck DJ, Mussalli GM, Avila C, Harnan C, Menticoglou S: Fetal death after normal biophysical profile score: An eighteen year experience. Am J Obstet Gynecol 181:1231, 1999

Devoe LD, Castillo RA, Sherline DM: The nonstress test as a diagnostic test: A critical reappraisal. Am J Obstet Gynecol 152:1047, 1986

Devoe LD, McKenzie J, Searle NS, Sherline DM: Clinical sequelae of the extended nonstress test. Am J Obstet Gynecol 151:1074, 1985

DeVries JIP, Visser GHA, Prechtl NFR: The emergence of fetal behavior. II. Quantitative aspects. Early Hum Dev 12:99, 1985

Druzin ML, Gratacos J, Keegan KA, Paul RH: Antepartum fetal heart rate testing, 7. The significance of fetal bradycardia. Am J Obstet Gynecol 139:194, 1981

Eller DP, Scardo JA, Dillon AE, Klein AJ, Stramm SL, Newman RB: Distance from an intrauterine hydrophone as a factor affecting intrauterine sound pressure levels produced by the vibroacoustic stimulation test. Am J Obstet Gynecol 173:523, 1995

Enkin M, Keirse MJNC, Renfrew M, Neilson JP: A Guide to Effective Care in Pregnancy and Childbirth, 2nd ed. New York, Oxford University Press, 1995, p 410

Frager NB, Miyazaki FS: Intrauterine monitoring of contractions during breast stimulation. Obstet Gynecol 69:767, 1987

Freeman RK: The use of the oxytocin challenge test for antepartum clinical evaluation of uteroplacental respiratory function. Am J Obstet Gynecol 121:481, 1975

Grant A, Elbourne D, Valentin L, Alexander S: Routine formal fetal movement counting and risk of antepartum late death in normally formed singletons. Lancet 2:345, 1989

Grubb DK, Paul RH: Amnionic fluid index and prolonged antepartum fetal heart rate decelerations. Obstet Gynecol 79:558, 1992

Guinn DA, Kimberlin KF, Wigton TR, Socol ML, Frederiksen MC: Fetal heart rate characteristics at 25 to 28 weeks gestation. Am J Perinat 15:507, 1998

Hage ML: Interpretation of nonstress tests. Am J Obstet Gynecol 153:490, 1985

Hammacher K, Hüter KA, Bokelmann J, Werners PH: Foetal heart frequency and perinatal condition of the foetus and newborn. Gynaecologia 166:349, 1968

Harrington K, Thompson O, Jorden L, Page J, Carpenter RG, Campbell S: Obstetric outcomes in women who present with a reduction in fetal movements in the third trimester of pregnancy. J Perinat Med 26:77, 1998

Hoskins IA, Frieden FJ, Young BK: Variable decelerations in reactive nonstress tests with decreased amniotic fluid index predict fetal compromise. Am J Obstet Gynecol 165:1094, 1991

Huddleston JF, Sutliff JG, Robinson D: Contraction stress test by intermittent nipple stimulation. Obstet Gynecol 63:669, 1984

Hykin J, Moore R, Duncan K, Clare S, Baker P, Johnson I, Botwell R, Mansfield P, Gowland P: Fetal brain activity demonstrated by functional magnetic resonance imaging. Lancet 354:645, 1999

Johnson MJ, Paine LL, Mulder HH, Cezar C, Gegor C, Johnson TRB: Population differences of fetal biophysical and behavioral characteristics. Am J Obstet Gynecol 166:138, 1992

Johnson T, Besigner R, Thomas R: New clues to fetal behavior and well-being. Contemp Ob/Gyn, May, 1988

Lee CY, DiLoreto PC, O'Lane JM: A study of fetal heart rate acceleration patterns. Obstet Gynecol 45:142, 1975

Leveno KJ, Williams ML, DePalma RT, Whalley PJ: Perinatal outcome in the absence of antepartum fetal heart rate acceleration. Obstet Gynecol 61:347, 1983

Magann EF, Chauhan SP, Kinsella MJ, McNamara MF, Whitworth NS, Morrisson JC: Antenatal testing among 1001 patients at high risk: The role of ultrasonographic estimates of amniotic fluid volume. Am J Obstet Gynecol 180:1330, 1999

Manning FA, Bondaji N, Harman CR, Casiro O, Menticoglou S, Morrison I, Berck DJ: Fetal assessment based on fetal biophysical profile scoring VIII: The incidence of cerebral palsy in tested and untested perinates. Am J Obstet Gynecol 178:696, 1998

Manning FA, Harman C, Menticoglou S: Fetal biophysical score and cerebral palsy at age 3 years. Am J Obstet Gynecol 174:319, 1996

Manning FA, Harman CR, Morrison I, Menticoglou SM, Lange IR, Johnson JM: Fetal assessment based on fetal biophysical profile scoring, IV. An analysis of perinatal morbidity and mortality. Am J Obstet Gynecol 150:245, 1984

Manning FA, Morrison I, Harman CR, Lange IR, Menticoglou S: Fetal assessment based on fetal biophysical profile scoring: Experience in 19,221 referred high-risk pregnancies, 2. An analysis of false-negative fetal deaths. Am J Obstet Gynecol 157:880, 1987

Manning FA, Platt LD, Sipos L: Antepartum fetal evaluation: Development of a fetal biophysical profile. Am J Obstet Gynecol 136:787, 1980

Manning FA, Snijders R, Harman CR, Nicolaides K, Menticoglou S, Morrison I: Fetal biophysical profile score, 6. Correlation with antepartum umbilical venous fetal pH. Am J Obstet Gynecol 169:755, 1993

Mari G, Deter RL: Middle cerebral artery flow velocity waveforms in normal and small-for-gestational-age fetuses. Am J Obstet Gynecol 166:1262, 1992

Matsuura M, Murata Y, Hirano T, Nagati N, Doi S, Suda K: The effects of developing autonomous nervous system on FHR variabilities determined by the power spectral analysis. Am J Obstet Gynecol 174:380, 1996

Meis PJ, Ureda JR, Swain M, Kelly RT, Penry M, Sharp P: Variable decelerations during nonstress tests are not a sign of fetal compromise. Am J Obstet Gynecol 154:586, 1986

Miller DA, Rabello YA, Paul RH: The modified biophysical profile: Antepartum testing in the 1990s. Am J Obstet Gynecol 174:812, 1996

Miller F, Miller D, Paul R, Rabello Y: Is one fetal heart rate acceleration during a non-stress test as reliable as two in predicting fetal status? Am J Obstet Gynecol 174:337, 1996

Mohide P, Keirse MJNC: Biophysical assessment of fetal well-being. In Chambers I, Erkin M, Kierse MJNC (eds): Effective Care Pregnancy and Childbirth, Vol I. Pregnancy. New York, Oxford University Press, 1991, p 477

Moore TR, Piaquadio K: A prospective evaluation of fetal

movement screening to reduce the incidence of antepartum fetal death. Am J Obstet Gynecol 160:1075, 1989

Nageotte MP, Towers CV, Asrat T, Freeman RK: Perinatal outcome with the modified biophysical profile. Am J Obstet Gynecol 170:1672, 1994

National Institute of Child Health and Human Development Research Planning Workshop. Electronic fetal heart rate monitoring: Research guidelines for interpretation. Am J Obstet Gynecol 177:1385, 1997

Neldam S: Fetal movements as an indicator of fetal well being. Dan Med Bull 30:274, 1983

Nijhuis JG, Prechtl HFR, Martin CB Jr, Bots RS: Are there behavioural states in the human fetus? Early Hum Dev 6:177, 1982

Oasin SM, Sachder R, Trias A, Senkowski K, Kemmann E: The predictive value of first-trimester embryonic heart rates in infertility patients. Obstet Gynecol 89:934, 1997

Oosterhof H, vd Stege JG, Lander M, Prechtl HFR, Aarnoudse JG: Urine production rate is related to behavioural states in the near term human fetus. Br J Obstet Gynaecol 100:920, 1993

Ott WJ, Mora G, Arias F, Sunderji S, Sheldon G: Comparison of the modified biophysical profile to a "new" biophysical profile incorporating the middle cerebral artery to umbilical artery velocity flow systolic/diastolic ratio. Am J Obstet Gynecol 178:1346, 1998

Patrick J, Campbell K, Carmichael L, Natale R, Richardson B: Patterns of gross fetal body movements over 24-hour observation intervals during the last 10 weeks of pregnancy. Am J Obstet Gynecol 142:363, 1982

Patrick J, Campbell K, Carmichael L, Natale R, Richardson B: Patterns of human fetal breathing during the last 10 weeks of pregnancy. Obstet Gynecol 56:24, 1980

Pazos R, Vuolo K, Aladjem S, Lueck J, Anderson C: Association of spontaneous fetal heart rate decelerations during antepartum nonstress testing and intrauterine growth retardation. Am J Obstet Gynecol 144:574, 1982

Pillai M, James D: Behavioral states in normal mature human fetuses. Arch Dis Child 65:39, 1990a

Pillai M, James D: The development of fetal heart rate patterns during normal pregnancy. Obstet Gynecol 76:812, 1990b

Platt LD, Paul RH, Phelan J, Walla CA, Broussard P: Fifteen years of experience with antepartum fetal testing. Am J Obstet Gynecol 156:1509, 1987

Ray M, Freeman R, Pine S, Hesselgesser R: Clinical experience with the oxytocin challenge test. Am J Obstet Gynecol 114:1, 1972

Rayburn WF: Clinical significance of perceptible fetal motion. Am J Obstet Gynecol 138:210, 1980

Read JA, Miller FC: Fetal heart rate acceleration in response to acoustic stimulation as a measure of fetal well-being. Am J Obstet Gynecol 129:512, 1977

Richards DS, Frentzen B, Gerhardt KJ, McCann ME, Abrams RM: Sound levels in the human uterus. Obstet Gynecol 80:186, 1992

Romero R, Mazor M, Hobbins JC: A critical appraisal of fetal acoustic stimulation as an antenatal test for fetal well-being. Obstet Gynecol 71:781, 1988

Rutherford SE, Phelan JP, Smith CV, Jacobs N: The four-quadrant assessment of amniotic fluid volume: An adjunct to antepartum fetal heart rate testing. Obstet Gynecol 70:353, 1987

Sadovsky E, Evron S, Weinstein D: Daily fetal movement recording in normal pregnancy. Riv Obstet Ginecol Practica Med Perinatal 59:395, 1979a

Sadovsky E, Laufer N, Allen JW: The incidence of different types of fetal movement during pregnancy. Br J Obstet Gynaecol 86:10, 1979b

Sadovsky E, Yaffe H: Daily fetal movement recording and fetal prognosis. Obstet Gynecol 41:845, 1973

Salvesen DR, Freeman J, Brudenell JM, Nicolaides KJ: Prediction of fetal acidemia in pregnancies complicated by maternal diabetes by biophysical scoring and fetal heart rate monitoring. Br J Obstet Gynaecol 100:227, 1993

Schellpfeffer MA, Hoyle D, Johnson JWC: Antepartum uterine hypercontractility secondary to nipple stimulation. Obstet Gynecol 65:588, 1985

Schucker JC, Mercer BM, Audibert F, Lewis RL, Friedman SA, Sibai BM: Serial amniotic fluid index in severe preeclampsia: A poor predictor of adverse outcome. Am J Obstet Gynecol 175:1018, 1996

Sherer DM, Spong CY, Ghidini A, Salafia CM, Minior RK: In preterm fetuses decreased amniotic fluid volume is associated with decreased fetal movements. Am J Obstet Gynecol 174:344, 1996

Smith CV, Nguyen HN, Kovacs B, McCart D, Phelan JP, Paul RH: Fetal death following antepartum fetal heart rate testing: A review of 65 cases. Obstet Gynecol 70:18, 1987

Smith JH, Anand KJ, Cotes PM, Dawes GS, Harkness RA, Howlett TA, Rees LH, Redman CW: Antenatal fetal heart rate variation in relation to the respiratory and metabolic status of the compromised human fetus. Br J Obstet Gynaecol 95:980, 1988

Sontag LW, Wallace RF: The movement response of the human fetus to sound stimuli. Child Dev 6:253, 1935

Soronkin Y, Bottoms SF, Dierker CJ, Rosen MG: The clustering of fetal heart rate changes and fetal movements in pregnancies between 20 and 30 weeks gestation. Am J Obstet Gynecol 143:952, 1982

Thacker SB, Berkelman RL: Assessing the diagnostic accuracy and efficacy of selected antepartum fetal surveillance techniques. Obstet Gynecol Surv 41:121, 1986

Timor-Tritsch IE, Dierker LJ, Hertz RH, Deogan NC, Rosen MG: Studies of antepartum behavioral state in the human fetus at term. Am J Obstet Gynecol 132:524, 1978

Todd AL, Tridinger BJ, Cole MJ, Cooney GH: Antenatal tests of fetal welfare and development at age 2 years. Am J Obstet Gynecol 167:66, 1992

Todros T, Sciarrone A, Piccoli E, Guiot C, Kaufmann P, Kingdom J: Umbilical Doppler waveforms and placental villous angiogenesis in pregnancies complicated by fetal growth restriction. Obstet Gynecol 93:499, 1999

Vindla S, James D: Fetal behavior as a test of fetal well-being. Br J Obstet Gynaecol 102:597, 1995

Visser GHA, Redman CWG, Huisjes HJ, Turnbull AC: Nonstressed antepartum heart rate monitoring: Implications of decelerations after spontaneous contractions. Am J Obstet Gynecol 138:429, 1980

Weiner Z, Divon MY, Katz N, Minior VK, Nasseri A, Girz B: Multi-variant analysis of antepartum fetal test in predicting neonatal outcome of growth retarded fetuses. Am J Obstet Gynecol 174:338, 1996

Williams JW: Obstetrics, 1st ed. New York, Appleton, 1903, p 158

Williams K, Farquharson D, Bebbington M, Dansereau J, Galeneau F, Wilson RD, Shaw D, Kent N: A randomized controlled clinical trial comparing nonstress test versus Doppler velocimetry as a screening test in a high risk population. (Abstract 315.) Am J Obstet Gynecol 182:S109, 2000

Zelop CM, Richardson DK, Heffner LJ: Outcomes of severely abnormal umbilical artery Doppler velocimetry in structurally normal singleton fetuses. Obstet Gynecol 87:434, 1996

41

Ultrasound and Doppler

The impact of ultrasonography on the practice of obstetrics has been profound. Ultrasonic methods for evaluating the fetus are now employed widely for the many reasons summarized in this chapter and cited frequently throughout the book. A carefully performed ultrasound examination reveals vital information about fetal anatomy, as well as fetal environment, growth, and well-being with no confirmed biological hazards. Ultrasound technology has evolved from producing images of the pregnancy to methods for measurement of both maternal and fetal circulatory function. The phenomenon of Doppler shift forms the technical basis for acquisition of information about the maternal–fetal hemodynamic circulations.

ULTRASONOGRAPHY

Since the first obstetrical application of ultrasound imaging by Donald and co-workers (1958), ultrasonic evaluation of the pregnant uterus has become indispensible. By 1989, 45 percent of pregnancies in the United States were evaluated sonographically (National Center for Health Statistics, 1992). The percentage continued to increase, which led the National Institutes of Health to commission the Routine Antenatal Diagnostic Imaging with Ultrasound (RADIUS) trial in an effort to determine whether all pregnant women should undergo ultrasound examinations. Their findings have sparked a lively debate within obstetrics and radiology as to the necessity for routine prenatal sonographic screening.

TECHNOLOGY. The picture displayed on the ultrasound screen is produced by sound waves reflecting back from the fetus or imaged structure. When alternating current is applied to a transducer made of a piezoelectric material, intermittent high-frequency sound waves exceeding 20,000 cps are generated. Applying a coupling agent, such as a water-soluble gel, diminishes the loss of ultrasound waves at the transducer-skin interface. The transducer emits a pulse of sound waves that passes through the layers of soft tissue. When an interface between structures of different tissue densities is encountered, some of the energy is reflected back to the transducer. The amount of energy reflected is proportional to the difference in densities at the interface. The reflected energy generates a small electrical voltage that is amplified and displayed on a screen, and appears as a shade of color or brightness somewhere on the continuum between white and black. Bone, for example, is dense (echogenic) and generates a voltage that appears white on the screen, while fluid (anechoic) appears black. Soft tissues appear as varying shades of gray.

Transabdominal scanning is most commonly performed with a 3.5- to 7-mHz curvilinear transducer which uses sequential firing of multiple crystals and generates an image so fast (more than 40 frames/sec) that the picture on the screen appears to be moving in "real-time." Higher frequency transducers yield better image resolutions; however, lower frequencies afford better tissue penetration.

SAFETY. No confirmed biological effects in mammalian tissue have been demonstrated in the frequency range of medical ultrasound (American Institute of Ultrasound in Medicine, 1991). In the low-intensity range of gray-scale imaging, no fetal risks have been demonstrated in over 30 years of use (Chap 42, p. 1153).

CLINICAL APPLICATIONS. Sonography has proved valuable for monitoring pregnancy in a variety of ways as shown in Table 41–1. The already widespread use of

TABLE 41–1. Some Indications for Obstetrical Ultrasonic Examinations

Estimation of gestational age with uncertain dates or verification of dates for women undergoing repeat cesarean delivery, labor induction, or elective abortion

Evaluation of fetal growth

Vaginal bleeding of undetermined etiology

Determination of fetal presentation

Suspected multiple gestation

Adjunct to amniocentesis

Significant uterine size/clinical dates discrepancy

Pelvic mass

Suspected molar pregnancy

Suspected ectopic pregnancy

Adjunct to special procedures, e.g., cerclage

Suspected fetal death

Suspected uterine abnormality

Intrauterine contraceptive device localization

Biophysical evaluation of fetal well-being

Observation of intrapartum events

Suspected polyhydramnios or oligohydramnios

Suspected abruptio placentae

Adjunct to external version from breech to vertex presentation

Estimation of fetal weight and/or presentation in preterm prematurely ruptured membranes and/or preterm labor

Abnormal serum alpha-fetoprotein value

Follow-up observation of identified fetal anomaly

Follow-up evaluation of placental location for identified placenta previa

History of previous congenital anomaly

Serial evaluation of fetal growth in multifetal gestation

Evaluation of fetal condition in late registrants for prenatal care

As adapted from the National Institutes of Health (1984) by the American College of Obstetricians and Gynecologists (1993).

sonography in obstetrics and its potential for identification of fetal abnormalities and for providing reassurance of fetal well-being have stimulated several questions that are difficult to answer:

1. Should sonography be used in all pregnancies and, if so, when should it be initiated, how often should it be repeated, and how vigorous an examination for possible fetal abnormalities should be carried out?
2. Who should perform the examination, and who should interpret the results?
3. What should be the responsibilities of the obstetrician?
4. In what circumstances should sonography be performed by a certified obstetrical or radiological specialist highly trained in sonography?

Some of these questions have been addressed and partially answered. The American College of Obstetricians and Gynecologists (1993) recommends that basic ultrasound examinations be performed by or reviewed by an appropriately trained operator. Shown in Table 41–2 are the guidelines recommended for a basic obstetrical ultrasound examination in both the first and second trimesters. Vaginal sonography may be necessary during the first trimester if abdominal scanning is insufficient to identify these specified components. A fetal anatomical survey is included in a basic second trimester examination. When a complete second- or third-trimester fetal anatomical survey cannot be completed—for example, when visualization is impaired due to oligohydramnios, fetal position, engaged fetal head, or maternal obesity—it should be noted in the report.

Targeted examinations, including a detailed evaluation of all fetal anatomy, are performed when an abnormality is suspected. These should be performed by an operator with especial expertise in such scanning.

A third type of ultrasound procedure is the "limited examination," in which many components of a basic examination are not done. Examples include estimation of amnionic fluid volume, placental localization, determination of fetal presentation, confirmation of fetal life or death, as an adjunct to amniocentesis or external cephalic version, or as part of fetal biophysical profile testing. Each examination should be labeled as limited, basic, or comprehensive, and any missing data should be addressed in the report.

The American Institute of Ultrasound in Medicine (1994) has provided similar guidelines for the performance of antepartum ultrasound examinations. The Institute specifically recommends evaluation of the cerebral ventricles and cerebellum, thorax and four-chamber view of the heart, spine, stomach, kidneys and bladder, umbilical cord insertion on the abdominal wall, and extremities.

SELECTED VERSUS ROUTINE ULTRASONIC SCANNING. Whether all pregnant women should undergo ultrasound screening remains unclear, but is the subject of lively debate by those for and against. Advantages of routine screening have included more accurate pregnancy dating, less frequent labor induction for postterm pregnancy, detection of multiple gestation and fetal growth restriction, and identification of fetal malformations.

Several researchers have demonstrated that ultrasonic estimated gestational age is more accurate than using the last menstrual period, and thus reduces the number of postterm pregnancy inductions. Waldenstrom and colleagues (1988), performed a single scan at approximately 15 weeks in nearly 2500 Swedish women. They found that the incidence of labor inductions for postterm pregnancy was 5.9 percent in screened compared with 9.1 percent in control women. Likewise, Tunon and colleagues (1996) compared the estimated de-

TABLE 41–2. Components of Basic Ultrasound Examination According to Trimester of Pregnancy

First Trimester	Second and Third Trimester
1. Gestational sac location	1. Fetal number
2. Embryo identification	2. Presentation
3. Crown-rump length	3. Fetal heart motion
4. Fetal heart motion	4. Placental location
5. Fetal number	5. Amnionic fluid volume
6. Uterus and adnexal evaluation	6. Gestational age
	7. Survey of fetal anatomy
	8. Evaluation for maternal pelvic masses

Modified from American College of Obstetricians and Gynecologists (1993), with permission.

livery date by both an 18-week ultrasound and by the last period in 15,241 unselected Norwegian women. They reported the postterm delivery rate to be 10 percent according to the menstrual data but only 4 percent with ultrasound dating. Olsen and Clausen (1997), however, have made a statistical argument that overestimation of postterm pregnancy could be prevented by simply adding 283 days to the last period instead of 280 days.

Another argument for routine ultrasound evaluation is that identifying fetal anomalies allows either pregnancy termination or optimization of delivery. Several studies are in conflict concerning this, and at least two support universal screening. Saari-Kemppainen and colleagues (1990) randomized over 9300 Finnish women to routine ultrasound between 16 and 20 weeks or to routine care with sonography if indicated. Perinatal mortality was significantly lower in the sonography group, largely because of pregnancy terminations for malformed fetuses and early detection and appropriate care of twin pregnancies. Routine ultrasound also resulted in improved pregnancy dating and a reduced rate of postterm pregnancy. Similarly, Luck (1992) performed routine ultrasound scanning at 19 weeks in over 8800 British women and concluded that this approach reduced perinatal morbidity and mortality because of pregnancy termination in 25 fetuses with crippling or lethal malformations.

By way of contrast, Bucher and Schmidt (1993) performed a meta-analysis of four trials in which nearly 16,000 women were randomized to routine versus selected scanning. They concluded that routine scanning may be effective and useful for malformation screening, but that it did not significantly improve pregnancy outcome as measured by live births or reduced perinatal mortality. Conflicting data such as these stimulated the larger RADIUS trial described next.

THE RADIUS TRIAL. This investigation was named the Routine Antenatal Diagnostic Imaging with Ultrasound trial. It was sponsored by the National Institute of Child Health and Human Development and results reported by Ewigman and colleagues (1993). It involved over 15,000 women at low risk for perinatal problems. Women assigned to universal screening underwent ultrasonic evaluation at 15 to 22 weeks and again at 31 to 35 weeks, while control-group women had indicated sonography only. A mean number of 0.6 procedures was performed in the control group, compared with 2.2 in the universally screened group. The rate of adverse perinatal outcomes was about 5 percent in each group. There were no significant differences in the incidence or outcomes of preterm delivery, postterm pregnancy, multifetal gestation, or growth-restricted infants. Moreover, ultrasonic detection of congenital anomalies had no effect on perinatal outcome. The RADIUS trialists

concluded that routine ultrasound screening for low-risk women did not improve perinatal outcome and thus did not justify routine ultrasound screening, which would increase the cost of perinatal care by $1 billion.

The RADIUS trial and its conclusions have been widely criticized. The trial included only "low-risk" women who were so rigorously defined that by one estimate only 0.8 percent of pregnancies would qualify (American Institute of Ultrasound in Medicine, 1994). Berkowitz (1993), in his review of these data, rightfully emphasized that because women in this study were of the lowest risk, if universal screening is not chosen, then health-care providers will have to be extremely vigilant in searching for problems or conditions that would be indicators for scanning.

Another criticism was the below average detection of fetal anomalies. Only 17 percent of major anomalies were detected before 24 weeks in the routine screening group. In other studies, as many as half of anomalies were reported to be identified. This is thought to be why identification of anomalies had such little impact on outcome. Specifically, only a third of affected fetuses could be terminated compared with two thirds in the Finnish trial reported by Saari-Kemppainen and co-workers (1990).

Finally, selection of perinatal morbidity and mortality as primary outcome measures are considered inappropriate for the very low-risk population studied. Thus, cost estimates for routine ultrasound are unjustified. In a financial analysis based on the results of the Helsinki trial, DeVore (1996) concluded that routine ultrasound would save the United States health-care system at least $280 million.

For all these reasons, the RADIUS trial has not settled the controversy over routine ultrasonic screening in pregnancy. Although it is not currently recommended for low-risk women, this is defined rigorously and the physician must be vigilant for any changes in risk status. Finally, the yield of a routine ultrasound examination appears to be directly related to the skill of the operator and possibly the quality of the equipment.

FETAL MEASUREMENTS. There are many tables and nomograms that describe the normal growth of various fetal structures. Shown in Tables 41–3 and 41–4 are commonly used gestational age nomograms for crown-rump length, biparietal diameter, head circumference, abdominal circumference, and femur length. There also are nomograms for dimensions of other fetal structures such as cerebellum, kidney, spleen, liver, humerus, ulna, tibia, fibula, clavicle, foot, and intraocular and binocular distances. For determining gestational age in the first trimester, the crown-rump length is accurate to within 3 to 5 days. In the second trimester, the biparietal diame-

TABLE 41–3. Predicted Menstrual Age in Weeks from Crown-Rump Length Measurements (in cm)[a]

CRL	MA	CRL	MA	CRL	MA	CRL	MA	CRL	MA	CRL	MA
0.2	5.7	2.2	8.9	4.2	11.1	6.2	12.6	8.2	14.2	10.2	16.1
0.3	5.9	2.3	9.0	4.3	11.2	6.3	12.7	8.3	14.2	10.3	16.2
0.4	6.1	2.4	9.1	4.4	11.2	6.4	12.8	8.4	14.3	10.4	16.3
0.5	6.2	2.5	9.2	4.5	11.3	6.5	12.8	8.5	14.4	10.5	16.4
0.6	6.4	2.6	9.4	4.6	11.4	6.6	12.9	8.6	14.5	10.6	16.5
0.7	6.6	2.7	9.5	4.7	11.5	6.7	13.0	8.7	14.6	10.7	16.6
0.8	6.7	2.8	9.6	4.8	11.6	6.8	13.1	8.8	14.7	10.8	16.7
0.9	6.9	2.9	9.7	4.9	11.7	6.9	13.1	8.9	14.8	10.9	16.8
1.0	7.2	3.0	9.9	5.0	11.7	7.0	13.2	9.0	14.9	11.0	16.9
1.1	7.2	3.1	10.0	5.1	11.8	7.1	13.3	9.1	15.0	11.1	17.0
1.2	7.4	3.2	10.1	5.2	11.9	7.2	13.4	9.2	15.1	11.2	17.1
1.3	7.5	3.3	10.2	5.3	12.0	7.3	13.4	9.3	15.2	11.3	17.2
1.4	7.7	3.4	10.3	5.4	12.0	7.4	13.5	9.4	15.3	11.4	17.3
1.5	7.9	3.5	10.4	5.5	12.1	7.5	13.6	9.5	15.3	11.5	17.4
1.6	8.0	3.6	10.5	5.6	12.2	7.6	13.7	9.6	15.4	11.6	17.5
1.7	8.1	3.7	10.6	5.7	12.3	7.7	13.8	9.7	15.5	11.7	17.6
1.8	8.3	3.8	10.7	5.8	12.3	7.8	13.8	9.8	15.6	11.8	17.7
1.9	8.4	3.9	10.8	5.9	12.4	7.9	13.9	9.9	15.7	11.9	17.8
2.0	8.6	4.0	10.9	6.0	12.5	8.0	14.0	10.0	15.9	12.0	17.9
2.1	8.7	4.1	11.0	6.1	12.6	8.1	14.1	10.1	16.0	12.1	18.0

CRL = crown-rump length; MA = menstrual age.
[a] The 90% interval is ±8 percent of the predicted age.
From Hadlock and associates (1992), with permission.

ter and femur length are most accurate, while a combination of measurements is usually used to estimate the fetal weight.

Between 14 and 26 weeks, a combination of measurements is used to most accurately estimate gestational age. In most cases, the biparietal diameter is the easiest and most reproducible measurement to obtain accurately, and has a variation of only ± 7 to 10 days (Mongelli and colleagues, 1996; Tunon and co-workers, 1996). If there is brachycephaly or dolichocephaly, the biparietal diameter frequently is inaccurate so the head circumference usually is more reliable after 14 weeks. Femur and humerus lengths correlate strongly with both the biparietal diameter and gestational age; the variation in femur length measurement is 7 to 11 days in the second trimester. The abdominal circumference has a wider variation (± 2.8 weeks) than either the biparietal diameter or the femur length, and thus it may not be useful for determining gestational age if the fetus is not growing appropriately.

After 26 weeks, all measurements are less accurate for estimating gestational age. In the third trimester, the variation in both biparietal diameter and femur measurements increases to ± 14 to 21 days. If a third-trimes-

ter ultrasound determination must be used to estimate gestational age, serial examinations may be helpful to confirm normal fetal growth.

Using sonographic measurements to determine gestational age employs a wide range of measurements that are cited by percentiles. For example, a biparietal diameter of 40 mm could represent a 16-week fetus (90th percentile), a 19-week fetus (10th percentile), or a 17-week fetus (50th percentile). From a thorough review, Jeanty (1991) determined that a combination of measurements is superior to a single measurement. Thus, the inherent inaccuracy in each measurement is reduced by averaging several different measurements. It is important, however, that each dimension be assessed individually before it is averaged with the others. If one measurement is significantly different from the rest, it might not be appropriate to include it in the gestational age calculation. Various fetal anomalies and certain genetic conditions can influence the growth of the biparietal diameter, abdominal circumference or femur length as well.

AMNIONIC FLUID MEASUREMENT. This has become an important method of fetal assessment (Chap. 40).

TABLE 41–4. Average Predicted Fetal Measurement at Specific Menstrual Ages

Menstrual Age (wk)	Biparietal Diameter (cm)	Head Circumference (cm)	Abdominal Circumference (cm)	Femur Length (cm)
12.0	1.7	6.8	4.6	0.7
12.5	1.9	7.5	5.3	0.9
13.0	2.1	8.2	6.0	1.1
13.5	2.3	8.9	6.7	1.2
14.0	2.5	9.7	7.3	1.4
14.5	2.7	10.4	8.0	1.6
15.0	2.9	11.0	8.6	1.7
15.5	3.1	11.7	9.3	1.9
16.0	3.2	12.4	9.9	2.0
16.5	3.4	13.1	10.6	2.2
17.0	3.5	13.8	11.2	2.4
17.5	3.8	14.4	11.9	2.5
18.0	3.9	15.1	12.5	2.7
18.5	4.1	15.8	13.1	2.8
19.0	4.3	16.4	13.7	3.0
19.5	4.5	17.0	14.4	3.1
20.0	4.6	17.7	15.0	3.3
20.5	4.8	18.3	15.6	3.4
21.0	5.0	18.9	16.2	3.5
21.5	5.1	19.5	16.8	3.7
22.0	5.3	20.1	17.4	3.8
22.5	5.5	20.7	17.9	4.0
23.0	5.6	21.3	18.5	4.1
23.5	5.8	21.9	19.1	4.2
24.0	5.9	22.4	19.7	4.4
24.5	6.1	23.0	20.2	4.5
25.0	6.2	23.5	20.8	4.6
25.5	6.4	24.1	21.3	4.7
26.0	6.5	24.6	21.9	4.9

There are various definitions of diminished amnionic fluid volume (oligohydramnios) and excessive fluid (hydramnios). These definitions depend on the method used to quantify fluid volume. The volume can also be assessed subjectively, and oligohydramnios is defined by obvious crowding of the fetus and absence of any significant fluid pockets, while hydramnios is an obvious excess of fluid and multiple areas containing sufficient fluid to accommodate a cross section of the fetal abdomen (Williams, 1993). Indeed, some believe that a subjective assessment by an experienced examiner is more accurate than other measurement schemes. One such method is measurement of the **maximum vertical fluid pocket** in which less than 2 cm indicates oligohydramnios, 2 to 8 cm is considered normal, and more than 8 cm signifies hydramnios (Chamberlain and colleagues, 1984; Manning and associates, 1980). Phelan and coworkers (1987) introduced the now-popular technique termed the **amnionic fluid index.** This technique is described in detail in Chapter 31, and normal values are shown in Table 31–3, p. 816, and Figure 31–2, p. 817.

FIRST TRIMESTER. Early pregnancy may be evaluated with abdominal or vaginal ultrasonography. All the components listed in Table 41–2 should be assessed. Using abdominal scanning, the gestational sac is reliably seen by 6 weeks menstrual age and fetal echoes and heart activity by 7 weeks. With transvaginal scanning, these are seen about 1 week earlier. When the serum β-hCG is 1800 mIU/mL, the gestational sac should be visible.

TABLE 41–4. Average Predicted Fetal Measurement at Specific Menstrual Ages (Continued)

Menstrual Age (wk)	Biparietal Diameter (cm)	Head Circumference (cm)	Abdominal Circumference (cm)	Femur Length (cm)
26.5	6.7	25.1	22.4	5.0
27.0	6.8	25.6	23.0	5.1
27.5	6.9	26.1	23.5	5.2
28.0	7.1	26.6	24.0	5.4
28.5	7.2	27.1	24.6	5.5
29.0	7.3	27.5	25.1	5.6
29.5	7.5	28.0	25.6	5.7
30.0	7.6	28.4	26.1	5.8
30.5	7.7	28.8	26.6	5.9
31.0	7.8	29.3	27.1	6.0
31.5	7.9	29.7	27.6	6.1
32.0	8.1	30.1	28.1	6.2
32.5	8.2	30.4	28.6	6.3
33.0	8.3	30.8	29.1	6.4
33.5	8.4	31.2	29.5	6.5
34.0	8.5	31.5	30.0	6.6
34.5	8.6	31.8	30.5	6.7
35.0	8.7	32.2	30.9	6.8
35.5	8.8	32.5	31.4	6.9
36.0	8.9	32.8	31.8	7.0
36.5	8.9	33.0	32.3	7.1
37.0	9.0	33.3	32.7	7.2
37.5	9.1	33.5	33.2	7.3
38.0	9.2	33.8	33.6	7.4
38.5	9.2	34.0	34.0	7.4
39.0	9.3	34.2	34.4	7.5
39.5	9.4	34.4	34.8	7.6
40.0	9.4	34.6	35.3	7.7

From Hadlock and co-workers (1984), with permission.

Early sonography is valuable in diagnosing anembryonic gestation or missed abortion. Visualization of an intrauterine pregnancy excludes ectopic pregnancy unless there is a heterotopic pregnancy (Chap. 34, p. 892). Multifetal gestation can be identified and the number of chorions determined. Indeed, the first trimester may be the most accurate time to evaluate this. A limited assessment of fetal anatomy may also be possible.

FETAL ANATOMY. Most attempts to survey fetal anatomy using ultrasound take place during the early second trimester or later. Green and Hobbins (1988) generally were unable to identify fetal structures transabdominally before 9 weeks; their success rate improved remarkably, however, as gestation progressed. By 12 weeks, they were able to visualize the stomach in 95 percent, the anterior abdominal wall in 80 percent, the adrenal glands in 100 percent, the kidneys in 100 percent, and the bladder in 60 percent. Similarly, Timor-Tritsch and associates (1990) reported consistent success at imaging the skull, brain, spine, limbs, and anterior abdominal wall in 35 fetuses examined transvaginally between 9 and 14 weeks. By 11 weeks, they were able to visualize the fingers and feet.

Although there are increasing numbers of case reports that describe detection of a variety of fetal anomalies during the first trimester, and in spite of the obvious potential for identifying congenital fetal malformations at this point, caution is recommended for several reasons:

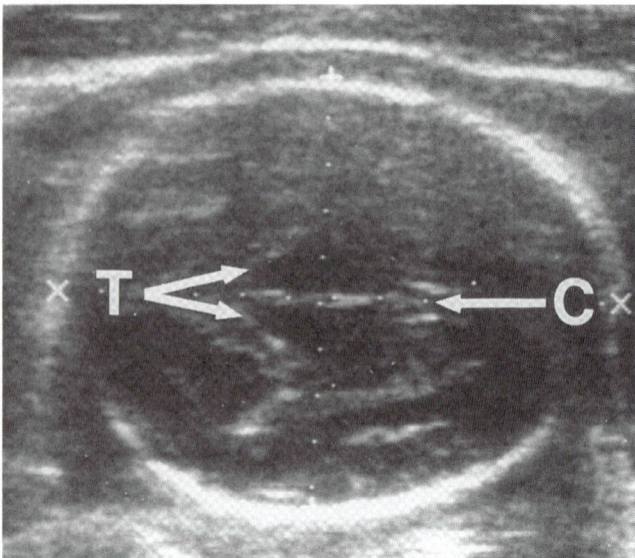

FIGURE 41–1. Transthalamic view in a 23-week fetus showing thalami (T) and cavum pellucidum (C). (From Lowe and colleagues, 1990.)

1. Normal first-trimester embryological development may mimic pathological changes typically seen in the second and third trimesters; for example, physiological anterior wall herniation may mimic an omphalocele.
2. Grossly abnormal embryos may appear normal, as with anencephaly.
3. Some abnormal embryos may manifest only with a crown-rump length that is less than expected for their gestational age (Levi and associates, 1990).

The American College of Obstetricians and Gynecologists (1993) cautions that whichever method is used, and regardless of the stage of pregnancy evaluated, it is unrealistic and unreasonable to expect detection of all fetal anomalies even with the most expert and thorough scanning. Gonçalves and colleagues (1994) reported that the overall sensitivity of sonography in detecting fetal defects was 53 percent. Overall specificity was 99 percent. Although the technique was about 90 percent sensitive for detecting lethal malformations, it missed serious cardiac defects, microcephaly, and many musculoskeletal deformities.

CENTRAL NERVOUS SYSTEM. Prenatal sonography has proven an excellent method to detect and characterize fetal central nervous system abnormalities. This is especially important because of the frequency of these abnormalities as well as their potential for causing severe disability or death. By adopting a systematic approach to the ultrasound evaluation of the central nervous system, it may be possible to identify virtually all

fetuses with major abnormalities (Filly and colleagues, 1989). Early identification allows timely consideration of prognosis and therapeutic options.

Three transverse (axial) sonographic views are recommended to depict the fetal brain and cranium (Nyberg, 1989). The transthalamic view (Fig. 41–1), which is used to measure biparietal diameter and head circumference, includes the thalami, cavum septi pellucidae, and the frontal horns of the lateral ventricles. Moving superiorly yields the transventricular view (Fig. 41–2) of the atria of the lateral ventricles which contain the echogenic choroid plexus. It also allows visualization of cranial contour. The transcerebellar view (Fig. 41–3) is obtained by angling through the posterior fossa and demonstrates the cerebellum, cisterna magna, and nuchal fold. Normal transverse cerebellar diameters for fetuses between 13 and 40 weeks have been described (Goldstein and associates, 1987). Between 15 and 22 weeks, the cerebellar diameter in millimeters is roughly equivalent to gestational age in weeks. The combined use of these three views has led to relatively sophisticated antenatal diagnoses, including aqueductal stenosis, holoprosencephaly, hydranencephaly, cerebral atrophy, porencephalic cysts, and intracranial tumors.

Filly and colleagues (1989) reported their experiences with 137 fetuses between 15 and 39 weeks who had sonographically diagnosed central nervous system abnormalities. Of these, 25 had an obvious neural-tube defect and 99 had hydrocephalus. Seven of the remaining 13 fetuses had a cisterna magna either smaller than 2 mm or larger than 11 mm in anterior–posterior diameter. While 6 of 137 fetuses with abnormalities were not identified, there were other apparent abnormalities in three. Thus, using this relatively simple sequence of

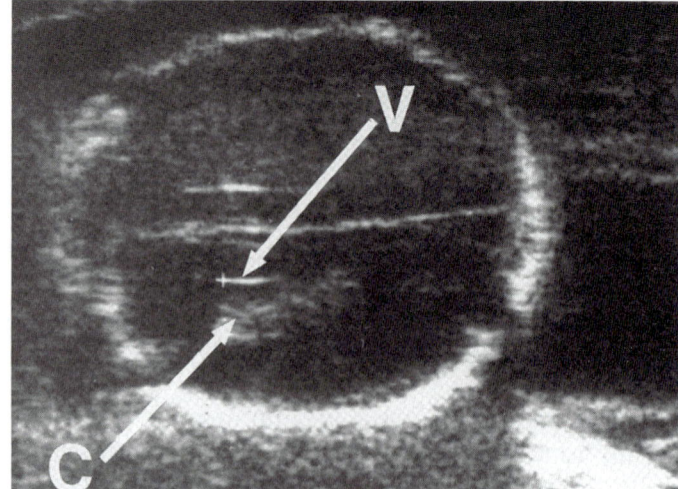

FIGURE 41–2. Transventricular view in a 20-week fetus showing choroid plexus (C) in the ventricular atrium (V). (From Lowe and associates, 1990.)

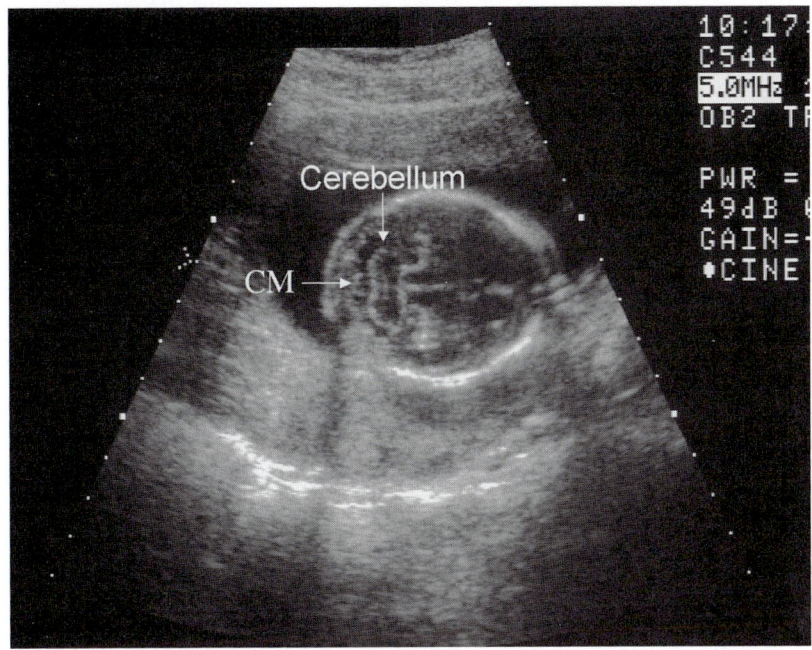

FIGURE 41-3. Transcerebellar view in an 18-week fetus showing the cisterna magna (cm) and cerebellum. (Courtesy of Dr. Jodi Dashe.)

evaluation, 134 of 137 fetuses with central nervous system abnormalities would have been identified. This same group also studied 150 normal fetuses between 15 and 40 weeks and found that the ventricular atrium could be identified and measured in 99 percent and the cisterna magna in 90 percent.

Monteagudo and associates (1991) found that transvaginal ultrasonography in the second and third trimesters may help refine the diagnosis in fetuses with central nervous system abnormalities. Using this approach, they improved their diagnosis in 5 of 13 fetuses. Recent reports such as that by Levine and colleagues (1999) suggest that in selected cases, fetal magnetic resonance imaging may improve prenatal diagnosis of central nervous system abnormalities (Chap. 42, p. 1156).

HYDROCEPHALUS. This is defined as the presence of excessive cerebrospinal fluid within the intracranial cavity. Its incidence is 0.3 to 0.8 per 1000 births (Romero and associates, 1988). On ultrasound, the excess fluid is reflected by ventriculomegaly, an enlargement of the ventricles. Some authors use the terms *hydrocephalus* and *ventriculomegaly* interchangeably. Others reserve hydrocephalus for cases in which the intracranial pressure is increased and the cranium enlarged.

The lateral ventricle is commonly measured at the atria, which is the confluence of the temporal and occipital horns (Fig. 41–4). In the past, hydrocephalus was diagnosed based on the lateral ventricular width—hemispheric width ratio, for which gestational-age specific nomograms have been developed (Jeanty, 1991). More recently, it has been established that the atrial

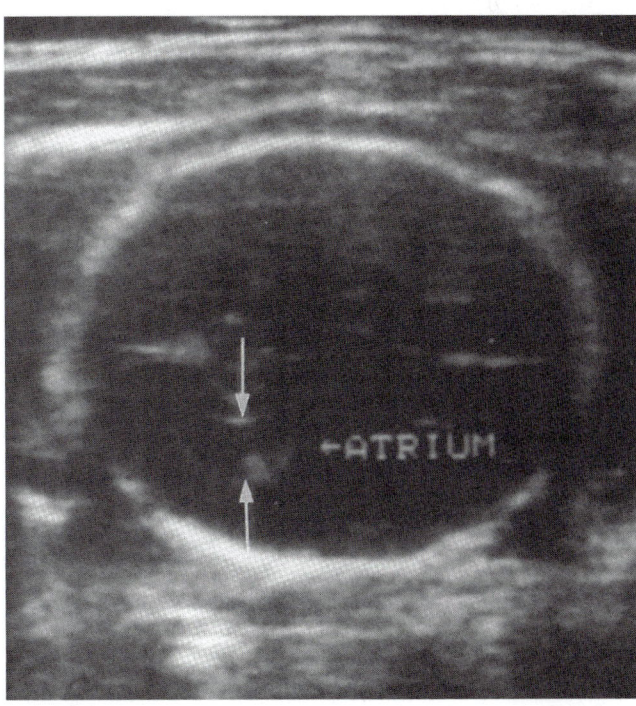

FIGURE 41-4. The ventricular atrium, with the echogenic choroid plexus and arrows defining the medial and lateral walls, is seen in this 23-week fetus. (From Twickler, 1996.)

measurement is relatively constant—between 6 and 9 mm—from 15 weeks until term (Cardoza and co-workers, 1988b). Mild ventriculomegaly, diagnosed when the atrial measurement is 10 to 15 mm, has been associated with developmental delay in up to 25 percent of affected infants (Bloom and colleagues, 1997). As the atrial measurement increases further (hydrocephalus), so does the likelihood of abnormal outcome. "Dangling" of the choroid plexus within the lateral ventricle is a characteristic finding in such cases (Cardoza and associates, 1988a; Mahony and colleagues, 1988).

Hydrocephalus is caused by a wide variety of genetic and environmental insults. The three most common associated anomalies are aqueductal stenosis (43 percent), Dandy–Walker syndrome (12 percent), and communicating hydrocephalus (38 percent). Each of these has multiple causes and prognosis is determined by the etiology. For example, mild to moderate hydrocephalus due to a spinal neural-tube defect generally has a good prognosis because brain development is often normal. Conversely, hydrocephalus caused by aqueductal stenosis generally has a poor prognosis, probably because it reflects abnormal brain development. It also is commonly associated with systemic fetal infection and aneuploidy. In a review of 53 consecutive cases of hydrocephalus caused by aqueductal stenosis, Levitsky and colleagues (1995) reported a mortality of 40 percent and normal development in only 10 percent of survivors. Dandy–Walker syndrome also is associated with single-gene and chromosomal disorders. Conversely, communicating hydrocephalus frequently is idiopathic and has a better prognosis. Although prenatal identification of the cause of hydrocephalus may be difficult, in some cases it may be inferred by the presence of associated malformations. For example, the finding of additional malformations other than a neural-tube defect implies a genetic etiology and an increased risk of intrinsic brain pathology. Almost three fourths of cases have associated malformations (Drugan and colleagues, 1989).

If hydrocephalus is isolated, the rate of progression of ventriculomegaly also strongly influences outcome. Relatively mild ventricular dilatation and slow progression usually has a good prognosis because enlargement is due to delayed parenchymal and cerebrospinal fluid pathway development and not necessarily a major cerebral malformation (Bannister and associates, 2000). Bloom and colleagues (1997) found that 25 percent of such infants had a developmental delay. Gupta and co-workers (1994) reviewed the outcomes of 276 cases of isolated hydrocephalus and found that 70 percent survived. Of these survivors, the 60 percent with normal developmental quotients were those with stable, non-progressive ventriculomegaly. Fetuses with progressive pathology generally have an unfavorable outcome, most likely because the initial infectious, hemorrhagic, chromosomal, or genetic insult was catastrophic.

Initial evaluation of hydrocephalus includes a thorough survey of fetal anatomy, karyotyping, and evaluation for congenital viral infection. With apparent isolated ventriculomegaly, serial ultrasound examinations to monitor the degree and rate of dilatation are recommended. Unfortunately, prognostic information is generally not available when decisions about pregnancy termination must be made.

NEURAL-TUBE DEFECTS. These are the second most common class of congenital anomalies after cardiac defects. Their incidence is about 1.6 per 1000 live births in the United States, and it approaches 8 per 1000 in the United Kingdom. Neural-tube defects result from failure of tube closure by the sixth gestational week (embryonic age 26 to 28 days). A more detailed account of the etiology of neural-tube anomalies is found in Chapter 36 (p. 958), and their diagnosis and management is discussed in Chapter 37 (p. 984).

Anencephaly can theoretically be diagnosed as early as 8 weeks; however, it can be missed in the first trimester (Levi and associates, 1990). In the second trimester, if an adequate ultrasound examination can be performed, anencephaly is diagnosed with virtually 100 percent accuracy (see Fig. 37–6, p. 982). It is characterized by absence of the cranial vault and brain above the base of the skull and orbits. Failure to obtain an adequate view of the biparietal diameter in the second trimester should raise suspicion. Hydramnios from impaired fetal swallowing commonly accompanies anencephaly but is typically a late finding. Goldstein and Filly (1988) reported increased amnionic fluid in 85 percent of anencephalic fetuses after 25 weeks, but in only about 10 percent before this time. Associated fetal anomalies are common but have not been extensively described because anencephaly itself is uniformly fatal.

Encephalocele is when the meninges and brain herniate through a cranial defect. A **meningocele** is when only meninges herniate. This lesion most commonly results from an occipital midline defect. Sonographically, these lesions vary in size and may have a cystic or solid appearance. If the cerebellum herniates into the defect, it is termed a *Chiari III malformation*. Encephaloceles are commonly associated with either hydrocephaly or microcephaly and there is a high incidence of mental impairment. An encephalocele is an important feature of *Meckel–Gruber syndrome* and frequently accompanies *amnionic band syndrome*. An occipital encephalocele can usually be detected using transthalamic and transcerebellar views. If a skull defect cannot be seen, the differential diagnosis should include cystic hygroma (see later discussion).

Spina bifida consists of a hiatus in the vertebrae,

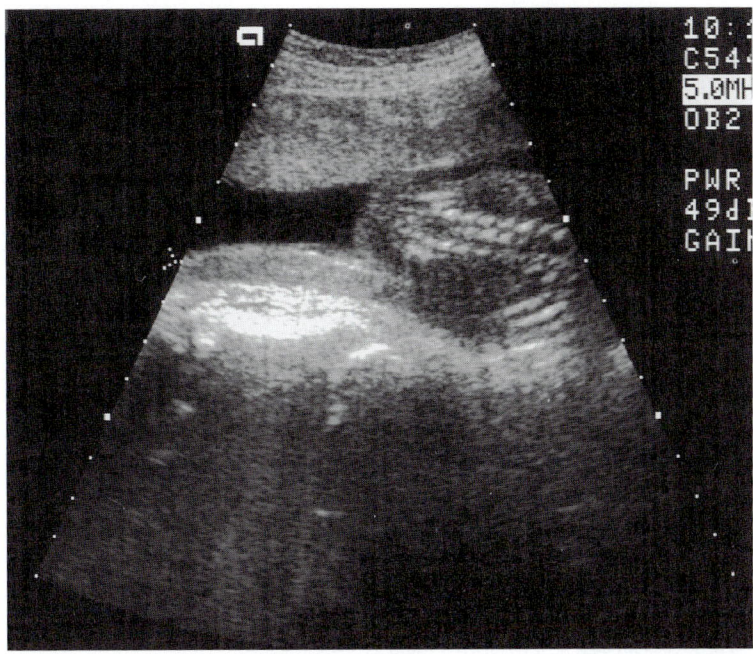

FIGURE 41–5. Coronal view of the lumbosacral spine in an 18-week fetus. (Courtesy of Dr. Jodi Dashe.)

through which a meningeal sac may protrude, forming a *meningocele.* If the sac contains neural elements, as it does in 90 percent of cases, the anomaly is called a *meningomyelocele* (see Fig. 36–11, p. 960). Spine defects can usually be visualized sonographically if the fetal spine is examined with sagittal, transverse, and coronal views (Fig. 41–5). Transverse images provide the best opportunity to detect the presence and extent of defects in the spine and overlying soft tissues. Movement of the lower extremities and urination may be seen despite the presence of neurologically significant spina bifida, and do not predict normal function after birth.

Some spine defects cannot be visualized directly. However, 99 percent of fetuses with spina bifida have one or more of five cranial signs on targeted sonography:

1. Small biparietal diameter.
2. Ventriculomegaly.
3. Frontal bone scalloping (*lemon sign,* see Fig. 37–7, p. 982).
4. Abnormal curvature of the cerebellum (*banana sign*) or cerebellum that cannot be visualized.
5. Effacement or obliteration of the cisterna magna.

These sonographic signs indicate the presence of the *Arnold–Chiari II* malformation, in which the medulla and fourth ventricle are elongated and, in combination with a portion of the cerebellum, extend through the foramen magnum into the upper cervical spinal canal. When a cranial sign is present, but a spine defect cannot be visualized, targeted ultrasound and amniocentesis for amnionic fluid alpha-fetoprotein and acetylcholinesterase measurement may be diagnostic.

CHOROID PLEXUS CYSTS. These cysts form when neuroepithelial folds in the choroid plexus of the lateral ventricle fill with cerebrospinal fluid. They vary in size from 2 to 20 mm and are usually transient, resolving by 24 weeks (Fig. 41–6). They do not interfere with normal brain development and are not associated with functional abnormalities. Because choroid plexus cysts are identified in 70 percent of fetuses with trisomy 18, in the past their presence often prompted genetic amniocentesis. It is now known, however, that these cysts are

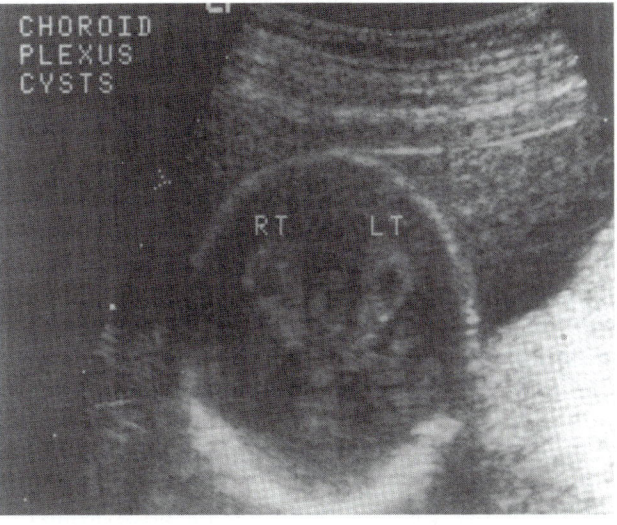

FIGURE 41–6. Bilateral small choroid plexus cysts seen in the lateral ventricles. (From Twickler, 1996.)

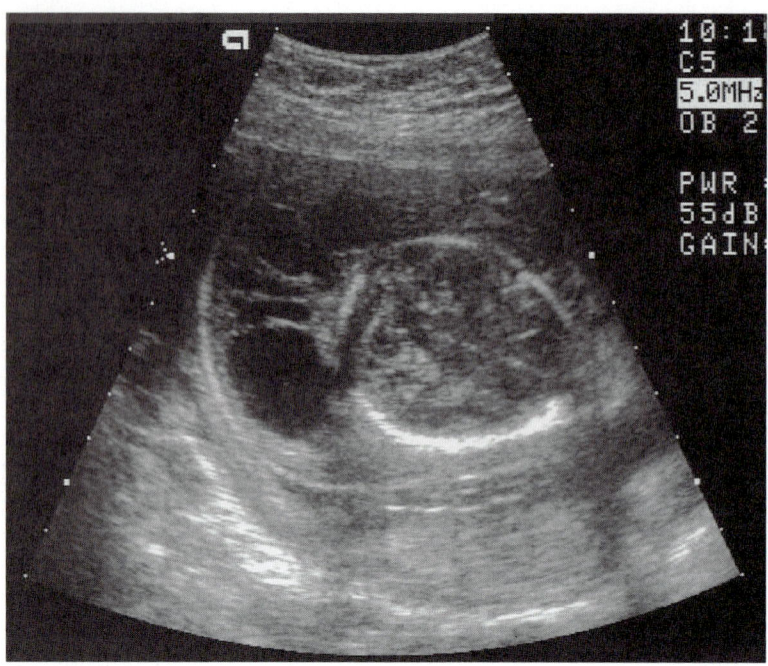

FIGURE 41-7. Large, septated cystic hygromas in a 17-week fetus with Turner syndrome. (Courtesy of Dr. Jodi Dashe.)

found in 1 to 3 percent of normal fetuses (Benacerraf and co-workers, 1990a; Chinn and associates, 1990). As discussed in Chapter 37 (p. 988), identification of choroid plexus cysts should prompt a targeted examination to search for other fetal anomalies. In most cases, if other anomalies are present, the risk of aneuploidy is high enough to warrant genetic amniocentesis (Leonardi and colleagues, 1996).

In the absence of associated findings, genetic amniocentesis likely is not warranted, especially if the age-related risk of aneuploidy is low and maternal serum screening does not indicate increased risk. Benacerraf and co-workers (1990b) calculated that if all second-trimester fetuses with isolated choroid plexus cysts underwent genetic amniocentesis, then 478 procedures would be done to identify each case of trisomy 18. From their meta-analysis, they identified only two cases among 478 such fetuses. Gupta and colleagues (1997) reviewed results from over 200,000 ultrasound examinations to determine the final trisomy 18 risk with isolated cyst according to maternal age. They concluded that invasive genetic testing might be indicated when an isolated cyst is identified in women over age 32.

CYSTIC HYGROMAS. This is a congenital malformation of the lymphatic system that appears as a large, often multiseptated, fluid-filled sac extending off the back or to the sides of the fetal neck (Fig. 41–7). Cystic hygromas usually develop as part of lymphatic obstruction sequence. Lymphatic fluid from the head ordinarily drains into the jugular vein near the heart. If this connection fails to develop by 40 days of gestation, lymph collects in the jugular lymphatic sac, which causes formation of a cystic hygroma in the cervical region. Lymphatic obstruction can also cause cardiac defects. The enlarged thoracic duct impinges on the developing heart, altering blood flow and in some cases leading to the development of hypoplastic left heart, coarctation of the aorta, or other flow-related anomalies.

Cystic hygromas may be identified during routine sonography. They are also detected by abnormal multiple marker screening tests, either because of the associated fetal aneuploidy or because of hydropic changes which lead to elevated hCG and alpha-fetoprotein levels (Saller and colleagues, 1992; Wenstrom and co-workers, 1996). Hygromas may be an isolated finding, part of a genetic syndrome such as Noonan syndrome, or in association with a chromosome anomaly. Approximately 60 to 70 percent are associated with fetal aneuploidy; 45, X (Turner syndrome) accounting for 75 percent, and trisomies 21, 18, 13, and mosaic aneuploidies for the remainder (Johnson, 1993; Romero, 1988; Shulman, 1992, and their colleagues).

Small, simple hygromas identified in the first trimester sometimes resolve. Resolution, however, does not reduce the risk of aneuploidy, and a full diagnostic workup is still performed. Johnson and colleagues (1993) evaluated 68 first-trimester fetuses with simple nuchal cystic hygromas and found that 60 percent were aneuploid. If the karyotype is normal, the prognosis depends largely on whether there is an accompanying heart defect or another genetic syndrome. Fetuses with normal karyotypes and cardiac anatomy and in whom there is spontaneous resolution of the hygroma usually have a good prognosis

(Shulman and co-workers, 1994; Trauffer and collaborators, 1994). These infants may have redundant nuchal tissue (pterygium colli), which can be surgically corrected.

Large, multiseptated lesions virtually never resolve, and have a worse prognosis than those without septations. Brumfield and colleagues (1996) described 61 fetuses with cystic hygroma and reported that those with septated lesions were more likely to have an abnormal karyotype or to develop hydrops, and their survival was significantly diminished. In a similar study of 150 fetuses, Bronshtein and co-workers (1993) found that 94 percent of fetuses with nonseptated hygromas were live born, compared with only 12 percent among fetuses with septated lesions.

THORAX. The fetal lungs develop between 20 and 25 weeks, and are usually visualized after this period. A variety of thoracic malformations can develop. Some of the more common include cystic adenomatoid malformation, bronchopulmonary sequestration, bronchogenic cysts, and chylothorax (Crane and colleagues, 1994; Gonçalves and associates, 1994). Prenatal diagnosis and therapy of these lesions is discussed in Chapter 37 (p. 995). Treadwell and associates (1996) have provided experiences that support a better prognosis than previously reported.

DIAPHRAGMATIC HERNIA. These congenital hernias result from incomplete fusion of the pleuroperitoneal membrane. They occur more frequently on the left, and have a frequency of 1 in 2000 to 5000 births (Callen, 1994; Romero and associates, 1988). The diagnosis and treatment of congenital diaphragmatic hernia is discussed in Chapter 37 (p. 995). Classically, with a left-sided hernia, the four-chamber cardiac view shows the heart pushed to the middle or to the right of the thorax by the stomach or bowel, which appear as cystic structures behind the left atrium. With a right-sided lesion, the liver is visualized in the right thorax, displacing the heart to the far left. Associated findings include absence of an intra-abdominal stomach bubble, a small abdominal circumference, and peristalsis in the fetal chest. Hydramnios is also common and was identified in 75 percent of affected fetuses studied by Adzick and co-workers (1985). Because diaphragmatic hernia is associated with other major anomalies or aneuploidy in almost half of all cases, a thorough evaluation of all fetal structures should be performed and amniocentesis offered.

HEART. As a group, cardiac malformations are the most common congenital anomalies, with an incidence of about 8 in 1000 live births (Chap. 36, p. 960). Almost 90 percent of cardiac defects are multifactorial or polygenic. Another 1 to 2 percent occur as part of a monogenic syndrome such as Holt Oram, Noonan, or a gene-deletion syndrome, which may be suspected after identification of specific associated anomalies. About 1 to 2 percent result from exposure to a teratogen such as isotretinoin or hydantoin or to maternal diabetes. Postnatal data suggest that about 5 percent of infants with congenital cardiac malformations have chromosomal abnormalities; however, this is 30 to 40 percent when a cardiac defect is diagnosed prenatally (Abuhammad, 1997). Approximately 50 to 70 percent of such fetuses will have other (extracardiac) anomalies identifiable sonographically. Nonetheless, the likelihood of aneuploidy or a deletion syndrome with an isolated cardiac malformation is believed to be at least 15 percent. For these reasons, fetal karyotype is indicated in affected fetuses. The most frequently encountered aneuploidies are trisomies 21, 18, and 13, and 45, X (Turner syndrome).

A general examination of the heart—four-chamber view, rate, and rhythm—should be included in the basic ultrasound examination. A more detailed targeted examination should be performed if any of the following risk factors are present: suspected cardiac abnormality seen on the four-chamber view; arrhythmia; presence of extracardiac anomalies; parent or sibling with heart defect; maternal diabetes; teratogen exposure; and nonimmune hydrops. If the fetus is known to have Down or Turner syndrome, or any other genetic syndrome that includes a cardiac defect, the cardiac examination may influence parental decisions.

Heart motion can be visualized sonographically by 6 to 7 weeks, and the four chambers become visible in the second trimester. A detailed cardiac evaluation, however, is usually not possible until at least 18 weeks. Even at this time, adequate anatomical cardiac assessment is dependent on fetal position and activity, maternal size, amnionic fluid volume, and availability of proper equipment and expertise. The study is often time consuming and may require collaboration with a pediatric cardiologist.

The four-chamber view is central to fetal cardiac assessment (Fig. 41–8). This view is obtained by imaging a transverse plane through the fetal thorax at a level just above the diaphragm. This view allows evaluation of the size, location, and orientation of the fetal heart. The atrial and ventricular chambers can be evaluated, the septum primum, foramen ovale, and interventricular septum viewed, and the atrioventricular valves observed. The moderator band is noted in the apex of the right ventricle and the foramen ovale flap in the left atrium. In addition, in some cases, the pulmonary veins and descending aorta are seen. Normally, the two atria and the two ventricles are similar in size, and the apex of the heart forms a 45-degree angle with the left anterior chest wall. The sensitivity of the four-chamber view for the detection of cardiac malformations averages about 50 percent in low-risk women (Abuhammad,

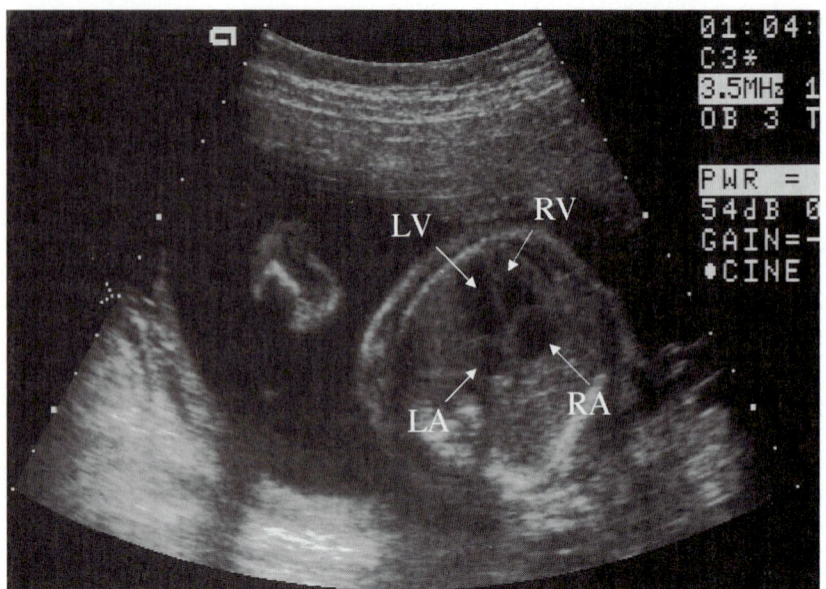

FIGURE 41–8. Transverse sonogram through the thorax of a 24-week fetus demonstrating a four-chamber cardiac view showing the right atrium (RA), left atrium (LA), right ventricle (RV), and left ventricle (LV). (Courtesy of Dr. Jodi Dashe.)

1997). In high-risk women undergoing targeted examination, it is as high as 90 percent (Bromley and associates, 1992; Copel and colleagues, 1987).

The four-chamber view allows evaluation of the cardiac axis, another good screening tool. The apex of the heart should be oriented along an imaginary line 45 degrees (± 15 degrees) to the left of the anterior–posterior dimension (Fig. 41–9). Deviation from that axis, usually to the left, indicates a high risk of cardiac and associated anomalies. Smith and colleagues (1995) evaluated 41,500 second- and third-trimester fetuses and found that 75 percent of those with congenital cardiac malformations had a cardiac axis greater than 75 degrees to the left. In a case-control study of 75 fetuses with congenital heart defects, Shipp and co-workers (1995) found that 45 percent of fetuses with abnormal hearts had left axis deviation, compared with none of the controls.

A complete cardiac evaluation should include examination of the ventricular outflow tracts and blood flow patterns through the heart. Starting with the four-chamber view, slight rotation of the transducer toward the right fetal shoulder shows the aortic outflow tract (long-axis view). In this view, the interventricular septum is visualized to be continuous with the anterior wall of the aorta, and the mitral valve continuous with the posterior aortic wall. Lack of continuity could indicate a ventricular septal defect. Once the aortic outflow tract has been identified, rotating the transducer in the opposite direction will allow visualization of the pulmonary outflow tract, as these two arteries appear to cross each other (Fig. 41–10). The aortic arch is best seen longitudinally (Fig. 41–11). Pulse Doppler and real-time Doppler color-flow mapping can then be used to evaluate blood flow through the fetal cardiovascular system (DeVore and associates, 1987; Shenker and colleagues, 1988). In addition, M-mode echocardiography is essential for arrhythmia evaluation and to measure chamber size, wall thickness, and wall and valve motion.

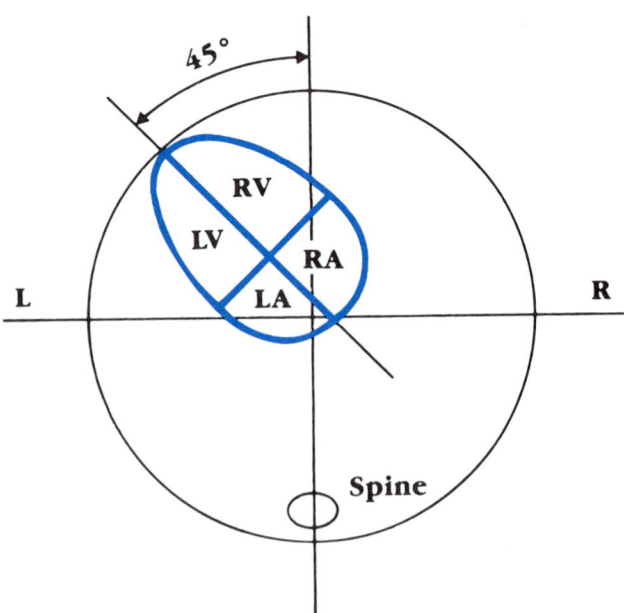

FIGURE 41–9. Measurement of the cardiac axis from the four-chamber view of the fetal heart. (LA = left atrium; LV = left ventricle; RA = right atrium; RV = right ventricle.) (From Comstock, 1987, with permission.)

ACCURACY. Ultrasound examination to detect fetal cardiac disease is imperfect, and its accuracy depends on the operator and the population studied. Crawford and colleagues (1988) reported their experiences with

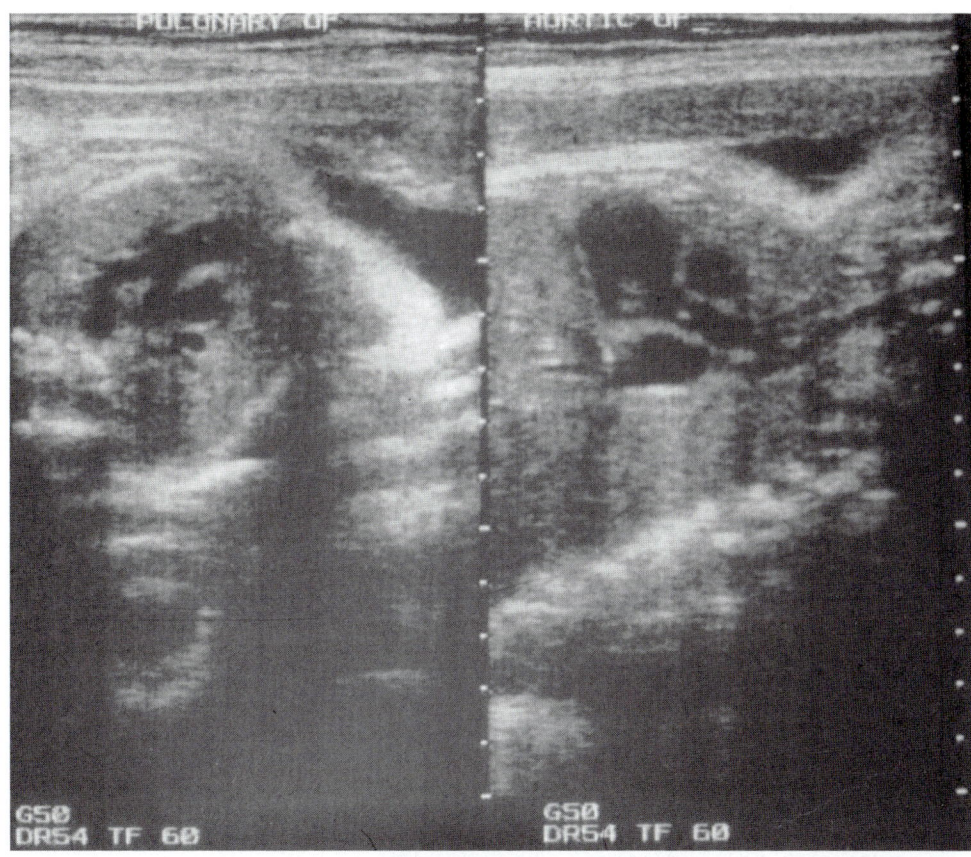

FIGURE 41–10. Views of the pulmonary and aortic outflow tracts from the four-chamber views of fetal heart showing right ventricular outflow (pulmonary artery) on left and left ventricular (aorta) on right.

almost 1000 women at high risk for having children with cardiac abnormalities. They performed over 1750 fetal echocardiograms and successfully identified 74 of 91 anomalies (80 percent). In almost half of those with cardiac anomalies, chromosomal or extracardiac structural defects were also found. They emphasized that heart disease diagnosed prenatally is often severe and is associated with a poor long-term prognosis.

By way of contrast, Benacerraf and associates (1987) studied a group of women who underwent ultrasonic studies for multiple reasons. Although 49 fetuses were subsequently found to have 66 cardiac defects, only 33 (50 percent) of these were detected antenatally. According to both of these reports, ventricular septal defects, anomalous pulmonary venous return, and aortic or pulmonic stenosis were especially likely to be missed by fetal ultrasound evaluation. Additionally, those cardiac defects characterized by inadequate growth—for example, hypoplastic left heart or aortic stenosis—may not have fully developed at the time of the midtrimester examination.

Ott (1995) reported a 14 percent sensitivity for detection of congenital heart disease in a low-risk population,

compared with 63 percent in the high-risk group. Lanouette and co-workers (1996) correctly emphasized that routine cardiac views are not consistently available for each routine ultrasound examination. They calculated the adjusted positive-predictive value to be about 55 percent. Berghella and associates (1996) found that collaboration with pediatric cardiologists significantly improved characterization of lesions in some cases. All women undergoing targeted ultrasound examination should be counseled about its limitations to detect fetal abnormalities, particularly certain types of cardiac malformations.

GASTROINTESTINAL TRACT. Using high-resolution diagnostic sonography, the integrity of the abdominal wall, umbilical cord insertion, and intraabdominal organs can be assessed with confidence (Fig. 41–12). The liver, spleen, gallbladder, and bowel can be identified in most fetuses. The stomach should be clearly identified during all examinations, as it is visible in 98 percent of fetuses after 14 weeks. Nonvisualization of the stomach is associated with an abnormal outcome in about half of fetuses studied after 14 weeks and 100 percent after

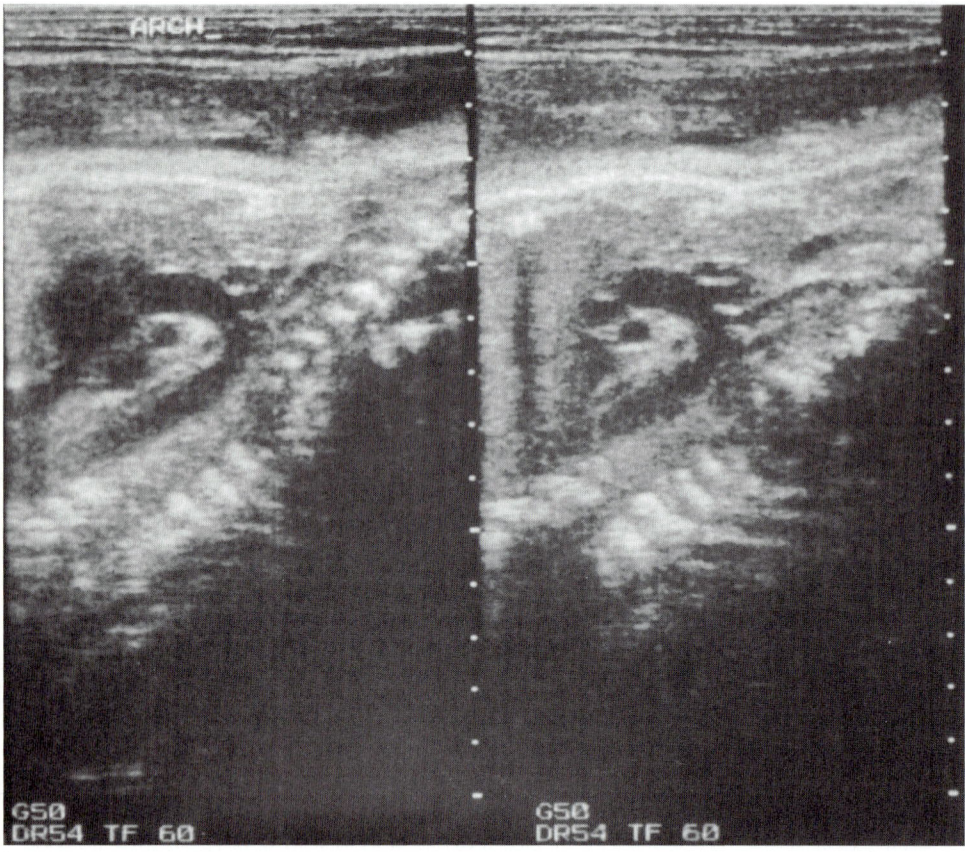

FIGURE 41–11. Longitudinal view of the aortic arch.

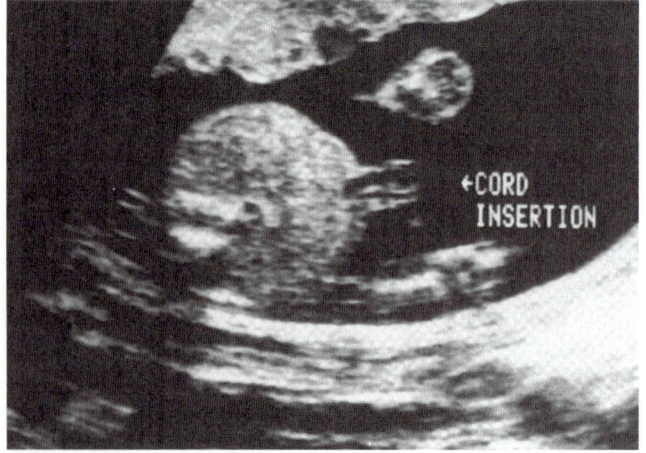

FIGURE 41–12. Transverse sonogram of a second-trimester fetus with an intact anterior abdominal wall and normal cord insertion. (From Lowe and associates, 1990.)

19 weeks (Millener and colleagues, 1993; Pretorius and co-workers, 1988). Associated abnormalities include tracheoesophageal fistula, esophageal atresia, diaphragmatic hernia, abdominal wall defects, and neurological abnormalities that inhibit fetal swallowing. Repeat sonograms should be performed for all cases of stomach nonvisualization, although subsequent visualization does not guarantee a normal outcome. Millener and co-workers (1993) evaluated 7200 sonograms performed after 14 weeks' gestation and found that a third of cases in which the stomach was seen on a subsequent examination had an abnormal outcome.

Normally, the appearance of the fetal bowel changes with gestational age, and considerable overlap exists between the sonographic appearance of normal and pathological conditions (Hertzberg, 1994). A common finding is **hyperechogenic bowel,** which has been associated with fetal aneuploidy and other genetic syndromes such as cystic fibrosis. Hyperechogenic bowel is generally defined as having a brightness equivalent to or greater than that of bone. The appearance of hyperechogenicity is affected by the transducer frequency, as it is much more likely to be visualized using a frequency of

8 MHz than 5 MHz (Vincoff and associates, 1999). One way to confirm hyperechogenicity is to isolate a view in which both bowel and bone (iliac crest) can be clearly visualized. Then, using a frequency of 5 MHz, gradually turn down the gain. If the bowel echogenicity disappears before the bone, it is not truly hyperechogenic (Slotnick and Abuhamad, 1996). Truly hyperechogenic bowel indicates an increased risk for aneuploidy, cystic fibrosis, congenital infection, and associated malformations (Berlin and collaborators, 1999; Yaron and co-workers, 1999). Some clinicians believe this should prompt a complete fetal evaluation, but others believe that as an isolated finding that only targeted ultrasonography is indicated. Hyperechogenic bowel has also been associated with bleeding into the amnionic fluid and unexplained fetal death (Nyberg and associates, 1993).

ABDOMINAL WALL DEFECTS. These defects as a group are relatively common malformations. The two most common are omphalocele and gastroschisis, and each has a frequency of approximately 1 in 5000 live births. Because of maternal serum alpha-fetoprotein screening programs and the performance of routine sonograms, these two defects are usually ascertained early in pregnancy. Although they have many similarities, it is important to recognize that they differ markedly in developmental pathology, association with other major abnormalities, and prognosis.

Gastroschisis is the result of an early vascular accident causing occlusion of either the right umbilical vein (the left vein persists in the cord) or the terminal segment of the right omphalomesenteric artery. The resulting localized ischemia produces a full-thickness defect in the abdominal wall to the right of the umbilical cord insertion, through which bowel can herniate into the amnionic cavity (Fig. 41–13). Because it occurs as the result of a vascu-

lar accident, it does not have the same associations with aneuploidy as does omphalocele. However, associated bowel defects have been reported in 10 to 30 percent of cases (Hoyme and co-workers, 1983). They usually have a good prognosis with survival of 80 to 90 percent (Callen, 1994). In rare cases the defect can be large enough to permit liver herniation, in which case the necessary reconstructive surgery is more complex and the outcome less sure. Gastroschisis is identified by the presence of extra-abdominal bowel floating free in the amnionic fluid, with the umbilical cord inserting in the usual place on the fetal abdomen.

An **omphalocele** occurs when there is failure of the lateral ectomesodermal folds to meet in the midline of the abdomen between the third and fourth weeks. As a result, the abdominal contents are covered only by a thin, two-layered sac composed of amnion and peritoneum, and the umbilical cord inserts into the apex of the sac (Fig. 41–14). It is associated with aneuploidy in 35 to 60 percent of cases—particularly trisomy 13, 18, and 20. It may occur as part of a genetic syndrome such as Beckwith–Weidemann syndrome or pentalogy of Cantrell (Callen, 1994). Omphalocele is also associated with other major anomalies in 50 to 70 percent of cases. Romero and colleagues (1988) described cardiac anomalies (45 percent), genitourinary anomalies (40 percent), and neural-tube defects (40 percent). The prognosis is thus determined not only by the size of the defect, but by the etiology and accompanying abnormalities. Recognition of an omphalocele mandates a complete fetal evaluation, including karyotype.

GASTROINTESTINAL ATRESIA. Most atresias are characterized by obstruction with proximal bowel dilatation.

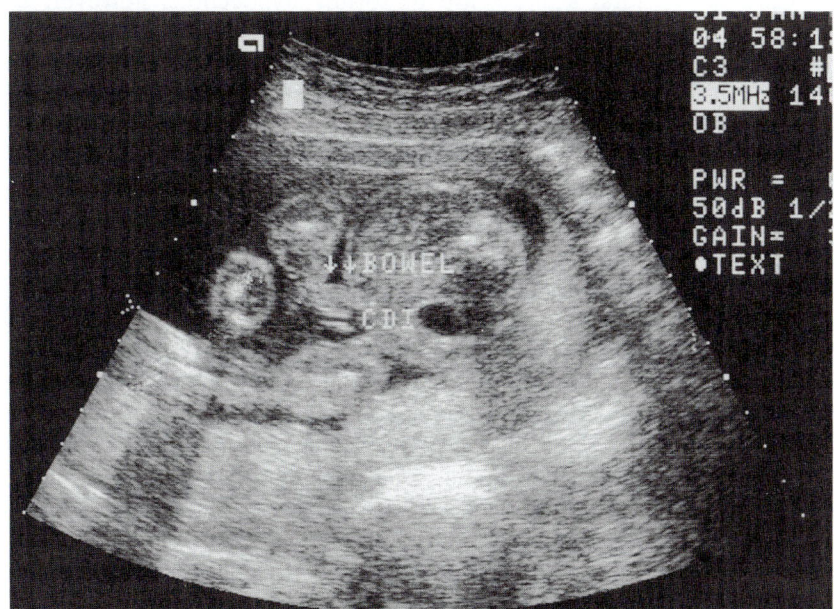

FIGURE 41–13. Transverse view of the abdomen showing gastroschisis with normal cord insertion (CDI), and exteriorized bowel protruding through a defect just lateral to the cord.

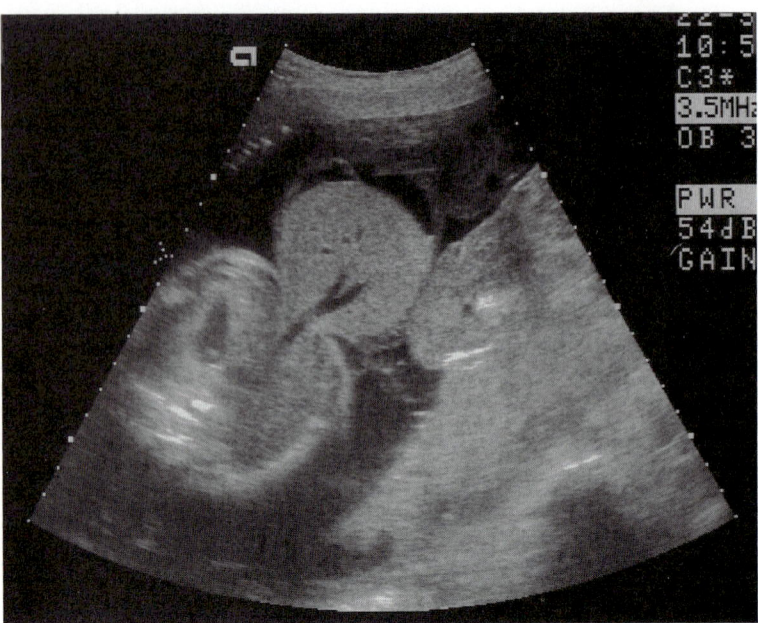

FIGURE 41–14. Transverse view of the abdomen showing an omphalocele as a large abdominal wall defect with exteriorized liver covered by a thin membrane. (Photograph courtesy of Dr. Jodi Dashe.)

In general, the more proximal the obstruction, the more likely it is to be associated with hydramnios. **Esophageal atresia** is one of the most common gastrointestinal anomalies, and is encountered in about 1 in 3000 births (Robertson and colleagues, 1994). The diagnosis is suspected when hydramnios is found in the absence of a fluid-filled stomach. This is an uncommon presentation, however, because up to 90 percent of cases are associated with a **tracheoesophageal fistula.** The latter cannot be diagnosed reliably in utero because the fistula permits fluid to enter the stomach (Pretorius and colleagues, 1987a). About half of fetuses with esophageal atresia have associated anomalies, including aneuploidy in 20 percent and growth restriction in 40 percent. Cardiac malformations are especially common.

Duodenal atresia occurs in about 1 in 10,000 live births (Robertson and colleagues, 1994). The lesion may be diagnosed prenatally by the demonstration of the *double-bubble sign,* which represents distention of the stomach and the first part of the duodenum (Fig. 41–15). Demonstrating continuity between these two structures will differentiate duodenal atresia from other causes of cystic structures in the fetal abdomen. The diagnosis of duodenal atresia generally is difficult before 24 weeks, although it has been made as early as 19 weeks (Romero and associates, 1988). About 30 percent of cases diagnosed antenatally have trisomy 21 and more than half have other associated anomalies. Obstructions in the lower small bowel usually result in multiple dilated loops, which may have increased peristaltic activity.

Large bowel obstructions and **anal atresia** are less readily diagnosed in utero because hydramnios is not a typical feature and the bowel may not be significantly dilated. The transverse view through the pelvis may reveal a fluid-filled structure (the enlarged rectum) between the bladder and the sacrum.

GENITOURINARY TRACT. Using transabdominal sonography, the fetal kidneys are visualized as paraspinous masses frequently as early as 14 weeks, and routinely by 18 weeks (Patten and co-workers, 1990). Using transvaginal sonography, the kidneys are visible before 14 weeks (Bronshtein and colleagues, 1990). Normal kidneys appear elliptical in parasagittal planes (Fig. 41–16) and circular in transverse planes (Fig. 41–17). Initially, fetal kidneys are uniformly hypoechoic; however, as pregnancy advances, more detail is visualized. The renal cortex, which is echogenic, surrounds the hypoechoic medullary pyramids and is outlined by perinephric fat and the renal capsule. The renal pelvis is centrally located and anechoic. An adrenal gland sits atop each kidney like a cap covering the upper pole, and appears very hypoechoic. They may be overlooked under ordinary circumstances, but become more visible when there is renal agenesis.

Nomograms have been developed that describe fetal kidney dimensions throughout pregnancy (Sagi and associates, 1987). In general, the kidney length in millimeters is roughly equivalent to the menstrual age in weeks (Callen, 1994). In general, the anterior–posteior (AP) dimension of the renal pelvis should be less than half of the entire kidney AP dimension.

Urine production normally begins late in the first trimester, and consequently the fetal bladder can be observed as an anechoic area in the pelvis early in the

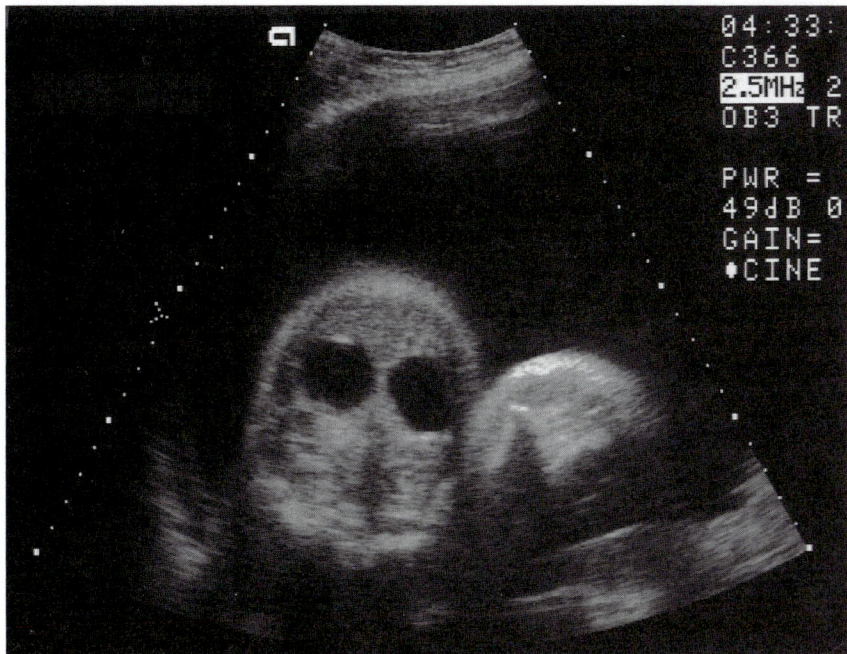

FIGURE 41–15. "Double bubble" of duodenal atresia is seen on this axial abdominal image of the fetus. (Photograph courtesy of Dr. Jodi Dashe.)

second trimester. Fetal urine production increases from 5 mL/hr at 20 weeks to about 50 mL/hr at 40 weeks (Rabinowitz and co-workers, 1989). In the normal fetus, the bladder fills and empties every 20 to 45 minutes. The placenta and membranes can produce normal amounts of amnionic fluid early in gestation. After 16 to 20 weeks, most of the fluid is produced by the kidneys, and otherwise unexplained oligohydramnios suggests a urinary abnormality. Conversely, normal amnionic fluid volume in the second half of pregnancy suggests urinary tract patency with at least one functioning kidney.

The overall incidence of fetal renal anomalies is cited as 0.2 to 1.4 percent. Several large prospective screening programs have reported that the incidence and type of anomaly identified depends on gestational age. For example, before 24 weeks, the detection of urinary tract anomalies is reported to be relatively low, and identified lesions tend to be serious or lethal. After 24 weeks, their detection increases, but identified lesions are less severe. Importantly, various forms of obstruction tend to develop over time. As shown in Table 41–5, obstruction accounts for the majority of urinary tract defects identified at birth.

Fugelseth and colleagues (1994) performed ultrasound examination at 17 and 32 weeks on 22,310 women. They identified 47 (0.18 percent) urinary tract abnormalities, of which 62 percent were found only at the second screening. Approximately half the anomalies were hydronephrosis and 20 percent were multicystic kidney, both of which develop over time. Gunn and co-workers (1995) prospectively evaluated 3856 fetuses after 28 weeks for obstetrical indications. Significant renal tract anomalies were identified prenatally and confirmed at birth in 55 fetuses (1.4 percent). These lesions included renal agenesis, multicystic dysplasia, and various types of reflux.

OBSTRUCTIVE UROPATHY. Renal agenesis, multicystic dysplasia, and various urinary tract abnormalities all result from obstruction. Timing of insult determines the outcome. Obstruction at the ureteropelvic junction is most common. It affects males twice as often as females. Renal function is likely to be preserved even with promi-

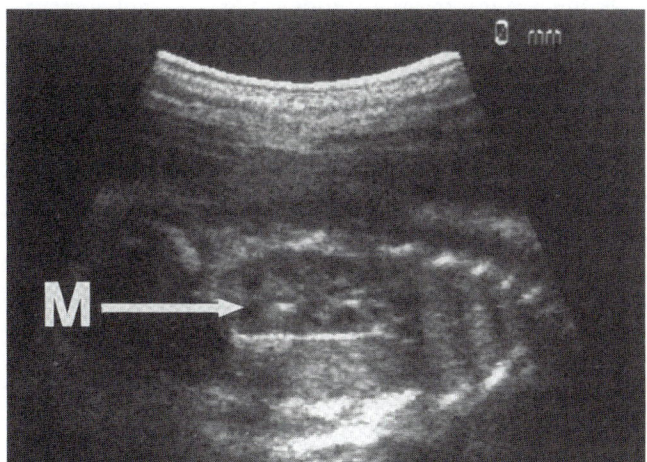

FIGURE 41–16. Longitudinal sonogram of a fetal kidney. The hypoechoic medullary pyramids (M) are depicted. (From Lowe and associates, 1990.)

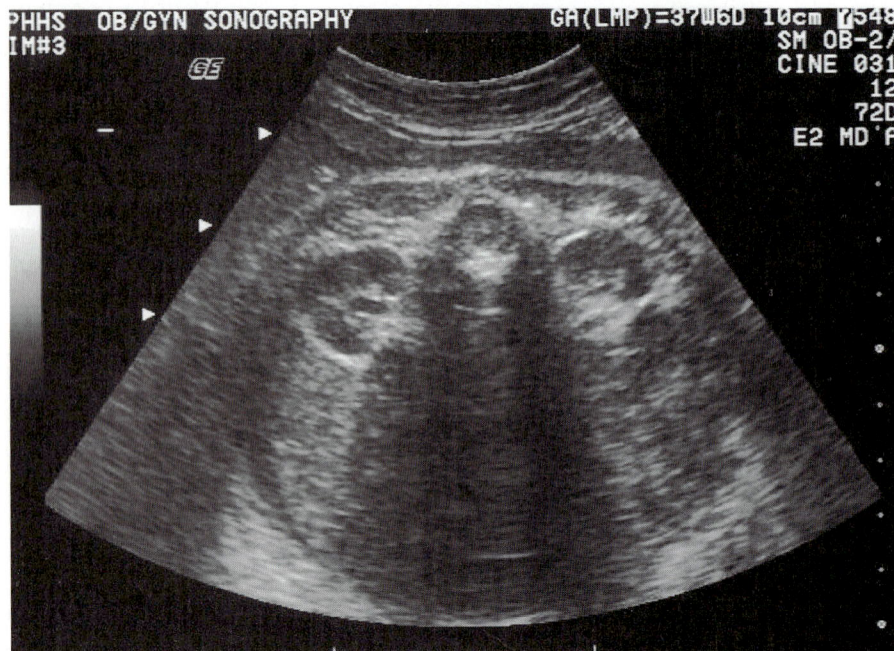

FIGURE 41–17. Transverse sonogram of a fetus demonstrating kidneys with anechoic renal pelves. (Photograph courtesy of Dr. Jodi Dashe.)

nent pelvic dilatation, because the obstruction is most often a functional one, unlike urethral obstructions, which are more often anatomical. Obstruction is bilateral in a third of cases, and when unilateral, there is an increased likelihood of anomalies involving the contralateral kidney, particularly multicystic dysplasia (see later discussion).

Obstruction can also occur at the ureterovesical junction or at the urethra. The severity and location of the obstruction can be determined by assessing amnionic fluid volume and the location of dilatation within the urinary tract. Renal pelvis dilatation usually indicates obstruction at the ureteropelvic junction or possibly at the ureterovesical junction. As a general rule, normal fetal ureters cannot be visualized, and thus their identi-

fication indicates hydroureter due to a lower block; for example, posterior urethral valves. Bladder outlet obstruction is usually accompanied by enlargement of the bladder and hydroureter.

Mild hydronephrosis (up to 4 to 5 mm) occurs in 2 to 3 percent of normal fetuses in the second trimester, but in as many as 25 percent with trisomy 21. In the absence of other risk factors, the likelihood that a fetus with isolated mild pyelectasis will have trisomy 21 is estimated to be only 1 in 340. Thus, amniocentesis is not usually performed for this finding alone (Benacerraf and colleagues, 1990b).

After 20 weeks the fetal renal pelves may be easily visible, and by convention, they are measured in the AP dimension. Based on studies that included postnatal follow-up, upper limits of the normal pelvis is 4 mm before 33 weeks and 7 mm after 33 weeks (Corteville, 1991; Mandell, 1991; Wilson, 1997, and their colleagues). Alternatively, Grignon and colleagues (1986) reported that dilatation less than 10 mm is usually physiological. While the size of the pelvis increases along with maternal hydration, it returns to normal (Robinson and co-workers, 1998).

Diagnosis of renal pelvis dilatation is important because it may identify those fetuses who require neonatal intervention to preserve kidney function. Ghidini and cohorts (1990) reported results from 70 fetuses with ureteropelvic junction obstruction. Those with renal pelvis dilatation less than 1 cm uniformly did well, whereas three fourths of those with dilatation more than 2 cm required postnatal pyeloplasty. Surprisingly, those with dilatation of 1 to 2 cm—about half of the total—did well if

TABLE 41–5. Frequency of Selected Urinary Tract Abnormalities in 72 Neonates

Abnormality	No.	Percent
Hydronephrosis and hydroureter	27	38
Renal cystic disease	13	18
Vesicoureteric reflux	9	12
Unilateral renal agenesis or hypoplasia	5	7
Duplication of collecting system	4	6
Urethral valves	3	4
Bilateral renal agenesis	2	3
Others	9	12

Adapted from Helin and Persson (1986) and Livera and co-workers (1989).

the findings were bilateral. Conversely, about 10 percent with unilateral dilatation of this magnitude eventually required pyeloplasty. Similarly, Adra and colleagues (1995) followed 84 cases of fetal pyelectasis and found that two thirds of those with renal pelves greater than 8 mm had renal pathology at birth, including ureteropelvic junction obstruction in 37 percent, vesicoureteral reflux in 33 percent, and problems such as malformations of the ureters or collecting system in the remainder.

RENAL AGENESIS. This has an incidence of about 1 in 4000 births. No kidneys are visualized sonographically at any point during gestation. The adrenal glands typically enlarge and occupy the renal fossae, and can be mistaken for kidneys. Without kidneys there is no urine production and the severe oligohydramnios that develops leads to pulmonary hypoplasia, limb contractures, a distinctive compressed face (Fig. 41–18), and ultimately death. When this combination of abnormalities is caused by renal agenesis, it is called *Potter syndrome,* after

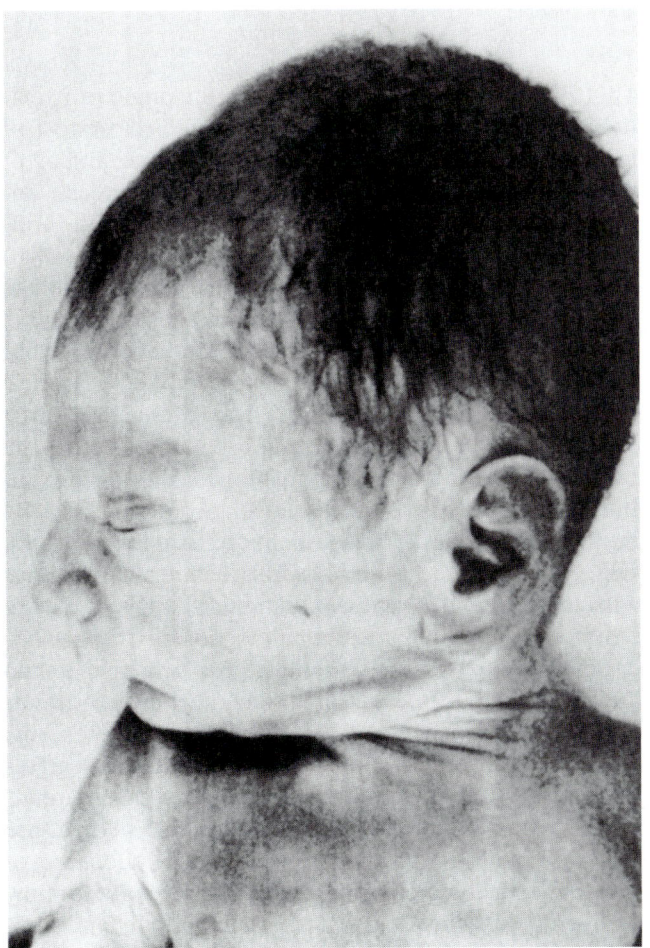

FIGURE 41–18. Infant with typical "Potter face," which is characteristic of renal agenesis and early oligohydramnios. (From Zerres and colleagues, 1984, with permission.)

E. L. Potter who described it in 1946. When these abnormalities result from oligohydramnios of some other etiology, it is called *oligohydramnios sequence.*

The recurrence risk for isolated bilateral renal agenesis is generally quoted as 3 percent, but a fetal autopsy is essential to rule out a mendelian syndrome, which could have a recurrence risk as high as 50 percent. The diagnosis of fetal renal agenesis should also prompt sonographic evaluation of the kidneys of parents and siblings. Roodhooft and colleagues (1984) showed that 13 percent of the first-degree relatives of fetuses with isolated bilateral renal agenesis had unilateral agenesis or other asymptomatic renal malformations. If a parent or sibling is discovered to be affected, the recurrence risk is much higher.

POLYCYSTIC KIDNEY DISEASE. Of the hereditary polycystic diseases, only autosomal recessive infantile polycystic kidneys may be reliably diagnosed antenatally. The autosomal dominant condition usually does not manifest until adulthood, but prenatal diagnosis has been described (Pretorius and associates, 1987b). Infantile polycystic kidney disease is characterized by abnormally large kidneys that fill the fetal abdomen and appear to have a solid, ground-glass texture. The abdominal circumference is enlarged, and there is usually severe oligohydramnios. The polycystic changes of these kidneys can only be identified microscopically.

MULTICYSTIC DYSPLASTIC KIDNEYS. These result from complete obstruction or atresia at the level of the renal pelvis or proximal ureter prior to 10 weeks (Callen, 1994). An affected kidney is partially or completely nonfunctional, and the diagnosis can usually be made antenatally. Sonographically there is abnormally dense renal parenchyma with multiple peripheral cysts of varying sizes that do not communicate with each other or the renal pelvis. This distinguishes them from obstructive pelviectasis, in which the fluid-filled areas do connect. If the insult occurred very early, the kidneys may simply be abnormally small—less than the fifth percentile in all three dimensions—and dense. Later insults can produce abnormally large dimensions.

Most often, segmental dysplasia is unilateral. Contralateral renal anomalies occur in 40 percent of cases; the most common is ureteropelvic junction obstruction (Callen, 1994; Kleiner and colleagues, 1986). The prognosis is generally good if findings are unilateral and amnionic fluid volume is normal, although occasionally the normal-appearing kidney may have segmental dysplastic changes that cannot be visualized sonographically. If multicystic dysplasia is bilateral, this generally has an extremely poor prognosis. Even if amnionic fluid volume remains adequate, antenatal destruction of renal tissue may result in neonatal renal failure.

DOPPLER VELOCIMETRY

The Doppler shift is a physical principle that states that when a source of light or sound waves is moving relative to an observer, the observer detects a shift in the wave frequency. Thus, when sound waves strike a moving target, the frequency of the sound waves reflected back is shifted proportionate to the velocity and direction of the moving target. Because the magnitude and direction of the frequency shift depend on the relative motion of the moving target, their velocity and direction can be determined.

Important to obstetrics, the Doppler principle is used to determine the volume and rate of blood flow through maternal and fetal vessels. In this situation the sound source is the ultrasound transducer, the moving target is the red blood cells flowing through the circulation, and the reflected sound waves are observed by the ultrasound transducer. Two kinds of Doppler are used in medicine. The continuous wave Doppler machine has two crystals—one that transmits a high-frequency sound wave, and another that continuously receives signals. It can record high frequencies using low power output and is easy to use. Unfortunately, it is nonselective, recognizing all signals along its path, and does not allow visualization of the blood vessel(s). In M-mode echocardiography, continuous wave Doppler is used to evaluation motion through time. It defines the blood flow through the heart, but because the cardiac structures are not visualized it requires the correlation with the sequence of waveforms produced with the sequence of structures interrogated by the sound wave.

The other type, pulse wave Doppler, has equipment that uses only one crystal, which transmits the signal and then waits until the returning signal is received before transmitting another one. It is more expensive and requires higher power, but allows precise targeting and visualization of the vessel of interest. Pulse wave Doppler can also be configured to allow color-flow mapping, in which computer software makes blood flowing away from the transducer look blue and blood flowing toward the transducer look red.

Various combinations of continuous Doppler, pulse wave Doppler, color-flow Doppler, and real-time ultrasound are commercially available, and are loosely referred to as duplex Doppler. Doppler is generally used in two ways to estimate circulatory hemodynamics:

1. Direct measurement of the volume of blood flow.
2. Indirect estimation of flow velocity using waveform analysis.

BLOOD FLOW MEASUREMENT. Doppler-shifted sound frequencies depend on a number of factors (Fig.

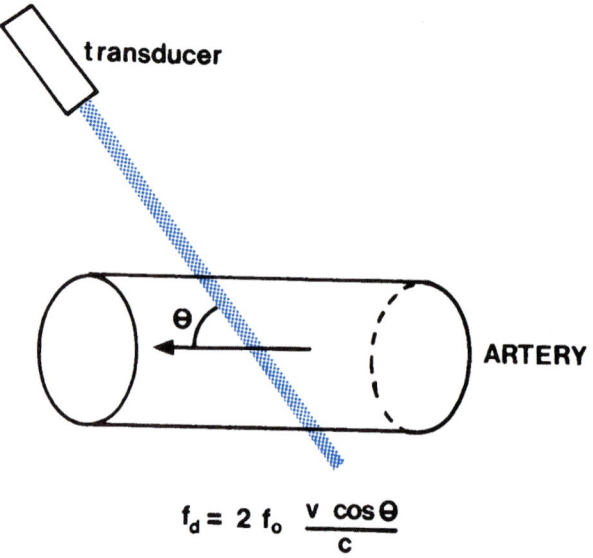

$$f_d = 2 f_o \frac{v \cos \Theta}{c}$$

FIGURE 41–19. Doppler equation: ultrasound emanating from transducer with initial frequency f_o strikes blood moving at velocity (v). Reflected frequency f_d is dependent on angle Θ between beam of sound and vessel. (From Copel and associates, 1988b.)

41–19). Pragmatic concerns include the angle of isonation (Θ). The cosine of this angle remains close to 1 as long as the angle is kept low, but at higher angles of insonance, especially those more than 60 degrees, considerable error in measurement is introduced. Thus measurements are better if flow is directed "head on" to the transducer, a feat sometimes difficult to accomplish.

The equation in Figure 41–19 includes a factor (v) for the velocity of blood in the vessel studied. The equation is used to estimate the velocity of red cells and derivatives from that factor. Because volume flow (mL/min) is simply velocity times cross-sectional area of the blood vessel (area equals pi times the square of the radius), it is possible to calculate volume flow by measuring the blood vessel diameter using ultrasound. Unfortunately, there are several technical difficulties with measurement of vessel diameters. The vessels are dynamic with changing diameters during the cardiac cycle, and their measurement is very sensitive to the angle of insonation. The many technical difficulties inherent in Doppler blood volume flow measurements result in high error rates for this methodology. Estimates of error up to 15 percent have been reported even under the best circumstances, and errors up to 50 percent are not uncommon (Burns, 1987; Gill, 1985). Because of these methodological problems, blood volume flow measurements have been largely abandoned in clinical applications.

BLOOD VELOCITY WAVEFORM ANALYSIS. Errors encountered in direct measurement of the volume of blood flow have led to development of several indirect indices of flow that compare different parts of the waveform. Because the indices are independent of the angle of insonation and do not require measurement of the diameter of the vessel, they provide useful information about flow without engendering excessive errors.

Doppler waveforms of vessels have been described in a variety of ways, but all the calculated indices are based upon the relationship between systole and diastole. The simplest of these indices to compute is the ratio of the maximal systolic flow velocity to the minimal end-diastolic flow velocity, or S/D ratio (Fig. 41–20). By evaluating blood flow during diastole, the S/D ratio provides an estimation of downstream resistance. In nonpregnant individuals, S/D ratios can be obtained only from the carotid and renal arteries, because only these arteries maintain continuous diastolic blood flow visible on waveform analysis. During pregnancy, the uterine and umbilical arteries normally maintain diastolic blood flow and the normal placental bed is characterized by low resistance and high blood flow. Thus the most useful S/D ratios are obtained from the maternal uterine or fetal umbilical arteries, and provide an indirect estimate of the adequacy of blood flow to the fetus. Blood flow velocity has also been studied in the umbilical vein and fetal cerebral circulation. Because of the low diastolic velocities seen in more central fetal vessels, such as the descending aorta, the S/D ratio is not useful elsewhere in the fetal circulation. Figure 41–21 illustrates several of the vessels in which S/D ratios have

been studied, as well as the corresponding S/D waveforms for blood velocity in these vessels.

The resistance to umbilical artery blood flow during diastole is initially high but decreases as gestation progresses; the S/D ratio decreases from about 4.0 at 20 weeks to about 2.0 at 40 weeks. An easy-to-remember rule is that the S/D ratio is generally less than 3.0 after 30 weeks (Fleischer and associates, 1985). Increases in S/D ratio can be found with maternal hypertension, lupus, and poorly controlled insulin-dependent diabetes. Elevated S/D ratios have been associated with fetal growth restriction and have been used as a screen for "fetal stress." Because there is a fair amount of variation in the S/D ratio, however, it is generally not used alone to direct pregnancy management. One exception to this rule concerns absent or reversed diastolic flow. This is a particularly ominous finding indicating extreme downstream resistance, placental dysfunction, and fetal compromise (Fig. 41–22). Absent diastolic flow should prompt a complete fetal evaluation, because almost half of cases may be due to fetal aneuploidy or a major congenital abnormality (Wenstrom and associates, 1991). In the absence of a fetal anomaly or a reversible maternal medical complication, absent or reversed end-diastolic flow should prompt consideration for delivery.

Another measure of resistance to blood flow is provided by the Pourcelot index, or resistance index (Fig. 41–20). This index is the difference between the systolic and diastolic values, divided by the systolic value ([S − D]/S, also expressed as 1 − [D/S]). This ratio is also applicable only to the umbilical and the uterine arteries, as low diastolic values limit its usefulness in the fetal aorta or other central vessels. The most complicated index to measure is the pulsatility index (systolic–diastolic/time-averaged velocity). It requires a digitized waveform for calculating the mean of the maximal frequencies represented. Because of the mean value in the denominator, this index can be computed using flow data from the fetal descending aorta without encountering the excessive variation that can be caused by division by small numbers as with the other two indices.

TECHNIQUES FOR SPECIFIC VESSELS

UTERINE AND ARCUATE ARTERIES. Uterine blood flow increases from 50 mL/min shortly after conception, to 500 to 750 mL/min by term. Its Doppler waveform shape is unique, characterized by high diastolic velocities similar to those in systole and highly turbulent flow, with many different velocities apparent (Fig. 41–21). The diastolic velocity increases and thus the indices decrease as term approaches (Hendricks and co-workers, 1989). A failure of this pattern to appear or the presence of a notch in the waveform at end-systole has

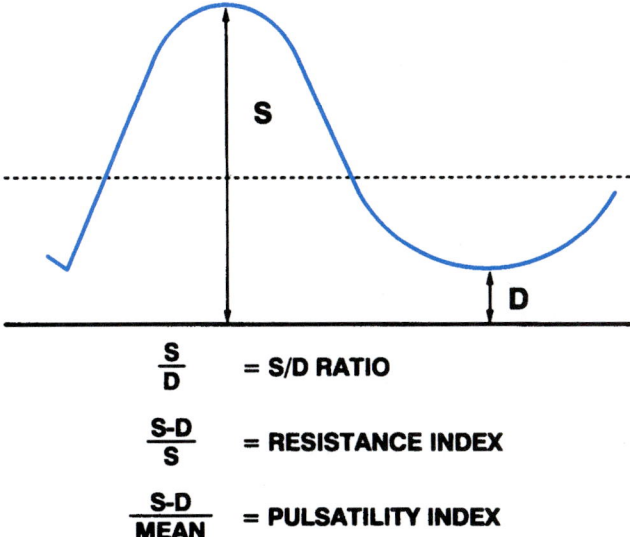

$$\frac{S}{D} = \text{S/D RATIO}$$

$$\frac{S-D}{S} = \text{RESISTANCE INDEX}$$

$$\frac{S-D}{\text{MEAN}} = \text{PULSATILITY INDEX}$$

FIGURE 41–20. Doppler systolic-diastolic waveform indices of blood flow velocity. Mean is calculated from computer digitized waveforms. (D = diastole; S = systole.) (From Low, 1991, with permission.)

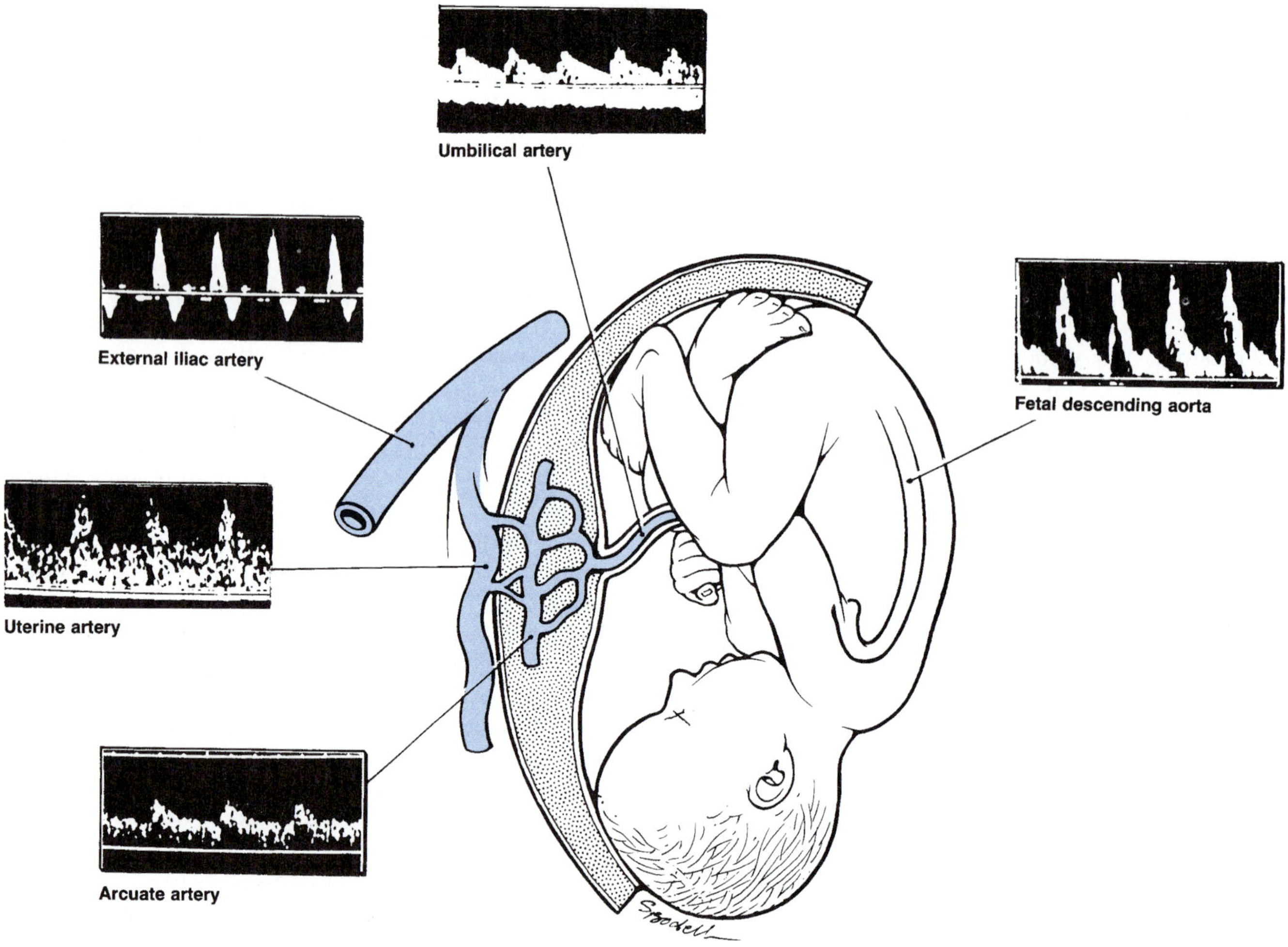

Umbilical artery

External iliac artery

Uterine artery

Arcuate artery

Fetal descending aorta

FIGURE 41–21. Doppler waveform from normal pregnancy. Shown clockwise are normal waveform from the maternal arcuate, uterine, and external iliac arteries, and from the fetal umbilical artery and descending aorta. Reversed end-diastolic flow velocity is apparent in the external iliac artery, whereas continuous diastolic flow characterizes the uterine and arcuate vessels. Finally, note the greatly diminished end-diastolic flow in the fetal descending aorta. (From Copel and colleagues, 1988b.)

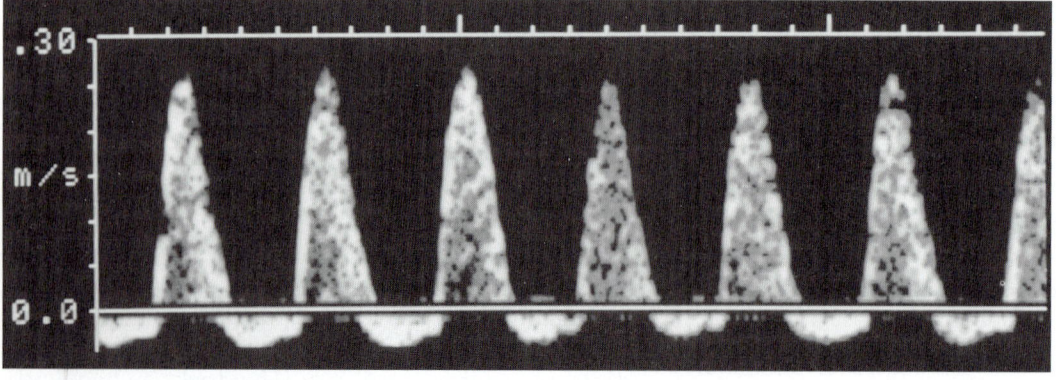

FIGURE 41–22. Doppler velocimetry demonstrating reversed diastolic flow. (Courtesy of Dr. Diane Twickler.)

been reported with fetal growth restriction (Schulman and associates, 1986). The external iliac arteries can be distinguished from the uterine arteries because they normally do not have diastolic flow (Fig. 46–21).

UMBILICAL VEIN. The intra-abdominal portion of the umbilical vein is relatively straight and the flow tends to be constant rather than pulsating. Therefore, the umbilical vein is a reasonable vessel for measuring volume flow rather than indexed flow. Umbilical vein blood flow measurements range from 108 to 153 mL/kg per minute, with decreasing flows as gestation advances (Gerson and co-workers, 1987).

FETAL DESCENDING AORTA. The descending aorta receives the majority of right-ventricular output via the ductus arteriosus, while the majority of left-ventricular output supplies the fetal head and upper arms. Flow in the descending aorta is highly pulsatile, with little diastolic flow. The straight course of the aorta also makes it amenable to volume flow studies. Waveform flow measurement is limited to the pulsatility index because of the lack of diastolic flow. Measurements of fetal descending aorta blood flow range from 185 to 246 mL/kg per minute (Eik-Nes and co-workers, 1982; Griffin and associates, 1985).

CEREBRAL BLOOD FLOW. Fetal heart rate testing evaluates the central nervous system control of cardiac function, which can be altered by cerebral hypoxemia. It has been hypothesized that Doppler evaluation of blood flow through cerebral vessels might allow detection of altered cerebral circulation before hypoxemia significant enough to change the fetal heart rate has occurred. The carotid arteries can be identified reliably, but they are too narrow to measure accurately. The middle cerebral artery is the most accessible vessel, and has been reported to demonstrate reductions in the pulsatility index at the onset of hypoxemia (Wladimiroff and co-workers, 1987). Chandran and colleagues (1993) compared middle cerebral artery pulsatility indices with fetal heart rate analysis in 27 growth-restricted fetuses. They found that Doppler was a more sensitive predictor of hypoxemia at birth than fetal heart rate testing (100 versus 82 percent) but had a lower specificity (50 versus 75 percent).

Middle cerebral artery (MCA) Doppler has been used to assess fetuses with anti-D isoimmunization. Mari and colleagues (1997) studied MCA blood velocity in 135 fetuses, and reported that the velocity increases at a predictable rate with advancing gestational age. Interestingly, they found that anemic fetuses have higher velocities than normal. This same group then studied 17 isoimmunized pregnancies and found that MCA Doppler correlated directly with fetal hematocrit

(d'Ancona and associates, 1997). They postulated that it could be used to noninvasively identify anemic fetuses.

FETAL CARDIAC FUNCTION. The measurement of fetal cardiac function may have immediate clinical importance as well as research implications.

CARDIAC OUTPUT. Doppler techniques that measure fetal cardiac output are extremely difficult to apply because of fetal movement, cardiac movement, and the technical factors discussed earlier. Combined use of two-dimensional ultrasound and Doppler echocardiography, however, does allow an assessment of blood flow through the heart. Normal flow patterns have been studied. Reed and colleagues (1986a, 1986b) reported that the normal mean right-ventricular output was 307 mL/kg/min and left-ventricular output was 232 mL/kg/min (right-to-left ventricular output ratio 55:45). DeSmedt and associates (1987) reported a slightly higher value for combined ventricular output. Abnormal flow patterns can be detected by calculating the ratio of right and left cardiac outputs (thus minimizing the effects of measurement errors, which would likely affect both ventricles equally), and by performing serial studies over a short time interval. Abnormal flow patterns suggest the presence of a congenital defect, which can then be studied with two-dimensional images.

DUCTUS ARTERIOSUS. Doppler evaluation of the ductus can be used to monitor fetal status and response to specific medications. Indomethacin is a prostaglandin synthase inhibitor used for tocolysis which has been implicated in premature (antenatal) closure of the ductus arteriosus. Premature closure leads to retrograde blood flow through the tricuspid valve or into the pulmonary arteries. Resulting increased pulmonary flow then causes reactive hypertrophy of the pulmonary arterioles and eventually pulmonary hypertension. Huhta and colleagues (1987) first observed reversible ductal constriction in three fetuses whose mothers received indomethacin for treatment of preterm labor. They subsequently confirmed ductus constriction in exposed lamb and human fetuses but not in 25 normal pregnancies. Vermillion and colleagues (1997) studied 61 indomethacin-treated women and reported that half of exposed fetuses developed ductal constriction. Fortunately, ductal constriction is largely reversible if medication is discontinued before 32 weeks (Moise, 1993).

FETAL ARRHYTHMIAS. Using several techniques, a variety of fetal cardiac arrhythmias can be diagnosed, and many can be treated antenatally. Most commonly, diagnosis requires a two-dimensional, real-time ultrasound examination to evaluate cardiac anatomy, followed by an M-mode echocardiographic evaluation to characterize the arrhythmia. An electrocardiogram (ECG), which documents the electrical depolarizing events in the heart, cannot be obtained in a fetus. M-mode echocardiography, however, measures the mechanical response to the depolarizing events, and thus can provide similar information indirectly. It is useful for diagnosing fetal cardiac arrhythmias, and in assessing ventricular wall function and functional atrial and ventricular outputs as well as the timing of these events. Precise diagnosis of a fetal arrhythmia is important because some, for example, supraventricular tachycardia, require pharmacological treatment to prevent or treat heart failure. Others, for example, premature atrial contractions, resolve spontaneously and need not be treated. The antenatal treatment of fetal arrhythmias is discussed in Chapter 37.

FETAL WELL-BEING. A recurring goal for Doppler ultrasound is that it could somehow be used to distinguish normal from abnormal pregnancies. It has been investigated as a means to predict fetal growth restriction, hypoxia, and distress. It has also been proposed that abnormal uteroplacental waveforms may identify women at risk for preeclampsia. Applications of this technology are discussed in relation to its use in the diagnosis and management of a variety of pregnancy complications, and their management is presented throughout this book. Doppler velocimetry has been proposed as a method of fetal surveillance, as discussed in Chapter 40. According to the American College of Obstetricians and Gynecologists (1999), Doppler velocimetry is not recommended for screening to detect fetuses at risk. It may have benefits in surveillance for suspected fetal growth restriction. Finally, the College considers fetal middle cerebral artery velocimetry to be investigational.

REFERENCES

Abuhammad A: Genetic aspects of congenital disease. In: A Practical Guide to Fetal Echocardiography. Philadelphia, Lippincott-Raven, 1997, p 1

Adra AM, Mejides AA, Dennaoui MS, Beydoun SN: Fetal pyelectasis: Is it always "physiologic"? Am J Obstet Gynecol 173:1263, 1995

Adzick NS, Harrison MR, Glick PL, Nakayama DK, Manning FA, deLorimier AA: Diaphragmatic hernia in the fetus: Prenatal diagnosis and outcome in 94 cases. J Pediatr Surg 20:357, 1985

American Institute of Ultrasound in Medicine: Guidelines for Performance of the Antepartum Obstetrical Ultrasound Examination. Rockville, MD, AIUM, 1994

American Institute of Ultrasound in Medicine: AIUM Bioeffects Committee: Safety Considerations for Diagnostic Ultrasound. Rockville, MD, AIUM, 1991

American College of Obstetricians and Gynecologists: Ante-

partum fetal surveillance. Practice Bulletin No. 9, October 1999

American College of Obstetricians and Gynecologists: Ultrasonography in pregnancy. Technical Bulletin No. 187, December 1993

Bannister CM, Russell SA, Rimmer S, Arora A: Pre-natal ventriculomegaly and hydrocephalus. Neurol Res 22:37, 2000

Benacerraf BR, Harlow B, Frigoletto F: Should amniocentesis be done for second trimester choroid plexus cysts? Abstract 1602, Official Proceedings of the 34th Annual Convention, American Institute of Ultrasound in Medicine, New Orleans, March 1990a

Benacerraf BR, Mandell J, Estroff JA, Harlow BL, Frigoletto FD Jr: Fetal pyelectasis: A possible association with Down syndrome. Obstet Gynecol 76:58, 1990b

Benacerraf BR, Pober BR, Sanders SP: Accuracy of fetal echocardiography. Radiology 165:847, 1987

Berghella V, Kaufman M, Huhta J, Wapner R: Accuracy of prenatal diagnosis of congenital heart defects. Am J Obstet Gynecol 174:419, 1996

Berkowitz RL: Should every pregnant woman undergo ultrasonography? N Engl J Med 329:874, 1993

Berlin BM, Norton ME, Sugarman EA, Tsipis JE, Allitto BA: Cystic fibrosis and chromosome abnormalities associated with echogenic fetal bowel. Obstet Gynecol 94:135, 1999

Bloom SL, Bloom DD, DellaNebbia C, Martin LB, Lucas MJ, Twickler DM: The developmental outcome of children with antenatal mild isolated ventriculomegaly. Obstet Gynecol 90:93, 1997

Bromley B, Estroff JA, Sanders SP, Parad R, Frigoletto FD, Benacerraf BR: Fetal echocardiography: Accuracy and limitations in a population of high and low risk for heart defects. Am J Obstet Gynecol 166:1473, 1992

Bronshtein M, Bar-Have I, Blumenfeld I, Bejar J, Toder V, Blumenfeld Z: The difference between septated and nonseptated nuchal cystic hygroma in the early second trimester. Obstet Gynecol 81:683, 1993

Bronshtein M, Yoffe N, Brandes JM, Blumenfeld Z: First and early second-trimester diagnosis of fetal urinary tract anomalies using transvaginal sonography. Prenat Diagn 10:653, 1990

Brumfield, Wenstrom KD, Davis RO, Owen J, Cosper P: Fetal cystic hygroma—prognosis of septated versus nonseptated lesions. Am J Obstet Gynecol 174:439, 1996

Bucher HC, Schmidt JG: Does routine ultrasound scanning improve outcome in pregnancy? Meta-analysis of various outcome measures. BMJ 307:13, 1993

Burns PN: Doppler flow estimations in the fetal and maternal circulations: Principles, techniques and some limitation. In Maulik D, McNellis D (eds): Reproductive and Perinatal Medicine. Doppler Ultrasound Measurement of Maternal–Fetal Hemodynamics, Vol VIII. Ithaca, NY, Perinatology Press, 1987, p 43

Callen PW: Ultrasonography in Obstetrics & Gynecology. Philadelphia, Saunders, 1994

Cardoza JD, Filly RA, Podrasky AE: The dangling choroid plexus: A sonographic observation of value in excluding ventriculomegaly. AJR 151:767, 1988a

Cardoza JD, Goldstein RB, Filly RA: Exclusion of fetal ventriculomegaly with a single measurement: The width of the lateral ventricular atrium. Radiology 169:711, 1988b

Chamberlain PF, Manning FA, Morrison I, Harmon CR, Lange IR: Ultrasound evaluation of amniotic fluid volume. I. The relationship of marginal and decreased amniotic fluid volumes to perinatal outcome. Am J Obstet Gynecol 150:245, 1984

Chandran R, Serra-Serra V: Middle cerebral artery flow velocity waveforms and fetal compromise [letter; comment]. Am J Obstet Gynecol 168:1335, 1993

Chinn D, Worthy L, Towers C, Miller E: Fetal choroid plexus cysts: Incidence and prediction of trisomy 18. Abstract 1621, Official Proceedings of the 34th Annual Convention of the American Institute of Ultrasound in Medicine, New Orleans, March 1990

Comstock CH: Normal fetal heart axis and position. Obstet Gynecol 70:255, 1987

Copel JA, Grannum PA, Hobbins JC, Cunningham FG: Doppler ultrasound in obstetrics. Williams Obstetrics, 17th ed (Suppl 16). Norwalk, CT, Appleton & Lange, 1988b

Copel JA, Pilu G, Green J, Hobbins JC, Kleinman CS: Fetal echocardiographic screening for congenital heart disease: The importance of the four-chamber view. Am J Obstet Gynecol 157:648, 1987

Corteville J, Gray D, Crane J: Congenital hydronephrosis: Correlation of fetal ultrasonographic findings with infant outcome. Am J Obstet Gynecol 165:384, 1991

Crane JP, LeFevre ML, Winborn RC, Evans JK, Ewigman BG, Bain RP, Frigoletto FD, McNellis D: A randomized trial of prenatal ultrasonographic screening: Impact on the detection, management, and outcome of anomalous fetuses. The RADIUS Study Group. Am J Obstet Gynecol 172:392, 1994

Crawford DC, Chita SK, Allan LD: Prenatal detection of congenital heart disease: Factors affecting obstetric management and survival. Am J Obstet Gynecol 159:352, 1988

d'Ancona RL, Rahman F, Ozcan T, Copel JA, Mari G: The effect of intravascular blood transfusion on the flow velocity waveform of the portal venous system of the anemic fetus. Ultrasound Obstet Gynecol 10:333, 1997

DeSmedt MCH, Visser GHA, Meijboom EJ: Fetal cardiac output estimated by Doppler echocardiography during mid- and late gestation. Am J Cardiol 60:338, 1987

DeVore GR: Financial implications of routine screening ultrasound. Ultrasound Obstet Gynecol 7:307, 1996

DeVore GR, Horenstein J, Siassi B, Platt LD: Fetal echocardiography, 7. Doppler color flow mapping: A new technique for the diagnosis of congenital heart disease. Am J Obstet Gynecol 156:1054, 1987

Donald I, MacVicar J, Brown TG: Investigation of abdominal masses by pulsed ultrasound. Lancet 7032:1188, 1958

Drugan A, Krause B, Canady A, Zador IE, Sacks AJ, Evans MI: The natural history of prenatally diagnosed cerebral ventriculomegaly. JAMA 261:1785, 1989

Eik-Nes SH, Marsal K, Brubakk AO, Kristofferson K, Ulstein M: Ultrasonic measurement of human fetal blood flow. J Biomed Eng 4:28, 1982

Ewigman BG, Crane P, Frigoletto FD, LeFevre ML, Bain RP, McNellis D, and the RADIUS Study Group: Effect of prenatal ultrasound screening on perinatal outcome. N Engl J Med 329:821, 1993

Filly RA, Cardoza JD, Goldstein RB, Barkovich AJ: Detection of fetal central nervous system anomalies: A practical level of effort for a routine sonogram. Radiology 172:403, 1989

Fleischer A, Schulman H, Farmakides G, Bracero L, Blattner P, Randolph G: Umbilical artery velocity waveforms and intrauterine growth retardation. Am J Obstet Gynecol 151:502, 1985

Fugelseth D, Lindemann R, Sande HA, Refsum S, Nordshus T: Prenatal diagnosis of urinary tract anomalies. The value of two ultrasound examinations. Acta Obstet Gynecol Scand 73:290, 1994

Gerson AG, Wallace DM, Stiller RJ, Paul D, Weiner S, Bolognese RJ: Doppler evaluation of umbilical venous and arterial flow in the second and third trimester of normal pregnancy. Obstet Gynecol 70:672, 1987

Ghidini A, Sirtori M, Bergani P, Orsenigo E, Tagliabue P, Parravicini E: Ureteropelvic junction obstruction in utero and ex utero. Obstet Gynecol 75:805, 1990

Gill RW: Measurement of blood flow by ultrasound accuracy and source of error. Ultrasound Med Biol 11:625, 1985

Goldstein I, Reece EA, Pilu G, Bovicelli L, Hobbins JC: Cerebellar measurements with ultrasonography in the evaluation of fetal growth and development. Am J Obstet Gynecol 156:1065, 1987

Goldstein RB, Filly RA: Prenatal diagnosis of anencephaly: Spectrum of sonographic appearances and distinction from the amniotic band syndrome. AJR 151:547, 1988

Gonçalves LF, Jeanty P, Piper JM: The accuracy of prenatal ultrasonography in detecting congenital anomalies. Am J Obstet Gynecol 171:1606, 1994

Green JJ, Hobbins JC: Abdominal ultrasound examination of first-trimester fetus. Am J Obstet Gynecol 159:165, 1988

Griffin DR, Teague MJ, Tallet P, Wilson K, Bilardo C, Massin L, Campbell S: A combination ultrasonic linear array scanner and pulsed Doppler velocimeter for the estimation of blood flow in the foetus and adult abdomen, 2. Clinical evaluation. Ultrasound Med Biol 11:37, 1985

Grignon A, Filiatrault D, Homsy Y, Robitaille P, Filion R, Boutin H, Leblond R: Ureteropelvic junction stenosis: Antenatal ultrasonographic diagnosis, postnatal investigation, and follow-up. Radiology 160:649, 1986

Gunn TR, Mora JD, Pease P: Antenatal diagnosis of urinary tract abnormalities by ultrasonography after 28 weeks' gestation: Incidence and outcome. Am J Obstet Gynecol 172:479, 1995

Gupta JK, Bryce FC, Lilford RJ: Management of apparently isolated fetal ventriculomegaly [review]. Obstet Gynecol Surv 49:716, 1994

Gupta JK, Khan KS, Thornton JG, Lilford RJ: Management of fetal choroid plexus cysts. Br J Obstet Gynaecol 104:881, 1997

Hadlock FP, Deter RL, Harrist RB, Park SK: Estimating fetal age: Computer-assisted analysis of multiple fetal growth parameters. Radiology 152:497, 1984

Hadlock FP, Shah YP, Kanon DJ, Lindsey JF: Fetal crown-rump length: Reevaluation of relation to menstrual age (5–18 weeks) with high-resolution real-time US. Radiology 182:501, 1992

Helin I, Persson PH: Prenatal diagnosis of urinary tract abnormalities by ultrasound. Pediatrics 78:879, 1986

Hendricks SK, Sorensen TK, Wang KY, Breshnell JM, Seguin EM, Zingheim RW: Doppler umbilical artery waveform indices—Normal values from fourteen to forty-two vessels. Am J Obstet Gynecol 161:761, 1989

Hertzberg BS: Sonography of the fetal gastrointestinal tract: Anatomic variants, diagnostic pitfalls, and abnormalities. AJR Am J Roentgenol 162:1175, 1994

Hoyme HE, Jones MC, Jones KL: Gastroschisis: Abdominal wall disruption secondary to early gestational interruption of the omphalomesenteric artery. Semin Perinatol 7:294, 1983

Huhta JC, Moise KJ, Fisher DJ, Sharif DS, Wasserstrum N, Martin C: Detection and quantitation of constriction of the fetal ductus arteriosus by Doppler echocardiography. Circulation 75:406, 1987

Jeanty P: Fetal biometry. In Fleischer AC, Romero R, Manning FA, Jeanty PJ, James AE (eds): The Principles and Practice of Ultrasonography in Obstetrics and Gynecology, 4th ed. Norwalk, CT, Appleton & Lange, 1991, p 93

Johnson MP, Johnson A, Holzgreve W, Isada NB, Wapner RJ, Treadwell MC, Heeger S, Evans MI: First-trimester simple hygroma: Cause and outcome. Am J Obstet Gynecol 168:156, 1993

Kleiner B, Filly RA, Mack L, Callen PW: Multicystic dysplastic kidney: Observations of contralateral disease in the fetal population. Radiology 161:27, 1986

Lanouette JM, Wolfe HM, DeVries KL, Puder KS, Gurczynski J: Adjusted positive predictive value of routine views for the detection of congenital heart disease (CHD). Am J Obstet Gynecol 174:420, 1996

Leonardi MR, Wolfe HM, Greb A, Johnson MP, Lanouette JM, Landwehr JB, Evans MI: Choroid plexus cysts and risk of aneuploidy. Am J Obstet Gynecol 174:435, 1996

Levi CS, Lyons EA, Lindsay DJ: Ultrasound in the first trimester of pregnancy. Radiol Clin North Am 28:19, 1990

Levine D, Barnes PD, Madsen JR, Abbott J, Mehta T, Edelman RR: Central nervous system abnormalities assessed with prenatal magnetic resonance imaging. Obstet Gynecol 94:1011, 1999

Levitsky DB, Mack LA, Nyberg DA, Shurtleff DB, Shields LA, Nghiem HV, Cyr DR: Fetal aqueductal stenosis diagnoses sonographically: How grave is the prognosis? AJR Am J Roentgenol 164:725, 1995

Livera LN, Brookfield DSK, Egginton JA, Hawnaur JM: Antenatal ultrasonography to detect fetal renal abnormalities: A prospective screening programme. BMJ 298:1421, 1989

Low JA: The current status of maternal and fetal blood flow velocimetry. Am J Obstet Gynecol 164:1049, 1991

Lowe TW, Peters MT, Twickler D, Cunningham FG: Obstetrical sonography update, 1990. Williams Obstetrics, 18th ed (Suppl 6). Norwalk, CT, Appleton & Lange, 1990

Luck CA: Value of routine ultrasound scanning at 19 weeks: A four-year study of 8,849 deliveries. BMJ 304:1474, 1992

Mahony BS, Nyberg DA, Hirsch JH, Petty CN, Hendricks SK, Mack LA: Mild idiopathic lateral cerebral ventricular dilatation in utero: Sonographic evaluation. Radiology 169:715, 1988

Mandell J, Blyth B, Peters C, Retik A, Estroff J, Benacerraf B: Structural genitourinary defects detected in utero. Radiology 178:193, 1991

Manning FA, Platt LD, Sipos L: Antepartum fetal evaluation: Development of fetal biophysical profile. Am J Obstet Gynecol 136:787, 1980

Mari G, Rahman F, Olofsson P, Ozcan T, Copel JA: Increase of fetal hematocrit decreases the middle cerebral artery peak systolic velocity in pregnancies complicated by rhesus alloimmunization. J Matern Fetal Med 6:206, 1997

Millener PB, Anderson NG, Chisholm RJ: Progonostic significance of nonvisualization of the fetal stomach by sonography. AJR Am J Roentgenol 160:827, 1993

Moise KJ Jr: Effect of advancing gestational age on the frequency of fetal ductal constriction in association with maternal indomethacin use. Am J Obstet Gynecol 168:1350, 1993

Mongelli M, Wilcox M, Gardosi J: Estimating the date of confinement: Ultrasonographic biometry versus certain menstrual dates. Am J Obstet Gynecol 174:278, 1996

Monteagudo A, Reuss ML, Timor-Tritsch IE: Imaging the fetal brain in the second and third trimesters using transvaginal sonography. Obstet Gynecol 77:27, 1991

National Center for Health Statistics: Advance report of new data from the 1989 birth certificate. In U.S. Public Health Service: Monthly Vital Statistics Report, Publication No. (PHS) 92-1120, Vol 40, No. 12 (S), April 1992, p. 1

National Institutes of Health: Diagnostic Ultrasound Imaging in Pregnancy, 1984. U.S. Department of Health and Human Services, No. 84-667, 1984

Nyberg DA: Recommendations for obstetric sonography in the evaluation of the fetal cranium. Radiology 172:309, 1989

Nyberg DA, Dubinsky T, Resta RG, Mahony BS, Hickok DE, Luthy DA: Echogenic fetal bowel during the second trimester: Clinical importance. Radiology 188:527, 1993

Olsen O, Clausen JA: Routine ultrasound dating has not been shown to be more accurate than the calendar method. Br J Obstet and Gynaecol 104:1221, 1997

Ott WJ: The accuracy of antenatal fetal echocardiography screening in high- and low-risk patients. Am J Obstet Gynecol 172:1741, 1995

Patten RM, Mack LA, Wang KY, Cyr DR: The fetal genitourinary tract. Radiol Clin North Am 28:115, 1990

Phelan JP, Ahn MO, Smith CV, Rutherford SE, Anderson E: Amnionic fluid index measurements during pregnancy. J Reprod Med 32:601, 1987

Potter EL: Bilateral renal agenesis. J Pediatr 29:68, 1946

Pretorius DH, Drose JA, Dennis MA, Manchester DK, Manco-Johnson ML: Tracheoesophageal fistula in utero: Twenty-two cases. J Ultrasound Med 6:509, 1987a

Pretorius DH, Gosink BB, Clautice-Engle T, Leopold GR, Minnick CM: Sonographic evaluation of the fetal stomach: Significance of nonvisualization. AJR Am J Roentgenol 151:987, 1988

Pretorius DH, Lee ME, Manco-Johnson ML, Weingast GR, Sedman AB, Gabow PA: Diagnosis of autosomal dominant polycystic kidney disease in utero and in the young infant. J Ultrasound Med 6:249, 1987b

Rabinowitz R, Peters MT, Vyas S, Campbell S, Nicolaides KH: Measurement of fetal urine production in normal pregnancy by real-time ultrasonography. Am J Obstet Gynecol 161:1264, 1989

Reed KL, Meijboom EJ, Sahn DJ, Scagnelli SA, Valdez-Cruz LM, Shenker L: Cardiac Doppler flow velocities in human fetuses. Circulation 73:41, 1986a

Reed KL, Sahn DJ, Scagnelli S, Anderson CF, Shenker L: Doppler echocardiographic studies of diastolic function in the human fetal heart: Changes during gestation. J Am Coll Cardiol 8:391, 1986b

Robertson FM, Crombleholme TM, Paidas M, Harris BH: Prenatal diagnosis and management of gastrointestinal disorders. Semin Perinatol 18:182, 1994

Robinson J, Tice K, Kolm P, Abuhamad A: Effects of maternal hydration on fetal renal pyelectasis. Obstet Gynecol 92:137, 1998

Romero R, Ghidini A, Costigan K, Touloukian R, Hobbins JC: Prenatal diagnosis of duodenal atresia: Does it make any difference? Obstet Gynecol 71:739, 1988

Roodhooft AM, Birnholz JC, Holmes LB: Familial nature of congenital absence and severe dysgenesis of both kidneys. N Engl J Med 310:1341, 1984

Saari-Kemppainen A, Karjalainen O, Ylostalo P, Heinonen OP: Ultrasound screening and perinatal mortality: Controlled trial of systematic one-stage screening in pregnancy. Lancet 336:387, 1990

Sagi J, Vagman I, David MP, Van Dongen LGR, Goudie E, Butterworth A, Jacobson MJ: Fetal kidney size related to gestational age. Gynecol Obstet Invest 23:1, 1987

Saller DN, Canick JA, Schwartz S, Blitzer MG: Multiple-maker screening in pregnancies with hydropic and nonhydropic Turner syndrome. Am J Obstet Gynecol 167: 1021, 1992

Schulman H, Fleischer A, Farmakides G, Bracero L, Rochelson B, Grunfeld L: Development of uterine artery compliance in pregnancy as detected by Doppler ultrasound. Am J Obstet Gynecol 155:1031, 1986

Shenker L, Reed KL, Marx GR, Donnerstein RL, Allen HD, Anderson CF: Fetal cardiac Doppler flow studies in prenatal diagnosis of heart disease. Am J Obstet Gynecol 158:1267, 1988

Shipp TD, Bromley B, Hornberger LK, Nadel A, Benacerraf BR: Levorotation of the fetal cardiac axis: A clue for the presence of congenital heart disease. Obstet Gynecol 85:97, 1995

Shulman LP, Emerson DS, Felker RE, Phillips OP, Simpson JL, Elias S: High frequency of cytogenetic abnormalities in fetuses with cystic hygroma diagnosed in the first trimester. Obstet Gynecol 80:80, 1992

Shulman LP, Emerson DS, Grevengood C, Felker RE, Gross SJ, Phillips OP, Elias S: Clinical course and outcome of fetuses with isolated cystic nuchal lesions and normal karyotypes detected in the first trimester. Am J Obstet Gynecol 171:1278, 1994

Slotnick RN, Abuhamad AZ: Prognostic implications of fetal echogenic bowel. Lancet 347:85, 1996

Smith RS, Comstock CH, Kirk JS, Lee W: Ultrasonographic left cardiac axis deviation: A marker for fetal anomalies. Obstet Gynecol 85:187, 1995

Timor-Tritsch IE, Monteagudo A, Peisner DB: High frequency transvaginal sonographic examination and malformation workup of the 9–14 week fetus. Abstract 374, 10th annual meeting of the Society of Perinatal Obstetricians, Houston, January 1990

Trauffer PML, Anderson CE, Johnson A, Heeger S, Morgan P, Wapner RJ: The natural history of euploid pregnancies with first-trimester cystic hygromas. Am J Obstet Gynecol 170:1279, 1994

Treadwell MC, Tomlinson MW, Wolfe HM, Flake A: Prenatal course of congenital cystic adenomatoid malformations. Am J Obstet Gynecol 174:441, 1996

Tunon K, Eik-Nes SH, Grottom P: A comparison between ultrasound and a reliable last menstrual period as predictors of the day of delivery in 15,000 examinations. Ultrasound Obstet Gynecol 8:178, 1996

Twickler DM: Obstetrical ultrasonography, part 1. Williams Obstetrics, 19th ed (Suppl 18). Stamford, CT, Appleton & Lange, April/May 1996

Vermillion ST, Scardo JA, Lashus AG, Wiles HB: The effect of indomethacin tocolysis on fetal ductus arteriosus constriction with advancing gestational age. Am J Obstet Gynecol 177:256, 1997

Vincoff NS, Callen PW, Smith-Bindman R, Goldstein RB: Effect of ultrasound transducer frequency on the appearance of the fetal bowel. J Ultrasound Med 18:799, 1999

Waldenstrom U, Nilsson S, Fall O, Axelsson O, Eklund G, Lindeberg S, Sjodin Y: Effects of routine one-stage ultrasound screening in pregnancy: A randomized controlled trial. Lancet 2:585, 1988

Wenstrom KD, Boots LR, and Cosper PC: Multiple marker screening test: Identification of fetal cystic hygroma, hydrops, and sex chromosome aneuploidy. J Matern Fetal Med 5:31, 1996

Wenstrom KD, Weiner CP, Williamson RA: Diverse maternal and fetal pathology associated with absent diastolic flow in the umbilical artery of high-risk fetuses. Obstet Gynecol 77:374, 1991

Williams K: Amniotic fluid assessment. Obstet Gynecol Surv 48:795, 1993

Wilson R, Lynch S, Lessoway V: Fetal pyelectasis: Comparison of postnatal renal pathology with unilateral and bilateral pyelectasis. Prenat Diagn 17:451, 1997

Wladimiroff JW, vd Wijngaard JA, Degani S, Noordam MJ, van Eyck J, Tonge HM: Cerebral and umbilical arterial blood flow velocity waveforms in normal and growth-retarded pregnancies. Obstet Gynecol 69:705, 1987

Yaron Y, Hassan S, Geva E, Kupferminc MJ, Yavetz H, Evans MI: Evaluation of fetal echogenic bowel in the second trimester. Fetal Diagn Ther 14:176, 1999

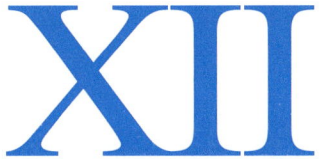

SECTION

Medical and Surgical Complications in Pregnancy

42

General Considerations and Maternal Evaluation

Medical and surgical illnesses complicating pregnancy require collaboration between obstetrician, internist, surgeon, anesthesiologist, and frequently other specialists. Because pregnancy does not make a woman immune to any disease, obstetricians must have a working knowledge of medical and surgical diseases common to childbearing-age women. Likewise, nonobstetricians should be familiar with effects that these diseases have on the pregnant woman, or vice versa. Importantly, normal pregnancy-induced physiological changes must be interpreted in relation to their effects on underlying nonobstetrical disorders. Finally, changes induced by pregnancy in many laboratory tests must be considered.

The purpose of this chapter is to review generalizations concerning the rational approach to management of pregnancy when complicated by medical or surgical diseases. One axiom to consider is: **A woman should never be penalized because she is pregnant.** Put another way: If a proposed medical or surgical regimen is altered simply because the woman is pregnant, can it be justified? This approach still allows individualization of care for women with most medical and surgical disorders that complicate pregnancy. Importantly, it may be especially helpful when dealing with consultants asked to see these women.

PHYSIOLOGICAL ALTERATIONS AND CHANGES IN LABORATORY VALUES

Pregnancy induces profound physiological changes in most organ systems and these may amplify or obfuscate evaluation of coincidental medical and surgical disorders. The wide ranges of pregnancy effects on normal physiology are discussed in Chapter 8 and are reviewed in the various chapters that follow.

Along with the marked physiological changes induced by pregnancy, a number of standard laboratory evaluations are also altered. Some of these would, in the nonpregnant woman, suggest marked aberrations or conversely, normalcy, at a time when the woman was either completely normal or actually quite ill. Many normal laboratory values for pregnancy are discussed both in Chapter 8 as well as in the following chapters in which the effects of superimposed disease are considered.

MEDICATIONS DURING PREGNANCY

Consideration for antepartum management of medical and surgical disorders always includes administration of a variety of drugs. Fortunately, the vast majority of medications necessary for management of the most commonly encountered complications can be used with

relative safety. There are, however, a few notable exceptions. These are considered in detail in Chapter 38 as well as in individual chapters in this section.

SURGERY DURING PREGNANCY

EFFECT OF SURGERY AND ANESTHESIA ON PREGNANCY OUTCOME. The risk of an adverse pregnancy outcome does not appear to be increased in women undergoing most uncomplicated surgical or anesthetic procedures. This risk may be increased, however, when surgical disorders or procedures are associated with complications. For example, complications from perforative appendicitis with feculent peritonitis are associated with increased maternal and perinatal morbidity and mortality even if surgical and anesthetic techniques are flawless. Conversely, if there are complications from these procedures, pregnancy outcome may be adversely affected. By way of example, if the woman who undergoes uncomplicated surgery for nonperforative appendicitis suffers vomiting with aspiration of acidic gastric contents, then resulting respiratory failure may cause fetal death, preterm labor, or both, as well as significant maternal morbidity and even mortality.

The most extensive experiences regarding anesthetic and surgical risks to pregnancy are from the Swedish Birth Registry and reported by Mazze and Källén (1989). These investigators studied the effects of 5405 nonobstetrical surgical procedures performed in 720,000 pregnant women from 1973 to 1981 (Table 42–1). Surgery was performed most commonly in the first trimester—41 percent—compared with 35 percent in the second trimester and 24 percent in the third. Abdominal surgery comprised a fourth of all operations, and another 19 percent were gynecological and urological procedures. Laparoscopic procedures were done in 16 percent of the women, and the vast majority were performed in the first trimester. Although laparoscopy was the most commonly performed first-trimester operation, appendectomy was the most commonly done procedure in the second trimester.

The types of anesthesia administered to the 5405 women in the Swedish report are shown in Table 42–2. Over half of these procedures were done using general anesthesia, and in 98 percent of these, nitrous oxide supplemented by another inhalation agent or intravenous medication was used.

PERINATAL OUTCOMES. Mazze and Källén (1989) concluded that excessive perinatal morbidity associated with nonobstetrical surgery during pregnancy was attributable to the disease itself, rather than to adverse effects of surgery and anesthesia. They compared preg-

TABLE 42–1. Nonobstetrical Operations in 5405 Swedish Women

| Type of Operation | Percent of Procedures by Trimester | | | Total (n = 5405) |
	First (n = 2252)	Second (n = 1881)	Third (n = 1272)	No. (%)
Central nervous system	7	6	6	323 (6)
Head and neck	8	6	10	419 (8)
Heart and lung	0.7	0.8	0.6	40 (0.7)
Abdominal	20	30	23	1331 (25)
Gynecological and urological	11	23	24	1008 (19)
Laparoscopy	34	1.2	6	868 (16)
Orthopedic	9	9	14	558 (10)
Endoscopy	4	11	9	406 (8)
Skin	4	3	4	202 (4)
Others	4	4	6	250 (5)

Adapted from Mazze and Källén (1989).

nancy outcomes for the 5405 women undergoing surgery with those in the total database of 720,000 pregnancies. As shown in Table 42–3, there was a significantly increased incidence of low-birthweight and preterm infants as well as neonatal deaths by 7 days in women who had undergone surgery.

An important observation from the Swedish study is that stillbirth and congenital malformation rates were not increased significantly. The latter observation is strengthened by the report from Czeizel and colleagues (1998) that anesthetic agents are not teratogenic. In another report, however, Källén and Mazze (1990) scrutinized 572 operations performed on the Swedish women at 4 to 5 weeks' gestation. They found a possible causal relationship with increased neural-tube defects. Sylvester and co-workers (1994) analyzed first-trimester outcomes in the Metropolitan Atlanta Congenital De-

fects Program. In a case-control study, they found a significantly increased risk of hydrocephaly associated with other major defects—especially eye anomalies—in women exposed to general anesthesia. Thus, as Rosen (1999) concluded, we cannot state categorically that anesthetic agents are not teratogenic.

LAPAROSCOPIC SURGERY DURING PREGNANCY. Over the past decade, the use of laparoscopic techniques has become common for diagnosis and management of a number of surgical disorders complicating pregnancy. The obvious application is diagnosis and management of ectopic pregnancy (Chap. 34, p. 894). With established pregnancy, in most studies laparoscopy has been used for exploration and treatment of adnexal masses (Chap. 35, p. 930), or for cholecystectomy or appendectomy (Chap. 48, pp. 1296 and 1281). Lachman and colleagues

TABLE 42–2. Anesthesia for Surgery in 5405 Pregnant Women

| Anesthesia | Percent by Trimester | | | Total (n = 5405) |
	First (n = 2252)	Second (n = 1881)	Third (n = 1272)	No. (%)
General	65	51	41	2929 (54)
Spinal or epidural	3	5	6	255 (5)
Infiltration	4	6	6	278 (5)
Nerve block	1	2	3	114 (2)
Topical	1	2	3	55 (1)
Unknown	25	34	41	1732 (32)

Adapted from Mazze and Källén (1989).

TABLE 42–3. Birth Outcomes in 5405 Pregnant Women Undergoing Nonobstetrical Surgery

Birth Outcome	Trimester (Observed/Expected)			Total	Significance (Total Outcomes)
	First	Second	Third		
Stillborn	1.1	1.7	1.5	1.4	NS
Death by 7 days	1.4	3.2	1.9	2.1	$P < .05$
Congenital malformation	1.0	0.9	1.5	1.1	NS
Birthweight < 1500 g	1.7	3.2	1.5	2.2	$P < .05$
Birthweight < 2500 g	1.4	1.8	2.2	2.0	$P < .05$

NS = not significant.
Adapted from Mazze and Källén (1989).

(1999) recently reviewed 518 reported procedures that were performed during pregnancy. Cholecystectomy was the most common (45 percent), followed by adnexal surgery (34 percent), and appendectomy (15 percent).

The precise effects of laparoscopy in the human fetus are currently unknown. Studies of pregnant ewes have been reported by Barnard and associates (1995) and Hunter and colleagues (1995). Using carbon dioxide insufflation for pneumoperitoneum, they found that uteroplacental blood flow falls when pressure exceeds 15 mm Hg. This was due to decreased perfusion pressure and increased placental vessel resistance. In some, but not all of the fetuses, acidemia developed. Reedy and colleagues (1995) studied these effects in baboons at the human equivalent gestation of 22 to 26 weeks. While there were no substantive changes at 10 mm Hg insufflation, pressure of 20 mm Hg caused significant maternal cardiovascular and respiratory changes by 20 minutes. Some of these include increased respiratory rate, respiratory acidosis, diminished cardiac output, and increased pulmonary artery pressure with concomitantly increased wedge pressure.

To study the impact of laparoscopy on perinatal outcomes, Reedy and colleagues (1997b) used the updated Swedish Birth Registry described earlier. From 1973 to 1993, the database contained outcomes from slightly over 2 million deliveries. During this same time, 2181 laparoscopies and 1522 laparotomies were performed during pregnancy in these women. As shown in Figure 42–1, laparoscopy was used primarily in the first trimester. These investigators compared perinatal outcomes with surgery versus those in the overall database. While they found an increased risk of low birthweight, preterm delivery, and fetal growth restriction in the operative group, there were no differences in outcome when laparoscopy and laparotomy were compared. The risk for congenital malformations also was not different in any of the comparisons.

Risks inherent to laparoscopy do not appear in-

creased compared with those in nonpregnant women. These risks appear to be uncommon, and indeed Nezhat and associates (1997) found no complications in their literature review. Conversely, Reedy and co-workers (1997a) surveyed 192 laparoscopic surgeons by mail and reported a number of complications, including those inherent to laparoscopy as well as one case of intrauterine placement of the Veress needle.

Many clinicians recommend **gasless laparoscopy** during pregnancy. This accomplishes two goals: it avoids cardiovascular changes with pneumoperitoneum and it decreases the risk of uterine perforation with the trocar or Veress needle. Akira and co-workers (1999) compared this technique with laparotomy in 35 women undergoing ovarian cystectomy at 12 to 16 weeks. They

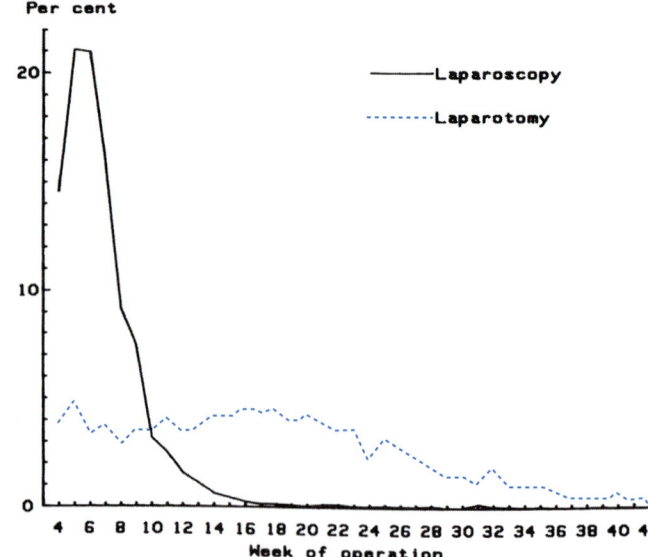

FIGURE 42–1. Distribution of laparoscopic procedures and laparotomies during pregnancy by weeks of gestation. (From Reedy and colleagues, 1997a, with permission.)

TABLE 42–4. Comparative Aspects of Various Forms of Radiation

Type	Physical Characteristics	Biological Effects
X-rays, γ-rays	Short-wavelength electromagnetic waves, highly penetrating, with the capacity of producing ionization with tissues and subsequent electrochemical reactions.	Electrochemical reaction. Can result in tissue damage with high exposures that result in cell death, mutation, cancer, and developmental defects. Effects are dose related.
Ultrasound	Sound waves with a frequency above the audible range, which produce mechanical compression and rarefactions in matter, and with *no* capability of producing ionization.	If the energy is high enough, sound waves can cause tissue disruption by cavitation and streaming hyperthermia. None of these effects occur with energies used in diagnostic ultrasonography.
Microwaves (radio frequency), radar, diathermy	Longer electromagnetic waves with variable ability to penetrate, but no ability to produce ionization within tissues.	The primary biological effect is hyperthermia, although possible nonthermal effects are being investigated. Cataract development is the most widely known complication of extensive microwave or radar exposure.
Electromagnetic waves	Very long waves which readily traverse tissue but with insignificant capacity to produce hyperthermia or cytotoxicity.	Electrical and magnetic fields in tissue with no consequences.

From Brent (1999), with permission.

reported significant benefits with laparoscopy. For a detailed discussion of techniques, the reader is referred to Chapter 26 in the second edition of *Operative Obstetrics* by Gilstrap and colleagues (2001).

IMAGING TECHNIQUES

A number of imaging modalities are used as an adjunct for both diagnosis and therapy during pregnancy. These include ultrasound, magnetic resonance imaging, and x-ray. Of these, x-ray is the most worrisome to both the obstetrician and the patient with regard to fetal safety. Although now less common, some radiological procedures are performed prior to recognition of early pregnancy. These procedures are usually undertaken because of emergencies such as trauma or life-threatening illness. Fortunately, most diagnostic x-ray procedures are associated with little or no known significant fetal risks. As with drugs and medications, however, radiological procedures during pregnancy may lead to litigation if there is an adverse pregnancy outcome, including therapeutic abortion because of either patient or physician anxiety.

IONIZING RADIATION. Radiation is a poorly understood term that often is applied not only to x-rays, but also to microwaves, ultrasound, diathermy, and radiowaves. The latter four energy forms have rather long wavelengths and are of low energy (Brent, 1999). Conversely, x-rays and gamma rays have short wavelengths with very high energy, and are forms of ionizing radiation. The types of radiation and their biological effects are summarized in Table 42–4.

Ionizing radiation from x-rays and gamma rays, with their high energy, is of primary concern from a biological standpoint. Ionizing radiation refers to waves or particles (photons) of significant energy that can break chemical bonds, such as those in DNA, or create free radicals or ions capable of causing tissue damage (Hall, 1991). Methods of measuring x-ray effects are summarized in Table 42–5. The standard terms used are the exposure (in air), the dose (to tissue), and the relative effective dose (to tissue). In the range of energies for diagnostic x-rays, the dose, expressed in rad, and the relative effective dose, expressed in rem, are the same and these units can be used interchangeably. For the sake of consistency, all doses to follow will be expressed in rad, the

TABLE 42–5. Some Measures of Ionizing Radiation

Exposure	The number of ions produced by x-rays per kg of air
	Unit: roentgen (R)
Dose	The amount of energy deposited per kg of tissue
	Traditional unit: rad[a]
	Modern unit: gray (Gy) (1 Gy = 100 rad)
Relative effective dose	The amount of energy deposited per kg of tissue normalized for biological effectiveness
	Traditional unit: rem[a]
	Modern unit: sievert (Sv) (1 Sv = 100 rem)

[a]For diagnostic x-rays, 1 rad = 1 rem.

traditional unit, or in gray (Gy), the modern unit (1 Gy = 100 rad).

X-RAY DOSE ESTIMATION. When calculating the dose of ionizing radiation such as that from x-ray, several factors are considered:

1. Type of study.
2. Type and age of equipment.
3. Distance of the organ in question from the source of radiation.
4. Thickness of the body part penetrated.
5. Method or technique used for the study (Wagner and colleagues, 1997).

When evaluating dose estimates, consideration is given not only to the mathematical model used but also to when the data were compiled. The use of faster screen film combinations, higher-frequency x-ray generators, and other technical improvements have contributed significantly to reduce radiation exposures in recent years.

Estimates of dose to the uterus and embryo for a variety of commonly used radiological examinations (plain film) are summarized in Table 42–6. Radiological studies of maternal body parts at the greatest distances from the uterus—for example, the head—result in a very small dose of scattered radiation to the developing embryo or fetus. The specific anthropometric features of the woman, x-ray techniques used, and performance parameters of the equipment should all be considered. Thus, data presented in the tables should serve only as a guideline. When the radiation dose for a specific individual is required, a medical physicist can be consulted.

POTENTIAL ADVERSE FETAL EFFECTS. The harmful effects of radiation exposure according to Brent (1999) are direct or indirect:

1. Cell death, which affects embryogenesis.
2. Growth restriction.
3. Congenital malformation.
4. Carcinogenesis (controversial).
5. Microcephaly and neonatal mental retardation.
6. Sterility.

TABLE 42–6. **Dose to Uterus for Common Radiological Procedures of Concern in Obstetrics**

Study	View	Dose[a]/View (mrad)	Films/Study[b]	Dose/Study (mrad)
Skull[c]	AP, PA	< 0.01		
	Lat	< 0.01	4.1	< 0.05
Chest	AP, PA[c]	0.01–0.05		
	Lat[d]	0.01–0.03	1.5	0.02–0.07
Mammogram[d]	CC	0.01–0.05		
	Lat	3–5	4.0	7–20
Lumbar spine	AP[e] (7 × 17″)	30–58		
	(14 × 17″)	33–65		
	Lat[d]	11–32	2.9	51–126
Lumbosacral spine	AP[c]	92–187		
	PA[d]	40–97		
	Lat[d]	12–33	3.4	168–359
Abdomen	AP[c]	80–163		
	PA[d]	23–55		
	Lat[d]	29–82	1.7	122–245
Intravenous pyelogram[b]	AP	130–264		
	PA	43–104		
	Lat	13–37	5.5	686–1398
Hip[b] (single)	AP	72–140		
	Lat	18–51	2.0	103–213

AP = anterior–posterior; CC = cranial–caudal; Lat = lateral; PA = posterior–anterior.
[a]Calculated for x-ray beams with half-value layers ranging from 2 to 4 mm Al equivalent using the methodology of Rosenstein (1988).
[b]Based on data and methods reported by Laws and Rosenstein (1978).
[c]Entrance exposure data from Conway (1989).
[d]Authors' estimates based on compilation of above data.
[e]Based on NEXT data reported in National Council on Radiation Protection and Measurements (1989).

The harmful fetal effects of ionizing radiation have been extensively studied in the case of cell damage with resultant dysfunction of embryogenesis, both in the animal model as well as from human studies of Japanese atomic bomb survivors.

ANIMAL STUDIES. Interestingly, adverse radiation effects in animals appear to be somewhat different than in humans. A number of animal studies have addressed these potential embryopathological effects (Brent, 1971, 1999; Wilson and colleagues, 1953). Several conclusions can be drawn:

1. High-dose ionizing radiation is most likely to be lethal to the preblastocyst during the preimplantation stage—the embryo is very insensitive to teratogenic or other effects of radiation at this time.
2. During the period of organogenesis, high-dose radiation is more likely to cause teratogenic changes, growth restriction, or lethal effects.
3. During the fetal period, the fetus will more likely manifest growth restriction and central nervous system effects.

In animal studies, various organs manifest teratogenic effects, whereas in humans, growth restriction and central nervous system anomalies are the most common following high-dose ionizing radiation. Most studies involved large doses—100 to 200 rad (1 to 2 Gy)—and a threshold phenomenon has been demonstrated (Brent, 1999). Unfortunately, as with drugs and medications, it is not always possible to extrapolate animal data directly to the human.

HUMAN DATA. Possible adverse human fetal effects of high-dose ionizing radiation are principally derived from two sources. One includes earlier reports of large-dose radiation given to treat women for malignancy, menorrhagia, and uterine myomas (Brent, 1989). Goldstein and Murphy (1929) reported that adverse effects of estimated radiation exposure of over 100 rad were either microcephaly or hydrocephaly in 19 of 75 exposed embryos. Other adverse effects included mental retardation, abnormal genitalia, growth restriction, microphthalmia, and cataracts. Dekaban (1968) reported 22 infants with microcephaly, mental retardation, or both following exposure to an estimated 250 rad in the first half of pregnancy. In both of these studies, other organ malformations were not found unless there was microcephaly, eye abnormalities, or growth restriction (Brent, 1999).

The second and most often quoted human data are derived from multiple studies of atomic bomb survivors from Hiroshima and Nagasaki (Miller and Mulvihill, 1982; Otake and co-workers, 1987). Adverse effects from in utero exposure to fallout from the atomic bomb

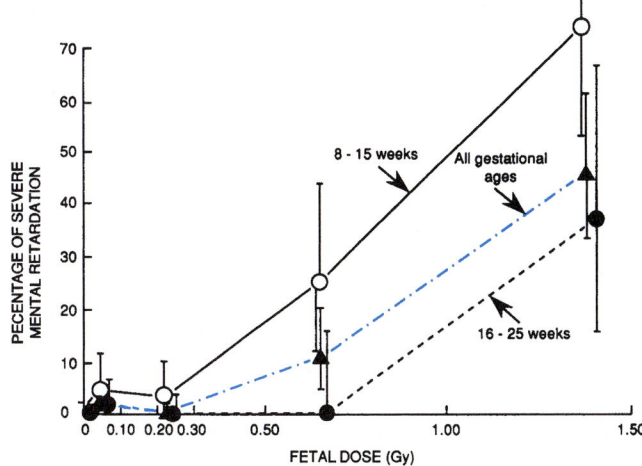

FIGURE 42–2. Effects of ionizing radiation on severe mental retardation in fetuses exposed at various gestational ages to the atomic bomb in Hiroshima and Nagasaki (1 Gy = 100 rad). The bar lines represent 90 percent confidence levels. (Data from Otake and associates, 1987, with permission.)

in these two cities was summarized by Yamazaki and Schull (1990). As shown in Figure 42–2, there is an increased risk of microcephaly and severe mental retardation with high exposure beginning at certain gestational ages. The risk is greatest at 8 to 15 weeks, and larger doses were necessary at 16 to 25 weeks to cause an equivalent proportion of mental retardation. Another important observation is the suggestion of a nonthreshold linear relationship of radiation dose at 8 to 15 weeks, so that even very low doses will cause a slight increase in mental retardation compared with the general population (Hall, 1991). There is no documented increased risk of mental retardation in humans at gestational ages less than 8 weeks or greater than 25 weeks, even with doses exceeding 50 rad (Committee on Biological Effects, 1990).

The effect of ionizing radiation on intelligence quotient (IQ) scores in children who were exposed in utero is also dependent on gestational age as well as radiation dose. The highest risk again is at 8 to 15 weeks, followed by 16 to 25 weeks for doses greater than 50 rad.

The implications of these findings seem straightforward. At 8 to 15 weeks, the embryo is most susceptible to radiation-induced mental retardation. This risk is probably a nonthreshold linear function of dose, with the risk of severe mental retardation being as low as 4 percent for 10 rad and as high as 60 percent for 150 rad (Committee on Biological Effects, 1990). These doses are many hundreds of times higher than from diagnostic radiation. Cumulative doses from multiple procedures may enter that harmful range, however, especially at 8 to 15 weeks' gestation. At 16 to 25 weeks, the risk is less, and there is no proven risk at 0 to 8 weeks or after 25 weeks.

Current evidence suggests that there is no increased fetal risk of malformations, growth restriction, or abortion from a radiation dose of less than 5 rad (Brent, 1999). In fact, the risk of spontaneous abortion, malformations, and fetal growth restriction in the general population not exposed to diagnostic radiation is much greater than that which can be theorized from exposure to 1 to 5 rad. According to Brent (1999) gross congenital malformations will not be increased in a human pregnant population exposed to less than 20 rad (0.2 Gy).

ONCOGENIC EFFECTS OF IONIZING RADIATION. It is controversial whether there is an association between in utero diagnostic radiation exposure and an increased risk of childhood cancers. According to some investigators, these cancers, and especially leukemia are increased (Diamond and colleagues, 1973; Shu and associates, 1994; Stewart and Kneale, 1970). Conversely, Brent (1999) and others have questioned such an association, and according to the National Radiological Protection Board (1993) of the United Kingdom, the risk barely exceeds threshold for diagnostic studies. The relative risk of childhood leukemia from fetal exposure of 1 to 2 rad has been estimated from several studies to be 1.5 to 2.0, or from 1 in 3000 in the general population to about 1 in 2000 after exposure (Chap. 18, p. 438). Brent (1999) emphasizes that if elective abortion is chosen based on this, 2000 exposed normal fetuses would be aborted for each case of leukemia prevented—a risk much lower than that for a sibling of a leukemic child, which is approximately 1 in 700.

In another study, two cases of childhood cancer were detected among 1630 atomic bomb survivors, each of whom had high exposure (Committee on Biological Effects, 1990). The data are not yet available on whether atomic bomb survivors are at risk for adult cancers, but late-occurring carcinogenic effects have been observed in laboratory mice exposed to high radiation doses.

THERAPEUTIC RADIATION. According to the Radiation Therapy Committee Task Group of the American Association of Physics in Medicine, about 4000 pregnant women annually undergo cancer therapy in the United States (Stovall and colleagues, 1995). They emphasize careful individualization of radiotherapy as a chosen alternative (Chap. 55, p. 1440). For example, shielding of the fetus can be done for many procedures, and the Task Group has detailed some of those in its report. Despite these precautions, the fetus may be exposed to unacceptable doses of radiation, and thus a carefully designed plan, including dosimetry calculation, must be considered.

DIAGNOSTIC RADIATION. As previously discussed, therapeutic abortion is not indicated because of fetal exposure to a single diagnostic x-ray procedure (Brent, 1999). To put fetal risk into perspective, it is important to know the dosimetry of x-ray procedures, realizing that averages are crude estimates. **According to the American College of Radiology (Hall, 1991), no single diagnostic procedure results in a radiation dose significant enough to threaten the well-being of the developing embryo and fetus.**

PLAIN FILMS. Doses for standard plain film x-rays are presented in Table 42–6. The most commonly used is the chest x-ray. Fetal exposure is exceptionally small (0.07 mrad), even for two views, and it is far below any significant risk for any gestational age. The single abdominal film has a higher dose because the embryo or fetus is directly in the x-ray beam. Its average exposure is approximately 100 mrad. Three films taken for a lumbosacral spine series increase the exposure to 300 mrad. The intravenous pyelogram may exceed 1 rad because of the number of films taken. For this reason, as discussed in Chapter 47 (p. 1259), the one-shot pyelogram may be useful when urolithiasis or other causes of urinary obstruction are suspected but unproven by ultrasound. Most "trauma series," such as x-rays of an extremity, skull, or rib series, deliver low doses because of the fetal distance from the target area. The single hip film is the highest of these, at 200 mrad.

Fetal indications for plain film studies are very limited; the most common is evaluation of the bony pelvis with breech presentation. As discussed in Chapter 22 (p. 512), this is usually done by computed tomographic scanning. Another example is a suspected fetal skeletal anomaly when the ultrasonic diagnosis is unclear, such as with caudal regression syndrome and sirenomelia.

FLUOROSCOPY AND ANGIOGRAPHY. Dosimetry calculations for fluoroscopy and angiography are much more difficult because of variations in the number of x-ray films obtained, fluoroscopy time, and the amount of fluoroscopy time the fetus is in the radiation field. As shown in Table 42–7, the range is quite variable. Although the Food and Drug Administration limits exposure rate for conventional fluoroscopy such as barium studies, special-purpose systems such as angiography units have potential for much higher exposure.

Commonly performed studies involving routine fluoroscopy are the upper gastrointestinal series and barium enema. Frequently, these are done early in pregnancy during the period of preimplantation or early organogenesis and most often before the woman is aware that she is pregnant. As expected, the upper gastrointestinal series has significantly less exposure to the fetus than a barium enema. Because of this exposure,

TABLE 42–7. Representative Doses to Uterus/Embryo from Common Fluoroscopic Procedures

Procedure	Total Dose to Uterus (mrad)	Fluoroscopic Exposure Time (sec)	Cinegraphic Exposure Time (sec)
Cerebral angiography[a]	< 10	—	—
Cardiac angiography[b,c]	65	223 (SD = 118)	49 (SD = 9)
Single vessel PTCA[b,c]	60	1023 (SD = 952)	32 (SD = 7)
Double vessel PTCA[b,c]	90	1186 (SD = 593)	49 (SD = 13)
Upper gastrointestinal series[d]	56	136	—
Barium swallow[b,e]	6	192	—
Barium meal[b,e]	8	228	—
Barium enema[b,f,g]	1945–3986	289–311	—
Small bowel series with upper gastrointestinal series[b,h]	2132 (SD = 2700)	684 (SD = 282)	—

PTCA = percutaneous transluminal coronary angioplasty.
[a]Wagner and associates, (1997).
[b]Calculations based on data of Gorson and colleagues, Table 18 (1984). Doses calculated for 168 cm² radiation field at tabletop with beam quality 3.5 mm aluminum equivalent half-value layer. Thickness of mother = 22 cm, depth of embryo 6 cm from anterior surface.
[c]Finci and co-workers (1987).
[d]Suleiman and colleagues (1991).
[e]Based on female data from Rowley and associates (1987).
[f]Assumes embryo in radiation field from entire examination.
[g]Bednarek and co-workers (1983).
[h]Thoeni and Gould (1991).

gastrointestinal endoscopy is commonly used when a pregnant woman needs evaluation (Chap. 48, p. 1296).

Angiography may occasionally be necessary in pregnancy for some maternal complications. As in the case of plain film x-rays, the farther the distance from the embryo or fetus, the less the exposure risk. Angiographic procedures should be performed when the information obtained alters pregnancy management.

COMPUTED TOMOGRAPHY. Scanning using computed tomography has become an important imaging modality for evaluation of all organ systems. In simple terms, it involves multiple exposures of very thin x-ray beams in a 360-degree circle with computerized interpretations of these exposures. The result is an axial (and occasionally sagittal) image of a body portion, referred to as a slice. Multiple slices of the target body part are obtained along the length of the entire organ or area in question.

Newer-generation tomography equipment is increasingly sensitive; however, higher resolution may be associated with higher radiation exposure. Conversely, because there is less scatter with newer equipment, areas not directly scanned have less exposure. For example, skin exposure from a head tomographic scan will typically be as high as 5 to 6 rad along the area scanned. In the body, doses typically range from approximately 5 rad at the skin surface to 2 rad in the center of the slice.

Spiral computed tomography is a recent advance in tomographic imaging which allows for continuous acquisition of images in a spiral with image reformatting in multiple planes compared with the conventional axial images. The exposure then becomes dependent on the pitch, which is the degree of stretching or tightening of the spiral. The less the pitch, the tighter the spiral, and the greater the exposure. At the present time, a typical pitch (range 1.0 to 2.0) results in radiation from spiral computed tomography exposure that is similar or less than that for conventional computed tomography (Jurik and colleagues, 1996). Because of its ease and brevity, there is a tendency to increase the number of acquisitions, and this increases radiation exposure (Zoetelief and Geleijns, 1998).

Many variables in each study affect calculation of radiation doses, especially slice thickness and number of cuts obtained. If a study is performed with and without contrast, twice as many images will be obtained, and the dose to the target area is therefore doubled. Fetal radiation exposure is also dependent on factors such as the size of the mother and the size and position of the fetus (Ragossino and colleagues, 1986). Finally, the closer the target area is to the fetus, the greater the

TABLE 42–8. Estimated Maximum Fetal Doses from Computed Tomographic Scans

Study[a]	Fetal Dose[b] (rad) at Gestational Age (wk)[c]									
	0–14		15–24		25–29		30–34		35–42	
	Head	Abdomen	Head	Abdomen	Head	Abdomen	Head	Abdomen	Head	Abdomen
Head (10 slices × 10 mm thick)	< 0.05	< 0.05	< 0.05	< 0.05	< 0.05	< 0.05	< 0.05	< 0.05	< 0.05	< 0.05
Chest (10 slices × 10 mm thick)	< 0.10	< 0.10	< 0.10	< 0.10	< 0.10	< 0.10	< 0.10	< 0.10	< 0.10	< 0.10
Abdomen (10 slices × 10 mm [5 mm gaps])	2.6	2.6	2.2	2.4	2.3	2.3	2.1	2.0	1.7	1.7
Lumbar spine (5 slices × 10 mm thick)	3.5	3.5	2.8	3.2	3.0	3.0	2.7	2.6	2.3	2.3
Pelvimetry[d] (1 slice × 10 mm thick, including lateral scout)	—	—	—	—	—	—	—	—	0.25	0.25

[a]Calculations based on conventional computed tomography. Spiral exposure will be the same or less than conventional computed tomography, depending on pitch (Zoetelief and Geleijns, 1998).
[b]Doses based on calculations derived from computed tomography dose index measurements (CTDI) as described in Shope and colleagues (1981). Doses are derived from the average of the CTDI values reported by the manufacturers of the GE 8800, Picker 1200SX, Toshiba TCT-900S, and Philips Tomoscan LX-models of computed tomographic scanners.
[c]Thickness of mother and position of fetus at gestational intervals based on measurements of Ragossino and co-workers (1986).
[d]Radiographic technique and dose for GE 9800 computed tomographic scanner, adapted from Moore and Shearer (1989).

fetal radiation exposure. Estimated maximal fetal doses from computed tomographic scans are summarized in Table 42–8.

Cranial computed tomographic scanning is the most commonly requested study in pregnant women. Nonenhanced computed tomographic scanning is the preferred imaging technique to detect acute hemorrhage within the epidural, subdural, or subarachnoid spaces, and is usually the initial procedure performed in emergency situations. A contrast scan should not be performed first, because it may mask identification of acute hemorrhage. Cranial computed tomography in women with eclampsia is discussed in Chapter 24 (p. 581).

Computed tomography pelvimetry is performed to evaluate maternal pelvic bony dimension for breech vaginal delivery (Chap. 18, p. 438). Depending on exposure parameters, fetal dose may approach 1.5 rad, but using a low-exposure technique, this dose can be reduced to 250 mrad (Moore and Shearer, 1989).

NUCLEAR MEDICINE STUDIES. Ventilation-perfusion lung scans, thyroid scans, and thallium heart scans require the intravenous injection of a radioisotope, which in turn emits radiation that is detected by sensitive cameras. Nuclear medicine studies are performed by "tagging" a radioactive element to a chemical agent. For instance, technetium[99m] is a radioisotope that can be tagged to red blood cells, sulphur colloid, or pertechnetate, as well as other agents. The method used to tag the agent will determine fetal radiation exposure, particularly if it crosses the placenta, or if it is excreted into urine, whereby fetal proximity to the maternal bladder increases exposure. The measurement of this radioactive substance is based on its decay, and the units used are the curie (Ci) or the becquerel (Bq). Doses usually are expressed in millicurie (mCi).

Depending on the physical and biochemical properties of a radioisotope, an average fetal exposure can be calculated (Wagner and co-workers, 1997; Zanzonico, 2000). Commonly used radiopharmaceuticals and the estimated absorbed fetal doses are given in Table 42–9. Recent studies show the exposures will vary with gestational ages and are greatest earlier in pregnancy for most radiopharmaceuticals; an exception is the effect of iodine[131] on the thyroid. (Wagner and associates, 1997). Also, the dose of radionuclide can be kept as low as possible (Adelstein, 1999).

For ventilation-perfusion lung scanning, perfusion is measure with injected ^{99}Tc-macroaggregated albumin

TABLE 42–9. **Radiopharmaceuticals Used in Nuclear Medicine Studies**

Study	Estimated Activity Administered per Examination (mCi)	Weeks' Gestation	Dose to Uterus/Embryo per Pharmaceutical (mrad)
Brain	20 mCi ^{99m}Tc DTPA	< 12[a]	880
		12	700[b]
Hepatobiliary	5 mCi ^{99m}Tc sulfur colloid		45
	5 mCi ^{99m}Tc HIDA		150
Bone	5 mCi ^{99m}Tc phosphate	< 12	460
Respiratory			
Perfusion	5 mCi ^{99m}Tc-macroaggregated albumin	< 12	50
Ventilation	10 mCi ^{133}Xe gas		20
Renal	20 mCi ^{99m}Tc DTPA	< 12	880
Abscess or tumor	3 mCi ^{67}Ga citrate	< 12	750
Cardiovascular	20 mCi ^{99m}Tc labeled red blood cells	< 12	500
	3 mCi [210]Tl chloride	< 12	1100
		12	640
		24	520
		36	300
Thyroid	5 mCi [99m]Tc O$_4$	< 8	240
	0.3 mCi [123]I (whole body)	1.5–6	10
	0.1 mCi [131]I[c]		
	Whole body	2–6	15
	Whole body	7–9	88
	Whole body	12–13	160
	Whole body	20	300
	Thyroid–fetal	11	72,000
	Thyroid–fetal	12–13	130,000
	Thyroid–fetal	20	590,000

[a]Exposures are generally greater prior to 12 weeks' gestation compared with greater gestational age.
[b]Some measurements account for placental transfer.
[c][131]I is the exception to this rule as its uptake and exposure increases with greater gestational age.
Based on data from Wagner and colleagues (1997).

and ventilation with inhaled xenon[127] or xenon[133]. Fetal exposure with either is negligible (Ginsberg and associates, 1989; Mountford, 1997).

Thyroid scanning with iodine[123] or iodine[131] seldom is indicated in pregnancy. With trace doses used for this, however, fetal risk is minimal. Therapeutic radioiodine in doses to treat Graves disease or thyroid cancer may cause fetal thyroid ablation (Green and colleagues, 1971).

The sentinel lymphoscintigram for detecting the axillary lymph node most likely to have tumor in the case of breast cancer has emerged as a popular preoperative study to replace lymph node dissection (DeAngelis and co-workers, 1999). The calculated dose is low and should not preclude its use during pregnancy.

ULTRASOUND. Diagnostic ultrasonography employs sound wave transmission at certain frequencies. At very high intensities, there is a potential for human tissue damage from heat and cavitation (Dakins, 1991; Merritt, 1989). In the low-intensity range of real-time imaging,

however, no fetal risks have been demonstrated in more than 35 years of use (Maulik, 1997; Miller and colleagues, 1998). Naumburg and associates (2000) recently performed a case-control study of 578 children with leukemia. When compared with healthy controls, a third of each cohort was found to have been exposed to ultrasound in utero.

Recent advances in technology have introduced Doppler-shift imaging coupled with gray-scale imaging to localize spectral waveforms and superimpose color mapping. Higher-energy intensities are used with this duplex Doppler imaging.

As of 1992 ultrasound equipment allows video displays of the thermal index and mechanical index. At the present time, unless ultrasound contrast is employed or temperature increases to the fetus exceed 0.5°C, then no potential risk is expected (Miller and associates, 1998). The thermal index applies to the Doppler evaluation, most commonly employed to evaluate the fetal heart and in the case of suspected growth restriction. In the case of Doppler, adverse effects reflected in thermal index changes have not been demonstrated in clinical situations (Maulik, 1997).

There is no contraindication to ultrasound imaging of maternal organs during pregnancy. To date, no documented harmful fetal effects have been reported from ultrasound imaging, nor would such effects be predicted from this nonionizing imaging modality. The wide range of clinical uses of ultrasound in pregnancy are further discussed in Chapter 41 as well as in most other sections of this book.

MAGNETIC RESONANCE IMAGING. Magnetic resonance imaging (MRI) has emerged as a major imaging modality in recent years because of high soft-tissue contrast, ability to characterize tissue, and ability to acquire images in any plane—particularly axial, sagittal, and coronal. Rather than ionizing radiation, magnetic resonance imaging employs powerful magnets to temporarily alter the state of hydrogen protons and molecules, especially water. Through a series of acquisitions, information about the location and characteristics of these hydrogen protons can be obtained as they are returned to their normal state. Because of these established attributes, magnetic resonance imaging has become a useful tool in both obstetrical and gynecological imaging. Technological advances have significantly reduced scan times—and thus cost—and they have improved image quality.

PRINCIPLES. Images are based on the radiofrequency signal emitted by hydrogen nuclei after they have been "excited" by radiofrequency pulses in the presence of a strong magnetic field. The radiofrequency signal emitted has characteristics called *relaxation times.* These include the T_1-relaxation time (longitudinal) and the T_2-relaxation time (transverse). In a magnetic field, protons will align themselves in the same direction as the field running through the bore of the magnet. If a radiofrequency pulse is applied, these protons are forced out of alignment and rotate in phase with one another. The T_1-relaxation is the time it takes for protons to realign with the magnetic field after a radiofrequency pulse is applied. T_2-relaxation is the time it takes for the protons to dephase from each other after a radiofrequency pulse is applied. Because these properties vary among tissues, they are the factors principally responsible for contrast among tissues. The signal intensity of one tissue compared with another—contrast—can be manipulated by varying the elapsed time between application of radiofrequency pulses, which is called the *repetition time.* Further manipulation by the time between a radiofrequency pulse and a sampling of the emitted signal is called the *echo-delay time.* The strength of the magnetic field within the bore of the magnet is measured in tesla (T) (1 tesla = 10,000 gauss).

TECHNIQUE. Tomograms are generated by application of radiofrequency pulse sequences in the presence of different external gradient magnetic fields that determine spatial encoding. The signals are interpreted and constructed into a digital image by a computer. Manipulations of the pulse sequence parameters and gradient fields can yield tomograms with different information in any plane through the entire body. Multiple sequences are employed with magnetic resonance imaging to define anatomy, pathology, and physiological properties of tissues. T_1- and T_2- weighted sequences are often part of a magnetic resonance imaging study, yielding tissue characteristics, anatomical detail, and abnormalities such as edema.

SAFETY. There have been three major areas examined concerning the potential effect of magnetic resonance imaging at field strengths used clinically, that is, those less than 2 tesla. These areas include the effects from static magnetic fields, gradient magnetic fields, and radiofrequency magnetic fields (Wagner and associates, 1997). To date, there are no reported harmful human effects from its use, including any mutagenic effects (American College of Radiology, 1998; Elster, 1994; Wagner and colleagues, 1997). In the study by Vadeyar and associates (2000), there were no demonstrable fetal heart rate pattern changes during imaging.

Absolute safety cannot be assured until larger studies are available for outcome analysis. The 1998 Standards of the American College of Radiology recommend that each request for a magnetic resonance imaging scan of a pregnant patient should be approved by the attending radiologist who will make the final decision. Indicated magnetic resonance imaging should be performed at any gestational age if no other imaging studies can be performed (American College of Radiology, 1998; Wagner and colleagues, 1997).

Contraindications to the use of magnetic resonance imaging include internal cardiac pacemakers, neurostimulators, implantable cardiac defibrillators, implantable electronic infusion pumps, cochlear implants, and some other devices. Certain intracranial aneurysm clips and any metallic foreign body in the globe of the eye contraindicate scanning.

MATERNAL INDICATIONS. Magnetic resonance imaging pelvimetry has been performed and is quite accurate in providing appropriate measurements of the pelvic inlet and midpelvis in the case of breech presentation (Chap. 22, p. 512). Its advantage over computed tomography is the improved resolution of the sagittal plane. Computed tomographic pelvimetry can be performed much more rapidly, however, which is a key advantage for women in labor.

Magnetic resonance imaging in maternal disorders unrelated to pregnancy has the advantage over computed tomography because of the lack of ionizing radiation. In some cases, it may be complementary to computed tomographic imaging, and in others it is preferable. For example, central nervous system abnormalities, such as brain tumors or spinal trauma, are clearly seen with magnetic resonance imaging (Mantello and associates, 1993). Evaluation of lumbar disc pathology is preferably with magnetic resonance imaging (LaBan and co-workers, 1995). Due to its greater accessibility, however, cranial computed tomography is the procedure of choice with trauma or if acute hemorrhage is suspected. Magnetic resonance imaging in eclampsia with T_1- and T_2-spin echo acquisitions and magnetic resonance angiography with phase-control imaging has given valuable insights into pathophysiology (Cunningham and Twickler, 2000; Morriss and colleagues, 1997). T_2-weighted images such as that shown in Figure 42–3 thus far demonstrate edema predominantly of the occipital lobes in eclampsia, typically confined to the gray-white matter junction (Digre and colleagues, 1993). *Magnetic resonance angiography* such as that shown in Figure 42–4, can be used to calculate flow of middle-sized vessels such as the middle and posterior cerebral

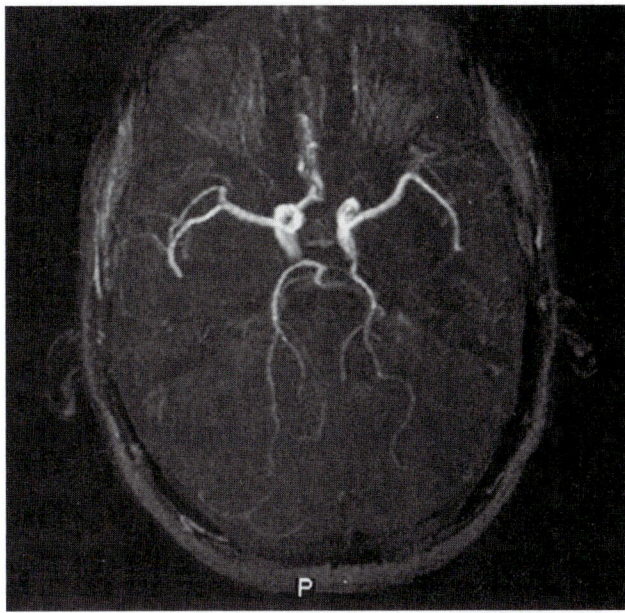

FIGURE 42–4. Magnetic resonance angiography done without contrast is used to locate vessels for orthogonal images. The middle cerebral arteries are seen as prominent lateral branches in this view. (From Nurenberg and Twickler, 1995.)

arteries. This has been useful to measure blood flow alterations induced by vasospasm.

Magnetic resonance imaging is particularly useful to evaluate the abdomen and retroperitoneal space during pregnancy. In this regard, it is preferable to computed tomography, which involves fetal radiation. Some examples include detection and localization of adrenal tumors including pheochromocytoma (Chap. 50), some gastrointestinal lesions (Chap. 48), as well as a number of intra-abdominal malignancies, including lymphoma, renal cell carcinoma, and hepatic tumors (Chap. 55).

Magnetic resonance imaging has been employed as an adjunct to transabdominal and transvaginal sonography in the characterization of uterine and ovarian masses in pregnancy (Curtis and colleagues, 1993; Kier and co-workers, 1990). Resolution obtained with its use is superior to ultrasonic imaging; however, improved resolution does not alter diagnosis or management in most cases (Fernandez and colleagues, 1995). As shown in Figure 42–5, magnetic resonance imaging clearly delineates myomas that are associated with pregnancy.

Postpartum complications of infection that include parametrial phlegmon, abscess, uterine dehiscence, and ovarian vein thrombosis can be imaged using either computed tomography or magnetic resonance imaging (Brown and associates, 1999; Twickler and colleagues, 1997; Woo and co-workers, 1993). Because of the ability of magnetic resonance imaging to project in the sagittal plane, it may provide better visualization of the bladder flap following cesarean section (Twickler and associates,

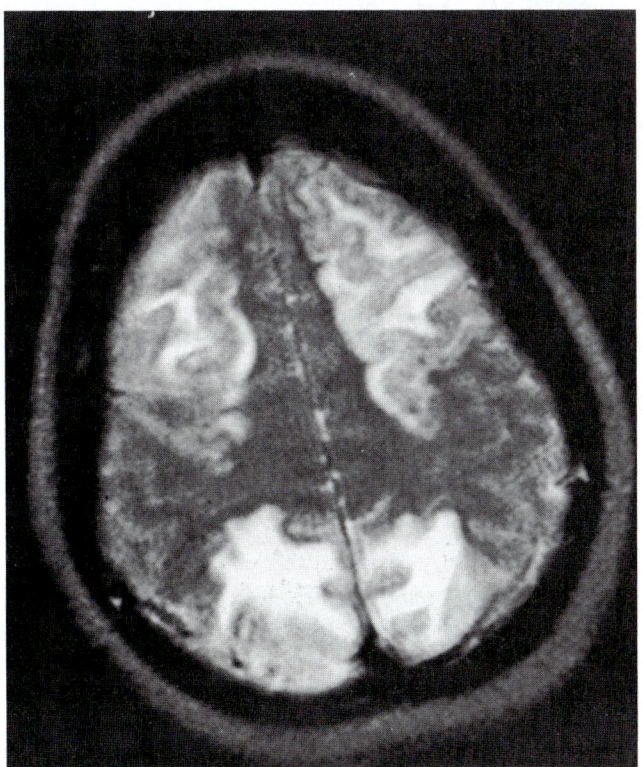

FIGURE 42–3. Edema of the brain in eclampsia is best demonstrated on T_2-weighted magnetic resonance images as bright signals in the frontal and occipital lobes. (From Nurenberg and Twickler, 1995.)

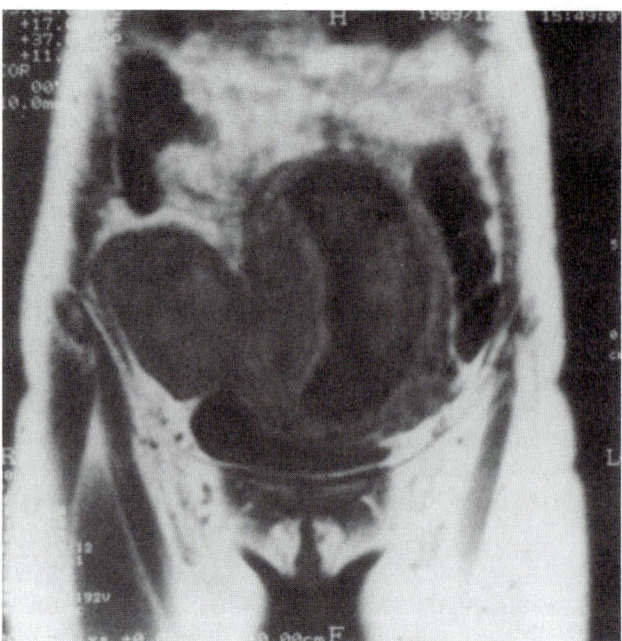

FIGURE 42–5. Coronal T_1-weighted image of right-sided uterine myoma in a pregnant woman. The coronal plane identifies the right pelvic mass arising from the myometrium. There are no cleavage planes separating the mass and uterus, thus confirming its uterine origin. (From Curtis and associates, 1993.)

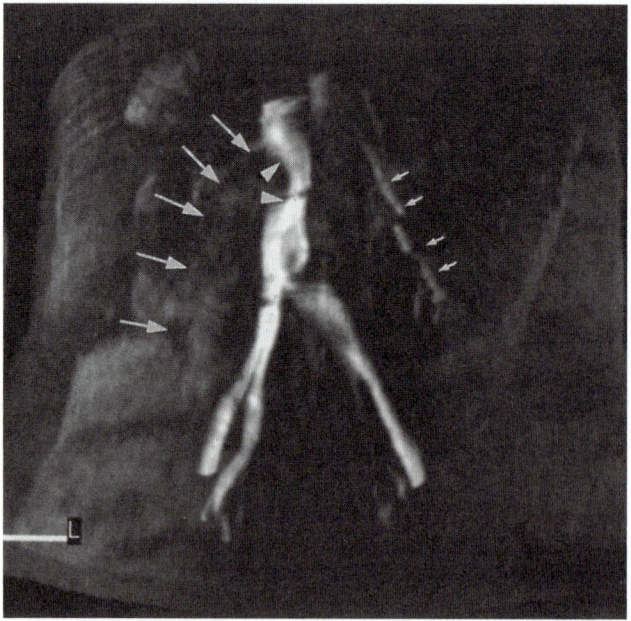

FIGURE 42–6. Reconstructed magnetic resonance venogram of the abdomen 6 days after cesarean section demonstrates normal flow in the left ovarian vein (*small arrows*). The thrombosed right ovarian vein (*large arrows*) has no flow, and the clot produces a mass effect at its confluence with the inferior vena cava (*arrowheads*). (From Nurenberg and Twickler, 1995.)

1991). A further advantage of magnetic resonance imaging may be the computerized reconstruction of the abdominal venogram (Fig. 42–6). Magnetic resonance imaging can also be used to further characterize a bladder flap mass, differentiating hematoma from abscess.

FETAL INDICATIONS. Although magnetic resonance imaging has some role in fetal evaluation, ultrasonic imaging remains the mainstay for fetal evaluation. Fast-acquisition sequencing with magnetic resonance imaging now allows it to overcome some of the problems with fetal movement and improved imaging, especially in cases of central nervous system and thoracic abnormalities. This is referred to as **HASTE**—*H*alf-Fourier *A*cquisition *S*ingle slow *T*urbo spin *E*cho. Levine and co-workers (1999) found that magnetic resonance images altered the diagnosis in 20 of 66 (40 percent) fetuses with central nervous system abnormalities. In some cases, magnetic resonance, imaging may be used to answer very specific questions of fetal anatomy and complex dysmorphology (Coakley and co-workers, 1999). Recently, a lecithin peak has been observed with magnetic resonance spectroscopy in three term fetuses, raising the possibility of in vivo analysis of lung maturity (Fenton and associates, 2000).

GUIDELINES FOR DIAGNOSTIC IMAGING DURING PREGNANCY. The American College of Obstetricians and Gynecologists (1995) has reviewed the effects of

TABLE 42–10. Guidelines for Diagnostic Imaging During Pregnancy

1. Women should be counseled that x-ray exposure from a single diagnostic procedure does not result in harmful fetal effects. Specifically, exposure to less than 5 rad has not been associated with an increase in fetal anomalies or pregnancy loss.

2. Concern about possible effects of high-dose ionizing radiation exposure should not prevent medically indicated diagnostic x-ray procedures from being performed on the mother. During pregnancy, other imaging procedures not associated with ionizing radiation, such as ultrasonography and magnetic resonance imaging, should be considered instead of x-rays when possible.

3. Ultrasonography and magnetic resonance imaging are not associated with known adverse fetal effects. However, until more information is available, magnetic resonance imaging is not recommended for use in the first trimester.

4. Consultation with a radiologist may be helpful in calculating estimated fetal dose when multiple diagnostic x-rays are performed on a pregnant woman.

5. The use of radioactive isotopes of iodine is contraindicated for therapeutic use during pregnancy.

From the American College of Obstetricians and Gynecologists (1995), with permission.

x-ray, ultrasonography, and magnetic resonance exposure during pregnancy. It has suggested the guidelines given in Table 42–10.

REFERENCES

Adelstein SJ: Administered radionuclides in pregnancy. Teratology 59:236, 1999

Akira S, Yamanaka A, Ishihara T, Takeshita T, Araki T: Gasless laparoscopic ovarian cystectomy during pregnancy: Comparison with laparotomy. Am J Obstet Gynecol 180:554, 1999

American College of Obstetricians and Gynecologists: Guidelines for diagnostic imaging during pregnancy. Committee Opinion No. 158, September 1995

American College of Radiology: MR Safety and Sedation. In 1998 American College of Radiology Standards, p. 457, 1998

Barnard JM, Chaffin D, Droste S, Tierney A, Phernetton T: Fetal response to carbon dioxide pneumoperitoneum in the pregnant ewe. Obstet Gynecol 85:669, 1995

Bednarek DR, Rudin S, Wong R, Andres ML: Reduction of fluoroscopic exposure for the air-contrast barium enema. Br J Radiol 56:823, 1983

Brent RL: Utilization of developmental basic science principles in the evaluation of reproductive risks from pre- and postconception environmental radiation exposures. Teratology 59:182, 1999

Brent RL: The effect of embryonic and fetal exposure to x-ray, microwaves, and ultrasound: Counseling the pregnant and nonpregnant patient about these risks. Semin Oncol 16:347, 1989

Brent RL: The response of the 9½ day old rat embryo to variations in exposure rate of 150 R x-irradiation. Radiat Res 45:127, 1971

Brown CE, Stettler RW, Twickler D, Cunningham FG. Puerperal septic pelvic thrombophlebitis: Incidence and response to heparin therapy. Am J Obstet Gynecol 181:143, 1999

Coakley FV, Hricak H, Filly RA, Barkovich AJ, Harrison MR: Complex fetal disorders: Effect of MR imaging on management—preliminary experience. Radiology 213:691, 1999

Committee on Biological Effects of Ionizing Radiation, National Research Council: Other somatic and fetal effects. In Beir V: Effects of Exposure to Low Levels of Ionizing Radiation. Washington, National Academy Press, 1990

Conway BJ: Nationwide evaluation of x-ray trends: Tabulation and graphical summary of surveys 1984 through 1987. Frankfort, KY, Conference of Radiation Control Program Directors, 1989

Cunningham FG, Twickler D: Cerebral edema complicating eclampsia. Am J Obstet Gynecol 182:94 2000

Curtis M, Hopkins MP, Zarlingo T, Martino C, Graciansky-Lengyl M, Jenison EL: Magnetic resonance imaging to avoid laparotomy in pregnancy. Obstet Gynecol 82:833, 1993

Czeizel AE, Pataki T, Rockenbauer M: Reproductive outcome after exposure to surgery under anesthesia during pregnancy. Arch Gynecol Obstet 261:193, 1998

Dakins DR: US output deliberations hinge on thermal effects. Diag Imaging May:91, 1991

DeAngelis GA, Gizienski T, Moore MM: Axillary sentinel node biopsy in breast cancer staging. Appl Radiol, 6:8, 1999

Dekaban AS: Abnormalities in children exposed to x-irradiation during various stages of gestation: Tentative timetable of radiation injury to the human fetus. J Nucl Med 9:471, 1968

Diamond EL, Schmerler H, Lilienfeld AM: The relationship of intrauterine radiation to subsequent mortality and development of leukemia in children: A prospective study. Am J Epidemiol 97:283, 1973

Digre KB, Varner MW, Osborn AG, Crawford S: Cranial magnetic resonance imaging in severe preeclampsia vs eclampsia. Arch Neurol 50:399, 1993

Elster AD: Questions and answers to the editor. AJR 162:1493, 1994

Fenton BW, Lin C-S, Ascher S, Macedonia C: Magnetic resonance spectroscopy to detect lecithin in amniotic fluid and fetal lung. Obstet Gynecol 95:457, 2000

Fernandez CO, Nurenberg P, Santos-Ramos R, Farrish T, Twickler D: A prospective comparison of ultrasound versus magnetic resonance imaging for evaluating ovarian masses in pregnancy. Presented at the annual meeting of the Society of Perinatal Obstetricians, Atlanta, January 1995

Finci L, Meier B, Steffenino G, Roy P, Rutishauser W: Radiation exposure during diagnostic catheterization and single- and double-vessel percutaneous transluminal coronary angioplasty. Am J Cardiol 60:1401, 1987

Gilstrap LC, Van Dorsten P, Cunningham FG: Diagnostic and surgical laparoscopy. In: Operative Obstetrics, 2nd ed. New York, McGraw-Hill, 2001

Ginsberg JS, Hirsh J, Rainbow AJ, Coates G: Risks to the fetus of radiologic procedures used in the diagnoses of maternal venous thromboembolic disease. Thromb Haemost 61:189, 1989

Goldstein L, Murphy DP: Etiology of the ill-health in children born after maternal pelvic irradiation, 2. Defective children born after postconception pelvic irradiation. Am J Roentgenol 22:322, 1929

Gorson RO, Lassen M, Rosenstein M: Patient dosimetry in diagnostic radiology. In Waggener RG, Kereiakes JG, Shalek R (eds): Handbook of Medical Physics, Vol II. Boca Raton, FL, CRC Press, 1984

Green HG, Gareis FJ, Shepard TH, Kelley VC: Cretinism associated with maternal sodium iodine[131] therapy during pregnancy. Am J Dis Child 122:247, 1971

Hall EJ: Scientific view of low-level radiation risks. Radiographics 11:509, 1991

Hunter JG, Swanstrom L, Thornburg K: Carbon dioxide pneumoperitoneum induces fetal acidosis in a pregnant ewe model. Surg Endosc 9:272, 1995

Jurik AG, Jensen LC, Hansen J: Total effective radiation dose from spiral CT and conventional radiography of the pelvis with regard to fracture classification. Acta Radiologica 37:651, 1996

Källén B, Mazze RI: Neural tube defects and first trimester operations. Teratology 41:717, 1990

Kier R, McCarthy SM, Scoutt LM, Viscarello R, Schwartz PE: Pelvic masses in pregnancy: MR imaging. Radiology 176:709, 1990

LaBan MM, Viola S, Williams DA, Wang AM: Magnetic resonance imaging of the lumbar herniated disc in pregnancy. Am J Phys Med Rehabil 74:59, 1995

Lachman E, Schienfeld A, Voss E, Gino G, Boldes R, Levine S, Borstein M, Stark M: Pregnancy and laparoscopic surgery. J Am Assoc Gynecol Laparosc 6:347, 1999

Laws PW, Rosenstein M: A somatic index for diagnostic radiology. Health Phys 35:629, 1978

Levine D, Barnes PD, Madsen JR, Abbott J, Mehta T, Edelman RR: Central nervous system abnormalities assessed with prenatal magnetic resonance imaging. Obstet Gynecol 94:1011, 1999

Mantello MT, Schwartz RB, Jones KM, Ahn SS, Tice HM: Imaging of neurologic complications associated with pregnancy. AJR 160:843, 1993

Maulik D: Biosafety of diagnostic Doppler ultrasonography. In: Doppler Ultrasound in Obstetrics and Gynecology. New York, Springer Verlag, 1997

Mazze RI, Källén B: Reproductive outcome after anesthesia and operation during pregnancy: A registry study of 5405 cases. Am J Obstet Gynecol 161:1178, 1989

Merritt CRB: Ultrasound safety: What are the issues? Radiology 173:304, 1989

Miller MW, Brayman AA, Abramowicz JS: Obstetric ultrasonography: a biophysical consideration of patient safety—the "rules" have changed. Am J Obstet Gynecol 179:241, 1998

Miller RW, Mulvihill JJ: Small head size after atomic radiation. Teratology 14:355, 1982

Moore MM, Shearer DR: Fetal dose estimates for CT pelvimetry. Radiology 171:265, 1989

Morriss MC, Twickler DM, Hatab MR, Clarke GD, Peshock RM, Cunningham FG: Cerebral blood flow and cranial magnetic resonance imaging in eclampsia and severe preeclampsia. Obstet Gynecol 89:561, 1997

Mountford PJ: Risk assessment of the nuclear medicine patient. Br J Radiol 100:671, 1997

National Council on Radiation Protection and Measurements: Exposure of the US Population from Diagnostic Medical Radiation. Bethesda, National Council on Radiation Protection, Report No. 100, 1989, p 26

National Radiological Protection Board: Board Statement on Diagnostic Medical Exposures to Ionizing Radiation During Pregnancy. Documents of the NRPB 4(4). London, HMSO, 1993

Naumburg E, Bellocco R, Cnattingius S, Hall P, Ekbom A: Prenatal ultrasound examinations and risk of childhood leukaemia: Case-control study. BMJ 320:282, 2000

Nezhat FR, Tazuke S, Nezhat CH, Seidman DS, Philips DR, Nezhat CR: Laparoscopy during pregnancy: A literature review. JSLS 1:17, 1997.

Nurenberg P, Twickler DM: Magnetic resonance imaging in obstetrics and gynecology. Williams Obstetrics, 19th ed (Suppl 11). Norwalk, CT, Appleton & Lange, February/March 1995

Otake M, Yoshimaru H, Schull WJ: Severe mental retardation among the prenatally exposed survivors of the atomic bombing of Hiroshima and Nagasaki: A comparison of the old and new dosimetry systems. Radiation Effects Research Foundation, Technical Report No. 16-87, 1987

Ragossino MW, Breckle R, Hill LM, Gray JE: Average fetal depth in utero: Data for estimation of fetal absorbed radiation dose. Radiology 158:513, 1986

Reedy MB, Galan HL, Bean-Lijewski JD, Carnes A, Knight AB, Keuhl TJ: Maternal and fetal effects of laparoscopic insufflation in the gravid baboon. J Am Assoc Gynecol Laparosc 2:399, 1995

Reedy MB, Galan HL, Richards WE, Preece CK, Wetter PA, Kuehl TJ: Laparoscopy during pregnancy. A survey of laparoendoscopic surgeons. J Reprod Med 42:33, 1997a

Reedy MB, Källén B, Kuehl TJ. Laparoscopy during pregnancy: A study of five fetal outcome parameters with use

of the Swedish Health Registry. Am J Obstet Gynecol 177:673, 1997b

Rosen MA: Management of anesthesia for the pregnant surgical patient. Anesthesiology 91:1159, 1999

Rosenstein M: Handbook of selected tissue doses for projections common in diagnostic radiology. Rockville, MD, Department of Health and Human Services, Food and Drug Administration. DHHS Pub No. (FDA) 89–8031, 1988

Rowley KA, Hill SJ, Watkins RA, Moores BM: An investigation into the levels of radiation exposure in diagnostic examinations involving fluoroscopy. Br J Radiol 60:167, 1987

Shope TG, Gagne RM, Johnson GC: A method for describing the doses delivered by transmission x-ray computed tomography. Med Phys 8:488, 1981

Shu XO, Jin F, Lnet MS, Zheng W, Clemens J, Mills J, Gao YT: Diagnostic x-ray and ultrasound exposure and risk of childhood cancer. Br J Cancer 70:531, 1994

Stewart A, Kneale GW: Radiation dose effects in relation to obstetric x-rays and childhood cancers. Lancet 1:1185, 1970

Stovall M, Blackwell CR, Cundif J, Novack DH, Palta JR, Wagner LK, Webster EW, Shalek RJ: Fetal dose from radiotherapy with photon beams: Report of AAPM radiation therapy Committee Task Group No. 36. Med Phys 22:63, 1995

Suleiman OH, Anderson J, Jones B, Rao GUV, Rosenstein M: Tissue doses in the upper gastrointestinal examination. Radiology 178:653, 1991

Sylvester GC, Khoury MJ, Lu X, Erickson JD: First-trimester anesthesia exposure and the risk of central nervous system defects: A population-based case-control study. Am J Public Health 84:1757, 1994

Thoeni RF, Gould RG: Enterolysis and small bowel series: Comparison of radiation dose and examination time. Radiology 178:659, 1991

Twickler DM, Setiawan AT, Evans R, Erdman W, Stettler R, Brown C: Imaging of puerperal septic thrombophlebitis: A prospective comparison of MR imaging, CT, and sonography. AJR 169:1039, 1997

Twickler DM, Setiawan AT, Harrell RS, Brown CEL: CT appearance of the pelvis after cesarean section. AJR 156:523, 1991

Vadeyar SH, Moore RJ, Strachan BK, Gowland PA, Shakespeare SA, James DK, Johnson IR, Baker PN: Effect of fetal magnetic resonance imaging on fetal heart rate patterns. Am J Obstet Gynecol 182:666, 2000

Wagner LK, Lester RG, Saldana LR: Exposure of the Pregnant Patient to Diagnostic Radiation. Philadelphia, Medical Physics Publishing, 1997, p 26

Wilson JG, Brent RL, Jordan HC: Differentiation as a determinant of the reaction of rat embryos on x-irradiation. Proc Soc Exp Biol Med 82:67, 1953

Woo GM, Twickler DM, Stettler RW, Erdman WA, Brown CEL: The pelvis after cesarean section and vaginal delivery: Normal MR findings. AJR 161:1249, 1993

Yamazaki JN, Schull WJ: Perinatal loss and neurological abnormalities among children of the atomic bomb: Nagasaki and Hiroshima revisited, 1949 to 1989. JAMA 264:605, 1990

Zanzonico PB: Internal radionuclide radiation dosimetry: A review of basic concepts and recent developments. 2000.

Zoetelief J, Geleijns J: Patient doses in spiral CT. Br J Radiol 71:584, 1998

43

Critical Care and Trauma

Women with a broad spectrum of pathophysiological conditions, some of which may have previously precluded pregnancy, may benefit from technology and expertise in *critical care obstetrics*. Examples include women with structural cardiac lesions or prosthetic heart valves and with functional class III or IV heart disease, women with acute or chronic pulmonary injuries, or those with complications of severe preeclampsia or septic shock syndrome. The pregnant woman is also at risk for trauma, including automobile accidents, attempted suicide, burns, physical abuse, and sexual assaults which may include gunshot and knife wounds. She and her fetus pose unique considerations for critical care, and it is imperative that obstetricians and other members of the health-care team have a working knowledge of these areas.

Because the pregnant woman is usually young and in good health until she suffers from some acute injury, her prognosis will hopefully be better than that of most patients admitted to an intensive care unit. For example, Lewinsohn and colleagues (1994) described 58 obstetrical patients admitted to an intensive care unit with a mean Apache II score of 11 with a mortality risk of 17 percent. Their actual mortality ratio—the ratio between actual and predicted mortality rate—was 0.42, significantly different from the expected 1.0 mortality ratio.

OBSTETRICAL INTENSIVE CARE

In a majority of cases, obstetrical patients who will need intensive care are those with complications specifically related to pregnancy. For example, hemorrhage, along with hypovolemic shock, is a frequent life-threatening complication in a busy obstetrical unit. Uterine atony or lacerations may require hysterectomy to stop hemorrhage (Chap. 25). It is not unusual for women delivered vaginally to require a surgical procedure to stop bleeding. Examples include vaginal repair of lacerations or laparotomy. Severe preeclampsia and eclampsia are also common obstetrical complications and intensive care is needed antepartum as well as postpartum. Finally, infections with sepsis syndrome are also common in obstetrics.

In many cases, critically ill women will be intensively managed in the obstetrical unit to include the recovery room. In some institutions, there are specialized rooms in the obstetrical suite where necessary equipment and experienced personnel are available. Triage to another specialized unit depends on the acuity of care needed and ability of the facility to provide it. Because of limitations of volume as well as expertise, women who require ventilatory support, invasive monitoring, or pharmacological support of circulation may be better served by transfer to a medical or surgical intensive care unit. The

type of unit necessary will be reflected by the medical, surgical, or obstetrical conditions of each patient.

Mabie and Sibai (1990) reported that 0.9 percent of women delivered at the University of Tennessee were admitted to the obstetrical intensive care unit. Kilpatrick and Matthay (1992) reported that only 0.4 percent of obstetrical patients were transferred to the medical-surgical intensive care unit at the University of California, San Francisco. At the University of North Carolina from 1983 through 1990, only 1 of every 400 pregnant or postpartum women required admission to the intensive care unit (Monaco and colleagues, 1993). At the Medical University of South Carolina only one obstetrical patient was admitted to the intensive care unit every 2 months (Collop and Sahn, 1993). At Parkland Hospital, 1.7 percent of almost 22,000 women delivered over an 18-month period were admitted to an obstetrical intensive care unit within the labor and delivery unit (Table 43–1). Only 11, or 3 percent, of these 376 women were transferred to a medical or surgical intensive care unit, usually for intubation and ventilatory support.

For the woman who is undelivered, ideal care is best provided by specially trained obstetricians and obstetrical nurses with experience in critical care medicine. In their absence, a team of physicians and nurses should be assembled to include those with special expertise sufficient to deal with all problem areas. Team members may include obstetricians, anesthesiologists, pulmonologists, cardiologists, and other intensivists.

ORGANIZATION. Patient care standards that have been established for obstetrical as well as intensive care areas must be met. Proper equipment is a basic prerequisite and standard critical care equipment is necessary. Any equipment that may be needed in the obstetrical suite may also be needed in the intensive care unit. The flow-directed pulmonary artery catheter, arterial lines,

TABLE 43–1. Indications for 376 Admissions to the Obstetrical Intensive Care Unit at Parkland Memorial Hospital over an 18-Month Period

Diagnosis	Number (%)
Hypertensive disorders	150 (40)
Obstetrical hemorrhage	56 (15)
Pulmonary insufficiency	34 (9)
Cardiac complications	19 (5)
Diabetes complications	15 (4)
Other medical complications	49 (13)
Surgical complications	26 (7)
Transfers to/from medical or surgical ICU	27 (7)

Data courtesy of Drs. Gerda Zeeman and George Wendel.

and ventilators are some mainstays of critical care units. Provisions must also be made for initial neonatal resuscitation and stabilization should delivery occur outside the obstetrical area.

Use of data flow sheets common to intensive care units is recommended. These facilitate quick assessment of the clinical condition. Key components of such flow sheets include hemodynamic parameters, ventilator settings, blood gas analyses, temperature, medications, intake to include specific fluids infused, output, daily weight, and basic laboratory values.

PULMONARY ARTERY CATHETER. In our experiences, invasive hemodynamic monitoring is seldom necessary for the critically ill obstetrical patient. In most of these patients, such monitoring seldom changes management. Some of these women, however, have multiple and complex problems that may be better solved with such monitoring. Pulmonary artery catheterization has been used to diagnose or manage a number of cardiac or pulmonary conditions complicating pregnancy, including myocardial infarction, cardiomyopathy, and mitral stenosis; acute respiratory distress syndrome; amnionic fluid embolism; and severe preeclampsia–eclampsia (Clark, 1988, 1995, 1997; Cunningham, 1986, 1987; Hankins, 1984, 1985, and all of their co-workers). Of equal importance, the information provided by these studies allows for an understanding of the pathophysiology of these as well as other conditions unique to obstetrics. Examples include pulmonary edema associated with the use of β-agonists and hemodynamic alterations of preeclampsia–eclampsia. **With improved understanding of this pathophysiology, the need for invasive monitoring is reduced.** The decision to use invasive monitoring is based on the condition and individual needs of the patient (Table 43–2).

Invasive monitoring is usually initiated through the internal or external jugular vein or the subclavian vein. The femoral and antecubital veins are used less frequently because of greater difficulty in positioning the catheter. In the woman with a coagulopathy, however, the antecubital approach may be prudent. The method is described in detail by Clark and colleagues (1997).

DATA COLLECTION. Continuous central venous and pulmonary artery pressures and intermittent pulmonary capillary wedge pressure measurements are obtained with the pulmonary artery catheter. Cardiac output can be measured by thermodilution. Heart rate and rhythm are monitored and may be continuously recorded. Systemic arterial pressure can be measured noninvasively by manual or automatic sphygmomanometers or by arterial catheterization.

Several mean pressures are measured: *filling pressures* include central venous and pulmonary capillary

wedge pressures; arterial pressures are those of the pulmonary and systemic circulations. Formulas for deriving various cardiopulmonary parameters are shown in Table 43–3. Cardiac output, stroke volume, and systemic and pulmonary vascular resistance can be corrected for

TABLE 43–2. Some Indications for Invasive Hemodynamic Monitoring

Sepsis with refractory hypotension or oliguria

Unexplained or refractory pulmonary edema, heart failure, or oliguria

Severe pregnancy-induced hypertension with persistent pulmonary edema or oliguria

Unexplained intraoperative or intrapartum cardiovascular decompensation

Selected cases with massive blood and volume loss or replacement

Acute respiratory distress syndrome

Persistent shock of undefined etiology

Amnionic fluid embolism

Some chronic conditions, particularly when associated with labor or major surgery

   NYHA class III or IV cardiac disease

   Peripartum or perioperative coronary artery disease

   Pulmonary hypertension

NYHA = New York Heart Association.
Modified from American College of Obstetricians and Gynecologists (1992).

TABLE 43–3. Formulas for Deriving Various Cardiopulmonary Parameters

Mean arterial pressure (MAP) (mm Hg) = [systolic pressure + 2 (diastolic pressure)] ÷ 3

Cardiac output (CO) (L/min) = heart rate × stroke volume

Stroke volume (SV) (mL/beat) = CO/HR

Stroke index (SI) (mL/beat/m²) = stroke volume/BSA

Cardiac index (CI) (L/min/m²) = CO/BSA

Systemic vascular resistance (SVR) (dynes × sec × cm⁻⁵) = [(MAP − CVP)/CO] × 80

Pulmonary vascular resistance (PVR) (dynes × sec × cm⁻⁵) = [(MPAP − PCWP)/CO] × 80

Lung compliance:

$$\text{Static} = \frac{\text{Tidal volume}}{\text{Plateau inspiratory pressure}}$$

$$\text{Dynamic} = \frac{\text{Tidal volume}}{\text{Peak inspiratory pressure}}$$

BSA = body surface area (m²); CO = cardiac output (L/min); CVP = central venous pressure (mm Hg); HR = heart rate (beats/min); MAP = mean systemic arterial pressure (mm Hg); MPAP = mean pulmonary artery pressure (mm Hg); PCWP = pulmonary capillary wedge pressure (mm Hg).

TABLE 43–4. **Central Hemodynamic Changes Induced by Pregnancy**

Measurement	Nonpregnant	Term Pregnant	Change (%)
Cardiac output (L/min)	4.3 ± 0.9	6.2 ± 1.0	+ 44
Heart rate (beats/min)	71 ± 10.0	83 ± 10.0	+ 17
Mean arterial pressure (mm Hg)	86.4 ± 7.5	90.3 ± 5.8	+ 4
Systemic vascular resistance (dynes/cm/sec^{-5})	1530 ± 520	1210 ± 266	− 21
Pulmonary vascular resistance (dynes/cm/sec^{-5})	119 ± 47	78 ± 22	− 35
Pulmonary capillary wedge pressure (mm Hg)	6.3 ± 2.1	7.5 ± 1.8	+ 18
Central venous pressure (mm Hg)	3.7 ± 2.6	3.6 ± 2.5	− 2
Left ventricular stroke work index (g/m/m^{-2})	41 ± 8	48 ± 6	+ 17
Colloid oncotic pressure (mm Hg)	20.8 ± 1.0	18.0 ± 1.5	− 14
Colloid oncotic/wedge pressure gradient (mm Hg)	14.5 ± 2.5	10.5 ± 2.7	− 28

From Clark and colleagues (1989), with permission.

body size by division of the values by body surface area to obtain **index values.** Specific body surface area nomograms have not been developed for pregnant women; thus nomograms for nonpregnant adults are used. Clark and colleagues (1989) have determined hemodynamic parameters for healthy nonpregnant and pregnant women at term (Table 43–4 and Fig. 43–1). Increased blood volume and cardiac output are accommodated by decreased vascular resistance and increased pulse rate.

As emphasized by Van Hook and Hankins (1997), hemodynamic information gained by pulmonary artery monitoring does not always reflect uteroplacental perfusion. Assessment of fetal heart rate pattern is more reliable for this purpose.

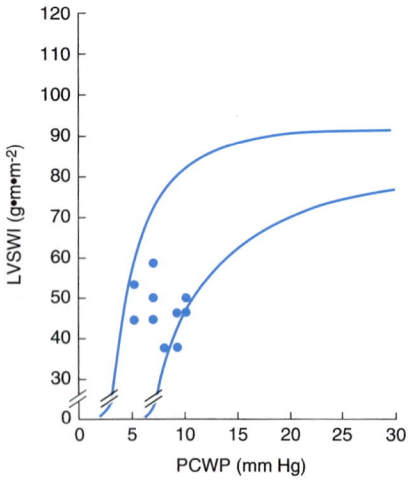

FIGURE 43–1. Normal ventricular function in term healthy women. (LVSWI = left ventricular stroke work index; PCWP = pulmonary capillary wedge pressure.) (Data from Clark and colleagues, 1989.)

DATA INTERPRETATION. Cardiac function is assessed in four areas: **Preload** is determined by intraventricular pressure and volume, thus setting the initial myocardial muscle fiber length. Clinically, the right and left ventricular end-diastolic filling pressures are assessed by central venous pressure and pulmonary capillary wedge pressure, respectively. Cardiac output plotted against central venous or pulmonary capillary wedge pressure constructs a cardiac function curve for the respective ventricle. The ventricular function curve demonstrates that a failing heart requires a higher preload or filling pressure to achieve the same cardiac output as a normally functioning heart (Fig. 43–1). Therapeutic manipulation of ventricular filling pressures and simultaneous measurement of cardiac output allows calculation of optimal preload at the bedside. Preload can be increased by the administration of crystalloid, colloid, or blood, and it can be decreased by the use of a diuretic or a vasodilator or by phlebotomy.

Afterload is defined as ventricular wall tension during systole and is dependent on end-diastolic ventricular radius, aortic diastolic pressure, and ventricular wall thickness. The extent to which right or left intraventricular pressures rise during systole depends primarily on the pulmonary or systemic vascular resistance (Fig. 43–2). With heart failure, increases in afterload such as with preeclampsia worsen failure by decreasing both stroke volume and cardiac output. Afterload, like preload, can be increased or decreased therapeutically. Increases are mediated through α-adrenergic stimulation, for example, with phenylephrine. Decreases in afterload or systemic vascular resistance can be achieved with numerous agents. The intermittent intravenous administration of small incremental doses of hydralazine with intermittent arterial pressure monitoring has been proven safe for both mother and fetus. Sodium nitroprusside by

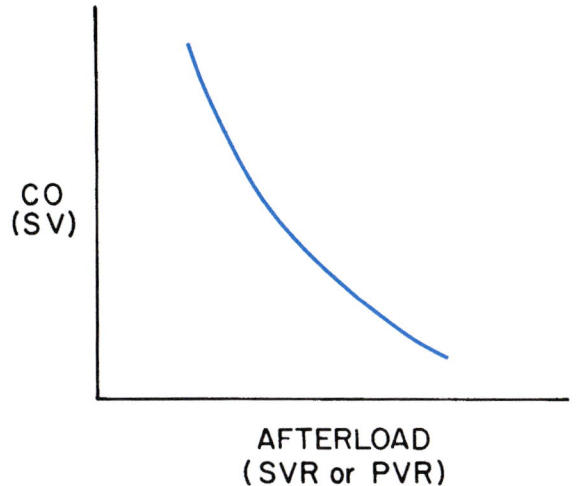

FIGURE 43–2. Relationship of afterload—either systemic vascular resistance (SVR) or pulmonary vascular resistance (PVR)—to cardiac output (CO) or stroke volume (SV) at a constant preload. (From Hankins and colleagues, 1983, with permission.)

continuous intravenous infusion is commonly used in medical intensive care units.

The **inotropic state** of the heart is defined as the force and velocity of ventricular contractions when preload and afterload are held constant. In low-output cardiac failure, both preload and afterload should be optimized. If this fails to restore cardiac output to an acceptable level, attention should be directed to improving myocardial contractility. Beta-agonists such as dopamine, dobutamine, and isoproterenol are effective in improving cardiac output acutely. Digitalis may be used either short term or long term.

Heart rate is important, and either tachycardia or bradycardia may cause problems. If cardiac output is compromised because of bradycardia, treatment either with atropine or cardiac pacing is indicated. Sustained tachycardia can lead to congestive heart failure because of shortened systolic ejection and diastolic filling times or myocardial ischemia, especially with valvar heart disease (Clark and colleagues, 1985). The pathophysiological basis of tachycardia should be determined and corrected; common causes include fever, hypovolemia, and pain.

COMPLICATIONS. An all-important risk of invasive monitoring is over-interpretation or misinterpretation of data. As emphasized by Van Hook and Hankins (1997), mere placement of the catheter is not beneficial, and it may be harmful. Other complications arise from gaining venous access and can be reduced by attention to detail and by experience. The most common is **pneumothorax,** which complicates 5 percent of subclavian and 0.01 percent of internal jugular vein insertions. Le-

thal **intrathoracic bleeding** has been reported during attempts at subclavian vein cannulation with injuries to either arteries or veins. The pulmonary artery catheter itself may incite a variety of ventricular and supraventricular **arrhythmias** as it passes through the right side of the heart. Disconnection of the catheter or introducer from the associated intravenous lines causes massive **hemorrhage.** Rare complications include pulmonary artery rupture, pulmonary infarction, sepsis, knotting of the catheter, thromboembolism, and balloon rupture. Given a broad range of medical and surgical patients with conditions necessitating invasive monitoring, 3 percent will sustain a major complication, including death.

CONTROVERSIES. There are no data from large studies in nonpregnant patients that pulmonary arterial catheterization improves outcome. In one of several studies of myocardial infarction, Connors and colleagues (1996) found excessive mortality in patients undergoing catheterization, despite adjusting for severity of disease. In 1997, the Pulmonary Artery Catheter Consensus Conference was convened by the National Institutes of Health and the Food and Drug Administration. Although this committee did not call for a moratorium on the use of pulmonary arterial catheterization, it acknowledged the need for randomized, controlled trials.

ARTERIAL LINES. Indwelling arterial catheters allow continuous monitoring of systemic blood pressure as well as provide easy access for arterial blood gas samples. Cannulation may be complicated by hematoma, infection, and vessel thrombosis. Serious complications from use of arterial lines, viz., gangrene and loss of a digit or extremity, develop in less than 1 percent of cases.

ACUTE PULMONARY EDEMA

There are two general causes of acute pulmonary edema. Alveolar flooding is caused by either heart failure or permeability edema from alveolar–capillary injury. In many obstetrical cases, a combination of the two is present. In a review of 45,000 pregnancies at the Medical Center of Delaware, Largoza and colleagues (1997) found 40 pregnant women with acute pulmonary edema. Of these, 11 were due to cardiac failure, 11 to tocolytic therapy, 10 to iatrogenic fluid overload, four to preeclampsia, two to infection, and two to renal or hepatic failure. From the University of California, San Francisco, DiFederico and associates (1998) reported that pulmonary edema complicated 0.5 percent of 16,810 deliveries. Commonly associated conditions were preeclampsia (28 percent), preterm labor (24 percent), fetal surgery (17 percent), and infection (14 percent). Karetzky and Ramirez (1998) described 19 cases in 10,852 deliveries, and noncardiogenic pulmonary edema predominated.

In our experiences at Parkland Hospital, in which tocolytic therapy is not used and intravenous crystalloid is administered conservatively in preeclampsia, most cases of pulmonary edema develop in older, usually obese women with chronic hypertension that is further complicated by preeclampsia. These cases often are precipitated by operative delivery with acute blood loss, anemia, and infection (Cunningham and associates, 1986; Sibai and colleagues, 1987). Of 376 women admitted over an 18-month period to the Obstetrical Intensive Care Unit at Parkland Hospital and shown in Table 43–1, less than 5 percent had pulmonary edema.

A number of disorders that have been associated with acute pulmonary injury and permeability edema in pregnancy are listed in Table 43–5. Although most of these are coincidental, some are unique to pregnancy. For example, pulmonary complications, including aspiration pneumonia and pulmonary edema, are common with eclampsia (Bhagwanjee and associates, 2000; Mattar and Sibai, 2000). Although questionably a sole cause, the use of β-agonists to forestall labor is associated with pulmonary edema. Occult chorioamnionitis and sepsis may be the primary cause with amplification by β-mimetics. Amon and associates (2000) described a 5 percent incidence of pulmonary edema with tocolytic therapy given to 257 women.

ACUTE RESPIRATORY DISTRESS SYNDROME. This syndrome is the worst form of respiratory failure. It has a mortality rate of 40 to 50 percent in nonpregnant

TABLE 43–5. Some Causes of Acute Lung Injury and Respiratory Failure in Pregnant Women

Pneumonia	Embolism
Aspiration	Amnionic fluid
Bacterial	Trophoblastic disease
Viral	Air
Sepsis	Connective-tissue disease
Chorioamnionitis	Substance abuse
Pyelonephritis	Heroin
Puerperal infection	Placidyl
Septic abortion	Methadone
Hemorrhage	Irritant inhalation and burns
Shock	Pancreatitis
Massive transfusion therapy	Pheochromocytoma
Arsenic poisoning	
Preeclampsia	

From Bolliger (1992), Clark (1997), Cunningham (1987), Davis (1992), Gottlieb (1991), Ridgway (1991), and their associates.

patients, and this increases to 90 percent if acute respiratory insufficiency was triggered or complicated by sepsis. In a series of 31 pregnant women with acute respiratory failure, Perry and colleagues (1996) reported a maternal mortality rate of 25 percent. There is no evidence that delivery improves maternal oxygenation (Tomlinson and associates, 1998).

Acute respiratory distress syndrome (ARDS) is a pathophysiological diagnosis. It includes both pulmonary alveolar epithelial injuries sustained via the airways and endothelial injuries sustained via the pulmonary vasculature. After recruitment to the site of inflammation by chemokines, neutrophils accumulate and initiate tissue injury by secretion of cytokines. This results in increased pulmonary capillary permeability, loss of lung volume, and shunting with resultant arterial hypoxemia. This has been reviewed recently by Luster (1998) and Ware and Matthay (2000).

Physiological criteria required for diagnosis of the syndrome differ, but it is important to remember that respiratory failure is a continuum from mild pulmonary insufficiency to total mechanical ventilatory dependence. For research purposes, most investigators define acute respiratory distress syndrome as diffuse pulmonary infiltrates on chest x-ray, ratio of arterial oxygen tension to the fraction of inspired oxygen (Pao_2:FiO_2) of less than 200 to 250, and no evidence for heart failure (Ware and Matthay, 2000; Weg and colleagues, 1998).

In nonpregnant patients, sepsis and diffuse infectious pneumonia are the most common single-agent causes of pulmonary failure. In pregnancy, infection, preeclampsia–eclampsia, and hemorrhage are commonly found (Catanzarite and Willms, 1997; Clark and associates, 1997). Perry and colleagues (1996) reported that almost 40 percent of obstetrical cases were caused by infection or sepsis. Importantly, more than 70 percent of women with pulmonary insufficiency have some combination of sepsis, shock, trauma, and fluid overload. Thus, multiplicity of causes is the rule with acute and severe lung injury.

CLINICAL COURSE. With pulmonary injury, the clinical condition depends largely on the magnitude of the insult, the ability to compensate for it, and the stage of the disease. For example, if the woman presents soon after the initial injury, there commonly are no physical findings except hyperventilation, and arterial oxygenation usually is adequate. Normal pregnancy-induced metabolic alkalosis may be accentuated because of hyperventilation. With continued insult, or with time, auscultatory and radiological evidence for pulmonary disease becomes more obvious. There will usually be decreased lung compliance and increased intrapulmonary blood shunting. There is progressive alveolar and

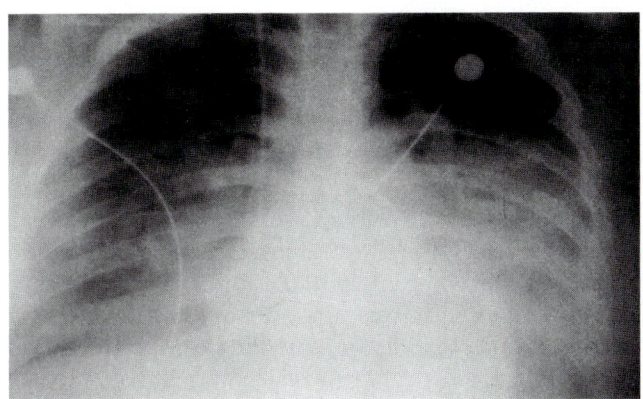

FIGURE 43–3. Severe acute respiratory distress syndrome with diffuse infiltrates. (Courtesy of Dr. Michael Landay.)

interstitial edema along with extravasation of inflammatory cells and erythrocytes.

Ideally, pulmonary injury will be identified at this early stage, the insult terminated, and specific therapy directed at the injury. If not, then further progression results in acute respiratory failure characterized by marked dyspnea, tachypnea, and hypoxemia. Further loss of lung volume results in worsening of both pulmonary compliance and increasing intrapulmonary shunts. There are diffuse abnormalities by auscultation, and the chest radiograph characteristically demonstrates bilateral lung involvement (Fig. 43–3). At this phase, injury has progressed to a point that ordinarily will be lethal in the absence of treatment with high inspired oxygen concentrations. Positive airway pressure, whether by mask or by intubation, is frequently necessary at this stage for airspace recruitment.

During the final phase of the respiratory distress syndrome, **intrapulmonary shunts** in excess of 30 percent result in severe and refractory hypoxemia. The marked increase in dead space, often exceeding 60 percent of tidal volume, leads to hypercapnia and an inability to provide ventilation and oxygenation. Metabolic and respiratory acidosis can result in myocardial irritability and dysfunction, which often leads to cardiac arrest. Microscopically, during end-stage disease, intra-alveolar fibrosis and fibroblastic infiltration of the alveolar septum combine to form massive tissue plates that completely mask the original architecture of the lung parenchyma.

MANAGEMENT. In acute and severe lung injury, attempts are made to provide adequate oxygenation of peripheral tissues while ensuring that therapeutic maneuvers do not further aggravate lung injury. While, at least intuitively, increasing oxygen delivery should produce a corresponding increase in tissue uptake, this

is difficult to measure (Evans and Smithies, 1999). Support of systemic perfusion with intravenous crystalloid and blood is imperative (Chap. 25, p. 653). Because sepsis is so commonplace in lung injury, empirical antimicrobial therapy is considered.

Three critical points merit emphasis:

1. Oxygen delivery is directly proportional to cardiac output.
2. The overwhelming majority of transported oxygen is bound to hemoglobin and is *not* in solution. Accordingly, oxygen delivery can be greatly improved by correction of anemia because each gram of hemoglobin carries 1.25 mL of oxygen when 90 percent saturated.
3. Increasing the arterial P_{O_2} from 100 to 200 mm Hg will result in the transport of only 0.1 mL of additional oxygen for each 100 mL of blood.

Reasonable goals in caring for the woman with severe lung injury are to obtain a Pa_{O_2} of 60 mm Hg or 90 percent oxyhemoglobin saturation at an inspired oxygen content of less than 50 percent, and with positive endexpiratory pressures of less than 15 mm Hg. According to Tomlinson and colleagues (1998), delivery of the fetus does not improve maternal oxygenation.

OXYHEMOGLOBIN DISSOCIATION CURVE. The propensity of the hemoglobin molecule to release oxygen is described by the oxyhemoglobin dissociation curve. Simplistically, the curve can be divided into an upper oxygen association curve representing the alveolar–capillary environment, and a lower oxygen dissociation portion representing the tissue capillary environment (Fig. 43–4). Shifts of the curve have their greatest impact at the steep portion because they affect oxygen delivery. A rightward shift is associated with decreased hemoglobin affinity for oxygen and hence increased tissue–capillary oxygen interchange. Rightward shifts are produced by hypercapnia, metabolic acidosis, increased body temperature, and increased 2,3-diphosphoglycerate levels. During pregnancy, the erythrocyte concentration of 2,3-diphosphoglycerate is increased by approximately 30 percent. This favors oxygen delivery to both the fetus and peripheral maternal tissues (Rorth and Bille-Brahe, 1971).

Fetal hemoglobin has a higher oxygen affinity than adult hemoglobin and its curve is positioned to the left of the adult curve (Fig. 43–4). At a level of 50 percent hemoglobin saturation, the maternal Pa_{O_2} is 27 mm Hg compared with 19 mm Hg in the fetus. Under normal physiological conditions, the fetus is constantly on the dissociation, or tissue, portion of the curve. Even with severe maternal lung disease with very low Pa_{O_2} levels, oxygen displacement to fetal tissues is favored. This has been confirmed by

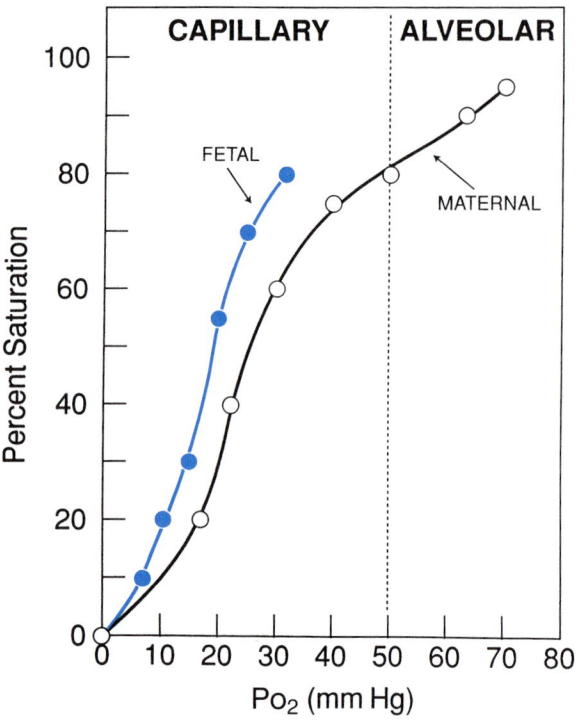

FIGURE 43–4. Oxyhemoglobin dissociation curve. With higher oxygen tension (Pao₂) in the pulmonary alveoli, adult hemoglobin is maximally saturated compared with the lower oxygen tension at the tissue capillary level. Note that at a given oxygen tension, fetal hemoglobin carries more oxygen than adult hemoglobin, as indicated by percent saturation.

studies of pregnant women and their fetuses at high altitude, where despite a maternal Pao₂ of only 60 mm Hg, the fetal Pao₂ is equivalent to that at sea level (Subrevilla and colleagues, 1971).

MECHANICAL VENTILATION. In some patients, positive pressure ventilation by face mask may be effective in early stages of pulmonary insufficiency (Wyncoll and Evans, 1999). In an attempt to maximize the fetal environment, however, early intubation and assisted ventilation is indicated in the pregnant woman if respiratory failure appears to be imminent. Mechanical ventilation usually requires a volume-cycled ventilator. The ventilator is adjusted to obtain a Pao₂ greater than 60 mm Hg, or a hemoglobin saturation of 90 percent and a Paco₂ of 35 to 45 mm Hg. This is the normal Paco₂ for pregnancy, and lower levels should be avoided because they can lower placental perfusion (Levinson and co-workers, 1974).

POSITIVE END-EXPIRATORY PRESSURE. With severe lung injury and high intrapulmonary shunt fractions, it may not be possible to provide adequate oxy-

genation with usual pressures, even with 100 percent oxygen. Positive end-expiratory pressure (PEEP) is usually successful in decreasing the shunt by recruiting collapsed alveoli. At low levels—for example, 5 to 15 mm Hg—positive pressure can usually be employed safely without invasive cardiovascular monitoring. At the higher levels, however, right-sided venous return can be impaired, resulting in decreased cardiac output and decreased uteroplacental circulation. Because positive pressure ventilation raises pulmonary capillary wedge pressure, it must be discontinued during such measurements. High levels can also result in overdistention of alveoli, falling compliance, and barotrauma.

FLUID THERAPY. Treatment of critically ill women with acute respiratory failure requires assiduously detailed attention to fluid balance because fluid overload further compromises pulmonary status (Wyncoll and Evans, 1999). In the intensive care setting, intake and output records should be supplemented with daily weights. A mechanically ventilated patient retains an extra liter of fluid daily. Because respiratory distress syndrome is characterized by a pulmonary permeability defect, fluid leaks into the interstitium, even at normal pressures. Thus, it is best to maintain the lowest pulmonary capillary wedge pressure possible while avoiding decreased cardiac output.

Some pregnancy-induced physiological changes may predispose the woman to greater risk of lung injury from fluid therapy. Robertson (1969) demonstrated a continuous decline in the colloid oncotic pressure (COP) across pregnancy; it fell from 28 mm Hg in the nonpregnant woman to 23 mm Hg at term. Benedetti and Carlson (1979) reported a further decline to 17 mm Hg in the puerperium. In women with preeclampsia, oncotic pressure was 16 mm Hg antepartum and 14 mm Hg postpartum (Zinaman and co-workers, 1985). The importance of these changes is their impact on the **colloid oncotic pressure/wedge pressure gradient.** Under normal conditions, this gradient exceeds 8 mm Hg; however, reductions to 4 mm Hg or less are associated with increased risks for pulmonary edema.

OTHER THERAPY. After promising preliminary data of **artificial or replacement surfactant therapy,** Anzueto and colleagues (1996) performed a prospective study of 725 patients with sepsis-induced lung failure. Continuous administration of aerosolized surfactant had no significant effect on 30-day survival or duration of mechanical ventilation. In another study, inhalation of **nitric oxide** caused early improvement, but mortality was unchanged (Wyncoll and Evans, 1999). In a small preliminary study, **prolonged methylprednisolone** therapy begun in patients with no improvement on day 7 demonstrated improved lung injury and reduced mortality (Meduri and associates, 1998).

Other specific therapies to include **immunotherapy** with anti-CD blocking antibodies, **lipid mediator antagonists** to arachidonic acid, and **antioxidants** are under current investigation (Clark and colleagues, 1997).

BACTEREMIA AND SEPTICEMIC SHOCK

Infections that most commonly cause bacteremia and septicemic shock in obstetrical patients are antepartum pyelonephritis (Chap. 47 p. 1255), chorioamnionitis and puerperal sepsis (Chap. 26), septic abortion (Chap. 33 p. 877), and necrotizing fasciitis (Chap. 26, p. 678). At least in nonpregnant patients, and regardless of etiology of septic shock, mortality is high. In two recent multicenter studies totaling nearly 2400 patients, the mortality rate at 28 days was 35 to 40 percent with severe sepsis and shock (Abraham and colleagues, 1997, 1998). Annane and co-workers (2000) recently published interesting observations in 189 nonpregnant patients with sepsis admitted to two French hospitals. Serum cortisol levels before and after corticotropin administration were predictive of survival. In the largest study of septic shock in pregnancy, Mabie and associates (1997) reported a 28 percent mortality in 18 women.

ETIOLOGY AND PATHOGENESIS. Because pelvic infections are polymicrobial, septic shock may be caused by any of a number of pathogens. Most commonly, bacteria that cause shock are from members of the endotoxin-producing *Enterobacteriaceae* family, especially *Escherichia coli*. Pathogens that less often cause shock are aerobic and anaerobic streptococci and *Bacteroides* and *Clostridium* species. Group A β-hemolytic streptococci, as well as *Staphylococcus aureus,* produce virulent exotoxins that cause all features of the sepsis syndrome (Chap. 26, p. 674). In pyelonephritis, *E coli* and *Klebsiella* species most likely cause bacteremia or septicemia (Cunningham and associates, 1987; Mabie and colleagues, 1997).

Sepsis is caused by an inflammatory response to a trigger—most often microbial endotoxins and exotoxins. These and other toxins stimulate inflammatory cytokine production by vascular endothelium. These cytokines include tumor necrosis factor and interleukin-1 and -8. Neutrophil adherence to endothelium follows, and leukocytes produce a number of toxic substances including proteases and cytokines (Wheeler and Bernard, 1999).

Endotoxin is a lipopolysaccharide that is released upon lysis of the cell wall of gram-negative bacteria. There are probably other bacterial substances that result

in mediator release with activation of complement, kinins, or the coagulation system (Chap. 25, p. 657). According to Levi and ten Cate (1999), 30 to 50 percent of nonpregnant patients with gram-negative sepsis have **disseminated intravascular coagulation.**

Bacterial **exotoxins** released by organisms can also cause shock and death. Examples include exotoxin A from *Pseudomonas aeruginosa* or toxic-shock-syndrome-toxin from *S aureus*. We, as well as others, have encountered a virulent toxic-shock-like syndrome caused by group A streptococcal infection (Nathan and colleagues, 1993). Extensive tissue necrosis and gangrene, especially of the postpartum uterus, may cause profound cardiovascular collapse and maternal death (Chap. 26, p. 685).

Release of vasoactive mediators produces selective vasodilation with maldistribution of blood flow. Leukocyte and platelet aggregation cause capillary plugging. Vascular endothelial injury causes profound capillary leakage and interstitial fluid accumulation. Depending on the injury and inflammatory response, there is a spectrum of clinical disease that is schematically depicted in Figure 43–5. Thus, sepsis is a clinical as well as pathophysiological continuum. The end results of this cascade of pathophysiological events cause the **septic shock syndrome.** In its early stages, clinical shock results primarily from decreased systemic vascular resistance that is not compensated fully by increased cardiac output. Hypoperfusion results in lactic acidosis, decreased tissue oxygen extraction, and end-organ dysfunction. This is also referred to as **multiple organ failure syndrome** (Table 43–6).

HEMODYNAMIC CHANGES IN SEPTIC SHOCK. A greater understanding of the septic shock syndrome has been made possible by direct hemodynamic measurements. The pathophysiology of sepsis has been elucidated by the elegant clinical studies of Parker (1987) and Parrillo (1990) and their colleagues from the National Institutes of Health. If circulating volume is initially restored, then septic shock can be characterized as a high cardiac output, low systemic vascular resistance condition. This is often referred to as the *warm phase* of septic shock. Concomitantly, pulmonary hypertension develops. Paradoxically, patients with severe sepsis are likely to have myocardial depression despite high cardiac output (Ognibene and co-workers, 1988). An elevated cardiac index with decreased systemic vascular resistance are the most common cardiovascular manifestations of septic shock and often have prognostic significance.

Most previously healthy women with sepsis complicating obstetrical infections respond well to fluid resuscitation, given along with intensive antimicrobial therapy and, if indicated, removal of infected tissue. If hypoten-

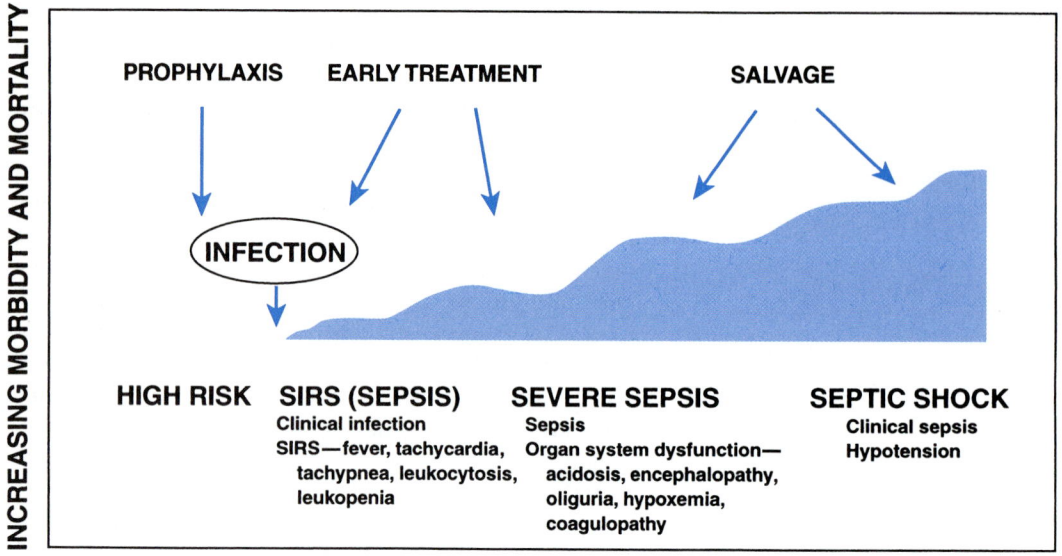

FIGURE 43–5. Systemic inflammatory response syndrome (SIRS). Graph depicts a continuum from infection to septic shock. (Courtesy Dr. Robert S. Munford.)

sion is not corrected following vigorous fluid infusion, then the prognosis is guarded. If there is no response to β-adrenergic inotropic agents, then there is severe and unresponsive vascular insufficiency or overwhelming myocardial depression. Oliguria and continued peripheral vasoconstriction characterize a secondary, *cold phase* of septic shock, from which survival is uncommon. Another poor prognostic sign with sepsis is continued end-organ dysfunction; that is, renal, pulmonary, and cerebral failure once hypotension has been corrected.

The average risk of death increases by 15 to 20 percentage points with failure of each organ system (Wheeler and Bernard, 1999).

DIAGNOSIS AND TREATMENT. Whenever serious bacterial infection is suspected, blood pressure and urine flow should be monitored closely. Septic shock, as well as hemorrhagic shock, should be considered whenever there is evidence of hypotension or oliguria.

TABLE 43–6. Multiple Organ Effects with Sepsis and Shock

Central nervous system	
Cerebral	Confusion, somnolence, coma, combativeness
Hypothalamic	Fever, hypothermia
Cardiovascular	
Blood pressure	Hypotension (vasodilation)
Cardiac	Increased cardiac output (early), myocardial depression (late), tachyarrhythmias
Pulmonary	Shunting with hypoxemia, diffuse infiltrates (capillary leak)
Renal	Hypoperfusion (oliguria), acute tubular necrosis
Hematological	Thrombocytopenia, leukocytosis, consumptive coagulopathy

Modified from American College of Obstetricians and Gynecologists (1995).

When shock from sepsis is suspected, prompt and aggressive treatment includes:

1. Careful monitoring of vital signs and urinary output.
2. Vigorous intravenous fluid infusion to restore circulating volume.
3. Administration of empirical antimicrobial drugs selected to provide coverage that includes all suspected pathogens.
4. Oxygen and ventilatory support if needed.
5. And, if indicated, surgical intervention after the clinical condition has been stabilized.

Shown in Table 43–7 is a scheme for treatment of sepsis syndromes. Rapid infusion with 2 L and sometimes as many as 4 to 6 L of crystalloid fluids may be required to restore renal perfusion in severely affected women. Because of the vascular leak, these women usually are hemoconcentrated, and if the hematocrit is 30 volume percent or less, then blood is given along with

TABLE 43–7. Management of Obstetrical Sepsis Syndromes

Suspected sepsis
  Determine site if possible
  Rapid crystalloid infusion—2 L Ringer solution
  Antimicrobial therapy
  Oxygen therapy

Sepsis with hypotension
  Continue crystalloid infusion
  Correct acidosis
  Excise infected tissue
    Curettage for septic abortion
    Debride wound infection
    Drain abscesses
  Monitor for organ dysfunction
    Urine output
    Mental status
    Respiratory insufficiency
    Skin perfusion
    Blood pressure
    Myocardial dysfunction
    Coagulopathy

Severe sepsis
  Mechanical ventilation
  Support circulation
    Inotropics
    Vasopressors
  Consider pulmonary artery catheter

From Cunningham (1998).

crystalloid to maintain the hematocrit at about 30 volume percent or perhaps slightly higher (Chap. 25, p. 653). The use of colloid solution, for example, 5 percent human albumin, is controversial (Clark and colleagues, 1997; Ware and Matthay, 2000). If aggressive volume replacement is not promptly followed by urinary output of at least 30 and preferably 50 mL/hr, as well as other indicators of improved perfusion, then consideration is given for insertion of a pulmonary artery catheter. Mortality is high when sepsis is further complicated by renal failure (Alexopoulos and colleagues, 1993). In women who are seriously ill, pulmonary capillary endothelium is also likely damaged, with alveolar leakage and pulmonary edema occurring even with low or normal pulmonary capillary wedge pressures—the **acute respiratory distress syndrome** described earlier (pp. 1164 to 1165). This must be differentiated from circulatory overload from overly vigorous fluid therapy, with which wedge pressures will be abnormally high.

Broad-spectrum antimicrobials are administered in maximal doses after appropriate cultures are taken. These include blood cultures, along with specimens of exudates that are not contaminated by normal flora. For women with infected abortions or those with deep fascial infections, a Gram-stained smear may be helpful in identifying *Clostridium perfringens* or group A streptococcal organisms. Generally, empirical coverage with regimens such as ampicillin plus gentamicin plus clindamycin suffices.

SURGICAL TREATMENT. Continuing sepsis may prove fatal, and debridement of necrotic tissue or drainage of purulent material is crucial. Of 18 pregnant women with septic shock, Mabie and colleagues (1997) reported that eight required surgical therapy to control the source of infection. A meticulous search is made for such foci. For women with an infected abortion, the uterine contents must be removed promptly by curettage. Hysterectomy is seldom indicated unless the uterus has been lacerated or is obviously intensely infected (Fig. 43–6). Bacterial shock may become clinically apparent several hours after evacuation of infected products from the uterus.

For women with pyelonephritis, continuing sepsis usually is from urinary obstruction caused by calculi or a perinephric abscess or phlegmon. With obstruction, ureteral catheterization or percutaneous nephrostomy may be lifesaving, and flank exploration with debridement may be indicated (Chap. 47, p. 1258). In some cases, end-stage pyonephrosis is found as a source of continuing sepsis and nephrectomy must be performed.

Puerperal infections causing sepsis that may be amenable to surgical treatment are those in which there are appreciable amounts of infected or devitalized tissue, or both. In addition to clostridial infections, there have

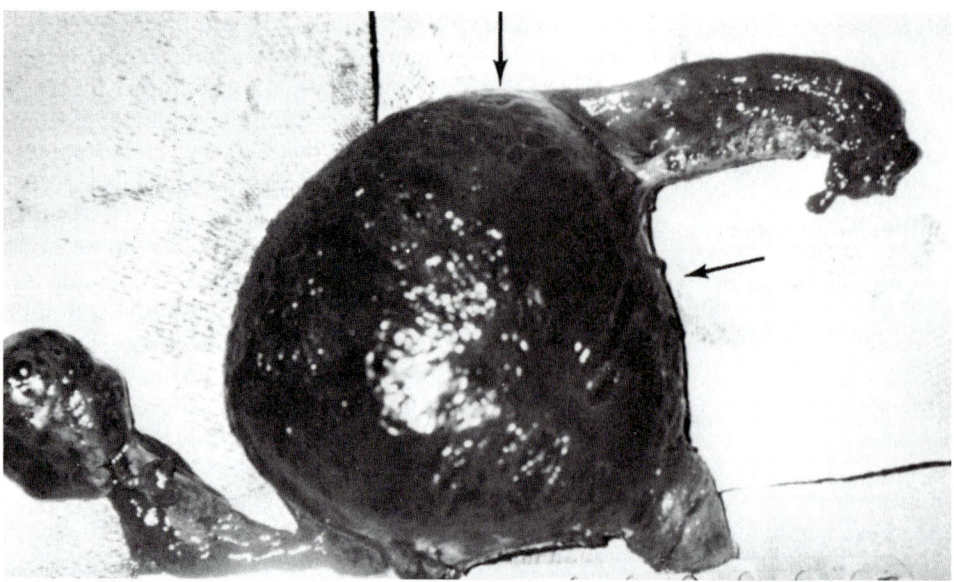

FIGURE 43–6. The numerous rents in the uterine serosa (*arrows*) were the consequence of gas formation plus intensive necrosis from *Clostridium perfringens*.

been reports in the past 10 years of women with massive uterine myonecrosis from group A β-hemolytic streptococci. The mortality rate in these women has been high (Mabie and co-workers, 1997; Nathan and colleagues, 1993). Other causes of sepsis are deep myofascial infections of the episiotomy site or abdominal surgical incision (see necrotizing fasciitis in Chap. 26, p. 684). These infections must be promptly recognized and aggressively treated (Feinberg and colleagues, 1996). In women with persistent infections following cesarean delivery, the uterine incision may undergo necrosis and dehiscence with subsequent peritonitis. Hysterectomy has been necessary following overwhelming sepsis due to a gas-forming *E coli* chorioamnionitis (Catanzarite and associates, 1994). Another source may be from a ruptured parametrial or intra-abdominal abscess. **Any woman with a puerperal infection who is suspected of developing peritonitis should be carefully evaluated for uterine incisional necrosis and separation or for bowel perforation.**

ADJUNCTIVE THERAPY

PRESSOR AGENTS. Vasoactive drugs are not given unless aggressive fluid treatment fails to correct hypotension and perfusion abnormalities. One commonly used agent is dopamine hydrochloride, which when given in doses of 2 to 10 μg/kg/min stimulates cardiac α-receptors to increase cardiac output. Doses of 10 to 20 μg/kg/min cause β-receptor stimulation, an increase in systemic vascular resistance, and an increase in blood pressure. At doses of more than 20 μg/kg/min, α-receptor

stimulation predominates, but dopamine is seldom needed at these higher doses. If there is no response to dopamine, then dobutamine, 5 to 15 μg/kg/min or norepinephrine, 5 to 20 μg/min, may be of benefit (Wheeler and Bernard, 1999).

OXYGENATION AND VENTILATION. Oxygen is administered in an attempt to improve tissue oxygenation. As the septic shock syndrome progresses and intravascular volume is restored, there may be substantive pulmonary capillary endothelial damage with leakage into alveoli. Resultant pulmonary edema causes hypoxemia, which worsens tissue hypoxia and acidosis. When this is severe and adequate oxygenation cannot be maintained by increased oxygen delivered via a nonrebreathing mask or by a continuous positive airway pressure mask, then tracheal intubation and mechanical ventilation that delivers positive pressure may prove to be lifesaving (see p. 1165).

ANTI-INFLAMMATORY AGENTS. Methylprednisolone given in large doses within a few hours of sepsis does not improve early or late morbidity or mortality (Bone and colleagues, 1987; Veterans Administration Systemic Sepsis Cooperative Study Group, 1987). Similarly, in 455 patients given intravenous ibuprofen or placebo for sepsis, there was no improvement in prevention of shock, respiratory failure, or mortality (Bernard and co-workers, 1997).

IMMUNOTHERAPY. There have been several studies using **antiendotoxin antibody** serum for gram-negative sepsis or septic shock. Although preliminary results were promising with a human monoclonal IgM antibody to lipid A, the observations of the French National Registry of HA-1A in Septic Shock (1994) were not. This cohort study of 600 patients showed that mortality was not decreased with treatment and suggested excess mortality in patients with non–gram-negative bacteremia.

A number of studies with **E5 murine monoclonal IgM antiendotoxin antibody** for gram-negative sepsis showed no improvement of mortality (Angus and associates, 2000; Bone and colleagues, 1995). E5 antibodies did result in prevention of acute respiratory distress syndrome and greater resolution of organ failure in patients with sepsis—an important finding because patients with suspected sepsis can be identified without waiting for culture results.

Because certain cytokines have been shown to mediate the inflammatory response in sepsis, **anticytokine antibodies** have been used in clinical trials. Abraham and colleagues (1998) used murine monoclonal antibody against tumor necrosis factor-α (TNF-α Mab) in 948 patients with septic shock. While the incidence of coagulopathy in the treated group was significantly decreased (19 versus 27 percent), there were no other benefits, including the 28-day mortality rate of about 40 percent in both groups.

Abraham and co-workers (1997) studied a recombinant **fusion protein of p55 tumor necrosis factor receptor** to competitively block TNF-α binding with cell-associated receptors. They treated 498 patients with severe sepsis and found a similar 28-day mortality in treated (35 percent) versus placebo-group patients (39 percent).

TRAUMA IN PREGNANCY

Trauma, homicide, and similar violent events are a leading cause of death in young women. According to the American College of Obstetricians and Gynecologists (1998), 1 in 12 pregnancies is associated with physical trauma. Indeed, injury-related deaths are the most commonly identified cause of maternal morbidity in Cook County, Illinois; New York City; Massachusetts; Utah; and North Carolina (Dannenberg, 1995; Fildes, 1992; Jacob, 1998; Sachs, 1987, and all their colleagues; Harper and Parsons, 1997). Although motor vehicle accidents, falls, and homicides are clearly sources of significant trauma in pregnancy, by far the most frequent form of trauma involves physical or sexual abuse. In many cases, trauma arises from domestic abuse or battering (Eisenstat and Bancroft, 1999; Kurzel and associates, 2000). Interestingly, Dietz and associates (1999) reported that women who were psychologically and physically abused in childhood frequently had an unintended first pregnancy.

BLUNT TRAUMA

PHYSICAL ABUSE. It is estimated that 5 million women each year are physically assaulted by their male partners (American College of Obstetricians and Gynecologists, 1999). Even more appalling is that pregnant women are not immune to such physical violence. In a recent mail survey, Horan and colleagues (1998) ascertained that ACOG Fellows routinely screen 27 percent of nonpregnant women for domestic violence at the first office visit. For pregnant women, 39 percent routinely screened at the first prenatal visit. While only a third of these physicians had received instruction on domestic violence during residency, two thirds learned through continuing education.

Most data concerning this subject are from public institutions. For example, a third of injuries to pregnant women cared for at the University of Mississippi Medical Center were intentionally inflicted (Poole and colleagues, 1996). McFarlane and colleagues (1992) and Berenson and co-workers (1991) questioned women attending public clinics and reported that almost a fourth had been physically or sexually abused during pregnancy. Cokkinides and colleagues (1999) found that 11 percent of 6000 pregnant women reported physical violence. Importantly, this was linked to poverty, poor education, and use of tobacco and alcohol. Kurzel and associates (2000) reported that drug use was associated with half of instances of battered pregnant women. Similar risk factors were reported from two multicenter emergency department studies of nonpregnant women (Grisso and co-workers, 1999; Kyriacou and associates, 1999).

The woman who is physically abused tends to present late, if at all, for prenatal care. Her risk of preterm labor and of chorioamnionitis is twice that of control women (Berenson and co-workers, 1994). Women abused during pregnancy are also at increased risk for low-birthweight infants as well as a higher cesarean delivery rate (Curry and colleagues, 1998; Parker and associates, 1994).

Risk factors for physical abuse in pregnancy have been generally subdivided into three categories (Stewart and Cecutti, 1993). *Social instability* includes such factors as young age; unmarried, divorced, or separated; lower level of education or unemployment; and unplanned pregnancy. *Unhealthy lifestyle* includes poor diet; substance abuse including alcohol, tobacco, and illicit drugs; and emotional problems. *Physical health problems* include acute and chronic medical conditions and use of prescription medications. Unfortunately, the abused pregnant woman tends to stay with the abuser, and 60 percent report two or more episodes of physical assault during pregnancy (McFarlane and colleagues, 1992). The woman who is physically or sexually abused in pregnancy should also be considered to be emotionally abused. Finally, Stewart (1994) observed the tendency for physical abuse to increase in the first several months following delivery.

SEXUAL ASSAULT. According to the Federal Bureau of Investigation (1998), there were nearly 100,000 forcible rapes of women reported in 1997. It generally is held that only 10 to 20 percent of sexual assaults are reported. Satin and co-workers (1991) reviewed over 5700 sexual assaults against women committed in Dallas County over 6 years, and found that 2 percent of the victims were pregnant. Associated physical trauma was less common than in nonpregnant rape victims, and only a third of assaults took place after 20 weeks. From a forensic standpoint, evidence collection was not altered.

Satin and co-workers (1992) also interviewed 2404 women postpartum and found that the lifetime prevalence of forced sexual contact was 5 percent. Compared with nonvictims, rape victims had a higher incidence of sexually transmitted diseases, urinary infections, vaginitis, drug use, and multiple hospitalizations. Berenson and colleagues (1992) reported that 8 percent of pregnant adolescents had been sexually assaulted. A member of their family was the perpetrator in 46 percent of cases, and a spouse or boyfriend in 33 percent.

The importance of psychological counseling for the rape victim and her family cannot be overemphasized. In addition to attention to physical and psychological injuries, exposure to sexually transmitted diseases must be considered. Shown in Table 43–8 are the current recommendations for prophylaxis recommended by the Centers for Disease Control and Prevention (1998).

AUTOMOBILE ACCIDENTS. According to the National Highway Traffic Safety Administration (1998), vehicular deaths are the leading cause of deaths in females 8 to 28 years old. Most cases of significant blunt trauma during pregnancy are caused by vehicle accidents, falls, and direct assault (Connolly and co-workers, 1997; Pak and colleagues, 1998). Car accidents account for the majority of these deaths, which might be prevented with the use of three-point restraints (American College of Obstetricians and Gynecologists, 1998; Crosby, 1996). Indeed, Pearlman and associates (2000) found that proper seatbelt use and crash severity were the best predictors of maternal-fetal outcomes. Despite this, Pearlman and Phillips (1996) found that a third of women did not use seat restraints or used them incorrectly during pregnancy. Similarly, Tyroch and associates (1999) reported that while 86 percent used restraints while pregnant, almost half used them incorrectly.

Effects of deployment of airbags in pregnant drivers or passengers have not been widely reported. Sims and associates (1996) reported three third-trimester women whose driver-side airbag deployed in 10 to 25 mph collisions. They reported no injuries. Schultze and colleagues (1998) reported a 20 percent placental abruption that caused a stillborn 28-week fetus in a woman whose airbag deployed in a 40 mph collision. Even less is known concerning passenger-side bags or doorbags.

TABLE 43–8. Guidelines for Prophylaxis of Sexually Transmitted Disease in Victims of Sexual Assault

Prophylaxis	Regimen	Alternative
N gonorrhoeae	Ceftriaxone, 125 mg IM, single dose	Cefixime, 400 mg po, single dose; or
		Spectinomycin, 2 g IM, single dose
C trachomatis	Azithromycin, 1 g po, single dose	Erythromycin-base, 500 mg po qid × 7 days; or
		Amoxicillin, 500 mg po tid × 7 days
T vaginalis	Metronidazole, 2 g po, single dose	
Hepatitis B	First dose hepatitis vaccine, repeated at 1–2 and 4–6 months	
Human immunodeficiency virus	Consider testing and possible retroviral prophylaxis	

From Centers for Disease Control and Prevention (1998).

OTHER BLUNT TRAUMA. Some other common causes of blunt trauma are falls and aggravated assaults (Luger and associates, 1995). Less common forms of blunt trauma include blast injury or crush injury (Awwad and co-workers, 1994a; Schoenfeld and colleagues, 1995). Serious intra-abdominal injuries are of particular concern and, probably related to the markedly increased pelvic and abdominal vascularity, retroperitoneal hemorrhage is encountered more commonly compared with nonpregnant women. Conversely, bowel injuries are less frequent because of the protective effect of the large uterus. Diaphragmatic, splenic, liver, and kidney injuries may also be sustained (Flick and colleagues, 1999; Icely and Chez, 1999).

TRAUMATIC PLACENTAL ABRUPTION. Placental separation is likely caused by deformation of the elastic myometrium around the relatively inelastic placenta (Crosby and associates, 1968). Abruption complicates 1 to 6 percent of "minor" injuries and up to 50 percent of major injuries (Goodwin and colleagues, 1990; Pearlman and co-workers, 1990). Reis and colleagues (2000) found that abruption was more likely in car accidents occurring at over 30 mph.

In many cases, findings with traumatic abruption are similar to those discussed in Chapter 25 (p. 624). Stettler and associates (1992) reviewed our experiences with 13 such women at Parkland Hospital and reported that although 11 had uterine tenderness, only five had vaginal bleeding. Other common findings are uterine contractions; evidence for fetal compromise such as fetal tachycardia, late decelerations, and acidosis; and fetal death. Because placental abruption associated with trauma may be concealed, the incidence of associated severe coagulopathy is probably higher than with nontraumatic abruption.

Kettel and co-workers (1988) emphasize that abruption may be occult and not associated with uterine pain, tenderness, and bleeding. According to Pearlman and associates (1990), detection of uterine contractile activity using electronic monitoring is suggestive of abruption. If tocolytics are used, they may obfuscate clinical findings of placental abruption.

UTERINE RUPTURE. This is uncommon with blunt trauma and is found in less than 1 percent of severe cases (American College of Obstetricians and Gynecologists, 1998). It is usually associated with a direct impact of substantive force. Findings may be identical to those for placental abruption, and maternal and fetal deterioration are soon inevitable. Dash and Lupetin (1991) described a 24-week pregnancy in which traumatic uterine rupture was confirmed using computed tomography.

FETAL–MATERNAL HEMORRHAGE. If there is considerable abdominal force associated with trauma, and especially if the placenta is lacerated, life-threatening fetal–maternal hemorrhage may be encountered (Pritchard and associates, 1991). Some degree of bleeding from the fetal to maternal circulation is found in 10 to 30 percent of trauma cases (Goodwin and Breen, 1990; Pearlman and associates, 1990). In 90 percent of these cases, however, hemorrhage is less than 15 mL. We encountered three cases of massive fetal–maternal hemorrhage in eight women with a traumatic abruption (Stettler and associates, 1992). It seems likely that this is not due to placental separation because there usually is no fetal bleeding into the intervillous space. More likely fetal hemorrhage is associated with a placental tear or "fracture" caused by stretching. In the three cases of massive fetal bleeding described above, two were associated with a placental laceration and the infants were stillborn (Fig. 43–7).

FETAL INJURY. According to Kissinger and co-workers (1991), the risk of fetal death with trauma is significant when there is direct fetoplacental injury, maternal shock, pelvic fracture, maternal head injury, or hypoxia. Although fetal injury and death are uncommon, there are many interesting case reports that describe it. Fetal skull and brain injury are most common. These injuries are more likely if the head is engaged, and the maternal pelvis is fractured on impact (Palmer and Sparrow, 1994). Conversely, fetal head injuries, presumably from a *contrecoup* effect, may be sustained in unengaged vertex or nonvertex presentations. Weyerts and colleagues (1992) described a newborn with paraplegia and contractures associated with a motor vehicle accident sustained several months before birth.

PENETRATING TRAUMA. Knife and gunshot wounds are the most common penetrating injuries and may be associated with aggravated assaults, suicide attempts, or attempts to cause abortion. The incidence of visceral injury with penetrating trauma is only 15 to 40 percent compared with 80 to 90 percent in nonpregnant individuals (Stone, 1999). When the uterus sustains penetrating wounds, the fetus is more likely than the mother to be seriously injured (Fig. 43–8). Indeed, although the fetus sustains injury in two thirds of such cases, visceral injuries to the mother are seen in only 20 percent (Buchsbaum, 1979). Awwad and colleagues (1994b) reported unique experiences with high-velocity penetrating wounds of the pregnant uterus collected over 16 years of civil war in Lebanon. Among 14 women, two died, but neither was as a direct result of intra-abdominal injury. Three observations were made:

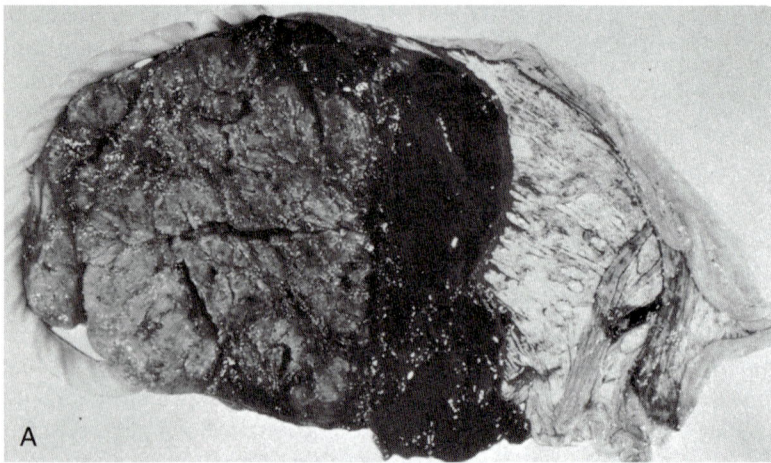

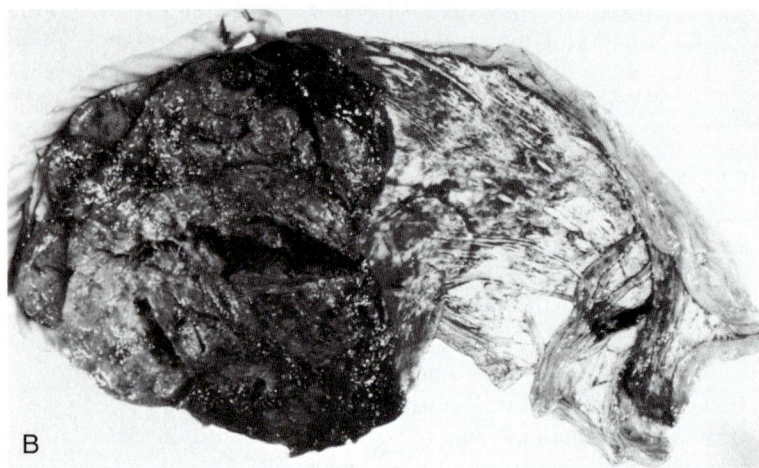

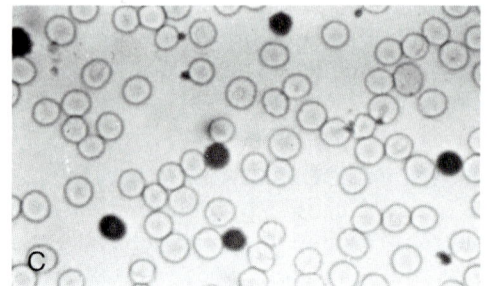

FIGURE 43–7. A. Partial placental abruption with adherent blood clot. The fetus died from massive hemorrhage, chiefly into the maternal circulation. **B.** The adherent blood clot has been removed. Note the laceration of the placenta. **C.** Kleihauer–Betke stain of a smear of maternal blood after fetal death. The dark cells(4.5 percent) are fetal red cells, whereas the empty cells are maternal in origin.

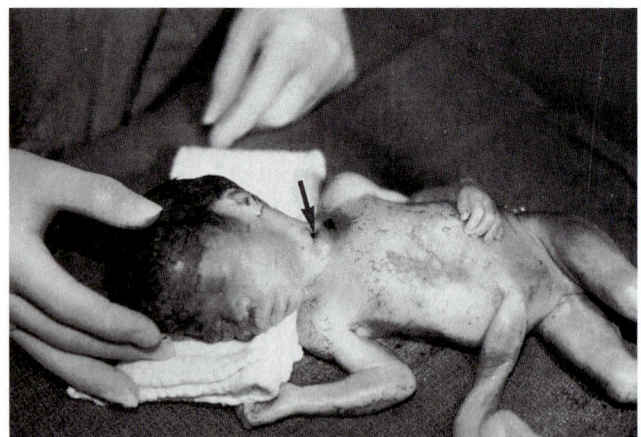

FIGURE 43–8. This 25-week fetus was killed by a gunshot wound to neck. The .22-caliber bullet entered the uterine fundus anteriorly and exited posteriorly in the lower uterine segment just underneath the serosa. (Photograph courtesy of Dr. R. Santos.)

1. Visceral injuries were present when the entrance wound was in either the upper abdomen or back.
2. When the entry wound site was anterior and below the uterine fundus, visceral injuries were absent in all six women.
3. Perinatal death ensued in half and was due to either maternal shock, uteroplacental injury, or direct fetal injury.

MANAGEMENT OF TRAUMA. With few exceptions, treatment priorities are directed toward the injured pregnant woman as they are for nonpregnant patients. Primary goals are evaluation and stabilization of maternal injuries. Attention to fetal assessment during the acute evaluation may divert attention from life-threatening maternal injuries (American College of Obstetricians and Gynecologists, 1998). Basic rules are applied to resuscitation, including establishing ventilation and arrest of hemorrhage along with treatment for hypovolemia with crystalloid and blood products. **An important aspect of management is deflection of the large uterus**

away from the great vessels to diminish their effect on decreased cardiac output. Hoff and associates (1991), as well as Scorpio and colleagues (1992), documented that fetal death is related to the severity of maternal injury. They found close correlation of low maternal serum bicarbonate level with fetal demise. Biester and co-workers (2000) did not find the Revised Trauma Score predictive of adverse pregnancy outcome.

Following emergency resuscitation, evaluation is continued for fractures, internal injuries, bleeding sites, as well as uterine and fetal injuries. If indicated, open peritoneal lavage should be performed in the pregnant woman (Scorpio and colleagues, 1992). Penetrating injuries in most cases must be evaluated using radiography (Chap. 42). Because clinical response to peritoneal irritation is blunted during pregnancy, an aggressive approach to exploratory laparotomy is pursued for abdominal trauma. Whereas exploration is mandatory for abdominal gunshot wounds, some advocate close observation for selected stab wounds (Grubb, 1992).

CESAREAN DELIVERY. The necessity for cesarean delivery of a live fetus depends on several factors. Laparotomy itself is not an indication for hysterotomy. Some considerations include gestational age, fetal condition, extent of uterine injury, and whether the large uterus hinders adequate treatment or evaluation of other intra-abdominal injuries (Awwad and colleagues, 1994a).

ELECTRONIC MONITORING. As for many other acute or chronic maternal conditions, fetal well-being may reflect the status of the mother, and thus fetal monitoring is another "vital sign" to help evaluate the extent of maternal injuries. Even if the mother is stable, the use of electronic monitoring may be predictive of placental abruption. Pearlman and associates (1990) reported no abruptions if uterine contractions were less often than every 10 minutes within 4 hours after trauma was sustained. **Importantly, 20 percent of women who had more frequent contractions had an associated placental abruption.** In these cases, abnormal tracings were common and included fetal tachycardia and late decelerations. Connolly and co-workers (1997) reported no adverse outcomes in women who had normal monitor tracings.

Because placental abruption usually develops early following trauma, fetal monitoring is begun as soon as the maternal condition is stabilized. The duration that post-trauma monitoring should be performed is not precisely known. According to Goodwin and Breen (1990), an observation period of 2 to 6 hours is sufficient if there are no other ominous signs such as contractions, uterine tenderness, or bleeding. It seems reasonable to continue monitoring as long as there are uterine contractions, a nonreassuring fetal heart pattern, vaginal bleed-ing, uterine tenderness or irritability, serious maternal injury, or ruptured membranes (American College of Obstetricians and Gynecologists, 1998). In very rare cases, abruptio placentae has developed days after trauma (Higgins and Garite, 1984).

FETAL–MATERNAL HEMORRHAGE. Routine use of the Kleihauer–Betke or an equivalent test in pregnant trauma victims is controversial (Pak and associates, 1998). It is unclear if their routine use will modify adverse outcomes associated with fetal anemia, cardiac arrhythmias, and death. In a retrospective review of 125 pregnant women with blunt injuries admitted to a level I trauma center, the Kleihauer–Betke test had a sensitivity of 56 percent, a specificity of 71 percent, and an accuracy of 27 percent (Towery and co-workers, 1993). These investigators concluded that the test was of little use in the setting of acute trauma, and electronic fetal monitoring or ultrasound, or both, are more useful in detecting fetal or pregnancy-associated complications. Dupre and associates (1993) reached similar conclusions, and while they found evidence for fetal–maternal hemorrhage in 22 percent of women studied, it was of no prognostic significance. Likewise, Connolly and co-workers (1997) performed 289 Kleihauer–Betke tests in traumatic injuries in pregnant women and in only one case was management affected.

For the woman who is D-negative, administration of anti-D immunoglobulin should be considered. This may be omitted if the test for fetal bleeding is negative. Isoimmunization may still develop if the fetal–maternal hemorrhage exceeds 15 mL of fetal cells.

Another important aspect of care for the pregnant trauma patient is to ensure that her tetanus immunization is current.

THERMAL INJURY. Although Parkland Hospital is a major burn center for the United States, we have not seen a large number of pregnant women with severe burns. Fetal prognosis is poor with severe burns. Usually the woman enters labor spontaneously within a few days to a week, and often delivers a stillborn infant. Contributory factors are hypovolemia, pulmonary injury, septicemia, and the intensely catabolic state associated with burns.

PROGNOSIS. From their review, Polko and McMahon (1998) concluded that pregnancy does not alter maternal outcome compared with nonpregnant women of similar age. A number of investigators have reported that maternal and fetal survival parallels the percentage of burned surface area (Table 43–9). In general, prognosis worsens when burns exceed 40 to 50 percent of body surface area. For instance, there was a 50 percent maternal and fetal loss in the 40 to 60 percent burn group

TABLE 43–9. Maternal and Fetal Mortality in 170 Pregnancies Complicated by Burns

Study	Burn (% TBSA)	Perinatal Outcomes	
		Maternal Deaths	*Fetal Deaths*
Rayburn et al (1984) (n = 30)	< 40	2/20	2/20
	40–60	3/6	3/6
	> 60	3/4	4/4
Amy et al (1985) (n = 30)	< 40	0/17	2/17
	40–50	0/3	2/3
	> 50	10/10	9/10
Rode et al (1990) (n = 33)	< 20	1/16	2/16
	20–50	1/8	3/8
	> 50	6/9	8/9
Akhtar et al (1994) (n = 50)	< 40	0/12	1/12
	40–60	3/6	3/6
	> 60	32/32	32/32
Mabrouk and el-Feky (1997) (n = 27)	< 25	0/19	9/19
	> 25	5/8	5/8

TBSA = total body surface area.

compared with 11 percent fetal and no maternal losses with a 20 to 40 percent area burn. In the 170 pregnant burned women reported in Table 43–9, as the total burned body surface area reaches or exceeds 50 percent, both maternal and fetal morbidity invariably exceeds 50 percent.

SKIN CONTRACTURES. Following serious abdominal burns, skin contractures that develop may be painful during a subsequent pregnancy and may even necessitate surgical decompression and split skin autografts (Matthews, 1982). Widgerow and colleagues (1991) described two women in whom surgical release without covering the resulting defect was sufficient. McCauley and colleagues (1991) followed seven women with severe circumferential truncal burns sustained at a mean age of 7.7 years. All of 14 subsequent pregnancies were delivered at term without major complications. Loss or distortion of nipples may cause problems in breast feeding.

ELECTRIC SHOCK. Earlier case reports were suggestive of a high fetal mortality with electric shock (Fatovich, 1993). In a prospective cohort study, however, Einarson and colleagues (1997) showed similar perinatal outcomes in 31 exposed women compared with normal pregnant controls. They concluded that traditional 110-volt North American electric current likely is less dan-

gerous than 220-volt currents available in Europe. Fish (2000) has described neurological and vascular effects of lightning injury.

CARDIOPULMONARY RESUSCITATION

Cardiac arrest fortunately is rare during pregnancy. There are special considerations for cardiopulmonary resuscitation (CPR) conducted in the second half of pregnancy. In nonpregnant women, external chest compression results in a cardiac output of only 30 percent of normal (Clark and colleagues, 1997). Cardiac output is even less in advanced pregnancy, when aortocaval compression from the enlarged uterus may impede resuscitative efforts by diminishing forward flow as well as venous return. **Thus, uterine displacement is paramount to accompany other resuscitative efforts.** Left lateral displacement can be accomplished manually by a member of the team, by tilting the operating table laterally, by placing a wedge under the right hip, or by using the Cardiff resuscitation wedge. Rees and Willis (1988) showed with a manikin that resuscitation with the Cardiff wedge was as efficient as resuscitation in the supine position.

Over the past few years, the recommendation by many authors is to perform cesarean delivery within 4 to 5 minutes of beginning cardiopulmonary resuscitation if the fetus is viable (Moise and Belfort, 1997). Certainly there is an inverse correlation between neurologically intact neonatal survival and the cardiac arrest-to-delivery interval in women delivered by perimorten cesarean. According to Clark and co-workers (1997) 98 percent of infants delivered before 5 minutes will be neurologically intact. From 6 to 15 minutes it is 83 percent; from 16 to 25 minutes, 33 percent; and 26 to 35 minutes, 25 percent. Based on theory and a few anecdotal case reports, delivery may also enhance maternal resuscitative efforts, which must be continued throughout surgery. For all of these reasons, the American College of Obstetricians and Gynecologists (1998) advises consideration for cesarean delivery in third-trimester pregnancy within 4 minutes of cardiac arrest. Unfortunately, as emphasized by Clark and associates (1997), these goals rarely can be met in actual practice. Whitten and Irvine (2000) recently reviewed indications for postmortem and perimortem cesarean delivery.

REFERENCES

Abraham E, Anzueto A, Gutierrez G, Tessler S, Pedro G, Wunderink R, Dal Nogare A, Nasraway S, Berman S, Cooney R, Levy H, Baughman R, Rumbak M, Light RB, Poole L, Allred R, Constant J, Pennington J, Porter S: Double-blind randomised controlled trial of monoclonal antibody to human tumour necrosis factor in treatment of septic shock. Lancet 351:929, 1998

Abraham E, Glauser MP, Butler T, Garbino J, Gelmont D, Laterre PF, Kudsk K, Bruining HA, Otto C, Tobin E, Zwingelstein C, Lesslauer W, Leighton A: p55 tumor necrosis factor receptor fusion protein in the treatment of patients with severe sepsis and septic shock. JAMA 277:1531, 1997

Akhtar MA, Mulawkar PM, Kulkarni HR: Burns in pregnancy: Effect on maternal and fetal outcomes. Burns 20:351, 1994

Alexopoulos E, Tambakoudis P, Bili H, Sakellariou G, Mantalenakis S, Papadimitriou M: Acute renal failure in pregnancy. Ren Fail 15:609, 1993

American College of Obstetricians and Gynecologists: Domestic violence. Educational Bulletin No. 257, December 1999

American College of Obstetricians and Gynecologists: Obstetric aspects of trauma management. Educational Bulletin No. 251, September 1998

American College of Obstetricians and Gynecologists: Septic shock. Technical Bulletin No. 204, April 1995

American College of Obstetricians and Gynecologists: Invasive hemodynamic monitoring in obstetrics and gynecology. Technical Bulletin No. 175, December 1992

Amon E, Midkiff C, Winn H, Holcomb W, Shumway J, Artal R: Tocolysis with advanced cervical dilatation. Obstet Gynecol 95:358, 2000

Amy BW, McManus WF, Goodwin CW, Mason A, Pruitt BA: Thermal injury in the pregnant patient. Surg Gynecol Obstet 161:209, 1985

Angus DC, Birmingham MC, Balk RA, Scannon PJ, Collins D, Kruse JA, Graham DR, Dedhia HV, Homann S, Mac-

Intyre N: E5 murine monoclonal antiendotoxin antibody in gram-negative sepsis. A randomized controlled trial. JAMA 283:1723, 2000

Annane D, Sébille V, Troché G, Raphaël JC, Gajdos P, Bellissant E: A 3-level prognostic classification in septic shock based on cortisol levels and cortisol response to corticotropin. JAMA 283:1038, 2000

Anzueto A, Baughman RP, Guntupalli KK, Weg JG, Wiedemann HP, Raventós AA, Lemarie F, Long W, Zaccardelli DS, Pattishall EN: Aerosolized surfactant in adults with sepsis-inducted acute respiratory distress syndrome. N Engl J Med 334:1417, 1996

Awwad JT, Azar GB, Aouad AT, Raad J, Karam KS: Postmortem cesarean section following maternal blast injury: Case report. J Trauma 36:260, 1994a

Awwad JT, Azar GB, Seoud MA, Mroueh AM, Karam KS: High-velocity penetrating wounds of the gravid uterus: Review of 16 years of civil war. Obstet Gynecol 83:259, 1994b

Benedetti TJ, Carlson RW: Studies of colloid osmotic pressure in pregnancy-induced hypertension. Am J Obstet Gynecol 135:308, 1979

Berenson AB, San Miguel VV, Wilkinson GS: Prevalence of physical and sexual assault in pregnant adolescents. J Adolesc Health 13:466, 1992

Berenson AB, Stiglich NJ, Wilkinson GS, Anderson GD: Drug abuse and other risk factors for physical abuse in pregnancy among white non-Hispanic, black and Hispanic women. Am J Obstet Gynecol 164:1491, 1991

Berenson AB, Wiemann CM, Wilkinson GS, Jones WA, Anderson GD: Perinatal morbidity associated with violence experienced by pregnant women. Am J Obstet Gynecol 170:1760, 1994

Bernard GR, Wheeler AP, Russell JA, Schein R, Summer WR, Steinberg KP, Fulkerson WJ, Wright PE, Christman BW, Dupont WD, Higgins SB, Swindell BB: The effects of ibuprofen on the physiology and survival of patients with sepsis. N Engl J Med 336:912, 1997

Bhagwanjee S, Paruk F, Moodley J, Muckart DJ: Intensive care unit morbidity and mortality from eclampsia: An evaluation of the Acute Physiology and Chronic Health Evaluation II score and the Glasgow Coma score. Crit Care Med 28:120, 2000

Biester EM, Tomich PG, Esposito TJ, Weber L: Trauma in pregnancy: Normal Revised Trauma Score in relation to other markers of maternofetal status—A preliminary study. Am J Obstet Gynecol 176:1206, 1997

Bolliger CT, van Zijl P, Louw JA: Multiple organ failure with the adult respiratory distress syndrome in homicidal arsenic poisoning. Respiration 59:57, 1992

Bone RC, Balk RA, Fein AM, Perl TM, Wenzel RP, Reines HD, Quenzer RW, Iberti TJ, Macintyre N, Schein RMH, the E5 Sepsis Study Group: A second large controlled clinical study of E5, a monoclonal antibody to endotoxin: Results of a prospective, multicenter, randomized, controlled trial. Crit Care Med 23:994, 1995

Bone RC, Fisher CJ Jr, Clemmer TP, Slotman GJ, Metz CA, Balk RA: A controlled clinical trial of high-dose methylprednisolone in the treatment of severe sepsis and septic shock. N Engl J Med 317:653, 1987

Buchsbaum HJ: Trauma in Pregnancy. Philadelphia, Saunders, 1979

Catanzarite V, Schibanoff JM, Chinn R, Mendoza A, Weiss R: Overwhelming maternal sepsis due to a gas-forming *Escherichia coli* chorioamnionitis. Am J Perinatol 11:205, 1994

Catanzarite VA, Willms D: Adult respiratory distress syndrome in pregnancy: Report of three cases and review of the literature. Obstet Gynecol Surv 52:381, 1997

Centers for Disease Control and Prevention: Treatment of sexually transmitted diseases. MMWR 47:1, 1998

Clark SL, Cotton DB, Hankins GDV, Phelan JP: Critical Care Obstetrics, 3rd ed. Boston, Blackwell Science, 1997

Clark SL, Cotton DB: Clinical indications for pulmonary artery catheterization in the patient with severe pregnancy-induced hypertension. Am J Obstet Gynecol 158:453, 1988

Clark SL, Cotton DB, Lee W, Bishop C, Hill T, Southwick J, Pivarnik J, Spillman T, DeVore GR, Phelan J, Hankins GDV, Benedetti TJ, Tolley D: Central hemodynamic assessment of normal term pregnancy. Am J Obstet Gynecol 161:1439, 1989

Clark SL, Hankins GDV, Dudley DA, Dildy GA, Porter TF: Amniotic fluid embolism. Analysis of a national registry. Am J Obstet Gynecol 172:1158, 1995

Clark SL, Phelan JP, Greenspoon J, Aldahl D: Labor and delivery in the presence of mitral stenosis: Central hemodynamic observations. Am J Obstet Gynecol 152:948, 1985

Cokkinides VE, Coker AL, Sanderson M, Addy C, Bethea L: Physical violence during pregnancy: Maternal complications and birth outcomes. Obstet Gynecol 93:661, 1999

Collop NA, Sahn SA: Critical illness in pregnancy. An analysis of 20 patients admitted to a medical intensive care unit. Chest 103:1548, 1993

Connolly AM, Katz VL, Bash KL, McMahon MJ, Hansen WF: Trauma and pregnancy. Am J Perinatol 14:331, 1997

Connors AF Jr, Speroff T, Dawson NV, Thomas C, Harrell FE Jr, Wagner D, Desbiens N, Goldman L, Wu AW, Califf RM, Fulkerson WJ Jr, Vidaillet H, Broste S, Bellamy P, Lynn J, Knaus WA: The effectiveness of right heart catheterization in the initial care of critically ill patients. JAMA 276:889, 1996

Crosby WM: Automobile trauma in pregnancy: Prevention and treatment. Prim Care Update Ob/Gyn 3:6, 1996

Crosby WM, Snyder RG, Snow CC, Hanson PG: Impact injuries in pregnancy, 1. Experimental studies. Am J Obstet Gynecol 101:100, 1968

Cunningham FG: Sepsis syndromes. Contemp Ob/Gyn 43:13, 1998

Cunningham FG, Lucas MJ, Hankins GDV: Pulmonary injury complicating antepartum pyelonephritis. Am J Obstet Gynecol 156:797, 1987

Cunningham FG, Pritchard JA, Hankins GDV, Anderson P, Lucas J, Armstrong K: Peripartum heart failure: A specific pregnancy-induced cardiomyopathy or the consequence of coincidental compounding cardiovascular events? Obstet Gynecol 67:157, 1986

Curry MA, Perrin N, Wall E: Effects of abuse on maternal complications and birth weight in adult and adolescent women. Obstet Gynecol 92:530, 1998

Dannenberg AL, Carter DM, Lawson HW, Ashton DM, Dorfman SF, Graham EH: Homicide and other injuries as causes of maternal death in New York City, 1987 through 1991. Am J Obstet Gynecol 172:1557, 1995

Dash N, Lupetin AR: Uterine rupture secondary to trauma: CT findings. J Comput Assist Tomogr 15:329, 1991

Davis RD, Burke JP, Wright LJ: Relapsing fever associated with ARDS in a parturient woman. A case report and review of the literature. Chest 102:630, 1992

Dietz PM, Spitz AM, Anda RF, Williamson DF, McMahon PM, Santelli JS, Nordenberg DF, Felitti VJ, Kendrick JS: Unintended pregnancy among adult women exposed to abuse or household dysfunction during their childhood. JAMA 282:1359, 1999

DiFederico EM, Burlingame JM, Kilpatrick SJ, Harrison M, Matthay MA: Pulmonary edema in obstetric patients is rapidly resolved except in the presence of infection or of nitroglycerine tocolysis after open fetal surgery. Am J Obstet Gynecol 179:925, 1998

Dupre AR, Morrison JC, Martin JN Jr, Floyd RC, Blake PG: Clinical application of the Kleihauer–Betke test. J Reprod Med 38:621, 1993

Einarson A, Bailey B, Inocencion G, Ormond K, Koren G: Accidental electric shock in pregnancy: A prospective cohort study. Am J Obstet Gynecol 176:678, 1997

Eisenstat SA, Bancroft L: Domestic violence. N Engl J Med 341:886, 1999

Evans, TW, Smithies M: ABC of intensive care. Organ dysfunction. BMJ 318:1606, 1999

Fatovich DM: Electric shock in pregnancy. J Emerg Med 11:175, 1993

Federal Bureau of Investigation: Crime in the United States, uniform crime reports, 1997. Washington, DC, US Department of Justice, 26:22 Nov 1998

Feinberg EB, Diaz CJ, Currie JL: Prompt recognition and aggressive treatment needed for necrotizing fasciitis of vulva. Contemp Ob/Gyn 41:81, 1996

Fildes J, Reed L, Jones N, Martin M, Barrett J: Trauma: The leading cause of maternal death. J Trauma 32:643, 1992

Fish RM: Electric injury, part III: Cardiac monitoring indications, the pregnant patient, and lightning. J Emerg Med 18:181, 2000

Flick RP, Bofill JA, King JC: Pregnancy complicated by traumatic diaphragmatic rupture. J Reprod Med 44:137, 1999

French National Registry of HA-1A (Centoxin) in Septic Shock: A cohort study of 600 patients. The National Committee for the Evaluation of Centoxin. Arch Intern Med 154:2393, 1994

Goodwin TM, Breen MT: Pregnancy outcome and fetomaternal hemorrhage after noncatastrophic trauma. Am J Obstet Gynecol 162:665, 1990

Gottlieb JE, Darby MJ, Gee MH, Fish JE: Recurrent noncardiac pulmonary edema accompanying pregnancy-induced hypertension. Chest 100:1730, 1991

Grisso JA, Schwarz DF, Hirschinger N, Sammel M, Brensinger C, Santanna J, Lowe RA, Anderson E, Shaw LM, Bethel CA, Teeple L: Violent injuries among women in an urban area. N Engl J Med 341:1899, 1999

Grubb DK: Nonsurgical management of penetrating uterine trauma in pregnancy: A case report. Am J Obstet Gynecol 166:583, 1992

Hankins GD, Wendel GD, Cunningham FG, Leveno KJ: Longitudinal evaluation of hemodynamic changes in eclampsia. Am J Obstet Gynecol 150:506, 1984

Hankins GD, Wendel GD, Leveno KJ, Stoneham J: Myocardial infarction during pregnancy. A review. Obstet Gynecol 65:139, 1985

Hankins GD, Wendel GD Jr, Whalley PJ, Quirk JG Jr: Cardiovascular monitoring in the high risk pregnancy. Perinatol Neonatol 7:29, 1983

Harper M, Parsons L: Maternal deaths due to homicide and other injuries in North Carolina: 1992–1994. Obstet Gynecol 90:920, 1997

Higgins SD, Garite TJ: Late abruptio placentae in trauma patients: Implications for monitoring. Obstet Gynecol 63:10S, 1984

Hoff WS, D'Amelio LF, Tinkoff GH, Lucke JF, Rhodes M, Diamond DL, Indeck M, Smith SJ Jr: Maternal predictors of fetal demise in trauma during pregnancy. Surg Gynecol Obstet 172:175, 1991

Horan DL, Chapin J, Klein L, Schmidt LA, Schulkin J: Domestic violence screening practices of obstetrician-gynecologists. Obstet Gynecol 92:785, 1998

Icely S, Chez RA: Traumatic liver rupture in pregnancy. Am J Obstet Gynecol 180:1030, 1999

Jacob S, Bloebaum L, Shah G, Varner MW: Maternal mortality in Utah. Obstet Gynecol 91:187, 1998

Karetzky M, Ramirez M: Acute respiratory failure in pregnancy. An analysis of 19 cases. Medicine 77:41, 1998

Kettel LM, Branch DW, Scott JR: Occult placental abruption after maternal trauma. Obstet Gynecol 71:449, 1988

Kilpatrick SJ, Matthay MA: Obstetric patients requiring critical care: A five-year review. Chest 101:1407, 1992

Kissinger DP, Rozycki GS, Morris JA Jr, Knudson MM, Copes WS, Bass SM, Yates HK, Champion HR: Trauma in pregnancy: Predicting pregnancy outcome. Arch Surg 126:1079, 1991

Kurzel RB, Cavens P, Lampley C, Blankstein J: Battery of the pregnant women. Obstet Gynecol 95:145, 2000

Kyriacou DN, Anglin D, Taliaferro E, Stone S, Tubb T, Linden JA, Muelleman R, Barton E, Kraus JF: Risk factors for injury to women from domestic violence. N Engl J Med 341:1892, 1999

Largoza MN: Acute pulmonary edema complicating pregnancy. Presented at the Annual Clinical Meeting of the American College of Obstetricians and Gynecologists, Las Vegas, NV, May 1997

Levi M, ten Cate H: Disseminated intravascular coagulation. N Engl J Med 341:586, 1999

Levinson G, Shnider SM, DeLorimier AA, Steffenson JL: Effects of maternal hyperventilation on uterine blood flow and fetal oxygenation and acid–base status. Anesthesiology 40:340, 1974

Lewinsohn G, Herman A, Leonov Y, Klinowski E: Critically ill obstetrical patients: Outcome and predictability. Crit Care Med 22:1412, 1994

Luger EJ, Arbel R, Dekel S: Traumatic separation of the symphysis pubis during pregnancy: A case report. J Trauma 38:255, 1995

Luster AD: Chemokines—chemotactic cytokines that mediate inflammation. N Engl J Med 338:436, 1998

Mabie WC, Barton JR, Sibai BM: Septic shock in pregnancy. Obstet Gynecol 90:553, 1997

Mabie WC, Sibai BM: Treatment in an obstetric intensive care unit. Am J Obstet Gynecol 162:1, 1990

Mabrouk AR, el-Feky AEH: Burns during pregnancy: A gloomy outcome. Burns 23:596, 1997

Mattar F, Sibai BM: Eclampsia. VIII. Risk factors for maternal morbidity. Am J Obstet Gynecol 182:307, 2000

Matthews RN: Old burns and pregnancy. Br J Obstet Gynaecol 89:610, 1982

McCauley RL, Stenberg BA, Phillips LG, Blackwell SJ, Robson MC: Long-term assessment of the effects of circumferential truncal burns in pediatric patients on subsequent pregnancies. J Burn Care Rehabil 12:51, 1991

McFarlane J, Parker B, Soeken K, Bullock L: Assessing for abuse during pregnancy. Severity and frequency of injuries and associated entry into prenatal care. JAMA 267:3176, 1992

Meduri GU, Headley AS, Golden E, Carson SJ, Umberger RA, Kelso T, Tolley EA: Effect of prolonged methylprednisolone therapy in unresolving acute respiratory distress syndrome. JAMA 280:159, 1998

Moise KJ Jr, Belfort MA: Damage control for the obstetric patient. Surg Clin North Am 77:835, 1997

Monaco TJ Jr, Spielman FJ, Katz VL: Pregnant patients in the intensive care unit: A descriptive analysis. South Med J 86:414, 1993

Nathan L, Peters MT, Ahmed AM, Leveno KJ: The return of life-threatening puerperal sepsis caused by group A streptococci. Am J Obstet Gynecol 169:571, 1993

National Highway Traffic Safety Administration: Motor vehicle crashes as a leading cause of death in 1994. 1998, www.nhtsa.dot.gov

Ognibene FP, Parker MM, Natanson C, Shelhamer JH, Parrillo JE: Depressed left ventricular performance. Response to volume infusion in patients with sepsis and septic shock. Chest 93:903, 1988

Pak LL, Reece EA, Chan L: Is adverse pregnancy outcome predictable after blunt abdominal trauma? Am J Obstet Gynecol 179:1140, 1998

Palmer JD, Sparrow OC: Extradural haematoma following intrauterine trauma. Injury 25:671, 1994

Parker B, McFarlane J, Soeken K: Abuse during pregnancy: Effects on maternal complications and birth weight in adult and teenage women. Obstet Gynecol 84:323, 1994

Parker MM, Shelmamer JH, Natanson C, Alling DW, Parrillo JE: Serial cardiovascular variables in survivors and non-survivors of human septic shock: Heart rate as an early predictor of prognosis. Crit Care Med 15:923, 1987

Parrillo JE, Parker MM, Natanson C, Suffredini AF, Danner RL, Cunnion RE, Ognibene FP: Septic shock in humans: Advances in the understanding of pathogenesis, cardiovascular dysfunction, and therapy. Ann Intern Med 113:227, 1990

Pearlman MD, Phillips ME: Safety belt use during pregnancy. Obstet Gynecol 88:1026, 1996

Pearlman MD, Klinich KD, Schneider LW, Rupp J, Moss S, Ashton-Miller J: A comprehensive program to improve safety for pregnant women and fetuses in motor vehicle crashes: A preliminary report. Am J Obstet Gynecol 182:1554, 2000.

Pearlman MD, Tintinalli JE, Lorenz RP: A prospective controlled study of outcome after trauma during pregnancy. Am J Obstet Gynecol 162:1502, 1990

Perry KG Jr, Martin RW, Blake PG, Roberts WE, Martin JN Jr: Maternal outcome associated with adult respiratory distress syndrome. Am J Obstet Gynecol 174:391, 1996

Polko LE, McMahon MJ: Burns in pregnancy. Obstet Gynecol Surv 53:50, 1998

Poole GV, Martin JN, Perry KG Jr, Griswold JA, Lambert CJ, Rhodes RS: Trauma in pregnancy: The role of interpersonal violence. Am J Obstet Gynecol 174:1873, 1996

Pritchard JA, Cunningham G, Pritchard SA, Mason RA: On reducing the frequency of severe abruptio placentae. Am J Obstet Gynecol 165:1345, 1991

Pulmonary Artery Catheter Consensus Conference: Consensus statement. Crit Care Med 25:910, 1997

Rayburn W, Smith B, Feller I, Varner M, Cruiskshank D: Major burns during pregnancy: Effects on fetal well being. Surg Gynecol Obstet 63:392, 1984

Rees GAD, Willis BA: Resuscitation in late pregnancy. Anaesthesia 43:347, 1988

Reis PM, Sander CM, Pearlman MD: Abruptio placentae after auto accidents. A case control study. J Reprod Med 45:6, 2000

Ridgway LE 3rd, Martin RW, Hess LW, Buchanan J, Whitworth NS, Martin JN Jr: Acute gestational pyelonephritis: The impact of colloid osmotic pressure, plasma fibronectin, and arterial oxygen saturation. Am J Perinatol 8:222, 1991

Robertson EG: Edema in normal pregnancy. J Reprod Fertil 9:27, 1969

Rode H, Millar AJW, Cywes S, Bloch CE, Boes EGM, Theron EJ, Lodder JV, van der Merwe AE, deKock M: Thermal injury in pregnancy—the neglected tragedy. S Afr Med J 77:346, 1990

Rorth M, Bille-Brahe NE: 2, 3-Diphosphoglycerate and creatine in the red cells during pregnancy. Scand J Clin Lab Invest 28:271, 1971

Sachs BP, Brown DAJ, Driscoll SG, Schulman E, Acker D, Ransil BJ, Jewett JF: Maternal mortality in Massachusetts. N Engl J Med 316:667, 1987

Satin AJ, Hemsell DL, Stone IC Jr, Theriot S, Wendel GD Jr: Sexual assault in pregnancy. Obstet Gynecol 77:710, 1991

Satin AJ, Ramin JM, Paicurich J, Millman S, Wendel GD Jr: The prevalence of sexual assault: A survey of 2404 puerperal women. Am J Obstet Gynecol 167:973, 1992

Schoenfeld A, Warchaizer S, Royburt M, Rosenblatt M, Friedman S, Ovadia J: Crush injury in pregnancy: An unusual experience in obstetrics. Obstet Gynecol 86:655, 1995

Schultze PM, Stamm CA, Roger J: Placental abruption and fetal death with airbag deployment in a motor vehicle accident. Obstet Gynecol 92:719, 1998

Scorpio RJ, Esposito TJ, Smith LG, Gens DR: Blunt trauma during pregnancy. Factors affecting fetal outcome. J Trauma 32:213, 1992

Sibai BM, Mabie BC, Harvey CJ, Gonzalez AR: Pulmonary edema in severe preeclampsia–eclampsia: Analysis of thirty-seven consecutive cases. Am J Obstet Gynecol 156:1174, 1987

Sims CJ, Boardman CH, Fuller SJ: Airbag deployment following a motor vehicle accident in pregnancy. Obstet Gynecol 88:726, 1996

Stettler RW, Lutich A, Pritchard JA, Cunningham FG: Traumatic placental abruption: A separation from traditional thought. Presented at the annual clinical meeting of American College of Obstetricians and Gynecologists, Las Vegas, May 1992

Stewart DE: Incidence of postpartum abuse in women with a history of abuse during pregnancy. Can Med Assoc J 151:1601, 1994

Stewart DE, Cecutti A: Physical abuse in pregnancy. Can Med Assoc J 149:1257, 1993

Stone IK: Trauma in the obstetric patient. Obstet Gynecol Clin North Am 26:459, 1999

Subrevilla LA, Cassinelli MT, Carcelen A, Malaga JM: Human fetal and maternal oxygen tension and acid-base status during delivery at high altitude. Am J Obstet Gynecol 111:1111, 1971

Tomlinson MW, Caruthers TJ, Whitty JE, Gonik B: Does delivery improve maternal condition in the respiratory-compromised gravida? Obstet Gynecol 91:108, 1998

Towery R, English TP, Wisner D: Evaluation of pregnant women after blunt injury. J Trauma 35:731, 1993

Tyroch AH, Kaups KL, Rohan J, Song S, Beingesser K: Pregnant women and car restraints: Beliefs and practices. J Trauma 46:241, 1999

Van Hook JW, Hankins GDV: Invasive hemodynamic monitoring. Prim Care Update Ob/Gyn 4:39, 1997

Veterans Administration Systemic Sepsis Cooperative Study Group: Effect of high-dose glucocorticoid therapy on mortality in patients with clinical signs of systemic sepsis. N Engl J Med 317:659, 1987

Ware LB, Matthay MA: The acute respiratory distress syndrome. N Engl J Med 342:1334, 2000

Weg JG, Anzueto A, Balk RA, Wiedemann HP, Pattishall EN, Schork MA, Wagner LA: The relation of pneumothorax and other air leaks to mortality in the acute respiratory distress syndrome. N Engl J Med 338:341, 1998

Weyerts LK, Jones MC, James HE: Paraplegia and congenital contractures as a consequence of intrauterine trauma. Am J Med Genet 43:751, 1992

Wheeler AP, Bernard GR: Treating patients with severe sepsis. N Engl J Med 340:207, 1999

Whitten M, Irvine LM: Postmortem and perimortem caesarean section: what are the indications? J R Soc Med 93:6, 2000

Widgerow AD, Ford TD, Botha M: Burn contracture preventing uterine expansion. Ann Plast Surg 27:269, 1991

Wyncoll DLA, Evans TW: Acute respiratory distress syndrome. Lancet 354:497, 1999

Zinaman M, Rubin J, Lindheimer MD: Serial plasma oncotic pressure levels and echoencephalography during and after delivery in severe preeclampsia. Lancet 1:1245, 1985

44

Cardiovascular Diseases

Heart disease is the third leading cause of death in 25- to 44-year-old women (Martin and colleagues, 1999). Because it is relatively common in women of childbearing age, heart disease of varying severity complicates about 1 percent of pregnancies. In the past, **rheumatic heart disease** accounted for the majority of cases, but over the past three decades, it has almost disappeared in this country. Meyer and colleagues (1994) described 74 pregnancies over 10 years complicated by cardiac disease, and only a few were caused by rheumatic fever. Similarly, Tan and de Swiet (1998) reported that only 12 percent of 73 women had cardiac disease caused by rheumatic lesions. Better medical management, together with a number of newer surgical techniques, has enabled more girls with **congenital heart disease** to reach childbearing age (Brickner and co-workers, 2000). Congenital heart lesions now constitute at least half of all cases of heart disease encountered during pregnancy (Bitsch and colleagues, 1989; McFaul and associates, 1988). **Hypertensive heart disease,** frequently complicated by heart disease of obesity, has become a relatively common cause of peripartum heart failure at Parkland Hospital (Cunningham and co-workers, 1986). Other varieties are even less common and include coronary, thyroid, syphilitic, and kyphoscoliotic cardiac disease, as well as idiopathic cardiomyopathy, cor pulmonale, constrictive pericarditis, various forms of heart block, and isolated myocarditis.

Maternal mortality related to heart disease has decreased remarkably over the past 50 years. Sachs and associates (1988) reported that maternal mortality from cardiac disease fell from 5.6 to 0.3 per 100,000 live births in Massachusetts from 1954 through 1985. Unfortunately, heart disease still contributes significantly to maternal mortality, both in the United States and throughout the world. Koonin and colleagues (1997) reported that heart disease was responsible for 5.6 percent of 1459 pregnancy-related deaths in the United States from 1987 to 1990. In the United Kingdom from 1994 through 1996, cardiac disease accounted for 40 of 105 indirect maternal deaths (de Swiet, 2000). Dorfman (1990) reported that 8 percent of maternal deaths in New York City from 1981 through 1983 were caused by cardiac disease. Similarly, Jacob and associates (1998) found that heart disease accounted for 15 percent of maternal mortality in Utah from 1982 through 1994.

PHYSIOLOGICAL CONSIDERATIONS WITH HEART DISEASE IN PREGNANCY

The marked hemodynamic changes stimulated by pregnancy have a profound effect on underlying heart disease in the pregnant woman. These physiological changes are detailed in Chapter 8 (p. 183). The most important consideration is that during pregnancy cardiac output is increased by as much as 30 to 50 percent. Capeless and Clapp (1989) have shown that almost half of the total increase has occurred by 8 weeks, and it is maximized by midpregnancy. The early increase can be attributed to augmented stroke volume that apparently results from decreased vascular resistance and is accompanied by diminished blood pressure. Later in pregnancy there is also an increased resting pulse, and stroke volume increases even more, presumably related to increased diastolic filling from augmented blood volume. These changes were reviewed by van Oppen and colleagues (1996) and McLaughlin and Roberts (1999).

An important study by Clark and colleagues (1989) contributed to the understanding of cardiovascular physiology during pregnancy. Using right-sided heart catheterization, these investigators measured hemodynamic function in 10 healthy primigravid women. Pregnancy values were compared with values measured again 11 to 13 weeks postpartum (Table 44–1). At or near term, cardiac output in the lateral recumbent position was increased 43 percent by virtue of elevated pulse rate and stroke volume. Systemic and pulmonary vascular resistance concomitantly decreased, and no change was observed in intrinsic left-ventricular contractility. As shown in Figure 44–1, pregnancy is characterized by normal left-ventricular function, and not hyperdynamic function as once thought. The investigators concluded that maintenance of normal left-ventricular filling pressures comes about as the result of ventricular dilatation.

Because significant hemodynamic alterations are apparent early in pregnancy, women with severe cardiac dysfunction may experience worsening of heart failure before midpregnancy. In others, heart failure develops when hypervolemia of pregnancy is maximal after 28 weeks. In the majority, heart failure develops peripartum when there are additional hemodynamic burdens.

TABLE 44–1. Hemodynamic Changes in 10 Normal Pregnant Women at Term Compared with Postpartum Values

Parameter	Change (%)
Cardiac output	+43
Heart rate	+17
Left ventricular stroke work index	+17
Vascular resistance	
Systemic	−21
Pulmonary	−34
Mean arterial pressure	+ 4
Colloid osmotic pressure	−14

Data from Clark and colleagues (1989).

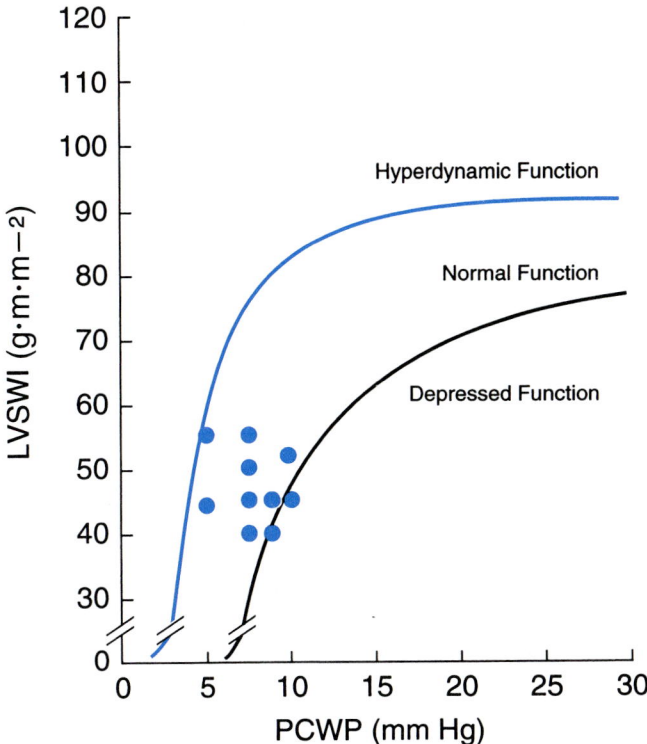

FIGURE 44-1. Left-ventricular function in late pregnancy in 10 healthy primigravid women. (LVSWI = left ventricular stroke work index; PCWP = pulmonary capillary wedge pressure.) (Data from Clark and colleagues, 1989.)

This is when the physiological capability for rapid changes in cardiac output is frequently overwhelmed in the presence of structural cardiac disease. For example, in 542 women whose pregnancies were complicated by heart disease, 8 of 10 maternal deaths were during the puerperium (Etheridge and Pepperell, 1977).

PROGNOSIS. The likelihood of a favorable outcome for the mother with heart disease depends upon the functional cardiac capacity, other complications that further increase cardiac load, and quality of medical care provided. Psychological and socioeconomical factors may also assume great importance, because for some women, bed rest may be required throughout pregnancy.

CONGENITAL HEART DISEASE IN OFFSPRING. Many congenital heart lesions appear to be inherited as polygenic characteristics (Chap. 36, p. 957). Thus, it might be expected that some women with congenital lesions would give birth to similarly affected infants. Whittemore and co-workers (1982) found a 10 percent incidence of fetal congenital heart disease in women born with cardiac anomalies. Only half of mother–fetus pairs were concordant for the same anomaly. Shime and col-

leagues (1987) found congenital cardiovascular lesions, including Marfan syndrome, in 3 percent of 87 infants born to women with congenital heart lesions.

DIAGNOSIS OF HEART DISEASE

Many of the physiological changes of normal pregnancy tend to make the diagnosis of heart disease more difficult (Chap. 8, p. 181). For example, in normal pregnancy, functional systolic heart murmurs are quite common. Respiratory effort in normal pregnancy is accentuated, at times suggesting dyspnea. Edema is generally present in the lower extremities during the latter half of pregnancy. It is important not to diagnose heart disease during pregnancy when none exists, and at the same time not fail to detect and appropriately treat heart disease when it does exist. Listed in Table 44–2 are a number of symptoms and clinical findings that may indicate heart disease. Pregnant women who have none of these findings rarely have serious heart disease.

DIAGNOSTIC STUDIES. Most diagnostic cardiovascular studies are noninvasive and can be conducted safely in pregnant women. In most cases, conventional testing including electrocardiography, echocardiography, and chest radiography will provide necessary data. If indicated, right-heart catheterization can be performed with limited x-ray fluoroscopy. On rare occasions, it may be necessary to perform left-heart catheterization. Technetium[99]-labeled albumin or red cells are often used to

TABLE 44–2. Some Clinical Indicators of Heart Disease During Pregnancy

Symptoms
  Progressive dyspnea or orthopnea
  Nocturnal cough
  Hemoptysis
  Syncope
  Chest pain
Clinical Findings
  Cyanosis
  Clubbing of fingers
  Persistent neck vein distention
  Systolic murmur grade 3/6 or greater
  Diastolic murmur
  Cardiomegaly
  Persistent arrhythmia
  Persistent split-second sound
  Criteria for pulmonary hypertension

evaluate ventricular function. The estimated fetal radiation exposure for a 20-mCi dose study is 120 mrad, well below the accepted level for significant teratogenic or oncogenic effect (Chap. 42, p. 1153). Thallium[201], used to evaluate regional coronary perfusion, yields a fetal exposure of 300 to 1100 mrad, depending on the stage of gestation. In cases with clear indications, any minimal theoretical risk will be outweighed by maternal benefits.

ELECTROCARDIOGRAPHY. As the diaphragm is elevated in advancing pregnancy, there is an average 15-degree left-axis deviation in the electrocardiogram, and mild ST changes may be seen in the inferior leads. Atrial and ventricular premature contractions are relatively frequent (Carruth and colleagues, 1981). Pregnancy does not alter voltage findings.

CHEST X-RAY. Anterior–posterior and lateral chest radiographs may be very useful when heart disease is suspected clinically. When used with a lead apron shield, fetal radiation exposure is minimized (Chap. 42, p. 1148). Slight heart enlargement cannot be detected accurately by x-ray because the heart silhouette normally is larger in pregnancy; however, gross cardiomegaly can be excluded.

ECHOCARDIOGRAPHY. The widespread use of echocardiography has allowed accurate diagnosis of most heart diseases during pregnancy. It allows noninvasive evaluation of structural and functional cardiac factors. Its use has also provided data on normal pregnancy-induced hemodynamic and cardiovascular changes. Some normal pregnancy-induced changes include tricuspid regurgitation and significantly increased left-atrial size and left-ventricular outflow cross-sectional area (Limacher and co-workers, 1985).

CLINICAL CLASSIFICATION. There is no clinically applicable test for accurately measuring functional cardiac capacity. A helpful clinical classification was first published in 1928 by the New York Heart Association, and was revised for the eighth time in 1979. One important change was the addition of an assessment of cardiac status after all data have been reviewed. Thus, the classification is no longer based only on clinical symptoms. The following is based on past and present disability and is uninfluenced by physical signs.

- **Class I.** Uncompromised: Patients with cardiac disease and *no limitation of physical activity.* They do not have symptoms of cardiac insufficiency, nor do they experience anginal pain.
- **Class II.** Slightly compromised: Patients with cardiac disease and *slight limitation of physical activity.* These women are comfortable at rest, but if ordinary physical

activity is undertaken, discomfort results in the form of excessive fatigue, palpitation, dyspnea, or anginal pain.
- **Class III.** Markedly compromised: Patients with cardiac disease and *marked limitation of physical activity.* They are comfortable at rest, but less than ordinary activity causes discomfort by excessive fatigue, palpitation, dyspnea, or anginal pain.
- **Class IV.** Severely compromised: Patients with cardiac disease and *inability to perform any physical activity without discomfort.* Symptoms of cardiac insufficiency or angina may develop even at rest, and if any physical activity is undertaken, discomfort is increased.

PRECONCEPTIONAL COUNSELING. The woman with significant heart disease may benefit from counseling before the decision to become pregnant (see also Chap. 9, p. 213). Maternal mortality generally varies directly with functional classification at pregnancy onset; however, this relationship may change as pregnancy progresses. Siu and colleagues (1997) observed a 10 percent incidence of heart failure in 250 women with class I or II disease. Their experiences, as well as those of McFaul and co-workers (1988), were that there were no maternal deaths in over 700 women in classes I or II. In some women, life-threatening cardiac abnormalities can be reversed by corrective surgery and subsequent pregnancy is less dangerous. In other cases, fetal considerations predominate. For example, women with a mechanical prosthetic valve generally take warfarin compounds, which are known to be teratogenic. Therefore, during pregnancy, heparin is usually substituted for warfarin.

The American College of Obstetricians and Gynecologists (1992a) had adopted the three-tiered classification according to risks for death during pregnancy. These risks, shown in Table 44–3, were developed to aid in counseling the woman regarding advisability of conception or continuation of pregnancy. As emphasized by Clark and colleagues (1997), common contemporaneous cardiac causes of maternal mortality are pulmonary complications, cardiomyopathy, infective endocarditis, coronary artery disease, and sudden arrhythmias.

GENERAL MANAGEMENT

Although a number of generalizations regarding management may be drawn, in clinical practice few women actually fit any "classic" pattern of structural cardiac disease. Siu and associates (1997) studied outcomes of 276 pregnancies involving 221 women with a variety of heart disorders. They found that poor maternal functional class or cyanosis, myocardial dysfunction, left-heart obstructive lesions, prior arrhythmia, and prior cardiac events were prognostic of complications during

TABLE 44–3. Risks for Maternal Mortality Caused by Various Heart Disease

Cardiac Disorder	Mortality (%)
Group 1—Minimal Risk	0–1
Atrial septal defect	
Ventricular septal defect	
Patent ductus arteriosus	
Pulmonic or tricuspid disease	
Fallot tetralogy, corrected	
Bioprosthetic valve	
Mitral stenosis, NYHA[a] classes I and II	
Group 2—Moderate Risk	5–15
2A:	
Mitral stenosis, NYHA classes III and IV	
Aortic stenosis	
Aortic coarctation without valvar involvement	
Fallot tetralogy, uncorrected	
Previous myocardial infarction	
Marfan syndrome, normal aorta	
2B:	
Mitral stenosis with atrial fibrillation	
Artificial valve	
Group 3—Major Risk	25–50
Pulmonary hypertension	
Aortic coarctation with valvar involvement	
Marfan syndrome with aortic involvement	

NYHA = New York Heart Association.
From the American College of Obstetricians and Gynecologists (1992a), with permission.

pregnancy. The likelihood of cardiac complications during pregnancy was 3, 30, and 66 percent when none, one, or more than one of these were present. Thus, individualization is essential in assuring optimal outcome. In most instances, management is with a team approach, involving obstetrician, cardiologist, anesthesiologist, and other specialists. Cardiovascular changes likely to be poorly tolerated by an individual woman are identified, and a plan is formulated to minimize such changes.

Four concepts that affect management are emphasized by the American College of Obstetricians and Gynecologists (1992a):

1. The 50 percent increase in blood volume and cardiac output by the early third trimester.
2. Further fluctuations in volume and cardiac output in the peripartum period.
3. A decline in systemic vascular resistance, reaching a nadir in the second trimester, and then rising to 20 percent below normal by late pregnancy.

4. Hypercoagulability, of special importance in women requiring anticoagulation in the nonpregnant state with coumarin derivatives.

Within this framework, both prognosis and management are influenced by the nature and severity of the specific lesion, in addition to the functional classification.

MANAGEMENT OF CLASSES I AND II. With rare exceptions, women in class I and most in class II go through pregnancy without morbidity. Throughout pregnancy and the puerperium, however, special attention should be directed toward both prevention and early recognition of heart failure. While infrequent today, in the past when severe mitral stenosis was common, heart failure developed in a third of these women (Sugrue and colleagues, 1981). By contrast, in nearly 250 pregnancies in women with class I or II heart disease in Toronto, only 10 percent developed failure (Siu and co-workers, 1997). Maternal mortality is low in classes I and II. Indeed, McFaul and co-workers (1988) and Siu and associates (1997) reported no maternal deaths in 726 pregnancies.

Infection has proved to be an important factor in precipitating cardiac failure. Each woman should receive instructions to avoid contact with persons who have respiratory infections, including the common cold, and to report at once any evidence for infection. Bacterial endocarditis is a deadly complication of valvar heart disease. Pneumococcal and influenza vaccines are recommended.

Cigarette smoking is prohibited, both because of its cardiac effects as well as the propensity to cause upper respiratory infections. Illicit drug use may be particularly harmful, as with the cardiovascular effects of cocaine or amphetamines, in addition to the propensity for intravenous use of any illegal substance to cause infective endocarditis.

The onset of congestive heart failure is generally gradual. The first warning sign is likely to be persistent basilar rales, frequently accompanied by a nocturnal cough. A sudden diminution in ability to carry out usual duties, increasing dyspnea on exertion, or attacks of smothering with cough are symptoms of serious heart failure. Clinical findings may include hemoptysis, progressive edema, and tachycardia.

LABOR AND DELIVERY. In general, delivery should be accomplished vaginally unless there are obstetrical indications for cesarean delivery. In some women with severe heart disease, **pulmonary artery catheterization** may be indicated for continuous hemodynamic monitoring (American College of Obstetricians and Gynecologists, 1992b). This may be performed electively when labor begins or planned cesarean delivery is performed.

In our experiences, such monitoring is rarely indicated in women who have remained in functional class I or II throughout pregnancy.

Relief from pain and apprehension is especially important. While intravenous analgesics provide satisfactory pain relief for some women, continuous epidural analgesia is recommended for most situations. The major danger of conduction analgesia is maternal hypotension (Chap. 15, p 372). This is especially dangerous in women with intracardiac shunts, in whom flow may be reversed with blood passing from the right-to-left within the heart or aorta, thereby bypassing the lungs. Hypotension can be very hazardous with pulmonary hypertension or aortic stenosis because ventricular output is dependent upon adequate preload. In women with these conditions, narcotic conduction analgesia or general anesthesia may be preferable.

During labor, the mother with significant heart disease should be kept in a semirecumbent position with lateral tilt. Vital signs should be taken frequently between contractions. Increases in pulse rate much above 100 per minute or in the respiratory rate above 24, particularly when associated with dyspnea, may suggest impending ventricular failure. With any evidence of cardiac decompensation, intensive medical management must be instituted immediately. It is essential to remember that delivery itself will not necessarily improve the maternal condition. Moreover, emergency operative delivery may be particularly hazardous. Clearly, both maternal and fetal conditions must be considered in the decision to hasten delivery under these circumstances.

For vaginal delivery in women with only mild cardiovascular compromise, epidural analgesia given along with intravenous sedation often suffices. This has been shown to minimize intrapartum cardiac output fluctuations and allows forceps or vacuum-assisted delivery. Subarachnoid blockade—spinal analgesia or saddle block—is not generally recommended in women with significant heart disease. For cesarean delivery, epidural analgesia is preferred by most clinicians with caveats for its use with pulmonary hypertension. Spinal analgesia is contraindicated with some lesions. Finally, general endotracheal anesthesia with thiopental, succinylcholine nitrous oxide, and at least 30 percent oxygen has also proved satisfactory (Chap. 15, p. 362).

INTRAPARTUM HEART FAILURE. Cardiovascular decompensation during labor may manifest as pulmonary edema and hypoxia, hypotension, or both. The proper therapeutic approach will depend upon the specific hemodynamic status and the underlying cardiac lesion. For example, decompensated mitral stenosis with pulmonary edema due to absolute or relative fluid overload is often best approached with aggressive diuresis, or if precipitated by tachycardia, by heart rate control

with β-blocking agents. On the other hand, the same treatment in a woman suffering decompensation and hypotension due to aortic stenosis could prove fatal. **Unless the underlying pathophysiology is understood and the cause of the decompensation clear, empirical therapy is hazardous.**

PUERPERIUM. Women who have shown little or no evidence of cardiac distress during pregnancy, labor, or delivery may still decompensate after delivery. Therefore, it is important that meticulous care be continued into the puerperium. Postpartum hemorrhage, anemia, infection, and thromboembolism are much more serious complications with heart disease. Indeed, these factors frequently act in concert to precipitate postpartum heart failure in women with underlying disease (Cunningham and associates, 1986).

If tubal sterilization is to be performed after vaginal delivery, it may be best to delay the procedure until it is obvious that the mother is afebrile, not anemic, and has demonstrated that she can ambulate without evidence of distress. Women who do not undergo tubal sterilization should be given detailed contraceptive advice. There are special considerations for contraception in women with various types of cardiac disorders. These are discussed in some of the following sections and in Chapter 58. The American College of Obstetricians and Gynecologists (2000) has also recently considered some of these specific situations.

MANAGEMENT OF CLASSES III AND IV. These severe cases are uncommon today. In the Toronto study cited earlier, only 2 percent of 221 women had class III or IV heart disease (Siu and associates, 1997). In their experiences with 445 pregnant women with heart disease, McFaul and colleagues (1988) reported 4 percent with class III and 7 percent with class IV. The important question in these women is whether pregnancy should be undertaken. If women choose to become pregnant, they must understand the risks and cooperate fully with planned care. If seen early enough, women with some types of severe cardiac disease should consider pregnancy interruption. If the pregnancy is continued, prolonged hospitalization or bed rest will often be necessary.

As for less severe disease, epidural analgesia for labor and delivery is usually recommended. Vaginal delivery is preferred in most cases, and cesarean delivery is limited to obstetrical indications. The decision for cesarean delivery must take into account the specific cardiac lesion, overall maternal condition, availability and experience of anesthetic support, as well as physical facilities. These women often tolerate major surgical procedures poorly, and should be delivered in a facility with experience with complicated cardiac disease.

SURGICALLY CORRECTED HEART DISEASE

The majority of clinically significant lesions are repaired during childhood. Morris and Menashe (1991) reviewed mortality statistics for over 2700 children having corrective cardiac surgery in Oregon from 1958 through 1989. At 25 years, more than 75 percent were still alive. In referral centers for congenital heart disease in adults, only 15 to 20 percent have not had previous surgical intervention (Perloff, 1997). Examples of defects not diagnosed until adulthood include atrial septal defects, pulmonic stenosis, bicuspid aortic valve, and aortic co-arctation (Brickner and colleagues, 2000). In some cases, the defect is mild and surgery is not required. In others a significant structural anomaly is amenable to surgical correction. With successful repair, many women will attempt pregnancy. In some instances, surgical corrections have been performed during pregnancy.

VALVE REPLACEMENT. A number of reproductive-age women have had a cardiac valvar prosthesis implanted to replace a severely damaged mitral or aortic valve. Reports of subsequent pregnancy outcomes are now quite numerous, and indeed, successful pregnancies have followed prosthetic replacement of even three heart valves (Nagorney and Field, 1981).

EFFECT ON PREGNANCY. Pregnancy is to be undertaken in these women only after serious consideration. Women with a **mechanical valve prosthesis** must be anticoagulated, and when not pregnant, warfarin is recommended. As shown in Table 44–4, a number of serious complications can develop, especially with mechanical valves. Thromboembolism involving the prosthesis and hemorrhage from anticoagulation are of extreme concern. Also, there may be deterioration in cardiac function. Maternal mortality is 3 to 4 percent with mechanical valves and fetal loss is common. The critical issue is anticoagulation, and there is a suggestion that heparin may be less effective than warfarin in preventing thromboembolic events. Unfortunately, there are known adverse fetal effects of warfarin (Caulin-Glaser and Setaro, 1999). Spontaneous abortions, stillbirths, and malformed fetuses are more common if warfarin is used (Chap. 38, p. 1014).

The results shown in Table 44–4 are similar to those reported by Chan and colleagues (2000) in their review of 28 studies published through 1997. They concluded that better maternal outcomes were achieved with continuation of warfarin throughout pregnancy; however, the embryopathy rate was 6.4 percent. While heparin substitution from 6 to 12 weeks eliminated embryopa-

TABLE 44–4. Perinatal Outcomes in 793 Women Who Had a Heart Valve Replaced Prior to Pregnancy

Type of Valve	No.	Maternal	Perinatal
Mechanical Valves (N = 528)			
Iturbe-Alessio et al (1986)	72	3 thromboses; 2 deaths	10/35 embryopathy; 1 stillborn
Ismail et al (1986)	76	4 deaths	5% embryopathy
Sareli et al (1989)	50	2 heart failure in labor	9 abortions; 7 stillborns; 2 neonatal deaths; 2 embryopathy
Hanania et al (1994)	108	10 thromboses with 3 emboli; 6 emboli; 4 deaths	30 abortions; 4 stillborns
Sbarouni and Oakley (1994)	151	13 thromboses; 8 emboli; 7 hemorrhage; 6 deaths	9 stillborns; 3 neonatal deaths
Suri et al (1999)	21	1 thrombosis with death; 2 hemorrhage	2 stillborns; 4 growth restricted
Sadler et al (2000)	50	4/14 thromboses with heparin; 1 death	70% pregnancy loss with warfarin; 25% pregnancy loss with heparin; 57% preterm delivery; 4 stillborns with warfarin
Porcine Xenograft (N = 265)			
Lee et al (1994)	95	4 valve dysfunction	—
Hanania et al (1994)	74	7 valve failure	9 abortions; 1 stillborn
Sbarouni and Oakley (1994)	63	17 valve deterioration	2 stillborns
Sadler et al (2000)	33	4 valve deterioration	1 neonatal death

thy, it was associated with significantly increased thromboembolic complications. Low-dose heparin is definitely inadequate and in the study by Iturbe-Alessio and colleagues (1986), 3 of 35 women taking low-dose heparin suffered massive thrombosis of a mitral prosthesis, and two of them died. Overall, Chan and co-workers (2000) found a 2.9 percent maternal mortality rate.

Porcine tissue valves are much safer during pregnancy (Table 44–4). This is primarily because anticoagulation is not required. Deviri and colleagues (1985) reported no thrombi in 22 pregnancies in 11 unanticoagulated women with porcine xenografts. Lee and associates (1994) described generally good outcomes in 95 pregnancies in 57 women with a porcine graft. Four of these developed valve dysfunction. Unfortunately, although less thrombogenic, such bioprostheses are not as durable as mechanical prostheses. Their use necessitates the acceptance of additional open-heart surgery at a future date. Fortunately, pregnancy does not appear to shorten this interval (North and colleagues, 1999; Salazar and co-workers, 1999).

MANAGEMENT. Full anticoagulation throughout pregnancy is recommended with either warfarin or heparin after the woman is counseled regarding respective risks. Most authors recommend full heparinization as described in Chapter 46 (p. 1238) to prolong the partial thromboplastin time by 1.5 to 2.5 times baseline values. Just before delivery, heparin is stopped. If delivery supervenes while the anticoagulant is still effective, and extensive bleeding is encountered, protamine sulfate is given. Anticoagulant therapy with warfarin or heparin may be restarted 6 hours following vaginal delivery, usually with no problems. Following cesarean delivery, however, full anticoagulation should be withheld for at least 24 hours. Clark and colleagues (2000) reviewed the use of coumarin derivatives in breast-feeding women and concluded that warfarin can be safely given as it has minimal transfer to milk.

CONTRACEPTION. Because of their possible thrombogenic action, oral contraceptives containing estrogen and a progestin are relatively contraindicated in women with prosthetic valves (Chap. 58, p. 1528). Such women are generally fully anticoagulated, and thus any increased risk is speculative. Sterilization should be considered because of serious problems during pregnancy.

VALVE REPLACEMENT DURING PREGNANCY. Although usually postponed, valve replacement during pregnancy occasionally may be lifesaving. A number of reviews and small series all confirm that surgery on the heart or great vessels is associated with major maternal

and fetal morbidity and mortality. Westaby and associates (1992) reviewed 115 cardiac surgeries using cardiopulmonary bypass from 1959 through 1990. They reported two maternal deaths and 17 percent fetal deaths. Weiss and colleagues (1998a) reviewed published cases from 1984 through 1996. In a total of 70 women, 59 of whom had cardiopulmonary bypass, maternal mortality was 6 percent and perinatal mortality was 30 percent. Valvar surgery was associated with a 9 percent maternal death rate.

Strickland and colleagues (1991) reported the Mayo Clinic experience in 10 women undergoing cardiopulmonary bypass with pump times ranging from 18 to 154 minutes. The fetal response to bypass was usually bradycardia, and they recommended that high-flow, normothermic perfusion be used if possible. Khandelwal and associates (1996) meticulously recorded fetal and uterine blood flow velocity patterns during a 74-minute bypass procedure at 19 weeks for aortic valve replacement. Despite high peak flow rates and sustained mean arterial pressures, uterine and umbilical artery resistances rose greatly, and fetal hydrocephalus and ascites were apparent within 2 days. Tripp and co-workers (1999) described use of pulsatile perfusion during aortic valve replacement at 14 weeks.

MITRAL VALVOTOMY. This operation is less common because the incidence of rheumatic mitral stenosis has declined. Schenker and Polishuk (1968) reported a total of 325 pregnancies in 182 women who previously had undergone mitral valvotomy. Despite this, heart failure developed in 42 percent of these women at some point during their first pregnancy following surgery. This percentage increased with successive pregnancies, and women suffering heart failure in one pregnancy inevitably had recurrence in subsequent pregnancies. Coexisting atrial fibrillation was especially ominous and commonly was associated with heart failure, thromboembolic disease, and death.

MITRAL VALVOTOMY DURING PREGNANCY. In the past, tight mitral stenosis that required intervention during pregnancy usually was treated surgically by closed mitral valvotomy (Pavankumar and associates, 1988). Following surgery, functional classification was usually downgraded from class III or IV to class I. There were no maternal deaths, and the fetal death rate was 7 percent. Birincioglu and co-workers (1999) described six women in whom mitral valve replacement was done in conjunction with cesarean delivery.

Within the past 20 years, percutaneous transcatheter balloon dilatation of the mitral valve has largely replaced surgical valvuloplasty during pregnancy (Caulin-Glaser and Setaro, 1999; Gupta and associates, 1998).

HEART TRANSPLANTATION. By 1994, the registry of the International Society for Heart and Lung Transplantation had compiled data from more than 30,000 heart and heart–lung transplant operations (Hosenpud and associates, 1994). The 3-year survival rate is 75 percent and it was inevitable that some of these women would become pregnant. Löwenstein and associates (1988) reported the first successful pregnancy in a transplant recipient. Key and associates (1989) as well as Kim and colleagues (1996) provided detailed data to show that the transplanted heart responded normally to pregnancy-induced changes.

Complications are common during pregnancy. Branch and collaborators (1998) analyzed 47 pregnancies in 35 women entered into the National Transplantation Pregnancy Registry. Almost half delivered before 37 weeks, and 40 percent had maternal complications. At follow-up, 20 percent of these women had died. Troché and co-workers (1998) reported 10 pregnancies from the France Transplant Association. Hypertension complicated nine, half were delivered by cesarean, and half the fetuses had growth restriction. Dashe and associates (1998) reviewed 32 pregnancies reported in heart or heart–lung transplant recipients. Almost half had hypertension, 25 percent had preeclampsia, and 38 percent were delivered preterm. A third underwent cesarean delivery. About 20 percent experienced rejection episodes in pregnancy, and in 40 percent cyclosporine doses were increased. Although there were no direct maternal deaths, three women had died within 6 months to 3 years after delivery.

VALVAR HEART DISEASE

Rheumatic fever is uncommon in the United States because of less crowded living conditions, availability of penicillin, and evolution of nonrheumatogenic streptococcal strains. Still, it remains the chief cause of serious mitral valvar disease in women. During epidemics of streptococcal pharyngitis, as many as 3 percent of untreated young adults may develop rheumatic fever.

MITRAL STENOSIS. Rheumatic endocarditis causes three fourths of cases of mitral stenosis. The contracted valve impedes blood flow from the left atrium to the ventricle. With tight mitral stenosis, the left atrium is dilated, as shown in Figure 44–2. As shown in Table 44–5, left-atrial pressure is chronically elevated and may result in significant passive pulmonary hypertension and a fixed cardiac output (Carabello and Crawford, 1997). The increased preload of normal pregnancy, as well as other factors that require increased cardiac output, may cause ventricular failure with pulmonary edema in these women with relatively fixed cardiac output. Indeed, 25 percent of women with mitral stenosis have cardiac failure for the first time during pregnancy (Caulin-Glaser and Setaro, 1999). In some cases, this is confused with idiopathic peripartum cardiomyopathy (Cunningham and colleagues, 1986).

The normal mitral-valve surface area is $4.0 \, cm^2$. When stenosis narrows this to less than $2.5 \, cm^2$, symptoms usually develop (Desai and colleagues, 2000). The most prominent complaint is dyspnea due to pulmonary venous hypertension and pulmonary edema. Other common symptoms are fatigue, palpitations, cough, and hemoptysis.

TABLE 44–5. Major Cardiac Valve Disorders

Type	Cause	Pathophysiology	Pregnancy
Mitral stenosis	Rheumatic	LA dilatation and pulmonary hypertension Atrial fibrillation	Heart failure from fluid overload, tachycardia
Mitral insufficiency	Rheumatic Mitral-valve prolapse LV dilatation	LV dilatation and eccentric hypertrophy	Ventricular function improves with afterload decrease
Aortic stenosis	Congenital Bicuspid valve	LV concentric hypertrophy, decreased cardiac output	Moderate stenosis tolerated, severe is life-threatening with decreased preload, e.g., hemorrhage, regional analgesia
Aortic insufficiency	Rheumatic heart disease Connective-tissue disease Congenital	LV hypertrophy and dilatation	Ventricular function improves with afterload decrease

LA = left atrium; LV = left ventricle.

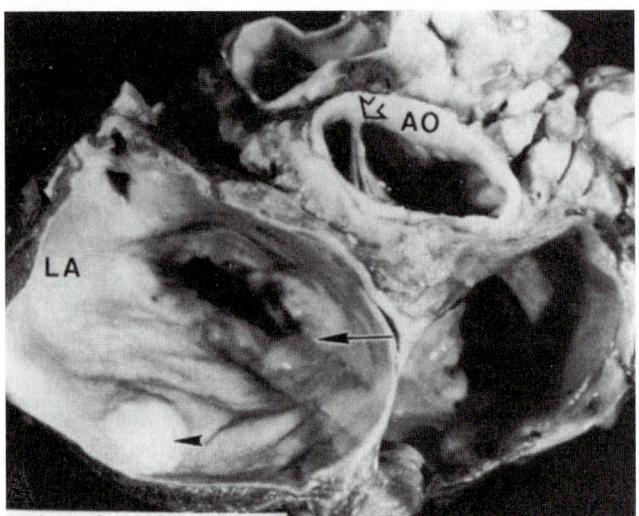

FIGURE 44–2. Superior view of heart of a patient with rheumatic mitral stenosis showing fibrous adhesions and narrowing of mitral valve (*arrow*). The left atrium (LA) is dilated. The *arrowhead* points to focal endocardial fibrosis and the open *arrow* shows mild fibrosis of the aortic valve (AO). (From Brady and Duff, 1989, with permission.)

In patients with significant mitral stenosis, tachycardia of any etiology shortens ventricular diastolic filling time and increases the mitral gradient, which raises left atrial and pulmonary venous and capillary pressures and may result in pulmonary edema (Ramin and Gilstrap, 1999). Thus, sinus tachycardia is often treated prophylactically with β-blocking agents. Atrial tachyarrhythmias, including fibrillation, are common in mitral stenosis and are treated aggressively with cardioversion if necessary. Atrial fibrillation also predisposes to mural thrombus formation and aortic embolization, which may lead to a thrombotic cerebrovascular accident.

MANAGEMENT. Limited physical activity is generally recommended. If symptoms of pulmonary congestion develop, activity is restricted even more, dietary sodium is restricted, and diuretic therapy started. A β-blocker drug is often given to slow heart rate response to activity and anxiety. Al Kasab and associates (1990) treated 25 pregnant women with mitral stenosis with either propranolol or atenolol. Their mean heart rate was decreased from 86 to 78 beats/min, and 92 percent had significant symptomatic improvement as measured by reassignment to a lower New York Heart Association classification. If new-onset atrial fibrillation develops, intravenous verapamil, 5 to 10 mg, is given, or electrocardioversion is performed. For chronic fibrillation, digoxin or a β- or calcium-channel blocker is given to slow ventricular response. Anticoagulation with heparin is also indicated.

Labor and delivery are particularly stressful for women with tight mitral stenosis. Pain, work, and anxiety cause tachycardia, with increasing chances of rate-related heart failure. Epidural analgesia for labor, with strict attention to avoid intravenous fluid overload, is ideal. As shown in Figure 44–3, pulmonary capillary wedge pressures usually increase even more immediately postpartum. Clark and colleagues (1985) hypothesize that this is likely due to loss of the low-resistance placental circulation as well as "autotransfusion" from the lower extremities and pelvic veins and the now empty uterus. Abrupt increases in preload may lead to increased pulmonary capillary wedge pressure and pulmonary edema. Thus, care must be taken to avoid fluid overload (Ramin and Gilstrap, 1999).

Vaginal delivery is preferable, and some authors recommend elective induction so that labor and delivery can be monitored and attended by the most knowledgeable team. In cases of severe stenosis with chronic heart failure, insertion of a pulmonary artery catheter may help guide management decisions. Intrapartum endocarditis prophylaxis is required.

MITRAL INSUFFICIENCY. Mitral regurgitation develops when there is improper coaptation of mitral-valve leaflets during systole, and this is eventually followed by left-ventricular dilatation and eccentric hypertrophy (Table 44–5). Chronic mitral regurgitation may be due to a number of causes, including rheumatic fever, mitral-valve prolapse, or left-ventricular dilatation of any etiology—for example, dilated cardiomyopathy. Mitral-valve vegetation, known as *Libman-Sacks endocarditis,* is relatively common in women with antiphospholipid antibodies which may co-exist with systemic lupus erythematosus (Roldan and colleagues, 1996; see Chap. 52, p. 1391). Less common causes include a calcified mitral annulus, possibly some appetite suppressants, and in older women, ischemic heart disease. Acute mitral insufficiency is caused by rupture of a chordae tendineae, infarction of papillary muscle, or by leaflet perforation from infective endocarditis.

In nonpregnant patients, symptoms from mitral-valve incompetence are rare, and valve replacement is seldom indicated, except for infective endocarditis. Likewise, mitral regurgitation is well tolerated during pregnancy, probably due to decreased systemic vascular resistance, which actually results in less regurgitation. Heart failure only rarely develops during pregnancy, and occasionally tachyarrhythmias need to be treated. Prophylaxis against bacterial endocarditis is given intrapartum.

AORTIC STENOSIS. Stenosis of the aortic valve is a disease of aging, and in a woman less than 30 years old, it is most likely due to a congenital lesion. This is the result of the decline in incidence of rheumatic diseases. The most common stenotic lesion is a bicuspid valve.

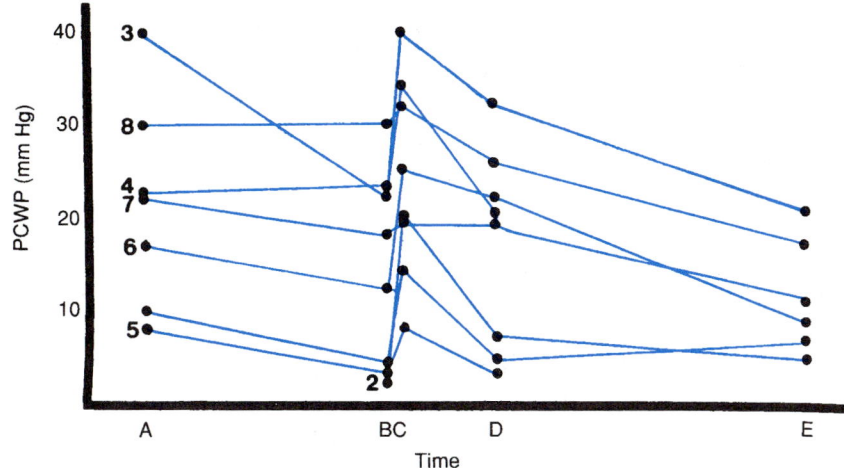

FIGURE 44–3. Intrapartum alterations in pulmonary capillary wedge pressure (PCWP) in eight women with mitral valve stenosis. **A.** First-stage labor. **B.** Second-stage labor, 15 to 30 minutes before delivery. **C.** Postpartum 5 to 15 minutes. **D.** Postpartum 4 to 6 hours. **E.** Postpartum 18 to 24 hours. (From Clark and colleagues, 1985, with permission.)

Stenosis reduces the normal 2- to 3-cm^2 aortic orifice and creates resistance to ejection. A systolic pressure gradient develops between the left ventricle and the systemic arterial outflow tract. Concentric left-ventricular hypertrophy follows, and if severe, end-diastolic pressures become elevated, ejection fraction declines, and cardiac output is reduced (Table 44–5). Characteristic clinical manifestations develop late and include chest pain, syncope, heart failure, and sudden death from arrhythmias. Life expectancy after exertional chest pain develops averages only 5 years, and valve replacement is indicated for symptomatic patients.

Clinically significant aortic stenosis is uncommonly encountered during pregnancy. Mild to moderate degrees of stenosis are well tolerated, but severe disease is life threatening. The principal underlying hemodynamic problem is the fixed cardiac output associated with severe stenosis. During pregnancy, a number of factors may be encountered that commonly decrease preload further and thus aggravate the fixed cardiac output. Some examples include blood loss, regional analgesia, and vena caval occlusion. Importantly, all of these factors decrease cardiac, cerebral, and uterine perfusion. Because of these considerations, severe aortic stenosis may be extremely dangerous during pregnancy. Reports after 1975 describe a collective mortality of 7 percent (Lao and colleagues, 1993b). Patients with valve gradients exceeding 100 mm Hg appear to be at greatest risk.

MANAGEMENT IN PREGNANCY. For the asymptomatic pregnant woman, no treatment except close observation is required. Management of the symptomatic woman includes strict limitation of activity and prompt treatment of infections. If symptoms persist despite bed rest, valve replacement or valvotomy using cardiopulmonary bypass must be considered. In general, balloon valvotomy for aortic valve disease is avoided because of a serious complication rate of over 10 percent. Some of these complications include stroke, aortic rupture, aortic valve insufficiency, and death (Carabello and Crawford, 1997). In rare cases, however, it may be preferable to perform valve replacement during pregnancy (Angel and colleagues, 1988; Lao and associates, 1993a).

For women with critical aortic stenosis, intensive monitoring during labor is important. Pulmonary artery catheterization may be helpful because of the narrow margin separating fluid overload from hypovolemia. Patients with aortic stenosis are dependent upon adequate end-diastolic ventricular filling pressures to maintain cardiac output and systemic perfusion. Abrupt decreases in end-diastolic volume may result in hypotension, syncope, myocardial infarction, and sudden death. Thus the key to the management of these women is the avoidance of decreased ventricular preload and maintenance of cardiac output. During labor and delivery, such women should be managed on the "wet" side, maintaining a margin of safety in intravascular volume in anticipation of unexpected hemorrhage. In women with a competent mitral valve, pulmonary edema is rare, even with moderate volume overload.

During labor, narcotic epidural analgesia seems ideal, thus avoiding potentially hazardous hypotension, which may be encountered with standard conduction analgesia techniques. Easterling and colleagues (1988) used standard epidural analgesia for five women with severe stenosis and demonstrated immediate and profound effects of decreased filling pressures. Thus, as emphasized by Thornhill and Camann (1994), slow administration of dilute local anesthetics into the epidural space allows for a safe block. Lao and associates (1993b) used this routinely in 20 such women. Forceps or vacuum delivery are used for standard obstetrical indications in hemodynamically stable women. Bacterial endocarditis prophylaxis is given at delivery.

AORTIC INSUFFICIENCY. Aortic regurgitation is the diastolic flow of blood from the aorta into the left ventricle. Common causes of aortic valvar incompetence are rheumatic fever, connective tissue abnormalities, and congenitally acquired lesions. With Marfan syndrome, the aortic root may dilate, resulting in aortic insufficiency (see p. 1201). Acute insufficiency may develop with bacterial endocarditis or aortic dissection. Aortic as well as mitral-valve insufficiency have been linked to the appetite suppressants fenfluramine and dexfenfluramine (Gardin, 2000; Jick, 1998; Khan, 1998, and all of their associates). These lesions (usually mild) are duration related and aortic regurgitation develops in 9 to 14 percent of exposed patients compared with 4 percent of nonexposed controls (Jick, 2000).

With chronic disease, left-ventricular hypertrophy and dilatation develop (Table 44–5). This is followed by slow-onset fatigue, dyspnea, and edema, although rapid deterioration usually follows. Aortic insufficiency is generally well tolerated during pregnancy. Like mitral-valve incompetence, diminished vascular resistance is thought to improve the lesion (Mendelson and Lang, 1995). Symptoms necessitate therapy for heart failure, including bed rest, sodium restriction, and diuretics. Epidural analgesia is used for labor as well as vaginal or cesarean delivery. Bacterial endocarditis prophylaxis is given at delivery.

CONGENITAL HEART DISEASE

The incidence of congenital heart disease in the United States is approximately 8 per 1000 live-born infants. About a third of these have critical disease that requires cardiac catheterization or surgery, or they die within the first year. Others will require surgery in childhood, and 85 percent survive to adulthood (Moodie, 1994). Estimates of incidence and distribution of specific lesions will depend on the age group surveyed—for example newborns versus autopsy studies. According to Nugent and associates (1990), the more common lesions at birth are ventricular septal defect (28 percent), pulmonary stenosis (10 percent), patent ductus (8 percent), atrial septal defect (7 percent), aortic stenosis (4 percent), and aortic coarctation (4 percent). Most adults—80 to 85 percent—with significant disease have

had some type of surgical intervention in childhood (Perloff, 1997).

Mendelson and Lang (1995) divide congenital heart lesions that complicate pregnancy into three groups:

1. Volume overload or left-to-right shunts, examples of which include atrial or ventricular septal defects.
2. Pressure overload, such as aortic and pulmonary stenosis, aortic coarctation, and hypertrophic subaortic stenosis.
3. Cyanotic lesions or right-to-left shunts that include Fallot tetralogy and Eisenmenger syndrome.

SEPTAL DEFECTS. After bicuspid aortic valve, **atrial septal defects** are the most commonly encountered congenital cardiac lesion in adults. They comprise a third of cases in adults (Brickner and colleagues, 2000). Many of these cases are asymptomatic until the third or fourth decade. The secundum-type defect accounts for 70 percent of all cases, and associated mitral-valve myxomatous abnormalities with prolapse are common. Most clinicians recommend repair if discovered in adulthood. Pregnancy is well tolerated unless pulmonary hypertension has developed, but this is rare because pulmonary artery pressures are low with an atrial septal defect (Zuber and associates, 1999). If congestive heart failure or an arrhythmia develops, treatment is given. Bacterial endocarditis prophylaxis is controversial, unless the defect was repaired with a patch. The risk is higher with associated mitral-valve pathology. The risk of atrial septal defect for the fetus is 5 to 10 percent.

Ventricular septal defects spontaneously close in 90 percent of patients during childhood. In adults the lesion follows bicuspid aortic valve, atrial septal defect, and pulmonic stenosis in frequency. Almost 75 percent of defects are paramembraneous, and physiological derangements are related to their size. In general, if the defect is less than 1.25 cm^2, pulmonary hypertension and heart failure do not develop. When the effective size of the defect is greater than the aortic valve orifice, symptoms rapidly develop, and most children undergo surgical repair before pulmonary hypertension develops. In contrast, adults with unrepaired large defects develop left-ventricular failure and pulmonary hypertension, as well as a high incidence of bacterial endocarditis (Brickner and colleagues, 2000).

Pregnancy is well tolerated with small to moderate left-to-right shunts. When pulmonary arterial pressures reach systemic levels, however, there is reversal or bidirectional flow or **Eisenmenger syndrome.** When this develops, maternal mortality is 30 to 50 percent. Jackson and colleagues (1993) described two women who had severe pulmonary hypertension despite early repair of septal defects in childhood. One pregnancy was aborted and the second woman died 5 days following preterm delivery. Thus, pregnancy is contraindicated, and therapeutic abortion is advised if contraception fails. Bacterial endocarditis is common with unrepaired defects, and antibiotic prophylaxis is recommended. Unless repair is associated with residual septal defect, the risk of endocarditis is low. About 5 to 10 percent of offspring will have a ventricular septal defect.

PERSISTENT DUCTUS ARTERIOSUS. Like other shunts, the physiological consequences of this lesion are related to its size. Most significant lesions are repaired in childhood. In those not undergoing repair, mortality is high beginning in the fifth decade (Brickner and coworkers, 2000). Thus, some women with an unrepaired persistent ductus will have developed pulmonary hypertension. Heart failure may develop in these women, and if systemic blood pressure falls, reversal of blood flow from the pulmonary artery into the aorta causes cyanosis. Sudden drops in blood pressure at delivery, as with conduction analgesia or hemorrhage, may lead to fatal collapse. Therefore, hypotension should be avoided whenever possible and treated vigorously if it develops. Prophylaxis for bacterial endocarditis should be given at delivery. The incidence of inheritance is about 5 percent.

CYANOTIC HEART DISEASE. When congenital heart lesions are associated with right-to-left shunting of blood past the pulmonary capillary bed, then cyanosis develops. The classical and most commonly encountered lesion in pregnancy is the **Fallot tetralogy.** This is characterized by a large ventricular septal defect, right ventricular hypertrophy, and an overriding aorta. The magnitude of the shunt varies inversely with systemic vascular resistance. Hence, during pregnancy, when peripheral resistance decreases, the shunt increases and cyanosis worsens. Women who have undergone repair, and in whom cyanosis did not reappear, do well in pregnancy.

Some women with **Ebstein anomaly** of the tricuspid valve may reach reproductive age. Right-ventricular failure from volume overload and appearance or worsening of cyanosis are common during pregnancy. If there is no cyanosis, these women usually tolerate pregnancy well.

EFFECT ON PREGNACY. Women with cyanotic heart disease do poorly during pregnancy. With uncorrected Fallot tetralogy, for example, maternal mortality approaches 10 percent. Any disease complicated by severe maternal hypoxemia is likely to lead to miscarriage, preterm delivery, or fetal death. There is a relationship between chronic hypoxemia and the polycythemia it causes with the outcome of pregnancy. When hypoxemia is intense enough to stimulate a rise in hematocrit

above 65 percent, pregnancy wastage is virtually 100 percent.

Sawhney and colleagues (1998) reported stillborn infants in 14 percent and fetal growth restriction in 36 percent of 24 pregnancies in women with cyanotic heart disease. Shime and associates (1987) reported that 13 of 23 women with cyanotic heart disease developed functional deterioration during pregnancy, and seven had cardiac failure. Three of these 23 infants (13 percent) died, and low birthweight was common. While Zuber and co-workers (1999) reported good outcomes in 19 women with Fallot tetralogy, they emphasized that prepregnancy functional class and systolic ventricular function were good in all of them.

PREGNANCY AFTER SURGICAL REPAIR. With satisfactory surgical correction prior to pregnancy, maternal risks are decreased dramatically, and fetal environment is improved. Singh and associates (1982) described 40 pregnancies in 27 women with surgically corrected tetralogy. They concluded that in women with no major residual defects after surgery, that pregnancy is usually well tolerated. Lao (1994), Megerian (1994), Lynch-Salamon (1993), and their colleagues described a total of 14 pregnancies in 10 women following successful *Mustard repair* for **transposition of the great vessels.** Two women developed cardiac failure during pregnancy and two others developed worrisome arrhythmias. Connolly and co-workers (1999) reported 60 pregnancies in 22 women who had transposition corrected in childhood. Maternal complications were uncommon and only two women developed heart failure, there was one case of endocarditis, and a woman with a single coronary artery had a myocardial infarction. All 50 live-born infants survived.

Labor and Delivery. Vaginal delivery is preferred unless there is an obstetrical indication for cesarean delivery. **Pulmonary artery catheter monitoring has limitations because of the sometimes bizarre anatomical abnormalities.** Care must be taken to avoid sudden blood pressure decreases. For labor pain, epidural opiates may suffice. There is controversy regarding epidural analgesia versus general anesthesia for cesarean delivery (Thornhill and Camann, 1994).

EISENMENGER SYNDROME. This syndrome is secondary pulmonary hypertension that develops with any cardiac lesion in which pulmonary vascular resistance becomes greater than systemic vascular resistance and in which there is some right-to-left shunting. The most common underlying defects are atrial or ventricular septal defects and persistent ductus arteriosus. Patients usually are asymptomatic, but eventually pulmonary hypertension is severe enough to cause right-to-left shunting.

The prognosis for pregnancy depends on the severity of pulmonary hypertension. In a review of 44 cases through 1978, Gleicher and associates (1979) reported maternal and perinatal mortality rates to be about 50 percent. There has been little improvement since then (Table 44–6). Yentis and colleagues (1998) reported a 40 percent maternal death rate from the United Kingdom from 1991 through 1995. Weiss and co-workers (1998b) cited 36 percent maternal deaths in a review of 73 pregnancies. Of 26 deaths, only three were antepartum and 23 occurred during delivery or within a month postpartum. These women tolerate hypotension poorly, and the cause of death usually is right-ventricular failure with cardiogenic shock. Management is discussed later in this chapter.

OTHER CARDIOVASCULAR CONDITIONS

PULMONARY HYPERTENSION. High pulmonary blood pressure is generally secondary to cardiac or pulmonary disease, and common causes are persistent and prolonged left-to-right shunting with development of Eisenmenger syndrome as previously discussed. Other causes are chronic lung disease, hemoglobinopathies, cocaine use, human immunodeficiency virus (HIV) infection, and appetite suppressants (Rubin, 1997). According to Edenborough and colleagues (2000), pulmonary hypertension and cor pulmonale complicating cystic fibrosis has an especially poor pregnancy prognosis (Chap. 46, p. 1243).

Primary pulmonary hypertension, characterized by medial hypertrophy and plexiform lesions, is usually idiopathic, but some previously unexplained cases may be due to antiphospholipid antibodies (Chap. 52, p. 1391). It has also been seen in young women who took certain appetite suppressants (Gaine and Rubin, 1998). The prognosis is bad and the mean survival from diagnosis is about 2 years. Long-term therapy with epoprostenol (prostacyclin) given intravenously by continuous infusion significantly lowers pulmonary vascular resistance (McLaughlin and colleagues, 1998). Easterling and associates (1999) recommend that response to nifedipine and prostacyclin be documented for at least a year before pregnancy is advised.

EFFECTS ON PREGNANCY. Maternal mortality is appreciable, whether pulmonary hypertension is primary or secondary. Torres and associates (1994) documented diminished pulmonary vascular resistance during pregnancy in a woman with primary disease. Kiss and colleagues (1995) reviewed literature since 1956 and reported a maternal mortality rate of 7 of 11 (65 percent) women with primary pulmonary hypertension. Weiss

and associates (1998b) reviewed 27 cases reported from 1978 through 1996 and found a 30 percent mortality rate. As discussed, women with Eisenmenger syndrome also have formidable mortality (Table 44–6).

While pregnancy is contraindicated with severe disease, milder degrees of secondary pulmonary hypertension probably go unnoticed. For example, with the more common use of pulmonary artery catheterization in women with heart disease, we have identified women with mild to moderate pulmonary hypertension who tolerated pregnancy, labor, and delivery quite well. Boggess and colleagues (1995) described nine women with interstitial and restrictive lung disease who ostensibly had varying degrees of pulmonary hypertension. Three women had severe disease, and all nine tolerated pregnancy reasonably well.

Treatment of symptomatic pregnant women includes limitation of activity and avoidance of the supine position in late pregnancy. Diuretics, supplemental oxygen, and vasodilator drugs are standard therapy for symptoms. Goodwin (1999) and Robinson (1999) and their colleagues have described both chronic and acute therapy with inhaled nitric oxide in two pregnant women. Easterling and associates (1999) successfully used nifedipine and prostacyclin during pregnancy, and Badalian and co-workers (2000) described continued epoprostenol (prostacyclin) infusion throughout a twin pregnancy.

Management of labor and delivery is particularly problematic. **These women are at greatest risk when there is diminished venous return and right ventricular filling which is associated with most maternal deaths.**

TABLE 44–6. Pregnancy Complications in 70 Women During 98 Pregnancies Complicated by Eisenmenger Syndrome

Mortality Factor	No. (%)
Maternal mortality	31/70 (44)
Atrial septal defect	6/16 (38)
Ventricular septal defect	18/40 (45)
Patent ductus arteriosus	8/29 (42)
Mortality by delivery	
Vaginal	20/60 (33)
Cesarean	7/15 (47)
Cause of death	
Thromboembolism	14 (44)
Hypovolemia	8 (26)
Preeclampsia	6 (18)

Data courtesy of Dr. Richard Lange (1999).

Regional analgesia is problematic because of possible hypotension. Careful attention is given to blood loss at delivery and avoidance of standard (non-narcotic) epidural analgesia. Pollack and colleagues (1990), as well as others, have reported successful labor analgesia without significant cardiovascular effects from morphine administered intrathecally. Thornhill and Camann (1994) recommend intrathecal morphine, which can be supplanted by careful administration of epidural local anesthetics. They also argue against the use of pulmonary artery catheterization for a number of technical and safety issues, not the least of which is that data are usually not clinically useful. Weiss and co-workers (2000) described a woman with severe primary pulmonary hypertension who was successfully delivered by cesarean using epidural analgesia and while inhaling 20 mg of aerosolized iloprost.

MITRAL-VALVE PROLAPSE. This diagnosis implies the presence of a pathological connective-tissue disorder—often termed *myxomatous degeneration*—which may involve the valve leaflets themselves, the annulus, or the chordae tendinae. Until recently, this condition was thought to have a prevalence as high as 15 percent in otherwise normal young women. Community-based studies, however, indicate the incidence to be only 2 to 3 percent (Freed and colleagues, 1999). For referred cases, it is commonly associated with a wide variety of other cardiac disorders, including atrial septal defect, Marfan syndrome, Epstein anomaly, and hypertrophic cardiomyopathy. The etiology of isolated myxomatous degeneration is unknown.

Most women with mitral-valve prolapse are asymptomatic and are diagnosed by routine physical examination or as an incidental finding at echocardiography. The small percentage of women with symptoms have anxiety, palpitations, dyspnea, atypical chest pain, and syncope. Nishimura and colleagues (1985) identified only those patients with redundant mitral-valve leaflets to be at increased risk of sudden death, infective endocarditis, or cerebral embolism. Still, of 213 young women with documented ischemic strokes, only 1.9 percent had mitral-valve prolapse compared with 2.7 percent of controls (Gilon and co-workers, 1999).

DIAGNOSIS. Mitral-valve prolapse implies the presence of a pathological condition and should be diagnosed with great caution and precision. Reliance upon strict diagnostic criteria is essential before assigning a pathological diagnosis or administration of endocarditis prophylaxis (Nishimura and McGoon, 1999).

EFFECTS ON PREGNANCY. Pregnant women with mitral-valve prolapse rarely have cardiac complications. In fact, pregnancy-induced hypervolemia may improve alignment of the mitral-valve (Rayburn and colleagues, 1987). For women who are symptomatic, β-blocking drugs are given to decrease sympathetic tone, relieve chest pain and palpitations, and reduce the risk of life-threatening arrhythmias. In general, mitral-valve prolapse has not been deleterious to pregnancy. We manage these women as if not pregnant and prescribe β-blocker drugs for symptoms. Mitral-valve prolapse with regurgitation is considered to be a significant risk factor for development of bacterial endocarditis. Women should be given antibiotic prophylaxis if there is regurgitation, valvular damage, or any of the risk factors discussed. Patients without evidence of pathological myxomatous change may in general expect excellent pregnancy outcome (Chia and associates, 1994).

PERIPARTUM CARDIOMYOPATHY. This is a diagnosis of exclusion and is similar to idiopathic dilated cardiomyopathy that occurs in nonpregnant adults. A relationship of pregnancy with dilated cardiomyopathy was cited by Virchow and Porak in 1870. While the term peripartum cardiomyopathy has been used widely to describe women with peripartum heart failure with no readily apparent etiology, it is doubtful that there is a pregnancy-induced cardiomyopathy. The National Heart, Lung, and Blood Institute convened a review panel which concluded that the disease is an acute condition rather than a preexisting one preceding pregnancy (Pearson and colleagues, 2000).

Because other causes must be excluded, careful evaluation of new-onset ventricular dysfunction is essential. According to Fatkin and collaborators (1999), a third of cases of idiopathic dilated cardiomyopathy are inherited. Felker and colleagues (2000) performed endomyocardial biopsy in 1230 nonpregnant patients who had unexplained cardiomyopathy. In exactly half of these, a cause for cardiomyopathy was found and the most common was myocarditis. Feldman and McNamara (2000) recently reviewed this association. Dilated cardiomyopathy is also found in HIV infection (Barbaro and associates, 1998). We carefully evaluated 28 women at Parkland Hospital with peripartum heart failure of obscure etiology who were initially thought to have idiopathic cardiomyopathy. In 21 of these, heart failure was ultimately attributed to hypertensive heart disease, clinically silent mitral stenosis, obesity, or viral myocarditis (Cunningham and associates, 1986). In the study by Felker and co-workers (2000), 26 of 51 women with peripartum cardiomyopathy had histological incidence of myocarditis on endomyocardial biopsy.

Chronic hypertension with superimposed preeclampsia is a common cause of heart failure during pregnancy (Chap. 45, p. 1212). In some cases, mild antecedant hypertension is undiagnosed, and when superimposed preeclampsia develops, it may cause otherwise inexplicable peripartum heart failure. Obesity is a common co-factor with chronic hypertension, and it can cause or contribute to underlying ventricular hypertrophy (Fig. 44–4). In the Framingham Heart Study, obesity alone was correlated with increased left-ventricular mass (Lauer and colleagues, 1991).

Regardless of the underlying condition that causes cardiac dysfunction, women who develop peripartum heart failure often have obstetrical complications that either contribute to or precipitate heart failure. For ex-ample, preeclampsia is common and may precipitate afterload failure. Acute anemia from blood loss magni-fies the physiological effects of compromised ventricular function. Similarly, infection and accompanying fever increase cardiac output and oxygen utilization.

IDIOPATHIC CARDIOMYOPATHY IN PREGNANCY. After a thorough search excludes an underlying cause for heart failure, idiopathic cardiomyopathy may be con-sidered (Brown and Bertolet, 1998; Hibbard and associ-

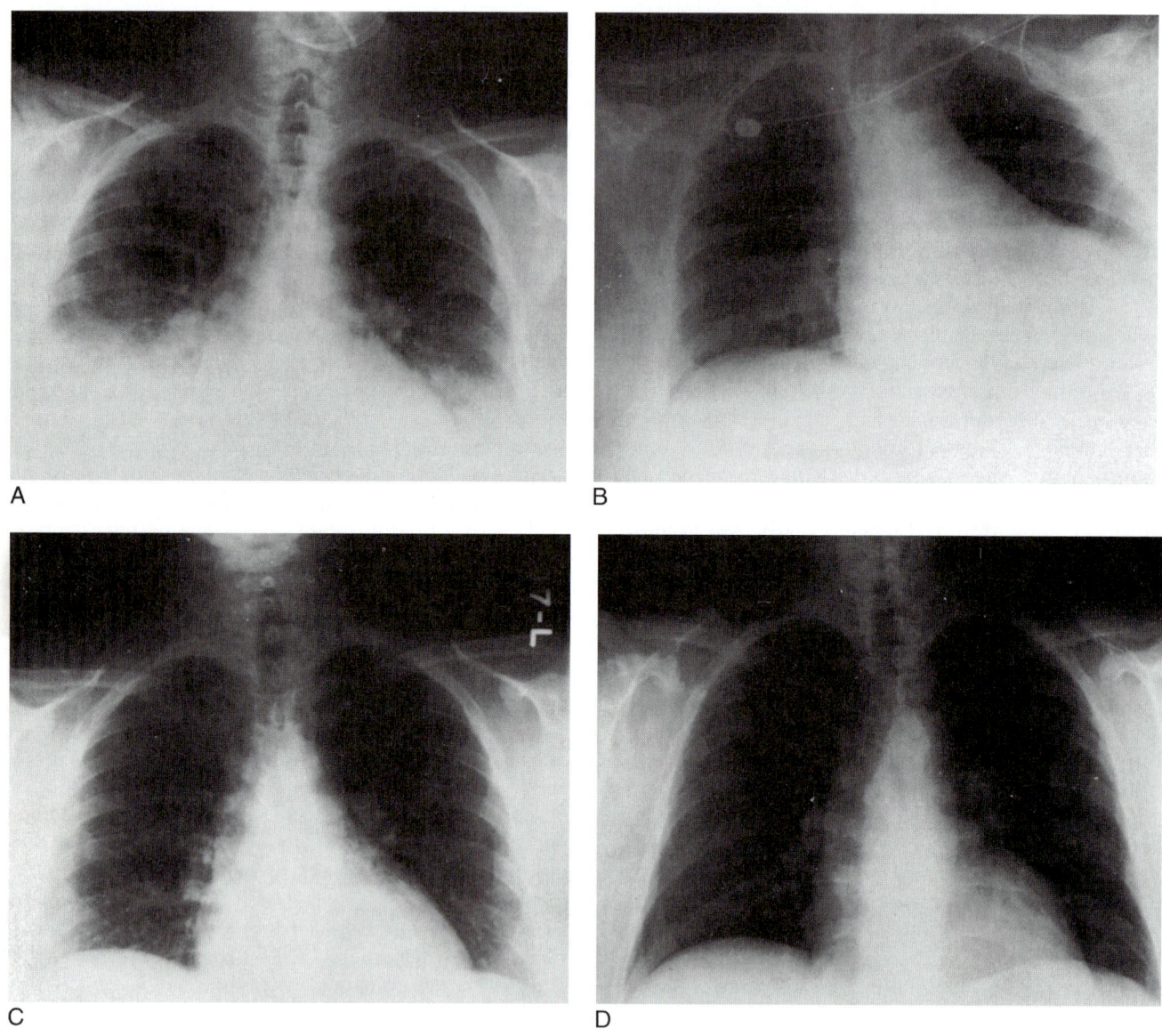

FIGURE 44–4. An obese 36-year-old Hispanic multipara with heart failure. **A.** She presented at term with severe preeclampsia, cardiomegaly, and pulmonary edema. **B.** One day later, pulmonary edema resolved but cardiomegaly persisted. Cardiomegaly improved in 2 days **(C)**, and almost completely resolved in 3 days **(D)**. (From Cunningham and associates, 1986, with permission.)

ates, 1999). We identified this in about 1 in 15,000 deliveries and this incidence is not different from that of idiopathic cardiomyopathy in young nonpregnant women (Cunningham and colleagues, 1986). Lampert (1993) and Mabie (1993) and their associates have implicated prolonged **β-mimetic tocolysis** with terbutaline as provoking cardiomyopathy. As previously discussed, clinically undetected **myocarditis** is found in up to half of these women if biopsy is done. O'Connell and colleagues (1986) found that a third of pregnant women with idiopathic cardiomyopathy had biopsy evidence of myocarditis compared with only 10 percent of nonpregnant patients.

Women with cardiomyopathy present with signs and symptoms of congestive heart failure. Dyspnea is universal, and other symptoms include orthopnea, cough, palpitations, and chest pain (Sheffield and Cunningham, 1999). The hallmark finding usually is impressive cardiomegaly (Fig. 44–5). Echocardiographic and Doppler studies confirm increased end-diastolic dimensions, an ejection fraction less than 45 percent, and/or fractional shortening of less than 30 percent (Hibbard and coworkers, 1999).

Therapy consists of treatment for heart failure (Brown and Bertolet, 1998). Sodium intake is limited and diuretics are given to reduce preload. Afterload

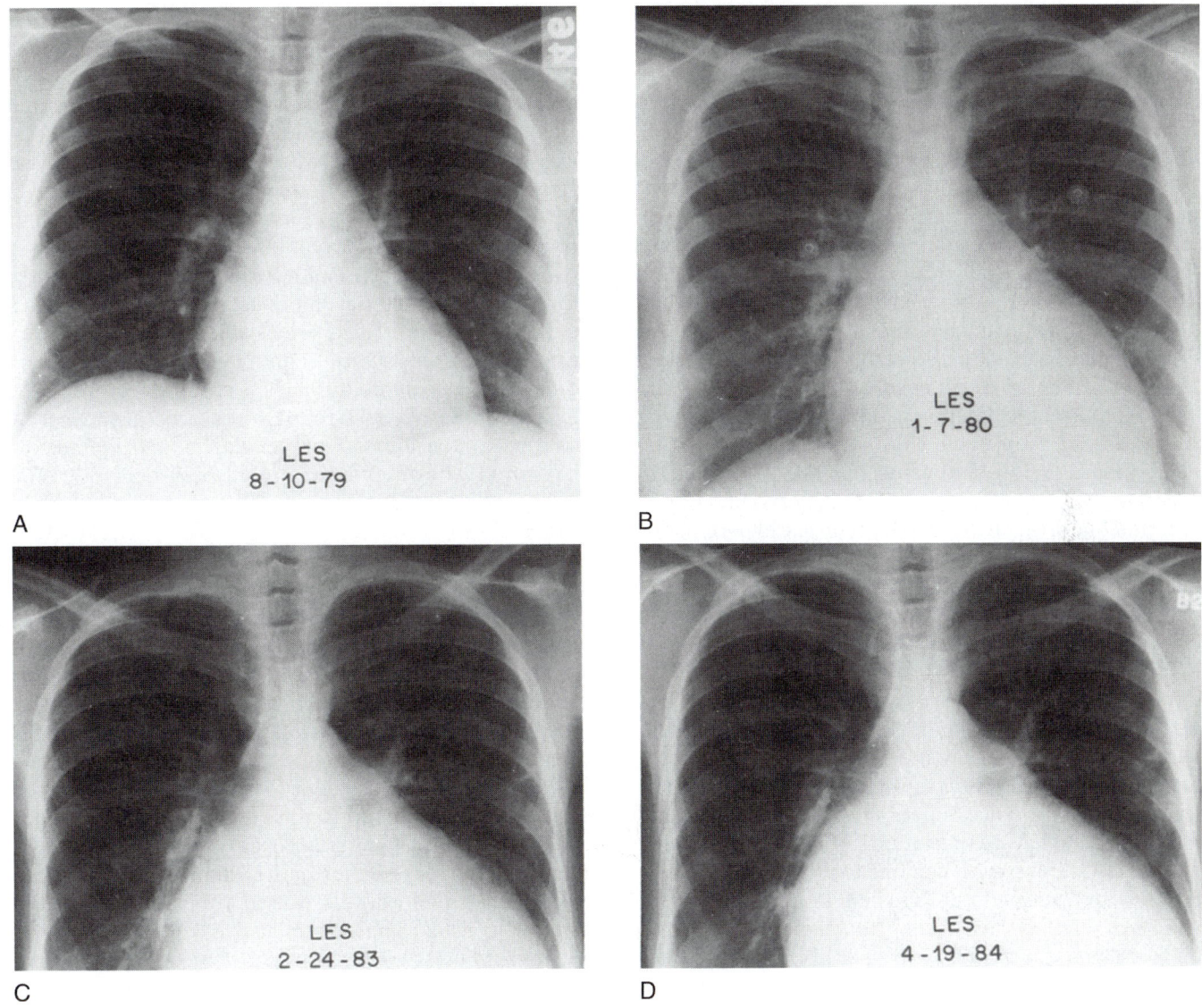

FIGURE 44–5. Idiopathic peripartum cardiomyopathy. Peripartum heart failure developed without any identifiable underlying cardiac disease. Despite an initially good symptomatic response and clearing of pulmonary edema, mild cardiomegaly persisted 3 months postpartum **(A)**. Over the ensuing 5 years **(B–D)** cardiomegaly worsened, and the woman died of end-stage heart failure at age 23. (From Cunningham and colleagues, 1986, with permission.)

reduction with hydralazine or another vasodilator is accomplished; however, angiotensin-converting enzyme inhibitors should be avoided if the woman is undelivered (Chap. 38, p. 1014). Digoxin is given for its inotropic effects unless complex arrhythmias are identified. Because there is a high incidence of associated pulmonary embolism, "low-dose" heparin is often recommended. Carlson and co-workers (2000) described a woman who presented postpartum with a lower-extremity arterial thromboembolism.

PROGNOSIS. The distinction between peripartum heart failure from an identifiable cause versus idiopathic cardiomyopathy is important. This distinction is somewhat artificial because, if biopsy is done, recall that at least half of women with peripartum cardiomyopathy will be found to have histological myocarditis. As shown in Figure 45–6, the 5- and 10-year survival rates are substantially lower with idiopathic disease. Ford and co-workers (2000) found better prognoses in women with idiopathic disease not complicated by underlying disease. According to Lampert and associates (1997), half of all women with peripartum cardiomyopathy regain left-ventricular function within 6 months, and they have a good prognosis. Conversely, the other half have high morbidity and mortality rates. Even women who regain normal ventricular function may have evidence for underlying pathology when dobutamine challenge testing is done (Lampert and colleagues, 1993).

It is important to determine the severity of underlying heart disease in women with new-onset peripartum heart failure. Witlin and associates (1997) studied 28 such women without an antecedent history of heart disease and found that two thirds had chronic hypertension. Their outcomes were dismal: five died, three underwent heart transplantation, and 18 had continued cardiac impairment. From their review, Heider and co-workers (1999) also concluded that the long-term prognosis is poor.

SUBSEQUENT PREGNANCY. Women with persistent ventricular dysfunction do not tolerate subsequent pregnancy very well. Even those with recovered ventricular function may have deterioration when pregnant again. Already discussed are the findings of Lampert and associates (1993, 1997) who demonstrated ventricular dysfunction to occur with dobutamine infusion in women with recovered normal resting function. Albanesi and da Silva (1999) described a propensity for ventricular dysfunction in 3 of 12 women in subsequent pregnancy.

INFECTIVE ENDOCARDITIS. This infection involves cardiac endothelium and produces vegetations that usually deposit on a valve. Infective endocarditis can involve a native or a prosthetic valve, or it may be associ-

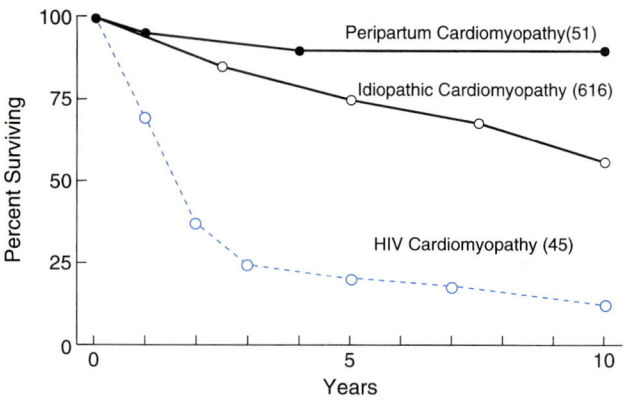

FIGURE 44–6. Survival according to underlying cause of cardiomyopathy. (Data from Felker and colleagues, 2000.)

ated with intravenous drug abuse. Children and adults who survive corrective surgery for congenital heart disease are at greatest risk (Morris and co-workers, 1998). About 75 percent of adults have a known preexisting heart lesion. The relative risks of endocarditis with some lesions are listed in Table 44–7.

Subacute bacterial endocarditis usually is due to a low-virulence bacterial infection superimposed on an underlying lesion. These are usually native valve infections. Organisms that cause indolent bacterial endocarditis are most commonly viridans group streptococci, or *Enterococcus* species. Group B streptococcal endocarditis can be subacute or acute. Gallagher and Watanakunakorn (1986) observed that almost 10 percent of the latter cases reported since 1962 were in pregnant women.

Acute endocarditis is usually caused by coagulase-positive staphylococci. *S. aureus* is the predominant organism in a third of native valve infections, and it causes half of those in intravenous drug abusers (Kaye, 1998). In those not associated with drug use, the left side is involved in 80 percent of cases, and mortality is nearly 50 percent (Røder and colleagues, 1999). *S. epidermis* commonly causes prosthetic valve infections. *Streptococcus pneumoniae* and *Neisseria gonorrheae* may cause acute, fulminating disease. Bataskov and colleagues (1991) described fatal gonococcal endocarditis complicating pregnancy. Deger and Ludmir (1992) reported antepartum endocarditis caused by *N. sicca,* and we have had a maternal death due to endocarditis from *N. mucosa* (Cox and associates, 1988). Although group B streptococcal infections are common in pregnant women and newborns, very few cases of endocarditis have been described (Kangavari and co-workers, 2000).

Symptoms of endocarditis are variable and often develop insidiously. Fever is virtually universal, and a murmur is heard in over 85 percent of cases (Kaye, 1998).

Anorexia, fatigue, and other constitutional symptoms are common, and the illness is frequently described as "flu-like." Other findings are anemia, proteinuria, and manifestations of embolic lesions, including petechiae, focal neurological manifestations, chest or abdominal pain, and ischemia in an extremity. In some cases, heart failure develops. In the usual case, symptoms usually persist for several weeks before the diagnosis is made. Thus, a high index of suspicion is necessary to consider endocarditis. Diagnosis is confirmed by excluding other causes of febrile illnesses and recovering positive blood cultures for typical organisms. Echocardiography and two-dimensional sector scanning are useful, but lesions only 3 to 4 mm in size or those on the tricuspid valve may be missed. **A negative echocardiographic study does not exclude endocarditis.**

Treatment is primarily medical with appropriate timing of surgical intervention if this becomes necessary. Knowledge of the infecting organism is imperative for sensible antimicrobial selection. Most viridans streptococci are sensitive to penicillin G given intravenously along with gentamicin for 2 weeks (Kaye, 1998). Complicated infections are treated longer, and women allergic to penicillin are either desensitized or given intravenous ceftriaxone or vancomycin for 4 weeks. Staphylococci, enterococci, and other organisms are treated according to microbial sensitivity for 4 to 6 weeks. Prosthetic valve infections are treated for 6 to 8 weeks. Persistent native valve infection may require replacement, and this is even more commonly indicated with an infected prosthetic valve.

ENDOCARDITIS IN PREGNANCY. Infective endocarditis is uncommon during pregnancy and the puerperium. Over a 7-year period, the incidence of endocarditis at Parkland Hospital was about 1 in 16,000 deliveries (Cox and associates, 1988). Two of seven women died. Treatment is the same as that described earlier. From their review, Seaworth and Durack (1986) and Cox and Leveno (1989) cited maternal mortality of about 25 to 35 percent.

ANTIMICROBIAL PROPHYLAXIS. The efficacy of antimicrobial prophylaxis to prevent bacterial endocarditis is questionable. Only 13 percent of cases arising in patients with high-risk cardiac lesions do so after a procedure (van der Meer and associates, 1992). The American Heart Association recommends prophylaxis based on risk stratification, and its 1997 recommended regimens are shown in Table 44–8.

OBSTETRICAL PROCEDURES. The 1997 guidelines include a long list of invasive procedures for which prophylaxis is recommended. Importantly, most dental procedures are included. Cesarean delivery constitutes an indication, but prophylaxis is optional with vaginal delivery. The incidence of transient bacteremia at delivery is about 5 to 10 percent (Boggess and colleagues, 1996). Although there is meager evidence that a significant number of cases of bacterial endocarditis have been prevented with antimicrobial prophylaxis given for uncomplicated delivery, its risk and costs are not great (McFaul and associates, 1988; Seaworth and Durack, 1986). Individualization seems appropriate. For example, with premature or prolonged membrane rupture, manual placental removal, or fourth-degree perineal lacerations in women with high- or moderate-risk lesions, prophylaxis is reasonable.

In the current guidelines shown in Table 44–8, prophylaxis for high-risk patients includes an initial dose

TABLE 44–7. Estimates of Relative Risks for Infective Endocarditis with Various Types of Cardic Lesions

High Risk	Moderate Risk	Not Recommended
Prosthetic heart valves	Most other congenital malformations not in high- or low-risk categories	Atrial septal defect
Previous endocarditis		Surgically corrected lesions without prosthesis (ASD, VSD, PDA)
Complex congenital cyanotic heart disease	Acquired valvar dysfunction, e.g., rheumatic heart disease	Coronary artery disease with previous bypass surgery
Surgically constructed systemic pulmonary shunts	Hypertrophic cardiomyopathy	Mitral-valve prolapse without regurgitation
	Mitral-valve prolapse with valvar regurgitation and/or thickened leaflets	Physiological murmurs
		Previous rheumatic fever without valvar dysfunction
		Pacemakers

ASD = atrial septal defect; PDA = patent ductus arteriosus; VSD = ventricular septal defect.
From Dajani and colleagues (1997), with permission.

TABLE 44–8. **1997 American Heart Association Guidelines for Bacterial Endocarditis Prophylaxis for Genitourinary and Gastrointestinal Procedures**

High-risk patients[a]—ampicillin plus gentamicin:

Intravenous or intramuscular ampicillin, 2 g, plus gentamicin, 1.5 mg/kg (not to exceed 120 mg), within 30 min before the procedure, then ampicillin 1 g, intramuscularly or intravenously, or amoxicillin, 1 g orally, 6 hours after the initial dose.

Penicillin-allergic patients—vancomycin and gentamicin:

Intravenous vancomycin, 1 g over 1–2 h, plus intravenous or intramuscular gentamicin, 1.5 mg/kg (not to exceed 120 mg); infusion to be completed within 30 min before the procedure.

Moderate-risk patients[a,b]—amoxicillin or ampicillin:

Oral amoxicillin, 2 g orally, 1 h before the procedure, or ampicillin, 2 g either intravenously or intramuscularly within 30 min of beginning the procedure.

[a]High- and moderate-risk lesions are listed in Table 44–7.
[b]Recommended regimen for dental procedures.
From Danjani and colleagues (1997), with permission.

of antimicrobial(s) to be completed within 30 minutes before the procedure is begun. Another dose is given 6 hours later. Obviously, accurate prediction of delivery time is problematic to timely administration of the first dose.

ARRHYTHMIAS. Cardiac arrhythmias are commonly encountered during pregnancy, labor and delivery, and the puerperium. It is debated whether arrhythmias are more common during pregnancy, but in our experiences, their detection is probably increased because of more frequent visits during prenatal care. Perhaps the normal but mild hypokalemia of pregnancy induces arrhythmias (Chap. 8, p. 177). Most arrhythmias in young women are not associated with organic heart disease, and most often their treatment is not different from that for nonpregnant patients.

Bradyarrhythmias, including complete heart block, are compatible with a successful pregnancy outcome. Some women with complete heart block will have syncope during labor and delivery and occasionally temporary cardiac pacing is necessary. Women with permanent artificial pacemakers usually tolerate pregnancy well (Jaffe and associates, 1987). With fixed-rate devices, cardiac output apparently is increased by augmented stroke volume.

Tachyarrhythmias are relatively common. Whenever these arrhythmias are encountered, underlying cardiac disease should be considered. *Wolff–Parkinson–White*

syndrome may first appear during pregnancy, but some women with previously diagnosed arrhythmias have an increased incidence of tachycardia during pregnancy (Widerhorn and co-workers, 1992). **Paroxysmal supraventricular tachycardia** is encountered most frequently. Siu and associates (1997) followed 25 women who had supraventricular tachycardia diagnosed before pregnancy. Half of these women had Wolff–Parkinson–White syndrome. Six of 13 women without Wolff–Parkinson–White Syndrome and 3 of 12 with the condition had supraventricular tachycardia during pregnancy. If vagal maneuvers do not stimulate conversion, treatment consists of digoxin, adenosine, or calcium-channel blocking drugs. Experience is accruing that adenosine is effective for cardioversion in hemodynamically stable pregnant women (Chakhtoura and co-workers, 1998). Although these drugs cross the placenta, they do not appear to harm the fetus. Dunn and Brost (2000), however, reported fetal bradycardia in response to adenosine given intravenously for maternal supraventricular tachycardia. Electrical cardioversion also is not contraindicated in pregnancy.

Ventricular tachycardia is uncommon in healthy young women without underlying heart disease. Brodsky and associates (1992) described seven pregnant women with new-onset ventricular tachycardia and reviewed 23 previously published reports. Most of these women were not found to have structural heart disease, and in 60 percent, arrhythmias were stimulated by physical exercise or psychological stress. Of those remaining, two had myocardial infarction, two had a prolonged QT interval, and anesthesia provoked tachycardia in another. In 6 of 26, no precipitating event was found. The investigators concluded that pregnancy events probably precipitated tachycardia and recommended β-blocker therapy for control.

Atrial flutter or fibrillation are more likely associated with underlying disease, such as thyrotoxicosis. Major complications include stroke (Ezekowitz and Levine, 1999). Thus, heparin is recommended by some authors if fibrillation is chronic, was identified before pregnancy, and persists during pregnancy. If atrial fibrillation is associated with mitral stenosis, pulmonary edema may develop in late pregnancy if the ventricular rate is increased. Digitalis is given to diminish ventricular response, and quinidine may prevent its recurrence.

DISEASES OF THE AORTA. Marfan syndrome and co-arctation of the aorta are two aortic diseases that place the pregnant woman at increased risk for **aortic dissection.** Other risk factors are bicuspid aortic valve and Turner or Noonan syndrome. Pepin and colleagues (2000) reported a high rate of aortic dissection or rupture in patients with *Ehlers–Danlos syndrome* (Chap. 52, p. 1399). Although the mechanism(s) involved are unclear, the initiating event in aortic dissection is an aortic intimal tear, and following medial hemorrhage, rupture may occur. It is taught that half of all aortic dissections in women under age 40 develop during late pregnancy (Simpson and D'Alton, 1997). Oskoui and Lindsay (1994), however, disputed this. They reviewed 196 consecutive aortic dissections and found nine in women less than 40, and none were pregnant. Easterling and colleagues (1991) found that aortic diameter increased significantly in normal women over the course of pregnancy. This increase was even greater for women who developed preeclampsia.

In most cases, women with aortic dissection present with severe chest pain described as ripping, tearing, or stabbing in nature. Diminution or loss of peripheral pulses in conjunction with a recently acquired murmur of aortic insufficiency are important physical findings. The differential diagnosis of aortic dissection includes myocardial infarction, pulmonary embolism, pneumothorax, and aortic valve rupture. Lang and Borow (1991) rightfully add obstetrical catastrophes to the list, especially placental abruption and uterine rupture.

Over 90 percent of patients have an abnormal chest x-ray. Although aortic angiography is the most definitive method for confirming the diagnosis, noninvasive imaging with sonography, computed tomography, and magnetic resonance imaging are being used more frequently. The urgency of the clinical situation frequently will dictate which procedure is best. Initial medical treatment is given to lower blood pressure. Proximal dissections most often need to be resected, along with aortic valve replacement if indicated. Distal dissections are more complex, and many may be treated medically.

MARFAN SYNDROME. This syndrome is usually inherited as an autosomal dominant trait with a high degree of penetrance. It is caused by an abnormal *fibrillin* produced by a mutation in the FBN1 gene located on chromosome 15q21. Fibrillin is a constituent of elastin, and thus this is a systemic connective-tissue disorder which is characterized by generalized weakness that can result in dangerous cardiovascular complications. Because all tissues are involved, other defects are frequent and include joint laxity and scoliosis. Progressive aortic dilatation causes aortic valve insufficiency, and there may be infective endocarditis, and mitral-valve prolapse with insufficiency. Aortic dilatation and dissecting aneurysm are the most serious abnormalities. Early death is due either to valvar insufficiency and heart failure or to a dissecting aneurysm. Long-term benefits from β-blocker therapy have been described for nonpregnant adults (Shores and colleagues, 1994).

EFFECT OF PREGNANCY. Deaths due to dissecting aortic aneurysm during pregnancy are frequent in women with Marfan syndrome. The previous grave concerns of the effects of pregnancy seem to have been overestimated. For example, from their review of published cases, Elkayam and associates (1995) found that 20 of 32 women had aortic dissection or rupture and 16 of these died. In a prospective longitudinal evaluation of 21 women during 45 pregnancies from the Johns Hopkins Hospital, only two had dissection and one died postpartum from graft infection (Rossiter and colleagues, 1995). They concluded that aortic dilatation more than 40 mm in diameter or mitral-valve dysfunction are high-risk factors for life-threatening cardiovascular complications during pregnancy. Conversely, women with minimal or no dilatation, and those with normal cardiac function by echocardiography, are counseled regarding the small but serious potential risk of aortic dissection.

Elkayam and colleagues (1995) also concluded that pregnancy was safer in women with Marfan syndrome who had no cardiovascular manifestations or aortic arch dilatation. They recommended β-blocker prophylactic therapy during pregnancy. The aortic root usually measures about 20 mm, and if dilatation reaches 40 mm, then dissection is more likely (Simpson and D'Alton, 1997). If it reaches 50 to 60 mm, then elective surgery should be considered before pregnancy (Gott and collaborators, 1999; Prêtre and Von Segesser, 1997). Aortic root replacement during pregnancy has been associated with hypoxic–ischemic cerebral damage in a 29-week fetus (Mul and co-workers, 1998). While Marfan syndrome itself is not an indication, they recommended cesarean delivery if there is aortic involvement. Otherwise, obstetrical indications for delivery are followed.

The condition is autosomally dominant and thus half of offspring are affected. Prenatal diagnosis is usually possible using linkage analysis (Chap. 36).

AORTIC COARCTATION. This is a relatively rare lesion often accompanied by lesions of other large arteries. For example, a bicuspid aortic valve is seen with echocardiography in a fourth of affected patients, and another 10 percent have cerebral artery aneurysms. Other associated lesions are persistent ductus arteriosus, septal defects, and Turner syndrome. The collateral circulation arising above the level of the coarctation expands, often to a striking extent, to cause localized erosion of rib margins by hypertrophied intercostal arteries. Typical findings on physical examination are hypertension in the upper extremities but normal or reduced blood pressures in the lower extremities. Dizon-Townson and colleagues (1995) described diagnosis during pregnancy using magnetic resonance imaging.

EFFECTS ON PREGNANCY. The major complications of coarctation are congestive heart failure after longstanding severe hypertension, bacterial endocarditis of the **bicuspid aortic valve,** and aortic rupture. Maternal mortality rates average about 3 percent (McAnulty and co-workers, 1990). Because hypertension may worsen in pregnancy, antihypertensive therapy using β-blocking drugs is usually required. Aortic rupture is more likely to occur late in pregnancy or early in the puerperium. Rupture may be associated with changes in the media that are histologically similar to those of Erdheim idiopathic medial cystic necrosis. Cerebral hemorrhage from **circle of Willis aneurysms** may also develop.

Congestive heart failure demands vigorous efforts to improve cardiac function and may warrant pregnancy interruption. Some authors have recommended that resection of the coarctation be undertaken during pregnancy to protect against the possibility of a dissecting aneurysm and aortic rupture. This has significant risks, especially for the fetus, because all the collaterals must be clamped for variable periods of time.

Some authors recommend cesarean delivery to prevent transient arterial blood pressure elevations that commonly accompany labor. It is feared that such blood pressure increases might lead to rupture of either the aorta or coexisting cerebral aneurysms. Available evidence, however, suggests that cesarean delivery should be limited to obstetrical indications. Bacterial endocarditis prophylaxis is given at delivery. About 2 percent of infants born to an affected patient will have the lesion.

ISCHEMIC HEART DISEASE. Coronary artery disease, which may lead to **myocardial infarction,** is a rare complication of pregnancy. While Mendelson and Lang (1995) cite the collective incidence of myocardial infarction complicating pregnancy to be 1 in 10,000, it probably is much lower than this. Frequently, women with coronary artery disease have classical risk factors such as cigarette smoking, familial hyperlipidemia, obesity, or hypertension. Bagg and colleagues (1999) reviewed 22 diabetic pregnant women with ischemic heart disease or class H diabetes (Chap. 51, p. 1361). They as well as Reece and associates (1986) and Pombar and colleagues (1995) documented unusually high mortality in pregnant diabetics who suffered myocardial infarction. Sutaria and collaborators (2000) and Mousa and associates (2000) each documented coronary artery occlusion in two pregnant smokers with hypercholesterolemia following a routine 500-mg ergometrine intramuscular injection. Schulte-Sasse (2000) described myocardial ischemia with prostaglandin E_1 vaginal suppositories. Thorp and colleagues (1994) described a 22-year-old woman with antiphospholipid antibodies who suffered a myocardial infarction 10 days postpartum.

Diagnosis during pregnancy is not different than in the nonpregnant patient. Measurement of serum levels of the cardiac-specific contractile protein, *troponin I,* is accurate for diagnosis. Shivvers and colleagues (1999) showed that troponin was undetectable across normal pregnancy.

PREGNANCY WITH PRIOR MYOCARDIAL DISEASE. The advisability of pregnancy after a myocardial infarction is unclear. Ischemic heart disease is characteristically progressive, and because it is usually associated with hypertension or diabetes, pregnancy seems inadvisable. Certainly, pregnancy increases cardiac workload; therefore, symptoms as well as adequacy of ventricular function prior to conception will determine outcome.

Vinatier and associates (1994) reviewed the 30 reported cases of pregnancy in women who had sustained an *infarction remote from pregnancy.* Although none of these women died, four had congestive heart failure and four had worsening angina during pregnancy. Pombar and co-workers (1995) reviewed outcomes of women with diabetes-associated ischemic heart disease and infarction. Three had undergone coronary artery bypass grafting before pregnancy. Of 17 women, eight died during pregnancy. All of these investigators concluded that ventricular performance should be assessed prior to conception using ventriculography, radionuclide studies, echocardiography, and coronary angiography. If there is no significant ventricular dysfunction, pregnancy will likely be tolerated. For the woman who becomes pregnant before these studies are performed, echocardiography should be done. Exercise tolerance testing may be indicated, and radionuclide ventriculography results in very little radiation exposure for the fetus (Chap. 42, p. 1153).

MYOCARDIAL INFARCTION DURING PREGNANCY. Treatment is similar to that of nonpregnant patients. Hankins and co-workers (1985) reviewed pregnancy outcomes in 68 cases and reported an overall maternal mortality rate of 30 to 35 percent. Hands and colleagues (1990) found an overall mortality of 30 percent. Of 50 women who sustained infarction in the third trimester, 40 percent died, compared with only 20 percent of the other 35 women who had an infarction earlier in pregnancy. Women who sustain an infarction less than 2 weeks prior to labor are at especially high risk of death (Esplin and Clark, 1999).

Acute management is similar to that in nonpregnant patients. Nitroglycerin and morphine are given with close blood pressure monitoring (Esplin and Clark, 1999). Lidocaine is given to suppress malignant arrhythmias. Calcium-channel or β-blockers are given if indicated. *Tissue plasminogen activator* has been used in pregnant women remote from delivery (Schumacher and associates, 1997). If the infarct has healed sufficiently, cesarean delivery is reserved for obstetrical indications, and most authors recommend epidural analgesia to reduce pain during labor (Esplin and Clark, 1999). Epidural analgesia or general anesthesia may be used for cesarean delivery. Thornhill and Camann (1994) recommend pulmonary artery catheter monitoring with an infarction within 6 months or when there is ventricular dysfunction. Others, including us, recommend such monitoring only if there is cardiac dysfunction.

In some women, invasive or surgical procedures may be indicated because of unrelenting disease. Hands and associates (1990) reported successful use of percutaneous transluminal coronary angioplasty in a 36-week pregnant woman. Sanchez-Ramos and co-workers (1994) and Craig and Ilton (1999) described percutaneous balloon angioplasty and transluminal intracoronary stenting. Garry and colleagues (1996) used an intra-aortic balloon pump in a woman who sustained an infarction at 25 weeks. They then performed bypass grafting at 32 weeks.

HYPERTROPHIC CARDIOMYOPATHY. Although concentric left-ventricular hypertrophy commonly develops after long-standing hypertension, there is a familial as well as a sporadic form not related to hypertension termed **idiopathic hypertrophic subaortic stenosis.** It is commonly associated with pheochromocytoma, Friedreich ataxia, Turner syndrome, and neurofibromatosis. In the half of cases that are inherited, about 50 percent are autosomally dominant disorders (Baughman, 1992). The abnormality is in the myocardial muscle, and it is characterized by idiopathic left-ventricular myocardial hypertrophy that may provide a pressure gradient to left-ventricular outflow (Lang and Borow, 1991). Diagnosis is confirmed by Doppler echocardiography.

The majority of affected women are asymptomatic, but dyspnea, anginal or atypical chest pain, syncope, and arrhythmias may develop. Complex arrhythmias may progress to sudden death, which is the most common form of death. Asymptomatic patients with runs of ventricular tachycardia are especially prone to sudden death. Symptoms are usually worsened by exercise.

MANAGEMENT IN PREGNANCY. Although limited reports suggest that pregnancy is well tolerated, congestive heart failure may develop. Benitez (1996) reviewed 109 pregnancies in 52 women with hypertrophic cardiomyopathy. Worsening of symptoms, including heart failure, angina, or arrhythmias developed in 40 percent, and two women died. Strenuous exercise is prohibited during pregnancy. Abrupt positional changes are avoided to prevent reflex vasodilation and decreased preload. Likewise, drugs that evoke diuresis or diminish vascular resistance are not used. If symptoms develop, especially angina, β-adrenergic or calcium-channel blocking drugs are given. The route of delivery is determined by obstetrical indications. Spinal analgesia is contraindicated, and even carefully administered epidural analgesia is controversial (Thornhill and Camann, 1994). Endocarditis prophylaxis is given at delivery. Infants rarely demonstrate inherited lesions at the time of birth.

REFERENCES

Albanesi FM, da Silva TT: Natural course of subsequent pregnancy after peripartum cardiomyopathy. Arq Bras Cardiol 73:47, 1999

Al Kasab SM, Sabag T, Al Zaibag M, Awaad M, Al Bitar I, Halim MA, Abdullah MA, Shahed M, Rajendran V, Sawyer W: Beta-adrenergic receptor blockade in the management of pregnant women with mitral stenosis. Am J Obstet Gynecol 163:37, 1990

American College of Obstetricians and Gynecologists: Cardiac disease in pregnancy. Technical Bulletin No. 168, June 1992a

American College of Obstetricians and Gynecologists: Invasive hemodynamic monitoring in obstetrics and gynecology. Technical Bulletin No. 175, December 1992b

American College of Obstetricians and Gynecologists: The use of hormonal contraception in women with coexisting medical conditions. Practice Bulletin No. 18, July 2000

Angel JL, Chapman C, Knuppel RA, Morales WJ, Sims CJ: Percutaneous balloon aortic valvuloplasty in pregnancy. Obstet Gynecol 72:438, 1988

Badalian SS, Silverman RK, Aubry RH, Longo J: Twin pregnancy in a woman on long-term epoprostenol therapy for primary pulmonary hypertension. J Repro Med 45:149, 2000

Bagg W, Henley PG, Macpherson P, Cundy TF: Pregnancy in women with diabetes and ischemic heart disease. Aust N Z J Obstet Gynaecol 39:99, 1999

Barbaro G, di Lorenzo G, Grisorio B, Barbarini G: Incidence of dilated cardiomyopathy and detection of HIV in myocardial cells of HIV-positive patients. N Engl J Med 339:1093, 1998

Bataskov KL, Hariharan S, Horowitz MD, Neibart RM, Cox MM: Gonococcal endocarditis complicating pregnancy: A case report and literature review. Obstet Gynecol 78:494, 1991

Baughman KL: Hypertrophic cardiomyopathy. JAMA 267:846, 1992

Benitez RM: Hypertrophic cardiomyopathy and pregnancy: Maternal and fetal outcomes. J Matern Fetal Invest 6:51, 1996

Birincioglu CL, Kucuker SA, Yapar EG, Yildiz U, Ulus AT, Yamak B, Katircioglu SF, Tasdemir O: Perinatal mitral valve interventions: A report of 10 cases. Ann Thorac Surg 67:1312, 1999

Bitsch M, Johansen C, Wennevold A, Osler M: Maternal heart disease: A survey of a decade in a Danish university hospital. Acta Obstet Gynecol Scand 68:119, 1989

Boggess KA, Easterling TR, Raghu G: Management and outcome of pregnant women with interstitial and restrictive lung disease. Am J Obstet Gynecol 173:1007, 1995

Boggess KA, Watts H, Hillier SL, Krohn MA, Benedetti TJ, Eschenback DA: Bacteremia shortly after placental separation during cesarean delivery. Obstet Gynecol 87:779, 1996

Brady K, Duff P: Rheumatic heart disease in pregnancy. Clin Obstet Gynecol 32:21, 1989

Branch KR, Wagoner LE, McGrory CH, Mannion JD, Radomski JS, Mortiz MH, Ohler L, Armenti VT: Risks of subsequent pregnancies on mother and newborn in female heart transplant recipients. J Heart Lung Transplant 17:698, 1998

Brickner ME, Hillis LD, Lange RA: Congenital heart disease in adults. First of two parts. N Engl J Med 342:256, 2000

Brodsky M, Doria R, Allen B, Sato D, Thomas G, Sada M: New-onset ventricular tachycardia during pregnancy. Am Heart J 123:933, 1992

Brown CS, Bertolet BD: Peripartum cardiomyopathy: A comprehensive review. Am J Obstet Gynecol 178:409, 1998

Capeless EL, Clapp JF: Cardiovascular changes in early phase of pregnancy. Am J Obstet Gynecol 161:1449, 1989

Carabello BA, Crawford FA: Valvular heart disease. N Engl J Med 337:32, 1997

Carlson KM, Browning JE, Eggleston MK, Gherman RB: Peripartum cardiomyopathy presenting as lower extremity arterial thromboembolism. J Reprod Med 45:351, 2000

Carruth JE, Mivis SB, Brogan DR, Wenger NK: The electrocardiogram in normal pregnancy. Chest 102:1075, 1981

Caulin-Glaser T, Setaro JF: Pregnancy and cardiovascular disease. In Burrow GN, Duffy TP (eds): Medical Complications During Pregnancy, 5th ed. Philadelphia, Saunders, 1999, p 111

Chakhtoura N, Angioli R, Yasin S: Use of adenosine for pharmacological cardioversion of SVT in pregnancy. Prim Care Update Ob/Gyns 5:154, 1998

Chan WS, Anand S, Ginsberg JS: Anticoagulation of pregnant women with mechanical heart valves: A systematic review of the literature. Arch Intern Med 160:191, 2000

Chia YT, Yeoh SC, Lim MCL, Viegas OA, Ratnam SS: Pregnancy outcome and mitral valve prolapse. Asia-Oceania J Obstet Gynaecol 20:383, 1994

Clark SL, Cotton DB, Hankins GDV, Phelan JP: Cardiac disease. In: Critical Care Obstetrics, 3rd ed. Boston, Blackwell Science, 1997, p 290

Clark SL, Cotton DB, Lee W, Bishop C, Hill T, Southwick J, Pivarnik J, Spillman T, DeVore GR, Phelan J, Hankins GDV, Benedetti TJ, Tolley D: Central hemodynamic assessment of normal term pregnancy. Am J Obstet Gynecol 161:1439, 1989

Clark SL, Phelan JP, Greenspoon J, Aldahl D, Horenstein J: Labor and delivery in the presence of mitral stenosis: Central hemodynamic observations. Am J Obstet Gynecol 152:984, 1985

Clark SL, Porter TF, West FG: Coumarin derivatives and breast-feeding. Obstet Gynecol 95:938, 2000

Connolly HM, Grogan M, Warnes CA: Pregnancy among women with congenitally corrected transposition of great arteries. J Am Coll Cardiol 33:1692, 1999

Cox SM, Hankins GDV, Leveno KJ, Cunningham FG: Bacterial endocarditis: A serious pregnancy complication. J Reprod Med 33:671, 1988

Cox SM, Leveno KJ: Pregnancy complicated by bacterial endocarditis. Clin Obstet Gynecol 32:48, 1989

Craig S, Ilton M: Treatment of acute myocardial infarction in pregnancy with coronary artery balloon angioplasty and stenting. Aust N Z J Obstet Gynaecol 39:194, 1999

Cunningham FG, Pritchard JA, Hankins GDV, Anderson PL, Lucas MK, Armstrong KF: Idiopathic cardiomyopathy or compounding cardiovascular events. Obstet Gynecol 67:157, 1986

Dajani AS, Taubert KA, Wilson W, Bolger AF, Bayer A,

Ferrieri P, Gewitz MH, Shulman ST, Nouri S, Newburger JW, Hutto C, Pallasch TJ, Gage TW, Levison ME, Peter G, Zuccaro G Jr: Prevention of bacterial endocarditis. Recommendations of the American Heart Association. JAMA 277:1794, 1997

Dashe JS, Ramin KD, Ramin SM: Pregnancy following cardiac transplantation. Prim Care Update Ob/Gyns 5:257, 1998

de Swiet M: Maternal mortality: Confidential enquiries into maternal deaths in the United Kingdom. Am J Obstet Gynecol 182:760, 2000

Deger R, Ludmir J: Neisseria sicca. Endocarditis complicating pregnancy. J Reprod Med 37:473, 1992

Desai DK, Adanlawo M, Naidoo DP, Moodley J, Kleinschmidt I: Mitral stenosis in pregnancy: A four-year experience at King Edward VIII Hospital, Durban South Africa. Br J Obstet Gynaecol 107:953, 2000

Deviri E, Levinsky L, Yechezkel M, Levy MJ: Pregnancy after valve replacement with porcine xenograft prothesis. Surg Gynecol Obstet 160:437, 1985

Dizon-Townson D, Magee KP, Twickler DM, Cox SM: Coarctation of the abdominal aorta in pregnancy: Diagnosis by magnetic resonance imaging. Obstet Gynecol 85:817, 1995

Dorfman SF: Maternal mortality in New York City, 1981–1983. Obstet Gynecol 76:317, 1990

Dunn JS Jr, Brost BC: Fetal bradycardia after IV adenosine for maternal PSVT. Am J Emerg Med 18:234, 2000

Easterling TR, Benedetti TJ, Schmucker BC, Carlson K, Millard SP: Maternal hemodynamics and aortic diameter in normal and hypertensive pregnancies. Obstet Gynecol 78:1073, 1991

Easterling TR, Chadwick HS, Otto CM, Benedetti TJ: Aortic stenosis in pregnancy. Obstet Gynecol 72:113, 1988

Easterling TR, Ralph DD, Schmucker BC: Pulmonary hypertension in pregnancy: Treatment with pulmonary vasodilators. Obstet Gynecol 93:494, 1999

Edenborough FP, Mackenzie WE, Stableforth DE: The outcome of 72 pregnancies in 55 women with cystic fibrosis in the United Kingdom 1977–1996. Br J Obstet Gynaecol 107:254, 2000

Elkayam U, Ostrzega E, Shotan A, Mehra A: Cardiovascular problems in pregnant women with Marfan syndrome. Ann Intern Med 123:117, 1995

Esplin S, Clark SL: Ischemic heart disease and myocardial infarction during pregnancy. Contemp OB/Gyn 44:27, 1999

Etheridge MJ, Pepperell RJ: Heart disease and pregnancy at the Royal Women's Hospital. Med J Aust 2:277, 1977

Ezekowitz, MD, Levine JA: Preventing stroke in patients with atrial fibrillation. JAMA 281:1830, 1999

Fatkin D, MacRae C, Sasaki T, Wolff MR, Porcu M, Frenneaux M, Atherton H, Vidaillet HJ, Spudich S, de Girolami U, Seidman JG, Seidman CE: Missense mutations in the rod domain of the lamin a/c gene as causes of dilated cardiomyopathy and conduction-system disease. N Engl J Med 341:1715, 1999

Feldman AM, McNamara D: Myocarditis. N Engl J Med 343:1388, 2000

Felker GM, Thompson RE, Hare JM, Hruban RH, Clemetson DE, Howard KL, Baughman KL, Kasper EK: Underlying causes and long-term survival in patients with initially unexplained cardiopathy. N Engl J Med 342:1077, 2000

Ford RF, Barton JR, O'Brien JM, Hollingsworth PW: Demographics, management, and outcome of peripartum cardiomyopathy in a community hospital. Am J Obstet Gynecol 182:1036, 2000

Freed LA, Levy D, Levine RA, Larson MG, Evans JC, Fuller

DL, Lehman B, Benjamin EJ: Prevalence and clinical outcome of mitral-valve prolapse. N Engl J Med 341:1, 1999

Gaine SP, Rubin LJ: Primary pulmonary hypertension. Lancet 352:719, 1998

Gallagher PG, Watanakunakorn C: Group B streptococcal endocarditis: Report of seven cases and review of the literature, 1962–1985. Rev Infect Dis 8:175, 1986

Gardin J, Schumacher D, Constantine G, Davis KD, Leung C, Reid CL: Valvular abnormalities and cardiovascular status following exposure to dexfenfluramine or phentermine/fenfluramine. JAMA 283:1703, 2000

Garry D, Leikin E, Fleisher AG, Tejani N: Acute myocardial infarction in pregnancy with subsequent medical and surgical management. Obstet Gynecol 87:802, 1996

Gilon D, Buonanno FS, Joffe MM, Leavitt M, Marshall JE, Kistler JP, Levine RA: Lack of evidence of an association between mitral-valve prolapse and stroke in young patients. N Engl J Med 341:8, 1999

Gleicher N, Midwall J, Hochberger D, Jaffin H: Eisenmenger's syndrome and pregnancy. Obstet Gynecol Surv 34:721, 1979

Goodwin TM, Gherman RB, Hameed A, Elkayam U: Favorable response of Eisenmenger syndrome to inhaled nitric oxide during pregnancy. Am J Obstet Gynecol 180:64, 1999

Gott VL, Greene PS, Alejo DE, Cameron DE, Naftel DC, Miller DC, Gillinov AM, Laschinger JC, Pyeritz RE: Replacement of the aortic root in patients with Marfan's syndrome. N Engl J Med 340:1307, 1999

Gupta A, Lokhandwala YY, Satoskar PR, Salvi VS: Balloon mitral valvotomy in pregnancy: Maternal and fetal outcomes. J Am Coll Surg 187:409, 1998

Hanania G, Thomas D, Michel PL, Garbarz E, Age C, Millaire A, Acar J: Pregnancy and prosthetic heart valves: A French cooperative retrospective study of 155 cases. Eur Heart J 15:1651, 1994

Hands ME, Johnson MD, Saltzman DH, Rutherford JD: The cardiac, obstetric, and anesthetic management of pregnancy complicated by acute myocardial infarction. J Clin Anesth 2:258, 1990

Hankins GD, Wendel GD Jr, Leveno KJ, Stoneham J: Myocardial infarction during pregnancy: A review. Obstet Gynecol 65:138, 1985

Heider AL, Kuller JA, Strauss RA, Wells SR: Peripartum cardiomyopathy: A review of the literature. Obstet Gynecol Surv 54:526, 1999

Hibbard JU, Lindheimer M, Lang RM: A modified definition for peripartum cardiomyopathy and prognosis based on echocardiography. Obstet Gynecol 94:311, 1999

Hosenpud JD, Novick RJ, Breen TJ, Daily OP: The registry of the International Society for Heart and Lung Transplantation: Eleventh official report—1994. J Heart Lung Transplant 13:561, 1994

Ismail MB, Abid F, Trabelsi S, Taktak M, Fekih M: Cardiac valve prostheses, anticoagulation, and pregnancy. Br Heart J 55:101, 1986

Iturbe-Alessio I, Fonseca MDC, Mutchinik O, Santos MA, Zajarias A, Salazar E: Risks of anticoagulant therapy in pregnant women with artificial heart valves. N Engl J Med 315:1390, 1986

Jackson GM, Dildy GA, Varner MW, Clark SL: Severe pulmonary hypertension in pregnancy following successful repair of ventricular septal defect in childhood. Obstet Gynecol 82:680, 1993

Jacob S, Bloebaum L, Shah G, Varner MW: Maternal mortality in Utah. Obstet Gynecol 91:187, 1998

Jaffe R, Gruber A, Fejgin M, Altaras M, Ben-Aderet N: Pregnancy with an artificial pacemaker. Obstet Gynecol Surv 42:137, 1987

Jick H: Heart valve disorders and appetite-suppressant drugs. JAMA 283:1738, 2000

Jick H, Vasilakis C, Weinrauch LA, Meier CR, Jick SS, Derby LE: A population-based study of appetite-suppressant drugs and the risk of cardiac-valve regurgitation. N Engl J Med 339:719, 1998

Kahn MA, Herzog CA, St. Peter JV, Hartley GG, Madlon-Kay R, Dick CD, Asinger RW, Vessey JT: The prevalence of cardiac valvular insufficiency assessed by transthoracic echocardiography in obese patients treated with appetite-suppressant drugs. N Engl J Med 339:713, 1998

Kangavari S, Collins J, Cercek B, Atar S, Siegel R: Tricuspid valve group B streptococcal endocarditis after an elective termination of pregnancy. Clin Cardiol 23:301, 2000

Kaye D: Infective endocarditis. In Fauci AS, Braunwald E, Isselbacher KJ, Wilson JD, Martin JB, Kasper DL, Hauser SL, Longo DL (eds): Harrison's Principles of Internal Medicine, 14th ed. New York. McGraw-Hill, 1998, p 785

Key TC, Resnik R, Kittrich HC, Reisner LS: Successful pregnancy after cardiac transplantation. Am J Obstet Gynecol 160:367, 1989

Khandelwal M, Rasanen J, Ludormirski A, Addonizio P, Reece EA: Fetal and uterine hemodynamics during and after maternal cardiopulmonary bypass (CPB). Am J Obstet Gynecol 174:460, 1996

Kim KM, Sukhani R, Slogoff S, Tomich PG: Central hemodynamic changes associated with pregnancy in a long-term cardiac transplant recipient. Am J Obstet Gynecol 174:1651, 1996

Kiss H, Egarter C, Asseryanis E, Putz D, Kneussl M: Primary pulmonary hypertension in pregnancy: A case report. Am J Obstet Gynecol 172:1052, 1995

Koonin LM, MacKay AP, Berg CJ, Atrash HK, Smith JC: Pregnancy-related mortality surveillance—United States, 1987–1990. MMWR 46:17, 1997

Lampert MB, Hibbard J, Weinert L, Briller J, Lindheimer M, Lang RM: Peripartum heart failure associated with prolonged tocolytic therapy. Am J Obstet Gynecol 168:493, 1993

Lampert MB, Weinert L, Hibbard J, Korcarz C, Lindheimer M, Lang RM: Contractile reserve in patients with peripartum cardiomyopathy and recovered left ventricular function. Am J Obstet Gynecol 176:189, 1997

Lang RM, Borow KM: Heart disease. In Barron WM, Lindheimer MD (eds): Medical Disorders During Pregnancy. St. Louis, Mosby Yearbook, 1991, p 148

Lange RA: Eisenmenger syndrome in adults. Internal Medicine Grand Rounds. University of Texas Southwestern Medical Center at Dallas. May 6, 1999, p 21

Lao TT, Adelman AG, Sermer M, Colman JM: Balloon valvuloplasty for congenital aortic stenosis in pregnancy. Br J Obstet Gynaecol 100:1141, 1993a

Lao TT, Sermer M, Colman JM: Pregnancy following surgical correction for transposition of the great arteries. Obstet Gynecol 83:655, 1994

Lao TT, Sermer M, MaGee L, Farine D, Colman JM: Congenital aortic stenosis and pregnancy—a reappraisal. Am J Obstet Gynecol 169:540, 1993b

Lauer MS, Anderson KM, Kannel WB, Levy D: The impact of obesity of left ventricular mass and geometry: The Framingham Heart Study. JAMA 266:231, 1991

Lee CN, Wu CC, Lin PY, Hsieh FJ, Chen HY: Pregnancy following cardiac prosthetic valve replacement. Obstet Gynecol 83:353, 1994

Limacher MC, Ware JA, O'Meara ME, Fernandez GC, Young JB: Tricuspid regurgitation during pregnancy: Two-dimensional and pulsed Doppler echocardiographic observations. Am J Cardiol 55:1059, 1985

Löwenstein BR, Vain NW, Perrone SV, Wright DR, Boullón FJ, Favaloro RG: Successful pregnancy and vaginal delivery after heart transplantation. Am J Obstet Gynecol 158:589, 1988

Lynch-Salamon DI, Maze SS, Combs CA: Pregnancy after Mustard repair for transposition of the great arteries. Obstet Gynecol 82:676, 1993

Mabie WC, Hackman BB, Sibai BM: Pulmonary edema associated with pregnancy: Echocardiographic insights and implications for treatment. Obstet Gynecol 81:227, 1993

Martin JA, Smith BL, Matthews TJ, Ventura SJ: Births and deaths: Preliminary data for 1998. Natl Vital Stat Rep 47:1, 1999

McAnulty JH, Metcalfe J, Ueland K: Heart disease and pregnancy. In Hurst JW, Schlant RC, Rackley CE, Sonnenblick EH, Wenger NK (eds): The Heart, 7th ed. New York, McGraw-Hill, 1990, p 1465

McFaul PB, Dornan JC, Lamki H, Boyle D: Pregnancy complicated by maternal heart disease. A review of 519 women. Br J Obstet Gynaecol 95:861, 1988

McLaughlin VV, Genthner DE, Panella MM, Rich S: Reduction in pulmonary vascular resistance with long-term epoprostenol (prostacyclin) therapy in primary pulmonary hypertension. N Engl J Med 338:273, 1998

McLaughlin MK, Roberts JM: Hemodynamic changes. In Lindheimer MD, Roberts JM, Cunningham FG (eds): Chesley's Hypertensive Disorders in Pregnancy, 2nd ed. Stamford, CT, Appleton & Lange, 1999

Megerian G, Bell JG, Huhta JC, Bottalico JN, Weiner S: Pregnancy outcome following a Mustard procedure for transposition of the great arteries: A report of five cases and review of the literature. Obstet Gynecol 83:512, 1994

Mendelson MA, Lang RM: Pregnancy and Heart Disease. In Barron WM, Lindheimer MD (eds): Medical Disorders During Pregnancy, 2nd ed. St. Louis, Mosby Yearbook, 1995, p 129

Meyer NL, Mercer B, Khoury A, Sibai B: Pregnancy complicated by cardiac disease: Maternal and perinatal outcome. J Mat Fetal Med 3:31, 1994

Moodie DS: Adult congenital heart disease. Curr Opin Cardiol 9:137, 1994

Morris CD, Menashe VD: 25-year mortality after surgical repair of congenital heart defect in childhood. JAMA 266:3447, 1991

Morris CD, Reller MD, Menashe VD: Thirty-year incidence of infective endocarditis after surgery for congenital heart defect. JAMA 279:599, 1998

Mousa HA, McKinley CA, Thong J: Acute postpartum myocardial infarction after ergometrine administration in a woman with familial hypercholesterolaemia. Br J Obstet Gynaecol 107:939, 2000

Mul TFM, van Herwerden LA, Coohen-Overbeck TE, Catsman-Berrevoets CE, Lotgering FK: Hypoxic–ischemic fetal insult resulting from maternal aortic root replacement, with normal fetal heart rate at term. Am J Obstet Gynecol 179:825, 1998

Nagorney DM, Field CS: Successful pregnancy 10 years after triple cardiac valve replacement. Obstet Gynecol 57:386, 1981

Nishimura RA, McGoon MD: Perspectives on mitral-valve prolapse. N Engl J Med 341:48, 1999

Nishimura RA, McGoon MD, Shub C, Miller FA, Ilstrup DM, Tajik AJ: Echocardiographically documented mitral-valve prolapse: Long-term follow-up of 237 patients. N Engl J Med 313:1305, 1985

North RA, Sadler L, Stewart AW, McCowan LM, Kerr AR, White HD: Long-term survival and valve-related complications in young women with cardiac valve replacements. Circulation 99:2669, 1999

Nugent EW, Planter WH, Edwards JE, Williams WH: The pathology, abnormal physiology, clinical recognition, and medical and surgical treatment of congenital heart disease. In Hurst JW, Schlant RC, Rackley CE, Sonnenblick EH, Wenger NK (eds): The Heart, 7th ed. New York, McGraw-Hill, 1990, p 655

O'Connell JB, Costanzo-Nordin MR, Subramanian R, Robinson JA, Wallis DE, Scanlon PJ, Gunnar RM: Peripartum cardiomyopathy: Clinical, hemodynamic, histologic and prognostic characteristics. J Am Coll Cardiol 8:52, 1986

Oskoui R, Lindsay J Jr: Aortic dissection in women < 40 years of age and the unimportance of pregnancy. Am J Cardiol 73:821, 1994

Pavankumar P, Venugopal P, Kaul U, Iyer KS, Das B, Sampathkumar A, Airon B, Rao IM, Sharma ML, Bhatia ML, Gopinath N: Closed mitral valvotomy during pregnancy: A 20 year experience. Scand J Thorac Cardiovasc Surg 22:11, 1988

Pearson GD, Veille JC, Rahimtoola S, Hsia J, Oakley CM, Hosenpud JD, Ansari A, Baughman KL: Peripartum cardiomyopathy. National Heart, Lung, and Blood Institute and Office of Rare Diseases (National Institutes of Health) Workshop Recommendations and Review). JAMA 283:1183, 2000

Pepin M, Schwarze U, Superti-Furga A, Byers PH: Clinical and genetic features of Ehlers–Danlos syndrome type IV, the vascular type. N Engl J Med 342:673, 2000

Perloff JK: Congenital heart disease in adults. In Braunwald E (ed): Heart Disease: A Textbook of Cardiovascular Medicine, 5th ed. Philadelphia, Saunders, 1997, p 964

Pollack KL, Chestnut DH, Wenstrom KD: Anesthetic management of a parturient with Eisenmenger's syndrome. Anesth Analg 70:212, 1990

Pombar X, Strassner HT, Fenner PC: Pregnancy in a woman with class H diabetes mellitus and previous coronary artery bypass graft: A case report and review of the literature. Obstet Gynecol 85:825, 1995

Prêtre R, Von Segesser LK: Aortic dissection. Lancet 349:1461, 1997

Ramin SM, Gilstrap LC III: Mitral-valve disease in pregnancy. Prim Care Update Ob/Gyns 6:106, 1999

Rayburn WF, LeMire MS, Bird JL, Buda AJ: Mitral valve prolapse: Echocardiographic changes during pregnancy. J Reprod Med 32:185, 1987

Reece EA, Egan JFX, Coustan DR, Tamborlane W, Bates SE, O'Neill TM, Fitzpatrick JG: Coronary artery disease in diabetic pregnancies. Am J Obstet Gynecol 154:150, 1986

Robinson JN, Banerjee R, Landzberg MJ, Thiet MP: Inhaled nitric oxide therapy in pregnancy complicated by pulmonary hypertension. Am J Obstet Gynecol 180:1045, 1999

Røder BL, Wandall DA, Frimodt-Møller N, Esperson F, Skinhøj P, Rosdahl VT: Clinical features of *Staphylococcus aureus* endocarditis. A 10-year experience in Denmark. Arch Intern Med 159:462, 1999

Roldan CA, Shively BK, Grawford MH: An echocardiographic study of valvular heart disease associated with systemic lupus erythematosus. N Engl J Med 335:1424, 1996

Rossiter JP, Repke JT, Morales AJ, Murphy EA, Pyeritz RE: A Prospective longitudinal evaluation of pregnancy in the Marfan syndrome. Am J Obstet Gynecol 173:1599, 1995

Rubin LJ: Primary pulmonary hypertension. N Engl J Med 336:111, 1997

Sachs BP, Brown DAJ, Driscoll SG, Schulman E, Acker D, Ransil BJ, Jewett JF: Hemorrhage, infection, toxemia, and cardiac disease, 1954–85: Causes for their declining role in maternal mortality. Am J Public Health 78:671, 1988

Sadler L, McCowan L, White H, Stewart A, Bracken M, North R: Pregnancy outcomes and cardiac complications in women with mechanical, bioprosthetic and homograft valves. Br J Obstet Gynaecol 107:245, 2000

Salazar E, Espinola N, Roman L, Casanova JM: Effect of pregnancy on the duration of bovine pericardial bioprostheses. Am Heart J 137:714, 1999

Sanchez-Ramos L, Chami YG, Bass TA, DelValle GO, Adair CD: Myocardial infarction during pregnancy: Management with transluminal coronary angioplasty and metallic intracoronary stents. Am J Obstet Gynecol 171:1392, 1994

Sareli P, England MJ, Berk MR, Marcus RH, Epstein M, Driscoll J, Meyer T, McIntyre J, van Gelderen C: Maternal and fetal sequelae of anticoagulation during pregnancy in patients with mechanical heart valve protheses. Am J Cardiol 63:1462, 1989

Sawhney H, Suri V, Vasishta K, Gupta N, Devi K, Grover A: Pregnancy and congenital heart disease—maternal and fetal outcome. Aust N Z J Obstet Gynaecol 38:266, 1998

Sbarouni E, Oakley CM: Outcome of pregnancy in women with valve prostheses. Br Heart J 71:196, 1994

Schenker JG, Polishuk WZ: Pregnancy following mitral valvotomy—A survey of 182 patients. Obstet Gynecol 32:214, 1968

Schulte-Sasse, U: Life threatening myocardial ischaemia associated with the use of prostaglandin E_1 to induce abortion. Brit J Obstet Gynaecol 107:700, 2000

Schumacher B, Belfort MA, Card RJ: Successful treatment of acute myocardial infarction during pregnancy with tissue plasminogen activator. Am J Obstet Gynecol 176:716, 1997

Seaworth BJ, Durack DT: Infective endocarditis in obstetric and gynecologic practice. Am J Obstet Gynecol 154:180, 1986

Sheffield JS, Cunningham FG: Diagnosing and managing peripartum cardiomyopathy. Contemp Ob/Gyn 44:74, 1999

Shime J, Mocarski EJM, Hastings D, Webb GD, McLaughlin PR: Congenital heart disease in pregnancy: Short- and long-term implications. Am J Obstet Gynecol 156:313, 1987

Shivvers SA, Wians FH, Keffer JH, Ramin SM: Maternal cardiac troponin I levels during normal labor and delivery. Am J Obstet Gynecol 180:122, 1999

Shores J, Berger KR, Murphy EA, Pyeritz RE: Progression of aortic dilatation and the benefit of long-term β-adrenergic blockade in Marfan's syndrome. N Engl J Med 330:1335, 1994

Simpson LL, D'Alton ME: Marfan syndrome: An update on pregnancy. Prim Care Update Ob/Gyns 4:1, 1997

Singh H, Bolton PJ, Oakley CM: Pregnancy after surgical correction of tetralogy of Fallot. BMJ 285:168, 1982

Siu SC, Sermer M, Harrison DA, Grigoriadis E, Liu G, Sorensen S, Smallhorn JF, Farine D, Amankwah KS, Spears JC, Colman JM: Risk and predictors for pregnancy-related complications in women with heart disease. Circulation 96:2789, 1997

Strickland RA, Oliver WC, Chantigian RC, Ney JA, Danielson GK: Anesthesia, cardiopulmonary bypass, and the pregnant patient. Mayo Clin Proc 66:411, 1991

Sugrue D, Blake S, MacDonald D: Pregnancy complicated by maternal heart disease at the National Maternity Hospital, Dublin, Ireland, 1969 to 1978. Am J Obstet Gynecol 139:1, 1981

Suri V, Sawhney H, Vasishta K, Renuka T, Grover A: Pregnancy following cardiac valve replacement surgery. Int J Gynaecol Obstet 64:239, 1999

Sutaria N, O'Toole L, Northridge D: Postpartum acute MI following routine ergometrine administration treated successfully by primary PTCA. Heart 83:97, 2000

Tan J, de Swiet M: Prevalence of heart disease diagnosed *de novo* in pregnancy in a West London population. Br J Obstet Gynaecol 105:1185, 1998

Thornhill ML, Camann WR: Cardiovascular disease. In Chestnut DH (ed): Obstetric Anesthesia. Mosby, St. Louis, 1994, p 746

Thorp JM Jr, Chescheir NC, Fann B: Postpartum myocardial infarction in a patient with antiphospholipid syndrome. Am J Perinatol 11:1, 1994

Torres PJ, Gratacós E, Magriñá J, Martinez-Crespo JM, Cardrach V: Primary pulmonary hypertension and preeclampsia: A successful pregnancy. Br J Obstet Gynaecol 101:163, 1994

Tripp HF, Stiegel RM, Coyle JP: The use of pulsatile perfusion during aortic valve replacement in pregnancy. Ann Thorac Surg 67:1169, 1999

Troché V, Ville Y, Fernandez H: Pregnancy after heart or heart–lung transplantation: A series of 10 pregnancies. Br J Obstet Gynaecol 105:454, 1998

Van der Meer JTM, Van Wijk W, Thompson J, Vandenbroucke JP, Valkenburg HA, Michel MF: Efficacy of antibiotic prophylaxis for prevention of native-valve endocarditis. Lancet 339:135, 1992

Van Oppen ACC, Stigter RH, Bruinse HW: Cardiac output in normal pregnancy: A critical review. Obstet Gynecol 87:310, 1996

Vinatier D, Virelizier S, Depret-Mosser S, Dufour Ph, Prolongeau JF, Monnier JC, Decoulx E, Theeten G: Pregnancy after myocardial infarction. Eur J Obstet Gynecol Reprod Biol 56:89, 1994

Weiss BM, Maggiorini M, Jenni R, Lauper U, Popov V, Bombeli T, Spahn DR: Pregnant patient with primary pulmonary hypertension: Inhaled pulmonary vasodilators and epidural anesthesia for cesarean delivery. Anesthesiology 91:1191, 2000

Weiss BM, von Segesser LK, Alon E, Seifert B, Turnia MI: Outcome of cardiovascular surgery and pregnancy: A systematic review of the period 1984–1996. Am J Obstet Gynecol 179:1643, 1998a

Weiss BM, Zemp L, Seifert B, Hess OM: Outcome of pulmonary vascular disease in pregnancy: A systematic overview from 1978 through 1996. J Am Coll Cardiol 31:1650, 1998b

Westaby S, Parry AJ, Forfar JC: Reoperation for prosthetic valve endocarditis in the third trimester of pregnancy. Ann Thorac Surg 53:263, 1992

Whittemore R, Hobbins JC, Engle MA: Pregnancy and its outcome in women with and without surgical treatment of congenital heart disease. Am J Cardiol 50:641, 1982

Widerhorn J, Widerhorn ALM, Rahimtoola SH, Elkayam U: WPW syndrome during pregnancy: Increased incidence after supraventricular arrhythmias. Am Heart J 123:796, 1992

Witlin AG, Mabie WC, Sibai BM: Peripartum cardiomyopathy: An ominous diagnosis. Am J Obstet Gynecol 176:182, 1997

Yentis SM, Steer PJ, Plaat F: Eisenmenger's syndrome in pregnancy: Maternal and fetal mortality in the 1990s. Br J Obstet Gynecol 105:921, 1998

Zuber M, Gautschi N, Oechslin E, Widmer V, Kiowski W, Jenni R: Outcome of pregnancy in women with congenital shunt lesions. Heart 81:271, 1999

45

Chronic Hypertension

Hypertension that antedates pregnancy is one of the most common medical complications encountered during pregnancy. Its variable incidence and severity, along with the well-known proclivity for pregnancy to induce or aggravate hypertension, has caused much confusion concerning the management of pregnant hypertensive women. For example, the majority of women with underlying chronic hypertension demonstrate improved blood pressure control during pregnancy and have largely uneventful pregnancies. Some, however, experience dangerous worsening of hypertension that is frequently accompanied by proteinuria, pathological edema, and convulsions. These latter women—except that chronic hypertension antedated pregnancy—are indistinguishable from an otherwise normotensive young nullipara who develops severe preeclampsia–eclampsia.

DEFINITIONS

There is a wide range of blood pressures in normal adults. The range in those with abnormally high pressures is also wide. Categorization therefore primarily relates to acute or long-term adverse effects associated with the sustained level of those blood pressures. Associations with normal or various levels of abnormal blood pressure are based on morbidity and mortality primarily in adult men. A useful categorization from the latest Joint National Committee (1997) on the Detection, Evaluation, and Treatment of High Blood Pressure is shown in Table 45–1. Within these categories, morbidity or mortality is further influenced by age, gender, race, and personal behaviors including smoking, excessive alcohol intake, obesity, and physical activity.

In adults, proven benefits accrue with treatment of chronic hypertension at sustained diastolic blood pressures of 90 mm Hg or greater (Korotkoff phase V) and/or systolic pressures of 160 mm Hg or more. Benefits are apparent even in otherwise healthy adults and treatment at even lower levels may benefit patients who are elderly, who have appreciable underlying atherosclerotic disease and/or postmyocardial infarction; or who have evidence of renal or cardiac dysfunction; or who have had a cerebrovascular thrombosis or hemorrhage.

DIAGNOSIS

A diagnosis of chronic hypertension complicating pregnancy is made whenever hypertension precedes pregnancy, or hypertension occurs prior to 20 weeks (Chap. 24, p. 569). Infrequently, women without chronic hypertension have repeated pregnancies in which hypertension appears only late in pregnancy. This is classified as *transient hypertension,* and likely is evidence of latent hypertensive vascular disease. The results of long-term follow-up studies of Chesley and co-workers (1976), as well as those of Sibai and colleagues (1986b, 1991, 1992), are supportive of this view.

In most women with hypertensive vascular disease, increased blood pressure is the only demonstrable finding. Some, however, have complications that increase the risk not only of pregnancy but also of life expectancy. These include hypertensive or ischemic cardiac disease,

TABLE 45–1. **Classification of Blood Pressure for Adults Ages 18 Years and Older**

Category	Systolic Pressure[a] (mm Hg)	Diastolic Pressure[a] (mm Hg)
Normal[b]	< 130	< 85
High normal	130–139	85–89
Hypertension[c]		
Stage 1 (mild)	140–159	90–99
Stage 2 (moderate)	160–179	100–109
Stage 3 (severe)	180–209	110–119
Stage 4 (very severe)	≥ 210	≥ 120

[a] When systolic and diasatolic pressures fall into different categories, the higher category is used to classify blood pressure status.
[b] Optimal blood pressure with respect to cardiovascular risk is < 120/80 mmHg. Used only for adults aged 18 years and older not taking antihypertensive drugs and not acutely ill.
[c] Based on the average of two or more readings taken at each of two or more visits after an initial screening.
From the Joint National Committee (1997).

renal insufficiency, prior cerebrovascular event, or retinal hemorrhages and exudates. Hypertensive vascular disease in pregnancy is encountered more frequently in older women. Obesity is another important predisposing factor, and as discussed in Chapter 48 (p. 1298), chronic hypertension may be increased as much as tenfold in obese compared with nonobese women. Moreover, obese women with chronic hypertension are more likely to develop superimposed preeclampsia (Rey and Couturier, 1994). As perhaps expected in older and usually obese women, diabetes mellitus is also prevalent. Finally, heredity, which includes racial factors, plays an important role in the development of chronic hypertension. Disease is common in African Americans and Mexican Americans, and frequently many members of the same family are hypertensive (Centers for Disease Control and Prevention, 1995).

In most women with chronic hypertension, the blood pressure falls by the second trimester, but the decrement is usually temporary (Ayala and associates, 1997; Cunningham and Lowe, 1991; Sibai and colleagues, 1990a). In most cases, the blood pressure rises during the third trimester to levels somewhat above those in early pregnancy (Fig. 45–1). Adverse outcomes in these women are dependent largely upon whether superimposed preeclampsia develops.

TREATMENT IN NONPREGNANT ADULTS

Even at the mildest end of the spectrum of abnormal blood pressures categorized in Table 45–1, therapy to

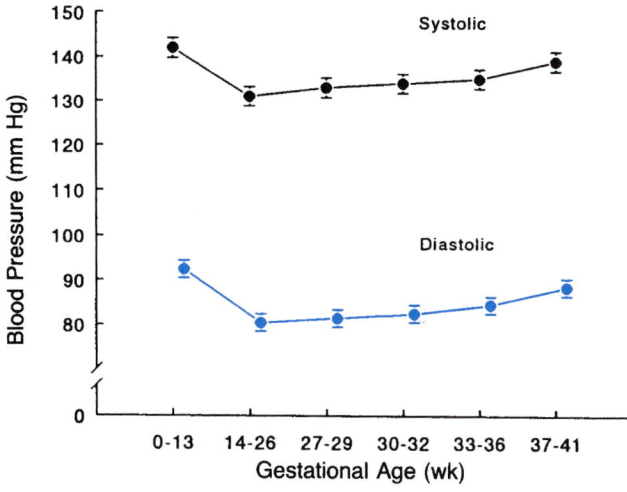

FIGURE 45–1. Systolic and diastolic blood pressure changes during pregnancy in 90 chronically hypertensive women who were given no antihypertensive treatment. (Mean ± SEM.) (Taken from Cunningham and Lowe, 1991; data from Sibai and colleagues, 1990a.)

reduce pressure is beneficial. Ferrer and associates (2000) have analyzed evidence from randomized trials of nonpregnant women aged 30 to 54 years. They computed that about 250 such women with mild to moderate hypertension would need to be treated for 5 years to prevent one cardiovascular event such as stroke or myocardial infarction. More than 20 large trials involving over 50,000 participants have established that antihypertensive treatment in adults with mild to moderate hypertension decreases mortality, stroke, and major cardiac events (Collins and MacMahon, 1994; Gueyffier and collaborators, 1997). Thus, regardless of pregnancy status, many such women would likely have been placed on antihypertensive medications as well as institution of behavioral lifestyle modifications prior to pregnancy. Nonpharmacological interventions include weight loss, prescribed physical activity, dietary adjustment, and cessation of smoking, excessive alcohol, and caffeine usage.

In women diagnosed with presumed chronic hypertension prior to midpregnancy, the benefits and safety of instituting antihypertensive therapy are less clear because of largely hypothetical concerns regarding their effect on fetal growth. Clearly, antihypertensive therapy in nonpregnant adult women with sustained diastolic pressures of 90 mm Hg or greater would not be considered harmful.

PRECONCEPTIONAL AND EARLY PREGNANCY EVALUATION

Evaluation of women with chronic hypertension is of great importance for either counseling or management during pregnancy. Ideally, they should be counseled prior to undertaking pregnancy (Chap. 9, p. 212). The duration of chronic hypertension, level of blood pressure control, and antihypertensive therapy is ascertained. Their general health, daily activities, diet, and adverse personal behaviors should be determined. Adverse events such as cerebrovascular accident, myocardial infarction, cardiac failure, or renal dysfunction are especially pertinent. These women are at marked increase risk for a recurrence or worsening of these outcomes during pregnancy. Women who require multiple antihypertensives for control of hypertension, or those who are poorly controlled, are also at increased risk for adverse pregnancy outcomes.

Evaluation also includes assessment of renal, hepatic, and cardiac function. Cardiac assessment should be targeted toward ascertainment of any dysrhythmias and/or evidence of left ventricular hypertrophy indicating either long-standing or poorly controlled hypertension, or both. Women with appreciable left-ventricular hypertrophy are at increased risk for cardiac dysfunction and congestive heart failure during pregnancy. In women with any prior adverse outcome, or in long-term hypertension, echocardiography is indicated.

Renal function is assessed by serum creatinine and quantification of proteinuria. If either is abnormal, these women are at further increased risk for adverse effects on pregnancy. The Working Group Report on Hypertension in Pregnancy (2000) of the National Heart, Lung, and Blood Institute concluded that the risks of fetal loss and accelerated deterioration of renal disease are increased if serum creatinine is above 1.4 mg/dL at conception. It can be difficult, however, to separate the effects of the pregnancy from inevitable progression of renal disease (Cunningham and associates, 1990; Jones and Hayslett, 1996). As a general principle, while not precisely linear, renal insufficiency is inversely proportional to increased risk of hypertensive complications on pregnancy outcome. Pregnancy is relatively contraindicated in women who, despite therapy, maintain persistent diastolic pressures of 110 mm Hg or greater, require multiple antihypertensives, or whose serum creatinine is greater than 2 mg/dL. Stronger contraindications include women who have had prior cerebrovascular thrombosis or hemorrhage, myocardial infarction, or cardiac failure.

Assessment of functional physical capabilities in regard to symptoms at rest and with mild or moderate activity should be determined. In women with prior cardiac dysfunction, baseline pulmonary function testing and longitudinal vital capacity testing throughout pregnancy may provide early identification of decreasing cardiac function and early pulmonary congestion. Ophthalmological evaluation is of importance for women with longstanding chronic hypertension.

EFFECTS OF CHRONIC HYPERTENSION ON PREGNANCY

MATERNAL EFFECTS. Most women taking monotherapy and whose hypertension is well controlled prior to pregnancy will do well. However, even these women have an increased risk of abruptio placentae, superimposed preeclampsia, and increased hospitalization. In addition, Jain (1997) reported a maternal mortality of 230 per 100,000 live births in women with hypertension compared with about 10 per 100,000 for normotensive women. The more severe the baseline maternal disease, and especially with documented end-organ damage, the more likely these complications.

Pregnancy-aggravated hypertension typically becomes manifest by a sudden rise in blood pressure that frequently is eventually complicated by substantial proteinuria. Extreme hypertension—systolic pressure greater than 200 mm Hg and diastolic pressure of 130

mm Hg or more—may rapidly result in oliguria and renal dysfunction. With the development of superimposed severe preeclampsia or eclampsia, the outlook for both infant and mother is serious unless the pregnancy is terminated. A number of common adverse pregnancy outcomes that are increased in women with chronic hypertension are considered next.

ABRUPTIO PLACENTAE. Premature placental separation is discussed in detail in Chapter 25 (p. 621). The incidence of abruptio placentae in a number of investigations is about 1 in 150 (Ananth and associates, 1999). This incidence is appreciably increased in women with hypertension. Sibai and colleagues (1998) reported placental abruption in 1.5 percent of 776 women with hypertension preceding pregnancy. Caritis and associates (1998) reported that 1 to 2 percent of 2539 women at high risk for preeclampsia enrolled in a low-dose aspirin trial had placental abruption. Hauth and co-workers (1995) performed meta-analysis of low-dose aspirin trials in women at high and low risk for preeclampsia, and reported that abruptio placentae occurred in about 1.4 percent. Thus, the risk of abruptio placentae in women with chronic hypertension is two- to threefold greater than for normotensive women. Ananth and colleagues (1999) observed that smoking increased these risks even further.

SUPERIMPOSED PREECLAMPSIA. The incidence of superimposed preeclampsia in women with chronic hypertension is variable because there is no precise definition. August and Lindheimer (1999) reported that superimposed preeclampsia developed in from 4 to 40 percent of these women. The incidence is higher in women with severe hypertension in early pregnancy (Sibai, 1991). Clearly, the occurrence of superimposed preeclampsia is directly related to the severity of baseline hypertension, as well as the need for treatment to achieve control. In the randomized Maternal Fetal Medicine Network study, Caritis and co-workers (1998) employed predefined criteria for preeclampsia in 774 women with chronic hypertension. They identified superimposed preeclampsia in 25 percent of these women. In another analysis of these same women, Sibai and co-workers (1998) reported that the incidence of superimposed preeclampsia was similar whether or not there was proteinuria at baseline. The incidence significantly increased, however, in those who had hypertension for at least 4 years or who had preeclampsia during a prior pregnancy.

Studies of low-dose aspirin therapy to reduce the incidence of superimposed preeclampsia in women with chronic hypertension have shown little benefit. In an early study, Beaufils and colleagues (1985) reported that therapy with low-dose aspirin and the antiplatelet agent

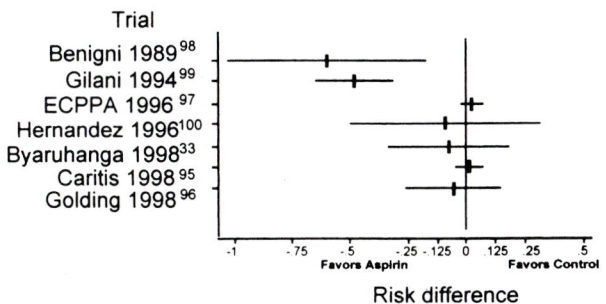

FIGURE 45-2. Effects of low-dose aspirin treatment compared with placebo controls and the incidence of preterm delivery. (Data from Mulrow and colleagues, 2000.)

dipyridamole was beneficial in reducing the incidence of superimposed preeclampsia and fetal growth restriction. In a European multicenter trial (EPREDA), Uzan and co-workers (1991) found that these same drugs were associated with significantly increased birthweight and a decreased incidence of fetal growth restriction in high-risk women. In the Network study reported by Caritis and associates (1998), the incidence of superimposed preeclampsia or fetal growth restriction were similar in women assigned to low-dose aspirin or placebo. In this same trial, maternal serum thromboxane B_2 reduction was not predictive of improved pregnancy outcomes with low-dose aspirin (Hauth and colleagues, 1998). As shown in Figure 45-2, a summary of randomized trials of low-dose aspirin in women with chronic hypertension suggests that the only benefit is fewer preterm deliveries.

MATERNAL ECONOMIC AND LIFESTYLE DEMANDS. There is little quantitative data to relate these issues to outcomes in pregnant women with chronic hypertension. As a group, these women require more time with their physicians to include office visits, fetal–maternal assessment in the third trimester, and increased hospitalization. Home rest affects economic stability as well as family dynamics. They require more time off from work, which is especially burdensome if they are self-employed or must care for children or other family members. These realities are discussed during preconceptional or early pregnancy counseling (Chap. 9, p. 212).

FETAL/NEWBORN EFFECTS. A number of adverse perinatal outcomes are substantively increased in pregnancy complicated by chronic hypertension.

FETAL GROWTH RESTRICTION. This incidence is in direct relation to the severity of hypertension. Its precise incidence and severity varies dependent upon other maternal factors, the choice of growth chart used in making this diagnosis, and certainly of confirmed gestational age. Maternal factors include age; the severity and control of hypertension, including need for additional antihypertensive medications; and presence of end-organ damage such as renal or cardiac dysfunction. Because of these factors, there is no data regarding safety or efficacy of treatment of women with mild chronic hypertension predating pregnancy. While such treatment is not harmful for the mother, the potential benefits or adverse fetal-neonatal effects have not been determined.

In the Network trial described above, Sibai and colleagues (1998) reported that only 10.7 percent of 763 women with chronic hypertension had small-for-gestational age newborns. Women with chronic hypertension and proteinuria early in pregnancy had 23 percent of infants who weighed less than the 10th percentile compared with 10 percent in women without baseline proteinuria. Von Dadelszen and co-workers (2000) employed meta-analysis to investigate the relation between fetal growth and oral antihypertensives to treat mild to moderate pregnancy hypertension. They concluded that a treatment-induced mean arterial pressure decrease was associated with significantly increased small-for-gestational age infants. This review is greatly confounded by inclusion of women with gestational and/or pregnancy-induced hypertension treated later in pregnancy as compared with women whose chronic hypertension was treated throughout pregnancy.

OTHER ADVERSE PERINATAL OUTCOMES. Preterm birth is increased in women with chronic hypertension (McCowan and colleagues, 1996; Meis and co-workers, 1998). From The Network, Sibai and colleagues (1998) reported that 33 percent of 763 women with chronic hypertension delivered before 37 weeks, and 18 percent before 35 weeks. They cited a perinatal death rate of 46 per 1000, which is markedly increased over healthy nulliparas. Rey and Couturier (1994) found a similar incidence of perinatal loss.

MANAGEMENT DURING PREGNANCY

The goal in women whose pregnancy is complicated by chronic hypertension is to minimize or prevent any of the adverse maternal or perinatal outcomes previously discussed. In general, management is targeted toward prevention of moderate or severe hypertension as well as prevention of severe pregnancy-aggravated hypertension. To some extent, these goals can be achieved pharmacologically with special attention to assure medication compliance. Personal health behavioral modifications include dietary counseling and reduction of behaviors such as smoking, alcohol, cocaine, or other substance abuse. It is accepted that women with severe hypertension must always be treated for maternal indications regardless of pregnancy status. This includes pregnant women with prior adverse outcomes, including cerebrovascular events, myocardial infarction, and cardiac or renal dysfunction. We agree with the philosophy of beginning antihypertensive treatment in an otherwise healthy woman with persistent diastolic pressures of 100 mm Hg or greater (August and Lindheimer, 1999). With end-organ dysfunction, treatment of pregnant women with diastolic pressures of 90 mm Hg or higher should be considered. Other than simply lowering blood pressure, there are no data indicating salutary effects in pregnancy outcomes. Specifically, the incidence of superimposed preeclampsia is not lowered. Moreover, there is no evidence that perinatal outcomes are improved by such treatment. As emphasized by the Working Group Report (2000), there is a need for further trials of treatment or observation in women with chronic hypertension and their possible benefits on pregnancy outcomes.

ANTIHYPERTENSIVE DRUGS. The following summary of antihypertensive drugs is categorized by their primary mode of action (Table 45–2) and as abstracted from several sources, including the *2000 Physician's Desk Reference.* In adults with chronic hypertension, initial pharmacological therapy is generally one of four agents: a diuretic, a low-dose of an angiotensin-converting enzyme inhibitor, a β-blocking agent, or a long-acting calcium-channel antagonist.

DIURETICS. Commonly used drugs include thiazide diuretics and loop-acting diuretics such as furosemide (Brater, 1998). In the short term, diuretics lower blood pressure by sodium and water diuresis and intravascular volume depletion. With time, there is "sodium escape" and intravascular volume depletion is corrected. Some aspect of lowered peripheral vascular resistance may contribute to the effectiveness of these agents. Diuretics have been shown to reduce long-term morbidity and mortality in adult men with chronic hypertension (Williams, 1998). Largely for theoretical concerns, diuretics are usually not instituted as first-line therapy during pregnancy, particularly after 20 weeks (Working Group Report, 2000).

ADRENERGIC BLOCKING AGENTS. These agents can act *centrally* by reducing nervous system sympathetic outflow and effect generalized decreased vascular tone. Central-acting agents include clonidine and α-methyldopa. *Beta-adrenergic receptor blockers* are also included in this category, and they also cause a generalized decrease in sympathetic tone. Examples are propranolol, metoprolol, and atenolol. The α/β-*adrenergic blocker,* labetalol is a commonly used agent in this category. Peripheral blockers are thought to have more potential for postural hypotension than the centrally acting agents. Based on clinical experience, the most commonly used drugs in pregnancy to treat hypertension are methyldopa or a β- or α/β-receptor blocker.

VASODILATORS. Hydralazine directly relaxes arterial smooth muscle and is used parenterally for treatment of acute severe intrapartum or immediate postpartum hypertension (Chap. 24, p. 592). Use of oral hydralazine as a sole oral agent for chronic hypertension is not recommended because of its relatively weak antihypertensive effects and because of resultant tachycardia. It may be effective for long-term use as an adjunct to other antihypertensives.

CALCIUM-CHANNEL ANTAGONISTS. These agents are divided into three subclasses based on modification of calcium entry into cells and interference with binding sites on voltage-dependent calcium channels. Common agents in these categories include the dihydropyridine nifedipine and the phenylalkyl amine derivative, verapamil. These agents have negative inotropic affects and thus can worsen cardiac dysfunction and congestive cardiac failure. Pahor and associates (2000) concluded that these agents were inferior to other first-line drugs in nonpregnant hypertensives. There is little published experience with these agents during pregnancy (Smith and colleagues, 2000).

ANGIOTENSIN-CONVERTING ENZYME INHIBITORS. These agents inhibit the conversion of angiotensin-I to the potent vasoconstrictor angiotensin-II. They are associated with serious fetal effects and are not used during pregnancy (Chap. 38, p. 1014). Angiotensin-receptor antagonists have effects similar to angiotensin-converting enzyme inhibitors, albeit instead of blocking the production of angiotensin-II, they inhibit binding to its receptor.

DRUG TREATMENT DURING PREGNANCY. As discussed, continued antihypertensive treatment for preg-

TABLE 45–2. Antihypertensives Categorized by Primary Mode of Action

Diuretics
Antiadrenergic blocking agents
  Central acting
  β-receptors
  α/β-receptors
Vasodilators
Calcium-channel antagonists
Angiotensin-converting enzyme (ACE) inhibitors
Angiotensin-receptor antagonists

nant women with chronic hypertension is debated. While beneficial to the mother to reduce her blood pressure, theoretically the lower pressure would decrease uteroplacental perfusion and possibly jeopardize her fetus. There is little experience, but some observational studies are shown in Table 45–3.

Sibai and colleagues (1983) reported their experience with chronic hypertension in 211 consecutive women with mild hypertension. Treatment was either not given or antihypertensive drugs were discontinued at the first prenatal visit. Only 13 percent of these 211 women required antihypertensive therapy later in pregnancy for diastolic pressures exceeding 110 mm Hg, and the perinatal mortality was 28 per 1000. Antihypertensive treatment was prescribed for 82 women whose diastolic pressure exceeded 90 mm Hg, while 82 women whose diastolic pressures remained less than 90 mm Hg were given no treatment. The perinatal mortality in each group was similar, but fetal growth restriction was increased fourfold in the treated group, presumably because of worse hypertension.

To summarize the studies presented in Table 45–3, all investigators found that superimposed preeclampsia or pregnancy-aggravated hypertension was associated with a worse prognosis. Importantly, treatment did not decrease the incidence of this complication. Most pregnancy outcomes were good without treatment. Perinatal mortality rates were low unless superimposed preeclampsia developed.

Some randomized trials of antihypertensive drug therapy in pregnant women with mild chronic hypertension are shown in Table 45–4. Only three trials were conducted during the 1990s, and only two were of appreciable size. Thus, data are not sufficient to provide a definitive answer regarding whether to treat women with mild or even moderate hypertension in pregnancy. One important observation of the two large and more contemporaneous studies was that no adverse outcomes

TABLE 45–3. Observational Studies of the Effects of Treatment of Chronic Hypertension During Pregnancy

Study and Treatment	No.	Superimposed Preeclampsia (%)	Perinatal Mortality (per 1000)
Chesley (1978)			
Chronic hypertension[a] (1972–1974), no antihypertensives	593	6	32
Superimposed preeclampsia[b] (1960–1974), hydralazine + α-methyldopa	196	—	214
Redman (1980)[c]			
Chronic hypertension	184	25	16
Superimposed preeclampsia	69	—	145
Sibai and associates (1983)			
Chronic hypertension, no antihypertensives	193	10	5
Superimposed preeclampsia, α-methyldopa and/or hydralazine	22	—	227
Mabie and associates (1986)			
Chronic hypertension, diastolic pressure < 90 mm Hg, no treatment	137	29	29
Chronic hypertension, diastolic pressure 90–100 mm Hg, α-methyldopa	26	46	0
Sibai and associates (1986a)			
Severe chronic hypertension, 170/100 mm Hg or greater, α-methyldopa + hydralazine	44	52	250
Rey and Couturier (1994)			
Chronic hypertension, treat if diastolic pressure > 100 mm Hg	337	21	45

[a] Three maternal deaths due to stroke, pulmonary embolus, and aspiration pneumonia.
[b] Two deaths due to stroke and postoperative infection.
[c] Data from Ounsted and associates (1983), reporting on long-term follow-up of children from the original and continuing study of treatment of chronic hypertension in pregnancy by Redman (1980).

TABLE 45–4. Randomized Trials of Drug Therapy in Pregnancies Complicated by Mild Chronic Hypertension

Reference	No.	Mean Gestation at Entry (weeks)	Mean DBP at Entry (mm Hg)	Treatment	Principal Findings
Leather et al (1968)	47	< 20	107	Methyldopa ± diuretics ± hydralazine versus no drug	Longer gestation and fewer perinatal deaths
Redman (1976)	208	21 and 22	88–90	Methyldopa ± hydralazine versus no drug	Fewer midpregnancy losses in treated women
Arias and Azmora (1979)	58	15 and 16	90–99	Methyldopa, diuretics, or hydralazine versus no drug	Compromised infants born to mothers in whom severe hypertension developed despite treatment
Butters et al (1990)	29	16	86	Double-blind; atenolol versus placebo	Poor fetal growth in treated women
Sibai et al (1990a)	263	< 11	91–92	Methyldopa versus labetalol versus no drug	No differences in outcomes
ECPPA (1996)	283	24	95–96	Slow-release nifedipine versus no drug	No differences in outcomes

DBP = diastolic blood pressure.
Adapted from Haddad and Sibai (1999), with permission.

were found in the treatment group. Thus, it is not unreasonable to treat women with uncomplicated mild or moderate sustained chronic hypertension who would otherwise be prescribed antihypertensive therapy when they were not pregnant.

The theoretical concern of fetal growth restriction due to reduced placental perfusion by lowering maternal blood pressure is confounded in that worsening blood pressure itself is associated with abnormal fetal growth. Breart and colleagues (1982) found that women with chronic hypertension whose diastolic pressure was less than 90 mm Hg had a 3 percent risk of fetal growth restriction, those with 90 mm Hg had a 6 percent risk, and those with 110 mm Hg or more had a 16 percent risk. Growth restriction from maternal treatment was not supported by the two large randomized trials shown in Table 45–4.

Results of the carefully done study of chronic hypertension in pregnant women reported by the Memphis group are summarized in Table 45–5. In this trial, Sibai and colleagues (1990a) randomized 263 women with mild to moderate chronic hypertension at 6 to 13 weeks to no treatment, or to receive either labetalol or α-methyldopa. The aim of therapy was to maintain the blood pressure less than 140/90 mm Hg. Women treated throughout pregnancy had significantly lower blood pressures than women randomized to no treatment, and the incidence of adverse outcomes was not altered by treatment. As perhaps expected, more women not initially given treatment eventually required antihypertensive therapy for serious hypertension, defined as blood pressure greater than 160/110 mm Hg.

A more recent randomized trial of women with mild to moderate hypertension in pregnancy was reported by the Gruppo di Studio Ipertensione in Gravidanza (1998). In this multicenter study, 283 women were randomized to treatment with slow-release nifedipine, 10 mg twice daily until delivery, or to no treatment. Women given no treatment were given nifedipine if diastolic pressure exceeded 110 mm Hg. These investigators also found no apparent benefit but also no harm in the nifedipine versus expectant management groups. Preterm delivery was high in both groups—45 percent in treated and 37 percent nontreated. There was no difference between the two groups in mean birthweight or growth-restricted infants.

SEVERE CHRONIC HYPERTENSION. As discussed, the prognosis for pregnancy outcomes with chronic hypertension is related to the severity of the disease before pregnancy. Many women with severe hypertension also have underlying renal disease (Cunningham and colleagues, 1990). Sibai and co-workers (1986a) described 44 pregnancies in women whose blood pressure at 6 to 11 weeks was 170/110 mm Hg or higher (Table 45–3). They were given treatment with α-methyldopa and oral hydralazine to maintain blood pressures less than 160/110 mm Hg, and they were hospitalized for treatment with parenteral hydralazine if blood pressures exceeded 180/120 mm Hg. Half developed superimposed preeclampsia, and all adverse perinatal outcomes were in this group. Specifically, all infants in the women with superimposed preeclampsia were preterm, nearly 80 percent were growth restricted,

TABLE 45-5. Maternal and Perinatal Outcomes in 263 Chronically Hypertensive Women Randomized to No Treatment or Treatment with Methyldopa or Labetalol During Pregnancy

		Treatment Group	
Factor	No Treatment (n = 90)	Methyldopa (n = 87)	Labetalol (n = 86)
Additional drugs for hypertension (%)	11	6	6
Superimposed preeclampsia	16	18	16
Abruptio placentae (%)	2	1	2
Preterm delivery (%)	10	12	12
Fetal growth restriction (%)	9	7	8
Perinatal mortality (per 1000)	11	11	12
Gestational age at delivery (wks)	39 ± 0.2	38.6 ± 0.2	38.7 ± 0.2
Birthweight (g)	3123 ± 69	3051 ± 73	3068 ± 71
Placental weight (g)	723 ± 33	716 ± 33	755 ± 69

From Sibai and co-workers (1990a), with permission.

and the perinatal mortality rate was 48 percent. By contrast, in the women with severe hypertension who did not develop superimposed preeclampsia, only 5 percent of fetuses were growth restricted and all survived.

ANTIHYPERTENSIVE DRUG SELECTION. Despite the relatively good results obtained with α-methyldopa, and the comparable results obtained without antihypertensive drugs, adrenergic-blocking drugs have been used extensively in England, Scotland, and Australia (Redman, 1982; Rubin and colleagues, 1983; Walker and associates, 1983). The results of treatment with labetalol are consistent with the view that the drug offers no advantages over α-methyldopa (Sibai and colleagues, 1990a). Rey (1992) observed that α-methyldopa significantly reduced uterine pulsatility indexes in chronically hypertensive women and in women with mild preeclampsia. Indexes were decreased in most, but not all, fetuses. Rubin and colleagues (1983) reported salutary results from a prospective study in which they compared placebo with the β-blocker atenolol given to 120 women with hypertension first apparent early in the third trimester. Because nearly 60 percent of their subjects were nulliparous, it was difficult to separate women with chronic hypertension from those with preeclampsia. The placebo group had worse perinatal outcomes, but there were more nulliparas assigned (67 versus 50 percent), and thus presumably more women had preeclampsia at the onset of the study. The same group (Butters and colleagues, 1990) reported that atenolol treatment of chronically hypertensive women resulted in a higher

incidence of growth-restricted neonates compared with untreated controls.

More recently, Lydakis and colleagues (1999) studied 223 women attending an antenatal hypertension clinic and who had 312 pregnancies. They concluded that atenolol treatment was associated with lower birthweight and ponderal indices as well as a trend toward more preterm births when compared with other antihypertensive monotherapy or to no treatment. Finally, ominous fetal heart rate patterns during labor were reported in 20 percent of women receiving β-blocker therapy for hypertension (Montan and Ingemarsson, 1989). The incidence of ominous patterns was increased even more in growth-restricted fetuses and in half of women given epidural analgesia.

Smith and colleagues (2000) reviewed the use of nifedipine to treat hypertension or for tocolysis in pregnancy. They summarized data reported from 1975 to 1997. They concluded that nifedipine is an effective drug to treat severe hypertension in pregnancy or for preterm labor. The studies of chronic nifedipine use in pregnancy, however, are too small to make recommendations about its routine use for women with chronic hypertension.

Vermillion and associates (1999) reported a randomized clinical trial of oral nifedipine compared with intravenous labetalol to treat 50 women with a hypertensive emergency of pregnancy. They reported that blood pressure control was significantly quicker with nifedipine but that both drugs were effective. Scardo and colleagues (1999) performed noninvasive hemodynamic evaluation in women within this same trial and found that women given nifedipine had a significantly increased cardiac index compared with women given labetalol. This accompanied a significantly decreased systemic vascular resistance in women given nifedipine.

Mulrow and colleagues (2000) performed a review for the Agency for Healthcare Research and Quality and summarized the risks and benefits of antihypertensive agents given to pregnant women (Table 45–6).

THERAPY RECOMMENDATIONS. The National High Blood Pressure Education Program Working Group on High Blood Pressure in Pregnancy (2000) stresses the limited data from which to draw conclusions concerning whether to treat mild chronic hypertension in pregnant women. The group did, however, recommend therapy to prevent hypertensive vascular damage when maternal diastolic blood pressure reached 100 mm Hg. They also concluded that early treatment of hypertension would probably reduce the need for subsequent hospitalization during pregnancy. In the study by Sibai and associates (1990a), subsequent treatment was needed for danger-

ous hypertension in 11 percent of women not given initial treatment, compared with only 6 percent in women given either α-methyldopa or labetalol beginning earlier in pregnancy. Methyldopa has been more extensively studied during pregnancy (Montan and colleagues, 1992, 1993). Indeed, Cockburn and co-workers (1982) reported no adverse effects in children up to 7½ years old whose mothers were treated with methyldopa for hypertension during pregnancy. Haddad and Sibai (1999) concluded that methyldopa is the initial agent of choice for treatment of pregnant women with mild to moderate chronic hypertension.

FETAL ASSESSMENT. Women with well-controlled chronic hypertension with no prior complicating factors can generally be expected to have a good pregnancy outcome. Because even otherwise healthy women with mild hypertension have an increased risk of abruptio placentae, superimposed preeclampsia, preterm delivery, and fetal growth restriction, serial antepartum assessment of fetal well-being is recommended (American

TABLE 45–6. Benefits and Risks of Antihypertensive Agents Given to Pregnant Women

Agent or Class	Benefits	Adverse Effects	Clinical Experience in Pregnancy
Methyldopa	*Fetal:* Insufficient evidence to rule out large effect on perinatal morbidity or mortality.	*Fetal:* Evidence of no major adverse events.	Large
	Maternal: Insufficient evidence to rule out large effect on maternal morbidity.	*Maternal:* Evidence of no major adverse events.	
β-blockers	Fetal: Insufficient evidence to rule out large effect of perinatal morbidity or mortality.	*Fetal:* Limited evidence of possible fetal growth restriction with atenolol used early in pregnancy.	Large
α/β-blockers	*Maternal:* Insufficient evidence to rule out large effect on maternal morbidity.	*Maternal:* Evidence of no major adverse events.	Small
Diuretics	*Fetal:* Insufficient evidence to rule out large effect on perinatal morbidity or motality.	*Fetal:* Evidence of no major adverse events.	Large
	Maternal: Insufficient evidence to rule out large effect on maternal morbidity.	*Maternal:* Evidence of no major adverse events.	
Calcium-channel blockers	*Fetal:* Insufficient evidence to rule out large effect on perinatal morbidity or mortality.	*Fetal:* Very limited evidence of no major adverse events.	Small
	Maternal: Insufficient evidence to rule out large effect on maternal morbidity.	*Maternal:* Very limited evidence of no major adverse events.	
Hydralazine	*Fetal:* Insufficient evidence to rule out large effect on perinatal morbidity or mortality.	*Fetal:* Evidence of no major adverse events.	Moderate (for chronic hypertension).
	Maternal: Insufficient evidence to rule out large effect on maternal morbidity.	*Maternal:* Evidence of no major adverse events.	
ACE inhibitors and ARBs	*Fetal:* No evidence.	*Fetal:* Risk of fetal renal failure if used in second or third trimester.	Small
	Maternal: No evidence.	*Maternal:* No evidence.	None

ACE = angiotensin-converting enzyme; ARB = angiotensin-receptor blocker.
From Mulrow and colleagues (2000), with permission.

College of Obstetricians and Gynecologists, 1999). The gestational age at which to initiate such testing varies with the severity of the disease and the overall clinical course. This is discussed in detail in Chapter 40. According to the Agency for Healthcare Research and Quality (Ferrer and colleagues, 2000), there are no data to address either the benefits or harm of various monitoring strategies for pregnant women with chronic hypertension.

PREGNANCY-AGGRAVATED HYPERTENSION OR SUPERIMPOSED PREECLAMPSIA. From the aforementioned studies, an incidence of superimposed preeclampsia of 25 percent would be commonly accepted for women with chronic hypertension (Caritis and co-workers, 1998). The diagnosis of superimposed preeclampsia may be difficult to make in these women. It is most difficult to be assured of the diagnosis in women with hypertension and underlying renal disease with proteinuria (Cunningham and associates, 1990).

In women with uncomplicated chronic hypertension, criteria that support the diagnosis of superimposed preeclampsia include the development of proteinuria; neurological symptoms, including severe headaches and visual disturbances; generalized pathological edema; oliguria; and certainly, convulsions or pulmonary edema. Laboratory abnormalities that support the diagnosis include increasing serum creatinine, thrombocytopenia, or appreciable serum hepatic transaminase elevations.

Some women with chronic hypertension have a worsening during pregnancy with no other findings of superimposed preeclampsia. This is most common near the end of the second trimester. In the absence of other supporting criteria for superimposed preeclampsia, including normal fetal growth and amnionic fluid volume, these women likely represent the higher end of the normal blood pressure curve shown in Figure 45–1. It is reasonable in such patients to either begin or increase the dose of antihypertensive therapy.

DELIVERY. The decision to effect delivery of women with chronic hypertension is viewed in the context of the clinical course, including severity of the underlying condition. In women with uncomplicated well-controlled chronic hypertension with an otherwise normal pregnancy course and with normal fetal growth and amnionic fluid volume, it is the practice at our institutions to await labor at term. In women with complications or in whom fetal testing becomes abnormal, or both, induction is considered. Thus, even markedly preterm pregnancies with superimposed severe preeclampsia or appreciable fetal growth restriction or abruptio placentae will prompt delivery. Special consideration for delivery of women with multifetal gestation and chronic hypertension is also warranted, and delivery is usually initiated prior to term. Women with a multifetal gestation and preeclampsia have greater incidence of adverse outcomes, including placental abruption and poor neonatal outcomes, than do those with singleton pregnancy and preeclampsia (Sibai and colleagues, 2000).

In general, vaginal delivery is usually attempted. This includes women with severe aggravated hypertension or superimposed preeclampsia. Most women, including those with preterm severe superimposed preeclampsia, can be induced successfully and have vaginal delivery (Alexander and colleagues, 1999; Atkinson and associates, 1995). Epidural analgesia for labor pain is appropriate in these women with chronic hypertension and superimposed preeclampsia. Lucas and colleagues (2001) randomized 738 women with pregnancy-induced hypertension to either epidural analgesia or to patient-controlled intravenous meperidine. Although more women assigned to epidural analgesia required ephedrine to correct hypertension (11 versus 0 percent) neonatal and maternal outcomes were similar. In a retrospective analysis of 327 women with severe hypertensive disease, Hogg and associates (1999) reported that epidural analgesia was safe in women with high-risk pregnancies complicated by superimposed severe preeclampsia. Hogg and co-workers (2000) reported preliminary data from a randomized trial of 105 women with severe preeclampsia. They found similar maternal and fetal outcomes in women assigned to epidural analgesia or to a patient-controlled intravenous analgesia (Table 45–7). Finally, Wallace and co-workers (1995) randomized 80 women with severe preeclampsia who were to undergo cesarean delivery. They were given either general anesthesia or epidural or spinal–epidural analgesia. Although a fourth of women in the latter two groups developed hypotension, neonatal outcomes were all good (Chap. 15, p. 379).

TABLE 45–7. Intrapartum Analgesia in 105 Women with Severe Preeclampsia

Outcome	Epidural (n = 53)	PCA Pump (n = 52)	P Value
Cesarean delivery (%)	9 (17)	6 (12)	.43
Maternal ephedrine (%)	5 (10)	0 (0)	.03
Neonatal naloxone (%)	5 (10)	28 (54)	.001
Average pain score[a]	4.2 ± 3.6	6.8 ± 2.7	.0001
Satisfaction score[b]	2.8 ± 1	2.2 ± 1	.01

PCA = patient controlled analgesia.
[a] 0 = none to 10 = worst possible.
[b] 1 = poor to 4 = excellent.
From Hogg and co-workers (2000), with permission.

POSTPARTUM CONSIDERATIONS. In many respects, postpartum observation and prevention and management of adverse complications are similar in women with severe chronic hypertension and those with severe preeclampsia–eclampsia. The development of cerebral edema, heart failure or pulmonary edema, or renal dysfunction is especially high within 24 to 36 hours following delivery (Benedetti and colleagues, 1980, 1985; Cunningham and associates, 1986; Sibai and co-workers, 1990b). Following delivery, maternal peripheral resistance may increase as early as 6 hours postpartum. Thus, left-ventricular workload is acutely increased and further aggravated at the same time that appreciable amounts of interstitial fluid are mobilized for excretion. Prompt treatment of severe hypertension, with or without diuretic therapy, is of great importance.

Many women with chronic hypertension and superimposed severe preeclampsia have contracted blood volumes compared with normal pregnant women (Pritchard and colleagues, 1984; Silver and associates, 1998). These women have marked vasoconstriction and, in general, have increased blood loss which may cause oliguria postpartum. It may be difficult and hazardous to attempt to maintain intravascular volume and renal perfusion solely with intravenous crystalloid or colloid solutions. In such women, blood transfusion may be necessary to maintain intravascular volume to ensure tissue perfusion.

REFERENCES

Alexander JM, Bloom SL, McIntire DD, Leveno KJ: Severe preeclampsia and the very low birth weight infant: Is induction of labor harmful? Obstet Gynecol 93:485, 1999

American College of Obstetricians and Gynecologists: Antepartum fetal surveillance. Practice Bulletin No. 9, October 1999

Ananth CV, Smulian JC, Vintzileos AM: Incidence of placental abruption in relation to cigarette smoking and hypertensive disorders during pregnancy: A meta-analysis of observational studies. Obstet Gynecol 93:622, 1999

Arias F, Zamora J: Antihypertensive treatment and pregnancy outcome in patients with mild chronic hypertension. Obstet Gynecol 53:489, 1979

Atkinson MW, Guinn D, Owen J, Hauth JC: Does magnesium sulfate affect the length of labor induction in women with pregnancy-associated hypertension? Am J Obstet Gynecol 173:1219, 1995

August P, Lindheimer MD: Chronic hypertension in pregnancy. In Lindheimer MD, Roberts JM, Cunningham FG (eds): Chesley's Hypertensive Disorders in Pregnancy, 2nd ed. Appleton & Lange, Stamford, CT, 1999, p 605

Ayala DE, Hermida RC, Mojón A, Fernandez JR, Silva I, Ucieda R, Iglesias M: Blood pressure variability during gestation in healthy and complicated pregnancies. Hypertension 30:611, 1997

Beaufils M, Uzan S, Donsimoni R, Colau JC: Prevention of preeclampsia by early antiplatelet therapy. Lancet 1:840, 1985

Benedetti TJ, Kates R, Williams V: Hemodynamic observations in severe preeclampsia complicated by pulmonary edema. Am J Obstet Gynecol 152:330, 1985

Benedetti TJ, Quilligan EJ: Cerebral edema in severe pregnancy-induced hypertension. Am J Obstet Gynecol 137:860, 1980

Brater DC: Diuretic therapy. N Engl J Med 339:387, 1998

Breart G, Rabarison Y, Plouin PF, Sureau C, Rumeau-Rouquette C: Risk of fetal growth retardation as a result of maternal hypertension: Preparation to a trial on antihypertensive drugs. Dev Pharmacol Ther 4:116, 1982

Butters L, Kennedy S, Rubin PC: Atenolol in essential hypertension during pregnancy. BMJ 301:587, 1990

Byaruhanga RN, Chipato T, Rusakaniko S: A randomized controlled trial of low-dose aspirin in women at risk from pre-eclampsia. Intl J Gynaecol Obstet 60:129, 1998

Caritis S, Sibai B, Hauth J, Lindheimer MD, Klebanoff M, Thom E, Van Dorsten P, Lando M, Paul R, Miodovnik M, Meis P, Thurnau G: Low-dose aspirin to prevent preeclampsia in women at high risk. N Engl J Med 338:701, 1998

Centers for Disease Control and Prevention: Hypertension among Mexican Americans—United States. 1982–1984 and 1988–1991. MMWR 44:635, 1995

Chesley LC: Superimposed preeclampsia or eclampsia. In Chesley LC (ed): Hypertensive Disorders in Pregnancy. New York, Appleton-Century-Crofts, 1978, pp 14, 302, 482

Chesley LC, Annitto JE, Cosgrove RA: Long-term follow-up study of eclamptic women: Sixth periodic report. Am J Obstet Gynecol 124:446, 1976

Cockburn J, Moar VA, Ounsted M, Redman CW: Final report of study on hypertension during pregnancy: The effects of specific treatment on the growth and development of the children. Lancet 1:647, 1982

Collins R, MacMahon S: Blood pressure, antihypertensive drug treatment and the risks of stroke and of coronary heart disease. Br Med Bull 50:272, 1994

Cunningham FG, Cox SM, Harstad TW, Mason RA, Pritchard JA: Chronic renal disease and pregnancy outcome. Am J Obstet Gynecol 163:453, 1990

Cunningham FG, Lowe TW: Cardiovascular diseases complicating pregnancy. In Williams Obstetrics, 18th ed (Suppl 14). Norwalk, CT, Appleton & Lange, 1991

Cunningham FG, Pritchard JA, Hankins GDN, Anderson PL, Lucas MK, Armstrong KF: Idiopathic cardiomyopathy or compounding cardiovascular events? Obstet Gynecol 67:157, 1986

ECPPA: Randomized trial of low dose aspirin for the prevention of maternal and fetal complications in high risk pregnant women. ECPPA (Estudo Colaborativo para Prevencao da Pre-eclampsia com Aspirina) Collaborative Group. Br J Obstet Gynaecol 103:39, 1996

Ferrer RL, Sibai BM, Mulrow CD, Chiquette E, Stevens KR, Cornell J: Management of mild chronic hypertension during pregnancy: A review. Obstet Gynecol 96:849, 2000

Gruppo di Studio Ipertensione in Gravidanza: Nifedipine versus expectant management in mild to moderate hypertension in pregnancy. Br J Obstet Gynaecol 105:718, 1998

Gueyffier F, Boutitie F, Boissel JP, Pocock S, Coope J, Cutler J, Ekbom T, Fagard R, Friedman L, Perry M, Prineas R, Schron E: Effect of antihypertensive drug treatment on cardiovascular outcomes in women and men. A meta-analysis of individual patient data from randomized controlled trials. The INDANA Investigators. Ann Intern Med 126:761, 1997

Haddad B, Sibai BM: Chronic hypertension in pregnancy. Ann Med 31:246, 1999

Hauth JC, Goldenberg RL, Parker CR Jr, Cutter GR, Cliver SP: Low-dose aspirin: Lack of association with an increase in abruptio placentae or perinatal mortality. Obstet Gynecol 85:1055, 1995 (Notice of correction 87:931, 1996)

Hauth JC, Sibai B, Caritis S, Van Dorsten P, Lindheimer M, Klebanoff M, MacPherson C, Landon M, Paul R, Miodovnik M, Meis P, Dombrowski M, Thurnau G, Walsh S, McNellis D, Roberts JM: Maternal serum thromboxane B$_2$ concentrations do not predict improved outcomes in high risk pregnancies in a low-dose aspirin trial. Am J Obstet Gynecol 179:1193, 1998

Hogg B, Hauth JC, Caritis SN, Sibai BM, Lindheimer M, Van Dorsten JP, Klebanoff M, MacPherson C, Landon M, Paul R, Miodovnik M, Meis PJ, Thurnau GR, Dombrowski MP, McNellis D, Roberts JM: Safety of labor epidural anesthesia for women with severe hypertensive disease. Am J Obstet Gynecol 181:1096, 1999

Hogg B, Owen J, Shih G, et al: A randomized trial of intrapartum analgesia in women with severe preeclampsia. Am J Obstet Gynecol 182:S148, 2000

Hou S: Pregnancy in chronic renal insufficiency and end-stage renal disease. Am J Kidney Dis 33:235, 1999

Jain L: Effect of pregnancy-induced and chronic hypertension on pregnancy outcome. J Perinatol 17:425, 1997

Joint National Committee: Sixth report of the Joint National Committee on prevention, detection, evaluation, and treatment of high blood pressure. Arch Intern Med 157:2413, 1997

Jones DC, Hayslett JP: Outcome of pregnancy in women with moderate or severe renal insufficiency. N Engl J Med 335:226, 1996

Leather HM, Humphreys DM, Baker P, Chadd MA: A controlled trial of hypotensive agents in hypertension in pregnancy. Lancet 2:488, 1968

Lucas MK, Sharma S, McIntire D, Sidawi JE, Ramin SM, Leveno KJ, Cunningham FG: A randomized trial of the effects of epidural analgesia on pregnancy-induced hypertension. Obstet Gynecol 2001 (in press)

Lydakis C, Lip GYH, Beevers M, Beevers DG: Atenolol and fetal growth in pregnancies complicated by hypertension. Am J Hypertension 12:541, 1999

Mabie WC, Pernoll ML, Biswas MK: Chronic hypertension in pregnancy. Obstet Gynecol 67:197, 1986

McCowan LME, Buist RG, North RA, Gamble G: Perinatal morbidity in chronic hypertension. Br J Obstet Gynaecol 103:123, 1996

Meis PJ, Goldenberg RL, Mercer BM, Iams JD, Moawad AH, Miodovnik M, Menard MK, Caritis SN, Thuranu GR, Bottoms SF, Das A, Roberts JM, McNellis D: The preterm prediction study: Risk factors for indicated preterm births. Am J Obstet Gynecol 178:562, 1998

Montan S, Anandakumar C, Arulkeurnaran S, Ingemarsson I, Ratnam SS: Effects of methyldopa on uteroplacental and fetal hemodynamics in pregnancy-induced hypertension. Am J Obstet Gynecol 168:152, 1993

Montan S, Ingemarsson I: Intrapartum fetal heart rate patterns in pregnancies complicated by hypertension. Am J Obstet Gynecol 160, 283, 1989

Montan S, Ingemarsson I: Marsal K, Sjoberg N: Randomized controlled trial of atenolol and pindolol in human pregnancy: Effects on fetal hemodynamics. BMJ 304:946, 1992

Mulrow CD, Chiquette E, Ferrer RL, Sibai BM, Stevens KR, Harris M, Montgomery KA, Stamm K: Evidence Report/ Technology Assessment No. 14 (Prepared by the San Antonio Evidence-based Practice Center based at the University of Texas Health Science Center at San Antonio under contract no. 2909-97-0012). AHRQ publication No. 00-E011. Rockville, MD: Agency for Healthcare Research and Quality. August 2000

Ounsted M, Cockburn J, Moar VA, Redman CW: Maternal hypertension with superimposed preeclampsia: Effects on child development at 7 years. Br J Obstet Gynaecol 90:644, 1983

Owen J, Hauth JC, Williams G, Davis RO, Goldenberg RL, Brumfield CG: A comparison of perinatal outcome in patients undergoing contraction stress testing performed by nipple stimulation versus spontaneously occurring contractions. Am J Obstet Gynecol 160:1081, 1989

Pahor M, Psaty BM, Alderman MH, Applegate WB, Williamson JD, Cavazzini C, Furberg CD: Health outcomes associated with calcium antagonists compared with other first-line antihypertensive therapies: A meta-analysis of randomised controlled trials. Lancet 356:1949, 2000

Pritchard JA, Cunningham G, Pritchard SA: The Parkland Memorial Hospital protocol for treatment of eclampsia: Evaluation of 245 cases. Am J Obstet Gynecol 148:951, 1984

Redman CWG: Controlled trials of treatment of hypertension during pregnancy. Obstet Gynecol Surv 37:523, 1982

Redman CWG: Treatment of hypertension in pregnancy. Kidney Int 18:267, 1980

Redman CWG: Fetal outcome in trial of antihypertensive treatment in pregnancy. Lancet 2:753, 1976

Rey E: Effects of methyldopa on umbilical and placental artery blood flow velocity waveforms. Obstet Gynecol 80:783, 1992

Rey E, Couturier A: The prognosis of pregnancy in women with chronic hypertension. Am J Obstet Gynecol 171:410, 1994

Rubin PC, Butters L, Clark DM, Reynolds B, Sumner DJ, Steedman D, Low RA, Reid JL: Placebo-controlled trial of atenolol in treatment of pregnancy-associated hypertension. Lancet 1:431, 1983

Scardo JA, Vermillion ST, Newman RB, Chauhan SP, Hogg BB: A randomized, double-blind, hemodynamic evaluation of nifedipine and labetalol in preeclamptic hypertensive emergencies. Am J Obstet Gynecol 181:862, 1999

Sibai BM: Diagnosis and management of chronic hypertension in pregnancy. Obstet Gynecol 78:451, 1991

Sibai BM, Abdella TN, Anderson GD: Pregnancy outcome in 211 patients with mild chronic hypertension. Obstet Gynecol 61:571, 1983

Sibai BM, Anderson GD: Pregnancy outcome of intensive therapy in severe hypertension in first trimester. Obstet Gynecol 67:517, 1986a

Sibai BM, El-Nazer A, Gonzalez-Ruiz A: Severe preeclampsia–eclampsia in young primigravid women: Subsequent pregnancy outcome and remote prognosis. Am J Obstet Gynecol 155:1011, 1986b

Sibai BM, Hauth J, Caritis S, Lindheimer MD, MacPherson C, Klebanoff M, Van Dorsten JP, Landon M, Miodovnik M, Paul R, Meis P, Thurnau G, Dombrowski M, Roberts J, McNellis D: Hypertensive disorders in twin versus singleton pregnancies. Am J Obstet Gynecol 182:938, 2000

Sibai BM, Lindheimer M, Hauth JC, Caritis S, Van Dorsten P, Klebanoff M, MacPherson C, Landon M, Miodovnik M, Paul R, Meis P, Dombrowski M: Risk factors for preeclampsia, abruptio placentae, and adverse neonatal outcomes among women with chronic hypertension. N Engl J Med 339:667, 1998

Sibai BM, Mabie WC, Shamsa F, Villar MA, Anderson GD: A comparison of no medication versus methyldopa or labetalol in chronic hypertension during pregnancy. Am J Obstet Gynecol 162:960, 1990a

Sibai BM, Mercer B, Sarinoglu C: Severe preeclampsia in the second trimester: Recurrence risk and long-term prognosis. Am J Obstet Gynecol 165:1408, 1991

Sibai BM, Sarinoglu C, Mercer BM: Eclampsia, VII. Pregnancy outcome after eclampsia and long-term prognosis. Am J Obstet Gynecol 166:1757, 1992

Sibai BM, Villar MA, Mabie BC: Acute renal failure in hypertensive disorders of pregnancy. Pregnancy outcome and remote prognosis in thirty-one consecutive cases. Am J Obstet Gynecol 162:777, 1990b

Silver HM, Seebeck M, Carlson R: Comparison of total blood volume in normal, preeclamptic, and nonproteinuric gestational hypertensive pregnancy by simultaneous measurement of red blood cell and plasma volumes. Am J Obstet Gynecol 179:87, 1998

Smith P, Anthony J, Johanson R: Nifedipine in pregnancy. Br J Obstet Gynaecol 107:299, 2000

Uzan S, Beaufils M, Breart G, Bazin B, Capitant C, Paris J: Prevention of fetal growth retardation with low-dose aspirin: Findings of the EPREDA trial. Lancet 337:1427, 1991

Vermillion ST, Scardo JA, Newman RB: A randomized, double-blind trial of oral nifedipine and intravenous labetalol in hypertensive emergencies of pregnancy. Am J Obstet Gynecol 181:858, 1999

von Dadelszen P, Ornstein MP, Bull SB, Logan AG, Koren G, Magee LA: Fall in mean arterial pressure and fetal growth restriction in pregnancy hypertension: A meta-analysis. Lancet 355:87, 2000

Walker JJ, Bonduelle M, Greer I: Antihypertensive therapy in pregnancy. Lancet 1:932, 1983

Wallace DH, Leveno KJ, Cunningham FG, Giesecke AH, Sherer VE, Sidawi JE: Randomized comparison of general and regional anesthesia for cesarean delivery in pregnancies complicated by severe preeclampsia. Obstet Gynecol 86:193, 1995

Williams GH: Hypertensive vascular disease. In Fauci AS, Braunwald E, Isselbacher KJ, et al (eds): Harrison's Principles of Internal Medicine, 14th ed. New York, McGraw-Hill, 1998, p 1390

Working Group Report on High Blood Pressure in Pregnancy. National Institute of Health. NIH Publication No. 00-3029, 2000

46

Pulmonary Disorders

During pregnancy, there are a number of important adaptations of the respiratory system and changes in pulmonary function. Physiologically these changes are necessary so that the increased oxygen demands of the hyperdynamic circulation and the fetus can be satisfied. There is no evidence that pulmonary function is impaired because of pregnancy, but inferential data suggest that advanced pregnancy may intensify the pathophysiological effects of many acute and chronic lung diseases. An example for acute disease is the disparate number of adult deaths in pregnant women that were observed during the influenza pandemics of 1918 to 1919 and 1957 to 1958. An example for chronic disease is the poor tolerance to pregnancy of women with severe chronic lung disease and especially cor pulmonale.

From 1 to 4 percent of pregnancies are complicated by asthma. During winter months, both viral as well as bacterial pneumonitis are frequent in young adults. Tuberculosis is more frequent now than it has been in many years and, more worrisome, mycobacterial infections are becoming resistant to contemporaneous tuberculostatic medications. Finally, a number of chronic pulmonary disorders—albeit uncommon—may precede pregnancy and present special management problems.

PULMONARY PHYSIOLOGY

The important and sometimes marked changes in the respiratory system induced by pregnancy are discussed in detail in Chapter 8 (p. 185). Because of their importance to the clinical approach of lung disease complicating pregnancy, some of these are now reiterated. There are four lung volumes and four lung capacities that are used commonly to describe pulmonary physiology. Except for residual volume and lung capacities derived therefrom, these can be measured using direct spirometric techniques. The physiological changes induced by pregnancy have been summarized by de Swiet (1991):

1. **Vital capacity** may be increased by 100 to 200 mL.
2. **Inspiratory capacity** increases by about 300 mL by late pregnancy.
3. **Expiratory reserve volume** decreases from a total of 1300 mL to about 1100 mL.
4. **Residual volume** decreases from a total of 1500 mL to about 1200 mL.
5. **Functional residual capacity,** the sum of expiratory reserve and residual volumes, is reduced considerably, by about 500 mL.
6. **Tidal volume** increases considerably from about 500 to 700 mL.
7. **Minute ventilation** increases 40 percent, from 7.5 L to a total of 10.5 L/min; this is primarily due to increased tidal volume because the respiratory rate is unchanged.

The sum of these changes is substantively increased ventilation due to deeper but not more frequent breathing. Presumably these changes are induced to help supply increased basal oxygen consumption, which increases incrementally by 20 to 40 mL/min in the second half of pregnancy. As a result, arterial P_{O_2} falls very slightly, P_{CO_2} averages 28 mm Hg, plasma pH is slightly alkalotic at 7.45, and bicarbonate decreases to about 20 mEq/L.

DYSPNEA DURING PREGNANCY. Pregnant women are frequently aware of the need to breathe. The common complaint of "shortness of breath" is not associated with exercise, and frequently is worse when the woman is sitting down. Milne and associates (1978) reported that about half of women notice dyspnea at rest by midpregnancy, and three fourths complained of this by 31 weeks. Although its exact mechanisms are unclear, dyspnea has been attributed to alveolar hyperventilation and a response to substantively decreased P_{CO_2}, as well as a consequence of normal anatomical changes in the thorax.

PNEUMONIA

According to the National Center for Health Statistics (Hoyert and colleagues, 1998), in the United States in 1997, pneumonia and influenza were the tenth leading cause of death in persons aged 25 to 44 years. Mortality from community-acquired pneumonia may be as high as 5 percent in the elderly and chronically ill; however, in young and healthy women the rate is much less.

Pneumonia is inflammation affecting the lung parenchyma distal to the larger airways and involving the respiratory bronchioles and alveolar units. Bronchopneumonia refers to patchy and diffuse areas of involvement, and at least implies a less severe form of pneumonitis because there is no consolidation seen radiographically. Pneumonitis causing an appreciable loss of ventilatory capacity is tolerated less well by women during pregnancy. This generalization seems to hold true regardless of the etiology of the pneumonia. Moreover, hypoxemia and acidosis are poorly tolerated by the fetus, and they frequently lead to preterm labor after midpregnancy. Because many cases of pneumonia follow common viral upper respiratory illnesses, worsening or persistence of symptoms should prompt consideration for the diagnosis of pulmonary parenchymal infection. **Any pregnant woman suspected of having pneumonia should undergo anteroposterior and lateral chest radiography.**

BACTERIAL PNEUMONIA. Bacteria usually reach the lung by inhalation or by aspiration of nasopharyngeal secretions. Some bacterial organisms that cause community-acquired pneumonia, such as *Streptococcus pneumoniae,* are part of the normal resident flora. Viruses usually are not present in normal flora. There are a number of factors that can upset the symbiotic relationship between colonizing bacteria and the mucosal and phagocytic defenses of the nasopharynx and bronchial tree. For example, there may be acquisition of a new virulent and invasive strain, or infection may follow a viral infection. Importantly, cigarette smoking and chronic bronchitis favor colonization with *S pneumoniae, Haemophilus influenzae,* and *Legionella.* Other risk factors include smoking, asthma, binge drinking, and human immunodeficiency virus (HIV) infection (Munn and colleagues, 1999; Yost and associates, 2000).

INCIDENCE AND CAUSES. According to Bartlett and Mundy (1995), the attack rate for all adults is 12 per 1000. It is much lower for young healthy women, and over the 5-year period from 1993 to 1997, the incidence of pneumonia complicating nearly 75,000 pregnancies at Parkland Hospital was about 1 in 600 (Yost and associates, 2000).

At least two thirds of adult pneumonias are bacterial, and *S pneumoniae* causes many of these. Brown and Lerner (1998) reviewed six studies totalling 1500 patients with community-acquired pneumonia. About a third were caused by *S pneumoniae* and in another third the etiological agent was not identified. Other common causes were *Mycoplasma pneumoniae, H influenzae,* and viruses, especially influenza A. *Chlamydia pneumoniae* likely is a significant cause of pneumonia during pregnancy as it is responsible for 5 to 10 percent of pneumonia in hospitalized adults (Bartlett and Mundy, 1995). *Legionella pneumophilia* occasionally causes outbreaks or sporadic cases in young adults, and it has been reported with pregnancy (Eisenberg and colleagues, 1997; Evenson, 1998). In one case, it was associated with septic shock (Tewari and co-workers, 1997). Gherman and associates (1995) described a 32-week pregnant woman in whom *Chlamydia psittaci* caused both pneumonia and fetal–placental infection.

DIAGNOSIS. Typical symptoms of pneumonia include productive cough, fever, chest pain, and dyspnea. Mild upper respiratory symptoms and malaise usually precede these symptoms. There usually is mild leukocytosis. Chest x-ray is essential for diagnosis, although its appearance does not accurately predict the etiology (Fig. 46–1).

As discussed, the responsible pathogen is identified in perhaps only half of cases. Although some recommend examination of Gram-stained sputum to search for pneumococci or possibly staphylococci, the American Thoracic Society (1993) stresses that its sensitivity and

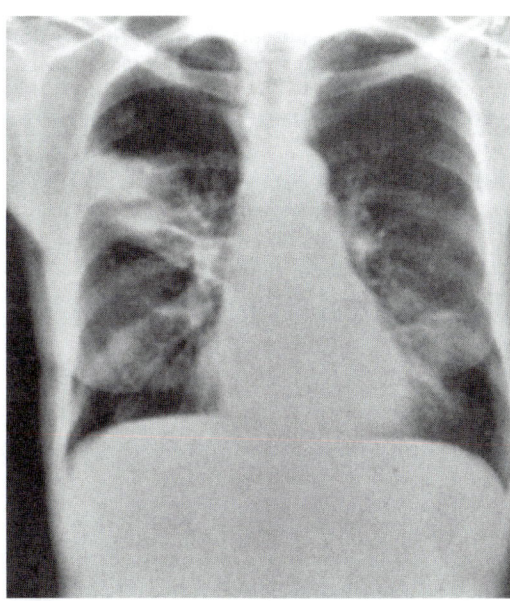

FIGURE 46–1. Posteroanterior chest radiograph shows right lobar pneumonia caused by pneumococcal infection. (From Bennett, 1994, with permission.)

specificity vary widely. Likewise, although routine sputum cultures often demonstrate pathogenic organisms, they too have poor predictability. Bartlett and Mundy (1995) reported that half of sputum samples show likely pathogens. Invasive techniques such as transtracheal aspiration are seldom indicated. Serological testing and cold agglutinin measurements are not routinely recommended. Finally, there are no currently available tests for bacterial antigens that are useful in evaluation of most of these patients.

MANAGEMENT. According to the American Thoracic Society (1993), the decision for hospitalization is perhaps the single most important decision for management of community-acquired pneumonia. Although it is the policy at Parkland Hospital to hospitalize all pregnant women with radiographically confirmed pneumonia, this is probably not necessary with appropriate home health care. At the least, risk factors—especially if multiple—that are shown in Table 46–1 should prompt consideration for hospitalization. Initial hospitalization can serve to allow close observation for the first day or so to be sure that infection is responsive to therapy. Pneumonia is a common cause if acute respiratory distress syndrome (Ware and Matthay, 2000). In some pregnant women, respiratory failure requires assisted ventilation (Chap. 43, p. 1164).

Because of factors cited, antimicrobial treatment must be empirical. Given that the majority of adult pneumonias are caused by pneumococci, mycoplasmas, or chlamydia, erythromycin therapy is the logical choice

TABLE 46–1. Factors That Increase the Risk of Death or Complications with Community-acquired Pneumonia

Coexisting Conditions

Chronic lung disease, diabetes, renal failure, heart failure, chronic liver disease, postsplenectomy states, neurological disease, neoplastic disease, or chronic alcohol abuse

Previous Hospitalization within 1 Year

Suspicion of aspiration

Altered mental states

Physical Findings

Respiratory rate > 30/min, hypotension, hypothermia or temperature > 38.3°C (101°F)

Extrapulmonary disease, or confusion

Laboratory Findings

Leukopenia (< 4000/μL), P_{O_2} 60 mm Hg or CO_2 retention, bacteremia, elevated serum creatinine, anemia, or evidence for sepsis or organ dysfunction

Radiological Findings

More than 1-lobe involvement, cavitation, rapid spreading, or pleural effusion

Modified from the American Thoracic Society (1993) and Fine and colleagues (1996).

in the uncomplicated case (American Thoracic Society, 1993). The usual dose is 500 to 1000 mg every 6 hours, and this can be given intravenously, at least initially. Yost and colleagues (2000) reported that erythromycin monotherapy was effective in all but one of 99 pregnant women hospitalized with uncomplicated pneumonia. The newer erythromycin analogs are acceptable.

For women with the complications listed in Table 46–1, or in those in whom staphylococcal or *Haemophilus* pneumonia is suspected, then cefotaxime, ceftizoxime, or cefuroxime is given instead. A β-lactam antimicrobial with a β-lactamase inhibitor is also suitable. Erythromycin added to either of these latter two regimens is recommended by some clinicians, and this is our practice at Parkland Hospital (Yost and associates, 2000). Of concern is the emergence of pneumococcal resistance. The Centers for Disease Control and Prevention (1999a) performed sentinel surveillance and found that 25 percent of strains were resistant to penicillin in 1997 compared with 14 percent for 1993–1994. Multidrug resistance is about 10 percent (Whitney and co-workers, 2000). Recently, the Food and Drug Administration (2000) has approved *levofloxacin* for treatment of adults with penicillin-resistant pneumococcal pneumonia. The drug is a fluoroquinolone and is classified as category C (Briggs and colleagues, 1998).

Clinical improvement is usually evident by 48 to 72 hours. Fever typically lasts 2 to 4 days. If fever persists, follow-up radiography should be considered. It is common for radiographic findings to worsen initially, and there may be progression of infiltrates or development of a pleural effusion. About 20 percent of cases of pneumococcal pneumonia have associated effusion; however, with mild clinical disease that is improving, such findings are inconsequential. Conversely, radiographic deterioration in the setting of *severe* community-acquired pneumonia is a poor prognostic feature and highly predictive of mortality.

PREVENTION. Pneumococcal vaccine has been shown to be 60 to 70 percent protective against the 23 vaccine-related serotypes. Its use may help decrease emergence of drug-resistant pneumococci. The vaccine is not given to otherwise healthy pregnant women. It is recommended by the Advisory Committee on Immunization Practices (1997) for immunocompromised adults including those with HIV infection. It is also given to those who have underlying diabetes, or cardiac, pulmonary, or renal disease. Another example is the pregnant woman with asplenia, for example, sickle-cell disease, who is especially susceptible to these infections.

EFFECT OF PNEUMONIA ON PREGNANCY. There is no doubt that maternal mortality from pneumonia was considerable during the preantibiotic era. In 1939, Finland and Dublin reported a 32 percent maternal mortality rate in 212 women. Since then, an overall downward trend in maternal and fetal morbidity and mortality has been emphasized. In five recent studies shown in Table 46–2, the overall maternal (1.6 percent) and perinatal (2.2 percent) mortality rates are still formidable. Preterm birth rates are increased over baseline. Importantly, 7 percent of these 323 women required intubation. These outcomes underscore the severity of pneumonia and also serve to emphasize the need for prompt diagnosis, close observation, and effective treatment.

VIRAL PNEUMONIA

INFLUENZA PNEUMONIA. Influenza is an acute respiratory infection caused by viruses of the *Orthomyxoviridae* family. Influenza A and B form one genus of these RNA viruses, and they are identified by nucleoprotein antigenic reactions. Some of their serological characteristics are reviewed in Chapter 56 (p. 1463). Outbreaks occur virtually every year, with global pandemics every 10 to 15 years. The virus is spread by aerosolized droplets and quickly infects ciliated columnar epithelium, alveolar cells, mucus gland cells, and macrophages. If uncomplicated, the usual clinical course is 2 to 5 days.

Influenza A is more serious than type B, and it is epidemic in the winter months. The onset of epidemics vary

TABLE 46-2. Maternal and Perinatal Outcomes with Pneumonia Complicating 317 Pregnancies

Series	Incidence	Adverse Maternal Outcomes	Adverse Perinatal Outcomes
Berkowitz and LaSala (1990) (n = 26)	1:275	2 intubations No deaths	No preterm births No perinatal deaths
Richey et al (1994) (n = 71)	1:850	5 intubations 2 deaths	1 preterm birth 4 stillbirths
Briggs et al (1996) (n = 34)		7 intubations 2 deaths	1 neonatal death 1 stillbirth
Munn et al (1997) (n = 59)	1:525	6 intubations 1 death	13 preterm births 20 low-birthweight
Yost et al (2000) (n = 133)	1:700	2 intubations No deaths	1 stillbirth 14 preterm births
Total (n = 323)		7% intubated 1.6% mortality rate	2.2% perinatal mortality

Expanded from Bloom and colleagues (1997).

annually as do their duration and peak periods (Centers for Disease Control and Prevention, 2000b). In most healthy adults, infection is self-limited, but pneumonia is the most common complication. Clinically, it is difficult to distinguish from bacterial pneumonia, especially infection caused by pneumococci. Primary pneumonitis is the most severe form, and it is characterized by sparse sputum production and radiographic interstitial infiltrates (Fig. 46-2). Secondary bacterial pneumonia is more common and usually is caused by streptococci or staphylo-

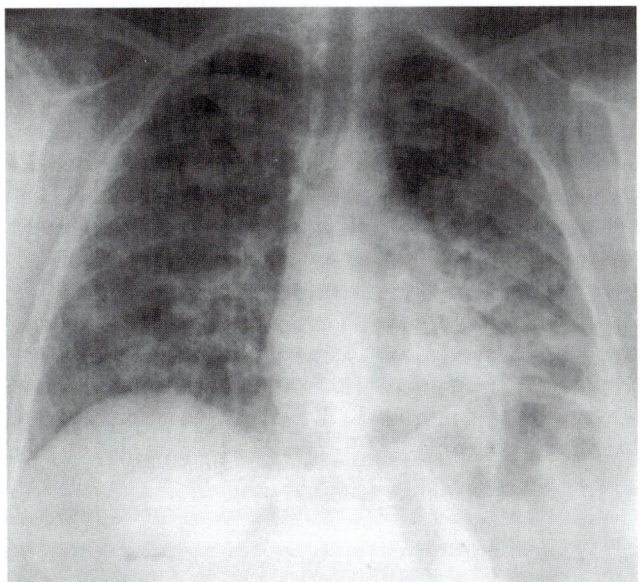

FIGURE 46-2. Chest radiograph taken at admission in a 27-week pregnant woman with presumed viral pneumonia. Diffuse infiltrates are seen. These worsened and she died a week later. (Richey and associates, 1994, with permission.)

cocci. Secondary infection usually manifests after 2 to 3 days of clinical improvement.

PREVENTION. For all of the previously discussed reasons, beginning in 1998, the Centers for Disease Control and Prevention (2000c) has recommended vaccination for all pregnant women after the first trimester. **Regardless of the stage of pregnancy, women who are at high risk because of underlying disease such as diabetes or heart disease should be vaccinated against influenza.** There is no evidence that influenza vaccine is teratogenic (Chap. 10, p. 240). Also, as Munoz and Englund (2000) indicated, some childhood protection against influenza will accrue.

TREATMENT. Generally, supportive treatment with antipyretics and bed rest is recommended for uncomplicated influenza (Apuzzio, 1999). The first class of drugs that has been available since 1976 for influenza treatment block ion-channel activity of viral M2 protein. **Amantadine** or **rimantadine,** 200 mg daily, are effective in reducing severity of infection if begun within 48 hours of symptoms. These may also be given prophylactically to high-risk nonimmunized exposed women and will prevent 50 to 90 percent of clinical infections (Couch, 2000). Both drugs are category C and while teratogenic in high doses given to animals, it is unclear if they are teratogenic to humans (Briggs and colleagues, 1998). Thus, after the first trimester, consideration should be given to their use depending on the clinical situation.

A new class of antiviral drugs—**neuraminidase inhibitors**—are highly effective to treat early influenza in adults (Centers for Disease Control and Prevention, 1999d, 2000c; Gubareva and associates, 2000). **Oseltami-**

vir for oral use and **zanamivir** by inhalation were approved in 1999. Neither drug is approved for use in children or pregnant women. When given to nonpregnant patients for long-term prophylaxis, oseltamivir was 80 to 85 percent effective in preventing symptomatic influenza (Hayden and colleagues, 1999). Inhaled zanamivir has been found effective for early treatment and prevention of complications in high-risk nonpregnant patients (MIST Study Group, 1998).

EFFECTS ON PREGNANCY. In the influenza pandemic of 1918–1919, pneumonia was a grave complication of pregnancy (Cox and Subbarao, 1999). In a study of 1350 cases, Harris (1919) reported a maternal mortality rate of 27 percent, which increased to 50 percent when pneumonia developed. The 1957–1958 pandemic was also severe, and half of childbearing-age women who died of influenza in Minnesota were pregnant (Freeman and Barno, 1959). Fortunately, during the last decade mortality rates have been substantially reduced. Despite this, Neuzil and colleagues (1998) reported that hospitalization for influenza was increased fivefold in third-trimester women compared with nonpregnant controls.

Irving and colleagues (2000) found no evidence of transplacental infection in 138 cord samples from pregnancies with second- or third-trimester influenza. Also, there is no firm evidence that the virus causes congenital malformations (Apuzzio, 1999). Saxén and associates (1990) identified no association between first-trimester influenza in 248 mothers of anencephalic fetuses. Conversely, in a case-control study, Lynberg and associates (1994) found a threefold risk of neural-tube defects if there was maternal influenza early in pregnancy. These may be related to associated hyperthermia (Kashyap and Gruslin, 2000).

Schizophrenia is more common in individuals born in late winter and early spring. Although some have provided epidemiological evidence that midpregnancy fetal exposure to influenza A increases the risks for schizophrenia, McGrath and Castle (1995), as well as Kashyap and Gruslin (2000), concluded from their reviews that the association is weak (Chap. 53, p. 1420).

VARICELLA PNEUMONIA. Varicella-zoster virus is a member of the DNA herpesvirus family, and almost 95 percent of adults are immune (Glantz and Mushlin, 1998). Primary infection causes **chickenpox,** which has an attack rate of 90 percent in seronegative individuals. In the healthy patient, the typical maculopapular and vesicular rash is accompanied by constitutional symptoms and fever for 3 to 5 days.

Although secondary skin infection with streptococci or staphylococci is the most common complication of chickenpox, varicella pneumonia is the most serious. It develops in about 10 percent of adults (Nathwani and colleagues, 1998). It usually appears 3 to 5 days into the course of the illness and is characterized by tachypnea, a dry cough, dyspnea, fever, and pleuritic chest pain. Chest x-ray discloses characteristic nodular infiltrates and interstitial pneumonitis (Fig. 46–3). In fatal cases, the lungs show scattered areas of necrosis and hemorrhage. Although resolution of pneumonitis parallels that of the skin lesions, fever and compromised pulmonary function may persist for weeks.

PREGNANCY. There is no convincing evidence that pregnant women are more likely to develop pneumonitis (Nathwani and associates, 1998). Although, retrospective studies cited disparate mortality in pregnancy, more recent descriptive studies indicate a mortality rate similar to nonpregnant persons. Still, this is about 10 percent, which makes the disease quite formidable. Paryani and Arvin (1986) reported that 4 of 43 pregnant women with chickenpox developed pneumonia, and one of the two who required ventilatory support died.

Serious infection with sepsis or pneumonia is associated with preterm delivery. If infection develops before 20 weeks, the fetus can be infected and permanent sequela may result (Chap. 56, p. 1464).

MANAGEMENT. Although its efficacy has yet to be proved, most authors recommend treatment for varicella pneumonitis with intravenous acyclovir, 10 mg/kg every 8 hours. In one retrospective study, nonpregnant patients with pneumonia who were given acyclovir within 36 hours of admission had improved oxygenation by the sixth day compared with untreated controls (Haake and co-workers, 1990). Smego and Asperilla

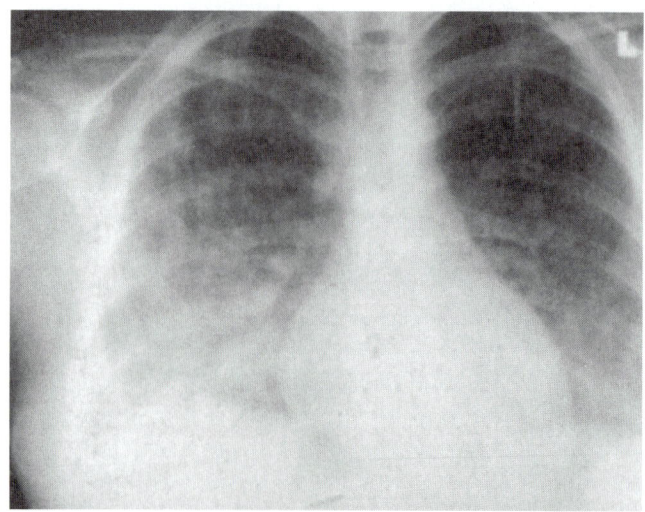

FIGURE 46–3. Varicella pneumonia with typical radiographic changes of diffuse, nodular peribronchial infiltrates. (From Chapman and Duff, 1993, with permission.)

(1991) reviewed acyclovir treatment for varicella pneumonia and found an average 15 percent maternal mortality rate.

PROPHYLAXIS. Administration of **varicella-zoster immunoglobulin** (**VZIG**) will either prevent or attenuate varicella infection in exposed susceptible individuals if given within 96 hours. The dose is 125 units per 10 kg given intramuscularly with a maximum dose of 625 units or 5 vials. Immunoglobulin is recommended by the Centers for Disease Control (1984) for immunocompromised susceptible adults who are exposed. Because of the severity of varicella during pregnancy, some clinicians recommend immunoglobulin administration for otherwise healthy but seronegative pregnant women (Chapman, 1998; Chapman and Duff, 1993). Up to 80 to 90 percent of adults are immune from prior symptomatic or asymptomatic infection; thus antibody testing with enzyme-linked immunosorbent assay (ELISA) or fluorescent antibody to membrane antigen (FAMA) should be done, if possible, prior to immune globulin therapy (Rouse and associates, 1996). Demonstration of antibodies by complement fixation indicates relatively recent infection. A rising complement-fixation titer is evidence for current or very recent disease.

PREVENTION. An attenuated varicella live-virus vaccine (Varivax) was licensed in 1995 by the Food and Drug Administration. It is recommended as one 0.5-mL dose for children 12 months to 12 years of age. For susceptible adults, two doses, 4 to 8 weeks apart, are recommended. Glantz and Mushlin (1998) concluded that routine prenatal serological testing of women with a negative varicella history is not cost-effective.

The vaccine is contraindicated in pregnancy. The vaccine virus can infect the fetus, with the highest risk between 13 and 20 weeks (Stallings, 2000). Huang and colleagues (1999) described a woman at term who ostensibly developed acute varicella after exposure to her two children who had been vaccinated 8 days previously. The manufacturer, Merck & Co., Inc. (West Point, Pennsylvania, 800-986-8999), has established a registry to follow outcomes when women are vaccinated within 3 months before pregnancy or at any time during pregnancy (Centers for Disease Control and Prevention, 1996).

FUNGAL AND PARASITIC PNEUMONIA. Fungal and parasitic pulmonary infections are usually of greatest consequence in the immunocompromised host, especially the woman with acquired immunodeficiency syndrome (AIDS).

PNEUMOCYSTIS PNEUMONIA. The most common infectious complication in women with AIDS is interstitial pneumonia caused by the parasite *Pneumocystis carinii.* Prior to the 1980s, this infection had last been prevalent during epidemics in World War II, when it was associated with opportunistic infection in malnourished individuals. In immunocompromised patients, this is a life-threatening infection, and since the AIDS epidemic began in the 1980s, it is a common complication (Chap. 57, p. 1493). Symptoms include dry cough, tachypnea, and dyspnea, and the characteristic radiographic finding is a diffuse infiltrate. Although the organism can be identified by sputum culture, bronchoscopy with lavage or biopsy may be necessary. Maternal mortality may be quite high, but this may represent bias for reporting severe cases (Saade, 1997).

Stratton and colleagues (1992) described 35 pregnant women with pneumocystis pneumonia enrolled in the AIDS Clinical Trials Centers. Treatment is with trimethoprim-sulfamethoxazole or pentamidine. Both drugs are category C. In some cases, tracheal intubation and mechanical ventilation may be required (Albino and Shapiro, 1994; Saade, 1997).

For some immunodeficiency virus–positive patients, the Centers for Disease Control (1999c) recommends prophylaxis against pneumocystis infection with once-daily double-strength oral trimethoprim-sulfamethoxazole. These include women with CD4+ T-lymphocyte counts less than $200/\mu$L, those with a history of oropharyngeal candidiasis, or those in whom CD4+ cells constitute less than 20 percent of lymphocytes.

FUNGAL PNEUMONIA. Any of a number of fungi can cause pneumonia during pregnancy. These are usually seen in women with HIV infection or those who are otherwise immunocompromised. Infections include histoplasmosis, coccidioidomycosis, cryptococcosis, and blastomycosis (Chap. 56, p. 1479). Their spores are found in soil, and although infection is common, it usually is mild and self-limited. Infection is characterized by cough and fever; only rarely is there dissemination.

Histoplasmosis and **blastomycosis** are not believed to be more common or more severe during pregnancy. Conversely, many have considered that **coccidioidomycosis** more commonly undergoes dissemination during pregnancy when compared with nonpregnant women (Stevens, 1995). This may be related to a stimulatory effect of the organism by estradiol-17β (Powell and associates, 1983). Wack and colleagues (1988) analyzed 10 cases among more than 47,000 pregnant women and concluded that the disease was rare. Arsura and associates (1998) reported 61 pregnant women with symptomatic infection. Half had associated *erythema nodosum,* which indicated a better overall prognosis. Most cases of **cryptococcal infection** reported during pregnancy are meningitis. Ely and co-workers (1998) described four otherwise healthy pregnant women who had cryptococccal pneumonia. Diagnosis is difficult because clinical presentation is similar to other community-acquired pneumonias.

Treatment of pregnant women with disseminated fungal infections has been successful using intravenous *amphotericin B* (category B) or *ketoconazole* (category C) (McGregor and associates, 1986; Wack and colleagues, 1988). Other anti-fungals effective against these infections include *flucytosine* and *fluconazole,* both category C (Briggs and colleagues, 1998).

ASTHMA

Asthma affects about 3 to 4 percent of the general population. The mortality rate from asthma ranges from 1 to 3 percent, and it causes nearly 5000 deaths annually in the United States. There are also long-term chronic sequelae that include reduced ventilatory function (Lange and colleagues, 1998). The National Asthma Education Program (1993) estimates that 1 to 4 percent of pregnancies are complicated by asthma. Status asthmaticus complicates about 0.2 percent of pregnancies (Mabie and associates, 1992).

PATHOPHYSIOLOGY. Asthma is a chronic inflammatory airway disorder with a major hereditary component. According to Lemanske and Busse (1997), increased airway responsiveness and inflammation have been linked to chromosomes 11q13 (high-affinity IgE receptor), 5q (cytokine gene cluster), and 14q (T-cell antigen receptor). There must also be an environmental stimulant in susceptible individuals. The hallmarks of asthma are reversible airway obstruction from bronchial smooth muscle contraction, mucus hypersecretion, and mucosal edema. There is airway inflammation and responsiveness to a number of stimuli, including irritants, viral infections, aspirin, cold air, and exercise. Mast cells and eosinophils are stimulated by stem-cell factor, cytokines, and kinases (Holgate, 1997). Mast-cell activation mediates bronchoconstriction by release of histamines, prostaglandin D_2, and leukotrienes. **Because**

F-series prostaglandins and ergonovine exacerbate asthma, these commonly used obstetrical drugs should be avoided if possible.

CLINICAL COURSE. Clinically, asthma represents a broad spectrum of illness ranging from mild wheezing to severe bronchoconstriction capable of causing respiratory failure, severe hypoxemia, and death. The functional result of acute bronchospasm is airway obstruction and decreased air flow. The work of breathing progressively increases and patients present with chest tightness, wheezing, or breathlessness. Subsequent alterations in oxygenation primarily reflect ventilation–perfusion mismatching as the distribution of airway narrowing is uneven.

The clinical stages of asthma are summarized in Table 46–3. With mild disease, hypoxia initially is well compensated by hyperventilation, as reflected by a normal arterial oxygen tension and decreased carbon dioxide tension with resultant respiratory alkalosis. As airway narrowing worsens, ventilation–perfusion defects increase and arterial hypoxemia ensues. With severe obstruction, ventilation becomes impaired sufficiently because of respiratory muscle fatigue to result in early CO_2 retention. Because of hyperventilation, this may only be seen initially as an arterial CO_2 tension returning to the normal range. Finally, with critical obstruction, respiratory failure follows, characterized by hypercapnia and acidemia.

Although these changes are generally reversible and well tolerated in the healthy nonpregnant individual, early stages of asthma may be dangerous to the pregnant woman and her fetus. The smaller functional residual capacity and the increased effective shunt render her more susceptible to develop hypoxia and hypoxemia.

EFFECTS OF PREGNANCY ON ASTHMA. There is no evidence that pregnancy has a predictable effect on underlying asthma. Schatz and colleagues (1988) prospectively studied both symptoms and spirometry measurements throughout pregnancy and the puerperium in 366 asthmatic women. They reported that about a third each

TABLE 46–3. Clinical Stages of Asthma

Stage	P_{O_2}	P_{CO_2}	pH	FEV$_1$ (% predicted)
Mild respiratory alkalosis	Normal	↓	↑	65–80
Respiratory alkalosis	↓	↓	↑	50–64
Danger zone	↓	Normal	Normal	35–49
	↓	↑	↓	< 35

Modified after Barth and Hankins (1991), with permission.

of these women improved, remained unchanged, or clearly worsened. In another prospective study of 198 pregnancies by Stenius-Aarniala and associates (1988), almost 40 percent of women required more intensive therapy for their asthma at some time during the pregnancy. **Thus, about one third of asthmatic women can expect worsening of disease at some time during pregnancy.**

Women beginning pregnancy with severe asthma are more likely to experience worsening disease than are those with mild disease. In about 60 percent of women, asthma behaves similarly with successive pregnancies. Although Schatz and colleagues (1988) reported a 10 percent asthma exacerbation during labor and delivery, Wendel and associates (1996) found this to be only 1 percent. Importantly, Mabie and associates (1992) reported an 18-fold increased risk of exacerbation following cesarean delivery compared with vaginal delivery.

EFFECTS OF ASTHMA ON PREGNANCY. Asthma, especially when severe, can affect pregnancy outcome substantively. Shown in Table 46–4 are maternal and perinatal outcomes in 3858 pregnancies complicated by asthma. In most studies, increased incidences of preeclampsia, preterm labor, low-birthweight infants, and perinatal mortality are noted. Although unproven, it seems logical that better perinatal outcomes would result from well-controlled asthma (Schatz, 1999). Maternal deaths may occur from **status asthmaticus.** Life-threatening complications include pneumothorax, pneumomediastinum, acute cor pulmonale, cardiac arrhythmias, and muscle fatigue with respiratory arrest. Mortality rates are substantively increased when asthma requires mechanical ventilation.

FETAL EFFECTS. Both animal and human studies are suggestive that maternal alkalosis may cause fetal hypoxemia well before maternal oxygenation is compromised (Rolston and associates, 1974). Fetal compromise is hypothesized to result from a combination of factors to include decreased uterine blood flow, decreased maternal venous return, and an alkaline-induced leftward shift of the oxyhemoglobin dissociation curve. Once the mother can no longer maintain normal oxygen tension and hypoxemia develops, the fetus responds with decreased umbilical blood flow, increased systemic and pulmonary vascular resistance, and finally decreased cardiac output. Realization that the fetus may be seriously compromised before maternal disease is severe underscores the need for aggressive management of all pregnant women with acute asthma. Monitoring the fetal response, in effect, becomes an indicator of maternal compromise.

CLINICAL EVALUATION. The subjective impression by the patient of the severity of asthma frequently does not correlate with objective measures of airway function or ventilation. Clinical examination also is inaccurate to predict severity, but useful signs include labored breathing, tachycardia, pulsus paradoxus, prolonged expiration, and use of accessory respiratory muscles. Signs of a potentially fatal attack include central cyanosis and altered level of consciousness.

Arterial blood gas analysis provides objective assessment of maternal oxygenation, ventilation, and acid–base status. With this information, the severity of an acute attack can be assessed (Table 46–3). In a prospective evaluation, however, Wendel and associates (1996) did not find routine blood gas analysis to help direct care in most pregnant women. In addition, care must be taken to interpret the results in relation to normal values for pregnancy. For example, a P_{CO_2} greater than 35 mm Hg with a pH less than 7.35 is consistent with hyperventilation and CO_2 retention in a pregnant woman.

TABLE 46–4. Maternal and Perinatal Outcomes of Pregnancies Complicated by Asthma

Study	No.	Perinatal Outcomes (%)			
		Pregnancy Hypertension	Growth Restriction	Preterm Delivery	Gestational Diabetes
Jana et al (1995)	182	18	NS	13	1.6
Schatz et al (1995)	486	10	6	4.8	1.2
Wendel et al (1996)	84	17	1	11	11
Alexander et al (1998)	817	~15	~5	~6	~
Demissie et al (1998)	2289	8	15	18	NS
Estimated average	3858	10.4	11.3	6.8	2.2

NS = not stated.

Pulmonary function testing has become routine in the management of chronic and acute asthma. Sequential measurements of the forced expiratory volume in one second (FEV$_1$) from maximum expiration is the single best measure to reflect severity of disease. The peak expiratory flow rate (PEFR) correlates well with the FEV$_1$, and it can be measured reliably with inexpensive portable peak flow meters. Brancazio and associates (1997) showed that the PEFR did not change over pregnancy in normal women. These two measurements are the most useful tests to monitor airway obstruction. An FEV$_1$ less than 1 L or less than 20 percent of predicted correlates with severe disease as manifest by hypoxia, poor response to therapy, and a high relapse rate (Noble and colleagues, 1988).

MANAGEMENT OF CHRONIC ASTHMA. According to the National Asthma Education Program (1993), effective management of asthma during pregnancy includes:

1. Objective assessment of pulmonary function and fetal well-being.

2. Avoidance or control of environmental precipitating factors.

3. Pharmacological therapy.

4. Patient education.

In general, women with moderate to severe asthma are instructed to measure and record PEFRs twice daily. Predicted values range from 380 to 550 L/min, and each woman has her own baseline value. Recommendations for therapy adjustments can be made using these measurements.

Outpatient treatment depends on the severity of disease. Shown in Tables 46–5 and 46–6 are drugs and suggested doses for home management of asthma in the pregnant woman. For mild asthma, *β*-agonists given by inhalation as needed are usually sufficient (Drazen and colleagues, 1996). **Inhaled corticosteroids** are the preferred treatment for persistent asthma (Lipworth, 1999; National Institutes of Health, 1997). Inhalations are administered every 3 to 4 hours as needed. The goal is to reduce the use of *β*-agonists for symptomatic relief. A case-control study from Canada with a cohort of over

TABLE 46–5. Long-term Control Medications for Asthma

Medication	Dose	Comments
Systemic corticosteroids		
Methylprednisolone	a. 7.5–60 mg PO daily or every other day	For long-term treatment of severe asthma
Prednisolone		
Prednisone	b. "Burst" of 40–60 mg PO daily for 3–10 days	Effective for initiating therapy or with gradual deterioration—use until 80% PEFR personal best, taper not necessary
Inhaled corticosteroids		
Beclomethasone		
42 μg/puff	4–20 puffs/day	Low-dose 4–12 puffs/day; High-dose 20+ puffs/day
84 μg/puff	2–10 puffs/day	Low-dose 2–6 puffs/day; High-dose 10+ puffs/day
Budesonide		
200 μg/dose	1–3+ inhalations/day	Low-dose 1–2 inhalations/day; High-dose 3+ inhalations/day
Triamcinolone		
100 μg/puff	4–20 puffs/day	Low-dose 4–10 puffs/day; High-dose 20+ puffs/day
Cromolyn		
MDI 1 mg/puff	2–4 puffs tid–qid	One dose prior to exercise or allergen exposure good for 1–2 hr
Nebulizer 20-mg solution	1 ampule tid–qid	
Theophylline	Starting dose 10 mg/kg/day with 300 mg maximum	Adjust dose for serum level 5–15 μg/mL
	Maintenance dose maximum is 800 mg/day	

MDI = metered-dose inhaler; PEFR = peak expiratory flow rate.
Modified from National Institutes of Health (1997).

TABLE 46-6. Adrenergic Drugs Used for Treatment of Asthma

Drug	Administration	Recommended Dosages
Short-acting		
Epinephrine (α, β_1, β_2)	Subcutaneous	0.3–0.5 mL of 1:1000 solution q 20 min × 3
	Inhaled	200–300 μg/puff; 1–2 puffs q 4 h
Isoetharine (β_2)	Inhaled	
	Metered dose	340 μg/puff; 3–7 puffs q 3–4 h
	Aerosolized	0.5 mL of 1% solution, diluted 1:3 with saline
Isoproterenol (β_1, β_2)	Inhaled	1:100 solution, 3–7 inhalations q 4–6 h
		1:200 solution, 5–15 inhalations q 4–6 h
	Intravenous	0.05–5 μg/min by infusion
Metaproterenol (β_2)	Inhaled	
	Metered dose	650 μg/puff; 2–3 puffs q 3–4 h
	Nebulizer	0.3 mL of 5% solution q 4 h
Terbutaline (β_2)	Subcutaneous	250 μg q 15 min × 3
	Oral	2.5 mg q 4–6 h
Long-acting		
Salmeterol inhaled	Metered	21 μg/puff; 2 puffs q 12 h
	Blister	50 μg/blister; 1 q 12 h
Albuterol SR	Oral	4 mg q 12 h

SR = sustained release.

15,600 nonpregnant asthmatics showed that inhaled corticosteroids reduced hospitalizations by 80 percent (Blais and associates, 1998). Wendel and colleagues (1996) reported a 55 percent reduction in readmissions for severe asthma exacerbations in pregnant women maintained on inhaled corticosteroids along with β-agonist therapy.

Cromolyn sodium (category B) and **nedocromil** inhibit mast-cell degranulation. They are ineffective for acute asthma and are taken chronically for prevention.

Theophylline is a methylxanthine, and its various salts are bronchodilators and possibly anti-inflammatory. Some of its derivatives are considered useful for oral maintenance therapy of outpatients who do not respond optimally to inhaled corticosteroids and β-agonists. Sustained-release theophylline preparations may also be helpful for use before bedtime in women with nocturnal symptoms.

Leukotriene modifiers are new drugs that inhibit leukotriene synthesis. Some examples include *zileuton, zafirinkast,* and *montelukast* (Medical Letter, 1999). Their pharmacology and mechanisms of action were reviewed recently by Drazen and colleagues (1999). They are given either orally or by inhalation for prevention and are not effective with acute disease. Their role in asthma treatment is currently unclear, and there is very little experience with their use in pregnancy.

MANAGEMENT OF ACUTE ASTHMA. Treatment of acute asthma during pregnancy is similar to that for the nonpregnant asthmatic. An exception is a significantly lowered threshold for hospitalization for the pregnant woman. Most will benefit from intravenous hydration to help clear pulmonary secretions. Supplemental oxygen is given by mask after a blood gas sample is obtained. The therapeutic aim is to maintain the P_{O_2} greater than 60 mm Hg, and preferably normal, along with 95 percent oxygen saturation. Baseline pulmonary function testing includes FEV_1 or PEFR. Continuous pulse oximetry and electronic fetal monitoring may provide useful information.

First-line pharmacological therapy of acute asthma includes use of a **β-adrenergic agonist,** either epinephrine, isoproterenol, terbutaline, albuterol, isoetharine, or metaproterenol (National Heart, Lung and Blood Institute, 1991; Nelson, 1995). The more commonly used short-acting agents, their dosages, and routes of administration are listed in Table 46–6. These drugs bind to specific cell-surface receptors and activate adenylyl cyclase, which increases intracellular cyclic AMP to modulate bronchial smooth muscle relaxation. They are given subcutaneously, by inhalation, or orally and are also used for maintenance therapy of outpatients. The long-acting preparations are used preferentially for maintenance.

It is now recommended that **corticosteroids** be given early to all patients in the course of severe acute asthma (National Heart, Lung and Blood Institute, 1991). Most recommended doses are probably higher than necessary. Still, in the United States, intravenous methylprednisolone, 40 to 60 mg, is usually given every 6 hours. Equipotent doses of hydrocortisone by infusion or prednisone orally can be given instead. **Because their onset of action is several hours, it is emphasized that steroids, whether given intravenously or by aerosol, are given along with β-agonists for treatment of acute asthma.**

Further management depends on the response to therapy. If initial therapy with β-agonists is associated with return of the PEFR to above 70 percent of baseline, then discharge is considered. Some women may benefit from 23-hour observation. Alternatively, for the woman with obvious respiratory distress or if the PEFR is less than 70 percent predicted after three doses of β-agonist, admission is advisable. She is given intensive therapy to include inhaled β-agonists, intravenous corticosteroids, and close observation for worsening respiratory distress or fatigue in breathing (Wendel and colleagues, 1996).

STATUS ASTHMATICUS AND RESPIRATORY FAILURE. Severe asthma of any type not responding after 30 to 60 minutes of intensive therapy is termed status asthmaticus. For nonpregnant patients with status asthmaticus, Braman and Kaemmerlen (1990) have shown that management in an intensive care unit will result in a good outcome in almost all cases. During pregnancy, consideration should be given to early intubation when the maternal respiratory status continues to decline despite aggressive treatment (see Table 46–3). Fatigue, carbon dioxide retention, or hypoxemia are indications for intubation and mechanical ventilation.

MANAGEMENT OF LABOR AND DELIVERY. Regularly scheduled medications are continued through labor and delivery. Stress-dose corticosteroids are administered to any woman given systemic steroid therapy within the preceding 4 weeks. The usual drug is 100 mg of hydrocortisone given intravenously every 8 hours. The peak expiratory flow rate should be determined on admission. If asthma symptoms develop, then serial measurements are made after treatments.

In choosing an analgesic for labor, a non–histamine-releasing narcotic, such as fentanyl, may be preferable to meperidine or morphine. Epidural analgesia for labor is ideal. For surgical delivery, conduction analgesia is preferred because tracheal intubation can trigger severe bronchospasm. In the event of refractory postpartum hemorrhage, prostaglandin E_2 and other uterotonics should be used instead of prostaglandin $F_{2\alpha}$, which has been associated with significant bronchospasm in asthmatic patients. Moreover, oxygen desaturation following 15-methyl $PGF_{2\alpha}$ given for postpartum hemorrhage has been reported in women without reactive airway disease (Hankins and colleagues, 1988).

THROMBOEMBOLIC DISEASE

Pregnancy and the puerperium traditionally are considered as one of the highest risks for otherwise healthy women to develop venous thrombosis and pulmonary embolism. Certainly, these remain a major cause of maternal death in the United States. From the Centers for Disease Control and Prevention, Koonin and colleagues (1997) reported that thrombotic pulmonary embolism caused 20 percent of 1459 pregnancy-related deaths in the United States from 1987 through 1990. Jacob and co-workers (1998) reported a similar incidence for Utah from 1982 through 1994. It was also the leading cause of direct maternal deaths in the United Kingdom from 1994 through 1996 (de Swiet, 2000).

INCIDENCE. The apparent decrease in the frequency of thromboembolism complicating pregnancy likely is related to more sophisticated diagnostic tests used to confirm the clinical diagnosis (American College of Obstetricians and Gynecologists, 1997). Also, the frequency of venous thromboembolic disease during the puerperium decreased remarkably when early ambulation became practiced widely. Stasis is probably the strongest single predisposing event to deep vein thrombosis and, therefore, should be minimized. Shown in Table 46–7 are reported incidences of thromboembolism—both deep venous thrombosis and pulmonary embolism—in almost 1 million pregnancies. From these reports, the incidence of all thromboembolism is 1 per 1000 pregnancies. About half are identified antepartum and the other half in the puerperium. In about 15 percent, pulmonary embolism either accompanies deep venous thrombosis or occurs de novo. Risk factors cited in some of these studies included cesarean delivery, which had a fivefold risk. Smoking also increased the risk, and postpartum thrombosis occurrence amplified with preeclampsia. Bernstein and Weiss (2000) described a risk scoring system to predict thromboembolism in pregnancy or postpartum.

More recently, attention has been directed to a number of isolated deficiencies of proteins involved either in coagulation inhibition or in the fibrinolytic system. These deficiencies—collectively referred to as *thrombophilias*—can lead to hypercoagulability and recurrent venous thromboembolism (Gherman and Goodwin, 2000; Lockwood, 1999). They are discussed in more detail in Chapter 52 (p. 1390). Principal thrombophilias

TABLE 46–7. Incidence of Thromboembolism in Pregnancy

Study	Pregnancies	Deep Vein Thrombosis and Thromboembolism Incidence (per 1000)				Pulmonary Embolism		
		No.	Total	Antepartum	Postpartum	No.	Rate	AP/PP
Cunningham et al (1993)	35,000	20	0.57	0.48	0.09	4	1:9000	50/50
Andersen et al (1998)	63,300	78	1.23	0.75	0.50	2	1:31,000	NS
Gherman et al (1999)	268,500	165	0.61	0.35	0.26	38	1:7000	40/60
McColl et al (1999)	72,000	62	0.86	0.57	0.29	11	1:6500	50/50
Lindqvist et al (1999)	479,400	608	1.27	0.64	0.63	90	1:5300	50/50
Witlin et al (1999)	88,000	38	0.43	0.26	0.17	11	1:8000	50/50
Estimated averages	1,006,200	971	0.97	0.52	0.45	156	1:6400	50/50

AP/PP = antepartum/postpartum incidence in percent; NS = not stated.

arise from mutations that cause quantitative or qualitative deficiencies of antithrombin III, proteins S and C, factors V and IX, prothrombin, and homozygosity for an abnormal methylenetetrahydrofolate reductase (MTHFR) gene. Additionally, double heterozygosity for factor V Leiden and G20210A prothrombin mutations—and presumably others—appears to increase the risk for recurrent thromboembolism (De Stefano and associates, 1999).

According to Greer (1999), the most common inherited thrombophilia known at this time is due to the **factor V Leiden** mutation that causes **resistance to activated protein C**—a natural anticoagulant. In a case-control study of 119 women who had thromboembolism during pregnancy, Gerhardt and colleagues (2000) found that 44 percent (7.7 percent controls) had factor V Leiden mutation with a subsequent ninefold risk for thrombosis. This risk was even higher if another mutation co-existed. McColl and co-workers (1999) found a fivefold increased incidence of prothrombin or factor V Leiden mutations in pregnancy complicated by thromboembolism.

The risk for antepartum thromboembolism with these inherited defects is not precisely known. In a small study, Hough and colleagues (1996) attributed a 15 percent risk to pregnancy-related thrombosis with the factor V Leiden mutation. The risk of thrombosis with protein C deficiency is estimated to be 3 to 10 percent, and for protein S deficiency it may be up to 6 percent. These risks are increased postpartum and are estimated to be 7 to 19 percent and 7 to 22 percent for proteins C and S deficiencies respectively (Greer, 1999).

SUPERFICIAL VENOUS THROMBOSIS. Thrombosis limited strictly to the superficial veins of the saphenous system is treated with analgesia, elastic support, and rest. If it does not soon subside, or if deep venous involvement is suspected, appropriate diagnostic measures are taken; and heparin is given if deep vein involvement is confirmed. Superficial thrombophlebitis is typically seen in association with superficial varicosities or as a sequela to intravenous catheterization.

DEEP VENOUS THROMBOSIS. Most cases in pregnancy are confined to the deep veins of the lower extremity. In the study from Memphis, two thirds involved the extremity only (Witlin and colleagues, 1999). In the study from Los Angeles, three fourths involved the extremities (Gherman and associates, 1999). In the Parkland experience, 16 of 20 women had deep venous thrombosis without embolism.

CLINICAL PRESENTATION. The signs and symptoms of deep venous thrombosis involving the lower extremity vary greatly, depending in large measure upon the degree of occlusion and the intensity of the inflammatory response. Ginsberg and colleagues (1992) reported that 58 of 60 antepartum women had thromboses in the left leg, and it was bilateral in the other two. Gherman and associates (1999) described an 80 percent occurrence in the left leg. Classical puerperal thrombophlebitis involving the lower extremity, sometime called **phlegmasia alba dolens** or **milk leg,** is abrupt in onset, with severe pain and edema of the leg and thigh. The thrombus typically involves much of the deep venous system from the foot to the iliofemoral region. Occasionally, reflex arterial spasm causes a pale, cool extremity with diminished pulsations. More likely, there may be appreciable volume of clot yet little reaction in the form of pain, heat, or swelling. Importantly, calf pain, either spontaneous or in response to squeezing, or to stretching the Achilles tendon (Homans sign), may be caused by a strained muscle or a contusion. The latter may be common during the early puerperium as the consequence of inappropriate contact between the calf and the delivery table leg holders.

DIAGNOSIS. Although **venography** or **phlebography** remains the standard for confirmation of deep venous thrombosis, noninvasive methods have largely replaced this test to confirm the clinical diagnosis. Venography is time-consuming, expensive, cumbersome, and has serious complications. Likewise, **impedance plethysmography,** which was used for some time as a noninvasive screening method, is seldom used today.

Real-time ultrasonography, used along with duplex and color Doppler ultrasound, is currently the procedure of choice to detect proximal deep vein thrombosis (American College of Obstetricians and Gynecologists, 2000). Lensing and colleagues (1989) evaluated 220 consecutive nonpregnant patients with clinically suspected deep venous thrombosis. They compared contrast venography with real-time ultrasonography and evaluated the **common femoral** and **popliteal veins** for full compressibility (no thrombosis) and noncompressibility (thrombosis). Both of these vessels were fully compressible in 142 of 143 patients with normal venograms (specificity, 99 percent). All 66 patients with proximal-vein thrombosis had noncompressible femoral or popliteal veins, or both (sensitivity, 100 percent).

According to Goldhaber (1998), a third of patients with negative findings on compression sonography will have an associated pulmonary embolism. This can happen either because the thrombosis has embolized, or because it arose from deep pelvic veins inaccessible to ultrasound evaluation. **In pregnant women, thrombosis associated with pulmonary embolism frequently originates in the iliac veins.**

Magnetic resonance imaging is reserved for specific cases in which the ultrasound findings are equivocal, or with negative ultrasound findings but strong clinical suspicion. This technique allows for excellent delineation of anatomical detail above the inguinal ligament, and phase images can be used to diagnose the presence or absence of pelvic vein flow (Fig. 46-4). An additional advantage is the ability to image in coronal and sagittal planes. Erdman and co-workers (1990) reported that magnetic resonance imaging was 100 percent sensitive and 90 percent specific for detection of venographically proven deep venous thrombosis in nonpregnant patients. Furthermore, in 44 percent of patients without deep venous thrombosis, they were able to demonstrate nonthrombotic conditions to explain the clinical findings that originally had suggested venous thrombosis. Some examples include cellulitis, edema, hematomas, or superficial phlebitis.

Computed tomographic scanning also may be used to assess the lower extremities. It is widely available but requires contrast agents and ionizing radiation. As

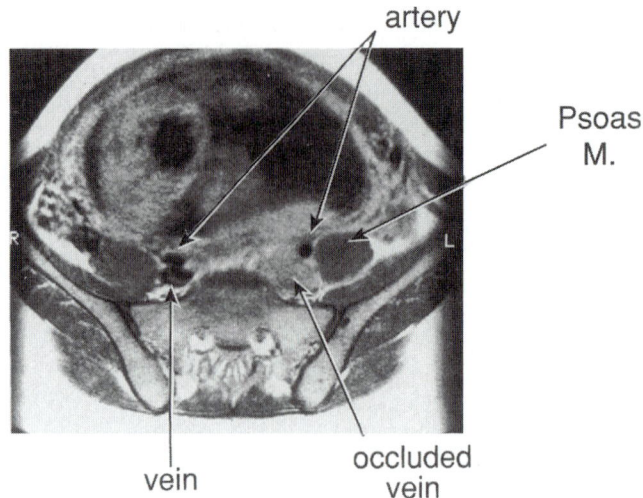

FIGURE 46-4. Magnetic resonance image through the pelvis of a 26-week pregnant woman who presented with symptoms of pulmonary embolism but without clinically apparent deep venous thrombosis of the lower extremities. The T_1-weighted image shows occlusion of left common iliac vein. Note normal absence of signal in the right iliac vein and both iliac arteries. (Photograph courtesy of Dr. Diane Twickler.)

discussed in Chapter 42 (p. 1151), radiation exposure to the fetus is negligible unless the pelvic veins are imaged.

PULMONARY EMBOLISM. Although it causes about 10 percent of maternal deaths, pulmonary embolism is relatively uncommon during pregnancy and the puerperium. From reports in the past 10 years of nearly 1 million pregnancies, the incidence averages about 1 in 6400 (Table 46-7). These reports indicate an almost equal prevalence for antepartum and postpartum embolism, but those developing postpartum have a higher mortality. In many cases, but certainly not all, clinical evidence for deep venous thrombosis of the legs precedes pulmonary embolization. In others, especially those that arise from deep pelvic veins, the woman usually is asymptomatic until symptoms of embolization develop (Figs. 46-4 and 46-5).

CLINICAL PRESENTATION. Findings from the International Cooperative Pulmonary Embolism Registry (ICOPER) were recently described by Goldhaber and colleagues (1999). Over a 2-year period, almost 2500 nonpregnant patients with a proven pulmonary embolism were enrolled. The most common symptoms were dyspnea (82 percent), chest pain (49 percent), cough (20 percent), syncope (14 percent), and hemoptysis (7 percent). According to the American College of Obstetricians and Gynecologists (1997), predominant clinical findings included tachypnea (89 percent), dyspnea (81 percent), pleuritic pain (72 percent), apprehension (59

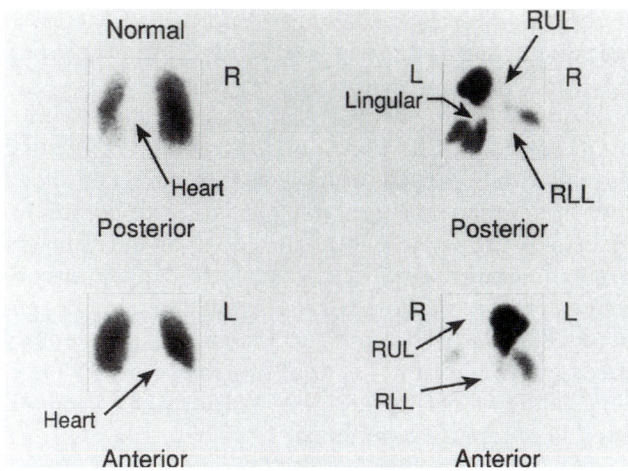

FIGURE 46–5. Abnormal ventilation–perfusion scintigraphy showing pulmonary emboli in a 26-week pregnant woman compared with a normal scan. Left anterior–posterior view of normal ventilation scan showing homogenous distribution of ^{133}Xe. Right, anterior–posterior view of perfusion scan showing large nonperfused areas (*arrows*). There is virtually no perfusion of the right upper (RUL) and lower lobes (RLL), and very little perfusion of the right middle lobe. The absence of lingular lobe perfusion is evident on the left side. (Photographs courtesy of Dr. Diane Twickler.)

percent), cough (54 percent), tachycardia (43 percent), and hemoptysis (34 percent). In some cases there is an accentuated pulmonic closure sound, rales, or friction rub. Right axis deviation may or may not be evident on the electrocardiogram. Even with massive pulmonary embolism, signs, symptoms, and laboratory data to support the diagnosis of pulmonary embolism may be deceivingly nonspecific.

DIAGNOSIS. In most centers, **ventilation–perfusion scintigraphy** is used because it is the least invasive technique that can accurately diagnose pulmonary embolism. These scans utilize a small dose of a radioactive agent, usually technetium (^{99m}Tc) macroaggregated albumin, which is administered intravenously. There is negligible fetal radiation exposure (Chap. 42, p. 1153). The scan may not provide a definite diagnosis because many other conditions—for example, pneumonia or local bronchospasm—can cause perfusion defects. Ventilation scans with inhaled xenon 133 or ^{99m}Tc were added to perfusion scans in the hope that ventilation would be abnormal, but perfusion normal, in areas of pneumonia or hypoventilation. Thus, while ventilation scanning increased the probability of an accurate diagnosis of pulmonary embolus in patients with **large perfusion defects** and **ventilation mismatches,** such as that shown in Figure 46–5, normal ventilation–perfusion does not rule out pulmonary embolism.

Because of these uncertainties, the National Heart,

Lung and Blood Institute commissioned the Prospective Investigation of Pulmonary Embolism Diagnosis (PIOPED, 1990). This study was designed to determine the sensitivities and specificities of ventilation–perfusion scans to diagnose pulmonary embolism. This investigation included 933 patients of whom 931 underwent scintigraphy and 755 pulmonary angiography; 33 percent of the 755 patients studied angiographically had pulmonary embolism. While almost all patients with an embolism had abnormal scans of high, intermediate, or low probability, so did most without embolism (sensitivity, 98 percent; specificity, 10 percent). Of 116 patients with high-probability scans, 88 percent had an embolism seen on angiography, but only a minority of those with a pulmonary embolism had a high-probability scan (sensitivity, 41 percent; specificity, 97 percent). Of 322 with intermediate-probability scans, 33 percent had an embolism on angiography, and for those with low-probability scan, the figure was 12 percent. **Importantly, 4 percent of patients with a near-normal to normal scan had pulmonary embolism detected by angiography.**

The PIOPED investigators concluded that a high-probability scan usually indicates pulmonary embolism, but that only a small number of patients with emboli have a high-probability scan. A low-probability scan combined with a strong clinical impression that embolism is unlikely makes the possibility of pulmonary embolism remote. Similarly, near-normal or normal scans make the diagnosis very unlikely. Finally, an intermediate-probability scan is of no help in establishing the diagnosis. Thus, the scan combined with clinical assessment permits a noninvasive diagnosis or exclusion of pulmonary embolism for only a minority of patients.

Because of these inaccuracies, most investigators recommend an integrated diagnostic approach for women with intermediate or low-probability scan results. For example, Goldhaber (1998) recommends continuation of workup if there is a high D-dimer serum level because normal levels have excellent negative predictive value. In patients with an elevated D-dimer level, he recommends noninvasive studies of the deep leg veins or pulmonary angiography. **Spiral computed tomography** has been used to noninvasively diagnose pulmonary embolism. It shows promise in identifying large vessel emboli but is less accurate for multiple small emboli. Finally, as discussed earlier and shown in Figure 46–4, magnetic resonance imaging can be used to visualize thromboses arising in pelvic veins (Erdman and colleagues, 1990).

MANAGEMENT OF THROMBOEMBOLISM

DEEP VENOUS THROMBOSIS. Treatment of deep venous thrombosis consists of anticoagulation, bed rest, and analgesia. For all women, during either pregnancy or postpartum, initial anticoagulation is with either unfractionated heparin or with low-molecular-weight heparin. For women still pregnant, heparin therapy is continued, and for those postpartum, warfarin therapy is given.

Most often, pain soon is relieved by these measures. After symptoms have completely abated, graded ambulation should be started with the legs fitted with elastic stockings, and anticoagulation continued. Recovery to this stage usually takes about 7 to 10 days.

HEPARIN. Intravenous heparin is given initially. The dosage schedule recommended by the American College of Obstetricians and Gynecologists (2000) includes a loading dose of 80 U/kg (minimum 5000 U). This is followed by a continuous infusion of heparin, 15 to 25 U/kg/hr. After 4 hours, the activated partial thromboplastin time (aPTT) is determined and adjusted as shown in Table 46–8. Once a steady state is achieved, then the aPTT is measured daily.

Deep venous thrombosis may also be treated with subcutaneous adjusted-dose heparin to maintain the aPTT at 1.5 times the control value as determined at 6 hours after the last injection (Hull and colleagues, 1992). Alternately, treatment with one of the low-molecular-weight heparin compounds is suitable (American College of Obstetricians and Gynecologists, 1998).

The ideal duration of therapy for pregnant women is uncertain. The American College of Obstetricians and Gynecologists (1997) recommends therapeutic subcutaneous heparinization for 3 to 4 months, followed by prophylactic or "mini-dose" heparin throughout pregnancy and for 6 to 12 weeks postpartum. Kearon and colleagues (1999) recently reported findings from a study of 162 nonpregnant patients with thromboses and a variety of underlying illnesses. Anticoagulation carried out for 6 months prevented 95 percent of recurrences from 3 to 6 months. Specifically, patients continuing

therapeutic heparin had a recurrence rate 1.3 percent per patient year compared with 27 percent in the group in which heparin was stopped at 3 months.

WARFARIN. Postpartum venous thrombosis is treated initially with heparin as described. Heparin is continued until oral anticoagulation with warfarin can be accomplished. If intravenous heparin and oral warfarin are initiated simultaneously, then heparin can be discontinued safely after 5 days. These women are anticoagulated with warfarin for at least 3 months. As previously discussed, data from Kearon and colleagues (1999) indicate that 6 months is preferable. **Warfarin is contraindicated in antepartum patients.**

LOW-MOLECULAR-WEIGHT HEPARIN. Clinical experience with low-molecular-weight heparin has accrued over the past decade (Ginsberg and Hirsh, 1998). This is a family of derivatives of commercial heparin that average about 4000 to 5000 daltons compared with about 12,000 to 16,000 daltons for conventional heparin. One such preparation, *logipram,* was shown to be safe and effective for treatment of proximal vein thrombosis in nonpregnant patients (Hull and co-workers, 1992). Simmoneau and colleagues (1997) showed equivalent efficiency and major complications in 612 nonpregnant patients with a pulmonary embolism randomized to either subcutaneous *tinzaprin* or intravenous heparin. The Columbus Investigators (1997) compared *reviparin* with unfractionated heparin to treat 1021 patients with venous thromboembolism, a third of whom had pulmonary embolism. The study drug was as safe and effective as standard heparin.

Thus, a number of preparations, all of which are pharmacologically unique, have been shown to be effective in preventing and treating deep vein thrombosis, but with fewer bleeding complications. Other advantages are once- or twice-daily administration, and most authors recommend that these subcutaneously administered drugs do not have to be monitored (American College of Obstetricians and Gynecologists, 1998; Lensing and associates, 1999). Their use in pregnant women has been limited and was reviewed recently by Bates (1999) and Chan (1999).

MANAGEMENT OF PULMONARY EMBOLISM. Treatment for pulmonary embolism is similar to that for deep venous thrombosis, but with less well-documented results. In general, heparin is given initially in a fashion similar to that for deep venous thrombosis. The American College of Obstetricians and Gynecologists (2000) recommends an intravenous loading dose of 80 U/kg with management otherwise as given for deep venous thrombosis.

Other methods are acceptable, and most authors rec-

TABLE 46–8. Adjusted Heparin Dose for Continuous Infusion Therapy for Venous Thrombosis

aPTT (sec)	Bolus (U/kg)	Hold Infusion (min)	Rate Change (U/hr)	Repeat aPTT (hr)
< 50	70	0	+200	4
50–59	0	0	+10	4
60–80	0	0	0	Next A.M.
81–99	0	0	−100	4
> 100	0	60	−200	4

aPTT = activated partial thromboplastin time.
From the American College of Obstetricians and Gynecologists (1997), with permission.

ommend starting with a dose of 1000 U/hour after an initial bolus dose of 5000 to 10,000 U given intravenously. The dose is maintained to produce a twofold prolongation of the activated partial thromboplastin time. Other methods include either intermittent intravenous injections of 5000 U heparin every 4 hours or 7500 U every 6 hours. Finally, heparin may be given subcutaneously in doses of 10,000 U every 8 hours or 20,000 U every 12 hours. The common theme in these regimens is that the total daily heparin dose is between 25,000 and 40,000 U.

In nonpregnant patients, the most common cause of death is recurrent pulmonary embolism (Goldhaber, 1998). To prevent this, most authors recommend therapeutic anticoagulation for 4 to 6 months. For women who develop thromboembolism postpartum, or for those who were given heparin antepartum and are now delivered, warfarin therapy is usually given.

VENA CAVAL FILTERS. Routine placement of a vena caval filter has no added advantage to heparin given alone to prevent pulmonary embolism in patients with deep vein thrombosis (Decousus and associates, 1998). In the very infrequent circumstances where heparin therapy fails to prevent recurrent pulmonary embolism from the pelvis or legs, or when embolism develops from these sites despite heparin given for their treatment, then a vena caval filter is indicated. The device is inserted through either the jugular or femoral vein. Greenfield and Michna (1988) recommend suprarenal placement during pregnancy. Hux and colleagues (1986) described the use of the Greenfield filter in five pregnant women and another who was 3 days postpartum. Thomas and associates (1997) described successful use of the Greenfield filter in eight pregnant women with complications of venous thromboembolism.

Retrievable filters may be used as short-term protection against embolism. These may be removed before they become endothelialized by 10 days, or they can be left permanently. Neill and colleagues (1997) described use of a **Gunther Tulip filter** placed at 37 weeks in a woman with recurrent embolization despite adequate anticoagulation. She underwent cesarean delivery at 38 weeks, and the filter removed 5 days postpartum.

COMPLICATIONS OF ANTICOAGULATION. The most serious complication with any of these regimens is hemorrhage, which is more likely if there has been recent surgery or lacerations, such as with delivery. Troublesome bleeding also is more likely if the heparin dosage is excessive. Unfortunately, many management schemes using laboratory testing to identify whether heparin dosage is sufficient to inhibit further thrombosis, yet not cause serious hemorrhage, have been discouraging.

Other complications include heparin-induced thrombocytopenia and osteoporosis (Toglia and Weg, 1996). Thrombocytopenia usually manifests within 2 to 3 weeks of initial therapy. Its incidence is 3 to 6 percent of patients given porcine heparin. Osteoporosis develops with long-term administration and is associated with heparin doses of 15,000 to 20,000 U/day for more than 6 months and is more prevalent in cigarette smokers (American College of Obstetricians and Gynecologists, 1997, 2000). Heparin-induced osteopenia is considered further in Chapter 50 (p. 1349).

ANTICOAGULATION AND ABORTION. The treatment of deep venous thrombosis with heparin does not preclude termination of pregnancy by careful curettage (Chap. 33, p. 871). After the products of conception are removed without trauma to the reproductive tract, heparin can be restarted in several hours in therapeutic doses without undue risk.

ANTICOAGULATION AND DELIVERY. Neither unfractionated nor low-molecular-weight heparins cross the placenta. The effects on blood loss at delivery will depend upon a number of variables, including:

1. Dose, route, and time of administration.
2. Magnitude of incisions and lacerations.
3. Intensity of postpartum myometrial contraction and retraction.
4. Presence of other coagulation defects.

Measured blood loss is not greatly increased with vaginal delivery if the midline episiotomy is modest in depth, there are no lacerations of the genital tract, and the uterus promptly becomes firmly contracted. Such ideal circumstances do not always prevail during and after vaginal delivery. For example, Mueller and Lebherz (1969) described 10 women with antepartum thrombophlebitis treated with heparin. Three who continued to receive heparin during labor and delivery bled remarkably and developed large hematomas.

In general, therapeutic heparin therapy should be stopped during the time of labor and delivery. If the uterus is well contracted and there has been negligible trauma to the lower genital tract, it can be restarted within several hours. Otherwise, a delay of 1 or 2 days may be prudent. Protamine sulfate administered slowly intravenously will generally reverse the effect of heparin promptly and effectively. Protamine sulfate should not be given in excess of the amount needed to neutralize the heparin, because it has an anticoagulant effect.

The woman who has very recently suffered a pulmonary embolism and who must be delivered by cesarean presents a serious problem. Reversal of anticoagulation may be followed by another embolus, and surgery while she is fully anticoagulated frequently results in life-threatening hemorrhage or troublesome hematomas. In this situation, consideration should be given before surgery for placement of a vena caval filter.

Serious bleeding is likely when heparin in usual therapeutic doses is administered to a woman who has undergone cesarean delivery within the previous 48 to 72 hours. Again, preexisting defects in the hemostatic mechanism, such as thrombocytopenia, or impaired platelet function as induced by aspirin, enhance the likelihood of hemorrhage with heparin.

THROMBOEMBOLISM ANTEDATING PREGNANCY.

Optimal management of women with firm evidence of a prior thromboembolism is unclear. The National Institutes of Health Consensus Conference (1986) concluded that the woman with either deep venous thrombosis or pulmonary embolism in a *prior* pregnancy should be given prophylactic subcutaneous heparin in doses of 5000 U, either two or three times daily throughout pregnancy. Similar recommendations were made in 1992 by the American College of Chest Physicians. The American College of Obstetricians and Gynecologists (2000) recommends 5000 to 10,000 units every 12 hours throughout pregnancy.

The study by Tengborn and colleagues (1989) suggests that such prophylaxis is not effective. They reported outcomes in 87 pregnant Swedish women who had prior thromboembolic disease. Despite heparin prophylaxis, usually 5000 U twice daily, 3 of 20 (15 percent) women developed antepartum recurrence, compared with 8 of 67 (12 percent) not given heparin.

The use of low-molecular-weight heparin has been reported to be efficacious for prophylaxis in high-risk pregnant women. Nelson-Piercy and co-workers (1997) gave enoxaparin, 40 mg subcutaneously once daily, during 69 pregnancies during which no thromboemboli were identified antepartum. One woman receiving only 20 mg subcutaneously daily developed a pulmonary embolus postpartum. Another concern was that a third of these women developed osteopenia. Hunt and associates (1997) gave Fragmin subcutaneously and monitored anti-Xa activity. None of 34 treated women had thromboembolism, but one had osteoporotic vertebral collapse postpartum. More recently, Brill-Edwards and associates (2000) withheld antepartum heparin prophylaxis in 125 such women. Only 3 (2.4 percent) had recurrence and they concluded that prophylaxis was unnecessary.

Our practice at Parkland Hospital for many years for women with a history of prior thromboembolism has been to administer subcutaneous heparin, 5000 to 7500 units two to three times daily. With this regimen, the recurrence of documented deep venous thrombosis embolization has been rare. More recently, we have successfully used 40 mg enoxaparin subcutaneously daily.

TUBERCULOSIS

Although still a major worldwide concern, tuberculosis has become less common in the United States in recent decades. In 1998, the rate was 6.8 per 100,000 persons (Centers for Disease Control and Prevention, 1999b). The number of cases of tuberculosis in women of childbearing age increased 40 percent in the United States between 1985 and 1992 (Cantwell and colleagues, 1994).

Importantly, tuberculosis in foreign-born persons has increased by 50 percent and in 1998 comprised 40 percent of the estimated 18,000 cases in the United States (Centers for Disease Control and Prevention, 1999b). Indeed, the disease in this country is one of the elderly, the urban poor, minority groups, and patients with acquired immunodeficiency syndrome (McKenna and colleagues, 1995).

Cure rates with directly observed 6-month short-course therapy approaches 90 percent for new infections (China Tuberculosis Control Collaboration, 1996). Of special concern is the recent emergence of drug-resistant tuberculosis. In the United States, 12 percent of 13,500 strains isolated from 1994 to 1997 were resistant to at least one drug (Pablos-Mendez and colleagues, 1998). The Global Tuberculosis Program of the World Health Organization showed in 1997 that there was variable drug resistance in 35 countries. Importantly, multidrug-resistant strains, defined as combined resistance to isoniazid and rifampin, averaged 1.4 percent but were as high as 14 percent in some countries. More recently, the World Health Organization published expanded data from 58 countries and cited similar findings (Brown, 2000). Moreover, 6-month chemotherapy with first-line drugs is inadequate in many cases caused by resistant strains (Espinal and associates, 2000). In the United States, there have been documented outbreaks of multidrug-resistant tuberculosis (MDR-TB) in persons with HIV-infections. In some of these cases, tuberculosis was transmitted to health-care workers.

CLINICAL COURSE.
Infection is via inhalation of *Mycobacterium tuberculosis,* which incites a granulomatous pulmonary reaction. In over 90 percent of patients, infection is contained and lies dormant for long periods. In some patients, especially those who are immunocompromised or who have other diseases, tuberculosis becomes reactivated to cause clinical disease. Clinical manifestations usually include cough with minimal sputum production, low-grade fever, hemoptysis, and weight loss. A variety of infiltrative patterns are seen on chest x-ray, and there may be associated cavitation or mediastinal lymphadenopathy. Acid-fast bacilli are seen on repeated stained smears of sputum in about two thirds of culture-positive patients. Extrapulmonary tuberculosis

may occur in any organ, and almost 40 percent of HIV-positive patients have disseminated disease (Weinberger and Weiss, 1999).

TUBERCULOSIS AND PREGNANCY. The considerable influx of women into the United States from Asia, Africa, Mexico, and Central America has been accompanied by an increased frequency of tuberculosis in pregnant women. Additionally, pregnant women who are HIV-positive are at greater risk. Margono and colleagues (1994) described their experiences from New York City. At Kings County and Saint Vincent's Hospitals from 1985 through 1990, the rate for tuberculosis during pregnancy was 12 cases per 100,000 deliveries. During 1991 and 1992 this rate rose to 95 per 100,000. There were 16 pregnant women with active tuberculosis, and 7 of 11 tested were HIV-positive.

PREGNANCY OUTCOMES. Prior to antituberculosis therapy, pregnancy was thought to have an adverse effect on the course of tuberculosis (Anderson, 1997). Contemporaneous experiences are sparse because chemotherapy has diminished adverse effects from severe disease. Jana and colleagues (1994) reported outcomes of 79 pregnancies from India complicated by active pulmonary tuberculosis. There were increased incidences of preterm delivery and low-birthweight and growth-restricted infants, as well as a sixfold increased perinatal mortality rate. Adverse outcomes correlated with late diagnosis, incomplete or irregular treatment, and advanced pulmonary lesions. They also studied outcomes in 33 pregnancies complicated by extrapulmonary tuberculosis (Jana and co-workers, 1999). While lymphadenitis did not affect outcomes, a third of women with renal, intestinal, and skeletal injections had low-birthweight infants. Figueroa-Damian and Arrendondo-Garcia (1998) reported similar outcomes in 25 pregnant women from Mexico City. In a recent prospective study from London, Llewelyn and associates (2000) reported that 9 of 13 pregnant women had extrapulmonary disease concomitant with delayed diagnoses.

DIAGNOSIS. Current guidelines include skin testing of only women in high-risk groups as shown in Table 46–9. The preferred antigen is purified protein derivative (PPD) in the intermediate strength of 5 tuberculin units. If the intracutaneously applied test is negative, no further evaluation is needed. A positive skin test is interpreted according to risk factors (American Thoracic Society/Centers for Disease Control, 1990). For *very high-risk* patients—that is, those who are HIV-positive, those with abnormal chest radiography, or those who have a recent contact with an active case—5 mm is considered positive. For those at *high risk*—foreign born, intravenous drug users who are HIV-negative,

TABLE 46–9. High-risk Groups Recommended for Tuberculosis Screening by the Advisory Committee for Elimination of Tuberculosis

1. Persons infected with the human immunodeficiency virus.
2. Close contacts of persons known or suspected to have tuberculosis, sharing the same household or other closed environment.
3. Persons with medical risk factors known to increase the risk of disease if infection has occurred.
4. Foreign-born persons from countries with a high tuberculosis prevalence.
5. Medically underserved low-income populations, including high-risk racial or ethnic minority population—for example, African, Hispanic, and Native Americans.
6. Alcoholics and intravenous drug users.
7. Residents of long-term-care facilities, correctional institutions, mental institutions, nursing homes/facilities, and other long-term residential facilities.

From Centers for Disease Control (1990).

low-income populations, or those with medical conditions that increase the risk for tuberculosis—10 mm is considered positive. For persons with none of these risk factors, 15 mm is defined as positive. If the chest radiograph is negative, then no treatment is necessary until after delivery, when isoniazid chemoprophylaxis is usually given for 1 year. Patients who have been vaccinated with *bacille Calmette-Guérin* (*BCG*) pose special problems with interpretation of skin testing.

TREATMENT. In nonpregnant tuberculin-positive patients who are younger than 35, and who have no evidence of active disease, isoniazid, 300 mg daily, is given for 1 year. Isoniazid is a category C drug that is considered safe in pregnancy. In pregnant women who are HIV-negative, however, most authors recommend that therapy be delayed until after delivery. Because of possibly increased isoniazid-induced hepatitis in postpartum women, some recommend withholding treatment until 3 to 6 months postpartum. Neither postpartum method is as effective as antepartum treatment to prevent active infection (Boggess and colleagues, 2000).

There are exceptions to delayed treatment in pregnancy. Known recent skin-test convertors are treated because the incidence of active infection is 3 percent in the first year. Skin-test positive women exposed to active infection are treated because the incidence of infection is 0.5 percent per year. Finally, HIV-positive women are treated because they have an 8 percent annual risk for active disease (Brost and Newman, 1997). An alternative is to withhold therapy until after 12 weeks in these asymptomatic women. Isoniazid toxicity includes hepatitis, which is more common in patients younger than 35. Although monitoring of liver enzymes indicates that 10 to 20 percent of patients have transient elevation, therapy is not discontinued unless their elevation is five-fold times normal (Weinberger and Weiss, 1999). Currently, the Centers for Disease Control and Prevention (1999b) do not recommend routine monitoring.

Because of emerging drug resistance, the Centers for Disease Control (1993) now recommends a four-drug regimen for the initial empirical treatment of nonpregnant patients with symptomatic tuberculosis. These are isoniazid, rifampin, and pyrazinamide with ethambutol or streptomycin given until susceptibility studies are done. Drug susceptibility testing is performed on all first isolates. Fortunately, most first-line tuberculostatic drugs do not appear to affect the fetus adversely. An exception is streptomycin, which may cause congenital deafness. Moreover, the safety of pyrazinamide given in early pregnancy has not been established.

The Centers for Disease Control (1993) recommend that the orally prescribed regimen for pregnant women should include:

1. **Isoniazid,** 5 mg/kg, not to exceed 300 mg daily, along with **pyridoxine,** 50 mg daily.
2. **Rifampin,** 10 mg/kg daily, not to exceed 600 mg daily.
3. **Ethambutol,** 5 to 25 mg/kg daily, not to exceed 2.5 g daily.

These drugs are given for a minimum of 9 months. For HIV-infected women, the use of rifampin or rifabutin may be contraindicated if certain nucleoside reverse transcriptase inhibitors are being administered (Centers for Disease Control and Prevention, 2000a). If there is resistance to these drugs, then pyrazinamide therapy is considered.

NEONATAL TUBERCULOSIS. Tubercle bacillemia during pregnancy can infect the placenta. The fetus may also be infected, and although **congenital tuberculosis** is rare, it can prove fatal. Its incidence likely will increase with concomitant HIV infection (Pillay and Jeena, 1999). In half of cases, infection is acquired hematogenously in the liver or lungs via the umbilical vein. In the other half, infants are infected by aspiration of infected secretions at delivery. In their review, Cantwell and associates (1994) found only 29 cases of congenital tuberculosis reported in the English literature since 1980. Only 12 of the mothers had active infection. Genital tuberculosis was common in these women, and all 14 who had endometrial biopsy performed showed active infection. Adhikari and colleagues (1997) described 11 culture-positive cases over 1 year from South Africa. Six neonates had congenital tuberculosis, and one died within 3 months. Six mothers were HIV-positive, and one died within 3 months.

Neonatal infection is unlikely if the mother with active disease has been treated before delivery, or if her sputum culture is negative. Because the newborn is quite susceptible to tuberculosis, most authors recommend isolation from the mother suspected of having active disease. If untreated, the risk of disease in the infant born to a woman with active infection is 50 percent in the first year (Jacobs and Abernathy, 1988). It is not known whether isoniazid chemoprophylaxis is efficacious for the infant. It may be given with or without BCG vaccination. For the symptomatic infant, the treatment regimen is essentially the same as for adults.

SARCOIDOSIS

Sarcoidosis is a chronic, multisystem disease of unknown etiology characterized by an accumulation of T lymphocytes and phagocytes within noncaseating granulomas. Disease appears to be mediated by an exaggerated response for T-helper lymphocytes. Pulmonary involvement is most common, followed by the skin, eyes, and lymph nodes. Its prevalence in the United States is 10 to 40 per 100,000, with equal sex distribution but a 10- to 20-fold predilection for African Americans (Crystal, 1998). Most patients are between 20 and 40 years old. Their clinical presentation varies, but most commonly dyspnea and a dry cough without constitutional symptoms develop insidiously over months. In about a fourth of patients, disease onset is abrupt, and 10 percent are asymptomatic at discovery.

Over 90 percent of patients have an abnormal chest x-ray. **Interstitial pneumonitis** is the hallmark of pulmonary involvement. About half of affected patients develop permanent radiological changes. **Lymphadenopathy,** especially of the mediastinum, is present in 75 to 90 percent of cases; 25 percent have **uveitis;** and 25 percent have skin involvement, usually manifest as **erythema nodosum.** Any other organ system can be involved. Confirmation of diagnosis is not possible without biopsy, and because the lung may be the only involved organ, tissue acquisition is often difficult.

The overall prognosis for sarcoidosis is good, and in half of patients it resolves without treatment. In the other half, permanent organ dysfunction persists, albeit mild and nonprogressive. About 10 percent die because of their disease. Glucocorticoids are the most widely used treatment; however, permanent organ derangement is seldom reversed by their use. Thus, the decision to treat is based on symptoms, physical findings, chest x-ray, and pulmonary function tests. Unless respiratory symptoms are prominent, therapy is usually withheld for a several-month observation period, and if inflammation does not subside, then prednisone, 1 mg/kg, is given daily for 4 to 6 weeks (Crystal, 1998).

SARCOIDOSIS AND PREGNANCY. Sarcoidosis uncommonly complicates pregnancy. De Regt (1987) described 14 cases over a 12-year period at Downstate Medical Center, during which time nearly 20,000 women were delivered. Reported beneficial effects of pregnancy are questionable because of the tendency of sarcoidosis to improve spontaneously. Available evidence is suggestive that sarcoidosis seldom affects pregnancy adversely unless there is severe preexisting disease (Selroos, 1990). De Regt (1987) reported two fatal cases due to extensive disease, one with multiple lung abscesses and the other with severe interstitial fibrosis. Seballos and associates (1994) described a woman with peripartum heart failure from pulmonary and cardiac sarcoidosis. Boggess and colleagues (1995) described two pregnancies in a woman with severe restrictive lung disease from sarcoidosis. Maisel and Lynam (1996) reported a 16-week pregnant woman who died suddenly from granulomatous meningitis with brain stem involvement and obstructive hydrocephaly.

Selroos (1990) reviewed 655 patients with sarcoidosis referred to the Mjölbolsta Hospital District in southern Finland. Of 252 women between 18 and 50 years old, 15 percent had sarcoidosis during pregnancy or within 1 year postpartum. There was no evidence for disease progression in the 26 pregnancies with active disease; three aborted spontaneously and the other 23 women were delivered at term. In 18 pregnancies in 12 women with inactive disease, pregnancy outcome was good and there was no evidence of disease activation. These experiences are similar to those reported by Agha and colleagues (1982) for 35 pregnancies cared for at the University of Michigan Hospital.

Active sarcoidosis is treated using the same guidelines as for the woman who is not pregnant. Severe disease warrants serial determination of pulmonary function. Symptomatic uveitis, constitutional symptoms, and pulmonary symptoms are treated with prednisone, 1 mg/kg per day.

CYSTIC FIBROSIS

Cystic fibrosis is one of the most common serious genetic disorders in Caucasians. It is caused by one of over 800 point mutations on the long arm of chromosome 7 that affect the chloride-ion channel—the *cystic fibrosis transmembrane conductance receptor regulator* (*CFTR*) (Chap. 37, p. 986). Its frequency is estimated to be 1 per 1500 Caucasian births and 1 per 17,000 African-American births. Median survival has increased from 14 years in 1969 to 30 years in 1995 (Ramsey, 1996). Because of improvements in diagnosis and treatment, nearly 80 percent of females with cystic fibrosis now survive to adulthood. Although many are infertile because of delayed sexual development and perhaps abnormal cervical mucus production, pregnancy is not uncommon. The North American Cystic Fibrosis Foundation estimated that 4 percent of cystic fibrosis patients become pregnant each year (Edenborough and colleagues, 1995). Males who survive to adulthood often have aspermia.

Mutations that result in cystic fibrosis cause altered epithelial cell membrane transport of electrolytes. The disorder is characterized by exocrine gland dysfunction with production of thick, viscid secretions. Eccrine sweat gland abnormalities provide the basis for the diagnostic **sweat test,** characterized by elevated sodium, potassium, and chloride levels in sweat.

Almost all affected patients have lung involvement, which is also the most common cause of death. Bronchial gland hypertrophy with mucous plugging and small-airway obstruction leads to subsequent infection that ultimately causes chronic bronchitis and bronchiectasis. Bacteria that colonize the respiratory tract include *Pseudomonas aeruginosa* in over 90 percent; *Staphylococcus aureus* and *H influenzae* are recovered in a minority of instances. Acute and chronic parenchymal inflammation ultimately causes extensive fibrosis, and along with airway obstruction, there is a ventilation–perfusion mismatch. Pulmonary insufficiency is the end result. Lung or heart–lung transplantation has a 5-year survival rate of 33 percent (Aurora and associates, 1999).

CYSTIC FIBROSIS AND PREGNANCY. Pulmonary involvement with chronic lung disease, hypoxia, and frequent infections may prove deleterious to pregnancy. **Cor pulmonale** is common, and Cohen and associates (1980) reported that 13 percent of pregnant women with cystic fibrosis developed heart failure. **Pancreatic dysfunction** also can contribute significantly to poor maternal nutrition.

While early reports suggested a deleterious effect of pregnancy on the course of cystic fibrosis, this may have been related to severe disease (Olson, 1997). Cohen and colleagues (1980) surveyed cystic fibrosis centers and reported information from 129 pregnancies. They found that increased maternal and perinatal mortality was related to severe pulmonary infection. They used the **Schwachman–Kulezycki** or **Taussig** scores of severity, which are based on radiological and clinical criteria. These range from 0 to 100, and a score of 50 or less in nonpregnant patients portends an overall bad prognosis, while a score of 90 or more predicts a good outcome. They concluded that pregnancy should be discouraged unless the score was at least 80. The long-term prognosis should also be considered—in this study, 18 percent of women had died within 2 years.

Kent and Farquharson (1993) reviewed outcomes in 215 pregnancies in 160 women with cystic fibrosis published from 1960 to 1991. Over 80 percent of the pregnancies progressed to 20 weeks. One fourth of these delivered preterm, and the perinatal death rate was 14 percent. The three maternal deaths were in women with the worst pulmonary function. Another 10 women with moderately severe pulmonary function died less than 6 months after delivery. Within 2 years of delivery, 14 percent of the women died.

Canny and co-workers (1991) reported their experiences with 38 pregnancies in 25 women with cystic fibrosis. Prepregnancy treatment was continued, including pancreatic enzyme replacement in the 12 women with pancreatic insufficiency, oral antibiotics, aerosolized bronchodilators, chest physiotherapy, and nutritional support. Admission was required for pulmonary complications during 30 percent of pregnancies. Three women developed gestational diabetes, and another had postpartum pancreatitis. Of 34 completed pregnancies, there were two preterm deliveries, and one growth-restricted term infant was delivered to a woman with severe obstructive lung disease. Only one mother died within 2 years of delivery, in contrast to 18 percent reported in the survey by Cohen and colleagues (1980). They stressed that the women they described were not as ill as many patients with cystic fibrosis. For example, they had a relatively late age at diagnosis and a high incidence of pancreatic sufficiency, both good prognostic factors.

Subsequent reports support that prognosis for both mother and fetus is dependent on lung involvement. Edenborough and colleagues (1995, 2000) described 69 pregnancies in women cared for in 11 cystic fibrosis centers in the United Kingdom. Excluding abortions, all 48 pregnancies resulted in live-born infants, but half were delivered preterm. They reported that if prepregnancy forced expiratory volume in 1 second was less than 60 percent predicted, there was substantive risk of preterm and cesarean delivery, respiratory complications, and early death of the mother. Gilljam and associates (2000) reported only six preterm births of 74 viable pregnancies in 54 women. Frangolias and colleagues (1997) described seven women with stable lung function during pregnancy. Jankelson and associates (1998) reported 13 pregnancies in 11 women, and five of six had normal lung function defined by an FEV_1 of over 80 percent. While these did well, four of five with an FEV_1 of less than 80 percent had worsening pulmonary function and were delivered preterm. Three of these five were dead within 7 years.

MANAGEMENT IN PREGNANCY. Prepregnancy counseling is imperative, and genetic counseling is discussed in Chapter 39 (p. 1076). Women who choose to become pregnant should be followed closely with serial pulmonary function testing and surveillance for superimposed infection, development of diabetes, and heart failure. Women who have a Schwachman–Kulezycki score of over 75, good nutritional status, and an FEV_1 of at least 70 percent usually tolerate pregnancy well. Careful attention is given to postural drainage and bronchodilator therapy. Inhaled recombinant human deoxyribonuclease I improves lung function by reducing sputum viscosity (Olson, 1997). Pancreatic insufficiency is treated by oral pancreatic enzyme replacement. Immediate hospitalization is recommended if complications develop, especially pulmonary infection. For labor and delivery, epidural analgesia is recommended, especially for operative delivery. Treatment of cor pulmonale consists of bronchodilators, oxygen, and diuretics.

CARBON MONOXIDE POISONING

Carbon monoxide is ubiquitous, and most nonsmoking adults have a carbon monoxyhemoglobin saturation of 1 to 3 percent. In cigarette smokers, levels may be as high as 5 to 10 percent. Toxic levels are frequently encountered in inadequately ventilated areas warmed by space heaters. Carbon monoxide is an odorless, tasteless gas that has a high affinity and binding for hemoglobin, thus displacing oxygen and impeding its transfer.

Pregnant women, and especially their fetuses, do not tolerate excessive carbon monoxide inhalation. Symptoms usually appear when carboxyhemoglobin concentration is 20 to 30 percent. Concentrations over 50 to 60 percent produce severe symptoms and may be fatal for the mother; presumably, lesser concentrations are fatal for the fetus. Because hemoglobin F has a higher affinity for carbon monoxide, fetal carboxyhemoglobin levels are 10 to 15 percent higher than those in the mother (Longo, 1977).

When a patient is breathing room air, the half-life of carboxyhemoglobin is 4 to 6 hours, but in 100 percent oxygen it is about 1 hour. **Hyperbaric oxygen** at 3 atmospheres of pressure decreases this to about 20 minutes. Treatment of carbon monoxide poisoning is supportive along with administration of inspired 100 percent oxygen (Tomaszewski, 1999). Hyperbaric oxygen is generally recommended in pregnancy, and Elkharrat and colleagues (1991) reported successful treatments in 44 pregnant women. Silverman and Montano (1997) also reported successful management of a woman whose abnormal neurological and cardiopulmonary findings abated in a parallel fashion with the associated fetal heart rate variable decelerations.

REFERENCES

Adhikari M, Pillay T, Pillay DG: Tuberculosis in the newborn: An emerging disease. Pediatr Infect Dis J 16:1108, 1997

Advisory Committee on Immunization Practices: Prevention of pneumococcal disease. MMWR 46:1, 1997

Agha FP, Vade A, Amendola MA, Cooper RF: Effects of pregnancy on sarcoidosis. Surg Gynecol Obstet 155:817, 1982

Albino JA, Shapiro JM: Respiratory failure in pregnancy due to Pneumocystis carinii: Report of a successful outcome. Obstet Gynecol 83:823, 1994

Alexander S, Dodds L, Armson BA: Perinatal outcomes in women with asthma during pregnancy. Obstet Gynecol 92:435, 1998

American College of Obstetricians and Gynecologists. Thromboembolism in pregnancy. Practice Bulletin No. 19, August 2000

American College of Obstetricians and Gynecologists: Anticoagulation with low-molecular-weight heparin during pregnancy. Committee on Obstetric Practice, Committee Opinion No. 211, November 1998

American College of Obstetricians and Gynecologists Thromboembolism in pregnancy. Educational Bulletin No. 234, March 1997

American Thoracic Society: Medical Section of the American Lung Association: Guidelines for the initial management of adults with community-acquired pneumonia: Diagnosis, assessment of severity, and initial antimicrobial therapy. Am Rev Respir Dis 148:1418, 1993

American Thoracic Society/Centers for Disease Control: Diagnostic standards and classification of tuberculosis. Am Rev Respir Dis 142:725, 1990

Andersen BS, Steffensen FH, Sørensen HT, Nielsen GL, Olsen J: The cumulative incidence of venous thromboembolism during pregnancy and puerperium. Acta Obstet Gynecol Scand 77:170, 1998

Anderson GD: Tuberculosis in pregnancy. Semin Perinatol 21:328, 1997

Apuzzio JJ: Viral influenza in pregnancy. Contemp Ob/Gyn 44:15, 1999

Arsura EL, Kilgore WB, Ratnayake SN: Erythema nodosum in pregnant patients with coccidioidomycosis. Clin Infect Dis 27:1201, 1998

Aurora P, Whitehead B, Wade A, Bowyer J, Whitmore P, Rees PG, Tsang VT, Elliot MJ, de Leval M: Lung transplantation and life extension in children with cystic fibrosis. Lancet 354:1594, 1999

Barbour LA, Pickard J: Controversies in thromboembolic disease during pregnancy: A critical review. Obstet Gynecol 86:621, 1995

Barth WH, Hankins GDV: Severe acute asthma in pregnancy. In Clark SL, Cotton DB, Hankins GDV, Phelan JP (eds): Critical Care Obstetrics, 2nd ed. Oxford, Blackwell, 1991, p 371

Bartlett JG, Mundy LM: Community-acquired pneumonia. N Engl J Med 333:1618, 1995

Bates SM: Optimal management of pregnant women with acute venous thromboembolism. Haemostasis 29:107, 1999

Bennett BB: Community-acquired pneumonia. Prim Care Update Ob/Gyn 1:139, 1994

Berkowitz K, LaSala A: Risk factors associated with the increasing prevalence of pneumonia during pregnancy. Am J Obstet Gynecol 163:981, 1990

Bernstein PS, Weiss N: Risk factor scoring for predicting venous thromboembolism in obstetric patients. Obstet Gynecol 95:S11, 2000

Blais L, Suissa S, Boivin JF, Ernst P: First treatment with inhaled corticosteroids and the prevention of admissions to hospital for asthma. Thorax 53:1025, 1998

Bloom SL, Ramin S, Cunningham FG: A prediction rule for community-acquired pneumonia. N Engl J Med 336:1913, 1997

Boggess KA, Myers ER, Hamilton CD: Antepartum or postpartum isoniazid treatment of latent tuberculosis infection. Obstet Gynecol 96:747, 2000

Boggess KA, Easterling TR, Raghu G: Management and outcome of pregnant women with interstitial and restrictive lung disease. Am J Obstet Gynecol 173:1007, 1995

Braman SS, Kaemmerlen JT: Intensive care of status asthmaticus. A 10-year experience. JAMA 264:366, 1990

Brancazio LR, Laifer SA, Schwartz T: Peak expiratory flow rate in normal pregnancy. Obstet Gynecol 89:383, 1997

Briggs GG, Freeman RK, Yaffe SJ (eds): Drugs in Pregnancy and Lactation, 5th ed. Baltimore, Williams & Wilkins, 1998

Briggs RG, Mabie WC, Sibai BM: Community-acquired pneumonia in pregnancy. Am J Obstet Gynecol 174:389, 1996

Brill-Edwards P, Ginsberg JS, Gent M, Hirsh J, Burrows R, Kearon C, Geerts W, Kovacs M, Weitz JI, Robinson S, Whittom R, Couture G, for the Recurrence of Clot in This Pregnancy Study Group: Safety of withholding heparin in pregnant women with a history of venous thromboembolism. N Engl J Med 343:1439, 2000

Brost BC, Newman RB: The maternal and fetal effects of tuberculosis therapy. Obstet Gynecol Clin North Am 24:659, 1997

Brown P: Drug resistant tuberculosis can be controlled, says WHO. BMJ 320:821, 2000

Brown PD, Lerner SA: Community-acquired pneumonia. Lancet 352:1295, 1998

Canny GJ, Corey M, Livingstone RA, Carpenter S, Green L, Levison H: Pregnancy and cystic fibrosis. Obstet Gynecol 77:850, 1991

Cantwell MF, Shehab ZM, Costello AM, Sands L, Green WF, Ewing Jr EP, Valway SE, Onorato IM: Congenital tuberculosis. N Engl J Med 330:1051, 1994

Centers for Disease Control: Initial therapy for tuberculosis in the era of multidrug resistance: Recommendations of the Advisory Council for Elimination of Tuberculosis. MMWR 42:1, 1993

Centers for Disease Control: Screening for tuberculosis and tuberculous infection in high-risk populations. Recommendations of the Advisory Committee for Elimination of Tuberculosis. MMWR 39:1, 1990

Centers for Disease Control: Varicella-zoster immune globulin distribution-United States and other countries, 1981–1983. MMWR 33:81, 1984

Centers for Disease Control and Prevention: Establishment of VARIVAX(r) Pregnancy Registry. MMWR 45:239, 1996

Centers for Disease Control and Prevention: Geographic variation in penicillin resistance in *Streptococcus pneumoniae*—selected sites, United States, 1997. MMWR 48:656, 1999a

Centers for Disease Control and Prevention: Tuberculosis elimination revisited: Obstacles, opportunities, and a renewed commitment: Advisory Council for the Elimination of Tuberculosis (ACET). MMWR 48:1, 1999b

Centers for Disease Control and Prevention: 1999 USPHS/IDSA guidelines for the prevention of opportunistic infections in persons infected with human immunodeficiency virus. MMWR 48:1, 1999c

Centers for Disease Control and Prevention: Neuraminidase inhibitors for treatment of influenza A and B infections. MMWR 48:1, 1999d

Centers for Disease Control and Prevention: Updated guidelines for the use of rifabutin or rifampin for the treatment and prevention of tuberculosis among HIV-infected patients taking protease inhibitors or nonnucleoside reverse transcriptase inhibitors. MMWR 49:185, 2000a

Centers for Disease Control and Prevention: Update: Influenza activity—United States, 1999–2000 season. MMWR 49:53, 2000b

Centers for Disease Control and Prevention: Prevention and control of influenza. MMWR 49:1, 2000c

Chan WS, Ray JG: Low molecular weight heparin use during pregnancy: Issues of safety and practicality. Obstet Gynecol Surv 54:649, 1999

Chapman S, Duff P: Varicella in pregnancy. Semin Perinatol 17:403, 1993

Chapman SJ: Varicella in pregnancy. Semin Perinatol 22:339, 1998

China Tuberculosis Control Collaboration: Results of directly observed short-course chemotherapy in 112,842 Chinese patients with smear-positive tuberculosis. Lancet 347:358, 1996

Cohen LF, di Sant Agnese PA, Friedlander J: Cystic fibrosis and pregnancy: A national survey. Lancet 2:842, 1980

Columbus Investigators: Low-molecular-weight heparin in the treatment of patients with venous thromboembolism. N Engl J Med 337:657, 1997

Couch RB: Prevention and treatment of influenza. N Engl J Med 343:1778, 2000

Cox NJ, Subbarao K: Influenza. Lancet 354:1277, 1999

Crystal RG: Sarcoidosis. In Fauci AS, Braunwald E, Isselbacher KJ, Wilson JD, Martin JB, Kasper DL, Hauser SL, Longo DL: (eds): Harrison's Principles of Internal Medicine, 14th ed. New York, McGraw-Hill, 1998, p 1922

Cunningham FG, MacDonald PC, Gant NF, Leveno KJ, Gilstrap LC: Williams Obstetrics, 19th ed. Norwalk, CT, Appleton & Lange, 1993

Decousus H, Leizorovicz A, Parent F, Page Y, Tardy B, Girard P, Laporte S, Faivre R, Charbonnier B, Barral FG, Huet Y, Simonneau G: A clinical trial of vena caval filters in the prevention of pulmonary embolism in patients with proximal deep-vein thrombosis. N Engl J Med 338:409, 1998

Demissie K, Breckenridge MB, Rhoads GG: Infant and maternal outcomes in the pregnancies of asthmatic women. Am J Respir Crit Care Med 158:1091, 1998

De Regt RH: Sarcoidosis and pregnancy. Obstet Gynecol 70:369, 1987

De Stefano V, Martinelli I, Mannucci PM, Paciaroni K, Chiusolo P, Casorelli I, Rossi E, Leone G: The risk of recurrent deep venous thrombosis among heterozygous carriers of both factor V Leiden and the G20210A prothrombin mutation. N Engl J Med 341:801, 1999

De Swiet M: Maternal mortality: Confidential enquiries into maternal deaths in the United Kingdom. Am J Obstet Gynecol 182:760, 2000

De Swiet M: The respiratory system. In Hytten F, Chamberlain G (eds): Clinical Physiology in Obstetrics, 2nd ed. London, Blackwell, 1991, p 83

Drazen JM, Israel E, Boushey HA, Chinchilli VM, Fahy JV, Fish JE, Lazarus SC, Lemanske RF, Martin RJ, Peters SP, Sorkness CS, Szefler SJ: Comparison of regularly scheduled with as-needed use of albuterol in mild asthma. N Engl J Med 335:841, 1996

Drazen JM, Israel E, O'Bryne PM: Treatment of asthma with drugs modifying the leukotriene pathway. N Engl J Med 340:197, 1999

Edenborough FP, Mackenzie WE, Stableforth DE: The outcome of 72 pregnancies in 55 women with cystic fibrosis

in the United Kingdom 1977–1996. Br J Obstet Gynaecol 107:254, 2000

Edenborough FP, Stableforth DE, Webb AK, Mackenzie WE, Smith DL: The outcome of pregnancy in cystic fibrosis. Thorax 50:170, 1995

Eisenberg VH, Eidelman LA, Arbel R, Ezra Y: Legionnaire's disease during pregnancy: A case presentation and review of the literature. Eur J Obstet Gynecol Rep Biol 17:15, 1997

Elkharrat D, Raphael JC, Korach JM, Jars-Guincestre MC, Chastang C, Harboun C, Gajdos P: Acute carbon monoxide intoxication and hyperbaric oxygen in pregnancy. Int Care Med 17:289, 1991

Ely EW: Peacock JE, Haponik EF, Washburn RG: Cryptococcal pneumonia complicating pregnancy. Medicine 77:153, 1998

Erdman WA, Jayson HT, Redman HC, Miller GL, Parkey RW, Peshock RW: Deep venous thrombosis of extremities: Role of MR imaging in the diagnosis. Radiology 174:425, 1990

Espinal MA, Kim SJ, Suarez PG, Kam KM, Khomenko AG, Migliori GB, Baéz K. Kochi A, Dye C, Raviglione MC: Standard short-course chemotherapy for drug-resistant tuberculosis. JAMA 283:2537, 2000

Evenson LJ: Legionnaires' disease. Prim Care Update Ob/Gyn 5:286, 1998

Figueroa-Damian R, Arrendondo-Garcia JL: Pregnancy and tuberculosis: Influence of treatment on perinatal outcome. Am J Perinatol 15:303, 1998

Fine MJ, Smith MA, Carson CA, Mutha SS, Sankey SS, Sankey SS, Weissfeld LA, Kapoor WN: Prognosis and outcomes of patients with community-acquired pneumonia: A meta-analysis. JAMA 275:134, 1996

Finland M, Dublin TD: Pneumococcic pneumonias complicating pregnancy and the puerperium. JAMA 112:1027, 1939

Food and Drug Administration: First drug for penicillin-resistant community-acquired pneumonia. JAMA 283:1679, 2000

Frangolias DD, Nakielna EM, Wilcox PG: Pregnancy and cystic fibrosis. Chest 111:963, 1997

Freeman DW, Barno A: Deaths from Asian influenza associated with pregnancy. Am J Obstet Gynecol 78:1172, 1959

Gerhardt A, Scharf RE, Beckmann MW, Struve S, Bender HG, Pillny M, Sandmann W, Zota RB: Prothrombin and factor V mutations in women with a history of thrombosis during pregnancy and the puerperium. N Engl J Med 10:374, 2000

Gherman RB, Goodwin TM: Obstetric implications of activated protein C resistance and factor V Leiden mutation. Obstet Gynecol Surv 55:117, 2000

Gherman RB, Goodwin TM, Leung B, Byrne JD, Hethumumi R, Montoro M: Incidence, clinical characteristics, and timing of objectively diagnosed venous thromboembolism during pregnancy. Obstet Gynecol 94:730, 1999

Gherman RB, Leventis LL, Miller RC: Chlamydial psittacosis during pregnancy: A case report. Obstet Gynecol 86:648, 1995

Gilljam M, Antoniou M, Shin J, Dupuis A, Corey M, Tullis DE: Pregnancy in cystic fibrosis: Fetal and maternal outcome. Chest 118:85, 2000

Ginsberg JS, Brill-Edwards P, Burrows RF, Bona R, Prandoni P, Büller HR, Lensing A: Venous thrombosis during pregnancy: Leg and trimester of presentation. Thromb Haemost 67:519, 1992

Ginsberg JS, Hirsh J: Use of antithrombotic agents during pregnancy. Chest 114:524S, 1998

Glantz JC, Mushlin AI: Cost-effectiveness of routine antenatal varicella screening. Obstet Gynecol 91:519, 1998

Goldhaber SZ: Pulmonary embolism. N Engl J Med 339:93, 1998

Goldhaber SZ, Visani L, De Rosa M: Acute pulmonary embolism: Clinical outcomes in the International Cooperative Pulmonary Embolism Registry (ICOPER). Lancet 353:1386, 1999

Greenfield LJ, Michna BA: Twelve-year clinical experience with the Greenfield vena caval filter. Surgery 104:706, 1988

Greer IA: Thrombosis in pregnancy: Maternal and fetal issues. Lancet 353:1258, 1999

Gubareva LV, Kaiser L, Hayden FG: Influenza virus neuraminidase inhibitors. Lancet 355:827, 2000

Haake DA, Zakowski PC, Haake DL, Bryson YJ: Early treatment with acyclovir for varicella pneumonia in otherwise healthy adults: Retrospective controlled study and review. Rev Infect Dis 12:788, 1990

Hankins GDV, Berryman GK, Scott RT, Hood D: Maternal arterial desaturation with 15-methyl prostaglandin F2 alpha for uterine atony. Obstet Gynecol 72:367, 1988

Harris JW: Influenza occurring in pregnant women. JAMA 72:978, 1919

Hayden FG, Atmar RL, Schilling M, Johnson C, Poretz D, Paar D, Huson L, Ward P, Mills RG: Use of the selective oral neuraminidase inhibitor oseltamivir to prevent influenza. N Engl J Med 341:1336, 1999

Holgate ST: The cellular and mediator basis of asthma in relation to natural history. Lancet 350:5, 1997

Hough R, Makris M, Preston F: Pregnancy in women with thrombophilia: Incidence of thrombosis and pregnancy outcome. Br J Haematol 93:1, 1996

Hoyert DL, Kochanek KD, Murphy SL: Deaths: Final data for 1997. Natl Vital Stat Rep 47(19):1, 1998

Huang W, Hussey M, Michel F: Transmission of varicella to a gravida via close contacts immunized with varicella-zoster vaccine. J Reprod Med 44:905, 1999

Hull RD, Raskob GE, Pineo GF, Green D, Trowbridge AA, Elliott CG, Lerner RG, Hall J, Sparling T, Brettell HR, Norton J, Carter CJ, George R, Merli G, Ward J, Mayo W, Rosenbloom D, Brant R: Subcutaneous low-molecular-weight heparin compared with continuous intravenous heparin in the treatment of proximal-vein thrombosis. N Engl J Med 326:975, 1992

Hunt BJ, Dought HA, Majumdar G, Copplestone A, Kerslake S, Buchanan N, Hughes G, Khamashta M: Thromboprophylaxis with low molecular weight heparin (Fragmin) in high risk pregnancies. Thromb Haemost 77:39, 1997

Hux CH, Wapner RJ, Chayen B, Rattan P, Jarrell B, Greenfield L: Use of the Greenfield filter for thromboembolic disease in pregnancy. Am J Obstet Gynecol 155:734, 1986

Irving WL, James DK, Stephenson T, Laing P, Jameson C, Oxford JS, Chakraverty P, Brown DW, Boon AC, Zambon MC: Influenza virus infection in the second and third trimesters of pregnancy: A clinical and seroepidemiological study. Br J Obstet Gynaecol 107:1282, 2000

Jacob S, Bloebaum L, Shah G, Varner MW: Maternal mortality in Utah. Obstet Gynecol 91:187, 1998

Jacobs RF, Abernathy RS: Management of tuberculosis in pregnancy and the newborn. Clin Perinatol 15:305, 1988

Jana N, Vasishta K, Jindal SK, Khunnu B, Ghosh K: Perinatal outcome in pregnancies complicated by pulmonary tuberculosis. Int J Gynecol Obstet 44:119, 1994

Jana N, Vasishta K, Saha SC, Ghosh K: Obstetrical outcomes among women with extrapulmonary tuberculosis. N Engl J Med 341:645, 1999

Jana N, Vasishta K, Saha SC, Khunnu B: Effect of bronchial asthma on the course of pregnancy, labour and perinatal outcome. J Obstet Gynaecol 21:227, 1995

Jankelson D, Robinson M, Parsons S, Torzillo P, Peat B, Bye P: Cystic fibrosis and pregnancy. Aust NZ J Obstet Gynaecol 38:180, 1998

Kashyap S, Gruslin A: Influenza vaccination during pregnancy. Prim Care Update Ob/Gyns 7:7, 2000

Kearon C, Gent M, Hirsh J, Weitz J, Kovacs MJ, Anderson DR, Turpie AG, Green D, Ginsberg JS, Wells P, MacKinnon B, Julian JA: A comparison of three months of anticoagulation with extended anticoagulation for a first episode of idiopathic venous thromboembolism. N Engl J Med 340:901, 1999

Kent NE, Farquharson DF: Cystic fibrosis in pregnancy. Can Med Assoc J 149:809, 1993

Koonin LM, MacKay AP, Berg CJ, Atrash HK, Smith JC: Pregnancy-related mortality surveillance—United States, 1987–1990. MMWR 46:17, 1997

Lange P, Parner J, Vestbo J, Schnohr P, Jensen G: A 15-year follow-up study of ventilatory function in adults with asthma. N Engl J Med 339:1194, 1998

Lemanske RF, Busse WW: Asthma. JAMA 278:1855, 1997

Lensing AWA, Prandoni P, Brandjes D, Huisman PM, Vigo M, Tomasella G, Krekt J, Wouter TCJ, Huisman MV, Büller HR: Detection of deep-vein thrombosis by real-time B-mode ultrasonography. N Engl J Med 320:342, 1989

Lensing AWA Prandoni P, Prins MH, Büller HR: Deep-vein thrombosis. Lancet 353:479, 1999

Lindqvist P, Dahlbäck B, Marŝál K: Thrombotic risk during pregnancy: A population study. Obstet Gynecol 94:595, 1999

Lipworth BJ: Modern drug treatment of chronic asthma. BMJ 318:380, 1999

Llewellyn M, Cropley I, Wilkinson RJ, Davidson RN: Tuberculosis diagnosed during pregnancy: A prospective study from London. Thorax 55:129, 2000

Lockwood CJ: Heritable coagulopathies in pregnancy. Obstet Gynecol Surv 54:754, 1999

Longo L: The biologic effects of carbon monoxide on the pregnant woman, fetus and newborn infant. Am J Obstet Gynecol 129:69, 1977

Lynberg MC, Khoury MJ, Lu X, Cocian T: Maternal flu, fever, and the risk of neural tube defects: A population-based case-control study. Am J Epidemiol 14C:244, 1994

Mabie WC, Barton JR, Wasserstrum N, Sibai BM: Clinical observations on asthma in pregnancy. J Matern Fetal Med 1:45, 1992

Margono F, Mroueh J, Garely A, White D, Duerr A, Minkoff HL: Resurgence of active tuberculosis among pregnant women. Obstet Gynecol 83:911, 1994

Maisel JA, Lynam T: Unexpected sudden death in a young pregnant woman: Unusual presentation of neurosarcoidosis. Ann Emerg Med 28:94, 1996

McColl MD, Walker ID, Greer IA: The role of inherited thrombophilia in venous thromboembolism associated with pregnancy. Br J Obstet Gynaecol 106:756, 1999

McGrath J, Castle D: Does influenza cause schizophrenia? A five year review. Aust NZ J Psychiatry 29:23, 1995

McGregor JA, Burns JC, Levin MJ, Burlington B, Meiklejohn G: Transplacental passage of influenza A/Bangkok (H3N2) mimicking amniotic fluid infection syndrome. Am J Obstet Gynecol 148:856, 1984

McGregor JA, Kleinschmidt-DeMasters BK, Ogle J: Meningoencephalitis caused by *Histoplasma capsulatum* complicating pregnancy. Am J Obstet Gynecol 154:925, 1986

McKenna MT, McCray E, Onorato I: The epidemiology of tuberculosis among foreign-born persons in the United States, 1986 to 1993. N Engl J Med 332:1071, 1995

Medical Letter on Drugs and Therapeutics: Drugs for asthma. 41:5, 1999

Milne JA, Howie AD, Pack AI: Dyspnea during normal pregnancy. Br J Obstet Gynaecol 85:260, 1978

MIST (Management of influenza in the Southern Hemisphere Trialists) Study Group: Randomized trial of efficacy and safety of inhaled zanamivir in treatment of influenza A and B virus infections. Lancet 352:1877, 1998

Mueller MJ, Lebherz TB: Antepartum thrombophlebitis. Obstet Gynecol 34:867, 1969

Munn MB, Groome LJ, Atterbury JL, Baker SL, Hoff C: Pneumonia as a complication of pregnancy. J Matern Fet Med 8:151, 1999

Munoz FM, Englund JA: A step ahead. Infant protection through maternal immunization. Pediatr Clin North Am 47:449, 2000

Nathwani D, Maclean A, Conway S, Carrington D: Varicella infections in pregnancy and the newborn. J Infect 36:59, 1998

National Asthma Education Program: Report of the Working Group on Asthma and Pregnancy: Executive Summary: Management of Asthma During Pregnancy. National Heart, Lung and Blood Institute. NIH publication 93-3279A, March 1993

National Heart, Lung and Blood Institute: National Asthma Education Program, expert panel report. Guidelines for the diagnosis and management of asthma. Pediatr Asthma Allergy Immunol 5:57, 1991

National Institutes of Health: Practical Guide for the Diagnosis and Management of Asthma. NIH Publication No. 97-4053, October 1997

National Institutes of Health Consensus Development Conference: Prevention of venous thrombosis and pulmonary embolism. JAMA 256:744, 1986

Neill AM, Appleton DS, Richards P: Retrievable inferior vena caval filter for thromboembolic disease in pregnancy. Br J Obstet Gynecol 104:1416, 1997

Nelson HS: Beta-adrenergic bronchodilators. N Engl J Med 333:499, 1995

Nelson-Piercy C, Letsky EA, de Swiet M: Low-molecular-weight heparin for obstetric thromboprophylaxis: Experience of sixty-nine pregnancies in sixty-one women at high risk. Am J Obstet Gynecol 176:1062, 1997

Neuzil KM, Reed GW, Mitchel EF, Simonsen L, Griffin MR: Impact of influenza on acute cardiopulmonary hospitalizations in pregnant women. Am J Epidemiol 148:1094, 1998

Noble PW, Lavee AE, Jacobs NM: Respiratory diseases in pregnancy. Obstet Gynecol Clin North Am 15:391, 1988

Olson GL: Cystic fibrosis in pregnancy. Semin Perinatol 21:307, 1997

Pablos-Mendez A, Raviglione MC, Laszlo A, Binkin N, Rieder HL, Bustreo F, Cohn DL, Lambregts-van Weezenbeek CSB, Kim SJ, Chaulet P, Nunn P: Global surveillance for antituberculosis-drug resistance, 1994–1997. N Engl J Med 338:1641, 1998

Paryani SG, Arvin AM: Intrauterine infection with varicella-zoster virus after maternal varicella. N Engl J Med 314:1542, 1986

Pillay T, Jeena PM: A neonate with hemorrhagic ascites. Lancet 354:914, 1999

PIOPED Investigators: Value of the ventilation/perfusion scan in acute pulmonary embolism: Results of the Prospec-tive Investigation of Pulmonary Embolism Diagnosis (PIOPED). JAMA 263:2753, 1990

Powell BL, Drutz DJ, Huppert M, Sun SH: Relationship of progesterone- and estradiol-binding proteins in Coccidioides immitis to coccidioidal dissemination in pregnancy. Infect Immun 40:478, 1983

Ramsey BW: Management of pulmonary disease in patients with cystic fibrosis. N Engl J Med 335:179, 1996

Richey SD, Roberts SW, Ramin KD, Ramin SM, Cunningham FG: Pneumonia complicating pregnancy. Obstet Gynecol 84:525, 1994

Riley P: Pneumococcal infections. Prim Care Update Ob/Gyns 7:22, 2000

Rolston DH, Shnider SM, de Lorimer AA: Uterine blood flow and fetal acid–base changes after bicarbonate administration to the pregnant ewe. Anesthesiology 40:348, 1974

Rouse DJ, Gardner M, Allen SJ, Goldenberg RL: Management of the presumed susceptible varicella (chickenpox)–exposed gravida: A cost-effectiveness/cost-benefit analysis. Obstet Gynecol 87:932, 1996

Saade GR: Human immunodeficiency virus (HIV)–related pulmonary complications in pregnancy. Semin Perinatol 21:336, 1997

Saxén L, Holmberg PC, Kurppa K, Kuosma E, Pyhälä R: Influenza epidemics and anencephaly. Am J Public Health 80:473, 1990

Schatz M: Asthma and pregnancy. Lancet 353:1202, 1999

Schatz M, Harden K, Forsythe A, Chilingar L, Hoffman C, Sperling W, Zeiger RS: The course of asthma during pregnancy, postpartum, and with successive pregnancies: A prospective analysis. J Allergy Clin Immunol 81:509, 1988

Schatz M, Zeiger RS, Hoffman CP, Harden K, Forsythe A, Chilingar L, Saunders B, Porreco R, Sperling W, Kagnoff M, Benenson AS: Perinatal outcomes in the pregnancies of asthmatic women: A prospective controlled analysis. Am J Respir Crit Care Med 151:1170, 1995

Seballos RJ, Mendel SG, Mirmiran-Yazdy A, Khoury W, Marshall JB: Sarcoid cardiomyopathy precipitated by pregnancy with cocaine complications. Chest 105:303, 1994

Selroos O: Sarcoidosis and pregnancy: A review with results of a retrospective survey. J Int Med 227:221, 1990

Silverman RK, Montano J: Hyperbaric oxygen treatment during pregnancy in acute carbon monoxide poisoning. A case report. J Reprod Med 42:309, 1997

Simmoneau G, Sors H, Charbonnier B, Page Y, Laaban JP, Azarian R, Laurent M, Hirsch JL, Ferrari E, Bosson JL, Mottier D, Beau B. For the THÉSÉ Group. A comparison of low-molecular-weight heparin with unfractionated heparin for acute pulmonar embolism. N Engl J Med 337:663, 1997

Smego RA, Asperilla MO: Use of acyclovir for varicella pneumonia during pregnancy. Obstet Gynecol 78:1112, 1991

Stallings SP: Varicella virus vaccine. Prim Care Update Ob/Gyns 7:16, 2000

Stenius-Aarniala B, Pririla P, Teramo K: Asthma and pregnancy: A prospective study of 198 pregnancies. Thorax 43:12, 1988

Stevens DA: Coccidioidomycosis. N Engl J Med 332:1077, 1995

Stratton P, Mofenson LM, Willoughby AD: Human immunodeficiency virus infection in pregnant women under care at AIDS Clinical Trials Centers in the United States. Obstet Gynecol 79:364, 1992

Tengborn L, Bergqvist D, Matzsch T, Bergqvist A, Hedner U: Recurrent thromboembolism in pregnancy and puerperium: Is there a need for thromboprophylaxis? Am J Obstet Gynecol 160:90, 1989

Tewari K, Wold SM, Asrat T: Septic shock in pregnancy associated with legionella pneumonia: Case report. Am J Obstet Gynecol 176:706, 1997

Thomas LA, Summers RR, Cardwell MS: Use of Greenfield filters in pregnant women at risk for pulmonary embolism. South Med J 90:215, 1997

Tomaszewski C: Carbon monoxide poisoning. Early awareness and intervention can save lives. Postgrad Med 105:39, 1999

Wack EE, Ampel NM, Galgiani JN, Bronnimann DA: Coccidioidomycosis during pregnancy: An analysis of ten cases among 47,120 pregnancies. Chest 94:376, 1988

Ware LB, Matthay MA: The acute respiratory distress syndrome. N Engl J Med 342:1334, 2000

Weinberger SE, Weiss ST: Pulmonary diseases. In Duffy TP Burrow GN, (eds): Medical Complications During Pregnancy, 5th ed. Philadelphia, Saunders, 1999, p 363

Wendel PJ, Ramin SM, Hamm CB, Rowe TF, Cunningham FG: Asthma treatment in pregnancy: A randomized controlled study. Am J Obstet Gynecol 175:150, 1996

Whitney CG, Farley MM, Hadler J, Harrison LH, Lexau C, Reingold A, Lefkowitz L, Cieslak PR, Cetron M, Zell ER, Jorgensen JH, Schuchat AS, for the Active Bacterial Core Surveillance Program of the Emerging Infections Program Network: Increasing prevalence of multidrug-resistant *Streptococcus pneumoniae* in the United States. N Engl J Med 343:1917, 2000

Witlin AG, Mattar FM, Saade GR, Van Hook JW, Sibai BM: Presentation of venous thromboembolism during pregnancy. Am J Obstet Gynecol 181:1118, 1999

Yost NP, Bloom SL, Richey SD, Ramin SM, Cunningham FG: An appraisal of treatment guidelines for antepartum community-acquired pneumonia. Am J Obstet Gynecol 183:131, 2000

47

Renal and Urinary Tract Disorders

Although some diseases of the kidney and urinary tract may be associated with pregnancy by chance, pregnancy often predisposes to the development of urinary tract disorders, an example being acute pyelonephritis. In other cases, pregnancy may predispose to worsening of renal disease and its sequelae, as with lupus nephritis complicated by hypertension. In the not too distant past, obstetrical dogma was that pregnancy was contraindicated in the woman with significant underlying renal disease. As experience was gained, however, it became apparent that most women with these disorders will go through pregnancy without serious sequelae.

URINARY TRACT CHANGES DURING PREGNANCY

Significant changes in both structure and function take place in the urinary tract during normal pregnancy (Chap. 8, p. 186). Urinary tract dilatation is one of the most significant anatomical alterations induced by pregnancy. It involves dilatation of the renal calyces and pelves, as well as the ureters. Faúndes and co-workers (1998) used ultrasound to measure the renal calyces during pregnancy and confirmed dilatation in about half with the right side more frequently and severely affected (Fig. 47–1). Some of the women demonstrated dilata-

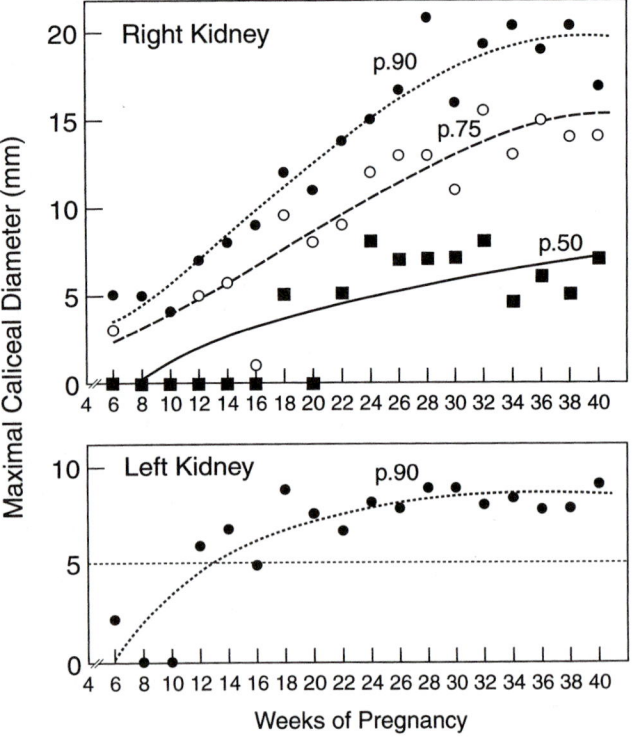

FIGURE 47–1. The 50th, 75th, and 90th percentiles for renal caliceal diameters measured using ultrasound in 1395 pregnant women from 4 to 42 weeks. (From Faúndes and co-workers, 1998, with permission.)

tion before the uterus reached the pelvic brim at about 14 weeks, implicating hormonal relaxation of the muscular layers of the urinary tract. There was further dilatation at 21 weeks due to mechanical compression of the ureters, especially on the right side. Most—all but 6 percent—of the women with pregnancy-induced dilatation of the urinary tract demonstrated resolution within 2 to 4 days of delivery. Interestingly, the fetal urinary tract mimics the maternal dilatation (Graif and colleagues, 1992).

An important consequence of dilatation and obstruction is potentially serious upper urinary infections. Another factor predisposing to infection is increased vesicoureteral reflux. These normal changes associated with pregnancy also may lead to erroneous interpretation of studies done to evaluate suspected pathological obstruction.

Evidence for hypertrophy of renal function is apparent very soon after conception. It appears to be mediated by pregnancy-induced intrarenal vasodilatation. Effective renal plasma flow and glomerular filtration are increased on the average by 40 and 65 percent, respectively. These changes have clinical relevance when interpreting renal function studies; for example, serum concentrations of creatinine and urea are decreased substantively. Other alterations include those related to maintaining normal acid–base homeostasis, osmoregulation, and fluid and electrolyte retention.

ASSESSMENT OF RENAL DISEASE DURING PREGNANCY

Interpretation of the **urinalysis** is essentially unchanged during pregnancy, except for the occasional glucosuria that is discovered. Although protein excretion normally is increased, it seldom reaches levels to be detected by usual screening methods. Higby and colleagues (1994) reported 24-hour protein excretion to be 115 mg with the 95 percent confidence level at 260 mg/day. There were no significant differences by trimester. They also showed that albumin excretion is minimal and ranges from 5 to 30 mg/day. Most investigators agree that proteinuria must exceed 300 to 500 mg/day to be considered abnormal for pregnancy. Unless precautions are taken to prevent contamination, there usually is an admixture of vaginal secretions when the specimen is collected; thus, a clean-catch specimen should be taken to verify any pathological proteinuria detected.

If the serum creatinine persistently exceeds 0.9 mg/dL (75 μmol/L), then intrinsic renal disease should be suspected. A carefully collected, timed urine specimen can be used to estimate the glomerular filtration rate by creatinine clearance. **Ultrasonography** provides imaging of renal size and relative consistency, as well as elements of obstruction (Fig. 47–1). Full-sequence **intravenous pyelography** is not done routinely, but injection of contrast media with one or two abdominal x-rays may be indicated by the clinical situation. The usual clinical indications for **cystoscopy** are followed. Although Packham and Fairley (1987) reported **renal biopsy** to be safe and helpful in guiding treatment in 111 pregnant women with renal disease, we agree with others that this procedure can usually be postponed until pregnancy is completed (Lindheimer and colleagues, 2000). If therapy would be changed by biopsy results, then it should be considered.

ORTHOSTATIC PROTEINURIA. Abnormal amounts of protein are sometimes detectable in urine formed while the pregnant woman is ambulatory but not when recumbent. No other evidence for renal disease is apparent. Such orthostatic or *postural proteinuria* has been observed in up to 5 percent of normal young adults. The pregnant woman with orthostatic proteinuria should be evaluated for bacteriuria, abnormal urinary sediment, reduced glomerular filtration rate, and hypertension. In the absence of these abnormalities, especially if protein excretion is not constant, orthostatic proteinuria is probably inconsequential.

PREGNANCY AFTER UNILATERAL NEPHRECTOMY. Because the excretory capacity of two kidneys is much in excess of ordinary needs, and because the surviving kidney usually undergoes hypertrophy with increased excretory capacity, women with one normal kidney most often have no difficulty in pregnancy. Indeed, pregnancy in these women is associated with significant augmentation of renal hemodynamics (Baylis and Davison, 1991). Before advising a woman with one kidney about the risk of future pregnancy, a thorough functional evaluation of the remaining organ is essential.

URINARY TRACT INFECTIONS

These are the most common bacterial infections encountered during pregnancy. Although **asymptomatic bacteriuria** is usual, symptomatic infection may involve the lower tract to cause **cystitis,** or it may involve the renal calyces, pelvis, and parenchyma to cause **pyelonephritis.**

Organisms that cause urinary infections are those from the normal perineal flora. There is now evidence that some strains of *Escherichia coli* have pili that enhance their virulence (Svanborg-Eden, 1982). Also called *adhesins* or *P-fimbriae,* these appendages allow bacterial attachment to glycoprotein receptors on uroepithelial cell membranes. Other markers for virulence include strains that produce hemolysin and have the papG gene that encodes the P-fimbriae tip adhesin

(Hooton and co-workers, 2000). Although pregnancy itself does not seem to enhance these virulence factors, urinary stasis apparently does, and along with vesicoureteral reflux in some women, it predisposes to symptomatic upper urinary infections.

In the early puerperium, bladder sensitivity to intravesical fluid tension is often decreased as a consequence of the trauma of labor as well as epidural or spinal analgesia. Sensations of bladder distention are also likely diminished by discomfort caused by a large episiotomy, periurethral lacerations, or vaginal wall hematomas. Following delivery, especially when oxytocin infusion is stopped, diuresis follows with copious urine production and bladder distention. Overdistention, coupled with catheterization to provide relief, commonly leads to urinary infection.

ASYMPTOMATIC BACTERIURIA. This refers to persistent, actively multiplying bacteria within the urinary tract without symptoms. The reported prevalence of bacteriuria in nonpregnant women is 5 to 6 percent (Hooton and colleagues, 2000). The incidence during pregnancy varies from 2 to 7 percent, and depends on parity, race, and socioeconomic status. The highest incidence has been reported in African-American multiparas with sickle-cell trait, and the lowest incidence has been found in affluent white women of low parity.

Bacteriuria is typically present at the time of the first prenatal visit, and after an initial negative urine culture, 1 percent or less of women develop urinary infection (Whalley, 1967). A clean-voided specimen containing more than 100,000 organisms per mL is considered evidence for infection. Although smaller numbers of bacteria may represent contamination, lower colony counts may sometimes represent active infection, especially in the presence of symptoms. Thus, it seems prudent to treat lower concentrations, because pyelonephritis may occur with counts of only 20,000 to 50,000/mL of a single uropathogen (Lucas and Cunningham, 1993).

SIGNIFICANCE. If asymptomatic bacteriuria is not treated, about 25 percent of infected women subsequently develop acute symptomatic infection during that pregnancy. Eradication of bacteriuria with antimicrobial agents has been shown to prevent most of these clinically evident infections. Although it is reasonable to perform routine screening for bacteriuria in women at high risk, screening via urine culture may not be cost effective when the prevalence is low. Less expensive tests such as the leukocyte esterase-nitrite dipstick have been shown to be cost effective with prevalences of 2 percent (Rouse and colleagues, 1995). Millar and associates (2000) reported that screening using enzymatic detection of catalase activity in the urine was ineffective.

Another approach for the low-risk population is to perform screening cultures selected by historical factors.

Covert bacteriuria has been associated in some studies with a number of adverse pregnancy outcomes. In early studies by Kass (1962), the incidence of preterm births and perinatal mortality was increased among bacteriuric women given placebo compared with treated 84 women. Kincaid-Smith and Bullen (1965) also reported an increased incidence of low-birthweight infants among untreated bacteriuric women, but were unable to reduce this with antimicrobial therapy. Other investigators did not corroborate a relationship between bacteriuria and low-birthweight infants (Table 47–1). From evidence currently available it seems unlikely that asymptomatic bacteriuria is a prominent factor in the genesis of low-birthweight or preterm infants.

In other studies, bacteriuria has been linked to an increased incidence of pregnancy hypertension and anemia. Using multivariate analysis for a perinatal registry cohort of 25,746 mother–infant pairs, Schieve and colleagues (1994) reported increased risks for low birthweight, preterm delivery, hypertension or preeclampsia, and maternal anemia. These findings are at variance with those shown in Table 47–2. Gilstrap and colleagues (1981b) compared pregnancy outcomes in 248 pregnant woman in whom bacteriuria was localized to the bladder or kidney and found no association with anemia, hypertension, or low-birthweight infants.

Bacteriuria persists after delivery in many of these women, and there is also a significant number with pyelographic evidence of chronic infection, obstructive lesions, or congenital urinary abnormalities (Kincaid-Smith and Bullen, 1965; Whalley and associates, 1965). Recurrent symptomatic infections are common.

TREATMENT. Women with asymptomatic bacteriuria may be given treatment with any of several antimicrobial regimens. Selection can be on the basis of in vitro susceptibilities, but most often it is empirical. Treatment for 10 days with nitrofurantoin macrocrystals, 100 mg

daily, has proved effective in most women. Other regimens include ampicillin, amoxicillin, a cephalosporin, nitrofurantoin, or a sulfonamide given four times daily for 3 days (Table 47–3). Single-dose antimicrobial therapy for bacteriuria has also been used with success (Andriole and Patterson, 1991). The recurrence rate for all of these regimens is about 30 percent. Failure of single-dose regimens may be an indication of upper tract infection and the need for more protracted therapy such as nitrofurantoin, 100 mg at bedtime for 21 days (Lucas

TABLE 47–2. Adverse Pregnancy Outcomes in Comparison of 248 Women with Asymptomatic Renal or Bladder Bacteriuria

| Complication | Bacteriuric Women (%)[a] | | Control Women (%)[a] (n = 248) |
	Renal (n = 114)	Bladder (n = 134)	
Anemia[b]	2.6	3.7	2.1
Hypertension	12	15	14
Low-birthweight infants	10	13	13
Fetal growth restriction	8	8	8
Preterm delivery	4	8	5

[a] All values not significant when compared for each group.
[b] Hematocrit less than 30.
Modified after Gilstrap and colleagues (1981b).

TABLE 47–1. Incidence of Low-birthweight Infants Born to Women with and without Asymptomatic Bacteriuria

	Bacteriuria No. (%)	Uninfected No. (%)
Gilstrap and colleagues (1981b)	248 (12)	248 (13)
Little (1966)	141 (9)	4735 (8)
Norden and Kilpatrick (1965)	114 (15)	109 (13)
Whalley (1967)	176 (15)	176 (12)
Wilson and associates (1966)	230 (11)	6216 (10)
Total and average	909 (12)	11,484 (9)

TABLE 47–3. Antimicrobial Agents Used for Treatment of Pregnant Women with Asymptomatic Bacteriuria

Single Dose
Amoxicillin, 3g
Ampicillin, 2 g
Cephalosporin, 2 g
Nitrofurantoin, 200 mg
Sulfonamide, 2 g
Trimethoprim-sulfamethoxazole, 320/1600 mg

Three-day Course
Amoxicillin, 500 mg three times daily
Ampicillin, 250 mg four times daily
Cephalosporin, 250 mg four times daily
Nitrofurantoin, 50–100 mg four times daily; 100 mg twice daily
Sulfonamide, 500 mg four times daily

Other
Nitrofurantoin, 100 mg four times daily for 10 days
Nitrofurantoin, 100 mg at bedtime for 10 days

Treatment Failures
Nitrofurantoin, 100 mg four times daily for 21 days

Suppression for Bacterial Persistence or Recurrence
Nitrofurantoin, 100 mg at bedtime for remainder of pregnancy

and Cunningham, 1994). For women with persistent or frequent bacteriuria recurrences, suppressive therapy for the remainder of pregnancy may be indicated. One regimen that has been successful is nitrofurantoin, 100 mg at bedtime.

CYSTITIS AND URETHRITIS. There is evidence that bladder infection during pregnancy develops without antecedent covert bacteriuria (Harris and Gilstrap, 1981). Typically, cystitis is characterized by dysuria, urgency, and frequency. There are few associated systemic findings. Usually there is pyuria as well as bacteriuria. Microscopic hematuria is common, and occasionally there is gross hematuria from hemorrhagic cystitis (Fakhoury and co-workers, 1994). Although asymptomatic infection is associated with renal bacteriuria in half of cases, more than 90 percent of the cases of cystitis are limited to the bladder (Harris and Gilstrap, 1981). Although cystitis is usually uncomplicated, the upper urinary tract may become involved by ascending infection. Certainly, 40 percent of pregnant women with acute pyelonephritis have preceding symptoms of lower-tract infection (Gilstrap and associates, 1981a).

TREATMENT. Women with cystitis respond readily to any of several regimens. Harris and Gilstrap (1981) reported a 97 percent cure rate with a 10-day ampicillin regimen. Sulfonamides, nitrofurantoin, or a cephalosporin also are effective when given for 10 days. Recently, as with covert bacteriuria, there has been a trend to use a 3-day course of therapy. The regimens summarized in Table 47–3 will generally prove satisfactory for cystitis. Single-dose therapy as described for asymptomatic bacteriuria has been shown effective for both nonpregnant and pregnant women, but concomitant pyelonephritis must be confidently excluded.

Frequency, urgency, dysuria, and pyuria accompanied by a "sterile" urine culture may be the consequence of urethritis caused by *Chlamydia trachomatis,* a common pathogen of the genitourinary tract. Mucopurulent cervicitis usually coexists and erythromycin therapy is effective (Chap. 57, p. 1493).

ACUTE PYELONEPHRITIS. Renal infection is the most common serious medical complication of pregnancy, occurring in approximately 2 percent of pregnant women. The potential seriousness of acute pyelonephritis during pregnancy can be underscored by the observation of Mabie and associates (1997) that acute pyelonephritis was the leading cause of septic shock during pregnancy. The population incidence varies and depends on the prevalence of covert bacteriuria and whether it is treated. For example, at Parkland Hospital, more than 95 percent of women attend prenatal clinics where bacteriuria screening is performed and treatment given for

the 8 percent who are infected. Gratacos and associates (1994) reported a significant reduction in the incidence of pyelonephritis after they instituted a screening program.

Renal infection is more common after midpregnancy. It is unilateral and right-sided in more than half of cases, and bilateral in a fourth. In most women, infection is caused by bacteria that ascend from the lower tract. Between 75 and 90 percent of renal infections are caused by bacteria that have P-fimbriae adhesins (Stenqvist and associates, 1987).

CLINICAL FINDINGS. The onset of pyelonephritis is usually rather abrupt. Symptoms include fever, shaking chills, and aching pain in one or both lumbar regions. There may be anorexia, nausea, and vomiting. The course of the disease may vary remarkably with fever to as high as 40°C or more and hypothermia to as low as 34°C. Tenderness usually can be elicited by percussion in one or both costovertebral angles. The urinary sediment frequently contains many leukocytes, frequently in clumps, and numerous bacteria. In a survey of 190 women admitted to Parkland Hospital, *E coli* was isolated from the urine in 77 percent, *Klebsiella pneumoniae* in 11 percent, and *Enterobacter* or *Proteus* each in 4 percent (Cunningham, 1988). Culture results were similar from 391 women with antepartum pyelonephritis treated at Los Angeles County–University of Southern California Medical Center (Wing and colleagues, 2000). **Importantly, about 15 percent of women with acute pyelonephritis also have bacteremia.**

Although the diagnosis usually is apparent, pyelonephritis may be mistaken for labor, chorioamnionitis, appendicitis, placental abruption, or infarcted myoma, and in the puerperium, for metritis with pelvic cellulitis.

Almost all clinical findings in these women are ultimately caused by endotoxemia, and so are the serious complications of acute pyelonephritis (Chap. 43). A frequent and sometimes dramatic finding is thermoregulatory instability characterized by high spiking fever as high as 42°C followed by hypothermia as low as 34°C (Fig. 47–2). Twickler and associates (1994) have shown a significantly decreased systemic vascular resistance and increased cardiac output in women with acute infection. These changes are mediated by *cytokines* elaborated by macrophages that include *interleukin-1,* previously termed *endogenous pyrogen,* or *tumor necrosis factor* (Parrillo, 1993).

Plasma creatinine should be measured early in the course of therapy. As shown in Figure 47–3, acute pyelonephritis in some pregnant women causes a considerable reduction in the glomerular filtration rate that is reversible. From 1 to 2 percent of women with antepartum pyelonephritis develop varying degrees of respiratory insufficiency caused by endotoxin-induced alveolar in-

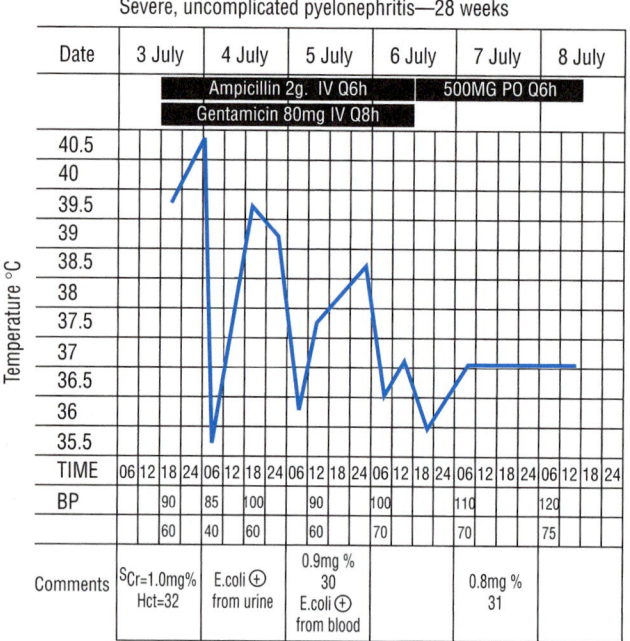

SD
Severe, uncomplicated pyelonephritis—28 weeks

Date	3 July	4 July	5 July	6 July	7 July	8 July

Ampicillin 2g. IV Q6h   500MG PO Q6h
Gentamicin 80mg IV Q8h

Temperature °C: 40.5, 40, 39.5, 39, 38.5, 38, 37.5, 37, 36.5, 36, 35.5

TIME: 06 12 18 24 | 06 12 18 24 | 06 12 18 24 | 06 12 18 24 | 06 12 18 24 | 06 12 18 24

BP: 90/60 | 85/40 100/60 | 90/60 | 100/70 | 110/70 | 120/75

Comments:
SCr=1.0mg%
Hct=32 | E.coli ⊕ from urine | 0.9mg % 30 E.coli ⊕ from blood | | 0.8mg % 31

FIGURE 47–2. Vital signs graphic chart from a 25-year-old primigravida with acute pyelonephritis at 28 weeks' gestation. (From Cunningham and colleagues, 1987, with permission.)

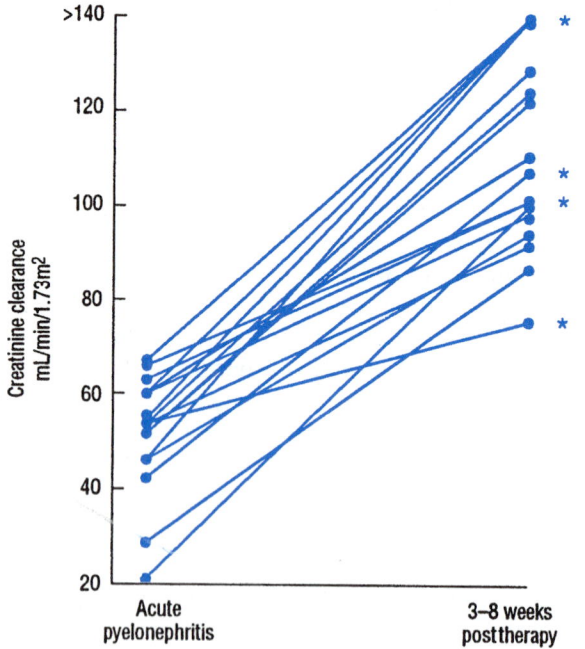

FIGURE 47–3. Endogenous creatinine clearance values in 18 pregnant women during and 3 to 8 weeks after an attack of acute pyelonephritis. Asterisk indicates patients reevaluated while still pregnant. (From Whalley and colleagues, 1975, with permission.)

jury and pulmonary edema (Cunningham and associates, 1987; Sanchez-Ramos and colleagues, 1995). In some women, pulmonary injury is severe with resultant **acute respiratory distress syndrome.** Occasionally, tracheal intubation with mechanical ventilation is lifesaving (Fig. 47–4).

Graham and associates (1993) confirmed that institution of antimicrobial treatment in these women was followed by increased uterine activity. This likely is due to endotoxin release. **Towers and co-workers (1991) reported that 8 percent of women with acute pyelonephritis who were given β-agonist tocolysis, developed respiratory insufficiency.** This is related to plasma colloid osmotic pressure decrease, alveolar capillary membrane injury, and sodium and fluid retaining properties of β-agonists (Lamont, 2000).

Endotoxin-induced **hemolysis** is also common, and about one third of these women develop acute anemia (Cox and colleagues, 1991). Recent evidence is indicative that acute pyelonephritis does not affect erythropoietin production either acutely or during the next several days of infection (Cavenee and colleagues, 1994).

MANAGEMENT. One scheme for management of the pregnant woman with acute pyelonephritis is shown in Table 47–4. Although we routinely obtain cultures of urine and blood, Wing and co-workers (2000) have recently shown in prospective trials that they are of limited clinical utility. **Intravenous hydration to ensure adequate urinary output is essential.** Because bacteremia and endotoxinemia are common, these women should be watched carefully to detect symptoms of endotoxin shock or its sequelae. Urinary output, blood pressure, and temperature are monitored closely. High fever should be treated, usually with a cooling blanket. Routine renal ultrasonography has not been shown to be useful and should be reserved for those women unresponsive to initial treatment (Seidman and colleagues, 1998).

These serious urinary infections usually respond quickly to intravenous hydration and antimicrobial therapy. The choice of drug is empirical, and ampicillin, plus gentamicin, cefazolin, or ceftriaxone have been shown to be 95 percent effective in randomized trials (Wing and colleagues, 1998, 2000). Ampicillin resistance of *E coli* has become common and only half of strains are sensitive in vitro to ampicillin, but most are sensitive to cefazolin (Millar and Cox, 1997; Wing and associates, 2000). For these reasons, many clinicians prefer to give gentamicin or another aminoglycoside with ampicillin. Serial determinations of serum creatinine are important if nephrotoxic drugs are given. Finally, some prefer a cephalosporin or extended-spectrum penicillin, which have been shown to be effective in 95 percent of infected

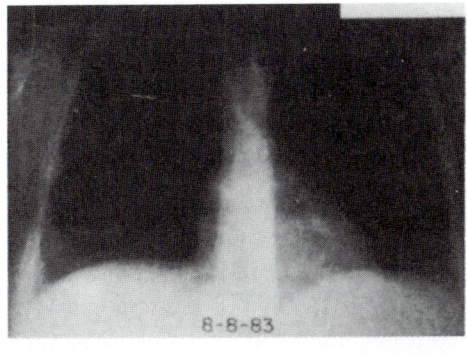
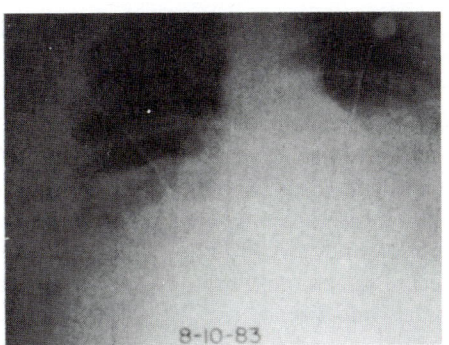
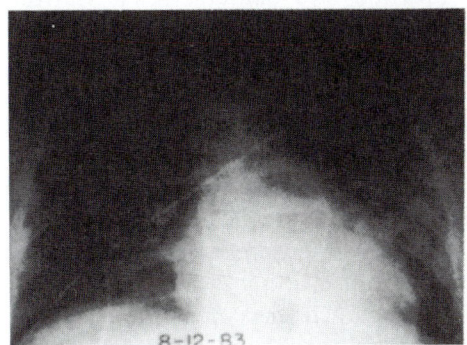
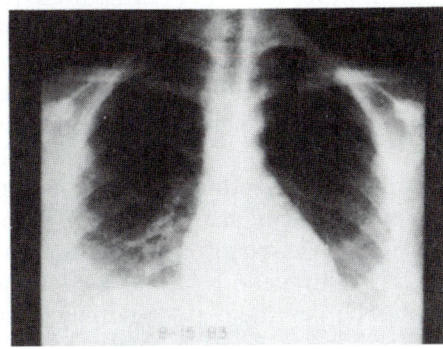

FIGURE 47–4. An 18-year-old multipara with acute pyelonephritis at 20 weeks had a normal radiograph when admitted 8-8-83. Respiratory distress 20 hours later was accompanied by a left-sided pulmonary infiltrate, which progressed to bilateral infiltrates by 8-10-83. The infiltrates improved, and she had a normal x-ray by 8-15-83. (From Cunningham and colleagues, 1987, with permission.)

women (Millar and Cox, 1997; Sanchez-Ramos and associates, 1995).

Clinical symptoms for the most part resolve during the first 2 days of therapy; but even though the symptoms promptly abate, many authors recommend therapy for a total of 7 to 10 days. Cultures of urine usually become sterile within the first 24 hours. Because changes in the urinary tract induced by pregnancy persist, reinfection is possible. If subsequent cultures of the urine are positive, we give nitrofurantoin, 100 mg at bedtime, for the remainder of pregnancy.

OUTPATIENT MANAGEMENT. Wing and associates (1999) described a randomized clinical trial in which they compared oral versus intravenous antimicrobial therapy for 92 highly selected women with antepartum pyelonephritis. They reported no significant differences in clinical responses or pregnancy outcomes between inpatients and outpatients. Importantly, two thirds of women were not considered candidates for outpatient therapy. Of those treated as outpatients, 30 percent were unable to adhere to their treatment regimen. All women in this trial received in-hospital intramuscular ceftriaxone, two 1-g doses 24 hours apart, before those randomized to early discharge were permitted to leave the hospital. Studies such as this suggest that outpatient management of pregnant women with acute pyelonephritis is applicable to very few women and it mandates close evaluation both before and after hospital discharge.

MANAGEMENT OF NONRESPONDERS. Almost 95 percent of pregnant women will be afebrile by 72 hours (Cunningham and associates, 1973; Wing and col-

TABLE 47–4. Management of the Pregnant Women with Acute Pyelonephritis

1. Hospitalization
2. Urine and blood cultures
3. Hemogram, serum creatinine, and electrolytes
4. Monitor vital signs frequently, including urinary output (place indwelling bladder catheter if necessary)
5. Intravenous crystalloid to establish urinary output to at least 30 mL/hr
6. Intravenous antimicrobial therapy
7. Chest x-ray if there is dyspnea or tachypnea
8. Repeat hematology and chemistry studies in 48 hours
9. Change to oral antimicrobials when afebrile
10. Discharge when afebrile 24 hours; consider antimicrobial therapy for 7–10 days
11. Urine culture 1–2 weeks after antimicrobial therapy completed

Modified from Lucas and Cunningham (1994).

leagues, 2000). If clinical improvement is not obvious by 48 to 72 hours, then the woman should be evaluated for urinary tract obstruction. A search is made for abnormal ureteral or pyelocaliceal distention. Most women with continuing infection and serious sequelae will have no evidence for obstruction, but some are found to have obstruction from calculi. Many investigators prefer renal sonography to detect underlying lesions, but its sensitivity is decreased in pregnancy and stones may not be visualized (Butler and associates, 2000; Maikranz and colleagues, 1987). Pyelocaliceal dilatation, urinary calculi, and possibly an intrarenal or perinephric abscess or phlegmon may be visualized (Cox and Cunningham, 1988). Sonar is not always successful in localizing these lesions; thus a negative examination should not prompt cessation of the workup in a woman with continuing urosepsis.

In some cases, a plain abdominal radiograph is indicated, because nearly 90 percent of renal stones are radiopaque. Possible benefits far outweigh any minimal fetal risk from radiation. If negative, then intravenous pyelography, modified to limit the number of radiographs taken after contrast injection, is recommended. The "one-shot pyelogram," in which a single radiograph is obtained 30 minutes after contrast injection, usually provides adequate imaging of the collecting system so that stones or structural anomalies can be detected (Butler and colleagues, 2000).

Passage of a double-J ureteral stent will relieve the obstruction in most cases (Rodriguez and Klein, 1988). If unsuccessful, then percutaneous nephrostomy is done. If this fails, surgical removal of renal stones is required for resolution of infection. Retrograde pyelography may disclose an end-stage obstructed kidney with pyonephrosis as a cause of continuing sepsis. In these cases, calculi frequently coexist, and nephrectomy may be lifesaving.

FOLLOW-UP. Recurrent infection, both covert and symptomatic, is common and can be demonstrated in 30 to 40 percent of women following completion of treatment for pyelonephritis (Cunningham and associates, 1973). Unless measures are taken to ensure urine sterility, then nitrofurantoin, 100 mg at bedtime, is given for the remainder of the pregnancy. Van Dorsten and co-workers (1987) reported that this regimen reduces recurrence of bacteriuria to 8 percent.

CHRONIC PYELONEPHRITIS. This disease is chronic interstitial nephritis thought to be caused by bacterial infection. In many cases, classical radiological scarring is accompanied by ureteral reflux with voiding; thus the term **reflux nephropathy.** Chronic infection is frequently not symptomatic, and in advanced cases, symptoms are those of renal insufficiency. Fewer than half of women

with chronic pyelonephritis have a clear history of preceding cystitis, acute pyelonephritis, or obstructive disease. The pathogenesis of this disease therefore is obscure, but it is doubtful that it is simply from persistent bacterial infection. Certainly, very few individuals with recurrent clinical episodes of urinary infections develop chronic infections or progressive renal involvement.

Maternal and fetal prognosis depends on the extent of renal destruction. El-Khatib and colleagues (1994) and Jungers and colleagues (1996) reported outcomes in 697 pregnancies in 290 women with reflux nephropathy. Impaired renal function and bilateral renal scarring were associated with increased maternal complications. When chronic pyelonephritis or any other chronic renal lesion is complicated by bacteriuria during pregnancy, there is an associated risk of superimposed acute pyelonephritis, which may lead to further deterioration. Martinell and colleagues (1990) found that almost half of women with renal scarring following childhood urinary infection had bacteriuria when pregnant. Renal injury as a consequence of chronic urinary tract infection beginning in childhood is much less common than it was early in the 20th century, probably as a result of improved health care (Hellerstein, 1999).

NEPHROLITHIASIS

Urinary stones are more common in men than women, and their average age of onset is in the third decade. Calcium salts make up about 80 percent of renal stones, and in half of these, idiopathic hypercalciuria is the most common predisposing cause (Asplin and colleagues, 1998). Hyperparathyroidism should be excluded. Familial occurrence is frequent, and patients with a previous stone form another stone every 2 to 3 years. Struvite stones are associated with infection, and often *Proteus* is cultured from the urine. Uric acid stones are even less common. Stones of the calcium oxalate variety are the most common encountered during pregnancy (Maikranz and colleagues, 1994).

Patients with calcium stones caused by hypercalciuria frequently respond to thiazide diuretics, with diminished stone formation. Patients with stone disease should be advised to keep well hydrated. In general, obstruction, infection, intractable pain, or heavy bleeding are indications for stone removal. Placing a flexible basket via cystoscopy to ensnare the calculus has been used with the greatest frequency, and this method is reasonable for use in pregnant women. **Lithotripsy** has replaced surgical therapy in many cases. This can be employed by extracorporeal means, percutaneous ultrasonic lithotripsy, or by ureteroscopic laser ablation of stones. Understandably, there is little information concerning its use during pregnancy.

STONE DISEASE DURING PREGNANCY. Because of their predilection for men and older patients, renal and ureteral lithiasis are relatively uncommon complications of pregnancy. From their review of 14 series, Hendricks and co-workers (1991) cite an incidence of about 1 per 2000 pregnancies. Butler and colleagues (2000) found a 1 per 3300 incidence in over 186,000 deliveries at Parkland Hospital. Presumably, pregnant women have fewer symptoms when they pass stones because of urinary tract dilatation (Hendricks and colleagues, 1991). These were not our findings in 73 episodes of nephrolithiasis in 57 pregnant women in whom the most common presenting symptom in 90 percent was pain. Most of these had flank pain, and only 23 percent had gross hematuria (Butler and co-workers, 2000).

Although women who have formed renal stones previously are at risk of doing so again, Maikranz and associates (1994) found no evidence that pregnancy increased this risk. Moreover, stone disease does not appear to have any adverse effects on pregnancy outcome except for an increased frequency of urinary infections. **Although urinary calculi seldom cause severe symptomatic obstruction during pregnancy, persistent pyelonephritis despite adequate antimicrobial therapy should prompt a search for renal obstruction, which most frequently is due to nephrolithiasis.**

DIAGNOSIS AND MANAGEMENT. Sonography may be helpful to confirm a suspected renal stone, but pregnancy hydronephrosis may obscure these findings (Fig. 47–5). Butler and colleagues (2000) reported that 21 of 35 (60 percent) renal sonograms done initially were positive in pregnant women with stone disease. If there is abnormal dilatation without stone visualization, then x-rays may be useful to identify stones. We prefer the one-shot pyelogram. Transabdominal color Doppler ultrasonography to detect absence of ureteral "jets" into the bladder has been suggested in the workup of suspected urolithiasis in pregnant women (Asrat and colleagues, 1998).

Treatment depends on the symptoms and the duration of pregnancy. Intravenous hydration and analgesics are always given. Almost half of pregnant women with symptomatic stones have associated infection which is treated vigorously. In 75 percent of the cases, there is improvement with conservative therapy and the stone usually passes spontaneously. The other 25 percent will need an invasive procedure such as ureteral stenting, percutaneous nephrostomy, laser lithotripsy, basket extraction, or occasionally surgical exploration (Butler and colleagues, 2000; Maikranz and colleagues, 1994). Carlan and associates (1995) and Scarpa and colleagues (1996) used transurethral laser in seven pregnant women and a ballistic lithotriptor in another two women to fragment stones.

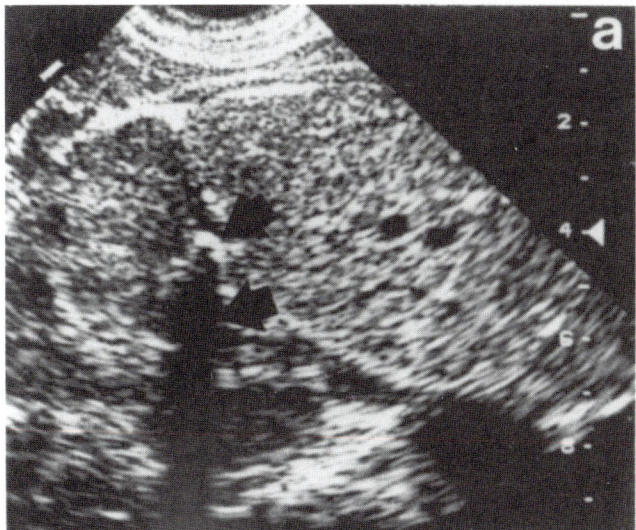

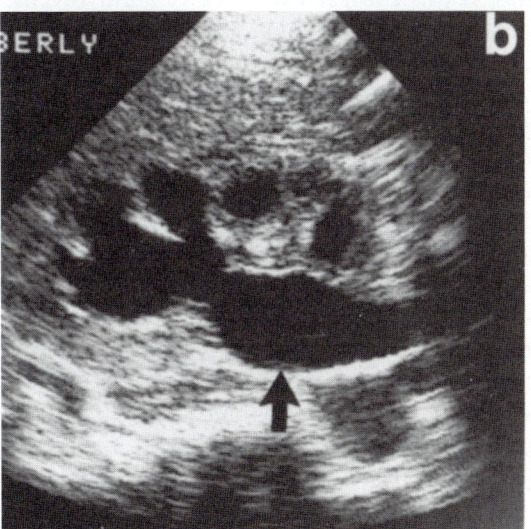

FIGURE 47–5. This 23-year-old multipara had a history of recurrent urinary infections and hypertension. **a.** At 6 weeks, ultrasound shows a right renal calculus (*upper arrow*) with typical acoustic shadowing (*lower arrow*). **b.** At 24 weeks, she presented with right flank pain, nausea and vomiting. Repeat ultrasonography demonstrated right hydronephrosis (*arrow*), but the previously identified calculus was no longer visible, suggesting that it had descended into the ureter. (From Hendricks and associates, 1991, with permission.)

GLOMERULOPATHIES

The kidney, especially the glomerulus and its capillaries, is subject to a large number and variety of acute and chronic diseases. They may result from a single stimulus such as poststreptococcal glomerulonephritis, or from a multisystem disease such as systemic lupus erythematosus. According to Brady and colleagues, (1998), there are five major clinical glomerulopathic syndromes: acute rapidly progressive glomerulonephritis, nephrotic syndrome, asymptomatic abnormalities of the urinary sediment, and chronic glomerulonephritis. The majority of these diseases are encountered in young women of childbearing age, and thus they may complicate pregnancy. Many of these disorders first become apparent because of chronic renal insufficiency.

ACUTE GLOMERULONEPHRITIS. This disorder may result from any of several causes, including those following infectious diseases, multisystem diseases, or primary disorders unique to the glomerulus (Table 47–5). All are characterized by an abrupt onset of hematuria and proteinuria accompanied by varying degrees of renal insufficiency and salt and water retention causing edema, hypertension, and circulatory congestion.

Acute poststreptococcal glomerulonephritis is prototypical of these syndromes and is of obstetrical interest because it was confused with the renal involvement of eclampsia up until the mid-19th century. Lever (1843) discovered then that the proteinuria of eclampsia was different from that due to "Brights disease" because it disappeared after delivery (Purkerson and Vekerdy, 1999).

Although poststreptococcal glomerulonephritis rarely develops acutely during pregnancy, its management is similar to acute glomerulonephritis from any cause. If it arises during the second half of pregnancy, in most cases it is clinically indistinguishable from preeclampsia. There are insufficient data to predict fetal or maternal prognosis. The prognosis and treatment of the other causes of acute glomerulonephritis listed in Table 47–5 depend on their etiology. Renal biopsy may be necessary in determining etiology as well as to direct

TABLE 47–5. Causes of Acute Glomerulonephritis

Immune complex (70%)
Idiopathic
Postinfectious (streptococcal, viral)
Lupus
Bacterial endocarditis
IgA nephropathy (uncommon)
Visceral abscesses
Pauci-immune (30%)
Wegener granulomatosis
Polyarteritis nodosa
Antiglomerular basement membrane disease (<1%)
Goodpasture syndrome (pulmonary hemorrhage)
Mimickers
Malignant hypertension
Thrombotic microangiopathies
Interstitial nephritis
Scleroderma
Preeclampsia–eclampsia

From Brady and colleagues (1998).

management (Lindheimer and Cunningham, 1994). For example, Yankowitz and colleagues (1992) reported successful management of a pregnancy complicated by *Goodpasture syndrome,* characterized by autoantibodies to basement membrane antigens, pulmonary hemorrhage, and glomerulonephritis.

Women with a history of poststreptococcal glomerulonephritis that has healed may undergo additional pregnancies without any appreciable increase in the incidence of complications. Some patients with acute glomerulonephritis never completely recover, and **rapidly progressive glomerulonephritis** leads to end-stage renal failure. Up to half of adults with sporadic poststreptococcal disease develop **chronic glomerulonephritis** with slowly progressive renal disease.

EFFECT OF GLOMERULONEPHRITIS ON PREGNANCY. Most cases of glomerulonephritis are not caused by poststreptococcal infection. In some cases, the underlying etiology is not found. Whatever the cause, glomerulonephritis has a profound effect on pregnancy outcome. Packham and colleagues (1989) reported the results of 395 pregnancies in 238 women who had been previously diagnosed with *primary* glomerulonephritis. The most common lesions on biopsy were membranous glomerulonephritis, IgA glomerulonephritis, and diffuse mesangial glomerulonephritis. Most of these women had normal renal function before becoming pregnant. The overall fetal loss was 26 percent; the perinatal mortality rate after 28 weeks was 80 per 1000. One fourth were delivered preterm, and 15 percent of fetuses were growth restricted. Overall, about half of these women developed hypertension; one quarter did so before 32 weeks, and it was severe in three fourths that did. Proteinuria worsened in 60 percent of these women. Factors that portended the worst perinatal prognosis included impaired renal function, early or severe hypertension, and nephrotic-range proteinuria.

RAPIDLY PROGRESSIVE GLOMERULONEPHRITIS. In some cases, acute glomerulonephritis does not resolve, and rapidly progressive glomerulonephritis progresses to end-stage renal failure within weeks to months. Patients with this form of disease may have a positive test for antineutrophil cytoplasmic antibody (ANCA) and demonstrate extensive extracapillary crescents within the glomerulus on renal biopsy (Lindheimer and Cunningham, 1994). Because extensive extracapillary or **crescenteric glomerulonephritis** is commonly identified, the two terms are often used interchangeably. Common causes of rapidly progressive disease are the same as those listed in Table 47–5. About 45 percent of cases are caused by immune-complex disease, 45 percent by pauci-immune glomerulonephritis, and 10 percent by antiglomerular basement membrane disease.

CHRONIC GLOMERULONEPHRITIS. In many cases the cause is unknown, but it may follow any of the primary lesions shown in Table 47–5. Chronic glomerulonephritis is characterized by progressive renal destruction over a period of years or decades, eventually producing the **end-stage kidney.** Usually, persistent proteinuria and hematuria accompany a gradual decline in renal function. Microscopically, the renal lesions are categorized as proliferative, sclerosing, or membranous.

According to Brady and associates (1998), chronic glomerulopathies may be detected in any of several ways:

1. Proteinuria or abnormal urinary sediment are detected by screening.
2. Routine blood screening shows anemia or elevated creatinine.
3. Bilaterally small kidneys are discovered on imaging.
4. During the course of evaluation for chronic hypertension.
5. If it exacerbates.

In some cases, women with symptoms and signs of preeclampsia–eclampsia, but without resolution postpartum, are found to have chronic glomerulonephritis.

The evolution, management, and prognosis of chronic glomerulonephritis depends on its etiology. In some patients, 10 to 20 years may elapse before end-stage renal failure supervenes. Renal biopsy may be helpful to establish prognosis.

NEPHROTIC SYNDROME. The nephrotic syndrome, or **nephrosis,** is a spectrum of renal disorders of many causes. Some of these are shown in Table 47–6, and the overlap with causes of acute glomerulonephritis in Table 47–5 is obvious. Nephrotic syndrome is characterized by proteinuria in excess of 3 g/day, hypoalbuminemia, hyperlipidemia, and edema. Most patients have microscopic renal abnormalities and may have accompanying evidence for renal dysfunction. The defects in the barriers of the glomerular capillary wall that allow excessive filtration of plasma proteins are caused by primary glomerular disease, or they may follow immunological or toxic injury or metabolic (diabetes) or vascular diseases.

Management of the nephrotic syndrome depends on its etiology. Edema is managed cautiously, especially during pregnancy. Jakobi and associates (1995) have described problems associated with massive vulvar edema that may complicate the nephrotic syndrome (Fig. 47–6). Dietary protein of high biological value is encouraged; however, high-protein diets only increase proteinuria. Thromboembolism occurs with some frequency, and includes arterial as well as venous thrombo-

ses. Renal vein thrombosis is particularly worrisome. The value, if any, of prophylactic anticoagulation is unclear. Some cases of nephrosis from primary glomerular disease will respond to corticosteroid or cytotoxic drug therapy. In most of those cases caused by infection or drugs, proteinuria recedes when the underlying cause is corrected.

TABLE 47–6. Causes of the Nephrotic Syndrome in Adults

Minimal change disease (20%)
  Idiopathic (majority)
  Drug-induced
  HIV infection
  Diabetes

Focal and segmental glomerulosclerosis (20%)
  Idiopathic (majority)
  HIV infection
  Diabetes
  Reflux nephropathy
  Sickle cell disease

Membranous glomerulopathy (35%)
  Idiopathic (majority)
  Hepatitis B, C, syphilis, malaria, endocarditis
  Amnioimmune disease—systemic lupus erythematosus, rheumatoid arthritis
  Drugs

Membranoproliferative glomerulonephritis (MPGN)
  Autoimmune disease—systemic lupus erythematosus
  Chronic hepatitis B, C, HIV infection, endocarditis

Diabetic nephropathy

Amyloidosis

From Brady and colleagues (1998).

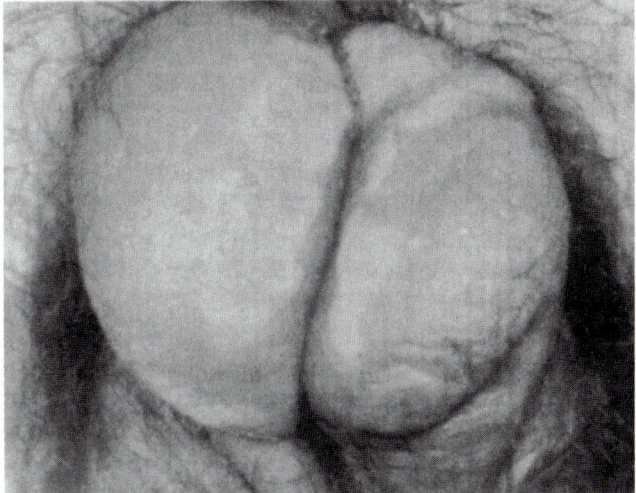

FIGURE 47–6. Massive vulvar edema at 32 weeks in a woman with the nephrotic syndrome secondary to diabetic nephropathy. (From Jakobi and colleagues, 1995, with permission.)

***NEPHROTIC SYNDROME COMPLICATING PREG-
NANCY.*** When the nephrotic syndrome complicates pregnancy, the maternal and fetal prognosis, as well as the appropriate treatment, depend on the underlying cause of the disease and the extent of renal insufficiency. Whenever possible, the specific cause should be ascertained and renal function assessed. In this regard, when the cause is not apparent, percutaneous renal biopsy may be of value.

Chronic proteinuria usually increases during pregnancy. Katz and associates (1980) observed that nearly half of women with chronic renal disease either developed proteinuria, or it worsened. In two thirds of their patients, as well as a similar number described by Stettler and Cunningham (1992), protein excretion exceeded 3 g/day. Similarly, Packham and colleagues (1989) reported that 60 percent of women with one of the primary glomerulopathies had increased proteinuria during pregnancy. Despite this, women without appreciably diminished renal function will usually have some augmentation of renal function (Cunningham and colleagues, 1990).

A review of reported cases of nephrosis indicates that the majority of women who are not hypertensive and do not have severe renal insufficiency will usually have a successful pregnancy outcome, particularly since glucocorticoids have been available. In other cases, however, in which there is evidence for renal insufficiency, moderate to severe hypertension, or both, the prognosis for mother and fetus is poor. Our experiences from Parkland Hospital with women who had proteinuria antecedent to pregnancy indicate that it is not a benign association (Stettler and Cunningham, 1992). Protein excretion in 65 pregnancies averaged 4 g/day, and a third of these women had classical nephrotic syndrome. Some degree of renal insufficiency was found in 75 percent of the women, 40 percent had chronic hypertension, and 25 percent had persistent anemia. Importantly, preeclampsia developed in 60 percent, and 45 percent of infants were delivered preterm. When abortions were excluded, however, 53 of 57 infants were born alive. In all 21 women who subsequently underwent renal biopsy, histological evidence of renal disease was found. Long-term follow-up indicated that at least 20 percent of women had progressed to end-stage renal disease, requiring dialysis or transplantation. Hemmelder and associates (1995) provided data that disease is accelerated during pregnancy in women with substantive proteinuria.

POLYCYSTIC KIDNEY DISEASE

In the adult this is an autosomally dominant disease linked to the alpha-hemoglobin gene complex and the phosphoglycerate kinase genes on the short arm of chromosome 16. The condition is genetically heterogeneous, and prenatal diagnosis is now available. The disease is found in 1 in 500 autopsies, accounts for 1 in 3000 hospital admissions, and causes 10 percent of all end-stage renal disease.

Symptoms usually appear in the third or fourth decade. Flank pain, hematuria, nocturia, proteinuria, and associated calculi and infection are common findings. Hypertension develops in three fourths of patients, and progression to end-stage renal disease is a major problem. Superimposed acute renal failure results from infection or obstruction from ureteral angulation by cyst displacement.

Asymptomatic **hepatic cysts** coexist in 30 percent of patients with polycystic kidneys. Hossack and colleagues (1988) studied 163 nonpregnant patients and reported substantively increased **cardiac valvar lesions** detected by echocardiography. The incidence of **mitral valve prolapse** was increased 13-fold over that of the control group, and there was excessive mitral, aortic, and tricuspid incompetence. Importantly, about 10 percent of patients die from an associated **intracranial berry aneurysm.**

POLYCYSTIC KIDNEY DISEASE AND PREGNANCY.

As with most chronic renal diseases, pregnancy outcome in women with polycystic kidney disease will depend on the degree of associated hypertension and renal insufficiency. Upper urinary tract infections are common. An in-depth study of the apparent effects of this disease on pregnancy and vice versa was provided by Chapman and co-workers (1994). A total of 235 affected women had 605 pregnancies. Pregnancy outcomes were compared with 108 unaffected family members during 244 pregnancies. Overall perinatal complication rates were similar (33 versus 26 percent), but hypertension, including preeclampsia, was more common in the affected women. Perinatal complications were more common in affected women who were over 30 years of age, and in those who developed preeclampsia. Pregnancy does not seem to accelerate the natural disease course (Lindheimer and colleagues, 2000).

CHRONIC RENAL DISEASE

A number of kidney diseases listed in Tables 47–5 and 47–6 may become chronic. When counseling the woman with chronic renal disease regarding fertility and the risk of a complicated pregnancy, it is important to determine the degree of functional impairment and the presence or absence of hypertension. The prognosis for a successful pregnancy outcome in general is not related to the underlying disorder. Some projection of pregnancy prognosis can be made by arbitrarily considering patients in one of three categories of functional impairment (Lindheimer and associates, 2000). These include those women with normal or *mild impairment* of renal function, defined by serum creatinine of less than 1.5 mg/dL and minimal hypertension; *moderate impairment* of renal function, defined as a serum creatinine of 1.5 to 3.0 mg/dL; and *severe renal insufficiency,* defined as a serum creatinine of greater than 3.0 mg/dL.

According to Lazarus and Brenner (1998), from 1982 through 1991, the most common causes of end-stage renal disease were diabetes and hypertension. Glomerulonephritis was the third most common. In many cases of chronic renal disease, biopsy will be necessary to determine the underlying cause. In some cases, this is done before pregnancy. Packham and Fairley (1987) performed 111 percutaneous biopsies in 104 pregnant women before the third trimester and reported a 5 percent complication rate. Lindheimer and colleagues (2000) believe that biopsy is usually best reserved until after pregnancy, unless it is perceived that biopsy results will significantly alter the management of renal disease.

PREGNANCY COMPLICATED BY CHRONIC RENAL DISEASE.

Most women with chronic renal disease complicating pregnancy have reasonably normal renal function. Importantly, preexisting hypertension along with the degree of renal insufficiency are predictive of pregnancy outcome. **However, in women with chronic renal disease, even if renal function is normal and the woman normotensive, pregnancy outcome is still not always good.** Despite the high incidence of hypertension and preeclampsia, preterm and growth-restricted infants, and other problems, the National High Blood Pressure Education Working Group (2000) concluded that the prognosis has substantively improved.

PHYSIOLOGICAL CHANGES.

In women with mild renal insufficiency, pregnancy is usually accompanied by a rise in renal plasma flow and glomerular filtration rate (Katz and colleagues, 1980). These changes are thought to be induced by renal vasodilation, and because this already is maximal with advanced renal disease, they are less evident in women with more severe renal dysfunction. In pregnant women studied at Parkland Hospital, only half of those with moderate renal insufficiency demonstrated augmented glomerular filtration rate (Cunningham and colleagues, 1990). None of those with severe disease showed augmentation of renal function.

Nonpregnant women with chronic renal insufficiency have normal blood volumes. During pregnancy, blood volume expansion is dependent on the severity of their disease, and it is proportional to the serum creatinine (Fig. 47–7). In women with mild to moderate dysfunction, there is normal pregnancy-induced hypervolemia

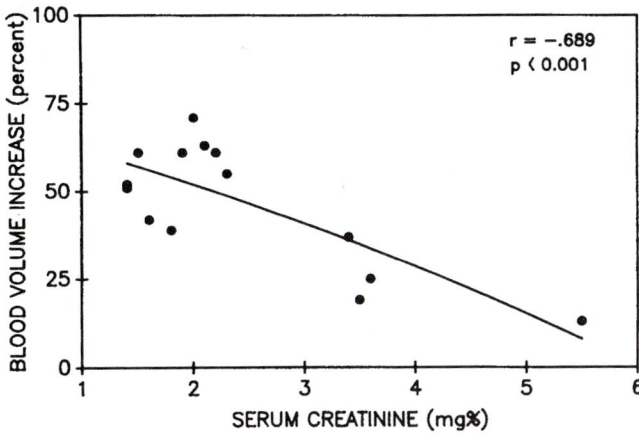

FIGURE 47–7. Blood volume expansion during pregnancy plotted as function of serum creatinine concentration. As renal insufficiency worsens (i.e., serum creatinine increases), the percent of blood volume expansion during pregnancy is less. (From Cunningham and colleagues, 1990, with permission.)

that averages 50 percent (Cunningham and associates, 1990). However, in women with severe renal insufficiency, volume expansion is attenuated, and averages only about 25 percent. Finally, although there is some degree of pregnancy-induced erythropoiesis in these women, it is not proportional to the plasma volume increase; thus, preexisting anemia is intensified.

PREGNANCY AND CHRONIC RENAL DISEASE WITH PRESERVED FUNCTION.

There are a number of studies that allow an estimation of risk of pregnancy for the woman with chronic renal disease. Katz and associates (1980) reviewed pregnancy outcomes in 89 women who had chronic renal disease but generally good renal function. Excluding abortions, of 121 pregnancies, perinatal mortality was 11 percent, 20 percent of infants were delivered preterm, and 24 percent were growth restricted. Importantly, superimposed preeclampsia was common and abruptio placentae developed in three instances. Surian and colleagues (1984) described the clinical course of 123 pregnancies in 86 women with biopsy-proven glomerular disease. Only a few of these women had renal dysfunction. In 40 percent there were obstetrical or renal complications, or both. Hypertension developed in 20 percent, and it persisted in half of these postpartum. In 8 percent of the women, renal function deteriorated, and this persisted in one half.

Packham and co-workers (1989), in a study cited previously, described their large experience from Melbourne with 238 women and 395 pregnancies complicated by preexisting primary glomerulonephritis. Only a few had preexisting renal insufficiency. All had undergone biopsy, and diffuse mesangial proliferative disease and IgA nephritis comprised 70 percent of the lesions.

During pregnancy, 15 percent of these women had impaired renal function and 60 percent had worsening proteinuria. Although only 12 percent had hypertension antedating pregnancy, over half became hypertensive during pregnancy. Hypertension before 20 weeks complicated 25 percent of these pregnancies, and 20 percent of all pregnancies had severe hypertension. About 5 percent developed irreversible worsening of renal function during pregnancy. The overall fetal loss was 26 percent. The overall perinatal mortality rate was 140 per 1000, and after 28 weeks, it was 80 per 1000. Factors associated with increased perinatal mortality and preterm delivery were impaired renal function, early or severe hypertension, and nephrotic-range proteinuria. In their absence, perinatal mortality was still 50 per 1000.

Other retrospective studies from Japan (Abe, 1991) and France (Jungers and colleagues, 1991) of large numbers of pregnancies in women with chronic primary glomerulonephritis substantiate these conclusions.

PREGNANCY WITH CHRONIC RENAL INSUFFICIENCY. Hou and colleagues (1985) described the outcomes of 25 pregnancies in 23 women studied because of moderate renal insufficiency defined by baseline serum creatinine ranging from 1.2 to 1.7 mg/dL. Pregnancy-induced or aggravated hypertension developed in slightly more than half of these women, and because of this nearly 60 percent were delivered preterm.

Cunningham and associates (1990) described the outcomes of 25 pregnancies in 23 women studied because of moderate renal insufficiency defined by baseline serum creatinine ranging from 1.2 to 1.7 mg/dL. Pregnancy-induced or aggravated hypertension developed in slightly more than half of these women, and because of this nearly 60 percent were delivered preterm. They also

reported their experience with 37 pregnancies complicated by moderate (serum creatinine 1.4 to 2.5 mg/dL) or severe (serum creatinine greater than 2.5 mg/dL) renal insufficiency. Common complications in these women included chronic hypertension (70 percent), anemia (75 percent), preeclampsia (60 percent), preterm delivery (35 percent), and fetal growth restriction (30 percent). Perinatal outcome was surprisingly good, and of 31 pregnancies reaching 26 weeks, 30 resulted in liveborn infants and all survived. Birthweight correlated inversely with serum creatinine concentration.

Jones and Hayslett (1996) described similar outcomes in 82 pregnancies in 67 women with moderate to severe chronic renal insufficiency. Hypertension complicated half of the pregnancies and 40 percent developed nephrotic-range proteinuria. Although 93 percent of the infants survived, 60 percent were preterm and 37 percent were growth restricted. Davison and Lindheimer (1999) have summarized perinatal outcomes in over 4100 pregnancies in more than 3000 women from 1954 to 1997. These women had mild, moderate, or severe renal insufficiency. Although the rate of preterm delivery remained high, there was a marked improvement in perinatal mortality over the five decades (Table 47–7).

MANAGEMENT. Women with chronic renal disease should have frequent prenatal visits to determine blood pressure. Serial measurements, the intervals determined by severity of findings, are done to estimate renal function, and protein excretion is monitored if indicated. Women should be screened and treated for bacteriuria to decrease the risk of pyelonephritis. Although protein-restricted diets are prescribed for nonpregnant patients with chronic renal disease, these are not recommended during pregnancy (Lindheimer

TABLE 47–7. Chronic Renal Disease and Pregnancy: Improvements in Perinatal Mortality over Five Decades[a]

Renal Disease Category	Pregnancy Outcome	Incidence (%)				
		1950s	1960s	1970s	1980s	1990s
Mild	Preterm delivery	8	10	19	25	25
	Perinatal mortality	18	15	7	<5	<3
Moderate	Preterm delivery	15	21	40	52	57
	Perinatal mortality	58	45	23	10	10
Severe	Preterm delivery	100	100	100	100	100
	Perinatal mortality	100	91	58	53	10

[a] Estimates are based on 3049 women with 4136 pregnancies (1954 to 1997) and do not include cases of connective-tissue disorders.
Modified from Davison and Lindheimer (1999), with permission.

and colleagues, 2000). Anemia associated with chronic renal insufficiency responds to recombinant erythropoietin given subcutaneously; however, hypertension is a well-documented side effect (Chap. 49). The appearance of hypertension is managed as described in Chapter 24, and suspected fetal growth restriction as in Chapter 29.

Except for an increased risk of hypertension and superimposed preeclampsia, women with relatively normal renal function and no hypertension before pregnancy usually have a relatively normal pregnancy. As renal impairment worsens, so does the likelihood of pregnancy complications. At least half of women with renal insufficiency will develop hypertension. Worsening of hypertension or superimposed preeclampsia develops in 80 percent of those with moderate insufficiency and 86 percent who have severe disease (Cunningham and co-workers, 1990; Packham and associates, 1989).

FOLLOW-UP. A long-standing unresolved issue is whether pregnancy accelerates chronic renal insufficiency. Jungers and associates (1995) found no adverse effect of pregnancy on actuarial survival in 360 women with chronic glomerulonephritis. Conversely, Abe (1991) concluded that pregnancy may accelerate antecedent disease in women with moderate dysfunction. It seems reasonable to conclude that, at least in most women, **in the absence of superimposed preeclampsia or severe placental abruption,** pregnancy does not appreciably accelerate deterioration in renal function. Importantly, because of the inevitable likelihood of long-term progression of the chronic disease, the ultimate maternal prognosis is guarded. In the study by Cunningham and associates (1990), at least 20 percent of women with moderate to severe disease had developed end-stage renal failure by a mean of 4 years. Similarly, Stettler and Cunningham (1992) reported that at least 20 percent of women with chronic proteinuria discovered during pregnancy had progressed to end-stage renal failure when followed for several years.

PREGNANCY AFTER RENAL TRANSPLANTATION

Between 1988 and 1996, almost 94,000 renal transplantations were performed in the United States (Hariharan and co-workers, 2000). The half-life for grafts from living donors is now 36 years and that for cadaveric grants is 20 years. These survival rates approximately doubled between 1988 and 1996, due in large part to the introduction of cyclosporine for the prevention of acute and chronic rejection and the introduction of muromonab-CD3 (OKT3 monoclonal antibody) for the treatment of acute rejection. In recent years, use of newer immunosuppressive drugs such as mycophenolate mofetil and tacrolimus has been associated with further reduction in the incidence of acute rejection episodes, although experience with these newer drugs is very limited (Hou, 1999). Importantly, resumption of renal function after transplantation promptly restores fertility to reproductive-age women.

Davison (1994) reviewed the outcomes in 3382 pregnancies in 2409 women, 80 percent of whom had had cadaveric transplants. Most were treated with azathioprine and prednisone. The incidence of spontaneous and therapeutic abortion was 35 percent. Of pregnancies that continued beyond the first trimester, over 90 percent had a successful outcome. Beginning early in pregnancy, the glomerular filtration rate in these women usually increased in proportion to that seen in normal women. Although proteinuria developed in 40 percent of these women, it was not significant in the absence of hypertension.

In pregnancies reviewed by Davison (1994), preeclampsia developed in 30 percent and signs of kidney rejection were observed in about 10 percent. Without renal biopsy, however, rejection may be difficult to distinguish from acute pyelonephritis, recurrent glomerulopathy, or severe preeclampsia. Serious infections, most likely related to immunosuppressive therapy, complicated some pregnancies. Urinary infections were diagnosed in 40 percent and the incidence of viral infections was increased. Prematurely ruptured membranes and preterm labor were common, and about half of live-born infants were delivered preterm. Fetal growth restriction averaged 20 percent. Fortunately, although respiratory distress syndrome was common among the preterm infants, it was seldom fatal. Fetal malformations were not increased. The newborns, as well as the mothers, were at increased risk of infection because of maternal immunosuppressive therapy.

Armenti and colleagues (1998), in observations from the National Transplantation Pregnancy Registry (NTPR), reported an excess of preterm and low-birthweight infants, as well as hypertension and cesarean deliveries, although fetal outcomes were generally satisfactory. From these experiences, Davison and Lindheimer (2000) recommend that these women satisfy a number of requisites before attempting pregnancy:

1. They should be in good general health without severe hypertension for at least 2 years after transplantation, because graft rejection is more common during this period.
2. There should be stable renal function without severe renal insufficiency and no evidence of graft rejection or persistent proteinuria.
3. Drug therapy is reduced to maintenance levels; that is, prednisone dosage of 15 mg/day or less; azathio-

prine at 2 mg/kg/day or less; and cyclosporine at 5 mg/kg/day or less.

Cyclosporine, now given routinely to renal transplantation recipients, decreases glomerular filtration rate and also may cause hypertension. In nonpregnant patients, cyclosporine may be associated with loss of renal function, hyperkalemia, hyperuricemia, hypertension, and rarely, a hemolytic uremic–type syndrome (Lindheimer and Cunningham, 1994). Thomas and associates (1997) reported that cyclosporine blood levels declined during pregnancy, although this was not associated with rejection episodes. Concern persists over the possibility of late effects in offspring subjected to immunosuppressive therapy in utero. These include malignancy, germ cell dysfunction, and malformations in the offsprings' children.

Finally, although pregnancy-induced renal hyperfiltration theoretically may impair long-term graft survival, Sturgiss and Davison (1995) found no evidence for this in a case-controlled study of 34 allograft recipients followed for a mean of 15 years.

MANAGEMENT. Close surveillance is necessary. Covert bacteriuria must be treated, and if recurrent, suppressive treatment for the remainder of pregnancy is given. Serial serum hepatic enzyme concentrations and blood counts are monitored for toxic effects of azathioprine and cyclosporine. Gestational diabetes is more common if corticosteroids are taken and glucose tolerance testing is done at about 26 weeks. Overt diabetes must be excluded.

Renal function is monitored, at first with serum creatinine determinations, but if abnormal, determination of glomerular filtration rate is preferable. According to Davison and Lindheimer (1999), a decline of less than 30 percent in the glomerular filtration rate during the third trimester is normal. If a significant decline is detected, then its cause must be determined. Possibilities include acute rejection, cyclosporine toxicity, preeclampsia, and urinary tract obstruction. Imaging studies and possibly kidney biopsy may be indicated.

Throughout pregnancy, the woman is carefully monitored for development or worsening of underlying hypertension, and especially superimposed preeclampsia. Management of hypertension during pregnancy is the same as for nontransplanted patients. The kidney dilates minimally to moderately as do normal kidneys (Levine and colleagues, 1995). Evidence for graft infection or rejection should prompt admission for aggressive management. Because of the significantly increased incidences of fetal growth restriction and preterm delivery, vigilant fetal surveillance is indicated (Chap. 40). Although cesarean delivery is reserved for obstetrical indications, occasionally the transplanted kidney will ob-

struct labor. The cesarean delivery rate approaches 50 percent (Armenti and co-workers, 1999).

DIALYSIS DURING PREGNANCY

Most often, significantly impaired renal function is accompanied by infertility. With chronic hemodialysis or peritoneal dialysis, however, fertility may be restored. Okundaye and associates (1998) surveyed dialysis units listed by the Health Care Financing Administration to determine the frequency and course of pregnancies in women receiving dialysis between 1992 and 1995. Approximately 40 percent of the units responded, and 241 women were identified who conceived either after starting or during dialysis. Hemodialysis was used in approximately 60 percent of these women and the remainder received peritoneal dialysis. Almost 80 percent of the women had some degree of hypertension, and it was severe in 13 percent. Over 95 percent of the women were anemic, defined as a hematocrit less than 30 percent. There were 11 infants with congenital malformations. Pregnancy outcomes are shown in Table 47–8. Early pregnancy losses and preterm births were common. Infant survival appeared to be worse in women who conceived after starting dialysis (40 percent) compared with those who commenced dialysis during an already established pregnancy (74 percent). These investigators, as well as Bagon and colleagues (1998), suggest that increased dialysis time may improve pregnancy outcome. The type of dialysis—hemodialysis versus peritoneal—did not appear to significantly influence pregnancy outcome.

ACUTE RENAL FAILURE

The incidence of renal failure associated with pregnancy has decreased substantively over the past 30 years. Nzerue and colleagues (1998) identified 21 cases of acute

TABLE 47–8. Pregnancy Outcomes in 241 Women Treated with Hemodialysis or Peritoneal Dialysis

Pregnancy Outcome	Conception and Dialysis (%)	
	Prior	During
Spontaneous abortion	14	42
Preterm delivery (≤32 weeks)	25	26
Stillbirths	1.8	8.1
Surviving infants	74	40

From Okundaye and associates (1998).

renal failure in pregnancy at Grady Memorial Hospital between 1986 and 1996. The incidence was 2 per 10,000 women delivered. Diseases and conditions associated with renal failure are shown in Table 47–9. Preeclampsia–eclampsia was the most common associated condition and was diagnosed in 38 percent of the women. Maternal mortality was 16 percent and maternal morbidity was common. The latter included end-stage kidney disease, seizures, hyponatremia, disseminated intravascular coagulation, and pulmonary edema. The stillbirth rate was 38 percent and a third of live-born infants were delivered preterm.

Data from the Renal Unit in Leeds, England, underscore the changing indications for dialysis for acute renal failure in obstetrical patients (Turney and colleagues, 1989). Whereas in earlier years obstetrical cases comprised 35 percent of patients requiring dialysis, more recently they accounted for only 10 percent. Almost all of the 142 obstetrical cases were contributed to or caused by abortion (25 percent), hemorrhage (35 percent), or preeclampsia (50 percent). The immediate mortality rate with acute renal failure was 20 percent. Importantly, after legalization of abortion in England in 1968, cases of obstetrical acute renal failure decreased by 30 percent.

Sibai and associates (1990) reported experiences from the University of Tennessee in 31 women with acute renal failure complicating hypertensive disorders of pregnancy. While 18 had "pure" preeclampsia, the remainder had antecedent chronic hypertension, parenchymal renal disease, or both. Half required dialysis, and three of these women died as a direct result of renal failure. About half of the women had suffered placental abruption and almost 90 percent had postpartum hemorrhage. Frangieh and co-workers (1996) reported that 3.8 percent of eclamptic women from the same institution had acute renal failure. This same group also reported that 3 percent of 69 women with *HELLP syndrome* (syndrome of hemolysis, elevated liver enzymes, and low platelet count) developed renal failure (Audibert and colleagues, 1996). Early identification and proper management of renal failure in women with pure preeclampsia does not result in residual renal damage.

MANAGEMENT. Identification of acute renal failure and its cause(s) is important (Thadhani and colleagues, 1996). In most women, renal failure develops postpartum so management is not complicated by fetal considerations. Oliguria is an important sign of acutely impaired renal function. Unfortunately, potent diuretics such as furosemide can increase urine flow without correcting but rather intensifying some causes of oliguria. In obstetrical cases, both prerenal and intrarenal factors are commonly operative. For example, with total placental abruption, severe hypovolemia is common from massive concealed hemorrhage. Superimposed preeclampsia may cause oliguria. Intense consumptive coagulopathy commonly triggered by an abruption might impede intrarenal microcirculation. More likely, however, consumptive coagulopathy causes even more blood loss from lacerations and surgical incisions, resulting in further renal hypoperfusion.

When azotemia is evident and severe oliguria persists, hemodialysis should be initiated before marked deterioration of general well-being occurs. Early dialysis appears to reduce appreciably mortality and may enhance the extent of recovery of renal function. After healing has taken place, renal function usually returns to normal or near normal.

PREVENTION. Acute tubular necrosis may often be prevented by the following means:

1. Prompt and vigorous replacement of blood in instances of massive hemorrhage, as in placental abruption, placental previa, uterine rupture, and postpartum uterine atony.
2. Termination of pregnancies complicated by severe preeclampsia and eclampsia with careful blood replacement if loss is excessive.
3. Close observation for early signs of septic shock in women with pyelonephritis, septic abortion, amnionitis, or sepsis from other pelvic infections.
4. Avoidance of potent diuretics to treat oliguria before initiating appropriate efforts to assure cardiac output adequate for renal perfusion.
5. Avoidance of vasoconstrictors to treat hypotension, unless pathological vasodilation is unequivocally the cause of the hypotension.

TABLE 47–9. Factors Associated with Acute Renal Failure During Pregnancy at Grady Memorial Hospital, 1986–1996

Factor	Percent
Preeclampsia–eclampsia	38
Drug abuse	29
Human immunodeficiency virus infection	14
Systemic lupus erythematosus	14
Abortion	14
Nephrotic syndrome	14
Sepsis	10
Postpartum hemorrhage	10
Sickle cell disease	10
Placental abruption	4
Obstructive uropathy	4
Other	33

From Nzerue and colleagues (1998), with permission.

Bilateral necrosis of the renal cortex is uncommon. It complicates between 15 and 30 percent of all cases of acute renal failure associated with obstetrical causes (Grünfeld and Pertuiset, 1987; Turney and colleagues, 1989). Most of the reported cases have followed such complications as placental abruption, preeclampsia–eclampsia, or endotoxin-induced shock. Histologically, the lesion appears to result from thrombosis of segments of the renal vascular system. The lesions may be focal, patchy, confluent, or gross. Clinically, renal cortical necrosis follows the course of acute renal failure with oliguria or anuria, uremia, and generally death within 2 to 3 weeks unless dialysis is initiated. Differentiation from acute tubular necrosis during the early phase is not possible. The prognosis depends on the extent of the necrosis, because recovery is a function of the amount of renal tissue spared.

OBSTRUCTIVE RENAL FAILURE. Rarely, bilateral ureteral compression by a very large pregnant uterus is greatly exaggerated, causing ureteral obstruction and, in turn, severe oliguria and azotemia. Brandes and Fritsche (1991) reviewed 13 cases that were the consequence of a markedly overdistended gravid uterus. They described a woman with twins who developed anuria and a serum creatinine level of 12.2 mg/dL at 34 weeks. After amniotomy, urine flow at 500 mL/hr was followed by rapid return to normal of the serum creatinine. Eckford and Gingell (1991) described 10 women in whom ureteral obstruction was relieved by stenting. The stents were left in place for a mean of 15.5 weeks and removed 4 to 6 weeks postpartum. Sadan and associates (1994) reported a similar experience in eight women who underwent ureteral stent placement during pregnancy for moderate to severe hydronephrosis. Mean gestational age at insertion was 29 weeks, and the stents remained in situ for a mean of 9 weeks. Renal function remained normal.

We have observed this phenomenon on several occasions (Satin and colleagues, 1993). Partial ureteral obstruction may be accompanied by fluid retention and significant hypertension. When the obstructive uropathy is relieved, diuresis ensues and hypertension dissipates. In one woman with massive hydramnios (9.4 L) and an anencephalic fetus, amniocentesis and removal of some of the amnionic fluid was followed promptly by diuresis, lowering of the plasma creatinine concentration, and improvement of hypertension. In our experiences, women with previous urinary tract surgery are more likely to have such obstructions. Austenfeld and Snow (1988) and Mansfield and colleagues (1995) also emphasized the high incidence of urinary infections in women who have undergone ureteral reimplantation. Conversely, Vordermark and associates (1990) reviewed published experiences with pregnancy following major urinary reconstruction, and found minimal complications.

IDIOPATHIC POSTPARTUM RENAL FAILURE. In 1968, Robson and associates described what they believed to be a new syndrome of **acute irreversible renal failure** that developed within the first 6 weeks postpartum. Pregnancy and delivery appeared to have been normal in the seven cases reported, and none of the known causes of renal failure was found. The pathological changes identified by renal biopsy were necrosis and endothelial proliferation in glomeruli, plus necrosis, thrombosis, and intimal thickening of the arterioles. No vascular abnormalities were demonstrated in the other visceral organs in the four cases in which autopsy was performed. Morphological changes in the erythrocytes consistent with microangiopathic hemolysis and thrombocytopenia were usually present. These findings are similar to those reported for the **postpartum hemolytic uremic syndrome.** Moreover, they are also similar to those in which renal failure is identified as part of the syndrome of **thrombotic thrombocytopenic purpura.** These syndromes are collectively termed **thrombotic microangiopathies,** and are considered in detail in Chapter 49.

REFERENCES

Abe S: An overview of pregnancy in women with underlying renal disease. Am J Kidney Dis 17:112, 1991

Andriole VT, Patterson TF: Epidemiology, natural history, and management of urinary tract infections in pregnancy. Med Clin North Am 75:359, 1991

Armenti VT, McGrory CH, Cater JR, Radomski JS, Moritz MJ: Pregnancy outcomes in female renal transplant recipients. Transplant Proc 30:1732, 1998

Asplin JR, Coe FL, Favus MJ: Nephrolithiasis. In Fauci AS, Braunwald E, Isselbacher KJ, Wilson JD, Martin JB, Kasper DL, Hauser SL, Longo DL (eds): Harrison's Principles of Internal Medicine, 14th ed. New York, McGraw-Hill, 1998, p 569

Asrat T, Roossin M, Miller EI: Ultrasonographic detection of ureteral jets in normal pregnancy. Am J Obstet Gynecol 178:1194, 1998

Audibert F, Friedman SA, Frangieh AY, Sibai BM: Diagnostic criteria for HELLP syndrome: Tedious or "helpful"? Am J Obstet Gynecol 174:454, 1996

Austenfeld MS, Snow BW: Complications of pregnancy in women after reimplantation for vesicoureteral reflux. J Urol 140:1103, 1988

Bagon JA, Vernaeve H, DeMuylder X, LaFontaine JJ, Martens J, Van Roost G: Pregnancy and dialysis. Am J Kidney Dis 31:756, 1998

Baylis C, Davison J: The urinary system. In Hytten F, Chamberlain G (eds): Clinical Physiology in Obstetrics, 2nd ed. London, Blackwell, 1991, p 245

Brady HR, O'Meara YM, Brenner BM: The major glomerulopathies. In Fauci AS, Braunwald E, Isselbacher KJ, Wilson JD, Martin JB, Kasper DL, Hauser SL, Longo DL (eds):

Harrison's Principles of Internal Medicine, 14th ed. New York, McGraw-Hill, 1998, p 1536

Brandes JC, Fritsche C: Obstructive acute renal failure by a gravid uterus: A case report and review. Am J Kidney Dis 18:398, 1991

Butler EL, Cox SM, Eberts E, Cunningham FG: Symptomatic nephrolithiasis complicating pregnancy. Obstet Gynecol 96:753, 2000

Carlan SJ, Schorr SJ, Ebenger MF, Danna PA, Anibarro GB: Laser lithotripsy in pregnancy. A case report. J Reprod Med 40:74, 1995

Cavenee MR, Cox SM, Mason R, Cunningham FG: Erythropoietin in pregnancies complicated by pyelonephritis. Obstet Gynecol 84:252, 1994

Chapman AB Johnson AM, Gabow PA: Pregnancy outcome and its relationship to progression of renal failure in autosomal dominant polycystic kidney disease. J Am Soc Nephrol 5:1178, 1994

Cox SM, Cunningham FG: Acute focal pyelonephritis (lobar nephronia) complicating pregnancy. Obstet Gynecol 71:510, 1988

Cox SM, Shelburne P, Mason R, Guss S, Cunningham FG: Mechanisms of hemolysis and anemia associated with acute antepartum pyelonephritis. Am J Obstet Gynecol 164:587, 1991

Cunningham FG: Urinary tract infections complicating pregnancy. Clin Obstet Gynecol 1:891, 1988

Cunningham FG, Cox SM, Harstad TW, Mason MT, Pritchard JA: Chronic renal disease and pregnancy outcome. Am J Obstet Gynecol 163:453, 1990

Cunningham FG, Lucas MJ, Hankins GDV: Pulmonary injury complicating antepartum pyelonephritis. Am J Obstet Gynecol 156:797, 1987

Cunningham FG, Morris GB, Mickal A: Acute pyelonephritis of pregnancy: A clinical review. Obstet Gynecol 42:112, 1973

Davison JM: Pregnancy in renal allograft recipients: Problems, prognosis, and practicalities. Baillieres Clin Obstet Gynecol 8:501, 1994

Davison JM, Lindheimer MD: Renal disorders. In Creasy RK, Resnick R (eds): Maternal–Fetal Medicine, 4th ed. Philadelphia, Saunders, 1999, p 873

Eckford SD, Gingell JC: Ureteric obstruction in pregnancy—diagnosis and management. Br J Obstet Gynaecol 98:1137, 1991

El-Khatib M, Packham DK, Becker GJ, Kincaid-Smith P: Pregnancy-related complications in women with reflux nephropathy. Clin Nephrol 41:50, 1994

Fakhoury GF, Daikoku NH, Parikh AR: Management of severe hemorrhagic cystitis in pregnancy. A report of two cases. J Reprod Med 39:485, 1994

Faúndes A, Bricola-Filho M, Pinto e Silva JC: Dilatation of the urinary tract during pregnancy: Proposal of a curve of maximal caliceal diameter by gestational age. Am J Obstet Gynecol 178:1082, 1998

Frangieh SA, Friedman SA, Audibert F, Usta I, Sibai BM: Maternal outcome in women with eclampsia. Am J Obstet Gynecol 174:453, 1996

Gilstrap LC III, Cunningham FG, Whalley PJ: Acute pyelonephritis in pregnancy: An anterospective study. Obstet Gynecol 57:409, 1981a

Gilstrap LC III, Leveno KJ, Cunningham FG, Whalley PJ, Roark ML: Renal infection and pregnancy outcome. Am J Obstet Gynecol 141:708, 1981b

Graham JM, Oshiro BT, Blanco JD, Magee KP: Uterine contractions after antibiotic therapy for pyelonephritis in pregnancy. Am J Obstet Gynecol 168:577, 1993

Graif M, Kessler A, Hart S, Daitzchman M, Mashiach S, Boichis H, Itzchak Y: Renal pyelectasis in pregnancy: Correlative evaluation of fetal and maternal collecting systems. Am J Obstet Gynecol 167:1304, 1992

Gratacos E, Torres PJ, Vila J, Alonso PL, Cararach V: Screening and treatment of asymptomatic bacteriuria in pregnancy to prevent pyelonephritis. J Infect Dis 169:1390, 1994

Grünfeld JP, Pertuiset N: Acute renal failure in pregnancy: 1987. Am J Kidney Dis 9:359, 1987

Hariharan S, Johnson CP, Bresnahan BA, Taranto SE, McIntosh MJ, Stablein D: Improved graft survival after renal transplantation in the United States, 1988 to 1996. N Engl J Med 342:605, 2000

Harris RE, Gilstrap LC III: Cystitis during pregnancy: A distinct clinical entity. Obstet Gynecol 57:578, 1981

Hellerstein S: The long-term consequences of urinary tract infections: A historic and contemporary perspective. Pediatr Ann 28:695, 1999

Hemmelder MH, de Zeeuw D, Fidler V, de Jong PE: Proteinuria: A risk factor for pregnancy-related renal function decline in primary glomerular disease? Am J Kidney Dis 26:187, 1995

Hendricks SK, Ross SO, Krieger JN: An algorithm for diagnosis and therapy of management and complications of urolithiasis during pregnancy. Surg Gynecol Obstet 172:49, 1991

Higby K, Suiter CR, Phelps JY, Siler-Khodr T, Langer O: Normal values of urinary albumin and total protein excretion during pregnancy. Am J Obstet Gynecol 171:984, 1994

Hooton TM, Scholes D, Stapleton AE, Roberts P, Winter C, Gupta K, Samadpour M, Stamm WE: A prospective study of asymptomatic bacteriuria in sexually active young women. N Engl J Med 343:992, 2000

Hossack KF, Leddy CL, Johnson AM, Schrier RW, Gabow PA: Echocardiographic findings in autosomal dominant polycystic kidney disease. N Engl J Med 319:907, 1988

Hou S: Pregnancy in chronic renal insufficiency and end-stage renal disease. Am J Kidney Dis 33:235, 1999

Hou SH, Grossman SD, Madias NE: Pregnancy in women with renal disease and moderate renal insufficiency. Am J Med 78:185, 1985

Jakobi P, Friedman M, Goldstein I, Zaidise I, Itskovitz-Eldor J: Massive vulvar edema in pregnancy: A case report. J Reprod Med 40:479, 1995

Jones DC, Hayslett JP: Outcome of pregnancy in women with moderate or severe renal insufficiency. N Engl J Med 335:226, 1996

Jungers P, Houillier P, Chauveau D, Choukroun G, Moynot A, Skhiri H, Labrunie M, Descamps-Latscha B, Grunfeld JP: Pregnancy in women with reflux nephropathy. Kidney Int 50:593, 1996

Jungers P, Houillier P, Forget D, Henry-Amar M: Specific controversies concerning the natural history of renal disease in pregnancy. Am J Kidney Dis 17:116, 1991

Jungers P, Houillier P, Forget D, Labrunie M, Skhiri H, Giatras I, Descamps-Latscha B: Influence of pregnancy on the course of primary chronic glomerulonephritis. Lancet 346:1122, 1995

Kass EH: Pyelonephritis and bacteriuria. Ann Intern Med 56:46, 1962

Katz AI, Davison JM, Hayslett JP, Singson E, Lindheimer MD: Pregnancy in women with kidney disease. Kidney Int 18:192, 1980

Kincaid-Smith P, Bullen M: Bacteriuria in pregnancy. Lancet 1:395, 1965

Lamont RF: The pathophysiology of pulmonary oedema with the use of beta-agonists. Br J Obstet Gynaecol 107:439, 2000

Lazarus JM, Brenner BM: Chronic renal failure. In Fauci AS, Braunwald E, Isselbacher KJ, Wilson JD, Martin JB, Kasper DL, Hausea SL, Lonso DL (eds): Harrison's Principles of Internal Medicine, 14th ed. New York, McGraw-Hill, 1998 p 1513

Levine D, Filly RA, Graber M: The sonographic appearance of renal transplants during pregnancy. J Ultrasound Med 14:291, 1995

Lindheimer MD, Cunningham FG: Renal disease complicating pregnancy. Williams Obstetrics, 19th ed (Suppl 6). Norwalk, CT, Appleton & Lange, April/May 1994

Lindheimer MD, Grünfeld JP, Davison JM. Renal disorders. In Barron WM, Lindheimer MD (eds): Medical Disorders During Pregnancy, 3rd ed. St. Louis, Mosby, 2000, p 39

Little PJ: The incidence of urinary infection in 5000 pregnant women. Lancet 2:925, 1966

Lucas MJ, Cunningham FG: Urinary tract infections complicating pregnancy. Williams Obstetrics, 19th ed (Suppl 5). Norwalk, CT, Appleton & Lange, Feb/March 1994

Lucas ML, Cunningham FG: Urinary infection in pregnancy. Clin Obstet Gynecol 36:855, 1993

Mabie WC, Barton JR, Sibai B: Septic shock in pregnancy. Obstet Gynecol 90:553, 1997

Maikranz P, Coe FL, Parks J, Lindheimer MD: Nephrolithiasis in pregnancy. Am J Kidney Dis 9:354, 1987

Maikranz P, Lindheimer MD, Coe FL: Nephrolithiasis in pregnancy. Baillieres Clin Obstet Gynecol 8:375, 1994

Mansfield JT, Snow BW, Cartwright PC, Wadsworth K: Complications of pregnancy in women after childhood reimplantation for vesicoureteral reflux: An update with 25 years of followup. J Urol 154:787, 1995

Martinell JF, Jodel U, Lidin-Janson G: Pregnancies in women with and without renal scarring after urinary infections in childhood. BMJ 300:840, 1990

Millar LK, Cox SM: Urinary tract infections complicating pregnancy. Infect Dis Clin North Am 11:13, 1997

Millar L, Debuque L, Leialoha C, Grandinetti A, Killeen J: Rapid enzymatic urine screening test to detect bacteriuria in pregnancy. Obstet Gynecol 95:601, 2000

National High Blood Pressure Education Program Working Group on High Blood Pressure in Pregnancy: Report of the National High Blood Pressure Education Program Working Group on High Blood Pressure in Pregnancy. Am J Obstet Gynecol 183:S1, 2000

Norden CW, Kilpatrick WH: Bacteriuria of pregnancy. In Kass EH (ed): Progress in Pyelonephritis. Philadelphia, Davis, 1965, p 64

Nzerue CM, Hewan-Lowe K, Nwawka C: Acute renal failure in pregnancy: A review of clinical outcomes at an inner city hospital from 1986–1996. J Natl Med Assoc 90:486, 1998

Okundaye I, Abrinko P, Hou S: Registry of pregnancy in dialysis patients. Am J Kidney Dis 31:766, 1998

Packham D, Fairley KF: Renal biopsy: Indications and complications in pregnancy. Br J Obstet Gynaecol 94:935, 1987

Packham DK, North RA, Fairley KF, Kloss M, Whitworth JA, Kincaid-Smith A: Primary glomerulonephritis and pregnancy. Q J Med 71:537, 1989

Parrillo JE: Pathogenetic mechanisms of septic shock. N Engl J Med 328:1471, 1993

Purkerson ML, Vekerdy L: The history of eclampsia, toxemia and the kidney in pregnancy. Am J Nephrol 19:313, 1999

Ridgway LE III, Martin RW, Hess LW, Buchanan J, Whitworth NS, Martin JN Jr: Acute gestational pyelonephritis: The impact on colloid osmotic pressure, plasma fibronectin, and arterial oxygen saturation. Am J Perinatol 8:222, 1991

Robson JS, Martin AM, Ruckley VA, MacDonald MK: Irreversible postpartum renal failure. Q J Med 37:423, 1968

Rodriguez PN, Klein AS: Management of urolithiasis during pregnancy. Surg Gynecol Obstet 166:103, 1988

Rouse DJ, Andrews WW, Goldenberg RL, Owen J: Screening and treatment of asymptomatic bacteriuria of pregnancy to prevent pyelonephritis. A cost-effectiveness and cost-benefit analysis. Obstet Gynecol 86:119, 1995

Sadan O, Berar M, Sagiv R, Dreval D, Gewurtz G, Korczak D, Zakut H, Bernstein D: Ureteric stent in severe hydronephrosis of pregnancy. Eur J Obstet Gynecol Reprod Biol 56:79, 1994

Sanchez-Ramos L, McAlpine KJ, Adair CD, Kaunitz AM, Delke I, Briones DK: Pyelonephritis in pregnancy: Once-a-day ceftriaxone versus multiple doses of cefazolin. A randomized double-blind trial. Am J Obstet Gynecol 172:129, 1995

Satin AJ, Seiken GL, Cunningham FG: Reversible hypertension in pregnancy caused by obstructive uropathy. Obstet Gynecol 81:823, 1993

Scarpa RM, de Lisa A, Usai E: Diagnosis and treatment of ureteral calculi during pregnancy with rigid ureteroscopes. J Urol 155:875, 1996

Schieve LA, Handler A, Hershow R, Persky V, Davis F: Urinary tract infection during pregnancy: Its association with maternal morbidity and perinatal outcome. Am J Public Health 84:405, 1994

Seidman DS, Soriano D, Dulitzki M, Heyman Z, Mashiach S, Barkai G: Role of renal ultrasonography in the management of pyelonephritis in pregnant women. J Perinatol 18:98, 1998

Sibai BM, Villar MA, Mabie BC: Acute renal failure in hypertensive disorders of pregnancy. Pregnancy outcome and remote prognosis in thirty-one consecutive cases. Am J Obstet Gynecol 162:777, 1990

Stenqvist K, Sandberg T, Lidin-Janson G, Orskov F, Orskov I, Svanborg-Eden C: Virulence factors of *Escherichia coli* in urinary isolates from pregnant women. J Infect Dis 156:870, 1987

Stettler RW, Cunningham FG: Natural history of chronic proteinuria complicating pregnancy. Am J Obstet Gynecol 167:1219, 1992

Sturgiss SN, Davison JM: Effect of pregnancy on long-term function of renal allografts. Am J Kidney Dis 26:54, 1995

Surian M, Imbasciati E, Cosci P, Banfi G, di Belgiojoso B, Brancaccio D, Minetti L, Ponticelli C: Glomerular disease and pregnancy: A study of 123 pregnancies in patients with primary and secondary glomerular diseases. Nephron 36:101, 1984

Svanborg-Eden C, Hagberg L, Leffler H, Lonberg H: Recent progress in the understanding of the role of bacterial adhesion in the pathogenesis of urinary tract infection. Infection 10:327, 1982

Thadhani R, Pascual M, Bonventre JV: Acute renal failure. N Engl J Med 334:1448, 1996

Thomas AG, Burrows L, Knight R, Panico M, Lapinski R, Lockwood CJ: The effect of pregnancy on cyclosporine levels in renal allograft patients. Obstet Gynecol 90:916, 1997

Towers CV, Kaminskas CM, Garite TJ, Nageotte MP, Dorchester W: Pulmonary injury associated with antepartum pyelonephritis: Can patients at risk be identified? Am J Obstet Gynecol 164:974, 1991

Turney JH, Ellis CM, Parsons FM: Obstetric acute renal failure 1956–1987. Br J Obstet Gynaecol 96:679, 1989

Twickler DM, Lucas MJ, Bowe L, McIntire DD, Barron J, Cunningham FG: Ultrasonographic evaluation of central and end-organ hemodynamics in antepartum pyelonephritis. Am J Obstet Gynecol 170:814, 1994

Van Dorsten JP, Lenke RR, Schifrin BS: Pyelonephritis in pregnancy: The role of in-hospital management and nitrofurantoin suppression. J Reprod Med 32:897, 1987

Vordermark JS, Deshon GE, Agee RE: Management of pregnancy after major urinary reconstruction. Obstet Gynecol 75:564, 1990

Whalley PJ: Bacteriuria of pregnancy. Am J Obstet Gynecol 97:723, 1967

Whalley PJ, Cunningham FG, Martin FG: Transient renal dysfunction associated with acute pyelonephritis of pregnancy. Obstet Gynecol 46:174, 1975

Whalley PJ, Martin FG, Peters PC: Significance of asymptomatic bacteriuria detected during pregnancy. JAMA 198:879, 1965

Wilson MG, Hewitt WL, Monzon OT: Effect of bacteriuria on the fetus. N Engl J Med 274:1115, 1966

Wing DA, Hendershott CM, Debuque L, Millar LK: Outpatient treatment of acute pyelonephritis in pregnancy after 24 weeks. Obstet Gynecol 94:683, 1999

Wing DA, Hendershott CM, Debuque L, Millar LK: A randomized trial of three antibiotic regimens for the treatment of pyelonephritis in pregnancy. Am J Obstet Gynecol 92:249, 1998

Wing DA, Park AS, DeBuque L, Millar LK: Limited clinical utility of blood and urine cultures in the treatment of acute pyelonephritis during pregnancy. Am J Obstet Gynecol 182:1437, 2000

Yankowitz J, Kuller JA, Thomas RL: Pregnancy complicated by Goodpasture syndrome. Obstet Gynecol 79:806, 1992

48

Gastrointestinal Disorders

During normal pregnancy, the gastrointestinal tract and its appendages undergo changes, both anatomical and functional, that can appreciably alter the criteria for diagnosis and treatment of several diseases to which they are susceptible. For example, nausea and vomiting are frequent symptoms early in normal pregnancy, but if these symptoms are erroneously attributed to normal physiological changes, then gastrointestinal disease may be overlooked. Conversely, persistent nausea and vomiting in late pregnancy should always prompt a search for underlying pathology. In another example, most obstetricians, but not most internists or gastroenterologists, are aware that upper abdominal pain—epigastric or right upper quadrant—can be an ominous sign of severe preeclampsia. During advanced pregnancy, gastrointestinal symptoms become more difficult to assess, and physical findings are often obscured by the large uterus which displaces abdominal organs and alter the location of pain and tenderness.

LAPAROTOMY AND LAPAROSCOPY

Laparotomy and surgical treatment may be lifesaving for certain conditions, acute appendicitis being the most common. Citing data from the Swedish Registry through 1981, Mazze and Källén (1989) reported that abdominal exploration by laparotomy or laparoscopy was performed in 1331 of 720,000 pregnancies—about 1 in every 500 pregnancies. Kort and associates (1993) reported that a total of 78 women in over 49,500 births had nonobstetrical surgery during pregnancy, an incidence of 1 in 635. The most common indications for surgery were appendicitis, adnexal masses, and cholecystitis.

During the past decade, laparoscopy has been shown safe during at least the first half of pregnancy. Reedy and associates (1997) updated the Swedish Registry which through 1993 had data from slightly over 2 million pregnancies. Of these, 2181 underwent laparoscopy and 1522 laparotomy for nonobstetrical indications—about 1 in every 800 pregnancies. As expected, laparoscopic procedures were mostly performed before 20 weeks (Chap. 42, p. 1145 and Fig. 42–1). The most common nongynecological procedures include cholecystectomy and appendectomy (Reedy and colleagues, 1998). For more details, as well as surgical technique, see Chapter 26 in *Operative Obstetrics* by Gilstrap and colleagues (2001).

DIAGNOSTIC TECHNIQUES

Fiberoptic endoscopic instruments have revolutionized the diagnosis and management of many gastrointestinal conditions. These instruments are particularly well-suited for use during pregnancy. Endoscopy permits evaluation of the esophagus, stomach, and duodenum (Van Dam and Brugge, 1999). With specialized instruments, the proximal jejunum can be studied, and the ampulla of Vater can be cannulated to perform *endoscopic retrograde cholangiopancreatography (ERCP)*. Cappell and Sidhom (1993) described experiences using panendoscopy in 20 pregnant women. These women were evenly distributed by trimester and in 14 (70 percent) a lesion was diagnosed—seven had esophagitis, two duodenal ulcers, three gastritis, and two had Mallory–Weiss tears. No significant complications of endoscopy were encountered. In another study, Cappell and Sidhom (1995) described successful use of *flexible sigmoidoscopy* in 24 pregnant women. *Colonoscopy* is used to view the entire colon and the distal ileum, and is invaluable in diagnosis and management of inflammatory bowel disease.

There are a number of noninvasive imaging techniques, and of these, abdominal ultrasonography has a crucial role in evaluation of some of these diseases, especially the gallbladder. Computed tomography must be limited in its application because of radiation exposure (Chap 42, p. 1151). Because of its safety and resolution, magnetic resonance imaging commonly is used instead for evaluating the abdomen and retroperitoneal space during pregnancy.

NUTRITIONAL SUPPORT

Specialized nutritional support can be delivered by enteral feedings, usually via a nasogastric tube, or parenterally, by peripheral or central venous access. When possible, enteral alimentation is preferable because is has few dangerous complications. In obstetrical patients, there are very few conditions that prohibit enteral nutrition as a first effort to prevent catabolism.

The purpose of parenteral feeding, or hyperalimentation, is to provide nutrition when the intestinal tract must be kept quiescent. Peripheral venous access may be adequate for short-term supplemental nutrition, which derives calories from isotonic fat solutions. Jugular or subclavian venous catheterization is necessary for total parenteral nutrition, because its hyperosmolarity requires rapid dilution in a high-flow system. These solutions provide up to 24 to 40 kcal/kg, principally as a hypertonic glucose solution. Heyland and colleagues (1998) reviewed 26 randomized trials with over 2200 nonpregnant patients who were given parenteral nutrition or standard therapy. In critically ill or postoperative patients, overall mortality was not influenced by parenteral nutrition.

TABLE 48–1. **Some Conditions in Which Parenteral Nutrition Has Been Used During 81 Pregnancies**

Anorexia nervosa	Inflammatory bowel disease
Appendiceal rupture	Intracranial hemorrhage
Bowel obstruction	Jejunoileal bypass
Burns	Leukemia
Cholecystitis	Pancreatic cancer
Diabetic complications	Short bowel syndrome
Esophageal injury	Small bowel obstruction
Hyperemesis gravidarum	

Data from Kirby (1988) and Russo-Stieglitz (1999) and their colleagues.

PARENTERAL NUTRITION DURING PREGNANCY. Shown in Table 48–1 are some reported uses of total parenteral nutrition for a variety of indications in 81 pregnant women. Gastrointestinal disorders were the most common indication, and the duration of parenteral feeding averaged 33 days. Complications are frequent and may be severe. Major mechanical complications include pneumothorax, hemothorax from injury to subclavian vessels, brachial plexus injury, and catheter malpositions. Greenspoon and colleagues (1989) described a maternal death from cardiac tamponade 7 days after successful placement of a subclavian venous catheter for hyperalimentation in a woman with hyperemesis gravidarum.

Russo-Stieglitz and associates (1999) reported results from parenteral nutrition during 26 pregnancies. Mean duration of therapy was 31 days with a range of 2 to 105 days. They observed a 50 percent complication rate with central catheters, and sepsis accounted for half of these complications. Early metabolic complications may be avoided by slowly increasing the dietary prescription to avoid fluid overload, osmotic diuresis, and massive electrolyte shifts due to insulin secretion. Late metabolic complications include gallstones and hepatic cholestasis.

DISORDERS OF THE UPPER GASTROINTESTINAL TRACT

HYPEREMESIS GRAVIDARUM. Nausea and vomiting of moderate intensity are especially common until about 16 weeks (Chap. 10, p. 242). Klebanoff and colleagues (1985) reported that slightly over half of 9000 women had vomiting in early pregnancy. Jewell and Young (2000) surveyed the Cochrane Database System and confirmed a salutary effect of antiemetics. When severe and unresponsive to simple therapy, the condition is termed *hyperemesis gravidarum,* which fortunately has become uncommon. This syndrome is defined loosely as vomiting sufficiently severe to produce weight loss, dehydration, acidosis from starvation, alkalosis from loss of hydrochloric acid in vomitus, and hypokalemia. In some cases, transient hepatic dysfunction develops (p. 1283). Hyperemesis appears to be related to high or rapidly rising serum levels of chorionic gonadotropin or estrogens (Goodwin and associates, 1994; van de Ven, 1997). An association with seropositivity to *Helicobacter pylori*—the causative agent of peptic ulcer disease—has been described by Frigo and co-workers (1998).

Godsey and Newman (1991) studied 140 women admitted for hyperemesis to the Medical University of South Carolina Hospital. In 27 percent of these women, multiple admissions were necessary. Vomiting may be prolonged, frequent, and severe. We have encountered women with severe prerenal azotemia with serum creatinine as high as 5 mg/dL. Serious complications include **Mallory–Weiss tears** and **esophageal rupture.** Schwartz and Rossoff (1994) described a woman whose retching led to bilateral pneumothoraces and pneumomediastinum. Robinson and colleagues (1998) described serious epistaxis caused by vitamin K deficiency coagulopathy in a woman with refractory hyperemesis at 15 weeks. A number of cases complicated by **Wernicke encephalopathy** from thiamine deficiency have been reported. Complications from this have included blindness, convulsions, and coma (Hillbom, 1999; Rees, 1997; Tesfaye, 1998, and their associates).

MANAGEMENT. First-line methods of outpatient treatment are discussed in Chapter 10 (p. 242). Murphy and Chez (2000) recently reviewed alternative therapies. When these fail, intravenous crystalloid solutions are used to correct dehydration, electrolyte deficits, and acid–base imbalances. This requires appropriate amounts of sodium, potassium, chloride, lactate or bicarbonate, glucose, and water, all of which should be administered parenterally until vomiting has been controlled.

Antiemetics such as promethazine, prochlorperazine, and chlorpromazine are given to alleviate nausea and vomiting. Nageotte and colleagues (1996) reported success with intravenous droperidol-diphenhydramine. For severe disease, metoclopramide may be given parenterally. This stimulates motility of the upper intestinal tract without stimulating gastric, biliary, or pancreatic secretions. Its antiemetic properties apparently result from central antagonism of dopamine receptors. Safari and co-workers (1998) conducted a randomized trial comparing oral methylprednisolone with promethazine. Immediate salutary effects were apparent in both groups, but the group receiving this steroid had significantly fewer readmissions. More recently, serotonin antagonists have been used to treat severe nausea in nonpregnant patients, but their use in pregnancy is limited (Briggs and colleagues, 1998).

With persistent vomiting, appropriate steps should be taken to diagnose and treat other diseases, such as gastroenteritis, cholecystitis, pancreatitis, hepatitis, peptic ulcer, pyelonephritis, and fatty liver of pregnancy. In some instances, social and psychological factors contribute to the illness (Deuchar, 1995). With correction of these latter circumstances, the woman usually improves remarkably while hospitalized, only to relapse after discharge. Positive assistance with psychological and social problems is beneficial.

With prolonged vomiting, consideration is given for nutritional support. As previously discussed, nutrition is best provided by the enteral route if possible. Hsu and colleagues (1996) described enteral nutrition utilizing a Dobbhoff nasogastric feeding tube after acute nausea and vomiting had subsided. In some women with persistent and severe disease, parenteral nutrition may be necessary (van de Ven, 1997).

REFLUX ESOPHAGITIS. Heartburn, also called pyrosis, is a common symptom in late pregnancy. The retrosternal burning sensation is caused by esophagitis from gastroesophageal reflux related to relaxation of the lower esophageal sphincter (Hytten, 1991). Common heartburn is seldom severe enough to warrant diagnostic investigation. Raising the head of the bed and ingestion of oral antacids usually suffices to relieve symptoms. If severe symptoms persist despite these simple measures, an H_2-receptor antagonist is prescribed. Both cimetidine and ranitidine are considered safe (Briggs and associates, 1998). If there is then no relief, endoscopy should be considered.

HIATAL HERNIA. Rigler and Eneboe (1935) performed upper gastrointestinal x-ray series in 195 unselected pregnant women in the last trimester. Almost 20 percent of 116 multiparas compared with 5 percent of 79 nulliparas had a hiatal hernia. When 10 women with a pregnancy-associated hernia were reexamined 1 to 18 months postpartum, only three had a persistent hernia. Such hernias may be produced by an intermittent but prolonged increase in intra-abdominal pressure.

The relationship of hiatal hernia with reflux esophagitis, and thus symptoms, is not clear. Cohen and Harris (1971) demonstrated no relationship between reflux and hernia, and showed that the lower esophageal sphincter functioned effectively even when displaced intrathoracically. Nevertheless, during pregnancy these hernias may cause vomiting, epigastric pain, and even bleeding from ulceration. Curran and colleagues (1999) described a 30-week pregnancy complicated by gastric outlet obstruction from a paraesophageal hernia that they successfully repaired.

DIAPHRAGMATIC HERNIA. Symptomatic diaphragmatic hernias rarely complicate pregnancy. These are herniations of abdominal contents through either the foramen of Bochdalek or the foramen of Morgagni. Kurzel and associates (1988) reviewed 18 symptomatic cases reported during pregnancy. All of these women had acute obstruction, and maternal mortality was 45 percent. They recommend repair during pregnancy even if the woman is asymptomatic. Flick and associates (1999) reported a case in which a woman had sustained a car accident several months before pregnancy. At 23 weeks she experienced symptomatic bowel herniation into the chest through a traumatic diaphragmatic defect. Ortega-Carnicer (1998) and Watkin (1993) and their colleagues described women with spontaneous rupture of the diaphragm during delivery.

ACHALASIA. This is a motor disorder of esophageal smooth muscle in which the lower sphincter does not relax properly with swallowing, and there are abnormal esophageal contractions. The cause is defective innervation of the smooth muscle of the esophagus and lower esophageal sphincter. Symptoms are dysphagia, chest pain, and regurgitation. Diagnosis is usually confirmed by demonstrating a bird's beak narrowing at the distal esophagus via barium esophagogram. Endoscopy may reveal esophageal dilatation, and manometry is confirmatory. Endoscopy is used to exclude secondary causes, particularly gastric carcinoma.

Surprisingly, pregnancy does not seem to worsen this condition. Mayberry and Atkinson (1987) described 20 pregnant women and reported no excessive reflux esophagitis compared with nonpregnant women with achalasia. Of 16 women who became pregnant after symptoms developed, 11 had no change in symptomatology, two improved, and three worsened. Kalish and associates (1999) described a 32-week pregnant woman whose achalasia was worsened by severe *Candida* esophagitis.

MANAGEMENT. Soft foods and anticholinergic drugs are prescribed. If symptoms persist, balloon dilatation is used, which may be complicated by perforation or hemorrhage. Almost 85 percent of nonpregnant patients respond to such treatment. Satin and colleagues (1992) and Fiest and associates (1993) reported successful outcomes with the use of pneumatic dilatation in two women with achalasia in pregnancy.

PEPTIC ULCER. In young women, peptic ulcer disease more often involves the duodenum rather than stomach. Ulcers may be caused by chronic gastritis induced by *Helicobacter pylori* and peptic ulcer disease (de Boer and Tytgat, 2000). They may also arise from use of aspirin and other nonsteroidal anti-inflammatory drugs. Acid secretion is also important, thus explaining the temporary efficacy of antisecretory agents.

During pregnancy, gastric secretion is reduced, motility is decreased, and there is considerably increased mucus secretion (Hytten, 1991). It is thus not surprising that active peptic ulcer disease is uncommon during pregnancy. In the past 30 years at Parkland Hospital, during which time we have cared for over 300,000 pregnant women, we have encountered very few women with symptomatic peptic ulcers. Even women with symptomatic ulcers antedating pregnancy most often note considerable improvement during pregnancy. Clark (1953) studied 313 pregnancies in 118 women with proven ulcer disease and reported a clear remission in almost 90 percent. These benefits were short lived, and within 3 months of delivery, symptoms recurred in over half. By the end of 2 years, almost every woman had suffered a recurrence.

Antacids are first-line therapy and H_2-receptor blockers are prescribed for those who do not respond. Proton-pump inhibitors such as omeprazole are not recommended during pregnancy (Briggs and colleagues, 1998). Sucralfate is the aluminum salt of sulfated sucrose that provides a protective coating at the ulcer base. Only about 10 percent of the aluminum salt is absorbed, and it is considered safe. If antibacterial therapy for *H pylori* is indicated, there are a number of treatment regimens that do not include tetracycline (de Boer and Tytgat, 2000). Endoscopy is performed if indicated.

UPPER GASTROINTESTINAL BLEEDING. Occasionally, persistent vomiting may be accompanied by worrisome upper gastrointestinal bleeding. The obvious concern is that there is a bleeding peptic ulceration; however, most of these women have minute linear mucosal tears near the gastroesophageal junction, or so-called *Mallory–Weiss tears.* These women usually respond promptly to conservative measures that include iced-saline irrigations, topical antacids, and intravenously administered H_2-blockers. In some instances, blood transfusions are needed. If indicated, endoscopy is used for diagnosis and perhaps hemostasis (Van Dam and Brugge, 1999). It should not be withheld because of pregnancy. It may be important to distinguish this from the more dangerous *Boerhaave syndrome,* which is esophageal rupture caused by greatly increased esophageal pressure from retching.

DISORDERS OF THE SMALL BOWEL AND COLON

PHYSIOLOGY. The small bowel has diminished motility during pregnancy. Lawson and colleagues (1985) showed that small bowel transit time was significantly prolonged in pregnant women (125 to 140 minutes) compared with nonpregnant controls (75 to 90 minutes). The colon undergoes muscular relaxation as well, and this is accompanied by increased absorption of water and sodium. Both of these predispose to constipation.

CONSTIPATION. The incidence of constipation during pregnancy is related to dietary fiber intake (Everson, 1992). In women with low-fiber diets, almost 40 percent complain of constipation at some time during pregnancy, and 20 percent do so in the third trimester. Such symptoms are usually only mildly bothersome, but we have on several occasions encountered pregnant women who developed megacolon from impacted stool. These women almost invariably had abused stimulatory laxatives. Preventative measures include a high-fiber diet along with bulk-forming laxatives.

INFLAMMATORY BOWEL DISEASE. These disorders include at least two forms of intestinal inflammation, ulcerative colitis and Crohn disease. The latter also is known as regional enteritis, Crohn ileitis, and granulomatous colitis. As shown in Table 48–2, these two diseases share common factors, and sometimes it is impossible to distinguish the two if Crohn disease involves the colon. In general, however, the salient clinical and laboratory features shown in Table 48–2 permit a confident diagnostic differentiation between these two. The etiology of both is enigmatic, but their pathogenesis has been partially elucidated. There appears to be a genetic predisposition toward both diseases with increased incidence in twins and first-degree relatives. An association with inflammatory bowel disease has been found with certain HLA alleles. Although suspected, neither an infectious nor an immune-mediated etiology has been proven.

ULCERATIVE COLITIS. Disease is confined to the superficial layers of the colon, typically beginning at the rectum and extending proximally for a variable distance. Sigmoidoscopic findings include mucosal granularity and friability, which are interspersed with mucosal ulcerations and a mucopurulent exudate. The extent of inflammation is proportional to symptoms, and bloody diarrhea is the cardinal presenting finding. The disease is characterized by exacerbations and remissions. *Toxic megacolon* is a particularly dangerous complication that necessitates colectomy in half of cases (Sheth and LaMont, 1998). *Extraintestinal manifestations* include arthritis, uveitis, and erythema nodosum. The risk of cancer is high and approaches 1 percent per year.

Management of ulcerative colitis is medical, and sulfasalazine is used for maintenance as well as active colitis (Glickman, 1998). One active metabolite is 5-aminosali-

TABLE 48–2. Some Differentiating Characteristics of Ulcerative Colitis and Crohn Disease

Characteristic	Ulcerative Colitis	Crohn Disease
Prevalence	70–150/100,000	20–40/100,000 (increasing)
Peak incidence	20–40 years	15–30 years
Genetic factors		
Twin concordance	~50% (monozygous)	High
Family history	~25%	~25%
HLA association	HLA-Bw35, HLA-B27	HLA-A2, HLA-B27
Natural history		
Bowel involvement	Large bowel mucosa and sub-mucosa	Small and large bowel mucosa and deeper layers; transmural involvement common
	Continuous involvement beginning at rectum (40% ulcerative proctitis only)	Small or large bowel only, or both; segmental involvement
Colonoscopy	Mucosal granularity and friability with superficial ulceration	Patchy involvement
	Rectal involvement	Perianal disease
Symptoms	Bloody diarrhea	Cramping abdominal pain and watery diarrhea
	Tenesmus	Vomiting, malnutrition, weight loss
Clinical course	Exacerbations and remission (60–75% acute intermittent; 15–20% continuous chronic unremitting)	Exacerbations and remission; surgery commonly required
Extraintestinal manifestations	Arthritis, pyoderma, erythema nodosum (about 10%)	Same
Complications	Toxic megacolon (2%)	Fistula formation
	Reactive arthritis	Reactive arthritis
	Sclerosing cholangitis	Toxic megacolon
	Cancer (3–5%)	Cancer risk less
Management	Medical	Medical
	Proctocolectomy curative	Segmental resection if indicated

From Farmer (1994), Glickman (1998), and Kodner and colleagues (1999).

cylic acid, which inhibits prostaglandin synthase. Wahl and colleagues (1998) have also shown that the parent compound inhibits activation of nuclear factor kappa B (NF-κB), which is a control mediator of the immune response. Prednisone is used for more severe active disease that does not respond to 5-aminosalicylic derivatives. Immunosuppressive drugs including azathioprine and cyclosporine have been used in conjunction with prednisone in nonpregnant patients with success. Finally, cyclosporine is beneficial to treat severely ill patients who otherwise would have a colectomy. Proctocolectomy is performed for recalcitrant disease, with permanent ileostomy or an ileoanal anastomosis with one of the newly devised continent ileal pouches.

CROHN DISEASE. This inflammatory disease has more protean manifestations than ulcerative colitis. It involves not only the bowel mucosa but also the deeper layers and, sometimes, there is transmural involvement (Table 48–2). The disease is typically segmental. About 30 percent of patients have small bowel involvement, 25 percent have isolated colon involvement, and 40 percent have both, usually with the terminal ileum and colon involved.

Complaints include abdominal pain and diarrhea, and obstructive symptoms are common. The disease is chronic and marked by exacerbations and remissions. Almost 30 percent of patients require surgery during the first year after the diagnosis is made; thereafter, 5 percent per year require surgery. Indeed, Crohn disease is the most common surgical disease of the small bowel (Evers and associates, 1999). Complications include fistula formation and perineal communications that interfere with vaginal delivery (Forsnes and co-workers, 1999; Ilnyckji and colleagues, 1999). Reactive arthritis is common, and the risk of cancer, while not as great as with ulcerative colitis, is increased substantively.

No regimen is universally effective for maintenance of asymptomatic periods. Sulfasalazine is effective for symptomatic disease in some patients. The newer 5-aminosalicylate formulations are better tolerated (Rampton, 1999). Prednisone therapy controls active disease but is less effective for small bowel involvement (Glickman, 1998). Thomsen and colleagues (1998) reported promising results with oral budesonide. Immunosuppressive drugs, including azathioprine and 6-mercaptopurine, are used more successfully than with ulcerative colitis. Brynskov and colleagues (1989) reported that oral cyclosporine was effective to control corticosteroid-resistant active disease in nonpregnant patients. Methotrexate is used successfully in steroid-dependent cases, and low-dose methotrexate maintains a remission (Feagan and associates, 2000). Belluzzi and associates (1996) reported a salutary effect of fish-oil capsules in preventing recurrences. Exciting new research centers around monoclonal antibodies directed against tumor necrosis factor, a proinflammatory cytokine (Present and colleagues, 1999). Also, growth hormone, which stimulates intestinal growth and repair may be beneficial (Slonim and co-workers, 2000).

Because cure is unlikely with resection of affected bowel, conservative surgery is indicated for complications, including no response to medical therapy. Unfortunately, resection is associated with a 50 percent recurrence requiring further surgery within 10 years (Rampton, 1999).

INFLAMMATORY BOWEL DISEASE AND PREGNANCY.
Chronic inflammatory bowel disease, either ulcerative colitis or Crohn disease, is relatively common in women of childbearing age. Donaldson (1985) concluded the following:

1. Pregnancy does not increase the likelihood of an attack of inflammatory bowel disease. If the disease is quiescent in early pregnancy, then flares are uncommon, but if they develop, they may be severe.
2. Active disease at conception increases the likelihood of poor pregnancy outcome.
3. Diagnostic evaluations, including limited radiological studies, should not be postponed if their results are likely to affect management.
4. Many of the usual treatment regimens, including corticosteroids, may be continued during pregnancy, and, if indicated, surgery should be performed.

Pregnancy outcomes were recently described by Kornfeld and co-workers (1997) in a population-based cohort study of 756 Swedish women with preexisting inflammatory bowel disease. Preterm birth, low birthweight, fetal growth restriction, and cesarean delivery were all increased 1.5- to 2-fold in affected women. Perinatal mortality, however, was not increased. Previously, Fedorkow and colleagues (1989) and Baird and associates (1990) reported similar findings from retrospective controlled studies. These findings are in contrast to those described subsequently.

ULCERATIVE COLITIS. In an extensive review of more than 1000 cases, Miller (1986) reported that ulcerative colitis quiescent at conception was worsened during pregnancy in about a third of cases (Table 48–3). Women with active disease at the time of conception had a worse prognosis, and almost half worsened during pregnancy. Therapy is the same as for nonpregnant patients. Maintenance is continued with 5-aminosalicylic acid derivatives and flares can be treated with corticosteroids. Habal and associates (1993) described the successful use of 5-aminosalicylic acid for 17 pregnant women during 19 pregnancies.

Ulcerative colitis seems to have few adverse effects on pregnancy outcome. Modigliani (2000) reviewed 2398 pregnancy outcomes published since 1965. He concluded that pregnancy outcomes were not substantively different from the general obstetrical population. The incidences of spontaneous abortion, preterm delivery, and stillbirths were remarkably low. These findings contradict those of Kornfeld and colleagues (1997) described earlier for both types of inflammatory bowel disease.

When colitis worsens during pregnancy, the cause may be psychogenic. Reassurance is therefore an important part of management. Parenteral nutrition can be employed in women with severe and prolonged exacerbations. Watson and Gaines (1987) and Boulton and colleagues (1994) reported two women in whom colectomy was performed during the third trimester for corticosteroid-resistant disease. According to Farouk and colleagues (2000), long-term function of an ileal pouch–anal anastomosis is not impaired by childbirth.

CROHN DISEASE. Pregnancy does not have adverse effects on the course of Crohn disease. Miller (1986) reported findings very similar to those described previously with ulcerative colitis—that is, disease quiescent at conception carries a good prognosis (Table 48–3). Woolfson and colleagues (1990) reported similar results, and they found that abdominal surgery was required during pregnancy in 5 percent of the women. Forsnes and associates (1999) have described diagnosis of an

TABLE 48–3. Effect of Pregnancy on Inflammatory Bowel Disease

Condition	Course During Pregnancy (%)		
	Improved	No Change	Worse
Inactive disease at conception			
Ulcerative colitis (n = 528)	—	66	34
Crohn disease (n = 186)	—	73	27
Active disease at conception			
Ulcerative colitis (n = 227)	27	24	45
Crohn disease (n = 93)	34	32	33

From Miller (1986).

enterovesical fistula diagnosed in a 15-week pregnant woman.

Crohn disease does not seem to have an overwhelmingly deleterious effect on pregnancy outcome. In their 20-year literature review, Korelitz (1998) reviewed the literature and found that there were good perinatal outcomes in the absence of active disease. While active disease is associated with adverse outcomes, an important factor is response to therapy. These findings are in contrast to those described earlier by Kornfeld and associates (1997). In a Danish study of 510 infants born to women with Crohn disease, Fonager and colleagues (1998) also found a twofold risk of low-birthweight infants and preterm birth.

Parenteral hyperalimentation has been used successfully for women with severe recurrences of inflammatory bowel disease during pregnancy (Kirby and associates, 1988; Russo-Stieglitz and colleagues, 1999).

OSTOMY AND PREGNANCY. Women with a colostomy or an ileostomy may develop complications during pregnancy. Gopal and colleagues (1985) described 82 pregnancies in 66 women following ostomy, usually done for inflammatory bowel disease. Although stomal dysfunction was common, it responded to conservative management in all cases. Bowel obstruction developed in six women, and in three, surgery was necessary. Ileostomy prolapse was surgically corrected in three women during pregnancy or at cesarean delivery, and in a fourth woman during the puerperium. The cesarean delivery rate was 37 percent, and a third of these were done because of prior abdominoperineal resection.

Over the past decade, colectomy with mucosal proctectomy and ileal pouch–anal anastomosis has become the surgical procedure of choice for ulcerative colitis and familial colonic polyposis. Disadvantages include frequent bowel movements, nocturnal fecal soilage in almost half of patients, and *pouchitis* (Kodner and colleagues, 1999). Juhasz and co-workers (1995) described subsequent pregnancies in women who had this anasto-

mosis. While stool frequency, pad soilage, and incontinence temporarily worsened during pregnancy, these abated postpartum. Farouk and associates (2000) found that childbirth did not worsen long-term function. These investigators as well as others have concluded that vaginal delivery is acceptable in these women.

INTESTINAL OBSTRUCTION. Bowel obstruction during pregnancy is probably not more common than in the general population. Meyerson and colleagues (1995) reported an incidence of 1 in 17,000 deliveries in over 150,000 women delivered over a 20-year period at two Detroit hospitals. From their review, Perdue and associates (1992) found incidences that varied from 1 in 1500 to 1 in 66,500 deliveries. As shown in Table 48–4, most cases—probably 60 to 70 percent—are due to adhesions from previous pelvic surgery, including cesarean deliv-

TABLE 48–4. Causes of Intestinal Obstruction During Pregnancy and the Puerperium in 216 Women

Cause	No	(%)
Adhesions	118	(55)
First trimester	8	
Second trimester	32	
Third trimester	53	
Postpartum	25	
Volvulus	53	(25)
Midgut	6	
Cecal	19	
Sigmoid	23	
Other	5	
Intussusception	11	(5)
Hernia, carcinoma, appendicitis	12	(5)
Other	22	(10)

Adapted from Connolly and colleagues (1995).

eries. Volvulus is another common cause, and in a third of the cases reported by Harer and Harer (1958), cesarean delivery was necessary to obtain proper exposure. Volvulus of the cecum and small bowel have been reported in late pregnancy or early in the puerperium (Carral and colleagues, 1998; Ranjan and Boulton, 1993). Woywodt and Kiss (1999) described a woman with severe geophagia who developed sigmoid obstruction with perforation, sepsis, and death. Spontaneous small bowel obstruction may also develop during pregnancy (Ventura-Braswell and associates, 1998; Wax and Christie, 1993).

Intestinal obstruction is a grave complication of pregnancy and results most frequently from pressure of the growing uterus on intestinal adhesions. According to Davis and Bohon (1983), there are three times when obstruction is more likely: around midpregnancy, when the uterus becomes an abdominal organ; at term, when the fetal head descends; and immediately postpartum, when there is an acute change in the uterine size. From their review, Perdue and colleagues (1992) found that 80 percent of pregnant women had nausea and vomiting. Importantly, abdominal pain, either continuous or colicky, was found in 98 percent. Abdominal tenderness was encountered in 70 percent. They reported abnormal bowel sounds in only 55 percent.

Limited x-ray examinations, including plain abdominal films, and those following administration of soluble contrast medium should be performed if obstruction is suspected. Perdue and associates (1992) reported that 38 of 42 pregnant women in whom x-rays were performed had radiographic evidence of obstruction.

The mortality rate with intestinal obstruction can be very high, principally because of errors in diagnosis, delayed diagnosis, reluctance to operate during pregnancy, and inadequate preparation for surgery (Firstenberg and Malangoni, 1998). Of 66 pregnancies, Perdue and associates (1992) described a 6 percent maternal mortality rate and a 26 percent fetal mortality rate. Two of the four women who died had adhesive obstruction late in pregnancy; one each had sigmoid or cecal volvulus.

Colonic pseudo-obstruction, or *Ogilvie syndrome,* is caused by adynamic colonic ileus, and about 10 percent of all reported cases follow delivery. The syndrome is characterized by massive abdominal distention with cecal dilatation. Although unusual, the large bowel may rupture, and decompression is recommended when the bowel becomes distended to 10 to 12 cm. In most cases, colonoscopy for decompression is effective but if peritonitis is suspected, laparotomy may be indicated. We have had success with colonic decompression by colonoscopy, and Moore and associates (1986) have described this in a woman 2 days following cesarean delivery. Ponec and associates (1999) reported that slow intravenous infusion of 2 mg neostigmine resulted in prompt decompression. Subsequently, Amaro and Rogers (2000) confirmed that 17 of 18 patients responded immediately to this treatment.

APPENDICITIS. Suspected appendicitis is one of the most common indications for surgical abdominal exploration during pregnancy. Mazze and Källén (1991) described findings from 720,000 Swedish registry deliveries and reported that 778 (about 1 in 1000 pregnancies) of these women underwent appendectomy during pregnancy. Appendicitis was confirmed in 65 percent, or about 1 in 1500 pregnancies.

Pregnancy often makes the diagnosis of appendicitis more difficult because:

1. Anorexia, nausea, and vomiting that accompany normal pregnancy are also common symptoms of appendicitis.
2. As the uterus enlarges, the appendix commonly moves upward and outward toward the flank, so that pain and tenderness may not be prominent in the right lower quadrant (Fig. 48–1).
3. Some degree of leukocytosis is the rule during normal pregnancy.
4. During pregnancy especially, other diseases may be confused with appendicitis, such as pyelonephritis, renal colic, placental abruption, and degeneration of a uterine myoma.
5. Pregnant women, especially those late in gestation,

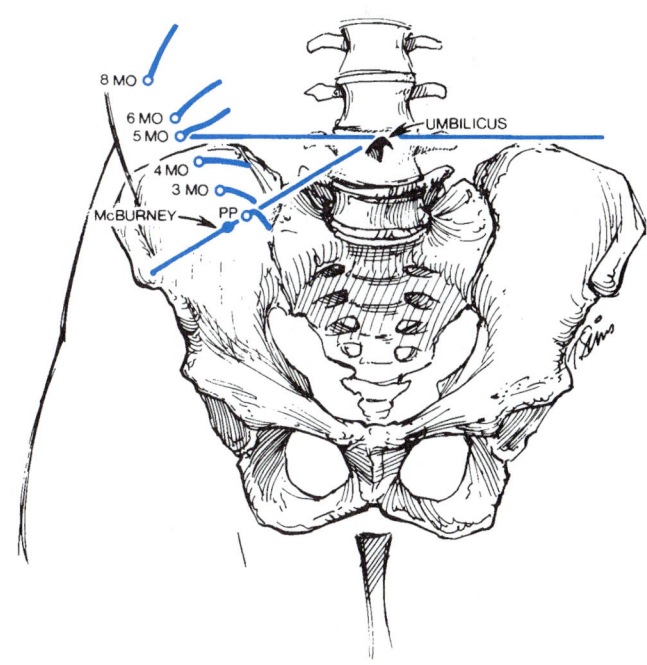

FIGURE 48–1. Changes in position of the appendix as pregnancy advances (MO = month, PP = postpartum). (Modified from Baer and associates, 1932.)

frequently do not have symptoms considered "typical" for nonpregnant patients with appendicitis.

As the appendix is pushed progressively higher by the growing uterus, containment of infection by the omentum becomes increasingly unlikely, and appendiceal rupture is more likely to cause generalized peritonitis. In the recent report by Tracey and Fletcher (2000), over half of pregnant women had perforative appendicitis. Acute appendicitis in late pregnancy has the worst prognosis, and indeed, in some older series maternal mortality approached 5 percent (Sharp, 1994). Increased fetal and maternal morbidity and mortality is almost invariably due to surgical delay.

DIAGNOSIS AND MANAGEMENT. Persistent abdominal pain and tenderness are the most reproducible findings. While most investigators have reported that pain migrates upward with appendiceal displacement with progressing pregnancy, Mourad and associates (2000) did not find this. They reported that 80 percent of 45 pregnant women had pain in the right lower quadrant regardless of trimester.

Graded compression using ultrasound imaging was effective in the diagnosis of appendicitis in nonpregnant patients (Puylaert and colleagues, 1987). While Landwehr and associates (1996) correctly diagnosed appendicitis in four of five pregnant women using this method, we have found that cecal displacement and uterine imposition makes precise examination difficult. Rao and colleagues (1998) performed appendiceal computed tomography in 100 consecutive nonpregnant patients with suspected appendicitis and found the technique to be 98 percent accurate (Fig. 48–2). Tomography needs to be evaluated in pregnant women before its widespread application.

If appendicitis is suspected, treatment is immediate surgical exploration. Even though diagnostic errors sometimes lead to removal of a normal appendix, it is better to operate unnecessarily than to postpone intervention until generalized peritonitis has developed.

In most reports, the diagnosis is verified in about half of women who undergo surgical exploration (Sharp, 1994). In the Swedish study of 778 women with suspected appendicitis, the diagnosis was confirmed in 65 percent (Mazze and Källén, 1991). In the first trimester, 77 percent of diagnoses were correct; however, in the latter two trimesters, only 57 percent of diagnoses were confirmed at surgery.

In nonpregnant patients, laparoscopy is done routinely for suspected acute appendicitis. Hellberg and colleagues (1999) randomized 500 nonpregnant patients with suspected acute appendicitis to either method. They concluded that the laparoscopic approach was safe and associated with faster postoperative recovery. Cer-

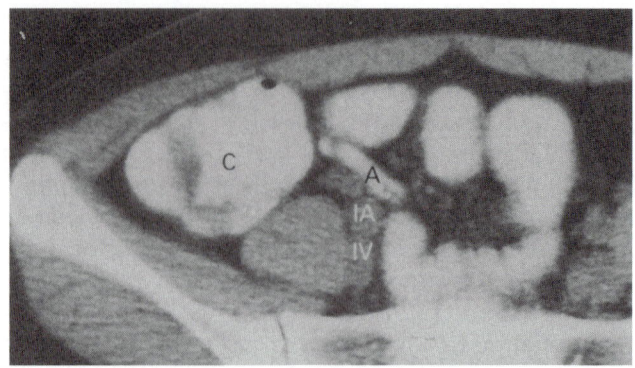
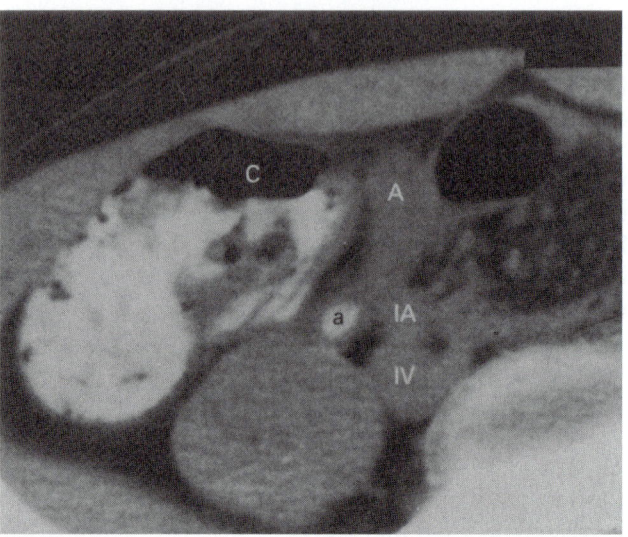

FIGURE 48–2. Appendiceal computed tomography. **Top.** Normal appendix (A), cecum (C), and internal iliac artery (IA) and vein (IV). **Bottom.** An inflamed, unopacified appendix (A) which is 15 mm in diameter and has a proximal fecolith in the appendix (a). (From Rao and colleagues, 1998, with permission.)

tainly in the first half of pregnancy, laparoscopy for suspected appendicitis is acceptable (Affleck and co-workers, 1999). Others have questioned the safety of creating a pneumoperitoneum with carbon dioxide, which may cause fetal acidosis and adversely affect fetal cardiovascular function (Amos and associates, 1996). As discussed on page 1274, the experiences with laparoscopy of Reedy and colleagues (1997) from the Swedish Registry are reassuring (see also Chap. 42, p. 1145). They found similar perinatal outcomes in nearly 2000 laparoscopic procedures compared with over 1500 laparotomies in women less than 20 weeks.

Intravenous antimicrobials are given, and Firstenberg and Malangoni (1998) recommend a second-generation cephalosporin or third-generation penicillin. Unless there is gangrene, perforation, or a periappendiceal phlegmon, antimicrobial therapy can be discontinued after surgery. If generalized peritonitis does not develop, then the prognosis is quite good. Seldom is cesarean delivery indicated at the time of appendectomy. Uterine contractions are common with peritonitis and, although some authors recommend tocolytic agents, we do not. De Veciana and colleagues (1994) reported that increased intravenous fluid administration and tocolytic use increased the risk for pulmonary injury with antepartum appendicitis.

Undiagnosed appendicitis often stimulates labor. The large uterus frequently helps to contain infection locally, but after delivery when the uterus rapidly empties, the walled-off infection is disrupted with spillage of free pus into the peritoneal cavity. In these cases, an acute surgical abdomen is encountered within a few postpartum hours.

Simply because it is coincidental, appendicitis during the early puerperium is rare. In some cases, especially with early appendicitis, diagnosis is particularly difficult because of the normally robust leukocytosis as well as the frequency of other puerperal disorders with similar signs and symptoms. Anorexia with any evidence of peritoneal irritation, such as distention and adynamic ileus, should suggest appendicitis. Puerperal pelvic infections typically do not cause peritonitis.

EFFECTS ON PREGNANCY. Appendicitis increases the likelihood of abortion or preterm labor, especially if there is peritonitis. Mazze and Källén (1991) found that spontaneous labor ensued with greater frequency if surgery for appendicitis was performed after 23 weeks. In the 45 cases described by Mourad and associates (2000), uterine contractions were reported in 19 of 23 women who were 24 weeks or greater. Fetal loss is increased in most series, and overall it is about 15 percent. In the Swedish study, fetal loss was 22 percent if surgery was performed after 23 weeks. Mays and colleagues (1995) have suggested a link between maternal–fetal sepsis and neonatal neurological injury in pregnancy complicated by appendicitis. In another long-term study, Viktrup and Hée (1998) found that appendicitis during pregnancy was not associated with subsequent infertility.

DISEASES OF THE LIVER

It is customary to divide liver diseases into those coincidental to pregnancy, those specifically related to pregnancy, and chronic liver disease that antedates pregnancy. Many disorders complicating pregnancy are coincidental, for example, acute viral hepatitis or drug-induced hepatic failure. There are some diseases that are induced by pregnancy that resolve following delivery. These include intrahepatic cholestasis of pregnancy, acute fatty liver of pregnancy, hepatocellular damage

due to severe preeclampsia, and hepatic dysfunction from hyperemesis gravidarum. Finally, pregnancy may be superimposed on chronic hepatitis or cirrhosis, esophageal varices, or liver transplantation.

HEPATIC PHYSIOLOGY. Pregnancy normally induces appreciable changes in some of the tests as well as physical findings that are usually employed to assess liver function (Table 48–5). Palmar erythema and spider angiomas may develop. Histological findings of liver biopsy specimens taken from normal pregnant women were not different when compared with nonpregnant subjects (Ingerslev and Teilum, 1945).

HYPEREMESIS GRAVIDARUM. Pernicious nausea and vomiting are discussed on page 1275. The liver may be involved, and biopsy findings are either normal or show some fatty changes (Knox and Olans, 1996). There may be mild hyperbilirubinemia, and serum hepatic transaminase levels are elevated in up to half of women who are hospitalized. Enzyme levels seldom exceed 200 U/L.

INTRAHEPATIC CHOLESTASIS OF PREGNANCY. Cholestasis of pregnancy also has been referred to as recurrent jaundice of pregnancy, cholestatic hepatosis, and icterus gravidarum. It is characterized clinically by pruritus, icterus, or both. The major histological lesion is intrahepatic cholestasis with centrilobular bile staining without inflammatory cells or proliferation of mesen-

TABLE 48–5. Results of Some Tests of Liver Function During Pregnancy

Test	Pregnancy Effects
Enzymes	
Alkaline phosphatase	Markedly increased
Aminotransferases	Unchanged
Lactic acid dehydrogenase	Unchanged
Bilirubin	Unchanged
Proteins	
Albumin	Decreased 1 g/dL
Globulin	Slightly increased
Hormone-binding proteins	Elevated
Transferrin	Elevated
Lipids	
Triglycerides	Elevated
Cholesterol	Doubled
Clotting factors	
Fibrinogen	Elevated
Factors VII, VIII, X	Elevated
Clotting times	Unchanged

chymal cells. The cause is unknown, and it was assumed to be stimulated in susceptible persons by high estrogen concentrations. Leslie and colleagues (2000), however, recently reported that maternal plasma estrogens are decreased in affected women compared with matched controls. Reyes and Sjovall (2000) have proposed that there is a defect in secretion of sulfated progesterone metabolites. There is evidence that obstetrical cholestasis is related to the many gene mutations that control hepatocellular-transport systems (Trauner and associates, 1998). Because of these genetic influences, the incidence of cholestasis varies. It is common in Chile and Sweden, and according to Reyes (1997), it complicated 4 percent of pregnancies in Chile in 1995. In other countries, its incidence is probably about 1 in 500 to 1000 pregnancies.

PATHOGENESIS. Presumably, a number of estrogen-induced changes account for cholestasis in susceptible women. Some drugs that similarly decrease the canalicular transport maximum for bile acids will aggravate the disorder. For example, we have encountered cholestatic jaundice in several pregnant women who were taking azathioprine following renal transplantation.

Bile acids are cleared incompletely by the liver and accumulate in plasma of women with cholestasis. Serum concentration of total bile acids may be elevated 10- to 100-fold (Lunzer and associates, 1986). Hyperbilirubinemia results from retention of conjugated pigment, but total plasma concentrations rarely exceed 4 to 5 mg/dL. The serum alkaline phosphatase is usually elevated more so than for normal pregnancy. Serum transaminase activities are normal to moderately elevated, and seldom exceed 250 U/L. Liver biopsy shows mild cholestasis with intracellular bile pigments and canalicular bile plugging without necrosis. These changes disappear after delivery, but often recur in subsequent pregnancies or when an oral estrogen-containing contraceptive is taken.

CLINICAL PRESENTATION. Most women with cholestasis develop pruritus in late pregnancy although the syndrome occasionally occurs in the second trimester. Kirkinen and Ryynänen (1995) reported a woman at 13 weeks with typical cholestasis who had hyperplacentosis associated with a triploid fetus. Generalized pruritus is usually the presenting symptom, but there are no accompanying skin changes unless there are excoriations from scratching. The differential diagnosis of skin eruptions is considered in Chapter 54 (p. 1431). A minority of women—perhaps 10 percent—develop jaundice within several days following pruritus. There are no constitutional symptoms.

Several other disorders should be considered. The absence of hypertension and proteinuria militate against liver disease associated with preeclampsia. Ultrasound examination will often serve to exclude biliary obstruction by gallstones. If serum transaminase levels are not appreciably elevated and the woman is asymptomatic, then viral hepatitis is not likely. However, as discussed subsequently, Locatelli and colleagues (1999) have shown a significantly higher rate of cholestasis in otherwise asymptomatic women seropositive for hepatitis C (16 percent) compared with seronegative controls (0.8 percent).

MANAGEMENT. Pruritus associated with cholestasis is caused by elevated serum bile salts, and may be quite troublesome. Orally administered *antihistamines* may provide some relief. *Cholestyramine* may be effective; however, our observations as well as those of Fisk and colleagues (1988) do not support this. Absorption of fat-soluble vitamins, already impaired, is worsened with cholestyramine. Thus, impaired coagulation from vitamin K deficiency may develop unless supplemented. Sadler and associates (1995) described spontaneous intracranial hemorrhage in a 29-week fetus whose mother—and presumably the fetus—developed hypoprothrombinemia with cholestyramine therapy. Matos and colleagues (1997), however, described a 37-week stillbirth from the same cause in an untreated woman with mild disease.

Retrospective observations showed that *ursodeoxycholic acid* quickly relieved pruritus and lowered serum hepatic enzyme levels in women with obstetric cholestasis (Kilby and associates, 1998). Palma and colleagues (1997) subsequently found it safe and effective in a small blinded placebo trial. Nicastri and co-workers (1998) reaffirmed these findings and further reported that addition of S-adenosylmethionine improved results with ursodeoxycholic acid.

Hirvioja and colleagues (1992) reported prompt relief of pruritus in 10 women given **dexamethasone,** 12 mg daily for 7 days. They postulated that associated diminished estrogen synthesis caused relief of pruritus as well as lowered serum transaminase levels.

EFFECT OF CHOLESTASIS ON PREGNANCY. Most observations indicate that adverse pregnancy outcomes are increased in women with cholestatic jaundice. Rioseco and co-workers (1994) retrospectively compared outcomes in 320 affected pregnancies with normal controls. Although meconium-stained amnionic fluid (25 versus 16 percent) and preterm delivery (12 versus 4 percent) were increased significantly, they attributed equivalent perinatal mortality to close pregnancy surveillance. Conversely, Alsulyman and associates (1996) retrospectively studied 79 women followed with weekly nonstress testing and amnionic fluid assessment. Compared with controls, women with cholestasis more often had abnormal testing that prompted delivery (25 versus 8 percent). They also had more frequent meconium passage (44 versus 8 percent), and the two fetal deaths were associated with thick meconium and a normal antepartum test within 5 days.

ACUTE FATTY LIVER OF PREGNANCY.
Acute liver failure may be caused by fulminant viral hepatitis, drug-induced hepatic toxicity, or acute fatty liver of pregnancy. The latter is also called **acute fatty metamorphosis** or **acute yellow atrophy,** and it is an uncommon complication that often has proved fatal for both mother and fetus. In its worst form, the incidence is probably about 1 in 10,000 pregnancies. Reyes and associates (1994) reported the incidence to be 1 in 15,000 in Santiago, Chile, while Castro and colleagues (1996a) found it to be 1 in 7000 in Los Angeles.

Gross examination of the liver in fatal cases shows a small, soft, yellow, and greasy organ. The prominent histological abnormalities consist of swollen hepatocytes in which the cytoplasm is filled with microvesicular fat with central nuclei and periportal sparing and minimal hepatocellular necrosis (Fig. 48–3).

ETIOLOGY AND PATHOGENESIS.
Current evidence suggests that recessively inherited mitochondrial abnormalities of fatty acid oxidation predispose a woman to fatty liver in pregnancy. From some reports, if the fetus is homozygous, the mother manifests liver failure. Sims and co-workers (1995) described a familial deficiency of long-chain 3-hydroxyacyl-CoA dehydrogenase (LCHAD) caused by a single codon mutation. Affected homozygous children had Reye-like syndromes, and some of these heterozygous women suffered fatty liver of pregnancy. There are other less common single-gene mutations that cause deficiency of β-oxidation enzymes. Isaacs and colleagues (1996) described a compound heterozygous fetus associated with maternal fatty liver in a heterozygous woman.

It would also appear that heterozygous LCHAD-deficient mothers are at risk for obstetrical complications even if their fetus is heterozygous or normal. Tyni and colleagues (1998) reviewed 79 pregnancies in 18 mothers with abnormal LCHAD heterozygosity. In 29 pregnancies, there was a homozygous LCHAD-deficient fetus, and preeclampsia and HELLP syndrome (hemolysis, elevated liver enzymes, and low platelets) were confined to this group. Almost half of LCHAD-deficient fetuses were growth restricted compared with only 10 percent of LCHAD-normal or carrier fetuses. In some of these there was growth restriction with no other complications. Earlier, Minakami and co-workers (1988) had linked biopsy-proven fatty metamorphosis in Japanese women with preeclampsia, with and without liver dysfunction. These women were studied before recognition of the gene mutations for β-oxidation enzymes.

Recurrent fatty liver in subsequent pregnancy is uncommon, but a few cases have been described (MacLean and co-workers, 1994; Reyes and associates, 1994; Usta and colleagues, 1994). This is more likely if the woman has a homozygously affected fetus (Treem and associates, 1994; Tyni and colleagues, 1998).

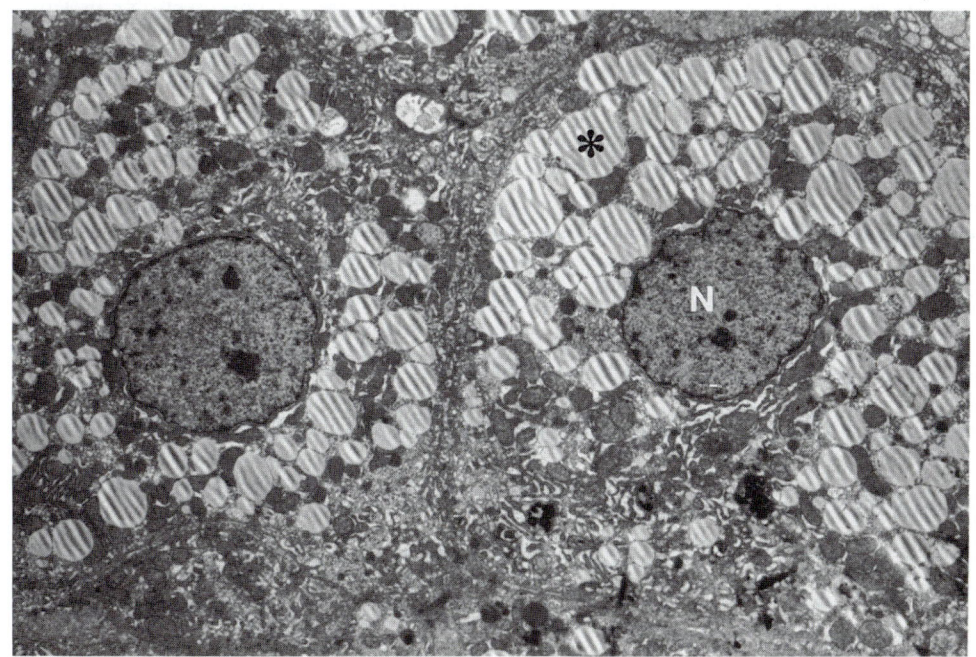

FIGURE 48–3. Fatty liver of pregnancy. Electron photomicrograph of two hepatocytes containing numerous microvesicular fat droplets (*). The nuclei (N) remain centered within the cells, unlike with the case of macrovesicular fat deposition. (Courtesy of Dr. Don Wheeler.)

CLINICAL FINDINGS. Acute fatty liver usually manifests late in pregnancy, although Monga and Katz (1999) described a typical case that began at 22 weeks. Castro and colleagues (1996a) reported a mean gestational age of 37.5 weeks (range 31 to 42) in 28 women with the syndrome. For inexplicable reasons, the disease is more common in nulliparas. It likely is more common with a male fetus, and 15 percent of cases have a multifetal gestation (Davidson and associates, 1998). Typically, there is onset over several days to weeks of malaise, anorexia, nausea and vomiting, epigastric pain, and progressive jaundice. In many women, vomiting is the major symptom. In perhaps half of these women, there is hypertension, proteinuria, and edema—signs suggestive of preeclampsia. Laboratory abnormalities include hypofibrinogenemia and prolonged clotting studies, hyperbilirubinemia of usually less than 10 mg/dL, and serum transaminase levels of 300 to 500 U/L (Table 48–6). Peripheral blood shows hemoconcentration and leukocytosis, frequently mild thrombocytopenia, and evidence for hemolysis. Castro and associates (1996a) also described markedly reduced antithrombin III levels.

Various imaging techniques have been purported to confirm the clinical diagnosis of acute fatty metamorphosis (Watson and Seeds, 1990). Castro and associates (1996b) found poor sensitivity with sonography (3/11), computed tomographic scanning (5/10), and magnetic resonance imaging (0/5). Usta and colleagues (1994) also observed that only 2 of 10 women studied with computed tomography had positive findings.

In many women, the syndrome worsens after diagnosis. Marked hypoglycemia is common, and obvious hepatic coma develops in 60 percent, severe coagulopathy in 55 percent, and evidence for renal failure in about half. Fetal death is common at this severe stage. Fortunately, either the disease is self-limited, or as generally accepted, delivery arrests rapid deterioration of liver function. During recovery, evidence for transient diabetes insipidus and acute pancreatitis is common and ascites is almost universal. Recovery usually is complete.

We have encountered a number of women with what appears to be a **forme fruste** of this disorder. Clinical involvement is relatively minor and laboratory aberrations—usually hemolysis and decreased fibrinogen levels—call attention to an abnormality. It is unlikely that there is a spectrum of liver involvement, and that liver failure is not universal and only represents the most extensive involvement. Probably many milder cases go unnoticed or they are attributed to preeclampsia.

COAGULOPATHY. The pathogenesis of the coagulopathy that complicates fatty liver of pregnancy results from increased consumption of procoagulants as well as impaired production by the liver. Shown in Table 48–6 are laboratory data suggestive of consumptive coagulopathy in 62 women with acute fatty liver. Almost all had low plasma fibrinogen levels. These are accompanied by variable elevations of fibrin split products or D-dimers. In a few cases, profound thrombocytopenia develops (Table 48–6). There usually is evidence for hemolysis, which can be severe. Echinocytes are the predominant red cell abnormality, presumably caused by impaired hepatic synthesis of various lipid components of the erythrocyte membrane (Cunningham and colleagues, 1985).

EFFECTS ON PREGNANCY. When there is severe hepatic dysfunction, there is frequently severe maternal hypovolemia and acidosis. Four of 14 women with acute fatty liver described by Usta and associates (1994) had encephalopathy. In the past, maternal mortality approached 75 percent, however, the contemporaneous outlook is much better. In the 62 women shown in Table 48–6, there were only two maternal deaths. Also in the past, fetal mortality was reported to be nearly 90 percent, but this now is about 15 to 20 percent.

TABLE 48–6. Laboratory Findings in 62 Women with Acute Fatty Liver of Pregnancy

Series	Patients	Laboratory Values—Mean ±1 SD (range)				
		Plasma Fibrinogen (mg/dL)	Fibrin Split Products (µg/mL)	Platelets (10³/µL)	Creatinine (mg/dL)	AST (U/L)
Usta et al (1994)	14	139 ± 79 (37–110)	ND	126 ± 96	2.4 ± 1.0 (1.1–3.6)	1067 ± 1098 (200–3670)
Castro et al (1996a)	28	125 (32–446)	ND	113 (11–186)	2.5 (1.1–5.2)	210 (45–1200)
Parkland Hospital	20	134 (35–380)	50 (16–256)	131 (9–300)	2.2 (0.9–4.3)	430 (53–1160)

AST = aspartate aminotransferase; ND = not done.

MANAGEMENT. Because spontaneous resolution usually follows delivery, many clinicians assume that delivery is essential for cure. Because of maternal acidosis that develops from liver failure in severe cases, some fetuses are dead when the diagnosis is made, and many others tolerate the stresses of even normal labor poorly. Procrastination in effecting delivery can increase the risk of coma and death from hyperammonemia, which is often further complicated by hypoglycemia, renal failure, acidosis, and severe hemorrhage.

Some authors recommend cesarean delivery to minimize the time until restoration of hepatic function begins. Cesarean delivery in the presence of a severe coagulopathy, however, may prove dangerous for the mother. Other problems might be encountered with an abdominal incision in circumstances in which severe hypoproteinemia and ascites are likely complications. Transfusions with variable amounts of fresh-frozen plasma, cryoprecipitate, whole blood, packed red cells, and platelets are usually necessary if surgery is performed or if lacerations complicate vaginal delivery (Chap. 25, p. 653).

Following delivery, hepatic dysfunction resolves. In the interim, intensive medical support is required. Maternal deaths are reported to be caused by sepsis, hemorrhage, aspiration, renal failure, pancreatitis, and gastrointestinal bleeding. Therapy is directed toward these complications. If hepatic failure does not resolve, liver transplantation is an alternative (Franco and colleagues, 2000; Ockner and associates, 1990). According to Kennedy and co-workers (1994), diabetes insipidus, presumably due to elevated vasopressinase concentrations, is common, and in our experiences, it develops in over half of affected women.

THE LIVER IN PREECLAMPSIA-ECLAMPSIA. The liver may be involved in women with severe preeclampsia and eclampsia (Chap. 24, p. 579). The lesion is unique and consists of periportal hemorrhage, fibrin deposition, and hepatocyte disruption with necrosis (Riely and Fallon, 1999). Both the degree of dysfunction and the histological changes that develop can vary considerably. Typically, upper abdominal pain—epigastric or right upper quadrant—signals potentially dangerous liver involvement. Thrombocytopenia commonly accompanies elevations in serum transaminase levels. Although aspartate aminotransferase levels vary from 50 to 3000 U/L, typically they are less than 500 U/L. Serum bilirubin levels sometimes are mildly elevated. Intrahepatic and subcapsular hemorrhage may develop and become so intense as to rupture the liver and produce extensive and fatal hemorrhage.

These complications were first described by Pritchard and colleagues in 1954. Weinstein (1982) later named this the *HELLP syndrome* to describe hemolysis (H),

elevated liver enzymes (EL), and low platelets (LP). There is clinical evidence that this syndrome may overlap with that of acute fatty liver of pregnancy.

PATHOGENESIS. Like other organs, most pathological lesions of liver involvement with preeclampsia are explicable on the basis of ischemia. This is perhaps enigmatic because the liver receives only a third of its blood supply from the hepatic artery, which can even be ligated without major sequelae (Stain and co-workers, 1996). The portal venous system is the major source of blood to the liver.

The exact incidence of liver involvement with preeclampsia is unknown, but it seems to be related to the severity of disease. For example, elevated serum transaminase levels are more common if thrombocytopenia is also identified. In some cases, however, the liver may be the only organ with obvious major involvement. Certainly, as illustrated by data shown in Table 48–7, liver involvement is common in fatal cases. Rolfes and Ishak (1986) reviewed findings in 97 women who died from preeclampsia–eclampsia and who were autopsied at the Armed Forces Institute of Pathology. There were hepatic histological abnormalities in 72 percent and 13 percent had infarctions. Other findings were periportal fibrin deposition, hemorrhage, and hepatocellular necrosis (Fig. 48–4).

CLINICAL PRESENTATION. In most women with preeclamptic liver disease, there will be obvious pregnancy-induced hypertension. Although the liver is more likely to be affected if there is epigastric pain, most women have no symptoms relating to the liver, and laboratory assessment discloses elevated serum transaminase lev-

TABLE 48–7. Laboratory and Anatomical Hepatic Findings in 97 Women Who Died from Preeclampsia–Eclampsia

Findings	Prevalence (%)
Hepatic symptoms	42/97 (43)
Serum transaminases (n = 26)	350–3720 U/L
Gross appearance	
Normal	28/97 (29)
Infarction	13/97 (13)
Hematoma	2/97 (2)
Histological appearance	
Pure fibrin deposition	33/97 (34)
Primary hemorrhage	9/97 (9)
Fibrin deposition and hemorrhage	31/97 (32)
Bile inspissation	10/97 (10)

Data from Rolfes and Ishak (1986).

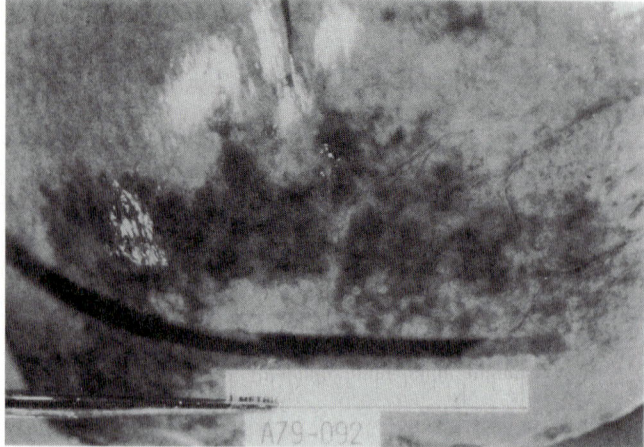

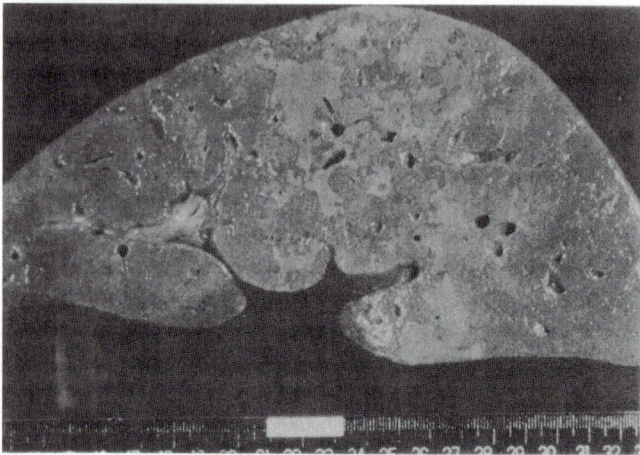

FIGURE 48–4. Top. Liver from a woman who died from eclampsia. Dark mottled surface is from numerous large hepatic infarctions similar to those seen in the lower photograph. **Bottom.** Liver of a second woman who died from eclampsia. There are multiple regions of hepatic infarction seen as serpiginous pale zones. (From Knox and Olans, 1996, with permission).

els. In most cases, these seldom exceed 200 to 500 U/L (Watson and Seeds, 1990). Similarly, serum bilirubin levels seldom exceed 2 to 4 mg/dL. Hepatic failure with encephalopathy and consumptive coagulopathy are not usual features of preeclamptic liver disease. Indeed, in the 97 fatal cases described by Rolfes and Ishak (1986), hepatic failure was diagnosed in only four.

When the diagnosis of pregnancy-induced hypertension is equivocal, preeclamptic liver involvement must be differentiated from fatty liver and hepatitis. As discussed, women with fatty liver of pregnancy often have hypertension and proteinuria, and the degree of liver dysfunction is the differentiating factor. Women with hepatitis usually do not have hypertension.

Management of women with preeclampsia and liver involvement almost always includes prompt delivery. Laboratory abnormalities usually peak by 24 to 48 hours postpartum, and hepatic enzyme abnormalities, lactic dehydrogenase, and platelet counts begin to normalize typically within about 2 to 3 days (Martin and colleagues, 1991).

HEPATIC HEMATOMA AND RUPTURE. Hemorrhage from hepatic and subcapsular hematomas are two feared complications of liver involvement with preeclampsia. Smith and colleagues (1991) reported an incidence of 1 in 45,000 pregnancies at Baylor College of Medicine. Our experiences from Parkland Hospital are similar. Stain and co-workers (1996) reported an incidence of 1 in 15,000 at Los Angeles County—University of Southern California Medical Center. Although liver rupture may develop spontaneously in an otherwise normal pregnant woman, the majority of cases are associated with preeclampsia and eclampsia (Ralston and Schwaitzberg, 1998; Rolfes and Ishak, 1986). As discussed in Chapter 24 (p. 579), women with HELLP syndrome are at much higher risk (Sheikh and associates, 1999). Moen and associates (1993) described a case associated with cocaine abuse in a woman at 30 weeks.

In typical cases, the hematoma usually develops on the diaphragmatic surface of the right lobe. Intrahepatic hematomas may also develop. It is likely that many of these go unrecognized. In other cases, there are right upper quadrant pain and tenderness, and the diagnosis can be confirmed by computed tomography (Fig. 48–5).

If the hematoma is intrahepatic and intact, close observation is reasonable. In some cases, however, liver rupture stimulates further bleeding which causes hemorrhagic shock and a distended abdomen that prompt surgical intervention before diagnostic studies can be

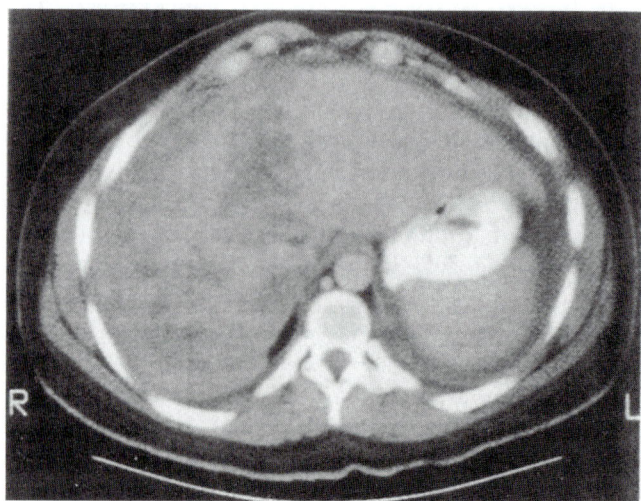

FIGURE 48–5. Computed tomography in severely preeclamptic woman at term shows intrahepatic and subcapsular hemorrhage in right lobe of liver. (From Howard and Jones, 1993, with permission.)

performed. In these cases, management includes resuscitation and correction of associated coagulopathy along with surgical exploration. Hysterotomy is done if the woman is undelivered. Local hemostasis may be attempted with suture, cautery, or Argon laser. If unsuccessful, temporary packing, hepatic artery ligation, or partial hepatic resection are performed (Ralston and Schwaitzberg, 1998). Bleeding usually is severe. Smith and associates (1991) reported that packing was associated with an overall 80 percent survival compared with 25 percent if lobectomy was done. Conversely, Stain and colleagues (1996) reported that arterial ligation was preferable. We managed an eclamptic woman with hepatic rupture who required many surgical procedures for hemostasis and was given over 200 units of blood products; fortunately, she survived. Hunter and colleagues (1995) resorted to liver transplantation in a woman with uncontrollable hemorrhage following hematoma rupture.

Maternal mortality is high with overt rupture. Of eight cases reported by Stain and co-authors (1996), three died. Ralston and Schwaitzberg (1998) cited about 60 percent mortality from their review.

VIRAL HEPATITIS. Hepatitis is the most common serious liver disease encountered in pregnant women. There are at least five distinct types of viral hepatitis: hepatitis A; hepatitis B; hepatitis D caused by the hepatitis B–associated delta agent; hepatitis C; and hepatitis E. Hepatitis C is transmitted by serum and hepatitis E is enterically transmitted. A sixth agent, hepatitis G virus, also called GBV-C, is transmitted by blood transfusion, detected serologically, but may not cause liver disease. All but hepatitis B are RNA viruses.

During their acute phases, these forms of hepatitis are often clinically similar. Interestingly, the viruses are not actually hepatotoxic; it is the immune response to them that causes hepatocellular necrosis (Dienstag and Isselbacher, 1998). In many cases, infections are subclinical, but if clinically apparent, symptoms may precede jaundice by 1 to 2 weeks. Symptoms include nausea and vomiting, headache, and malaise. Low-grade fever is more common with hepatitis A. When jaundice develops, symptoms usually improve, but there may be pain and tenderness over the liver. Serum aminotransferase levels vary, and their peaks do not correspond with disease severity. Peak levels of 400 to 4000 U/L are usually reached by the time jaundice develops (Dienstag and Isselbacher, 1998). Serum bilirubin levels usually peak at 5 to 20 mg/dL, and they typically continue to rise despite falling aminotransferase levels. There usually is complete clinical and biochemical recovery within 1 to 2 months in all cases of hepatitis A and most cases of hepatitis B.

The Centers for Disease Control have issued guidelines to minimize infectivity of patients hospitalized for viral hepatitis. It recommends that feces, secretions, and bedpans and other articles in contact with the intestinal tract be handled with glove-protected hands. These precautions need not be continued once hepatitis A is excluded. Extra precautions, such as double gloving during delivery and surgical procedures, are wise in cases of hepatitis B and C.

COMPLICATIONS. The case fatality rate for nonpregnant patients with acute hepatitis is 0.1 percent, and for those ill enough to be hospitalized, it is as high as 1 percent. Most fatalities are due to *fulminant hepatic necrosis,* which in later pregnancy must be distinguished from acute fatty liver. About half of patients with fulminant hepatitis have infection with the B virus, and many of these are associated with the delta agent. Hepatic encephalopathy is the usual presentation of patients with fulminant hepatitis, and mortality is 80 percent.

A small number of patients with hepatitis A infection have *relapsing hepatitis,* in which there is recurrence of symptoms and biochemical abnormalities weeks to months after recovery from acute infection. Some form of chronic hepatitis B infection follows acute disease in 5 to 10 percent of cases. Most of these patients will be asymptomatic carriers, but others have low-grade chronic persistent hepatitis or chronic active hepatitis with or without cirrhosis. Hepatitis C infection is associated with a high incidence of persistently abnormal biochemical tests, chronic active hepatitis, and cirrhosis.

HEPATITIS A. Previously called infectious hepatitis, this infection is caused by a 27-nm RNA picornavirus. It is transmitted by the fecal–oral route. Individuals developing this disease shed virus in their feces, and during the relatively brief period of viremia their blood is also infectious. The infection is usually spread by ingestion of contaminated blood or water, and the incubation period is about 2 to 7 weeks. The signs and symptoms are not very specific, and it may go undiagnosed. The majority of cases are anicteric. Although usually mild, occasionally fulminant hepatitis develops. This is more common if there is underlying chronic hepatitis C (Vento and colleagues, 1998).

Serological confirmation can be done even when serum transaminase levels are still elevated. Early detection is by identification of IgM antibody (Table 48–8). Although this indicates acute infection, it may persist for several months. During convalescence, IgG antibody predominates; it persists and is responsible for immunity from subsequent hepatitis A infection. The formalin-inactivated vaccine is reported to be over 90 percent effective. The Centers for Disease Control and Prevention (1999) recommends consideration for vaccination of susceptible persons traveling to high-risk countries,

TABLE 48–8. Simplified Diagnostic Approach in Patients with Hepatitis

Diagnosis	Serological Test			
	HB$_s$Ag	IgM Anti-HAV	IgM Anti-HB$_c$	Anti-HCV
Acute hepatitis A	−	+	−	−
Acute hepatitis B	+	−	+	−
Chronic hepatitis B	+	−	−	−
Acute hepatitis A with chronic B	+	+	−	−
Acute hepatitis A and B	+	+	+	−
Acute hepatitis C	−	−	−	+

HAV = hepatitis A virus; HB$_c$ = hepatitis B core; HB$_s$Ag = hepatitis B surface antigen; HCV = hepatitis C virus.
Modified from Dienstag and Isselbacher (1998).

illicit drug users, those with chronic liver disease or clotting-factor disorders, and food handlers. Duff and Duff (1998) recently reviewed its use.

HEPATITIS A AND PREGNANCY. In developed countries, the effects of hepatitis A on pregnancy are not dramatic. At least in some underprivileged populations, however, both perinatal and maternal deaths are substantively increased. Treatment consists of a balanced diet and diminished activity. We have long followed the policy of hospitalizing all pregnant women with hepatitis until it is clear that they are able to eat and drink, and that liver function is improving, or at least not continuing to deteriorate. Women with less severe illness may be managed as outpatients (American College of Obstetricians and Gynecologists, 1998).

There is no evidence that hepatitis A virus is teratogenic. Risk of transmission to the fetus is negligible, but vertical transmission at the time of delivery was documented to cause an outbreak of hepatitis A in a neonatal intensive care unit (Watson and colleagues, 1993). The risk of preterm birth appears to be increased somewhat for pregnancies complicated by hepatitis A.

The pregnant woman recently exposed by close personal or sexual contact to a person with hepatitis A should be given prophylaxis with 1 mL immune globulin.

HEPATITIS B. Once referred to as serum hepatitis, this infection is found worldwide but is endemic in some regions, especially in Asia and Africa. Hepatitis B is a DNA hepadnavirus that is a major cause of acute hepatitis and its serious sequelae, namely chronic hepatitis, cirrhosis, and hepatocellular carcinoma. The latter is so common that the World Health Organization considers hepatitis B to be second only to tobacco among human carcinogens. The most serious consequences are the result of chronic infection, which occurs in 5 to 10 percent of infected adults and 70 to 90 percent of infected in-

fants. According to the Centers for Disease Control and Prevention (1998b), reported cases decreased by 50 percent from 1990 to 1998. Only half of cases are icteric and symptomatic. There are an estimated 1 million chronic carriers.

A variety of immunological markers to hepatitis B have been identified in patients with acute or chronic disease, in those who have had the disease and now are immune, and in chronic carriers. The hepatitis B virus (Dane particle), core antigen (HB$_c$Ag), surface antigen (HB$_s$Ag), e antigen (HB$_e$Ag), and their corresponding antibodies are all detectable by various techniques. The virus is unique in that concentrations of viral antigen and particles in serum and other body fluids may reach 10 trillion per milliliter.

Hepatitis B infections are found most often among intravenous drug abusers, homosexuals, health-care personnel, and patients who have been treated often with blood products, such as hemophiliacs. It is transmitted by infected blood or blood products, and in saliva, vaginal secretions, and semen; thus, it is a sexually transmitted disease. The e antigen correlates with infectivity and the presence of intact viral particles.

After infection with hepatitis B, the first virological marker is HB$_s$Ag (Fig. 48–6). Infection is diagnosed by detection of HB$_s$Ag in serum. Although HB$_e$Ag invariably is present during early acute hepatitis, its persistence indicates chronic infection. Approximately 90 percent of persons with hepatitis B infections recover completely. Of the 10 percent who are chronically infected, about a fourth develop chronic liver disease.

HEPATITIS B AND PREGNANCY. Neither the prevalence nor the clinical course of hepatitis B infection in the mother, including fulminant hepatitis, is altered by pregnancy, at least in developed countries. Treatment is supportive, and as with hepatitis A, the likelihood for preterm delivery is increased.

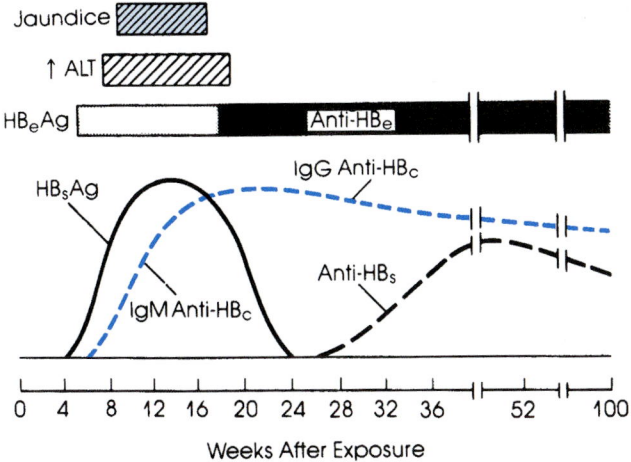

FIGURE 48–6. Acute hepatitis B—Appearance of various antigens and antibodies. (ALT = alanine aminotransferase.) (From Dienstag and Isselbacher, 1998, with permission.)

Transplacental viral transfer from the mother to the fetus is associated with acute hepatitis but not chronic seropositivity. With acute infection in the first trimester, 10 percent of fetuses are infected, and in the third trimester this number is 80 to 90 percent (American College of Obstetricians and Gynecologists, 1998). With chronic maternal infection, perinatal transmission is by ingestion of infected material during delivery or exposure subsequent to birth, for example, breast feeding. Some infected infants are asymptomatic, others develop fulminant disease, and nearly 85 percent become chronic carriers. Vertical transmission correlates closely with maternal HB$_e$Ag status. Mothers with hepatitis B surface and e antigens are very likely to transmit the disease to their infants, whereas those who are negative for e antigen but positive for anti-HB$_e$ antibody do not appear to transmit the infection.

PREVENTION OF NEONATAL INFECTION. The Centers for Disease Control (1990) estimate that about 18,000 infants were born in the United States in 1987 to HB$_s$Ag-positive women. Without immunoprophylaxis given at delivery, nearly 4000 will become chronically infected with hepatitis B. Infection of the newborn whose mother chronically carries the virus can usually be prevented by the administration of hepatitis B immune globulin very soon after birth, followed promptly by hepatitis B vaccine. As discussed in Chapter 10 (p. 240), concern for adverse effects of this vaccine appear to be unfounded according to the U.S. Food and Drug Administration (Niu and colleagues, 1999).

The Centers for Disease Control (1991), as well as the American College of Obstetricians and Gynecologists (1998), recommend hepatitis B serological screening for all prenatal patients. For inner-city lower socioeconomic

groups, the prevalence of seropositivity for hepatitis B virus is about 1 percent. It is somewhat lower for military populations and private patients. In a study of over 7700 pregnant women, Webb and associates (1996) reported a prevalence of 0.85 percent for hepatitis B. Rindfusz and colleagues (1996), in a seroprevalence study of immunodeficiency virus, hepatitis B, and hepatitis C, found a rate of 2 percent. As emphasized by Duff (1994), selective screening will identify only 30 to 50 percent of seropositive women.

For high-risk mothers who test antigen negative, vaccine can be provided during pregnancy. Ingardia and colleagues (1999) observed that seroprotection in pregnant women (45 percent) was lower than the 60 to 70 percent cited for nonpregnant individuals. For women who test positive, offspring should be given hepatitis B immune globulin and recombinant vaccine. A second and third dose of vaccine are given to the child at 1 and 6 months of age.

HEPATITIS D. Also called delta hepatitis, this is a defective RNA virus that is a hybrid particle with a hepatitis B surface antigen coat and a delta core. The virus must co-infect with hepatitis B and cannot persist in serum longer than hepatitis B virus. Transmission is similar to hepatitis B viral infection. Chronic infection with B and D hepatitis produces more severe disease and up to 75 percent of those affected develop cirrhosis. Neonatal transmission has been reported, but hepatitis B vaccination usually prevents delta hepatitis.

HEPATITIS C. This is a single-stranded RNA virus of the family Flaviviridae. Transmission of hepatitis C infection appears to be identical to hepatitis B. While it is more prevalent in intravenous drug abusers, hemophiliacs, and those with high-risk sexual behavior, only half of anti-HCV positive persons have risk factors (Alter and co-workers, 1999). The Centers for Disease Control and Prevention (1998a) cites a seroprevalence of 1.8 percent, or 4 million infected Americans. After acute infection, anti-C antibody is not detected for an average of 15 weeks, and in some cases it is not detectable for a year. Antibody does not prohibit transmission, and Conry-Cantilena and colleagues (1996) found that 86 percent of 213 anti-HCV positive persons had hepatitis C virus RNA and thus were infective.

The incidence of persistent disease is common after hepatitis C infection. About half of patients have abnormal liver tests for more than a year. In two thirds of these, biopsy shows chronic active hepatitis, which in 20 to 30 percent will progress to cirrhosis within 20 to 30 years.

Screening of blood donors for hepatitis C virus has markedly decreased the incidence of post-transfusion hepatitis. According to Dienstag and Isselbacher (1998), the incidence of transfusion-related hepatitis has fallen to imperceptible levels since screening has been done with second-generation anti-HCV assays.

EFFECT ON PREGNANCY. There is no reason to believe that antepartum hepatitis C infection is different compared with nonpregnant women. Importantly, 75 percent of anti-HCV positive individuals have chronic disease. Bohman and colleagues (1992) reported a 2.3 percent seroprevalence rate in pregnant women at Parkland Hospital. Risk factors included intravenous drug use, sexually transmitted diseases, increased age and parity, history of transfusions, multiple sex partners, and sex partners who used intravenous drugs. In a similar population from San Juan, Puerto Rico, Deseda and associates (1995) found a 1.9 percent prevalence. Silverman and colleagues (1993) found a seroprevalence of 4.3 percent in pregnant women from a university hospital in Philadelphia. Women attending public clinics had an incidence of 5.2 percent whereas only 1.5 percent of private patients were anti-HCV positive. In another serosurvey of high-risk prenatal patients, Leikin and co-workers (1994) reported a seroprevalence rate of 4.6 percent.

Perinatal outcome is not adversely affected in anti-HCV positive women compared with seronegative controls. Importantly, however, hepatitis C infection is transmitted vertically to the fetus–infant. There have now been a number of studies that have addressed this, and the vertical transmission rate varies between 3 and 6 percent (Conte, 2000; Hillemanns, 2000; Ohto, 1994; Resti, 1998, and all their colleagues). As in adult-to-adult transmission, antibody is not protective, and Floreani and co-workers (1996) found that 65 percent of anti-HCV positive mothers also had hepatitis C virus RNA.

Currently, there are no methods to prevent transmission at birth (American College of Obstetricians and Gynecologists, 1998). Because of this, the Centers for Disease Control and Prevention (1998a) do not recommend screening in pregnant women; however, neonates of known anti-HCV-positive mothers should be tested and provided follow-up. Burns and Minkoff (1999) recommend selective screening based on risk factors. Women found to be anti-HCV-positive are offered counseling and identified for long-term follow-up.

HEPATITIS E. This is a waterborne RNA virus that is enterically transmitted. Epidemiologically it has features resembling hepatitis A; for example, it causes epidemic outbreaks in undeveloped countries. Serological confirmation is currently not widely available. Most cases are transmitted by contaminated water supplies, and the disease is not easily communicable by person-to-person contact. Preliminary evidence in infected pregnant women suggests a high incidence of vertical transmission, including transplacentally (Khuroo and colleagues, 1995). There is some evidence that it is more severe in pregnancy, especially when acquired late (Baker, 2000).

HEPATITIS G. Bloodborne infection with this flavivirus-like RNA virus is usually with hepatitis C co-infection. It does not increase the severity of infection, and while it can cause chronic infection, its contribution to acute or chronic liver disease requires better definition (Dienstag and Isselbacher, 1998). In a Scottish study, 0.08 percent of over 180,000 nonremunerated blood donors were seropositive (Jarvis and associates, 1996). Infant transmission has been described by Feucht (1996) and Inaba (1997) and their colleagues.

CHRONIC HEPATITIS. This is a disorder of varying etiology that is characterized by continuing hepatic necrosis, active inflammation, and fibrosis that may lead to cirrhosis and ultimately liver failure. It has only been in the last decade that the extent of chronic liver disease due to acute viral hepatitis has been appreciated. By far, most cases are due to chronic infection with either hepatitis B or C viruses. Another cause is autoimmune chronic hepatitis, characterized by high serum titers of homogeneous antinuclear antibodies. In both forms, there is evidence that a cellular immune reaction is interactive with a genetic predisposition.

As discussed earlier, most cases of acute viral hepatitis B and C go clinically unnoticed. Similarly, most cases of chronic hepatitis are asymptomatic and frequently are suspected from elevated serum transaminase levels done for screening, for example, during blood donation or life insurance application. When present, symptoms are nonspecific and usually include fatigue. Diagnosis is made by liver biopsy. In some patients, cirrhosis with liver failure or bleeding varices is the presenting finding.

There is now considerable experience with treatment of chronic viral hepatitis with one of the *interferons.* These are cytokines with antiviral, antiproliferative, and immunoregulatory effects. Treatment for 6 months has been shown to decrease viremia and improve histological findings in about 40 percent of patients, but the relapse rate is 20 percent. The synthetic nucleoside *ribavirin,* while not very effective alone, improves the efficacy of interferon therapy (Davis and associates, 1998; McHutchinson and co-workers, 1998). The nucleoside analog *lamivudine* was also found to be effective in about 50 percent of patients (Dienstag and colleagues, 1999; Lai and associates, 1998).

CHRONIC HEPATITIS AND PREGNANCY. Pregnancy is uncommon when disease is severe because anovulation is common. Most young women, however, are either asymptomatic or have only mild liver disease. For the seropositive, asymptomatic woman, there usually is no problem with pregnancy. With known (symptomatic) chronic active hepatitis, interaction with pregnancy will depend primarily on the intensity of the disease and whether there is portal hypertension (Lee, 1992). The few women whom we have managed have done well, but because their long-term prognosis is poor, they should be counseled regarding abortion and sterilization. As discussed on page 1284, Locatelli and co-workers (1999) have observed a higher incidence of cholestatic jaundice in hepatitis C seropositive women (16 percent) compared with negative controls (0.8 percent).

In women with autoimmune chronic hepatitis, corticosteroids, alone or combined with azathioprine, have increased fertility and survival. Their pregnancy outcome is also related to severity of disease (Levine, 2000).

CIRRHOSIS. Hepatic cirrhosis is characterized by irreversible chronic injury to the liver parenchyma with extensive fibrosis and regenerative nodules. In all patients, *Lannec cirrhosis* from chronic exposure to alcohol is the most common cause. In young women, however, and thus most pregnant women, *postnecrotic cirrhosis* from chronic B or C viral hepatitis is the most common cause. Other causes include biliary cirrhosis from long-standing obstruction and cardiac cirrhosis from chronic right-sided heart failure. Fung and Li (1999) described a pregnant woman with biliary cirrhosis from recurrent pyogenic cholangitis. Although cirrhosis is the final common pathway for a variety of hepatic injuries, the clinical manifestations are inseparable. These include jaundice, edema, coagulopathy, metabolic abnormalities, and portal hypertension along with its sequela of gastroesophageal varices and splenomegaly.

CIRRHOSIS AND PREGNANCY. Women with cirrhosis are very likely to be infertile. Traditionally, perinatal loss is high, and maternal prognosis grave. Esophageal varices were prone to bleed, with fatal hemorrhage as the consequence. Schreyer and associates (1982) reviewed 69 pregnancies in 60 women with cirrhosis without shunts and 28 pregnancies in another 23 women with cirrhosis who had undergone portal decompression shunting. Severe variceal hemorrhage was increased sevenfold in nonshunted women compared with those who had undergone such procedures (24 versus 3 percent). Pajor and Lehoczky (1994) cared for 11 cirrhotic women during pregnancy. Although all survived, transient hepatic failure developed in six, variceal hemorrhage in six, and 6 of 12 infants were growth restricted. Aggarwal and associates (1999) reported nine pregnancies in seven women with cirrhosis. Half were delivered preterm, and one woman died.

ESOPHAGEAL VARICES. Portal venous hypertension that results from cirrhosis or from extrahepatic portal vein obstruction is associated with esophageal varices. Postnecrotic hepatitis and chronic alcoholism with cirrhosis and hepatic sinusoidal resistance account for almost all cases of portal hypertension in young women. A seemingly equal number of cases of esophageal varices, at least in pregnant women, are caused by extrahepatic portal hypertension in which there is resistance to flow in portal or splenic veins. About half of these are idiopathic, but a number arise as a complication of thrombosis from umbilical vein catheterization when the woman was a neonate.

Whatever its underlying cause, portal vein pressure rises from its normal value of 10 to 15 mm Hg to exceed 30 mm Hg. This leads to formation of a collateral circulation, which carries blood to the systemic circulation. Drainage is via the gastric, intercostal, and other veins ultimately to the esophageal system, where varices develop. Bleeding is usually from varices near the gastroesophageal junction. About a third of patients bleed, and the mortality is 50 percent with the first episode. Most bleed again, with a 30 percent mortality. Bleeding can be torrential. Acute therapy consists of early endoscopy for diagnosis with *band ligation* for control of hemorrhage (Stanley and Hayes, 1997). In some cases, *sclerotherapy* by intravariceal injection may facilitate banding. *Balloon tamponade* of severe bleeding using a triple-lumen tube can be lifesaving. Emergency shunting is used in 10 to 20 percent of patients in whom hemorrhage is not controlled by endoscopy. This interventional radiology procedure, known as *transjugular intrahepatic portosystemic stent shunting (TIPSS)*, can also control bleeding from gastric varices.

VARICES AND PREGNANCY. Bleeding from esophageal varices causes much of the maternal mortality associated with cirrhosis. Hillemanns and colleagues (1996) described a maternal death at 20 weeks when portal hypertension caused rupture of a splenic artery aneurysm. There is concern that vaginal delivery with increased portal pressures from Valsalva maneuvers will increase the risk of bleeding (Lee, 1992). Britton (1982) reviewed outcomes in 160 pregnancies complicated by cirrhosis, varices, or both (Table 48–9). Bleeding was common when pregnancy was complicated by varices, regardless of whether these were associated with cirrhosis. Mortality, however, was higher if varices were associated with cirrhosis. Specifically, maternal mortality from bleeding in women with cirrhosis was 18 percent, but it was only 2 percent in those without cirrhosis. Perinatal mortality was high in both groups.

MANAGEMENT. Treatment during pregnancy is the same as for the nonpregnant patient. For the woman

TABLE 48–9. Outcomes in 160 Pregnancies Complicated by Cirrhosis, Esophageal Varices, or Both

Outcome	Cirrhosis (n = 53)	Varices without Cirrhosis (n = 38)
Varices	35/53 (66%)	38/38 (100%)
Pregnancies	83	77
Bleeding during pregnancy at risk	13/21 (62%)	25/54 (46%)
Operation during pregnancy	5	2
Pregnancy outcome		
Losses		
Abortions	14	10
Stillborn	4	5
Neonatal death	3	2
Vaginal delivery	59	43
Cesarean	11	11
Maternal mortality	7	2

Modified from Britton (1982), with permission.

with known varices, β-blocking drugs such as propranolol are given to reduce portal pressure and hence the risk of bleeding. Endoscopic band ligation can be done for acute bleeding (Starkel and associates, 1998). It also can be done prophylactically, and Zeeman and Moise (1999) described a woman who underwent banding at 15, 26, and 31 weeks to prevent bleeding. Sclerotherapy has also been successfully used during pregnancy (Iwase and colleagues, 1994; Pauzner and associates, 1991). There is little experience in pregnancy with TIPSS.

ACUTE ACETAMINOPHEN OVERDOSAGE. Acetaminophen is commonly used during pregnancy. Overdosage from suicidal attempts may lead to acute liver failure. Early symptoms of overdosage are nausea, vomiting, diaphoresis, malaise, and pallor. After a latent period of 24 to 48 hours, liver failure begins to develop, and usually begins to resolve in 5 days.

The antidote is N-acetylcysteine, and it must be given promptly. The drug is thought to act by increasing glutathione levels, which facilitates metabolism of the toxic metabolite. The need for treatment is based on projections of possible plasma hepatotoxic levels as a function of the time of acute ingestion. Many clinicians use the nomogram established by Rumack and Matthew (1975). Plasma levels are obtained 4 hours after ingestion, and if greater than 120 μg/mL, treatment is given. If plasma determinations are not available, empirical treatment is given if the dose exceeded 7.5 g. An oral loading dose of 140 mg/kg of N-acetylcysteine is followed by 17 maintenance doses of 70 mg/kg every 4 hours for 72 hours total treatment time.

After 14 weeks, the fetus has some cytochrome

P-450 activity, which is necessary for metabolism of acetaminophen to the toxic metabolite. Riggs and colleagues (1989) reported data from the Rocky Mountain Poison and Drug Center and described follow-up experiences in 60 such women. The likelihood of maternal and fetal survival was better if the antidote was given soon after overdosage. At least one 33-week fetus appears to have died as a direct result of hepatotoxicity 2 days after ingestion. The case reported by Wang and associates (1997) describes similar acetaminophen levels in maternal and cord blood of about 41 μg/mL, which confirms placental transfer. Both mother and infant died from hepatorenal failure within 1½ to 3 days after ingestion.

LIVER TRANSPLANTATION. The first successful pregnancy in a liver transplantation recipient was reported by Walcott and associates (1978). Since then, a number of women with successful pregnancies following transplantation have been described. The Pittsburgh group reported experiences with 12 pregnancies in 11 women (Laifer and colleagues, 1990). While most had stable serum hepatic transaminase levels, three women had acute or chronic rejection or hepatitis. Pregnancy complications included hypertension in half the women, anemia in 25 percent, and preterm delivery in 80 percent. Neuropsychiatric complications were also common. Ville and co-workers (1993) described pregnancy outcomes in 19 French women after liver transplantation. Of 11 viable pregnancies, all were delivered at term, although hypertension developed in three and liver dysfunction in one. Skannal and associates (1995) described a successful outcome in a woman with a combined liver–kidney transplant.

Radomski and associates (1995) presented results from the National Transplantation Pregnancy Registry. They described outcomes in 38 pregnancies in 29 transplantation recipients. More than 80 percent of infants were live-born, and only 40 percent were preterm. Rayes (1998) described 19 pregnancies in 16 German women who underwent liver transplantation. There were six abortions, 12 term babies, and one preterm. Three term infants were growth restricted. Of 13 viable infants, five had hypertension and two had transient serum transaminase level increases.

DISEASES OF THE GALLBLADDER AND PANCREAS

CHOLELITHIASIS AND CHOLECYSTITIS. In the United States, 20 percent of women over 40 have gallstones. Most stones contain cholesterol, and its oversecretion into bile is thought to be a major factor in the pathogenesis. Biliary sludge, which may increase during pregnancy, is an important precursor to gallstone formation. The cumulative risk of a patient with silent gallstones to require surgery for symptoms or complications is about 1 to 2 percent per year; it is 10 percent at 5 years, and 18 percent at 15 years (Greenberger and Isselbacher, 1998). For these reasons, prophylactic cholecystectomy is not warranted for asymptomatic stones.

A number of nonsurgical approaches have been used for gallstone disease. These include oral bile acid therapy with chenodeoxycholic acid, extracorporeal shock wave lithotripsy, and contact dissolution with methyl tertbutyl ether placed directly into the gallbladder. There is no experience with any of these methods during pregnancy, and they are currently not recommended.

Acute cholecystitis usually develops when there is obstruction of the cystic duct. Bacterial infection plays a role in 50 to 85 percent of these acute inflammatory conditions. In over half of patients with acute cholecysti-

tis, a history of previous right-upper-quadrant pain from cholelithiasis is elicited. With acute disease, pain is accompanied by anorexia, nausea and vomiting, low-grade fever, and mild leukocytosis. Ultrasonography can be used to visualize stones as small as 2 mm, and false-positive and false-negative rates for diagnosing gallstones are about 2 to 4 percent (Greenberger and Isselbacher, 1998). Ultrasonic examination confirms gallstones in up to 90 percent of patients (Fig. 48–7).

Symptomatic gallbladder diseases include acute cholecystitis, biliary colic, jaundice, and acute pancreatitis. In most of these cases, cholecystectomy is warranted (Bateson, 1999). Whereas acute cholecystitis responds to medical therapy, contemporary consensus is that early cholecystectomy is indicated (Greenberger and Isselbacher, 1998). In acute cases, medical therapy consisting of nasogastric suction, intravenous fluids and antimicrobials, and analgesics is instituted before surgical therapy. According to a National Institutes of Health Consensus Conference (1993), laparoscopic cholecystectomy has become the treatment of choice for most patients. Data from most centers indicate a twofold increased incidence of major biliary, vascular, and bowel complications when the laparoscopic technique is compared with open cholecystectomy (Fletcher and co-workers, 1999).

GALLBLADDER DISEASE DURING PREGNANCY. Most findings are supportive of the view that pregnancy increases the risk of gallstones. After the first trimester, both gallbladder volume during fasting and residual volume after contracting in response to a test meal are twice as great as in nonpregnant subjects (Braverman and colleagues, 1980). Incomplete emptying may result in retention of cholesterol crystals, a prerequisite for cholesterol gallstones. Biliary sludge, probably a forerunner to gallstones, was immediately seen ultrasonically in one fourth of nearly 300 postpartum women. Maringhini and co-workers (1987) used similar tech-

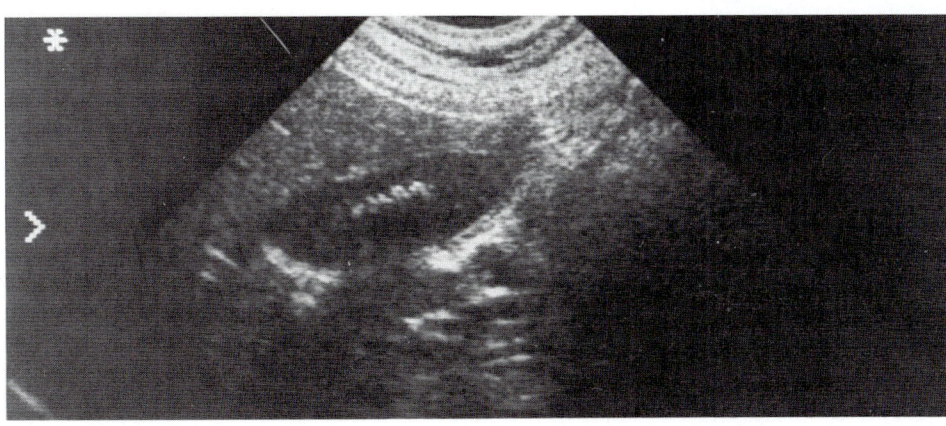

FIGURE 48–7. Multiple floating gallstones visualized in a 26-week pregnant woman. (Photograph courtesy of Dr. Diane Twickler.)

niques and showed that 30 percent of women developed sludge during pregnancy. In many cases this resolves within a year.

MANAGEMENT. Acute cholecystitis during pregnancy or the puerperium is initially managed in a manner similar to that for nonpregnant women. In the past, most practitioners favored medical therapy. Landers and colleagues (1987) at the University of California, San Francisco, first reported their experiences with 30 women with cholecystitis for an incidence of about 1 in 1000 deliveries. Gallstones were found in 96 percent of women, and although most presented for care before the third trimester, 25 women were treated conservatively, but four of these failed such therapy. Glasgow and co-workers (1998) from the same institution later reported experiences with another 47 pregnant women with symptomatic gallstones. Conservative therapy was attempted in all, but 36 percent required surgery.

Dixon and colleagues (1987) performed cholecystectomies in 18 of 44 women with acute cholecystitis or cholelithiasis with biliary colic. The women treated surgically did well; however, 15 of the 26 managed medically had recurrent symptoms during pregnancy. Multiple hospitalizations were common in the latter group, and two women required prolonged parenteral nutrition during late pregnancy. Davis and co-workers (1995) and Lee and associates (2000) described a total of 77 cases of cholecystitis and cited better outcomes with primary surgical management.

Because of these factors—namely, cholecystitis is a surgical disease; it has a high recurrence rate during the same pregnancy; and when it recurs later in gestation, preterm labor is more likely and cholecystectomy technically more difficult—our management at Parkland Hospital has evolved to a more aggressive surgical approach. This is particularly true for the woman with concomitant biliary pancreatitis (see later discussion).

LAPAROSCOPIC CHOLECYSTECTOMY. Uncomplicated laparoscopic cholecystectomy in a 31-week pregnant woman was first described by Pucci and Seed (1991). Subsequently, reasonable experiences have been reported from several centers that indicate this to be as equally acceptable as open cholecystectomy before the third trimester (Barone, 1999; Cosenza, 1999; Glasgow, 1998, and their colleagues). Graham and co-workers (1998) reviewed 105 cases reported through 1997 and added six of their own. They concluded that laparoscopic cholecystectomy was safe throughout pregnancy.

ENDOSCOPIC RETROGRADE CHOLANGIOPAN-CREATOGRAPHY. Treatment during pregnancy of biliary duct obstruction by gallstones has been greatly facilitated by their removal with endoscopic retrograde

cholangiopancreatography (ERCP) (Nesbitt and co-workers, 1996). Because these patients have more morbidity and mortality, especially with associated biliary pancreatitis, it has become commonplace to perform endoscopic sphincterotomy and gallstone extraction to be followed in a few days with laparoscopic cholecystectomy. In most cases, it will also obviate the need for intraoperative cholangiography, which some feel is contraindicated in pregnancy (Graham and colleagues, 1998).

ASYMPTOMATIC GALLSTONES DURING PREGNANCY. Gallstones are relatively common in asymptomatic pregnant women. An incidence of ultrasonically visualized asymptomatic stones of 2.5 to 10 percent during pregnancy or the puerperium has been reported in over 1500 women (Maringhini and colleagues, 1987; Valdivieso and co-workers, 1993). Cholecystectomy is not indicated for silent stones during pregnancy.

PANCREATITIS. Acute pancreatic inflammation is triggered by activation of pancreatic trypsinogen followed by autodigestion characterized by cellular membrane disruption and proteolysis, edema, hemorrhage, and necrosis. In nonpregnant patients, acute pancreatitis is most likely associated with gallstones (45 percent) and alcohol abuse (35 percent), but during pregnancy, cholelithiasis is almost always the predisposing condition. It also is encountered in the postoperative patient and is associated with trauma, drugs, certain metabolic conditions including acute fatty liver of pregnancy, familial hypertriglyceridemia, and some viral infections. More recently, pancreatitis has been linked to the more than 800 mutations of the cystic fibrosis transmembrane conductance regulator gene (Durie, 1998).

Clinically, acute pancreatitis is characterized by mild to incapacitating epigastric pain, nausea and vomiting, and abdominal distention. Patients are usually in distress and have low-grade fever and tachycardia; hypotension is common. Findings include abdominal tenderness, and up to 10 percent of patients have associated pulmonary findings. Serum amylase levels three times upper normal values are confirmatory, but there is no correlation with their degree of elevation and severity of disease. In fact, usually by 48 to 72 hours, serum amylase levels return to normal despite evidence for continuing pancreatitis. Measurement of serum lipase activity increases the diagnostic yield. There is usually leukocytosis, and 25 percent of patients have hypocalcemia. Serum bilirubin and aspartate aminotransferase levels are usually somewhat elevated.

A number of prognostic factors may be used to predict severity of the disease. These include respiratory failure, shock, need for massive colloid replacement, hypocalcemia of less than 8 mg/dL, or dark hemorrhagic fluid on paracentesis. If three of the first four features are documented, survival is only 30 percent.

MANAGEMENT. Therapy is medical and includes analgesics for pain, intravenous hydration, and measures to decrease pancreatic secretion by ceasing oral intake. Nasogastric suction has not been shown to improve the outcome in mild to moderate disease. Antimicrobials have been shown to improve outcome in necrotizing pancreatitis (Sainio and colleagues, 1995). In most patients, acute pancreatitis is self-limited, and in 90 percent, inflammation subsides within 3 to 7 days after treatment. For patients with severe necrotizing pancreatitis, ERCP and papillotomy is usually done and intensive supportive therapy is given. In some patients, laparotomy with debridement and drainage may be lifesaving.

PANCREATITIS DURING PREGNANCY. The predisposition of pregnancy toward gallstone formation may indirectly link pregnancy with pancreatitis. At Parkland Hospital, pancreatitis complicates about 1 in 3300 pregnancies (Ramin and colleagues, 1995). Swisher and associates (1994) reported an incidence of 1 in 1500 at UCLA Medical Center. Legro and Laifer (1995) found an incidence of 1 in 4000 at Magee Women's Hospital. In most of these women, cholelithiasis commonly coexists. In a small number of pregnant women with pancreatitis, there is an associated familial hyperlipidemic syndrome, usually hypertriglyceridemia (Nies and Dreiss, 1990; Sanderson and colleagues, 1991). Watts and associates (1992) described two pregnant women with hypertriglyceridemia due to familial lipoprotein lipase deficiency.

DIAGNOSIS. Pancreatitis is diagnosed during pregnancy using the same criteria as in nonpregnant patients. Legro and Laifer (1995) reported 11 cases of pancreatitis complicating early pregnancy. Only a third were diagnosed correctly initially; another third were thought to have hyperemesis gravidarum. Ramin and colleagues (1995) reported that all but 1 of 43 pregnant women with pancreatitis had nausea, vomiting, and abdominal pain as presenting complaints. Ordorica and associates (1991) confirmed earlier studies that serum amylase and lipase levels are not changed during pregnancy. Serial determinations of serum amylase and lipase activity remain the best methods to confirm the clinical diagnosis of pancreatitis. Block and Kelley (1989) reported that in all 21 pregnant women, serum amylase values exceeded 1500 IU/L. As shown in Table 48–10, the mean amylase value in 43 pregnant women with pancreatitis was about 1400 IU/L, and the mean lipase value, about 7000 IU/L. Amylase values do not correlate with the severity of disease.

MANAGEMENT. Therapy is the same as for nonpregnant patients described earlier. In pregnant women, mild inflammation usually subsides in response to conservative therapy. In the Parkland Hospital series, all 43 women responded to conservative treatment and were hospitalized for a mean of 8.5 days (Ramin and colleagues, 1995). In 30 women described by Swisher and associates (1994), three women with associated gallstones underwent laparotomy for diagnostic uncertainty or unrelenting pain. In women with severe disease, fetal loss is high because of associated hypovolemia, hypoxia, and acidosis. Because more than half of cases are associated with gallstone disease, ERCP for common duct stones will likely be helpful (Nesbitt and colleagues, 1996). Cholecystectomy should be considered after inflammation subsides (see p. 1296).

PANCREATIC TRANSPLANTATION. According to the United Network for Organ Sharing (UNOS), the 3-year graft survival for pancreatic transplantation is almost 70 percent (Lin and associates, 1998). Because there is improved survival when a combined pancreas and kidney are grafted, most operations include both organs. Diabetes accounts for about a fourth of cases of renal failure leading to kidney transplantation.

Tydén and colleagues (1989) described four women in whom pancreatic–kidney transplantation was fol-

TABLE 48–10. Selected Laboratory Values in 43 Pregnant Women with Pancreatitis

Value	Mean	Range	Normal
Serum amylase (IU/L)	1392	111–4560	30–110
Serum lipase (IU/L)	6929	36–41,824	23–208
Total bilirubin (mg/dL)	1.7	0.1–4.9	0.2–1.3
Aspartate transferase (U/L)	120	11–498	3–35
Leukocytes (per μL)	12,000	7000–14,600	4100–10,900

From Ramin and colleagues (1995), with permission.

lowed in 1 to 2 years by pregnancy. Because of pelvic placement of the pancreatic graft, there was concern that the enlarging uterus or labor might cause pancreatitis, but this did not occur. Moreover, glucose homeostasis was well-maintained throughout pregnancy. Of concern is the one woman who suffered acute pancreatic graft rejection postpartum. Successful vaginal deliveries have been described by Allenby and colleagues (1998). Notification of the National Transplantation Pregnancy Registry is encouraged by Armenti and co-workers (1997). At least two successful pregnancies have followed pancreatic islet autotransplantation (Teuscher and colleagues, 1994; Wahoff and associates, 1995).

OBESITY

Excessive weight has become one of the major health problems in the United States as well as other "advanced" societies. Its etiology is multifactorial, and although it certainly is not simply a gastrointestinal disorder, it is considered here. In the National Health and Nutrition Examination Surveys from 1960 to 1991, an alarming increase was found in the prevalence of excessive weight among adults over the past decade (Kuczmarski and colleagues, 1994). It was estimated at that time that approximately a third of all adults in the United States were overweight. Indeed, Allison and co-workers (1999) attributed around 300,000 excessive deaths to obesity in this country in 1991. Because of this, a stated national health care goal of Healthy People 2000 was to reduce the prevalence of obesity to 20 percent or less (Public Health Service, 1990). Unfortunately, this was not achieved, and at the beginning of 2000, over half of the of the of the population was now overweight (see also Chap. 1, p. 11).

RISKS OF OBESITY. Individuals who are overweight are at increased risk for diabetes, hypertension, dyslipidemia, cardiovascular disease, stroke, liver and gallbladder disease, sleep apnea, osteoarthritis, colon cancer, as well as a number of obstetrical complications (Must and colleagues, 1999). Although the exact contribution of excessive weight and excess mortality has been controversial, in their prospective study, Calle and associates (1999) found that the mortality risk increased along with increasing body mass index (Fig. 48–8).

DEFINITION OF OBESITY. A variety of classifications have been used to define obesity. The most commonly used method is the body mass index (BMI) shown in Figure 48–9. It is calculated as weight in kilograms divided by height in meters squared (kg/m^2). This is also known as *Quetelet's index.* The 1985 National Institutes of Health Consensus Panel on Obesity defined obesity

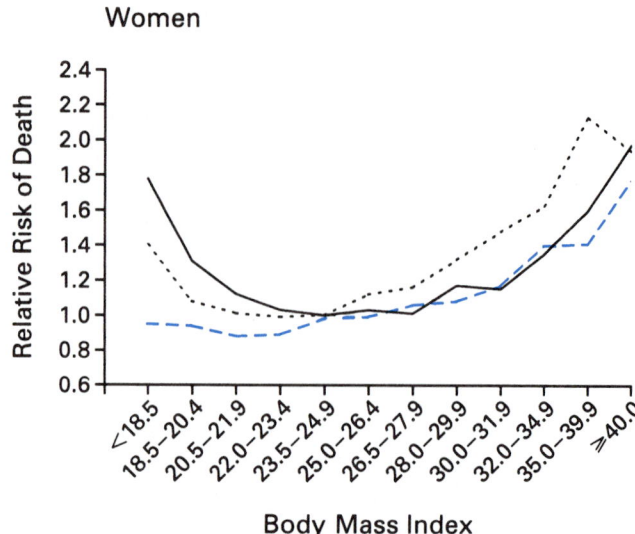

Women

FIGURE 48–8. Body mass index and multivariate relative risk of death from cardiovascular disease (· · · ·), cancer (----), and all other causes (——) among women who had never smoked and who had no history of disease at enrollment. The reference category was made up of subjects with a body mass index of 23.5 to 24.9. (From Calle and associates, 1999, with permission.)

as a 20 percent increase in body weight or a body mass index greater than the 85th percentile, which is 27.3 for women between 20 and 29 years old (Burton and Foster, 1985). Using this definition, nearly 40 percent of young adult women in the United States are obese.

EFFECTS OF OBESITY ON PREGNANCY. Marked obesity is unequivocally a hazard to the pregnant woman and her fetus. Because there have been no standardized definitions of obesity, in the past investigators have used a variety of classifications. For example, Garbaciak and associates (1985) defined morbid obesity as greater than 150 percent of ideal weight. They reported that chronic hypertension was increased about tenfold and gestational diabetes was found in about 10 percent of these women. Johnson and colleagues (1987) described the pregnancy outcomes of 588 women who weighed more than 250 pounds. Hypertension, diabetes, and postterm pregnancy were more frequent when compared with a group of control women who weighed less than 200 pounds. Cunningham and associates (1986) described obesity as a common co-factor along with hypertension in causing peripartum heart failure.

Isaacs and associates (1994) compared pregnancy outcomes in 103 women weighing more than 300 pounds with 69 control women whose weight averaged 160 pounds. Obese women had an increased incidence of chronic hypertension and diabetes. The primary cesarean delivery rate was increased threefold, and postpar-

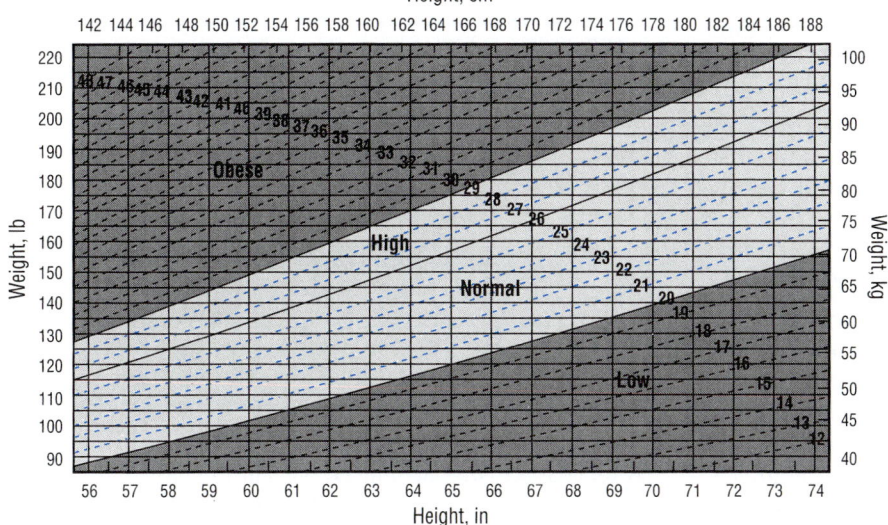

FIGURE 48–9. Chart for estimating body mass index (BMI) and weight category. To find BMI category (e.g., obese) find the point where the height and weight intersect. To estimate BMI, read the bold number on the dashed line that is closest to this point. (From the National Academy of Sciences, 1992.)

tum complications were also increased in obese women. Finally, infants were larger in obese women, and 10 percent weighed more than 4000 g. Bianco and colleagues (1998) reported similar findings in over 600 morbidly obese women as shown in Table 48–11.

Fetal and neonatal complications are increased in obese women. Wolfe and colleagues (1990) reported difficulty in sonographic fetal visualization in women whose body mass index was greater than the 90th percentile. Several investigators then reported that obese women had a two- to threefold risk for neural-tube defects as well as other anomalies (Mikhail, 1996; Waller, 1994; Werler, 1996, and their collaborators). Subsequently, Shaw and colleagues (1996, 2000) found a significant twofold increased incidence of neural-tube defects in women whose body mass index was 30 or higher.

TABLE 48–11. Pregnancy Complications in 613 Morbidly Obese Women[a]

Factor	Obese[a] (n = 613)	Controls (n = 11,313)	p
Weight (mean ± SD)	105 ± 16 kg	59 ± 7 kg	< .05
Age (mean)	27.5 years	28.7 years	NS
Preexisting complications			
Diabetes	7.3%	1.6%	< .01
Hypertension	5.4%	0.3%	< .01
Asthma	17%	6.6%	< .01
Antepartum complications			
Gestational diabetes	14%	4.3%	< .01
Preeclampsia	14%	3.2%	< .01
Placental abruption	1.8%	0.9%	< .05
Intrapartum complications			
Fetal distress	12%	8.7%	< .05
Cesarean delivery	31%	16%	< .01
Neonatal outcomes			
Birthweight (mean ± SD)	3350 ± 600 g	3270 ± 530 g	< .05
Large-for-gestational-age	18%	12%	< .01
Neonatal ICU admission	13%	8.7%	< .01

NS = not significant.
[a] Body mass index (BMI) > 35.
Data from Bianco and colleagues (1998).

MANAGEMENT. Management of obesity during pregnancy is a challenge. The usual net caloric increase during normal pregnancy ranges from 20,000 to 40,000 kcal and about 3.6 kg of gained weight is fat (Kliegman and Gross, 1985). A program of weight reduction is probably unrealistic, but if such a regimen is chosen, it is mandatory that the quality of the diet be monitored closely and that ketosis be avoided.

SURGICAL PROCEDURES FOR OBESITY. Various means to surgically decrease gastric volume have been devised to treat morbid obesity (Yanovski and Yanovski, 1999). A number of women have had pregnancies following such therapy. *Gastroplasty* creates a narrow channel through the stomach by using stapling devices. Bilenka and colleagues (1995) described 14 pregnancies in nine women who had undergone *vertical banded gastroplasty*. These women lost a mean of about 80 pounds and had fewer complications in subsequent pregnancies. Martin and co-workers (2000) described 23 pregnancies in women after *adjustable gastric banding*. For three women with excessive nausea and vomiting, band adjustment to decrease obstruction was successful.

Gastric bypass excludes the lower 90 percent of stomach by creating an upper gastrojejunostomy. Printen and Scott (1982) described their experiences with 51 pregnancies in 45 women who underwent gastric bypass surgery because of morbid obesity. Of the 46 infants delivered, fetal growth restriction was not a problem. Richards and colleagues (1987) reported similar experiences from 57 pregnancies cared for at the University of Utah. These women weighed an average of 194 pounds before and 147 pounds after surgery. Using pregnancies before gastric bypass as controls, they reported that the mean birthweight decreased from 3600 to 3200 g. Only 16 percent of the women had large-for-gestational-age infants compared with 37 percent before surgery. Impressively, the incidence of hypertension complicating pregnancy fell from 46 to 9 percent in women who had lost weight. Wittgrove and co-workers (1998) reported similar findings in 43 women.

Jejunoileal bypass has been followed by significant long-term morbidity and mortality, and the operation has been abandoned by most. Knudsen and Källén (1986) reported results from the Danish–Swedish registry concerning 77 pregnancies after intestinal bypass. They described a lower mean birthweight, shorter gestations, and more small-for-gestational-age infants in these women when compared with nonobese control women. Of the 10 or so pregnant women with a jejunoileal bypass cared for at Parkland Hospital, most did well. They were given supplemental iron, folic acid, vitamin B_{12}, and a commercially available prenatal vitamin–mineral preparation. All but one infant were appropriately grown and in good health.

REFERENCES

Affleck DG, Handrahan DL, Egger MJ, Price RR: The laparoscopic management of appendicitis and cholelithiasis during pregnancy. Am J Surg 178:523, 1999

Aggarwal SH, Suril V, Vasishta K, Jha M, Dhiman RK: Pregnancy and cirrhosis of the liver. Aust N Z J Obstet Gynaecol 39:503, 1999

Allenby K, Campbell DJ, Lodge JPA: Vaginal delivery following combined pelvic renal and pancreatic transplant. Br J Obstet Gynaecol 105:1036, 1998

Allison DB, Fontaine KR, Manson JE, Stevens J, VanItallie TB: Annual deaths attributable to obesity in the United States. JAMA 282:1530, 1999

Alsulyman OM, Ouzounian JG, Ames-Castro M, Goodwin TM: Intrahepatic cholestasis of pregnancy: Perinatal outcome associated with expectant management. Am J Obstet Gynecol 175:957, 1996

Alter MJ, Kruszon-Moran D, Nainan OV, McQuillan GM, Gao F, Moyer LA, Kaslow RA, Margolis HS: The prevalence of hepatitis C virus infection in the United States, 1988 through 1994. N Engl J Med 341:556, 1999

Amaro R, Rogers AI: Neostigmine infusion: New standard of care for acute colonic pseudo-obstruction? Am J Gastroenterol 95:304, 2000

American College of Obstetricians and Gynecologists: Viral hepatitis in pregnancy. Educational Bulletin No. 248, July 1998

Amos JD, Schorr SJ, Norman PF: Laparoscopic surgery during pregnancy. Am J Surg 171:435, 1996

Armenti VT, McGrory CH, Cater J, Radomski JS, Jarrell BE, Moritz MJ: The National Transplantation Pregnancy Registry: Comparison between pregnancy outcomes in diabetic cyclosporine-treated female kidney recipients and CyA-treated female pancreas–kidney recipients. Transplant Proc 29:669, 1997

Baer JL, Reis RA, Arens RA: Appendicitis in pregnancy with changes in position and axis of normal appendix in pregnancy. JAMA 98:1359, 1932

Baird DD, Narendranathan M, Sandler RS: Increased risk of preterm birth for women with inflammatory bowel disease. Gastroenterology 99:987, 1990

Baker AL: Liver and biliary tract diseases. In Barron WM, Lindeimer MD (eds): Medical Disorders During Pregnancy, 3rd ed. St. Louis, Mosby, 2000, p 330

Barone JE, Bears S, Chen S, Tsai J, Russell JC: Outcome study of cholecystectomy during pregnancy. Am J Sur 177:232, 1999

Bateson MC: Gallbladder disease. BMJ 318:1745, 1999

Belluzzi A, Brignola C, Campieri M, Pera A, Boschi S, Migliolo M: Effect of an enteric-coated fish-oil preparation on relapses in Crohn's disease. N Engl J Med 334:1557, 1996

Bianco AT, Smilen SW, Davis Y, Lopez S, Lapinski R, Lockwood CJ: Pregnancy outcome and weight gain recommendations for the morbidly obese woman. Obstet Gynecol 91:97, 1998

Bilenka B, Ben-Shlomo I, Cozacov C, Gold CH, Zohar S: Fertility, miscarriage and pregnancy after vertical banded gastroplasty operation for morbid obesity. Acta Obstet Gynecol Scand 74:42, 1995

Block P, Kelley TR: Management of gallstone pancreatitis during pregnancy and the postpartum period. Surg Gynecol Obstet 168:426, 1989

Bohman V, Stettler RW, Little BB, Wendel G, Sutor LJ, Cunningham FG: Seroprevalence and risk factors for hepatitis C virus antibody in pregnant women. Obstet Gynecol 80:609, 1992

Boulton R, Hamilton M, Lewis A, Walker P, Pounder R: Fulminant ulcerative colitis in pregnancy. Am J Gastroenterol 89:931, 1994

Braverman DZ, Johnson ML, Kern F Jr: Effects of pregnancy and contraceptive steroids on gallbladder function. N Engl J Med 302:362, 1980

Briggs GG, Freeman RK, Yaffee SJ: Drugs in Pregnancy and Lactation, 5th ed. Baltimore, Williams & Wilkins, 1998

Britton RC: Pregnancy and esophageal varices. Am J Surg 143:421, 1982

Brynskov J, Freund L, Rasmussen SN, Lauritsen K, de Muckadell OS, Williams N, MacDonald AS, Tanton R, Molia F, Campanini MC, Bianchi P, Ranzi T, Di Palo FQ, Malchow-Moller A, Thomsen OO, Tage-Jensen U, Binder V, Riis P: A placebo-controlled, double-blind, randomized trial of cyclosporin therapy in active chronic Crohn's disease. N Engl J Med 321:845, 1989

Burns DN, Minkoff H: Hepatitis C: Screening in pregnancy. Obstet Gynecol 94:1044, 1999

Burton BT, Foster WR: Health implications of obesity: An NIH Consensus Development Conference. J Am Diet Assoc 85:1117, 1985

Calle EE, Thun MJ, Petrelli JM, Rodriguez C, Heath CW Jr: Body-mass index and mortality in a prospective cohort of US adults. N Engl J Med 341:1097, 1999

Cappell MS, Sidhom O: Multicenter, multiyear study of safety and efficacy of flexible sigmoidoscopy during pregnancy in 24 females with follow-up of fetal outcome. Dig Dis Sci 40:472, 1995

Cappell MS, Sidhom O: A multicenter, multiyear study of the safety and clinical utility of esophagogastroduodenoscopy in 20 consecutive pregnant females with follow-up of fetal outcome. Am J Gastroenterol 88:1900, 1993

Carral JML, Chandrashekar MV, Rogers IM, Olajide F: Volvulus of the right colon in pregnancy. Int J Clin Prac 52:270, 1998

Castro MA, Goodwin TM, Shaw KJ, Ouzounian JG, McGehee WG: Disseminated intravascular coagulation and antithrombin III depression in acute fatty liver of pregnancy. Am J Obstet Gynecol 174:211, 1996a

Castro MA, Ouzounian JG, Colletti PM, Shaw KJ, Stein SM, Goodwin TM: Radiologic studies in acute fatty liver of pregnancy. A review of the literature and 19 new cases. J Reprod Med 41:839, 1996b

Centers for Disease Control: Public health service interagency guidelines for screening donors of blood, plasma, organs, tissues, and semen for evidence of hepatitis B and hepatitis C. MMWR 40:1, 1991

Centers for Disease Control: Protection against viral hepatitis. Recommendations of the Immunization Practices Advisory Committee. MMWR 39:1, 1990

Centers for Disease Control and Prevention: Prevention of hepatitis A through active or passive immunization. MMWR 48:1, 1999

Centers for Disease Control and Prevention: Recommendations for prevention and control of hepatitis C virus (HCV) infection and HCV-related chronic disease. MMWR 47:1, 1998a

Centers for Disease Control and Prevention: Summary of notifiable diseases, United States 1998. MMWR 47:1, 1998b

Clark DH: Peptic ulcer in women. BMJ 2:1254, 1953

Cohen S, Harris LD: Does hiatus hernia affect competence of the gastroesophageal sphincter? N Engl J Med 284A:1053, 1971

Connolly MM, Unti JA, Nora PF: Bowel obstruction in pregnancy. Surg Clin North Am 75:101, 1995

Conry-Cantilena C, VanRaden M, Gibble J, Melpolder J, Shakil AO, Viladomiu L, Cheung L, DiBisceglie A, Hoofnagle J, Shih JW, Kaslow R, Ness P, Alter HJ: Routes of infection, viremia, and liver disease in blood donors found to have hepatitis C virus infection. N Engl J Med 334:1691, 1996

Conte D, Fraquelli M, Prati D, Colucci A, Minola E: Prevalence and clinical course of chronic hepatitis C virus (HVC) infection and rate of HCV vertical transmission in a cohort of 15,250 pregnant women. Hepatology 31:751, 2000

Cosenza CA, Saffari B, Jabbour N, Stain SC, Garry D, Parekh D, Selby RR: Surgical management of biliary gallstone disease during pregnancy. Am J Surg 178:545, 1999

Cunningham FG, Lowe TW, Guss S, Mason R: Erythrocyte morphology in women with severe preeclampsia and eclampsia. Am J Obstet Gynecol 153:358, 1985

Cunningham FG, Pritchard JA, Hankins GVD, Anderson PL, Lucas MK, Armstrong KF: Idiopathic cardiomyopathy or compounding cardiovascular events? Obstet Gynecol 67:157, 1986

Curran D, Lorenz R, Czako P: Gastric outlet obstruction at 30 weeks' gestation. Obstet Gynecol 93:851, 1999

Davidson KM, Simpson LL, Knox TA, D'Alton ME: Acute fatty liver of pregnancy in triplet gestation. Obstet Gynecol 91:806, 1998

Davis A, Katz VL, Cox R: Gallbladder disease in pregnancy. J Reprod Med 40:759, 1995

Davis GL, Esteban-Mur R, Rustgi V, Hoefs J, Gordon SC, Trepo C, Shiffman ML, Zeuzem S, Craxi A, Ling MH, Albrecht J: Interferon alfa-2b alone or in combination with ribavirin for the treatment of relapse of chronic hepatitis C. N Engl J Med 339:1493, 1998

Davis MR, Bohon CJ: Intestinal obstruction in pregnancy. Clin Obstet Gynecol 26:832, 1983

de Boer WA, Tytgat GNJ: Treatment of Helicobacter pylori infection. BMJ 320:31, 2000

Deseda CC, Sweeney PA, Woodruff BA, Lindegren ML, Shapiro CN, Onorato IM: Prevalence of hepatitis B, hepatitis C, and human immunodeficiency virus infection among women attending prenatal clinics in San Juan, Puerto Rico, from 1989–1990. Obstet Gynecol 85:75, 1995

Deuchar N: Nausea and vomiting in pregnancy: A review of the problem with particular regard to psychological and social aspects. Br J Obstet Gynaecol 102:6, 1995

De Veciana M, Towers CV, Major CA, Lien JM, Toohey JS: Pulmonary injury associated with appendicitis in pregnancy: Who is at risk? Am J Obstet Gynecol 171:1008, 1994

Dienstag JL, Isselbacher KJ: Acute viral hepatitis. In Braunwald E, Fauci AS, Hauser SL, Isselbacher JK, Kasper DL, Martin JB, Wilson JD (eds): Harrison's Principles of Internal Medicine, 14th ed. New York, McGraw-Hill, 1998, p 1677

Dienstag JL, Schiff ER, Wright TL, Perrillo RP, Hann HWL, Goodman Z, Growther L, Condreay LD, Woessner M, Rubin M, Brown NA: Lamivudine as initial treatment for chronic hepatitis B in the United States. N Engl J Med 341:1256, 1999

Dixon NF, Faddis DM, Silberman H: Aggressive management of cholecystitis during pregnancy. Am J Surg 154:294, 1987

Donaldson RM: Management of medical problems in pregnancy—inflammatory bowel disease. N Engl J Med 312:1618, 1985

Duff B, Duff P: Hepatitis A vaccine: Ready for prime time. Obstet Gynecol 91:468, 1998

Duff P: Viral hepatitis. Prim Care Update Ob/Gyn 1:58, 1994

Durie PR: Pancreatitis and mutations of the cystic fibrosis gene. N Engl J Med 339:687, 1998

Evers BM, Townsend CM, Thompson JC: Small intestine. In Schwartz SI, Shires GT, Spencer FC, Daly JM, Fischer JE, Galloway AC (eds): Principles of Surgery. New York, McGraw-Hill, 1999, p 1229

Everson GT: Gastrointestinal motility in pregnancy. Gastroenterol Clin North Am 21:751, 1992

Farmer RG: Crohn's Disease. In Gitnick G, Hollander D, Samloff IM, Schoenfield LJ, Vierling JM (eds): Principles and Practice of Gasteroenterology and Hepatology. Norwalk, CT, Appleton & Lange, 1994, p 395

Farouk R, Pemberton JH, Wolff BG, Dozois RR, Browning S, Larson D: Functional outcomes after ileal pouch–anal anastomosis for chronic ulcerative colitis. Ann Surg 231:919, 2000

Feagan BG, Fedorak RN, Irvine EJ, Wild G, Sutherland L, Steinhart AH, Greenberg GR, Koval J, Wong CJ, Hopkins M, Hanauer SB, McDonald JWD: A comparison of methotrexate with placebo for the maintenance of remission in Crohn's disease. N Engl J Med 342:1627, 2000

Fedorkow DM, Persaud D, Nimrod CA: Inflammatory bowel disease: A controlled study of late pregnancy outcome. Am J Obstet Gynecol 160:998, 1989

Feucht HH, Zollner B, Polywka S, Laufs R: Vertical transmission of hepatitis G. Lancet 347:615, 1996

Fiest TC, Foong A, Chokhavatia S: Successful balloon dilation of achalasia during pregnancy. Gastrointest Endosc 39:810, 1993

Firstenberg MS, Malangoni MA: Gastrointestinal surgery during pregnancy. Gastroenterol Clin North Am 27(1):73, 1998.

Fisk NM, Bye WB, Storey GNB: Maternal features of obstetric cholestasis: 20 years experience at King George V Hospital. Aust N Z J Obstet Gynecol 28:172, 1988

Fletcher DR, Hobbs MST, Tan P, Valinsky LJ, Hockey RL, Pikora TJ, Knuiman MW, Sheiner HJ, Edis A: Complications of cholecystectomy: Risks of the laparoscopic approach and protective effects of operative cholangiography. Ann Surg 229:449, 1999

Flick RP, Bofill JA, King JC: Pregnancy complicated by traumatic diaphragmatic rupture. A case report. J Reprod Med 44:127, 1999

Floreani A, Paternoster D, Zappalà, Cusinato R, Bombi G, Grella P, Chiaramonte M: Hepatitis C virus infection in pregnancy. Br J Obstet Gynaecol 103:325, 1996

Fonager K, Sorensen HT, Olsen J, Dahlerup JF, Rasmussen SN: Pregnancy outcome for women with Crohn's disease: A follow-up study based on linkage between national registries. Am J Gastroenterol 93:2426, 1998

Forsnes LT EV, Eggleston MK, Heaton JO: Enterovesical fistula complicating pregnancy: A case report. J Reprod Med 44:297, 1999

Franco J, Newcomer J, Adams M, Saeian K: Auxiliary liver transplant in acute fatty liver of pregnancy. Obstet Gynecol 95:1042, 2000

Frigo P, Lang C, Reisenberger K, Heinz K, Hirschl AM: Hyperemesis gravidarum associated with *Helicobacter pylori* seropositivity. Obstet Gynecol 91:615, 1998

Fung TY, Li CY: Successful pregnancy in a woman with secondary biliary cirrhosis with portal hypertension from recurrent pyogenic cholangitis. A case report. J Reprod Med 44:475, 1999

Garbaciak JA Jr, Richter M, Miller S, Barton JJ: Maternal weight and pregnancy complications. Am J Obstet Gynecol 152:238, 1985

Gilstrap LC, Van Dorsten PV, Cunningham FG (eds): Diagnostic and operative laparoscopy. In: Operative Obstetrics, 2nd ed. New York, McGraw-Hill, 2001, in press

Glasgow RE, Visser BC, Harris HW, Patti MG, Kilpatrick SJ, Mulvihill SJ: Changing management of gallstone disease during pregnancy. Surg Endosc 12:241, 1998

Glickman RM: Inflammatory bowel disease. Ulcerative colitis and Crohn's disease. In Fauci AS, Braunwald E, Isselbacher KJ, Wilson JD, Martin JB, Kasper DL, Hauser SL, Longo DL (eds): Harrison's Principles of Internal Medicine, 1998, 14th ed. New York, McGraw-Hill, 1998, p 1633

Godsey RK, Newman RB: Hyperemesis gravidarum: A comparison of single and multiple admissions. J Reprod Med 36:287, 1991

Goodwin TM, Hershman JM, Cole L: Increased concentration of the free β-subunit of human chorionic gonadotropin in hyperemesis gravidarum. Acta Obstet Gynecol Scand 73:770, 1994

Gopal KA, Amshel AL, Shonberg IL, Levinson BA, Vanwert M, Vanwert J: Ostomy and pregnancy. Dis Colon Rectum 28:912, 1985

Graham G, Baxi L, Tharakan T: Laparoscopic cholecystectomy during pregnancy: A case series and review of the literature. Obstet Gynecol Surv 53:566, 1998

Greenberger NJ, Isselbacher KJ: Diseases of the gallbladder and bile ducts. In Fauci AS, Braunwald E, Isselbacher KJ, Wilson JD, Martin JB, Kasper DL, Hauser SL, Longo DL (eds): Harrison's Principles of Internal Medicine 14th ed. New York, McGraw-Hill, 1998, p 1633

Greenspoon JS, Masaki DI, Kurz CR: Cardiac tamponade in pregnancy during central hyperalimentation. Obstet Gynecol 73:465, 1989

Habal FM, Hui G, Greenberg GR: Oral 5-aminosalicylic acid for inflammatory bowel disease in pregnancy: Safety and clinical course. Gastroenterology 105:1057, 1993

Harer WB Jr, Harer WB Sr: Volvulus complicating pregnancy and the puerperium: A report of three cases and review of the literature. Obstet Gynecol 12:399, 1958

Hellberg A, Rudberg C, Kullman E, Enochsson L, Fenyo G, Graffner H, Hallerback B, Johansson B, Anderberg B, Wenner J, Ringqvist I, Sorensen S: Prospective randomized multicentre study of laparoscopic versus open appendicectomy. Br J Surg 86:48, 1999

Heyland DK, MacDonald S, Keefe L, Drover JW: Total parenteral nutrition in the critically ill patient. JAMA 280:2013, 1998

Hillbom M, Pyhtinen J, Pylvänen V, Sotaniemi K: Pregnant, vomiting, and coma: A case report. Lancet 353:1584, 1999

Hillemanns P, Dannecker C, Kimmig R, Hasbargen U: Obstetric risks and vertical transmission of hepatitis C virus infection in pregnancy. Acta Obstet Gynecol Scand 79:543, 2000

Hillemanns P, Knitza R, Müller-Höcker J: Rupture of splenic artery aneurysm in a pregnant patient with portal hypertension. Am J Obstet Gynecol 174:1665, 1996

Hirvioja ML, Tuimala R, Vuori J: The treatment of intrahepatic cholestasis of pregnancy by dexamethasone. Br J Obstet Gynaecol 99:109, 1992

Howard EW, Jones HL: Massive hepatic necrosis in toxemia of pregnancy. Tex Med 9:74, 1993

Hsu JJ, Clark-Glena R, Nelson DK, Kim CH: Nasogastric enteral feeding in the management of hyperemesis gravidarum. Obstet Gynecol 88:343, 1996

Hunter SK, Martin M, Benda JA, Zlatnik FJ: Liver transplant after massive spontaneous hepatic rupture in pregnancy complicated by preeclampsia. Obstet Gynecol 85:819, 1995

Hytten FE: The alimentary system. In Hytten F, Chamberlain G (eds): Clinical Physiology in Obstetrics. London, Blackwell, 1991, p 137

Ilnyckyji A, Blanchard JF, Rawsthorne P, Bernstein CN: Perianal Crohn's disease and pregnancy: Role of the mode of delivery. Am J Gastroenterol 94:3274, 1999

Inaba N, Okajima Y, Kang XS, Ishikawa K, Fukasawa I: Maternal–infant transmission of hepatitis G virus. Am J Obstet Gynecol 177:1537, 1997

Ingardia CJ, Kelley L, Steinfeld JD, Wax JR: Hepatitis B vaccination in pregnancy: Factors influencing efficacy. Obstet Gynecol 93:983, 1999

Ingerslev M, Teilum G: Biopsy studies on the liver in pregnancy, 2. Liver biopsy on normal pregnant women. Acta Obstet Gynaecol Scand 25:352, 1945

Isaacs JD, Magann EF, Martin RW, Chauhan SP, Morrison JC: Obstetric challenges of massive obesity complicating pregnancy. J Perinatol 14:10, 1994

Isaacs JD, Sims HF, Powell CK, Bennett MJ, Hale DE, Treem WR, Strauss AW: Maternal acute fatty liver of pregnancy associated with fetal trifunctional protein deficiency: Molecular characterization of a novel maternal mutant allele. Pediatr Res 40:393, 1996

Iwase H, Morise K, Kawase T, Horiuchi Y: Endoscopic injection sclerotherapy for esophageal varices during pregnancy. J Clin Gastroenterol 18:80, 1994

Jarvis LM, Davidson F, Hanley JP, Yap PL, Ludlam CA, Simmonds P: Infection with hepatitis G virus among recipients of plasma products. Lancet 348:1352, 1996

Jewell D, Young G: Interventions for nausea and vomiting in early pregnancy. Cochrane Database Syst Rev 2: CD000145, 2000

Johnson SR, Kolberg BH, Varner MW, Railsback LD: Maternal obesity and pregnancy. Surg Gynecol Obstet 164:431, 1987

Juhasz ES, Fozard B, Dozois RR, Ilstrup DM, Nelson H: Ileal pouch–anal anastomosis function following childbirth: An extended evaluation. Dis Colon Rectum 38:159, 1995

Kalish RB, Garry D, Figueroa R: Achalasia with *Candida* esophagitis during pregnancy. Obstet Gynecol 94:850, 1999

Kennedy S, Hall PM, Seymour AE, Hague WM: Transient diabetes insipidus and acute fatty liver of pregnancy. Br J Obstet Gynaecol 101:387, 1994

Khuroo MS, Kamili S, Jameel S: Vertical transmission of hepatitis E virus. Lancet 345:1025, 1995

Kilby MD, Weaver JB, Penn R, Eggington E, Chambers J, Ellas E: A retrospective observational study of patients with pregnancies complicated by obstetric cholestasis. Br J Obstet Gynaecol 105:Suppl 17, 1998

Kirby DF, Fiorenza V, Craig RM: Intravenous nutritional support during pregnancy. JPEN 12:72, 1988

Kirkinen P, Ryynänen M: First-trimester manifestation of intrahepatic cholestasis of pregnancy and high fetoplacental hormone production in a triploid fetus. J Reprod Med 40:471, 1995

Klebanoff MA, Koslowe PA, Kaslow R, Rhoads GG: Epidemiology of vomiting in early pregnancy. Obstet Gynecol 66:612, 1985

Kliegman RM, Gross T: Perinatal problems of the obese mother and her infant. Obstet Gynecol 66:299, 1985

Knox TA, Olans LB: Liver disease in pregnancy. N Engl J Med 335:568, 1996

Knudsen LB, Källen B: Intestinal bypass operation and pregnancy outcome. Acta Obstet Gynecol Scand 65:831, 1986

Kodner IJ, Fry RD, Fleshman JW, Birnbaun EH, Read TE: Colon, rectum, and anus. In Schwartz SI, Shires GT, Spencer FC, Daley JM, Fischer JE, Galloway AC (eds): Principles of Surgery, 7th ed. New York, McGraw-Hill, 1999, p 1311

Korelitz BI: Inflammatory bowel disease and pregnancy. Gastroenterol Clin North Am 27:214, 1998

Kornfeld D, Cnattingius S, Ekbom A: Pregnancy outcomes in women with inflammatory bowel disease—A population-based cohort study. Am J Obstet Gynecol 177:942, 1997

Kort B, Katz VL, Watson MJ: The effect of nonobstetric operation during pregnancy. Surg Gynecol Obstet 177:371, 1993

Kuczmarski RJ, Flegal KM, Campbell SM, Johnson CL: Increasing prevalence of overweight among US adults: The National Health and Nutrition Examination Surveys, 1960 to 1991. JAMA 272:205, 1994

Kurzel RB, Naunheim KS, Schwartz RA: Repair of symptomatic diaphragmatic hernia during pregnancy. Obstet Gynecol 71:869, 1988

Lai CL, Chien RN, Leung NWY, Chang TT, Guan R, Tai DI, Ng KY, Wu PC, Dent JC, Barber J, Stephenson SL, Gray DF: A one-year trial of lamivudine for chronic hepatitis B. N Engl J Med 339:61, 1998

Laifer SA, Darby MJ, Scantlebury VP, Harger JH, Caritis SN: Pregnancy and liver transplantation. Obstet Gynecol 76:1083, 1990

Landers D, Carmona R, Crombleholme W, Lim R: Acute cholecystitis in pregnancy. Obstet Gynecol 69:131, 1987

Landwehr JG, Leonardi MR, Bryant DR, Johnson SC, Bottoms SF: Graded-compression ultrasound (GCUS) for early recognition of appendicitis in pregnancy. Am J Obstet Gynecol 147:389, 1996

Lawson M, Kern F, Everson GT: Gastrointestinal transit time in human pregnancy: Prolongation in the second and third trimesters followed by postpartum normalization. Gastroenterology 89:996, 1985

Lee S, Bradley JP, Mele MM, Sehdev HM, Ludmir J: Cholelithiasis in pregnancy: Surgical versus medical management. Obstet Gynecol 95:S70, 2000

Lee WM: Pregnancy in patients with chronic liver disease. Gastroenterol Clin North Am 21:889, 1992

Legro RS, Laifer SA: First trimester pancreatitis: Maternal and neonatal outcome. J Reprod Med 40:689, 1995

Leikin EL, Reinus JF, Schmell E, Tejani N: Epidemiologic predictors of hepatitis C virus infection in pregnant women. Obstet Gynecol 84:529, 1994

Leslie KK, Reznikov L, Simon FR, Fennessey PV, Reyes H, Ribalta J: Estrogens in intrahepatic cholestasis of pregnancy. Obstet Gynecol 95:372, 2000

Levine AB: Autoimmune hepatitis in pregnancy. Obstet Gynecol 95:1033, 2000

Lin HM, Kauffman HM, McBride MA, Davies DB, Rosendale JD, Smith CM, Edwards EB, Daily OP, Kirklin J, Shield CF, Hunsicker LG: Center-specific graft and patient survival rates. 1997 United Network for Organ Sharing (UNOS) report. JAMA 280:1153, 1998

Locatelli A, Roncaglia N, Arreghini A, Bellini P, Vergani P, Ghidini A: Hepatitis C virus infection is associated with a higher incidence of cholestasis of pregnancy. Br J Obstet Gynaecol 106:498, 1999

Lunzer M, Barnes P, Byth K, O'Halloran M: Serum bile acid concentrations during pregnancy and their relationship to obstetric cholestasis. Gastroenterology 91:825, 1986

MacLean MA, Cameron AD, Cumming GP, Murphy K, Mills P, Hilan KJ: Recurrence of acute fatty liver of pregnancy. Br J Obstet Gynaecol 101:453, 1994

Maringhini A, Marcenò MP, Lanzarone F, Caltagirone M, Fusco G, Di-Cuonzo G, Cittadini E, Pagliaro L: Sludge and stones in gallbladder after pregnancy: Prevalence and risk factors. J Hepatol 5:218, 1987

Martin JN Jr, Blake PG, Perry KG Jr, McCaul JF, Hess LW, Martin RW: The natural history of HELLP syndrome: Patterns of disease progression and regression. Am J Obstet Gynecol 164:1500, 1991

Martin LF, Finigan KM, Nolan TE: Pregnancy after adjustable gastric banding. Obstet Gynecol 94:927, 2000

Matos A, Bernardes J, Ayres-de-Campos D, Patricio B: Antepartum fetal cerebral hemorrhage not predicted by current surveillance methods in cholestasis of pregnancy. Obstet Gynecol 89:803, 1997

Mayberry JF, Atkinson M: Achalasia and pregnancy. Br J Obstet Gynaecol 94:855, 1987

Mays J, Verma U, Klein S, Tejani N: Acute appendicitis in pregnancy and the occurrence of major intraventricular hemorrhage and periventricular leukomalacia. Obstet Gynecol 86:650, 1995

Mazze RI, Källén B: Appendectomy during pregnancy: A Swedish registry study of 778 cases. Obstet Gynecol 77:835, 1991

Mazze RI, Källén B: Reproductive outcome after anesthesia and operation during pregnancy: A registry study of 5405 cases. Am J Obstet Gynecol 161:1178, 1989

McHutchison JG, Gordon SC, Schiff ER, Shiffman ML, Lee WM, Rustgi VK, Goodman ZD, Ling MH, Cort S, Albrecht JK: Interferon alfa-2b alone or in combination with ribavirin as initial treatment for chronic hepatitis C. N Engl J Med 339:1485, 1998

Meyerson S, Holtz T, Ehrinpresis M, Dhar R: Small bowel obstruction in pregnancy. Am J Gastroenterol 90:299, 1995

Mikhail LN, Mittendorf R, Walker CK: The association of maternal obesity and isolated major fetal congenital cardiac anomalies in African-American women. Am J Obstet Gynecol 174:446, 1996

Miller JP: Inflammatory bowel disease in pregnancy: A review. J Roy Soc Med 79:221, 1986

Minakami H, Oka N, Sato T, Tamada T, Yasuda Y, Hirota N: Preeclampsia: A microvesicular fat disease of the liver? Am J Obstet Gynecol 159:1043, 1988

Modigliani RM: Gastrointestinal and pancreatic disease. In Barron WM, Lindheimer MD, Davison JM (eds): Medical Disorders of Pregnancy, 3rd ed. St. Louis, Mosby, 2000, p 316

Moen MD, Caliendo MJ, Marshall W, Uhler ML: Hepatic rupture in pregnancy associated with cocaine use. Obstet Gynecol 82:687, 1993

Monga M, Katz AR: Acute fatty liver in the second trimester. Obstet Gynecol 93:811, 1999

Moore JG, Gladstone NS, Lucas GW, Ravry MJR, Ansari AH: Successful management of post-cesarean-section acute pseudoobstruction of the colon (Ogilvie's syndrome) with colonoscopic decompression. A case report. J Reprod Med 31:1001, 1986

Mourad J, Elliott JP, Erickson L, Lisboa L: Appendicitis in pregnancy: New information that contradicts long-held clinical beliefs. Am J Obstet Gynecol 185:1027, 2000

Murphy P, Chez RA: Management of nausea and vomiting in pregnancy: Alternative therapies. Contemp Ob/Gyn 45:55, 2000

Must A, Spadano J, Coakley EH, Field AE, Colditz G, Dietz WH: The disease burden associated with overweight and obesity. JAMA 282:1523, 1999

Nageotte MP, Briggs GG, Towers CV, Asrat T: Droperidol and diphenhydramine in the management of hyperemesis gravidarum. Am J Obstet Gynecol 174:1801, 1996

National Institutes of Health Consensus Development Conference Statement on Gallstones and Laparoscopic Cholecystectomy. Am J Surg 165:390, 1993

Nesbitt TH, Kay HH, McCoy MC, Herbert WNP: Endoscopic management of biliary disease during pregnancy. Obstet Gynecol 87:806, 1996

Nicastri PL, Diaferia A, Tartagni M, Loizzi P, Fanelli M: A randomised placebo-controlled trial of ursodeoxycholic acid and S-adenosylmethionine in the treatment of intrahepatic cholestasis of pregnancy. Br J Obstet Gynaecol 105:1205, 1998

Nies BM, Dreiss RJ: Hyperlipidemic pancreatitis in pregnancy: A case report and review of the literature. Am J Perinatol 7:166, 1990

Niu MT, Salive ME, Ellenberg SS: Neonatal deaths after hepatitis B vaccine: The vaccine adverse event reporting system, 1991–1998. Arch Pediatr Adolesc Med 153:1279, 1999

Ockner SA, Brunt EM, Cohn SM, Krul ES, Hanto DW, Peters MG: Fulminant hepatic failure caused by acute fatty liver of pregnancy treated by orthotopic liver transplantation. Hepatology 11:59, 1990

Ohto H, Terazawa S, Sasaki N, Sasaki N, Hino K, Ishiwata C, Kako M, Ujiie N, Endo C, Matsui A, Okamoto H, Mishiro S, Vertical Transmission of Hepatitis C Virus Collaborative Study Group: Transmission of hepatitis C virus from mothers to infants. N Engl J Med 330:744, 1994

Ordorica SA, Frieden FJ, Marks F, Hoskins IA, Young BK: Pancreatic enzyme activity in pregnancy. J Reprod Med 36:359 1991

Ortega-Carnicer J, Ambrós A, Alcazar R: Obstructive shock due to labor-related diaphragmatic hernia. Crit Care Med 26:616, 1998

Pajor A, Lehoczky D: Pregnancy in liver cirrhosis—assessment of maternal and fetal risks in eleven patients and review of the management. Gynecol Obstet Invest 38:45, 1994

Palma J, Reyes H, Ribalta J, Hernandez I, Sandoval L, Almuna R, Liepins J, Lira F, Sedano M, Silva O, Tohá D, Silva JJ: Ursodeoxycholic acid in the treatment of cholestasis of pregnancy: A randomized, double-blind study controlled with placebo. J Hepatol 27:1022, 1997

Pauzner D, Wolman I, Niv D, Ber A, David MP: Endoscopic sclerotherapy in extrahepatic portal hypertension in pregnancy. Am J Obstet Gynecol 164:152, 1991

Perdue PW, Johnson HW Jr, Stafford PW: Intestinal obstruction complicating pregnancy. Am J Surg 164:384, 1992

Ponec RJ, Saunders MD, Kimmey MB: Neostigmine for the treatment of acute colonic pseudo-obstruction. N Engl J Med 341:137, 1999

Present DH, Rutgeerts P, Targan S, Hanauer SB, Mayer L, van Hogezend RA, Podolsky DK, Sands BE, Braakman T, DeWoody KL, Schaible TF, van Deventer SJ: Infliximab for the treatment of fistulas in patients with Crohn's disease. N Engl J Med 340:1398, 1999

Printen KJ, Scott D: Pregnancy following gastric bypass for the treatment of morbid obesity. Am Surg 48:363, 1982

Pritchard JA, Weisman R, Ratnoff OD, Vosburgh G: Intravascular hemolysis, thrombocytopenia and other hematologic abnormalities associated with severe toxemia of pregnancy. N Engl J Med 250:87, 1954

Public Health Service: Healthy People 2000: National Health Promotion and Disease Prevention Objectives. Washington, DC: US Department of Health and Human Services, Public Health Service, DHHS Publication No. (PHS) 90-50212, 1990

Pucci RO, Seed RW: Case report of laparoscopic cholecystectomy in the third trimester of pregnancy. Am J Obstet Gynecol 165:401, 1991

Puylaert JBCM, Rutgers PH, Lalisang RI: A prospective study of ultrasound in the diagnosis of appendicitis. N Engl J Med 317:666, 1987

Radomski JS, Ahlswede BA, Jarrell BE, Mannion J, Cater J,

Moritz JM, Armenti VT: Outcomes of 500 pregnancies in 335 female kidney, liver, and heart transplant recipients. Transplant Proc 27:1089, 1995

Ralston SJ, Schwaitzberg SD: Liver hematoma and rupture in pregnancy. Semin Perinatol 22:141, 1998

Ramin KD, Ramin SM, Richey SD, Cunningham FG: Acute pancreatitis in pregnancy. Am J Obstet Gynecol 173:187, 1995

Rampton DS: Management of Crohn's disease. BMJ 319:1480, 1999

Ranjan V, Boulton JM: Primary volvulus of the small bowel following normal delivery. Br J Obstet Gynaecol 100:860, 1993

Rao PM, Rhea JT, Novelline RA, Mostafavi AA, McCabe CJ: Effect of computed tomography of the appendix on treatment of patients and use of hospital resources. N Engl J Med 338:141, 1998

Reedy MB, Källén B, Kuehl TJ: Laparoscopy during pregnancy: A study of five fetal outcome parameters with use of the Swedish Health Registry. Am J Obstet Gynecol 177:673, 1997

Reedy M, Uy K, Thompson E, Rayburn WL: Laparoscopy during pregnancy: A safe alternative to laparotomy? Contemp Ob/Gyn 43:75, 1998

Rees JH, Ginsberg L, Schapira AHV: Two pregnant women with vomiting and fits. Am J Obstet Gynecol 177:1539, 1997

Resti M, Azzari C, Mannelli F, Moriondo M, Novembre E, de Martino M, Vierucci A, Tuscany Study Group on Hepatitis C virus infection in children: Mother to child transmission of hepatitis C virus: Prospective study of risk factors and timing of infection in children born to women seronegative for HIV-1. BMJ 317:437, 1998

Rayes N, Neuhaus R, David M, Steinmuller T, Bechstein WO, Neuhaus P: Pregnancies following liver transplantation—how safe are they? A report of 19 cases under cyclosporine A and tacrolimus. Clin Transplant 12:396, 1998

Reyes H: Intrahepatic cholestasis. A puzzling disorder of pregnancy [Review]. J Gastroenterol Hepatol 12:211, 1997

Reyes H, Sandoval L, Wainstein A, Ribalta J, Donoso S, Smok G, Rosenberg H, Meneses M: Acute fatty liver of pregnancy: A clinical study of 12 episodes in 11 patients. Gut 35:101, 1994

Reyes H, Sjovall J: Bile acids and progesterone metabolites in intrahepatic cholestasis of pregnancy. Ann Med 32:94, 2000

Richards DS, Miller DK, Goodman GN: Pregnancy after gastric bypass for morbid obesity. J Reprod Med 32:172, 1987

Riely CA, Fallon HJ: Liver diseases. In Burrow GN, Duffy TP (eds): Medical Complications During Pregnancy, 5th ed. Philadelphia, Saunders, 1999, p 269

Riggs BS, Bronstein AC, Kulig K, Archer PG, Rumack BH: Acute acetaminophen overdose during pregnancy. Obstet Gynecol 74:247, 1989

Rigler LG, Eneboe JB: Incidence of hiatus hernia in pregnant women and its significance. J Thorac Surg 4:262, 1935

Rindfusz D, Seydel F, Pezzullo J, Peters S, Pinckert T: The seroprevalence rate of HIV, hepatitis B, hepatitis C and syphilis in a large urban population—a five year analysis. Am J Obstet Gynecol 174:406, 1996

Rioseco AJ, Ivankovic MB, Manzur A, Hamed F, Kato SR, Parer JT, Germain AM: Intrahepatic cholestasis of pregnancy: A retrospective case-control study of perinatal outcome. Am J Obstet Gynecol 170:890, 1994

Robinson JN, Banerjee R, Thiet MP: Coagulopathy secondary to vitamin K deficiency in hyperemesis gravidarum. Obstet Gynecol 92:673, 1998

Rolfes DB, Ishak KG: Liver disease in toxemia of pregnancy. Am J Gastroenterol 81:1138, 1986

Rumack BH, Matthew H: Acetaminophen poisoning and toxicity. Pediatrics 55:871, 1975

Russo-Stieglitz KE, Levine AB, Wagner BA, Armenti VT: Pregnancy outcome in patients requiring parenteral nutrition. J Matern–Fetal Med 8:164, 1999

Sadler LC, Lane M, North R: Severe fetal intracranial haemorrhage during treatment with cholestyramine for intrahepatic cholestasis of pregnancy. Br J Obstet Gynaecol 102:169, 1995

Safari HR, Fassett MJ, Souter IC, Alsulyman OM, Goodwin TM: The efficacy of methylprednisolone in the treatment of hyperemesis gravidarum: A randomized, double-blind, controlled study. Am J Obstet Gynecol 179:921, 1998

Sainio V, Kemppainen E, Puolakkainen P, Taavitsainen M, Kivisaari L, Valtonen V, Haapiainen R, Schröder T, Kivilaakso E: Early antibiotic treatment in acute necrotizing pancreatitis. Lancet 346:663, 1995

Sanderson SL, Iverius PH, Wilson DE: Successful hyperlipemic pregnancy. JAMA 265:1858, 1991

Satin AJ, Twickler D, Gilstrap LC: Esophageal achalasia in late pregnancy. Obstet Gynecol 79:812, 1992

Schreyer P, Caspi E, El-Hindi JM, Eschar J: Cirrhosis—Pregnancy and delivery: A review. Obstet Gynecol Surv 37:304, 1982

Schwartz M, Rossoff L: Pneumomediastinum and bilateral pneumo-thoraces in a patient with hyperemesis gravidarum. Chest 106:1904, 1994

Sharp HT: Gastrointestinal surgical conditions during pregnancy. Clin Obstet Gynecol 37:306, 1994

Shaw GM, Todoroff K, Schaffer DM, Selvin S: Maternal height and prepregnancy body mass index as risk factors for selected congenital anomalies. Paediatr Perinat Epidemiol 14:234, 2000

Shaw GM, Velie EM, Schaffer D: Risk of neural tube defect–affected pregnancies among obese women. JAMA 275:1093, 1996

Sheikh RA, Yasmeen S, Pauly MP, Riegler JL: Spontaneous intrahepatic hemorrhage and hepatic rupture in the HELLP syndrome: Four cases and a review. J Clin Gastroenterol 28:323, 1999

Sheth SG, LaMont JT: Toxic megacolon. Lancet 351:509, 1998

Silverman NS, Jenkin BK, Wu C, McGillen P, Knee G: Hepatitis C virus in pregnancy: Seroprevalence and risk factors for infection. Am J Obstet Gynecol 169:583, 1993

Sims HF, Brackett JC, Powell CK, Treem WR, Hale DE, Bennett MJ, Gibson B, Shapiro S, Strauss AW: The molecular basis of pediatric long chain 3-hydroxyacyl-CoA dehydrogenase deficiency associated with maternal acute fatty liver of pregnancy. Proc Natl Acad Sci USA 92:841, 1995

Skannal DG, Dungy-Poythress LJ, Miodovnik M, First MR: Pregnancy in a combined liver and kidney transplant recipient with type 1 primary hyperoxaluria. Obstet Gynecol 86:641, 1995

Slonim AE, Bulone L, Damore MB, Goldberg T, Wingertzahn MA, McKinley MJ: A preliminary study of growth hormone therapy for Crohn's disease. N Engl J Med 342:1633, 2000

Smith LG, Moise KJ Jr, Dildy GA III, Carpenter RJ Jr: Spontaneous rupture of liver during pregnancy: Current therapy. Obstet Gynecol 77:171, 1991

Stain SC, Woodburn DA, Stephens AL, Katz M, Wagner WH, Donovan AJ: Spontaneous hepatic hemorrhage associated with pregnancy. Treatment by hepatic arterial interruption. Ann Surg 224:72, 1996

Stanley AJ, Hayes PC: Portal hypertension and variceal haemorrhage. Lancet 350:1235, 1997

Starkel P, Horsman Y, Geubel A: Endoscopic bank ligation: A safe technique to control bleeding esophageal varices in pregnancy. Gastrointest Endosc 48:212, 1998

Swisher SG, Hunt KK, Schmit PJ, Hiyama DT, Bennion RS, Thompson JE: Management of pancreatitis complicating pregnancy. Am Surg 60:759, 1994

Tesfaye S, Achari V, Yang YC, Harding S, Bowden A, Vora JP: Pregnant, vomiting, and going blind: A case report. Lancet 352:1594, 1998

Teuscher AU, Sutherland DER, Robertson RP: Successful pregnancy after pancreatic islet autotransplantation. Transplant Proc 26:3520, 1994

Thomsen OO, Cortot A, Jewell D, Wright JP, Winter T, Veloso FT, Vatn M, Persson T, Pettersson E: A comparison of budesonide and mesalamine for active Crohn's disease. N Engl J Med 339:370, 1998

Tracey M, Fletcher HS: Appendicitis in pregnancy. Am Surg 66:555, 2000

Trauner M, Meier PJ, Boyer JL: Molecular pathogenesis of cholestasis. N Engl J Med 339:1217, 1998

Treem WR, Rinaldo P, Hale DE, Stanley CA, Millington DS, Hyams JS, Jackson S, Turnbull DM: Acute fatty liver of pregnancy and long-chain 3-hydroxyacyl-coenzyme A dehydrogenase deficiency. Hepatology 19:339, 1994

Tydén G, Brattström C, Björkman U, Landgraf R, Baltzer J, Hillebrand G, Land W, Calne R, Brons GM, Squifflet JP, Ghysen J, Alexandre GPJ: Pregnancy after combined pancreas–kidney transplantation. Diabetes 38:43, 1989

Tyni T, Ekholm E, Pihko H: Pregnancy complications are frequent in long-chain 3-hydroxyacyl-coenzyme A dehydrogenase deficiency. Am J Obstet Gynecol 178:603, 1998

Usta IM, Barton JR, Amon EA, Gonzalez A, Sibai BM: Acute fatty liver of pregnancy: An experience in the diagnosis and management of fourteen cases. Am J Obstet Gynecol 171:1342, 1994

Valdivieso V, Covarrubias C, Siegel F, Cruz F: Pregnancy and cholelithiasis: Pathogenesis and natural course of gallstones diagnosed in early puerperium. Hepatology 17:1, 1993

Van Dam J, Brugge WR: Endoscopy of the upper gastrointestinal tract. N Engl J Med 341:1738, 1999

van de Ven CJM: Nasogastric enteral feeding in hyperemesis gravidarum. Lancet 349:445, 1997

Vento S, Garofano T, Renzini C, Cainelli F, Casali F, Ghironzi G, Ferraro T, Concia E: Fulminant hepatitis associated with hepatitis A virus superinfection in patients with chronic hepatitis C. N Engl J Med 338:286, 1998

Ventura-Braswell AM, Satin AJ, Higby K: Delayed diagnosis of bowel infarction secondary to maternal midgut volvulus at term. Obstet Gynecol 91:808, 1998

Viktrup L, Hée P: Fertility and long-term complications four to nine years after appendectomy during pregnancy. Acta Obstet Gynecol Scand 77:746, 1998

Ville Y, Fernandez H, Samuel D, Bismuth H, Frydman R: Pregnancy in liver transplant recipients: Course and outcome in 19 cases. Am J Obstet Gynecol 168:896, 1993

Wahl C, Liptay S, Adler G, Schmid RM: Sulfasalazine: A potent and specific inhibitor of nuclear factor kappa B. J Clin Invest 101:1163, 1998

Wahoff DC, Leone JP, Farney AC, Teuscher AU, Sutherland DER: Pregnancy after total pancreatectomy and autologous islet transplantation. Surgery 117:353, 1995

Walcott WO, Derick DE, Jolley JJ, Synder DL, Schmid R: Successful pregnancy in a liver transplant patient. Am J Obstet Gynecol 132:340, 1978

Waller DK, Mills JL, Simpson JL, Cunningham GC, Conley MR, Lassman MR, Rhoads GC: Are obese women at higher risk for producing malformed offspring? Am J Obstet Gynecol 170:541, 1994

Wang PH, Yang MJ, Lee WL, Chao HT, Yang ML, Hung JH: Acetaminophen poisoning in late pregnancy. A case report. J Reprod Med 42:367, 1997

Watkin DS, Hughes S, Thompson MH: Herniation of colon through the right diaphragm complicating the puerperium. J Laparoendoscopic Surg 3:583, 1993

Watson JC, Fleming DW, Borella AJ, Olcott ES, Conrad RE, Baron RC: Vertical transmission of hepatitis A resulting in an outbreak in a neonatal intensive care unit. J Infect Dis 167:567, 1993

Watson WJ, Gaines TE: Third-trimester colectomy for severe ulcerative colitis. J Reprod Med 32:869, 1987

Watson WJ, Seeds JW: Acute fatty liver of pregnancy. Obstet Gynecol Surv 45:585, 1990

Watts GF, Morton K, Jackson P, Lewis B: Management of patients with severe hypertriglyceridaemia during pregnancy: Report of two cases with familial lipoprotein lipase deficiency. Br J Obstet Gynaecol 99:163, 1992

Wax JR, Christie TL: Complete small-bowel volvulus complicating the second trimester. Obstet Gynecol 82:689, 1993

Webb G, Huddelston J, Vroom D, Gohr A: Neither universal screening for hepatitis B or repeat screening of high-risk patients is cost effective. Am J Obstet Gynecol 174:406, 1996

Weinstein L: Syndrome of hemolysis, elevated liver enzymes, and low platelet count: A severe consequence of hypertension in pregnancy. Am J Obstet Gynecol 142:159, 1982

Werler MM, Louik C, Shapiro S, Mitchell AA: Prepregnant weight in relation to risk of neural tube defects. JAMA 275:1089, 1996

Wittgrove AC, Jester L, Wittgrove P, Clark GW: Pregnancy following gastric bypass for morbid obesity. Obes Surg 8:461, 1998

Wolfe HM, Sokol RJ, Martier SM, Zador IE: Maternal obesity: A potential source of error in sonographic prenatal diagnosis. Obstet Gynecol 76:339, 1990

Woolfson K, Cohen Z, McLeod RS: Crohn's disease and pregnancy. Dis Colon Rectum 33:869, 1990

Woywodt A, Kiss A: Perforation of the sigmoid colon due to geophagia. Arch Surg 134:88, 1999

Yanovski JA, Yanovski SZ: Recent advances in basic obesity research. JAMA 282:1504, 1999

Zeeman GG, Moise KJ: Prophylactic banding of severe esophageal varices associated with liver cirrhosis in pregnancy. Obstet Gynecol 94:842, 1999

49

Hematological Disorders

ANEMIAS

Iron-deficiency Anemia
Anemia from Acute Blood Loss
Anemia Associated with Chronic Disease
Megaloblastic Anemia
Acquired Hemolytic Anemias
Hemolytic Anemias Caused by Inherited Erythrocyte
   Defects
Aplastic and Hypoplastic Anemia

HEMOGLOBINOPATHIES

Sickle-cell Hemoglobinopathies
Other Hemoglobinopathies
Thalassemias
Polycythemia

THROMBOCYTOPENIAS

Gestational Thrombocytopenia
Inherited Thrombocytopenias
Immune Thrombocytopenic Purpura
Thrombocytosis
Thrombotic Microangiopathies
Inherited Coagulation Defects
Thrombophilias

Pregnancy induces physiological changes that often confuse the diagnosis of several hematological disorders and the assessment of their treatment. This is especially true for anemia. A number of marked pregnancy-induced hematological changes are discussed in detail in Chapter 8 (p. 177). One of the most significant changes is that of blood volume expansion with a disproportionate plasma volume increase, resulting in normally decreased hematocrit.

Pregnant women are susceptible to any of a variety of hematological abnormalities that may affect any woman of childbearing age. These include chronic disorders diagnosed before pregnancy such as hereditary anemias, immunological thrombocytopenia, and even malignancies to include leukemias and lymphomas. In other cases disorders arise during pregnancy because of pregnancy-induced demands such as iron-deficiency anemia and megaloblastic anemia of folate deficiency. In yet other cases pregnancy may unmask underlying hematological disorders such as compensated hemolytic anemias caused by hemoglobinopathies or red cell membrane defects. Finally, any hematological disease may first arise during pregnancy such as autoimmune hemolysis or aplastic anemia.

ANEMIAS

A precise definition of anemia in women is complicated by normal differences in the concentrations of hemoglobin between women and men, between white and black women, between women who are pregnant and those who are not, and between pregnant women who receive iron supplements and those who do not.

Extensive hematological measurements have been made in healthy nonpregnant women, none of whom were iron deficient because each had histochemically proven iron stores, and none were folate deficient because marrow erythropoiesis remained normoblastic. On the basis of data presented in Table 49–1, anemia

in nonpregnant women is defined as hemoglobin concentration less than 12 g/dL and less than 10 g/dL during pregnancy or the puerperium. The hemoglobin concentration is lower in midpregnancy, as shown in Figure 49–1. Early in pregnancy and again near term, the hemoglobin level of most healthy women with iron stores is 11 g/dL or higher. For these reasons, the Centers for Disease Control (1990) defined anemia as less than 11 g/dL in the first and third trimesters, and less than 10.5 g/dL in the second trimester.

The modest fall in hemoglobin levels observed during pregnancy in healthy women not deficient in iron or folate is caused by a relatively greater expansion of plasma volume compared with the increase in hemoglobin mass and red cell volume. The disproportion between the rates at which plasma and erythrocytes are added to the maternal circulation is normally greatest during the second trimester. The long-used term **physiological anemia** to describe this process is an oxymoron and should be discarded. Late in pregnancy, plasma expansion essentially ceases while hemoglobin mass continues to increase (Chap. 8, p. 177).

During the puerperium, in the absence of excessive blood loss, hemoglobin concentration is not appreciably less than predelivery. After delivery the hemoglobin level typically fluctuates to a modest degree around the predelivery value for a few days and then rises to the higher nonpregnant level. The rate and magnitude of increase early in the puerperium are the result of the amount of hemoglobin added during pregnancy and the amount lost by blood loss at delivery and modified by a puerperal decrease in plasma volume.

TABLE 49–1. Hemoglobin Concentrations in 85 Healthy Women with Proven Iron Stores

Hemoglobin (g/dL)	Nonpregnant	Midpregnancy	Late Pregnancy
Mean	13.7	11.5	12.3
Less than 12.0	1%	72%	36%
Less than 11.0	None	29%	6%
Less than 10.0	None	4%	1%
Lowest	11.7	9.7	9.8

From Scott and Pritchard (1967), with permission.

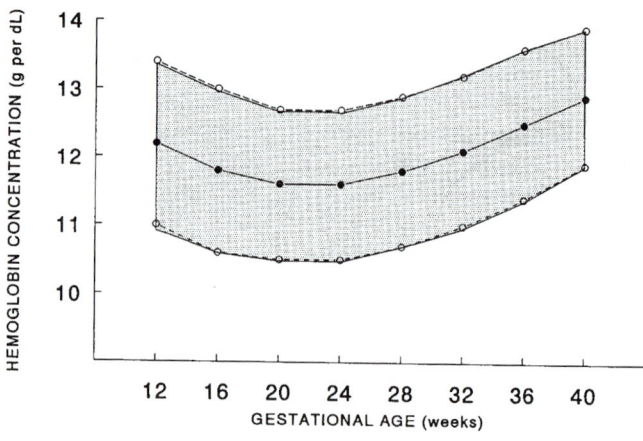

FIGURE 49–1. Mean hemoglobin concentrations (●—●) and 5th and 95th (○—○) percentiles for healthy pregnant women taking iron supplements. (Data from Centers for Disease Control, 1989a).

FREQUENCY OF ANEMIA. Although anemia is somewhat more common among indigent pregnant women, it is by no means restricted to them. The frequency of anemia during pregnancy varies considerably, depending primarily upon whether supplemental iron is taken during pregnancy. For example, Taylor and associates (1982) reported that hemoglobin levels at term averaged 12.7 g/dL among women who took supplemental iron compared with 11.2 g/dL for women who did not.

ETIOLOGY OF ANEMIA. Any disorder causing anemia encountered in childbearing-age women may complicate pregnancy. A classification based primarily on etiology and including most of the common causes of anemia in pregnant women is shown in Table 49–2.

EFFECTS OF ANEMIA ON PREGNANCY. The etiology of anemia is important when evaluating its effects on pregnancy outcome. For example, maternal and perinatal outcomes are altered markedly in women with sickle-cell anemia. Currently, there is no evidence that adverse outcomes are related to the anemia itself but rather to the vascular complications of sickling. According to Bennett and colleagues (1998), anemia per se, was seldom a cause for pregnancy-associated hospitalizations in the 1991–1992 National Hospital Discharge Data.

Most studies of the effects of anemia on pregnancy, such as those discussed in Chapter 10 (p. 235), describe large populations, and at least ostensibly deal with nutritional anemias, specifically those due to iron deficiency. Klebanoff and co-workers (1991) studied nearly 27,000 women and found a slightly increased risk of preterm birth with midtrimester anemia. Lieberman and collaborators (1987) found a positive association with low hematocrit and preterm birth in black women, and suggested that anemia was a marker for nutritional deficiencies. Anemia may be associated with fetal growth restriction. According to Barker and colleagues (1990), this may lead to adult cardiovascular disease (Chap. 29, p. 757). Kadyrov and co-workers (1998) have provided evidence that maternal anemia influences placental vascularization by altering angiogenesis during early pregnancy.

According to the World Health Organization, anemia has been implicated as contributory in up to 40 percent of maternal deaths in third-world countries (Viteri, 1994). Ironically, in otherwise healthy women, higher hemoglobin concentrations are more likely associated with adverse pregnancy outcome. In these cases, the normal blood volume expansion of pregnancy appears to have been curtailed. Murphy and colleagues (1986) reported findings from the Cardiff Birth Survey of over 54,000 singleton pregnancies and described excessive perinatal mortality with high hemoglobin concentrations. Specifically, women whose hemoglobin concentration exceeded 13.2 g/dL at 13 to 18 weeks had excessive perinatal mortality, low-birthweight infants, and preterm delivery, as well as preeclampsia in nulliparas. Scanlon and associates (2000) studied the relationship between maternal hemoglobin and preterm or growth-restricted infants in 173,031 pregnancies. Low hemoglobin (< 3 SD) at 12 weeks was associated with a 1.7-fold risk for preterm birth whereas high hemoglobin (> 3 SD) at 12 or 18 weeks had 1.3- to 1.8-fold increases in fetal growth restriction.

IRON-DEFICIENCY ANEMIA. The two most common causes of anemia during pregnancy and the puerperium are iron deficiency and acute blood loss. Not infrequently, the two are intimately related, because excessive blood loss with its concomitant loss of hemoglobin iron and exhaustion of iron stores in one pregnancy can be an important cause of iron-deficiency anemia in the next pregnancy.

Iron deficiency is common in women, and the Centers for Disease Control and Prevention (1989) estimate that about 8 million American women of childbearing age are iron deficient. Poor nutritional status frequently is associated with iron-deficiency anemia (Scholl, 1998). In a typical gestation with a single fetus, the maternal need for iron induced by pregnancy averages close to 800 mg; about 300 mg for the fetus and placenta and about 500 mg, if available, for maternal hemoglobin mass expansion. Approximately 200 mg more are shed through the gut, urine, and skin. This total amount—1000 mg—considerably exceeds the iron stores of most women. Unless the difference between the amount of stored iron available to the mother and the iron requirements of normal pregnancy cited is compensated for by absorption of iron from the gastrointestinal tract, iron-deficiency anemia develops.

With the rather rapid expansion of blood volume during the second trimester, iron lack is often manifested by an appreciable drop in hemoglobin concentra-

TABLE 49–2. Causes of Anemia During Pregnancy

Acquired
Iron-deficiency anemia
Anemia caused by acute blood loss
Anemia of inflammation or malignancy
Megaloblastic anemia
Acquired hemolytic anemia
Aplastic or hypoplastic anemia
Hereditary
Thalassemias
Sickle-cell hemoglobinopathies
Other hemoglobinopathies
Hereditary hemolytic anemias

tion. Although the rate of expansion of blood volume is not so great in the third trimester, the need for iron is still increased because augmentation of maternal hemoglobin mass continues, and considerable iron is now transported to the fetus. Because the amount of iron diverted to the fetus from an iron-deficient mother is not much different from the amount normally transferred, the newborn infant of a severely anemic mother does not suffer from iron-deficiency anemia. Neonatal iron stores are related to maternal iron status (Blot and co-workers, 1999). They are also influenced by when and how the cord is clamped (Chap. 13, p. 319).

DIAGNOSIS. Classical morphological evidence of iron-deficiency anemia—erythrocyte hypochromia and microcytosis—is less prominent in the pregnant woman compared with the nonpregnant woman with the same hemoglobin concentration. Moderate iron-deficiency anemia during pregnancy—for example, a hemoglobin concentration of 9 g/dL—usually is not accompanied by obvious morphological changes in erythrocytes. With this degree of anemia from iron deficiency, however, serum ferritin levels are lower than normal, and there is no stainable bone marrow iron. The serum iron-binding capacity is elevated, but by itself this is of little diagnostic value because it also is elevated during normal pregnancy in the absence of iron deficiency. Moderate normoblastic hyperplasia of the bone marrow also is found to be similar to that in normal pregnancy. **Thus, iron-deficiency anemia during pregnancy is the consequence primarily of expansion of plasma volume without normal expansion of maternal hemoglobin mass.**

The initial evaluation of a pregnant woman with moderate anemia should include measurements of hemoglobin, hematocrit, and red cell indices; careful examination of a peripheral blood smear; a sickle-cell preparation if the woman is of African origin; and measurement of serum iron concentration or ferritin, or both. Serum ferritin levels normally decline during pregnancy (Goldenberg and colleagues, 1996). Levels less than 15 μg/L confirm iron-deficiency anemia (Centers for Disease Control and Prevention, 1989). Alternatively, van den Broek and colleagues (1998) provided evidence that a cutoff point of 30 μg/L has an 85 percent positive-predictive value and a 90 percent negative-predictive value. Pragmatically, the diagnosis of iron deficiency in moderately anemic pregnant women usually is presumptive and based largely on the exclusion of other causes of anemia.

When the pregnant woman with moderate iron-deficiency anemia is given adequate iron therapy, a hematological response is detected by an elevated reticulocyte count. The rate of increase of hemoglobin concentration or hematocrit varies considerably, but usually it is slower than in nonpregnant women. The reason is

related largely to the differences in blood volumes, and during the latter half of pregnancy, newly formed hemoglobin is added to the characteristically much larger volume.

TREATMENT. The objectives of treatment are correction of the deficit in hemoglobin mass and eventually restitution of iron stores. Both of these objectives can be accomplished with orally administered, simple iron compounds—ferrous sulfate, fumarate, or gluconate—that provide a daily dose of about 200 mg of **elemental iron.** If the woman cannot or will not take oral iron preparations, then parenteral therapy is given (Andrews, 1999; Hallak and associates, 1997). To replenish iron stores, oral therapy should be continued for 3 months or so after the anemia has been corrected.

Transfusions of red cells or whole blood seldom are indicated for the treatment of iron-deficiency anemia unless hypovolemia from blood loss coexists or an emergency operative procedure must be performed on a *severely* anemic woman.

ANEMIA FROM ACUTE BLOOD LOSS. Anemia resulting from recent hemorrhage is more likely to be evident during the puerperium. Both abruptio placentae and placenta previa may be sources of serious blood loss and of anemia before as well as after delivery. Earlier in pregnancy, anemia caused by acute blood loss is common in instances of abortion, ectopic pregnancy, and hydatidiform mole. Massive hemorrhage demands immediate treatment to restore and maintain perfusion of vital organs (Chap. 25, p. 635). Even though the amount of blood replaced commonly does not completely repair the hemoglobin deficit created by the hemorrhage, in general, once dangerous hypovolemia has been overcome and hemostasis has been achieved, the residual anemia should be treated with iron. For the moderately anemic woman whose hemoglobin is more than 7 g/dL, whose condition is stable, who no longer faces the likelihood of further serious hemorrhage, who can ambulate without adverse symptoms, and who is not febrile, iron therapy for at least 3 months rather than blood transfusions is the best treatment.

ANEMIA ASSOCIATED WITH CHRONIC DISEASE. Weakness, weight loss, and pallor have been recognized since antiquity as characteristics of chronic disease. A wide variety of disorders—chronic infections and neoplasms, especially—result in moderate and sometimes severe anemia, usually with slightly hypochromic and microcytic erythrocytes. In the past, infections—especially tuberculosis, endocarditis, or osteomyelitis—were common causes, but antimicrobial therapy has decreased their incidences significantly. Today, chronic renal failure, cancer and chemotherapy, human immunodeficiency virus (HIV) infection, and chronic inflammation are the most common causes of this form of anemia. The common denominator is increased production of cytokines that mediate the immune or inflammatory response (Means, 1999).

In nonpregnant patients with chronic inflammatory diseases, the hemoglobin concentration is rarely less than 7 g/dL. Typically, bone marrow cellular morphology is not altered markedly. Serum iron concentration is decreased, and serum iron-binding capacity, while lower than in normal pregnancy, is not much below the normal nonpregnant range. Serum ferritin levels usually are elevated. Thus, although slightly different from each other mechanistically, these anemias share similar features which include varying degrees and combinations of alterations in reticuloendothelial function, iron metabolism, and decreased erythropoiesis (Andrews, 1999).

During pregnancy, a number of chronic diseases may cause anemia. Some of these are chronic renal disease, suppuration, inflammatory bowel disease, systemic lupus erythematosus, granulomatous infections, malignant neoplasms, and rheumatoid arthritis. Anemia is typically intensified as plasma volume expands out of proportion to red cell mass expansion. Women with severe **acute pyelonephritis** often develop overt anemia. This appears to result from increased red cell destruction but with normal erythropoietin production (Cavenee and colleagues, 1994).

CHRONIC RENAL DISEASE. Any type of chronic renal insufficiency can be accompanied by anemia of variable severity, usually due to erythropoietin deficiency. There is also an element of anemia of chronic disease. During pregnancy, red cell mass is augmented in some of these women, but less so than in normal pregnancy (Cunningham and associates, 1990). The degree of red cell mass expansion corresponds to the degree of renal impairment, and because total blood volume expansion usually is normal in these women, preexisting anemia is intensified.

TREATMENT. Anemia of chronic disorders responds to treatment with **recombinant erythropoietin.** It has been used successfully to treat anemia associated with chronic renal insufficiency, chronic inflammation, and malignancy (Goodnough and associates, 1997). From their review, Vora and Gruslin (1998) found only a few reports of its use during pregnancy. Braga and colleagues (1996) treated five women with severe anemia from chronic renal insufficiency. We have treated only a few pregnant women whose anemia was due to chronic renal insufficiency. While red cell mass usually increased over several weeks, a worrisome side effect is hypertension, which is already prevalent in these women (Chap. 47,

p. 1264). In the study by Braga and co-workers (1996) cited earlier, one of five treated women developed placental abruption.

MEGALOBLASTIC ANEMIA. Megaloblastic anemias are a family of hematological disorders whose characteristic blood and bone marrow abnormalities are caused by impaired DNA synthesis. The prevalence of megaloblastic anemia during pregnancy varies considerably throughout the world, and it is now rare in the United States.

FOLIC ACID DEFICIENCY. In the United States, megaloblastic anemia beginning during pregnancy almost always results from folic acid deficiency, and in the past was referred to as **pernicious anemia of pregnancy.** It usually is found in women who do not consume fresh green leafy vegetables, legumes, or animal protein. Women with megaloblastic anemia may have developed troublesome nausea, vomiting, and anorexia during pregnancy. As the folate deficiency and anemia worsen, anorexia often becomes more intense, further aggravating the dietary deficiency. In some instances, excessive ethanol ingestion is either the cause or contributes to its development.

In normal nonpregnant women, the daily folic acid requirement is 50 to 100 μg/day. During pregnancy, requirements for folic acid are increased, and as discussed in Chapter 10 (p. 237), 400 μg/day is recommended. The earliest biochemical evidence is low folic acid activity in plasma. The earliest morphological evidence usually is hypersegmentation of neutrophils. As anemia develops, the newly formed erythrocytes are macrocytic. With preexisting iron deficiency, macrocytic erythrocytes cannot be detected by measurement of the mean corpuscular volume. Careful examination of a smear of peripheral blood, however, usually will demonstrate some macrocytes. As the anemia becomes more intense, an occasional nucleated erythrocyte appears in the peripheral blood. At the same time, examination of the bone marrow discloses megaloblastic erythropoiesis. Anemia may then become severe, and thrombocytopenia, leukopenia, or both also may develop.

The fetus and placenta extract folate from maternal circulation so effectively that the fetus is not anemic even when the mother is severely anemic from folate deficiency. Cases have been recorded in which newborn hemoglobin levels were 18 g/dL or more, while maternal values were as low as 3.6 g/dL (Pritchard and Scott, 1970).

TREATMENT. The treatment of pregnancy-induced megaloblastic anemia should include folic acid, a nutritious diet, and iron. As little as 1 mg of folic acid administered orally once daily produces a striking hematological response. By 4 to 7 days after beginning treatment, the reticulocyte count is increased appreciably, and leukopenia and thrombocytopenia are corrected promptly. Sometimes the rate of increase in hemoglobin concentration or hematocrit is disappointing, especially when compared with the usual exuberant reticulocytosis that starts soon after therapy has been initiated.

PREVENTION. A diet sufficient in folic acid prevents megaloblastic anemia. A great deal of attention has been devoted to the role of folate deficiency in the genesis of neural-tube defects (Chap. 10, p. 237; Chap. 36, p. 958). These findings led the Centers for Disease Control (1992) and the American College of Obstetricians and Gynecologists (1996) to recommend that all childbearing-age women consume at least 0.4 mg of folic acid daily. Additional folic acid is given in circumstances where folate requirements are unusually excessive, as in multifetal pregnancy or hemolytic anemia, such as sickle-cell disease. Other indications include Crohn disease, alcoholism, and some inflammatory skin disorders. There is evidence that women who previously have had infants with neural-tube defects have a lower recurrence rate if folic acid, 4 mg daily, is given prior to and through early pregnancy.

VITAMIN B$_{12}$ DEFICIENCY. Megaloblastic anemia caused by lack of vitamin B$_{12}$ during pregnancy is exceedingly rare. **Addisonian pernicious anemia** is characterized by the failure to absorb vitamin B$_{12}$ because of lack of intrinsic factor. It is an extremely uncommon autoimmune disease in women of reproductive age, and typically has its onset in women over 40. Moreover, unless women with this disease are treated with vitamin B$_{12}$, infertility may be a complication. In our limited experience, vitamin B$_{12}$ deficiency in pregnant women is more likely encountered following partial or total gastric resection. Other causes are Crohn disease, ileal resection, and bacterial overgrowth in the small bowel.

Serum vitamin B$_{12}$ levels are measured by radioimmunoassay. During pregnancy, these normally are lower than nonpregnant values because of decreased serum concentrations of B$_{12}$-carrier proteins, the **transcobalamins** (Zamorano and colleagues, 1985). Women who have had a total gastrectomy should be given 1000 mg of cyanocobalamin (vitamin B$_{12}$) intramuscularly at monthly intervals. Those with a partial gastrectomy usually do not need such therapy, but vitamin B$_{12}$ levels during pregnancy should be measured. There is little reason for withholding folic acid during pregnancy simply out of fear of jeopardizing the neurological integrity of women who might be pregnant and simultaneously have unrecognized, and therefore untreated, Addisonian pernicious anemia.

ACQUIRED HEMOLYTIC ANEMIAS

AUTOIMMUNE HEMOLYTIC ANEMIA. This is an uncommon condition and the cause for aberrant antibody production is unknown. Anemias caused by these factors may be due to warm-active autoantibodies (80 to 90 percent), cold-active antibodies, or a combination. These syndromes also may be classified as primary or idiopathic, and half are secondary to underlying diseases or other factors. Examples of the latter include lymphomas and leukemias, connective-tissue diseases, some infections, chronic inflammatory diseases, or drug-induced factors (Provan and Weatherall, 2000). In some cases classified initially as idiopathic, careful follow-up may allow detection of an underlying disease.

With autoimmune hemolytic anemia, typically both the direct and indirect antiglobulin (Coombs) tests are positive. Hemolysis and the positive antiglobulin tests may be the consequence of either IgM or IgG antierythrocyte antibodies. Spherocytosis and reticulocytosis are characteristic of the peripheral blood smear. **Cold-agglutinin disease** may be induced by *Mycoplasma pneumoniae* or infectious mononucleosis.

Women with autoimmune hemolytic anemia sometimes demonstrate marked acceleration of hemolysis during pregnancy. Glucocorticoids usually are effective as in the nonpregnant state, and treatment is with prednisone, 1 mg/kg per day, or its equivalent. Coincidental thrombocytopenia usually is corrected by therapy.

IgM antibodies do not cross the placenta and thus fetal red cells are not affected; however, IgG antibodies, especially subclasses IgG$_1$ and IgG$_3$, do cross. The most common example of adverse fetal effects from maternally produced IgG antibodies is maternal D isoimmunization with hemolytic disease in the fetus and neonate (Chap. 39, p. 1057). Transfusion of red cells for the mother with severe autoimmune hemolytic disease is complicated by the presence of circulating antierythrocyte antibodies. Warming the donor cells to body temperature decreases their destruction by cold agglutinins.

DRUG-INDUCED HEMOLYTIC ANEMIA. Drug-induced hemolysis encountered during pregnancy must be differentiated from other forms of autoimmune hemolytic anemia. Hemolysis typically is mild; it resolves upon withdrawing the drug, and it can be prevented by avoidance of the drug. Mechanisms of actions differ, but generally they are mechanisms of drug-mediated immunological injury to red cells. The drug acts as a high-affinity hapten with a red cell protein to which antidrug antibodies attach, for example IgM antipenicillin antibodies. It may act as a low-affinity hapten and adhere to cell membrane proteins. Some drugs that may induce antierythrocyte antibodies that might be used during pregnancy are shown in Table 49–3.

The severity of symptoms depends on the degree of hemolysis. Usually there is mild to moderate chronic hemolysis, but some drugs that act as low-affinity haptens may precipitate severe acute hemolysis. Garratty and associates (1999) recently described seven cases of severe hemolytic anemia caused by cefotetan prophylaxis for obstetrical procedures. The direct antiglobulin test is positive; there is spherocytosis and reticulocytosis; and there may be thrombocytopenia and leukopenia. In most cases, withdrawing the offending drug results in reversal of symptoms. Corticosteroids are of questionable efficacy, and transfusions are given only if there is severe anemia. Especially in African-American women, drug-induced hemolysis is much more often related to a congenital erythrocyte enzymatic defect, such as severe **glucose-6-phosphate dehydrogenase (G6PD) deficiency** (p. 1314).

PREGNANCY-INDUCED HEMOLYTIC ANEMIA. Unexplained hemolytic anemia during pregnancy is a rare but apparently distinct entity in which severe hemolysis develops early in pregnancy and resolves within months after delivery. It is characterized by no evidence for an immune mechanism or for any intraerythrocytic or extraerythrocytic defects (Starksen and associates, 1983). Because the fetus-infant also may demonstrate transient hemolysis, an immunological cause is suspected. Maternal corticosteroid treatment usually is effective. We have observed one woman with recurrent hemolysis during several pregnancies, and in each instance, intense severe hemolytic anemia was controlled by prednisone given until delivery. Her children appear to be normal.

TABLE 49–3. Some Drugs Associated with Positive Red Cell Antiglobulin Tests

Drug	Immune Injury
Acetaminophen	Uncertain
Cephalosporins	High-affinity hapten
Chlorpromazine	Uncertain
Erythromycin	Uncertain
Ibuprofen	Uncertain
Isoniazid	Uncertain
Methyldopa	Autoantibody induction
Penicillins	Hapten
Probenecid	Low-affinity hapten
Quinidine	Low-affinity hapten
Rifampin	Low-affinity hapten
Thiopental	Low-affinity hapten

PAROXYSMAL NOCTURNAL HEMOGLOBINURIA. Although commonly regarded as a hemolytic anemia, this is a hemopoietic stem cell disorder characterized by formation of defective platelets, granulocytes, and erythrocytes. Paroxysmal nocturnal hemoglobinuria is acquired and arises from one abnormal clone of cells, much like a neoplasm (Packham, 1998). One mutated X-linked gene responsible for this condition is termed **PIG-A** for phosphatidylinositol glycan protein A. Resultant abnormal anchor proteins of erythrocyte and granulocyte membrane makes them unusually susceptible to lysis by complement (Provan and Weatherall, 2000).

Its clinical manifestation is that of acquired hemolytic anemia that has an insidious onset and a chronic course. Hemoglobinuria develops at irregular intervals and is not necessarily nocturnal. Hemolysis may be initiated by transfusions, infections, or surgery. The severity of disease ranges from mild to lethal. Complications include those from chronic anemia, which is exacerbated by iron deficiency from urinary loss of iron. Almost 40 percent of patients suffer venous thromboses, and the Budd–Chiari syndrome caused by hepatic vein thrombosis has been observed. Renal abnormalities and hypertension also are common. Median survival after diagnosis is 10 years but 15 percent undergo spontaneous long-term remission (Hillmen and colleagues, 1995). Except possibly for marrow transplantation, no definitive treatment exists.

EFFECTS ON PREGNANCY. Paroxysmal nocturnal hemoglobinuria is a serious and unpredictable disease and pregnancy may be dangerous. Greene and colleagues (1983) reviewed 31 cases in pregnancy and found that complications developed in over three fourths. Maternal mortality was 10 percent and almost half of the women had postpartum venous thrombosis, including Budd–Chiari syndrome or cerebral vein thrombosis. Solal-Céligny and co-workers (1988) reported eight pregnancies of which only half resulted in surviving infants. In a multicenter study, De Gramont and colleagues (1987) reported complications during two thirds of 38 pregnancies. Although they observed no maternal deaths, life-threatening complications were common, especially from hemolysis and hemorrhage.

OTHER ACQUIRED ANEMIAS. As described by Pritchard and associates (1976), overt fragmentation (microangiopathic) hemolysis with visible hemoglobinemia infrequently complicates **preeclampsia–eclampsia.** This commonly is referred to as **HELLP syndrome,** from *H*emolysis, *EL*evated liver enzymes, and *L*ow *P*latelets (Chap. 24, p. 579). The most fulminant acquired hemolytic anemia encountered during pregnancy is caused by the exotoxin of *Clostridium perfringens* (Chap. 33,

p. 877) or that of group A β-hemolytic streptococcus (Chap. 26, p. 678). Finally, Gram-negative bacterial endotoxin, or lipopolysaccharide, especially with severe acute pyelonephritis, may be accompanied by evidence of hemolysis and mild to moderate anemia (Cox and colleagues, 1991).

HEMOLYTIC ANEMIAS CAUSED BY INHERITED ERYTHROCYTE DEFECTS The normal erythrocyte is shaped like a biconcave disc, and there is a redundancy of membrane surface area relative to volume. This allows numerous cycles of reversible deformations as the erythrocyte withstands shearing forces created in arteries and negotiates through splenic slits a fraction of its cross-sectional diameter. A number of inherited red cell membrane defects or enzyme deficiencies result in destabilization of the membrane lipid bilayer. Subsequent loss of lipids from the erythrocyte membrane, surface area deficiency, and poorly deformable cells that undergo hemolysis results in varying degrees of anemia. Some of these inherited membrane defects that will cause accelerated destruction are hereditary spherocytosis, pyropoikilocytosis, and ovalocytosis.

HEREDITARY SPHEROCYTOSIS. There are several inherited erythrocyte membrane protein deficiencies that give rise to the syndrome of hereditary spherocytosis. Although most are due to autosomally dominant variably penetrant **spectrin** deficiency, others are autosomally recessive and may be caused by **ankyrin** or **protein 4.2** deficiency or combinations thereof (Rosse and Bunn, 1994). These disorders are characterized clinically by varying degrees of anemia and jaundice as the consequence of hemolysis of microspherocytic red cells (Fig. 49–2). Confirmation of diagnosis is by documentation of spherocytes on peripheral smear, reticulocytosis, and increased osmotic fragility.

Hemolysis with corresponding anemia is dependent upon an intact spleen, which is usually enlarged. Splenectomy, although not correcting the membrane defect, spherocytosis, or increased osmotic fragility, does greatly reduce hemolysis, anemia, and jaundice. So-called **crisis,** characterized by severe anemia from accelerated red cell destruction or more likely failure of production, or both, may develop in the woman with a functioning spleen. Infection must be detected and vigorously treated.

PREGNANCY. In general, women with hereditary spherocytosis do well during pregnancy. Folic acid supplementation is recommended. Maberry and associates (1992) reported our experiences from Parkland Hospital with 50 pregnancies in 23 women with spherocytosis. In late pregnancy, hematocrits varied from 23 to 41 percent (mean 31) and reticulocyte counts ranged from 1 to 23

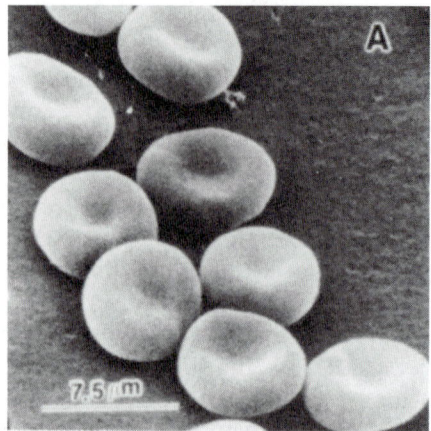

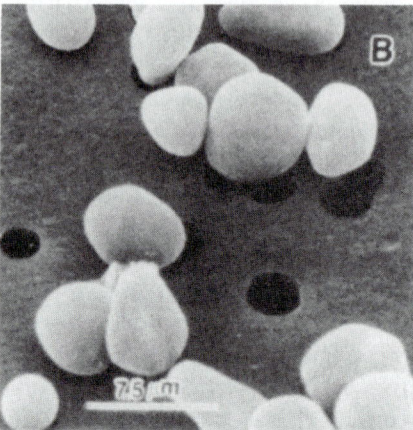

FIGURE 49–2. Scanning electron micrograph showing normal-appearing erythrocytes from a heterozygous carrier of recessive spherocytosis (**A**) and her daughter, a homozygote with severe anemia (**B**). (From Agre, 1989, with permission.)

percent. There was minimal maternal morbidity. There were eight abortions, and four of 42 infants were born preterm but none were growth retarded. Infection in four women intensified hemolysis and three required transfusions. Similar results were reported by Pajor and colleagues (1993) in 19 pregnancies in eight Hungarian women.

The newborn infant who has inherited hereditary spherocytosis may or may not demonstrate hyperbilirubinemia and anemia during the neonatal period. We observed the hemoglobin level to fall to as low as 5.0 g/dL by 5 weeks of age in the daughter of a woman with hereditary spherocytosis.

RED CELL ENZYME DEFICIENCIES. A number of erythrocyte enzymes are necessary for its anaerobic utilization of glucose. A deficiency of many but certainly not all of these enzymes may cause **hereditary nonspherocytic anemia.** Most of are inherited as autosomal recessive traits. **Glucose-6-phosphate dehydrogenase deficiency,** by far the most commonly identified enzyme deficiency, is a well-known exception that is X-linked. There are over 400 variants of this enzyme (Beutler, 1991). In the A variant, inherited by about 2 percent of African-American women, erythrocytes are markedly deficient in normal enzyme activity. In this, the deficient or homozygous state, both X chromosomes are affected. The heterozygous state, with one deficient and one normal X chromosome, is identified in 10 to 15 percent of African-American women. The defect probably confers some degree of protection against malarial infection. Random X-chromosome inactivation results in a variable deficiency of enzyme activity. Infections or several oxidant drugs may induce hemolysis in some heterozygous as well as homozygous women. Thus, anemia is episodic, although some variants induce chronic nonspherocytic hemolysis. Because young erythrocytes contain more enzyme activity than do older erythrocytes, in the absence of bone marrow depression, anemia ultimately stabilizes and is corrected soon after the drug is discontinued.

Pyruvate kinase deficiency, although unusual, is probably the next most common enzyme deficiency. It is inherited as an autosomal recessive trait. Ghidini and Korker (1998) described conservative management without transfusions in a woman whose hemoglobin reached a nadir of 6.8 g/dL at midpregnancy. Gilsanz and colleagues (1993) described recurrent hydrops fetalis, due to homozygously affected fetuses. In a fourth pregnancy, they diagnosed fetal anemia and lack of pyruvate kinase deficiency using funipuncture.

There are a number of other very rare enzyme abnormalities that may cause hemolysis, and some that do not. Although the degree of chronic hemolysis varies, most episodes of severe anemia with all of these enzyme deficiencies are induced by drugs or infections as previously discussed. During pregnancy, iron and folic acid are given. Oxidant drugs are avoided, and bacterial infections are treated promptly. Transfusions with red cells are given only if the hematocrit falls below 20, unless there is evidence for heart failure or hypoxia.

APLASTIC AND HYPOPLASTIC ANEMIA. Although rarely encountered during pregnancy, aplastic anemia is a grave complication. The diagnosis is made when anemia, usually with thrombocytopenia, leukopenia, and markedly hypocellular bone marrow, is demonstrated (Marsh and colleagues, 1999). In about a third of cases, anemia is induced by drugs and other chemicals, infection, irradiation, leukemia, and immunological disorders. *Fanconi anemia* and *Diamond–Blackfan syndrome* are inherited. In the other two thirds of cases, a cause cannot be determined (Provan and Weatherall, 2000). The basic functional defect appears to be a marked decrease in committed marrow stem cells. There

is considerable evidence that the condition is immunologically mediated (Young and Maciejewski, 1997). With severe disease, defined as bone marrow hypocellularity of less than 25 percent, the 1-year survival rate is only 20 percent.

APLASTIC ANEMIA DURING PREGNANCY. In most cases, aplastic anemia and pregnancy appear to have been a chance association. Because about a third of women improved following termination of pregnancy, it has been postulated that pregnancy induces erythroid hypoplasia in some way (Aitchison and colleagues, 1989). Certainly, in a few women, hypoplastic anemia has been identified first during a pregnancy and then improved or even resolved when the pregnancy terminated, only to recur with a subsequent pregnancy (Bourantas and associates, 1997; Snyder and colleagues, 1991).

Rijhsinghani and Wiechert (1994) described two pregnancies in a woman with *Diamond–Blackfan anemia*. This rare form of pure red cell aplasia may be inherited as autosomally recessive. Some patients respond to glucocorticoid therapy, but most are transfusion-dependent. Our experiences with two such women are similar. *Gaucher disease* is an autosomally recessive lysosomal enzyme deficiency that has multisystem involvement. Anemia and thrombocytopenia are worsened by pregnancy (Granovsky-Grisaru and associates, 1995). Subsequently, this same Israeli group showed that *alglucerase* enzyme replacement improved pregnancy outcomes in six women (Elstein and colleagues, 1997).

The two great risks to the pregnant woman with aplastic anemia are hemorrhage and infection (Ascarelli and co-workers, 1998). In cases reported since 1960, mortality during or after pregnancy has been 50 percent, and almost invariably, mortality is due to bleeding or sepsis. *Fanconi anemia* appears to be associated with a better prognosis. Alter and colleagues (1991) reviewed the literature and concluded that women who become pregnant had less severe disease.

MANAGEMENT. None of the erythropoietic agents that predictably produce remission in other anemias are effective. The treatment for severe aplastic anemia that is most likely to be effective is **bone-marrow or stem-cell transplantation.** For patients with less severe disease, or those for whom a donor cannot be found, **antithymocyte globulin** is the best available therapy (Marsh and associates, 1999). Immunosuppressive therapy with cyclosporine improves the response to antithymocyte globulin. Corticosteroids are possibly of value, as are large doses of testosterone or other androgenic steroids. Treated women almost certainly become virilized. The female fetus may develop the stigmata of androgen excess (pseudohermaphroditism), depending upon the compound, dose, and capacity of the placenta to aromatize the androgen (Chap. 7, p. 121).

A continuous search for infection should be made, and when found, specific antimicrobial therapy should be started promptly. Granulocyte transfusions are given only during actual infection. Red cell transfusions are given for symptomatic anemia, and we transfuse routinely to maintain the hematocrit at about 20. If the platelet count is very low, platelet transfusions may be needed to control hemorrhage. Vaginal delivery performed so as to minimize incisions and lacerations will lessen blood loss if the uterus is stimulated to contract vigorously after delivery. Even when thrombocytopenia is intense, the risk of severe hemorrhage can be minimized by vaginal delivery performed to avoid lacerations and an extensive episiotomy.

BONE MARROW TRANSPLANTATION. This requires immunosuppressive therapy for some months after transplantation. Previous blood transfusions, and even pregnancy, enhance the risk of graft rejection. For patients who are disease free at 2 years, survival rates of 90 percent accrue with transplantation (Deeg and colleagues, 1998). Acute and chronic graft-versus-host disease is the most common serious complication and causes two thirds of deaths within the first two years (Socié and co-workers, 1999). This same group reported that half of 95 women patients subsequently became pregnant.

There have been a number of case reports of successful pregnancies in women who previously had undergone bone marrow transplantation (Borgna-Pignatti and associates, 1996; Eliyahu and Shalev, 1994). We have followed only two women with prior marrow transplantation, and both demonstrated a normal pregnancy-induced hematological response to pregnancy and had uneventful courses. Sanders and colleagues (1996) reviewed outcomes in 41 women with 72 pregnancies following bone marrow transplantation. Excluding 20 early pregnancy losses and terminations, the remaining 52 were productive of live-born infants. Almost half of these pregnancies were complicated—25 percent of the total had preterm delivery and 15 percent had hypertension.

HEMOGLOBINOPATHIES

SICKLE-CELL HEMOGLOBINOPATHIES. Sickle hemoglobin (hemoglobin S) results from a single β-chain substitution of glutamic acid by valine because of an A for T substitution at codon 6 of the β-globin gene. Sickle-cell anemia (SS disease), sickle cell–hemoglobin C disease (SC disease), and sickle cell–β-thalassemia disease

(S–β-thalassemia disease) are the most common of the sickle hemoglobinopathies. Maternal morbidity and mortality, abortion, and perinatal mortality are all increased with these hemoglobinopathies.

PATHOPHYSIOLOGY. Red cells with hemoglobin S undergo sickling when they are deoxygenated and the hemoglobin aggregates. Constant sickling and de-sickling causes membrane damage, and the cell may become irreversibly sickled. Clinically, the hallmark of sickling episodes are periods during which there is ischemia and infarction within various organs. These changes produce clinical symptoms, predominately pain, and are called "sickle crisis." There often is severe pain with sickle-cell disease, and there may be aplastic, megaloblastic, sequestration, and hemolytic crises. In a study of 392 infants with sickle-cell disease diagnosed before 6 months, Miller and associates (2000) reported that 18 percent had severe morbidity when followed for a mean of 10 years.

Chronic and acute changes from sickling include bony abnormalities such as osteonecrosis of femoral and humeral heads, renal medullary damage, autosplenectomy in homozygous SS patients and splenomegaly in other variants, hepatomegaly, ventricular hypertrophy, pulmonary infarctions, cerebrovascular accidents, leg ulcers, and a propensity to infection and sepsis with Gram-positive as well as Gram-negative organisms (Serjeant, 1997; Weatherall and Provan, 2000). The median age at death is 42 years for men and 48 years for women (Platt and associates, 1994).

INHERITANCE OF SICKLING SYNDROMES. The inheritance of the gene for S hemoglobin from each parent results in sickle-cell anemia (SS disease). In the United States, 1 of 12 African Americans has the sickle-cell trait, which results from inheritance of one gene for the production of S hemoglobin and one for normal hemoglobin A. The theoretical incidence of sickle-cell anemia among African Americans is 1 in 576 ($1/12 \times 1/12 \times 1/4 = 576$), but the disease is less common during pregnancy because of earlier mortality, especially during early childhood.

About 1 in 40 African Americans has the gene for hemoglobin C. Therefore, the probability of hemoglobin S and C traits in a black couple is about 1 in 500 ($1/40 \times 1/12$), and the probability of their child co-inheriting the gene for hemoglobin S and an allelic gene for hemoglobin C is 1 in 4. As the consequence of these genetic frequencies, about 1 of 2000 ($1/12 \times 1/40 \times 1/4$) pregnant African-American women is expected to have SC disease.

The inheritance of the gene for hemoglobin S from one parent and the allelic gene for β-thalassemia from the other results in sickle cell–β-thalassemia disease.

Because the incidence of β-thalassemia minor is about 1 in 40 to 50, S–β-thalassemia occurs about 1 in 2000 (1/12 × 1/40 × 1/4).

PREGNANCY AND SICKLE-CELL SYNDROME. Pregnancy is a serious burden to women with sickle hemoglobinopathies, especially hemoglobin SS disease. Ischemic necrosis of multiple organs, but especially bone marrow causes severe pain—so-called **sickle-cell crisis**—usually becoming more frequent, and infections and pulmonary complications are more common. Powars and colleagues (1986), in an extensive review, compared maternal and perinatal outcomes from before and after 1972. They reported that maternal mortality fell from 6 to 1 percent in these two periods. Poddar and colleagues (1986) reported a maternal mortality rate of 7 per 644 (1.1 percent) in pregnant women with hemoglobin SS disease. In some Nigerian studies, maternal mortality rates ranged from 2 to 9 percent.

As shown in Table 49–4, in addition to excessive maternal mortality, more than a third of pregnancies in women with sickle syndromes terminated in abortion, stillbirth, or neonatal death. Smith and associates (1996) provided data from the National Institutes of Health Cooperative Study of Sickle Cell Disease. Of 155 women with SS disease, there were 320 pregnancies. A third were terminated either by elective or spontaneous abortions, the stillbirth rate was 9 per 1000, and 63 percent of infants were born alive.

HEMOGLOBIN SC. In nonpregnant women, morbidity and mortality from sickle cell–hemoglobin C disease are appreciably lower than from sickle-cell anemia. Indeed, fewer than half of women with SC disease have ever been symptomatic prior to pregnancy. During pregnancy and the puerperium, however, attacks of severe bone pain and episodes of pulmonary infarction and embolization become more common (Cunningham and

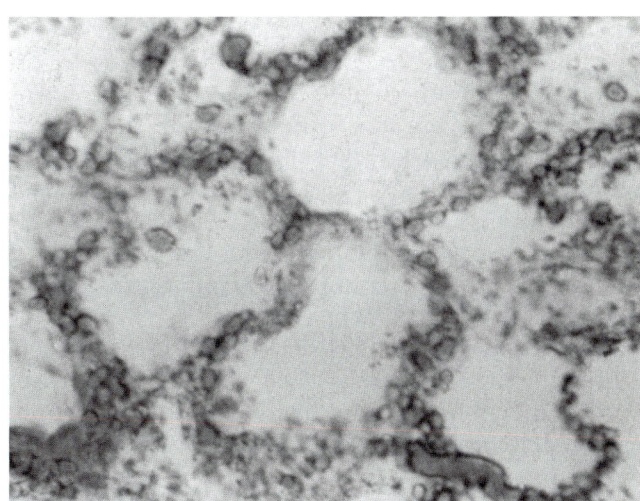

FIGURE 49–3. Photomicrograph from the lung of a 21-year-old primipara who died 36 hours postpartum after developing acute dyspnea. There was massive fat and bone marrow embolized to both lungs. (From Maberry and Cunningham, 1993.)

associates, 1983). A particularly worrisome pulmonary complication is related to embolization of necrotic bone marrow, both fat and cellular, and acute respiratory insufficiency may develop (Fig. 49–3). In an 18-year anterospective study at Parkland Hospital, the maternal mortality rate for women with hemoglobin SC disease was close to 2 percent (Pritchard and coworkers, 1973). As shown in Table 49–4, maternal deaths with hemoglobin SC disease were as common as with SS disease. The perinatal mortality rate is somewhat greater than that of the general population but nowhere as great as with sickle-cell anemia. In 39 women with SC hemoglobin who had 77 pregnancies, Smith and colleagues (1996) reported no maternal or fetal deaths.

MANAGEMENT OF SICKLING SYNDROMES. Adequate management of pregnant women with sickle-cell anemia or other sickle-cell hemoglobinopathies necessitates close observation with careful evaluation of all symptoms, physical findings, and laboratory studies. In the absence of infection or nutritional deficiency, the hemoglobin concentration usually does not fall below 7 g/dL. Because these women maintain their hemoglobin concentration by intense hemopoiesis to compensate for the markedly shortened erythrocyte life span, any factor that impairs erythropoiesis or increases red cell destruction, or both, aggravates the anemia. The folic acid requirements during pregnancy complicated by sickle-cell anemia are considerable and supplementary folic acid of 1 mg/day is given.

One rather common danger is that the symptomatic woman may categorically be considered to be suffering

TABLE 49–4. Pregnancy Outcomes Reported Since 1956 for Women with Sickle-cell Anemia and Hemoglobin SC Disease

	Sickle-cell (SS) Disease	Hemoglobin SC Disease
Women	1144	293
Pregnancies	2145	740
Maternal deaths (per 100,000)	~2500	~2300
Spontaneous abortions (%)	20	16
Perinatal mortality (per 1000)	~180	~75

Data from Carache (1980), El-Shafei (1992), Howard (1995), Milner (1980), Morris (1994), Poddar (1986), Powars (1986), Seoud (1994), Smith (1996), and their colleagues.

from a sickle-cell crisis. As a result, ectopic pregnancy, placental abruption, pyelonephritis, appendicitis, cholecystitis, or other serious obstetrical or medical problems that cause pain, anemia, or both may be overlooked. **The term "sickle-cell crisis" should be applied only after all other possible causes of pain or fever or reduction in hemoglobin concentration have been excluded.**

The cause of pain is intense sequestration of sickled erythrocytes with infarction in various organs. These episodes may develop acutely, especially late in pregnancy, during labor and delivery, and early in the puerperium. Acute infarction is usually accompanied by severe pain, and because the bone marrow is frequently involved, intense bone pain is common. Relief of pain from intravascular sickling is not afforded by heparinization or dextran. To maintain blood volume, intravenous hydration is given, along with meperidine or morphine administered parenterally for severe pain. Many of these women frequently are dehydrated due to diminished oral intake secondary to pain and they often have fever, which exacerbates hypovolemia. Oxygen given via nasal cannula may increase oxygen tension and decrease the intensity of sickling at the capillary level. We have found that red cell transfusions after the onset of severe pain do not dramatically improve the intensity of the pain and may not shorten its duration. Conversely, as discussed later, prophylactic red cell transfusions almost always eliminate pain episodes by preventing vasoocclusive episodes.

There are special circumstances during pregnancy that increase appreciably the morbidity of these women. Covert bacteriuria and acute pyelonephritis are increased substantively, and careful surveillance for bacteriuria and its eradication is important to prevent most urinary symptomatic infections. If pyelonephritis develops, these erythrocytes are extremely susceptible to endotoxin, which can cause dramatic and rapid red cell destruction while simultaneously suppressing erythropoiesis. As described in Chapter 56 (p. 1466), parvovirus B19 can destroy erythrocyte precursors and cause reversible hypoplastic anemia (Weatherall and Provan, 2000). Pneumonia, especially due to *Streptococcus pneumoniae*, is common. The Advisory Committee on Immunization Practices (1997) recommends polyvalent pneumococcal vaccine for these women. Influenza vaccine should be given annually. In addition, vaccination against *Haemophilus influenzae* type B is recommended by some for asplenic states (Association of Professors of Gynecology and Obstetrics, 1999).

As many as 40 percent of patients suffer from a serious and frequent complication known as **acute chest syndrome** (Vichinsky and colleagues, 2000). It is characterized by pleuritic chest pain, fever, cough, lung infiltrates, and hypoxia. There is a spectrum of pathology that includes infection, infarction, pulmonary sequestra-

tion, and fat embolization. Recurrent episodes may lead to restrictive chronic lung disease associated with arteriolar vasculopathy (Powars and co-workers, 1988). Van Erk and associates (1992) reported a maternal death in a woman with sickle-cell disease thought to be a result of pulmonary hypertension secondary to vasculopathy.

Women with sickle-cell anemia rarely die of heart disease, but almost all of these women eventually have some degree of **cardiac dysfunction.** In most cases, ventricular dysfunction from hypertrophy is compensated by increased preload and decreased afterload with a normal ejection fraction and a high cardiac output. Chronic hypertension will worsen this (Gandhi and colleagues, 2000). During pregnancy, the basal hemodynamic state characterized by high cardiac output and increased blood volume is further aggravated (Veille and Hanson, 1994). Although most of these women tolerate changes of pregnancy without problems, when complications such as severe preeclampsia or serious infections develop, ventricular failure may ensue (Cunningham and associates, 1986).

ASSESSMENT OF FETAL HEALTH. Because of the high incidence of fetal growth restriction and perinatal mortality, serial fetal assessment is necessary. The American College of Obstetricians and Gynecologists (1999) recommends weekly antepartum fetal surveillance beginning at 32 to 34 weeks. Serial ultrasonography is usually done to monitor fetal growth and amnionic fluid volume. Anyaegbunam and colleagues (1991) reported observations of fetal well-being obtained during 39 sickling crisis in 24 women. In almost 60 percent, they demonstrated reversible nonreactive stress tests, and all had an increased uterine artery systolic–diastolic (S/D) ratio. They found no changes in the umbilical artery S/D ratios, however, suggesting that transient effects of sickle-cell crisis do not compromise umbilical and hence fetal blood flow. At Parkland Hospital, we serially assess these women with ultrasound to determine amnionic fluid volume and follow fetal growth. Nonstress or contraction stress tests are not done routinely unless fetal movement is reported to be diminished or other significant complications develop that prompt admission.

DELIVERY. Labor and delivery in women with hemoglobin SS disease should be managed the same way as for women with cardiac disease (Chap. 44, p. 1185). The woman should be kept confortable but not oversedated. Epidural analgesia is ideally suited for labor and delivery. Compatible blood should be available. If a difficult vaginal or cesarean delivery is contemplated, and the hematocrit is less than 20 percent, the hemoglobin concentration should be increased by packed erythrocyte transfusions. At the same time, care must be taken to prevent circulatory overload from ventricular failure and pulmonary edema.

PROPHYLACTIC RED CELL TRANSFUSIONS. In a number of conditions, prophylactic transfusions decrease morbidity in sickle-cell syndromes. An example is perioperative transfusion. Another is transfusions to prevent strokes in high-risk children (Adams and coworkers, 1998). There currently is controversy over the use of prophylactic transfusions during pregnancy for women with sickle-cell syndromes (American College of Obstetricians and Gynecologists, 2000d). The most dramatic impact of prophylactic transfusion has been on maternal morbidity. In a 10-year study at Parkland Hospital, we offered prophylactic transfusions to all pregnant women with sickle-cell syndromes. Red cell transfusions were given throughout pregnancy to maintain the hematocrit above 25 percent and hemoglobin S at no greater than 60 percent (Cunningham and associates, 1979). There was minimal maternal morbidity such as pain, fever, and suppression of erythropoiesis. In a later study, we compared these and additional women with historical controls not given blood (Cunningham and associates, 1983). When pregnancy outcomes were compared with historical controls not routinely transfused, there was a significant reduction in maternal morbidity and hospitalizations. A comparative study by Howard and colleagues (1995) showed similar data.

In a multicenter study, Koshy and colleagues (1988) randomized 72 pregnant women with sickle-cell disease to be given either prophylactic transfusions or to be transfused only if indicated. They reported that the incidence of painful sickle-cell crises was decreased significantly in women transfused prophylactically, but there were no differences in perinatal outcomes. They observed a nonsignificant decrease in cumulative complications in women given prophylactic transfusions compared with controls (19 versus 42 percent). Because they did not find any improvement in survival of the mother or fetus, coupled with risks inherent in blood transfusions, they concluded that prophylactic red cell transfusions were not necessary.

Current consensus is that either management plan may be appropriate for a particular woman. Thus, management is individualized, and some choose prophylactic transfusions in women with a history of multiple vaso-occlusive episodes and poor obstetrical outcomes. Unfortunately, these are not always predictive of complications for the current pregnancy, especially in women with SC hemoglobin (Cunningham and colleagues, 1983).

COMPLICATIONS. Hazards of multiple transfusions are not insignificant, and morbidity from transfusions has proved troublesome. Delayed hemolytic transfusion re-

actions occur in as many as 10 percent of patients (Garratty, 1997). Hepatitis and red cell isoimmunization are major problems. At Parkland Hospital, the incidence of isoimmunization per unit of blood transfused was 3 percent in patients with sickle-cell disease (Cox and associates, 1988). In 12 studies, a mean of 25 percent of chronically transfused sickle-cell patients were isoimmunized (Garratty, 1997). Finally, although the spectre of iron overload and transfusion hemochromatosis is worrisome, we found no evidence of this in liver biopsies performed in 40 such women transfused during pregnancy (Yeomans and co-workers, 1990). There also was no evidence of acute or chronic hepatitis in these biopsy specimens.

EXPERIMENTAL THERAPY. Increasing the production of hemoglobin S may be harmful to patients with sickle-cell anemia because blood viscosity increases with hematocrit. Conversely, induction of hemoglobin F by stimulating gamma-chain synthesis appears to be a promising form of chronic treatment for sickling and some thalassemia syndromes. Gamma chains of hemoglobin F inhibit polymerization of hemoglobin S and therefore inhibit sickling. Combined regimens of **hydroxyurea** and **5-azacytidine** as well as **recombinant erythropoietin** and **hydroxyurea** increase fetal hemoglobin production with less sickling (Schechter and Rodgers, 1995). In addition, hydroxyurea reduces sickle erythrocyte adherence to endothelium (Steinberg, 1999). While the drug decreases yearly sickle-cell crises by about half, its long-term safety is unknown (Charache and associates, 1995). Experience with hydroxyurea in pregnancy is limited, but it is teratogenic in animals (Briggs and colleagues, 1998). Perrine and colleagues (1993) have given **butyric acid** as a means of increasing hemoglobin F.

A promising treatment for severe symptomatic sickle-cell anemia is **bone marrow transplantation** as discussed on page 1315. Because there is a basic defect in bone marrow stem cells in hemoglobinopathies, introduction of normal hemoglobin A erythrocyte precursors may be curative (Walters and associates, 1996). According to Steinberg (1999), about 100 sickle-cell patients—mostly children—have undergone transplantation. Mortality is 10 percent and most survivors were symptom free.

Prenatal diagnosis of sickle-cell disease may allow for in utero **stem cell therapy** with normal hemoglobin A stem cells (Eddleman, 1998; Shaaban and Flake, 1999). The immunological immaturity of the second-trimester fetus may dampen rejection of foreign cells and thus allow a higher success rate for transplantation.

Finally, transgenic "knock-out" mice that make only human globin chains have been developed (Paszty and colleagues, 1997; Ryan and co-workers, 1997). A sickle-cell mouse has also been developed, and although not a perfect human model, a more thorough understanding of the disease should evolve (Nagel, 1998).

CONTRACEPTION AND STERILIZATION. Because of chronic debility, the further complications caused by pregnancy, and the predictably shortened life span of women with sickle-cell anemia, contraception and possibly sterilization are important considerations. According to the American College of Obstetricians and Gynecologists (2000b), estrogen–progesterone oral contraceptives have not been assessed well in women with sickle hemoglobinopathies. Many authors, however, do not recommend their use because of potential adverse vascular and thrombotic effects (Chap. 58, p. 1525). Progesterone has been long known to prevent painful sickle-cell crises. Thus, low-dose oral progesterone or progesterone implants may be used, although some investigators feel that the safety issue is unclear. Conversely, de Abood and associates (1997) reported significantly fewer as well as less intense pain crises in women given depot medroxyprogesterone intramuscularly. Intrauterine devices probably are contraindicated in women with sickle-cell anemia because of increased risk of infection. The safest contraceptives for these women are unfortunately those with the highest failure rates—condoms/foam and diaphragms. Permanent sterilization is obviously an option for women with sickle-cell hemoglobinopathies.

SICKLE-CELL TRAIT. The inheritance of the gene for hemoglobin S from one parent and for hemoglobin A from the other results in sickle-cell trait. The amount of S hemoglobin is distinctly less than the amount of A hemoglobin. The frequency of red cell sickling among African Americans is reported to be about 8 percent. We tested almost 50,000 black women attending Parkland Maternal Health and Family Planning Clinics and also determined that 8 percent had sickle trait.

Extensive studies of the effect, or lack of effect, of sickle-cell trait on pregnancy have been reported (Pritchard and associates, 1973; Tuck and co-workers, 1983). Sickle-cell trait did not influence unfavorably the frequency of abortion, perinatal mortality, low birthweight, or pregnancy-induced hypertension. Urinary infection, however, was about twice as common in the group with sickle-cell trait. Subsequent investigations disclosed that twice as many pregnant women with sickle-cell trait had asymptomatic bacteriuria as did black women whose erythrocytes did not sickle (Whalley, 1967). Tollin and Seely (1994) have described a woman with hypopituitarism who they speculate suffered an intrapartum pituitary infarction related to sickle-cell trait.

Sickle-cell trait should not be considered a deterrent to pregnancy on the basis of increased risks to the mother. The probability, however, for a serious sickle-cell hemoglobinopathy in her offspring is 1 in 4 whenever the father carries a gene for an abnormal hemoglobin or for β-thalassemia. Prenatal diagnosis of sickle-cell disease through amniocentesis or chorionic villus sampling is now available (Chap. 37, p. 989). Xu and colleagues (1999) recently described single-blastomere DNA analysis and successful in-vitro fertilization of a couple with sickle-cell trait. The ethics associated with prenatal screening for hemoglobinopathies have been summarized by Bowman (1991).

OTHER HEMOGLOBINOPATHIES

HEMOGLOBIN C AND C–β-THALASSEMIA. Hemoglobin C results from a single β-chain substitution of glutamic acid by lysine at position 6. It is quite common in West Africa, but only about 2 percent of African Americans have the mutant gene for hemoglobin C. Hemoglobin C trait does not cause anemia, nor does it predispose to adverse pregnancy outcomes. When coinherited with sickle-cell trait, the resultant hemoglobin SC causes the problems previously discussed.

Pregnancy and homozygous hemoglobin C disease or hemoglobin C–β-thalassemia appear to be relatively benign associations. Maberry and colleagues (1990) reported our experiences with 72 pregnancies complicated by C-hemoglobinopathies. The degree of anemia was usually mild to moderate, and the mean third-trimester hematocrit was 27 percent (range 21 to 33) for 49 pregnancies complicated by hemoglobin CC disease and 30 percent (range 28 to 33) for 23 pregnancies complicated by C–β-thalassemia. Blood volume expansion in these women averaged about 35 percent compared with their nonpregnant volumes.

Pregnancy outcomes (Table 49–5) were not different in women with C hemoglobin syndromes compared with the general obstetrical population. When severe anemia is identified, iron or folic acid deficiency or some other superimposed cause should be suspected. Supplementation with folic acid and iron, unless blood is transfused, is likely to prove of value in pregnant women with any hemoglobinopathy.

HEMOGLOBIN E. Hemoglobin E is the second most common hemoglobin variant worldwide. Hemoglobin E results from a single β-chain substitution of lysine for glutamic acid at codon 26. The hemoglobin is susceptible particularly to oxidative stress. The prevalence of hemoglobin E trait is common in Southeast Asia and is very close to that for hemoglobin S in the United States. Homozygous inheritance gives rise to **hemoglobin E disease.** This hemoglobinopathy has become more prevalent in the United States since the influx of a large

TABLE 49–5. Outcomes in 72 Pregnancies Complicated by Hemoglobin CC and C–β-Thalassemia

	Hemoglobin CC	C–β-thalassemia
Women	15	5
Pregnancies	49	23
Maternal complications[a]	0	0
Spontaneous abortions	7	1
Birthweight (g)		
Mean	2990	2960
Range	1145–4770	2320–3980
Stillbirths	0	2
Neonatal deaths	1	0
Surviving infants	42	20

[a] Excluding mild to moderate anemia.
From Maberry and colleagues (1990), with permission.

number of Southeast Asians after 1970. Hurst and co-workers (1983) identified homozygous hemoglobin E, hemoglobin E plus α-thalassemia, or hemoglobin E trait in 36 percent of Cambodian children and 25 percent of Laotians, but in only 1 percent of Vietnamese. Alpha- and β-thalassemia traits were prevalent in all groups.

The homozygous state for hemoglobin E is associated with little or no anemia, hypochromia, marked microcytosis, and erythrocyte targeting. In our limited experience, pregnancies in women homozygous for hemoglobin E do not appear to be at increased risk. Iron-deficiency anemia as the consequence of intestinal parasites, repeated pregnancies, or both, may co-exist with E hemoglobinopathy.

Hemoglobin E–β-thalassemia is a common cause of childhood anemia in Southeast Asia (Fucharoen and Winichagoon, 2000). It has been reported to cause severe anemia that may require transfusion during pregnancy (Hsia, 1991). Hemoglobin SE is usually considered benign, but Eichhorn and colleagues (1999) reported a sickle-like crisis in a patient that was precipitated by B19 parvovirus infection. It is not clear if hemoglobin SE disease is as ominous during pregnancy as hemoglobin SC or S–β-thalassemia disease (Ramahi and colleagues, 1988).

HEMOGLOBINOPATHY IN THE NEWBORN. Infants with sickle-cell anemia, sickle cell–hemoglobin C disease, and homozygous hemoglobin C disease can be identified accurately at birth by electrophoresis performed on hemoglobin obtained from uncontaminated cord blood. The Agency for Health Care Policy and Research (1993) of the United States Public Health Service has recommended that all newborn babies be tested for sickle-cell disease regardless of their race or ethnic background. In most states, such screening is performed routinely on blood submitted for phenylketonuria and hypothyroidism testing. The Texas Department of Health performs hemoglobin electrophoresis using a specific technique called **isoelectric focusing.** The benefit of screening for sickle hemoglobinopathies is that there is clearly decreased mortality in children with sickle-cell disease who are recognized at birth and given monthly prophylactic injections of penicillin G and assessed closely for risk factors for strokes (Adams and colleagues, 1998; Centers for Disease Control and Prevention, 2000).

PRENATAL DIAGNOSIS. Using polymerase chain reaction (PCR), prenatal diagnosis of sickle-cell anemia is currently relatively simple, accurate, and rapid (Chap. 36, p. 966). The DNA used can be obtained by either amniocentesis or chorionic villus sampling. Hemoglobin C and most instances of β-thalassemia can be identified by analysis of DNA polymorphism or by identifying in vitro the kinds of globin chains synthesized by fetal red cells obtained from the fetus or placenta.

THALASSEMIAS. The genetically determined hemoglobinopathies termed thalassemias are characterized by impaired production of one or more of the normal globin peptide chains. Abnormal synthesis rates may result in ineffective erythropoiesis, hemolysis, and varying degrees of anemia. The different forms of thalassemia are classified according to the globin chain that is deficient in amount compared with its partner chain. Several hundred thalassemia syndromes have been described. The two major forms involve either impaired production of α-peptide chains causing α-thalassemia, or of β-chains to cause β-thalassemia. The incidence of these traits during pregnancy for all races is probably 1 in 300 to 500 (Gehlbach and Morgenstern, 1988).

ALPHA-THALASSEMIAS. Because there are two α-globin genes, the inheritance of α-thalassemia is more complicated than for β-thalassemia. Four clinical syndromes, the consequence of impaired α-globin chain synthesis, have been identified. For each syndrome, a close correlation has been established between clinical severity and the degree of impairment of synthesis of α-globin chains. In most populations, the α-globin chain "cluster" or gene loci are duplicated on chromosome 16. Thus, the normal genotype for diploid cells can be expressed as αα/αα. There are two main groups of α-thalassemia determinants: α⁰-thalassemia is characterized by the deletion of both loci from one chromosome (−/αα), whereas α⁺-thalassemia is characterized by the loss of a single locus from one chromosome (−α/αα heterozygote) or both (−α/−α, homozygote).

There are two major phenotypes. The deletion of all four α-globin chain genes (−/−) characterizes **homozy-**

gous α-thalassemia. Because α-chains make up fetal hemoglobin, the fetus is affected. Without α-globin chains, hemoglobin Bart (γ_4) and hemoglobin H (β_4) are formed as abnormal tetramers. Hemoglobin Bart has an appreciably increased affinity for oxygen. The fetus dies either in utero or very soon after birth, and demonstrates the typical clinical features of nonimmune hydrops fetalis shown in Figure 49–4 (see also Chap. 39, p. 1068). Lam and associates (1999) found that sonography at 12 to 13 weeks was 100 percent sensitive and specific for identifying affected fetuses by measuring the cardiothoracic ratio. Carr and colleagues (1995) transfused a fetus with α-thalassemia at 25, 26, and 32 weeks and reversed its ascites. The transfusion-dependent infant was delivered at 34 weeks. **Hemoglobin Bart disease** is a common cause of stillbirths in Southeast Asia. Hsieh and associates (1989) studied 20 such hydropic fetuses by funipuncture at 17 to 35 weeks and reported that blood contained 65 to 98 percent Bart hemoglobin.

The compound heterozygous state for α^o- and α^+-thalassemia results in the deletion of three of four genes ($-/-\alpha$), leaving only one functional α-globin gene per diploid genome. This is referred to as **hemoglobin H disease** (β_4), and it is compatible with extrauterine life. The abnormal red cells at birth contain a mixture of hemoglobin Bart (γ_4), hemoglobin H (β_4), and hemoglobin A. The neonate appears well at birth, but after early infancy, hemolytic anemia develops. Most, if not all, of the 20 to 40 percent of hemoglobin Bart present at birth is replaced postnatally by hemoglobin H. In the adult, 7 to 16 percent of hemoglobin is H (Chen and colleagues, 2000). The disease is char-acterized by hemolytic anemia of varying severity and, in some patients, disease severity is similar to β-thalassemia major. Anemia in these women usually is worsened during pregnancy.

A deletion of two genes results clinically in **α-thalassemia minor,** which is characterized by minimal to moderate hypochromic microcytic anemia. These may be due to α^o- or α^+-thalassemia traits. Thus, genotypes may be $-\alpha/-\alpha$ or $-/\alpha\alpha$. Differentiation is only by DNA analysis (Weatherall and Provan, 2000). Because there is no associated clinical abnormality with α-thalassemia minor, it often goes unrecognized. Hemoglobin Bart is present at birth, but as it dissipates, it is not replaced by hemoglobin H. Red cells are hypochromic and microcytic, and the hemoglobin concentration is normal to slightly depressed. Women with α-thalassemia minor appear to tolerate pregnancy quite well.

The single gene deletion ($-\alpha/\alpha\alpha$) is the **silent carrier state.** No clinical abnormality is evident in the individual with a single gene deletion.

FREQUENCY. The relative frequency of α-thalassemia minor, hemoglobin H disease, and hemoglobin Bart disease varies remarkably among racial groups. All of these variants are encountered in Asians. In individuals of African descent, however, even though α-thalassemia minor is demonstrated in about 2 percent, hemoglobin H disease is extremely rare and hemoglobin Bart disease is unreported. The reason for the discrepancy is that Asians usually have α^o-thalassemia minor with both

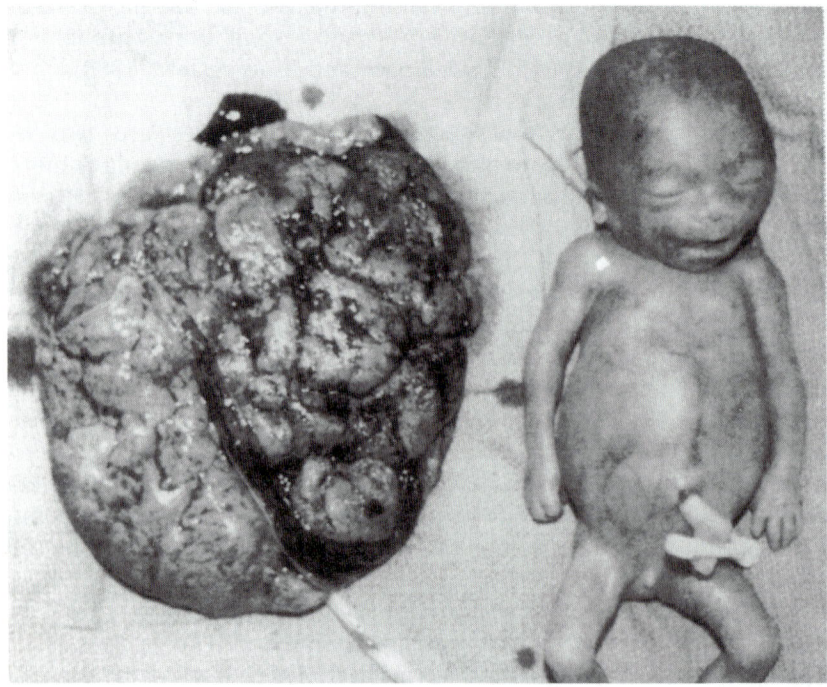

Figure 49–4. Stillborn hydropic fetus with extremely large placenta caused by homozygous α-thalassemia. (From Hsia, 1991, with permission.)

gene deletions typically from the same chromosome ($-/\alpha\alpha$), whereas in blacks with α^+-thalassemia minor, one gene is deleted from each chromosome ($-\alpha/-\alpha$). The α-thalassemia syndromes appear sporadically in other racial and ethnic groups. Diagnosis of α-thalassemia minor, as well as α-thalassemia major in the fetus, can be accomplished by DNA analysis using molecular techniques (American College of Obstetricians and Gynecologists, 2000c).

BETA-THALASSEMIAS. The β-thalassemias are the consequence of impaired production of β-globin chains, and the molecular pathology for the defective production is quite complex. Over 150 point mutations in the β-globin gene have been described (Weatherall, 2000). Most are single nucleotide substitutions that produce transcription defects, RNA splicing or modification, translation, or highly unstable hemoglobins. Thus, deletional and nondeletional mutations affect the transcription, processing, or translation of β-globin RNA. The $\delta\gamma\beta$-gene "cluster" is on chromosome 11.

With β-thalassemia there is decreased β-chain production and excess α-chains precipitate to cause cell membrane damage. These basic defects lead to the panorama of pathology that characterizes homozygous β-thalassemia, so-called β-thalassemia major or **Cooley anemia.** With heterozygous β-thalassemia minor, hypochromia, microcytosis, and slight to moderate anemia develop without the intense hemolysis that characterizes the homozygous state. The hallmark of the common β-thalassemias is an elevated hemoglobin A_2 level.

In the typical case of **thalassemia major,** the neonate is healthy at birth, but as the hemoglobin F level falls, the infant becomes severely anemic and fails to thrive. If children are entered into an adequate transfusion program, they develop normally until the end of the first decade when effects of iron loading become apparent. Prognosis is improved by iron-chelation therapy with deferoxamine (Olivieri and associates, 1998). Females who survive beyond childhood usually are sterile, and life expectancy even with transfusion therapy is shortened. Lucarelli and associates (1993) reported a 3-year survival rate of 94 percent with bone marrow transplantation for 151 patients.

In the past, pregnancy in women with severe thalassemia was rare. As therapy with iron-chelation and transfusions has become standardized, a number of centers have reported encouraging pregnancy outcomes. In two studies from Athens, Aessopos (1999) and Daskalakis (1998) and their colleagues reported a total of 31 pregnancies without severe complications. Kumar and associates (1997) from Manipur, India, described 32 women who had successful pregnancies. All of these investigators stress that underlying cardiomyopathy

should be excluded and that intensive surveillance is needed throughout pregnancy.

With **β-thalassemia minor,** A_2 hemoglobin—composed of two α- and two δ-globin chains—is increased to more than 3.5 percent. Simultaneously, hemoglobin F, composed of two α- and two γ-globin chains, is usually increased to more than 2 percent. The red cells are hypochromic and microcytic but anemia is mild. The hemoglobin concentration typically is 8 to 10 g/dL late in the second trimester, with an increase to between 9 and 11 g/dL near term, compared with a hemoglobin level of 10 to 12 g/dL in the nonpregnant state. There is usually pregnancy-induced augmentation of erythropoiesis and, using ^{51}chromium-tagged erythrocytes, we have documented normal blood volume expansion with slightly subnormal red cell mass expansion.

There is no specific therapy for β-thalassemia minor during pregnancy. Most often, the outcomes for the mother and fetus are satisfactory (Jensen and colleagues, 1995). Blood transfusions are seldom indicated except for hemorrhage. Prophylactic iron and folic acid in daily doses of about 60 mg and 1 mg, respectively, are given.

The potential exists for the fetus to inherit β-thalassemia major or sickle cell—β-thalassemia. Prenatal diagnosis of β-thalassemia using chorionic villus sampling can be carried out at 9 to 13 weeks (Weatherall and Provan, 2000). This may be difficult and is not always successful. Techniques include a combination of site-specific restriction endonuclease analysis, restriction fragment polymorphism linkage analysis, polymerase chain reaction, and oligonucleotide probes (Monni and co-workers, 1993). Galvani (2000) and Kanavakis (1999) and their associates have described preimplantation blastomere biopsy to select unaffected embryos for in vitro fertilization.

POLYCYTHEMIA. Erythrocytosis during pregnancy is usually of the secondary type related to chronic hypoxia, most often from congenital cardiac disease or a pulmonary disorder (Chap. 44, p. 1193). Occasionally it follows heavy cigarette smoking. We have encountered otherwise healthy young pregnant women who were heavy smokers with chronic bronchitis and a hematocrit of 55 to 60 percent! If polycythemia is severe, the probability of a successful pregnancy outcome is remote.

Brewer and colleagues (1992) described a woman with persistent erythrocytosis associated with a placental site tumor. The hematocrit remained around 55 to 60 percent until hysterectomy was done. Serum erythropoietin concentration was normal.

Polycythemia vera is a myeloproliferative hemopoietic stem cell disorder characterized by excessive proliferation of erythroid, myeloid, and megakaryocytic precursors. It likely is an acquired genetic disorder of stem cells (Provan and Weatherall, 2000). Symptoms are related to increased blood viscosity, and thrombotic complications are common. It is a condition of older patients and rarely co-exists with pregnancy. Ruch and Klein (1964) described a woman whose nonpregnant hematocrit was as high as 63. During each of two pregnancies, however, her hematocrit ranged from a low of 35 during the second trimester to 44 at term. Fetal loss seems to be high in women with polycythemia vera.

Measurement of serum erythropoietin by radioimmunoassay will differentiate polycythemia vera (low values) from secondary polycythemia (high values). There is evidence that erythroid precursors in this disorder will respond to erythropoietin and may even be hypersensitive.

THROMBOCYTOPENIAS

Low platelet counts in pregnancy may appear clinically to be idiopathic or, more often, to be associated with one of the following disorders: acquired hemolytic anemia, severe preeclampsia or eclampsia, severe obstetrical hemorrhage with blood transfusions, consumptive coagulopathy from placental abruption or similar hypofibrinogenemic states, septicemia, lupus erythematosus, antiphospholipid antibodies, megaloblastic anemia caused by severe folate deficiency, drugs, viral infections, allergies, aplastic anemia, or excessive irradiation. Some forms are inherited (George, 2000). An enormous number of drugs and naturally occurring foods can cause platelet dysfunction (George and Shattil, 1991). Aspirin is a prototype. Kain and associates (1995) observed that cocaine use was associated with a 6 percent incidence of thrombocytopenia in pregnant women.

GESTATIONAL THROMBOCYTOPENIA. Normal pregnancy may be accompanied by a physiological drop in platelet concentration, usually evident in the third trimester. There is no evidence that platelet lifespan is decreased or that platelet activation occurs in normal pregnancy (Baker and Cunningham, 1999; Star and colleagues, 1997). Thus, it is thought that decreased platelet counts occur from hemodilution as well as platelet trapping. Gestational thrombocytopenia is a diagnosis of exclusion. In addition to the usual secondary causes of thrombocytopenia, a number of platelet alterations are commonly associated with preeclampsia–eclampsia. These are discussed in Chapter 24 (p. 576) and include mild to very severe thrombocytopenia as well as increased platelet activation, adherence, and platelet dysfunction.

The definition used for thrombocytopenia is important. From their review, Rouse and associates (1998) cite an incidence of gestational thrombocytopenia—defined as less than $150,000/\mu L$—of 4 to 7 percent. Burrows and Kelton (1993a) reported that 6.6 percent of 15,471 pregnant women had a platelet count of less than $150,000/\mu L$, but in only 1.2 percent was it less than $100,000/\mu L$. Almost three fourths of 1027 women whose platelet counts were less than $150,000/\mu L$ were healthy and found to have incidental thrombocytopenia. The other fourth had either a hypertensive disorder of pregnancy (21 percent) or an immunological disorder (4 percent). Boehlen and associates (2000) found that 11.6 percent of 6770 pregnant women had platelet counts of less than $150,000/\mu L$, and that $116,000/\mu L$ was 2.5 standard deviations below the mean.

INHERITED THROMBOCYTOPENIAS. The **Bernard–Soulier syndrome** is characterized by lack of platelet membrane glycoprotein (GPIb/IX) and severe dysfunction. Maternal antibodies against fetal GPIb/IX antigen can cause isoimmune fetal thrombocytopenia. Peng and colleagues (1991) described an affected woman who during four pregnancies had episodes of postpartum hemorrhage, gastrointestinal hemorrhage, and fetal thrombocytopenia. Fujimori and associates (1999) described a similarly affected woman whose neonate died from intracranial hemorrhage from thrombocytopenia.

Chatwani and associates (1992) described a woman with autosomally dominant **May–Hegglin anomaly.** Because fetal inheritance could not be excluded, they performed cesarean section at term. The infant was not affected. Urato and Repke (1998) described a women diagnosed 2 years before pregnancy. Vaginal delivery was allowed, and despite a platelet count of $16,000/\mu L$, she did not bleed excessively. The neonate inherited the anomaly, but also had no bleeding despite a platelet count of $35,000/\mu L$.

IMMUNE THROMBOCYTOPENIC PURPURA. The entity long referred to as **idiopathic thrombocytopenic purpura (ITP)** is usually the consequence of an immune process in which antibodies are directed against platelets. Antibody-coated platelets are destroyed prematurely in the reticuloendothelial system, especially the spleen. The mechanism of production of these platelet-associated immunoglobulins—PAIgG, PAIgM, and PAIgA—is not known, but most investigators consider them to be autoantibodies.

The American Society of Hematology convened a panel to develop clinical practice guidelines for diagnosis and management of immune thrombocytopenic purpura (George and colleagues, 1996). Acute ITP is most often a childhood disease that follows a viral infection. Most cases resolve spontaneously, although perhaps 10 percent become chronic. Conversely, in adults ITP is primarily a chronic disease of young women and rarely resolves spontaneously. Secondary forms of chronic thrombocytopenia must be ruled out to include systemic lupus erythematosus, lymphomas, leukemias, or a number of systemic diseases. For example, up to 10 percent of HIV-positive patients have associated thrombocytopenia (Glantz and Roberts, 1994). About 2 percent have positive serological tests for lupus, and some cases are associated with high titers of anticardiolipin antibodies.

Outcomes for adults with primary ITP are shown in Table 49–6. A small number recover spontaneously, and for those who do not, platelet counts usually range from 10,000 to 100,000/μL. In those whose platelet counts remain less than 30,000/μL, or those with significant bleeding at higher levels, treatment with prednisone, 1 to 2 mg/kg, will raise the platelet count in about two thirds, but relapse is exceedingly common (George and associates, 1996). Glucocorticoids exert their action by suppressing phagocytic activity of the splenic monocyte–macrophage system.

For patients with no response to corticosteroid therapy in 2 to 3 weeks, those in whom massive doses are needed to sustain remission, or those with frequent recurrences, splenectomy is indicated. In about 60 percent, there is substantive improvement as the consequence of decreased removal of platelets by the spleen and reduced antibody production. Massive doses—400 mg/kg—of gamma globulin given intravenously over 5 days results in satisfactory platelet count elevation in two thirds of patients. Such therapy may be useful in patients with life-threatening thrombocytopenia refractory to other therapy, or preoperatively before splenectomy.

Therapy is problematic for the 30 percent of adults who do not respond to corticosteroids or splenectomy.

TABLE 49–6. Outcome of Immune Thrombocytopenic Purpura in 1761 Adults from 12 Studies

Outcome	Number	Percent
Complete remission		
Spontaneous (no therapy)	27	1.5
Following therapy	1027	64
Hemorrhagic complications		
Acute deaths		
Intracerebral hemorrhage	36	2
Other hemorrhage	7	<1
Other deaths	35	2
Persistent thrombocytopenia	465	26
Later spontaneous recovery	22	5
Later hemorrhagic death	25	5

Data from George and colleagues (1996).

Immunosuppressive drugs, including azathioprine, cyclophosphamide, and cyclosporine, have been used with some success. Danazol, vinca alkaloids, plasma exchange, and high-dose dexamethasone pulse therapy have been described.

IMMUNE THROMBOCYTOPENIA AND PREGNANCY. There is no evidence that pregnancy increases the risk of relapse in women with previously diagnosed immune thrombocytopenia. Nor does it make the condition worse in women with active disease. It is certainly not unusual for women who have been in clinical remission for several years to have recurrent thrombocytopenia during pregnancy; however, this may be because of closer surveillance. Hyperestrogenemia has also been suggested as a cause.

Treatment is considered if the platelet count is less than 50,000/μL (George and associates, 1996). Corticosteroids in a dose of 1 mg/kg per day may be required for improvement, and most likely treatment will have to be continued throughout pregnancy. Corticosteroid therapy usually produces amelioration, but in refractory disease, high-dose immunoglobulin is given intravenously. Clark and Gall (1997) reviewed 16 case reports of 21 pregnancies in which ITP was treated with immunoglobulin. All but four responded with post-treatment platelet counts of over 50,000/μL; in 11 of these, it exceeded 100,000/μL. Such therapy is expensive, and in 2000, hospital costs for a 5-day course of treatment ranged from $5500 to $8000 for a 70-kg person. Also, shortages of immunoglobulin for high-dose infusion are not uncommon (Centers for Disease Control and Prevention, 1999).

In women with no response to steroid or immunoglobulin therapy, splenectomy may be effective. Late in pregnancy, the procedure technically is more difficult and cesarean delivery may be necessary to improve exposure.

FETAL AND NEONATAL EFFECTS. Platelet-associated IgG antibodies can cross the placenta and cause thrombocytopenia in the fetus-neonate. The severely thrombocytopenic fetus is at increased risk for intracranial hemorrhage as the consequence of labor and delivery. This fortunately is unusual. Payne and colleagues (1997) reviewed studies of maternal ITP published since 1973 and added their experiences with 55 cases. Of a total of 601 newborns, 12 percent had severe thrombocytopenia (< 50,000/μL). Only six infants had intracranial hemorrhage, and in three of these the initial platelet count was 50,000/μL or greater.

Considerable attention has been directed at identifying the fetus with potentially dangerous thrombocytopenia. All investigators have concurred that there is not a strong correlation between fetal and maternal platelet

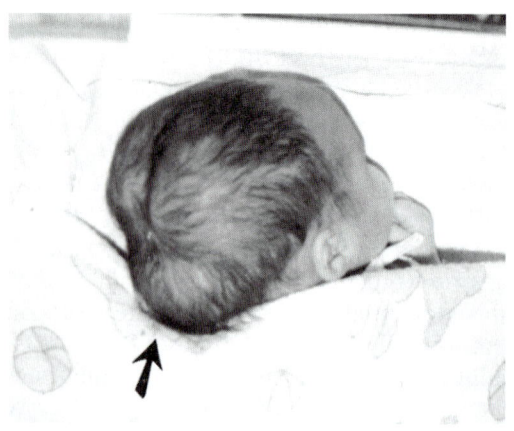

Figure 49–5. Newborn with extensive cephalohematomas, especially over the occipital bone (*arrow*). The mother had chronic immune thrombocytopenic purpura for which splenectomy had been performed years earlier. Severe thrombocytopenia developed in this pregnancy and she was treated with prednisone. Her platelet count at cesarean section was 115,000/μL and in cord blood it was 17,000/μL. The infant was treated with corticosteroids and platelet transfusions and did well.

counts (Fig. 49–5) (George and associates, 1996; Payne and co-workers, 1997). Because of this, several investigators have attempted to quantify the relationship between maternal IgG circulating platelet antibody, platelet-associated antibody, and fetal platelet count. Unfortunately, there is little concurrence. Kaplan and associates (1990) and Samuels and colleagues (1990) reported conflicting results in using indirect platelet immunoglobulin for identification of high-risk neonates. In both studies, however, historical information was useful. Specifically, a history of ITP remote from pregnancy increased the likelihood of neonatal thrombocytopenia.

Burrows and Kelton (1993a) detected neonatal thrombocytopenia (cord platelets < 50,000/μL) in 19 of 15,932 newborns (0.12 percent). Only 1 of 756 mothers with gestational thrombocytopenia had an affected infant. Of 1414 hypertensive women with thrombocytopenia, five infants had thrombocytopenia. Conversely, of 46 mothers with immune thrombocytopenic purpura, four infants had thrombocytopenia. Importantly, isoimmune thrombocytopenia was associated with profound thrombocytopenia, with cord platelet counts less than 20,000/μL, and there was one fetal death and two other cases of intracranial hemorrhage (see later discussion). In a similar population study, Boehlen and associates (1999) determined antiplatelet antibodies in pregnant women whose platelet counts were less than 150,000/μL. This included 12 percent of almost 6800 women. Of 430 thrombocytopenic women, 9 percent had antibodies detected, but these were of no predictive value. Sainio and co-workers (2000) performed cord platelet counts in almost 4500 neonates. About 2 percent were less than

150,000/μL but only 0.2 percent (1 in 410) were less than 50,000/μL. All cases with bleeding were due to isoimmune thrombocytopenia.

DETECTION OF FETAL THROMBOCYTOPENIA. Scott and co-workers (1983) concluded earlier that no clinical characteristic or laboratory test would accurately predict fetal platelet count. They recommended intrapartum platelet determinations made on blood obtained from the fetal scalp once the cervix was 2 to 3 cm dilated and the membranes ruptured. Whenever the platelet count in scalp blood was identified to be less than 50,000/μL, they performed immediate cesarean delivery. Daffos and colleagues (1985) subsequently reported percutaneous umbilical cord blood sampling for platelet quantification in fetuses whose mothers had immune thrombocytopenia (Chap. 37, p. 991). This was associated with a high complication rate. Berry and associates (1997) reported no complications but found only a high negative-predictive value. Payne and colleagues (1997) summarized six such studies reported since 1988. Of 195 cases, severe neonatal thrombocytopenia (< 50,000/μL) was found in 7 percent; however, the serious complication rate of cordocentesis was 4.6 percent.

Because of the low incidence of severe neonatal thrombocytopenia and morbidity, Burrows and Kelton (1993b), as well as Silver and colleagues (1995) concluded that fetal platelet determinations and cesarean delivery are not necessary. Payne and associates (1997) as well as the American Society of Hematology (George and co-workers, 1996) concur. Peleg and Hunter (1999) recently surveyed members of the Society of Maternal–Fetal Medicine and received a 60 percent response. Only a third recommended fetal testing with chronic ITP, and a fourth would do fetal testing in women with new-onset ITP during pregnancy.

ISOIMMUNE THROMBOCYTOPENIA. Platelet isoimmunization can develop in a manner identical to erythrocyte antigen isoimmunization. Its incidence may be as high as 1 in 2000 to 3000 births. If fetal platelet antigens for which maternal platelets are negative gain access to her circulation, the mother then may produce antibodies in subsequent pregnancies that will destroy fetal platelets that have this antigen. The most common antibody is against PL^{A1} platelet-specific antigen. About 2 percent of Caucasians are homozygous for PL^{B1} antigen (Jaegtvik and associates, 2000). The first pregnancy is affected in about half of cases. This disorder is discussed in Chapter 39 (p. 1072).

THROMBOCYTOSIS. Thrombocytosis, or thrombocythemia, generally is defined as platelets persisting in numbers greater than 450,000/μL. Common causes of **secondary** or **reactive thrombocytosis** are malignant tumors, iron deficiency, hemorrhage, inflammatory diseases, and connective-tissue disorders. Platelet counts seldom exceed 800,000/μL in these secondary disorders, and prognosis depends on the underlying disease. On the other hand, **essential thrombocytosis** is a myeloproliferative disorder that accounts for most cases in which platelet counts exceed 1 million/μL. Thrombocytosis usually is asymptomatic, but arterial and venous thromboses may develop. Cortelazzo and colleagues (1995) reported that myelosuppression with hydroxyurea for nonpregnant patients with essential thrombocytosis decreased thrombotic episodes from 24 to 4 percent compared with untreated controls.

PREGNANCY. While case reports indicate that pregnancies associated with thrombocytosis have excessive spontaneous abortions, placental infarctions, and preterm delivery, this likely is not the case. Beard and co-workers (1991) described nine pregnancies in six women whose mean platelet count was 1.25 million/μL. One woman aborted and eight pregnancies were delivered at term. Randi and colleagues (1994) reported that six pregnancies in five women with essential thrombocytosis (mean platelets 1.5 million/μL) were normal. Treatment that has been suggested during pregnancy includes aspirin, dipyridamole, heparin, plateletpheresis, or combinations thereof. Delage and co-workers (1996) reviewed 11 cases in which interferon-α was given with successful outcomes. They also described a woman at midpregnancy who had platelets of 2.3 million/μL and had transient blindness. Thrombocytapheresis was performed and interferon-α was used to keep the platelets at around 1 million/μL until delivery.

THROMBOTIC MICROANGIOPATHIES. The original description in 1925 by Moschcowitz of **thrombotic thrombocytopenic purpura** was characterized by the pentad of thrombocytopenia, fever, neurological abnormalities, renal impairment, and hemolytic anemia. In 1955, Gasser and colleagues described the **hemolytic uremic syndrome,** which was similar to thrombotic thrombocytopenic purpura but with more profound renal involvement and fewer neurological aberrations. In 1968, Robson and co-workers described **postpartum renal failure** characterized by uremia associated with microangiopathic hemolytic anemia and thrombocytopenia (Chap. 47, p. 1268).

Although it is likely that there are different etiologies to account for the variable findings within these syndromes, they are clinically indistinguishable in adults (Moake, 1998). There is, however, a pure form of the hemolytic uremic syndrome in children, incited by viral or bacterial infection. Kincaid-Smith and co-workers (1988) reported an association between the lupus anticoagulant and thrombotic microangiopathy. There is no evidence that postpartum renal failure differs remarkably from the hemolytic uremic syndrome except that the woman recently had been pregnant. It seems likely that these syndromes account for the occasional case of severe preeclampsia accompanied by hemolysis and thrombocytopenia that does not respond to delivery (Kahra and associates, 1998; Magann and colleagues, 1994).

PATHOGENESIS. Microthrombi, consisting of hyaline material made up of platelets and small amounts of fibrin, develop within arterioles and capillaries. These aggregates produce ischemia or infarctions in various organs. The general consensus is that intravascular platelet aggregation stimulates the cascade of events leading to end-organ failure, and although there is evidence for endothelial damage, it is unknown whether this is a consequence or a cause. For over 20 years, unusually large multimers of von Willebrand factor have been identified with active disease. Recently, it was shown that the metalloprotease responsible for cleaving von Willebrand factor secreted by endothelial cells is neutralized by antibodies during an acute episode (Furlan and colleagues, 1998; Tsai and associates, 1998). Because these resulting large multimers bind platelets and cause aggregation, they likely are the inciting agents of thrombotic thrombocytopenic purpura, but not hemolytic uremic syndrome (Moake, 1998).

CLINICAL PRESENTATION. Thrombotic microangiopathies are characterized by thrombocytopenia, fragmentation hemolysis, and variable organ dysfunction. A viral prodrome may precede up to 40 percent of cases. Neurological symptoms are present or develop in up to 90 percent of patients and include headache, altered consciousness, convulsions, or stroke. Because renal involvement is common, the two syndromes are difficult to separate (Moake, 1998). Renal failure is thought to be more severe with the hemolytic uremic syndrome, and in half of the cases, dialysis is required.

HEMATOLOGICAL ABNORMALITIES. Thrombocytopenia is usually severe. Fortunately, even with very low platelet counts, spontaneous severe hemorrhage is uncommon. Microangiopathic hemolysis is associated with moderate to marked anemia, and transfusions are frequently necessary. The blood smear is characterized by erythrocyte fragmentation with schizocytosis. The reticulocyte count is high, and nucleated red blood cells are numerous. Consumptive coagulopathy, although common, is usually subtle and clinically insignificant.

TREATMENT. Plasmapheresis and exchange transfusion with normal plasma has remarkably improved the outcome for these formerly commonly fatal diseases.

Transfusions with red blood cells are imperative for life-threatening anemia. Rock and colleagues (1991) found plasma exchange to be superior to plasma infusion in nonpregnant patients; however, overall mortality was still 30 percent. Bell and co-workers (1991) reported their experiences with 108 patients treated at Johns Hopkins Hospital; 10 percent of these patients were pregnant. Those with minimal neurological symptoms were given prednisone, 200 mg daily, but if there were neurological abnormalities or rapid clinical deterioration, plasmapheresis and plasma exchange were performed daily. About a fourth of patients with mild disease responded to prednisone alone. Of those requiring plasmapheresis, relapses were common but overall survival was 91 percent. As emphasized by Hayward (1994) and Shumak (1995) and their associates, relapses (20 to 30 percent) are common and include long-term sequelae such as renal impairment.

PREGNANCY AND THROMBOTIC MICROANGIOPATHY.
Evidence is lacking that pregnancy predisposes women to develop thrombotic microangiopathies. Over a 25-year period, Dashe and co-workers (1998) encountered 11 pregnancies complicated by these syndromes or their presumed variants among nearly 275,000 women from our well-defined catchment area who were delivered at Parkland Hospital. This frequency of 1 in 25,000 is not greater than that in our general hospital population.

It is not surprising that severe preeclampsia and eclampsia complicated further by thrombocytopenia and overt hemolysis have been confused with thrombotic thrombocytopenic purpura and vice versa (Hsu and colleagues, 1995; Magann and co-workers, 1994). Differentiating between preeclampsia, especially atypical preeclampsia, and these syndromes can be difficult, especially at the outset. One constant feature of thrombotic microangiopathies is hemolytic anemia, which is rarely severe with preeclampsia, even when the syndrome of hemolysis, elevated liver enzymes, and low platelets (HELLP) is present. While deposition of hyaline microthrombi within the liver is seen with thrombotic microangiopathy, hepatocellular necrosis characteristic of preeclampsia has not been described. Whereas delivery leads to resolution of preeclampsia with HELLP syndrome, there is no evidence that thrombotic microangiopathy is improved by delivery (Letsky, 2000). Importantly, seven of 11 women described by Dashe and colleagues (1998) had recurrent disease either when not pregnant or within the first trimester of a subsequent pregnancy.

Unless the diagnosis is unequivocally one of these thrombotic microangiopathies, rather than severe preeclampsia or eclampsia, the response to pregnancy termination should be evaluated before resorting to plasmapheresis and exchange transfusion, massive-dose glucocorticoid therapy, or other therapy. **Plasmapheresis is not indicated for preeclampsia–eclampsia complicated by hemolysis and thrombocytopenia.**

In the past, maternal and fetal outcomes in reported cases have been dismal. Weiner (1987) reviewed 65 cases in which he tried carefully to exclude women with preeclampsia. Perinatal mortality was 80 percent. With plasma therapy, maternal salvage was excellent, but without such therapy, mortality was 68 percent. Egerman and co-workers (1996) described 11 women whom they treated with plasmapheresis from 1988 through 1996. There were two maternal and three fetal deaths. In our experiences from Parkland Hospital, five of eight women treated by plasmapheresis had a dramatic salutary response (Dashe and associates, 1998).

LONG-TERM PROGNOSIS. Recent observations indicate that pregnant women with thrombotic microangiopathy have a number of long-term complications. In the Parkland study by Dashe and associates (1998), 9-year follow-up disclosed multiple recurrences; renal disease requiring dialysis and/or transplantation; severe hypertension; and blood-borne infectious diseases. Two women died remote from pregnancy—one from dialysis complications and one from acquired immunodeficiency syndrome (AIDS) transmitted by blood therapy. Egerman and colleagues (1996) reported similar observations. Although it is not possible to ascertain if the guarded prognosis in these women is different from the natural history, clearly, development of thrombotic microangiopathy during pregnancy has severe immediate and long-term mortality.

INHERITED COAGULATION DEFECTS. Obstetrical hemorrhage, a common event, is rarely the consequence of an inherited defect in the coagulation mechanism. There are a number of syndromes, however, that are particularly important.

HEMOPHILIAS. Hemophilia A is an X-linked recessively transmitted disease characterized by a marked deficiency of *small component* antihemophilic factor (factor VIII:C). The heterozygous state is responsible for the disease. It is rare among women compared with men. With few exceptions, the homozygous state that results from the inheritance of two abnormal X chromosomes is the requisite for hemophilia A in women. In a few instances, it appears in women spontaneously, as a newly mutant gene.

The genetic and clinical features of severe deficiency of factor IX—Christmas disease or hemophilia B—are quite similar to those for hemophilia A. Guy and associates (1992) reviewed five cases in pregnancy, all with a favorable outcome. They recommended administration of factor IX where levels are below 10 percent.

The degree of risk is influenced markedly by the level of circulating factor VIII:C or factor IX. If the level is at or very close to zero, the risk is major. In female carriers, activity is expected to average 50 percent, but there is a range due to lyonization (Letsky, 2000). If levels fall below 10 to 20 percent, hemorrhage may occur. These clotting factors increase appreciably during normal pregnancy and in carriers of hemophilia A and B. Desmopressin may also stimulate factor VIII:C release. The risk of hemorrhage is reduced by avoiding lacerations, minimizing episiotomy, and maximizing postpartum myometrial contractions and retraction. Kadir and co-workers (1997) reported that 20 percent of carriers had postpartum hemorrhage; in two it was massive.

Affected male fetuses may develop hematomas with either vaginal or cesarean delivery (Kadir and associates, 1997). After delivery the risk of hemorrhage in the neonate increases, especially if circumcision is attempted.

Whenever the mother has hemophilia A or B, all of her sons will have the disease, and all of her daughters will be carriers. If she is a carrier, half of her sons will inherit the disease and half of her daughters will be carriers. Prenatal diagnosis of hemophilia is possible in some families using chorionic villus biopsy (Chap. 37, p. 989). The confirmation of a male fetus also identifies a 50 percent risk of inheriting hemophilia.

FACTOR VIII INHIBITOR. Rarely, antibodies directed against factor VIII are acquired and may lead to life-threatening hemorrhage. This phenomenon has been identified in women during the puerperium. The prominent clinical feature is severe, protracted, repetitive hemorrhage from the reproductive tract starting a week or so after an apparently uncomplicated delivery (Reece and associates, 1988). The activated partial thromboplastin time is markedly prolonged. Treatment has included multiple transfusions of whole blood and plasma, huge doses of cryoprecipitate, large volumes of an admixture of activated coagulation factors including porcine factor VIII, immunosuppressive therapy, and attempts at various surgical procedures, especially curettage and hysterectomy.

VON WILLEBRAND DISEASE. Clinically, von Willebrand disease is a heterogenous group of about 20 functional disorders involving aberrations of factor VIII complex and platelet dysfunction. These abnormalities are the most commonly inherited bleeding disorders, and their prevalence is about 1 percent (Mannucci, 1998). Most of the variants of von Willebrand disease are inherited as autosomal dominant traits. Examples are types I and II disease which are the most common

variants. Type III, which is the most severe, is phenotypically recessive.

The **von Willebrand factor** (vWF) is a large, multimeric glycoprotein that forms part of the factor VIII complex. It is essential for normal platelet adhesion to subendothelial collagen and formation of a primary hemostatic plug at the site of blood vessel injury. It also plays a major role in the stabilization of the coagulant properties of factor VIII. The procoagulant component is the antihemophilic factor or factor VIII:C, which is a glycoprotein synthesized by the liver. Conversely, von Willebrand factor, which is present in platelets as well as plasma, is synthesized by endothelium and megakaryocytes under the control of autosomal genes on chromosome 12. The von Willebrand factor antigen (vWF:Ag) is the antigenic determinant measured by immunoassays.

CLINICAL PRESENTATION. Symptomatic patients usually present with evidence of a platelet defect. The possibility of von Willebrand disease is usually considered in women with bleeding suggestive of a chronic disorder of coagulation. The classical autosomal dominant form usually is symptomatic in the heterozygous state. The less common but clinically more severe autosomal recessive form is manifest when inherited from both parents, both of whom demonstrate little or no disease. Type I, which accounts for 75 percent of variants of von Willebrand disease, is characterized clinically by easy bruising, epistaxis, mucosal hemorrhage, and excessive bleeding with trauma, including surgery. Its laboratory features are usually a prolonged bleeding time, prolonged partial thromboplastin time, decreased von Willebrand factor antigen, decreased factor VIII immunological as well as coagulation-promoting activity, and inability of platelets in plasma from an affected person to react to a variety of stimuli.

EFFECT OF PREGNANCY. During pregnancy, women with von Willebrand disease often develop normal levels of factor VIII coagulant activity as well as von Willebrand factor antigen, although the bleeding time still may be prolonged. These levels may double or triple by term. If factor VIII activity is very low, or if there is bleeding, then treatment is recommended. With significant bleeding, 15 or 20 units of cryoprecipitate are given every 12 hours. Alternatively, factor VIII concentrates may be given that contain high-molecular-weight vWF multimers (Koate-HS, Hemate-P). These concentrates are highly purified and are heat treated to destroy human immunodeficiency virus. Lubetsky and associates (1999) have described continuous infusion with Hemate-P during nine surgical procedures and one vaginal delivery.

There have been a number of studies describing pregnancy outcomes in women with von Willebrand disease. Conti and associates (1986) summarized 38 cases, and in a fourth bleeding was reported with abortion, delivery, or the puerperium. Similarly, Greer and colleagues (1991) reported that eight of 14 pregnancies were complicated by postpartum hemorrhage. Kadir and co-workers (1998) reported their experiences from the Royal Free Hospital in London with 84 pregnancies in women with von Willebrand disease. There was a 20 percent incidence of primary postpartum hemorrhage and another 20 percent had late hemorrhage. Most cases were associated with low vWF levels in untreated women. No woman given prophylactic peripartum treatment had hemorrhage.

INTERITANCE. Although most patients with von Willebrand disease are heterozygous variants with a mild bleeding disorder, the disease can be severe. Certainly when both parents have the disorder, their homozygous offspring will develop a serious bleeding disorder. Mullaart and colleagues (1991) documented evidence for periventricular hemorrhage in a 32-week fetus who inherited type IIa von Willebrand disease from her father. Sherer and associates (1998) reviewed these and other predisposing causes of fetal intracranial hemorrhage. Chorionic villus biopsy with DNA analysis to detect the missing genes has been accomplished (Chap. 37, p. 989). Some authorities recommend cesarean delivery to avoid trauma to a possibly affected fetus if the mother has had severe disease.

OTHER INHERITED COAGULATION FACTOR DEFICIENCIES. A number of rare coagulopathies may result in a manner similar to the hemophilias. **Factor VII deficiency** is a rare autosomal recessive disorder, the gene for which is on chromosome 13. Normally, factor VII increases during pregnancy, but it may do so only mildly in factor VII–deficient patients (Fadel and Krauss, 1989).

Factor X or **Stuart–Prower factor** deficiency is extremely rare and is inherited as an autosomal recessive trait. Factor X levels typically rise during normal pregnancy by 50 percent. Konje and colleagues (1994) described a woman with 2 percent activity who was given prophylactic treatment with plasma-derived factor X, which raised plasma levels to 37 percent; however, she suffered an intrapartum placental abruption. Bofill and co-workers (1996) gave intrapartum fresh-frozen plasma to a woman with less than 1 percent factor X activity, and she delivered spontaneously without incident.

Factor XI (plasma thromboplastin antecedent) deficiency probably is the consequence of an autosomal trait that is manifest as severe disease in the homozygous individuals but a minor defect in the heterozygote. This deficiency state is most prevalent in Ashkenazi Jews, and it seldom is encountered in pregnancy. Musclow and colleagues (1987) described 41 deliveries in 17 women with factor XI deficiency, and in none were transfusions required. They also described a 37-week pregnant woman who developed a spontaneous hemarthrosis. Kadir and associates (1998) described 29 pregnancies in 11 women. In none of these did factor XI levels increase; 15 percent had primary postpartum hemorrhage, and 25 percent had delayed hemorrhage. Peripartum treatment with factor XI concentrate at the time of delivery prevents hemorrhage (Letsky, 2000).

Factor XII deficiency is another autosomal recessive disorder that rarely complicates pregnancy. An increased incidence of thromboembolism is encountered in nonpregnant patients with this deficiency. Lao and colleagues (1991) reported an affected pregnant woman in whom placental abruption developed at 26 weeks.

Factor XIII deficiency is autosomal recessive and it may be associated with maternal intracranial hemorrhage (Letsky, 2000). Treatment is given with fresh-frozen plasma.

Autosomally inherited abnormalities of fibrinogen usually involve the formation of a functionally defective fibrinogen, commonly referred to as **dysfibrinogenemia** (Edwards and Rijhsinghani, 2000). Familial **hypofibrinogenemia**—sometimes **afibrinogenemia**—are infrequent recessive disorders. Our experiences suggest that hypofibrinogenemia represents a heterozygous autosomal dominant state with 50 percent of the offspring affected. Typically, thrombin-clottable protein has ranged from 80 to 110 mg/dL when nonpregnant, and this increases by 40 or 50 percent in normal pregnancy. Those pregnancy complications that give rise to acquired hypofibrinogenemia, that is, placental abruption, are more common in fibrinogen deficiency, but the existence of such conditions provided the impetus for study. Goodwin (1989) reviewed the literature and reported a high incidence of placental abruption and postpartum hemorrhage. Trehan and Fergusson (1991) and Funai and associates (1997) described successful outcomes in two women in whom fibrinogen or plasma infusions were given weekly or biweekly throughout pregnancy.

THROMBOPHILIAS. A number of important regulatory proteins inhibit clotting. There are physiological antithrombotic proteins that act as inhibitors at strategic sites in the coagulation cascade to maintain blood fluidity under normal circumstances. Examples include **antithrombin III** and **protein C** and its co-factor, **protein S.** Inherited deficiencies of these inhibitory proteins are caused by mutations of genes influencing their control. Because they may be associated with recurrent thromboembolism, they are collectively referred to as *thrombophilias*. Other inherited coagulopathies arise from mutations that include **activated protein C resistance** from factor V single-gene mutations of which the most common is the factor V Leiden mutation. There is also a function-enhancing mutation in the **prothrombin gene (G20210A)** and also **hyperhomocystinemia.**

Taken in toto, these mutations are common. For each syndrome there are many different single-gene point mutations that may be responsible (see discussion that follows). The aggregate prevalence of the six aforementioned coagulants is nearly 20 percent. Their inheritance is usually associated in nonpregnant patients with increased risk of deep-vein thrombosis and pulmonary embolism, sagittal sinus thrombosis, and portal vein thrombosis. Heijboer and colleagues (1990) studied the prevalence of isolated abnormal coagulation-inhibiting proteins in 277 nonpregnant patients with venographically proven deep-vein thrombosis. Their incidence combined was 8.3 percent compared with 2.2 percent for normal controls. In some of these patients, environmental provocation such as surgery or oral contraceptive use will enhance the likelihood of thromboembolism.

Pregnancy is also an inciting factor in many of these thrombophilias. Pregnancy-related complications include, in addition to thromboembolism, increased risk for severe early-onset preeclampsia, placental infarction and abruption, fetal growth restriction, and stillbirths. Some of these are listed in Table 49–7. De Stefano and co-workers (1994) cited pregnancy as a common triggering event for thrombosis in 238 patients with inherited thrombophilia.

In general, venous thrombosis and pulmonary embolism are treated as for any case (Chap. 46, p. 1237). Patients with prior episodes are given heparin prophylaxis. Routine screening for thrombophilia is not warranted in asymptomatic women with no history of thrombosis (American College of Obstetricians and Gynecologists, 2000a; Lockwood, 1999). It is uncertain if prophylaxis is

necessary in women without prior adverse outcomes but who are incidentally found to have thrombophilia.

ANTITHROMBIN III DEFICIENCY. These are rare mutations but the most thrombogenic (Table 49–7). Most are point mutations (Lockwood, 1999). Conard and co-workers (1990) reported that half of 63 pregnancies with antithrombin III deficiency were complicated by thrombosis either antepartum or postpartum. From their review, Swain and Gilstrap (1999) cite a risk of 45 to 70 percent of thromboembolism during pregnancy. Seguin and colleagues (1994) reviewed 23 cases of neonatal antithrombin III deficiency. There were 11 cases of thrombosis and 10 deaths. Heparin therapy is indicated throughout pregnancy (Toglia and Weg, 1996).

PROTEIN C DEFICIENCY. This deficiency is autosomal dominant, and there are a number of mutations. They are characterized by various combinations of reduced immunological and functional protein C levels (Lockwood, 1999). The heterozygous trait for protein C results in plasma levels of 55 to 65 percent of normal, and has an incidence of about 1 in 300 (Allaart and associates, 1993). Diagnosis during pregnancy has been problematic because some investigators have reported that pregnancy changes circulating levels. In a prospective cross-sectional study, however, Faught and colleagues (1995) reported that protein C levels were unchanged during pregnancy. Most authorities recommend that the diagnosis be established in the nonpregnant state.

About half of heterozygotes will suffer venous thrombotic episodes by adulthood. Homozygotes, or double heterozygotes, have severe deficiency usually manifest as *purpura fulminans* in the neonate. Conard and colleagues (1990) reported that 25 percent of 93 pregnancies complicated by protein C deficiency had deep-vein thrombosis. Puerperal thromboembolism is twice as

TABLE 49–7. Inherited Coagulopathies or Thrombophilias and Their Influence on Adverse Pregnancy Outcomes

Factor	Incidence (%)	Adverse Pregnancy Event (Relative Risk)				
		Thrombosis–Embolism	Pregnancy Wastage	Stillborn	Placental Infarction/ Abruption	Preeclampsia
Anti-thrombin III deficiency	0.1	50–250	2–5	5	?	Rare
Protein C deficiency	0.35	100	?	2–3	?	?
Protein S deficiency	0.01	90	?	3–4	?	Increased
Resistance to activated protein C	3–7	5–20	1–3	2–5	8–20	1–8
Prothrombin gene mutation	2–3	3–15	?	?	9	Increased
Hyperhomocystinemia	1–10	Increased	Increased	5	2–3	3

Includes data from Dizon-Townson and co-workers (1996), Gerdhart and associates (2000), Gherman and Goodwin (2000), Greer (1999), Kupferminc and colleagues (1999), Lockwood (1999), and van der Molen and associates (2000).

common as antepartum occurrence. Roos and co-workers (1990) described a woman with functional protein C deficiency who suffered a sagittal sinus thrombosis 10 days postpartum.

PROTEIN S DEFICIENCY. This is a cofactor for protein C activity, and its deficiency is caused by one of several autosomal dominant mutations. There are three types depending on free, functional, and total antigenically determined levels (Lefkowitz and colleagues, 1996). According to Comp and colleagues (1986), total protein S plasma concentrations, as well as functional protein S activity, are diminished substantively during normal pregnancy. Faught and associates (1995) observed that while total protein S concentration did not differ across pregnancy, there was a significant fall in free protein S levels after early pregnancy. Lefkowitz and co-workers (1996) reported a striking decline in protein S functional levels; thus diagnosis during pregnancy is difficult.

The lifetime risk of thromboembolism in patients with protein S deficiency is about 50 percent (Allaart and colleagues, 1993). Conard and associates (1990) described thrombosis in five of 29 pregnancies with this deficiency. One woman had a cerebral vein thrombosis. While the incidence of antepartum thromboembolism is increased, thrombosis is even more likely in the puerperium in a manner similar to protein C (Lockwood, 1999). Because of this, most authorities recommend that anticoagulation with heparin be given during pregnancy. Likely because many of these women already are receiving warfarin when they conceive, the disorder is associated with several fetal anomalies (Chap. 38, p. 1014).

ACTIVATED PROTEIN C RESISTANCE. This currently is the most prevalent thrombophilic syndrome. It is characterized by resistance of plasma to the anticoagulant effect of activated protein C. It is much more common than protein S, C, and antithrombin III deficiencies combined, with a frequency in the normal population of 3 to 7 percent (Svensson and Dahlback, 1994). The most common mutation is *factor V Leiden,* which is a G → A substitution in nucleotide 1691 that results in substitution of glutamine for arginine at position 506. This single missense gene mutation is autosomal dominant. Inheritance causes a thromboembolic risk because the Arg506 cleavage site is now resistant to the naturally occurring anticoagulant, activated protein C. Factor V Leiden is extremely common in Europeans (5 to 9 percent), intermediate in Hispanic Americans (2 percent), and rare in African Americans and Asians (Fassett and colleagues, 2000; Rees and co-workers, 1995).

As discussed earlier, functional protein S levels normally decline during pregnancy. This causes resistance to activated protein C which is amplified by normal increased factor VIII levels during pregnancy. The combination appears to exacerbate the prethrombotic effects of the factor V Leiden mutation (Walker and co-workers, 1997). As shown in Table 49–7, the risk for thromboembolism during pregnancy is increased 50-fold and is as high as 30 percent (Dizon-Townson and colleagues, 1997). Pregnancy wastage is only slightly increased, and the risk for preeclampsia is increased from two- to eightfold. Importantly, 10 percent of affected pregnancies have placental infarctions on the fetal side (Dizon-Townson and associates, 1996). The risk for abruptio placentae is increased up to eightfold (Wiener-Megnagi and co-workers, 1998). It also appears that fetuses heterozygous for factor V Leiden mutation can suffer cerebrovascular infarctions with resultant cerebral palsy (Thorarensen and colleagues, 1997).

HYPERHOMOCYSTINEMIA. A number of enzymes can affect plasma levels of homocysteine. When these are deficient, hyperhomocystinemia develops and increases the risk for atherosclerosis, thromboembolism, fetal neural-tube defects, and recurrent miscarriage (Lockwood, 1999). The most common cause is the C667T thermolabile mutation of 5,10-methylene tetrahydrofolate reductase (MTHFR). This is autosomal recessive, and Kupferminc and associates (1999) found a prevalence of 8 percent of homozygotes in women with normal pregnancies.

Fortunately, because it is so common, complications are uncommon even with MTHFR homozygosity. Lockwood (1999) cites a 10 percent lifetime incidence of thromboembolism, which is increased only 2.5-fold over normal. Thromboembolism is probably also more likely in pregnancy, as are other adverse pregnancy outcomes (Table 49–7). Laivuori and associates (2000) did not find an excessive incidence of preeclampsia. In a number of placentas examined because of bad perinatal outcomes, Khong and Hague (1999) found acute atherosis, intraluminal endovascular trophoblast, and infarctions. None of these was specific.

PROTHROMBIN G20210A MUTATION. This mutant gene is found in about 2 to 3 percent of the population and is associated with a three- to fourfold lifetime risk of thromboembolism (Margaglione and associates, 1998). As shown in Table 49–7, the risk of thromboembolism in pregnancy is increased 15-fold (Gerhardt and collaborators, 2000). It is also associated with an increased incidence of abruptio placentae and fetal growth restriction (Kupferminc and co-workers, 1999).

REFERENCES

Adams RJ, McKie VC, Hsu L, Files B, Vichinsky E, Pegelow C, Abboud M, Gallagher D, Kutlar A, Nichols FT, Bonds

DR, Brambilla D: Prevention of a first stroke by transfusions in children with sickle-cell anemia and abnormal results on transcranial doppler ultrasonography. N Engl J Med 339:5, 1998

Advisory Committee on Immunization Practices: Prevention of pneumococcal diseases. MMWR 46:1, 1997

Aessopos A, Karabatsos F, Farmakis D, Katsantoni A, Hatziliami A, Youssef J, Karagiorga M: Pregnancy in patients with well-treated β-thalassemia: Outcome for mothers and newborn infants. Am J Obstet Gynecol 180:360, 1999

Agency for Health Care Policy and Research, Sickle Disease Guideline Panel: Sickle Cell Disease: Comprehensive Screening and Management in Newborns and Infants. Rockville, MD, US Public Health Service, Department of Health and Human Services, April 1993

Agre P: Hereditary spherocytosis. JAMA 262:2887, 1989

Aitchison RGM, Marsh JCW, Hows JM, Russel NH, Gordon-Smith EC: Pregnancy associated aplastic anaemia: A report of five cases and review of current management. Br J Haematol 73:541, 1989

Allaart CF, Poort SR, Rosendaal FR, Reitsma PH, Bertina RM, Briet E: Increased risk of venous thrombosis in carriers of hereditary protein C deficiency defect. Lancet 341:134, 1993

Alter BP, Frissora CL, Halpérin DS, Freedman MH, Chitkara U, Alvarez E, Lynch L, Adler-Brecher B, Auerbach AD: Fanconi's anaemia and pregnancy. Br J Haematol 77:410, 1991

American College of Obstetricians and Gynecologists: Thromboembolism in pregnancy. Practice Bulletin No. 19, August 2000a

American College of Obstetricians and Gynecologists: The use of hormonal contraception in women with coexisting medical conditions. Practice Bulletin No. 18, July 2000b

American College of Obstetricians and Gynecologists: Genetic screening for hemoglobinopathies. Committee on Genetics. Committee Opinion No. 238, July 2000c

American College of Obstetricians and Gynecologists: Precis: An update in obstetrics and gynecology. Obstetrics, 2nd ed. Washington, DC, ACOG, 2000d, p 82

American College of Obstetricians and Gynecologists: Antepartum fetal surveillance. Practice Bulletin No. 9, October 1999

American College of Obstetricians and Gynecologists: Nutrition and women. Educational Bulletin No. 229, October 1996

Andrews NC: Disorders of iron metabolism. N Engl J Med 341:1986, 1999

Anyaegbunam A, Morel M-I G, Merkatz IR: Antepartum fetal surveillance tests during sickle cell crisis. Am J Obstet Gynecol 165:1081, 1991

Ascarelli MH, Emerson ES, Bigelow CL, Martin JN: Aplastic anemia and immune-mediated thrombocytopenia: Concurrent complications encountered in the third trimester of pregnancy. Obstet Gynecol 91:803, 1998

Association of Professors of Gynecology and Obstetrics: Immunization for women's health. APGO Educational Series on Women's Health Issues. Washington, DC, 1999

Baker PN, Cunningham FG: Platelet and coagulation abnormalities. In Lindheimer MD, Roberts JM, Cunningham FG (eds): Chesley's Hypertensive Disorders in Pregnancy, 2nd ed. Stamford, CT, Appleton & Lange, 1999, p 349

Barker DJP, Bull AR, Osmond C, Simmonds SJ: Fetal and placental size and risk of hypertension in adult life. BMJ 301:259, 1990

Beard J, Hillmen P, Anderson CC, Lewis SM, Pearson TC: Primary thrombocythaemia in pregnancy. Br J Haematol 77:371, 1991

Bell WR, Braine HG, Ness PM, Kickler TS: Improved survival in thrombotic thrombocytopenic purpura–hemolytic uremic syndrome. Clinical experience in 108 patients. N Engl J Med 325:398, 1991

Bennett TA, Kotelchuck M, Cox CE, Tucker MJ, Nadeau DA: Pregnancy-associated hospitalization in the United States in 1991 and 1992: A comprehensive view of maternal morbidity. Am J Obstet Gynecol 178:346, 1998

Berry SM, Leonardi MR, Wolfe HM, Dombrowski MP, Lanouette JM, Cotton DB: Maternal thrombocytopenia. Predicting neonatal thrombocytopenia with cordocentesis. J Reprod Med 42:276, 1997

Beutler E: Glucose-6-phosphate dehydrogenase deficiency. N Engl J Med 324:169, 1991

Blot I, Diallo D, Tchernia G: Iron deficiency in pregnancy: Effects on the newborn. Curr Opin Hematol 6:65, 1999

Boehlen F, Hohlfeld P, Extermann P, De Moerloose P: Maternal antiplatelet antibodies in predicting risk of neonatal thrombocytopenia. Obstet Gynecol 93:169, 1999

Boehlen F, Hohlfeld P, Extermann P, Perneger TV, De Moerloose P: Platelet count at term pregnancy: A reappraisal of the threshold. Obstet Gynecol 95:29, 2000

Bofill JA, Young RA, Perry KG Jr: Successful pregnancy in a woman with severe factor X deficiency. Obstet Gynecol 88:723, 1996

Borgna-Pignatti C, Marradi P, Rugolotto S, Marcolongo A: Successful pregnancy after bone marrow transplantation for thalassaemia. Bone Marrow Transplant 18:235, 1996

Bourantas K, Makrydimas G, Georgiou I, Repousis P, Lolis D: Aplastic anemia: Report of a case with recurrent episodes in consecutive pregnancies. J Reprod Med 42:672, 1997

Bowman JE: Prenatal screening from hemoglobinopathies. Am J Hum Genet 48:433, 1991

Braga J, Marques R, Branco A, Goncalves J, Lobato L, Pimentel JP, Flores MM, Goncalves E, Jorge CS: Maternal and perinatal implications of the use of human recombinant erythropoietin. Acta Obstet Gynecol Scan 75:449, 1996

Brewer CA, Adelson MD, Elder RC: Erythrocytosis associated with a placental-site trophoblastic tumor. Obstet Gynecol 79:846, 1992

Briggs GG, Freeman RK, Yaffe SJ: Drugs in Pregnancy and Lactation, 5th ed. Baltimore, Wilkins and Waverly, 1998, p 517

Burrows RF, Kelton JG: Fetal thrombocytopenia and its relation to maternal thrombocytopenia. N Engl J Med 329:1463, 1993a

Burrows RF, Kelton JG: Pregnancy in patients with idiopathic thrombocytopenic purpura: Assessing the risks for the infant at delivery. Obstet Gynecol Surv 48:781, 1993b

Carache S, Scott J, Niebyl J, Bonds D: Management of sickle cell disease in pregnant patients. Obstet Gynecol 55:407, 1980

Carr S, Dixon D, Star J, Dailey J: Intrauterine therapy for homozygous α-thalassemia. Obstet Gynecol 85:876, 1995

Cavenee MR, Cox SM, Mason R, Cunningham FG: Erythropoietin in pregnancies complicated by pyelonephritis. Obstet Gynecol 84:252, 1994

Centers for Disease Control: Recommendations for the use of folic acid to reduce the number of cases of spina bifida and other neural tube defects. MMWR 41 (RR-14), 1992

Centers for Disease Control: Anemia during pregnancy in low-income women—United States, 1987. MMWR 39:73, 1990

Centers for Disease Control: CDC criteria for anemia in children and childbearing-aged women. MMWR 38:400, 1989

Centers for Disease Control and Prevention: Availability of immune globulin intravenous for treatment of immune deficient patients—United States, 1997–1998. MMWR 48:159, 1999

Centers for Disease Control and Prevention: Recommendations to prevent and control iron deficiency in the United States. MMWR 38:400, 1989

Centers for Disease Control and Prevention: Update: Newborn screening for sickle cell disease—California, Illinois, and New York, 1998. MMWR 49:729, 2000

Charache S, Terrin ML, Moore RD, Dover GJ, Barton FB, Eckert SV, McMahon RP, Bonds DR, the Investigators of the Multicenter Study of Hydroxyurea in Sickle Cell Anemia: Effect of hydroxyurea on the frequency of painful crises in sickle cell anemia. N Engl J Med 332:1317, 1995

Chatwani A, Bruder N, Shapiro T, Reece A: May–Hegglin anomaly: A rare case of maternal thrombocytopenia in pregnancy. Am J Obstet Gynecol 166:143, 1992

Chen FE, Ooi C, Ha SY, Cheung BMY, Todd D, Liang R, Chan TK, Chan V: Genetic and clinical features of hemoglobin H disease in Chinese patients. N Engl J Med 343:544, 2000

Clark AL, Gall SA: Clinical uses of intravenous immunoglobulin in pregnancy. Am J Obstet Gynecol 176:241, 1997

Comp PC, Thurnau GR, Welsh J, Esmon CT: Functional and immunologic protein S levels are decreased during pregnancy. Blood 68:881, 1986

Conard J, Horellou MH, Van Dreden P, Lecompte T, Samama M: Thrombosis and pregnancy in congenital deficiencies in AT III, protein C or protein S: Study of 78 women. Thromb Haemost 63:319, 1990

Conti M, Mari D, Conti E, Muggiasca L, Mannucci PM: Pregnancy in women with different types of von Willebrand disease. Obstet Gynecol 68:282, 1986

Cortelazzo S, Finazzi G, Ruggeri M, Vestri O, Galli M, Rodeghiero F, Barbui T: Hydroxyurea for patients with essential thrombocythemia and a high risk of thrombosis. N Engl J Med 332:1132, 1995

Cox JV, Steane E, Cunningham G, Frenkel EP: Risk of alloimmunization and delayed hemolytic transfusion reactions in patients with sickle cell disease. Arch Intern Med 148:2485, 1988

Cox SM, Shelburne P, Mason R, Guss S, Cunningham FG: Mechanisms of hemolysis and anemia associated with acute antepartum pyelonephritis. Am J Obstet Gynecol 164:587, 1991

Cunningham FG, Cox SM, Harstad TW, Mason RA, Pritchard JA: Chronic renal disease and pregnancy outcome. Am J Obstet Gynecol 163:453, 1990

Cunningham FG, Pritchard JA: Prophylactic transfusions of normal red blood cells during pregnancies complicated by sickle cell hemoglobinopathies. Am J Obstet Gynecol 135:994, 1979

Cunningham FG, Pritchard JA, Hankins GDV, Anderson PL, Lucas MK, Armstrong KF: Idiopathic cardiomyopathy or compounding cardiovascular events. Obstet Gynecol 67:157, 1986

Cunningham FG, Pritchard JA, Mason R: Pregnancy and sickle hemoglobinopathy: Results with and without prophylactic transfusions. Obstet Gynecol 62:419, 1983

Daffos F, Capella-Pavlovsky M, Forestier F: Fetal blood sampling during pregnancy with the use of a needle guided by ultrasound: A study of 606 consecutive cases. Am J Obstet Gynecol 153:655, 1985

Dashe JS, Ramin SM, Cunningham FG: The long-term consequences of thrombotic microangiopathy (thrombotic thrombocytopenic purpura and hemolytic uremic syndrome) in pregnancy. Obstet Gynecol 91:662, 1998

Daskalakis GJ, Papageorgiou IS, Antsaklis AJ, Michalas SK: Pregnancy and homozygous beta thalassaemia major. Br J Obstet Gynaecol 105:1028, 1998

de Abood M, de Castillo Z, Guerrero F, Espino M, Austin KL: Effect of Depo-Provera® or Microgynon® on the painful crises of sickle cell anemia patients. Contraception 56:313, 1997

Deeg HJ, Leisenring W, Storb R, Nims J, Flowers MED, Witherspoon RP, Sanders J, Sullivan KM: Long-term outcome after marrow transplantation for severe aplastic anemia. Blood 91:3637, 1998

De Gramont A, Krulik M, Debray J: Paroxymal nocturnal haemoglobinuria and pregnancy. Lancet 1:868, 1987

De Stefano V, Leone G, Mastrangelo S, Tripodi A, Rodeghiero F, Castaman G, Barbui T, Finazzi G, Bizzi B, Mannucci PM: Clinical manifestations and management of inherited thrombophilia: Retrospective analysis and follow-up after diagnosis of 238 patients with congenital deficiency of antithrombin III, protein C, protein S. Throm Haemost 72:352, 1994

Delage R, Demers C, Cantin G, Roy J: Treatment of essential thrombocythemia during pregnancy with interferon-α. Obstet Gynecol 87:814, 1996

Dizon-Townson DS, Nelson LM, Easton K, Varner MW, Ward K: The factor V Leiden mutation may predispose women to severe preeclampsia. Am J Obstet Gynecol 175:902, 1996

Dizon-Townson DS, Nelson LM, Jang H, Varner MW, Ward K: The incidence of the factor V Leiden mutation in an obstetric population and its relationship to deep vein thrombosis. Am J Obstet Gynecol 176:833, 1997

Eddleman KA: Stem cells: What the obstetrician needs to know. Contemp Ob/Gyn 43:141, 1998

Edwards RZ, Rijhsinghani A: Dysfibrinogenemia and placental abruption. Obstet Gynecol 95:1043, 2000

Egerman RS, Witlin AG, Friedman SA, Sibai BM: Thrombotic thrombocytopenic purpura and hemolytic uremic syndrome in pregnancy: Review of 11 cases. Am J Obstet Gynecol 195:950, 1996

Eichhorn RF, Buurke EJ, Blok P, Berends MJ, Jansen DL: Sickle cell-like crisis and bone marrow necrosis associated with parvovirus B19 infection and heterozygosity for haemoglobins S and E. J Intern Med 245:103, 1999

Eliyahu S, Shalev E: A successful pregnancy after bone marrow transplantation for severe aplastic anaemia with pretransplant conditioning of total lymph-node irradiation and cyclophosphamide. Br J Haematol 86:649, 1994

El-Shafei AM, Dhaliwal JK, Sandhu AK: Pregnancy in sickle cell disease in Bahrain. Br J Obstet Gynaecol 99:101, 1992

Elstein D, Granovsky-Grisaru S, Rabinowitz R, Kanai R, Abrahamov A, Zimran A: Use of enzyme replacement therapy for Gaucher disease during pregnancy. Am J Obstet Gynecol 177:1509, 1997

Fadel HE, Krauss JS: Factor VII deficiency and pregnancy. Obstet Gynecol 73:453, 1989

Fassett MJ, Bohn YC, Kuo J, Wing DA: Longitudinal evaluation of activated protein C resistance among normal pregnancies of Hispanic women. Am J Obstet Gynecol 182:1433, 2000

Faught W, Garner P, Johnes G, Ivey B: Changes in protein C and protein S levels in normal pregnancy. Am J Obstet Gynecol 172:147, 1995

Fucharoen S, Winichagoon P: Clinical and hematologic aspects of hemoglobin E beta-thalassemia. Curr Opin Hematol 7:106, 2000

Fujimori K, Ohto H, Honda S, Sato A: Antepartum diagnosis of fetal intracranial hemorrhage due to maternal Bernard–Soulier syndrome. Obstet Gynecol 94:817, 1999

Funai EF, Klein SA, Lockwood CJ: Successful pregnancy outcome in a patient with both congenital hypofibrinogenemia and protein S deficiency. Obstet Gynecol 90:858, 1997

Furlan M, Robles R, Galbusera M, Remuzzi G, Kyrle PA, Brenner B, Krause M, Scharrer I, Aumann V, Mittler U, Solenthaler M, Lämmle B: Von Willebrand factor–cleaving protease in thrombotic thrombocytopenic purpura and the hemolytic-uremic syndrome. N Engl J Med 339:1578, 1998

Galvani DW, Jayakumar KS, Jordan A, Dasgupta R, Deeble TJ: Antenatal testing for haemoglobinopathies [letter]. Br J Haematol 108:198, 2000

Gandhi SK, Powers JC, Nomeir A-M, Fowle K, Kitzman DW, Rankin KM, Little WC: The pathogenesis of acute pulmonary edema associated with hypertension. N Engl J Med 344:17, 2000

Garratty G: Severe reactions associated with transfusion of patients with sickle cell disease. Transfusion 37:357, 1997

Garratty G, Leger RM, Arndt PA: Severe immune hemolytic anemia associated with prophylactic use of cefotetan in obstetric and gynecologic procedures. Am J Obstet Gynecol 181:103, 1999

Gasser C, Gautier E, Steck A, Siebenmann RE, Dechslin R: Haemolytisch-uramisch Syndrome: Bilaterale Nierenrindennekrosen bei akuten erworbenin haemolytischen Anamien. Schweiz Med Wochenschr 85:905, 1955

Gehlbach DL, Morgenstern LL: Antenatal screening for thalassemia minor. Obstet Gynecol 71:801, 1988

George JV: Platelets. Lancet 355:1531, 2000

George JN, Shattil SJ: The clinical importance of acquired abnormalities of platelet function. N Engl J Med 324:27, 1991

George JN, Woolf SH, Raskob GE, Wasser JS, Aledort LM, Ballem PJ, Blanchette VS, Bussel JB, Cines DB, Kelton JG, Lichtin AE, McMillan R, Okerbloom JA, Regan DH, Warrier I: Idiopathic thrombocytopenic purpura: A practice guideline developed by explicit methods for The American Society of Hematology. Blood 88:3, 1996

Gerhardt A, Scharf RE, Beckmann MW, Struve S, Bender HG, Pillny M, Sandmann W, Zotz RB: Prothrombin and factor V mutations in women with a history of thrombosis during pregnancy and the puerperium. N Engl J Med 342:374, 2000

Gherman RB, Goodwin TM: Obstetric implications of activated protein C resistance and factor V Leiden mutation. Obstet Gynecol Surv 2000 55:117, 2000

Ghidini A, Korker VL: Severe pyruvate kinase deficiency anemia. A case report. J Reprod Med 43:713, 1998

Gilsanz F, Vega MA, Gomez-Castillo E, Ruiz-Balda JA, Omenaca F: Fetal anaemia due to pyruvate kinase deficiency. Arch Dis Child 69:523, 1993

Glantz JC, Roberts DJ: Pregnancy complicated by thrombocytopenia secondary to human immunodeficiency virus infection. Obstet Gynecol 83:825, 1994

Goldenberg RL, Tamura T, DuBard M, Johnston KE, Copper RL, Neggers Y: Plasma ferritin and pregnancy outcome. Am J Obstet Gynecol 175:1356, 1996

Goodnough LT, Monk TG, Andriole GL: Erythropoietin therapy. N Engl J Med 336:933, 1997

Goodwin TM: Congenital hypofibrinogenemia in pregnancy. Obstet Gynecol Surv 44:157, 1989

Granovsky-Grisaru S, Aboulafia Y, Diamant YZ, Horowitz M, Abrahamov A, Zimran A: Gynecologic and obstetric aspects of Gaucher's disease: A survey of 53 patients. Am J Obstet Gynecol 172:1284, 1995

Greene MF, Frigoletto FD Jr, Claster SZ, Rosenthal D: Pregnancy and paroxysmal nocturnal hemoglobinuria: Report of a case and review of the literature. Obstet Gynecol Surv 38:591, 1983

Greer IA: Thrombosis in pregnancy: Maternal and fetal issues. Lancet 353:1258, 1999

Greer IA, Lowe GDO, Walker JJ, Forbes CD: Haemorrhagic problems in obstetrics and gynaecology in patients with congenital coagulopathies. Br J Obstet Gynaecol 98:909, 1991

Guy GP, Baxi LV, Hurlet-Jensen A, Chao CR: An unusual complication in a gravida with factor IX deficiency: Case report with review of the literature. Obstet Gynecol 80:502, 1992

Hallak M, Sharon A-S, Diukman R, Auslender R, Abramovici H: Supplementing iron intravenously in pregnancy: A way to avoid blood transfusions. J Reprod Med 42:99, 1997

Hayward CPM, Sutton DMC, Carter WH, Campbell ED, Scott JG, Francombe WH, Shumak KH, Baker MA: Treatment outcomes in patients with adult thrombotic thrombocytopenic purpura–hemolytic uremic syndrome. Arch Intern Med 154:982, 1994

Heijboer H, Brandjes DPM, Büller HR, Sturk A, ten Cate JW: Deficiencies of coagulation-inhibiting and fibrinolytic proteins in outpatients with deep-vein thrombosis. N Engl J Med 323:1512, 1990

Hillmen P, Lewis SM, Bessler M, Luzzatto L, Dacie JV: Natural history of paroxysmal nocturnal hemoglobinuria. N Engl J Med 333:1253, 1995

Howard RJ, Tuck SM, Pearson TC: Pregnancy in sickle cell disease in the UK: Results of a multicentre survey of the effect of prophylactic blood transfusion on maternal and fetal outcome. Br J Obstet Gynaecol 102:947, 1995

Hsia YE: Detection and prevention of important α-thalassemia variants. Semin Perinatol 15:35, 1991

Hsieh FJ, Chang FM, Ko TM, Kuo PL, Chang DY, Chen HY: The antenatal blood gas and acid–base status of normal fetuses and hydropic fetuses with Bart hemoglobinopathy. Obstet Gynecol 74:722, 1989

Hsu HW, Belfort MA, Vernino S, Moake JL, Moise KJ: Postpartum thrombotic thrombocytopenic purpura complicated by Budd–Chiari syndrome. Obstet Gynecol 85:839, 1995

Hurst D, Little B, Kleman KM, Emburg SH, Lubin GH: Anemia and hemoglobinopathies in Southeast Asian refugee children. J Pediatr 102:692, 1983

Jaegtvik S, Husebekk A, Aune B, Øian P, Dahl LB, Skogen B: Neonatal alloimmune thrombocytopenia due to anti-HPA 1a antibodies; the level of maternal antibodies predicts the severity of thrombocytopenia in the newborn. Br J Obstet Gynaecol 107:691, 2000

Jensen CE, Tuck SM, Wonke B: Fertility in β-thalassaemia major: A report of 16 pregnancies, preconceptual evaluation and a review of the literature. Br J Obstet Gynaecol 102:625, 1995

Kadir RA, Economides DL, Braithwaite J, Goldman E, Lee CA: The obstetric experience of carriers of haemophilia. Br J Obstet Gynaecol 104:803, 1997

Kadir RA, Lee CA, Sabin CA, Pollard D, Economides DL: Pregnancy in women with von Willebrand's disease or factor XI deficiency. Br J Obstet Gynaecol 105:314, 1998

Kadyrov M, Kosanke G, Kingdom J, Kaufmann P: Increased

fetoplacental angiogenesis during first trimester in anaemic women. Lancet 352:1747, 1998

Kahra K, Draganov B, Sund S, Hovig T: Postpartum renal failure: A complex case with probable coexistence of hemolysis, elevated liver enzymes, low platelet count, and hemolytic uremic syndrome. Obstet Gynecol 92:698, 1998

Kain ZN, Mayes LC, Pakes J, Rosenbaum SH, Schottenfeld R: Thrombocytopenia in pregnant women who use cocaine. Am J Obstet Gynecol 173:885, 1995

Kanavakis E, Vrettou C, Palmer G, Tzetis M, Mastrominas M, Traeger-Synodinos J: Preimplantation genetic diagnosis in 10 couples at risk for transmitting beta-thalassaemia major: Clinical experience including the initiation of six singleton pregnancies. Prenat Diagn 19:1217, 1999

Kaplan C, Daffos F, Forestier F, Tertain G, Catherine N, Pons JC, Tchernia G: Fetal platelet counts in thrombocytopenic pregnancy. Lancet 336:979, 1990

Khong TY, Hague WM: The placenta in maternal hyperhomocysteinaemia. Br J Obstet Gynaecol 106:273, 1999

Kincaid-Smith P, Fairley KF, Kloss M: Lupus anticoagulant associated with renal thrombotic microangiopathy and pregnancy-related renal failure. Q J Med 69:795, 1988

Klebanoff MA, Shiono PH, Selby JV, Trachtenberg AI, Graubard BI: Anemia and spontaneous preterm birth. Am J Obstet Gynecol 164:59, 1991

Konje JC, Murphy P, de Chazal R, Davidson A, Taylor D: Severe factor X deficiency and successful pregnancy. Br J Obstet Gynaecol 101:910, 1994

Koshy M, Burd L, Wallace D, Moawad A, Baron J: Prophylactic red-cell transfusions in pregnant patients with sickle cell disease: A randomized cooperative study. N Engl J Med 319:1447, 1988

Kumar RM, Rizk DEE, Khuranna A: β-thalassemia major and successful pregnancy. J Reprod Med 42:294, 1997

Kupferminc MJ, Eldor A, Steinman N, Many A, Bar-Am A, Jaffa A, Fait G, Lessing J: Increased frequency of genetic thrombophilia in women with complications of pregnancy. N Engl J Med 340:9, 1999

Laivuori H, Kaaja R, Ylikorkala O, Hiltunen T, Kontula K: 677 C→T polymorphism of the methylenetetrahydrofolate reductase gene and preeclampsia. Obstet Gynecol 96:277, 2000

Lam YH, Tang MHY, Lee CP, Tse HY: Prenatal ultrasonographic prediction of homozygous type 1 α-thalassemia at 12 to 13 weeks of gestation. Am J Obstet Gynecol 180:148, 1999

Lao TT, Lewinsky RM, Ohlsson A, Cohen H: Factor XII deficiency and pregnancy. Obstet Gynecol 78:491, 1991

Lefkowitz JB, Clarke SH, Barbour LA: Comparison of protein S functional and antigenic assays in normal pregnancy. Am J Obstet Gynecol 175:657, 1996

Letsky EA: Hematologic disorders. In Barron WM, Lindheimer MD (eds): Medical Disorders During Pregnancy, 3rd. St. Louis, Mosby, 2000, p 267

Lieberman E, Ryan KJ, Monson RR, Schoenbaum SC: Risk factors accounting for racial differences in the rate of premature birth. N Engl J Med 317:743, 1987

Lockwood CJ: Heritable coagulopathies in pregnancy. Obstet Gynecol Surv 54:754, 1999

Lu ZM, Goldenberg RL, Cliver SP, Cutter G, Blankson M: The relationship between maternal hematocrit and pregnancy outcome. Obstet Gynecol 77:190, 1991

Lubetsky A, Schulman S, Varon D, Martinowitz U, Kenet G, Gitel S, Inbal A: Safety and efficacy of continuous infusion of a combined factor VIII–von Willebrand factor (vWF)

concentrate (Haemate-P) in patients with von Willebrand disease. Thromb Haemost 81:229, 1999

Lucarelli G, Angelucci E, Giardini C, Baronciani D, Galimberti M, Polchi P, Bartolucci M, Muretto P, Albertini F: Fate of iron stores in thalassaemia after bone-marrow transplantation. Lancet 342:1388, 1993

Maberry MC, Cunningham FG: Sickle cell hemoglobinopathies complicating pregnancy. In Williams Obstetrics, 19th ed. Norwalk, CT, Appleton & Lange, Suppl 2, August/September, 1993

Maberry MC, Mason RA, Cunningham FG, Pritchard JA: Pregnancy complicated by hereditary spherocytosis. Obstet Gynecol 79:735, 1992

Maberry MC, Mason RA, Cunningham FG, Pritchard JA: Pregnancy complicated by hemoglobin CC and C–β-thalassemia disease. Obstet Gynecol 76:324, 1990

Magann EF, Bass D, Chauhan SP, Sullivan DL, Martin RW, Martin JN Jr: Antepartum corticosteroids: Disease stabilization in patients with the syndrome of hemolysis, elevated liver enzymes, and low platelets (HELLP). Am J Obstet Gynecol 171:1148, 1994

Mannucci PM: Treatment of von Willebrand disease. Haemophilia 4:661, 1998

Margaglione M, Brancaccio V, Guiliani N: Increased risk for venous thrombosis in carriers of the prothrombin G (A20210 gene variant). An Intern Med 129:89, 1998

Marsh J, Schrezenmeier H, Marin P, Ilhan O, Ljungman P, McCann S, Socié G, Tichelli A, Passweg J, Hows J, Raghavachar A, Locasciulli A, Bacigalupo A: Prospective randomized multicenter study comparing cyclosporin alone versus the combination of antithymocyte globulin and cyclosporin for treatment of patients with non-severe aplastic anemia: A report from the European Blood and Marrow Transplant (EBMT) Severe Aplastic Anaemia Working Party. Blood 93:2191, 1999

Means RT: Advances in the anemia of chronic disease. Int J Hematol 70:7, 1999

Miller ST, Sleeper LA, Pegelow CH, Enos LE, Wang WC, Weiner SJ, Wethers DL, Smith J, Kinney TR: Prediction of adverse outcomes in children with sickle-cell disease. N Engl J Med 342:83, 2000

Milner PF, Jones BR, Döbler J: Outcome of pregnancy in sickle cell anemia and sickle cell–hemoglobin C disease. Am J Obstet Gynecol 138:239, 1980

Moake JL: Moschcowitz, multimers, and metalloprotease. N Engl J Med 339:1629, 1998

Monni G, Ibba RM, Lai R, Cau G, Mura S, Olla G, Rosatelli C, Cao A: Early transabdominal chorionic villus sampling in couples at high genetic risk. Am J Obstet Gynecol 168:170, 1993

Morris JS, Dunn DT, Poddar D, Serjeant GR: Haematological risk factors for pregnancy outcome in Jamaican women with homozygous sickle cell disease. Br J Obstet Gynaecol 101:770, 1994

Mullaart RA, Van Dongen P, Gabreëls FJM, van Oostrom C: Fetal periventricular hemorrhage in von Willebrand's disease: Short review and first case presentation. Am J Perinatol 8:190, 1991

Murphy JF, O'Riordan J, Newcombe RG, Coles EC, Pearson JF: Relation of haemoglobin levels in first and second trimester to outcome of pregnancy. Lancet i:992, 1986

Musclow CE, Goldenberg H, Bernstein EP, Abbot D: Factor XI deficiency presenting as hemarthrosis during pregnancy. Am J Obstet Gynecol 157:178, 1987

Nagel RL: A knockout of a transgenic mouse—animal models of sickle cell anemia. N Engl J Med 339:194, 1998

Olivieri NF, Brittenham GM, McLaren CE, Templeton DM, Cameron RG, McClelland RA, Burt AD, Fleming DA: Long-term safety and effectiveness of iron-chelation therapy with deferiprone for thalassemia major. N Engl J Med 339:417, 1998

Packham CH: Pathogenesis and management of paroxysmal nocturnal haemoglobinuria. Blood Reviews 12:1, 1998

Pajor A, Lehoczky D, Szakács Z: Pregnancy and hereditary spherocytosis. Arch Gynecol Obstet 253:37, 1993

Paszty C, Brion CM, Manci E, Witowska HE, Stevens ME, Mohandas N, Rubin EM: Transgenic knockout mice with exclusively human sickle hemoglobin and sickle cell disease. Science 278:876, 1997

Payne SD, Resnik R, Moore TR, Hedriana HL, Kelly TF: Maternal characteristics and risk of severe neonatal thrombocytopenia and intracranial hemorrhage in pregnancies complicated by autoimmune thrombocytopenia. Am J Obstet Gynecol 177:149, 1997

Peleg D, Hunter SK: Perinatal management of women with immune thrombocytopenic purpura: Survey of United States perinatologists. Am J Obstet Gynecol 180:645, 1999

Peng TC, Kickler TS, Bell WR, Haller E: Obstetric complications in a patient with Bernard–Soulier syndrome. Am J Obstet Gynecol 165:425, 1991

Perrine SP, Ginder GD, Fuller DV, Dover GH, Ikuta T, Wikowska HE, Cai S-P, Vichinsky EP, Olivieri NF: A short-term trial of butyrate to stimulate fetal-globin-gene expression in the β-globin disorders. N Engl J Med 328:81, 1993

Platt OS, Brambilla DJ, Rosse WF, Milner PF, Castro O, Steinberg MH, Klug PP: Mortality in sickle cell disease—life expectancy and risk factors for early death. N Engl J Med 330:1639, 1994

Poddar D, Maude GH, Plant MJ, Scorer H, Serjeant GR: Pregnancy in Jamaican women with homozygous sickle cell disease: Fetal and maternal outcome. Br J Obstet Gynaecol 93:927, 1986

Powars D, Weidman JA, Odom-Maryon T, Niland JC, Johnson C: Sickle cell chronic lung disease: Prior morbidity and the risk of pulmonary failure. Medicine 67:66, 1988

Powars DR, Sandhu M, Niland-Weiss J, Johnson C, Bruce S, Manning PR: Pregnancy in sickle cell disease. Obstet Gynecol 67:217, 1986

Pritchard JA, Cunningham FG, Mason RA: Coagulation changes in eclampsia: Their frequency and pathogenesis. Am J Obstet Gynecol 124:855, 1976

Pritchard JA, Scott DE: Iron demands in pregnancy. In Hallberg L, Harwerth HG, Vanotti A (eds): Iron Deficiency Pathogenesis, Clinical Aspects, Therapy. New York, Academic Press, 1970

Pritchard JA, Scott DE, Whalley PJ, Cunningham FG, Mason RA: The effects of maternal sickle cell hemoglobinopathies and sickle cell trait on reproductive performance. Am J Obstet Gynecol 117:662, 1973

Provan D, Weatherall D: Red cells II: Acquired anaemias and polycythaemia. Lancet 355:1260, 2000

Ramahi AJ, Lewkow LM, Dombrowski MP, Bottoms SF: Sickle cell E hemoglobinopathy and pregnancy. Obstet Gynecol 71:493, 1988

Randi ML, Barbone E, Rossi C, Girolami A: Essential thrombocythemia and pregnancy. A report of six normal pregnancies in five untreated patients. Obstet Gynecol 83:915, 1994

Reece EA, Coustan DR, Hayslett JP, Holford T, Coulehan J, O'Connor TZ, Hobbins JC: Diabetic nephropathy: Pregnancy performance and fetomaternal outcome. Am J Obstet Gynecol 159:56, 1988

Rees DC, Cox M, Clegg JB: World distribution of factor V Leiden. Lancet 346:1133, 1995

Rijhsinghani A, Wiechert RJ: Diamond–Blackfan anemia in pregnancy. Obstet Gynecol 83:827, 1994

Robson JS, Martin AM, Ruckley VA, MacDonald MK: Irreversible postpartum renal failure. Q J Med 37:423, 1968

Rock GA, Shumak KH, Buskard NA, Blanchette VS, Kelton JG, Nair RC, Spasoff RA, Canadian Apheresis Study Group: Comparison of plasma exchange with plasma infusion in the treatment of thrombotic thrombocytopenic purpura. N Engl J Med 325:393, 1991

Roos KL, Pascuzzi RM, Kuharik MA, Shapiro AD, Manco-Johnson MJ: Postpartum intracranial venous thrombosis associated with dysfunctional protein C and deficiency of protein S. Obstet Gynecol 76:492, 1990

Rosse W, Bunn HF: Hemolytic anemias. In Isselbacher KJ, Braunwald E, Wilson JD, Martin JB, Fauci AS, Kasper DL (eds): Harrison's Principles of Internal Medicine, 13th ed. New York, McGraw-Hill, 1994, p 1743

Rouse DJ, Owen J, Goldenberg RL: Routine maternal platelet count: An assessment of a technologically driven screening practice. Am J Obstet Gynecol 179:573, 1998

Ruch WA, Klein RL: Polycythemia vera and pregnancy. Obstet Gynecol 23:107, 1964

Ryan TM, Ciavatta DJ, Townes TM: Knockout-transgenic mouse model of sickle cell disease. Science 278:873, 1997

Sainio S, Järvenpää AL, Renlund M, Riikonen S, Teramo K, Kekomäki R: Thrombocytopenia in term infants: A population-based study. Obstet Gynecol 95:441, 2000

Samuels P, Bussel JB, Braitman LE, Tomaski A, Druzin ML, Mennuti MT, Cines DB: Estimation of the risk of thrombocytopenia in the offspring of pregnant women with presumed immune thrombocytopenic purpura. N Engl J Med 323:229, 1990

Sanders JE, Hawley J, Levy W, Gooley T, Buckner CD, Deeg HJ, Doney K, Storb R, Sullivan K, Witherspoon R, Appelbaum FR: Pregnancies following high-dose cyclophosphamide with or without high-dose busulfan or total-body irradiation and bone marrow transplantation. Blood 87:3045, 1996

Scanlon KS, Yip R, Schieve LA, Cogswell ME: High and low hemoglobin levels during pregnancy: Differential risk for preterm birth and small for gestational age. Obstet Gynecol 96:741, 2000

Schechter AN, Rodgers GP: Sickle cell anemia—basic research reaches the clinic. N Engl J Med 332:1372, 1995

Scholl TO: High third-trimester ferritin concentration: Associations with very preterm delivery, infection, and maternal nutritional status. Obstet Gynecol 92:161, 1998

Scott DE, Pritchard JA: Iron deficiency in healthy young college women. JAMA 199:147, 1967

Scott JR, Rote NS, Cruikshank DP: Antiplatelet antibodies and platelet counts in pregnancies complicated by autoimmune thrombocytopenic purpura. Am J Obstet Gynecol 145:932, 1983

Seguin J, Weatherstone K, Nankervis C: Inherited antithrombin III deficiency in the neonate. Arch Pediatr Adolesc Med 48:389, 1994

Seoud MA, Cantwell C, Nobles G, Levy DL: Outcome of pregnancies complicated by sickle cell and sickle C hemoglobinopathies. Am J Perinatol 11:187, 1994

Serjeant GR: Sickle-cell disease. Lancet 350:725, 1997

Shaaban AF, Flake AW: Fetal hematopoietic stem cell transplantation. Semin Perinatol 23:515, 1999

Sherer DM, Anyaegbunam A, Onyeije C: Antepartum fetal intracranial hemorrhage, predisposing factors and prenatal sonography: A review. Am J Perinatol 15:431, 1998

Shumak KH, Rock GA, Nair RC: Late relapses in patients successfully treated for thrombotic thrombocytopenic purpura. Ann Intern Med 122:569, 1995

Silver RM, Branch W, Scott JR: Maternal thrombocytopenia in pregnancy: Time for a reassessment. Am J Obstet Gynecol 173:479, 1995

Smith JA, Espeland M, Bellevue R, Bonds D, Brown AK, Koshy M: Pregnancy in sickle cell disease: Experience of the Cooperative Study of Sickle Cell Disease. Obstet Gynecol 87:199, 1996

Snyder TE, Lee LP, Lynch S: Pregnancy-associated hypoplastic anemia: A review. Obstet Gynecol Surv 46:264, 1991

Socié G, Stone JV, Wingard JR, Weisdorf D, Henslee-Downey PJ, Bredeson C, Cahn JY, Passweg JR, Rowlings PA, Schouten HC, Kolb HJ, Klein JP: Long-term survival and late deaths after allogeneic bone marrow transplantation. N Engl J Med 341:14, 1999

Solal-Céligny P, Tertian G, Fernandez H, Pons J-C, Lambert T, Na-jean Y, Clauvel JP, Papiernik E, Tchernia G: Pregnancy and paroxysmal nocturnal hemoglobinuria. Arch Intern Med 148:593, 1988

Star J, Rosene K, Ferland J, Dileone G, Hogan J, Kestin A: Flow cytometric analysis of platelet activation throughout normal gestation. Obstet Gynecol 90:562, 1997

Starksen NF, Bell WR, Kickler TS: Unexplained hemolytic anemia associated with pregnancy. Am J Obstet Gynecol 146:617, 1983

Steinberg MH: Management of sickle cell disease. N Engl J Med 340:1021, 1999

Svensson PJ, Dahlback B: Resistance to activated protein C as a basis for venous thrombosis. N Engl J Med 330:517, 1994

Swain LS, Gilstrap LC: Antithrombin III deficiency in pregnancy. Prim Care Update Ob/Gyns 6:111, 1999

Taylor DJ, Mallen C, McDougal N, Lind T: Effect of iron supplementation on serum ferritin levels during and after pregnancy. Br J Obstet Gynaecol 89:1011, 1982

Thorarensen O, Ryan S, Hunter J, Youkin DP: Factor V Leiden mutation: An unrecognized cause of hemiplegic cerebral palsy, neonatal stroke, and placental thrombosis. Ann Neurol 42:372, 1997

Toglia MR, Weg JG: Venous thromboembolism during pregnancy. N Engl J Med 335:108, 1996

Tollin SR, Seely EW: Case report: Postpartum hypopituitarism in a patient with sickle cell trait. Am J Med Sci 308:35, 1994

Trehan AK, Fergusson ILC: Congenital afibrinogenaemia and successful pregnancy outcome. Case report. Br J Obstet Gynaecol 98:722, 1991

Tsai HM, Lian ECY: Antibodies to Von Willebrand factor–cleaving protease in acute thrombotic thrombocytopenic purpura. N Engl J Med 339:1585, 1998

Tuck SM, Studd JWW, White JM: Pregnancy in women with sickle cell trait. Br J Obstet Gynaecol 90:108, 1983

Urato AC, Repke JT: May–Hegglin anomaly: A case of vaginal delivery when both mother and fetus are affected. Am J Obstet Gynecol 179:260, 1998

van den Broek NR, Letsky EA, White SA, Shenkin A: Iron status in pregnant women: Which measurements are valid? Br J Haematol 103:817, 1998

van der Molen AF, Arends GE, Nelen W, van der Put NJM, Heil SG, Eskes TKAB, Blom HJ: A common mutation in the 5, 10-methylenetetrahydrofolate reductase gene as a new risk factor for placental vasulopathy. Am J Obstet Gynecol 182:1258, 2000

Van Erk A, Visschers G, Jansen W, Statius Van Eps L: Maternal death due to sickle cell chronic lung disease. Br J Obstet Gynaecol 99:162, 1992

Veille J, Hanson R: Left ventricular systolic and diastolic function in pregnant patients with sickle cell disease. Am J Obstet Gynecol 170:107, 1994

Vichinsky EP, Neumayr LD, Earles AN, Williams R, Lennette ET, Dean D, Nickerson B, Orringer E, McKie V, Bellevue R, Daeschner C, Manci EA: Causes and outcomes of the acute chest syndrome in sickle cell disease. N Engl J Med 342:1855, 2000

Viteri FE: The consequences of iron deficiency and anemia in pregnancy. Adv Exp Med Biol 352:127, 1994

Vora M, Gruslin A: Erythropoietin in obstetrics. Obstet Gynecol Surv 53:500, 1998

Walker MC, Garner PR, Keely EJ, Rock GA, Reis MD: Changes in activated protein C resistance during normal pregnancy. Am J Obstet Gynecol 177:162, 1997

Walters MC, Patience M, Leisenring W, Eckman JR, Scott JP, Mentzer WC, Davies SC, Ohene-Frempong K, Bernaudin F, Matthews DC, Storb R, Sullivan KM: Bone marrow transplantation for sickle-cell disease. N Engl J Med 335:369, 1996

Weatherall DJ: Single gene disorders or complex traits: Lessons from the thalassaemias and other monogenic diseases. BMJ 321:1117, 2000

Weatherall DJ: The thalassaemias. BMJ 314:1675, 1997

Weatherall DJ, Provan AB: Red cell I: Inherited anaemias. Lancet 355:1169, 2000

Weiner CP: Thrombotic microangiopathy in pregnancy and the postpartum period. Semin Hematol 24:119, 1987

Wiener-Megnagi Z, Ben-Shalomo I, Goldberg Y, Shalev E: Resistance to activated protein C and the Leiden mutation: High prevalence in patients with abruptio placentae. Am J Obstet Gynecol 179:1565, 1998

Whalley PJ: Bacteriuria of pregnancy. Am J Obstet Gynecol 97:723, 1967

Xu K, Shi ZM, Veeck LL, Hughes MR, Rosenwaks Z: First unaffected pregnancy using preimplantation genetic diagnosis of sickle cell anemia. JAMA 281:1701, 1999

Yeomans E, Lowe TW, Eigenbrodt EH, Cunningham FG: Liver histopathologic findings in women with sickle cell disease given prophylactic transfusion during pregnancy. Am J Obstet Gynecol 163:958, 1990

Young NS, Maciejewski J: The pathophysiology of acquired aplastic anemia. N Engl J Med 336, 1365, 1997

Zamorano AF, Arnalich F, Sánchez Casas E, Sicilia A, Solis C, Vázquez JJ, Gasalla R: Levels of iron, vitamin B_{12}, folic acid and heir binding proteins during pregnancy. Acta Haematol 74:92, 1985

50

Endocrine Disorders

THYROID DISEASES

Hyperthyroidism
Subclinical Thyrotoxicosis
Hypothyroidism
Subclinical Hypothyroidism
Nodular Thyroid Disease
Postpartum Thyroiditis

PARATHYROID DISEASE

Hyperparathyroidism
Hypoparathyroidism
Pregnancy-associated Osteoporosis

ADRENAL GLAND DISORDERS

Pheochromocytoma
Cushing Syndrome
Addison Disease
Primary Aldosteronism

PITUITARY DISEASES

Prolactinomas
Acromegaly
Diabetes Insipidus
Sheehan Syndrome
Lymphocytic Hypophysitis

A variety of endocrine disorders can complicate pregnancy and vice versa. The most common of these, diabetes mellitus, is discussed in Chapter 51. Because thyroid disorders are also common in young women, they are encountered with some frequency during pregnancy. Other endocrinopathies, although less common, may have devastating effects on pregnancy outcome if unrecognized and untreated, for example, pheochromocytoma.

The pathogenic basis of most endocrine disorders is disordered autoimmunity. A number of autoantigens, autoantibodies, and cellular immune elements have been identified to cause destruction or stimulation of thyroid, pancreatic, or adrenal glandular tissue (Baker, 1997). Usually a nonspecific event—for example, viral infection—initiates an antigen and organ-specific response with subsequent immune-mediated glandular destruction. Frequently there is a genetic predisposition also, and inheritance of major histocomptibility complex antigens or increased target organ susceptibility plays a role. Finally, environmental factors predispose to development of some of these autoimmune endocrinopathies.

THYROID DISEASES

A number of thyroid disorders are common in the general population, especially in young women. The incidence of sporadic nontoxic goiter is estimated to be as much as 5 percent of the North American population. The incidence of hyperthyroidism, hypothyroidism, and thyroiditis probably approaches 1 percent for each condition.

The interactions between pregnancy and the thyroid gland are fascinating from at least three aspects. First, there are the now well-known and seemingly aberrant changes in tests of thyroid function induced by pregnancy; and indeed, there may be actual functional changes. Second, there is an intimate relationship between maternal and fetal thyroid function. Although the latter is largely autonomous even early in pregnancy, drugs that affect the maternal thyroid also affect the fetal gland. Third, there are a number of related abnormal pregnancy and thyroid conditions that at least appear to interact. For example, clinical thyrotoxicosis may be caused by gestational trophoblastic disease. Thyroid autoantibodies have been associated with increased early pregnancy wastage, and uncontrolled thyrotoxicosis and untreated hypothyroidism are both associated with adverse pregnancy outcomes. Finally, there is evidence that although the severity of some autoimmune thyroid disorders is ameliorated during pregnancy, these same disorders may be exacerbated postpartum.

THYROID PHYSIOLOGY. The impact of pregnancy on maternal thyroid physiology is substantial. There are changes in the structure and function of the gland that can cause confusion in the diagnosis of thyroid abnormalities. Consequently, evaluation of thyroid disorders and proper interpretation of thyroid function tests during pregnancy requires an understanding of these changes. These are discussed in detail in Chapter 8 (p. 192) and are now summarized.

Anatomically, there is moderate thyroid enlargement as a result of glandular hyperplasia and increased vascularity. Histologically, the appearance of the gland is consistent with active formation and secretion of thyroid hormone. Thyroid gland volume determined ultrasonographically increases during pregnancy, although its echostructure and echogenicity remain unchanged (Rasmussen and colleagues, 1989). Importantly, pregnancy does not cause impressive thyromegaly, and thus any goiter or nodule should be approached as if pathological.

During pregnancy, there is increased uptake of radioiodine by the maternal thyroid gland. Beginning as early as the second month, total serum thyroxine and triiodothyronine concentrations rise sharply. Daily thyroxine secretion is probably increased, perhaps due to increased placental degradation. Contrary to previous teaching, substantial amounts of thyroxine are transferred from mother to fetus, at least in those cases of fetal hypothyroidism due to enzyme defects or thyroid agenesis (Vulsma and colleagues, 1989). During pregnancy, the serum concentration of the major thyroid hormone carrier protein, *thyroid-binding globulin* (*TBG*), is increased considerably. This is due to a combination of estrogen-stimulated hepatocyte production as well as altered glycosylation of the protein that inhibits degradation. *Thyrotropin-releasing hormone* (*TRH*) is undetectable in maternal serum, and its secretion does not appear to be altered during normal pregnancy. Beginning at mid-pregnancy, fetal serum TRH is detectable, but does not increase. Injected TRH shows minimal placental transfer (Bajoria and co-workers, 1998).

Thyrotropin or *thyroid-stimulating hormone* (*TSH*) is a 28- to 30-kDa glycoprotein related to follicle-stimulating hormone (FSH), luteinizing hormone (LH), and chorionic gonadotropin (hCG). It is not bound by carrier proteins, its concentration is unchanged during pregnancy, and it does not cross the placenta. It appears that the thyrotropic substance isolated from human placenta, previously called *chorionic thyrotropin*, is in reality chorionic gonadotropin which has a very small crossover activity of 0.1 percent, but it is produced in prodigious quantities (Grossman and associates, 1997). Thus, in early pregnancy, coincidental with maximum chorionic gonadotropin levels, serum free thyroxine levels increase while thyrotropin levels decrease. Despite this, they usually are within the normal range. During most of pregnancy, however, levels of free thyroxine and tri-iodothyronine, as well as thyrotropin, are maintained within a narrow normal range, and thus there is not overt functional hyperthyroidism.

HYPERTHYROIDISM. Thyrotoxicosis, or hyperthyroidism, complicates about 1 in 2000 pregnancies (Mestman and colleagues, 1995). As perhaps expected, mild thyrotoxicosis is difficult to diagnose during pregnancy. Some helpful signs include:

1. Tachycardia that exceeds the increase associated with normal pregnancy.
2. An abnormally elevated sleeping pulse rate.
3. Thyromegaly.
4. Exophthalmos.
5. Failure in a nonobese woman to gain weight despite normal or increased food intake.

Confirmation has been made easier by assays to determine elevated serum free thyroxine levels along with the recent development of assays that reliably measure thyrotropin levels less than 0.1 mU/L. In fact, such accuracy has led to discovery of *subclinical hyperthyroidism* (Utiger, 1994). In younger persons, exogenous thyroxine replacement sometimes causes thyrotoxicosis, but as many as 5 percent of older persons may be affected spontaneously. Rarely, hyperthyroidism may be associated with normal serum thyroxine values but abnormally high serum triiodothyronine levels, so-called **T₃-toxicosis.**

THYROTOXICOSIS AND PREGNANCY. The overwhelming cause of thyrotoxicosis in pregnancy is **Graves disease,** an organ-specific autoimmune process usually associated with thyroid-stimulating antibodies. These autoantibodies mimic thyrotropin in its ability to stimulate thyroid function, and they appear to be responsible for both thyroid hyperfunction and growth in Graves disease. In an earlier classical study, Amino and colleagues (1982) reported that thyroid-stimulating antibody activity declined during pregnancy in 41 women with Graves disease. This was associated with chemical remission during almost all pregnancies. Between 1 and 4 months postpartum, many women had recurrence of antithyroid antibodies along with hyperthyroxinemia. Recently, Kung and Jones (1998) confirmed that the decline in antibody levels during pregnancy was accompanied by a mirror-image increase in thyroid stimulating–blocking antibody levels (Fig. 50–1). These changes were associated with corresponding decreased free thyroxine levels during pregnancy with a return to baseline at 4 months postpartum. Thus, it appears that any ameliorative effects of pregnancy on thyroid-stimulating antibodies is from production of blocking antibodies.

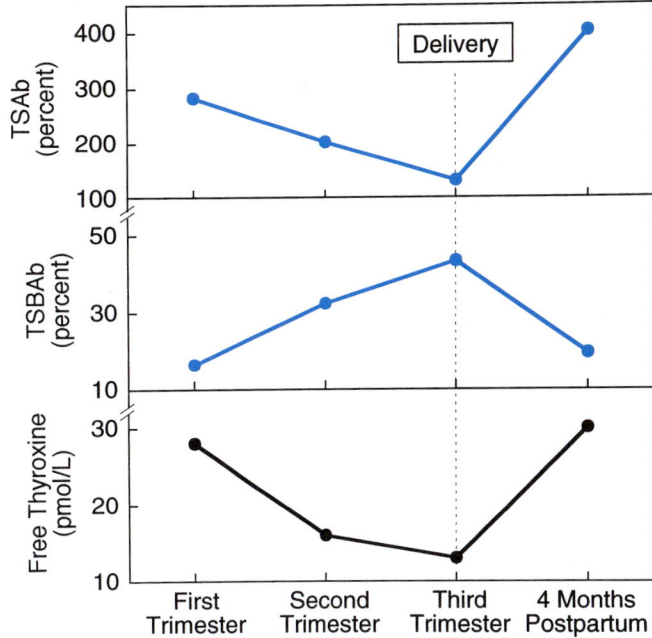

FIGURE 50–1. Change across pregnancy and at 4 months postpartum in maternal serum thyroid-stimulating antibody (TSAb), thyroid stimulating-blocking antibody (TSBAb) and free thyroxine. (Data from Kung and Jones, 1998.)

TREATMENT. Thyrotoxicosis during pregnancy is generally treated medically. Hyperthyroidism can nearly always be controlled by thioamide drugs (Weetman, 2000). Some prefer *propylthiouracil* because it partially inhibits the conversion of T_4 to T_3, it crosses the placenta less readily then *methimazole,* and it is not associated with **aplasia cutis,** which has been attributed to methimazole. Wing and associates (1994) have provided evidence in 185 pregnant thyrotoxic women that both drugs are effective and safe. Transient leukopenia manifests in about 10 percent of patients given thioamide drugs, but this does not require cessation of therapy. In about 0.2 percent, agranulocytosis develops suddenly and mandates discontinuance of the drug. It is not dose related, and because of its acute onset, serial leukocyte counts during therapy are not helpful (Franklyn, 1994; Mestman and colleagues, 1995). If fever or sore throat develop, patients are instructed to discontinue medication immediately and to report for a complete blood count (Vanderpump and associates, 1996). Although either thioamide has the potential for causing fetal complications, it is difficult to ascribe all cases of neonatal thyroid abnormalities to them because thyrotropin-blocking antibodies also cross the placenta and may bind to the fetal thyroid gland.

A regimen employing propylthiouracil without replacement thyroid hormone has been followed at Parkland Hospital for four decades with very satisfactory pregnancy outcomes for women who become euthyroid (Davis and associates, 1989). The dose of propylthiouracil is empirical, and for nonpregnant patients, the American Thyroid Association recommends an initial dose of 100 to 600 mg for propylthiouracil or 10 to 40 mg for methimazole (Singer and colleagues, 1995). In pregnant women, the American College of Obstetricians and Gynecologists (1993) recommends a starting dose of 300 to 450 mg daily for propylthiouracil. Reinwein and associates (1993) randomized 509 nonpregnant thyrotoxic patients to therapy with either 10 or 40 mg of methimazole. Of these, 68 and 83 percent, respectively, were euthyroid by 3 weeks. At 6 weeks, these numbers were 85 and 92 percent. In pregnant women, Wing and colleagues (1994) reported the median time to normalization of the free thyroxine index was 7 to 8 weeks with either methimazole or propylthiouracil.

In our experiences, metabolic control requires higher doses than most authorities recommend for pregnant women (Davis and colleagues, 1989). Of 52 women with thyrotoxicosis given an initial propylthiouracil dose that averaged 600 mg, about half underwent remission, and the dose was decreased to less than 300 mg within 8 weeks. In a third, however, it was necessary to increase the dose. In only 10 percent of these women could the dose be decreased to 150 mg by delivery. Kriplani and colleagues (1994) similarly found that the initial dose of carbimazole could be decreased in only a fourth of 32 pregnant thyrotoxic women. These clinical experiences are at variance with observations discussed earlier suggesting that remission is commonly induced by pregnancy.

Thyroidectomy may be carried out after thyrotoxicosis has been brought under medical control. Because of the increased vascularity of the thyroid gland during pregnancy, such surgery is more complicated than in the nonpregnant state. For women who cannot adhere to medical treatment or in whom drug therapy proves toxic, thyroidectomy may be appropriate. Miccoli and co-workers (1996) cite an incidence of about 2 percent for vocal cord palsy and 3 percent for hypoparathyroidism.

PREGNANCY OUTCOME. Pregnancy outcomes in thyrotoxic women depend upon whether metabolic control is achieved. In women who remain hyperthyroid despite therapy, and in those whose disease is untreated, there is a higher incidence of preeclampsia and heart failure, as well as adverse perinatal outcomes (Table 50–1). Sherif and colleagues (1991) reported perinatal mortality of 8 percent in 92 women with thyrotoxicosis, and Kriplani and associates (1994) reported 12 percent fetal mortality in 32 such women.

TABLE 50–1. Pregnancy Outcomes in 239 Women with Overt Thyrotoxicosis

Factor	Treated and Euthyroid (n = 149)	Uncontrolled Thyrotoxicosis (n = 90)
Maternal Outcome		
Preeclampsia	17 (11%)	15 (17%)
Heart failure	1	7 (8%)
Death	—	1
Perinatal Outcome		
Preterm delivery	12 (8%)	29 (32%)
Growth restriction	11 (7%)	15 (17%)
Stillborn	0/59	6/33 (18%)
Thyrotoxicosis	1	2
Hypothyroid	4	0
Goiter	2	0

Data from Davis (1989), Kriplani (1994), and Millar (1994), and all of their colleagues.

THYROID STORM OR HEART FAILURE. Thyroid storm is encountered only rarely in untreated women with Graves disease (Davis and associates, 1989). In some, storm is caused by a large functioning tumor (Tewari and co-workers, 1998). Heart failure is much more likely than thyroid storm, and it is caused by the profound myocardial effects of thyroxine (Klein and Ojamaa, 1998). This is characterized by a high-output state similar to constant exercising. Ironically, normal pregnancy causes a similar effect. Thus, it is not surprising that all of these effects are additive or even synergistic. In 239 women shown in Table 50–1, heart failure developed in 3 percent. If thyrotoxicosis was not controlled, this rate was 8 percent and pulmonary edema commonly was precipitated by preeclampsia, anemia, or sepsis. In our experiences, and as shown in Figure 50–2, thyroxine-induced cardiomyopathy is reversed with treatment over several weeks to months.

If thyroid storm develops, or if there is heart failure in the face of untreated or incompletely treated thyrotoxicosis, the woman should be managed in an intensive care unit. Specific treatment consists of 1 g of propylthiouracil given orally or crushed through a nasogastric tube. Propylthiouracil is continued in 200-mg doses every 6 hours. An hour later, iodide is given to inhibit the release of T_3 and T_4 from the thyroid gland. It is administered orally as 5 drops of supersaturated solution of potassium iodide (SSKI) every 8 hours; or Lugol solution, 10 drops every 8 hours. In the woman with a history of iodine-induced anaphylaxis, lithium carbonate, 300 mg every 6 hours, is given instead of iodide solution (Burch and Wartofsky, 1993). Blood levels of

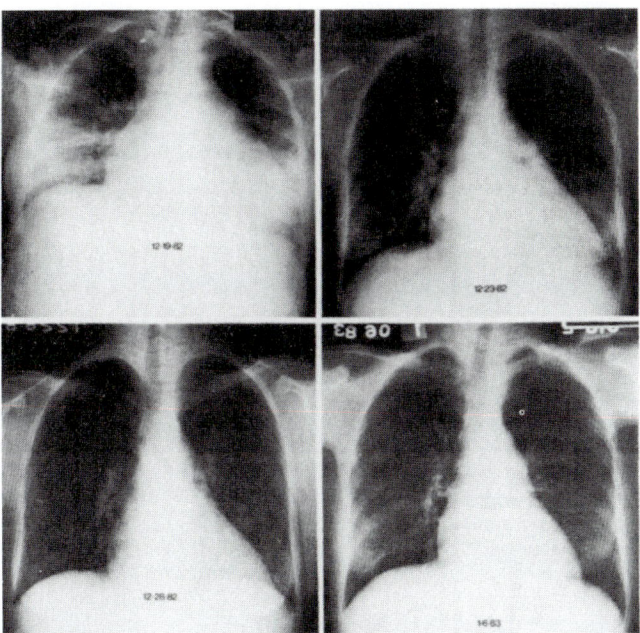

FIGURE 50–2. Serial chest radiographs demonstrating the 18-day resolution of pulmonary edema and cardiomegaly in a 27-year-old thyrotoxic woman with septic abortion and heart failure at 20 weeks' gestation. (From Hankins and colleagues, 1984, with permission.)

lithium should be monitored and kept within the range of 0.5 to 1.5 mmol/L. In addition, most authorities recommend dexamethasone, 2 mg intravenously every 6 hours for four doses, to further block peripheral conversion of T_4 to T_3. Some recommend intravenous administration of a β-blocker drug, but this should be approached cautiously if there is heart failure. Propranolol, labetalol, and esmolol have all been used intrapartum (Bowman and colleagues, 1998). A principal directive of therapy is supportive treatment and aggressive management of serious hypertension, infection, and anemia.

EFFECTS OF THYROTOXICOSIS ON THE NEONATE.
The neonate may manifest transient thyrotoxicosis, which sometimes requires antithyroid drug treatment. Conversely, long-standing exposure in utero to these drugs may cause neonatal hypothyroidism. In either case, the fetus may develop a goiter (Fig. 50–3). Earlier estimates of adverse fetal effects induced by thiourea drugs were exaggerated, and their use during pregnancy carries an extremely small risk (Momotani and associates, 1997; O'Doherty and colleagues, 1999). Of the 239 thyrotoxic women treated with thiourea shown in Table 50–1, there was evidence for hypothyroidism in only four infants. Davidson and colleagues (1991) described a case of Graves disease in which the mother was overtreated with propylthiouracil, and the fetus devel-

oped a goiter by 28 weeks. Fetal blood sampling confirmed hypothyroidism, and thyroxine injected intraamnionically at 35, 36, and 37 weeks caused rapid resolution of the goiter.

Finally, at least four long-term studies have been done to evaluate intellectual and physical development of children born to thyrotoxic mothers treated with thiourea drugs during pregnancy (Mestman, 1998a). No adverse effects on subsequent growth and development were found when compared with age-matched controls.

NEONATAL THYROTOXICOSIS AFTER MATERNAL THYROID ABLATION. Even after being rendered euthyroid by surgery or radiation, women with Graves disease occasionally give birth to infants with manifestations of thyrotoxicosis, including goiter and exophthalmos. Watson and Fiegen (1995) described nonimmune hydrops from fetal thyrotoxicosis. Neonatal thyrotoxicosis results from the transplacental passage of maternal thyroid-stimulating antibodies (Wallace and collaborators, 1995). Such fetal thyrotoxicosis can cause fetal demise (Houck and associates, 1988; Page and co-workers, 1988). Fetal thyrotoxicosis is diagnosed by tachycardia in the appropriate clinical setting. Although this is adequate evidence to begin treatment, some have advocated cord blood sampling to assess fetal thyroid status (Hatjis, 1993; Wenstrom and colleagues, 1990).

SUBCLINICAL THYROTOXICOSIS. This is defined as a low serum concentration of thyrotropin along with

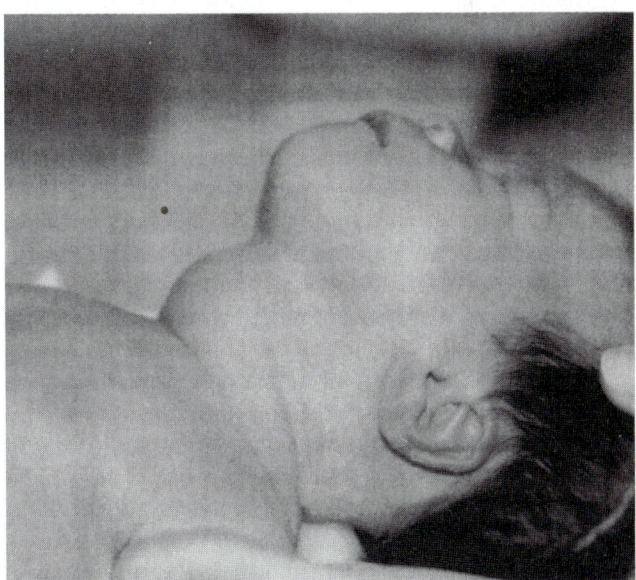

FIGURE 50–3. Term neonate delivered vaginally to a woman with a 3-year history of thyrotoxicosis that recurred at 26 weeks' gestation. The mother was given methimazole, 30 mg daily, and was euthyroid at delivery. The infant chemically was hypothyroid.

normal serum levels of T_3 and T_4. The overall prevalence in nine studies of community or clinic populations was about 4 percent (Marqusee and colleagues, 1998). About half of these patients were taking excessive thyroxine replacement therapy that suppressed thyrotropin. In the other half, the course of subclinical hyperthyroidism is variable, but many patients do not progress to overt thyrotoxicosis. Indeed, 40 percent of this half eventually have normal thyrotropin concentrations.

Long-term effects from subclinical thyrotoxicosis are for the most part currently unclear. It may cause cardiac arrhythmias and hypertrophy as well as osteopenia. Certainly, adverse effects on pregnancy have not been studied. Thus if there is no obvious cause of persistently depressed serum thyrotropin in an otherwise asymptomatic young woman, it seems reasonable at this time to periodically monitor for overt disease (Marqusee and co-workers, 1998).

THYROID DYSFUNCTION WITH GESTATIONAL TROPHOBLASTIC DISEASE.
Serum thyroxine levels in women with molar pregnancy usually are elevated appreciably. Because many of these tumors are diagnosed early, clinically apparent hyperthyroidism is less common than in the past. In their review of earlier studies, Goodwin and Hershman (1997) estimate this was about 20 percent (Chap. 32, p. 840).

HYPOTHYROIDISM.
Clinical hypothyroidism is diagnosed if free thyroxine levels are low and the thyrotropin level is elevated. Overt hypothyroidism complicating pregnancy is uncommon, probably because it is often associated with infertility. Glinoer and colleagues (1994) reported that euthyroid women with thyroid antibodies early in pregnancy go on to develop overt hypothyroidism in 40 percent of cases.

The experiences of Davis and colleagues (1988), as well as those of Leung and associates (1993), indicate that hypothyroid women who do become pregnant have a high incidence of preeclampsia and placental abruption with a correspondingly inordinate number of low-birthweight and stillborn infants (Table 50–2). Wasserstrum and Anania (1995) observed an inordinately high incidence of fetal distress (14 percent) during labor in 43 hypothyroid pregnancies. Heart failure is also encountered with increased frequency in hypothyroid women.

Replacement therapy is with thyroxine, 50 to 100 μg daily. Serum thyrotropin is measured at 4 to 6 week intervals and thyroxine adjusted by 25- to 50-μg increments. The goal is to keep the thyrotropin level at or slightly below normal. During pregnancy, thyrotropin is measured each trimester. Mandel and colleagues (1990), as well as Tamaki and associates (1990), presented evidence that pregnancy is associated with a

TABLE 50–2. Pregnancy Complications in 96 Women with Overt or Subclinical Hypothyroidism

Complications	Hypothyroidism	
	Overt N = 39 (%)	Subclinical N = 57 (%)
Preeclampsia	12 (31)	9 (16)
Abruptio placentae	3 (8)	0 (0)
Anemia	5 (13)	1 (2)
Postpartum hemorrhage	4 (10)	2 (4)
Cardiac dysfunction	1 (3)	1 (2)
Birthweight less than 2000 g	10 (26)	6 (11)
Stillbirths	3[a] (8)	1[b]

[a] One due to eclampsia.
[b] Due to syphilis.
Modified from Davis and colleagues (1988) and Leung and associates (1993).

50-μg increase in thyroxine requirements. Despite this, Girling and de Swiet (1992) reported that doses were unchanged in 80 percent of 35 pregnancies.

SUBCLINICAL HYPOTHYROIDISM.
This condition is defined by an abnormally elevated serum thyrotropin and normal serum thyroxine in an asymptomatic patient. Its incidence in women between 18 and 45 is about 5 percent (Canaris and colleagues, 2000; Woeber, 1997). Between 10 and 20 percent progress to overt hypothyroidism within 1 to 4 years. High-risk factors include thyrotropin levels over 10 mU/L and antimicrosomal antibodies. The American Thyroid Association (Singer and associates, 1995) recommends that most patients be given treatment before they become symptomatic.

Jovanovic-Peterson and associates (1988) reported a high incidence of subclinical hypothyroidism in 51 pregnant women with type I diabetes, all of whom had normal thyroxine levels before conception. Effects of subclinical hypothyroidism on pregnancy outcome are not clear, but thyroxine replacement is recommended by most. There is a suggestion that these women are at greater risk for pregnancy-induced hypertension and preterm delivery (Table 50–2).

As discussed next, recent preliminary observations by Haddow and colleagues (1999) and Pop and associates (1999a) suggest diminished intelligence quotients (IQ) in children born to women with untreated subclinical hypothyroidism.

EFFECT OF HYPOTHYROIDISM ON THE FETUS AND INFANT.
In the past, because most infants of hypothyroid mothers appeared healthy and without clinical evidence of thyroid dysfunction, it was presumed that they were euthyroid with normal fetal development. This is

despite the fact that thyroid hormones are a known prerequisite for mental development (Utiger, 1999a). More recently, however, information is accruing that maternal hypothyroidism—either overt or subclinical—may cause subnormal mental development. Pop and associates (1999a) showed that maternal 12-week serum-free thyroxine levels below the 10th percentile were a significant risk factor for impaired psychomotor development. Haddow and colleagues (1999) evaluated children of 48 untreated women whose maternal serum thyrotropin values were above the 99.6th percentile. Serum samples had been stored following maternal serum alpha-fetoprotein screening in the early second trimester. As shown in Table 50–3, elevated maternal thyrotropin values were associated with offspring with diminished school performance, reading recognition, and IQ scores when compared with matched controls.

It seems likely that the majority of women with hypothyroidism of this degree have antithyroid antibodies and impending autoimmune thyroid failure. For example, in the study by Haddow and co-workers (1999), at the time of follow-up 65 percent of the 48 untreated women had developed clinical hypothyroidism. In another study, Dussault and Fisher (1999) assessed thyroid function in mothers who had given birth to 259 hypothyroid newborns detected by the Quebec screening program. They found an increased incidence of maternal thyroid dysfunction in these women compared with controls (20 versus 13 percent).

These findings have led the Endocrine Society (2000) to recommend development of cost-effective screening programs for all pregnant women. Others emphasize the unknowns concerned with population screening (Davies, 2000). Moreover, it seems unlikely that effects of treatment given after the period of early cerebral development would be efficacious (Pop and colleagues, 1999b; Utiger, 1999a). Because of this, the American Association of Clinical Endocrinologists (Gharib and

co-workers, 1999) does not recommend routine antepartum thyrotropin screening. It does, however, recommend screening and appropriate treatment in women *considering* pregnancy. The American Thyroid Association (1999) recommends that the individual patient and her physician decide.

RADIOIODINE TREATMENT DURING PREGNANCY. If maternal hypothyroidism was caused by ablative radioiodine therapy (not tracer doses) during pregnancy, destruction of the fetal thyroid gland may have also resulted. Any exposed infant must be carefully evaluated and probably treated prophylactically for hypothyroidism (Berg and colleagues, 1998). Abortion should be considered. There is no evidence that therapeutic radioiodine causes fetal anomalies if pregnancy occurs after radiation effects have dissipated, and the woman is euthyroid. Casara and colleagues (1993) described outcomes in 70 pregnant women treated 2 to 10 years previously with radioiodine for thyroid cancer. Only 1 of 73 infants had an anomaly, and three were low birthweight. Ayala and associates (1998) reported three anomalous fetuses of 39 born to 26 women treated for thyroid cancer 2 months to 14 years before conception. They found no relationship to radioiodine but cautioned against pregnancy for 1 year after treatment.

IODIDE DEFICIENCY. Adequate iodide ingestion is extremely important for normal fetal thyroid and neurological development. Iodide deficiency may result in **endemic cretinism,** and the World Health Organization estimated in 1990 that 20 million people worldwide have varying degrees of preventable brain damage due to fetal iodide deficiency (Hetzel, 1994).

Thilly and associates (1978) studied a group of women from a region in Africa where severe endemic goiter is common because of iodine deficiency. Women whose iodine deficiency was corrected prenatally had

TABLE 50–3. Neuropsychological Evaluation of 7- to 9-Year-Old Children Born to Untreated Women with Elevated Second-Trimester Serum Thyrotropin Levels Compared with Normal Controls

Factor	Untreated Hypothyroidism (n = 48)	Control Women (n = 124)	P Value
Serum TSH concentration (mU/L)	13.2	1.4	< .001
Serum free T$_4$ concentration (ng/dL)	0.71	0.97	< .001
Elevated serum antithyroid antibodies	77%	14%	< .001
WISC-III full-scale IQ score	100	107	.005
PIAT-R reading-recognition score	95	100	.05
School-learning problems	21%	11%	.09

Data from Haddow and co-workers (1999).

significantly higher thyroxine levels and lower thyrotropin levels at delivery compared with nonsupplemented women. Mean cord serum thyrotropin levels in infants born to mothers not receiving supplementation was 19.6 mU/mL, compared with 9.4 mU/mL in newborns of treated mothers. Cao and co-workers (1994) studied these effects in a severely iodine-deficient region of China. They found that women given iodine supplementation in the first or second trimester had a 2 percent incidence of infants with moderate or severe neurological abnormalities. This was in contrast to an incidence of 9 percent in women not supplemented until the last trimester. Thus, iodine supplementation is necessary for pregnant women in areas of endemic iodine deficiency found in Latin America, Asia, and Africa (Hetzel, 1994). As emphasized by Delange (1996), iodide supplementation should ideally be given before conception.

CONGENITAL HYPOTHYROIDISM. The clinical diagnosis of hypothyroidism in neonates is difficult to make and is missed in nearly all cases. Because of this, newborn mass screening was introduced in 1974 and is now mandatory in all states. Early and aggressive thyroxine replacement therapy is critical for these infants. According to various reports based on these mass screening programs, congenital hypothyroidism is found in about 1 in 4000 to 7000 infants. The most common cause is thyroid agenesis (75 percent), followed by thyroid dyshormonogenesis (10 percent), and about another 10 percent have transient hypothyroidism (Lindsay and Toft, 1997). There are now 5- to 7-year follow-up data from infants identified by early screening programs who were treated promptly and adequately with thyroid hormone. Most, if not all, sequelae of congenital hypothyroidism—including intellectual impairment—were found to be preventable (Burrow and colleagues, 1994). Unfortunately, Grant and colleagues (1992) reported that 8 percent of 449 infants with congenital hypothyroidism also had other major associated anomalies.

PRETERM INFANTS. Transient hypothyroxinemia is common in preterm infants. It has been assumed that treatment was not necessary, and recently, Van Wassenaer and colleagues (1997) evaluated 157 infants born before 30 weeks and randomized to 8 μg/kg of thyroxine or placebo given daily. Follow-up at 6, 12, and 24 months with careful psychomotor and neurological testing showed no differences in the groups.

NODULAR THYROID DISEASE. Evaluation and management of a thyroid nodule during pregnancy depends on the stage of gestation. The likelihood that a solitary nodule will be malignant is from 5 to 30 percent. Even if malignant, the majority are low-grade neoplasms. Most authorities recommend against radioiodine scanning, although tracer doses used are associated with minimal fetal irradiation (Chap. 42, p. 1153). *Ultrasound* examination reliably detects nodules greater than 0.5 cm, and their solid or cystic nature also can be determined.

Fine-needle aspiration of thyroid nodules is an excellent method for assessment during pregnancy. Mestman (1999) recommends biopsy for nonfunctional solitary nodules before midpregnancy. This is performed for solid lesions over 2 cm and cystic lesions over 4 cm. In other cases, biopsy is done only if there is cervical lymphadenopathy or the nodule is growing. Rosen and Walfish (1986) and Doherty and colleagues (1995) provided data from a total of 53 pregnant women assessed for neoplasia because of nodular disease. Many of these underwent fine-needle aspiration, and 40 percent were found to have a malignancy.

Because most thyroid carcinomas are well differentiated and pursue an indolent course, some recommend that surgery be postponed until after delivery. Moosa and Mazzaferri (1997) studied 61 women with thyroid cancer diagnosed during pregnancy. In 75 percent, thyroidectomy was delayed until postpartum. In a long-term follow-up, these women had outcomes similar to nonpregnant control patients. In their review, Driggers and co-workers (1998) and Morris (1998) found minimal fetal loss related to thyroid cancer surgery. We are of the view that if pregnancy is less than about 24 to 26 weeks, that is, the time before surgery *might* stimulate preterm labor, then thyroidectomy surgery can be safely performed.

POSTPARTUM THYROIDITIS. The propensity for thyroiditis likely antedates pregnancy, and like other autoimmune endocrinopathies, a precipitating event such as a viral illness interplays with genetic and other factors. For example, Pacini and associates (1998) found serum thyroid antibodies in 30 percent of preadolescent girls exposed to radioactive fallout from the Chernobyl disaster, compared with 3 percent of a nonexposed control group.

Transient postpartum hypothyroidism or thyrotoxicosis associated with autoimmune thyroiditis is common. When women are carefully scrutinized postpartum, clinical and biochemical evidence of thyroid dysfunction has been found consistently in 5 to 10 percent regardless of their geographic locale (Dayan and Daniels, 1996; Lucas and colleagues, 2000). In women with type I diabetes, up to 25 percent develop postpartum thyroid dysfunction (Alvarez-Marfany and associates, 1994). Nevertheless, postpartum thyroiditis is diagnosed infrequently, largely because it typically develops after the traditional postpartum examination and because it results in vague and nonspecific symptoms. These factors should not lead to an underestimation of its clinical importance. Hayslip and colleagues (1988) reported that such women were significantly more likely than euthyroid women to manifest depression, carelessness, and memory impairment 3 to 5 months after delivery. Lucas and co-workers (2000) documented a 9 percent incidence of depression at 6 months in women with thyroiditis.

PATHOGENESIS. Thyroiditis is thought to be caused by an initiating inflammatory event followed by a specific autoreaction from the immune system (Baker, 1997). It is characterized histologically as a destructive, lymphocytic thyroiditis. Many women who develop this disorder have antithyroid antibodies earlier during pregnancy. When postpartum thyroiditis develops, the majority of women are found to have a positive assay for microsomal autoantibodies (Jansson and co-workers, 1988). Other women at increased risk for postpartum thyroid dysfunction include those who have experienced it before and those who have a personal or family history of autoimmune disease. Iodine deficiency may also play a role (Glinoer and associates, 1992).

THYROID AUTOANTIBODIES. Thyroid microsomal autoantibodies have been identified in 7 to 10 percent of women either early in pregnancy or shortly following delivery (Jansson and associates, 1988; Kuijpens and co-workers, 1998). Stagnaro-Green and collaborators (1990) found that the incidence was 20 percent in 552 consecutive women studied before 13 weeks' gestation. Although 17 percent of these autoantibody-positive women aborted, only 8 percent of control women did so. Singh and co-workers (1995) reported similar observations.

When microsomal autoantibody titers are followed sequentially in seropositive women during pregnancy and the puerperium, a characteristic pattern emerges. As shown in Figure 50–4, titers decrease somewhat dur-

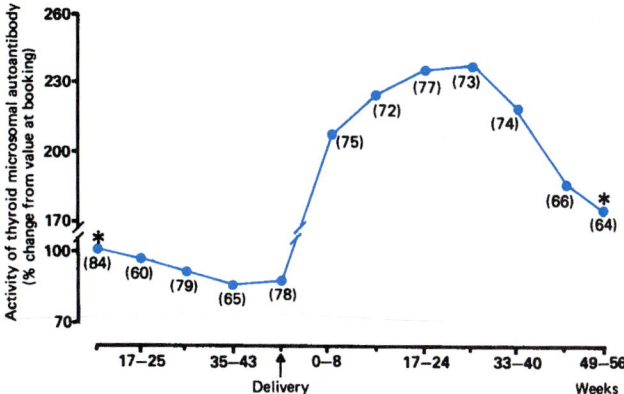

FIGURE 50–4. Changes in serum activity of thyroid microsomal autoantibody during pregnancy and up to 12 months postpartum in 84 women. Numbers in parentheses indicate women assessed at each time point. ($P < .001$ when compared with values at delivery.) (From Fung and colleagues, 1988, with permission.)

ing pregnancy, rise to a peak 4 to 6 months after delivery, and then decline to early pregnancy levels by 10 to 12 months postpartum. Detection of microsomal autoantibodies either early in pregnancy or shortly after delivery helps to identify women at high risk for developing postpartum thyroid dysfunction (Hidaka and associates, 1994). Premawardhana and co-workers (2000) have shown that thyroid peroxidase antibodies are also associated with a high incidence of long-term thyroid dysfunction.

An association between maternal serum thyroid autoantibodies and fetal **Down syndrome** has long been suspected. Cuckle and colleagues (1988) identified both types of thyroid autoantibodies more frequently in pregnancies with Down syndrome versus normal controls, but the differences were not significant.

CLINICAL MANIFESTATIONS. There are two recognized clinical phases of postpartum thyroiditis (Table 50–4). Between 1 and 4 months after delivery, approximately 4 percent of all women develop transient **thyrotoxicosis** (Lucas and colleagues, 2000; Walfish and Chan, 1985). The onset is abrupt and a small, painless goiter is commonly found. Although there may be many symptoms, only fatigue and palpitations are more frequent in these thyrotoxic women compared with euthyroid postpartum controls

In these cases, thyrotoxicosis results from excessive release of preformed hormone because of glandular disruption—*destruction-induced thyrotoxicosis*—rather than excessive hormone. Thus, antithyroid medications such as propylthiouracil and methimazole are ineffective, and they may even hasten the development of a subsequent hypothyroid phase. Treatment usually is not necessary, but if symptoms due to excessive thyroid hormone are severe, a β-adrenergic blocker may be useful. Approximately two thirds of these women return directly to a euthyroid state, but the other third subsequently experience hypothyroidism.

Between 4 and 8 months postpartum, 2 to 5 percent of all women develop **hypothyroidism** (Jansson and co-workers, 1988; Lucas and associates, 2000). At least a third of such women will previously have experienced the thyrotoxic phase of postpartum thyroid dysfunction. Goiters, as well as clinically significant symptoms, are common and are more prominent than during the thyrotoxic phase. Hypothyroidism can develop rapidly, sometimes within a month. Thus, women at risk for postpartum hypothyroidism should be evaluated regularly, and at least in selected situations, thyroid function tests should be performed. If hypothyroidism develops and the severity of symptoms warrants, thyroxine replacement is initiated. It has been suggested that thyroxine be continued for 6 to 12 months and then gradually withdrawn (Jansson and colleagues, 1988).

TABLE 50–4. Comparison of Two Phases of Postpartum Thyroiditis

	Postpartum Thyroiditis	
Manifestation	1–4 Months	4–8 Months
Condition	Thyrotoxicosis	Hypothyroidism
Incidence	4%	2–5%
Mechanism	Destruction-induced hormone release	Thyroid failure
Symptoms	Small, painless goiter; fatigue, palpitations	Goiter, fatigue, inability to concentrate
Treatment	β-blockers for symptoms	Thyroxine 6–12 months
Sequelae	2/3 become euthyroid 1/3 develop hypothyroidism	1/3 permanently hypo-thyroid

Women who experience postpartum thyroiditis are at high risk of developing permanent hypothyroidism. This incidence is about 25 percent (Dayan and Daniels, 1996; Lucas and colleagues, 2000; Premawardhana and associates, 2000). The incidence may be even greater if subclinical disease is considered. Permanent hypothyroidism is much more common in women with antiperoxidase antibodies (Kuijpens and colleagues, 1998). Premawardhana and co-workers (2000) found that almost half of women with postpartum thyroiditis associated with thyroid peroxidase antibodies developed hypothyroidism when followed for 6 to 7 years. The importance of long-term follow up in these women is apparent.

PARATHYROID DISEASE

The function of **parathyroid hormone (PTH)** is to maintain extracellular fluid calcium concentration. This 115 amino-acid hormone acts directly on bone and kidney and indirectly on small intestine through its effects on synthesis of vitamin D (1,25 $(OH)_2D$) to increase serum calcium. Parathyroid hormone secretion is regulated by serum ionized calcium concentration through a negative feedback system. **Calcitonin** is a potent hypocalcemic hormone produced by the thyroid gland. It acts in many ways as a physiological parathyroid hormone antagonist. The interrelationships between these hormones and calcium metabolism, as well as **PTH-related protein** produced by fetal tissue, are discussed in Chapter 8 (p. 193).

Because of substantive fetal calcium needs—300 mg/day in late pregnancy and a total of 30 g—and increased renal calcium loss from augmented glomerular filtration, parathyroid hormone levels were thought to be increased in pregnant women. With newer assay methods, however, Seely and co-workers (1997) observed a significant decrease in intact 1-84 parathyroid hormone longitudinally during pregnancy. They also demon-strated a twofold increase in serum concentrations of 1,25-dihydroxyvitamin D—presumably of placental and decidual origin. They speculate that this hormone increases gastrointestinal absorption to meet the needs of pregnancy. At the same time, total serum calcium levels decline during pregnancy, paralleling the decrease in serum albumin concentration (Power and associates, 1999). Ionized calcium levels, however, are unchanged in pregnancy (Dahlman and colleagues, 1994).

HYPERPARATHYROIDISM. Hypercalcemia is caused by hyperparathyroidism or cancer in 90 percent of cases. Primary hyperparathyroidism is relatively common with a prevalence rate of 0.15 percent, and its incidence peaks between the third and fifth decades (Potts, 1998). Because many automated laboratory systems include measurement of serum calcium, cases of hyperparathyroidism that previously would have been undiagnosed are being detected. Almost 80 percent of cases are caused by a solitary adenoma and another 15 percent by generalized chief cell hyperplasia. In most tumor-related cases, the malignancy and the cause of increased serum calcium are obvious. Parathyroid hormone produced by tumors is similar but not identical to the natural hormone and therefore is usually not detected by routine assays.

About half of patients with hyperparathyroid-induced hypercalcemia have minimal symptoms. Findings include fatigue, depression, and confusion; anorexia, nausea, and vomiting; constipation; nephrolithiasis; and peptic ulcer disease. Generally, symptoms are not apparent until the serum calcium exceeds 12 mg/dL in the nonpregnant person. **Hypercalcemic crisis** manifests as stupor, nausea, vomiting, weakness, fatigue, and dehydration.

There is controversy regarding management in nonpregnant patients. Silverberg and colleagues (1999) compared surgical excision with observation in 121 patients with primary hyperparathyroidism. Half of these were cured by parathyroidectomy, and bone density improved. Of the half observed, about a fourth had progression of disease, for example, six of eight had recurrence of nephrolithiasis. These findings led Utiger (1999b) to recommend surgical therapy for all patients.

HYPERPARATHYROIDISM IN PREGNANCY. This situation is uncommon, and reviews cite only about 100 pregnant women reported with this disease (Carella and Gossain, 1992; Kelly, 1991). It is presumed that many hypercalcemic pregnant women with hyperparathyroidism are either not detected or not reported. As in nonpregnant patients, hyperparathyroidism is usually caused by a parathyroid adenoma, but it can be due to ectopic parathyroid hormone production, or rarely to parathyroid carcinoma (Montoro and colleagues, 2000). Symptoms include hyperemesis, generalized weakness, renal calculi, pancreatitis, and psychiatric disorders.

Pregnancy will theoretically improve hyperparathyroidism because of significant calcium shunting to the fetus as well as augmented renal excretion (Power and colleagues, 1999). When the "protective effects" of pregnancy are withdrawn, however, there is significant danger of postpartum hypercalcemia and possible crisis.

Ludwig (1962) first described adverse pregnancy outcomes with hyperparathyroidism. He reported excessive stillbirths, preterm deliveries, and neonatal tetany. With earlier detection and better management, the incidence of adverse effects is much lower (Carella and Gossain, 1992; Shangold and associates, 1982). Certainly, if asymptomatic hypercalcemic women are included, adverse perinatal outcomes are less common.

MANAGEMENT. Surgical removal of the parathyroid adenoma has become preferable management during pregnancy (Mestman, 1998b). Elective neck exploration is well tolerated by pregnant women (Graham and associates, 1998; Kort and colleagues, 1999). In one woman, a mediastinal adenoma was removed at 23 weeks (Rooney and co-workers, 1998). An alternative is to treat the asymptomatic women with oral phosphate, 1 to 1.5 g daily in divided doses. This may lower serum calcium, thus allowing parathyroidectomy to be postponed until after delivery.

For women with dangerously elevated serum calcium levels, or in those who are mentally obtunded—*hypercalcemic crisis*—emergency treatment is instituted. Intravenous hydration with normal saline to evoke diuresis is the first step. Urine flow should exceed 150 mL/hr. *Furosemide* given in conventional doses will block tubular reabsorption of calcium. Careful attention to prevent hypokalemia and hypomagnesemia is important. Adjunctive therapy includes *mithramycin,* which inhibits bone resorption; *calcitonin,* which decreases skeletal calcium release; and oral phosphorus.

NEONATAL EFFECTS. In the normal infant, cord blood calcium levels are higher than maternal levels. With hyperparathyroidism, abnormally elevated maternal levels further suppress fetal parathyroid function, resulting in a fall in newborn serum calcium levels, which reach a nadir at 24 to 48 hours. Accordingly, 15 to 25 percent of these infants develop severe hypocalcemia with or without tetany (Molitch, 1992). At times, neonatal tetany alone has led to a search that identified a maternal parathyroid adenoma (Beattie and co-workers, 2000).

HYPOPARATHYROIDISM. The most common cause of hypocalcemia is hypoparathyroidism that usually follows parathyroid or thyroid surgery. Chronically hypocalcemic pregnant women may have a fetus with skeletal demineralization. Treatment usually prevents symptomatic hypocalcemia. The woman is given 1,25-dihydroxyvitamin D_3 (calcitriol), dihydrotachysterol, or large doses of vitamin D (50,000 to 150,000 U/day); together with calcium gluconate or calcium lactate (3 to 5 g/day); and a diet low in phosphates. The fetal risks from large doses of vitamin D have not been established. Caplan and Beguin (1990) reported their experiences with treatment of five pregnant women and observed that whereas the calcitriol dose was increased during the second half of pregnancy, it was reduced during lactation.

PREGNANCY-ASSOCIATED OSTEOPOROSIS. In some women during pregnancy or lactation, idiopathic osteoporosis develops. The condition was first described in 1948 by Albright and Reifenstein. While its cause is controversial, most believe that pregnancy unmasks preexisting bone disease (Black and co-workers, 2000; Henderson and collaborators, 2000). Dunne and colleagues (1993) and Smith and associates (1995) described a total of 59 women with symptomatic osteoporosis during pregnancy. The most common symptom was back pain in late pregnancy or postpartum. Other symptoms were hip pain, either unilateral or bilateral, and difficulty in weight bearing. In 29 women, there was no apparent reason for osteopenia except pregnancy. Some known causes include long-term heparin or corticosteroid therapy during pregnancy. In a few cases, overt hyperparathyroidism or thyrotoxicosis eventually develop (Khovidhunkit and Epstein, 1996). Although overt osteonecrosis of the femoral head during normal pregnancy has been described (Chang and associates, 1993), we have seen this only as a complication of known causes. Examples include corticosteroid therapy as described by Spencer and colleagues (1999), sickle-cell disease, or heparin therapy.

Treatment is problematical, but most recommend calcium and vitamin D supplementation. Long-term follow-up indicates that while bone density improves, these women, as well as their offspring, may have chronic osteopenia (Blanch and co-workers, 1994; Carbone and colleagues, 1995).

ADRENAL GLAND DISORDERS

Pregnancy has profound effects on adrenal gland cortical secretion and its control or stimulation. These interrelationships are discussed in detail in Chapter 8 (p. 194). Serum corticotropin levels increase after a marked reduction in early pregnancy, undoubtedly related to corticotropin-releasing hormone synthesized by the placenta (Carr and Rainey, 1994). The considerable increase in plasma cortisol is explained by increased transcortin production and binding. In addition, plasma renin increases, which increases angiotensin II and in turn aldosterone secretion. Baseline adrenal medullary hormone secretion is probably unaffected. Although there is no evidence that pregnancy causes any adrenal-specific disorders, a number of adrenal disorders may coexist with pregnancy.

PHEOCHROMOCYTOMA. These are chromaffin tumors that secrete catecholamines. Most are located in the adrenal medulla, but 10 percent are located in the sympathetic ganglia. In adults, they are called the *10-percent tumor* because 10 percent are bilateral, 10 percent are extra-adrenal, and about 10 percent are malignant. There is an association with medullary thyroid carcinoma and hyperparathyroidism in some of the autosomally dominant or recessive **multiple endocrine neoplasia syndromes (MENS),** as well as neurofibromatosis and von Hippel–Lindau disease. Pheochromocytomas are common findings at autopsy but are frequently not diagnosed. Only 0.1 percent of hypertensive patients have a pheochromocytoma.

Symptoms are usually paroxysmal and manifest as hypertensive crisis, seizure disorders, or anxiety attacks. Hypertension is sustained in 60 percent of patients, but half of these also have paroxysmal crises. Other symptoms during paroxysmal attacks are headaches, profuse sweating, palpitations, and apprehension. Chest pain, nausea and vomiting, and pallor or flushing are also common. There is usually severe hypertension and tachycardia.

The standard screening test is quantification of catecholamine metabolites in a 24-hour urine specimen (Keely, 1998). Diagnosis is established by measurement of 24-hour urine vanillylmandelic acid (VMA), metanephrines, or unconjugated catecholamines. Determination of plasma catecholamine levels is not recommended.

Adrenal localization is usually successful with computed tomography or magnetic resonance imaging.

Extra-adrenal tumors may be localized using these, but often abdominal arteriography (after α-blockade is accomplished) or ^{131}I-metaiodobenzylguanidine (MIBG) scanning is necessary for localization.

PHEOCHROMOCYTOMA COMPLICATING PREGNANCY.
These tumors are rare but dangerous complications of pregnancy. Geelhoed (1983) cited an earlier review of 89 cases in which 43 mothers died. Maternal death was much more common if the tumor was not diagnosed antepartum—58 versus 18 percent. With modern diagnostic methods and management, maternal survival has improved. Ahlawat and colleagues (1999) reviewed 42 cases reported from 1988 through 1999. Shown in Table 50–5 are their results compared with the earlier review by Harper and co-workers (1989). Maternal mortality most recently had decreased from 16 to 4 percent, but **there were no maternal deaths when the diagnosis was made antepartum.** In more recent years, this proportion has increased. Botchan and associates (1995) reviewed available literature and stressed a team approach to management of these tumors.

Grimbert and colleagues (1999) described 56 pregnancies in 30 women with **von Hippel–Lindau disease.** Only two pregnancies were complicated by a pheochromocytoma.

There are several methods of tumor localization during pregnancy. From their review, Ahlawat and colleagues (1999) reported that 21 of 22 tumors were found using sonography, 10 of 11 with computed tomographic scanning, and 10 of 10 using magnetic resonance imaging (Fig. 50–5).

In some cases, the principal challenge is to differentiate preeclampsia from the hypertensive crises caused by a pheochromocytoma. Onset in early pregnancy may be a clue, and the lack of proteinuria with episodic hypertension may point to a pheochromocytoma.

TABLE 50–5. Outcomes of Pregnancies Complicated by Pheochromocytoma

Factor	Incidence in Percent	
	1980–1987[a] (n = 48)	1988–1997[b] (n = 42)
Diagnosis		
Antepartum	51	83
Postpartum	36	14
Autopsy	12	2
Maternal mortality	16	4
Fetal wastage	26	11

[a]Data from Harper and colleagues (1989).
[b]Data from Ahlawat and associates (1999).

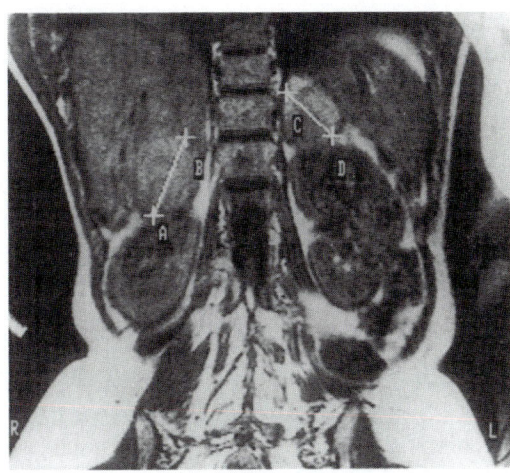

FIGURE 50–5. Magnetic resonance imaging in a 34-week pregnant woman shows bilateral pheochromocytomas **(A, B** and **C, D).** (From van der Vaart and colleagues, 1993, with permission.)

Combs and colleagues (1989) have shown that during paroxysmal hypertension, cardiac output falls substantively. They expressed appropriate concerns for adverse fetal effects of hypertensive paroxysms. Bassoon-Zaltzman and associates (1995) described a normotensive 20-week pregnant woman with intermittent ventricular tachycardia. Although pheochromocytoma was diagnosed by elevated catecholamine levels, the tumor was not found in the bladder until 4 months after uncomplicated delivery.

MANAGEMENT. Management of hypertension and symptoms with an α-adrenergic blocker such as *phenoxybenzamine* is imperative. The dose is 10 to 30 mg, two to four times daily. After α-blockade is achieved, β-blockers may be given for tachycardia if necessary. In some cases, surgical exploration and tumor removal may be performed during pregnancy. Janetschek and associates (1998) described laparoscopic surgical removal of an adrenal pheochromocytoma in 16- and 20-week pregnancies. Favorable outcomes were described for 10 of 26 women in whom the diagnosis was made in pregnancy and blood pressure controlled pharmacologically during cesarean delivery done along with tumor resection (Ahlawat and colleagues, 1999).

Recurrent tumors are troublesome. We have cared for three women in whom recurrent pheochromocytoma was identified during pregnancy. Hypertension was managed with phenoxybenzamine in all three. Two infants were healthy, but a third was stillborn in a mother with a massive tumor load who was receiving phenoxybenzamine, 100 mg daily. In all three women, tumor resection was done postpartum. One woman died of persistent metastases several years later. Other case reports suggest that even with good blood pressure control, dangerous peripartum hypertension may develop (Lyons and Colmorgen, 1988; Sweeney and Katz, 1994).

CUSHING SYNDROME. Long-term exposure to glucocorticoids leads to Cushing syndrome, which may be corticotropin-dependent or independent (Williams and Dluhy, 1998). The most common cause is iatrogenic from corticosteroid treatment. Endogenous Cushing syndrome is caused by increased adrenal cortisol production. Most cases are due to bilateral adrenal hyperplasia stimulated by corticotropin-producing pituitary adenomas, and these cases are known as *Cushing disease.* Most of these are microadenomas less than 1 cm. Occasionally, abnormal secretion of hypothalamic corticotropin-releasing factor may cause corticotrophic hyperplasia. Hyperplasia may also be caused by nonendocrine tumors that produce polypeptides similar to either corticotropin-releasing factor or corticotropin. About a fourth of cases of Cushing syndrome are corticotropin independent. Most are caused by an adrenal adenoma, which is usually bilateral, and half are malignant.

The typical body habitus is caused by adipose tissue deposition, which characteristically results in *moon facies,* a *buffalo hump,* and truncal obesity. Fatiguability and weakness, hypertension, hirsutism, amenorrhea, cutaneous striae, and easy bruisability are each encountered in 70 to 80 percent of cases. Diagnosis is made by elevated plasma cortisol that cannot be suppressed by dexamethasone. Free cortisol excretion in a 24-hour urine specimen is also elevated. Neither test is totally accurate, and both are harder to interpret in obese patients.

PREGNANCY AND CUSHING SYNDROME. Because most women with Cushing syndrome have amenorrhea, associated pregnancy is rare. Buescher and co-workers (1992) found only 70 or so cases in their review. Kamiya and colleagues (1998) cite 97 cases from the Japanese literature. Most cases were caused by adrenal tumors, of which 80 percent were benign. These reports stressed difficulties in diagnosis because of pregnancy-induced increases in plasma cortisol, corticotropin, and corticotropin-releasing factor.

Pregnant women usually have the classical findings of Cushing syndrome. In some, symptoms may be exacerbated. Maternal complications include hypertension in 60 to 90 percent and gestational diabetes in about half. Heart failure is common during pregnancy, and Buescher and associates (1992) reported three maternal deaths in 65 pregnancies. Perinatal morbidity and mortality are correspondingly high. Preterm delivery was reported in 60 percent, and perinatal mortality in about 25 percent.

MANAGEMENT. Long-term medical therapy for Cushing syndrome usually is ineffective. Ketoconazole blocks steroid production and it has been used successfully. Definitive therapy is resection of the pituitary or adrenal adenoma. Unfortunately, recurrences are difficult to manage. During pregnancy, management of hypertension in mild cases may suffice until delivery. Although pituitary adenomas are encountered less commonly during pregnancy, successful transsphenoidal resection at midpregnancy has been described (Mellor and associates, 1998). Removal of an adrenal adenoma can be curative (Kamiya and colleagues, 1998). Direct attempts to treat Cushing syndrome were reported in 16 cases summarized by Aron and associates (1990). In six women, unilateral adrenalectomy was done for an adenoma; in five, bilateral resection was done for hyperplasia; four were treated with *metyrapone, aminoglutethimide,* or *cyproheptadine;* and one underwent pituitary irradiation. A few cases during pregnancy have been successfully treated with oral *ketoconazole* (Berwaerts and co-workers, 1999). The drug also blocks testicular steroidogenesis; therefore, treatment of a woman with a male fetus is worrisome.

ADDISON DISEASE. Primary adrenocortical insufficiency, or Addison disease, is rare. More than 90 percent of the glands must be destroyed for symptoms to develop. Whereas in the past chronic granulomatous diseases such as tuberculosis and histoplasmosis caused most cases, **idiopathic autoimmune adrenalitis** is now responsible for the majority. There is an increased incidence of concurrent Hashimoto thyroiditis, premature ovarian failure, type 1 diabetes, and Graves disease. These **polyglandular autoimmune syndromes** also include pernicious anemia, vitiligo, alopecia, nontropical sprue, and myasthenia gravis.

ADDISON DISEASE AND PREGNANCY. Before 1953, only 50 published cases of Addison disease in pregnancy had been identified, suggesting that untreated adrenal hypofunction caused infertility. With the synthesis of cortisone and related compounds, pregnancy has become much more common in these women. Fetal prognosis in general parallels maternal health. Because serum cortisol levels are increased during pregnancy, evaluation should include documentation of a lack of response to infused corticotropin (O'Shaughnessy and Hackett, 1984). Seaward and colleagues (1989) found only five cases published since 1972. They reported a woman with unrecognized Addison disease who suffered a placental abruption and fetal death associated with addisonian crisis. Albert and associates (1989) reported six successful pregnancy outcomes in six women in whom adrenal insufficiency had been diagnosed before conception.

The woman with adrenal insufficiency is observed for evidence of either inadequate or excessive steroid replacement. Except at times of stress, replacement therapy need not be greater than in the nonpregnant state. There may be little need during pregnancy for potent mineralocorticoid compounds. During labor and after delivery or after a surgical procedure, steroid replacement must be increased appreciably to approximate the normal adrenal response. Hydrocortisone, 100 mg, is usually given intravenously every 8 hours. It is important that shock from causes other than adrenocortical insufficiency—for example, hemorrhage or sepsis—be recognized and treated promptly.

PRIMARY ALDOSTERONISM. Hyperaldosteronism is caused by an adrenal aldosteronoma in about 75 percent of cases, and idiopathic bilateral adrenal hyperplasia in the remainder (Ganguly, 1998). In view of the very high levels of aldosterone in normal pregnancies, it is not surprising that there may be amelioration of symptoms as well as electrolyte abnormalities during pregnancy (Biglieri and Slaton, 1967; Murakami and associates, 2000). Unless there is an unequivocal adrenal adenoma localized by computed tomography or magnetic resonance imaging, medical therapy is given. In many cases, hypertension responds to *spironolactone,* but β-blockers or calcium-channel blockers also may be required.

PREGNANCY AND HYPERALDOSTERONISM. From their review, Webb and Bayliss (1997) reported 15 cases of primary aldosteronism associated with pregnancy. Most presented with hypertension and hypokalemia. Of the 12 with known causes, an adrenal adenoma was identified in 10. Baron and associates (1995) diagnosed an adrenal adenoma in a 14-week pregnant woman with mild hypertension and hypokalemia. Adrenalectomy was performed at 17 weeks with no further hypertension. Nezu and co-workers (2000) described two women found to have an aldosteronoma postpartum. Both were normotensive throughout pregnancy, but they developed severe hypertension 3 to 4 weeks postpartum. Tumor resection is curative, and as with other adrenal tumors, laparoscopic adrenalectomy is widely used in nonpregnant patients (Ganguly, 1998). This technique may prove to be useful during pregnancy.

PITUITARY DISEASES

The normal pituitary enlarges in pregnancy, predominately from lactotropic cellular hyperplasia. These effects arise from estrogen stimulation, as discussed in Chapter 8 (p. 191).

PROLACTINOMAS. With the advent of serum prolactin assays in the 1970s, the relative common frequency of prolactinomas was appreciated. Almost simultaneously, the ergot derivative, *bromocriptine*—a dopamine-receptor stimulator—was developed as a powerful prolactin inhibitor. Amenorrhea, galactorrhea, and hyperprolactinemia caused by pituitary microadenomas were found to be amenable to bromocriptine therapy. Many pregnancies have resulted from bromocriptine treatment, which does not appear to affect the fetus.

PROLACTINOMAS AND PREGNANCY. Prolactinomas are classified arbitrarily by their size determined by computed tomography or magnetic resonance imaging. By convention, a microadenoma is 10 mm or less, and a macroadenoma is greater than 10 mm. Because symptoms caused by pregnancy-induced pituitary enlargement are much more frequent with macroadenomas, most authorities recommend definitive therapy with surgery or irradiation before pregnancy (Molitch, 1998).

Molitch (1985) analyzed outcomes in almost 250 women with previously untreated **microadenomas** who became pregnant. Only four women developed symptomatic enlargement during pregnancy, and another 11, who were asymptomatic, had radiographic evidence for enlargement. In a review of 352 pregnancies, Albrecht and Betz (1986) reported 2.3 percent with visual disturbances, 4.8 percent with headaches, and 0.6 percent with diabetes insipidus.

Symptomatic tumor enlargement during pregnancy is more common with **macroadenomas.** According to Molitch (1985), 15 percent of 45 such women developed headaches or visual field defects during pregnancy. Albrecht and Betz (1986) reported that 15 percent of 144 women had visual disturbances, 15 percent had headaches, and 1.4 percent developed diabetes insipidus. Kupersmith and colleagues (1994) described visual loss during pregnancy in six of eight women with macroadenomas.

Molitch (1998) recommends that pregnant women with microadenomas be assessed regularly for headaches and visual symptoms. Those with macroadenomas should also have visual field testing during each trimester. Serial serum prolactin concentrations are not recommended because prolactin normally increases during pregnancy. Computed tomography or magnetic resonance imaging during pregnancy is recommended only if symptoms develop. Symptomatic tumor enlargement during pregnancy is treated immediately with bromocriptine. Relative resistance of macroprolactinomas has been described during pregnancy (Shanis and Check, 1996). Surgery is undertaken for women with no response. More than 6000 pregnant women have taken bromocriptine at some time during pregnancy and there have been no adverse effects (Molitch, 1995).

ACROMEGALY. Acromegaly is caused by excessive growth hormone, usually from an acidophilic or a chromophobic pituitary adenoma. In normal pregnancy, pituitary growth hormone levels decrease as placental epitopes are secreted. Diagnosis is confirmed by the failure of an oral glucose-tolerance test to suppress pituitary growth hormone (Molitch, 1998). Pregnancy is rare in acromegalic women, possibly because half are hyperprolactinemic. Management is similar for prolactinomas, with close monitoring for symptoms of tumor enlargement. From their review, Prager and Braunstein (1995) recommend that symptomatic tumor enlargement during pregnancy be treated with bromocriptine or surgery. Herman-Bonert and associates (1998) reported successful treatment of three pregnant women with *octreotide.*

DIABETES INSIPIDUS. Vasopressin deficiency is usually due to a hypothalamic or stalk disorder, rather than a pituitary lesion (Lamberts and associates, 1998). True diabetes insipidus is a rare complication of pregnancy. Only a few cases have been cared for in the last 45 years at Parkland Hospital, during which time there were nearly 350,000 deliveries. This incidence is remarkably close to that cited by Hime and Richardson (1978). As long as the woman takes vasopressin replacement therapy, there should be no serious pregnancy complications. Preferable therapy is intranasal administration of *desmopressin,* the synthetic analog of vasopressin, which is 1-deamino-8-D-arginine vasopressin (DDAVP). Most women require increased doses during pregnancy, likely because of an increased metabolic clearance rate stimulated by placental vasopressinase (Lindheimer and Barron, 1994). In a literature review, Ray (1998) found 53 cases in which DDAVP was used during pregnancy with no adverse sequelae. Because of this same mechanism, **subclinical diabetes insipidus** may become symptomatic during pregnancy. Krege and associates (1989) reviewed 17 such cases. Iwasaki and colleagues (1991) showed that pregnancy unmasked subclinical forms of both nephrogenic as well as central diabetes insipidus.

Diabetes insipidus during pregnancy has been described as arising from a hemorrhage into a macroadenoma (Freeman and co-workers, 1992). One case followed an occluded ventriculoperitoneal shunt (Goolsby and Harlass, 1996). Another case that manifest during pregnancy as oligohydramnios, did not resolve postpartum (Hanson and colleagues, 1997).

In a few instances of diabetes insipidus, there appeared to have been an impairment of labor, possibly caused by diminished or absent endogenous oxytocin (Hime and Richardson, 1978). Sende and associates

(1975) were unable to detect oxytocin by radioimmunoassay in plasma of a pregnant woman with diabetes insipidus before labor, but during labor and the puerperium there was an oxytocin surge. A woman described by Chau and associates (1969) lactated normally, with normal milk ejection pressures.

In our experience, transient secondary diabetes insipidus is more likely encountered with **acute fatty liver of pregnancy** (Chap. 48, p. 1285). This association was described by Cammu and colleagues (1987) as being nephrogenic; however, the syndrome may be due to altered vasopressinase clearance because of hepatic dysfunction. Thus, this type of diabetes insipidus should respond to DDAVP. Harper and associates (1987) described transient disease in a 38-week pregnant woman with biopsy-proven viral hepatitis.

SHEEHAN SYNDROME. Pituitary ischemia and necrosis associated with obstetrical blood loss may cause hypopituitarism, referred to as Sheehan syndrome (Chap. 25, p. 638). Acutely, women may have persistent hypotension, tachycardia, hypoglycemia, and failure of lactation. Subsequent deficiencies of some or all pituitary-responsive hormones may develop. Diabetes insipidus with or without anterior pituitary deficiency has been described following massive obstetrical hemorrhage and prolonged shock (Kan and Calligerous, 1998). Ammini and Mathur (1994) described 12 cases seen from New Delhi. The average duration of onset of symptoms was 5 years.

LYMPHOCYTIC HYPOPHYSITIS. This autoimmune pituitary disorder is characterized by massive infiltration by lymphocytes and plasma cells with parenchymal destruction. The majority of cases have been associated with pregnancy (Madsen, 2000; Patel and associates, 1995; Thodou and colleagues, 1995). There are varying degrees of hypopituitarism or symptoms of mass effect, including headaches and visual field defects. Associated hypothyroidism is common. Pressman and colleagues (1995) reviewed 44 cases and found that 25 percent had other autoimmune diseases. Treatment is problematic, but the disease may be self-limited (Gagneja and associates, 1999). Surgery during pregnancy is warranted only in cases of severe chiasmal compression unresponsive to corticosteroid therapy. In nonpregnant women with disease, spontaneous pregnancies have been reported, and ovulation induction has also been successful (Verdú and colleagues, 1998).

REFERENCES

Ahlawat SK, Jain S, Kumari S, Varma S, Sharma BK: Pheochromocytoma associated with pregnancy: Case report and review of the literature. Obstet Gynecol Surv 54:728, 1999

Albert E, Dalaker K, Jorde R, Berge LN: Addison's disease and pregnancy. Acta Obstet Gynecol Scand 68:185, 1989

Albrecht BH, Betz G: Prolactin-secreting pituitary tumors and pregnancy. In Olefshy JM, Robinson RJ (eds): Contemporary Issues in Endocrinology and Metabolism: Prolactinomas, Vol II. New York, Churchill Livingston, 1986, p 195

Albright F, Reifenstein EC: The Parathyroid Glands and Metabolic Bone Disease. Baltimore, Williams & Wilkins, 1948.

Alvarez-Marfany M, Roman SH, Drexler AJ, Robertson C, Stagnaro-Green A: Long-term prospective study of postpartum thyroid dysfunction in women with insulin dependent diabetes mellitus. J Clin Endocrinol Metab 79:10, 1994

American College of Obstetricians and Gynecologists: Thyroid disease in pregnancy. Technical Bulletin No. 181, June 1993

American Thyroid Association: Haddow study of maternal hypothyroidism during pregnancy. Public Health Committee Statement 1999. Thyroid 9:971, 1999

Amino N, Mori H, Iwatani Y, Tanizawa O, Kawashima M, Tsuge I, Ibaragi K, Kumahara Y, Miyai K: High prevalence of transient postpartum thyrotoxicosis and hypothyroidism. N Engl J Med 306:849, 1982

Ammini AC, Mathur SK: Sheehan syndrome: An analysis of possible aetiological factors. Aust N Z J Obstet Gynaecol 34:534, 1994

Aron DC, Schnall AM, Sheeler LR: Cushing's syndrome and pregnancy. Am J Obstet Gynecol 162:244, 1990

Ayala C, Navarro E, Rodríguez JR, Silva H, Venegas E, Astorga R: Conception after iodine-131 therapy for differentiated thyroid cancer. Thyroid 8:1009, 1998

Bajoria R, Peek MJ, Fisk NM: Maternal-to-fetal transfer of thyrotropin-releasing hormone in vivo. Am J Obstet Gynecol 178:264, 1998

Baker JR Jr: Autoimmune endocrine disease. JAMA 278:1931, 1997

Baron F, Sprauve ME, Huddleston JF, Fisher AJ: Diagnosis and surgical treatment of primary aldosteronism in pregnancy: A case report. Obstet Gynecol 86:644, 1995

Bassoon-Zaltzman C, Sermer M, Lao TT, Drucker D: Bladder pheochromocytoma in pregnancy without hypertension. J Reprod Med 40:149, 1995

Beattie GC, Ravi NR, Lewis M, Williams H, Blair AW, Campbell IW, Browning GG: Rare presentation of maternal primary hyperparathyroidism. BMJ 321:223, 2000

Berg GEB, Nyström EH, Jacobsson L, Lindberg S, Lindstedt RG, Mattsson S, Niklasson CA, Norén AH, Westphal OGA: Radioiodine treatment of hyperthyroidism in a pregnant woman. J Nucl Med 39:357, 1998

Berwaerts J, Verhelst J, Mahler C, Abs R: Cushing's syndrome in pregnancy treated by ketoconazole: Case report and review of the literature. Gynecol Endocrinol 13:175, 1999

Biglieri EG, Slaton PE Jr: Pregnancy and primary aldosteronism. J Clin Endocrinol Metab 27:1628, 1967

Black AJ, Topping J, Durham B, Farquharson RG, Fraser WD: A detailed assessment of alterations in bone turnover, calcium homeostasis, and bone density in normal pregnancy. J Bone Miner Res 15:557, 2000

Blanch J, Pacifici R, Chines A: Pregnancy-associated osteoporosis: Report of two cases with long-term bone density follow-up. Br J Rheum 33:269, 1994

Botchan A, Hauser R, Kupferminc M, Grisaru D, Peyser MR, Lessing JB: Pheochromocytoma in pregnancy: Case report and review of the literature. Obstet Gynecol Surv 50:321, 1995

Bowman ML, Bergmann M, Smith JF: Intrapartum labetalol for the treatment of maternal and fetal thyrotoxicosis. Thyroid 8:795, 1998

Buescher MA, McClamrock HD, Adashi EY: Cushing syndrome in pregnancy. Obstet Gynecol 79:130, 1992

Burch HB, Wartofsky L: Life-threatening thyrotoxicosis. Endocrinol Metab Clin North Am 22:263, 1993

Burrow GN, Fisher DA, Larsen PR: Maternal and fetal thyroid function. N Engl J Med 331:1072, 1994

Cammu H, Velkeniers B, Charels K, Vincken W, Amy JJ: Idiopathic acute fatty liver of pregnancy associated with transient diabetes insipidus. Br J Obstet Gynaecol 94:173, 1987

Canaris GJ, Manowitz NR, Mayor G, Ridgway C: The Colorado Thyroid Disease Prevalence Study. Arch Intern Med 160:526, 2000

Cao XY, Jiang XM, Dou ZH, Rakeman MA, Zhang ML, O'Donnell K, Tai M, Amette K, Delong N, Delong GR: Timing of vulnerability of the brain to iodine deficiency in endemic cretinism. N Engl J Med 331:1739, 1994

Caplan RH, Beguin EA: Hypercalcemia in a calcitriol-treated hypoparathyroid woman during lactation. Obstet Gynecol 76:485, 1990

Carbone LD, Palmieri GMA, Graves SC, Smull K: Osteoporosis of pregnancy: Long-term follow-up of patient and their offspring. Obstet Gynecol 86:664, 1995

Carella MJ, Gossain VV: Hyperparathyroidism and pregnancy: Case report and review. J Gen Intern Med 7:448, 1992

Carr BR, Rainey WE: The adrenal. Infert Reprod Med Clin North Am 5:749, 1994

Casara D, Rubello D, Saladini G, Piotto A, Pelizzo MR, Girelli ME, Busnardo B: Pregnancy after high therapeutic doses of iodine[131] in differentiated thyroid cancer: Potential risks and recommendations. Eur J Nucl Med 20:192, 1993

Chang CC, Greenspan A, Gershwin ME: Osteonecrosis: Current perspectives on pathogenesis and treatment. Semin Arthritis Rheum 23:47, 1993

Chau SS, Fitzpatrick RJ, Jamieson B: Diabetes insipidus and parturition. Br J Obstet Gynaecol 76:444, 1969

Combs CA, Easterling TR, Schmucker BC, Benedetti TJ: Hemodynamic observations during paroxysmal hypertension in a pregnancy with pheochromocytoma. Obstet Gynecol 74:439, 1989

Cuckle H, Wald N, Stone R, Densem J, Haddow J, Knight G: Maternal serum thyroid antibodies in early pregnancy and fetal Down's syndrome. Prenat Diag 8:439, 1988

Dahlman T, Sjberg, Bucht E: Calcium homeostasis in normal pregnancy and puerperium. Acta Obstet Gynecol Scand 73:393, 1994

Davidson KM, Richards DS, Schatz DA, Fisher DA: Successful in utero treatment of fetal goiter and hypothyroidism. N Engl J Med 324:543, 1991

Davies TF: The ATA, the Endocrine Society, and AACE confuse endocrinologists on thyroid disease in pregnancy. Thyroid 10:107, 2000

Davis LE, Leveno KL, Cunningham FG: Hypothyroidism complicating pregnancy. Obstet Gynecol 72:108, 1988

Davis LE, Lucas MJ, Hankins GDV, Roark ML, Cunningham FG: Thyrotoxicosis complicating pregnancy. Am J Obstet Gynecol 160:63, 1989

Dayan CM, Daniels GH: Chronic autoimmune thyroiditis. N Engl J Med 335:99, 1996

Delange F: Administration of iodized oil during pregnancy: A summary of the published evidence. Bull World Health Org 74:101, 1996

Doherty CM, Shindo ML, Rice DH, Montero M, Mestman JH: Management of thyroid nodules during pregnancy. Laryngoscope 105:251, 1995

Driggers RW, Kopelman JN, Satin AJ: Delaying surgery for thyroid cancer in pregnancy. A case report. J Reprod Med 43:909, 1998

Dunne F, Walters B, Marshall T, Heath DA: Pregnancy-associated osteoporosis. Clin Endocrinol 39:487, 1993

Dussault JH, Fisher DA: Thyroid function in mothers of hypothyroid newborns. Obstet Gynecol 93:15, 1999

Endocrine Society: News and facts. Recommendations in response to major hypothyroidism study. www.endo-society.org/maternalthyroiddeficiency, February 2000

Franklyn JA: The management of hyperthyroidism. N Engl J Med 330:1731, 1994

Freeman R, Wezenter B, Silverstein M, Kuo D, Weiss KL, Kantrowitz AB, Schubart UK: Pregnancy-associated subacute hemorrhage into a prolactinoma resulting in diabetes insipidus. Fertil Steril 58:427, 1992

Fung HY, Kologln M, Collison K, John R, Richards CJ, Hall R, McGregor AM: Postpartum thyroid dysfunction in Mid Glamorgan. BMJ 296:241, 1988

Gagneja H, Arafah B, Taylor HC: Histologically proven lymphocytic hypophysitis: Spontaneous resolution and subsequent pregnancy. Mayo Clin Proc 74:150, 1999

Ganguly A: Primary aldosteronism. N Engl J Med 339:1828, 1998

Geelhoed GW: Surgery of the endocrine glands in pregnancy. Clin Obstet Gynecol 26:865, 1983

Gharib H, Cobin RH, Dickey RA: Subclinical hypothyroidism during pregnancy: Position statement from the American Association of Clinical Endocrinologists. Endocr Pract 5:367, 1999

Girling JC, de Swiet M: Thyroxine dosage during pregnancy in women with primary hypothyroidism. Br J Obstet Gynaecol 99:368, 1992

Glinoer D, Lemone M, Bourdoux P, DeNayer P, Delange F, Kinthaert J, Lejeune B: Partial reversibility during late postpartum of thyroid abnormalities associated with pregnancy. J Clin Endocrinol Metab 74:453, 1992

Glinoer D, Riahi M, Grun JP, Kinthaert J: Risk of subclinical hypothyroidism in pregnant women with asymptomatic autoimmune thyroid disorders. J Clin Endocrinol Metab 79:197, 1994

Goodwin TM, Hershman JM: Hyperthyroidism due to inappropriate production of human chorionic gonadotropin. Clin Obstet Gynecol 40:32, 1997

Goolsby L, Harlass F: Central diabetes insipidus: A complication of ventriculoperitoneal shunt malfunction during pregnancy. Am J Obstet Gynecol 174:1655, 1996

Graham EM, Freedman LJ, Forouzan I: Intrauterine growth retardation in a woman with primary hyperparathyroidism. J Reprod Med 43:451, 1998

Grant DB, Smith I, Fuggle PW, Tokar S, Chapple J: Congenital hypothyroidism detected by neonatal screening: Relationship between biochemical severity and early clinical features. Arch Dis Child 67:87, 1992

Grimbert P, Chauveau D, Richard S, Rémy P, Grünfeld JP: Pregnancy in von Hippel–Lindau disease. Am J Obstet Gynecol 180:110, 1999

Grossman M, Weintraub BD, Szkudlinski MW: Novel insights into the molecular mechanisms of human thyrotropin action: Structural, physiological, and therapeutic implications for the glycoprotein hormone family. Endocr Rev 18:476, 1997

Haddow JE, Palomaki GE, Allan WC, Williams JR, Knight

GJ, Gagnon J, O'Heir C, Mitchell ML, Hermos RJ, Waisbren SE, Faix JD, Klein RZ: Maternal thyroid deficiency during pregnancy and subsequent neuropsychological development of the child. N Engl J Med 341:549, 1999

Hankins GDV, Lowe TW, Cunningham FG: Dilated cardiomyopathy and thyrotoxicosis complicated by septic abortion. Am J Obstet Gynecol 149:85, 1984

Hanson RS, Powrie RO, Larson L: Diabetes insipidus in pregnancy: Treatable cause of oligohydramnios. Obstet Gynecol 89:816, 1997

Harper M, Hatjis CG, Appel RG, Austin WE: Vasopressin-resistant diabetes insipidus, liver dysfunction, and hyperuricemia and decreased renal function. J Reprod Med 32:862, 1987

Harper MA, Murnaghan GA, Kennedy L, Hadden DR, Atkinson AB: Pheochromocytoma in pregnancy. Five cases and a review of the literature. Br J Obstet Gynaecol 96:594, 1989

Hatjis CG: Diagnosis and successful treatment of fetal goitrous hyperthyroidism caused by maternal Graves' disease. Obstet Gynecol 81:837, 1993

Hayslip CC, Fein HG, O'Donnell VM, Friedman DS, Klein TA, Smallridge RC: The value of serum antimicrosomal antibody testing in screening for symptomatic postpartum thyroid dysfunction. Am J Obstet Gynecol 159:203, 1988

Henderson PH, Sowers MF, Kutzko KE, Jannausch ML: Bone mineral density in grand multiparous women with extended lactation. Am J Obstet Gynecol 182:1371, 2000

Herman-Bonert V, Seliverstov M, Melmed S: Pregnancy in acromegaly: Successful therapeutic outcome. J Clin Endocrinol Metab 83:727, 1998

Hetzel BS: Iodine deficiency and fetal brain damage. N Engl J Med 331:1770, 1994

Hidaka Y, Tamaki H, Iwatani Y, Tada H, Mitsuda N, Amino N: Prediction of postpartum Graves thyrotoxicosis by measurement of thyroid stimulating antibody in early pregnancy. Clin Endocrinol 41:15, 1994

Hime MC, Richardson JA: Diabetes insipidus and pregnancy: Case report, incidence, and review of literature. Obstet Gynecol Surv 3:375, 1978

Houck JA, Davis RE, Sharma HM: Thyroid-stimulating immunoglobulin as a cause of recurrent intrauterine fetal death. Obstet Gynecol 71:1018, 1988

Iwasaki Y, Oiso Y, Kondo K, Takagi S, Takatsuki K, Hasegawa H, Ishikawa K, Fujimura Y, Kazeto S, Tomita A: Aggravation of subclinical diabetes insipidus during pregnancy. N Engl J Med 324:522, 1991

Janetschek G, Finkenstedt G, Gasser R, Waibel UG, Peshel R, Bartsch G, Neumann HPH: Laparoscopic surgery for pheochromocytoma: Adrenalectomy, partial resection, excision of paragangliomas. J Urol 150:330, 1998

Jansson R, Dahlberg PA, Karlsson FA: Postpartum thyroiditis. Bailliores Clin Endocrinol Metab 2:619, 1988

Jovanovic-Peterson L, Peterson CM: De novo clinical hypothyroidism in pregnancies complicated by type I diabetes, subclinical hypothyroidism, and proteinuria: A new syndrome. Am J Obstet Gynecol 159:442, 1988

Kamiya Y, Okada M, Yoneyama A, Jin-No Y, Hibino T, Watanabe O, Kajitura S, Suzuki Y, Iwata H, Kobayashi S: Surgical successful treatment of Cushing's syndrome in a pregnant patient complicated with severe cardiac involvement. Endocr J 45:499, 1998

Kan AKS, Calligerous D: A case report of Sheehan syndrome presenting with diabetes insipidus. Aust N Z J Obstet Gynaecol 38:224, 1998

Keely E: Endocrine causes of hypertension in pregnancy—when to start looking for zebras. Semin Perinatol 22:471, 1998

Kelly TR: Primary hyperparathyroidism during pregnancy. Surgery 110:1028, 1991

Khovidhunkit W, Epstein S: Osteoporosis in pregnancy. Osteoporosis Int 6:345, 1996

Klein I, Kaie O: Thyrotoxicosis and the heart. Endocrinol Metab Clin North Am 27:51, 1998

Kort KC, Schiller HJ, Numann PJ: Hyperparathyroidism and pregnancy. Am J Surg 177:66, 1999

Krege J, Katz VL, Bowes WA Jr: Transient diabetes insipidus of pregnancy. Obstet Gynecol Surv 44:789, 1989

Kriplani A, Buckshee K, Bhargava VL, Takkar D, Ammini AC: Maternal and perinatal outcome in thyrotoxicosis complicating pregnancy. Eur J Obstet Gynecol Reprod Biol 54:159, 1994

Kuijpens JL, de Haan-Meulman M, Vader HL, Pop VJ, Wiersinaga WM, Drexhage HA: Cell-mediated immunity and postpartum thyroid dysfunction: A possibility for the prediction of disease? J Clin Endocrinol Metab 83:1959, 1998

Kung AWC, Jones BM: A change from stimulatory to blocking antibody activity in Graves' disease during pregnancy. J Clin Endocrinol Metab 83:514, 1998

Kupersmith MJ, Rosenberg C, Kleinberg D: Visual loss in pregnant women with pituitary adenomas. Ann Intern Med 121:473, 1994

Lamberts SWJ, de Herder WW, van der Lely AJ: Pituitary insufficiency. Lancet 352:127, 1998

Leung AS, Millar LE, Koonings PP, Montoro M, Mestman JH: Perinatal outcome in hypothyroid pregnancies. Obstet Gynecol 81:349, 1993

Lindheimer MD, Barron WM: Water metabolism and vasopressin secretion during pregnancy. Bailliores Clin Obstet Gynaecol 8:311, 1994

Lindsay RS, Toft AD: Hypothyroidism. Lancet 349:413, 1997

Lucas A, Pizarro E, Granada ML, Salinas I, Foz M, Sanmarti A: Postpartum thyroiditis: Epidemiology and clinical evolution in a nonselected population. Thyroid 10:71, 2000

Ludwig GD: Hyperparathyroidism in relation to pregnancy. N Engl J Med 267:637, 1962

Lyons CW, Colmorgen GHC: Medical management of pheochromocytoma in pregnancy. Obstet Gynecol 72:450, 1988

Madsen JR: Case records of the Massachusetts General Hospital. Case 34-2000. N Engl J Med 343:1399, 2000

Mandel SJ, Larsen PR, Seely EW, Brent GA: Increased need for thyroxine during pregnancy in women with primary hypothyroidism. N Engl J Med 323:91, 1990

Marqusee E, Haden ST, Utiger RD: Subclinical thyrotoxicosis. End Metab C 27:37, 1998

Mellor A, Harvey RD, Pobereskin LH, Sneyd JR: Cushing's disease treated by transsphenoidal selective adenomectomy in mid-pregnancy. Br J Anaesth 80:850, 1998

Mestman JH: Management of thyroid nodules in pregnancy. Contemp Obstet Gynecol 43:27, 1999

Mestman JH: Hyperthyroidism in pregnancy. Endocrinol Metab Clin North Am 27:127, 1998a

Mestman JH: Parathyroid disorders of pregnancy. Semin Perinatol 22:485, 1998b

Mestman JH, Goodwin TM, Montoro MM: Thyroid disorders of pregnancy. Endocrinol Metab Clin North Am 24:41, 1995

Miccoli P, Vitti P, Rago T, Iacconi P, Bartalena L, Bogazzi F, Fiore E, Valeriano R, Chiovato L, Rocchi R, Pinchera A: Surgical treatment of Graves' disease: Subtotal or total thyroidectomy? Surgery 120:1020, 1996

Millar LK, Wing DA, Leung AS, Koonings PP, Montoro MN,

Mestman JH: Low birth weight and preeclampsia in pregnancies complicated by hyperthyroidism. Obstet Gynecol 84:946, 1994

Molitch ME: Pituitary diseases in pregnancy. Semin Perinatol 22:457, 1998

Molitch ME: Endocrine emergencies in pregnancy. Baillieres Clin Endocrinol Metab 6:167, 1992

Molitch ME: Pregnancy and the hyperprolactinemic woman. N Engl J Med 312:1364, 1985

Momotani N, Noh JH, Ishikawa N, Ito K: Effects of propylthiouracil and methimazole on fetal thyroid status in mothers with Graves' hyperthyroidism. J Clin Endocrinol Metab 82:3633, 1997

Montoro MN, Paler RJ, Goodwin TM, Mestman JH: Parathyroid carcinoma during pregnancy. Obstet Gynecol 96: 841, 2000

Moosa M, Mazzaferri EL: Outcome of differentiated thyroid cancer diagnosed in pregnant women. J Clin Endocrinol Metab 82:2862, 1997

Morris PC: Thyroid cancer complicating pregnancy. Obstet Gynecol Clin North Am 25:401, 1998

Murakami T, Ogura EW, Tanaka Y, Yamamoto M: High blood pressure lowered by pregnancy. Lancet 356:1980, 2000

Nezu M, Miura Y, Noshiro T, Inoue M: Primary aldosteronism as a cause of severe postpartum hypertension in two women. Am J Obstet Gynecol 182:745, 2000

O'Doherty MJ, McElhatton PR, Thomas SHL: Treating thyrotoxicosis in pregnant or potentially pregnant women. BMJ 318:5, 1999

O'Shaughnessy RW, Hackett KJ: Maternal Addison's disease and fetal growth retardation. J Repord Med 29:752, 1984

Pacini F, Vorontsova T, Molinaro E, Kuchinskaya E, Agate L, Shavrova E, Astachova L, Chiovato L, Pinchera A: Prevalence of thyroid autoantibodies in children and adolescents from Belarus exposed to the Chernobyl radioactive fallout. Lancet 352:763, 1998

Page DV, Brady K, Mitchell J, Pehrson J, Wade G: The pathology of intrauterine thyrotoxicosis: Two case reports. Obstet Gynecol 72:479, 1988

Patel MC, Guneratne N, Haq N, West TET, Weetman AP, Clayton RN: Peripartum hypopituitarism and lymphocytic hypophysitis. Q J Med 88:571, 1995

Pop VJ, Kujipens JL, van Baar AL, Verkerk G, van Son MM, de Vijlder JJ, Vulsma T, Wiersinga WM, Drexhage HA, Vader HL: Low maternal free thyroxine concentrations during early pregnancy are associated with impaired psychomotor development in infancy. Clin Endocrinol 50:149, 1999a

Pop VJ, van Baar AL, Vulsma T: Should all pregnant women be screened for hypothyroidism? Lancet 354:1224, 1999b

Potts JT: Disease of the parathyroid gland and other hyper- and hypocalcemic disorders. In Fauci AS, Braunwald E, Isselbacher KJ, Wilson JD, Martin JB, Kasper DL, Hauser SL, Longo DL (eds): Harrison's Principles of Internal Medicine, 14th ed. New York, McGraw-Hill, 1998, p 2227

Power ML, Heaney RP, Kalkwarf HJ, Pitkin RM, Repke JT, Tsang RC, Schulkin J: The role of calcium in health and disease. Am J Obstet Gynecol 181:1560, 1999

Prager D, Braunstein GD: Pituitary disorders during pregnancy. Endocrinol Metab Clin North Am 24:1, 1995

Premawardhana LD, Parkes AB, Ammari F, John R, Darke C, Adams H, Lazarus JH: Postpartum thyroiditis and long-term thyroid status: Prognostic influence of thyroid peroxidase antibodies and ultrasound echogenicity. J Clin Endocrinol Metab 85:71, 2000

Pressman EK, Zeidman SM, Reddy UM, Epstein JI, Brem H: Differentiating lymphocytic adenohypophysitis from pituitary adenoma of the peripartum patient. J Reprod Med 40:251, 1995

Rasmussen NG, Hornnes PJ, Hegedüs L: Ultrasonographically determined thyroid size in pregnancy and postpartum: The goitrogenic effect of pregnancy. Am J Obstet Gynecol 160:1216, 1989

Ray JG: DDAVP use during pregnancy: An analysis of its safety for mother and child. Obstet Gynecol Surv 53:450, 1998

Reinwein D, Benker G, Lazarus JH, Alexander WD, the European Multicenter Study Group on Antithyroid Drug Treatment: A prospective randomized trial of antithyroid drug doses in Graves' disease therapy. J Clin Endocrinol Metab 76:1516, 1993

Rooney DP, Traub AI, Russell CFJ, Hadden DR: Cure of hyperparathyroidism in pregnancy by sternotomy and removal of a mediastinal parathyroid adenoma. Postgrad Med J 74:233, 1998

Rosen IB, Walfish PG: Pregnancy as a predisposing factor in thyroid neoplasia. Arch Surg 121:1287, 1986

Seaward PGR, Guidozzi F, Sonnendecker EWW: Addisonian crisis in pregnancy: Case report. Br J Obstet Gynaecol 96:1348, 1989

Seely EW, Brown EM, DeMaggio DM, Weldon DK, Graves SW: A prospective study of calciotropic hormones in pregnancy and postpartum: Reciprocal changes in serum intact parathyroid hormone and 1,25-dihydroxyvitamin D. Am J Obstet Gynecol 176:214, 1975

Sende P, Pantelakis N, Suzuki K, Bashore R: Plasma oxytocin level in pregnancy with diabetes insipidus. Clin Res 23:242A, 1975

Shangold MM, Dor N, Welt SI, Fleischman AR, Crenshaw MC Jr: Hyperparathyroidism and pregnancy: A review. Obstet Gynecol Surv 37:217, 1982

Shanis BS, Check JH: Relative resistance of a macroprolactinoma to bromocriptine therapy during pregnancy. Gynecol Endocrinol 10:91, 1996

Sherif IH, Oyan WT, Bosairi S, Carrascal SM: Treatment of hyperthyroidism in pregnancy. Acta Obstet Gynecol Scand 70:461, 1991

Silverberg SJ, Shane E, Jacobs TP, Siris E, Bilezikian JP: A 10-year prospective study of primary hyperparathyroidism with or without parathyroid surgery. N Engl J Med 341:1249, 1999

Singer PA, Cooper DS, Levy EG, Ladenson PW, Braverman LE, Daniels G, Greenspan FS, McDougall IR, Nikolai TF: Treatment guidelines for patients with hyperthyroidism and hypothyroidism. JAMA 273:808, 1995

Singh A, Dantas ZN, Stone SC, Asch RH: Presence of thyroid antibodies in early reproductive failure: Biochemical versus clinical pregnancies. Fertil Steril 63:277, 1995

Smith R, Athanasou NA, Ostlere SJ, Vipond SE: Pregnancy-associated osteoporosis. Q J Med 88:865, 1995

Spencer C, Smith P, Rafla N, Weatherell R: Corticosteroids in pregnancy and osteonecrosis of the femoral head. Obstet Gynecol 94:848, 1999

Stagnaro-Green A, Roman SH, Cobin RH, El-Harazy E, Alvarez-Marfany M, Davies TF: Detection of at-risk pregnancy by means of highly sensitive assays for thyroid autoantibodies. JAMA 264:1422, 1990

Sweeney WJ, Katz VL: Recurrent pheochromocytoma during pregnancy. Obstet Gynecol 83:820, 1994

Tamaki H, Amino N, Takeoka K, Mitsuda N, Miyai K, Tanizawa O: Thyroxine requirement during pregnancy for replacement therapy of hypothyroidism. Obstet Gynecol 76:230, 1990

Tewari K, Balderston KD, Carpenter SE, Major CA: Papillary thyroid carcinoma manifesting as thyroid storm of pregnancy: Case report. Am J Obstet Gynecol 179:818, 1998

Thilly CH, Delange F, Lagasse R, Bourdoux P, Ramioul L, Berquist H, Ermans AM: Fetal hypothyroidism and maternal thyroid status in severe endemic goiter. J Clin Endocrinol Metab 47:354, 1978

Thodou E, Asa SL, Kontogeorgos G, Kovacs K, Horvath E, Ezzat S: Clinical case seminar: Lymphocytic hypophysitis: Clinicopathological findings. J Clin Endocrinol Metab 80:2302, 1995

Utiger RD: Maternal hypothyroidism and fetal development. N Engl J Med 341:601, 1999a

Utiger RD: Treatment of primary hyperparathyroidism. N Engl J Med 341:1301, 1999b

Utiger RD: Subclinical hyperthyroidism: Just a low serum thyrotropin concentration, or something more? N Engl J Med 331:1302, 1994

Vanderpump MPJ, Ahlquist JAO, Franklyn JA, Clayton RN: Consensus statement for good practice and audit measures in the management of hypothyroidism and hyperthyroidism. BMJ 313:539, 1996

Van der Vaart CH, Heringa MP, Dullaart RPF: Multiple endocrine neoplasia presenting as phaeochromocytoma during pregnancy. Br J Obstet Gynaecol 100:1144, 1993

Van Wassenaer AG, Kok JH, de Vijlder JJM, Briët JM, Smit BJ, Tamminga P, van Baar A, Dekker FW, Vulsma T: Effects of thyroxine supplementation on neurologic development in infants born at less than 30 weeks' gestation. N Engl J Med 336:21, 1997

Verdú LI, Martin-Caballero C, García-López G, Cueto MJ: Ovulation induction and normal pregnancy after panhypopituitarism due to lymphocytic hypophysitis. Obstet Gynecol 91:850, 1998

Vulsma T, Gons M, De Vijilder JJM: Maternal–fetal transfer of thyroxine in congenital hypothyroidism due to a total organification defect or thyroid agenesis. N Engl J Med 321:13, 1989

Walfish PG, Chan JYC: Postpartum hyperthyroidism. J Clin Endocrinol Metab 14:417, 1985

Wallace C, Couch R, Ginsbert J: Fetal thyrotoxicosis: A case report and recommendations for prediction, diagnosis, and treatment. Thyroid 5:125, 1995

Wasserstrum N, Anania CA: Perinatal consequences of maternal hypothyroidism in early pregnancy and inadequate replacement. Clin Endocrinol 42:353, 1995

Watson WJ, Fiegen MM: Fetal thyrotoxicosis associated with nonimmune hydrops. Am J Obstet Gynecol 172:1039, 1995

Webb JC, Bayliss MP: Pregnancy complicated by primary aldosteronism. South Med J 90:243, 1997

Weetman AP: Graves' disease. N Engl J Med 343:1236, 2000

Wenstrom KD, Weiner CP, Williamson RA, Grant SS: Prenatal diagnosis of fetal hyperthyrodism using funipuncture. Obstet Gynecol 76:513, 1990

Williams DH, Dluhy RG: Diseases of the adrenal cortex. In Fauci AS, Braunwald E, Isselbacher KJ, Wilson JD, Martin JB, Kasper DL, Houser SL, Longo DL (eds): Harrison's Principles of Internal Medicine, 14th ed. New York, McGraw-Hill, 1998, p 2042

Wing DA, Millar LK, Koonings PP, Montoro MN, Mestman JH: A comparison of propylthiouracil versus methimazole in the treatment of hyperthyroidism in pregnancy. Am J Obstet Gynecol 170:90, 1994

Woeber KA: Subclinical thyroid dysfunction. Arch Int Med 157:1065, 1997

51

Diabetes

This and the preceding 20 editions of *Williams Obstetrics* provide witness that the 20th century has been a remarkable time for the diabetic woman who becomes pregnant. At the beginning of the century, diabetic women suffered from infertility, and the rare woman achieving pregnancy faced a dismal prognosis. Maternal death was a real threat, and perinatal survival a mere 40 percent. The availability of insulin, beginning in 1922, restored fertility and virtually abolished maternal mortality. At the same time, perinatal survival did not change appreciably.

To improve this dismal perinatal mortality, obstetricians increasingly focused on both timing and mode of delivery, so that by the 1930s, awareness of fetal macrosomia and intrapartum deaths led to frequent cesarean delivery (White and colleagues, 1939). Some improvement followed, but unexplained late antepartum deaths continued to be a problem and led to early delivery with resultant neonatal immaturity and its consequences. The development of the White Classification in 1949, by which fetal risk was shown to be proportional to the severity of maternal diabetes, permitted individualized timing of delivery and helped reduce perinatal mortality. These management landmarks improved perinatal survival to about 85 percent by the late 1950s (White, 1978b). In the ensuing years, up to the present, several refinements in management of diabetic women and their fetuses or infants have resulted in a perinatal mortality rate, excluding malformations, nearly equivalent to that observed in normal pregnancies.

CLASSIFICATION

Diabetes is classified as type 1 (insulin dependent) or type 2 (noninsulin dependent) according to whether the patient requires exogenous insulin to prevent ketoacidosis. Some differentiating characteristics between types 1 and 2 are shown in Table 51–1.

Type 1 diabetes is immune mediated and develops in genetically susceptible persons. This predisposition is permissive rather than causal and disease presumably is triggered by a viral infection. There is inflammatory *insulitis* with lymphocytic infiltration of islets. Subsequently, there is immune stimulation of antibodies against the β-cell. The cell membrane then becomes susceptible to autoimmune cytotoxic antibodies, which leads to eventual cellular destruction and resultant diabetes. The genetics of type 1 diabetes is complex, but there is general agreement that there is an association with the HLA-D histocompatibility complex located on chromosome 6. There is a low vertical transmission rate in type 1 disease. Moreover, the concordance rate for diabetes in monozygous twins, rather than being nearly 100 percent if diabetes were solely genetic in origin, is less than 50 percent (Foster, 1998).

Type 2, noninsulin-dependent diabetes has no HLA association. The disease has a familial occurrence and concordance in monozygotic twins is 100 percent. Nearly 40 percent of siblings and a third of offspring develop abnormal glucose tolerance or obvious diabetes (Foster, 1998). Its pathophysiology is abnormal insulin secretion and insulin resistance in target tissues. Most patients are overtly obese, and there is speculation that peripheral insulin resistance induced by obesity leads to β-cell exhaustion.

Diabetes is the most common medical complication of pregnancy. Patients can be separated into those who were known to have diabetes before pregnancy (overt) and those diagnosed during pregnancy (gestational). In 1998, a total of 103,691 American women had pregnancies complicated by diabetes, representing 2.6 percent

TABLE 51–1. Some General Characteristics of Insulin-dependent (Type 1) and Noninsulin-dependent (Type 2) Diabetes Mellitus

Characteristics	Type 1 (Insulin Dependent)	Type 2 (Noninsulin Dependent)
Genetic locus[a]	Chromosome 6	Unknown
Age at onset	Usually < 40[b]	> 40
Habitus	Normal to wasted	Obese
Plasma insulin	Low to absent	Normal to high
Plasma glucagon	High, suppressible	High, resistant
Acute complication	Ketoacidosis	Hyperosmolar coma
Insulin therapy	Responsive	Responsive/resistant
Sulfonylurea	Unresponsive	Responsive

[a] Both are polygenic.
[b] Most cases appear before age 20.
From Foster (1998), with permission.

of all live births (Ventura and colleagues, 2000). It is estimated that 90 percent of all pregnancies complicated by diabetes are due to gestational diabetes. Thus, in 1998, approximately 10,000 American women with overt diabetes, and 90,000 with gestational diabetes, delivered live births.

CLASSIFICATION DURING PREGNANCY. Table 51–2 gives a classification recommended by the American College of Obstetricians and Gynecologists in 1986. This was replaced in 1994 because, according to the American College of Obstetricians and Gynecologists, "a single classification based on the presence or absence of good maternal metabolic control and the presence or absence of maternal diabetic vasculopathy is more helpful." In the 1986 classification, women diagnosed to have gestational diabetes are subdivided according to their degree of glycemia. Specifically, those with fasting hyperglycemia (105 mg/dL or greater) are placed into class A_2. Approximately 15 percent of women with gestational diabetes will exhibit fasting hyperglycemia (Sheffield and co-workers, 2000). Women in classes B to H, corresponding to the White classification (1978a), have overt diabetes antedating pregnancy. The White system emphasizes that end-organ derangements, especially involving the eyes, kidneys, and heart, have significant effects on pregnancy outcome.

DIAGNOSIS OF OVERT DIABETES DURING PREGNANCY. The woman with high plasma glucose levels, glucosuria, and ketoacidosis presents no problem in diagnosis. Similarly, women with a random plasma glucose level greater than 200 mg/dL plus classical signs and symptoms such as polydipsia, polyuria, and unexplained weight loss or fasting glucose of 126 mg/dL or higher, should be considered to have overt diabetes (American Diabetes Association, 1999b). The new diagnostic cutoff value for overt diabetes of a fasting plasma glucose of 126 mg/dL or higher is based on data that indicate the risk of retinopathy rises dramatically at that fasting level. The woman at the opposite end of the spectrum, with only minimal metabolic derangement, may be difficult to identify. The likelihood of impaired carbohydrate metabolism is increased appreciably in women who have a strong familial history of diabetes, have given birth to large infants, demonstrate persistent glucosuria, or have unexplained fetal losses.

Reducing substances are commonly found in the urine of pregnant women. Commercially available dipsticks may be used to identify glucosuria while avoiding a positive reaction from lactose. Even then, glucosuria most often does not reflect impaired glucose tolerance, but rather augmented glomerular filtration (Chap. 8). Nonetheless, the detection of glucosuria during pregnancy warrants further investigation (Gribble and co-authors, 1995).

DETECTION OF GESTATIONAL DIABETES. Gestational diabetes mellitus is defined as carbohydrate intolerance of variable severity with onset or first recognition during pregnancy. This definition applies regardless of whether or not insulin is used for treatment. Undoubtedly, some women with gestational diabetes have previously unrecognized overt diabetes. Sheffield and co-workers (2000) studied outcomes in 1190 diabetic women delivered at Parkland Hospital between 1991 and 1995. They found that women with fasting hyperglycemia diagnosed before 24 weeks had pregnancy out-

TABLE 51–2. Classification of Diabetes Complicating Pregnancy

Class	Onset	Fasting Plasma Glucose	2-hour Postprandial Glucose	Therapy
A_1	Gestational	< 105 mg/dL	< 120 mg/dL	Diet
A_2	Gestational	> 105 mg/dL	> 120 mg/dL	Insulin

Class	Age of Onset (yr)	Duration (yr)	Vascular Disease	Therapy
B	Over 20	< 10	None	Insulin
C	10–19	10–19	None	Insulin
D	Before 10	> 20	Benign retinopathy	Insulin
F	Any	Any	Nephropathy[a]	Insulin
R	Any	Any	Proliferative retinopathy	Insulin
H	Any	Any	Heart	Insulin

[a] When diagnosed during pregnancy: 500 mg or more proteinuria per 24 hours measured before 20 weeks' gestation.
From American College of Obstetricians and Gynecologists (1986).

comes similar to those for women in classes B through FR. This finding indicates that fasting hyperglycemia early in pregnancy likely represents overt diabetes rather than gestational diabetes. Bartha and colleagues (2000) also found that women diagnosed to have gestational diabetes early in pregnancy are a high-risk subgroup.

SCREENING. Despite more than 30 years of research, there is lack of consensus regarding the optimal approach to screening for gestational diabetes. The major issues include whether universal or selective screening should be used, as well as which 50-g glucose test threshold is best to identify women at risk for gestational diabetes (Bonomo and colleagues, 1998; Danilenko-Dixon and colleagues, 1999).

Since 1980 there have been four international workshop–conferences on gestational diabetes held in Chicago, and these have attempted to provide consensus statements on screening for diabetes (Metzger and Coustan, 1998). At the most recent workshop, in 1997, prior recommendations for universal screening were changed to selective screening using the guidelines shown in Table 51–3. It was recommended that screening for gestational diabetes should be performed between 24 and 28 weeks in those women not known to have glucose intolerance earlier in pregnancy. This evaluation may be done in one or two steps. In the two-step procedure, a 50-g oral glucose challenge test is followed by a diagnostic 100-g oral glucose tolerance test if results exceed a predetermined plasma glucose concentration. In the one-step approach, the diagnostic 100-g test is administered without the preceding 50-g test.

When the two-step method is used, plasma glucose is measured 1 hour after a 50-g glucose load without regard to the time of day or time of last meal. A value of 140 mg/dL (7.8 mmol/L) or higher will identify 80 percent of all women with gestational diabetes. Using a value of 130 mg/dL (7.2 mmol/L) or higher will increase the yield to over 90 percent; however, 20 to 25 percent of women will have positive tests compared with 14 to 18 percent when the 140 mg/dL or greater threshold is used. The recommended criteria for interpretation of the 100-g diagnostic glucose tolerance test are shown in Table 51–4.

Gabbe and co-authors (1998) surveyed practicing obstetricians in the United States and found that 96 percent screened all pregnant women for gestational diabetes, usually between 25 and 29 weeks. Similarly, Owen and colleagues (1995) surveyed Obstetrics and Gynecology residency programs and found that 97 percent were using universal screening between 24 and 28 weeks. The American College of Obstetricians and Gynecologists (1994) has concluded that selective screening may be appropriate in some clinical settings and universal screening in other circumstances.

The day-to-day reproducibility of the 50-g screening test has also been tested (Espinosa de los Monteros and co-workers, 1993). While 90 percent of normal results

TABLE 51–3. Fourth International Workshop–Conference on Gestational Diabetes: Recommended Screening Strategy Based on Risk Assessment for Detecting Gestational Diabetes (GDM)

Low Risk

    Blood glucose testing not routinely required if all of the following characteristics are present:

        Member of an ethnic group with a low prevalence of gestational diabetes

        No known diabetes in first-degree relatives

        Age less than 25 years

        Weight normal before pregnancy

        No history of abnormal glucose metabolism

        No history of poor obstetrical outcome

Average Risk

    Perform blood glucose testing at 24–28 weeks using one of the following:

        Average risk—women of Hispanic, African, Native American, South or East Asian origins

        High risk—women with marked obesity, strong family history of type 2 diabetes, prior gestational diabetes, or glucosuria

High Risk

    Perform blood glucose testing as soon as feasible: If gestational diabetes is not diagnosed, blood glucose testing should be repeated at 24–28 weeks or at any time a patient has symptoms or signs suggestive of hyperglycemia

From Metzger and Coustan (1998), with permission.

TABLE 51–4. American College of Obstetricians and Gynecologists 1994 Criteria for Diagnosis of Gestational Diabetes Using 100 G of Glucose Taken Orally

Timing of Measurement	Plasma Glucose (mg/dL)[a]	
	National Diabetes Data Group (1979)	Carpenter and Coustan (1982)
Fasting	105	95
1 hr	190	180
2 hr	165	155
3 hr	145	140

[a] Gestational diabetes is diagnosed when any two values are met or exceeded.
Adapted from the American College of Obstetricians and Gynecologists (1994), with permission.

were reproducible the next day, only 83 percent of abnormal tests were reproducible. Murphy and colleagues (1994) studied the accuracy and precision of reflectance photometers (Accu-Check III) for screening. Use of the glucometer required redefining the circumstances for testing as well as threshold values for abnormal results. It seems best to avoid these devices for screening.

DIAGNOSTIC CRITERIA. There is not international agreement as to the optimal glucose tolerance test for the definitive diagnosis of gestational diabetes. The World Health Organization (1985) recommends the 75-g 2-hour oral glucose tolerance test and this approach is often used in Europe (Weiss and colleagues, 1998). In the United States, the *100-g 3-hour oral glucose tolerance test* performed after an overnight fast remains the standard (American College of Obstetricians and Gynecologists, 1994). Catalano and co-workers (1993) found that the 100-g 3-hour test was not reproducible in 25 percent of women when repeated 1 week after the initial test. They attributed this to increased norepinephrine-mediated gluconeogenesis due to maternal stress at initial testing.

Thus, there is not a consensus as to which glucose threshold values to use for diagnosis of gestational diabetes. Plasma values suggested by the American College of Obstetricians and Gynecologists (1994) are shown in Table 51–4. These permit use of normative data suggested by the National Diabetes Data Group (1979) as well as those of Carpenter and Coustan (1982). Diagnosis of gestational diabetes is generally made in either set of criteria when any two values are met or exceeded. Schwartz and colleagues (1999), however, suggest that replacing the National Diabetes Data Group criteria with the Carpenter and Coustan criteria would increase by 54 percent the number of pregnant women with a diagnosis of gestational diabetes. This would increase

costs, while only minimally affecting the prevalence of macrosomia, which is the outcome of greatest importance. According to the survey by Owen and colleagues (1995), 77 percent of residency programs use the National Diabetes Data Group (1979) criteria, and 96 percent require two or more abnormal values. These are the diagnostic criteria in use at Parkland Hospital. The American Diabetes Association (1999) appears to endorse any of these approaches for screening or diagnosis of gestational diabetes.

GESTATIONAL DIABETES

"Gestational" diabetes implies that this disorder is induced by pregnancy, perhaps due to exaggerated physiological changes in glucose metabolism (Chap. 8, p. 174). An alternative explanation is that gestational diabetes is maturity-onset or type 2 diabetes unmasked or discovered during pregnancy. For example, Harris (1988) found that the prevalence of undiagnosed glucose intolerance in nonpregnant women between the ages of 20 and 44 years was virtually identical to the prevalence of gestational diabetes. Catalano and colleagues (1999) evaluated the longitudinal changes in insulin sensitivity, insulin response, and endogenous glucose production in women with normal glucose tolerance and in those with gestational diabetes before and during pregnancy. They found that women with gestational diabetes had abnormalities in glucose metabolism that are hallmarks of type 2 diabetes.

Use of the diagnostic term **gestational diabetes** has been encouraged in order to communicate the need for increased surveillance and to convince women of the need for further testing postpartum. The likelihood of fetal death with appropriately treated gestational diabetes has been found no different than in the general population (Metzger and Coustan, 1998). The most important perinatal concern is excessive fetal growth, which may result in birth trauma. **Importantly, more than half of women with gestational diabetes ultimately develop overt diabetes in the ensuing 20 years, and there is mounting evidence for long-range complications that include obesity and diabetes in their offspring.** Because of its strong link with obesity, prevention efforts are difficult.

MATERNAL AND FETAL EFFECTS. There has been an important shift in focus concerning adverse fetal consequences of gestational diabetes. Importantly, unlike in women with overt diabetes, fetal anomalies are not increased (Reece and Hobbins, 1986). Similarly, whereas pregnancies in women with overt diabetes are at greater risk for fetal death, this danger is not apparent for those with postprandial hyperglycemia only; that is, class A$_1$ (Lucas and co-workers, 1993). In contrast, gestational diabetes with elevated fasting glucose (class A₂), has been associated with unexplained stillbirth similar to overt diabetes (Johnstone and colleagues, 1990). The American Diabetes Association (1999a) has concluded that fasting hyperglycemia (> 105 mg/dL) may be associated with an increased risk of fetal death during the last 4 to 8 weeks of gestation. Adverse maternal effects include an increased frequency of hypertension and the need for cesarean delivery.

MACROSOMIA. The perinatal focal point is avoidance of difficult delivery due to macrosomia, with concomitant birth trauma due to shoulder dystocia. Except for the brain, most fetal organs are affected by macrosomia that commonly (but not always) characterizes the fetus of a diabetic woman. Modanlou and colleagues (1982) as well as McFarland and associates (2000) observed that macrosomic infants of diabetic mothers were anthropometrically different from other large-for-age infants. Specifically, those whose mothers had diabetes had excessive fat deposition on the shoulders and trunk (Fig. 51–1), predisposing these fetuses to shoulder dystocia. Similarly, Bernstein and Catalano (1994), using measurements of subscapular and triceps skinfold thickness, found that fat infants of diabetic women more often required cesarean delivery for cephalopelvic disproportion. Fortunately, shoulder dystocia is uncommon, even in women with gestational diabetes. For example, Magee and colleagues (1993) diagnosed shoulder dystocia in 3 percent of women with class A₁ diabetes. None of these infants sustained brachial plexus injuries.

Macrosomia in these infants is compatible with the long-recognized association between fetal hyperinsulinemia resulting from maternal hyperglycemia, which in turn stimulates excessive somatic growth. Similarly, neonatal hyperinsulinemia may provoke hypoglycemia within minutes of birth. The incidence varies greatly depending on the threshold used to define significant neonatal hypoglycemia. According to the American Diabetes Association (1995), values less than 35 mg/dL at term are abnormal. A lower value is considered abnormal in preterm infants, because glycogen stores have not reached term levels. Magee and co-workers (1993) reported that 4 percent of infants of women with gestational diabetes required intravenous glucose therapy for hypoglycemia.

There is extensive evidence that insulin and the insulin-like growth factors I (IGF-I) and II (IGF-II) have a role in the regulation of fetal growth (Chap. 29, p. 744). Insulin is secreted by fetal pancreatic β-cells primarily during the second half of gestation, and is believed to stimulate somatic growth and adiposity. These growth factors, which structurally are proinsulin-like polypeptides, are produced by virtually all fetal

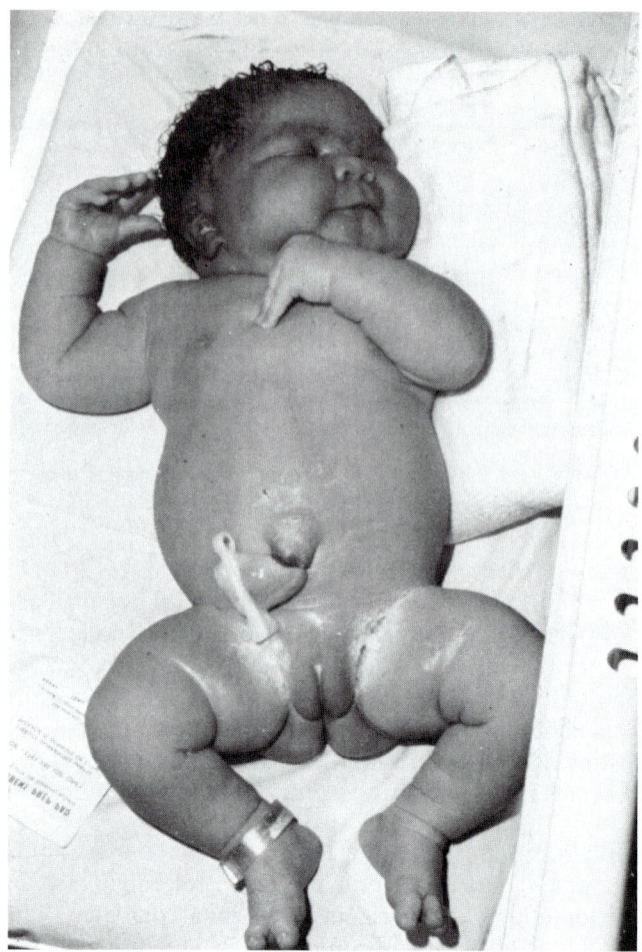

FIGURE 51–1. This macrosomic infant who weighed 6050 g was born to a woman with gestational diabetes.

organs and are potent stimulators of cell differentiation and division. Verhaeghe and co-workers (1993) measured cord serum insulin-like growth factors and insulin (C-peptide) concentrations throughout gestation in women without diabetes and found that levels correlated with birthweight. Large-for-age infants had significantly increased levels of these factors.

Maternal obesity is an independent and more important risk factor for large infants in women with gestational diabetes than is glucose intolerance (Leonardi and Bottoms, 1996; Lucas and colleagues, 1993). Moreover, maternal obesity is itself an important confounding factor in the diagnosis of gestational diabetes. Johnson and colleagues (1987) reported that 8 percent of 588 women who weighed more than 250 pounds had gestational diabetes compared with less than 1 percent of women who weighed less than 200 pounds. Landon and colleagues (1994) and Zhang and co-workers (1995) found that the risk of gestational diabetes was increased in women with truncal obesity.

MANAGEMENT. Women with gestational diabetes can be divided into two functional classes depending on their level of fasting glucose. Insulin therapy is usually recommended when standard dietary management does not consistently maintain the fasting plasma glucose at less than 105 mg/dL or the 2-hour postprandial plasma glucose at less than 120 mg/dL (American College of Obstetricians and Gynecologists, 1994). Whether insulin should be used in women with lesser degrees of fasting hyperglycemia, that is, 105 mg/dL or less, is unclear because there are no controlled trials to identify ideal glycemia targets for prevention of fetal risks. The Fourth International Workshop Conference on Gestational Diabetes (Metzger and Coustan, 1998), however, recommended that maternal capillary glucose levels be kept 95 mg/dL or less in the fasting state. The American Diabetes Association (1999) has recommended insulin therapy when nutritional management fails to maintain fasting blood glucose at or below 95 mg/dL or 2-hour postprandial blood glucose levels at or below 120 mg/dL.

DIET. Nutritional counseling is a cornerstone in management. The goals of such therapy are:

1. To provide the necessary nutrients for the mother and fetus.
2. To control glucose levels.
3. To prevent starvation ketosis.

Proposed daily caloric intakes and pregnancy weight gain for women with gestational diabetes are shown in Table 51–5. These recommendations pertain to women treated with insulin as well as dietary restrictions. Significant caloric restriction to 1200 to 1800 kcal/day has been studied in overweight women with gestational diabetes (Dornhorst and colleagues, 1991). For obese women, an intake of about 1800 kcal/day has been

shown to reduce hyperglycemia and plasma triglycerides with no increase in ketonuria (Franz and co-authors, 1994). Major and colleagues (1998) studied carbohydrate restriction in women weighing approximately 185 pounds at delivery and reported that this approach resulted in improved glucose control, less need for insulin, and a decreased incidence of macrosomia. Although maternal weight gain and fetal macrosomia may be decreased, the safety of this approach has not been established, and it is not recommended by the American College of Obstetricians and Gynecologists (1994).

EXERCISE. A liberal exercise program is encouraged. Jovanovic-Peterson and associates (1989) have shown that a program of cardiovascular-conditioning exercise improves glycemic control when compared with diet alone. Appropriate exercises are those that use the upper-body muscles or place little mechanical stress on the trunk region during exercise (Durak and co-workers, 1990). It is proposed that when the lower body is kept from an excessive weight-bearing load, the work effort can be increased safely, permitting a cardiovascular workout without fear of fetal distress. Jovanovic-Peterson and Peterson (1990) reported that such upper body cardiovascular training resulted in lower glucose levels. The effects of exercise on glucose levels only become apparent after 4 weeks of exercise.

INSULIN. Most practitioners—93 percent according to Owen and colleagues (1995)—initiate insulin therapy in women with gestational diabetes if fasting hyperglycemia greater than 105 mg/dL persists despite diet therapy. Usually, institution of insulin therapy requires hospitalization to safely titrate the dosage and educate the woman on self-administration and measurement of capillary glucose levels.

Experts differ in their approach to insulin therapy in gestational diabetes. A total dose of 20 to 30 units given once daily, before breakfast, is commonly used to initiate therapy. The total dose is usually divided into two thirds intermediate-acting insulin and a third short-acting insulin.

Once insulin therapy has been initiated, it must be recognized that the level of glycemia necessary to reduce fetal and neonatal complications of gestational diabetes has not been established. DeVeciana and colleagues (1995) randomized 66 women with fasting hyperglycemia (class A_2 gestational diabetes) and treated with insulin to glucose surveillance using either preprandial or postprandial (1-hour after each meal) capillary blood glucose concentrations measured by glucometer. Postprandial surveillance was shown to be superior to preprandial because blood glucose control was significantly improved with less neonatal hypoglycemia (3 versus 21 percent), less macrosomia (12 versus 42 percent), and

TABLE 51–5. Recommended Daily Caloric Intake and Pregnancy Weight Gain in Women with Gestational Diabetes with and without Concomitant Insulin Therapy

Current Weight in Relation to Ideal Body Weight[a]	Daily Caloric Intake (kcal/kg)[b]	Recommended Pregnancy Weight Gain (lb)
< 80–90%	36–40	28–40
80–120% (ideal)	30	25–35
120–150%	24	15–25
> 150%	12–18	15–25

[a] Ideal weight based on desirable weight before pregnancy (American Diabetes Association, 1995).
[b] Caloric intake for current pregnancy weight.
Adapted from the American College of Obstetricians and Gynecologists (1994) and the American Diabetes Association (1995).

fewer cesarean deliveries for dystocia (24 versus 39 percent). Bansal and co-authors (1996), however, have challenged these conclusions, because the women analyzed had prestudy fasting glucose values consistent with overt diabetes.

Prophylactic insulin given to decrease complications related to macrosomia in women with fasting euglycemia (class A₁) has not been proven to be beneficial. Langer and co-authors (1994) reviewed 23 reports from 1979 through 1993 and found that none demonstrated improved perinatal outcomes related to any management approach, including prophylactic insulin given to the mother. There have been only three randomized studies to date. Thompson and colleagues (1990) randomized 108 women with gestational diabetes to diet alone or diet plus insulin and showed a significant birthweight reduction in the insulin-treated group. In contrast, Nordlander and co-workers (1989) randomized 261 gestational diabetics to diet or diet plus insulin and found no neonatal benefits from insulin therapy. Garner and colleagues (1997) randomized 300 gestational diabetics to strict glucose control versus routine obstetrical care. Intensive therapy had little effect on birthweight, birth trauma, operative delivery or neonatal complications.

Langer and colleagues (1994) managed 1145 women with gestational diabetes using an "intensified" approach guided by glucometer measurements seven times each day. Goals included fasting glucose levels between 60 and 90 mg/dL and postprandial levels less than 120 mg/dL. In contrast, another 1316 women in the "conventional" management group had the same glucose control goals, but without glucometers because there were insufficient instruments available. Women in both groups underwent glucose surveillance for an average of 12 weeks and a similar number of glucose measurements were performed in each study group—approximately 350 per patient. Although mean glucose values were not different between the "intensive" and "conventional" management groups, macrosomia, cesarean delivery, and shoulder dystocia were significantly reduced in women managed intensively.

ORAL HYPOGLYCEMIC AGENTS. Oral glucose-lowering agents are not recommended during pregnancy by the American Diabetes Association (1999a). Langer and colleagues (1999) randomized 257 women with gestational diabetes to insulin or glyburide therapy. Near normoglycemic levels were achieved equally well with either insulin or glyburide. There were no apparent neonatal complications attributable to the oral hypoglycemic agent.

OBSTETRICAL MANAGEMENT. In general, women with gestational diabetes who do not require insulin

seldom require early delivery or other interventions (American College of Obstetricians and Gynecologists, 1994). There is no consensus regarding whether antepartum fetal testing is necessary, and if so, when to begin such testing in women without severe hyperglycemia (Metzger and Coustan, 1998). This is based on the low risk of fetal death. Elective induction, compared with spontaneous labor, is controversial in women with sonographic diagnosis of fetal macrosomia to prevent shoulder dystocia. Conway and Langer (1996) found that elective delivery reduced the rate of shoulder dystocia from 2.2 to 0.7 percent. In contrast, Combs and colleagues (1993b) and Adasheck and associates (1996) found no advantages. Women who require insulin therapy for fasting hyperglycemia, however, typically receive fetal testing and are managed as if they had overt diabetes.

POSTPARTUM CONSEQUENCES. The Fourth Workshop-Conference recommended that women diagnosed to have gestational diabetes undergo evaluation with a 75-g oral glucose tolerance test at 6 to 12 weeks after delivery. The criteria for interpretation of this test are shown in Table 51–6. Women whose 75-g test is normal should be reassessed at a minimum of 3-year intervals (American Diabetes Association, 1999b). Although postpartum follow-up of women diagnosed to have gestational diabetes has been recommended throughout the 1990s, reports on compliance have only recently become available. Kaufmann and colleagues (1999) measured physician and patient compliance rates during a 5-year postpartum follow-up period in 66 women with gestational diabetes. Compliance was poor and only 30 percent of the women reported receiving a yearly 2-hour glucose tolerance test although the risk of developing diabetes was 60 percent in others tested on an annual basis.

These recommendations for postpartum follow-up are based on the 50-percent likelihood of women with gestational diabetes developing overt diabetes within 20 years of delivery (O'Sullivan, 1982). If fasting hyperglycemia develops during pregnancy, diabetes is more likely to persist postpartum. For example, in women with fasting glucose levels of 105 to 130 mg/mL, 43 percent were found to be overtly diabetic (Metzger and colleagues, 1985). When fasting glucose exceeded 130 mg/dL during pregnancy, 86 percent of women became overtly diabetic. Similarly, Dacus and co-workers (1994) and Greenberg and colleagues (1995) have also concluded that insulin therapy during pregnancy, and especially before 24 weeks, is a powerful predictor of diabetes after the pregnancy.

Women with gestational diabetes are at risk not only for postpartum development of type 2 diabetes, but also for cardiovascular complications associated with

TABLE 51-6. Postpartum Evaluation for Glucose Intolerance in Women with Gestational Diabetes

Time Tested	2-hr, 75-g Oral Glucose Tolerance Test Plasma Glucose (mg/dL)		
	No Diabetes	Impaired Glucose Tolerance	Diabetes
Fasting	< 115	< 140	≥ 140[a]
½, 1, 1½ hr	All < 200	1 value ≥ 200	1 value ≥ 200
2 hr	< 140	140-199	≥ 200

[a] Fasting plasma glucose determination of ≥ 140 on two occasions establish the diagnosis.
From the American College of Obstetricians and Gynecologists (1994), with permission.

abnormal serum lipids, and hypertension and abdominal obesity. Pallardo and colleagues (1999) evaluated cardiovascular disease risk factors in 788 women with gestational diabetes 3 to 6 months postpartum. The degree of postpartum glucose intolerance was significantly associated with obesity, plasma triglyceride levels, and hypertension. These results imply that identification of women with gestational diabetes also identifies those with risk factors for cardiovascular disease.

Recurrence of gestational diabetes in subsequent pregnancies was documented in 20 of 30 women reported by Philipson and Super (1989). Obese women were more likely to have impaired glucose intolerance in subsequent pregnancies. Thus, lifestyle behavioral changes, including weight control and exercise between pregnancies, could be a valuable strategy to prevent recurrence of gestational diabetes as well as type 2 diabetes later in life (Pan, 1997). Interestingly, perinatal outcomes in women with previous gestational diabetes but with normal glucose tolerance tests during a subsequent pregnancy were not improved with regard to birthweight, macrosomia, route of delivery, and neonatal complications (Danilenko-Dixon and colleagues, 2000).

Low-dose oral contraceptives may be used safely by women with recent gestational diabetes (Chap. 58, p. 1526). The rate of subsequent diabetes in oral contraceptive users is not significantly different than in those who did not use hormonal contraception (Kjos and colleagues, 1990a).

GESTATIONAL DIABETES AT PARKLAND HOSPITAL. Universal glucose screening was not performed at Parkland until recently. Selective screening was instead based on many of the risk factors previously enumerated. A standard 50-g oral glucose tolerance test was performed between 24 and 28 weeks without regard to recent meal status. The National Diabetes Data Group

(1979) criteria shown in Table 51-4 were used. Women diagnosed to have class A₁ gestational diabetes were seen weekly in a specific clinic designed to provide dietary counseling. Fasting plasma glucose measurements were obtained at each visit. Women without other complications such as hypertension or postterm gestation were permitted to enter spontaneous labor and antepartum testing was not used. Women diagnosed to have class A₂ gestational diabetes were managed as overt diabetics, as described later.

Beginning January 1997, universal screening for gestational diabetes was performed between 24 and 28 weeks using a standard 1-hour, 50-g oral glucose challenge test. All obstetrical management practices previously used during selective screening were continued during universal screening. The practice of universal screening doubled the number of women tested in one year from approximately 4300 to 8200 women. Despite this, the number of women actually diagnosed with gestational diabetes remained unchanged at approximately 225 per year. Importantly, universal screening for gestational diabetes did not increase or decrease obstetrical outcomes attributable to this diagnosis (Casey and colleagues, 1999).

OVERT DIABETES

Unlike gestational diabetes, it is unquestioned that overt diabetes has a significant impact on pregnancy outcome. Even the embryo, as well as the fetus and the mother, can experience serious complications directly attributable to diabetes. The likelihood of successful outcomes for the fetus-infant and the overtly diabetic mother are related somewhat to the degree of diabetes control, but more importantly, to the intensity of any underlying maternal cardiovascular or renal disease. Therefore, as the alphabetic classification shown in Table 51-2 ad-

TABLE 51–7. Outcomes in Percent of Pregnancies Complicated by Type 1 Diabetes Compared with National Data in Sweden, 1983–1985

Factor	Type 1 Diabetes (n = 491)	National Data (n = 279,000)	P value
Preeclampsia	21	5	< .001
Preterm birth	25	6	< .001
Macrosomia	20	4	< .001
Growth restriction	1	3	< .05
Stillbirths	2	0.4	< .01
Perinatal mortality	3	0.7	< .0001

Adapted from Hanson and Persson (1993), with permission.

vances, the likelihood of a good pregnancy outcome lessens.

Hanson and Persson (1993) prospectively chronicled the effects of overt diabetes on pregnancy outcomes in Sweden. Their unique analysis included all deliveries between 1983 and 1985, during which period 491 insulin-dependent women in classes B or more advanced were identified. Their outcomes were compared with 279,000 pregnancies in nondiabetic women and are shown in Table 51–7. Women with diabetic pregnancies experience significantly increased adverse pregnancy outcomes. As shown in Table 51–8, Swedish women in the more advanced classes of overt diabetes increasingly developed preeclampsia. This complication occurred in 54 percent of women with diabetic nephropathy (class F). Similarly, Sibai and colleagues (2000) reported the risk of preeclampsia to be 11 percent in class B, 22 percent in class C, 21 percent in class D, and 36 percent in classes F-R.

FETAL EFFECTS. Improved fetal surveillance, neonatal intensive care, and maternal metabolic control have reduced perinatal losses with overt diabetes to 2 to 4

TABLE 51–8. Frequency of Preeclampsia in Pregnancies Complicated by Type 1 Diabetes—Sweden, 1983–1985

White Classification	Pregnancies (%)	Preeclampsia (%)
B	164 (33)	12
C	129 (26)	22
D	172 (35)	23
F	26 (5)	54
Total	491 (100)	21

From Hanson and Persson (1993), with permission.

percent. These rates have seemingly plateaued because the two major causes of fetal death—congenital malformations and "unexplained" fetal death—remain unchanged by medical intervention (Garner, 1995a).

ABORTION. Several studies have shown that spontaneous abortion is associated with poor glycemic control during the first trimester (Greene and colleagues, 1989; Mills and associates, 1988b). Rosenn and colleagues (1994) enrolled 215 women with type 1 diabetes for prenatal care before 9 weeks, and 24 percent experienced spontaneous abortions. Only those type 1 diabetic women with initial glycohemoglobin A_1 concentrations above 12 percent or persistent preprandial glucose concentrations above 120 mg/dL were at increased risk for abortion.

PRETERM DELIVERY. Overt diabetes antedating pregnancy is a risk factor for preterm birth. Sibai and co-workers (2000) from the Maternal–Fetal Medicine Units Network of the National Institute of Child Health and Development analyzed pregnancy outcomes in 461 women with pregestational diabetes and found that 9 percent of these women spontaneously delivered at 34 weeks or less compared with 4.5 percent of nondiabetic women. Moreover, 7 percent of diabetic women compared with 2 percent of normal women underwent indicated preterm delivery.

MALFORMATIONS. The incidence of major malformations in women with type 1 diabetes is 5 to 10 percent (Rosenn and co-workers, 1994). These account for almost half of perinatal deaths in diabetic pregnancies. Specific types of anomalies linked to maternal diabetes and their relative incidence are summarized in Table 51–9. Diabetes is not associated with increased risk for fetal chromosomal abnormalities (Henriques and colleagues, 1991).

TABLE 51–9. Congenital Malformations in Infants of Women with Overt Diabetes

Anomaly	Ratios of Incidence[a]
Caudal regression	252
Situs inversus	84
Spina bifida, hydrocephaly, or other central nervous system defect	2
Anencephaly	3
Heart anomalies	4
Anal/rectal atresia	3
Renal anomalies	5
Agenesis	4
Cystic kidney	4
Duplex ureter	23

[a] Ratio of incidence is in comparison with the general population. Heart anomalies include transposition of the great vessels, ventricular septal defect, and atrial septal defect.
Adapted from Mills and colleagues (1979) and the American Diabetes Association (1995), with permission.

It is generally believed that increased severe malformations are the consequence of poorly controlled diabetes both preconceptionally as well as early in pregnancy (see Chaps. 9 and 36). The retrospective study of Miller and co-workers (1981) suggested that women with lower glycosylated hemoglobin values at conception had fewer anomalous fetuses compared with women with abnormally high values. Lucas and colleagues (1989) found that fetal anomalies correlated with high levels of glycosylated hemoglobin as well as diabetic vasculopathy and with duration of disease greater than 10 years. Data from Mills and colleagues (1988a) from the Diabetes in Early Pregnancy Study did not totally corroborate these findings. This investigation enrolled over 600 diabetic women, and it was concluded that a normal glycosylated hemoglobin did not guarantee that diabetes-associated anomalies would be avoided. Conversely, an elevated level did not necessarily indicate an increased risk. Despite this, these investigators observed that women in whom periconceptional glucose control was optimized had 5 percent fetal malformations compared with 9 percent in the group who did not present for care until after organogenesis was complete.

Schaefer-Graf and associates (2000) analyzed the pattern of congenital anomalies in pregnancies complicated by pregestational as well as gestational diabetes. The initial fasting glucose level was significantly higher in pregnancies with fetal malformations. Moreover, those with multiple organ system fetal anomalies had significantly higher initial fasting glucose levels (166 ± 64 mg/dL) compared with pregnancies in which only a single organ system was affected (141 ± 55 mg/dL) or with those with no anomalies (115 ± 38 mg/dL). The most common single-organ system anomalies were cardiac (38 percent), musculoskeletal (15 percent), and central nervous system (10 percent). The frequency of these specific organ system malformations was unrelated to the degree of glycemia.

Kitzmiller and associates (1991) tested the effectiveness of intensive periconceptional glycemic management by comparing pregnancy outcomes in 84 women with well-controlled diabetes before conception with 110 diabetics who presented for care between 6 and 30 weeks. Only 1.2 percent of the preconceptionally controlled women had a fetus with a major anomaly compared with 11 percent of those who enrolled late.

ANIMAL STUDIES. Many investigators are conducting animal experiments to elucidate molecular mechanisms by which diabetes and/or hyperglycemia during embryogenesis induces fetal malformations. Sivan and colleagues (1996) and Wiznitzer and associates (1996) have found that the antioxidants vitamin E and lipoic acid, when given to pregnant diabetic rats, prevent fetal malformations. They hypothesize that hyperglycemia induces oxidative free-radical molecules that are embryotoxic and that antioxidants inhibit this process. Alternatively, Reece and colleagues (1996) demonstrated that hyperglycemia induces reduced specific gene activity, producing a state of arachidonic acid deficiency causally related to the development of neural-tube defects in rats.

"UNEXPLAINED" FETAL DEMISE. Stillbirths without identifiable cause are a phenomenon peculiar to pregnancies complicated by overt diabetes. They are declared "unexplained" because no factors such as obvious placental insufficiency, abruption, fetal growth restriction, or oligohydramnios are apparent. These infants are typically large for age and die before labor, usually at about 35 weeks or later (Garner, 1995b). The incidence of unexplained stillbirths in the Swedish study shown in Table 51–7 was 1 percent.

Recent investigations using cordocentesis have provided new insights into acid–base metabolism in fetuses of diabetic mothers. Salvesen and colleagues (1992, 1993) reported decreased fetal pH, and increased P_{CO_2}, lactate, and erythropoietin in diabetic pregnancies. Such findings lend credence to the long-held hypothesis that hyperglycemia-mediated chronic aberrations in transport of oxygen and fetal metabolites may account for these unexplained fetal deaths (Pedersen, 1977).

Between 1984 and 1993, Richey and co-workers (1995) were at the bedside in two pregnancies at Parkland Hospital where "unexplained" fetal deaths were seemingly in progress. In both of these rare clinical instances, the fetus was macrosomic and there was excessive amnionic fluid. Both fetuses were acidemic before labor and both placentae were hydropic due to edema of the chorionic villi. These features were linked to maternal hyperglycemia, and it was hypothesized that osmotically induced villous edema led to impaired fetal oxygen transport.

Explicable stillbirths due to placental insufficiency also occur with increased frequency in women with overt diabetes, usually in association with severe preeclampsia. This, in turn, is increased in women with advanced diabetes and vascular complications. Similarly, ketoacidosis can cause fetal death.

HYDRAMNIOS. Although diabetic pregnancies are often complicated by hydramnios, the cause is unclear. A likely, although unproven explanation is fetal polyuria resulting from fetal hyperglycemia (Chap. 31, p. 819). Dashe and co-authors (2000), in a study performed at Parkland Hospital, found that the amnionic fluid index parallels the amnionic fluid glucose level among women with diabetes. This finding suggests that the hydramnios associated with diabetes is a result of increased amnionic fluid glucose concentration.

NEONATAL EFFECTS. Before tests of fetal health and maturity became available, preterm delivery was deliberately effected to avoid unexplained fetal deaths. Although this practice has been abandoned, there is still an increased frequency of preterm delivery in women with diabetes. As shown in Table 51–7, Hanson and Persson (1993) reported that 25 percent of Swedish women with classes B to F diabetes were delivered at 36 weeks or less. Most preterm births are associated with advanced diabetes and superimposed preeclampsia.

Modern neonatal care has largely eliminated neonatal deaths due to immaturity. Cnattingius and colleagues (1994) reported only one infant death due to immaturity in 914 singleton births to B to F diabetic women. However, neonatal *morbidity* due to preterm birth continues to be a serious consequence. Indeed, some of the morbidities in these infants of diabetic women are considered to be uniquely related to aberrations in maternal glucose metabolism.

RESPIRATORY DISTRESS. Conventional obstetrical teaching, at least until the late 1980s, generally held that fetal lung maturation was delayed in diabetic pregnancies, thus placing these infants at increased risk for respiratory distress (Gluck and Kulovich, 1973). Subsequent observations have challenged the concept of diabetes-altered fetal lung function. Gestational age, rather than overt diabetes, is likely the most significant factor governing the development of respiratory distress (Berko-

witz and colleagues, 1996; Fadel and associates, 1988; Kjos and colleagues, 1990b).

HYPOGLYCEMIA. A rapid decrease in plasma glucose concentration after delivery is characteristic of the infant of a diabetic mother. This is attributed to hyperplasia of the fetal β-islet cells induced by chronic maternal hyperglycemia. Prompt recognition and treatment of the hypoglycemic infant has minimized sequelae.

HYPOCALCEMIA. Defined as serum calcium less than 7 mg/dL, hypocalcemia is one of the major metabolic derangements in infants of diabetic mothers. Its cause has not been explained. Theories include aberrations in magnesium–calcium economy unique to diabetic pregnancy, asphyxia, and preterm birth (Cruikshank and co-workers, 1980). DeMarini and colleagues (1994) randomized 137 pregnant women with insulin-dependent diabetes to strict glucose control versus customary control to test the effect of maternal glucose levels on neonatal hypocalcemia. Almost a third of infants in the customary control group developed hypocalcemia whereas this developed in only 18 percent of infants in the strict glucose control group. Gestational age and preeclampsia were also implicated.

HYPERBILIRUBINEMIA. The pathogenesis of hyperbilirubinemia in infants of diabetic mothers is uncertain. Factors implicated have included preterm birth and polycythemia with hemolysis. Venous hematocrits of 65 to 70 vol percent have been observed in as many as 40 percent of these infants (Salvesen and associates, 1992). Renal vein thrombosis has also been reported to result from polycythemia.

CARDIAC HYPERTROPHY. Infants of diabetic pregnancies may have hypertrophic cardiomyopathy that occasionally progresses to congestive heart failure (Gandhi and co-authors, 1995; Reller and Kaplan, 1988). These infants are typically macrosomic and fetal hyperinsulinemia has been implicated in the pathogenesis of heart disease. Way (1979) reported that the cardiomyopathy in infants of diabetic mothers generally disappears by 6 months of age.

LONG-TERM COGNITIVE DEVELOPMENT. Rizzo and colleagues (1995) used multiple tests of intelligence and psychomotor development to assess 196 children of diabetic women up to 9 years of age. They concluded that maternal diabetes had a negligible impact on cognitive development.

INHERITANCE OF DIABETES. Offspring of women with overt diabetes have a low risk of developing insulin-dependent diabetes, with surveys suggesting an incidence of 1 to 3 percent (Garner, 1995a). The risk is 6 percent if only the father has overt diabetes. If both parents have type 1 diabetes, the risk is 20 percent. McKinney and colleagues (1999) studied 196 children with insulin-dependent diabetes and found older maternal age and maternal type 1 diabetes to be important risk factors.

ALTERED FETAL GROWTH. The incidence of macrosomia rises significantly when mean maternal blood glucose concentrations exceed 130 mg/dL (Willman and co-authors, 1986). Some authors have objected to classification of these infants as either "macrosomic" or "non-macrosomic," because this ignores the observation that virtually all are *growth promoted* (Bradley and associates, 1988). This is discussed in Chapter 29 (p. 744). As shown in Figure 51–2, the birthweight distribution of infants of diabetic mothers is skewed toward consistently heavier birthweights compared with normal pregnancies.

When in gestation macrosomia commences is of some interest. Landon and co-workers (1989) performed serial ultrasound examinations during the third trimester in 79 women with diabetes and observed that excessive fetal abdominal circumference growth was detectable by 32 weeks (Fig. 51–3), suggesting that excessive weight accrues primarily during the third trimester. Keller and colleagues (1990), however, reported that some macrosomic fetuses can be recognized before 24 weeks. Similarly, Rey and co-authors (1999) and Raychaudhuri and Maresh (2000) concluded that macrosomia was determined primarily by early pregnancy diabetes control.

MATERNAL EFFECTS. Diabetes and pregnancy interact significantly such that maternal welfare can be seriously jeopardized. With the possible exception of diabetic retinopathy, however, the long-term course of diabetes is not affected by pregnancy.

Maternal deaths have become rare in women with diabetes, although as emphasized by Cousins (1987), mortality is increased 10-fold, most often as a result of ketoacidosis, underlying hypertension, preeclampsia, and pyelonephritis. The rare woman with coronary artery disease (class H) is at particular risk of dying as a result of pregnancy (Chap. 44, p. 1202). Pombar and colleagues (1995) reviewed 17 women with class H diabetes and only half survived pregnancy.

DIABETIC NEPHROPATHY. As discussed in Chapter 47 (p. 1263), diabetic nephropathy is the leading cause of end-stage renal disease in the United States (American Diabetes Association, 1999b). The incidence of renal failure is nearly 30 percent with type 1 diabetes, and ranges from 4 to 20 percent in those with type 2 disease. Importantly, the incidence of nephropathy in individuals with type 1 disease declined during the 1980s, probably as a result of improved glucose control (Bojestig and colleagues, 1994). Indeed, Krolewski and associates (1995) have identified that subclinical diabetic nephropathy increases abruptly when hemoglobin A_1 values exceed 10 percent. The natural history of clinically detectable nephropathy in type 1 disease begins with microalbuminuria—30 to 300 mg of albumin per 24 hours. This may manifest as early as 5 years after the onset of diabetes (Nathan, 1993). After another 5 to 10

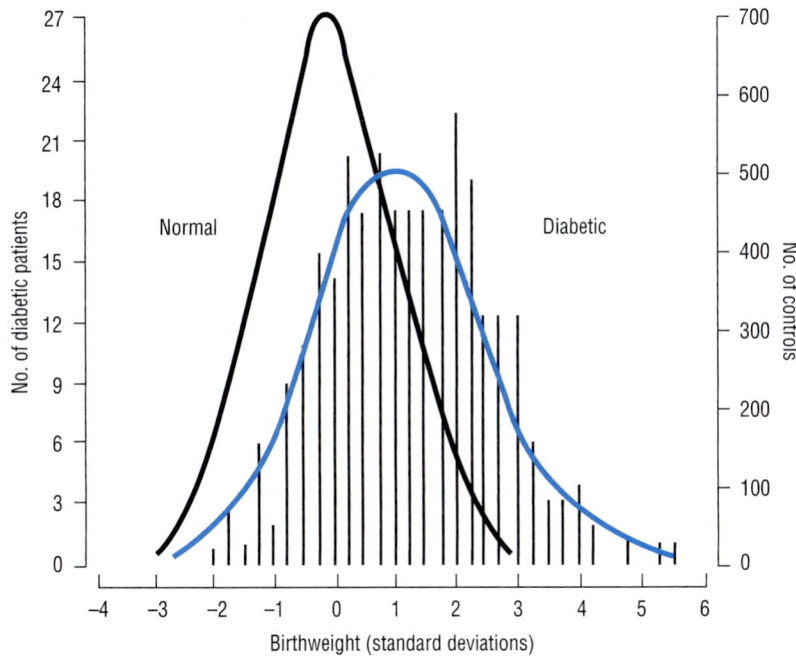

Figure 51–2. Distribution of birthweights (standard deviation from the normal mean for gestational age) for 280 infants of diabetic mothers and 3959 infants of normal mothers. (From Bradley and co-workers, 1988, with permission.)

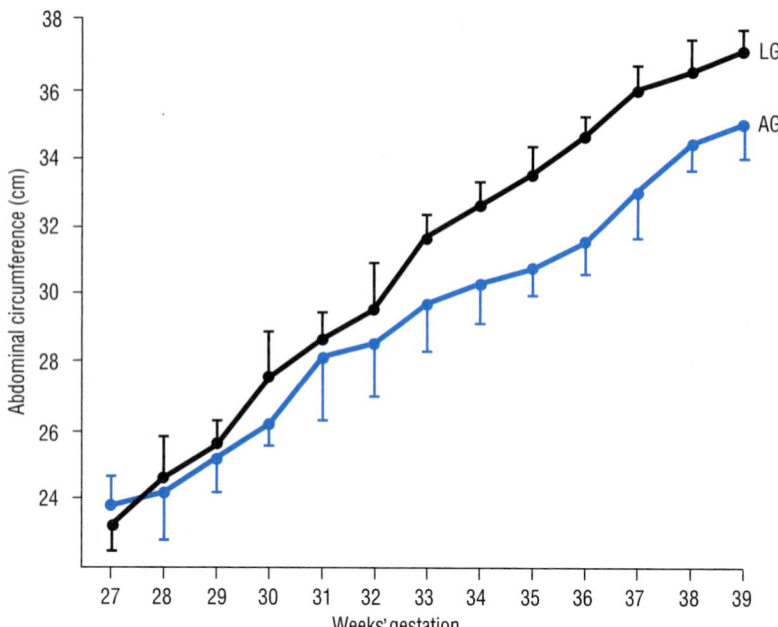

FIGURE 51–3. Comparison of abdominal circumference growth curve for appropriate-for-gestational age (AGA) and large-for-gestational age (LGA) fetuses of diabetic mothers. Growth is accelerated at 32 weeks in the LGA group. (From Landon and co-workers, 1989, with permission.)

years, overt proteinuria—more than 300 mg of albumin per 24 hours—develops in patients destined to have end-stage renal disease. Hypertension invariably develops during this period, and renal failure ensues typically in the next 5 to 10 years.

The incidence of class F diabetes in recent large reports is approximately 5 percent (Hanson and Persson, 1993; Siddiqi and associates, 1991). With nephropathy, preeclampsia and indicated preterm delivery increase substantially. As shown in Table 51–8, approximately half of women in class F develop preeclampsia. Combs and associates (1993a) measured urinary protein excretion before 20 weeks in 311 diabetic women and preeclampsia developed in 38 percent with proteinuria exceeding 500 mg/day. Women with microproteinuria—defined as 190 to 500 mg/day—also had an increased risk of preeclampsia. Conversely, How and colleagues (2000) in an analysis of 460 women with classes B through F-R diabetes, did not find an increased rate of preeclampsia in women with 30 to 500 mg of proteinuria per day. Chronic hypertension with diabetic nephropathy increased the risk of preeclampsia to 60 percent. Gordon and associates (1996) have reported 100 percent perinatal survival in 46 pregnancies complicated by class F diabetes. Plasma creatinine values of 1.5 mg/dL or greater and protein excretion of 3 g per 24 hours or greater before 20 weeks were predictive for preeclampsia.

Chaturvedi and associates (1995) studied the relationship between pregnancy and long-term maternal complications in 1358 European women with type 1 diabetes, of whom 582 had been pregnant. The incidence of either microalbuminuria or macroalbuminuria was not increased in women with prior pregnancies compared with nulliparas. They concluded that pregnancy did not exacerbate or modify diabetic nephropathy. Miodovnik and colleagues (1996) found that a fourth of 46 class F diabetic women developed end-stage renal failure at a mean of 6 years after pregnancy.

DIABETIC RETINOPATHY. Retinal vascular disease is a highly specific complication of both type 1 and type 2 diabetes. The prevalence of retinopathy is related to duration of diabetes. After 20 years of diabetes, nearly all patients with type 1 diabetes have some degree of retinopathy and more than 60 percent of patients with type 2 diabetes have some degree of retinopathy (American Diabetes Association, 1999b). Diabetic retinopathy is now the most important cause of visual impairment in the United States in persons under 60 years of age (Clark and Lee, 1995).

The first and most common visible lesions are small microaneurysms followed by blot hemorrhages when erythrocytes escape from the aneurysms. These areas leak serous fluid that forms hard exudates. These features are termed *benign* or *background* or *nonproliferative retinopathy*. These findings would place a pregnant woman into class D (Table 51–2) regardless of the duration of diabetes. With increasingly severe retinopathy, the abnormal vessels of background eye disease become occluded, leading to retinal ischemia with infarctions that appear as *cotton wool exudates*. These are considered *preproliferative retinopathy*. In response to ischemia, there is neovascularization on the retinal surface (Fig. 51–4A) and out into the vitreous cavity, and these obscure vision when there is hemorrhage. Laser photo-

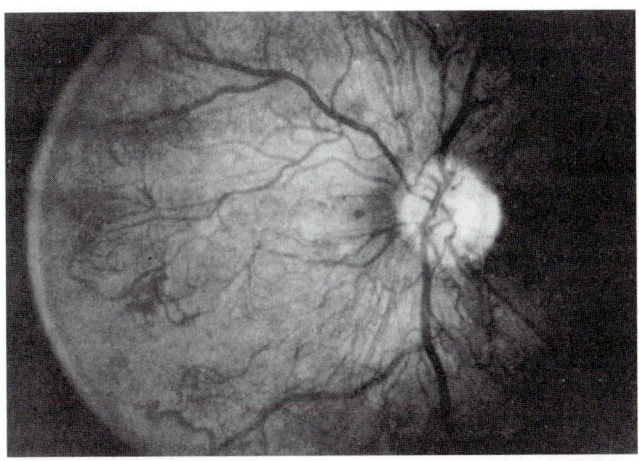

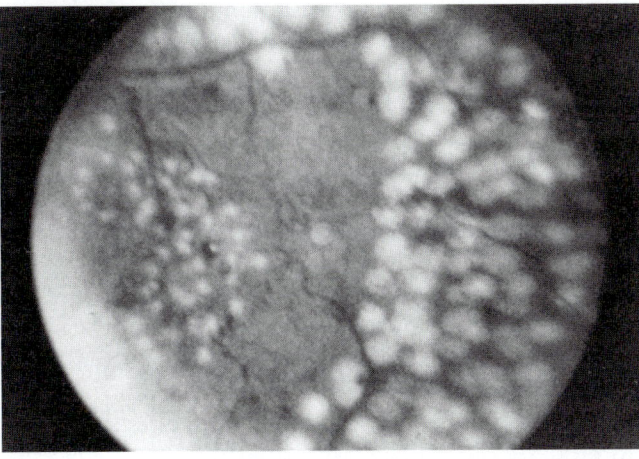

FIGURE 51–4. Retinal photographs from a 30-year-old diabetic woman. **A.** Optic nerve head showing severe proliferative retinopathy characterized by extensive networks of new vessels surrounding the optic disc. **B.** A portion of the acute photocoagulation full "scatter" pattern following argon laser treatment. (From Elman and colleagues, 1990, with permission.)

coagulation (Fig. 51–4B) before these vessels hemorrhage reduces by half the rate of progression of visual loss and blindness and is indicated during pregnancy for affected women. Siddiqi and colleagues (1991) reported that almost a third of 175 insulin-dependent pregnant women examined by 10 weeks had background retinal changes (class D) or proliferative retinopathy (class R). Puza and Malee (1996) reviewed routine ophthalmological surveillance during pregnancy.

There is continuing debate about the effect of pregnancy on proliferative retinopathy (Garner, 1995a). This complication is the one exception in which pregnancy is thought to possibly exert a detrimental effect on the long-term outcome of diabetes. Klein and co-workers (1990) concluded that pregnancy worsened proliferative

retinopathy, but Chaturvedi and co-authors (1995) found equivalent prevalence of both background and proliferative retinopathy in women with prior pregnancies compared with nulliparous women. Most authors agree that laser photocoagulation and good glycemic control during pregnancy minimize the potential for deleterious effects of pregnancy (Garner, 1995a). There are case reports that link sudden institution of rigorous metabolic control during pregnancy to acute worsening of retinopathy (Dahl-Jørgensen and colleagues, 1985; Van Ballegooie and associates, 1984). Wang and co-workers (1993) have observed that although retinopathy worsened during the critical months of rigorous glucose control, in the longer term, the rate of deterioration of eye disease was slowed. Lauszus and colleagues (1998) reported that proliferative retinopathy, in the absence of nephropathy, did not endanger the fetus or newborn infant. In contrast, McElvy and colleagues (2000) found that a fourth of 253 women with retinopathy at the beginning of their pregnancies suffered progression of eye disease during pregnancy despite intensive glucose control. Moreover, progression of retinopathy was associated with reduced fetal weight.

In a preliminary report, Kitzmiller and colleagues (1999) implicated insulin lispro in the development of proliferative retinopathy during pregnancy. Conversely, Buchbinder and associates (2000), in a study of 13 pregnant women treated with insulin lispro, found no evidence that such therapy was linked to the development or progression of diabetic retinopathy.

DIABETIC NEUROPATHY. Although uncommon, some pregnant women will demonstrate peripheral symmetrical sensorimotor neuropathy due to diabetes. Another form, **diabetic gastropathy,** is very troublesome in pregnancy because it causes nausea and vomiting, nutritional problems, and difficulty with glucose control. Treatment with metoclopramide and H_2-receptor antagonists is sometimes successful.

PREECLAMPSIA. Hypertension induced or exacerbated by pregnancy is the major complication that most often forces preterm delivery in diabetic women. According to Garner (1995a), the perinatal mortality rate is increased 20-fold for preeclamptic diabetic women compared with those who are normotensive. Especial risk factors for preeclampsia include any vascular complications, preexisting proteinuria, and/or chronic hypertension. Interestingly, the occurrence of preeclampsia does not seem to be related to glucose control (Garner and co-authors, 1990). Preeclampsia is discussed in Chapter 24.

KETOACIDOSIS. Although ketoacidosis affects only about 1 percent of diabetic pregnancies, it remains one of the most serious complications (Garner, 1995a). Diabetic ketoacidosis may occur as a result of hyperemesis gravidarum, use of β-sympathomimetic drugs for tocolysis, infections, and use of corticosteroids to induce fetal lung maturation. Fetal loss is about 20 percent with ketoacidosis.

Kent and colleagues (1994) found that only half of young women with recurrent ketoacidosis had successful pregnancies compared with 95 percent of women without ketoacidosis. A prominent factor implicated in recurrent ketoacidosis was noncompliance. Indeed, ketoacidosis and poor patient compliance have long been considered prognostically bad signs in pregnancy (Pedersen and colleagues, 1974).

INFECTIONS. According to Stamler and co-authors (1990), approximately 80 percent of insulin-dependent diabetics develop at least one episode of infection during pregnancy compared with 25 percent in nondiabetic women. Common infections include candida vulvovaginitis, urinary infections, puerperal pelvic infections, and respiratory tract infections. Cousins (1987) observed that antepartum pyelonephritis developed in 4 percent of women with type 1 diabetes compared with 1 percent in nondiabetics. They also reported that renal infection was associated with increased preterm delivery. Fortunately, these latter infections can be minimized by screening for asymptomatic bacteriuria (Chap. 47, p. 1253).

MANAGEMENT. The goals of management are tailored somewhat uniquely for pregnant women. Management preferably should begin before pregnancy and include specific goals during each trimester.

PRECONCEPTION. To prevent early pregnancy loss as well as congenital malformations in infants of diabetic mothers, optimal medical care and patient education are recommended before conception (American Diabetes Association, 1999a). This is also discussed in Chapter 9. Unfortunately, unplanned pregnancies, thus preempting preconceptional care, continue to occur in approximately 60 percent of women with diabetes (Holing and co-authors, 1998). Thus, diabetic women begin pregnancy with suboptimal glucose control (Casele and Laifer, 1998). The American Diabetes Association (1999a) has defined optimal preconceptional glucose control using insulin to include self-monitored preprandial glucose levels of 70 to 100 mg/dL and postprandial values of less than 140 mg/dL and less than 120 mg/dL at 1 and 2 hours, respectively. Hemoglobin A_1 or A_{1c} measurement, which expresses an average of circulating glucose for the past 4 to 8 weeks, is useful to assess early metabolic control. Optimal preconceptional glycated hemoglobin values have been defined as those within or near the upper limit of normal for a specific

laboratory or within three standard deviations of the normal mean (American Diabetes Association, 1999a). The most significant risk for malformations is with levels exceeding 10 percent (American College of Obstetricians and Gynecologists, 1994). Folate, 400 μg/day, given periconceptually and during early pregnancy, decreases the risk of neural-tube defects (Milunsky and co-workers, 1989).

FIRST TRIMESTER. Careful monitoring of glucose control is essential to management. For this reason, many clinicians hospitalize these women during early pregnancy to institute an individualized glucose control program and to provide education concerning the ensuing months of pregnancy. It also provides an opportunity to assess the extent of vascular complications of diabetes and to precisely establish gestational age.

Maternal glycemic control can usually be achieved with **multiple daily insulin injections** and adjustment of dietary intake. Oral hypoglycemic agents are not used because they may cause fetal hyperinsulinemia. Piacquadio and colleagues (1991) demonstrated increased rates of congenital malformations in infants of Mexican-American women treated during early pregnancy with oral hypoglycemic drugs.

Subcutaneous insulin infusion by a calibrated pump may be used during pregnancy. The pump has both advantages and disadvantages, and as emphasized by Kitzmiller and associates (1985) and Leveno and colleagues (1988), any salutary pregnancy effects have yet to be determined. The risk of nocturnal hypoglycemia is increased during pregnancy and, therefore, great care should be taken in selecting patients for this therapy (American College of Obstetricians and Gynecologists, 1994).

The goals of self-monitored capillary blood glucose control recommended during pregnancy are shown in Table 51–10. Self-monitoring of capillary glucose levels using glucometers is strongly recommended as this involves the woman in her own care. Campbell and co-workers (1994) measured maternal glucose responses to standardized meals throughout normal pregnancies to better characterize plasma glucose goals for manage-

TABLE 51–10. Patient-monitored Capillary Blood Glucose Goals During Pregnancy in Diabetic Women

Specimen	Blood Glucose (mg/dL)
Fasting	60–90 (3.3–5.0 mmol)
Premeal	60–105 (3.3–5.8 mmol)
Postprandial 1 hr	100–120 (5.5–6.7 mmol)
0200–0600	60–120 (3.3–6.7 mmol)

Adapted from the American Diabetes Association (1995).

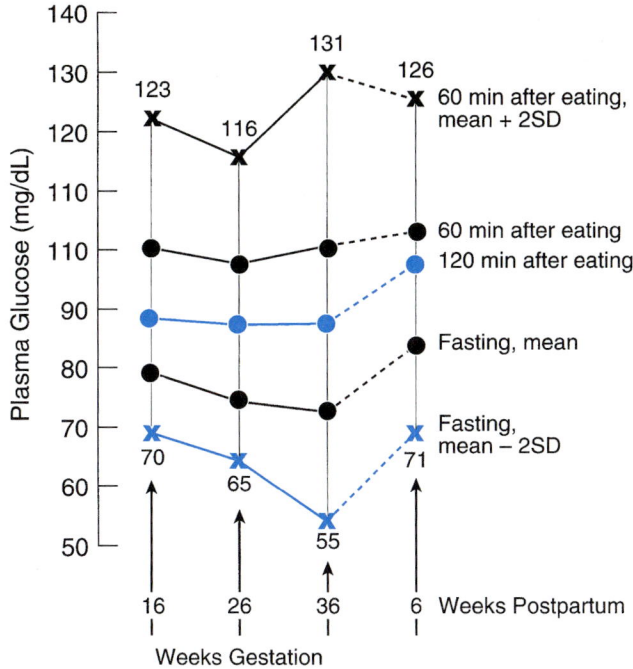

FIGURE 51–5. Maternal glucose response to a standardized meal throughout normal pregnancy in 45 healthy primiparous women. (Adapted from Campbell and co-workers, 1994.)

ment of diabetic women (Fig. 51–5). These results correspond remarkably to the recommendations shown in Table 51–10.

New technology is under development that offers the future possibility of noninvasive glucose monitoring. Such an automatic and painless means to obtain blood glucose information would undoubtedly greatly facilitate patient compliance with glucose control during pregnancy. Tamada and colleagues (1999) reported clinical results with such a monitoring device (Cygnus, Inc., Redwood City, California). The device extracts glucose through the skin using electrical potentials—a process known as iontophoresis. It then measures glucose concentrations in the extracted sample. The device provides up to three glucose readings per hour and causes only transient mild skin irritation at the sensor site. Tamada and colleagues (1999) found close agreement between these noninvasive glucose measurements and those obtained using repeated fingersticks to obtain blood samples.

The Committee on Maternal Nutrition of the National Research Council has recommended a total caloric intake of 30 to 35 kcal/kg of ideal body weight, given as three meals and three snacks daily (Garner, 1995a). An ideal dietary composition is 55 percent carbohydrate, 20 percent protein, and 25 percent fat with less than 10 percent saturated fat. There are no studies to support or refute these guidelines. Obese women may

be managed with lower caloric intake as long as weight loss and ketonuria are avoided.

Although achieving euglycemia based on normal pregnancy blood glucose values is the goal in management of overtly diabetic women, achieving this goal is not always possible. Thus, individualized programs are often necessary to avoid both excessive hyperglycemia as well as frequent episodes of hypoglycemia. Diabetes tends to be unstable in the first trimester, followed by a stable period, and then by an increase in insulin requirement from about 24 weeks (Steel and co-workers, 1994). This rise is due to the increased production of pregnancy hormones, which are insulin-antagonists (Chap. 6, p. 113 and Chap. 8, p. 174). The absolute increase in mean insulin requirement was 52 units in 237 women with type 1 diabetes, but there was wide variation (Steel and associates, 1994). The magnitude of increase was directly related to maternal weight and inversely related to diabetes duration.

Rosenn and colleagues (1995) assessed the impact of maternal hypoglycemia in 84 pregnant women with overt diabetes. Clinically significant hypoglycemia with glucometer values less than 35 mg/dL were documented in 70 percent of the women with a peak incidence between 10 and 15 weeks. Almost a fourth of these 84 women experienced unconsciousness and 15 percent developed seizures as a result of hypoglycemia. These investigators recommended caution in attempting euglycemia in women with recurrent episodes of hypoglycemia.

We have reported that good pregnancy outcomes can be achieved in women with mean preprandial plasma glucose values up to 143 mg/dL (Leveno and associates, 1979). Interestingly, the Diabetes Control and Complications Trial Research Group (1993) found that similar glucose values—intensive control was defined as mean values less than 155 mg/dL—delayed and slowed diabetic retinopathy, nephropathy, and neuropathy in nonpregnant patients. Thus, overtly diabetic women with glucose values considerably above those defined as normal both during and after pregnancy can except good outcomes.

SECOND TRIMESTER. As discussed in Chapter 36, maternal serum alpha-fetoprotein concentration at 16 to 20 weeks is used in association with targeted ultrasound at 18 to 20 weeks in an attempt to detect neural-tube defects and other anomalies (American College of Obstetricians and Gynecologists, 1994). Maternal serum alpha-fetoprotein values may be lower in diabetic pregnancies, and interpretation is altered accordingly (Martin and associates, 1990). Albert and colleagues (1996) used sonography to identify

72 percent of 29 fetal anomalies in 289 diabetic pregnancies.

THIRD TRIMESTER. Weekly visits to monitor glucose control and to evaluate for preeclampsia are a typical recommendation. Serial ultrasonography at 3- to 4-week intervals is performed to evaluate both excessive and insufficient fetal growth as well as amnionic fluid volume. A program of fetal surveillance using some of the antepartum tests described in Chapter 40 is usually begun between 26 and 32 weeks depending on clinical risk factors for fetal death (Lagrew and co-workers, 1993). According to the American College of Obstetricians and Gynecologists (1999), antepartum testing is recommended at least weekly. Some testing protocols in women with overt diabetes stipulate at least twice weekly testing (Kjos and colleagues, 1995).

Hospitalization is recommended for women whose diabetes is poorly controlled and for those with hypertension. Because of increased hospitalization costs, as well as reluctance of third-party payers, routine antepartum hospitalization for the overt diabetic woman is no longer commonly practiced. With a predominately indigent population at Parkland Hospital, conversion to outpatient management was associated with a doubling of the perinatal mortality rate. This doubling of mortality was due solely to unexplained fetal deaths that typically occurred at about 36 weeks. Consequently, most women with insulin-dependent diabetes currently accept hospitalization from 34 weeks until delivery.

Anecdotal reports of decreased insulin requirement during the last weeks of pregnancy have long been considered a warning sign of uteroplacental insufficiency. There is little objective evidence to support this concern. Berria and colleagues (2000) observed that decreased insulin requirement after 35 weeks was encountered in 5 percent of overtly diabetic women, and this was not associated with increased perinatal risks.

DELIVERY. Ideally, delivery of the diabetic woman should be accomplished near term. When the gestational age is certain, tests to determine fetal pulmonary maturation are not done, and delivery is planned after 38 completed weeks. For others, the lecithin–sphingomyelin ratio is measured at about 38 weeks and, if 2.0 or greater, delivery is effected. If severe hypertension develops, delivery is carried out even though the ratio is less than 2.0.

According to the American College of Obstetricians and Gynecologists (1994), if preterm labor occurs, tocolytic therapy with β-sympathomimetic drugs is best avoided in women with diabetes. These medications may significantly worsen maternal glucose control, causing ketoacidosis. Similarly, they advise caution in the use of corticosteroids to promote lung maturation.

In the overtly diabetic woman within class B or C White classification, cesarean delivery has commonly been used to avoid traumatic birth of a large infant at or near term. In women with more advanced diabetes, especially those with vascular disease, the reduced likelihood of successfully inducing labor remote from term has also contributed appreciably to an increased cesarean rate. Labor induction may be attempted when the fetus is not excessively large, and the cervix is considered favorable (Chap. 20). In the reports cited earlier with low perinatal mortality, the cesarean rate was more than 50 percent in Melbourne (Martin and colleagues, 1987), 55 percent in Los Angeles (Gabbe and colleagues, 1977), 69 percent in Boston (Kitzmiller and colleagues, 1978), 70 percent in a midwestern multicenter study (Schneider and co-workers, 1980), and 81 percent in Dallas (Leveno and associates, 1979). At Parkland Hospital, the cesarean delivery rate for overtly diabetic women has remained at about 80 percent for the past 20 years.

It is important to considerably reduce or delete the dose of long-acting insulin given on the day of delivery. Regular insulin should be used to meet most or all of the insulin needs of the mother at this time, because insulin requirements typically drop markedly after delivery. We have found that constant insulin infusion by calibrated pump is most satisfactory (Table 51–11). During labor and after either cesarean or vaginal delivery, the woman should be hydrated adequately intravenously as well as given glucose in sufficient amounts to maintain normoglycemia. Capillary or plasma glucose levels should be checked frequently, and regular insulin administered accordingly. It is not unusual for the woman to require virtually no insulin for the first 24 hours or so and then for insulin requirements to fluctuate markedly during the next few days. Infection must be promptly detected and treated.

TABLE 51–11. Low-dose Insulin Infusion for the Diabetic Woman During the Intrapartum Period

Blood Glucose (mg/dL)	Insulin Dosage[a] (U/hr)	Fluids (125 mL/hr)
< 100	0	D$_5$ lactated Ringer
100–140	1.0	D$_5$ lactated Ringer
141–180	1.5	Normal saline
181–220	2.0	Normal saline
> 220	2.5	Normal saline

[a] Dilution is 25 U of regular insulin in 250 mL of normal saline with 25 mL flushed through line administrated intravenously. A fingerstick glucose test is performed every 1 to 2 hours. The insulin pump and intravenous solution are adjusted accordingly. From the American College of Obstetricians and Gynecologists (1994), with permission.

CONTRACEPTION

There is no single contraceptive method appropriate for all women with diabetes (see also Chaps. 58 and 59). Diabetes carries a risk of vascular disease, and the estrogens in oral contraceptives statistically increase the risk of thromboembolism, stroke, and myocardial infarction. Although many clinicians are reluctant to prescribe oral contraceptives for overtly diabetic women, recent investigations on their safety have yielded conflicting results. Lidegaard (1995) cautioned against use of oral contraceptives because of increased risk of strokes, whereas Petersen and colleagues (1994) concluded that contemporaneous low-dose pills did not increase cardiovascular risks in these women. The American College of Obstetricians and Gynecologists (1994) advises that use of low-dose oral contraceptives should probably be restricted to women without vasculopathy or additional risk factors such as a strong history of ischemic heart disease. The lowest dose of estrogen and progesterone should be prescribed. Low-dose combination oral contraceptive preparations do not increase the risk of type 2 diabetes in postpartum women with recent gestational diabetes (Kjos and colleagues, 1990a).

Progestin-only oral or parenteral contraceptives may also be used because of minimal effects on carbohydrate metabolism. Unfortunately, fear of litigation has largely removed the *progestin implant* system (Norplant) from current use.

Physicians have also been reluctant to recommend intrauterine devices in diabetic women, primarily because of a possible increased risk of pelvic infections. The Food and Drug Administration package insert for the Copper T 380A IUD (Paragard) lists diabetes as one of the contraindications. However, Kjos and colleagues (1994), based on their investigations and review of the literature, concluded that diabetic women are often ideal candidates for intrauterine devices.

For all of the reasons cited, many overtly diabetic women elect puerperal sterilization, and this should be made readily available.

REFERENCES

Adashek JA, Lagrew DC, Iriye BK, Carr MH, Porto M, Freeman RK: The influence of ultrasound examination at term on the rate of cesarean section. Am J Obstet Gynecol 174:328, 1996

Albert TJ, Landon MB, Wheller JJ, Samuels PS, Cheng RF, Gabbe S: Prenatal detection of fetal anomalies in pregnancies complicated by insulin-dependent diabetes mellitus. Am J Obstet Gynecol 174:1424, 1996

American College of Obstetricians and Gynecologists: Antepartum fetal surveillance. Practice Bulletin No. 9, October 1999

American College of Obstetricians and Gynecologists: Diabe-

tes and pregnancy. Technical Bulletin No. 200, December 1994

American College of Obstetricians and Gynecologists: Management of diabetes mellitus in pregnancy. Technical Bulletin No. 92, May 1986

American Diabetes Association: Clinical practice recommendations, 1999. Diabetes Care 23:S10, 1999a

American Diabetes Association: Report of the Expert Committee on the Diagnosis and Classification of Diabetes Mellitus. Diabetes Care 22(Suppl 1): 512, 1999b

American Diabetes Association: Medical Management of Pregnancy Complicated by Diabetes, 2nd ed. Jovanovic-Peterson L (ed). Alexandria, VA, ADA, 1995

Bansal RK, Ecker JL, Laros RK: Blood glucose monitoring in gestational diabetes (letter). N Engl J Med 334:598, 1996

Bartha JL, Martinez-Del-Fresno P, Comino-Delgado R: Gestational diabetes mellitus diagnosed during early pregnancy. Am J Obstet Gynecol 182:346, 2000

Berkowitz K, Reyes C, Sadaat P, Kjos S: Comparison of fetal lung maturation in well dated diabetic and non-diabetic pregnancies. Am J Obstet Gynecol 174:373, 1996

Bernstein IM, Catalano PM: Examination of factors contributing to the risk of cesarean delivery in women with gestational diabetes. Obstet Gynecol 83:462, 1994

Berria R, Villarreal JA, Conway DI, Langer O: Is there an association between decreased insulin requirements and perinatal outcome in late pregnancy? Am J Obstet Gynecol 182:S81, 2000

Bojestig M, Arnqvist HJ, Hermansson G, Karlberg BE, Ludvigsson J: Declining incidence of nephropathy in insulin-dependent diabetes mellitus. N Engl J Med 330:15, 1994

Bonomo M, Gandini ML, Mastropasqua A, Begher C, Valentini U, Faden D, Morabito A: Which cutoff level should be used in screening for glucose intolerance in pregnancy? Am J Obstet Gynecol 179:179, 1998

Bradley RJ, Nicolaides KH, Brudenell JM: Are all infants of diabetic mothers "macrosomic"? BMJ 297:1583, 1988

Buchbinder A, Miodovnik M, McElvy S, Rosenn B, Kranias G, Khoury J, Siddiqui TA: Is insulin lispro associated with the development or progression of diabetic retinopathy during pregnancy? Am J Obstet Gynecol 183:1162, 2000

Campbell DM, Sutherland HW, Pearson DMW: Maternal glucose response to a standardized test meal through pregnancy and postnatally. Am J Obstet Gynecol 171:143, 1994

Carpenter MW, Coustan DR: Criteria for screening tests for gestational diabetes. Am J Obstet Gynecol 144:768, 1982

Casele HL, Laifer SA: Factors influencing preconception control of glycemia in diabetic women. Arch Intern Med 158:1321, 1998

Casey BM, Lucas MJ, McIntire DD, Leveno KJ: Population impact of universal screening for gestational diabetes. Am J Obstet Gynecol 180:536, 1999

Catalano PM, Avallone DA, Drago BS, Amini SB: Reproducibility of the oral glucose tolerance test in pregnant women. Am J Obstet Gynecol 169:874, 1993

Catalano PM, Huston L, Amini SB, Kalhan SC: Longitudinal changes in glucose metabolism during pregnancy in obese women with normal glucose tolerance and gestational diabetes mellitus. Am J Obstet Gynecol 180:903, 1999

Chaturvedi N, Stephenson JM, Fuller JH: The relationship between pregnancy and long-term maternal complications in the EURODIAB IDDM complications study. Diabetic Med 12:494, 1995

Clark CM Jr, Lee DA: Prevention and treatment of the complications of diabetes mellitus. N Engl J Med 332:1210, 1995

Cnattingius C, Berne C, Nordstrom ML: Pregnancy outcome and infant mortality in diabetic patients in Sweden. Diabetic Med 11:696, 1994

Combs CA, Rosenn B, Kitzmiller JL, Khoury JC, Wheeler BC, Miodovnik M: Early-pregnancy proteinuria in diabetes related to preeclampsia. Obstet Gynecol 82:802, 1993a

Combs CA, Singh NB, Khoury JC: Elective induction versus spontaneous labor after sonographic diagnosis of fetal macrosomia. Obstet Gynecol 81:492, 1993b

Conway D, Langer O: Elective delivery for macrosomia in the diabetic pregnancy: A clinical cost-benefit analysis. Am J Obstet Gynecol 174:331, 1996

Cousins L: Pregnancy complications among diabetic women: Review 1965–1985. Obstet Gynecol Surv 42:140, 1987

Cruikshank DP, Pitkin RM, Reynolds WA, Williams GA, Hargis GK: Altered maternal calcium homeostasis in diabetic pregnancy. J Clin Endocrinol Metab 50:264, 1980

Dacus JV, Meyer NL, Muram D, Stilson R, Phipps P, Sibai BM: Gestational diabetes: Postpartum glucose tolerance testing. Am J Obstet Gynecol 171:927, 1994

Dahl-Jørgensen K, Brinchmann-Hansen O, Hanssen KF, Sandvik L, Aagenaes ø, Aker Diabetes Group: Rapid tightening of blood glucose control leads to transient deterioration of retinopathy in insulin-dependent diabetes mellitus: The Oslo study. BMJ 290:811, 1985

Danilenko-Dixon D, Annamalai A, Mattson L, Lesnick T, Ogburn P: Perinatal outcomes in consecutive pregnancies discordant for gestational diabetes. Am J Obstet Gynecol 182:S80, 2000

Danilemoko-Dixon DR, Van Winter JT, Nelson RL, Ogburn PL: Universal versus selective gestational diabetes screening: Application of 1997 American Diabetes Association recommendations. Am J Obstet Gynecol 181:798, 1999

Dashe JS, Nathan L, McIntire DD, Leveno KJ: Correlation between amniotic fluid glucose correlation and amniotic fluid volume in pregnancy complicated by diabetes. Am J Obstet Gynecol 182:901, 2000

DeMarini S, Mimouni F, Tsang RC, Khoury J, Hertzberg V: Impact of metabolic control of diabetes during pregnancy on neonatal hypocalcemia: A randomized study. Obstet Gynecol 83:918, 1994

DeVeciana M, Major CA, Morgan M, Asrat T, Toohey JS, Lien JM, Evans AT: Postprandial versus preprandial blood glucose monitoring in women with gestational diabetes mellitus requiring insulin therapy. N Engl J Med 333:1237, 1995

Diabetes Control and Complications Trial Research Group: The effect of intensive treatment of diabetes on the development and progression of long-term complications in insulin-dependent diabetes mellitus. N Engl J Med 329:977, 1993

Dornhorst A, Nicholls JSD, Probst F, Paterson CM, Hollier KL, Elkeles RS, Beard RW: Calorie restriction for treatment of gestational diabetes. Diabetes 40:161, 1991

Durak EP, Jovanovic-Peterson L, Peterson CM: Comparative evaluation of uterine response to exercise on five aerobic machines. Am J Obstet Gynecol 162:754, 1990

Elman KD, Welch RA, Frank RN, Goyert GL, Sokol RJ: Diabetic retinopathy in pregnancy: A review. Obstet Gynecol 75:119, 1990

Espinosa de los Monteros A, Parra A, Carino N, Ramirez A: The reproducibility of the 50-g, 1-hour glucose screen for diabetes in pregnancy. Obstet Gynecol 82:515, 1993

Fadel HE, Saad SA, Davis H, Nelson GH: Fetal lung maturity in diabetic pregnancies: Relation among amniotic fluid,

insulin, prolactin, and lecithin. Am J Obstet Gynecol 159:457, 1988

Foster DW: Diabetes mellitus. In Fauci AS, Braunwald E, Isselbacher KJ, Wilson JD, Martin JB, Kasper DL, Hauser SL, Longo DL (eds): Harrison's Principles of Internal Medicine, 14th ed. New York, McGraw-Hill, 1998, p 2060

Franz MJ, Horton ES, Bantle JP, Beebe CA, Brunzell JD, Coulston AM, Henry RR, Hoogwerf BJ, Stacpoole PW: Nutrition principles for the management of diabetes and related complications. Diabetes Care 17:490, 1994

Gabbe S, Hill L, Schmidt L, Schulkin J: Management of diabetes by obstetrician-gynecologists. Obstet Gynecol 91:643, 1998

Gabbe SG, Mestman JH, Freeman RK, Goebelsmann UT, Lowensohn RI, Nochimson D, Cetrulo C, Quilligan EJ: Management and outcome of diabetes mellitus, classes B–R. Am J Obstet Gynecol 129:723, 1977

Gandhi JA, Zhang Y, Maidman JE: Fetal cardiac hypertrophy and cardiac function in diabetic pregnancies. Am J Obstet Gynecol 173:1132, 1995

Garner P: Type 1 diabetes mellitus and pregnancy. Lancet 346:157, 1995a

Garner P, Okun N, Keely E, Wells G, Perkins S, Sylvain J, Belcher J: A randomized controlled trial of strict glycemic control and tertiary level obstetric care versus routine obstetric care in the management of gestational diabetes: A pilot study. Am J Obstet Gynecol 177:190, 1997

Garner PR: Type 1 diabetes and pregnancy. Correspondence. Lancet 346:966, 1995b

Garner PR, D'Alton ME, Dudley DK, Huard P, Hardie M: Preeclampsia in diabetic pregnancies. Am J Obstet Gynecol 163:505, 1990

Gluck L, Kulovich MV: Lecithin:sphingomyelin ratios in amniotic fluid in normal and abnormal pregnancy. Am J Obstet Gynecol 115:539, 1973

Gordon M, Lawdon MB, Samuels P, Hissrich S, Gabbe SG: Perinatal outcome and long-term follow-up associated with modern management of diabetic nephropathy. Obstet Gynecol 87:401, 1996

Greenberg LR, Moore TR, Murphy H: Gestational diabetes mellitus: Antenatal variables as predictors of postpartum glucose intolerance. Obstet Gynecol 86:97, 1995

Greene MF, Hare JW, Cloherty JP, Benacerraf BR, Soeldner JS: First-trimester hemoglobin A_1 and risk for major malformation and spontaneous abortion in diabetic pregnancy. Teratology 39:225, 1989

Gribble RK, Meier PR, Berg RL: The value of urine screening for glucose at each prenatal visit. Obstet Gynecol 86:405, 1995

Hanson U, Persson B: Outcome of pregnancies complicated by type 1 insulin-dependent diabetes in Sweden: Acute pregnancy complications, neonatal mortality and morbidity. Am J Perinatol 10:330, 1993

Harris MI: Gestational diabetes may represent discovery of preexisting glucose intolerance. Diabetes Care 11:402, 1988

Henriques CU, Damm P, Tabor A, Goldstein H, Mølstsed-Pedersen L: Incidence of fetal chromosome abnormalities in insulin dependent diabetic women. Acta Obstet Gynecol Scand 70:295, 1991

Holing EV, Brown ZA, Beyer CS, Connell FA: Why don't women with diabetes plan their pregnancies? Diabetes Care 21:889, 1998

How H: Is "incipient nephropathy" associated with an increased rate of preeclampsia in women with pregestational diabetes? Am J Obstet Gynecol 182:S79, 2000

Johnson SR, Kolberg BH, Vance MW, Railsback LD: Maternal obesity and pregnancy. Surg Gynecol Obstet 164:431, 1987

Johnstone FD, Nasrat AA, Prescott RJ: The effect of established and gestational diabetes on pregnancy outcome. Br J Obstet Gynaecol 97:1009, 1990

Jovanovic-Peterson L, Durak EP, Peters CM: Randomized trial of diet versus diet plus cardiovascular conditioning on glucose levels in gestational diabetes. Am J Obstet Gynecol 161:415, 1989

Jovanovic-Peterson L, Peterson CM: Dietary manipulation as a primary treatment strategy for pregnancies complicated by diabetes. J Am Coll Nutr 9:320, 1990

Kaufmann RC, Smith T, Bochantin T, Khardori R, Evans MS, Steahly L: Failure to obtain follow-up testing for gestational diabetic patients in a rural population. Obstet Gynecol 93:734, 1999

Keller JD, Metzger BE, Dooley SL, Tamura RK, Sabbagha RE, Freinkel N: Infants of diabetic mothers with accelerated fetal growth by ultrasonography: Are they all alike? Am J Obstet Gynecol 163:893, 1990

Kent LA, Gill GV, Williams G: Mortality and outcome of patients with brittle diabetes and recurrent acidosis. Lancet 344:778, 1994

Kitzmiller JL, Main E, Ward B, Theiss T, Peterson DL: Insulin lispro and the development of proliferative diabetic retinopathy during pregnancy [letter]. Diabetes Care 22:874, 1999

Kitzmiller JL, Cloherty JP, Younger MD, Tabatabaii A, Rothchild SB, Sosenkol I, Epstein MF, Singh S, Neff RK: Diabetic pregnancy and perinatal outcome. Am J Obstet Gynecol 131:560, 1978

Kitzmiller JL, Gavin LA, Gin GD, Jovanovic-Peterson L, Main EK, Zigrang WD: Preconception care of diabetes: Glycemic control prevents congenital anomalies. JAMA 265:731, 1991

Kitzmiller JL, Younger MD, Hare JW, Phillippe M, Vignati L, Fargnoli B, Grause A: Continuous subcutaneous insulin therapy during early pregnancy. Obstet Gynecol 65:606, 1985

Kjos SL, Leung A, Henry DA, Victor MR, Paul RH, Medearis AL: Antepartum surveillance in diabetic pregnancies: Predictors of fetal distress in labor. Am J Obstet Gynecol 173:1532, 1995

Kjos SL, Shoupe D, Donyou S, Friedman RL, Bernstein GS, Mestman JH, Mishell DR Jr: Effect of low-dose oral contraceptives on carbohydrate and lipid metabolism in women with recent gestational diabetes: Results of a controlled, randomized, prospective study. Am J Obstet Gynecol 163:1822, 1990a

Kjos SL, Walther FJ, Montoro M, Paul RH, Diaz F, Stabler M: Prevalence and etiology of respiratory distress in infants of diabetic mothers: Predictive value of fetal lung maturation tests. Am J Obstet Gynecol 163:898, 1990b

Klein BEK, Moss SE, Klein R: Effect of pregnancy on progression of diabetic retinopathy. Diabetes Care 13:34, 1990

Krolewski AS, Laffel LMB, Krolewski M, Quinn M, Warran JH: Glycosylated hemoglobin and the risk of microalbuminuria in patients with insulin-dependent diabetes mellitus. N Engl J Med 332:1251, 1995

Lagrew DC, Pircon RA, Towers CV, Dorchester W, Freeman RK: Antepartum fetal surveillance in patients with diabetes: When to start? Am J Obstet Gynecol 168:1820, 1993

Landon MB, Mintz MC, Gabbe SG: Sonographic evaluation of fetal abdominal growth: Predictor of the large-for-gestational-age infant in pregnancies complicated by diabetes mellitus. Am J Obstet Gynecol 160:115, 1989

Landon MB, Osei K, Platt M, O'Dorisio T, Samuels P, Gabbe SG: The differential effects of body fat distribution on insulin and glucose metabolism during pregnancy. Am J Obstet Gynecol 171:875, 1994

Langer O, Conway D, Berkus M, Xenakis EMJ: Oral hypoglycemic agent is comparable to insulin in GDM management: A randomized study. Am J Obstet Gynecol 180:65, 1999

Langer O, Rodriquez DA, Xenakis EMJ, McFarland MB, Berkus MD, Arrendondo F: Intensified versus conventional management of gestational diabetes. Am J Obstet Gynecol 170:1036, 1994

Lauszus FF, Gron PL, Klebe JG: Pregnancies complicated by diabetic retinopathy. Acta Obstet Gynecol Scand 77:814, 1998

Leonardi MR, Bottoms SF: Increased incidence of large for gestational age infants not attributable to gestational diabetes. Am J Obstet Gynecol 174:393, 1996

Leveno KJ, Fortunato SJ, Raskin P, Williams ML, Whalley PJ: Continuous subcutaneous insulin infusion during pregnancy. Diabetes Res Clin Pract 4:257, 1988

Leveno KJ, Hauth JC, Gilstrap LC III, Whalley PJ: Appraisal of "rigid" blood glucose control during pregnancy in the overtly diabetic woman. Am J Obstet Gynecol 135:853, 1979

Lidegaard O: Oral contraceptives, pregnancy, and risk of cerebral thromboembolism: The influence of diabetes, hypertension, migraine, and previous thrombotic disease. Br J Obstet Gynaecol 102:153, 1995

Lucas MJ, Leveno KJ, Williams ML, Raskin P, Whalley PJ: Early pregnancy glycosylated hemoglobin, severity of diabetes, and fetal malformations. Am J Obstet Gynecol 161:426, 1989

Lucas MJ, Lowe TW, Bowe L, McIntire DD: Class A_1 gestational diabetes: A meaningful diagnosis? Obstet Gynecol 82:260, 1993

Magee MS, Walden CE, Benedetti TJ, Knopp RH: Influence of diagnostic criteria on the incidence of gestational diabetes and perinatal mortality. JAMA 26:609, 1993

Major CH, Henry J, DeVeciona M, Morgan MA: The effects of carbohydrate restriction in patients with diet-controlled gestational diabetes. Obstet Gynecol 91:600, 1998

Martin AO, Dempsey LM, Minogue J, Liu K, Keller J, Tamura R, Frienkel N: Maternal serum α-fetoprotein levels in pregnancies complicated by diabetes: Implications for screening programs. Am J Obstet Gynecol 163:1209, 1990

Martin FR, Health P, Mountain KR: Pregnancy in women with diabetes. Fifteen years' experience: 1973–1985. Med J Aust 146:187, 1987

McElvy S, Demarini S, Miodovnik M, Khoury J, Rosenn B, Kranias G, Tsang R: Progression of diabetic retinopathy: Association with pregnancy and reduced fetal weight. Am J Obstet Gynecol 182:S77, 2000

McFarland MB, Langer O, Fazioni E, Trylovich CG, Kobes CG: Anthropometric and body composition differences in large-for-gestational age, but not appropriate-for-gestational age infants of mothers with and without diabetes mellitus. J Soc Gynecol Invest 7:231, 2000

McKinney PA, Parslow R, Gurney KA, Law GR, Bodansky HJ, Williams R: Perinatal and neonatal determinants of childhood type 1 diabetes: A case-control study in Yorkshire, U.K. Diabetes Care 22:928, 1999

Metzger BE, Bybee DE, Freinkel N, Phelps RL, Radvany RM, Vaisrub N: Gestational diabetes mellitus: Correlations between the phenotypic and genotypic characteristics of the mother and abnormal glucose tolerance during the first year postpartum. Diabetes 34:111, 1985

Metzger BE, Coustan DR: Summary and recommendations of the fourth international workshop-conference on gestational diabetes mellitus. Diabetes Care 21:B161, 1998

Miller E, Hare JW, Cloherty JP, Dunn PJ, Gleason RE, Soeldner JS, Kitzmiller JL: Elevated maternal hemoglobin A_{1c} in early pregnancy and major congenital anomalies in infants of diabetic mothers. N Engl J Med 304:1331, 1981

Mills JL, Baker L, Goldman AS: Malformations in infants of diabetic mothers occur before the seventh gestational week. Implications for treatment. Diabetes 28:292, 1979

Mills JL, Knopp RH, Simpson JL, Jovanovic-Peterson L, Metzger BE, Holmes LB, Aarons JH, Brown Z, Reed GF, Bieber FR, Van Allen M, Holzman I, Ober C, Peterson CM, Witham JM, Duckles A, Mueller-Heubach E, Polk BF, National Institute of Child Health and Human Development Diabetes in Early Pregnancy Study: Lack of relation of increased malformation rates in infants of diabetic mothers to glycemic control during organogenesis. N Engl J Med 318:671, 1988a

Mills JL, Simpson JL, Driscoll SG, Jovanovic-Peterson L, Van Allen M, Aarons JH, Metzger B, Bieber FR, Knopp RH, Holmes LB, Peterson CM, Witham-Wilson M, Brown Z, Ober C, Harley E, MacPherson TA, Duckles A, Mueller-Heubach E, National Institute of Child Health and Human Development Diabetes in Early Pregnancy Study: Incidence of spontaneous abortion among normal women and insulin-dependent diabetic women whose pregnancies were identified within 21 days of conception. N Engl J Med 319:1617, 1988b

Milunsky A, Jick H, Bruell CL, MacLaughlin DS, Rothman FJ, Willett W: Multivitamin/folic acid supplementation in early pregnancy reduces the prevalence of neural tube defects. JAMA 262:2847, 1989

Miodovnik M, Rosenn BM, Khoury JC, Grigsby JL, Siddiqi TA: Does pregnancy increase the risk for development and progression of diabetic nephropathy? Am J Obstet Gynecol 174:1180, 1996

Modanlou HD, Komatsu G, Dorchester W, Freeman RK, Bosu SK: Large-for-gestational-age neonates: Anthropometric reasons for shoulder dystocia. Obstet Gynecol 60:417, 1982

Murphy NJ, Meyer BA, O'Kell RT, Hogard ME: Screening for gestational diabetes mellitus with a reflectance photometer: Accuracy and precision of a single-operator model. Obstet Gynecol 83:1038, 1994

Nathan DM: Long-term complications of diabetes mellitus. N Engl J Med 328:1676, 1993

National Diabetes Data Group: Classification and diagnosis of diabetes mellitus and other categories of glucose intolerance. Diabetes 28:1039, 1979

Nordlander E, Hanson U, Persson B: Factors influencing neonatal morbidity in gestational diabetic pregnancy. Br J Obstet Gynaecol 96:671, 1989

O'Sullivan JB: Body weight and subsequent diabetes mellitus. JAMA 248:949, 1982

Owen J, Phelan ST, Landon MP, Gabbe SG: Gestational diabetes survey. Am J Obstet Gynecol 172:615, 1995

Pallardo F, Herranz L, Garcia-Ingelmo T, Grande C, Martin-Vaquero P, Janez M, Gonzalez A: Early postpartum metabolic assessment in women with prior gestational diabetes. Diabetes Care 22:1053, 1999

Pan XR, Li GW, Hu YH, Wang JX, Yang WY, An ZX, Hu ZX, Lin J, Xiao JZ, Cao HB, Liu PA, Jiang XG, Jiang YY, Wang JP, Zheng H, Zhang H, Bennett PH, Howard BV: Effects of diet and exercise in preventing NIDDM in people with impaired glucose tolerance. The Da Qing IGT and Diabetes Study. Diabetes Care 20:537, 1997

Pedersen J: The Pregnant Diabetic and Her Newborn, 2nd ed. Baltimore, Williams & Wilkins, 1977, p 211

Pedersen J, Mølsted-Pedersen L, Andersen B: Assessors of fetal perinatal mortality in diabetic pregnancy. Analysis of 1332 pregnancies in the Copenhagen series, 1946–1972. Diabetes 23:302, 1974

Petersen KR, Skouby SO, Sidelmann J, Pedersen LM, Jespersen J: Effects of contraceptive steroids on cardiovascular risk factors in women with insulin-dependent diabetes mellitus. Am J Obstet Gynecol 171:400, 1994

Philipson EH, Super DM: Gestational diabetes mellitus: Does it recur in subsequent pregnancy? Am J Obstet Gynecol 160:1324, 1989

Piacquadio K, Hollingsworth DR, Murphy H: Effects of in-utero exposure to oral hypoglycemic drugs. Lancet 338:866, 1991

Pombar X, Strassner HT, Fenner PC: Pregnancy in a woman with class H diabetes mellitus and previous coronary artery bypass graft: A case report and review of the literature. Obstet Gynecol 85:825, 1995

Puza SW, Malee MP: Utilization of routine ophthalmologic examinations in pregnant diabetic patients. J Mat Fet Med 5:7, 1996

Raychaudhuri K, Maresh MJ: Glycemic control throughout pregnancy and fetal growth in insulin-dependent diabetes. Obstet Gynecol 95:190, 2000

Reece EA, Hobbins JC: Diabetic embryopathy: Pathogenesis, prenatal diagnosis, and prevention. Obstet Gynecol Surv 41:325, 1986

Reece EA, Wu YK, Ait-Allah A, Salameh W: Altered expression of PLA_2 gene implicated in molecular mechanism of diabetes-induced neural tube defects (NTDs): A new revelation. Am J Obstet Gynecol 174:311, 1996

Reller MD, Kaplan S: Hypertrophic cardiomyopathy in infants of diabetic mothers: An update. Am J Perinatol 5:353, 1988

Rey E, Attie C, Bonin A: The effects of first-trimester diabetes control on the incidence of macrosomia. Am J Obstet Gynecol 181:202, 1999

Richey SD, Sandstad JS, Leveno KJ: Observations concerning "unexplained" fetal demise in pregnancy complicated by diabetes mellitus. J Mat Fet Med 4:169, 1995

Rizzo AA, Dooley SL, Metzger BE, Cho NH, Ogata ES, Silverman BL: Prenatal and perinatal influences on long-term psychomotor development in offspring of diabetic mothers. Am J Obstet Gynecol 173:1753, 1995

Rosenn B, Miodovnik M, Combs CA, Khoury J, Siddiqi TA: Glycemic thresholds for spontaneous abortion and congenital malformations in insulin-dependent diabetes mellitus. Obstet Gynecol 84:515, 1994

Rosenn BM, Miodovnik M, Holcberg G, Khoury JC, Siddiqi TA: Hyperglycemia: The price of intensive insulin therapy for pregnant women with insulin-dependent diabetes mellitus. Obstet Gynecol 85:417, 1995

Salvesen DR, Brudenell MJ, Nicolaides KH: Fetal polycythemia and thrombocytopenia in pregnancies complicated by maternal diabetes mellitus. Am J Obstet Gynecol 166:1287, 1992

Salvesen DR, Brudenell MJ, Snijders JM, Ireland RM, Nicolaides KH: Fetal plasma erythropoietin in pregnancies complicated by maternal diabetes mellitus. Am J Obstet Gynecol 168:88, 1993

Schaefer-Graf UM, Buchanan TA, Xiang A, Songster G, Montoro M, Kjos SL: Patterns of congenital anomalies and relationship to initial maternal fasting glucose levels in pregnancies complicated by type 2 and gestational diabetes. Am J Obstet Gynecol 182:313, 2000

Schneider JM, Curet LB, Olson RW, Shay G: Ambulatory care of the pregnant diabetic. Obstet Gynecol 56:144, 1980

Schwartz ML, Ray WN, Lubarsky SL: The diagnosis and classification of gestational diabetes mellitus: Is it time to change our tune? Am J Obstet Gynecol 180:1560, 1999

Sheffield JS, Casey BM, Lucas MJ, Rezai K, McIntire DD, Leveno KJ: Gestational diabetes: Effects of the degree of hyperglycemia and the gestational age at diagnosis. Soc Gyn Inv 6:6A, 1999

Sibai BM, Caritis S, Hauth J, Lindheimer M, VanDorsten JP, MacPherson C, Klebanoff M, Landon M, Miodovnik M, Paul R, Meis P, Dombrowski M, Thurnau G, Roberts J, McNellis D, for the National Institute of Child Health and Human Development Network of Maternal–Fetal Medicine Units: Risks of preeclampsia and adverse neonatal outcomes among women with pregestational diabetes mellitus. Am J Obstet Gynecol 182:364, 2000

Siddiqi T, Rosenn B, Mimouni F, Khoury J, Miodovnik M: Hypertension during pregnancy in insulin-dependent diabetic women. Obstet Gynecol 77:514, 1991

Sivan E, Wu YK, Homko C, Reece EA: Dietary vitamin E prophylaxis and diabetic embryopathy: Morphological, biochemical, and molecular analyses. Am J Obstet Gynecol 174:303, 1996

Stamler EF, Cruz ML, Mimouni F, Rosenn B, Siddiqi T, Khoury J, Miodovnik M: High infectious morbidity in pregnant women with insulin-dependent diabetes: An understated complication. Am J Obstet Gynecol 163:1217, 1990

Steel JM, Johnstone FD, Hume R, Mao JH: Insulin requirements during pregnancy in women with type 1 diabetes. Obstet Gynecol 83:253, 1994

Tamada JA, Garg S, Jovanovic L, Pitzer KR, Fermi S, Potts RO and the Cygnus Research Team: Non-invasive glucose monitoring; Comprehensive clinical results. JAMA 282:1839, 1999

Thompson DJ, Porter KB, Gunnells DJ, Wagner PC, Spinnato JA: Prophylactic insulin in the management of gestational diabetes. Obstet Gynecol 75:960, 1990

Van Ballegooie E, Hooymans JMM, Timmerman Z, Reitsma WD, Sluiter WJ, Schweitzer NMJ, Doorenbos H: Rapid deterioration of diabetic retinopathy during treatment with continuous subcutaneous insulin infusion. Diabetes Care 7:236, 1984

Ventura SJ, Martin JA, Curtin SC, Mathews TJ, Park MS: Births: Final data for 1998. National Vital Statistics Reports, Vol 48, No. 3. Hyattsville, MD, 2000

Verhaeghe J, Van Bree B, Van Herck E, Laureys J, Bouillon R, Van Assche FA: C-peptide, insulin-like growth factor I and II, and insulin-like growth factor binding protein-1 in umbilical cord serum: Correlations with birthweight. Am J Obstet Gynecol 169:89, 1993

Wang Ph, Lau J, Chalmers TC: Meta-analysis of effects of intensive blood-glucose control on late complications of type 1 diabetes. Lancet 341:1306, 1993

Way GL: The natural history of hypertrophic cardiomyopathy in infants of diabetic mothers. J Pediatr 95:1020, 1979

Weiss PAM, Haeusler M, Kainer F, Purstner P, Haas J: Toward universal criteria for gestational diabetes: Relationships between seventy-five and one hundred gram glucose loads and between capillary and venous concentrations. Am J Obstet Gynecol 178:830, 1998

White P: Classification of obstetric diabetes. Am J Obstet Gynecol 130:228, 1978a

White P: Pregnancy complicating diabetes. Am J Obstet Gynecol 130:1127, 1978b

White P, Titus RS, Joslin EP: Prediction and prevention of late pregnancy accidents in diabetes. Am J Med Sci 198:487, 1939

Willman SP, Leveno KJ, Guzick DS, Williams LM, Whalley PJ: Glucose threshold for macrosomia in pregnancy complicated by diabetes. Am J Obstet Gynecol 154:470, 1986

Wiznitzer A, Hershkovitz R, Mimon E, Mazor M, Leiberman JR, Bashan N, Reece EA: The antioxidant lipoic acid prevents malformations in offspring of diabetic rats. Am J Obstet Gynecol 174:310, 1996

World Health Organization: Diabetes Mellitus: Report of a WHO Study Group. Geneva: WHO; 1985. Technical Report Series No. 727

Zhang S, Folsom AR, Flack JM, Lin K: Body fat distribution before pregnancy and gestational diabetes: Findings from coronary artery risk development in young adults (CARDIA) study. BMJ 311:1139, 1995

52

Connective-Tissue Disorders

IMMUNE-MEDIATED CONNECTIVE-TISSUE DISEASES

Systemic Lupus Erythematosus
Antiphospholipid Antibodies
Rheumatoid Arthritis
Systemic Sclerosis (Scleroderma)
Vasculitis Syndromes
Dermatomyositis and Polymyositis (Idiopathic
   Inflammatory Myositis)

INHERITED CONNECTIVE-TISSUE DISORDERS

Marfan Syndrome
Ehlers–Danlos Syndrome

Connective-tissue disorders, also referred to as collagen-vascular disorders, are a group of diseases that are not organ specific and thus cause generalized clinical findings. They are principally characterized by connective-tissue abnormalities that are immunopathologically mediated as the consequence of a variety of autoantibodies. These are also called *immune-complex disease* because many are mediated by deposition of immune complexes in specific organ or tissue sites, including the glomerulus and blood vessel walls. Some disorders that are characterized by sterile inflammation, especially of the skin, joints, blood vessels, and kidney, are referred to as *rheumatic diseases*. For inexplicable reasons, many of these rheumatic diseases mostly affect women.

Another major category of connective-tissue diseases includes inherited disorders of bone, skin, cartilage, blood vessels, and basement membranes. Examples of these are Marfan syndrome, osteogenesis imperfecta, and Ehlers–Danlos syndrome.

IMMUNE-MEDIATED CONNECTIVE-TISSUE DISEASES

Although the pathogenesis for all of these disorders has not been elucidated, they can be separated into those clearly associated with autoantibody formation and those without evidence of the rheumatoid factor, the so-called seronegative spondyloarthropathies (Hahn, 1997). The former category includes systemic lupus erythematosus, rheumatoid arthritis, Sjögren syndrome, progressive systemic sclerosis (scleroderma), mixed-connective tissue disease, dermatomyositis, polymyositis, and a variety of vasculitis syndromes. The seronegative spondyloarthropathies all are strongly associated with the presence of the HLA-B27 antigen but not the rheumatoid factor (Benjamin and Parkham, 1992; Moll, 1994). These include ankylosing spondylitis, psoriatic arthritis, Reiter disease, and likely the arthritis syndromes associated with ulcerative colitis and Crohn disease.

Because renal involvement is common with many of these syndromes, and because pregnancy is adversely affected by glomerulopathic syndromes, a search for co-existing renal involvement is paramount to evaluation. Hypertension likewise is common, and exacerbation during pregnancy frequently forces early delivery. In some of these immune-mediated diseases, *antiphospholipid antibodies* are formed that can cause injury to maternal vasculature and to the placenta. Conversely, they can arise de novo and do similar damage.

IMMUNOLOGICAL ASPECTS. The immune system basically protects cells, tissues, and organs perceived as *self* and attacks and destroys foreign or nonself antigenic material by the production of antibodies directed against foreign or *nonself* antigens. For some as yet unknown reason, the immune system may be stimulated to begin producing antibodies directed against self or normal tissues. These "misdirected" antibodies are called **autoantibodies** and are increased in many connective-tissue disorders. The stimulus responsible for their production is unknown, but a variety of inciting reasons are suspected that include bacterial or viral injury to genetically susceptible tissues.

Autoantibodies induce tissue destruction in susceptible tissues by at least two mechanisms, singly or in combination. The **cytotoxic mechanism** involves direct antibody attachment to a specific surface antigen, which results in cell injury or destruction. The **immune complex mechanism** results in tissue damage when the antigen–antibody complex itself attaches to a susceptible tissue. The complex is then believed to incite a complement response or "cascade," which results in the release of chemotactic substances that attract a variety of polymorphonuclear cells. The combination of any or all of the immune complexes, chemotactic substances, and leukocytes, either intra- or extracellularly, causes release of a variety of substances such as cytokines and lysosomal enzymes that attack tissues.

Both normal and abnormal immune responses are mediated through thymus-derived (T) and bone-marrow derived (B) lymphocyte production. Principal mediators are T, B, and large lymphocytes as well as monocytes-macrophages. *Cytokines* are soluble proteins that are stimulated by immune system activation. Such activation is regulated by the ordered production of a myriad of cytokines that control gene activation and functional cell surface molecule expression (Winchester, 1992). The large number of lymphocyte surface molecules is classified by their *cluster differentiation (CD)* antigens. Probably the best known of these is CD4, which is a 59-kd member of the immunoglobulin G superfamily. It is the receptor for the human immunodeficiency virus envelope gp120.

The **major histocompatibility complex (MHC)** is a series of 40 to 50 genes located on the short arm of chromosome 6, and it is known as the **human leukocyte-associated (HLA)** complex. These genetic loci code for distinct cell-surface glycoproteins, including transplantation antigens, and they are involved in self and nonself recognition. Class I antigens include HLA-A, -B, and -C. Class II antigens include HLA-DR, -DQ, and -DP. Through a variety of complex interactions, including T- and B-cell stimulation and interaction with immunoglobulins and the complement system, nonself antigens or, in the abnormal state, self antigens (normal tissue), are destroyed.

IMMUNE-MEDIATED DISEASE AND PREGNANCY. Very few immune disorders are definitely proven to arise only during pregnancy. Maternal isoimmunization from fetal red cell or platelet antigens is the most common (Chap. 39, p. 1057). Some theories of the cause of preeclampsia–eclampsia implicate an immunological basis (Chap. 24, p. 569). Some cases of recurrent abortion are also attributed to immunological causes (Chap. 33, p. 859).

There are some pregnancy-induced immunological alterations that potentially modulate connective-tissue disorders (Chap. 8, p. 179). They include depression of cell-mediated immunity and some antibody responses, increased immunoglobulin-secreting cells, decreased inflammatory response, abnormal lymphocyte stimulation, decreased T/B lymphocyte ratio, and increased levels of circulating immune complexes. Complement levels during pregnancy normally may be elevated, and there may be low-grade activation of the classical pathway. Serum levels of autoantibodies are not increased appreciably during normal pregnancy (Kutteh, 1996).

Although it is generally thought that these immunological changes have negligible effects on immune-mediated collagen-vascular disorders, the effects of large amounts of estrogen, progesterone, and prolactin cannot be ignored. For example, estrogens upregulate and androgens downregulate T-cell response, and a number of cytokines are regulated by sex hormones (Lockshin and Druzin, 1995). Also, recall that autoimmune rheumatic diseases mostly affect women. Lockshin (1998) postulates a modulating effect of hormones rather than a causative role.

SYSTEMIC LUPUS ERYTHEMATOSUS. Lupus is a disease(s) of unknown etiology in which tissues and cells are damaged by autoantibodies and immune complexes directed at one or more components of cell nuclei (Mills, 1994). Almost 90 percent of cases are in women, and its prevalence in childbearing-aged women is about 1 in 500 (Lockshin and Sammaritano, 2000). The 10- and 20-year survival rates are 75 and 50 percent (Jacobsen and colleagues, 1999). Infection, lupus flares, end-organ failure, and cardiovascular disease account for most deaths.

Some autoantibodies produced in patients with lupus are shown in Table 52–1. A number of genetic, environmental, and sex hormonal factors result in abnormal hormonal and cellular immune responses and inadequate clearing of antibodies and immune complexes. Genetic influences are indicated by a higher concordance with monozygotic compared with dizygotic twins and a 10 percent frequency in patients with one affected family member. The relative risk of disease is increased threefold if HLA-DR2 or -DR3 genes are found (Arnett, 1997). The lupus anticoagulant is associated with HLA class II-DQB genes inherited with HLA-DR4 or DR7. In general, estrogens enhance disease and testosterone reduces antibody response. Thus, some individuals are genetically predisposed to lupus. Under the influence of multiple genes, often triggered by environmental stimuli and highly influenced by gender, a number of clinical syndromes may develop, fulfilling diagnostic criteria for lupus.

CLINICAL FINDINGS. Lupus is notoriously variable in its presentation, course, and outcome (Gladman and Urowitz, 1997). Clinical manifestations may be confined initially to one organ system, with other systems becoming involved as the disease progresses; or the

TABLE 52–1. Some Autoantibodies Produced in Patients with Systemic Lupus Erythematosus

Antibody	Incidence (%)	Clinical Associations
Antinuclear	98	Multiple antibodies; repeat negative test makes lupus unlikely
Anti-DNA	70	Associated with nephritis and clinical activity
Anti-Sm	30	Specific for lupus
Anti-RNP	40	Polymyositis, scleroderma, lupus, mixed-connective tissue disease
Anti-Ro (SS-A)	30	Sjögren syndrome, cutaneous lupus, neonatal lupus, ANA-negative lupus, congenital heart block
Anti-La (SS-B)	10	Always with anti-Ro; Sjögren syndrome
Antihistone	70	Common in drug-induced lupus (95%)
Antiphospholipid	50	Lupus anticoagulant and anticardiolipin associated with thrombosis, fetal loss, thrombocytopenia, valvar heart disease; false-positive test for syphilis
Antierythrocyte	60	Overt hemolysis uncommon
Antiplatelet	—	Thrombocytopenia

ANA = antinuclear antibody.
Modified from Hahn (1998), with permission.

disease may be manifested initially by multi-system involvement (Table 52–2). Common findings are malaise, fever, arthritis, rash, pleuropericarditis, photosensitivity, anemia, and cognitive dysfunction. At least half of patients have renal involvement. *Libman-Sacks endocarditis* was described with lupus, but likely is due to anticardiolipin antibodies (Hojnik and associates, 1996).

LABORATORY FINDINGS. Identification of antinuclear antibodies (ANA) is the best screening test; however, a positive test is not specific for lupus. For example, low titers are found in some normal individuals, other autoimmune diseases, acute viral infections, and chronic inflammatory processes; several drugs can also cause a positive reaction. Almost all patients with lupus have a positive test. Antibodies to double-stranded DNA (dsDNA) and to Sm (Smith) antigens are relatively specific for lupus, whereas other antibodies shown in Table 52–1 are not.

Anemia is common, and there may be leukopenia and thrombocytopenia. Proteinuria and casts are found in the half of patients with glomerular lesions, and there may be renal insufficiency. Other laboratory findings include false-positive syphilis serology, prolonged partial thromboplastin time, and rheumatoid factors.

DIAGNOSIS. The recently revised criteria of the American Rheumatism Association for diagnosis of systemic lupus are shown in Table 52–3. If any four or more of these 11 criteria are present, serially or simultaneously, the diagnosis of lupus is made.

DRUG-INDUCED LUPUS. Numerous drugs have been reported to induce a lupus-like syndrome. This syndrome is rarely associated with glomerulonephritis, and disease usually regresses when the medication is discontinued (Rubin, 1997). Drugs associated with this syndrome include procainamide, quinidine, hydralazine, α-methyldopa, phenytoin, and phenobarbital. Combination estrogen and progestin oral contraceptives have been implicated, but this has not been proven.

LUPUS AND MATERNAL OUTCOME. A number of factors apparently determine the effects of lupus on pregnancy outcome. Some that are important include the disease state at the beginning of pregnancy, age and parity, co-existence of other medical or obstetrical disorders, and antiphospholipid antibodies.

A number of investigators have attempted to ascertain the effects of lupus on maternal outcome. Their reports indicate lupus improved in a third of women followed during pregnancy; a third remained unchanged, and a third worsened. Importantly, in all their series, at least some of the women had disease that worsened. Thus, in any given pregnancy, the clinical condition can worsen or a flare can occur rapidly and often without biochemical or clinical warning (Khamashta and colleagues, 1997; Ruiz-Irastorza and co-workers, 1996). Petri (1998) observed a 7 percent major morbidity during pregnancy and estimates a 1 in 20 chance of a life-threatening event. Generally these are due to renal impairment, myocarditis, or serositis, but complications associated with preeclampsia and antiphospholipid antibody syndrome are worrisome.

TABLE 52–2. Clinical Manifestations of Systemic Lupus Erythematosus

Organ System	Clinical Manifestations	Percent
Systemic	Fatigue, malaise, fever, weight loss	95
Musculoskeletal	Arthralgias, myalgias, polyarthritis, myopathy	95
Hematological	Anemia, hemolysis, leukopenia, thrombocytopenia, lupus anti-coagulant	85
Cutaneous	Malar (butterfly) rash, discoid rash, photosensitivity, oral ulcers, alopecia, skin rashes	80
Neurological	Cognitive dysfunction, organic brain syndromes, psychosis, seizures	60
Cardiopulmonary	Pleuritis, pericarditis	60
Renal	Proteinuria, casts, nephrotic syndrome	60
Gastrointestinal	Anorexia, nausea, pain, diarrhea	45
Thrombosis	Venous (10%), arterial (5%)	15
Ocular	Conjunctivitis	15
Fetal loss	Recurrent abortion, early preeclampsia, stillbirths	30

Modified from Hahn (1998), with permission.

TABLE 52–3. **1997 Revised Criteria of the American Rheumatism Association for Systemic Lupus Erythematosus**[a]

Criteria	Comments
Malar rash	Malar erythema
Discoid rash	Erythematous patches, scaling, follicular plugging
Photosensitivity	
Oral ulcers	Usually painless
Arthritis	Nonerosive involving two or more peripheral joints
Serositis	Pleuritis or pericarditis
Renal disorders	Proteinuria > 0.5 g/day or > 3+ dipstick, or cellular casts
Neurological disorders	Seizures or psychosis without other cause
Hematological disorders	Hemolytic anemia, leukopenia, lymphopenia, or thrombocytopenia
Immunological disorders	Anti-dsDNA or anti-Sm antibodies, or false-positive VDRL, abnormal level of IgM or IgG anticardiolipin antibodies, or lupus anticoagulant
Antinuclear antibodies	Abnormal titer of ANAs

ANAs = antinuclear antibodies; dsDNA = double-stranded DNA; Sm = Smith antigens; VDRL = Venereal Disease Research Laboratories test for syphilis.
[a] If four criteria are present at any time during course of disease, systemic lupus can be diagnosed with 98 percent specificity and 97 percent sensitivity.
From Hochberg (1997), with permission.

In studies in which women served as their own non-pregnant controls, investigators have universally reported increased disease activity during pregnancy (Petri, 1991; Ruiz-Irastorza, 1996; Zulman, 1980, and all their co-workers). In a review of her extensive experiences at Johns Hopkins, Petri (1998) reported an increased incidence of renal and hematological flares during pregnancy. Despite this, there was not an increase in the overall severity of flares measured using several indices. **One fact is certain: lupus can be life threatening to both mother and her fetus-infant.** The clinician must remain vigilant about the development of such life-threatening dangers.

In general, pregnancy outcome is better if:

1. Lupus activity has been quiescent for at least 6 months.
2. There is no active renal involvement manifest by proteinuria or renal dysfunction.
3. Superimposed preeclampsia does not develop.
4. There is no evidence of antiphospholipid antibody activity.

LUPUS NEPHROPATHY. Women with nephropathy whose disease stays in remission usually have a good pregnancy outcome. Packham and associates (1992) described their experiences in 41 women and found similar outcomes in 64 pregnancies before and after nephritis was diagnosed. Hypertension developed during almost half of pregnancies, and it was frequently early and severe. Likewise, proteinuria worsened in half of these women during pregnancy. Julkunen and colleagues (1993b) reported similar findings. Of the 125 pregnancies reported by Lockshin (1989), 63 percent of women with preexisting renal disease developed preeclampsia compared with only 14 percent of those without underlying renal disease. The World Health Organization has identified six classes of lupus glomerulonephritis. While proliferative lesions generally are associated with a more severe clinical course than membranous or mesangial lesions, 5-year survival of the former is now over 80 percent with cytotoxic drugs (Austin and Balow, 1999).

Although most authorities recommend continuation of immunosuppressive therapy during pregnancy in women with nephritis, it is not clear whether the dosage should be increased peripartum. While it is often stated that this is the time that activation or exacerbations are most likely to develop, firm evidence for this is not conclusive.

LUPUS VERSUS PREECLAMPSIA–ECLAMPSIA. Preeclampsia is common in all women with lupus, and superimposed preeclampsia is encountered even more often in those with nephropathy. It may be difficult, if not impossible, to differentiate lupus nephropathy from severe preeclampsia (Repke, 1998). Central nervous system involvement with lupus may culminate in convulsions similar to those of eclampsia. Thrombocytopenia, with or without hemolysis, may further confuse the diagnosis. It has not been proven if decreased complement values or increased anti-DNA titers are useful to identify worsening lupus activity. If identified, these laboratory features support the diagnosis of a renal flare. According to Petri (1998), most women with renal flares during pregnancy do not develop hypertension. In such problem cases, management is identical as for preeclampsia–eclampsia described in Chapter 24. Corticosteroid therapy is continued. The most common causes of death in these women when not pregnant are malignant hypertension with glomerulonephritis and neurological catastrophes such as seizures, strokes, and coma.

MANAGEMENT DURING PREGNANCY. Current management consists primarily of monitoring the clinical conditions of both maternal and fetal patients and a number of laboratory values in the mother. Monitoring of lupus activity and the identification of pending lupus flares by a variety of laboratory techniques has been recommended by some clinicians. The sedimentation rate is uninterpretable because of pregnancy-induced hyperfibrinogenemia. Although falling or low levels of complement components C_3, C_4, and CH_{50} are more likely to be associated with active disease, higher levels provide no assurance against disease activation. Varner and co-workers (1983) found no correlation between clinical manifestations of disease and C_3 and C_4 complement levels in half of their pregnant patients. Our experiences, as well as those of Lockshin and Druzin (1995), have been similar.

Frequent hematological evaluation and assessment of renal and hepatic functions are done to detect changes in disease activity during pregnancy and the puerperium. Hemolysis is characterized by a positive Coombs test, anemia, reticulocytosis, and unconjugated hyperbilirubinemia. Thrombocytopenia, leukopenia, or both, may develop. According to Lockshin and Druzin (1995), chronic thrombocytopenia in early pregnancy may be due to **antiphospholipid antibodies.** It also may be caused by lupus activity. Finally, thrombocytopenia may indicate the onset of preeclampsia.

Increased serum transaminase activity reflects hepatic involvement, as does a rise in serum bilirubin. Azathioprine therapy also may induce enzyme elevations. Urine is tested frequently to detect new-onset or worsening proteinuria. Overt proteinuria that persists is an ominous sign and is even more ominous if accompanied by other evidence for the nephrotic syndrome or abnormal serum creatinine.

The fetus should be closely observed for adverse effects imposed by a hostile intrauterine environment. Fetal growth is monitored closely and careful attention is given to the development of hypertension. Singsen and colleagues (1985) and Petri (1998) recommend screening for anti-SS-A and anti-SS-B antibodies, and if found, a search for fetal cardiac dysfunction and arrhythmias should be made (see p. 1385). Although we routinely evaluate the fetus for an arrhythmia, we do not screen for these antibodies. Antepartum fetal surveillance is done as outlined by the American College of Obstetricians and Gynecologists (1999) and as discussed in Chapter 40 (p. 1107). Farine and associates (1998) reported an 11 percent incidence of absent end-diastolic umbilical artery velocity in 56 fetuses. Unless hypertension develops, or there is evidence for fetal compromise or retarded growth, pregnancy is allowed to progress to term. Delivery decisions are made using obstetrical criteria. Peripartum corticosteroids in "stress doses" are given to women who are taking these drugs or who recently have done so.

PHARMACOLOGICAL TREATMENT. There is no cure and complete remissions are rare. Approximately a fourth of patients have mild disease, which is not life-threatening, but may be disabling because of pain and fatigue. Arthralgia and serositis are managed by **nonsteroidal anti-inflammatory drugs,** including aspirin. Because of the risk of premature closure of the fetal ductus arteriosus, therapeutic doses probably should not be used after 24 weeks. Low-dose aspirin, however, can be used safely throughout gestation in the management of the antiphospholipid syndrome (see p. 1394). Life-threatening and severely disabling manifestations are managed with **corticosteroids** such as prednisone, 1 to 2 mg/kg per day. After the disease is controlled, this is tapered to a daily dose of 10 to 15 mg given each morning. Corticosteroid therapy can result in the development of gestational or even insulin-dependent diabetes.

Immunosuppressive and cytotoxic agents such as *azathioprine* and *cyclophosphamide* are beneficial in controlling active disease (Hahn, 1998). In nonpregnant patients, they are usually reserved for lupus nephritis or disease that is steroid resistant. Azathioprine is less toxic and recommended daily oral doses are 2 to 3 mg/kg. It is avoided during pregnancy unless life-threatening complications develop. Although Ramsey-Goldman and associates (1993) found that women exposed to either drug did not have more adverse pregnancy outcomes, Enns and associates (1999) reported that cyclophosphamide is teratogenic. **Antimalarials** help control skin disease, and Parke and Rothfield (1996) and Petri (1998) recommend their continuation if in use.

For **severe lupus flares,** Petri (1998) recommends pulse therapy consisting of methylprednisolone, 1000 mg per 24 hours for 3 days, then return to maintenance doses if possible.

LONG-TERM PROGNOSIS AND CONTRACEPTION. In general, women with lupus and chronic vascular or renal disease should limit family size because of morbidity associated with the disease as well as increased adverse perinatal outcomes. Tubal sterilization may be advantageous. It is performed with greatest safety postpartum or any other time when the disease is quiescent. Oral contraceptives must be used with caution in women with lupus because vascular disease is a relatively common component. Progestin-only implants and injections provide effective contraception with no known effects on lupus flares. Intrauterine devices probably should not be prescribed if the woman is receiving immunosuppressive therapy (Chap. 58, p. 1539).

EFFECTS OF LUPUS ON THE FETUS AND NEONATE. There is no doubt that fetal growth restriction and perinatal mortality and morbidity are increased significantly in pregnancies complicated by lupus (Table 52–4). Prognosis is worsened with a lupus flare, significant proteinuria, renal impairment, and with associated hypertension and/or the development of preeclampsia (Aggarwal, 1999; Carmona, 1999; Rahman, 1998, and their associates).

The reasons at least partially responsible for adverse fetal consequences include decidual vasculopathy with placental infarction and decreased perfusion (Hanly and colleagues, 1988; Lubbe and Liggins, 1984). Magid and associates (1998) reported that these effects occur in the absence of antiphospholipid antibodies. Anti-SS-A (Ro) and anti-SS-B (La) antibodies may damage the fetal heart and conduction system causing neonatal

death (Alexander and co-workers, 1992; Tseng and Buyon, 1997).

NEONATAL LUPUS. This unusual syndrome is characterized by skin lesions—*lupus dermatitis*—and a variable number of hematological and systemic derangements, and occasionally congenital heart block (Tseng and Buyon, 1997). The incidence is about 5 to 10 percent. Lockshin and colleagues (1988) prospectively followed 91 infants born to women with lupus; four had definite neonatal lupus and four had possible disease.

Cutaneous lupus, thrombocytopenia, and autoimmune hemolysis are transient and clear within a few months (Lee and Weston, 1984). Weston and colleagues (1999) stress that thrombocytopenia and hepatic involvement are present as frequently as cardiac disease and therefore should be investigated.

CONGENITAL HEART BLOCK. This is the consequence of diffuse myocarditis and fibrosis in the region between the atrioventricular node and bundle of His. Miyagawa and associates (1997) reported that in Japanese women, some maternal HLA-DR5 haplotypes (DRB1*1101, DQA1*0501, and DQB1*0301) were associated with neonatal cutaneous lupus and others with congenital heart block (HLA-DQB1*062). Buyon and colleagues (1993) reported that congenital heart block occurred almost exclusively in infants of women with antibodies to the SS-A or SS-B antigens. Even in the

TABLE 52–4. Maternal and Perinatal Effects of Systemic Lupus Erythematosus

Outcome	Description
Maternal	
Lupus flare	Overall a third flare during pregnancy
Preeclampsia	Controversial if incidence is increased
	Flare can be life threatening (1 in 20 chance)
	Flares associated with worse perinatal outcomes
	Prognosis worse if antiphospholipid antibodies
	Increased incidence common with nephritis
Preterm labor	Increased
Perinatal	
Preterm delivery	Increased with preeclampsia
Growth restriction	Increased
Stillbirth	Increased, especially with antiphospholipid antibodies
Neonatal lupus	About 10 percent incidence—transient except for heart block

Data from Lockshin and Sammaritano (2000), Petri and Albritton (1993), and Yasmeen and co-workers (2000).

presence of such antibodies, however, the incidence of arrhythmia is only 3 percent (Lockshin and associates, 1988). The cardiac lesion is permanent and a pacemaker is generally necessary. Long-term outlook is not good, with a third of affected infants dying within 3 years (Waltuck and Buyon, 1994). The recurrence risk for neonatal cutaneous lupus is 25 percent and for congenital heart block it is 10 to 15 percent (Julkunen and colleagues, 1993a).

Maternal corticosteroid administration to treat fetal heart block is controversial. Richards and associates (1990) described such a fetus whose ascites cleared promptly with maternal corticosteroid therapy even though heart block and bradycardia persisted. Shinohara and colleagues (1999) reported no heart block in 26 neonates whose mothers received corticosteroid maintenance therapy before 16 weeks. By contrast, 15 of 61 neonates with heart block were born to women in whom corticosteroid therapy was begun after 16 weeks. Saleeb and colleagues (1999) recommend fluorinated steroids if therapy is given.

ANTIPHOSPHOLIPID ANTIBODIES. A number of antibodies directed against negatively charged phospholipids have been described and studied in detail over the past 25 years. These antiphospholipid antibodies include **lupus anticoagulant (LAC)** and **anticardiolipin antibod-** ies **(ACAs).** They may be of IgG, IgM, and IgA classes, alone or in combination. Although they may be found in normal persons, they also are associated with the **antiphospholipid antibody syndrome.** This is characterized by recurrent arterial and/or venous thromboses, thrombocytopenia, and fetal losses—especially stillbirths, during the second half of pregnancy (Meng and Lockshin, 1999; Oshiro and associates, 1996). The syndrome may occur alone or in association with systemic lupus erythematosus or other autoimmune disorders.

Feinstein and Rapaport (1972) introduced the term *lupus anticoagulant* in a review of acquired inhibitors of coagulation. This was based on the early recognition that certain patients with lupus had some tests of coagulation that were prolonged and thus suggested anticoagulant activity. Paradoxically, the so-called anticoagulant is powerfully thrombotic in vivo. This is despite that the lupus anticoagulant prolongs all phospholipid-dependent coagulation tests including the prothrombin time, partial thromboplastin time, and Russell viper venom time. Each of these tests requires a phospholipid surface to which other clotting factors attach and combine (Fig. 52–1).

Thus, detection of the lupus anticoagulant is based indirectly upon the prolongation of in vitro tests by this circulating antiphospholipid antibody. Anticardiolipin antibody usually is detected serologically using enzyme-

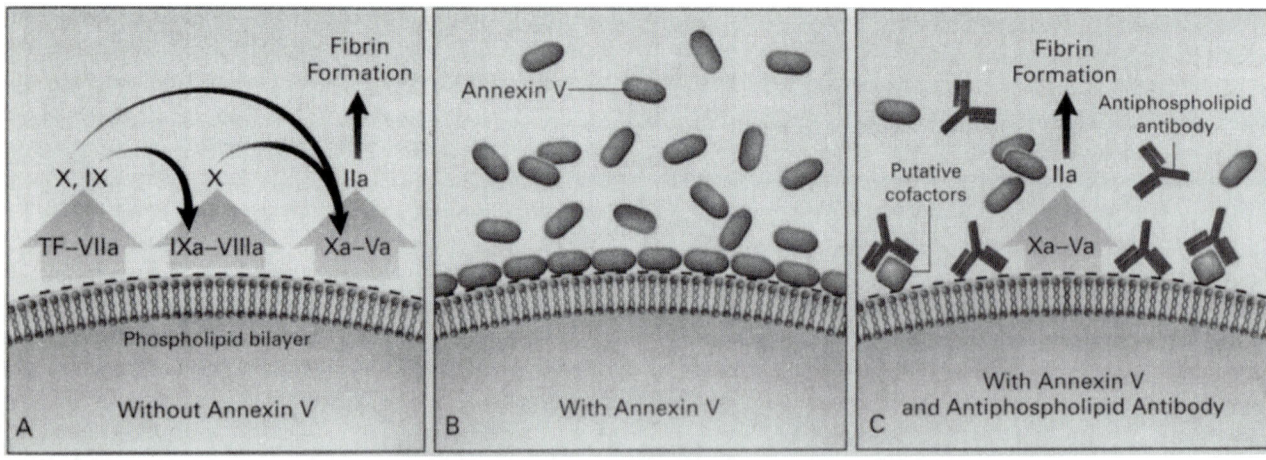

FIGURE 52–1. Mechanisms of the reduction of annexin V levels and acceleration of coagulation associated with antiphospholipid antibodies. **A.** Anionic phospholipids ($-$) on the surface of the cell-membrane bilayer serve as potent co-factors for assembly of three coagulation complexes: tissue-factor-VIIa (TF-VIIa) complex, IXa-VIIIa complex, and Xa-Va complex. The phospholipids thus accelerate blood coagulation by generating factors IXa and Xa. Factor Xa yields factor IIa (thrombin) and in turn cleaves fibrinogen to form fibrin. **B.** When antiphospholipid antibodies are absent, annexin V forms clusters that bind to the surface of anionic phospholipids and inhibit coagulation. **C.** Directly or through an interaction with protein-phospholipid co-factors, antiphospholipid antibodies disrupt the ability of annexin V to cluster on the phospholipid surface. This reduces binding affinity of annexin V, which permits more anionic phospholipid to be available to form complexes with coagulation proteins. Coagulation is thus accelerated and thrombosis promoted. (From Rand and colleagues, 1997a, with permission.)

linked immunoabsorbent assays (ELISA). Most often IgM anticardiolipin antibodies found alone are stimulated by infections or drugs and are innocuous (Silver and colleagues, 1996).

PATHOPHYSIOLOGY. Many patients with lupus have circulating antibodies either specifically directed against cardiolipin(s) or against phospholipid binding proteins such as β_2-glycoprotein I (apolipoprotein H). Anticardiolipin antibodies apparently bind directly to β_2-glycoprotein I, and these proteins act as a co-factor in this antigen–antibody reaction (Chamley, 1997).

The major activity of β_2-glycoprotein I appears to be its phospholipid-dependent anticoagulant inhibition of prothrombinase activity of platelets and adenosine diphosphate–induced platelet aggregation (Shi and colleagues, 1993). This results from the binding of this protein to negatively charged phospholipid surfaces such as activated platelets. Thus, β_2-glycoprotein I competitively inhibits the binding of coagulation factors, especially factor XII and the prothrombinase complex to negatively charged phospholipid surfaces and prevents activation of the coagulation cascade (Schousboe and Rasmussen, 1995). An antibody directed against β_2-glycoprotein I would bind and prevent it from acting as a phospholipid-dependent anticoagulant. This may not apply in all cases, because Laszlo and colleagues (1992) reported a patient with homozygous β_2-glycoprotein I deficiency who had no evidence of thrombotic episodes.

Beta$_2$-glycoprotein I is found in high concentrations on the surface of the syncytiotrophoblast. This might be expected, because it is a critical area to ensure that coagulation does not occur. Beta$_2$-glycoprotein I also may be involved in implantation, because it is known that this protein binds heparin. Moreover, trophoblastic cells have heparin-like binding sites. Thus, a local loss of β_2-glycoprotein I by an antibody directed against it might prevent implantation or result in intervillous-space thrombosis, or both (Chamley, 1997).

Lupus anticoagulant appears to require a co-factor for its in vitro anticoagulant function. Specifically, it does not bind directly to negatively charged phospholipids, but instead, it binds to phospholipid-bound prothrombin (Bevers and associates, 1991).

There are other phospholipid-binding proteins that may be involved in the pathophysiology of the antiphospholipid antibody syndrome. These include **protein C** and **protein S,** both endogenous anticoagulants, and **annexin V.** The latter is also known as placental anticoagulant protein I or lipocortin V, and it coats the syncytiotrophoblast in high concentration (Chamley, 1997). Thus, an antibody that binds protein C or S would result in venous, arterial, or decidual thrombosis, while binding of annexin V would result in coagulation and thrombosis in the intervillous space (Fig. 52–1).

Rand and co-workers (1997b) reported that placental tissue from pregnancy complicated by the antiphospholipid antibody syndrome had significantly less apical membrane-associated annexin V than a normal placenta. Exposure of placental villous cultures to five different antiphospholipid IgGs also resulted in a significant reduction in apical membrane annexin V. In another study, Rand and colleagues (1997a) found a reduction in annexin V in endothelial cell tissue cultures exposed to antiphospholipid antibodies. The pathophysiology of this sequence of events is illustrated in Figure 52–1.

These discoveries led to the development of direct assays to measure antibodies against β_2-glycoprotein I and prothrombin. The latter are increased in and associated with pregnancies complicated by the antiphospholipid antibody syndrome (Faden, 1997; Falcón, 1997; Forastiero, 1997; Ogasawara, 1996, and their co-workers). Conversely, others have not observed a clinically significant association with these antibodies (Caruso, 1999; Cuadrado, 1998; Lee, 1999; Leroy, 1998; Lynch, 1999, and all their associates).

ASSOCIATION OF ANTIPHOSPHOLIPID ANTIBODIES WITH LUPUS. There is considerable cross-reactivity with anticardiolipin and lupus anticoagulant antibodies and lupus. Love and Santoro (1990) reviewed 29 series that included over 1000 patients with lupus and reported an average frequency of 34 percent for lupus anticoagulant and 44 percent for anticardiolipin antibodies. In nearly half, both antibodies were found.

In general, patients with the lupus anticoagulant have higher levels of anticardiolipin antibodies, and about a third of those with biological false-positive tests for syphilis have anticardiolipin antibodies (Branch, 1990). Conversely, only about 20 percent of patients with identifiable anticardiolipin have the lupus anticoagulant. Importantly, in patients with lupus, documentation of either anticardiolipin or lupus anticoagulant is a risk factor for thrombosis, neurological disorders, or thrombocytopenia (Love and Santoro, 1990). As discussed in Chapter 33 (p. 834), these antibodies have also been associated with pregnancy loss (Kutteh and colleagues, 1999). Hojnik and colleagues (1996) reported that *Libman–Sacks endocarditis* is much more prevalent in lupus patients who have antiphospholipid antibodies. There is also an association with antiphospholipid antibodies and dilated postpartum cardiomyopathy and giant cell (temporal) arteritis (Airoldi and colleagues, 1996; Duhaut and associates, 1998). Finally, the association of these antibodies with the development of "primary" vaso-occlusive disease involving numerous different organs, but especially the kidney, has been documented by renal biopsy (Nochy and colleagues, 1999).

ANTIPHOSPHOLIPID ANTIBODIES IN NORMAL PREGNANCY.

Nonspecific antiphospholipid antibodies in low titers have been found in 3 to 6 percent of all otherwise healthy nonpregnant populations screened. Lockwood and colleagues (1989) studied 737 normally pregnant women without a history of recurrent pregnancy loss. They found that two (0.27 percent) had a lupus anticoagulant and 16 (2.2 percent) had elevated concentrations of either IgM- or IgG-anticardiolipin antibodies. Harris and Spinnato (1991) studied 1449 consecutive pregnant women and found 1.8 percent positive for IgG-anticardiolipin and 4.3 percent for IgM-anticardiolipin antibodies. Most assays were low positive (see later discussion) and did not correlate with adverse outcome. Pattison and co-workers (1993) studied 933 consecutive prenatal patients and found nine (0.1 percent) with anticardiolipin antibody, 11 (1.2 percent) with lupus anticoagulant, and two women with both. Yasuda and associates (1995) found that 7 percent of 860 pregnant Japanese women had anticardiolipin antibodies, and they had an increased risk of abortion, preeclampsia, and fetal growth restriction.

DIAGNOSIS.

A number of indications for testing are listed in Table 52–5. Lockshin and Druzin (1995) recommend a conservative interpretation of results to be based on repeated tests from a reliable laboratory that are consistent with each clinical case. Because only approximately 20 percent of patients with the antiphospholipid antibody syndrome have a positive lupus anticoagulant reaction alone, both the clotting test to identify the lupus anticoagulant and the anticardiolipin ELISA test must be performed.

Efforts have been made to standardize the anticardiolipin antibody by using ELISA. By agreement reached at the 1987 International Anti-Cardiolipin Workshop, values are reported in units and expressed as either *negative* or *low, medium,* or *high positive* (Harris and colleagues, 1987).

Tests for the lupus anticoagulant are nonspecific coagulation tests. The *partial thromboplastin time* is generally prolonged because the anticoagulant interferes with conversion of prothrombin to thrombin in vitro. Tests considered most specific are the *dilute Russell viper venom test (dRVVT)* and the *platelet neutralization procedure* (Lockwood and Rand, 1994). There is currently disagreement as to which of these is best for screening; but if any of the tests are positive after adding normal plasma, the diagnosis is confirmed.

Harris and co-workers (1998) developed two tests that they describe as more sensitive and specific for identifying the antiphospholipid antibody syndrome. These include an ELISA using β_2-glycoprotein I, which has a sensitivity from 40 to 90 percent and a specificity of 82 percent. The other is the APHL Phospholipid Mixture (Louisville APL Diagnostics), which is a kit with sensitivity of 98 percent and specificity of more than 99 percent (Merkel and colleagues, 1999). The kit may serve as a follow-up study in patients identified to have a positive anticardiolipin ELISA.

ANTIPHOSPHOLIPID ANTIBODIES AND PREGNANCY.

There is a strong association between the lupus anticoagulant and anticardiolipin antibodies with decidual vasculopathy, placental infarction, fetal growth restriction, early-onset preeclampsia, and recurrent fetal death. Some of these women, like those with lupus, also have a high incidence of venous and arterial thromboses, cerebral thrombosis, hemolytic anemia, thrombocytopenia, and pulmonary hypertension (Khamashta and colleagues, 1997; Silver and associates, 1994).

MECHANISM OF ACTION.

Although it is not precisely known how these act, a number of mechanisms have been proposed. It seems reasonable to conclude that the actions of antiphospholipid antibodies are multifactorial. According to Chamley (1997), platelets may be damaged directly by antiphospholipid antibody, or indirectly by binding β_2-glycoprotein I, which causes platelets to be susceptible to aggregation. Rand and colleagues (1997a, 1997b, 1998) propose that phospholipid-containing endothelial cell or syncytiotrophoblast membranes may be damaged directly by the antiphospholipid antibody or indirectly by antibody binding to either β_2-glycoprotein I or annexin V (see Fig. 52–1). This prevents the cell membranes from protecting the syncytiotrophoblast and endothelium and results in exposure of basement membrane. It is known that damaged platelets adhere to exposed basement membrane of endothelium and syncytiotrophoblast and

TABLE 52–5. Indications to Identify Lupus Anticoagulant and Antiphospholipid Antibodies

Recurrent pregnancy loss
Unexplained second- or third-trimester loss
Early-onset severe preeclampsia
Venous or arterial thrombosis
Unexplained fetal growth restriction
Autoimmune or connective-tissue disease
False-positive serological test for syphilis
Prolonged coagulation studies
Positive autoantibody tests

From Kutteh (1995), with permission.

result in thrombus formation (Lubbe and colleagues, 1983; Lubbe and Liggins, 1984).

There are other proposed mechanisms. Pierro and co-investigators (1999) reported that antiphospholipid antibodies decreased decidual production of the vasodilating prostaglandin E_2. Decreased fibrinolytic activity due to prekallikrein inhibition by lupus anticoagulant has been described (Sanfelippo and Drayna, 1981). Decreased protein C or S activity, as well as subtle increases in activation of prothrombin have been reported (Ogunyemi and associates, 2001; Zangari and colleagues, 1997). Amengual and co-workers (1998) presented evidence that thrombosis with the antiphospholipid syndrome is due to activation of the tissue factor pathway.

ADVERSE PREGNANCY OUTCOMES. Although there is no doubt that these antibodies are associated with increased fetal wastage, it is unclear as to the extent of these adverse sequelae. In most studies in which recurrent abortions and fetal deaths are described, women were usually included because they had repeated adverse outcomes. In the previously cited studies, the incidence of antiphospholipid antibodies in the general obstetrical population is about 3 to 5 percent. Data are too limited to draw conclusions concerning the impact of these antibodies on bad outcomes. According to the Utah group, fetal deaths are now more characteristic of these antibodies than first-trimester miscarriages (Ariel, 2001; Oshiro, 2000; Roque, 2001, and all their associates).

Looking at the issue another way, the incidence of these antibodies may be increased in adverse obstetrical outcomes associated with the syndromes. Polzin and colleagues (1991) identified antiphospholipid antibodies in a fourth of 37 women with growth-restricted fetuses. None had evidence for lupus anticoagulant. Branch and co-workers (1989) found a 16 percent incidence of antiphospholipid antibodies in 43 women with severe preeclampsia before 34 weeks. Six of the seven women with antibodies also had lupus anticoagulant, and one woman had multiple cerebral infarctions. Similarly, Moodley and associates (1995) observed an incidence of antibodies in 11 percent of 34 women with severe preeclampsia before 30 weeks.

When otherwise unexplained fetal deaths are examined, anticardiolipin antibodies do not appear to play a significant role. Haddow and co-workers (1991) measured anticardiolipin antibodies in 309 pregnancies with fetal death and found no differences when compared with 618 viable pregnancies. Similarly, Infante-Rivard and associates (1991) did not find an increased incidence of lupus anticoagulant or IgG anticardiolipin antibodies in a case-control study of 331 women with spontaneous abortion or fetal death.

TREATMENT GUIDELINES. Women with high-titer anticardiolipin antibody or with the presence of the lupus anticoagulant and a previous second- or third-trimester fetal death not attributable to other causes should be treated (Branch, 1998; Lockshin and Druzin, 1995). Similarly, some women with recurrent early-pregnancy loss and high titers of antibodies may benefit from therapy (Kutteh, 1996). A number of treatments for women with antiphospholipid antibodies have been evaluated, including low-dose aspirin, prednisone, heparin, and immunoglobulin (Coulam, 1995). These are thought to counteract the adverse action of antiphospholipid antibodies by affecting both the immune and coagulation systems.

Once daily **low-dose aspirin** (60 to 80 mg) blocks the conversion of arachidonic acid to thromboxane A_2 while allegedly sparing prostacyclin production (Kaaja and co-workers, 1993; Lellouche and colleagues, 1991). This would result in reduced thromboxane A_2—which aggregates platelets and causes vasoconstriction—while sparing prostacyclin, which has the opposite effect. There appear to be no major side effects from low-dose aspirin other than a slight risk of small vessel bleeding during surgical procedures.

Heparin most often is used in doses of 5000 to 10,000 units administered subcutaneously every 12 hours. Some authors recommend measurement of heparin levels because clotting tests may be altered by lupus anticoagulant. According to Cowchock (1998), preinjection levels are monitored to ensure protection of patients most at risk of thromboembolism. The rationale for heparin therapy is to prevent thrombotic episodes in both venous and arterial circulations, especially in women with a history of such events. Heparin therapy also prevents thrombosis in the microcirculation, including the decidual–trophoblastic interface (Toglia and Weg, 1996). As discussed, heparin binds to β_2 glycoprotein I, which covers the syncytiotrophoblast. This prevents binding of anticardiolipin and anti–β_2-glycoprotein I antibodies to their surfaces, which likely prevents cellular damage (Chamley, 1997; Schousboe and Rasmussen, 1995). Heparin also binds to antiphospholipid antibodies in vitro, and likely in vivo as well (Ermel and associates, 1995).

Heparin therapy is associated with a number of complications. These are discussed in detail in Chapter 46 (p. 1237) and include bleeding, thrombocytopenia, osteopenia, and osteoporosis. Although **low-molecular weight heparin** preparations have fewer adverse effects, Cowchock (1998) does not recommend their use. This is because activated partial thromboplastin tests (APTT) are not prolonged by these heparins and thus factor Xa inhibition tests are mandatory for monitoring anticoagulation effectiveness. Also, each preparation has a different molecular weight, renal clearance, and most importantly, biological consequences.

Glucocorticoids likely should not be used in the so-called primary antiphospholipid antibody syndrome; that is, those conditions without associated connective-tissue disorders. Even so, some patients with these conditions can be expected to develop over time an associated disorder such as lupus (Carbone and colleagues, 1999). In instances of "secondary" antiphospholipid syndromes, the dose of prednisone should be maintained at the lowest effective level to prevent flares (Kutteh, 1997). Steroid therapy has significant adverse effects, including osteopenia, osteoporosis, and pathological fractures (Shilletto and associates, 1996). Steroids also impede wound healing, and they induce gestational and overt diabetes (Laskin and co-workers, 1997).

Immunoglobulin therapy has usually been reserved for women with overt disease or heparin-induced thrombocytopenia, or both. It is also used when other first-line therapies have failed, especially when preeclampsia and fetal growth restriction were associated with these failures (Cowchock 1996, 1998; Petri, 1997; Silver and Branch, 1997). Immunoglobulin is administered intravenously in doses of 0.4 g/kg daily for 5 days (total dose of 2 g/kg). This is repeated monthly, or it is given as a single dose of 1 g/kg each month. Immunoglobulin has been evaluated in a preliminary placebo-controlled study by Branch and colleagues (2000), who showed that a definitive study was feasible. The drug costs the provider $5000 to $8000 for each 5-day course, and it may cause anaphylactic reactions, especially in women who have IgA deficiency due to anti-IgA antibodies. Aseptic meningitis also has been reported (Sekul and colleagues, 1994).

Immunosuppressive therapy has also not been well evaluated, but azathioprine and cyclosporine do not appear to improve standard therapies (Silver and Branch, 1997). Methotrexate and cyclophosphamide are contraindicated because of teratogenic potential (Enns and associates, 1999; Silver and Branch, 1997).

RESULTS WITH TREATMENT. Although improved outcomes are reported with some of the preceding treatments, Branch and associates (1985) caution that fetal growth restriction and preeclampsia still are common. Low-dose aspirin and corticosteroid therapy are not universally successful, and some women with lupus and antiphospholipid antibodies have normal pregnancy outcomes without treatment (Stafford-Brady and colleagues, 1988). Similarly, women with lupus anticoagulant and prior bad pregnancy outcomes have had liveborn infants without treatment (Trudinger and associates, 1988). Lockshin and co-workers (1989) reported that 23 of 32 women with a prior fetal death and antiphospholipid antibody greater than 40 IgG units, had a

recurrent fetal death despite treatment with prednisone or aspirin, or both.

Current data suggests the most efficacious therapy to be low-dose heparin—7500 to 10,000 units administered subcutaneously, twice daily—given along with low-dose aspirin, 60 to 80 mg once daily. If active lupus also is present, then prednisone is usually also given.

RHEUMATOID ARTHRITIS. This is a chronic multisystem disease characterized by a variety of systemic manifestations. Its cause is unknown, but the pathogenesis is immunologically mediated. Infiltrating T cells secrete cytokines that mediate inflammation and systemic symptoms. Its prevalence is about 0.8 percent, and women are affected three times more often than men. The cardinal feature is inflammatory synovitis that usually involves the peripheral joints. It has a propensity for cartilage destruction, bony erosions, and joint deformities. Disease onset is generally between ages 35 and 50.

There is a genetic predisposition, and 20 percent of monozygous twins and 5 percent of dizygous twins are concordant (Lipsky, 1998). There is also an association with the class II major histocompatibility complex molecules (HLA-DR4), which are important in the immune response. A prolonged duration of cigarette smoking also appears to increase the risk of rheumatoid arthritis in women (Karlson and colleagues, 1999). Hazes and colleagues (1990) reported a protective effect of pregnancy in the development of rheumatoid arthritis. An excellent review of its pathophysiology was provided by Firestein (1997).

CLINICAL MANIFESTATIONS. Rheumatoid arthritis is a chronic polyarthritis. In addition to symptoms of synovitis, the majority of patients have fatigue, anorexia, weakness, weight loss, and vague musculoskeletal symptoms. The hands, wrists, knees, and feet are commonly involved. Pain, aggravated by movement, is accompanied by swelling and tenderness. Extra-articular manifestations include rheumatoid nodules, vasculitis, and pleuropulmonary symptoms. Fortunately, the kidney usually is spared. The 1987 revised criteria of the American Rheumatism Association have approximately a 90 percent specificity and sensitivity for the diagnosis (Arnett and colleagues, 1988).

MANAGEMENT. Treatment is directed at pain relief, reduction of inflammation, protection of articular structures, and preservation of function. Treatment is important before cartilage loss is irreversible. Physical and occupational therapy and self-management instructions are essential. Aspirin or another one of the nonsteroidal anti-inflammatory drugs are the cornerstone of therapy. Aspirin therapy for nonpregnant patients consists of 3 to 4 g per day contained in enteric coated capsules. A blood level of 15 to 20 mg/dL is the desired therapeutic level. Tinnitus develops with blood levels of approximately 25 mg/dL. While other nonsteroidal agents are not more effective, their gastrointestinal tolerance may make them a better choice.

Glucocorticoid therapy may be added, and 7.5 mg of prednisone daily for the first 2 years of active disease substantively reduces progressive joint erosions (Kirwan and colleagues, 1995). Otherwise, corticosteroids are avoided if possible, but low-dose therapy is used by some along with salicylates. A variety of disease-modifying drugs and immunosuppressive therapy are used for more severe disease. Some have considerable toxicity and include hydroxychloroquine, sulfasalazine, low-dose methotrexate, gold compounds, and penicillamine. High-dose cyclosporine is reserved for the most severe cases. Orthopedic surgery for joint deformities, including replacement, is commonly performed.

EFFECTS OF PREGNANCY. In 1938, Hench reported marked improvement in the inflammatory component of rheumatoid arthritis during pregnancy. Conversely, postpartum exacerbation is common (Lockshin and Druzin, 1995). Because cortisol levels in plasma were considered to be markedly increased in pregnancy, Hench used cortisone to treat rheumatoid arthritis, and there was a favorable effect. It was subsequently demonstrated that increased secretion of cortisol did not account for all of the remissions. Sex hormones supposedly interfere with a number of putative processes involved in arthritis pathogenesis, including immunoregulation and interactions with the cytokine system (Masi and associates, 1999; Østensen, 1999; Wilder and Elenkov, 1999).

Unger and associates (1983) reported that amelioration of rheumatoid arthritis correlated with serum levels of **pregnancy-associated α_2-glycoprotein.** This compound has immunosuppressive properties and likely suppresses at least one mediator of an inflammatory response, interleukin-2 (Nicholas and colleagues, 1985). Nelson and co-workers (1993) later reported that amelioration of disease was associated with a disparity in HLA class II antigens between mother and fetus. They suggested that the maternal immune response to paternal HLA antigens may have a role in pregnancy-induced remission of arthritis.

Silman and associates (1992) performed a case-control study with 88 women with rheumatoid arthritis and reported that pregnancy had a "protective effect" for disease onset. Conversely, there was a sixfold increased likelihood of new-disease onset in the first 3 months postpartum. Iijima and associates (1998) observed only two new cases in 2547 postpartum women.

Barrett and co-workers (2000a) reported that a flare was more common if women were breast feeding.

In a prospective study, Østensen and Husby (1983) confirmed the amelioration of symptoms during early pregnancy in women with rheumatoid arthritis. They also described exacerbations within 3 months postpartum in 11 of 12 women. In a study from Leiden, van der Horst-Bruinsma and colleagues (1998) found that a favorable outcome was related to maternal–fetal MHC class II incompatibility. Conversely, Barrett and co-workers (2000b) performed a prospective study of 140 pregnant women recruited nationally in the United Kingdom and followed during the last trimester and at 1 and 6 months postpartum. There was only a modest fall in objectively assessed disease activity. Only 16 percent had complete remission. At least 25 percent had substantive levels of disability. Thus, while overall disease actually did not exacerbate postpartum, the mean number of inflamed joints increased significantly. Thus, most women with rheumatoid arthritis improve during pregnancy, some women develop disease during pregnancy, and others become worse (Nelson and Østensen, 1997).

Østensen (1991) reviewed outcomes of 76 pregnancies in 51 women with **juvenile rheumatoid arthritis.** Pregnancy had no effects on presentation of disease, but disease activity became quiescent or remained so during pregnancy. Postpartum flares were common, as discussed for rheumatoid arthritis. Joint deformities were common in these women, and 15 of 20 cesarean deliveries were done for contracted pelves or joint prostheses. These observations are supported by the summary of similar results in 39 Polish women with a history of juvenile rheumatoid arthritis (Musiej-Nowakowska and Ploski, 1999).

PERINATAL OUTCOME. There are no obvious adverse effects of rheumatoid arthritis on pregnancy outcome, including preterm labor (Klipple and Cecere, 1989). Although Kaplan (1986) reported that women who go on to develop the disease have had a higher than expected incidence of spontaneous abortion, Nelson and colleagues (1992) did not observe this.

MANAGEMENT DURING PREGNANCY. In most instances, women with rheumatoid arthritis can be reassured that successful pregnancy outcome is likely. Large doses of aspirin or other nonsteroidal anti-inflammatory drugs typically used for nonpregnant patients might adversely affect the fetus and neonate (Chap. 38, p. 1027). Concerns include impaired hemostasis, prolonged gestation, and premature closure of the ductus arteriosus (Briggs and colleagues, 1998). Nonetheless, these drugs remain appropriate for treatment of symptomatic women during pregnancy. Corticosteroids are also used as indicated. Gold compounds have been used in pregnancy, but their fetal effects are largely unknown. Immunosuppressive therapy with azathioprine, cyclophosphamide, or methotrexate is not routinely used during pregnancy. Of these, only azathioprine should be considered for use during pregnancy because the other agents are teratogenic (Buckley and co-workers, 1997; Enns and associates, 1999; Ramsey-Goldman and Shilling, 1997).

If cervical spine involvement exists, particular attention is warranted during pregnancy. Subluxation is common with such involvement, and pregnancy, at least theoretically, predisposes to this because of joint laxity, as discussed in Chapter 8 (p. 170). Intense involvement of certain joints may interfere with delivery; for example, severe hip deformities may preclude vaginal delivery.

CONTRACEPTION. Combination oral contraceptives are a logical choice because of their effectiveness, and the possibility they might improve rheumatoid arthritis (Bijlsma and associates, 1992). In fact, all reversible methods of contraception discussed in Chapter 58 are appropriate except that the intrauterine device should not be used in women receiving immunosuppressive therapy.

SYSTEMIC SCLEROSIS (SCLERODERMA). This is a multisystem disorder of unknown etiology characterized by fibrosis of skin, blood vessels, and visceral organs. Its prevalence averages 1 in 10,000, with a 3 to 1 female dominance. This strong prevalence for women and the increased incidence in the years following childbirth has led to the hypothesis that microchimerism may be involved in the pathogenesis of systemic sclerosis (Maloney and associates, 1999; Nelson and colleagues, 1998). Artlett and co-workers (1998) demonstrated Y-chromosomal DNA in 32 of 69 women (46 percent) with systemic sclerosis compared with 4 percent of controls. These investigators showed that low concentrations of male DNA may normally remain in the maternal circulation for decades after birth of a male infant (Chap. 37, p. 992). The reverse of this may occur in which maternal cells have been observed to engraft and persist in some immunodeficient infants. Maloney and colleagues (1999) have shown persistent maternal microchimerism in six of nine immunocompetent women with systemic sclerosis. Whether this contributes to the development of systemic sclerosis currently is unresolved (Russo-Stieglitz and colleagues, 2001).

CLINICAL COURSE. Symptoms in systemic sclerosis involve its attacks upon the gastrointestinal tract, heart, lungs, and kidneys. **Overlap syndrome** refers to the presence of systemic sclerosis with features of other connective-tissue disorders. **Mixed connective-tissue disease** is a term used for the syndrome involving features of lupus, systemic sclerosis, polymyositis, rheumatoid arthritis, and high titers of anti-RNP antibodies (see Table 52–1).

The hallmark of the disease is overproduction of normal collagen. This results in fibrosis of skin and the gastrointestinal tract, especially the distal esophagus. Pulmonary interstitial fibrosis along with vascular changes may cause pulmonary hypertension. Antinuclear antibodies are found in 95 percent of patients, and immunoincompetence is common. Common symptoms are Raynaud phenomenon (95 percent) and swelling of the distal extremities and face. Half of patients have symptoms from esophageal involvement, especially fullness and epigastric burning pain. Pulmonary involvement is common and causes dyspnea. Renal failure causes half of the deaths caused by systemic sclerosis. Mortality is high with renal or pulmonary involvement, and 10-year survival is less than 50 percent. There is, however, a small subset of patients who have a better prognosis. Women with CREST—calcinosis, Raynaud phenomenon, esophageal involvement, sclerodactyly, and telangiectasia—have milder disease.

There is no effective treatment. Therapy is symptomatic and directed at end-organ involvement. Corticosteroids are helpful only for inflammatory myositis and hemolytic anemia. The use of **angiotensin converting enzyme (ACE) inhibitors,** however, can be lifesaving (Steen, 1997, 1999). These agents should always be considered in the face of developing renal compromise or severe unresponsive hypertension. Steen (1999) reported the use of ACE inhibitors under such conditions during pregnancy without fetal effects, but these agents have been associated with severe fetal consequences.

The use of **recombinant human relaxin** in patients with systemic sclerosis was reported by Seibold and co-workers (1998). The results of this initial study, however, were inconclusive.

EFFECTS ON PREGNANCY. Pregnancy outcome with scleroderma probably is related to the severity of underlying disease. From their review of 94 cases, Maymon and Fejgin (1989) found that a third of women had exacerbations of symptoms during pregnancy; 15 percent died of hypertension, renal failure, or cardiopulmonary complications; and there was a 20 percent fetal mortality rate. The majority of maternal deaths have been case reports and do not accurately reflect the risks involved.

Steen and colleagues (1989, 1999) reported more optimistic outcomes in 214 women with scleroderma, 45 percent of whom had had diffuse disease. Major complications included *renal crisis* in three women characterized by malignant hypertension and renal failure. One woman died at 25 weeks; another was delivered preterm and died during hemodialysis 3 years later. The incidence of renal crisis was not considered different from that of nonpregnant women over the same period. They did not find an increased incidence of preeclampsia or hypertension. Infertility also was not a problem (Steen and Medsger, 1999).

In these studies by Steen and associates (1989, 1999), the risks for preterm delivery, fetal growth restriction, and perinatal mortality were increased, but not dramatically so. As some have reported for rheumatoid arthritis, a higher incidence of prediagnosis early pregnancy wastage was observed in these women in a case-controlled study (Silman and Black, 1988).

As perhaps expected, dysphagia and reflux esophagitis are aggravated by pregnancy (Steen, 1999). Treatment is described in Chapter 48 (p. 1276). Chin and colleagues (1995) described a woman with scleroderma who developed a Mallory–Weiss tear at 28 weeks from persistent vomiting despite therapy. Women with diffuse scleroderma or with hypertension, renal or cardiac involvement, or pulmonary fibrosis do poorly. Women with renal insufficiency and malignant hypertension have an increased incidence of superimposed preeclampsia. In the presence of rapidly worsening renal or cardiac disease, pregnancy termination should be considered.

Vaginal delivery may be anticipated, unless the soft-tissue changes wrought by scleroderma produce dystocia requiring abdominal delivery. Tracheal intubation for general anesthesia has special concerns because these women typically have limited ability to open their mouths (Black and Stevens, 1989). Because of esophageal dysfunction, aspiration is also more likely, and epidural analgesia is preferable.

Steen and Medsger (1999) emphasized that with careful timing of pregnancy in women without renal, pulmonary, or cardiac disease and with careful monitoring, successful pregnancy outcomes are achievable for both mother and fetus.

CONTRACEPTION. Due to the progressive and often unrelenting nature of this disease, permanent sterilization should be considered. Other forms of reversible contraception are acceptable, but hormonal agents, especially combination oral contraceptives, probably should not be used especially in women with pulmonary, cardiac, or renal involvement.

VASCULITIS SYNDROMES. Inflammation and damage to blood vessels may be primary or due to another disease. Most cases are presumed to be caused by immunopathogenetic mechanisms, specifically, immune-complex deposition. These syndromes are difficult to classify because of overlap. One current classification includes polyarteritis nodosa, hypersensitivity angiitis, Wegener granulomatosis, giant cell arteritis, and arteritis of collagen disease or miscellaneous arteritis (Valente and associates, 1997). Sneller and Fauci (1997) have presented a more extensive classification along with a scholarly review of the role of adhesion molecules and cytokines in the pathogenesis of these diffuse syndromes.

POLYARTERITIS NODOSA. Polyarteritis (periarteritis) nodosa is a rare disease with protean manifestations. The pathological lesion is necrotizing vasculitis of small- and medium-sized arteries. The classical variety is one of the progressive vasculitis syndromes characterized clinically by myalgia, neuropathy, gastrointestinal disorders, hypertension, and renal disease. Up to a third of cases are associated with hepatitis B antigenemia.

Symptoms are nonspecific and vague. Fever, weight loss, and malaise are present in over half of cases. Renal failure, hypertension, and arthralgias are common (Rao and associates, 1998). The diagnosis of polyarteritis nodosa is from classical findings of vasculitis on biopsy material of involved organs.

Treatment is largely ineffective and currently consists of high-dose prednisone and possibly cytotoxic medications (Allen and Bressler, 1997). Even with corticosteroid and immunosuppressive treatment, almost half of patients die within a year of diagnosis.

PREGNANCY. Only a few documented cases of polyarteritis nodosa in association with pregnancy have been reported. While definitive conclusions are unclear, certainly if active arteritis is identified during pregnancy, mortality is high. Owen and Hauth (1989) reviewed the courses of 12 pregnant women. In seven, polyarteritis first manifested during pregnancy, and it was rapidly fatal by 6 weeks postpartum. The diagnosis was not made until autopsy in six of the seven women. Five other women were in remission at conception. Four of these women continued pregnancy, resulting in one stillborn and three successful outcomes. Aya and co-workers (1996) described a woman with hepatitis B–associated polyarteritis who developed severe preeclampsia at 31 weeks.

WEGENER GRANULOMATOSIS. This is a necrotizing granulomatous vasculitis of the upper and lower respiratory tract and kidney. According to Sneller (1995), common lesions include sinusitis and nasal disease (90 percent), pulmonary infiltrates or nodules (85 percent), glomerulonephritis (75 percent), and musculoskeletal lesions (65 percent). It is uncommon and usually encountered after age 50. There have been only a few cases reported in association with pregnancy (Fields and colleagues, 1991; Palit and Clague, 1990). Pauzner and associates (1994) reviewed 15 pregnancies in 10 women with Wegener granulomatosis. In eight women with known disease preceding pregnancy, five had a relapse and two died. Luisiri and associates (1997) reviewed 13 cases associated with pregnancy and reported similar results.

ARTERITIS SYNDROMES. These uncommon syndromes involve medium- and large-sized arteries.

TEMPORAL OR GIANT CELL ARTERITIS. The diagnosis is usually established by biopsy of the temporal artery, but more recently, Schmidt and associates (1997) have reported that by utilizing color duplex ultrasonography of the temporal artery, a diagnosis can be made. They describe the specific image to be a dark halo that likely is due to edema of the artery wall. This sign was present in 73 percent of 30 patients with temporal arteritis.

TAKAYASU ARTERITIS. This is so-called *pulseless disease,* which is most prevalent in young women. When compared with temporal arteritis, the onset of Takayasu arteritis occurs almost exclusively in patients younger than 40 years of age. This form of arteritis also is associated with abnormal angiography of the upper aorta and its main branches, resulting in upper extremity vascular impairment (Michel and co-workers, 1996). Today, noninvasive methods, including computed tomography or magnetic resonance angiography, or both, can be used to detect this disorder prior to the development of severe vascular compromise (Numano and Kobayashi, 1999). There is no known serological test specific for Takayasu arteritis (Hoffman and Ahmed, 1998).

Takayasu arteritis may respond to corticosteroid therapy; however, surgical bypass sometimes is required to reestablish circulation. Severe renovascular hypertension, cardiac involvement, and pulmonary hypertension frequently preclude a good pregnancy outcome. Conversely, from their review of 14 cases, Nagey and colleagues (1983) reported good pregnancy outcomes. Other case reports and one series of four patients reported by Railton and Allen (1988) substantiate this optimism.

Most authors advise that blood pressure be taken in the lower extremity. Hemodynamic monitoring may be helpful if severe hypertension is identified (Winn and associates, 1988). Epidural analgesia has been advocated for labor and delivery (Crofts and Wilson, 1991).

DERMATOMYOSITIS AND POLYMYOSITIS (IDIOPATHIC INFLAMMATORY MYOSITIS). These are uncommon acute, subacute, or chronic inflammatory diseases of unknown cause involving skin and muscle, in particular. Prevailing theories are that the syndromes are caused by either viral infections or autoimmune disorders. At least a third of cases are associated with one of the connective-tissue disorders, including rheumatoid arthritis, lupus, mixed connective-tissue disease, or scleroderma. The disease may manifest as a severe generalized myositis with a cutaneous eruption, fever, and a fatal outcome within a few days or weeks. It may also assume a chronic form, characterized by the gradual development of paresis with little, if any, cutaneous or systemic involvement. Laboratory manifestations include elevated muscle enzymes in serum, and an abnormal electromyogram. Confirmation is by biopsy. The disease usually responds to high-dose corticosteroid therapy, and cytotoxic drugs such as azathioprine, cyclophosphamide, and methotrexate are reserved for refractory cases (Kofteridis and colleagues, 1999; Solomon and D'Alton, 1996).

About 15 percent of adults developing dermatomyositis have an associated malignant tumor. The time of appearance of the two diseases may be separated by several years. Extirpation of the malignant lesion sometimes is followed by a permanent remission of the dermatomyositis. The most common sites of associated cancer are breast, lung, stomach, and ovary. The uterus and cervix also have been reported as primary sites.

There are only a few reports of dermatomyositis complicating pregnancy. King and Chow (1985) reported five uneventful pregnancies in three women with dermatomyositis. In four of these, disease was inactive. Gutierrez and colleagues (1984) reviewed outcomes in 10 pregnancies among seven women with active disease. They reported three abortions, three perinatal deaths, and five preterm deliveries. Rosenzweig and colleagues (1989) reviewed 24 pregnancy outcomes in 18 women with primary polymyositis-dermatomyositis. In half, the diagnosis preceded pregnancy. Although they were in remission at conception, one fourth had an exacerbation in the second or third trimester. Excluding abortions, there were two perinatal deaths and two growth-restricted neonates. In the other half in whom disease became manifest first during pregnancy, outcomes were less favorable. One woman died 6 weeks postpartum when she suffered a severe exacerbation. Excluding abortions, half of the eight pregnancies resulted in perinatal death. Two fetuses developed ascites, and two were growth restricted. Ohno and associates (1992) described two women with established dermatomyositis who had evidence of disease activity during pregnancy but with good maternal and fetal outcomes. Papapetropoulos and co-workers (1998) reported two successful pregnancies and a therapeutic abortion in one of their patients. The therapeutic abortion was performed during an acute exacerbation.

The best form of contraception for these women is not known. Contraceptives containing hormones probably should not be used, especially combination estrogen–progestin contraceptives. Unfortunately, little data are available. While sterilization might seem at first to be an obvious choice, some women have mild chronic disease, and others may experience a permanent remission if an associated malignancy is identified and cured.

INHERITED CONNECTIVE-TISSUE DISORDERS

MARFAN SYNDROME. Marfan syndrome is an autosomal dominant connective-tissue disorder that affects both sexes equally. There appears to be no racial or ethnic basis for the syndrome. There are many mild cases in which the intrinsic connective tissue lesion is subclinical with no effect on longevity. Although the specific defect is still controversial, there is a degeneration of the elastic lamina in the media of the aorta. The cardiovascular lesion is the most serious abnormality, involving most of the ascending aorta and predisposing to aortic dilatation or dissecting aneurysm. Early death in Marfan syndrome is ultimately caused by either valvar insufficiency and congestive heart failure or rupture of a dissecting aneurysm. Mor-Yosef and colleagues (1988) report an increased frequency of dissecting and ruptured aneurysms during pregnancy. These were more likely in the last trimester. The syndrome was recently reviewed by Elkayam and associates (1995) and is discussed in detail in Chapter 44, (p. 1201).

EHLERS–DANLOS SYNDROME. This disease is characterized by a variety of changes in connective tissue, including hyperelasticity of the skin. In the more severe types of the syndrome, there is a strong tendency for fatal rupture of any of several arteries, causing strokes or bleeding. Rupture of the colon or uterus has been described. There are at least 11 types of disease based on skin, joint, or other tissue involvement. They include some autosomal dominant, some recessive, and some X-linked types. Their estimated aggregate prevalence is about 1 in 5000 (Prockop and colleagues, 1998). There is overlap between these types, and in most, the underlying molecular defect of collagen or procollagen is unknown. Types I, II, and III are autosomally dominant, and each accounts for about 30 percent of cases.

Women with Ehlers–Danlos syndrome have an increased frequency of preterm rupture of membranes and preterm delivery. There is also increased antepartum and postpartum hemorrhage, and tissue fragility makes episiotomy repair and cesarean delivery difficult. Multiple musculoskeletal abnormalities may develop or worsen during pregnancy, and back pain may be exacerbated (Klipple and Riordan, 1989). Sorokin and colleagues (1994) surveyed women members of the Ehlers–Danlos National Foundation, who reported a stillbirth rate of 3 percent, preterm delivery rate of 23 percent, cesarean delivery rate of 8 percent, and postpartum bleeding problems in 15 percent. Case reports and literature reviews have been provided by Hordnes (1994) and Sakala and Harding (1991).

REFERENCES

Aggarwal N, Sawhney H, Vasishta K, Chopra S, Bambery P: Pregnancy in patients with systemic lupus erythematosus. Aust N Z J Obstet Gynaecol 39:28, 1999

Airoldi ML, Eid O, Tosetto C, Meroni PL: Case report: Postpartum dilated cardiomyopathy in anti-phospholipid positive women. Lupus 5:247, 1996

Alexander E, Buyon JP, Provost TT, Guarnieri T: Anti-Ro/SSA antibodies in the pathophysiology of congenital heart block in neonatal lupus syndrome: An experimental model. Arthritis Rheum 35:176, 1992

Allen NB, Bressler PB: Diagnosis and treatment of the systemic and cutaneous necrotizing vasculitis syndromes. Med Clin N Am 81:243, 1997

Amengual O, Atsumi T, Khamashta MA, Hughes GRV: The role of the tissue factor pathway in the hypercoagulable state in patients with the antiphospholipid syndrome. Thromb Haemost 79:276, 1998

Ariel M, Elad R, Yaron Y, Amiram E, Lessing J, Kuperminc M: Third-trimester unexplained intrauterine fetal death is associated with inherited thrombophilia. Am J Obstet Gynecol 184:S10, 2001

Arnett FC: The genetics of human lupus. In Wallace DJ, Hahn BH (eds): Dubois' Lupus Erythematosus, 5th ed. Baltimore, Williams & Wilkins, 1997, p. 77

Arnett FC, Edworthy SM, Bloch DA, McShane DJ, Fries JF, Cooper NS, Healy LA, Kaplan SR, Liang MH, Luthra HS: The American Rheumatism Association 1987 revised criteria for the classification of rheumatoid arthritis. Arthritis Rheum 31:315, 1988

Artlett CM, Smith B, Jimenez SA: Identification of fetal DNA and cells in skin lesions from women with systemic sclerosis. N Engl J Med 338:1186, 1998

Austin HA, Balow JE: Natural history and treatment of lupus nephritis. Semin Nephrol 19:2, 1999

Aya AGM, Hoffet M, Mangin R, Balducchi JP, Eledjam JJ: Severe preeclampsia superimposed on polyarteritis nodosa. Am J Obstet Gynecol 174:1659, 1996

Barrett JH, Brennan P, Fiddler M, Silman A: Breast-feeding and postpartum relapse in women with rheumatoid and inflammatory arthritis. Arthritis Rheum 43:1010, 2000a

Barrett JH, Brennan P, Fiddler M, Silman AJ: Does rheumatoid arthritis remit during pregnancy and relapse postpartum? Results from a nationwide study in the United Kingdom performed prospectively from late pregnancy. Arthritis Rheum 42:1219, 2000b

Benjamin R, Parham P: HLA-B27 and diseases: A consequence of inadvertent antigen presentation. Rheum Dis Clin North Am 18:11, 1992

Bevers EM, Galli M, Barbui T, Comfurius P, Zwaal RF: Lupus anticoagulant IgG's (LA) are not directed to phospholipids only, but to a complex of lipid-bound human prothrombin. Thromb Haemost 66:629, 1991

Bijlsma JWJ, Van Den Brink HR: Estrogens and rheumatoid arthritis. Am J Reprod Immunol 28:231, 1992

Black CM, Stevens WM: Scleroderma. Rheum Dis Clin North Am 15:193, 1989

Branch DW: Antiphospholipid antibodies and reproductive outcome: The current state of affairs. J Reprod Immunol 38:75, 1998

Branch DW: Antiphospholipid antibodies and pregnancy. Semin Perinatol 14:139, 1990

Branch DW, Andres R, Digre KB, Rote NS, Scott JR: The association of antiphospholipid antibodies with severe pre-eclampsia. Obstet Gynecol 73:541, 1989

Branch DW, Peaceman AM, Druzin M, Silver RK, El-Sayed Y, Silver RM, Esplin MS, Spinnato J, Harger J: A multicenter, placebo-controlled pilot study of intravenous immune globulin treatment of antiphospholipid syndrome during pregnancy. The Pregnancy Loss Study Group. Am J Obstet Gynecol 182:122, 2000

Branch DW, Scott JR, Kochenour NK, Hershgold E: Obstetric complications associated with lupus anticoagulant. N Engl J Med 313:1322, 1985

Briggs GG, Freeman RK, Yaffee SJ: Drugs in Pregnancy and Lactation, 5th ed. Baltimore, Williams & Wilkins, 1998

Buckley LM, Bullaboy CA, Leichtman L, Marquez M: Multiple congenital anomalies associated with weekly low-dose methotrexate treatment of the mother. Arthritis Rheum 40:971, 1997

Buyon JP, Winchester RJ, Slade SG, Arnett F, Copel J, Friedman D, Lockshin MD: Identification of mothers at risk for congenital heart block and other neonatal lupus syndromes in their children. Comparison of enzyme-linked immunoabsorbent assay and immunoblot for measurement of anti SSA/Ro and anti SSB/La antibodies. Arthritis Rheum 36:1263, 1993

Carbone J, Orera M, Rodriguez-Mahou M, Rodriguez-Perez C, Sanchez-Ramon S, Seoane E, Rodriguez JJ, Zabay JM, Fernandez-Cruz E: Immunological abnormalities in primary APS evolving into SLE: 6 years' follow-up in women with repeated pregnancy loss. Lupus 8:274, 1999

Carmona F, Font J, Cervera R, Muñoz F, Cararach V, Balasch J: Obstetrical outcome of pregnancy in patients with systemic lupus erythematosus. A study of 60 cases. Euro J Obstet Gynecol Reprod Biol 83:137, 1999

Caruso A, DeCarolis S, DiSimone N: Antiphospholipid antibodies in obstetrics: New complexities and sites of action. Human Reprod Update 5:267, 1999

Chamley LW: Antiphospholipid antibodies or not? The role of β_2 glycoprotein I in autoantibody-mediated pregnancy loss. J Reprod Immunol 36:123, 1997

Chin KAJ, Kaseba CM, Weaver JB: Mallory–Weiss syndrome complicating pregnancy in a patient with scleroderma: Diagnosis and management. Br J Obstet Gynaecol 102:498, 1995

Coulam CB: Immunotherapy for recurrent spontaneous abortion: Early pregnancy. Bio Med 1:13, 1995

Cowchock S: Treatment of antiphospholipid syndrome in pregnancy. Lupus 7 (Suppl 2):S95, 1998

Cowchock S: Prevention of fetal death in the antiphospholipid antibody syndrome. Lupus 5:467, 1996

Crofts SL, Wilson E: Epidural analgesia for labour in Takayasu's arteritis: Case report. Br J Obstet Gynaecol 98:408, 1991

Cuadrado MJ, Tinahones F, Camps MT, DeRamon E, Gómez-Zumaquero JM, Mujic F, Khamashta MA, Hughes GRV: Antiphospholipid, anti-β_2 glycoprotein I and anti-oxidized-low-density-lipoprotein antibodies in antiphospholipid syndrome. Q J Med 91:619, 1998

Duhaut P, Berruyer M, Pinede L, Demolombe-Rague S, Loire R, Seydoux D, Dechavanne M, Ninet J, Pasquier J, Groupe de Recherché sur L'Artérite á Cellules Géantes: Anticardiolipin antibodies and giant cell arteritis. Arthritis Rheumatol 41:701, 1998

Elkayam U, Ostrzega E, Shotan A, Mehra A: Cardiovascular problems in pregnant women with the Marfan syndrome. Ann Intern Med 123:117, 1995

Enns GM, Roeder E, Chan RT, Catts ZA-K, Cox VA, Golabi M: Apparent cyclophosphamide (Cytoxan) embryopathy: A distinct phenotype? Am J Med Genet 86:237, 1999

Ermel LD, Marshburn PB, Kutteh WH: Interaction of heparin with antiphospholipid antibodies (APA) from the sera of women with recurrent pregnancy loss (RPL). Am J Reprod Immunol 33:14, 1995

Faden D, Tincani A, Tanzi P, Spatola L, Lojacono A, Tarantini M, Balestieri G: Anti-beta 2 glycoprotein I antibodies in a general obstetric population: Preliminary results on the prevalence and correlation with pregnancy outcome. Anti-β_2 glycoprotein I antibodies are associated with some obstetrical complications, mainly preeclampsia–eclampsia. Euro J Obstet Gynecol Reprod Biol 73:37, 1997

Falcón CR, Martinuzzo ME, Forastiero RR, Cerrato GS, Carreras LO: Pregnancy loss and autoantibodies against phospholipid-binding proteins. Obstet Gynecol 89:975, 1997

Farine D, Granovsky-Grisaru S, Ryan G, Seaward GR, Teoh TG, Laskin C, Ritchie JWK: Umbilical artery blood flow velocity in pregnancies complicated by systemic lupus erythematosus. J Clin Ultrasound 26:379, 1998

Feinstein DI, Rapaport SI: Acquired inhibitors of blood coagulation. In Spaet TH (ed): Progress in Hemostasis and Thrombosis, Vol 1. New York, Grune and Stratton, 1972, p 75.

Fields GL, Ossorio MA, Roy TM, Bunke CM: Wegener's granulomatosis complicated by pregnancy: A case report. J Reprod Med 36:463, 1991

Firestein G: Etiology and pathogenesis of rheumatoid arthritis. In Kelley WN, Harris ED, Ruddy S, Sledge CB (eds): Textbook of Rheumatology, Vol 1, 5th ed. Philadelphia, Saunders, 1997, p 851

Forastiero RR, Marinuzzo ME, Cerrato GS, Kordich LC, Carreras LO: Relationship of anti-β_2 glycoprotein I and anti-prothrombin antibodies to thrombosis and pregnancy loss in patients with antiphospholipid antibodies. Thromb Haemost 78:1008, 1997

Gladman DD, Urowitz MB: Systemic lupus erythematosus—clinical features. In Klippel JH, Dieppe PA (eds): Rheumatology. St. Louis, Mosby, 1997, p 7.1

Gutierrez G, Dagnino R, Mintz G: Polymyositis/dermatomyositis and pregnancy. Arthritis Rheum 27:291, 1984

Haddow JE, Rote NS, Dostal-Johnson D, Palomaki GE, Pulkkinen AJ, Knight GJ: Lack of an association between late fetal death and antiphospholipid antibody measurements in the second trimester. Am J Obstet Gynecol 165:1308, 1991

Hahn BH: Systemic lupus erythematosus. In Braunwald E, Fauci AS, Hauster SL, Isselbacher KJ, Kasper DL, Longo DL, Martin JB, Wilson JD (eds): Harrison's Principles of Internal Medicine, 14th ed. New York, McGraw-Hill, 1998, p 1874

Hann BH: Pathogenesis of systemic lupus erythematosus. In Kelley WN, Harris ED, Ruddy S, Sledge CB (eds): Textbook of Rheumatology, Vol 2, 5th ed. Philadelphia, Saunders, 1997, p 1015

Hanly JG, Gladman DD, Rose TH, Laskin CA, Urowitz MB:

Lupus pregnancy: A prospective study of placental changes. Arthritis Rheum 31:358, 1988

Harris EN, Gharavi AE, Patel SP, Hughes GVR: Evaluation of the anti-cardiolipin antibody test: Report of an international workshop. Clin Exp Immunol 68:215, 1987

Harris EN, Pierangeli SS, Gharavi AE: Diagnosis of the antiphospholipid syndrome: A proposal for use of laboratory tests. Lupus 7(Suppl 2): S144, 1998

Harris EN, Spinnato JA: Should anticardiolipin tests be performed in otherwise healthy pregnant women? Am J Obstet Gynecol 165:1272, 1991

Hazes JMW, Dijkmans BAC, Vandenbroucke JP, De Vries RRP, Cats A: Pregnancy and the risk of developing rheumatoid arthritis. Arthritis Rheum 33:1770, 1990

Hench PG: Ameliorating effect of pregnancy on chronic atrophic (infectious rheumatoid) arthritis, fibrositis and intermittent hydrarthrosis. Proc Mayo Clin 13:161, 1938

Hochberg MC: Updating the American College of Rheumatology revised criteria for the classification of systemic lupus erythematosus. Arthritis Rheum 40:1725, 1997

Hoffman GS, Ahmed AE: Surrogate markers of disease activity in patients with Takayasu arteritis: A preliminary report from the International Network for the study of the systemic vasculitides (INSSYS). Int J Cardiol 66 (Suppl 1):S191, 1998

Hojnik M, George J, Ziporen L, Shoenfeld Y: Heart valve involvement (Libman–Sacks endocarditis) in the antiphospholipid syndrome. Circulation 93:1579, 1996

Hordnes K: Ehlers–Danlos syndrome and delivery. Acta Obstet Gynecol Scand 73:671, 1994

Iijima T, Tada H, Hidaka Y, Yagoro A, Mitsuda N, Kanzaki T, Murata Y, Amino N: Prediction of postpartum onset of rheumatoid arthritis. Ann Rheum Dis 57:460, 1998

Infante-Rivard C, David M, Gauthier R, Rivard GE: Lupus anticoagulants, anticardiolipin antibodies, and fetal loss: A case-control study. N Engl J Med 325:1063, 1991

Jacobsen S, Petersen J, Ullman S, Junker P, Voss A, Rasmussen JM, Tarp U, Poulsen LH, van Overeem Hansen G, Skaarup B, Hansen TM, Pødenphant J, Halberg P: Mortality and causes of death of 513 Danish patients with systemic lupus erythematosus. Scand J Rheumatol 28:75, 1999

Julkunen H, Jouhikainen T, Kaaja R, Leirisalo-Repo M, Stephansson E, Palosuo T, Teramo K, Friman C: Fetal outcomes in lupus pregnancy: A retrospective case control study of 242 pregnancies in 112 patients. Lupus 2:125, 1993a

Julkunen H, Kaaja R, Palosuo T, Grönhagen-Riska C, Teramo K: Pregnancy in lupus nephropathy. Acta Obstet Gynecol Scand 72:258, 1993b

Kaaja R, Julkunen H, Viinikka L, Ylikorkala O: Production of prostacyclin and thromboxane in lupus pregnancies: Effect of small dose of aspirin. Obstet Gynecol 81:327, 1993

Kaplan D: Fetal wastage in patients with rheumatoid arthritis. J Rheumatol 13:875, 1986

Karlson EW, Lee I-M, Cook NR, Manson JE, Buring JE, Hennekens CH: A retrospective cohort study of cigarette smoking and risk of rheumatoid arthritis in female health professionals. Arthritis Rheum 42:910, 1999

Khamashta MA, Ruiz-Irastorza G, Hughes GRV: Systemic lupus erythematosus flares during pregnancy. Rheum Dis Clin North Am 23:15, 1997

King CR, Chow S: Dermatomyositis and pregnancy. Obstet Gynecol 66:589, 1985

Kirwan JR, the Arthritis and Rheumatism Council Low-Dose Glucocorticoid Study Group: The effect of glucocorticoids on joint destruction in rheumatoid arthritis. N Engl J Med 333:142, 1995

Klipple GL, Cecere FA: Rheumatoid arthritis and pregnancy. Rheum Dis Clin North Am 15:213, 1989

Klipple GL, Riordan KK: Rare inflammatory and hereditary connective tissue diseases. Rheum Dis Clin North Am 15:383, 1989

Kofteridis DP, Malliotakis PI, Sotsiou F, Vardakis NK, Vamvakas LN, Emmanouel DS: Acute onset of dermatomyositis presenting in pregnancy with rhabdomyolysis and fetal loss. Scand J Rheumatol 28:192, 1999

Kutteh WH: Antiphospholipid antibodies and reproduction. J Reprod Immunol 35:151, 1997

Kutteh WH: Antiphospholipid antibody–associated recurrent pregnancy loss: Treatment with heparin and low-dose aspirin is superior to low-dose aspirin alone. Am J Obstet Gynecol 174:1584, 1996

Kutteh WH: Recurrent pregnancy loss. Williams Obstetrics, 19th ed (Suppl 15). Stamford, CT, Appleton & Lange, October/November 1995

Kutteh WH, Rote NS, Silver R: Antiphospholipid antibodies and reproduction: The antiphospholipid antibody syndrome. AJRI 41:133, 1999

Laskin CA, Bombardier C, Hannah M, Mandel FP, Ritchie JW, Farewell V, Farine D, Spitzer K, Fielding L, Solonninka CA, Yeung M: Prednisone and aspirin in women with autoantibodies and unexplained recurrent fetal loss. N Engl J Med 337:148, 1997

Laszlo FJM, Bansci M, van der Linden IK, Bertina RM: β2 glycoprotein 1 deficiency and the risk of thrombosis. Thromb Haemost 67:649, 1992

Lee LA, Weston WL: New findings in neonatal lupus syndrome. Am J Dis Child 138:233, 1984

Lee RM, Emlen W, Scott JR, Branch DW, Silver RM: Anti-β2 glycoprotein I antibodies in women with recurrent spontaneous abortion, unexplained fetal death, and antiphospholipid syndrome. Am J Obstet Gynecol 181:642, 1999

Lellouche F, Martinuzzo M, Said P, Maclouf J, Carreras LO: Imbalance of thromboxane/prostacyclin biosynthesis in patients with lupus anticoagulant. Blood 78:2894, 1991

Leroy V, Arvieux J, Jacob M-C, Maynard-Muet M, Baud M, Zarski J-P: Prevalence and significance of anticardiolipin, anti-β2 glycoprotein I and anti-prothrombin antibodies in chronic hepatitis C. Br J Haematol 101:468, 1998

Lipsky PE: Rheumatoid arthritis. In Braunwald E, Fauci AS, Hauser SL, Isselbacher DJ, Longo DL, Martin JB, Kasper DL, Wilson JD (eds): Harrison's Principles of Internal Medicine, 14th ed. New York, McGraw-Hill, 1998, p 1880

Lockshin MD: Why do women have rheumatic disease? Scan J Rheumatol 107:5, 1998

Lockshin MD: Pregnancy does not cause systemic lupus erythematosus to worsen. Arthritis Rheum 32:665, 1989

Lockshin MD, Bonfa E, Elkon K, Druzin ML: Neonatal lupus risk to newborns of mothers with systemic lupus erythematosus. Arthritis Rheum 31:697, 1988

Lockshin MD, Druzin ML: Rheumatic disease. In Barron WM, Lindheimer JD (eds): Medical Disorders During Pregnancy, 2nd ed. St. Louis, Mosby, 1995, p 307

Lockshin MD, Druzin ML, Qamar T: Prednisone does not prevent recurrent fetal death in women with antiphospholipid antibody. Am J Obstet Gynecol 160:439, 1989

Lockshin MD, Sammaritano LR: Rheumatic disease. In Barron WM, Lindheimer MD (eds): Medical Disorders During Pregnancy, 3rd ed. St. Louis, Mosby, 2000, p 355

Lockwood CJ, Rand JH: The immunobiology and obstetrical

consequences of antiphospholipid antibodies. Obstet Gynecol Surv 49:432, 1994

Lockwood CJ, Romero R, Feinberg RF, Clyne LP, Coster B, Hobbins JC: The prevalence and biologic significance of lupus anticoagulant and anticardiolipin antibodies in a general obstetric population. Am J Obstet Gynecol 161:369, 1989

Love PE, Santoro SA: Antiphospholipid antibodies: Anticardiolipin and the lupus anticoagulant in systemic lupus erythematosus (SLE) and in non-SLE disorders. Ann Intern Med 112:682, 1990

Lubbe WF, Liggins GC: The lupus-anticoagulant: Clinical and obstetric complications. N Z Med J 97:398, 1984

Lubbe WFF, Palmer SJ, Butler WS, Liggins GC: Fetal survival after prednisone suppression of maternal lupus anticoagulant. Lancet 2:1361, 1983

Luisiri P, Lance NJ, Curran JJ: Wegener's granulomatosis: Time to change the standard of care. Arthritis Rheum 40:2099, 1997

Lynch A, Byers T, Emlen W, Rynes D, Shetterly SM, Hamman RF: Association of antibodies to Beta$_2$-glycoprotein 1 with pregnancy loss and pregnancy-induced hypertension: A prospective study in low-risk pregnancy. Obstet Gynecol 93:193, 1999

Magid MS, Kaplan C, Sammaritano LR, Peterson M, Druzin ML, Lockshin MD: Placental pathology in systemic lupus erythematosus: A prospective study. Am J Obstet Gynecol 179:226, 1998

Maloney S, Smith A, Furst DE, Myerson D, Rupert K, Evans PC, Nelson JL: Microchimerism of maternal origin persists into adult life. J Clin Invest 104:41, 1999

Masi AT, Chatterton RT, Aldag JC: Perturbations of hypothalamic–pituitary–gonadal axis and adrenal androgen functions in rheumatoid arthritis: An odyssey of hormonal relationships to the disease. Ann NY Acad Sci 876:53, 1999

Maymon R, Fejgin M: Scleroderma in pregnancy. Obstet Gynecol Surv 44:530, 1989

Meng C, Lockshin M: Pregnancy in lupus. Curr Opin Rheumatol 11:348, 1999

Merkel PA, Chang Y, Pierangeli SS, Harris EN, Polisson RP: Comparison between the standard anticardiolipin antibody test and a new phospholipid test in patients with connective tissue diseases. J Rheumatol 26:591, 1999

Michel BA, Arend WP, Hunder GG: Clinical differentiation between giant cell (temporal) arteritis and Takayasu's arteritis. J Rheumatol 23:106, 1996

Mills JA: Systemic lupus erythematosus. N Engl J Med 330:1871, 1994

Miyagawa S, Shinohara K, Kidoguchi K, Fujita T, Fukumoto T, Yamashina Y, Hashimoto K, Yoshioka A, Sakurai S, Nishihara O, Shirai T: Neonatal lupus erythematosus: HLA-DR and -DQ distributions are different among the groups of anti-Ro/SSA-positive mothers with different neonatal outcomes. J Invest Dermatol 108:881, 1997

Moll JMH: The place of psoriatic arthritis in the spondarthritides. Baillière's Clin Rheumatol 8:395, 1994

Moodley J, Bhoola V, Duursma J, Pudifin D, Byrne S, Kenoyer DG: The association of antiphospholipid antibodies with severe early-onset preeclampsia. S Afr Med J 85:105, 1995

Mor-Yosef S, Younis J, Granat M, Kedari A, Milgalter A, Schenker JG: Marfan's syndrome in pregnancy. Obstet Gynecol Surv 43:382, 1988

Musiej-Nowakowska E, Ploski R: Pregnancy and early onset pauciarticular juvenile chronic arthritis. Ann Rheum Dis 58:475, 1999

Nagey DA, Fortier KJ, Hayes BA, Linder J: Takayasu's arteri-

tis in pregnancy: A case presentation demonstrating the absence of placental pathology. Am J Obstet Gynecol 147:463, 1983

Nelson JL, Furst DE, Maloney S, Gooley T, Evans PC, Smith A, Bean MA, Ober C, Bianchi DW: Microchimerism and HLA-compatible relationships of pregnancy in scleroderma. Lancet 351:559, 1998

Nelson JL, Hughes KA, Smith AG, Nisperos BB, Branchaud AM, Hansen JA: Maternal–fetal disparity in HLA class II alloantigens and the pregnancy-induced amelioration of rheumatoid arthritis. N Engl J Med 329:466, 1993

Nelson JL, Østensen M: Pregnancy and rheumatoid arthritis. Rheum Dis Clin North Am 23:195, 1997

Nelson JL, Voigt LF, Koepsell TD, Dugowson CE, Daling JR: Pregnancy outcome in women with rheumatoid arthritis before disease onset. J Rheumatol 19:18, 1992

Nicholas NS, Panayi GS, Nouri AME: Human pregnancy serum inhibits interleukin-2 production. Clin Exp Immunol 58:587, 1985

Nochy D, Daugas E, Droz D, Beaufils H, Grünfeld J-P, Piette J-C, Bariety J, Hill G: The intrarenal vascular lesions associated with primary antiphospholipid syndrome. J Am Soc Nephrol 10:507, 1999

Numano F, Kobayashi Y: Takayasu arteritis—beyond pulselessness. Intern Med 38:226, 1999

Ogasawara M, Aoki K, Matsuura E, Sasa H, Yagami Y: Anti-β_2 glycoprotein I antibodies and lupus anticoagulant in patients with recurrent pregnancy loss: Prevalence and clinical significance. Lupus 5:587, 1996

Ogunyemi D, Francisco C: Venous thromboembolism and associated thrombophilias in pregnancy. Am J Obstet Gynecol 184:S192, 2001

Ohno T, Imai A, Tamaya T: Successful outcomes of pregnancy complicated with dermatomyositis. Gynecol Obstet Invest 33:187, 1992

Oshiro BT, Silver RM, Scott JR, Yu H, Branch W: Antiphospholipid antibodies and fetal death. Obstet Gynecol 87:489, 1996

Østensen M: Sex hormones and pregnancy in rheumatoid arthritis and systemic lupus erythematosus. Ann NY Acad Sci 876:131, 1999

Østensen M: Pregnancy in patients with a history of juvenile rheumatoid arthritis. Arthritis Rheum 34:881, 1991

Østensen M, Husby G: A prospective clinical study of the effect of pregnancy on rheumatoid arthritis and ankylosing spondylitis. Arthritis Rheum 26:1155, 1983

Owen J, Hauth JC: Polyarteritis nodosa in pregnancy: A case report and brief literature review. Am J Obstet Gynecol 160:606, 1989

Packham DK, Lam SS, Nicholls K, Fairley KF, Kincaid-Smith PS: Lupus nephritis and pregnancy. QJM 83:315, 1992

Palit J, Clague RB: Wegener's granulomatosis presenting during first trimester of pregnancy. Br J Rheumatol 29:389, 1990

Papapetropoulos T, Kanellakopoulou N, Tsibri E, Paschalis C: Polymyositis and pregnancy: Report of a case with three pregnancies. J Neurol Neurosurg Psychiatry 64:406, 1998

Parke AL, Rothfield NF: Antimalarial drugs in pregnancy—the North American experience. Lupus 5(Suppl 1):S67, 1996

Pattison NS, Chamley LW, McKay EJ, Liggins GC, Butler WS: Anti-phospholipid antibodies in pregnancy: Prevalence and clinical associations. Br J Obstet Gynaecol 100:909, 1993

Pauzner R, Mayan H, Hershko E, Alcalay M, Farfel Z: Exacerbation of Wegener's granulomatosis during pregnancy: Report of a case with tracheal stenosis and literature review. J Rheumatol 21:1153, 1994

Petri M: Pregnancy in SLE. Baillière's Clin Rheumatol 12:449, 1998

Petri M: Hopkins lupus pregnancy center: 1987–1996. Rheum Dis Clin North Am 23:1, 1997

Petri M, Allbritton J: Fetal outcome of lupus pregnancy: A retrospective case-control study of the Hopkins Lupus Cohort. J Rheumatol 20:650, 1993

Petri M, Howard D, Repke J: Frequency of lupus flare in pregnancy: The Hopkins lupus pregnancy center experience. Arthritis Rheum 34:1538, 1991

Pierro E, Cirino G, Bucci MR, Lazzarin N, Andreani CL, Mancuso S, Lanzone A, Navarra P: Antiphospholipid antibodies inhibit prostaglandin release by decidual cells of early pregnancy: Possible involvement of extracellular secretory phospholipase A_2. Fertil Steril 71:342, 1999

Polzin WJ, Kopelman JN, Robinson RD, Read JA, Brady K: The association of antiphospholipid antibodies with pregnancies complicated by fetal growth restriction. Obstet Gynecol 78:1108, 1991

Prockop DJ, Kuivaniemi H, Tromp G: Inherited disorders of connective tissue. In Braunwald E, Fauci AS, Hauser SL, Isselbacher KJ, Kasper DL, Longo DL, Martin JB, Wilson JD (eds): Harrison's Principles of Internal Medicine, 14th ed. New York, McGraw-Hill, 1998, p 2183

Rahman P, Gladman DD, Urowitz MB: Clinical predictors of fetal outcome in systemic lupus erythematosus. J Rheumatol 25:1526, 1998

Railton A, Allen DG: Takayasu's arteritis in pregnancy. A report of 4 cases. S Afr Med J 73:123, 1988

Ramsey-Goldman R, Mientus MJ, Kutzer JE, Mulvihill J, Medsger TA Jr: Pregnancy outcome in women with systemic lupus erythematosus treated with immunosuppressive drugs. J Rheumatol 20:1152, 1993

Ramsey-Goldman R, Schilling E: Immunosuppressive drug use during pregnancy. Rheum Dis Clin N Am 23:149, 1997

Rand JH: Antiphospholipid antibody syndrome: New insights on thrombogenic mechanisms. Am J Med Sci 316:142, 1998

Rand JH, Wu X-X, Andree HAM, Lockwood CJ, Guller S, Scher J, Harpel PC: Pregnancy loss in the antiphospholipid-antibody syndrome—A possible thrombogenic mechanism. N Engl J Med 337:154, 1997a

Rand JH, Wu X-X, Guller S, Scher J, Andree HAM, Lockwood CJ: Antiphospholipid immunoglobulin G antibodies reduce annexin-V levels on syncytiotrophoblast apical membranes and in culture media of placental villi. Am J Obstet Gynecol 177:918, 1997b

Rao JK, Allen NB, Pincus T: Limitations of the 1990 American College of Rheumatology classification criteria in the diagnosis of vasculitis. Ann Intern Med 129:345, 1998

Repke JT: Hypertensive disorders of pregnancy: Differentiating preeclampsia from active systemic lupus erythematosus. J Reprod Med 43:350, 1998

Richards DS, Wagman AJ, Cabaniss ML: Ascites not due to congestive heart failure in a fetus with lupus-induced heart block. Obstet Gynecol 76:957, 1990

Roque H, Paidas M, Rebarber A, Maturi J, O'Neill L, Kuczynski E, Lockwood C: Maternal thrombophilia is associated with second- and third-trimester fetal death. Am J Obstet Gynecol 184:S27, 2001

Rosenzweig BA, Rotmensch S, Binette SP, Phillippe M: Primary idiopathic polymyositis and dermatomyositis complicating pregnancy: Diagnosis and management. Obstet Gynecol Surv 44:162, 1989

Rubin RL: Drug induced lupus. In Wallace DJ, Hahn BH (eds): Dubois' Lupus Erythematosus, 5th ed. Baltimore, Williams & Wilkins, 1997, p 871

Ruiz-Irastorza G, Lima F, Alves J, Khamashta MA, Simpson J, Hughes GR, Buchanan NM: Increased rate of lupus flare during pregnancy and the puerperium: A prospective study of 78 pregnancies. Br J Rheumatol 35:133, 1996

Russo-Stieglitz K, Rasheed M, Artlett C, Jimenez S, Jefferson T: Influence of prior pregnancies on disease course and mortality in systemic sclerosis. Am J Obstet Gynecol 184:S190, 2001

Sakala EP, Harding MD: Ehlers–Danlos syndrome type III and pregnancy. J Reprod Med 36:622, 1991

Saleeb S, Copel J, Friedman D, Buyon JP: Comparison of treatment with fluorinated glucocorticoids to the natural history of autoantibody-associated congenital heart block. Arthritis Rheum 42:2335, 1999

Sanfelippo MJ, Drayna CJ: Prekallikrein inhibition associated with the lupus anticoagulant. Am J Clin Pathol 77:275, 1981

Schmidt WA, Kraft HE, Vorpahl K, Völker L, Gromnica-Ihle EJ: Color duplex ultrasonography in the diagnosis of temporal arteritis. N Engl J Med 337:1336, 1997

Schousboe I, Rasmussen MS: Synchronised inhibition of the phospholipid mediated autoactivation of factor XII in plasma by β_2 glycoprotein I and anti-β_2 glycoprotein I. Thromb Haemost 73:798, 1995

Seibold JR, Clements PJ, Furst DE, Mayes MD, McCloskey DA, Moreland LW, White B, Wigley FM, Rocco S, Erikson M, Hannigan JF, Sanders ME, Amento EP: Safety and pharmacokinetics of recombinant human relaxin in systemic sclerosis. J Rheumatol 25:302, 1998

Sekul EA, Cupler E, Dalakas MC: Aseptic meningitis associated with high-dose intravenous immunoglobulin therapy: Frequency and risk factors. Ann Int Med 121:259, 1994

Shi W, Chong BH, Hogg P, Chesterman CN: Anticardiolipin antibodies block the inhibition by β_2 glycoprotein I of the factor Xa generating activity of platelets. Thromb Haemost 70:324, 1993

Shilletto N, Granovsky-Grisaru S, Teoh TG, Spitzer K, Farine D, Laskin C: Vertebral compression fractures in pregnancies complicated by prolonged heparin and corticosteroid therapy. Am J Obstet Gynecol 174:392, 1996

Shinohara K, Miyagawa S, Fujita T, Aono T, Kidoguchi K: Neonatal lupus erythematosus: Results of maternal corticosteroid therapy. Obstet Gynecol 93:952, 1999

Silman A, Black CM: Increased incidence of spontaneous abortion and infertility in women with scleroderma before disease onset: A controlled study. Ann Rheum Dis 47:441, 1988

Silman A, Kay A, Brennan P: Timing of pregnancy in relation to the onset of rheumatoid arthritis. Arthritis Rheum 35:152, 1992

Silver RM, Branch DW: Autoimmune diseases in pregnancy: Systemic lupus erythematosus and antiphospholipid syndrome. Clin Perinatol 24:291, 1997

Silver RM, Draper ML, Scott JR, Lyon JL, Reading J, Branch DW: Clinical consequences of antiphospholipid antibodies: An historic cohort study. Obstet Gynecol 83:372, 1994

Silver RM, Porter TF, Van Leeuween I, Jeng G, Scott JR, Branch DW: Anticardiolipin antibodies: Clinical consequences of "low titers." Obstet Gynecol 87:494, 1996

Singsen BH, Akhter JE, Weinstein MM, Sharp GC: Congenital complete heart block and SSA antibodies: Obstetric implications. Am J Obstet Gynecol 153:495, 1985

Sneller MC: Wegener's granulomatosis. JAMA 273:1288, 1995

Sneller MC, Fauci AS: Pathogenesis of vasculitis syndromes. Med Clin N Am 81:221, 1997

Solomon JE, D'Alton ME: Dermatomyositis in pregnancy. Curr Opin Obstet Gynecol 8:83, 1996

Sorokin Y, Johnson MP, Rogowski N, Richardson DA, Evans MI: Obstetric and gynecologic dysfunction in the Ehlers–Danlos syndrome. J Reprod Med 39:281, 1994

Stafford-Brady FJ, Gladman DD, Urowitz MB: Successful pregnancy in systemic lupus erythematosus with an untreated lupus anticoagulant. Arch Intern Med 148:1647, 1988

Steen VD: Pregnancy in women with systemic sclerosis. Obstet Gynecol 94:15, 1999

Steen VD: Scleroderma and pregnancy. Rheum Dis Clin North Am 23:133, 1997

Steen VD, Conte C, Day N, Ramsey-Goldman R, Medsger TA: Pregnancy in women with systemic sclerosis. Arthritis Rheum 32:151, 1989

Steen VD, Medsger Jr TA: Fertility and pregnancy outcome in women with systemic sclerosis. Arthritis Rheum 42:763, 1999

Toglia MR, Weg JG: Venous thromboembolism during pregnancy. N Engl J Med 335:108, 1996

Trudinger BJ, Stewart GJ, Cook CM, Connelly A, Exner T: Monitoring lupus anticoagulant-positive pregnancies with umbilical artery flow velocity waveforms. Obstet Gynecol 72:215, 1988

Tseng CE, Buyon JP: Neonatal lupus syndrome. Rheum Dis Clin North Am 23:31, 1997

Unger A, Kay A, Griffin AJ, Panayi GS: Disease activity and pregnancy associated α_2-glycoprotein in rheumatoid arthritis. BMJ 286:750, 1983

Valente RM, Hall S, O'Duffy JD, Conn DL: Vasculitis and related disorders. In Kelly WN, Harris ED, Ruddy S, Sledge CB (eds): Textbook of Rheumatology, Vol II, 5th ed. Philadelphia, Saunders, 1997, p 1079

Van der Horst-Bruinsma IE, de Vries RRP, de Buch PDM, van Schendel PW, Breedveld FC, Schreuder GMTh, Hazes JMW: Influence of HLA-class II incompatibility between mother and fetus on the development and course of rheumatoid arthritis of the mother. Ann Rheum Dis 57:286, 1998

Varner MW, Meehan RT, Syrop CH, Strottman MP, Gopelrud CP: Pregnancy in patients with systemic lupus erythematosus. Am J Obstet Gynecol 145:1025, 1983

Waltuck J, Buyon JP: Autoantibody-associated congenital heart block: Outcome in mothers and children. Ann Intern Med 120:544, 1994

Weston WL, Morelli JG, Lee LA: The clinical spectrum of anti-Ro-positive cutaneous neonatal lupus erythematosus. J Am Acad Mermatol 40:675, 1999

Wilder RL, Elenkov IJ: Hormonal regulation of tumor necrosis factor-α, interleukin-12 and interleukin-10 production by activated macrophages. Ann NY Acad Sci 876:14, 1999

Winchester R: Genetic susceptibility to systemic lupus erythematosus. In Lahita RG (ed): Systemic Lupus Erythematosus, 2nd ed. New York, Churchill Livingstone, 1992, p 65

Winn HN, Setaro JF, Mazor M, Reece A, Black HR, Hobbins JC: Severe Takayasu's arteritis in pregnancy: The role of central hemodynamic monitoring. Am J Obstet Gynecol 159:1135, 1988

Yasmeen S, Eby-Wilkens EM, Gilbert WM, Department of Ob/Gyn, Center for Health Services Research in Primary Care, University of California, Davis, Sacramento, CA: Pregnancy outcomes in women with systemic lupus erythematosus (SLE). SMFM Abstracts S165. Am J Obstet Gynecol 182:533, 2000

Yasuda M, Takakuwa K, Tokunaga A, Tanaka K: Prospective studies of the association between anticardiolipin antibody and outcome of pregnancy. Obstet Gynecol 86:555, 1995

Zangari M, Lockwood CJ, Scher J, Rand JH: Prothrombin activation fragment (F1.2) is increased in pregnancy patients with antiphospholipid antibodies. Thromb Research 85:177, 1997

Zulman JI, Talal N, Hoffman GS, Epstein WV: Problems associated with the management of pregnancies in patients with systemic lupus erythematosus. J Rheumatol 7:37, 1980

53

Neurological and Psychiatric Disorders

NEUROLOGICAL DISORDERS

Neurological diseases are relatively common in women of childbearing age. Many of these disorders are physically and mentally disabling, and in the past precluded childbearing. Therapeutic advances have changed that, however, and currently many women with chronic neurological disease become pregnant. Although the majority of such conditions are compatible with successful pregnancy outcome, most also require special therapies and entail specific risks with which the clinician should be familiar.

DIAGNOSIS OF NEUROLOGICAL DISEASE DURING PREGNANCY. Most women with chronic neurological disease have been diagnosed before pregnancy. Occasionally, however, new neurological symptoms arise during gestation and must be distinguished from complications of pregnancy. Because neurological symptoms are complex and may involve cognitive as well as neuromuscular functions, they must also be distinguished from psychiatric disorders. In general, the pregnant woman should receive the same evaluation as anyone else, and should not be penalized for her pregnancy. If indicated, the techniques discussed subsequently should not be withheld from the pregnant woman.

CENTRAL NERVOUS SYSTEM IMAGING. Various imaging techniques have been developed during the past 30 years that have revolutionized the visualization of anatomical lesions responsible for neurological disease. Computed-tomography scanning and magnetic resonance imaging have opened new vistas for the diagnosis, classification, and management of many neurological and psychiatric disorders.

Cranial computed tomography is safe during pregnancy (see Table 42–8). In some diseases, it is used preferentially to magnetic resonance imaging, while in others it is complementary. Certainly it is more widely available, and is commonly used whenever rapid diagnosis is necessary to differentiate between medical and surgical management of an acute neurological catastrophe. In hemorrhagic lesions, tomography may be superior to magnetic resonance imaging.

Magnetic resonance imaging is also believed to be safe in pregnancy and, in fact, may be the imaging modality of choice because of its low associated risk. It is helpful in diagnosing demyelinating diseases, screening for arteriovenous malformations, evaluating congenital and developmental nervous system abnormalities, identifying posterior fossa lesions, and diagnosing spinal cord diseases. A relative disadvantage is the limited space available within the scanner, which makes it difficult to monitor critically ill patients. Because the claustrophobic conditions of the scanner may be difficult for some pregnant women to tolerate, premedication may be beneficial. For both magnetic resonance imaging and computed tomographic scanning, the woman should be positioned in left lateral tilt with a wedge under her right hip to avoid hypotension and aortic pulsations, which can degrade the image.

Cerebral angiography with contrast injection, usually via femoral artery access, is a valuable adjunct to the diagnosis and treatment of some cerebrovascular diseases. Careful abdominal shielding may be used to limit x-ray exposure during fluoroscopy and film exposure (see Table 42–7).

HEADACHE. Table 53–1 lists the prevalence of the most common neurological disorders, and headache is by far the most common neurological complaint during pregnancy.

TENSION HEADACHES. More than 90 percent of headaches are caused by tension, or they are migraine headaches (Paulson, 1995). Tension headaches are characterized by tightness and pain in the back of the neck and head that can persist for hours. There are no associated neurological disturbances, and the pain usually responds to rest, massage, application of heat or ice, anti-inflammatory medications, or a mild tranquilizer. The patient with recurrent tension headaches may benefit from counseling about stress management. Headaches may also be a symptom of depression.

MIGRAINE HEADACHES. The term *migraine* describes periodic, hemicranial, throbbing headaches that are often accompanied by nausea and vomiting. There are four types of migraine headaches. *Common migraine* is often familial and it is characterized by a usually unilateral headache, nausea and vomiting, and scalp tenderness of several hours duration. *Classical migraine* has similar symptoms but is preceded by premonitory neurological phenomena such as visual scotoma or halluci-

TABLE 53–1. Prevalence of Neurological Disorders

Disorder	Prevalence
Migraine	2000
Epilepsy	650
Cerebral palsy	250
Multiple sclerosis	100
Spinal cord injury	50
Subarachnoid hemorrhage	50
Myasthenia gravis	4
Genetic disorders (excluding malformations)	< 10

From Kurtzke (1982), with permission.

nations. This type of migraine can sometimes be averted if medication is taken at the first premonitory sign. *Basilar migraine* includes vertigo, dysarthria, and diplopia. *Complicated migraine* includes more severe transient neurological symptoms, and thus may mimic an ischemic event. Because migraine is frequently a diagnosis of exclusion, the initial attack should prompt a full neurological workup to rule out other more serious pathology.

Migraines may begin in childhood, adolescence, or young adulthood and tend to diminish both in frequency of recurrence as well as severity with advancing years. Stewart and colleagues (1992) reported that 18 percent of women and 6 percent of men suffer from migraine headaches at some time. Such headaches are especially common in young women, and several studies have indicated an as yet unclear relationship between hormone levels and migraine. The exact pathophysiology is uncertain, but prodromal neurological symptoms are believed to be caused by cerebral artery vasoconstriction and decreased blood flow. Presumably, vasodilation follows and is responsible for the headache. Serotonin has been implicated in this mechanism (Olesen, 1994). In some cases, migraines are associated with stroke (Tietjen, 2000). Tzourio and colleagues (1995) have shown a three- to sixfold increase in ischemic stroke in young women with migraines, although the absolute risk is small, from 10 to 20 per 100,000. Migraineurs who smoked or used oral contraceptives, however, were particularly vulnerable and had a 10- to 14-fold increased risk.

EFFECTS OF PREGNANCY. Several studies in which over 1500 pregnant women were surveyed indicate that approximately 70 percent of women with migraines experience a dramatic improvement during pregnancy (Uknis and Silberstein, 1991; Welch, 1994). Menstrual migraines typically improve, most likely because they are provoked by the drop in estrogen levels just before menstruation and are thus relieved by the high estrogen levels of pregnancy (Aube, 1999; Fettes, 1997). Women with menstrual migraines can expect a relapse postpartum. The remainder perceive either no change or worsening of symptoms.

About 15 percent of migraine headaches appear for the first time during pregnancy. These migraines are more likely to be preceded by an aura than not, and often appear in the first trimester when hormone levels are rising (Aube, 1999). Because migraine symptoms are similar to those of other more serious disorders, a complete evaluation, including neuroimaging as necessary, should be performed.

MANAGEMENT. Most migraine headaches respond to simple analgesics such as aspirin or acetaminophen, with or without caffeine or butalbital, especially if given early. Antiemetics frequently are needed. For severe headaches, codeine or meperidine is given along with promethazine for its antiemetic and sedative effects. Although almost half of classical migraines can be aborted by ergotamine taken in the prodromal period, ergotamine preparations are potent vasoconstrictors that should be avoided in pregnancy because of concerns about their effect on uteroplacental blood flow and vasoconstriction of fetal vessels. Ergotamine-induced uterine hypertonicity may also be responsible for fetal demise (Au and colleagues, 1985). Moreover, several case reports have described anomalies in exposed infants (Graham, 1983; Hughes, 1988; Verloes, 1990, and their colleagues). Ergotamine may be associated with maternal myocardial infarction, pulmonary edema, bronchospasm, bowel infarction, and stroke when given peripartum (Reprotox, 1998).

Sumatriptan is an agonist for a specific vascular serotonin receptor found in the cranial arteries and dura mater. It relieves headaches by causing vasoconstriction and is highly effective in the treatment of migraine attacks (Bateman, 1993). According to Welch (1993), a 6-mg subcutaneous dose results in improvement of over 80 percent of patients within 2 hours. The drug also relieves nausea and vomiting and greatly reduces the need for analgesics. Although previously administered only by injection, it is now available as a nasal spray and in pill form. Whether or not sumatriptan can be given safely in pregnancy is controversial, and some authors consider it to be contraindicated (Pfaffenrath and Rehm, 1998). It causes embryo lethality when given to animals at doses toxic to the mother, but does not appear to cause structural abnormalities. Sumatriptan has not been studied extensively in pregnancy, but a registry of 150 cases and two series totaling 162 exposures have not shown any teratogenic effects (Eldridge, 1997; O'Quinn, 1999; Shuhaiber, 1998, and their colleagues).

For women with frequent migraine attacks, prophylactic therapy is indicated (Welch, 1993). Amitriptyline, 10 to 150 mg/day, propranolol, 20 to 80 mg three times daily, or atenolol, 50 to 100 mg/day, are safe in pregnancy and have been used with success.

SEIZURE DISORDERS. Approximately 0.5 to 2.0 percent of the population—including as many as 1.1 million American women of childbearing-age—have epilepsy, which complicates 1 in 200 pregnancies (Brodie and Dichter, 1996; Yerby, 1994). Convulsive disorders are the second most prevalent and certainly the most serious common neurological conditions encountered in pregnant women. Epilepsy can affect the course of pregnancy, labor, and delivery and can alter fetal development, and pregnancy can exacerbate epilepsy. The metabolism of antiepileptic medications during pregnancy is changed, and teratogenetic effects of several anticonvulsant medications are unquestioned.

PATHOPHYSIOLOGY. A seizure is defined as a paroxysmal disorder of the central nervous system characterized by an abnormal neuronal discharge with or without a loss of consciousness. Epilepsy is defined as a condition characterized by a tendency for two or more recurrent seizures unprovoked by any known proximate insult. This excludes seizures due to acute systemic metabolic derangement or to an acute central nervous system insult.

A standard classification of seizures is shown in Table 53–2. Partial seizures originate in one localized area of the brain, and affect a correspondingly localized area of neurological function. They are believed to result from a lesion caused by trauma, abscess, tumor, or perinatal factors, although a specific lesion is rarely demonstrated. Simple motor seizures start in one region of the body and progress toward other areas on the same side, producing tonic and then clonic movements. Simple seizures can also affect sensory function or produce autonomic dysfunction or psychological changes. Consciousness is usually not lost and recovery is rapid. Partial seizures can secondarily generalize, producing loss of consciousness and convulsions. Complex partial seizures, also called temporal lobe or psychomotor seizures, usually involve clouding of the consciousness and a feeling of disassociation or a dyscognitive state.

Generalized seizures involve both hemispheres of the brain simultaneously, and may be preceded by an aura before an abrupt loss of consciousness. In grand mal seizures, loss of consciousness is followed by tonic contraction of the muscles and rigid posturing, and then by clonic contractions of all extremities while the muscles gradually relax. Loss of bowel or bladder control is common. Return to consciousness is gradual, and the patient may be confused and disoriented for some time.

Absence seizures, also called petit mal, involve a loss of consciousness without muscle activity, are very brief, and are characterized by immediate recovery of consciousness and orientation. Appropriate selection of an anticonvulsant is based on accurate seizure classification (Table 53–3).

SPECIFIC CAUSES. Some identifiable causes of convulsive disorders in adolescents and young adults include trauma, alcohol and other drug-induced withdrawals, brain tumors, or arteriovenous malformations. A search for all of these, including biochemical abnormalities, is necessary when a new-onset seizure disorder is encountered in a pregnant woman. The diagnosis of idiopathic seizures is one of exclusion. Lumbar puncture, skull x-rays, and arteriography have been largely replaced by evaluation with computed tomography, magnetic resonance imaging, or both. The pregnant woman should receive the same evaluation as a nonpregnant individual.

EPILEPSY DURING PREGNANCY. The major pregnancy-related threats to women with epilepsy are an increase in seizure frequency and risk of congenital malformations in their offspring. Hollingsworth and Resnik (1988) reviewed studies including 2385 pregnancies and found increased seizure frequency in 35 percent, decreased frequency in 15 percent, and no change in 50 percent. Increased seizure frequency is often associated with subtherapeutic anticonvulsant levels, a lower seizure threshold, or both. Subtherapeutic levels are caused by a variety of factors, some of which are amenable to therapeutic intervention. Nausea and vomiting leads to skipped doses; decreased gastrointestinal motility and the use of antacids reduces drug absorption; expanded intravascular volume lowers serum drug levels; the induction of hepatic, plasma, and placental enzymes increases drug metabolism; and increased glomerular filtration hastens drug clearance. These changes are offset somewhat by the fact that decreased protein binding increases free drug levels. An important factor that can be averted by appropriate counseling is that women often self-discontinue medication because they think it can harm the fetus. The seizure threshold can also be affected by various factors, including exhaustion from sleep deprivation and hyperventilation during labor. Women with the most severe disease are most susceptible to increased seizure frequency during preg-

TABLE 53–2. International Classification of Epileptic Seizures

Partial Seizures
Simple partial seizures—with motor, sensory, autonomic or psychic symptoms
Complex partial seizure—simple partial onset followed by impairment of consciousness or impairment of consciousness at onset
Partial seizures evolving to secondarily generalized seizures

Generalized Seizures
Absence seizures—typical or atypical
Myoclonic seizures
Clonic seizures
Tonic seizures
Tonic–clonic seizures
Atonic seizures

Unclassified Epileptic Seizures

Adapted from the Commission on Classification and Terminology of the International League Against Epilepsy (1989).

TABLE 53–3. Treatment with Antiepileptic Drugs, According to Type of Seizure and Epileptic Syndrome

Type of Seizure and Epileptic Syndrome	First-Line Drug	Second-Line Drug
Primary generalized		
Absence seizures[a]	Ethosuximide, valproic acid[b]	Lamotrigine
Myoclonic seizures[a]	Valproic acid[b]	Acetazolamide, clonazepam, lamotrigine, primidone
Tonic–clonic seizures	Valproic acid,[b] carbamazepine, phenytoin	Lamotrigine, phenobarbital, primidone
Absence epilepsy with onset in childhood[a]	Ethosuximide	Valproic acid,[b] lamotrigine
Absence epilepsy with onset in adolescence[a]	Valproic acid[b]	Ethosuximide, lamotrigine
Juvenile myoclonic epilepsy[a]	Valproic acid[b]	Acetazolamide, clonazepam, primidone, lamotrigine
Infantile spasms (West syndrome)	Corticotropin[c]	Clonazepam, valproic acid[b]
Lennox–Gastaut syndrome	Valproic acid,[b] lamotrigine	Carbamazepine[d]
Partial		
Simple partial seizures, complex partial seizures, secondarily generalized tonic–clonic seizures, and partial epileptic syndromes	Carbamazepine, phenytoin	Gabapentin, lamotrigine, phenobarbital, primidone, tiagabine, topiramate, valproic acid[b,e]

[a] Carbamazepine and phenytoin are contraindicated.
[b] Divalproex sodium may be better tolerated than valproic acid.
[c] Vigabatrin, which is not marketed in the United States, may be an alternative first-line drug where available.
[d] Clonazepam, felbamate, phenobarbital, primidone, or vigabatrin may be used alternatively.
[e] Methsuximide may be used alternatively for any of the partial seizures or partial epilepsy syndromes.
From Devinsky (1999), with permission.

nancy, probably because their seizure control is more difficult and thus susceptible to minor changes.

The offspring of epileptic women are at increased risk to have certain congenital malformations caused by the epilepsy itself, the anticonvulsant medications, or a combination of both. On average, 7 percent of the offspring of epileptic women have major congenital abnormalities compared with 3 percent of the general population. Some seizure disorders are inheritable, and almost 10 percent of children develop a seizure disorder later in life. The specific drug-related risks are discussed in Chapter 38 (p. 1007).

Older data suggested that epileptic women were at increased risk to have a variety of pregnancy complications other than seizures. This is controversial, however, because of ascertainment bias, and because these findings did not address the confounding effects of alcohol and drug abuse and socioeconomic factors. Nelson and Ellenberg (1982), using data from the Collaborative Perinatal Project, reported an increased incidence of preeclampsia, perinatal mortality, cesarean delivery, and preterm birth among epileptic women, as well as increased low birthweight, congenital malformations, cerebral palsy, seizures, and mental retardation in the offspring. In contrast, Olafsson and colleagues (1998) performed a population-based study of all epileptic women delivered in Iceland over a 19-year period. Although these women had a twofold increased cesarean delivery rate, the risk of other adverse obstetrical events was similar to that for the general population. While the risk of major congenital malformations was increased 2.7-fold in the offspring of epileptic women, mean birthweight and perinatal mortality were not different.

MANAGEMENT DURING PREGNANCY. For a number of reasons, epileptic women will benefit from counseling prior to pregnancy.

PRECONCEPTIONAL COUNSELING. As discussed in Chapter 9 (p. 205), preconceptional counseling is preferable for optimal anticonvulsant management. In addition to issues addressed in that chapter, postpartum contraception should be discussed. Co-administration of oral contraceptives and anticonvulsants such as phenobarbital, primidone, phenytoin, and carbamazepine may cause breakthrough bleeding and contraceptive failure because they induce hepatic P_{450} microsomal enzyme systems, which in turn increase estrogen metabolism. Although an increased failure rate is speculative, the American College of Obstetricians and Gynecologists (1990) recommends that oral contraceptives containing 50 μg of estrogen be used in epileptic women taking anticonvulsants. Oral contraceptives are not associated with exacerbation of seizures (Table 58–6).

PRENATAL CARE. The major goal of pregnancy management is to keep the woman seizure free. To accomplish this, she may need treatment for nausea and vomiting, she should avoid seizure-provoking stimuli, and compliance is urged for medication. In general, antiepileptic medication should be maintained at the lowest dose associated with seizure control. While some clinicians routinely monitor serum drug levels during pregnancy, we recommend that they be measured only when seizures occur, or if noncompliance is suspected. Altered protein binding of antiepileptic drugs during pregnancy makes standard values for therapeutic serum levels unreliable in pregnancy. Lander and Eadie (1991) reported that seizure control was not improved by routine monitoring. While determination of free or unbound drug levels may be more helpful, it currently is not widely available and has not been studied.

Women taking antiepileptic medication should take folic acid as most of these agents deplete this nutrient. Some investigators recommend vitamin K for women ingesting phenytoin because it has been implicated in functionally defective neonatal vitamin K–dependent clotting factors II, VII, IX, and X. Cornelissen and associates (1993) demonstrated diminished levels in half of cord blood samples in women taking anticonvulsants compared with 20 percent of control infants. It is unclear, however, whether vitamin K crosses the placenta. Moreover, hemorrhage in the newborn is usually prevented by prompt parenteral administration of vitamin K. For these reasons, we do not administer vitamin K to the epileptic mothers.

A midpregnancy targeted ultrasound examination may identify anomalies. Other than this, fetal monitoring because of epilepsy may not be necessary. Tests of fetal well-being might be indicated if there is poor fetal growth, inadequate seizure control, or co-morbid maternal conditions.

CEREBROVASCULAR DISEASES. In the United States, cerebrovascular disease is the eighth leading cause of death in women 25 to 44 years old. Cerebrovascular disease refers to disorders of one or more blood vessels of the brain, with the majority of lesions in the arterial system. The resultant pathological lesion is a stroke, which is an acute neurological injury due to ischemia caused by embolization, occlusion, or rupture of a vessel (Easton and colleagues, 1998). Although distinctly uncommon in young women, disorders of cerebral circulation have continued to be a prominent cause of maternal deaths in the United States. The Maternal Mortality Collaborative (Rochat and associates, 1988) reported that 10 percent of 507 direct maternal deaths from 1980 to 1985 were caused by strokes.

Fortunately, stroke and intracranial thrombosis are relatively rare complications of pregnancy. Lanska and Kryscio (1998) used the National Hospital Discharge Survey to identify all pregnancy-related strokes and intracranial thromboses in the United States from 1979 to 1991. They reported 17.7 cases of stroke and 11.4 cases of intracranial venous thrombosis per 100,000 deliveries. Kittner and co-workers (1996) reported similar rates when they analyzed data from a regional hospital-based registry of strokes in the Baltimore–Washington area. They found 11 cerebral infarctions and 9 hemorrhages per 100,000 deliveries.

Some causes of stroke in young women are listed in Table 53–4. There is evidence that inherited thrombophilias also contribute to cerebrovascular disease, although the appropriate prophylaxis or therapy for these conditions is as yet unknown. The postpartum period is a time of greatest risk. Kittner and colleagues (1996) reviewed records of all women aged 15 to 44 in the Central Maryland and Washington, D.C., area who had the diagnosis of stroke between 1988 and 1991. Among 254 cases, there were 31 associated with pregnancy. The relative risk of 0.7 for cerebral infarction during pregnancy was increased to 8.7 postpartum. The relative risk of intracerebral hemorrhage was significantly increased 2.5-fold during pregnancy and increased to 28-fold postpartum. Causes of strokes included preeclampsia–eclampsia, carotid dissection, thrombotic thrombocyto-

TABLE 53–4. Types of Strokes During Pregnancy or the Puerperium in 93 Women

Type	Number
Ischemic Strokes (53)	
Preeclampsia–eclampsia	11
Arterial thrombosis	9
Venous thrombosis	10
Arterial embolism	4
Vasculopathy	5
Amnionic fluid embolism	1
Arterial dissection	2
Other	2
Unknown	10
Hemorrhagic Strokes (40)	
Hypertensive	12
Arteriovenous malformation	7
Saccular aneurysm	3
Cocaine	3
Cavernous angioma	2
Vasculopathy	2
Unknown	8

From Kittner (1996), Sharshar (1995), Simolke (1991), Witlin and associates (2000), and their colleagues.

penic purpura, cortical vein thrombosis, postherpetic vasculitis, arteriovenous malformation, primary central nervous system vasculopathy, and cocaine use.

ISCHEMIC STROKES. These strokes may result from thrombosis of an artery or vein, or from arterial embolism.

CEREBRAL ARTERY THROMBOSIS. The vast majority of strokes afflict older individuals, result from cerebral artery thrombosis caused by atherosclerosis, and are preceded by transient ischemic attacks. The patient usually presents with sudden onset of severe headache, hemiplegia or other neurological deficits, or seizures. A thorough workup should be performed, that includes serum lipid profile, echocardiography, and cranial computed tomographic scanning or angiogram as necessary. Therapy includes rest, analgesia, and aspirin. There is evidence that prompt treatment with low-molecular-weight heparin or tissue plasminogen activator (t-PA) may improve outcomes with acute ischemic stroke (Kay and colleagues, 1995; National Institute of Neurological Disorders and Stroke Study Group, 1995).

Unfortunately, the Multicenter Acute Stroke Trial Europe Study Group (1996) reported that early streptokinase for ischemic stroke resulted in increased mortality from hemorrhage. To be effective, t-PA must be given without delay, and this can result in its being given before radiological evaluation confirms arterial occlusion. Caplan and colleagues (1997) estimate that among every 100 patients who are eligible for thrombolysis according to current guidelines, 25 or more will not have arterial occlusions, and they have a 5 to 10 percent risk of hemorrhage from the therapy. Accurate diagnosis is thus essential before initiating therapy, and the evaluation of pregnant women should not be delayed if they are to be candidates for thrombolysis.

Arterial thrombosis during pregnancy is probably not more common than stroke from cerebral embolism or intracranial hemorrhage (Table 53–4). In over 29,000 consecutive births at the Mayo Clinic, Wiebers and Whisnant (1985) identified only one case each of cerebral thrombosis and intracranial hemorrhage. In almost 90,000 pregnant women, Simolke and colleagues (1991) identified only two cases of cerebral artery thrombosis. One of these women had other features of connective-tissue disease. Cerebral thrombosis and other thrombotic complications occur more frequently in women who have antiphospholipid antibodies. According to Branch (1990), as many as a third of ischemic strokes in otherwise healthy patients under 50 years of age are caused by these antibodies (Chap. 52, p. 1391). Conversely, Voetsch and colleagues (2000) found no relationship with arterial ischemic strokes and inherited thrombophilias in young Brazilian women.

CEREBRAL VENOUS THROMBOSIS. Lateral or superior sagittal venous sinus thromboses usually occur in the puerperium. There appears to be an association with preeclampsia, sepsis, and thrombophilias. Symptoms include severe headache, drowsiness, confusion, convulsions, and focal neurological deficits, along with hypertension and papilledema. As discussed in Chapter 46 (p. 1234), venous thrombosis is more common in patients with inherited thrombophilias. These include factor V Leiden mutation (activated protein C resistance), methylene tetrahydrofolate reductase deficiency, deficiencies of proteins C and S, antithrombin III, and plasminogen, as well as lupus anticoagulant and antiphospholipid antibodies.

Cerebral venous thrombosis is not common in the United States and Europe. Cross and colleagues (1968) reported the incidence to be 1 in 20,000 pregnancies in Scotland. In the series from Parkland Hospital, two women with sagittal sinus thrombosis were identified, for an incidence of 1 in 45,000 deliveries (Simolke and co-workers, 1991). Likely because of the link with sepsis and preeclampsia, cerebral venous thrombosis remains common in undeveloped countries. Srinivasan (1984) reported its incidence in Madurai, India, to be 1 in 250 deliveries.

Venous thrombosis of the cerebral circulation is more common in the puerperium. Cantú and Barinagarrementeria (1993) described 72 cases associated with pregnancy from Mexico City over a 20-year period. All but five occurred postpartum. Headaches were the most common presenting symptom (73 percent) and 10 percent had convulsions. Magnetic resonance is the imaging procedure of choice (Cartlidge, 2000). Management includes anticonvulsants to control seizures and antimicrobials if septic thrombophlebitis is suspected. Heparin anticoagulation is controversial because bleeding may develop spontaneously. Donaldson and Lee (1994) recommend that heparin be risked, especially if there is no hemorrhagic infarction demonstrated by tomography. In a small randomized study, Einhäupl and associates (1991) described improved outcomes in nonpregnant patients given heparin therapy. In all cases the prognosis is guarded.

CEREBRAL EMBOLISM. This most commonly involves the middle cerebral artery. This type of stroke is more common during the latter half of pregnancy or early puerperium. The source of arterial occlusion may be unclear at first, but a diligent search may determine that emboli are associated with heart disease.

Management of embolic stroke consists of supportive measures and consideration for anticoagulation once hemorrhage or infarction has been excluded. Because infarction follows cerebral embolization, it is sometimes confused with cerebral artery thrombosis. Many cases of cerebral embolism in young women never are found to have an underlying cause, and the risk of recurrence therefore is speculative. On the other hand, if an underlying cause is identified, recurrence is more common unless treatment or prophylaxis can be given. Thus, it is important to aggressively pursue an etiology when these lesions are identified during pregnancy. The most commonly found origin of emboli is a cardiac arrhythmia, especially atrial fibrillation associated with rheumatic valvular disease. They also may arise from rheumatic heart disease without arrhythmia or mitral valve prolapse. Finally, emboli from infective endocarditis must be considered (Cox and associates, 1988).

HEMORRHAGIC STROKES. Hemorrhagic and ischemic strokes occur with about equal frequency during pregnancy (Table 53–4). *Intracerebral hemorrhage* into the substance of the brain may complicate chronic essential hypertension (often in older women), hypertension with superimposed preeclampsia, or may be associated with pure preeclampsia. It can also be caused by crack cocaine abuse (Mercado and colleagues, 1989; Witlin and associates, 2000). This is in contrast to *subarachnoid hemorrhage,* which is more likely to be due to an underlying malformation and associated with an otherwise normal pregnancy. According to Cartlidge (2000), intracerebral hemorrhage has a high mortality rate because of its location (Fig. 53–1). In 13 women shown in Table

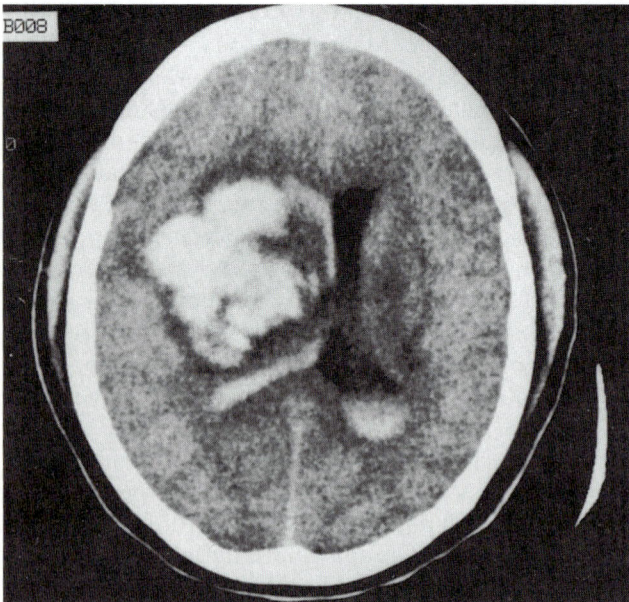

FIGURE 53–1. Cranial computed tomograph showing a massive, ultimately fatal, right-sided intracerebral hemorrhage with associated contralateral hydrocephaly. The 23-year-old primigravid woman refused hospitalization for pregnancy-induced hypertension and she next was seen comatose with blood pressures as high as 260/160 mm Hg.

53–4, six died and most of the others suffered permanent neurological sequelae. These experiences underscore the importance of proper management for acute hypertension to prevent cerebrovascular pathology (Lanska and Kryscio, 2000).

SUBARACHNOID HEMORRHAGE. Intracranial vascular anomalies can become symptomatic during pregnancy. Rupture of a cerebral aneurysm or angioma or bleeding from an arteriovenous malformation occurs in 1 in 75,000 gestations. The cardinal feature is sudden severe headache, along with visual changes, cranial nerve abnormalities, focal neurological deficits, or altered consciousness. The patient typically has signs of meningeal irritation, tachycardia, hypertension, slight fever, leukocytosis, and proteinuria. According to Dias and Sekhar (1990), bleeding from aneurysms is more common than from arteriovenous malformations, with a ratio of 3 to 1 during pregnancy. The incidence during pregnancy supposedly does not differ from that in the general nonobstetrical population (Minielly and associates, 1979). The mortality rate is reported to be as high as 35 percent (Dias and Sekhar, 1990).

RUPTURED ANEURYSM. Bleeding from a ruptured aneurysm reportedly is more common during the second half of pregnancy, but about 20 percent bleed before midpregnancy (Dias and Sekhar, 1990). There likely is a relationship between pregnancy-associated hypertension and ruptured aneurysms. Henderson and Torbey (1988) described a case temporally related to crack cocaine smoking.

Prompt evaluation is important because re-bleeding can be fatal and early neurosurgical clip ligation can prevent this. If the computed tomographic scan of the head is normal, but the clinical picture strongly suggests intracranial hemorrhage, the cerebrospinal fluid can be examined to confirm the presence of blood and this is followed by angiography to locate the lesion. We agree with Giannotta and colleagues (1986) who recommend that the workup be pursued as aggressively as if these women were not pregnant.

Treatment includes bed rest, analgesia, and sedation. Whether to attempt repair of potentially accessible vascular lesion during pregnancy is controversial. The risk of recurrent hemorrhage is difficult to estimate, but appears to depend on the rate of aneurysm growth. Kamitani and co-workers (1999) reported that four of six fast-growing aneurysms (more than 8 percent increase in size per year) bled again, while none of the 14 slow-growing aneurysms had recurrent bleeding. Immediate surgical correction obviates the need to monitor growth and thus has clear advantages. The potential for adverse fetal effects from the surgery is real. While the fetus generally tolerates hypothermia well, hypotension is problematic and should be avoided. If the woman requires surgery near term, cesarean delivery followed by craniotomy is a consideration. If remote from term, there appears to be no advantage to pregnancy termination.

Vaginal delivery is not prohibited following surgical repair, although some authorities perform vaginal delivery only after 2 months from the event. A major obstetrical problem concerns the management of delivery in women who survive intracranial hemorrhage, but in whom repair is not done. Some authorities, but certainly not all, recommend against bearing down, and thus favor cesarean delivery. On the basis of a review of 142 cases of intracranial aneurysms that ruptured before or during pregnancy, Hunt and co-workers (1974) concluded that there is no contraindication to vaginal delivery. With an unrepaired aneurysm, Wiebers (1988) recommends cesarean delivery only if bleeding occurred in the third trimester. We agree with Cartlidge (2000) who recommends cesarean delivery if the aneurysm has not been repaired.

ARTERIOVENOUS MALFORMATIONS. Vascular malformations causing subarachnoid hemorrhage are uncommon. According to Horton and co-workers (1990), the incidence of bleeding from cerebral arteriovenous malformations is not increased during pregnancy. Simolke and associates (1991) encountered only one case in nearly 90,000 deliveries cared for at Parkland Hospital (Fig. 53-2). Conversely, bleeding from these lesions caused 8 percent of strokes listed in Table 53-4. Although it is commonly accepted that bleeding from these malformations occurs with similar frequency throughout gestation, Dias and Sekhar (1990) reported an increased frequency with advancing gestational age.

There is no general agreement in nonpregnant patients about whether all of these lesions should be resected, even if they are accessible. However, the risk of recurrent hemorrhage in unoperated lesions is high. Without surgical therapy, about 5 to 7 percent will bleed again within the first year, and perhaps 2 to 3 percent per year thereafter (Itoyama and associates, 1989). In nonpregnant patients, the mortality rate is 10 percent after the first hemorrhage, 13 percent after the second hemorrhage, and approximately 20 percent after subsequent hemorrhages (Wilkins, 1985). Dias and Sekhar (1990) reported a mortality rate of 28 percent after the first bleeding event in pregnant women.

In pregnancy, management decisions to operate should be based on neurosurgical considerations (Finnerty and associates, 1999). Because of the high risk of recurrent hemorrhage, the conduct of labor and delivery following a bleeding episode during pregnancy from an inoperable lesion is critical. Although Dias and Sekhar (1990) found no evidence to support better maternal outcome with cesarean delivery, it seems best to avoid

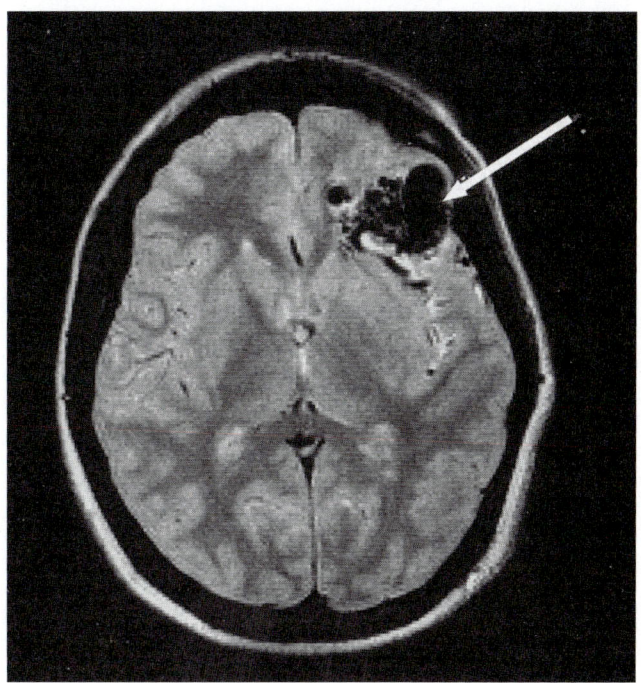

FIGURE 53-2. Magnetic resonance image of a left-sided frontal lobe atriovenous malformation. The lesion caused subarachnoid bleeding at 29 weeks in a 24-year-old primigravida who presented with severe headache, nausea, and vomiting. (From Simolke and colleagues, 1991, with permission.)

vaginal delivery if the malformation was not corrected surgically.

DEMYELINATING AND DEGENERATIVE DISEASES. Demyelinating diseases comprise a group of neurological disorders that involve focal or patchy destruction of central nervous system myelin sheaths accompanied by an inflammatory response. The degenerative diseases frequently are inherited, and are characterized by gradually evolving and progressive neuronal death from unknown causes.

MULTIPLE SCLEROSIS. This disease is the most common chronic demyelinating neurological disorder. Multiple sclerosis (MS) usually begins in young adults and is most common in 20- to 40-year-old white women. The etiology in unknown, but it likely involves a combination of heredity and environmental factors. One theory is that it is caused by a virally triggered autoimmune phenomenon in genetically susceptible individuals. There are four forms of the disease which are recognized primarily for research classification (Confavreux and colleagues, 2000; Lublin and Reingold, 1996). *Relapsing-remitting MS* is characterized clinically by unpredictable recurrent attacks of focal or multifocal neurological dysfunction. Early in the disease, attacks typically last 2 to 3 days, followed by complete recovery over several weeks. As attacks become more frequent, recovery may not be complete, and permanent deficits can accrue. In *secondary progressive MS,* the disease pursues a progressive downhill course after each relapse. *Primary progressive MS* is characterized by gradual progression of disability from the initial diagnosis. *Progressive-relapsing MS* refers to primary progressive MS with apparent relapses.

Classical symptoms include loss of vision and diplopia, and over 40 percent of patients have optic neuritis during the course of disease. In fact, 75 percent of women who have isolated optic neuritis will go on to develop multiple sclerosis within 15 years. Other common symptoms are weakness, hyperreflexia, spasticity, paresthesia, ataxia and intention tremor, nystagmus, dysarthria, diminished vibratory sense, and bladder dysfunction. The diagnosis is one of exclusion, and is confirmed by cerebrospinal fluid analysis and magnetic resonance imaging. The characteristic multifocal white matter lesions, termed plaques, are present in more than 90 percent of patients and represent discrete areas of demyelination (Hauser and Goodkin, 1998).

The goal of treatment is to arrest the disease or its symptoms. Corticosteroids may diminish the severity of acute flares, but they have no effect on permanent disability. Symptomatic relief can be provided by analgesics; carbamazepine, phenytoin, or amitriptyline (for neurogenic pain); baclofen (for spasticity); α-adrenergic blockade (to relax the bladder neck); and cholinergic and anticholinergic drugs (to stimulate or inhibit bladder contractions). Immunosuppressive therapy with cyclosporine, azathioprine, and cyclophosphamide is often prescribed for aggressive cases but has not been accepted by all as efficacious (Ebers, 1994).

Both interferon-β 1a and 1b have been shown to favorably modify the course of disease (McDonald, 1995). The PRISMS (Prevention of Relapses and Disability by Interferon beta-1a Subcutaneously in Multiple Sclerosis) Study Group (1998) prospectively randomized 560 patients with MS from 22 centers to one of two different doses of interferon or placebo. They found that both doses of interferon significantly lowered the relapse rate, prolonged the time to first relapse, and delayed both the progression to disability and the accumulated disability. Because depression, thrombotic thrombocytopenic purpura, and various autoimmune reactions are side effects of treatment, patients receiving interferon-β should be closely monitored (Walther and Hohlfeld, 1999).

EFFECTS OF PREGNANCY. There is no evidence that pregnancy precipitates MS, and in most cases pregnancy has no deleterious effect on its course. In fact, several studies indicate that women who have been pregnant have less deterioration than those who have not (Damek and Shuster, 1997). However, acute exacerbation during the first few months postpartum is common, possibly

due to the reversal of the relative immune suppression of pregnancy (Cartlidge, 2000; Schneider and associates, 1996). Abramsky (1994) summarized eight retrospective studies of over 1000 pregnancies and found that the disease worsened during pregnancy in only 10 percent, but 30 percent had worsening in the puerperium. In a prospective study of 125 women, Roullet and associates (1993) confirmed a 43 percent postpartum exacerbation rate. Conversely, in a prospective investigation of 58 pregnancies, Sadovnick and co-workers (1994) found that postpartum relapses were no more common than in nonpregnant controls.

If uncomplicated, MS usually has no adverse effects on pregnancy outcome. Schneider and colleagues (1996) reported increased preterm delivery and a slight increase in the rate of congenital malformations. Women may become fatigued more easily, and those with bladder dysfunction are prone to urinary infection. Labor is unaffected, and the indications for cesarean delivery are obstetrical. Women with lesions at or above T_6 are at risk for autonomic dysreflexia, and they should receive epidural anesthesia accordingly. Although spinal analgesia has anecdotally been associated with exacerbations, some authorities consider epidural analgesia to be safe (Weinreb, 1994). Bader (1994) rightfully emphasizes the high incidence of postpartum exacerbation regardless of analgesia or anesthesia.

Perinatal outcome is not altered significantly, but the incidence of multiple sclerosis in offspring is increased nearly 15-fold. Although breast feeding is not associated with an increased risk of postpartum exacerbation, such an exacerbation may prevent the woman from breast feeding. Exacerbation may also limit a woman's ability to provide general infant care, and the need for assistance during this period should be anticipated (Nelson and colleagues, 1988).

HUNTINGTON DISEASE. This degenerative disease of the cerebral cortex and basal ganglia is characterized by a combination of choreoathetotic movements and progressive dementia. Since the mean age of onset is 40 years, Huntington disease rarely complicates pregnancy. Because it is inherited as an autosomal dominant trait, a family history of the disease does arouse interest during pregnancy. With the development of several DNA probes, as well as the use of the polymerase chain reaction, prenatal diagnosis is now possible (Chap. 36, p. 966). Prenatal diagnosis is highly controversial because termination is often not considered in view of the late age of disease onset. Also, prenatal diagnosis could prejudice health insurance carriers and others against the child.

MYASTHENIA GRAVIS. This disease is an immune-mediated neuromuscular disorder that affects about 1 in 10,000 persons and has a predilection for women of childbearing age. The etiology is unknown, but genetic factors play a role as it is more common in those with the HLA-B8 antigen. The disease is characterized by weakness resulting from IgG-mediated destruction of postsynaptic striated muscle acetylcholine receptors. Even though acetylcholine is released normally, without adequate receptors it produces diminished endplate action potentials that do not always trigger muscle action potentials and thus results in weakened muscle contractions.

Myasthenia gravis is characterized by easy fatigability of facial, oropharyngeal, extraocular, and limb muscles. Cranial muscles are involved early and disparately, and diplopia and ptosis are common. Facial muscle weakness causes difficulty in smiling, chewing, and speech. In 85 percent of patients the weakness becomes generalized. The course of the disease is variable, but it tends to be marked by exacerbations and remissions, especially when it first becomes clinically apparent. Remissions seldom are complete or permanent. Systemic diseases, concurrent infections, and even emotional upset may precipitate myasthenic crises, of which there are three types: myasthenic crises, characterized by severe muscle weakness, inability to swallow, and respiratory muscle paralysis; refractory crises, characterized by the same symptoms but unresponsive to the usual therapy; and cholinergic crises, in which excessive cholinergic medication leads to nausea, vomiting, muscle weakness, abdominal pain, and diarrhea. All three crisis types can be life threatening, but a refractory crisis is a medical emergency. Women with bulbar myasthenia are at particular risk during a crisis because they may be unable to swallow or even ask for help.

Myasthenia is manageable but not curable. About 75 percent of patients have thymic hyperplasia or a thymoma. Young women are more likely to respond to thymectomy with remission (Cartlidge, 2000). Anticholinesterase medications bring about improvement by impeding degradation of acetylcholine, but seldom produce normal muscle function. Pyridostigmine, an analog of neostigmine, is the most commonly used preparation. Ironically, the side effects of overdosage are increased weakness, which is sometimes difficult to differentiate from myasthenic symptoms. Nearly all patients respond to immunosuppressive therapy with corticosteroids, azathioprine, and cyclosporine (Cartlidge, 2000). Cyclophosphamide is used for refractory cases. Short-term clinical improvement has been reported following intravenously administered immunoglobulin or plasmapheresis.

EFFECTS OF PREGNANCY. Pregnancy does not appear to affect the course of myasthenia gravis, which may be marked by exacerbations and remissions just like any other 9-month period. The enlarging uterus may compromise respiration, and diminished energy levels common to most pregnancies may be tolerated poorly. Plauché (1991) found that 30 percent of women improve, 30 percent are unchanged, and 40 percent worsen during pregnancy. Although the disease has no adverse general effects on pregnancy outcome, he reported nine maternal deaths among 322 pregnancies. Most of these were due to complications of myasthenia or its treatment. Because the greatest period of risk is within the first year following diagnosis, Cartlidge (2000) recommends that pregnancy be postponed until there is sustained symptomatic improvement.

Management during pregnancy includes close observation with liberal bed rest and prompt treatment of infection. Most patients respond well to pyridostigmine administered every 3 to 4 hours. Those in remission who become pregnant while taking corticosteroids or azathioprine should continue these medications. Acute onset of myasthenia or its exacerbation demands prompt admission and supportive care. Plasmapheresis should be used for emergency situations, taking care not to provoke maternal hypotension or hypovolemia (Drachman, 1994). There is at least one report of thymectomy performed in a 17-week pregnant woman (Ip and colleagues, 1986).

Most women with myasthenia gravis tolerate labor without difficulty. Because the disease does not affect smooth muscle, labor usually proceeds normally. Oxytocin can be administered as necessary. Careful observation and prompt respiratory support are essential. Narcotics must be used with care, and any drug with a curare-like effect must be avoided—examples include magnesium sulfate, muscle relaxants used with general anesthesia, and aminoglycoside antibiotics. Amide-type local anesthetic agents are used for epidural analgesia for labor (Bader, 1994). Cesarean delivery is for obstetrical indications, with regional analgesia preferred unless there is significant bulbar involvement or respiratory compromise. During second-stage labor, some women may have impairment of voluntary expulsive efforts, and forceps delivery may be necessary

NEONATAL EFFECTS. Acetylcholine-receptor antibodies have been detected in most myasthenic patients, and these IgG antibodies can be transferred to the fetus. Fortunately, only about 10 to 20 percent of neonates develop symptoms. Vernet-der Garabedian and colleagues (1994) have shown that newborns are more likely to have symptoms if their mothers produce autoantibodies directed against embryonic rather than adult acetylcholine receptors. Transient symptomatic myasthenia gravis in the affected infant is typically demonstrated by a feeble cry, poor suckling, and respiratory distress, which are corrected by parenteral neostigmine or small doses of edrophonium. Although symptoms resolve within 2 to 6 weeks as the antibodies are cleared, the perinatal death rate among offspring of myasthenic mothers was considerably higher than the background rate at 68 per 1000 (Plauché, 1991).

NEUROPATHIES. Peripheral neuropathy is a general term used to describe a disorder of peripheral nerve(s) due to a variety of causes. Its discovery should prompt a search for an etiology. Polyneuropathies are often associated with systemic diseases, such as diabetes and drugs, environmental toxins, and an imposing list of genetic diseases. Mononeuropathies signify focal involvement of a single nerve trunk and imply local causation such as trauma, compression, or entrapment.

GUILLAIN–BARRÉ SYNDROME. This is an acute demyelinating polyradiculoneuropathy. In over two thirds of cases, it follows clinical or serological evidence for viral infections, especially cytomegalovirus and Epstein-Barr virus. Approximately 10 percent of cases develop within weeks following a surgical procedure. In 1977, there was an epidemic of Guillain–Barré syndrome following immunization against swine influenza. The disease is thought to be immune mediated, but its pathogenesis is unclear. The pathological finding is a primary T-cell lymphocytic infiltration of cranial nerves, ventral and dorsal roots, dorsal root ganglia, peripheral nerves, lymph nodes, and liver, heart, spleen, and other organs, apparently occurring aberrantly in response to a precipitating infection (Ropper, 1992).

Clinical features include areflexic paralysis with mild sensory disturbances, and sometimes evidence of autonomic dysfunction. The full syndrome takes 1 to 3 weeks to develop. Management is supportive, but patients should be hospitalized because about 25 percent will need ventilatory assistance, and the mortality rate for this complication is high. Corticosteroids have not been effective, although plasmapheresis or intravenous high-dose immunoglobulin (2 g/kg over 5 days) have been shown to be of benefit if begun within 1 to 2 weeks of symptoms (van der Meché and colleagues, 1992). Almost 85 percent of patients will have full recovery, but about 3 percent will die from complications of the acute condition.

EFFECTS OF PREGNANCY. There does not appear to be an increased incidence of Guillain–Barré syndrome during pregnancy; however, the incidence is significantly increased postpartum. Cheng and co-workers (1998) reviewed all cases of Guillain–Barré occurring in Swedish reproductive-age women between 1978 and 1993 and found that the age-adjusted rate ratio was unchanged during pregnancy but was significantly increased three-fold in the first 30 days after delivery. The first 2 weeks postpartum was a time of particularly increased risk.

Management is not changed by pregnancy. Hurley and colleagues (1991) described three pregnancies complicated by this syndrome and reviewed 31 others. As in nonpregnant patients, after an insidious onset, paresis and paralysis most often continued to ascend, and respiratory insufficiency then became a common and serious problem. About a third ultimately required ventilatory support, and overall maternal mortality was 13 percent. Bravo and associates (1982) successfully ventilated a mother for 5 weeks before delivery of a healthy infant. Kuller and associates (1995) and Rockel and co-workers (1994) described successful outcomes in pregnant women in whom plasmapheresis was performed. High-dose immunoglobulin may also be administered safely in pregnancy.

BELL PALSY. This is an acute idiopathic peripheral facial paralysis of unknown etiology. It is thought to be a viral-induced mononeuropathy and is relatively common, especially in reproductive-age women. Women are affected two to four times more often than men of the same age, and pregnant women are affected three to four times more commonly than nonpregnant women (Cohen and colleagues, 2000). Falco and Eriksson (1989) reported an incidence of 1 in 2500 births at Brigham and Women's Hospital. Increased extracellular fluid, viral inflammation, and the relative immune suppression of pregnancy are thought to be predisposing factors. The onset is usually abrupt and painful, with maximum weakness within 48 hours. In some cases, hyperacusis and loss of taste accompany varying degrees of facial muscle paralysis. Electromyography may be helpful in determining prognosis—if denervation extends beyond 10 days, healing will be delayed and likely incomplete.

EFFECTS OF PREGNANCY. Pregnancy does not alter the overall good prognosis for spontaneous recovery from Bell palsy, and nearly 90 percent of affected women will recover function within a few weeks to months. Poor prognostic markers for incomplete recovery are bilateral disease and recurrence in a subsequent pregnancy (Cohen and associates, 2000). Shapiro and co-workers (1999) noted that hypertension or preeclampsia was present in over 20 percent of cases of Bell palsy, compared to only 5 percent in the general population. Treatment with short-term corticosteroids remains controversial, but the bulk of evidence suggests that these drugs do not hasten resolution. Surgical decompression is seldom indicated. Supportive care includes prevention of injury to the constantly exposed cornea, facial muscle massage, and reassurance. Dorsey and Camann (1993) have provided evidence that regional analgesia does not exacerbate the neuropathy.

CARPAL TUNNEL SYNDROME. This syndrome is characterized by hand and wrist pain extending into the forearm and sometimes into the shoulder. It is caused by compression of the median or (less frequently) ulnar nerve, which are especially vulnerable to compression within the carpal tunnel at the wrist. Typically, the woman awakens with burning, numbness, or tingling in the inner half of one or both hands, and the fingers feel numb and useless. Symptoms are bilateral in 80 percent of cases, and often exhibit a diurnal pattern (Seror, 1998). Although some symptoms of carpal tunnel syndrome are experienced by a fourth of pregnant women, new onset of the full syndrome is much less frequent. Stolp-Smith and colleagues (1998) made the diagnosis in less than 1 percent of nearly 11,000 pregnant women. Ekman-Ordeberg and colleagues (1987) verified carpal tunnel syndrome in 2.3 percent of almost 2400 pregnant women.

Carpal tunnel syndrome is self-limited, and treatment is symptomatic. A splint applied to the very slightly flexed wrist and worn during sleep usually provides relief. Ekman-Ordeberg and colleagues (1987) and Courts (1995) reported that this relieved pain in 80 percent of 132 women. Only three required surgical decompression. The signs and symptoms most often regress after delivery, although surgical decompression and corticosteroid injections are occasionally necessary (Dammers and associates, 1999). In the report by Stolp-Smith and co-workers (1998), 11 percent of women underwent surgery postpartum. In rare instances, symptoms may recur long after pregnancy and surgical release is necessary (Al Qatten and colleagues, 1994).

The syndrome should be distinguished from De Quervain tendinitis caused by swelling of the conjoined tendons and sheaths near the distal radius. Schumacher and colleagues (1985) described six women with tendinitis during pregnancy, and two also had carpel tunnel syndrome. Nerve conduction studies may be helpful in distinguishing these entities. Seror (1998) reported that two thirds of women with carpal tunnel syndrome had evidence of an acute median nerve lesion at the wrist with motor or sensory conduction blocks, or both, and approximately 10 percent had signs of severe denervation.

SPINAL CORD INJURY. Trauma, especially motor vehicle accidents, accounts for most spinal cord injuries. With well-organized trauma systems, almost 95 percent of patients with cord injuries survive the initial hospitalization (Ditunno and Formal, 1994). Most patients are young adults, who typically injure the cervical or thoracic spine. Lesions caused by trauma or tumor do not

prevent conception, and pregnancy outcome is usually good. In a survey of 472 reproductive-age women with spinal cord injury, Jackson and Wadley (1999) found that approximately 67 percent of affected women had intercourse after the injury, and almost 14 percent became pregnant. Women with spinal cord injury had lower birthweight infants and experienced more pregnancy complications than unaffected women. Complications included urinary tract infections, anemia, pressure necrosis of skin, and aggravation of constipation (Baker and associates, 1992; Hughes and colleagues, 1991). Over half of women have significant bowel dysfunction (Glickman and Kamm, 1996). Westgren and co-workers (1993) described 49 pregnancies in 29 women with traumatic cord injuries. Three fourths developed urinary infections, there was a 20 percent preterm delivery rate, and perinatal mortality was 3.8 percent.

There are two serious and life-threatening complications that can develop. If the lesion is above T_{10}, the cough reflex will be impaired and respiratory function may be compromised. Pulmonary function should be determined before or early in pregnancy, and carefully monitored throughout gestation. In some cases, women with high lesions may need ventilatory support in late pregnancy or in labor. In women with lesions above T_{5-6}, autonomic hyperreflexia can occur. In this potentially life-threatening event, splanchnic nerves are excited by some stimulus and are not dampened because of lack of central inhibition. The resultant sudden sympathetic stimulation of nerves below the cord lesion causes a throbbing headache, facial flushing, sweating, bradycardia, and paroxysmal hypertension. A variety of stimuli including urethral, bladder, rectal, or cervical distention, catheterization, cervical dilatation, uterine contractions, or examination of pelvic structures may precipitate dangerous hypertension, which must be treated immediately. In the report by Westgren and colleagues (1993), 12 of 15 women at risk suffered at least one episode of autonomic hyperreflexia. Spinal or epidural analgesia can prevent or avert dysreflexia, and should be instituted at the start of labor. General anesthesia is not preferred because the depth of anesthesia necessary to control the spasms and dysreflexia can cause hypotension and respiratory dysfunction (Hambly and Martin, 1998).

Uterine contractions are not affected by cord lesions. Indeed, labor is often easy, even precipitous, and comparatively painless. If the lesion is below T_{12}, then contractions are felt normally. There is great concern that women with lesions above T_{12} may deliver at home unattended before they realize that labor has begun. However, these women can be taught to palpate uterine contractions, or home tocodynamometry can be used. Serial examinations with admission for advanced cervical dilatation or effacement may also be helpful, and some authorities recommend weekly cervical examinations beginning at about 28 weeks. Hughes and associates (1991) recommend elective admission between 36 and 37 weeks.

Delivery is preferably vaginal. The American College of Obstetricians and Gynecologists (1993b) recommends continuous cardiac rhythm monitoring along with intra-arterial pressure monitoring. Epidural or spinal analgesia is used to minimize autonomic hyperreflexia. In some cases, second-stage labor may be prolonged due to diminished expulsive efforts. Westgren and colleagues (1993) cited a cesarean rate of 63 percent, but concluded that this was because of inexperience of the health-care providers.

SHUNTS FOR MATERNAL HYDROCEPHALUS. Many cases of pregnancy have been described in women with ventriculoperitoneal, ventriculoatrial, or ventriculopleural shunts for hydrocephalus. Pregnancy outcomes have usually been satisfactory. Although Landwehr and colleagues (1994) reported no shunt complications during eight pregnancies in four women with ventriculoperitoneal shunts, others have reported shunt obstruction, typically late in pregnancy. Wisoff and associates (1991) described 21 pregnancies in 18 women with various shunts. Neurological complications developed in 13 of 17 pregnancies in women with preexisting shunts, including headaches (60 percent), nausea and vomiting (35 percent), lethargy (30 percent), ataxia (20 percent), and gaze paresis (20 percent). Most responded to conservative management. Computed tomography discloses acute hydrocephaly, which can be relieved by tapping the shunt or pumping it several times daily. Surgical revision may be necessary.

In women with shunts, vaginal delivery is preferred, and unless there is a meningomyelocele, epidural analgesia is permitted (Bader, 1994). Subarachnoid block is felt by some authorities to be contraindicated, but others support its use (Littleford and colleagues, 1999). Antimicrobial prophylaxis is indicated if the peritoneal cavity is entered for cesarean delivery or tubal sterilization.

BRAIN DEATH. A few instances of maternal brain death during pregnancy have been described in which life support systems and parenteral alimentation were used for extended periods of time while the fetus achieved maturity (Dillon and associates, 1982; Field and colleagues, 1988). In the case described by Bernstein and co-workers (1989), life support was begun at 15 weeks for a brain-dead woman and continued until 32 weeks. Catanzarite and colleagues (1997) described a case of brain death at 25 weeks in which aggressive tocolysis and antibiotic therapy were required to continue the pregnancy another 25 days. Such therapy is not always successful (Vives and collaborators, 1996).

The ethical, financial, and legal implications, both civil and criminal, that may arise from attempting or not attempting such care are profound.

BENIGN INTRACRANIAL HYPERTENSION (PSEUDOTUMOR CEREBRI). This condition is characterized by headache, stiff neck, visual disturbances, and papilledema from increased intracranial pressure in an otherwise healthy individual. Its cause is thought to be overproduction or underabsorption of cerebrospinal fluid. It is commonly found in young women, especially those who are obese or who recently have gained weight. It is probably not more prevalent during pregnancy, as once believed (Ireland and associates, 1990). Criteria for diagnosis include elevated cerebrospinal fluid pressure, normal cerebrospinal fluid composition, and normal cranial computed tomography or magnetic resonance imaging. In some patients, spinal fluid protein concentration may be low. Interestingly, Bates and associates (1982) reported that men and nonpregnant women with this condition had significantly increased cerebrospinal fluid prolactin concentrations.

Pseudotumor is usually self-limited; however, permanent visual impairment may develop in a significant number of patients, and optic atrophy can cause blindness. Treatment is aimed at prevention of visual defects by lowering the elevated pressure. Repetitive lumbar punctures to remove cerebrospinal fluid will lower pressure, and can be performed safely without brainstem herniation if there is no ventriculomegaly. Drugs that can be given safely during pregnancy to lower pressure include acetazolamide, furosemide, or dexamethasone. In rare cases, lumboperitoneal shunting of spinal fluid is necessary.

EFFECTS OF PREGNANCY. Benign intracranial hypertension is usually detected by midpregnancy, is self-limited, and resolves postpartum. Headache is the presenting symptom in 95 percent of women, and almost 75 percent have blurred vision. It is arguable whether the incidence of pseudotumor is increased in pregnancy. Katz and colleagues (1989) reported it in about 1 in 1000 pregnancies. They described 11 such pregnancies and concluded that pregnancy increased the likelihood of symptoms in women who already had intracranial hypertension. They also reported a 30 percent recurrence rate. In our experiences, the incidence is not nearly so high.

Treatment of benign intracranial hypertension during pregnancy is identical to that for nonpregnancy. Any perceived increased risk of pregnancy complications is probably due to the associated obesity, and not to the pseudotumor. From their review of 54 pregnancies, Katz and associates (1989) did not report increased adverse perinatal outcomes. Labor is permitted, the route of delivery is decided by obstetrical indications, and epidural analgesia is not contraindicated. Landwehr and colleagues (1994) have described four women in whom lumboperitoneal shunting was performed.

CHOREA GRAVIDARUM. Any chorea that develops during pregnancy is known as chorea gravidarum (Golbe, 1994). Because cases in the past were linked to rheumatic fever, chorea is now rare. It can still occur in association with streptococcus A infection, but more often may be caused by collagen-vascular disease (Prasher and Barrett, 1993). Up to 2 percent of patients with systemic lupus erythematosus exhibit chorea (Branch, 1990). Most of these patients have antiphospholipid antibodies (Chap. 52, p. 1391). Omdal and Roalsø (1992) described a woman with chorea gravidarum who had a recurrence while taking steroidal contraceptives 20 years later.

PSYCHIATRIC DISORDERS

Pregnancy and the puerperium are at times sufficiently stressful to provoke mental illness. Such illness may represent recurrence or exacerbation of a preexisting psychiatric disorder, or it may be the onset of a new disorder. The Department of Health and Human Services has reported that 1 of every 8 persons will suffer from a depressive disorder and that the rate is almost doubled for women (Depression Guideline Panel, 1993). Unfortunately, depression is appropriately treated in fewer than a fourth of affected women (American College of Obstetricians and Gynecologists, 1993a). The under-recognition of depression frequently occurs in primary care settings where most medical care is obtained. Similarly, women who suffer with postpartum depression are often not properly identified and treated.

PSYCHOLOGICAL ADJUSTMENT TO PREGNANCY. While pregnancy often evokes overwhelming joy, it is also stressful for most women. In some women with ambivalent feelings about the pregnancy, stress may be appreciably increased. Response to stress may be seen in a variety of subtle or not so subtle ways. For example, many women express concerns about whether their baby is normal. For those whose fetus is at higher risk for a congenital malformation, stress is increased (Tunis and Golbus, 1991). Throughout pregnancy, and especially toward term, anxiety develops about child care and the lifestyle changes that will ensue after delivery. In a number of women, the fear of childbirth pain is particularly stressful. Pregnancy experiences may be altered by medical and obstetrical complications that may ensue. Burger and colleagues (1993) have shown that women who suffer complicated pregnancies are twice

as likely to have fear for their fetus or to become depressed.

For those women with a history of psychiatric illness, pregnancy is often a time of general well-being. Indeed, mood disorders with their initial onset during pregnancy tend to be milder (O'Hara and colleagues, 1984). However, for women who have serious forms of mental disorders that predate pregnancy—in particular bipolar illness, schizoaffective disorder, or schizophrenia—the illness may not remain quiescent.

By contrast, the puerperium has long been recognized as a time of increased risk for mental illness. According to Weissman and Olfson (1995), 10 to 15 percent of recently delivered women will develop a nonpsychotic postpartum depressive disorder. In some, severe, psychotic depressive or manic illness follows delivery. Although puerperal psychoses is not a separate diagnosis, a woman is at least 30 times more likely to require admission for a psychotic or severe mental illness in the month following delivery than she is in the previous 2 years (Kendell and colleagues, 1987). Importantly, preexisting mental illness has a high recurrence rate in the puerperium. Despite this predilection, suicide is uncommon during pregnancy and the year following delivery (Appleby, 1991).

PRENATAL EVALUATION. Issues concerning mental health should be addressed. Screening for mental illness should be performed during the first prenatal examination. This involves obtaining a history of any prior psychiatric disorders, including hospitalizations, outpatient care, and prior or current use of psychoactive medications. Current symptoms that might indicate mental dysfunction should be investigated. According to Oates (1989), 15 to 20 percent of pregnant women will have mental health issues that need to be considered in their management. Certain conditions such as anxiety and depression may be associated with an increased risk of preterm delivery (Paarlberg and associates, 1996).

Risk factors for mental illness should also be carefully evaluated. A history of sexual abuse increases the risk for depressive illness. Benedict and co-workers (1999), in a study involving 357 high-risk pregnant women, reported that women with a past history of sexual abuse were significantly more likely to report depressive symptomology, negative life events, and physical and verbal abuse before and during pregnancy. Substance abuse, violence, and depression also appear to be linked. Horrigan and colleagues (2000) found that women who reported a history of substance abuse were highly likely to have severe depression or to be a victim of physical or sexual abuse, or both. They recommended that women who report one of these factors be carefully monitored for evidence of the other two (also Chap. 9, p. 210). Because eating disorders are exacerbated by pregnancy, evidence of such a disorder should also prompt careful follow-up during pregnancy.

CLASSIFICATION OF MENTAL DISORDERS. The American Psychiatric Association last revised its Diagnostic and Statistical Manual (DSM-IV) in 1993. Its purpose is to classify mental disorders and specify criteria required for their diagnosis.

MAJOR MOOD DISORDERS. These disorders include major depression, considered a unipolar disorder, and bipolar disorder or manic-depressive illness, which includes manic and depressive episodes. Primary mood disorders occur de novo, while both depressive and manic disorders are significantly influenced by genetic factors. First-degree relatives of individuals with manic depression are at 15 percent risk of being similarly affected (McInnis and DePaulo, 1996). A number of provocative conditions can also lead to mood disorders. For depression, these include grief reactions, substance abuse, use of certain medications, and other medical disorders (Depression Guideline Panel, 1993). Potential causes of mania or manic symptoms include substance abuse such as cocaine, hyperthyroidism, and central nervous system tumors. The importance of detecting major mood disorders is underscored when one considers that they are a predisposing factor in up to two thirds of suicides in the United States.

SCHIZOPHRENIA. This is a common major form of mental illness, with a 6-month prevalence rate of about 1 percent (Myers and colleagues, 1984). Its morbidity is higher than for any other psychiatric disorder. Its hallmarks include delusions, hallucinations, incoherence, and inappropriate affect. Four major subtypes of schizophrenia are recognized: catatonic, disorganized, paranoid, and undifferentiated. Schizophrenia has a major genetic component, with 50 percent concordance with monozygotic twins. If one parent is schizophrenic, the empirical risk to offspring is 5 to 10 percent. The onset of illness is around age 20 and commonly, work and psychosocial functioning deteriorate over time. Women have a slightly later onset than men, and may occasionally marry and become pregnant before they fall ill. With appropriate treatment, patients may experience a decrease or cessation of symptoms such that the 5-year social recovery is 60 percent. For all patients at 5 years, half are employed, 30 percent are mentally handicapped, and 10 percent require continued hospitalization.

Patients with a schizoaffective disorder have a chronic deteriorating psychotic disorder similar to schizophrenia, but combined with prominent mood symptoms. Although the psychosis rarely abates, the mood symptoms often improve with therapy, giving this condition a better prognosis than schizophrenia.

ANXIETY DISORDERS. These disorders involve paroxysmal and persistent psychological feelings of dread, irritability, and ruminations that are accompanied by physiological changes such as sweating, dyspnea, insomnia, and trembling. Anxiety disorders are commonly encountered in everyday medical practices, and they are more easily recognized when subdivided into panic disorder, obsessive-compulsive disorder, post-traumatic stress disorder, and phobic disorder.

PERSONALITY DISORDERS. These disorders are characterized by the chronic use of certain coping mechanisms in an inappropriate, stereotyped, and maladaptive manner. The Diagnostic and Statistical Manual recognizes three clusters of personality disorders:

1. Paranoid, schizoid, and schizotypal personality disorders, which are characterized by oddness or eccentricity.
2. Histrionic, narcissistic, antisocial, and borderline disorders, which are all characterized by dramatic presentations along with self-centeredness and erratic behavior.
3. Avoidant, dependent, compulsive, and passive/aggressive personalities, which are characterized by underlying fear and anxiety.

Genetic and environmental factors are important in the genesis of these disorders, whose prevalence may be as high as 20 percent. Management is through psychotherapy; however, only about 20 percent of affected individuals recognize their problems and seek psychiatric help.

EFFECTS OF PREGNANCY ON MENTAL ILLNESS. It is difficult to differentiate biochemical factors from life stressors as a primary cause of mental illness in pregnancy. Hormones are known to affect mood, as evidenced by premenstrual syndrome and menopausal depression. The absolute level of hormone appears to be important. Estrogen modulates serotonergic function, has been used therapeutically to treat depression, and may be a factor in the mood elevation experienced by many women during pregnancy (Joffe and Cohen, 1998). Conversely, corticotropin-releasing hormone, which is usually elevated in pregnancy, is present at lower levels in women with pregnancy-related depression (Schmeelk and colleagues, 1999). The rate of change of hormone levels also appears to be influential. Women who experience postpartum depression often have higher predelivery estrogen and progesterone levels, and experience a greater drop to lower levels postpartum (Ahokas and co-workers, 1999; Harris and associates, 1994).

It is also true, however, that pregnancy is a major life stressor that can unmask or exacerbate depressive tendencies. According to Weissman and Olfson (1995), almost 10 percent of pregnant women meet diagnostic criteria for major depression. It is more likely with marital problems, unwanted pregnancy, and a personal or family history of depression. Séguin and co-workers (1995) further showed that women of low socioeconomic status are more depression prone. Bergant and colleagues (1999) correlated pregnancy-related depression to low socioeconomic status as well as increased burden from children, diminished life satisfaction, and increased anxiety. Bryan and co-workers (1999), in a study that included the population of Olmstead County Minnesota, found that pregnancy-related depression was associated with young maternal age, single marital status, tobacco or illegal drug use during pregnancy, hyperemesis gravidarum, high utilization of emergency services, and previous affective disorder.

POSTPARTUM DISORDERS.

MATERNITY BLUES. Also called *postpartum blues,* this is a mood disturbance experienced by approximately 50 percent of women within 3 to 6 days after parturition (Kendell and colleagues, 1987). There is evidence that blues are precipitated by progesterone withdrawal (Harris and co-workers, 1994).

Although a variety of symptoms have been assessed, core features include insomnia, weepiness, depression, anxiety, poor concentration, irritability, and affective lability. Obviously, these are common symptoms present in minor or even major depressive episodes. Affective lability describes the changeable mood experienced by many of these women. They may be transiently tearful for several hours and then recover completely, only to be tearful again the next day. Importantly, symptoms are mild and usually only last between a few hours to a few days. Supportive treatment is indicated, and mothers can be reassured that the dysphoria is transient and most likely due to the biochemical changes. They should be monitored for development of more severe psychiatric disturbances including postpartum depression or psychosis.

POSTPARTUM DEPRESSION. In nearly all respects, postpartum depression is similar to other major and minor depressions that develop at any time. Typically, depression is considered postpartum if it begins within 3 to 6 months after childbirth. Criteria for diagnosis of major depression are given in Table 53–5.

Depressive disorders with an onset within 2 to 3 months of delivery develop in approximately 8 to 15 percent of postpartum women. This incidence is only slightly higher than the usual 6-month prevalence for depression among women in the general population. Certain groups of women have a much higher likelihood of developing depression during the puerperium. Adolescents and women with a history of a depressive illness each have a risk of postpartum depression of about 30

TABLE 53–5. Criteria for Major Depressive Episode

At least five[a] of the following symptoms for a 2-week period; one symptom must be either depressed mood or loss of interest or pleasure nearly every day:

1. Depressed mood most of the day
2. Markedly diminished interest or pleasure in all, or almost all, activities most of the day
3. Significant weight loss or weight gain when not dieting, or decrease or increase in appetite
4. Insomnia or hypersomnia
5. Psychomotor agitation or retardation
6. Fatigue or loss of energy
7. Feelings of worthlessness or excessive or inappropriate guilt
8. Diminished ability to think or concentrate
9. Recurrent thoughts of death, recurrent suicidal ideation without a specific plan or a suicide attempt

The symptoms cause clinically significant distress or impairment in social, occupational, or other important areas of functioning.

Symptoms are not due to the direct effects of a substance or general medical condition.

Symptoms are not within 2 months of the loss of a loved one.

In severe cases, may be accompanied by psychosis (bizarre or paranoid thought).

[a] Minor depression requires 2 weeks of depressed mood and fewer than five symptoms.
Adapted from American Psychiatric Association (1993).

percent (Weissman and Olfson, 1995). Up to 70 percent of women with previous postpartum depression will have a subsequent episode. Finally, if a woman has both a previous puerperal depression and current episode of blues, her chances of developing a major depression increase to 85 percent (Hannah and associates, 1992).

COURSE AND TREATMENT. The natural course is one of gradual improvement over the 6 months after delivery (Fleming and colleagues, 1992). The prospects for full recovery are generally good. Pfuhlmann and colleagues (1999) reexamined 39 women 6 to 26 years after they suffered from a postpartum psychiatric illness. They reported that although half of the women relapsed in a subsequent delivery, only 10 percent never recovered completely. Almost 15 percent had a monophasic course with full recovery, and half had a multiphasic course with an average of 2.5 depressive episodes per patient with eventual full recovery.

Because in some cases the woman may remain symptomatic for months to years, maternal depressive illness may affect the quality of her relationship with her child. Depressed mothers have shown less social interaction and play facilitation with their children (Stein and associates, 1991).

Supportive treatment alone is not sufficient for major postpartum depression. Pharmacological intervention is needed in most instances, and affected women should be managed in conjuction with a psychiatrist. Treatment options include antidepressants, anxiolytic agents, and electroconvulsive therapy. As discussed in Chapter 38 (p. 1026), some psychotropic medications pass into breast milk and can cause neonatal sedation, and lithium toxicity has been reported (Chaudron and Jefferson, 2000; Ito, 2000). Bottle feeding should therefore be considered.

Treatment also includes monitoring for thoughts of suicide or infanticide, emergence of psychosis, and response to treatment. Psychotherapy focuses on the woman's fears and concerns regarding her new responsibilities and roles. For some women, the course of illness is severe enough to warrant hospitalization.

POSTPARTUM PSYCHOSIS. This is the most worrisome and severe puerperal mental disorder. It is estimated to occur in 1 to 4 of 1000 births (Weissman and Olfson, 1995). In our experiences, it is not nearly so common. Women with postpartum psychosis lose touch with reality. They have stretches of lucidity alternating with psychosis. Also frequently noted are symptoms of confusion and disorientation that are often seen in toxic states or delirium.

Two types of women seem to be susceptible: women with an underlying depressive, manic, schizophrenic, or schizoaffective disorder, and women who have had a

history of depression or a severe life event in the preceding year (Kumar and associates, 1993). Women with preexisting psychotic illness are at highest risk, with bipolar disorder and schizoaffective disorder being the most strongly associated. A brief interval between the earlier psychiatric episode and parturition increases the likelihood of relapse. Other risk factors are biologically related and include younger age, primiparity, and family history of psychiatric illness. Marks and co-workers (1991) studied 88 high-risk women after childbirth. Of these, 45 women had no previous psychiatric disorder and 43 had a history of psychosis. A fourth developed postpartum psychosis, and all these cases occurred in women with a history of bipolar or schizoaffective disorder. Another fourth had a nonpsychotic postpartum depression, and all these cases were in women with a history of a severe life event.

Approximately a quarter of women who have had one episode of postpartum psychosis will have a recurrence in the next pregnancy. This statistic emphasizes the need to identify women with a prior history and to monitor them closely. The peak onset of psychotic symptoms is 10 to 14 days after parturition, but the risk remains high for months after delivery (Brockington and colleagues, 1981). Even though rare, the risk of a psychotic episode during the postpartum period is still 10 to 15 times greater than at other times during a woman's life. In most instances, women with this disorder will go on to develop a relapsing psychotic illness that recurs during times unrelated to pregnancy or parturition.

COURSE AND TREATMENT. The course is variable and depends upon the type of underlying illness. For those with manic-depressive and schizoaffective psychoses, the time to recovery is about 6 months (Sneddon, 1992). The clinical course of bipolar illness or schizoaffective disorder in puerperal women is comparable to that of nonpuerperal women. The most impaired level of functioning at follow-up is among those suffering from schizophrenia. These women should be referred for psychiatric care. The severity of postpartum psychosis mandates pharmacological treatment and, in most cases, hospitalization. The woman who is psychotic usually will have difficulty in caring for her infant, and may have delusions leading to thoughts of self-harm or harm of the infant. Fortunately, reports from mother–baby psychiatric units claim few incidents of infant harm.

TREATMENT OF MENTAL DISORDERS. A large number of psychotropic medications are now available for management of mental disorders (Kuller and colleagues, 1996). The fetal risks are discussed in Chapter 38 (p. 1026). Most pregnant women requiring pharmacotherapy have preexisting severe psychiatric illnesses such as bipolar disorder, schizoaffective disorder, schizophrenia, or recurrent major depression. Other women requiring treatment are those who have an emotional disorder that evolves during pregnancy.

ANTIDEPRESSANTS. Ethical considerations for managing depressed pregnant women have been reviewed by Coverdale and colleagues (1996). Severe depression requires treatment and, in most cases, the benefits of therapies outweigh the risks. Tricyclic antidepressants such as amitriptyline, doxepin, imipramine, and nortriptyline are commonly used for depressive disorders. Maternal side effects include orthostatic hypotension, and constipation. Sedation is also common, making these medications particularly helpful with depression-associated sleep problems. Monoamine oxidase inhibitors (MAOIs) are very effective antidepressants that are used less frequently because they cause orthostatic hypotension. Also, simultaneous administration of meperidine and some anesthetic agents can stimulate a life-threatening hyperthermic crisis (Mortola, 1989). Experience with selective serotonin reuptake inhibitors (SSRIs), including fluoxetine and sertraline, has made them the primary treatment for most depressive illnesses. They do not cause orthostatic hypotension, constipation, or sedation, which makes them preferable to other antidepressants.

ANTIPSYCHOTICS. Women with severe psychiatric syndromes such as schizophrenia, schizoaffective disorder, or bipolar disorder have a high likelihood of requiring antipsychotic treatment during pregnancy. Typical anti-psychotics are dopamine antagonists. Clozapine is the only available atypical antipsychotic, and it has a different but unknown action. Antipsychotics differ by potency and side-effect profile. The lower-potency agents, chlorpromazine and thioridazine, have greater anticholinergic properties and are sedating.

LITHIUM. The safety of lithium during pregnancy is controversial (Chap. 38, p. 1027). In addition to concerns about teratogenicity, there are considerations of its narrow therapeutic index. Lithium toxicity in the breast-feeding newborn has been reported.

BENZODIAZEPINES. These may be required during pregnancy for women who have severe and debilitating anxiety disorders or for assaultive or agitated psychotic patients. Diazepam may be associated with prolonged neonatal neurological depression when given close to delivery.

ELECTROCONVULSIVE THERAPY. Treatment of depression with electroshock during pregnancy is occasionally necessary for the woman with a major mood disorder unresponsive to pharmacological therapy. Griffiths and colleagues (1989) reported results obtained in a woman who underwent 11 such treatments from 23 to 31 weeks. They used thiamylal and succinylcholine, intubation, and assisted ventilation during each treatment. They found that plasma levels of epinephrine, norepinephrine, and dopamine were elevated two- to threefold within minutes of electroshock. Despite this, the fetal heart rate tracing and maternal heart rate,

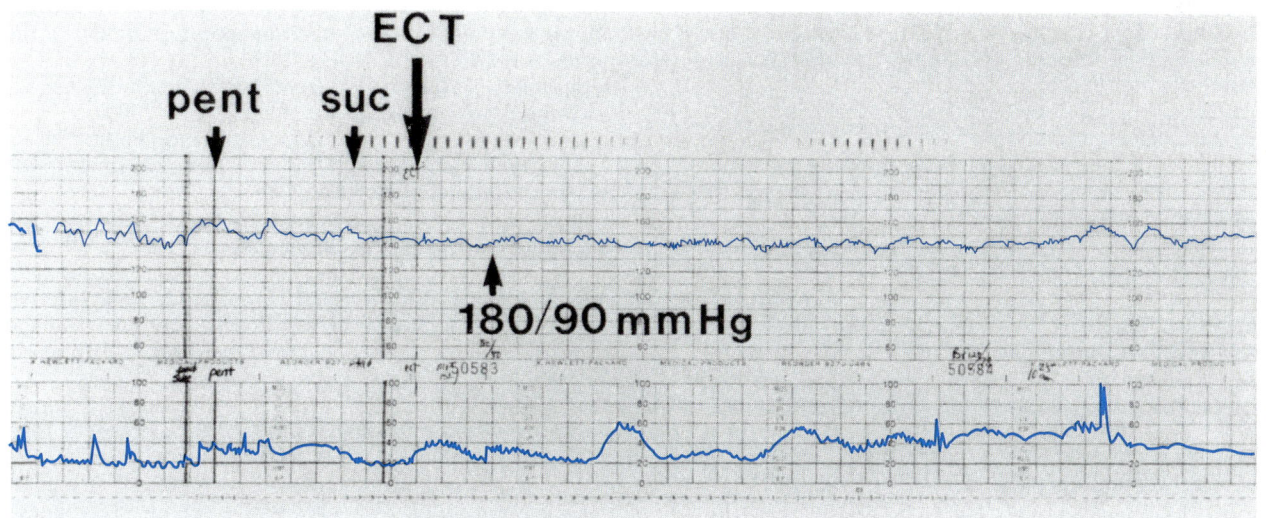

FIGURE 53–3. Continuous fetal cardiotocography during electroconvulsive therapy at 34 weeks. Note regular uterine contractions and postshock subsequent hypertonic–tetanic contractions. Medications before electroconvulsive therapy (ECT) and blood pressure after therapy are noted. (pent = thiopental sodium; suc = succinylcholine; paper speed, 3 cm/ min.) (From Sherer and colleagues, 1991, with permission.)

blood pressure, and oxygen saturation remained normal. Varan and co-workers (1985) described a variable fetal heart rate deceleration characteristic of cord compression during electroconvulsive therapy. Sherer and associates (1991) described a woman who underwent seven weekly antepartum electroconvulsive treatments beginning at 30 weeks. Each treatment was followed by hypertension, uterine hypertonicity, and uterine bleeding (Fig. 53–3). Subsequently, placental abruption was shown to be the cause. Miller (1994) reviewed 300 published case reports of electroconvulsive therapy during pregnancy, and found that complications occurred in about 10 percent. These included transient benign fetal arrhythmias, mild vaginal bleeding, abdominal pain, and self-limited uterine contractions. Women who were not adequately prepared also had an increased risk for aspiration, aortocaval compression, and respiratory alkalosis. Important preparatory steps include cervical assessment, discontinuation of nonessential anticholinergic medication, uterine and fetal heart rate monitoring, intravenous hydration, administration of a nonparticulate antacid, and positioning in left lateral tilt. During the procedure, excessive hyperventilation should be avoided and the airway should be protected.

REFERENCES

Abramsky O: Pregnancy and multiple sclerosis. Ann Neurol 36:S38, 1994

Ahokas A, Kaukoranta J, Aito M: Effect of oestradiol on postpartum depression. Psychopharmacology 146:108, 1999

Al Qattan MM, Manktelow RT, Bowen CVA: Pregnancy-induced carpal tunnel syndrome requiring surgical release longer than 2 years after delivery. Obstet Gynecol 84:249, 1994

American College of Obstetricians and Gynecologists: Depression in women. Technical Bulletin no. 182, July 1993a

American College of Obstetricians and Gynecologists Committee on Obstetrics: Obstetric management of patients with spinal cord injury. ACOG Committee Opinion no. 121, April 1993b

American College of Obstetricians and Gynecologists: Precis IV. Fertility Control. Washington, DC: American College of Obstetricians and Gynecologists, 1990, p 8

American Psychiatric Association. DSM-IV Draft Criteria. Washington, DC, APA, 1993

Appleby L: Suicide during pregnancy and in the first postnatal year. BMJ 302:137, 1991

Au KL, Woo JS, Wong VC: Intrauterine death from ergotamine overdosage. Eur J Obstet Gynecol Reprod Biol 19:313, 1985

Aube M: Migraine in pregnancy. Neurology 53:S26, 1999

Bader AM: Neurological and neuromuscular disease. In Chestnut DH (eds): Obstetric Anesthesia: Principles and Practice. St. Louis, Mosby, 1994, p 920

Baker ER, Cardenas DD, Benedetti TJ: Risks associated with pregnancy in spinal cord-injured women. Obstet Gynecol 80:428, 1992

Bateman DN: Sumatriptan. Lancet 341:221, 1993

Bates GW, Whitworth NS, Parker JL, Johnson MP: Elevated cerebrospinal fluid prolactin concentration in women with pseudotumor cerebri. South Med J 75:807, 1982

Benedict MI, Paine LL, Paine LA, Brandt D, Stallings R: The association of childhood sexual abuse with depressive symptoms during pregnancy, and selected pregnancy outcomes. Child Abuse Negl 23:659, 1999

Bergant AM, Heim K, Ulmer H, Illmensee K: Early postnatal depressive mood: Associations with obstetric and psychosocial factors. J Psychosom Res 46:391, 1999

Bernstein IM, Watson M, Simmons GM, Catalano PM, Davis G, Collins R: Maternal brain death and prolonged fetal survival. Obstet Gynecol 74:434, 1989

Branch DW: Antiphospholipid antibodies and pregnancy: Maternal implications. Semin Perinatol 14:139, 1990

Bravo RH, Katz M, Inturisi M, Cohen NH: Obstetric management of Landry Guillain–Barré syndrome. Am J Obstet Gynecol 142:714, 1982

Brockington IF, Cernik KF, Schofield EM, Downing AR, Francis AF, Keelan C: Puerperal psychosis. Phenomena and diagnosis. Arch Gen Psychiatry 38:829, 1981

Brodie MJ, Dichter MA: Antiepileptic drugs. N Engl J Med 334:168, 1996

Bryan TL, Georgiopoulos AM, Harms RW, Huxsahl JE, Larson DR, Yawm BP: Incidence of postpartum depression in Olmsted County, Minnesota. A population-based, retrospective study. J Reprod Med 44:352, 1999

Burger J, Horwitz SM, Forsyth BWC, Leventhal JM, Leaf PJ: Psychological sequelae of medical complications during pregnancy. Pediatrics 91:566, 1993

Cantú C, Barinagarrementeria F: Cerebral venous thrombosis associated with pregnancy and puerperium. Stroke 24:1880, 1993

Caplan LR, Mohr JP, Kistler JP, Koroshetz W: Should thrombolytic therapy be the first-line treatment for acute ischemic stroke? N Engl J Med 337:1309, 1997

Cartlidge NEF: Neurologic disorders. In Barron WM, Lindheimer MD (eds): Medical Disorders During Pregnancy, 3rd ed. St. Louis, Mosby, 2000, p 516

Catanzarite VA, Willms DC, Holdy KE, Gardner SE, Ludwig DM, Cousins LM: Brain death during pregnancy: Tocolytic therapy and aggressive maternal support on behalf of the fetus. Am J Perinatol 14:431, 1997

Chaudron LH, Jefferson JW: Mood stabilizers during breastfeeding: A review. J Clin Psychiatry 61:79, 2000

Cheng Q, Jiang GX, Fredrikson S, Link H, de Pedro-Cuesta J: Increased incidence of Guillain–Barre syndrome postpartum. Epidemiology 9:601, 1998

Cohen Y, Lavie O, Granoxsky-Grisaru S, Aboulafia Y, Diamant YZ: Bell palsy complicating pregnancy: A review. Obstet Gynecol Surv 55:184, 2000

Commission on Classification and Terminology of the International League Against Epilepsy: Proposal for the classification of epilepsy and epileptic syndromes. Epilepsia 30:389, 1989

Confavreux C, Vukusic S, Moreau T, Adeleine P: Relapses and progression of disability in multiple sclerosis. N Engl J Med 343:1430, 2000

Cornelissen M, Steegers-Theunissen R, Kollée L, Eskes T, Vogels-Mentink G, Motohara K, De Abreu R, Monnens L: Increased incidence of neonatal vitamin K deficiency resulting from maternal anticonvulsant therapy. Am J Obstet Gynecol 168:923, 1993

Courts RB: Splinting for symptoms of carpal tunnel syndrome during pregnancy. J Hand Ther 8:31, 1995

Coverdale JH, Chervenak FA, McCullough LB, Bayer T: Ethically justified clinically comprehensive guidelines for the management of the depressed pregnant patient. Am J Obstet Gynecol 174:169, 1996

Cox SM, Hankins GDV, Leveno KJ, Cunningham FG: Bacterial endocarditis: A serious pregnancy complication. J Reprod Med 33:671, 1988

Cross JN, Castro PO, Jennett WB: Cerebral strokes associated with pregnancy and the puerperium. BMJ 3:214, 1968

Damek DM, Shuster EA: Pregnancy and multiple sclerosis. Mayo Clin Proc 72:977, 1997

Dammers JWHH, Veering MM, Vermeulen M: Injection with methylprednisolone proximal to the carpal tunnel: Randomised double blind trial. BMJ 319:884, 1999

Depression Guideline Panel: Depression in Primary Care, Vol I. Detection and Diagnosis. Clinical Practice Guideline No. 5. Rockville, MD, US Department of Health and Human Services, Public Health Service, Agency for Health Care Policy and Research (AHCPR Pub. No. 93-0550), April 1993

Devinsky O: Patients with refractory seizures. N Engl J Med 340:1566, 1999

Dias MS, Sekhar LN: Intracranial hemorrhage from aneurysms and arteriovenous malformations during pregnancy and the puerperium. Neurosurgery 27:855, 1990

Dillon WP, Lee RV, Tronolone MJ, Buckwald S, Foote RJ: Life support and maternal death during pregnancy. JAMA 248:1089, 1982

Ditunno JF Jr, Formal CS: Chronic spinal cord injury. N Engl J Med 330:550, 1994

Donaldson JO, Lee NS: Arterial and venous stroke associated with pregnancy. Neurol Clin 12:583, 1994

Dorsey DL, Camann WR: Obstetric anesthesia in patients with idiopathic facial paralysis (Bell's palsy): A 10-year survey. Anesth Analg 77:81, 1993

Drachman DB: Myasthenia gravis. N Engl J Med 330:1797, 1994

Easton HD, Hauser SK, Martin JB: Cerebrovascular diseases. In Fauci AS, Braunwald E, Isselbacher KJ, Wilson JD, Martin JB, Kasper DL, Hauser SL, Longo DL (eds): Harrison's Principles of Internal Medicine, 14th ed. New York, McGraw-Hill, 1998, p 2325

Ebers GC: Treatment of multiple sclerosis. Lancet 343:275, 1994

Einhäupl KM, Villringer A, Meister W, Mehraein S, Garner C, Pellkofer M, Haberl RL, Pfister HW, Schmiedek P: Heparin treatment in sinus venous thrombosis. Lancet 338:597, 1991

Ekman-Ordeberg G, Sälgeback S, Ordeberg G: Carpal tunnel syndrome in pregnancy. A prospective study. Acta Obstet Gynecol Scand 66:233, 1987

Eldridge RE, Ephross SA, and the Sumatriptan Registry Advisory Committee: Monitoring birth outcomes in the sumatriptan pregnancy registry. Teratology 55:48, 1997

Falco NA, Eriksson E: Idiopathic facial palsy in pregnancy and the puerperium. Surg Gynecol Obstet 169:337, 1989

Fettes I: Menstrual migraine. Methods of prevention and control. Postgrad Med 101:67, 1997

Field DR, Gates EA, Creasy RK, Jonsen AR, Laros RK Jr: Maternal brain death during pregnancy. JAMA 260:816, 1988

Finnerty JJ, Chisholm CA, Chapple H, Login IS, Pinkerton JV: Cerebral arteriovenous malformation in pregnancy: Presentation and neurologic, obstetric, and ethical significance. Am J Obstet Gynecol 181:296, 1999

Fleming AS, Klein E, Corter C: The effects of a social support group on depression, maternal attitudes and behavior in new mothers. J Child Psychol Psychiatry 33:685, 1992

Giannotta SL, Daniels J, Golde SH, Zelman V, Bayat A: Ruptured intracranial aneurysms during pregnancy. A report of four cases. J Reprod Med 31:139, 1986

Glickman S, Kamm MA: Bowel dysfunction in spinal-cord-injury patients. Lancet 347:1651, 1996

Golbe LI: Pregnancy and movement disorders. Neurol Clin 12:497, 1994

Graham JM, Mavin-Padilla M, Hoefnagel D: Jejunal atresia associated with Cafergot ingestion during pregnancy. Clin Pediatr 22:226, 1983

Griffiths EJ, Lorenz RP, Baxter S, Talon NS: Acute neurohumoral response to electroconvulsive therapy during pregnancy. A case report. J Reprod Med 34:907, 1989

Hambly PR, Martin B: Anaesthesia for chronic spinal cord lesions. Anaesthesia 53:273, 1998

Hannah P, Adams D, Lee A, Glover V, Sandler M: Links between early post-partum mood and post-natal depression. Br J Psychiatry 160:777, 1992

Harris B, Lovett L, Newcombe RG, Read GF, Walker R, Riad-Fahmy D: Maternity blues and major endocrine changes: Cardiff puerperal mood and hormone study II. BMJ 308:949, 1994

Hauser HL, Goodkin DE: Multiple sclerosis and other demyelinating diseases. In Fauci AS, Braunwald E, Isselbacher KJ, Wilson JD, Martin JB, Kasper DL, Hauser SL, Longo DL (eds): Harrison's Principles of Internal Medicine, 14th ed. New York, McGraw-Hill, 1998, p 2409

Henderson CE, Torbey M: Rupture of intracranial aneurysm associated with cocaine use during pregnancy. Am J Perinatol 5:142, 1988

Hollingsworth DR, Resnik R (eds): Medical Counseling Before Pregnancy. New York, Churchill Livingstone, 1988, p 415

Horrigan TJ, Schroeder AV, Schaffer RM: The triad of substance abuse, violence, and depression are interrelated in pregnancy. J Subst Abuse Treat 18:55, 2000

Horton JC, Chambers WA, Lyons SL, Adams RD, Kjellberg RN: Pregnancy and the risk of hemorrhage from cerebral arteriovenous malformations. Neurosurgery 27:867, 1990

Hughes HE, Goldstein DA: Birth defects following maternal exposure to ergotamine, beta-blockers, and caffeine. J Med Genet 25:396, 1988

Hughes SJ, Short DJ, Usherwood MMcD, Tebbutt H: Management of the pregnant women with spinal cord injuries. Br J Obstet Gynaecol 98:513, 1991

Hunt HB, Schrifin BS, Suzuki K: Ruptured berry aneurysms and pregnancy. Obstet Gynecol 43:827, 1974

Hurley TJ, Brunson AD, Archer RL, Lefler SF, Quirk JG: Landry Guillain–Barré Strohl syndrome in pregnancy: Report of three cases treated with plasmapheresis. Obstet Gynecol 78:482, 1991

Ip MSM, So SY, Lam WK, Tang LCH, Mok CK: Thymectomy in myasthenia gravis during pregnancy. Postgrad Med J 62:473, 1986

Ireland B, Corbett JJ, Wallace RB: The search for causes of idiopathic intracranial hypertension. A preliminary case-control study. Arch Neurol 47:315, 1990

Ito S: Drug therapy for breast-feeding women. N Engl J Med 343:118, 2000

Itoyama Y, Uemura S, Ushio Y, Kuratsu J, Nonaka N: Natural course of unoperated intracranial arteriovenous malformation: Study of 50 cases. J Neurosurg 71:805, 1989

Jackson AB, Wadley V: A multicenter study of women's self-reported reproductive health after spinal cord injury. Arch Phys Med Rehabil 80:1420, 1999

Joffe H, Cohen LS: Estrogen, serotonin, and mood disturbance: Where is the therapeutic bridge? Biol Psychiatry 44:798, 1998

Kamitani H, Masuzawa H, Kanazawa I, Kubo T: Bleeding risk in unruptured and residual cerebral aneurysms—angiographic annual growth rate in nineteen patients. Acta Neurochir 141:153, 1999

Katz VL, Peterson R, Cefalo RC: Pseudotumor cerebri and pregnancy. Am J Perinatol 6:442, 1989

Kay R, Wong KS, Yu YL, Chan YW, Tsoi TH, Ahuja AT, Chan FL, Fong KY, Law CB, Wong A, Woo J: Low-molecular-weight heparin for the treatment of acute ischemic stroke. N Engl J Med 333:1588, 1995

Kendell RE, Chalmers JC, Platz C: Epidemiology of puerperal psychoses. Br J Psychiatry 150:662, 1987

Kittner SJ, Stern BJ, Feeser BR, Hebel R, Nagey DA, Buchholz DW, Early CJ, Johnson CJ, Macko RF, Sloan MA, Wityk RJ, Wozniak MA: Pregnancy and the risk of stroke. N Engl J Med 335:768, 1996

Kuller JA, Katz VL, McCoy MC, Hansen WF: Pregnancy complicated by Guillain Barré syndrome. South Med J 88:987, 1995

Kuller JA, Katz VL, McMahon MJ, Wells SR, Bashford RA: Pharmacologic treatment of psychiatric disease in pregnancy and lactation: Fetal and neonatal effects. Obstet Gynecol 87:789, 1996

Kumar R, Marks M, Wieck A, Hirst D, Campbell I, Checkley S: Neuroendocrine and psychosocial mechanisms in postpartum psychosis. Prog Neuropsychopharmacol Biol Psychiatry 17:571, 1993

Kurtzke JF: The current neurologic burden of illness and injury in the United States. Neurology 32:1207, 1982

Lander CM, Eadie MJ: Plasma antiepileptic drug concentrations during pregnancy. Epilepsia 32:257, 1991

Landwehr JB, Isada NB, Pryde PG, Johnson MP, Evans MI, Canady AI: Maternal neurosurgical shunts and pregnancy outcome. Obstet Gynecol 83:134, 1994

Lanska DJ, Kryscio RJ: Risk factors for peripartum and postpartum stroke and intracranial venous thrombosis. Stroke 31:1274, 2000

Lanska DJ, Kryscio RJ: Stroke and intracranial venous thrombosis during pregnancy and puerperium. Neurology 53:1162, 1998

Littleford JA, Brockhurst NJ, Bernstein EP, Georgoussis SE: Obstetrical anesthesia for a parturient with a ventriculoperitoneal shunt and third ventriculostomy. Can J Anaesth 46:1057, 1999

Lublin FD, Reingold SC: Defining the course of multiple sclerosis: Results of an international survey. National Multiple Sclerosis Society (USA) Advisory Committee on Clinical Trials of New Agents for Multiple Sclerosis. Neurology 46:907, 1996

Marks MN, Wieck A, Checkley SA, Kumar R: Life stress and post-partum psychosis: a preliminary report. Br J Psychiatry Suppl 10:45, 1991

McDonald WI: New treatments for multiple sclerosis. BMJ 310:345, 1995

McInnis MG, DePaulo JR Jr: Major mood disorders. In: Emery and Rimoin's Principles and Practice of Medical Genetics, Vol II. New York, Churchill Livingstone, 1996, p 1843

Mercado A, Johnson G Jr, Calver D, Sokol RJ: Cocaine, pregnancy, and postpartum intracerebral hemorrhage. Obstet Gynecol 73:467, 1989

Miller LJ: Use of electroconvulsive therapy during pregnancy. Hosp Commun Psychiatry 45:444, 1994

Minielly R, Yuzpe AA, Drake CG: Subarachnoid hemorrhage secondary to ruptured cerebral aneurysm in pregnancy. Obstet Gynecol 53:64, 1979

Mortola JF: The use of psychotropic agents in pregnancy and lactation. Psychiatr Clin North Am 12:69, 1989

Multicenter Acute Stroke Trial Europe Study Group: Thrombolytic therapy with streptokinase in acute ischemic stroke. N Engl J Med 335:145, 1996

Myers JK, Weissman MM, Tischler GL, Holzer CE, Leaf PJ, Orvaschel H, Anthony JC, Boyd JH, Burke JD, Kramer M, Stoltzman R: Six-month prevalence of psychiatric disorders in three communities. Arch Gen Psychiatry 41:959, 1984

National Institute of Neurological Disorders and Stroke Study Group: Tissue plasminogen activator for acute ischemic stroke. N Engl J Med 333:1581, 1995

Nelson KB, Ellenberg JH: Maternal seizure disorder, outcome of pregnancy, and neurologic abnormalities in the children. Neurology 32:1247, 1982

Nelson LM, Franklin GM, Jones MC, the Multiple Sclerosis Study Group: Risk of multiple sclerosis exacerbation during pregnancy and breast-feeding. JAMA 259:3441, 1988

Oates M: Management of major mental illness in pregnancy and the puerperium. Baillieres Clin Obstet Gynaecol 3:905, 1989

O'Hara MW, Neunaber DJ, Zekoski EM: Prospective study of postpartum depression: Prevalence, course, and predictive factors. J Abnorm Psychol 93:158, 1984

Olafsson E, Hallgrimsson JT, Hauser WA, Ludvigsson P, Gudmundsson G: Pregnancies of women with epilepsy: A population-based study in Iceland. Epilepsia 39:887, 1998

Olesen J: Understanding the biologic basis of migraine. N Engl J Med 331:1713, 1994

Omdal R, Roalsø S: Chorea gravidarum and chorea associated with oral contraceptives diseases due to antiphospholipid antibodies? Acta Neurol Scand 86:219, 1992

O'Quinn S, Ephross SA, Williams V, Davis RL, Gutterman DL, Fox AW: Pregnancy and perinatal outcomes in migraineurs using sumatriptan: A prospective study. Arch Gynecol Obstet 263:7, 1999

Paarlberg KM, Vingerhoets AJJM, Passchier J, Dekker GA, Heinen AGJJ, van Geijn HP: Psychosocial factors as predictors of low birthweight and preterm delivery. Am J Obstet Gynecol 174:381, 1996

Paulson GW: Headaches in women, including women who are pregnant. Am J Obstet Gynecol 173:1734, 1995

Pfaffenrath V, Rehm M: Migraine in pregnancy: What are the safest treatment options? Drug Safety 19:383, 1998

Pfuhlmann B, Franzek E, Beckmann H, Stober G: Long-term course and outcome of severe postpartum psychiatric disorders. Psychopathology 32:192, 1999

Plauché WC: Myasthenia gravis in mothers and their newborns. Clin Obstet Gynecol 34:82, 1991

Prasher VP, Barrett K: Neuropsychiatric aspects of Sydenham's chorea: A case report. J Psychosom Obstet Gynecol 14:159, 1993

PRISMS (Prevention of Relapses and Disability by Interferon beta-1a Subcutaneously in Multiple Sclerosis) Study Group: Randomised double-blind placebo-controlled study of interferon beta-1a in relapsing/remitting multiple sclerosis. Lancet 352:1498, 1998

Reprotox Database: Ergotamine. RTC: 1396; CAS Registry: 113-15-5; October 1, 1998

Rochat RW, Koonin LM, Atrash HK, Jewett JJ and the Maternal Mortality Collaborative: Maternal mortality in the United States: Report from the Maternal Mortality Collaborative. Obstet Gynecol 72:91, 1988

Rockel A, Wissel J, Rolfs A: Guillain–Barré syndrome in pregnancy: An indication for caesarean section? J Perinat Med 22:393, 1994

Ropper AH: The Guillain–Barré syndrome. N Engl J Med 326:1130, 1992

Roullet E, Verdier-Taillefer MH, Amarenco P, Gharbi G, Alperovitch A, Marteau R: Pregnancy and multiple sclerosis: A longitudinal study of 125 remittent patients. J Neurol Neurosurg Psychiatry 56:299, 1993

Sadovnick AD, Eisen K, Hashimoto SA, Farquhar R, Yee IML, Hooge J, Kastrukoff L, Oger JJF, Paty DW: Pregnancy and multiple sclerosis. A prospective study. Arch Neurol 51:1120, 1994

Schmeelk KH, Granger DA, Susman EJ, Chrousos GP: Maternal depression and risk for postpartum complications: Role of prenatal corticotropin-releasing hormone and interleukin-1 receptor antagonist. Behav Med 25:88, 1999

Schneider J, Blea C, Hendricks SK: Increased familial incidence of multiple sclerosis: Genetics and epidemiology in pregnancy. Am J Obstet Gynecol 174:445, 1996

Schumacher HR Jr, Dorwart BB, Korzeniowski OM: Occurrence of de Quervains tendinitis during pregnancy. Arch Intern Med 145:2083, 1985

Séguin L, Potvin L, St. Denis M, Loiselle J: Chronic stressors, social support, and depression during pregnancy. Obstet Gynecol 85:583, 1995

Seror P: Pregnancy-related carpal tunnel syndrome. J Hand Surg [Br] 23:98, 1998

Shapiro JL, Yudin MH, Ray JG: Bell's palsy and tinnitus during pregnancy: Predictors of pre-eclampsia? Three cases and a detailed review of the literature. Acta Otolaryngol 119:647, 1999

Sharshar T, Lamy C, Mas JL: Incidence and causes of strokes associated with pregnancy and puerperium. A study in public hospitals of Île de France. Stroke 26:930, 1995

Sherer DM, DAmico ML, Warshal DP, Stern RA, Grunert HF, Abramowicz JS: Recurrent mild abruptio placenta occurring immediately after repeated electroconvulsive therapy in pregnancy. Am J Obstet Gynecol 165:652, 1991

Shuhaiber S, Pastuszak A, Schick B, Matsui D, Spivey G, Brochu J, Koren G: Pregnancy outcome following first trimester exposure to sumatriptan. Neurology 15:581, 1998

Simolke GA, Cox SM, Cunningham FG: Cerebrovascular accidents complicating pregnancy and the puerperium. Obstet Gynecol 78:37, 1991

Sneddon J: The mother and baby unit: An important approach. In Hamilton JA, Harberger PN (eds): Postpartum Psychiatric Illness. Philadelphia, University of Pennsylvania Press, 1992

Srinivasan K: Ischemic cerebral vascular disease in the young. Two common causes in India. Stroke 15:733, 1984

Stein A, Gath DH, Bucher J, Bond A, Day A, Cooper PG: The relationship between postnatal depression and mother–child interaction. Br J Psychiatry 158:46, 1991

Stewart WF, Lipton RB, Celentano DD, Reed ML: Prevalence of migraine headache in the United States: Relation to age, income, race and other sociodemographic factors. JAMA 267:64, 1992

Stolp-Smith KA, Pascoe MK, Ogburn PL Jr: Carpal tunnel syndrome in pregnancy: Frequency, severity, and prognosis. Arch Phys Med Rehabil 79:1285, 1998

Tietjen GE: The relationship of migraine and stroke. Neuroepidemiology 19:13, 2000

Tunis SL, Golbus MS: Assessing mood states in pregnancy. Survey of the literature. Obstet Gynecol Surv 46:340, 1991

Tzourio C, Tehindrazanarivelo A, Iglésias S, Alpérovitch A, Chedru F, d'Anglejan-Chatillon J, Bousser MG: Case-control study of migraine and risk of ischemic stroke in young women. BMJ 310:830, 1995

Uknis A, Silberstein SD: Migraine and pregnancy. Headache 31:372, 1991

Van der Meché FGA, Schmitz PIM, The Dutch Guillain–Barré Study Group: A randomized trial comparing intravenous immune globulin and plasma exchange in Guillain–Barré syndrome. N Engl J Med 326:1123, 1992

Varan LR, Gillieson MS, Skene DS, Sarwer-Foner GJ: ECT in an acutely psychotic pregnant woman with actively aggressive (homicidal) impulses. Can J Psychiatry 30:363, 1985

Vernet-der Garabedian B, Lacokova M, Eymard B, Morel E, Faltin M, Zajac J, Sadovsky O, Dommergues M, Tripon P, Bach JF: Association of neonatal myasthenia gravis with antibodies against the fetal acetylcholine receptor. J Clin Invest 94:555, 1994

Verloes A, Emonts P, Dubois M, Rigo J: Paraplegia and arthrogryposis multiplex of the lower extremities after intrauterine exposure to ergotamine. J Med Genet 27:213, 1990

Vives A, Carmona F, Zabala E, Fernandez C, Cararach V, Iglesias X: Maternal brain death during pregnancy. Int J Gynaecol Obstet 52:67, 1996

Voetsch B, Damasceno BP, Camargo EC, Massaro A, Bacheshi LA, Scaff M, Annichino-Bizzacchi JM, Arruda VR: Inherited thrombophilia as a risk factor for the development of ischemic stroke in young adults. Thromb Haemost 83:229, 2000

Walther EU, Hohlfeld R: Multiple sclerosis: Side effects of interferon beta therapy and their management. Neurology 53:1622, 1999

Weinreb HJ: Demyelinating and neoplastic diseases in pregnancy. Neurol Clin 12:509, 1994

Weissman MM, Olfson M: Depression in women: Implications for health care research. Science 269:799, 1995

Welch KMA: Migraine and pregnancy. Adv Neurol 64:77, 1994

Welch KMA: Drug therapy of migraine. N Engl J Med 329:1476, 1993

Westgren N, Hultling C, Levi R, Westgren M: Pregnancy and delivery in women with a traumatic spinal cord injury in Sweden, 1980–1991. Obstet Gynecol 81:926, 1993

Wiebers DO: Subarachnoid hemorrhage in pregnancy. Semin Neurol 8:226, 1988

Wiebers DO, Whisnant JP: The incidence of stroke among pregnant women in Rochester, Minn, 1955 through 1979. JAMA 253:3055, 1985

Wilkins RH: Natural history of intracranial vascular malformations: A review. Neurosurgery 16:421, 1985

Wisoff JH, Kratzert KJ, Handwerker SM, Young BK, Epstein F: Pregnancy in patients with cerebrospinal fluid shunts: Report of a series and review of the literature. Neurosurgery 29:827, 1991

Witlin AG, Mattar F, Sibai BM: Postpartum stroke: A twenty-year experience. Am J Obstet Gynecol 183:83, 2000

Yerby MS: Pregnancy, teratogenesis, and epilepsy. Neurol Clin 12:749, 1994

54

Dermatological Disorders

Most skin diseases are encountered with similar frequency in pregnant and nonpregnant women. There are, however, a number of skin changes induced by the hormonal influences of pregnancy. For example, episodes of pruritus are common during pregnancy, and in many instances, itching is not accompanied by a skin eruption. A common etiology is intrahepatic cholestasis and bile salt retention, commonly known as *pruritus gravidarum* (Chap. 48, p. 1283). There also are a number of pregnancy-specific dermatoses that usually are symptomatic and thus may be alarming. Importantly, some of these may be associated with adverse pregnancy outcomes.

PHYSIOLOGICAL SKIN CHANGES IN PREGNANCY

Hormonal changes induced by normal pregnancy may have rather remarkable influences on the skin. As discussed in Chapters 6 and 8, fetoplacental hormone production, stimulation, or alteration of clearance may increase the plasma availability of estrogens, progesterone, and a variety of androgens. Similarly, there are profound changes in the availability or concentrations of some adrenal steroids, including cortisol, aldosterone, and deoxycorticosterone. Presumably related to enlargement of the intermediate lobe of the pituitary gland, plasma levels of melanocyte-stimulating hormone (MSH) become remarkably elevated by 8 weeks' gestation. Production of pro-opiomelanocortin has been demonstrated in placental extracts, and this ultimately is a source of $\alpha-$ and $\beta-$melanocyte-stimulating hormone. In their review, Paus and Cotsarelis (1999) describe hair-growth modulation by estrogens, androgens, thyroid hormones, glucocorticords, and prolactin.

HYPERPIGMENTATION. According to Vaughan Jones and Black (1999), some degree of skin darkening is observed in 90 percent of all pregnant women. Its exact cause is not known, but it is doubtful that elevated serum levels of melanocyte-stimulating hormone are responsible. Estrogens play a role in melanogenesis in mammals and may be the inciting factor. Hyperpigmentation is evident beginning early in pregnancy, and this is more marked in dark-skinned women. These effects are more pronounced in naturally hyperpigmented areas such as the areolae, perineum, and umbilicus. Areas prone to friction, including the axillae and inner thighs, also may become darkened. When the *linea alba* becomes pigmented, it is renamed the *linea nigra*.

Pigmentation of the face, referred to as the mask of pregnancy, is also called *chloasma* or *melasma*. This is seen in at least half of pregnant women. Melasma is aggravated by sunlight or other ultraviolet light expo-

sure; its severity may be altered by avoiding excessive exposure and using sunscreens. It is caused by melanin deposition into epidermal or dermal macrophages, and although the former usually regresses postpartum, dermal melanosis may persist up to 10 years in a third of women. Oral contraceptives may aggravate melasma and should be avoided in susceptible women. If particularly disfiguring, topical application of 2 to 5 percent hydroxyquinone or 0.1 percent tretinoin ointment or cream may provide some improvement (Griffiths and colleagues, 1993; Kimbrough-Green and co-workers, 1994). Sunscreen use should be continued.

NEVI. All persons have some form of benign or melanocytic nevi. It has been taught that these pigmented cutaneous tumors commonly enlarge and darken during pregnancy, and they may be confused with malignant melanomas. Recently, however, Pennoyer and colleagues (1997) carefully observed these benign lesions and found that only 6 percent of 129 nevi changed in diameter over pregnancy. Four of these increased by 1 mm, and four decreased by 1 mm. They concluded that the more striking changes were in nonmelanocytic lesions. Thus, although nevi are shown histologically to have enlarged melanocytes and increased melanin deposition, there is no evidence that they undergo malignant transformation during pregnancy. According to the study by the World Health Organization Melanoma Program, the average malignant tumor is slightly but significantly thicker when discovered during pregnancy (MacKie and colleagues, 1991). These authors concluded that this represents either a delay in identification or pregnancy-induced melanoma stimulation. Malignant melanoma is discussed in detail in Chapter 55 (p. 1447).

CHANGES IN HAIR GROWTH. During pregnancy, there is an increased proportion of *anagen*—growing hairs, to that of *telogen*—resting hairs (Lynfield, 1960; Randall, 1994). Estrogens prolong the anagen state and androgens enlarge hair follicles in dependent areas such as the beard (Paus and Cotsarelis (1999). Postpartum, these effects are lost and shedding of hair becomes prominent. *Telogen effluvium* describes the rather abrupt hair loss that is seen beginning approximately 1 to 4 months postpartum. This process is sometimes characterized by alarming amounts of hair shedding, usually associated with brushing or washing. Fortunately, the process is self limited, and the woman may be reassured that normal hair growth is usually restored by 6 to 12 months (Headington, 1993; Kois and Phelan, 1994).

Mild hirsutism is common during pregnancy, and this may be most noticeable on the face. Women who are predisposed genetically to coarse hair growth are affected most profoundly. More severe degrees of hirsutism are unusual, and if accompanied by other evidence for masculinization, this should prompt consideration for another androgen source. We have cared for several pregnant women at Parkland Hospital who had virilization caused by adrenal tumors or pregnancy luteomas (Chap. 8, p. 171).

VASCULAR CHANGES. Augmented cutaneous blood flow in pregnancy is associated with marked decreases in peripheral vascular resistance (Spetz, 1964). This is thought to serve to dissipate excess heat generated by increased metabolism. There are a number of presumably estrogen-induced changes in the small vessels that are encountered with some frequency. Spider angiomas are found in two thirds of white women and about 10 percent of African Americans during pregnancy (Wong and Ellis, 1984). Most of these vascular lesions regress postpartum. Palmar erythema is likewise more commonly noticed in whites—two thirds, than in blacks—one third. Capillary hemangiomas, especially of the head and neck, are seen in about 5 percent of women during pregnancy.

One vascular condition that may be distressing is *pregnancy gingivitis,* which is caused by growth of the gum capillaries. This so-called *epulis of pregnancy* may become more severe as gestation progresses, but it may be controlled by proper dental hygiene and avoidance of trauma. Epulis should not be confused with *pyogenic granuloma of pregnancy,* which is also called *granuloma gravidarum.* These lesions are typical pyogenic granulomas, which are found in the oral cavity and often arise from the gingival papillae. Powell and colleagues (1994) described laser excision of a large granuloma in a 37-week pregnant woman.

DERMATOSES OF PREGNANCY

A number of dermatological conditions have been identified as unique to pregnancy, or if not unique, they are encountered with a greater frequency during gestation. Terminology has been confusing. Shornick (1998) concluded that only three conditions are universally accepted as unique to pregnancy: cholestasis, pruritic urticarial papules and plaques of pregnancy, and herpes gestationis (Table 54–1). Pruritus during pregnancy is common, but the incidence is obviously subject to subjective reporting. In nearly 3200 pregnant women who were carefully studied over one year, Roger and colleagues (1994) found that 1.6 percent had significant pruritus by their protocol.

CHOLESTASIS OF PREGNANCY. This syndrome includes *pruritus gravidarum* and *cholestatic jaundice of pregnancy.* In the study of 3200 pregnant women by

Roger and associates (1994), 51 (1.6 percent) women had pruritus, and 22 women (0.6 percent of the total) had pruritus gravidarum. The disorder is considered to be a mild variant of intrahepatic cholestasis of pregnancy (Chap. 48, 1283). Bile salts deposited in the dermis cause pruritus, and skin lesions develop with scratching and excoriation. The gross appearances and clinical presentation of these dermatoses may be confusing (Table 54–1).

PRURITIC URTICARIAL PAPULES AND PLAQUES OF PREGNANCY. Pruritic urticarial papules and plaques of pregnancy (PUPPP), referred to as *polymorphic eruption of pregnancy* in the United Kingdom, is the most common pruritic dermatosis of pregnancy. In the study by Roger and co-workers (1994) cited previously, 25 of nearly 3200 women (0.8 percent) had this dermatosis during pregnancy. It is characterized by an intensely pruritic cutaneous eruption that usually appears late during pregnancy (Table 54–1). Shown in Figure 54–1 are the erythematous urticarial papules and plaques that first develop on the abdomen, usually around striae. The lesions then are likely to spread to the buttocks, thighs and extremities (Alcalay and associates, 1987; Aronson and colleagues, 1998).

Pruritus may be severe with these lesions. In about 40 percent of women, the urticarial component predominates; in 45 percent, the erythematous pattern is prominent; and in 15 percent, a combination is seen (Aronson and associates, 1998). The erythematous patches are widespread. The face is usually spared, and seldom is there excoriation. The disease is more common in nulliparas and seldom recurs in subsequent pregnancies. It may resemble herpes gestationis, but there are no vesicles or bullae.

PATHOPHYSIOLOGY. The pathogenetic mechanism is unknown. Because of diverse clinical findings, classification can be confusing. On biopsy, there is a mild nonspecific lymphohistiocytic perivasculitis with an eosinophilic component. Importantly, there is no immunoglobulin or complement deposition seen using immunofluorescent staining of dermis (Aronson and colleagues, 1998). The absence of a linear band of C_3 in the basement membrane differentiates this dermatosis from herpes gestationis. Aractingi and associates (1998) have reported provocative evidence that this disorder may be stimulated by fetal cells that have invaded maternal skin.

TREATMENT. Some women obtain relief from oral antihistamines and skin emollients, but most require topical corticosteroid creams or ointments for relief. Oral corticosteroids are given if these fail to relieve severe itching. The rash disappears quickly either before or within several days following delivery. In 15 to 20 percent of

TABLE 54–1. Dermatological Disorders Unique to Pregnancy

Disorder	Frequency	Clinical Characteristics	Histopathology	Perinatal Outcome	Treatment	Comments
Cholestasis of pregnancy	Common (1–2%)	Onset third trimester; intense pruritus; generalized; excoriations common	Noncharacteristic; excoriations common	Perinatal morbidity increased	Antipruritics, cholestyramine	Considered a mild form of cholestatic jaundice; recurs in subsequent pregnancies
Pruritic urticarial papules and plaques of pregnancy (PUPPP)	Common (0.25–1%)	Onset second or third trimester; intense pruritus; patchy or generalized; abdomen, thighs, arms, buttocks; erythematous papules, urticarial papules and plaques	Lymphocytic perivascular infiltrate; negative immunofluorescence	No adverse effects	Antipruritics, emollients, topical corticosteroids, oral corticosteroids if severe	Common in nulliparas; seldom recurs in subsequent pregnancies
Prurigo of pregnancy (prurigo gestationis and papular dermatitis)	Uncommon (1:300–1:2400)	Onset second or third trimester; localized or generalized; 1–5 mm pruritic papules; excoriations common	Lymphocytic perivascular infiltrate; parakeratosis; acanthosis; negative immunofluorescence	Probably unaffected	Antipruritics, topical corticosteroids, oral corticosteroids if severe	Prurigo gestationis localized to forearms and trunk; papular dermatitis is generalized; does not recur in subsequent pregnancies
Herpes gestationis (pemphigoid gestationis)	Rare (1:10,000)	Onset second or third trimester, sometimes 1–2 weeks postpartum; severe pruritus; abdomen, extremities, or generalized; urticarial papules and plaques, erythema, vesicles, and bullae	Edema; infiltrate of lymphocytes, histiocytes, and eosinophils; C_3 and IgG deposition at basement membrane	Possibly increased preterm birth; transient neonatal lesions (5–10%)	Antipruritics, topical corticosteroids, oral corticosteroids if severe	Also associated with gestational trophoblastic disease; exacerbations and remissions during pregnancy are common; postpartum exacerbations are very common; recurrence in subsequent pregnancies is more severe
Impetigo herpetiformis	Rare	Onset third trimester; local, then generalized; erythema with marginal sterile pustules; mucous membranes involved; systemic symptoms	Microabscesses; spongioform pustules of Kogoj; neutrophils	Maternal sepsis common from secondary infection	Antibiotics, oral corticosteroids	Possible pustular psoriasis; persists for weeks to months postpartum; may recur with subsequent pregnancies

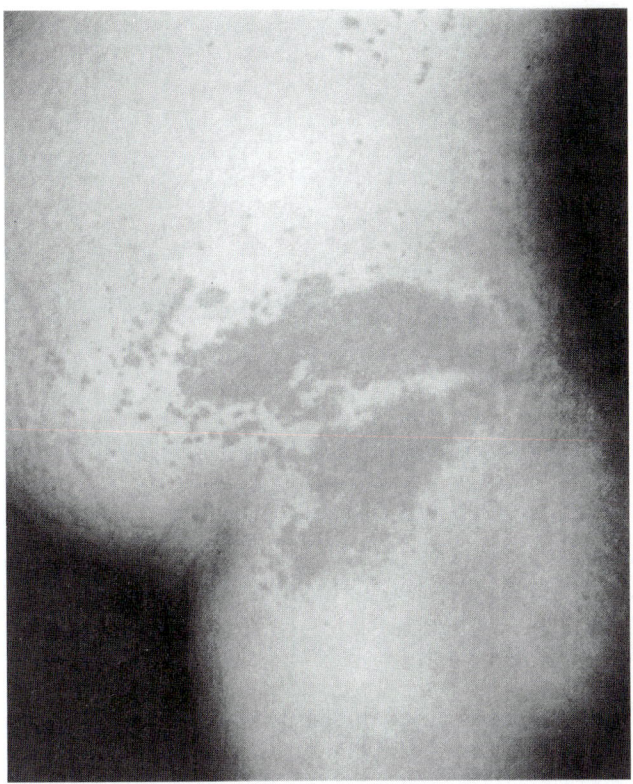

FIGURE 54–1. Pruritic urticarial papules and plaques of pregnancy on the left hip. (From Aractingi and colleagues, 1998, with permission.)

women, symptoms persist for 2 to 4 weeks postpartum (Vaughan Jones and co-workers, 1999). There is no evidence that perinatal morbidity is increased (Aronson and colleagues, 1998).

PRURIGO OF PREGNANCY. These lesions have been described by a multitude of names. According to Shornick (1998), the disorder includes *prurigo gestationis* and *papular dermatitis,* which likely are variants of the same disease and are not specific to pregnancy. The mild and more common variant, prurigo gestationis, is characterized by small, pruritic, rapidly excoriated lesions on the forearms and trunk. Lesions typically have their onset at 25 to 30 weeks, and vesicles or bullae do not develop. Papular dermatitis, described by Spangler and colleagues in 1962, is a rare dermatitis of late pregnancy. It is characterized by generalized pruritic eruptions. These lesions appear as soft, red to violet to red-brown papules, some of which have a centrally hemorrhagic crust.

Pruritus is usually controlled with antihistamines and topical corticosteroid creams. Perinatal outcome does not appear to be adversely affected with these syndromes (Vaughan Jones and Black, 1999).

HERPES GESTATIONIS. This pruritic blistering skin eruption usually presents in multiparous women in late pregnancy, but it may begin early in pregnancy or up to a week postpartum. It occasionally may accompany gestational trophoblastic disease. Also called *pemphigoid gestationis,* herpes gestationis is similar to bullous pemphigoid seen in elderly patients (Fine, 1995). Immunologically, it is indistinguishable from bullous pemphigoid (Nousari and Anhalt, 1999; Triffet and colleagues, 1999). Thus, it is an autoimmune organ-specific blistering skin disease (Engineer and associates, 2000).

Severe herpes gestationis can be serious, but fortunately it is rare. The previously reported incidence of about 1 in 50,000 pregnancies may have been an underestimate. Roger and colleagues (1994) reported an incidence of 1 in 1700 pregnancies, and Zurn and associates (1992) reported an incidence of 1 in 7000.

Herpes gestationis is characterized by an extremely pruritic widespread eruption with lesions that vary from erythematous and edematous papules to large, tense vesicles and bullae (Figs. 54–2 and 54–3). Common sites of involvement are the abdomen and the extremities. Exacerbations and remissions throughout pregnancy are common, and up to 75 percent of women suffer intrapartum exacerbations (Shornick, 1998). In subsequent pregnancies, the disease invariably recurs, and it usually does so earlier and is more severe. Baxi and colleagues (1991) reported a woman in whom recurrence was documented in five pregnancies; however, in each pregnancy, the disease was less severe. Although morphological changes may develop in the small intestinal mucosa similar to those of adult celiac disease, they do not appear to cause significant malabsorption.

ETIOPATHOGENESIS. This autoimmune disease is caused by development of an antibody to the basement membrane zone (anti-BMZ) in the epidermis. There is an inherited predisposition with a markedly increased incidence of HLA-DR3 and HLA-DR4 antigens in affected women (Baker, 1997). Although over half of women with herpes gestationis have these antigens, they are found in only 3 percent of unaffected women. These antigens are also associated with Graves disease and Hashimoto thyroiditis. For example, Shornick and Black (1992) reported that 10 percent of 75 women with herpes gestationis also had Graves disease.

Autoantibodies are common in women with herpes gestationis, and Shornick and associates (1993) demonstrated anti-HLA antibodies in all 39 women with biopsy-proven disease. The incidence of these antibodies in normal nulliparas is only 20 percent. This antibody is a thermostable immunoglobulin G that reacts with bullous pemphigoid antigen 2 (BPAG2) in the epidermis. BPAG2 is a 180-kD protein that is integral to adhesion structures that anchor basal cells to their basement

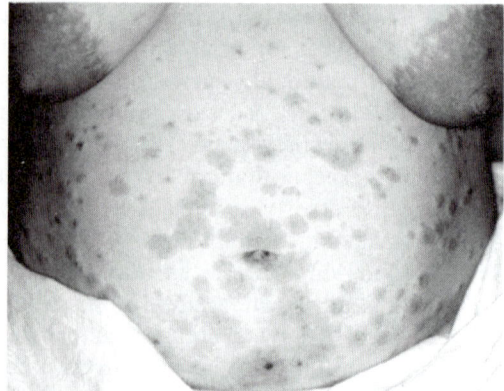

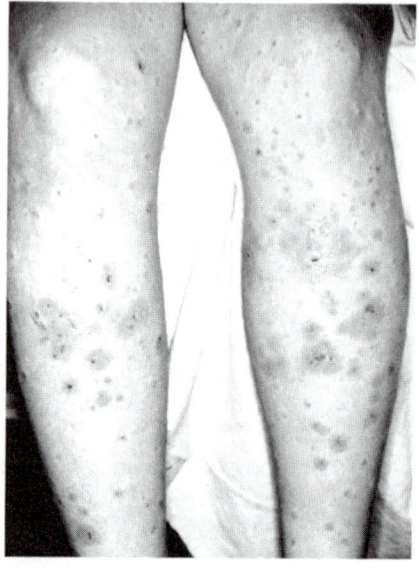

FIGURE 54–2. Herpes gestationis at 30 weeks' gestation. Subsequently, remarkable relief from the intense pruritus, as well as considerable decrease in the intensity of the skin reaction, was provided by corticosteroid treatment.

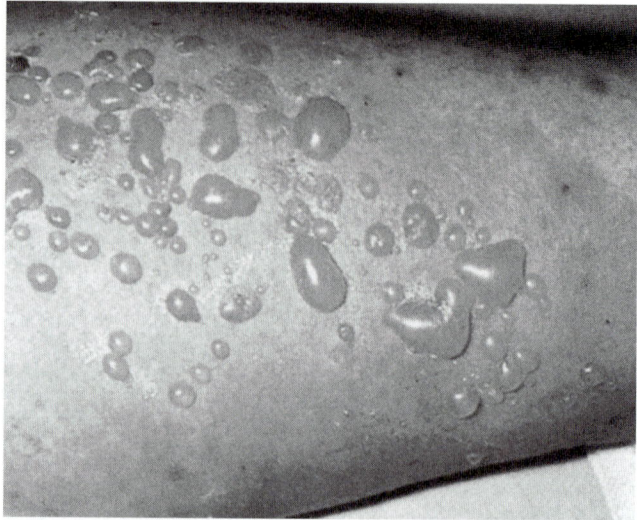

FIGURE 54–3. Herpes gestationis with large, tense bullae located on the thigh. (From Holmes and Black, 1983, with permission.)

membrane (Nousari and Anhalt, 1999). It is also called *herpes gestationis serum factor,* and it reacts with amnionic tissue. Finally, this antibody is passively transferred to the fetus.

Histologically, the classical finding in herpes gestationis is subepidermal edema with infiltrates of lymphocytes, histocytes, and eosinophils. Direct immunofluorescent techniques applied to a skin biopsy are of value for confirming the diagnosis, and C_3 complement and sometimes IgG are deposited along the basement membrane zone.

TREATMENT. Pruritus may be quite severe. Only a few women obtain relief from topical corticosteroids and antihistamines. Orally administered prednisone, 1 mg/kg daily, usually brings relief promptly and inhibits formation of new lesions. The healed sites usually are not scarred but frequently are hyperpigmented. Dapsone

and cyclosporine have been used to treat women who cannot tolerate corticosteroid therapy (Fine, 1995; Paternoster and colleagues, 1997). Castle and associates (1996) used cyclophosphamide successfully to treat a woman whose herpes gestationis persisted postpartum despite high-dose corticosteroid therapy.

EFFECT ON PREGNANCY. It is unclear if herpes gestationis causes adverse fetal outcomes. Shornick and Black (1992) reviewed 74 pregnancies and reported an increased incidence of preterm delivery and growth-restricted infants. Perinatal mortality, however, was not increased.

Lesions similar to those of the mother develop in up to 10 percent of neonates (Chen and colleagues, 1999). These usually clear spontaneously within a few weeks. C_3 complement deposited at the basement membrane of the newborn's skin and herpes gestationis factor in cord serum were described by Katz and associates (1976).

IMPETIGO HERPETIFORMIS. This is a rare pustular eruption that may be seen in late pregnancy. Some authors consider it to be a form of pustular psoriasis that occurs coincidental to pregnancy, while others consider it to be a distinct pregnancy dermatosis (Aronson and Halaska, 1995). Oumeish and associates (1982) described a woman in whom this dermatosis recurred in nine successive pregnancies. In three pregnancies, there was fetal hydrocephaly. There also were two unexplained perinatal deaths. This woman also developed characteristic skin lesions when taking estrogen–progesterone oral contraceptives.

The hallmark lesions of impetigo herpetiformis are sterile pustules that form around the margin of erythematous patches (Fig. 54–4). The erythematous lesions characteristically begin at flexures and extend peripherally. Mucous membranes are usually involved. The char-

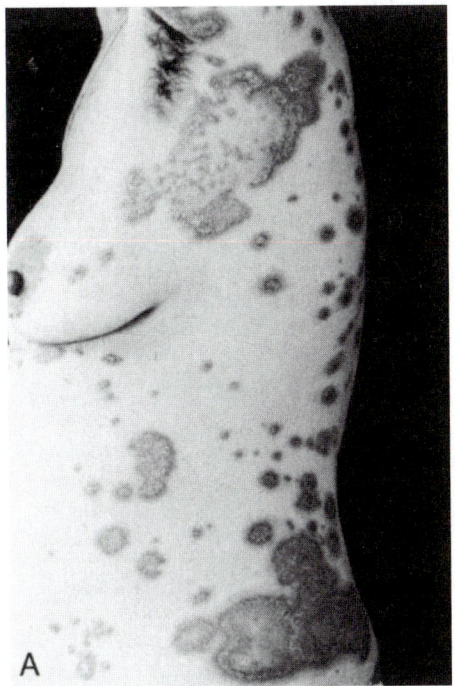

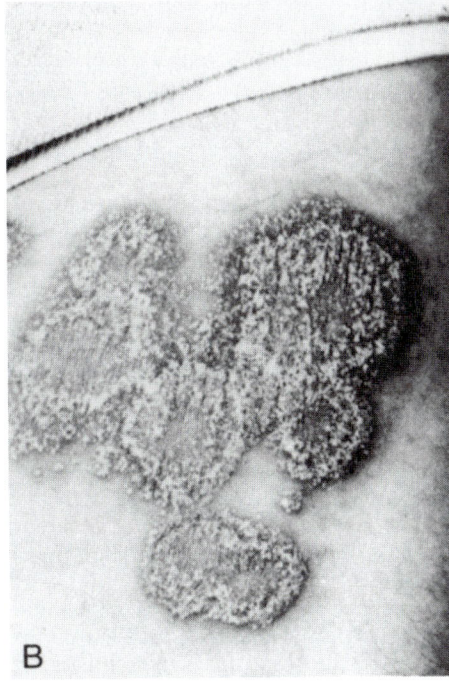

FIGURE 54–4. Impetigo herpetiformis. **A.** Round polycyclic patches over sides of the trunk at the time of admission. **B.** Patches over the thigh, with fresh pustules in the periphery encircling crusted older lesions. (From Lotem and associates, 1989, with permission.)

acteristic histological lesion is a microabscess. The spongelike epidermal cavity, which is filled with neutrophils, has been termed the *spongioform pustule of Kogoj.*

Pruritus is not severe, but constitutional symptoms are common. In addition to nausea, vomiting, diarrhea, and chills and fever, hypoalbuminemia and hypocalcemia are common. Although the pustules are initially sterile, they may become secondarily infected after rupture, and sepsis is a serious concern.

Treatment is given with systemic corticosteroids along with antimicrobials to treat secondary infection and sepsis. The disease may persist for several weeks to months after delivery. Fetal morbidity and mortality are related to the severity of maternal infection, but may be seen even with controlled disease (Vaughan Jones and Black, 1999; Wolf and colleagues, 1995).

PREEXISTING SKIN DISEASE

A number of chronic dermatological disorders may complicate pregnancy. These may antedate pregnancy or manifest for the first time during pregnancy. Many of these diseases are like other chronic disorders, which usually have no predictable course during pregnancy.

ACNE. An oral cogener of retinoic acid, *isotretinoin* (Accutane), is commonly prescribed for severe cystic acne, but it has proven to be highly teratogenic (Chap. 38, p. 1015). Lammer and colleagues (1985) reported a 26-fold risk for craniofacial, cardiac, and central nervous system malformations in fetuses exposed to isotretinoin. Likewise, *etretinate,* a similar compound utilized for the treatment of psoriasis, has been classified as category X because of associated major anomalies. Oral *tretinoin* is an antineoplastic drug that also is teratogenic.

Retinoic acid derivatives have prolonged biological activity, and Nulman and colleagues (1998) found the elimination half-life of isotretinoin to be nearly 40 hours. Wiegand and Chou (1998) demonstrated complete clearance by 2 weeks. Etretinate may be detected in the serum of women for as long as 2 years after cessation of therapy (DiGiovanna and associates, 1989). Fortunately, the Pregnancy Prevention Program implemented in 1988 has been successful in avoiding most pregnancies in women taking isotretinoin (Mitchell and colleagues, 1995). The program calls for serum pregnancy testing 2 weeks before therapy is begun. According to Chan and associates (1995), this program was not as effective in Australia because of lack of compliance with use of effective contraception.

For the pregnant woman with severe acne, topically applied benzoyl peroxide appears to be safe, and along with either clindamycin or erythromycin gel, may suffice to control the disease. **Topical tretinoin** is thought to pose no significant teratogenic risk; however, it is class C_m (Briggs and colleagues, 1998).

HIDRADENITIS SUPPURATIVA. A chronic, progressive inflammatory and suppurative disorder of skin and supporting structures, hidradenitis suppurativa is characterized by apocrine gland plugging that leads to anhidrosis and bacterial infection. Subcutaneous extension causes scarring and sinus formation. In most cases, skin involvement is in multiple apocrine gland sites, but it may be seen only in the axillae, groin, perineum, perirectal area, or under the breasts.

The disease is hormonally responsive and thus not seen until puberty. It has been said to be improved by pregnancy, but postpartum exacerbations may occur. In our experiences, it is not appreciably changed by pregnancy. Treatment is control of acute infections with either systemic antimicrobials or clindamycin ointment. Low-dose isotretinoin for 4 to 6 months has been used with good long-term results in a retrospective study by Boer and van Gemert (1999). **Isotretinoin is a category X drug contraindicated during pregnancy.** Definitive treatment is wide surgical excision, but this most often should be postponed until after pregnancy.

OTHER CONDITIONS. Boyd and colleagues (1996) noted that 65 percent of women reported improvement of *psoriasis* with pregnancy. Almost 90 percent, however, reported a postpartum flare. If *pemphigus* appears during pregnancy for the first time, it may be confused with herpes gestationis (Vaughan Jones and Black, 1999). Even with corticosteroid therapy, mortality is 10 percent secondary to sepsis caused by infection of denuded skin. Daniel and colleagues (1995) reviewed 17 immunopathologically confirmed cases and reported four stillborn infants. Lesions of *neurofibromatosis* may increase in size and number as a result of pregnancy. As discussed in Chapter 56 (p. 1475), *Hansen disease* likely worsens during pregnancy (Aronson and Halaska, 1995).

REFERENCES

Alcalay J, Ingber A, David M, Hazaz B, Sandbank M: Pruritic urticarial papules and plaques of pregnancy: A review of 21 cases. J Reprod Med 32:315, 1987

Aractingi S, Berkane N, Bertheau P, Le Goue C, Dausset J, Uzan S, Carosella ED: Fetal DNA in skin of polymorphic eruptions of pregnancy. Lancet 352:1898, 1998

Aronson IK, Bond S, Fiedler VC, Vomvouras S, Gruber D, Ruiz C: Pruritic urticarial papules and plaques of pregnancy: Clinical and immunopathologic observations in 57 patients. J Am Acad Dermatol 39:933, 1998

Aronson IK, Halaska BN: Dermatologic disease. In Barron

WM, Lindheimer MD (eds): Medical Disorders During pregnancy. St Louis, Mosby, 1995, p 451

Baker JR: Autoimmune endocrine disease. JAMA 278:1931, 1997

Baxi LV, Kovilam OP, Collins MH, Walther RR: Recurrent herpes gestationis with postpartum flare: A case report. Am J Obstet Gynecol 164:778, 1991

Boer J, van Gemert MJ: Long-term results of isotretinoin in the treatment of 68 patients with hidradenitis suppurativa. J Am Acad Dermatol 40:73, 1999

Boyd AS, Morris LF, Phillips CM, Menter MA: Psoriasis and pregnancy: Hormone and immune system interaction. Int J Dermatol 35:169, 1996

Briggs GG, Freeman RK, Yaffe SJ: Drugs in Pregnancy and Lactation, 5th ed. Baltimore, Williams & Wilkins, 1998

Castle SP, Mather-Mondrey M, Bennion S, David-Bajar K, Huff C: Chronic herpes gestationis and antiphospholipid antibody syndrome successfully treated with cyclophosphamide. J Am Acad Dermatol 34:333, 1996

Chan A, Keane RJ, Hanna M, Abbott M: Terminations of pregnancy for exposure to oral retinoids in South Australia, 1985–1993. Aust N Z J Obstet Gynaecol 35:4:422, 1995

Chen SH, Chopra K, Evans TY, Raimer SS, Levy ML, Tyring SK: Herpes gestationis in a mother and child. J Am Acad Dermatol 40:847, 1999

Daniel Y, Shenhav M, Botchan Am, Peyser MR, Lessing JB: Pregnancy associated with pemphigus. Br J Obstet Gynaecol 102:667, 1995

DiGiovanna JJ, Zech LA, Ruddel ME, Gantt G, Peck GL: Etretinate. Persistent serum levels after long-term therapy. Arch Dermatol 125:246, 1989

Engineer L, Bhol K, Ahmed AR: Pemphigoid gestationis: A review. Am J Obstet Gynecol 183:483, 2000

Fine JD: Management of acquired bullous skin diseases. N Engl J Med 333:1475, 1995

Griffiths CEM, Finkel LJ, Ditre CM, Hamilton TA, Ellie CN, Voorhees JJ: Topical tretinoin (retinoic acid) improves melasma. A vehicle-controlled, clinical trial. Br J Dermatol 129:415, 1993

Headington JT: Telogen effluvium: New concepts and review. Arch Dermatol 129:356, 1993

Holmes RC, Black MM: Dermatosis of pregnancy. J Am Acad Dermatol 8:406, 1983

Katz SI, Hertz KC, Yaoita H: Immunopathology and characterization of the HG factor. J Clin Invest 57:1434, 1976

Kimbrough-Green CK, Griffiths CEM, Finkel LJ, Hamilton TA, Bulengo-Ransby SM, Ellis CN, Voorhees JJ: Topical retinoic acid (tretinoin) for melasma in black patients. A vehicle-controlled clinical trial. Arch Dermatol 130:727, 1994

Kois JM, Phelan ST: Hair loss in women. Prim Care Update ob/Gyns 1:130, 1994

Lammer EJ, Chen DT, Hoar RM, Agnish ND, Benke PJ, Braun JT, Curry CJ, Fernhoff PM, Grix AW, Lott IT, Richard JM, Sun SC: Retinoic acid embryopathy. N Engl J Med 313:837, 1985

Lotem M, Katzenelson V, Rotem A, Hod M, Sandbank M: Impetigo herpetiformis: A variant of pustular psoriasis or a separate entity? J Am Acad Dermatol 20:338, 1989

Lynfield VL: Effect of pregnancy on the human hair cycle. J Invest Dermatol 35:323, 1960

MacKie RM, Bufalina R, Morabito A, Sutherland C, Cascinelli N: Lack of effect of pregnancy on outcome of melanoma. Lancet 337:653, 1991

Mitchell AA, Van Bennekom CM, Louik C: A pregnancy-prevention program in women of childbearing age receiving isotretinoin. N Engl J Med 333:101, 1995

Nousari HC, Anhalt GJ: Pemphigus and bullous pemphigoid. Lancet 354:667, 1999

Nulman I, Berkovitch M, Klein J, Pastuszak A, Lester RS, Shear N, Koren G: Steady-state pharmacokinetics of isotretinoin and its 4-oxo metabolite: Implications for fetal safety. J Clin Pharmacol 38:926, 1998

Oumeish OY, Farraj SE, Bataineh AS: Some aspects of impetigo herpetiformis. Arch Dermatol 118:103, 1982

Paternoster DM, Bruno G, Grella PV: New observations on herpes gestationis therapy. Int J Gynaecol Obstet 56:277, 1997

Paus R, Cotsarelis G: The biology of hair follicles. N Engl J Med 341:491, 1999

Pennoyer JW, Grin CM, Driscoll MS, Dry SM, Walsh SJ, Gelineau JP, Grant-Kels JM: Changes in size of melanocytic nevi during pregnancy. J Am Acad Dermatol 36:378, 1997

Powell JL, Bailey CL, Coopland AT, Otis CN, Frank JL, Meyer I: Nd:YAG laser excision of a giant gingival pyogenic granuloma of pregnancy. Laser Surg Med 14:178, 1994

Randall VA: Androgens and human hair growth. Clin Endocrinol 40:439, 1994

Roger D, Vaillant L, Fignon A, Pierre F, Bacq Y, Brechot JF, Grangeponte MC, Lorette G: Specific pruritic diseases of pregnancy: A prospective study of 3192 pregnant women. Arch Dermatol 130:734, 1994

Shornick JK: Dermatoses of pregnancy. Semin Cutan Med Surg 17:172, 1998

Shornick JK, Black MM: Fetal risks in herpes gestationis. J Am Acad Dermatol 26:63, 1992

Shornick JK, Jenkins RE, Briggs DC, Welsh KI, Kelly SE, Garvey MP, Black MM: Anti-HLA antibodies in pemphigoid gestationis (herpes gestationis). Br J Dermatol 129:257, 1993

Spangler AS, Reddy W, Bardawil WA, Roby CC, Emerson K: Papular dermatitis of pregnancy: A new clinical entity. JAMA 181:577, 1962

Spetz S: Peripheral circulation during normal pregnancy. Acta Obstet Gynecol Scand 43:309, 1964

Triffet MK, Gibson LE, Leiferman KM: Severe subepidermal blistering disorder with features of bullous pemphigoid and herpes gestationis. J Am Acad Dermatol 40:797, 1999

Vaughan Jones SA, Black MM: Pregnancy dermatoses. J Am Acad Dermatol 40:233, 1999

Vaughan Jones SA, Hern S, Nelson-Piercy C, Seed PT, Black MM: A prospective study of 200 women with dermatoses of pregnancy correlating clinical findings with hormonal and immunopathological profiles. Br J Dermatol 141:71, 1999

Wiegand U-W, Chou RC: Pharmacokinetics of oral isotretinoin. J Am Acad Dermatol 39:S8, 1998

Wolf Y, Groutz A, Walman I, Luxman D, David MP: Impetigo herpetiformis during pregnancy: Case report and review of the literature. Acta Obstet Gynecol Scand 74:229, 1995

Wong RC, Ellis CN: Physiologic skin changes in pregnancy. J Am Acad Dermatol 10:929, 1984

Zurn A, Celebi CR, Bernard P, Didierjean L, Saurat JH: A prospective immunofluorescence study of 111 cases of pruritic dermatoses of pregnancy: IgM anti-basement membrane zone antibodies as a novel finding. Br J Dermatol 126:474, 1992

55

Neoplastic Diseases

Cancer during pregnancy is uncommon but not rare. In a survey of 2.7 million births in Sweden, Lambe and Ekbom (1995) found an incidence of 1 in 6000 pregnancies. According to Martin and associates (1999) from the National Center for Health Statistics, malignancies are the second leading cause of death in women 25 to 44 years of age, and the most common are those of the hemopoietic and lymphatic systems, thyroid, breast, cervix, ovary, and colon, and melanoma. Sachs and colleagues (1990) reviewed 886 maternal deaths in Massachusetts from 1954 to 1985, and reported that 5 percent were cancer related. The most common malignancies associated with pregnancy are those of the genital tract and breast, and malignant melanoma (Buekers and Lallas, 1998; Kaiser and associates, 2000; Nevin and colleagues, 1995).

Although the approach to the pregnant woman with cancer may need to be modified compared with that of a nonpregnant patient, *the woman should not be **penalized** for being pregnant.* Specific questions to be asked include:

1. Does pregnancy adversely affect maternal cancer?
2. What risk does cancer or its treatment pose to the fetus?
3. Should the pregnancy be terminated because it represents a significant obstacle for effective cancer therapy?
4. Should the pregnancy be allowed to continue under a very carefully defined regimen?
5. If the neoplasm exists before conception, how should the woman be counseled regarding birth control and advisability of pregnancy?
6. Is pregnancy advisable following cancer treatment?
7. How should the woman be counseled preconceptionally regarding risk of chemotherapy to future offspring?

PRINCIPLES OF CANCER THERAPY DURING PREGNANCY

SURGERY. Surgical intervention for suspected or proven malignancies may be indicated for diagnostic, staging, or therapeutic purposes. Extra-abdominal procedures are usually well tolerated by both mother and fetus, as are most intraperitoneal operations that do not interfere with the reproductive tract. If indicated, however, the ovaries may be removed safely after about 8 weeks' gestation because placental progesterone production is adequate (Chap. 6, p. 123). Ovariectomy before this time may cause abortion, which often can be prevented by progesterone administration.

Although diagnostic and staging operations have classically been deferred until the second trimester so as to minimize abortion risks, this probably is not necessary. Documenting fetal life by ultrasound between 9 and 11 weeks indicates that 95 percent of fetuses will reach viability. Therapeutic surgery should be performed regardless of gestational age if maternal well-being is imperiled.

RADIATION THERAPY. Unlike diagnostic x-ray procedures, therapeutic radiation may result in significant fetal exposure to ionizing radiation. The amount of radiation exposure will depend on the dose, tissue being treated, and field size. The potential adverse effects of diagnostic radiation include cell deaths, carcinogenesis, and genetic effects on future generations (Brent, 1989, 1999; Hall, 1991). As discussed in Chapter 42 (p. 1149), the characteristic adverse fetal effects of high-dose radiation are microcephaly and mental retardation. For example, children born to pregnant women exposed to atomic bomb explosions had a 2.4 percent incidence of mental retardation with 10 to 50 rad exposure, and this was increased to nearly 18 percent if exposure was 50 to 100 rad (Otake and Schull, 1984). The most critical time appeared to be between 8 and 15 weeks' gestation.

The National Council on Radiation Protection and Measurements (Brent, 1987) concluded that exposure of the embryo to less than 5 rad is associated with negligible risk for major malformations. It was further suggested that the threshold for radiation effects may be 15 to 20 rad. Although the most susceptible period appears to be during organogenesis, there is no gestational age that is considered safe for therapeutic radiation exposure, because late exposure can cause fetal growth restriction and brain damage. Diagnostic x-ray procedures have very low exposure and should not be delayed if the information gained will directly affect therapy (Chap 42, p. 1150).

The necessity for therapeutic radiation raises issues such as abortion, teratogenesis, and fetal sequelae. Therapeutic radiation to the abdomen is contraindicated because of a high risk of fetal death or damage, unless of course abortion induction is one of its purposes. In some cases, such as the head and neck, radiation therapy to supradiaphragmatic areas can be given relatively safely with abdominal shielding; however, in others, such as the breasts, significant scatter doses can accrue to the fetus. Lippman and colleagues (1988) calculated fetal doses of up to 100 rad during radiotherapy for breast cancer if the uterus reached the xiphoid.

CHEMOTHERAPY

EFFECT ON PREGNANCY OUTCOME. Chemotherapy is now recommended for a variety of malignancies such as those of the hemopoietic and lymphatic systems, ovarian cancer, and breast cancer—not only as palliative therapy but also as potentially curative therapy. Chemotherapeutic agents are often recommended as adjunctive therapy along with surgery or radiation in an attempt to provide optimal therapy in women of reproductive age. Although such therapy with these agents may be associated with either increased rates of cure or at least remission, there is a general reluctance to use chemotherapy in the pregnant woman because of the concern for potential malformations, growth retardation, and the risk of malignancy in future offspring. The risk of adverse fetal effects is dependent primarily on the gestational age at the time of chemotherapy. Most antineoplastic drugs should be considered potentially harmful to the fetus, especially if given between 5 and 10 weeks' gestation, and thus during organogenesis—the period of maximal susceptibility. Most antineoplastic drugs given after the first trimester are without obvious adverse sequelae, although long-term effects have not been evaluated thoroughly. In a review of the reproductive toxicology of alkylating agents, Glantz (1994) concluded that these agents could be employed after the first tri-

mester as necessary. As expected, most of the antineoplastic drugs shown in Table 55–1 are classified as category D.

Zemlickis and associates (1992b) reported four spontaneous abortions and two of five fetuses with major malformations when chemotherapy was given to nine women during the first trimester. Eight women treated later in pregnancy had lower-birthweight infants than controls, but no malformations. Doll and collaborators (1988) reviewed chemotherapy-induced teratogenesis, and their findings are shown in Table 55–2. These investigators noted six instances (25 percent) of fetal malformations during 24 first-trimester exposures to combination chemotherapy compared with 24 of 139 (17 percent) exposed to single-agent therapy. Many of these women had been given folate antagonists and some were given concomitant radiation. If these women were excluded, the incidence of malformations with single-agent therapy was only 6 percent. In contrast, during the second and third trimesters there was no evidence for increased risk of teratogenesis, and of 131 cases there were only

TABLE 55–1. **Some Drugs Used for Treatment of Neoplasms**

Class/Drug	Risk Category	Common Uses for Cancer Therapy
Alkylating Agents		
Busulfan	D	Leukemias
Chlorambucil	D	Lymphomas, leukemias
Cyclophosphamide	D	Breast, ovary, lymphomas, leukemias
Melphalan	D	Ovary, leukemia, myeloma
Procarbazine	D	Lymphomas
Antimetabolites		
5-Fluorouracil	D	Breast, gastrointestinal
6-Mercaptopurine	D	Leukemias
Methotrexate	D	Trophoblastic disease, lymphomas, leukemias, breast
6-Thioguanine	D	Leukemias
Antibiotics		
Bleomycin	D	Cervix, lymphomas
Daunorubicin	D	Leukemias
Doxorubicin	D	Leukemias, lymphomas, breast
Other Agents		
All-trans-retinoic acid	X	Leukemia
L-Asparaginase	C	Leukemia
Cisplatin	D	Ovary, cervix, sarcoma
Hydroxyurea	D	Leukemias
Prednisone	B	Lymphomas, leukemias, breast
Tamoxifen	D	Breast, uterus
Taxol	D	Breast, ovary
Vinblastine	D	Breast, lymphomas, choriocarcinoma
Vincristine	D	Leukemias, lymphomas

TABLE 55–2. Frequency of Fetal Malformations Associated with Chemotherapy During Pregnancy

Class	First Trimester		Second/Third Trimester	
	No.	(%)	No.	(%)
Alkylating agents	6/44	(14)	1/26	(4)
Antimetabolites	15/77	(19)	0/38	
Plant alkaloids	1/14	(7)	0/6	
Antibiotics	0/1		0/1	
Combinations	7/45	(16)	1/79	(1.3)
Total	24/139	(17)	2/150	(1.3)

Modified from Doll and colleagues (1988).

two fetal malformations. From their review, Koren and colleagues (1990) estimate the major malformation rate at 10 percent for first-trimester exposure.

Because the magnitude of secretion of chemotherapeutic agents in breast milk has not been established, breast feeding is not recommended. There is also concern for exposure of health-care workers to chemotherapeutic agents. Selevan and colleagues (1985) reported a twofold increased risk of fetal loss in nurses exposed during the first trimester, and they recommended caution during mixing and administration of antineoplastic drugs. Currently, guidelines from the Occupational Safety and Health Administration are that all antineoplastic drugs be mixed in biological safety cabinets with laminar flow hoods.

Late effects on offspring of women treated for cancer during pregnancy have also been analyzed. Li and associates (1979) found only two childhood malignancies in offspring of 146 women treated during 286 pregnancies. Similarly, Avilés and colleagues (1991) found no adverse sequelae in 43 children exposed to antineoplastic drugs in utero, and who were evaluated 3 to 19 years later.

OVARIAN FUNCTION AND FERTILITY AFTER CANCER THERAPY. Treatment of advanced Hodgkin lymphoma with multiple-drug regimens may result in azoospermia (Waxman, 1985). In women there is depressed follicular maturation as well as ovarian fibrosis. Ovarian susceptibility depends on the woman's age and the drug dose given. Interestingly, the prepubertal ovary is more resistant to effects of chemotherapy.

If fertility is not lost, there does not appear to be an increased incidence of abortion, fetal chromosomal damage, or fetal anomalies (Rustin and colleagues, 1984). Gershenson (1988) reviewed subsequent outcomes in women successfully treated with chemotherapy for germ cell ovarian tumors, and although 68 percent had regular menses, the remainder had total or

partial ablation of ovarian function. Affected women were significantly older at diagnosis.

Following bone marrow transplantation, either for aplastic anemia or malignant disease, long-term mortality is excessive even for patients free of disease at 2 years (Socié and co-workers, 1999). This was found to be due to late-recurring leukemia or graft-versus-host disease.

BREAST CARCINOMA

Breast cancer is the most common malignancy of women of all age groups. Almost 1 of every 10 American women will eventually be afflicted. Thus, it is not surprising that breast cancer is one of the three most common malignancies encountered during pregnancy (Berry and colleagues, 1999; Sorosky and Scott-Conner, 1998). Its incidence has been estimated to be 10 to 30 women per 100,000 pregnancies (Isaacs, 1995). Nulliparity is a risk factor for breast cancer.

A number of obstetrical outcomes may influence the risk for breast cancer. Term pregnancy increases the short-term risk, and this amplifies the effects of carriers of BRCA1 and BRCA2 mutations (Jernström and co-workers, 1999). Conversely, preterm delivery, preeclampsia, and induced abortion have no effect (Ekbom, 1997; Hsieh, 1999; Melbye, 1997, and all of their colleagues). Women with breast cancer and their controls are equally likely to report induced abortions (Tang and associates, 2000). Breast feeding also seems to have no association with breast cancer occurrence (Michels and colleagues, 1996).

EFFECTS OF PREGNANCY ON BREAST CANCER. Pregnancy does not have dramatic influences on the course of mammary cancer. Melbye and colleagues (2000) have presented intriguing evidence that higher serum levels of alpha-fetoprotein are associated with a lower incidence of breast cancer. It is, however, undisputed that regional nodes are more likely involved with microscopic metastases. Hochman and Schreiber (1953), and others since then, contend that the 5-year survival rate in breast cancer coexisting with pregnancy is primarily dependent on the stage of the disease at the time of diagnosis, and that interruption of pregnancy has no influence on the course. Thus, survival in pregnant women is comparable with the rates expected with similar disease stages in nonpregnant women (King and colleagues, 1985; Nugent and O'Connell, 1985; Zemlickis and associates, 1992a).

Past pregnancy may adversely affect the survival of young women with breast cancer. For example, in a review of 407 women aged 20 to 29 years, Guinee and colleagues (1994) reported that the risk of dying from breast malignancy was significantly greater in women whose cancer was first diagnosed during pregnancy compared with those who had never been pregnant. Korzeniowski and Dyba (1994), in a review of the survival of 1885 women with operable breast cancer, reported that the survival rates decreased with the number of pregnancies, and the prognosis was best in women who had never been pregnant. Thus, almost paradoxically, the reproductive factors reported to decrease the risk of breast cancer may actually have an adverse effect on the prognosis.

Although survival is stage-dependent, there may be serious delays in clinical assessment, diagnostic procedures, and treatment of pregnant women with breast tumors (Berry and colleagues, 1999). Delays in diagnosis may be greater than 1 year in some women (Marchant, 1994). Although most women undergo examination during pregnancy, hormonally induced physiological breast changes tend to obscure breast masses. This is particu-

larly evident during lactation when there is lobular hyperplasia and galactostasis. This observation at least partially explains the more advanced stages of cancer at diagnosis, which consequently have a worse prognosis (Sorosky and Scott-Conner, 1998). According to Jacob and Stringer (1990), about 30 percent of pregnant women with breast cancer have stage I disease; 30 percent, stage II; and 40 percent, stages III and IV. Souadka and colleagues (1994) reported that a fourth of 43 pregnant women with breast cancer had metastatic disease apparent at the outset. Bonnier and associates (1997) found an inordinately and significantly higher incidence of inflammatory cancer in 154 pregnant women compared with 308 age-matched nonpregnant controls (26 versus 9 percent). As shown in Table 55–3, about two thirds of pregnant women have concomitant axillary node involvement. This is substantively higher than the 40 to 50 percent reported for nonpregnant women (Hoover, 1990).

King and colleagues (1985) described experiences with 63 pregnant women treated for breast carcinoma at the Mayo Clinic. They reported that 63 percent of these women had axillary nodal metastases compared with only 38 percent of similar-age nonpregnant women described by others. Zemlickis and associates (1992a) reported that pregnant women with breast cancer had a 2.5-fold risk of metastatic disease compared with nonpregnant control women. Utilizing a mathematical model, Nettleton and colleagues (1996) have estimated that a delay in diagnosis of 6 months increases the chance of nodal metastasis by more than 10 percent.

PLACENTAL METASTASES. Occasionally, malignant breast cells are found upon placental microscopic examination (Dunn and co-workers, 1999). These have been

TABLE 55–3. Axillary Node Involvement in Pregnancy-associated Breast Cancer

Investigators	Number	Positive Nodes	
		No.	(%)
Haagensen (1971)	48	33	(69)
Ribeiro and Palmer (1977)	88	78	(89)
Clark and Reid (1978)	121	100	(83)
Donegan (1979)	24	17	(71)
Petrek et al (1991)	56	34	(61)
Ishida et al (1992)	192	111	(58)
Souadka et al (1994)	43	34	(80)
Bonnier et al (1997)	114	64	(56)
Berry et al (1999)	22	14	(67)
Total	708	485	(68)[a]

[a] Compared with 40–50% in nonpregnant women.

confined to the intervillous space, and fetal disease has not been reported (Chap. 32, p. 849).

DIAGNOSIS AND TREATMENT. The diagnostic approach in the pregnant woman with a breast tumor should not differ significantly from that for a nonpregnant woman. **Any suspicious breast mass found during pregnancy should prompt an aggressive plan to determine its cause, whether by fine-needle aspiration or by open biopsy.** Fine-needle aspiration is often the preferred procedure for the initial evaluation of a breast mass detected in pregnancy or during lactation, and breast biopsy is usually reserved for masses in which fine-needle aspiration is not diagnostic (Sorosky and Scott-Conner, 1998). The risk of mammography is negligible for the fetus if appropriate shielding is used, and the amount of radiation exposure is less than 100 mrad. (Chap. 42, p. 1150). The dense breast tissue of pregnancy makes this test less reliable. In the review by Liberman and colleagues (1994), of 23 cases of pregnancy-associated invasive breast carcinoma, there were mammographic findings in only 18 (78 percent). Using fine-needle aspiration, it is possible to differentiate a cyst or galactocele from solid tumors. Excisional biopsy should be done if cytological results are not diagnostic. According to Barnavon and Wallack (1990), aspiration is 66 percent sensitive and 95 percent specific. Collins and co-workers (1995) biopsied masses in 17 pregnant women and found only one cancer. Thirteen of these had a lactating adenoma.

Once the breast malignancy is diagnosed, chest x-ray and limited metastatic search is performed. Whereas computerized tomography bone and liver scans are both sensitive and specific, they are probably contraindicated during pregnancy because of the ionizing radiation (Pelsang, 1998). Magnetic resonance imaging and ultrasonography are reasonable alternatives to assess for liver involvement. Magnetic resonance imaging is not only sensitive but has the added advantage of multiplanar images and excellent contrast resolution. Ultrasound has been reported to be more sensitive than magnetic imaging for detection of liver metastases (Pelsang, 1998). Clarke and colleagues (1989) have reported that the sensitivity of ultrasound in detecting liver metastasis is 76 percent.

Surgical treatment should not be delayed because of pregnancy. In the absence of metastatic disease, wide excision, modified radical mastectomy, or total mastectomy with axillary node staging can be performed (Isaacs, 1995). Berry and colleagues (1999) performed modified radical mastectomy followed by chemotherapy in 18 of 22 pregnant women. Risks from these procedures are minimal, and the incidence of abortion is negligible. Because breast-conserving surgery usually requires adjunctive radiotherapy, this technique is usually

not recommended for pregnant women unless the malignancy is diagnosed in the late third trimester (Sorosky and Scott-Conner, 1998).

Radiotherapy is not recommended during pregnancy because abdominal scatter is considerable even with shielding. The fetus receives at least 100 to 150 rad when the maternal radiation dose to the breast is 5000 rad (Sorosky and Scott-Conner, 1998).

Data indicate that nonpregnant women with node-positive cancer should be given adjuvant **chemotherapy** without delay. It therefore seems advisable to give chemotherapy for node-positive disease if delivery is not anticipated soon. Chemotherapy with cyclophosphamide, doxorubicin, and 5-fluorouracil is currently recommended by most (Berry and colleagues, 1999). After the first trimester, methotrexate can be substituted for doxorubicin (Sorosky and Scott-Conner, 1998). Surgical ablation of the ovaries would appear to have no place in the management of pregnant women with breast cancer (Isaacs, 1995).

Berry and colleagues (1999) have recently described their experience with 24 pregnant women with primary or recurrent carcinoma of the breast. Of the 22 women with primary cancer of the breast, 18 had modified radical mastectomies—14 during pregnancy and four during the postpartum period. Each woman had a central venous catheter placed, and all of the women were given combination chemotherapy with cyclophosphamide, doxorubicin, and fluorouracil every 3 to 4 weeks during the second and third trimester of pregnancy. The median gestational age at delivery was 38 weeks with a range of 33 to 40 weeks. Only one newborn had a birthweight less than the 10th percentile for gestational age, and none of the 24 infants had congenital malformations.

PREGNANCY FOLLOWING BREAST CANCER. About 10 percent of women treated for breast cancer subsequently become pregnant, and 70 percent of these do so within the first 5 years (Harvey and colleagues, 1981; Hornstein and colleagues, 1982). There is little evidence to suggest that pregnancy after mastectomy for breast cancer adversely affects survival (Averette and colleagues, 1999). Dow and colleagues (1994) found no differences in recurrences or distant metastasis with or without subsequent pregnancies. More recent investigations by Kroman (1997) and Velentgas (1999) and their colleagues confirmed these findings. Similarly, there are no data to suggest that lactation adversely affects the course of breast cancer. Moreover, successful lactation and breast feeding is possible after conservative surgery and radiation for breast cancer, even from the side of the treated breast (Higgins and Haffty, 1994). Recommendations for future pregnancies in women successfully treated for breast malignancy are based on several factors, including consideration for recurrence. It seems reasonable to advise a delay of 2 to 3 years, which is the most critical observation period.

LYMPHOMAS AND LEUKEMIAS

LYMPHOMAS

HODGKIN DISEASE. The lymphatic tumor of Hodgkin disease constitutes approximately 40 percent of malignant lymphomas. Hodgkin disease is the most common lymphoma encountered in childbearing-age women. It has a bimodal peak incidence in ages 18 to 30 and again after 50. Its concurrence with pregnancy has been estimated to be about 1 in 6000 (DiSaia and Creasman, 1993), although our experience indicates that it is much less common. The most common finding is peripheral adenopathy, and neck and supraclavicular nodes are commonly involved. Patients may be asymptomatic or they may present with fever, night sweats, malaise, weight loss, and pruritus (Peleg and Ben-Ami, 1998). Diagnosis is established by histological examination of involved nodes. In more than 70 percent of cases of Hodgkin disease, patients present with painless enlargement of lymph nodes above the diaphragm—axillary, cervical, or submaxillary (Peleg and Ben-Ami, 1998).

The pregnant woman with Hodgkin disease presents special management considerations. A tenet of treatment is that careful staging is essential, and either local radiotherapy or systemic chemotherapy is indicated. The *Ann Arbor staging system,* shown in Table 55–4, was designed for Hodgkin lymphomas but is also used for other lymphomas. Some use its revision, termed the *Cotswold classification* (Urba and Longo, 1992). Pregnancy limits the widespread application of some radiographic studies of the chest, abdomen, pelvis, and lower extremities. Spiral chest computed tomography can be used with the "pitch" set so that radiation dosage approaches that of conventional chest scanning. Magnetic resonance imaging is a reasonable alternative to computed tomographic scanning for evaluating thoracic and abdominal para-aortic lymph nodes. Radionuclide gallium scanning is used more frequently and has about 750 to 1000 mrad (see Table 42–9, p. 1153). Routine staging laparotomy is controversial but is considered essential for those patients in whom radiotherapy alone is chosen, and thus documentation of unsuspected abdominal disease would significantly alter treatment. Although this may be done in early pregnancy, it does not seem advisable in later pregnancy.

Treatment is individualized depending upon the suspected disease stage and pregnancy duration. Whereas radiotherapy is preferable for isolated neck adenopathy, it is not recommended if the fields to be used will deliver significant radiation scatter to the fetus. Wong and Strassner (1990) estimated fetal exposure from maternal therapy with 4400 rad delivered to the midline of the central supradiaphragmatic axis. Fetal dosage was calculated to be 63, 88, and 220 rad in early, mid-, and late pregnancy, respectively. Because of this, Ward and Weiss (1989) recommend dose and field modification. Nisce and colleagues (1986) temporarily modified their radiotherapeutic regimen to deliver only 1500 to 2000 rad to supradiaphragmatic sites in seven women with a second- or third-trimester pregnancy. Despite this reduction to what were considered subcurative doses, fetal radiation exposure ranged from 2 to 50 rad and averaged about 20 rad. When evaluated at 6 to 11 years of age, all seven children were normal, but two mothers had died.

Because of data shown in Table 55–2, chemotherapy is probably best avoided during the first trimester, but it is a relatively safe option later. With obvious widespread disease, chemotherapy is given at diagnosis. Postponement of therapy until fetal maturity is achieved is considered reasonable by some if the diagnosis is made late in pregnancy and the mother is asymptomatic.

There are no convincing data that pregnancy itself adversely affects Hodgkin lymphoma, and the disease does not cause increased pregnancy wastage. Because aggressive radiation and chemotherapy are often necessary to affect cure, pregnancy termination may be a

TABLE 55–4. Ann Arbor Staging System for Lymphomas

Stage	Findings
I	Involvement in single lymph node region or single extralymphatic site.
II	Involvement of two or more lymph node regions on the same side of the diaphragm. Includes localized involvement of extralymphatic site (stage IIE).
III	Involvement of lymph node regions or extralymphatic sites on both sides of diaphragm.
IV	Disseminated involvement of one or more extralymphatic organs, with or without lymph node involvement.

Substage A = asymptomatic patient; substage B = patients with fever, sweats, or weight loss.

reasonable option when the diagnosis of Hodgkin disease is made in the first half of pregnancy. Holmes and Holmes (1978) analyzed 93 pregnancy outcomes when either the pregnant woman or the father had Hodgkin disease, and the great majority were satisfactory. Jacobs and associates (1981) reported their experiences from Stanford University and found that neither chemotherapy during the second and third trimesters, nor irradiation to the mediastinum and neck, appeared to adversely affect the fetus or neonate. **Pregnant women with Hodgkin disease are inordinately susceptible to infections and sepsis, and both radiotherapy and chemotherapy increase this susceptibility.**

FERTILITY AFTER TREATMENT. Horning and co-workers (1981) evaluated the reproductive potential of women after treatment for Hodgkin disease. They reported that 55 percent of women resumed normal menses after chemotherapy. No birth defects or developmental abnormalities were evident in 24 infants subsequently born to these women. The risk of second cancers, especially leukemia, is substantively increased in patients with Hodgkin disease. Tucker and colleagues (1988) reported this to be almost 20 percent within 15 years. When compared with radiotherapy given alone, Kaldor and associates (1990) reported that the risk for leukemia was increased almost ninefold following chemotherapy.

Other complications of therapy for Hodgkin disease include myocardial damage and infarction, pulmonary fibrosis, hypothyroidism, and marrow suppression (Peleg and Ben-Ami, 1998).

NON-HODGKIN LYMPHOMAS. Non-Hodgkin lymphomas have recently become the most common neoplasms among persons aged 20 to 40. Their incidence has risen sharply because of their relationship to the acquired immunodeficiency syndrome. Indeed, 5 to 10 percent of persons infected with human immunodeficiency virus (HIV) will develop a lymphoma. Pollack and colleagues (1993) described a case of non-Hodgkin lymphoma of B-cell origin, with metastasis to the placenta, in a woman with HIV infection. Burkitt lymphoma is an aggressive tumor usually of B-cell origin. Barnes and associates (1998) reviewed 19 pregnancies complicated by this lymphoma; 17 women did not survive one year.

The concurrence of non-Hodgkin lymphoma with pregnancy has been rare, although its incidence is expected to increase because of the rising incidence of HIV infection. In a 50-year literature review, Ward and Weiss (1989) described only 75 cases associated with pregnancy. Avilés and colleagues (1990) reported their experiences with 16 pregnant women with these malignancies. Although half of the cases of lymphoma were discovered in the first trimester, these investigators be-

gan cytotoxic drug therapy and observed no fetal malformations. All but one offspring were healthy at 3 to 11 years. Eight of the 16 mothers who had remissions were alive 4 to 9 years later. Catlin and co-workers (1999) described a fascinating case in which a maternal natural-killer-cell lymphoma metastasized transplacentally and engrafted the fetus. Both mother and infant succumbed from the malignancy.

Extensive staging is required for non-Hodgkin lymphomas, and the Ann Arbor system shown in Table 55–4 is used. Radiotherapy typically is used for stage I disease, whereas chemotherapy is recommended for most stage II and all stage III and IV tumors. Unfortunately, the disease is often widespread when the peripheral nodes are involved and staging laparotomy is of little or no benefit (Peleg and Ben-Ami, 1998).

LEUKEMIAS. Except for acute lymphocytic leukemia, which is a childhood disorder, leukemias are more prevalent after age 40. Despite this, acute leukemias are among the most common malignant neoplasms of young women, but paradoxically, their incidence complicating pregnancy is cited to be about 1 case per 100,000 (Harrison and colleagues, 1994). This has also been our experience at Parkland Hospital, and we have encountered about 10 women with leukemia in nearly 300,000 pregnancies. Caligiuri and Mayer (1989) reviewed 350 reports of pregnancy complicated by leukemia. Of 72 newly diagnosed cases during pregnancy and reported since 1975, 44 had acute myelogenous leukemia, 20 acute lymphocytic leukemia, and eight had one of the chronic leukemias.

EFFECT ON PREGNANCY. Most pregnant women with acute leukemia will have pancytopenia. The survival of untreated acute leukemia may be extremely short, with the median survival of acute myelogenous leukemia being 3 months or less (Peleg and Ben-Ami, 1998). In more recent times, there is an improved survival rate with these malignancies, and in three fourths of women who develop **acute leukemia** during pregnancy, remission can usually be induced with chemotherapy. Thus, maternal and fetal outcomes have improved substantively in recent years (Reynoso and colleagues, 1987). For example, McLain (1974) reported that the maternal mortality rate was 100 percent and perinatal mortality was 34 percent in 256 women with acute leukemia treated before 1970. According to Lewis and Laros (1986), maternal death from acute leukemia has become negligible since 1970, although many of these unfortunate women die months to years following pregnancy. Survival has also improved for women with **chronic myelogenous** and **lymphocytic leukemias.** The rare chronic **hairy-cell leukemia** has been reported in only six pregnancies (Stiles and colleagues, 1998).

Despite being improved, perinatal outcomes are generally poor for leukemic women. Reynoso and colleagues (1987) analyzed 58 reported cases of acute leukemia during pregnancy in a 10-year period. Nearly 75 percent of these were diagnosed during the second and third trimesters. Half of the women had acute myelogenous leukemia, and most cases were treated with chemotherapy, with a reported remission rate of 75 percent. Only 40 percent of pregnancies in these women resulted in live-born infants. Similarly, Caligiuri and Mayer (1989) reported preterm delivery in about 50 percent of women diagnosed during pregnancy. The stillbirth rate was also increased.

Several cases of **congenital leukemia** in infants of nonleukemic mothers have been recorded, although no case of transmission of maternal leukemia to the fetus has been authenticated. Conversely, a third of tumors metastatic to the placenta are leukemias and lymphomas (Chap. 32, p. 849).

MANAGEMENT. In general, multiagent chemotherapy is given as soon as the diagnosis of leukemia is established, even if in the first trimester. Rare cases of spontaneous remission of acute leukemia after pregnancy have been reported (Antunez-de-Mayolo and colleagues, 1989). These observations perhaps implicate a hormonal influence, but hormone receptors were not studied. Because there is no evidence that pregnancy has a deleterious effect on leukemia, termination is not recommended to improve the prognosis, but it is a consideration in early pregnancy to avoid potential teratogenesis from chemotherapy. Morishita and colleagues (1994) described the use of umbilical blood sampling to monitor the fetus of a woman receiving combination chemotherapy for acute myelogenous leukemia. Fetal hemopoiesis was not adversely affected, and there were no apparent developmental abnormalities.

The use of all-trans-retinoic-acid (tretinoin) has been described for treatment of acute promyelocytic leukemia, a subset of acute myelogenous leukemia (Celo and colleagues, 1994). Harrison and associates (1994) reported successful treatment of this leukemia with tretinoin in the second trimester without adverse fetal effects. Currently, it would seem prudent to avoid this vitamin A derivative during pregnancy. As discussed in Chapter 38 (p. 1015), the teratogenic effects of vitamin A and two of its derivatives, isotretinoin and etretinate, have been well described (American College of Obstetricians and Gynecologists, 1995). Claahsen and colleagues (1998) have recently reported a woman with acute myeloid leukemia who was treated with idarubicin and cytosine-arabinoside during the second and third trimesters of pregnancy. The newborn had growth restriction and was preterm, but had no structural abnormalities.

Significant complications in pregnancy that include infection and hemorrhage should be anticipated at the time of delivery in women with active disease. Manifestations include anemia, neutropenia, and thrombocytopenia. Vaginal delivery is preferable, and cesarean section is reserved for obstetrical indications.

MALIGNANT MELANOMA

Melanomas are relatively common in women of childbearing age, and a significant proportion of women may have the diagnosis made during pregnancy (MacKie, 1999). The incidence of melanoma in general has been increasing over the last several decades (Dennis, 1999; Squartrito and Harlow, 1998). Its incidence in pregnancy is not known exactly, but has been estimated to range from 0.14 to 2.8 per 1000 live births (Derek and Strassner, 1990). As emphasized by Salopek and colleagues (1995), melanomas are underreported because many are treated on an outpatient basis and are not entered into a tumor registry. Melanomas are most common in light-skinned Caucasians, and over 90 percent originate in the skin from pigment-producing melanocytes, usually arising from a preexisting nevus. Any suspicious behavior in a pigmented cutaneous lesion such as changes in contour, surface elevation, discoloration, itching, bleeding, or ulceration warrants a biopsy.

Melanomas are clinically staged: stage I has no palpable lymph nodes, stage II has palpable nodes, and in stage III there are distant metastases. Approximately 85 percent of cases are stage I disease (Squartrito and Harlow, 1998). Tumor thickness is the single most important predictor of survival in stage I patients. The Clark classification is most widely used and includes five levels of involvement by depth into the epidermis, dermis, and subcutaneous fat.

EFFECT OF PREGNANCY. Earlier reports that pregnancy stimulates growth of malignant melanoma have not been substantiated. Pregnancy is associated with increased melanocyte-stimulating hormones, and some melanomas contain sex steroid hormone receptors. Ellis (1991) has shown that pregnancy and estrogen-containing oral contraceptives probably increase dysplastic nevus changes, a forerunner to melanoma development. More recent data would suggest that oral contraceptives are not etiological in the development of melanoma (Gefeller and colleagues, 1998; Pfahlberg, 1997). In his review of 11 studies, however, Holly (1986) concluded that there was no adverse effect on survival if melanoma was first diagnosed during pregnancy, or if pregnancy developed in a woman with previously recognized melanoma. Findings from the World Health

Organization (WHO) Melanoma Programme (MacKie and colleagues, 1991) indicate that women in whom melanoma was diagnosed during pregnancy had significantly greater tumor thickness when compared with women diagnosed before or after pregnancy.

Primary surgical treatment for melanoma is determined by the stage of the disease and includes wide local resection sometimes with extensive regional lymph node dissection. In a study from the WHO Melanoma Programme, Cascinelli and co-workers (1998) reported that routine regional node dissection improved survival in nonpregnant patients with microscopic node metastases. Prophylactic chemotherapy or immunotherapy is usually avoided during pregnancy; however, chemotherapy for active disease is given if indicated by tumor stage, maternal prognosis, and gestational age. In most cases of metastatic melanoma, treatment is at best palliative. Therapeutic abortion does not appear to improve survival in women with melanoma (Dipaola and colleagues, 1997).

Prognosis is determined by the stage of the lesion, and patients with deep cutaneous invasion or regional node involvement have a much poorer prognosis. As discussed earlier, women who are pregnant when melanoma is diagnosed have thicker skin tumors. As shown in Figure 55–1, these women have a higher mortality rate when compared with women whose melanoma was diagnosed before or after pregnancy. Survival is equivalent, however, stage-for-stage, when pregnancy is compared with nonpregnancy. Kjems and Krag (1993) summarized the survival rate from five studies of 338 pregnant and 1360 nonpregnant women with stage I melanoma. They found no significant differences in 5-year survival rates between the two groups. Because most recurrences manifest by 2 (60 percent) to 5 (90 percent) years, most authorities recommend that future pregnancies be avoided for 3 to 5 years after treatment.

PLACENTAL METASTASES. According to their review, Dildy and colleagues (1989) found that a third of reported cases of malignancies metastatic to the fetus or placenta have been malignant melanoma (Chap. 32, p. 848). Ferreria and co-workers (1998) described a case of melanoma metastatic to the placenta that reacted with melanoma-specific anti-S-100 protein and HMB-45 antibodies. Although in some cases, the tumor undergoes regression in the neonate, many infants have succumbed to disease (Anderson and colleagues, 1989).

GENITAL CANCER

Genital tract cancer is the most common form of cancer encountered during pregnancy. The distribution of various malignancies is summarized in Table 55–5.

CERVICAL NEOPLASIA. Pregnancy provides an opportune time for screening for cervical neoplasia and premalignant disease, especially for women who do not seek or have access to routine health care. Incidence

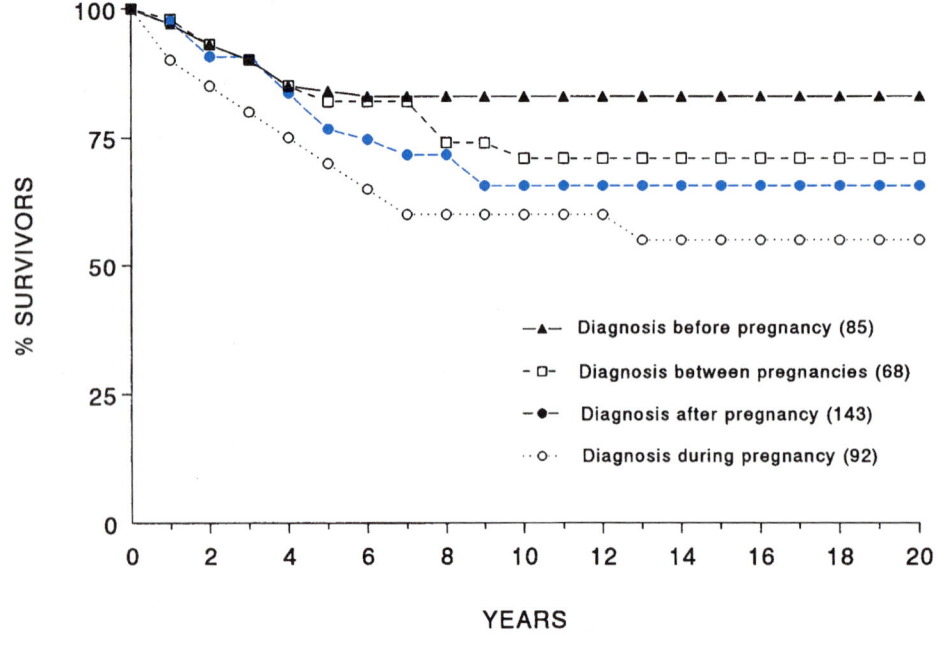

FIGURE 55–1. Disease-free survival in 388 women with malignant melanoma. Decreased survival in women diagnosed during pregnancy is due to increased thickness of tumors. (Modified from MacKie and colleagues, 1991, with permission.)

—▲— Diagnosis before pregnancy (85)
- ▫- Diagnosis between pregnancies (68)
—●— Diagnosis after pregnancy (143)
··○·· Diagnosis during pregnancy (92)

TABLE 55–5. Frequency of Genital Malignancies Associated with Pregnancy

Study	Primary Site (%)				
	Cervix	Ovary	Corpus	Vulva/Vagina	Other
Barber and Brunschwig (1963) (n = 62)	76	16	3	5	—
Phelan (1968) (n = 27)	96	4	—	—	—
Lutz et al (1977) (n = 40)	75	10	—	15	—
Haas (1984) (n = 261)	88	8	1	—	3
Total (n = 390)	85	9	1	3	1

Adapted from Nevin and associates (1995).

data for cervical neoplasia complicating pregnancy varies widely. Cervical dysplasia is quite common; Jolles (1989) cited an incidence in reproductive-age women of 26 per 1000. The incidence of carcinoma-in-situ was about 5 per 1000 women. According to Hacker and associates (1982), the average incidence of carcinoma-in-situ during pregnancy is about 1.3 per 1000, and for invasive carcinoma it is about 1 per 2200 pregnancies. Nevin and colleagues (1995) reported that approximately 1 in 2000 pregnancies is associated with cervical carcinoma and approximately 3 percent of women with cervical cancer were pregnant. Method and Brost (1999) cite the incidence to range from 0.1 to 1.3 per 1000 pregnancies. In our experiences, invasive cervical cancer is not nearly so common as these higher figures. Certain types of human papillomavirus are associated with both high-grade intraepithelial lesions as well as invasive cancer. Routine human papillomavirus testing is not recommended except for research studies (Kaufman and Adam, 1999).

INTRAEPITHELIAL NEOPLASIA. The effects of pregnancy and delivery on premalignant and malignant epithelial cervical lesions are not understood completely. In the study by Kiguchi and co-workers (1981), progression from dysplasia to invasive carcinoma after delivery (0.4 percent) was almost half that for nonpregnant women (1 percent). Moreover, the regression rates of moderate and marked dysplasia within 6 months after delivery were higher than those for the general population. Fife and colleagues (1996) found an increased incidence of high-cancer risk viruses—human papillomavirus types 16, 18, 31, 35, 45, 51, 52, and 56—when they compared pregnant with nonpregnant women.

According to Talebian and co-workers (1976), the incidence of abnormal cytology during pregnancy is about 3 percent, which is similar to that reported for nonpregnant women. Evaluation of the Papanicolaou smear can, however, be more difficult during pregnancy (Connor, 1998). Evaluation of an abnormal cytological smear is the same as for nonpregnant women with minor modifications (Economos and associates, 1993). During pregnancy, colposcopic evaluation is easier to perform because the transformation zone is better exposed due to physiological eversion. Colposcopically directed biopsies are used liberally to assess any suspicious lesions (Palle and co-workers, 2000). Biopsy sites may actively bleed because of hyperemia, and this can usually be stopped easily with Monsel solution, silver nitrate, vaginal packing, or occasionally a suture. Multiple biopsies need not all be taken on one occasion but rather may be obtained over a period of time. The diagnostic accuracy of colposcopy is 99 percent, and complications arise in fewer than 1 percent of uses (Economos and associates, 1993; Hacker and co-workers, 1982).

During pregnancy, endocervical curettage is omitted to avoid risks of hemorrhage and membrane rupture. Cone biopsy usually is reserved to exclude invasive cancer. If possible, conization is avoided because of an increased incidence of hemorrhage, abortion, and preterm labor (Table 55–6). Indeed, conization during pregnancy is less than satisfactory for at least three reasons:

1. The epithelium and underlying stroma within the cervical canal cannot be excised extensively because of the risk of membrane rupture. Of 376 conizations during pregnancy reviewed by Hacker and colleagues (1982), residual neoplasia was found in 43 percent of subsequent specimens.

2. Blood loss is common during and after conization and Averette and colleagues (1970) reported that nearly 10 percent of 180 pregnant women required transfusion.

3. There is increased relative risk of 1.6-fold for preterm delivery (El-Bastawissi and colleagues, 1999). Of interest, laser vaporization of the cervix for intraepithelial neoplasia before pregnancy does not appear to be associated with preterm delivery (van Rooijen and Persson, 1999).

TABLE 55–6. Complications Associated with Cervical Conization During Pregnancy

Study	Complication (%)			
	Immediate Bleeding	Delayed Bleeding	Abortion	Perinatal Deaths
Rogers and Williams (1967)	14	0	—	4
Daskal and Pitkin (1968)	5	5	17	6
Horowitz and associates (1969)	8	—	0	3
Averette and colleagues (1970)	7	4	27	5
Hannigan and co-workers (1982)	12	4	18	4
Average	9	4	18	5

Modified from Hannigan and colleagues (1982).

If cytological changes of mild cervical intraepithelial neoplasia are identified and subsequently confirmed, further follow-up during pregnancy may consist of colposcopic evaluation. In the absence of lesions detected by a satisfactory colposcopy, simply repeating the cervical smears later in pregnancy is usually adequate. Cytological changes that are suggestive of moderate or severe dysplasia or invasive disease require colposcopically directed biopsies to identify the responsible lesion. Women with histologically confirmed intra-epithelial neoplasia may be followed with cytology and colposcopically directed biopsies, allowed to deliver vaginally, and given definitive treatment after delivery. In a recent study by Yost and colleagues (1999), there was regression postpartum in 68 percent of women with grade II and 70 percent of those with grade III neoplasia. Although 7 percent of women with grade II lesions progressed to grade III lesions, none of the lesions progressed to invasive carcinoma.

INVASIVE CARCINOMA OF THE CERVIX. Pregnancy co-existing with invasive cervical carcinoma complicates both staging and treatment. Accurate identification of the extent of cancer is more difficult during pregnancy because induration of the base of the broad ligaments—which in nonpregnant women characterizes tumor spread beyond the cervix—may be less prominent during pregnancy. Thus, the extent of the tumor is more likely to be underestimated in the pregnant woman. Limited computed tomography of the pelvis is acceptable, but to avoid ionizing radiation, magnetic resonance imaging is a useful adjunct to ascertain extent of disease, including urinary tract involvement (Gilstrap and colleagues, 2001; Hannigan, 1990). Cystoscopy and sigmoidoscopy can be performed as necessary to rule out mucosal involvement.

Because cervical carcinoma is relatively uncommon during pregnancy, only a few institutions have had ex-tensive experience with its management. Some generalizations, however, can be made. The survival rate for invasive carcinoma has not been profoundly different for pregnant and nonpregnant women within a given stage of disease, although these descriptive studies have been small. Van Der Vange and colleagues (1995), in a review of 44 women with cervical cancer associated with pregnancy who were matched with 44 controls, reported an overall 5-year survival rate of 80 percent among pregnant subjects and 82 percent among controls. The mode of delivery has not been shown to affect maternal survival significantly, although experiences are limited because most women were delivered by hysterotomy or cesarean section (Hacker and colleagues, 1982). In general, when frankly invasive carcinoma is identified, most clinicians favor abdominal delivery, if for no other reason than that the cervix would not lacerate during dilatation.

MANAGEMENT. Treatment of cervical cancer varies according to its stage and pregnancy duration. Treatment for microinvasive disease diagnosed by cone biopsy to exclude frankly invasive disease follows guidelines similar to those for intraepithelial disease. Thus, continuation of pregnancy and vaginal delivery are considered safe, with therapy given postpartum.

Invasive cancer demands relatively prompt therapy. In general, during the first half of pregnancy, immediate treatment is advised, whereas during the latter half a reasonable option is to await not only fetal viability, but fetal maturity (Greer and colleagues, 1989). In a report of 12 pregnant women with invasive cervical carcinoma along with a review of the literature, van Vliet and colleagues (1998) concluded that delayed treatment to allow greater fetal maturity was reasonable in women with nonbulky lesions, lesions less than stage IIB, and gestation past 20 weeks. Preferred treatment for selected patients with stage I and early stage IIA small-diameter (less than 3 cm) invasive carcinoma is **radical hysterectomy plus pelvic lymphadenectomy.** Surgical treatment allows ovarian conservation and vaginal function, and minimizes exposure at an early age to the adverse effects of radiation on the intestinal and urinary tracts. Nisker and Shubat (1983) described 49 cases of stage IB cervical cancer complicating pregnancy, and reported a 30 percent severe complication rate from radiation therapy compared with only 7 percent in those treated by radical surgery. Surgical dissection during pregnancy actually may be facilitated by softening of uterine supportive structures. Before 20 weeks, hysterectomy is usually performed with the fetus in situ. In later pregnancy, however, hysterotomy may first be necessary.

Radiotherapy is given for more extensive cancer. Early in pregnancy, external irradiation is given and if spontaneous abortion does not ensue, then curettage is performed. During the second trimester, spontaneous abortion may be delayed, and hysterotomy may be necessary in up to a fourth of cases. About a week following abortion, external radiation is begun, followed by intracavitary radium application. After 24 weeks, the risk of delay to allow fetal maturity is unknown, but allowing pulmonic maturity seems reasonable, especially for early lesions (i.e., stage I disease).

PROGNOSIS. The overall prognosis for all stages of cervical cancer during pregnancy is probably similar to that for nonpregnant women (Sood and Sorosky, 1998). The results from several published reports are shown in Table 55–7. These aggregate results suggest no difference in survival when pregnant women are compared with nonpregnant women. Included are 49 cases of stage IB cancer and reported by Nisker and Shubat (1983). These investigators found a 5-year survival of only 70 percent compared with 87 percent in nonpregnant women with similar stages. This difference might be due to understaging of the disease during pregnancy.

It is unknown if vaginal delivery through a cancerous cervix worsens the prognosis; however, most oncologists favor abdominal delivery based on theoretical considerations. Moreover, recurrence in the episiotomy scar after vaginal delivery has been reported (Cliby and colleagues, 1994). Direct implantation of tumor cells is likely the mechanism of recurrence in these cases.

ENDOMETRIAL CARCINOMA. Because endometrial carcinoma characteristically develops in women past the reproductive age, it is seen only rarely in association with pregnancy. Schammel and colleagues (1998) reviewed 14 cases reported in the literature and described an additional five cases. The majority of cases reported thus far have been well-differentiated adenocarcinomas. Although treatment consists primarily of abdominal hysterectomy and bilateral salpingo-oophorectomy, Schammel and colleagues (1998) reported conservative therapy consisting of curettage with or without progestational therapy in four women. Interestingly, there have been at least four viable infants reported out of these 19 cases. Kowalczyk and co-workers (1999) described a 28-year-old woman with well-differentiated carcinoma who conceived after successful treatment with megestrol for 6 months.

TABLE 55–7. Five-year Survival Rates of Pregnant and Nonpregnant Women Treated for Cervical Cancer

Study	Pregnant No.	(%)	Nonpregnant No.	(%)
Sablinska et al (1977)				
Stage I	114	(72)	208	(76)
Stage II	116	(54)	270	(56)
Lee et al (1981)				
Stage IA	3	(100)	30	(100)
Stage IB–surgery	17	(93)	156	(91)
Stage IB–radiation	4	(80)	32	(88)
Nisker and Shubat (1983)				
Stage IB	49	(70)	NS	(87)
Van Der Vange et al (1995)				
Stages IA, IB, IIA	21	(85)	18	(85)

NS = not stated.

OVARIAN CARCINOMA. Malignant ovarian neoplasms are the fourth most common cause of death from cancer and the leading cause of death from genital tract cancers in North American women. Their incidence during pregnancy is not accurately known, but it has been reported to average about 1 per 25,000 deliveries (Jacob and Stringer, 1990; Jolles, 1989). According to the American College of Obstetricians and Gynecologists (1990), about 1 of every 1000 pregnant women will undergo surgical exploration for an adnexal mass. Most adnexal masses encountered during pregnancy will be either mature teratomas or cystadenomas (Boulay and Podczaski, 1998; Whitecar and colleagues, 1999). According to several reviews, only about 5 percent of adnexal neoplasms diagnosed during pregnancy are malignant, compared with 15 to 20 percent in nonpregnant women (Jacob and Stringer, 1990; Whitecar and associates, 1999). This is likely due to the younger age of pregnant women, and because of the disparate number of corpus luteum cysts.

Pregnancy apparently does not alter the prognosis of most ovarian malignancies, but complications such as torsion and rupture may develop. Most pregnant women who have ovarian cancer are asymptomatic. Prior to widespread use of ultrasonic evaluation of pregnancy, most pelvic masses were detected by routine prenatal examination during early pregnancy. Diagnosis afterward is more difficult because an adnexal tumor is usually obscured by the enlarging uterus. In many centers, universal sonography is performed during pregnancy, and the detection of adnexal masses has increased concomitantly. Certainly, sonography is indicated for women in whom there is a palpable adnexal mass, and it is helpful to differentiate functional cystic masses from solid or multiseptated masses. With the former, expectant management is acceptable, but the latter require surgery for diagnosis. Evaluation of pelvic masses is discussed in detail in Chapter 35 (p. 930).

MANAGEMENT. If ovarian cancer is discovered at laparotomy, treatment is similar to that for the nonpregnant woman, and this depends on gestational age as well as the stage, histological type, and grade of the tumor. After frozen section verifies malignancy, complete surgical staging with careful inspection of all peritoneal and visceral surfaces is performed. **Malignant ovarian tumors apparently confined to one ovary require complete surgical staging, and this is recommended also in tumors of low malignant potential** (Yazigi and associates, 1988). Procedures include peritoneal washings for cytological examination, multiple biopsies of the diaphragmatic undersurface and pelvic and parietal peritoneum, wedge resection of the opposite ovary, partial omentectomy, and excisional biopsies of pelvic and aortic lymph nodes. Whereas in most advanced stages hysterectomy and bilateral adnexectomy are indicated, in certain circumstances it can be justified to remove the tumor and await fetal maturity. In some cases, chemotherapy is given while awaiting pulmonary maturation. Maternal CA-125 serum levels are too variable during pregnancy to monitor for response to therapy (Aslam and associates, 2000; Spitzer and colleagues, 1998).

PROGNOSIS. According to Jolles (1989), two thirds of ovarian cancers found during pregnancy are of the common epithelial types. The remainder are germ-cell tumors, and occasionally a stromal-cell tumor. There does not appear to be an adverse influence of pregnancy on these malignancies. About 70 cases of invasive **epithelial cell tumors** coexistent with pregnancy have been reported (Dgani and colleagues, 1989; Van Dessel and coworkers, 1988). Foersterling and Blythe (1999) have recently described a woman with both an ovarian serous cystadenocarcinoma (stage IC) and a stage IA endometrial adenocarcinoma. Epithelial tumors are the most frequent ovarian malignancies in nonpregnant as well as pregnant women. Because of the relatively young age of the pregnant population, there is a higher proportion of less-advanced tumors. Thus, tumors with low-malignant potential and stage IA are seen more often compared with nonpregnant women. In some cases, borderline tumors will have been diagnosed before pregnancy and treated conservatively (Gotlieb and colleagues, 1998).

Karlen and associates (1979) reviewed 27 cases of **dysgerminomas** during pregnancy. They found significant obstetrical complications in nearly half of the women and reported a 30 percent recurrence in apparent stage IA cases. Buller and colleagues (1992) described conservative surgical management to allow pregnancy progression in three women with dysgerminomas. They recommended follow-up with magnetic resonance imaging and tumor markers to monitor for recurrences. Young and associates (1984) reviewed 36 cases of **gonadal stromal tumors** that accounted for 4 percent of reported ovarian malignancies complicating pregnancy. All of these tumors were stage I and they had an excellent prognosis. An **endodermal sinus tumor** has been diagnosed because of persistently elevated maternal serum alpha-fetoprotein levels (van der Zee and colleagues, 1991). This tumor has an overall bad prognosis (Farahmand and associates, 1991; Malhotra and Sood, 2000). Elit and colleagues (1999) reported on the use of bleomycin, cisplatin, and etoposide in a woman with this malignancy at 24 weeks. The newborn had ventriculomegaly and cerebral atrophy, the etiology of which was unclear. Maymon and co-workers (1998) described a woman with primary ovarian **hepatoid carcinoma** who also had elevated alpha-fetoprotein levels. Kalir and Friedman (1998) have described a **gynandroblastoma**—sex cord and stromal cells of both ovarian and testicular types—in a 32-year-old pregnant woman.

VULVAR CANCER

Invasive **squamous cell carcinoma** of the vulva is primarily a disease of postmenopausal women, and thus is only rarely associated with pregnancy. Regan and Rosenzweig (1993) found 17 cases in their review. Heller and associates (2000) more recently found 23 cases to review and described a 28-year-old with a 4-cm vulvar lesion noted near term. They concluded that radical surgery for stage I disease was feasible during pregnancy even in the last trimester. **Vulvar intraepithelial neoplasia** is seen more often in young women, and it is associated with human papillomavirus in most. Its potential for progression to invasive disease is unclear. Interestingly, the association with invasive disease and papillomavirus infection is not as closely linked as it is with cervical carcinoma (American College of Obstetricians and Gynecologists, 1994). Despite this, Messing and Gallup (1995) reported a trend toward younger women with vulvar carcinoma, which more frequently has a papillomavirus association. Kuller and colleagues (1990) reviewed five cases of **vulvar sarcoma** discovered during pregnancy. In four of these, cure was obtained by a variety of therapies.

Any suspicious vulvar lesion should be biopsied. Treatment of invasive disease is individualized according to the clinical stage and depth of invasion. Vaginal delivery is not contraindicated if the vulvar incisions are well healed.

UTERINE LEIOMYOMAS

Benign uterine leiomyomas are common in older pregnant women, and especially in black women. Because they are seldom malignant, leiomyomas complicating pregnancy are considered in Chapter 35 (p. 926).

LEIOMYOMATOSIS PERITONEALIS DISSEMINATA.
Rarely at cesarean section or puerperal tubal ligation, numerous subperitoneal smooth muscle tumors are found that at first appear to be disseminated carcinomatosis. Leiomyomatosis peritonealis disseminata results from stimulation, probably by estrogen, of multicentric subcoelomic mesenchymal cells to become smooth muscle cells. According to the review by Lashgari and colleagues (1994), about half of the 45 reported cases were discovered during pregnancy. Although surgical exci-

sion has been recommended, there is evidence that these tumors regress after pregnancy. Marom and associates (1998) as well as Ling and colleagues (2000) have described women who had tumors extending up the vena cava into the heart. Bekkers and colleagues (1999) have reported a rare malignant leiomyoblastoma during pregnancy.

GASTROINTESTINAL TRACT CANCER

COLORECTAL CARCINOMA. Cancer of the colon and rectum are the second most frequent malignancies in women of all age groups in the United States. These tumors seldom complicate pregnancy because they are uncommon before age 40 (Cappell, 1998). The majority—80 percent or more—of colorectal carcinomas in pregnant women arise from the rectum (Skilling, 1998). Fewer than 250 cases of colon cancer have been reported in pregnant women (Walsh and Fazio, 1998).

The most common symptoms of colorectal cancer are abdominal pain, distention, nausea and vomiting, constipation, and rectal bleeding. The diagnosis may be delayed because these symptoms may be ascribed to the pregnancy. Gonsoulin and colleagues (1990) described a woman with colon carcinoma and hepatic metastases in whom maternal serum alpha-fetoprotein levels were elevated persistently after first being measured at 16 weeks. Certainly, if symptoms suggestive of colon disease persist, digital rectal examination, tests for occult blood, and flexible sigmoidoscopy followed by colonoscopy are done if indicated. Seidman and colleagues (1992) described a woman in whom an intussuscepted colon cancer was diagnosed using magnetic resonance imaging.

From limited information available, it appears that the segmental distribution of colon cancer lesions is the same as in nonpregnant women. Importantly, 60 to 70 percent of lesions are palpable by rectal examination. Tumors above the peritoneal reflection are uncommon, and Chan and associates (1999a) described only 41 cases in their review of the English-language literature. Van Voorhis and Cruikshank (1989) reported two additional women with colon cancer who had persistent microcytic, hypochromic anemia from occult bleeding.

MANAGEMENT. Treatment of colorectal cancer follows the same general guidelines as for nonpregnant patients, and when there is no evidence for metastatic disease, surgery is performed. During the first half of the pregnancy, hysterectomy is not necessary in order to perform colon or rectal resection, and thus therapeutic abortion is not mandated. During later pregnancy, as well as in the presence of metastatic disease, delaying therapy to allow fetal maturation is considered. Vaginal delivery is usually permitted if obstetrical conditions are favorable, but rectal lesions below the pelvic brim may cause dystocia. Hemorrhage, obstruction, or perforation may force surgical intervention (Donegan, 1983).

There is no evidence that pregnancy influences the usual course of colorectal cancer. Thus, prognosis is similar to that for identical stages in nonpregnant patients. Unfortunately, pregnant women usually present with advanced disease (Walsh and Fazio, 1998). Carcinoembryonic antigen (CEA), a useful tumor marker for colon cancer, may be elevated during pregnancy and therefore is of little value.

OTHER GASTROINTESTINAL NEOPLASMS. Gastric cancer is rarely associated with pregnancy, and most reported cases are from Japan. Hirabayashi and collaborators (1987) reviewed outcomes in 60 pregnant women with this malignancy seen over a 70-year period from 1916 to 1985. Delay in diagnosis during pregnancy was unfortunately common, and the prognosis was consistently poor—88 percent of women were dead within one year of diagnosis. As discussed in Chapter 48 (p. 1274), persistent upper gastrointestinal symptoms should be evaluated by endoscopy. Davis and Chen (1991) and Chan and colleagues (1999b) each described a woman with gastric cancer who attributed her continued epigastric pain during pregnancy to preexisting peptic ulcer disease.

Stewart and colleagues (1997) reviewed their experiences with seven pregnancies in five women with **Zollinger–Ellison syndrome.** They advise surgical resection of the tumor before pregnancy is undertaken, but in women with metastatic disease or in those with pre-

viously undiagnosed tumors, antiacid and antisecretory treatment usually suffices.

At least 21 cases of **carcinoid tumors** complicating pregnancy have been reported. In his review, Durkin (1983) found that most cases were of gastrointestinal origin, and some were incidentally diagnosed at cesarean section. **Pancreatic cancer** is very rare during pregnancy (Gamberdella, 1984). Bondeson and colleagues (1990) described an endocrine pancreatic malignancy in which the diagnosis was confused because of chorionic gonadotropin produced by an early pregnancy. Primary **hepatic cancer** during pregnancy also is rare (Gisi and Floyd, 1999; Purtilo and associates, 1975). Balderston and co-workers (1998) described a 23-year-old woman at 26 weeks who had a massive intrahepatic cholangiocarcinoma masquerading as the HELLP syndrome (syndrome of hemolysis, elevated liver enzymes, and low platelet count). She died 3 weeks postpartum.

RENAL TUMORS

Walker and Knight (1986) reviewed 71 cases of primary renal neoplasms associated with pregnancy. Half were **renal cell carcinoma,** and a palpable abdominal mass was the presenting finding in almost 90 percent of these women. Pain was the second most common presenting symptom (50 percent), and hematuria was found in half the cases. Only a fourth of these women had the classical triad of hematuria, pain, and a palpable mass. Diagnosis has been improved by contemporaneous imaging studies (Fig. 55–2). Smith and co-workers (1994) added nine new cases since 1986 in their updated review. They suggest that earlier diagnosis is common now because

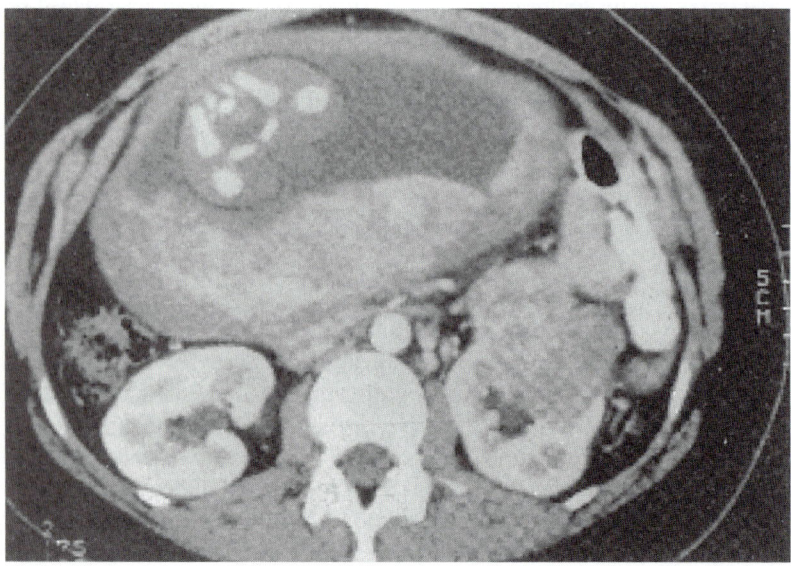

FIGURE 55–2. Computed tomographic scan of a pregnant woman with large renal mass on left side. (From Gross and associates, 1995, with permission.)

of ultrasonography. We have encountered only six pregnant women with this malignancy during the past 30 years at Parkland Hospital. They either presented because of painless hematuria, or the tumor was found by abdominal palpation done routinely in conjunction with cesarean deliveries. If suspected antepartum, the diagnosis can be confirmed by intravenous pyelography, ultrasonic-directed needle biopsy, magnetic resonance imaging, or limited computed tomographic scanning as shown in Figure 55–2. Fazeli-Matin and co-workers (1998) described partial nephrectomy in a woman with renal carcinoma at 14 weeks.

OTHER TUMORS

Thyroid cancers are the most common endocrine malignancies, and it has been estimated that approximately 10 percent of those cases occurring during the reproductive years are diagnosed during pregnancy or within the first year after birth (Morris, 1998). Tewari and associates (1998) described a woman with Graves thyrotoxicosis and thyroid storm who was subsequently found to also have papillary adenocarcinoma involving the cervical nodes. Rossing and colleagues (2000) have presented intriguing findings that suggest that thyroid stimulation during pregnancy and lactation may result in a transient increase in papillary thyroid cancer. Diagnosis is usually by fine-needle aspiration. Treatment consists primarily of surgery performed during the second trimester or after delivery (Chap. 50, p. 1346). Most thyroid cancers are well-differentiated and follow an indolent course.

Brain tumors are uncommon. Isla and colleagues (1997) described seven cases in over 126,000 deliveries from Hospital La Paz in Madrid. Two women died, one from intrapartum hemorrhage into a meningioma. Tewari and co-workers (2000) described eight women with malignant brain tumors associated with pregnancy. Another two women had postpartum gestational choriocarcinoma metastatic to the brain. These cases were from a 20-year survey of five California hospitals with about 312,000 deliveries during the 20-year study period. Maternal outcomes were horrific—five women died, two who lived had significant neurological defects, and only three are in remission.

REFERENCES

American College of Obstetricians and Gynecologists: Committee on Obstetrics: Vitamin A supplementation during pregnancy. Committee Opinion No. 157, September 1995

American College of Obstetricians and Gynecologists: Genital human papillomavirus infections. Technical Bulletin No. 193, June 1994

American College of Obstetricians and Gynecologists: Cancer of the ovary. Technical Bulletin No. 141, May 1990

Anderson JF, Kent S, Machin GA: Maternal malignant melanoma with placental metastasis: A case report with literature review. Pediatr Pathol Lab Med 9:35, 1989

Antunez-de-Mayolo J, Ahn YS, Temple JD, Harrington WJ: Spontaneous remission of acute leukemia after the termination of pregnancy. Cancer 63:1621, 1989

Aslam N, Ong C, Woelfer B, Nicolaides K, Jurkovic D: Serum CA125 at 11–14 weeks of gestation in women with morphologically normal ovaries. Br J Obstet Gynaecol 107:689, 2000

Averette HE, Mirhashemi R, Moffat FL: Pregnancy after breast carcinoma. Cancer 85:2301, 1999

Averette HE, Nasser N, Yankow SL, Little WA: Cervical conization in pregnancy. Am J Obstet Gynecol 106:543, 1970

Avilés A, Diaz-Maqueo JC, Talavera A, Guzmán R, Garcia EL: Growth and development of children of mothers treated with chemotherapy during pregnancy: Current status of 43 children. Am J Hematol 36:243, 1991

Avilés A, Diaz-Maqueo JC, Torras V, Garcia EL, Guzmán R: Non-Hodgkin lymphomas and pregnancy: Presentation of 16 cases. Gynecol Oncol 37:335, 1990

Balderston KD, Tewari K, Azizi F, Yu JK: Intrahepatic cholangiocarcinoma masquerading as the HELLP syndrome (hemolysis, elevated liver enzymes, and low platelet count) in pregnancy: Case report. Am J Obstet Gynecol 179:823, 1998

Barber HRK, Brunschwig A: Gynecologic cancer complicating pregnancy. Am J Obstet Gynecol 85:156, 1963

Barnavon Y, Wallack MK: Management of the pregnant patient with carcinoma of the breast. Surg Gynecol Obstet 171:347, 1990

Barnes MN, Barrett JC, Kimberlin DF, Kilgore LC: Burkitt lymphoma in pregnancy. Obstet Gynecol 91:675, 1998

Bekkers RL, Massuger LF, Berg PP, Haelst UG, Bulten J: Uterine malignant leiomyoblastoma (epithelioid leiomyosarcoma) during pregnancy. Gynecol Oncol 72:433, 1999

Berry DL, Theriault RL, Holmes FA, Parisi VM, Booser DJ, Singletary SE, Buzdar AU, Hortobagyi GN: Management of breast cancer during pregnancy using a standardized protocol. J Clin Oncol 17:855, 1999

Bondeson AG, Bondeson L, Thompson NW: Early pregnancy masquerading as a marker for malignancy in a young woman with curable neoplasm of the pancreas. Br J Surg 77:108, 1990

Bonnier P, Romain S, Dilhuydy JM, Bonichon F, Julien JP, Charpin C, Lejeune C, Martin PM, Piana L: Influence of pregnancy on the outcome of breast cancer: A case-control study. Int J Cancer 72:720, 1997

Boulay R, Podczaski E: Ovarian cancer complicating pregnancy. Obstet Gynecol Clin North Am 25:386, 1998

Brent RL: Underutilization of developmental basic science principles in the evaluation of reproductive risks from pre- and postconception environmental radiation exposures. Teratology 59:182, 1999

Brent RL: The effect of embryonic and fetal exposure to x-ray, microwaves and ultrasound: Counseling the pregnant and nonpregnant patient about these risks. Semin Oncol 16:347, 1989

Brent RL: Ionizing radiation. Contemp Ob/Gyn 30:20, 1987

Buekers TE, Lallas TA: Chemotherapy in pregnancy. Obstet Gynecol Clin North Am 25:323, 1998

Buller RE, Darrow V, Manetta A, Porto M, DiSaia PJ: Conservative surgical management of dysgerminoma concomitant with pregnancy. Obstet Gynecol 78:887, 1992

Caligiuri MA, Mayer RJ: Pregnancy and leukemia. Semin Oncol 16:388, 1989

Cappell MS: Colon cancer during pregnancy: The gastroenterologist's perspective. Gastroenterol Clin 27:225, 1998

Cascinelli N, Morabito A, MacKie RM, Belli F: Immediate or delayed dissection of regional nodes in patients with melanoma of the trunk: A randomised trial. Lancet 351:793, 1998

Catlin EA, Roberts JD, Erana R, Preffer FI, Ferry JA, Kelliher AS, Atkins L, Weinstein HJ: Transplacental transmission of natural-killer-cell lymphoma. N Engl J Med 341:85, 1999

Celo JS, Kim HC, Houlihan C, Canavan BF, Manzullo GP, Saidi P: Acute promyelocytic leukemia in pregnancy: All trans retinoic acid as a newer therapeutic option. Obstet Gynecol 83:808, 1994

Chan YM, Ngai SW, Lao TT: Colon cancer in pregnancy. A case report. J Reprod Med 44:733, 1999a

Chan YM, Ngai SW, Lao TT: Gastric adenocarcinoma presenting with persistent, mild gastrointestinal symptoms in pregnancy. J Reprod Med 44:986, 1999b

Claahsen HL, Semmekrot BA, Van Dongen PW, Mattijssen V: Successful fetal outcome after exposure to idarubicin and cytosine-arabinoside during the second trimester of pregnancy—a case report. Am J Perinatol 15:295, 1998

Clark RM, Reid J: Carcinoma of the breast in pregnancy and lactation. Int J Radiat Oncol Biol Phys 4:693, 1978

Clarke MP, Kane RA, Steele G Jr: Prospective comparison of preoperative imaging and intraoperative ultrasonography in the detection of liver tumors. Surgery 106:849, 1989

Cliby WA, Dodson MK, Podratz KC: Cervical cancer complicated by pregnancy: Episiotomy site recurrences following vaginal delivery. Obstet Gynecol 84:179, 1994

Collins JC, Liou S, Wile AG: Surgical management of breast masses in pregnant women. J Reprod Med 40:785, 1995

Connor JP: Noninvasive cervical cancer complicating pregnancy. Obstet Gynecol Clin North Am 25:331, 1998

Davis JL, Chen MD: Gastric carcinoma presenting as an exacerbation of ulcers during pregnancy. A case report. J Reprod Med 36:450, 1991

Dennis LK: Analysis of the melanoma epidemic, both apparent and real. Data from the 1973 through 1994 surveillance, epidemiology, and end results program registry. Arch Dermatol 135:275, 1999

Derek JW, Strassner HT: Melanoma in pregnancy. Clin Obstet Gynecol 33:782, 1990

Dgani R, Shoham Z, Atar E, Zosmer A, Lancet M: Ovarian carcinoma during pregnancy: A study of 23 cases in Israel between the years 1960 and 1984. Gynecol Oncol 33:326, 1989

Dildy GA Jr, Moise KJ Jr, Carpenter RJ Jr, Klima T: Maternal malignancy metastasis to the products of conception: A review. Obstet Gynecol Surv 44:535, 1989

Dipaola RS, Goodin S, Ratzell M, Florczyk M, Karp G, Ravikumar TS: Chemotherapy for metastatic melanoma during pregnancy. Gynecol Oncol 66:526, 1997

DiSaia PJ, Creasman WT: Cancer in pregnancy. In: Clinical Gynecologic Oncology, 4th ed. St. Louis, Mosby Year Book, 1993, p 533

Doll DC, Ringenberg S, Yarbro JW: Management of cancer during pregnancy. Arch Intern Med 148:2058, 1988

Donegan WL: Cancer and pregnancy. CA Cancer J Clin 33:194, 1983

Donegan WL: Mammary carcinoma and pregnancy. Major Prob Clin Surg 5:448, 1979

Dow KH, Harris JR, Roy C: Pregnancy after breast-conserving surgery and radiation therapy for breast cancer. Monogr Natl Cancer Inst 16:131, 1994

Dunn JS, Anderson CD, Brost BC: Breast carcinoma metastatic to the placenta. Obstet Gynecol 94:846, 1999

Durkin JW: Carcinoid tumor and pregnancy. Am J Obstet Gynecol 145:757, 1983

Economos K, Veridiano NP, Delke I, Collado ML, Tancer L: Abnormal cervical cytology in pregnancy: A 17-year experience. Obstet Gynecol 81:915, 1993

Ekbom A, Hsieh C, Lipworth L, Adami H, Trichopoulos D: Intrauterine environment and breast cancer risk in women: A population-based study. J Natl Cancer Inst 88:71, 1997

El-Bastawissi AY, Becker TM, Daling JR: Effect of cervical carcinoma in situ and its management on pregnancy outcome. Obstet Gynecol 93:207, 1999

Elit L, Bocking A, Kenyon C, Natale R: An endodermal sinus tumor diagnosed in pregnancy: Case report and review of the literature. Gynecol Oncol 72:123, 1999

Ellis DL: Pregnancy and sex steroid hormone effects on nevi of patients with the dysplastic nevus syndrome. J Am Acad Dermatol 25:467, 1991

Farahmand SM, Marchetti DL, Asirwatham JE, Dewey MR: Case report ovarian endodermal sinus tumor associated with pregnancy: Review of the literature. Gynecol Oncol 41:156, 1991

Fazeli-Matin S, Goldfarb DA, Novick AC: Renal and adrenal surgery during pregnancy. Urology 52:510, 1998

Ferreira CMM, Maceira JMP, Coelho JMCdO: Melanoma and pregnancy with placental metastases. Am J Dermatopathol 20:403, 1998

Fife KH, Katz BP, Roush J, Handy VD, Brown DR, Hansell R: Cancer-associated human papillomavirus types are selectively increased in the cervix of women in the first trimester of pregnancy. Am J Obstet Gynecol 174:1487, 1996

Foersterling DL, Blythe JG: Ovarian carcinoma, endometrial carcinoma, and pregnancy. Gynecol Oncol 72:425, 1999

Gamberdella FR: Pancreatic carcinoma in pregnancy: A case report. Am J Obstet Gynecol 149:15, 1984

Gefeller O, Hassan K, Willie L: Cutaneous malignant melanoma in women and the role of oral contraceptives. Br J Dermatol 138:122, 1998

Gershenson DM: Menstrual and reproductive function after treatment with combination chemotherapy for malignant ovarian germ cell tumors. J Clin Oncol 6:270, 1988

Gilstrap LG, Van Dorsten PV, Cunningham FG (eds): Cancer in pregnancy. In: Operative Obstetrics, 2nd ed. New York, McGraw-Hill, 2001.

Gisi P, Floyd R: Hepatocellular carcinoma in pregnancy. A case report. J Reprod Med 44:65, 1999

Glantz JC: Reproductive toxicology of alkylating agents. Obstet Gynecol Surv 49:709, 1994

Gonsoulin W, Mason B, Carpenter RJ Jr: Colon cancer in pregnancy with elevated maternal serum α-fetoprotein level at presentation. Am J Obstet Gynecol 163:1172, 1990

Gotlieb WH, Flikker S, Davidson B, Korach Y, Kopolovic J, Ben-Baruch G: Borderline tumors of the ovary. Cancer 82:141, 1998

Greer BE, Easterling TR, McLennan DA, Benedetti TJ, Cain JM, Figge DC, Tamimi HK, Jackson JC: Fetal and maternal considerations in the management of stage I-B cervical cancer during pregnancy. Gynecol Oncol 34:61, 1989

Gross AJ, Zoller G, Hermanns M, Ringert RH: Renal cell carcinoma during pregnancy. Br J Urol 75:254, 1995

Guinee VF, Olsson H, Moller T, Hess KR, Taylor SH, Fahey

T: Effect of pregnancy on prognosis for young women with breast cancer. Lancet 343:1587, 1994

Haagensen CD: Diseases of the Breast, 2nd ed. Philadelphia, Saunders, 1971, p 660

Haas JF: Pregnancy in association with newly diagnosed cancer: A population-based epidemiologic assessment. Int J Cancer 34:229, 1984

Hacker NF, Berek JS, Lagasse LD, Charles EH, Savage EW, Moore JG: Carcinoma of the cervix associated with pregnancy. Obstet Gynecol 59:735, 1982

Hall EJ: Scientific view of low-level radiation risks. Radiographics 11:509, 1991

Hannigan EV: Cervical cancer in pregnancy. Clin Obstet Gynecol 33:837, 1990

Harrison P, Chipping P, Fothergill GA: Successful use of all trans retinoic acid in acute promyelocytic leukemia presenting during the second trimester of pregnancy. Br J Haematol 86:681, 1994

Harvey JC, Rosen PP, Ashikari R, Robbins GF, Kinne DW: The effect of pregnancy on the prognosis of carcinoma of the breast following radical mastectomy. Surg Gynecol Obstet 153:723, 1981

Heller DS, Cracchiolo B, Hameed M, May T: Pregnancy-associated invasive squamous cell carcinoma of the vulva in a 28-year-old, HIV-negative woman. A case report. J Reprod Med 45:659, 2000

Higgins S, Haffty BG: Pregnancy and lactation after breast-conserving therapy for early stage breast cancer. Cancer 73:2175, 1994

Hirabayashi M, Ueo H, Okudaira Y, Matsumata T, Hanawa S, Sugimachi K: Early gastric cancer and a concomitant pregnancy. Am Surg 53:730, 1987

Hochman A, Schreiber H: Pregnancy and cancer of the breast. Obstet Gynecol 2:268, 1953

Holly EA: Melanoma and pregnancy. Recent results. Cancer Res 102:118, 1986

Holmes GE, Holmes FF: Pregnancy outcomes of patients treated for Hodgkin's disease: A controlled study. Cancer 41:1317, 1978

Hoover HC Jr: Breast cancer during pregnancy and lactation. Surg Clin North Am 70:1151, 1990

Horning SJ, Hoppe RT, Kaplan HS, Rosenberg SA: Female reproductive potential after treatment for Hodgkin's disease. N Engl J Med 304:1377, 1981

Hornstein E, Skornick Y, Rozin R: The management of breast carcinoma in pregnancy and lactation. J Surg Oncol 21:179, 1982

Hsieh CC, Wuu J, Lambe M, Trichopoulos D, Adami HO, Ekbom A: Delivery of premature newborns and maternal breast-cancer risk. Lancet 353:1239, 1999

Isaacs JH: Cancer of the breast in pregnancy. Surg Clin North Am 75:47, 1995

Ishida T, Yoko T, Kasumi F: Clinical pathological characteristics and progress of breast cancer patients associated with pregnancy and lactation. Analysis of case-control study in Japan. Jpn J Cancer Res 83:1143, 1992

Isla A, Alvarez F, Gonzalez A, Garcia-Grande A, Perez-Alvarez M, Garcia-Blazquez M. Brain tumor and pregnancy. Obstet Gynecol 89:19, 1997

Jacob JH, Stringer CA: Diagnosis and management of cancer during pregnancy. Semin Perinatol 14:79, 1990

Jacobs C, Donaldson SS, Rosenberg SA, Kaplan HS: Management of the pregnant patient with Hodgkin's disease. Ann Intern Med 95:669, 1981

Jernström H, Lerman C, Ghadirian P, Lynch HT, Weber B, Garber J, Daly M, Olopade OI, Foulkes WD, Warner E,

Brunet JS, Narod SA: Pregnancy and risk of early breast cancer in carriers of BRCA1 and BRCA2. Lancet 354:1846, 1999

Jolles CJ: Gynecologic cancer associated with pregnancy. Semin Oncol 16:417, 1989

Kaiser HE, Nawab E, Nasir A, Chmielarczyk W, Krenn M: Neoplasms during the progression of pregnancy. In Vivo 14:277, 2000

Kaldor JM, Day NE, Clarke A, Van Leeuwen FE, Henry-Amar M, Fiorentino MV, Bell J, Pedersen D, Band P, Assouline D, Koch M, Choi W, Prior P, Blair V, Langmark F, Kirn VP, Neal F, Peters D, Pfiffer R, Karjalainen S, Cuzick J, Sutcliffe SB, Somers R, Pellae-Cosset B, Pappagallo GL, Fraser P, Storm H, Stoval M: Leukemia following Hodgkin's disease. N Engl J Med 322:7, 1990

Kalir T, Friedman F Jr: Gynandroblastoma in pregnancy: Case report and review of literature. Mt Sinai J Med 65:292, 1998

Karlen JR, Akbari A, Cook WA: Dysgerminoma associated with pregnancy. Obstet Gynecol 53:330, 1979

Kaufman RH, Adam E: Is human papillomavirus testing of value in clinical practice? Am J Obstet Gynecol 180:1049, 1999

Kiguchi K, Bibbo M, Hasegawa T, Kurihara S, Tsutsui F, Wied G: Dysplasia during pregnancy: A cytologic follow-up study. J Reprod Med 26:66, 1981

King RM, Welch JS, Martin JK, Coulam CB: Carcinoma of the breast associated with pregnancy. Surg Gynecol Obstet 160:228, 1985

Kjems E, Krag C: Melanoma and pregnancy. Acta Oncologia 32:371, 1993

Koren G, Weiner L, Lishner M, Zemlickis D, Finegen J: Cancer in pregnancy: Identification of unanswered questions on maternal and fetal risks. Obstet Gynecol Surv 45:509, 1990

Korzeniowski S, Dyba T: Reproductive history and prognosis in patients with operable breast cancer. Cancer 74:1591, 1994

Kowalczyk CL, Malone J, Peterson EP, Jacques SM, Leach RE: Well-differentiated endometrial adenocarcinoma in an infertility patient with later conception. J Reprod Med 44:57, 1999

Kroman N, Jensen MB, Melbye M, Wohlfahrt J, Mouridsen HT. Should women be advised against pregnancy after breast-cancer treatment? Lancet 350:319, 1997

Kuller JA, Zucker PK, Peng TCC: Vulvar leiomyosarcoma in pregnancy. Am J Obstet Gynecol 162:164, 1990

Lambe M, Ekbom A: Cancers coinciding with childbearing: Delayed diagnosis during pregnancy? BMJ 311:1607, 1995

Lashgari M, Behmaram B, Ellis M: Leiomyomatosis peritonealis disseminata. A report of two cases. J Reprod Med 39:652, 1994

Lee RB, Neglia W, Park RC: Cervical carcinoma in pregnancy. Obstet Gynecol 58:584, 1981

Lewis BJ, Laros RK Jr: Leukemia and lymphoma. In Laros RK Jr (ed): Blood Disorders in Pregnancy. Philadelphia, Lea & Febiger, 1986, p 85

Li FP, Fine W, Jaffe N, Holmes GE, Holmes FF: Offspring of patients treated for cancer in childhood. J Natl Cancer Inst 62:1193, 1979

Liberman L, Giess CS, Dershaw DD, Deutch BM, Petrek JA: Imaging of pregnancy-associated breast cancer. Radiology 191:245, 1994

Ling FT, David TE, Merchant N, Yu E, Butany JW: Intracardiac extension of intravenous leiomyomatosis in a pregnant woman: A case report and review of the literature. Can J Cardiol 16:73, 2000

Lippman ME, Lichter AS, Danforth DN Jr: Diagnosis and

Management of Breast Cancer. Philadelphia, Saunders, 1988, p 415

Lutz MH, Underwood PB Jr, Rozier JC, Putney FW: Genital malignancy in pregnancy. Am J Obstet Gynecol 129:536, 1977

MacKie RM: Pregnancy and exogenous hormones in patients with cutaneous malignant melanoma. Curr Opin Oncol 11:129, 1999

MacKie RM, Bufalino R, Morabito A, Sutherland C, Cacsinelli N: Lack of effect of pregnancy on outcome of melanoma. Lancet 337:653, 1991

Malhotra N, Sood M: Endodermal sinus tumor in pregnancy. Gynecol Oncol 78:265, 2000

Marchant DJ: Breast cancer in pregnancy. Clin Obstet Gynecol 37:993, 1994

Marom D, Pitlik S, Sagie A, Ovadia Y, Bishara J: Intravenous leiomyomatosis with cardiac involvement in a pregnant woman. Am J Obstet Gynecol 178:620, 1998

Martin JA, Smith BL, Mathews TJ, Ventura SJ: Births and deaths: Preliminary data for 1998. Natl Vital Stat Rep 47:1, 1999

Maymon E, Piura B, Mazor M, Bashiri A, Silberstein T, Yanai-Inbar I: Primary hepatoid carcinoma of ovary in pregnancy. Am J Obstet Gynecol 179:820, 1998

McLain CR Jr: Leukemia in pregnancy. Clin Obstet Gynecol 17:185, 1974

Melbye M, Wohlfahrt J, Lei U, Norgaard-Pedersen B, Mouridsen HT, Lambe M, Michels KB: Alpha-fetoprotein levels in maternal serum during pregnancy and maternal breast cancer incidence. J Natl Cancer Inst 92:1001, 2000

Melbye M, Wohlfahrt J, Olsen JH, Frisch M, Westergaard T, Helweg-Larsen K, Andersen PK: Induced abortion and the risk of breast cancer. N Engl J Med 336:81, 1997

Messing MJ, Gallup DG: Carcinoma of the vulva in young women. Obstet Gynecol 86:51, 1995

Method MW, Brost BC: Management of cervical cancer in pregnancy. Semin Surg Oncol 16:251, 1999

Michels KB, Willett WC, Rosner BA, Manson JE, Hunter DJ, Colditz GA, Hankins SE, Speizer FE: Prospective assessment of breastfeeding and breast cancer incidence among 89,887 women. Lancet 347:431, 1996

Morishita S, Imai A, Kawabata I, Tamaya T: Acute myelogenous leukemia in pregnancy: Fetal blood sampling and early effects of chemotherapy. Int J Gynecol Obstet 44:273, 1994

Morris PC: Thyroid cancer complicating pregnancy. Obstet Gynecol Clin North Am 25:401, 1998

Nettleton J, Long J, Kuban D, Wu R, Shaeffer J, El-Mahdi A: Breast cancer during pregnancy: Quantifying the risk of treatment delay. Obstet Gynecol 87:414, 1996

Nevin J, Soefers R, Dahaeck K, Bloch B, van Wyk L: Cervical carcinoma associated with pregnancy. Obstet Gynecol Surv 50:228, 1995

Nisce LZ, Tome MA, Shaoqin H, Lee BJ, Kutcher GJ: Management of coexisting Hodgkin's disease and pregnancy. Am J Clin Oncol 9:146, 1986

Nisker JA, Shubat M: Stage IB cervical carcinoma and pregnancy: Report of 49 cases. Am J Obstet Gynecol 145:203, 1983

Nugent P, O'Connell TX: Breast cancer and pregnancy. Arch Surg 120:1221, 1985

Otake M, Schull WJ: In utero exposure to A-bomb radiation and mental retardation: A reassessment. Br J Radiol 57:409, 1984

Palle C, Bangsboll S, Andreasson B: Cervical intraepithelial neoplasia in pregnancy. Acta Obstet Gynecol Scand 79:306, 2000

Peleg D, Ben-Ami M: Lymphoma and leukemia complicating pregnancy. Obstet Gynecol Clin North Am 25:365, 1998

Pelsang RE: Diagnostic imaging modalities during pregnancy. Obstet Gynecol Clin North Am 25:287, 1998

Petrek JA, Dukoff R, Rogatko A: Prognosis of pregnancy-associated breast cancer. Cancer 67:869, 1991

Pfahlberg A: Systematic review of case control studies: Oral contraceptives show no effect on melanoma risk. Public Health Rev 25:309, 1997

Phelan JT: Cancer and pregnancy. NY State J Med 68:3011, 1968

Pollack RN, Sklavin WT, Rao S, Divon MY: Metastatic placental lymphoma associated with maternal human immunodeficiency virus infection. Obstet Gynecol 81:856, 1993

Purtilo DT, Clark JV, Williams R: Primary hepatic malignancy in pregnant women. Am J Obstet Gynecol 121:41, 1975

Regan MA, Rosenzweig BA: Vulvar carcinoma in pregnancy: A case report and literature review. Am J Perinatol 10:334, 1993

Reynoso EE, Shepherd FA, Messner HA, Farquharson HA, Garvey MB, Baker MA: Acute leukemia during pregnancy: The Toronto leukemia study group experience with long-term follow-up of children exposed in utero to chemotherapeutic agents. J Clin Oncol 5:1098, 1987

Ribeiro GG, Palmer MK: Breast carcinoma associated with pregnancy: A clinician's dilemma. BMJ 2:1524, 1977

Rossing MA, Voigt LF, Wicklund KG, Daling JR: Reproductive factors and risk of papillary thyroid cancer in women. Am J Epidemiol 151:765, 2000

Rustin GJ, Booth M, Dent J, Salt S, Rustin F, Bagshawe KD: Pregnancy after chemotherapy for gestational trophoblastic tumours. BMJ 288:103, 1984

Sablinska R, Tarlowska L, Stelmachow J: Invasive carcinoma of the cervix associated with pregnancy: Correlation between patient age, advancement of cancer and gestation, and result of treatment. Gynecol Oncol 5:363, 1977

Sachs BP, Penzias AS, Brown DAJ, Driscoll SG, Jewett JF: Cancer-related maternal mortality in Massachusetts, 1954–1985. Gynecol Oncol 36:395, 1990

Salopek TG, Marghoob AA, Slade M, Ro B, Rigel DS, Kopf AW, Bart RS: An estimate of the incidence of malignant melanoma in the United States. Dermatol Surg 21:301, 1995

Schammel DP, Mittal KR, Kaplan K, Deligdisch L, Tavassoli FA: Endometrial adenocarcinoma associated with intrauterine pregnancy: A report of five cases and a review of the literature. Int J Gynecol Pathol 17:327, 1998

Seidman DS, Heyman Z, Ben-Ari GY, Mashiach S, Barkai G: Use of magnetic resonance imaging in pregnancy to diagnose intussusception induced by colonic cancer. Obstet Gynecol 79:822, 1992

Selevan SG, Lindbohm ML, Hornung RW, Hemminki K: A study of occupational exposure to antineoplastic drugs and fetal loss in nurses. N Engl J Med 313:1173, 1985

Skilling JS: Colorectal cancer complicating pregnancy. Obstet Gynecol Clin North Am 25:417, 1998

Smith DP, Goldman SM, Beggs DS, Lanigan PJ: Renal cell carcinoma in pregnancy. Report of three cases and review of the literature. Obstet Gynecol 83:818, 1994

Socié G, Stone JV, Wingard JR, Weisdorf D, Henslee-Downey PJ, Bredeson C, Cahn JY, Passweg JR, Rowlings PA, Schouten HC, Kolb HJ, Klein JP: Long-term survival and late deaths after allogeneic bone marrow transplantation. N Engl J Med 341:14, 1999

Sood AK, Sorosky JI: Invasive cervical cancer complicating

pregnancy: How to manage the dilemma. Obstet Gynecol Clin North Am 25:343, 1998

Sorosky JI, Scott-Conner CEH: Breast disease complicating pregnancy. Obstet Gynecol Clin North Am 25:353, 1998

Souadka A, Zouhal A, Souadka F, Jalil N, Benjelloun S, Benjaafar B, Mansouri M, El Gueddari B: Breast cancer and pregnancy: Forty-three cases reported in the National Oncology Institute between 1985 and 1988. Rev Fr Gynecol Obstet 89:67, 1994

Spitzer M, Kaushal N, Benjamin F: Maternal CA-125 levels in pregnancy and the puerperium. J Reprod Med 43:387, 1998

Squartrito RC, Harlow SP: Melanoma complicating pregnancy. Obstet Gynecol Clin North Am 25:407, 1998

Stewart CA, Termanini B, Sutliff VE, Corleto VD, Weber C, Gibril F, Jensen RT: Management of the Zollinger–Ellison syndrome in pregnancy. Am J Obstet Gynecol 176:224, 1997

Stiles GM, Stanco LM, Saven A, Hoffmann KD: Splenectomy for hairy cell leukemia in pregnancy. J Perinatol 18:200, 1998

Talebian F, Krumholz BA, Shayan A, Mann LI: Colposcopic evaluation of patients with abnormal cytologic smears during pregnancy. Obstet Gynecol 47:693, 1976

Tang MT, Weiss NS, Daling JR, Malone KE: Case-control differences in the reliability of reporting a history of induced abortion. Am J Epidemiol 151:1139, 2000

Tewari K, Balderston KD, Carpenter SE, Major CA: Papillary thyroid carcinoma manifesting as thyroid storm of pregnancy: Case report. Am J Obstet Gynecol 179:818, 1998

Tewari K, Cappuccini F, Asrat T, Flamm BL, Carpenter SE, DiSaia P, Quilligan EJ: Obstetric emergencies precipitated by malignant brain tumors. Am J Obstet Gynecol 182:1215, 2000

Tucker MA, Coleman CN, Cox RS, Varghese A, Rosenberg SA: Risk of second cancers after treatment for Hodgkin's disease. N Engl J Med 318:76, 1988

Urba WJ, Longo DL: Hodgkin's disease. N Engl J Med 326:678, 1992

Van Der Vange N, Weverling GJ, Ketting BW, Ankum WM, Samlal R, Lammes FB: The prognosis of cervical cancer associated with pregnancy. A matched cohort study. Obstet Gynecol 85:1022, 1995

Van Der Zee AGJ, de Bruijin HWA, Bouma J, Aalders JG, Oosterhuis JW, de Vries EGE: Endodermal sinus tumor of the ovary during pregnancy: A case report. Am J Obstet Gynecol 164:504, 1991

Van Dessel T, Hameeteman TM, Wagenaar SS: Mucinous cystadenocarcinoma in pregnancy. Case report. Br J Obstet Gynaecol 95:527, 1988

Van Rooijen M, Persson E: Pregnancy outcome after laser vaporization of the cervix. Acta Obstet Gynecol Scand 78:346, 1999

Van Vliet W, van Loon AJ, ten Hoor KA, Boonstra H: Cervical carcinoma during pregnancy: Outcome of planned delay in treatment. Eur J Obstet Gynecol Reprod Biol 79:153, 1998

Van Voorhis B, Cruikshank DP: Colon carcinoma complicating pregnancy. J Reprod Med 34:923, 1989

Velentgas P, Daling JR, Malone KE, Weiss NS, Williams MA, Self SG, Mueller BA: Pregnancy after breast carcinoma. Cancer 85:2424, 1999

Walker JL, Knight EL: Renal cell carcinoma in pregnancy. Cancer 58:2343, 1986

Walsh C, Fazio VW: Cancer of the colon, rectum, and anus during pregnancy. The surgeon's perspective. Gastroenterol Clin North Am 27:257, 1998

Ward FT, Weiss RB: Lymphoma and pregnancy. Semin Oncol 16:397, 1989

Waxman J: Cancer, chemotherapy and fertility. BMJ 290:1096, 1985

Whitecar P, Turner S, Higby K: Adnexal masses in pregnancy: A review of 130 cases undergoing surgical management. Am J Obstet Gynecol 181:19, 1999

Wong DJ, Strassner HT: Melanoma in pregnancy. Clin Obstet Gynecol 33:782, 1990

Yazigi R, Sandstad J, Munoz A: Primary staging in ovarian tumors of low malignant potential. Gynecol Oncol 31:402, 1988

Yost NP, Santoso JT, McIntire DD, Iliya FA: Postpartum regression rates of antepartum cervical intraepithelial neoplasia II and III lesions. Obstet Gynecol 93:359, 1999

Young RH, Dudley AG, Scully RE: Granulosa cell, Sertoli–Leydig cell, and unclassified sex cord-stromal tumors associated with pregnancy: A clinicopathological analysis of thirty-six cases. Gynecol Oncol 18:181, 1984

Zemlickis D, Lishner M, Degendorfer P, Panzarella T, Burke B, Sutcliffe SB, Koren G: Maternal and fetal outcome after breast cancer in pregnancy. Am J Obstet Gynecol 166:781, 1992a

Zemlickis D, Lishner M, Degendorfer P, Panzarella T, Sutcliffe SB, Koren G: Fetal outcome after in utero exposure to cancer chemotherapy. Arch Intern Med 152:573, 1992b

56

Infections

The pregnant woman and her fetus are susceptible to many infections and infectious diseases. Some of these may be quite serious and life-threatening for the mother, whereas others may have a profound impact on neonatal outcome by virtue of a high likelihood of fetal infection.

IMMUNOLOGICAL CHANGES OF PREGNANCY

There is much speculation concerning possible effects of decreased immune surveillance during pregnancy. These effects are engendered by maternal tolerance for the foreign-tissue antigens of the semiallogeneic fetal "graft" (Chap. 2, p. 21). Although there are subtle changes in circulating immunoglobulin levels in pregnancy, these appear to be of no consequence. Polymorphonuclear leukocyte chemotaxis and adherence may be depressed beginning in midpregnancy. Assessment of cell-mediated immunity is difficult, but available evidence suggests that maternal lymphocytes are as fully competent as paternal and unrelated cells in producing a cytotoxic response (Stirrat, 1991).

FETAL AND NEWBORN IMMUNOLOGY. The active immunological capacity of the fetus and neonate is compromised compared with that of older children and adults. According to Stirrat (1991), fetal cell-mediated and humoral immunity begin to develop by 9 to 15 weeks. Despite the ability to synthesize immunoglobulin G (IgG), the primary fetal response to infection is immunoglobulin M (IgM) production. Conversely, passive immunity is provided by IgG transferred actively across the placenta. By 16 weeks, transfer begins to increase rapidly, and by 26 weeks fetal concentrations are equivalent to those of the mother. After birth, breastfeeding is protective against some infections. But this begins to decline at 2 months of age (WHO Collaborative Study Team, 2000).

Neonatal infection, especially in its early stages, may be difficult to diagnose because of failure to respond in a classical fashion. If the fetus was infected in utero, there may be depression and acidosis at birth for no apparent reason. The infant may suck poorly, vomit, or develop abdominal distention. Respiratory insufficiency may develop, which is similar in many ways to idiopathic respiratory distress syndrome. The neonate may be lethargic or jittery. The response to sepsis may be hypothermia rather than hyperthermia, and the total leukocyte count and neutrophil counts may be depressed or not influenced by sepsis.

Bacteria, viruses, or parasites may gain access transplacentally during the viremic, bacteremic, or parasitemic stage of maternal infection (Newton, 1999). They may also cross the intact membranes (Table 56–1). Fetal infections may develop early in pregnancy to produce obvious stigmata at birth. Conversely, organisms may colonize and infect the fetus during labor and delivery. Thus, preterm rupture of membranes, prolonged labor, and manipulations may increase the risk of neonatal infection (Yancey and colleagues, 1996). Infections

---

TABLE 56–1. Some Causes of Fetal and Neonatal Infections

Intrauterine
Transplacental
  Viruses: varicella-zoster, coxsackie, parvovirus, rubella, cytomegalovirus, human immunodeficiency virus, others
  Bacteria: listeria, syphilis
  Protozoa: toxoplasmosis, malaria
Ascending infection
  Bacteria: group B streptococcus, coliforms, others
  Viruses: herpes simplex
Intrapartum
Maternal exposure
  Bacteria: gonorrhea, chlamydia, group B streptococcus, tuberculosis
  Viruses: herpes simplex, papillomavirus, human immunodeficiency virus, hepatitis B
External contamination
  Bacteria: staphylococcus, coliforms, others
  Viruses: herpes simplex
Neonatal
  Human transmission: staphylococcus, herpes simplex virus
  Respirators and catheters: staphylococcus, coliforms

occurring at less than 72 hours of age usually are caused by bacteria acquired in utero or during delivery, whereas infections after that time most likely have been acquired after birth.

A major mechanism for postnatal infection is from those caring for the infant. Indwelling venous and arterial umbilical catheters may cause infection. Ventilatory systems can be the source of life-threatening infection. **The very-low-birthweight infant who survives the first few days is at considerable risk of dying later from infection acquired in the intensive-care nursery.**

Bacteria most often responsible for sepsis in the newborn have varied during the past several decades. For example, in the 1930s and 1940s, group A β-hemolytic streptococci were involved principally. With the widespread use of penicillin, these infections decreased, to be replaced by staphylococcus in the 1950s, and coliforms and group B streptococcus beginning in the 1970s and predominating today.

VIRAL INFECTIONS

VARICELLA-ZOSTER. This is a DNA herpesvirus that remains latent in the dorsal root ganglia after primary infection. It may be reactivated years later to cause herpes zoster or shingles (Gilden and co-workers, 2000). Most adults have had chickenpox acquired during childhood and 95 percent have serological evidence of immunity (Glantz and Mushlin, 1998). Varicella infection in adults tends to be much more severe than in children. Approximately half of all varicella deaths occur in the 5 percent of adult population that are susceptible, a mortality 23 times greater than that from childhood varicella (Preblud, 1986).

Although disputed, there is evidence that varicella infection is especially severe during pregnancy. Paryani and Arvin (1986) reported that 4 of 43 of infected pregnant women, or about 10 percent, developed pneumonitis. Two of these women required ventilatory support, and one died. Despite this, successful pregnancy outcomes can follow complicated varicella pneumonia (Chandra and colleagues, 1998). Treatment is described in Chapter 46 (p. 1228) and usually consists of oxygenation, assisted ventilation when necessary, and treatment with acyclovir given intravenously (Cox and colleagues, 1990).

Maternal herpes zoster infection is more common in older or immunocompromised patients. There is no evidence that zoster is more frequent or more severe in pregnant women. Eyal and associates (1983), in a review of 15 cases of zoster during pregnancy, concluded that there was little evidence that zoster caused congenital malformations.

PREVENTION. Administration of **varicella-zoster immunoglobulin (VZIG)** will either prevent or attenuate varicella infection in exposed susceptible individuals if given within 96 hours. The dose is 125 U per 10 kg given intramuscularly with a maximum dose of 625 units or five vials. Immunoglobulin is recommended by the Centers for Disease Control and Prevention (1996b) for immunocompromised susceptible adults who are exposed, but it is not recommended routinely for pregnant women. Because of the severity of varicella during pregnancy, some authors do recommend immunoglobulin administration for exposed but otherwise healthy pregnant women (McGregor and colleagues, 1987; Paryani and Arvin, 1986). Up to 80 to 90 percent of adults are immune from prior symptomatic or asymptomatic infection, and thus antibody testing with enzyme-linked immunosorbent assay (ELISA) or fluorescent antibody to membrane antigen (FAMA) is done, if possible, prior to immune globulin therapy. Rouse and colleagues (1996) performed decision analysis and found such an approach to be cost effective.

An attenuated live-virus vaccine (Varivax) was approved for use in 1995 (American College of Obstetricians and Gynecologists, 2000). One dose is recommended routinely for all children between 1 and 12 years old. This successfully results in 97 percent seroconversion. Two doses, 4 to 8 weeks apart, are recommended for adolescents and adults with no history of varicella. **The vaccine is not recommended for pregnant women.** Using a decision analytic model, Glantz and Mushlin (1998) concluded that routine antenatal screening of all pregnant women with negative or indeterminate varicella histories was not cost effective. Smith and colleagues (1998), utilizing an analytic cost-effectiveness model, concluded that selective serotesting of all pregnant women with a negative or uncertain history of varicella, followed by postpartum vaccination, would prevent almost 50 percent of cases of chickenpox and was cost effective.

FETAL EFFECTS. Maternal chickenpox during the first half of pregnancy may cause congenital malformations by transplacental infection. Some of these include chorioretinitis, cerebral cortical atrophy, hydronephrosis, and cutaneous and bony leg defects (Fig. 56–1). Pastuszak and co-workers (1994) described 106 women with varicella infection before 20 weeks and computed the absolute risk of embryopathy to be about 2 percent. In a prospective study by Enders and colleagues (1994), a total of 1373 women had varicella infection during pregnancy. There was no clinical evidence of congenital varicella infection after 20 weeks. Only 2 of 472 pregnancies (0.4 percent) in which there was maternal infection before 13 weeks had infants with congenital varicella. The highest risk was between 13 and 20 weeks, during which time 7 of 351 exposed fetuses (2 percent) had

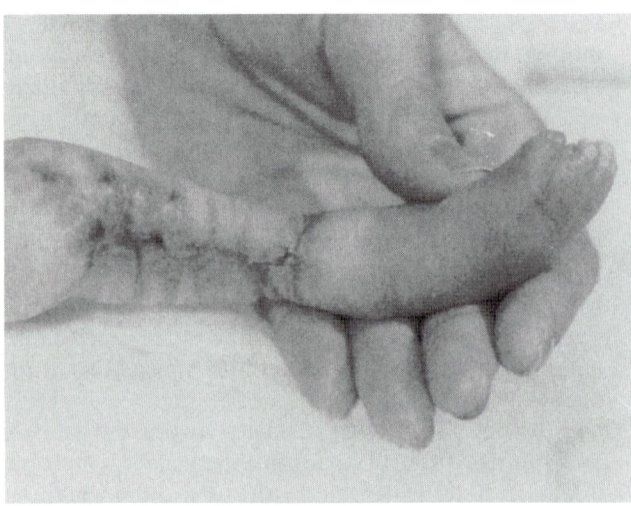

FIGURE 56–1. Atrophy of the lower extremity with bony defects and scarring in a fetus infected during the first trimester by varicella. (From Paryani and Arvin, 1986, with permission.)

evidence of congenital varicella. Jones and associates (1994) likewise observed a 1.4 percent incidence of fetal varicella syndrome in 146 live-born infants exposed before 20 weeks.

Fetal exposure later in pregnancy is associated with congenital varicella lesions, and zoster occasionally develops at several months of age (Chiang and colleagues, 1995). Fetal exposure to the virus just before or during delivery, and therefore before maternal antibody has been formed, poses a serious threat to the newborn. Friedman and associates (1994) described an epidemic outbreak in a neonatal intensive care unit. The incubation period for varicella infection is short and usually less than 2 weeks. In some instances, the infant will develop disseminated visceral and central nervous system disease, which is commonly fatal. Varicella-zoster or zoster immunoglobulin (ZIG) is administered to the neonate whenever the onset of maternal disease is within about 5 days before or after delivery. Perinatal mortality at other times is minimal because passive maternal antibody is protective. Despite passive immunoglobulin therapy, however, Miller and colleagues (1989) reported that 15 percent of infants developed severe infection.

INFLUENZA. These infections are caused by members of the *Orthomyxoviridae* family. Influenza A and B form one genus of these RNA viruses and are identified by nucleoprotein antigenic reactions. These are subclassified further by hemagglutinin (H) and neuraminidase (N) antigenic makeup. The viral strain then is characterized by its origin and the year isolated. For example, one component in the 1995–1996 trivalent vaccine was A/Johannesburg/33/94-like (H_3N_2), the 33rd influenza A virus isolated from a patient in Johannesburg, South Africa, in 1994 and having antigens of the H_3 hemagglutinin and N_2 neuraminidase subtypes.

Influenza A is more serious than influenza B and usually develops during winter epidemics. Infection usually is not life-threatening for otherwise healthy adults. If pneumonia develops, the prognosis becomes serious. In a statistical study based on 1350 cases, Harris (1919) found a gross maternal mortality rate of 27 percent, which increased to 50 percent when pneumonia developed. In August and September 1957, 50 percent of childbearing-age women who died of influenza in Minnesota were pregnant (Freeman and Barno, 1959).

PREVENTION. Vaccination against influenza is recommended by the Centers for Disease Control and Prevention (1998b) for all pregnant women after the first trimester. Regardless of gestational age, women who have chronic underlying medical disorders such as diabetes or heart disease are vaccinated. There is no evidence of teratogenicity (Chap. 10, p. 240).

Amantadine is an antiviral agent with specific activity against influenza A viruses. Given prophylactically during epidemics, it is 70 to 90 percent effective in preventing influenza (Centers for Disease Control and Prevention, 1994a). If therapy is begun within 48 hours of onset of symptoms, amantadine reduces the duration of fever and systemic symptoms. It is reserved for nonimmunized women at high risk for influenza complications (Chap. 46, p. 1227).

A new class of antiviral drugs—**neuraminidase inhibitors**—is highly effective to treat early influenza in adults (Centers for Disease Control and Prevention, 1999a; Gubareva and colleagues, 2000). There are now two approved agents for nonpregnant individuals. **Oseltamivir** is taken orally and **zanamivir** is inhaled. They are discussed further in Chapter 46 (p. 1227).

FETAL EFFECTS. There is no firm evidence that influenza A virus causes congenital malformations (Korones, 1988). Saxén and associates (1990) identified no association with increased first-trimester influenza in 248 mothers of anencephalic children. Conversely, Lynberg and associates (1994) reported increased neural-tube defects in children born to women with influenza early in pregnancy. This may be related to associated hyperthermia (Kashyap and Gruslin, 2000). McGregor and colleagues (1984) have convincingly demonstrated that the virus can infect the fetus, at least late in pregnancy. There is controversial evidence that fetal exposure to influenza A may predispose to schizophrenia in later life (Kunugi and associates, 1995; McGrath and Castle, 1995).

MUMPS. Mumps is an uncommon adult infectious disease caused by an RNA paramyxovirus. Up to 80 to 90 percent of adults are seropositive. The virus primarily infects the salivary glands, but may involve the gonads, meninges, pancreas, and other organs. Treatment is symptomatic. Mumps during pregnancy is no more severe than in nonpregnant adults and there is no evidence for its teratogenicity (Ouhilal, 2000).

The live attenuated Jeryl–Lynn vaccine strain is contraindicated in pregnant women. Likewise, **MMR vaccine**—measles, mumps, and rubella—is composed of live-attenuated viruses and contraindicated in pregnancy (Association of Professors of Gynecology and Obstetrics, 1999).

FETAL EFFECTS. Infection has been confirmed in a 10-week fetus (Kurtz and colleagues, 1982). Attenuated Jeryl–Lynn virus has been recovered from placental tissue of women given the vaccine 7 to 10 days before elective abortion (Yamauchi and co-workers, 1974). Despite this, there is no firm evidence that mumps infection causes increased fetal wastage. We agree with Miller and Hager (2000) that mumps infection is not an indication for termination of pregnancy. Manson and associates (1960) described 501 cases complicating pregnancy and reported that major fetal anomalies were not increased. Siegel (1973) confirmed this in a cohort study. Congenital mumps is very rare.

RUBEOLA (MEASLES). Most adults are immune to measles. Unfortunately, when measles becomes epidemic, as it did from 1989 to 1991, unvaccinated women may develop measles pneumonia with adverse maternal and perinatal outcomes (Eberhart-Phillips and colleagues, 1993; Stein and Greenspoon, 1991). About 3 percent of nonpregnant adults with measles develop clinical pneumonia.

The virus does not appear to be teratogenic, but there is an increased frequency of abortion and low-birthweight infants with maternal measles (Siegel, 1973; Siegel and Fuerst, 1966). Moroi and colleagues (1991) reported that placental infection caused death in a 25-week uninfected fetus. If the woman develops measles shortly before birth, there is considerable risk of serious infection developing in the neonate, especially in preterm infants. Passive immunization can be achieved by administering immune serum globulin, 5 mL given intramuscularly within 3 days of exposure. Active vaccination is not done during pregnancy, but susceptible women are vaccinated routinely postpartum (Association of Professors of Gynecology and Obstetrics, 1999). Periodic "catch-up" vaccination campaigns that target children age 9 months to 14 years have been successful in control of measles (de Quadros and colleagues, 1996).

RESPIRATORY VIRUSES. Approximately three fourths of acute viral respiratory infections are caused by more than 200 antigenetically distinct viruses. Respiratory viruses cause the common cold, pharyngitis, laryngotracheobronchitis, bronchitis, and pneumonia. Rhinovirus, coronavirus, and adenovirus are major causes of the common cold. The first two are RNA viruses and usually produce a trivial, self-limited illness characterized by rhinorrhea, sneezing, and congestion. There are 100 distinct serotypes. The DNA-containing adenovirus is more likely to produce cough and lower respiratory tract involvement, including pneumonia. Pneumonia complicating pregnancy is often preceded by an acute upper respiratory viral infection.

Mothers suffering from common cold had a four- to fivefold increased risk of fetal anencephaly when a 393-woman cohort of the Finnish Register of Congenital Malformations was analyzed (Kurppa and associates, 1991). These investigators further found that fever—a commonly quoted possible cause of anencephaly—was not found to be a factor. Adenoviral infection is a common cause of childhood myocarditis, and Towbin and colleagues (1994) used polymerase chain reaction to document fetal myocarditis at 29 weeks.

HANTAVIRUS. An outbreak in western states caused by the virulent respiratory hantavirus had an overall 60 percent case-fatality rate (Centers for Disease Control and Prevention, 1993). Pneumonitis that progresses to adult respiratory distress syndrome is characteristic. Gilson and colleagues (1994) described two pregnant women with the *Four Corners* strain who survived.

ENTEROVIRUS INFECTIONS. These viruses are a major subgroup of RNA picornaviruses that include poliovirus, coxsackievirus, and echovirus. Even though they are trophic for intestinal epithelium, they can cause widespread infections that may include the central nervous system, skin, heart, and lungs. Most infections are subclinical. Occasionally, fulminant newborn disease is caused by enteroviral infections. Hepatitis A is an enterovirus 72 that is discussed in Chapter 48 (p. 1289). These viruses may cause fetal infection. Dahlquist and colleagues (1995) found that maternal enteroviral infection is a risk factor for childhood-onset diabetes.

COXSACKIEVIRUS. Most of these infections are clinically inapparent, but the virus may cause aseptic meningitis, a polio-like illness, rashes, respiratory disease, or pleuritis, pericarditis, and myocarditis. The virus can be fatal to the fetus-infant, although causing only minor symptoms in the mother.

Brown and Karunas (1972) reported that congenital malformations were increased slightly in pregnant women who had serological evidence of coxsackievirus, but not echovirus infections. Viremia may cause hepatitis, myocarditis, and encephalomyelitis, which can cause fetal death. Garcia and associates (1991) reported that histological placentitis was common following maternal enteroviral infection. Strong and Young (1995) described clinical chorioamnionitis associated with maternal coxsackie viremia. The virus was grown from amnionic fluid as well as from neonatal spinal fluid in both twins. Dommergues and colleagues (1994) described fetal ventriculomegaly and cardiomyopathy in a stillborn infant whose amnionic fluid contained enterovirus.

POLIOVIRUS. Most of these infections are subclinical or mild. The virus is trophic for the central nervous system and symptomatic infections can cause paralytic disease—poliomyelitis. Siegel and Goldberg (1955), in a carefully controlled study in New York City, demonstrated that pregnant women not only were more susceptible to polio but also had a higher death rate. With the widespread use of vaccination during childhood, polio has become rare in the United States. Inactivated subcutaneous polio vaccine is recommended for susceptible pregnant women who must travel to endemic areas or in other high-risk situations. Live oral polio vaccine has been used for mass vaccination during pregnancy without harmful fetal effects (Harjulehto and associates, 1989).

PARVOVIRUS. Human B19 parvovirus causes **erythema infectiosum, or fifth disease.** This is a trivial maternal infection but occasionally causes fetal death. B19 is a small, single-stranded DNA virus that replicates in rapidly proliferating cells, such as erythroblast precursors. It is the only known human parvovirus (Rodis, 1999). Viremia occurs during the prodrome, which is followed by clinical features, including a bright red macular rash and erythroderma that affects the face giving a *slapped cheek* appearance. The rash, with accompanying arthralgias, may be due to immune-complex disease. In most women, the disease is asymptomatic. Confirmation of infection is by IgM-specific antibody. There is no evidence that the mild infection is altered by pregnancy (Valeur-Jensen and colleagues, 1999).

The attack rate of susceptible adults in school outbreaks is 20 to 30 percent (Young, 1995). In a study of 30,946 pregnant women, Valeur-Jensen and colleagues (1999) reported that having children aged 6 to 7 years was associated with a fourfold rate of seroconversion. Harger and colleagues (1998) as well as Jensen and associates (2000) reported that B19 infection in pregnancy was significantly higher if the woman was exposed to her own children. Interestingly, being a schoolteacher was not the highest risk factor in either of these two studies.

B19 parvovirus is trophic for erythroid cells and only those persons with the erythrocyte membrane P antigen are susceptible (Brown and colleagues, 1994). In women with hemolytic anemia—for example, sickle-cell disease—parvovirus infection may cause an aplastic crisis. Ville and associates (1995) described a **mirror syndrome** or **maternal hydrops syndrome**—preeclampsia-like disease related to placentomegaly—in a 25-week pregnancy with fetal hydrops caused by anemia from parvovirus infection.

FETAL EFFECTS. Maternal infection may be associated with abortion and fetal death. Rogers and co-workers (1993) found B19 parvovirus in two of 80 spontaneous abortuses, but there were no associated pathological changes. Tiessen and associates (1994) described a fetus with congenital anomalies possibly caused by first-trimester parvovirus infection. Shilleto and colleagues (1996) found evidence for fetal myocardial damage by measuring creatine kinase levels obtained by cordocentesis. During an outbreak in Connecticut, the fetal loss rate was 5 percent in 39 infected women (Rodis and colleagues, 1990). In London, the Public Health Laboratory Service Working Party on Fifth Disease (1990) prospectively followed 190 women infected during pregnancy. The transplacental infection rate was 33 percent. The overall risk of fetal death was 9 percent, and midpregnancy infection was associated with 12 percent fetal loss. Early fetal death is not usually associated with hydropic changes but is common in fetuses dying after midpregnancy (Wright and colleagues, 1996). Pustilnik and Cohen (1994) described discordant infection at 20 weeks in diamnionic–dichorionic twins.

Diagnosis is confirmed by parvovirus-specific IgM antibodies. Viral DNA may be detectable in serum during the prodrome but not after the rash develops. Use of polymerase chain reaction to detect viral DNA has been described (Rogers and colleagues, 1993; Yamakawa and associates, 1995). For women with positive serology, ultrasonic examination is indicated. If there is hydrops, then fetal transfusion is recommended by some authors (Peters and Nicolaides, 1990; Sahakian and associates, 1991; Thorp and colleagues, 1994). The technique is described in Chapter 37 (p. 993). Conversely, Morey (1991) and Fairley (1995) and their co-workers have described spontaneous resolution. Rodis and colleagues (1998a) did a survey and reported that approximately a third of fetuses with hydrops had spontaneous resolution and almost 85 percent of hydropic fetuses who received intrauterine transfusions survived. In another report, Rodis and colleagues (1998b) described the long-term outcome of children following maternal B19 parvovirus infection. They concluded that developmental delay was not apparently increased from fetal exposure.

RUBELLA. Also called **German measles,** rubella virus typically causes infections of minor import in the absence of pregnancy. During pregnancy, however, it has been directly responsible for inestimable wastage, and even more importantly, for severe congenital malformations. This relationship was first recognized by Gregg (1942), an Australian ophthalmologist.

PREVENTION. Although large epidemics of rubella have virtually disappeared in the United States because of immunization, the disease, with its horrific teratogenic potential, persists. From 1992 to 1997, 65 percent of reported cases were in persons older than 20 (Association of Professors of Gynecology and Obstetrics, 1999). From 6 to 25 percent of women are susceptible, and the Centers for Disease Control and Prevention (1994b) reported that outbreaks in 1993 and 1994 involved colleges, work settings, and prisons. In a review of 350 women from a cohort of high-risk pregnant women, 53 (15 percent) were found to be nonimmune (McElhaney and colleagues, 1999).

To eradicate the disease completely, the following approach is recommended for immunizing the adult population, particularly women of childbearing age:

1. Education of health-care providers and the general public on the dangers of rubella infection.
2. Vaccination of susceptible women as part of routine medical and gynecological care, including college health services.
3. Vaccination of susceptible women visiting family planning clinics.
4. Identification and vaccination of unimmunized women immediately after childbirth or abortion.
5. Vaccination of nonpregnant susceptible women identified by premarital serology.
6. Vaccination of all susceptible hospital personnel who might be exposed to patients with rubella or who might have contact with pregnant women.

Rubella vaccination should be avoided shortly before or during pregnancy because the vaccine contains attenuated live virus (Association of Professors of Gynecology and Obstetrics, 1999). The Centers for Disease Control (1990) has maintained a registry since 1971 to monitor the fetal effects of vaccination. Through 1989, 321 susceptible women who were immunized within 3 months of conception had been followed to term. Fortunately, there is no evidence that the vaccine induces malformations.

DIAGNOSIS. Confirmation of rubella infection is often difficult. Not only are the clinical features of other illnesses quite similar, but about a fourth of rubella infections are subclinical despite viremia that may infect the embryo and fetus. Absence of rubella antibody indicates susceptibility. Antibody signifies an immune response to viremia. If maternal antibody is demonstrated at the time of exposure to rubella or before, it is exceedingly unlikely that the fetus will be affected. Despite native or vaccine-induced immunity, subclinical rubella infections may develop during outbreaks. Although asymptomatic **reinfection** in early pregnancy has been described without fetal effects (Morgan-Capner and colleagues, 1985), fetal infection has been documented in five seropositive mothers (Best and associates, 1989). In two, therapeutic abortion was performed, and the other three term infants had aspects of congenital rubella syndrome.

Viremia precedes clinically evident disease by about 1 week. The nonimmune person who acquires rubella viremia demonstrates peak antibody titers 1 to 2 weeks after the onset of the rash, or 2 to 3 weeks after the onset of viremia. The promptness of the antibody response, therefore, may complicate serodiagnosis unless serum is collected initially within a few days after the onset of the rash. If, for example, the first specimen was obtained 10 days after the rash, detection of antibodies would fail to differentiate between very recent disease or pre-existing immunity to rubella. Specific IgM antibody by radioimmunoassay can be detected from early after onset of clinical disease. It peaks at 7 to 10 days, and persists for 4 weeks after appearance of the rash (American College of Obstetricians and Gynecologists, 1992). Using very sensitive radioimmunoassays, it may persist for up to a year. Importantly, rubella reinfection can give rise to transient low levels of IgM. The use of immunoglobulin is not recommended for exposure.

CONGENITAL RUBELLA SYNDROME. Rubella is one of the most teratogenic agents known (Chap 38, p. 1006). **With rubella, as with any fetal infection, the concept of an infected versus an affected infant must be understood.** Only about half of women with affected infants give a history of a rash during pregnancy. Miller and colleagues (1982) have shown that 80 percent of women with rubella infection and a rash during the first 12 weeks have a fetus with congenital infection (Fig. 56–2). At 13 to 14 weeks this incidence was 54 percent, and it was 25 percent by the end of the second trimester. As the duration of pregnancy increases, fetal infections are less likely to cause congenital malformations. For example, rubella defects were seen in all infants with evidence of intrauterine infections before 11 weeks, but only in 35 percent of those infected at 13 to 16 weeks. Although no defects were found in 63 children infected after 16 weeks, they were followed only 2 years. Hwa and associates (1994) reported a much lower incidence of infection in 103 fetuses whose mothers had serologically confirmed rubella infection prior to 29 weeks.

Thus, clinical manifestations of congenital rubella correlate with the timing of maternal infection and fetal

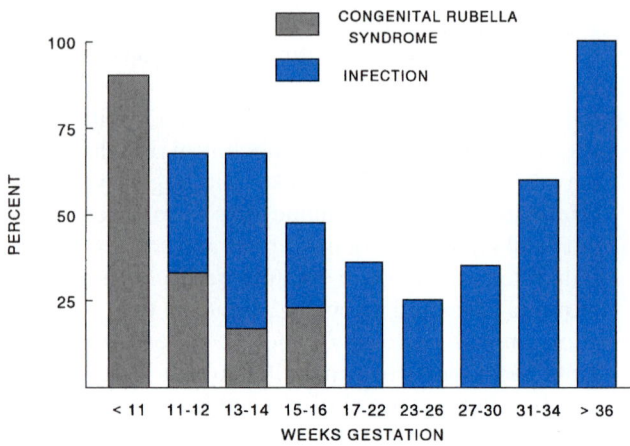

FIGURE 56–2. Proportion of fetuses with evidence for rubella infection but no stigmata (dark bars) compared with fetuses born with congenital rubella syndrome (hatched bars). (Data from Miller and colleagues, 1982.)

organ development. Congenital rubella syndrome includes one or more of the following:

- Eye lesions, including cataracts, glaucoma, microphthalmia, and other abnormalities
- Heart disease, including patent ductus arteriosus, septal defects, and pulmonary artery stenosis
- Sensorineural deafness
- Central nervous system defects, including meningoencephalitis
- Fetal growth restriction
- Thrombocytopenia and anemia
- Hepatitis, hepatosplenomegaly, and jaundice
- Chronic diffuse interstitial pneumonitis
- Osseous changes
- Chromosomal abnormalities

Infants born with congenital rubella may shed the virus for many months and thus be a threat to other infants, as well as to susceptible adults who come in contact with them.

The **extended rubella syndrome,** with progressive panencephalitis and type I diabetes, may not develop clinically until the second or third decade of life. Perhaps as many as a third of infants who are asymptomatic at birth may manifest such developmental injury (American College of Obstetricians and Gynecologists, 1993). Webster (1998) recently reviewed the teratogenic effects of the rubella virus.

CYTOMEGALOVIRUS. This is a ubiquitous DNA herpesvirus that eventually infects most humans. It is the most common cause of perinatal infection, and evidence for fetal infection is found in from 0.5 to 2 percent of

all neonates. The virus is transmitted horizontally by droplet infection and contact with saliva and urine, vertically from mother to fetus-infant, and as a sexually transmitted disease. Day-care centers are a common source of infection. Usually by 2 to 3 years of age, children acquire the infection from one another and then transmit it to their parents (Demmler, 1991; Pass, 1991).

Following primary infection, the virus becomes latent, and like other herpesvirus infections, there is periodic reactivation with viral shedding despite the presence of serum antibody. Humoral antibody is produced, but cell-mediated immunity appears to be the primary mechanism for recovery. Immunosuppressed states, whether naturally acquired or drug-induced, increase the propensity for serious cytomegalovirus infection. Presumably, decreased cell-mediated immune surveillance places the fetus-infant at high risk for sequelae of these infections.

The public health importance concerning morbidity of perinatal cytomegalovirus infection was first emphasized in 1971. According to Yow and Demmler (1992), in the ensuing 20 years, over 800,000 fetuses were infected and 50,000 were born with symptomatic disease. Many have died, and most of the survivors have severe handicaps, including mental retardation, blindness, and deafness. Collectively, the annual cost for their care is nearly $2 billion (American College of Obstetricians and Gynecologists, 2000). Another 120,000 infected children who were asymptomatic at birth have neurological impairments.

MATERNAL INFECTION. There is no evidence that pregnancy increases the risk or clinical severity of maternal cytomegalovirus infection. Most infections are asymptomatic, but about 15 percent of adults have a mononucleosis-like syndrome characterized by fever, pharyngitis, lymphadenopathy, and polyarthritis. As shown in Figure 56–3, the risk of seroconversion among susceptible women during pregnancy is from 1 to 4 percent. Immunity from previous infection can be demonstrated in up to 85 percent of pregnant women from lower socioeconomic backgrounds, whereas only half of women in higher income groups are seropositive. Primary infection, which is transmitted to the fetus in approximately 40 percent of cases, more often is associated with severe morbidity (Fowler and co-workers, 1992; Liesnard and associates, 2000). Although transplacental infection is not universal, an infected fetus is more likely with maternal infection during the first half of pregnancy.

As with other herpesviruses, maternal immunity to cytomegalovirus does not prevent recurrence (reactivation), nor unfortunately does it prevent congenital infection. In fact, because most infections during pregnancy are recurrent, the majority of congenitally infected neonates are born to these women. Fortunately, congenital

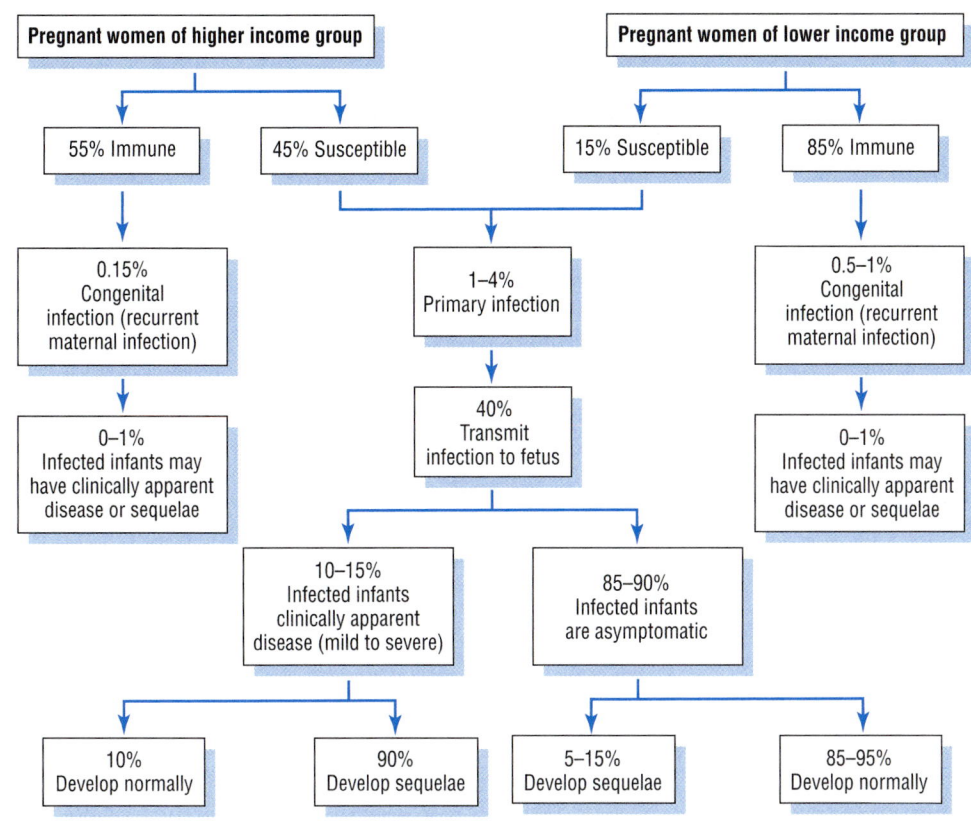

FIGURE 56–3. Characteristics of cytomegalovirus infection in pregnancy. (From Stagno and Whitley, 1985, with permission.)

infections that result from recurrent infection are less often associated with clinically apparent sequelae than are those from primary infections.

CONGENITAL INFECTION. This causes **cytomegalic inclusion disease,** a syndrome that includes low birthweight, microcephaly, intracranial calcifications, chorioretinitis, mental and motor retardation, sensorineural deficits, hepatosplenomegaly, jaundice, hemolytic anemia, and thrombocytopenic purpura. Many of these features are also common with rubella. Perlman and Argyle (1992) emphasized the need to consider cytomegaloviral infection in preterm infants with neurological findings, and suggest that such an encephalopathic process is progressive. Fortunately, of the estimated 40,000 infants born infected in the United States each year, only approximately 10 percent demonstrate this syndrome, which is more prevalent in neonates born to women with primary infection during the first half of pregnancy.

Fowler and colleagues (1992) reported long-term results from 197 newborns with congenital cytomegalovirus viremia followed at the University of Alabama at Birmingham. About 20 percent of infants in the primary-infection group had symptomatic infection at birth; none in the recurrent-infection group were symptomatic at birth. After a mean of 4.7 years, morbidity

was identified in 25 percent of the primary-infection group and 8 percent of the recurrent-infection group. Overall, 13 percent of primarily infected mothers had children whose intelligence quotients (IQs) were less than 70, whereas none of the other children had mental impairment. Sensorineural hearing loss was found in 15 versus 5 percent of primary- and recurrent-infection groups, respectively.

MANAGEMENT. Currently, there is no effective therapy. Serological screening is not recommended by the American College of Obstetricians and Gynecologists (2000):

1. There is no accurate predictability of the sequelae of primary infection.
2. There is no vaccine.
3. 1 to 2 percent of all infants excrete cytomegalovirus, and attempts to identify and isolate them are expensive and impractical (Demmler, 1991; Hagay and colleagues, 1996).

The predictive value of a positive maternal genitourinary culture or cervical cytology in assessing fetal risk for infection is likewise minimal. Asymptomatic cytomegalovirus excretion can be shown in up to 10 percent of pregnant women, and the majority have recurrent infections that are low-risk for their fetuses.

Primary infection is diagnosed by fourfold-increased IgG titers in paired acute and convalescent sera measured simultaneously, or preferentially by detecting maternal IgM cytomegalovirus antibody. Recurrent infection usually is not accompanied by IgM antibody production. Unfortunately, neither of these methods is totally accurate.

Counseling regarding fetal outcome depends on the stage of gestation during which primary infection is documented. Even with a high infection rate with primary infection in the first half of pregnancy, the majority of infants develop normally.

PRENATAL DIAGNOSIS. In some cases, effects of fetal infection are detected by sonography, computed tomography, or magnetic resonance imaging. Microcephaly, ventriculomegaly, or cerebral calcifications may be seen (Fig. 56–4). Hyperechoic bowel has also been described as a sequela (Forouzan, 1992; Muller and colleagues, 1995; Peters and associates, 1995). Nearly 30 years ago, fetal cytomegalovirus infection was confirmed by amnionic fluid culture. As risks became better known for fetal involvement, a number of investigators reported the efficacy of confirming suspected primary infections by amniocentesis for viral culture or by cordocentesis to detect IgM. More recently, polymerase chain reaction has been used to detect viral DNA in amnionic fluid and fetal blood.

Lynch and colleagues (1991) reported that viral isola-

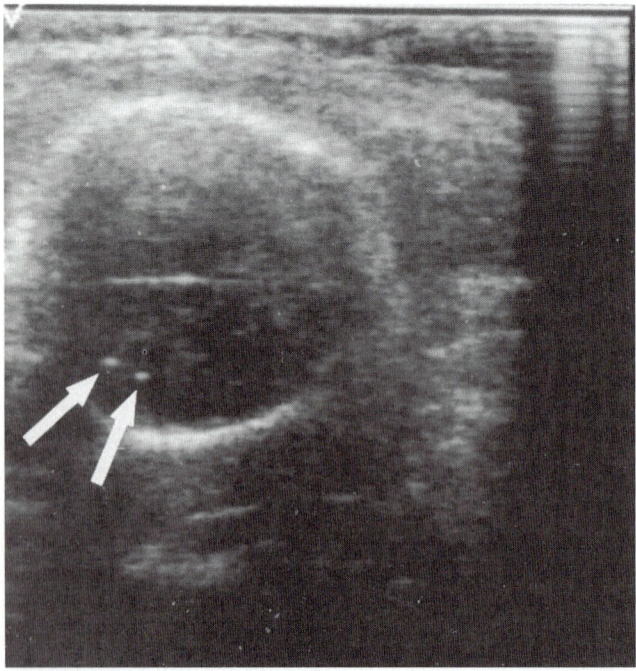

FIGURE 56–4. Intracranial calcifications (*arrows*) seen by ultrasonography in a microcephalic fetus at about 30 weeks. (Courtesy of Dr. R. Santos.)

tion from amnionic fluid and elevated cord-blood total IgM were helpful to confirm infection. Hohlfeld and co-workers (1991) confirmed fetal infection using the **shell vial assay** for viral antigen in amnionic fluid and fetal blood. Donner and co-workers (1993) measured cord blood IgM antibodies, viral culture, and polymerase chain reaction to diagnose fetal infections. In all of these studies, amniocentesis provided diagnostic results, but fetal blood analysis provided further information concerning fetal condition—anemia, thrombocytopenia, elevated hepatic enzymes, and total IgM.

Lamy and colleagues (1992) prospectively evaluated fetal cytomegalovirus transmission in nearly 1800 Belgian women. At their initial prenatal visit, about half (861) were seronegative. They were tested at each prenatal visit and 20 (2.3 percent) seroconverted before 22 weeks. Only seven allowed evaluation and two were uninfected. In the other five, amnionic fluid cultures were positive for cytomegalovirus; abortions were performed and histopathological evaluation disclosed brain involvement in all five.

Bodeus and colleagues (1999) described 98 pregnancies with congenital infection and emphasize that a negative culture or polymerase chain reaction of amnionic fluid does not always exclude fetal infection. Antsaklis and associates (2000) also observed this.

In another study from Belgium, Liesnard and co-workers (2000) described 210 fetuses born to women with suspected primary cytomegaloviral infection. Of these, at least 60 percent were proven to have primary infection while the other 40 percent had IgG and IgM antibodies when first studied. All women underwent amniocentesis and in most cases fetal cord blood was also obtained. These samples were tested with polymerase chain reaction, viral culture, and anticytomegalovirus IgM as well as nonspecific tests. The results of these are shown in Table 56–2. The overall fetal transmission rate was about 25 percent. Combined culture and polymerase chain reaction results allowed diagnosis in 44 of 55 infected fetuses (80 percent). Polymerase chain reaction of amnionic fluid was 78 percent sensitive and superior to culture techniques. Importantly, the false-negative rate in samples taken before 21 weeks was 70 percent. The authors concluded that sampling had been done too close to maternal infection (seroconversion) and recommend amniocentesis after this time. Antsaklis and colleagues (2000) also concluded that polymerase chain reaction to amplify amnionic fluid viral DNA was the most accurate test.

BACTERIAL INFECTIONS

GROUP A STREPTOCOCCUS. Infection caused by *Streptococcus pyogenes* is rarely encountered today.

TABLE 56–2. Fetal Cytomegalovirus Infection According to Gestational Age at Diagnosis

First Positive Serology	Primary Infection		Cytomegalovirus IgM Positive[a]	
	Infected Fetus-Infant	Missed[b]	Infected Fetus-Infant	Missed[b]
≤ 8 wk	5/14	1	0/24	0
> 8 to ≤ 20 wk	18/67	4	15/46	2
> 20 wk	16/52	4	1/7	0
Total	39/133 (29%)	9	16/77 (21%)	2

[a] First testing showed IgM and IgG antibodies.
[b] Newborns found to be infected but not diagnosed antenatally.
Adapted from Liesnard and co-workers (2000), with permission.

These infections are particularly virulent, and the organism produces a number of toxins and enzymes. More recently, sporadic puerperal infections from group A streptococci have been observed. Postoperative or postpartum infection outbreaks may be nosocomial from asymptomatic carriage in health-care workers (Centers for Disease Control and Prevention, 1999b; Kolmos and colleagues, 1997). The organism produces a **toxic shock-like syndrome** that is highly fatal. We encountered three cases at Parkland Hospital in 1992, and two caused maternal deaths (Nathan and colleagues, 1993). Prompt penicillin treatment, sometimes combined with surgical debridement, may be lifesaving (Chap. 26, p. 678). A less virulent exotoxin causes **scarlet fever,** and treatment is also given with penicillin. **Erysipelas** is an acute streptococcal skin infection, and bacteremia is common.

GROUP B STREPTOCOCCUS. Asymptomatic carriage of group B streptococcus—*S agalactiae*—is common, especially in the vagina and rectum. The Vaginal Infections and Prematurity Study Group (Regan and co-workers, 1991) reported that 15 to 20 percent of over 8000 pregnant women from five clinical centers were culture positive for group B streptococci between 23 and 26 weeks. The organism has been implicated in several adverse pregnancy outcomes, including preterm labor, prematurely ruptured membranes, covert and overt chorioamnionitis, and puerperal sepsis, as well as in fetal and neonatal infections. There also have been case reports of postpartum maternal osteomyelitis and mastitis caused by group B infection (Berkowitz and McCaffrey, 1990; Rench and Baker, 1989).

EPIDEMIOLOGY. Half of newborns of carrier women become colonized almost immediately at birth. Serious neonatal infections with group B streptococci are at least as prevalent as those from coliform organisms. During the 1970s, neonatal group B infections increased remarkably in frequency. For example, in Victoria, Australia, group B infection caused one third of perinatal deaths due to infection (Fliegner and Garland, 1990).

It is clear that intrapartum fetal transmission from the colonized mother may lead to severe neonatal sepsis soon after birth. The overall attack rate of early-onset sepsis is about 1 to 2 per 1000 of all births. In a multicenter case-control study of over 50,000 births, early-onset sepsis from all organisms was 3.5 per 1000 live births (Schuchat and colleagues, 2000). Group B streptococcus caused 1.4 per 1000 and *Escherichia coli* 0.6 per 1000. Although preterm or low-birthweight infants are at highest risk, more than half of the cases of neonatal sepsis are in term neonates. In the study by Schuchat and associates (2000), group B streptococcal sepsis was found less often in preterm neonates than sepsis from other organisms such as *E coli.*

NEONATAL SEPSIS. Infection in infants before 7 days is defined as **early-onset disease** (Schrag and colleagues, 2000). In some cases, the infant is born acidemic and depressed. We have even encountered a number of "unheralded" intrapartum stillbirths. In many neonates, septicemia includes signs of serious illness that usually develop within 6 to 12 hours of birth. These include respiratory distress, apnea, and shock. At the outset, therefore, the illness must be differentiated from idiopathic respiratory distress syndrome. The mortality rate with early-onset disease is about 25 percent, and preterm infants fare less well. Unfortunately, it is not uncommon for surviving infants to exhibit neurological sequelae apparently sustained during hypotension from the sepsis syndrome.

Late-onset disease usually manifests as meningitis a week or more (7 days to 3 months) after birth. These cases are most often caused by serotype III organisms. The mortality rate, although appreciable, is less for late-onset meningitis than for early-onset sepsis. Here again, neurological sequelae are common in survivors.

EVOLUTION OF PREVENTION STRATEGIES. Steigman and associates (1978) reported an absence of early-onset group B streptococcal sepsis in 130,000 newborn infants given 50,000 units of aqueous penicillin G intramuscularly at birth as prophylaxis against gonococcal ophthalmia neonatorum. A prospective study of nearly 19,000 infants was then carried out by Siegel and co-workers (1980) at Parkland Hospital. About half of these infants were randomized to receive aqueous procaine penicillin G intramuscularly within 1 hour of birth as prophylaxis against ophthalmia neonatorum and also to evaluate its impact on group B infections. The incidence of streptococcal disease was significantly lowered in those given penicillin. It was worrisome, however, that the incidence of infection and mortality caused by penicillin-resistant nonstreptococcal organisms increased. In another study of almost 11,000 neonates, Patel and colleagues (1999) gave postnatal penicillin prophylaxis and reported a reduction in the incidence of neonatal group B infection from 9 per 1000 to 4 per 1000. Death from sepsis was also decreased from 3 per 1000 to 1 per 1000.

Earlier, Pyati and co-workers (1983) reported that penicillin prophylaxis at birth was of little benefit in preventing early-onset group B disease in low-birthweight neonates. Many infants who did poorly were subsequently found to have positive cord blood cultures when single-dose penicillin was given for ophthalmic prophylaxis. Thus, in these already covertly infected fetuses, single-dose penicillin was inadequate to treat established neonatal infection.

Emphasis was next placed on intrapartum treatment of mothers found to be colonized near the time of delivery. Boyer and Gotoff (1986) randomized intrapartum and neonatal ampicillin treatment of colonized mothers. They observed decreased neonatal colonization (9 versus 51 percent) and early-onset sepsis (none versus 6 percent) in infants born to treated women. Garland and Fliegner (1991) screened over 30,000 Australian clinic patients at 32 weeks and treated asymptomatic carriers intrapartum with intravenous penicillin. Nearly 27,000 private patients admitted to their hospital were not screened. Although there were no group B infections in neonates of clinic patients, by contrast, there were 27 infections and eight deaths in the unscreened private control group. Tuppurainen and Hallman (1989) reported similar results with almost 9000 women screened for heavy colonization using a rapid test on arrival to the delivery unit.

Gibbs and colleagues (1994) and Pylipow and associates (1994) performed screening cultures at around 28 weeks. They treated culture-positive women in labor only if they developed risk factors. Using this approach, they prevented half to two thirds of cases of neonatal sepsis. Choice of antimicrobials may prove to be important. In the earlier study from Parkland, Siegel and asso-

ciates (1980) documented penicillin-resistant neonatal infections. McDuffie and colleagues (1993) reported ampicillin-resistant enterobacterial infection in four neonates whose mothers were given intrapartum ampicillin. For these reasons, Amstey and Gibbs (1994) recommended consideration for penicillin G intrapartum prophylaxis. Bloom and colleagues (1996) found that bactericidal concentrations of ampicillin were achieved in amnionic fluid and cord blood within 5 minutes of administration.

RECOMMENDED PREVENTION STRATEGIES. Although there is not a consensus regarding the most efficacious prevention strategy, there are now guidelines. These consensus opinions were published by the American College of Obstetricians and Gynecologists (1996), the Centers for Disease Control and Prevention (1996a), and the American Academy of Pediatrics and American College of Obstetricians and Gynecologists (1997). Either a risk-based or a screening-based approach should be utilized to identify women to be given intrapartum prophylaxis.

With the risk-based approach, intrapartum antibiotic prophylaxis is given to women with preterm labor (less than 37 weeks), preterm premature rupture of the membranes, rupture of membranes 18 hours or longer, previous sibling with group B streptococcal disease, or with intrapartum fever (38°C or greater). Prior identification of group B bacteriuria is also considered a risk factor.

With the culture-based approach, all women are screened for group B streptococcal colonization at 35 to 37 weeks and intrapartum antibiotics given to carriers. Because of the concern of ampicillin-resistant organisms, especially *E coli,* penicillin G is recommended by many authorities for intrapartum prophylaxis (Schuchat and colleagues, 2000). Ampicillin is an acceptable alternative, and continues to be widely used during penicillin G shortages that occurred in 1999 (Osmon, 2000). Either clindamycin or erythromycin may be utilized in the penicillin-allergic woman.

In 1997, the Centers for Disease Control and Prevention (Factor and associates, 2000) surveyed 165 hospitals in its Active Bacterial Core Surveillance system and found that 58 percent had group B prevention policies. This is up from 35 percent in 1994. Importantly, hospitals that adopted a policy showed a significantly decreased neonatal infection rate. In another surveillance study involving eight states, Schrag and colleagues (2000) reported a significant decrease in group B streptococcal disease with incorporation of strategies for intrapartum antibiotic prophylaxis—from 1.7 per 1000 births to 0.6 per 1000 in 1998.

In a study of over 5000 consecutive deliveries, Towers and colleagues (1999a) reported that if the risk-based strategy was utilized, 20 percent of women would be candidates for intrapartum prophylaxis. In another study, Towers and colleagues (1999b) identified 49 cases of early-onset group B streptococcal sepsis in 47,000 deliveries. Of these 49 babies, 40 were delivered at term and only 12 (30 percent) were delivered with an intrapartum risk factor.

The screening-based Centers for Disease Control protocol was implemented at McGee Women's Hospital in 1995 and Brozanski and associates (2000) studied its effect on neonatal group B sepsis. Nearly 29,000 deliveries occurred during the 4-year period from 1995 to 1999 when screening was codified. The prevalence of early-onset group B sepsis was 0.14 per 1000 compared with 1.16 per 1000 in 31,000 women delivered from 1992 through 1995 when there was no policy in place.

In early 1995 at Parkland Hospital we adopted the American College of Obstetricians and Gynecologists (1996) risk-based approach for intrapartum antimicrobial treatment for high-risk pregnancies. In addition, all neonates whose mothers were not given intrapartum antibiotic prophylaxis are treated in the delivery room with aqueous procaine penicillin G, 50,000 units intramuscularly. This approach was chosen because surveillance studies from 1972 through 1994 showed the lowest infection rates from 1981 through 1986 when universal neonatal penicillin prophylaxis was utilized (Siegel and Cushion, 1996). As shown in Figure 56–5, in the first year, early-onset group B infection was decreased from 1.6 per 1000 to 0.4 per 1000 (Wendel and associates, 2000).

Thus, implementation of either the screening-based or risk-based protocol is associated with diminished group B neonatal sepsis. There are still major concerns about antimicrobial resistance, and we are continuing to monitor this approach to determine its effect on neonatal sepsis, maternal morbidity, and resistant infections in the nursery. Bergeron and colleagues (2000) have provided preliminary data that a rapid-detection polymerase chain reaction method is accurate and reliable to identify women in labor with group B colonization. Schuchat (2000) cautioned that this labor-intensive test, even if proven in clinical trials, is not a panacea for the overall problem.

VACCINATION. Because some protection against serious neonatal infection is conferred by maternal antibody, it is logical that vaccination with capsular polysaccharide antigen may prove efficacious. Baker and colleagues (1988) reported that maternal immunization to type III antigen produces antibody in about 60 percent of women. Coleman and co-workers (1992) as well as the Institute of Medicine (1985) have cited vaccine development as attainable and as a priority.

LISTERIOSIS. *Listeria monocytogenes* is an uncommon but probably underdiagnosed cause of neonatal sepsis. The Centers for Disease Control and Prevention (2001) estimates that nearly 2500 individuals in the United States annually are ill with listeriosis and over 500 will die. In a recent multistate outbreak, 50 cases were caused by a rare strain that resulted in six deaths in adults and spontaneous abortion in two pregnant women (Centers for Disease Control and Prevention, 1999d). This Gram-positive aerobic motile bacillus can be isolated from soil, water, and sewage. From 1 to 5 percent of adults carry listeria in their feces. Food-borne transmission is important, and outbreaks of listeriosis have been reported from manure-contaminated cabbage, pasteurized milk, and fresh Mexican-style cheese.

Listerial infections are more common in very old or young, pregnant, or immunocompromised patients. Because cell-mediated immunity is important in defense, some authors have speculated that pregnant women are susceptible. Tappero and colleagues (1995)

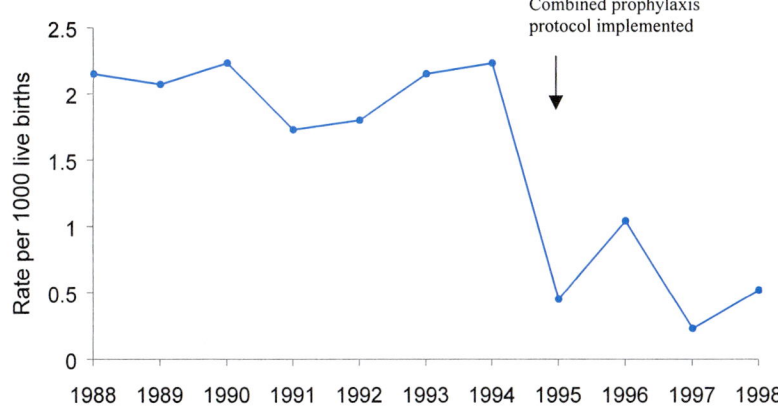

FIGURE 56–5. Effect of implementation of risk-based protocol for prevention of early-onset group B streptococcal infections in the neonate. Graph shows incidence of group B neonatal infections per 1000 live births at Parkland Hospital from 1988 through 1998. (From Wendel and colleagues, 2000, with permission.)

from the Listeriosis Study Group surveyed culture results from 29 million persons from 1989 through 1992. The incidence of infection had declined by 40 percent compared with the previous 4-year surveillance period. Although perinatal listeriosis infection rates declined by 50 percent, almost a third of reported culture-proven cases were in pregnant women. In the epidemic in Los Angeles County in 1985, which was caused by contaminated Mexican-style cheese, 65 percent of cases were in pregnant women or their fetus-neonates. Interestingly, Mascola and associates (1994) observed that women with multifetal gestation were at a fourfold risk for infection.

Listeriosis during pregnancy may be asymptomatic or cause a febrile illness that is confused for influenza, pyelonephritis, or meningitis (Silver, 1998; Sirry and colleagues, 1994). The diagnosis usually is not apparent until blood cultures are reported as positive. Occult or clinical infection also may stimulate labor (Boucher and Yonekura, 1986). Meconium passage is common with fetal infection. Maternal listeremia causes fetal infection that characteristically produces disseminated granulomatous lesions with microabscesses. Topalovski and colleagues (1993) demonstrated macroabscesses in seven infected placentas (Fig. 56–6).

The neonate is particularly susceptible to infection, and mortality approaches 50 percent. Early-onset neonatal sepsis is a common manifestation, whereas late-onset listeriosis manifests after 3 to 4 weeks of age as

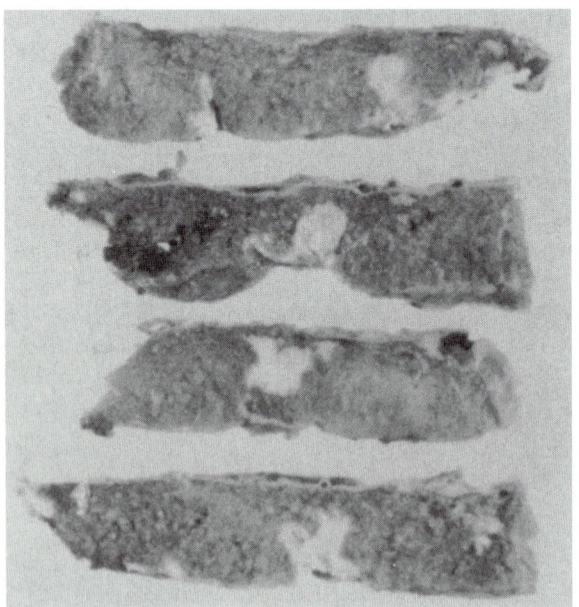

FIGURE 56–6. Listeriosis: multiple cut surfaces of placenta show several well-demarcated, grayish-white macroabscesses that appear solid and are indistinguishable from ischemic infarcts. (From Topalovski and colleagues, 1993, with permission.)

meningitis. In this regard, these infections are very similar to those caused by group B streptococci, discussed previously.

TREATMENT. There are no clinical trials concerning efficacy, but a combination of ampicillin and gentamicin is usually recommended because of proven laboratory synergism. The efficacy of trimethoprim-sulfamethoxazole has been documented, and it should be given to penicillin-allergic women. There is evidence that maternal antimicrobial treatment may be effective for fetal infection (Linnan and colleagues, 1988).

SALMONELLA AND SHIGELLA

SALMONELLOSIS. Infections from *Salmonella* and *Shigella* species continue to be a major cause of food-borne illness. There are from 800,000 to 4 million cases of salmonella infections each year in the United States, which result in 500 deaths (Centers for Disease Control and Prevention, 1999c). The organisms are ubiquitous in warm-blooded animals and almost all of more than 2200 serovars cause human illness (Baird-Parker, 1990). Enteritis is contracted through contaminated food, and symptoms include diarrhea, abdominal pain, fever, chills, nausea, and vomiting. Scialli and Rarick (1992) described a woman with enteritis and bacteremia from group C1 salmonella infection. Amnionic fluid cultures also were positive, and infection caused fetal death at 15 weeks. Management is usually by intravenous fluid rehydration. Antimicrobials prolong the carrier state and are not given in uncomplicated infections.

TYPHOID FEVER. Uncommonly seen in the United States, this disease is caused by *Salmonella typhi,* which is spread by oral ingestion of contaminated food, water, or milk. In pregnant women, the disease is more likely to be encountered during epidemics or in those who are infected with human immunodeficiency virus (HIV) (Duff and Engelsgjerd, 1983; Hedriana and colleagues, 1995). From their review, Dildy and associates (1990) reported that antepartum typhoid fever in former years resulted in abortion or preterm labor in up to 80 percent of cases, with a fetal mortality rate of 60 percent and a maternal mortality rate of 25 percent. Subsequent experiences fortunately were much more favorable.

Chloramphenicol remains the most effective treatment, but many clinicians give intravenous trimethoprim-sulfamethoxazole, ampicillin, ciprofloxacin, ofloxacin, or cefotaxime. Antityphoid vaccines appear to exert no harmful effects when administered to pregnant women. Typhoid and cholera vaccine should be given in an epidemic or before travel to endemic areas (Association of Professors of Obstetrics and Gynecology, 1999).

SHIGELLOSIS. Bacillary dysentery caused from *Shigella* infection is a relatively common cause of inflammatory exudative diarrhea in adults. Bloody stools are common. Shigellosis is more common in children attending day-care centers. It is highly contagious with primary attack rates up to 75 percent, and exposed family members may be infected in over half of cases (Guerrant and Bobak, 1991). Clinical manifestations range from mild diarrhea to severe dysentery, abdominal cramping, tenesmus, fever, and systemic toxicity. Although shigellosis is self-limited, careful attention to treatment of dehydration is essential in severe cases. We have encountered women in whom secretory diarrhea exceeded 10 L/day! In severely ill women, the treatment of choice is trimethoprim-sulfamethoxazole.

HANSEN DISEASE. This disease, which was in the past termed leprosy, is caused by *Mycobacterium leprae.* From their review, Lockwood and Sinha (1999) reported that type I or reversal reactions tend to occur postpartum. Type II reactions—erythema nodosum leprosum—occurred throughout pregnancy and during lactation. Dapsone and clofazimine for treatment appear to be safe for use during pregnancy (Farb and associates, 1982). Rifampin therapy is also effective. Duncan (1980) reported an excessive incidence of low-birthweight infants born to infected women. Duncan and associates (1984) were unable to demonstrate any morphological evidence of placental infection in 82 infected pregnant women. Neonatal infection apparently is acquired from skin-to-skin or droplet transmission.

LYME DISEASE. This disease is caused by the spirochete *Borrelia burgdorferi.* It is the most commonly reported vector-borne illness in the United States. Lyme borreliosis results from the bite of ticks of the genus *Ixodes.* Early local infection causes a distinctive skin lesion, **erythema migrans,** which may be accompanied by a flu-like syndrome and regional adenopathy. If untreated, disseminated infection may develop in days to weeks after inoculation. Multisystem involvement is common, but skin lesions, arthralgia and myalgia, carditis, and meningitis predominate. If still untreated after several weeks to months, late infection manifests in perhaps half of patients. Native immunity is acquired and the disease enters a chronic phase. Whereas some patients remain asymptomatic, others develop a variety of dermatological, rheumatic, or neurological manifestations.

Serological diagnosis has pitfalls and clinical diagnosis is important. Although positive in about half of patients with early disease, most with late untreated Lyme disease have a positive enzyme-linked immunosorbent assay. Optimal treatment has not been established. In early infection, treatment with doxycycline or ampicillin is recommended. Pregnant women are given oral amoxicillin or penicillin V for 3 weeks (American College of Obstetricians and Gynecologists, 1993). Cefuroxime is preferred but erythromycin can be given for penicillin-allergic women. In a study of 58 pregnant Slovenian women with erythema migrans, 14-day treatment with penicillin V, penicillin G, or ceftriaxone were all effective (Maraspin and colleagues, 1996). For later infection manifested by meningitis or carditis, high-dose intravenous penicillin G is recommended. Chronic arthritis is treated with amoxicillin and probenecid orally for 30 days, or with ceftriaxone or penicillin G intravenously for 14 days (Smith and co-workers, 1991).

NEONATAL INFECTION. There is concern that infection may have fetal effects because other spirochetes, viz., *Treponema pallidum,* cause congenital infection. Schlesinger and colleagues (1985) documented the persistence of spirochetes in fetal spleen, kidney, and bone marrow at 35 weeks in a woman who had Lyme disease during early pregnancy. Weber and associates (1988) demonstrated the organism in brain and liver of a term infant who died suddenly and unexpectedly at 1 day of age. The mother had responded to oral penicillin for erythema migrans at 8 weeks. Markowitz and associates (1986) reviewed 19 cases complicating pregnancy, and reported that 25 percent had preterm labor, fetal death, or rash-like illness in the newborn. Strobino and colleagues (1993) serologically evaluated 2000 pregnant women in an endemic area of New York state. Although the number of infected women was small, they reported that maternal exposure to Lyme disease was not associated with fetal death, preterm delivery, or malformations. In a review of 105 pregnant women with erythema migrans, 93 had normal pregnancies at term (Maraspin and colleagues, 1999). Two spontaneously aborted and six were delivered of preterm infants of which two died. Four others had congenital anomalies, and Strobino and colleagues (1999) found no association with Lyme disease and heart malformations when they compared 704 children with cardiac anomalies to 796 controls.

PROTOZOAL INFECTIONS

TOXOPLASMOSIS. Infection with *Toxoplasma gondii* is transmitted through encysted organisms by eating infected raw or undercooked beef or pork and through contact with oocytes in infected cat feces, or the fetus can be infected transplacentally. Maternal immunity appears to protect against fetal infection; thus, for congenital toxoplasmosis to develop, the mother must have acquired the infection during pregnancy. About a third of North American women acquire protective antibodies before pregnancy, and this is higher in those keeping cats as pets (Freij and Sever, 1996). In Europe, undercooked meat products are the main risk factor (Cook and associates, 2000). The Centers for Disease Control and Prevention (Lopez and colleagues, 2000) estimates that there are between 400 and 4000 cases of congenital toxoplasmosis each year in the United States.

Acute toxoplasmosis complicates about 1 to 5 per 1000 pregnancies (American College of Obstetricians and Gynecologists, 1993). Symptoms include fatigue, muscle pains, and sometimes lymphadenopathy, but most often infection is subclinical. Infection in pregnancy may cause abortion or result in a live-born infant with evidence of disease. The risk of fetal infection increases with duration of pregnancy, but overall it approaches 50 percent (Wong and Remington, 1994). Fetal infection is more virulent the earlier that infection is acquired, but fortunately infection is less common earlier in pregnancy. With third-trimester infection, 60 percent of infants will have evidence of perinatal infection. Conversely, only 10 percent of those infected in the first trimester have congenital toxoplasmosis. Overall, less than a fourth of newborns with congenital toxoplasmosis have evidence for clinical illness at birth. Later, however, most go on to develop some sequela of infection. Clinically affected infants at birth usually have evidence of generalized disease with low birthweight, hepatosplenomegaly, icterus, and anemia. Some primarily have neurological disease with convulsions, intracranial calcifications (see Fig. 56–4), mental retardation, and hydrocephaly or microcephaly. Almost all infected infants eventually develop chorioretinitis.

SCREENING. In the past decade, serological screening for toxoplasmosis has become feasible. In some European countries *prenatal screening* is done routinely. Despite this, a multidisciplinary committee of the Royal College of Obstetricians and Gynaecologists (1992) recommended against instituting universal prenatal screening in the United Kingdom. The American College of Obstetricians and Gynecologists (2000) does not recommend routine screening except for pregnant women with HIV infection.

If anti-toxoplasma IgG antibody is confirmed before pregnancy, then the woman is not at risk for a congenitally infected fetus. In most cases, however, serological testing is not done until the woman is pregnant. If antibody, usually determined by the Sabin Feldman dye test or indirect fluorescence on enzyme-linked immunosorbent assay, is present in low titers, it probably represents previously acquired immunity. It could also be IgM from recent infection, although IgM may persist for years (Freij and Sever, 1996; Wong and Remington, 1994). The Centers for Disease Control and Prevention recommends that all IgM-positive samples be confirmed by a reference laboratory (Lopez and co-workers, 2000).

The most accurate confirmation of active infection is a rise in IgG titer in two appropriately spaced but simultaneously tested serum samples. Very high titers—that is, greater than 1:512—more likely indicate recent or current illness. Sever and colleagues (1988) reported increased microcephaly, deafness, and mental retardation in children born to women whose titers were 1:256 or higher.

A polymerase chain reaction assay with high specificity and sensitivity has been developed (Hohlfeld and colleagues, 1994). The technique permits prenatal diagnosis within a day by assay of amnionic fluid. It also can be used to document fetal infection prior to 20 weeks. In a multicenter study of 122 women from six European Toxoplasma Centers, Foulon and colleagues (1999a) reported that amnionic fluid polymerase chain reaction had an 81 percent sensitivity and 96 percent specificity.

MANAGEMENT. For the woman thought to have active disease, Wong and Remington (1994) recommend antimicrobial treatment. There is evidence that **spiramycin,** a macrolide antibiotic used widely in Europe, reduces the incidence of fetal infection, but it may not modify its severity. It is available through the Food and Drug Administration (301-443-4280), or the manufacturer, Rhône-Poulenc Rover in Valley Forge, PA. Treatment may also be given with **pyrimethamine plus sulfadiazine.**

Daffos and colleagues (1988) obtained amnionic fluid and fetal blood samples by cordocentesis in 746 French women with proven infection up to 25 weeks. Maternal infection was diagnosed by toxoplasma-specific IgM antibody. All women with presumed infection were treated with spiramycin, 3 g daily throughout pregnancy. Of the 42 (6 percent) of their fetuses found to have infection, 39 were already infected before treatment by demonstrating IgM-specific antibody by cordocentesis. For these women, pyrimethamine and either sulfadoxine or sulfadiazine were added to the spiramycin regime.

Foulon and co-workers (1990b) reported a 12 percent incidence of congenital toxoplasmosis in 50 Belgian women infected before midpregnancy. They concluded that serological screening with invasive fetal diagnosis was safe and feasible. Foulon and associates (1990a) described a case in which prenatal diagnosis was confirmed by tissue culture of a chorionic villus biopsy. Hohlfeld and co-workers (1994) showed the risk of fetal infection to be 7.4 percent using the polymerase chain reaction test on amnionic fluid. The negative-predictive value for this test was 99.7 percent. Berrebi and colleagues (1994) studied 163 women with acute toxoplasmosis before 26 weeks. All were treated with spiramycin and some also were given pyrimethamine and sulfadiazine. All 27 of 162 live-born infants with proven congenital infection had normal development at 15 to 71 months of age. Pratlong and associates (1996) reported that antenatal diagnosis of fetal infection was 77 percent effective using ultrasound examination and fetal blood sampling for IgM, IgA, and nonspecific markers.

Guerina and associates (1994) screened 635,000 infants born in Massachusetts and New Hampshire. In 100 of these, cord blood was positive for IgM toxoplasma antibodies. Congenital infection was confirmed in 52, and treatment was given for 1 year. Although not proven, there is some evidence that early treatment may reduce long-term sequelae.

In a review of studies of treatment of toxoplasmosis during pregnancy, Wallon and colleagues (1999) concluded that the efficacy of antenatal treatment in reducing congenital toxoplasmosis was unclear. Foulon and colleagues (1999b), in a study of 144 women from five reference centers, concluded that antenatal antibiotics did not reduce the maternal–fetal transmission rate, but did reduce the sequelae of such infection. Moreover, the earlier the antibiotics were given, the least likely sequelae were to occur.

MALARIA. There are four species of *Plasmodium* that cause human malaria: *vivax, ovale, malariae,* and *falciparum.* Organisms are transmitted by the bite of a female *Anopheles* mosquito. Nearly 300 to 500 million persons worldwide are infected at any given time and the disease causes from 1 to 3 million deaths annually (Murray and colleagues, 2000). Almost 40 percent of the world population—2 billion people—are at risk of contracting the disease. Malaria has been effectively eradicated in Europe and most of North America except for parts of Mexico.

The disease is characterized by fever and flu-like symptoms including chills, headaches, myalgia, and malaise, which may occur at intervals. Symptoms are less severe in immune patients. Malaria may be associated with anemia and jaundice, and falciparum infections may cause kidney failure, coma, and death.

EFFECTS ON PREGNANCY. Malarial episodes increase significantly by 3- to 4-fold during the latter two trimesters of pregnancy and 2 months postpartum (Diagne and associates, 2000). Pregnancy enhances the severity of falciparum malaria, especially in nonimmune nulliparous women (Nathwani and colleagues, 1992; Robier and co-workers, 1999). The incidence of abortion and preterm labor is increased with malaria (Menendez and associates, 2000).

Increased fetal loss may be related to placental and fetal infection. Fifty years ago, Jones (1950) found that parasites have an affinity for decidual vessels and may involve the placenta extensively without affecting the fetus. Ismail and colleagues (2000) studied 1179 placentas from an endemic area in Tanzania. Of these, 35 percent showed parasites, and half of women with in-

fected placentas had negative blood film testing for malaria. Despite heavy placental involvement, neonatal infection is uncommon. Covell (1950) studied this extensively in Africa and cited an incidence of neonatal malaria of only 0.3 percent. In nonimmune women, congenital malaria may develop in up to 7 percent of neonates (Hulbert, 1992). Cot and colleagues (1992) showed that chloroquine chemoprophylaxis decreased placental infection in asymptomatic infected women to 4 percent compared with 19 percent of untreated controls; however, mean birthweight was not different.

TREATMENT. Commonly used antimalarial drugs are not contraindicated during pregnancy. Some of the newer antimalarial agents have antifolic acid activity, and may theoretically contribute to the development of megaloblastic anemia. In actual practice, this does not appear to be the case. In at least one study by Keuter and co-workers (1990), nulliparas were more likely to remain parasitemic after therapy for falciparum infection. The maternal outcome is worse if falciparum malaria is drug resistant (Alecrim and colleagues, 2000).

Chloroquine is the treatment of choice for all forms of malaria except chloroquine-resistant *P falciparum* and newly emerging strains of resistant *P vivax*. For severe malaria, chloroquine is given intravenously. For the woman with chloroquine-resistant infection, **mefloquine** is given orally. For severe resistant malaria, quinine or quinidine is given parenterally. Wong and associates (1992) report a successful outcome in a 31-week pregnant woman treated with intravenous quinine and exchange transfusion. At high doses, mefloquine is teratogenic and embryotoxic for some laboratory animals. Despite this, sparse data from the World Health Organization (1995) and other reports indicate the drug to be safe and effective in pregnancy (Briggs and colleagues, 1998).

PROPHYLAXIS. This is recommended for travel to endemic areas. If chloroquine-resistant falciparum or vivax malaria has not been reported, prophylaxis is initiated 1 to 2 weeks before the endemic area is entered. Chloroquine, 300 mg of base, is given orally once a week, and this is continued until 4 weeks after return to nonendemic areas (Bradley and Warhurst, 1995; Wyler, 1993). Travel to areas endemic for chloroquine-resistant strains is discouraged during early pregnancy, after which mefloquine prophylaxis is given (Briggs and associates, 1998). The drug was evaluated for prophylaxis in 339 pregnant women after 20 weeks and found to be 85 percent effective in preventing falciparum malaria and 100 percent for vivax infections (Nosten and associates, 1994; Nosten and Price, 1995). In nonpregnant persons, doxycycline is recommended for chemoprophylaxis.

Several vaccines are currently under evaluation. Almost all vaccine trials have focused on two of nearly 6000 estimated falciparum proteins. One chimeric protein vaccine, SPF 66, has been field-tested and is perhaps 10 to 30 percent effective (Olliaro and colleagues, 1996). Murray and co-authors (2000) predict a licensed vaccine in about 5 years.

AMEBIASIS. Most persons infected with *Entamoeba histolytica* are asymptomatic cyst-passers. Amoebic dysentery may take a fulminant course during pregnancy. Prognosis is worse if complicated by a hepatic abscess, which may be quite serious during pregnancy, and rupture has been reported (Constantine and colleagues, 1987). Therapy is similar to that for the nonpregnant woman, and metronidazole is the drug of choice.

MYCOTIC INFECTIONS. Disseminated infection during pregnancy is uncommon with coccidiomycosis, blastomycosis, cryptococcosis, or histoplasmosis. Their identification and management are considered in Chapter 46 (p. 1229).

REFERENCES

Alecrim WD, Espinosa FE, Alecrim MG: *Plasmodium falciparum* infection in the pregnant patient. Infect Dis Clin North Am 14:83, 2000

American Academy of Pediatrics and American College of Obstetricians and Gynecologists: Perinatal infections. In: Guidelines for Perinatal Care, 4th ed. Washington, DC, AAP and ACOG, 1997

American College of Obstetricians and Gynecologists: Prevention of Early-onset Group B Streptococcus Disease in Newborns. Committee on Obstetric Practice. Committee Opinion No. 173, June 1996

American College of Obstetricians and Gynecologists: Perinatal Viral and Parasitic Infections. Practice Bulletin No. 20, September 2000

American College of Obstetricians and Gynecologists: Rubella and Pregnancy. Technical Bulletin No. 171, August 1992

Amstey MS, Gibbs RS: Is penicillin G a better choice than ampicillin for prophylaxis of neonatal group B streptococcal infections? Obstet Gynecol 84:1058, 1994

Antsaklis AJ, Daskalakis GJ, Mesogitis SA, Koutra PT, Michalas SS: Prenatal diagnosis of fetal primary cytomegalovirus infection. Br J Obstet Gynaecol 107:84, 2000

Association of Professors of Gynecology and Obstetrics: Immunization for women. APGO Educational Series on Women's Health Issues. Washington, DC, APGO, 1999

Baird-Parker AC: Foodborne illness: Foodborne salmonellosis. Lancet 336:1231, 1990

Baker CJ, Rench MA, Edwards MS, Carpenter RJ, Hays BM, Kasper DL: Immunization of pregnant women with a polysaccharide vaccine of group B streptococcus. N Engl J Med 319:1180, 1988

Bergeron MG, Ke D, Ménard C, Picard FJ, Gagnon M,
Bernier M, Ouellette M, Roy PH, Marcoux S, Fraser WD: Rapid detection of group B streptococci in pregnant women at delivery. N Engl J Med 343:175, 2000

Berkowitz K, McCaffrey R: Postpartum osteomyelitis caused by group B streptococcus. Am J Obstet Gynecol 163:1200, 1990

Berrebi A, Kobuch WE, Bessieres MH, Bloom MC, Rolland M, Sarramon MF, Roques C, Fournié A: Termination of pregnancy for maternal toxoplasmosis. Lancet 344:36, 1994

Best JM, Banatvala JE, Morgan-Capner P, Miller E: Fetal infection after maternal reinfection with rubella: Criteria for defining reinfection. BMJ 299:773, 1989

Bloom SL, Leveno KJ, Gilstrap LC, Cox SM: Timing of intrapartum ampicillin infusion for group B streptococcus (GBS) prophylaxis. Am J Obstet Gynecol 174:407, 1996

Bodeus M, Hubinont C, Bernard P, Bouckaert A, Thomas K, Goubau P: Prenatal diagnosis of human cytomegalovirus by culture and polymerase chain reaction: 98 pregnancies leading to congenital infection. Prenat Diagn 19:314, 1999

Boucher M, Yonekura ML: Perinatal listeriosis (early onset): Correlation of antenatal manifestations and neonatal outcome. Obstet Gynecol 68:593, 1986

Boyer KM, Gotoff SP: Prevention of early-onset neonatal group B streptococcal disease with selective intrapartum chemoprophylaxis. N Engl J Med 314:1665, 1986

Bradley DJ, Warhurst DC: Malaria prophylaxis: Guidelines for travelers from Britain. BMJ 310:709, 1995

Briggs GG, Freeman RK, Yaffe SJ (eds): Drugs in Pregnancy and Lactation, 5th ed. Baltimore, Williams & Wilkins, 1998

Brown GC, Karunas RS: Relationship of congenital anomalies and maternal infection with selected enteroviruses. Am J Epidemiol 95:207, 1972

Brown KE, Hibbs JR, Gallinella G, Anderson SM, Lehman ED, McCarthy P, Young NS: Resistance to parvovirus B19 infection due to lack of virus receptor (erythrocyte P antigen). N Engl J Med 330:1192, 1994

Brozanski BS, Jones JG, Krohn MA, Sweet RL: Effect of a screening-based prevention policy on prevalence of early-onset group B streptococcal sepsis. Obstet Gynecol 95:496, 2000

Centers for Disease Control: Rubella prevention: Recommendations of the Immunization Practices Advisory Committee (ACIP). MMWR 39:1, 1990

Centers for Disease Control and Prevention: Multistate outbreak of Listeriosis—United States, 2000. MMWR 49:1129, 2001

Centers for Disease Control and Prevention: Neuraminidase inhibitors for treatment of influenza A and B infections. MMWR 48:1, 1999a

Centers for Disease Control and Prevention: Nosocomial group A streptococcal infections associated with asymptomatic health-care workers—Maryland and California, 1997. MMWR 48:163, 1999b

Centers for Disease Control and Prevention: Salmonella. Fact Sheets. July 16, 1999c

Centers for Disease Control and Prevention: Update: Multistate outbreak of listeriosis—United States, 1998–1999. MMWR 47:1117, 1999d

Centers for Disease Control and Prevention: Listeriosis. Fact Sheets. December 25, 1998a

Centers for Disease Control and Prevention: Prevention and control of influenza. Recommendations of the Advisory Committee on Immunization Practices (ACIP). MMWR 47:1, 1998b

Centers for Disease Control and Prevention: Prevention of

neonatal group B streptococcal disease: A public health perspective. 45:RR-7:1, 1996a

Centers for Disease Control and Prevention: Prevention of varicella: Recommendations of the Advisory Committee on Immunization Practices (ACIP) MMWR 45:1, 1996b

Centers for Disease Control and Prevention: Prevention and control of influenza, 2. Antiviral agents. Recommendations of the Immunization Practices Advisory Committee (ACIP). MMWR 43:1, 1994a

Centers for Disease Control and Prevention: Rubella and congenital rubella syndrome—United States, January 1, 1991–May 7, 1994. MMWR 43:391, 1994b

Centers for Disease Control and Prevention: Update: Hantavirus pulmonary syndrome—United States, 1993. MMWR 42:816, 1993

Chandra PC, Patel H, Schiavello HJ, Briggs SL: Successful pregnancy outcome after complicated varicella pneumonia. Obstet Gynecol 92:680, 1998

Chiang CP, Chiu CH, Huang YC, Lin TY: Two cases of disseminated cutaneous herpes zoster in infants after intrauterine exposure to varicella-zoster virus. Pediatr Infect Dis J 14:395, 1995

Coleman RT, Sherer DM, Maniscalco WM: Prevention of neonatal group B streptococcal infections: Advances in maternal vaccine development. Obstet Gynecol 80:301, 1992

Constantine G, Menon V, Luesley D: Amoebic peritonitis in pregnancy in the United Kingdom. Postgrad Med J 63:495, 1987

Cook AJC, Gilbert RE, Buffolano W, Zufferey J, Petersen E, Jenum PA, Foulon W, Semprini AE, Dunn DT on behalf of the European Research Network on Congenital Toxoplasmosis. Sources of toxoplasma infection in pregnant women: European multicentre case-control study. BMJ 321:142, 2000

Cot M, Roisin A, Barro D, Yada JP, Verhave P, Carnevale P, Breart G: Effect of chloroquine chemoprophylaxis during pregnancy on birth weight: Results of a randomized trial. Am J Trop Med Hyg 46:21, 1992

Covell G: Congenital malaria. Trop Dis Bull 47:1174, 1950

Cox SM, Cunningham FG, Luby J: Management of varicella pneumonia complicating pregnancy. Am J Perinatol 7:300, 1990

Daffos F, Forestier F, Capella-Pavlovsky M, Thulliez P, Aufrant C, Valenti D, Cox W: Prenatal management of 746 pregnancies at risk for congenital toxoplasmosis. N Engl J Med 381:271, 1988

Dahlquist GG, Ivarsson S, Lindberg B, Forsgren M: Maternal enteroviral infection during pregnancy as a risk factor for childhood IDDM. A population-based case-controlled study. Diabetes 44:408, 1995

Demmler GJ: Summary of a workshop on surveillance for congenital cytomegalovirus disease. Rev Infect Dis 13:315, 1991

De Quadros CA, Olivé JM, Hersh BS, Strassburg MA, Henderson DA, Brandling-Bennett D, Alleyne GAO: Measles elimination in the Americas. JAMA 275:224, 1996

Diagne N, Rogier C, Sokhna CS, Tall A, Fontenille D, Roussilhon C, Spiegel A, Trape J-F: Increased susceptibility to malaria during the early postpartum period. N Engl J Med 343:598, 2000

Dildy GA III, Martens MG, Faro S, Lee W: Typhoid fever in pregnancy: A case report. J Reprod Med 35:273, 1990

Dommergues M, Petitjean J, Aubry MC, Delezoide AL, Narcy F, Fallet-Bianco C, Freymuth F, Dumez Y, Lebon P: Fetal enteroviral infection with cerebral ventriculomegaly and cardiomyopathy. Fetal Diagn Ther 9:77, 1994

Donner C, Liesnard C, Content J, Busine A, Aderca J, Rodesch F: Prenatal diagnosis of 52 pregnancies at risk for congenital cytomegalovirus infection. Obstet Gynecol 82:481, 1993

Duff P, Engelsgjerd B: Typhoid fever on an obstetrics–gynecology service. Am J Obstet Gynecol 145:113, 1983

Duncan ME: Babies of mothers with leprosy have small placentae, low birth weights and grow slowly. Br J Obstet Gynaecol 87:461, 1980

Duncan ME, Fox H, Harkness RA, Rees RJW: The placenta in leprosy. Placenta 5:189, 1984

Eberhart-Phillips JE, Frederick PD, Baron RC, Mascola L: Measles in pregnancy: A descriptive study of 58 cases. Obstet Gynecol 82:797, 1993

Enders G, Miller E, Cradock-Watson J, Bolley I, Ridehalgh M: Consequences of varicella and herpes zoster in pregnancy: Prospective study of 1739 cases. Lancet 343:1548, 1994

Eyal A, Friedman M, Peretz BA, Paldi E: Pregnancy complicated by herpes zoster: A report of two cases and literature review. J Reprod Med 28:600, 1983

Factor SH, Whitney CG, Zywicki SS, Schuchat A: Effects of hospital policies based on 1996 group B streptococcal disease consensus guidelines. Obstet Gynecol 95:377, 2000

Fairley CK, Smoleniec JS, Caul OE, Miller E: Observational study of effect of intrauterine transfusions on outcome of fetal hydrops after parvovirus B19 infection. Lancet 346:1335, 1995

Farb H, West DP, Pedvis-Leftick A: Clofazimine in pregnancy complicated by leprosy. Obstet Gynecol 59:122, 1982

Fliegner JR, Garland SM: Perinatal mortality in Victoria, Australia: Role of group B streptococcus. Am J Obstet Gynecol 163:1609, 1990

Forouzan I: Fetal abdominal echogenic mass: An early sign of intrauterine cytomegalovirus infection. Obstet Gynecol 80:535, 1992

Foulon W, Naessens A, de Catte L, Amy JJ: Detection of congenital toxoplasmosis by chorionic villus sampling and early amniocentesis. Am J Obstet Gynecol 163:1511, 1990a

Foulon W, Naessens A, Mahler T, de Waele M, de Catte L, de Meuter F: Prenatal diagnosis of congenital toxoplasmosis. Obstet Gynecol 76:769, 1990b

Foulon W, Pinon JM, Stray-Pedersen B, Pollak A, Lappalainen M, Decoster A, Villena I, Jenum PA, Hayde M, Naessens A: Prenatal diagnosis of congenital toxoplasmosis: A multicenter evaluation of different diagnostic parameters. Am J Obstet Gynecol 181:843, 1999a

Foulon W, Villena I, Stray-Pedersen B, Decoster A, Lappalainen M, Pinon JM, Jenum PA, Hedman K, Naessens A: Treatment of toxoplasmosis during pregnancy: A multicenter study of impact on fetal transmission and children's sequelae at age 1 year. Am J Obstet Gynecol 180:410, 1999b

Fowler KB, Stagno S, Pass RF, Britt WJ, Boll TJ, Alford CA: The outcome of congenital cytomegalovirus infection in relation to maternal antibody status. N Engl J Med 326:663, 1992

Freeman DW, Barno A: Deaths from Asian influenza associated with pregnancy. Am J Obstet Gynecol 78:1172, 1959

Freij BJ, Sever JL: What do we know about toxoplasmosis? Contemp Ob/Gyn 41:41, 1996

Friedman CA, Temple DM, Robbins KK, Rawson JE, Wilson JP, Feldman S: Outbreak and control of varicella in a neonatal intensive care unit. Pedriatr Infect Dis J 13:152, 1994

Garcia AGP, Basso NG, Fonseca MEF, Zuardi JAT, Outanni

HN: Enterovirus associated placental morphology: A light, virological, electron microscopic and immunohistologic study. Placenta 12:53, 1991

Garland SM, Fliegner JR: Group B streptococcus (GBS) and neonatal infections: The case for intrapartum chemoprophylaxis. Aust NZ J Obstet Gynaecol 31:2, 1991

Gibbs RS, McDuffie RS Jr, McNabb F, Fryer GE, Miyoshi T, Merenstein G: Neonatal group B streptococcal sepsis during 2 years of a universal screening program. Obstet Gynecol 84:496, 1994

Gilden DH, Kleinschmidt-DeMasters BK, LaGuardia JJ, Mahalingam R, Cohrs RJ: Neurologic complications of the reactivation of varicella-zoster virus. N Engl J Med 342:635, 2000

Gilson GJ, Maciulla JA, Nevils BG, Izquierdo LE, Chatterjee MS, Curet LB: Hantavirus pulmonary syndrome complicating pregnancy. Am J Obstet Gynecol 171:550, 1994

Glantz JC, Mushlin AI: Cost-effectiveness of routine antenatal varicella screening. Obstet Gynecol 91:519, 1998

Gregg NM: Congenital cataract following German measles in the mother. Trans Ophthalmol Soc Aust 3:35, 1942

Gubareva LV, Kaiser L, Hayden FG: Influenza virus neuraminidase inhibitors. Lancet 355:827, 2000

Guerina NG, Hsu HW, Meissner C, Maguire JH, Lynfield R, Stechenberg B, Abroms I, Pasternack MS, Hoff R, Eaton RB, Grady GF, and the New England Regional Toxoplasma Working Group: Neonatal serologic screening and early treatment for congenital Toxoplasma gondii infection. N Engl J Med 330:1858, 1994

Guerrant RL, Bobak DA: Bacterial and protozoal gastroenteritis. N Engl J Med 325:327, 1991

Hagay ZJ, Biran G, Ornoy A, Reece EA: Congenital cytomegalovirus infection: A long-standing problem still seeking a solution. Am J Obstet Gynecol 174:241, 1996

Harger JH, Adler SP, Koch WC, Harger GF: Prospective evaluation of 618 pregnant women exposed to parvovirus B19: Risks and symptoms. Obstet Gynecol 91:413, 1998

Harjulehto T, Aro T, Hovi T, Saxén L: Congenital malformations and oral poliovirus vaccination during pregnancy. Lancet 1:771, 1989

Harris JW: Influenza occurring in pregnant women. JAMA 72:978, 1919

Hedriana HL, Mitchell JL, Williams SB: Salmonella typhi chorioamnionitis in a human immunodeficiency virus–infected pregnant woman. J Reprod Med 40:157, 1995

Hohlfeld P, Daffos F, Costa JM, Thulliez P, Forestier F, Vidaud M: Prenatal diagnosis of congenital toxoplasmosis with a polymerase-chain reaction test on amniotic fluid. N Engl J Med 331:695, 1994

Hohlfeld P, Vial Y, Maillard-Brignon C, Vaudaux B, Fawer CL: Cytomegalovirus fetal infection: Prenatal diagnosis. Obstet Gynecol 78:615, 1991

Hulbert TV: Congenital malaria in the United States: Report of a case and review. Clin Infect Dis 14:922, 1992

Hwa HL, Shyu MK, Lee CN, Wu CC, Kao CL, Hsieh FJ: Prenatal diagnosis of congenital rubella infection from maternal rubella in Taiwan. Obstet Gynecol 84:415, 1994

Institute of Medicine, Committee on Issues and Priorities for New Vaccine Development: Prospects for immunizing against streptococcal group B. In: New Vaccine Development: Establishing priorities, Vol I. Diseases of Importance in the United States. Washington, DC, National Academy Press, 1985, p 424

Ismail MR, Ordi J, Menendez C, Ventura PJ, Aponte JJ, Kahigwa E, Hirt R, Cardesa A, Alonso PL: Placental pathology in malaria: A histological, immunohistochemical, and quantitative study. Hum Pathol 31:85, 2000

Jensen IP, Thorsen P, Jeune B, Møller BR, Vestergaard BF: An epidemic of parvovirus B19 in a population of 3596 pregnant women: a study of sociodemographic and medical risk factors. Br J Obstet Gynaecol 107:637, 2000

Jones BS: Congenital malaria: 3 cases. BMJ 2:439, 1950

Jones KL, Johnson KA, Chambers CD: Offspring of women infected with varicella during pregnancy: A prospective study. Teratology 49:29, 1994

Kashyap S, Gruslin A: Influenza vaccination during pregnancy. Prim Care Update Ob/Gyns 7:7, 2000

Keuter M, van Eijk A, Hoogstrate M, Raasveld M, van de Ree M, Ngwawe WA, Watkins WM, Were JBO, Brandling-Bennett AD: Comparison of chloroquine, pyrimethamine and sulfadoxine, and chlorproguanil and dapsone as treatment for falciparum malaria in pregnant and non-pregnant women, Kakamega district, Kenya. BMJ 301:466, 1990

Kolmos HJ, Svendsen RN, Nielsen SV: The surgical team as a source of postoperative wound infections caused by Streptococcus pyogenes. J Hospital Infection 35:207, 1997

Korones SB: Uncommon virus infections of the mother, fetus, and newborn: Influenza, mumps and measles. Clin Perinatol 15:259, 1988

Kunugi H, Nanko S, Takei N, Saito K, Hayashi N, Kazamatsuri H: Schizophrenia following in utero exposure to the 1957 influenza epidemics in Japan. Am J Psychiatry 152:450, 1995

Kurppa K, Holmberg PC, Kuosma E, Aro T, Saxén L: Anencephaly and maternal common cold. Teratology 44:51, 1991

Kurtz JB, Tomlinson AH, Pearson J: Mumps virus isolated from a fetus. BMJ 284:471, 1982

Lamy ME, Mulongo KN, Gadisseux JF, Lyon G, Gaudy V, Van Lierde M: Prenatal diagnosis of fetal cytomegalovirus infection. Am J Obstet Gynecol 166:91, 1992

Liesnard C, Donner C, Brancart F, Gosselin F, Delforge ML, Rodesch F: Prenatal diagnosis of congenital cytomegalovirus infection: Prospective study of 237 pregnancies at risk. Obstet Gynecol 95:881, 2000

Linnan MJ, Mascola L, Lou XD, Goulet V, May S, Salminen C, Hird DW, Yonekura ML, Hayes P, Weaver R, Audurier A, Plikaytis BD, Fannin SL, Kleks A, Broome CV: Epidemic listeriosis associated with Mexican-style cheese. N Engl J Med 319:823, 1988

Lockwood DN, Sinha HH: Pregnancy and leprosy: A comprehensive literature review. Int J Lepr Other Mycobact Dis 67:6, 1999

Lopez A, Dietz VJ, Wilson M, Navin TR, Jones JL: Preventing congenital toxoplasmosis. MMWR 49(RR02):57, 2000

Lynberg MC, Khoury MJ, Lu X, Cocian T: Maternal flu, fever, and the risk of neural tube defects: A population-based case-control study. Am J Epidemiol 140:244, 1994

Lynch L, Daffos F, Emanuel D, Giovangrandi Y, Meisel R, Forestier F, Cathomas G, Berkowitz RL: Prenatal diagnosis of fetal cyto-megalovirus. Am J Obstet Gynecol 165:714, 1991

Manson MM, Logan WPD, Loy RM: Rubella and other virus infections during pregnancy. London, Her Majesty's Stationery Office, 1960

Maraspin V, Cimperman J, Lotric-Furlan S, Pleterski-Rigler D, Strle F: Erythema migrans in pregnancy. Wien Klin Wochenschr 111:933, 1999

Maraspin V, Cimperman J, Lotric-Furlan S, Pleterski-Rigler D, Strle F: Treatment of erythema migrans in pregnancy. Clin Infect Dis 22:788, 1996

Markowitz LE, Steere AC, Benach JL, Slade JD, Broome CV: Lyme disease during pregnancy. JAMA 255:3394, 1986

Mascola L, Ewert DP, Eller A: Listeriosis: A previously unreported medical complication in women with multiple gestations. Am J Obstet Gynecol 170:1328, 1994

McDuffie RS Jr, McGregor JA, Gibbs RS: Adverse perinatal outcome and resistant enterobacteriaceae after antibiotic usage for premature rupture of the membranes and group B streptococcus carriage. Obstet Gynecol 82:487, 1993

McElhaney RD Jr, Ringer M, DeHart DJ, Vasilenko P: Rubella immunity in a cohort of pregnant women. Infect Control Host Epidemiol 20:64, 1999

McGrath J, Castle D: Does influenza cause schizophrenia? A five year review. Aust N Z J Psychiatry 29:23, 1995

McGregor JA, Burns JC, Levin MJ, Burlington B, Meiklejohn G: Transplacental passage of influenza A/Bangkok (H_3N_2) mimicking amniotic fluid infection syndrome. Am J Obstet Gynecol 148:856, 1984

McGregor JA, Mark S, Crawford GP, Levin MJ: Varicella zoster antibody testing in the case of pregnant woman exposed to varicella. Am J Obstet Gynecol 157:218, 1987

Menendez C, Ordi J, Ismail MR, Ventura PJ, Aponte JJ, Kahigwa E, Font F, Alonso PL: The impact of placental malaria on gestational age and birthweight. J Infect Dis 181:1740, 2000

Miller E, Cradock-Watson JE, Pollock TM: Consequences of confirmed maternal rubella at successive stages of pregnancy. Lancet 2:781, 1982

Miller E, Cradock-Watson JE, Ridehalgh MKS: Outcome in newborn babies given anti-varicella-zoster immunoglobulin after perinatal maternal infection with varicella-zoster virus. Lancet 2:371, 1989

Miller RD, Hager WD: Mumps in pregnancy. Contemp Ob/Gyn 45:119, 2000

Morey AL, Nicolini U, Welch CR, Economides D, Chamberlain PF, Cohen BJ: Parvovirus B19 infection and transient fetal hydrops. Lancet 337:496, 1991

Morgan-Capner P, Hambling MH, Coleman TJ, Watkins RP, Stern H, Hodgson J, Dulake C, Boswell PA, Booth J, Best JM: Detection of rubella-specific IgM in subclinical rubella reinfection in pregnancy. Lancet 1:246, 1985

Moroi K, Saito S, Kurata T, Sata T, Yanagida M: Fetal death associated with measles virus infection of the placenta. Am J Obstet Gynecol 164:1107, 1991

Muller F, Dommergues M, Aubry MC, Simon-Bouy B, Gautier E, Oury JF, Narcy F: Hyperechogenic fetal bowel: An ultrasonographic marker for adverse fetal and neonatal outcome. Am J Obstet Gynecol 173:508, 1995

Murray HW, Pépin J, Nutman TB, Hoffman SL, Mahmoud AAF: Tropical medicine. BMJ 320:490, 2000

Nathan L, Peters MT, Ahmed AM, Leveno KJ: The return of life-threatening puerperal sepsis caused by group A streptococci. Am J Obstet Gynecol 169:571, 1993

Nathwani D, Currie PF, Douglas JG, Green ST, Smith NC: Plasmodium falciparum malaria in pregnancy: A review. Br J Obstet Gynaecol 99:118, 1992

Newton ER: Diagnosis of perinatal TORCH infections. Clin Obstet Gynecol 42:59, 1999

Nosten F, Price RN: New antimalarials. A risk-benefit analysis. Drug Saf 12:264, 1995

Nosten F, ter Kuile F, Maelankiri L, Chongsuphajaisiddhi T, Nopdonrattakoon L, Tangkitchot S, Boudreau E, Bunnag D, White NJ: Mefloquine prophylaxis prevents malaria during pregnancy: A double-blind, placebo-controlled study. J Infect Dis 169:595, 1994

Olliaro P, Cattani J, Wirth D: Malaria, the submerged disease. JAMA 275:230, 1996

Osmon DR: Antimicrobial prophylaxis in adults. Mayo Clin Proc 75:98, 2000

Ouhilal S: Viral diseases in pregnancy: A review of rubella, chickenpox, measles, mumps and 5th disease. Prim Care Update Ob/Gyns 7:31, 2000

Paryani SG, Arvin AM: Intrauterine infection with varicella-zoster virus after maternal varicella. N Engl J Med 314:1542, 1986

Pass RF: Day-care centers and the spread of cytomegalovirus and parvovirus B19. Pediatr Ann 20:419, 1991

Pastuszak AL, Levy M, Schick B, Suber C, Feldkamp M, Gladstone J, Bar-Levy F, Jackson E, Donnenfeld A, Meschino W, et al: Outcome after maternal varicella infection in the first 20 weeks of pregnancy. N Engl J Med 330:901, 1994

Patel DM, Rhodes PG, LeBlanc MH, Graves GR, Glick C, Morrison J: Role of postnatal penicillin prophylaxis in prevention of neonatal group B streptococcus infection. Acta Paediatr 88:874, 1999

Perlman JM, Argyle C: Lethal cytomegalovirus infection in preterm infants: Clinical, radiological, and neuropathological findings. Ann Neurol 31:64, 1992

Peters MT, Lowe TW, Carpenter A, Kole S: Prenatal diagnosis of congenital cytomegalovirus infection with abnormal triple-screen results and hyperechoic fetal bowel. Am J Obstet Gynecol 173:953, 1995

Peters MT, Nicolaides KH: Cordocentesis for the diagnosis and treatment of human fetal parvovirus infection. Obstet Gynecol 75:501, 1990

Pratlong F, Boulot P, Villena I, Issert E, Tamby I, Cazenave J, Dedet J-P: Antenatal diagnosis of congenital toxoplasmosis: Evaluation of the biological parameters in a cohort of 286 patients. Br J Obstet Gynaecol 103:552, 1996

Preblud SR: Varicella: Complications and cost. Pediatrics 785:728, 1986

Public Health Laboratory Service Working Party on Fifth Disease: Prospective study of human parvovirus (B19) infection in pregnancy. BMJ 300:1166, 1990

Pustilnik TB, Cohen AW: Parvovirus B19 infection in a twin pregnancy. Obstet Gynecol 83:834, 1994

Pyati SP, Pildes RS, Jacobs NM, Ramamurthy RS, Yeh TF, Raval DS, Lilien LD, Amma P, Metzger WI: Penicillin in infants weighing two kilograms or less with early-onset group B streptococcal disease. N Engl J Med 308:1383, 1983

Pylipow M, Gaddis M, Kinney JS: Selective intrapartum prophylaxis for group B streptococcus colonization: Management and outcome of newborns. Pediatrics 93:631, 1994

Regan JA, Klebanoff MA, Nugent RP, The Vaginal Infections and Prematurity Study Group: The epidemiology of group B streptococcal colonization in pregnancy. Obstet Gynecol 77:604, 1991

Rench MA, Baker CJ: Group B streptococcal breast abscess in a mother and mastitis in her infant. Obstet Gynecol 73:875, 1989

Robier C, Tall A, Diagne N, Fontenille D, Spiegel A, Trape JF: Plasmodium falciparum clinical malaria: Lessons from longitudinal studies in Senegal. Parassitologia 41:255, 1999

Rodis JF: Parvovirus infection. Clin Obstet Gynecol 42:107, 1999

Rodis JF, Borgida AF, Wilson M, Egan JF, Leo MV, Odibo AO, Campbell WA: Management of parvovirus infection in pregnancy and outcomes of hydrops: A survey of members of the Society of Perinatal Obstetricians. Am J Obstet Gynecol 179:985, 1998a

Rodis JF, Quinn DL, Gary GW Jr, Anderson LJ, Rosengren S, Cartter ML, Campbell WA, Vintzileos AM: Management and outcomes of pregnancies complicated by human B19 parvovirus infection: A prospective study. Am J Obstet Gynecol 163:1168, 1990

Rodis JF, Rodner C, Hansen AA, Borgida AF, Deoliveira I, Shulman Rosengren S: Long-term outcome of children following maternal human parvovirus B19 infection. Obstet Gynecol 91:125, 1998b

Rogers BB, Singer DB, Mak SK, Gary GW, Fikrig MK, McMillan PN: Detection of human parvovirus B19 in early spontaneous abortuses using serology, histology, electron microscopy, in situ hybridization, and the polymerase chain reaction. Obstet Gynecol 81:402, 1993

Rouse DJ, Gardner M, Allen S: Varicella-zoster immune globulin (VZIG) for the at-risk gravida? A decision analysis. Am J Obstet Gynecol 174:410, 1996

Royal College of Obstetricians and Gynaecologists: Multidisciplinary Working Group: Prenatal screening for toxoplasmosis in the UK. London, RCOG, 1992

Sahakian V, Weiner CP, Naides SJ, Williamson RA, Scharosch LL: Intrauterine transfusion treatment of nonimmune hydrops fetalis secondary to human parvovirus B19 infection. Am J Obstet Gynecol 164:1090, 1991

Saxén L, Holmberg PC, Kurppa K, Kuosma E, Pyhälä R: Influenza epidemics and anencephaly. Am J Public Health 80:473, 1990

Schlesinger PA, Duray PH, Burke BA, Steere AC, Stillman MT: Maternal–fetal transmission of Lyme disease spirochete, *Borrelia burgdorferi*. Ann Intern Med 103:67, 1985

Schrag SJ, Zywicki S, Farley MM, Reingold AL, Harrison LH, Lefkowitz LB, Hadler JL, Danila R, Cieslak PR, Schuchat A: Group B streptococcal disease in the era of intrapartum antibiotic prophylaxis. N Engl J Med 342:15, 2000

Schuchat A: Neonatal group B streptococcal disease—screening and prevention. N Engl J Med 343:209, 2000

Schuchat A, Zywicki SS, Dinsmoor MJ, Mercer B, Romaguera J, O'Sullivan MJ, Patel D, Peters MT, Stoll B, Levine OS: Risk factors and opportunities for prevention of early-onset neonatal sepsis: A multicenter case-control study. Pediatrics 105:21, 2000

Scialli AR, Rarick TL: Salmonella sepsis and second-trimester pregnancy loss. Obstet Gynecol 79:820, 1992

Sever JL, Ellenberg JH, Ley AC, Madden DL, Fuccillo DA, Tzan NR, Edmonds DM: Toxoplasmosis: Maternal and pediatric findings in 23,000 pregnancies. Pediatrics 82:181, 1988

Shilleto N, Barrett JR, Allen L, Ryan G, Morrow RJ, Farine D: Human parvovirus B19 related hydrops and elevated fetal creatine kinase. Am J Obstet Gynecol 174:403, 1996

Siegel JD, Cushion NB: Prevention of early onset group B streptococcal disease: Another look at single dose penicillin at birth. Obstet Gynecol 87:692, 1996

Siegel JD, McCracken GH Jr, Threlkeld N, Milvenan B, Rosenfeld CR: Single-dose penicillin prophylaxis against neonatal group B streptococcal infections. N Engl J Med 303:769, 1980

Siegel M: Congenital malformations following chickenpox, measles, mumps, and hepatitis: Results of a cohort study. JAMA 226:1521, 1973

Siegel M, Fuerst HT: Low birth weight and maternal virus diseases: A prospective study of rubella, measles, mumps, chickenpox, and hepatitis. JAMA 197:88, 1966

Siegel M, Goldberg M: Incidence of poliomyelitis in pregnancy. N Engl J Med 253:841, 1955

Silver HM: Listeriosis during pregnancy. Obstet Gynecol Surv 53:737, 1998

Sirry HW, George RH, Whittle MJ: Meningo-encephalitis due to listeria monocytogenes in pregnancy. Br J Obstet Gynaecol 101:1083, 1994

Smith LG, Pearlman M, Smith LG, Faro S: Lyme disease: A review with emphasis on the pregnant woman. Obstet Gynecol Surv 46:125, 1991

Smith WJ, Jackson LA, Watts DH, Koepsel TD: Prevention of chickenpox in reproductive-age women: Cost-effectiveness of routine prenatal screening with postpartum vaccination of susceptibles. Obstet Gynecol 92:535, 1998

Stagno S, Whitley RJ: Herpesvirus infections of pregnancy, 2. Herpes simplex virus and varicella-zoster virus infections. N Engl J Med 313:1327, 1985

Steigman AJ, Bottone EJ, Hanna BA: Control of perinatal group B streptococcal sepsis: Efficacy of single injection of aqueous penicillin at birth. Mt Sinai J Med 45:685, 1978

Stein SJ, Greenspoon JS: Rubeola during pregnancy. Obstet Gynecol 78:925, 1991

Stirrat G: The immune system. In Hytten F, Chamberlain G (eds): Clinical Physiology in Obstetrics. London, Blackwell, 1991, p 101

Strobino B, Abid S, Gewitz M: Maternal Lyme disease and congenital heart disease: A case-control study in an endemic area. Am J Obstet Gynecol 180:711, 1999

Strobino BA, Williams CL, Abid S, Chalson R, Spierling P: Lyme disease and pregnancy outcome: A prospective study of two thousand prenatal patients. Am J Obstet Gynecol 169:367, 1993

Strong BS, Young SA: Intrauterine coxsackie virus, group B type 1, infection: Viral cultivation from amniotic fluid in the third trimester. Am J Perinatol 12:78, 1995

Tappero JW, Schuchat A, Deaver KA, Mascola L, Wenger JD: Reduction in the incidence of human listeriosis in the United States. Effectiveness of prevention efforts? JAMA 273:1118, 1995

Thorp JA, Yeast JD, Cohen GR, Meyer BA, Mitchell C: Severe nonimmune hydrops caused by parvovirus B19 infection and treated with intravascular transfusion of blood and platelets. J Matern Fetal Invest 4:111, 1994

Tiessen RG, Van Elsacker-Niele AMW, Vermeij-Keers CHR, Oepkes D, Van Roosmalen J, Gorsira MCB: A fetus with a parvovirus B19 infection and congenital anomalies. Prenat Diagn 14:173, 1994

Topalovski M, Yang SS, Boonpasat Y: Listeriosis of the placenta: Clinicopathologic study of seven cases. Am J Obstet Gynecol 169:616, 1993

Towbin JA, Griffin LD, Martin AB, Nelson S, Siu B, Ayres NA, Demmler G, Moise KJ Jr, Zhang YH: Intrauterine adenoviral myocarditis presenting as nonimmune hydrops fetalis: Diagnosis by polymerase chain reaction. Pediatr Infect Dis J 13:144, 1994

Towers CV, Rumney PJ, Minkiewicz SF, Asrat T: Incidence of intrapartum maternal risk factors for identifying neonates at risk for early-onset group B streptococcal sepsis: A prospective study. Am J Obstet Gynecol 181:1197, 1999a

Towers CV, Suriano K, Asrat T: The capture of at-risk term newborns for early-onset group B streptococcal sepsis determined by a risk factor approach. Am J Obstet Gynecol 181:1243, 1999b

Tuppurainen N, Hallman M: Prevention of neonatal group B streptococcal disease: Intrapartum detection and chemoprophylaxis of heavily colonized parturients. Obstet Gynecol 73:583, 1989

Valeur-Jensen AK, Pedersen CB, Westergaard T, Jensen IP,

Lebech M, Andersen PK, Aaby P, Pedersen BN, Melbye M: Risk factors for parvovirus B19 infection in pregnancy. JAMA 281:1099, 1999

Ville Y, de Gayffier A, Brivet F, Leruez M, Marchal P, Morinet F, Troalen F, Fernandez H, Frydman R: Fetal–maternal hydrops syndrome in human parvovirus infection. Fetal Diagn Ther 10:204, 1995

Wallon M, Liou C, Garner P, Peyron F: Congenital toxoplasmosis: Systematic review of evidence of efficacy of treatment in pregnancy. BMJ 318:1511, 1999

Weber K, Bratzke H-J, Neubert U, Wilske B, Duray PH: *Borrelia burgdorferi* in a newborn despite oral penicillin for Lyme borreliosis during pregnancy. Pediatr Infect Dis J 7:286, 1988

Webster WS: Teratogen update: Congenital rubella. Teratology 58:13, 1998

Wendel GD, McIntire DJ, Leveno KJ: Reducing neonatal group B streptococcal disease (letter). N Engl J Med 342:1366, 2000

WHO Collaborative Study Team on the Role of Breastfeeding on the Prevention of Infant Mortality: Effect of breastfeeding on infant and child mortality due to infectious diseases in less developed countries: a pooled analysis. Lancet 355:451, 2000

Wong RD, Murthy ARK, Mathisen GE, Glover N, Thornton PJ: Treatment of severe falciparum malaria during pregnancy with quinidine and exchange transfusion. Am J Med 92:561, 1992

Wong SY, Remington JS: Toxoplasmosis in pregnancy. Clin Infect Dis 18:853, 1994

World Health Organization: Control of tropical diseases (CTD): Malaria control. Geneva, WHO Office of Information, 1995

Wright C, Hinchliffe SA, Taylor C: Fetal pathology in intrauterine death due to parvovirus B19 infection. Br J Obstet Gynaecol 103:133, 1996

Wyler DJ: Malaria chemoprophylaxis for the traveler. N Engl J Med 329:31, 1993

Yamakawa Y, Oka H, Hori S, Arai T, Izumi R: Detection of human parvovirus B19 DNA by nested polymerase chain reaction. Obstet Gynecol 86:126, 1995

Yamauchi T, Wilson C, St Geme JW: Transmission of live, attenuated mumps virus to the human placenta. N Engl J Med 290:710, 1974

Yancey MK, Duff P, Kubilis P, Clark P, Frentzen BH: Risk factors for neonatal sepsis. Obstet Gynecol 87:188, 1996

Young NS: B19 parvovirus. Ballieres Clin Haematol 8:25, 1995

Yow MD, Demmler GJ: Congenital cytomegalovirus disease—20 years is long enough. N Engl J Med 326:703, 1992

57

Sexually Transmitted Diseases

Sexually transmitted diseases are relatively common during pregnancy, especially in indigent, urban populations plagued by drug abuse and prostitution. Screening, identification, education, and treatment are important components of prenatal care for women at increased risk for these infections. Consequently, as a part of routine prenatal care, common sexually transmitted diseases that are often sought include syphilis, gonorrhea, chlamydia, hepatitis B virus, human immunodeficiency virus, and human papillomavirus.

In the following treatment protocols for sexually transmitted diseases, we attempt to adhere to the intensive, but frequently modified, treatment schedules provided periodically by the Centers for Disease Control and Prevention (1998b).

SYPHILIS

Through the 1980s, there was an increase in the incidence of syphilis in the United States that peaked in 1990, but since then, rates have declined 85 percent to 1998 (Centers for Disease Control and Prevention, 1999d). Shown in Figure 57–1 are the incidences for adult-acquired as well as congenital syphilis. The rate of syphilis in the United States in 1998 was a record low of 2.6 cases per 100,000 persons, which is very near the goal set for the National Health Objective for 2000. The South, with 6.6 cases per 100,000 is the only region not meeting this goal. Likewise, a record low incidence of congenital syphilis, 20.6 cases per 100,000 live births, was recorded in 1998 by the Centers for Disease Control and Prevention (1999a). These declines continued through 1999 (Vastag, 2001). The results are so promising that the Centers for Disease Control and Prevention

have created the National Plan for Syphilis Elimination (Mitka, 2000).

Minkoff and colleagues (1990) reported associations with maternal syphilis and drug abuse, particularly crack cocaine, and lack of prenatal care. Klass and colleagues (1994), in a study of prenatal syphilis at the Boston City Hospital over four decades, reported a prevalence of syphilis in women either before or during pregnancy of 2.4 percent in 1951 compared with 3.9 percent in 1991. They concluded that the continued prevalence of syphilis at delivery was associated with substance abuse, human immunodeficiency virus infection, lack of prenatal care, treatment failures, and reinfection. Antepartum syphilis can profoundly affect pregnancy outcome by causing preterm labor, fetal death, and neonatal infection by transplacental or perinatal infection (Gilstrap and Wendel, 1999; Vaules and associates, 2000). Fortunately, of the many congenital infections, syphilis is not only the most readily prevented but also the most susceptible to therapy.

CLINICAL MANIFESTATIONS. Primary syphilis follows an incubation period of 10 to 90 days (average 3 weeks), but usually less than 6 weeks. During pregnancy, the primary genital lesion, or sometimes multiple lesions, may be of such small size or be so located as to go unnoticed. For example, a **cervical chancre** is more common in pregnant women, probably because of inoculation of the friable cervix. The primary chancre is characterized by a painless firm ulcer with raised edges and a granulation base. It persists for 2 to 6 weeks and then heals spontaneously but is often accompanied by nontender, enlarged inguinal lymph nodes.

Approximately 4 to 10 weeks after healing of the chancre, secondary syphilis usually appears in the form

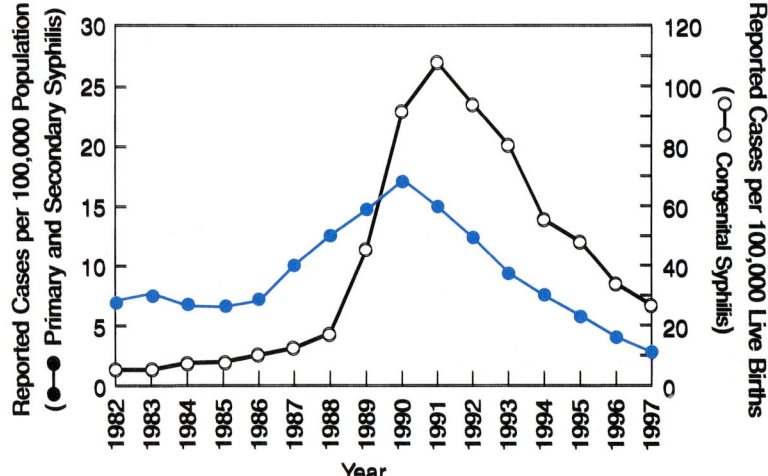

FIGURE 57–1. Rates of primary and secondary syphilis in women and congenital syphilis for the United States, 1982–1997. (From Centers for Disease Control and Prevention, 1997a.)

of a highly variable skin rash. About 15 percent of women still have a chancre. The lesions of secondary syphilis may be mild and go unnoticed in 25 percent of patients. In some, lesions are limited to the genitalia, where they appear as elevated areas, or **condylomata lata,** which occasionally cause vulvar ulcerations (Fig. 57–2). Secondary syphilis may also cause alopecia. At times the first and only suggestion of the disease is the delivery of a stillborn infant or a live-born infant severely afflicted with congenital syphilis.

FETAL AND NEONATAL INFECTION. In the past, syphilis accounted for nearly a third of stillbirths. Today syphilis has a smaller but persistent role in fetal death. For example, at Parkland Hospital from 1988 to 1995, congenital syphilis accounted for 6.3 percent of stillbirths (Cunningham and Hollier, 1997). The number of cases of congenital infection in black women from Baltimore for 1996 was 550 per 100,000 births compared with that for the United States of 30 per 100,000 births (Centers for Disease Control and Prevention, 1998a). Many of these mothers have inadequate prenatal care, and Southwick and colleagues (1999) reported an outbreak of congenital syphilis associated with inadequate prenatal testing for syphilis. McFarlin and co-workers (1994) reported that the serological titer and unknown duration of infection were major risk factors for congenital syphilis. In a review of 322 cases of congenital syphi-

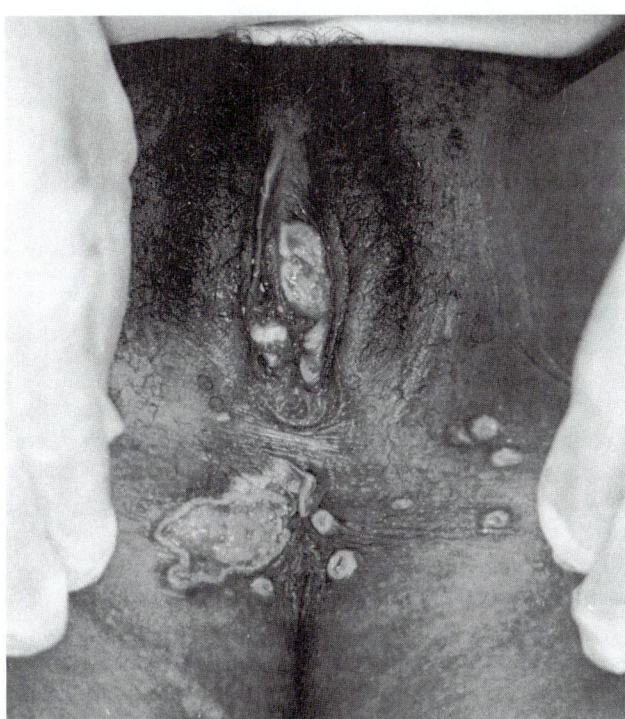

FIGURE 57–2. Genital condylomata lata of secondary syphilis. (From Wendel and Cunningham, 1991.)

lis, Coles and associates (1995) reported that only 20 percent of the newborns had a complete laboratory workup, including long-bone radiographs and spinal fluid analysis. Of the 80 women treated for syphilis during pregnancy, only 30 percent were treated appropriately for their stage of infection.

Spirochetes readily cross the placenta and can result in congenital infection. Because of relative immunoincompetence prior to about 18 weeks, the fetus generally does not manifest clinical disease if infected before this time (Silverstein, 1962). The frequency of congenital syphilis varies with both the stage and duration of maternal infection. The highest incidence is in neonates born to mothers with early syphilis—primary or secondary—and the lowest incidence with late latent disease—greater than 1-year duration (Centers for Disease Control, 1988; Fiumara and colleagues, 1952). As expected, early latent disease is associated with a higher rate of congenital infection because spirochetemia is greater in proximity to primary infection. **Importantly, any stage of maternal syphilis may result in fetal infection.**

PATHOLOGY. Syphilis is a chronic infection, and the spirochete causes lesions in the internal organs that include interstitial changes in the lungs (*pneumonia alba of Virchow*), liver (*hypertrophic cirrhosis*), spleen, and pancreas. Recently acquired infections are more likely to be associated with fetal morbidity and mortality. Syphilitic infection also causes *osteochondritis* in the long bones, which is most readily recognizable radiographically in the femur, tibia, and radius.

With syphilitic infection, the placenta becomes large and pale. Microscopically, villi appear to have lost their characteristic arborescent appearance and to have become thicker and club shaped. Rogers and colleagues (1999) described large villi in 70 percent of placentas from 34 stillborn infants with congenital syphilis. In 23 live-born infants with congenital syphilis, half had placentas with large villi. There is a marked decrease in the number of blood vessels, which in advanced cases almost entirely disappear as a result of endarteritis and proliferation of stromal cells. Perhaps related to this, Lucas and colleagues (1991) demonstrated increased vascular resistance in uterine and umbilical arteries of infected pregnancies. Spirochetes are sparsely scattered throughout the placenta even when they are present in large numbers in fetal organs. They may be demonstrated by examination under the darkfield microscope of scrapings from the intima of the vessels of the fresh umbilical cord. In a study of 25 untreated women, Schwartz and associates (1995) reported that necrotizing funisitis was the most frequent pathological lesion, occurring in a third of cases. Spirochetes were detected in 89 percent of these cords using silver and immunofluorescent staining.

SEROLOGICAL DIAGNOSIS. A suitable serological screening test such as the *Venereal Disease Research Laboratory* (*VDRL*) *slide test* or the *rapid plasma reagin* (*RPR*) *test* is performed at the first prenatal visit. Testing is required by law in all 50 states. Fortunately, these serological tests will be positive in the majority of women with primary syphilitic lesion and in all of those with secondary syphilis. They will almost always be positive 4 to 6 weeks after infection. Because such reagin tests lack specificity, a treponemal test such as the *fluorescent treponemal antibody absorption test* (*FTA-ABS*) or the *microhemagglutination assay for antibodies to Treponema pallidum* (*MHA-TP*) is used to confirm a positive result. A new treponemal specific test that is intended to replace the MHA-TP test is the *Treponema pallidum passive particle agglutination* (*TP-PA*) *test* (Pope and Fears, 2000).

Cord blood screening is an insensitive test to detect early congenital syphilis. Thus, and especially for women at high risk for syphilis, a second nontreponemal screening test should be done at the time of delivery (Centers for Disease Control and Prevention, 1998b).

FETAL DIAGNOSIS. Wendel and colleagues (1989) have shown that motile spirochetes can be seen in amnionic fluid obtained transabdominally in women with syphilis and fetal death. They later reported that the polymerase chain reaction was 100 percent specific for detection of *Treponema pallidum* in amnionic fluid and neonatal serum and spinal fluid (Wendel and colleagues, 1991). Because of myriad pathological changes in the fetus, ultrasound examination may be suggestive or even diagnostic. For example, the infant shown in Figure 57–3 has a large abdomen due to marked hepatosplenomegaly from congenital syphilis. The placenta weighed almost as much as the infant! The fetus may also have edema, ascites, and hydrops. The newborn may be jaundiced with petechiae or purpuric skin lesions, lymphadenopathy, rhinitis ("snuffles"), pneumonia, myocarditis, and nephrosis (Gilstrap and Wendel, 1999).

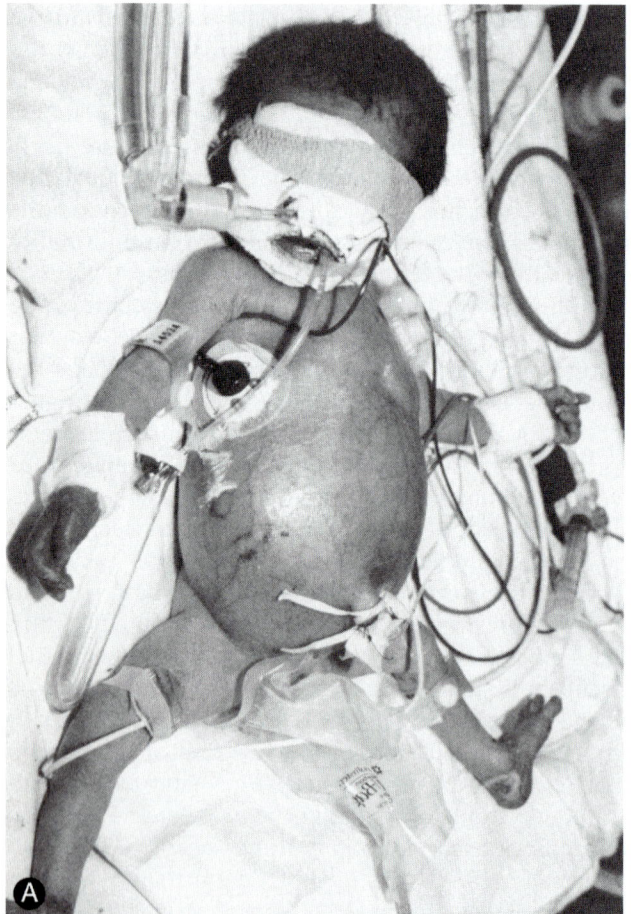
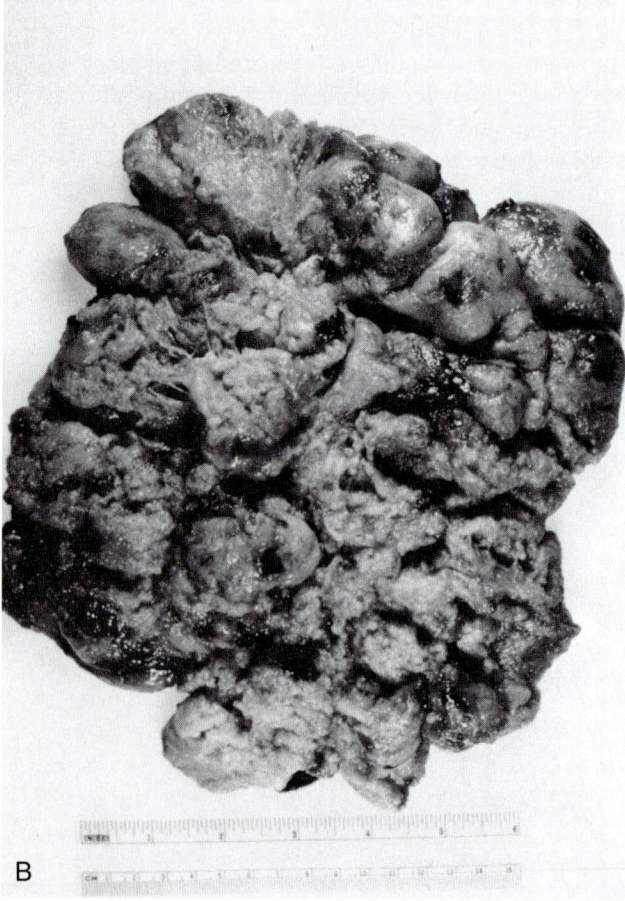

FIGURE 57–3. Congenital syphilis. **A.** A 29-week-old, severely ill infant with an enlarged abdomen caused by marked hepatosplenomegaly plus ascites. **B.** The large syphilitic placenta of the same infant weighed 1200 g, almost the birthweight of the infant. (Photographs courtesy of Dr. G. Wendel.)

TREATMENT. Penicillin remains the treatment of choice; however, treatment of syphilis during pregnancy has not been evaluated rigorously. In a survey, Rolfs (1995) concluded that there are no useful comparative data available for ascertaining optimal therapy. Syphilis therapy during pregnancy is dual; it is given to eradicate maternal infection and to prevent congenital syphilis. The principal difficulty in defining successful treatment has been because fetal syphilis could not be confirmed. Although the prenatal diagnosis of severe fetal syphilis can be made by funipuncture, its clinical utility is not yet clear (Wendel and associates, 1991).

In retrospective analyses, benzathine penicillin G has been shown to cure early maternal infection and prevent neonatal syphilis in 98 percent of cases (Zenker and Rolfs, 1990). In a recent study of 340 pregnant women with syphilis, Alexander and colleagues (1999) reported six (1.8 percent) fetal treatment failures with maternal benzathine penicillin G therapy. Four of these six were in 75 women with secondary syphilis and the other two were in 102 women with early latent syphilis. Conover and colleagues (1998) reported a case of congenital syphilis with a penicillin regimen "exceeding CDC guidelines." Thus, although the Centers for Disease Control guidelines may be up to 98 percent effective in prevention of congenital syphilis, there will be some treatment failures.

As shown in Table 57–1, the current Centers for Disease Control and Prevention guidelines for treatment of syphilis in pregnancy include the same dosage schedule of benzathine penicillin G as for nonpregnant adults. Some authorities recommend a second dose of benzathine penicillin, 2.4 million units intramuscularly, 1 week after the initial dose, especially for women in the third trimester or for pregnant women with secondary syphilis. Pregnant women with a history of penicillin allergy can be skin tested to confirm the risk of immuno-globulin E (IgE)–mediated anaphylaxis. If skin tests are reactive, penicillin desensitization as described by Wendel and associates (1985) is recommended and is followed by benzathine penicillin G treatment. Chisholm and colleagues (1997) reported 16 pregnant women who underwent penicillin desensitization (11 oral and six intravenous procedures) prior to syphilis treatment. Both regimens were effective, but the oral route was easier to administer and was less expensive ($144 versus $319).

Unfortunately, there are no proven alternatives to penicillin therapy during pregnancy. Erythromycin, which may be curative in the mother, may not prevent congenital syphilis (Fenton and Light, 1976; Hashisaki and colleagues, 1983; Wendel, 1988). It is not currently recommended as a penicillin alternative. The cephalo-sporins, such as ceftriaxone, and the newer macrolide antibiotic, azithromycin, may prove useful but have not been adequately evaluated (Rolfs, 1995). Tetracyclines, including doxycycline, are effective for treatment of syphilis in the nonpregnant woman, but are generally not recommended during pregnancy because of the risk of yellow-brown discoloration of the fetal deciduous teeth.

There is concern that despite recommended treatment during pregnancy, some newborns still have obvious clinical stigmata of congenital syphilis. This of course depends on the duration of untreated syphilis to which the fetus is exposed. For example, in 1988, the Centers for Disease Control reported that up to 20 percent of newborns had stigmata despite maternal therapy.

TABLE 57–1. Recommended Treatment for Pregnant Women with Syphilis

Category	Treatment
Early syphilis[a]	Benzathine penicillin G, 2.4 million units intramuscularly as a single injection; some authorities recommend a second dose 1 week later
Syphilis of more than 1-year duration[b]	Benzathine penicillin G, 2.4 million units intramuscularly weekly for 3 doses
Neurosyphilis[c]	Aqueous crystalline penicillin G, 3–4 million units intravenously every 4 hours for 10–14 days *or* Aqueous procaine penicillin, 2.4 million units intramuscularly daily, plus probenecid 500 mg orally four times daily, both for 10–14 days

[a] Primary, secondary, and latent syphilis of less than 1-year duration.
[b] Latent syphilis of unknown or more than 1-year duration; cardiovascular or late benign syphilis.
[c] Some experts administer benzathine penicillin, 2.4 million units intramuscularly, after completion of the neurosyphilis treatment regimens.
From the Centers for Disease Control and Prevention (1998b).

As expected, half of these method failures were in mothers not given treatment until the third trimester. In a recent study of 334 women with antepartum syphilis treated at Parkland Hospital, Alexander and colleagues (1999) showed that a treatment failure rate of 0.8 percent was generally confined to women treated after 26 weeks. It seems likely that fetal infections that fail therapy are of such duration and severity that there is already irreversible damage.

In all women with primary syphilis and about half with secondary infection, penicillin treatment is followed by the *Jarisch–Herxheimer reaction*. Uterine contractions frequently develop with this reaction, and they may be followed by evidence of fetal distress manifested as late fetal heart rate decelerations (Klein and colleagues, 1990). In a study of 50 pregnant women who received benzathine penicillin for syphilis, Myles and colleagues (1998) report a 40 percent incidence of the Jarisch–Herxheimer reaction. Of the 31 women monitored electronically, 42 percent developed regular uterine contractions (median onset 10 hours) and 39 percent developed variable decelerations (median onset 8 hours). All contractions resolved within 24 hours of therapy. Lucas and co-workers (1991) used Doppler velocimetry and demonstrated associated acute vascular-resistance changes. Obvious fetal involvement, characterized by ultrasonic evidence for ascites, is associated with almost universally adverse fetal outcome despite therapy.

Hill and Maloney (1991) and Satin and colleagues (1992) have described fetuses with hepatosplenomegaly, gastrointestinal tract obstruction, and placentomegaly. Barton and co-workers (1992) found that delivery and neonatal treatment may be the best option for near-term hydropic fetuses with congenital syphilis.

Prior to syphilotherapy, all women should be offered counseling and testing for antibody to human immunodeficiency virus (HIV). Both treponemal and nontreponemal tests are felt to be accurate for the diagnosis of syphilis in HIV-infected patients. For these women, the Centers for Disease Control and Prevention (1998b) recommend the same treatment as for HIV-negative persons; that is, benzathine penicillin G, 2.4 million units intramuscularly for primary and secondary syphilis. Additional multiple doses of benzathine penicillin G—as given for late syphilis—are recommended by some authorities. Women with latent syphilis and HIV infection should be treated with three weekly doses of 2.4 million units of benzathine penicillin G. Clinical and serological follow-up to detect treatment failures is also recommended at 3, 6, 9, 12, and 24 months.

LUMBAR PUNCTURE. Whether to perform routine cerebrospinal fluid analysis has been controversial. Many asymptomatic patients have spinal fluid abnormalities with primary, secondary, and early latent syphilis, but most do not develop neurosyphilis after appropriate treatment. The Centers for Disease Control and Prevention (1998b) recommend lumbar puncture in latent syphilis of more than 1-year duration if there are neurological or ophthalmological symptoms, treatment failures, evidence of active tertiary syphilis—aortitis, gamma, or iritis—or if there is concomitant HIV infection.

FOLLOW-UP. Any patient treated for syphilis needs conscientious follow-up. Sexual contacts within the last 3 months should be evaluated for syphilis and treated presumptively, even if seronegative. Maternal serological titers should be determined monthly and at delivery to confirm a serological response to treatment or to document reinfection in this high-risk group.

TREATMENT OF CONGENITAL SYPHILIS. Every infant with suspected or proven congenital syphilis should have a cerebrospinal fluid examination prior to treatment. After therapy, they should be followed at monthly intervals until nontreponemal serological tests become negative or serofast. The Centers for Disease Control and Prevention (1998b) recommend that symptomatic infants or those with abnormal spinal fluid examination be treated initially with aqueous penicillin G, 100,000 to 150,000 U/kg administered as 50,000 U/kg intravenously every 12 hours for the first 7 days of life. This is followed by similar intravenous treatment every 8 hours for a total of 10 days, or aqueous procaine penicillin G, 50,000 U/kg intramuscularly each day to complete a total of 10 days of penicillin treatment. Asymptomatic seropositive infants with a normal spinal fluid examination can be treated with a single dose of benzathine penicillin G, 50,000 U/kg intramuscularly. **Infants born to mothers treated with erythromycin for syphilis during pregnancy should be retreated as though they have congenital syphilis.**

GONORRHEA

The incidence of gonorrhea in the United States decreased by 70 percent from 1981 to 1996. The rate for 1998 was 133 cases per 100,000 population (Centers for Disease Control and Prevention, 2000). A similar rate was reported for 1999 (Vastag, 2001). The highest rate in women of all races was in the 15- to 19-year age group.

The prevalence of gonorrhea during pregnancy varies but may be as high as 7 percent and reflects the risk status of the population (Wendel and Wendel, 1993). Risk factors include being single, adolescence, poverty, drug abuse, prostitution, other sexually transmitted diseases, and lack of prenatal care. Gonococcal infection is also a marker for concomitant chlamydial infection in about 40 percent of infected pregnant women (Christmas and associates, 1989).

In most pregnant women, gonococcal infection is limited to the lower genital tract, including the cervix, urethra, and periurethral and vestibular glands. Acute salpingitis is rare, and Yip and colleagues (1993) found only 15 cases reported since 1950. They reviewed possible mechanisms, and a likely one is that salpingitis develops if cervical infection ascends before obliteration of the uterine cavity through fusion of the chorion and decidua at 12 weeks. Reactivated or persistent preexisting infection can cause tubo-ovarian abscess, but this seems unlikely.

There is some evidence that pregnancy alters the clinical presentation of gonorrhea. For example, some investigators have reported increased rates of oropharyngeal and anal infections during pregnancy (Campos-Outcalt and Ryan, 1995). Increased noncervical infection may be from altered sexual practices because of pregnancy, cultural customs, or both. Finally, pregnant women may account for a disproportionate amount of disseminated gonococcal infection in women (Ross, 1996). These observations may reflect heightened medical attention during pregnancy, increased gonococcal dissemination from engorged pelvic vasculature, or possibly the altered immunostatus of pregnancy.

Because of all of these factors, a screening test for gonorrhea is recommended at the first prenatal visit or prior to an induced abortion. In high-risk populations, the Centers for Disease Control and Prevention (1998b) recommend that a repeat culture be obtained after 28 weeks.

EFFECT ON PREGNANCY. Gonococcal infection may have deleterious effects on pregnancy outcome in any trimester. There is an association between untreated gonococcal cervicitis and septic spontaneous abortion, or infection after induced abortion (Burkman and associates, 1976). Preterm delivery, prematurely ruptured membranes, chorioamnionitis, and postpartum infection are more common in women with *Neisseria gonorrhoeae* detected at delivery (Alger and associates, 1988). Maxwell and Watson (1992) reported that expectant management of the culture-positive woman was reasonable even with prematurely ruptured membranes as long as antimicrobial treatment was given promptly.

Sheffield and colleagues (1999) recently reviewed clinical outcomes of 25 pregnant women admitted to Parkland Hospital for disseminated gonococcal infection. Their mean gestational age at presentation was 25 weeks, and all promptly responded to appropriate antimicrobial therapy. One stillborn infant and one spontaneous abortion were attributed to gonococcal sepsis.

TREATMENT. In many areas, antimicrobial-resistant *N gonorrhoeae*, particularly penicillinase-producing strains, have rendered some β-lactam drugs ineffective for therapy. Also disconcerting are the reports of quinolone-resistant *N gonorrhoeae* in several parts of the world (Ehret and Judson, 1998; Centers for Disease Control and Prevention, 1998b). As shown in Table 57–2, ceftriaxone is recommended for uncomplicated gonococcal infection during pregnancy. Spectinomycin as an initial treatment followed by erythromycin is recommended for women allergic to penicillin or β-lactam antibiotics (American College of Obstetricians and Gynecologists, 1994b). Ramus and associates (1996), in a study of 62 pregnant women with probable endocervical gonorrhea, reported that the regimens recommended by the Centers for Disease Control for the treatment of gonorrhea in pregnancy were effective. Intramuscular ceftriaxone (125 mg) and oral cefixime (400 mg) resulted in a cure rate of 93 percent and 97 percent, respectively.

Screening for syphilis and *Chlamydia trachomatis* should precede treatment, if possible. If chlamydial testing is unavailable, presumptive therapy is given. Treatment for sexual contacts and maternal test-of-cure cultures help to ensure efficacy of therapy. Because gonococcal reinfection is common, repeat screening in late pregnancy should be considered for women treated earlier during pregnancy (American College of Obstetricians and Gynecologists, 1994b).

DISSEMINATED GONOCOCCAL INFECTIONS. Gonococcal bacteremia may lead to petechial or pustular skin lesions, arthralgias, septic arthritis, or tenosynovitis. The Centers for Disease Control and Prevention (1998b) recommend ceftriaxone, 1000 mg intramuscularly or intravenously every 24 hours. Alternative initial regimens include cefotaxime or ceftizoxime, 1000 mg intravenously every 8 hours. Spectinomycin, 2 g every 12 hours, may be used in women allergic to β-lactam drugs. All of the preceding regimens should be continued for 24 to 48 hours after improvement and then therapy changed to cefixime, 400 mg orally two times daily, to

TABLE 57–2. Treatment of Uncomplicated Gonococcal Infections During Pregnancy

Ceftriaxone, 125 mg intramuscularly as a single dose
or
Cefixime, 400 mg orally in a single dose
or
Spectinomycin, 2 g intramuscularly
For possible concomitant chlamydial infection, use erythromycin (see Table 57–4)

From the Centers for Disease Control and Prevention (1998b).

complete a week of therapy. Ciprofloxacin is a recommended alternative to cefixime in the nonpregnant patient, but is contraindicated for pregnant and lactating women (Chap. 38, p. 1021).

For gonococcal *endocarditis,* therapy should be continued for at least 4 weeks, and for *meningitis,* 10 to 14 days (Centers for Disease Control and Prevention, 1998b). Endocarditis rarely complicates pregnancy, but it may be fatal (Bataskov and colleagues, 1991). Pantanowitz and colleagues (1998) recently reported a case of gonococcal arthritis and endocarditis in a 22-year-old woman with a threatened abortion.

Varady and colleagues (1998) reported on an unusual case of a gonococcal scalp abscess in a neonate delivered by cesarean. Membranes had been ruptured for 14 hours, and a scalp electrode had been in place for 2 hours before delivery.

TREATMENT OF NEONATES. All infants are given prophylaxis against eye infection (Chap. 16, p. 396). Infants born to untreated infected women are given ceftriaxone, 25 to 50 mg/kg, either intravenously or intramuscularly for one dose. Those who develop gonococcal ophthalmia should be hospitalized and evaluated for disseminated infection (Erdem and Schleiss, 2000). Gonococcal ophthalmia may be treated with the same single-dose ceftriaxone regimen as given for asymptomatic infants born to culture-positive women (Centers for Disease Control and Prevention, 1998b). Some pediatricians prefer to continue antibiotics until cultures have been negative for 48 to 72 hours. The mother and infant should also be evaluated for concomitant chlamydial infection. Isolation is recommended until treated for 24 hours. Topical antibiotic preparations are not appropriate. Both parents also should be treated for gonorrhea.

CHLAMYDIAL INFECTIONS

Chlamydia trachomatis is an obligate intracellular bacterium that has several serotypes, including those that cause *lymphogranuloma venereum.* The most commonly encountered strains are those that attach only to columnar or transitional cell epithelium and cause cervical infection.

MATERNAL INFECTIONS. Genital infection with *C trachomatis* is one of the most common sexually transmitted bacterial diseases in women of reproductive age in the United States. According to Macmillan and colleagues (1999), this is also true for the United Kingdom and Europe. *C trachomatis* infection is also common in pregnant women, and its incidence depends on the demographic makeup of the population. For example,

the prevalence of symptomatic and asymptomatic genital infections in private obstetrical patients is below 2 percent, but is up to 25 percent in some groups of young, unmarried, inner-city women attending public clinics (McGregor and French, 1991; Ryan and colleagues, 1990). In a review of nearly 2500 women who initiated prenatal care prior to 20 weeks, Allaire and colleagues (1998) reported a 15 percent prevalence of *C trachomatis.* Risk factors for chlamydial infection in pregnant women include age less than 25 years, presence or history of other sexually transmitted disease, multiple sexual partners, and a new sexual partner within 3 months (American College of Obstetricians and Gynecologists, 1994b).

DIAGNOSIS. Cultures are expensive and less accurate than newer methods. The direct fluorescent antibody (DFA) test has 90 percent sensitivity and 98 percent specificity compared with culture (Korn, 2000). Enzyme immunoassay (EIA) is less specific. DNA detection tests include polymerase chain reaction (PCR). Witkin and associates (1996) evaluated this test for identification of chlamydia from introital samples and found 97 percent sensitivity and 100 percent specificity. Andrews and associates (1996) reported that a ligase chain reaction assay (LCR) was both sensitive and specific for genitourinary infection in pregnant women.

SYMPTOMATIC INFECTION. Most pregnant women have subclinical or asymptomatic chlamydial infection. The organism may cause several clinical syndromes that include **urethritis, mucopurulent cervicitis,** and **acute salpingitis** (Table 57–3). Mucopurulent cervicitis is difficult to classify during pregnancy. It may be secondary to either chlamydial or gonococcal infection, or it may represent the normally stimulated cervical mucus.

TABLE 57–3. Symptomatic Chlamydial Infections

Maternal
Acute urethral syndrome
Bartholinitis
Mucopurulent cervicitis
Salpingitis
Perihepatitis
Conjunctivitis
Reactive arthritis

Neonatal
Conjunctivitis
Pneumonitis

Adapted from American College of Obstetricians and Gynecologists (1994b).

***ASYMPTOMATIC INFECTION AND PREGNANCY OUT-
COME.*** There is no doubt that perinatal transmission is
associated with neonatal **conjunctivitis** and **pneumonia**
(Hammerschlag and colleagues, 1989; Salpietro and colleagues, 1999; Schachter and co-workers, 1986). There is
vertical transmission to at least half of infants delivered
vaginally to infected women (McGregor and French,
1991). While eye prophylaxis for gonococcal infection
with silver nitrate, erythromycin, or tetracycline is effective, none of these prevent chlamydial conjunctivitis
(Centers for Disease Control and Prevention, 1998b).
When eye infection is identified, oral erythromycin,
50 mg/kg/day in four divided doses, is given for 10 to
14 days.

Although many investigators have examined the effects of asymptomatic chlamydial infection on pregnancy outcome, its role remains controversial. In one
recent study, Sozio and Ness (1998) found no association
with increased abortion. Some investigators have found
that untreated maternal cervical chlamydial infection
increases the risk for preterm delivery, prematurely ruptured membranes, and perinatal mortality (Alger, 1988;
Claman, 1995; Gravett, 1986; Martius, 1988; Ngassa,
1994, and their colleagues). Conversely, others have
found that only women with recent chlamydial infection,
confirmed by antichlamydial IgM antibody testing, are
at risk for these adverse outcomes (Berman and co-
workers, 1987; Sweet and associates, 1987). Because of
this confusion, the effects of treatment are also understandably controversial. For example, while Cohen and
colleagues (1990) and Ryan and associates (1990) reported a reduction in adverse perinatal events in women
treated with erythromycin, data from the Vaginal Infections and Prematurity Study Group demonstrated no
such improvement (Martin, 1990). This latter study was
a large, multicenter, randomized, placebo-controlled,
blinded investigation carried out under the auspices of
the National Institutes of Health.

Sweet and colleagues (1987) prospectively studied
270 pregnant women with untreated cervical infection
and compared outcomes with chlamydia-negative controls. There were no differences in the incidences of
preterm labor, prematurely ruptured membranes,
chorioamnionitis, neonatal sepsis, or postpartum uterine infections. In women with IgM antibody to *C trachomatis,* however, preterm labor or prematurely ruptured
membranes were more likely. Berman and colleagues
(1987) also reported this association. Andrews and colleagues (2000) reported a carefully done case-control
study from the Maternal-Fetal Medicine Units Network.
They found that chlamydial infection at 24 weeks was
associated with a two- to threefold increased risk for
preterm birth.

Chlamydial infection does not appear to be associated with an increased risk of chorioamnionitis nor with

pelvic infection after cesarean delivery (Blanco and colleagues, 1985; Gibbs and Schachter, 1987). Conversely,
delayed postpartum uterine infection with *C trachomatis*
has been described by Hoyme and associates (1986).
The syndrome, which develops 2 to 3 weeks postpartum,
is distinct from early postoperative metritis. It is characterized by vaginal bleeding or discharge, low-grade fever, lower abdominal pain, and uterine tenderness.

NEONATAL INFECTIONS

CONJUNCTIVITIS. Ophthalmic chlamydial infections
are one of the most common causes of preventable
blindness in undeveloped countries. Inclusion conjunctivitis develops in as many as a third of neonates born to
mothers with cervical infection. Salpietro and colleagues
(1999) recently reported that 40 percent of cases of
neonatal conjunctivitis in Italy were caused by *C trachomatis.* Symptomatic conjunctivitis tends to appear later
than disease caused by *N gonorrhoeae,* and the two must
be differentiated because treatment is not the same.
According to Crombleholme (2000), the highest sensitivity and specificity is found with DNA amplification
techniques discussed earlier.

PNEUMONITIS. *C trachomatis* is a relatively common
cause of afebrile pneumonia in infants at 1 to 3 months
of age (Centers for Disease Control and Prevention,
1998b). Bilateral pulmonary infiltrates and chronic
cough are often associated with poor weight gain.

SCREENING. The role for routine screening tests for
C trachomatis during pregnancy remains unclear. Currently, universal prenatal screening is not considered
cost effective. Newer DNA probes and polymerase
chain reaction may make detection cheaper and quicker.
The American College of Obstetricians and Gynecologists (1994b) recommends targeted screening of high-
risk populations. The Centers for Disease Control and
Prevention (1998b) recommends screening for pregnant
women less than 25 years old or those who have new or
multiple sex partners. They also suggest that "periodic
prevalence surveys" of chlamydial infection might be
helpful. In a study of 149 pregnant women with lower
genital tract chlamydia, Miller (1998) found that 17 percent had recurrent chlamydial colonization after treatment. Repeat culture in the third trimester would seem
reasonable in women with positive initial cultures or for
those at high risk.

TREATMENT. Currently recommended regimens for
treatment of chlamydial infection in pregnant women
are shown in Table 57–4. Erythromycin base, 500 mg
orally four times a day for 7 days is the primarily recommended regimen during pregnancy. For women who
cannot tolerate erythromycin, the dosage is reduced by

TABLE 57–4. Treatment of *Chlamydia trachomatis* During Pregnancy

Regimens	Dosage
First choice	Erythromycin base, 500 mg orally four times daily for 7 days
	or
	Amoxicillin, 500 mg orally three times daily for 7 days
Alternatives	Erythromycin ethylsuccinate, 800 mg orally four times daily for 7 days
	or
	Erythromycin base, 250 mg orally four times daily for 14 days
	or
	Erythromycin ethylsuccinate, 400 mg orally four times daily for 14 days
	or
	Azithromycin, 1 g orally as a single dose

From the Centers for Disease Control and Prevention (1998b).

half and the duration of therapy doubled. Alternatively, the amoxicillin regimen may be given. In a randomized trial of treatment of *C trachomatis* in pregnancy, Silverman and colleagues (1994) reported cure rates of 82 percent for amoxicillin and 85 percent for erythromycin. Side effects were less frequent with amoxicillin (13 versus 32 percent). In another randomized trial during pregnancy, Wehbeh and colleagues (1998) reported that the cure rate for single-dose azithromycin was 95 percent. Only 7 percent of women receiving azithromycin had significant side effects compared with 39 percent of those given erythromycin. From their review of 11 randomized trials, Brocklehurst and Rooney (2000) concluded that erythromycin and amoxicillin were equally effective. Once again, amoxicillin was far better tolerated.

Erythromycin estolate and tetracyclines should not be used during pregnancy. Sex partners within the prior 30 days should be examined and treated for chlamydial infection.

LYMPHOGRANULOMA VENEREUM

There are several serovars of *C trachomatis* that cause lymphogranuloma venereum (LGV). The primary genital infection is transient and seldom recognized. Inguinal adenitis may follow and at times lead to suppuration. It may be confused with chancroid. Ultimately, the lymphatics of the lower genital tract and perirectal tissues may be involved, with sclerosis and fibrosis, which can cause vulvar elephantiasis and especially severe rectal stricture. Fistula formation involving the rectum, perineum, and vulva also may be quite troublesome.

For treatment during pregnancy, erythromycin, 500 mg four times daily, is given for 21 days (Centers for

Disease Control and Prevention, 1998b). Although data regarding efficacy are scarce, some authorities recommend azithromycin given in multiple doses over 2 to 3 weeks. Some of these infections that we have encountered at Parkland Hospital have been long-standing, and there was little response to multiple antimicrobial regimens that in one case included erythromycin, sulfamethoxazole, tetracycline, and chloramphenicol.

HERPES SIMPLEX VIRUS

Management of pregnancy complicated by maternal herpesvirus genital infection, while much simplified compared with previous recommendations, remains problematic. There are currently no available rapid diagnostic tests that reliably document contemporary infection. Moreover, there are minimal data to estimate risks for the neonate exposed to recurrent maternal infection.

VIROLOGY. Two types of herpes simplex virus (HSV) have been distinguished based on immunological as well as clinical differences. Type 1 is responsible for most nongenital herpetic infections. In adults, however, HSV-1 primary infection involves the genital tract in a third of cases (Langenberg and colleagues, 1999). Type 2 virus is recovered almost exclusively from the genital tract and is transmitted in the great majority of instances by sexual contact. The incidence of antibodies specific for type 2 herpes increases with age and varies considerably with the population studied. It has been estimated that as many as 45 million people in the United States have been diagnosed with genital HSV-2 infection (Centers for Disease Control and Prevention, 1998b). In the absence of antibody, exposure to a sexual partner with active herpetic lesions will in the majority of instances result in clinical disease.

ANTIBODIES. Several assay systems are available commercially and in research settings to detect serum anti-HSV antibody. While there currently is no reliable commercially available assay to differentiate HSV-1 from HSV-2 antibody, premarket testing of at least one assay is ongoing in early 2000. In a national seroepidemiological survey from 1976 to 1994, 25 percent of women had antibody to HSV-2 (Fleming and colleagues, 1997). The risks for type 2 antibody were greatest among black and previously married women. Kulhanjian and colleagues (1992) have proposed that serological screening of couples during pregnancy for HSV-2 antibodies would stimulate the need for sexual precautions if discordancy were found, that is, a seronegative woman with a positive partner.

CLINICAL INFECTION. Symptoms vary depending on whether there has been previous infection. Importantly, prior HSV-1 infection may modify a primary HSV-2 genital infection because of cross-reacting antibodies. According to the American College of Obstetricians and Gynecologists (1999), these HSV-2 infections clinically may be divided into three groups: **Primary infection** indicates no prior antibodies to HSV-1 or HSV-2. **Nonprimary first episode** defines newly acquired HSV-2 infection with preexisting HSV-1 cross-reacting antibodies. **Recurrent infection** is reactivation of prior HSV-2 infection in the presence of antibodies to HSV-2.

PRIMARY INFECTION. Only a third of newly acquired HSV-2 genital infections are symptomatic (Langenberg and colleagues, 1999). Other first episodes are mild or asymptomatic, because of some immunity from cross-reacting antibody from childhood-acquired type 1 infection. With primary infection, the typical incubation period of 3 to 6 days is followed by a papular eruption with itching or tingling which then becomes painful and vesicular, with multiple vulvar and perineal lesions that may coalesce (Fig. 57–4). Inguinal adenopathy may be severe. Transient systemic influenza-like symptoms are common and are presumably caused by viremia. Occasionally, hepatitis, encephalitis, or pneumonia may develop. Frieden and colleagues (1990) reported six cases of maternal encephalitis complicating pregnancy; only two women lived.

The vulvar and perineal vesicles are traumatized easily, eventually ulcerate, but usually do not become secondarily infected. Vulvar lesions are likely to be extremely painful and may cause considerable debility. Urinary retention may develop because of the pain induced by micturition or because of sacral nerve involvement. In 2 to 4 weeks, all signs and symptoms of infection

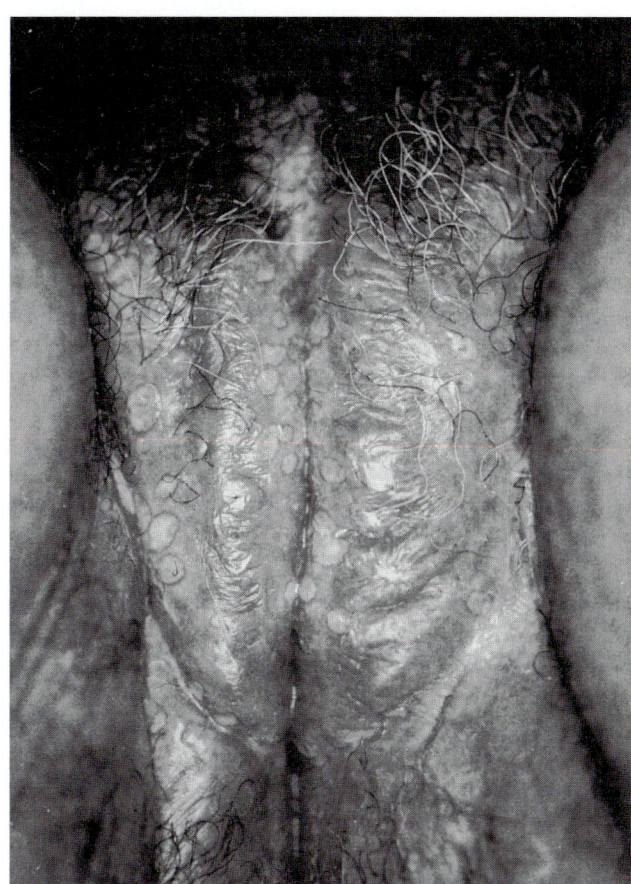

FIGURE 57–4. First-episode primary genital herpes simplex virus infection. (From Wendel and Cunningham, 1991.)

disappear. Cervical involvement is common and may be inapparent clinically. Some cases are severe enough as to require hospitalization.

NONPRIMARY FIRST EPISODE. In some women, there is not full protection from previously existing HSV-1 antibody. These cases may present as a first clinical infection that does not behave like the primary infection described earlier. In general, these infections are characterized by fewer lesions, less systemic manifestations, less pain, and briefer duration of lesion and viral shedding. In some cases, it may be impossible to differentiate clinically between the two types of first infection. Serological diagnosis is possible but of little clinical benefit.

RECURRENT INFECTIONS. During the latency period in which viral particles reside in nerve ganglia, reactivation is common and mediated through variable but poorly understood stimuli. Reactivation is termed recurrent infection and results in herpesvirus shedding. Most recurrent genital herpes is caused by type 2 virus (Centers for Disease Control and Prevention, 1998b). These lesions generally are fewer in number, less tender, and shed virus for shorter periods (2 to 5 days) than those of primary infection. Typically they recur at the same sites. Although commonly involved in primary disease, cervical involvement is less frequent with recurrent infections (Brown and colleagues, 1985).

In a study of 110 women with genital herpes infection, Wald and associates (1995) reported that 55 percent had subclinical shedding of HSV-2 at some time during a mean follow-up of 105 days. Subclinical shedding lasted for a mean of 1.5 days. Subclinical shedding often followed symptomatic recurrence, was more frequent in women with frequent symptomatic recurrences, and accounted for approximately a third of the total days of reactivation of infection. Wald and colleagues (2000) more recently reported that HSV-2 seropositive patients with no history of lesions had subclinical shedding in 3 percent of cases compared with 2.7 percent in seropositive individuals with a history of lesions. Undoubtedly, such subclinical shedding of virus is responsible for many sexually transmitted cases to partners who are seronegative (American College of Obstetricians and Gynecologists, 1999).

DIAGNOSIS. Recovery of virus by *tissue culture* is most optimal for confirmation of clinically apparent infection and asymptomatic recurrences. The sensitivity of culture is nearly 95 percent before the lesions undergo crusting. There are virtually no false positives. With symptomatic recurrences, about half of the cultures will be positive after 48 hours.

Cytological examination after alcohol fixation and Papanicolaou staining—the *Tzanck smear*—has a maximum sensitivity of 70 percent. False-positive cervical smears may be due to cytomegalovirus infection, which is common. The *polymerase chain reaction* has been prospectively studied as a method of detection of genital herpes DNA. Cone and associates (1994) found that the frequency of newborn exposure to herpesvirus secretions from seropositive mothers was almost eight times higher when polymerase chain reaction was used to identify viral DNA compared with culture techniques.

TREATMENT. Antiviral therapy with acyclovir, famciclovir, and valacyclovir has been utilized for treatment of first-episode genital herpes in nonpregnant women. Suppressive therapy with these agents has also been utilized for treatment of recurrent infections. Oral or parenteral preparations attenuate clinical infection as well as the duration of viral shedding. Valacyclovir results in higher plasma acyclovir levels than acyclovir when given in late pregnancy (Kimberlin and colleagues, 1998). For intense discomfort, analgesics and topical anesthetics may provide some relief, and severe

urinary retention is treated with an indwelling bladder catheter.

Acyclovir appears to be safe for use in pregnant women. The manufacturer of acyclovir and valacyclovir, in cooperation with the Centers for Disease Control and Prevention, maintains a registry for exposure to these drugs during pregnancy (1.888.825.5249). More than 700 infants have been exposed to acyclovir during the first trimester, and there does not appear to be an increase in adverse fetal or neonatal effects (Scott, 1999).

Many women with *HIV infection* also have genital herpes, and treatment failures with recommended doses of acyclovir have been reported. Higher dosages of acyclovir may be beneficial for immunoincompetent women with HIV infection and severe recurrent genital herpes (Stone and Whitington, 1990).

RECURRENT INFECTION. Other than suppression, acyclovir is of little benefit in recurrent genital herpes. It has been evaluated as suppressive therapy during pregnancy to prevent recurrences near term. Scott and associates (1996) randomized 46 women who had earlier first-episode infection to acyclovir (400 mg orally three times daily) or placebo beginning at 36 weeks. None of the 21 women given acyclovir compared with 9 of 25 (36 percent) given placebo had recurrent herpes at delivery. The incidence of asymptomatic viral shedding was not increased with acyclovir. Thus, prophylactic acyclovir treatment may decrease the frequency of cesarean delivery in women with recurrent herpes. In a randomized study of 63 pregnant women with recurrent genital herpes, Brocklehurst and associates (1998) reported that suppressive acyclovir significantly reduced the number of clinical recurrences but not the cesarean delivery rate. Scott and Alexander (1998) reported that acyclovir suppression in late pregnancy was cost effective. Suppressive therapy given orally reduces the signs and symptoms of recurrent infection but does not completely eliminate asymptomatic viral shedding (Brocklehurst and colleagues, 1998; Haddad and associates, 1993).

In the pharmacokinetics study by Kimberlin and colleagues (1998), acyclovir was concentrated in the amnionic fluid but there was no evidence of preferential fetal drug accumulation. The drug readily crosses the placenta by passive transfer (Gilstrap and colleagues, 1994; Henderson and associates, 1993).

CLINICAL COURSE DURING PREGNANCY. Approximately 80 percent of young women with recently acquired genital herpes infection will have an average of 2 to 4 **symptomatic** recurrences during pregnancy (Brown, 1985; Harger, 1989; Vontver, 1982, and their colleagues). Concomitant cervical shedding is identified in about 15 percent of women with clinically evident vulvar recurrences.

Brown (1985) and Arvin (1986) and their co-workers found that about 10 percent of the recurrences in pregnancy will be **asymptomatic,** and these more frequently involve the perineum rather than the cervix. The incidence of positive cultures at any time during pregnancy or at delivery for nonpregnant women who had herpes is only 1 to 2 percent. Although clinical recurrences appear to be slightly more common in late pregnancy, asymptomatic cervical shedding of herpesvirus is unaffected by the duration of pregnancy. Additionally, **remote recurrences**—those on the buttocks, back, thigh, and anus—have low rates of concomitant cervical virus shedding, and this allows consideration for vaginal delivery (Harger and colleagues, 1989; Wittek and co-workers, 1984).

VIRUS SHEDDING AT DELIVERY. The reported prevalence rates for isolation of genital tract herpesvirus vary considerably depending on the population studied, but equally important is whether women were included (or excluded) because of prior symptomatic infection. Prober and colleagues (1988) obtained specimens for culture from mothers and infants at the time of nearly 7000 deliveries without regard to the maternal history of genital herpes. Only 14 (0.2 percent) were positive for herpesvirus, and 12 of these women had recurrent infections. In a similar study, Brown and associates (1991) cultured nearly 16,000 women in early labor. Only 56 (0.35 percent) were positive, and a third of these had serological evidence for a recently acquired but subclinical first infection. Although a third of these infants developed neonatal infection, only 1 of 34 infants became infected when born to women with recurrent infection.

Cone and associates (1994), in a prospective study of 100 asymptomatic women with a negative culture, reported that herpes simplex virus was identified in nine women using polymerase chain reaction. None of the neonates born to these women manifested herpes infection. They concluded that newborn exposure to herpesvirus during labor and delivery in seropositive women is more frequent than previously thought.

FETAL AND NEONATAL DISEASE. First-episode infection in early pregnancy is probably not associated with an increased rate of spontaneous abortion. Fagnant and Monif (1989) reviewed the literature and described 15 cases of congenital herpetic infection acquired during early pregnancy. Brown and Baker (1989) found that late-pregnancy primary infection results in an increased incidence of preterm labor.

Infection is transmitted only rarely across the placenta or intact membranes. The fetus almost always becomes infected by virus shed from the cervix or lower genital tract. The virus either invades the uterus following membrane rupture or contacts the fetus at delivery. Newborn infection has three forms:

1. Disseminated, with involvement of major viscera (Fig. 57–5).
2. Localized, with involvement confined to the central nervous system, eyes, skin, or mucosa.
3. Asymptomatic.

Nearly half of infected neonates are preterm, and their risk of infection correlates with whether there is primary or recurrent maternal infection. Nahmias and colleagues (1971) reported a 50 percent risk of neonatal infection with primary maternal infection, but only 4 to 5 percent with recurrent infection. Prober and associates (1987) reported that none of 34 neonates exposed to recurrent viral shedding at delivery became infected. This is thought to be due to a smaller viral load in maternal secretions with recurrent infection. It also likely is related to transplacentally acquired antibody, which decreases the incidence and severity of neonatal disease.

Localized infection is usually associated with a good outcome. Conversely, even with treatment with acyclovir or vidarabine, disseminated neonatal infection is associated with a mortality rate of at least 60 percent (Whitley and colleagues, 1991). Importantly, serious ophthalmic and central nervous system damage has been identified in at least half of survivors.

ANTEPARTUM MANAGEMENT. Because of the severity of neonatal infection, cesarean delivery has been used

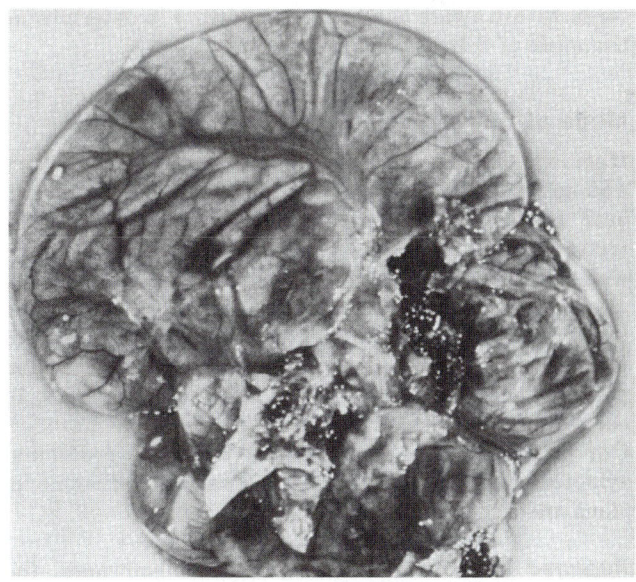

FIGURE 57–5. Cross-section showing necrotic brain tissue in a newborn infant who died from disseminated herpesvirus infection.

widely in instances when genital herpetic lesions are suspected. The premise that all neonatal infections can be avoided by carefully screening the obstetrical population has not been proven correct. As discussed earlier, a number of asymptomatic women will secrete virus at the time of delivery. While most have asymptomatic recurrent infection with correspondingly low virulence, some have nonprimary, first-episode infection without HSV-2 antibody. It seems reasonable to give acyclovir or valacyclovir suppressive therapy beginning at 36 weeks in women who have had herpetic lesions during pregnancy. Virological monitoring is not recommended.

According to the American College of Obstetricians and Gynecologists (1999), cesarean delivery is indicated in women with an active genital lesion or in those with a typical prodrome of an impending outbreak. Thus, cesarean delivery is performed only if primary or recurrent lesions are visualized near the time of labor or when the membranes are ruptured. Roberts and colleagues (1995) reported a decrease in the cesarean section rate in women with herpes during pregnancy from 59 percent to 37 percent after adoption of the 1988 guidelines of American College of Obstetricians and Gynecologists, which succinctly stated is, "no lesions, no cesarean."

RUPTURED MEMBRANES. In the absence of previous examination or instrumentation, there is no evidence that external lesions cause ascending membrane and fetal infection in the presence of ruptured membranes. The recommendation is to disregard the duration of membrane rupture in formulating a plan of delivery for women with perineal lesions. Unless there are other contradictory factors—for example, gross immaturity— then cesarean delivery is performed.

CARE OF THE NEONATE. An exposed infant of a mother known or suspected of having genital herpes should be isolated and cultures taken for herpes. It is not necessary to separate baby and mother when the mother has herpetic lesions. Instead, she is instructed in hand washing and to avoid any contact between her lesions, her hands, and the baby. Breast feeding is allowed under these conditions. Family members with oral herpetic lesions should avoid kissing the newborn and should use careful hand-washing techniques.

ACQUIRED IMMUNODEFICIENCY SYNDROME

Acquired immunodeficiency syndrome (AIDS) was first described in 1981 when a cluster of patients was found to have defective cellular immunity and *Pneumocystis carinii* pneumonia. Infections in women are increasing overall, and the proportion of women and adolescent girls tripled from 7 to 23 percent from 1985 to 1998. Since that time, worldwide prevalence of this devastating disease has progressed almost geometrically. In the United States through 1998, Fauci (1999) quotes estimates of 650,000 to 900,000 infected individuals and almost a half million deaths. By 1994, death caused by HIV infection became the leading cause of death in persons aged 25 to 44 years (Fig. 57–6). As expected, perinatally acquired infection has also increased. Through 1993, the Centers for Disease Control and Prevention (1997b) estimated that 15,000 HIV-infected children were born to HIV-positive women in the United States.

Black women have a disparately increased infection rate, and in 1997, it was estimated that 1 in 160 African-American women were infected. In 1997 there were more cases of AIDS in African-American men and women in the United States than any other racial/ethnic group (Centers for Disease Control and Prevention, 1998d). Haverkos and colleagues (1999) reported the

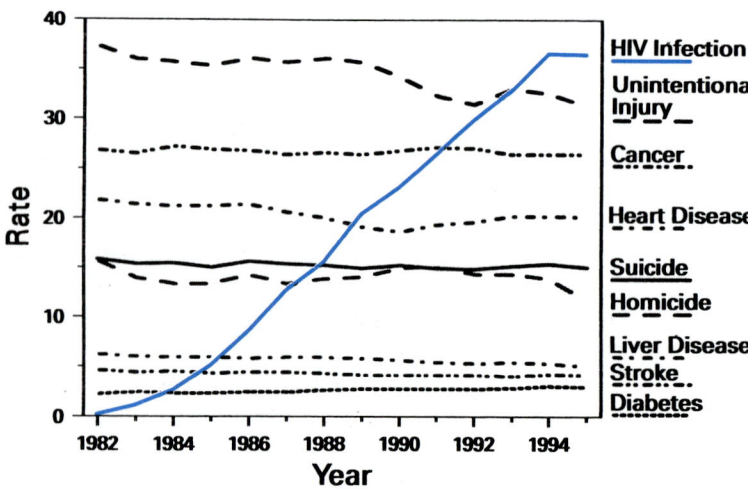

FIGURE 57–6. Death rates per 100,000 population for leading causes of death in persons aged 25 to 44 years in the United States through 1995. (From Centers for Disease Control and Prevention, 1997c.)

relative risk for AIDS was 4.7 for African Americans compared with 1.0 for whites, 3.0 for Hispanics, 0.5 for Native Americans, and 0.4 for Asian/Pacific Islanders.

ETIOLOGY. Causative agents of the immunodeficiency syndrome are DNA retroviruses termed **human immunodeficiency viruses,** HIV-1 and HIV-2. Most cases worldwide in 1992 were caused by HIV-1 infection. While HIV-2 infection is endemic in West Africa, it is uncommon in the United States. Currently, the Centers for Disease Control and Prevention (1998b) does not recommend routine testing for HIV-2 except in blood donors and persons exposed to high-risk practices in HIV-2 endemic countries.

Retroviruses have genomes that encode *reverse transcriptase,* which allows DNA to be transcribed from RNA. The virus thus can make DNA copies of its own genome in host cells. Transmission is similar to hepatitis B virus, and sexual intercourse, especially among male homosexuals, is the major mode of transmission. The virus also is transmitted by blood or blood-contaminated products, and mothers may infect their infants.

The Centers for Disease Control and Prevention (1996a) reported that in 1994, women accounted for the most rapid increases in the number of cases. About half of cases among women are secondary to injected-drug use and a third are attributed to heterosexual contact. Chirgwin and associates (1999) found that two significant risk factors were nonparenteral drug use and anal intercourse. The pregnancy rate for this group was 55 per 100 person-years of follow-up. In a seven-city study of HIV seroconversions among patients attending sexually transmitted disease clinics, Weinstock and colleagues (1998) reported that most infections are now transmitted heterosexually and are associated with drug use. There is also an increasing proportion of children with perinatally acquired AIDS born to women with heterosexually acquired infection. In 1994, The Centers for Disease Control (1994a) estimated a prevalence of HIV seropositivity among childbearing women in 1992 to be 1 to 2 per 1000.

PATHOGENESIS. The common denominator of clinical illness with AIDS is profound immunosuppression, principally of cell-mediated immunity, which gives rise to a variety of opportunistic infections and neoplasms. Thymus-derived lymphocytes—*T lymphocytes*—defined phenotypically by the CD4 surface antigen, are the principal targets. The CD4 site serves as a receptor for the virus. Co-receptors are necessary for infection, and two chemokine receptors—CCR5 and CXCR4—have been identified to fill this role (Kahn and Walker, 1998). After attachment, the virus is internalized and uses *reverse transcriptase* to transcribe its genomic RNA and DNA.

Viral DNA thus is integrated into cellular DNA for the life of the cell, which is shortened by infection. At the same time, viremia can be detected and quantified using the viral-RNA assay. After initial infection, the level of viremia usually decreases to a *set-point,* and patients with the highest viral burden progress more rapidly to AIDS and death (Kahn and Walker, 1998). After infection, over time the number of T cells drops insidiously and progressively, resulting eventually in profound immunosuppression. Monocyte-macrophages may also be infected, and microglial brain cell infection may cause neuropsychiatric abnormalities. HIV-infected persons also have an increased incidence of neoplasms, notably Kaposi sarcoma, B-cell and non-Hodgkin lymphomas, and some carcinomas.

CLINICAL MANIFESTATIONS. The incubation period from exposure to clinical disease is usually within days to weeks. Figure 57–7 illustrates the natural history of HIV-1 infection. Acute illness is similar to many other viral syndromes and usually lasts less than 10 days. Common symptoms include fever and night sweats, fatigue, rash, headache, lymphadenopathy, pharyngitis, myalgias, arthralgias, nausea, vomiting, and diarrhea (Kahn and Walker, 1998). After symptoms abate, the set-point of chronic viremia begins. Stimuli that cause further progression from asymptomatic viremia to the immunodeficiency syndrome are presently unclear, but the median time is about 10 years (Fauci and Lane, 1994).

When HIV-positivity is associated with any number of clinical findings, then AIDS is diagnosed. Generalized lymphadenopathy, oral hairy leukoplakia, aphthous ulcers, and thrombocytopenia are common. A number of opportunistic infections that may herald AIDS include esophageal or pulmonary candidiasis, persistent herpes simplex or zoster, condyloma acuminata, tuberculosis, cytomegalovirus, molluscum contagiosum, pneumocystis, toxoplasmosis, and others. Neurological disease is common, and about half of patients have central nervous system symptoms. A CD4+ count of less than $200/\mu L$ is also considered definitive for the diagnosis of AIDS.

SEROLOGICAL TESTING. The enzyme immunoassay assay (EIA) is used as a screening test for HIV antibodies. A positive screening test has a sensitivity of over 99.5 percent. A positive test is confirmed with either the Western blot or immunofluorescence assay (IFA). Although highly specific, the Western blot is less sensitive than immunoassay because more antibody is required for a positive result. Thus, immunofluorescence assay can be used to resolve an EIA-positive, Western blot-indeterminate sample. According to the Centers for Disease Control and Prevention (1998b), antibody can be detected in 95 percent of patients within 6 months

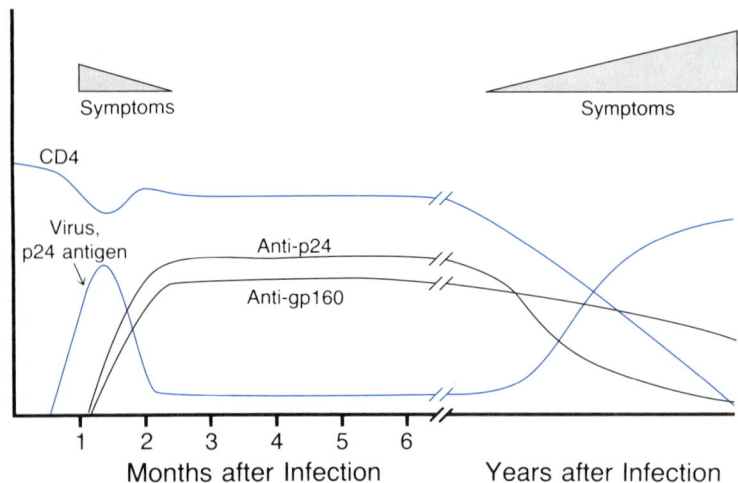

FIGURE 57–7. Schematic model of the natural history of HIV-1 infection. (From Clark and colleagues, 1991, with permission.)

of infection, and thus, antibody serotesting does not exclude earlier infection. For acute primary HIV infection, identification of viral p24 core antigen or viral RNA is necessary.

False-positive confirmatory results are rare, and in one study of almost 300,000 blood donors, no false-positive Western blot results were detected by using viral culture (Centers for Disease Control and Prevention, 1995). An indeterminate Western blot test can result from factors that include:

1. Recently infected individuals who are seroconverting.
2. End-stage HIV disease.
3. Perinatally exposed infants who are seroconverting.
4. Nonspecific reactions of uninfected current or past pregnant women.

SCREENING. There is disagreement as to who should be screened, and more importantly, how positive results should be managed. Certainly it is reasonable to test all blood products, and this has been done since mid-1983. Lackritz and associates (1995) reported that the risk of HIV transmission was one case for every 450,000 to 660,000 donations of screened blood. In 1992, the Food and Drug Administration mandated HIV-2 testing for all blood donors.

In 1991, the Institute of Medicine recommended universal, but voluntary, prenatal screening. The Centers for Disease Control and Prevention (1998b) as well as the American Academy of Pediatrics and the American College of Obstetricians and Gynecologists (1997) also recommend this approach. Ecker (1996) calculated that such testing was cost-effective in pregnant populations with an HIV prevalence exceeding 9 per 1000. Patrick and colleagues (1998), however, in a retrospective study

done in British Columbia, concluded that prenatal screening was cost-effective even in a low-prevalence setting.

Grimes and associates (1999) recently reviewed legal considerations of HIV screening for pregnant women. They concluded that the best way to avoid liability is to offer HIV testing to all and to document such counseling. For women who initially decline testing, they recommend offering testing at each visit, and documenting such counseling.

MATERNAL AND FETUS-INFANT INFECTION. To determine maternal HIV seroprevalence, Gwinn and colleagues (1991) tested nearly 2 million newborns from 38 states born in 1988 and 1989. They estimated that 1.5 women per 1000 were infected nationwide; for New York City it was 5.8 per 1000; and for the District of Columbia it was 5.5 per 1000. Lindsay and associates (1991) showed that inner-city prenatal patients in Atlanta were more likely seropositive if they had not registered for prenatal care. Importantly, although in all of these studies women were from an inner-city minority population, only half were considered at high risk. These studies underpin recommendations that serological testing and counseling be offered to all pregnant women.

It is now well established that mother-to-infant transmission accounts for most HIV infections among children. Transplacental transmission can occur early, and the virus has been identified in early pregnancies terminated by elective abortion (Lewis and co-workers, 1990). In most cases, however, transmission occurs at birth, and 15 to 25 percent of infants born to untreated HIV-infected mothers will be infected (Centers for Disease Control and Prevention, 1998b).

Vertical transmission is more common in preterm

births, especially those associated with prolonged membrane rupture. Analyzing data from the Perinatal AIDS Collaborative Transmission Study, Kuhn and colleagues (1999) reported a 3.7 relative risk for intrapartum HIV transmission with preterm delivery. Landesman and associates (1996) reported that HIV-1 transmission at birth was increased from 14 to 25 percent in women whose membranes were ruptured for more than 4 hours. Concurrent syphilis infection is also strongly associated with vertical perinatal HIV transmission (Lee and colleagues, 1998). Finally, there is evidence that breast feeding increases postnatal HIV-1 transmission by 10 to 20 percent (Dunn and colleagues, 1992). In a randomized clinical trial from Kenya, Nduati and associates (2000) reported a 16 percent transmission from breast feeding.

During the past several years, it has been found that perinatal HIV transmission can be most accurately correlated with measurement of plasma viral-RNA burden (Dickover and associates, 1996). As shown in Figure 57–8, in two studies, neonatal infection is around 5 percent with less than 1000 copies/mL and over 40 percent with levels greater than 100,000 copies/mL. Mofenson and colleagues (1999) reported findings from 480 pregnancies studied by the Pediatric AIDS Clinical Trials Group. Using multivariate analysis, they found that plasma HIV-1 RNA level was the best predictor of risk for perinatal transmission. Importantly, zidovudine therapy that reduced these levels to below 500 copies/mL minimized the risk. They also observed that infusions of HIV-1 hyperimmune globulin did not alter the risk of transmission.

Many women who are delivered of infants who subsequently develop AIDS were asymptomatic during pregnancy. According to the Centers for Disease Control and Prevention (1998b), maternal morbidity and mortality are not increased by pregnancy in seropositive but otherwise asymptomatic women. Conversely, adverse fetal outcomes may be increased with maternal HIV infection. For example, in a review of 634 women who delivered after 24 weeks, Stratton and colleagues (1999) reported that adverse pregnancy outcomes are common in HIV-infected women and are associated with CD4 proportion of less than 14 percent. The rate of preterm birth was 20 percent, and fetal growth restriction was identified in 24 percent. Langston and associates (1995) reported increased stillbirths with maternal HIV infection.

MANAGEMENT DURING PREGNANCY. Counseling is mandatory for the HIV-positive woman. This is preferable early in pregnancy, and if she chooses to continue pregnancy, ongoing counseling for psychological support is important. The evolution of management during pregnancy has followed advances made in treatment of nonpregnant persons with HIV infection. Current standards dictate that the pregnant woman and her fetus are entitled to the most efficacious therapy available. Because of the devastating consequences of this infection if untreated, a shift has occured from an exclusive focus on fetal protection to a more balanced approach to treatment of mother and fetus (Kass and co-workers, 2000).

In just a short time, major advances in HIV therapy have been made. A number of investigations have shown that a combination of **nucleoside analogs**—zidovudine, didanosine, zalcitabine, or lamivudine—given along with a **protease inhibitor**—indinavir, rito-

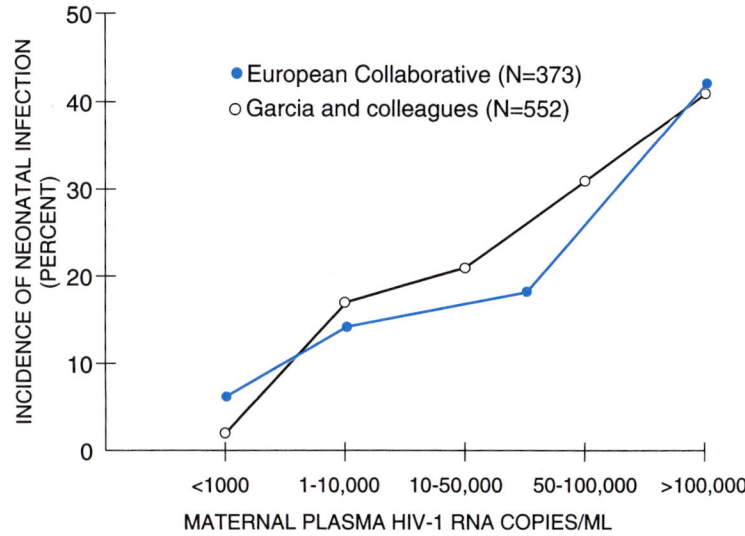

FIGURE 57–8. Incidence of perinatal human immunodeficiency infection plotted against maternal plasma HIV-1 RNA levels in 925 neonates. (Data are from the European Collaborative Study, 1999, and Garcia and colleagues, 1999.)

navir, or saquinavir—is highly effective in suppressing HIV-RNA levels (Carpenter and associates, 1996). Short-term survival is improved and morbidity is reduced in asymptomatic HIV-infected patients given triple chemotherapy (Cameron, 1998; Collier, 1996; Gulick, 1997; Hammer, 1997; Hogg, 1999; Montaner, 1998, and their colleagues). Triple chemotherapy in 2001 is standard first-line therapy for nonpregnant adults in the United States.

Although multidrug regimens are efficacious for treatment of HIV-infected patients, there are few studies regarding their use during pregnancy. Considering the high mortality and morbidity associated with this disease, however, the Centers for Disease Control and Prevention (1998d) recommends that combination antiretroviral therapy be offered to pregnant women. These guidelines were updated for the United States Public Health Service by the Perinatal HIV Guidelines Working Group (2000, 2001). They undoubtedly will be updated frequently to keep pace with use of new antiretroviral drugs.

The earliest studies documented the efficacy of perinatal zidovudine in decreasing HIV transmission (Connor and colleagues, 1994). Although having no known maternal advantages, the Protocol 076 regimen decreased perinatal infection from 25 to 8 percent. Regimens now known to have maternal benefits have been combined with zidovudine prophylaxis intrapartum and are shown in Table 57–5.

The Working Group recommends measurement of CD4+ T-lymphocyte counts and HIV-1 RNA levels approximately each trimester, or about every 3 to 4 months. These are used to make decisions to begin antiretroviral therapy, to alter therapy, to decide route of delivery, or to begin prophylaxis for *Pneumocystis carinii* pneumonia.

TABLE 57–5. Antiretroviral Therapy Regimens

Timing	Regimens

Antepartum—combination therapy with two nucleoside analog reverse transcriptase inhibitors plus either a non-nucleoside analog or a protease inhibitor.
   The regimen should include:
 	
   Zidovudine, 100 mg five times daily, beginning at 14–34 wk and continued throughout pregnancy
 	
               plus
Another nucleoside analog and either a non-nucleoside analog or a protease inhibitor
	Nucleoside analogs
	   Zidovudine (ZDU)
	   Zalcitabine
	   Didanosine
	   Stavudine
	   Lamivudine (3TC)
	   Abacavir
	
	Non-nucleoside analogs
	   Nevirapine
	   Delavirdine
	   Efavirenz
	Protease inhibitors
	   Indinavir
	   Ritonavir
	   Saquinavir
	   Nelfinavir
	   Amprenavir

Intrapartum—chemoprophylaxis
   1. Woman has taken above regimen(s) during pregnancy
 	
   2. No prior therapy
	
	Zidovudine, 2 mg/kg given intravenously over 1 hour, followed by continuous infusion of 1 mg/kg/hr until delivery
	Nevirapine, single dose and another dose for infant at 48 h
	Zidovudine orally plus lamivudine during labor; 1 week ZDU/3TC for newborn
	Zidovudine intravenous regimen plus 6-wk ZDU for newborn
	Nevirapine plus zidovudine regimens

Postpartum—no antiretroviral therapy during pregnancy or intrapartum	Infant: zidovudine 6-week regimen Mother: evaluation for combination therapy

From Perinatal HIV Guidelines Working Group (2000, 2001).

Even with treatment, noninfectious maternal complications are increased in these women and their infants. Lorenzi and colleagues (1998) reported that 29 of 37 (78 percent) pregnant women treated with two reverse transcriptase inhibitors, with or without protease inhibitors, had one or more adverse events. Almost half of their infants (14 of 30) had adverse events and preterm delivery was frequent. At least two follow-up studies of children from the Pediatric AIDS Clinical Trial Group 076 Study found no adverse effects in children at 18 months and up to a mean of 5.6 years after zidovudine exposure (Culnane and associates, 1999; Sperling and colleagues, 1998).

Testing for other sexually transmitted diseases and for tuberculosis is done. Vaccination is given for hepatitis B, influenza, and perhaps pneumococcal infection. If the CD4+ count is below $200/\mu L$, primary prophylaxis for *P carinii* pneumonia is recommended with either sulfamethoxazole-trimethoprim or aerosolized pentamidine. Pneumonia is treated with oral or intravenous sulfamethoxazole-trimethoprim or pentamidine. Other symptomatic opportunistic infections that may develop include toxoplasmosis, herpesvirus infections, and candidiasis.

The Centers for Disease Control and Prevention, and the Infectious Disease Society of America (1999b) have published a symposium on guidelines for prevention of opportunistic infections in persons infected with HIV.

PREVENTION OF TRANSMISSION. Precautions for antepartum, peripartum, and pediatric care of infected mothers and infants are similar to those for hepatitis B, with avoidance of exposure to blood and body fluids. **If heightened awareness of these precautions is reserved for women known to be seropositive, a large number of women with incubating infection or who are asymptomatic but undiagnosed will pose a larger threat to medical personnel.**

The Centers for Disease Control (1987b) emphasize that because medical history and examination cannot identify reliably all patients infected with immunodeficiency virus or other blood-borne pathogens, blood and body-fluid precautions should be used consistently in all patients. These precautions are as follows:

1. All health-care workers who participate in invasive procedures, including surgical or obstetrical procedures, must use appropriate barrier precautions to prevent skin and mucous-membrane contact with blood and other body fluids of all patients. Gloves, surgical masks, and protective eyewear (goggles) must be worn for all invasive procedures that commonly result in the generation of droplets, splashing of blood or other body fluids, or the generation of bone chips. Fluid-resistant gowns or aprons that pro-

vide an effective barrier should be worn during invasive procedures that are likely to result in the splashing of blood or other body fluids. Those who perform or assist in vaginal or cesarean deliveries should wear gloves and gowns when handling the placenta or the infant until blood and amniotic fluid have been removed from the infant's skin, and should wear gloves during care of the cord. Mouth-suction devices for clearing the airway should be avoided.

2. If a glove is torn or there is a needle-stick or other injury, the glove should be removed and a new glove used as promptly as patient safety permits. The needle or instrument involved in the incident also should be removed from the sterile field.

These "universal precautions" were soon followed by "standard precautions," which added a body substance isolation policy. Such substances include:

1. Blood.
2. All body fluids, secretions, and excretions (except sweat) regardless of whether they contain visible blood.
3. Nonintact skin and mucous membranes (Garner, 1996; West and Cohen, 1997).

Somewhat disconcerting is a recent report by Ganguly and Sinnott (1999) involving a survey of 150 medical students and exposure to body fluids. Although most of the students followed universal guidelines, 62 reported 101 exposures to body fluids and nine were with HIV-positive specimens!

For health-care workers exposed significantly to contaminated fluids—for example, a needle-stick injury—postexposure prophylaxis is recommended by the Centers for Disease Control and Prevention (1996b). Treatment is given with zidovudine, 200 mg three times a day, and lamivudine, 150 mg twice a day for 4 weeks. If the source patient has advanced AIDS, a high load of HIV, or has been treated with nucleoside analogs, a protease inhibitor such as indinavir, 800 mg three times daily, is added.

PREVENTION OF VERTICAL TRANSMISSION. The two principal approaches suggested for prevention of maternal–infant transmission of HIV infection are antiretroviral therapy and cesarean delivery. Use of treatment regimens shown in Table 57–5 and discussed earlier will substantively lower vertical transmission of virus (Boucher, 1996; Connor, 1994; Matheson, 1995, and all their colleagues). Mauskopf and colleagues (1996) have calculated that the method is cost-effective.

In a study regarding the efficacy of abbreviated regimens of zidovudine prophylaxis on perinatal transmission, Wade and colleagues (1998) reported that perinatal transmission rate was 6 percent if zidovudine was begun in the prenatal period, 10 percent if given only intrapartum, 9 percent if given to the newborn within the first 48 hours, and 19 percent if started on day 3 or later. Lallemant and co-workers (2000) also confirmed the efficacy of maternal treatment beginning at 28 weeks. Stiehm and colleagues (1999), reporting for the Pediatric AIDS Clinical Trials Group Study 185 Team, found that zidovudine prophylaxis is also highly effective in reducing perinatal transmission in women with advanced disease.

CESAREAN DELIVERY.

In a retrospective study, the European Collaborative Study Group (1994) reported that elective cesarean delivery decreased the risk of vertical transmission by approximately 50 percent. The European Mode of Delivery Collaboration (1999) was a randomized trial of cesarean versus vaginal delivery for HIV-positive women. Of 436 women initially randomized, infection status was available from 370 infants. HIV-infection developed in 3 of 170 newborns (1.8 percent) of mothers assigned cesarean delivery versus 21 of 200 newborns (10.5 percent) of mothers assigned vaginal delivery ($P < .001$). Importantly, when analyzed according to antiretroviral therapy, there was a nonsignificant difference in the rate of transmission in women given zidovudine and comparing cesarean with vaginal delivery (2.1 versus 3.3 percent).

A recent meta-analysis of 15 prospective cohort studies was published by the International Perinatal HIV Group (1999). A total of 8533 mother–infant pairs were available for analysis. Vertical HIV transmission was reduced significantly to less than half when cesarean was compared with other modes of delivery. When antiretroviral therapy was given in the prenatal, intrapartum, and neonatal periods along with cesarean delivery, the likelihood of vertical transmission was reduced by 87 percent compared with other modes of delivery and without antiretroviral therapy.

Based on these findings, as well as others not cited, the American College of Obstetricians and Gynecologists (2000) concluded that scheduled cesarean delivery should be discussed and recommended for HIV-infected women with an HIV-1 RNA load of greater than 1000 copies/mL. This is whether or not antiretroviral therapy is ongoing. Scheduled delivery may be done as early as 38 weeks to lessen the chances of membrane rupture.

Others have expressed concern that morbidity may be significantly increased in HIV-infected women undergoing cesarean delivery. Stringer and colleagues (1999) as well as Star and co-workers (1999) made a plea for restraint regarding routine prophylactic cesarean delivery for prevention of vertical transmission. They concluded that combination antiretroviral therapy may reduce the risk of vertical transmission to as low as 2 percent or less. Indeed, Morris and associates (1999) reported no perinatal transmission in 76 women receiv-

ing highly active antiretroviral therapy (HAART). Our experiences at Parkland Hospital are similar, and perinatal transmission in women taking HAART has been less than 2 percent. Accordingly, prophylactic cesarean delivery would be of benefit for only a small number of treated women.

BREAST FEEDING.

Breast milk increases the risk of neonatal transmission and in general is not recommended in HIV-positive women. Cited previously was the randomized trial from Ghana by Nduati and co-workers (2000). Transmission of HIV-1 infection was found to be 16 percent. It has been estimated that one to two thirds of maternal transmission in breast-fed infants is from breast milk (Van de Perre, 1999). Despite this, in underdeveloped countries, formula feeding may be impractical and associated with increased mortality from diarrheal and respiratory infections (De Cock and colleagues, 2000). The World Health Organization and United Nations Children's Fund (1998) have recommended continuing breast-feeding promotion for women living in settings where infectious diseases and malnutrition are the primary causes of infant deaths, such as in many developing countries.

HUMAN PAPILLOMAVIRUS

Genital papillomavirus infection, either symptomatic or asymptomatic, is common (Hagensee and colleagues, 1999). Of 2597 high-risk pregnant women enrolled in the New Orleans Center of the Vaginal Infections and Prematurity Study, 28 percent were seropositive for HPV-16 capsid antibodies. The most important sequela is development of cervical, vaginal, and vulvar neoplasia, which is discussed in Chapter 55 (p. 1448). Several types of human papillomaviruses (HPV) cause mucocutaneous warts or **condylomata acuminata.** Genital warts, are usually caused by HPV types 6 and 11, but may also be caused by 16, 18, and 30s, 40s, 50s, and 60s groups (Ferenczy, 1995). Cervical intraepithelial neoplasia and cancer risk is highest with 16, 18, 45, and 56, and intermediate with 31, 33, 35, 39, 51, 52, 58, and 66 (American College of Obstetricians and Gynecologists, 1994a). The epidemiology and pathophysiology of condylomata acuminata has been extensively reviewed by the Centers for Disease Control and Prevention (1999c).

Viral types 6 and 11 can cause **laryngeal papillomatosis** in children, and evidence is consistent that in some cases the virus may be transmitted by aspiration of infected material at delivery. The rate of perinatal vital transmission is unclear, but all agree that symptomatic disease in children is rare. For example, Watts and associates (1998) found evidence of virus in only 5.3 percent of specimens from neonatal oral or nasopharyngeal, anal, and genital areas. Tseng and associates (1998), in a study of 301 pregnant women with papillomavirus, reported that the overall transmission for 16/18-type virus was 40 percent (27 of 68 newborns). The rate was significantly higher for those delivered vaginally compared with cesarean deliveries (51 versus 27 percent). Tenti and co-workers (1999) documented a 30 percent transmission rate of virus to the neonatal oropharynx. Importantly, they showed that the virus was cleared by 5 weeks. Manns and collaborators (1999) documented that only 3 percent of infants were seropositive to HPV-16 by 1 to 2 years.

CONDYLOMATA ACUMINATA. For unknown reasons, genital warts frequently increase in number and size during pregnancy, sometimes filling the vagina or covering the perineum, making it difficult to perform vaginal delivery or episiotomy (Fig. 57–9). In women without grossly visible lesions, Snyder and co-workers (1990), but not Goldaber and associates (1993), found an association with papillomavirus infection and episiotomy breakdown. Certainly, the mucorrhea throughout pregnancy offers ideal moist conditions for viral growth. Accelerated viral replication with advancing pregnancy was hypothesized earlier to explain the growth of peri-

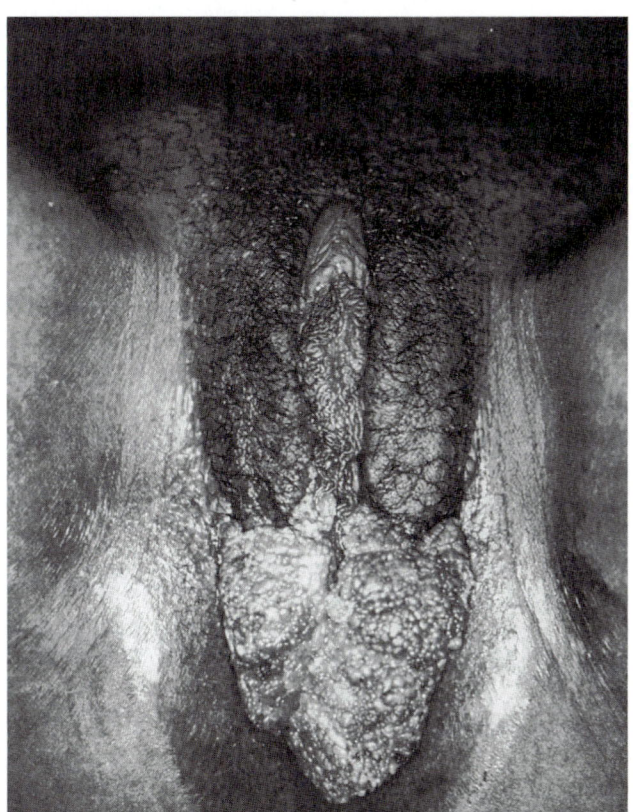

FIGURE 57–9. Extensive vulvar condylomata acuminata in a woman near term. (From Wendel and Cunningham, 1991.)

neal lesions, progression of some to cervical neoplasm, and increased detection of cervical viral DNA in some studies (Gary and Jones, 1985; Rando and co-workers, 1989). More recent data from Fife and colleagues (1999) substantiates this. They studied 232 women and found 31 percent were positive for papillomavirus DNA in the first trimester and 36 percent positive in late pregnancy. In paired samples from 83 women comparing first-trimester viral identification with postpartum specimens, there was a significant decline in positivity from 40 to 27 percent.

Because papillomavirus infection can be subclinical and multifocal, most women with vulvar lesions also have cervical infection, and vice versa (Spitzer and colleagues, 1989). Vulvar lesions often improve rapidly or disappear postpartum, possibly related to loss of either vascularity, excessive moisture, or the alleged immunosuppression of pregnancy.

TREATMENT. While treatment during pregnancy may be very unsatisfactory, it is usual for these lesions to clear rapidly following delivery. During pregnancy, washing of the external genitalia, plus cleansing of the vagina by gentle douching, followed by thorough drying of the external genitalia, performed at least once daily, may inhibit proliferation of the warts as well as minimize discomfort.

Because lesions commonly regress after delivery, it is not always necessary to try to eradicate them during pregnancy. If they produce discomfort, then they are treated. Therapy is directed toward minimizing toxicity to the mother and fetus and debulking the genital warts in the late second or third trimester so that recurrence is less likely prior to delivery. While there are several agents available for use in nonpregnant women, pregnancy limits their use.

Trichloroacetic or **bichloracetic acid,** 80 to 90 percent, applied topically once a week, is an effective regimen for external warts. Some clinicians prefer **cryotherapy** or **laser ablation** of lesions in pregnancy (Bergman and colleagues, 1984; Ferenczy, 1984). Schwartz and associates (1988) reported good results in 31 of 32 women treated with combination laser and 85 percent trichloroacetic acid therapy.

Podophyllin resin, 5-fluorouracil cream, imiquimod cream, and **interferon** therapy should not be used in pregnancy because of concerns about maternal and fetal toxicity (American College of Obstetricians and Gynecologists, 1994a; Centers for Disease Control and Prevention, 1998b).

Occasionally, condylomata acuminata attain enormous size, as shown in Figure 57–9, and these may even necessitate cesarean section. If the woman is seen several weeks before delivery, the large lesions sometimes can be removed by excision, electrocautery, cryosurgery, or laser ablation. Matsunaga and colleagues (1987) reported successful results in 51 women with rather extensive cervical or labial lesions. Enthusiasm has been expressed for use of the carbon-dioxide laser during pregnancy to remove large lesions under anesthesia (Ferenczy, 1984).

NEONATAL INFECTION. An indeterminate, but probably small, number of infants and children born to women with genital papillomavirus lesions will become infected and develop **laryngeal papillomatosis.** In one study, over 44,000 children were followed for 7 years, and there were no cases of laryngeal papillomatosis identified (Shah and colleagues, 1986). When they do develop, these papillomas are usually found on the true vocal cords, and HPV-6 or -11 was identified in 92 percent of 57 cases (Abramson and colleagues, 1987). They are persistent, recurrent, and disfiguring. The question has been posed whether cesarean section might avoid infection of the fetus-infant, but this is not recommended currently (American College of Obstetricians and Gynecologists, 1994a; Centers for Disease Control and Prevention, 1998e). In at least one case, elective repeat cesarean section was done at term; however, the child developed extensive respiratory papillomatosis at 7 months (Shah and associates, 1986). Puranen and associates (1996), in a study of 98 children of infected mothers, found that a third of these children had positive oral scrapings for papillomavirus DNA. One child developed papilloma caused by HPV-16, which was the same type found in the birth canal at delivery.

CHANCROID

Haemophilus ducreyi can cause painful, nonindurated genital ulcers, or soft chancre, at times accompanied by painful inguinal lymphadenopathy. While common in some developing countries, it had become rare in the United States. In 1987, however, its incidence was increased tenfold over the previous 10 years, and drug use and sex-for-drugs were shown to be important risk factors for infection (Schmid and co-workers, 1987). Importantly, the infection is a high-risk cofactor for HIV and syphilis transmission (Centers for Disease Control and Prevention, 1998e).

Diagnosis by culture is difficult because appropriate media is not widely available. Instead, clinical diagnosis is made when typical painful genital ulcer(s) are dark-field negative and herpesvirus tests are negative. Recommended treatment is erythromycin base, 500 mg orally four times daily for 7 days; ceftriaxone, 250 mg in a single intramuscular dose; or azithromycin, 1 g orally as a single dose (Centers for Disease Control and Prevention, 1998b).

TRICHOMONAS INFECTIONS

Trichomonas vaginalis was identified in 13 percent of nearly 14,000 women cultured at midpregnancy by the Vaginal Infections and Prematurity Study Group (Cotch and colleagues, 1991). Race-specific prevalence was 23 percent for blacks, 6.6 percent for Hispanics, and 6.1 percent for white women. Using polymerase chain reaction, Witkin and co-workers (1996) detected trichomonas in 10 percent of 300 prenatal patients. Symptomatic infection is much less common, and vaginitis is characterized by symptoms of a yellow discharge, abnormal odor, and vulvar pruritus. These women usually have a purulent vaginal discharge, vulvovaginal erythema, and *colpitis macularis* or "strawberry cervix."

Trichomonads are demonstrated readily in a wet mount of vaginal secretions as flagellated, ovoid, motile organisms that are somewhat larger than leukocytes. The sensitivity of this technique depends on the concentration of organisms, the degree of dilution, and the experience of the examiner, but is generally considered to be about 85 percent. Trichomonads are identified most accurately by culture using Diamond medium; however, DeMeo and associates (1996) have shown that a DNA probe test was 90 percent sensitive and 99.8 percent specific.

The Vaginal Infections and Prematurity Study Group (Cotch and associates, 1997) used multivariate analysis and reported significant associations between trichomoniasis and preterm prematurely ruptured membranes, preterm delivery, and low-birthweight infants. According to Goldenberg and colleagues (1997), the association of preterm delivery with antepartum colonization with *T vaginalis* is difficult to assess because of commonly associated risk factors. Further prospective investigation is warranted before adopting widespread screening and treatment to eradicate this organism in hope of decreasing its possible deleterious effects on pregnancy outcome.

TREATMENT. Metronidazole, the only trichomonacidal drug available in the United States, is quite effective in eradicating *T vaginalis*. Oral administration is the preferred route. Lossick (1990) reviewed clinical experiences with metronidazole and found that 250 mg given three times daily for 7 days, or 2 g as a single dose, had median cure rates of 92 and 96 percent, respectively. Unfortunately, there are few data regarding efficacy of any regimen in pregnancy. According to the Centers for Disease Control and Prevention (1998b), pregnant women can be treated with a 2-g single dose of oral metronidazole.

Men apparently have transient infection with *T vaginalis*. Although the need for concomitant treatment is uncertain, most investigators have found higher relapse rates in women whose partners were not treated. Lossick (1990) recommends that steady sex partners be treated, and the Centers for Disease Control (1998b) recommends that all partners be treated.

OTHER SEXUALLY TRANSMITTED DISEASES

There are many more infections and infestations that can be acquired as the consequence of sexual intercourse. Among others, these include hepatitis B and C, *Candida vulvovaginitis, scabies,* and *pediculosis pubis.* These infections are discussed elsewhere. Sexual partners at risk of fecal–oral transmission may acquire any of a number of enteric infections.

REFERENCES

Abramson AL, Steinberg BM, Winkler B: Laryngeal papillomatosis: Clinical histopathologic and molecular studies. Laryngoscope 87:678, 1987

Alexander JM, Sheffield JS, Sanchez PJ, Mayfield J, Wendel GD Jr: Efficacy of treatment for syphilis in pregnancy. Obstet Gynecol 93:5, 1999

Alger LS, Lovchik JC, Hebel JR, Blackmon LR, Crenshaw MC: The association of *Chlamydia trachomatis, Neisseria gonorrhoeae,* and group B streptococci with preterm rupture of the membranes and pregnancy outcome. Am J Obstet Gynecol 159:397, 1988

Allaire AD, Huddleston JF, Graves WL, Nathan L: Initial and repeat screening for *Chlamydia trachomatis* during pregnancy. Infect Dis Obstet Gynecol 6:116, 1998

American Academy of Pediatrics and American College of Obstetricians and Gynecologists: Guidelines for Perinatal Care, 4th ed. Washington, DC, AAP and ACOG, 1997, p 218

American College of Obstetricians and Gynecologists: Scheduled cesarean delivery and the prevention of vertical transmission of HIV infection. Committee Opinion No. 234, May 2000

American College of Obstetricians and Gynecologists: Management of herpes in pregnancy. Practice Bulletin No. 8, October 1999

American College of Obstetricians and Gynecologists: Genital human papillomavirus infections. Technical Bulletin No. 193, June 1994a

American College of Obstetricians and Gynecologists: Gonorrhea and chlamydial screening. Technical Bulletin No. 190, March 1994b

Andrews WW, Goldenberg RL, Mercer B, Iams J, Meis P, Moawad A, Das A, VanDorsten JP, Caritis SN, Thurnau G, Miodovnik M, Roberts J, McNillis D, for the National Institute of Child Health and Human Development Maternal-Fetal Medicine Units Network: The Preterm Prediction Study: Association of second-trimester genitourinary chlamydia infection with subsequent spontaneous preterm birth. Am J Obstet Gynecol 183:662, 2000

Andrews WW, Lee H, Toden WJ, Mott CW: Detection of genitourinary tract chlamydia infection in pregnant women by ligase chain reaction assay. Am J Obstet Gynecol 174:410, 1996

Arvin AM, Hensleigh PA, Prober CG, Au DS, Yasukawa LL, Wittek AE, Palumbo PE, Paryani SG, Yeager AS: Failure of antepartum maternal cultures to predict the infant's risk of exposure to herpes simplex virus at delivery. N Engl J Med 315:796, 1986

Barton JR, Thorpe EM Jr, Shaver DC, Hager WD, Sibai BM: Nonimmune hydrops fetalis associated with maternal infection with syphilis. Am J Obstet Gynecol 167:56, 1992

Bataskov KL, Hariharan S, Horowitz MD, Neibart RM, Cox MM: Gonococcal endocarditis complicating pregnancy: A case report and literature review. Obstet Gynecol 78:494, 1991

Bergman A, Bhatia NN, Broen EM: Cryotherapy for treatment of genital condyloma during pregnancy. J Reprod Med 29:432, 1984

Berman SM, Harrison HR, Boyce WT, Haffner WJJ, Lewis M, Arthur JB: Low birth weight, prematurity, and postpartum endometritis. JAMA 257:1189, 1987

Blanco JD, Diaz KC, Lipscomb KA, Bruun D, Gibbs RS: *Chlamydia trachomatis* isolation in patients with endometritis after cesarean section. Am J Obstet Gynecol 152:278, 1985

Boucher M, Lapointe N, Samson J, Fauvel M, Tran T, Hankins C: HIV-1 transmission from mother to child: Analysis of obstetrical, medical, and immunological determinants. Am J Obstet Gynecol 174:411, 1996

Brocklehurst P, Kinghorn G, Carney O, Helsen K, Ross E, Ellis E, Shen R, Cowan F, Mindel A: A randomized placebo controlled trial of suppressive acyclovir in late pregnancy in women with recurrent genital herpes infection. Br J Obstet Gynaecol 105:275, 1998

Brocklehurst P, Rooney G: Intervention for treating genital *Chlamydia trachomatis* infection in pregnancy. Cochrane Database Syst Rev 2:CD000054, 2000

Brown ZA, Baker DA: Acyclovir therapy during pregnancy. Obstet Gynecol 73:526, 1989

Brown ZA, Benedetti J, Ashley R, Burchett S, Selke S, Berry S, Vontver LA, Corey L: Neonatal herpes simplex virus infection in relation to asymptomatic maternal infection at the time of labor. N Engl J Med 324:1247, 1991

Brown ZA, Vontver LA, Benedetti J, Critchlow CW, Hickok DE, Sells CJ, Berry S, Corey L: Genital herpes in pregnancy: Risk factors associated with recurrences and asymptomatic shedding. Am J Obstet Gynecol 153:24, 1985

Burkman RT, Tonascia JA, Atienza MF, King TM: Untreated endocervical gonorrhea and endometritis following elective abortion. Am J Obstet Gynecol 126:648, 1976

Cameron DW, Heath-Chiozzi M, Danner S, Cohen C, Kravcik S, Maurath C, Sun E, Henry D, Rode R, Potthoff A, Leonard J: Randomized placebo-controlled trial of ritonavir in advanced HIV-1 disease. The Advanced HIV Disease Ritonavir Study Group. Lancet 351:543, 1998

Campos-Outcalt D, Ryan K: Prevalence of sexually transmitted diseases in Mexican-American pregnant women by country of birth and length of time in the United States. Sex Trans Dis 22:78, 1995

Carpenter CC, Fischl MA, Hammer SM, Hirsch MS, Jacobsen DM, Katzenstein DA, Montaner JSG, Richman DD, Saag MS, Schooley RT, Thompson MA, Vella S, Yeni PG, Volberding PA: Antiretroviral therapy for HIV infection in 1996. JAMA 276:146, 1996

Centers for Disease Control: National HIV seroprevalence summary: Results through 1992. Atlanta, US Department of Health and Human Services, Public Health Service, CDC, 1994a

Centers for Disease Control: Recommendations of the US

Public Health Service Task Force on the use of zidovudine to reduce perinatal transmission of human immunodeficiency virus. MMWR 43:1, 1994b

Centers for Disease Control: Guidelines for the prevention and control of congenital syphilis. MMWR 37:1, 1988

Centers for Disease Control: Recommendations for prevention of HIV transmission in healthcare settings. MMWR 36:1s, 1987b

Centers for Disease Control and Prevention: Summary of notifiable diseases, United States, 1998. MMWR 48:1, 2000

Centers for Disease Control and Prevention: Congenital syphilis—United States, 1998. MMWR 48:757, 1999a

Centers for Disease Control and Prevention: 1999 USPHS/IDSA guidelines for the prevention of opportunistic infections in persons infected with human immunodeficiency virus. MMWR 48/RR-10:1, 1999b

Centers for Disease Control and Prevention: Prevention of genital HPV infection and sequelae: Report of an external consultants' meeting. Atlanta, Centers for Disease Control and Prevention (CDC), December 1999c

Centers for Disease Control and Prevention: Primary and secondary syphilis—United States, 1998. MMWR 48:873, 1999d

Centers for Disease Control and Prevention: Epidemic of congenital syphilis, Baltimore, 1996–1997. MMWR 47:904, 1998a

Centers for Disease Control and Prevention: 1998 Guidelines for treatment of sexually transmitted diseases. MMWR 47:1, 1998b

Centers for Disease Control and Prevention: Update: Critical need to pay attention to HIV prevention for African Americans. National Center for HIV, STD & TB, Division of HIV/AIDS Prevention, November 13, 1998c

Centers for Disease Control and Prevention: Public Health Service Task Force recommendations for the use of antiretroviral drugs in pregnant women infected with HIV-1 for maternal health and for reducing perinatal HIV-1 transmission in the United States. MMWR 47/RR-2:1, 1998d

Centers for Disease Control and Prevention: Summaries of notifiable diseases in the United States. MMWR 46:61, 1997a

Centers for Disease Control and Prevention: Update: Perinatally acquired HIV/AIDS—United States, 1997. MMWR 46:1086, 1997b

Centers for Disease Control and Prevention: Update: Trends in AIDS incidence, deaths, and prevalence—United States, 1996. MMWR 46:165, 1997c

Centers for Disease Control and Prevention: Update: Mortality attributable to HIV infection among persons age 25–44 years—United States, 1994. MMWR 45:1, 1996a

Centers for Disease Control and Prevention: Update: Provisional public health service recommendations for chemoprophylaxis after occupational exposure to HIV. MMWR 45:468, 1996b

Centers for Disease Control and Prevention: USPHS/Division of STD Prevention: Sexually transmitted disease surveillance. September 1995

Chirgwin KD, Feldman J, Dehovitz JA, Minkoff H, Landesman SH: Incidence and risk factors for heterosexually acquired HIV in an inner-city cohort of women: Temporal association with pregnancy. J Acquir Immune Defic Syndr Hum Retrovirol 20:295, 1999

Chisholm CA, Katz VL, McDonald TL, Bowes WA Jr: Penicillin desensitization in the treatment of syphilis during pregnancy. Am J Perinatol 14:553, 1997

Christmas JT, Wendel GD, Bawdon RE, Farris R, Cartwright G, Little BB: Concomitant infection with *Neisseria gonorrhoeae* and *Chlamydia trachomatis* in pregnancy. Obstet Gynecol 74:295, 1989

Claman P, Toye B, Peeling RW, Jessamine P, Belcher J: Serologic evidence of *Chlamydia trachomatis* infection and risk of preterm birth. Can Med Assoc J 153:259, 1995

Clark SJ, Saag MS, Decker WD, Campbell-Hill S, Roberson JL, Veldkamp PJ, Kappes JC, Hahn BH, Shaw GM: High titers of cytopathic virus in plasma of patients with symptomatic primary HIV-1 infection. N Engl J Med 324:954, 1991

Cohen I, Veille JC, Calkins BM: Improved pregnancy outcome following successful treatment of chlamydial infection. JAMA 263:3160, 1990

Coles FB, Hipp SS, Silberstein GS, Chen JH: Congenital syphilis surveillance in upstate New York, 1989–1992: Implications for prevention and clinical management. J Infect Dis 171:732, 1995

Collier AC, Coombs RW, Schoenfeld DA, Bassett RL, Timpone J, Baruch A, Jones M, Facey K, Whitacre C, McAuliffe VJ, Friedman HM, Merigan TC, Reichman RD, Hooper C, Corey L: Treatment of human immunodeficiency virus infection with saquinavir, zidovudine, and zalcitabine. AIDS Clinical Trials Group. N Engl J Med 334:1011, 1996

Cone RW, Hobson AC, Brown Z, Ashley R, Berry S, Winter C, Corey L: Frequent detection of genital herpes simplex virus DNA by polymerase chain reaction among pregnant women. JAMA 272:792, 1994

Connor EM, Sperling RS, Gelber R, Kiselev P, Scott G, O'Sullivan MJ: Reduction of maternal–infant transmission of human immunodeficiency virus type 1 with zidovudine treatment. N Engl J Med 331:1173, 1994

Conover CS, Rend CA, Miller GB Jr, Schmid GP: Congenital syphilis after treatment of maternal syphilis with a penicillin regimen exceeding CDC guidelines. Infect Dis Obstet Gynecol 6:134, 1998

Cotch MF, Pastorek JG II, Nugent RP, Hillier SL, Gibbs RS, Martin DH, Eschenbach DA, Edelman R, Carey JC, Regan JA, Krohn MA, Klebanoff MA, Rao AV, Rhoads G: *Trichomonas vaginalis* associated with low birth weight and preterm delivery. Sex Transm Dis 24:353, 1997

Cotch MF, Pastorek JG II, Nugent RP, Yerg DE, Martin DH, Eschenbach EA, for the Vaginal Infections and Prematurity Study Group: Demographic and behavioral predictors of *Trichomonas vaginalis* infection among pregnant women. Obstet Gynecol 78:1087, 1991

Crombleholme WR: Neonatal chlamydial infections. Contemp Ob/Gyn 45:76, 2000

Culnane M, Fowler M, Lee SS, McSherry G, Brady M, O'Donnell K, Mofenson L, Gortmaker SL, Shapiro DE, Scott G, Jimenez E, Moore EC, Diaz C, Flynn PM, Cunningham B, Oleske J: Lack of long-term effects of in utero exposure to zidovudine among uninfected children born to HIV-infected women. Pediatric AIDS Clinical Trials Group Protocol 219/076 Teams. JAMA 13:281, 1999

Cunningham FC, Hollier LM: Fetal death. In: Williams Obstetrics, 20th ed. (Suppl 4). Norwalk, CT, Appleton & Lange, August/September 1997

De Cock KM, Fowler MG, Mercier E, de Vincenzi I, Saba J, Hoff E, Alnwick DJ, Rogers M, Shaffer N: Prevention of mother-to-child HIV transmission in resource-poor countries. JAMA 283:1175, 2000

DeMeo LR, Draper DL, McGregor JA, Moore DF, Peter CR, Kapernick PS, McCormack WM: Evaluation of a deoxyribonucleic acid probe for the detection of *Trichomonas vaginalis* in vaginal secretions. Am J Obstet Gynecol 174:1339, 1996

Dickover RE, Garratty EM, Herman SA, Sim MS, Plaeger S, Boyer PJ, Keller M, Deveikis A, Stiehm ER, Bryson YJ: Identification of levels of maternal HIV-1 RNA associated with risk of perinatal transmission. JAMA 275:599, 1996

Dunn DT, Newell ML, Ades AE, Peckham CS: Risk of human immunodeficiency virus type 1 transmission through breast-feeding. Lancet 340:585, 1992

Ecker JL: The cost-effectiveness of human immunodeficiency virus screening in pregnancy. Am J Obstet Gynecol 174:716, 1996

Ehret JM, Judson FN: Quinolone-resistant *Neisseria gonorrhoeae:* the beginning of the end? Report of quinolone-resistant isolates and surveillance in the southwestern United States, 1989 to 1997. Sex Transm Dis 25:522, 1998

Erdem G, Schleiss MR: Gonococcal bacteremia in a neonate. Clin Pediatr 39:43, 2000

European Collaborative Study: Maternal viral load and vertical transmission of HIV-1: An important factor but not the only one. AIDS 13:1377, 1999

European Collaborative Study: Cesarean section and risk of vertical transmission on HIV-1 infection. Lancet 343:1464, 1994

European Mode of Delivery Collaboration: Elective caesarean-section versus vaginal delivery in prevention of vertical HIV-1 transmission: A randomized clinical trial. Lancet 353:1035, 1999

Fagnant RJ, Monif GRG: How rare is congenital herpes simplex? A literature review. J Reprod Med 34:417, 1989

Fauci AS: The AIDS epidemic: Considerations for the 21st century. N Engl J Med 341:1046, 1999

Fauci AS, Lane HC: Human immunodeficiency virus (HIV) disease: AIDS and related disorders. In Isselbacher KJ, Braunwald E, Wilson JD, Martin JB, Fauci AS, Kasper DL (eds): Harrison's Principles of Internal Medicine, 13th ed. New York, McGraw-Hill, 1994, p 1566

Fenton LJ, Light IJ: Congenital syphilis after maternal treatment with erythromycin. Obstet Gynecol 47:492, 1976

Ferenczy A: Epidemiology and clinical pathophysiology of condylomata acuminata. Am J Obstet Gynecol 172:1331, 1995

Ferenczy A: Treating genital condyloma during pregnancy with the carbon dioxide laser. Am J Obstet Gynecol 148:9, 1984

Fife KH, Katz BP, Brizendine EJ, Brown DR: Cervical human papillomavirus deoxyribonucleic acid persists throughout pregnancy and decreases in the postpartum period. Am J Obstet Gynecol 180:1110, 1999

Fiumara NJ, Fleming WL, Downing JG, Good FL: The incidence of prenatal syphilis at the Boston City Hospital. N Engl J Med 247:48, 1952

Fleming DT, McQuillan GM, Johnson RE, Nahmias AJ, Aral SO, Lee FK, St. Louis ME: Herpes simplex virus type 2 in the United States, 1976 to 1994. N Engl J Med 337:1105, 1997

Frieden FJ, Ordorica SA, Goodgold AL, Hoskins IA, Silverman F, Young BK: Successful pregnancy with isolated herpes simplex virus encephalitis: Case report and review of the literature. Obstet Gynecol 75:511, 1990

Ganguly R, Holt DA, Sinnott JT: Exposure of medical students to body fluids. J Am Coll Health 47:207, 1999

Garcia PM, Kalish LA, Pitt J, Minkoff H, Quinn TC, Burchett SK, Kornegay J, Jackson B, Moye J, Hanson C, Zorrilla C, Lew JF: Maternal levels of plasma human immunodefi-

ciency virus type 1 RNA and the risk of perinatal transmission. N Engl J Med 341:394, 1999

Garner JS: Guideline for isolation precautions in hospitals. The Hospital Infection Control Practices Advisory Committee. Infect Control Hosp Epidemiol 17:53, 1996

Gary R, Jones R: Relationship between cervical condylomata, pregnancy and subclinical papillomavirus infection. J Reprod Med 30:393, 1985

Gibbs RS, Schachter J: Chlamydial serology in patients with intra-amniotic infection and controls. Sex Trans Dis 14:213, 1987

Gilstrap LC, Bawdon RE, Roberts SW, Sobhi S: The transfer of the nucleoside analog ganciclovir across the perfused human placenta. Am J Obstet Gynecol 170:967, 1994

Gilstrap LC, Wendel GD Jr: Syphilis in pregnancy. Contemp Obstet Gynecol 44:96, 1999

Goldaber KG, Wendel PJ, McIntire DD, Wendel GD Jr: Postpartum perineal morbidity after fourth degree perineal repair. Am J Obstet Gynecol 168:489, 1993

Goldenberg RL, Andrews WW, Yuan AC, MacKay HT, St. Louis ME: Sexually transmitted disease and adverse outcomes of pregnancy. Clin Perinatol 24:23, 1997

Gravett MG, Nelson HP, DeRouen T, Critchlow C, Eschenbach DA, Holmes KK: Independent associations of bacterial vaginosis and *Chlamydia trachomatis* infection with adverse pregnancy outcome. JAMA 256:1899, 1986

Grimes RM, Richards EP, Helfgott AW, Eriksen NL: Legal considerations in screening pregnant women for human immunodeficiency virus. Am J Obstet Gynecol 180:259, 1999

Gulick RM, Mellors JW, Havlir D, Eron JJ, Gonzalez C, McMahon D, Richmond DD, Valentine FT, Jonas L, Meibohm A, Emini EA, Chodakewitz JA: Treatment with indinavir, zidovudine, and lamivudine in adults with human immunodeficiency virus infection and prior antiretroviral therapy. N Engl J Med 337:779, 1997

Gwinn M, Pappaioanou M, George JR, Hannon WH, Wasser SC, Redus MA: Prevalence of HIV infection in childbearing women in the United States: Surveillance using newborn blood samples. JAMA 265:1704, 1991

Haddad J, Langer B, Astruc D, Messer J, Lokiec F: Oral acyclovir and recurrent genital herpes during late pregnancy. Obstet Gynecol 82:102, 1993

Hagensee ME, Slavinsky J 3rd, Gaffga CM, Suros J, Kissinger P, Martin DH: Seroprevalence of human papillomavirus type 16 in pregnant women. Obstet Gynecol 94:653, 1999

Hammer SM, Squires KE, Hughes MD, Grimes JM, Demeter LM, Currier JS, Eron JJ Jr, Feinberg JE, Balfour HH Jr, Deyton LR, Chodakewitz JA, Fischl MA: A controlled trial of two nucleoside analogues plus indinavir in persons with human immunodeficiency virus infection and CD4 cell counts of 200 per cubic millimeter or less. N Engl J Med 337:725, 1997

Hammerschlag MR, Cummings C, Roblin PM, Williams TH, Delke I: Efficacy of neonatal ocular prophylaxis for the prevention of chlamydial and gonococcal conjunctivitis. N Engl J Med 320:769, 1989

Harger JH, Amortegui AJ, Meyer MP, Pazin GJ: Characteristics of recurrent genital herpes simplex infections in pregnant women. Obstet Gynecol 73:367, 1989

Hashisaki P, Wertzberger GG, Conrad GL, Nichols CR: Erythromycin failure in the treatment of syphilis in a pregnant woman. Sex Transm Dis 10:36, 1983

Haverkos HW, Turner JF Jr, Moolchan ET, Cadet JL: Relative

rates of AIDS among racial/ethnic groups by exposure categories. J Natl Med Assoc 91:17, 1999

Henderson GI, Hu ZQ, Perez TB, Devi BG, Frosto TA, Schenker S: Ganciclovir transfer by human placenta and its effects on rat fetal cells. Am J Med Sci 306:151, 1993

Hill LM, Maloney JB: An unusual constellation of sonographic findings associated with congenital syphilis. Obstet Gynecol 78:895, 1991

Hogg RS, Yip B, Kully C, Craib KJP, O'Shaughnessy MV, Schechter MT, Montaner JSG: Improved survival among HIV-infected patients after initiation of triple-drug antiretroviral regimens. CMAJ 160:659, 1999

Hoyme UB, Kiviat N, Eschenbach DA: The microbiology and treatment of late postpartum endometritis. Obstet Gynecol 68:226, 1986

Institute of Medicine, Committee on Prenatal and Newborn Screening for HIV Infection: HIV Screening of Pregnant Women and Newborns. Washington, DC, National Academy Press, 1991

International Perinatal HIV Group: The mode of delivery and the risk of vertical transmission of human immunodeficiency virus type 1: A meta-analysis of 15 prospective cohort studies. N Engl J Med 340:977, 1999

Kahn JO, Walker BD: Acute human immunodeficiency virus type 1 infection. N Engl J Med 339:33, 1998

Kass NE, Taylor HA, Anderson J: Treatment of human immunodeficiency virus during pregnancy: The shift from an exclusive focus on fetal protection to a more balanced approach. Am J Obstet Gynecol 182:856, 2000

Kimberlin DF, Weller S, Whitley RJ, Andrews WW, Hauth JC, Lakeman F, Miller G: Pharmacokinetics of oral valacyclovir and acyclovir in late pregnancy. Am J Obstet Gynecol 179:846, 1998

Klass PE, Brown ER, Pelton SI: The incidence of prenatal syphilis at the Boston City Hospital: A comparison across four decades. Pediatrics 94:24, 1994

Klein VR, Cox SM, Mitchell MD, Wendel GD: The Jarisch–Herxheimer reaction complicating syphilotherapy in pregnancy. Obstet Gynecol 75:375, 1990

Korn AP: *Chlamydia trachomatis* infections in pregnancy. Contemp Ob/Gyn 45:65, 2000

Kuhn L, Steketee RW, Weedon J, Abrams EJ, Lambert G, Bamji M, Schoenbaum E, Farley J, Nesheim SR, Palumbo P, Simonds RJ, Thea DM: Distinct risk factors for intrauterine and intrapartum human immunodeficiency virus transmission and consequences for disease progression in infected children. Perinatal AIDS Collaborative Transmission Study. J Infect Dis 179:52, 1999

Kulhanjian JA, Soroush V, Au DS, Bronzan RN, Yasukawa LL, Weylman LE, Arvin AM, Prober CG: Identification of women at unsuspected risk of primary infection with herpes simplex virus type 2 during pregnancy. N Engl J Med 326:916, 1992

Lackritz EM, Satten GA, Aberele-Grasse J, Dodd RY, Raimondi VP, Lajseen RS, Lewis WR, Notari EP, Petersen LR: Estimated risk of transmission of the human immunodeficiency virus by screened blood in the United States. N Engl J Med 333:1721, 1995

Lallemant M, Jourdain G, LeCoeur S, Kim S, Koetsawang S, Comeau AM, Phoolcharoen W, Essex M, McIntosh K, Vithayasai V: A trial of shortened zidovudine regimens to prevent mother-to-child transmission of human immunodeficiency virus type 1. N Engl J Med 343:982, 2000

Landesman SH, Kalish LA, Burns DN, Minkoff H, Fox HE, Zorrilla C, Garcia P, Fowler MG, Mofenson L, Tuomala R: Obstetrical factors and the transmission of human immu-

nodeficiency virus type 1 from mother to child. N Engl J Med 334:1617, 1996

Langenberg AGM, Corey L, Ashley RL, Leong WP, Straus SE: A prospective study of new infections with herpes simplex virus type 1 and type 2. N Engl J Med 341:1432, 1999

Langston C, Lewis DE, Hammill HA, Popek EJ, Kozinetz CA, Kline MW, Hanson IC, Shearer WT: Excess intrauterine fetal demise associated with maternal human immunodeficiency virus infection. J Infect Dis 172:1451, 1995

Lee MJ, Hallmark RJ, Frenkel LM, Del Priore G: Maternal syphilis and vertical perinatal transmission of human immunodeficiency virus type-1 infection. Int J Gynaecol Obstet 63:247, 1998

Lewis SH, Reynolds-Kohler C, Fox HE, Nelson JA: HIV-1 in trophoblastic and villous Hofbauer cells, and haematological precursors in eight-week fetuses. Lancet 335:565, 1990

Lindsay MK, Feng TI, Peterson HB, Slade BA, Willis S, Klein L: Routine human immunodeficiency virus infection screening in unregistered and registered inner-city parturients. Obstet Gynecol 77:599, 1991

Lorenzi P, Spicher VM, Laubereau B, Hirschel B, Kind C, Rudin C, Irion O, Kaiser L: Antiretroviral therapies in pregnancy: Maternal, fetal and neonatal effects. Swiss HIV Cohort Study, the Swiss Collaborative HIV and Pregnancy Study, and the Swiss Neonatal HIV Study. AIDS 12:F241, 1998

Lossick JG: Treatment of sexually transmitted vaginosis/vaginitis. Rev Infect Dis 12:S665, 1990

Lucas MJ, Theriot SK, Wendel GD: Doppler systolic–diastolic ratios in pregnancies complicated by syphilis. Obstet Gynecol 77:217, 1991

Macmillan S, Walker R, Oloto E, Fitzmaurice A, Templeton A: Ignorance about chlamydia among sexually active women—a two centre study. Hum Reprod 14:1131, 1999

Manns A, Strickler HD, Wiktor SZ, Pate EJ, Gray R, Waters D: Low incidence of human papillomavirus type 16 antibody seroconversion in young children. Pediatr Infect Dis J 18:833, 1999

Martin DH, Vaginal Infections and Prematurity Study Group: Erythromycin treatment of *Chlamydia trachomatis* infections during pregnancy. Abstract 683 presented at 30th Interscience Conference on Antimicrobial Agents and Chemotherapy, Atlanta, October 1990

Martius J, Krohn MA, Hillier SL, Stamm WE, Holmes KK, Eschenbach DA: Relationships of vaginal *Lactobacillus* species, cervical *Chlamydia trachomatis*, and bacterial vaginosis to preterm birth. Obstet Gynecol 71:89, 1988

Matheson PB, Abrams EJ, Thomas PA, Hernan MA, Thea DM, Lambert G, Krasinski K, Bamji M, Rogers MF, Heagarty M: Efficacy of antenatal zidovudine in reducing perinatal transmission of human immunodeficiency virus type 1. The New York City Perinatal HIV Transmission Collaborative Study Group. J Infect Dis 172:353, 1995

Matsunaga J, Bergman A, Bhatia NN: Genital condylomata acuminata in pregnancy: Effectiveness, safety and pregnancy outcome following cryotherapy. Br J Obstet Gynaecol 94:168, 1987

Mauskopf JA, Paul JE, Wichman DS, White AD, Tilson HH: Economic impact of treatment of HIV-positive pregnant women and their newborns with zidovudine. JAMA 276:132, 1996

Maxwell GL, Watson WJ: Preterm premature rupture of membranes: Results of expectant management in patients with cervical cultures positive for group B streptococcus or *Neisseria gonorrhoeae*. Am J Obstet Gynecol 166:945, 1992

McFarlin BL, Bottoms SF, Dock BS, Isada NB: Epidemic syphilis: Maternal factors associated with congenital infection. Am J Obstet Gynecol 170:535, 1994

McGregor JA, French JI: *Chlamydia trachomatis* infection during pregnancy. Am J Obstet Gynecol 164:1782, 1991

Miller JM Jr: Recurrent chlamydial colonization during pregnancy. Am J Perinatol 15:307, 1998

Minkoff HL, McCalla S, Delke I, Stevens R, Salwen M, Feldman J: The relationship of cocaine use to syphilis and human immunodeficiency virus infections among inner-city parturient women. Am J Obstet Gynecol 163:521, 1990

Mitka M: US effort to eliminate syphilis moving forward. JAMA 283:1555, 2000

Mofenson LM, Lambert JS, Stiehm ER, Bethel J, Meyer WA III, Whitehouse J, Moye J, Reichelderfer P, Harris DR, Fowler MG, Mathieson B, Nemo GJ: Risk factors for perinatal transmission of human immunodeficiency virus type 1 in women treated with zidovudine. N Engl J Med 341:385, 1999

Montaner JS, Reiss P, Cooper D, Vella S, Harris M, Conway B, Wainberg MA, Smith D, Robinson P, Hall D, Myers M, Lange JM: A randomized, double-blind trial comparing combinations of nevirapine, didanosine, and zidovudine for HIV-infected patients: The INCAS Trial. Italy, The Netherlands, Canada and Australia Study. JAMA 279:957, 1998

Morris A, Zorrilla C, Vajarant M, Dobles A, Cu-Uvin S, Jones T: A review of protease inhibitor use in pregnancy. Presented at Sixth Conference on Retroviruses and Opportunistic Infections, Chicago, January 31–February 4, 1999

Myles TD, Elam G, Park-Hwang E, Nguyen T: The Jarisch–Herxheimer reaction and fetal monitoring changes in pregnant women treated for syphilis. Obstet Gynecol 92:859, 1998

Nahmias AJ, Josey WE, Naib ZM, Freeman MG, Fernandez RJ, Wheeler JH: Perinatal risk associated with maternal genital herpes simplex virus infection. Am J Obstet Gynecol 110:825, 1971

Nduati R, John G, Mbori-Ngacha D, Richardson B, Overbaugh J, Mwatha A, Ndinya-Achola J, Bwayo J, Onyango FE, Hughes J, Kreiss J: Effect of breastfeeding and formula feeding on transmission of HIV-1. A randomized clinical trial. JAMA 283:1167, 2000

Ngassa PC, Egbe JA: Maternal genital *Chlamydia trachomatis* infection and the risk of preterm labor. Int J Gynaecol Obstet 47:241, 1994

Pantanowitz L, Hodkinson J, Zeelie R, Jones N: Gonococcal endocarditis after a threatened abortion. A case report. J Reprod Med 43:1043, 1998

Patrick DM, Money DM, Forbes J, Dobson SR, Rekart ML, Cook DA, Middleton PJ, Burdge DR: Routine prenatal screening for HIV in a low-prevalence setting. CMAJ 159:942, 1998

Perinatal HIV Guidelines Working Group Members: U.S. Public Health Service Task Force recommendations for the use of antiretroviral drugs in pregnant women infected with HIV-1 for maternal health and for reducing perinatal HIV-1 transmission in the United States. USPHS, February 25, 2000. http://www.hivatis.org?list, January 24, 2001

Pope V, Fears MB: Serodia *Treponema pallidum* passive particle agglutination (TP-PA) test. In Larsen SA, Pope V, Jonnson RE, Kennedy EJ (eds): Supplement to A Manual of Tests for Syphilis, 9th ed. Washington, DC, American Public Health Association, 2000, p 365

Prober CG, Hensleigh PA, Boucher FD, Yasukawa LL, Au DS, Arvin AM: Use of routine viral cultures at delivery to identify neonates exposed to herpes simplex virus. N Engl J Med 318:887, 1988

Prober CG, Sullender WM, Yasukawa LL, Au DS, Yeager AS, Arvin AM: Low risk of herpes simplex virus infections in neonates exposed to the virus at the time of vaginal delivery to mothers with recurrent genital herpes simplex virus infections. N Engl J Med 316:240, 1987

Puranen M, Yliskoski M, Saarikoski S, Syränen S: Vertical transmission of human papillomavirus from infected mothers to their newborn babies and persistence of the virus in childhood. Am J Obstet Gynecol 174:694, 1996

Ramus R, Mayfield J, Wendel G: Evaluation of the current CDC recommended treatment guidelines for gonorrhea in pregnancy. Am J Obstet Gynecol 174:409, 1996

Rando RF, Lindheim S, Hasty L, Sedlacek TV, Woodland M, Eder C: Increased frequency of detection of human papillomavirus deoxyribonucleic acid in exfoliated cervical cells during pregnancy. Am J Obstet Gynecol 161:50, 1989

Roberts SW, Cox SM, Dax J, Wendel GD Jr, Leveno KJ: Genital herpes during pregnancy: No lesions, no cesarean. Obstet Gynecol 85:261, 1995

Rogers B, Sheffield J, Margraf L, Fong D, McIntire D, Zeray F, Sanchez P, Wendel G: Placental villous enlargement correlates with poor pregnancy outcome in congenital syphilis. Presented at the annual meeting of the Society for Pediatric Pathology, 1999

Rolfs RT: Treatment of syphilis in 1993. Clin Infect Dis 20:23, 1995

Ross JDC: Systemic gonococcal infection. Genitourin Med 72:404, 1996

Ryan GM, Abdella TN, McNeeley SG, Baselski V, Drummond DE: *Chlamydia trachomatis* infection in pregnancy and effect of treatment on outcome. Am J Obstet Gynecol 162:34, 1990

Salpietro CD, Bisigano G, Fulia F, Mariono A, Barberi I: *Chlamydia trachomatis* conjunctivitis in the newborn. Arch Pediatr 6:317, 1999

Satin AJ, Twickler DM, Wendel GD Jr: Congenital syphilis associated with dilation of fetal small bowel: A case report. J Ultrasound Med 11:49, 1992

Schachter J, Grossman M, Sweet RL, Holt J, Jordan C, Bishop E: Prospective study of perinatal transmission of *Chlamydia trachomatis*. JAMA 255:3374, 1986

Schmid GP, Sanders LL, Blount JH, Alexander ER: Chancroid in the United States: Reestablishment of an old disease. JAMA 258:3265, 1987

Schwartz DA, Larsen SA, Beck-Sague C, Fears M, Rice RJ: Pathology of the umbilical cord in congenital syphilis: Analysis of 25 specimens using histochemistry and immunofluorescent antibody to *Treponema pallidum*. Hum Pathol 26:784, 1995

Schwartz DB, Greenberg MD, Daoud Y, Reid R: Genital condylomas in pregnancy: Use of trichloroacetic acid and laser therapy. Am J Obstet Gynecol 158:1407, 1988

Scott LL: Prevention of perinatal herpes: Prophylactic antiviral therapy? Clin Obstet Gynecol 42:134, 1999

Scott LL, Alexander J: Cost-effectiveness of acyclovir suppression to prevent recurrent genital herpes in term pregnancy. Am J Perinatol 15:57, 1998

Scott LL, Sanchez PJ, Jackson GL, Zeray F, Wendel GD: Acyclovir suppression to prevent cesarean section after first episode genital herpes in pregnancy. Obstet Gynecol 87:69, 1996

Shah K, Kashima H, Polk BF, Shah F, Abbey H, Abramson

A: Rarity of cesarean delivery in cases of juvenile-onset respiratory papillomatosis. Obstet Gynecol 68:795, 1986

Sheffield JS, Sigman A, McIntire D, Cunningham FG, Wendel GD Jr.: Disseminated gonococcal infection in women: A 24-year experience. Abstract No. 522: Presented at thirteenth annual meeting of the International Society for Sexually Transmitted Diseases Research, Denver, July 11–14, 1999

Silverman NS, Sullivan M, Hochman M, Womack M, Jungkind DL: A randomized, prospective trial comparing amoxicillin and erythromycin for the treatment of *Chlamydia trachomatis* in pregnancy. Am J Obstet Gynecol 170:829, 1994

Silverstein AM: Congenital syphilis and the timing of immunogenesis in the human fetus. Nature 194:196, 1962

Snyder RR, Hammond TL, Hankins GDV: Human papillomavirus associated with poor healing of episiotomy repairs. Obstet Gynecol 76:664, 1990

Southwick KL, Guidry HM, Weldon MM, Mert KJ, Berman SM, Levine WC: An epidemic of congenital syphilis in Jefferson County, Texas, 1994–1995: Inadequate prenatal syphilis testing after an outbreak in adults. Am J Public Health 89:557, 1999

Sozio J, Ness RB: Chlamydial lower genital tract infection and spontaneous abortion. Infect Dis Obstet Gynecol 6:8, 1998

Sperling RS, Shapiro DE, McSherry GD, Britto P, Cunningham BE, Culnane M, Coombs RW, Scott G, Van Dyke RB, Shearer WT, Jimenez E, Diaz C, Harrison DD, Delfraissy JF: Safety of the maternal–infant zidovudine regimen utilized in the Pediatric AIDS Clinical Trial Group 076 Study. AIDS 12:1805, 1998

Spitzer M, Krumholz BA, Seltzer VL: The multicentric nature of disease related to human papillomavirus infection of the female lower genital tract. Obstet Gynecol 73:303, 1989

Star J, Powrie R, Cu-Uvin S, Carpenter CCJ: Should women with human immunodeficiency virus be delivered by cesarean? Obstet Gynecol 94:799, 1999

Stiehm ER, Lambert JS, Mofenson LM, Bethel J, Whitehouse J, Nugent R, Moye J Jr, Glenn Fowler M, Mathieson BJ, Reichelderfer P, Nemo GJ, Korelitz J, Meyer WA 3rd, Sapan CV, Jimenez E, Gandia J, Scott G, O'Sullivan MJ, Kovacs A, Stek A, Shearer WT, Hammill H: Efficacy of zidovudine and human immunodeficiency virus (HIV) hyperimmune immunoglobulin for reducing perinatal HIV transmission from HIV-infected women with advanced disease: Results of Pediatric AIDS Clinical Trials Group protocol 185. J Infect Dis 179:567, 1999

Stone DM, Whitington WL: Treatment of genital herpes. Rev Infect Dis 12:S610, 1990

Stratton P, Tuomala RE, Abboud R, Rodriguez E, Rich K, Pitt J, Diaz C, Hammill H, Minkoff H: Obstetric and newborn outcomes in a cohort of HIV-infected pregnant women: A report of the women and infants transmission study. J Acquir Immune Defic Syndr Hum Retrovirol 20:179, 1999

Stringer JSA, Rouse DJ, Goldenberg RL: Prophylactic cesarean delivery for the prevention of perinatal human immunodeficiency virus transmission. JAMA 281:1946, 1999

Sweet RL, Landers CV, Walker C, Schachter J: *Chlamydia trachomatis* infection and pregnancy outcome. Am J Obstet Gynecol 156:824, 1987

Tenti P, Zappatore R, Migliora P, Spinillo A, Belloni C, Carnevali L: Perinatal transmission of human papillomavirus from gravidas with latent infections. Obstet Gynecol 93:475, 1999

Tseng CJ, Liang CC, Soong YK, Pao CC: Perinatal transmission of human papillomavirus in infants: Relationship between infection rate and mode of delivery. Obstet Gynecol 91:92, 1998

United Nations Children's Fund: The state of the world's children 1998—breastmilk and transmission of HIV—Panel 6—UNICEF home information participation organization activities. Source: http://www.unicef.org/sowc98/panel6.htm, 1998

Van de Perre P: Transmission of human immunodeficiency virus type 1 through breast-feeding: How can it be prevented? J Infect Dis 179:S405, 1999

Varady E, Nsanze H, Slattery T: Gonococcal scalp abscess in a neonate delivered by cesarean section. Sex Transm Infect 74:451, 1998

Vastag B: CDC says rates are up for gonorrhea, down for syphilis. JAMA 285:155, 2001

Vaules MB, Ramin KD, Ramsey PS: Syphilis in pregnancy: A review. Prim Care Update Ob/Gyns 7:26, 2000

Vontver LA, Hickok DE, Brown Z, Reid L, Corey L: Recurrent genital herpes simplex virus infection in pregnancy: Infant outcome and frequency of asymptomatic recurrences. Am J Obstet Gynecol 143:75, 1982

Wade NA, Birkhead GS, Warren BL, Charbonneau TT, French PT, Wang L, Baum JB, Tesoriero JM, Savicki R: Abbreviated regimens of zidovudine prophylaxis and perinatal transmission of the human immunodeficiency virus. N Engl J Med 339:1409, 1998

Wald A, Zeh J, Selke S, Ashley RL, Corey L: Virologic characteristics of subclinical and symptomatic genital herpes infections. N Engl J Med 333:770, 1995

Wald A, Zeh J, Selke S, Warren T, Ryncarz AJ, Ashley R, Krieger JN, Corey L: Reactivation of genital herpes simplex virus type 2 infection in asymptomatic seropositive persons. N Engl J Med 342:844, 2000

Watts DH, Koutsky LA, Holmes KK, Goldman D, Kuypers J, Kiviat NB, Galloway DA: Low risk of perinatal transmission of human papillomavirus: Results from a prospective cohort study. Am J Obstet Gynecol 178:365, 1998

Wehbeh HA, Ruggeirio RM, Shahem S, Lopez G, Ali Y: Single-dose azithromycin for *Chlamydia* in pregnant women. J Reprod Med 43:509, 1998

Weinstock H, Sweeney S, Satten GA, Gwinn M: HIV seroincidence and risk factors among patients repeatedly tested for HIV attending sexually transmitted disease clinics in the United States, 1991 to 1996. STD Clinic HIV Seroincidence Study Group. J Acquir Immune Defic Syndr Hum Retrovirol 19:506, 1998

Wendel GD: Gestational and congenital syphilis. Clin Perinatol 15:287, 1988

Wendel GD, Cunningham FG: Sexually transmitted diseases in pregnancy. In: Williams Obstetrics, 18th ed. (Suppl 13). Norwalk, CT, Appleton & Lange, August/September 1991

Wendel GD, Maberry MC, Christmas JT, Goldberg MS, Norgard MV: Examination of amniotic fluid in diagnosing congenital syphilis with fetal death. Obstet Gynecol 74:967, 1989

Wendel GD, Sanchez PJ, Peters MT, Harstad TW, Potter LL, Norgard MV: Identification of *Treponema pallidum* in amniotic fluid and fetal blood from pregnancies complicated by congenital syphilis. Obstet Gynecol 78:890, 1991

Wendel GD, Stark RJ, Jamison RR, Molina RD, Sullivan TJ: Penicillin allergy and desensitization in serious infections during pregnancy. N Engl J Med 312:1229, 1985

Wendel PJ, Wendel GD: Sexually transmitted disease in pregnancy. Semin Perinatol 17:443, 1993

West KH, Cohen ML: Standard precautions—a new approach to reducing infection transmission in the hospital setting. J Intraven Nurs 20:S7, 1997

Whitley R, Arvin A, Prober C, Corey L, Burchett S, Plotkin S, the National Institute of Allergy and Infectious Diseases Collaborative Antiviral Study Group: Predictors of morbidity and mortality in neonates with herpes simplex virus infections. N Engl J Med 324:450, 1991

Witkin SS, Inglis SR, Polaneczky M: Detection of *Chlamydia trachomatis* and *Trichomonas vaginalis* during pregnancy by introital sampling. Am J Obstet Gynecol 174:409, 1996

Wittek AE, Yeager AS, Au DS, Hensleigh PA: Asymptomatic shedding of herpes simplex virus from the cervix and lesion site during pregnancy: Correlation of antepartum shedding with shedding at delivery. Am J Dis Child 138:439, 1984

Yip L, Sweeny PJ, Bock BF: Acute suppurative salpingitis with concomitant intrauterine pregnancy. Am J Emerg Med 11:476, 1993

Zenker PN, Rolfs RT: Treatment of syphilis, 1989. Rev Infect Dis 12:S590, 1990

Family Planning

58

Contraception

The practice of obstetrics in the United States has been influenced by forces from outside the medical community more than any other specialty. In no other branch of medicine are social, religious, and political forces more obvious than in family planning. Although the majority of fertile American women would prefer to avoid pregnancy in any one given year, they and their physicians are confronted continuously by these forces. Women's health-care providers must continue to counsel and prescribe in an area in which confusion is common, change seems continual, and scientific evidence is all too often ignored by legal, legislative, and judicial communities. To add to this, unbalanced media coverage of contraceptive technologies has been detrimental (Entwistle and colleagues, 2000).

Even in some affluent industrialized countries, women are denied access to family planning services. In the United States, access for indigent women to these services is frequently a political and not medical decision. To correct these inequities, women must make their opinions known to legislators, to the judiciary, and to the news media. Such efforts can be effective, as exemplified by the recent approval of oral contraceptives by the Japanese government after a 35-year delay

TABLE 58–1. Voluntary Risks in Perspective

Activity	Chance of Death (per Year)
Risks for Men and Women of All Ages	
Motorcycling	1 in 1000
Automobile driving	1 in 5900
Power boating	1 in 5900
Playing football	1 in 25,000
Canoeing	1 in 100,000
Risks for Women Aged 15–44 Years	
Using tampons	1 in 350,000
Having sexual intercourse (PID)	1 in 50,000
Risks for Women Preventing Pregnancy	
Using oral contraceptives	
Nonsmoker	1 in 67,000
Age < 35	1 in 200,000
Age 35–44	1 in 29,000
Heavy smoker (25 or more cigarettes per day)	1 in 1700
Age < 35	1 in 5300
Age 35–44	1 in 700
Using IUDs (per year)	1 in 10 million
Using diaphragm, condom, or spermicides	None
Using fertility awareness methods	None
Undergoing sterilization:	
Laparoscopic tubal ligation	1 in 38,500
Hysterectomy	1 in 1,600
Vasectomy	1 in 1,000,000
Risk per Pregnancy from Continuing Pregnancy	1 in 10,000
Risk from Terminating Pregnancy	
Legal abortion	
Before 9 weeks	1 in 263,000
Between 9–12 weeks	1 in 100,000
Between 13–15 weeks	1 in 35,000
After 15 weeks	1 in 10,000

IUDs = intrauterine devices; PID = pelvic inflammatory disease.
Sources: Berg (1996), Cates (1980), Dinman (1980), Escobedo (1989), Harlap (1991), Lawson (1994), Lee (1981), and all their colleagues. From Hatcher and colleagues (1998), with permission.

(American College of Obstetricians and Gynecologists, 1999b).

There currently are powerful and effective methods of regulating fertility. None is completely without side effects and some danger—for example, latex condoms can initiate anaphylactic reactions. **Thus, while there is no totally safe contraceptive method, and the lack of contraception is even more dangerous, both are less dangerous than driving an automobile for 1 year.** Some of these risks are shown in Table 58–1. Those who prescribe contraceptives must be familiar with currently available drugs and methods and their side effects. We must strive to reduce these side effects and risks to a minimum, to recognize and manage them, and we must be aware that one of the major risks of contraception failure is unplanned pregnancy.

WHO NEEDS CONTRACEPTION?

When no contraception is used by presumably fertile sex partners, about 90 percent of women will conceive within 1 year. Young women, regardless of age, who do not want to be pregnant are best advised to use contraception whenever they begin sexual activity. Some girls—perhaps the majority—ovulate before their first menstrual period.

Contraceptive advice for the woman nearing menopause is a more difficult question because it is impossible to predict when fertility has ended. Results of a study by Metcalf (1979) indicate that *when menstruation remained regular, there was evidence of ovulation in almost every cycle.* Oligomenorrhea or increasing cycle length was associated with a diminished frequency, but not complete cessation of ovulation. Even the presence of hot flushes, amenorrhea, and elevated gonadotropin levels do not absolutely guarantee against subsequent ovulation. Primordial follicles with apparently normal oocytes have been observed in ovaries from women over 50 years of age.

Even so, pregnancies are rare in women over 50. Therefore, older women are probably best advised that regular menstrual periods imply recurrent ovulation irrespective of age. A woman younger than 50 who has not menstruated for 2 years is very unlikely to ovulate spontaneously, although there are reported instances (Szlachter and co-workers, 1979).

CONTRACEPTIVE METHODS

Methods of variable effectiveness currently employed include:

1. Oral steroidal contraceptives.
2. Injected or implanted steroidal contraceptives.
3. Intrauterine devices.
4. Physical, chemical, or barrier techniques.
5. Withdrawal.
6. Sexual abstinence around the time of ovulation.
7. Breast feeding.
8. Permanent sterilization.

Current contraceptive use by men and women is presented in Figure 58–1. Estimates of the failure rate *during the first year of use* with each of these techniques are given in Table 58–2. Effective education, as well as motivation, undoubtedly would have appreciably reduced the cited failure rates (Vessey and co-workers, 1982). Mature women who continued to use one technique for a long time typically experienced very low failure rates.

Elective abortion is not a contraceptive technique. It serves, at times, as a less than ideal remedy for contraceptive failure or neglect (Chap. 33, p. 869).

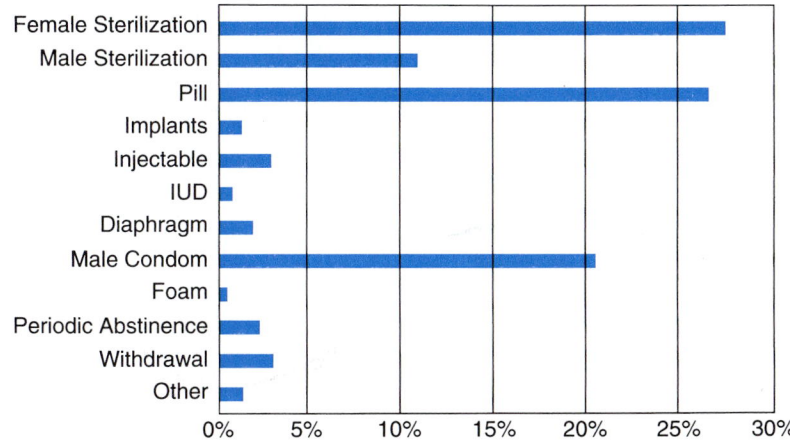

FIGURE 58–1. Contraceptive use in the United States circa 1995 for users aged 15 to 44. Data from Piccinino and Mosher (1998a, 1998b). (IUD = intrauterine device.) (From the Association of Professors of Obstetrics and Gynecology, 1999, with permission.)

TABLE 58–2. **Failure and Continuation Rates at 1 Year for Various Methods of Birth Control**

Method	Percent of Women with Accidental Pregnancy within the First Year		Percent of Women Continuing Use at 1 Year[c]
	Typical Use[a]	*Perfect Use*[b]	
Chance[d]	85	85	
Spermicides[e]	26	6	40
Periodic abstinence	25		63
Calendar		9	
Ovulation method		3	
Symptothermal[f]		2	
Postovulation		1	
Cervical cap[g]			
Parous women	40	26	42
Nulliparous women	20	9	56
Diaphragm[g]	20	6	56
Withdrawal	19	4	
Condom[h]			
Female (Reality)	21	5	56
Male	14	3	61
Pill	5		71
Progestin only		0.5	
Combined		0.1	
Emergency contraception	Reduces risk by at least 75 percent[i]		
Intrauterine device (IUD)			
Progestasert	2.0	1.5	81
Copper T 380A	0.8	0.6	78
Depo-Provera	0.3	0.3	70
Norplant and Norplant-II	0.05	0.05	88
Lactation	Highly effective, temporary[j]		
Female sterilization	0.4	0.4	100
Male sterilization	0.15	0.10	100

[a] Among typical couples who initiate use of a method (not necessarily for the first time), the percentage who experience an accidental pregnancy during the first year if they do not stop use for any other reason.

[b] Among couples who initiate use of a method (not necessarily for the first time) and who use it *perfectly* (both consistently and correctly), the percentage who experience an accidental pregnancy during the first year if they do not stop use for any other reason.

[c] Among couples attempting to avoid pregnancy, the percentage who continue to use a method for 1 year.

[d] The percentages becoming pregnant in the typical use and perfect use columns are based on data from populations where contraception is not used and from women who cease using contraception in order to become pregnant. Among such populations, about 89% become pregnant within 1 year. This estimate was lowered slightly (to 85%) to represent the percentage who would become pregnant within 1 year among women now relying on reversible methods of contraception if they abandoned contraception altogether.

[e] Foams, creams, gels, vaginal suppositories, and vaginal film.

[f] Cervical mucus (ovulation) method supplemented by calendar in the preovulatory and basal body temperature in the postovulatory phases.

[g] With spermicidal cream or jelly.

[h] Without spermicides

[i] For treatment schedules, see Table 58–13.

[j] To maintain effective protection against pregnancy, another method of contraception must be used as soon as menstruation resumes, the frequency or duration of breast feeding is reduced, bottle feeding is introduced, or the baby reaches 6 months of age.

Modified with permission from Hatcher and colleagues (1998).

HORMONAL CONTRACEPTIVES

When introduced in 1960, hormonal contraceptives represented a dramatic departure from previous traditional methods. These contraceptives are available in a variety of oral, injectable, and implantable forms. Oral contraceptives are a combination of estrogen and progestin or a progestin only—the *mini pill.* Injectable or implantable contraceptives contain progestins alone or a combination of estrogen and progestin. In 1995, 10.4 million women in the United States used an oral contraceptive for fertility control (Piccinino and Mosher, 1998a, 1998b).

ESTROGEN PLUS PROGESTIN CONTRACEPTIVES. Combined estrogen–progesterone contraceptives may be given orally, by intramuscular injection, or by patch. The oral contraceptives are used most commonly and often consist of a combination of an estrogen and a progestational agent taken daily for 3 weeks and omitted for 1 week, during which time there is withdrawal uterine bleeding. Injectable combined agents are discussed on page 1535. Currently under testing in the United States is a contraceptive patch (EVRA) containing 17-deacetylnorgestimate and ethinyl estradiol (Creasy and associates, 2000).

MECHANISMS OF ACTION. The contraceptive actions of steroidal medications are multiple, but the most important effect is to prevent ovulation by suppression of hypothalamic gonadotropin-releasing factors. This prevents pituitary secretion of follicle-stimulating and luteinizing hormones.

Estrogen alone in sufficient dose will inhibit ovulation by suppressing gonadotropins. It also likely inhibits implantation by altering normal endometrial maturation. Estrogen accelerates ovum transport; however, progestins cause slowing. Thus, their possible role in altered tubal and uterine motility is unclear.

Progestins produce thick, scanty, cellular cervical mucus that impairs sperm transport. Also, sperm capacitation is likely inhibited. Similar to estrogens, progestins produce an endometrium that is unfavorable to blastocyst implantation. Finally, progestins also can inhibit ovulation by suppressing gonadotropins.

The net or combined effect of estrogen and progestin with respect to contraception is extremely effective ovulation suppression, sperm penetration blockage by cervical mucus, and unfavorable endometrium for implantation if the first two mechanisms fail. Estrogen plus progestin combined oral contraceptives, *if taken daily for 3 weeks out of every 4,* provide virtually absolute protection against conception.

PHARMACOLOGY

ESTROGENS. In the United States, the only estrogens available are *ethinyl estradiol* and its 3-methyl ether, *mestranol* (Fig. 58–2). To be bioactive, the methyl group at carbon 3 of mestranol must be removed by hepatic conversion into ethinyl estradiol. The exact conversion factor for potency of ethinyl estradiol to mestranol is not known, but it probably is 1.2 to 1.5. The vast majority of all prescriptions for combined oral contraceptives in the United States are for 35-μg doses or less of estrogen, and *all of these contain ethinyl estradiol.*

PROGESTINS. Only 19-nortestosterone derivatives are currently used for progestins because derivatives of 17α-acetoxyprogesterone in high doses produce breast tumors in female beagles. Of the compounds currently available in the United States (Fig. 58–2), only norgestrel has two isomers. Levonorgestrel is the bioactive isomer; *Nordette* contains 0.15 mg of this compound and Alesse contains 0.1 mg. *Lo/Ovral* contains 0.3 mg of dl-norgestrel (a combination of dextro and levo forms), of which only half is in the active levo form. Two newer progestins, *desogestrel* and *norgestimate,* are now available (Fig. 58–2). A third progestin, *gestodene,* is used in Europe. Even low doses of these compounds are associated with minimal metabolic changes but excellent cycle control (Åkerlund and colleagues, 1993). Several new progestins with low androgenic properties and minimal effects on lipids are in the process of approval and subsequent marketing in the United States.

All progestins were initially chosen because of their progestational potencies, but now they are compared for estrogenic, antiestrogenic, and androgenic effects. These actions for each are generally considered when prescribing for a specific woman (Table 58–3). For example, if a low androgenic effect were desired for a woman because of acne, a good choice would be one containing 35 μg of ethinyl estradiol and 0.4 to 0.5 mg of norethindrone. Another would be *Ortho-Cyclen;* it contains 0.25 mg of norgestimate, which has less androgenic effect than any other currently available progestin. This is followed closely by desogestrel-containing agents, which have low affinity for testosterone receptors and high affinity for progesterone receptors (Burkman 1993; Collins, 1993; Phillips and colleagues, 1992).

It is apparent that these progestins also have profound effects on plasma lipids, lipoproteins, clotting factors, vessel disease, diabetes, and a variety of nonendocrine effects, which are discussed later.

A. Estrogens

B. Progestins

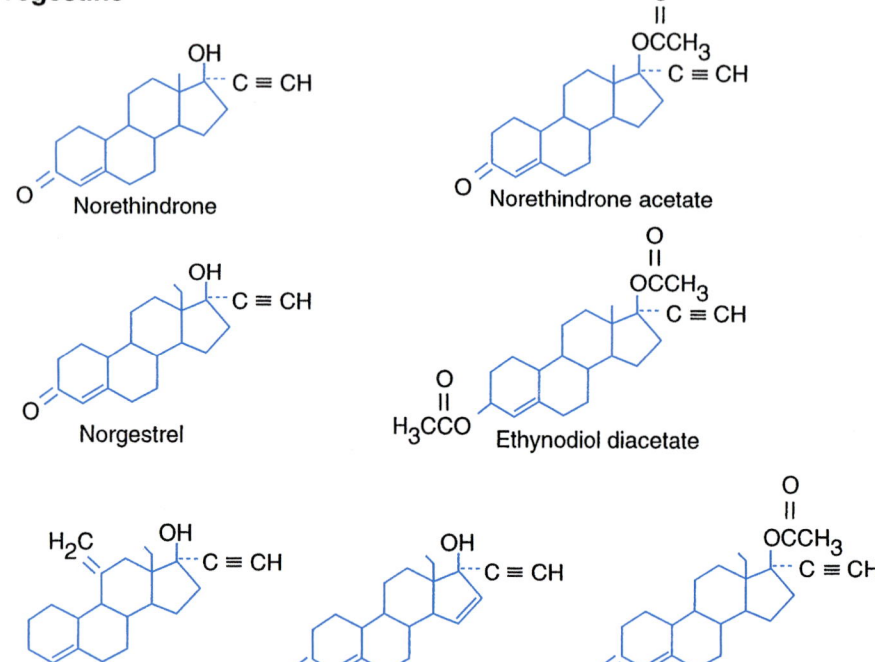

FIGURE 58–2. Structural formulas of contraceptive steroids currently in use in the United States.

DOSAGE AND ADMINISTRATION. Since oral contraceptives have come into use, the amounts of estrogen and progestin have been reduced remarkably. This is important, because most adverse effects are dose related. The lowest acceptable dose is governed by the ability to prevent unacceptable breakthrough bleeding. Daily estrogen content is usually 20 to 35 μg of ethinyl estradiol. None of the products sold in the United States contains more than 50 μg. The amount of progestin varies in two ways:

1. Among older, now well-evaluated formulations, progestin dose remains constant during the cycle (monophasic).
2. In some newer preparations, progestin and estrogen dosage varies during the cycle (biphasic and triphasic).

To prevent ovulation induction, and to help recognize preexisting early pregnancy, it is generally recommended that women begin oral contraceptives within the first 7 days of the menstrual cycle. Many women, however, start their use after delivery or abortion, before return of menses. If their use is initiated at any time other than during or immediately after a normal menstrual cycle, or within 3 weeks of delivery, another means of birth control should be used throughout the first week to avoid the risk of pregnancy due to induced ovulation.

To obtain maximum protection and promote regular use of oral contraceptives, most suppliers offer dispensers that provide 21 sequentially and individually wrapped, color-coded tablets containing hormones, followed by seven usually inert tablets of another color (Fig. 58–3). It is important for maximum contraceptive efficiency and for peace of mind that each woman adopt an effective scheme for assuring daily (or nightly) self-administration. One technique is to keep a pill supply and toothbrush close to each other and to swallow a pill at tooth brushing time, either in the morning or in the eve-

TABLE 58-3. Some Oral Contraceptives Currently Available in the United States Grouped by Androgenic Activity, Steroid Content, and Phasic Type

Type	Name	EE (μg)	Progestin (mg)
Low Androgenic Activity of Progestin Component[a]			
Monophasic	Modicon, Brevicon, Nelova 0.5/35, NEE 0.5/35	35	Norethindrone 0.5
	Ovcon 35	35	Norethindrone 0.4
	Ortho-Cyclen	35	Norgestimate 0.25
	Ortho-Cept, Desogen	30	Desogestrel 0.15
	Mircette[b]	20	Desogestrel 0.15
Triphasic	Ortho Tri-Cyclen	35/35/35	Norgestimate 0.18/0.215/0.25
Medium Androgenic Activity of Progestin Component			
Monophasic	Norlestrin 1/50	50	Norethindrone acetate 1.0
	Ovcon 50, Genora 1/50, Norethin 1/50M	50	Norethindrone 1.0
	Demulen	50	Ethynodiol diacetate 1.0
	Demulen 1/35	35	Ethynodiol diacetate 1.0
	Ortho-Novum 1/35, Norinyl 1 + 35, Genora 1/35, Norethin 1/35E, Norcept-E 1/35, Nelova 1/35, NEE 1/35	35	Norethindrone 1.0
	Loestrin 1/20	20	Norethindrone acetate 1.0
	Alesse	20	Levonorgestrel 0.1
Biphasic	Ortho-Novum 10/11, NEE 10/11, Jenest-28	35/35	Norethindrone 0.5/1.0
Triphasic	Ortho-Novum 7/7/7	35/35/35	Norethindrone 0.5/0.75/1.0
	Tri-Norinyl	35/35/35	Norethindrone 0.5/1.0/0.5
	Triphasil, Tri-Levlen	30/40/30	Levonorgestrel 0.5/0.075/0.125
	Estrostep	20/30/35	Norethindrone acetate 1.0
High Androgenic Activity of Progestin Component			
Monophasic	Ovral	50	Norgestrel 0.5
	Norlestrin 2.5/50	50	Norethindrone acetate 2.5
	Loestrin 1.5/30	30	Norethindrone acetate 1.5
	Lo-Ovral	30	Norgestrel 0.3
	Nordette	30	Levonorgestrel 0.15
	Levlen	30	Levonorgestrel 0.15
Progestin Only			
Monophasic	Micronor	None	Norethindrone 0.35
	Nor-QD	None	Norethindrone 0.35
	Ovrette	None	Norgestrel 0.075

EE = ethinyl estradiol.
[a] All these compounds have a favorable high-density lipoprotein (HDL)/low-density lipoprotein (LDL) cholesterol ratio, but the compounds containing desogestrel appear to have a more favorable effect by virtue of not decreasing the HDL$_2$-cholesterol fraction (Godsland and Wynn, 1984; Krauss, 1988).
[b] On days 22 and 23 an inert tablet is taken and on days 24-28 a tablet containing 10 μg of ethinyl estradiol is taken.
Modified by Mishell and colleagues (1997), with permission.

ning. If one dose is missed, nothing serious is likely to happen if higher dose monophasic estrogen and progestin pills are used. It may be desirable to double the next dose to minimize breakthrough bleeding and to stay on schedule. If several doses are missed or lower dose pills are used, another form of effective contraception (a barrier technique) should be used. The pill can be restarted after withdrawal bleeding. Without bleeding, the possibility of pregnancy must be considered and excluded prior to resumption of oral contraceptive use.

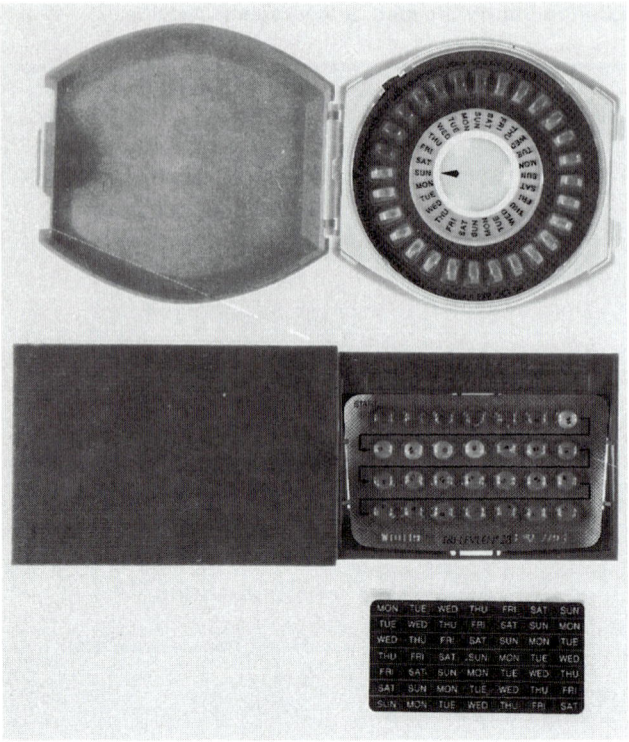

FIGURE 58–3. Oral contraceptive tablets in different containers.

PHASIC PILLS. These preparations were developed in an effort to reduce the amount of total progestin per cycle without sacrificing contraceptive efficacy or cycle control. The reduction is achieved by beginning the contraceptive cycle with a low dose of progestin, and increasing this later in the cycle. For example, a monophasic combined pill containing 35 μg of ethinyl estradiol plus 1.0 mg of norethindrone (*Ortho 1/35; Norinyl 1/35*) supplies 21 mg of progestin per cycle versus a similar triphasic combination (*Ortho 7/7/7*), which supplies 15.75 mg of norethindrone per cycle (Table 58–3). Another nonphasic formulation (*Ovcon 35*), however, supplies only 8.4 mg of norethindrone per cycle.

Triphasic formulations are highly effective in preventing pregnancy (Ellis, 1987; Toews and colleagues, 1987). The theoretical advantage is a reduction in metabolic changes attributable to progestin, and thereby a reduction in adverse effects. Unfortunately, beneficial effects of oral progestins may also be reduced. Estrogen dose may be kept constant, or it may be increased temporarily later in the cycle. Examples include Triphasil and Estrostep, where ethinyl estradiol doses are 30/40/30 and 20/30/35 μg per each 7-day period, respectively. In all such preparations, however, estrogens are kept between 20 and 40 μg of ethinyl estradiol.

Despite the cited advantages, both theoretical and actual, there are distinct disadvantages to triphasic formulations (Hatcher and colleagues, 1990; Woods and associates, 1992). These include:

1. Confusion due to multicolored pills.
2. Breakthrough bleeding (spotting), which almost is doubled compared with nonphasic pills.
3. Loss of flexibility due to difficulty in ''doubling up'' if a pill is missed.

Still, compliance has been good even in teenaged women.

The problem of breakthrough bleeding has been addressed by the use of Mircette, which provides 21 days of pills containing ethinyl estradiol (20 μg) and desogestrel (150 μg). These 21 tablets are followed for 2 days with inert tablets, then for 5 days with tablets containing 10 μg of ethinyl estradiol. This schedule appears to decrease breakthrough bleeding.

DRUG INTERACTIONS. Oral contraceptives interfere with the actions of some drugs (Tables 58–4 and 58–5). Conversely, some drugs decrease the contraceptive effectiveness of combination oral contraceptives (Table 58–6). Phenytoin and rifampin are believed to increase breakthrough bleeding and reduce contraceptive effectiveness of pills containing less than 50 μg of ethinyl estradiol (Hatcher and colleagues, 1998). The mecha-

TABLE 58–4. Drugs Whose Effectiveness is Decreased by Combination Oral Contraceptives

Interacting Drug	Adverse Effect
Acetaminophen and aspirin	Possibly decreased pain relief
Benzodiazepine tranquilizers	Possibly increased or decreased tranquilizer effectiveness and psychomotor function
Methyldopa	Decreased hypotensive effect
Oral anticoagulants	Decreased anticoagulant effect
Oral hypoglycemics	Possibly decreased hypoglycemic effects

Modified from Rizack and Hillman (1985).

TABLE 58–5. Drugs Whose Effectiveness Is Increased by Oral Contraceptives

Interacting Drug	Adverse Effect
Alcohol	Possibly increased effect
Aminophylline	Increased effect
Antidepressants	Possibly an increased effect
Benzodiazepines	Possibly increased or decreased tranquilizer effectiveness and psychomotor function
Beta-blockers	Possibly increased blocker effect
Caffeine	Increased effect
Corticosteroids	Possibly increased toxicity
Theophylline	Increased effect

Modified from Rizack and Hillman (1985).

nism is not entirely clear, but phenytoin stimulates hepatic enzymes that might accelerate the enzymatic degradation of these synthetic hormones. Other agents, such as barbiturates, are known to induce hepatic hydroxylases (Aronson, 1993; Shenfield, 1993). Some broad-spectrum antibiotics such as ampicillin and tetracycline are still listed in labelings as reducing the efficacy of oral contraceptives; however, this likely is not true. Because vitamin C competes for active sulfate in the intestinal wall and increases the bioavailability of ethinyl estradiol, erratic use of vitamin C can result in breakthrough bleeding (Kubba and Guillebaud, 1993).

SAFETY. In general, oral contraceptives, when appropriately monitored, as outlined later in this discussion, have proven to be relatively safe for most women (Table 58–1). The possibility of adverse effects from "The Pill" has received so much attention for so long that the major adverse effect among users may be the anxiety created by almost incessant publicity! Unfortunately, physicians as well as the public are frequently confused by the many and often conflicting reports.

BENEFICIAL EFFECTS. The combined estrogen plus progestin pill is the most effective **reversible** form of contraception available. Failure rates of 0.32 per 100 woman-years or lower have been documented (Vessey and co-workers, 1982). Other reported beneficial effects include increased bone density; reduced menstrual blood loss with less anemia; fewer ectopic pregnancies; less dysmenorrhea associated with endometriosis; fewer functional ovarian cysts and salpingitis; fewer premenstrual complaints; less endometrial and ovarian cancer; reduction in various benign breast diseases; improvement in hirsutism; improvement of acne; prevention of atherogenesis; decreased incidence and severity of pelvic inflammatory disease; and improvement in rheumatoid arthritis (Burkman and colleagues, 2000; Guillebaud, 1997; Hatcher and associates, 1998; Rosenfield and Broholm, 1994; Sulak and Kaunitz, 1999).

BONE MASS DENSITY. Most studies show a small positive effect on bone mass in women who use oral contraceptives (Burkman, 1994; Sulak and Kaunitz, 1999). In a cross-sectional international study, Petitti and co-

TABLE 58–6. Drugs Known and Suspected to Decrease Contraceptive Effectiveness of Combination Oral Contraceptives and Recommended Management

Drugs	Recommended Management
Barbiturates	Use back-up or higher dose contraceptive
Carbamazepine[a]	Use back-up or higher dose contraceptive
Felbamate	Use back-up or higher dose contraceptive
Griseofulvin	Use back-up or higher dose contraceptive
Ketoconazole/Itraconazole	Use back-up or higher dose contraceptive
Phenytoin	Use back-up or higher dose contraceptive; monitor phenytoin concentration because of possible enhancement of phenytoin effect
Primidone	Use alternative contraceptive
Rifampin	Use back-up or higher dose contraceptive
Topiramate	Use back-up or higher dose contraceptive

[a] Possible decreased contraceptive effect.
Modified from American College of Obstetricians and Gynecologists (2000), Association of Professors of Gynecology and Obstetrics (1999), and Frederiksen (1998).

workers (2000) showed significantly increased bone mass after only 6 months of use. In a population-based Australian study, Pasco and colleagues (2000) found a cumulative increase in bone density with duration of use. Berenson and associates (2000) performed a prospective study and showed a slight increase at 1 year with two agents.

POSSIBLE ADVERSE EFFECTS

METABOLIC EFFECTS. Oral contraceptives have a wide range of metabolic effects that are often combined and overlapping. Metabolic changes, often qualitatively similar to those of pregnancy, have been identified in women taking oral contraceptives. For example, plasma thyroxine and thyroid-binding proteins are elevated. Plasma cortisol concentration increases with a nearly comparable increase in transcortin. It is extremely important, therefore, that these pregnancy-like effects be considered when evaluating laboratory tests.

LIPOPROTEINS AND LIPIDS. The combination oral contraceptives increase triglycerides and total cholesterol. Estrogen decreases concentration of low-density lipoprotein (LDL) cholesterol and increases high-density lipoprotein (HDL) cholesterol. Some progestins cause the reverse (Stadel, 1981). The importance of such changes in the genesis of *arterial vascular disease* such as myocardial infarction or stroke is not clear but is cause for concern (Knopp, 1988; Mishell, 1988). The adverse changes noted in HDL–LDL ratios are the consequences of the 19-nortestosterone progestins, and these changes are likely related to the specific progestin and its dose (Kauppinen-Mäkelin and colleagues, 1992). Progestins can alter relative amounts of total HDL, HDL_2, and HDL_3, and it is the HDL_2 fraction that provides cardiovascular protection (Miller and co-workers, 1982; Tikkanen and associates, 1982). Therefore, estrogen and progestin effects on specific HDL_2 fraction may be of special importance because these drugs may alter cardiovascular risks even though total HDL cholesterol values are increased or unchanged.

The lipid effects of combination contraceptives are time and dose dependent. Maximal effects of progestins are usually best measured after 6 months of use (Åkerlund and associates, 1994; Burkman, 1993). The use of monophasic contraceptives containing 150 μg desogestrel and 30 μg of ethinyl estradiol (Desogen, Ortho-Cept) reduced LDL cholesterol 15 percent while levonorgestrel preparations caused no significant changes. No significant change in LDL cholesterol resulted from the use of triphasic and high-dose monophasic compounds containing norethindrone (Burkman, 1993).

Desogestrel-containing compounds do not decrease HDL_2 cholesterol while they increase total HDL cholesterol. If lipoproteins are a concern, compounds containing desogestrel or possibly norgestimate can be used.

Lipoprotein (a) or Lp(a) has been identified as an atherogenic lipoprotein (Bartens and Wanner, 1994). Estrogens appear to exert a favorable response by reducing circulatory levels of lipoprotein (a). Its atherogenic action appears to be mediated by reduction of plasminogen activation. Decreased plasmin then results in reduced activation of transforming growth factor-beta (TGF-β), which is a powerful inhibitor of smooth muscle cell proliferation. If TGF-β were reduced in arteries with intimal injury, smooth muscle would proliferate, resulting in a narrowing of the artery.

CARBOHYDRATE METABOLISM. Oral contraceptives decrease glucose tolerance in a significant percentage of users, apparently as a direct consequence of the estrogen dose used (Wynn and Godsland, 1986). Progestins usually are observed to increase insulin secretion and create insulin resistance (Wynn and Niththyananthan, 1982). Because of these effects, contraceptive steroids may intensify preexisting *diabetes* or may prove sufficiently diabetogenic to induce clinically apparent disease in susceptible women. The risk of the latter appears low because in the great majority of women the effect on carbohydrate metabolism is slight (Phillips and Duffy, 1973). As with pregnancy, diabetogenic effects are often reversible when oral contraceptives are terminated. Speroff (2000a) has provided an excellent review of this subject.

Estrogen–progestin oral contraceptive use by women who had *gestational diabetes* has been discouraged by some. Concern centers around the possible acceleration of the appearance of insulin-dependent diabetes. According to Kalkhoff (1980), the incidence of diabetes among normal women taking these contraceptives is almost identical to that in a general population. Conversely, the incidence of diabetes among women with previous gestational diabetes taking these contraceptives is increased tenfold. Whether oral contraceptives hasten the onset of permanent disease in gestational diabetics is still an important unanswered question.

There is also concern about contraceptive use in women with previous gestational diabetes and possible associations between mild hyperglycemia or hyperinsulinemia and increased cardiovascular risk. Skouby and associates (1985) studied a small group of women with previous gestational diabetes who were using a triphasic pill containing levonorgestrel (Triphasil, Tri-Levlen). They found that glucose, insulin, and glucagon response, as well as serum cholesterol, high-density lipoproteins, and low-density lipoproteins were unchanged compared with pretreatment values. In contrast, Wynn and Godsland (1986), in a long-term study of women taking 30 μg of ethinyl estradiol and 0.15 mg of levonorgestrel (*Nordette*), reported that there was a progressive deterioration of glucose tolerance. There was less effect when 1 mg norethindrone was given. Thus, norgestrel appears to have the greatest antagonizing effect on insulin and glucose metabolism, and this effect becomes more pronounced over time. If combination oral contraceptives are used in women with a history of gestational diabetes, compounds containing low-dose estrogen (20 μg) and desogestrel should be considered.

PROTEIN METABOLISM. Estrogens increase hepatic production of a variety of *globulins*. Increased *angiotensinogen* production appears to be dose related, and its conversion by renin to angiotensin I has been suspected to be associated with so-called "pill-induced" hypertension (p. 1529). *Fibrinogen,* and likely factors II, VII, IX, X, XII, and XIII, are increased in direct proportion to estrogen dose (Comp, 1996; Kaunitz, 1999b). The relationship of these increased clotting factors to venous and arterial thrombosis is discussed on page 1528, but the incidence of both forms of thrombosis appear to be estrogen dose related (Mann, 1982).

LIVER DISEASE. *Cholestasis* and *cholestatic jaundice* are uncommon complications in users of oral contraceptives; the signs and symptoms clear when the medication is stopped. It appears that oral contraceptives may accelerate the development of gallbladder disease in women who are susceptible, but there is no overall increased long-term risk (Royal College of General Practitioners, 1982; Strom and colleagues, 1986). There is no reason to withhold oral contraceptives from women recovered from viral hepatitis.

NEOPLASIA. Hormonal contraception as a cause of cancer appears to be unlikely (Cancer and Steroid Hormone Study, 1986, 1987a, 1987b; Prentice and Thomas, 1987; Schlesselman and colleagues, 1988). In fact, a protective effect against ovarian and endometrial cancer has been shown in these studies. There are, however, conflicting reports concerning the risks of premalignant and malignant changes of the liver, pituitary, cervix, and breast.

HEPATIC HYPERPLASIA AND CANCER. Use of estrogen plus progestin contraceptives has been linked circumstantially with the development of *hepatic focal nodular hyperplasia* and actual tumor formation that most often, but not always, is benign. This association has been observed in women using high-dose estrogen-containing formulations (usually mestranol) for prolonged periods. Neuberger and associates (1986) reported an association between prolonged oral contraceptive use and *hepato-*

cellular carcinoma in women younger than age 50. In contrast, conclusions derived from a multicenter World Health Organization study (1989a) support the view that there is no increased risk of hepatic cancer.

Benign hepatic nodules have extensive proliferation of large and small thin-walled blood vessels. The lesions on rupture can be complicated by bleeding, hemoperitoneum, and shock, which proved fatal in 8 of 24 cases cited by Antoniades and colleagues (1975). The liver may become enlarged to palpation, and imaging studies disclose a space-occupying lesion(s). If identified before rupture, stopping the oral contraceptives and resection of the lesion has been recommended. Some liver lesions appear to disappear spontaneously after discontinuing oral contraceptives. Increased growth and vascularity during pregnancy or the puerperium, leading to rupture and death, have occurred (Kent and co-workers, 1978). The use of newer, low-dose combination oral contraceptives appears to have reduced the incidence of this unusual condition (Waetjen and Grimes, 1996).

PITUITARY ADENOMAS. According to the Pituitary Adenoma Study Group (1983), oral contraceptives do not increase the risk of pituitary *prolactinomas*. Awareness that these neoplasms may cause menstrual irregularities, along with imaging technology to visualize them, has resulted in their diagnosis before steroidal contraceptives are given.

CERVIX. There is a correlation between the risk of preinvasive cervical cancer and oral contraceptive use, and the risk of invasive cancer increases after 5 years of use (Thomas and Ray, 1996; Vessey and associates, 1983b; Zondervan and co-workers, 1996). It is unclear if these associations are causally related. For example, oral contraceptive users do not have the benefit of barrier or spermicidal protection from the human papillomavirus, and they more frequently are screened cytologically for cervical cancer (Butterworth and associates, 1992).

BREAST CANCER. It is unclear whether oral contraceptives contribute to the development of *breast cancer.* In the largest study, no increased risk for breast cancer among oral contraceptive users was demonstrated (Cancer and Steroid Hormone Study, 1986). Moreover, risk did not vary according to preparation or duration of use. Whereas a New Zealand study (Paul and colleagues, 1986) confirmed these findings, a Swedish study (Meirik and associates, 1986) suggested a slightly increased risk of breast cancer among women who used oral contraceptives for 12 or more years. Gabrick and co-workers (2000) reported a higher risk in women with a strong family history, but this was with older preparations with high-dose estrogens. The Collaborative Group on Hormonal Factors in Breast Cancer (1996) studied more than 53,000 women with breast cancer. They found a small but significantly increased relative risk of breast cancer in women taking combined oral contraceptives or within 10 years of stopping. For current users, the risk was 1.24, it was 1.16 for those 1 to 4 years after stopping, and 1.07 for those 5 to 9 years after stopping.

When breast tumors were discovered in the 1996 collaborative study, the tumors were reported to be less aggressive and to be detected at an earlier stage. Moreover, the risk was not influenced by early use, duration of use, use prior to pregnancy, the dose or type of hormone used. Because oral contraceptives did not appear to alter risk factors in women with and without a family history of breast cancer.

Long-term studies of the newer, low-dose oral contraceptives have not yet been performed. The 1 in 9 attack rate of breast cancer would make it difficult for a small increased risk to be detected. The Food and Drug Administration (1984) has not changed its recommendations regarding oral contraceptive prescribing and the risks for breast cancer. Speroff (2000b) performed a scholarly evidence-based review of 54 epidemiological studies that addressed this problem. He concluded that there was no evidence that oral contraceptives, including high-estrogen or high-progesterone dose, increased breast cancer risk even with prolonged use.

NUTRITION. Aberrations in the levels of several *nutrients,* similar to changes induced by normal pregnancy, have been described for women who use oral contraceptives. Lower plasma levels in users compared with nonusers have been described by some investigators for ascorbic acid, folic acid, vitamin B_{12}, niacin, riboflavin, and zinc.

PYRIDOXINE DEFICIENCY. Biochemical changes compatible with vitamin B_6 (pyridoxine) deficiency have been documented with oral contraceptive use. These are similar to those of normal pregnancy (Wynn, 1975). Estrogens induce the rate-limiting liver enzyme, *tryptophan oxygenase,* which enhances tryptophan metabolism in a way that suggests pyridoxine deficiency (also see discussion of *depression,* p. 1530). The similarity of changes in tryptophan and pyridoxine metabolism to those of normal pregnancy strongly implies that estrogen–progestin contraceptives do not induce clinically significant pathological changes.

CARDIOVASCULAR EFFECTS. There are a number of uncommon but significant cardiovascular risks associated with hormonal contraceptive use.

THROMBOEMBOLISM. The risk of *deep vein thrombosis* and *pulmonary embolism* has been estimated to be increased by 3- to 11-fold in women who use oral contraceptives

(Realini and Goldzieher, 1985; Stadel, 1981). Contraceptive use during the month before an operative procedure appears to significantly increase the risk of postoperative thromboembolism. These risks clearly are estrogen-dose related, and the risk decreases with the use of formulations containing 20 to 35 μg of ethinyl estradiol (Westhoff, 1998).

In the mid-1990s, there was a 1.5- to 2-fold increased risk reported for venous thromboembolism associated with contraceptives containing either desogestrel or gestodene when compared with those containing levonorgestrel or norethindrone (Bloemenkamp and colleagues, 1995; Jick and associates, 1995; Spitzer and co-workers, 1996; World Health Organization, 1995). These findings were not confirmed in subsequent reports, which show that desogestrel, gestodene, levonorgestrel, and norgestimate all have similar low risks of association with venous thromboembolism (Association of Professors of Obstetrics and Gynecology, 1999; Farmer and associates, 1998; Kaunitz, 1999b; Speroff, 1998; Westhoff, 1998).

Mishell (2000) performed a scholarly evidence-based review of the risks of venous thromboembolism in oral contraceptive users. After analyzing six epidemiologically sound studies, he considered that the risk is increased three- to fourfold in users (but not former users). Importantly, the baseline risk is low—about 1 per 10,000 woman-years—and thus the incidence with oral contraceptives of 1.0 to 3.0 per 10,000 woman-years is small. Moreover, it is half that of the 5.7 per 10,000 woman-years incidence estimated for pregnancy.

The mechanism by which estrogen–progestin contraceptives enhance the risk of venous thrombosis and thromboembolism is unclear. Development of distinctive vascular intimal and medial lesions with associated occlusive thrombi has been described (Irey and co-workers, 1970). Moreover, platelet aggregation may be accelerated, and both plasma antithrombin III activity and endothelial plasminogen activator are likely to be reduced. The enhanced risk of thromboembolism appears to decrease rapidly once the contraceptive is stopped. Women who develop thromboembolism while taking estrogen-containing contraceptives, however, also appear to be at increased risk during pregnancy and the early puerperium. Those most at risk for venous thrombosis and embolism include women with the factor V Leiden mutation and those with protein C and S deficiencies (Comp, 1996). Other clinical factors that increase the risk of venous thrombosis and embolism are hypertension, obesity, diabetes, smoking, and a sedentary lifestyle (Hatcher and associates, 1998).

STROKE AND ARTERIAL THROMBOSIS. According to the World Health Organization Collaborative Study (1998), ischemic and hemorrhagic strokes are uncommon in nonsmoking women younger than 35. The incidence is 10 and 24 events per 1 million woman years, respectively. The earlier reports by Lidegaard (1993, 1998) that the risk of cerebral thromboembolism was increased in women using low-dose estrogen contraceptives stimulated a number of focused studies. At least five subsequent studies concluded that the use of such compounds by healthy, nonsmoking women is not associated with an increased risk of thrombotic or hemorrhagic strokes (Mishell, 2000; Petitti and co-workers, 1996; Schwartz and associates, 1998; World Health Organization Collaborative Study, 1996). Importantly, women who have hypertension, or who smoke, or have migraine headaches have an increased risk of hemorrhagic and thrombotic strokes (Mishell, 2000; Schwartz and colleagues, 1998).

HYPERTENSION. An association between oral contraceptives and hypertension was apparent by the late 1960s. Several reports appeared of the occasional woman who, while using an estrogen–progestin contraceptive, became overtly hypertensive. Usually blood pressure returned to normal when the medication was stopped. Oral contraceptives, presumably in response to estrogen, were shown to increase plasma angiotensinogen (renin substrate) to levels near those found in normal pregnancy. Although the great majority of women using oral contraceptives demonstrate these changes, most do not become hypertensive. Progestin appears to contribute to the hypertension. Weir (1982) observed that women who developed hypertension while taking estrogen–progestin oral contraceptives and who become normotensive after stopping the contraceptive, redeveloped hypertension when oral contraception was reinstituted, even if the contraceptive employed contained no estrogen.

Unfortunately, normotensive women who are destined to become hypertensive in response to oral contraceptives usually cannot be identified in advance. The development of hypertension during pregnancy does not preclude subsequent use of oral contraceptives.

MYOCARDIAL INFARCTION. Oral contraceptives containing low-dose estrogen and low-androgenic progestins are not associated with an increased risk of myocardial infarction in nonsmokers (Lewis, 1996; Petitti, 1998; Sidney, 1996, 1998, and their colleagues; Mishell, 2000; World Health Organization Collaborative Study, 1997a). The American College of Obstetricians and Gynecologists (1994) cited no contraindication for oral contraceptives in nonsmoking women past age 35. Finally, the Food and Drug Administration revised their labeling of oral contraceptives to remove restrictions for nonsmoking women past age 40 (Contraception Report, 1992).

It must not be forgotten that smoking is an independent risk factor for myocardial infarction, which is enhanced synergistically by oral contraceptives. The two critical points with respect to smoking and oral contraceptives appear to be more than 15 cigarettes per day for current and past smokers and age over 35 (Craft and Hannaford, 1989).

MIGRAINE HEADACHES. The frequency and intensity of attacks of *migraine headaches* may improve or worsen. Most clinicians prefer to avoid these contraceptives in such women, not only because they are likely to be unacceptable but also because some migraines are indistinguishable from mild or impending stroke. Moreover, it appears likely that even a history of migraine headaches is associated with an increased risk of thrombotic and hemorrhagic strokes (American College of Obstetricians and Gynecologists, 2000; Schwartz and co-workers, 1998).

EFFECTS ON REPRODUCTION

POSTPILL AMENORRHEA. When combination contraception is discontinued, ovulation usually resumes promptly. Similar to the postpartum period, within 3 months after discontinuance, at least 90 percent of women who previously ovulated regularly will have done so again. Bracken and associates (1990) observed a reduced conception rate for at least six cycles after stopping these contraceptives.

CONGENITAL DEFECTS. In earlier studies, fetal limb-reduction deformities were reported in pregnancies conceived while taking, or soon after taking, combination oral contraceptives (Janevich and co-workers, 1974). Subsequently, Rothman and Louik (1978) and Savolainen and associates (1981) found no increased major malformations in infants whose mothers recently had used oral contraceptives. Similarly, Lammer and Cordero (1986) found no association between major malformations and contraceptive exposure in early pregnancy (Chap. 38, p. 1017). Even so, the woman who thinks that she may be pregnant should be advised to stop the oral contraceptive–*but use another contraceptive technique*—until it can be established whether or not she is pregnant.

LACTATION. Use of combined oral contraceptive hormones by nursing mothers reduces the amount of *breast milk*. Only very small quantities of the hormones are excreted in milk. Because progestin-only oral contraceptives have little effect on lactation and provide excellent contraception, they are preferred for up to 6 months in women who are using breast feeding exclusively (p. 1531). After 6 months, a backup barrier technique should be added (Kaunitz, 1997). A woman who is only breast feeding intermittently should have effective contraception beginning as soon as 3 weeks postpartum (Kaunitz, 1997).

OTHER EFFECTS. *Cervical mucorrhea,* likely due to cervical ectopy, is fairly common in response to the estrogen component (Critchlow and colleagues, 1995). The mucus at times may be irritating to the vagina and vulva. *Vaginitis* or *vulvovaginitis,* especially that caused by *Candida,* also may develop. Antibiotic therapy in pill users increases the frequency of such infections.

Hyperpigmentation of the face and forehead (*chloasma*) is more likely in women who demonstrated such a change during pregnancy (Chap. 54, p. 1430). Almost all women using combination contraceptives have increased pigmentation of breast areola and perineum. Acne may improve or, at times, be aggravated, often dependent on the androgenic property of the progestin used (Table 58–3). Combined contraceptives suppress gonadotropins and thus diminish ovarian androstenedione secretion and resultant testosterone production. If a low androgenic progestin such as desogestrel or norgestimate is used in the combination pill, overall androgen effect is reduced and acne will likely improve.

Uterine *myomas* most likely are not increased in size by oral contraceptives (Parazzini and colleagues, 1992).

Weight gain has been a troublesome complaint from women who use oral contraceptives, although an increase in weight is far from uniform. Some of the weight may be caused by fluid retention, but it is likely to be a consequence of increased dietary intake.

Low-dose estrogen formulations are not associated with *depression,* but oral contraceptives containing 50 μg or more of estrogen were associated with depression (Kay, 1984). Goldzeiher and Zamah (1995) reported that depression is more likely to improve with low-dose oral contraceptives.

Preliminary studies from the Centers for Disease Control and Prevention have not shown a significantly increased rate of human immunodeficiency virus (HIV) infection in women using hormonal contraceptives (National Institute of Child Health and Human Development, 1996). Clearly, hormonal contraception does not prevent the transmission of the virus that causes acquired immunodeficiency syndrome (AIDS) or any other known viral infection.

RISK OF DEATH. The risk of death from oral contraceptives is very low if the woman is younger than 35, has no systemic illness, and does not smoke (Table 58–7). Porter and associates (1987) reported their experiences with nearly 55,000 woman-years of oral contraceptive use in the Group Health Cooperative of Puget Sound and attributed only one death to their use. The risk of dying as the consequence of using an oral contraceptive certainly is less than that of pregnancy, even though the risk with the latter is quite low (Tables 58–1 and 58–7).

Similar results have been reported from England. Vessey and colleagues (1989), in a 20-year follow-up study of over 17,000 women, reported that the overall relative risk of death in women taking oral contraceptives was 0.9 compared with women of similar age using barrier methods. Deaths due to cancer and their relative risk were breast, 0.9; cervix, 3.3; and ovary, 0.4. The death risk from cardiovascular disease was 1.5, and most cardiovascular deaths were in smokers.

POSTPARTUM USE. Women who do not breast feed, and especially those who have undergone abortions,

TABLE 58–7. Annual Number of Birth-related or Method-related Deaths Associated with Fertility Control per 100,000 Women According to Age

Category	Age (yr)					
	15–19	*20–24*	*25–29*	*30–34*	*35–39*	*40–44*
Method-related Deaths						
OCP nonsmoker	0.3	0.5	0.9	1.9	13.8	31.6
OCP smoker	2.2	3.4	6.6	13.5	51.1	117.2
IUD	0.8	0.8	1.0	1.0	1.4	1.4
Birth-related Deaths						
No contraception	7.0	7.4	9.1	14.8	25.7	28.2
Condom (failure)	1.1	1.6	0.7	0.2	0.3	0.4
Diaphragm/spermicide (failure)	1.9	1.2	1.2	1.3	2.2	2.8
Rhythm method (failure)	2.5	1.6	1.6	1.7	2.9	3.6

IUD = intrauterine device; OCP = oral contraceptive pill.
Modified from Ory (1983), with permission.

may ovulate before 6 to 7 weeks after pregnancy (Chap. 17, p. 418). There is an advantage, therefore, to starting oral contraceptives before the traditional "6-weeks postpartum check." On the other hand, increased risks of adverse effects, especially venous thromboembolism, might be anticipated from use of estrogen–progestin contraceptives earlier in the puerperium. The use of 35-μg or smaller estrogen doses has reduced this risk greatly, and thus far, in our now extensive experience in which oral contraceptives have been started during the third week postpartum, there has been no evidence of increased morbidity or mortality.

COST. The price of oral contraceptives has increased remarkably, and this likely does not reflect the cost of the ingredients. The typical cost of oral contraceptives and other forms of contraception are listed in Table 58–8. Fixed dose estrogen–progestin contraceptives containing norethindrone and either 35 or 50 μg of estrogen are available as *generic products*. Because regulations allow a 25 percent variance in bioavailability, poor cycle control might follow their use in women as they change from one generic manufacturer to another.

CONTRAINDICATIONS. If a contraindication is listed, combined oral contraceptive pills should probably never be used for contraception (Table 58–9).

PROGESTATIONAL CONTRACEPTIVES

ORAL PROGESTINS. So-called *mini-pills* (Table 58–3) consist solely of 350 μg or less of a progestin used daily. They have not achieved widespread popularity because of a much higher incidence of irregular bleeding and a higher pregnancy rate. They impair fertility without always inhibiting ovulation. This likely results from inducing cervical mucus that impedes sperm penetration and from altering endometrial maturation sufficiently to thwart successful blastocyst implantation. Contraceptive effectiveness is greatest if there is ovulation suppression that paradoxically results in an increased incidence of abnormal uterine bleeding. Therefore, if menses are not disturbed, or only minimally disturbed, ovulation is likely not suppressed, and the pregnancy risk is greater. Actual pregnancy rates with progestin-only pills range from 1.1 to 9.6 pregnancies per 100 women in the first year (Trussell and Kost, 1987). Guillebaud (1985) reported a lower rate of 0.9 pregnancies per 100 married women with a decreasing rate observed with advancing age (25 to 29 years, 3.1; 30 to 34 years, 2.0; 35 to 39 years, 1.0; 40 or older, 0.3 pregnancies per 100 married women).

The contraceptive effectiveness of oral progestin-only contraceptives is decreased by barbiturates, rifampin, and likely by carbamazepine. Phenytoin also

decreases the contraceptive effectiveness of progestin-only pills, and the phenytoin anticonvulsant effect also may be increased. The best management is to use backup contraceptives or increase the dose for women taking carbamazepine and phenytoin. For women taking barbiturates or rifampin, oral progestin-only pills should not be used, and these women should use an alternate method of contraception (Frederiksen, 1998).

Women taking carbamazepine, phenytoin or rifampin should not use levonorgestrel implants (Norplant). In such cases an alternate method of contraception must be used (Frederiksen, 1998). Finally, depot medroxy-progesterone contraceptive effectiveness is decreased in women taking aminoglutethimide. An alternate contraceptive method also must be used in these women.

BENEFITS. Benefits are similar to those described earlier for the combined oral contraceptives. In addition, these formulations have not been shown to increase the risk of cardiovascular disease or malignancy (Guillebaud, 1985). They are less likely to increase blood pressure or cause headaches (Vessey and colleagues, 1985). They have minimal effects on carbohydrate metabolism and allegedly cause less depression, dysmenorrhea, and premenstrual symptoms. When used by lactating women, these agents are virtually 100 percent effective for up to 6 months, and they have little effect on milk production (Betrabet and colleagues, 1987; Shikary and associates, 1987). Smokers who cannot use combined oral contraceptives after age 35 can use these agents. Finally, they can be used in women with altered glucose tolerance and, **with caution,** in women who had hypertension or headaches while taking combination oral contraceptives.

DISADVANTAGES. The major disadvantages are contraceptive failure and an increased incidence of ectopic pregnancy when contraception fails. Irregular uterine bleeding is a distinct disadvantage and can consist of amenorrhea, spotting, breakthrough bleeding, and prolonged periods of amenorrhea or menorrhagia. Ovarian functional cysts develop with a greater frequency in women using these agents. Another disadvantage is that they must be taken at the same or nearly the same time daily (Guillebaud, 1985). *If a progestin-only pill is taken even 3 hours late, a backup form of contraception must be used for the next 2 days* (American College of Obstetricians and Gynecologists, 1994).

CONTRAINDICATIONS. Progestin-only pills are contraindicated in women, especially older women, with unexplained uterine bleeding. A history of a previous ectopic pregnancy or previous functional ovarian cysts should also be considered a relative contraindication. The Food and Drug Administration has required the

TABLE 58–8. Unit Costs for Contraceptive Drugs, Methods, and Associated Services

Method	Unit Cost in US Dollars	
	Managed Payment Model	Public Payer Model
Tubal ligation[a]	2465	1190
Vasectomy[a]	755	353
Oral contraceptives		
Drug	21/cycle	17/cycle
Office visit[a]	38	16
Implant		
Drug[a]	365	365
Insertion[a]	333	48
Removal	100	80
Injectable contraceptive		
Drug	30/quarter	30/quarter
Office visit	38/quarter	17/quarter
Progesterone-T IUD		
Device	82	82
Insertion	207	62
Removal	70	11
Copper-T IUD		
Device[a]	184	109
Insertion[a]	207	62
Removal	70	11
Diaphragm[b]		
Device (1st and 3rd year)	18	15
Office visit (device fitting)	38	16
Spermicidal jelly[c]	12	8
Male condom[b]	1	0.33
Female condom[b]	4	1.25
Spermicides[b, c]	12	9
Cervical cap[b]		
Device (1st and 3rd year)	31	19
Office visit (device fitting)	38	16
Spermicidal jelly[c]	12	9
Withdrawal	0	0
Periodic abstinence	0	0
No method	0	0

IUD = intrauterine device.
[a] First year only.
[b] Method costs were calculated on 83 acts of intercourse per year. Diaphragm and cap users were assumed to replace their devices during the third year.
[c] Used for 10 acts of intercourse.
Adapted with permission from Trussell and colleagues (1995) and Association of Professors of Gynecology and Obstetrics (1999).

TABLE 58-9. Contraindications and a Warning About the Use of Combination Oral Contraceptives

Oral contraceptives should not be used in women with any of the following conditions:

Thrombophlebitis or thromboembolic disorders

A past history of deep-vein thrombophlebitis or thromboembolic disorders

Cerebrovascular or coronary-artery disease

Known or suspected breast carcinoma

Endometrial carcinoma or other known or suspected estrogen-dependent neoplasia

Undiagnosed abnormal genital bleeding

Cholestatic jaundice of pregnancy or jaundice with prior pill use

Hepatic adenomas or carcinomas

Known or suspected pregnancy

Warnings:

Cigarette smoking increases the risk of serious cardiovascular side effects from oral contraceptive use. This risk increases with age and with heavy smoking (15 or more cigarettes per day) and is quite marked in women over 35 years of age. Women who use oral contraceptives should be strongly advised not to smoke.

From *Physician's Desk Reference* (2000).

same package insert labeling of contraindications for both combination and progestin-only oral contraceptives.

INJECTABLE PROGESTIN CONTRACEPTIVES. The advantages of injected progestins include a contraceptive effectiveness comparable with or better than combined oral contraceptives, long-lasting action with injections required only 4 to 6 times a year, and minimal impairment of lactation (American College of Obstetricians and Gynecologists, 1994). Depot medroxyprogesterone acetate (*Depo-Provera*) and norethindrone ethanthate (*Norgest*) have been used effectively world wide for many years. *Depo-Provera* was approved for contraceptive use in the United States in 1992, however, Norgest is not yet available. The mechanisms of action of both drugs appear to be multiple and include ovulation inhibition, increased cervical mucus viscosity, and production of an endometrium unfavorable for ovum implantation (Mishell, 1996).

BENEFITS AND DISADVANTAGES. These are similar to those for oral progestins. Cushman and associates (1996) reported that women attending urban family planning clinics rated injectable contraceptives as less convenient and thought them to be less effective than pill or Norplant users. The disadvantages include pro-

longed amenorrhea, uterine bleeding during and after use, and prolonged anovulation after discontinuation. Return of fertility is delayed but not prevented. Triglycerides and HDL cholesterol are both reduced in long-term users, but LDL cholesterol is not increased (Deslypere and associates, 1985). These agents modify glucose metabolism only slightly in long-term users. As might be expected, the incidence of iron-deficiency anemia is decreased in long-term users, likely as a result of prolonged amenorrhea. The reported risks of breast cancer are conflicting. Skegg and colleagues (1995) pooled the results of the New Zealand and World Health Organization case-control studies, which included almost 1800 women with breast cancer and 14,000 controls. Within the first 5 years of use, the contraceptive was associated with a twofold risk of cancer, but overall the risk was not increased. Cervical and hepatic malignancy do not appear to be increased, and the risk of ovarian and endometrial cancers is decreased in women using this contraception (Earl and David, 1994; Kaunitz, 1996). The risk of cervical carcinoma-in-situ may be increased (Thomas and colleagues, 1995). Weight gain is a real and predictable problem. There is an average gain of 5.4 pounds for the first year, 8.1 pounds after 2 years, and 13.8 pounds after 4 years of use (World Health Organization, 1990). In small studies, Mainwaring and colleagues (1995) and Moore and associates (1995) reported no weight gain in the first year of use. Headaches, breast tenderness, and depression have been reported to be associated with these injections.

In long-term users of depot medroxyprogesterone, loss of bone mineral density is a potential problem in women 18 to 39 years of age (Scholes and colleagues, 1999). This may be even a greater problem for teenagers because bone density is increased most rapidly from age 10 to 30 (Cromer and colleagues, 1996; Sulak and Kaunitz, 1999). This is a particularly worrisome problem, but bone loss appears to be reversible after discontinuation of therapy (Cundy and colleagues, 1994). It is unknown if "add-back" estrogen therapy during depot contraception will reduce or reverse bone density loss during therapy.

Depot medroxyprogesterone is injected deeply into the upper outer quadrant of the buttock without massage to ensure that the drug is released slowly. The usual dose is 150 mg every 90 days. Within days, this results in plasma levels of approximately 1.5 to 3 ng/mL, which gradually decline to 0.2 ng/mL at 6 months and become undetectable by 7 to 9 months (Ortiz and colleagues, 1977). An additional contraceptive method should be used for at least 2 weeks after the initial injection. Berenson and Wiemann (1996) reported that 12 percent of adolescents who chose this method failed to obtain a second injection within 4 months of the initial injection.

Norethindrone ethanthate is injected in a similar manner in a dose of 200 mg, but it must be reinjected every 60 days (World Health Organization, 1983). Within a week of injection, plasma levels of norethindrone plateau at 10 to 17 ng/mL and remain at these values for about 3 to 4 weeks. After this time, the levels fall to approximately 4 ng/mL for 30 to 60 days (Goebelsmann and colleagues, 1979).

PROGESTIN IMPLANTS (NORPLANT SYSTEM). The *Norplant System* provides levonorgestrel in six silastic containers that are implanted subdermally. Each is 34 mm long, 2.4 mm in diameter, and contains 36 mg of levonorgestrel. The combined 216-mg dose results in an almost immediate plasma release of about 85 μg/day for the first 6 to 8 weeks, resulting in immediate contraceptive effectiveness. By 9 months after insertion, the release rate is about 50 μg/day, gradually decreasing to 25 to 30 μg/day by 60 months, when it should be removed (Hatcher and colleagues, 1998).

EFFECTIVENESS. During 18,530 woman-months of use, 19 pregnancies were reported in women using levonorgestrel implants; 11 of these were in years 6 to 8 (Diaz and colleagues, 1987). Data from the Population Council (Sivin, 1988), based on more than 12,000 woman-years of experience, indicates a failure rate in the first year of 0.04 per 100 woman-years. The rate was 0.2 in the second year, and rates of 0.9, 0.5, and 1.1 were reported in the third, fourth, and fifth years. Thus, this form of contraception is one of the most effective available. Importantly, after termination of use, normal fertility is promptly restored (Sivin and colleagues, 1992).

MODE OF ACTION. Up to a third of cycles may be ovulatory based on serum progesterone determinations of 3 ng/mL (Brache and associates, 1990). This estimate is likely overestimated by a factor of two; however, with progestin-induced changes in cervical mucus and endometrium, the contraceptive effect is extremely good. Despite early reports that contraceptive effectiveness was inversely proportional to body weight in excess of 70 kg, the development of a thinner silastic tube has partially eliminated this concern.

ADVANTAGES AND DISADVANTAGES. These are almost identical to those for oral progestins (described earlier), except for the effect on carbohydrate metabolism. Konje and associates (1992) reported that after 6 months of use, glucose and insulin values were altered even in nondiabetic women. They cautioned that these changes were not significant in normal women, but there were concerns in potential diabetics. It also appears that bone density loss does not occur with use of the Norplant System (Cromer and associates, 1996; Naessen and co-

workers, 1995). In a cross-sectional study of 103 users, Alvarez-Sanchez and colleagues (2000) demonstrated an 18 percent incidence of enlarged (> 25 mm) ovarian follicles compared with only 4 percent in a copper–intrauterine device control group. The longest time to resolution was 4 weeks.

Because of minor surgery involved, there are also problems associated with local infection. If the capsules are not inserted as directed, removal is more difficult. Finally, it should be remembered that barbiturates, carbamazepine, phenytoin and rifampin reduce the contraceptive effectiveness of Norplant (p. 1531). Some side effects of Norplant are listed in Table 58–10.

CONTRAINDICATIONS. These are the same as those for oral progestins. Importantly, as emphasized by the American Medical Association Board of Trustees (1992), these agents are not to be used by governmental agencies to coerce women into using contraception in return for receipt of benefits.

LEGAL DIFFICULTIES. Despite the effectiveness, safety, and patient satisfaction with this excellent contraceptive, it has become the target of personal injury lawyers. They have found "a new area to litigate" based upon the alleged but totally unproven accusation that the silicone content of the rods is producing illness. The *New York Times* on May 28, 1995, published a lead article entitled "Will the Lawyers Kill Off Norplant?" The story noted that in Dallas a woman stated she was "very happy with her Norplant but was having it out on the advice of her lawyer." She went on to say, "Once

TABLE 58–10. Side Effects of Norplant During the First Year of Use

Side Effects	Frequency (%)
Headache	17–19
Ovarian enlargement	3–12
Dizziness	5–8
Breast tenderness	6
Nervousness	6
Nausea	5–8
Acne	4–7
Dermatitis	4–8
Breast discharge	3–5
Change in appetite	3–6
Weight gain	3–6
Hair loss or growth	2–3

Data from Hatcher and associates (1998).

I get my money, can I get a second Norplant put in?" In our own clinics, Norplant insertions have decreased from approximately 150 to less than 5 per month since the litigation assault began, and requests for Norplant removals have soared.

According to the American College of Obstetricians and Gynecologists (1995), Wyeth-Ayerst Laboratories has announced that it will "offer health care providers legal defense and indemnification for lawsuits associated with the Norplant contraceptive implant." We agree with Dr. Wayne Barden, vice president of the Population Council, who was quoted in the *New York Times* article as saying, "I guess we could have expected it . . . You'd think women would say, wait a minute—isn't this a little too much?" Despite this being "a little too much," it appears that in the United States personal injury lawyers have effectively reduced the use of this safe and highly effective contraceptive. Moreover, a 3-year, two-rod implant system (Norplant II) has been approved by the Food and Drug Administration, but it has not been marketed (Berenson and colleagues, 1998).

INJECTABLE MEDROXYPROGESTERONE ACETATE/ESTRADIOL CYPIONATE.
A new contraceptive for use by monthly injection has been approved by the Food and Drug Administration. The agent contains 25 mg of medroxyprogesterone acetate plus 5 mg of estradiol cypionate and will be marketed under the name Lunelle or Cyclo-Provera (Kaunitz, 1999a).

MECHANISM OF ACTION.
The drug inhibits ovulation and suppresses endometrial proliferation (Aedo and co-workers, 1985). Estradiol values reach a peak level by 3 to 4 days postinjection at values comparable to those associated with preovulatory surges in a normal ovulatory menstrual cycle. The values of estradiol remain at this level for approximately 10 to 14 days (Oriowo and colleagues, 1980). The subsequent decrease in estradiol values results in estrogen-induced withdrawal bleeding 10 to 20 days after the injection (Oriowo and colleagues, 1980; World Health Organization, Special Program on Research, 1989b).

EFFECTIVENESS.
Only six method failures in 70,000 woman-years of use have been reported (Hall and co-workers, 1994). This is an effectiveness similar to that seen following female sterilization procedures.

ADVANTAGES AND DISADVANTAGES.
The frequency of injection is an obvious problem, but the drug likely will be marketed in a nonreusable sterile device that will allow self-injection and ease of use by medical and nursing staffs. After 3 months use, bleeding irregularities appear to be less common than with depot medroxy-progesterone acetate injections (Kaunitz, 1999a). Fully two thirds of long-term users have regular menses (World Health Organization, 1989b). Return to fertility after discontinuation is rapid, with up to 83 percent of women conceiving within 12 months of discontinuation (Kaunitz, 1999a). The rate of return to fertility was much more rapid than after discontinuing depot medroxy-progesterone acetate injections. The other effects of this new agent are similar to those for medroxyprogesterone injections for hypertension, headaches, dizziness, mastalgia, malaise, cervical changes, and weight gain (Cuong and co-workers, 1996; Sang and colleagues, 1995; World Health Organization, 1988, 1993).

METABOLIC EFFECTS.
Procoagulant factors were not increased in women using this agent, and only slight decreases in factors VII and X activities were noted. Tissue plasminogen factor was increased while antithrombin III activity and protein C concentrations were slightly decreased (Hall, 1998). No instances of stroke, thromboembolic events, anaphylaxis or myocardial infarction have been reported (Kaunitz, 1999a). Lipid changes do not appear to be clinically important, but slight variations have been reported within days following injection and at 1 year of use (Nelson, 2000; Shulman, 2000). Glucose response was increased slightly, and insulin response to glucose challenges was also increased slightly during use. Liver transaminases and bilirubin were also increased slightly while alkaline phosphatase values were decreased (World Health Organization, 1997b). No studies of bone density have as yet been reported.

PROPOSED CONTRAINDICATIONS.
These are similar to those for combined oral contraceptives, which are listed in Table 58–9 (Kaunitz, 1999a).

MECHANICAL METHODS OF CONTRACEPTION

INTRAUTERINE CONTRACEPTIVE DEVICES.
At one time in the United States, approximately 7 percent of sexually active women used an intrauterine device (IUD) for contraception. The two devices currently approved for use in the United States are shown in Figure 58–4. The levonorgestrel-containing device (LNg-IUD) has not been approved for use. The percentages of unwanted pregnancies during the first year of perfect use associated with each IUD are 0.6 percent for the Copper T (Cu T), 1.5 percent for the Progestasert, and 0.1 percent for the LNg 20. Typical failure rates are 0.8 percent, 2.0 percent, and 0.1 percent respectively.

By 1986, the two most popular intrauterine devices used by American women had been withdrawn vol-

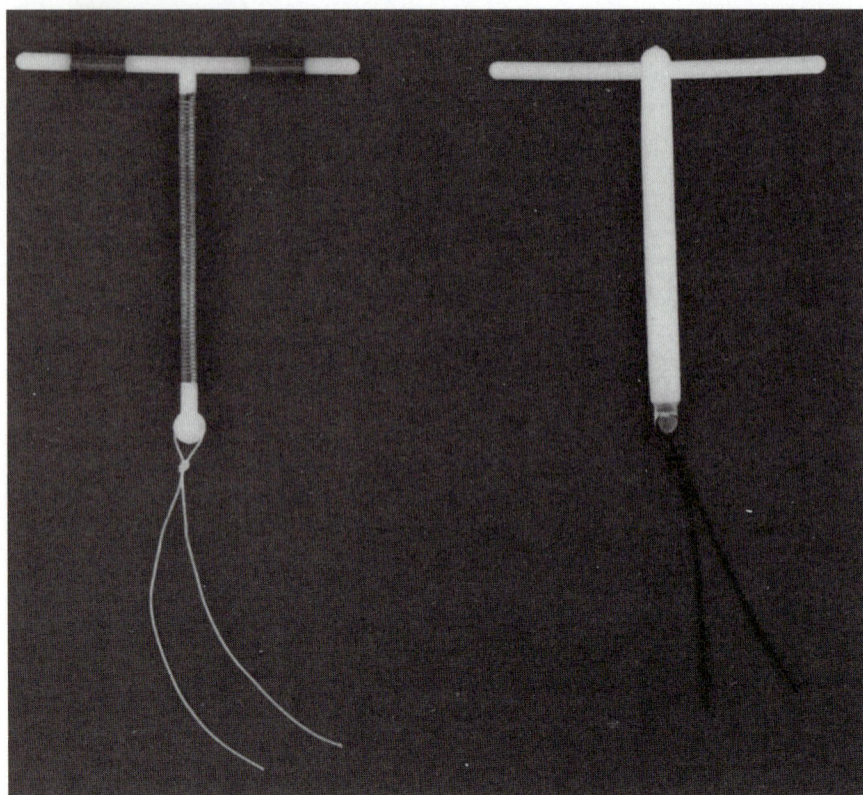

FIGURE 58–4. Two intrauterine contraceptive devices available in 2001: Copper T 380A (*left*) and Progestasert (*right*). (Courtesy of GynoPharma, Somerville, NJ, and ALZA Corp., Palo Alto, CA.)

untarily from the market by their manufacturers. The Lippes Loop and Copper 7 (Cu 7) were withdrawn because of the financial burden of defense in liability cases. At that time, about half of the 2 million women in the United States wearing these devices were acceptable candidates for oral contraceptive therapy. Some of the remaining women continued to use the inert plastic devices, which could be left in place indefinitely. Many women, however, had to choose between alternative, albeit less effective, contraceptive measures and permanent sterilization. Fortunately, the Progestasert (Fig. 58–4) continued to be marketed in the United States in limited quantities but at a very high cost. By 1988, the Cu T model 380A (Fig. 58–4) became available, but it too is very expensive.

With new information on safety, the IUD is once again gaining in popularity for several reasons. The most likely reason is that the Cu T and LNg 20 are "use and forget" effective reversible methods of contraception that do not have to be replaced for 10 and 5 years, respectively. It is now established that the major actions of IUDs are not as abortifacients but as contraceptives. The risk of pelvic infections is markedly reduced with the current use of a monofilament string and newer techniques to ensure safer insertion. The risk of an associated ectopic pregnancy also has been clarified. Specifically, the contraceptive effect of the IUDs actually

decreases the number of ectopic pregnancies (World Health Organization, 1985, 1987). If a pregnancy does occur, however, that pregnancy is more likely to be ectopic, especially in a woman using the Progestasert (Mishell and Sulak, 1997). Finally, the legal liability appears to be less since the Food and Drug Administration now classifies the Cu T and Progestasert as drugs. As such, the manufacturers must provide product information to be read by patients prior to insertion. This, plus signed consent forms which include a reasonable listing of risks and benefits, should reduce legal liability (Mishell and Sulak, 1997).

TYPES OF INTRAUTERINE DEVICES. In general, devices are one of two varieties. Those that are **chemically inert** are composed of a nonabsorbable material, most often polyethylene, and impregnated with barium sulfate for radiopacity. In those that are **chemically active,** there is continuous elution of copper or a progestational agent. At the present time only chemically active IUDs are available.

PROGESTASERT. This is a T-shaped ethylene vinyl acetate co-polymer with a vertical stem containing 38 mg of progesterone and barium sulfate in a silicone base. The progesterone source supplies approximately 65 μg/

day into the uterine cavity for 1 year. This does not alter plasma progesterone values. The device is 36 mm long and 32 mm wide, and has a single dark blue to black string attached to the base of the stem (Fig. 58–4). For insertion, the withdrawal technique must be used (Fig. 58–5).

LEVONORGESTREL DEVICE (LNg-IUD). This device is similar to the Progestasert, but contains levonorgestrel. It is currently in use in Europe and being tested in the United States. Its major advantage is the need to replace it only once every 5 years, compared with yearly for the Progestasert. This device releases levonorgestrel into the uterus at a relatively constant rate of 20 μg/ day, which markedly reduces the systemic effects of the progestin. It is a T-shaped polyethylene structure that has its stem wrapped with a cylinder of polydimethylsiloxane/levonorgestrel mixture. A permeable membrane surrounds the mixture to regulate the rate of hormone release.

COPPER T 380A. This device is composed of polyethylene and barium sulfate. The stem is wound with 314 mm^2 of fine copper wire, and the arms each have 33-mm^2 copper bracelets, thus totalling 380 mm^2 of copper. Two strings extend from the base of the stem (Fig. 58–4). Originally, the strings were blue, but they now are an off-white color. **This device should not be "loaded" into its inserter tube more than 5 minutes before it is inserted.** The malleable arms tend to retain the "memory" of the inserter.

MECHANISMS OF ACTION. These mechanisms have not been defined precisely. Interference with successful implantation of the fertilized ovum, which at one time was

believed to be the mode of action, is the least important action (Mishell and Sulak, 1997). The intense local inflammatory response that is induced, especially by copper-containing devices, in turn leads to lysosomal activation and other inflammatory actions that are spermicidal (Alvarez and associates, 1988; Ortiz and Croxatto, 1987). In the unlikely event that fertilization does occur, the same inflammatory actions are directed against the blastocyst. The report by Lippes and co-workers (1978) that insertion of a Cu T or Cu 7 device up to 7 days after coitus effectively prevented pregnancy strongly supports the concept that copper-bearing devices can also compromise the blastocyst. For the chemically inert devices, contraceptive effectiveness generally increases with increased size and extent of contact with endometrium.

Another possible mechanism includes accelerated tubal motility likely induced by the intrauterine inflammatory response. Also, the endometrium is an extremely hostile site for implantation even if fertilization and successful tubal transport have occurred. The endometrium is atrophic in long-time Progestasert users.

The action of these devices may very well be outside the uterus (Sivin, 1989). There may be a major effect in preventing fertilization by spermicidal action or speeding ovum transport through the fallopian tube, or both (Alvarez and co-workers, 1988; Ortiz and Croxatto, 1987). Finally, progestin-containing devices may interfere with sperm penetration through thickened cervical mucus.

EFFECTIVENESS. Intrauterine devices have 1-year and long-term continuation rates second only to implantable contraceptives (p. 1520). One-year continuation rates are equal to those of oral contraceptives. This almost

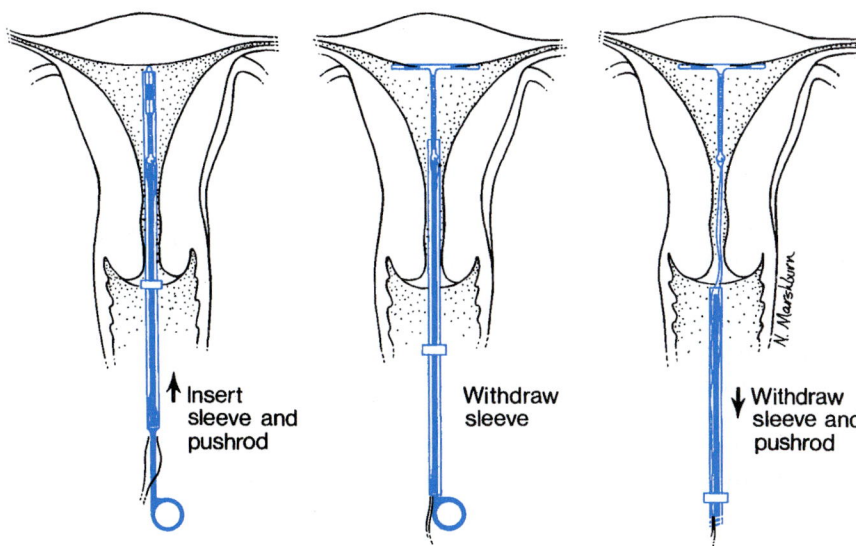

Insert sleeve and pushrod

Withdraw sleeve

Withdraw sleeve and pushrod

FIGURE 58–5. Insertion of Copper T 380A using the withdrawal technique. (Redrawn from Porter and associates, 1983, with permission.)

certainly is due to their effectiveness and a once-only approach to contraception.

The effectiveness of the devices is similar to overall effectiveness of oral contraceptives. Even so, the typical first-year failure rate with a Progestasert is double that with the Cu T 380A (2.0 versus 0.8 percent). The Cu T 380A is one of the most effective contraceptive means available. Importantly, the unintended pregnancy rate decreases progressively after the first year of use (Vessey and associates, 1983a). This must in part be due to true method failures and not user failures. The LNg-IUD appears to be even more effective than the Cu T 380A (Rowe, 1992) with perfect and typical user failure rates of 0.1 percent.

BENEFICIAL EFFECTS. Progesterone and the newer levonorgestrel-containing devices reduce menstrual blood loss and can even be used to treat menorrhagia. Moreover, the reduced menstrual blood loss is often associated with a reduction in dysmenorrhea. Despite the initial high cost of the device and insertion, the overall extended use of the Cu T 380A and the LNg-IUD make them both very cost effective. Women with contraindications to combination oral contraceptives and Norplant can often use these devices. Even the LNg-IUD can be used because it releases very small amounts of localized hormone. The LNg-IUD also is reported to reduce the incidence of pelvic infections and to be useful in women with uterine fibroids (Toivonen and associates, 1991; van den Hurk and O'Brien, 1999). With discontinuation, fertility is not impaired (Sivin and colleagues, 1992).

ADVERSE EFFECTS. Numerous complications have been described with use of various intrauterine devices. For the most part, however, common side effects have not been serious, and the serious side effects have not been common. Moreover, with progressive use and advancing user age, unintended pregnancy, expulsion, and bleeding complications decrease in frequency.

UTERINE PERFORATION AND ABORTION. The earliest adverse effects are those associated with insertion. They include clinically apparent or silent *uterine perforation,* either while sounding the uterus or during insertion of the device, and *abortion of an unsuspected pregnancy.* The frequency of these complications depends on operator skill and the precautions taken to avoid interrupting a pregnancy. The incidence of perforations with the Cu T 380A is 0.6 per 1000 insertions, and for the Progestasert the incidence is 1.1 per 1000 insertions (World Health Organization, 1987). Although devices may migrate spontaneously into and through the uterine wall, most perforations occur, or at least begin, at the time of insertion.

UTERINE CRAMPING AND BLEEDING. Uterine *cramping* and some *bleeding* are likely to develop soon after insertion, and they persist for variable periods. Cramping can be minimized by administering a nonsteroidal anti-inflammatory agent approximately 1 hour prior to insertion. The occasional increase in cramping with menses also can be controlled in a similar manner.

MENORRHAGIA. *Blood loss* with menstruation is commonly doubled with the use of the Cu T 380A, and it may be so great as to cause iron-deficiency anemia. Most providers measure hemoglobin or hematocrit annually in women with IUDs as well as any time they complain of heavy menstruation. This is a troubling side effect, and approximately 10 to 15 percent of women using the copper device have it removed for this problem (Hatcher and associates, 1998).

Progestasert, because of its localized progesterone action, is associated with a low incidence of menorrhagia and anemia. For example, normal menstruation results in blood loss of about 35 mL. Mean blood loss with most copper-containing devices is approximately 50 to 60 mL per cycle, but can be more (Guillebaud and colleagues, 1979). Mean blood loss with the Progestasert is about 25 mL per cycle. Blood loss with the LNg-IUD may be even less than with the Progestasert.

INFECTION. *Pelvic infections,* including septic abortion, have developed with a variety of intrauterine devices. *Tubo-ovarian abscesses,* which may be unilateral, have been described. With suspected infection, the device should be removed, and the woman treated with effective antibiotics. Deaths from sepsis have been reported with these devices. Because of the risk of severe pelvic infections with sterility, IUD use is usually discouraged for women under the age of 25 or those of low parity. According to Vessey and associates (1983a), there is not prolonged impairment of fertility after removing the devices from parous women.

Daling (1985) and Cramer (1985) and their associates reported that IUDs are associated with increased infertility due to tubal factors. These effects were negligible with copper-bearing devices, but more apparent in nulliparous women, especially if they had multiple sexual partners and used the now-discontinued Dalkon shield. Interestingly, Lee and Rubin (1988) reported that married women and those with only one sexual partner had no higher risk of developing pelvic infection than controls **after** the first 4 months of use.

Following insertion of an IUD, bacteria can be recovered from the uterine cavity for several days, but at appreciably lower rates after the first 24 hours (Mishell and colleagues, 1966). There is a small increased risk of pelvic infection for up to the first 20 days following insertion (Farley and associates, 1992). There currently is no consensus whether antibiotic administration at the time of insertion reduces the incidence of postinsertion infections (Ladipo, 1991; Sinei, 1990; Walsh, 1998, and their associates). Thus, the major risk of infection is due to insertion and does not increase with long-term use. In fact, long-term use of copper- and hormonal-containing devices results in pelvic infection rates comparable to those of oral contraceptive users. Any infection after 45 to 60 days should be considered sexually transmitted and appropriately treated (Lee and associates, 1983). The newer copper- and progestin-releasing devices also may reduce the incidence of pelvic infection (Toivonen and co-workers, 1991).

Women with intrauterine devices may be at greater risk for HIV infection than women using other forms of contraception (Musicco and associates, 1996). IUDs should not be used in HIV-positive women (Hatcher and colleagues, 1998).

Actinomyces-like structures identified in Papanicolaou smears and the prolonged use of an IUD have been linked. In his scholarly review, Fiorino (1996) cited an incidence of 7 percent of *Actinomyces* seen on cytology smears in women with these devices, compared with less than 1 percent of nonusers. The clinical importance of this finding is not clear, but it is worrisome. In most studies, an increased prevalence of *Actinomyces israelii* or actinomyces-like organisms was apparent only after several years of use. Moreover, women who developed a pelvic abscess caused by this organism had used the device for a mean of 8 years before symptoms developed. Keebler and co-workers (1983) showed that once the smear became positive for actinomyces, all subsequent smears remained positive until the device was removed.

In the absence of symptoms, the incidental finding of actinomyces by cytology is problematic. Penicillin therapy is not effective; therefore, some clinicians chose to remove the device, although there is no evidence that this will prevent infection (Fiorino, 1996). Most agree, however, that if signs or symptoms of infection develop in women who harbor actinomyces, the device should be removed and antibiotic therapy instituted.

PREGNANCY WITH A DEVICE IN UTERO. As emphasized in Chapter 10 (p. 227), it is important to identify all pregnant women who might be using an IUD. A device within the pregnant uterus may be dangerous for the woman and her fetus. A device residing beyond the uterus may be dangerous for the woman. Appropriate steps should be taken at delivery to identify and ensure removal of the device.

When pregnancy is recognized and the tail of the device is visible through the cervix, it should be removed. This will help reduce subsequent complications such as late abortion, sepsis, and preterm birth. Tatum

and co-workers (1976) observed the abortion rate to be 54 percent with the device left in situ compared with 25 percent if promptly removed. Moreover, with the device remaining in situ, the frequency of low birthweight, chiefly from preterm delivery, was 20 percent, compared with about 5 percent if the device was removed early. Vessey and associates (1979) confirmed these observations. If the tail is not visible, attempts to locate and remove the device may result in abortion. Some practitioners have successfully used sonographically assisted removal of devices without visible strings.

Second-trimester abortion with an IUD in place is more likely to be septic (Lewit, 1970; Vessey and associates, 1974). Sepsis is at times fulminant and often fatal, and because of these risks, the woman should be offered the option of pregnancy termination (American College of Obstetricians and Gynecologists, 1992). Women pregnant with a device in utero who demonstrate any evidence of uterine infection must have intensive antibiotic therapy and prompt uterine evacuation.

Fetal malformations have not been reported to be increased with pregnancies complicated by the presence of any intrauterine device.

ECTOPIC PREGNANCIES. Although most intrauterine pregnancies are prevented, the device provides less protection against extrauterine nidation. With a contraceptive failure, the risk for an ectopic pregnancy increases significantly and may be increased even more in women using Progestasert (Chap. 34, p. 884). Because the device does not prevent extrauterine pregnancy reliably, women already at high risk for an ectopic pregnancy—those with previous salpingitis, ectopic pregnancy, or tubal surgery—are poor candidates for an IUD.

CONTRAINDICATIONS. Contraindications to the use of the Cu T 380A and Progestasert are listed in Table 58–11.

PROCEDURES FOR INSERTION. The Food and Drug Administration requires that before an intrauterine device is inserted, the woman must be given a brochure detailing the side effects and apparent risks from its use. Most devices have a special inserter, usually a sterile graduated plastic tube into which the device is withdrawn just before insertion (Fig. 58–5). Timing of insertion influences the ease of placement as well as the pregnancy and expulsion rates. Insertion near the end of normal menstruation, when the cervix is usually softer and the canal somewhat more dilated, may facilitate insertion and at the same time exclude early pregnancy. Insertion, however, need not be limited to this time. For the woman who is sure she is not pregnant and does not want to be pregnant, insertion may be carried out anytime during the ovulation cycle.

TABLE 58–11. Contraindications to Use of an Intrauterine Device

Copper T 380A

Pregnancy or suspicion of pregnancy

Abnormalities of the uterus resulting in distortion of the uterine cavity

Acute pelvic inflammatory disease (PID) or a history of PID

Postpartum endometritis or infected abortion in the past 3 months

Known or suspected uterine or cervical malignancy, including unresolved abnormal Pap smear

Genital bleeding of unknown etiology

Untreated acute cervicitis or vaginitis, including bacterial vaginosis, until infection is controlled

Wilson disease

Allergy to copper

Patient or her partner has multiple sex partners

Conditions associated with increased susceptibility to infections with microorganisms including, but not limited to leukemia, acquired immunodeficiency syndrome (AIDS), and intravenous drug abuse

Genital actinomycosis

A previously inserted intrauterine device (IUD) that has not been removed

Progestasert

Pregnancy or suspected pregnancy

History of ectopic pregnancy or a condition that predisposes to ectopic pregnancy

Presence or history of PID or factors that predispose to PID

Patient or her partner has multiple sex partners

Presence or history of one or more sexually transmitted infections, including but not limited to gonorrhea or chlamydial infections

Postpartum endometritis or infected abortion

Incomplete involution of uterus following abortion or childbirth

A previously inserted IUD still in place

History of pelvic surgery that may be associated with an increased risk of ectopic pregnancy, eg, surgery of the fallopian tubes or surgery for pelvic adhesions or endometriosis

Abnormalities of the uterus resulting in distortion of the uterine cavity or uteri that measure < 6 cm or > 10 cm by sounding

Known or suspected uterine or cervical malignancy including an unresolved, abnormal Pap smear

Genital bleeding of unknown etiology

Vaginitis or cervicitis unless and until infection has been eradicated and has been shown to be nongonococcal and nonchlamydial

Genital actinomycosis

Conditions or treatments associated with increased susceptibility to infections with microorganisms including but not limited to leukemia, diabetes, a history of endocarditis or certain types of heart disease that are associated with an increased risk of endocarditis, AIDS, and conditions requiring chronic corticosteroid therapy

Intravenous drug abuse

Contraindications from ParaGard Prescribing Information, Raritan, NJ: Ortho-McNeil Pharmaceutical Corporation, January 1996; and Progestasert System Prescribing Information, Palo Alto, CA: ALZA Pharmaceuticals, June 1994.

Insertion at the time of delivery or very soon thereafter is followed by an unsatisfactorily high expulsion rate. The recommendation has been made, therefore, to withhold insertion for at least 8 weeks to reduce expulsion as well as to minimize the risk of perforation. In our extensive experiences, however, earlier insertion has not led to perforation or expulsion rates significantly higher than for insertion remote from pregnancy. In the absence of infection, the device may be inserted immediately after early abortion.

A satisfactory technique for insertion and a plan for follow-up is as follows:

1. Determine if there are contraindications, counsel the woman regarding various problems associated with device use, and obtain consent.
2. Administer preinsertion aspirin or codeine to allay cramps.
3. Perform a pelvic examination to identify the position and size of the uterus and adnexa. If abnormalities are found, a device is often contraindicated.
4. Visualize the cervix and grasp it with a tenaculum. Use sterile instruments and a sterile intrauterine device. Wipe the cervix and the vaginal walls with an antiseptic solution. The cervical canal and uterine cavity are first straightened by applying gentle traction on the tenaculum, and the uterus is sounded to identify the direction and depth of the uterine cavity. The movable flange on the barrel of the inserter should be adjusted to the depth to which the device should be inserted. As shown in Figure 58–5, the inserter, with the device contained within its most distal portion, is then gently inserted to the fundus. After rotating the inserter so that the device is positioned high in the transverse plane of the uterus, the inserter is removed while the device is held in the fundus by the plastic rod within the inserter. **Thus, the device is not pushed out of the tube, but rather it is held in place by the rod while the inserter tube is withdrawn.**
5. Cut the marker tail 2 cm from the external os, remove the tenaculum, observe for bleeding from the tenaculum puncture sites, and if there is no bleeding, remove the speculum.
6. Advise the woman to report promptly any apparent adverse effects.

EXPULSION. Loss of the device from the uterus is most common during the first month after insertion. The woman should be instructed to palpate the strings protruding from the cervix by either sitting on the edge of a chair or squatting down and then advancing the middle finger into the vagina until the cervix is reached. The woman should be checked in 1 month, usually after menses, for appropriate placement by identifying the tail protruding from the cervix. Barrier contraception may be desirable during this time, especially if a device has been expelled previously.

LOCATING A LOST DEVICE. When the tail of a device cannot be visualized, the device may have been expelled, or it may have perforated the uterus. In either event, pregnancy is possible. Conversely, the tail simply may be in the uterine cavity along with a normally positioned device. Often, gentle probing of the uterine cavity with a Randall stone clamp or a rod with a terminal hook will retrieve the string. **Never assume that the device has been expelled unless it was seen.**

When the tail is not visible and the device is not felt by gentle probing of the uterine cavity, sonography is done to ascertain if the device is within the uterine cavity. If these findings are negative or inconclusive, then a plain x-ray of the abdomen and pelvis is taken with a sound inserted into the uterine cavity. Instillation of radiocontrast for hysterography may be done, and hysteroscopy is yet another alternative. Obviously none of these maneuvers except sonography should be performed during early pregnancy.

An open device of inert material, such as the Lippes Loop, located outside the uterus may or may not do harm. Perforations of large and small bowel and bowel fistulas, with attendant morbidity, have been reported remote from the time of insertion. An extrauterine copper-bearing device induces an intense local inflammatory reaction and adherence to the inflamed structure. Chemically inert devices usually are removed easily from the peritoneal cavity by laparoscopy or posterior colpotomy. Copper-bearing devices are more firmly adherent and laparotomy may be necessary.

A device may penetrate the uterine wall in varying degrees. At times, part of the device may extend into the peritoneal cavity while the remainder is firmly fixed in the myometrium. Devices also can penetrate into the cervix and actually protrude into the vagina.

REPLACEMENT. Chemically inert devices may be left in the uterus indefinitely. In some cases, the polyethylene compound becomes encrusted with calcium salts, and endometrial erosion causes bleeding that prompts replacement. Copper-bearing devices have to be replaced periodically. The Copper T 380 A is approved for 10 years of continuous use. The Progestasert device should be replaced annually, and the LNg-IUD has been used effectively for 5 years.

BARRIER METHODS. For many years, condoms, vaginal spermicidal agents, and vaginal diaphragms have been used for contraception with variable success (Table 58–2).

MALE CONDOM. These products provide effective contraception, and their failure rate with experienced and strongly motivated couples has been as low as 3 or 4 per 100 couple-years of exposure (Vessey and co-workers, 1982). Generally, and during the first year of use especially, the failure rate is much higher (Table 58–2). Trussell and colleagues (1990) also reported that women older than 30 years of age had fewer unintended pregnancies than those younger than 25.

When used properly, condoms provide considerable but not absolute protection against a broad range of sexually transmitted diseases, including HIV infection, gonorrhea, syphilis, herpes, chlamydia, and trichomoniasis. They also possibly prevent and ameliorate premalignant changes in the cervix (Population Reports, 1982). Because the Centers for Disease Control and Prevention recommend condoms for couples at risk for HIV infection, including those with multiple sex partners, their use has escalated exponentially since the mid-1980s.

The contraceptive effectiveness of the male condom is enhanced appreciably by the use of a condom with a reservoir tip and with spermicidal lubricant added to the condom. The contraceptive and antibacterial and antiviral effectiveness is improved even more with the addition of an intravaginal spermicidal agent. Such vaginal agents as well as those used only for lubrication should be water-based products. Oil-based products will destroy latex condoms and diaphragms (Waldron, 1989).

LATEX SENSITIVITY. Some individuals are extremely sensitive to latex. Because latex provides protection against sexually transmitted diseases, and natural membrane condoms do not, this created a dilemma until recently. A nonallergenic condom has been developed of synthetic thermoplastic elastomer usually used in surgical gloves (Mason, 1992). A polyurethane condom is also currently available in the United States (Table 58–12). Both products are effective against sexually transmitted diseases, including HIV (Waldron, 1991). Unfortunately, the polyurethane condom has a significantly higher breakage rate than latex condoms, 7.2 and 1.1 percent, respectively (Frezieres and colleagues, 1998).

FEMALE CONDOM (VAGINAL POUCH). The Food and Drug Administration refers to female condoms as vaginal pouches. Before approval for marketing, a vaginal pouch must be proven to prevent pregnancy and sexually transmitted diseases, including HIV. Only one device is available, and it is marketed as the *Reality* condom. It is a polyurethane sheath with one flexible polyurethane ring at each end. The open ring remains outside the vagina, and the closed internal ring is fitted under the symphysis like a diaphragm (Fig. 58–6). In vitro tests have shown the female condom to be impermeable to human immunodeficiency virus, cytomegalovirus, and hepatitis B virus. It has a 0.6 percent breakage rate. The slippage and displacement rate is about 3 percent compared with an 8 percent rate for male condoms. Overall, acceptability has been about 60 percent for women and 80 percent for men. Unfortunately, the pregnancy rate is higher than with the male condom (Table 58–2).

SPERMICIDAL CONTRACEPTIVES. These contraceptives are marketed variously as creams, jellies, suppositories, film, and foam in aerosol containers (Fig. 58–7). They are used widely in this country, especially by women who find oral contraceptives or an IUD unacceptable. They are useful especially for women who need temporary protection, for example, during the first week after starting oral contraceptives or while nursing.

Most agents can be purchased without a prescription. Typically, they work by providing a physical barrier to sperm penetration as well as a chemical spermicidal action. The active spermicidal ingredient is nonoxynol-9 or octoxynol-9. **To be highly effective, the spermicides must be deposited high in the vagina in contact with**

TABLE 58–12. Characteristic Male Condoms

Type	Latex	Natural Membrane	Plastic
Brand names	Numerous	Fourex, Naturalamb	Avanti, Reality
Material	Natural rubber	Lamb cecum	Polyurethane[a]
Lubricant use	Water based only	Any	Any
Cost	Low	Moderate	Moderate/high
Pregnancy prevention	Yes	Yes	Yes
STD prevention	Yes	No	Likely

STD = sexually transmitted disease.
[a] Nonpolyurethane plastic condoms may become available soon.
From Hatcher and colleagues (1998), with permission.

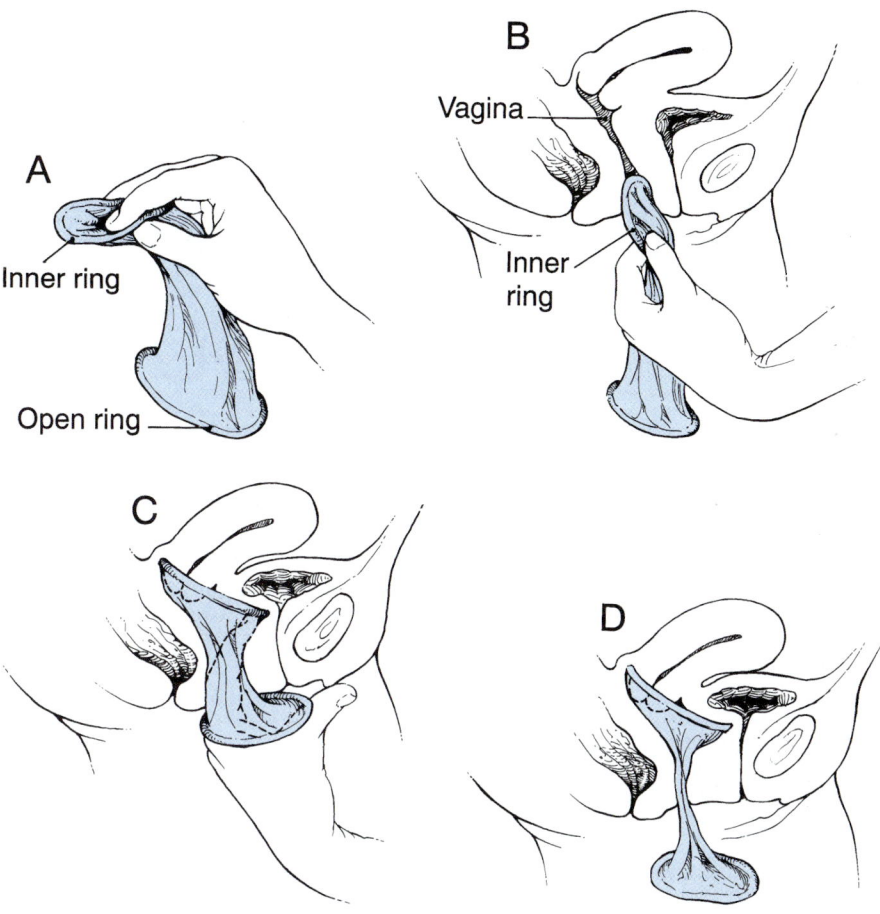

FIGURE 58–6. *Reality* female condom insertion and positioning. **A.** Inner ring is squeezed for insertion. **B.** Sheath is inserted similarly to a diaphragm. **C.** Inner ring is pushed up as far as it can go with index finger. **D.** Vaginal pouch is in place. (Figure from Wisconsin Pharmacal Company, Jackson, WI, and Contraception Report, 1992, with permission.)

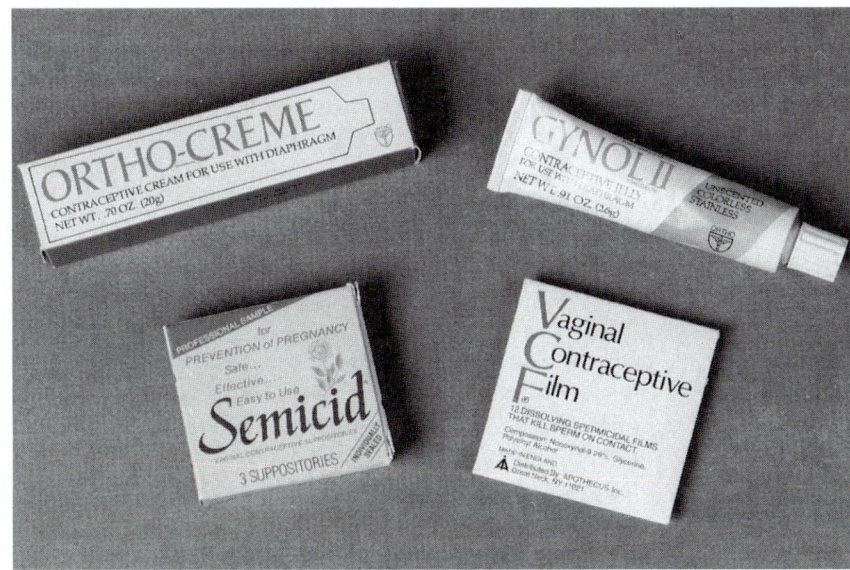

FIGURE 58–7. Vaginal contraceptive agents; cream, jelly, suppository, and film.

1544 SECTION XIV FAMILY PLANNING

the cervix shortly before intercourse. Their duration of maximal spermicidal effectiveness is usually no more than 1 hour. Thereafter they must be reinserted before repeat intercourse. Douching should be avoided for at least 6 hours after intercourse.

High pregnancy rates are primarily attributable to inconsistent use rather than to method failure. If inserted regularly and correctly, foam preparations probably result in 5 to 12 pregnancies per 100 woman-years of use (Trussell and associates, 1990). Spermicides in current use appear to provide at least partial protection against some sexually transmitted diseases, including gonorrhea and probably papillomavirus and HIV (Feldblum and Fortney, 1988).

LEGAL DIFFICULTIES. Although a preliminary study suggested that vaginal spermicides might be associated with an increased frequency of fetal malformations, well-designed studies by Mills and co-workers (1982) and Shapiro and associates (1982) found no such association. In fact, the Food and Drug Administration (1986) concluded that evidence *did not* support an association between spermicide use and congenital malformations. Despite this scientific evidence, a court decision in *Wells v Ortho Pharmaceutical* was rendered in favor of the plaintiff in a suit alleging that congenital malformations were caused by maternal spermicide exposure. The decision was upheld by an appellate court. Subsequently, Louik and colleagues (1987) reported results from their case-controlled surveillance system and found no association with spermicide use and Down syndrome, hypospadias, limb-reduction defects, neoplasms, or neural-tube defects. Strobino and colleagues (1988) also did not identify increased congenital malformations in a cohort study. Thus, evidence indicates that spermicide use is not teratogenic (Briggs and colleagues, 1998).

DIAPHRAGM PLUS SPERMICIDE. The vaginal diaphragm, consisting of circular rubber dome of various diameters supported by a circumferentially placed metal spring, can be very effective when used in combination with spermicidal jelly or cream. The spermicide is applied to the superior surface both along the rim and centrally. The device is then placed in the vagina so that the cervix, vaginal fornices, and anterior vaginal wall are partitioned effectively from the remainder of the vagina and the penis. At the same time, the centrally placed spermicidal agent is held against the cervix by the diaphragm. When appropriately positioned, the rim is lodged superiorly deep in the posterior vaginal fornix, and inferiorly the rim lies in close proximity to the inner surface of the symphysis immediately below the urethra (Fig.

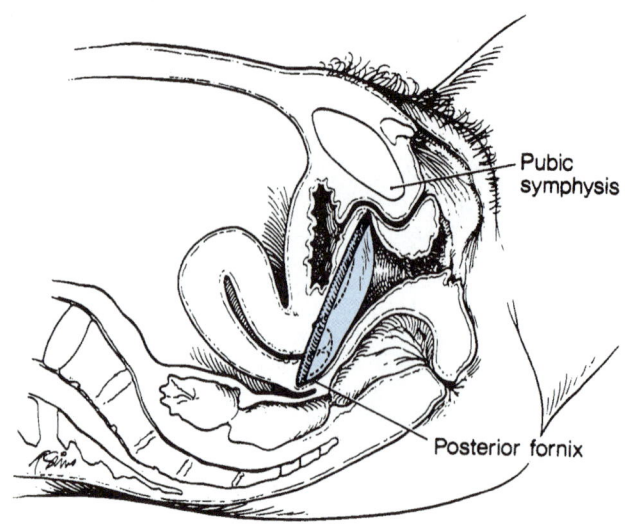

FIGURE 58–8. A diaphragm in place creates a physical barrier between the vagina and cervix and, importantly, provides for intimate contact between the contraceptive jelly or cream and the cervix.

58–8). If the diaphragm is too small, it will not remain in place. If too large, it will be uncomfortable when it is forced into position. A cystocele or uterine prolapse is very likely to result in instability and therefore expulsion. Because the variables of size and spring flexibility must be specified, the diaphragm is available only by prescription.

The diaphragm and spermicidal agent can be inserted hours before intercourse, but if more than 2 hours elapse, additional spermicide should be placed in the upper vagina for maximum protection and be reapplied before each coital episode. The diaphragm should not be removed for at least 6 hours after intercourse. Because toxic shock syndrome has been described following its use, it may be worthwhile to remove the diaphragm at the end of 6 hours, or at least the next morning, to minimize this uncommon event (Alcid and associates, 1982).

The diaphragm requires a high level of motivation for proper use that, when expended, is accompanied by a low pregnancy rate. Vessey and colleagues (1982) reported a pregnancy rate of only 1.9 to 2.4 per 100 woman-years for established users. Bounds and associates (1995), in a small study, reported a much higher failure rate of 12.3 per 100 women-years. The unintended pregnancy rate is lower in women past 35 than in those younger than 30. Finally, diaphragm use results in a decreased incidence in sexually transmitted diseases compared with condom use (Rosenberg and colleagues, 1992). There is a slight but real increase in urinary infections associated with diaphragm use (Hatcher and associates, 1998).

CONTRACEPTIVE SPONGE. This device is no longer marketed.

CERVICAL CAP. The *Prentif* cavity-rim cervical cap was approved for use by the Food and Drug Administration in 1988. The flexible, cuplike device, made of natural rubber, is fitted around the base of the cervix. It can be self-inserted and allowed to remain in place for no more than 48 hours. It should be used with a spermicide applied once at insertion. According to trials conducted by the National Institutes of Health, the cap is comparable in effectiveness to the diaphragm. Unfortunately, the cost is high, and the fitting is critical for the device to be successful. Moreover, user misplacement of the cap makes it a less effective method overall than the diaphragm and a spermicidal agent.

PERIODIC (RHYTHMIC) ABSTINENCE. Ideally, sexual abstinence during and around the time of ovulation should prevent pregnancy; unfortunately, this is not always the case. For example, pregnancy rates with various methods of periodic abstinence—rhythm, natural family planning, or fertility awareness methods—have been estimated from 5 to 40 per 100 woman-years (Population Reports, 1981). In other words, this is an unwanted pregnancy rate of 25 percent during the first year of use (Table 58–2).

The human ovum is probably susceptible to successful fertilization for only about 12 to 24 hours after ovulation. Motile sperm, however, have been identified in cervical mucus as many as 7 days after coitus or artificial insemination, and in oviducts of women undergoing laparotomy as long as 85 hours after coitus (Ahlgren, 1975). It is unlikely, however, that sperm retain the capability for successful fertilization for this long a period.

CALENDAR RHYTHM METHOD. Ovulation most often occurs about 14 days before the onset of the next menstrual period, but unfortunately, not necessarily 14 days after the onset of the last menstrual period. Therefore, the *calendar rhythm method* is not reliable. In 1982, the International Planned Parenthood Federation concluded that "couples electing to use periodic abstinence should, however, be clearly informed that the method is not considered an effective method of family planning."

TEMPERATURE RHYTHM METHOD. The temperature rhythm method relies on *slight* changes—sustained 0.4 degree Fahrenheit increase—in the morning basal body temperature that usually occur just before ovulation. This method is much more likely to be successful if, during each menstrual cycle, intercourse is avoided until

well after the ovulatory temperature rise. For this method to be most effective, the woman must abstain from intercourse from the first day of menses through the third day after the increase in temperature. For obvious reasons, this is not a popular method of contraception! With excellent compliance, however, unwanted pregnancies occur at about 2 percent during the first year of use (Table 58–2).

CERVICAL MUCUS RHYTHM METHOD. The *cervical mucus rhythm method,* or so-called *Billings method,* depends on awareness of vaginal "dryness" and "wetness" as the consequence of changes in the amount and kind of cervical mucus formed at different times in the menstrual cycle. Abstinence is required from the beginning of menses until 4 days after slippery mucus is identified. This method has not achieved popularity. A small, handheld device that detects small variations in electrolyte concentrations in vaginal or oral secretions is also claimed to be capable of predicting ovulation 5 to 7 days in advance. Roumen and Dieben (1988) found that this device was not accurate in predicting the day of ovulation. When the cervical mucus method is used accurately, the first year failure rate is approximately 3 percent (Table 58–2).

SYMPTOTHERMAL METHOD. The symptothermal method combines the use of changes in cervical mucus (onset of fertile period), changes in basal body temperature (end of fertile period), and calculations to estimate the time of ovulation. This is a more complex system to learn and apply, and it does not appreciably improve reliability (Table 58–2). The use of home kits to detect luteal hormone increases which appear in the urine on the day prior to ovulation may improve the accuracy of periodic abstinence methods (Hatcher and associates, 1998).

For the interested reader, the December 1991 supplement to the *American Journal of Obstetrics and Gynecology* was devoted to the subject of natural family planning. It included 27 papers on this subject, as well as a final discussion and recommendations (Queenan and associates, 1991).

CONTRACEPTIVE CHOICES FOR ADOLESCENTS. A discussion of the biological antecedents of teenage pregnancy has been presented in Chapter 4. Briefly stated, menarche has decreased from approximately age 17 in the mid-1800s to near 12 years of age in the year 2001. Unfortunately, this means that reproductive function is established sooner than the psychological understanding of the consequences of sexual activity. This far too often results in intermittent spontaneous sexual encounters and unrealistic perception of the risks for pregnancy and sexually transmitted diseases (Cromer and associates, 1996; Sulak and Haney, 1993). Contraception is most often sought more than a year after sexual activity has begun (Mosher and McNally, 1991).

COMBINED ORAL CONTRACEPTIVES. As a method, these agents are the best choice for this age group because they provide effective contraception, increased bone density, and can be used to improve acne and regulate irregular menses. The obvious disadvantage is the daily requirement of taking a pill.

LONG-ACTING METHODS OF CONTRACEPTION. The **Norplant System** is an obvious choice because it provides effective contraception for 5 years with a "use and forget" system. The implants do not result in bone loss at a critical time when bone mass should be increasing (Sulak and Kaunitz, 1999). The disadvantages for an adolescent woman include menstrual irregularities and an insertion site inside the upper arm.

Injectable depot medroxyprogesterone is an effective contraceptive that also may be considered a "use and forget" method for 3 months. The disadvantages include the injections every 3 months, menstrual irregularities, and loss of bone mass (Sulak and Kaunitz, 1999).

The newly approved injectable medroxyprogesterone acetate plus estradiol cypionate also provides an effective contraception with better control of menses and, **it is hoped,** little or no bone mass loss. This compound, however, is not a true "use and forget" method because monthly injections are required.

Barrier techniques despite their obvious advantage of providing some protection against sexually transmitted diseases are not good choices for adolescents. These methods obviously require preplanning and motivation for their proper use. Such methods, especially vaginal spermicides and male condoms, should be considered primarily as backup contraceptives and protective methods directed against sexually transmitted diseases.

CONTRACEPTIVE CHOICES FOR WOMEN PAST 35. Although fertility decreases beginning at age 35 to 40 years, these women are still at risk for unwanted pregnancy and for sexually transmitted diseases. Henshaw (1998) reported that half of all pregnancies in women in their 40s are unintended, and that 65 percent of this half are terminated.

COMBINED ORAL CONTRACEPTIVES. These agents, especially the newer, low-dose estrogen compounds, when used by nonsmokers without systemic disease, are highly effective, well tolerated, provide many health benefits, and are associated with minimal risk (Beck, 1995; Speroff and Sulak, 1995). As discussed, these agents can be used until the menopause.

INJECTABLE DEPOT MEDROXYPROGESTERONE. This is a highly effective hormonal contraceptive, and it can also be used by some women who cannot for medical reasons take combination oral contraceptives (Speroff and Sulak, 1995).

INJECTABLE MEDROXYPROGESTERONE PLUS ESTRADIOL CYPIONATE. This product at first glance appears to be an excellent product for women in this age group except for the requirement of monthly injections. It may prove to be superior to implants and depot medroxyprogesterone injections if abnormal bleeding is less troublesome. Certainly, abnormal uterine bleeding in older women might be the result of a genital malignancy (Sulak and Haney, 1993).

PROGESTIN IMPLANTS (NORPLANT SYSTEM). These are exceedingly effective, well tolerated, and should be considered for women past 35 (Speroff and Sulak, 1995). The only apparent disadvantage for use in older women is the possible adverse effects of levonorgestrel on glucose tolerance and lipoproteins.

INTRAUTERINE DEVICES. This method is a logical choice for an older woman who has completed her family and is in a monogamous relationship.

BARRIER TECHNIQUES AND SPERMICIDAL AGENTS. These methods can be used either as primary or backup contraception. Their effectiveness improves with advancing age after 40, likely because fertility also decreases appreciably after age 40. This method also provides additional protection against sexually transmitted diseases (Speroff and Sulak, 1995; Sulak, 1996).

POSTCOITAL CONTRACEPTION

ESTROGENS AND PROGESTINS. The first *morning-after pill* was stilbestrol which, according to Kuchara (1971), prevented pregnancies in 1000 women who had inadequate contraception at the time of intercourse. Stilbestrol is no longer recommended, but pregnancy prevention is reported with other hormonal regimens as well as with insertion of copper-containing IUDs. A number of oral contraceptive regimens—known as the *Yuzpe method*—were approved in 1997 by the Food and Drug Administration for use as postcoital emergency contraception (Table 58–13). This was followed in 1998 by FDA approval of the first emergency contraceptive kit. The *Preven Emergency Contraceptive Kit* contains a pregnancy test and four oral contraceptive tablets each containing 50 μg of ethinyl estradiol and 0.25 mg of levonorgestrel. Two tablets are taken within 72 hours of intercourse followed 12 hours later by the second dose. Best results are obtained if the steroidal agents are

TABLE 58–13. Oral Contraceptives Used for Emergency Contraception in the United States

Brand	Manufacturer	Pills per Dose[a] and Color	Ethinyl Estradiol (μg per dose)	Levonorgestrel (mg per dose)[b]
Preven[c]	Gynétics	2 blue	100	0.50
Ovral[a]	Wyeth-Ayerst	2 white	100	0.50
Alesse[d]	Wyeth-Ayerst	5 pink	100	0.50
Levlite[d]	Berlex	5 pink	100	0.50
Nordette[d]	Wyeth-Ayerst	4 light-orange	120	0.60
Levlen[d]	Berlex	4 light-orange	120	0.60
Levora[d]	Watson	4 white	120	0.60
Lo/Ovral[d]	Wyeth-Ayerst	4 white	120	0.60
Plan B	Wyeth-Ayerst	1 white	0	0.75
Triphasil[d]	Wyeth-Ayerst	4 yellow	120	0.50
Tri-Levlen[d]	Berlex	4 yellow	120	0.50
Trivora[d]	Watson	4 pink	120	0.50
Ovrette	Wyeth-Ayerst	20 yellow	0	0.75

[a] The treatment schedule is one dose within 72 hours after unprotected intercourse, and another dose 12 hours later.
[b] The progestin in Ovral, Lo/Ovral, and Ovrette is norgestrel, which contains two isomers, only one of which (levonorgestrel) is bioactive; the amount of norgestrel in each tablet is twice the amount of levonorgestrel.
[c] Preven is the only dedicated product specifically marketed for emergency contraception.
[d] Declared safe and effective for use as emergency contraception by the Food and Drug Administration.
Modified from Hatcher and colleagues (1998), with permission.

taken within 72 hours of intercourse. All oral hormone regimens shown in Table 58–13 follow the same dosage schedule.

Access to emergency contraception is not universal. Trussell and colleagues (2000) found that only 75 percent of attempts to access care through the Emergency Contraception Hotline were successful. Physicians can register to be included as a resource and patients can call for referrals on the Hotline at 1-888-NOT-2-LATE (888.668.2528). The Emergency Contraception Website is not-2-late.com.

MECHANISM OF ACTION. The major mechanism is inhibition or delay of ovulation (Food and Drug Administration, 1997). Other mechanisms include alteration of the endometrium, sperm penetration, and tubal motility. **Established pregnancies are not harmed.**

Combined estrogen and progestin regimens are highly effective and have been reported to decrease the risk of pregnancy by 75 percent (Trussell and associates, 1996, 1998b). Thus, if 100 women had unprotected intercourse during the second to third week of their menstrual cycle, eight would be expected to conceive. With appropriate use of one of the regimens shown in Table 58–13, only two would actually conceive.

Due to the estrogen in these compounds, nausea and vomiting remain major problems. Trussell and associates (1998a) reported nausea in 50 percent of women and vomiting in 20 percent. For this reason, we routinely

prescribed an oral antiemetic at least 1 hour before each dose. Raymond and colleagues (2000) conducted a randomized trial and found that 1-hour pretreatment with 50-mg meclizine given orally decreased nausea from 64 to 47 percent compared with placebo. If vomiting occurs within 2 hours of a dose, the dose must be repeated.

PROGESTINS ONLY. The use of progestin-only pills results in markedly less nausea and vomiting. According to the Task Force on Postovulatory Methods of Fertility Regulation (1998), progestins are more effective than combination estrogen and progestin pills.

OVRETTE METHOD. The use of this agent, consisting of 20 pills within 72 hours of unprotected intercourse followed in 12 hours by a second dose of 20 pills, has proven to be effective and is less likely to cause nausea and vomiting. Each dose of 20 pills contains 0.75 mg of levonorgestrel.

PLAN B METHOD. In 1998, the Food and Drug Administration approved a new progestin-only regimen, marketed as Plan B, which consists of two tablets each containing 0.75-mg levonorgestrel (American College of Obstetricians and Gynecologists, 1999a). The first dose is taken within 72 hours of unprotected coitus and the second dose 12 hours later. This new regimen resulted in a crude pregnancy rate of 1.1 percent versus

3.2 percent in a similar group of women treated with the Yuzpe regimen.

COPPER-CONTAINING INTRAUTERINE DEVICES.

Fasoli and co-workers (1989) summarized nine studies that included results from 879 women who accepted some type of copper-containing IUD as a sole method of postcoital contraception. Only one pregnancy was reported, and it aborted spontaneously. More recently, Trussell and Stewart (1998) reported that when the IUD was inserted up to 5 days after unprotected coitus, the failure rate was 1 percent. A secondary advantage is that an effective 10-year method of contraception is already in place.

MIFEPRISTONE (RU 486) AND EPOSTANE.

These methods are discussed in Chapter 33 (p. 874). They should be ideal for postcoital contraception by their action to block progesterone production (epostane) or its action (mifepristone). Implantation would be prevented by either mechanism to produce so-called *menstrual induction*. Glasier and colleagues (1991, 1992) reported that a single, 600-mg oral dose of mifepristone prevented pregnancy in 402 women at risk compared with four pregnancies in 398 women given two doses of 100 μg of ethinyl estradiol and 1 mg of norgestrel 12 hours apart.

Progestin and combination estrogen and progestin agents must be used within 72 hours of unprotected intercourse to be effective. A single, 600-mg dose of mifepristone is effective up to 17 days after intercourse (Weiss, 1993). Grimes and Cook (1992) propose that mifepristone for postcoital contraception will lower the induced abortion rate.

METHOTREXATE AND MISOPROSTOL.

Hausknecht (1995) reported that intramuscular methotrexate, 50 mg/m², plus vaginally administered misoprostol, 800 mg, 5 to 7 days later, was highly effective in inducing abortion up to 63 days menstrual age. The methotrexate dose is the same used to treat ectopic pregnancies; misoprostol is commonly used for cervical ripening and induction (Chap. 20, p. 472). Of the 178 women enrolled in the study, 96 percent had a successful medical abortion. If postcoital contraception fails, this regimen is a logical next choice if an abortion is chosen.

FAILURE OF POSTCOITAL CONTRACEPTION.

Any postcoital contraceptive method is associated with failures. This can likely be reduced by employing a barrier technique until the next menses to prevent fertilization after use of the postcoital method. It must be remembered that estrogen administration prior to ovulation may induce ovulation. Finally, if menses are delayed for more than 3 weeks past their expected onset, pregnancy is likely.

CONTRACEPTIVE CHOICES FOR WOMEN WITH MEDICAL CONDITIONS.

Pregnancies in women with medical complications often result in dangers that far exceed those seen with most forms of contraception. The choice of the most effective and safest method of contraception, however, is dependent on the physician's understanding of the basic pathophysiology of the disease and how this is modified by pregnancy. Only with such knowledge can the appropriate contraceptive or recommendation for sterilization be made. For these reasons, such recommendations are made throughout this book as individual diseases are discussed.

LACTATION

Breast feeding is important to infant health and to child-spacing. For mothers who are nursing, ovulation during the first 10 weeks after delivery is unlikely (Pérez, 1981). Nursing is not a reliable method of family planning, however, for women whose infants are on a 3- to 4-hour, daytime-only feeding schedule and are receiving other food. **Waiting for first menses involves a risk of pregnancy because ovulation may antedate menstruation.** Certainly, after the first menses, contraception is essential unless the woman desires another pregnancy. Estrogen–progestin contraceptives may reduce both the rate and the duration of milk production. The benefits from prevention of pregnancy by the use of combined oral contraceptives would appear to outweigh the risks in selected patients, but progestin-only oral contraceptives appear to be the best choice in most cases (p. 1531). In a retrospective cohort study, Kjos and colleagues (1998) reported that for women with gestational diabetes, use of a progestin-only oral contraceptive increased the risk of insulin-dependent diabetes threefold.

Intrauterine devices have been recommended for the lactating, but potentially ovulating, sexually active woman. An increased rate of uterine perforation has been identified in lactating women with an IUD, perhaps as the consequence of vigorous myometrial contractions and involution brought about by the release of oxytocin in response to suckling (Heartwell and Schlesselman, 1983). The risk is not so great, however, that intrauterine devices should not be used.

REFERENCES

Aedo AR, Landgren BM, Johannisson E, Diczfalusy E: Pharmacokinetic and pharmacodynamic investigations with monthly injectable contraceptive preparations. Contraception 31:453, 1985

Ahlgren M: Sperm transport to and survival in the human fallopian tube. Gynecol Invest 6:206, 1975

Åkerlund M, Almström E, Högstedt S, Nabrink M: Oral contraceptive tablets containing 20 and 30 μg desogestrel. Acta Obstet Gynecol Scand 73:136, 1994

Åkerlund M, Røde A, Westergaard J: Comparative profiles of reliability, cycle control and side effects of two oral contraceptive formulations containing 150 μg desogestrel and either 30 μg or 20 μg ethinyl oestradiol. Br J Obstet Gynaecol 100:832, 1993

Alcid DV, Kothari N, Quinn EP, Geismar L, Glowinsky LZ: Toxic-shock syndrome associated with diaphragm use for only nine hours. Lancet 1:1363, 1982

Alvarez F, Brache V, Fernandez E, Guerrero B, Guiloff E, Hess R, Salvatierra AM, Zacharias S: New insights on the mode of action of intrauterine contraceptive devices in women. Fertil Steril 49:768, 1988

Alvarez-Sanchez F, Brache V, de Oca VM, Cochon L, Faundes A: Prevalence of enlarged ovarian follicles among users of levonorgestrel subdermal contraceptive implants (Norplant). Am J Obstet Gynecol 182:535, 2000

American College of Obstetricians and Gynecologists: The use of hormonal contraception in women with coexisting medical conditions. Practice Bulletin No. 18, July 2000

American College of Obstetricians and Gynecologists: FDA approves new emergency contraception drug. ACOG Today 43:7, 1999a

American College of Obstetricians and Gynecologists: Japan approves birth control pill. ACOG Today 43:6, 1999b

American College of Obstetricians and Gynecologists: ACOG Newsletter 39(5):5, 1995

American College of Obstetricians and Gynecologists: Hormonal contraception. ACOG Technical Bulletin No. 198, October 1994

American College of Obstetricians and Gynecologists: The intrauterine device. ACOG Technical Bulletin No. 164, February 1992

American Medical Association Board of Trustees: Requirements or incentives by government for the use of long-acting contraceptives. JAMA 267:1818, 1992

Antoniades K, Campbell WN, Hecksher RH, Kessler WB, McCarthy GE Jr: Liver cell adenoma and oral contraceptives. JAMA 234:628, 1975

Aronson J: Serious drug interactions. Practitioner 234:789, 1993

Association of Professors of Gynecology and Obstetrics: Educational Series on Women's Health Issues: Contraception. February, 1999

Bartens W, Wanner C: Lipoprotein(a): New insights into an atherogenic lipoprotein. Clin Invest 72:558, 1994

Beck WW: Use of oral contraceptives in women in their 40s. Clin Obstet Gynecol Postgrad Ob-Gyn 15:46, 1995

Berenson AB, Rickert VI, Grady JJ: A prospective study of the effects of oral and injectable contraception on bone mineral density. Obstet Gynecol 95:S6, 2000

Berenson AB, Wiemann CM: Contraceptive use among adolescent mothers at 6 months postpartum. Paper presented at the 44th Annual Clinical Meeting of the American College of Obstetricians and Gynecologists, Denver, April 27–May 1, 1996

Berenson AB, Wiemann CM, McCombs SL, Somma-Garcia A: The rise and fall of levonorgestrel implants: 1992–1996. Obstet Gynecol 92:790, 1998

Berg CJ, Atrash HK, Koonin LM, Tucker M: Pregnancy-related mortality in the United States, 1987–1990. Obstet Gynecol 88:161, 1996

Betrabet SS, Shikary ZK, Toddywalla VS, Toddywalla SP, Patel D, Saxena BN: ICMR Task Force Study on hormonal contraception. Transfer of norethindrone (NET) and levo-norgestrel (LNG) from a single tablet into the infant's circulation through the mother's milk. Contraception 35:517, 1987

Bloemenkamp KWM, Helmerhorst FM, Büller HR, Vandenbroucke JP: Enhancement by factor V Leiden mutation of risk of deep-vein thrombosis associated with oral contraceptives containing a third-generation progestogen. Lancet 346:1593, 1995

Bounds W, Guillebaud J, Dominik R, Dalberth BT: The diaphragm with and without spermicide. A randomized, comparative efficacy trial. J Reprod Med 40:764, 1995

Brache V, Alvarez-Sanchez F, Faundes A, Tejada AS, Cochon L: Ovarian endocrine function through 5 years of continuous treatment with Norplant subdermal contraceptive implants. Contraception 41:169, 1990

Bracken MB, Hellenbrand KG, Holford TR: Conception delay after oral contraceptive use: The effect of estrogen dose. Fertil Steril 53:21, 1990

Briggs GG, Freeman RK, Yaffe SJ: Drugs in Pregnancy and Lactation, 5th ed. Baltimore, Williams & Wilkins, 1998

Burkman RT Jr: Non-contraceptive effects of hormonal contraceptives: Bone mass, sexually transmitted disease and pelvic inflammatory disease, cardiovascular disease, menstrual function, and future fertility. Am J Obstet Gynecol 170:1569, 1994

Burkman RT: Lipid metabolism effects with desogestrel-containing oral contraceptives. Am J Obstet Gynecol 168:1033, 1993

Burkman RT, Kaunitz AM, Shulman LP, Sulak PJ: Oral contraceptives and noncontraceptive benefits: Summary and application of data. Int J Fertil 45:134, 2000

Butterworth CE Jr, Hatch KD, Macaluso M, Cole P, Sauberlich HE, Soong SJ, Borst M, Baker V: Folate deficiency and cervical dysplasia. JAMA 267:528, 1992

Cancer and Steroid Hormone Study of the Centers for Disease Control and the National Institute of Child Health and Development: Combination oral contraceptive use and the risk of endometrial cancer. JAMA 257:796, 1987a

Cancer and Steroid Hormone Study of the Centers for Disease Control and the National Institute of Child Health and Development: The reduction in risk of ovarian cancer associated with oral-contraceptive use. N Engl J Med 316:650, 1987b

Cancer and Steroid Hormone Study of the Centers for Disease Control and the National Institute of Child Health and Development: Oral-contraceptive use and the risk of breast cancer. N Engl J Med 315:405, 1986

Cates W: Putting the risks in perspective. Contracept Tech Update 1:111, 1980

Collaborative Group on Hormonal Factors in Breast Cancer: Breast cancer and hormonal contraceptives: Collaborative reanalysis of individual data on 53,297 women with breast cancer and 100,239 women without breast cancer from 54 epidemiological studies. Lancet 347:1713, 1996

Collins D: Selectivity information on desogestrel. Am J Obstet Gynecol 168:1010, 1993

Comp PC: Coagulation and thrombosis with OC use: Physiology and clinical relevance. Dialogues in Contraception 5(1):1, 1996

Contraception Report 3:4, May 1992

Craft P, Hannaford PC: Risk factors for acute myocardial infarction in women: Evidence from the Royal College of General Practitioners' Oral Contraceptive Study. BMJ 298:165, 1989

Cramer DW, Schiff I, Schoenbaum SC, Gibson M, Belisle S, Albrecht A, Stillman RJ, Berger MJ, Wilson E, Stadel BV,

Seibel M: Tubal infertility and the intrauterine device. N Engl J Med 312:941, 1985

Creasy G, Hall N, Shangold G: Patient adherence with the contraceptive patch dosing schedule versus oral contraceptives. Obstet Gynecol 95:S60, 2000

Critchlow CW, Wölner-Hanssen P, Eschenback DA, Kiviat NB, Koutsky LA, Stevens CE, Holmes KK: Determinants of cervical ectopia and of cervicitis: Age, oral contraception, specific cervical infection, smoking, and douching. Am J Obstet Gynecol 173:534, 1995

Cromer BA, Blair JM, Mahan JD, Zibners L, Naumovski Z: A prospective comparison of bone density in adolescent girls receiving depot medroxyprogesterone acetate (Depo-Provera), levonorgestrel (Norplant), or oral contraceptives. J Pediatr 129:671, 1996

Cundy T, Cornish J, Evans MC, et al: Recovery of bone density in women who stop using medroxyprogesterone acetate. BMJ 308:247, 1994

Cuong DT, My Huong NT: Comparative phase III clinical trial of two injectable contraceptive preparations, depot-medroxyprogesterone acetate and Cyclofem, in Vietnamese women. Contraception 54:169, 1996

Cushman LF, Kalmuss D, Davidson AR, Heartwell S, Rulin M: Beliefs about Depo-Provera among three groups of contraceptors. Adv Contracept 12:43, 1996

Daling JR, Weiss NS, Metch BJ, Chow WH, Soderstrom RM, Moore DE, Spadoni LR, Stadel BV: Primary tubal infertility in relation to the use of an intrauterine device. N Engl J Med 312:937, 1985

Deslypere JP, Thiery M, Vermenulen A: Effect of long-term hormonal contraception on plasma lipids. Contraception 31:633, 1985

Diaz S, Pavez M, Miranda P, Johansson ED, Croxatto HB: Long-term followup of women treated with Norplant implants. Contraception 35:551, 1987

Dinman BD: The reality and acceptance of risk. JAMA 244:1226, 1980

Earl DT, David DJ: Depo-Provera: An injectable contraceptive. Am Fam Physician 49:891, 1994

Ellis JW: Multiphasic oral contraceptives: Efficacy and metabolic impact. J Reprod Med 32:38, 1987

Entwistle VA, Watt IS, Johnson F: The case of Norplant as an example of media coverage over the life of a new health technology. Lancet 355:1633, 2000

Escobedo LG, Peterson HB, Grubb GS, Franks AL: Case-fatality rates for tubal sterilization in U.S. hospitals, 1979–1980. Am J Obstet Gynecol 160:147, 1989

Farley TMM, Rosenberg MJ, Rowe PJ, Chen JH, Meirik O: Intrauterine devices and pelvic inflammatory disease: An international perspective. Lancet 339:785, 1992

Farmer RDT, Todd JC, Lewis MA, MacRae KD, Williams TJ: The risks of venous thromboembolic disease among German women using oral contraceptives: A database study. Contraception 57:67, 1998

Fasoli M, Parazzini F, Cecchetti G, La Vecchia C: Post-coital contraception: An overview of published studies. Contraception 39:459, 1989

Feldblum PJ, Fortney JA: Condoms, spermicides and the transmission of human immunodeficiency virus: A review of the literature. Am J Public Health 78:52, 1988

Fiorino AS: Intrauterine contraceptive device–associated actinomycotic abscess and Actinomyces detection on cervical smear. Obstet Gynecol 87:142, 1996

Food and Drug Administration: Prescription Drug Products. Certain combined oral contraceptives for use as postcoital emergency contraception: notice. Federal Register, February 25, 62:8609, 1997

Food and Drug Administration: Drug Bull 18:18, 1988

Food and Drug Administration: Drug Bull 16:21, 1986

Food and Drug Administration: Drug Bulletin 14:2, 1984

Frederiksen MC: Contraceptive counseling for increased acceptance. Dialogues in Contraception 5(6):6, 1998

Frezieres RG, Walsh TL, Nelson AL, Clark VA, Coulson AH: Breakage and acceptability of a polyurethane condom: A randomized, controlled study. Fam Plan Perspect 30:73, 1998

Glasier A, Thong KJ, Dewar M, Mackie M, Baird DT: Mifepristone (RU 486) compared with high-dose estrogen and progestogen for emergency postcoital contraception. N Engl J Med 327:1041, 1992

Glasier A, Thong KJ, Dewar M, Mackie M, Baird DT: Postcoital contraception with mifepristone. Lancet 337:1414, 1991

Godsland IF, Wynn V: Does the new progestagen desogestrel have metabolic advantages? Lancet 2:359, 1984

Goebelsmann U, Stanczyk FZ, Brenner PF, Goebelsmann AE, Gentzschein EK, Mishell DR Jr: Serum norethindrone (NET) concentrations following intramuscular NET enanthate injection. Effect upon serum LH, FSH, estradiol and progesterone. Contraception 19:283, 1979

Goldzieher JW, Zamah NM: Oral contraceptive side effects: Where's the beef? Contraception 52:327, 1995

Grabrick DM, Hartmann LC, Cerhan JR, Vierkant RA, Therneau TM, Vachon CM, Olson JE, Couch FJ, Anderson KE, Pankratz VS, Sellers TA: Risk of breast cancer with oral contraceptive use in women with a family history of breast cancer. JAMA 284:1791, 2000

Grimes DA, Cook RJ: Mifepristone (RU 486)—an abortifacient to prevent abortion? N Engl J Med 327:1088, 1992

Guillebaud J: Contraception Today: A Pocket Book for General Practitioners, 3rd ed. London, Martin Dunitz, 1997

Guillebaud J: Contraception: Your Questions Answered. New York, Pitman, 1985

Guillebaud J, Barnett MD, Gordon YB: Plasma ferritin levels as an index of iron deficiency in women using intrauterine devices. Br J Obstet Gynaecol 86:51, 1979

Hall PE: New once-a-month injectable contraceptives with particular reference to Cyclofem®/Cyclo-Provera™. Int J Gynecol Obstet 62:S43, 1998

Hall PE, Task Force on Research on Introduction and Transfer of Technologies for Fertility Regulation, Special Programme of Research, Development and Research Training in Human Reproduction, World Health Organization, Geneva, Switzerland: The introduction of Cyclofem into national family planning programmes: Experience from studies in Indonesia, Jamaica, Mexico, Thailand and Tunisia. Contraception 49:489, 1994

Harlap S, Kost K, Forrest JD: Preventing Pregnancy, Protecting Health: A New Look at Birth Control Choices in the United States. New York, The Alan Guttmacher Institute, 1991

Hatcher RA, Stewart F, Trussell J, Kowal P, Guest F, Stewart GK, Cates W: Contraceptive Technology, 15th ed, New York, Irvington, 1990, p 370

Hatcher RA, Trussell J, Stewart F, Cates Jr W, Stewart GK, Guest F, Kowal P: Contraceptive Technology, 17th ed. New York, Ardent Media, 1998, pp 230, 278, 322, 327, 384, 409–414, 424–425, 439, 449–450, 467, 494, 520, 800–801

Hausknecht RU: Methotrexate and misoprostol to terminate early pregnancy. N Engl J Med 333:537, 1995

Heartwell SF, Schlesselman S: Risk of uterine perforation

among users of intrauterine devices. Obstet Gynecol 61:31, 1983

Henshaw SK: Unintended pregnancy in the United States. Fam Plan Perspect 30:24, 1998

International Planned Parenthood Federation, International Medical Advisory Panel: Statement on periodic abstinence for family planning. IPPF Med Bull 18:2, 1982

Irey NS, Nanion WC, Taylor HB: Vascular lesions in women taking oral contraceptives. Arch Pathol 89:1, 1970

Janevich DT, Piper JM, Glebatis DM: Oral contraceptives and congenital limb reduction defects. N Engl J Med 291:697, 1974

Jick H, Jick SS, Gurewich V, Myers MW, Vasilakis C: Risk of idiopathic cardiovascular death and nonfatal venous thromboembolism in women using oral contraceptives with differing progestogen components. Lancet 346:1589, 1995

Kalkhoff RK: Relative sensitivity of postpartum gestational diabetic women to oral contraceptive agents and other metabolic stress. Diabetes Care 3:421, 1980

Kaunitz AM: Considering postpartum contraception and the role of lactation. Dialogues in Contraception 5(3):5, 1997

Kaunitz AM: Depot medroxyprogesterone acetate contraception and the risk of breast and gynecologic cancer. J Reprod Med 45:419, 1996

Kaunitz AM: Medroxyprogesterone acetate/Estradiol cypionate: Overview of a new contraceptive. Dialogues in Contraception 6(1):1, 1999a

Kaunitz AM: Oral contraceptive use and venous thromboembolism: Translating epidemiologic data into clinical practice. ACOG Clin Rev 4:1, 1999b

Kauppinen-Mäkelin R, Kuusi T, Ylikorkala O, Tikkanen MJ: Contraceptives containing desogestrel or levonorgestrel have different effects on serum lipoproteins and post-heparin plasma lipase activities. Clin Endocrinol 36:203, 1992

Kay CR: The Royal College of General Practitioners' Oral Contraception Study: Some recent observations. Clin Obstet Gynaecol 11:759, 1984

Keebler C, Chatwani A, Schwartz R: Actinomyces infection associated with intrauterine contraceptive devices. Am J Obstet Gynecol 145:596, 1983

Kent DR, Nissen ED, Nissen SE, Ziehm DJ: Effect of pregnancy on liver tumor associated with oral contraceptives. Obstet Gynecol 51:148, 1978

Kjos SL, Peters RK, Xiang A, Thomas D, Schaefer U, Buchanan TA: Contraception and the risk of type 2 diabetes mellitus in Latina women with prior gestational diabetes mellitus. JAMA 280:533, 1998

Knopp RH: Cardiovascular effects of endogenous and exogenous sex hormones over a woman's lifetime. Am J Obstet Gynecol 158:1630, 1988

Konje JC, Otolorin EO, Ladipo OA: The effect of continuous subdermal levonorgestrel (Norplant) on carbohydrate metabolism. Am J Obstet Gynecol 166:15, 1992

Krauss RM: The effects of oral contraceptives on plasma lipids and lipoproteins. Int J Fertil 1988:33 (Suppl 2):35–42.

Kubba A, Guillebaud J: Combined oral contraceptives: Acceptability and effective use. BMJ 49:140, 1993

Kuchara LK: Postcoital contraception with diethylstilbestrol. JAMA 218:562, 1971

Ladipo OA, Farr G, Otolorin E, Konje JC, Sturgen K, Cox P, Champion CV: Prevention of IUD-related pelvic infection: The efficacy of prophylactic doxycycline at IUD insertion. Adv Contracept 7:43, 1991

Lammer EJ, Cordero JF: Exogenous sex hormone exposure and the risk for major malformations. JAMA 255:3128, 1986

Lawson HW, Frye A, Atrash HK, Smith JC, Schulman HB, Ramick M: Abortion mortality, United States, 1972 through 1987. Am J Obstet Gynecol 171:1365, 1994

Lee BW: Risk assessment. JAMA 246:1196, 1981

Lee NC, Rubin GL: The intrauterine device and pelvic inflammatory disease revisited: New results from the woman's health study. Obstet Gynecol 72:1, 1988

Lee NC, Rubin GL, Ory HW, Burknan RT: Type of intrauterine device and the risk of pelvic inflammatory disease. Obstet Gynecol 62:1, 1983

Lewis MA, Spitzer WO, Heinemann LAJ, MacRae KD, Bruppacher R, Thorogood M: Third generation oral contraceptives and risk of myocardial infarction: An international case-control study. BMJ 312:88, 1996

Lewit S: Outcome of pregnancy with an intrauterine device. Contraception 2:47, 1970

Lidegaard Ø: Oral contraception and risk of a cerebral thromboembolic attack: Results of a case-control study. BMJ 306:956, 1993

Lidegaard Ø, Edström B, Kreiner S: Oral contraceptives and venous thromboembolism. Contraception 57:291, 1998

Lippes J, Tatum HJ, Maulid D, Zielezny M: A continuation of the study of postcoital IUDs. Paper presented at the annual meeting of the Association of Planned Parenthood Physicians, San Diego, October 25, 1978

Louik C, Mitchell AA, Werler MM, Hanson JW, Shapiro S: Maternal exposure to spermicides in relation to certain birth defects. N Engl J Med 317:474, 1987

Mainwaring R, Hales HA, Stevenson K, Hatasaka HH, Pouson AM, Jones KP, Peterson CM: Metabolic parameter, bleeding, and weight changes in U.S. women using progestin only contraceptives. Contraception 51:149, 1995

Mann JI: Progestogens in cardiovascular disease: An introduction to the epidemiologic data. Am J Obstet Gynecol 142:752, 1982

Mason V (ed): New contraceptive methods: The good, the bad, and the ugly. Contracept Tech Update 13:101, 1992

Meirik O, Lund E, Adami H, Bergstrom R, Christoffersen T, Bergsö P: Oral contraceptive use and breast cancer in young women: A joint national case-control study in Sweden and Norway. Lancet 1:650, 1986

Metcalf MG: Incidence of ovulatory cycles in women approaching the menopause. J Biosoc Sci 11:39, 1979

Miller NE, Hammett F, Saltissi S, Rao S, van Zeller H, Coltart J, Lewis B: Relation of angiographically defined coronary artery disease to plasma lipoprotein subfractions and apolipoproteins. BMJ 282:1741, 1982

Mills JL, Harley EE, Reed GF, Berendes HW: Are spermicides teratogenic? JAMA 248:2148, 1982

Mishell DR Jr: Oral contraceptives and cardiovascular events: Summary and application of data. Int J Fertil 45:121, 2000

Mishell DR Jr: Pharmacokinetics of depot medroxyprogesterone acetate contraception. J Reprod Med 41:381, 1996

Mishell DR Jr: Use of oral contraceptives in women of older reproductive age. Am J Obstet Gynecol 158:1652, 1988

Mishell DR Jr, Bell JH, Good RG, Moyer DL: The intrauterine device: A bacteriologic study of the endometrial cavity. Am J Obstet Gynecol 96:119, 1966

Mishell DR Jr, Darney PD, Burkman RT, Sulak PJ: Practice guidelines for OC selection: Update. Contraception 5:7, 1997

Mishell DR Jr, Sulak PJ: The IUD: Dispelling the myths and assessing the potential. Dialogues in Contraception 5(2):1, 1997

Moore LL, Valuck R, McDougall C, Fink W: A comparative study of one-year weight gain among users of medroxy-progesterone acetate, levonorgestrel implants, and oral contraceptives. Contraception 52:215, 1995

Mosher WD, McNally JW: Contraceptive use at first premarital intercourse: United States, 1965–1988. Fam Plan Perspect 23:108, 1991

Musicco M, Nicolosi A, Saracco A, Lazzarin A: IUD use and man to woman sexual transmission of HIV-1. In Bardin CW, Mishell DR Jr (eds): A New Look at IUDs—Advancing Contraceptive Choices. Stoneham, Butterworth-Heineman, 1996

Naessen T, Olsson SE, Gudmundson J: Differential effects on bone density of progestogen-only methods for contraception in premenopausal women. Contraception 52:35, 1995

National Institute of Child Health and Human Development: NICHD News Notes, May 6, 1996

Nelson AL: Selecting a contraceptive method: Role of MPA/E_2C. J Reprod Med 45:879, 2000

Neuberger J, Forman D, Doll R, Williams R: Oral contraceptives and hepatocellular carcinoma. BMJ 292:1355, 1986

New York Times: Will the lawyers kill off Norplant? May 28, 1995, section 3, p 1

Oriowo MA, Landgren BM, Stenstrom B, Diczfalusy E: A comparison of the pharmacokinetic properties of three estradiol esters. Contraception 21:415, 1980

Ortiz ME, Croxatto HB: The mode of action of IUDs. Contraception 36:37, 1987

Ortiz A, Hirol M, Stanczyk FZ, Goebelsmann U, Mishell DR: Serum medroxyprogesterone acetate (MPA) concentrations and ovarian function following intramuscular injection of Depo-MPA. J Clin Endocrinol Metab 44:32, 1977

Ory HW: Mortality associated with fertility and fertility control: 1983. Fam Plan Perspect 15:57, 1983

Parazzini F, Negri E, La Vecchia C, Fedele L, Rabaiotti M, Luchini L: Oral contraceptive use and risk of uterine fibroids. Obstet Gynecol 79:430, 1992

Pasco JA, Kotowicz MA, Henry MJ, Panahi S, Seeman E, Nicholson GC: Oral contraceptives and bone mineral density: A population-based study. Am J Obstet Gynecol 182:265, 2000

Paul C, Skegg DCG, Spears GFS, Kaldor JM: Oral contraceptives and breast cancer: A national study. BMJ 293:723, 1986

Pérez A: Natural family planning: Postpartum period. Int J Fertil 26:219, 1981

Petitti DB, Piaggio G, Mehta S, Cravioto MC, Meirik O: Steroid hormone contraception and bone mineral density: A cross-sectional study in an international population. Obstet Gynecol 95:736, 2000

Petitti DB, Sidney S, Bernstein A, Wolf S, Quesenberry C, Ziel HK: Stroke in users of low-dose oral contraceptives. N Engl J Med 335:8, 1996

Petitti DB, Sidney S, Quesenberry CP: Oral contraceptive use and myocardial infarction. Contraception 57:143, 1998

Phillips A, Hahn DW, McGuire JL: Preclinical evaluation of norgestimate, a progestin with minimal androgenic activity. Am J Obstet Gynecol 167:1191, 1992

Phillips N, Duffy T: One-hour glucose tolerance in relation to the use of oral contraceptive drugs. Am J Obstet Gynecol 116:91, 1973

Piccinino LJ, Mosher WD: Trends in contraceptive use in the United States: 1982–1995. Fam Plan Perspect 30:4, 1998a

Piccinino LJ, Mosher WD: Trends in contraceptive use in the United States: 1982–1995. Fam Plan Perspect 30:46, 1998b

Pituitary Adenoma Study Group: Pituitary adenomas and oral contraceptives: A multi-center case controlled study. Fertil Steril 39:753, 1983

Population Reports: Periodic Abstinence: How Well Do New Approaches Work? Series L, No. 3, September 1981, p 33

Population Reports: Update on Condoms—Products, Protection, Promotion. Series H, No. 6, September–October 1982, p 121

Porter CW, Waife RS, Holtrap HR: The Health Provider's Guide to Contraception, International ed. Watertown, MA, Pathfinder Fund, 1983

Porter JB, Jick H, Walker AM: Mortality among oral contraceptive users. Obstet Gynecol 70:29, 1987

Prentice RL, Thomas DB: On the epidemiology of oral contraceptives and disease. Adv Cancer Res 49:285, 1987

Queenan JT, Jennings VH, Spieler JM, von Hertzen H, (eds): Natural family planning: Current knowledge and new strategies for the 1990s. Am J Obstet Gynecol (Suppl) 165:1977, 1991

Raymond EG, Creinin MD, Barnhart KT, Lovvorn AE, Rountree RW, Trussell J: Meclizine for prevention of nausea associated with use of emergency contraceptive pills: A randomized trial. Obstet Gynecol 95:271, 2000

Realini JP, Goldzieher JW: Oral contraceptives and cardiovascular disease: A critique of the epidemiologic studies. Am J Obstet Gynecol 152:729, 1985

Rizack MA, Hillman CDM: The Medical Letter handbook of adverse drug interactions. New Rochelle NY: The Medical Letter, 1985

Rosenberg MJ, Davidson AJ, Chen JH, Judson FN, Douglas JM: Barrier contraceptives and sexually transmitted diseases in women: A comparison of female-dependent methods and condoms. Am J Pub Health 82:669, 1992

Rosenfield A, Broholm C: The safety of modern contraceptives. Aust N Z J Obstet Gynaecol 34:305, 1994

Rothman KJ, Louik C: Oral contraceptives and birth defects. N Engl J Med 299:522, 1978

Roumen FJME, Dieben TOM: Ovulation prediction by monitoring salivary electrical resistance with the Cue fertility monitor. Obstet Gynecol 71:49, 1988

Rowe PJ: Research on Intrauterine Devices. Annual Technical Report 1991. Geneva, Switzerland, Special Programme of Research, Development and Research Training in Human Reproduction, World Health Organization, 1992, p 127

Royal College of General Practitioners' Oral Contraceptive Study: Oral contraceptives and gallbladder disease. Lancet 2:957, 1982

Sang GW, Shao QX, Ge RS, Ge JL, Chen JK, Song S, Fang KJ, He ML, Luo SY, Chen SF, et al: A multi-centered phase III comparative clinical trial of Mesigyna, Cyclofem and Injectable No. 1 given by intramuscular injection to Chinese women. II: The comparison of bleeding patterns. Contraception 51:185, 1995

Savolainen E, Saksela E, Saxen L: Teratogenic hazards of oral contraceptives analyzed in a national malformation register. Am J Obstet Gynecol 140:521, 1981

Schlesselman JJ, Stadel BV, Murray P, Lai S: Breast cancer in relation to early use of oral contraceptives: No evidence of latent effect. JAMA 259:1828, 1988

Scholes D, Lacroix AZ, Ott SM, Ichikawa LE, Barlow WE: Bone mineral density in women using depot medroxyprogesterone acetate for contraception. Obstet Gynecol 93:233, 1999

Schwartz SM, Petitti DB, Siscovick DS, Longstreth WJ Jr, Sidney S, Raghunathan TE, Quesenberry CP Jr, Kelaghan J: Stroke and use of low-dose oral contraceptives in young women. A pooled analysis of two US studies. Stroke 29:2277, 1998

Shapiro S, Slone D, Heinonin OP, Kaufman DW, Rosenberg L, Mitchell AA, Helmrich SP: Birth defects and vaginal spermicides. JAMA 247:2381, 1982

Shenfield GM: Oral contraceptives: Are drug interactions of clinical significance? Drug Saf 9:21, 1993

Shikary ZK, Betrabet SS, Patel ZM, Patel S, Joshi JV, Toddywala VS, Toddywala SP, Patel DM, Jhaveri K, Saxena BN: ICMR Task Force Study on hormonal contraception. Transfer of levonorgestrel (LNG) administered through different drug delivery systems from the maternal circulation via breast milk. Contraception 35:477, 1987

Sidney S, Petitti DB, Quesenberry CP Jr, Klaatsky AL, Ziel HK, Wolf S: Myocardial infarction in users of low-dose oral contraceptives. Obstet Gynecol 88:939, 1996

Sidney S, Siscovick DS, Petitti DB, Schwartz SM, Quesenberry CP, Psaty BM, Raghunathan TE, Kelaghan J, Koepsell TD: Myocardial infarction and use of low-dose oral contraceptives. A pooled analysis of 2 US studies. Circulation 98:1058, 1998

Sinei SKA, Schulz KF, Lamptey PR, Grimes DA, Mati JKG, Rosenthal SM, Rosenberg MJ, Riara G, Mjage PN, Bhullar VB, Ogembo HV: Preventing IUD-related pelvic infection: The efficacy of prophylactic doxycycline at insertion. Br J Obstet Gynaecol 97:412, 1990

Sivin I: IUDs are contraceptives, not abortifacients: A comment on research and belief. Stud Fam Plan 20:355, 1989

Sivin I: International experience with Norplant and Norplant-2 contraceptives. Stud Fam Plan 19:81, 1988

Sivin I, Stern J, Diaz S, Pavéz M, Alvarez F, Brache V, Mishell DR Jr, Lacarra M, McCarthy T, Holma P, Darney P, Klaisle C, Olsson SE, Odlind V: Rates and outcomes of planned pregnancy after use of Norplant capsules, Norplant II rods, or levonorgestrel-releasing or copper-T Cu 380 Ag intrauterine contraceptive devices. Am J Obstet Gynecol 166:1208, 1992

Skegg DCG, Noonan EA, Paul C, Spears GFS, Meirik O, Thomas DB: Depot medroxyprogesterone acetate and breast cancer. JAMA 273:10, 1995

Skouby SO, Kühl C, Mølsted-Pedersen L, Petersen K, Christensen MS: Triphasic oral contraception: Metabolic effects in normal women and those with previous gestational diabetes. Am J Obstet Gynecol 153:495, 1985

Speroff L: Oral contraceptives and carbohydrate metabolism. Dialogues in Contraception 6:1, 2000a

Speroff L: Oral contraceptives and breast cancer risk: Summary and application of data. Int J Fertil 45:113, 2000b

Speroff L: Oral contraceptives and arterial and venous thrombosis: A clinician's formulation. Am J Obstet Gynecol 179:S25, 1998

Speroff L, Sulak PJ: Contraception in the later reproductive years: A valid aspect of preventive health care. Dialogues in Contraception 4:1, 1995

Speroff L, Westhoff CL: Breast disease and hormonal contraception: Resolution of a lasting controversy. Dialogues in Contraception 5(3):1, 1997

Spitzer WO, Lewis MA, Heinemann LAJ, Thorogood M, MacRae KD: Third generation oral contraceptives and risk of venous thromboembolic disorders: An international case-control study. BMJ 312:83, 1996

Stadel BV: Oral contraceptives and cardiovascular disease. N Engl J Med 305:612, 1981

Strobino B, Kline J, Warburton D: Spermicide use and pregnancy outcome. Am J Public Health 78:260, 1988

Strom BL, Tamragouri RN, Morse ML, Lazar EL, West SL, Stolley PD, Jones JK: Oral contraceptives and other risk factors for gallbladder diseases. Clin Pharmacol Ther 39:335, 1986

Sulak PJ: The perimenopause: A critical time in a woman's life. Int J Fertil 41:85, 1996

Sulak PJ, Haney AF: Unwanted pregnancies: Understanding contraceptive use and benefits in adolescents and older women. Am J Obstet Gynecol 168:2042, 1993

Sulak PJ, Kaunitz AM: Hormonal contraception and bone mineral density. Dialogues in Contraception 6(2):1, 1999

Szlachter BN, Nachtigall LE, Epstein J, Young BK, Weiss G: Premature menopause: A reversible entity? Obstet Gynecol 54:396, 1979

Task Force on Postovulatory Methods of Fertility Regulation: Randomized controlled trial of levonorgestrel versus the Yuzpe regimen of combined oral contraceptives for emergency contraception. Lancet 352:428, 1998

Tatum HJ, Schmidt FH, Jain AK: Management and outcome of pregnancies associated with Copper-T intrauterine contraceptive device. Am J Obstet Gynecol 126:869, 1976

Thomas DB, Ray RM, and the World Health Organization Collaborative Study of Neoplasia and Steroid Contraceptives: Oral contraceptives and invasive adenocarcinomas and adenosquamous carcinomas of the uterine cervix. Am J Epidemiol 144:281, 1996

Thomas DB, Ye Z, Ray RM, WHO Collaborative Study of Neoplasia and Steroid Contraceptives: Cervical carcinoma in situ and use of Depo-medroxyprogesterone acetate (DMPA). Contraception 51:25, 1995

Tikkanen MJ, Nikkilä EA, Kuusi T, Sipinen SU: High density lipoprotein$_2$ and hepatic lipase: Reciprocal changes produced by estrogen and norgestrel. J Clin Endocrinol Metab 54:1113, 1982

Toews M, Boone S, Watson M, Whillans J: A multicenter phase IV study of Ortho 7/7/7 tablets in previous users of oral contraceptives. Curr Ther Res 41:509, 1987

Toivonen J, Luukkainen T, Allonen H: Protective effect of intrauterine release of levonorgestrel on pelvic infections: Three years' comparative experience of levonorgestrel and copper-releasing intrauterine devices. Obstet Gynecol 77:261, 1991

Trussell J, Duran V, Shochet T, Moore K: Access to emergency contraception. Obstet Gynecol 95:267, 2000

Trussell J, Ellertson C, Stewart F: The effectiveness of the Yuzpe regimen of emergency contraception. Fam Plan Perspect 28:58, 1996

Trussell J, Ellertson C, Stewart F: Emergency contraception. A cost-effective approach to preventing pregnancy. Women Health Primary Care 1:52, 1998a

Trussell J, Hatcher RA, Cates W Jr, Stewart FH, Kost K: Contraceptive failure in the United States: An update. Stud Fam Plan 21:51, 1990

Trussell J, Kost K: Contraceptive failure in the United States: A critical review of the literature. Stud Fam Plan 18:237, 1987

Trussell J, Leveque JA, Koenig JD, London R, Boarden S, Henneberry J, LaGuardia KD, Stewart F, Wilson TG, Wysocki S, et al: The economic value of contraception: A comparison of 15 methods. Am J Publ Health 85:494, 1995

Trussell J, Rodriguez G, Ellertson C: New estimates of the effectiveness of the Yuzpe regimen of emergency contraception. Contraception 57:363, 1998b

Trussell J, Stewart F: An update on emergency contraception. Dialogues in Contraception 5(6):1, 1998

van den Hurk PJ, O'Brien S: Non-contraceptive use of the

levonorgestrel-releasing intrauterine system. Obstetrician and Gynaecologist 1:13, 1999

Vessey MP, Johnson B, Doll R, Peto R: Outcome of pregnancy in women using intrauterine devices. Lancet 1:495, 1974

Vessey MP, Lawless M, McPherson K, Yeates D: Fertility after stopping use of intrauterine contraceptive device. BMJ 286:106, 1983a

Vessey MP, Lawless M, Yeates D, McPherson K: Progestin-only oral contraception: Findings in a large prospective study with special reference to effectiveness. Br J Fam Plan 10:117, 1985

Vessey MP, Lawless M, Yeates D: Efficacy of different contraceptive methods. Lancet 1:841, 1982

Vessey MP, McPherson K, Lawless M, Yeates D: Neoplasia of the cervix uteri and contraception: A possible adverse effect of the pill. Lancet 2:930, 1983b

Vessey MP, Meisler L, Flavel R, Yeates D: Outcome of pregnancy in women using different methods of contraception. Br J Obstet Gynaecol 86:548, 1979

Vessey MP, Villard-Mackintosh L, McPherson K, Yeates D: Mortality among oral contraceptive users: 20 year follow up of women in a cohort study. BMJ 299:1487, 1989

Waetjen LE, Grimes DA: Oral contraceptives and primary liver cancer: Temporal trends in three countries. Obstet Gynecol 88:945, 1996

Waldron T: Newer, innovative condoms may help increase compliance. Contracept Tech Update 12:171, 1991

Waldron T: Tests show commonly used substances harm latex condoms. Contracept Tech Update 10:20, 1989

Walsh T, Grimes D, Frezieres R, Nelson A, Bernstein L, Coulson A, Benstein G: Randomized controlled trial of prophylactic antibiotics before insertion of intrauterine devices. Lancet 351:1005, 1998

Weir RJ: Effect on blood pressure of changing from high to low dose steroid preparations in women with oral contraceptive induced hypertension. Scott Med J 27:212, 1982

Weiss BD: RU 486: The progesterone antagonist. Arch Fam Med 2:63, 1993

Westhoff CL: Oral contraceptives and thrombosis: An overview of study methods and recent results. Am J Obstet Gynecol 179:S38, 1998

Woods ER, Grace E, Havens KK, Merola JL, Emans SJ: Contraceptive compliance with a levonorgestrel triphasic and a norethindrone monophasic oral contraceptive in adolescent patients. Am J Obstet Gynecol 166:901, 1992

World Health Organization: Facts about once-a-month injectable contraceptives: Memorandum from a WHO meeting. Bull WHO 71:677, 1993

World Health Organization: Injectable contraceptives: Their role in family planning, monograph. Geneva, WHO, 1990

World Health Organization: Combined oral contraceptives and liver cancer. Int J Cancer 43:254, 1989a

World Health Organization: Mechanism of action, safety and efficacy of intrauterine devices. Technical Report No. 753. Geneva, Switzerland, WHO, 1987

World Health Organization Collaborative Study of Cardiovascular Disease and Steroid Hormone Contraception: Cardiovascular disease and use of oral and injectable progestogen-only contraceptives and combined injectable contraceptives. Results of an international, multicenter, case-control study. Contraception 57:315, 1998

World Health Organization Collaborative Study of Cardiovascular Disease and Steroid Hormone Contraception: Acute myocardial infarction and combined oral contraceptives: Results of an international multi-center case-control study. Lancet 349:1202, 1997a

World Health Organization United Nations Development Programme/United Nations Population Fund/World Health Organization/World Bank, Special Programme of Research, Development and Research Training in Human Reproduction, Task Force on Long-Acting Systemic Agents for Fertility Regulation: Comparative study of the effects of two once-a-month injectable steroidal contraceptives (Mesigyna® and Cyclofem®) on lipid and lipoprotein metabolism. Contraception 56:193, 1997b

World Health Organization Collaborative Study of Cardiovascular Disease and Steroid Hormone Contraception: Ischaemic stroke and combined oral contraceptives: Results of an internation, multi-center case-control study. Lancet 348:498, 1996

World Health Organization Collaborative Study of Cardiovascular Disease and Steroid Hormone Contraception: Effect of different progestogens in low estrogen oral contraceptives on venous thromboembolic disease. Lancet 246:1582, 1995

World Health Organization Special Programme of Research, Development and Research Training in Human Reproduction Task Force on Long-Acting Systemic Agents for Fertility Regulation. A multi-centered phase III comparative study of two hormonal contraceptive preparations given one-a-month by intramuscular injection. II: The comparison of bleeding patterns. Contraception 40:531, 1989b

World Health Organization Task Force on Long-Acting Systemic Agents for Fertility Regulation, Special Programme of Research, Development and Research Training on Human Reproduction: A multi-centered phase III comparative study of two hormonal contraceptive preparations given once-a-month by intramuscular injection. I: Contraceptive efficacy and side effects. Contraception 37:1, 1988

World Health Organization Special Programme of Research, Development and Research Training in Human Reproduction, Task Force on Intrauterine Devices for Fertility Regulation: A multinational case-control study of ectopic pregnancy. Clin Reprod Fertil 3:131, 1985

World Health Organization, Special Programme of Research, Development and Research Training in Human Reproduction, Task Force on Long-acting Systemic Agents for the Regulation of Fertility: Multinational comparative clinical evaluation of two long-acting injectable contraceptive steroids: Norethindrone enanthate and medroxyprogesterone acetate-final report. Contraception 28:1, 1983

Wynn V: Vitamins and oral contraceptive use. Lancet 1:561, 1975

Wynn V, Godsland I: Effects of oral contraceptives on carbohydrate metabolism. J Reprod Med 31:892, 1986

Wynn V, Niththyananthan R: The effect of progestin in combined oral contraceptives on serum lipids with special reference to high-density lipoproteins. Am J Obstet Gynecol 142:766, 1982

Zondervan KT, Carpenter LM, Painter R, Vessey MP: Oral contraceptives and cervical cancer—further findings from the Oxford Family Planning Association Contraceptive Study. Brit J Cancer 73:1291, 1996

59

Sterilization

FEMALE STERILIZATION

Puerperal Tubal Sterilization
Nonpuerperal (Interval) Tubal Sterilization
Hazards from Tubal Sterilization
Restoration of Fertility
Hysterectomy
Hysteroscopy

MALE STERILIZATION

Cardiovascular Disease
Prostatic and Testicular Carcinoma

Surgical sterilization is the most popular form of contraception among couples of reproductive age (Fig. 59–1). According to the Association for Voluntary Surgical Contraception (1989), 66 percent of 976,000 sterilization procedures performed in the United States in 1987 were in women.

With approximately 700,000 women a year currently choosing voluntary sterilization, it is obvious that this is a procedure that women not only want, but demand. Despite this clear mandate, there are still an excessive number of federal rules and regulations that mainly serve to discourage voluntary sterilization among financially underprivileged women. This is done by threatening to sever federal funding to the organizations that provide service. These restrictive practices will likely appear as ridiculous to future generations as will the men (certainly not women) who devised and promulgated them.

FEMALE STERILIZATION

From a medical standpoint, sterilization can be performed at any time and often is done at cesarean delivery. For women who deliver vaginally, the early puerperium is a particularly convenient time. The oviducts are accessible at the umbilicus directly beneath the abdominal wall for several days after delivery. Thus, the operation is technically simple, and hospitalization need not be prolonged. All these factors collectively make this a less dangerous procedure than an interval sterilization.

Some prefer to perform sterilization in the immediate puerperium (Bucklin and Smith, 1999). This has some disadvantages, and some clinicians prefer to wait for 12 to 24 hours. For example, at Parkland Hospital, puerperal tubal ligation is performed in the obstetrical surgical suite the morning after delivery to minimize hospital stay. The likelihood of postpartum hemorrhage in multiparous women subsides remarkably 12 hours after delivery. In addition, the status of the newborn can be ascertained much more precisely several hours after birth.

PUERPERAL TUBAL STERILIZATION. The first tubal sterilization reported in the United States 120 years ago consisted of ligating the oviducts with a silk ligature about 1 inch from their uterine attachment following a

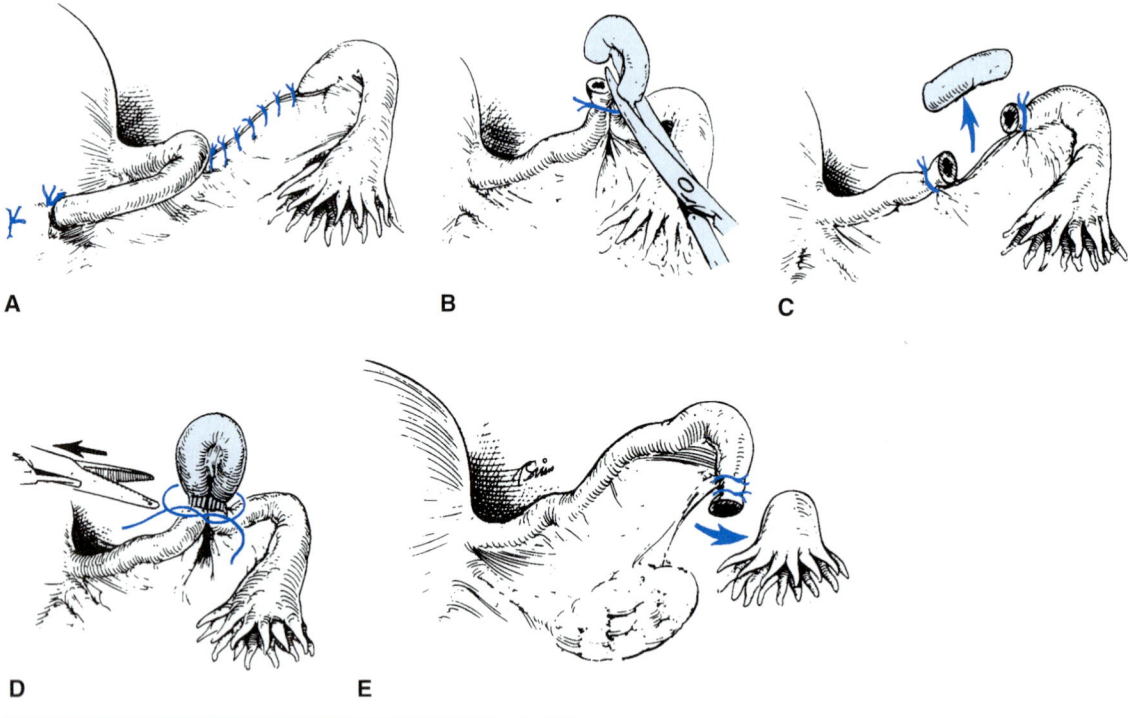

FIGURE 59–1. Various techniques for tubal sterilization. **A.** Irving procedure: the medial cut end of the oviduct is buried in the myometrium posteriorly, and the distal cut end is buried in the mesosalpinx. **B.** Pomeroy procedure: a loop of oviduct is ligated, and the knuckle of tube above the ligature is excised. **C.** Parkland procedure: a midsegment of tube is separated from the mesosalpinx at an avascular site, and the separated tubal segment is ligated proximally and distally and then excised. **D.** Madlener procedure: a knuckle of oviduct is crushed and then ligated without resection. **E.** Kroener procedure: the tube is ligated across the ampulla; and the distal portion of the ampulla, including all of the fimbriae, is resected.

second cesarean delivery (Lungren, 1881). Literally, the woman had her tubes tied. Subsequently, it became apparent that an unacceptably high failure rate followed ligation without tubal resection. A variety of techniques are now employed to disrupt tubal patency.

IRVING PROCEDURE.

This procedure is least likely to fail. The procedure involves severing the oviduct and separating it from the mesosalpinx sufficiently to create a medial segment of tube (Fig. 59–1A). The distal stump of the proximal tubal segment is buried within a tunnel in the myometrium posteriorly, and the proximal end of the distal tubal segment is buried within the mesosalpinx. The procedure requires considerable exposure.

POMEROY PROCEDURE.

This is the simplest, reasonably effective method of dividing the tube (Fig. 59–1B). It generally has been considered important that plain catgut be used to ligate the knuckle of tube, because the rationale of this procedure is based on prompt absorption of the ligature and subsequent separation of the severed tubal ends.

PARKLAND PROCEDURE.

The Parkland procedure, shown in Figure 59–1C, was developed in the 1960s and was designed to avoid the initial intimate approximation of the cut ends of the oviduct inherent with the Pomeroy procedure. A small infraumbilical abdominal wall incision is made. The oviduct is identified by grasping the midportion with a Babcock clamp and confirming by direct identification of distal fimbriae. This prevents confusing the round ligament with the midportion of the oviduct. **Whenever the oviduct is inadvertently dropped, it is mandatory to repeat completely the identification procedure just described.**

An avascular site (Fig. 59–2A) in the mesosalpinx adjacent to the oviduct is then perforated with a small hemostat, and the jaws are opened to separate the oviduct from the adjacent mesosalpinx for about 2.5 cm. The freed oviduct is ligated proximally and distally with 0 chromic suture, and the intervening segment of about 2 cm is excised and inspected for hemostasis (Fig. 59–2B). Both resected segments are labeled and submitted for histological confirmation. The failure rate has been approximately 1 in 400 procedures.

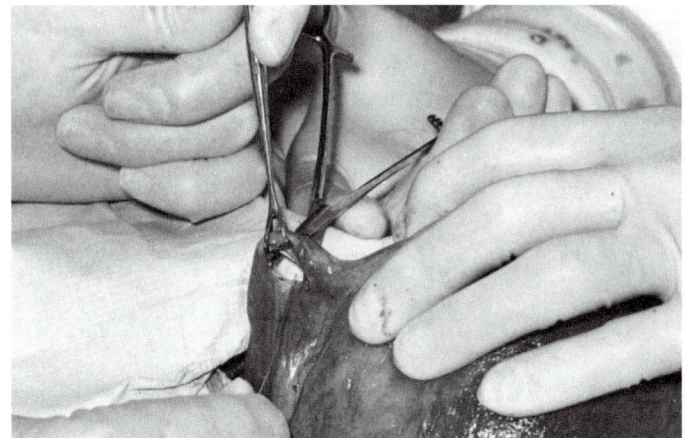

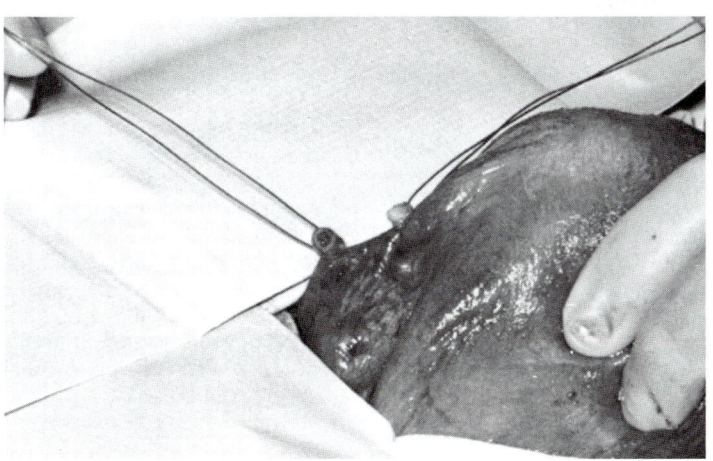

FIGURE 59–2. Sterilization at cesarean delivery. **Top.** An avascular site in the mesosalpinx adjacent to the midportion of the oviduct has been identified, and a small hemostat inserted through the avascular site. The jaws of the clamp have been opened to separate mesosalpinx from tube for about 2.5 cm. A ligature is being inserted. **Bottom.** The segment of oviduct separated from mesosalpinx has been ligated and resected.

MADLENER PROCEDURE. This procedure is similar to the Pomeroy operation, except that a knuckle of tube is crushed and ligated with nonabsorbable suture but not resected (Fig. 59–1D). **This procedure is mentioned only to discourage its use because of a failure rate of about 7 percent.**

FIMBRIECTOMY. Removal of all of the distal tube to effect sterilization was recommended by Kroener (1969) and others. Kroener doubly ligated the oviduct with silk suture and then excised the fimbriated end (Fig. 59–1E). Although he reported no failures, others have, and in some instances, the rate has been as high as 3 percent (Metz, 1977; Taylor, 1972). Failures are usually due to a small amount of fimbrial tissue being left, or from recanalization of the proximal portion of the tube.

NONPUERPERAL (INTERVAL) TUBAL STERILIZA-TION. The techniques of nonpuerperal tubal sterilization, including modifications that have been recommended to accomplish sterilization through tubal occlusion, are almost bewildering in number. Basically, they consist of:

1. Ligation and resection at laparotomy, as described earlier for puerperal sterilization.
2. The permanent application of a variety of rings or clips to the fallopian tubes, usually by laparoscopy.
3. Electrocoagulation of a segment of the oviducts, again usually through a laparoscope.

LAPAROTOMY. Once the uterus has involuted completely and returned to the true pelvis postpartum, exposure is enhanced if the uterus and adnexa are pushed out of the true pelvis to beneath the abdominal wall using a manipulator inserted into the uterus. Using this technique, "minilaparotomies" can be performed through a 3-cm incision made suprapubically, and tubal sterilization can be effected.

COLPOTOMY. *Vaginal tubal sterilization* can usually be performed as an interval procedure once the uterus has involuted and pregnancy-induced hyperemia has subsided. The peritoneal cavity is entered through the posterior vaginal fornix—colpotomy or culdotomy—the oviducts are grasped, and either a Parkland or Pomeroy-type resection or fimbriectomy is performed. This approach has a higher infection rate and often a higher failure rate.

LAPAROSCOPY. An article in *Life* magazine on July 28, 1972 referred to the laparoscopic technique as "Band-Aid" surgery (Fig. 59–3). Laparoscopic tubal ligation is the leading method of family planning for women desiring sterlization (Filshie, 1999). The woman is usually cared for in an ambulatory surgical setting. Anesthesia, usually general with tracheal intubation, is induced. After producing a pneumoperitoneum with carbon dioxide, the sterilization procedure is accomplished. Most often the woman can be discharged several hours later. The actual disruption of tubal contin-

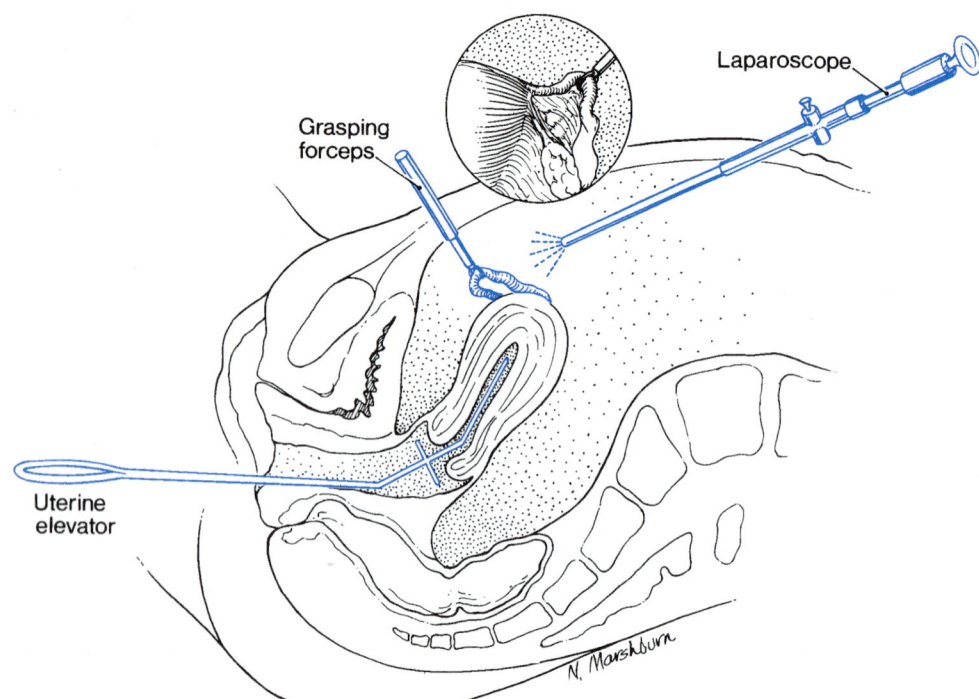

FIGURE 59–3. Tubal sterilization using laparoscopic technique. Note pneumoperitoneum to ensure adequate visualization and exposure for surgery, and the laparoscopically directed instrument grasping one fallopian tube prior to cauterization or application of a clip or ring. A uterine elevator is used to move the uterine fundus toward the anterior abdominal wall.

uity has been accomplished using loops, clips, and electrocauterization with and without transection of the tube. Because electrocauterization destroys a large segment of tube, surgical reversal, most often, is not possible, and this procedure is not generally recommended for women under 25, or those of low parity.

HAZARDS FROM TUBAL STERILIZATION. Principal hazards are anesthetic complications, inadvertent injury of adjacent structures, the rare occurrence of pulmonary embolism, and failure to produce sterility with subsequent development of an ectopic pregnancy (Chap. 34).

Because of improved safety with anesthetic and laparoscopic techniques, the case-fatality rates for tubal sterilization have diminished appreciably over the past 2 decades. For example, from 1977 to 1981, Peterson and co-workers (1983) estimated the case-fatality frequency to be 8 per 100,000 procedures. More recently, Hatcher and colleagues (1998) reported mortality rates of approximately 1.5 per 100,000 for laparoscopic sterilizations. This compares favorably with maternal mortality rates of approximately 8 per 100,000 live births (Chap. 1, p. 6).

DeStefano and co-workers (1983) identified intraoperative or postoperative complications in 1.7 percent of a large number of women who underwent nonpuerperal laparoscopic tubal electrocoagulation for sterilization. Factors identified to increase morbidity were previous abdominal or pelvic surgery, a history of previous pelvic infection, obesity, diabetes, and general anesthesia.

TUBAL STERILIZATION FAILURES. No method of tubal sterilization is without failure. Either uterine or ectopic pregnancies may result from such failures.

INTERVAL TUBAL FAILURE. The reasons for interval tubal failures are not always apparent, but some reasons are:

1. Surgical errors likely account for 30 to 50 percent of cases.
2. The patient was already pregnant at the time of the surgery, a so-called luteal phase pregnancy.
3. An occlusion method failure may be due to fistula formation, which may follow electrocautery procedures. Faulty clips may not be occlusive enough, or the fallopian tube may spontaneously undergo reanastomosis.
4. Equipment failure, such as a defective electric current for the electrocautery, also may be a causative factor.

PUERPERAL STERILIZATION FAILURE. Although an increased failure rate for sterilization at the time of cesarean delivery has been reported by some, with the technique for tubal sterilization used at Parkland Hospital (Figs. 59–1C and 59–2), we have identified no difference. Two major reasons account for the failure of puerperal sterilizations. These are:

1. Surgical errors, which include transection of the round ligament instead of the oviduct or partial transection of the oviduct.
2. Formation of a fisula tract between the severed tubal stumps, or spontaneous reanastomosis.

Soderstrom (1985) concluded that most sterilization failures were not preventable. A similar conclusion was reached by the American College of Obstetricians and Gynecologists (1996), which stated, "pregnancies after sterilization may occur without any technical errors."

METHOD-ASSOCIATED STERILIZATION FAILURES. It is apparent that certain sterilization methods are associated with lower failure rates than others. For example, from review of the data listed in Table 59–1, puerperal sterilization and interval unipolar coagulation appear to have the lowest failure rates. When less than three tubal sites are coagulated, the 5-year cumulative probability of pregnancy is about 12 per 1000 procedures. This compares with only 3 per 1000 if three or more sites are coagulated (Peterson and associates, 1999). Finally, the lifetime increased cumulative failure rates over time are supportive that failures after 1 year are not likely due to technical errors.

ECTOPIC PREGNANCY. Approximately half of the pregnancies that occur after a failed electrocoagulation procedure are ectopic, compared with 10 percent following failure of a ring, clip, or tubal resection method (Hatcher and colleagues, 1990). These must be compared with an ectopic pregnancy rate in nonsterilized women of about 1 percent (Chap. 34, p. 885). **Any symptoms of pregnancy in a woman after tubal sterilization must be investigated, and an ectopic pregnancy must be excluded.**

POSTTUBAL LIGATION SYNDROME. This syndrome is variably characterized by pelvic discomfort, ovarian cyst formation, and especially menorrhagia. It remains to be established that tubal ligation induces any of these changes. Kasonde and Bonnar (1976) measured menstrual blood loss before and for 6 to 12 months after tubal sterilization. They found no significant changes in menstrual blood loss. They also reported that women who presented with menorrhagia soon after sterilization usually had the problem beforehand, or they had been using oral contraceptives, which reduced blood loss. DeStefano and co-workers (1983)

TABLE 59–1. Life-table Cumulative Probability (per 1000 Procedures) of Pregnancy Among Women Undergoing Tubal Sterilization by Method

Method	Years Since Sterilization		
	One	Five	Ten
Puerperal partial salpingectomy	0.6	6.3	7.5
Interval procedure			
Unipolar coagulation	0.7	2.3	7.5
Bipolar coagulation	2.3	16.5	24.8
Silicone rubber band	5.9	10.0	17.7
Partial salpingectomy	7.3	15.1	20.1
Spring clip	18.2	31.7	36.5

Modified from Peterson and colleagues (1996), with permission.

followed nearly 2500 women for 2 years after tubal sterilization and reported that, except for menstrual pain, there was no increase in the prevalence of adverse menstrual function. In fact, half or more of women with adverse menstrual function before sterilization had an improvement over 2 years following sterilization. DeStefano and colleagues (1985) and Shy and associates (1992) included a control group of women whose partners had undergone vasectomy. They reported that abnormal menstrual bleeding seldom developed unless it was reported before sterilization. Interestingly, women with menstrual irregularities before sterilization were less likely than controls to revert spontaneously to normal cyclic menses later. Vessey and associates (1983) compared the frequency of gynecological and psychological disorders among women who had undergone tubal sterilization with those in women whose husbands had undergone vasectomy, and found little difference between the two groups.

Recent observations reported by Peterson and colleagues (2000) for the U.S. Collaborative Review of Sterilization Working Group are important. They showed that tubal sterilization is not followed by increased risks for menstrual abnormalities. This was concluded after study of 9514 women who had undergone tubal sterilization and who were compared with a cohort of 573 women whose partners had undergone vasectomy. Neither increased volume of menstrual flow nor intermenstrual bleeding were different in the two groups. In fact, women who had tubal sterilization were more likely to report decreased duration of bleeding, amount of bleeding, and dysmenorrhea.

Some women who had undergone tubal sterilization were reported by Hargrove and Abraham (1981) to have high serum estradiol and low serum progesterone levels compared with controls. Other investigators have failed to identify luteal phase dysfunction after tubal sterilization, except possibly after techniques that can cause obstruction of the utero-ovarian artery (Alvarez-Sanchez and colleagues, 1981; Donnez and associates, 1981).

Although complete transection of the oviduct is mandatory, it is desirable at the same time to preserve blood supply through the adjacent mesosalpinx. This likely minimizes the possibility of "postligation" abnormalities attributed by some to tubal sterilization. Interestingly, El-Minawi and associates (1983), by means of venography, commonly identified uterovaginal and ovarian varicosities after the Pomeroy and some other procedures, but not following the Parkland technique.

RESTORATION OF FERTILITY. No woman should undergo tubal sterilization believing that her fertility can be restored by either surgery or assisted reproductive techniques that include in-vitro fertilization and ovum transfer. These procedures are costly, difficult, and uncertain. Success rates vary greatly depending upon the age of the woman and the technology utilized.

HYSTERECTOMY. For the woman who desires no more children, hysterectomy has many theoretical advantages. In the absence of uterine or other pelvic disease, however, hysterectomy for sterilization at the time of cesarean delivery, early in the puerperium, or even remote from pregnancy is difficult to justify. Mortality rates for hysterectomy for benign diseases vary from 5 to 25 per 100,000 in women aged 35 to 44 (Wingo and colleagues, 1985). With cesarean hysterectomy, blood loss is greater than with cesarean plus tubal sterilization, and urinary tract injury is appreciable (Gilstrap and colleagues, 2001).

HYSTEROSCOPY. Sterilization utilizing hysteroscopy to visualize the tubal ostia and somehow obliterate them is a worthy goal and has received considerable attention. To date, the failure rate and other problems limit the clinical utility of this approach (Zatuchni and colleagues, 1983).

MALE STERILIZATION

It is estimated that more than 400,000 men annually undergo vasectomy in the United States. Through a small incision in the scrotum, the lumen of the vas deferens is disrupted to block the passage of sperm from the testes (Fig. 59–4). The procedure is usually performed within 20 minutes using local analgesia. Techniques generally are either traditional or no-scapel vasectomy (Clenney and Higgins, 1999). According to Hendrix and colleagues (1999) in their review, compared with vasectomy, female tubal sterilization has a 20-fold increased complication rate, 10- to 37-fold failure, and a 3-fold higher cost. In Dallas in 2000, total charges for a vasectomy were $700 compared with $5500 for an outpatient laparoscopic tubal ligation.

A disadvantage of vasectomy is that sterility is not immediate. Complete expulsion of sperm stored in the reproductive tract beyond the interrupted vas deferens takes about 3 months or 20 ejaculations (American College of Obstetricians and Gynecologists, 1996). Semen should be checked until two consecutive sperm counts are zero. During this period, another form of contraception must be used. The failure rate for vasectomy is much less than 1 percent, but is dependent on several factors. These include failure from unprotected intercourse too soon after ligation, failure to occlude the vas deferens, or recanalization. Hendrix and colleagues

(1999) reported that female tubal sterilization is 10 to 37 times more likely to fail than vasectomy.

Restoration of fertility after a successful vasectomy does not always succeed. A review of several reports suggests that odds for success are about 50 percent, with somewhat higher rates following microsurgical reanastomosis. As with women, the risks of regret after sterilization appear to relate primarily to immaturity at the time of sterilization (Howard, 1982). Three factors that appear to be important in restoration of fertility after previous vasectomy are:

1. The application of meticulous microsurgical techniques for reanastomosis.
2. The length of time after vasectomy.
3. The presence of sperm granulomas.

CARDIOVASCULAR DISEASE. Antibodies directed at spermatozoa can be identified frequently after vasectomy. Concern was raised over the possibility that the immune response might cause harmful systemic changes. Carefully made observations on a very large number of men who had undergone vasectomy several years before have not identified an increase in cardiovascular disease, circulating immune complexes, or damage to retinal blood vessels (Giovannucci and colleagues, 1992; Goldacre and co-workers, 1983). More recently, Manson and associates (1999) provided data from the U.S. Physicians' Health Study that included a 15-year follow-up of 1159 physicians who had undergone vasectomy. Compared with controls, there was no difference in occurrence of myocardial infarction or stroke.

PROSTATIC AND TESTICULAR CARCINOMA. There is no convincing evidence of an increased incidence of testicular cancer following vasectomy (Giovannucci and colleagues 1992). Although Giovannucci and associates (1993a, 1993b) reported a weak positive correlation between vasectomy and prostatic carcinoma, Hayes and co-workers (1993) did not. The consensus report from the 1993 National Institutes of Health Conference on Vasectomy and Prostate Cancer concluded that data were insufficient to alter recommendations for the procedure. A subsequent study by Lesko and colleagues (1999) of 1216 vasectomized men and 1400 controls indicated an almost twofold risk of prostatic cancer in men less than 55 years old but no increased risk thereafter.

REFERENCES

Alvarez-Sanchez F, Segal SJ, Brache V, Adejuwon CA, Leon P, Faundes A: Pituitary–ovarian function after tubal ligation. Fertil Steril 36:606, 1981

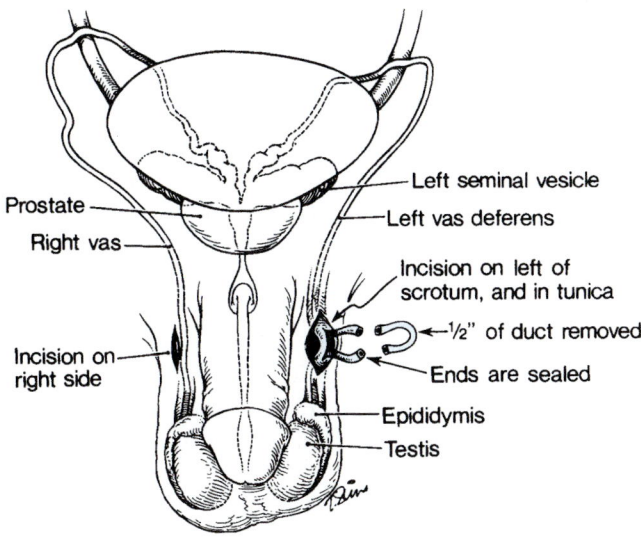

FIGURE 59–4. Male reproductive system showing the site of vasectomy.

Prostate
Right vas
Incision on right side
Left seminal vesicle
Left vas deferens
Incision on left of scrotum, and in tunica
½" of duct removed
Ends are sealed
Epididymis
Testis

American College of Obstetricians and Gynecologists: Sterilization. ACOG Technical Bulletin No. 222, April, 1996

Association for Voluntary Surgical Contraception News 27:1, 1989

Bucklin BA, Smith CV: Postpartum tubal ligation: Safety, timing and other implications for anesthesia. Anesth Analg 89:1269, 1999

Clenney TL, Higgins JC: Vasectomy techniques. Am Fam Physician 60:137, 1999

DeStefano F, Greenspan JR, Dicker RC, Peterson HB, Strauss LT, Rubin GL: Complications of interval laparoscopic tubal sterilization. Obstet Gynecol 61:153, 1983

DeStefano F, Perlman JA, Peterson HB, Diamond EL: Long-term risk of menstrual disturbances after tubal sterilization. Am J Obstet Gynecol 152:835, 1985

Donnez J, Wauters M, Thomas K: Luteal function after tubal sterilization. Obstet Gynecol 57:65, 1981

El-Minawi MF, Masor N, Reda MS: Pelvic venous changes after tubal sterilization. J Reprod Med 28:641, 1983

Filshie M: Laparoscopic sterilization. Semin Laparosc Surg 2:112, 1999

Gilstrap LC, Van Dorsten P, Cunningham FG (eds): Obstetric hysterectomy. In: Operative Obstetrics, 2nd ed, New York, McGraw-Hill, 2001

Giovannucci E, Ascherio A, Rimm EB, Colditz GA, Stampfer MJ, Willett WC: A prospective study of vasectomy and prostate cancer in U.S. men. JAMA 269:876, 1993a

Giovannucci E, Tosteson TD, Speizer FE, Ascherio A, Vessey MP, Colditz GA: A retrospective cohort study of vasectomy and prostate cancer in U.S. men. JAMA 269:878, 1993b

Giovannucci E, Tosteson TD, Speizer FE, Vessey MP, Colditz GA: A long-term study of mortality in men who have undergone vasectomy. N Engl J Med 326:1392, 1992

Goldacre JM, Holford TR, Vessey MP: Cardiovascular disease and vasectomy. N Engl J Med 308:805, 1983

Hargrove JT, Abraham GE: Endocrine profile of patients with post-tubal ligation syndrome. J Reprod Med 26:359, 1981

Hatcher RA, Stewart F, Trussel J, Kowal P, Guest F, Stewart GK, Cates W: Contraceptive Technology, 15th ed. New York, Irvington, 1990, pp 391, 403, 416

Hatcher RA, Trussell J, Stewart F, Cates W, Steward GK, Guest F, Kowal D: Contraceptive Technology, 17th ed. New York, Ardent Media, 1998, p 548

Hayes RB, Pottern CM, Greenberg R, Schoenberg J, Swanson GM, Liff J: Vasectomy and prostate cancer in US blacks and whites. Am J Epidemiol 137:263, 1993

Hendrix NW, Chauhan SP, Morrison JC: Sterilization and its consequences. Obstet Gynecol Surv 54:766, 1999

Howard G: Who asks for vasectomy reversal and why? BMJ 285:490, 1982

Kasonde JM, Bonnar J: Effect of sterilization on menstrual blood loss. Br J Obstet Gynaecol 83:572, 1976

Kroener WF Jr: Surgical sterilization by fimbriectomy. Am J Obstet Gynecol 104:247, 1969

Lesko SM, Louik C, Vezina R, Rosenberg L, Shapiro S: Vasectomy and prostate cancer. J Urol 161:1848, 1999

Lungren SS: A case of cesarean twice. Am J Obstet Dis Women Child 14:78, 1881

Manson JE, Ridker PM, Spelsberg A, Ajani U, Lotufo PA, Hennekens CH: Vasectomy and subsequent cardiovascular disease in US physicians. Contraception 59:181, 1999

Metz KGP: Failures following fimbriectomy. Fertil Steril 28:66, 1977

National Institutes of Health: Vasectomy and Prostate Cancer Conference. Department of Health and Human Services. The National Institute of Child Health and Human Development, National Cancer Institute, and National Institute of Diabetes and Digestive and Kidney Diseases, March 2, 1993

Peterson HB, DeStefano F, Rubin GL, Greenspan JR, Lee NC, Ory HW: Deaths attributed to tubal sterilization in the United States, 1977 to 1981. Am J Obstet Gynecol 146:131, 1983

Peterson HB, Jeng G, Folger SG, Hillis SA, Marchbanks PA, Wilcox LS for the U.S. Collaborative Review of Sterilization Working Group: The risk of menstrual abnormalities after tubal sterilization. N Engl J Med 343:1681, 2000

Peterson HB, Xia Z, Hughes JM, Wilcox LS, Tylor LR, Trussel J: The risk of pregnancy after tubal sterilization: Findings from the U.S. Collaborative Review of Sterilization. Am J Obstet Gynecol 174:1161, 1996

Peterson HB, Xia Z, Wilcox LS, Tylor LR, Trussel J: Pregnancy after tubal sterilization with bipolar electrocoagulation. U.S. Collaborative Review of Sterilization Working Group. Obstet Gynecol 94:163, 1999

Shy KK, Stergachis A, Grothaus LG, Wagner EH, Hecht J, Anderson G: Tubal sterilization and risk of subsequent hospital admission for menstrual disorders. Am J Obstet Gynecol 166:1698, 1992

Soderstrom RM: Sterilization failures and their causes. Am J Obstet Gynecol 152:395, 1985

Taylor TS: Editorial comment. Obstet Gynecol Surv 27:168, 1972

Vessey MP, Huggins G, Lawless M, Yeates D: Tubal sterilization: Findings in a large prospective study. Br J Obstet Gynaecol 90:203, 1983

Wingo PA, Huezo CM, Rubin GL, Ory HW, Peterson HB: The mortality risk associated with hysterectomy. Am J Obstet Gynecol 152:803, 1985

Zatuchni GI, Shelton JD, Goldsmith A, Sciarra JJ (eds): Female transcervical sterilization. In: PARFR Series on Fertility Regulation. Philadelphia, Harper & Row, 1983

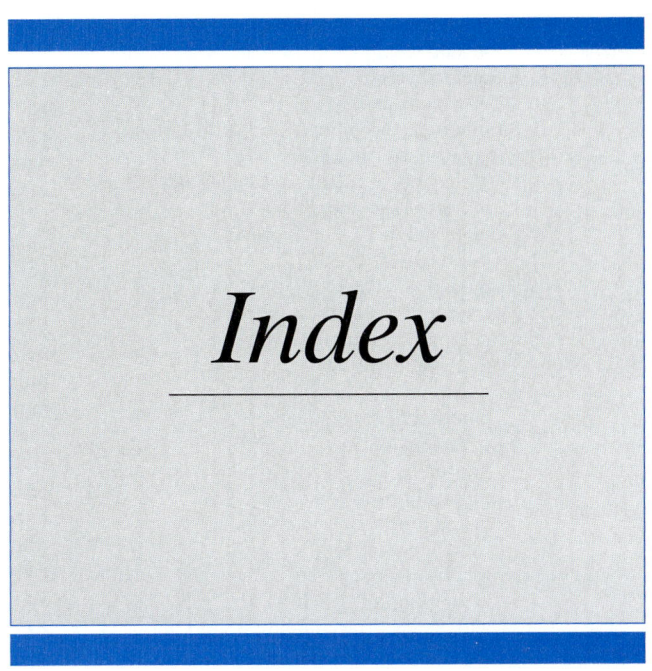

Index

Page numbers followed by *f* indicate figures; page numbers followed by *t* indicate tables.

ISBN 0-07-112195-1

90000

9 780071 121958

CUNNINGHAM/
WILLIAM'S OBSTET IE

ISBN 0-8385-9647-9

90000

9 780838 596470

CUNNINGHAM/
WILLIAM'S OSTET